GERALD E. SWANSON, M.D.
9601 UPTON ROAD
MINNEAPOLIS, MN 55431
TELE: 881-6869

(1390⁰⁰)

The High Risk Patient: Management of the Critically Ill

The High Risk Patient: Management of the Critically Ill

Edited by

EDWARD D. SIVAK, M.D., F.A.C.P., F.C.C.P., F.C.C.M.

Chief, Section of Critical Care Medicine
Meridia Huron Hospital
Assistant Clinical Professor of Medicine
Case Western Reserve University, School of Medicine
University Hospital of Cleveland
Cleveland, Ohio

THOMAS L. HIGGINS, M.D., F.A.C.P., F.C.C.P., F.C.C.M., F.A.C.C.

Director, Cardiothoracic Intensive Care Unit
Cleveland Clinic Foundation
Associate Professor of Anesthesiology
Cleveland Clinic Foundation Health Science Center of the Ohio State University
Cleveland, Ohio

ADAM SEIVER, M.D., Ph.D., F.A.C.S., F.C.C.M.

Clinical Assistant Professor of Surgery
Division of Trauma and Critical Care
Stanford University School of Medicine
Stanford, California
Senior Consultant
Strategic Decisions Group
Menlo Park, California

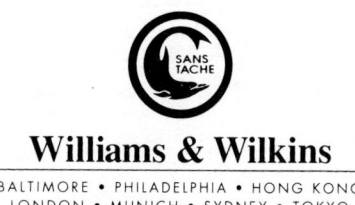

Williams & Wilkins
BALTIMORE • PHILADELPHIA • HONG KONG
LONDON • MUNICH • SYDNEY • TOKYO

A WAVERLY COMPANY

1995

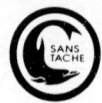

Executive Editor: Carroll C. Cann
Developmental Editor: Susan Hunsberger
Production Manager: Laurie Forsyth
Project Editor: Rebecca Krumm

Copyright © 1995
Williams & Wilkins
Rose Tree Corporate Center
1400 North Providence Rd., Suite 5025
Media, PA 19063-2043 USA

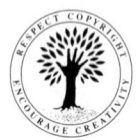

All rights reserved. This book is protected by copyright. No part of this book may be reproduced in any form or by any means, including photocopying, or utilized by any information storage and retrieval system without written permission from the copyright owner.

Accurate indications, adverse reactions, and dosage schedules for drugs are provided in this book, but it is possible they may change. The reader is urged to review the package information data of the manufacturers of the medications mentioned.

Printed in the United States of America

Library of Congress Cataloging-in-Publication Data

The high risk patient : management of the critically ill / edited by
  Edward D. Sivak, Thomas L. Higgins, Adam Seiver.
     p.   cm.
  Includes index.
  ISBN 0-683-07785-6
  1. Critical care medicine.   2. Intensive care units.   I. Sivak,
Edward D.   II. Higgins, Thomas L.   III. Seiver, Adam.
     [DNLM: 1. Critical Illness. 2. Critical Care—methods.   WX 218
H6385 1994]
RC86.7.H54   1994
616′.028—dc20
DNLM/DLC
for Library of Congress
                                          94-28870
                                             CIP

                              94 95 96 97 98
                        1 2 3 4 5 6 7 8 9 10

TO THE PAST, THE PRESENT AND THE FUTURE

To Michael V. Sivak, Sr., M.D.
(Teacher, Role Model, and Visionary)

To Barbara
(Gratitude and love)

To Eddie, Anna, Mike, and Tom
(With pride and affection)
(May you always benefit from the past and the present)

Edward D. Sivak, M.D.

**TO MY WIFE SUZANNE AND TO MY CHILDREN,
AMY, MATTHEW, AND WILLIAM**

(For the reminder that a balanced life is worth the occasional missed deadline)

Thomas L. Higgins, M.D.

FOR MY WIFE, ANA, AND MY SON, MILES

Adam Seiver, M.D., Ph.D.

PREFACE

Critical illness defines the focal point in the pathogenesis of various disease processes where action must be taken to avoid significant morbidity and mortality during the ICU phase of illness. Antecedent to the focal point are certain risk factors and events that influence the subsequent course of the illness. We have referred to these circumstances as the pre-ICU phase throughout the text. If particular emphasis is not placed on follow-up rehabilitation in the post-ICU phase, a patient may return to the ICU because of relapse or the development of other co-morbid conditions, which again may result in increased mortality. Whenever possible, we have requested all contributors to couch their discussions around this three-compartment model, as illustrated in Figure 1. The pre-ICU phase of illness should be viewed as a potentially high risk phase for certain patients. Certain factors such as age, co-morbid conditions, generalized debilitation, and misdiagnosis can predispose a patient to a more severe illness if the clinician does not recognize such risk factors. The caregiver should constantly strive to minimize risk factors by prevention or early intervention in the hope of preventing critical illness. Although ICU admission is not always preventable, early recognition of the high risk situation may limit morbidity and mortality.

Critical illness does not always neatly manifest as discrete entities. On the contrary, clinical presentations occur in manifestations of coma, pulmonary edema, hypotension, and other symptoms. The approach to the critically ill patient is the development of a differential diagnosis while simultaneous stabilizing hemodynamic, respiratory and neurologic systems. Organ system derangement is the usual presentation. For this reason, we have divided our text into discussions by organ system. In addition, we have further divided each section into subsections by major clinical entities that occupy significant amounts of time for the critical care practitioner. When a patient is seen for evaluation of coma, the evaluation is that of coma—not encephalopathy, not stroke, and so forth. The differential diagnosis later unfolds into a specific disease entity for which treatment, intervention, and long-range plans of rehabilitation, no matter how brief, are instituted. Specific disease entities are reviewed from the pre-ICU phase, where an understanding of these risks helps one to focus on therapeutic intervention. Following the ICU phase, long-term plans for rehabilitation are in order. Often, the caregiver is asked about the post-ICU phase of illness. We have attempted to answer some of these questions in the form of outcome, predictions, and probabilities.

When reading specific portions of the text, the reader is directed to cross references. For example, the chapter on weaning of the ventilator-dependent patient contains pointers to other chapters such as nutritional support, altered mental function, and fluid and electrolyte balance. Wherever possible and appropriate, we have included sections on important components of physiology by devoting entire chapters to the subject. The chapters on increased intracranial pressure, respiratory failure, the respiratory muscles and the work of breathing, the determinants of cardiac function, and disorders of hepatic function and are specific examples. An entire section has been devoted to the integument, frequently overlooked and misunderstood as an organ system of the body. To emphasize the care of the entire patient, we have included general support considerations. In this section, topics such as preoperative assessment, fluid and electrolyte replacement, and utilization of blood and blood products are discussed. In this section we have also grouped multiple organ System failure, discussions about adrenergic receptors and pharmacology of vasoactive drugs, and antibiotic pharmacokinetics and antibiotic selection because of their interdependence in the care of the critically il patient.

Beyond the care of the critically ill patient is another component of ICU management—the requirements for the patient care team to work together. In the section on managerial and quality assurance issues, topics such as the team concept of patient care, psychologic stress and the patient caregiver, quality assurance, infection control, and standards for procedures and complications are reviewed. We have also included issues such as pitfalls in hemodynamic and respiratory monitoring, the role of the biomedical engineer, and computerization of the ICU because of our increasing dependence on new technology in the assessment and management of our patients. Rounding out this section are practical discussions on minimizing the risks of liability and defining the limits of therapeutic intervention. We have also included an appendix on the application of statistics in the ICU to remind the reader that we must constantly strive to understand that there is also a statistical basis for the art of critical care medicine. This addition is intended to supplement the information contained in the chapter on predictive indices and severity of illness indicators.

No preface is complete without proper recognition of

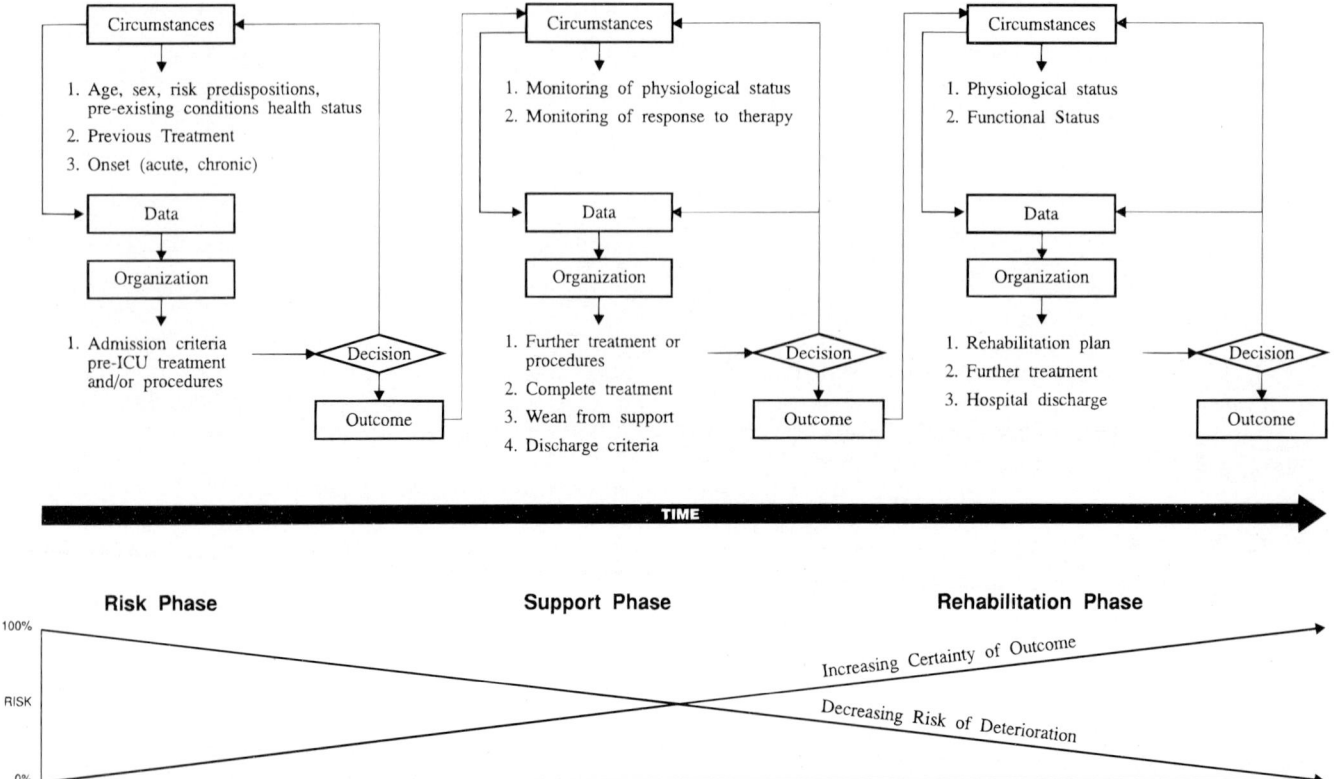

Figure 1. The high risk patient: management of the critically ill. (Courtesy of George Morrison, CDI.)

those individuals who have provided substance and encouragement, which cannot be quantitated by accolades or number of pages. First and without a doubt we owe the success of this text to the experience, perseverance, and unrelenting efforts of our contributors. Behind the scene, Mr. Carroll Cann was one of the unsung heroes of the battle to complete all the manuscripts. Regardless of deadlines, he was always correct in estimating the necessary time, reminding us that there would be a few late details and manuscripts, and constantly keeping us on track without one discouraging word or hint of dismay at our requests for a bit more time. As we moved closer to production, Mrs. Susan Hunsberger performed what seemed to be a task of major magnitude by reading the text and finding all the overlooked details that we thought were insignificant, and taking care of them, too! Carroll reminded us of schedules, but Susan reminded us that the clock was ticking. Mr. Keith Stincic from the library of Meridia Huron Hospital provided invaluable last minute reference checks. In the final phases of production was the task of copy editing. For this, we thank Mrs. Holly Lukens. She and her team added the finishing touches, which only true experts can provide.

Special thanks to the countless numbers of nurses, respiratory therapists, resident physicians, our colleagues, patients, and their families from whom we have learned invaluable lessons, which are contained within, and to Dr. Leo Pozuelo for the final reading of the proof pages.

Finally, and without any in-depth discussion, we thank our spouses and families for their patience of saints, their love, wisdom, wit, humor, and sometimes gentle sarcasm—all necessary elements required for the completion of this text.

Cleveland, Ohio   Edward D. Sivak
Cleveland, Ohio   Thomas L. Higgins
Stanford, California   Adam Seiver

CONTRIBUTORS

David J. Adelstein, M.D.
Staff Physician
Department of Hematology and Medical Oncology
Cleveland Clinic Foundation
Cleveland, Ohio

John C. Alverdy, M.D.
Associate Professor of Surgery
University of Chicago
Chicago, Illinois

Steven W. Andresen, D.O.
Staff Physician
Department of Hematology and Medical Oncology
Cleveland Clinic Foundation
Cleveland, Ohio

Tatsuo Araida, M.D.
Assistant Clinical Professor of Surgery
University of California, Davis Medical Center
Sacramento, California

Andrea P. Baldyga, M.D.
Department of Cardiothoracic Anesthesia and Cardiovascular Surgery
Cleveland Clinic Foundation
Cleveland, Ohio

Gene H. Barnett, M.D.
Vice Chairman of Neurosurgery
Head, Section of Neurosurgical Oncology and Stereotaxis
Cleveland Clinic Foundation
Cleveland, Ohio

Richard C. Becker, M.D.
Associate Professor of Medicine
Director, Thrombosis Research Center
Director, Coronary Care Unit
University of Massachusetts Medical School
Worcester, Massachusetts

Philip F. Binkley, M.D.
Assistant Professor of Medicine
Division of Cardiology
Ohio State University College of Medicine
Columbus, Ohio

Blaise F. D. Bourgeois, M.D.
Professor of Neurology and Pediatrics
Washington University School of Medicine
St. Louis, Missouri

Eric P. Brass, M.D., Ph.D.
Chair, Department of Medicine
Harbor-UCLA Medical Center
Torrance, California

Thomas A. Broughan, M.D.
Associate Professor of Surgery
Surgical Director, Liver Transplant Program
Alonzo Alverly Ross, M.D. Centennial Chair in General Surgery
University of Texas Medical Branch at Galveston
Galveston, Texas

Earl Z. Browne, Jr., M.D.
Department of Plastic Surgery
Cleveland Clinic Foundation
Cleveland, Ohio

Ronald M. Bukowski, M.D.
Director Experimental Therapeutic Program
Staff Physician Department of Hematology and Medical Oncology
Cleveland Clinic Foundation
Cleveland, Ohio

Carolyn P. Cacho, M.D.
Assistant Professor of Medicine
Division of Nephrology
Case Western Reserve University School of Medicine
Cleveland, Ohio

William D. Carey, M.D., F.A.C.P., F.A.C.G.
Head, Section of Hepatology
Cleveland Clinic Foundation
Cleveland, Ohio
Associate Professor of Medicine
Ohio State University College of Medicine
Columbus, Ohio
Associate Professor of Medicine
Pennsylvania State University
Hershey, Pennsylvania

CONTRIBUTORS

John J. Caronna, M.D.
Professor and Vice Chairman of Neurology
Cornell University Medical College
Attending Neurologist
New York Hospital-Cornell Medical Center
New York, New York

Paul N. Casale, M.D., F.A.C.C.
Staff Physician
Lancaster General Hospital
Lancaster, Pennsylvania

Germaine M. Casmishion, M.D.
Clinical Assistant Professor of Medicine (Dermatology)
Brown University Program in Medicine
Associate Director, Division of Dermatology
Rhode Island Hospital
Providence, Rhode Island

Bart Chernow, M.D., F.A.C.P.
Professor of Medicine, Anesthesia, and Critical Care
Johns Hopkins University School of Medicine
Physician-in-chief
Sinai Hospital of Baltimore
Baltimore, Maryland

John W. Christman, M.D.
Assistant Professor of Medicine
Division of Pulmonary Medicine
Director, Medical Intensive Care Unit
Nashville Veterans Administration Medical Center
Nashville, Tennessee

Raphael S. Chung, M.D., F.A.C.S.
Staff Surgeon
Cleveland Clinic Foundation
Cleveland, Ohio

Suzanne Clark, M.S.N., M.A., R.N.
Clinical Nurse Specialist
Consultant and Liaison Service
Kaiser Permanente
Assistant Clinical Professor
University of California, Los Angeles School of Nursing
Los Angeles, California

Robert J. Cody, M.D., F.A.C.P., F.A.C.C.
James Hay and Ruth Jansson Wilson Professor of Medicine
Assistant Division Director, Research Affairs
Cardiology Division
Ohio State University College of Medicine
Columbus, Ohio

Edward M. Cordasco, Jr., D.O.
Private Practitioner
Riverside Pulmonary Associates, Inc.
Columbus, Ohio

Joseph P. Coyle, M.D.
Director, Cardiac Anesthesia and Cardiovascular Recovery Unit
Carolinas Medical Center
Charlotte, North Carolina

James Dougherty, M.D., F.A.C.E.P.A.
Associate Professor of Emergency Medicine
Northeastern Ohio University School of Medicine
Research Director, Emergency Medicine Residency
Akron General Medical Center
Akron, Ohio

Kathleen Dracup, D.N.Sc., F.A.A.N.
Professor of Nursing
University of California, Los Angeles School of Nursing
Los Angeles, California

Mary Lynn Droughton, M.S.N., R.N.
Clinical Nurse Specialist
Department of Head and Neck Oncology
Cleveland Clinic Foundation
Cleveland, Ohio

George L. Drusano, M.D.
Professor of Medicine and Pharmacology
Director, Division of Clinical Pharmacology
Albany Medical College
Albany, New York

Isaac Eliachar, M.D., F.A.C.S., F.I.C.S.
Head, Section of Laryngastracheal Reconstruction
Department of Otolaryngology and Communicative Disorders
Cleveland Clinic Foundation
Cleveland, Ohio

Fawzy G. Estafanous, M.D.
Chairman of Anesthesiology
Cleveland Clinic Foundation
Cleveland, Ohio

Mary Jo Fitzpatrick, M.S., R.N., C, CCRN
Quality Improvement Specialist
Patient Care Services at Grant Medical Center
Manager of Nursing Education, Critical Care
Riverside Methodist Hospital
Columbus, Ohio

Charles F. Frey, M.D.
Professor and Vice Chairman of Surgery
University of California, Davis Medical Center
Sacramento, California

Dennis K. Giles, R.R.T.
Supervisor, Respiratory Therapy Section
Department of Pulmonary and Critical Care Medicine
Cleveland Clinic Foundation
Cleveland, Ohio

Inderjit S. Gill, M.B.B.S., F.R.C.S. (Ire), F.R.C.S. (C)
Cardiac Surgeon
University of Ottawa Heart Institute
Ottawa, Ontario, Canada

CONTRIBUTORS

Joel S. Gochberg
Chief Technical Officer
Clinical Dimentions, Inc.
Subsidiary of Micro Health Systems
West Orange, New Jersey

Peter Goldberg, M.D.
Associate Professor of Medicine and Anesthesiology
McGill University
Director, Intensive Care Unit
Montreal Chest Hospital Centre
Associate Physician, Intensive Care Unit
Royal Victoria Hospital
Montreal, Quebec, Canada

Joseph A. Golish, M.D., F.A.C.P., F.C.C.P.
Staff Physician
Department of Pulmonary and Critical Care Medicine
Cleveland Clinic Foundation
Cleveland, Ohio
Clinical Assistant Professor of Medicine
Ohio State University College of Medicine
Columbus, Ohio

Steven A. Gould, M.D., F.A.C.S.
Chief of Service
Department of Surgery
Michael Reese Hospital and Medical Center
Professor of Surgery
University of Illinois College of Medicine
Chicago, Illinois

Barth A. Green, M.D., F.A.C.S.
Professor of Neurological Surgery, Orthopaedics, and Rehabilitation
University of Miami School of Medicine
Director, Neurosurgery Services
University of Miami/Jackson Memorial Medical Center
Director of Clinical Research
The Miami Project
Miami, Florida

Cyril M. Grum, M.D.
Associate Professor of Internal Medicine
Division of Pulmonary and Critical Care Medicine
University of Michigan Medical Center
Ann Arbor, Michigan

Gabriel P. Haas, M.D.
Assistant Professor and Chief
Section of Urologic Oncology
Wayne State University School of Medicine
Detroit, Michigan

Edward F. Haponik, M.D.
Professor of Internal Medicine
Section on Pulmonary and Critical Care Medicine
Bowman Gray School of Medicine
Winston-Salem, North Carolina

Marcus T. Haug, III, Pharm. D., M.Sc.
Pharmacokinetics Pharmacist
Department of Hospital Pharmacy and Lung Transplant Team
Cleveland Clinic Foundation
Cleveland, Ohio

Darell Heiselman, D.O., F.C.C.M., F.A.C.P., F.A.C.C., F.C.C.P.
Professor of Medicine
Northeastern Ohio University School of Medicine
Chief, Critical Care Medicine
Akron General Medical Center
Akron, Ohio

Dan J. Hendrickson, M.D., F.C.C.P.
Private Practitioner
Odesa, Texas

Thomas L. Higgins, M.D., F.A.C.P., F.C.C.P., F.C.C.M., F.A.C.C.
Director, Cardiothoracic Intensive Care Unit
Cleveland Clinic Foundation
Cleveland, Ohio

Katherine Hodge, M.D.
Senior Resident
Department of General Surgery
University of Hawaii
Honolulu, Hawaii

James W. Holcroft, M.D., F.A.C.S.
Professor of Surgery
University of California, Davis Medical Center
Sacramento, California

Byron J. Hoogwerf, M.D.
Staff Endocrinologist
Department of Endocrinology
Cleveland Clinic Foundation
Cleveland, Ohio

Russell D. Hull, M.B.B.S., M.Sc., F.R.A.C.P., F.R.C.P.(C), F.A.C.P., F.C.C.P.
Professor of Medicine
Head, Division of General Internal Medicine
University of Calgary
Calgary, Alberta, Canada

Conrad Iber, M.D., F.A.C.P.
Assistant Professor of Medicine
University of Minnesota
Minneapolis, Minnesota

Charles Lee Jackson, M.D.
Chairman of Urology
Cleveland Clinic Florida
Fort Lauderdale, Florida

Bryan E. Jewett, M.D., F.A.C.S.
Assistant Professor of Surgery
Uniformed Services University of Health Sciences
Bethesda, Maryland

CONTRIBUTORS

Mani S. Kavuru, M.D.
Director, Pulmonary Function Laboratory, Department of Pulmonary and Critical Care Medicine
Cleveland Clinic Foundation
Cleveland, Ohio

Lucy Kester, M.B.A., R.R.T.
Educational Coordinator, Respiratory Therapy
Department of Pulmonary and Critical Care Medicine
Cleveland Clinic Foundation
Cleveland, Ohio

Thomas F. Keys, M.D., F.A.C.P.
Director, Office of Quality Management
Staff Physician
Department of Infectious Diseases
Cleveland Clinic Foundation
Cleveland, Ohio

Thomas J. Kirby, M.D., F.A.C.S., F.R.C.S. (C)
Head, Pulmonary Transplantation
Cleveland Clinic Foundation
Cleveland, Ohio

Allan L. Klein, M.D.
Department of Cardiology
Cleveland Clinic Foundation
Cleveland, Ohio

Donna Guinn Klein, R.N., J.D.
Head, Health Care Section
McGlinchey, Staffort, and Lang
New Orleans, Louisiana

Russell C. Klein, M.D.
Assistant Dean, Alumni Affairs and Continuing Medical Education
Professor of Medicine
Louisiana State University School of Medicine
New Orleans, Louisiana

William A. Knaus, M.D., F.A.C.P.
Director, ICU Research
George Washington University School of Medicine
Washington, D.C.

John J. Komara, Jr., R.R.T.
Supervisor, Respiratory Therapy Section
Department of Pulmonary and Critical Care Medicine
Cleveland Clinic Foundation
Cleveland, Ohio

Pierre Lavertu, M.D., F.R.C.S.(C), F.A.C.S.
Vice Chairman and Head, Section of Head and Neck Surgery
Department of Otolaryngology and Communicative Disorders
Cleveland Clinic Foundation
Cleveland, Ohio

James W. Leatherman, M.D.
Assistant Professor of Medicine
University of Minnesota
Division of Pulmonary and Critical Care Medicine
Hennepin County Medical Center
Minneapolis, Minnesota

Gail S. Lebovic, M.A., M.D.
Chief Surgical Resident
Stanford University Hospital
Stanford, California

Kerry H. Levin, M.D.
Department of Neurology Staff Neurologist
Cleveland Clinic Foundation
Cleveland, Ohio

Edward Levine, M.D.
Assistant Professor of Surgery
Division of Surgical Oncology
Louisiana State University School of Medicine
New Orleans, Louisiana

Alan E. Lichtin, M.D.
Staff Physician
Department of Hematology and Medical Oncology
Cleveland Clinic Foundation
Cleveland, Ohio
Clinical Assistant Professor
Ohio State University College of Medicine
Columbus, Ohio

David L. Longworth, M.D.
Chairman of Infectious Diseases
Cleveland Clinic Foundation
Cleveland, Ohio
Associate Professor of Medicine
Ohio State University College of Medicine
Columbus, Ohio

Floyd D. Loop, M.D., F.A.C.S., F.A.C.C.
Chairman
Board of Governors
Staff Physician
Department of Thoracic and Cardiovascular Surgery
Cleveland Clinic Foundation
Cleveland, Ohio

Melvin Lopata, M.D.
Professor and Vice-Head of Medicine
Chief, Section of Respiratory and Critical Care Medicine
University of Illinois College of Medicine
Chicago, Illinois

Bruce W. Lytle, M.D., F.A.C.S., F.A.C.C.
Staff Surgeon
Department of Thoracic and Cardiovascular Surgery
Cleveland Clinic Foundation
Cleveland, Ohio

CONTRIBUTORS

Kenneth Maiese, M.D.
Assistant Professor of Neurology
Cornell University Medical College
Assistant Attending Neurologist
New York Hospital-Cornell Medical Center
New York, New York

Lionel A. Mandell, M.D., F.R.C.P.(C)
Professor of Medicine
Chief, Division of Infectious Diseases
McMaster University
Hamilton, Ontario, Canada

John J. Marini, M.D., F.A.C.P., F.C.C.P.
Professor of Medicine
University of Minnesota
Director, Pulmonary and Critical Care Medicine
St. Paul-Ramsey Medical Center
St. Paul, Minnesota

Paul L. Marino, M.D., Ph.D., F.C.C.M.
Director, Critical Care
Presbyterian Medical Center of Philadelphia
Philadelphia, Pennsylvania

John C. Marshall, M.D., F.R.C.S.(C), F.A.C.S.
Department of Surgery
University of Toronto
Toronto Hospital
Toronto, Ontario, Canada

Richard J. Martin, M.D., F.C.C.P.
Senior Faculty Member
Jewish Center for Immunology and Respiratory Medicine
Professor of Medicine
University of Colorado Health Sciences Center
Denver, Colorado

Laura E. Matarese, M.S., R.D., L.D., C.N.S.D.
Nutritional Support Coordinator
Cleveland Clinic Foundation
Cleveland, Ohio

Richard Menzies, M.D.
Assistant Professor of Medicine and Epidemiology and Biostatistics
McGill University
Associate Physician-in-Chief
Montreal Chest Hospital Centre
Montreal, Quebec, Canada

Moulay A. Meziane, M.D., F.C.C.P.
Head, Section of Thoracic Imaging
Department of Radiology
Cleveland Clinic Foundation
Cleveland, Ohio

Stephen L. Moore, D.O.
Director, Cardiac Electrophysiology and Pacing
Elyria Memorial Hospital and Medical Center
North Ohio Heart Center
Lorain, Ohio

Lori J. Morgan, M.D.
Research Fellow
Department of Surgery
Stanford University Medical Center
Stanford, California

Harold H. Morris, III, M.D.
Head, Section of Epilepsy and Sleep Disorders
Department of Neurology
Cleveland Clinic Foundation
Cleveland, Ohio

Eric D. Morse, M.D.
General Surgeon
Private Practice
Carmichael, California

Avery B. Nathans, M.D.
Resident in General Surgery
Department of Surgery
University of Toronto
Toronto, Ontario, Canada

Andrew C. Novick, M.D.
Chairman of Urology
Cleveland Clinic Foundation
Cleveland, Ohio

James P. Orlowski, M.D., F.A.A.P., F.C.C.P., F.C.C.M.
Director, Pediatric Intensive Care
University Community Hospital
Professor of Pediatrics
University of South Florida
Tampa, Florida

John T. Owings, M.D.
Chief Resident
Department of Surgery
University of California, Davis Medical Center
Sacramento, California

Emil P. Paganini, M.D., F.A.C.P.
Associate Professor of Clinical Medicine
Head, Section of Dialysis and Extracorporeal Therapy
Department of Nephrology and Hypertension
Cleveland Clinic Foundation
Cleveland, Ohio

Sherri J. Patchen, R.N., M.S.N.
Neurological Nurse Clinician
Department of Neurosurgery
University of Miami School of Medicine
Miami, Florida

John H. Petre, Ph.D.
Director, Clinical Engineering
Division of Anesthesia
Cleveland Clinic Foundation
Cleveland, Ohio

CONTRIBUTORS

Melinda S. Phinney, M.D.
Chief Resident
Department of Medicine
Northeastern Ohio University College of Medicine
Akron City Hospital
Akron, Ohio

Joseph F. Pietrolungo, D.O.
Fellow in Cardiology
Department of Cardiology
Cleveland Clinic Foundation
Cleveland, Ohio

Edson J. Pontes, M.D.
Professor and Chairman of Urology
Wayne State University School of Medicine
Detroit, Michigan

Gary E. Raskob, M.Sc.
Assistant Professor of Medicine
Assistant Professor of Biostatistics and Epidemiology
University of Oklahoma Health Sciences Center
Oklahoma City, Oklahoma

Susan J. Rehm, M.D., F.A.C.P.
Staff Physician
Department of Infectious Diseases
Vice Chairman, Division of Education
Director, Medical Student Education
Cleveland Clinic Foundation
Cleveland, Ohio

Thomas W. Rice, M.D., F.A.C.S.
Head, Section of General Thoracic Surgery
Cleveland Clinic Foundation
Cleveland, Ohio

Jean E. Rinaldo, M.D., F.C.C.P.
Professor of Medicine
Division of Pulmonary Medicine
Chief, Pulmonary/Critical Care
Nashville Veterans Administration Medical Center
Nashville, Tennessee

Benjamin Robalino, M.D.
Fellow in Cardiology
Cleveland Clinic Foundation
Cleveland, Ohio

Herbert J. Rogove, D.O., FCCM
Director, Critical Care Services
Riverside Methodist Hospital
Clinical Associate Professor of Medicine
Ohio State University College of Medicine
Columbus, Ohio

Coleman Rotstein, M.D.
Associate Professor of Medicine
Division of Infectious Diseases
McMaster University
Hamilton, Ontario, Canada

Frank Rutledge, M.D., F.R.C.P.(C), F.C.C.P.
Associate Coordinator, Critical Care Trauma Centre
Victoria Hospital
London, Ontario, Canada

J. Dean Sandham, M.D., F.R.C.P.(C)
Chief, Division of Critical Care Medicine
University of Calgary
Director, Intensive Care Unit
Foothills Hospital
Calgary, Alberta, Canada

Robert M. Savage, M.D., F.A.C.C.
Staff Physician
Department of Cardiothoracic Anesthesia and Cardiology
Cleveland Clinic Foundation
Cleveland, Ohio

Adam Seiver, M.D., Ph.D., F.A.C.S., F.C.C.M.
Clinical Assistant Professor of Surgery
Division of Trauma and Critical Care
Stanford University School of Medicine
Stanford, California
Senior Consultant
Strategic Decisions Group
Menlo Park, California

Kathleen M. Shannon, M.D.
Assistant Professor of Neurological Sciences
Rush-Presbyterian-St. Luke's Medical Center
Chicago, Illinois

Leslie R. Sheeler, M.D.
Head, Section of Pituitary and Adrenal Disorders
Department of Endocrinology
Cleveland Clinic Foundation
Cleveland, Ohio

William J. Sibbald, M.D., F.R.C.P.(C), F.A.C.P., F.C.C.P., F.C.C.M.
Professor of Medicine
University of Western Ontario
Coordinator, Critical Care/Trauma Unit
Victoria Hospital
London, Ontario, Canada

Carl A. Sirio, M.D.
Assistant Professor of Anesthesiology and Critical Care Medicine
University of Pittsburgh School of Medicine
Pittsburgh, Pennsylvania

Edward D. Sivak, M.D., F.A.C.P., F.C.C.P., F.C.C.M.
Chief, Section of Critical Care Medicine
Meridia Huron Hospital
Assistant Clinical Professor of Medicine
University Hospitals of Cleveland
Cleveland, Ohio

Peter H. Slugg, M.D., F.A.C.P.
Associate Director, Human Pharmacology
Bristol-Myers Squibb Pharmaceutical Research Institute
Princeton, New Jersey

CONTRIBUTORS

David L. Snook, M.D.
Dermatologist
Shrewsbury, Massachusetts

Ezra Steiger, M.D., F.A.C.S.
Vice Chairman of General Surgery
Head, Section of Surgical Nutrition
Cleveland Clinic Foundation
Cleveland, Ohio

Theodore A. Stern, M.D.
Psychiatrist and Director, Residents' Division
Avery D. Weisman Psychiatry Consultation Service
Massachusetts General Hospital
Associate Professor of Psychiatry
Harvard Medical School
Boston, Massachusetts

Robert W. Stewart, M.D.
Director, Cardiac Transplantation
Department of Thoracic and Cardiac Surgery
Cleveland Clinic Foundation
Cleveland, Ohio

George E. Tesar, M.D.
Chairman of Psychiatry and Psychology
Cleveland Clinic Foundation
Cleveland, Ohio

George E. Thibault, M.D.
Professor of Medicine
Harvard Medical School
Chief, Medical Services
Brocton/West Roxbury Veterans Affairs Medical Center
West Roxbury, Massachusetts

J. Walton Tomford, M.D.
Staff Physician
Cleveland Clinic Foundation
Clinical Assistant Professor of Medicine
Case Western Reserve University School of Medicine
Cleveland, Ohio
Assistant Professor of Medicine
Ohio State University College of Medicine
Columbus, Ohio
Clinical Assistant Professor of Medicine
Pennsylvania State University
Hershey, Pennsylvania

Philip A. Villanueva, M.D.
Assistant Professor of Neurological Surgery
University of Miami School of Medicine
Co-Director, Neurosurgery Intensive Care Unit
University of Miami/Jackson Memorial Medical Center
Miami, Florida

David P. Vogt, M.D.
Staff Surgeon
Department of General and Liver Transplant Surgery
Cleveland Clinic Foundation
Cleveland, Ohio

Stephen J. Voyce, M.D.
Clinical Assistant Professor of Medicine
Hahnemann University
Scranton, Pennsylvania

Burton C. West, M.D., F.A.C.P.
Clinical Professor of Medicine
Case Western Reserve University School of Medicine
Chairman of Medicine
Meridia Huron Hospital
Cleveland, Ohio

Bruce L. Wilkoff, M.D., F.A.C.C.
Director, Cardiac Pacing and Electrophysiology Research
Director, Cardiovascular Computing
Associate Professor of Internal Medicine
Ohio State University College of Medicine
Columbus, Ohio

Eugene I. Winkelman, M.D., F.A.C.P.
Emeritus Consultant
Department of Gastroenterology
Cleveland Clinic Foundation
Cleveland, Ohio

Jay B. Wish, M.D.
Associate Professor of Medicine
Case Western Reserve University School of Medicine
Director, Hemodialysis Unit
University Hospitals of Cleveland
Cleveland, Ohio

William Witcik, M.D.
Fellow in Cardiology
Department of Cardiology
Cleveland Clinic Foundation
Cleveland, Ohio

Jean-Pierre Yared, M.D.
Associate Staff Physician
Department of Cardiothoracic Anesthesia
Cleveland Clinic Foundation
Cleveland, Ohio

Joseph Zarconi, M.D., F.A.C.P.
Assistant Professor of Medicine
Northeastern Ohio University College of Medicine
Staff Physician
Akron City Hospital
Akron, Ohio

CONTENTS

SECTION ONE. THE NERVOUS SYSTEM

1. Coma ... *Kenneth Maiese and John J. Caronna* 3
2. Neuropsychiatric Disturbance in the Critically Ill Patient ... *George E. Tesar and Theodore A. Stern* 29
3. Disorders of Temperature Regulation ... *Kathleen M. Shannon* 51
4. Intensive Care Management of Intracranial Hypertension ... *Gene H. Barnett* 65
5. Intensive Care Management of Nonischemic Brain Injuries ... *Gene H. Barnett* 76
6. Management of Seizures in the Intensive Care Unit ... *Harold H. Morris, III, and Blaise F. D. Bourgeois* 94
7. Infections of the Intracranial Central Nervous System ... *J. Walton Tomford* 102
8. Neuromuscular Disorders ... *Kerry H. Levin* 127
9. Spinal Cord Injury: An ICU Challenge for the 1990s ... *Philip A. Villanueva, Sherri J. Patchen, and Barth A. Green* 146

SECTION TWO. THE RESPIRATORY SYSTEM

10. Respiratory Failure, Respiratory Muscles, and the Work of Breathing ... *John J. Marini* 163
11. Disorders of Control of Ventilation ... *Melvin Lopata* 178
12. Management of the Upper Airway in the Critically Ill Patient ... *Mani S. Kavuru, Isaac Eliachar, and Edward D. Sivak* 189
13. Postoperative Management following Head and Neck Surgery ... *Pierre Lavertu and Mary Lynn Droughton* 212
14. Bronchospastic Disease ... *Dan J. Hendrickson and Richard J. Martin* 228
15. Management of Chronic Obstructive Pulmonary Disease ... *Richard Menzies and Peter Goldberg* 242
16. Mechanical Ventilation ... *Cyril M. Grum* 280
17. The Adult Respiratory Distress Syndrome ... *John W. Christman and Jean E. Rinaldo* 302
18. Acute Inhalation Injury ... *Edward F. Haponik* 315
19. Life-Threatening Pulmonary Hemorrhage ... *James W. Leatherman and Conrad Iber* 341
20. Management of the General Thoracic Surgical Patient ... *Thomas W. Rice, Thomas L. Higgins, and Thomas J. Kirby* 356

CONTENTS

21. Pneumonia in the Noncompromised Host ... *David L. Longworth* 385

22. Pneumonia in the Compromised Host ... *Lionel A. Mandell and Coleman Rotstein* 399

23. Pulmonary Embolism: Prevention, Diagnosis, and Management in the Critically Ill ... *Gary E. Raskob, J. Dean Sandham, and Russell D. Hull* 417

24. Rehabilitation of the Ventilator-Dependent Patient ... *Edward D. Sivak* 438

25. Utilization of Respiratory Care Services and Related Technology in the High Risk Patient ... *John J. Komara, Jr., Lucy Kester, and Dennis K. Giles* 461

Section Three. The Cardiovascular System

26. Determinants of Cardiac Function ... *Philip F. Binkley* 507

27. Common Disorders of Cardiac Rhythm and Conduction in the Critically Ill Patient ... *Bruce L. Wilkoff and Stephen L. Moore* 530

28. Cardiopulmonary Resuscitation ... *James P. Orlowski* 553

29. Acute Myocardial Infarction ... *Paul N. Casale and Benjamin Robalino* 570

30. Surgical Intervention in Myocardial Ischemia and Infarction ... *Thomas L. Higgins, Inderjit S. Gill, and Floyd D. Loop* 587

31. Nonischemic Alteration of Myocardial Function ... *Richard C. Becker and Stephen J. Voyce* 610

32. Intensive Care Aspects of Cardiac Transplantation ... *Robert W. Stewart* 640

33. Acute Valvular Regurgitation ... *Joseph F. Pietrolungo, William Witcik, and Allan L. Klein* 656

34. Management of a Hypertensive Emergency ... *Robert J. Cody* 686

35. Thoracic Aortic Dissections and Aneurysms ... *Bruce W. Lytle* 700

36. Postoperative Care of the Vascular Surgery Patient ... *Eric D. Morse and James W. Holcroft* 713

37. Postoperative Hypertension ... *Robert M. Savage, Fawzy G. Estafanous, and Thomas L. Higgins* ... 728

Section Four. The Renal System

38. Acid/Base and Electrolyte Disorders ... *Jay B. Wish and Carolyn P. Cacho* 755

39. Acute Renal Failure in the Intensive Care Setting: Prevention, Diagnosis, Treatment, and Follow-up ... *Emil P. Paganini* 783

40. Special Considerations in the Patient with Chronic Renal Failure in the Intensive Care Unit ... *Joseph Zarconi and Melinda S. Phinney* 802

41. Renal Transplantation, Revascularization, and the Hypertensive Adrenal Patient ... *Charles Lee Jackson and Andrew C. Novick* 825

42. Management of the Urologic Patient ... *Gabriel P. Haas and Edson J. Pontes* 839

Section Five. The Hematologic System and Oncologic Considerations

43. Thrombotic Thrombocytopenic Purpura and Variants ... *Steven W. Andresen and Ronald M. Bukowski* 859

44. Oncologic Toxicities and Emergencies ... *David J. Adelstein and Alan E. Lichtin* 866

45. Hematologic Disorders in the Intensive Care Unit ... *Andrea P. Baldyga* 899

Section Six. The Integument

46. Serious Gram-positive Bacterial Infections with Cutaneous Manifestations ... *David L. Snook* 925

47. Serious Gram-negative Bacterial, Ricksettsial, and Viral Infections with Cutaneous Manifestations ... *Germaine M. Camishion* 939

48. Life-Threatening Cutaneous Reactions ... *David L. Snook and Germaine M. Camishion* 958

49. Skin Problems of the Critically Ill Patient ... *Earl Z. Browne, Jr.* 976

Section Seven. The Gastrointestinal System

50. Gastrointestinal Bleeding ... *Raphael S. Chung* 989

51. Severe Intra-abdominal Infection ... *Gail S. Lebovic, Lori J. Morgan, Katherine Hodge, and Adam Seiver* 1000

52. Acute Pancreatitis ... *Charles F. Frey and Tatsuo Araida* 1015

53. Biliary Sepsis ... *Thomas A. Broughan* 1046

54. Disorders of Hepatic Function ... *Eugene I. Winkelman* 1058

55. Intensive Care Aspects of Liver Transplants ... *David P. Vogt and William D. Carey* 1134

Section Eight. The Endocrine System

56. The Diabetic Patient ... *Byron J. Hoogwerf* 1157

57. The Pituitary-Endocrine Axis ... *Leslie R. Sheeler* 1173

58. Calcium and Magnesium in Serious Illness: A Practical Approach ... *Paul L. Marino* 1183

Section Nine. General Support Considerations

59. Surgical Risks, Preoperative Assessment, and Preventive Strategies for the Critically Ill Patient ... *Edward M. Cordasco, Jr., and Joseph A. Golish* 1199

60. Fluid Resuscitation of the Critically Ill Patient ... *John T. Owings and James W. Holcroft* 1226

61. Principles of Blood Replacement ... *John C. Alverdy, Edward Levine, and Steven A. Gould* 1240

62. Nutrition Support in the Management of the Critically Ill ... *Laura E. Matarese, Ezra Steiger, and Bryan E. Jewett* 1249

63. Sedation, Pain Relief, and Neuromuscular Blockade in the Critically Ill ... *Thomas L. Higgins and Joseph P. Coyle* 1278

64. Multiple Organ System Failure: A Spectrum of Risk and of Disease ... *Frank S. Rutledge and William J. Sibbald* 1291

65. Receptor Physiology and Pharmacology in Circulatory Shock ... *Thomas L. Higgins and Bart Chernow* 1313

66. Antibiotic Pharmacokinetics ... *Marcus T. Haug, III, and Peter H. Slugg* 1338

67. Critical Care Antimicrobials: Choice and Use ... *Burton C. West and George L. Drusano* 1365

68. Acquired Immunodeficiency Syndrome ... *Susan J. Rehm* 1399

69. Substance Abuse and Overdose ... *James Dougherty and Darell Heiselman* 1424

70. Toxins and Poisonings ... *Eric P. Brass* 1454

71. Imaging Techniques in the Intensive Care Unit ... *Moulay A. Meziane* 1473

SECTION TEN. MANAGERIAL AND QUALITY ASSURANCE ISSUES

72. The Team Concept of Patient Care ... *Kathleen Dracup and Bart Chernow* 1555

73. Psychologic Stress in the Critically Ill Patient ... *Suzanne Clark* 1566

74. Quality Assessment and Assurance in the Intensive Care Unit ... *Carl A. Sirio and William A. Knaus* 1576

75. Infection Control ... *Thomas F. Keys* 1587

76. Procedures: Standards, Indications, and Quality ... *Herbert J. Rogove and Mary Jo Fitzpatrick* 1599

77. Pitfalls in Hemodynamic and Respiratory Monitoring ... *Jean-Pierre Yared* 1630

78. The Role of the Biomedical Engineer ... *John H. Petre* 1651

79. Disease Classification, Severity of Illness, Quantitation of Therapeutic Intervention, and Prediction of Outcome of Patient Care ... *Edward D. Sivak and George E. Thibault* 1664

80. Computerized Patient Management Systems for the Intensive Care Unit ... *Joel S. Gochberg and Edward D. Sivak* 1697

81. Minimizing the Risk of Liability ... *Russell C. Klein and Donna Guinn Klein* 1718

82. Foregoing Life-Supporting or Death-Prolonging Therapy ... *James P. Orlowski* 1727

Appendix: Clinical Epidemiology and Biostatistics for the Intensive Care Physician ... *John C. Marshall and Avery B. Nathens* 1739

Index 1753

Section One

THE NERVOUS SYSTEM

Chapter 1

COMA

KENNETH MAIESE
JOHN J. CARONNA

Twenty-five percent of all patients admitted to intensive care units in the United States die.[1] Individuals admitted in coma suffer a much higher mortality rate: those in coma for more than 48 hours have a 77% mortality rate. By contrast, individuals not in coma have an 11% mortality rate.[2] If one also considers the economic burden of intensive care management for high mortality patients which is estimated to exceed 40 billion dollars per year, it becomes increasingly clear that coma is one of the most important neurologic conditions. Furthermore, coma demands rapid patient assessment and treatment by the examining physician to avert death or permanent disability.

Altered states of consciousness vary in degree from mild to severe, and in kind, depending on whether the content of consciousness is impaired (as in delirium) or whether the level of consciousness is affected (as in coma).

Confusional state describes patients with altered content of consciousness manifested by poor attention span, altered sensory perception, disorientation in time and place, and impaired memory. **Delirium** occurs when a subject loses contact with the environment. Lucid periods alternate with states of disorientation, delusions, hallucinations, and agitation. **Obtundation** refers to a reduced state of alertness, and is the mildest degree of impaired level of consciousness. The obtunded patient is drowsy and spends most of the time asleep. Patients in stupor are unresponsive if not stimulated, but can be aroused by vigorous stimuli. Arousal rarely outlasts the application of the stimulus.

Coma is a state of pathologic sleep from which the patient cannot be aroused. Eye opening does not occur, and there is no comprehensive speech or purposeful movement. Reflex movements such as flexor (decorticate) or extensor (decerebrate) posturing may be present. In some cases, after a period of coma lasting hours to days, wakefulness returns without evidence of purposeful behavior or cognition. Sleep wake cycles can be preserved. This functionally decorticate state is distinct from coma and is termed the **vegetative state.**

PATHOPHYSIOLOGY OF COMA
Structural Mechanisms

Both arousal and conscious behavior define level of consciousness. The activities of the upper brain stem, reticular formation, hypothalamus, and thalamus maintain arousal (wakefulness). The ability to interact with one's environment (conscious behavior) requires intact cerebral hemispheres functioning in concert with the reticular activating system.

Cerebral Hemispheres

Damage to both cerebral hemispheres, to the diencephalon, or to the brain stem can result in coma. Studies suggest that damage, such as an infarct, to the language-dominant hemisphere produces coma.[3] In addition, sodium amobarbital injected into the carotid artery of the language-dominant hemisphere produces transient unresponsiveness. Simultaneous recordings of the electroencephalogram (EEG) may document only unilateral slowing on the side of injection. These results indicate that the dominant hemisphere plays a physiologic role in controlling state of consciousness and language function. Nevertheless, unilateral lesions to the dominant hemisphere produce only temporary coma. Unilateral lesions in either hemisphere can decrease alertness acutely, but bilateral dysfunction of the cerebral hemispheres is necessary to yield persistent coma.

Frontal Limbic System

Coma has been linked to lesions in the frontal limbic system, especially lesions due to abrupt vascular occlusions of the anterior cerebral arteries or hemorrhage into the frontal lobes. After several days of coma, patients may progress to the vegetative state, also called akinetic mutism. This state consists of preserved sleep/wake cycles, but without external evidence of mental activity or spontaneous motor activity. Coma secondary to damage to the frontal limbic system usually involves bilateral dysfunction of the cingulate gyri and portions of the septal area, frontal lobes, thalamus, or hypothalamus. An EEG usually reveals diffuse slowing over the hemisphere convexities. Thus, coma of frontal lobe origin reflects bilateral involvement of the cerebral hemispheres.

Thalamus

Bilateral lesions of the thalamus can produce coma. Medial thalamic ischemia can arise from occlusion of the basilar artery at its apex or at the origin of a perforating vessel from the basilar communicating artery. Anterior bilateral thalamic lesions are secondary to occlusion of the anterior thalamosubthalamic artery. Patients have an abrupt onset of coma that eventually progresses to an extended course of hypersomnia.

Hypothalamus

Anterior hypothalamic lesions produce behavioral manifestations consistent with sleep. Bilateral paramedian involvement of the posterior hypothalamus yields a depressed consciousness with eventual coma. It is believed that the hypothalamic lesions yielding coma also involve the adjacent midbrain reticular formation.

Midbrain and Pons

The midbrain and pons play a crucial role in maintaining consciousness. Isolated bilateral lesions of the midbrain that extend into the pontine tegmentum have resulted in coma,[4] but it is rare for unilateral lesions to do so.

Cellular Mechanisms

Coma caused by cellular neuronal damage is multifactorial in origin. Some clinical examples include:

- Ischemia
- Abnormal glucose metabolism
- Altered ionic gradients
- Excessive neurotransmitter
- Neuropeptide release

During periods of ischemia of less than 5 minutes, cell death is limited to the susceptible neurons of the hippocampus and cerebellum. Pyramidal neurons in the CA1 zone of the hippocampus are the most sensitive of all brain cells to even brief ischemia. The hippocampus is associated with memory processing, and thus, an amnestic syndrome may follow recovery from ischemic/anoxic coma.[5] Necrosis of hippocampal neurons is evident in animal models, as well as in humans, 24 hours or more following prolonged cardiac arrest with coma.[6,7] The mechanism that delays cell death in the hippocampal neurons is unknown, but may be related to calcium ion influx and excitatory neurotransmitter release.[8,9] Such disturbances may result in the death of neurons.[10-12] During the onset of cerebral ischemia, extracellular calcium rapidly flows into neurons and intracellular calcium concentrations increase 1000-fold.[13] Calcium-activated stimulation of phospholipid breakdown can initiate the release of free fatty acid products, which can yield further membrane peroxidation and free radical release.[14] Therefore, calcium-channel antagonists are under investigation as possible therapeutic agents in the treatment of cerebral ischemia.[15,16]

Following the resolution of focal or global ischemia, cerebral blood flow returns with the resumption of oxygen delivery, restoration of metabolism, and removal of toxins. Although restored cerebral blood flow prevents further neuronal death from ischemia, reperfusion can result in cell death.[17] Endothelium, which normally functions as an antithrombotic surface, can become an active procoagulant during reperfusion with clot formation resulting in subsequent ischemic neuronal death.[18] Endothelial cells also can produce superoxide, which may contribute to reperfusion.[19] Both ischemia and hypertension can result in enzymatic hydrolysis of membrane-bound phospholipids releasing arachidonic acid and other free fatty acids into the extracellular space.[20] The release of free fatty acids and the production of free radicals during postischemic recirculation can result in diffuse damage to cerebral tissue and blood vessels. The relative significance of fatty acids and free radicals in the pathogenesis of ischemic brain injury is currently under investigation.

Evidence suggests that release of excitatory neurotransmitters such as glutamate during ischemia can result in postanoxic brain damage.[21] Studies have reported central nervous system (CNS) necrosis following peripheral administration of glutamate.[22] Although exposure to glutamate results in dendritic swelling,[23] the toxic mechanism has not been established but may be a result of calcium influx into cells. During global ischemia, cell death occurs in regions dense with glutamate receptors, such as the cerebral cortex and hippocampus.[24,25] In animal experiments, glutamate antagonists have reduced or eliminated ischemic neuronal death.[26,27]

Neuropeptides have been implicated in the pathogenesis of ischemia.[28] Investigations have examined the role of opiate antagonists in animal models of ischemia.[29] Although some groups have reported improved neurologic outcome following opiate antagonist administration,[30,31] others have documented the opposite.[32,33] The mechanism of ischemic tissue preservation by opiate antagonists is currently unknown.

Modulation of adrenergic, as well as imidazole, receptors may play a role in the pathogenesis of cell death during prolonged ischemia with coma. Idazoxan, an alpha-2 adrenergic antagonist, has reduced neuronal death during global ischemia[34] and rilmenidine, an alpha-2 adrenergic agonist, has prevented cell death during focal ischemia.[35] These two agents are similar in that both occupy imidazole receptor sites, which may represent the possible mechanism for neuronal preservation and may thus provide a target for possible therapy during coma.

PRE-ICU PHASE

Risk Factors of Coma

When evaluating a patient in coma in the intensive care unit (ICU), the clinician should consider all premorbid circumstances including those which are operative in the pre-ICU phase of illness. The clinical situation prior to coma would in a sense define the risk of coma. Ultimately, one would try to intervene prior to the onset of coma, but alternatively, knowledge of the pre-ICU situation may lead to expedient diagnosis and appropriate therapeutic intervention. Risk factors can be broadly classified into structural and metabolic categories. The pathophysiologic mechanisms responsible for progressive deterioration in neurologic functions vary, but the final common pathway is coma.

Structural Lesions (Supratentorial)

Coma secondary to structural disease can arise from three different mechanisms:

- Bilateral impairment of the cortices without lesions in the brain stem will impair consciousness.
- Lesions selectively involving the rhinencephalic structures will produce coma.
- Hemispheric mass lesions that alter diencephalic structures will produce coma.

Acute or subacute destructive hemisphere lesions, such as strokes or invasive neoplasms, alter consciousness by involving the cerebrum, thalamus, or hypothalamus.

Pathophysiology of Structural Lesions

Supratentorial structural lesions displace adjacent and remote brain tissue to produce coma. Subsequent glial proliferation, inflammatory cell invasion, and vascular engorgement from the initial insult provide additional mass effect. The cerebral vascular bed influences the effect of intracranial lesions. The cerebral arterial and arteriolar bed attempt to maintain a constant cerebral perfusion with changes in systemic arterial pressure through mechanical constriction and dilation. This vascular bed is also sensitive to carbon dioxide and oxygen tensions. Intracranial insults can alter the mechanical and chemical regulation of the vascular bed resulting in passive dilatation of the vessels. This contributes to the progression of the supratentorial mass effect, and subsequent deterioration of consciousness. Intracranial lesions such as hemorrhage, abscess, and metastatic tumors produce more mass effect with edema than extra-axial lesions such as dural-based meningioma.

Intracranial hypertension secondary to obstruction of venous outflow or rise in spinal fluid pressure does not directly contribute to coma. Patients with cerebrospinal fluid (CSF) pressures of 1000 mm H_2O remain asymptomatic. Raised intracranial pressure usually produces no adverse effects secondary to the intrinsic mechanism and chemical regulation of the vascular bed. Confusion, obtundation, and coma can occur, however, when raised intracranial pressure results in increased pressure gradients. Mass lesions that obstruct CSF or venous outflow prevent even distribution of blood and spinal fluid. Volume changes thus produce gradients in intracranial pressure, yielding subsequent mass effect and coma. During the advanced stages of intracranial hypertension, episodic arterial dilatation develops, sometimes at intervals of 15 to 30 minutes, that produces transient neurologic dysfunction. Plateau waves of elevated CSF pressure may be precipitated by a rise in carbon dioxide pressure, such as during periods of sleep, postural changes, or increase in intrathoracic pressure such as during bronchospasm or coughing (Fig. 1-1). The central issue in the pathology of coma secondary to structural lesions relates consistently to abnormal intracranial compartmentation.

Mass Effect

Supratentorial herniation from mass effect results in progressive deterioration of neurologic function initially of the cerebral hemispheres and subsequently of the brain stem. There are, however, some exceptions to this rule. Acute cerebral hemorrhage can rapidly flood the ventricular system, compress the fourth ventricle, and result in acute

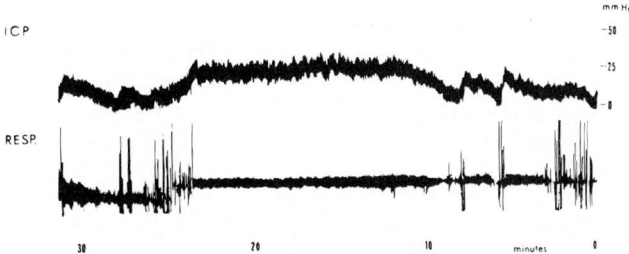

Fig. 1-1. A plateau wave shown with associated respiratory changes. (Redrawn from Hanlon, K.: Description and uses of intracranial pressure monitoring. Heart Lung, 5:281, 1976.)

medullary failure with resultant respiratory failure and death. Withdrawal of CSF during a lumbar puncture in a patient with incipient transtentorial herniation from a supratentorial mass can produce similar effects. Therefore, cranial computed tomography should precede lumbar puncture in patients with coma and focal findings. Supratentorial mass effect can be described as cingulate, central (transtentorial), or uncal herniation. These are considered to be the end result of a mass lesion (Fig. 1-2). **Cingulate herniation** refers to the displacement of the cingulate gyrus under the falx cerebri with subsequent compression of the internal cerebral vein. A mass in the cerebral hemisphere that produces cingulate herniation can compress the ipsilateral anterior cerebral artery producing subsequent vascular ischemia, edema, and mass effect. **Central**

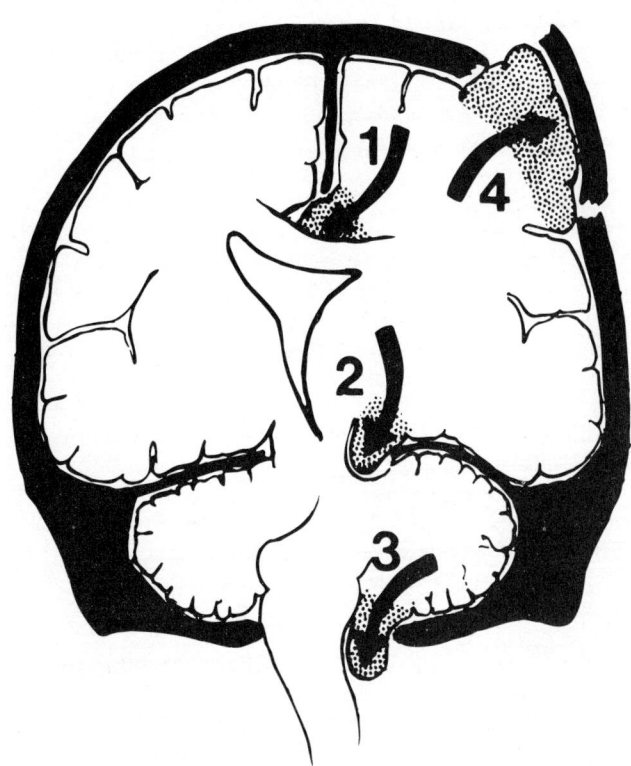

Figure 1-2. Brain herniation: cingulate (1), temporal/uncal (2), cerebellar (3), and transcalvarial (4). (Redrawn from Fishman, R. A.: N. Engl. J. Med., *293*:706, 1975.)

herniation refers to downward displacement of the hemisphere with compression of the diencephalon and midbrain through the tentorial notch. Lesions of the frontal, parietal, and occipital lobes can initially precipitate cingulate herniation and can progress to central herniation. Displacement of the diencephalon against the midbrain can produce hemorrhage in the pretectal region and thalamus. The medial perforating branches of the basilar artery become ruptured during herniation of the midbrain and pons. **Uncal herniation** involves the temporal lobe shift of the uncus and hippocampal gyrus toward the midline, which compresses the adjacent midbrain. During this process, the ipsilateral third cranial nerve and the posterior cerebral artery are compressed by the uncus and edge of the tentorium. Both central and uncal herniation can compress the posterior cerebral artery yielding occipital lobe ischemia. Further increased intracranial pressure can result from compression of the aqueduct. In this instance, CSF cannot drain from the supratentorial ventricular system, and so the pressure gradient on structures below the obstruction increases. The associated expansion of the supratentorial volume can produce pressure necrosis of the parahippocampal gyrus.

Extracerebral versus Intracerebral Lesions

Supratentorial lesions can be further classified as either extracerebral or intracerebral. Extracerebral lesions include neoplasms, infections, and trauma-related injuries such as hematomas. As a rule, however, headaches, seizures, motor/sensory deficits, and cranial nerve dysfunction usually represent the initial symptoms of neoplasms rather than an altered state of consciousness. At times, slowly progressing frontal lobe lesions can produce behavior changes prior to coma. Subdural empyema, a process secondary to otorhinologic infection, meningitis, or intracerebral abscess, can present as an extracerebral lesion. Initial presentation includes subdued consciousness, sinusitis, headaches, focal skull tenderness, and fever. Further deterioration can lead to language dysfunction, provided the dominant hemisphere is involved, hemiparesis, seizures, and eventual coma. Intracerebral lesions include neoplasms, cerebral vascular diseases, and abscesses. Initially, intracerebral disease produces focal neurologic deficits involving functions of motor, sensation, or language prior to altering consciousness. Yet, frontal lobe lesions as well as intraventricular masses may present only with changes in personality before progressing to coma.

Hemorrhage into the cerebral parenchyma is the most common cause of altered consciousness among supratentorial vascular lesions with at least 25% of all cerebral hemorrhages resulting in coma.[36] The causes of cerebral hemorrhage include:

- Intracerebral blood vessel rupture into the parenchyma
- Arterial aneurysm rupture
- Leakage of arteriovenous malformations
- Metastatic tumor hemorrhage

Primary cerebral hemorrhages secondary to hypertension usually involve the putamen, internal capsule, or thalamus and can result in coma. With involvement of these structures, patients can present initially with motor/sensory deficits, headache, or loss of language function. The size of the hemorrhage also correlates with the neurologic deficit.[37] Hemorrhage occupying one hemisphere invariably results in coma.

Intraventricular hemorrhage may result from extension of a parenchymal cerebral bleed producing little more than a chemical meningitis. Coma secondary to intraventricular hemorrhage occurs with a rapid flooding of blood into the ventricles resulting in a pressure gradient between the anterior and posterior fossae and subsequent medullary failure.

Large cerebral infarcts may present initially with obtundation that seldom progresses to coma. Loss of cardiac output and cerebral blood flow in patients suffering cerebral infarcts commonly produces coma. Systemic hypotension can be secondary to myocardial infarction, cardiac arrhythmias, or pulmonary failure. Cerebral vascular congestion and edema reach a maximum within 4 days following the cerebral infarct, however. At this point, patients are at risk of coma with transtentorial herniation.

Embolization sometimes causes coma. The pathophysiology of this process is unclear, but it may be secondary to a large hemisphere infarct that involves the hemisphere or diencephalon. Alternately, embolization may involve a "virgin area" that is opposite a previously infarcted hemisphere yielding bilateral cerebral dysfunction. Bilateral hemisphere infarcts as well as insults to the diencephalon or brain stem may arise from dissemination of the emboli.

Bilateral medial thalamic infarction with extension into the paramedian mesencephalic region acutely produces coma. This uncommon syndrome results from occlusion of the thalamosubthalamic perforating arteries arising from the posterior cerebral artery. After the abrupt onset of coma, the patient progresses to hypokinesia and apathy. Eventually, in several days, the patient is able to verbalize but suffers deficits in memory and cognition. Insults to the posteromedial thalamus yield duration of coma with eventual arousal to a vegetative state.

Cerebral vein or venous sinus occlusion can present with headache, nausea, vomiting, and eventual stupor or coma. Bacterial infections may be complicated by cavernous sinus occlusion or cortical thrombophlebitis. Venous sinus occlusion may also result from epidural tumor compression of a hypercoagulable state induced by pregnancy, contraceptive agents, collagen-vascular disease, carcinomatous meningitis or dehydration. Approximately 20% of venous sinus occlusions are idiopathic. The presentation of venous thrombosis usually depends on the site of occlusion, such as cavernous sinus lesion initially presenting with deficits of cranial nerves III, IV, V, VI. Superior sagittal sinus thrombosis may have a nonspecific course of headache, as well as seizures, before resulting in hemiparesis and coma, however. Cranial magnetic resonance imaging (MRI) is the study of choice to diagnose sagittal sinus thrombosis. Recently, combined pentobarbital coma and intraventricular drainage have been advocated prior to instituting anticoagulation therapy.[38]

Intracerebral lesions such as neoplasms or abscesses impair consciousness via the mass effect that they exert.

As the lesions enlarges, the brain parenchyma is displaced, resulting in central or uncal herniation. Hemorrhage into a tumor may follow the course of a cerebral bleed. Pituitary apoplexy represents one example of this course. The acute expansion of a pituitary tumor from infarction of hemorrhage is not completely understood. It may represent the tumor exhausting its blood supply, mass effect of the tumor comprising its vascular source, or tumor necrosis secondary to cholesterol emboli. In any event, patients present with headache, retro-orbital pain, visual field deficits from chiasmal involvement, and extraocular cranial nerve palsies. Coma ensues secondary to eventual diencephalon and brain stem compression or increase in intracranial pressure from the cerebral hemorrhage.

Miscellaneous Causes of Coma from Supratentorial Defects

Intracerebral lesions may produce coma by other mechanisms. Convulsions alter consciousness with a postictal state. Lateral or third ventricle obstruction can produce ventricular hypertension with displacement of the brain stem. Transient obstruction of ventricular outflow such as by third ventricle cysts can produce intermittent loss of consciousness. Neoplasms may also infiltrate the thalamus and hypothalamus. The involvement of the diencephalon may yield changes in cognition and behavior that progress to coma.

Structural Lesions (Subtentorial)

Lesions below the tentorium may involve the brain stem directly or impair its function by compression. Coma arises from intrinsic brain stem lesions secondary to central destruction of the paramedian midbrain or impairment of the vascular supply of the brain stem. Subtentorial brain stem ischemia rapidly produces coma secondary to reticular formation destruction (Table 1-1). Pupillary and respiratory abnormalities accompany this process. Hypoventilation should prompt intubation and mechanical ventilation. In contrast, supratentorial infarction does not abruptly alter consciousness and does not begin with pontine or midbrain dysfunction.

Lesions with mass effect may alter consciousness by exerting direct pressure on the pons and midbrain with resultant ischemia and necrosis. Upward transtentorial herniation of the cerebellum and mesencephalon occurs with enlarging masses of the posterior fossa.[39] During this process, the posterior third ventricle is compressed, obstructing CSF flow and contributing to raised intracranial pressure. Upward herniation also distorts the vasculature of the mesencephalon, compresses the veins of Galen and Rosenthal, and produces superior cerebellar infarction from occlusion of the superior cerebellar arteries. Downward herniation of the cerebellar tonsils from a posterior fossa mass occurs either as an isolated process or in conjunction with upward herniation and direct brain stem compression. It is normal for the cerebellar tonsils to extend 2 cm into the cervical canal. Downward compression of the tonsils into the foramen magnum produces ischemia of the cerebellar tonsils, medulla, and upper cervical cord (Fig. 1-3).

The differential diagnostic possibilities of causes of coma from subtentorial lesions include:

- Infarction
- Hemorrhage with hematoma formation (venous or arterial)
- Vascular malformations
- Abscesses
- Granulomas
- Neoplasm

Occlusion of the basilar artery with subsequent midbrain pontine infarction and coma can result from:

- Syphilis
- Collagen vascular disease
- Atherosclerosis
- Hypotension
- Emboli

Vertebral artery occlusion, which can lead to basilar artery ischemia, may result from vigorous cervical spine manipulation or a collagen vascular disease, such as cranial arteritis.

Approximately 75% of subtentorial, subdural, and extradural hematomas follow trauma. Veins are commonly the source of hemorrhage which can account for a subacute presentation. Occipital headache can present initially followed by vertigo, vomiting, ataxia, meningismus, and subsequent coma.

Intracranial hemorrhages in the pons can result in coma. Cerebral vascular disease is the most common risk factor for pontine hemorrhage.[40] Hemorrhage from the paramedian arterioles or from rupture of brain stem vascular malformations can extend into the fourth ventricle. Coma usually does not result from hemorrhage confined to the basis pontis. In these cases, patients lose motor function of all extremities and lower cranial nerves, but cognition remains intact, producing a "locked-in" syndrome. The common sequelae of pontine hemorrhage includes acute

Table 1-1. Clinical Findings with Subtentorial Lesions

Lesion	Clinical Syndrome
Rupture of veins due to trauma to cerebellar area	Occipital headache, followed by vertigo, ataxia, meningismus
Pontine hemorrhage	Loss of motor function of all extremities and lower cranial nerves ("Locked-in" Syndrome)
	Acute coma, ataxic breathing, pinpoint, nonreactive pupils, loss of oculocephalic response, quadriplegia
Intra-cerebellar hemorrhage	Progressive occipital headache, vomiting, vertigo, dysarthria, ataxia, oculomotor dysfunction, lower extremity paralysis, altered consciousness
Vertebral and cerebellar artery ischemia-cerebellar infarction	Vertigo, nystagmus, ataxia, dysarthria headaches
Posterior fossa abscess	Fever, meningismus, occipital headache

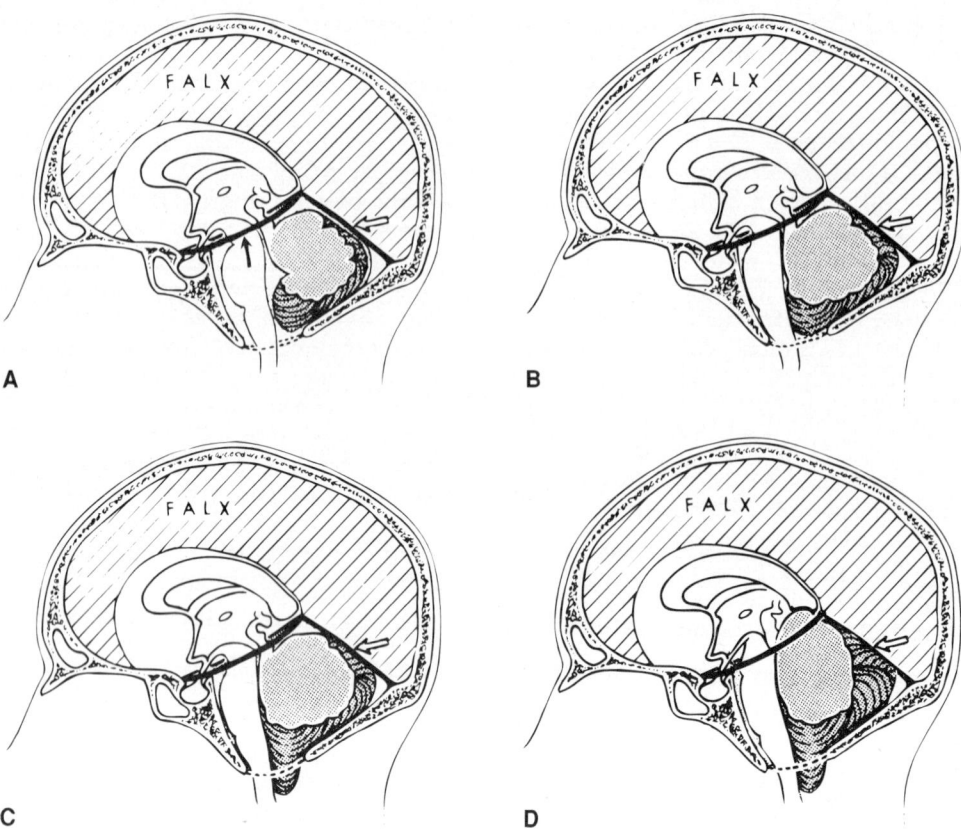

Fig. 1-3. Midsagittal sections of the brain. A, Normal anatomy; open arrow indicates tentorium and closed arrow indicates free margin of tentorium. B, Direct brain stem compression. C, Downward cerebellar herniation. D, Upward and downward cerebellar herniation. (Redrawn from Cuneo, R. A., et al.: Upward transtentorial herniation: seven cases and a literature review. Arch. Neurol., 36:619, 1979.)

coma, ataxic breathing, pinpoint, nonreactive pupils, loss of oculocephalic response, and quadriplegia.[41]

One tenth of subtentorial parenchymal intracranial hemorrhages occur in the cerebellum. Hemorrhages less than 2-3 cm usually result in focal dysfunction. Occipital headache, oculomotor dysfunction, and unilateral cerebellar disturbance represent the degree of impairment. Larger hemorrhages can infiltrate the brain stem to produce coma. Patients with progressive occipital headache, vomiting, vertigo, dysarthria, ataxia, oculomotor dysfunction, lower extremity paralysis, and altered consciousness require immediate surgical decompression. Patients that have progressed to the level of pontine hemorrhage with coma have a poor prognosis.[42] Hypertension is the cause of cerebellar hemorrhage in most patients. The disorder is also seen with posterior fossa angiomas and anticoagulant therapy.

Vertebral and cerebellar artery ischemia can result in acute cerebellar infarction. Following the insult, cerebellar edema acts as a posterior fossa mass lesion resulting in brain stem compression and coma. Clinical onset includes vertigo, nystagmus, ataxia, dysarthria, and headache. If surgical decompression is not performed, the course progresses to quadriplegia, stupor, and coma. Atherosclerotic disease of the vertebral or inferior cerebellar arteries and hypertension appear to be risk factors for cerebellar infarction.

Abscesses of the cerebellum and of the pontine and midbrain tegmentum that destroy the reticular system produce coma. Usually, plegia and extraocular dysfunction gradually develop prior to coma. The diagnosis of a posterior fossa abscess becomes suspect with fever, meningismus, and occipital headache. One quarter of cases have a middle ear source.

Granulomas and neoplasms may also involve the posterior fossa. Progressive loss of integrity of the brain stem will eventually result in coma. Lethargy and dementia are observed prior to this, especially with obstructive hydrocephalus of the fourth ventricle. Table 1-1 summarizes some of the common clinical findings in subtentorial lesions that can progress to coma.

Metabolic Disease

Alteration in cognitive function is the earliest presentation of metabolic encephalopathy, and if allowed to proceed unchecked, it progresses to coma.[43] Although levels of attention and alertness are affected in metabolic coma, each disease process also yields an agitated state while subclinical deficits directly result in coma. For example, severe anoxic ischemia following cardiac arrest reproduces coma, whereas alcohol withdrawal initially results in an agitated delirium. Metabolic encephalopathy is often reversible if the underlying systemic disorder is corrected. The anatomic locus of metabolic brain disease has not been clearly defined.

Hypoxia

Lack of oxygen to the brain can be divided into anoxic anoxia, anemic anoxia, and ischemia. Anoxic anoxia consists of low arterial oxygen content and tension, possibly secondary to decreased oxygen in the environment or inability for oxygen to enter the circulatory system, as in pulmonary disease. Anemic anoxia consists of low oxygen content in the blood secondary to decreased hemoglobin content. Ischemic anoxia is a state of insufficient cerebral blood flow. "Low flow states" may result from cardiovascular collapse or conditions of increased vascular resistance such as stroke or migraine. The brain normally consumes approximately 3.5 ml of oxygen for each 100 g of brain tissue per minute. Delirium supervenes when this rate declines to 2.5 ml. Rates of cerebral oxygen metabolism below 2 ml/100 g per minute are incompatible with a conscious state.

Organs vary in their tolerance to ischemia. Renal tubular cells and myocardial cells can tolerate periods of circulatory arrest of up to 30 minutes; liver cells up to 1 to 2 hours; and lung tissue more than 2 hours. Because the brain uses oxygen to metabolize glucose and cannot store oxygen, it survives only for minutes after its oxygen supply is reduced below critical levels.[44] Pyramidal cells in Sommer's sector of the hippocampus, Purkinje cells of the cerebellum, and pyramidal cells of the third and fifth layers of the cerebral cortex are vulnerable to even moderate degrees of anoxia. Widespread necrosis of the cortex with the brain stem intact produces a vegetative state. More profound anoxia affecting the cortex, basal ganglia, and brain stem results in coma and subsequent death.[45]

Ninety percent of the cerebral energy required to maintain nerve transmission and regulate ionic gradients across cell membranes is derived from the oxidation of glucose. During hypoxia, aerobic metabolism of glucose fails, and glycolysis, the anaerobic degradation of glucose to lactate and pyruvate, is accelerated. Lactate, the end product of anaerobic glycolysis, appears in increased concentrations in the brain, CSF, and cerebral venous blood. This cerebral acidosis leads to cerebral arteriolar dilatation and an increase in cerebral blood flow. The energy produced during hypoxia is insufficient to meet normal metabolic requirements thereby yielding confusion, agitation, and coma. With acute anoxia, consciousness is lost within 15 seconds. The EEG slows with arterial oxygen pressure below 35 mm Hg or with cerebral blood flow less than 40% of normal. Loss of the EEG tracing occurs when cerebral oxygen pressure reaches 20 mm Hg or following 20 seconds of complete anoxia.

Conditions that reduce cerebral blood flow or blood oxygen content can also result in secondary depression of the myocardium. Hypoxia complicated by hypotension is more severe than uncomplicated hypoxia because, in the former, delivery of oxygen and glucose is diminished as is the removal of metabolic degradation products. In any event, several disease states can result in coma as a result of cessation of circulation or prolonged hypoxia.

Occlusion of the pulmonary arteries, which occurs with **pulmonary embolism,** produces an abrupt drop in cardiac output and cerebral blood flow. Approximately two thirds of patients have alterations in consciousness. With a large embolus, diffuse cerebral ischemia with coma is accompanied by cardiovascular collapse. In addition to disorders of cognition, individuals may also suffer from chest pain, dyspnea, syncope, or focal neurologic dysfunction.

Fat embolism in which pulmonary and cerebral vessels become occluded with lipid and fibrin debris can produce cerebral ischemia.[46] Ischemia can result from respiratory failure with multiple pulmonary microemboli yielding hypoxia or intrinsic involvement of the cerebral vasculature. Diffuse neurologic signs of lethargy, stupor, and coma can occur in conjunction with focal deficits such as monoplegia.[47] A cutaneous petechial hemorrhage on the upper torso and neck also develops. The syndrome is seen in association with musculoskeletal trauma, steroid therapy, burns, pancreatic inflammation, and alcoholic hepatic disease.

Coma also occurs in association with **cardiac surgery.** Emboli, as well as episodes of hypotension during surgery, can lead to diffuse cerebral ischemia. Although patients may survive the initial insult, cognitive deficits may be present in approximately one third of such patients.

Severe degrees of **anemia,** myocardial infarction, congestive heart failure, and pulmonary disease can lead to coma. One may witness neurologic deterioration with lethargy, small reactive pupils, myoclonus, and hemiplegia with progressive cerebral hypoperfusion. Coma is seen with isolated anemia in patients with 50% reduction of blood oxygen-carrying capacity.

Hypertensive encephalopathy leads to diffuse cerebral ischemia. Alterations of the blood-brain barrier, arteriole necrosis, and diffuse infarcts and hemorrhages are present in this syndrome. Some patients may suffer from chronic hypertension with acute increases in blood pressure. These acute rises in systolic pressure are transient but recurrent and can cause headache, agitation, cortical blindness, delirium, seizures, and coma. These attacks can last from minutes to days. Reduction of systemic blood pressure resolves these symptoms; however, a decrease in systolic pressure markedly below baseline for an individual may yield cerebral ischemia or infarction.

Disseminated intravascular coagulation involves platelet aggregation, fibrin deposition in arterioles, venules, and capillaries. Patients may suffer from altered cognition, speech, delirium, or in some cases, coma. The syndrome is secondary to disorders of sepsis, malignancy, and collagen vascular disease. Complications include dermal and fundoscopic hemorrhage, as well as subdural and intracerebral bleeding. Serum blood evaluation reveals thrombocytopenia, hypofibrinogenemia, and increased fibrin split products. Similar alteration in mental status can occur from platelet consumption in thrombotic thrombocytopenia purpura (see Chap. 44).

Migraine headaches can result in coma. The mechanism is believed secondary to vascular insufficiency of the tributaries of the basilar artery. Symptoms range from confusion, fever, meningismus, ataxia, syncope, and amnesia to coma. Most episodes of coma resolve within 24 hours, but they can persist for days and may be precipitated by head trauma, work, and angiography.[48] Approximately 80% of patients have a positive family history.

Fifty percent of the fatal poisonings in the United States are secondary to **carbon monoxide.** Elevated blood levels of carbon monoxide that result in hypoxia can lead to coma. Complications can include residual disease, pulmonary edema, and psychiatric disease.[49] Neither clinical presentation nor level of carboxyhemoglobin predicts patient outcome. Hyperbaric oxygen has been advocated over normobaric oxygen as the preferred treatment.[50,51]

Hypoxemia with coma can be secondary to **near drowning.** The hypoxemia results from either diffuse atelectasis induced by surfactant inactivation from freshwater aspiration or physiologic shunting from diffuse alveolar flooding of salt water. Near drowning complicated by coma can result in permanent neurologic sequelae. Aggressive pulmonary management with positive end-expiratory pressure (PEEP) of continuous positive airway pressure (CPAP) can reduce the incidence of permanent neurologic injury.[52]

Hypoglycemia

Under physiologic conditions, glucose is the brain's only substrate and crosses the blood-brain barrier by facilitated transport. The normal brain uses about 5.5 mg (31 μmol) of glucose per 100 g tissue each minute. If there is hypoglycemia, which is defined in adults as a blood glucose concentration of less than 40 mg/dl, signs and symptoms of encephalopathy result secondary to cerebral cortex and/or brain stem dysfunction. The cerebral cortex is more vulnerable to the effects of hypoglycemia however, whereas the brain stem and basal ganglia exhibit less histologic damage during periods of reduced serum glucose.

Neurologic presentation during hypoglycemia can vary from focal motor or sensory deficits to coma. Acute symptoms of hypoglycemia are better correlated with the rate at which blood glucose levels decrease than with the degree of hypoglycemia. The blood glucose level at which cerebral metabolism fails and symptoms develop varies among individuals, but, in general, confusion occurs at levels below 30 mg/dl and coma at levels below 10 mg/dl. The brain stores approximately 2 g of glucose and glycogen. For this reason, a patient in hypoglycemic coma may survive 90 minutes without suffering irreversible brain damage.

The etiology of metabolic coma from hypoglycemia is not well defined. Brain energy reserves are well maintained during the first 90 minutes of hypoglycemic coma. Thus, the disorder cannot solely be attributed to lack of cerebral energy. During hypoglycemia, amino acids such as gamma-aminobutyric acid (GABA), glutamate, glutamine, and alanine as well as acetylcholine synthesis are suppressed. Whether reduction of these agents or alteration in nerve synaptic transmission significantly contributes to the onset of coma associated with severe hypoglycemia is unknown.

Infection

Severe cases of **bacterial meningitis** can lead to significant cerebral edema and coma.[53] The edema can result in transtentorial as well as cerebellar tonsillar herniation. In addition, meningitis may lead to vasculitis with subsequent occlusion of cerebral vessels, as well as both communicating and noncommunicating hydrocephalus.

Both subacute **bacterial endocarditis** and nonbacterial thrombotic endocarditis can lead to widespread cerebral infarction. Usually, a focal deficit occurs with release of emboli. In severe cases, however, patients present with an encephalopathic picture of depressed cognition and delirium that progresses to coma.

Plasmodium falciparum can extend to involve the central nervous system (CNS). Focal neurologic signs are reported, but most patients present with confusion, lethargy, and sometimes coma. Chills and fever follow the course of the systemic illness. Theories concerning the etiology of the cerebral ischemia from malaria include occlusion of vessels from parasite-infected erythrocytes, perivascular hemorrhage, reduced oxygen from infected erythrocytes, and disseminated intravascular coagulation.

The most common viral agents that cause **encephalitis** and coma are the arboviruses such as Eastern equine, Western equine, and St. Louis encephalitis and herpes simplex virus type 1 and type 2. One must also be familiar with less prominent viral causes of coma. Infection with the Epstein-Barr virus (EBV), which has been implicated in multiple systemic disorders, can present as coma. Clinical signs include mydriasis, nystagmus, respiratory insufficiency, and decerebrate posturing. Treatment with intravenous acyclovir can reverse the process if therapy is instituted early in the course of infection.[54] Disseminated herpes zoster infection is another rare cause of coma. As many as 30% of patients have asymptomatic meningitis. Coma usually occurs only in immunocompromised individuals and is preceded by a cutaneous dermatomal rash, headache, confusion, and sometimes, hemiplegia.

Herpes simplex encephalitis presents with a variety of signs including coma. Genital herpes simplex virus type 2 presents with acute meningitis even without genital lesions.[55] Prognosis has been good in 50% of survivors. Hemiplegia and aphasia usually resolve within months. Nevertheless, 33% of the patients with "favorable outcome" suffer from permanent neurologic sequelae, which include the Korsakoff syndrome. Good prognosis has been attributed to early treatment with acyclovir. Those patients who lapse into prolonged coma suffer from respiratory dysfunction and die usually within 4 months.[56]

Drugs

At least 10% of patients with acute drug intoxication require admission to an ICU. Complications of any drug overdose include hypotension, hypertension, anemia, neuropathies, renal failure, cardiac arrest, and coma. Approximately 50% of patients use multiple drugs.[57] Proper diagnosis relies heavily on the physical examination since an accurate or complete history may be unobtainable from the patient. Screening of blood and urine for toxins aids in the diagnosis, but it has limitations because the interactions among multiple drugs and the different rates of gastric absorption alter subsequent serum and urine drug levels. Some common drugs that can produce an overdose include:

- Barbiturate
- Alcohol
- Glutethimide
- Benzodiazepines

- Opiates and heroin
- Cocaine
- Tricyclic antidepressants
- Lithium
- Valproate

Excessive **barbiturate consumption** results in hypothermia, hypotension, and in extreme cases, apnea. Initially, vestibular and cerebellar function are affected by the drug, resulting in dysarthria, nystagmus, and ataxia. Pupils remain small and reactive with ciliospinal reflexes. In coma, the oculocephalic and oculovestibular responses are depressed or even absent. Hyporeflexia and flaccid tone usually accompany barbiturate overdose except in cases of rapid ingestion where hyperreflexia and extensor plantar responses are temporarily evident.

Alcohol ingestion can be indistinguishable from other encephalopathies such as depressant drug intoxication or hypoglycemia. In addition, progressive loss of consciousness may be complicated by underlying cerebral trauma such as a subdural hematoma. Evidence of "alcohol on the breath" provides insight into the cause of the coma, but it does not enable one to distinguish between intoxication by pure alcohol and that caused by a "cocktail" of alcohol, sedative, and hypnotic drugs. As the blood alcohol level rises the following sequelae are seen:

- At blood alcohol levels above 100 mg/dl, individuals become confused, ataxic, and dysarthric.
- Levels above 200 mg/dl can result in diplopia and lethargy.
- Levels greater than 300 mg/dl lead to reactive, midposition pupils, hypothermia, hypoventilation, tachycardia, and coma.

Determinations of serum alcohol levels have been recommended for patients in whom such determinations are necessary to guide treatment. The alcohol level should be determined in individuals who have used alcohol and have abused multiple drugs who present with trauma, seizures, psychosis, or coma.[58]

The presentation of glutethimide poisoning is similar to that of excessive barbiturate consumption. Although individuals can experience prolonged coma, subjects may regain partial consciousness of oculocephalic responses with repetitive tactile noxious stimuli. Glutethimide poisoning differs from barbiturate overdose in that pupils are mid-position, unequal and sometimes fixed with loss of ciliospinal reflexes. Ingestion of greater than 10 g or plasma concentrations exceeding 30 μg/ml are usually associated with coma. In addition to high levels of plasma concentration, predictors of poor outcome include advanced age and coingestion of barbiturates.[59]

Benzodiazepines can yield stupor as well as coma; however, limited or no cardiovascular or respiratory depression occurs. Large amounts of these agents depress oculocephalic and oculovestibular responses. Pupils are small but reactive. Recent clinical trials have studied the efficacy of the benzodiazepines antagonist flumazenil. Resolution of coma was noted as rapidly as 2 minutes following injection and consciousness was maintained up to 45 minutes. No evidence of withdrawal symptoms was present. In addition, flumazenil was considered to have a diagnostic value in cases of mixed drug intoxications.[60,61,62]

Opiate and heroin overdoses occur by either parenteral injection or sniffing of the agent. Systemic complications include hypothermia, hypotension, bradycardia, respiratory slowing, and pulmonary edema. The onset of coma does not require long-term opiate administration and can result following an initial injection of the opiate. Patients in opiate coma characteristically have pinpoint pupils sluggishly reactive to bright light.

Toxicity from **cocaine administrative** has systemic, psychiatric, and neurologic manifestations. Cocaine has been shown to induce coronary artery constriction,[63] myocardial infarction,[64] sinus tachycardia, premature ventricular contractions, ventricular fibrillation and asystole,[65] aortic artery rupture,[66] and intestinal ischemia.[67] Psychiatric manifestations of cocaine use include anxiety, agitation, depression, paranoia, and visual and auditory hallucinations. Suicidal ideation can be the initial presentation.[68,69] The causes of behavior disturbances secondary to cocaine use are unknown, but they are believed to be related to the agent's effect on norepinephrine, serotonin, and dopamine levels. Neurologic complications of cocaine use range from benign headaches to coma. Seizures are the most common presentation and are usually generalized and self-limited. Status epilepticus can occur and can result in persistent cognitive disturbance.[68] Seizures are believed to be related to cocaine's direct convulsant properties as well as its ability to generate seizure activity.[70] Focal neurologic manifestations from cocaine ingestion include:

- Subarachnoid hemorrhage[71]
- Anterior spinal artery syndrome
- Lateral medullary syndrome
- Transient ischemic attacks[72]
- Cerebral infarction[73]

Tachycardia and blood pressure elevation occur within minutes of intranasal administration of cocaine.[71] Although the exact mechanism of cocaine-related cerebral vascular disease is unknown, adrenergic stimulation and surges in blood pressure may play a significant role. In addition, cerebral vasculitis has been associated with cocaine abuse.[74]

Individuals with a headache following cocaine use usually have a benign course. Headaches often occur in association with nausea, arthralgia, and chest pain.[68] Although the intensity and focality of the headaches can vary, symptoms usually resolve within 1 week. More severely, individuals can succumb to transient loss of consciousness. The unresponsiveness can resolve over several minutes and is usually attributed to syncope, although patients can suffer from prolonged coma with increased mortality if coma is accompanied by systemic complications of hyperthermia,[75] renal failure, or cardiac failure.

Overmedication with **tricyclic antidepressant** (TCA) agents leads to cardiovascular and neurologic dysfunction. In one study, amitriptyline accounted for 70% of the cases of self-poisoning with antidepressant agents. Half the patients had taken more than one agent, and one third had ethanol in their blood.[76] Approximately 20% of such patients have cardiac manifestations including supraventricular tachycardia. The most common electrocardiographic (ECG) abnormalities include alterations of the T waves, right bundle branch block, and left bundle branch block. Ventricular dysrhythmia resulting in cardiac arrest also can occur.[77] A QRS interval greater than or equal to 100 msec is predictive of seizures of ventricular arrhythmias.[78] A Glasgow coma scale of less than 8 has been reported to be a more sensitive predictor of eventual complications than a QRS interval prolongation and mandates intensive care monitoring.[79] Desipramine has the highest incidence of seizures (17.9%) when compared to other tricyclic antidepressants. Seizures were also more common with overdosage of the cyclic antidepressants amoxapine and maprotiline.[80] Because toxicity with TCA occurs soon after ingestion of the drug, complete digestive evacuation is required in addition to ventilatory and hemodynamic assistance.[81] Recently, prenalterol, a cardioselective beta agonist, has been reported as efficacious in the treatment of bradycardia and hypotension following TCA poisoning.[82]

Lithium toxicity can present with tremors, akathisia, and inattention. The toxicity may be delayed by several days following initial ingestion and may progress to seizures, lethargy, and coma. Treatment consists of supportive care with artificial ventilation and fluid and electrolyte infusions in conjunction with hemodialysis.[83]

Valproate intoxication can occur if drug levels are not closely monitored or during suicide attempts. It has also been reported with carnitive insufficiency.[84] Elevated serum concentrations can result in prolonged coma and permanent neurologic sequelae following resolution of the coma.[85] Significant cerebral edema has been noted with valproate intoxication with levels of 2300 μmol/L. Treatment in these cases should be directed toward the prevention or reduction of diffuse cortical edema.[86]

Several agents can cause metabolic acidosis either by direct action or through by-products of the original agents. These drugs usually produce confusion, stupor, and subsequent coma. On ingestion, **methanol** is degraded into formaldehyde, which affects retinal ganglion cells. Toxicity can occur abruptly or over several days. **Ethylene glycol** is metabolized to glycolaldehyde, oxalic acid, and hippuric acid. Significant metabolic acidosis rapidly occurs with subsequent disorientation, seizures, and coma. An examination is significant for papilledema, nystagmus, and oxalic acid crystals in the urine. **Salicylates** can yield initially tinnitus, dyspnea, and seizures that progress to coma. The agent causes a metabolic acidosis in the tissues, but this is compensated by a respiratory alkalosis. The urine remains acidotic. During stupor or coma, pupillary responses, and oculocephalics remain intact, but extensor plantar responses may be present. **Potassium cyanide** poisoning also results in severe metabolic acidotic. **Sodium nitroprusside,** an agent used in low-output congestive heart failure, is metabolized into cyanide and is excreted by the kidney as thiocyanate. Cyanide toxicity may develop during bolus infusion, after administration for longer than 72 hours, or during periods of renal insufficiency. Cardiopulmonary arrest and coma are frequent in patients with severe intoxication.[87] Treatment consists of assisted ventilation, gastric lavage, and sodium bicarbonate administration. Administration of beta stimulants and hydrocobalamin has also been advocated.[88] **Ibuprofen,** a popular "over-the-counter" analgesic agent, is rarely associated with CNS toxicity, although this agent, which can result in metabolic acidosis, can produce lethargy as well as coma.[89] Treatment of the underlying acidemia, renal dysfunction, and gastric bleeding is advocated.[90,91]

Blockade of central cholinergic neurotransmission during anesthesia or intensive care management may be induced by opiates, benzodiazepines, pheothiazines, butyrophenones, ketamine, etomidate, nitrous oxide, and cimetidine. This central anticholinergic syndrome mimics atropine intoxication and consists of hallucinations, confusion, seizures, respiratory depression, and coma. Postanesthetic central anticholinergic syndrome can be avoided by administrating physostigmine during the anesthesia. Central anticholinergic syndrome during intensive care management can be also treated with physostigmine, which has proved efficacious in the treatment of cholinergic blockade agitation during mechanical ventilation.[92]

Demyelinating Disease

Diffuse demyelination of the CNS can progress to coma. **Adrenoleukodystrophy,** a disorder of diffuse demyelination in the CNS, is a sex-linked recessive trait that affects male adolescents. Initial symptoms involve changes in behavior, gout, and loss of vision. Many individuals are not clinically adrenal insufficient. As the disease progresses, seizures become subsequent coma. **Progressive multifocal leukoencephalopathy** is a disorder of diffuse multifocal demyelination of white matter secondary to infection with the papovavirus. Immunocompromised individuals with neoplasms (lymphomas), collagen vascular disease (sarcoid), or acquired immunodeficiency syndrome (AIDS) are at greatest risk. Over several months, this disease results in hemiparesis, visual loss, and ataxia, with eventual progression to coma. **Focal demyelination** of the CNS, such as in multiple sclerosis, usually does not result in coma. One must be aware of prior evidence of localized demyelination when evaluating patients in coma, however. Individuals with bilateral internuclear ophthalmoplegia and cervical myelopathy who suffer cardiac or pulmonary arrest may clinically appear to have a poor chance of recovery or even complete loss of brain stem function. In fact, some of these individuals experience "reversible coma" with rapid recovery to baseline if their clinical presentation was primarily a result of focal demyelinating disease.[93]

Endocrine Disease

Diabetes mellitus can result in coma through several mechanisms. **Diabetic ketoacidosis** results in dehydration, hyperosmolality, hypotension, and metabolic acidosis. Each of these factors contributes to a depressed level of consciousness. Patients who eventually become comatose also suffer from hypothermia. **Nonketotic hyperglycemic hyperosmolality** alone can result in coma. Patients at risk are the elderly with adult-onset noninsulin-dependent diabetes, those individuals receiving diuretic agents such as mannitol or drugs that lead to hyperglycemia such as corticosteroids, and patients undergoing cardiac surgery.[94] Individuals who become symptomatic have blood glucose levels higher than 800 mg/dl, are severely dehydrated, and may have moderate lactic acidosis.

Patients can present with focal or general seizures, cerebral ischemic infarction, or lethargy progressing to coma. Diabetic lactic acidosis also causes dehydration, significant hypotension, and metabolic acidosis similar to diabetic ketoacidosis; however, the syndrome differs in that ketone bodies are not evident in the serum and lactic acidosis usually occurs in patients using oral hypoglycemic agents. Diabetes can lead to coma by several other mechanisms. Autonomic neuropathy can cause orthostatic hypotension, ventricular arrhythmias, and subacute myocardial ischemia. Rapid reversal of a hyperosmolar state can result in significant cerebral edema with coma. Chronic diabetes can be complicated by renal insufficiency, uremic coma, hypertension, and increased risk of cerebral vascular secondary to the elevated blood pressure and in association with diabetic arteriosclerosis.

Hypothyroidism occurs in approximately 2% of the population over 65 years old. Most cases of hypothyroidism are secondary to primary thyroid dysfunction, but the syndrome can also result from radioiodine therapy, thyroidectomy, and autoimmune thyroiditis.[95] Initial clinical symptoms include fatigue, inattentiveness, and memory loss. Progression of the disease results in ataxia, peripheral neuropathy, sensorineural hearing loss, vestibular disease, seizures, and eventually myxedema coma. Myxedema coma may be precipitated by phenobarbital, narcotic, or phenothiazine use secondary to decreased rates of metabolism of these agents. Myxedema is also characterized by hypothermia, pleural and pericardial effusions, bradycardia, ventricular arrhythmia, respiratory acidosis, hypoxia, and hypoglycemia. In light of the immediate respiratory risk with myxedema coma, patients are to be managed in an ICU. An individual's cardiovascular status is most predictive of eventual outcome.[96] Because initial large loading doses have been reported to precipitate tissue hypoxia and myocardial ischemia, low dose triiodothyronine replacement has been proposed.[97]

Thyrotoxicosis can be precipitated by infection, surgery, or levothyroxine overdosage. Initial presentation includes tremor, anxiety, and confusion. During thyroid storm, symptoms progress with fever, tachycardia, pulmonary edema, cardiac dysrhythmia, congestive heart failure, and coma. Some elderly patients with thyrotoxicosis may initially present with apathy and depression and may progress to coma if left untreated. Patients in thyroid storm require acute intensive care management. Plasma extraction has recently been proposed for treatment of thyroxine intoxication.[98]

Hypoadrenalism (Addison's disease), in the untreated state, can produce delirium and coma. Addisonian crisis is associated with hypotension, hyponatremia, hyperkalemia, and hypoglycemia. Affected individuals develop flaccid tone, loss of deep tendon reflexes, seizures, and occasionally papilledema from cerebral edema secondary to glucocorticoid deficiency. Hypoadrenalism may be secondary to acute infections such as cytomegalovirus, may follow surgical procedures, or may be introduced iatrogenically by sudden withdrawal of exogenous steroids following long-term use.

Hyperadrenalism (Cushing's syndrome) infrequently results in coma. Excess glucocorticoids usually yield an encephalopathy with either euphoria or depression. Chronic elevation of steroids may result in metabolic alkalosis with hypokalemia. Eventual coma may ensue secondary to increased P_{CO_2} and decreased P_{O_2} from compensatory respiratory depression.

Pituitary disease is also an uncommon cause of coma. A pituitary tumor that quickly exceeds its blood supply may hemorrhage during pituitary apoplexy. The subsequent mass lesion with possible subarachnoid hemorrhage may result in coma. Hypopituitarism may also lead to thyroid and adrenal insufficiency secondary to loss of trophic hormones to these organs. Coma in this instance would be a result of hypothyroidism and/or hypoadrenalism.

Systemic Disease

Coma may be a manifestation of hepatic, renal, pancreatic, and pulmonary disease. These disorders are briefly highlighted because they are discussed more extensively in later chapters.

Hepatic encephalopathy may initially present as an agitated, as well as an apathetic, delirium. Lateral gaze nystagmus and ocular bobbing have been noted. Oculomotor paralysis usually occurs only in association with Wernicke's disease. Asterixis is present in the jaw, hands, and feet. The etiology of hepatic coma is unclear, but ammonia elevations in blood and brain appear to play a role. Ammonia can halt energy metabolism of neurons, as well as be directly neurotoxic. A reduction in systemic ammonia levels can resolve the coma; however, ammonia levels do not correlate directly with the extent of mental impairment.

Current theories of the neurochemical cause for hepatic encephalopathy implicate the activation of the neurotransmitter GABA. Some animal models of hepatic encephalopathy have shown increased GABA receptors.[94] Because benzodiazepines can modulate GABA activity, the benzodiazepine antagonist flumazenil can also correct mental impairment in individuals with hepatic encephalopathy.[100] In addition, diazepam binding inhibitor, a neuropeptide that may regulate GABA transmission, is preferentially increased in the CSF of patients with hepatic encephalopathy.[101]

Renal failure, if untreated with dialysis, can lead to uremic encephalopathy. Similar to other metabolic disorders, uremia can produce confusion, agitation, delirium, tremor, asterixis, and seizures that eventually progress to coma. Uremia is also characterized by metabolic acidosis, aseptic meningitis with elevated CSF protein, multifocal myoclonus, and tetany. Papilledema does not usually occur. Although the condition resolves with correction of serum electrolytes and blood urea nitrogen, the mechanism of the disorder is unknown. Elevated concentrations of urea alone do not result in coma. The factors believed to account for uremic encephalopathy include increased permeability of the blood-brain barrier, metabolic acidosis, altered potassium and serum levels, and increased cerebral calcium levels.

During the first week of **pancreatitis,** individuals may experience abdominal pain with delirium, hallucinations, seizures, and coma. The etiology of the disorder is unknown, but cerebral edema, fat and fibrin thrombi, and areas of demyelination have been noted in autopsy.

Hypoventilation in conjunction with disorders such as obstructive pulmonary disease, pulmonary edema, obesity, and neuromuscular disease can subsequently lead to coma. Patients may initially complain of headache and may become lethargic. Asterixis and myoclonus are common, and some patients may have evidence of increased intracranial pressure with papilledema secondary to carbon dioxide retention. Although patients experience hypoxia as well as hypercapnia during pulmonary disease, the hypercapnia corresponds best with the degree of mental impairment. In fact, levels of carbon dioxide in excess of 95 mm Hg are anesthetic. Treatment involves mechanical respiratory assistance in severe cases to ensure adequate oxygenation and resolution of carbon dioxide retention; however, rapid correction of hypercapnia with subsequent metabolic alkalosis of serum pH greater than 7.60 can lead to seizures and coma.

Seizures

Although epilepsy is discussed in Chapter 6, seizures in relation to coma is discussed here. Seizures alter consciousness during both ictal and postictal periods. Coma is usually a result of a generalized seizure, although petit mal status and complex partial status may infrequently produce stupor and coma. The postictal period is defined as a period of depressed consciousness without active epileptic activity. Clinical presentation during this period may range from delirium to stupor. The postictal period can last greater than 24 hours but usually resolves within 15 to 30 minutes following a convulsion. Pupillary function and oculovestibular responses remain intact. Individuals are usually hyperpneic secondary to metabolic acidosis by muscular production of lactic acid. Approximately 50% of patients during the postictal period have bilateral extensor plantar responses.

Status epilepticus is characterized by repetitive seizures during which the patient never regains consciousness. Untreated patients suffer anoxic brain damage. The individual may require general anesthesia if anticonvulsants do not control the seizures. Seizures, including status epilepticus, as well as myoclonus, frequently follow cerebral anoxia, as occurs in cardiac arrest. Approximately 40% of survivors of cardiac arrest in one study experienced residual seizures or myoclonus.[102] Status epilepticus and myoclonic status epilepticus following encephalopathy were suggestive of poor outcome with inability to regain consciousness.[102,103] In addition, electrographic status without somatic motor manifestations was also suggestive of poor outcome.[104]

Seizures may be the result of underlying metabolic disorders, destructive lesions such as those secondary to cerebrovascular disease, invasive neoplasms, anoxia, collagen vascular disease, infection, or prior cerebral surgery with subsequent scar tissue. Experimentally, amino acid transmitters have been implicated in the pathogenesis of focal epilepsy.[105] Intraoperative measurements of epileptic patients have revealed elevated concentrations of glutamate, aspartate, and glycine.[106]

THE ICU PHASE

Management of the Comatose Patient

The objective in managing the comatose patient is to discern the cause of the altered state of consciousness and to correct or halt the disorder. Because proper diagnosis and treatment of the underlying disease process may require an extended period of time, basic principles to stabilize the patient in coma should be instituted. Initial evaluation can be incorporated into the initial management (Table 1-2).

Ventilation

The respiratory rate and its pattern should be documented prior to therapeutic measures such as intubation and mechanic ventilation. Alterations in respiration correlate with brain dysfunction.[43] An adequate airway should be obtained following an initial examination of the respiratory rate. If intubation is required, as in a comatose patient, the existence of a neck fracture must be ruled out prior to hyperextension of the head for endotracheal tube insertion. Arterial blood gases (ABGs) should be obtained to ensure adequate oxygenation (oxygen saturation greater than 90%) and to monitor serum acid/base status.

Spontaneous hyperventilation represents either compensation for metabolic acidosis or a response to primary stimulation. In metabolic acidosis, the arterial blood pH is usually less than 7.3 and the serum bicarbonate concentration is usually below 10 mEq/L. In respiratory acidosis, a lactic acidosis in the CSF stimulates medullary receptors in the absence of any systemic acidosis to maintain the arterial pH greater than 7.45. The serum bicarbonate concentration remains normal or slightly reduced. In metabolic acidosis and respiratory alkalosis, the P_{CO_2} is usually below 30 mm Hg. Mixed metabolic acidosis and respiratory alkalosis can occur concurrently, such as in hepatic coma and excessive salicylate ingestion. Hyperventilation with metabolic acidosis is usually a result of uremia, diabetic ketoacidosis, anoxic or spontaneous lactic acidosis, or ingestion of acidic agents. Diabetes and uremia are diagnosed by appropriate laboratory tests. If diabetes, uremia and anoxia can be ruled out, the metabolic acidosis is secondary to spontaneous lactic acidosis or poisoning with exogenous toxins such as methyl alcohol or ethyl alcohol. Metabolic acidosis secondary to exogenous agents can be treated through intravenous infusions of sodium bicarbonate to restore the blood pH to normal.

Respiratory alkalosis occurs secondary to salicylate ingestion, hepatic coma, gram negative sepsis, pulmonary disease, and psychogenic hyperventilation. These disorders can be distinguished by clinical examination and the appropriate laboratory tests. Salicylate poisoning causes a combined respiratory alkalosis and metabolic acidosis that depresses the serum bicarbonate disproportionately to the degree of serum pH elevation. Hepatic coma is usually accompanied by evidence of liver dysfunction. Hyperventilation is seen with gram-negative sepsis and may be a result

Table 1–2. Coma Decision Tree

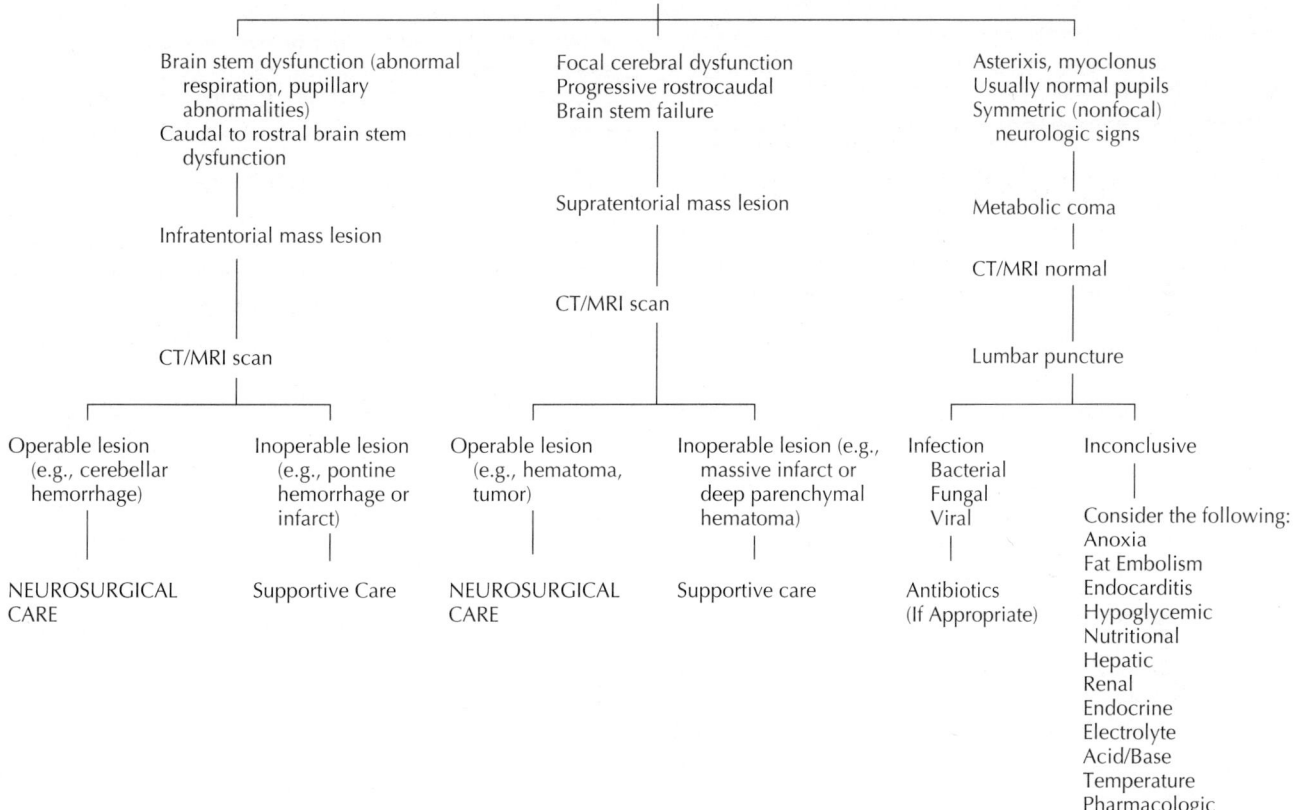

of a direct endotoxin effect on the CNS. Respiratory alkalosis as a result of pulmonary edema or pneumonia rarely decreases the serum bicarbonate level. Psychogenic hyperventilation does not result in coma, but may present a symptom in an individual with psychogenic unresponsiveness.

Hypoventilation represents either respiratory compensation for metabolic alkalosis or respiratory depression with consequent acidosis. In metabolic alkalosis, the arterial pH and the serum bicarbonate are elevated. The arterial P_{CO_2} is elevated but is usually less than 50 mm Hg. In untreated respiratory acidosis, the arterial pH is low and the serum bicarbonate level is either normal or high depending on renal compensation and the rapidity of onset of respiratory failure. The arterial P_{CO_2} is usually above 55 mm Hg.

Metabolic alkalosis results from either excessive ingestion of alkali or excessive loss of acid through gastrointestinal and renal routes. Respiratory acidosis is caused by either peripheral respiratory failure, such as pulmonary or neuromuscular disease, or central respiratory failure such as damage to the brain stem medulla, which controls respiration. Severe respiratory acidosis of any origin is best treated by artificial respiration.

Metabolism

Once adequate ventilation has been established, blood should be obtained for determination of serum glucose, routine chemistries, and toxicology. Because patients in coma may have poor nutrition and are susceptible to Wernicke's encephalopathy, thiamine, 100 mg intravenously, should be given initially. Immediate bedside glucose determinations should be made to identify hypoglycemia. If present, 50 mg of 50% dextrose should be administered. Although administration of 1 ampule of dextrose is not detrimental in cases of hyperosmolar coma, identification of hyperglycemic states is important because elevated serum glucose levels may promote ischemic damage in cases of anoxic coma.[107] Naloxone, 0.4 to 0.8 mg, should also be administered intravenously regardless of whether opiate overdosage is suspected.

Hemodynamics

Blood pressure can provide a vital clue to the cause of coma. Hypertension may be secondary to Cushing's reflex with increased intracranial pressure or brain stem ischemia. Hypertension also is associated with intracranial hemorrhage. Elevated blood pressure may also produce coma as in hypertensive encephalopathy. Hypotension may be indicative of myocardial infarction, hemorrhagic shock, sepsis, or sedative-hypnotic drug overdose. The pulse rate and rhythm may be additional clues to the cause of coma. Bradycardia associated with an elevated blood pressure may be suggestive of brain stem compression or raised intracranial pressure; however, elevated intracranial pressure does not decrease the heart rate in all instances.[108] Reversible causes of transtentorial herniation, such as subdural hematoma, should be immediately considered before cardiovascular collapse ensues.

ECG abnormalities may be associated with intracerebral disease. The triad of QT prolongation, U waves, and T-wave inversion is seen in 8% of patients after ischemic or hemorrhagic stroke.[109] The morphology of the ECG is also significant in other diseases. Repolarization changes, T-wave notching, and prolongation of the QT interval can occur with meningitis.[110] One study was able to correlate QT prolongation and T-wave abnormalities with left frontal hematomas.[111] In addition, subarachnoid hemorrhage has been associated with multiple dysrhythmia, which includes multifocal ventricular premature beasts, couplets, nonsustained ventricular tachycardia, sinus bradycardia, and atrial fibrillation.[112] Other investigators have noted that dysrhythmia usually occurs in the initial 48 hours following subarachnoid hemorrhage.[113] Prolongation of the QRS interval as well as dysrhythmia can occur in comatose patients after administration of ethanol, pesticides, tricyclic antidepressants, anticonvulsants, sedatives, trichloroethylene, and chlorpropamide.[114] A shortened or prolonged QT interval may indicate hypercalcemia or hypocalcemia, respectively.

Seizure Control

Status epilepticus can result in permanent anoxic brain damage and as a result requires immediate attention. Once the patient's airway has been stabilized, generalized convulsions can initially be treated with diazepam, up to 10 mg total dose intravenously. This is to be followed by phenytoin, at a loading dose of 1000 mg (50 mg/min), but the dose may be raised to 1500 mg if required. If status epilepticus continues, phenobarbital, 20 mg/kg intravenously, should be administered. Persistent convulsions at this point require general anesthesia. In the case of generalized convulsions that are inconsistent with status epilepticus, phenytoin, 300 mg orally once a day, should be maintained in individuals with EEG or CT/MRI evidence of a persistent epileptic focus (hemorrhage, neoplasm, large ischemic infarct, abscess, etc.). Patients convulsing from ethanol withdrawal and who do not have evidence of an epileptic focus should not be maintained on long-term anticonvulsant therapy. Cessation of alcohol consumption will resolve their seizures. In addition, individuals with severe alcohol abuse are rarely compliant with daily medication administration.

Temperature Regulation

Measurement of the patient's rectal temperature is a vital component of the initial evaluation. Hypothermia can be secondary to environmental exposure, near drowning, sedative drug overdose, hypothyroidism, and Wernicke's disease. Hypothermic patients with temperatures below 34°C (93.2°F) should be slowly warmed to maintain body temperature above 36°C (96.8°F). Because hypothermia below 80°F results in coma, resuscitative measures are indicated in all hypothermic patients even if all vital signs are absent. Hypothermic patients have recovered following cardiac arrest presumably because of the protective effects of low body temperature and depressed cerebral oxygen requirements.[115,116] The exception is patients who are both hypothermic and hyperkalemic.[117] Hypothermia has also been shown to reduce neuronal death in the hippocampus and caudate putamen in animal models with forebrain ischemia.[118]

The presence of fever in a comatose patient demands an investigation for an underlying infection. When head trauma is a possible cause of coma, the presence of cervical spine injury should be assumed until the cervical spine can be examined radiologically. Thus, the neck should not be flexed, but should be stabilized immediately by a headboard to prevent movement during physical and radiologic examination.

The presence of meningismus may indicate bacterial meningitis or subarachnoid hemorrhage; however, up to 12 hours may elapse before subarachnoid hemorrhage has produced significant chemical meningeal irritation to be detected by neck flexion. Meningismus may be present in coma, despite the presence of bacterial or chemical meningitis. Alternate causes of fever include intracranial abscess and subdural empyema, but individuals may be afebrile with encapsulated abscesses. If meningitis is suspected in a comatose patient, lumbar puncture should be performed, provided the neurologic examination and cranial CT/MRI reveal no evidence of increased intracranial pressure. The CSF should be examined for cell count, protein, glucose, culture, and xanthochromia. If no organism can be identified, a third-generation cephalosporin such as ceftriaxone, which penetrates the meninges, should be used until final CSF cultures are available.

Gastrointestinal Aspiration

Placement of a nasogastric tube with subsequent charcoal lavage is indicated in patients with suspected oral drug overdose. This procedure places the patient at risk for aspiration because the nasogastric tube dilates the gastroesophageal sphincter and permits regurgitation of gastric contents around the tube. Although not completely preventive, a cuffed endotracheal tube reduces the risk of aspiration and should be placed in comatose individuals prior to gastric lavage.

Urologic Care

As part of the initial critical care management, comatose patients require indwelling urine catheters to assess fluid output; however, the urinary catheter is a significant source of sepsis. Approximately 80% of patients catheterized for longer than 10 days develop sepsis.[119] In addition, antibiotic therapy during maintenance of a Foley catheter may increase bacterial resistance.[120] Spontaneous micturition is possible in comatose individuals, however.[121] Therefore, to limit the complications of infection, spontaneous micturition should be attempted in patients with coma when continual follow-up of diuresis is no longer required.

General Physical Examination

During the initial assessment of the patient in coma, the individual's general physical examination should not be overlooked. The patient should be evaluated for evidence of head trauma such as scalp laceration, hemotympani, otorrhea, and rhinorrhea. Blisters of the skin during coma may be suggestive of barbiturate overdose.[122] Biopsy reveals eccrine sweat duct necrosis. The blisters are not secondary to infection and do not contraindicate the continued therapeutic use of barbiturates. Patients in coma may also suffer from peripheral nerve injuries.[123] Compartment syndromes and compression neuropathies have been described in comatose individuals of duration ranging from 4 to 48 hours.[124]

Neurologic Examination

The neurologic examination that follows is derived from the Glasgow Coma Scale developed by Teasdale and Jennett for head injury and the techniques for evaluating brain stem function described by Plum and Posner (Tables 1–3 and 1–4). The neurologic examination consists of an as-

Table 1–3. Clinical Examination Correlation with CNS Structure

Clinical Signs	CNS Structure
Speech	Cerebral structure
Purposeful movement	
Eye opening, Sleep/Wake cycles	Brain stem sensory pathways (reticular activating system)
Decorticate posturing, decerebrate posturing	Brain stem motor pathways
Pupillary reactivity	Midbrain: third cranial nerve
Corneal reflex—Sensory	Upper pons
	Fifth cranial nerve
Corneal reflex—Motor response	Seventh cranial nerve
	Lower pons
Doll's eyes, caloric responses	Eighth cranial nerve (vestibular portion) connects via brain stem pathways with third, fourth, sixth cranial nerves
Spontaneous breathing, maintained blood pressure	Medulla
Deep tendon reflexes	Spinal cord

Table 1–4. Glasgow Coma Scale

Eye Opening Response	
Spontaneous	4
To voice	3
To pain	2
None	1
Best Verbal Response	
Oriented	5
Confused	4
Inappropriate words	3
Incomprehensible sounds	2
None	1
Best Motor Response	
Obeys commands	6
Localizes pain	5
Withdraws to pain	4
Flexion to pain	3
Extension to pain	2
None	1
Total Coma Score (sum of individual scores)	3–15

sessment of the level of consciousness as determined by eye opening, verbal responses, and reflex or purposive movements in response to noxious stimulation of the face, arms, and legs; neuro-ophthalmologic function as indicated by pupillary size and response to light, spontaneous eye movements, oculocephalic (doll's eyes), and oculovestibular (ice water caloric) responses; and vegetative function as reflected mainly by the respiratory pattern. This approach considers the brain in terms of its hierarchical, longitudinal organization into cortical and brain stem functions. Clinical neurologic signs can be correlated with specific anatomic sites to establish the severity and extent of CNS dysfunction.

Level of consciousness is best determined by the ease and degree, if any, of behavioral arousal. Attempts should be made to elicit a behavioral motor response by verbal stimulation alone. If there is no response after shouted commands, noxious stimulation can be applied to the face by digital supraorbital pressure and individually to the arms and legs by compression of distal interphalangeal joints with a tongue blade or pen. Eye opening indicates activity of the reticular activating system; verbal responses indicate hemispheric function. (See the introductory comments of this chapter for definition of states of consciousness.)

The absence of motor response, especially if flaccidity and areflexia are also present, indicates severe brain stem depression and is frequently found in terminal coma or in severe sedative intoxication.

Decerebrate or extensor responses correlate with destructive lesions of the midbrain and upper pons, but also may be present in reversible metabolic states such as anoxia encephalopathy. Decorticate or flexor responses occur after damage to the hemispheres, as well as in metabolic depression of brain function. Withdrawal and localizing responses imply purposeful or voluntary behavior. Obeying commands is the best response and marks the return of consciousness.

Generalized or focal repetitive movements that are not affected by stimuli usually represent seizure activity. Focal seizures usually indicate a focal cortical lesion but may also occur in hypoglycemia, hyperosmolality, and some drug intoxications (e.g., with aminophylline and tricyclic antidepressants).

Neuro-Ophthalmologic Examination

Fundi. The fundus of each eye should be examined for signs of increased intracranial pressure (papilledema and hemorrhage). Subhyaloid hemorrhage indicates the presence of subarachnoid or intracerebral hemorrhage but may follow severe head trauma.

Pupils. In coma due to metabolic brain disease, the pupils are generally small but reactive to light. Small, reactive pupils are present in normal persons during sleep and are a common finding in elderly persons because of degenerative changes in the iris and ciliary muscles. Small, sluggishly reactive pupils that respond to naloxone are characteristic of an overdose of opiates. Pinpoint pupils occur in pontine hemorrhage. Bilateral dilated, fixed pupils indicate sympathetic nervous system overactivity either from an endogenous sympathetic discharge (e.g., during anoxia/ischemia) or from exogenous catecholamine (e.g., dopamine). Similar pupils, dilated or mid-dilated, are seen in glutethimide-induced coma and overdosage with tricyclic antidepressant or other atropine-like agents. The pupils are large but reactive in coma due to amphetamine, cocaine, and LSD overdosage. Midposition, fixed pupils indicate midbrain failure and loss of both sympathetic and parasympathetic pupillary tone, whether caused by structural or metabolic disease. Such fixed and midposition, rather than dilated, pupils are seen in death. A unilateral dilated fixed pupil usually means damage to parasympathetic fibers of the third cranial nerve as described in the section on uncal herniation. If the patient has suffered head trauma, an ipsilateral epidural or subdural hematoma is probably present. If there is no evidence of trauma, an intrahemispheric mass lesion (hematoma, tumor, or abscess) is the probable cause of herniation.

Eye Movements. Deeply comatose patients may have no spontaneous eye movements. In such cases, doll's eyes responses and the ice water caloric test can be used to determine the integrity of the eighth, sixth, and third cranial nerves and their interconnecting brain stem pathways. When the cortical influences are depressed but brain stem gaze mechanisms are intact, if the head is rotated horizontally to one side, the eyes deviate conjugately to the opposite side. Brisk back-and-forth eye movements, like those of a doll in response to rocking the head to and fro, are characteristic of metabolic coma. Doll's eyes indicate the integrity of proprioceptive fibers from the neck structures, the vestibular nuclei, and the nuclei of the third and sixth cranial nerves. Unilateral lesions of the brain stem eliminate the doll's eyes response to the side of the lesion. When the doll's eyes are absent, it becomes necessary to perform the ice water caloric test. In deep coma, the doll's eyes disappear before the ice water caloric responses because the latter are produced by a stronger stimulus. The caloric response is elicited in comatose patients by irrigating the tympanum with 30 to 50 ml of ice water. When the patient is supine with the head elevated 30°, cold water produces convection currents in the lateral semicircular canal that inhibit the firing of the ipsilateral vestibular nerve. In the absence of cortical influence on the oculovestibular pathways, cold water produces tonic deviation of the eyes to the side of irrigation. Metabolic factors (sedative-hypnotic coma, phenytoin overdosage) and structural (brain stem) lesions eliminate the caloric response, as does labyrinthine disease. Disconjugate ocular deviation implies unilateral lesions or metabolic depression of brain stem pathways. If one or both eyes fail to abduct, the lesion is in the medial longitudinal fasciculus or third cranial nerve. The distinction between the two eyes can be made by examining the pupillary size and reaction to light. Failure of abduction indicates a lesion of the sixth cranial nerve.

Further Diagnostic and Therapeutic Management

Radiologic Imaging

Cranial CT or MRI consists of one of the first lines of investigation in determining an etiology for coma. Approximately 50% of patients receiving a CT scan for coma in one study had an abnormal scan. More than 80% of these patients presented with an intracerebral hemorrhage.[125] CT within 72 hours of onset of intracerebral hemorrhage usually provides greater resolution than MRI.

In acute anoxic coma, CT usually is unremarkable. Approximately 48 hours following a prolonged anoxic episode, hypodensities in the cerebral and cerebellar cortices and in the caudate and lenticular nuclei can occur.[126,127] Days to weeks later, focal infarcts, edema, and diffuse and focal atrophy may be evident. Clinical state or progression of deficits will indicate the necessity for further radiologic imaging. A CT without contrast dye is helpful in suspected cases of cerebral hemorrhage. Contrast CTs are necessary to visualize the cerebral vasculature following the exclusion of a cerebral hemorrhage.

Patients in coma who present with cranial nerve deficits and posturing are most likely to suffer from a significant mass lesion involving the cortices or the brain stem; however, others have reported that patients in coma with unilateral masses may not initially suffer from transtentorial herniation. CT and MRI in this group have demonstrated horizontal displacement at the level of the pineal body.[128,129]

Elevated Intracranial Pressure

Raised Intracranial Pressure (ICP) must be rapidly treated to avoid cerebral damage secondary to compression of tissue or loss of cerebral blood flow. Once the cause of elevated ICP is known, treatment can be focused to resolve the underlying disorder. For example, focal lesions such as acute subdural hematoma can be surgically treated to return ICP to within normal limits. Measurement of ICP can be performed through the use of epidural monitoring or through intraventricular pressure measurements. The latter requires puncture of the brain and is susceptible to infection. ICP monitoring has enabled one to differentiate between active hydrocephalus and cerebral atrophy and can define the need for surgery in progressive subdural effusions.[130] ICP monitoring has also been linked to prognosis. Most patients with a maximum ICP increase of less than 30 mm Hg experience good recovery; however, a pressure rise above 30 mm Hg represents a great risk for brain tamponade.[131,132] Other investigators have noted that aggressive treatment based on ICP monitoring can significantly reduce mortality when this treatment is applied to patients in coma secondary to head injury.[133]

Medical treatment for elevated ICP relies on several methods. The goal is to normalize elevated ICP by restricting cerebral blood flow or fluid to the brain tissue. Treatments that are currently used include:

- Hyperventilation
- Diuresis
- Fluid restriction
- Blood pressure control
- Steroids
- Drug therapy

Hyperventilation produces a state of hypocapnia. Hypocapnia, in turn, decreases cerebral blood flow globally through vasoconstriction. Reduction in P_{CO_2} from 40 to 30 mm Hg can reduce ICP by approximately 30%. It is recommended to maintain a P_{CO_2} of 25 to 30 mm Hg. Aggressive hypoventilation below 25 mm Hg may significantly reduce cerebral blood flow and may result in cerebral ischemia. Over a course of 24 to 48 hours, the cerebral vasculature reequilibrates during the hypocapnic state, and no further reduction in ICP is attained by this method.

Fluid restriction and fluid elimination are both used in treating elevated ICP. Normal saline is administered to maintain normal serum osmolality and to prevent systemic intravascular depletion. Restriction of normal saline infusion to half the maintenance level can help to reduce ICP. In addition to fluid restriction, osmotic agents can be administered on a short-term basis to control ICP. These drugs do not cross the blood-brain barrier and therefore pull water from cerebral tissue across an osmotic gradient into plasma. Long-term therapy with osmotic agents may not be as efficacious as short-term use. Equilibrium with cerebral tissue is eventually established with these drugs.

Mannitol has successfully been used as an osmotic agent to reduce ICP. Recommended doses are 0.50 to 1.0 g/kg with higher doses effective for up to 6 hours. Mannitol has been shown to consistently reduce ICP and increase cerebral perfusion pressure and cerebral blood flow approximately 10 to 20 minutes after infusion.[134] Low flows correlate with the most damaged cerebral tissue. Diuretics have also been used to produce an osmotic diuresis. They decrease formation of CSF by removing sodium and water from brain tissue. The renal loop diuretics such as furosemide and ethacrynic acid are usually employed in conjunction with osmotic agents when a single agent does not sufficiently reduce ICP.

Excessive use of osmotic agents can result in intravascular volume depletion and hypotension. Rapid osmotic diuresis can also produce large fluid shifts out of the brain and rupture cortical veins which results in subdural hematomas. Electrolyte disturbances can also result from the use of osmotic drugs. Hypernatremia, hypocalcemia, and hypokalemia do occur with chronic osmotic diuresis. Coma aggravated by the syndrome of inappropriate secretion of antidiuretic hormone (SIADH) can further complicate serum electrolyte abnormalities. Strict monitoring of fluid intake and output as well as regular measurement of serum osmolality, electrolytes, and glucose are vital to avoid the complications of osmotic diuresis.

In conjunction with reduction of ICP, it is important to monitor systemic mean arterial blood pressure (MAP) and cerebral perfusion pressure (CPP) (CPP = MAP − ICP). CPP is proportional to cerebral blood flow (CBF) when either MAP or ICP is altered.[135] In one study, a CPP less than 60 mm Hg was associated with eventual death, whereas a CPP of 90 mm Hg or greater correlated with eventual recovery.[136] Other investigators have reported that CPP greater than or equal to 30 mm Hg is well tolerated, however.[137] As noted, variations in MAP can affect CBF and CPP. With loss of autoregulation in impaired areas of the brain, systemic hypotension can adversely lower CBF and CPP while systemic hypertension can increase ICP by promoting transudation of fluid across sections of "leaky" blood-brain barrier in damaged tissue (see Chap. 4).

As a general guide, systemic blood pressure should be controlled to maintain a systolic pressure of at least 100 to 110 mm Hg, to allow a CPP of greater than 60 mm Hg to be maintained. Periods of hypotension should be controlled with volume expansion and pressor administration, whereas excessive blood pressure should be countered with antihypertensives.

Analgesics, inhalation anesthetics, and muscle relaxants all have been recommended to reduce ICP in patients "agitated" by mechanical ventilation. Sedatives such as benzodiazepines and butyrophenones reduce CBF as well as ICP. Narcotics have been promoted as being able to reduce ICP, but studies with agents such as phenoperidine report reductions in MAP but no change in ICP.[138] Halogenated anesthetics such as halothane, isoflurane, and enflurane reduce cerebral metabolism but raise ICP by elevating CBF through direct cerebrovasodilation. Neuromuscular blockade can prevent elevations in ICP by blocking increases in intrathoracic venous pressure secondary to mechanical ventilation. The drawbacks to muscle relaxants include the inability to evaluate motor function and eventual recovery, as well as the complications of pressure necrosis and corneal abrasions. Although pupillary responses remain unaltered, these agents are recommended for only short-term use.

Conflicting evidence has existed concerning the use of **steroids** to reduce elevated ICP. Steroids are efficacious in reducing edema from brain neoplasms and for treating such conditions as pseudotumor cerebri; however, a prospective double-blind controlled trial found no advantage to high dose dexamethasone versus control in ICP management, as well as clinical outcome in severe head injury.[139] Postanoxic cerebral edema is resistant to treatment. Corticosteroids have not proved beneficial in the treatment of global brain ischemia.[140] In addition, steroids may also elevate serum glucose and worsen cerebral ischemia.[141]

Barbiturate administration can reduce CBF and cerebral metabolic requirements, although the efficacy of barbiturates to reduce elevated ICP is controversial. In patients suffering cardiac arrest with coma, a single intravenous loading dose of thiopental produced no improvement in outcome.[142] In addition, prophylactic use of pentobarbital following severe head injury did not decrease the incidence of elevated ICP or the duration of ICP hypertension.[143] Yet, other investigators report adequate control of raised ICP and improved outcome following severe head injury with high dose barbiturate coma therapy.[144]

Hypotension is the most notable complication of barbiturate administration. Animal studies have revealed that less cardiovascular instability occurs with continuous barbiturate infusion than with intermittent bolus injections.[145] Barbiturates may also result in dysrhythmia, as well as myocardial depression.

Calcium-channel antagonists are currently under investigation in the treatment of CBF and ICP following coma. Nimodipine in the rat model has been shown to improve CBF and reduce brain edema following middle cerebral artery occlusion.[146] In clinical trials, patients treated with nimodipine that suffered prolonged cardiac arrests appeared to have an improved survival rate over the control group.[147] Calcium-influx blockers have also increased survival in individuals following severe head injury in which the mechanism is believed to be a reduction in cerebral vasospasm.[148]

Electrophysiologic Monitoring

The EEG can be a sensitive indicator of cerebral function. Recent advances have employed compressed spectral array EEG for continuous monitoring of comatose patients. With this method, hours of EEG activity are compressed into a pictorial representation that reveals time distribution and temporal characteristics of frequencies, as well as the intensity of total electrical activity (Fig. 1-4). The early detection of these parameters permits rapid assessment of the comatose state and can direct therapy.[149]

In animal studies, EEG activity becomes abnormal when CBF falls below 16 ml/100g per minute and is isoelectric with CBF less than 12 ml/100g per minute. Clinically, the EEG is classified in terms of increasing severity in five categories. Grade I represents normal alpha with theta-delta activity; grade II is theta-delta activity with some normal alpha activity; grade III is dominant theta-delta activity with no normal alpha activity; grade IV is low voltage delta activity with alpha coma (nonreactive alpha activity); and grade V represents an isoelectric tracing. In individuals suffering postanoxic or metabolic coma, grade I is compatible with a good prognosis, grades II and III have no definitive predictive value, and grades IV and V are compatible with a poor prognosis and infrequent recovery.[150,151] Alpha coma is frequently associated with cardiac arrest and usually suggests a poor prognosis (Fig. 1-5). Yet, other investigators have reported that this electrical pattern can lack prognostic significance.[152] Periodic lateralizing epileptiform discharges (PLEDs) may occur following focal cerebral insults such as infarction, but do not necessarily indicate active epileptic activity (Fig. 1-6). In general, the EEG is useful in assessing cortical dysfunction and identifying the presence of occult seizure activity.

Evoked potentials can provide information regarding the functional state of the cerebral cortex during coma. Somatosensory evoked potentials (SEPs) determine the functional integrity of the spinal cord posterior columns, brain stem medial lemniscus, thalamus, and frontoparietal sensorimotor cortex. When bilateral absence of cortical responses exists despite the origin of the coma, individuals

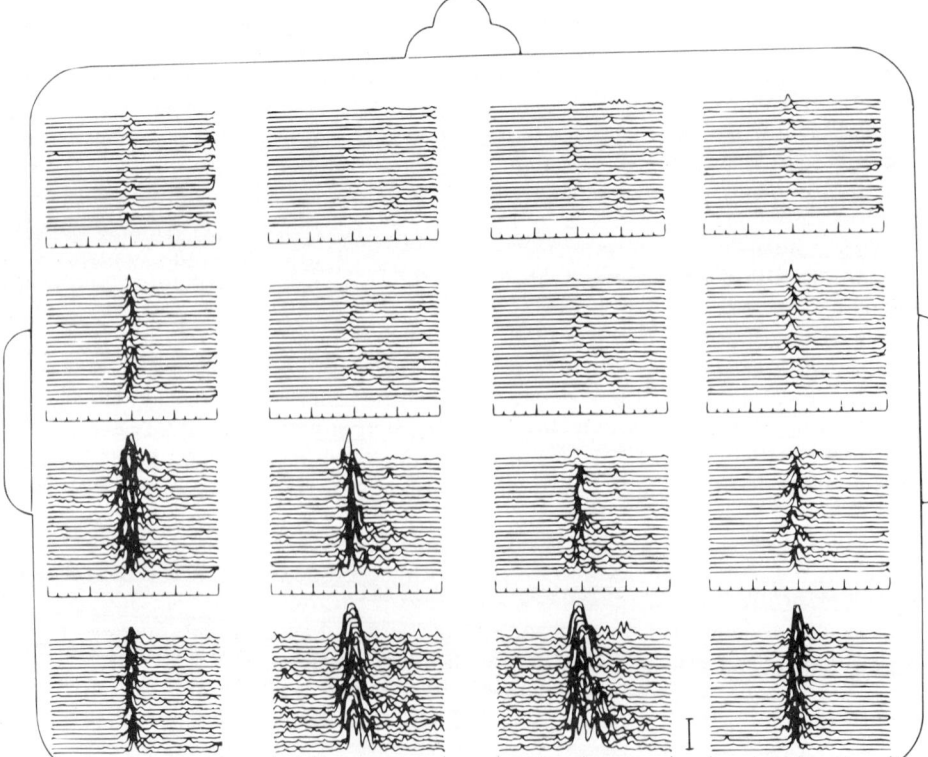

Figure 1-4. Compressed spectral array from parasagittal and temporal leads in a normal subject. (Redrawn from Klass, D. W., and Daley, D. D. (Eds.): Current Practice of Clinical EEG. New York, Raven Press, 1979, p. 471.)

COMA

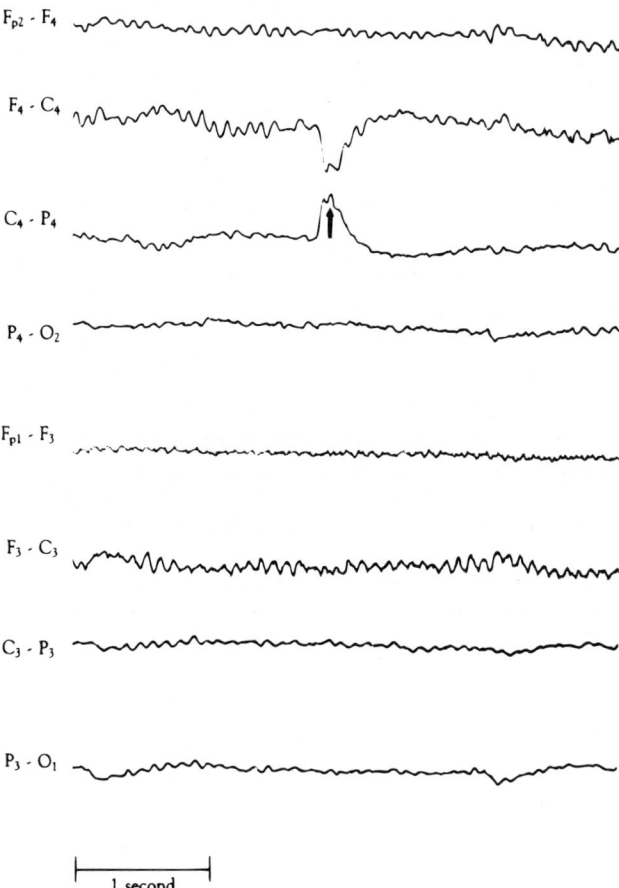

Figure 1-5. Example of alpha coma. The arrow represents a respirator artifact. (Redrawn from Dyro, F. M.: The EEG Handbook. Boston, Little, Brown, 1989, p. 61.)

experience a mortality rate as high as 98%.[153-156] With the exception of those in anoxic coma, patients who maintain normal responses throughout their illness maintain a good prognosis.[157] In anoxic coma, recovery remains favorable, but patients may have permanent neurologic sequelae.[158] In one study, normal SEPs were associated with a survival rate of 74%.[154] Others have emphasized that SEPs remain superior to motor evoked potentials in assessing outcome of comatose individuals.[157]

Brain stem auditory evoked potentials (BAEPs) can correlate with brain stem dysfunction during coma. Simultaneous latency increase of all components can be consistent with progressive ischemia of the posterior fossa and a decrease in CPP. Mechanical distortion of the brain stem is usually represented by loss of waves III, IV and V with preservation of wave I. Although BAEPs are not usually modified by exogenous factors,[159] BAEPs can be falsely altered by hypothermia.[160] In addition, combined use of anesthetics and barbiturates can induce latency and eventual abolition of BAEPs.[161]

Gastrointestinal Complications

Gastric stress ulcers may occur as a result of raised ICP. Upper gastrointestinal tract bleeding usually occurs 48 hours after the elevated ICP and requires correction of the cerebral hypertension, as well as stabilization of the systemic hemodynamic status. During prolonged periods of coma while patients are maintained on ventilatory assistance, digestive tract ulcers can result in irreversible gastrointestinal hemorrhage.[162]

Prevention of gastric ulcers in comatose individuals requires regular administration of H_2 blockers or antacids. Both forms of therapy are equally effective in limiting gastric bleeding; however, antacids are more effective in raising the pH of gastric contents than H_2 blockers such as cimetidine.[163] Antacid administration is not completely benign. Magnesium tricilicate mixtures administered in large doses over extended periods have resulted in hyperosmolality and coma.[164]

Nutrition

Patients in coma with functional gastrointestinal tracts should receive daily enteral nutrition, of between 3000 and 4500 calories per day. Small caliber silicone tubes should be used to avoid gastric reflux, aspiration, and naso-

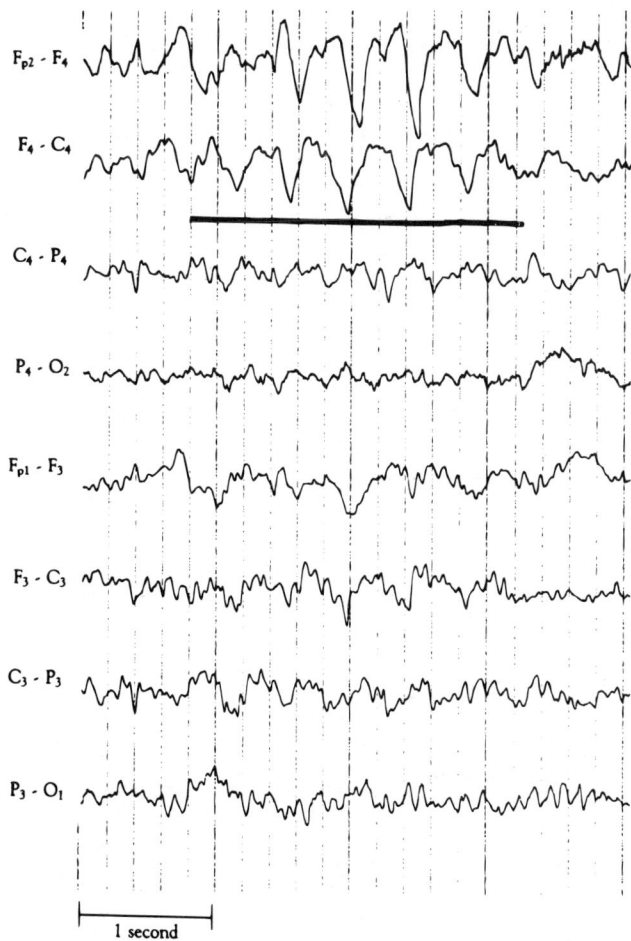

Figure 1-6. Periodic lateralizing epileptiform discharges (PLEDs) (underlined) are seen in acute insults, such as the result of infarct, trauma, neoplasm, cellulitis, or abscess. (Redrawn from Dyro, F. M.: The EEG Handbook. Boston, Little, Brown, 1989, p. 68.)

pharyngeal complications. Refrigerated nutritional solutions check bacterial proliferation to avoid diarrhea.[165] Continuous administration of enteral nutrition has no advantage over intermittent nutritional support. No significant differences have been noted in factors such as aspiration, total caloric intake, or dysentery.[166] Jejunal hyperalimentation had been advocated in comatose patients secondary to traumas with clinically silent abdomens. This method has been reported to increase caloric and nitrogen intake while reducing infection and duration of intensive care unit management.[167] In patients with impaired gastric function such as high tube reflux, however, total parenteral nutrition is preferred.[168]

Establishment of Brain Death

Although aggressive diagnosis and management of the comatose patient can reduce mortality, individuals may still suffer from significant morbidity. Unfortunately, "high-tech" medical care can sustain individuals with overwhelming and critical cerebral damage by mechanical supports. Brain death is declared with the documentation of loss of function of the entire cortex and brain stem.[164] The following criteria should be considered in a brain-dead individual:

- Lack of response to noxious stimulation
- Absence of brain stem reflexes
- Fixture of pupils to light stimulation
- Absence of corneal blink reflex, doll's eyes, and cold water caloric responses
- Lack of spontaneous respirations (apnea)

Drug poisoning, hypothermia, electrolyte abnormalities, or extensive neuromuscular paralysis must be excluded before proceeding to an apnea test.

The documentation of apnea is vital to the determination of brain death. Although multiple methods exist to establish apnea, we recommend using apneic oxygenation to determine brain death.[170] The patient's P_{CO_2} is adjusted to approximately 40 mm Hg in the setting of a normal serum bicarbonate and P_{O_2} greater than 90% saturation. The respirator is disconnected, 100% O_2 is administered, and the chest is observed for evidence of spontaneous respiratory activity. Preoxygenation is not required prior to respirator disconnection.[171] Individuals who breathe should be replaced on mechanical ventilation. Arterial blood gases are monitored to detect a rise in P_{CO_2} to 60 mm Hg. This level of hypercapnia is sufficient to produce a degree of CSF acidosis that maximally stimulates medullary respiratory receptors. If no respirations are noted at this point, the patient is connected to the respirator and the test is repeated within 12 to 24 hours. Failure of the patient to exhibit spontaneous respirations during the second examination with a P_{CO_2} of 60 mm Hg represents brain death.

We believe that the clinical criteria of brain death are sufficiently conservative that when properly applied they will never lead to the diagnosis of brain death in an individual who would otherwise recover. Nevertheless, some centers have found it useful to use supplementary tests such as absence of electrocerebral activity to support the clinical diagnosis. In addition, such tests are required in specific cases, as with patients receiving neuromuscular blocking agents. CBF is lost in brain-dead individuals. Xenon-enhanced computed tomography (CT) has been applied to brain death. Xenon-enhanced CT scanning combines the noninvasive anatomical information of the CT scan with an analysis of local CBF. Serial CT scans are performed during xenon inhalation to map CBF. The technique is then able to quantitate CBF from brain regions.[172,173]

Transcranial Doppler imaging of cerebral arteries has been used as an adjunct to determine brain death. The pattern consistent with loss of brain function is one sharply contoured systolic flow but absent or reduced flow during diastole.[174] This pattern reveals increased distal vascular resistance. An absent signal is difficult to interpret, however, because it occurs in 3 to 6% of patients without cerebrovascular disease. Yet, a normal transcranial Doppler imaging pattern probably excludes brain death in patients clinically without brain stem reflexes.[175]

Measurement of esophageal motility has been advocated as a supplementary test of brain death in patients on neuromuscular blocking agents.[176] Spontaneous lower esophageal motility persists in paralyzed patients. An intact pathway between the brain and esophagus is required for lower esophageal contractions; however, these contractions are lost in brain death.

THE POST-ICU PHASE

Prognosis Following Coma

Nontraumatic Coma

Prediction of outcome following coma has been the subject of multiple clinical studies. Duration of coma has been cited as one vital factor. Earlier reports have noted that postarrest coma longer than 3 days carried an unfavorable prognosis.[177] Although occasional case reports document recovery following prolonged coma,[178] several studies even report some permanent neurologic sequelae if coma duration is greater than 6 hours.[178,180] Others have correlated outcome with the pattern of motor responses and the presence or absence of particular brain stem reflexes. Comatose patients with epilepsy or myoclonus did not recover. Increased numbers of brain stem reflex abnormalities were associated with reduced survival;[181-184] however, these studies were undertaken on a relatively small number of patients.

Earnest et al.[185,186] documented early and late improvement in more than 100 individuals following out-of-hospital cardiac arrest. Absence of pupillary light reactions, oculocephalic reflexes, and purposeful movements to pain were each associated with reduced chance of recovery. Neurologic signs noted on hospital admission did not correlate with eventual outcome. Patients who remained in coma at discharge failed to regain independence. The inability to regain response to painful stimuli or pupillary light reflex during extensive periods of hospitalization has also been noted as consistent with an unfavorable outcome.[187]

As part of a multicenter study to establish guidelines for prognosis in comatose patients, Levy et al.[188] examined 210 patients in whom cardiopulmonary failure was the cause of coma and correlated clinical signs with outcome at 1 year. Only patients in coma for 6 hours were included and each individual underwent serial neurologic examination. Coma was defined as those individuals who failed to open their eyes spontaneously or in response to noise, no comprehensible words were expressed, commands were not obeyed, and purposeful movement to painful stimuli did not exist. Most patients destined to recover awakened within a short period. After 3 days, 25 patients had regained consciousness and by 2 weeks, the number of conscious patients increased to only 28. Only one of the 17 patients still in coma at 1 week subsequently regained consciousness. The patient's age and sex, the location of the initial insult, the cause of the coma, and the presence of generalized seizures did not influence the degree of recovery; however, the clinical examination did correlate with recovery. Individuals without pupillary light reflexes at the initial examination never regained independence. Absence of corneal reflexes following the first day was also a poor prognosis. Others have also noted the absence of brain stem vestibulaocular reflex following coma to be indicative of a poor prognosis.[189] Individuals with the best chance of recovery had preserved brain stem function following the initial insult.

Several findings on examination correlated with a good outcome. During the initial examination, the most favorable sign was incomprehensible speech, such as moaning, but this was rare. At day 1, the following signs were each associated with at least a 50% chance of regaining independent function:

- Any form of speech
- Orienting spontaneous eye movements
- Intact oculocephalic or oculovestibular responses
- Ability to follow commands
- Normal skeletal tone

Other clinical signs were suggestive of poor likelihood of meaningful recovery. As previously noted, the absence of specific brain stem reflexes were consistent with a poor prognosis. In addition, after 3 days, absent or posturing motor responses were incompatible with eventual independent living.

Toxic/Metabolic Coma

Coma can be a complication in almost 70% of acute drug intoxications.[190] Fortunately, coma secondary to sedative drug intoxications carries a mortality rate of less than 1%.[191] If sufficient ventilatory and hemodynamic support are supplied in a timely fashion, most individuals experience no residual neurologic impairment. Complications can include cardiovascular collapse secondary to hypothermia, hypotension, dysrhythmia, myocardial infarction, or pulmonary edema. In cases of cardiac arrest, prognosis is more consistent with survival data following anoxic coma.

Traumatic Coma

Prediction of outcome for traumatic coma parallels the criteria used for nontraumatic coma (Table 1–5). Coma of prolonged duration rarely results in recovery of independent function. A favorable prognosis relies on such characteristics as youth, intact pupillary reflex, and the presence of spontaneous eye movements.[192] Others have noted that moderate to severe closed-head injury leading to coma uniformly impairs verbal intellectual functioning. This verbal impairment is independent of duration of coma, age, and premorbid intelligence.[193]

Additional factors play a role in the eventual outcome from traumatic coma. Specific lesions, such as subdural hematoma, that result in coma can have less than a 10% recovery rate.[194] In studies with blunt trauma, comatose patients with increased plasma glucose, hypokalemia, or elevated serum leukocyte counts were associated with lower Glasgow coma scale scores and an increased probability of death.[195]

The foregoing prognostic guidelines for nontraumatic coma, toxic/metabolic coma, and traumatic coma should be used cautiously. One must be certain that the evaluation of clinical signs is correct. In addition, the effects of anticholinergic agents on pupillary reactivity and the effect of paralytic drugs on motor response must be excluded.

The ability to predict prognosis following coma can benefit the patient, family, and physician. Families can be spared both the emotional and financial burdens of caring for individuals with an insignificant chance of independent function. Physicians can then properly allocate limited resources to patients with the potential to profit from advanced medical care.

Table 1–5. Trauma Scale

Glasgow Coma Scale Total	
14–15	5
11–13	4
8–10	3
5–7	2
3–4	1
Respiratory Rate	
10–24/min	4
25–35/min	3
>35/min	2
1–9/min	1
None	0
Respiratory Expansion	
Normal	1
None	0
Systolic Blood Pressure	
>89 mm Hg	4
70–89 mm Hg	3
50–69 mm Hg	2
0–49 mm Hg	1
No pulse	0
Peripheral Perfusion (Capillary refill)	
Normal	2
Delayed	1
None	0
Total Trauma Score (sum of the individual scores)*	1–16

* Scores less than 10 represents a less than 60% chance of survival.

REFERENCES

1. Raffin, T. A.: Intensive care unit survival of patients with systemic illness. Am. Rev. Respir., Dis. *140:*528, 1989.
2. Teres, D., Brown, R. B., and Lemeshow, S.: Predicting mortality of intensive care coma. Crit. Care Med., *10:*86, 1982.

3. Albert, M. L., et al.: Cerebral dominance for consciousness. Arch. Neurol., 33:453, 1976.
4. Obrador, S., et al.: Comatose state maintained during eight years following a vascular pontomesencephalic lesion. Electroencephalog. Clin. Neurophysiol., 38:21, 1975.
5. Volpe, B. T., and Hirst, W.: The characterization of an amnesic syndrome following hypoxic ischemic injury. Arch. Neurol., 40:436, 1983.
6. Pulsinelli, W. A., and Petito, C. K.: Delayed neuronal recovery and neuronal death in rat hippocampus following severe cerebral ischemia: possible relationship to abnormalities in neuronal processes. J. Cereb. Blood Flow Metab., 4: 194, 1984.
7. Petito, C. K., Feldman, E., Pulsinelli, W. A., and Plum, F.: Delayed hippocampal damage in humans following cardiorespiratory arrest. Neurology, 37:1281, 1987.
8. Simon, R. P., et al.: Calcium overload in selectively vulnerable neurons of the hippocampus during and after ischemia: an electron microscopy study in the rat. J. Cereb. Blood. Flow. Metab., 4:350, 1984.
9. Jorgensen, M. B., and Diemer, N. H.: Selective neuronal loss after cerebral ischemia in the rat: possible role of transmitter glutamate. Acta Neurol. Scand., 66:536, 1982.
10. White, B. C., et al.: Possible role of calcium blockers in cerebral resuscitation: a review of the literature and synthesis for future studies. Crit. Care Med., 11:202, 1983.
11. Siesjo, B. K., and Bengtsson, F.: Calcium fluxes, calcium antagonists, and calcium-related pathology in brain ischemia, hypoglycemia, and spreading depression: a unifying hypothesis. J. Cereb. Blood Flow Metab., 9:127, 1989.
12. Nakayami, H., Ginsberg, M. D., and Dietrich, W. D.: (Semapamil), a novel calcium channel blocker and serotonin 52 antagonist, markedly reduces infarct size following middle cerebral artery occlusion in the rat. Neurology, 38:1667, 1988.
13. Krause, G. S., et al.: Ischemia, resuscitation, and reperfusion: mechanics of tissue injury and prospects for protection. Am. Heart J., 111:368, 1986.
14. Siesjo, B. K., and Wieloch, T.: Molecular mechanisms of ischemic brain damage Cal+ related events. In Cerebrovascular Diseases: Thirteenth Research Conference. Edited by M. Reivich and H. Hurtig. New York, Raven Press, 1985.
15. Alps, B. J., and Hass, W. K.: The potential beneficial effect of nicardipine in a rat model of transient forebrain ischemia. Neurology, 37:809, 1987.
16. Vibulsresth, S., et al.: Failure of nimodipine to prevent ischemic neuronal damage in rats. Stroke, 18:210, 1987.
17. Weisfeldt, M. L.: Reperfusion and repefusion injury. Clin. Res., 35:13, 1987.
18. Rosenblum, W. I.: Biology of disease: aspects of endothelial malfunction and function in cerebral microvessels. Lab. Invest., 55:252, 1986.
19. Matsubara, T., and Ziff, M.: Superoxide anion release by human endothelial cells: synergism between a phorbol ester and a calcium ionophore. J. Cell. Physiol., 127:207, 1986.
20. Kontos, H. A.: Oxygen radicals in cerebral vascular injury. Circ. Res., 57:508, 1985.
21. Rothman, S. M., and Olney, J. W.: Glutamate and the pathophysiology of hypoxic-ischemic brain damage. Ann. Neurol., 19:105, 1986.
22. Olney, J. W.: Glutamate-induced neuronal necrosis in the infant mouse hypothalamus: an electron microscopic study. J. Neuropath. Exp. Neurol., 30:75, 1971.
23. Olney, J. W., Fuller, T., and DeGubareff, T.: Acute dendiotoxic changes in the hippocampus of kainate-treated rats. Brain Res., 176:91, 1979.
24. Monaghan, D. T., et al.: Anatomical distributions of four pharmacologically distinct H-L glutamate binding sites. Nature, 306:176, 1983.
25. Brierly, J. B., and Graham, D. I.: Hypoxia and vascular disorders of the central nervous system. In Greenfield's Neuropathology. Edited by J. H. Adams, J. A. N. Corsellis, L. W. Duchen. New York, John Wiley and Sons, 1984.
26. Simon, R. P., et al.: Blockage of N-methyl-D-aspartate receptors may protect against ischemic damage in the brain. Science, 226:850, 1984.
27. Rothman, S.: Synaptic release of excitatory amino acid neurotransmitter mediates anoxic neuronal death. J. Neurosci., 4:1884, 1984.
28. Faden, A. I.: Endogenous opioids: physiologic and pathophysiologic actions. J. Am. Osteopath. Assoc., 84(Suppl): 129, 1984.
29. Faden, A. I.: Opiate antagonists in the treatment of stroke. Curr. Concepts Cerebrovasc. Dis., 18:27, 1983.
20. Hosobuchi, Y., Baskin, D. S., and Woo, S. K.: Reversal of induced ischemic neurologic deficit in gerbils by the opiate antagonist naloxone. Science, 215:69, 1982.
31. Wexler, B. C.: Naloxone ameliorates the pathophysiologic changes which lead to and attend an acute stroke in stroke-prone/SHR. Stroke, 15:30, 1984.
32. Holaday, J. W., and D'Amato, R. J.: Naloxone or TRH fails to improve neurological deficits in gerbil models of "stroke." Life Sci., 31:385, 1982.
33. Cutler, J. R., et al.: Failure of naloxone to reverse vascular neurologic deficits. Neurology, 33:1517, 1983.
34. Gustafson, I., Yoshitayo, M., and Wieloch, T. W.: Postischemic administration of idazoxan, and alpha-2 adrenergic receptor antagonist, decreases neuronal damage in the rat brain. J. Cereb. Blood Flow Metab., 9:171, 1989.
35. Maiese, K., Pek, L., Berger, S. B., and Reis, D. J.: Reduction in focal cerebral ischemia by agents acting at imidazole receptors. J. Cereb. Blood Flow Metab., 12:53, 1992.
36. Tuhrin, S., et al.: Prediction of intracerebral hemorrhage survival. Ann. Neurol., 24:258, 1988.
37. Douglas, M. A., and Haerer, A. F.: Long term prognosis of hypertensive intracerebral hemorrhage. Stroke, 3:488, 1982.
38. Hanley, D. F., et al.: Treatment of sagittal sinus thrombosis associated with cerebral hemorrhage and intracranial hypertension. Stroke, 19:903, 1988.
39. Cuneo, R. A., et al.: Upward transtentorial herniation: seven cases and a literature review. Arch. Neurol., 36:618, 1979.
40. Bewermeyer, H., et al.: Spontaneous pontine hemorrhage. An analysis of 38 cases. Nervenarzt., 59:640, 1988.
41. Bewermeyer, H., Neveling, M., Ebhardt, G., and Heiss, W. D.: Spontaneous pontine hemorrhage. Fortschr. Neurol. Psychiatr., 52:259, 1984.
42. Dunne, J. W., Chakera, T. W., and Kermode, S.: Cerebellar hemorrhage-diagnosis and treatment: a study of 75 consecutive cases. Q. J. Med., 64:739, 1987.
43. Plum, F., and Posner, J. B.: The diagnosis of stupor and coma. 3rd Ed, Philadelphia, F. A. Davis, 1980.
44. Seisjo, B. K., and Plum, F.: Pathophysiology of anoxic brain damage. In Biology of Brain Dysfunction. Edited by G. E. Gaul. Vol. 1. New York, Plenum, 1972.
45. Sevestre, H., et al.: Anoxic encephalopathy after cardiocirculatory insufficiency: neuropathological study apropos of 16 cases. Ann. Med. Interne (Paris), 139:245, 1988.
46. Jacobsson, D. M., Terrence, C. F., and Reinmuth, D. M.: The neurologic manifestations of fat embolism. Neurology, 36:847, 1986.
47. Findlay, J. M., and DeMajo, W.: Cerebral fat embolism Can. Med. Assoc. J., 131:755, 1984.

48. Munte, T. F., and Muller-Vahl, H.: Familial migraine coma: a case study. Dtsch. J. Neurol., 237:59, 1990.
49. Naeije, R., Peretz, A., and Cornil, A.: Acute pulmonary edema following carbon monoxide poisoning. Intensive Care Med., 6:189, 1980.
50. Mathieu, D., et al.: Acute carbon monoxide poisoning: risk of late sequelae and treatment by hyperbaric oxygen. J. Toxicol. Clin. Toxicol., 23:315, 1985.
51. Grim, P. S., Gottlieb, L. J., Broddie, A., and Batson, E.: Hyperbaric oxygen therapy. JAMA, 263:2216, 1990.
52. Gonzalez-Rothi, R. J.: Near drowning: consensus and controversies in pulmonary and cerebral resuscitation. Heart Lung, 16:474, 1987.
53. Romer, F. K.: Bacterial meningitis: a 15 year review of bacterial meningitis from departments of internal medicine. Dan. Med. Bull., 24:35, 1977.
54. Demey, H. E., et al.: Coma as a presenting sign of Epstein-Barr encephalitis. Arch. Intern. Med., 148:1459, 1988.
55. Boucquey, D., et al.: Herpes simplex virus type 2 meningitis without genital lesions: an immunoblot study. J. Neurol., 237:285, 1990.
56. Buge, A., Chamouard, J. M., and Rancurel, G.: Prognosis of herpes simplex encephalitis: retrospective study of 19 cases. Presse Med., 17:13, 1988.
57. Stewart, R. B., et al.: Epidemiology of acute drug intoxications: patient characteristics, drugs and medical complications. Clin. Toxicol., 7:513, 1974.
58. Gibb, K.: Serum alcohol levels, toxicology screens, and use of the breath alcohol analyzer. Ann. Emerg. Med., 15:349, 1986.
59. Greenblatt, D. J., et al.: Correlates of outcome following acute glutethimide overdosage. J. Forensic. Sci., 24:76, 1979.
60. Ritz, R., Zuber, M., Elasasser, S., and Scollo-Lavizzari, G.: Use of flumazenil in intoxicated patients with coma: a double-blind placebo-controlled study in ICU. Intensive Care Med., 16:242, 1990.
61. Kulka, P. J., Lauven, P. M., Schwilden, H., and Rommelscheim, K.: The efficacy of the benzodiazepine antagonist flumazenil (Ro 15-1788) based on the EEG of mechanically ventilated intensive care patients. Anaesthesist, 38:424, 1989.
62. Geller, E., et al.: The use of flumazenil in the treatment of 34 intoxicated patients. Resuscitation, 16(Suppl):557, 1988.
63. Lange, R. A., et al.: Cocaine-induced coronary-artery vasoconstriction. N. Engl. J. Med., 321:1557, 1989.
64. Isner, J. M., et al.: Acute cardiac events temporally related to cocaine abuse. N. Engl. J. Med., 315:1438, 1986.
65. Nanji, A. A., and Filipenko, J. D.: Asystole and ventricular fibrillation associated with cocaine intoxication. Chest, 85:132, 1984.
66. Barth, C. W. III, Bray, M., and Roberts, W. C.: Rupture of the ascending aorta during cocaine intoxication. Am. J. Cardiol., 57:496, 1986.
67. Nalbandian, H., Sheth, N., Dietrich, R., and Georgiou, J.: Intestinal ischemia caused by cocaine ingestion: report of two cases. Surgery, 97:374, 1985.
68. Lowenstein, D. H., et al.: Acute neurologic and psychiatric complications associated with cocaine abuse. Am. J. Med., 83:841, 1987.
69. Wetti, C. V., and Wright, R. K.: Death caused by recreational cocaine use. JAMA, 241:2519, 1979.
70. Stripling, J. S., and Hendricks, C.: Effect of cocaine and lidocaine on the expression of kindled seizures in the rat. Pharmacol. Biochem. Behav., 14:379, 1980.
71. Lichtenfeld, P. J., Rubin, D. B., and Feldman, R. S.: Subarachnoid hemorrhage precipitated by cocaine snorting. Arch. Neurol., 41:223, 1984.
72. Mody, C. K., et al.: Neurologic complications of cocaine abuse. Neurology, 38:1189, 1988.
73. Levine, S. R., et al.: "Crack" cocaine-associated stroke. Neurology, 37:1849, 1987.
74. Krendel, D. A., Ditter, S. M., Frankel, M. R., and Ross, W. K.: Biopsy-proven cerebral vasculitis associated with cocaine abuse. Neurology, 40:1092, 1990.
75. Roberts, J. R., Quattrocchi, E., and Howland, M. A.: Severe hyperthermia secondary to intravenous drug above. Am. J. Emerg. Med., 2:373, 1984.
76. Hulten, B. A., and Heath, A.: Clinical aspects of tricyclic antidepressant poisoning. Acta Med. Scand., 213:275, 1983.
77. Boffard, V., Palmier, B., Bouletreau, B., and Motin, J.: Acute tricyclic antidepressant intoxication: evaluation of severity and treatment. A study of 165 patients with cardiovascular manifestations. Ann. Med. Interne (Paris), 133:256, 1982.
78. Boehnert, M. T., and Lovejoy, F. H.: Value of the QRS duration versus the serum drug level in predicting seizures and ventricular arrhythmias after an acute overdose of tricyclic antidepressants. N. Engl. J. Med., 313:474, 1985.
79. Emerman, C. L., Connors, A. F., and Burma, G. M.: Level of consciousness as a predictor of complications following tricyclic overdose. Ann. Emerg. Med., 16:326, 1987.
80. Wedin, G. P., Oderda, G. M., Klein-Schwartz, W., and Gorman, R. L.: Relative toxicity of cyclic antidepressants. Ann. Emerg. Med., 15:979, 1986.
81. Callaham, M., and Kassel, D.: Epidemiology of fatal tricyclic antidepressant ingestion: implications for management. Ann. Emerg. Med., 14:1, 1985.
82. Heath, A., Marin, P., and Sjostrand, I.: Inotropic effect of prenalterol in amitriptyline poisoning. Intensive Care Med., 10:209, 1984.
83. Jaeger, A., Saunder, P., Kopferschmitt, J., and Jaegle, M. L.: Toxicokinetics of lithium intoxication treated by hemodialysis. J. Toxicol. Clin. Toxicol., 23:501, 1985.
84. Triggs, J. W., Bohan, T. P., Lin, S. N., and Willmore, L. J.: Valproate-induced coma with ketosis and carnitine insufficiency. Arch. Neurol., 47:1131, 1990.
85. Bigler, D.: Neurological sequelae after intoxication with sodium valproate. Acta Neurol. Scand., 72:351, 1985.
86. Hintze, G., Klein, H. H., Prange, H., and Kreuzer, H.: A case of valproate intoxication with excessive brain edema. Klin. Wochenschr., 65:424, 1987.
87. Bismuth, C., et al.: Cyanide poisoning: priority of symptomatic treatment, 25 cases. Presse Med., 13:2493, 1984.
88. Tassan, H., et al.: Potassium cyanide poisoning treated with hydroxocobalamin. Ann. Fr. Anesth. Reanim., 9:383, 1990.
89. Chelluri, L., and Jastremski, M. S.: Coma caused by ibuprofen overdose. Crit. Care Med., 14:1078, 1986.
90. Bennett, R. R., Dunkelberg, C. C., and Marks, E. S.: Acute oliguric renal failure due to ibuprofen overdose. South. Med. J., 78:430, 1985.
91. Danza, F. L.: Endoscopic studies of gastric and duodenal injury after the use of ibuprofen, aspirin, and other nonsteroidal anti-inflammatory agents. Am. J. Med., 77:19, 1984.
92. Schneck, H. J., and Rupreht, J.: Central anticholinergic syndrome (CAS) in anesthesia and intensive care. Acta. Anaesthesiol. Belg., 40:219, 1989.
93. Ringel, R. A., Riggs, J. E., and Brick, J. F.: Reversible coma with prolonged absence of pupillary and brainstem reflexes: an unusual response to a hypoxic-ischemic event in MS. Neurology, 38:1275, 1988.
94. Seki, S.: Clinical features of hyperosmolar hyperglycemic nonketoic diabetic coma associated with cardiac operations. J. Thorac. Cardiovasc. Surg., 91:867, 1986.

95. Mazzaferri, E. L.: Adult hypothyroidism. Part 1. Postgrad. Med., *79*:64, 1986.
96. Feinichel, P., et al.: Myxedematous coma: prognostic and therapeutic re-evaluation. Presse Med., *17*:1345, 1988.
97. McCulloch, W., Price, P., Hinds, C. J., and Wass, J. A.: Effects of low dose oral triiodothyronine in myxoedema coma. Intensive Care. Med., *11*:259, 1985.
98. Binimelis, J., et al.: Massive thyroxine intoxication: evaluation of plasma extraction. Intensive Care Med., *13*:33, 1987.
99. Pappas, S. C.: Increased gamma-aminobutyric acid (GABA) receptors in the brain precede hepatic encephalopathy in fulminant hepatic failure. Hepatology, *4*:1051, 1984.
100. Scollo-Lavizzari, G.: Reversal of hepatic coma by benzodiazepine antagonist (RO 15-1788). Letter. Lancet, *1*:1324, 1985.
101. Rothstein, J. D., et al.: Cerebrospinal fluid content of diazepam binding inhibitor in chronic hepatic encephalopathy. Ann. Neurol., *26*:57, 1989.
102. Krumholz, A., Stern, B. J., and Weiss, H. D.: Outcome from coma after cardiopulmonary resuscitation: relation to seizures and myoclonus. Neurology, *38*:401, 1988.
103. Jumas-As, A., and Brenner, R. P.: Myoclonic status epilepticus: a clinical and electroencephalographic study. Neurology, *40*:1199, 1990.
104. Simon, R. P., and Aminoff, M. J.: Electrographic status epilepticus in fatal anoxic coma. Ann. Neurol., *20*:351, 1986.
105. Perry, T. L., and Hansen, S.: Amino acid abnormalities in epileptogenic foci. Neurology, *31*:872, 1981.
106. Sherwin, A., et al.: Excitatory amino acids are elevated in human epileptic cerebra cortex. Neurology, *38*:920, 1988.
107. Longstreth, W. T., et al.: Neurologic outcome and blood glucose levels during out-of-hospital cardiopulmonary resuscitation. Neurology, *36*:1186, 1986.
108. Leipzig, T. J., and Lowensohn, R. I.: Heart rate variability in neurosurgical patients. Neurosurgery, *19*:356, 1986.
109. Goldstein, D. S.: The electrocardiogram in stroke: relationship to pathophysiological type and comparison with prior tracings. Stroke, *10*:253, 1979.
110. Mehta, S. S., Kronzon, I., and Laniado, S.: Electrocardiographic changes in meningitis. Isr. J. Med. Sci., *10*:748, 1974.
111. Yamour, B. J., Sridharan, M. R., Rice, J. R., and Flowers, N. C.: Electrocardiographic changes in cerebrovascular hemorrhage. Am. Heart J., *99*:294, 1980.
112. Stober, T., et al.: Cardiac arrhythmias in subarachnoid hemorrhage. Acta Neurochir. (Wien), *93*:37, 1981.
113. DiPasquale, G., et al.: Holter detection of cardiac arrhythmias in intracranial subarachnoid hemorrhage. Am. J. Cardiol., *59*:596, 1987.
114. Durakovic, Z., and Bagic, A.: Changes in the electrocardiogram in patients with coma due to poisoning. Acta. Med. Iugosl., *43*:287, 1989.
115. Leonov, Y., et al.: Mild cerebral hypothermia during and after cardiac arrest improves neurologic outcome in dogs. J. Cereb. Blood Flow Metab., *10*:57, 1990.
116. Conn, A. W., and Barker, G. A.: Fresh water drowning and near-drowning: an update. Can. Anaesth. Soc. J., *31*:S38, 1984.
117. Schaller, M., Fischer, A. P., and Perrett, C. H.: Hyperkalemia: a prognostic factor during acute severe hypothermia. JAMA, *264*:1842, 1990.
118. Minamisawa, H., Smith, M., and Siesjo, B. K.: The effect of mild hyperthermia and hypothermia on brain damage following 5, 10, and 15 minutes of forebrain ischemia. Ann. Neurol., *28*:26, 1990.
119. de Jongh, C. A., Caplan, E. S., and Schimpff, S. C.: Infections in the critical care patient. *In* Textbook of Critical Care. Edited by W. C. Shoemaker, W. L. Thompson, and P. R. Holbrook. Philadelphia, W. B. Saunders, 1984.
120. Kass, E. H.: Chemotherapeutic and antibiotic drugs in the management of infections of the urinary tract. Am. J. Med., *18*:764, 1955.
121. Wyndaele, J. J.: Micturition in comatose patients. J. Urol., *135*:1209, 1986.
122. Dunn, C., et al.: Coma blisters: report and review. Cutis, *45*:423, 1990.
123. Mubarak, S. J., and Owen, C. A.: Compartment syndrome and its relation to the crush syndrome: a spectrum of disease. Clin. Orthop., *113*:81, 1975.
124. Shields, R. W., Root, K. E., and Wilbourn, A. J.: Compartment syndromes and compression neuropathies in coma. Neurology, *36*:1370, 1986.
125. Mills, M. L., Russo, L. S., Vines, F. S., and Ross, B. A.: High yield criteria for urgent cranial computed tomography scans. Ann. Emerg. Med., *15*:1167, 1986.
126. Tippin, J., Adams, H. P., and Smoker, W. R. K.: Early computed tomographic abnormalities following profound cerebral hypoxia. Arch. Neurol., *41*:1098, 1984.
127. Goldberg, H. I.: Stroke. *In* Cranial Computed Tomography. Edited by S. H. Lee and K. C. V. G. Rao. New York, McGraw-Hill, 1983.
128. Ropper, A. H.: Lateral displacement of the brain and level of consciousness in patients with an acute hemispheral mass. N. Engl. J. Med., *314*:953, 1986.
129. Ropper, A. H.: A preliminary MRI study of the geometry of brain displacement and level of consciousness with acute intracranial masses. Neurology, *39*:622, 1989.
130. Gaal, M. R.: Intracranial pressure recording. Principles, technics, results and possibilities. Fortschr. Med., *102*:957, 1984.
131. Moss, E., Gibson, J. S., McDowell, D. G., and Gibson, R. M.: Intensive management of severe head injuries. A scheme of intensive management of severe head injuries. Anaesthesia, *38*:214, 1983.
132. Nordby, H. K., and Gunnerd, N.: Epidural monitoring of the intracranial pressure in severe head injury characterized by non-localizing motor response. Acta Neurochir. (Wien), *74*:21, 1985.
133. Saul, T. G., and Ducker, T. B.: Effect of intracranial pressure monitoring and aggressive treatment on mortality in severe head injury. J. Neurosurg., *56*:498, 1982.
134. Mendelow, A. D., et al.: Effect of mannitol on cerebral blood flow and cerebral perfusion pressure in human head injury. J. Neurosurg., *63*:43, 1985.
135. Miller, J. D., Stanek, A., and Langfitt, T. W.: Concepts perfusion pressure and vascular compression during intracranial hypertension. Prog. Brain Res., *35*:411, 1972.
136. Changaris, D. G., et al.: Correlation of cerebral perfusion pressure and glasgow coma scale to outcome. J. Trauma, *27*:1007, 1987.
137. Williams, L. F.: Hemorrhagic shock as a source of unconsciousness. Surg. Clin. North Am., *48*:263, 1986.
138. Bingham, R. M., and Hinds, C. J.: Influence of bolus doses of phenoperidine on intracranial pressure and systemic arterial pressure in traumatic coma. Br. J. Anaesth., *59*:592, 1987.
139. Dearden, N. M., et al.: Effect of high-dose dexamethasone on outcome from severe head injury. J. Neurosurg., *64*:81, 1986.
140. Grafton, S. T., and Longstreth, W. T.: Steroids after cardiac arrest: a retrospective study with concurrent nonrandomized controls. Neurology, *38*:1315, 1988.
141. D'Alecy, L. G., Lundy, E. F., Barton, K. J., and Zelenack, G. B.: Dextrose containing intravenous fluid impairs outcome

141. and increases death after eight minutes of cardiac arrest and resuscitation in dogs. Surgery, *100*:505, 1986.
142. Brain Resuscitation Clinical Trial I Study Group: Randomized clinical study of theipental loading in comatose survivors of cardiac arrest. N. Engl. J. Med., *314*:397, 1986.
143. Ward, J. D., et al.: Failure of prophylactic barbiturate coma in the treatment of severe head injury. J. Neurosurg., *62*:383, 1985.
144. Nordby, H. K., and Nesbakken, R.: The effect of high dose barbiturate decompression after severe head injury: a controlled clinical trial. Acta Neurochir. (Wien), *72*:157, 1984.
145. Selman, W. R., Spetzler, R. F., Anton, A. H., and Crumrine, R. C.: Management of prolonged therapeutic barbiturate coma. Surg. Neurol., *15*:9, 1981.
146. Jacewicz, M., et al.: Nimodipine pretreatment improves cerebral blood flow and reduces brain edema in conscious rats subjected to focal cerebral ischemia. J. Cereb. Blood Flow Metab., *10*:903, 1990.
147. Roine, R. O., et al.: Nimodipine after resuscitation from out-of-hospital ventricular fibrillation: a placebo-controlled, double blind, randomized trial. JAMA, *264*:3171, 1990.
148. Kostron, H., et al.: Treatment of cerebral vasospasm following severe head injury with the calcium influx blocker nimodipine. Neurochirurgia (Stuttg.), *28(Suppl. 1)*:103, 1985.
149. Bricolo, A., et al.: Clinical application of compressed spectral array in long-term EEG monitoring of comatose patients. Electroencephalogr. Clin. Neurophysiol., *45*:211, 1978.
150. Synek, V. M.: Prognostically important EEG coma patterns in diffuse anoxic and traumatic encephalopathies in adults. J. Clin. Neurophysiol., *5*:161, 1988.
151. Bassetti, C., and Scollo-Lavizzari, G.: Value of the EEG in the prognosis of post-anoxic coma following cardiocirculatory arrest. EEG EMGZ., *18*:97, 1987.
152. Austin, E. J., Walkus, R. J., and Longstreth, W. T.: Etiology and prognosis of alpha coma. Neurology, *38*:773, 1988.
153. Haupt, W. F.: Prognostic value of multimodal evoked potentials in neurologic intensive care patients. Klin. Wochenshc., *66(Suppl.)*:53, 1988.
154. Firsching, R., and Frowein, R. A.: Multimodality evoked potentials and early prognosis in comatose patients. Neurosurg. Rev., *13*:141, 1990.
155. Ganes, T., and Lundar, T.: EEG and evoked potentials in comatose patients with severe brain damage. Electroencephalogr. Clin. Neurophysiol., *69*:6, 1988.
156. Brunko, E., and Zegers de Beyl, D.: Prognostic value of early cortical somatosensory evoked potentials after resuscitation from cardiac arrest. Electroencephalogr. Clin. Neurophysiol., *66*:15, 1987.
157. Zentner, J., and Ebner, A.: Somatosensory and motor evoked potentials in the prognostic assessment of traumatic and non-traumatic comatose patients. EEG EMGZ., *19*:267, 1988.
158. Ahmed, I.: Use of somatosensory evoked potentials in the prediction of outcome from coma. Clin. Electroencephalogr., *19*:78, 1988.
159. Drummond, J. C., Todd, M. M., and Sang U, H.: The effect of high dose sodium thiopental on brainstem auditory and median nerve somatosensory evoked responses in humans. Anesthesiology, *63*:249, 1985.
160. Hall, J. W., Bull, J. M., and Cronau, L. H.: Hypo and hyperthermia in clinical auditory brainstem response measurement: two case reports. Ear Hear., *9*:137, 1988.
161. Garcia-Larrea, L., et al.: Transient drug-induces abolition of BAEPs in coma. Neurology, *38*:1487, 1988.
162. Mucea, N., et al.: Stress ulcers in intensive care (etiology, symptomatology and therapy). Resuscitation, *12*:59, 1984.
163. Engelhardt, D., et al.: Comparison between cimetidine-pirenzepine and antacids for the prevention of stress hemorrhage in intensive care patients: a controlled clinical study on 125 patients. Dtsch. Med. Wochenschr., *110*:908, 1985.
164. Farcy, J. H.: Hyperosmolality due to antacid treatment. Anaesthesia, *44*:911, 1989.
165. Regnier, B., Fagniez, P. L., Amamou, M., and Carlet, J.: Artificial enteral nutrition: overview of the technics and their applications. Ann. Anesthesiol. Fr., *21*:29, 1980.
166. Kocan, M. J., and Hickisch, S. M.: A comparison of continuous and intermittent enteral nutrition in NICU patients. J. Neurosci. Nurs., *18*:333, 1986.
167. Grahm, T. W., Zadrozny, D. B., and Harrington, T.: The benefits of early jejunal hyperalimentation in the head-injured patient. Neurosurgery, *25*:729, 1989.
168. Hausmann, D., Mosebach, K. O., Caspari, R., and Rommelscheim, K.: Combined enteral-parenteral nutrition versus total parenteral nutrition in brain-injured patients. A comparative study. Intensive Care Med., *11*:80, 1985.
169. Walker, E. A.: A collaborative study 1977: an appraisal of the criteria of cerebral death: a summary statement. JAMA, *237*:982, 1977.
170. Schafer, J. A., and Caronna, J. J.: Duration of apnea needed to confirm brain death. Neurology, *28*:661, 1978.
171. Marks, S. J., and Zisfein, J.: Apneic oxygenation in apnea tests for brain death: a controlled trial. Arch. Neurol., *47*:1066, 1990.
172. Darby, J. M., Yonas, H., Gur, D., and Latchaw R. E.: Xenon-enhanced computed tomography in brain death. Arch. Neurol., *44*:551, 1987.
173. Darby, J. M., Yonas, H., and Brenner, R. P.: Brainstem death with persistent EEG activity: evaluation by xenon-enhanced computed tomography. Crit. Care Med., *15*:519, 1987.
174. Petty, G. W., et al.: The role of transcranial doppler in confirming brain death: sensitivity, specificity, and suggestions for performance and interpretation. Neurology, *40*:300, 1990.
175. Ropper, A. H., Kehne, S. M., and Wechler, L.: Transcranial doppler in brain death. Neurology, *37*:1733, 1987.
176. Sinclair, M. E., and Suter, P. M.: Lower esophageal contractility as an indicator of brain death in paralyzed and mechanically ventilated patients with head injury. Br. Med. J., *294*:935, 1987.
177. Bell, J. A., and Hodgson, H. J. F.: Coma after cardiac arrest. Braun, *97*:361, 1974.
178. Falk, R. H.: Physical and intellectual recovery following prolonged hypoxic coma. Postgrad. Med. J., *66*:384, 1990.
179. Thomassen, A., and Weinberg, M.: Prevalence and prognostic significance of coma after cardiac arrest outside intensive care and coronary units. Acta Anaesthesiol. Scand., *23*:143, 1979.
180. Maiese, K., et al.: Persistent cognitive impairment in cardiac arrest survivors. Ann. Neurol., *24*:131, 1988.
181. Snyder, B. D., Ramirez-Lassepas, M., and Lippert, D. M.: Neurologic status and prognosis after cardiopulmonary arrest: I. A retrospective study. Neurology, *27*:807, 1977.
182. Snyder, B. D., et al.: Neurologic prognosis after cardiopulmonary arrest: II. Level of consciousness. Neurology, *30*:52, 1980.
183. Snyder, B. D., et al.: Neurologic prognosis after cardiopulmonary arrest: III. Seizure activity. Neurology, *30*:1292, 1980.
184. Snyder, B. D., et al.: Neurologic prognosis after cardiopulmonary arrest: IV. Brainstem reflexes. Neurology, *31*:1092, 1981.
185. Earnest, M. P., et al.: Quality of survival after out-of-hospital

cardiac arrest: predictive value of early neurologic evaluation. Neurology, *29:*56, 1979.
186. Earnest, M. P., et al.: Long-term survival and neurologic status after resuscitation from out-of-hospital cardia arrest. Neurology, *30:*1298, 1980.
187. Bertini, G., et al.: Prognostic significance of early clinical manifestations in postanoxic coma: a retrospective study of 58 patients resuscitated after prehospital cardiac arrest. Crit. Care Med., *17:*627, 1989.
188. Levy, D. E., et al.: Predicting outcome from hypoxic-ischemic coma. JAMA, *253:*1420, 1985.
189. Mueller-Jensen, A., Neunzig, H. P., and Emskotter, T.: Outcome prediction in comatose patients: significance of reflex eye movement analysis. J. Neurol. Neurosurg. Psychiatry, *50:*389, 1987.
190. Stewart, R. B., et al.: Epidemiology of acute drug intoxications: patient characteristics, drugs, and medical complications. Clin. Toxicol., *7:*513, 1974.
191. Arieff, A. I., and Friedman, E. A.: Coma following non-narcotic drug overdosage: management of 208 adult patients. Am. J. Med., *266:*405, 1973.
192. Braakman, R., Jennett, W. B., and Minderhoud, J. M.: Prognosis of the posttraumatic vegetative state. Acta Neurochir. (Wien), *95:*49, 1988.
193. Mayes, S. D., Pelco, L. E., and Campbell, C. J.: Relationships among pre- and post-injury intelligence, length of coma and age in individuals with severe close head injuries. Brain Inj., *3:*301, 1989.
194. Gennarelli, T. A., et al.: Influence of the type of intracranial lesion on outcome from severe head injury. J. Neurosurg., *56:*26, 1982.
195. Kassum, D. A., Thomas, E. J., and Wang, C. J.: Early determinations of outcome in blunt injury. Can. J. Surg., *27:*64, 1984.

SUPPLEMENTAL READINGS

Ahmed, I.: Can somatosensory evoked potentials predict outcome from coma? Clin. Electroencephalogr., *23:*126, 1992.
Dawson, V. L., et al.: Nitric oxide mediates glutamate neurotoxicity in primary cortical cultures. Proc. Natl. Acad. Sci. U.S.A., *88:*6368, 1991.
Garcia-Larrea, L., et al.: The combined monitoring of brain stem auditory evoked potentials and intracranial pressure in coma: a study of 57 patients. J. Neurol. Neurosurg. Psychiatry, *55:*792, 1992.
Maiese, K., Boniece, I., DeMeo, D., and Wagner, J. A.: Peptide growth factors protect against ischemia in culture by preventing nitric oxide toxicity. J. Neurosci., *13:*3034, 1993.
Maiese, K., Boniece, I., Skurat, K., and Wagner, J. A.: Protein kinases modulate the sensitivity of hippocampal neurons to nitric oxide toxicity and anoxia. J. Neurosci. Res., *36:*77, 1993.
Mattson, M. P., Murrain, M., Guthrie, P. B., and Kater, S. B.: Fibroblast growth factor and glutamate: opposing roles in the generation and degeneration of hippocampal neuroarchitecture. J. Neurosci., *9:*3728, 1989.
Nowicki, J. P., Duval, D., Poigner, H., and Scatton, B.: Nitric oxide mediates neuronal death after focal cerebral ischemia in the mouse. Eur. J. Pharmacol., *204:*339, 1991.
Rothstein, T. L., Thomas, E. M., and Sumi, S. M.: Predicting outcome in hypoxic-ischemic coma: a prospective clinical and electrophysiologic study. Electroencephalogr. Clin. Neurophysiol., *79:*101, 1991.
Sazbon, L., et al.: Course and outcome of patients in vegetative state of nontraumatic aetiology. J. Neurol. Neurosurg. Psychiatry, *56:*407, 1993.
Verma, A., et al.: Carbon monoxide: a putative neural messenger. Science, *259:*381, 1993.
Winkler, E., et al.: Use of flumazenil in the diagnosis and treatment of patients with coma of unknown etiology. Crit. Care Med., *21:*538, 1993.

Chapter 2

NEUROPSYCHIATRIC DISTURBANCE IN THE CRITICALLY ILL PATIENT

GEORGE E. TESAR
THEODORE A. STERN

Disturbances of mentation and behavior commonly accompany critical illness and its treatment. Although a patient's mental state and behavior may reflect an expected psychologic reaction to having an illness or being in an ICU, mental status changes are usually caused by the primary illness or its treatment. Sometimes, the onset of neuropsychiatric disturbance signifies an important change in medical status. Therefore, whenever mental status changes occur in a critically ill patient, a thorough neuropsychiatric evaluation should follow. This evaluation should include a mental status examination (MSE) and psychologic profile, as well as investigation of systemic and metabolic abnormalities, drug toxicity, withdrawal states, and other reversible factors that can affect the central nervous system (CNS). Once a cause of neuropsychiatric disturbance has been established, specific medical, behavioral, psychotherapeutic, and/or pharmacologic treatment(s) can be instituted.

Common problems (e.g., anxiety, depression, confusion, agitation, interpersonal and behavioral disturbances, and noncompliance with care) and problems specific to critical care populations (e.g., patients undergoing cardiac surgery, those infected with the human immunodeficiency virus (HIV), those who require mechanical ventilation, and those who have overdosed) will be discussed in this review. Some attention will also be devoted to the recognition and management of neuropsychiatric problems that arise after transfer out of the ICU.

NEUROPSYCHIATRIC MENTAL STATUS EXAMINATION

A systematic bedside MSE is key for accurate diagnosis. Such an examination should be a routine part of the evaluation of each ICU patient, because critically ill patients commonly have abnormalities of affect, behavior, and cognition. The three factors that may interfere with the routine and systematic performance of the MSE are:

- The requirements for evaluation and treatment of the primary illness may occupy more of the physician's attention and time than secondary neuropsychiatric complications.
- The inability of the patient to communicate may make it difficult to perform the necessary examination and to interpret its results.
- Neuropsychiatric symptoms are often regarded as appropriate and understandable reactions to critical illness and, therefore, are not considered worthy of specific evaluation and treatment.

The format recommended for the neuropsychiatric evaluation of the ICU patient should include assessing the following:

- Appearance and behavior
- Speech and language
- Mood and affect
- Thinking
- Perceptions
- Sensorium
- Judgment

Appearance and Behavior

Simple observation with or without the patient's knowledge can provide diagnostic clues. Automatic movements (e.g., blepharospasm, twitching, picking at intravenous [IV] tubing or bed sheets) may indicate the presence of a delirium or of complex partial seizure activity. Disorganized or chaotic movements (e.g., restlessness, agitation) may be a manifestation of delirium. A paucity of movement may signify coma, paralysis, depression, the apathy of a frontal lobe syndrome, or muscular rigidity secondary to a number of disorders (e.g., neuroleptic malignant syndrome [NMS], a side effect of treatment of neuroleptic medication).

Observation of the patient's behavior and appearance should be accompanied by a brief neurologic examination involving assessment of cranial nerve function, neuromuscular tonus, gross motor movement, response to sensory stimuli; examination of deep tendon and cortical reflexes (e.g., glabella, suck, snout, rooting, palmomental, grasp, and plantar); and performance of a fundoscopic examination. Although these procedures are not a formal part of the MSE, their performance is essential to the diagnosis of CNS disorders that can be mistaken for functional (i.e., nonorganic) psychiatric disorders.

Speech and Language

Speech and language are often difficult to test in ICU patients who may be intubated, sedated, fatigued, inattentive, depressed, aphasic, or suffering from a sensory deficit (e.g., vision or hearing impairment). The nursing staff should be called on for their observations of the patient's communication skills and willingness to cooperate with verbal commands. The conscious patient unable to speak can be asked to respond in writing (or if physically unable to write, to use an alphabet board). Assessment of writing is diagnostically helpful since the ability to write, in general, indicates grossly normal cognitive function.[4] When the patient is manually dysfunctional, reliance on other intact motor functions (e.g., eye blink, head nod, foot or toe movement) will be necessary to indicate affirmative and negative responses.

Mood and Affect

Mood refers to the individual's prevailing emotional state and is ascertained by asking the patient how she or he feels. Affect is the more immediate, observable feeling state, (i.e., the visible expression of feeling), and is assessed in terms of its range (e.g., constricted, labile, normal), appropriateness (e.g., with regard to the stated mood), and quality (e.g., manic, depressed, euthymic). Although a paucity or delay of responsiveness suggests a depressed mood, these qualities can also be an indication of fatigue, apathy, or confusion. Further inquiry should be made about the presence of other signs and symptoms of clinical depression (e.g., sleep and appetite disturbances, impaired concentration, poor motivation, loss of interest, guilty rumination, and suicidal thinking). If the clinical state is characterized by heightened energy and four or more of the following symptoms (i.e., distractibility, talkativeness, reckless behavior, hypersexuality, racing ideas, grandiosity, and hyposomnia [mnemonic: DTR HIGH]), then a diagnosis of mania should be made. When mania presents in the ICU, it is likely to be secondary to one or more medical causes (e.g., seizures in the right temporal lobe, metabolic disturbance, infection, CNS neoplasm) or to medications (e.g., corticosteroids, isoniazid, procarbazine hydrochloride, levodopa).[5]

A depressed mood should also be distinguished from the apathetic state associated with dementia or a frontal lobe syndrome. Frontal lobe dysfunction, which frequently occurs in the absence of focal neurologic findings, can be assessed by having the patient perform one or more Luria maneuvers (e.g., fist-side-palm, fist-ring, and reciprocal movements tests) which are named after the Russian neuropsychologist.[6] Other tests of frontal lobe function include visual pattern completion tests and more sophisticated procedures such as the Wisconsin Card Sort and Trailmaking tests, parts A and B.[2] Each of these examinations assesses the patient's cognitive ability, mental flexibility (i.e., ability to change from one conceptual set to another), and ability to inhibit responses.

Thinking

The patient's thinking is evaluated according to its form, flow, and content.[3] The form of thought refers to its coherence and the quality of thought associations. A formal thought disorder is characteristic of psychosis and is manifest by a loosening of associations (i.e., the logical interconnectedness between thoughts is lost) and tangential thinking (i.e., thinking that becomes sidetracked and never reaches its goal). An increase in the rate (flow) of thought is common in mania and in some anxiety states. The term "flight of ideas" is used to describe a sequence of thoughts that are connected but spoken so rapidly that they are difficult for the observer to follow. Patients who exhibit flight of ideas usually will respond affirmatively to the question, "Are your thoughts moving so quickly that you can barely speak them?" Delusions (i.e., fixed, false ideas), obsessions, and destructive ideation (e.g., suicidal or homicidal thoughts) constitute abnormal thought content. Delusions are commonly paranoid, but may also be nihilistic, jealous, or grandiose.

The presence of a thought disorder is usually indicative of psychosis. In the most general terms, psychosis can be defined as a state of being out of touch with reality. Thinking is abnormal, and both delusions and hallucinations are usually present. Psychosis should be viewed as a symptom with a differential diagnosis and not as a diagnosis. If an individual is psychotic and has a clear sensorium, then the psychosis is generally functional (i.e., there is no identifiable organic basis) and represents one of the psychotic disorders listed in the *Diagnostic and Statistical Manual of the American Psychiatric Association,* third edition, revised (DSM III-R) (i.e., schizophrenia, delusional disorder).[7] If the psychotic patient's sensorium is abnormal, however, then a diagnosis of delirium (acute confusional state) must be considered. Delirium rather than functional psychosis is the most likely diagnosis in the critically ill patient whose thinking, behavior, and perceptions are disturbed. When delirium develops, a comprehensive search for an underlying organic or drug-related etiology is warranted.

An important part of the MSE is the evaluation of suicidal thinking. The evaluator should assess for suicidal ideation, particularly if the patient is depressed or is being treated for the sequelae of a drug overdose (OD). Not all ODs constitute a suicide attempt, but denial of an attempt by the patient who has overdosed must be evaluated thoroughly. The circumstances surrounding the OD, the lethality of the attempt (both the nature of the chosen method and the likelihood of being rescued from the attempt), the patient's attitude toward failure of the attempt, and the patient's desire to make further suicide attempts should be assessed. Psychiatric consultation should be ordered routinely if a suicide attempt is suspected; useful and often necessary information can be obtained from available family members and interested parties. The patient's right to confidentiality is waived in these instances since actual or suspected suicidality constitutes a medical and psychiatric emergency. Any psychiatric disorder, but particularly affective (i.e., mood) and psychotic disorders, increase the lifetime risk of suicide. Therefore, it is important to perform a thorough MSE that focuses on mood and affect, as well as on content and form of thinking.

Perceptions

Abnormal perceptions are classified as hallucinations, illusions, or distortions.[3] An hallucination is a false perception (e.g., auditory, visual, olfactory, gustatory, tactile, or

Table 2–1. Minimental State Examination

```
                                                          Patient _____
                                                          Examiner _____
                                                          Date _____
                              "MINI-MENTAL STATE"
Maximum
 score   Score                      Orientation
   5      ( )    What is the (year) (season) (date) (day) (month)?
   5      ( )    Where are we: (state) (county) (town) (hospital) (floor).
                                    Registration
   3      ( )    Name 3 objects: 1 second to say each. Then ask the patient all 3 after you have said them. Give 1 point for each correct
                 answer. Then repeat them until he learns all 3. Count trials and record.
                                                                                      Trials _____
                              Attention and Calculation
   5      ( )    Serial 7s. 1 point for each correct. Stop after 5 answers. Alternatively spell "world" backwards.
                                      Recall
   3      ( )    Ask for the 3 objects repeated above. Give 1 point for each correct.
                                     Language
   9      ( )    Name a pencil, and watch (2 points)
                 Repeat the following "No ifs ands or buts." (1 point)
                 Follow a 3-stage command:
                   "Take a paper in your right hand, fold it in half, and put it on the floor" (3 points)
                 Read and obey the following:
                                 Close your eyes (1 point)
                 Write a sentence (1 point)
                 Copy design (1 point)
                 Total score
                 ASSESS level of consciousness along a continuum        Alert    Drowsy    Stupor    Coma
```

(From Folstein, M. F., Folstein, S. E., and McHugh, P. R.: "Mini-mental state," a practical method for grading the cognitive state of patients for the clinician. J. Psychiatr. Res., *12*:189, 1975.)

---

somatosensory) that occurs in the absence of an external stimulus. Hallucinations associated with functional psychotic disorders are usually auditory; on occasion they may be visual. Hallucinations that are visual, olfactory, gustatory, tactile, or somatosensory are more likely to be caused by an underlying organic disturbance (e.g., metabolic encephalopathy, complex partial seizures), drug toxicity (e.g., due to lidocaine), or substance withdrawal (e.g., from alcohol or sedative-hypnotic agents). The presence of any type of hallucination, particularly if it is of recent onset, is an indication for a thorough medical and neurologic evaluation.

Illusions and distortions are almost always indicative of CNS dysfunction. An illusion is a misinterpretation of a stimulus arising from a real object (e.g., misperceiving a light bulb as a fire). A distortion is an altered perception of a real object (e.g., macropsia and micropsia occurring in the context of complex partial seizures).

Sensorium

Sensorium is comprised of the following intellectual functions:

- Attention
- Orientation
- Memory (immediate, recent, and long-term)
- Cognition (reasoning, calculation, and abstraction)
- Constructional ability

A valid and reliable assessment of a patient's sensorium depends on the presence of normal attention. If an individual is inattentive, it will be impossible to assess accurately the integrity of the other functions. Several tests are commonly used to test attention: subtracting serial sevens, spelling the word "world" backwards, repeating the names of the month in reverse order, and repeating digits. Digit repetition is perhaps the best test because educational level and the presence of dyslexia do not affect test performance. Most people with normal attention can repeat five to seven digits forward and four to five digits backward.[1]

The Mini-Mental State Examination (MMSE) of Folstein, Folstein, and McHugh (Table 2-1) is probably the best bedside tool to examine the components of a patient's sensorium.[8] It was developed to screen clinical populations for dementia. Although it is not sufficiently sensitive to detect subtle cases of dementia,[9] it is useful when screening for cognitive impairment. A perfect score is 30. A score of 24 or more suggests an intact sensorium, whereas scores of less than 24 suggest cognitive dysfunction. An abnormal MMSE should stimulate a more thorough investigation for treatable abnormalities.

Judgment

Judgment is the capacity to perceive, discern, or make reasonable decisions. An abnormal sensorium (e.g., due to delirium or dementia) obviously compromises judgment. When sensorium is normal, other factors (e.g., mood disorder, psychotic disorder, personality disorder, intense anxiety, or anger) can impair judgment. In general, any patient behavior that is inconsistent with caregivers' expectations may raise doubts about the patient's decision-making power. For example, a patient's wish to discontinue life-sustaining treatment almost always provokes concern about the patient's judgment unless it is clear that all efforts to sustain a meaningful life have failed and the patient's judgment is not clouded by neuropsychiatric disturbance (e.g., psychosis, depression).

Evaluation of judgment has traditionally been accomplished by asking the patient two questions: (1) What would you do if you were in a movie theater and saw smoke coming from an empty section of the theater? and (2) What would you do if you found a stamped, sealed, addressed envelope in the street? Responses to these questions are of questionable clinical value and are probably no more informative than other tests of sensorium and higher cognitive function. The kinds of judgments that the ICU physician will more likely be interested in range from a patient's process of reasoning about their current and future care, the likelihood of acting on hallucinatory perceptions and delusional beliefs, and their capacity for acting on suicidal or homicidal impulses.[3]

When the patient's judgment is considered abnormal, it is important to identify the cause (e.g., delirium, depression, psychosis), to correct the underlying abnormality when possible and to determine whether it is necessary to assume the patient's right to make independent decisions. If the patient's judgment is abnormal (i.e., the capacity to make reasonable decisions is impaired), then it may be necessary to appoint a guardian. In emergency situations, however, the physician has the right to make independent decisions that reflect sound medical judgment and are believed to be in the patient's best interest.

NEUROPSYCHIATRIC DISORDERS IN ICU PATIENTS

Common neuropsychiatric disorders encountered in ICU patients include:

- Anxiety
- Depression
- Delirium
- Agitation

Anxiety

Diagnostic and Clinical Characteristics

Anxiety is a universal human response to danger. It is an emotion difficult to describe, but familiar to most as an uncomfortable sense of inner tension and foreboding. Mild to moderate anxiety is adaptive to the extent that it alerts one to presence of danger and mobilizes the resources necessary for a quick and effective response. Anxiety that is severe, however, can disrupt attention and impair cognition.

It is not surprising that the conscious ICU patient experiences some degree of anxiety. The possibility of death, disability, disfigurement, or pain and the spectre of unforeseen circumstances are sufficient to produce anxiety in most critically ill patients. When the patient's anxiety becomes too intense, or begins to overwhelm the patient's ability to cope, it can interfere with patient management. Anxiety can result in unwanted consequences in the critically ill cardiac patient by elevating levels of serum catecholamine; it can interfere with the patient's ability to fol-

Table 2–2. Physical Signs and Symptoms of Anxiety

Anorexia	Lightheadedness
Butterflies in stomach	Muscle tension
Chest pain or tightness	Nausea
Diaphoresis	Pallor
Diarrhea	Palpitations
Dizziness	Paresthesias
Dyspnea	Sexual dysfunction
Dry mouth	Stomach pain
Faintness	Tachycardia
Flushing	Tremulousness
Headache	Urinary frequency
Hyperventilation	Vomiting

(From Rosenbaum, J. F.: The drug treatment of anxiety. N. Engl. J. Med., *306*:401, 1982.)

low directions by disturbing concentration; and it can be life-threatening in patients who must cooperate with the strict demands of life-support devices (e.g., use of mechanical ventilation and the intra-aortic balloon pump [IABP]).

Anxiety is evident to caretakers either because the patient reports it or because of its physical manifestations (Table 2–2). Psychologically minded patients may be aware of its presence and its causes. Others may be unable to identify their discomfort as anxiety. Typically, the anxious patient appears hypervigilant, exhibits muscular tension that results in restlessness or immobility, and has difficulty relaxing or falling asleep. Some anxious patients may avoid sleep for fear of death. In some patients, tension may contribute to blunted affect, and constricted range of emotion that can be mistaken for depression.

Etiologic and Predisposing Factors

Certain medical (Table 2–3) and psychiatric disorders predispose patients to anxiety in the ICU. Cardiac patients have been found to exhibit a high rate of anxiety in the first day or so after admission to a coronary care unit (CCU).[10] Anxiety has also been shown to increase significantly at the time of transfer from the CCU to a step-down unit.[11] Anxious patients, particularly those with psychiatric histories, may have difficulty weaning from the ventilator. In fact, a personal history of any psychiatric disorder in the ICU patient is likely to be associated with a higher than usual level of anxiety. Untreated anxiety and phobic disorders (e.g., panic disorder, agoraphobia, social phobia, generalized anxiety disorder, obsessive compulsive disorder, and post-traumatic stress disorder), a history of alcohol or sedative abuse, and personality disorders will all reduce the threshold for an anxious response.

Treatment

Orientation to the circumstances and treatment plan, anticipation and discussion of unexpressed fears and concerns, and reassurance are measures that are indicated and usually sufficient to allay most of the patient's anxiety.[12] Preoperative teaching helps to reduce postoperative anxiety because it prepares the patient for new and unexpected experiences. It may be necessary to repeat instructions or to provide repeated reassurance for the anxious patient. Repeated instructions of this type may also indicate the need for anxiolytic treatment.

Although anxiety is an expected and appropriate reaction to many circumstances encountered by the ICU patient, its consequences are potentially harmful (e.g., elevated heart rate and blood pressure, cardiac arrhythmias, trouble weaning from the ventilator) and should be treated.[13] The goals of treatment include control of emotional reactivity, autonomic responses to fear and conflict, circulating catecholamine levels (thereby reducing potential for cardiac arrhythmias in selected patients), and disruption of sleep patterns. Stern and colleagues found that despite these considerations, only two thirds of all patients admitted to a CCU had any anxiolytic or hypnotic medication prescribed during their entire course in the CCU.[14] Both patient and physician concerns about drug dependency and oversedation further limited the prescription of anxiolytic agents despite the staff's recognition of the patient's anxiety. Patients on fixed medication schedules were far more likely to receive their medication than those on an as needed basis. There is an understandable reluctance to prescribe medications with CNS depressant properties when the patient's mental state is already disrupted or the medical condition is tenuous. Careful clinical evaluation, close monitoring, and selection of an appropriate agent should minimize the risk of adverse consequences, however.

Benzodiazepines are the agents of choice for the pharmacologic treatment of anxiety, because they have few side effects. The choice of a particular agent depends on its pharmacologic and pharmacokinetic profile (Table 2-4), as well as the clinical circumstances. Diazepam, 5 to 10 mg orally, tid or qid, can be used in uncomplicated situations. In general, however, the short- to intermediate-lasting agents with half-lives in the range of 8 to 20 hours (e.g., lorazepam, 0.5 to 2 mg tid or qid; oxazepam, 10 to 30 mg orally, every 4 to 6 hours; and alprazolam, 0.25 to 1.0 mg orally, tid to qid) are preferred because they are excreted quickly, and in most patients their serum levels do not build up with repeated dosing.[15] Additionally, lorazepam, unlike other benzodiazepines whose intramuscular (IM) administration may be more problematic, can be administered safely and effectively by all routes. For example, IM injection of chlordiazepoxide has been associated with sterile abscess formation because of its tendency to crystalize at physiologic pH;[16] IM diazepam is absorbed erratically from areas with relatively poor perfusion (e.g., the gluteal area);[16] and parenteral midazolam is restricted in some hospitals because of its potent respiratory depressant effect.[17] Other benzodiazepines marketed in the United States are unavailable in the injectable form. The long-lasting agents, diazepam, chlordiazepoxide, and clorazepate, have as their metabolite the long-lasting, active agent, nordiazepam ($t\frac{1}{2}$ = 60 to 100 hours), which builds up with repeated dosing and can be the cause of prolonged and unwanted sedation.[15]

Depression

Diagnosis and Clinical Characteristics

The term depression is used to refer both to a diagnosis (syndrome) and also to an emotional state or mood (symptom). Depressed mood is a universally experienced emotion commonly referred to as sadness (melancholy), disappointment, dejection, despondency, or grief. It is however only one of the symptoms required to make a clinical diagnosis of **major depression.**

Major depression is defined in the DSM III-R as a disturbance of mood or interest occurring for a period of at least 2 weeks and associated with a minimum of five of the following eight neurovegetative symptoms:

- Disturbed sleep
- Loss of normal interest and motivation
- Guilty rumination that is excessive or inappropriate
- Loss of energy
- Impaired concentration
- Disturbed appetite
- Psychomotor agitation or retardation
- Hopelessness, suicidal rumination, or the wish to be dead[15]

A diagnosis of **adjustment disorder with depressed mood** is made when the onset of depressed mood follows an identifiable stressor and the necessary criteria for major depression are not met.[7] The diagnosis of major depression implicitly warrants a trial of antidepressant medication, whereas a solitary and transient symptom of depressed mood may not.

Table 2-3. Physical Causes of Anxiety-Like Symptoms

Type of Cause	Specific Cause
Cardiovascular	Angina pectoris, arrhythmias, congestive heart failure, hypertension, hypovolemia, myocardial infarction, syncope (of multiple causes), valvular disease, vascular collapse (shock)
Dietary	Caffeine, monosodium glutamate (Chinese restaurant syndrome), vitamin-deficiency diseases
Drug-related	Akathisia (secondary to antipsychotic drugs), anticholinergic toxicity, digitalis toxicity, hallucinogens, hypotensive agents, stimulants (amphetamines, cocaine, and related drugs), withdrawal syndromes (alcohol or sedative-hypnotics), bronchodilators (theophylline, sympathomimetics)
Hematologic	Anemias
Immunologic	Anaphylaxis, systemic lupus erythematosus
Metabolic	Hyperadrenalism (Cushing's disease), hyperkalemia, hyperthermia, hyperthyroidism, hypocalcemia, hypoglycemia, hyponatremia, hypothyroidism, menopause, porphyria (acute intermittent)
Neurologic	Encephalopathies (infectious, metabolic, and toxic), essential tremor, intracranial mass lesions, postconcussive syndrome, seizure disorders (especially of the temporal lobe), vertigo
Respiratory	Asthma, chronic obstructive pulmonary disease, pneumonia, pneumothorax, pulmonary edema, pulmonary embolism
Secreting tumors	Carcinoid, insulinoma, pheochromocytoma

(Adapted from Rosenbaum, J. F.: The drug treatment of anxiety. N. Engl. J. Med., *306*:401, 1982.)

Table 2-4. Benzodiazepines Commonly Used in the United States

Drug	Elimination Half-Life (hours)	Onset	Active Metabolites	Approximate Dose Equivalence (mg)	Possible Route(s) of Administration[b]
Diazepam[a]	30–60	Very fast	Yes[c]	5	PO, IM, IV
Chlordiazepoxide	20–50	Slow	Yes[c]	25	PO
Clorazepate[d]	30–100	Fast	Yes[c]	7.5	PO
Prazepam	50–80	Very slow	Yes	10	PO
Flurazepam[e]	50–100	Fast	Yes[f]	15	PO
Quazepam	30–100	Intermed.	Yes	15	PO
Clonazepam[g]	20–50	Slow	Yes	0.25	PO
Lorazepam[h,i]	10–18	Intermed.	No	1	PO, IM, IV
Temazepam[e]	10–12	Intermed.	No	15	PO
Oxazepam[h,i]	6–12	Slow	No	15	PO
Alprazolam[a]	8–14	Very fast	Minor[j]	0.5	PO
Triazolam[k]	1.5–3	Intermed.	No	0.25	PO
Midazolam[l]	1–4	Very fast	No	2.5	IM, IV

[a] High abuse liability
[b] For preparations available in the United States
[c] The principal active metabolite is nordiazepam ($t_{1/2}$ = 60–100 hr)
[d] Clorazepate itself is inactive, but is rapidly converted in gastric acid to its active metabolite, nordiazepam.
[e] Relatively low incidence of rebound insomnia, probably because of relatively long elimination half-life.
[f] Norflurazepam is the principle metabolite with half-life similar to that of nordiazepam.
[g] Labeled for the treatment of petit mal epilepsy, but has also been used successfully to treat panic disorder, mania, nocturnal myoclonus, and other sleep-related movement disorders.
[h] Inactivated by glucuronidation which (a) does not depend on hepatic microsomal activity, and (b) remains intact except in the most severe instances of hepatic dysfunction.
[i] Excreted principally in the urine.
[j] It is unclear to what extent metabolites contribute to alprazolam's activity, but, judging from its duration of clinical activity (i.e., 4–6 hr), probably not much at all.
[k] Its use is associated at times with profound anterograde amnesia, and its discontinuation with considerable rebound insomnia.
[l] Used principally for induction of anesthesia and sedation during procedures. The most lipophilic and the most potent of benzodiazepines currently available in the United States.

Accurate diagnosis, evaluation, and treatment of depression in patients with medical illness can be impeded in several ways. Failure to appreciate the symptom/syndrome distinction is one way, because mistaking the syndrome for a symptom may result in the withholding of treatment that is indicated. A closely related problem is the practice of withholding treatment for depression that is regarded as appropriate because it occurs in the context of a terminal or catastrophic illness. Debates about the value and indication for specific antidepressant treatment in these circumstances may take on a moral tone that probably reflects a common opposition to the prescription and use of mind-altering drugs. Instead, objective evaluation for the signs and symptoms of depression should guide treatment decisions. Unfortunately, the task of diagnosing depression is further complicated by the overlap of symptoms (e.g., sleep disturbance, appetite impairment, or fatigue) that can be due either to the medical illness or to the presence of an affective disorder. As a result, the diagnosis of depression in the medically ill patient often relies less on the presence of somatic symptoms and more on the presence of psychologic symptoms (e.g., hopelessness, thoughts of death, guilty rumination, and impaired motivation).[18] A personal history of depression and a family history of depression or alcoholism increase the likelihood that the symptoms are explained by a major depressive episode.

The diagnosis of depression may be particularly difficult to establish in elderly patients. In some, depression may impair cognition to the degree that dementia is erroneously diagnosed and in others it is mistaken for the apathy associated with frontal lobe dysfunction. Moreover, elderly depressed patients may not have classic presenting symptoms and instead manifest irritability, regressive behavior, and refusal to cooperate.

Incidence

Many medically ill individuals complain of a depressed mood.[18] It has been estimated that up to 36% of medically ill individuals suffer from depressive syndrome.[19] In one study of ICU patients at the Massachusetts General Hospital, major depression was the second most frequently diagnosed psychiatric disorder.[20] Among 340 ICU patients seen by psychiatric consultants, 15.3% were given a diagnosis of major depression, and an additional 6.8% received a diagnosis of adjustment disorder with depressed mood.[19] In another study, 5% of the admissions to a medical ICU were a direct result of drug overdose,[21] a condition frequently associated with major depression.

Differential Diagnosis

Depression is a nonspecific symptom of a wide range of affective disorders (e.g., major depression, dysthymia, bipolar affective disorder, cyclothymia, organic mood disorder), and other neuropsychiatric disorders (e.g., delirium, dementia, schizophrenia, and personality disorders), and neuromedical disorders (Table 2-5). It can also be a side effect of certain medications used in the ICU (Table 2-6).

As noted previously, major depression should be distinguished from adjustment disorder with depressed mood (also known as minor depression), and from dysthymia, a diagnosis made when the individual has suffered from depressed mood accompanied by fewer than five neurovegetative symptoms for approximately 2 years.[7] While antidepressant treatment may be indicated for either of these diagnoses, the likelihood of successful treatment is less than for dysthymia. When making the diagnosis of a major depressive episode, it is important to determine whether the episode is occurring in the context of bipolar affective disorder, because the use of antidepressants can trigger the onset of mania unless prophylaxis with lithium is implemented.

The diagnosis of major depression, particularly if it is atypical, should prompt the investigation for an underlying organic cause. The diagnosis of organic mood disorder is made when an alteration of mood can be attributed to a specific underlying organic disorder (e.g., hypothyroidism, stroke, Cushing's syndrome, or hyperparathyroidism).[7] Endocrine disturbances constitute the most frequent causes of organic mood disorders, but HIV-related disorders (e.g., HIV encephalopathy, acquired immunodeficiency syndrome [AIDS]) are contributing to an increasing proportion of both adjustment disorders and major depressive episodes with organic cause seen in ICU patients.

Organic mood disorder is distinct from delirium and dementia, which can manifest depressed mood. Hypoactive deliria, in particular, may be misdiagnosed as depression unless the physician performs a thorough MSE and detects the underlying confusion and fluctuating level of consciousness. Although demented patients may suffer from a superimposed depression, it is important to distinguish depressed mood from the apathy associated with degenerative changes in the frontal lobes. Specific tests of frontal lobe function (e.g., Luria maneuvers, visual pattern completion tests, Wisconsin card sorting) can help clarify the diagnosis.[1,2]

Evaluation

No specific laboratory test is pathognomonic of major depression. Therefore, laboratory evaluation should focus on the identification of metabolic and systemic factors that can cause depression. Most ICU patients will have undergone a thorough laboratory investigation on several occasions. The evaluating physician should check the patient's hematocrit and white blood cell count, thyroid function tests, recent electrolyte levels (including serum magnesium and calcium), blood urea nitrogen, creatinine, liver function tests, serum ammonia, ABG determinations, vitamin B_{12} and folate levels, and a Veneral Disease Research Laboratories (VDRL) test. Depending on the clinical circumstances, HIV testing may be recommended because HIV encephalopathy may present with features of a variety of psychiatric illnesses, including depression. A computed tomographic (CT) scan of the head is indicated in selected cases and an electroencephalogram (EEG) may help to rule out an underlying delirium.

Treatment

Resolution of depression depends on accurate diagnosis and then, frequently, the combination of both psychologic

Table 2–5. Medical Conditions Commonly Associated with Depressive Symptoms

Collagen vascular disorders
  Systemic lupus erythematosus
  Polyarteritis nodosa
Endocrine disorders
  Hyperadrenalism
  Hypoadrenalism
  Hyperparathyroidism
  Hypoparathyroidism
  Hyperthyroidism
  Hypothyroidism
Infections
  AIDS
  Post-influenza
  Hepatitis
  Mononucleosis
Neoplasms
  Pancreatic carcinoma
  Carcinoid
  Neurologic disorders
  Stroke (CVA)
  Subcortical dementia
  Multiple sclerosis
  Brain tumor
Vitamin deficiencies
  Vitamin B_{12} deficiency
  Wernicke's encephalopathy

(From Geringer, E. S., and Stern, T. A.: Anxiety and depression in critically ill patients. Probl. Crit. Care, 2:35, 1988.)

Table 2–6. Drugs Commonly Associated with Depressive Symptoms

Alcohol
Antihypertensives
  Reserpine
  Methyldopa
  Thiazides
  Clonidine
  Hydralazine
Antiparkinsonian agents
  Levodopa
  Carbidopa
  Amantadine
Barbiturates
Benzodiazepines
Beta blockers (especially propranolol)
Bromides
Carbon monoxide
Cimetidine
Cocaine
Digitalis (toxicity)
Disulfiram
Heavy metals (especially lead)
Metoclopromide
Opiates
Oral contraceptives
Steroids

(From Geringer, E. S., and Stern, T. A.: Anxiety and depression in critically ill patients. Probl. Crit. Care, 2:35, 1988.)

Table 2–7. Antidepressant Drugs Currently Available in the United States

Drug	Typical Daily Dose (mg)	Therapeutic Plasma Levels (ng/ml)	Anticholinergic Effects	Sedative Effects	Half-Life (hr)	Comments
Tricyclic Antidepressants[1]						
Amitriptyline	75–300		S[2]	S	22–26	Injectable form available
Trimipramine	75–300		I	S		
Imipramine	75–300	>225	I	I	30	Injectable form available
Doxepin	75–300	100–250(?)	S	S		
Protriptyline	15–60		S	W		
Nortriptyline	30–150	50–150	W	W	26	Least likely TCA to cause PH[3]
Desipramine	75–300	>125	W	W		
Other Polycyclic Antidepressants						
Maprotiline	75–200		W	I	51	Seizures and cardiac arrhythmias reported at doses >200 mg/day
Trazodone	150–400		W	S	3–9	Side effect: Priapism
Amoxapine	75–300		W	W	30	Side effect: tardive dyskinesia
Bupropion	150–450		W	W		Seizures reported at doses >450 mg/day
Serotonin-Selective Reuptake Inhibitors (SSRIs)						
Fluoxetine	10–60		W	W	7–9 days	Side effect: akathisia
Paroxetine	20–50		W	W	21	
Sertraline	50–200		W	W	26	
Monoamine Oxidase Inhibitors (MAOIs)[4]						
Isocarboxazid	20–50		W	W		
Phenelzine	30–60		W	W		Potent hypotensive effect
Tranylcypromine	20–50		W	W		
Psychostimulants[5]						
Dextroamphetamine	5–20		W	W	10–30	Half-life = 10–30 hr
Methylphenidate	5–30		W	W	4–12	Half-life = 4–12 hr

[1] All TCAs have quinidine-like effects on the cardiac conduction system. Their use is relatively contraindicated and should be monitored carefully in the presence of bundle branch block, QRS > 100 msec, and QTc > 440 msec.
[2] S = strong; I = intermediate; and W = weak
[3] PH = postural hypotension
[4] Hypertensive crisis can occur when used in combination with foods high in tyramine content and with sympathomimetic agents. Also, combined use with meperidine (Demerol) causes delirium and therefore is absolutely contraindicated.
[5] Maximum therapeutic effect is usually evident within 2 days of initiation.
(Adapted from Hyman, S. E., and Tesar, G. E.: Manual of Psychiatric Emergencies. 3rd Ed. Boston, Little, Brown, 1994.)

and pharmacologic treatments. In many cases where a diagnosis of adjustment disorder with depressed mood is made, appropriate reassurance and the opportunity for emotional ventilation may be sufficient to alleviate sadness, feelings of loss, and a sense of being defeated by the illness.[12]

When these efforts are unproductive, however, or if a diagnosis of major depression has been made, then a trial of antidepressant medication is indicated. The specific treatment selected depends on the patient's medical status and on the pharmacologic properties of the agent(s) being considered. When the risks of antidepressants are considered excessive, then the physician should consider the use of electroconvulsive therapy (ECT).

The antidepressant drugs currently available for use in the United States are listed in Table 2–7. Because most of these agents have comparable clinical efficacy when tested in controlled clinical trials, the choice of which agent to use depends largely on its side effect profile. In general, the task for the critical care physician is to select an agent that has relatively rapid onset of action with minimal side effects.

Tricyclic Antidepressants. The tricyclic antidepressants (TCAs) (Table 2–7) have been among the most widely prescribed and extensively studied of the available antidepressants. They have properties that limit their use in critical care patients, however, particularly patients with heart disease.[22] TCAs are known to affect central and peripheral adrenergic, cholinergic, histaminergic, and serotonergic activity, as well as the cardiac conduction system. These actions are believed to account for their therapeutic and adverse effects. The drug effects of particular concern to the ICU physician are central and peripheral anticholinergic effects (e.g., tachycardia, decreased intestinal motility, dry mouth, blurring of vision, mental confusion) and cardiovascular effects (e.g., tachycardia, orthostatic, hypotension, conduction delays, and arrhythmias). Of the TCAs, desipramine has the least anticholinergic activity and nortriptyline is least likely to produce orthostatic hypotension; however, all TCAs exert a quinidine-like effect and are equally capable of slowing conduction through the His-ventricular segment of the conduction system. Although clinically significant effects on conduction are unlikely to occur at therapeutic serum levels of TCAs, preexistent conduction defects (e.g., intraventricular conduction delay [IVCD], bundle branch block, and delayed repolarization) and coadministration of drugs that have quinidine-like, or type IA antiarrhythmic properties (e.g., quinidine, procainamide, disopyramide, phenothiazines) increase the risk of significant TCA-associated conduction and rhythm disturbances. Furthermore, the delayed onset of action of TCAs (i.e., 2 to 3 weeks from the time therapeutic serum levels are achieved) makes it difficult to assess their efficacy in the ICU, where multiple factors interact to produce a rapidly changing clinical situation. For all these reasons, the use of TCAs in the ICU should probably be limited to patients who require an antidepressant and one or more of the following:

- Preexisting treatment with a TCA at the time of ICU admission
- Requirement for parenteral antidepressants[23]
- A good response to a TCA in the past
- Lack of response to any of the other available antidepressants
- Refusal of ECT

Newer Antidepressants. The newest antidepressants, fluoxetine, sertraline, paroxetine, and bupropion (Table 2-7), have relatively benign side effects. Neither fluoxetine nor bupropion has substantial anticholinergic or cardiovascular toxicity, although both agents can cause gastrointestinal disturbances, headache, and psychomotor excitation (e.g., tremor, restlessness). Bupropion, in doses greater than 450 mg daily, has been reported to cause seizures in bulimic patients,[24] and there is anecdotal evidence that fluoxetine may precipitate suicidal ideation;[25] however, this has not been noted by all investigators.[26] Although fluoxetine is marketed as a 20-mg capsule, treatment may be started with as little as 5 mg per day; 20 mg is an average daily antidepressant dose. Bupropion is typically started at 50 mg bid and is increased toward a maximum of 450 mg orally per day. Other antidepressants (e.g., maprotiline, amoxapine, and trazodone) have not lived up to promising forecasts because of reports of unacceptable side effects, such as seizures (from maprotiline and amoxapine), cardiac arrhythmias (from maprotiline and trazodone), extrapyramidal symptoms (from amoxapine), and priapism (from trazodone) (Table 2-7). Like fluoxetine, sertraline and paroxetine are serotonin-selective reuptake inhibitors (SSRIs). Their side effect profiles are similar, however, unlike fluoxetine and its active metabolite norfluoxetine, which has a half-life of up to 9 days, both sertraline and paroxetine have no active metabolites and have half-lives of approximately 1 day.

Psychostimulants. Commonly overlooked but effective antidepressant agents are the psychostimulants, dextroamphetamine and methylphenidate (Table 2-7). Despite their reputation for abuse, they are particularly well suited for the treatment of depression in the ICU setting. These agents combine a rapid onset of action with relatively few side effects. They have been used safely and effectively to treat depression in geriatric and medically ill patients[27,28] and in those who have undergone cardiac surgery.[29] Prescription of either dextroamphetamine or methylphenidate, 2.5 to 10 mg orally once daily or up to three times per day, is usually effective within 1 to 2 days of administration.[30,31] The effective dose can be continued on a daily basis with little, if any, risk of habituation.[30,31] Hypertension and cardiac arrhythmias are relative contraindications to the use of psychostimulants. Mild elevations in blood pressure and heart rate may be stimulated by their use and patients should be monitored every 30 minutes for at least 1 to 2 hours following initial dosing. Nausea, vomiting, tremor, and mental confusion are other potential side effects.

Monoamine Oxidase Inhibitors (MAOIs). The MAOIs (Table 2-7) are a class of antidepressants whose use is generally reserved for treatment-resistant depression, atypical depression, or panic disorder. The side effect of hypotension and the risk of hypertensive crisis when MAOIs are used in combination with indirect-acting sympathomimetic agents (e.g., ephedrine, dopamine) are important contraindications to the initiation of an MAOI in the ICU setting.[32] Treatment of MAOI-induced hypertensive crisis can be acutely managed with administration of phentolamine, an alpha-1 antagonist. If a patient is already being treated with an MAOI (e.g., phenelzine, isocarboxazid, or tranylcypromine, it may as well be continued because inhibition of the enzyme, monoamine oxidase, persists up to 3 weeks after drug discontinuation.[32]

Lithium. Lithium is more of a mood stabilizing agent than an antidepressant, and it is prescribed to patients with underlying affective disorders, particularly bipolar (i.e., manic-depressive) disorder, and aggressivity. It is rare for lithium to be initiated in the ICU. One situation where it is indicated is prophylaxis of steroid-induced mania during corticosteroid treatment of a medical illness.[33] If a patient is already taking lithium, it is important to monitor serum lithium levels, fluid and electrolyte balance (being especially mindful of hyponatremia because of its tendency to be associated with elevated serum lithium levels), renal function, and medications that can elevate lithium levels (e.g., indomethacin, thiazide diuretics).[15] Lithium toxicity can be manifest by gastrointestinal symptoms (e.g., nausea, vomiting, diarrhea) and neurologic symptoms (e.g., tremors, seizures), and death. Dialysis (preferably hemodialysis) is indicated for patients with elevated serum lithium levels and signs of neurologic toxicity (e.g., tremors, confusion, seizures, coma).[34]

Delirium

Traditionally, the terms ICU psychosis or ICU syndrome have been used to designate abnormalities of affect, behavior, and cognition in ICU patients.[35,36] This terminology reflects early concerns about the psychologic hazards of being exposed to a highly sophisticated, impersonal environment designed to prevent death. Drawing on experimental data that suggested a relationship between sleep deprivation and subsequent psychosis, early theorists reasoned that ICU patients become psychotic because they were routinely deprived of sleep and exposed to sensory overload, deprivation, or monotony. Subsequently, it became clear that other factors, many having no specific relationship to the ICU setting, contribute to acute confusional states in ICU patients.[35,36]

A diagnosis of delirium more specifically and appropriately describes the disordered mentation and behavior that commonly occurs in ICU patients. Although some patients become psychotic in an ICU or have a psychotic condition that antedates admission to the ICU (e.g., schizophrenia), most ICU patients with mental status changes are delirious because of one or more factors that disrupt the integrity of the CNS. Toxic/metabolic encephalopathy, acute organic brain syndrome, and acute confusional state are terms often used in place of delirium.

Diagnostic and Clinical Features

The diagnosis of delirium is made on clinical grounds. Acute onset of confusion and an altered level of consciousness are the hallmarks of delirium, an organic mental disorder that is usually, though not always, reversible. Recovery generally occurs over a period of days to weeks, but some cases progress to irreversible brain failure.[37] The prompt recognition of delirium is important for timely treatment and prevention of untoward sequelae.

In addition to abnormal sensorium characterized by impaired attention, disorientation, and poor short-term memory, the delirious patient typically exhibits:

- Abnormalities of perception (e.g., illusions, hallucinations)
- Disordered thinking (e.g., loosening of associations)
- Abnormal thought content (e.g., paranoid delusions)
- Mood disturbance (e.g., depression or excitation)
- Disorganized behavior (e.g., picking at bed sheets or IV tubing)
- Disturbance of the sleep/wake cycle (i.e., the patient is often awake at night and drowsy during the day)

Typically, the delirious patient's level of consciousness fluctuates. If the patient is examined during a lucid interval, the diagnosis may be overlooked. Misdiagnosis can also occur when a corresponding disturbance of mood (e.g., irritability, depression) is the predominant feature; when the delirious patient is quiet, inactive, and apathetic (hypoactive delirium); or when the patient has some awareness of the dysfunction and attempts to conceal it by using defenses of denial, projection, and avoidance. Delirium may also be accompanied by other signs of CNS derangement (e.g., asterixis, tremor, dysgraphia, slurred or aphasic speech, trouble following commands, and abnormal cortical and deep tendon reflexes).

Numerous organic (Table 2–8) and drug-related (Table 2–9) disturbances have been implicated in the etiology of delirium, although certain of those conditions or factors (e.g., stroke, shock, drug toxicity, drug withdrawal, fluid disturbance and electrolyte imbalance) tend to occur more frequently than do others in the ICU setting. Those that require emergent attention and correction are identified by the mnemonic, WWHHHHIMP:

- Withdrawal from sedative-hypnotic or other drugs
- Wernicke's encephalopathy
- Hypertensive crisis
- Hypoxia
- Hypoglycemia
- Hypoperfusion of the brain
- Intracranial bleeding
- Meningitis/Encephalitis
- Poisoning (i.e., drug toxicity)

Table 2–8. Differential Diagnosis of Delirium

System/Problem	Etiologic Factors

PRIMARY INTRACRANIAL DISEASE	Infection
	  HIV encephalopathy
	  Meningitis/encephalitis
	  Neurosyphilis
	Neoplasm
	  Space-occupying lesion
	Seizure
	  Postictal state
	  Complex partial seizure/status
	Vascular
	  Hypertensive encephalopathy
	  Intracranial hemorrhage
	  Vasculitis
	  Stroke
	Miscellaneous
	  Normal pressure hydrocephalus

SYSTEMIC DISEASES THAT SECONDARILY AFFECT THE BRAIN	Cardiopulmonary
	  Cardiac arrest
	  Congestive heart failure
	  Respiratory failure
	  Shock
	Endocrine/metabolic
	  Acid-base disturbance
	  Adrenal dysfunction
	  Fluid/electrolyte imbalance
	  Diabetic ketoacidosis
	  Hypoglycemia
	  Hepatic failure (encephalopathy)
	  Renal failure (uremia)
	  Parathyroid dysfunction
	  Thyroid dysfunction
	  Porphyria
	Infection
	  Sepsis
	  Subacute bacterial endocarditis
	Neoplasm
	  Paraneoplastic syndromes
	Nutritional deficiency
	  Folic acid
	  Niacin (pellagra)
	  Thiamine (Wernicke's encephalopathy, Wernicke-Korsakoff psychosis)
	  Vitamin B_{12} (pernicious anemia)

EXOGENOUS TOXIC AGENTS	Drugs of abuse
	  Alcohol
	  Amphetamines
	  Cocaine
	  LSD
	  Phencyclidine
	Nonmedicinal
	  Carbon monoxide
	  Heavy metals
	Medications (See Table 2–9)

DRUG WITHDRAWAL	Alcohol
	Propanediols
	  Chloral hydrate
	  Meprobamate
	Sedative-hypnotic agents
	  Barbiturates
	  Benzodiazepines
	  Narcotics

(Adapted from Tesar, G. E., and Stern, T. A.: Evaluation and treatment of agitation in the intensive care unit. J. Intensive Care Med., 1:137, 1986.)

Table 2-9. Common Delirium-Inducing Drugs Used in the ICU

Drug Group	Agent
Antiarrhythmics	Lidocaine
	Mexiletine
	Procainamide hydrochloride
	Quinidine sulfate
Antibiotics	Penicillin
	Rifampin
Anticholinergics	Atropine sulfate
Antihistamines	Nonselective
	Diphenhydramine hydrochloride
	Promethazine hydrochloride
	H_2 blockers
	Cimetidine
	Ranitidine
Beta blockers	Propranolol hydrochloride
Narcotic analgesics	Meperidine hydrochloride
	Morphine sulfate
	Pentazocine

(Adapted from Tesar, G. E., and Stern, T. A.: Evaluation and treatment of agitation in the intensive care unit. J. Intensive Care Med., 1:137, 1986.)

Delirium is the most important psychiatric complication that develops after cardiac surgery. Multiple factors in the intervals before, during, and after cardiac surgery have been identified as potential causes of delirium (Table 2-10); however, a recent meta-analysis of studies investigating the relationship between delirium and cardiac surgery failed to identify an outstanding causative factor.[38]

Drug OD is a common cause of delirium in the medical ICU (MICU). Between 1977 and 1981, 5% of all admissions to an 18-bed MICU at Massachusetts General Hospital were a direct result of drug OD.[39] The most frequently ingested drugs were alcohol, TCAs, benzodiazepines, narcotics, neuroleptics, and barbiturates, in that order.[21] Drug OD is included in the differential diagnosis of delirium, and even though a patient may deny OD, physical signs and symptoms of OD (e.g., Kussmaul breathing from aspirin toxicity) should be heeded, and toxicologic analysis of the blood and urine should be performed.

As a group, the elderly are more susceptible to the development of postoperative delirium. Whereas the incidence of delirium following general surgery is 0.1% among all patients, approximately 10 to 15% of elderly postoperative patients become delirious.[40]

Evaluation

Delirium in the ICU patient is commonly a manifestation of multiple, concurrent features of critical illness such as fever, infection, hemodynamic instability, respiratory compromise, and/or toxicity from drugs used to treat the primary illness and its complications. Therefore, delirium may persist until the underlying illness is adequately treated, and toxic drugs and life-supporting devices (e.g., mechanical ventilation and the IABP) can be discontinued. Both the patient and the hospital chart should be thoroughly examined for all possible causes of delirium, and laboratory testing that is either incomplete or outdated should be performed so that specific abnormalities (e.g., fluid and electrolyte imbalance, acid/base disturbances, anemia, hypoxia, hypercarbia, and vitamin B_{12} or folic acid deficiency) can be identified and treated specifically whenever possible.

Although no laboratory test is diagnostic of delirium, an EEG can help to support the clinical impression and to potentially rule out nonorganic psychiatric disturbances. The EEG of the delirious patient is characteristically abnormal with diffuse, generalized slowing, the severity of which parallels the intensity of delirium.[41,42] In contrast, the EEG is normal in nonorganic psychiatric disorders (e.g., nonorganic psychoses, anxiety states, affective disorders, and psychogenic dissociative disorders), and may be normal or disclose a focal abnormality in a patient with complex partial seizures. In some cases of mild delirium, slowing seen on the EEG remains within normal limits and is only abnormal relative to fast baseline activity.[42,43]

Treatment

The treatment of delirium has three goals:

- To reverse the underlying cause(s) and thereby prevent potentially irreversible brain failure
- To ease psychic pain
- To control abnormal behavior that is disruptive and potentially dangerous both to the patient and to the staff

Drug Toxicity. Drug toxicity is an important cause of delirium in the ICU, and when suspected, can be treated by eliminating or reducing the offending agent(s) or by using a specific antidote. It has been suggested that the likelihood of delirium occurring in an ICU patient depends on the number of drugs with anticholinergic properties administered.[44] Anticholinergic toxicity is likely to be the

Table 2-10. Factors Contributing to the Development of Delirium Following Cardiac Surgery

Time Course	Factor
Preoperative	History of myocardial infarction
	Preexisting central nervous system dysfunction
	Psychiatric disorders/factors
	Panic-level anxiety
	Major depression
	Alcohol or drug abuse
	Poor understanding of or reluctance to undergo planned procedure
	Severe physical illness
Intraoperative	Body temperature ≤28°C
	Complexity of surgical procedure
	Systolic blood pressure ≤50–60 mm Hg
	Total anesthesia time
	Type of oxygenator used in the bypass device (?)
Postoperative	Complications during recovery
	Environment (e.g., sensory overload/deprivation)
	Intra-aortic balloon pump (?)
	Medications administered (e.g., excess anticholinergic agents, narcotics, sedative-hypnotics)

(From Tesar, G. E., and Stern, T. A.: Evaluation and treatment of agitation in the intensive care unit. J. Intensive Care Med., 1:137, 1986.)

source of delirium in a patient who exhibits dilated pupils, warm skin, erythema, dry mucous membranes, and diminished or absent bowel sounds. An antidote such as physostigmine, 1 to 2 mg, may be infused slowly IV on a one-time basis to confirm the diagnosis,[45] or as a continuous drip to maintain reversal of anticholinergic delirium.[46]

Narcotic-induced delirium can be reversed with naloxone hydrochloride, 0.4 mg subcutaneously or IV. One or two doses may be sufficient to reverse toxicity produced by short-lasting narcotics (e.g., morphine sulfate [$t\frac{1}{2}$ = 4 hours] or hydromorphone [$t\frac{1}{2}$ = 2 to 4 hours]), whereas repeated doses may be necessary to maintain reversal when long-lasting narcotics (e.g., methadone [$t\frac{1}{2}$ = 50 to 60 hours] or MS-Contin) have been responsible for the delirious state.

Normeperidine toxicity, an under-recognized cause of neuropsychiatric symptoms in ICUs, poses a more complex problem.[47] Although naloxone hydrochloride will reverse the effects of the short-lasting meperidine ($t\frac{1}{2}$ = 2 to 4 hours), it may have little effect on its long-lasting active CNS excitatory metabolite, normeperidine ($t\frac{1}{2}$ = 12 to 36 hours). High doses of meperidine (i.e., greater than or equal to 300 mg daily of parenteral meperidine given for 3 or more days) commonly produce confusion, auditory and visual hallucinations, psychomotor arousal, and neuromuscular irritability (e.g., tremors, myoclonus, twitching, generalized seizures). The optimal treatment of normeperidine toxicity depends on discontinuation of meperidine and judicious use of a benzodiazepine (e.g., lorazepam) or a barbiturate to control irritability. A standard toxicology reference should be consulted for the description, evaluation, and treatment of toxicity due to these and other agents.[48]

Drug Withdrawal. Drug withdrawal, an important cause of delirium in the ICU patient, is easily overlooked and difficult to identify. No laboratory test is available to confirm the diagnosis of drug withdrawal. Moreover, the ICU patient is frequently unable to communicate effectively to provide a relevant history, and the physical signs of drug withdrawal (e.g., fever, signs of autonomic arousal, and neuromuscular irritability) are nonspecific and may be manifestations of the primary illness, its complications, or its treatment. These circumstances necessitate a high index of suspicion for substance withdrawal in the delirious ICU patient. The emergency nature of many ICU admissions increases the likelihood that a substance will not be continued, either because of its inappropriate use outside the hospital, or because of an inadvertent failure to include it in the ICU orders following transfer from another unit in the hospital.

In hospitalized patients, severe alcohol withdrawal or delirium tremens (DTs), usually begins on the second hospital day, but may not begin until the fifth hospital day.[49] The DTs can be prevented if premonitory signs (e.g., fever, tremor, tachycardia, and elevated blood pressure) are treated with a cross-reacting sedative-hypnotic agent, the safest of which is an oral benzodiazepine. Any benzodiazepine will suffice (see Table 2-4), although chlordiazepoxide, 25 to 100 mg orally, three to four times daily, has been advocated as the standard treatment. In elderly patients and those with impaired hepatic function, either oxazepam, 10 to 30 mg orally, every 4 to 6 hours, or lorazepam, 1 to 2 mg orally, every 6 to 8 hours, is preferred. Oxazepam is excreted unchanged by the kidneys and has an elimination half life of 8 to 10 hours. Metabolic inactivation of lorazepam ($t\frac{1}{2}$ = 10 to 20 hours) depends on glucuronidation, a metabolic step that is relatively preserved in patients with hepatic dysfunction. Lorazepam offers the added advantage of being adequately absorbed after oral, IM, or IV administration. Once the DTs have commenced, the treatment of choice is IV diazepam in young patients without liver disease, or IV lorazepam in elderly patients and those with compromised liver function. In patients with hepatic insufficiency, repeated administration of a long half-life agent such as diazepam ($t\frac{1}{2}$ = 30 to 60 hours) can result in increasing serum levels of both the parent compound and its active metabolite (i.e., nordiazepam, $t\frac{1}{2}$ = 60 to 100 hours). When rapid control of intense agitation is mandatory, however, diazepam may be the treatment of choice because a single IV bolus of diazepam achieves peak activity more quickly than IV lorazepam. Diazepam, 10 to 20 mg IV, can be given during the induction phase of treatment, followed by 5-mg boluses every 5 minutes until behavioral calm is achieved.[50] In one study, the average dose of diazepam for induction was 89 mg in alcoholic patients with intercurrent illnesses and 46 mg in those without.[50] Total doses ranged from 50 to 780 mg.[50] In one reported case, as much as 2640 mg of IV diazepam over 48 hours was required to control severe DTs.[51] Beta blockers and clonidine have been used adjunctively to control autonomic arousal. The addition of a high-potency neuroleptic may also be helpful despite theoretic concerns about its ability to lower the seizure threshold.[12] Over the years, the mortality rate from DTs has dropped dramatically, from as high as 30% to about 4%.[49]

The course of withdrawal from sedative-hypnotics depends on the type of agent (i.e., barbiturate or barbiturate analogue versus a benzodiazepine), its elimination half-life, and the duration of its use. Untreated withdrawal from a barbiturate or any of its analogues (Table 2-11) can be lethal. Fever, autonomic arousal, sweating, neuromuscular irritability, paranoia, and frightening hallucinations typically precede the onset of seizures, coma, and death.[52] The withdrawal from benzodiazepines is usually less intense than from a barbiturate and rarely progresses to death.

In general, the interval from drug discontinuation to onset of withdrawal depends on the drug's elimination half-life. For example, withdrawal from diazepam may not begin for up to 5 days because of the gradual elimination of the parent compound and its active metabolite, nordiazepam ($t\frac{1}{2}$ up to 200 hours in patients with hepatic dysfunction). In contrast, withdrawal can occur within hours of the last dose of shorter-acting barbiturates (e.g., pentobarbital); the barbiturate analogues (e.g., meprobamate, ethchlorvynol, and chloral hydrate); and benzodiazepines (e.g., alprazolam, lorazepam, and oxazepam). Sudden discontinuation is more likely to result in withdrawal after prolonged (greater than 4 months) rather than short-term (less than 4 months) use.[53]

Successful treatment of delirium secondary to sedative-hypnotic withdrawal depends on adequate replacement of the same, or a cross-reactive substance (i.e., one with

Table 2–11. Nonbenzodiazepine Sedative-hypnotic Agents

Class	Drug	Half-life (h)	Comments
Barbiturate	Amobarbital	14–42	
	Butalbital		Contained in Fiornial, Fioricet, Esgic, and other analgesic compounds
	Methohexital	4–6	
	Pentobarbital	15–50	Used in barbiturate (pentobarbital) tolerance test
	Phenobarbital	24–96	
	Secobarbital	20–28	No longer available
	Thiopental	3–8	
Propanediol carbamate	Meprobamate	10	
Chloral derivatives	Chloral hydrate	8–10	
	Ethchlorvynol	6	
Piperidinediones	Glutethimide	10	Variable GI absorption can cause fluctuating levels of consciousness after overdose
	Methyprylon	4	

a similar mechanism of action). If the specific substance is known, then it can be resumed. If the substance is not known, however, or if it has a short-to-intermediate half-life, then it may be wise to substitute a long-lasting barbiturate, such as phenobarbital, which can be tapered more easily and safely than an agent with a short or intermediate duration of action. This procedure is best accomplished after performance of the **pentobarbital tolerance test** (a method to determine the patient's sedative-hypnotic requirement), followed by a program of phenobarbital replacement and gradual withdrawal (Table 2–12).

Opioid withdrawal may occur in addicts who have been abusing street drugs or have been in a methadone maintenance program, or in those who have been receiving high doses of narcotics to control pain. Autonomic arousal, psychomotor agitation, and neuromuscular irritability are nonspecific, but yawning and lacrimation are signs that may distinguish narcotic withdrawal from other types of drug withdrawal. Narcotic withdrawal is not lethal; delirium is less likely to occur from narcotic withdrawal than from sedative-hypnotic withdrawal. Replacement with narcotics, followed by gradual, measured dosage reduction is an accepted treatment for the opiate-withdrawal syndrome. Methadone is commonly used for the taper, because of its long half-life (approximately 36 hours). Tapering by 10% of the total daily dose every 1 to 2 days permits a gradual, steady reduction of serum opioid levels.[55] The addition of clonidine, often in doses of 0.1 mg orally, three times daily, has been reported to attenuate autonomic arousal associated with opioid withdrawal.[55]

Non-Specific Delirium and its Treatment with Neuroleptic Agents. Even when a thorough investigation fails to disclose a treatable cause of delirium, pharmacologic treatment may be required to maintain patient safety. Although there is little in the way of controlled scientific investigation to support its use, the high-potency neuroleptic agent, haloperidol, a butyrophenone, has an extensive record of safety and efficacy when used to treat delirium in ICU settings.[56,57] Unlike its older counterpart, the low-potency neuroleptic chlorpromazine, haloperidol in standard doses (i.e., 5 to 10 mg daily) has trivial effects on heart rate, blood pressure, pulmonary artery pressure, and cardiac conduction,[56] and unlike the benzodiazepines and narcotics that are frequently used to sedate confused patients, haloperidol does not depress central respiratory drive.[58] Haloperidol is believed to exert its clinical effect through blockade of central dopamine receptor activity, and does not seem to interfere with dopamine-mediated augmentation of renal blood flow.[12,56] Like other neuroleptic agents that block central dopamine receptor activity, however, haloperidol is capable of producing extrapyramidal symptoms (e.g., akathisia, acute dystonia, parkinsonism).

The starting dose of haloperidol depends on the patient's hemodynamic stability, integrity of the CNS, and the intensity of accompanying agitation.[12,36,59] Elderly individuals, in particular those with evidence of CNS disturb-

Table 2–12. Pentobarbital Tolerance Test and Phenobarbital Technique for Withdrawal from Barbiturates and Nonbarbiturate Analogues (e.g., Meprobamate, Glutethimide)

Pentobarbital tolerance test
1. Examine the patient for signs of sedative-hypnotic withdrawal (e.g., fever, irritability, tremor, hyperreflexia, and other signs of autonomic arousal).
2. Administer pentobarbital, 200 mg orally, and examine the patient 1 hour later for signs of barbiturate intoxication (e.g., nystagmus, slurred speech, or drowsiness).
3. If after one hour there are no signs of barbiturate effect, give an additional 100 mg pentobarbital every hour until there is evidence of intoxication.
4. The total amount of pentobarbital administered is equivalent to the patient's 6-hour pentobarbital requirement. This amount should be multiplied by four to calculate the 24-hour pentobarbital requirement.

Phenobarbital technique of withdrawal
1. Convert the 24-hour pentobarbital requirement to the phenobarbital equivalent:

    pentobarbital 100 mg = phenobarbital 30 mg

    and administer in three divided doses. For example, if the amount of pentobarbital administered is 400 mg (24-hour requirement, 1600 mg), then give phenobarbital 480 mg, or 160 mg every 8 hours.
2. After 24–48 hours, begin the tapering process and reduce the dose of phenobarbital by 30 mg per day.
3. If signs of withdrawal become apparent, administer phenobarbital 60–120 mg IM, and increase the total daily requirement accordingly.

(Adapted from Tesar, G. E., and Stern, T. A.: Evaluation and treatment of agitation in the intensive care unit. J. Intensive Care Med., 1:137, 1986.)

ance (e.g., stroke, dementia), tend to be less tolerant of haloperidol's side effects, particularly its extrapyramidal effects. In this group, the starting dose may be as little as 0.5 mg orally, two to three times per day. A low initial dose and gradual dosage escalation is also advised in patients with low or unstable blood pressure caused, for example, by volume depletion, hypotensive agents, low cardiac output, or sepsis. Patients receiving concurrent treatment with a beta-blocking drug should be watched carefully because the concurrent administration of propranolol and haloperidol has been reported to cause hypotension and complete heart block.[60] In otherwise stable patients, the starting dose of haloperidol is 2 to 5 mg orally, three to four times per day or more if agitation is intense. The frequency of administration depends on the patient's clinical response. Initially it may be necessary to administer haloperidol every 4 hours to calm a restless or agitated patient. Once calm is achieved, the total daily dose can be given at 8- or even 12-hour intervals, with one third given in the daytime and two thirds at night. The maintenance dose is generally lower than the dose necessary to produce a calming effect. Use of a neuroleptic should be maintained throughout the course of delirium. Sudden discontinuation of haloperidol after its short-term use is generally uneventful; however, haloperidol should be resumed if delirium recurs or it should be reinstituted and tapered gradually following the unlikely event of a withdrawal dyskinesia (i.e., reversible abnormal involuntary movements that may resemble those of tardive dyskinesia and develop after sudden discontinuation of a neuroleptic agent).

Parenteral administration of haloperidol is indicated when the oral route is unavailable, when malabsorption is evident, or when a more rapid onset of effect is desired. Peak blood levels of haloperidol are achieved within 2 to 3 hours of a single oral dose and 30 to 60 minutes after parenteral dosing.[61] The parenteral dose of haloperidol (both IM and IV) is approximately half the oral dose.[12,61] IM administration ensures absorption (given sufficient muscle mass and peripheral capillary perfusion), but repeated injections can be painful and may also produce secondary elevation of serum creatine phosphokinase (CPK) levels, which can obfuscate the evaluation of concurrent chest pain. As a result, IV rather than IM administration of haloperidol may be preferable, particularly in the ICU where IV access has been established and monitoring equipment is in place. Furthermore, extrapyramidal symptoms appear to be uncommon when haloperidol is administered IV,[62] although this point is controversial.[63] (For further discussion about IV haloperidol, see the section of this chapter on agitation.)

Extrapyramidal effects (e.g., acute dystonia, akathisia, parkinsonism) may occur during treatment with neuroleptic drugs, including haloperidol, and are best treated by reducing the neuroleptic dosage and/or adding an anticholinergic agent (e.g., benztropine mesylate), an antihistamine (e.g., diphenhydramine), a benzodiazepine (e.g., lorazepam), or a beta blocker (e.g., propranolol). If laryngeal dystonia is unresponsive to the recommended pharmacologic treatment(s), paralysis and intubation of the patient may be necessary. Akathisia (i.e., motor restlessness) can be indistinguishable from nonspecific agitation; it may be resistant to all treatments except discontinuation of the neuroleptic agent. Elderly individuals, particularly those with CNS impairment, are most susceptible to the development of parkinsonism. Treatment alternatives includes those mentioned, as well as conversion to a low-potency neuroleptic (e.g., chlorpromazine) (Table 2-13). Because both anticholinergic agents and low-potency neuroleptics can aggravate delirium as a result of their anticholinergic properties, however, amantadine hydrochloride, which presumably acts by augmenting dopaminergic rather than reducing cholinergic transmission, may be administered at a dose of 100 mg orally, 2 or 3 times daily.

Table 2-13. Relative Potencies of Neuroleptic Agents[a]

Potency	Generic	Approx. Dose Equivalent (mg)	Sedation	PH[b]	Anticholinergic	EPS[c]
Low	Chlorpromazine	100	3+[d]	4+	3+	1+
	Thioridazine	100	4+	4+	4+	1+
	Chlorprothixene	75	4+	4+	3+	1+
	Mesoridazine	50	4+	4+	3+	1+
Intermediate	Loxapine	10	3+	2+	2+	2+
	Molindone	10	3+	2+	2+	2+
	Perphenazine	8	2-3+	2+	2+	2+
High	Trifluoperazine	5	1-2+	1+	1+	3+
	Thiothixene	5	1+	1+	1+	4+
	Fluphenazine	2	1+	1+	1+	4+
	Droperidol	2	3+	2-3+	1+	3+
	Haloperidol	2	1+	1+	1+	4+
	Pimozide	1	2+	2+	1+	4+

[a] Neuroleptic agents not used for the treatment of agitation, delirium, or psychosis include prochlorperazine (Compazine), metochlopromide (Reglan), promethazine (Phenergan), and trimethobenzamide (Tigan). Each of these agents is capable of causing extrapyramidal symptoms (EPS).
[b] PH = postural hypotension
[c] EPS = extrapyramidal symptoms
[d] 1+ = weak; 2+ = mild–moderate; 3+ = strong; 4+ = very strong
(Adapted from Hyman, S. E., and Tesar, G. E.: Manual of Psychiatric Emergencies. 3rd Ed. Boston, Little, Brown, 1994.)

Nonpharmacologic Treatment. Behavioral and environmental interventions may offer further benefit when combined with drug treatments. Such measures include:

- Reassurance and explanation to the patient, relatives, and significant others about the nature of delirium, its usual course, and the available treatment
- Frequent orientation of the patient to time, date, place, and the circumstances
- Provision of a soft light and a clock in the patient's field of vision at all times
- Frequent contact with selected individuals who are familiar to the patient and who are involved in the patient's care

These measures should not be viewed as alternatives, but rather as helpful adjuncts to the pharmacologic treatment of delirium.

Agitation

Agitation is a common clinical ICU problem that must be treated promptly and effectively to prevent potential harm to the patient and the staff.[35,36] Appropriate management of the agitated patient requires the use of mechanical restraint and occasionally massive doses of sedating medication. When these measures fail or when rapid control of the patient is urgent, paralysis and intubation may be necessary.

Etiology

Delirium is probably the most common cause of agitation in the ICU, but many other factors that compromise a patient's ability to tolerate the demands of critical care can precipitate agitation. Panic-level anxiety, pain, personality style, and factors that limit one's ability to comprehend the nature and demands of intensive care (e.g., cognitive, language, and sensory impairment) are also sources of agitation that can be treated specifically. Panic or phobic anxiety should be treated with a high-potency benzodiazepine such as alprazolam, clonazepam, or lorazepam and should be distinguished from paranoia (i.e., a delusional belief that others are out to harm one); paranoia usually requires treatment with a neuroleptic agent. Pain, a common source of agitation, may remain undetected because of a patient's inability to communicate or because of a reluctance among physicians and nurses to administer sufficient analgesic medication for fear of promoting addiction.[64] Akathisia, a subjective sense of motor restlessness that can occur as a result of treatment with neuroleptic medication, can also be manifest as agitation. It is best treated by reducing the neuroleptic dosage and adjunctive treatment with a benzodiazepine or a beta blocker.[65] Individuals who have reduced capacity to exercise control over their behavior (e.g., those with frontal lobe damage or mental retardation) and those with an inability to fully comprehend the situation (e.g., because of a language barrier, sensory impairment, or intellectual impairment) are also at risk of becoming agitated in the ICU. Patients with CNS dysfunction are susceptible to further cognitive deterioration, and therefore, an enhanced risk of becoming agitated.

Pharmacologic Treatment

No single pharmacologic method has proved best for controlling intense agitation. When the cause of agitation is unknown, many clinicians begin treatment with a benzodiazepine (e.g., diazepam or lorazepam). Although there is a risk of further disinhibiting the agitated patient, the use of a benzodiazepine will cover for the possibility of withdrawal from alcohol, a barbiturate, a barbiturate analogue, or a benzodiazepine.

If the clinician is assured that alcohol and drug withdrawal do not account for the patient's agitated state, and other sources of agitation have been identified and are being treated specifically, treatment with haloperidol should be initiated. In practice, both haloperidol and a benzodiazepine are often used in combination to treat agitation. The use of these agents and alternative methods for the control of agitation will be discussed below.

IV Haloperidol. Although haloperidol is not approved for IV use by the United States Food and Drug Administration (FDA), administration of haloperidol by the IV route is expedient and particularly well suited to the treatment of the acutely agitated ICU patient. The mean distribution time of IV haloperidol in normal volunteers is 11 minutes, although it may be longer in critically ill patients.[61] Clinically, onset occurs in 15 to 20 minutes, and the peak effect occurs within 30 to 45 minutes.[61] After a steady state has been achieved, the elimination half-life is approximately 24 hours, or longer in patients with hepatic insufficiency.[61] Bolus infusion of IV haloperidol is acceptable, but should be extended over 5 minutes when the patient is hypotensive or volume depleted. Because IV haloperidol precipitates with phenytoin and heparin, the IV should be flushed with saline prior to infusion of haloperidol.[12,56]

IV haloperidol can be given as a series of bolus infusions or as a continuous drip. A protocol for the initiation and maintenance of IV haloperidol to treat the agitated patient is outlined in Table 2-14. If a calming effect has not oc-

Table 2-14. Protocol for Use of IV Haloperidol

INITIATION*	
Intensity of Agitation	Starting Dose
Mild	0.5–2.0 mg
Moderate	5.0–10.0 mg
Severe	10.0 mg or more

TITRATION AND MAINTENANCE
1. Allow 15 to 20 minutes before the next dose.
2. If agitation persists, administer double dose every 20 minutes until agitation subsides. Dose limit depends on clinician's appraisal of effectiveness.
3. If patient is calming, repeat last dose at next dosing interval.
4. Adjust dose and interval to patient's clinical course.
5. Regular, not prn, dosing is advised.

* Prior to IV infusion of haloperidol, flush line with normal saline if patient is receiving concurrent infusions of heparin or diphenylhydantoin (phenytoin). (See Chap. 3.)
(Adapted from Tesar, G. E., and Stern, T. A.: Evaluation and treatment of agitation in the intensive care unit. J. Intensive Care Med., 1:137, 1986.)

curred within 15 to 20 minutes of the initial infusion, doubling the dose has proved more effective than repeating the same dose. For example, if no calming is evident after a 5-mg bolus of IV haloperidol, the next dose should be 10 mg. If the 10-mg dose is equally unsuccessful, the next dose should be 20 mg, and so on. The optimal dose is followed by a period of calm for one or more hours. The duration of calm determines the dosing interval. Once a calming dose and a suitable dosing interval have been determined, the amount of each bolus can be reduced. In our experience, however, it has occasionally been necessary to repeat the same dose of IV haloperidol hourly to maintain a state of calm.[66,67] Although amounts greater than 50 mg are required uncommonly, an individual bolus of 150 mg[67] and as much as 1200 mg per day of IV haloperidol has been administered to control intense agitation.[68] The continuous infusion of haloperidol has been reported to control intense agitation that resisted treatment with hourly IV boluses of haloperidol.[69,70] An added benefit of the continuous infusion method is that it eliminates the extra staff work required to prepare the haloperidol for hourly administration (e.g., hourly preparation of a 50-mg aliquot of haloperidol will require multiple 5-mg vials).

Although haloperidol has a record of relative cardiac safety, two recent reports document torsades de pointes cardiac arrhythmia in medically ill patients who received IV haloperidol.[71,72] Metzger and Friedman proposed alcoholic cardiomyopathy as a risk factor, and two of the four patients presented by Wilt and colleagues had developed congestive heart failure before receiving IV haloperidol. Cardiac rhythm and the corrected QT interval (QTc) should be monitored in ICU patients receiving IV haloperidol. Intravenous use should be discontinued if the QTc increases by more than 25% of the baseline value.

Other Neuroleptics. Although haloperidol is the neuroleptic of choice in the ICU patient, other neuroleptics (see Table 2-13) have been used successfully. Droperidol, a butyrophenone neuroleptic, is similar to haloperidol, but is more sedating and more likely to produce hypotension. When compared with haloperidol in the treatment of agitated emergency room patients, droperidol produced more rapid control of agitation.[73] Chlorpromazine, an aliphatic phenothiazine neuroleptic, can cause severe orthostatic hypotension, has potent anticholinergic properties, and its quinidine-like properties increase the likelihood of cardiac arrhythmias. Therefore, chlorpromazine is not the neuroleptic of choice in the ICU setting. A survey documenting the safe and effective use of this agent in medical settings suggested that it be considered as a second-line agent when standard treatments of agitation have failed, however.[74] When chlorpromazine is used, oral or IM administration is recommended, because the risk of serious side effects is greater with IV administration.

Benzodiazepines. Benzodiazepines (see Table 2-4) do not have a specific antipsychotic effect, but they do help to control agitation in the psychotic or delirious patient when these drugs are administered alone or in combination with neuroleptic agents. Benzodiazepines are also the treatment of choice when agitation is due to panic and phobic anxiety. High-potency benzodiazepines such as alprazolam and clonazepam effectively control panic attacks.[75,76] Neither agent is available for parenteral use, however, and lorazepam, which can be given either orally or parenterally, is a suitable alternative for the treatment of panic anxiety when the oral route is unavailable. Midazolam, a water-soluble imidazolebenzodiazepine with a rapid onset of action, a short elimination half-life ($t_{1/2}$ = 1 to 4 hours), and a potency twice that of diazepam, has been used successfully to control agitation.[77,78] Its continuous infusion under carefully monitored circumstances has been reported to control agitation in ICU patients without causing respiratory depression.[78]

The combination of a benzodiazepine and a neuroleptic is frequently more effective than the use of either agent alone. Several lines of evidence support the combined use of a neuroleptic, usually haloperidol, and lorazepam for the treatment of agitation.[79-81] The addition of lorazepam to an existing neuroleptic regimen in chronically psychotic patients resulted in a statistically significant reduction of the mean neuroleptic dosage administered over a 6-month period.[79] Adams and colleagues have reported that doses of IV haloperidol greater than 10 mg seem to confer no extra advantage in the treatment of critically ill cancer patients who are delirious and agitated. They have found that alternating 10-mg doses of IV haloperidol with comparatively high doses of IV lorazepam (i.e., as high as 350 mg per day) produces a superior calming effect.[80,81]

Nondepolarizing Muscle Relaxants. When all other treatment methods fail to control agitation, it may be necessary to intubate, paralyze, and sedate the agitated patient. Metocurine iodide or pancuronium bromide can be used to paralyze the patient. Pancuronium has a tendency to increase heart rate, blood pressure, and cardiac output as a result of both its antimuscarinic activity and its ability to release norepinephrine and block its reuptake.[82] Metocurine, which can produce mild hypotension and a compensatory increase in heart rate due to rate (of infusion) dependent release of histamine,[83] is often the preferred agent because it produces less autonomic instability than pancuronium. Liberal use of morphine sulfate is indicated to ensure the tranquility of the paralyzed, but otherwise conscious, patient. Staff members should remember to speak in a professional and compassionate manner when they are in the presence of the patient. (See Chap. 64 for more detailed information.)

SELECTED PROBLEMS

Interpersonal and Behavioral Problems

Personality style has long been regarded as an important variable that determines a patient's responses to illness and hospitalization.[84] Response patterns that are rigid or unyielding suggest a personality disorder and can be a source of considerable disruption in the ICU, where the patient's cooperation is essential. The successful evaluation and management of certain behavioral problems will be aided by an appreciation of the concept of personality, as well as by the particular forms (or styles) that it takes.

Personality development occurs in a series of stages. The degree of success at each stage influences the person's ultimate ability to trust others, to separate comfortably from parents (providers), to tolerate ambiguity, to develop a stable identity, to form an adequate level of self-esteem, and to be productive. A failure to negotiate any of these developmental tasks successfully can result in an arrest of personality development, and therefore, in enduring behavior patterns that are abnormal and interpersonal relationships that are disturbed. For example, the individual who lacks a sense of basic trust in others will have difficulty forming a cooperative alliance with the ICU staff. Patients who stubbornly resist following commands because of rigid, controlling personality characteristics are likely to cause behavioral and interpersonal problems in the ICU.

When stress is extreme or prolonged, even patients with relatively intact personalities can become overwhelmed and regress to earlier, less mature patterns of coping (e.g., being excessively dependent, being unable to make decisions). Maladaptive responses can provoke conflict between the patient and the ICU staff and can be the source of patient anxiety, depression and anger. When these reactions are intense or prolonged, pharmacologic treatment of anxiety, depression, or agitation may be necessary. Intense anxiety, despondency, or anger can also be the cause of regressive and inappropriate behavior. In these circumstances, pharmacologic treatment of intense emotions can improve behavior. Both pharmacologic treatment and psychologic support (e.g., reassurance, helping the patient to recognize and express anger and frustration) allow the patient to cope more effectively. The type of support that will be most helpful depends to some extent on the patient's personality style.[84]

Some of the commonly encountered personality problems encountered in the ICU include:

- Paranoid personality
- Schizoidal personality
- Dependent character
- Hysterical personality
- Narcissistic patient
- Obsessive character

Paranoid personalities are suspicious and accusatory, and they sense danger as coming from outside themselves. Clear, simple, and frequently repeated explanations of their illness and its management are necessary to allay fears of being harmed, manipulated, or crossed by others.

The schizoidal personality is distant, cold, and uninvolved and may appear to be depressed. Illness is experienced by these individuals as an intrusion. To prevent an increase in anxiety, the patient's desire for privacy and distance must be respected.

The dependent character can be one of the most annoying for the ICU staff. Such patients tend to be clingy, needy, and demanding and repeatedly call for assistance with the bedside nursing call button. This behavior is a response to fear of abandonment or loss of health. If unaddressed, fear may beget anger. Dependent behavior can be managed by supportive reassurance, limit setting, and ventilation of unexpressed anger.

Patients with hysterical personality characteristics tend to be dramatic and anxious and respond to their illness as if it were an attack on their appearance or sense of self. They respond to attention, psychologic support, and the opportunity to ventilate their fears. Detailed or technical explanations of their illness and its management may only increase their anxiety and should be avoided.

The narcissistic patient experiences illness as a threat to self-esteem and integrity. The patient's sense of worthiness and accomplishment should be supported. When this does not occur, the narcissistic patient can become intensely angry and uncooperative.

Obsessive characters tend to be meticulous, organized individuals who experience illness as punishment for letting things get beyond their control. The obsessive person's need for control often interferes dramatically with care even when it becomes necessary for the patient to relinquish control (e.g., to life-supporting devices). Real or imagined loss of control can precipitate panic level anxiety. Provision of detailed explanations and clear instructions helps to reaffirm the patient's sense of control and to decrease anxiety.

Many individuals exhibit one or more of these traits. When these traits dominate a patient's character, or when stress is extreme or prolonged, however, abnormal behavior may ensue that requires the skills of a consulting psychiatrist.

Noncompliance and the Threat to Sign Out

When a patient threatens to sign out against medical advise, the clinician has two responsibilities: (1) to assess the safety of discontinuing the patient's care; and (2) to assess the patient's capacity to make an informed decision.

Fear and panic, the failure to communicate anger, and psychosis are the common causes of a patient's threat to sign out of the ICU.[12] Both paranoia and personality disturbance are also common factors. A firm but compassionate and reassuring discussion of the situation is indicated. If possible, it is always helpful to involve the patient's family or a significant other whom the patient trusts and respects. The patient can be offered a benzodiazepine (e.g., diazepam or lorazepam), or a neuroleptic (e.g., haloperidol) if prior use of a benzodiazepine agent has failed to control escalating anxiety or if the patient is psychotic.

The patient who insists on leaving should be allowed to do so if she or he demonstrates adequate comprehension of the situation and can satisfactorily weigh the risks and benefits of his or her decision. If the patient's judgment is impaired by the effects of psychosis (e.g., paranoid delusions), delirium, dementia, or a treatable psychiatric disorder (e.g., panic anxiety, severe depression), then the patient should be detained; however, the impact of detention on the patient's well being must also be assessed. For example, the hemodynamic consequences of combativeness or struggling against restraints may produce an unacceptably high risk of adverse cardiovascular consequences. In all such instances, careful documentation of the clinical circumstances, efforts to treat the patient, and the decisions that have been made should be recorded in the patient's chart.

Weaning from the Ventilator

Successful weaning from ventilator support depends not only on achievement of the important physiologic criteria for weaning, but also on the patient's neuropsychiatric status.

Anxiety or fear is common during mechanical ventilation[85] and is the principle neuropsychiatric factor that interferes with successful weaning.[12] The rapid, shallow respirations of the anxious patient prevent maximal inspiratory effort and also deplete energy stores. Intermittent mandatory ventilation (IMV) with combinations of pressure support and CPAP offer theoretical advantages over the traditional T tube or trial and error method of weaning. The latter method may exacerbate anxiety by forcing periods of spontaneous ventilation. In contrast, the presence of the ventilator with Pressure Support augmentation to reduce airway resistance may provide patients with some psychologic support[86] (see Chap. 24).

Depression and other psychiatric disturbances can also compromise the weaning process. It has been suggested that a recent loss or a history of psychiatric treatment increases the likelihood of failed attempts.[87] Fatigue, poor concentration, loss of interest, and impaired motivation can interfere with the well-coordinated effort necessary to wean the patient from the ventilator successfully.

Specific treatment of anxiety or depression may be necessary for successful weaning from the ventilator. Hypnosis and relaxation techniques have been useful in calming the patient and helping the patient to conserve energy; they also distract the patient and help the patient conserve energy; they also distract the patient from the weaning process itself.[12] Although the use of benzodiazepines is traditionally avoided in this population because of their respiratory depressant properties, a low dose of a short or intermediate half-life agent (e.g., alprazolam, lorazepam, or oxazepam) may be used without significantly compromising respiration. If the patient's anxiety achieves panic proportions and cannot be controlled by these measures, use of a neuroleptic agent such as haloperidol, 5 to 10 mg, is indicated. Care must be taken to avoid precipitation of extrapyramidal side effects that can reduce chest wall compliance. If the effects of a secondary depression interfere with weaning efforts, then the patient may benefit from the administration of a psychostimulant such as methylphenidate or dextroamphetamine. Psychologic support to help the patient deal with the effects of loss, worry about family matters, or fear of dying may be indicated.

HIV Infection and AIDS

Neuropsychiatric Manifestations

The neuropsychiatric manifestations of HIV infection and AIDS can be divided into two main categories: (1) the significant emotional responses that occur at various points in the course of the illness (e.g., at the times of initial diagnosis, disease progression, and failed treatments); and (2) organic brain syndromes that result from brain involvement by neoplasia, metabolic derangement, and infection with HIV or opportunistic organisms. Although the psychologic reactions of afflicted patients are similar to those that occur in response to other critical illnesses (e.g., burns, deforming trauma, and cancer), various medical, psychologic, social, and political factors result in a greater intensity of distress experienced by HIV-infected patients.[88] The medical team responsible for the care of these patients must be prepared to anticipate, recognize, and respond to the emotional reactions of HIV-infected patients, to distinguish "appropriate" reactions from treatable psychiatric disorders (e.g., anxiety disorders, major depression), and to identify organic mental disorders that mimic functional (i.e., nonorganic) psychiatric disturbances. Caretakers must also deal with their own reactions to patients whose lifestyles commonly involve homosexuality and drug abuse. Even if the patient does not belong to one of the aforementioned high-risk groups for HIV infection, caretakers are faced with the stress of their own reactions to death and dying and the potential for unwitting infection with HIV from the patient's body fluids.

Etiology of Neuropsychiatric Disturbances Related to HIV Infection

HIV type I infection may be accompanied by focal disorders (e.g., cerebral toxoplasmosis, primary CNS lymphoma, progressive multifocal leukoencephalopathy, cryptococcal abscess, varicella zoster encephalitis, tuberculous brain abscess or tuberculoma, neurosyphilis, and HIV-associated vasculopathy) or nonfocal disorders (e.g., AIDS dementia complex, cytomegalovirus encephalitis, metabolic encephalopathies, herpes simplex virus encephalitis, and acute HIV-1 related encephalitis).[89] AIDS patients with or without neurologic disturbance are also at high risk for secondary emotional distress precipitated by receiving the diagnosis, having their illness progress, losing function and support systems, or facing the ever present specter of inevitable death.

HIV Encephalopathy

HIV has direct neurotoxic effects referred to variously as subacute encephalitis, AIDS encephalopathy, AIDS dementia complex, and HIV encephalopathy. The onset is usually at a time when there is significant immunodeficiency and opportunistic infection.[89] Occasionally, however, the encephalopathy is the presenting feature of AIDS. Early on, forgetfulness, loss of concentration, and mental slowing are the most commonly reported symptoms. As the illness progresses, patients exhibit signs of a subcortical dementia involving short term memory deficits, reduced mental flexibility, a lack of spontaneity, impaired ability to manipulate acquired knowledge, and problems initiating, carrying out, and completing complex activities. Ultimately, global dementia accompanied by aphasia, amnesia, and parietal lobe syndromes develops late in the disease.[89] Apathy commonly accompanies this cognitive deterioration and can be mistaken for depression despite the absence of subjective dysphoria. Unlike depression, apathy tends not to respond to pharmacologic treatment.

The onset and progression of physical and mental changes may be a source of considerable distress to the patient who is experiencing a gradual, but inexorable loss of control. In some patients, worry can escalate towards panic-level anxiety, whereas in others, an early sense of loss can develop into abject hopelessness marked by suicidal thinking. In still other individuals, neuropsychiatric disorders (e.g., panic attacks, depression, mania, or an agitated psychosis) without an obvious precipitant may be the heralding signs of HIV encephalopathy and AIDS.[90] When clinically significant HIV encephalopathy is not evident, the presence of neuropsychiatric symptoms might be explained by the toxic effects of drugs used to treat AIDS (e.g., zidovudine [AZT], or 9-(1,3-dihydroxy-2-propoxymethyl)[guanine] or the effects of pathology in other organ systems (e.g., hypoxia secondary to Pneumocystis carinii pneumonia).

Treatment

The principles of treatment are the same as those discussed previously in reference to the major psychiatric disorders. Some measure of comfort and relief can be achieved by providing reassurance and support. Following discharge from the hospital the AIDS patient may need help acquiring public assistance and locating new lodging if she or he is unemployed and has dwindling or depleted savings. If unaccepting family members abandon the patient, then referral to a local support group may be helpful. Regular, on-going visits to a physician, either the primary physician or a psychiatrist, can provide stability within an otherwise chaotic situation.

Psychopharmacologic treatment is indicated when psychotherapeutic measures are inadequate to control mounting distress or when the patient's symptoms meet criteria for the diagnosis of a major psychiatric disorder.

Anxiolytic agents are particularly helpful in reducing intolerable levels of distress when the patient is frightened, shows evidence of autonomic arousal, or exhibits an attentional deficit because of intense anxiety. Those at risk for extreme anxiety are individuals with premorbid anxiety disorders and homosexual men, who as a group have been shown more likely to suffer from anxiety disorders.[91] In those individuals with anxiety, the benzodiazepines are the drugs of choice. The selection of a particular agent depends on the desired pharmacokinetic properties and the diagnosis. When the level of anxiety threatens to escalate to panic proportions and the patient appears to be on the verge of losing behavioral control, however, then a high-potency neuroleptic agent such as haloperidol may be needed.

The diagnosis of depression in HIV-infected individuals suffers from the same difficulties that attend the diagnosis of depression in other medically ill patients. Once the decision to treat has been made, the clinician must chose between the various antidepressant agents available. The TCAs are used commonly and successfully in patients with asymptomatic HIV infection.[92] They are perhaps less effective when prescribed to patients who are in the more advanced stages of AIDS.[92] If used, they should be initiated at low doses, starting at 10 to 25 mg orally at bedtime and increased by 10 to 25 mg every 1 or 2 nights, with adjustment of the dose according to the levels of side effects and depressive symptoms. Empirically, depressed HIV-infected patients respond to TCAs at lower than the usual antidepressant doses. Correspondingly, HIV patients exhibit a greater sensitivity to the anticholinergic, adrenergic, and hypotensive effects of the TCAs. As a result of these findings, the psychostimulants (i.e., dextroamphetamine, methylphenidate, and pemoline) have been given to the depressed HIV-infected patient when TCAs have been contraindicated, have proved ineffective, or when the patient is cognitively impaired. In addition to improved mood, appetite stimulation, and psychomotor activation, the prescription of psychostimulant drugs has been associated with qualitative and quantitative improvements in higher cortical function within hours of their administration.[93]

The management of delirium in HIV-infected patients is no different from the management of delirium in other patients. The physician should attend first to the identification and treatment of underlying organic and toxic causes of delirium. As these causes are eliminated and delirium persists, the use of a neuroleptic agent, such as haloperidol, is indicated. The recommendations regarding choice of agent, route and frequency of administration, and the management of side effects are similar to the recommendations for HIV-negative patients with the exception that those with HIV encephalopathy tend to require lower neuroleptic doses.

PROBLEMS THAT DEVELOP FOLLOWING TRANSFER OUT OF THE ICU

Common sense dictates that a patient's anxiety in the ICU will diminish as the time of transfer out of the ICU approaches; however, this is not always the case. Coronary patients, for example, have been shown to experience a high degree of anxiety on transfer from the CCU and have a surge of catecholamine secretion.[11] Ventilator-dependent patients also can be expected to experience escalating anxiety in anticipation of plans to transfer their care to the home environment.[94,95] In general, patients who have become psychologically dependent on monitoring devices and on the constant attention of the ICU staff will have the most difficulty separating from the ICU environment. Preparation for their departure should include reassurance, an opportunity for verbalization of concerns, and psychologic preparation for the ultimate date of discharge. Reassurance that intensive care is no longer necessary should be accompanied by informing the patient that monitoring will be less frequent and less intense. A visit by ICU nurses to a patient who has been transferred out of the ICU is both comforting to the patient and also rewarding for the nurses.

Although anxiety is often the first response to transfer from the ICU, depression may soon follow. Those who have had a myocardial infarction, who have been disfigured by trauma, or who have become disabled by their illness frequently enter the recovery period with a sense of loss, vulnerability, and depression that intensifies after discharge from the hospital.[96] Loss of function, the need to redefine family, social, and occupational roles, and the need to modify unhealthy behaviors (e.g., smoking, sedentary lifestyle) all contribute to the patient's sense of inadequacy and sometimes to a sense of hopelessness. In the majority, depressed mood is transient and adjustment is complete. In some patients, however, depression becomes chronic and interferes with both psychologic and physical recovery from the primary illness. Patients with either depressive symptoms or a depressive disorder tend to have worse physical, social, and role functioning, worse perceived current health, and greater bodily pain than nondepressed controls;[97] the combination of depression and a chronic medical condition has an even more profound effect on a patient's function.[96] For cardiac patients, cardiac rehabilitation may be indicated to improve functional capacity and mood. When a disturbance of mood persists and is associated with neurovegetative features of major depression, evaluation by a psychiatrist and/or treatment with antidepressant medication are indicated.

Recollection of the ICU experience varies among former critical care patients. In one study, 50% of critical care patients could not remember details of their admission 48 hours after discharge from the ICU.[98] In another study, approximately 50% of patients could not recall their experience with mechanical ventilation; only 37% of those with head injuries could recall the experience.[99] Other patients develop a post-traumatic stress disorder characterized by intrusive and unpleasant recollections of the ICU experience. Typically, these patients have been delirious in the ICU or have an anxiety disorder. At the time of follow-up, their unusual experience continues to be unprocessed and unresolved and some patients continue to be plagued by disconcerting recollections of paranoid delusions and frightening visual hallucinations. Some patients are too afraid and/or embarrassed to discuss these experiences and hesitate to speak about them spontaneously. Therefore, the physician should make a habit of inquiring routinely at follow-up visits about delirium and its psychologic aftermath. Discussion and reassurance are generally sufficient to allay patient concerns and to promote symptom relief. Persistence of symptoms, however, may be an indication for psychiatric referral.

The majority of patients recover uneventfully after acute cardiac illness and cardiac surgery. Only 5% continue to show substantial performance deficits at 6 months' follow-up.[100] Psychiatric and CNS disorders that are present prior to surgery predict a less favorable outcome.[101] Most patients will benefit from participation in some form of monitored physical activity (e.g., a program of cardiac rehabilitation). Early mobilization, physical reconditioning, and the resumption of normal sexual activity are probably the best antidotes to post-ICU anxiety and depression.[102,103]

In conclusion, neuropsychiatric disturbance is an important variable that can compromise the care of the ICU patient. Patients with premorbid neuropsychiatric disorders are more susceptible to cognitive, affective, and/or behavioral deterioration in the ICU setting either because of psychologic or CNS vulnerability, because of withdrawal from psychotropic medication that is discontinued at the time of ICU admission, or because of abnormal interactions between psychotropic medication and other medications prescribed in the ICU. Even those without prior neuropsychiatric disturbance, however, may develop abnormalities of mood, cognition, or behavior because of the individual or combined effects of medication, the patient's medical condition, life-support devices, or the stress of a prolonged stay in the ICU. The tasks for the intensive care physician are first to determine the cause(s) of these disturbances and then to institute the appropriate treatment. A comprehensive MSE, thorough chart review, and search for specific organic abnormalities are essential. Valuable information can be also gained from an assessment of the patient's personality style and habitual responses to stressful situations. Effective post-ICU follow-up can help to prevent behavioral regression and depression due to the effects of deconditioning. Follow-up visits should address potential patient concerns about problems that occurred during the ICU stay (e.g., delirium) and the impact of illness on usual activities (e.g., sex, work, and other physical activities).

REFERENCES

1. Strub, R. L., and Black, F. W.: The mental status examination in neurology. 2nd Ed. Philadelphia, F. A. Davis Co., 1987.
2. Mesulam, M. M.: Principles of behavior neurology. Philadelphia, F. A. Davis Co., 1988, p. 26.
3. Manschreck, T. C., and Keller, M. B.: The biologic mental status examination. In Outpatient Psychiatry: Diagnosis and Treatment. Baltimore, Williams & Wilkins, 1979.
4. Chedru, F., and Geschwind, N.: Writing disturbances in acute confusional states. Neuropsychologia, 40:343, 1972.
5. Krauthammer, C., and Klerman, G. L.: Secondary mania: manic syndromes associated with antecedent physical illness or drugs. Arch. Gen. Psychiatry, 35:1333, 1978.
6. Luria, A. R.: Higher Cortical Functions in Man. New York, Basic Books, 1966.
7. American Psychiatric Association: Diagnostic and Statistical Manual of Mental Disorders. 3rd Ed. Washington, D.C., American Psychiatric Association, 1987.
8. Folstein, M. F., Folstein, S. E., and McHugh, P. R.: Mini-mental state: a practical method for grading the cognitive state of patients for the clinician. J. Psychiatr. Res., 12:189, 1975.
9. Anthony, L., et al.: Limits of the "mini-mental state" as a screening test for dementia and delirium among hospital patients. Psychol. Med., 12:397, 1982.
10. Cassem, N. H., and Hackett, T. P.: Psychiatric consultation in coronary care unit. Ann. Intern. Med., 75:9, 1971.
11. Klein, R. F., et al.: Transfer from a coronary care unit: some adverse responses. Arch. Intern. Med., 122:104, 1968.
12. Cassem, N. H., and Hackett, T. P.: The setting of intensive care. In Massachusetts General Hospital Handbook of General Hospital Psychiatry. Littleton, MA, PSG Publishing, 1987.
13. Stern, T. A., and Tesar, G. E.: Anxiety and the cardiovascular system. Mt. Sinai J. Med., 55:230, 1988.
14. Stern, T. A., Caplan, R. A., and Cassem, N. H.: Use of benzodiazepines in a coronary care unit. Psychosomatics, 28:19, 1987.
15. Baldessari, R. J.: Chemotherapy in Psychiatry. Cambridge, Harvard University Press, 1985.
16. Greenblatt, D. J., Shader, R. I., and Abernathy, D. R.: Current status of benzodiazepines (first of two parts). N. Engl. J. Med., 309:354, 1983.
17. Abramowicz, M.: Midazolam. Med. Lett. Drugs Ther., 28: 73, 1986.
18. Cameron, O. G.: Guidelines for diagnosis and treatment of depression in patients with medical illness. J. Clin. Psychiatry, 51(Suppl):49, 1990.
19. Geringer, E. S., and Stern, T. A.: Anxiety and depression in critically ill patients. Probl. Crit. Care, 2:35, 1988.
20. Rundell, J. R., Murray, G. B., and Wise, M. G.: Psychiatric consultation in critical care medicine. Probl. Crit. Care, 2: 1, 1988.

21. Stern, T. A., Mulley, A. G., and Thibault, G. E.: Life-threatening drug overdose. JAMA, 251:1983, 1984.
22. Dec, G. W., and Stern, T. A.: Tricyclic antidepressants in the intensive care unit. J. Intensive Care Med., 5:69, 1990.
23. Massie, M. J., and Lesko, L.: Psychological Care of the Patient with Cancer. New York, Oxford University Press, 1989.
24. Horne, T. L., et al.: Treatment of bulimia with bupropion: a multicenter controlled trial. J. Clin. Psychiatry, 49:262, 1988.
25. Teicher, M. H., Glod, C., and Cole, J. O.: Emergence of intense suicidal preoccupation during fluoxetine treatment. Am. J. Psychiatry, 147:207, 1990.
26. Fava, M., and Rosenbaum, J. F.: Suicide and fluoxetine: is there a relationship? J. Clin. Psychiatry, 52:108, 1991.
27. Kaplitz, S. E.: Withdrawn, apathetic geriatric patients responsive to methylphenidate. J. Am. Geriatr. Soc., 27:467, 1975.
28. Kaufmann, M. W., Murray, G. B., and Cassem, N. H.: The use of D-amphetamine in medically ill depressed patients. J. Clin. Psychiatry, 43:463, 1982.
29. Kaufmann, M. W., Cassem, N. H., and Murray, G. B.: The use of methylphenidate in depressed patients after cardiac surgery. J. Clin. Psychiatry, 45:82, 1984.
30. Woods, S. W., Tesar, G. E., Murray, G. B., and Cassem, N. H.: Psychostimulant treatment of depressive disorders secondary to medical illness. J. Clin. Psychiatry, 47:12, 1986.
31. Masand, P., Pickett, P., and Murray, G. B.: Psychostimulants for secondary depression in medical illness. Psychosomatics, 32:203, 1991.
32. Lipson, R. E., and Stern, T. A.: Management of monoamine oxidase inhibitor-treated patients in the emergency and critical care setting. J. Intensive Care Med., 6:117, 1991.
33. Bernstein, J. G.: Handbook of Drug Therapy in Psychiatry. Boston, John Wright—PSG Inc, 1983.
34. Jefferson, J. W., Greist, J. H., and Ackerman, D. L.: Lithium: Encyclopedia for Clinical Practice. Washington, D.C., American Psychiatric Press, 1983.
35. Tesar, G. E., and Stern, T. A.: Evaluation and treatment of agitation in the intensive care unit. J. Intensive Care Med., 1:137, 1986.
36. Tesar, G. E., and Stern, T. A.: Rapid tranquilization of the agitated intensive care unit patient. J. Intensive Care Med., 3:195, 1988.
37. Lipowski, Z. J.: Delirium: acute brain failure in man. Springfield, IL, Charles C Thomas, 1980.
38. Smith, L. W., and Dimsdale, J. E.: Postcardiotomy delirium: conclusions after 25 years? Am. J. Psychiatry, 146:452, 1989.
39. Thibault, G. E., et al.: Medical intensive care: indications, interventions, and outcomes. N. Engl. J. Med., 302:938, 1980.
40. Seymour, G.: Medical Assessment of the Elderly Surgical Patient. Rockville, MD, Aspen Systems, 1986.
41. Romano, J., and Engle, G. L.: Studies of delirium. I. electroencephalograph data. Arch. Neurol. Psychiatry, 51:356, 1944.
42. Engel, G. L., and Romano, J.: Delirium, a syndrome of cerebral insufficiency. J. Chronic Dis., 9:260, 1959.
43. Lipowski, Z. J.: Delirium in the elderly patient. N. Engl. J. Med., 320:578, 1989.
44. Tune, L. E., et al.: Association of postoperative delirium with raised serum levels of anticholinergic drugs. Lancet, 2:651, 1981.
45. Granacher, R. P., and Baldessarini, R. J.: Physostigmine. Arch. Gen. Psychiatry, 32:375, 1975.
46. Stern, T. A.: Continuous infusion of physostigmine. J. Clin. Psychiatry, 44:463, 1983.
47. Shochet, R. B., and Murray, G. B.: Neuropsychiatric toxicity of meperidine. J. Intensive Care Med., 3:246, 1988.
48. Haddad, L. M., and Winchester, J. F. (Eds.): Clinical Management of Poisoning and Drug Overdose. Philadelphia, W. B. Saunders, 1983.
49. Cushman, P.: Delirium tremens: update on an old disorder. Postgrad. Med., 82:117, 1987.
50. Thompson, W. L., Johnson, A. D., and Maddrey, W. L.: Diazepam and paraldehyde for treatment of severe delirium tremens: a controlled trial. Ann. Intern. Med., 82:175, 1980.
51. Nolop, K. B., and Natow, A.: Unprecedented sedative requirements during delirium tremens. Crit. Care Med., 13:246, 1985.
52. Khantzzian, E. J., and McKenna, G. J.: Acute toxic and withdrawal reactions associated with drug use and abuse. Ann. Intern. Med., 90:361, 1979.
53. Task Force Report of the American Psychiatric Association: Benzodiazepine Dependence, Toxicity, and Abuse. Washington, D.C., American Psychiatric Press, 1990.
54. Renner, J. A.: Drug addiction. In Massachusetts General Hospital Handbook of General Hospital Psychiatry. 2nd Ed. Littleton, MA, PSG Publishing, 1987.
55. Gold, M. S., Pottach, A. C., and Sweeney, D. R., et al.: Opiate withdrawal using clonidine. JAMA, 243:343, 1980.
56. Sos, J., and Casem, N. H.: Managing postoperative agitation. Drug Ther., 10:103, 1980.
57. Settle, E. C., and Ayd, F. J.: Haloperidol: a quarter century of experience. J. Clin. Psychiatry, 44:440, 1983.
58. Shader, R. I.: Extrapyramidal and cardiovascular side effects of butyrophenones. In Butyrophenones in Psychiatry. New York, Raven Press, 1972.
59. Thompson, T. L., and Thompson, W. L.: Treating postoperative delirium. Drug Ther., 13:30, 1983.
60. Alexander, H. E., McCarthy, K., and Giffen, M. B.: Hypotension and cardiopulmonary arrest associated with concurrent haloperidol and propranolol therapy. JAMA, 252:87, 1984.
61. Forsman, A., and Ohman, R.: Pharmacokinetic studies of haloperidol in man. Curr. Ther. Res., 20:314, 1976.
62. Menza, M. A., Murray, G. B., and Holmes, V. F., et al.: Decreased extrapyramidal symptoms with intravenous haloperidol. J. Clin. Psychiatry, 48:278, 1987.
63. Moller, H. J., et al.: Efficacy and side effects of haloperidol in psychotic patients. Oral versus intravenous administration. Am. J. Psychiatry, 139:1571, 1982.
64. Marks, R. M., and Sachar, E. J.: Undertreatment of medical inpatients with narcotic analgesics. Ann. Intern. Med., 78:173, 1973.
65. Lipinski, J. F., and et al.: Propranolol in the treatment of neuroleptic-induced akathisia. Am. J. Psychiatry, 141:412, 1984.
66. Tesar, G. E., Murray, G. B., and Cassem, N. H.: Use of high-dose intravenous haloperidol in agitated cardiac patients. J. Clin. Psychopharmacol., 5:344, 1985.
67. Stern, T. A.: The management of depression and anxiety following myocardial infarction. Mt. Sinai J. Med., 52:623, 1985.
68. Sanders, K., Murray, G. B., and Cassem, N. H.: High-dose intravenous haloperidol for agitated delirium in a cardiac patient on intra-aortic balloon. J. Clin. Psychopharmacol., 11:146, 1991.
69. Fernandez, F., Holmes, V. F., Adams, F., and Kavanaugh, J. J.: Treatment of severe, refractory agitation with a haloperidol drip. J. Clin. Psychiatry, 49:239, 1988.

70. Dixon, D., and Craven, J.: Continuous infusion of haloperidol. Am. J. Psychiatry, *150:*673, 1993.
71. Metzger, E., and Friedman, R.: Prolongation of the corrected Qt and torsades de pointes cardiac arrhythmia associated with intravenous haloperidol in the medically ill. J. Clin. Psychopharmacol., *13:*128, 1993.
72. Wilt, J. L., Minnema, A. M., Johnson, R. F., and Rosenblum, A. M.: Torsade de pointes associated with the use of intravenous haloperidol. Ann. Intern. Med., *119:*391, 1993.
73. Resnick, M., and Burton, B. T.: Droperidol vs haloperidol in the initial management of acutely agitated patients. J. Clin. Psychiatry, *45:*298, 1984.
74. Muskin, P. R., Mellman, L. A., and Kornfeld, D. S.: A "new" drug for treating agitation and psychosis in the general hospital. chlorpromazine. Gen. Hosp. Psychiatry, *8:*404, 1986.
75. Ballenger, J. C., et al.: Alprazolam in panic disorder and agoraphobia: results from a multicenter trial. I. Efficacy in short-term treatment. Arch. Gen. Psychiatry, *45:*413, 1988.
76. Tesar, G. E., et al.: Double-blind, placebo-controlled comparison of clonazepam and alprazolam for panic disorder. J. Clin. Psychiatry, *52:*69, 1991.
77. Mendoza, R., Djenderedjian, A. H., Adams, J., and Ananth, J.: Midazolam in acute psychotic patients with hyperarousal. J. Clin. Psychiatry, *48:*291, 1987.
78. Shapiro, J. M., et al.: Midazolam infusion for sedation in the intensive care unit. Anesthesiology, *64:*394, 1986.
79. Salzman, C., Green, A. I., Rodriguez-Villa, F., and Jaskiw, G. I.: Benzodiazepines combines with neuroleptics for management of severe disruptive behavior. Psychosomatics, *27* (*Suppl.*):17, 1986.
80. Adams, F.: Neuropsychiatric evaluation and treatment of delirium in the critically ill cancer patient. Cancer Bull., *36:*156, 1984.
81. Adams, F., Fernandez, F., and Andersson, B. S.: Emergency pharmacotherapy of delirium in the critically ill cancer patient. Psychosomatics, *27* (*Suppl.*):33, 1986.
82. Miller, R. D., and Savarese, J. J.: Pharmacology of muscle relaxants. *In* Anesthesia. 2nd Ed. Vol. 2. New York, Churchill Livingstone, 1986.
83. Edwards, R. P., et al.: Cardiac responses to imipramine and pancuronium during anesthesia with halothane or enflurane. Anesthesiology, *50:*421, 1979.
84. Bibring, G. L., and Kahana, R. J.: Lectures in Medical Psychology: An Introduction to the Care of Patients. New York, International University Press, 1968.
85. Bergbom-Engberg, I., and Haljamae, H.: Assessment of patients' experience of discomforts during respiratory therapy. Crit. Care Med., *17:*1068, 1989.
86. Irwin, R. S., and Demers, R. R.: Mechanical ventilation. *In* Intensive Care Medicine. Boston, Little, Brown, 1985.
87. Mendel, J. G., and Khan, F. A.: Psychological aspects of weaning from mechanical ventilation. Psychosomatics, *21:*465, 1980.
88. Dilley, J. W., and Forstein, M.: Psychosocial aspects of the human immunodeficiency virus (HIV) epidemic. *In* Review of Psychiatry. Vol. 9. Washington, D.C., American Psychiatric Press, 1990.
89. Brew, B. J., Sidtis, J. J., Petito, C. K., and Price, R. W.: The neurologic complications of AIDS and human immunodeficiency virus infection. *In* Advances in Contemporary Neurology. Vol. 29. Philadelphia, F. A. Davis, 1988.
90. Beckett, A.: The neurobiology of human immunodeficiency virus infection. *In* Review of Psychiatry. Vol. 9. Washington, D.C., American Psychiatric Press, 1990.
91. Atkinson, J. H., et al.: Prevalence of psychiatric disorders among men infected with human immunodeficiency virus. Arch. Gen. Psychiatry, *45:*859, 1988.
92. Fernandez, F.: Psychiatric diagnosis and pharmacotherapy of patients with HIV infection. *In* Review of Psychiatry. Vol. 9. Washington, D.C., American Psychiatric Press, 1990.
93. Holmes, V. F., Fernandez, F., and Levy, J. K.: Psychostimulant response in AIDS-related complex patients. J. Clin. Psychiatry, *50:*5, 1989.
94. Sivak, E. D., Cordasco, E. M., Gipson, W. T., and Mehta, A.: Home care ventilation: the Cleveland Clinic experience from 1977 to 1985. Respir. Care, *31:*294, 1986.
95. Clark, K.: Psychosocial aspects of prolonged ventilator dependency. Respir. Care, *31:*329, 1986.
96. Wishnie, H. A., Hackett, T. P., and Cassem, N. H.: Psychological hazards of convalescence following myocardial infarction. JAMA, *215:*1292, 1971.
97. Wells, K. B., et al.: The functioning and well-being of depressed patients. JAMA, *262:*914, 1989.
98. Turner, J. S., et al.: Patients' recollection of intensive care unit experience. Crit. Care Med., *90:*966, 1990.
99. Bergbom-Engberg, I., and Haljamae, H.: Patient experiences during respiratory treatment: reason for intermittent positive-pressure ventilation treatment and patient awareness in the intensive care unit. Crit. Care Med., *89:*22, 1989.
100. Savageau, J. A., et al. Neuropsychological dysfunction following elective cardiac operations: II. A six-month reassessment. J. Thorac. Cardiovasc. Surg., *84:*595, 1982.
101. Bass, C.: Psychosocial outcome after coronary artery bypass surgery. Br. J. Psychiatry, *145:*526, 1984.
102. Hellerstein, H. K., and Friedman, E. H.: Sexual activity and the postcoronary patient. Arch. Intern. Med., *125:*987, 1970.
103. Wenger, N. K.: Early ambulation physical activity: myocardial infarction and coronary artery bypass surgery. Heart Lung, *13:*14, 1984.

Chapter 3

DISORDERS OF TEMPERATURE REGULATION

KATHLEEN M. SHANNON

BODY TEMPERATURE

Cells function best in a stable, unchanging environment. The more highly evolved the species, the more stringent are the cellular environment requirements. Body temperature regulation ensures that the temperature of the cellular environs is constant, providing the mechanisms for dissipation of excessive heat and for conservation or generation of heat. The optimum body temperature range for a given species depends on its size and degree of phylogenetic advancement; mean body temperature is inversely proportional to size, and the normal range of tolerated body temperatures is narrower for more advanced species. To allow for dissipation of excess heat, mean body temperature must exceed mean ambient earth temperature (22°C). The body temperature for any species is the highest possible, taking into account the body mass, metabolic rate and amount of thermal insulation.[1] In man, normal mean human body temperature is 36.7°C ($\pm$0.22°C)[2] and the human central nervous (CNS) system functions poorly when the core temperature falls outside the range of 35 to 40.5°C.

Humans are tropical homeotherms; in the nude, resting condition, they are in a state of thermoneutrality when the ambient temperature is 28°C.[1] At all other temperatures and under working conditions, a sophisticated system of autonomic and behavioral strategies functions to generate or dissipate heat, thus maintaining acceptable body temperature. The ability to dissipate heat far outweighs the ability to conserve and generate heat. Humans are thus considerably more susceptible to hypothermia than to hyperthermia.

Heat is transferred to and from the body by four mechanisms.[3] **Radiative heat transfer** is heat transfer which occurs by electromagnetic transfer between two objects not in contact with each other. An example of such heat transfer warming of the skin by the sun's rays. **Conductive heat transfer** is that between two objects which are in direct contact, and depends on the extent of contact, the relative temperatures of the two objects and the relative heat conductivity of the objects. A barefooted person loses a small amount of heat by conduction to the cold floor on which he or she stands. **Convective heat loss** occurs when heat is transferred to aliquots of air which then move away from the body to be replaced by new aliquots. The degree of convective heat loss depends on the relative temperatures of the skin and air, the amount of air movement, and the amount of skin exposed. The concept of "windchill" is based on properties of convective heat loss.

Evaporative heat loss results from vaporization of water or sweat on the skin. The amount of heat transfer depends on the amount of wet skin, the relative ambient humidity, and the presence of airflow across the skin.

BODY TEMPERATURE MEASUREMENT

Since the first use in 1776, of a mercury in glass thermometer to record sublingual temperature,[4] the ideal site to record temperature has been sought. Surface temperatures are poorly reflective of the core temperature, and their use should be discouraged. Temperature recordings from the rectum or oral cavity are commonly used for isolated or repeated measurements in the outpatient or inpatient setting. Sublingual temperatures can be affected by the level of cooperation, temperature of recent oral contents, and by mouth breathing, but are acceptable for routine temperature screening in cooperative, reasonably healthy individuals. Rectal temperature is a more accurate reflection of core temperature, and is well tolerated for repeated measurements.[5] Esophageal temperature probes are invaluable for continuous monitoring in the surgical suite and ICU setting. The most precise estimation of core temperature can be determined using an otic temperature probe; however, otic probes[5] carry a 20% risk of otic trauma.[5,6] Central venous or pulmonary artery temperatures may be altered by the temperature of inspired gases or of infused fluids; the risk associated with Swan-Ganz catheters countermands their use solely for the purpose of temperature monitoring. Catastrophic thermoregulatory disorders commonly produce temperatures outside the range of available thermometers. It is imperative that personnel in settings such as the operating room, ICU and emergency room have access to thermometers which register temperatures below 25 and above 42°C.

THERMOREGULATION

Anatomy and Physiology of Thermoregulation

The posterior hypothalamus is the site of the temperature "set point." Afferent impulses from peripheral receptors travel in the nervous system with somesthetic pain impulses. Peripheral temperature input from skin thermoreceptors is integrated with central temperature data from thermosensors in the anterior hypothalamus and possibly the medulla and spinal cord. This information is then compared to the "set point." Significant deviations from "set point" trigger autonomic (and behavioral) responses that restore the body temperature to normal. The efferent pathways involved are the sympathetic autonomic nervous system (peripheral blood flow regulation and sweating) and the peripheral motor system (shivering). In the less acute situation, behavioral adaptations and acclimatization provide additional protection against cold environment.

Thermoregulatory Response to Cold Stress

In a resting person, the major source of heat production is metabolic processes in the viscera.[7] When exposed to cold, the body first works to conserve as much of this basal heat production as possible (vasoconstriction and piloerection). When this is inadequate, thermogenetic processes (shivering and nonshivering thermogenesis) are brought into play.

Vasoconstriction reduces the volume of the thermal core increasing the insulative value of the peripheral tissues, and reducing radiant heat loss. Vasoconstriction occurs in response to decrease in core temperature, but also to cooling of the skin. Central thermosensors take precedence; local skin warming will not inhibit vasoconstriction if the core temperature is subnormal. In extreme cold, there may be cycles of vasoconstriction and vasodilation, originally thought to be a protective mechanism for the extremities. More recent thought is that cold-induced vasodilation reflects cold induced vasoregulatory dysfunction. The ability to conserve heat by vasoconstriction is limited by 2 major sources of continued heat loss. First, the brain demands 20% of cardiac output, and cerebral autoregulation is resistant to cold-induced vasoconstriction. Consequently, as much as 50% of basal heat production may be lost through the uncovered head. Second, there is no control over heat losses through expiration of warmed air.

Piloerection traps a thin layer of air next to the skin surface, increasing its insulation properties. In a relatively hairless person, it is not a significant help against cold exposure.

Shivering thermogenesis is the most important mechanism of heat generation. The stimulus for shivering is a drop in skin temperature. Early shivering is characterized by asynchronous fragmentary muscle contraction; as it progresses, it becomes violent and generalized, and may interfere with volitional motor activities and speech. Heat is produced because muscle contraction occurs without performance of external work. Unfortunately, the heat produced by shivering is partially offset by increased blood flow to skeletal muscles and by movement of the shivering limbs through the air, increasing convective heat loss. Prolonged shivering may lead to extreme muscle fatigue and eventually to muscle failure. Body temperature may fall precipitously once shivering ceases.[7]

Nonshivering thermogenesis is known to occur, and may be important in acclimatization to chronic cold temperatures. Metabolic processes mediated by catecholamines and hormones increase after exposure to chronic cold temperatures. Brown adipose tissue, found in neonates and in limited amounts in adult humans, when metabolized, produces heat. Metabolism of brown fat has been shown to produce significant body heat only in neonates, however.[8]

Behavioral adaptations to cold stress are essential to survival. Changing body posture (e.g., curling up) decreases the surface area available for heat loss, and may reduce heat loss by as much as 50%.[7] Warm, insulating clothing may markedly decrease heat loss; when clothing is bulky, however, the surface area for heat loss is actually increased, and when wet, it has no more insulating value than lightweight summer clothing.

Exposure to cold for more than 2 weeks induces cold **acclimatization.** Cold acclimatized subjects do not shiver when exposed to temperatures that make nonacclimatized persons shiver, yet they maintain normothermia. It is believed that cold acclimatization occurs because of increases in nonshivering thermogenesis, mediated by the sympathetic nervous system.[7]

Thermoregulatory Response to Heat Stress

The two naturally occurring causes of increase in core temperature are exposure to high ambient temperatures and physical exercise. The resulting increase in core body temperature triggers two major cooling mechanisms: vasodilation of skin blood vessels, and sweating. Over time, behavioral modification and acclimatization permit a greater degree of heat intolerance.

When in a thermoneutral environment, the cutaneous blood vessels of the hands and feet are in a state of vasoconstriction. Within 15 seconds of application of heat to the trunk, superficial blood vessels in the hand dilate. This **reflex vasodilation** is inhibited when the central temperature is subnormal, suggesting that central thermosensor input supersedes peripheral input.[9] Vasodilation increases the skin to environment temperature gradient, increasing heat transfer by convection, conduction and radiation. Heat is lost by vasodilation of skin blood vessels only when the environmental temperature is lower than the core temperature.

When environmental temperature exceeds core temperature, or when vasodilation alone does not sufficiently cool, **sweating** is called into play. Eccrine sweat glands, widely and symmetrically distributed over the body surface, are innervated by sympathetic cholinergic neurons. Sweating occurs over the entire body surface in response to an increase in core temperature of 1°C. Cooling results from evaporation of sweat, and is dependent on the percentage of body area covered by sweat, the relative humidity of the environment, and the presence or absence of airflow across wet skin. Evaporation of 1.7 ml of sweat produces 1 kcal of cooling. Maximal sweat production averages 1.5 L per hour, which could potentially relieve a heat load of 882 kcal per hour.[10] Unfortunately, when sweating is profuse, as much as 20% may drip from the skin, making it ineffective at cooling. It is often impossible to sustain such sweating rates, and the cooling ability of sweat decreases as the environmental humidity increases and the wind becomes still. Unrestricted access to water and electrolytes is essential to prevent dehydration and arrest of sweating.

Behavioral responses to heat include decreasing the level of exertion, removing warm clothing, seeking shelter from heat and sun, and drinking cool fluids.

Chronic exposure to high environmental temperatures leads to **heat acclimatization.** After 1-2 weeks of daily exposure to heat stress, sweating begins at a lower core temperature and is more exuberant. The sodium content in sweat and urine decreases. The cardiovascular system adapts, and heart rate slows. There may also be a decrease in basal metabolic rate in heat-acclimatized subjects.[11] Acclimatization occurs faster in physically fit individuals and those who work daily in heat.[12]

THERMOREGULATORY DISORDERS

General Mechanisms

There are 2 major mechanisms of serious thermoregulatory disturbance (Table 3-1). The first is exposure to overwhelming thermal stress in the presence of an intact thermoregulatory system. The precipitating stress may be endogenous such as environmental heat (heat stroke), or exogenous, such as excessive heat from skeletal muscle contraction (malignant hyperthermia). Alternatively, thermoregulatory systems themselves may be impaired leading to disorders of temperature regulation despite normal ambient temperatures. Such thermoregulatory dysfunction may be due to structural lesions involving one or more areas of the thermoregulatory pathway, or the intact thermoregulatory pathway may be rendered dysfunctional by an outside influence.

Structural lesions at any of a number of loci in the nervous system may impair thermoregulation. Afferent transmission of temperature information may be impaired by peripheral neuropathy or spinal cord transection. Hypothalamic function may be handicapped by tumor, stroke, infection, inflammation, or Wernicke's encephalopathy. Effector mechanisms may be affected by lesions in the brain stem, spinal cord, neuromuscular junction, or muscles.

Functional abnormalities of the thermoregulatory system may be due to age, drug exposure, or medical illness. For example, infants have heightened susceptibility to cold stress because they have a large surface area to mass ratio, and reduced ability to shiver. Conversely, the elderly are prone to both heat and cold stress because of reduced vascular reactivity, blunted perception of temperature, reduced shivering and sweating, and poor behavioral responses to thermal stress.

Table 3-1. Mechanisms of Thermoregulatory Disturbance

Overwhelming Stress
  exogenous
  endogenous
Failure of Thermoregulatory Mechanism
  Structural
    afferent stimuli
    hypothalamus
    efferent stimuli
  Functional
    age
    drugs (see Table 3-2)
    medical illness (see Table 3-3)

Table 3-2. Drug-Related Thermoregulatory Dysfunction

Causing Hypothermia
  Decreased vasoconstriction
    vasodilators
    ethanol
  Decreased cardiac output
    diuretics
    beta-blockers
  Hypothalamic depression
    phenothiazines
    butyrophenones
    alpha-blockers
    ethanol
  Behavioral dysfunction
    sedatives
    opioids
    cannabinoids
    ethanol
Causing Hyperthermia
  Increased heat production
    thyroid supplementation
    sympathomimetics
    tricyclic
  Decreased sweating
    anticholinergics
    tricyclic antidepressants
    antihistamines
    phenothiazines
  Decreased cardiac output
    diuretics
    beta blockers
  Decreased vasodilation
    sympathomimetics
    alpha-agonists
  Hypothalamic depression
    phenothiazines
    butyrophenones
    alpha blockers
  Behavioral dysfunction
    sedatives
    opioids
    ethanol
    cannabinoids

Many classes of drugs impair thermoregulatory mechanisms (Table 3-2). Phenothiazines have antihistaminic, anticholinergic and anticatecholaminergic properties. As such, they impair sweating and vasoregulation, and may have an effect on central systems in thermoregulation. Adaptation to extremes of temperature is blunted, and both hypothermia and hyperthermia have been reported to occur.[13] Tricyclic antidepressants have anticholinergic and catecholaminergic properties; they impair sweating and central mechanisms; in isolation, they usually produce hypothermia. When combined with monoamine oxidase inhibitors (MAOIs), severe hyperthermia may result.[13] Opiates cause cutaneous vasodilation; opiate withdrawal may cause profuse diaphoresis with piloerection; hyperthermia may be seen with acute withdrawal or when inadvertently administered to patients taking MAOIs. Amphetamines have multiple effects on catecholamine neurotransmitters; amphetamine overdose has been associated with life-threatening hyperthermia.[13] Ethanol is the most frequent predisposing factor in hypothermia in the young. It is believed to lower the hypothalamic set point, produce peripheral vasodilation, and alter both cold perception and behavioral response to cold. Cannabinoids make one less adaptable to thermal stress producing hyperthermia when ambient temperature is elevated and hypothermia with cold exposure. Anticholinergic drugs suppress sweating and predispose to hyperthermia when ambient temperature is elevated. Hypnosedatives may blunt perception of temperature extremes or may impair behavioral adjustments to ambient temperature.

Medical illnesses have multiple effects on thermoregulation (Table 3-3). Basal metabolic heat production and ability to generate excess heat are affected by changes in thyroid and adrenal function. Muscle wasting or weakness affect the ability to generate heat by muscular work or shivering. Involuntary muscle rigidity may cause increased heat production. Vasodilation may be impaired by cardio-

THE HIGH RISK PATIENT: MANAGEMENT OF THE CRITICALLY ILL

Table 3-3. Medical Illnesses Affecting Thermoregulation

Causing Hypothermia
  Decreased basal heat production
    hypothyroidism
    hypoadrenalism
    hypopituitarism
    hypoglycemia
    diabetic ketoacidosis
    cirrhosis
  Decreased vasoregulation
    congestive heart failure
    autonomic failure
    peripheral vascular disease
    sympathectomy
    arteritis
    Raynaud's phenomenon
    overwhelming infection
  Decreased shivering-thermogenesis
    muscle wasting/weakness
  Increased evaporative losses
    burns
    dermatoses
    idiopathic hyperhidrosis

Causing Hyperthermia
  Increased basal heat production
    hyperthyroidism
  Increased thermogenesis
    skeletal muscle rigidity
  Decreased evaporative losses
    congenital anhidrosis
    skin scarring

vascular disease, autoimmune arteritis or by Raynaud's phenomenon, or enhanced by local skin conditions, or sympathectomy. Sweating may be congenitally absent or impaired by extensive skin scarring; evaporative losses may be enhanced by skin burns or by pathologic hyperhidrosis. Acute, severe infections may present as hypothermia.[14] It may be impossible to distinguish the infected subpopulation of hypothermic patients by white blood cell count, blood pressure or pulse, or arterial pH. Hypothermia due to infection is associated with decreased systemic vascular resistance, however, the risks of right heart catheterization contraindicate routine use of this procedure. Empiric treatment of hypothermic patients with broad spectrum antibiotics is recommended until infection can be excluded.[15]

Although medical illness, drug exposure, and structural lesions may result in significant impairments of thermoregulation, they are frequently found to predispose patients to other more devastating disorders and rarely, in isolation, cause catastrophic thermoregulatory disorders which require intensive levels of therapy. The catastrophic thermoregulatory disorders which are likely to require intensive therapy include accidental hypothermia, malignant hyperthermia, neuroleptic malignant syndrome, and heat stroke.

Accidental Hypothermia

Hypothermia is defined as core temperature less than 35°C. Cold water immersion or exposure to excessive cold when clothing is wet or inadequate can make even the healthiest person hypothermic. Ill or elderly persons may be susceptible to hypothermia despite normal or only mildly decreased environmental temperatures. Annual mortality from hypothermia over the age of 74 is 23.1 per million, compared to 1.3 per million between the ages of 15 and 24.[16] Numerous systemic factors, including illness and drug exposure increase the likelihood of hypothermia (Table 3-4).

Pre-ICU Phase

Cold water immersion rapidly causes extreme hypothermia. There are few defenses under such circumstances. Subcutaneous fat has some insulative value, and persons with a higher amount of body fat are more resistant to immersion hypothermia. Unfortunately, shivering and thrashing about are poor heat generators in cold water for two reasons: (1) muscular activity causes vasodilation; and (2) moving continuously exposes the body to ever-changing layers of cold water, increasing conductive heat loss. Remaining still allows the development of a thin layer of relatively warmer water, which has insulating properties. The presence of a life vest which allows the victim to remain still may be life saving.

Hyperthermia may result from exposure to cold during hiking or other outdoor activity, when clothing is inadequate, or becomes wet. The temperature fall is more gradual than seen with cold water immersion. Shivering occurs until the subject becomes exhausted, or until a temperature below 30°C is reached, at which time it ceases and the fall in body temperature is accelerated.

When hypothermia develops in the absence of significant cold exposure, an underlying medical illness, advanced age, debility, or ethanol or drug exposure will nearly always be identified. The elderly are the most common victims of hypothermia in the home. Population stud-

Table 3-4. Causes of Hypothermia

Overwhelming Environmental Stress
  Accidental
    cold water immersion
    cold exposure
  Iatrogenic
    during anesthesia
    cardiopulmonary bypass

Failure of Thermoregulation
  Failure to maintain basal heat production
    hypothyroidism
    hypoglycemia
    hypopituitarism
    hypoadrenalism
  Absent or inadequate shivering
    skeletal muscle wasting
    skeletal muscle weakness
  Absent or inadequate vasoconstriction
    congestive heart failure
    medications
    overwhelming infection
  Failure of central mechanisms
    hypothalamic lesion
  Failure of behavioral strategies
    age
    dementia
    sedation
    psychiatric disease

Table 3–5. Clinical Features of Hypothermia (by Severity)

	Organ System	Features
MILD (32–35°C)	Central Nervous System	Confusion, Shivering
	Cardiovascular	Cold, cyanotic extremities
		Increased blood pressure, pulse and respiratory rate
		(Bradycardia—late)
		(Prolonged PR, QT intervals)
	Renal	"Cold diuresis"
	Gastrointestinal	Ileus, Pancreatic dysfunction (hyperglycemia)
	Hematological	Mild leukocytosis
MODERATE (28–32; dgC)	Central Nervous System	Obtundation (<30°C—coma)
		Absent shivering
		(Muscle rigidity)
		Apnea
	Cardiovascular	Depressed myocardial conduction and contractility
		Ventricular fibrillation
	Renal	"Cold diuresis"
	Hematological	Hemoconcentration, Leukopenia
	Metabolic	Hyperkalemia, Metabolic Acidosis
SEVERE (<28°C)	Central Nervous System	Coma—may resemble brain death
		(EEG—electrocerebral silence)
		Decreased cerebral metabolism
		Decreased CNS blood flow
	Cardiovascular	Bradycardia
		Profound vasoconstriction

ies of the elderly have demonstrated subnormal body temperature in 10 to 17%.[17,18] Basal metabolic rate, and the capacity for vasoconstriction,[19] shivering and nonshivering thermogenesis are all known to diminish with age.[20] Some elderly have paradoxic vasodilation at low temperatures.[21] Perception of cold is blunted in the elderly as well, leading to reduced behavioral adaptation.[20] Victims of indoor hypothermia are frequently found to have collapsed on the floor in light clothing; almost all have had at least one medical illness, usually cardiovascular disease, or they have fractured a hip.[22]

Clinical Features. Hypothermia is classified according to its severity as mild (32 to 35°C), moderate (28 to 32°C) or severe (below 28°C) (Table 3–5). Mild hypothermia is characterized by confusion, signs of peripheral vasoconstriction (i.e., weak pulse, cold, cyanotic extremities), and shivering. Blood pressure, heart, and respiratory rates are increased early. Bradycardia with prolongation of P-R and QT intervals are seen as core temperature drops.[23] "Cold diuresis" results from a defect in renal tubular reabsorption.[24] Adynamic ileus, pancreatic dysfunction with hyperglycemia, and mild hepatic dysfunction are also common.[25,26] The white blood count (WBC) may be slightly elevated. Coagulopathy is rare, and may be due to an underlying systemic illness rather than hypothermia.

Moderately hypothermic patients are more deeply obtunded with blunted or absent verbal responses. Below 30°C, patients may be comatose. Myocardial conduction and contractility are depressed with progressive slowing of conduction. In as many as 1 in 3 patients, electrocardiographic changes include an Osborn wave (J-point elevation).[27] Supraventricular arrhythmias are common above 30°C; below 30°C, ventricular fibrillation is frequent.[28] Muscle tone is increased, but shivering is absent. "Cold diuresis" continues, and hemoconcentration becomes more pronounced. WBC and platelet counts fall. Electrolyte and acid-base abnormalities include hyponatremia, hyperkalemia and metabolic acidosis. Hyponatremia and hyperkalemia are believed to result from depressed enzymatic activity of the cellular sodium-potassium ATPase. Metabolic acidosis results from poor perfusion of the extremities; with rewarming, return of acidotic blood increases metabolic acidosis and the resulting K^+/H^+ shift may exacerbate hyperkalemia.[22] Because serum hyperkalemia is often the result of redistribution of potassium ions, it is important to remember that total body potassium stores may be near normal.

Severe hypothermia may present as apparent death. There is marked bradycardia; profound vasoconstriction makes measurement of blood pressure extremely difficult. Apnea occurs around 24°C.[29] Cerebral metabolism is markedly decreased, and cerebral blood flow decreases to very low levels. Coma is profound, and may resemble clinical brain death.[30] Electroencephalogram (EEG) may show no apparent brain activity. Cardiac output falls precipitously below 30°C. There is widespread organ dysfunction. Extreme hyperkalemia (>10 mmol/L) portends a grave prognosis.[31]

Treatment. Therapy of hypothermia begins with prevention. Hikers and climbers should wear layers of clothing and should have dry clothing available for rapid clothing changes. Elderly and others who are at risk for hypothermia should be instructed to maintain dwelling temperature at 20°C and to dress according to weather reports rather than perceived level of thermal discomfort.

Emergency treatment of hypothermia begins in the field. Rewarming should begin immediately, and the victim should be transported to an emergency facility as soon as safely possible. The victim must be handled with utmost care to minimize the risk of myocardial irritability; when a hill is traversed, the patient's head must be kept down to prevent hypotension.

Rewarming. Rewarming is the mainstay of therapy. Rewarming may be passive or active. For passive rewarming, wet clothing is removed and replaced with warm, dry clothing or blankets and the head is covered. The victim is removed to a warm environment or placed in a sleeping bag with a normothermic heat donor. Passive rewarming is slow, averaging 0.38°C per hour,[25] and once shivering has ceased (below 30°C) is rarely sufficient to reverse hypothermia. Active rewarming may be external or internal. External rewarming with radiant lamps, warm water baths, or heat blankets may produce peripheral vasodilation, resulting in the return of cold, acidotic, hyperkalemic blood to the core. An afterdrop in temperature or rewarming shock may result.[32] There is considerable controversy whether active external rewarming should ever be used; clearly, it should not be used without intensive monitoring, and when used, active rewarming devices should be applied to the trunk rather than the extremities. Active internal rewarming techniques which can be applied in the field include warm intravenous (IV) fluids and warm, humidified oxygen. Ingestion of warm liquids may trigger a pharyngeal reflex which results in reflex vasodilation, and may no longer be recommended.[33] Warm gastric and rectal lavage is safe. When more rapid rewarming rates are desirable because of cardiovascular instability, thoracic or peritoneal lavage or partial cardiopulmonary bypass may be used. Peritoneal lavage with warm (around 40°C) saline or peritoneal dialysate raises the core temperature as much as 4°C per hour, and is safely performed in the emergency room or hospital setting. Moreover, it may detect occult intra-abdominal trauma. Profoundly hypothermic patients with marked hemodynamic instability are best treated with cardiopulmonary bypass which has the additional benefits of rapid control of oxygenation, and acid/base and electrolyte balance. The choice of a rewarming technique should be based on the severity of hypothermia and cardiovascular stability. Patients who have core temperature greater than 33°C, are able to shiver and are hemodynamically stable should be warmed by passive external rewarming with or without warm humidified oxygen and warm IV fluids. Patients who have moderate hypothermia and mild to moderate hemodynamic instability should be warmed in the field with the above techniques; on arrival to the hospital, if response has been judged to be inadequate, warm peritoneal lavage should be started. Severe hypothermia should be treated with cardiopulmonary bypass.

Other Therapy. The role of cardiopulmonary resuscitation (CPR) in the management of hypothermia has been controversial. It has been judged not likely effective when hypothermia is profound, and carries the risk of increasing myocardial irritability. However, prudence dictates that for pulseless patients, CPR should be instituted immediately at the scene and continued until the temperature exceeds 32°C, safely outside the window of highest risk of ventricular fibrillation.[3] It has been suggested that patients with severe hyperkalemia (>10 mmol/L) not be considered, since there then appears to be no chance of survival.[31] The use of antiarrhythmic drugs when temperature is low and circulation poor is also controversial, but recent evidence suggests that bretylium may be the drug of choice for hypothermic arrhythmia.[34] Bradycardia is atropine resistant.[3] When determining dose for all medications, account should be taken of reduced circulation and impaired hepatic metabolic function. Electrical defibrillation is unlikely to be successful until temperature returns to 30°C.[28] Nevertheless, it is recommended that one or two cardioversion attempts be made when ventricular fibrillation is encountered.[3] Hypotension should be treated with aggressive fluid support, guided by central venous or pressure. Swan-Ganz catheter insertion may exacerbate myocardial irritability, and should be avoided.[23] Dopamine may be used to supplement fluid resuscitation in treating hypotension.[3] Moderate to severe hypothermia is associated with profound respiratory depression. Endotracheal intubation and ventilation with warm (<43°C), humidified oxygen is nearly always required. Care should be taken to interpret arterial blood gases (ABGs); specimens taken from a hypothermic patient and analyzed at 37°C will yield falsely elevated Pco_2 and o_2 and falsely depressed pH.[3]

The following screening laboratories should be obtained: coagulation studies, blood count, platelets, ABGs, electrolytes, blood urea nitrogen (BUN) and creatinine, serum glucose, amylase, hepatic function studies, thyroid functions, serum cortisol and drug screen. The high incidence of underlying ethanol abuse dictates prophylactic thiamine administration (dose of 100 mg IM). Cardiac rhythm, oxygen saturation, arterial blood pressure, and core temperature should be monitored continuously.

Severely hypothermic patients, any who have required institution of CPB, and patients who have become normothermic, but have lingering multiple organ dysfunction require admission to the ICU setting. Patients with less severe hypothermia may be admitted to a general medical ward.

ICU Phase

In the absence of a continuing source of cold exposure or an ongoing medical process which presents lasting thermal stress, intensive care will focus on support of vital functions, control of myocardial irritability, fluid management, and normalization of acid/base status. Cardiac rhythm, core temperature, arterial blood pressure, and oxygenation should be monitored continuously. Electrolytes, renal and hepatic function, glucose, amylase, coagulation studies and blood count should be monitored frequently.

Pulmonary management should be directed to detect and treat adult respiratory distress syndrome and pneumonia. Intubation and assisted ventilation will usually have been initiated in the emergency room, and should be continued as indicated by clinical status. Abdominal ileus should be managed by nasogastric (NG) tube; feeding should be postponed until intestinal motility improves. Fluid support should be directed to prevent acute renal failure; cold diuresis is to be expected, and the absence of polyuria is a poor sign. Decreased circulating blood volume and hypofunction of the liver dictate prudence in dosing and monitoring drugs. Obtundation which progresses despite response of the temperature to treatment indicates the development of cerebral edema, which should be treated with cautious hyperventilation and osmotic diuresis. The failure to respond to these measures is an indication for monitoring the intracerebral pressure. Coagulation studies should be closely monitored. Infection is a common consequence of prolonged hypothermia, and therefore surveillance should be initiated in the ICU and continued until discharge. Specific therapy for underlying medical conditions should be begun. Therapy of frostbite should be delayed until temperature has returned to physiologic range; frostbite treatment includes rewarming of frozen tissue, tetanus prophylaxis and gentle debridement. A detailed discussion of treatment of thermal tissue injuries is outside the scope of this chapter. For more information, the reader is referred to Edlich et al.[23] Short-term survival estimates in accidental hypothermia range between 20 and 75%.[3] A proposed hypothermia outcome scoring system found death within 24 hours to be associated with need for CPR in the prehospital setting, tracheal intubation, NG tube placement, Foley catheter placement, elevated serum potassium, BUN and creatinine levels, low hemoglobin, low core temperature, hypotension, and bradycardia.[34]

Once temperature has returned to normal and respiratory, cardiovascular, and renal function have stabilized, the patient can be discharged to a step-down or general medical ward.

Post-ICU Phase

Following discharge from the ICU, therapy of residual organ dysfunction should be continued as indicated. Discharge planning should begin in earnest. Patients who have survived an acute episode of hypothermia are known to be more susceptible than normal to recurrent episodes of hypothermia. They have decreased perception of cold and decreased ability to generate heat by shivering and nonshivering thermogenesis.[19] They must be counseled to maintain a dwelling temperature of 20°C, and when leaving home to heed weather reports rather than perceived temperature when dressing. A hat should always be worn during cool temperatures. Alcohol and drug rehabilitation programs should be encouraged if appropriate. Family and community support systems should be arranged so that the patient can be monitored periodically.

Heat Stroke

Hyperthermic illnesses occur when the body is exposed to high levels of exogenous or endogenous heat and heat dissipation mechanisms are impaired by high environmental heat and humidity, underlying medical conditions, or drugs (Table 3-6). Sustained core temperature above 42°C causes permanent tissue damage.[35]

Heat syndromes related to environmental exposure have been described. "**Heat cramps**" are painful muscle cramps that occur during work in hot environments when water is taken for rehydration, but salt is not replenished. Resolution occurs with salt replacement.[10] "**Heat exhaustion**" occurs when salt and water are not replaced during exertion in hot weather. Heat exhaustion may be predominantly related to salt depletion, to water depletion or to

Table 3-6. Causes of Hyperthermia

Overwhelming Exogenous Stress
  environmental heat and humidity (classical heat stroke)
Overwhelming Endogenous Stress
  skeletal muscle activity (exertional heat stroke)
  hyperthyroidism
  malignant hyperthermia
Failure of thermoregulation
  Decreased sweating
    age
    dehydration
    drugs (see Table 3-2)
    medical illness (see Table 3-3)
  Decreased vasodilation
    age
    decreased cardiac reserve
    drugs (see Table 3-2)
    medical illness (see Table 3-3)
  Hypothalamic depression
    drugs (neuroleptic malignant syndrome)

Table 3-7. Features of Classical and Exertional Heat Stroke

	Classical	Exertional
Occurrence	epidemic	sporadic
Age	elderly	young
Sex	male/female	male
Health	underlying illness	healthy
Precipitant	environmental heat	strenuous exercise
Sweating	absent	often profuse
Acid-base	respiratory alkalosis	metabolic acidosis
CPK	slight increase	marked increase
Potassium	decreased	increased
Renal failure	rare	30%
Coagulopathy	rare	common

both. **Water-depletion heat exhaustion** presents as hyperthermia, marked thirst, fatigue, weakness and impaired judgement; when severe, there may be delirium or stupor. **Salt-depletion heat exhaustion** presents as headache, weakness, giddiness, anorexia, nausea, vomiting, diarrhea and muscle cramps.[36,37] "**Heat stroke**" is a catastrophic syndrome of extreme hyperpyrexia (generally >40°C) with central nervous and multiple organ system dysfunction.[38]

Pre-ICU Phase

Traditionally, heat stroke can be divided into two categories: classic and exertional (Table 3-7).

Classic heat stroke is a disease of elderly or infirm persons who are exposed to high ambient temperatures. Classic heat stroke occurs in epidemics when daily temperatures are very high or when extreme humidity accompanies less extreme temperatures; urban populations are more susceptible because temperatures do not fall at night.[10] In heat stroke epidemics, the majority of cases occur after 2 weeks of sustained temperatures near 38°C.[38] Sedentary life style, poor cardiac reserve, diminished capacity to sweat,[39] and underlying medical illness and medications make the elderly prone to classic heat stroke. Patients often are found to have predisposing medical conditions or to take multiple medications.

Exertional heat stroke is a disease of young, healthy males who become hyperthermic during work or exercise in extreme heat. The majority of cases have occurred in military recruits, long distance runners and football players. At least three factors are known to predispose normal persons to heat stroke: dehydration, lack of heat acclimation, and poor physical fitness.

Alcoholism, chronic illness, fatigue, sleep deprivation, obesity, and improper clothing increase risk of both classic and exertional heat stroke.[40]

Clinical Features (Table 3-8). In 80% of patients with heat stroke, the onset is acute. There may be brief prodromal symptoms such as lassitude, dizziness, confusion, drowsiness, nausea, anorexia, anxiety, and headache.[41] Core temperature may reach 47°C.[38]

In **classic heat stroke,** the skin is usually warm and dry. Tachypnea leads to respiratory alkalosis, sometimes with tetany.[35] Hypotension and tachycardia are nearly universal.[38] As long as the cardiac index is sufficient to meet

Table 3-8. Clinical Features of Heat Stroke

	Organ System	Features
CLASSICAL HEAT STROKE	Central Nervous System	Obtundation, cerebellar ataxia, miosis, seizures, warm, dry skin
	Cardiovascular	Tachypnea, respiratory alkalosis (tetany), hypotension, tachycardia, ST segment depression, T-wave changes, supraventricular arrhythmias
	Gastrointestinal	Increased transaminases
EXERTIONAL HEAT STROKE	Central Nervous System	Diaphoresis, cool, clammy skin
	Cardiovascular	Tachypnea, rapid pulse, hypotension, lactic acidosis
	Renal	Acute renal failure (rhabdomyolysis) (CPK elevated from rhabdomyolysis) hyperuricemia, hyperkalemia
	Gastrointestinal	Diarrhea, hyperbilirubinemia (rare)
	Hematological	Consumptive coagulopathy

circulatory demands (greater than 6L/m² per minute), the pulse is full and rapid; when cardiac index falls below 3 L/m² per minute, the skin becomes ashen and the pulse thready.[36,42] Electrocardiographic features include ST-segment depression, T-wave abnormalities, and supraventricular arrhythmias. Signs of nervous system dysfunction include obtundation, cerebellar ataxia, and small pupils. Focal neurologic deficits are uncommon.[43] Convulsions may occur immediately or during cooling.[38] Liver dysfunction is manifested by modest elevation in transaminases.

In **exertional heat stroke,** the patient may have intense diaphoresis with deceptively cool, clammy skin. Tachypnea and rapid pulse with hypotension are nearly universal. Exertional heat stroke is virtually always associated with rhabdomyolysis; lactic acidosis, hyperuricemia, hyperkalemia, increased CPK and myoglobinuria are also common. Acute renal failure is seen in as many as 30%. Thermal injury to blood vessels produces consumptive coagulopathy. Petechial and gross organ hemorrhage are seen at necropsy.[44] Severe dehydration is uncommon in acute heat stroke. Some degree of dehydration and sodium loss are universal, however. Clinically manifest hepatic dysfunction with hyperbilirubinemia is rare, occurring in less than 5%. Histologic changes of hepatocellular damage are present in less than 10%. Gastrointestinal dysfunction is most often characterized by diarrhea, which may be exacerbated by cooling.

Treatment. When the victim is discovered, clothing should be removed, an IV line should be placed and respiratory function supported if necessary. The victim should be removed to a cool environment, and transported to an emergency facility as soon as possible. Comatose patients should be intubated. A rectal probe for temperature should be inserted to a depth of 20 cm.[10] External cooling may be accomplished by wetting the skin thoroughly and briskly rubbing the skin with ice packs. Air flow should be directed across the body with a fan. Immersion in cold water and packing in ice will produce vasoconstriction; constant massage to stimulate circulation is required with these techniques. The temperature should be recorded continuously and external cooling discontinued when the core temperature falls below 40°C. An empirically developed cooling rate of 0.3°C in rectal temperature every 5 minutes the first half hour is strongly associated with survival.[40] Rarely, temperature will not respond to external cooling. In these cases, iced peritoneal lavage, iced gastric lavage or partial cardiopulmonary bypass with external cooling of blood may be required. Hypotension usually responds to cooling; aggressive fluid support is not often required. When treatment is instituted promptly, as many as 70% of patients are normothermic within 2 hours, and may be discharged from the hospital. Twenty to 30% of patients have delayed response to cooling with prolonged coma and hyperthermic complications, and require admission to the hospital.[43] Patients with persistent coma, hypotension, seizures, severely elevated serum CPK and myoglobinuria with hyperkalemia, or coagulopathy should be admitted to the ICU setting.

ICU Phase

In the absence of a continuing source of heat production, once the temperature has been controlled, no relapses can be expected. Comatose patients should be intubated, if not already intubated, and may require assisted ventilation. Temperature, cardiac rhythm, blood pressure, and urine output should be continuously monitored. An arterial line and Swan-Ganz catheter are required to adequately monitor blood pressure and fluid status. Electrolytes, urine myoglobin, BUN, creatinine, CPK, ABGs, coagulation and liver function studies should be monitored frequently. ABGs should be corrected for temperature. Hyperthermia, when present at admission to the ICU, should be treated as outlined above. Large amounts of bicarbonate may be required to correct acidosis; bicarbonate replacement should be directed by frequent ABGs. Coagulopathy can be treated with fresh frozen plasma; the role of low dose heparin is not yet clear. Fluid support and osmotic diuresis are usually necessary to prevent acute oliguric renal failure secondary to myoglobinuria. Once renal failure has occurred, conventional therapy, including dialysis if indicated, should be instituted. In the setting of oliguric renal failure, hyperkalemia should be aggressively treated with polystyrene sulfonate. Liver dysfunction dictates judicious use of drugs. Single seizures or flurries of brief seizures require no treatment except airway protection; prolonged seizures (5 minutes) or status epilepticus may be treated acutely with IV diazepam or lorazepam.[45] Subacute or chronic treatment of seizures with phenytoin is usually not required. Severe skeletal muscle necrosis may produce compartment syndromes.[46] The most common clinical presentation of compartment syndrome is a tight extremity with warm skin. An alert patient will usually complain of distal paresthesia. Because tissue pressures in compartment syndrome may be well below arterial pressure, the presence of peripheral pulse does not exclude the diagnosis. A typical clinical presentation should prompt measurement of tissue pressure and consideration of fasciotomy.[47]

Normothermia, normokalemia, normal or stable renal function, and normal coagulation should be present before discharge from the ICU. With rapid, directed therapy, mortality from exertional heat stroke should be less than 5%, and from classical heat stroke less than 20%.

Post-ICU Phase

Post-ICU care should focus on lingering organ dysfunction (renal and hepatic) and on rehabilitation from widespread skeletal necrosis. Underlying medical conditions should be identified and treated, and offending medications eliminated. Acute exertional heat stroke seems to confer on its survivors a lifelong sensitivity to recurrent episodes. It is difficult to discern whether these individuals have an unusual propensity to develop hyperthermia which is a primary defect or whether an acute episode of heat stroke causes secondary thermoregulatory abnormalities.[10] In any event, survivors must be counseled to avoid overexertion in high environmental heat and to take in adequate amounts of hydration and electrolyte when exposed to heat. Patients should be given lists of medications that predispose to hyperthermia and should be avoided. Elderly, urban residents should be instructed to seek shelter in community "cooling" centers when daily temperatures exceed 37°C.

Malignant Hyperthermia

Malignant hyperthermia (MH) was first described in 1960 by Denborough, who witnessed an episode in a patient with fear of anesthesia and a family history of 10 anesthetic deaths.[48] MH, which complicates 1 in 15,000 pediatric and 1 in 50,000 to 150,000 adult surgeries, is an explosive syndrome characterized by muscle rigidity with skeletal muscle necrosis, fever, and autonomic dysfunction.

Pre-ICU Phase

MH mostly occurs during induction with inhalational anesthetics and depolarizing skeletal muscle relaxants, but MH reactions can occur anytime during general anesthesia, during the first several postoperative hours or during operative procedures under regional or local anesthesia. Other drugs and chemicals have been linked to MH (Table 3-9), and episodes have been reported which were not associated with surgery or pharmacologic triggers, usually under conditions of extreme physical or emotional stress.[49] It is believed that there is a population of persons who are susceptible to MH in whom episodes of MH may be triggered by various exogenous and endogenous triggers.[50] Similar syndromes occur in various animals, most notably swine.[49]

The immediate cause of MH is a sudden increase in intracellular calcium because of excessive release from the sarcoplasmic reticulum.[49] Normal muscle contraction begins when the muscle membrane is depolarized by action of acetylcholine (ACh) at the neuromuscular junction. Depolarization extends to the sarcoplasmic reticulum membrane which then releases calcium into the sarcoplasm. Calcium binds to troponin which causes a conformational change in the calcium-binding protein, exposing myosin crossbridge binding sites on actin. Actin-myosin crossbridges form; there is sliding of filaments and the muscle contracts. Relaxation occurs when calcium is actively taken up into the sarcoplasmic reticulum. Both contraction and relaxation require energy which is provided by hydrolysis of ATP to ADP and phosphorus. Heat is produced during this reaction. It is believed that the MH sarcoplasmic reticulum is "leakier" than normal in response to certain "triggering agents." Excessive calcium influx into the sarcoplasm activates myosin ATP-ase; muscle contracture ensues and ATP stores are depleted. Muscle contraction without external work causes marked heat production. This muscle rigidity is profound and does not respond to nondepolarizing muscle relaxants.[51]

In humans, most cases occur between the ages of 3 and 30 years. Among teens, males are affected more frequently than females, but this may reflect their larger muscle mass and higher incidence of major trauma requiring surgical intervention.[49] Preoperative fever, strenuous muscle activity, anxiety and muscle trauma may increase MH risk.[52] Up to 50% of patients with MH have had prior anesthesia, which was uncomplicated in half.[49] MH susceptibility is an inherited trait. Although as few as 30% of patients with documented MH give a positive family history, formal testing of muscle biopsies reveals some members with MH susceptibility in up to 80% of families.[53] Initially thought to be an autosomal dominant trait, studies suggest variable patterns of inheritance. It has been suggested that certain muscle diseases (Duchenne's muscular dystrophy, myotonia, central core disease) predispose to MH. However, the

Table 3-9. Precipitants of Malignant Hyperthermia

Inhalation anesthetics
  halothane
  enflurane
  isoflurane
  diethyl ether
  divinyl ether
  fluroxene
  trichloroethylene
  ethyl chloride
  cyclopropane
  methoxyflurane
  seroflurane
Depolarizing skeletal muscle relaxants
  succinyl choline
  decamethonium
Nondepolarizing skeletal muscle relaxants*
  gallamine
  D-tubocurarine
Amide local anesthetics*
Nitrous oxide*
Common chemicals*
  carbon tetrachloride
Other drugs*
  ethanol
  caffeine
  anticholinergics
  monoamine oxidase inhibitors
  sympathomimetics

* Possible precipitants.

association between these muscle diseases and MH has not been proven,[54] and routine preoperative MH prophylactic techniques are not recommended.

Clinical Features. The most common clinical presentation of MH is the sudden development of muscle rigidity during induction of anesthesia. Masseter muscle rigidity which makes intubation difficult is said to be the hallmark of MH. However, obvious rigidity occurs in only 75% of MH cases, and when venous pH and end-tidal P_{CO_2} are recorded, it can be seen that the earliest manifestations of MH are venous acidosis and increased expired CO_2. Fever occurs within minutes to hours and is progressive, rising as fast as 0.5°C per minute to a temperature as high as 43°C (109.4°F).[54] Tachycardia is universal and is seen within 30 minutes of onset of anesthesia in 90% of patients.[55] Ventricular extrasystoles are frequent; malignant arrhythmias including ventricular tachycardia and fibrillation may supervene. Spontaneous respirations are rapid and deep, and the soda lime in the anesthesia breathing circuit becomes hot and discolored. There may be a transient phase of vasodilation associated with profuse diaphoresis and flushing of the skin. Later, there is persistent vasoconstriction, which when coupled with markedly increased venous oxygen extraction results in oxygen resistant cyanosis.[55] Blood pressure is labile. If muscle rigidity is not controlled, there may be widespread skeletal muscle edema and necrosis. Untreated MH is a multiorgan system disease. Noncardiogenic pulmonary edema may be seen; the liver, brain and kidneys become edematous. Widespread cellular damage leads to excessive release of tissue thromboplastin resulting in consumptive coagulopathy.[54] Excessive myoglobin release from injured muscle causes acute renal failure. In the terminal phases of the illness, hypotension portends circulatory failure. Brain function is profoundly depressed; brain death may occur.

Serum calcium and potassium are markedly increased early in the course of the syndrome; later, they are severely depleted. Increases in phosphorus, magnesium, and blood glucose are prolonged. Acid/base disturbance is common; usually, both metabolic acidosis and respiratory alkalosis are seen. The arteriovenous (A-V) O_2 difference is markedly increased and venous acidosis is profound with markedly elevated serum lactic acid levels. Skeletal muscle necrosis causes marked increases in serum CK (as high as 100,000 units); usually with myoglobinemia and myoglobinuria. BUN and creatinine values reflect prerenal azotemia. The ECG reveals sinus tachycardia with ventricular extrasystoles which progress to trigeminy or bigeminy, and eventually to ventricular tachycardia. Chest radiographs may reveal pulmonary edema. Liver enzymes are often elevated. Coagulation studies are compatible with consumptive coagulopathy.

Treatment. A careful preanesthetic history is the most vital preventative measure. In addition to personal anesthetic history, it is important to obtain family history of complications of anesthesia, and unexplained episodes of hyperthermia or severe stress reactions. Masseter spasm during anesthesia is thought to be a strong clinical sign of MH, although laboratory-proven MH susceptibility may be present in as few as 25 to 50% of patients with documented masseter spasm in the past.[56] A history of muscle cramps with exercise or mild hyperthermic reactions to extremes of temperature or vigorous exercise should be sought. Physical stigmata including ptosis, spinal or foot deformities, hernias, hypermobile joints, and dental anomalies have been described in some patients, but usually these are absent.[49] Screening serum CK values are abnormal in 40% of MH susceptible patients, but are also abnormal in 10% of normal patients. Therefore, most elevated preoperative CK values are seen in normal persons.[53] If one has a high index of suspicion for MH susceptibility, such as with a patient with a positive family history of anesthetic death, a prior episode of masseter muscle rigidity during induction of anesthesia, or a history of hyperthermic crisis during surgery of following emotional or physical stress, the operating room should be prepared for an MH crisis, and the anesthetic protocol should avoid triggering agents. Some have advocated obtaining muscle biopsy on all persons suspected by personal or family history of anesthesia reaction. These patients should undergo muscle biopsy for halothane or caffeine contracture testing.[49] It is costly and unnecessary to test all such persons; if a careful anesthetic history reveals possible MH susceptibility, anesthetists must be informed and must be prepared to manage an acute MH crisis.

Patients known to be MH susceptible may be anesthetized. Thirty-six vials of dantrolene (20 mg/60 ml) sodium should be on hand. An automatic cooling blanket should be placed under the patient and set to maintain the temperature at 37°C to prevent MH stress reaction secondary to shivering. When possible, inhalational anesthetics should be avoided; narcotics, barbiturates, diazepam, droperidol, nitrous oxide and ester class local anesthetics carry a lower risk, and can be used. Pancuronium is the preferred skeletal muscle relaxant. Routine monitoring of core temperature, ECG, blood pressure, end-expiratory CO_2 and venous blood gases should be performed during surgery, and temperature should be closely monitored in the postoperative period.[53,54] Core temperature should be monitored as long as the threat of MH or MH recurrence remains. Although pretreatment with dantrolene (4 to 7 mg/kg/day orally for 3 days or 2.5 mg/kg over 30 minutes IV) was recommended in the past,[54] prophylactic dantrolene causes generalized weakness, with increased dependence on artificial ventilation and increased risk of adverse effects, and is better avoided. Patients who are at high risk for MH should be monitored for several hours postoperatively in an ICU setting, even if anesthesia is uncomplicated, since onset of hyperthermia may occur hours after the triggering event.

At the first sign of MH, all triggering agents should be discontinued. Elective surgery should be interrupted. Should surgery be essential, it can be carried out using alternative anesthetics. A clean anesthesia machine should be obtained, and the patient hyperventilated at three times the normal respiratory rate to remove excess CO_2. Arterial and venous blood should be drawn immediately for electrolytes, calcium, magnesium, phosphorus, arterial and venous blood gases, and CPK. Two large bore IV lines should be inserted and the patient infused with cooled IV solution.[57] The skin should be wetted and cooled with fans or cooling blankets or massaged with ice packs. Dantrolene sodium, the preferred treatment for MH should be given as soon as possible. Dantrolene is a hydantoin derivative which inhibits the release of calcium from the sarcoplasmic reticulum by depressing the mechanism that couples the depolarization of sarcoplasmic reticulum with calcium release.[52] It appears to have its primary action in skeletal muscle. The rarity and severity of MH has made controlled trials of therapy in MH impractical. However, dantrolene has been shown to relieve halothane-induced malignant hyperthermia in susceptible swine, and has been shown in anecdotal reports to be effective in preventing MH reactions in MH susceptible patients and in relieving established MH reactions in humans.[52] In one study, all patients who were treated with Dantrolene within 24 hours of onset of MH survived.[52] Each 60-ml vial contains 20 mg of dantrolene. It is diluted with sterile, nonbacteriostatic distilled water and is administered IV at a rate not to exceed 1 mg/kg per minute. Up to 10 mg/kg may be given over 15 minutes. The average effective dose established in a prospective multicenter trial was 2.5 mg/kg.[57] The loading dose can be repeated every 15 minutes should the reaction remain uncontrolled. Once the reaction appears to be controlled, a maintenance infusion of 1 to 2 mg/kg IV every 3 to 4 hours should be begun. Acidosis should be partially corrected (to pH 7.2 to 7.3) with sodium bicarbonate.[55] The patient should be transferred to an ICU setting.

ICU Phase

The following should be monitored continuously: cardiac rhythm, core temperature (esophageal, rectal probe, or central venous temperature probe), and urine output. Until the clinical state has returned to normal, frequent samples should be obtained for arterial and venous blood gases, serum electrolytes, calcium, phosphorus and magnesium, urea nitrogen and creatinine, CPK, urine myoglobin, and coagulation profile.

The patient should be maintained on ventilatory support and hyperventilated as necessary. A central line or Swan-Ganz catheter may aid fluid support. A maintenance dantrolene infusion of 1 to 2 mg/kg every 3 to 4 hours should be continued until all signs of MH have resolved.[55] Dantrolene is a highly alkaline agent and is injurious to veins; therefore, once it is feasible to begin enteral medications, the drug should be given enterally. Surface cooling should be continued; should temperature not respond to surface cooling, iced peritoneal or gastric lavage, or partial CPB with external cooling should be begun. Cooling should be stopped when the core temperature reaches 38.3°C. Arrhythmias may be treated with procaine, procainamide or verapamil, but the blood pressure should be monitored if verapamil and dantrolene are given concomitantly because these agents may have a depressor effect.[49] Osmotic diuresis should be instituted with mannitol to ensure adequate urine output thus to prevent myoglobinuric renal failure. Calculation of the mannitol dose should include the 3 g of mannitol present in each vial of Dantrolene. Furosemide should be given to enhance diuresis and excretion of the sodium burden from sodium bicarbonate. Early hyperkalemia may be treated with glucose and insulin; late hypokalemia will require potassium administration as dictated by serum levels.

Seventy years ago, the mortality of MH approached 80%; however, with increased recognition and treatment of early MH reactions and improved prophylaxis in MH susceptible persons, recent mortality is less than 10%.[49] Mortality is correlated to the maximum temperature being less than 5% below 38.3°C and almost 90% over 42.8°C.[49]

Most patients require 24 to 48 hours intensive monitoring after onset of MH before they can be safely transferred out of the ICU setting. Patients with severe, refractory MH or with systemic complications may require prolonged ICU care. Criteria for discharge from the ICU include normal temperature, renal function, blood gases, muscle tone, and coagulation, stable cardiac rhythm, and improving mental state.

Post-ICU Phase

Generally, patients who have had rapid resolution of MH following appropriate therapy will have normal recovery and will not require prolonged hospitalization. It is imperative that these patients and their families be counseled about the nature of MH. They should be informed about the risk factors for MH reactions and anesthetics to be avoided. Patients should be issued an information card about MH and wear a medic-alert bracelet. Patients who have had extensive skeletal muscle necrosis will usually require extensive rehabilitative therapy, which is best carried out in a specialized rehabilitation setting. Other organ system residua, particularly renal impairment, may be present and should be managed in the conventional way.

Neuroleptic Malignant Syndrome

The neuroleptic malignant syndrome (NMS) is a triad of fever, extrapyramidal signs (movement disorder, muscle rigidity), and change in mentation that occurs in the context of treatment with neuroleptic medications. The incidence of this disorder approaches 1% in patients treated with neuroleptic agents (haloperidol, chlorpromazine, trifluoperazine, etc.).[58]

Pre-ICU Phase

Although it most commonly affects young, schizophrenic males who take high potency neuroleptic agents, the disorder has occurred in patients of all ages and both sexes after any duration exposure to virtually any dose of any medication in this class for any therapeutic indication.[59] Precipitating factors may often be identified, and include systemic illness, exertion, dehydration, and organic brain damage. Psychomotor agitation, rapid neuroleptization, and use of parenteral neuroleptics may also increase risk.[53] Physical exercise in heat has also been identified as a risk factor.[60] Most patients are taking other psychotropic agents, including lithium, tricyclic antidepressants, and benzodiazepines;[53] concomitant anticholinergic or other antiparkinsonian drug administration occurs with considerable frequency.

The pathogenesis of NMS is believed to be blockade of central hypothalamic thermoreceptors with loss of normal thermoregulatory control coupled with blockade of extrapyramidal dopamine receptors producing muscle rigidity with increased metabolic heat production and dysfunction of the reticular activating system with decreased level of consciousness.

Clinical Features. Onset of the syndrome relative to initiation of neuroleptic therapy is within 7 days in 67% and 30 days in 96% of patients.[58] The earliest signs may be extrapyramidal and include muscle hypertonicity, parkinsonism (tremor, rigidity, akinesia), chorea, or dystonia. Fever may be present concomitant with, shortly before or after extrapyramidal signs. The core temperature may exceed 41°C. The patient, unless dehydrated, sweats profusely. Other autonomic disturbances are prominent, notable among them tachycardia, labile blood pressure, skin pallor, tachypnea, and urinary incontinence. Rarely, autonomic disturbances may precede other manifestations. Mental status abnormalities range from agitation to sedation, stupor, obtundation, and coma. Other neurologic abnormalities are common, and include mutism, dysphagia, ataxia, involuntary posturing and changes in deep tendon reflexes.[61] Gastrointestinal motility is markedly decreased; ileus is common. While the initial symptoms may be insidious, the entire syndrome often develops over 24 to 72 hours. Biochemical abnormalities are frequent; most are nonspecific. Elevation of creatine phosphokinase is universal, and may be to levels exceeding 15,000.[61] Sixty-seven percent of patients have myoglobinuria.[57] Myoglobinuria and dehydration secondary to insensible losses predispose to acute oliguric renal failure and are seen in 30% of patients in some series.[62] Hepatic enzymes are elevated into the twice normal range.[62] Leukocytosis and thrombocytosis are common. Fifty percent of patients have hypocalcemia. Serum iron is frequently reduced, and has been suggested to be a marker for NMS.[62]

Treatment. The catastrophic nature of NMS and its relative infrequency have precluded controlled clinical trials of therapeutic agents. Therapy is largely empiric and is drawn from experience with treatment of dopamine deficiency syndromes as well as from treatment strategies used in malignant hyperthermia. The former approach addresses central dopamine blockade and uses dopaminergic drugs of three types: (1) indirect dopamine agonists (amantadine); (2) dopamine precursor (levodopa); and (3) direct-acting dopamine agonists (bromocriptine). The latter concerns using dantrolene to reduce the role of muscle metabolic heat production in temperature elevation.

Health care workers must maintain a vigilant attitude when treating patients with any medication that blocks dopamine receptors. Patients who are particularly at risk for developing NMS, and thus should be scrupulously followed, are agitated patients who are being treated with rapidly escalating doses of high potency parenteral neuroleptics. The routine use of prophylactic anticholinergic agents to prevent extrapyramidal symptoms in these patients may interfere with thermoregulatory sweating and is to be discouraged. Such patients should be closely monitored for signs of rigidity, fever, or autonomic instability. The development of any extrapyramidal sign or change in mental alertness or responsivity should prompt reevaluation and possible discontinuation of the offending medication. Parkinsonism which develops at this time should be cautiously treated with anticholinergic medications, or preferably amantadine. Dystonias should be carefully treated with anticholinergic medications. At the first sign of fever or autonomic dysfunction, the neuroleptic agent and any anticholinergic medications should be discontinued. Dehydration should be corrected if present, and underlying systemic illness should be sought. Vital signs should be monitored closely. Should temperature escalation be noted, outpatients should be hospitalized.

IV access should be established, and blood should be obtained for WBC count, electrolytes, muscle enzymes (LDH, CPK, aldolase), thyroid functions, culture, and ABGs. A chest radiograph and urinalysis should be obtained; cerebrospinal fluid should be sent for cell counts and culture.

External cooling with skin wetting and fan ventilation or cooling blankets should be started. Skin massage counteracts vasoconstriction. Vital signs should be monitored closely, and any deterioration, particularly autonomic dysfunction or continued fever escalation should prompt admission to the ICU.

ICU Phase

More than 30% of patients with NMS require intensive care. Most require assisted ventilation because of aspiration pneumonitis, noncardiogenic pulmonary edema, pulmonary embolism, decreased chest wall compliance or necrosis of respiratory muscles.[53,58] Cardiac rhythm, blood pressure, and respiratory and renal function should be monitored continuously. Arterial line and Swan-Ganz catheter placement are invaluable in monitoring. External cooling measures should be continued. When cooling measures are ineffective, they should be supplemented with invasive cooling with iced peritoneal lavage or CPB.

Although there are no controlled trials of medications in NMS, empiric dopaminergic treatment has been associated with favorable outcome.[63] For mild hyperthermia and extrapyramidal symptoms alone, amantadine, 200 mg daily in two divided doses, should suffice. For more pronounced hyperthermia or when hyperthermia is accompanied by moderate extrapyramidal signs or changes in mental status, levodopa, 200 mg, and carbidopa, 50 mg (2 Sinemet 25/100 tablets), should be administered tid. Alternatively, bromocriptine should be given, 45 mg daily in three divided doses. Both levodopa and bromocriptine may exacerbate psychosis; bromocriptine may exacerbate hypotension. Dopaminergic therapy should be closely monitored. The development of ileus prevents use of dopaminergic medications, because no parenteral preparations are available. Anecdotal reports suggest that dantrolene sodium, in doses similar to those outlined previously are beneficial in NMS.[63] Dantrolene is expensive, and dantrolene therapy is associated with generalized weakness with prolongation of ventilator dependence; IV dantrolene is injurious to veins. Dantrolene therapy should be reserved for patients who have prolonged or increasing therapy despite cooling measures and dopaminergic therapy, or in whom enteral dopaminergic therapy is prevented by ileus.

Fluid replacement and osmotic diuresis should be directed toward preventing acute renal failure. Oliguric renal failure should be managed in a conventional manner.

The duration of thermoregulatory instability in NMS averages 10 days; however, when NMS is secondary to parenteral neuroleptic medications, recovery may take as long as 30 days. Once temperature and autonomic functions appear normal, dopaminergic medications and dantrolene should be withdrawn and the patient monitored for relapse. Once the patient has been monitored for 48 hours, and has no relapse of hyperthermia or autonomic failure, he or she may be discharged from the ICU.

Although reported mortality is as high as 20%, more recent series report acute mortality at 10% or less.[62]

Post-ICU Phase

More than half the survivors of NMS have minor abnormalities of vital signs, muscle enzymes, or extrapyramidal function. They may have permanent neurologic sequelae including changes in mentation and memory, and ataxia. Physical therapy or rehabilitation may be necessary for those with prolonged or severe illness.

Should continued psychiatric therapy be indicated, the psychiatrist should explore options for non-neuroleptic therapy. When there is no alternative to neuroleptic therapy, a lower potency neuroleptic such as thioridazine should be used when possible. Patients who are restarted on neuroleptics may have recurrent NMS, and should be carefully monitored for early changes in muscle tone, temperature, and autonomic function. Most patients (87% in 1 series) who require neuroleptic agents are able to tolerate them when these drugs are reintroduced.

In conclusion, catastrophic thermoregulatory disorders are rare, but explosive in onset and dramatic in appearance. Delayed treatment results in high mortality and morbidity, but prompt specific therapy with physical and pharmacologic means accompanied by aggressive surveillance for and treatment of medical complications leads to acceptably low mortality. Thermoregulatory disturbances are often recurrent; continuity of care following discharge to medical wards and into the community may prevent repetition of these life-threatening disorders.

REFERENCES

1. Carbanac, M., and Brinnel, H.: The pathology of human temperature regulation. Thermiatrics. Experientia, 43:27, 1987.
2. Ivy, A. D.: What is normal or normality? Q. Bull. Northwestern Univ. Med. School, 18:22, 1944.
3. Elder, P. T.: Accidental hypothermia, In Textbook of Critical Care. Edited by W. C. Shoemaker et al. Philadelphia, W. B. Saunders, 1989.
4. Holdcroft, A.: Body Temperature Control in Anesthesia, Surgery and Intensive Care. London, Bailliere Tindall, 1980.
5. Cork, R. C., Vaughan, R. W., and Humphrey, L. S.: Precision and accuracy of intraoperative temperature monitoring. Anesth. Analg., 62:211, 1983.
6. Davis, F. M., Barnes, P. K., and Bailey, J. S.: Aural thermometry during profound hypothermia. Anesth. Intensive Care, 9:124, 1981.
7. Carlson, L. D., and Hsieh, A. C.: Temperature and humidity. Part A: Cold. In Environmental Physiology. Edited by N. B. Slonim. St. Louis, C. V. Mosby, 1974.
8. Cunningham, S., et al.: The characterization and energetic potential of brown adipose tissue in man. Clin. Sci., 69:343, 1985.
9. Johnson, R. H., and Park, D. M.: Intermittent hypothermia. J. Neurol. Neurosurg. Psychiatry, 36:411, 1973.
10. Knochel, J. P.: Heat stroke and related heat stress disorders. Dis. Mono., 35:301, 1989.
11. Galvao, P. E.: Human heat production in relation to body weight and body surface. J. Appl. Physiol., 3:21, 1950.
12. Robinson, S., and Wiegman, D. L.: Heat and humidity. In Environmental Physiology. Edited by N. B. Slonim. St. Louis, C. V. Mosby, 1974.
13. Lomax, P.: Neuropharmacological aspects of thermoregulation. In The Nature and Treatment of Hypothermia. Edited by R. S. Pozos, and L. E. Wittmers. Minneapolis, University of Minnesota Press, 1981.
14. Lewin, S., Brittman, L. R., and Holzman, R. S.: Infection in hypothermic patients. Arch. Intern. Med., 141:920, 1981.
15. Morris, D. L., Chambers, H. F., Morris, M. G., and Sande, M. A.: Hemodynamic characteristics of patients with hypothermia due to occult infection and other causes. Ann. Intern. Med., 102:153, 1985.
16. Lybarger, J. A., and Kilbourne, E. M.: Hyperthermia and hypothermia in the elderly: an epidemiologic review. In Homeostatic Function in Aging. Edited by B. B. Davis, and W. G. Wood. New York, Raven Press, 1985.
17. Fox, R. H., MacGibbon, R., Davies, L., and Woodward, P. M.: Problem of the old and the cold. Br. Med. J., 1:21, 1973.
18. Eddy, T. P., Payne, P. R., Salvosac, C., and Wheeler, E. F.: Body temperatures in the elderly. Lancet, 2:1088, 1970.
19. Collins, K. J., et al.: Accidental hypothermia and impaired temperature homeostasis in the elderly. Br. Med. J., 1:353, 1977.
20. Horvath, S. M., Radcliffe, C. E., Hatt, P. K., and Spurr, G. B.: Metabolic responses of old people to a cold environment. J. Appl. Physiol., 8:145, 1955.
21. Johnson, R. H., and Spalding, J. M. K. (Eds.): Disorders of the Autonomic Nervous System. Oxford, Blackwell Scientific, 1974.
22. Woodhouse, P., Keating, W. R., and Coleshaw, S. R. K.: Factors associated with hypothermia in patients admitted to a group of inner city hospitals. Lancet, 2:1201, 1989.
23. Edlich, R. F., et al.: Cold injuries. Compr. Ther., 15:13, 1989.
24. Rosenfeld, J. B.: Acid-base and electrolyte disturbances in hypothermia. Am. J. Cardiol., 12:678, 1963.
25. Maclean, D., Murison, J., and Griffiths, P. D.: Acute pancreatitis in diabetic ketoacidosis, accidental hypothermia and hypothermic myxoedema. Br. Med. J., 4:757, 1973.
26. Vandam, L. D., and Burnap, T. K.: Hypothermia. N. Engl. J. Med., 261:546, 1959.
27. Osborn, J. J.: Experimental hypothermia: respiratory and blood Ph changes in relationship to cardiac function. Am. J. Physiol., 75:389, 1953.
28. Mouritzen, C. V., and Anderson, M. N.: Myocardial temperature gradients and ventricular fibrillation during hypothermia. J. Thorac. Cardiovasc. Surg., 49:937, 1965.
29. Martyn, J. W.: Diagnosing and treating hypothermia. Can. Med. Assoc. J., 125:1089, 1981.
30. Plum, F., and Posner, J. B.: The Diagnosis of Stupor and Coma. 3rd Ed. Philadelphia, F. A. Davis Company, 1980.
31. Schaller, M., Fischer, A. P., and Perret, C. H.: Hyperkalemia: a prognostic factor during acute severe hypothermia. JAMA, 264:1842, 1990.
32. Miller, J. W., Danzl, D. F., and Thomas, D. M.: Urban accidental hypothermia 135 cases. Ann. Emerg. Med., 9:456, 1980.
33. Bangs, C. C.: Hypothermia and frostbite. Emerg. Med. Clin. North Am., 2:475, 1984.

34. Danzl, D. F., et al. Hypothermia outcome score: development and implications. Crit. Care Med., *17:*227, 1989.
35. Shibolet, S., et al.: Heat stroke: its clinical picture and mechanism in 36 cases. Q. J. Med., *36:*525, 1967.
36. Al-D'bbag, M., Khogali, M., and Ghallab, M.: Clinical picture and management of heat exhaustion. *In* Heat Stroke and Temperature Regulation. Edited by M. Khogali, and J. R. S. Hales. Sydney, Academic Press, 1983.
37. Clowes, G. H. A., and O'Donnell, T. F.: Heat Stroke. N. Engl. J. Med., *291:*564, 1974.
38. Hart, G. R., et al.: Epidemic classical heat stroke: clinical characteristics and course of 28 patients. Medicine (Baltimore), *61:*189, 1982.
39. Robbins, A. S.: Hypothermia and heat stroke: protecting the elderly patient. Geriatrics, *44:*73, 1989.
40. Khogali, M., and Mustafa, M. K. Y.: Physiology of Heat Stroke: A review. *In* Heat Stroke and Temperature Regulation. Edited by M. Khogali, and J. R. S. Hales. Sydney, Academic Press, 1983.
41. Bark, N.: Heat stroke in psychiatric patients. Two cases and a review. J. Clin. Psychiatry, *43:*377, 1982.
42. O'Donnell, T. F., Jr., and Clowes, G. H. A., Jr.: The circulatory abnormalities of heat stroke. N. Engl. J. Med., *287:*734, 1972.
43. Al-Khawashki, M. I., Mustafa, M. K. Y., Khogali, M., and El-Sayed, H.: Clinical presentation of 172 heat stroke cases seen at Mina and Arafat—September, 1982. *In* Heat Stroke and Temperature Regulation. Edited by M. Khogali, and J. R. S. Hales. Sydney, Academic Press, 1983.
44. Wright, D. O., Reppert, L. B., and Cuttino, J. T.: Purpuric manifestation of heat stroke. Arch. Intern. Med., *77:*27, 1946.
45. DeLorenzo, R. J.: Status epilepticus. *In* Current Therapy in Neurosurgical Disease, 3. Edited by R. R. Johnson. Philadelphia, B. C., Decker, 1990.
46. Amundson, D. E.: The spectrum of heat related injury with compartment syndrome. Mil. Med., *154:*450, 1989.
47. Moore, R. D., and Friedman, R. J.: Current concepts in pathophysiology and diagnosis of compartment syndromes. J. Emerg. Med., *7:*657, 1989.
48. Denborough, M. A., and Lovell, R. R. H.: Anaesthetic deaths in a family. Lancet, *2:*45, 1960.
49. Britt, B. A.: Malignant hyperthermia. *In* Complications in Anesthesiology. Edited by F. K. Orkin and L. H. Cooperman. Philadelphia, J. B. Lippincott, 1983.
50. Wingard, D. W.: A stressful situation. Anesth. Analg., *59:*321, 1980.
51. Muldoon, S. M., Boggs, S. D., and Freas, W.: Malignant hyperthermia. *In* Textbook of Critical Care. Edited by W. C. Shoemaker et al. Philadelphia, W. B. Saunders, 1989.
52. Ward, A., Chaffman, M. O., and Sorkin, E. M.: Dantrolene: a review of its pharmacodynamic and pharmacokinetic properties and therapeutic use in malignant hyperthermia, the neuroleptic malignant syndrome and an update of its use in muscle spasticity. Drugs, *32:*130, 1986.
53. Lazarus, A., Mann, S. C., and Caroff, S. N. (eds.): The Neuroleptic Malignant Syndrome and Related Conditions. Washington, D.C., American Psychiatric Press, 1989.
54. Gronert, G. A.: Malignant hyperthermia. Anesthesiology, *53:*395, 1980.
55. Tomarken, H. L., and Britt, B. A.: Malignant hyperthermia. Ann. Emerg. Med., *16:*1253, 1987.
56. Allen, G. C., and Rosenberg, H.: Malignant hyperthermia susceptibility in adult patients with masseter muscle rigidity. Can. J. Anaesth., *37:*31, 1990.
57. Kolb, M. E., Horne, M. L., and Martz, R.: Dantrolene in human malignant hyperthermia: a multicenter study. Anesthesiology, *56:*254, 1982.
58. Caroff, S. N.: The neuroleptic malignant syndrome. J. Clin. Psychiatry, *41:*79, 1980.
59. Kurlan, R., Hamill, R., and Shoulson, I.: Review: neuroleptic malignant syndrome. Clin. Neuropharmacol., *7:*109, 1984.
60. Shalev, A., Hermesh, H., and Munitz, H.: The role of external heat load in triggering the neuroleptic malignant syndrome. Am. J. Psychiatry, *145:*110, 1988.
61. Guze, B. H., and Baxter, L. R.: Neuroleptic malignant syndrome. N. Engl. J. Med., *313:*163, 1985.
62. Rosebush, P., and Stewart, T.: A prospective analysis of 24 episodes of neuroleptic malignant syndrome. Am. J. Psychiatry, *146:*717, 1989.
63. Granato, J. E., et al.: Neuroleptic malignant syndrome: successful treatment with dantrolene and bromocriptine. Ann. Neurol. *14:*89, 1983.

s
Chapter 4

INTENSIVE CARE MANAGEMENT OF INTRACRANIAL HYPERTENSION

GENE H. BARNETT

The principles that direct the management of raised intracranial pressure (ICP) are largely independent of the cause of increased ICP. This chapter focuses on the general approach for managing the patient with intracranial hypertension before, during and after intensive care unit (ICU) admission. Disease specific considerations are addressed in the chapters on non-ischemic brain injury.

PATHOPHYSIOLOGY OF RAISED ICP

The craniospinal cavity comprises a nearly rigid compartment bounded by the dura mater and is composed of the brain and spinal cord, cerebrospinal fluid (CSF), and blood. This modified **Monro-Kellie** doctrine forms the basis for both understanding the pathophysiology of raised ICP and its management. Normal ICP (<10 mm Hg) is maintained by the rates of CSF production and drainage as well as cerebral blood volume. The majority of CSF is produced within the ventricles by the choroid plexus. Fluid flows from the lateral ventricle to the third ventricle, then fourth ventricle through the foramina of Luschka and Magendie. It then passes over and under the brain in the subarachnoid space where it is absorbed largely by the arachnoid villi. Introduction of a "mass lesion" (either a true mass such as a blood clot or abscess, or expansion of the brain or fluid compartments such as from edema or hydrocephalus, respectively) results in a rise in ICP. Initially, an incremental increase in volume of the "mass" is accommodated by displacement of intravascular blood and CSF into the systemic circulation (Fig. 4-1), resulting in only small changes in ICP. Thereafter, an exponential rise in ICP occurs with the volume of the mass being accommodated by displacement and compression of neural tissue. As volume of the mass lesion increases, a situation of "high compliance" becomes one of "low compliance" where very small incremental changes in volume lead to large changes in ICP. (A slowly introduced mass is better accommodated and explains why some tumors that grow over many years but that have considerable volume may exist in the presence of normal ICP.) The pressure-volume curve can also be expressed in a linear fashion by the pressure-volume index (PVI) where PVI = dV/log Po/dP (Po = initial ICP, dV = changes in volume, dP = changes in pressure). A PVI of less than 15 ml is indicative of low compliance. Management of high ICP focuses on reducing the volume of the intracranial contents and therefore ICP or, more accurately, creating a more favorable pressure-volume curve (Fig. 4-2).

ICP itself is important for three reasons. First, ICP, when elevated, can set an **upper limit on cerebral blood flow** (CBF) as shown by the following equation:

$$CBF = (IMAP - ICP)/CVR$$

where:

CBF = Cerebral blood flow
IMAP = Intracranial mean arterial pressure
ICP = Intracranial pressure
CVR = Cerebrovascular resistance

As ICP (or dural sinus pressure) approaches the mean intracranial arterial pressure, blood flow decreases and eventually ceases when these two pressures become equal. A pressure difference of 45 to 50 mm Hg is generally regarded as the minimum allowable before cerebral ischemia may ensue. Preventing fatal global cerebral ischemia is a focus of therapy.

Second, changes in ICP may reflect expansion of a mass lesion even before "elevated levels" (typically > 15 to 20 mm Hg) have occurred. This is particularly important when the mass is in a small compartment of the cranial vault such as the temporal fossa. Here, an expanding temporal lobe lesion may lead to clinical brain herniation before compliance of the entire cranial vault becomes compromised and ICP becomes high. A gradual upward trend in ICP within the "normal range" usually heralds this clinical decompensation.

Lastly, ICP needs to be considered within the context of **pressure gradients** within the neuraxis. The consistency of the brain is such that in the presence of a pressure gradient the brain moves by the principle of bulk flow. Mass lesions generate local pressure elevations which generate local distortions in brain shape, size, and place. Flow ceases when pressures become equilibrated. When CSF moves freely throughout the craniospinal cavity, the opportunities for large pressure gradients to occur are minimized. Blockage of one or more CSF pathway may result in large gradients which is potentially fatal. Supratentorial brain swelling that blocks the subarachnoid space at the base of the brain can result in fatal rostro-caudal herniation after opposing spinal CSF pressure is released by lumbar puncture.

SIGNS OF RAISED ICP

Until elevated ICP causes global cerebral ischemia and alterations in the level of consciousness, ICP itself is rela-

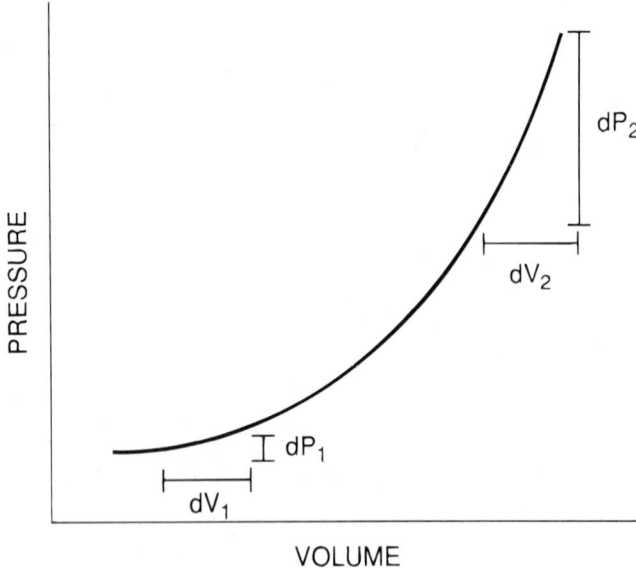

Fig. 4-1. Plot of intracranial pressure as a volume is introduced into the intracranial space. An incremental change in volume initially results in only small changes in pressure (dP₁).

tively silent. Loss of spontaneous venous pulsations or the presence of papilledema on funduscopic exam may be helpful, but the former is not always reliable and papilledema takes days to develop and may be mimicked by optic neuritis. **Systemic hypertension** is an ominous sign after brain injury with the exception of elevated blood pressure in the setting of focal cerebral ischemia where the response is a physiologic attempt to maintain CBF in a regionally deficient area. The so-called "Cushing response" (systolic hypertension, widened pulse pressure, bradycardia) is an unreliable sign of elevated ICP as bradycardia occurs no more frequently than tachycardia. Most of the other signs associated with high ICP are due to the direct effects of a mass lesion rather than ICP itself. The more common signs of raised ICP are:

- Changes in level of consciousness
- Altered respirations
- Oculomotor nerve palsy
- Abducens nerve palsy

Change in level of consciousness occurs as a result of bilateral dysfunction of the reticular activating system. A unilateral lesion of the cerebral hemisphere may cause sufficient shift of midline structures so as to impair function bilaterally and impair consciousness. Bilateral supratentorial masses, global cerebral ischemia, and brain stem lesions are among other causes.

Altered respirations often accompany such changes in consciousness. Normal respiration may deteriorate to Cheyne-Stokes, hyperventilation, irregular apneustic, and finally, agonal patterns. The reader is referred to the monograph by Plum and Posner[1] for a thorough discussion of mass lesions, altered consciousness, and associated clinical signs.

Pupillary dilatation with or without loss of ipsilateral ocular adduction is evidence of an **oculomotor nerve palsy.** Direct compression from mesial temporal lobe herniation (uncal herniation) and stretch from midbrain torsion are potential causes. This finding is classically associated with a mass lesion affecting the ipsilateral cerebral hemisphere and is considered the most accurate clinical sign for identifying the laterality of an acute intracranial mass. There are myriad other causes of oculomotor nerve palsies. A progressive syndrome characterized by a change in consciousness with hemiparesis (ipsilateral, contralateral, or bilateral) in the presence of a third nerve palsy is most suggestive of an underlying expansile mass lesion.

Unilateral or bilateral **abducens nerve palsy** (cranial nerve VI) is thought to result from stretch of these nerves because of rostro-caudal movement of the brain and brain stem. This is commonly referred to as a "false localizing sign" because the location of the lesion producing this palsy may be far removed (even contralateral) to the affected nerve.

PRE-ICU PHASE

Initial management of a patient with suspected intracranial hypertension requires the physician or emergency medical team to perform several tasks which, when the patient is seriously ill, may need to be done concurrently. Foremost among these are:

- Patient stabilization
- Institution of ICP therapy
- Neurologic and systemic assessment
- Triage

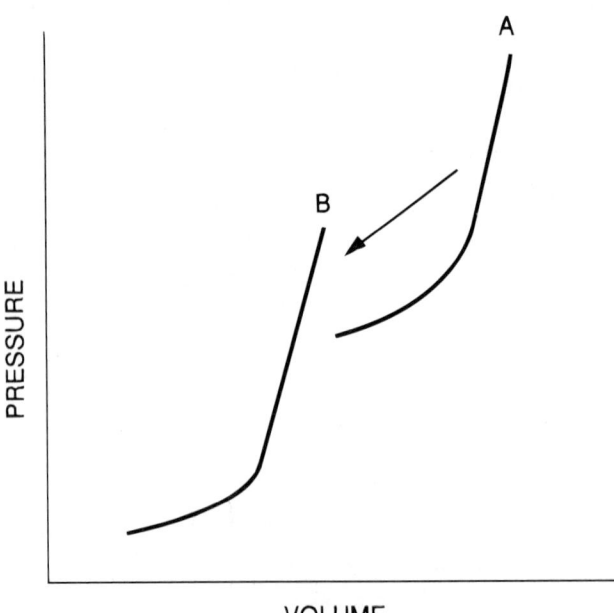

Fig. 4-2. Effect of some therapies for intracranial pressure is not to move down the pressure volume curve (A), but rather to generate a more favorable pressure volume curve (B).

Patient Stabilization

Patient assessment and stabilization should begin at the site of the accident or attack and continue in the emergency room. Traditional "field" measures include intravenous (IV) access and fluid administration, airway management, respiratory support and, in trauma, spinal immobilization.[2,3] Recent studies have supported the benefit of early aggressive actions such as intubation and administration of hyperosmolar agents by properly trained emergency medical technicians or paramedics. Pulse oximetry is likely also to become an important tool in the field to establish adequacy of oxygenation.[4] Air evacuation services providing rapid transport to specialized trauma centers are credited with reducing mortality and morbidity although results are less clear in urban settings.[5,6]

Emergency room measures focus on ventilation, normalization of systemic blood pressure, and reduction of elevated ICP. Protracted or even transient brain ischemia and/or hypoxia due to hypotension or respiratory failure occurring up to one week after the initial insult may substantially worsen neurologic outcome. The neurologic assessment should be repeated after sustained oxygen saturations of greater than 90% and systolic pressures of at least 90 mm Hg are attained.

Airway and Ventilation

Impaired consciousness from brain injury may cause airway obstruction, aspiration, and altered ventilatory patterns. Despite improvements in management in recent years, some studies suggest that airway protection and management is inadequate in up to 42% of patients undergoing transfer to a brain injury unit.[7,8] In cases of trauma, thoracic injuries such as hemo/pneumothorax, flail chest, and pulmonary contusions may also compromise pulmonary function in this setting and are associated with a poor outcome.[9]

Oral or nasal devices may be used to establish an airway. Oral airways are difficult to place in agitated patients and may induce gagging or vomiting. Nasal airways are usually better tolerated but they (and nasogastric tubes) should be used with caution after facial trauma unless basal skull fracture has been excluded. Patients with impending respiratory failure or obstruction, suspected intracranial hypertension (IH), or those requiring sedation or paralysis should be intubated. Specific considerations in patients with traumatic head injury are presented in Chapter 5.

If intracranial hypertension is suspected, pretreatment with IV 20% mannitol 0.5 to 1.0 g/kg, mask hyperventilation (except in the presence of an anterior skull fracture), and a short-acting barbiturate (e.g., methohexital) or nondepolarizing neuromuscular blocker (e.g., vecuronium) should be considered in an effort to avoid high ICP and possible brain herniation during the act of intubation.

Normalization of Systemic Blood Pressure

Hypotension is almost never due to raised ICP or other central nervous system injury unless: (1) there is a physiologic transection of the cervical or high thoracic spinal cord resulting in spinal shock, or (2) the patient has suffered massive lower brain stem damage such as with tonsilar herniation. Treatable causes of hypotension such as hypovolemia or myocardial infarction should be assessed.

Resuscitative measures in the setting of hypotension center on fluid administration. In patients with suspected intracranial injuries, hypotonic fluids are avoided so as to minimize the potentiation of brain swelling. Suitable solutions include 0.9% NaCl or lactate of Ringer's (with or without dextrose), 5% albumin, 25% albumin, high molecular weight dextran, plasma, or blood. Isotonic colloid solutions seem to have little advantage over isotonic crystalloids. Hyperosmolar agents such as hypertonic saline solutions may be superior to isotonic fluids at least in early resuscitation because they tend to lower ICP while repleting intravascular volume.[10,11] Clearly, blood and blood products should be considered in the presence of anemia or clotting factor deficiency. Pressor, inotropic, and chronotropic agents should not be used in lieu of appropriate fluid resuscitation but may be used in accordance with the general principles of shock management. A minimum systolic blood pressure of 90 mm Hg should be sought.

As noted earlier, systemic hypertension after brain injury is an ominous sign and may well indicate elevated ICP or brain stem compression. Efforts to reduce systemic hypertension may compromise cerebral perfusion pressure; however, spontaneous systolic pressures of greater than 200 mm Hg should be reduced as it may limit edema generation from hydrostatic pressure.

Neurologic Assessment

The aim of the history and neurologic examination is to assess the nature of brain injury and the likelihood and extent of elevated ICP (see Chap. 5). Radiologic studies may also provide important information on ICP after brain injury.

Radiographic Examination

Contemporary use of skull **x-ray studies** in the evaluation of ICP is limited even though they may provide evidence of a mass lesion by demonstrating midline shift of a calcified pineal gland or chronic ICP elevation (e.g., eroded sella, copper beaten inner table). Issues pertaining to radiographs and computerized neuroimaging (CT and MRI) after traumatic brain injury are presented in Chapter 71.

Computerized tomography (CT) has largely supplanted the use of radiographs in the evaluation of an intracranial disorder. Recent studies suggest that CT imaging may be a better indicator of impending clinical deterioration than the neurologic examination in certain instances. CT evidence of hemispheric swelling and obliteration of the basal subarachnoid cisterns suggest high ICP and are particularly ominous findings.[13,14,15] CT findings correlated with raised ICP are shown in Table 4-1. The significance of lateral midline shift in coma as being prognostic of reversibility is controversial.[14,16]

Magnetic resonance imaging (MRI) has opened up new dimensions in the diagnosis and prognostication of brain injury. MRI appears to be far more sensitive in demonstrating nonhemorrhagic, brain stem, or extra-axial le-

Table 4-1. CT Features Suggesting Raised ICP

Obliteration of basal CSF cisterns
Size of subdural hematoma*
Ventricular size
Presence of subarachnoid hemorrhage*
Severity of contusion*
Degree of midline shift
Ventricular index

* Applies in cases of head trauma.

sions than CT and may show some intraparenchymal contusions and tissue derangements that CT never shows.[17,18] CT and MRI are equally sensitive detectors of intraparenchymal hemorrhagic lesions but CT surpasses MRI for demonstration of subarachnoid hemorrhage. Although techniques of monitoring and supporting critically ill patients have been recently defined, the logistical considerations usually preclude MRI in the setting of severe head injury or multiple internal injuries.[19] MRI has proven very sensitive and reasonably practical in the evaluation of spinal injuries.

Cerebral angiography has been largely replaced by the aforementioned imaging techniques and adaptations such as magnetic resonance angiography. Specific uses of angiography are discussed in Chapter 5.

Triage

Patients with suspected acute high ICP require hospital admission and, depending on the underlying process, may require surgery and/or ICU care. Specific guidelines for various types of brain injury are presented in Chapter 5.

Institution of ICP Therapy

Suspected or documented intracranial mass lesions or high ICP elevations demand temporizing measures until the nature and severity of the intracranial disorder can be assessed and more definitively instituted. One protocol for emergency treatment of raised ICP in head injury is shown in Table 4-2. Steroids should be reserved for disorders known to have vasogenic brain edema or proven to be steroid responsive (e.g., tumor, abscess, intracerebral hemorrhage). Opiate antagonists, free radical scavengers, and a host of other agents have also proven ineffective. Despite many human clinical studies that found no benefit for the use of steroids after head injury, some recent animal studies suggest that very high doses of methylprednisolone analogues may enhance early recovery.[12]

Table 4-2. Emergency Management of Raised ICP

20 mg Furosemide IV push
20% Mannitol 1 g/kg IV
Lidocaine 2 mg/kg IV prior to intubation
Intubation with hyperventilation to Pco$_2$ no less than 25 mm Hg
Dexamethasone 20 mg IV push (if steroid-responsive etiology)
Neuroimaging to establish cause of deterioration
Ventricular drainage if hydrocephalus suspected/known

Criteria for ICP Monitoring

ICP monitoring is instituted in our unit in acutely brain injured patients with:

- CT evidence of focal or global brain edema or mass
- GCS < 10 or progressive decline in level of consciousness*
- Postcraniotomy for evacuation of intracranial clot
- Pharmacologic paralysis or heavy sedation required for control of agitation, etc.

The aim of these guidelines is to provide information that may warn us of an expanding mass lesion or global cerebral ischemia in the setting where the clinical examination may not be a reliable indicator.

ICU ISSUES

Evaluation and Treatment of Raised ICP

Role of ICP Monitoring

The role of ICP monitoring and therapy in many neurologic disorders remains controversial.[20,21,22] There is support for both empiric treatment of suspected raised ICP as well as therapy titrated to measured ICPs; studies claiming to support empiric therapy, however, have failed to match appropriate control populations. Most neurosurgical and neurologic ICUs in this country use ICP monitoring in selected brain injured patients because:

- It provides a rational basis of therapy.
- It has long-term prognostic value.
- An upward trend may indicate expansion of a mass lesion before clinical signs appear.

In addition, early detection and correction of large elevations (i.e., > 40 mm Hg) may prevent global cerebral ischemia and death.

When ICP trends are monitored over hours or days, episodic elevations known as **pressure waves** may be found.[23] Originally described by Lundberg, the only wave of prognostic significance was the "plateau wave" where ICP would rise from mildly elevated levels to values of 60 mm Hg or more for several minutes and then return to baseline (Fig. 4-3). Originally believed to be a sign of dysautoregulation, these phenomena are now believed to result from a physiologic attempt to maintain ICP by increasing cerebral blood flow and, hence, cerebral blood volume and ICP.[24]

The factors that lead to raised ICP were discussed earlier in this chapter. Maximum benefit from ICP measurements requires the practitioner to also have a thorough understanding of techniques of monitoring and treatment.

When there is a disruption in the integrity of this normally nearly sealed system, a marked expansion of a mass may result in little or no change in ICP until late in the process of expansion. As such, ICP monitoring may produce spuriously low results in the setting of CSF leakage (either traumatic, idiopathic, or postsurgical), or when ICP

* Glasgow coma scale

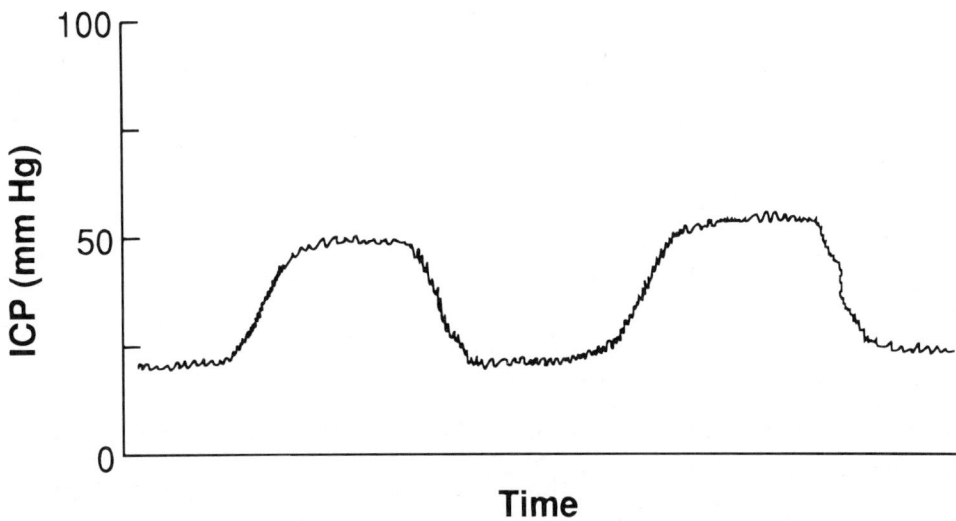

Fig. 4–3. Episodic sustained elevations of intracranial pressure (ICP) to more than 50 mm Hg are "plateau waves" and are a sign of decompensating intracranial hypertension.

is being monitored by a fluid coupled system (ventricular catheter or subarachnoid bolt) with a leak in the monitoring system. These scenarios are probably the most common reasons for failure of ICP monitoring to foretell brain herniation.

ICP Monitoring Techniques

The most commonly used techniques of ICP measurement are the ventricular catheter and subarachnoid screw (or bolt). Both of these systems use fluid columns to couple the CSF pressure to an external transducer. Fluid coupled systems require that they be "balanced" or "zeroed" to the atmosphere (because clinical ICP is really the difference between the absolute ICP and atmospheric pressure). This procedure is commonly performed with the transducer at midventricular level.

The **ventricular catheter** is commonly considered to be the gold standard of ICP recording. It is among the oldest techniques of directly measuring ICP. Most of the early work on the clinical significance of ICP is based on data derived from these devices, and the catheter may allow therapeutic drainage of CSF in the presence of high pressures.[25]

Placement requires moderate skill and is done using sterile technique. Frontal sites are more commonly selected than others. Typically a burr hole or twist drill hole is placed 1 to 2 cm anterior to the coronal suture and 3 cm lateral to the sagittal suture. A 5- to 6-cm length of catheter tubing is passed along a line perpendicular to the plane of the skull at the entry point. (A tripod-like guide has recently been introduced which is said to facilitate accurate placement of the catheter although we have not found this to be so.) The distal end of the tubing is tunneled subcutaneously several centimeters, using a trochar and attached to a drainage and transduction system. Risk of bacterial contamination of the system is minimized if the system is not manipulated and fluid is collected in a closed fashion.[26,27] We replace catheters every 5 days and monitor CSF for cell count, glucose, gram stain, and culture daily. A ventricular catheter allows ICP to be monitored while the patient is undergoing MRI.

The main disadvantages of ventricular drainage are that it is the most invasive method of ICP monitoring and, as such, carries the greatest risk of hemorrhage and infection. Also, obstruction of the catheter tip by blood, debris, or collapsed ventricles may lead to spurious readings.

The **subarachnoid bolt** is a less invasive method of measuring ICP than the ventricular catheter and its risk of hemorrhage and infection are also less. The bolt is widely used and relatively simple to place. Location is not critical, however, it is usually placed near the vertex so as not to become dislodged by head rotation. Some studies suggest that ICP may be higher on the side of an expanding mass lesion, therefore all systems other than ventricular catheters are placed on the side of the largest lesion.[28–30] After the skin is prepared and a small incision fashioned, a twist drill or burr hole is made. The dura and arachnoid are opened sharply, the bolt screwed in place, and tubing connected as with the ventricular catheter. New MR-compatible bolts are available, or a stopcock secured in a twist drill hole may serve as well. ICP recording can also be obtained using a Silastic catheter placed in the subdural space through a twist drill or burr hole.

Bolts are inexpensive, easily placed, and have a low risk of infection or hemorrhage. The main disadvantage of the subdural bolt or catheter is that they tend to fail when ICPs approach 22 to 25 mm Hg which is when accurate ICP monitoring is probably most important.[31] Failure is usually due to so-called microleaks that occur at connection sites. This situation results in brain or debris occluding the lumen of the bolt, dampening of the wave form, and spurious readings (usually too low). Continuous infusion of 0.1 ml per hour of nonbacteriostatic saline into the bolt may mitigate this problem. Because of the frequency of spuriously low ICPs, many institutions have abandoned using the subarachnoid bolt.

Nonfluid Coupled Systems

Several nonfluid filled systems that allow accurate recording of ICP have become popular in recent years. Potential problems with such systems include drift, inability to check the accuracy of the device once it is placed, high cost, and fragility. Modern nonfluid coupled ICP monitoring systems, however, have largely overcome these problems.

The Gaeltec ICP monitor may be used in either the subdural or epidural space. This monitor is one of the few nonfluid coupled devices allowing calibration and check of the balance in vivo. It uses a Wheatstone bridge in the transducer tip that directly measures the difference between the absolute ICP and atmospheric pressure. Wave form fidelity is very good and can be directly displayed on most physiologic monitors. Its disadvantages are, however, that it is a high cost device, pneumocephalus has been reported as a complication of its use, and fragility seriously limits the frequency of reuse.[32]

The Steritek ICP monitoring system is designed for epidural or subdural use. A counterbalance principle is employed; that is, an external pump generates and measures the pressure required to close a valve in the sensor. The status of the valve is transmitted to the external control box by means of a pneumatic cable. As the valve is kept open by a membrane exposed to the ICP, the external pump can accurately record ICP. Wave form analysis is not possible, and there are some theoretic concerns over the validity of ICP recordings from the epidural space.

The Camino ICP system uses fiberoptics to transmit reflected light from a mirror in the tip of the sensor. The amount of reflected light is related to the difference between absolute ICP and atmospheric pressure. Wave form fidelity is good and the device is reasonably priced and rugged.[33] It can be placed in the subdural space, directly in brain parenchyma to measure brain tissue pressures, or in a ventricle. Intraparenchymal placement using a bolt-like device is safe and rapid (Fig. 4–4). In our experience, drift is minimal, usually less than 1 to 2 mm Hg over a week or more (although we have had a few cases of a +6- and −6-mm Hg drift). The device should be replaced every 5 days or if drift is suspected. We routinely use the Camino system for ICP monitoring except when CSF drainage is required in which case we use a ventricular catheter.

Other monitoring techniques may provide some useful information regarding ICP. Visual and auditory evoked potentials, as well as transcranial Doppler monitoring may show characteristic abnormalities at ICPs of 30 to 40 mm Hg. At present, however, they are unable to reliably assess ICP elevations in the range of 15 to 20 mm Hg where therapeutic decisions are made. For now, these techniques should be viewed as useful adjuncts to invasive ICP monitoring.

Principles of Management

The focus of intracranial pressure management is to:

- Remove or halt the growth of the mass lesion
- Further reduce the volume of the blood compartment
- Reduce the volume of the CSF compartment
- Reduce the volume of the brain

Many brain disorders such as hemorrhage, infarction, and head injury result in the gradual development of intracranial hypertension over a period of 2 to 4 days. The focus of management in this setting is a gradual escalation in the intensity of treatment so as to maintain ICP at less than 15 or 20 mm Hg. Often, however, the specialist in intensive care is confronted with a patient who is in the midst of herniation and is having very high ICPs (>40 mm Hg) on presentation. This situation constitutes a true neurologic emergency and is addressed in the Pre-ICU section.

Gradual elevations of ICP should be treated so as to provide only that degree of medical management that is required to maintain ICP at below 15 to 20 mm Hg. More aggressive approaches may result in temporary reductions of ICP into the single digit range, but often at the price of systemic instability, secondary brain ischemia, or reduced therapeutic options if and when ICH recurs.

Our approach at the Cleveland Clinic Neurosurgical Intensive Care Unit is to manage the patient with raised ICP with three questions in mind:

- To what degree can or should this problem be treated surgically?
- What specific measures are required and appropriate for directly reducing the ICP?
- What measures are required to maintain systemic stability and to reduce the chance of secondary brain injury?

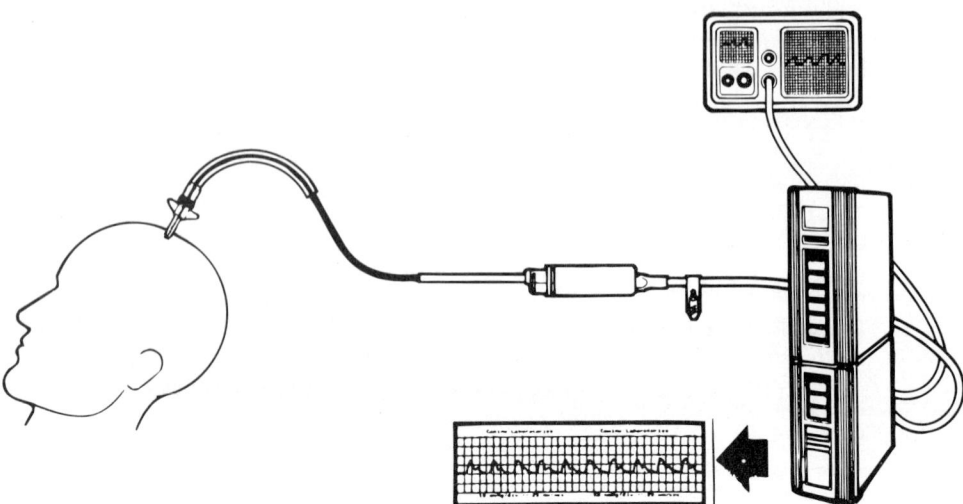

Fig. 4–4. Fiberoptic intracranial pressure bolt (Camino).

Table 4-3. Cleveland Clinic NICU Intracranial Hypertension Guidelines

I. Assess Need for Surgical Therapy
II. Medical Management
   A. **Basic Measures**
      1. Optimize head elevation (usually 30°–45°). Keep head in neutral rotation. Measure intracranial mean arterial pressure (IMAP) with transducer at head level. CPP = IMAP − ICP.
      2. Avoid overhydration/hypotonic fluids. Use 0.9% NaCl—modify to maintain serum Na < 160 mEq/L.
      3. Maintain Hematocrit 33–37%.
      4. Steroid treatment of vasogenic edema only (dexamethasone load 0.2–0.3 mg/kg, then 0.1–0.2 mg/kg). **Maintain normoglycemia.**
      5. Limit volume of intracranial CSF compartment.
         a. **Acetazolamide** (250–500 ml/mg. p.o. qid, then 125 mg IV qid).
         b. **Ventricular drainage.**
      6. Medullary suppressants and/or sedation. Consider paralysis.
         a. **Lidocaine** (0.7–1.5 mg/kg IV push).
         b. **Succinylcholine** (0.15–0.30 mg/kg IV push).
         c. **Methohexital** (1 mg/kg IV push).
         d. **Pentobarbital/phenobarbital** (0.5–1.0 mg/kg IV/IM tid). Agitation.
         e. **Benzodiazepines** lorazepam (0.007–0.03 mg/kg q 1–2 h prn). Agitation.
         f. **Morphine SO$_4$** (1–2 mg IV prn). Agitation due to pain.
         g. **Major tranquilizers** Haloperidol (1–2 mg IV q 1 h prn). Psychosis.
      7. Treat seizures aggressively.
         a. **Lorazepam** (0.035–0.07 mg/kg IV push).
         b. **Phenytoin** (Load 18 mg/kg, then 1.5 mg/kg q 8 h).
         c. **Phenobarbital** (Load 12–15 mg/kg, then 1 mg/kg tid).
      8. Maintain normothermia.
         a. Antipyretics: Acetaminophen/Aspirin (350 mg q 3–4 h prn) T. [core] > 38.5°C.
         b. Cooling blankets.
         c. Pharmacologic paralysis:
            i. **Pancuronium bromide** (Load 0.04–0.1 mg/kg, then 1–2 mg q 1–4 h).
            ii. **Vecuronium bromide** (0.08–0.1 mg/kg)
   B. **Aggressive Measures (Continue at least 24–48 hours after normal ICP, then taper off)**
      1. Hyperventilate to Paco$_2$ 15–27 torr (Acute effect).
      2. Diuretics
         a. **Mannitol** (0.25–1 g/kg) AVOID SYSTEMIC DEHYDRATION (bun > 20) and hypernatremia > 160 mEq/L.
         b. *Furosemide* (0.15–0.3 mg/kg) (Useful in absence of BBB).
         c. *25% Albumin* (0.25–1 g/kg) IN CONJUNCTION with furosemide.
      3. Maintain adequate MAP to maintain CPP > 45–50 torr.
         a. Volume Therapy
            i. **5% Albumin or 5% PPF** (0.5–1.0 g/kg) PAWP ≤ 10 or slow CVP and overall fluid balance even-near or negative.
            ii. **25% Albumin** (0.2–0.4 g/kg PCWP ≤ 10 or low CVP and overall fluid balance is positive.
            iii. **Dextran 40** (0.7 ml/kg, modified to maintain normovolemia by PCWP/CVP).
         b. Pressors to maintain CPP ≥ 45–55 torr:
            i. **Dopamine** (50–400 mg/100 ml).
            ii. **Phenylephrine** (5–20 mg/250 ml).
            iii. **Norepinephrine** (4–16 mg/250 ml).
      4. High dose barbiturates (uses only with PA line):
         a. **Pentobarbital** (Load 4–7 mg/kg, then 1–4 mg/kg^{-1}hr^{-1} to achieve and maintain EEG burst suppression [3 bursts/m]).
         b. **Thiopental** (Load 2–4 mg/kg, then 0.2–0.7 mg/kg^{-1}hr^{-1} to achieve and maintain EEG burst suppression [3 bursts/min]).
      5. Hypothermia: Paralyze and cool to 31°C. Requires use of PA catheter and ICP monitor.
III. Systemic Stabilization
   1. *Limit* systolic arterial pressure (SAP 100–130 torr while ensuring CCP of at least 45–55 torr).
      a. Beta-blockers (avoid in geriatrics):
         i. **Propranolol** (1–2 mg/q 4–6 hrs IV).
         ii. **Labetalol** (Load 0.2–1 mg/kg slow IV push, then infusion or boluses).
         iii. **Esmolol** (5 g/500 ml 0.9% NaCl).
      b. *Sodium Nitroprusside* (50–400 mg/100 ml 0.9% NaCl). Check thiocyanate levels.
      c. **Nitroglycerine** (50 mg/100 ml–400 mg/100 ml).
      d. *Others*: Hydralazine, nifedipine, captopril, enalapril.
   2. Maintain PAWP at 8–12 torr.
   3. Maintain renal output > 0.5 ml/kg (dopamine 1–2 μg/kg/m —N.B., ALSO INCREASES CEREBRAL BLOOD FLOW AND ICP).
   4. Maintain oxygen saturation > 95%. Use minimum of 3 mm Hg of PEEP or CPAP in intubated patient.
   5. Maintain normal oncotic pressures.
      a. TPN (start gradually on 2nd or 3rd day). Use with albumin solutions if serum albumin < 3.0 mg/dl.
   6. Maintain blood glucose 100–200 mg/dl.

(Courtesy of the Cleveland Clinic Foundation, Cleveland, OH.)

Stereotypical approaches and drug dosages for these measures are outlined in the attached Cleveland Clinic Neurosurgical Intensive Care Unit Intracranial Hypertension Guidelines (Table 4-3). As ICP control is a dynamic process, the patient must be constantly reassessed with these three questions in mind until ICP begins to diminish and these measures can be tapered.

ICP Reduction—Surgical. In general, the role for surgical treatment of raised ICP is limited. Hydrocephalus may require placement of internal or external CSF drainage devices. In head injury, hematomas and contusions that produce raised ICP or tissue shifts may warrant surgical resection. Posterior fossa subdural or extradural hematomas may be difficult to diagnose but may constitute neurosurgical emergencies. Early removal of posttraumatic hematomas is associated with improved outcome. Depressed skull fractures producing dural sinus obstruction may lead to raised ICP and surgical correction should be considered.[34] Also, in rare instances lobectomy or craniectomy may be warranted when medical therapies fail to control runaway ICP.

ICP Reduction—Medical. The direct medical treatment of intracranial pressure only constitutes a small part of the overall management of the patient. Nonetheless, this area is traditionally considered "ICP Management." Often, the most simple measures for reducing ICP are overlooked in favor of more aggressive modalities.

Basic Measures

Optimization of head elevation and position can substantially improve the ICP in patients who have poor intracranial compliance (see Table 4-3, section A). Minimum ICP usually occurs in the range of 30 to 45° of head elevation; however, one must bear in mind that, in some cases, having the patients flat or nearly upright is best. As head elevation increases, there is a tendency for the cerebral perfusion pressure (CPP = IMAP − ICP) to drop. As long as the CPP is greater than 45 mm Hg, it will likely not be of any consequence. In fact, high CPPs with their associated levels of high hydrostatic pressure in regions of damaged capillaries may promote brain edema and later deterioration. In order to accurately determine the CPP, we place the arterial transducer at head level so as to avoid unduly complex mathematical calculations.

The head should be kept in a neutral position, and this may require the use of some type of cervical collar. The neck should be kept free of any compressing structure, such as tracheostomy tapes, and internal jugular catheters should be avoided. These measures facilitate venous drainage from the dural venous sinuses, thereby reducing cerebral blood volume.

In general, patients need not be "fluid restricted." Rather, they should be "free water restricted." We initiate maintenance fluids that are 0.9% in NaCl. As serum osmolality and sodium increase, the fluid is modified so as to keep the serum sodium below 160 mEq/L. There is little evidence that hyperosmolality or hypernatremia has serious long-term consequences when the patient is kept normovolemic.

The hematocrit should be kept in the range of approximately 33 to 37%. Lower hematocrits result in reduced oxygen delivery with consequential vasodilatation and increased cerebral blood volume. Increased cerebral blood volume results in an elevation of the ICP. Higher hematocrits may result in sludging, particularly in zones of ischemia as would be expected as global ICP increases or in the "ischemia penumbra" around mass lesions.

Steroids may be used to treat vasogenic edema. Dexamethasone (24 to 60 mg/day in two to six divided doses) is our drug of choice because of its minimal mineralocorticoid effects. Tumors, abscesses, and intracerebral hematomas produce vasogenic edema and, as such, are candidates for steroid treatment. The use of steroids for the treatment of head injury or infarction is not rational and has not been proven to be of any benefit in many studies.

The volume of the CSF compartment may be primarily increased or raised secondary to outflow obstruction due to a mass lesion. Medical treatment for reducing CSF volume with acetazolamide has proven useful for the short-term reduction in CSF production in hydrocephalus. In cases where hydrocephalus is a major contributor to intracranial hypertension, external ventricular drainage is indicated.

Patient agitation and reaction to painful stimuli can result in substantial elevations in the ICP. Prior to suctioning (or placement of invasive lines), we routinely administer IV lidocaine. This has proven to be a powerful medullary suppressant with reduction of the gag reflex. Patients requiring a greater level of sedation may require treatment with methohexital (Brevital), or succinylcholine. Provisions for airway protection and ventilation must be available in nonintubated patients because of apnea when using the latter agents. We routinely use phenobarbital as a mild sedative for patients who are at risk of rehemorrhage. Benzodiazepines are used when patients are agitated, or to prevent alcohol withdrawal. Morphine sulfate is generally reserved for when patients are agitated due to pain. Major tranquilizers such as haloperidol are administered IV when patients are delirious or psychotic. Propofol, which may also be used for sedation, often results in increased CPP, and allows rapid recovery for assessment.[35]

Seizures should be treated aggressively as the resulting increase in cerebral blood flow and blood volume can produce ICP elevations that may be fatal. A bolus of IV lorazepam (Ativan) followed by phenytoin or phenobarbital will prove satisfactory in most cases. Focal or generalized status epilepticus may require a continuous infusion of lorazepam or induction of general anesthesia, such as with high dose barbiturate therapy.

Fever is another factor that can substantially raise ICP on the basis of increased cerebral blood flow. This situation is initially treated aggressively with antipyretics. Should these fail, cooling blankets with pharmacologic paralysis are required to keep the temperature below 38.5°C.

Aggressive Measures

These should be instituted in a gradual fashion appropriate for the degree of ICP elevation while basic measures are continued (see Table 4–3, section B). Hyperventilation should be used incrementally to help blunt temporary increases in ICP and may be used at the time of intubation so as to avoid ICP spikes during this process. Although hyperventilation only results in short-term reduction of ICP, it must be continued until ICP is once again under control as there is a profound rebound effect upon cessation.

The risk of hyperventilation-induced ischemia is controversial.[36] We do not believe that there is compelling evidence that hyperventilation to the recommended levels results in secondary brain ischemia. Hyperventilation may be useful beyond ICP reduction as its induced alkalosis may help buffer lactate production.

Diuretics are one of the mainstays of ICP management. Mannitol is one of the few hyperosmolar agents that does not result in ICP rebound because it does not pass the blood-brain barrier. Mannitol only works in regions where there is an intact blood-brain barrier, however, and in regions where the blood-brain barrier is disrupted there most likely will indeed be rebound swelling after a dose. For this reason we start at a small dosage, commonly 12.5 g every 4 hours and increase as required.[37] Concomitantly, we measure central venous or pulmonary artery wedge pressures to ensure that the patient is not becoming systemically hypovolemic.

Furosemide can be used as an adjunct or in place of mannitol. Furosemide's effects are to reduce CSF production and brain water by means of systemic dehydration. Furosemide is one agent that will work to reduce brain volume when there are widespread disruptions of the blood-brain barrier. We commonly use furosemide in conjunction with 25% albumin in an effort to shrink extravascular fluid volume while maintaining intravascular volume.

Concomitant with use of these brain diuretics is loss of systemic intravascular volume. Efforts are made to maintain an adequate volume and intracranial mean arterial pressure with colloid. While short-term fluid resuscitation issues are well understood (and addressed in the Pre-ICU section), there is little solid information on the long-term effects of crystalloid versus colloid in the setting of the brain edema. With crystalloid or total parenteral nutrition (TPN) used as maintenance fluids, we commonly supplement a low intravascular volume with colloid solutions. When fluid balance is near even or negative, then 5% albumin or purified plasma fraction are administered. When the patient is intravascularly depleted, but has an overall positive fluid balance, then 25% albumin may be useful. Dextran 40 may also be used, particularly when cerebral ischemia is a factor. We do not routinely use high molecular weight dextran because of problems with bleeding disorders. Similarly, pressors may be required to maintain an adequate perfusion pressure. Suggested agents and dosages are outlined in the accompanying guidelines.

When all these measures have failed (and one has reassessed the patient in terms of less drastic modes of reducing ICP), then high dose barbiturate therapy (barbiturate coma) should be considered. Pulmonary artery catheters should be placed so as to help maintain hemodynamic stability. After a loading dose of either pentobarbital or thiopental, the drug is continuously infused so as to maintain the patient in EEG burst suppression at a rate of approximately three bursts per minute. Higher doses are of no theoretical or clinical benefit. Pentobarbital is our drug of choice as it will clear faster than thiopental in this setting. These patients are at increased risk of sepsis, particularly pneumonia. Daily chest radiographs and frequent blood counts should be a part of routine management.

Last, when all else fails, systemic hypothermia can be instituted. This technique requires cooling the patient to approximately 31°C, use of a pulmonary artery catheter and systemic paralysis. Clinical assessment of the patient's neurologic status during this and barbiturate coma is essentially nil. Pupillary reflexes are commonly reserved in barbiturate coma, however, they may disappear in hypothermia. Midposition or dilated pupils in either case are ominous signs. The patient should be assessed not only with an ICP monitor but, when possible, with an EEG and evoked potential monitoring. Even if hypothermia can temporarily control ICP, often pressures return to pretreatment levels when normothermia is restored.

Systemic Stabilization. Aggressive management of ICP frequently results in systemic destabilization. Such cardiovascular or metabolic derangements may superimpose further injury on damaged cerebral tissue and lead to tissue destruction.

Although hypotension is more commonly a problem than hypertension, the latter can result in increased brain edema through capillary leakage induced by high hydrostatic pressures. Systolic or intracranial systolic arterial pressures of greater than 150 mm Hg should probably be avoided except in chronically hypertensive patients who may have altered autoregulatory responses.

Pulmonary artery wedge pressure should be maintained in the range of 8 to 14 mm Hg. Lower levels may result in systemic collapse and cerebral thrombosis. Higher levels can result in excessive right heart filling pressures that result in increased dural sinus pressures, increased cerebral blood volume, and elevations in the ICP.

Patients may develop mild azotemia consistent with a "pre-renal" state. Low dose dopamine infusions may ameliorate this; however, this dose may also result in increase cerebral flow and ICP.

The oxygen saturation should be 93% or more. Also, we routinely use 3 torr of PEEP or CPAP in intubated patients so as to prevent microatelectasis. Higher levels of PEEP may be used as required and generally are well tolerated unless the patient's intracranial compartment is particularly noncompliant or PEEP levels exceed 15 mm Hg.[38] When necessary, oxygen saturations may be allowed to drop to 90% so as to avoid further increases in PEEP which would result in systemic hypotension. It should be noted that the acceptable range of pulmonary artery wedge pressures may need to be increased in patients who are on a high level of PEEP.

Brain Death

When efforts to control ICP fail and global cerebral ischemia results, cerebral function ceases and the brain dies. The stereotypical pattern of slowly rising ICP that eventually reached the mean intracranial arterial pressure and lead to abrupt cardiovascular collapse is shown in Figure 4–5. Aggressive fluid resuscitation and, on occasion, pressors may be required to regain normotension. Diabetes insipidus due to cessation of vasopressin production commonly occurs a few hours later and leads to brisk diuresis that can rapidly lead to hypovolemia and hypernatremia. Intravenous desmopressin acetate (0.25 to 0.5 ml IV, bid, as needed) and hypotonic fluid administration is corrective.

Use of high dose barbiturates may preclude the clinical diagnosis of brain death. Cerebral circulatory arrest as documented by cerebral angiography or brain scan may prove diagnostic in appropriate clinical settings.[39] These tests should be performed under conditions of normotension. Angiography should be performed using injection of the aortic arch and document extracranial filling of the carotid and vertebral arteries with absence of the intracranial circulation. Brain scans may not adequately exclude posterior fossa blood flow.

Tapering Therapy

As ICP comes under control (i.e., < 15 or 20 mm Hg using a fixed treatment regimen), therapy should start to be tapered. As cessation of hyperosmolar, hyperventilation, and hypothermia therapies may induce ICP rebound it is important that they not be abruptly discontinued. Generally the most aggressive treatments are withdrawn first. I favor discontinuing treatments in the order shown in Table 4–4.

Table 4–4. Order of Withdrawal of Aggressive ICP Treatments after Attaining ICP Control

Hypothermia
High-dose barbiturates
Hyperventilation
Hyperosmolar/diuretic therapy

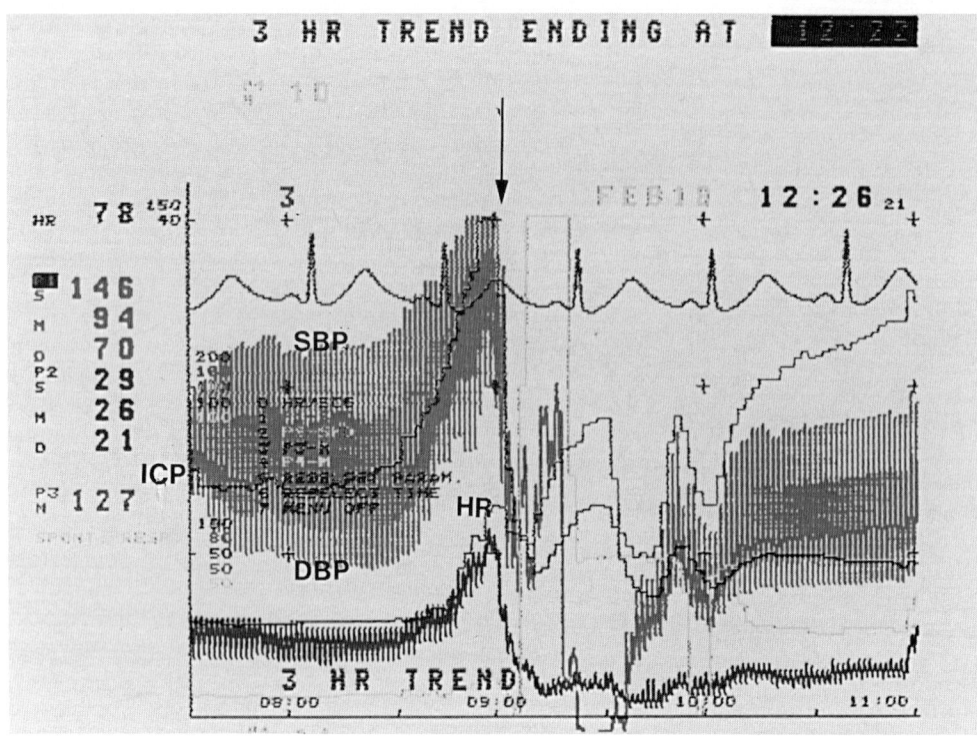

Fig. 4-5. Plot of blood pressure (SBP/DBP), heart rate (HR), and intracranial pressure (ICP) in setting of uncontrolled ICP. Arrow denotes time of hemodynamic collapse due to absence of cerebral perfusion pressure.

POST-ICU PHASE

Successful weaning of ICP medical therapy may be completed on a regular nursing floor without ICP monitoring once the patient's pressures are well controlled using only hyperosmolar/diuretic therapy. Excessive intake of free water or infection with fever may result in ICU readmission because of neurologic deterioration from brain swelling. Also, patients recovering from intracranial hypertension are, in general, subject to the same medical and rehabilitation considerations as discussed in Chapter 5. However, protracted intracranial hypertension itself may have resulted in sufficient global cerebral ischemia to result in prolonged, if not permanent, cognitive disorders. Integration of working memory into long-term memory is particularly susceptible to ICP-induced global ischemia and dysfunction of this process can cause serious problems with rehabilitation.

In conclusion, optimal management of intracranial hypertension requires an understanding of the pathophysiology of ICP, ICP monitoring techniques, and the principles of therapy. Recent insights into mechanisms of cellular injury in the CNS, development of new "cytoprotective" pharmacologic agents, and promising work in CNS tissue grafting may provide new treatments capable of further improving outcome.[40]

REFERENCES

1. Plum, F., and Posner, J. B., (Eds.): Diagnosis of Stupor and Coma. 2nd Ed. Philadelphia, F. A. Davis Co., 1972, pp. 1–286.
2. Ornato, J. P., Craren, E. J., Nelson, N. M., and Kimball, K. F.: Impact of improved emergency medical services and emergency trauma care on the reduction in mortality from trauma. J. Trauma, 25:575, 1985.
3. Pons, P. T., et al.: Prehospital advanced trauma life support critical penetrating wounds to the thorax and abdomen. Trauma, 25:828, 1985.
4. Silverston, P.: Pulse oximetry at the roadside: a study of pulse oximetry in immediate care. BMJ., 298:711, 1989.
5. Genoni, M., Bogen, M., Fritz, M., and Malcrida, R.: Utilization of helicopters for the prevention of secondary cerebral lesions in severe craniocerebral injuries. Z. Unfallchir. Versicherungsmed., 82:163, 1989.
6. Schwab, C. W., et al.: The impact of an air ambulance system on an established trauma center. J. Trauma, 25:580, 1985.
7. Gentleman, D., and Jennett, B.: Audit of transfer of unconscious head-injured patients to a neurosurgical unit. Lancet, 335:330, 1990.
8. Andrews, P. J., Piper, I. R., Dearden, N. M., and Miller, J. D.: Secondary insults during intrahospital transport of head-injured patients. Lancet, 335:327, 1990.
9. Hans, P., Albert, A., Franssen, C., and Born, J.: Improved outcome prediction based on CSF extrapolated creatine kinase BB isoenzyme activity and other risk factors in severe head injury. J. Neurosurg., 71:54, 1989.
10. Gunnar, W., Kane, J., and Barrett, J.: Cerebral blood flow following hypertonic saline resuscitation in an experimental model of hemorrhagic shock and head injury. Braz. J. Med. Biol. Res., 22:287, 1989.
11. Shackford, S. R.: Fluid resuscitation in head injury. J. Inten. Care. Med., 5:59, 1990.
12. Hall, E. D., and Yonkers, P. A.: Comparison of two ester prodrugs of methylprednisolone on early neurologic recovery in a murine closed head injury model. J. Neurotrauma, 6:163, 1989.
13. Colquhoun, I. R., and Burrows, E. H.: The prognostic significance of the third ventricle and basal cisterns in severe closed head injury. Clin. Radiol., 40:13, 1989.
14. Ross, D. A., et al.: Brain shift, level of consciousness in patients with acute intracranial hematoma. J. Neurosurg., 71: 4989, 1989.

15. Mizutani, T., Manaka, S., and Tsutsumi, H.: Estimation of intracranial pressure using computed tomography scan findings in patients with severe head injury. Surg. Neurol., *33:*178, 1990.
16. Ropper, A. H.: Lateral displacement of the brain and level of consciousness in patients with an acute hemispheral mass. N. Engl. J. Med., *314:*953, 1986.
17. Levin, H. S., et al.: Magnetic resonance imaging after "diffuse" nonmissile head injury: a neurobehavioral study. Arch. Neurol., *42:*963, 1985.
18. Snow, R. B., Zimmerman, R. D., Gandy, S. E., and Deck, M. D. F.: Comparison of magnetic resonance imaging and computed tomography in the evaluation of head injury. Neurosurgery, *18:*45, 1986.
19. Barnett, G. H., Ropper, A. H., and Johnson, K. A.: Physiologic support and monitoring of critically ill patients during magnetic resonance imaging. J. Neurosurg., *68:*246, 1988.
20. Ropper, A. H.: In favor of intracranial pressure monitoring and aggressive therapy in neurologic practice. Arch. Neurol., *42:*1194, 1985.
21. Saul, T. G., and Ducker, T. B.: Effect of intracranial pressure monitoring and aggressive treatment on mortality in severe head injury. J. Neurosurg., *56:*498, 1982.
22. Stuart, G. G., Merry, G. S., Smith, J. A., and Yelland, J. D.: Severe head injury managed without intracranial pressure monitoring. J. Neurosurg., *59:*601, 1983.
23. Lundber, N.: Continuous recording and control of ventricular fluid pressure in neurosurgical practice. Acta Psychiatr. Scand., *36(Suppl. 149)*:1, 1960.
24. Rosner, M. J., and Becker, D. P.: Origin and evolution of plateau waves. Experimental observations and a theoretical model. J. Neurosurg., *50:*312, 1961.
25. Lundber, N.: Continuous recording and control of ventricular fluid pressure in neurosurgical practice. Acta Psychiatr. Scand., *36(Suppl. 149)*:1, 1960.
26. Aucoin, P. J., et al.: Intracranial pressure monitors: epidemiologic study of risk factors and infections. Am. J. Med., *80:*369, 1986.
27. Mayhall, C. G., et al.: Ventriculostomy-related infections: a prospective epidemiologic study. N. Engl. J. Med., *310:*553, 1984.
28. Barlow, P., et al.: Clinical evaluation of two methods of subdural pressure monitoring. J. Neurosurg., *653:*578, 1985.
29. Gosch, H. H., and Kindt, G. W.: Subdural monitoring of acute increase intracranial pressure. Surg. Forum, *23:*405, 1972.
30. Mendelow, A. D., Rowan, J. O., Murray, L., and Kerr, A. E.: A clinical comparison of subdural screw pressure measurements with ventricular pressure. J. Neurosurg., *58:*45, 1983.
31. Miller, J. D., Bobo, H., and Kapp, J. P.: Inaccurate pressure readings for subarachnoid bolts. Neurosurgery, *19:*253, 1986.
32. Gentleman, D., and Mendelow, A. D.: Intracranial rupture of a pressure monitoring transducer. Technical note. Neurosurgery, *19:*91, 1986.
33. Levin, A. B.: The use of fiberoptic intracranial pressure monitor in clinical practice. Neurosurgery, *1:*266, 1977.
34. Indications for operative treatment and operative technique in closed head injury. *In* Textbook of Head Injury. Edited by S. K. Gudeman, et al. Philadelphia, W. B. Saunders, 1991, p. 138.
35. Farling, P. A., Johnston, J. R., and Coppel, D. L.: Propofol infusion for sedation of patients with head injury in intensive care: a preliminary report. Anaesthesia, *44:*222, 1989.
36. Darby, J. M., Yonas, H., Marion, D. W., and Latchaw, R. E.: Local "inverse steal" induced by hyperventilation in head injury. Neurosurgery, *23:*84, 1988.
37. Marshall, L. F., Smith, R. W., Rauscher, L. A., and Shapiro, H. M.: Mannitol dose requirements in brain-injured patients. J. Neurosurg., *48:*169, 1978.
38. Apuzzo, M. L. J., et al.: Effect of positive end expiratory pressure ventilation on intracranial pressure in man. J. Neurosurg., *46:*227, 1977.
39. Kaufman, H. H., et al.: Detection of brain death in barbiturate coma L—the dilemma of an intracranial pulse. Neurosurgery, *25:*275, 1989.
40. Foster, A. C., Gill, R., Iversen, L. L., and Woodruff, G. N.: Systemic administration of MK-801 protects against ischaemia-induced hippocampal neurodegeneration in the gerbil. Br. J. Pharmacol., *90(Suppl.)*:9, 1987.

Chapter 5

INTENSIVE CARE MANAGEMENT OF NONISCHEMIC BRAIN INJURIES

GENE H. BARNETT

The brain is subject to certain injuries, both acute and chronic, that may lead to admission to an ICU (Table 5-1). The principles of diagnosis and management of these neurologic disorders are often foreign to general intensivists, so much so that many institutions have dedicated neurologic or neurosurgical ICUs. This chapter aims to provide an introduction to neurologic critical care focusing on the management of common disorders that may present as masses, such as hemorrhages, trauma, tumors, and abscesses. Metabolic disorders, seizures, some infections, and issues pertaining to raised intracranial pressure (ICP) are discussed in other chapters.

The cornerstone of neurologic diagnosis is the neurologic history and examination. The differential diagnosis of disorders of the central nervous system (CNS) is often approached by using these symptoms and signs to determine the location of the lesion and the time course of onset as a guide to the nature of the lesion. The guidelines presented here are a gross oversimplification of neurologic differential diagnosis; however, they provide a foundation for the intensivist that may help with understanding the process by which neurologists and neurosurgeons diagnose and assess their patient and alert them to potentially serious changes in the neurologic condition of the patient. An in-depth understanding of the techniques of neurologic differential diagnosis is well beyond the scope of this chapter because it requires a thorough understanding of the anatomy and function of the nervous system as well as the range of possible presentations of any given brain disorder. The interested reader is referred to the texts of Adams and Victor,[1] Kandel and Schwartz,[2] and Patten.[3]

LOCALIZATION

The symptoms and signs of a brain lesion are often less related to the nature of the lesion than its location. A simplified outline of the functions mediated by various brain structures is presented in Table 5-2. By determining the overlap between possible sites of involvement for each symptom or sign, its location can often be deduced. For instance, the isolated loss of right limb strength implies a small lesion of the deep left hemisphere or pons. The same finding in conjunction with loss of production of speech content suggests a larger lesion situated in the left hemisphere. Right limb weakness with slurred speech and incoordination of the left limbs, however, localizes the lesion to the left brain stem or cerebellum.

PRESENTATION

The temporal onset of patient symptoms and signs can provide important clues to the neurologic diagnosis. The abrupt onset of symptoms (or worsening of existing symptoms) suggests a vascular event (ischemic, hemorrhagic, migrainous), seizure, or acute obstruction of the cerebrospinal fluid (CSF). An onset over hours is compatible with:

- Hemorrhage into the brain substance
- Infection
- Metabolic disorder
- Partial CSF obstruction
- Expanding mass lesion

Symptoms that have progressed over days to weeks are consistent with:

- Expanding lesion such as tumor
- Abscess
- Hydrocephalus
- Chronic subdural hematoma

For the examples cited, a sudden onset would suggest an infarction, whereas symptoms progressing over weeks or more would be more suggestive of a mass such as a tumor. A review of pertinent aspects of the neurologic examination is presented subsequently; stereotypic brain herniation syndromes are reviewed in Chapter 4.

ACUTE LESIONS

Traumatic Head Injury

There have been substantial advances in understanding the pathophysiology and management of traumatic brain injuries in the past three decades. Nonetheless, traumatic head injury remains a major cause of death and disability in the United States and throughout the industrialized world.[4] In the United States, head injury accounts for 2% of all deaths and 26% of all injury deaths and occurs at a yearly rate of 16.9 per 100,000.[5] Most are due to motor vehicle accidents (57%), gunshot wounds (14%), or falls (12%). The majority of patients with severe head injury also suffer from other injuries; conversely, many patients with multiple trauma also harbor brain injuries. In a series of patients admitted to a trauma unit, nearly 60% of deaths were in patients with head injuries. Among these, the head injury itself directly (68%) or indirectly (26%) led to the death in 94% of cases.[6]

Table 5–1. Common Neurologic Causes of ICU Admission

Traumatic head injury
Stroke
   Ischemic
    Hemorrhagic
Seizures
Metabolic encephalopathy
Hydrocephalus
Elevated intracranial pressure
Tumors
Infections
Perioperative care and monitoring

Prevention of head injury remains the most effective means of reducing associated mortality and morbidity. Areas with mandatory seat belt laws and high motorist compliance have seen substantial reductions in the number of fatal and operative head injuries.[7] Similarly, the use of helmets substantially reduces head injury deaths from motorcycle and bicycle accidents: Helmeted riders have one tenth the number of skull fractures than nonwearers and an 88% reduction in brain injuries.[8-10]

These prevention efforts, along with aggressive ICU management techniques,[11] led to a decline in the number of fatal head injuries in the United States during the 1960s and 1970s. Although this rate plateaued on a national level in the 1980s, certain head injury centers report further reductions in morbidity and mortality with new approaches to field and hospital care.[12] Specialized trauma and head injury units appear to have superior results, particularly with respect to patients with moderate or mild injuries.[13-17] This increase in head injury survival has not resulted in a proportionate rise in the number of vegetative survivors; rather, increased survival in moderate and patients with mild head injuries accounts for this change.[18,19]

One method of approaching the pathophysiology of common traumatic brain injuries is through the following groups:

- Concussive head injury
- Contusion
- Subdural hematoma (SDH)
- Extradural hematoma (EDH)
- Skull fracture

Concussive Head Injury

Rapid acceleration/deceleration events are often associated with changes in consciousness. In their mildest forms, concussive head injuries may produce amnesia for events leading up to the injury (**retrograde amnesia**) without loss of consciousness. Stronger blows may result in actual loss of consciousness with **anterograde amnesia** that extends beyond the return of consciousness and lucidity. Animal experiments and human postmortem studies suggest that these clinical syndromes are related to angular accelerations, perhaps resulting in impact of the midbrain on surrounding structures, such as the tentorium and clivus.[20] At its extreme, concussive head injury may result in permanent coma even without the development of contusions or frank hemorrhages (see later). Microscopic analysis demonstrates diffuse disruption of neural axons at the white matter–cortical junction—so-called **shear injuries**.[21] High resolution neuroimaging techniques often demonstrate small midbrain hemorrhages in this setting.

Contusion

In closed head injury, brain contusions typically result from impact of the brain substance with the inner skull, falx, or tentorium. Common sites of brain contusion include the frontal, temporal, and occipital poles. Although many contusions occur at the site of a blow (coup injuries), they may also occur opposing the external injury (contrecoup injuries). A rotational force may potentiate the likelihoods and magnitude of many brain contusions. Histologically contusions are characterized by microhemorrhages and edema. They may mature to zones of scar (gliosis) or progress to regions of infarction or hemorrhage. Early after injury, computed tomography (CT) scan is often normal but may develop into areas of low, high, or mixed density. Magnetic resonance imaging (MRI) is far more sensitive than CT and may show increased T2-weighted signal changes reflecting contusion both soon and long after head injury despite a normal CT appearance.

Table 5–2. Guide to the Functional Anatomy of the Brain

Structure	Function
Frontal lobe	Problem solving (D)
	Planning and initiation of task (D)
	Gaze to OS
	Movement of face and limbs on OS
	Speech production (D)
Parietal lobe	Appreciation of sensation on OS
	Understanding speech (D)
	Numerical functions (D)
	Spatial perception
Occipital lobe	Visual functions
Temporal lobe	Memory
	Sound and speech perception (D)
Hypothalamus	Temperatures, thirst, hunger, autonomic regulation
Thalamus	Major sensory and motor integration and relay for OS
Midbrain	Conduit of motor and sensory information for OS of head and body
	Some eye movements
Pons	Conduit of motor and sensory information for OS of body
	Relay for limb coordination for SS
	Mediates some eye movements and their coordination
	Receives facial sensation for SS
	Mediates facial movement for SS
	Receives hearing and balance input from SS
Midbrain	Conduit of motor and sensory information for opposite and SS of body
	Regulation of respiration
	Regulation of blood pressure
	Mediates swallowing and tongue movements
	Mediates vagal autonomic function
Cerebellum	Coordination of limbs, SS
	Posture
	Gait

D, Dominant hemisphere; OS, opposite side; SS, same side.

Subdural Hematoma

The brain surface is connected to dural and cranial vessels, predominantly by **bridging veins**. Abrupt acceleration/deceleration forces may cause the brain to glide in the cranial vault, tearing one or more of these vessels. Because the brain occupies most of the intracranial volume in younger patients, very large forces are required to tear these vessels compared with those required in the setting of brain atrophy, as seen in advanced age, Alzheimer's disease, and alcoholism. The presence of SDH in a younger patient is usually an ominous sign because the forces required to create the SDH usually result in a significant underlying brain injury, and the resulting SDH may be due to brain rupture rather than bridging vessel avulsion.[22] A direct blow to the head is not required to produce symptomatic SDH. Any injury that creates a sufficient acceleration/deceleration force may produce SDH. Anticoagulation is another potentiating factor of SDH at any age and may transform a minor injury. Subdural hemorrhage surrounding the brain stem and cerebellum (posterior fossa SDH) usually leads to rapidly developing coma and death. It is difficult to diagnose because it rarely produces localizing symptoms and is difficult to visualize on CT scans.

The typical clinical syndrome of **acute SDH** is a severe closed head injury with slowly progressive loss of consciousness and development of focal neurologic deficits. CT may be normal if the scan is obtained immediately after injury, but the image soon develops a crescent of high density over a broad expanse of brain with or without changes in the brain substance (Fig. 5-1). MRI scan often shows the clot to be more massive than apparent by CT but does not possess high T1-weighted signal until a few days after hemorrhage. Distortion of brain substance and herniation syndromes are described in Chapters 1 and 4.

The symptoms and signs of SDH may not occur for days to weeks after head injury. After initial hemorrhage, a membrane of neovascularization may form from the dural surface and extend to the brain, forming a lenticular cavity. Typically this region is filled with liquid blood degradation products resembling motor oil. Expansion of the **chronic SDH** is attributed to rehemorrhage from these fragile neovascular vessels. Chronic SDH is most commonly seen in the presence of brain atrophy or after shunting procedures for hydrocephalus.

Extradural Hematoma

A potential space exists between the dura and inner table of the skull. Skull fracture that results in tear of a dural vessel can cause hemorrhage into this space, producing an EDH.[23] A common clinical presentation is that of a severe head injury with a return to normal consciousness (the so-called **lucid interval**), complaint of severe headache, and delayed progressive onset of neurologic deterioration. Rupture of the middle meningeal artery owing to fracture of the thin squamous portion of the temporal bone is a common cause of EDH in children and young adults. Again the early CT image may be normal but later shows a lentiform area of high density (Fig. 5-2). Although EDH may

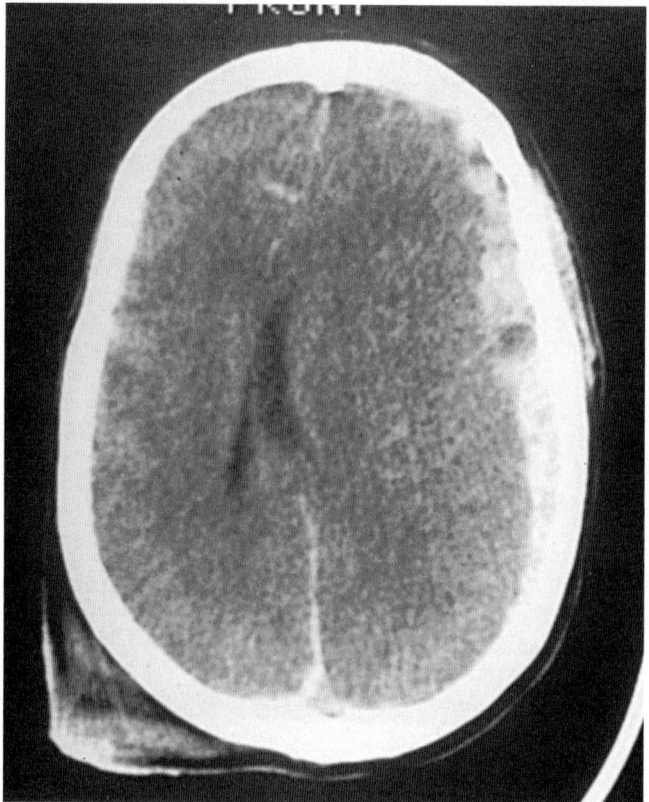

Fig. 5-1. CT of an acute subdural hematoma. Note the crescent-shaped region of high density.

be fatal, early recognition and treatment can lead to full recovery.

Skull Fracture

The forces required to produce skull fracture are often in excess of those required to result in underlying brain damage.[24] As such, the presence of a skull fracture may increase the likelihood of serious intracranial pathology by 200%, and more than 75% of intracranial hematomas are associated with skull fractures. Fractures may be linear, depressed, open, or closed, or they may affect the skull base.

A linear fracture through the base of the skull may result in disruption of important neural or vascular structures as well as loss of CSF containment. The symptoms and signs of **basilar skull fracture** are described later. Fracture through the cribriform plate may produce raccoon's eyes and CSF rhinorrhea. Disruption of the sphenoid bone may result in blindness owing to transection of the optic nerve, diplopia from injury to the nerves of extraocular movement, and vascular syndromes such as hemispheric infarction or carotocavernous fistula. Petrous bone fractures can produce facial paralysis, deafness and vertigo, CSF otorrhea, and fatal occlusion or rupture of major dural venous sinuses. The presence of basilar skull fracture can often be detected by careful clinical examination (see later).

Displacement of fractured skull below the surrounding surface can result in a meningeal tear, contusion or disruption of brain, or obstruction or disruption of underlying dural venous sinuses. These **depressed skull fractures** are generally well visualized on appropriate radiographs and CT with bone windows (Fig. 5-3). Leakage of CSF or displacement where the outer skull surface is depressed below the surrounding inner surface are usually grounds for urgent surgical intervention.

Disruption of tissues overlying and lining the skull in the region of the fracture may allow development of CSF leakage. Such **open skull fractures** create the opportunity for intracranial infectious complications, such as abscess or meningitis, and may render ICP monitoring techniques ineffective. Open fractures of the calvarium generally require surgical intervention, whereas many open fractures of the skull base heal spontaneously or with use of external CSF drainage devices.

Hemorrhagic Stroke

Nontraumatic rupture of intracranial vessels results in bleeding into:

- Brain substance (intracerebral hemorrhage [ICH])
- Ventricles (intraventricular hemorrhage)
- Subarachnoid space (subarachnoid hemorrhage [SAH])
- Combination of these compartments

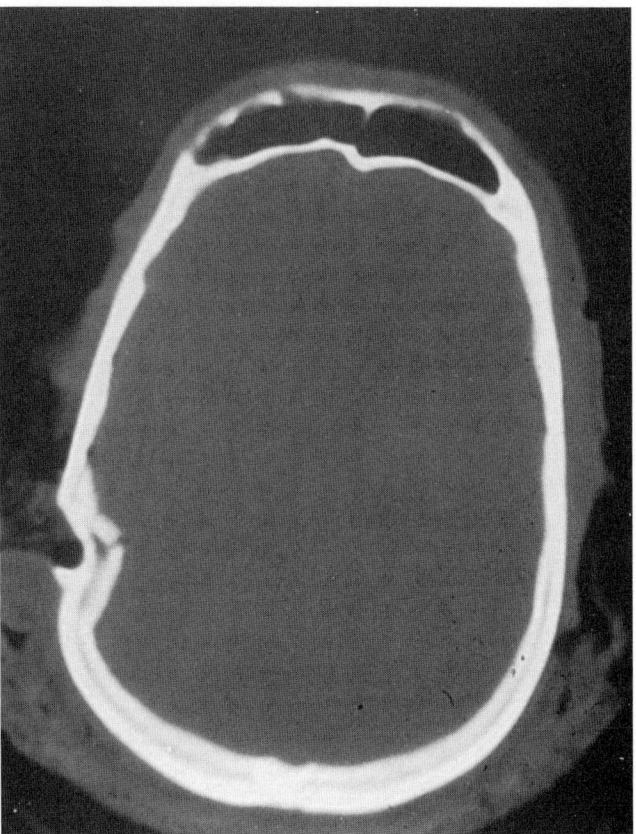

Fig. 5-3. Depressed skull fracture of the right parietal area. CT scan using bone windows.

Bleeding usually occurs at the site of a vessel anomaly, such as a congenital or acquired weakness of an otherwise normal artery, or in the presence of an abnormal vascular structure or malformation.

Intracerebral and Intraventricular Hemorrhage

Exposure to chronic elevations in blood pressure can result in fibrinoid degeneration of cerebral arteries leading either to vessel occlusion (hypertensive infarct) or development of microaneurysm resulting in **hypertensive ICH**. Small, perforating arteries are more commonly affected than larger surface vessels, resulting in preferential areas of hemorrhage, including the basal ganglia, thalamus, pons, and cerebellum.[25] Improved management of systemic hypertension has resulted in a marked reduction in the incidence of this type of ICH in recent decades in the United States, but hypertensive ICH remains a problem in certain regions, ethnic groups, and diseases associated with intractable hypertension as well as many other countries, including Japan.[26] Deposition of amyloid in the walls of cerebral arteries (**amyloid angiopathy**) is becoming increasingly recognized as a cause of nonhypertensive hemorrhage in the elderly, commonly affecting the white matter of the cerebral hemispheres. Vasculitis, coagulopathies, anticoagulation, or use of systemic thrombolytic agents are other causes of ICH.

Onset of symptoms of ICH are often gradual and usually

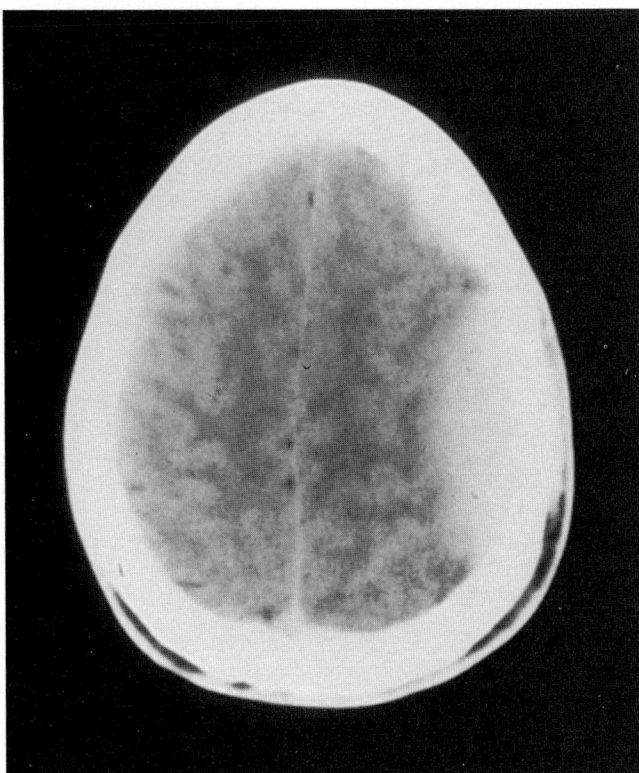

Fig. 5-2. Acute extradural hematoma. The lens-shaped area of high density represents an acute (as opposed to chronic) collection of blood in the potential space between the dura and the skull.

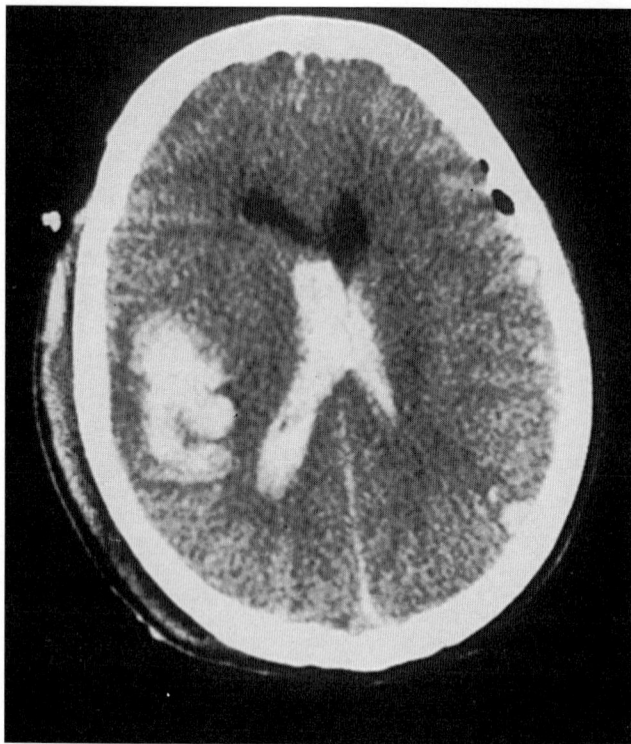

Fig. 5-4. CT scan of an intracerebral hemorrhage of the right parietal lobe associated with intraventricular hemorrhage.

painless. The jet of arterial blood may dissect between neural tracts but is often destructive as well. Symptoms may develop from direct neural destruction; clot expansion producing brain distortion, compression, or raised ICP; or edema in response to the clot. ICHs situated near the ventricular system may rupture into the ventricular system (Fig. 5-4). These **intraventricular hemorrhages** can limit local damage by reducing the size of the intraparenchymal bleed component but may lead to hydrocephalus by red cell-mediated blockage of CSF drainage. Peripherally located clots may also liberate blood into the subarachnoid space and CSF, regardless of the cause. An ICH may take weeks to months before it is totally resorbed. Hemoglobin degradation products are particularly neurotoxic and may engender ongoing damage via liberation of free radicals and other toxins. Early clot removal may therefore minimize chronic brain injury if it can be performed with sufficiently low risk.

Vascular malformations are abnormal arrangements of vessels that are common sources of ICH, particularly in young adults. Bleeding from cavernous angiomas and venous angiomas is generally under low pressure, rare, and an infrequent cause of ICU admission.[27] **Arteriovenous malformations** (AVMs), however, are typically high flow fistulas between the arterial and venous systems that often result in reduced arterial pressure in vessels feeding the malformation and impaired autoregulation of the brain surrounding the AVM.[28,29] They may present with seizures, progressive neurologic deficit, or hemorrhage. Bleeding occurs at a rate of 2 to 4% per year[30,31] and is associated with death in nearly 40% of cases.[32] As with other causes of ICH, the ventricular system or subarachnoid space may also harbor blood after AVM rupture.

Aneurysmal Subarachnoid Hemorrhage

Aneurysms of the cerebral arteries can occur in the setting of congenital anomalies of the vessels as found in polycystic kidney disease or at sites of acquired wall weakness owing to trauma, atherosclerosis, or mechanical stress found at vessel bifurcations or sharp bends.[33] Rupture of a cerebral aneurysm commonly results in SAH, which is associated with high mortality and morbidity. The likelihood of aneurysmal hemorrhage increases with aneurysm size, particularly those with angiographic diameters of greater than 5 to 10 mm, and occurs at a rate of 2 to 4% per year. The incidence of SAH is 11 per 100,000 and, in contrast to ischemic stroke and hypertensive hemorrhage, has not changed appreciably over the last three decades.[34,35]

After SAH, rehemorrhage, cerebral vasospasm, and hydrocephalus may further complicate ICU management and can prove fatal. **Rehemorrhage** occurs most frequently in the first 24 to 48 hours after initial SAH and is associated with a mortality of 60%.[36,37] **Cerebral vasospasm** typically occurs 1 to 2 weeks after SAH and is believed to be induced by degradation products of the subarachnoid clot.[38,39] Although angiographic vasospasm occurs in 60% of these patients, symptomatic vasospasm (new focal deficits or altered level of consciousness without other cause) is seen in only 20 to 40% of cases. Symptomatic vasospasm results from focal or global cerebral ischemia and may result in stroke or death. **Hydrocephalus** owing to obstruction of CSF drainage can occur abruptly after SAH, when it is associated with a poor prognosis, or more gradually over days to months, when symptoms usually respond favorably to CSF diversion procedures, such as ventriculostomy or shunt.[40,41] Various grading systems for SAH have been proposed (Table 5-3). An increasing grade implies decreasing likelihood of survival.[42,43]

PROGRESSIVE MASS LESIONS

Lesions that gradually enlarge over days to months often cause no symptom until they, or the surrounding zone of reactive edema, are large enough to distort or compress functionally important regions of the brain, induce elevated ICP or headache, or incite seizure activity. Brain abscesses and intracranial tumors behave in this fashion and, when symptoms are severe, acute, or those of herniation, prompt admission to the ICU is in order.

Abscesses

Brain Abscess

The most common cause of intracranial abscess has traditionally been extension of untreated or undertreated infections of the paranasal sinuses or otitis/mastoiditis.[44,45] The incidence of brain abscess has markedly declined over the last few decades, likely as a result of improved antibiotic treatment of predisposing disorders, yet mortality remains as high as 60%. Chronic immunosuppression, bacteremia, and iatrogenic infections are other common causes of this disorder.[44-46]

For most bacterial brain abscesses, the initial phase is a cerebritis in which the involved tissue is softened and infiltrated by bacteria and reactive cells.[47] Over a period of a few weeks, the infection is usually sequestered within a firm, avascular capsule, which inhibits entry of antibiotics and expands as the infection proceeds. A zone of vasogenic edema, often several times the volume of the abscess, usually surrounds the abscess and can directly cause neurologic dysfunction in addition to contributing to mass effect. At this time, neuroimaging studies generally show a ring-enhancing lesion that may be indistinguishable from tumor (Fig. 5-5). Fungal, parasitic, and other infectious mass lesions (e.g., tuberculomas) are comparatively rare but are increasing in frequency primarily as a result of human immunodeficiency virus infections.

Subdural Empyema

Purulent infections of the subdural space may result from direct extension of a parameningeal infection such

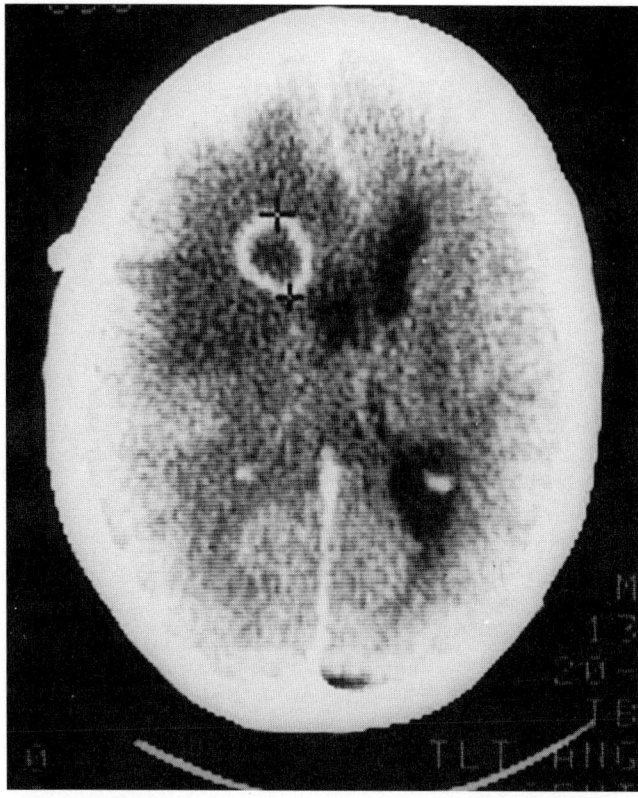

Fig. 5-5. Right frontal lobe abscess defined by ring-enhancing capsule. Note the exuberant area of surrounding edema and the midline shift.

Table 5-3. Commonly Used Subarachnoid Hemorrhage Grading Systems

Hunt-Hess Scale
  I. Asymptomatic or mild headache and slight nuchal rigidity
 II. Moderate to severe headache, nuchal rigidity, no neurologic deficit other than cranial nerve palsy
III. Confusion, drowsiness, or mild focal signs
 IV. Stupor, moderate to severe hemiparesis, possibly early decerebrate rigidity and vegetative disturbances
  V. Deep coma, decerebrated rigidity, moribund appearance
(Serious systemic disease such as hypertension, diabetes, or severe vasospasm seen on arteriography results in placement of the patient in the next less favorable category)

Cooperative Aneurysm Study Scale
  I. Free of symptoms
 II. Mildly ill, alert, and responsive, headache present
III. Moderately ill
    a. Lethargic, headache, no focal signs
    b. Alert, major focal signs present
 IV. Severely ill
    a. Stuporous, no focal signs
    b. Drowsy, major focal signs present
  V. Coma, moribund, and/or extensor posturing

World Federation of Neurological Surgeons Scale
  I. Glasgow Coma Scale score 15, no headache or focal signs
 II. Glasgow Coma Scale score 15, headache, nuchal rigidity, no focal signs
III. Glasgow Coma Scale score 13-14, can have headache or nuchal rigidity, no focal signs
 IV. a. Glasgow Coma Scale score 13-14, can have headache, nuchal rigidity, or focal signs
    b. Glasgow Coma Scale score 9-12, can have headache, nuchal rigidity, or focal signs
  V. Glasgow Coma Scale score 8 or less, can have headache, nuchal rigidity, or focal signs

(Data from Hunt, W. E., and Hess, R. M.: Surgical risk as related to time intervention in the repair of intracranial aneurysms. J. Neurosurg., 28: 14, 1968; and Torner, J. C., et al.: Reliability of neurological grading scales in subarachnoid hemorrhage: report of the Cooperative Aneurysm Study. In Cerebrovascular Diseases. Edited by F. Plum and W. Pulsinelli. New York, Raven Press, 1985, p. 77; and Adams, H. P., and Biller, J.: Hemorrhagic intracranial vascular disease. In Clinical Neurology. Vol. 2. Edited by R. J. Joynt. Philadelphia, J. B. Lippincott, 1992, p. 12.)

as sinusitis or as a result of trauma or neurosurgical procedures.[44-46] Untreated they spread over the cerebral surface, inciting an inflammatory reaction that often results in thrombophlebitis with seizures and stroke. CT and MRI show marked contrast enhancement of the meninges about a nonenhancing fluid collection (Fig. 5-6).

Tumors

A wide variety of tumors, both primary and metastatic, may affect the brain. Tumors within the substance of the brain are referred to as intraparenchymal or intra-axial, whereas tumors of the meninges, cranial nerves, and skull are called extra-axial. Brain tumors may cause symptoms in a variety of ways, including the mechanisms common to mass lesions (as discussed previously), seizures, and direct destruction of brain tissue. As with abscesses, exuberant vasogenic edema may be precipitated by some tumors. Although symptom progression is typically subacute and relentless, acute deterioration may prompt ICU admission owing to hemorrhage into the tumor; obstruction of CSF flow by the tumor; or seizure resulting in hypoventilation, hypercapnea, and herniation.

PRE-ICU PHASE

Initial management of the patient with suspected intracranial hypertension requires the physician or emergency medical team to perform several tasks, which when the

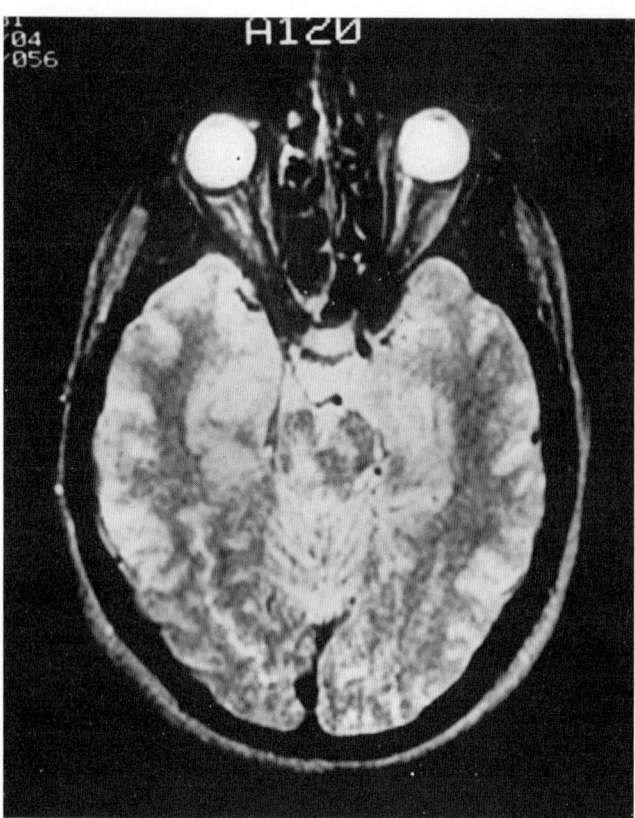

Fig. 5–6. The area of high signal on this T2-weighted MRI in right midbrain accounted for the patient's left hemiparesis. CT of this area was normal.

patient is seriously ill may need to be done concurrently. Foremost among these are:

- Patient stabilization
- Institution of brain therapy
- Neurologic and systemic assessment
- Triage

Patient Stabilization

Patient assessment and stabilization should begin at the site of the accident or attack and continue in the emergency room. Traditional "field" measures include intravenous access and fluid administration, airway management, respiratory support, and, in trauma, spinal immobilization.[48,49] Studies have supported the benefit of early aggressive actions, such as intubation, use of pulse oximetry to establish adequacy of oxygenation and administration of hyperosmolar agents. By reducing transport time to specialized trauma centers, air evacuation services are credited with reduced mortality and morbidity (although results are less clear in urban settings).[50,51] Emergency room measures focus on ventilation, normalization of systemic blood pressure, and, if present, reduction of elevated intracranial pressure. Protracted or even transient brain ischemia or hypoxia owing to hypotension or respiratory failure occurring up to 1 week after the initial insult may substantially worsen neurologic outcome. The neurologic assessment should not be considered valid until sustained oxygen saturations of greater than 90% and systolic pressures of at least 90 mm Hg are attained.

Airway and Ventilation

Impaired consciousness from brain injury may cause airway obstruction, aspiration, and altered ventilatory patterns. Despite improvements in management in recent years, some studies suggest that airway protection and management is inadequate in up to 42% of patients undergoing transfer to a brain injury unit.[52,53] In cases of trauma, thoracic injuries, such as hemothorax/pneumothorax, flail chest, and pulmonary contusions, may also compromise pulmonary function in this setting and are associated with a poor outcome.[54]

Oral or nasal devices may be used to establish an airway. Oral airways are difficult to place in agitated patients and may induce gagging or vomiting. Nasal airways are usually better tolerated, but they (and nasogastric tubes) should be used with caution after facial trauma unless basal skull fracture has been excluded. Patients with impending respiratory failure or obstruction, patients with suspected intracranial hypertension (IH), and those requiring sedation or paralysis should be intubated.

If IH is suspected, pretreatment with intravenous 20% mannitol 0.5 to 1.0 g/kg, mask hyperventilation (except in the presence of an anterior skull fracture), and a short-acting barbiturate (e.g., methohexital) or nondepolarizing neuromuscular blocker (e.g., vecuronium) should be considered in an effort to avoid high ICP and possible brain herniation during the act of intubation.

Normalization of Systemic Blood Pressure

Hypotension is almost never due to raised ICP or other CNS injury unless (1) there is a physiologic transection of the cervical or high thoracic spinal cord resulting in spinal shock or (2) the patient has suffered massive lower brain stem damage such as with tonsillar herniation. Treatable causes of hypotension, such as hypovolemia or myocardial infarction, should be assessed. Resuscitative measures in the setting of hypotension center on fluid administration. In patients with suspected intracranial injuries, hypotonic fluids are to be avoided so as to minimize potentiation of brain swelling. Suitable solutions include 0.9% sodium chloride or Ringer's lactate (with or without dextrose), 5% albumin, 25% albumin, high molecular weight dextran, plasma, or blood. Isotonic colloid solutions seem to have little advantage over isotonic crystalloids. Hyperosmolar agents such as hypertonic saline solutions may be superior to isotonic fluids, at least in early resuscitation because they tend to lower ICP while repleting intravascular volume.[55,56] Clearly blood and blood products should be considered in the presence of anemia or factor deficiency. Pressor, inotropic, and chronotropic agents should not be used in lieu of appropriate fluid resuscitation but may be used in accordance with the general principles of management of shock. A minimum systolic blood pressure of 90 mm Hg should be sought. Systemic hypertension after brain injury is an ominous sign and may indicate elevated ICP or brain stem compression. Efforts to reduce systemic

Table 5–4. Guidelines for Neurologic History Taking in Acute Brain Injury

Nature of Event
Symptoms and events leading to episode
Trauma
    Cause (e.g., MVA, fall, crush, gunshot)
    Severity (e.g., velocities/restraint, height/surface, what/weight, caliber/range)

Patient Condition
Alteration of consciousness? How long?
Hypotension or hypoxia
Interval between event and medical attention
Neurologic condition at first examination
Neurologic course

Past Medical History
Neurologic disorders (seizures, syncope, deficits)
Ethanol or substance abuse
Medications
Allergies

MVA, Motor vehicle accident.

---

hypertension may compromise cerebral perfusion pressure; however, spontaneous systolic pressures of greater than 200 mm Hg should be reduced because it may limit edema generation from hydrostatic pressure.

Assessment

The foundation of neurologic assessment is the history and the neurologic examination. Radiographic examinations are of ever-increasing importance in the diagnosis of cranial or spinal injuries. Indications for use of such studies are controversial; however, suggested guidelines are presented here.

History

When the patient is lucid and conscious, a detailed account of the accident or event and the patient's previous health may be determined. Under less ideal circumstances (which usually prevail whenever the injury is severe or the patient has suffered amnesia or loss of consciousness), information is generally sparse, must be quickly obtained, and is commonly provided by paramedical personnel. Data collection must be directed at determining the factors occurring either before or after the event that may influence outcome and, for trauma, the likelihood of severe head or systemic injury (Table 5-4).

Examination

Blunt traumatic head injury is commonly divided into three categories: mild, moderate, and severe. The criteria for these divisions may vary; however, they are usually determined by the patient's first neurologic evaluation after systemic stabilization in the emergency room as gauged by some variant of the Glasgow Coma Scale (GCS) (Table 5-5):[57] The scale was designed as a means to track the course of head-injured patients within each category. As subset scores are not equivalent (i.e., a 3 on the eye scale is not of the same significance as a 3 on the motor scale), it was not intended that the subset scores be added to produce a total GCS score. Nonetheless, total GCS scores do have some prognostic significance. A GCS score of 14 or greater is often designated a mild injury with a good prognosis, 9 to 13 as moderate with an indeterminate outcome, and 8 or lower as a severe head injury that will likely result in a poor outcome or death. Age, best motor response, and pupillary response are grossly accurate predictors of long-term outcome in 90% of head-injured patients in one series. GCS scores of head-injured children or adults with nonconcussive head injuries do not have the prognostic significance as those cited here.

Low total GCS scores are good at predicting the presence of diffuse CNS injuries, tract disruption, and intracranial mass lesions. This system does not take into account, however, other ominous findings, such as cranial nerve palsies or skull fractures, that may exist in cases with high GCS scores but may portend subsequent deterioration. Moreover, confounding factors such as intoxication, postictal states, and metabolic derangements may result in a falsely low GCS score. As such, the GCS score alone is an insufficient neurologic examination on which to make therapeutic and triage decisions.[58,59] Accurate neurologic assessment demands the most complete appropriate examination that the patient's condition allows. Suggestions for the examination in patients with mild and more severe cases are presented in Tables 5-6 and 5-7.

The neurologic examination may be substantially worsened by profound hypotension (i.e, systolic blood pressure less than 60 mm Hg). Although examinations performed under mild to moderate hypotension (60 to 90 mm Hg) are usually valid, it is recommended that judgment regarding the severity of neurologic damage be withheld until a sustained systolic pressure of greater than 90 mm Hg is obtained.

Neuroimaging

Skull radiographs can provide valuable information in the assessment of patients with traumatic head injuries. Their use in other acute brain disorders is limited largely to detection of raised ICP (see Chap. 4). Criteria for obtaining these studies are controversial because most skull x-ray

---

Table 5–5. Glasgow Coma Scale Score

Eyes
4 Spontaneously open
3 Open to command
2 Open to pain
1 No opening

Verbal
5 Coherent
4 Confused
3 Mumbles/garbled
2 Groans
1 No vocalization

Motor
6 Follows instructions
5 Localizes to pain
4 Normal flexion to pain
3 Abnormal flexion to pain
2 Extension to pain
1 No response

Table 5-6. Guidelines for Neurologic Examination after Brain Injury: All Patients

Level of consciousness (awake, drowy, stuporous, obtunded, coma)
Glasgow Coma Scale score
Cranial nerves II-X, including
    Pupillary responses
    Corneal reflexes
    Oculocephalic/caloric
    Gag
    ± ciliospinal
    Presence of retinal hemorrhages
Myotatic reflexes
Sensory examination to pain
Presence or absence of Babinski or Hoffman responses
Evidence of skull fracture (for trauma or syncope)
    Linear
    Depressed
    Basilar
        Raccoon's eyes
        CSF rhinorrhea
        CSF otorrhea
        Hemotympanum/CSF
        Blood in external auditory meatus
        Battles's sign
        Cranial nerve VII and/or VIII palsy
Evidence of facial fracture (for trauma or syncope)
Respiratory pattern (hyperventilation)
Cranial or neck bruit
Systemic examination (for trauma or syncope)
    Skin (e.g., lacerations, abrasions, contusions)
    Cardiopulmonary (e.g., blood pressure, breath sounds, rubs, ABGs)
    Spine (tenderness)
    Abdomen (tenderness, ecchymoses, rigidity, sounds, hematuria, ± lavage)
    Limbs (fractures, dislocations, hematomas, pulses)
    Laboratory tests—electrolytes, serum glucose, calcium, magnesium phosphate, complete blood count, toxicology screening

ABGs, Arterial blood gases; CSF, cerebrospinal fluid.

Table 5-7. Guidelines for Neurologic Examination after Brain Injury: Mild Injuries

Orientation (person, place, time)
Recollection of accident (anterograde, retrograde amnesia; loss of consciousness)
Recent memory, long-term memory
Cranial nerves I, XI, XII and confrontation visual fields
Strength, drift, coordination
Remainder of sensory examination
Gait (e.g., if spinal fracture excluded)

Table 5-8. Guidelines for Skull Radiographs after Head Trauma (anteroposterior, lateral, and Towne's views)

GCS score of 13 or less
GCS score of 14 or more with
    History of amnesia or loss of consciousness
    Suspected fracture by physical examination
    Complaint of severe headache

GCS, Glasgow Coma Scale.

or multiply injured patient is being stabilized in the emergency suite.

The presence of cervical spine injuries in conjunction with head injuries has been estimated to be as high as 10 to 15%.[60,61] Lateral **cervical spine radiographs** are therefore obtained in patients meeting the aforementioned criteria for skull radiographs. The area from C1 through the top of T1 must be assessed for fracture, retropharyngeal swelling, or malalignment. Adequate visualization of the cervicothoracic junction may require traction on the upper limbs during the exposure or a "swimmer's view." Complaints of neck pain should prompt more extensive studies, including anteroposterior, oblique, and open mouth odontoid views. (The physician should bear in mind that cervical collars or other restraints may temporarily align an unstable cervical fracture—particularly type II odontoid fractures—making radiographic diagnosis difficult.

CT has become the definitive radiographic means of assessing the cranial vault, base of skull, upper and lower cervical regions, and intracranial cavity after head injury. Practical and safety issues tend to restrict the use of CT after head injury. Most hospitals do not have a CT imager in the emergency room complex, and technicians are not necessarily "in-house" at all hours. Therefore transport of a potentially unstable patient or delay until a technician is available may be required to obtain this study. Also, certain early lesions such as developing EDHs, SDHs, and zones of contusion and ischemia may not be visible on an initial scan.[62,63] Our criteria for CT scanning after head injury in stabilized patients are summarized in Table 5-9.

There is usually sufficient time to get a limited CT examination (i.e., single slices through the brain stem, third ventricle, high lateral ventricles) to assess the need for neurosurgical intervention, even in unstable patients. Late

films after head injury are normal; yet the presence of a radiographically documented skull fracture increases the chances of significant intracranial pathology by 200%, and more than 75% of traumatic intracranial hematomas are associated with skull fractures. Our guidelines for obtaining skull radiographs are presented in Table 5-8. These x-ray films should be examined for linear or depressed fractures, indirect evidence of fracture such as intracranial air or air-fluid levels in the sphenoid sinus, foreign bodies, or evidence of mass lesions by shift in the position of a calcified pineal gland. Portable radiographs by experienced technicians are usually satisfactory, so these studies can almost always be obtained while the severely injured

Table 5-9. Guidelines for Computed Tomography Imaging after Head Trauma

GCS score of 13 or less in absence of intoxication
GCS score of 11 or less in presence of intoxication
Sustained deterioration of 2 GCS points or development of focal neurologic deficit
Presence of skull fracture (clinical or radiographic)
Inability to visualize a cervical spine structure adequately
Early use of general anesthesia for surgical repair of non-CNS injury after a concussive injury that produced altered consciousness

CNS, Central nervous system; GCS, Glasgow Coma Scale.

generation imagers can perform a complete intracranial study in virtually the same amount of scan time as older machines take to provide three slices. As such, the indications for diagnostic burr holes are limited to patients with very low GCS scores (8 or less) or lateralizing neurologic signs (e.g., pupillary dilatation) in the presence of severe hypotension that is refractory to medical management.

CT evidence of hemorrhage in the corpus callosum, third ventricle, and subarachnoid space are characteristic of so-called shear injuries. In contrast to patients with expanding mass lesions, these patients are usually immediately comatose, have low ICPs, and rarely harbor a skull fracture, and serial CT imaging shows dilation of the ventricular system over a period of weeks in response to loss of white matter.

One study suggests that CT imaging may be a better indicator of clinical deterioration than the neurologic examination in certain instances.[16] Hemispheric swelling and obliteration of the basal subarachnoid cisterns on CT imaging are particularly ominous findings after head trauma.[64-66] Penetrating injuries by nonmetallic foreign bodies may, however, not be accurately diagnosed by CT.

CT is recognized as the most sensitive and accurate imaging technique for the diagnosis of **acute intracranial hemorrhage**, including all forms of hemorrhagic stroke. The definitive diagnosis of acute intracerebral hemorrhage is made by the presence of high density within the brain parenchyma on CT. (Hemorrhage in the presence of anemia [hemoglobin less than 10 g/dl] may fail to demonstrate these findings.) Blood is visualized in 90% of SAH, the extent and persistence of which are correlated with the risk of developing vasospasm. Most benign intra-axial brain tumors appear as nonenhancing zones of low density (with or without mass effect), whereas most benign extra-axial lesions enhance after administration of intravenous contrast. Most malignant intra-axial tumors (both primary and metastatic) and abscesses enhance and are surrounded by zones of low density edema. Subdural empyemas demonstrate meningeal enhancement about a low density subdural collection of purulence.

MRI has opened up new dimensions in the diagnosis and prognostication of traumatic and nontraumatic brain injury. MRI appears to be far more sensitive in demonstrating nonhemorrhagic, brain stem, or extra-axial lesions than CT (Fig. 5-6), and images may show some intraparenchymal contusions and tissue derangements that CT never shows.[67,68] Although CT is superior to MRI for the detection of acute (less than 3 days old) intracerebral hemorrhage, the two techniques are nearly equal for subacute (3 days to 3 weeks) hemorrhages, and MRI is superior for detection of chronic bleeds. CT surpasses MRI for demonstration of SAH.

Although techniques of monitoring and supporting critically ill patients have been defined, the logistical considerations usually preclude MRI in the setting of severe head injury or multiple internal injuries.[69] MRI has proved sensitive and reasonably practical in the evaluation of spinal injuries. MRI provides several advantages over CT for the diagnosis of intracranial tumors and abscesses. MRI is more sensitive than CT and may demonstrate additional lesions than found by CT. Lesions of the posterior fossa, skull base, and proximate to the calvarium are difficult to visualize with CT because of bone artifact, which is absent on MRI. Further, many primary brain tumors extend well beyond CT boundaries, better correlating with certain types of MRI acquisition techniques. MRI is also more flexible than CT in terms of the planes of image presentation without the need for special medical image workstations.

Cerebral angiography has been largely replaced by the aforementioned imaging techniques and **magnetic resonance angiography** (MRA). Angiography may still prove useful after serious head injury if CT and MRI are unavailable or when vascular compromise is suspected, such as in the setting of delayed neurologic deficits or when intracranial or neck bruits are detected. Although MRA can demonstrate such lesions as well as intracranial aneurysms and vascular malformations, its sensitivity has not been fully established, and angiography remains the standard.

Triage

The emergency room disposition of patients with brain injuries ranges from discharge to ICU admission, at times requiring emergency craniotomy or other surgical intervention. Complicating the decision process is the fact that the full extent of the injury may not be initially apparent; this is particularly true of traumatic brain injury. Guidelines for allowing a patient to return home after traumatic brain injury are presented in Table 5-10. A responsible person accompanying the patient is typically given instructions for observation and a list of conditions for which the patient should be returned for medical evaluation or care.

All other patients with traumatic brain injury are usually admitted to a regular neurosurgical floor or the ICU for observation and care. Hospitals with large volumes of intoxicated patients with head injuries may have a special overnight area in the emergency room to avoid overwhelming regular inpatient facilities. Hospitalized patients are placed on frequent neurologic checks with monitoring of GCS score, pupillary symmetry, and limb strength. Patients requiring surgery or ICP monitoring or those risking neurologic deterioration are admitted to the ICU, and a neurosurgical consultation is obtained (Table 5-11). Patients with nontraumatic brain injuries are usually admitted to the hospital for observation or treatment in the setting of an acute or rapidly progressive focal neurologic deficit or loss of consciousness. Such symptoms and signs in the presence of a demonstrable or suspected intracranial mass lesion usually dictate ICU admission and neurosurgical consultation.

Table 5-10. Guidelines for Emergency Room Discharge to Home after Traumatic Brain Injury

Patient is neurologically normal, has been throughout the accident, and has no clinical or radiographic evidence of fracture
Patient is now neurologically normal (or baseline) but had suffered altered consciousness and has
  No evidence of skull fracture or other injury
  Close access to a neurosurgical center (< 15 min)
  Someone who can spend the next 24 hours with the patient and administer a head chart

Table 5–11. Guidelines for ICU Admission and Neurosurgical Assessment

Intracranial hemorrhage
Hydrocephalus
Large contusion amenable to decompression
Candidate for intracranial pressure monitoring
Cerebrospinal fluid rhinorrhea or otorrhea
Penetrating injuries or depressed fracture
Nontraumatic lesion associated with mass effect and altered consciousness
Neurologic deterioration suspected to be due to cerebral vasospasm

ICU PHASE

Intensive care management of the brain-injured patient is primarily directed toward prevention of secondary metabolic or ischemic brain injuries and toward preventing, detecting, and treating systemic complications. Even without direct traumatic injury to other organ systems, derangements of pulmonary, cardiac, coagulation, and gastrointestinal systems may occur that may lead to a worsening of the patient's neurologic condition or death.

Intracranial Pressure

The potential for elevations in ICP that may result in focal or global brain ischemia is a feature common to all the disorders discussed in this chapter. ICP management has traditionally been the thrust of ICU treatment of brain injury, often at the expense of the well-being of other organ systems. These principles of ICP measurement and management are presented in Chapter 4. Contemporary ICU approaches to brain injury commonly consider elevated ICP to be but one, albeit important, variable of the overall evaluation and treatment equation.

Systemic Management and Assessment

Cardiopulmonary Factors

Brain injuries are commonly associated with large abrupt elevations in **circulating catecholamine** levels.[70] These may lead to cardiac dysrhythmias, cardiac ischemia, and neurogenic pulmonary edema.[71] Post-traumatic hypokalemia may exacerbate arrhythmias.[72] Cardiac enzymes should be followed for several days after head injury and isoenzymes and electrocardiograms (ECGs) obtained for large elevations or changes in ECG monitor patterns. Arrhythmias and cardiac ischemia may be mitigated or prevented by early administration of beta-adrenergic blocking agents.

Blood pressure regulation is recommended so as to prevent acute brain ischemia in zones of edema or around mass lesions in response to hypotension. Also, excessive blood pressure (i.e., systolic pressures of greater than 170 to 180 mm Hg) should probably be avoided because this may promote edema generation. The severity of diencephalic fits (episodic abnormal posturing, diaphoresis, tachycardia, and hypertension) may be lessened by use of beta-adrenergic blocking agents.

Aspiration pneumonitis frequently complicates a severe head injury. A sputum culture followed by empiric use of a late-generation cephalosporin and aminoglycoside antibiotic is suggested for documented aspiration or the strong clinical suspicion of aspiration even before x-ray changes are apparent. The development of pulmonary edema requires placement of a pulmonary artery catheter and may necessitate use of positive pressure ventilation, positive end-expiratory pressure (PEEP), or continuous positive airway pressure (CPAP). PEEP and CPAP are usually well tolerated unless the levels of positive pressure are greater than 10 mm Hg and intracranial compliance poor.[73]

Neurogenic pulmonary edema can be distinguished from non-neurogenic causes by the high fluid protein and low pulmonary artery wedge pressure associated with the former. Electron microscopy has shown sphincterlike annular constrictions in pulmonary veins that constrict after head injury and may have a role in the development of this disorder.[74] Chlorpromazine may be useful in the treatment of neurogenic pulmonary edema.

Tracheostomy may be required in patients with prolonged intubation or in those who cannot protect an airway. Patients with GCS scores of 7 or less are so likely to need a tracheostomy that early tracheostomy is advocated in this group.[75]

Nutrition

Trauma patients of all ages have markedly elevated **nutritional requirements.** Acute brain injury alone may lead to elevations of the metabolic rate equal to those found after multiple systemic injury. Estimations of resting energy expenditure from standard formulas may grossly underestimate nutritional requirements.[76] Early nutrition may reduce the incidence and severity of multiorgan failure or wound complications. Administration of beta-adrenergic blockers or barbiturates can substantially reduce these metabolic demands.[77,78]

Hypoalbuminemia is common after acute brain injury and is associated with a poor prognosis in critically ill patients. The goal of meeting these requirements can usually be met with either enteral or parenteral feedings. It is our experience, however, that absorption from enteral sources is unreliable, can make fluid management difficult, and increases the risk of aspiration pneumonia. We typically begin parenteral feedings on the second or third day after severe head injury and give 25% albumin for patients with serum albumin levels of less than 3.0 g/dl.

Clinical reports assert that parenteral **hyperalimentation** does not contribute to raised ICP. Experimental evidence and our own experience suggest that it does; consequently we increase diuretic (mannitol or furosemide) dosage as required to maintain ICP less than 15 to 20 mm Hg.

Lastly, stress response, total parenteral nutrition, or steroids may result in **hyperglycemia.** This has proved to be detrimental to ischemic tissues. Frequent glucose checks and, if necessary, insulin infusions may be required to keep the blood glucose level in the range between 100 and 200 mg/dl.[79]

Stress Ulcer Prophylaxis

Hemorrhagic gastritis has long been recognized as a complication of head injury (Cushing's ulcer) that may lead to further morbidity.[80] Agents that raise the pH of gastric secretions substantially reduce the risk of serious upper gastrointestinal hemorrhage owing to stress. Although sucralfate may theoretically reduce the risk of developing an aspiration pneumonia, we have not found it to be as effective in preventing upper gastrointestinal bleeding as H_2 blocking agents (such as ranitidine or famotidine) or a magnesium-aluminum antacid. Pancreatitis is a frequently unrecognized gastrointestinal complication of HI.[81]

Coagulopathy

Disorders of coagulation occur with unsettling frequency after head injury and predispose the patient to further intracranial or systemic hemorrhagic complications.[82] The prothrombin time, activated partial thromboplastin time, and platelet count should be monitored daily. Prolongation of these coagulation tests, fall in the platelet count, or clinical evidence of bleeding should prompt acquisition of a fibrinogen level, review of the blood smear, and tests of fibrin degradation products to detect disseminated intravascular coagulation. We favor aggressive correction of even mildly abnormal coagulation values.

Multiple Organ Dysfunction and Sepsis

Nearly half of severely head-injured patients harbor serious internal injuries.[83] Even in the absence of trauma, brain injury itself and protracted intubation may predispose to sepsis or dysfunction of one or more organ systems. The development of such disorders seriously complicates patient management, in which fluid, blood pressure, and blood flow manipulations are the mainstays of therapy. Strategies to address these issues are discussed elsewhere in this book. In general, a balance between optimal brain and systemic treatments is sought when they are at odds, unless to do so would clearly lead to death or irreparable brain injury.

ACUTE LESIONS

Although certain general ICU management principles apply to the broad spectrum of acute brain injuries, there are often specific considerations for a given type of injury.

Traumatic Brain Injury

Physiologic Monitoring

The cornerstone of closed traumatic brain injury is detection and control of elevated ICP. Unfortunately ICP measurement provides information only on the potential upper limit of cerebral blood flow and oxygen delivery and no information on tissue metabolism and integrity. Xenon inhalation techniques, single-photon emission computed tomography, positron-emission tomography (PET), jugular bulb catheters, transcranial Doppler, and laser flowmetry may all provide information on **cerebral blood flow,** and some (PET and jugular bulb catheters) provide data on brain metabolism. These primarily investigational techniques suggest that some traditional therapies for traumatic brain injury are probably best avoided. For instance, hyperventilation to control ICP after traumatic brain injury may generate metabolic evidence of brain ischemia and result in poorer outcome when compared with some other methods of management, such as CSF drainage, and tight blood pressure regulation to minimize edema generation may sufficiently impair perfusion to result in ischemia-induced edema.[84,85]

Electrophysiologic Monitoring

Techniques such as electroencephalography (EEG) and evoked potential monitoring (EPM) are used for diagnostic, monitoring, and prognostic purposes because they frequently show abnormal results after HI and may herald clinical neurologic deterioration. Unilateral and, in particular, bilateral absence or loss of evoked potentials has a grave prognosis, as does absence of EEG activity on initial examination.[86] Frequent or continuous EPM may prove useful in detecting early changes in neurologic condition, although a practical system with adequate sensitivity remains elusive.[87,88]

Cerebral Protection

Agents that protect against or reverse neurologic injury after brain trauma remain elusive. Corticosteroids are generally considered not to be of benefit after traumatic brain injury.[89,90] Laboratory studies of methylprednisolone analogs in animal models of traumatic brain injury and two multicenter spinal cord injury studies showing significant benefit from early (less than 6 hours after injury) administration of high dose methylprednisolone suggest that these agents may be useful in minimizing the effects of CNS trauma.[91,92] Investigational agents such as lazaroids, calcium-channel blockers, and amino acid analogs may provide other routes of brain protection and resuscitation in the future.[93]

Traumatic Intracranial Hemorrhage

The management of these disorders is largely surgical. Acute EDH and SDH require craniotomy for surgical evacuation, the former having the better prognosis. Similarly, intracerebral clots may be removed in an open procedure or treated using ICP management techniques; however, stereotactic techniques, such as those using thrombolysis, may provide a less invasive means of effecting clot evacuation.

Open Brain Injury

Risk of infection associated with loss of CSF containment is a focal point of open brain injuries. **Penetrating wounds,** such as gun shots or stabbing, and depressed fractures (in which the degree of depression equals skull thickness) require urgent, if not emergent, surgical exploration and debridement unless the patient is moribund. The use of antibiotic prophylaxis is recommended. Skull base fractures can cause **CSF rhinorrhea** or **otorrhea** that may eventually lead to meningitis. Fortunately, most traumatic CSF leaks spontaneously resolve without surgical intervention. Antibiotic prophylaxis is not recommended because if meningitis does develop, it is likely to be due to a resistant organism.[94,95]

Delayed Neurologic Deterioration

The specialist in intensive care should be aware of several conditions that may lead to neurologic deterioration days to weeks after the initial brain injury. Foremost are metabolic derangements leading to encephalopathy. **Hyponatremia,** formerly attributed to syndrome of inappropriate antidiuretic hormone (SIADH), has been shown in many instances to be due to cerebral salt wasting, perhaps mediated by atrial natriuretic peptide.[96-98] Treatment is by replacement of salt and volume, with fluid restriction reserved for cases of SIADH in which reduced blood volume is demonstrable.

Delayed intracranial hemorrhage has become increasingly recognized after head injury in the CT era. SDH and EDH can develop hours to weeks after head injury in the presence of a normal CT scan shortly after injury and lead to a progressive neurologic deficit.[99,100] Intracerebral clots ("Spat-Apoplexie") may occur up to 2 weeks after head injury, but usually do so in the setting of a previously abnormal CT scan.[101-103] Cerebrovascular complications other than hemorrhage may also occur after head injury. CNS infarction occurring 1 to 14 days after head injury is rare (occurring in about 2% of cases), may involve any vascular territory, and is probably due to direct vascular compression from an intracranial mass.[104] Vasospasm, as determined by transcranial Doppler hypervelocity, may also develop after head injury. Although pharmacologic manipulation to reduce these flows is possible, a beneficial effect on outcome has not been demonstrated.[103] Delayed nonhemorrhagic encephalopathy and limb tremor are other rare complications of head injury.[106,107]

Hemorrhagic Stroke

Intracerebral Hemorrhage

Identification of the cause of hemorrhage, correction of factors predisposing to rehemorrhage, management of ICP, vigilance and treatment of hydrocephalus, and cerebral protection are important issues in the early management of ICH. Coagulation and bleeding abnormalities should be recognized and corrected if the patient is expected to survive the event. Systemic hypertension is brought under control, often with continuous infusions of hypotensive agents such as sodium nitroprusside, and widely fluctuating pressures are stabilized with attention toward adequacy of intravascular volume and sedatives.

The principles of management of ICP and hydrocephalus are discussed in Chapter 4. Vasogenic brain edema surrounding the clot may contribute substantially to ICP elevations and neurologic dysfunction in the days after hemorrhage. Although their use is controversial,[108] I favor the use of corticosteroids in the first week after hemorrhage or when brain edema is significant. The role of clot evacuation is also unclear. Removal of the hemorrhage would theoretically be of benefit by decreasing stretch on local structures, removing acute and chronic sources of tissue injury, and allowing better control of ICP. Surgical and solely medical therapies, however, are both associated with poor outcomes in this disorder.[109] Stereotactic evacuation of intracerebral hematomas by use of thrombolytic agents instilled into the clot has proved promising,[110] but its role and indications for use remain undefined.

Aneurysmal Subarachnoid Hemorrhage

The management of SAH is qualitatively similar to that of ICH, but because the risk of rehemorrhage is high and the consequences dire, therapy is far more rigid in this disorder. A detailed review of our principles of management is presented in the review by Whiting and colleagues.[111]

Blood pressure is strictly controlled at levels that are normotensive (often less than 110 mm Hg, systolic) or lower for that patient because as **rehemorrhage** is associated with a 40% mortality. Patients are kept in quiet, dimly illuminated rooms.[112] Liberal use of sedation and even anesthesia with mechanical ventilation may be required to calm certain individuals.[113] Steroids may help reduce headache from blood-induced aseptic meningitis. Antifibrinolytics, once commonly used to reduce the risk of rebleeding, have been shown not to improve outcome and are associated with thrombotic complications.[114] Despite sedation, frequent CT scans and monitoring with transcranial Doppler can usually detect early hydrocephalus and vasospasm, often before they become clinically evident.

Hydrocephalus developing in the first hours after SAH is an ominous prognostic sign suggesting obstruction of intracerebral CSF drainage and requires urgent external drainage. Overdrainage must also be avoided so as to minimize the risk of rehemorrhage and lumbar puncture contraindicated because of the potential for rostrocaudal herniation. Ventricular enlargement may slowly progress over days, weeks, or even months after SAH and is typically due to malabsorption. During the ICU stay, judicious use of lumbar drainage or spinal taps may obviate the need for placement of a permanent CSF shunting system.

Patients are begun on a cerebroselective vasodilator, nimodipine, on admission to minimize the ischemic complications of **cerebral vasospasm.** Management of cerebral vasospasm is greatly facilitated if the aneurysm has been surgically obliterated because induced hypertension can then be used to prevent ischemia without a significant risk of inducing aneurysmal rehemorrhage. Systolic blood pressures are elevated to levels that induce clinical improvement, often to levels as high as 200 mm Hg.[115] Cardiac hemodynamics are also optimized with pulmonary artery occlusion pressures (typically 14 to 18 mm Hg) selected to maximize cardiac output and hematocrits maintained in the range of 35 to 40%.[116] Patients with unclipped aneurysms are treated similarly except that blood pressure is rarely elevated above 150 mm Hg systolic.[117]

Postcraniotomy Care

Patients are admitted to the ICU after craniotomy for close neurologic monitoring to detect early deterioration, blood pressure control to prevent rehemorrhage, and prevention and control of brain swelling. **Neurochecks** are abbreviated neurologic examinations focused on the region of the nervous system of interest. They are performed frequently (often every 15 minutes) immediately after surgery, then less often as the patient stabilizes and risk of deterioration diminishes. The medical team may often be alerted to developing brain swelling, bleeding, or ischemia well before herniation or other permanent damage occurs, by these observations when carefully performed.

In the course of intracranial surgery, arteries and veins are often transected and the stumps cauterized or clipped. These hemostatic actions are most vulnerable to failure resulting in rupture and hemorrhage in the first hours and days after surgery. Neurosurgeons often impose strict **blood pressure limits** on postoperative patients in an effort to minimize the risk of postoperative bleeding. Although seemingly arbitrary, levels chosen often reflect the surgeon's opinion on the competency of intracranial hemostasis. If postoperative blood pressure seems excessively low and risks systemic ischemia, the intensivist should consult the surgeon before modifying the blood pressure parameters.

Maintenance of low postoperative blood pressure may be required after resection of AVMs or correction of chronic carotid stenosis to prevent **reperfusion hemorrhage,** also known as normal perfusion pressure breakthrough syndrome.[28,29] Chronic, critically low brain perfusion pressures found in these settings may result in low terminal cerebral artery blood pressures, resulting in chronic cerebral vasodilatation with loss of autoregulation. When normal pressures are reestablished, cerebral arterioles are unable to vasoconstrict sufficiently to protect cerebral capillaries, resulting in edema generation and capillary rupture with hemorrhage. This disorder is often fatal, although it has been successfully managed by induction of barbiturate coma. Prevention, by maintaining low postoperative blood pressures, is warranted in patients at risk.

Brain retraction, manipulation, and resection of lesions such as tumors may induce considerable brain swelling. Management of postoperative **brain edema** uses the principles discussed in Chapter 4. Free water is restricted, but systemic hypovolemia is to be avoided to prevent blood hyperviscosity complications, such as systemic or intracranial venous thrombosis. Steroids may be used even in the absence of typical causes of vasogenic edema (tumors, blood, abscesses), but their role is controversial and may predispose to infection and hyperglycemia. Excessive blood pressure should be avoided to minimize hydrostatic pressure on the capillaries, and nutrition should be optimized to maintain normal blood oncotic pressure. Hyperosmolar agents are usually reserved for treatment of documented brain edema.

Progressive Mass Lesions. Patients with progressive mass lesions are usually admitted to ICU management for assessment of acute neurologic or systemic deterioration, systemic support, treatment of ICP, or control of seizures. These subjects are addressed in Chapters 4 and 6.

Pulmonary embolus occurs frequently in those patients who are nonambulatory, especially those with brain tumors, and may be fatal. Treatment is limited in the immediate postcraniotomy period to vena cava filters because anticoagulation and thrombolytic therapy risk intracranial hemorrhage. These agents are relatively contraindicated for the first 10 to 14 days after intracranial surgery but may be used thereafter without substantial risk of intracranial complications even in patients with malignant brain tumors.

Dexamethasone and methylprednisolone are used commonly in the management of brain edema owing to **tumor** or **abscess** because they have minimal salt-retaining effects and are potent inhibitors of vasogenic edema. Despite the theoretic risk of potentiating the growth of brain abscesses, steroid use is warranted, especially in the first days to weeks, because brain edema itself may prove life-threatening. As always, systemic hypovolemia is to be avoided in the management of these disorders and should be corrected if present.

POST-ICU PHASE

Management of the brain-injured patient after leaving the ICU centers on preventing ICU readmission and formulating a plan for rehabilitation and reintegration into society.

ICU Readmission

Causes for ICU readmission include premature ICU discharge and delayed development of the complications cited previously. The clinician should have a high index of suspicion with regard to deep vein thrombosis resulting in pulmonary embolus. Pulmonary angiography or lower limb venography should be considered in the setting of unexplained fever, limb swelling, hypoxia, or hypotension. Other causes of delayed or persistent fever after head injury include aspiration pneumonia, sinusitis, pancreatitis, urinary tract infection, and drug reaction. "Central fever" is exceedingly rare and should be considered a diagnosis of exclusion.

Placement and Rehabilitation

Prognosis

Functional disability is common after brain injury, particularly in trauma patients.[118] A number of clinical and laboratory assessments may prove useful predictors of outcome. Several of these have been discussed previously. Among common ICU measures of acuity, GCS score, and injury severity score are the best predictors of outcome from head injury, whereas trauma injury severity score (TISS) is the best predictor of level of ICU care.[119-121] Other factors contributing to poor outcome include low preinjury vocational status, patient age, chronic alcohol abuse or intoxication at injury, and high physical or psychologic difficulties.[122,123] Curiously, high preinjury intelligence does not appear to lead to greater recovery potential. Instead this group suffers the greatest loss in after-injury; this group may have the largest postinjury reductions in IQ.[124] Laboratory tests that may be prognostic include CSF creatine kinase,[125] and depressed cerebral metabolic rate of oxygen and cerebral blood flow.[126]

Rehabilitation

Specialized head injury rehabilitation programs have been developed in an effort to improve and recovery after brain injury. The effects of these programs on comatose patients are controversial. Attempts to hasten arousal and therefore the cognitive rehabilitation of comatose patients by various forms of sensory stimulation have met with mixed results. Pierce et al. reported that vigorous multimodality stimulation failed to have any effect on levels of consciousness or time to obey a simple command despite favorable results in their pilot study.[127]

Cognitive and other neurologic disorders as well as social issues after mild to moderate brain injury may have a negative impact on the patient's rehabilitation potential. Moderately head-injured patients often have poor insight into the nature and extent of their deficits, and post-traumatic epilepsy limits recovery and social reintegration.[128] Denial of the severity and consequences of head injury may be practiced by both the patient and family. Health care workers may develop an adversarial relationship with them if they vigorously attempt to dismiss this psychologic defense mechanism.[129] A well-planned and well-implemented physical and cognitive rehabilitation program is critical for this group of patients. Although the majority of patients with minor brain injury fully recover, injury commonly results in cognitive defects that persist for a few weeks, but defects may persist for months.[130] PET imaging may confirm metabolic abnormalities in such patients.[131] Neuropsychologic testing may be required to document subtle although functionally significant deficits.[132] Last, a note of caution: The cognitive and physical gains made after brain injury may not be permanent. There is mounting evidence that brain injury can accelerate cognitive changes of aging or that previous focal neurologic deficits may recur as the patient ages.[133,134]

In conclusion, critical care management of brain-injured patients is generally complex, and effective therapy requires a comprehensive approach to early treatment. As a result, many patients with even moderate injury may return to productive lives when properly assessed, stabilized, and treated.

REFERENCES

1. Adams, R. D., and Victor, M. (eds.): Principles of Neurology. 2nd Ed. New York, McGraw-Hill, 1981.
2. Kandel, E. R., and Schwartz, J. H. (eds.): Principles of Neural Science. 2nd Ed. New York, Elsevier, 1985.
3. Patten, J.: Neurological Differential Diagnosis. New York, Springer-Verlag, 1980.
4. Lee, S. T.: Features of head injury in a developing country—Taiwan (1977–1987). J. Trauma, 30:194, 1990.
5. Sosin, D. M., Sacks, J. J., and Smith, S. M.: Head injury–associated deaths in the United States from 1979 to 1986. JAMA, 262:2251, 1989.
6. Gennarelli, T. A. et al.: Mortality of patients with head injury and extracranial injury treated in trauma centers. J. Trauma, 29:1193, 1989.
7. MacKilloop, H. I.: Effects of seatbelt legislation and reduction of highway speed limits in Ontario. Can. Med. Assoc., 119:1154, 1978.
8. Krantz, K. P. G.: Head and neck injuries to motorcycle and moped riders—with special regard to the effect of protective helmets. Injury, 16:253, 1985.
9. Wasserman, R. C., and Buccini, R. V.: Helmet protection from head injuries among recreational bicyclists. Am. J. Sports Med., 18:96, 1990.
10. Thompson, R. S., Rivara, F. P., and Thompson, D. C.: A case-controlled study of the effectiveness of bicycle safety helmets. N. Engl. J. Med., 320:1361, 1989.
11. Becker, D. P., et al.: The outcome from severe head injury with early diagnosis and intensive management. J. Neurosurg., 47:491, 1977.
12. MacKenzie, E. J., Edelstein, S. L., and Flynn, J. P.: Trends in hospitalized discharge rates for head injury in Maryland, 1976–86. Am. J. Public Health, 80:217, 1990.
13. Klauber, M. R., et al.: Determinants of head injury mortality: importance of the low risk patient. Neurosurgery, 24:31, 1989.
14. Colohan, A. R., et al.: Head injury mortality in two centers with different emergency medical services and intensive care. J. Neurosurg., 71:202, 1989.
15. Best, J. G., Cales, R. H., and Gazzaniga, A. B.: Impact of regionalization. The Orange County experience. Arch. Surg. 118:740, 1983.
16. Bowers, S. A., and Marshall, L. F.: Outcome in 200 consecutive cases of severe head injury treated in San Diego county: a prospective analysis. Neurosurgery, 6:237, 1980.
17. Lowe, D. K., et al.: Patterns of death, complication, and error in the management of motor vehicle accident victims: implications for a regional system of trauma care. J. Trauma, 23:503, 1983.
18. Miller, J. D., et al.: Further experience in the management of severe brain injury. J. Neurosurg., 54:289, 1981.
19. Miller, J. D., et al.: Significance of intracranial hypertension in severe head injury. J. Neurosurg., 47:503, 1977.
20. Ommaya, A. K., and Gennarelli, T. A.: Cerebral concussion and traumatic unconsciousness: correlation of experimental and clinical observations on blunt head injuries. Brain, 97:633, 1974.
21. Gennarelli, T. A., et al.: Diffuse axonal injury and traumatic coma in the primate. Ann. Neurol., 12:564, 1982.
22. Gennarelli, T. A., and Thibault, L. E.: Biomechanics of acute subdural hematoma. J. Trauma, 22:680, 1982.
23. Cordobes, F., et al.: Observations on 82 patients with extradural hematoma: comparison of results before and after the advent of computerized tomography. J. Neurosurg., 54:179, 1981.
24. Gurdjian, E. S., Webster, J. E., and Lissner, H. R.: The mechanism of skull fracture. J. Neurosurg., 7:106, 1950.
25. Cole, F. M., and Yates, P. O.: Pseudo-aneurysms in relationship to massive cerebral hemorrhage. J. Neurol. Neurosurg. Psychiatry, 30:61, 1967.
26. Weinfeld, F. D.: The national survey of stroke. Stroke, 12(Suppl. 1):1, 1981.
27. Voigt, K., and Yasargil, M. G.: Cerebral cavernous haemangiomas or cavernomas. Neurochirurgia (Stuttg.), 19:59, 1976.
28. Barnett, G. H., et al.: Cerebral circulation in AVM surgery. Neurosurgery, 20:836, 1987.
29. Spetzler, R. F., et al.: Normal perfusion pressure breakthrough theory. Clin. Neurosurg., 25:651, 1978.
30. Forster, D. M. C., Steiner, L., and Hakanson, S.: Arteriovenous malformation of the brain: a long-term clinical study. J. Neurosurg., 37:562, 1972.
31. Drake, C. G.: Cerebral arteriovenous malformations: considerations for and experience with surgical treatment in 166 cases. Clin. Neurosurg., 226:145, 1979.
32. Perret, G., and Nishioka, H.: Arteriovenous malformations: an analysis of 545 cases of cranio-cerebral arteriovenous malformations and fistulae reported to the cooperative study. J. Neurosurg., 25:467, 1966.
33. Crompton, M. R.: The pathogenesis of cerebral aneurysms. Brain, 89:797, 1966.
34. Sundt, T. M., Jr., and Whisnant, J. P.: Subarachnoid hemorrhage from intracranial aneurysms: surgical management

and natural history of disease. N. Engl. J. Med., 299:116, 1978.
35. Drake, C. G.: Management of cerebral aneurysm. Stroke, 12:273, 1981.
36. Kassell, N. F., and Torner, J. C.: Aneurysmal rebleeding: a preliminary report from the Cooperative Aneurysm Study. Neurosurgery, 13:479, 1983.
37. Locksley, H. B.: Report on the Cooperative Study of Intracranial Aneurysms and SAH; section V, part II: natural history of SAH, intracranial aneurysms and AVM. Based on 6368 cases in the cooperative study. J. Neurosurg., 25:321, 1966.
38. Kassell, N. F., Sasaki, T., Colohan, A. R., and Nazar, G.: Cerebral vasospasm following aneurysmal subarachnoid hemorrhage. Stroke, 16:562, 1985.
39. Fischer, C. M., Kistler, J. P., and Davis, J. M.: Relation of cerebral vasospasm to SAH visualized by computerized tomographic scanning. Neurosurgery, 6:1, 1980.
40. Ropper, A. H., and Zervas, N. T.: Outcome one year after SAH from cerebral aneurysm. J. Neurosurg., 56:753, 1984.
41. Youmans, J.: Special problems associated with subarachnoid hemorrhage. Neurol. Surg., 53:1807, 1982.
42. Hunt, W. A., and Hess, R. M.: Surgical risk as related to time intervention in the repair of intracranial aneurysms. J. Neurosurg., 28:14, 1968.
43. Adams, H. P., and Biller, J.: Hemorrhagic intracranial vascular disease. *In* Cranial Neurology. Vol. 2. Edited by R. J. Joynt. Philadelphia, J. B. Lippincott, 1992, p. 12.
44. van Alphen, H. A. M., and Dreissen, J. J. R.: Brain abscess and subdural empyema: factors influencing mortality and results of various surgical techniques. J. Neurol. Neurosurg. Psychiatry, 39:481, 1976.
45. Garfield, J.: Management of supratentorial intracranial abscess: a review of 200 cases. Br. Med. J., 2:7011, 1969.
46. Beller, A. J., Sahar, A., and Praiss, I.: Brain abscess: review of 89 cases over a period of 30 years. J. Neurol. Neurosurg. Psychiatry, 36:757, 1973.
47. Britt, R. H., Enzmann, D. R., and Yeager, A. S.: Neuropathological and computerized tomographic findings in experimental brain abscess. J. Neurosurg., 55:590, 1981.
48. Ornato, J. P., Craren, E. J., Nelson, N. M., and Kimball, K. F.: Impact of improved emergency medical services and emergency trauma care on the reduction in mortality from trauma. J. Trauma, 25:575, 1985.
49. Pons, P. T., et al.: Prehospital advanced trauma life support for critical penetrating wounds to the thorax and abdomen. Trauma, 25:828, 1985.
50. Genoni, M., Bogen, M., Fritz, M., and Malcrida, R.: Utilization of helicopters for the prevention of secondary cerebral lesions in severe craniocerebral injuries. Z. Unfallchir. Versicherungsmed. Berufskr., 82:163, 1989.
51. Schwab, C. W., et al.: The impact of an air ambulance system on an established trauma center. J. Trauma, 25:580, 1985.
52. Gentleman, D., and Jennett, B.: Audit of transfer of unconscious head-injured patients to a neurosurgical unit. Lancet, 335:330, 1990.
53. Andrews, P. J., Piper, I. R., Dearden, N. M., and Miller, J. D.: Secondary insults during intrahospital transport of head-injured patients. Lancet, 335:327, 1990.
54. Hans, P., Albert, A., Franssen, C., and Born, J.: Improved outcome prediction based on CSF extrapolated creatine kinase BB isoenzyme activity and other risk factors in severe head injury. J. Neurosurg., 71:54, 1989.
55. Gunnar, W., Kane, J., and Barrett, J.: Cerebral blood flow following hypertonic saline resuscitation in an experimental model of hemorrhagic shock and head injury. Braz. J. Med. Biol. Res., 22:287, 1989.
56. Shackford, S. R.: Fluid resuscitation in head injury. J. Intens. Care Med., 5:59, 1990.
57. Teasdale, G., and Jennett, B.: Assessment of coma and impaired consciousness: a practical scale. Lancet, 2:81, 1974.
58. Fisher, C. M.: The neurological examination of the comatose patient. Acta Neurol. Scand., 36(Suppl.):1, 1969.
59. Plum, F., and Posner, J. B.: The Diagnosis of Stupor and Coma. 3rd Ed. Philadelphia, F. A. Davis, 1980.
60. Michael, D. B., Guyot, D. R., and Darmody, W. R.: Coincidence of head and cervical spine injury. J. Neurotrauma, 6:177, 1989.
61. Bayless, P., and Ray, V. G.: Incidence of cervical spine injuries in association with blunt head trauma. Am. J. Emerg. Med., 7:139, 1989.
62. Deitch, D., and Kirshner, H. S.: Subdural hematoma after normal CT. Neurology, 39:985, 1989.
63. Kwan, A. L., Howng, S. L., Sun, Z. M., and Lin, C. N.: Delayed onset of traumatic epidural hematoma. Kao Hsiung I Hsueh Ko Hsueh Tsa Chich, 5:683, 1989.
64. Colquhoun, I. R., and Burrows, E. H.: The prognostic significance of the third ventricle and basal cisterns in severe closed head injury. Clin. Radiol., 40:13, 1989.
65. Ross, D. A., et al.: Brain shift, level of consciousness in patients with acute intracranial hematoma. J. Neurosurg., 71:498, 1989.
66. Miziutani, T., Manaka, S., and Tsutsumi, H.: Estimation of intracranial pressure using computed tomography scan findings in patients with severe head injury. Surg. Neurol., 33:178, 1990.
67. Snow, R. B., Zimmerman, R. D., Gandy, S. E., and Deck, M. D. F.: Comparison of magnetic resonance imaging and computed tomography in the evaluation of head injury. Neurosurgery, 18:45, 1986.
68. Levin, H. S., et al.: Magnetic resonance imaging after 'diffuse' nonmissile head injury: a neurobehavioral study. Arch. Neurol., 42:963, 1985.
69. Barnett, G. H., Ropper, A. H., and Johnson, K. A.: Physiologic support and monitoring of critically ill patients during magnetic resonance imaging. J. Neurosurg., 68:246, 1988.
70. Chiolero, R., et al.: Hormonal and metabolic changes following severe head injury or noncranial injury. JPEN J. Parenter. Enteral Nutr., 13:5, 1989.
71. Bashour, T. T., Morelli, R. L., Cunningham, T., and Budge, W. R.: Acute coronary thrombosis following head trauma in a young man. Am. Heart J., 199:676, 1990.
72. Pomeranz, S., Constantini, S., and Rappaport, Z. H.: Hypokalemia in severe head trauma. Acta Neurochir. (Wien), 97:62, 1989.
73. Burchiel, K. J., Steege, T. D., and Wyler, A. R.: Intracranial pressure changes in brain-injured patients requiring positive end-expiratory pressure ventilation. Neurosurgery, 8:443, 1981.
74. Schraufnagel, D. E., and Patel, K. R.: Sphincters in pulmonary veins: an anatomic study in rats. Am. Rev. Respir. Dis., 141:721, 1990.
75. Lanza, D. C., et al.: Predictive value of the Glasgow Coma Scale for tracheotomy in head injured patients. Ann. Otol. Rhinol. Laryngol., 99:38, 1990.
76. Moore, R. R., Najarian, M. P., and Konvolinka, C. W.: Measured energy expenditure in severe head trauma. J. Trauma, 29:1633, 1989.
77. Fried, R. C., et al.: Barbiturate therapy reduces nitrogen excretion in acute head injury. J. Trauma, 29:1558, 1989.
78. Chiolero, R. L., et al.: Effects of propranolol on resting metabolic rate after severe head injury. Crit. Care Med., 17:328, 1989.
79. Pulsinelli, W. A., et al.: Increased damage after ischemic

stroke in patients with hyperglycemia with or without established diabetes mellitus. Am. J. Med., 74:540, 1983.
80. Brown, T. H., Davidson, P. F., and Larson, G. M.: Acute gastritis occurring within 24 hours of severe head injury. Gastrointest. Endosc., 35:37, 1989.
81. Newby, L. K., Affronti, J., Baillie, J., and Cotton, P. B.: Post-traumatic pancreatitis [letter]. Gastrointest. Endosc., 36:79, 1990.
82. Kurokawa, Y., et al.: Enlarging of intracranial hemorrhagic lesions and coagulative-fibrinolytic abnormalities in multiple-injury patients. No Shinkei Geka, 17:335, 1989.
83. Baker, C. C., et al.: Epidemiology of trauma deaths. Am. J. Surg., 140:144, 1980.
84. Orbrist, W. D., et al.: Cerebral blood flow and metabolism in comatose patients with acute head injury. J. Neurosurg., 6:241, 1984.
85. Muizelaar, J. P., et al.: Adverse effects of prolonged hyperventilation in patients with severe head injury: a randomized clinical trial. J. Neurosurg., 75:731, 1991.
86. Judson, J. A., Cant, B. R., and Shaw, N. A.: Early prediction of outcome from cerebral trauma by somatosensory evoked potentials. Crit. Care Med., 18:363, 1990.
87. Nagao, S., et al.: Prediction and evaluation of brainstem function by auditory brainstem responses in patients with uncal herniation. Surg. Neurol., 27:81, 1978.
88. Synek, V. M.: Value of a revised EEG coma scale for prognosis after cerebral anoxia and diffuse head injury. Clin. Electroencephalogr., 21:25, 1990.
89. Cooper, P., et al.: Dexamethasone and severe head injury: a prospective double blind study. J. Neurosurg., 51:307, 1979.
90. Gudeman, S., Killer, J. D., and Becker, D.: Failure of high-dose steroid therapy to influence intracranial pressure in patients with severe head injury. J. Neurosurg., 51:301, 1979.
91. Hall, E. D., and Yonkers, P. A.: Comparison of two ester prodrugs of methylprednisolone on early neurologic recovery in a murine closed head injury model. J. Neurotrauma, 6:163, 1989.
92. Bracken, M. B., et al.: Methylprednisolone or naloxone treatment after acute spinal cord injury: 1-year follow-up data. Results of the second National Acute Spinal Cord Injury Study. J. Neurosurg., 76:23, 1992.
93. King, W. A., et al.: Tumor-associated neurological dysfunction prevented by lazaroids in rats. J. Neurosurg., 74:112, 1991.
94. Klastersky, J., Sadeghi, M., and Brihaye, J.: Antimicrobial prophylaxis in patients with rhinorrhea or otorrhea: A double blind study. Surg. Neurol., 6:111, 1976.
95. MacGee, E. E., Cauthen, J. C., and Brackett, C. E.: Meningitis following acute traumatic cerebrospinal fluid fistula. J. Neurosurg., 33:312, 1970.
96. Diringer, M., et al.: Plasma atrial natriuretic factor and subarachnoid hemorrhage. Stroke, 19:1119, 1988.
97. Nelson, P. B., et al.: Hyponatremia in intracranial disease; perhaps not the syndrome of inappropriate secretion of antidiuretic hormone (SIADH). J. Neurosurg., 55:938, 1981.
98. Rosenfeld, J. V., et al.: The effect of subarachnoid hemorrhage on blood and CSF atrial natriuretic factor. J. Neurosurg., 71:32, 1989.
99. Deitch, D., and Kirshner, H. S.: Subdural hematoma after normal CT. Neurology, 39:985, 1989.
100. Kwan, A. L., Howng, S. L., Sun, Z. M., and Lin, C. N.: Delayed onset of traumatic epidural hematoma. Kao Hsiung I Hsueh Ko Hsueh Tsa Chih, 5:683, 1989.
101. Gentleman, D., Nath, F., and Macpherson, P.: Diagnosis and management of delayed traumatic intracranial haematomas. Br. J. Neurosurg., 3:367, 1989.
102. Elsner, H., et al.: Delayed traumatic intracerebral hematomas: "Spat-Apoplexie:" report of two cases. J. Neurosurg., 72:813, 1990.
103. Okada, T.: Clinical aspects of traumatic intracerebral hematomas: pathogenesis of delayed traumatic intracerebral hematomas. Nippon Ika Daigaku Zasshi, 56:545, 1989.
104. Mirvis, S. E., et al.: Posttraumatic cerebral infarction diagnosed by CT: prevalence, origin, and outcome. AJNR, 11:355, 1990.
105. Compton, J. S., et al.: A double blind placebo controlled trial of the calcium entry blocking drug, nicardipine, in the treatment of vasospasm following severe head injury. Br. J. Neurosurg., 4:9, 1990.
106. Ram, Z., et al.: Delayed nonhemorrhagic encephalopathy following mild head trauma: case report. J. Neurosurg., 71:608, 1989.
107. Biary, N., Cleeves, L., Findley, L., Koller, W.: Post-traumatic tremor. Neurology, 39:103, 1989.
108. Poungvarin, N., et al.: Effects of dexamethasone in primary supratentorial intracerebral hemorrhage. N. Engl. J. Med., 316:1229, 1987.
109. Juvela, S., et al.: The treatment of spontaneous intracerebral hemorrhage: a prospective randomized trial of surgical and conservative treatment. J. Neurosurg., 70:755, 1989.
110. Matsumoto, K., and Hondo, H.: CT-guided stereotaxic evacuation of hypertensive intracerebral hematoma. J. Neurosurg., 61:440, 1984.
111. Whiting, D. M., Barnett, G. H., and Little, J. R.: Management of subarachnoid hemorrhage in the critical care unit. Cleve. Clin. J. Med., 56:775, 1989.
112. Nibblenik, D. W., Torner, J. C., and Henderson, W. G.: Intracranial aneurysms and SAH. Report of a randomized treatment study: IV-A regulated bed rest. Stroke, 8:202, 1977.
113. Kassell, N. F., et al.: Overall management of ruptured aneurysms: comparison of early and later operation. Neurosurgery, 9:120, 1981.
114. Kassell, N. F., Torner, J. C., and Adams, H. P.: Antifibrinolytics do not alter mortality following aneurysmal SAH. Stroke, 15:188, 1984.
115. Giannotta, S. L., McGillicuddy, J. E., and Kindt, G. W.: Diagnosis and treatment of postoperative cerebral vasospasm. Surg. Neurol., 8:286, 1977.
116. Pritz, M. B., et al.: Treatment of patients with neurological deficits associated with cerebral vasospasm by intravascular volume expansion. Neurosurgery, 3:364, 1978.
117. Kassell, N. F., et al.: Treatment of ischemic deficits from vasospasm with intravascular volume expansion and induced arterial hypertension. Neurosurgery, 11:337, 1982.
118. Tate, R. L., et al.: Psychosocial outcome for the survivors of severe blunt head injury: the results from a consecutive series of 100 patients. J. Neurol. Neurosurg. Psychiatry, 52:1128, 1989.
119. Rocca, B., et al.: Comparison of four severity scores in patients with head trauma. J. Trauma, 29:299, 1989.
120. Pal, J., Brown, R., and Fleiszer, D.: The value of the Glasgow Coma Scale and Injury Severity Score: predicting outcome in multiple trauma with head injury. J. Trauma, 29:746, 1989.
121. Gensemer, I. B., et al.: Psychological consequences of blunt head trauma and relation to other indices of severity of injury. Ann. Emerg. Med., 18:9, 1989.
122. Stambrook, M., et al.: Effects of mild, moderate and severe closed head injury on long-term vocational status. Brain Inj., 4:183, 1990.

123. Brooks, N., et al.: Alcohol and other predictors of cognitive recovery after severe head injury. Brain Inj., *3:*235, 1989.
124. Mayes, S. D., Pelco, L. E., and Campbell, C. J.: Relationships among pre- and post-injury intelligence, length of coma and age in individuals with severe closed-head injuries. Brain Inj., *3:*301, 1989.
125. Pasaoglu, A., and Pasaoglu, H.: Enzymatic changes in the cerebrospinal fluid as indices of pathological change. Acta Neurochir. (Wien), *97:*71, 1989.
126. Jaggi, J. L., et al.: Relationship of early cerebral blood flow and metabolism to outcome in acute head injury. J. Neurosurg., *72:*176, 1990.
127. Pierce, J. P., et al.: The effectiveness of coma arousal intervention. Brain Inj., *4:*191, 1990.
128. Allen, C. C., and Ruff, R. M.: Self-rating versus neuropsychological performance of moderate versus severe head-injured patients. Brain Inj., *4:*7, 1990.
129. Ridley, B.: Family response in head injury: denial . . . or hope for the future? Soc. Sci. Med., *29:*555, 1989.
130. Lowdon, I. M., Briggs, M., and Cockin, J.: Post-concussional symptoms following minor head injury. Injury, *20:*193, 1989.
131. Humayun, M. S., et al.: Local cerebral glucose abnormalities in mild closed head injured patients with cognitive impairments. Nucl. Med. Commun., *10:*335, 1989.
132. McSherryd, J. A.: Cognitive impairment after head injury. Am. Fam. Physician, *40:*186, 1989.
133. Geyde, A., et al.: Severe head injury hastens age of onset of Alzheimer's disease. Am. Geriatr. Soc., *37:*970, 1989.
134. Corkin, S., Rosen, T. J., Sullivan, E. V., and Clegg, R. A.: Penetrating head injury in young adulthood exacerbates cognitive decline in later years. J. Neurosci., *9:*3876, 1989.

Chapter 6

MANAGEMENT OF SEIZURES IN THE INTENSIVE CARE UNIT

HAROLD H. MORRIS, III
BLAISE F. D. BOURGEOIS

SEIZURES

Physicians working in ICUs are frequently confronted with patients who have epilepsy or seizures as a single problem or as one of a number of manifestations of underlying illness. The intensive care physician may also be involved in the care of an epileptic patient on long-term anticonvulsant therapy who is in the ICU for an unrelated problem. Epilepsy is the condition of recurrent seizures and the cause of the seizures cannot be cured. By this definition then, a patient with several seizures secondary to hyponatremia or tricyclic antidepressant overdose is not necessarily epileptic; a patient with recurrent seizures secondary to trauma may well be epileptic. The distinction is more than semantic because if a patient with seizures is not epileptic, an antiepileptic drug may be required only acutely, and long-term treatment may not be indicated.[1]

An epileptic may have different seizure types, such as generalized tonic clonic and absence seizures. A brief description of the classification of epileptic seizures is necessary to aid in proper diagnosis and treatment.[1] In brief, seizures are divided into three large groups (Table 6-1): partial seizures, or seizures beginning focally; generalized seizures, or seizures which are bilateral, symmetric, and begin without focal onset; and unclassified epileptic seizures, which are seizures in which the information required for classification is insufficient or incomplete. Common examples of partial seizures are focal motor seizures or complex partial seizures; examples of generalized seizures would be generalized tonic clonic and absence. Classification is most accurate when both clinical and electroencephalographic (EEG) information about the seizure is available; it is less reliable if only EEG or clinical data are at hand. One should keep in mind that the classification of seizures is not synonymous with the classification of the epilepsies. The reader who wishes to review the latter is referred to the International Classification of Epilepsies and Epileptic Syndromes.[2]

STATUS EPILEPTICUS

Status epilepticus has been defined by the World Health Organization as "a condition characterized by an epileptic seizure that is sufficiently prolonged or repeated at sufficiently brief intervals so as to produce an unvarying and enduring epileptic condition."[3] In the case of status epilepticus, many workers divide seizures into two large categories: convulsive status epilepticus and nonconvulsive status epilepticus (Table 6-2). Convulsive status epilepticus may be generalized (e.g., generalized tonic clonic status epilepticus) or focal (e.g., focal motor status epilepticus). Nonconvulsive status epilepticus may also be generalized (e.g., absence status) or focal (complex partial status epilepticus). The Epilepsy Foundation of America's Working Group on Status Epilepticus has defined status epilepticus as more than 30 minutes of (1) continuous seizure activity or (2) two or more sequential seizures without full recovery of consciousness between seizures.[4] This manner of classification is useful in that the convulsive forms have a greater medical urgency for treatment and are also easier to recognize clinically; the nonconvulsive forms may be correctly diagnosed only with EEG help.

Approximately 50,000 to 60,000 cases of status epilepticus occur each year in the United States. About one third of these patients are known epileptics, one third have an acute illness, and in one third, status epilepticus is the beginning of an epileptic condition. Mortality ranges from 2 to 25% but is almost always related to the underlying illness triggering the status; only 1 to 2% die from the seizures themselves.[5]

Most authors use a 30-minute seizure duration of recurrent seizures without full recovery in between for a 30-minute period as the practical definition of status epilepticus. When faced with a patient having a generalized tonic clonic seizure, however, the physician cannot delay intervention for this time period. We suggest that a patient be treated as though he or she were in status after two or three generalized tonic clonic seizures in a 24-hour period. The 30-minute seizure duration as a practical definition for the diagnosis of status does have a scientific rationale when therapeutic intervention is considered. Experimentally there is considerable evidence that respiratory and circulatory compromise begins and permanent damage to the central nervous system (CNS) may occur after this time interval.[6]

Generalized tonic clonic status epilepticus is the best known and most serious type of epilepsy that demands ICU admission. Because of the short time interval until permanent damage may occur, the physician should consider prompt admission to the ICU for vigorous treatment. Patients may have other types of status epilepticus, however, and a medical decision of how vigorously to treat and which anticonvulsant to use is of obvious importance and is directly related to proper classification. Even with

Table 6–1. International Classification of Seizures

Partial (focal)
  Simple partial (e.g., focal motor, sensorium is not impaired)
  Complex partial (e.g., psychomotor seizure, sensorium is impaired)
  Partial with secondary generalization (e.g., a focal motor seizure evolving into a generalized tonic clonic seizure)
Generalized (generalized from onset both clinically and by electroencephalogram)
  Tonic clonic (grand mal)
  Tonic
  Clonic
  Myoclonic
  Absence (petit mal)
Unclassified

partial status or nonconvulsive status, there is evidence that permanent CNS damage may occur after 30 minutes, and treatment should not be delayed.[6]

PRE-ICU PHASE

Logically, one would like to prevent the requirement for intensive care if at all possible. Frequently this can be done in patients with seizures if correct diagnosis is promptly made and effective treatment instituted. Many epileptics go through a stage of increasing seizure frequency before developing status epilepticus. This situation has been termed "serial seizures." If this increasing frequency is noted, prompt treatment may avoid a more serious illness and hospitalization. A known epileptic should have serum anticonvulsant levels done on an emergent basis if a significant increase in seizure frequency occurs. If the anticonvulsant level is low, the reason for the low level should be determined. One of the most common causes of increasing frequency of seizures in a known epileptic is poor compliance with medications. Forgetting or running out of drugs is the most common explanation given by the patient; less often, deliberate noncompliance occurs (e.g., the woman with a newly diagnosed pregnancy who thinks the anticonvulsants might harm her fetus). Loss of potency of anticonvulsants owing to age, heat, or humidity may occur but is rare. Similarly, mistakes in filling the prescription with the proper drug occur, and when no good explanation for a low anticonvulsant level is apparent, the physician should personally inspect the patient's medication.

Other than noncompliance, explanations for an unexpected low serum anticonvulsant level include an increased clearance of the drug (as with pregnancy or other physiologic changes), decreased absorption (e.g., taking phenytoin along with antacids or nasogastric feedings), or increased metabolism. Drug interactions may result in altered antiepileptic drug levels and increased seizure frequency. If the serum antiepileptic drug level is satisfactory, other explanations for increased seizure frequency must be sought. Intercurrent febrile illnesses, ethanol excess, or sleep deprivation may result in an increase in seizure frequency. Last, a progressive CNS illness (e.g., brain tumor or a degenerative disease) may result in an increasing frequency of seizures.

As a general rule, one should question the seizure diagnosis when faced with a patient with increasing seizure frequency. EEG is the only laboratory test that can help confirm and classify the diagnosis in this situation. On occasion, monitoring with simultaneous EEG and video recording is required to make a correct diagnosis. Epilepsy programs using prolonged EEG and video monitoring for diagnosis report that 10 to 20% of patients have had their seizures incorrectly classified or have had pseudoseizures.[7] Even neurologists and epilepsy monitoring unit personnel frequently have difficulty distinguishing epileptic seizures from pseudoseizures. Pseudoseizures are nonepileptic events that may closely resemble true epileptic seizures.[7-9] Not uncommonly, epileptic seizures and pseudoseizures coexist in the same patient. Pseudoseizures should be considered if the patient maintains awareness during generalized seizures. A synchronous clonic movement of arms or legs, opisthotonic posturing, and shaking of the head from side to side are other clinical clues that the patient may have pseudoseizures. Lack of an impaired sensorium immediately postictally and the occurrence of directed, purposeful behavior are other phenomena suggestive but not diagnostic of pseudoseizures. Commonly, an EEG is required to establish the correct diagnosis. Patients may, on occasion, be heavily medicated with antiepileptic drugs yet still exhibit pseudoseizures; one of us has seen at least two patients who allowed themselves to be heavily sedated, intubated, and admitted to ICUs because of serial pseudoseizures or "pseudoseizure status." Nonepileptic myoclonus, decerebrate posturing, tetanic spasms, and tetanus may resemble seizures and must be considered in a differential diagnosis.

As part of the diagnostic evaluation of a patient with frequent seizures, and in addition to EEG and antiepileptic drug levels, the physician should obtain a complete blood count; glucose, electrolytes, calcium, and magnesium levels; and measurements of renal and hepatic functions. Depending of the medical circumstances, determinations of serum osmolality, arterial blood gases, computed tomography or magnetic resonance imaging scan of the brain, cerebrospinal fluid (CSF) examination and toxicology screen may be required. In a frequently cited study of status epilepticus in a general hospital,[10] the most common precipitating cause in known epileptics was an inadequate anticonvulsant level; the second largest group consisted of patients whose status epilepticus was a complication of

Table 6–2. Classification of Status Epilepticus

Convulsive
  Generalized
    Tonic clonic
    Tonic
    Clonic
    Myoclonic
  Partial (e.g., epilepsia partialis continua, focal motor status)
Nonconvulsive
  Generalized (e.g., absence status or petit mal status)
  Partial
    Complex partial
    Simple partial (with no motor phenomena, e.g., focal sensory)

Table 6–3. Causes of Status Epilepticus

In Adults
Poor compliance with anticonvulsant
Idiopathic
Alcohol/drug related
Toxic-metabolic
Trauma
Tumor
CNS infection
Cerebrovascular disease

In Children
Poor compliance with anticonvulsant
Toxic-metabolic, especially sodium
CNS infection
Fever, no CNS infection
Idiopathic
CNS malformation

CNS, Central nervous system.

Table 6–5. Volume of Distribution of Major Antiepileptic Drugs

Drug	Volume of Distribution* (L/kg)
Phenytoin	0.75
Phenobarbital	0.50
Carbamazepine	1.50
Valproate	0.17
Ethosuximide	0.65

* Values in children, especially in young infants, may be as much as 1.5 times higher.

ethanol abuse (Table 6–3). In the case of a known epileptic with an increasing seizure frequency and an inadequate anticonvulsant level, it is probably unnecessary to order the full laboratory battery and neuroimaging as outlined here; good clinical judgment should be used to make the decision on a case-by-case basis. When presented with a patient who is not a known epileptic and is having frequent seizures, the physician's job is significantly more difficult. The primary objectives are to:

- Determine the cause of the patient's seizures
- Treat the underlying cause and the seizures simultaneously

The most common primary neurologic illnesses that include frequent seizures as a presenting sign are cerebral vascular disease trauma, stroke, tumor (primary or metastatic), infection (meningitis, encephalitis, and abscess), metabolic (hyponatremia, hypoglycemia, hyperosmolar coma, renal failure), and toxic (Table 6–4). In approximately 25 to 35% of patients in multiple series, no cause for the status epilepticus can be determined.[5] In children,

Table 6–4. Toxic and Metabolic Causes of Status Epilepticus

Metabolic Causes
  Hyponatremia
  Hypoglycemia
  Hyperosmolar coma
  Hypocalcemia
  Hypomagnesemia
  Anoxia
  Uremia
  Acute hepatic failure
Substance-Related Causes
  Ethanol abuse/withdrawal
  Barbiturate withdrawal
  Benzodiazepine withdrawal
  Cocaine and other stimulants
  Tricyclic antidepressant overdose
  PCP
  Strychnine
  Organophosphate poisoning

status epilepticus may be the first presentation of an epileptic disorder. In children younger than 3 years of age, the most common cause of status are meningitis, metabolic derangement (especially of sodium), and fever. In known epileptic children, inadequate serum antiepileptic drug levels are the most common factor associated with status epilepticus.[11,12]

As stated earlier, the necessity for an ICU admission of patients with increasing seizure frequency or even with status epilepticus can often be avoided through rapid diagnostic and therapeutic intervention. The patient with increasing seizure frequency is considered first. In many cases, there is enough time to gather historical and laboratory data pointing toward one of the causes listed in Table 6–3 and/or 6–4. If the seizure exacerbation is due to a relatively low serum anticonvulsant level, the condition usually responds promptly when the concentration of that particular drug is raised. Once there is an exacerbation of the seizures, however, it may be necessary to achieve initially higher levels than those at which the patient was previously controlled. The desired serum level can be achieved by administering a loading bolus of the corresponding drug, which can often be given orally depending on the degree of urgency. Patients who are on primidone maintenance therapy should receive a bolus of phenobarbital based on the phenobarbital level. The loading dose of the antiepileptic drug can be calculated based on the drug's volume of distribution (V_d in L/kg) (Table 6–5) multiplied by the difference between the desired level (C_d in mg/L) and the observed level (C_o in mg/L) or:

$$\text{Dose} = V_d\,(C_d - C_o)$$
$$\text{mg/kg} = \text{L/kg}\,(\text{mg/L} - \text{mg/L})$$

For example, if the phenytoin level is to be raised by 12 mg/L from 8 to 20 mg/L, a bolus of 0.75 L/kg × 12 mg/L = 9 mg/kg will be necessary. This needs to be followed by the first maintenance dose within 6 hours. The determination of the maintenance dose depends on the cause of the fall in the patient's serum drug concentration. If poor compliance was the cause, the patient should receive the dose that he or she was supposed to take originally. If compliance is not the problem, the maintenance dose should be increased approximately in proportion to the relative fall in serum level. For instance, if the measured lower level is two thirds of previous levels or of the desired level, the maintenance dose should be increased by approximately 50%, i.e., to 1.5 times the original dose. For phenytoin, the nonlinear relationship between dose and level (concentration dependent kinetics) should be taken into account, and the relative dosage increase should be less than the desired relative increase in steady-state level.

In cases of seizure exacerbations that are not due to a fall in serum concentration but to one of the other causes listed in Tables 6-3 and 6-4, the management should consist of three steps:

- Temporary intermittent administration of a benzodiazepine, such as lorazepam, clonazepam, diazepam, or clorazepate
- Increasing the level of the patient's regular antiepileptic drug above the usual values
- Appropriate diagnostic and therapeutic measures for the underlying cause, if there is one

The dose for lorazepam is 0.05 mg/kg intramuscularly or intravenously, up to a maximum of 4 mg/dose and 10 mg per 24 hours. In contrast to diazepam, lorazepam is well absorbed after intramuscular injection.[13] Diazepam can be given orally, intravenously, or rectally, and the dose is 0.2 to 0.5 mg/kg (the higher dose is for young children), up to a maximum of 20 mg/dose.[14] Clonazepam is not available for parenteral use in the United States. An oral dose of 1 to 2 mg can be used. Oral clorazepate can also be used, and this is particularly useful in patients in whom the exacerbation of the seizures is related to alcohol withdrawal. Following an initial dose of 30 mg, a total of 60 to 90 mg per day are administered during the first 2 days; this is then followed by a decrease to 30 mg per day in divided doses during the third and fourth days and then 7.5 to 15 mg per day until discontinuation when the patient is stable.

Once the patient is in true status epilepticus, the initial treatment is almost identical in all patients, and one often has to proceed before the information or the laboratory results indicating the underlying cause are available. This applies especially to convulsive status. Unless status epilepticus occurs as a complication in a patient already in an ICU, the initial treatment will almost invariably be administered outside of the ICU, and this treatment is therefore discussed here. The treatment of status epilepticus has been the subject of several excellent reviews.[15-17] The essential steps are summarized in Table 6-6.

Administration of an antiepileptic drug should never be the first step in the treatment of status epilepticus, but it should always be preceded by attention to the cardiorespiratory system, insertion of an intravenous line, obtaining blood for diagnostic purposes, and administration of concentrated glucose. If there is any question of the nutritional state of the patient or of alcohol abuse, thiamine, 100 mg intramuscularly, should also be administered. Even if ineffective, these last measures are nevertheless harmless. A minute-by-minute time frame for the suggestive steps is often recommended, but it can be difficult to apply practically.

As a general guideline, phenytoin infusion should be completed approximately 30 minutes after the onset of the intervention. The reason for the rate limit of 50 mg per minute for the phenytoin infusion is that the parenteral preparation contains propylene glycol, which is cardiotoxic. It is necessary therefore to monitor blood pressure and the electrocardiogram (ECG) during the infusion. The treatment of status should include an infusion of phenytoin or phenobarbital and should not be limited to the administration of a benzodiazepine even if the seizures are initially controlled by the benzodiazepine. Benzodiazepines are redistributed rapidly to fatty tissues other than brain and offer only short-term protection. The duration of action of lorazepam may exceed that of diazepam, and this is the main reason for its increasing use in the treatment of status epilepticus. Even after lorazepam, phenytoin or phenobarbital should be infused subsequently. If, after the phenytoin infusion is completed, the status is not controlled and it becomes necessary to administer phenobarbital, one should intubate the patient (if it has not been done earlier). The doses of phenytoin and phenobarbital indicated in Table 6-6 are based on average volumes of distribution and are intended to provide adequate blood levels immediately after infusion. Because of interpatient variability and of redistribution of the drug, it is advisable to measure serum levels within the next few hours and to reload if necessary. The first maintenance dose of the drug must be given within the first 6 hours following the last loading dose. Because cerebral edema is a possible complication of prolonged status epilepticus, treatment with steroids, such as dexamethasone, may be considered (see Chap. 4). Finally, if the seizure activity persists despite adequate loading with phenytoin and phenobarbital, the next step is either barbiturate coma or anesthesia, and this should be started within about 1 hour of the onset of the intervention.

The initial drug treatment of frequent seizures of status in the patient who is not a known epileptic does not differ basically from the treatment in the known epileptic. Until an underlying cause has been identified and can be treated specifically, it is necessary to apply the same treatment as to any patient in status. Of course, depending on the underlying cause, it may be more difficult or even impossible to control the seizures unless the primary cause has been successfully treated.

Table 6-6. Essential Steps in the Management of Generalized Convulsive Status Epilepticus

1. Assessment of cardiorespiratory function, insertion of oral airway, administration of oxygen
2. Insertion of intravenous catheter, blood for glucose (consider Dextrostix), BUN, electrolytes, antiepileptic drug levels, metabolic and drug screen
3. Infusion of 50 ml 50% glucose, saline infusion with B-vitamin complex
4. If convulsive activity present, lorazepam (0.1 mg/kg, maximum 2 mg/min, up to 4–8 mg) or diazepam (10–20 mg) IV, followed by infusion of phenytoin 20 mg/kg, at a rate of 50 mg/min or less. Two additional doses of phenytoin of 5 mg/kg each may be given
5. If seizures persist after the phenytoin infusion is completed, phenobarbital may be given at a rate of 100 mg/min until seizure control is achieved or up to a dose of 20 mg/kg
6. If seizures persist, transfer to ICU for barbiturate coma or general anesthesia

BUN, Blood urea nitrogen.

Table 6–7. Non–Central Nervous System Complications of Status Epilepticus

Cardiopulmonary
  Aspiration pneumonia
  Postictal pulmonary edema[17]
  Cardiac arrhythmia
  Myocardial infarction[18]
  Hypertension (early); hypotension (later)
Musculoskeletal
  Posterior fracture-dislocation of shoulder[19]
  Compression fracture of vertebra
  Rhabdomyolysis
Other Systemic Complications[5,9,17]
  Hyperpyrexia
  Hyperkalemia (e.g., secondary to rhabdomyolysis)
  Hypoglycemia
  Lactic acidosis
  Renal failure (e.g., secondary to hypotension, myoglobinuria)
  Death (not due to the underlying illness but to status itself)

ICU PHASE

Presumably much of the diagnostic evaluation will have been completed before the patient is admitted to the ICU. The blood studies will have already been obtained, and in the case of generalized tonic clonic status or focal motor status, treatment will have been initiated. As mentioned previously, an EEG is essential to diagnose either absence or complex partial status epilepticus. In addition to completing unfinished diagnostic studies and treating both the seizures and their underlying cause, the physician must watch for the common complications of status epilepticus and treat them if they occur (Table 6-7).

Complications of Status Epilepticus

Simon has reviewed the physiologic consequences of status epilepticus.[18] Relatively soon after the onset of the seizures, the patient may develop hyperglycemia, hypertension, and lactic acidosis. These findings do not necessarily explain the cause of the status, and in most patients, they are self-limited and do not require treatment.

Hyperthermia, leukocytosis, and CSF pleocytosis may all be seen in status epilepticus and do not themselves imply an infectious cause of the illness[10] (Table 6-8). Elevations of plasma prolactin, glucagon, growth hormone, and adrenocorticotropic hormone (ACTH) may occur transiently during and after status epilepticus.[21]

Aspiration pneumonia is relatively common in convulsive status epilepticus, and the diagnosis and treatment of that entity are discussed in Chapter 21. Suffice it, however, that early intubation in generalized status epilepticus is recommended both to prevent aspiration and because of the frequent occurrence of respiratory compromise as a result of treatment with barbiturates or benzodiazepines.

Rhabdomyolosis with myoglobinuria, renal failure, and hyperkalemia may occur as a result of the intense motor activity and should be watched for and treatment, if needed, instituted. Fractures of the thoracic and lumbar vertebrae are relatively common. Dislocation of the shoulder and fractures of long bones are infrequent. Broken (and aspirated) or loosened teeth and tongue lacerations are a common occurrence.

The neurologic complications of status epilepticus include both cerebral edema and neuronal death. Either or both of these entities may be seen diffusely or focally. Focal and selective neuronal death has been shown to occur in experimental animals who were well oxygenated and had good cardiovascular function during status epilepticus.[22-24] The areas most affected are in the hippocampus, especially CA4 and CA1, layers three and four of the cerebral cortex, and the ventral medial nuclei of the thalamus.[23] This distribution of injury is similar (but not absolutely identical) to the pathologic features of ischemia and hypoglycemia. It has been proposed that in these different entities there may be a process of neuronal injury that has a similar mechanism.[6,24-26] For example, glutamate and aspartate are both excitatory neurotransmitters; there are several types of glutamate receptors, but the N-methyl-d-aspartate (NMDA) receptor has received the most attention for its possible role in the production of injury during seizures. When the NMDA receptor is activated by glutamate released during a seizure, excessive amounts of both sodium and calcium enter the neuron. The large excess of intracellular calcium is partially responsible for cytotoxicity. Additional agents that may contribute to neuronal damage include free radicals, arachidonic acid, and free fatty acids.[24] Because of these and similar reports, there is a strong case for neuronal damage produced by the seizures themselves independent of systemic physiologic abnormalities. These findings strongly support the notion that aggressive treatment and prompt control are required in status epilepticus. As a corollary to these considerations, EEG monitoring is an absolute requirement in the treatment of the patient in status epilepticus who has received neuromuscular blocking agents. Stopping the peripheral manifestations of the convulsions by these means alone does not prevent neuronal injury. Only by EEG can the physician determine whether there is still ongoing ictal activity in the paralyzed patient.

Some findings on neuroimaging may lead the physician to believe erroneously that an underlying tumor or other structural pathologic feature is responsible for the patient's status epilepticus. During and after focal status epilepticus, one may find angiographic evidence of transiently increased regional blood flow.[27] Increased regional blood flow and glucose metabolism have been found in positron-emission tomography scans.[28] Finally, focal cerebral edema on computed tomography and magnetic resonance imaging scans of the brain may occur and may last from days to weeks.[29,30]

Table 6–8. Physiologic Changes Secondary to Status Epilepticus

Leukocytosis (WBCs >12,000) in 63% without infection
Cerebrospinal fluid pleocytosis (WBCs >5) in 18% without infection
Fever (rectal temperature >99.5°F) in 63% without infection

(From Aminoff, M. J., and Simon, R. P.: Status epilepticus: Causes, clinical features and consequences in 98 patients. Am. J. Med., 69:657, 1980.)

Table 6–9. Pentobarbital Coma

Loading dose: 5–15 mg/kg IV, over 1 hour, sufficient to achieve EEG burst suppression pattern
Maintenance IV infusion of 1–5 mg/kg/h for at least 12 hours
Infusion rate of pentobartibal for maintenance should be sufficient to maintain EEG burst suppression pattern

EEG, Electroencephalogram.

Barbiturate Coma

In cases of status epilepticus that cannot be controlled by the measures outlined in Table 6-6, one reason for transfer to the ICU may be the necessity to proceed with barbiturate coma. Every patient in whom this therapeutic modality is used needs to be intubated, to be on mechanical ventilation, and to have continuous EEG monitoring. Usually, pentobarbital is used (Table 6-9).[31,33] A loading bolus of 5 to 15 mg/kg is given initially by intravenous infusion over approximately an hour. At the end of this initial infusion, the EEG tracing should consist of a burst suppression pattern. The loading dose is followed by a maintenance infusion of 1 to 5 mg/kg per hour for at least 12 hours before discontinuation or tapering is attempted. The rate of the pentobarbital maintenance infusion may be sufficient to maintain the burst suppression EEG pattern (Fig. 6-1). Most patients develop hypotension with systolic blood pressure of 80 to 90 mm Hg, especially during the initial bolus. The blood pressure usually normalizes when the infusion rate is decreased, but an infusion of saline or dopamine may be necessary. Complete seizure control for 12 to 25 hours can be followed by abrupt discontinuation of the pentobarbital infusion. Tapering is usually not necessary because of the relatively slow elimination of the drug. After the pentobarbital infusion is discontinued, pentobarbital is often measurable in the blood for several days.

Pharmacokinetic Interactions

Patients who are in ICU following status epilepticus or who develop status in the ICU are likely to be receiving other medications in addition to the antiepileptic drugs. It is therefore always important to anticipate possible pharmacokinetic interactions, which can alter the maintenance dosage requirement of the antiepileptic drug or of the other drugs. Table 6-10 summarizes pharmacokinetic interactions.[34,35] In most cases, no dosage changes are necessary initially, but the levels should be monitored at least on a daily basis. In circumstances of renal failure, hypoproteinemia, or with concurrent usage of drugs that are highly protein bound, measurement of the free (unbound) antiepileptic drug level is suggested. This is of clinical relevance especially for phenytoin and valproate. Valproate almost invariably displaces phenytoin from serum albumin and thus increases the free fraction of phenytoin. If no drug levels are available for a particular drug that is potentially affected, a corresponding change in dosage is appropriate.

Because anoxic-ischemic encephalopathies and severe toxic-metabolic encephalopathies are common in ICUs, a brief discussion of generalized status myoclonicus is in order.[36,38] In this clinical entity, the patient is usually deeply comatose following a cardiopulmonary arrest and resuscitation. The patient may or may not have exhibited a few generalized tonic-clonic seizures. Myoclonic jerks of the face or extremities occur almost continuously; these may be obvious or subtle. Other subtle findings, such as epileptic nystagmoid eye movements, may be noted.[35] The EEG in these people is abnormal and demonstrates generalized epileptiform activity, which may be almost continuous; electrographic seizures commonly are found. The

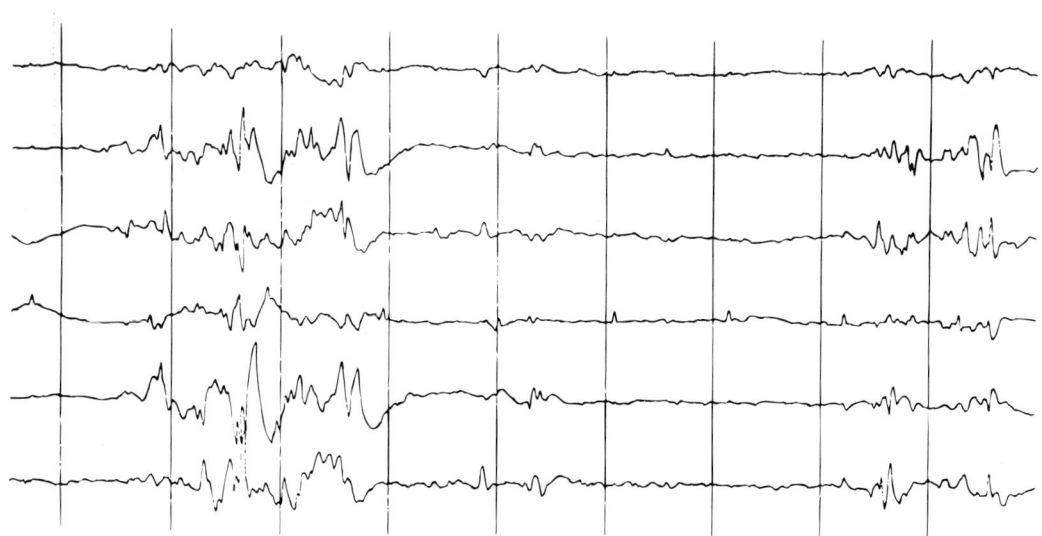

Fig. 6–1. Burst suppression EEG pattern of a patient under barbiturate anesthesia.

Table 6-10. Possible Pharmacokinetic Interactions between Antiepileptics and Other Drugs

Drug Causing Interaction (A)	Drug Affected (B)	Effect of (A) on Serum Concentration or Effect of (B)
Phenytoin, carbamazepine, phenobarbital, primidone	Carbamazepine, valproate	Decrease
Valproate	Phenobarbital	Increase
Carbamazepine	Phenytoin	Increase
Phenytoin, carbamazepine	Primidone	Increase of phenobarbital
Phenytoin	Cyclosporine	Decrease
Phenytoin, carbamazepine, phenobarbital, primidone	Digoxin, steroids, coumadin, chloramphenicol, doxycycline, theophylline	Decrease
Amiodarone, anticoagulants, azapropazone, chloramphenicol, cimetidine, disulfiram, sulfonamide	Phenytoin	Increase
Isoniazid, propoxyphene	Phenytoin, carbamazepine, primidone	Increase
Erythromycin, verapamil	Carbamazepine	Increase

prognosis of these patients is poor, and the majority die or develop a chronic vegetative state. The clinical and EEG manifestations are resistant to antiepileptic drugs. Because the prognosis of these unfortunate individuals depends more on the severity of the insult than on the neurologic or EEG picture, many neurologists do not believe that aggressive treatments such as barbiturate coma are worthwhile in this clinical setting.

Finally, one may be dealing with a patient requiring intensive care for a problem that is not related to seizures or even to the nervous system but who is a known epileptic on long-term antiepileptic therapy. Whether during the pre-ICU phase or in the ICU, the management of this patient should be similar to the management outlined previously for the patient with increasing seizure frequency. The reason is that many systemic illnesses, in particular infectious processes and metabolic derangements, tend to lower the seizure threshold and thus to put the patient at higher risk for clinical seizure activity. The focus of attention is first to maintain relatively high serum antiepileptic drug levels and secondly to anticipate and correct possible interactions between the antiepileptic drugs and the other drugs used for the intensive treatment of the patient. Third, two commonly used antiepileptic drugs, carbamazepine and valproate, are not currently available in a parenteral form. In a patient who is unable to take medications orally, both of these drugs can be given rectally, using the oral suspension form, or they can be temporarily substituted with phenytoin or phenobarbital, using the appropriate loading and maintenance regimen as described.

POST-ICU PHASE

When the patient is able to be discharged from the ICU and go to the open floor, one of the first decisions to be made is whether or not anticonvulsants should be continued. As mentioned at the beginning of this chapter, a judgment should be made as to whether or not the patient has epilepsy. If the answer is yes, of course an antiepileptic therapy must be continued. If the patient is not thought to be epileptic, no definite statement can be made. If the patient had a self-limiting acute illness, e.g., metabolic encephalopathy or drug overdose, the anticonvulsant may be discontinued over several days. If the patient has experienced a permanent CNS insult, e.g., cerebral infarct, hemorrhage, trauma, or tumor, long-term anticonvulsant treatment is appropriate. If the patient is seizure free for a year or two, one may consider tapering and discontinuing anticonvulsants. Unfortunately, a significant percentage of patients experience a seizure with anticonvulsant discontinuation. The history, examination, neuroimaging study, and EEG cannot accurately predict which patient can have medication successfully discontinued.

Because the most common cause of status epilepticus is inadequate antiepileptic drug blood level, most patients continue treatment. Patient education is the most important preventive measure that health care givers can administer at this point. The patient, or responsible adult, should know that long-term drug treatment is a requirement and that the patient is not "cured" by a brief course of treatment. They should know that for most antiepileptic drugs the patient is unprotected if he or she misses medication for more than 24 hours. They should be informed about the consequences of skipped doses and what to do if a dose is forgotten. The patient should be warned about drug interactions and instructed to ask about these any time another medication is prescribed. In addition, drugs administered in the ICU may be discontinued later, and the reversibility of an interaction may lead to yet another readjustment of the dose of the antiepileptic drug. Therefore, anticonvulsant levels should be monitored more closely during the post-ICU phase.

REFERENCES

1. Commission on Classification and Terminology of the International League Against Epilepsy: Proposal for revised clinical and electroencephalographic classification of epileptic seizures. Epilepsia, *22:*489, 1981.
2. Commission on Classification and Terminology of the International League Against Epilepsy: Proposal for revised classification of epilepsies and epileptic syndromes. Epilepsia, *30:*389, 1989.
3. Gastaut, H. (ed.): Dictionary of Epilepsy. Part I: Definitions. Geneva, World Health Organization, 1973.
4. Working Group on Status Epilepticus: Treatment of convulsive status epilepticus: recommendations of the Epilepsy Foundation of America's Working Group on Status Epilepticus. JAMA, *270:*854, 1993.
5. Hauser, W. H.: Status epilepticus: Epidemiologic considerations. Neurology, *40(Suppl. 2):*9, 1990.

6. Lothman, E.: The biochemical basis and pathophysiology of status epilepticus. Neurology, *40*(*Suppl. 2*):13, 1990.
7. King, D. W., et al.: Pseudoseizures: diagnostic evaluation. Neurology, *32*:18, 1982.
8. Gulick, T. A., Spinks, I. P., and King, D. W.: Pseudoseizures: ictal phenomena. Neurology, *32*:24, 1982.
9. Gates, J. R., et al.: Ictal characteristics of pseudoseizures. Arch. Neurol., *42*:1183, 1985.
10. Aminoff, M. J., and Simon, R. P.: Status epilepticus: causes, clinical features and consequences in 98 patients. Am. J. Med., *69*:657, 1980.
11. Dunn, D. W.: Status epilepticus in children: etiology, clinical features, and outcome. J. Child. Neurol., *3*:167, 1988.
12. Phillips, S. A., and Shanahan, R. J.: Etiology and mortality of status epilepticus in children, a recent update. Arch. Neurol., *46*:74, 1989.
13. Greenblatt, D. J., et al.: Pharmacokinetics and bio-availability of intravenous, intramuscular, and oral lorazepam in humans. J. Pharm. Sci., *68*:57, 1976.
14. Lombroso, C. T.: Intermittent home treatment of status and clusters of seizures. Epilepsia, *30*:S11, 1989.
15. Delgado-Escueta, A. V., et al.: Status Epilepticus. New York, Raven Press, 1983.
16. Leppik, I. E.: Status epilepticus. Neurol. Clin. North Am., *4*:633, 1986.
17. Treiman, D. M.: The role of benzodiazepines in the management of status epilepticus. Neurology, *40*:32, 1990.
18. Simon, R. P.: Physiologic consequences of status epilepticus. Epilepsia, *26*:S58, 1985.
19. Sechi, G. P., et al.: Myocardial infarction complicating status epilepticus. Epilepsia, *26*:572, 1985.
20. Pear, B. L.: Bilateral posterior-fracture dislocation of the shoulder—an uncommon complication of a convulsive seizure. N. Engl. J. Med., *283*:135, 1970.
21. Meldrum, B. S., et al.: Endocrine factors and glucose metabolism during prolonged seizures in baboon. Epilepsia, *20*:527, 1979.
22. Meldrum, B. S., Vigoroux, R. A., and Brierley, J. B.: Systemic factors and epileptic brain damage. Prolonged seizures in paralyzed, artificially ventilated baboons. Arch. Neurol., *29*:82, 1973.
23. Nevander, G., Ingvar, M., Auer, R., and Siesjo, B. K.: Status epilepticus in well-oxygenated rats causes neuronal necrosis. Ann. Neurol., *18*:281, 1985.
24. Siesjo, B. K., and Wieloch, T.: Epileptic brain damage: pathophysiology and neurochemical pathology. *In* Advances in Neurology. Vol. 44. Edited by A. V. Delgado-Escueta, A. A. Ward, D. M. Woodbury, and R. J. Porter. New York, Raven Press, 1986.
25. Olney, J. W., Collins, R. C., and Sloviter, R. V.: Excitotoxic mechanisms of epileptic brain damage. *In* Advances in Neurology. Vol. 44. Edited by A. V. Delgado-Escueta, A. A. Ward, D. M. Woodbury, and R. J. Porter. New York, Raven Press, 1986.
26. Meldrum, B. S.: Cell damage in epilepsy and the role of calcium in cytotoxicity. *In* Advances in Neurology. Vol. 44. Edited by A. V. Delgado-Escueta, A. A. Ward, D. M. Woodbury, and R. J. Porter. New York, Raven Press, 1986.
27. Lee, S. H., and Goldberg, H. I.: Hypervascular pattern associated with idiopathic focal status epilepticus. Radiology, *125*:159, 1977.
28. Franck, G. et al.: Regional cerebral blood flow and metabolic rates in human focal epilepsy and status epilepticus. *In* Advances in Neurology. Vol. 44. Edited by A. V. Delgado-Escueta, A. A. Ward, D. M. Woodbury, and R. J. Porter. New York, Raven Press, 1986.
29. Sammaritano, M., et al. Prolonged focal cerebral edema associated with partial status epilepticus. Epilepsia, *26*:334, 1985.
30. Kramer, R. E., et al.: Transient focal abnormalities of neuroimaging studies during focal status epilepticus. Epilepsia, *28*:528, 1987.
31. Rashkin, M. C., Youngs, C., and Penovich, P.: Pentobarbital treatment of refractory status epilepticus. Neurology, *37*:500, 1987.
32. Lowerstein, D. H., Aminoff, M. J., and Simon, R. P.: Barbiturate anesthesia in the treatment of status epilepticus: clinical experience with 14 patients. Neurology, *38*:395, 1988.
33. Van Ness, P. C.: Pentobarbital and EEG burst suppression in treatment of status epilepticus refractory to benzodiazepines and phenytoin. Epilepsia, *31*:61, 1990.
34. Kutt, H.: Interactions between anticonvulsants and other commonly prescribed drugs. Epilepsia, *25*:S118, 1984.
35. Levy, R. H., et al. (eds.): Antiepileptic Drugs. New York, Raven Press, 1989.
36. Celesia, G. G., Grigg, M. M., and Ross, E.: Generalized status myoclonicus in acute anoxic and toxic-metabolic encephalopathies. Arch. Neurol., *45*:781, 1988.
37. Simon, R. P., and Aminoff, M. J.: Electrographic status epilepticus in fatal anoxic coma. Ann. Neurol., *20*:351, 1986.
38. Krumholz, A., Stern, A. J., and Weiss, H. D.: Outcome from coma after cardiopulmonary resuscitation (CPR): relation to seizures and myoclonus. Neurology, *38*:401, 1988.

Chapter 7

INFECTIONS OF THE INTRACRANIAL CENTRAL NERVOUS SYSTEM

J. WALTON TOMFORD

Infections of the central nervous system (CNS) in adults can cause devastating clinical sequelae and substantial mortality. The classic CNS infection, acute community-acquired bacterial meningitis, is seen relatively infrequently by itself. Evaluation of adult patients with neurologic findings with symptoms and signs suggestive of infection, however, is a frequent clinical challenge. Parameningeal as well as parenchymal infections together with infectious meningitis result in a significant number of patients needing the ICU.

This chapter discusses the diagnosis and treatment of serious intracranial CNS infections. Mention is made of other disorders that can mimic primary intracranial infections and confuse the initial differential diagnosis.[1,2] Infectious myopathies, botulism, diphtheria, tetanus, rabies, and spinal infections are not covered. Enteroviral meningitis can initially be confused with acute bacterial meningitis, a true medical emergency. Acute viral meningitis, however, is not dwelled on here because prognosis for spontaneous recovery is almost uniformly excellent.[3]

A brief discussion of the unique anatomy, physiology, and immunology of the CNS indicates the critical importance of quick, accurate diagnosis and institution of therapy. Several important points need to be made with regard to managing these infections. CNS infections, particularly bacterial meningitis and herpes encephalitis, have significant mortality, and the morbidity and long-term sequelae of these infections, even when properly diagnosed, are high if the infection is not rapidly or adroitly managed. As in the case of cardiopulmonary resuscitation, delays in diagnosis and therapy can result in the patient being kept alive by heart and lung support systems in a persistently vegetative state.

The intracranial nervous system has little room to expand within the rigid skull. If brain tissues swell, they may do so by herniation through dural and skull openings.[4] The secondary neurologic insults that may occur as a result of such herniation are important to remember, not only in connection with diagnosis of diffuse and focal infections of the CNS, but also with regard to management of these infections.[5,6] In several specific situations, lumbar puncture (LP) is contraindicated, and skill must be exercised in alleviating increased intracranial pressure.[7]

The CNS has a unique arterial supply, a unique venous system, and its own unique fluid, cerebrospinal fluid (CSF), which it produces and reabsorbs. An understanding of these systems is important not only with regard to the pathology produced by infection, but also with regard to how treatment involves their function. In this chapter, infections of the arteries of the CNS, such as mycotic aneurysms, are discussed. In addition, focal infectious involvement of the intracranial venous system is detailed. Effects of infection on CSF physiology are also mentioned. Standard references give excellent discussions of the role of all three of these body fluid systems; their pathophysiology should be reviewed.[8,9]

The intracranial CNS is also unique with regard to the blood-brain and blood-CSF barriers, which play such important roles in the pathogenesis of CNS infections (especially acute meningitis) as well as in their therapy.[10] The CNS tolerates microbial invasion poorly. The concentration of immunoglobulin in the CSF is low, and complement is hardly existent. There is no lymphatic system per se, and the vasculature has unique properties that predispose it to poor tolerance of changes in pressure and oxygen levels. The skull's excellent blood supply and unique blood-brain and blood-CSF barriers help to prevent infections, but when infection does occur, the CNS has relatively weak immune defenses.[11] These factors undoubtedly form the basis for the clinical adage that antimicrobials used for therapy of CNS infection must be carefully selected and must be given in the highest doses clinically possible.[12] An important corollary is that operative drainage of localized infections is usually a top priority.

The number of patients seen each year with an individual type of infection is not usually large, but the sum of patients presenting to a hospital with potential CNS infections may be sizeable.[13] Serious infections of the CNS encompass a broad variety of types of microorganisms, including prions, viruses, spirochetes, rickettsiae, mycoplasma, bacteria, yeasts, fungi, mycobacteria, and parasites.[12] Infectious disorders of the cranial portion of the CNS can be usefully divided into three anatomic classes: parameningeal, meningeal, and parenchymal infections (Table 7-1). I believe that too much emphasis has been placed on classification schemes based mainly on CSF laboratory values. Alterations in CSF may be similar with different types of infection. The patient's history, the results of the physical examination, and certain key laboratory and radiographic tests are just as important in formulating the differential diagnosis of a CNS infection. As discussed subsequently, in some situations, such as a brain or subdural abscess, sampling the CSF is actually contraindicated.

Although CNS infections are often classified by organism, by the time the type of organism has been confirmed, many major diagnostic and therapeutic decisions have already been made. An anatomic approach with consideration of important subdivisions within each class is the more likely situation initially facing the clinician with such critically ill patients. Obviously organism-specific information is critical in the choice of the best antimicrobial regimen. In management of this whole group of infections, however, there is much more involved than choice of antimicrobials.[14-16] Correct anatomic localization of infection as well as likely organism(s) involved is critical in deciding the wisdom and usefulness of LP as well as neurosurgical intervention for diagnostic or therapeutic purpose. Thus anatomic classification seems to be a useful starting point for the clinician faced with such critically ill patients.

The following discussion begins with the initial approach (pre-ICU evaluation) to the acutely ill patient with symptoms and signs suggestive of a CNS infection. Diagnosis is the usual thrust of the pre-ICU stage. Then, medical and surgical aspects of treatment in the ICU phase are discussed, followed by prognostic as well as rehabilitative aspects of care (the post-ICU phase).

Rather than discussing management for each organism separately, in a comprehensive overview for the practicing clinician, it seems more important to mention differences in diagnosis and management: for example, cryptococcal meningitis can initially have a presentation similar to that of herpes encephalitis, and it may be critical to distinguish these two important different causes of CNS infection.[17] This approach is more practical than a discussion of the choice of antimicrobial therapy for acute community-acquired bacterial meningitis due to specifically Streptococcus pneumoniae, meningococcus, or Haemophilus influenzae.

Given the large number of microbes that can produce infection in the CNS, initial antimicrobial therapy is often chosen to combat the organism(s) most likely to cause that particular type of infection.[18,19] Pharmacologic therapies are then often adjusted several days later based on the results of blood cultures, CSF analysis (if appropriate), biopsy or examination of surgical specimens (if obtained), and response to therapy.

PRE-ICU EVALUATION

Parameningeal Infections

The first class of CNS infections we consider in detail are the parameningeal infections. These anatomically distinct infections not uncommonly produce meningeal signs and CSF pleocytosis, and they can easily mimic true meningitis due to a virus, bacteria, fungus, or other microbe. This group can be divided as follows:

- Skeletal and soft tissue infections
- Vascular infections including intracranial arteritis
- Septic dural venous sinus phlebitis
- Epidural and subdural empyema

Skeletal and Soft Tissue Infections

Skeletal and soft tissue infections of the head and neck are important clinical entities that may produce signs and symptoms referable to the CNS.[9,20,21] Such parameningeal infections can involve the intracranial arteries and veins, especially the veins that cross the dura, and can cause true bacterial meningitis and parenchymal brain infections. Head and neck infections can also directly invade the epidural and subdural spaces.

Because parameningeal infections can serve as a source for true intracranial infections, pre-ICU evaluation of a possible CNS infection must include a focused history and physical examination of the head and neck region. Attention must be paid to the scalp and skull to identify a history of past or recent trauma, surgery to the area, or infectious skin lesions. The history and physical examination should focus on the face; external and middle ear; mastoid area; visual systems; and air sinuses, particularly the frontal, ethmoid, and sphenoid sinuses. Although the maxillary sinus is the most commonly involved in sinusitis, it does not abut the dura, and CNS complications are rarely the result of isolated maxillary sinus infection. The sphenoid sinus cannot be directly examined, but when it becomes infected, serious CNS and eye infection can occur.[22] Historical and physical examination clues to sphenoid sinus involvement include:

- Boring, retro-orbital, or unilateral headache
- Pain, paresthesia in cranial nerves V1, V2, and V3
- Pus in middle or superior turbinates
- Orbital complications[22,20]

The physician should also inquire about midline skin defects (dermoid sinuses) and about recent furuncles on the scalp or face, especially the upper nasal and the intercanthal area. A thorough history and physical examination should also include the nares, eyes, teeth, throat, and cervical areas as well as the jugular and carotid vessels.[21]

In a discussion of the skeletal and soft tissue foci, rhinocerebral zygomycetes infection merits separate attention. This dramatic clinical entity is invariably seen in diabetics or patients receiving high doses of immunosuppressive medication. Its course illustrates how quickly and impressively infections in parameningeal areas can invade the CNS. Patients with zygomycetes infection often have a subacute onset of fever, disorientation, facial pain, and necrotic purulent lesions or discharge in the nasopharynx. When the entity is the initial presentation of diabetes, there is invariably diabetic ketoacidosis. Involvement of the eye and nares with neuropathies of cranial nerves I

Table 7–1. Anatomic Approach to Central Nervous System Infections

Parameningeal
   Skeletal and soft tissue infection
   Vascular infection
   Septic dural venous sinus phlebitis
   Epidural and subdural empyema
Meningeal
   Acute purulent meningitis
   Chronic meningitis
   Aseptic meningitis
Parenchymal
   Encephalitis
   Brain abscess

through VI frequently occurs, and the infection often crosses the dura to involve the meninges, brain parenchyma, and intracranial vasculature with cerebral arteritis, cavernous sinus thrombosis, and cerebral infarction. The course of zygomycetes infection can be halted, however, by early diagnosis and a combination of medical (amphotericin B) and surgical treatment.[23,24] When considering rhinocerebral zygomycosis, the clinician needs to perform a careful history to uncover risk factors and perform a thorough examination of the eyes, cranial nerves, nares, palate, and pharynx.

Given the propensity for skeletal and soft tissue infections to become parameningeal foci with additional spread within the CNS, after a thorough history and examination, the patient with signs and symptoms of CNS infection should undergo computed tomography (CT) scanning. A cost-effective way to delineate secondary intracranial complications as well as parameningeal foci such as sinusitis or mastoiditis is to order a high quality CT scan of the brain and do additional scans through the mastoid, orbits, paranasal sinuses, and skull. A few quick views of the mastoids, orbits, and paranasal sinuses are instrumental in evaluation and more accurate than plain films of this area as well as being easier to read. Such radiographic assistance does not (with the caveats to be discussed) waste precious time and can be invaluable in correct diagnosis.[25]

Vascular Infections

This group includes the clinical findings produced by three types of vascular infections:

- Sepsis
- Infective endocarditis
- Cerebral septic arteritis (including mycotic aneurysms)

Sepsis. Sepsis often produces a clinical picture of CNS deterioration without direct anatomic involvement of the CNS.[26] The reason for this is obvious: The organisms that most often produce the syndrome of true sepsis, Escherichia coli, pseudomonas, or enterobacter, rarely invade an intact CNS. This is an important point for the ICU physician to remember. Kaiser and McGee[19] have suggested that it is not often easy to separate the CNS signs of sepsis from primary CNS disease, particularly when the presentation is of acute meningitis, i.e., fulminant course less than 48 hours with fever, headache, meningismus, and an impaired sensorium.[19] Sepsis can also be confused with a subacute CNS infection syndrome of 1 to 7 days of illness with moderate fever, increasing headache with progressive impairment of higher integrative functions, and focal defects.[19] Usually, but not always, these can be separated based on clinical presentation; time course; historical aspects, such as fever and malaise; and CNS signs and symptoms, such as change of mental status and CNS focal defects. As a rule, if there are signs and symptoms of primary CNS involvement, rapid consideration should be given to LP or CT (or both) but only after the patient with altered mental status and the obvious sepsis syndrome has been stabilized in the ICU with antibiotics, fluids, and pressors.[5]

If there is any doubt about differentiating among sepsis syndrome, acute meningitis syndrome, and subacute CNS syndrome, the antimicrobial regimen chosen should be active against both gram-positive and gram-negative organisms and should penetrate the pharmacologic barrier at the blood-brain and brain-CSF interface. In adults, with the exception of Streptococcus pneumoniae, H. influenzae, meningococcus, and occasional streptococci, Staphylococcus aureus, and Listeria monocytogenes, most organisms that present with septicemia do not show a strong propensity for directly invading the CNS.[27,28] From experimental models of meningitis, it appears that bacteremia, specifically without necessarily initial manifestations of sepsis, is the manner by which these specific pathogens most commonly gain entrance into the CNS.[11,29] With the exception of these direct invaders of the CNS, most cases of bacteremia or septicemia produce CNS symptoms (delirium) without direct anatomic invasion.

Infective Endocarditis. One important exception to this general caveat is infective endocarditis. I consider endocarditis a major form of "parameningeal" CNS infection of great importance to the ICU physician. Neurologic manifestations of endocarditis are not uncommon and can be a clue to this otherwise occasionally difficult to diagnose disease.[30,31] These manifestations are also important to remember in the evaluation of CSF pleocytosis that is culture-negative. The following facts need emphasis:

- Blood cultures are positive in at least 50 to 60% of cases of acute bacterial meningitis.
- CNS abnormalities in endocarditis are frequently the initial clinical manifestation.
- In 5 to 10% of cases of infective endocarditis, the patient is afebrile.

I recommend drawing two to four blood cultures from every patient with an acute neurologic illness, particularly if there is the slightest suspicion of an inflammatory disorder or the cause is unknown. Blood cultures would be superfluous in an obvious case of multiple sclerosis; however, a strokelike presentation or a perplexing case of CSF pleocytosis may actually represent endocarditis.

Lerner[31] and others[12,30,32] have divided the neurologic complications of endocarditis into several categories:

- Septicemic presentation (almost exclusively in acute bacterial endocarditis)
- "Cerebritis" and meningitis
- Vascular events including stroke and intracerebral hemorrhage
- Mycotic aneurysms
- Brain abscess

True bacterial meningitis and brain abscess are infrequently associated with endocarditis, and these particular entities are covered elsewhere in this chapter. There are several infectious CNS complications, however, unique to endocarditis: diffuse cerebritis, strokelike presentation especially in the face of prosthetic valve endocarditis, and mycotic aneurysm of the CNS.

Diffuse meningoencephalitis (cerebritis) with abnormal

mental status, frequent meningismus, and parameningeal-type CSF abnormalities with occasional focal neurologic findings can occasionally be the presenting sign of endocarditis (usually acute) and is often due to S. aureus. This is not surprising if one considers that a significant percentage of blood flow across the aortic and mitral valve perfuses the brain. The CT scan of a patient with meningoencephalitis secondary to bacterial endocarditis often appears normal, and analysis of CSF often shows a moderate neutrophilic pleocytosis (5 to 500 cells), a protein level of 20 to 200 mg/dl, and glucose level in the 45 to 80 mg/dl range.[32] CSF cultures are rarely positive, and when they are positive, it is usually for S. aureus. Once this clinical entity is recognized, it is treated by an appropriately active antimicrobial agent that crosses the blood-brain, blood-CSF barrier. The physician needs to anticipate complications, such as increased intracranial pressure or cardiac complications of infective endocarditis, that may warrant transfer to the ICU. Magnetic resonance imaging (MRI) studies in such patients suggest that microemboli may cause much of the findings; control of the infection is the key to management.[32] Although controversial, anticoagulation is generally contraindicated in cases of native valve endocarditis.[32-34]

With prosthetic valve endocarditis, the clinical approach is different. Given the large number of prosthetic valve replacements per year, the continued need for anticoagulation for patients with mechanical valves or atrial fibrillation, and the low but significant percentage of prosthetic valve endocarditis cases (approximately 2% over the life of the prosthetic valve), the management of these patients is of great importance.[32,34-36] Current experience with this clinical conundrum would suggest that despite risk of hemorrhage associated with anticoagulation, such patients with valves requiring anticoagulation do better when anticoagulation is continued.[37] Acute management of these patients, however, is probably assisted by changing from oral to intravenous anticoagulation as well as titration to the lower end of full efficacy.

Cerebral Septic Arteritis. Mycotic aneurysm of the CNS, although rare, is usually due to prior or concomitant endocarditis. Infection occurring in an intracranial artery can have disastrous consequences and is often associated either with subacute bacterial endocarditis, usually streptococcus, or acute bacterial endocarditis usually due to S. aureus. These aneurysms tend to occur fairly distal to the circle of Willis and can be different to detect, either on magnetic resonance angiogram or standard contrast angiography. The management of mycotic aneurysms in the CNS is controversial because their true incidence is not well delineated, and at least 30% of those discovered and treated with appropriate antimicrobial agents appear to heal without sequelae.[31,32,38] Patients with focal findings as well as evidence of meningoencephalitis with abnormal CSF and emboli or unexplained neurologic deterioration should probably undergo angiography. Obviously, appropriate consultation should be obtained from neurologic, neurosurgical, and neuroradiology colleagues.

Septic Dural Venous Sinus Phlebitis

Septic thrombosis of the dural venous sinuses, although uncommon, may present dramatically as a parameningeal infection of the CNS. The three most important intracranial venous systems all interconnect, but each is nevertheless associated with unique clinical syndromes.[6,14]

First, septic thrombosis of the **cavernous sinus** is usually a secondary complication of midline or upper facial infection, sphenoid sinusitis, ethmoid sinusitis, otitis media, or dental infection. It often presents acutely with sharp, increasing frontal or retro-orbital headache with eye complaints and change in mental status suggestive of clinical toxicity. The classic findings include:

- Ptosis
- Proptosis
- Chemosis
- Paralysis of cranial nerves III, IV, and VI
- Involvement of cranial nerves V_1 and V_2

The majority of patients have an abnormal CSF pattern: meningeal (30%) or parameningeal (55%). A CT scan often shows associated sinusitis and can exclude venous infarction if therapy with anticoagulants is being considered (controversial). Carotid artery angiography can show luminal abnormalities in the intracavernous portion with direct involvement or secondary occlusion. Orbital venography has been mentioned in some reports but is technically difficult. Additional complications of septic cavernous sinus include associated true bacterial meningitis and spread to the other cavernous sinus or dural venous sinuses, pituitary involvement, and cortical venous thrombosis with infarction. S. aureus is the most common causative organism (70%), with streptococci accounting for another 20% of these infections.[39]

Septic lateral sinus thrombosis is an uncommon but important complication of acute and especially chronic otitis media with associated mastoiditis. These patients present subacutely with unilateral temporal headache, ear pain, and nausea and vomiting. There is obvious otitis media and fever. CSF pressure is usually elevated owing to interference with CSF reabsorption by arachnoid villi with frequent papilledema. There may be additional complications of cranial nerve VI palsy and retro-orbital and temporoparietal headache owing to cranial nerve V irritation, termed Gradenigo's syndrome. If there is pleocytosis, there is invariably an associated epidural, subdural, or brain abscess.[39]

CT scan in lateral sinus thrombosis invariably shows the associated mastoiditis and is helpful in delineating associated dural empyemas, brain abscesses, and venous infarctions. The organisms most commonly involved include those that cause chronic otitis media:

- Proteus mirabilis
- S. aureus
- E. coli
- Bacteroides fragilis
- Pseudomonas aeruginosa[39]

One report describes a case with associated polymicrobial anaerobic septicemia, although extracranial secondary involvement is rare.[40]

Septic thrombosis of the **superior sagittal sinus** is the

least common and most serious of this class of parameningeal infections. Meningitis remains the major infection predisposing to this syndrome, with rare cases associated with frontal sinusitis, mastoiditis with spread via the lateral sinus, pharyngitis, dental infection, or pelvic septic thrombophlebitis with spread via the vertebral veins. Although thrombosis of the posterior portion of the sagittal sinus may produce increased intracranial pressure, usually antecedent involvement of the anterior portion of the sagittal venous sinus produces the major clinical findings owing to venous infarction of the anterior and superior portions of the medial part of the cerebral hemispheres. Thus there is likely a combination of seizures, hemiparesis, hemianopia, aphasia, conjugate eye deviation, or weakness and numbness of the lower extremities. The CSF is invariably abnormal in this syndrome because the majority of cases are secondary complications of bacterial meningitis.[39] CT scans can show a "delta sign" owing to failure of contrast uptake in the venous phase of the sagittal sinus.[25] The MRI scan with gadolinium, however, appears to be a promising, better way to detect this severe complication and obviate the seldom indicated venous phase carotid angiogram. The organisms responsible for this syndrome are those associated with bacterial meningitis and frontal sinusitis. In one series, the majority of cases of sagittal sinus thrombophlebitis were due to S. pneumoniae (40%), S. aureus (20%), and streptococcal species (20%).[39]

Epidural and Subdural Empyema

Intracranial epidural and subdural empyemas frequently coexist and have a similar pathophysiology and microbiology. Because this chapter uses an anatomic classification, we consider them separately. In epidural empyemas, the inciting focus of infection is usually in the paranasal sinuses, middle ear, mastoid, orbit, craniotomy flap, or skull. Usually the adult patient with intracranial epidural empyema has several days of an unremitting headache and fever. Most of the other symptoms are due to the primary focus of infection (sinusitis; otitis; osteomyelitis; or associated complications of extension into the subdural space, meninges, or brain parenchyma). The dura is closely approximated to the inner surface of the cranium except where it invaginates to form the falces (cerebri and cerebelli), tentorium cerebelli, and diaphragma sella. Cranial epidural abscesses usually enlarge too slowly to produce clinical deterioration with focal signs; thus diagnosis is often delayed.[42]

The possible presence of an epidural empyema is considered by many to be a relative contraindication to a spinal tap. The lack of focal findings, seizures, or papilledema in uncomplicated cases, however, leads the clinician with few clues to the presence of this type of CNS empyema. If CSF is sampled in a patient with uncomplicated epidural empyema, it is invariably sterile and provides evidence only of a parameningeal type of response: elevated protein, normal glucose, and few to a moderate number of white cells, predominantly but not invariably polymorphonuclear leukocytes.[42]

Epidural abscesses are often associated with other dominant findings, such as subdural empyema, cortical venous thrombosis, meningitis, or brain abscess, and should be evaluated expeditiously by imaging. CT scan, however, is not 100% accurate: If there is high suspicion of an epidural abscess, contrast enhancement should be used in the CT scan, or an angiogram may be needed to confirm the diagnosis. Reports suggest that MRI offers advantages over CT in the diagnosis of epidural empyema, especially those occurring postoperatively.[25]

The organisms usually involved in epidural empyemas include those responsible for the primary focus of infection, such as streptococci, haemophilus species, gram-negative aerobic bacilli, and anaerobes such as bacteroides species including Bacteroides fragilis. If the primary focus of infection is an infected craniotomy flap or chronic sinusitis, S. aureus must be considered a likely sole or contributory pathogen.[42]

In contradistinction to isolated epidural pus collections, empyema below the dura has been termed "the most imperative of neurosurgical emergencies."[42] It is a more common entity than epidural empyema and is associated with a much higher mortality because of its clinical presentation and complications. Even in the modern antibiotic era, the mortality of subdural empyema is around 20%.[43] Although the arachnoid membrane is relatively impervious to direct invasion, subdural empyema is often complicated by purulent meningitis (around 15%), cortical venous thrombosis (around 30%), and brain abscess (around 25%).[42] Infection of the paranasal sinuses, especially the frontal sinuses, is the most common predisposing factor in 50 to 75% of cases of subdural empyema; chronic otitis media with associated mastoiditis, trauma, and neurosurgery are the other important predisposing factors. In adults, as opposed to infants, bacterial meningitis is invariably a complication as opposed to a predisposition in the development of subdural empyema. The potential subdural space is relatively free over and between the cerebral hemispheres but is restricted in the central basal regions by the tentorium cerebelli and the structures at the base of the brain. Most subdural empyemas occur over the cerebral convexities, but the 20% that occur in the parafalx region or posterior fossa can be more difficult to diagnose. Once infection is present in the subdural space, pus accumulates rapidly and spreads, either from the frontal sinus over the frontal and parietal portions of the convexities or to the temporal or posterior fossa from an ear infection.[44]

The patient with a subdural empyema has symptoms and signs associated with this inciting infection. In 80 to 90% of cases, there is also usually the rapid development of high fever, focal headache that becomes more generalized, vomiting, and focal neurologic findings. Hemiparesis or hemiplegia can be seen in more than 75% of patients with subdural empyema, and seizures can occur in more than half. All of these symptoms may progress rapidly. Prior antibiotic therapy may obscure the symptoms and signs of CNS infection by masking any associated sinusitis or otitis that might otherwise provide a clue to the cause of the rapidly developing neurologic findings. All of these symptoms and signs are usually due to understandable complications of:

- Increased intracranial pressure
- Meningeal irritation

- Focal cortical inflammation (corresponding to the associated empyema)

There is usually an associated brisk blood leukocytosis. The clinician may be tempted to perform LP, especially if there are associated signs and symptoms of true meningitis, but LP is relatively contraindicated given the numerous reports that have documented herniation occurring when LP is performed in patients with subdural empyema.[42,43] If CSF is obtained, it is usually sterile and indicative of nonspecific parameningeal disease (increased protein, polymorphonuclear pleocytosis, and normal glucose), which is another reason why LP is not recommended.[43] Elevated opening pressure may, however, be a helpful clue in diagnosis if LP is performed and pressure measured. Nuchal rigidity is often seen in patients with subdural empyema without meningitis, which makes differentiation between these two conditions difficult. If subdural empyema is suspected based on clinical presentation, especially in the presence of papilledema, focal neurologic findings, and seizures, it would be better to begin empiric therapy (discussed later), attempt to substantiate the diagnosis rapidly, and perform surgical drainage. CT scanning is the method of choice for confirming the diagnosis, and it helps to detect the site of head or neck infection responsible for the subdural empyema. CT scan also localizes the empyema and guides the surgical approach for drainage.

The usual CT appearance of subdural empyema is a crescent-shaped area of hypodensity adjacent to the cranium or falces cerebri with occasional loculations and mass effect. With administration of intravenous contrast material, there may be a fine line of enhancement between the subdural collection and the cortex with occasional patchy enhancement of brain substance adjacent to the empyema.

It is important to note that in some well-documented cases, the CT scan was done at the time when the subdural empyema was isodense with a resultant false-negative scan. This misinterpretation can lead to grave clinical errors. MRI or cerebral angiography may thus be indicated when the clinical picture is confusing and the CT scan in a patient with head and neck infection shows only cerebritis with a midline shift that could represent subdural empyema.[25]

The organisms that can cause subdural empyema are the same as those that cause epidural empyema. These usually include single organism or polymicrobial infections, which may consist of various types of streptococci, haemophilus, gram-negative enteric bacteria, S. aureus, and occasionally anaerobes.[42]

Meningitides

The second major anatomic class of CNS infections comprises the true meningitides. Meningitis is the classic form of intracranial infection. In contrast to the mostly bacterial entities so far considered, meningitis may be caused by a broad variety of types of organisms, from viruses to parasites. Strictly speaking, most forms of meningitis involve not only the subarachnoid space, but also the adjacent brain cortex.[19] We next consider, however, those infections that foremost and directly involve the meninges. In a similar manner, when we consider parenchymal brain infections, there is often meningeal involvement as well, but the primary pathology involves the brain parenchyma rather than the linings of the brain.[45]

In this section, we consider in detail only the pre-ICU phase of those infectious agents that predominantly and initially invade the subarachnoid space, either hematogenously or contiguously.

The acute "aseptic" meningitis syndrome can be caused by a broad range of infectious organisms.[46] Similar to acute bacterial meningitis, acute aseptic meningitis must be diagnosed rapidly. Certain diseases, such as sinusitis and otitis, can present as acute aseptic meningitis, and these have been previously discussed as parameningeal infections. Certain organisms are more important causes of chronic meningitis with chronic inflammation of the meninges, which include the yeasts (cryptococcus and candida), dimorphic fungi such as Histoplasma capsulatum and Coccidioides immitis, and Mycobacterium tuberculosis. These pathogens can cause great morbidity and mortality if diagnosis is not suspected early and treatment begun before the diagnosis is confirmed by culture. Yeasts, fungi, and mycobacteria classically produce a chronic form of true meningitis, but importantly they can present in a more acute form similar to acute purulent meningitis.[47,48] These topics, however, are beyond the scope of this chapter, and the reader is referred elsewhere for further discussion.[12,49]

Another type of meningitis that can be touched on only briefly is recurrent meningitis, which may be due to predisposing anatomic defects owing to trauma; surgery; congenital abnormalities; tumor invasion of the dura; or immunologic defects, such as asplenia, immunoglobulin deficiency, or complement deficiencies. Historical and physical evidence of these predisposing factors should be elicited in the evaluation of the initial bout of bacterial meningitis because meningitis is more than likely to recur if these defects are not corrected or managed during the initial infection.[50] Post-traumatic and postneurosurgical meningitis and acute bacterial meningitis in the presence of a CNS shunt are reviewed elsewhere.[51,52]

Four spirochetal diseases have been emphasized as potential treatable pathogens in acute meningitis.[53] Syphilis and leptospirosis have been recognized for years as potential causes of the acute aseptic meningitis syndrome, and relapsing fever and Lyme disease also have been cited as important causes of meningitis. These four spirochetal organisms have been discussed by Coyle and Dattwyler.[54] When the diagnosis of a meningeal infection remains in question in a patient with CSF pleocytosis, this particular class of organisms should be considered as well.

The first task for the clinician evaluating meningitis, however, is to exclude acute purulent bacterial meningitis. Despite the availability of new antibiotics that remain highly active against the 10 or fewer most common bacteria, bacterial meningitis continues to be associated with unacceptably high morbidity and mortality.[55-58] Many authors suggest that rapid, occasionally empiric initiation of antibacterial therapy is almost as important as history, physical examination, and results of CSF analysis, if not contraindicated based on clinical information available before and not after the CT scan has been done. Rapid high dose administration of the appropriate antimicrobial regimen is the key to successful management of this potentially, rapidly fatal disease.[59]

Even minimal delays are not acceptable in this clinical situation. Several points should be remembered: (1) The number of possible causative organisms and their antibiotic sensitivity patterns are relatively few; an effective empiric therapy regimen can easily be formulated; (2) if LP is believed to be indicated, it should be performed immediately, and two samples of blood should be drawn immediately for culture before beginning empiric therapy; in this situation, blood cultures are positive in at least 60% of the cases, and CSF Gram stain results are extremely useful in diagnosis and therapy; (3) if a LP cannot be done quickly owing to technical factors, i.e., a wildly delirious patient, profound coagulopathy, or infection at the LP site, or is contraindicated owing to suspicion of a mass lesion, such as brain abscess, subdural empyema, or papilledema, or evidence of increased intracranial pressure, empiric therapy should still be initiated before CT; (4) over the next 6 to 12 hours, the clinician can concentrate on management of increased intracranial pressure, obtain a CT scan or MRI scan if necessary to exclude a mass lesion, and monitor clinical response.

More patients have probably been harmed by inappropriate delay in LP and antimicrobial therapy than by adverse effects produced by LP. The following 6 to 24 hours, antimicrobial therapy can be adjusted based on the patient's early response, blood culture results, CT scan results, and CSF analysis. Multiple reports suggest that appropriate empiric therapy for the first 12 to 18 hours does not invalidate the usefulness of the Gram stain, may only slightly decrease the chance of a positive culture result, and is prudent clinical practice.[55,60,61]

In the differential diagnosis of meningitis, parameningeal infections that are close to the dura, local vascular infections such as microbial arteritis and phlebitis, and distal foci of infection in the heart and lung should be considered. For many adults, however, the source of the bacteria is not obvious. To clarify the pathogenesis of bacterial meningitis, investigators have looked to experimental models, which have provided studies of assistance to the clinician.[11] The results of studies using these models suggest that there are a limited number of bacteria that have tropism and virulence for the CNS by this route:

- S. pneumoniae
- Meningococcus
- H. influenzae
- Other streptococci
- S. aureus
- Listeria monocytogenes
- Gram-negative enteric bacilli (rarely)

In the pre-ICU phase, the clinical presentations of infection with these organisms are fairly similar, and only important differences are mentioned (Table 7-2). Antimicrobial therapy, of course, is different, and this is emphasized in the discussion of the ICU phase of patient care.

The first three of these organisms, S. pneumoniae, meningococcus, and H. influenzae, cause at least 65% of the

Table 7-2. Clinical Signs of Acute Meningitis

Fever and headache
Change in mental status
Nuchal rigidity
Seizures
Cranial nerve dysfunction (III, IV, V, VI, VII)
Focal weakness
Florid delirium
Petechial or purpuric rash

cases of bacterial meningitis in adults. The pathologic process usually appears to involve nasopharyngeal colonization with a virulent strain that the host cannot contain, infection of the nasopharynx, and primary bacteremia with rapid invasion of the subarachnoid space presumably through the choroid plexi and ventricles. Logarithmic proliferation of organisms within these areas of impaired host defense may lead to secondary bacteremia that serves as a locus for reseeding.

For organisms other than the three just discussed, the pathologic process is less well understood. For the classic three pathogens, however, the previous discussion fits with the clinical observation that in adult patients with bacterial meningitis there is often a preceding upper respiratory infection.

A change of mental status is the strongest and often the first indicator of bacterial meningitis. Approximately one-fourth of patients with bacterial meningitis experience rapid progression of headache, fever, and mental status change, leading to the need for hospitalization within 24 hours. In these patients, rapid recognition and treatment of disease is important because the mortality of this type of bacterial meningitis remains high. Other patients with bacterial meningitis experience a more protracted onset of complaints developing over 1 to 7 days, sometimes in conjunction with or after an upper respiratory tract infection. Mortality is lower in this group than among those with rapid presentation. The need for rapid recognition and treatment in this second group, however, is just as vital. As opposed to the specific symptoms of fever, headache, and mental status change seen in the acute group, those patients with subacute presentations often have a more confusing presentation with nausea, vomiting, rigors, sweats, myalgias, and the important symptom of photophobia.[19] In more than 80% of all cases of meningitis, there are meningeal signs, such as nuchal rigidity and Kernig's sign.[14]

The vast majority of patients with bacterial meningitis have fever, but advanced age, presence of uremia, immunosuppression, or developing hypothermia can alter this sign. About 50% of the patients in most series are comatose or obtunded at the time of presentation; only 5% or fewer are fully alert.[14] The clinical presentation in the elderly patient with bacterial meningitis may be decidedly different.[62] In older patients, there may be only low-grade or absent fever. Confusion is common, however, and these patients are more likely to present with severe mental status changes and concomitant pneumonia. Only 57% of older patients in one series, however, had meningismus, and fewer than one-fourth complained of headache.[59] Most noncomatose elderly patients have evidence of nuchal rigidity, but this clinical finding can be confused with degenerative joint disease or parkinsonism. Even for older patients, a spinal tap is virtually mandatory if there is suspicion of bacterial meningitis, unless LP is contraindicated by one of the circumstances discussed in this chapter.[18]

Particular attention in the initial evaluation of bacterial meningitis should be paid to the presence of seizures, which can occur in 20 to 30%, and true focal findings, which may be seen in 10 to 20%. Seizures with focal findings may also be present owing to Todd's paresis or false localizing signs. Bacterial meningitis should still be high in the differential diagnosis in the presence of fever, mental status change, seizures, and focal findings, but when the latter two are present, the clinician should entertain the diagnosis of epidural and subdural empyema, encephalitis, or brain abscess.[19]

Dysfunction of cranial nerves III, IV, VI, and VII, which is present in 10 to 20% of patients with bacterial meningitis, may be related to pressure phenomena, although one should also be concerned about herniation, especially in the presence of a third cranial nerve palsy. Hemiparesis and other focal findings may be seen in 15% of patients with bacterial meningitis. These signs may also represent Todd's paresis secondary to a seizure, although when this is the case, the focal findings usually clear in 24 hours. Nevertheless, the clinician cannot wait this long in the presence of such focal findings; a mass lesion should be considered. Increased intracranial pressure (180 mm H_2O) is almost universal and is due to a combination of cytotoxic, vasogenic, and interstitial cerebral edema. Opening CSF pressure sometimes is in the range of 400 to 450 mm H_2O, in which case the risk of herniation either related or unrelated to LP greatly increases. Papilledema in true bacterial meningitis, however, is uncommon, and if this sign is present, exclusion of a mass lesion is mandatory. Papilledema with the clinical picture of meningitis should be considered indicative of a brain abscess or subdural empyema until proved otherwise. The appropriate approach would be rapid evaluation, institution of empiric antimicrobial therapy, CT scan, and then LP if both of these entities can be safely excluded (see Chap. 71).

Other physical findings of importance include florid delirium and maniacal behavior, which may accompany pneumococcal or meningococcal meningitis as well as herpes simplex virus (HSV) encephalitis, other encephalitides, and temporal lobe abscess.[14]

A petechial or purpuric rash in the presence of fever, change of mental status, and meningismus usually indicates meningococcal meningitis. Similar skin lesions, however, can accompany neisseria gonorrheal meningitis, S. pneumoniae bacteremia, meningitis with disseminated intravascular coagulation, and staphylococcal endocarditis with meningitis. ECHO virus, especially type 9, can produce a similar rash, can occur in outbreaks such as meningococcal meningitis, and can produce a similar brisk CSF pleocytosis with up to 1000 polymorphonuclear leukocytes per mm^3. The rash of meningococcus infection, however, usually spreads to the face and neck from the rest of the body, whereas ECHO virus, especially type 9, involves the face and neck early in the development of the exanthem.[14]

To confuse matters further, the rickettsial disease, Rocky Mountain spotted fever (RMSF), which occurs most commonly in the Southeastern United States and eastern seaboard, can produce meningeal signs, CSF pleocytosis, and diffuse petechial rash. The rash of RMSF classically appears on the palms and soles first but then generalizes to the rest of the body, where it can mimic the rash seen in fulminant meningococcemia, which usually starts out on the trunk and spreads centrifugally.[63]

The organism causing the rash can usually be identified by bedside culture and biopsy or scraping a petechial lesion. The most prudent course is to treat the patient for bacterial meningitis while awaiting results of a CSF analysis, outcome of culture, response to therapy, and other data. RMSF is treated with tetracycline, in contrast to bacterial meningitis or viral meningitis. RMSF has a slower onset than meningococcemia, and the CSF changes of RMSF are more often lymphocytic and less impressive than those of meningococcus, although there is considerable overlap. These differences help the clinician distinguish the two so as to avoid inappropriate or delayed empiric therapy.[63]

In considering bacterial meningitis in adults, one final organism, L. monocytogenes, deserves attention. Although cases of listeria meningitis have been described with epidemics of consumption of contaminated food, most reported cases have occurred sporadically and have affected the elderly and those who are immunosuppressed because of human immunodeficiency virus (HIV) infection, pregnancy, or steroid therapy.[64] Listeria meningitis is in a class by itself because it has an increased tendency to produce seizures and focal defects early. It also can produce a peculiar type of brain stem meningoencephalitis with ataxia, cranial nerve palsies, and nystagmus (rhomboencephalitis). The CSF is invariably abnormal, usually with a predominance of neutrophils, but it is not uncommon for the CSF (but not the blood) to be sterile, especially when there is rhomboencephalitis. Blood cultures usually grow a profusion of organisms early on and are highly recommended when this disease is suspected.[65,66]

From the previous discussion, it is obvious that two quickly drawn blood cultures are extremely helpful in evaluating for bacterial meningitis. The diagnosis, however, ultimately rests on the overall clinical presentation plus expert analysis of the CSF. It is here that rapid assessment, competent nursing care (especially of a delirious patient), and expertise in performing bedside procedures are all essential. If there are no clinical contraindications, three to four tubes of CSF should be obtained by LP. Several important aspects of CSF analysis are to be emphasized. Besides measuring opening pressure (if possible) and noting the gross appearance of the CSF, the clinician must obtain enough fluid for cell count and differential, bacterial culture and Gram stain, measurement of glucose and protein, and a small amount (1 to 2 ml) for a bacterial antigen test and other tests as warranted. The clinician should assiduously avoid traumatic LPs because spurious red cells complicate the separation of subarachnoid hemorrhage from bacterial meningitis, an occasional clinical conundrum.[67] If the LP is traumatic, the two disorders may be difficult to separate: Subarachnoid hemorrhage can produce headache, fever, abnormal mental status, CSF pleocytosis, and occasional hypoglycorrhachia. When the CSF obtained at LP is clear, any of the tubes may be sent for analysis. When the tap is traumatic and there is blood in the first and perhaps subsequent tube, the two tubes sent for cell count should be any nonconsecutive tubes.

I believe that too much emphasis has been placed on bacterial antigen assays, such as those that use agglutination to detect S. pneumoniae, H. influenzae type B, and Neisseria meningitidis types A, B, C, W, and Y 135, and group B streptococcus. The latest data suggest that these tests have problems with reproducibility.[68] Bacterial antigen detection methods are most helpful in identifying cases of partial treatment of bacterial meningitis. Although antimicrobial therapy for 24 to 48 hours may shift the CSF response toward lymphocytes and decrease organisms identifiable by Gram stain, it does not so affect the bacterial antigen detection.[5,69,70]

When a LP has been traumatic and no blood-free specimen is obtained for evaluation, some authors have suggested using the ratio of peripheral red to white blood cells to estimate white blood cell count. Such an approach, however, is controversial. This is another reason why I believe that clinicians should practice LP skills so as to avoid traumatic taps.

A Gram stain is the most important immediately available test to aid in the diagnosis of meningitis. One member of the patient care team must develop expertise in the processing of CSF specimens for Gram staining, and this person must perform this task as rapidly as possible while other team members are caring for the patient. The CSF must be carried quickly to the laboratory for immediate culture, Gram stain preparation, and cell count. A tube of CSF must be centrifuged correctly, preferably in a machine used for cytologic preparation because this improves the yield in obtaining a pellet. The incidence of false-negative test results is high when this cannot be achieved, which compromises patient care. The spun specimen must be laid carefully on a glass slide, gently heat fixed, and carefully stained with particular attention to counterstaining. Then it is examined under an oil-immersion lens. For reasons that are unclear, there are occasionally artifacts in the CSF, and the decolorization step can be troublesome, even in the most experienced hands. The stained slide should be saved for review by expert colleagues. Given the logarithmic growth of organisms in bacterial meningitis, the Gram stain is positive in at least 50% of cases except when listeria is causing the infection; this organism's slower growth usually results in lower yield on Gram stain.

Typically the CSF of patients with acute bacterial meningitis has increased opening pressure (greater than 180 mm H_2O), elevated protein concentration (120 mg/dl or greater), and glucose level of 50 to 60% or less of that of the blood. There are usually 100 to 500 cells per mm^3 or greater and more than 80% are polymorphonuclear leukocytes. There are important, atypical presenting patterns, however, even when the CSF specimen has been handled rapidly to prevent spontaneous lysis of polymorphonuclear leukocytes or adherence of cells to the side of the tube. Several of these atypical CSF patterns deserve mention: (1) The CSF may be turbid yet contain few white blood cells. In this pattern of minimal pleocytosis, with turbidity owing to enormous numbers of organisms, i.e., greater than 10^3 to 10^5, the prognosis is poor. (2) In 9% of cases of bacterial meningitis, the CSF glucose level may be normal.[59] (3) In up to 15% of cases, lymphocytic pleocytosis may be seen.[71] This causes diagnostic confusion and may lead to errors in patient treatment unless attention is paid to the overall clinical situation as indicated by the history and physical examination. (4) A maximum of 3 to 5 cells per mm^3 may be considered normal.[70]

It has been stated that the presence of a single polymorphonuclear leukocyte in an otherwise normal CSF should be considered within normal limits if the patient is without signs of meningeal infection and levels of glucose and protein are normal; it has also been stated that seizures may produce pleocytosis.[72,73] Seizures, however, may well be the clue to the initial diagnosis of bacterial meningitis. I believe that the presence of one polymorphonuclear leukocyte in the CSF in this setting warrants consideration of intracranial infection, possibly bacterial meningitis, especially if seizure activity is present.

CSF cell count and protein may remain normal in some neonates and immunocompromised patients who are unable to mount a defense even several hours after the onset of meningitis. A published case illustrates this fact and points out the danger in relying too much on the results of CSF analysis without considering the entire clinical picture.[74]

CSF culture results may not be 100% predictive, even when obtained before institution of antimicrobial therapy. For example, Geisler et al.[75] noted in a series of patients with purulent meningitis of unknown origin that a certain percentage met clinical criteria for acute bacterial meningitis, and CSF samples from these patients were high in protein, low in glucose, and contained polymorphonuclear leukocytes in abundant numbers. Although these patients responded well to antimicrobial therapy, their blood culture and CSF culture results were negative for bacterial disease.[75] It might be argued that some of the patients in this series had early viral meningitis (up to two-thirds of viral meningitis cases have early polymorphonuclear leukocyte predominance, and some viruses, such as the one causing lymphocytic choriomeningitis and herpes simplex I and II, can cause hypoglycorrhachia), but more careful review of Geisler's patients does not support this contention.[75] If the suspicion of bacterial meningitis is high and a repeat LP fails to show the classic shift to lymphocytes seen in most cases of viral aseptic meningitis and CSF and blood cultures remain negative, the clinician should continue the antimicrobial regimen for intracranial infection while he or she continues to search for the causative organism(s).[76] In such clinical situations, the acute presentation of a classically chronic meningitis, such as tuberculosis or cryptococcosis, or another entity, such as leptospirosis, RMSF, or a free-living ameba infection, should also be considered.[59,77]

Swartz and O'Hanley[14] have differentiated common from uncommon CNS infections based on three CSF patterns:

- Neutrophilic low glucose
- Lymphocytic normal glucose
- Lymphocytic low glucose

Acute bacterial meningitis classically presents with neutrophilic, low-glucose CSF. Other rare infections that need to be considered include amebic meningoencephalitis caused by naegleria (associated with swimming in brackish waters) and acanthamoeba species (associated with disorders of immunosuppression). CSF wet mounts and cytology can be key in diagnosing some of these uncommon CNS pathogens. More traditional chronic CNS pathogens, such as M. tuberculosis, cryptococcus, and fungi, which usually are characterized by lymphocytic and normal glucose CSF early in their course and by low glucose CSF late in their course, can present early on with a CSF pattern similar to that of acute bacterial meningitis, i.e., neutrophilic normal or low glucose.[59,78] Finally, two parameningeal infections discussed earlier may also present with neutrophilic CSF with normal glucose: embolic cerebral infarction owing to bacterial endocarditis and subdural empyema. These infections usually are associated with lymphocytic normal glucose CSF but may present with neutrophilic low glucose CSF if there is associated true meningitis.[14]

In the early phase of viral meningitis, CSF occasionally may be neutrophilic, although the glucose level is usually normal.[46,79,80] Most cases of viral infection, however, present with a so-called aseptic meningitis CSF profile with lymphocytes and normal glucose level. The term aseptic meningitis was introduced in 1925 to describe an acute onset of meningitic signs similar to bacterial meningitis but with predominantly mononuclear cells, absence of bacteria on stains and culture, no known parameningeal infection, and a short and benign course. The diagnosis of aseptic meningitis in the premicrobial era when purulent meningitis was virtually 100% fatal implied an excellent prognosis. Currently an aseptic meningitis CSF profile alone, however, cannot assure a good prognosis and may be due to a variety of treatable serious disorders.[46] As just mentioned, this presentation can characterize many cases of meningitis due to common bacteria that have been only partially treated and in which case cessation of antibacterial therapy would be disastrous.[59]

Parenchymal Infections

Meningoencephalitis

Parenchymal infections of the CNS, which in presentation often mimic true bacterial meningitis, also have a poor prognosis unless rapidly diagnosed and treated.

Meningoencephalitis, which is often due to virulent viruses, may be suspected on clinical presentation, history, and physical examination. This disease, however, can exactly mimic acute purulent meningitis. Thus LP should be performed without delay. The benign CSF profile often seen with meningoencephalitis provides false reassurance, however: Aggressive diagnostic and therapeutic intervention must be instituted as rapidly as if acute bacterial meningitis were present if therapy is to be lifesaving. Because a lymphocytic, normal glucose CSF profile can represent partially treated bacterial meningitis due to common pathogens, viral meningoencephalitis, or brain abscess, a CT scan or MRI scan is indicated for full evaluation.[18]

The most common cause of treatable meningoencephalitis is HSV, and this disease is the focus of our discussion. HSV encephalitis can present with the same CSF profile (lymphocytes and normal glucose) as other CNS infections.[15,59] When HSV is under consideration, LP should be performed to exclude other diseases and radiographic studies reviewed to localize the infection, which is invariably in the temporal lobe. These tests may help the clinician select the appropriate therapy. In contrast, when a brain abscess or other focal mass infection is present except for the cerebritis phase of an early brain abscess, LP is contraindicated because of increased risk of herniation. LP may help in the exclusion of other diseases, which often show a different CSF profile. CT or MRI results also aid in the evaluation of parenchymal CNS infection and in detecting contraindications to LP.[25,81]

Patients presenting with meningoencephalitis caused by any of a variety of organisms tend to have subacute onset of mild fever; headache (which ranges from mild to severe); and, with later presentation, possibly focal defects, including focal seizures, hemiparesis, and cranial nerve deficits, and an altered level of consciousness. Meningismus is not as prominent in patients with meningoencephalitis as in those with bacterial meningitis, but when meningismus does occur, patients usually have fever and occasionally focal findings, such as positive Babinski sign. Papilledema is uncommon, but signs of increased intracranial pressure may be present. As opposed to many patients with brain abscess and bacterial meningitis, those with meningoencephalitis rarely have extracranial sites of infection.[82]

The presentation of meningoencephalitis has been described in landmark studies by Whitley et al. and the National Institute of Allergy and Infectious Disease (NIAID) collaborative antiviral study group,[17] which reviewed encephalitis presumed due to HSV over the last 20 years. Their data and clinical findings help us realize that HSV encephalitis, which is the prototype of these diseases, is difficult to diagnose definitely even when history, physical examination, and laboratory findings that some clinicians consider pathognomonic are present.[17]

The pathologic findings in HSV encephalitis are often said to be focal and limited to the temporal lobe. Whitley's data, however, suggest that this is not a particularly sensitive or specific finding. All patients in Whitley's series underwent open brain biopsy after enrollment based on clinical suspicion (Table 7-3). The morbidity from open brain biopsy in 432 patients was surprisingly low (2%), probably

Table 7-3. Clinical Findings in Suspected Herpes Simplex Encephalitis

Acute febrile encephalopathy
Temporal lobe signs
Evidence of localizing central nervous system disease (brain scan, EEG, CT scan, MRI scan)
Cerebrospinal fluid findings compatible with viral encephalitis

a reflection of the expertise of their neurosurgical teams. Despite good clinical suspicion, only 45% of the patients in the series had biopsies that were proved by culture or additional virologic studies to contain HSV.[17]

One-third of the encephalitides in this series remained undiagnosed despite evaluation by electroencephalogram (EEG) (before this study said to be highly sensitive for HSV encephalitis) CT, biopsy, and extensive clinical and serologic follow-up.

The other 22% of patients in Whitley's series had diseases that were proved by biopsy not to be HSV and identified by evaluation of brain tissue or other clinical criteria as something else. Among the 9% of Whitley's patients who had non-HSV diseases that were treatable, some had subdural abscesses, brain abscesses, or subdural empyema, which shows how closely these suppurative diseases can mimic HSV encephalitis. Several patients had chronic granulomatous infections, such as tuberculosis and cryptococcosis, and several had brain tumors.

Approximately 13% of the total patients in Whitley's series had nontreatable diseases that mimicked HSV encephalitis. The largest group included viral diseases caused by togaviruses, specifically arboviruses.[17] The largest group with a single virus that mimicked HSV had Epstein-Barr virus meningoencephalitis.[17] These are important findings for the bedside clinician to remember in initial evaluation.

Once the history and physical examination have been performed in an encephalitis case, the clinician is faced with the dilemma of what laboratory tests to order. EEG is one of the more sensitive ways to diagnose a focal meningoencephalitis, but this test is usually not available 24 hours a day and has a specificity of only 40% for HSV.[17] CT can be helpful in excluding a brain abscess when the clinical picture is of a focal meningoencephalitis.[14] When brain abscess is present, LP is relatively contraindicated, but a spinal tap can be helpful in diagnosis of focal meningoencephalitis.

Kaiser and McGee[19] have developed algorithms for management of parenchymal brain infections: (1) When the patient presents less than 48 hours after onset of symptoms and there are focal findings, one should begin broad-spectrum antimicrobial therapy (to be discussed shortly) and then proceed with a CT scan. With subacute illness of 2 to 7 days' duration, and focal findings CT can be performed before institution of antimicrobial therapy provided there is only a 1-to 2 hour delay.[19] If there is clinical concern that the patient might have bacterial meningitis, however, no harm would be done by performing a rapid evaluation with blood cultures and beginning appropriate antibiotics before the CT scan is obtained. If a CT scan or MRI scan shows a focal abnormality, the clinician must decide whether the findings are more compatible with brain abscess or meningoencephalitis.[18]

As is discussed subsequently, with many cases of brain abscess there may be localized infection in the head and neck area, heart, or lung. Such infection is usually rapidly identifiable as the source for bacteria causing a brain abscess. Thus, when baseline evaluation shows no evidence of a pulmonary infection, endocarditis, or another parameningeal focus, antiviral therapy for focal encephalitis should be begun quickly. Nevertheless, predictions based on clinical presentations, CT scan, or MRI findings are not 100% reliable, especially early on or when therapy with dexamethasone sodium phosphate (Decadron) has been instituted for cerebral edema. Repeat frequent clinical evaluations and laboratory and radiographic evaluation are in order after initiation of therapy, especially if the patient is not improving.

The earlier therapy for HSV encephalitis is started, the greater the chance of minimizing morbidity and mortality.[83] If biopsy is performed, the specimen must be examined to identify not only HSV, but also bacteria, including anaerobes, acid-fast bacilli, and yeast. These organisms can rarely cause disease that mimics HSV encephalitis.[17] Many clinicians would begin therapy with acyclovir (more efficacious than adenine arabinoside) before obtaining the results of biopsy. Initiating therapy with or without biopsy has been continuously debated, however.[84,85] Results of biopsy can be nondiagnostic (30%) or even erroneous. Two patients in the NIAID series (1%) had negative biopsy results and at postmortem were found to have HSV in brain tissue.[83]

Although arguments can be made for performing a biopsy before institution of acyclovir therapy, I believe that it is more appropriate to begin acyclovir therapy on suspicion of HSV encephalitis. This is analogous to rapid initiation of antibacterial therapy for acute bacterial meningitis. Unfortunately, from examination of Whitley's data, it is evident that roughly half of patients are overtreated, and a significant percentage of these (9%) may have other conditions potentially curable by entirely different forms of therapy.[17]

With this in mind, I propose that when the CT scan or MRI scan leads to a suspicion of HSV encephalitis and a brain abscess has been reasonably excluded but there are focal findings, LP should be performed. The results of CSF evaluation help exclude the rare cases of acute bacterial meningitis that mimic HSV encephalitis; more importantly, spinal tap results may identify one of the treatable entities other than HSV encephalitis. These other entities include tuberculosis and cryptococcal meningitis, rickettsial diseases, and other important syndromes such as listeriosis that have CSF patterns usually different from that of HSV encephalitis.

In addition, because Epstein-Barr virus infection appears to be the second most common, identifiable viral cause of encephalitis in Whitley's series, it is reasonable to obtain a peripheral blood smear to identify atypical lymphocytosis and to request an Epstein-Barr virus IgM level. If these were positive (blood smear examination takes less than an hour), acyclovir therapy might be theoretically discontinued.[86] If, after several days, the patient is not improving or continues to deteriorate and there is a definite focal finding on CT scan, brain biopsy should be considered.[85]

Two technical comments may be of help in managing HSV encephalitis. First, preliminary results indicate that MRI may be more sensitive than CT in detecting early signs of HSV encephalitis.[87] Second, stereotactic techniques for brain biopsy might be associated with less morbidity than open brain biopsy, particularly in patients with significant cerebral edema for whom brain biopsy is relatively more difficult. Stereotactic techniques appear to provide almost as much useful information as traditional biopsy and may be used more frequently in this setting.[88]

The classic CSF findings of HSV encephalitis include mildly elevated protein, normal glucose, mild pleocytosis (0 to 500 lymphocytes) and opening pressure in the range of 180 to 300 mm H_2O. This CSF pattern is similar to that of viral meningitis secondary to enteroviruses. In addition, in Whitley's encephalitis series, 12% of patients with identifiable diseases and 12% of patients without a final diagnosis had normal CSF findings, as did 5% of patients with HSV encephalitis.[83] These results support the author's contention that CSF profiles are not infallible diagnostic tools. Clearly the clinical picture of HSV encephalitis tends to worsen if not treated, whereas aseptic meningitis owing to enterovirus generally improves spontaneously within 1 to 2 days.[83]

In elderly patients, HSV encephalitis causes particularly high morbidity and mortality. Viral aseptic meningitis is uncommon in patients over the age of 40; any person over the age of 40 with CNS disease with an aseptic meningitis pattern is more likely to have a viral meningoencephalitis such as HSV encephalitis or arbovirus infection rather than a benign enteroviral infection.[59]

A review of encephalitis epidemiology by geographic region and season in the United States may be instructive. Arbovirus infections, especially St. Louis encephalitis and La Crosse encephalitis, are relatively common and can mimic HSV encephalitis.[89] These diseases tend to occur in the summer during outbreaks of enteroviral aseptic meningitis. The CSF patterns are the same, and the clinical picture may be similar. HSV encephalitis tends to show a different time distribution: It is more likely to occur in winter or spring. In the United States, the evaluation of patients in summer to fall is troublesome, however, because of the overlap in disease prevalence.[45]

Finally, initial serologic studies for HSV have no role in excluding or including HSV encephalitis in the differential diagnosis. Most cases of HSV encephalitis represent reactivation of the virus, but in the 25 to 30% that are probably primary infection, tests for antibody to herpes simplex I, the isolate in the vast majority of adult cases, may be negative.[83] Excluding HSV encephalitis based on negative antibody titer results is inappropriate.[90] Research reports have described the rapid diagnosis of HSV encephalitis by means of polymerase chain reaction assay and other antigen detection systems, but these assays are not clinically available and have had limited field trial.[83,91]

Brain Abscess

Brain abscess is a localized suppurative infection of CNS parenchyma with an incidence approximately one-fifth that of pyogenic meningitis.[13] Although brain abscesses are rare, if not diagnosed early or improperly treated, mortality is significant. Despite the use of modern antibiotic therapy and refined surgical techniques, the mortality rate of brain abscess remains high.[92] Data suggest, however, that CT and MRI can help in formulating an accurate diagnosis earlier with further decrease in mortality.[93]

A graphic self-description of the entire course of a brain abscess has been published.[94] A brain abscess is a dynamic lesion that begins as a localized area of nonsuppurative inflammation (cerebritis) and progresses over time to necrosis and frank suppuration. Its presentation depends on when in the abscess' time course the patient seeks treatment. Symptoms usually include headache that is mild to severe and occasionally focal deficits and seizures that progress over days to weeks. The typical headache of brain abscess is often more severe than that of meningoencephalitis, and the headache is usually present somewhat longer before treatment is sought, but these differences are not exclusive.[19]

Evidence of a contiguous focus of infection is much more suggestive of brain abscess. Thus a thorough head and neck examination and evaluation for parameningeal foci are important in evaluation of a potential brain abscess. For example, brain abscess in the frontal lobe may be a sequela of frontal or ethmoid sinusitis. Likewise, infection in the middle ear may give rise to an abscess in the temporal lobe, whereas infection in the mastoid may also give rise to a cerebellar abscess. Any part of the brain may be so affected, however, including the brain stem, parietal lobe, occipital lobe, and pituitary gland.[93] The diversity of anatomic presentations possible with brain abscess differentiates this entity from most forms of meningoencephalitis, which usually have focal characteristics mainly limited to the temporal lobe.[82]

A significant percentage of brain abscesses may arise from distal infections, including suppurative lung infections such as bronchiectasis, lung abscess, or pneumonia. In addition, a small minority are associated with right-to-left intracardiac shunts or endocarditis.[93] Most metastatic brain abscesses are either single or multiple areas of infection at the junction of the gray and white matter, which may help to differentiate the presentation of this type of brain abscess from meningoencephalitis.

On physical examination, the presence of a contiguous infection in the head and neck area or pulmonary area with fever, focal findings, and papilledema should lead the clinician to suspect brain abscess and move quickly to order a CT scan. As has been mentioned, papilledema is uncommon in bacterial meningitis and meningoencephalitis. Papilledema in this setting favors brain abscess. In addition, seizures are more commonly seen with brain abscess than with other entities we have discussed except for epidural and subdural empyemas and meningoencephalitis.[14]

When the clinician is in doubt about whether the diagnosis is brain abscess or meningoencephalitis, a radiographic study should be ordered first because LP as the initial diagnostic confirmatory test is relatively contraindicated. It should be emphasized again that the CSF findings in a brain abscess can be the same as those of meningoencephalitis. In both situations, culturing and examination of CSF mainly exclude other mimicking entities rather than providing the organism responsible for brain abscess or meningoencephalitis.[19]

With regard to radiographic criteria of a brain abscess, one should remember that multifocal lesions and ring-enhancing lesions are suggestive but not pathognomonic for brain abscess. The single criteria for radiographic confirmation of a brain abscess is the presence of air produced by the organisms. In the postoperative situation, however, this can be exceedingly difficult when air can be present for a long time secondary to the neurosurgical procedure alone.[25]

Furthermore, radiographic criteria always have to be coupled with the clinical findings. For example, an area of cerebritis identified in an isolated area of the temporal lobe of a patient could be either brain abscess or HSV encephalitis. Clinically the latter presentation would most likely represent brain abscess if there was an associated middle ear infection discovered by clinical examination and CT. Even ring enhancement by contrast material is not entirely specific for a brain abscess because it can also be seen in encephalitis as well as hematoma.[95]

The microbiology of brain abscesses caused by contiguous sites (60 to 70%) is as follows. Organisms causing temporal lobe abscesses are usually of middle ear origin and include anaerobic, streptococci, B. fragilis, and aerobic gram-negative rods. Infection in the frontal or parietal lobes may be due to paranasal sinus infection and usually involves anaerobic streptococci, various haemophilus species, pneumococcus, bacteroides, or S. aureus.[92] Fifteen percent of brain abscesses may be due to mastoid infection, in which case infection may be in the temporal lobe or cerebellum. The causative organisms are similar to those associated with middle ear infections.[93]

Approximately 5% of brain abscesses occur as a consequence of neurosurgery or brain trauma, and they are caused by S. aureus, anaerobic bacteria, or skin flora such as "low grade" organisms, including diphtheroids and coagulase-negative staphylococcus. Distinguishing healing changes after neurosurgery from postoperative brain abscess can be exceedingly difficult. Even low grade organisms, once they have caused purulent infection, can produce serious neurologic side effects from secondary edema.[93]

Approximately 25% of brain abscesses arise from distal sites of infection, and up to 10% of brain abscesses have no known site of origin. In such situations, it would be difficult to distinguish the early stage of these abscesses from meningoencephalitis because a distal or contiguous site of infection would much more likely favor a brain abscess. Pulmonary infection leads to 15% of brain abscesses, and right-to-left intracardiac shunts through the heart cause some 5% of the cases; abdominal infections and other distal infections rarely seed the brain. Organisms typically involved in these types of brain abscesses are streptococci, gram-negative rods, anaerobes, and S. aureus.[93]

The presentation of intracranial CNS infections in acquired immunodeficiency syndrome (AIDS) patients is beyond the scope of this chapter and is covered elsewhere in this text as well as the recent literature.[96] In the presence of other immunosuppressive disorders, particularly those associated with steroid use, when there are focal neurologic findings, such as headache and focal weakness, a concern is nocardia infection (usually due to silent pulmonary infections), progressing to the brain in a hematogenous manner. In an immunocompromised patient with a brain abscess, the most likely organism is nocardia.[93]

In the rapidly expanding population of persons with HIV infection and organ transplant patients, a mass lesion might also be toxoplasmosis associated with immunosuppression.[97] In such cases, stereotactic brain biopsy can be quite helpful in making the differential diagnosis. Another concern in immunosuppressed patients or those receiving steroid therapy is that steroid therapy can profoundly decrease the ring enhancement on CT suggestive of brain abscess.[25] When at all possible, one should try to perform CT before steroids are administered.

Other mass lesions of the brain, including tuberculoma, cryptococcoma, and parasitic infections such as cysticercosis, may mimic pyogenic brain abscess. These conditions are unusual enough, however, and are discussed elsewhere.[25]

ICU PHASE

Parameningeal Infections

Many patients with intracranial infections experience an alteration in mental status that necessitates transfer to an ICU for aggressive diagnosis and therapy, including cardiopulmonary monitoring and support as well as rapid institution of appropriate antimicrobial therapy, if not done already. Attention needs to be directed to electrolyte management, control of cerebral edema, and administration of antiseizure medications. Neurosurgical procedures, such as placement of an intracranial pressure monitoring device or burr holes to drain an epidural or subdural empyema, may be needed. An essential component of care of the patient with a CNS infection is immediate administration of antimicrobial agents. Because of the urgency to institute pharmacotherapy, I believe that one member of the patient care team should be personally responsible for rapid institution of the antimicrobial regimen once it has been chosen. Administration of antimicrobial agents alone, however, is not sufficient to treat patients with CNS infection.[16,98] The multidisciplinary approach may include the assistance of a neuroradiologist, infectious disease physician, otolaryngologist, ophthalmologist, intensive medicine specialist, neurologist, and neurosurgeon.

In the foregoing discussions of parameningeal, meningeal, and parenchymal CNS infections, we considered a broad variety of types of microbes, including viruses, rickettsiae, mycobacteria, mycoplasma, bacteria, yeasts, fungi, and parasites. The range of antimicrobial agents that may be used to treat these pathogens is too broad to be discussed in this chapter; the reader is referred to other sources for detailed discussions of drug penetration, pharmacokinetics, dosages, and adverse effects.[10,12] We discuss, however, general principles of their usage in this chapter.

In general, antimicrobial therapy for a CNS infection must not only be chosen rapidly and appropriately, but also administered in the highest doses possible. In making decisions about type and dosage of antimicrobial medication, the clinician needs to remember what has been mentioned about organisms likely responsible for CNS infections and the limited penetration of the CNS by antimicrobial agents (both the blood-brain barrier and the blood-CSF barrier). The limitations imposed by these barriers as well as aspects of lipid solubility, ionization coefficients, and protein binding are appropriately discussed in greater detail elsewhere.[10] In addition, several authors have also addressed pharmacologic problems that develop with the meningeal inflammation that occurs with infection and how to manage the problems that arise because of pressure phenomena such as hydrocephalus or brain edema. The reader is referred to additional references for more information on these topics.[12]

All antimicrobial agents can have significant side effects, such as skin rashes and hematologic toxicity. One side effect, true anaphylactic penicillin allergy, has probably been overemphasized. A thorough history usually elicits the needed information about true immediate penicillin hypersensitivity. When necessary, procedures such as penicillin skin testing and desensitization are available.[99,100] There is not enough time, however, to perform either one of these procedures when acute bacterial meningitis is present. The best alternative is to administer a third-generation cephalosporin because these agents have only a 10% cross reactivity at most, if there is suspicion of true anaphylaxis secondary to penicillin.[99]

Even under the best of circumstances, however, the clinician may at times be forced to make difficult choices. The best stance is to acknowledge that side effects are likely with any medication. Although chloramphenicol is usually an excellent choice for such CNS infections as meningitis due to haemophilus, pneumococcus, or meningococcus; complicated brain abscesses; and RMSF, the drug can cause irreversible bone marrow aplasia. Given the potential morbidity and mortality as a result of these infections, the 1:20,000 chance that chloramphenicol will cause aplasia seems a reasonable risk-to-benefit ratio in the correct clinical setting; for example a history of true penicillin anaphylaxis.

Skeletal and Soft Tissue Infections

Most parameningeal infections are bacterial. If a scalp or skin lesion has produced a CNS infection, the most likely choice for antibiotic therapy would be a semisynthetic penicillin such as nafcillin at a dosage of 2 g intravenously every 4 hours. For a parameningeal infection due to zygomycetes, high dose amphotericin B may be begun and rapidly escalated, usually over the first day after recognition of this syndrome, to at least 50 mg/day, even at the risk of substantial nephrotoxicity.[24] Strict control of diabetes mellitus is essential to management of this syndrome as well as debridement of the sinuses and occasionally intracranial structures by otolaryngology, ophthalmology, and neurosurgery colleagues.[23]

Later we consider the antibacterial regimens for parameningeal infections associated with the paranasal sinuses, middle ear, and mastoid and their associated CNS infections: septic thrombosis of the dural venous sinuses, epidural empyema, subdural empyema, true bacterial meningitis, and brain abscess.

Vascular Infections

The vascular type of parameningeal infections have been divided into sepsis, infective endocarditis, cerebral septic arteritis (usually associated with endocarditis), and septic dural venous phlebitis.

Sepsis. Sepsis is a large topic of current intense clinical interest.[26] Cytokine therapy may be able to reduce the current mortality of 30 to 50% from this disease, which is the best result currently achieved with antimicrobial therapy and ICU support.[101] Some patients with true bacterial meningitis, especially due to pneumococcus, H. influenzae, and meningococcus organisms, in addition to true CNS invasion also manifest the septic syndrome with profound hypotension, decreased renal output, and multiple organ failure.[18] We mentioned, however, that disorders of higher integrative function are common in sepsis of all kinds, including bloodstream infections due to S. epidermidis, enterococcus, and gram-negative bacilli, which rarely, if ever, invade an intact CNS. Nevertheless, if there is difficulty in differentiating the acute meningitis syndrome from sepsis, a reasonable initial antibiotic agent would be nafcillin added to a regimen of an aminoglycoside plus ceftazidime (the latter included for its activity against pseudomonas). If there is concern about methicillin-resistant S. aureus, which can be both community and hospital acquired, vancomycin should be used instead of nafcillin.

Infective Endocarditis. General therapeutic approaches to endocarditis have been discussed elsewhere.[102] The important factor in treatment of endocarditis-associated CNS infection is that the antimicrobial agent of choice be able to cross the blood-brain barrier. For example, cefazolin is a reasonable choice for methicillin-sensitive S. aureus endocarditis when the patient has a true penicillin allergy. If the patient has a CNS complication, however, such as cerebritis, stroke, meningitis, or cerebral abscess, cefazolin would be inappropriate; an alternative might be vancomycin or desensitization. Other aspects of the treatment of CNS complications of cerebral endocarditis are beyond the scope of this chapter. The reader is referred to a discussion of such problems as the advantages and disadvantages of anticoagulation, factors in the decision to replace the valve, and management of mycotic aneurysm of intracranial arteries.[32]

Septic Dural Venous Sinus Phlebitis

ICU management of septic cavernous sinus thrombosis includes antibacterial therapy for S. aureus, streptococcus, and oral anaerobes (more than 95% of cases are treated effectively by a regimen such as a semisynthetic penicillin [nafcillin] plus metronidazole). Surgical drainage of a facial infection, ethmoid sinusitis, sphenoid sinusitis, or dental infection, which are the usual sources for intracranial infection, aid diagnosis as well as therapy.[39] Additional therapy with heparin remains controversial owing to the risk of hemorrhage from sites of associated cortical venous infarction or from the intracavernous walls of the carotid artery, both of which are associated with this entity. The use of steroids is equally controversial except when thrombosis has spread to the pituitary gland and adrenal crisis has occurred. Surgical drainage of the cavernous sinus by itself is hazardous and is not recommended.[39]

ICU management of septic lateral sinus thrombosis should include antibacterial therapy for the bacterial species usually involved with chronic otitis media, including proteus species, S. aureus, E. coli, B. fragilis, and anaerobic streptococci.[39] A combination of nafcillin and chloramphenicol provides reasonable coverage. Concern about interaction between the beta-lactam bactericidal drug and a bacteriostatic drug (chloramphenicol) is probably not necessary with chloramphenicol because chloramphenicol is actually bactericidal to many CNS pathogens.[12] In addition, experience shows that there is little antagonism when the combination of a penicillin-type drug and chloramphenicol is used for other CNS infections, including true meningitis.[12] The combination of clavulanic acid and ticarcillin or imipenem-cilastatin seems reasonable to treat septic lateral sinus thrombosis because of polymicrobial primary infection, but there is less experience with these medications for CNS infections.[10] If there is no improvement after 12 to 24 hours of adequate doses of the antimicrobial agent, radical mastoidectomy should be performed with exploration of the area over the lateral sinus to search for an associated epidural phlegmon or abscess. A needle may be passed into the lateral sinus to document thrombosis, but the sinus should not be removed because it will recanalize over time with correct treatment. Cerebral edema usually occurs, partly because of interference with absorption of CSF, and this may be corrected with mannitol and steroids; some clinicians have advocated LP every 48 hours to relieve cerebral edema. If papilledema and decreased visual acuity do not improve, subtemporal decompression may be needed.[39]

Before antibiotic medications were available, septic lateral sinus thrombosis could spread to the jugular vein and then extracranially, often requiring jugular vein ligation. Blood cultures can help to identify organisms involved in CNS infection, especially bacterial meningitis, and may be helpful in evaluating lateral sinus thrombosis.[39] Anticoagulation is not recommended for patients with lateral sinus thrombosis because there is risk of hemorrhagic venous infarction. There is often epidural phlegmon or abscess identified and treated at the time of mastoidectomy.[21]

ICU management of septic thrombosis of the superior sagittal sinus is less frequently a problem than management of cavernous or lateral sinus suppurative thrombosis. Sagittal sinus thrombosis, however, can be catastrophic when it occurs in association with meningitis, and the clinician should be alert to its signs: refractory seizures, profound depression of mental status, and signs of brain stem herniation. Most cases are either associated with meningitis or rarely occur with sinusitis or mastoiditis with extension from the lateral dural sinus: Nafcillin plus cefotaxime is a reasonable combination of therapy. Even with antibiotic treatment and attention to associated cerebral edema (which often occurs owing to involvement of the CSF absorptive system), the mortality of this type of CNS thrombosis is great. Heparin is contraindicated because of the high rate of venous hemorrhagic infarction, and surgical procedures, except for draining an associated infected air sinus when it harbors primary infection, are of no avail and may actually worsen the already desperate neurologic situation. Complete occlusion of the superior sagittal sinus has often been viewed as a fatal complication in some cases of bacterial meningitis.[39]

Epidural and Subdural Empyema

Of the two parameningeal empyemas, the less common abscess of the epidural space is managed more straightforwardly in the ICU. In this situation, antibiotics have often been initiated to treat the primary focus of infection—usually post-traumatic or postneurosurgical or involving the skull, paranasal air sinuses, mastoids, or orbits. The most appropriate agents to treat nosocomially acquired S. aureus, including methicillin-sensitive and methicillin-resistant varieties, and gram-negative bacilli are vancomycin plus ceftriaxone, ceftizoxime or cefotaxime. The results of cultures and stains of surgically drained fluid can further guide antibiotic selection. Empiric therapy may need to be directed against aerobic streptococci as well as haemophilus species and bacteroides. Before Gram stain or culture results are available, an empiric regimen might include a combination of nafcillin and chloramphenicol because the third-generation cephalosporins do not treat bacteroides effectively.

Surgical therapy of epidural empyema is aimed at decompression, reduction of mass effect, and prevention of further epidural extension.[42] Should a postoperative craniotomy flap infection occur, craniotomy and even flap removal may be required because often the bone is also involved because of decreased blood supply. When epidural abscess is associated with a parameningeal or contiguous site of infection, burr holes may often suffice for drainage and for obtaining material for bacteriologic analysis and planning of therapy. Follow-up postoperative CT or MRI may play a significant role in directing further surgical drainage if antimicrobial therapy is not adequate to treat residual infection. Such infection is particularly likely to recur in parafalcine or subtemporal regions; superinfection from organisms acquired at the time of the original drainage may also occur.[42]

Subdural empyema is more common and its treatment far more urgent than managing epidural collections of pus. Subdural empyema may be suspected from the presence of a contiguous source of infection in the presence of fever, headache, altered mental status, and focal findings, such as hemiparesis with seizures (53%). CT and occasionally MRI may be used to help guide the neurosurgeon's approach to the treatment of subdural empyema.[44] As is the case with epidural empyemas, the cultures obtained at craniotomy are negative about one-third of the time, usually because partial treatment has been given. Given the urgency of the situation, this is not a particular problem because the Gram stain can usually still accurately guide therapy. An appropriate regimen for postneurosurgical patients, those who have had intracranial pressure monitoring, and head trauma patients who have subdural empyema associated with these conditions usually includes antibiotic agents active against S. aureus (methicillin-resistant and methicillin-sensitive S. aureus) and coagulase-negative staphylococci and occasionally nosocomial types of gram-negative enteric bacilli with multiple resistance patterns. For this type of subdural empyema, surgical drainage is imperative and should be arranged as soon as the empyema is recognized clinically, confirmed by CT or MRI, and antimicrobial therapy and prophylaxis for seizures begun.

Many authors suggest initial treatment with steroids to minimize cerebral edema if this effect is seen on CT, but steroid therapy in general is to be discouraged.[44]

The controversy as to whether subdural empyema should be managed surgically by burr holes or craniotomy is complicated by inadequate attention in comparative series to the patient's level of consciousness at the time of operation. Silverberg and DiNubile,[42] however, have argued that craniotomy is necessary in up to 20% of patients initially treated with trephination. In addition, they argue that in subdural empyema the pus is so tenacious that it cannot be suctioned or irrigated via the burr holes and that these holes may become clogged by brain substance because of the tremendous amount of acute cerebral edema. In addition, burr holes have no role in managing parafalcine or posterior fossa collections of infection. Craniotomy has the advantage of providing better decompression and allowing more extensive visualization and drainage of the infected area.[42]

Some neurosurgeons have suggested antibiotic irrigation of the subdural space, but most beta-lactam antibiotics and imipenem should be avoided because of their epileptogenic potential. Drains may be left in place for a day or two, but CNS defense mechanisms generally tolerate these poorly, and one should be alert to the danger of nosocomial superinfection.[42]

In adults, subdural empyema (similar to epidural empyema) is often associated with contiguous head and neck infection. Surgical drainage of the empyema and consultation with an otolaryngologist to drain the contiguous focus of infection simultaneously are equally important in such cases. The organisms causing subdural abscess are occasionally multiple and may include streptococcus, both aerobic and anaerobic; coagulase-positive staphylococcus, usually methicillin-sensitive S. aureus acquired from the community; anaerobes including B. fragilis; and rarely gram-negative enteric bacilli. For the types of infectious organisms involved in subdural empyema, empiric therapy is often the rule. A reasonable starting regimen is nafcillin, cefotaxime or ceftriaxone, and metronidazole; the number of antimicrobial agents can then be decreased when a specimen obtained at the time of neurosurgical decompression has been analyzed by culture and Gram stain.[43]

Meningitides

In the past several years, third-generation cephalosporins have proved to be particularly useful in the treatment of meningitis due to H. influenzae (accounting for 5% of infections) or gram-negative enteric bacilli. At least one-fifth of H. influenzae isolates have been found to be resistant to penicillin.[56,98] Although H. influenzae and especially gram-negative enteric bacilli are unusual causes of community-acquired meningitis in adults, they do occur, and their resistance pattern is significant to patient management.[103] The advent of third-generation cephalosporins decreased the frequency with which chloramphenicol was used, particularly for H. influenzae. For certain neurologic infections, however, chloramphenicol remains the drug of choice and may be even more efficacious than third-generation cephalosporins. Anaerobic meningitis acquired in a bacteremic fashion is uncommon, but this mode of pathogenesis is quite common for the six or seven major organisms involved in true bacterial meningitis.

Third-generation cephalosporins have an advantage over chloramphenicol because they lack the potential for irreversible aplastic anemia, as has been discussed. Gram-negative enteric bacilli causing postoperative or post-traumatic meningitis before the development of third-generation cephalosporins was exceedingly difficult to treat. Chloramphenicol has not performed well in the treatment of gram-negative enteric bacillary meningitis.[59] Intrathecal administration of aminoglycosides has been ineffective, which is not surprising given what we know today about CSF circulation. Intrathecal therapy probably plays little primary role in the treatment of such infections.[59] Instead third-generation cephalosporins, including ceftazidime, have been proved to be of great assistance for treatment of gram-negative bacillary meningitis.[19]

Acute bacterial meningitis is a relatively common CNS infection that must, as has been discussed, be treated quickly. I favor empiric administration of ampicillin (penicillin) and ceftriaxone. When results of blood culture and CSF confirm the responsible organisms, usually in 24 to 48 hours, the regimen can be adjusted. Gram stain often helps in rapid identification of the organisms likely to be involved. Gram stain of the CSF, however, requires at minimum 10 to 15 minutes, and if much longer, this is unacceptable. In addition, Gram stain differentiation in CSF of pneumococci from H. influenzae can be difficult, and not all gram-negative pleomorphic coccobacillary infections are necessarily due to H. influenzae. Finally, listeria meningitis appears to be on the increase, especially in the elderly, and as mentioned previously, a Gram stain of this organism is frequently negative. For all of these reasons, I favor administering 2 g ampicillin intravenously every 4 hours and ceftriaxone 2 g intravenously every 12 hours, so coverage is provided as additional information is gathered. This regimen should provide antibacterial concentration in CSF adequate to combat the organisms just discussed as well as the presumed causes of community-acquired purulent meningitis of unknown origin.[75]

The use of penicillin for listeria instead of ampicillin may not make a difference as long as high doses are used.[104] An important point to consider, however, is that in a patient older than age 50 with a negative Gram stain and certain clinical signs, listeria is high on the list of possibilities. Listeria is not treatable by a third-generation cephalosporin alone or chloramphenicol; thus in these patients, penicillin or ampicillin should be prescribed and given in addition to systemic and probably intrathecal gentamicin.[59] The initial regimen of penicillin plus ceftriaxone can be tapered according to the results of CSF culture and sensitivity testing performed during the first 2 days of therapy. If the results of culture, Gram stain, and the bacterial antigen detection test are negative, and the patient is improving clinically, I would urge continuation of that therapy for 10 to 14 days, as is standard for bacterial meningitis caused by the pathogens discussed in this chapter.

Some 10 to 25% of H. influenzae isolates are ampicillin resistant, and this is the important reason for administering ceftriaxone.[59] Before development of the third-generation cephalosporins, chloramphenicol was frequently used in bacterial meningitis. It is still a good alternative for treatment of patients with true penicillin or cephalosporin allergy. Initial concern about bacteriostatic problems with chloramphenicol have been dispelled as the drug shows excellent bactericidal activity against H. influenzae, pneumococcus, and N. meningitidis.[10] Use of the third-generation cephalosporins has been spurred by concern about the extremely rare hematologic toxicity reported with chloramphenicol. Another concern regarding antibiotic resistance is that in certain parts of the United States and abroad, 1 to 5% of pneumococcus isolates may be partially resistant to penicillin.[59,105] This resistance is why using penicillin or ampicillin as initial therapy for community-acquired bacterial meningitis in adults may have to be re-evaluated.

Fortunately these S. pneumoniae isolates have only intermediate resistance to penicillin, with minimal inhibitory concentrations (MIC) of 0.2 µ/ml, and ceftriaxone has demonstrated adequate activity to destroy these organisms.[105] High doses of vancomycin are effective in treating these forms of pneumococcal meningitis as well. The very high penicillin resistance patterns reported from South Africa a number of years ago have not become widespread yet.[59]

In addition to S. pneumoniae and H. influenzae, N. meningitidis may also show antibiotic resistance. There have been rare isolates, again in South Africa, that show increased resistance to penicillin, and such isolates should be watched for elsewhere in the world in the future.[59,105] Determination of the MIC of antibiotic agents for treating all isolates from the CSF should be standard in hospital bacteriology laboratories.

The third-generation cephalosporins have been proved effective in controlled trials using ceftriaxone, cefotaxime, and ceftizoxime in treating bacterial meningitis due to S. pneumoniae, H. influenzae and N. meningitides.[10] Moxalactam and cefoperazone are not appropriate in this clinical situation. Ceftazidime, a fourth-generation cephalosporin, has proved helpful in the management of P. aeruginosa meningitis, but its activity against S. pneumoniae is questionable, and this agent should not be part of initial therapy unless suspicion of pseudomonas is high.

Although not effective against listeria, the third-generation cephalosporins have also proved helpful in treating bacterial meningitis due to gram-negative enteric bacilli, such as E. coli, klebsiella, and enterobacter. These pathogens rarely cause community-acquired meningitis except with trauma or recent neurosurgery, but it is important to point out that researchers have noted increased occurrence of these pathogens, especially among immunocompromised, alcoholic, or elderly patients.[65] This finding provides additional support for using ceftriaxone, cefotaxime, or ceftizoxime in the initial regimen for acute bacterial meningitis.

The aminoglycoside agents such as gentamicin are active against enteric gram-negative bacilli and can be used in combination with other agents against CNS pathogens, such as listeria. On the rare occasions when CSF shows these types of infections, however, standard intravenous therapy does not deliver a high enough concentration of aminoglycoside to give effective CSF levels.[29,98] This problem was recognized many years ago and led to the use of intrathecal (lumbar) administration in such clinical situations. Before clinical use of third-generation cephalosporins, however, administering aminoglycoside intrathecally plus systemically provided unsatisfactory treatment.[59] There was some initial enthusiasm for placement of intraventricular reservoirs, which may improve efficacy, but this is not an easy therapeutic option for emergent acute bacterial meningitis. Despite the obvious problem of obtaining adequate intracranial and especially intraventricular levels of aminoglycoside agents, in cases of listeria as well as P. aeruginosa meningitis, the patient should receive beta-lactam drug therapy, high dose systemic intravenous aminoglycosides, and intrathecal dosages of 5 to 10 mg of preservative-free aminoglycoside every 24 hours.[98]

Overdiagnosis of penicillin allergy by the general population remains a problem. The true incidence of cephalosporin cross reactivity in the face of true penicillin allergy is at most 10%, and true anaphylaxis from cephalosporins is extremely uncommon.[99] In the face of community-acquired bacterial meningitis, a true medical emergency, once the patient is in the ICU and being monitored, the physician should administer the most appropriate antibiotic and be prepared to manage reactions.

Despite enthusiasm for the monobactams, carbapenems, and quinolones, there is less experience using these antibiotics to treat CNS infections, and they are not recommended in general. In addition, imipenem can increase the seizure threshold, and the quinolones are not appropriate for any of the community-acquired organisms.[10]

Chloramphenicol's penetration into the CNS remains exceptional, and studies show that it is indeed bactericidal to the three pathogens that most often cause meningitis as well as streptococcus and anaerobes (with the exception of the enterococcus).[12] There are four problems, however, with chloramphenicol: (1) 1 : 20,000 incidence of irreversible bone marrow aplasia; (2) the inadequacy of chloramphenicol therapy for infections caused by S. aureus, listeria, and gram-negative enteric bacilli (these organisms account for meningitis in 5 to 10% of most modern series);[27] (3) problems with the gray baby syndrome, which is exceedingly rare in adults; and (4) emergence of chloramphenicol-resistant strains of H. influenzae in certain parts of the world.[105] Nevertheless, this drug is an inexpensive alternative that is well tolerated and has excellent penetration; it can occasionally be useful as alternative therapy for beta-lactamase–positive H. influenzae or when rickettsial disease is under consideration.

Trimethoprim-sulfamethoxazole has good penetration in the CSF and has been used successfully in cases of listeria, gram-negative rod infection, pneumococcus, H. influenzae, and meningococcal meningitis, and it should be remembered as an alternative therapy in limited situations.[107]

Rapid evaluation, exclusion of conditions that mimic meningitis, and early institution of appropriate antimicrobial therapy remain the cornerstones of therapy for acute bacterial meningitis. Management of the frequent complication of brain edema, however, is also important, and this plays a key role in the ICU care of these patients. Swartz and O'Hanley[14] have pointed out that when CSF pressure is 500 mm H$_2$O, only enough CSF should be withdrawn to permit Gram stain and culture. Swartz also points out that increased intracranial pressure, which often accompanies brain edema, can be managed with mannitol (0.25 to 0.5 mg/kg over 20 to 30 minutes), cautious fluid restriction, and dexamethasone administered in 10-mg increments initially until an effect is achieved and repeated every 4 to 6 hours.[14] Dexamethasone takes several hours to have an effect, however. As well, the patient may be intubated (if not already) and hyperventilated to treat brain edema.

Standard ICU care for patients with acute bacterial meningitis includes management of the airway and oxygenation. Seizures are uncommon with acute bacterial meningitis but frequently occur with focal CNS infections. Initially seizures can be controlled with intravenous administration of diazepam and anticonvulsant medications. One should, however, be aware that hypotension can occur as a result of too rapid administration of phenytoin sodium.

Drug interactions may occur if phenytoin or phenobarbital are administered with chloramphenicol.[14] Finally, the syndrome of inappropriate antidiuretic hormone (SIADH) secretion is a frequent accompaniment of acute bacterial meningitis.[59] Hyponatremia should be managed such that hypotension is not produced or exacerbated and SIADH not corrected too rapidly.[98] Shock often accompanies CNS infection, especially meningococcemia and occasionally pneumococcemia. Shock in these cases is mainly due to the rebound bacteremia that occurs after initial invasion of the CNS; its management is discussed elsewhere in this book.

As has been discussed in this chapter, a parameningeal focus of infection, such as acute mastoiditis or other head and neck infection, should be sought in every case of acute bacterial meningitis. Surgical drainage of the parameningeal site should be considered 36 to 72 hours after initiation of therapy for the CNS infection. In such cases, consultations from otorhinolaryngology, ophthalmology, and neurosurgery colleagues can be invaluable.

There continues to be controversy about the use of steroids in treating acute bacterial meningitis.[98,108,109,110,111,113-115] Addisonian crisis and accompanying Waterhouse-Friderichsen syndrome occur infrequently when cortisol levels have been monitored.[116] A collaborative study in children appeared to show an advantage to administering high doses of dexamethasone along with antimicrobial therapy as initial therapy for acute bacterial meningitis.[114] The design of this study has been criticized, however, because the only variable shown to be improved by this therapy was the incidence of sensorineural hearing loss. Similar enthusiasm for the use of steroids in septic shock was followed by proof that steroids are relatively inefficacious and probably harmful in those circumstances.[101] The use of physiologic steroid doses in the unusual situation of addisonian crisis cannot be refuted nor can pharmacologic doses of dexamethasone in the presence of cerebral edema or herniation syndromes. Outside of these particular situations, however, the widespread use of high dose steroids as additional or even preantibiotic therapy (as some studies suggest) for acute bacterial meningitis awaits further study.

Regardless of the initial antimicrobial therapy chosen, the clinician must reassess the clinical situation frequently, especially if the patient fails to improve. For example, encephalitis, early cerebritis, and endocarditis can mimic acute bacterial meningitis, and the initial diagnosis may be in error. If the clinician believes that the correct diagnosis is in doubt, repeat LP is warranted. Durack and Spanos[117] pointed out that in most cases of proven bacterial meningitis, a repeat LP adds little to management decisions if the patient is improving.

Clinicians may also be concerned about the duration of therapy. In general, 7 days of antimicrobial therapy is sufficient to treat meningococcal meningitis and 10 days for H. influenzae. Antimicrobial therapy for pneumococcal meningitis should usually last 10 to 14 days.[118] Because of concerns about endocarditis, therapy for S. aureus meningitis should be continued for 4 weeks; for listeria and gram-negative bacillary meningitis, therapy should be continued for at least 3 or more weeks.[66,119]

Prophylaxis in meningococcal or H. influenzae meningitis is discussed in other articles.[120,121] In adults, prophylaxis is certainly indicated for meningococcal disease; rifampin usually suffices, although there has been some enthusiasm for the use of quinolones. The American College of Physicians has pointed out that meningococcal vaccination may also be useful for close contacts.[122]

Finally, adult patients with pneumococcal meningitis in particular should be cautioned that their condition could be the initial manifestation of an occult CSF leak, in which case the meningitis might recur. If meningitis should recur, the clinician would be obviated to search for a CSF leak as well as consider other predisposing conditions.[50]

Parenchymal Infections

Meningoencephalitis

In discussing therapy for acute CNS parenchymal infections, we concentrate first on the most common nonepidemic, focal brain parenchymal diseases, HSV encephalitis.

The incidence of HSV encephalitis is 1 per 250,000 to 500,000 population per year in the United States. This incidence is less than that of aseptic meningitis or bacterial meningitis and is about the same as that of brain abscess, which it can clinically mimic. Many diseases, both treatable and untreatable, can closely mimic HSV encephalitis; only about 30 to 50% of patients with a clinical picture compatible with HSV encephalitis are found actually to have this condition.[17] Nevertheless, the clinician must commit to the most likely diagnosis quickly and initiate therapy promptly. As an aid in diagnosis, some data suggest that MRI may play an important role in the early detection of herpes encephalitis.[25]

Trials of adenine arabinoside (the first agent to show clinical efficacy in treating this disease) versus acyclovir showed a significant advantage for acyclovir: 80% of those treated with acyclovir compared with 50% of those treated with adenine arabinoside survived.[123-125] Nevertheless, the mortality and morbidity of HSV encephalitis remain high, especially in the elderly. The need for early diagnosis and treatment still cannot be overemphasized.

The usual recommended dosage of acyclovir for HSV encephalitis is 10 mg/kg intravenously every 8 hours, with appropriate reduction of dosage for significant azotemia.[83] This dose is two times the dose for non-CNS HSV infections and should be continued for at least 10 to 14 days. Growing numbers of reports of relapse, however, including one patient I saw, suggest longer therapy. In the patient I treated who suffered relapse, a biopsy was performed after the second relapse and confirmed HSV encephalitis, so my own preference would be for a full 3 weeks of intravenous antibiotic therapy. I also recommend early institution of physical therapy to decrease the debilitating effects of this heretofore clinically devastating infection. During acyclovir therapy, renal function should be monitored carefully because at the recommended dose, there have been reports of crystalluria.[126] Cerebral edema is an all too common accompaniment of this disease, and its effects can be noted both clinically and on CT. Thus in fluid management, the clinician must carefully walk the line between dehydration with possible crystalluria and hypotension and overhydration with worsening of cerebral edema or exacerbation of SIADH (or both). Steroid therapy is not generally recommended in this situation, although if brain herniation occurs or neurologic signs worsen, the clinician may be forced to use them. With the difficulty of establishing an exact diagnosis without biopsy, I prefer to treat CNS pressure phenomena with methods other than steroids. If the true diagnosis is cerebral cryptococcosis or another viral disease, the well-known adverse effects of high dose steroids on such diseases might outweigh the possible benefit of steroid therapy for cerebral edema.[83]

Acyclovir has been reported to produce a CNS toxicity of its own, but fortunately such problems are rare.[127] Seizures, which are so important as a diagnostic clue in the presentation of HSV encephalitis, can usually be managed well with standard therapy, such as phenytoin and carbamazepine. As has been mentioned before, constant reassessment of the clinical situation is important, and if the patient continues to deteriorate, the clinician should not hesitate to consider an alternative diagnosis. One would then proceed with a repeat radiologic imaging, another LP, and consider performing brain biopsy. So far, there has been no known difficulties with acyclovir-resistant HSV causing encephalitis; if the diagnosis is correct, the patient usually stabilizes after several days of acyclovir therapy.[83]

Acyclovir at dosages of 15 mg/kg every 8 hours has been recommended to treat the unusual syndrome of varicella virus encephalitis. This disease is uncommon, is usually seen in the presence of immunosuppression, and is discussed elsewhere.[82] Mycoplasma has also been reported to cause encephalitis.[128] Some of the diseases that can mimic herpes encephalitis are either uncommon or not treatable and are beyond the scope of this text.[1,129] Other infectious causes include Epstein-Barr virus encephalitis, herpes B encephalitis associated with laboratory accidents as well as occasional epidemics of arthropod encephalitis, especially eastern equine encephalitis, St. Louis encephalitis, and La Crosse encephalitis with epidemics in the United States.[83,89,130] In addition, a Japanese encephalitis has been reported that may be of epidemiologic importance for travelers. Most of these forms of encephalitis are either self-limited or untreatable. The reader is referred to several references concerning their diagnosis and prognosis.[82,83]

Brain Abscess

A broad range of different types of microorganisms can cause brain abscess, and this must be taken into account in treatment planning. With the exception of immunocompromised patients and the occasional patient with a mass lesion owing to a parasite, tuberculosis, cryptococcosis, or a fungus such as aspergillus, brain abscesses are usually caused by bacteria. There will be an increasing role for stereotactic biopsy, a more advanced form of needle aspiration, to identify the likely causative organism(s) and thus guide the choice of antimicrobial therapy. Choosing the correct antimicrobial agent to treat a brain abscess is important because the patient will require prolonged therapy, and toxicity becomes an issue. The number of antibacterial agents that are useful in treating CNS parenchymal infections is limited.[93,131] When a blood culture is positive for an organism that has caused endocarditis or comes from a distant focus of infection, however, the clinician should have little trouble prescribing the appropriate antimicrobial agent for the associated brain abscess.

For the most common form of brain abscess, those associated with contiguous foci of infection, empiric treatment depends on the location of the abscess (Table 7-4). For temporal lobe and cerebellar abscesses, a reasonable choice of antimicrobial therapy would be penicillin 24 million units per day, ceftriaxone 2 g intravenously every 12 hours, and metronidazole 750 mg intravenously every 8 hours. For frontal and parietal lobe abscesses caused by anaerobic streptococci, bacteroides, haemophilus, pneumococcus, or S. aureus organisms, a reasonable choice of drug would be penicillin or nafcillin with ceftriaxone and metronidazole; this regimen could be changed after culture results are received, for example, if staphylococcus could be excluded. In patients with true anaphylactic penicillin allergy, the choice of antibiotic agent is more difficult. The clinician might consider chloramphenicol plus ceftriaxone in such cases, although these agents are less than optimal for treating an abscess due to S. aureus. Fortunately, data suggest that clindamycin has a good record against brain abscess due to S. aureus, streptococcus, and anaerobes.[131] A reasonable choice for the penicillin-allergic patient with a brain abscess might be clindamycin plus ceftriaxone, at least until gram-negative bacilli could be excluded. Alternatively, if the abscess was caused by methicillin-resistant S. aureus, vancomycin would be the obvious choice to cover this organism.[10]

Table 7-4. Therapy for Brain Abscess (Contiguous Focus)

Location/Origin	Antimicrobial Regimen
Frontal lobe	Nafcillin + ceftriaxone + metronidazole
Temporal lobe and cerebellum	Penicillin + ceftriaxone + metronidazole
Post-traumatic and postsurgical	Vancomycin + ceftriaxone + metronidazole

Table 7–5. Therapy for Brain Abscess (Distal Focus)

Origin	Antimicrobial Regimen
Lungs	Nafcillin + metronidazole or clindamycin (Trimethoprim-sulfamethoxazole if nocardia)
Intracardiac shunt	Nafcillin
Intrapulmonary shunt	
Endocarditis	
Unknown	Penicillin or ceftriaxone

Finally, postoperative brain abscesses and epidural empyemas caused by Staphylococcus epidermidis and fastidious organisms associated with the scalp such as Propionibacterium acnes are becoming more common. In such situations, vancomycin would provide excellent coverage if given at doses of 1.0 g intravenously every 12 hours.[12]

The 30% or more of brain abscesses caused by distal foci or unknown sites are often multiple and can occur in the frontal, temporal, parietal, and occipital lobe. These types of brain abscesses are most often caused by anaerobic streptococci, anaerobic gram-negative rods, and occasionally S. aureus (Table 7-5). S. aureus, however, is less likely than the others to cause brain abscess associated with right-to-left shunts. Penicillin and ceftriaxone are good antibiotic choices to treat these brain abscesses if S. aureus can be excluded.

The clinician choosing antimicrobial therapy for a brain abscess would do well to remember that abscesses range in size from an area of cerebritis to mature abscesses with capsules. Brain abscesses commonly are polymicrobial in origin, involving not only aerobic gram-positive and gram-negative rods, but also, as pointed out a number of years ago, a wide variety of anaerobes.[93]

Medical therapy alone may be sufficient to treat early cerebritis when the causative organism has been identified (by stereotactic biopsy, for example). Medical therapy alone may be the only option to treat multiple brain abscesses.[93] Controversy still surrounds the issue of neurosurgical intervention to treat brain abscess, and an increasing number of brain abscesses are being managed medically alone.[93] A surgical approach and often excision, however, are still highly recommended to treat abscesses in the posterior fossa, those abscesses that are not responding to therapy, and when the diagnosis is still in doubt and the patient's condition is continuing to deteriorate despite reasonable empiric therapy.[93] When contiguous foci of infection are present, surgical therapy is usually necessary for these foci. Procedures may be performed over the first several days of ICU care to drain infections in the middle ear, mastoid, or sinuses or associated with craniotomy wound infections. Such procedures are important adjuncts of management and may also, because they provide material for culture and Gram stain, aid in identification of organisms likely causing the contiguous brain abscess.

Because seizures are so often associated with brain abscesses, many authors have recommended primary seizure prophylaxis. The agents that have been recommended are the same anticonvulsive medications used to treat seizures in other CNS infections and are covered elsewhere.

Steroid therapy should be minimized in patients with brain abscesses because these agents delay the development of brain abscess capsules and may give falsely reassuring results on CT scans.[25] Steroid agents have obvious deleterious effects on the control of bacteria, and they may decrease brain penetration of antibiotics by their anti-inflammatory properties.[10]

When clinical and radiologic evidence points to a large mass effect with cerebral edema, steroid therapy for a brief period of time may be reasonable. Prolonged steroid therapy, such as dexamethasone administered for 3 or 4 weeks, can nevertheless predispose to secondary infections and gastrointestinal bleeding. When prolonged steroid therapy is being considered, continued reassessment is needed, as is consultation with intensive medicine specialists, infectious disease physicians, neurologists, and neurosurgeons.

Mention should be made of the relationship between meningitis and brain abscess. Brain abscess can accompany listeria meningitis, and in children with citrobacter or haemophilus meningitis, secondary brain abscesses can occur.[93] In adults, however, brain abscess on occasion can lead to meningitis and rarely follows it. The mechanism by which the former occurs is rupture of the brain abscess into the ventricular spaces or over the cerebellar convexities, leading to secondary meningitis. The mortality is great in such situations, and therapy is probably of little avail. The rarity and futility of this situation are another reason that LP is seldom indicated in establishing the microbial cause of a brain abscess.

Brain abscesses due to parasitic infections, such as cysticercosis, schistosomiasis, and amebiasis, are outside the scope of this chapter.[12] One parasitic infection of the brain parenchyma deserves mention because of its frequent occurrence and association with immunosuppressive therapy. Toxoplasmosis of the CNS has become much more frequent with the spread of HIV disease.[97] In fact, the most common form of toxoplasmosis brain abscess is seen in patients who are immunosuppressed by HIV. CNS toxoplasmosis, however, may also occur in patients whose immune system function has been suppressed by cancer, chemotherapy, high dose steroid therapy, or a variety of other conditions. Such abscesses are usually large and multifocal and can be difficult to distinguish from bacterial infections that can also occur in such situations.[97]

In patients who are immunosuppressed by cancer therapy, mass lesions associated with infection should probably be aspirated or biopsied stereotactically to exclude recurrence of the neoplasms as well as to obtain material for histologic and culture analysis. Antimicrobial therapy for a toxoplasmosis abscess is usually chosen based on the results of histologic analysis because culture is not readily available. Empiric therapy for toxoplasmosis is the procedure of choice in patients with HIV infection because toxoplasmosis is by far the most common cause of treatable mass lesions in such patients.[96] For patients with CNS toxoplasmosis, initial therapy includes high doses of pyrimethamine (25 to 100 mg orally every day) and a sulfonamide drug, preferably sulfadiazine. In the United States, however, there are no sulfonamide drugs available for intravenous administration, so alternative drugs such as clindamycin may be used.[96] Folinic acid, 1.0 to 5.0 mg orally every day may be added to the regimen to obviate potential hematologic toxicity without altering efficacy.

In addition to the hematologic toxicity just mentioned, for which daily monitoring is imperative, complications of therapy for toxoplasmosis brain abscesses include sulfa crystalluria. To manage these effects, hydration must be maintained with avoidance of overhydration and exacerbation of cerebral edema.

Surgical extirpation is usually not indicated for toxoplasmosis brain abscesses, provided that the condition is recognized early and therapy administered long enough (up to 6 months).

Aspergillus, cryptococcus, and other yeasts have been known to cause CNS infections in immunocompromised hosts.[23,49] Another organism, Nocardia asteroides, is also known to invade the CNS. Nocardiosis is a syndrome that should be readily recognized.[93] When a parenchymal brain infection or mass lesion is suspected in a patient receiving steroids, the clinician should consider a nocardia brain abscess first. Early recognition and treatment of this disorder are critical to patient survival. Traditionally sulfadiazine was given in high doses to treat nocardia infection, but data suggest that high dose trimethoprim-sulfamethoxazole (20 mg/kg intravenously every day in three or four divided doses) is the drug of choice for CNS nocardiosis.[93] Even this regimen is not immediately effective, and so concurrent steroid therapy should be tapered (slowly but definitively) to improve the antimicrobial regimen. High dose amikacin may be added for synergy. In the face of a parenchymal CNS infection, the ability of this drug to cross into the CSF is not necessarily the issue; it is more important that the drug cross the blood-brain barrier than the blood-CSF barrier. It is reasonable to add amikacin to trimethoprim-sulfamethoxazole, which has excellent penetration and in vitro activity for nocardia.

Actinomyces can mimic nocardia on initial Gram stain results, but nocardia is associated almost invariably with immunosuppression (owing to steroid therapy, diabetes, or cancer chemotherapy), whereas actinomycosis is usually associated with odontogenic sources of infection or pleuropulmonary or pelvic sources. The microbiology laboratory can be of great assistance in helping to identify nocardia brain abscess versus actinomycosis brain abscess because in both the Gram stain shows gram-positive branching rods in a characteristic pattern. Nocardia is often partially acid-fast staining, whereas actinomyces is not. This distinction is important because actinomyces infections necessitate an entirely different regimen of either penicillin or clindamycin.

POST ICU PHASE

We next consider the post-ICU phase of patient care for a CNS infection and briefly touch on prognosis (Table 7-6) and rehabilitation of these patients.[132]

Throughout this chapter, great morbidity and significant mortality of CNS infections are emphasized, particularly when the diagnosis is not made quickly, and therapy is inappropriate or started too late. The CNS usually tolerates microbial invasion poorly except for infection by viruses responsible for enteroviral forms of acute aseptic meningitis. This chapter focuses on those diseases that produce significant morbidity and mortality, and much work is needed in the area of better adjunctive therapy, for example, of acute bacterial meningitis.[98]

Table 7-6. Prognosis of Central Nervous System (CNS) Infection

CNS Infection Example	Average Mortality (%)
Mycotic aneurysm	20–30 (>80 if ruptured)
Septic dural venous sinus phlebitis	30 (>80 if sagittal sinus)
Subdural empyema	20–30
Acute bacterial meningitis	15
HSV encephalitis	25
Brain abscess	10

The post-ICU phase of patient care for all the anatomic classes of CNS infection—parameningeal, meningeal, and parenchymal—is generally similar. Further, the overall mortalities are generally equivalent for infections due to the organisms we have discussed.

The mortality of rhinocerebral mucor, a soft tissue parameningeal infection, is 10 to 30%, similar to figures reported for the CNS complications of sepsis, endocarditis, mycotic aneurysm, and most forms of dural venous sinus infectious phlebitis except for sagittal sinus thrombosis, which has a nearly 100% mortality.[23]

Epidural empyema, if detected early enough and unassociated with other invasive CNS infection, has a good prognosis. The mortality of subdural empyema, similar to that of many other infectious syndromes we have discussed, is 10 to 20%, and significant neurologic sequelae include seizures (incidence of 34%) and hemiparesis (incidence of 17%).[42]

The post-ICU phase of acute bacterial meningitis depends to some extent on the particular organism involved. Overall mortality is still about 20%, reflecting perhaps the outcome of patients with a fulminant presentation. In adults, the three organisms most often responsible for meningitis have mortality rates of 26% for pneumococcus, 10% for meningococcus, and 6% for haemophilus. For the rare cases of S. aureus meningitis, mortality is 5 to 10% and for listeria about 28%. Mortality in adults appears to be highest with community-acquired meningitis associated with immunosuppression or with gram-negative meningitis and in the elderly.[132] Neurologic sequelae of acute bacterial meningitis have been better studied in children. Much has been written about eighth cranial nerve damage in children, and this can occasionally occur in adult patients.[12,133]

The prognosis for adults surviving acute bacterial meningitis varies. Rehabilitation may take much time and effort on the part of the patient and family but can be rewarded by good recovery if higher integrative functions return within the first several days of therapy. Patients who appear comatose after a week of therapy for acute bacterial meningitis, however, often enter a persistent vegetative state, which is at the heart of the emphasis on institution of therapy immediately on suspicion of acute bacterial meningitis.

HSV encephalitis in adults has been associated with a

20% mortality, even with excellent care and when acyclovir was started early.[83] Further, of those older than 30 who survived, only 40% were normal, 15 to 20% had mild impairment, and 30 to 40% were left with severe neurologic sequelae such as near persistent vegetative state. These problems are not surprising given the necrosis of the brain associated with HSV encephalitis.[83,134]

Despite advances in monitoring and antimicrobial therapy, the mortality for brain abscess appears to have decreased only slightly over the past 30 years. It has been suggested, however, that CT has decreased the mortality of brain abscess by about two-thirds, from 30% in the pre-CT era to about 10% today, probably related to earlier diagnosis.[135] In adults, seizures are a common sequela of brain abscess, as are significant focal neurologic findings. As with recovery from HSV encephalitis, these and other sequelae in brain abscess patients can pose major rehabilitative problems.

In summary, this chapter examines reasons for the minimum of 10 to 30% mortality of serious CNS infections even in well-controlled large series. The morbidity of these diseases among survivors is also great, emphasizing the importance of astute diagnosis and treatment. A practical anatomic approach to CNS infections has been used to discuss management of parameningeal, meningeal, and parenchymal infections before, during, and after ICU care. We have emphasized that the overall clinical data—history, physical examination, pertinent laboratory findings, and radiographic studies—are important in rapid diagnosis and therapeutic attack. It was also noted that when acute bacterial meningitis presents with focal findings other than ophthalmoplegia, therapy needs to be instituted before a LP can be safely done.

We have mentioned that diseases do not necessarily correlate specifically with CSF profiles and that too much emphasis should not be placed on analysis of CSF culture, cell count with differential, glucose, and protein alone. Furthermore, of the entities we have emphasized, only in acute bacterial meningitis is the culture of CSF positive—as it is also in forms of cryptococcal and mycobacterial meningitis that may clinically mimic acute bacterial meningitis. In other words, the LP is only one aspect of diagnostic management and is contraindicated in some situations. After initial evaluation and after blood has been drawn for culture, it is crucial that the physician rapidly institute appropriate therapy and not always delay to secure a CT scan or MRI scan or risk cerebral herniation by performing a LP.

Finally, and most important, we discuss appropriate forms of antimicrobial and surgical therapy for these infections, based on the principles of minimizing morbidity and mortality of CNS infections as well as their therapy.

REFERENCES

1. Reik, L. Jr.: Disorders that mimic CNS infections. Neurol. Clin., *4:*223, 1986.
2. Scott, B. D., and Schmidt, J. H.: Pneumococcal meningitis due to psoas abscess. South. Med. J., *82:*1310, 1989.
3. Aseptic Meningitis—New York State and United States, Weeks 1-36, 1991. M.M.W.R., *40:*773, 1991.
4. Bleck, T. P., and Klawans, H. L.: Neurologic emergencies. Med. Clin. North Am., *70:*1167, 1986.
5. Lambert, H. P.: Meningitis: Diagnostic Problems. *In* Infections of the Central Nervous System. Edited by H. P. Lambert. Philadelphia, B. C. Decker, 1991.
6. Victor, M., and Adams, R. D. Textbook of Neurology. 4th Ed. New York, McGraw-Hill, 1989.
7. The diagnostic spinal tap. Health and Public Policy Committee, American College of Physicians. Ann. Intern. Med., *104:* 880, 1986.
8. Fishman, R.: Cerebrospinal Fluid in Diseases of the Nervous System. Philadelphia, W. B. Saunders, 1980.
9. Greenlee, J. E.: Anatomic considerations in central nervous system infections. *In* Principles and Practice of Infectious Diseases. 3rd Ed. Edited by G. L. Mandell, R. G. Douglas, and J. E. Bennett. New York, Churchill Livingstone, 1990.
10. Thea, D., and Barza, M.: Use of antibacterial agents in infections of the central nervous system. Infect. Dis. Clin. North Am., *3:*553, 1989.
11. Tunkel, A. R., and Scheld, W. M.: Bacterial meningitis: pathogenetic and pathophysiologic mechanisms. *In* Infections of the Central Nervous System. Edited by H. P. Lambert. Philadelphia, B. C. Decker, 1991.
12. Wood, M., and Anderson, M. (eds.): Neurological Infections. Philadelphia, W. B. Saunders, 1988.
13. Griffin, D. E.: Approach to the patient with infection of the central nervous system. *In* Infectious Diseases. Edited by S. L. Gorbach, J. G. Bartlett, and N. R. Blacklow. Philadelphia, W. B. Saunders, 1992, p. 1155.
14. Swartz, M. N., and O'Hanley, P.: Central nervous system infections. *In* Scientific American Medicine. Edited by E. Rubenstein and D. D. Federman. New York, Scientific American Medicine, Subsection 8, 1991, p. 1.
15. Hirsch, M. S., and Cutler, R. W. P.: Acute viral central nervous system diseases. *In* Scientific American Medicine. Edited by E. Rubenstein and D. D. Federman. New York. Scientific American Medicine, Subsection 27, 1990, p. 1.
16. Roos, K. L., and Scheld, W. M.: The management of fulminant meningitis in the intensive care unit. Infect. Dis. Clin. North Am., *3:*137, 1989.
17. Whitley, R. J., et al.: Diseases that mimic herpes simplex encephalitis: diagnosis, presentation and outcome. JAMA, *262:*234, 1989.
18. McGee, Z. A., and Baringer, J. R.: Acute meningitis. *In* Principles and Practice of Infectious Diseases. 3rd Ed. Edited by G. L. Mandell, R. G. Douglas, and J. E. Bennett. New York, Churchill Livingstone, 1990, p. 741.
19. Kaiser, A. B., and McGee, Z. A.: Central nervous system infections. *In* Textbook of Critical Care. 2nd Ed. Edited by W. C. Shoemaker, et al. Philadelphia, W. B. Saunders, 1989, p. 830.
20. Munford, R. S.: Orbital infections. *In* Current Clinical Topics in Infectious Diseases, 4. Edited by J. S. Remington, and M. N. Swartz. New York, McGraw-Hill, 1983, p. 111.
21. Kaplan, R. J.: Neurological complications of infections of the head and neck. Otolaryngol. Clin. North Am., *9:*729, 1976.
22. Lew, D., et al.: Sphenoid sinusitis: a review of 30 cases. N. Engl. J. Med., *309:*1149, 1983.
23. Sepkowitz, K., and Armstrong, D.: Space-occupying fungal lesions of the central nervous system. *In* Infections of the Central Nervous System. Edited by W. M. Scheld, R. J. Whitley, and D. T. Durack. New York, Raven Press, 1991, p. 741.
24. Terrell, C. L., Hughes, C. E.: Antifungal agents used for deep-seated mycotic infections. Mayo Clin. Proc., *67:*69, 1992.
25. Zimmerman, R. A.: Imaging of intracranial infections. *In*

Infections of the Central Nervous System. Edited by W. M. Scheld, R. J. Whitley, and D. T. Durack. New York, Raven Press, 1991.
26. Bone, R. C.: The pathogenesis of sepsis. Ann. Intern. Med., 115:45, 1991.
27. Wenger, J. D., and Broome, C. V.: Bacterial meningitis: Epidemiology. In Infections of the Central Nervous System. Edited by H. Lambert. Philadelphia, B. C. Decker, 1991, p. 16.
28. Schlech, W. F. III, et al.: Bacterial meningitis in the United States: 1978 through 1981. The National Bacterial Meningitis Surveillance Study. JAMA, 253:1749, 1985.
29. Tunkel, A. R., Wispelwey, B., and Scheld, W. M.: Bacterial meningitis: recent advances in pathophysiology and treatment. Ann. Intern. Med., 112:610, 1990.
30. Kanter, M. C., and Hart, R. G.: Neurologic complications of infective endocarditis. Neurology, 41:1015, 1991.
31. Lerner, P. I.: Neurologic complications of infective endocarditis. Med. Clin. North Am., 69:385, 1985.
32. Francioli, P.: Central nervous system complications of infective endocarditis. In Infections of the Central Nervous System. Edited by W. M. Scheld, R. J. Whitley, and D. T. Durack. New York, Raven Press, 1991, p. 515.
33. Delahaye, J. P., et al.: Cerebrovascular accidents in infective endocarditis: role of anticoagulation. Eur. Heart J., 11:1074, 1990.
34. Masuda, J., et al.: Histopathological analysis of the mechanisms of intracranial hemorrhage complicating infective endocarditis. Stroke, 23:843, 1992.
35. Bloomfield, P., Wheatley, P. J., Prescott, R. J., and Miller, H. C.: Twelve-year comparison of a Bjork-Shiley mechanical heart valve with porcine bioprosthesis. N. Engl. J. Med., 324:573, 1991.
36. Cowgill, L. D., Addonizio, V. P., Hopeman, A. R., and Harken, A. H.: Prosthetic valve endocarditis. Curr. Probl. Cardiol., 11:617, 1986.
37. Wilson, W. R., et al.: Anticoagulant therapy and central nervous system complications in patients with prosthetic valve endocarditis. Circulation, 57:1004, 1978.
38. Wilson, W. R., et al.: The management of patients with mycotic aneurysm. In Current Clinical Topics in Infectious Disease, 2. Edited by J. S. Remington and M. N. Swartz. New York, McGraw-Hill, 1981, p. 151.
39. Southwick, F. S., Richardson, E. P., Jr., and Swartz, M. N.: Septic thrombosis of the dural venous sinuses. Medicine, 65:82, 1986.
40. Pallares, R., Santamario, J., Ariza, X., and Gudiol, F.: Polymicrobial anaerobic septicemia due to lateral sinus thrombophlebitis. Arch. Intern. Med., 143:164, 1983.
41. Zimmerman, R. D., and Haines, A. B.: The role of MR imaging in the diagnosis of infections of the central nervous system. In Current Clinical Topics in Infectious Disease. Vol. 10. Edited by J. S. Remington and M. N. Swartz. McGraw-Hill, New York, 1989, p. 82.
42. Silverberg, A. L., and DiNubile, M. J.: Subdural empyema and cranial epidural abscess. Med. Clin. North Am., 69:361, 1985.
43. Kaufman, D. M., Miller, M. H., and Steigbigel, N. H.: Subdural empyema: Analysis of 17 recent cases and review of the literature. Medicine, 54:485, 1975.
44. Helfgott, D. C., Weingarten, K., and Hartmann, B. J.: Subdural empyema. In Infections of the Central Nervous System. Edited by W. M. Scheld, R. J. Whitley, and D. T. Durack. New York, Raven Press, 1991, p. 487.
45. Ho, D. D., and Hirsch, M. S.: Acute viral encephalitis. Med. Clin. North Am., 69:415, 1985.
46. Connolly, K. J., and Hammer, S. M.: The acute aseptic meningitis syndrome. Infect. Dis. Clin. North Am., 4:599, 1990.
47. Tucker, T., and Ellner, J. J.: Chronic meningitis. In Infections of the Central Nervous System. Edited by W. M. Scheld, R. J. Whitley, and D. T. Durack. New York, Raven Press, 1991, p. 703.
48. Karandanis, D., and Shulman, J. A.: Recent survey of infectious meningitis in adults: Review of laboratory findings in bacterial, tuberculous, and aseptic meningitis. South. Med. J., 69:449, 1976.
49. Perfect, J. R.: Diagnosis and treatment of fungal meningitis. In Infections of the Central Nervous System. Edited by W. M. Scheld, R. T. Whitley, and D. T. Durack. New York, Raven Press, 1991, p. 693.
50. Hermans, P. E., Goldstein, N. P., and Wellman, W. E.: Mollaret's meningitis and differential diagnosis of recurrent meningitis. Report of case, with review of the literature. Am. J. Med., 52:128, 1972.
51. Kaufman, B. A., Tunkel, A. R., Pryor, J. C., and Dacey, R. G., Jr.: Meningitis in the neurosurgical patient. Med. Clin. North Am., 4:677, 1990.
52. Mayhall, C. G., et al.: Ventriculostomy-related infections: a prospective epidemiologic study. N. Engl. J. Med., 310:553, 1984.
53. Pachner, A. R.: Spirochetal diseases of the CNS. Neurol. Clin. North Am., 4:207, 1986.
54. Coyle, P. K., and Dattwyler, R.: Spirochetal infection of the central nervous system. Infect. Dis. Clin. North Am., 4:731, 1990.
55. Lauter, C. B.: Antibiotic therapy of life-threatening infectious diseases in the emergency department. Ann. Emerg. Med., 18:1339, 1989.
56. Overturf, G. D.: Pyogenic bacterial infections of the CNS. Neurol. Clin., 4:69, 1986.
57. Kaplan, S. L.: Recent advances in bacterial meningitis. Adv. Pediatr. Infect. Dis., 4:83, 1989.
58. Bryan, C. S., Reynolds, K. L., and Crout, L.: Promptness of antibiotic therapy in acute bacterial meningitis. Ann. Emerg. Med., 15:544, 1986.
59. Swartz, M. N.: Acute bacterial meningitis. In Infectious Diseases. Edited by S. L. Gorbach, J. G. Bartlett, and N. R. Blacklow. Philadelphia, W. B. Saunders, 1992, p. 1160.
60. Talan, D. A., Hoffman, J. R., Yoshikawa, T. T., and Overturf, G. D.: Role of empiric parenteral antibiotics prior to lumbar puncture in suspected bacterial meningitis: state of the art. Rev. Infect. Dis., 10:365, 1988.
61. Bohr, V., et al.: 875 cases of bacterial meningitis: Diagnostic procedures and the impact of preadmission antibiotic therapy. Part III of a three-part series. J. Infect., 7:193, 1983.
62. Behrman, R. E., et al.: Central nervous system infections in the elderly. Arch. Intern. Med., 149:1596, 1989.
63. Kaplowitz, L. G., Fischer, J. J., and Sparling, P. F.: Rocky Mountain spotted fever: a clinical dilemma. In Current Clinical Topics in Infectious Diseases. 2nd Ed. Edited by J. S. Remington and M. N. Swartz. New York, McGraw-Hill, 1981, p. 89.
64. Update: Foodborne listeriosis—United States, 1988-1990. MMWR, 41:251, 1992.
65. Cherubin, C. E., Marr, J. S., Sierra, M. F., and Becker, S.: Listeria and gram-negative bacillary meningitis in New York City, 1972-1979: Frequent causes of meningitis in adults. Am. J. Med., 71:199, 1981.
66. Pollock, S. S., Pollock, T. M., and Harrison, M. J. G.: Infection of the central nervous system by Listeria monocytogenes: a review of 54 adult and juvenile cases. Q. J. Med., 53:331, 1984.

67. Leonard, J. M.: Cerebrospinal fluid formula in patients with central nervous system infection. Neurol. Clin., 4:3, 1986.
68. Wilson, C. B., and Smith, A. L.: Rapid tests for the diagnosis of bacterial meningitis. In Current Clinical Topics in Infectious Diseases. 7th Ed. Edited by J. S. Remington and M. N. Swartz. New York, McGraw-Hill, 1986, p. 134.
69. Ray, C. G., Wasilauskas, B. L., and Zabransky, R.: Laboratory diagnosis of central nervous system infections. Cumitech 14, American Society for Microbiology, Washington, D.C., 1982.
70. Greenlee, J. E.: Cerebrospinal fluid in central nervous system infections. In Infections of the Central Nervous System. Edited by W. M. Scheld, R. T. Whitley, and D. T. Durack. New York, Raven Press, 1991, p. 361.
71. Powers, W. J.: Cerebrospinal fluid lymphocytosis in acute bacterial meningitis. Am. J. Med., 79:216, 1985.
72. Aminoff, M. J., and Simon, R. P.: Status epilepticus: causes, clinical features and consequences in 98 patients. Am. J. Med., 69:657, 1980.
73. Schmidley, J. W., and Simon, R. P.: Postictal pleocytosis. Ann. Neurol., 9:81, 1981.
74. Bamberger, D. M., and Smith, O. J.: Haemophilus influenzae meningitis in an adult with initially normal cerebrospinal fluid. South. Med. J., 83:348, 1980.
75. Geiseler, P. J., Nelson, K. E., and Levin, S.: Community-acquired purulent meningitis of unknown etiology. A continuing problem. Arch. Neurol., 38:749, 1981.
76. Geiseler, P. J., et al.: Community-acquired purulent meningitis: a review of 1,316 cases during the antibiotic era, 1954-1976. Rev. Infect. Dis., 2:725, 1980.
77. Primary amebic meningoencephalitis—North Carolina, 1991. M.M.W.R., 41:437, 1992.
78. Sheller, J. R., and Des Prez, R. M.: CNS tuberculosis. Neurol. Clin., 4:143, 1986.
79. Varki, A. P., and Puthuvan, P.: Value of second lumbar puncture in confirming a diagnosis of aseptic meningitis. A prospective study. Arch. Neurol., 36:581, 1979.
80. Feigin, R. D., and Shackelford, P. G.: Value of repeat lumbar puncture in the differential diagnosis of meningitis. N. Engl. J. Med., 289:571, 1973.
81. Gower, D. J., Baker, A. L., Bell, W. O., and Ball, M. R.: Contraindications to lumbar puncture as defined by computed cranial tomography. J. Neurol. Neurosurg. Psychiatry, 50:1071, 1987.
82. Whitley, R. J.: Viral encephalitis. N. Engl. J. Med., 323:242, 1990.
83. Whitley, R. J., and Schlitt, M.: Encephalitis caused by herpes viruses including B virus. In Infections of the Central Nervous System. Edited by W. M. Scheld, R. T. Whitley, and D. T. Durack. New York, Raven Press, 1991, p. 41.
84. Barza, M., and Pauker, S. G.: The decision to biopsy, treat or wait in suspected herpes encephalitis. Ann. Intern. Med., 92:641, 1980.
85. Soong, S. J., et al.: Use of brain biopsy for diagnostic evaluation of patients with suspected herpes simplex encephalitis: a statistical model and its clinical implications. NIAID Collaborative Antiviral Study Group. J. Infect. Dis., 163:17, 1991.
86. Bhatti, N., et al.: Encephalitis due to Epstein-Barr virus. J. Infect., 20:69, 1990.
87. Schroth, G., et al.: Early diagnosis of herpes simplex encephalitis by MRI. Neurology, 37:179, 1987.
88. Chandrasoma, P. T., Smith, M. M., and Apuzzo, M. L.: Stereotactic biopsy in the diagnosis of brain masses: comparison of results of biopsy and resected surgical specimen. Neurosurgery, 24:160, 1989.
89. Tsai, T. F.: Arboviral infections in the United States. Infect. Dis. Clin. North Am., 5:73, 1991.
90. Nahmias, A. J., et al.: Herpes simplex virus encephalitis: laboratory evaluations and their diagnostic significance. J. Infect. Dis., 145:829, 1982.
91. Aurelius, E., et al.: Rapid diagnosis of herpes simplex encephalitis by nested polymerase chain reaction assay of cerebrospinal fluid. Lancet, 337:189, 1991.
92. Chun, C. H., Johnson, J. D., Hofstetter, M., and Raff, M. J.: Brain abscess: a study of 45 consecutive cases. Medicine, 65:415, 1986.
93. Wispelwey, B., Dacey, R. G., and Scheld, W. M.: Brain abscess. In Infections of the Central Nervous System. Edited by W. M. Scheld, R. T. Whitley, and D. T. Durack. New York, Raven Press, 1991, p. 457.
94. Frank, J.: Illness and invulnerability. N. Engl. J. Med., 308:1268, 1983.
95. Salzman, C., and Tuazon, C. U.: Value of the ring-enhancing sign in differentiating intracerebral hematomas and brain abscesses. Arch. Intern. Med., 147:951, 1987.
96. McArthur, J. C.: Neurologic complications of human immunodeficiency virus infection. In Infectious Diseases. Edited by S. L. Gorbach, J. G. Bartlett, and N. R. Blacklow. Philadelphia, W. B. Saunders, 1992, p. 956.
97. Dukes, C. S., Luft, B. S., and Durack, D. T.: Toxoplasmosis of the central nervous system. In Infections of the Central Nervous System. Edited by W. M. Scheld, R. T. Whitley, and D. T. Durack. New York, Raven Press, 1991, p. 801.
98. Tauber, M. G., and Sande, M. A.: General principles of therapy of pyogenic meningitis. Infect. Dis. Clin. North Am., 4:661, 1990.
99. Saxon, A., Beall, G. N., Rohr, A. S., and Adelman, D. C.: Immediate hypersensitivity reactions to beta-lactam antibiotics. Ann. Intern. Med., 107:204, 1987.
100. Sogn, D. D., et al.: Results of the National Institute of Allergy and Infectious Diseases Collaborative Clinical Trial to test the predictive value of skin testing with major and minor penicillin derivatives in hospitalized patients. Arch. Intern. Med., 152:1025, 1992.
101. Bone, R. C., et al.: A controlled clinical trial of high-dose methylprednisolone in the treatment of severe sepsis and septic shock. N. Engl. J. Med., 317:653, 1987.
102. Korzeniowski, O. M., and Kaye, D.: Endocarditis. In Infectious Diseases. Edited by S. L. Gorbach, J. G. Bartlett, and N. R. Blacklow. Philadelphia, W. B. Saunders, 1992, p. 548.
103. Spagnuolo, P. J., et al.: Hemophilus influenzae meningitis: The spectrum of disease in adults. Medicine, 61:74, 1982.
104. Gallagher, P. G., and Watanakunakorn, C.: Listeria monocytogenes endocarditis: a review of the literature 1950-1986. Scand. J. Infect. Dis., 20:359, 1988.
105. Baquero, F., and Loza, E.: Penicillin resistance in Spain. Infect. Dis. Clin. Pract., 1:147, 1992.
106. Roman-Campos, G., and Toro, G.: Herpetic brainstem encephalitis. Neurology, 30:981, 1980.
107. Levitz, R. E., and Quintiliani, R.: Trimethoprim-sulfamethoxazole for bacterial meningitis. Ann. Intern. Med., 100:881, 1984.
108. Schattner, A. M.: Should we add corticosteroids to the treatment of acute bacterial meningitis? Q. J. Med., 82:181, 1992.
109. Mustafa, M. M., et al.: Cerebrospinal fluid prostaglandins, interleukin 1 beta, and tumor necrosis factor in bacterial meningitis. Clinical and laboratory correlations in placebo-treated and dexamethasone-treated patients. Am. J. Dis. Child., 144:883, 1990.
110. McGowan, J. E., Jr., Chesney, P. J., Crossley, K. B., and LaForce, F. M.: Guidelines for the use of systemic glucocorti-

costeroids in the management of selected infections: Working Group on Steroid Use, Antimicrobial Agents Committee, Infectious Disease Society of America. J. Infect. Dis., *165:* 1, 1992.
111. Girgis, N. I., et al.: Dexamethasone treatment for bacterial meningitis in children and adults. Pediatr. Infect. Dis. J., *8:* 848, 1989.
112. Harbin, G. L., and Hodges, G. R.: Corticosteroids as adjunctive therapy for acute bacterial meningitis. South. Med. J., *72:*977, 1979.
113. Lebel, M. H., et al.: Dexamethasone therapy for bacterial meningitis: results of two double-blind, placebo-controlled study. N. Engl. J. Med., *319:*964, 1988.
114. Odio, C. M., et al.: The beneficial effects of early dexamethasone administration in infants and children with bacterial meningitis. N. Engl. J. Med., *324:*1525, 1991.
115. Tauber, M. G., and Sande, M. A.: Dexamethasone in bacterial meningitis: increasing evidence for a beneficial effect. Pediatr. Infect. Dis. J., *8:*842, 1989.
116. Bosworth, D. C.: Reversible adrenocortical insufficiency in fulminant meningococcemia. Arch. Intern. Med., *139:*823, 1979.
117. Durack, D. T., and Spanos, A.: End-of-treatment spinal tap in bacterial meningitis: is it worthwhile? JAMA, *248:*75, 1982.
118. Radetsky, M.: Duration of treatment in bacterial meningitis: a historical inquiry. Pediatr. Infect. Dis. J., *9:*2, 1980.
119. Schlesinger, L. S., Ross, S. C., and Schaberg, D. R.: Staphylococcus aureus meningitis: a broad-based epidemiologic study. Medicine, *66:*148, 1987.
120. Granoff, D. M., and Ward, J. I.: Current status of prophylaxis for Haemophilus influenza infections. *In* Current Clinical Topics in Infectious Disease. 5th Ed. Edited by J. S. Remington and M. N. Swartz. New York, McGraw-Hill, 1984, p. 290.
121. Lieberman, J. M., Greenberg, D. P., and Ward, J. I.: Prevention of bacterial meningitis: vaccines and chemoprophylaxis. Infect. Dis. Clin. North Am., *4:*703, 1990.
122. American College of Physicians Task Force on Adult Immunization and Infectious Disease Society of America: Guide to Adult Immunization. 2nd Ed. Philadelphia, American College of Physicians, 1990.
123. Skoldenberg, B., et al.: Acyclovir versus Vidarabine in herpes simplex encephalitis: randomized multicentre study in consecutive Swedish patients. Lancet, *2:*707, 1984.
124. Whitley, R. J., et al.: Herpes simplex encephalitis: vidarabine therapy and diagnostic problems. N. Engl. J. Med., *304:*313, 1981.
125. Whitley, R. J., et al.: Vidarabine versus acyclovir therapy in herpes simplex encephalitis. N. Engl. J. Med., *314:*144, 1986.
126. Keating, M. R.: Antiviral agents. Mayo Clin. Proc., *67:*160, 1992.
127. Feldman, S., Rodman, J., and Gregory, B.: Excessive serum concentrations of acyclovir and neurotoxicity. J. Infect. Dis., *157:*385, 1988.
128. Clyde, W. A.: Mycoplasmal diseases of the central nervous system. *In* Infections of the Central Nervous System. Edited by W. M. Scheld, R. T. Whitley, and D. T. Durack. New York, Raven Press, 1991, p. 283.
129. Calabrese, L. H., Furlan, A. J., Gragg, L. A., and Ropos, T. J.: Primary angiitis of the central nervous system: diagnostic criteria and clinical approach. Cleve. Clin. J. Med., *59:*293, 1992.
130. Eastern Equine Encephalitis—Florida, Eastern United States, 1991. M.M.W.R., *40:*533, 1991.
131. Kaplan, K.: Brain abscess. Med. Clin. North Am., *69:*345, 1985.
132. Evans, R. W., Baskin, D. B., and Yatsu, F. M. (Eds.): Prognosis in Neurological Disease. New York, Oxford University Press, 1992.
133. Pomeroy, S. L., Holmes, S. J., Dodge, P. R., and Feigin, R. D.: Seizures and other neurologic sequelae of bacterial meningitis in children. N. Engl. J. Med., *323:*1651, 1990.
134. Lilly, R., et al.: The human Kluver-Bucy syndrome. Neurology, *33:*1141, 1983.
135. Seydoux, C., and Francioli, P.: Bacterial brain abscesses: factors influencing mortality and sequelae. Clin. Infect. Dis., *15:*394, 1992.

SUPPLEMENTAL READINGS

Asensi, F., et al.: Imipenem cilastatin therapy in a child with meningitis caused by a multiply resistant pneumococcus. Pediatr. Infect. Dis. J., *8:*895, 1989.

Carithers, H. A., and Margileth, A. M.: Cat scratch disease: acute encephalopathy and other neurologic manifestations. Am. J. Dis. Child., *145:*98, 1991.

Domingo, P., et al.: Bacterial meningitis with "normal" cerebrospinal fluid in adults: a report on five cases. Scand. J. Infect. Dis., *22:*115, 1990.

Durand, M. L., et al.: Acute bacterial meningitis in adults: a review of 493 episodes. N. Engl. J. Med., *328:*21, 1993.

Feldman, M.: Southern Internal Medicine Conference: Whipple's disease. Am. J. Med. Sci., *291:*56, 1986.

Fishman, R. A.: Cerebrospinal Fluid in Diseases of Nervous System. 2nd Ed. Philadelphia, W. B. Saunders, 1992.

Jensen, A. G., et al.: Staphylococcus aureus meningitis. Arch. Intern. Med., *153:*1902, 1993.

Latchaw, R. E. (ed.): MR and CT Imaging of the Head, Neck, and Spine. 2nd Ed. St. Louis, C. V. Mosby, 1991.

Malone, D. G., et al.: Osteomyelitis of the skull base. Neurosurgery, *30:*426, 1992.

Nau, R., et al.: Meningoencephalitis with septic intracerebral infarction: a new feature of CNS listeriosis. Scand. J. Infect. Dis., *22:*101, 1990.

Power, C., et al.: Cytomegalovirus and Resmussen's encephalitis. Lancet, *336:*1282, 1990.

Righter, J.: Pneumococcal meningitis during intravenous ciprofloxacin therapy. Am. J. Med., *88:*548, 1990.

Siegman-Igra, Y., et al.: Nosocomial acinetobacter meningitis secondary to invasive procedures: report of 25 cases and review. Clin. Infect. Dis., *17:*843, 1993.

Weingarten, R. D., Mankiewicz, Z., and Gilbert, D. N.: Meningitis due to penicillin-resistant Streptococcus pneumoniae in adults. Rev. Infect. Dis., *12:*118, 1990.

Wenzel, R., et al.: Acute febrile cerebrovasculitis: a syndrome of unknown, perhaps rickettsial cause. Ann. Intern. Med., *104:* 606, 1986.

Chapter 8

NEUROMUSCULAR DISORDERS

KERRY H. LEVIN

Neuromuscular disorders include diseases of the motor unit and present primarily as weakness and dysfunction of motor control. The motor unit includes the anterior horn cells of the spinal cord, the spinal roots, peripheral nerve trunks, the neuromuscular junction, and the muscle fibers themselves. Clinical neurologic diagnosis and treatment often depend on identification of the anatomic site of the lesion. Therefore the disorders discussed in this chapter have been grouped by anatomic site. They all share in common, when disease is severe, the need for intensive medical care. The following entities are reviewed:

- Guillain-Barré syndrome (GBS)
- Neuromuscular transmission disorders
    Myasthenia gravis (MG)
    Lambert-Eaton myasthenic syndrome (LEMS)
    Botulism
- Motor neuron disease
    Amyotrophic lateral sclerosis (ALS)
    Polio
    Tetanus
- Primary muscle disease

GUILLAIN-BARRÉ SYNDROME

Guillain-Barré Syndrome (GBS), also referred to as acute inflammatory polyradiculoneuropathy, is an acute demyelinating peripheral neuropathy affecting motor and sensory roots and peripheral nerves, including myelinated nerves serving autonomic functions. It is one of the few neuromuscular emergencies in that rapidly progressive respiratory failure or airway obstruction may occur, requiring life support.

The annual incidence of GBS throughout the world appears to be between 1 and 1.5 cases per 100,000.[1] The earliest symptoms in GBS are often sensory: sensations of crawling under the skin (formications), numbness, or tingling. These may be first noted in the hands or feet. They seldom advance to significant sensory loss and rarely reach clinical significance. Aching muscular pain or muscle soreness may be an early feature in up to one half of patients.

The most prominent feature of GBS is weakness, progressive over hours to days. Symptoms usually begin in the legs but may be more prominent in the arms or hands at first. Many patients become severely disabled, unable to feed themselves or walk, whereas others never develop more than moderate motor deficits. Functional motor skills can be further compromised by involvement of large myelinated sensory fibers subserving joint position sense, with resultant ataxia owing to loss of proprioception. In this setting, severe motor disability may result even when objective weakness is only moderate. About 50% of patients reach maximum deficit within 2 weeks of onset; 90% do so within 4 weeks.[2]

The clinical neurologic examination varies widely from individual to individual, as would be expected from the wide spectrum of clinical presentations. Essentially all patients have decreased or absent deep tendon reflexes, although this need not be symmetric. Sensory abnormalities remain minimal in many cases, limited to blunting of pain sensation at toes and fingers. An uncommon variant presents with a profound, almost pure sensory dysfunction, especially severe in the realm of proprioception.[3]

Motor involvement ranges from minimal limb weakness to quadriplegia. In most patients, there is a mix of proximal and distal weakness, both in the legs and arms, usually symmetric. Cranial nerve involvement occurs less commonly. In patients with severe generalized weakness, there also tends to be bilateral facial weakness. Asymmetric cranial nerve VII involvement also occurs. Involvement of one or more extraocular nerves (cranial nerves III, IV, or VI) is less common, amounting to about 10% in one study.[4] In one specific presentation of GBS, the so-called Miller-Fisher variant,[5] major manifestations are limited to ophthalmoplegia, ataxia of gait, and areflexia. Only rarely has pupillary involvement been noted.[6,7] Weakness of respiratory muscles (diaphragmatic and intercostal as well as auxiliary muscles) is common.

Autonomic dysfunction is common and potentially life-threatening. Signs of sympathetic and parasympathetic failure and overactivity may alternate.[8,9] Sinus tachycardia occurs in more than 50% of severe cases. Reduced peripheral vascular tone may lead to orthostatic hypotension.[8] This likely occurs as a result of loss of sympathetic vascular reflexes, as it is unaccompanied by increased heart rate or diaphoresis.[10]

Hypertension is likewise common, although less well understood.[1] Different studies have shown catecholamine levels to be increased and also normal. Positive phentolamine test results in some patients have suggested denervation hypersensitivity,[11] raising the possibility that hypertension is due to abnormal sensitivity to normal levels of pressor amines.[1] Plasma renin levels have been noted to be markedly elevated in patients with hypertension.[12]

Episodes of parasympathetic overactivity may occur, being characterized by facial flushing, bradycardia, and tightness of the chest and abdomen.[8] Loss of sympathetic function may be manifested by loss of sweating, Horner's syndrome, reduced temperature regulation, gastric dilatation, loss of gastric acidity, and disturbances of urethral and anal sphincters.[1] In children, one can see vasomotor disturbances, acrodynia, and excessive sweating with peripheral vasoconstriction.[13]

The majority of patients have a monophasic course and spontaneous recovery, although up to 10% may be left with significant neurologic sequelae. Despite optimal medical care, mortality remains at 2 to 3%.[14]

Pathology

The pathologic features of GBS were first definitively studied by Asbury et al. in 1969[15] and subsequently by Prineas.[16] The predominant features are mononuclear cell infiltration of the endoneurium and demyelination. The endoneurial cellular infiltration tends to be perivenular and occurs in a segmental, patchy distribution from the root level to the intramuscular twigs. Macrophages participate in the removal of myelin off nerve axons and Schwann cells.

At the cellular level, the pathogenesis of GBS is not fully understood. Much evidence suggests that this process is immunologically mediated, the targets of immune attack being peripheral nerve myelin or Schwann cells. Sera of patients with acute phase GBS cause local demyelination after intraneural injection into rat sciatic nerve.[17] Antiperipheral nerve myelin antibodies have been detected in the sera of patients with GBS.[18] Cellular factors also appear to play a role in the immunologic pathogenesis.[19]

Although the primary process is demyelination, in severe cases, axonal degeneration occurs. Patients with primarily demyelinating lesions recover function relatively quickly because new myelin is laid down by surviving Schwann cells. Patients with significant superimposed axon loss have more protracted, less complete recoveries, owing to the slow axonal regeneration and failure of complete reinnervation, which leads to muscle atrophy.

Pathogenesis

Approximately 50% of individuals have some identifiable prodromal illness. Table 8-1 outlines the most com-

Table 8-1. Common Prodromal Illnesses Associated with Guillain-Barré Syndrome

Viral
  Cytomegalovirus
  Epstein-Barr virus
  Human immunodeficiency virus
  Vaccinia
  Variola
Bacterial
  Mycoplasma
  Campylobacter
Other
  Recent surgery
  Vaccination
  Lymphoma
  Collagen vascular disorders

Table 8-2. Clinical Features Strongly Supportive of Guillaine-Barré Syndrome

Progressive motor weakness over 3-4 weeks, with relative symmetry and only mild sensory symptoms or signs
Areflexia or marked hyporeflexia
Facial weakness (frequently bilateral) in almost 50%
Presence of autonomic dysfunction
Absence of fever at onset of neurologic symptoms

(From Asbury, A. K., et al.: Criteria for diagnosis of Guillain-Barré syndrome. Ann. Neurol., 3:565, 1978.)

mon causes. In many of these, this is a viral infection.[20] The most common prodrome appears to be the "glandular fever-like" syndrome caused by cytomegalovirus (CMV).[21,22] GBS has also been associated with Epstein-Barr virus (EBV) infection,[23] vaccinia, variola, and others.[1]

The leading nonviral pathogens appear to be Mycoplasma pneumoniae, and campylobacter.[24,25] A disorder that closely resembles GBS has been associated with seroconversion to and latent infection with the human immunodeficiency virus (HIV).[26] Other precipitating factors include surgery,[27] lymphomas, vaccinations, and collagen vascular diseases.[1]

Pre-ICU Phase

Accurate diagnosis of GBS rests on a combination of appropriate clinical, cerebrospinal fluid (CSF), and electromyographic (EMG) findings. As Arnason[1] pointed out, the problem is not with recognition of a typical case but with knowing the boundaries by which the core disorder is delimited. Criteria for diagnosis were established by an ad hoc committee under the aegis of the National Institute of Neurological and Communicative Disorders and Stroke (NINCDS) in 1978.[2] The clinical features required for or strongly supportive of the diagnosis are outlined in Table 8-2.

The CSF shows characteristic changes in almost all patients. CSF protein is not expected to rise until 48 hours after onset of symptoms.[3] Protein elevation is usually evident by 1 week[19] but may not reach its peak for 4 to 6 weeks.[28] Electrophoresis of protein constituents may show elevations of IgG concentration, and isoelectric focusing may show oligoclonal banding similar to patterns seen in multiple sclerosis.[29] Cells in the CSF are limited in number. Presence of more than 10 white cells/µl should raise the suspicion of an active infectious process: i.e., primary HIV infection, poliomyelitis, and Lyme disease.

Electromyography can be useful in the support of the diagnosis. A variety of EMG presentations may be seen, depending on the interval of time between onset of symptoms and performance of the study, the particular sites of demyelination, and the presence of superimposed axon loss. Evidence of segmental demyelination is present in about 50% of patients during the first 2 weeks of illness and in 85% by the third week. In about 10% of patients, involvement is so severe that segmental demyelination is never really appreciated because of the superimposed axonal degeneration.[30]

Rapid progressive weakness with limited sensory in-

Table 8-3. Differential Diagnosis of Guillain-Barré Syndrome

Poliomyelitis
Lyme disease
Botulism
Acute intermittent porphyria
Diphtheritic neuropathy
Malignant infiltration of meninges
Periodic paralysis
Cytosine arabinoside neuropathy[34]
Toxins
    Arsenic
    Gold
    Thallium
    Organophosphates
    Hexacarbons

volvement can be the presentation of other neuromuscular disorders. Table 8-3 outlines the major disorders that can present clinical pictures similar to GBS.

Poliomyelitis is often associated with a viral prodrome multiple days in length, is not associated with significant sensory symptoms, and demonstrates weakness that is often asymmetric, with a CSF formula suggesting acute infection (see discussion later). Acute intermittent porphyria can present with severe motor and autonomic neuropathy. The neuropathic presentation may mimic GBS closely. Distinguishing features favoring porphyria may include abdominal pain, mental disturbances, unusual "nonanatomic" sensory symptoms, preservation of ankle reflexes, and persistent marked tachycardia.[31] Botulism presents early with ocular and bulbar motor signs and then later with extremity weakness (see discussion later). The meningoradiculopathy of Lyme disease is often asymmetric and associated with severe radicular pain and significant sensory loss.

Acute intoxication with organophosphates, hexacarbons, arsenic, gold, and thallium can produce pictures similar to GBS.[32,33] Acute arsenic intoxication may present clinically and electromyographically in a manner indistinguishable from GBS but is usually associated with marked distal sensory loss and distal more than proximal weakness. Most arsenic intoxications, however, are chronic and present little resemblance to GBS. With heavy thallium intoxication, the onset of sensory and motor involvement can be rapid. These features as well as autonomic instability resemble GBS, but marked central nervous system (CNS) signs are often present as well. Neuropathy is a rare complication of gold therapy, but pain, sensory loss, and weakness may be sudden in onset, asymmetric, and rapidly progressive, resembling GBS.[34]

After establishing a working diagnosis of GBS, appropriate management depends on assessment of the degree of impairment, length of course, and tempo of progression. The patient with mild-to-moderate weakness for several weeks, without signs of progression, is likely at the nadir of illness and requires minimal observation and no specific treatment. Such patients need not be admitted to the hospital if the facts presented appear reliable and home support is available.

In contrast, the patient with symptoms for only several days may or may not show significant deficits, and prognosis is unknown. If any weakness exists, such patients should be admitted to the hospital for observation and workup. Patients can decompensate neurologically over hours, regardless of their clinical picture on presentation. If close nursing care and bedside respiratory surveillance are available on the general hospital floor, patients need not be admitted directly to the ICU. Bedside nursing care should include evaluation of ease of respiration, ability to swallow, changes in motor function, and stability of blood pressure and heart rate. Bedside respiratory monitoring should include forced vital capacity (FVC) and negative inspiratory force (NIF), performed on an every-4-hour basis while the patient is awake.

The initial laboratory workup for a patient with GBS should include routine blood counts, sedimentation rate, and electrolytes. CSF examination, as mentioned previously, can aid the diagnosis, although the findings may not be fully supportive until 2 weeks into the illness. EMG evaluation for electrophysiologic evidence of peripheral demyelination can yield supportive evidence at any stage of the illness, although the findings are more clear cut once the patient has developed maximum deficits or later.

Routine arterial blood gas determination is a useful means to document baseline arterial oxygen saturation and to determine the severity of respiratory failure, but it is insensitive in the identification of patients with early respiratory insufficiency of neuromuscular cause. Waiting for hypoxemia and hypercarbia to occur before undertaking intubation is unsafe and increases the morbidity from an emergency intubation.

The finding of hypoxemia by arterial blood gas determination is a later finding in neuromuscular respiratory failure, as are findings of clinical dyspnea and decreased tidal volume. These observations are therefore insensitive in the identification of patients with early respiratory insufficiency, who may shortly require ventilatory assistance. More sensitive indicators of progressive respiratory failure include the FVC and NIF.[36] As the FVC begins to fall, spontaneous cough weakens, and there is progressive difficulty in clearing secretions. The intrinsic sigh mechanism is lost, and peripheral alveoli remain collapsed. Finally, tidal volume falls and hypoxemia supervenes. When the FVC falls to less than 10 to 15 ml/kg, respiratory collapse is likely. When the vital capacity falls to 15 ml/kg, the patient should be monitored in an ICU.

ICU Phase

General Support

Patients are admitted to the ICU under the following circumstances:

- Rapid progression of weakness
- Progressive respiratory failure
- Serious risk of aspiration owing to incompetency of deglutition
- Autonomic instability

Although the first two indications are dealt with routinely with elective intubation, the management of autonomic instability remains a difficult process. Both the sympathetic and the parasympathetic systems may be involved, and overactivity may alternate with underactivity.

Paralysis of the smooth muscles of the bronchial tree has been reported.[13] Stiff bronchi lead to inability to dilate and constrict alternately, reducing the ability to clear secretions. There may also be increased secretory activity of the bronchial mucosa following denervation of the lung.

Sinus tachycardia can be seen in one half of severe cases.[8] This may respond to carotid sinus massage if the vagal system is intact. Bradycardia is sometimes seen in the setting of generalized parasympathetic overactivity[8] and may respond to atropine.

Orthostatic hypotension may occur as a result of reduced peripheral vascular tone, seen with loss of sympathetically mediated vascular reflexes. In this setting, pulse rate does not increase in the face of precipitous decrease of blood pressure. As fluids pool peripherally, cardiac output is lowered. Cardiac output can be further compromised by positive pressure assisted ventilator support. Minor dehydration can further compromise cardiac output and blood pressure. In such situations, plasma expanders may be more useful than pressor agents.[1] In fact, patients may be highly sensitive to pressors such as phenylephrine,[37] perhaps because of sympathetic denervation hypersensitivity.[11] Conversely, hypertension is also a frequent accompaniment of GBS. Its basis is uncertain. Denervation of the carotid sinus has been postulated.[38] There may be an abnormal sensitivity to normal levels of endogenous pressor amines, following along the lines of denervation hypersensitivity.[1] Plasma renin levels have also been found to be elevated in patients with hypertension, and propranolol has been suggested as treatment for that reason.[12,39] It has been recommended that an alpha-adrenergic inhibitor be added to propranolol in the presence of elevated levels of catecholamines because propranolol may enhance the pressor effect of norepinephrine.[39]

Plasmapheresis

The value of specific treatments for GBS has been clarified over the last several years. The use of corticosteroids in the treatment of acute GBS was shown to be without benefit in one cooperative trial.[40] It is now clear, based on the findings of the GBS Study Group,[14] that some patients are benefitted by a course of plasmapheresis treatments early in their illness. Patients who were begun on plasmapheresis before ventilatory support remained on ventilator support an average of 9 days, whereas those not given plasmapheresis remained on support 23 days. The difference was less striking if ventilator support was begun before plasmapheresis. Three to five exchanges were performed over 7 to 14 days. In a follow-up report, four factors were found to correlate with poorer outcomes with plasmapheresis:

- Reduced amplitude of the compound muscle action potential response on stimulation distally (20% of normal or less)
- Older age
- Time from onset of disease of 7 days or less
- Need for ventilator support[41]

The most important of these was the low amplitude compound muscle action potential, suggesting significant motor axon loss.

Plasmapheresis is in general well tolerated. Plasmapheresis-related reactions most commonly included fever, chills, urticaria, muscle cramps, and paresthesias, probably related to the plasma used for replacement in one study, in which these reactions accounted for 50% of all reactions.[42] Severe reactions, such as hypotension, cardiac arrhythmia, bronchospasm, convulsions, and respiratory arrest, accounted for 3% of all reactions. No deaths were directly related to the procedure. Other complications of plasmapheresis include immunoglobulin depletion and infection. In GBS patients, there is the added risk factor of autonomic instability. Because of this, many institutions prefer to initiate plasmapheresis in the setting of the ICU.

There have now been several reports of early relapse of GBS after completion of plasmapheresis treatments[43,44] within 2 to 6 weeks of the last treatment. In general, patients do not return to the nadir of their illness but may require second courses of plasmapheresis. This occurrence may be the result of cessation of plasmapheresis treatments before disease activity has ceased, thus allowing humoral factors related to pathogenesis to reaccumulate in the circulation.

Intravenous Immunoglobulin (IVIG) Treatment

Several studies have now clearly established the efficacy of IVIG in the treatment of GBS.[45,46] A recent study has shown that IVIG is as effective as plasmapheresis, with fewer complications. The normal dosage is 0.4 gram/kg per day for 5 days. Side effects are usually of the "transfusion reaction" type, including diaphoresis, dizziness, and hypotension, and are treated by slowing the infusion rate and using premedication. There is a higher relapse rate after IVIG treatment compared to plasmapheresis, perhaps because the treatment period is less than 1 week and the disease process may still be immunologically active when treatment is completed. Retreatment in such cases is usually successful. In my own practice, I have used plasmapheresis in otherwise healthy individuals and have reserved IVIG for the elderly and patients with significant underlying illness.

Post-ICU Phase

All patients who have reached levels of disability requiring transfer to the ICU require weeks to months of recovery.[19,47,48] This is accomplished by a comprehensive neurorehabilitation that may require admission to a rehabilitation facility. Patients with more severe weakness, whose EMG pictures suggest marked axon loss, have prolonged recovery periods and are left with permanent deficits. A combination of physical therapy, appropriate braces, and home health aids allows the patient to return home to continue convalescence. At 1 year, residual deficits may be seen in more than 20% of patients, but fewer than 10% of deficits are severe.[41,49] Late relapses occur in approximately 10% of patients, some of whom may go on to demonstrate a clinical picture of chronic inflammatory demyelinating polyradiculoneuropathy (CIDP).

NEUROMUSCULAR TRANSMISSION DISORDERS

The neuromuscular junction (NMJ) is the synapse between the motor nerve terminal and the muscle fiber innervated by it. After transmission of the chemical acetylcholine (ACh) across the synapse and after binding of ACh to its receptors at the muscle end plate, ion channels open and the muscle membrane is depolarized, producing a propagated action potential along the muscle fiber and muscle contraction. The most common disorder of NMJ transmission is myasthenia gravis (MG), which affects the postsynaptic acetylcholine receptors (AChRs). A less common disorder is the Lambert-Eaton myasthenic syndrome (LEMS), which affects the presynaptic release of ACh. A number of drugs and toxins alter NMJ transmission and can produce life-threatening weakness.

Myasthenia Gravis

MG is an autoimmune disorder associated with production of antibody against the postsynaptic skeletal muscle AChR. MG is a disorder of muscle weakness with a prevalence of 1:10,000 to 20,000. The onset of disease occurs primarily in two age groups: young women and elderly men (60 to 75 years of age). There is an increased incidence of other autoimmune syndromes in patients with MG. These include:

- Thyroiditis
- Graves' disease
- Rheumatoid arthritis
- Systemic lupus erythematosus
- Diabetes
- Pernicious anemia
- Pemphigus vulgaris

Many other patients may have circulating autoantibodies associated with these diseases, although they do not demonstrate the diseases themselves.[50] Although the disease is not hereditary, certain histocompatibility locus antigen (HLA) types are associated with MG,[51] and there is an increased incidence of autoimmune diseases of different types in family members.

Pre-ICU Phase

MG presents clinically as fatigability and weakness of voluntary skeletal muscle. A diagnostic cornerstone of the disease is the tendency for symptoms to be most apparent with physical activity and exercise and least apparent after rest. Cranial muscles are most likely to be involved first. Often patients present with complaints of ptosis and diplopia owing to weakness of the levator palpebrae and extraocular muscles. Later masseter, facial, and oropharyngeal muscles weaken, with resultant difficulty with chewing, facial expression, and swallowing. Subsequently there may be weakness of proximal muscles of the extremities as well as weakness of the diaphragm and intercostal muscles, leading to respiratory insufficiency. For staging pur-

Table 8–4. Osserman Classification of Adult Myasthenia Gravis (MG)

I.	Ocular MG
II.	A. Mild generalized MG
	B. Moderate generalized MG
III.	Acute fulminating MG
IV.	Late severe MG (severe symptoms developing 2 years or more after onset of group I or II symptoms)

(From Osserman, K. G., and Genkins, G.: Studies in myasthenia gravis: review of twenty-year experience in over 1200 patients. Mt. Sinai J. Med., 38:497, 1971.)

poses, MG has been classified into four categories,[52] (Table 8–4).

Early on in the disease process, symptoms tend to vary remarkably from hour to hour, day to day. Generally patients have fewest symptoms on arising in the morning and maximal symptoms late in the day. When symptoms are mild, no objective evidence of dysfunction can be found by examination, and variability of symptoms, such as blurry vision, fatigue, and trouble swallowing, often leads the physician to the erroneous diagnosis of hysteria or depression. Diagnosis is most difficult in those patients who do not progress rapidly enough to demonstrate a defined symptom complex or obvious findings.

The neurologic examination may be normal in patients with MG. In established disease, cranial findings may include asymmetric ptosis; dysconjugate gaze, which may not be classifiable into weakness of particular extraocular muscles; and bifacial weakness giving rise to a snarl rather than a smile. Speech may be nasal or frankly dysarthric, with worsening as the patient continues to speak. Subtle abnormalities can be elicited by fatiguing muscle groups. When the patient is asked to sustain upgaze for 1 minute, progressive ptosis or dysconjugate gaze (or both) may appear. Neck flexion may be weakened in patients before proximal muscles of the arms and legs show weakness.

The pathology of MG is seen in skeletal muscle and the thymus. There is no pertinent pathology identifiable by light microscopy of skeletal muscle preparations. Electron microscopy of the NMJ identifies the characteristic features of widening of the synaptic cleft, simplification of the postsynaptic junctional folds, and loss of AChRs.

About 75% of myasthenic patients have thymic abnormalities.[59] The vast majority show thymic hyperplasia, primarily of the germinal centers of the medulla of the gland. In about 10 to 15% of all abnormal thymus glands, there is evidence of thymoma. These tumors are usually of the mixed lymphoepithelial cell type, and they rarely metastasize but do invade tissues of the mediastinum.

Weakness in MG occurs as a result of loss of AChRs at the muscle end plate. Although ACh is released in normal amounts from the presynaptic nerve terminal, there are too few receptors at the postsynaptic site to accept it, and therefore less depolarization of the muscle membrane occurs. With exercise, there is a natural decline in the release of ACh from the nerve terminal, which compounds the problem of depolarization at the receptor site and makes weakness even worse.[54]

The diagnosis of MG depends on a combination of history, clinical features, and laboratory confirmatory studies. The oldest supportive test for MG is the edrophonium chloride (Tensilon) test. This powerful acetylcholinesterase inhibitor reduces ACh breakdown in the NMJ seconds after intravenous injection, increasing the concentration of ACh in the synapse and improving NMJ transmission briefly. This is identified clinically by improvement in diplopia, ptosis, or other myasthenic signs exhibited by the patient. Unfortunately, the test is much less useful when no objective deficits are present by which to judge improvement. Table 8-5 describes how the edrophonium test is performed.

The EMG assesses the response of the muscle to repetitive stimulation of the nerve trunk that innervates it. Repetitive stimulation studies are positive in about 95% of patients with generalized disease, but if all severities of disease are grouped together, the diagnosis is apparent by this technique in only 50%. A specialized needle electrode examination known as single-fiber EMG is more sensitive, yielding a positive result in 77% of patients with restricted ocular forms of MG and 92% of patients with mild generalized MG.[55]

Serologic testing can be helpful in supporting the diagnosis. The presence of antibody to AChR is extremely specific for the diagnosis of MG. Using a combination of assays to detect antibodies with differing binding characteristics, Howard et al.[56] found elevated concentrations of antibody in 80% of patients with restricted ocular MG, in 91% of patients with mild generalized MG, and 96% of patients with moderate-to-severe generalized MG. False-positive test results for antibody have been found in individuals exposed to the cobra venom alpha-bungarotoxin, which is used in the assay. Other false-positive results were seen in patients who had recently undergone anesthesia with muscle relaxants, such as suxamethonium chloride and dimethyltubocurarine iodide (Metubine). False-positive results have been found occasionally among patients with ALS, pernicious anemia, and those taking the drug D-penicillamine.[56]

Computed tomography (CT) or magnetic resonance imaging (MRI) of the thorax should be performed to identify evidence of thymic hyperplasia or possible thymoma. The presence of other autoimmune disorders should be assessed with thyroid functions, antithyroid antibody, vitamin B_{12} level, antiparietal cell antibodies, and antinuclear factor.

When considering the diagnosis of MG, one should keep in mind that many chemical agents have an adverse effect

Table 8-5. Edrophonium Chloride (Tensilon) Test

Record baseline heart rate
Identify observable myasthenic signs
Have 1.0 ml atropine IV ready at bedside
Administer 2 mg edrophonium IV bolus
Allow 30-60 sec to observe effect; check heart rate
If no adverse effects, give remaining 8 mg edrophonium IV bolus
Nonspecific symptoms, such as stomach contractions and light-headedness, indicate systemic effect
Check heart rate
Observe for change in myasthenic signs over 1-4 min

Table 8-6. Agents that Can Exacerbate Myasthenia Gravis

Type	Specific Agent
Metabolic states	Hypocalcemia
	Hypermagnesemia
Neuromuscular blockers	Curare
	Succinylcholine
Antibiotics	Aminoglycosides
	Lincomycin, clindamycin
	Polymyxins
	Tetracycline (?)
Antiarrhythmics	Procaine—procainamide
	Quinine—quinidine
	Lidocaine
	Beta-blockers
Psychotropics	Phenothiazines
	Lithium
Miscellaneous	Iodinated contrast agents
	Organophosphates
	Cholinesterase inhibitors
	Phenytoin (?)

on NMJ transmission. Table 8-6 lists the most commonly encountered agents likely to cause worsening of MG. These effects reach clinical significance when NMJ transmission is already impaired as in MG, although rarely these agents may cause weakness transiently in patients without MG. Some drugs, such as succinylcholine and curare, produce NMJ blockade by binding to the AChR, although the former drug acts by hyperdepolarizing the membrane, and the latter acts by preventing depolarization. Other agents such as organophosphates inactivate acetylcholinesterase and hyperdepolarize the membrane by flooding the synapse with ACh. Many drugs that interfere with NMJ transmission do so by affecting the calcium equilibrium of the nerve terminal. The release of ACh is aided by calcium influx into the nerve terminal. Reduction of calcium entry reduces the normal release of ACh. Iodinated contrast agents used in angiography reduce calcium availability by binding it. Most important in this process appears to be sodium citrate and sodium edetate, used as sequestering agents in the media.[57] Acute respiratory failure and myasthenic crisis have been reported when such agents have been used in the setting of MG or LEMS.[57,58]

Magnesium acts as a calcium antagonist at the NMJ by competing for entry into the nerve terminal. This competition reduces calcium entry and ACh release. Renal failure is essentially the only setting in which elevation of the body's magnesium concentration can produce weakness. In MG, however, heavy intake of magnesium-containing cathartics can cause weakness.[59] The effects of the aminoglycoside group of antibiotics on myasthenics may be compared with the effect of magnesium at the NMJ.[60,61] Of the group of aminoglycosides, neomycin appears to be the most toxic and tobramycin the least toxic.[60]

Other antibiotics have a negative effect on NMJ transmission. Polymyxin drugs (polymyxin B, polymyxin E, colistin) produce weakness by noncompetitive blockade of AChRs.[63] Monobasic amino acid antibiotics such as lincomycin and clindamycin also block NMJ transmission.[64]

Antiarrhythmic and anesthetic drugs of parent compounds such as procaine, lidocaine, and quinine also produce neuromuscular blockade. Their exact mechanism of action is unclear, but they are known to produce curariform blocks of AChRs, impair propagation of nerve terminal impulses, reduce ACh release, and hamper propagation of the muscle fiber action potential.[65] Beta-adrenergic blocking drugs have also been reported to affect NMJ transmission by a curariformlike action.[66]

Other drugs have been reported to worsen myasthenic states, including lithium[67] and phenothiazines.[68] Rare reports of tetracycline-related and phenytoin-related worsening have also been described.[69] In the treatment of drug-induced myasthenic worsening, no one agent is effective for all offenders. After discontinuation of the drug in question, baseline function is eventually reached. Calcium may be the most effective treatment for reversing antibiotic-induced weakness. In other cases, anticholinesterase may be useful.[64,70]

Only one drug, D-penicillamine, has been associated with pathogenesis of MG. This drug is associated with production of antibody against AChR, and the condition is reversed by cessation of the drug.[71]

General Management Considerations. The management of MG depends on many factors related to the extent of disease, age of the patient, and the presence or absence of thymoma. In general, patients who are optimally treated seldom require intensive care during the course of the disease, although some patients have particularly fulminant or fragile conditions easily tipped into decompensation by infection, pregnancy, or medication change.

There is no reliable information about the spontaneous remission rate of MG among adults. In children, a steadily progressive spontaneous remission rate of 22.4 per 1000 person years has been measured.[72] In that study, by 5 years, approximately 10% of the patients had undergone remission, by 15 years 30%, and by 20 years almost 40%.

The prognosis among patients with restricted ocular disease appears to be distinct from patients with bulbar and generalized MG. One study has shown that among patients with pure ocular MG for at least 2 years, only 15% subsequently developed generalized MG.[73] These patients should be managed differently because the risk of long-term life-threatening disease is low.

New-Onset Myasthenia Gravis. After diagnosis, patients with mild forms of MG benefit from oral anticholinesterase medication. Pyridostigmine (Mestinon) can be started at 30 or 60 mg every 6 hours and titrated up, as tolerated. The 4-hour half-life suggests that the drug should not be taken more frequently than every 3 to 4 hours. In my experience, a dosage greater than 120 mg every 3 to 4 hours provides no valuable increment in myasthenic management, places the patient at risk for cholinergic crisis, and overlooks the need to switch to more appropriate therapeutic agents (see discussion later).

In all patients with thymic enlargement, surgical removal should be considered. In older patients, such enlargement may indicate thymoma. In younger patients with thymic enlargement owing to hyperplasia, studies suggest that thymectomy has a positive effect on the course of disease.[54,74] A study of patients receiving transsternal thymectomy as the primary therapy before introduction of immunosuppressant therapy showed 92% of patients were improved, 80% were free of generalized weakness after a mean follow-up of 39 months, 55% were on no medication, and 38% had never received drugs.[75] Forty percent of patients had at least moderate generalized or bulbar dysfunction. Unfortunately, data comparing directly the effects of other therapeutic agents are not available. Grob and colleagues[76] studied two groups of patients between 1960 and 1980. One group of 121 had thymectomy (and were more seriously ill), whereas 355 received corticosteroids.[76] The results are given in Table 8–7. Because each investigating institution carries a treatment bias, patient selection for different arms of a comparative study is biased and difficult to compare with studies from other institutions. Although thymectomy is recommended because it is associated with a better prognosis, it is not the appropriate treatment for rapid reversal of severe myasthenic symptoms.

The use of corticosteroids is a highly personalized therapy. The time to begin steroids, the dosage schedule, and the amount of medication are highly subjective judgments. About 40% of patients experience an acute exacerbation in the early stage of daily high dose steroid therapy.[77,78] Onset can be any time within the first 3 weeks of therapy, and most patients experience mild-to-moderate deterioration, although some require respiratory support. It has been suggested that this exacerbation can be avoided by the gradual increase of steroids when given on an alternate-day schedule.[79] Such a schedule, however, is not appropriate for the patient with rapidly progressive or fulminant myasthenic symptoms. In these patients, a typical starting dose of prednisone would be between 60 and 100 mg each day. In my experience, little significant positive clinical effect occurs during the first 1 to 2 weeks, and as such some patients with marginally compensated respiratory function or progressive swallowing difficulty need other, more quickly-acting therapeutic maneuvers. To avoid the complications of long-term corticosteroid therapy, many physicians add azathioprine after it is clear that long-term steroid use will be necessary. Use of azathioprine in this setting permits more rapid steroid tapering.

Plasmapheresis may be the fastest way to stabilize rapidly progressive MG in those medical centers where this procedure is available. In each treatment, between 2 and 3 L of the patient's plasma is replaced with 5% albumin and saline. Although studies have suggested that improvement in strength may occur as quickly as 1 day after treat-

Table 8–7. Comparison of Patients with and without Thymectomy

	Thymectomy		Without Thymectomy	
	Male	Female	Male	Female
% Improvement	41	42	34	40
% Mortality	8	13	16	10

(Data from Grob, D., Brunner, N. G., and Namba, T.: The natural course of myasthenia gravis and effect of therapeutic measures. Ann. N.Y. Acad. Sci., *377*:652, 1981.)

Table 8-8. Predictive Factors for Prolonged Postoperative Mechanical Ventilation in Myasthenia Gravis

Duration of myasthenia gravis >6 years
History of chronic respiratory disease
Required dose of pyridostigmine >750 mg/day
Other factors:
    Pain from sternotomy[84]
    Intraoperative phrenic nerve damage[85]

(Data from references 85 to 87.)

ment,[80] most studies show significant change in myasthenic symptoms after about 7 days, with treatments on an alternate-day schedule.[81] When plasmapheresis is used alone, it is usually helpful only briefly.[82] The positive effects may linger 3 to 6 weeks after a course of plasmapheresis, but deterioration to the previous level of function is expected thereafter, attributed to rebound of antibody production. For this reason, simultaneous immunosuppression with prednisone or prednisone and azathioprine is often used in combination with long-term plasmapheresis.[83] In patients undergoing long-term immunosuppression without maximal effect, long-term plasmapheresis has been a useful adjunctive therapy.[83,84]

Preoperative Patient. Myasthenic patients are at increased risk for complications from surgery. Patients who are not optimally treated for MG are at the greatest risk for postoperative pulmonary complications. This pertains to patients preparing for thymectomy as well as other procedures.

For newly diagnosed patients, the consideration for upcoming thymectomy should influence therapeutic plans. If the patient's condition can be stabilized without corticosteroids, postoperative infectious complications are minimized and healing is faster. If anticholinesterase medication is inadequate, plasmapheresis should be used. Patients who are candidates include those whose respiratory status is marginal, whose ability to control secretions is abnormal, and whose general strength is poor. Plasmapheresis should be discontinued about 72 hours before surgery to allow recirculation of depleted immunoglobulins. Leventhal[85] studied multiple factors and their relative value in predicting the need for prolonged postoperative ventilatory support. The factors that correctly predicted prolonged ventilatory support are listed in Table 8-8.

In myasthenics, maximal control of MG is necessary preoperatively. Patients already on corticosteroids should be given extra corticosteroid directly before surgery. Patients on anticholinesterase medication do not need these drugs during surgery but may be given their usual dose preoperatively. Succinylcholine and other neuromuscular blocking agents should be avoided if at all possible during surgery because they prolong the need for postoperative assisted ventilation.

ICU Phase

Myasthenics who reach the ICU are in need of ventilatory support, airway protection, or close monitoring. Patients with unstable neuromuscular function fit into three main categories:

- Myasthenic crisis
- Cholinergic crisis
- Immediate postoperative state

Myasthenic Crisis. Patients with MG may experience acute deterioration of their condition for several reasons. Intercurrent infection is the most common cause. For well-controlled patients, the consequent fluctuation in their disease is mild, and intensive care is not needed. For poorly controlled patients, infection can precipitate severe myasthenic symptoms. The use of drugs that impede NMJ transmission can precipitate myasthenic worsening also (see Table 8-6). Pregnancy and the postpartum state have both been associated with myasthenic worsening, perhaps owing to the immunologic changes that occur during pregnancy.

Increasing pyridostigmine alone does not usually abort a myasthenic crisis.[88] Such anticholinesterase medications are most effective when used in the setting of mild disease or to "fine-tune" symptoms already treated by other means. They do not have the ability to improve NMJ transmission enough to have a significant impact on respiratory failure, marked dysphagia, or severe weakness. In fact, pushing pyridostigmine to high dose can precipitate toxicity and paradoxically worsen weakness (see later). Generally if the patient requires acute ventilatory support, it is not necessary to continue anticholinesterase over the short term.[89] Many specialists believe that time off anticholinesterase medication may enable the drug to be more effective when reintroduced several days later, at a lower dose. When using pyridostigmine in the ICU setting, it is often administered parenterally via the intramuscular or subcutaneous route, but at doses $\frac{1}{30}$ of the corresponding oral dose. In weaning the patient off mechanical ventilation, anticholinesterase medication may be useful in providing a small but significant increase in motor strength.

Patients with myasthenic crisis are often most helped over the short-term by a series of five to seven plasmapheresis treatments. If the patient is not yet under immunosuppressive treatment, the initiation of corticosteroids may also add to the long-term benefit, realizing that clinical effect may not be significant for at least 2 weeks.

Withdrawing ventilatory support too early may exhaust muscles of respiration. Establishing that the FVC is at least twice the expected tidal volume and the NIF is at least -25 cm H_2O helps ensure adequate pulmonary reserve in the direct postextubation period for patients with neuromuscular causes of hypoventilation.

Cholinergic Crisis. The known myasthenic may experience an acute clinical deterioration as a result of overdosage of anticholinesterase medication. This paradoxic worsening occurs because ACh floods the synapse, failing to detach from AChR binding sites and freezing the muscle fiber in a depolarized state, akin to the action of succinylcholine. This produces progressive muscle weakness. Although the patient may also show systemic effects of cholinergic excess (abdominal cramping, diarrhea, excessive bronchial secretions, sweating, salivation, bradycardia, hypotension), the appearance of this condition may be indistinguishable from myasthenic crisis.

Performance of an intravenous edrophonium chloride (Tensilon) challenge test is the only way to separate cholinergic from myasthenic crisis clearly (see Table 8-5). In the patient with anticholinesterase intoxication, challenge with an intravenous anticholinesterase such as edrophonium produces either no clinical change or worsening of weakness. In the undertreated myasthenic, however, the drug should produce improvement. The edrophonium should be given in small doses, beginning with 1 mg, adding 1 to 2 mg at a time every 2 to 3 minutes if there is no response, to a total dose of 10 mg. Equipment for emergency intubation should be at hand.

The treatment of cholinergic crisis is supportive, after discontinuation of the drug. Patients with this condition usually are already immunosuppressed and may report that their myasthenia had been in fact improving. In this situation, the previously required dosage of anticholinesterase has become unnecessarily high for the current level of myasthenic symptoms.

Postoperative Myasthenic Patient. The care of the postoperative myasthenic patient involves, above all, the proper support of pulmonary function. Not only must adequate oxygenation be guaranteed, but also maximum lung expansion must be provided to prevent atelectasis and subsequent pneumonia. The appropriate time for withdrawal of ventilatory support must be individualized for each patient. The most important indications are a strong cough reflex as well as those measurements that confirm adequate respiratory muscle function, the FVC and NIF. The competence and strength of the cough reflex indicate the patient's ability to clear the airway of secretions after extubation.

As mentioned previously, the study by Leventhal[83] identified risk factors for the need for prolonged postoperative ventilatory support (see Table 8-8). Whether the patient requires ventilatory support or not, anticholinesterase dosing should be individualized. Pyridostigmine reaches peak activity about 1 to 2 hours after oral dosage and thus can be restarted after the patient is alert or when efforts to withdraw ventilatory support begin.[90] Others believe that anticholinesterase should be reinstituted immediately postoperatively to improve ventilatory mechanics.[86,87] Although narcotic analgesics cause respiratory depression and can be detrimental in the marginally compensated myasthenic, morphine sulfate under close supervision can be administered safely for pain relief without risk of neuromuscular blockade. The use of antibiotics and antiarrhythmics may further complicate the postoperative course, and these drugs should be chosen carefully and monitored closely. Generally the successful care of the myasthenic undergoing surgery requires the coordinated efforts of a team of health care professionals that is experienced in the care of myasthenic patients.

Lambert-Eaton Myasthenic Syndrome

LEMS is a disorder of NMJ transmission related to impaired ACh release from the presynaptic terminals. Clinically patients demonstrate a picture primarily of proximal muscle weakness of the extremities. Significant involvement of ocular and bulbar musculature is uncommon. Remarkable advances have occurred in the understanding of the pathogenesis of LEMS. It is now established that LEMS is an autoimmune disorder in which IgG antibodies affect cell surface molecules of the motor nerve terminal, probably the voltage-gated calcium channels or related molecules of the active zones of ACh release. This impairs release of ACh, which blocks NMJ transmission.[91] This occurs at all cholinergic end plates and therefore produces a syndrome of muscle weakness and reduced cholinergic parasympathetic function, manifested by impotence, constipation, and dryness of the mouth and eyes. Some two thirds of patients have an associated malignancy, most often small cell carcinoma of the lung. Among patients without carcinoma, the incidence of thyroid and gastric (parietal cell) autoantibodies is equal to that in patients with MG.[92] The use of immunosuppressants such as prednisone[93] and plasmapheresis[94] has significantly aided the treatment of these patients.

Patients with LEMS seldom require intensive care for their neuromuscular disease. Occasionally, however, patients develop a fulminant course with progressive respiratory failure and dysphagia. Such patients should be treated as if they had MG because issues surrounding their intensive care are identical.

Botulism

Botulism is a life-threatening neuromuscular condition produced by neurotoxins elaborated by Clostridium botulinum. The disease occurs in three situations:

- Ingestion of toxin in foods
- Production of toxin in a traumatic wound infected by C. botulinum
- Production of toxin by colonized C. botulinum in the gastrointestinal tract of infants

Food-borne botulism is increasing because of renewed interest in home canning of foods.

Eight immunologically distinct toxin types have been described. Types A, B, and E are the most common in humans. The toxin acts by entering the motor nerve terminals, and preventing release of ACh. A cholinergic synapse may be blocked by as few as 10 molecules of toxin.[95] Recovery occurs through sprouting of new nerve fibers and reestablishment of new NMJs.[96]

Pre-ICU Phase

Generally botulism presents neurologically as symmetric descending weakness. Symptoms usually begin 12 to 36 hours (range 6 hours to 8 days) after ingestion of contaminated food.[97] Nausea and vomiting are present in only one third of patients with types A and B disease but are more common with type E intoxication. Early symptoms include weakness, lassitude, and dizziness. Interruption of cholinergic autonomic function causes dryness of mouth, sometimes to the point of complaints of sore throat. Ileus, constipation, and urinary retention may also occur.

Neurologic symptoms may occur concurrently or may

be delayed for up to 3 days.[97] Cranial nerves are affected first: Diplopia occurs as a result of paralysis of extraocular muscles, and blurred vision occurs as a result of fixed dilation of pupils. Bulbar involvement results in dysphonia, dysarthria, and dysphagia. Later weakness of extremity muscles and muscles of respiration occurs.

Physical findings may include somnolence in patients with type B intoxication.[98] Postural hypotension may be prominent. Ocular signs include ophthalmoplegia, ptosis, and fixed dilated pupils. The mucous membranes of the mouth are often red, dry, and crusted, at times leading to the erroneous diagnosis of streptococcal pharyngitis.[97] There may be generalized weakness. Deep tendon reflexes may be present or absent. The sensory examination is normal.

Recovery is gradual and occurs over weeks to months. The diagnosis can be difficult to make in the early stages. Findings of unexplained postural hypotension, dilated pupils, dry membranes, and weakness should raise suspicion of the diagnosis. In some patients, nausea, vomiting, and abdominal distention are prominent. An ileus pattern radiographically may be seen, and exploratory laparotomy may be performed mistakenly in search of intestinal obstruction.[97] Certain anticholinergic drug poisonings (atropine, belladonna, jimsonweed) can produce some features of this disorder. Other features may suggest GBS.

The diagnosis of botulism rests on clinical suspicion and special laboratory confirmatory tests. EMG examination can support the diagnosis if the typical features of a presynaptic defect of NMJ transmission are present, although in severe cases, no electrical motor responses may be obtainable. The diagnosis can be confirmed by demonstrating (1) toxin in the blood, (2) toxin or C. botulinum organisms in the stool or gastric contents, or (3) toxin in the food. Toxin is detected by bioassay in mice. Culture of the organism anaerobically is difficult.[97]

ICU Phase

Respiratory failure is the most common cause of death in these individuals. Careful evaluation of FVC is necessary, as in other neuromuscular disorders. In the acute stage, if ileus is not present, cleansing saline enemas can remove any unabsorbed toxin.

Antitoxin therapy is recommended. Treatment for types A and E intoxication is more clearly efficacious than for type B.[99] Antitoxin should be administered as soon as possible, although delayed use may still be beneficial, owing to the finding of toxin in the blood of some patients as long as 30 days after intoxication. All preparations of antitoxin are of equine origin. Up to 20% of patients have untoward reactions, requiring testing for hypersensitivity and desensitization before use if necessary. One vial of antitoxin should be administered intramuscularly and one intravenously. This should be repeated in 2 to 4 hours if symptoms persist. Antitoxin is available through the Centers for Disease Control (Atlanta).*

The use of penicillin to eradicate C. botulinum in the bowel is of uncertain value. Even in the case of wound infection by C. botulinum, use of antibiotic does not prevent intoxication.

Guanidine hydrochloride, a drug that enhances release of ACh from motor nerve terminals, has been shown to improve the neurologic status of patients, including respiratory function. About half the patients have failed to respond.[100,101] Serious complications from guanidine therapy include bone marrow suppression and renal toxicity, severely limiting the applicability of this therapy in standard care.

Post-ICU Care

Speed of recovery from botulism depends on the severity of neurologic damage sustained. In all cases, return of strength occurs as new nerve sprouts reach muscle fibers to reestablish NMJs that were lost during the acute stage of disease. This process can be measured in months in those patients rendered quadriplegic from the disease.

MOTOR NEURON DISORDERS

Motor neuron disorders comprise conditions that have in common the destruction or involvement of anterior horn cells in the spinal cord, leading to paralysis in the absence of sensory symptoms. In the United States, although poliomyelitis was by far the most common motor neuron disorder before the advent of the polio vaccines, the degenerative disorder ALS is now most common.

Amyotrophic Lateral Sclerosis (ALS)

ALS is confined to the motor system with sparing of the extraocular muscles and sphincters. Both lower motor neurons (anterior horn cells and cranial motor nuclei of the brain stem) and upper motor neurons (cortical motor neurons) are involved. Some patients present with primarily lower motor neuron involvement. In the bulbar form of this presentation, there is progressive dysarthria leading to anarthria and dysphagia leading to inability to swallow, with consequent aspiration. When limbs are involved first, there is progressive atrophy and weakness of the limb muscles associated with fasciculation of muscle. Other patients present with primarily upper motor neuron involvement. The bulbar picture includes choking on foods and spastic dysarthria. When limbs are involved, the upper motor neuron picture is characterized by spasticity and weakness of extremities.

The usual course of ALS is relentlessly progressive, ending in death by 3 years in 39 to 50% of patients.[102,103] Patients have been reported with unusually prolonged courses and with courses showing stabilization after years of progression.[104] Patients with later onset and those with predominantly bulbar or pseudobulbar involvement have been observed to demonstrate a more rapid rate of progression,[102] although a more recent study disagrees.[103] The prevalence of ALS ranges between 4 and 6 per 100,000 population, with an annual incidence of 0.4 to 1.8 per 100,000.[105] The mean age at onset is 56 years and at death 59 years, with a male-to-female ratio of 2:1.

Diagnosis is aided by the EMG, which shows active,

---
* Telephone number 404-639-3753 weekdays and 404-639-2888 at all other times.

Table 8–9. Treatable Disorders that Mimic Amyotrophic Lateral Sclerosis

Structural disorders of spinal cord
   Cervical or thoracic canal stenosis
   Anomalies of the foramen magnum or cord
   Tumors of the brain stem or cord
Metabolic disorders[103]
   Hypercalcemia—hyperparathyroidism
   Hyperthyroidism
Toxins
   Mercury
   Lead
Motor neuropathies
   Due to paraproteinenic states[105] (Waldenström's macroglobulinemia, myeloma)
   Associated with paraneoplastic states[104]
   Associated with GM_1 antibody[106]
   Due to unusual demyelinating disorders
Myopathy
   Polymyositis (subacute)
   Inclusion body myositis

chronic motor axon loss while sparing sensory axons. Mild creatine kinase elevations are common.

Potentially treatable disorders that can imitate ALS are listed in Table 8–9. Cervical myelopathy secondary to cervical spondylosis and canal stenosis is diagnosed by myelography or MRI. Tumors and anomalies of the region of the foramen magnum, tumors of the cervical or thoracic spinal cord, thyrotoxicosis, exposure to mercury, lead intoxication, and hypercalcemia can produce syndromes that are similar to various forms of ALS.[105] Paraneoplastic[106,107] and paraproteinemic[108] states have also produced lower motor neuron syndromes. Cramps and fasciculations seen in some normal individuals can be mistaken for ALS.[110] Other neuromuscular conditions can be confused with ALS in some situations. The pure bulbar presentation of ALS can be confused with MG. Slowly progressive limb weakness can be confused with inflammatory myopathies, such as polymyositis and inclusion body myositis.

Pre-ICU Phase

Optimal management of the patient with ALS is carried out with the multidisciplinary team work of the occupational therapist, physical therapist, speech therapist, social worker, and nutritionist. Physical rehabilitation programs promote maximum mobility and provide orthotic devices for ambulation. The speech therapist can assess the integrity of the swallowing mechanism and if necessary help perform a barium swallow esophagram to assess competency of the glottis. In patients who are no longer able to swallow safely, the placement of a percutaneous endoscopic gastrostomy (PEG) feeding tube is the least complicated, most easily tolerated procedure and allows for greatest ease in feeding at home. The nutritionist serves the important function of formulating appropriate diets to maximize protein and caloric intake, despite limitations owing to dysphagia. Even in the patient without significant dysphagia, weight loss is a constant problem and one that should be addressed before serious negative nitrogen balance has occurred.

Respiratory deterioration is usually gradual until the terminal phase of the disease. An abnormal maximum expiratory pressure can detect early respiratory muscle involvement.[111] Inspiratory muscle training may improve respiratory function in patients with chest wall and diaphragmatic weakness.[112] Rarely patients may have respiratory failure as their first or sole manifestation of ALS.[113,114] In some cases, this may be due to preferential involvement of phrenic anterior horn cells, leading to early diaphragmatic weakness. The appropriate management of the ALS patient mandates early discussions with the patient to determine his or her interest in life support for respiratory failure. Patients who have been denied the right to make an unhurried decision are likely to exhibit discontent and anger when involuntarily placed on a ventilator because of abrupt clinical deterioration.

ICU Phase

Patients with ALS are admitted to the ICU either for the purpose of elective intubation and ventilatory support or after having been emergently intubated elsewhere. The patient with weakening respiratory function is easily pushed into frank respiratory failure by events such as aspiration pneumonia, atelectasis, and heart failure.[105] Patients with impending respiratory failure should have all conservative measures performed before considering mechanical ventilation. Use of oxygen, digoxin, cardiac afterload reducing agents, and diuretics may avoid the need for intubation in some patients. A newly marketed device that delivers continuous positive air pressure by nasal mask may be a useful interim treatment (see Chapt. 24).

Many ALS patients intubated for acute pulmonary decompensation are unable to be weaned from mechanical ventilation, even though the immediate cause of acute exacerbation has been successfully treated. Chronic alveolar hypoventilation owing to diaphragmatic involvement is the likely reason for this. Alveolar hypoventilation owing to diaphragmatic weakness may occur during sleep, even when the general degree of respiratory muscle weakness would not be expected to cause respiratory failure.[115] This may be worsened by increased extracellular bicarbonate from hypercapnia, leading to blunting of respiratory drive, increased somnolence, and disturbed sleep.[116]

Weaning the patient from mechanical ventilation may be attempted using various techniques. As noted previously, the patient may maintain adequate ventilation during the day, although at night function deteriorates. A rocking bed has been useful in some patients for this purpose. Some patients may require only nighttime assisted ventilation and are otherwise able to maintain respiratory function independently.

Post-ICU Phase

Owing to technologic advances, ALS patients with respiratory failure can be offered home-based mechanical ventilation.[117-119] This approach may be most attractive to those without severe extremity weakness or generalized wasting, who continue to interact actively with others. The ultimate goal of home care ventilation is not only to support the respiratory system, but also to augment the emotional coping skills so social interaction between the patient and others can continue.[117] The use of such technology is predicated on the notion that even though physical ability will continue to deteriorate, intellectual interchange will not.

Once the patient has decided on home care ventilation, an evaluation of the psychosocial milieu of the patient is necessary. There is an assessment of the degree of home support available to the patient as well as the coping skills of the patient and family. Conflicts in the home predating the illness and arising from the illness must be assessed before home care is considered.[117]

In the hospital, the patient and family are trained to provide daily care to the ventilator-dependent patient. The goal is to provide the needed care without the support of health care professionals, thus increasing the sense of independence in patient care.[117]

The ethical issue raised by home mechanical ventilation is the advisability of providing life support to an individual facing progressive, incapacitating disease that is invariably fatal. Patients are usually given choices before their illness takes a serious turn and are asked to make a commitment to a complicated life support system before they have had the opportunity to know what is really involved. In one study, no patient recognized the full impact of the illness until sometime after ventilatory support was instituted.[117] This fact makes objective decision making about long-term ventilatory care difficult. Beyond psychosocial and psychiatric evaluations of the patient and family, long-term success also depends on the financial resources available for such an expensive undertaking. Successful home care requires a team approach consisting of the physician, nurse, social worker, psychiatrist, and respiratory therapist.[120]

Poliomyelitis

Poliomyelitis is an acute viral infectious illness characterized by selective destruction of motor neurons of the spinal cord and brain stem, causing flaccid, asymmetric weakness. Since the availability of the Salk and Sabin vaccines in 1954 and 1961, the incidence in the United States has been drastically reduced, although the virus remains ubiquitous in the environment. An increase in the incidence of poliomyelitis in the United States is likely due to a combination of failure to vaccinate all individuals and immigration of infected individuals from other regions of the world. Because of younger physicians' inexperience with this condition, the illness may go unrecognized or misdiagnosed.

Polioviruses are classified in the genus Enterovirus, within the family Picornaviridae, and are composed of types 1, 2, and 3. Rates of infection increase to maximum in late summer or early fall in temperate regions but are relatively constant in tropical regions. The virus is acquired by the oral route, where it replicates in the oral pharynx and lower gastrointestinal tract. Host-to-host transmission is via oral pharyngeal secretions and feces, not through its infection of the nervous system. Epidemiologically the neurologic disease can therefore be thought of as an accident of evolution of the poliovirus because it fails to contribute to its survival.[121]

Paralysis is an unusual complication of poliovirus infection. During an epidemic, 90 to 95% of infections are asymptomatic. Four percent to 8% of infections result in a nonspecific, minor illness, and 1 to 2% are associated with neurologic symptoms or signs.[122] Proportionately higher rates of paralysis and mortality, however, are seen in individuals beyond infancy and young childhood.

After exposure, the virus is released into the feces within 24 to 48 hours and continues for 2 to 6 weeks, although rarely excretion may persist for as long as several months.[123] Once the virus has gained entry into the CNS, high titers are present on the day before onset of paralysis and remain for 2 to 4 days afterward, reaching undetectable levels by the seventh day. It is unclear why poliovirus infection is specific for motor neurons of the spinal cord, brain stem, and selected other cells of the cerebrum and cerebellum, but a likely scenario is hematogenous entry into CNS, followed by involvement of particular neurons because of surface receptors recognized by the virus particles.[121]

The clinical picture of minor illness is often not recognized. When more apparent, there may be sore throat or abdominal discomfort, sometimes accompanied by low grade fever, malaise, and headache. The incubation period is usually 1 to 3 days, whereas the symptomatic period may last 1 to 4 days.

Major illness represents an extension of the minor illness in individuals so affected.[121] The total incubation period (including minor illness) ranges from 3 to 35 days but is usually 4 to 10 days. Two separate illnesses, minor and major, occur in about one third of children under age 10 years; for all others, the early nonspecific symptoms lead directly into the neurologic symptoms. Major illness begins with fever and malaise, followed by headache and vomiting. Within 1 day, neck and back stiffness develops. The patient may be drowsy but arousable and oriented. The illness may end there. If paralysis is to develop, it usually begins 2 to 5 days after onset of headache. In children, the preparalytic phase is shorter and better tolerated. In adults destined to develop weakness, the illness is more severe, with tremulousness and agitation. The muscles are sensitive and stiff and may demonstrate fasciculations. There may be transient hyperreflexia, followed by areflexia as weakness develops.

Large motor neurons are preferentially involved. Lumbar segments of the spinal cord are more involved than cervical segments, and the brain stem is less involved than the spinal cord. Autonomic and sensory neuronal populations are involved in the inflammatory process pathologically but rarely permanently, leaving few symptoms correlated with dysfunction of those pathways.

Bulbar involvement takes several forms. Involvement of nuclei of cranial nerves IX and X is most common, leading to paralysis of muscles of phonation and swallowing. Facial muscles can be involved either unilaterally or bilaterally. Disorders of extraocular muscles are rare. Involvement of the reticular formation leads to difficulties in cardiovascular equilibrium and integration of breathing and swallowing mechanisms. Irregular breathing patterns as well as loss of autonomic respiratory control during wakefulness have been described.[124] Other abnormalities that may arise include abnormal ECG patterns, hypertension, and cardiac arrhythmias. In the severest form of involvement of the reticular formation, known as polioencephalitis, including regions from the hypothalamus to the spinal cord, the acute illness is also characterized by a clouding of consciousness.[121] Other autonomic involvement includes urinary retention from bladder paralysis (especially in men with paraplegia), gastric atony, and constipation.

Sensory symptoms are not uncommon during the acute illness, such as shooting pains and paresthesias. Objective sensory loss is extremely rare.

In the fully expressed syndrome, poliomyelitis is a unique clinical entity. When symptoms and signs are fragmentary, however, the diagnosis may be confusing. GBS may show features similar to some of those in acute poliomyelitis. The neurologic complications of acute porphyria and botulism may also show similar findings. Other viral encephalitides have also been associated with mild paralysis, including coxsackie and echoviruses.[125]

The laboratory features of acute poliomyelitis include a white blood cell count ranging from 10,000 to 30,000. The CSF is almost always abnormal. Most white blood cell counts lie between 20 and 300/µl, although as few as 3 and as many as 3000 can be seen. Polymorphonuclear cells predominate for the first 48 to 72 hours, then shifting to mainly lymphocytes. The white blood cell count is usually normal by 2 weeks. CSF protein can be as high as 100 mg/dl initially and up to 200 mg/dl after 1 to 2 weeks. The CSF glucose is normal. Poliomyelitis usually produces a diagnostic four-fold increase in serum antibody titer between the acute and convalescent sera. A complement fixing antibody titer of greater than 32 is presumptive evidence of recent poliovirus infection.[126]

Pre-ICU Phase

The treatment of acute poliomyelitis rests on supportive care because no antiviral agent is useful. Passive administration of immune serum prevents hematogenous seeding of the nervous system, but by the time weakness has begun, the viremic stage has passed.[121] During epidemics, patients with nonspecific systemic symptoms should remain quiet because exercise during this period could worsen subsequent paralysis.[121] Patients have an urge to exercise aching, stiff muscles, but this should be discouraged. Diazepam can be used to treat restlessness and anxiety, and hot packs can be applied to sore muscles.

Patients with poliomyelitis should be hospitalized and kept at bed rest. Appropriately placed pillows can minimize neck and lumbar pain. Narcotics and sedatives may cloud the clinical picture and complicate the respiratory status and should be avoided if possible. Joints of paralyzed limbs should be moved passively through their full range of motion to prevent contractures, although physical therapy itself can be delayed until the convalescent period.

ICU Phase

Various factors act simultaneously to produce respiratory insufficiency and incompetence of the airway. Loss of neurons to intercostal muscles and the diaphragm produces peripheral alveolar hypoventilation. Involvement of the central respiratory regulatory center in the brain stem produces a central disorder of respiration. Weakness of pharyngeal and laryngeal musculature interferes with swallowing and the cough reflex. As in other neuromuscular conditions, following the FVC and NIF accurately predicts the need for assisted mechanical ventilation. Although peripheral and central disorders of respiration usually occur simultaneously, when peripheral (intercostal and diaphragmatic) function is relatively spared, spirometric assessments may give "false-negative" information concerning a central disorder of respiration. Patients at risk are those with other evidence of bulbar involvement. Early signs of respiratory distress include apprehension, anxiety, and insomnia. Pulse rate or blood pressure may increase, and the depth and rhythm of respirations may become irregular. Sleep apnea occurs late, as voluntary and reflex breathing become dissociated and the patient must remain awake to continue spontaneous respiration. Finally, automatic breathing is lost while awake.[121] It may not be until the last two features of central respiratory failure develop that arterial oxygen saturation falls appreciably.

Patients who do not reach this stage of severe respiratory impairment can benefit from pulmonary physiotherapy, frequent turning, and postural drainage. Most patients who require assisted ventilation during the acute illness can eventually be weaned from the respirator. Some patients may be left with limited pulmonary reserve and may need a rocking bed or nighttime assisted ventilation.[121]

The cardiovascular and autonomic complications, as mentioned previously, respond to supportive measures and are almost never a persistent problem after the acute illness subsides. Conventional therapies are appropriate for these complications, such as arrhythmias, congestive heart failure, hypertension, and hypotension.

Post-ICU Phase

The primary thrust of care after acute illness is rehabilitation. Aggressive physical therapy to maintain joint flexibility and begin an exercise program to strengthen weakened muscles is required for favorable outcomes. Orthopedic consultation should be sought to evaluate the need for tendon transplantation and heel cord lengthening as well as other procedures to maximize stability of the spinal column. Surgery should not be undertaken for 1 to 2 years after illness, however, to allow for the full extent of spontaneous recovery.[118] In the meantime, braces may be used to improve joint function.

Years after recovery from poliomyelitis, patients may slowly develop progressive weakness. This condition, known as "postpolio syndrome," usually does not become apparent to the patient for some 15 to 25 years after the initial illness. It is thought to represent the effects of normal dropout of motor neurons owing to the aging process.[127] To the polio victim, each surviving motor neuron contributes proportionately much more than normal to the total muscle innervation. Thus, the loss of a single motor neuron produces denervation of many muscle fibers, an event that could produce symptoms of weakness. Although there is no medical treatment, patients should remain in an active physical therapy program to promote flexibility and range of motion of joints, to maximize mobility.

Tetanus

Tetanus occurs as the result of infection by Clostridium tetani, which produces a neurotoxin specific for anterior horn cells of the spinal cord and brain stem. In contrast to other entities discussed in this section, tetanus does not produce weakness or muscle atrophy. Rather the clinical features are of generalized stiffness and spasm of muscles, including bulbar musculature. The result is a life-threatening illness, which, until the advent of intensive care, was associated with 50% mortality.

C. tetani is nearly ubiquitous in the human environment, being especially prevalent in dust, dirt, feces, and soil. Tetanus is an infective disease, requiring the presence of the toxin-producing bacteria within the body, as opposed to botulism, in which exogenous toxin can produce disease. Tetanus, however, is not contagious. The most common source of infection is through a skin wound, although a significant number of cases show no obvious wound source. The incidence of this illness is much higher in developing countries because of poor wound hygiene and care and lack of immunization of the population. In the United States, a study between 1970 and 1971 showed that 13% of all cases were in drug abusers, mainly "skin poppers" who injected drugs subcutaneously.[128] More recently, for the years 1987 and 1988, tetanus was a disease of older adults.[129] This finding emphasizes the necessity for health care practitioners to review immunization status of adolescent and adult patients.

After establishment of tetanus infection in a skin wound, the expressed toxin is thought to gain access to the nervous system both by hematogenous spread and by traveling up motor axons intraneurally until the spinal cord is reached.[130] The CNS contains high affinity acceptors for tetanus toxin gangliosides, which form the binding sites.[131] The clinical picture results from a blocking of the normal central inhibitory pathways influencing reflex and voluntary activity. This disinhibition of alpha and gamma motor neurons produces unchecked excitation and continuous efferent impulses to muscles. Autonomic disinhibition also occurs, especially along sympathetic pathways.

Pre-ICU Phase

Tetanus usually starts within 2 weeks of onset of a suspicious wound. The greater the amount of toxin present, the shorter the incubation period, the more severe and fulminant the manifestations, and the shorter the survival time. In humans, local tetanus is rare because the toxin probably gains access to the motor neurons via the bloodstream before it does through nerves close to the wound site. In generalized tetanus, muscles of the head and neck are involved first, probably because their distance from the spinal cord is short. Then symptoms extend throughout the body. Tetanus toxin itself does not permanently alter the nervous system, although the complications of hypoxia can.[130]

The clinical picture of tetanus resembles strychnine poisoning.

Table 8–10. Clinical Manifestations of Tetanus

Muscle pain and stiffness
Muscle rigidity: trismus, risus sardonicus, dysphagia
Spasms: respiratory and laryngeal/pharyngeal muscles
Autonomic fluctuations: blood pressure, heart rate and rhythm

The clinical manifestations are listed in Table 8–10. The first symptoms of tetanus are muscle pain and stiffness in the jaw, abdomen, or back. The patient may describe difficulty in swallowing. Rigidity replaces stiffness, with flexors and extensors equally involved. This is first seen in muscles of the head, characterized by a clenched jaw (trismus) and stiffness of facial muscles (risus sardonicus). Rigidity of pharyngeal muscles impairs swallowing and promotes aspiration. Tightening of muscles of the thorax can produce an opisthotonic posture. Reflexes are generally hyperactive.

Spinal convulsions are characterized by paroxysmal increases of the underlying rigidity. They are uncoordinated, in contrast to epileptic convulsions. Pharyngeal spasms may suddenly obstruct the airway. Spasms of the respiratory muscles may arrest respiration for as long as 10 to 20 seconds. Supervening hypoxia tends to end the convulsion.[130] Spinal convulsions can be elicited by mere touch or positioning of the patient and are a leading cause of morbidity and mortality. Acute pharyngeal/laryngeal spasm can lead to unexpected death from asphyxia or massive aspiration. Long-lasting or repeated spasms may give rise to cumulative effects of hypoxia on the brain and spinal cord. Pneumonia is a common complication. Fever may have a multifactorial origin in patients with tetanus: due to extreme muscular work, direct effect of toxin on central temperature regulation, or infectious complication. For these reasons, fever is a negative prognostic indicator.

Autonomic complications may also be life-threatening. Blood pressure may fluctuate between hypertension and hypotension. There may be tachycardia or other arrhythmias. These events may stem from acute hypoxia, central involvement by the tetanus toxin, or muscle stress.[130] With the use of muscle relaxants, however, it has become clear that hypertensive episodes may appear independently of muscle spasms.[132]

In developed countries, early tetanus may be misdiagnosed because of its rare occurrence. Early on, patients may be considered to have dystonic reactions to phenothiazines or may be thought to be suffering from meningitis or hypocalcemia.[130] Strychnine poisoning may manifest similar clinical features.

Treatment of the initiating wound is expected, although what good it does once the manifestations of tetanus have appeared is unclear. Penicillin G has been used to treat wounds infected with tetanus bacilli.

The use of human tetanus immune globulin (TIG) as an antitoxin during acute illness is of controversial benefit.[130] All studies taken into account, there has been negligible statistical benefit in lowering morbidity and mortality since its introduction in the early 1900s. From a pathophysiologic point of view, if tetanus is already clinically apparent, significant toxin will have either reached the CNS or is situated intraneurally, areas inaccessible to TIG. It remains standard of care, however, to provide this therapy. A total of 500 of 1000 units of human antitoxin should be administered parenterally. Animal sera should never be used.

ICU Phase

All patients with tetanus should be admitted to the hospital. In the presence of spinal convulsions of greater than mild degree, risk of death increases, and intensive care is required. One of the most effective methods of combating the rigidity and spinal convulsions is with muscle relaxants, most importantly the benzodiazepines. They act rapidly intravenously, provide sedation, and reduce anxiety. They inhibit polysynaptic spinal reflexes, which are exaggerated in tetanus. For a drug such as diazepam, the doses required are much higher than those used in other diseases. In adults, 6 mg/kg/day is often exceeded, with a report of as much as 9.3 mg/kg/day.[133] When toxic doses have been reached, addition of barbiturates may be useful. Longer-acting barbiturates may be useful for long-standing rigidity, whereas barbiturate anesthetics may be used in the setting of acute spinal convulsions.

General care of the tetanus patient is difficult. Movement should be minimized. Pain should be relieved by relaxation, not by opiates, which may aggravate tetanus. Owing to the severe workload of muscle, caloric requirements are high.

Respiratory embarrassment owing to spasms and large doses of sedatives often requires assisted ventilation and tracheostomy. Even with mechanical ventilation, high pressures may be required to counteract the rigidity of the thorax. For this reason, considerable attention has been drawn to the use of muscle paralysis and mechanical ventilation. Theoretically such a combination for the 2 weeks usually required for the illness to take its course would be ideal treatment. Sedation and paralysis are recommended until muscle spasm has ceased. Periodic cessation in paralysis allows for clinical assessment. Table 8–11 outlines states of tetanus according to clinical course and management.[134] These multimodality approaches to the treatment of tetanus have decreased the mortality rate in adults from 47 to 12%.[135] Obvious limitations of such long paralyzation include the increased complication rate coincident with the use of intensive technology, the difficulty in diagnosing complications, and the psychologic effect on the patient unable to move or communicate.[136] Improved management of tetanus in the ICU has resulted in decreased mortality, particularly from respiratory failure.[134] This advance has also replaced respiratory failure as a leading cause of mortality with cardiovascular failure.[134,137]

Post-ICU Phase

Tetanus toxin is eliminated slowly, with requirement for mechanical ventilation ranging from 10 to 14 days. If curarization has been used, another several days may be necessary. Because convalescence can be lengthy, long-term care involves ensuring adequate nutrition as well as continuing care of persisting complications (due to infection or cerebral ischemia). Physical rehabilitation plays an important role as well.

MUSCLE DISORDERS

Most muscle diseases are slowly progressive over years. Certain dystrophies may eventually be associated with respiratory muscle weakness, but only in the late stage of disease. Such patients are seldom candidates for intensive care. Adult onset acid maltase deficiency (AMD) is one progressive myopathy that can present early in its course with respiratory muscle weakness, necessitating ICU admission.

This myopathy, transmitted by autosomal recessive inheritance, is also known as type II glycogenosis because of the prominent storage of glycogen in muscle cells as a result of lack of one of the glycolytic enzymes, acid maltase. In infants, this condition is known as Pompe's disease and is rapidly fatal owing to marked enlargement of vital organs caused by the glycogenosis.

In adults, the onset of weakness is usually in the third or fourth decade of life, and progress of the predominantly proximal weakness is slow.[138] About 50% of patients with AMD develop significant respiratory muscle weakness. In one study, one third of patients presented with respiratory failure.[139] The variable phenotypic expression of this genetic disorder is not fully explained, even by hypothesizing heterogeneity owing to multiple allelic genes coding for the enzyme. In a given individual, different muscles and different muscle fibers in the same muscle show differing amounts of vacuolar change and glycogenosis pathologically, whereas all muscles show the enzymatic abnormality when measured by bioassay.

Respiratory failure may be abrupt, but the patient usually has a history of slowly progressive respiratory symptoms, marginally compensated. Patients may give a history of daytime somnolence and progressive dyspnea.[140,142] There may be clinical and fluoroscopic evidence of diaphragmatic weakness, but this has been shown to be an unreliable test of diaphragmatic function in neuromuscular disease.[115] Mild respiratory muscle weakness may be diffi-

Table 8–11. Stages of Tetanus According to Clinical Course and Management

Phase	Clinical Course	Management
1	Severe tetanospasms Autonomic overactivity	Ventilatory support Tracheostomy Curarization, sedation Beta-blockers, penicillin Wound excision, immunization Total enteral nutrition
2	Opportunistic infections	Add appropriate antibiotic therapy
3	Tonic muscle spasms Residual coma due to sedation	Add active physical therapy Wean curarization, sedation, and ventilatory support
4	Tonic muscle spasms Inadequate deglutition and management of secretions	Airway protection Continue physical therapy, early mobilization Wean tube feeding

(From Trujillo, M. H., et al.: Impact of intensive care management on the prognosis of tetanus: analysis of 641 cases. Chest, 92:63, 1987.)

cult to document. If lung compliance is normal, vital capacity may not be altered. With significant diaphragmatic weakness, measured volumes are reduced.[139]

These patients may be in frank respiratory failure. It has been our experience to receive patients dependent on mechanical ventilation from other hospitals, undiagnosed or unweanable. The significant hypoxemia likely results from a continuation of hypoventilation from respiratory muscle weakness as well as impaired ventilation-perfusion from compression atelectasis owing to hypoventilation and elevated diaphragms.[139] These patients usually have normal chest radiographs, making the diagnosis of chronic obstructive pulmonary disease untenable. Separating patients with nonpulmonary diseases from those with primary pulmonary disease can be difficult in this setting. In the patient with primary pulmonary disease, Pa_{O_2} and the Pa_{CO_2} rarely return to more normal values by voluntary hyperventilation, whereas this can occur in patients with either CNS respiratory center disorders or neuromuscular diseases.

Although respiratory muscle weakness is a common problem in many long-standing or generalized neuromuscular disorders, it is only rarely seen as the sole or primary manifestation of a neuromuscular disorder. Aside from AMD, there have been rare reports of ALS, spinal muscular atrophy, mild proximal myopathy, and peripheral neuropathy presenting with respiratory failure.[142-144] Such patients may present with isolated diaphragmatic paralysis as the sole clue to diagnosis. Peripheral nervous system causes for this may include involvement of the anterior horn cells supplying those muscles (syringomyelia, poliomyelitis, motor neuron diseases including ALS); trauma to the phrenic nerves by surgery, radiation, or malignant compression; or isolated myopathy.[140]

The patient with AMD and respiratory compromise need not require intensive care, unless there is precipitous deterioration owing to a complicating factor such as pneumonia. The use of a rocking bed can both stabilize a patient with progressive respiratory compromise and allow the intubated patient to be weaned.

Because AMD is a slowly progressive disease, attempts at weaning and rehabilitation are extremely important to the patient's continued independence. A respiratory muscle training program has been used in quadriplegic patients[145] and has been used with success in patients with dystrophy[146] and AMD.[112] This simple technique involves breathing against an inspiratory resistor for 15 minutes twice per day. Once a threshold of diaphragmatic fatigue at a given resistor setting has been established, that setting is used for a period of 6 weeks, at which time pulmonary function tests are rechecked and a higher resistor setting is used for the next training period. The patient described by Martin and colleagues[112] showed progressive improvement in supine pulmonary volumes and was eventually able to sleep flat without supplemental oxygen.

REFERENCES

1. Arnason, B. G. W.: Acute inflammatory demyelinating polyradiculoneuropathies. *In* Peripheral Neuropathy. 2nd Ed. Edited by P. J. Dyck, P. K. Thomas, E. H. Lambert, and R. Bunge. Philadelphia, W. B. Saunders, 1984.
2. Asbury, A. K., et al.: Criteria for diagnosis of Guillain-Barré syndrome. Ann. Neurol., *3:*565, 1978.
3. Asbury, A. K.: Diagnostic considerations in Guillain-Barré syndrome. Ann. Neurol., *9(Suppl.):*1, 1981.
4. Castaigne, P., Brunet, P., and Nouailhat, F.: Enquete clinique sur les polyradiculonevrites inflammatoires en France. Rev. Neurol. (Paris), *115:*849, 1966.
5. Fisher, C. M.: Unusual variant of acute idiopathic polyneuritis (syndrome of ophthalmoplegia, ataxia and areflexia). N. Engl. J. Med., *255:*57, 1956.
6. Keane, J. R.: Tonic pupils with acute ophthalmoplegic polyneuritis. Ann. Neurol., *2:*93, 1977.
7. Williams, D., et al.: Landry-Guillain-Barré syndrome with abnormal pupils and normal eye movements: a case report. Neurology, *29:*1033, 1979.
8. Lichtenfeld, P.: Autonomic dysfunction in the Guillain-Barré syndrome. Am. J. Med., *50:*772, 1971.
9. Tuck, R. R., and McLeod, J. G.: Autonomic dysfunction in the Landry-Guillain-Barré syndrome. Proc. Aust. Assoc. Neurol., *15:*197, 1978.
10. Goulon, M., Nouailhat, F., Grosbuis, S., and Gajdos, P.: Hypotension orthostatique a pouls invariable. Rev. Neurol. (Paris), *125:*257, 1971.
11. Mitchell, P. L., and Meilman, E.: The mechanism of hypertension in the Guillain-Barré syndrome. Am. J. Med. *42:*986, 1967.
12. Laufer, J., et al.: Raised plasma renin activity in the hypertension of the Guillain-Barré syndrome. Br. Med. J., *282:*1272, 1981.
13. Gecow, A., and Pawela, I.: Autonomic disturbances in the Guillain-Barré Strohl syndrome in children. Pol. Med. J., *10:*1230, 1971.
14. Guillain-Barré Syndrome Study Group: Plasmapheresis and acute Guillain-Barré syndrome. Neurology, *35:*1096, 1985.
15. Asbury, A. K., Arnason, B. G., and Adams, R. D.: The inflammatory lesion in idiopathic polyneuritis: its role in pathogenesis. Medicine, *48:*173, 1969.
16. Prineas, J. W.: Pathology of Guillain-Barré syndrome. Ann. Neurol., *9(Suppl.):*6, 1981.
17. Saida, T., et al.: In vivo demyelinating activity of sera from patients with Guillain-Barré syndrome. Ann. Neurol., *11:*69, 1981.
18. Koski, C. L., Gratz, E., Sutherland, J., and Mayer, R. F.: Clinical correlation with anti-peripheral-nerve myelin antibodies in Guillain-Barré syndrome. Ann. Neurol., *19:*573, 1986.
19. Loffel, N. B., et al.: The Landry-Guillain-Barré syndrome: complications, prognosis, and natural history in 123 cases. J. Neurol. Sci., *33:*71, 1977.
20. Dowling, P. C., and Cook, S. D.: Role of infection in Guillain-Barré syndrome: laboratory confirmation of herpes viruses in 41 cases. Ann. Neurol., *9(Suppl.):*44, 1981.
21. Klemola, E., et al.: The Guillain-Barré syndrome associated with acquired cytomegalovirus infection. Acta Med. Scand., *181:*603, 1967.
22. Leonard, J. C., and Tobin, J. O'H.: Polyneuritis associated with cytomegalovirus infections. Q. J. Med., *40:*435, 1971.
23. Smith, M. S., and Laguna, J. F.: Neurologic complications of infectious mononucleosis. Pediatr. Clin. North Am., *26:*315, 1979.
24. Goldschmidt, B., et al.: Mycoplasma antibody in Guillain-Barré syndrome and other neurological disorders. Ann. Neurol., *7:*108, 1980.
25. Griffin, J. W., and Ho, T.: The Guillain-Barré syndrome at 75: the campylobacter connection. Ann. Neurol., *34:*125, 1993.
26. Cornblath, D. R., et al.: Inflammatory demyelinating poly-

neuritis associated with human t-cell lymphotrophic virus type iii infection. Ann. Neurol., *21:*32, 1982.
27. Arnason, B. G., and Asbury, A. K.: Idiopathic polyneuritis after surgery. Arch. Neurol., *18:*500, 1968.
28. Wiederholt, W. C., and Mulder, D. W.: Cerebrospinal fluid findings in the Landry-Guillain-Barré-Strohl syndrome. Neurology, *15:*184, 1965.
29. Link, H.: Demonstration of oligoclonal immunoglobulin G in Guillain-Barré syndrome. Acta Neurol. Scand., *52:*111, 1978.
30. Albers, J. W., Donofrio, P. D., and McGonagle, T. K.: Sequential electrodiagnostic abnormalities in acute inflammatory demyelinating polyradiculoneuropathy. Muscle Nerve, *8:*528, 1985.
31. Ridley, A.: Porphyric neuropathy. In Peripheral Neuropathy, 2nd Ed. Edited by P. J. Dyck, P. K. Thomas, E. H. Lambert, and R. Bunge. Philadelphia, W. B. Saunders, 1984.
32. Senanayake, N., and Johnson, M. K.: Acute polyneuropathy after poisoning by a new organophosphate insecticide. N. Engl. J. Med., *306:*155, 1982.
33. Wilbourn, A. J.: Metal neuropathies. In Toxic Neuropathies, Course B-1. American Association of Electromyography and Electrodiagnosis, 1984.
34. Doyle, J. B., and Cannon, E. F.: Severe polyneuritis following gold therapy for rheumatoid arthritis. Ann. Intern. Med., *33:*1468, 1950.
35. Russell, J. A., and Powles, R. L.: Neuropathy due to cytosine arabinoside. Br. Med. J., *2:*652, 1974.
36. O'Donahue, W. J., Jr., et al.: Respiratory failure in neuromuscular disease. JAMA, *235:*733, 1976.
37. Birchfield, R. I., and Shaw, C. M.: Postural hypotension in Guillain-Barré syndrome. Arch. Neurol., *10:*149, 1964.
38. Hobday, J. D., and Baker, A. J.: Guillain-Barré syndrome complicated by hypertension and ileitis. Med. J. Aust., *2:*536, 1968.
39. Stapleton, F. B., Skoglund, R. R., and Daggett, R. B.: Hypertension associated with Guillain-Barré syndrome. Pediatrics, *62:*588, 1978.
40. Hughes, R. A. C., Newsom-Davis, J. M., and Perkins, G. D.: Controlled trial of prednisolone in acute polyneuropathy. Lancet, *2:*750, 1978.
41. McKhann, G. M., et al.: Plasmapheresis and Guillain-Barré syndrome: Analysis of prognostic factors and the effect of plasmapheresis. Ann. Neurol., *23:*347, 1988.
42. Sutton, D. M. C., et al.: Complications of plasma exchange. Transfusion, *29:*124, 1989.
43. Ropper, A. H., Albers, J. W., and Addison, R.: Limited relapse in Guillain-Barré syndrome after plasma exchange. Arch. Neurol., *45:*314, 1988.
44. Osterman, P. O., et al.: Early relapses after plasma exchange in acute inflammatory polyradiculoneuropathy. Lancet, *2:*116, 1986.
45. Kleyweg, R. P., van der Meche, F. G. A., and Meulstee, J.: Treatment of Guillain-Barré syndrome with high dose gammaglobulin. Neurology, *38:*1639, 1988.
46. Van der Meché, F. G. A., et al.: A randomized trial comparing intravenous immune globulin and plasma exchange in Guillain-Barré syndrome. N. Engl. J. Med., *326:*1123, 1992.
47. Kennedy, R. H., et al.: Guillain-Barré syndrome. A 42-year epidemiologic and clinical study. Mayo Clin. Proc., *53:*93, 1980.
48. Pleasure, D. E., Lovelace, R. E., and Duvoisin, R. C.: The prognosis of acute polyradiculoneuritis. Neurology, *18:*1143, 1968.
49. Truax, B. T.: Autonomic disturbances in the Guillain-Barré syndrome. Semin. Neurol., *4:*462, 1984.
50. Penn, A. S., Schotland, D. L., and Rowland, L. P.: Immunology of muscle disease. Res. Public Assoc. Res. Nerve Ment. Dis., *49:*25, 1971.
51. Piskanen, R., Tiilikainen, A., and Hokkanen, E.: Histocompatibility antigens associated with myasthenia gravis. Ann. Clin. Res., *4:*304, 1972.
52. Osserman, K. E., and Genkins, G.: Studies in myasthenia gravis: review of twenty-year experience in over 1200 patients. Mt. Sinai J. Med., *38:*497, 1971.
53. Castleman, B.: The pathology of the thymus gland in myasthenia gravis. Ann. N. Y. Acad. Sci., *135:*496, 1966.
54. Levin, K. H., and Richmond, D. P.: Myasthenia gravis. Clin. Aspects Immun., *4:*23, 1989.
55. Kelly, J. J., et al.: The laboratory diagnosis of mild myasthenia gravis. Ann. Neurol., *12:*238, 1982.
56. Howard, F. M., Jr., et al.: Clinical correlations of antibodies that bind, block, or modulate human acetylcholine receptors in myasthenia gravis. Ann. N. Y. Acad. Sci., *505:*526, 1987.
57. Van den Bergh, P., Kelly, J. J., Carter, V., and Munsat, T. L.: Intravascular contrast media and neuromuscular junction disorders. Ann. Neurol., *19:*206, 1986.
58. Canal, N., and Faranceschi, M.: Myasthenic crisis precipitated by iothalamic acid. Lancet, *1:*1288, 1983.
59. Swift, T. R.: Weakness from magnesium containing cathartics: electrophysiologic studies. Muscle Nerve, *2:*295, 1979.
60. Elmquvist, D., and Josefsson, J. O.: The nature of the neuromuscular block produced by neomycine. Acta Physiol. Scand., *54:*105, 1962.
61. Singh, Y. N., Marshall, I. G., and Harvey, A. L.: Some effects of the aminoglycoside antibiotic amikacin on neuromuscular and autonomic transmission. Br. J. Anaesth., *50:*109, 1978.
62. DeRosayro, M., and Healey, T. E. J.: Tobramycin and neuromuscular transmission in the rat-isolated phrenic nerve-diaphragm preparation. Br. J. Anaesth., *50:*251, 1978.
63. Singh, Y. N., Marshall, I. G., and Harvey, A. L.: Depression of transmitter release and postjunctional sensitivity during neuromuscular block produced by antibiotics. Br. J. Anaesth., *51:*1027, 1979.
64. Swift, T. R.: Disorders of neuromuscular transmission other than myasthenia gravis. Muscle Nerve, *4:*334, 1981.
65. Trackman, D. B., and Skom, J. H.: Procainamide—a hazard in myasthenia gravis. Arch. Neurol., *13:*316, 1965.
66. Herishanu, Y., and Rosenberg, P.: Beta-blockers and myasthenia gravis. Ann. Intern. Med., *83:*834, 1975.
67. Neil, J. R., Himmelhoch, J. M., and Licata, S. M.: Emergence of myasthenia gravis during treatment with lithium carbonate. Arch. Gen. Psychiatry, *33:*1090, 1976.
68. McQuillen, M. P., Gross, M., and Johns, R. T.: Chlorpromazine-induced weakness in myasthenia gravis. Arch. Neurol. *8:*286, 1963.
69. Argov, Z., and Mastaglia, F. L.: Disorders of neuromuscular transmission caused by drugs. N. Engl. J. Med., *301:*409, 1979.
70. Wright, E. A., and McQuillen, M. P.: Antibiotic-induced neuromuscular blockade. Ann. N. Y. Acad. Sci., *183:*358, 1971.
71. Masters, C. L., et al.: Penicillamine-associated myasthenia gravis, anti-acetylcholine receptor and anti-striational antibodies. Am. J. Med., *63:*689, 1977.
72. Rodriguez, M., Gomez, M. R., Howard, F. M., Jr., and Taylor, W. F.: Myasthenia gravis in children: long-term follow-up. Ann. Neurol., *13:*504, 1983.
73. Bever, C. T., Jr., et al.: Prognosis of ocular myasthenia. Ann. Neurol., *14:*516, 1983.
74. Buckingham, J. M., et al.: Value of thymectomy in myasthenia gravis: a computer-adjusted matched study. Ann. Surg., *184:*453, 1976.

75. Olanow, C. W., et al.: Thymectomy as primary therapy in myasthenia gravis. Ann. N. Y. Acad. Sci., 505:595, 1987.
76. Grob, D., Brunner, N. G., and Namba, T.: The natural course of myasthenia gravis and effect of therapeutic measures. Ann. N. Y. Acad. Sci., 377:652, 1981.
77. Mann, J. D., John, T. R., Campa, J. F., and Muller, W. H.: Long-term prednisone followed by thymectomy in myasthenia gravis. Ann. N. Y. Acad. Sci., 274:608, 1976.
78. Millkin, C., and Eaton, L. M.: Clinical evaluation of acth and cortisone with myasthenia gravis. Neurology, 1:145, 1951.
79. Seybold, M., and Drachman, D. B.: Gradually increasing doses of prednisone in myasthenia gravis. N. Engl. J. Med., 290:81, 1974.
80. Nielsen, V. K., et al.: Rapid improvement of myasthenia gravis after plasma exchange. Ann. Neurol., 11:160, 1982.
81. Tindall, R.: Scientific overview of myasthenia gravis and assessment of the role of plasmapheresis. In Therapeutic Apheresis and Plasma Profusion. New York, Alan R. Liss, 1982.
82. Kornfeld, P. E., et al.: Plasmapheresis in refractory generalized myasthenia gravis. Arch. Neurol., 38:478, 1981.
83. Seybold, M. E.: Plasmapheresis in myasthenia gravis. Ann. N. Y. Acad. Sci., 505:584, 1987.
84. Rodnitzky, R. L., and Bosch, E. P.: Chronic long-interval plasma exchange in myasthenia gravis. Arch. Neurol., 41:715, 1984.
85. Leventhal, S.: Prediction of the need for post-operative mechanical ventilation in myasthenia gravis. Anesthiology, 53:26, 1980.
86. Graham, T. R., Pearson, O. T., and Holden, M. P.: Letter to Editor. Cleve. Clin. Q., 53:115, 1986.
87. Sivak, E. D., et al.: Post-operative ventilatory dependency following thymectomy for myasthenia gravis. Cleve. Clin. Q., 51:585, 1984.
88. Rowland, L. P., et al.: Fatalities in myasthenia gravis: a review of 39 cases with 26 autopsies. Neurology, 6:307, 1956.
89. Rowland, L. P.: Controversies about the treatment of myasthenia gravis. J. Neurol. Neurosurg. Psychiatry, 43:644, 1980.
90. Gracy, D. R., Divertie, M. B., and Howard, F. M., Jr.: Mechanical ventilation for respiratory failure in myasthenia gravis. Mayo Clin. Proc., 58:597, 1983.
91. Lambert, E. H.: Disorders of the motor nerve terminal: The Lambert-Eaton myasthenic syndrome. Didactic Program, American Association of Electromyography and Electrodiagnosis, 1986.
92. Lennon, V. A., Lambert, E. H., Whittingham, S., and Fairbanks, V.: Autoimmunity in the Lambert-Eaton myasthenic syndrome. Muscle Nerve, 5:S21, 1982.
93. Streib, E. W., and Rothner, A. D.: Eaton-Lambert myasthenic syndrome: long-term treatment of three patients with prednisone. Ann. Neurol., 10:448, 1981.
94. Newsom-Davis, J., and Murray, N. M.: Plasma exchange and immunosuppressant drug treatment in Lambert-Eaton myasthenic syndrome. Neurology, 34:480, 1984.
95. Howard, B. D., and Gunderson, C. B., Jr.: Effects and mechanisms of polypeptide neurotoxins that act pre-synaptically. Ann. Rev. Pharmacol. Toxicol., 20:307, 1980.
96. Duchen, L. W.: An electron microscopic study of the changes induced by botulinum toxin in the motor end plates of slow and fast skeletal muscle fibers of the mouse. J. Neurol. Sci., 14:47, 1971.
97. Schaffner, W.: Clostridium botulinum (botulism). In Principles and Practice of Infectious Diseases. 3rd Ed. Edited by G. L. Mandell, R. G. Douglas, Jr., and J. E. Bennett. New York, Churchill Livingstone, 1990.
98. Koenig, M. G., et al.: Type B botulism in man. Am. J. Med., 42:208, 1967.
99. Tacket, C. O., et al.: Equine antitoxin use and other factors that predict outcome in type a food borne botulism. Am. J. Med., 76:794, 1984.
100. Cherington, M., and Ryan, D. W.: Treatment of botulism with guanidine: Early neurophysiologic studies. N. Engl. J. Med., 282:195, 1970.
101. Kaplan, J. E., et al.: Botulism type A and treatment with guanidine. Ann. Neurol., 6:69, 1979.
102. Mulder, D. W., and Howard, F. M.: Patient resistence and prognosis in amyotrophic lateral sclerosis. Mayo Clin. Proc., 51:537, 1976.
103. Juergens, S. M., Kurland, L. T., Okazaki, H., and Mulder, D. W.: ALS in Rochester, Minnesota, 1925–1977. Neurology, 30:463, 1980.
104. Norris, F. H., Denys, E. H., and U, K. S.: Differential diagnosis of adult motor neuron disease. In The Diagnosis and Treatment of Amyotrophic Lateral Sclerosis. Edited by D. W. Mulder. Boston, Houghton Mifflin, 1980.
105. Tandan, R., and Bradley, W. G.: Amyotrophic lateral sclerosis: Part 1. Clinical features, pathology and ethical issues in management. Ann. Neurol., 18:271, 1985.
106. Dhib-Jalbut, S., and Liwnicz, B. H.: Immunocytochemical binding of serum IgG from a patient with oat cell tumor and paraneoplastic motor neuron disease to normal human cerebral cortex and molecular layer of the cerebellum. Acta Neuropathol. (Berl.) 69:96, 1986.
107. Levin, K. H.: Paraneoplastic neuromuscular syndromes. In 1993 AAEM Course B: Neuromuscular Complications of Systemic Diseases. Rochester, MN, American Association of Electrodiagnostic Medicine, 1993, p. 47.
108. Latov, N.: Plasma cell dyscrasia and motor neuron disease. In Human Motor Neuron Diseases. Edited by L. P. Rowland. New York, Raven Press, 1982.
109. Pestronk, A., et al.: A treatable multifocal motor neuropathy with antibodies to GM-1 ganglioside. Ann. Neurol., 24:73, 1988.
110. Hudson, A. J., Brown, W. F., and Gilbert, J. J.: The muscular pain-fasciculation syndrome. Neurology, 28:1105, 1978.
111. Goldstein, R. L., et al.: Peripheral neuropathy presenting with respiratory insufficiency as the primary complaint: problem of recognizing alveolar hypoventilation due to neuromuscular disorders. Am. J. Med., 56:433, 1974.
112. Martin, R. J., et al.: Respiratory improvement by muscle training in adult-onset acid maltase deficiency. Muscle Nerve, 6:201, 1983.
113. Parhad, I. M., Clark, A. W., Barrow, K. D., and Staunton, S. B.: Diaphragmatic paralysis in motor neuron disease: report of two cases and a review of literature. Neurology, 28:18, 1978.
114. Sivak, E. D., and Streib, E. W.: Management of hypoventilation in motor neuron disease presenting with respiratory insufficiency. Ann. Neurol., 7:188, 1980.
115. Newsom-Davis, J., Goldman, M., Loh, L., and Casson, M.: Diaphragmatic function and alveolar hypoventilation. Q. J. Med., 45:87, 1976.
116. Heineman, N., and Ho Goldring, R. N.: Bicarbonate and the regulation of ventilation. Am. J. Med., 57:361, 1974.
117. Sivak, E. D., Gipson, W. T., and Hanson, M. R.: Long-term management of respiratory failure in amyotrophic lateral sclerosis. Ann. Neurol., 12:18, 1982.
118. Peters, S. G., and Viggianno, R. W.: Home mechanical ventilation. Mayo Clin. Proc., 63:1208, 1988.
119. Howard, R. S., Wiles, C. M., and Loh, L.: Respiratory complications and their management in motor neuron disease. Brain, 112:1155, 1989.

120. Sivak, E. D., Cordasco, E. M., Gipson, W. T., and Mehta, A.: Home care ventilation: the Cleveland Clinic experience from 1977–1985. Respir. Care, *31:*294, 1986.
121. Price, R. W., and Plum, F.: Poliomyelitis. *In* Handbook of Clinical Neurology. Vol. 34. Edited by P. J. Vinken and G. W. Bruyn. Amsterdam, Elsevier, 1978.
122. Horstman, D. M.: Epidemiology of poliomyelitis and allied diseases. Yale J. Biol. Med., *36:*5, 1963.
123. Horstman, D. M., Ward, R., and Melnick, J. L.: The isolation of poliomyelitis virus from human extraneural sources. III. Persistence of virus in stools after acute infection. J. Clin. Invest., *25:*278, 1946.
124. Plum, F.: Neurologic integration of behavioral and metabolic control of breathing. *In* Breathing: Hering-Bruer Centenary Symposium. Edited by R. Porter. London, J. & A. Churchill, 1970.
125. Magoffin, R. L., Lennette, E. H., Hollister, A. C., Jr., and Schmidt, N. J.: An etiologic study of clinical paralytic poliomyelitis. JAMA, *175:*269, 1961.
126. Melnick, J. L., and Wenner, H. A.: Entroviruses. *In* Diagnostic Procedures for Viral and Rickettsial Infection. Edited by E. H. Lennette, and N. J. Schmidt. New York, American Public Health Association, 1969.
127. Dalakas, M. C., et al.: A long-term follow-up study of patients with post-poliomyelitis neuromuscular symptoms. N. Engl. J. Med., *314:*959, 1986.
128. CDC Tetanus Surveillance Report #4. Atlanta, 1974.
129. Tetanus—United States, 1987 and 1988. JAMA, *263:*1192, 1990.
130. Habermann, E.: Tetanus. *In* Handbook of Clinical Neurology. Vol. 33. Edited by P. J. Vinken and G. W. Bruyn. Amsterdam, Elsevier, 1978.
131. VanHeyningin, W. E.: The fixation of tetanus toxin, strychnine, serotonin, and other substances by ganglioside. J. Gen. Microbiol., *31:*275, 1963.
132. Corbett, J. L., and Harris, P. J.: Studies on the sympathetic nervous system in tetanus. Naunyn-Schmiedebergs Arch. Exp. Pathol. Pharmakol., *276:*447, 1973.
133. Femi-Pearse, D.: Experience with diazepam in tetanus. Br. Med. J., *2:*862, 1966.
134. Trujillo, M. H., et al.: Impact of intensive care management on the prognosis of tetanus: analysis of 641 cases. Chest, *92:*63, 1987.
135. Cornil, A., Thys, I. P., Ectors, M., and Degoute, I.: Tetanos A Et Soins Intensif S. Proceedings of the Fourth International Conference on Tetanus, Lyon, Fondation Meriux, 1975.
136. Roth, F., and Stirnemann, H.: Some aspects in the treatment of severe tetanus. *In* Principles on Tetanus. Edited by L. Eckmann. Bern, Huber, 1967.
137. Wright, D. K., Lalloo, U. G., Naziager, S., and Govender, P.: Autonomic nervous system dysfunction in severe tetanus: current perspectives. Crit. Care Med., *17:*371, 1989.
138. Engel, A. G.: Acid maltase deficiency in adults: studies in four cases of a syndrome which may mimic muscular dystrophy or other myopathies. Brain, *93:*599, 1970.
139. Rosenow, E. G., III, and Engel, A. G.: Acid maltase deficiency in adults presenting as respiratory failure. Am. J. Med., *64:*485, 1978.
140. Sivak, E. D., et al.: Adult-onset acid maltase deficiency presenting as diaphragmatic paralysis. Ann. Neurol., *9:*613, 1981.
141. Sivak, E. D., et al.: Respiratory insufficiency in adult-onset acid maltase deficiency. South. Med. J., *80:*205, 1987.
142. Miller, R. D., et al.: Exertional dyspnea: primary complaint in unusual cases of progressive muscular atrophy and amyotrophic lateral sclerosis. Ann. Intern. Med., *46:*119, 1957.
143. Goldstein, R. L., et al.: Peripheral neuropathy presenting with respiratory insufficiency as the primary complaint: problem of recognizing alveolar hypoventilation due to neuromuscular disorders. Am. J. Med., *56:*443, 1974.
144. Bellamy, D., et al.: A case of primary alveolar hypoventilation associated with myoproximal myopathy. Am. Rev. Respir. Dis., *112:*867, 1975.
145. Gross, D., et al.: The effect of training on strength and endurance of the diaphram in quadriplegia. Am. J. Med., *68:*27, 1980.
146. DiMarco, A. F., et al.: Respiratory muscle training in muscular dystrophy. Clin. Res., *30:*427a, 1982.

Chapter 9

SPINAL CORD INJURY: AN ICU CHALLENGE FOR THE 1990s

PHILIP A. VILLANUEVA
SHERRI J. PATCHEN
BARTH A. GREEN

There are 10,000 to 20,000 new spinal cord injuries (SCIs) each year in the United States, with the prevalence estimated to be approximately 250,000 to 350,000.[1,2] When compared with the 125,000 severe brain injuries or 500,000 strokes occurring annually,[3] this appears to be a rare problem numerically. Because of the high morbidity, mortality, and economic impact, however, SCI, similar to severe burns, has been designated as a catastrophic disease by the United States government. Over the last 20 years, it has become apparent that the best outcome with regard to treatment of a catastrophic disease can be achieved with a systems approach. The ideal SCI system includes programs and protocols for the following:

- Prevention
- Prehospital management (emergency medical services [EMS])
- Acute in-hospital care
- Rehabilitation
- Lifelong follow-up phases[4]

The implementation of these systems has resulted in the fact that SCI victims who survive the first year following their injury can enjoy a relatively normal life expectancy. It must be kept in mind, however, that SCI remains one of the most devastating entities that may confront the ICU team.

Probably the most important component of the acute care phase that has impact on early morbidity and mortality involves intensive care management. In the past, SCI had been relatively restricted to the younger population because older SCI patients frequently did not survive the acute stage of injury, usually because of systemic complications. As emergency care systems have evolved and the acute phases of trauma care have improved, however, the disease may now be seen to affect the entire age spectrum from the newborn (owing to birth trauma) to the very elderly.[5] Consequently the ICU management must now be concerned with a much broader patient base than before and be prepared to deal with a potential multiplicity of preexisting medical problems, especially in the case of the older patient. (For purposes of discussion, this chapter does not deal with the pediatric age group, here taken to mean under 15 years of age.)

Although, as stated previously, the SCI patient may be of any age, the "typical" profile remains that of a man in the late second or third decade. The majority of injuries occur in the early morning hours or on weekends, and most are associated in some manner with the ingestion of drugs or alcohol, although not necessarily by the victim. The most common causes are motor vehicle accidents (MVAs); falls; penetrating wounds; and industrial, agricultural, and sporting injuries.[1] The cause and frequency may vary depending on the climate, geography, and population of the area studied, but MVAs are usually at the top or near the top of the list, although in metropolitan areas, gunshot wounds may frequently be the number one cause. Overall mortality in the first year ranges from 6 to 10%, depending on the center reporting, but morbidity is always 100% because of the development of secondary systemic complication(s).[4] This morbidity compounds the already tremendous economic impact of this problem, which has been estimated to be greater than $1,000,000 per case, which translates into a multibillion dollar annual health care problem. The recognition, treatment, and, it is hoped, prevention of the early complications of paralysis during the acute care ICU phase are stressed in this chapter.

PRE-ICU PHASE

This phase encompasses the prehospital and emergency room management of the patient. The key phrases in therapy during this phase are index of suspicion and prevention of secondary injury. The Advanced Trauma Life Support (ATLS) Program of the American College of Surgeons recognizes that the risk of a spinal injury is significantly increased in the case of a high-speed MVA or in the case of any injury above the clavicle. Indeed, it is stressed that such a spinal injury be assumed to exist and then ruled out. By doing so, the risk of converting a spinal column injury to a SCI may be reduced significantly. This is done by the proper extrication, stabilization, and immobilization of the patient at the accident scene and rapid transportation to a tertiary trauma center that can diagnose and treat spinal column injuries and SCIs. Evaluation of the patient's status at the accident scene should be performed so as at least to screen for some of the more obvious signs of SCI. These are:

- Weakness or paralysis of extremities
- Alteration or absence of sensory function in extremities or trunk

- Incontinence
- Superficial signs of trauma to head, neck, or back or deformities of the spine
- Pain on palpation of the neck or spine

Any unconscious patient must be considered to have a SCI unless proven otherwise.[5,6]

At the scene, the ABCs (airway, breathing, circulation) of trauma should be followed.

Airway

In the awake patient, a standard oral airway or tape-wrapped tongue depressor should be available but not inserted unless necessary. In the case of the unconscious patient, an oral or nasal airway should be inserted, and some patients may even require intubation. If the latter is required, blind nasotracheal intubation is preferred because the potential for secondary cervical cord injury is less. Oral intubation, however, may be necessary as a lifesaving measure if facial injuries or difficult anatomy obviates the nasotracheal approach. If so, it should be performed keeping the neck immobilized in as neutral a position as possible.

Breathing

If the patient has inadequate respiratory excursion, assistance in the form of ambu-bagging should be carried out.

Circulation

The principles here are threefold:

- Stop active bleeding.
- Support cardiac rhythm and tone, either pharmacologically or with external massage.
- Treat shock.

Acute SCI patients can experience two types of physiologic shock, hemorrhagic or neurogenic. A third syndrome "spinal shock," which should not be confused with neurogenic shock, is a neurologic state of apparent "short circuiting" of the spinal cord seen only in SCI patients with a complete lesion. Spinal shock is discussed in more detail later in this chapter. In most cases, hemorrhagic shock is associated with the multisystem injuries occurring in the majority of SCI victims. Treatment of hypovolemic hemorrhagic shock is, of course, replacement of volume.

Neurogenic shock, in contrast, occurs from injury to the cervical or upper thoracic spinal cord or brain stem and results in a loss of sympathetic control (i.e., a sympathectomy). Neurogenic shock can occur regardless of whether the lesion is complete or incomplete. These patients present with bradycardia, hypotension, and commonly with hypothermia from the loss of body heat from the dilated peripheral vasculature. Most of the quadriplegia remains with chronic hypotension and hypothermia. In neurogenic shock, it is not volume depletion but rather volume distribution that is the problem. For both types of shock, treatment is augmentation of venous return, via position (Trendelenburg), Military Anti-Shock Trousers (MAST) garment, or pharmacologic means. In neurogenic shock, a dose of 0.4 mg of atropine intravenously may be a useful adjunct at the accident scene.

Immobilization

All patients should be placed in the neutral supine position and splinted from head to hips. The entire spine must be immobilized owing to the risk (15%) of multiple levels of injury. The most efficient system remains a simple rigid spine board. The forehead should be securely held to the board by tape or straps, with sandbags on either side of the head. The chest is secured similarly but more loosely, and the pelvis, knees, and ankles are snugly secured. Care must be taken not to alter any prior anatomic deformity, such as a scoliotic or kyphotic deformity (i.e., especially in geriatric patients).

Transportation

Once baseline assessments are documented and physiologic stability is accomplished, two peripheral intravenous lines, a Foley catheter, and nasogastric tube should be inserted and the patient transported by ground or air. Careful neurologic and physiologic monitoring are essential en route. Telemetry and Doppler technology have made this transport safer. Cervical traction should never be applied at the accident scene or during transport from the accident scene because of the risk of increased secondary injury from overdistraction of severely disrupted cervical spine injuries.[5,6] A rigid but transparent Miami J collar (Jerome Medical, Philadelphia, PA) is ideal for head and neck immobilization during transport.

EMERGENCY ROOM MANAGEMENT

The emergency room marks a critical point in the management of the patient with acute SCI. Here the patient is usually first evaluated by the hospital-based SCI team. Likewise, it is the first opportunity for a thorough examination to be performed and other injuries assessed and treated. Appropriate intervention in the emergency room may prevent or minimize subsequent complications.

The emergency room management is essentially a continuation of the on-scene process. Physiologic homeostasis is established or maintained, with priority given to the same accident scene ABCs. At this time, the SCI team assesses the neurologic and spinal column status, while the trauma team evaluates and stabilizes the patient for other systemic problems.[7]

If the airway is inadequate, awake, nasal intubation is carried out while the head and neck remain immobilized in the neutral position on the backboard. If a nasal intubation is impossible blindly and fiberoptic scope guidance is likewise impossible or contraindicated (e.g., the presence of a basilar skull or multiple facial fractures), a surgical airway is created, usually via cricothyroidotomy, and a standard endotracheal tube, size 7.0 to 8.0, is inserted. Respiratory support is maintained if dictated by the patient's status. Because injuries to the C4 level and above impair phrenic nerve function, mechanical ventilatory support is necessary in patients with such an injury as well as those with systemic injuries that may indirectly impair respiration. Serial blood gas values are obtained regardless of whether the patient is intubated or not. For those patients not requiring airway, oxygen support via 40% humidified face mask is maintained. For the intubated patient, initial settings of F_{IO_2} of 45% IMV 8, tidal volume (V_T) of 15 ml/kg, and positive end-expiratory pressure (PEEP) +5 cm are set. Baseline goals are an arterial P_{O_2} greater than or equal to 100 torr, P_{CO_2} less than or equal to 45 torr, and pH 7.35 to 7.45. A question arises as to which patients with SCI need intubation and ventilatory support. The apneic patient or the one without an airway is, of course, easily identified. The patient who is breathing is evaluated as to respiratory rate and quality, room air P_{O_2} and P_{CO_2}. Criteria for intubation and ventilatory support are a respiratory rate greater than 30, P_{CO_2} greater than 45 torr, or P_{O_2} less than 70 torr. Increased respiratory work, evidenced by retraction of the accessory muscles, is a relative criterion. If supplemental oxygen does not relieve the problem, intubation is considered.

At the same time the aforementioned factors are considered, vascular access is initiated. Usually all that is necessary are two short, large-bore (14- or 16-gauge) peripheral catheters. An alternative, especially when fluid resuscitation may be required, is the insertion of a 7.5-French pulmonary catheter introducer sheath. If the "hub" is kept sterile and capped at the time of insertion, these may be used subsequently for inserting a pulmonary artery or other multilumen catheter. A Foley catheter is inserted to monitor urinary output. Blood is drawn for baseline chemistry, including cardiac enzymes, complete blood count, platelets, clotting studies, serum amylase, toxicology (if indicated), and type and screen (or type and cross if surgery is contemplated). Other initial diagnostic studies are as follows: electrocardiogram (ECG), anteroposterior and lateral survey of all spinal levels, and anteroposterior chest and abdominal views. Other x-ray studies, including skull series and extremity views, are obtained, if indicated. In the case of the multiple trauma patient, the physical examination of the abdomen may be negative owing to the lack of sensory functions associated with the SCI or owing to an overall lack of response as in a concomitantly head-injured patient. Therefore abdominal "clearance" is necessary, usually via diagnostic peritoneal lavage or abdominal computed tomography (CT). If a life-threatening systemic injury is present, priority is given to its treatment, while maintaining the spine immobilized. Similarly, if any other diagnostic test is urgently indicated, e.g., angiography, it, too, may be performed with the patient splinted.

As noted previously, the neurologic assessment is performed at this time. It must be stressed that the examination is a thorough one, evaluating cranial as well as spinal function, because a significant number of patients with spine injury have concomitant head trauma and vice versa. A brain CT scan may be indicated in the radiographic evaluation of the SCI patient.

Neurologic Evaluation

The neurologic evaluation of the acute spinal-cord-injured patient in the emergency room should focus on the following three categories of function:

- Voluntary motor function
- Sensory function (testing both lateral columns; pain or temperature; dorsal columns; crude touch, vibration, or position sense)
- Rectal examination, documenting volitional anal sphincter contraction and perianal lateral and dorsal column sensory function[8]

In our center, we define a **complete SCI** lesion as a patient who has no volitional motor function or sensory function below the level of injury. We find that reflexes are unreliable predictors of outcome and, in general, a poor assessment tool in these acutely injured patients.[7] In our experience and that of other large SCI centers, approximately 5 to 7% of complete injury patients end up significantly improving functionally or actually walking in many cases.[8] These patients who break the "golden rule" that complete injuries never get better are usually lower velocity accident victims. We further define **incomplete SCI** as the loss of some degree of voluntary motor function or testable sensory function below or distal to the level of injury; these patients make up the majority of the SCI patient population in the 1990s. The prognosis for the incomplete patients is much better, with most regaining at least some degree of neurologic function. It is much more significant prognostically, however, to be incomplete with regard to lateral column, i.e., pain and temperature preservation, than to dorsal column, i.e., touch, vibration, or position sense function.

A commonly misunderstood concept is the spinal shock syndrome. The spinal shock patient has a functional, not usually an anatomic, transection of the spinal cord with an associated flaccid paralysis, i.e., a lack of motor tone at and below the level of injury, and a lack of sensory and reflex function at the same levels.[9] Some time between 6 and 16 weeks after injury, spinal shock subsides. When complete SCI victims are transformed from a lower motor neuron into an upper motor neuron status, with trunk and extremity spasticity and hyperreflexia as well as increased tone, this signals the resolution of spinal shock. The bowel and bladder and sphincter functions follow suit, initially during the spinal shock phase, being lower motor neuron or flaccid and becoming upper motor neuron or spastic. Reflex erections often also herald the end of spinal shock. The confusion lies in the fact that many clinicians counsel patients that they cannot tell them for sure whether their injury is complete or incomplete until they are out of spinal shock, which is not a reasonable statement because by definition everyone in spinal shock has a complete injury; i.e. they have no volitional motor, sensory, or reflex function below the area of injury. The resolution of spinal shock does not change this status or their poor prognosis for further recovery.

Almost all patients with complete or incomplete injuries have what is considered a "zone of injury," where they have abnormal function at, below, and even at times slightly above the level of injury. This local zone of incompleteness of injury does not mean that the injury is incomplete with regard to prognosis. The only important parameter that defines a true incomplete lesion with regard to prognosis is distal, volitional motor function or sensory

Table 9-1. Incomplete Spinal Cord Injury Syndromes

Type of Injury	Deficit	Prognosis for Walking*
Central cord syndrome	Motor deficit more pronounced in upper extremities Variable sensory findings	Fair to good—able to ambulate with or without spastic gait Residual upper extremity deficit and painful dysesthesia May experience return of bowel and bladder control
Anterior cord syndrome	Motor deficit Pain/temperature deficit Preserved vibration/proprioception	Poor—usually no functional motor improvement
Brown-Sequard syndrome	Ipsilateral motor deficit Ipsilateral vibration/proprioception deficit Contralateral pain/temperature deficit	Fair—may ambulate with orthotic braces or a cane May experience return of bowel, bladder, and sexual function
Posterior cord syndrome	No motor deficit Preserved pain/temperature Vibration/proprioception deficit	Fair—preserved motor function, but difficult to ambulate due to loss of bilateral position sense
Conus medullaris syndrome	Symmetric motor and sensory deficits Bowel, bladder, and sphincter deficit Saddle sensation deficit	Fair to good—often able to ambulate, but bowel, bladder, & sexual deficits may persist
Cauda equina syndrome	Lower motor neuron injury (flaccid paresis) Painful lower extremities Motor and sensory deficits dependent on severity of injury	Fair to good—potential for motor, sensory, bowel, bladder, and sexual recovery dependent on severity of injury

* Prognosis varies with each syndrome with regard to level and severity of injury.

function, or what is termed sacral-sparing, which is determined by a rectal examination with voluntary anal sphincter contraction or lateral column sensory function in the anal or perianal area.[8] It is much more important prognostically to have lateral column sparing, i.e., pain or temperature sensation, rather than dorsal column, i.e., touch, vibration, or position sensation sparing. This is probably because the lateral columns have a different blood supply than the dorsal columns, and incompleteness in either of the major lateral column groups, i.e., motor or pain and temperature, provides a high probability of further recovery in the same distribution (i.e., motor), whereas dorsal column sensory sparing alone, which is associated with the anterior cord syndrome, does not necessarily precede an evolving clinical recovery.

Less than 1% of acute SCI patients develop a syndrome that is sometimes termed ascending cord necrosis or acute ascending cord syndrome. In this rare instance, patients with an initial neurologic level are characterized by an ascending motor and sensory deficit. Sometimes this ascending functional loss may be limited to one or a few segments, but at other times it can continue to evolve up into the brain stem and result in a fatal brain stem syndrome. No one is quite sure what causes this rare syndrome or how to treat it, but it is hypothesized that it probably represents a type of stuttering and extending vascular infarction picture. In rare cases, some of the lost function is reversible, but in the majority of cases, that is unfortunately not what transpires.

Because the majority of acute SCI patients present with incomplete lesions, it is useful to describe some of the more common clinical pictures presenting in the emergency room or ICU.[9] These include:

- Central cord syndrome
- Anterior cord syndrome
- Brown-Sequard syndrome
- Posterior cord syndrome
- Conus medullaris syndrome
- Cauda equina injury
- Hysterical conversion

Table 9-1 summarizes incomplete injury deficits and prognosis for walking.

The **central cord syndrome** usually occurs in middle-aged or elderly men and most often is associated with a hyperextension injury, usually without associated spinal column fracture or dislocation. These patients have a preexisting spinal canal stenosis, i.e., spondylosis and stenosis, which when combined with a whiplash or hyperextension injury results in a bruise to the spinal cord. This was initially thought to be due to a central gray matter hematoma or injury, although contemporary human autopsy tissue analysis has pointed to more of a diffuse white matter injury being responsible. Characteristically these patients have incomplete injury, with greater motor and sensory deficit in the upper than the lower extremities and the most marked deficit in the distal upper extremities, i.e., the hands and fingers. This deficit is often associated with painful dysesthesias and hypersensitivity, especially of the distal upper extremities. These patients often but not always recover sphincter function and most often plateau neurologically with at least some degree of residual deficit. If this is at an unacceptable level, the injuries are reclassified as myeloradiculopathies rather than acute injuries, and the patients are reimaged with CT and magnetic resonance imaging (MRI) in a varied way for a possible delayed surgical decompression.

The **anterior SCI syndrome** or anterior cord syndrome has usually been associated with hyperflexion injury with loss of volitional motor and pain and temperature function but with preservation of touch, vibration, and position sense, i.e., dorsal column function. These patients are much better off than those with a complete lesion because they have position sense and are able to transfer more independently and have crude touch and pressure sensation, which makes them less likely to suffer from certain systemic complications, such as decubitus ulcers. They do not, however, have the same good prognosis for recovery as those with sparing of lateral column function. They usually remain only with their sensation, with no further motor recovery.

The **Brown-Sequard syndrome** is a physiologic hemisection of the cord, which at times can be associated with an actual partial anatomic transection, such as is seen in penetrating wounds. It is usually associated, however, with rotational closed injuries. The patients present with ipsilateral loss of touch, vibration, and position sense and motor function and contralateral loss of pain and temperature sensation. Their greatest deficit is in the ipsilateral upper extremity, and they often present as mimicking a brachial plexis syndrome and may actually be associated with a brachial plexis injury. These patients are more likely to fall into the 1% of the ascending cord necrosis syndrome patients than the other incomplete lesions, but this is a rare occurrence. Most often these patients improve significantly enough that with minor orthotic assistance (i.e., cane), they are able to walk but still usually retain a significant ipsilateral upper extremity deficit over the long-term.

The **posterior cord syndrome** is a rare injury involving loss only of dorsal columns, which makes it difficult to use the preserved motor function because of the lack of proprioception. The patients usually recover at least some degree of lost dorsal column function but can remain with a significant disability.

The **conus medullaris syndrome** is an injury that usually occurs at the second most mobile level of the spinal column, i.e., the junction of the thoracic and lumbar spine. These injuries are interesting because they have the potential for a lower extremity functional recovery (walking) despite being a "complete spinal cord lesion" because of the ability of lower motor neurons (i.e., peripheral nerves) to regenerate and recover functionally.

A good prognosis is also true of most **cauda equina injuries** that occur in lumbar and supersacral spine injuries, with the recovery depending on the mechanism and velocity of injury and degree of neural element disruption as well as the adequacy and timeliness of decompression.

The **hysterical conversion** or malingering patient can be bothersome in the emergency room. These patients usually come in with a flaccid paraplegia from the umbilicus down, with no apparent sensation preserved. They may or may not have reflexes, and x-ray studies and MRI and CT scans are always negative. A clue is that they usually have good anal sphincter tone. Often, a skilled neurologic examiner can make the appropriate diagnosis initially, although medically and legally, as well as psychiatrically, these patients can be dangerous.

ICU PHASE

Not all patients who have suffered SCI require ICU management. In our institution, the criteria for ICU admission are as follows:

- SCI on ventilatory support
- SCI with concomitant intracranial injury with Glasgow Coma Scale score less than 12
- SCI with potential for cardiorespiratory, other systemic, or neurologic worsening
- Spinal traction with need for adjustment/manipulation

All other acute SCI patients are admitted to the intermediate care (step-down) unit.

The ICU management of the SCI patient is considered on a system-by-system protocol basis. The treatment modalities represent those at the University of Miami Medical Center, and although other approaches may undoubtedly be effective, these have proved to be valuable in the population treated in our center.

Pulmonary Management

The majority of systemic problems in acute SCI are related to the respiratory system. Likewise, they frequently contribute the most to prolonged ICU stay and delay of effective rehabilitation. There is an almost 100% incidence of pulmonary complications in quadriplegics if the following are considered: inability to clear airway, retained secretions, and development of atelectasis. These, in turn, may lead to significantly worse complications, such as pneumonia, loss of pulmonary compliance, and ventilation-perfusion (V/Q) mismatch (increased "shunt"), which significantly impair the patient's recovery. SCI patients may start out in the ICU with compromised respiratory function from many possible sources, such as paralysis of the intercostal muscles or diaphragm muscles, partial or complete paralysis of the vocal cords, pulmonary contusion, rib or clavicle fractures, pneumothorax, hemothorax, or aspiration. The best therapy for the foregoing problems is prevention, which is why all acute SCI patients in the ICU are treated with kinetic therapy.[10]

All patients are placed on a Rotorest treatment table (Kinetic Concepts, San Antonio, TX) on arrival in the ICU (Figs. 9-1 and 9-2). This apparatus allows cervical or extremity traction to be maintained while providing constant turning to mobilize pulmonary secretions as well as alter the V/Q dynamics, at least to some extent. The design of the bed allows access to all areas of the patient's thorax and can accommodate all respiratory or chest drainage systems. Chest tubes can be placed through the bed frame to obviate the risks of reflux contamination.

Oxygen saturation is measured and kept at or above 95%. All patients are given chest physiotherapy and twin jet nebulization with a bronchodilator every 4 hours. A mucolytic may be added if indicated. Intermittent positive-pressure breathing (IPPB) may be used if there is significant atelectasis in the unintubated patient, but the use of this modality is relatively infrequent in our center. Continuous positive airway pressure (CPAP) mask may also be used but again is relatively rarely indicated. All unintubated patients are given supplemental oxygen, usually via the 40% humidified mist mask route. Daily vital capacities as well as twice-daily spontaneous tidal volumes are measured. All patients are placed on incentive spirometry, also on an every-4-hour schedule. All patients are monitored with a finger applied oximeter system, and arterial blood gases are sent on a daily basis or more frequently as needed.

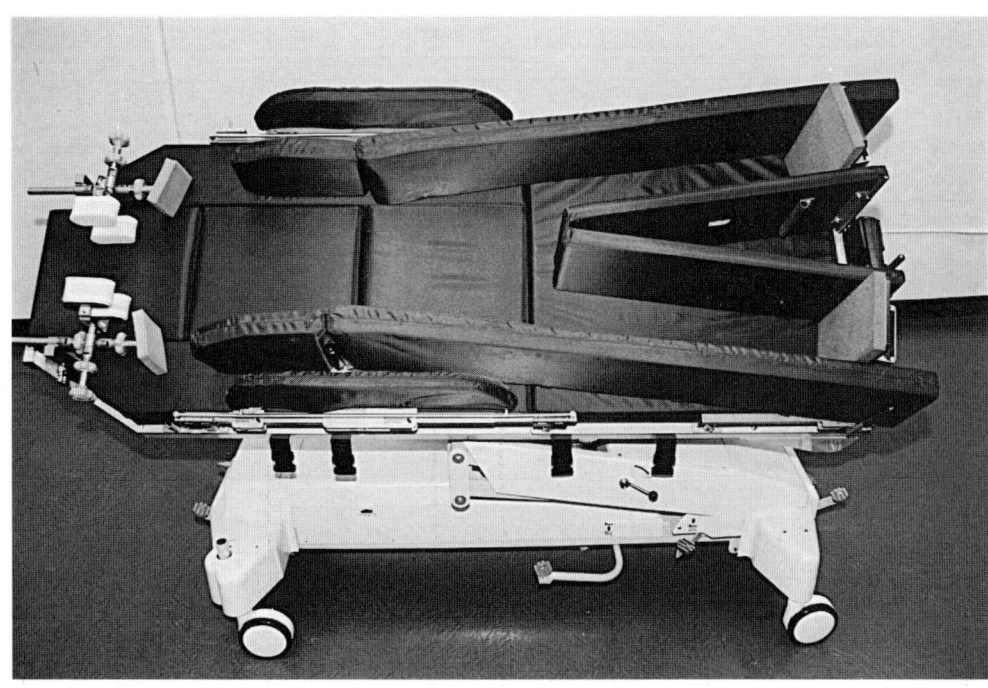

Fig. 9–1. Rotorest treatment bed. (Courtesy of Kinetic Concepts, San Antonio, TX.)

An arterial monitoring line is inserted for both blood gas sampling and blood pressure monitoring.

The indications for intubation have already been discussed. Once a patient has required intubation, therapy is directed toward resolving the problems that have required intubation. In the case of a pneumonic process, sputum cultures and a chest film are obtained daily. In the case of atelectasis, a slight increase in V_T is used, at least initially, to open collapsed small airways. This increment is usually between 2 and 4 ml/kg above the baseline. In general,

PEEP is used to provide optimum oxygenation. A baseline of +5 cm is used in all intubated patients. It is raised by increments of 2 to 3 cm to optimize oxygenation. Above 15 cm PEEP, especially in the case of adult respiratory distress syndrome (ARDS), or earlier if cardiac instability exists, an oximetric pulmonary artery catheter is placed. Generally it is our practice to use increased PEEP rather than increased F_{IO_2} above 45% to optimize oxygenation. If a pulmonary catheter is in place, PEEP is titrated to provide a Q_S/Q_T ratio between 15 and 20%. Alternatively, espe-

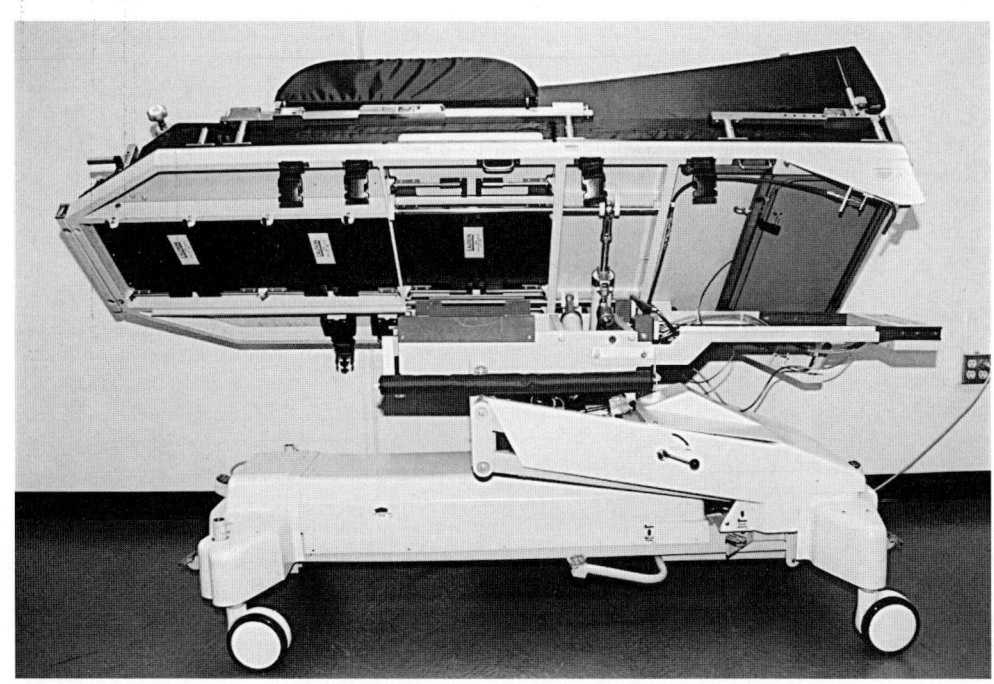

Fig. 9–2. Rotorest treatment bed (underside). (Courtesy of Kinetic Concepts, San Antonio, TX.)

cially in patients without a pulmonary artery catheter, the P_{O_2}/F_{IO_2} ratio may be used as a guideline, titrating to a ratio of 300:1. When necessary, of course, F_{IO_2} may be increased, but usually 60% is the maximum fraction needed except in the most resistant ARDS cases.

It is not infrequent for the SCI patient to develop mucous plugging, whether intubated or not. In the case of the latter, short-term intubation may be required to effect adequate pulmonary toilet. The presence of an endotracheal or nasotracheal tube also allows for fiberoptic bronchoscopy in these cases. This technique is invaluable for clearing small airways of mucous plugs as well as obtaining optimal sputum cultures if an infection is suspected.

The problem of ventilatory weaning is frequently encountered in the high level lesion SCI patient. In these cases, early investigation of portable ventilator usage is recommended because it may facilitate mobilization of the patient and allow rehabilitation to proceed. These patients often require a tracheostomy for long-term airway control. In other cases, we usually do not perform tracheostomies earlier than the twenty-first day postinjury. If the pulmonary status indicates that intubation will be prolonged beyond 3 weeks or airway control will be necessary, the tracheostomy is performed. Prolonged intubation may be associated with development of a tracheoesophageal fistula or tracheal stenosis. Another complication seen with prolonged nasotracheal intubation in SCI victims is a fever of unknown cause owing to an unsuspected sinusitis.

There is no universally accepted means of ventilatory wean in the SCI patient. Our experience has been first to reduce the PEEP by decrements of 2 to 3 cm down to a PEEP of +5 cm. Again a P_{O_2}/F_{IO_2} ratio greater than or equal to 300 or a shunt of less than 20% is used as a guideline. Next the F_{IO_2} is gradually reduced by 5% decrements to room air (21%), again monitoring arterial blood gases. Finally, the ventilatory rate is decreased to a point at which the patient is on a setting of PEEP +5 cm (actually CPAP +5 cm) and F_{IO_2} 21%. This point may be relatively difficult to achieve. Useful adjuncts have been an intravenous aminophylline drip, usually in the range of 0.5 to 1.0 mg/kg per hour, or the institution of the pressure support (PS) ventilatory mode, usually beginning at +15 cm and decreasing by 2 to 3 cm daily until the final setting is CPAP +5 cm, PS +5 cm, F_{IO_2} 21%. At this point, if the P_{O_2}/F_{IO_2} ratio is greater than 300, the respiratory rate is less than 30, P_{O_2} is greater than 70 torr, and P_{CO_2} is less than 45 torr; if there is no objective respiratory distress; and if the patient can protect his or her airway, consideration is given to extubation. If the patient has been intubated for more than 7 days, methylprednisolone, 500 mg intravenously, may be given before extubation to diminish vocal cord swelling. (This latter technique is empiric but has proven helpful in our experience.) After extubation, kinetic therapy, twin jet nebulization, chest physiotherapy, and incentive spirometry, as described previously, are used aggressively. Likewise, if spinal stability allows, the patient is mobilized to the point of being out of bed in a chair or tilting frame or table.

Two other topics may be considered under the heading of pulmonary management: deep vein thrombosis/pulmonary embolism (DVT/PE) and the halo orthosis. DVT/PE is a significant risk for the SCI patient at any level of involvement.[11] In our experience, the aggressive use of kinetic therapy has significantly reduced the incidence of DVT and virtually eliminated the incidence of fatal pulmonary emboli reported to be as high as 3 to 13% in SCI patients in the literature.[10] Once the patient is taken off of the Rotorest treatment table, however, prophylactic heparinization (5000 units subcutaneously every 12 hours) or coated aspirin therapy is initiated and maintained throughout the acute hospitalization and rehabilitation phases of care. The halo orthosis provides another potential pulmonary problem. Although undoubtedly this device enables early mobilization and rehabilitation, the jacket component, by its very design, impedes access for adequate chest physiotherapy and may indeed act as an externally restrictive device with regard to chest wall expansion.[12] Therefore, the patient in a halo brace requires close monitoring of pulmonary status, especially vital capacity and spontaneous tidal volume measurements. If these appear impaired, the jacket is adjusted to optimize respiratory function, and pulmonary toilet may be increased in frequency to minimize the negative effects of the orthosis.

Cardiovascular Management

Although pulmonary/respiratory problems frequently provide the most common source of ICU morbidity in the acute SCI patient, cardiovascular dysfunction may present the greatest threat to life in the early phase of care.[13] The concept of neurogenic shock has been discussed previously. This phenomenon may persist as long as 6 weeks after injury. In the ICU phase, the combination of hypotension and bradycardia may significantly impair other systems, specifically the pulmonary, renal, and central nervous systems. Acute left ventricular failure has become more frequently identified in the acute SCI population. The cause of this condition remains unclear, but a catecholamine outpouring at the time of injury or in the early acute phase has been implicated. The immediate repercussions are inadequate systemic perfusion as well as a congestive heart failure picture. No simple means of preventing this has been found to be effective in the human population, although the use of thyrotropin-releasing hormone (TRH) and naloxone have been shown to be of some benefit in controlled laboratory studies.[14,15] Therapy must therefore be directed toward correcting the hypotension and bradycardia.

As previously discussed, a baseline ECG and cardiac enzymes are usually sent as part of the emergency room workup. If they have not been obtained, they should be sent on admission to the ICU. Also, past cardiac history should be obtained, whenever possible, especially in the case of the older SCI patient (older than 40 years). The patient's cardiac rhythm and blood pressure are monitored via ECG and arterial line. A multilumen central line is inserted, allowing monitoring, fluid infusion, and venous sampling. In the case of a bradycardia with adequate blood pressure, therapy is initiated when the pulse drops below 50. Usually atropine, 0.4 to 1 mg intravenously as needed, is sufficient therapy. The bradycardia tends to resolve as the neurogenic shock picture subsides. If there is an associated hypotension, a pressor agent (usually dopamine) is added. The dose required is usually between 3 and 8 μg/kg per minute. Dopamine is usually our choice because of its inotropic and chronotropic (beta$_1$) effects at lower doses as well as its effect on increasing renal perfusion. If there is no need for increased splanchnic perfusion, dobutamine is selected, again in the same dose range. Rarely have we found it necessary to use a digitalis preparation to increase cardiac efficiency unless there was a premorbid cardiac condition that required its usage. Indeed the cardiac slowing effect of the digitalis drugs may aggravate the patient's tendency toward bradycardia.

The usage of cardiac pacemakers, temporary as well as permanent, is a consideration in the ICU phase of SCI management. If the patient has a preexisting cardiac condition (arrhythmia) that has been worsened by the SCI and it is thought that the condition will be permanent or at least long-term (i.e., more than 2 weeks' duration), consideration is given to at least temporary, transvenous pacing. Likewise, if the patient is refractory to the inotrope/chronotrope and is symptomatic (HR <50 with systolic BP <90), consideration for pacing is given. If, however, the patient is responsive to the intravenous medication(s), it is rare that we have found it necessary to use pacing. Rather, it has been our choice to maintain the dopamine/dobutamine drip until the cardiovascular impairment of the acute SCI has worn off.

As a rule, most acute SCI patients do not need volume expansion per se to augment blood pressure unless there has been associated hypovolemia. If present, this is usually due to blood loss from multisystem trauma, in which case therapy is directed to reestablish a normal circulating volume, i.e., "prime the pump." This is usually done with crystalloid, although packed red blood cells may be transfused if it is thought that the oxygen-carrying capacity needs to be increased. In general, packed red blood cells are not used unless the hematocrit is less than 24% or the hemoglobin is less than 7 mg/dl.

Of significant value in the cardiovascular management of the SCI patient is the use of the oximetric pulmonary artery catheter. This allows determination of the relative "fullness" of the "tank" (pulmonary wedge pressure [PWP]) as well as the efficiency of the "pump" (cardiac output index [CO/CI]) and mixed venous oxygen saturation (SVO$_2$). Cardiotonic drugs and fluids may be titrated against these parameters. As a rule, PWP is maintained between 12 and 16 mm Hg, CO/CI kept approximately 1.5 times the estimated baseline, and SVO$_2$ maintained between 65 and 75%. These ranges, of course, vary depending on the individual patient, but in general these parameters cover the needs of the majority of SCI patients.

The problem of hypothermia in the acute SCI patient should be mentioned briefly. Because of the physiologic sympathectomy that often occurs in patients with injuries about T5, temperature regulation may prove to be a serious problem. These patients are extremely sensitive to ambient temperature changes. If there is an acute change in mental status, the development of new arrhythmias, or a deterioration in cardiac status, and if these are unexplained by other factors, one should consider hypothermia as a potential cause. Body temperature in SCI patients should

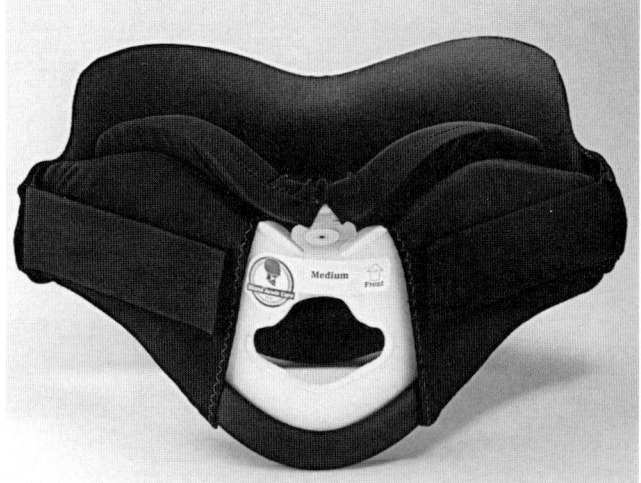

Fig. 9–3. Miami acute care collar.

be taken with a thermometer that registers below 94°F. Therapy is directed at restoring a normal core temperature, i.e., between 96 and 99°F. Blankets, both standard and hyperthermic, may be used, and warming the intravenous fluid via a blood warmer may also prove helpful.

Neurologic Management

The most important part of the nervous system ICU SCI management protocol involves close monitoring of the neurologic status. This means that neurologic assessments by the critical care nursing staff on each shift must be documented along with at least twice-daily neurologic assessments by the intensivist or responsible physician. This protocol is complicated in patients with a concomitant head injury. Patients with closed nonsurgical brain lesions or postoperative craniotomy patients may require ICP monitoring and treatment. Open lacerations or fractures or postoperative craniotomies provide an additional potential problem, with tong or halo ring placement interfering with the scalp and bone defects or flaps. If no external device can be applied, the patient should be maintained on the Rotorest bed in a rigid collar. The product used in our institution is a special MAC (Miami Acute Collar) designed for ICU patients with a soft posterior piece to avoid occipital scalp breakdown (Fig. 9–3). This cervical orthosis is a two-piece apparatus that has a precut opening in front for a tracheostomy tube, and the piece covering the neck is transparent to allow direct visualization of the skin and neck morphology. This feature eliminates the fear of a collar acting like a tourniquet in a swelling injured neck or of a progressive expanding hematoma or subcutaneous emphysema going unnoticed, with potentially devastating effects. Figure 9–4 is a Miami J collar. We use this collar once patients are out of the ICU. The posterior piece is rigid and gives the added support needed.

Another problem encountered in the patient who has undergone surgical decompression/stabilization or who has a penetrating spinal injury is that of a parameningeal infection. The clinical symptoms may vary from low grade

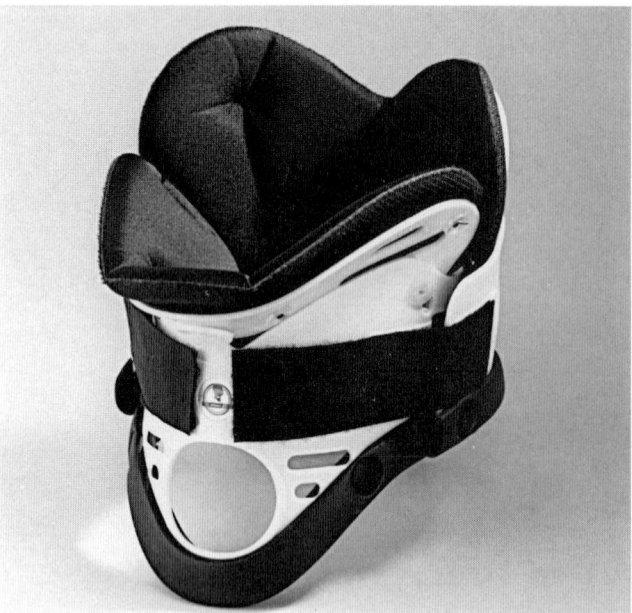

Fig. 9–4. Miami J collar.

temperature elevation and moderate leukocytosis to altered mental status, including seizures and coma. An elevated index of suspicion is necessary to pursue a diagnosis in the subtle cases. Cerebrospinal fluid examination (CSF) is usually necessary to confirm the diagnosis and identify the organism involved. Careful checks of traumatic and surgical wounds may also reveal the infection source. Treatment may require surgical debridement of infected sites as well as antibiotic coverage capable of bactericidal concentrations in CSF. In rare cases, direct intrathecal antibiotic therapy may become necessary.

Gastrointestinal and Nutritional Management

Most patients with acute SCI develop an immediate ileus.[16] Likewise, a significant number may have associated abdominal trauma. In the acute phase, most patients require total parenteral nutrition (TPN). It should be remembered that these patients have a surprisingly high resting energy expenditure as well as being markedly catabolic.[17] Therefore acute nutritional support needs to supply between 150 and 200% of the expected baseline calories during the acute phase. Care must be taken to supply a significant proportion as lipid and branched-chain amino acids as well as phosphate salts for adenosine triphosphate (ATP) production. The protein-calorie wasting seen in SCI may be devastating in terms of wound repair as well as eventual rehabilitation.[18] Baseline parameters obtained on ICU admission include, in addition to standard blood chemistries, liver enzymes, serum triglycerides, serum magnesium and transferrin levels, and a 24-hour urine urea nitrogen. These are followed on a weekly basis during the acute care stage. If available within the institution, calorimetry can be of significant help in estimating the patient's metabolic needs more accurately. There are a number of TPN formulas available, and each patient requires adjustment of the formula to fit his or her needs. Generally we have found that a formula of 21% dextrose/7% amino acids plus intravenous lipid infusion satisfies the requirements of most of our patients.

One of the most perplexing difficulties we have encountered is the development of acute pancreatitis and acalculous cholecystitis. The cause of the former remains unknown, although the relative parasympathetic dominance that occurs with cervical and high thoracic injuries remains a plausible explanation.[16] It has been suggested by detailed serum analyses that this may not be a true pancreatitis but rather an amylasemia, which is associated with spiking temperatures, ileus, and abdominal distention. Acakulous cholecystitis has become a more frequently recognized entity and may be related to the use of TPN insofar as the enteral tract is not used, and the gallbladder is not emptied. Diagnosis can be made in the ICU by ultrasonography. Prevention of pancreatitis is essentially impossible. Its therapy remains nasogastric suction, TPN, and following serum and urine amylase levels. Once the amylase levels have begun to subside, we begin enteral feedings, usually with Gatorade, and advance to commercial formulas as tolerated.

In the past, one of the worse morbidities with regard to the gastrointestinal system in patients with acute SCI in the ICU has been the development of stress ulcers. Although this problem has not totally been eliminated, it has become rare because of the practice of placing a sump tube in the patient's stomach as soon as the patient is admitted to the hospital and connecting it to a "low constant suction" system; the pH is checked every 4 hours and is titrated above 4.5 with antacids. These patients have the opposite of a vagotomy; they have a sympathectomy, especially in cervical and upper thoracic injuries, which creates an imbalance of the autonomic nervous system, with increased acid production. This status is further complicated by the stasis of acid in the paralyzed gut (i.e., ileus) and also by the relative gut ischemia from the stress associated with spinal cord and multisystem injuries. In addition to the pH protocol, in certain selected cases, the intravenous histamine blockers are used, although not nearly to the degree that they were before the implementation of this successful protocol.

Once the acute ileus has resolved and bowel sounds are present, feeding with nasogastric sump tube or nasogastric Silastic feeding tube is ideal for patients who cannot be fed orally for various reasons. In cases in which nasogastric feeding is not possible, a jejunostomy or percutaneous endoscopic gastrostomy (PEG) has also been used. The jejunostomy has the advantage of reduced risk of regurgitation and aspiration, whereas the PEG has the advantage of ease and rapidity of placement. Both are quite helpful, however, in allowing the patient to use the enteral feeding route during the time when he or she is suffering from paralysis and other multisystem injuries.

Once the enteral tract is working, the patient is placed on a bowel training program, including a combination laxative, stool softener, and suppositories every other day. At times, manual disimpaction may be necessary, especially as evidenced by patients alternating between a pattern of diarrhea and constipation. If diarrhea becomes intractable, especially as a result of systemic antibiotic therapy, gut flora can be replaced with acidophilus bacterial granules, 1 pack enterally three times a day or orally, and enteral yeast is controlled with nystatin 1 million units enterally, also three times a day.

Genitourinary Management

Genitourinary complications have traditionally been among the greatest problems regarding long-term morbidity and mortality within the SCI population. Only recently, however, has this surfaced as a major morbidity in ICU patients,[19] which has led to a more aggressive management protocol during the acute period. Most SCI patients with neurogenic or paralyzed bladders have significant urinary tract contamination or infarction the rest of their lives. At most times, however, they seem to live in symbiosis with the organisms in their bladder. In the acute care period, however, when they have multiple invasive lines, including tongs and central venous or arterial catheters and arterial lines, as well as fresh surgical wounds, bacteriuria is not acceptable and may lead to major problems with septicemia and seeding of secondary sites.

In our protocol, all patients with acute SCI have an indwelling Foley catheter while initially in the ICU. This catheter usually incorporates a temperature probe, and when possible Silastic catheters more resistant to infection and sediment formation are used. A urinary collection system must be in line with the catheter and be kept sterile and be capable of registering hourly and cumulative urinary outputs. These systems are of considerable value in monitoring renal function, especially when pressor support is necessary. The indwelling catheter is maintained until the hourly total intravenous fluid rate is below 100 ml per hour, allowing for discontinuation of the catheter and initiation of an intermittent catheterization program. Unless the patient can be managed with an acute 4-hour intermittent catheterization program, it is more traumatic and frustrating than useful to remove the Foley catheter. Simply, the input and output must be balanced to allow for reasonable volumes with each catheterization. Once the 4-hour program is in place in the ICU (this should be done sterilely), the interval may be increased to 6 hours, either because the patient tolerates the volumes or because the patient starts to void spontaneously, which usually heralds the end of spinal shock. It is beneficial, long-term, to initiate intermittent catheterization as early as possible to allow for more of a physiologic reexpansion of the bladder and maintenance of its volume capacity, which is severely jeopardized by a long-term indwelling Foley catheter or suprapubic catheter drainage. Also, the intermittent catheterization program is effective in reducing the incidence of urinary tract infections and autonomic dysreflexia.

Generally prophylactic antibiotics are not used while patients have indwelling catheters. The treatment for urinary tract infections, however, remains a topic of debate.[20] In our practice, a positive urine culture is treated if the quantitative count is greater than 100,000, if a single organism is identified, or if there are more than 5 white blood cells on microscopic examination, even if there is no significant temperature elevation in the ICU setting. In the case of a urinary tract infection that is due to a yeast organism, replacement of the catheter with a triple-lumen urinary catheter to allow bladder irrigation with an amphotericin or acetic acid solution has proved helpful. Urinary diversion procedures or those to facilitate bladder drainage, e.g., cystostomy and sphincterotomy, are usually not required during the ICU phase unless there is an obstructive process involving the bladder neck or urethra or a direct injury creating a fistula or fissure.

In the subacute and chronic phases of care, including rehabilitation and lifelong follow-up, renal or genitourinary system stones, infections, reflux, hydronephrosis, and renal failure remain a significant problem but have been so effectively treated that they no longer represent the major cause of death in the SCI population, as was the case in the 1970s and early 1980s. During the acute care phase, formation of these calculi can be prevented with a combination of kinetic therapy using the Rotorest treatment table and good hydration and adequate drainage of the bladder as well as keeping the urine sterile during this high risk period.

Musculoskeletal and Skin Protocol

The musculoskeletal system is at high risk early in the hospitalization of the patient with acute SCI. Decubitus ulcers not only involving the skin, but also the underlying subcutaneous tissue, muscles, and even bone may have started (although not superficially obvious) at the accident scene or during transport, from prolonged immobilization on a rigid spine board. It takes less than a few hours for the damage necessary for a significant decubitus ulcer to form, although it may be several weeks before it manifests itself with a superficial ulcer or skin lesion.

Decubitus prevention precautions in the early acute stage provide a better rehabilitation candidate for that phase of care. Early on in the ICU phase, the most effective way to deal with this problem is mobilization on a kinetic treatment table with oscillation of the patient to be interrupted only by important tests, feeding, hygiene, bowel/bladder care, or respiratory treatments.[10] Early after injury, the muscles begin to lose protein, and massive urea excretion follows, with both disuse and denervation atrophy occurring. The soft tissues in and around the joints begin to contract, as does the overlying skin, because of lack of movement as well as a general catabolic trend. In addition to kinetic therapy, these patients should be treated with an aggressive range of motion program to involve all joints in all four extremities and to be repeated by the nursing staff every shift. A daily bathing and lotion application protocol should include a careful inspection of all skin areas. This can be safely accomplished on the Rotorest treatment table because of the series of hatches and latches making skin access feasible without jeopardizing spinal column stability, a unique feature of this apparatus. Treatment of patients with acute SCI on Stryker frames or Circoelectric beds or any type of mud, sand, or air beds is inappropriate and dangerous, as has been shown in multiple articles in the medical literature.[21,22]

Although kinetic therapy is effective in preventing decubitus ulcers, it can also be used effectively to treat those that are preexisting. In these cases, keeping the decubitus ulcer clean and dry and serial appropriate debridement, both surgical and chemical, should be included with active kinetic therapy. Oscillation of the patient provides alternating pressure points and appears to improve circulation in the area of the sore. The systemic complications commonly experienced from the immobility of patients placed on an air or mud bed can be avoided by a combination of good nursing care and kinetic therapy.

Another major musculoskeletal problem is the rapid mobilization of calcium from the skeleton and its subsequent deposition in the soft tissues, especially in and around joints as heterotopic bone or in the genitourinary system in the form of calculi. In the long term, this process results in an advanced state of osteoporosis, which can be associated with pathologic fractures with even minor manipulation of the extremities. In the ICU, especially in the high lesion patients who have been immobilized for weeks or months, it is not unusual for patients to experience a fractured extremity or joint dislocation. There is no way to limit or reverse this osteoporotic process in acute SCI patients, although research in this area has intensified as better diagnostic tools have become available.

Heterotopic bone is the deposition of calcium in and around major joints most commonly seen in SCI and other paralysis victims. These calcified masses can result in a significant increase in disability by total or partial loss of range of motion, especially of the hip or knee joints. These patients often cannot sit in a wheelchair or lie flat in bed and are excluded from brace walking or computerized bicycle ergometry because of their frozen joints. Heterotopic bone, similar to pathologic fractures, is more common in the subacute rather than the hyperacute SCI victim but does occur in the ICU and can be a significant consideration in the differential diagnosis of the fever of unknown origin. Monitoring the sedimentation rate and a bone scan as well as plain x-ray films are all helpful in making this diagnosis, but usually the proof lies in ruling out deep venous thrombosis by venogram; i.e., diagnosis by elimination can often be made.

Significant controversy surrounds the initiation of etidronate disodium (Didronel) therapy in the ICU. Once heterotopic bone formation does occur, however, high dose intravenous Didronel has proven to be effective during the hyperacute phase of this process, i.e., when the extremity is red and swollen and hot, although it is of little benefit once the heterotopic bone has formed.[23]

Another ICU problem that is most common in quadriplegics is the development of painful shoulder joints. Most often this is due to a combination of immobility and lying in one position. Even in patients receiving good range-of-motion therapy, however, it occasionally occurs as an inflammatory bursitis or capsulitis. In addition to aggressive and frequent range of motion of the joint, nonsteroidal anti-inflammatory agents can be helpful in selected patients.

A major issue relating to the musculoskeletal system is the maintenance of spinal column immobility. In our experience, this is possible only in the Rotorest treatment table or Stoke-Mendeville bed. Both have contour surface frames that allow adjustment for snug and effective immobilization of the head, neck, chest, and pelvic areas to prevent secondary injury to the spinal cord and nerve roots owing to inadvertent loss of alignment. This problem was significant with the previously used devices, such as the Stryker frame and Circoelectric bed.[21,22] Kinetic therapy and the Rotorest treatment table offer the optimal environment for acutely paralyzed patients, especially considering that the majority of them have unstable spinal injuries and multisystem trauma as well. Patients can be rotated in varying degrees of Trendelenberg or reverse Trendelenberg and can be rotated to either side selectively as far as degree and frequency, i.e., adjusting to individual problems and characteristics of SCI patients. If one believes in postural reduction of thoracic and lumbar injuries, this can also be accomplished while the patient continues to rotate in a close manner using special attachments available for the treatment table. Extremity fractures can also be effectively maintained in traction during oscillation, minimizing the risks of fat emoli further complicating the patient's medical condition.

Psychologic Protocol

All patients with acute SCI experience a series of psychologic stages, to varying degrees and at different time intervals, depending on the nature of their injury and their premorbid status. The family or significant others experience the same psychologic sequelae, usually in a little delayed fashion chronologically, as compared with the SCI victim.[24] It is imperative that all nurses, allied health professionals, and physicians dealing with these patients in the ICU are aware of this problem and are able to act as an integral part of the solution.

The first stage is termed "denial." The paralysis patient denies that he or she is really paralyzed or that it is a significant and potentially permanent problem. Patients often relate to other persons they have known who have had spinal fractures or paralysis and have recovered or to articles in nonmedical publications such as the *National Enquirer* or *Reader's Digest* that describe cures for paralysis. Denial usually does not last long because after several days or a week at the most, SCI patients realize that they can no longer deny their paralysis and they are not getting up and walking out of the hospital as expected; this is when the second stage—"anger"—begins. This is the most destructive phase. Patients can become verbally or, in some cases, physically abusive. Patients may want to sue the physician, nurse, ambulance driver, or hospital. The family goes through an equally aggressive, hostile (often guilt-ridden) period, and it is important during this phase for the staff to be well trained not to react in a negative way to the patient or family but rather to try to educate them with regard to the fact that all SCI victims experience these feelings and that it is best to limit the damage to themselves or family or the people trying to care for them. Although quite destructive, the anger phase usually lasts only a short time, terminating once the patients or families realize that it does not do any good to be angry.

The next phase is the "depression" stage and can last anywhere from days to weeks, months, or even years. In some people, it actually never ends, and in rare cases it results in suicide. During this phase, the patient presents to the nurses and physicians with a withdrawn attitude and a refusal to eat, undergo tests, receive therapy, or medications. They often ask the staff to help them kill themselves or to end their misery. It is important during this stage to involve the rehabilitation psychologist on an active daily basis, not only with the patient, but also with the family or significant others. In addition, tricyclic antidepressant medications such as amitriptyline can be most helpful in getting the patients through this stage. The next, final psychologic phase is the "coping" stage. Once this change occurs, rehabilitation can really become effective. Often, this happens in the ICU setting. In the coping period, patients and most often family or significant others make the decision to cope as best as they can with their new disability on a day-to-day basis, although they never really accept their paralysis. At any time, they would be happy to exchange it for whatever monetary or psychologic benefits they have received. An important part of the realization of this phase is education of patients and significant others with regard to the expected prognosis, short-term and long-term, of their particular injury. Also, it should be emphasized that there is hope, not based on emotion alone but based on good neuroscientific research, that in the future there may be reasonable treatments to reactivate or reconnect injured nervous system tissue functionally. Research areas such as bioengineering and CNS regeneration have virtually exploded over the last decade and are actively being pursued by laboratories and research centers across the United States and around the world. An important part of patient and family indoctrination to their new status is the tour through the spinal cord rehabilitation center and any available research laboratories. This is also a phase in which, in addition to rehabilitation psychologist counseling, peer counseling can be most helpful.

POST-ICU PHASE

The ICU phase is the most critical in the SCI system with regard to morbidity and survival because the highest morbidity and mortality in these paralyzed patients, who most often have associated multisystem injuries, is experienced in the first weeks following their traumatic event. A well-organized, effectively implemented ICU/SCI Multisystem Protocol results in early physiologic stabilization and the potential for rapid mobilization (with or without surgery) into the subacute and rehabilitative phases of care, with minimum systemic complications. In the past, most of the major long-term complications in SCI patients originated in the pre-ICU or ICU phases of care and have often led to the poor life expectancy and long, frequent rehospitalizations experienced by these patients. Table 9–2 lists the various conditions and complications associated with spinal cord dysfunction that is seen in the acute as well as chronic SCI patient.

The determination of exactly when an acute SCI patient is transferred out of the ICU is focused primarily on two components: (1) cardiovascular and respiratory stability and (2) spinal column stability (surgery or orthosis). In a multisystem trauma patient with SCI, the other systemic complications often overshadow these determinants.

Table 9–2. Conditions and Complications Associated with Spinal Cord Dysfunction

Loss of motor power	Metabolic disturbances
Loss of sensation	Negative calcium balance
Pressure sores	Negative nitrogen balance
Urinary dysfunction	Hormonal imbalance
Bowel dysfunction	Circulatory disturbances
Sexual dysfunction	Orthostatic hypotension
Autonomic hyperreflexia	Edema
Pain	Deep vein thrombophlebitis
Spasticity	Respiratory disturbances
Joint contractures	Psychologic problems
Heterotopic ossifications	Social problems
	Vocational problems

In our neurosurgical ICU, the average length of stay for an uncomplicated cervical injury varies with the patient's age. For quadriplegic patients younger than 40 years of age, the average ICU stay is 4 to 6 weeks, and the stay is longer for patients older than 40 years of age, about 6 to 9 weeks. The total length of stay for all patients with a diagnosis of quadriplegia averages 6 weeks to 3 months. For ventilatory-dependent patients, the ICU and acute care stay averages 3 to 6 months. Patients with the diagnosis of paraplegia are usually admitted directly to the acute care floor rather than the ICU. The average length of stay on the acute floor care ranges from 3 weeks for patients younger than 40 years of age to 6 weeks in patients older than 40. The ICU physicians, nurses, and allied health professionals, including the rehabilitation psychologists, social services person, physical therapists, and occupational therapists, should all be involved in a team decision with regard to graduating the patient on to the next phase of care. Once the decision is made, it should be discussed with both the patient and the family with regard to the rationale of timing, logistics, and other significant issues. As part of this process, the patient and family or significant others should be prepared by visiting the facility responsible for the next phase of treatment as well as by counseling with regard to what to expect long-term and short-term.

Most patients are transported from the ICU not directly to rehabilitation but to an intermediate step-down unit or floor care program that normally in our center lasts only 1 week in uncomplicated cases of pure SCI, i.e., without multiple system problems. The purpose of this phase is to make sure the patient is physiologically and neurologically stable and can not only survive out of the ICU, but also function well with the decreased acuity of physician and nursing care. At the beginning of this phase, allied health professionals from the rehabilitation center play a larger role in the patient's daily activity schedule, although most of the programs should have been initiated while the patient was still in the ICU. The goal of this subacute phase of care includes getting patients out of bed into a wheelchair and getting them to the point, endurance-wise and with regard to the safety of all systems, that they can actively participate in the rehabilitation program. Ongoing evaluations and reevaluations from the rehabilitation team are frequent during this period, which can range from a week in uncomplicated cases to several months in the higher quadriplegics, especially those with ventilator dependence. Once it is determined by the SCI team that the patient is ready to move on to the next phase, logistical and medical arrangements are made for the transfer.

The rehabilitation phase is more than physical restoration. Equally important are the psychologic, social, recreational, sexual, educational, and all of the other holistic parts of a good rehabilitation experience. The overall goal of the rehabilitative phase is to return each patient to society with an optimal degree of independence and mobility. If a patient is taught only how to get in and out of bed and how to manage bowel and bladder programs, most likely the patient will go home and never leave the house again. The patient will most likely also remain a dependent, noncontributing member of society and a tremendous liability to his or her family as well as the tax-paying population. The newer scenario that has been made possible through the sophistication of the rehabilitation phase has been discharging a well-rounded, well-educated, and well-conditioned paralysis victim from the rehabilitation center. This rehabilitation graduate can reintegrate into society in a meaningful way with regard to his or her family and significant others as well as the work force. Rehabilitation for paraplegics used to average anywhere from 3 to 4 months and for quadriplegics anywhere from 6 to 8 months or even longer. Today most rehabilitation centers are able to accomplish the initial inpatient rehabilitation care in less than half of that time. This is made possible partially because of the availability of more sophisticated outpatient programs. These programs have been complemented by transitional living facilities and communal living facilities as well as more meaningful work evaluation and vocational rehabilitation programs. There has also been a significant evolution of technology available to improve the quality of life of quadriplegics and in certain cases to increase their functional capacities. At our center, outpatient SCI patients may benefit from computerized multichannel electromyography (EMG) biofeedback and functional electrical stimulation (FES) treatment modalities. EMG biofeedback is capable of identifying motor activity in some muscles that is beyond the ability of traditional motor testing methods to identify and is effective as a treatment adjunct to other interventions, such as FES and conventional physiotherapy. The closed loop FES cycle ergometry has been found to be a beneficial aerobic exercise for quadriplegic patients who are not able to achieve cardiopulmonary conditioning, such as able-bodied individuals or paraplegics with upper body functioning. This treatment involves the use of computer-controlled, low-voltage currents to stimulate the paralyzed lower limbs and generate muscle contractions, which enable the patient to pedal a cycle ergometer against resistance.

An important theme throughout the SCI system of care is prevention. Prevention of secondary complications in all phases has resulted in the fact that today the average SCI victim who survives the first year has a normal life expectancy. As a matter of fact, today paralysis victims who survive the first year die of the same causes as their able-bodied peers, i.e., cancer, stroke, and heart disease, rather than renal failure and decubitus ulcers, which, as recently as several years ago, were the major causes of death in this population. Among the most important aspects of the prevention of complications after hospitalization are the outpatient clinics, which are staffed by a multidisciplinary team of SCI physicians, nurses, and allied health professionals. These clinics should be visited by the SCI patient at least every 6 months. As recently as 10 years ago, quadriplegics were readmitted to a hospital with complications for an average of 3 weeks a year and paraplegics for 2 weeks a year. Today, rehospitalizations occur rarely and continue to be reduced owing to improvements in medical care and better compliance by a more educated SCI consumer population.

SCI patients continue to present one of the most complex and perplexing clinical challenges to critical care medicine in the 1990s. This challenge has been met head-on, however, and today owing to a combination of factors, including commitment to a systems approach to care and a higher level of sophistication of ICU staff and better technology and medications, not only is there reduced morbidity and mortality, but also a better prognosis for neurologic outcome and recovery. Today a reasonable quality of life can be a reality for patients with paralysis.

REFERENCES

1. Stover, S. L., and Fine, P. R. (Eds.): Spinal Cord Injury: The Facts and Figures. Birmingham, University of Alabama at Birmingham, 1986.
2. Young, J. S., and Northrup, N. E.: Statistical information pertaining to some of the most commonly asked questions about spinal cord injury. SCI Digest, 1:11, 1979.
3. Frankowski, R. F., Annagers, J. F., and Whitman, S.: Epidemiological and descriptive studies. Part 1: The descriptive epidemiology of head trauma in the US. In Central Nervous System Trauma Status Report. Edited by D. P. and J. T. Povlishock. Bethesda, MD, National Institutes of Health, 1985, p. 33.
4. Green, B. A., and Eismont, F. J.: Acute spinal cord injury: a systems approach. Centr. Nerv. Syst. Trauma, 1:173, 1984.
5. Green, B. A., Eismont, F. J., and O'Heir, J. T.: Pre-hospital management of spinal cord injuries. Paraplegia, 25:229, 1987.
6. Thal, E. R., and Ramenofsky, M. L. (Eds.): The Advanced Trauma Life Support Program, Instructor Manual. Chicago, American College of Surgeons, 1989.
7. Green, B. A., Klose, K. J., Eismont, F. J., and O'Heir, J. T.: Immediate management of the spinal cord injured patient. In The Spinal Cord Injured Patient: Comprehensive Management. Edited by B. Y. Lee, L. E. Ostrander, G. V. B. Cochran, and W. W. Shaw. Philadelphia, W. B. Saunders, 1991, p. 24.
8. Green, B. A., Eismont, F. J., and O'Heir, J. T.: Spinal cord injury—a systems approach: prevention, emergency medical services, and emergency room management. Crit. Care Clin., 3:471, 1987.
9. Green, B. A., Klose, J. K., and Goldberg, M. L.: Clinical and research considerations in spinal cord injury. In Central Nervous System Trauma Status Report. Edited by D. P. Becker and J. T. Povlishock. Bethesda, MD, National Institutes of Health, 1985, p. 341.
10. Green, B. A., Green, K. L., and Klose, K. J.: Kinetic therapy for spinal cord injury. Spine, 8:722, 1983.
11. Consensus Conference: Prevention of venous thrombosis and pulmonary embolism. JAMA, 256:744, 1986.

12. Lind, B., Bake, B., Lundqvist, C., and Nordwal, A.: Influence of halo vest treatment on vital capacity. Spine, *12:*449, 1987.
13. Gilbert, J.: Critical care management of the patient with acute spinal cord injury. Crit. Care Clin., *3:*549, 1987.
14. Faden, A. I., Jacobs, T. P., and Smith, M. T.: Thyrotropin releasing hormone in experimental spinal injury: dose response and late treatment. Neurology, *34:*11, 1984.
15. Flamm, E. S., et al.: Experimental spinal cord injury: treatment with naloxone. Neurosurgery, *10:*3, 1982.
16. Gore, R., Mintzer, R., and Calenoff, L.: Gastrointestinal complications of spinal cord injury. Spine, *6:*538, 1981.
17. Apelgren, K. N., and Wilmore, D. W.: Nutritional care of the critically ill patient. Surg. Clin. North Am., *63:*497, 1983.
18. Bildsten, C., and Lamid, S.: Nutritional management of a patient with brain damage and spinal cord injury. Arch. Phys. Med. Rehabil., *64:*382, 1983.
19. Thomas, J.: Spinal Cord Injury: The Facts and Figures, Medical Sciences Programs and Spinal Cord Injury Program. Washington, D.C., Department of Education, National Institute of Handicapped Research, 1986.
20. Owens, G. F., and Addonizio, J. C.: Urologic evaluation and management of the spinal cord injured patient. *In* The Spinal Cord Injured Patient: Comprehensive Management. Edited by B. Y. Lee, L. E. Ostrander, G. V. B. Cochran, and W. W. Shaw. Philadelphia, W. B. Saunders, 1991, p. 124.
21. Slabaugh, P. B., and Nickel, V. L.: Complications associated with the Stryker frame. J. Bone Joint Surg., *60A:*1111, 1978.
22. Smith, T. K., Whitaker, J., and Stauffer, E. S.: Complications associated with the use of the circular electric turning frame. J. Bone Joint Surg., *57:*711, 1975.
23. Stover, S. L.: Heterotopic ossification. *In* Management of Spinal Cord Injuries. Edited by R. F. Bloch and M. Basbaum. Baltimore, William & Wilkins, 1986, p. 284.
24. Woodbury, B., and Redd, C.: Psychological issues and approaches. *In* Spinal Cord Injury: Concepts and Management Approaches. Edited by L. E. Buchanan and D. A. Nawoczenski. Baltimore, Williams & Wilkins, 1987, p. 185.

Section Two

THE RESPIRATORY SYSTEM

Chapter 10

RESPIRATORY FAILURE, RESPIRATORY MUSCLES, AND THE WORK OF BREATHING

JOHN J. MARINI

The primary purpose of the lungs is to accomplish exchange of metabolically essential gases (O_2 and CO_2) with the environment. Given this overall objective, respiratory failure can be defined as the inability to maintain stable and homeostatically appropriate blood gas concentrations without intolerable dyspnea or external (usually mechanical) assistance. Respiratory failure is sometimes classified as acute or chronic, depending on the serum concentrations of bicarbonate, O_2 and CO_2 measured in the arterial blood. Yet, this distinction has limited utility, in that the blood gases can remain abnormal and the respiratory system seriously dysfunctional (but well compensated) on a long-term basis, without failing to achieve its primary purpose of taking in oxygen and eliminating CO_2 at metabolically appropriate rates. In a real sense, therefore, chronic hypoxemia or hypercapnia do not necessarily denote chronic **failure** of the system.

The metabolic output of CO_2 is linked to O_2 consumption in a ratio that varies little in the "steady state." Nonetheless, O_2 and CO_2 are transported by different mechanisms. Whereas the carrying capacity for oxygen is limited by the concentration and circulation rate of hemoglobin, the CO_2 content of blood is an essentially linear function of its partial pressure.[1] Because CO_2 is more tissue soluble than O_2, body stores of these two gases are vastly different. Consequently, changing the rate of ventilation produces different effects on the blood and tissue concentrations of O_2 and CO_2[2] (Fig. 10-1). Immediately following the abrupt onset of apnea, for example, O_2 plummets, whereas CO_2 rises only slowly (about 6 mm Hg in the first minute and 3 to 6 mm Hg every minute thereafter).

Concentration differences drive gases from the alveolar spaces to the pulmonary capillary blood. Alveolar concentrations of O_2 and CO_2 are functions of their relative rates of replenishment and depletion by the flows of alveolar gas and blood. The normally chosen rates of ventilation and perfusion achieve an oxygen tension that ensures full saturation of arterial hemoglobin and an arterial CO_2 concentration that guarantees a ventilatory reserve adequate for high levels of metabolic activity, a normally responsive ventilatory drive, and a modest work of breathing.

Although the gas exchanging functions of the lung often fail simultaneously, more often, dysfunction of one mechanism of gas exchange predominates. Respiratory failure can be subclassified as **parenchymal** failure due to injury to the lung tissue itself, and **pump** failure, due to the result of a disproportion between the ventilatory workload and the capability of the ventilatory musculature to meet it. Seriously dysfunctional O_2 exchange characterizes parenchymal failure, whereas hypercapnia is the hallmark of pump failure.

In a certain sense, the primary manifestations of respiratory failure relate to the abnormal gas concentrations themselves. Serious aberrancies of blood gas tensions and contents result in a spectrum of secondary changes, such as those mediated by intracellular acidosis and by the release of adrenergic and stress hormones.[3] Apart from the dyspnea that accompanies failure of the ventilatory process, dysfunction of oxygen-sensitive vital organs, alteration of right ventricular afterload, and redistribution of the pulmonary and systemic circulations are some of the most important of many well known consequences of acutely altered blood gases.

PARENCHYMAL FAILURE

Background and Pre-ICU Phase

To understand parenchymal failure requires comprehension of alveolar gas kinetics and the mechanisms by which hypoxemia can develop. As typically classified, hypoxemia can be the result of six fundamental mechanisms acting separately or together (Table 10-1):

Reduced Fraction of Inspired Oxygen

Although virtually never a problem in the intensive care setting, the very low inspired O_2 concentrations encountered at high altitudes or in fires occurring in closed spaces may be the proximate cause of hypoxemia.

Hypoventilation

When breathing atmospheric concentrations of O_2 under normobaric conditions, the concentrations of nitrogen in the blood and alveolus are relatively constant and unaffected by changes in ventilation. Therefore, the rise in alveolar CO_2 tension that results from hypoventilation produces a consequent reduction in P_{AO_2}. Immediately after the onset of hypoventilation, and before the steady state is established, O_2 is reabsorbed more quickly than the CO_2 concentration accumulates, accounting for disproportionate desaturation encountered during transient hypoventilation.[4] In the clinical setting, the shallow

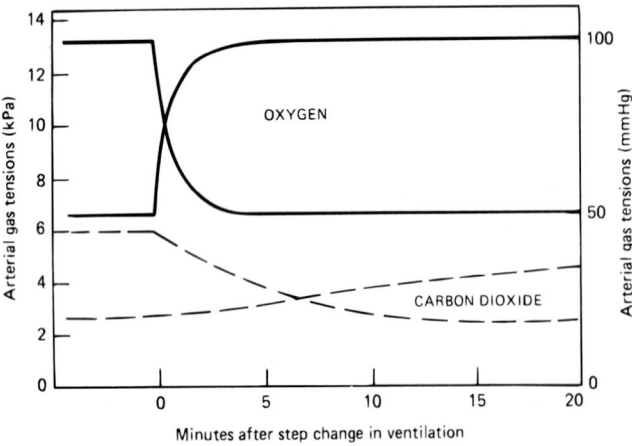

Fig. 10–1. Time course of the rates of change in arterial blood gas tensions following step changes in ventilation (normal subject). Because the body stores of O_2 are much smaller than those of CO_2, arterial PO_2 equilibrates at a much faster rate. Note that the $PaCO_2$ equilibration time following a step **increase** in the rate of ventilation is shorter than for a step decrease of equal magnitude. (From Nunn, J. F.: Applied Respiratory Physiology. 3rd Ed. Boston, Butterworths, 1987, p. 272.)

breathing of hypoventilation is often accompanied by microatelectasis (and shunting).

Diffusion Limitation

Because oxygen transfer depends on the gradient of PO_2 existing between alveolus and blood, the permeability of the alveolar membrane for O_2, and the duration of transit, it is theoretically possible that a limitation in the transfer capacity of the alveolus might develop, should the time available for transcapillary O_2 transfer prove inadequate. Reductions of alveolar surface area or increases of blood flow enhance the possibility of diffusion limitation, whereas diffusion limitation can be at least partially offset by an increase in FIO_2.

Shunt

Complete failure of ventilation relative to perfusion diverts mixed venous blood directly into the arterial circulation. Such admixture may be the result of lung infiltration, or of an abnormal intrapulmonary or intracardiac communication. Pulmonary hypertension may initiate or accentuate right to left transfer of systemic venous blood at the right atrial level.

Ventilation—Perfusion Mismatching

Because the tensions of alveolar PO_2 and PCO_2 are set by the relative rates of ventilation and perfusion, hypoxemia results whenever the rate of ventilation is insufficient to reload the suffusing venous blood with oxygen. Large regional discrepancies in V/Q matching lead to local O_2 desaturation and arterial hypoxemia. This mechanism virtually always contributes significantly to hypoxemia in the clinical setting.

Low Mixed Venous Oxygen Tension

Mixed venous O_2 tension can plummet when oxygen delivery to the systemic tissues fails to keep pace with oxygen consumption.[5] Such circumstances are likely to develop during states of pathologically depressed cardiac output or severe anemia. As desaturated blood perfuses alveoli with suboptimal ventilation, the capillary O_2 concentration reflects the deficit, contributing to arterial desaturation.

General Approach to Problems of Parenchymal Failure

Oxygenation failure can result from any process interfering with the transfer of oxygen across the alveolar capillary. Such problems include pneumonitis, atelectasis, congestive heart failure and the adult respiratory distress syndrome (ARDS). The underlying process must be reversed whenever possible. The adjunctive treatment of these problems includes the administration of supplementary oxygen, clearance of retained secretions, reversal of atelectasis or tissue edema, and improvement of the oxygen demand/delivery ratio (e.g., by cardiovascular support, or by reducing VO_2 with sedation, analgesia, or relief of an excessive breathing workload).

ICU PHASE OF PARENCHYMAL FAILURE

ARDS is the prototypical problem of parenchymal failure that requires support in an ICU environment. This condition, which is well covered elsewhere in this book, develops when the lung tissue sustains acute and generalized injury sufficient to breach the alveolar-capillary barrier to protein. Proteinaceous alveolar edema is soon followed by the formation of hyaline membranes, hemorrhagic infiltration, and alveolar microcollapse. Extensive regions of the lung become airless, as this process replaces all but 25 to 50% of the normal aerated lung volume with atelectasis, edema, or cellular infiltrate.

No treatment currently available is known to accelerate the process of recovery from ARDS. Hence, a rational approach to management of this problem is to provide adequate support while avoiding further organ injury or compromise of gas exchange. Unfortunately, most types of treatment leveled at ARDS have the potential for compromising tissue oxygen delivery or furthering tissue damage. For example, whereas it is appropriate to limit the hydrostatic forces applied across the permeable vascular endothelium, it is equally important not to compromise tissue

Table 10–1. Mechanisms of Hypoxemia

Mechanism	Clinical Example
Reduced FIO_2	High altitude exposure
Alveolar Hypoventilation	Sedative ingestion
Veno-arterial Shunting	Atelectasis
Ventilation/Perfusion Mismatching	Acute Bronchitis
*Low Mixed Venous O_2 Saturation	Circulatory insufficiency
*Diffusion Limitation	Exercise hypoxemia

* These mechanisms are secondary contributors to one or more primary causes of hypoxemia.

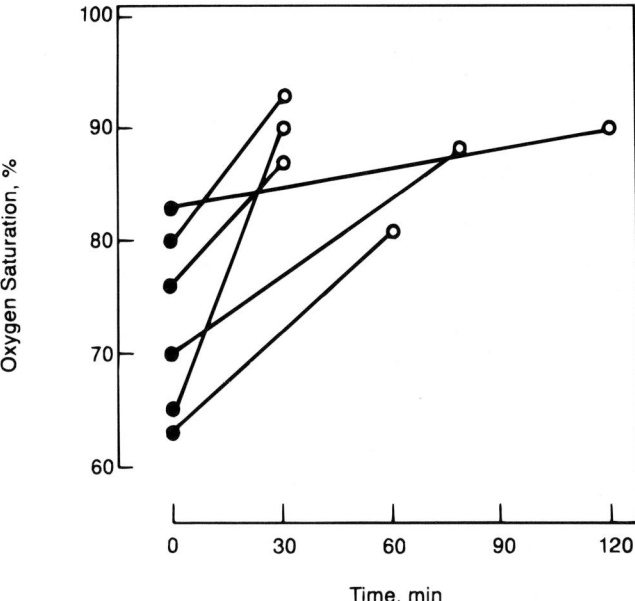

Fig. 10–2. Oxygen saturation recorded by oximetry in an intermittently agitated patient with the adult respiratory distress syndrome, before (closed circles) and after (open circles) bolus dosing of a paralytic agent (pancuronium). This patient, under treatment with positive end-expiratory pressure, was actively using the expiratory muscles and experienced a significant reduction in cardiac output during muscle relaxation. (From Coggeshall, J. W., Marini, J. J., and Newman, J. H.: Improved oxygenation after muscle relaxation in the adult respiratory distress syndrome. Arch. Intern. Med., 145:1718, 1985.)

oxygen delivery by overly aggressive diuresis. Sufficient hemoglobin should circulate to maximize tissue O₂ delivery. The appropriate hemoglobin concentration to realize this goal has not been determined; however, the appropriate concentration almost certainly lies within the range of 10 to 13 g/dl.[6] Cardiac output should be maintained at levels commensurate with normal urine flow, hepatic function, and nervous system operation.

By providing measurements of central vascular pressures (CVP and wedge) and cardiac output and mixed venous oxygen saturation, the Swan-Ganz (balloon flotation) catheter often provides data vital in adjusting fluids, end-expiratory lung volume, cardiovascular support, and inspired oxygen saturation to optimize O₂ delivery.[7] The mixed venous O₂ saturation often reflects the impact of agitation, anxiety, or the work of breathing on arterial oxygenation. A severely depressed Sv_{O_2} may be one indication of a disproportion between O₂ consumption and delivery. Sedation or paralysis may then prove to have a beneficial effect on both arterial O₂ saturation and systemic O₂ utilization (Fig. 10–2).[8] Mechanical ventilation not only assists the gas exchanging functions of the lung but also relieves the breathing workload which reduces the oxygen consumed by the ventilatory apparatus.[9] When cardiac reserves are marginal, relieving this burden may help improve the O₂ delivered to other vital organs.[10]

The question of what constitutes appropriate target values for the arterial blood gases that guide clinical decision making is currently a topic of intense debate.[11,12] Satisfactory resolution of this controversy has assumed increasing urgency with the recognition of the serious damage that can be inflicted by the use of the positive pressures required to "normalize" arterial pH, P_{CO_2}, and O₂ saturation. Blood gas normalization often requires the application of pressures significantly higher than those for which the healthy lung was designed. Recent data from several laboratories indicate that peak transalveolar tidal pressures that exceed approximately 35 cm H₂O risk not only overt rupture to the normal alveolus (with consequent radiographically definable barotrauma), but also increased permeability of the alveolar-capillary membrane (Fig. 10–3).[13,14] This latter damage, more subtle and less commonly recognized than the radiographically distinctive forms of alveolar rupture, may actually perpetuate the very type of injury that mechanical ventilation is attempting to treat.

The reason why pressures of this magnitude prove damaging may be found in recent observations of the radiographic appearance[15] and lung pathology[16] of ARDS. Most clinicians define ARDS as a process of diffuse lung injury and increased elastic recoil which is quite unlike lobar pneumonia, atelectasis, contusion, and other regional disorders. While the injury may indeed be widespread, its manifestations clearly are not, at least not from the viewpoint of lung mechanics. Radiographic studies have convincingly shown that most detectable consolidation occurs in dependent regions,[15,17] whereas nondependent areas tend to remain normally aerated (Fig. 10–4). Such observations strongly suggest that the injured lung is not so much stiff as it is functionally small. The alveoli that remain patent may be normally compliant, and perhaps unusually fragile. Therefore, pressures that apply unusual distending forces are likely to injure the viable tissue that remains.

Certain types of ventilator induced barotrauma, long recognized in children, have only recently been identified in adults. Interstitial emphysema,[18] tension cyst formation,[19] bronchopulmonary damage,[20] and perhaps even systemic gas embolism[21] are now known to be frequent, and perhaps unavoidable, consequences of prolonged exposure to transalveolar ventilatory pressures that exceed approximately 40 cm H₂O. It is intriguing to consider the possibility that such types of machine-related damage might produce the entrenched infections that serve as reservoirs driving the sepsis syndrome and multisystem organ failure later in the course of these illnesses.

Not all clinicians realize how intimately the provision of ventilatory support is linked to the need to apply pressure. For an identical impedance presented by the lung and chest wall, minute ventilation correlates linearly with mean alveolar pressure.[22] In addition, the efficiency of oxygen exchange across the alveolus in this setting also relates directly to mean alveolar pressure.[23] With conventional treatment, therefore, the primary therapeutic objective of safely achieving adequate gas exchange is inextricably linked to pressure application.

Although excessive pressures must not be applied during the tidal cycle, it is equally clear that a certain minimal level of transalveolar pressure must be maintained to keep the lung fully recruited. Studies conducted in animals, infants, and patients with acute lung injury have demon-

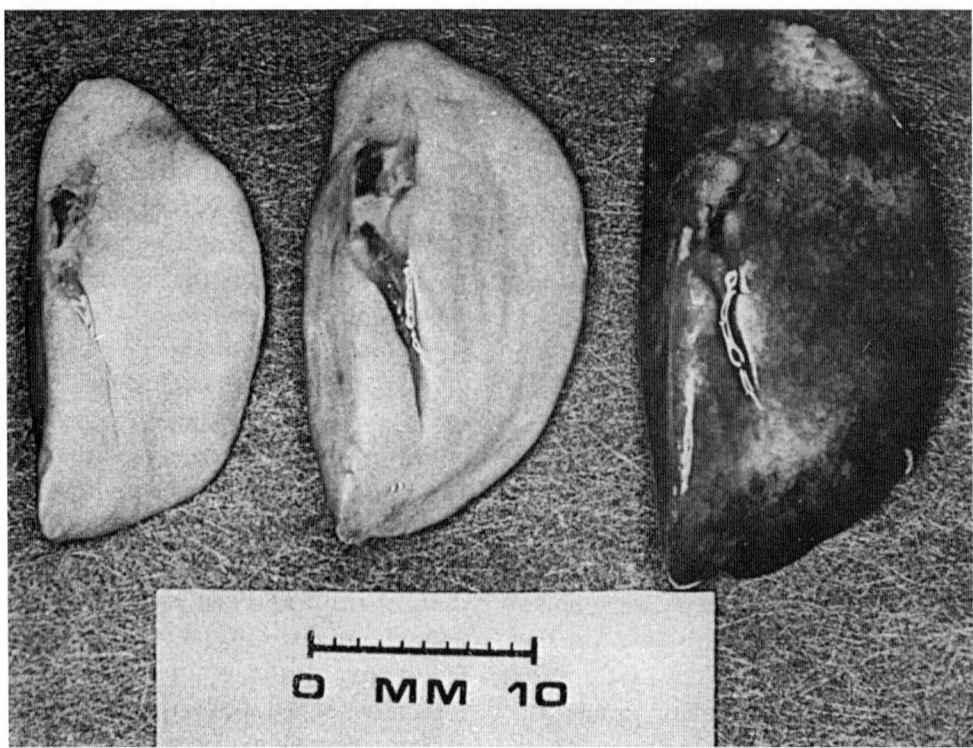

Fig. 10-3. Gross appearance of the left lungs of normal, anesthetized rats ventilated for 60 minutes or less with peak and end-expiratory airway pressures as designated. All animals exposed to peak airway pressures of 45 cm H_2O experienced perivascular edema. Those ventilated at high peak pressure without positive end-expiratory pressure also incurred alveolar hemorrhage and pulmonary edema (right). Transalveolar pressures were somewhat less than these values. (From Webb, H., and Tierney, D.: Experimental pulmonary edema due to intermittent positive pressure ventilation with high inflation pressures: protection by positive end-expiratory pressure. Am. Rev. Respir. Dis., 110:556, 1974.)

strated the need to maintain sufficient end-expiratory alveolar pressure to prevent transient or persistent closure of otherwise viable lung units (see Fig. 10-3).[24,25] Tidal closure and reopening of jeopardized alveoli may be an essential mechanism of ventilator-induced lung injury. In the setting of ARDS, there exist 3 general classes of alveoli: (1) those that remain open without the aid of an end-expiratory bias pressure; (2) those that are densely infiltrated and unlikely to aerate whatever pressure is applied to them; and (3) those that are potentially recruitable at modest end-expiratory biasing pressures, generally in the range of 10 to 15 cm H_2O. The alveoli of this last category may be very important to oxygen exchange because the perfusion to these units tends to be well preserved.

The mechanism of positive end-expiratory pressure (PEEP) has been extensively investigated. It now seems

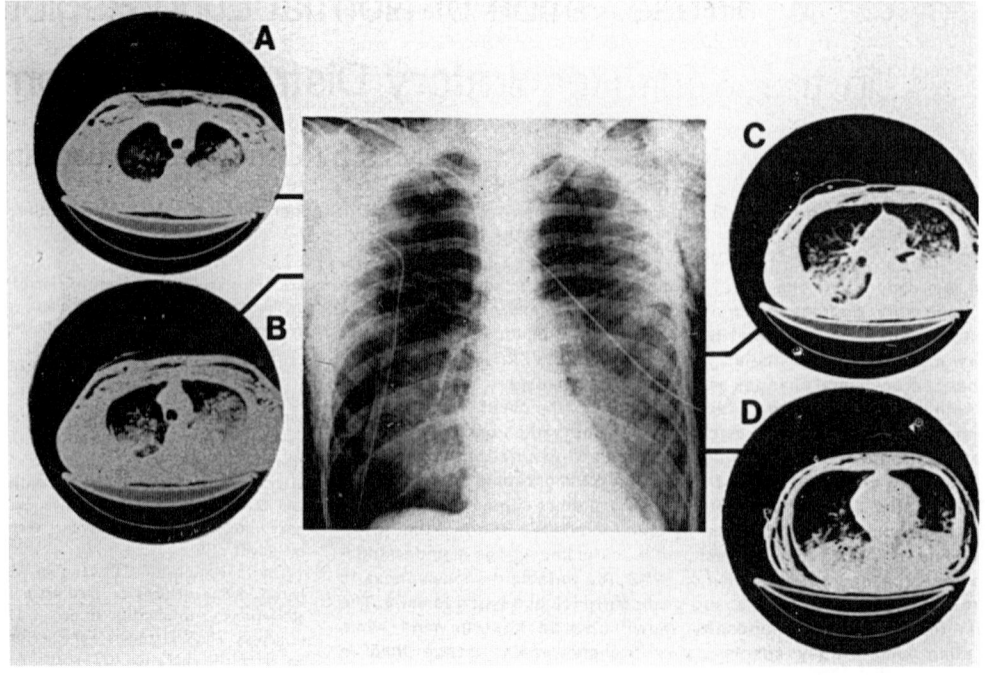

Fig. 10-4. Comparison of standard anteroposterior chest roentgenogram of adult respiratory distress syndrome with computed tomographic sections from four well-separated regions. Despite the appearance of diffuse involvement suggested by the chest film, infiltrates are actually distributed in an unbalanced fashion, with density most prominent in dependent regions. Anterior regions have nearly normal radiographic density. (From Maunder, R. J., et al.: Preservation of normal lung regions in the adult respiratory distress syndrome: analysis by computed tomography. JAMA, 255:2463, 1986.)

likely that recruitable alveoli are kept open at **transalveolar** pressures of 15 cm H$_2$O or less (which may correspond to PEEP levels as high as 20 or 25 cm H$_2$O in some instances, depending on the stiffness of the chest wall). Such pressures can be applied externally or created in the process of dynamic hyperinflation.[26] Once PEEP exceeds 15 cm H$_2$O, further increments tend to improve arterial oxygenation less impressively, and to act by different mechanisms. Redistribution of lung water from the alveolar spaces to the interstitium, a process already underway at lower PEEP levels, continues in this higher range. Perhaps more important, further improvement in the Pao$_2$ seems to depend on the simultaneous reduction of cardiac output and shunt fraction which accompany the increase in intrapleural pressure and right ventricular afterload that high PEEP entails.[27]

Duty Cycle and Inverse Ratio Ventilation

In recent years, a controversy has emerged regarding the value (or nonvalue) of inverse ratio ventilation, a ventilatory mode that extends the inspiratory duty cycle to > 0.5 (Fig. 10-5). Advocates believe that such a strategy improves oxygenation and diminishes the potential for barotrauma.[28,29] Critics question this view, suspecting that such methods are dangerous, uncomfortable, and unnecessary.[30,31] Whereas there is little evidence that ratio **inversion** per se offers "special" benefit, there is little doubt that **extending** the duty cycle can help improve gas exchange and help improve CO$_2$ exchange.[32] Actual inversion of the ratio may be unnecessary to realize such benefits.

Table 10-2. Pressure Targeted Therapeutic Strategy for Moderate to Severe ARDs

Control alveolar pressure, not Paco$_2$.
Minimize oxygen consumption.
Use low Vt & least Palv required for **unequivocal** therapeutic goals.
Hold **transalveolar** pressure (tmPalv) < 35 cm H$_2$O.
Use "permissive hypercapnia" as peak tmPalv approaches 30 cm H$_2$O.
Maintain end-expiratory Palv (PEEP + Auto-PEEP) > 7 but < 15 cm H$_2$O.
Make necessary increases of mean Paw by changing ti/ttot, not PEEP.
Consider adjunctive methods* to improve gas exchange and O$_2$ delivery.

* In addition to standard measures, such as skillful management of pulmonary vascular pressure, repositioning, use of cardiotonic agents, and minimizing O$_2$ demand, these might include (where available) such experimental methods as intravenous (IVOX) or intratracheal catheter assisted gas exchange and Ecco$_2$R.

Therapeutic Strategy for ARDS

Using the concepts just discussed, a rational approach can be formulated to the ventilatory support of patients with ARDS (Table 10-2).[33] Oxygen and ventilatory demands should be reduced to a functional minimum. It is imperative that peak alveolar pressures not rise to unsafe levels, and it is desirable that sufficient end-expiratory pressure be maintained to keep the lung near its full recruitment potential. This minimum end-expiratory alveolar pressure, the sum of PEEP and auto-PEEP, is rarely more than 7 to 15 cm H$_2$O and is usually greatest during the early phase of the disease. At the same time, the clinician should employ the least mean airway pressure needed to achieve adequate gas exchange. A strategy of "permissive hypercapnia" often proves helpful in this regard.[34] When mean airway pressure must be raised to ensure appropriate O$_2$ exchange, extending the duty cycle may be preferable to raising PEEP for at least two reasons. First, decelerating end-inspiratory flow modestly reduces the dead space fraction.[35] Second, raising PEEP forces either an increase in end-tidal alveolar pressure (when tidal volume is preserved), or a reduction in the delivered tidal volume (reducing ventilatory efficiency). Deep sedation or paralysis may be required when the duty cycle is inverted, especially during volume-controlled ventilation. On the basis of current information, reasonable target values might be: **transmural** Palvmax: ≤35 cm H$_2$O, PEEP: 7 to 15 cm H$_2$O, and inspiratory time fraction: 0.33 to 0.66, depending on the response of arterial O$_2$ saturation and the Pao$_2$/Fio$_2$ ratio.

POST-ICU PHASE OF PARENCHYMAL FAILURE

It has been my clinical experience that parenchymal failure often tends to reverse rather abruptly after weeks of little progress with gas exchange improving dramati-

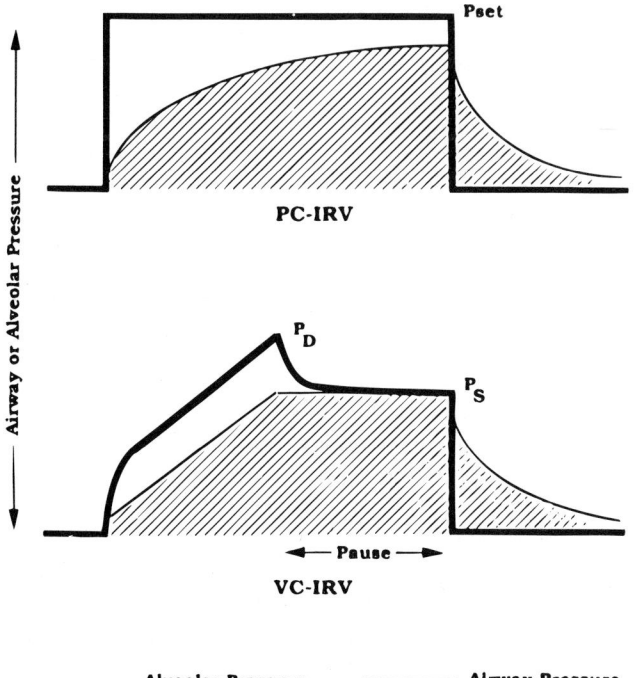

Fig. 10-5. Inverse ratio ventilation achieved by two methods. Both pressure controlled ventilation (PC-IRV) and flow controlled, volume cycled ventilation (VC-IRV) (here applied by constant flow with an end-inspiratory pause) allow for ratio inversion, with a consequent increase in mean alveolar pressure (hatched areas). Both methods also allow ventilation to distribute more evenly to compartments with different ventilatory time constants. Pset, P$_D$, and Ps are set level of airway pressure, and peak dynamic and peak static pressures, respectively. (From Marini, J. J.: Lung mechanics in the adult respiratory distress syndrome. In Clinics in Chest Medicine. Edited by H. P. Wieedemann, M. A. Matthay, and R. A. Matthay. Philadelphia, W. B. Saunders, 1990, p. 673.)

cally over a few days. This turnaround is signalled by a significant decline in the minute ventilation requirement, usually (but not invariably) occurring before oxygen exchange has improved greatly. Following weeks of therapy that has included, at various times, bed rest, sedation, and pharmacoparalysis, the ventilatory muscles are expected to be weak. However, in recent years it has become clear that many patients who experience sepsis may also be the victims of "critical illness neuromyopathy," a major cause of delayed recovery of muscle strength.[36] The combination of paralytic agents and corticosteroids can also induce myopathy and profound weakness,[37] retarding the recovery process. In these patients, tracheostomy, the use of a CPAP mask, or noninvasive ventilation with biphasic or bilevel airway pressure (Bi-Pap) may prove especially helpful after extubation. Although recuperation is often prolonged, many patients recover nearly normal lung function when tested one year later. In others, persistent restriction or obstruction can be demonstrated.[38]

VENTILATORY (PUMP) FAILURE

Background and ICU Phase

Ventilatory failure reflects a disproportion between ventilatory workload and capability. Many individuals compensate for chronic overloading of the ventilatory pump by allowing CO_2 to build to abnormal levels which improves the efficiency of each tidal breath. Hypercapnia is a necessary, but not sufficient condition; acidosis is a common, but not invariable sign.

The rate of discharge of CO_2 from the lung is a direct function of alveolar ventilation. Therefore, even though parenchymal disease impairs the efficiency of carbon dioxide elimination, such impediments can almost invariably be overcome by providing sufficient ventilation. Retention of CO_2 seldom results from infiltrative parenchymal disease alone. Rather, the proximate cause of hypercapnia and ventilatory failure is usually pump dysfunction because of a disproportion between workload and capability.

The ventilatory pumping mechanism is comprised of the controlling rhythm generator, (the ventilatory "control center"), the respiratory muscles, and the thoracic cage.[39] Serious dysfunction of any single component may be sufficient to precipitate ventilatory failure and CO_2 retention. Examples of such disorders are primary alveolar hypoventilation, myasthenia gravis, and flail chest, respectively. Frequently, a single disease process gives rise to dysfunction of more than one pump component. Morbid obesity, for example, may be accompanied by load-related dysfunction of the diaphragm and accessory inspiratory muscles, as well as by blunted chemosensitivity.[40] (The latter presumably relates to endogenous factors in combination with mass loading or sleep disturbance.)

Work of Breathing

The load that must be borne by the ventilatory pump is a function of the ventilation rate (l/min) and the energy expended per liter of tidal volume exchange. Normally, inspiration is the energetically costly process, and deflation occurs passively, powered by the elastic recoil energy stored during inspiration in the tissues of the expanded chest.[41] For this reason, and because inspiration and active exhalation are powered by different sets of muscles, it is customary to consider the energy cost of breathing only from the inspiratory side.

Oxygen Consumption

If it were possible to precisely quantify the rate of energy consumed by the ventilatory muscles during the act of breathing, such measurements would give an excellent indication of the strain experienced by the ventilatory apparatus. Attempts to quantify the energetic costs of breathing, however, are currently confined to one of several suboptimal indices: the oxygen cost to the entire body of imposing or relieving a breathing stress,[42] the magnitude of the integrated electromyographic signal recorded from a selected region,[43] and the pressure or work output of the ventilatory pump.[44,45]

For more than a half century the technique of measuring the difference in total body O_2 consumption (V_{O_2}) before and after a change in ventilatory stress has been used to estimate the O_2 cost associated with that intervention. Although such estimates attempt to quantify respiratory muscle activity at the metabolic level, such differences in O_2 consumption cannot be attributed solely to the muscles of inspiration; changes in VO_2 can result from any alterations in comfort or metabolism that occur in any organ system. Apart from the imprecision inherent in such measurements, by necessity, ΔV_{O_2} must be assessed intermittently, after some intervention has been undertaken. With these limitations in mind, it has been estimated that respiratory muscle O_2 consumption, normally <5% of V_{O_2}, may exceed 25% of the total resting V_{O_2} in the setting of acute respiratory failure.

Although seldom employed for this purpose in the clinical setting, the integrated electromyographic (EMG) signal correlates closely with the metabolic cost of muscular contraction. Theoretically, this correlation would enable "on line" monitoring of metabolic energy cost. Unfortunately, although this technique is superficially attractive, unresolved problems abound. The electrical activity of a single muscle does not necessarily reflect the global activity of the entire muscular pump, and it is difficult to maintain effective contact of a surface electrode for an extended time. These problems notwithstanding, the EMG of certain accessory muscles (e.g., sternocleidomastoid) may yet prove a useful indicator of ventilatory stress.[46]

Mechanical Output

Given the extraordinary difficulty of obtaining accurate, representative, and continuous estimates of respiratory muscle metabolic activity, assessing the **mechanical** output of the ventilatory pump poses an attractive option. The mechanical power of the ventilatory pump during inspiration is the product of minute ventilation and the average inspiratory pressure (P) it must develop (Fig. 10-6). At any instant, the pressure cost of inspiration relevant to breathing effort is specified by a simplified inspiratory

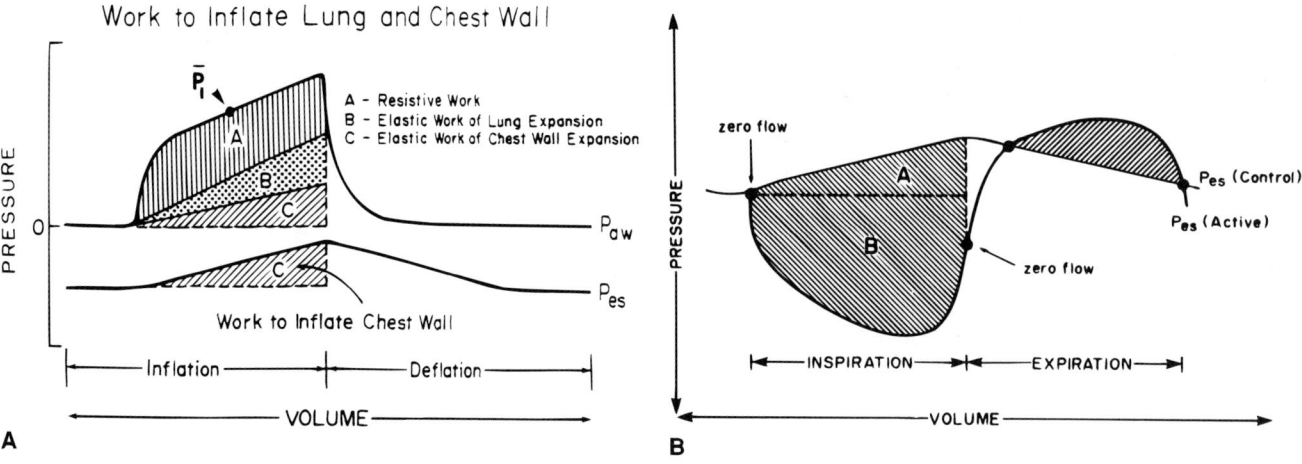

Fig. 10-6. Work required to inflate the total respiratory system during passive inflation at a constant rate of inspiratory flow (A) and during spontaneous ventilation (B). Because the product of tidal volume and mean inflation pressure (PI) quantifies the inspiratory work/breath under passive conditions, PI reflects the inspiratory work per liter of ventilation. The subcomponents of the workload can be quantified as the airway (Paw) or esophageal (Pes) pressure-volume areas indicated. During spontaneous breathing a Pes-volume area (B) reflects the work done across the lung and external circuit; the work done in expanding the passive chest wall (A) is added to estimate the total work of chest expansion. (Adapted from Marini, J. J., Smith, T. C., and Lamb, V. J.: External work output and force generation during synchronized intermittent mechanical ventilation: effect of machine assistance on breathing effort. Am. Rev. Respir. Dis., *138*:1169, 1988; and Marini, J. J.: Strategies to Minimize Breathing Effort during Mechanical Ventilation. Philadelphia, W. B. Saunders, 1990.)

"equation of motion" of the ventilatory system, which in modified form can be expressed:

$$P = Pr + Pelt + Pap$$

Here, the pressure applied across the respiratory system can be viewed as the sum of three components:

- The flow resistive pressure (Pr)
- The tidal elastic pressure (Pelt)
- The end-expiratory residual pressure (auto-PEEP, Pap) in excess of any PEEP already applied at the airway opening (Fig. 10-7)

Pr is the product of flow rate ($\dot{V}$) and inspiratory airflow resistance (Ri). Tidal elastic pressure (Pelt) is the ratio of the volume (Vi) inspired in excess of the end-expiratory value and the compliance of the respiratory system (C). When PEEP is in use, the **total** residual end-expiratory alveolar pressure (Pex) is the sum of two pressures, one externally applied at the level of the airway opening (PEEP), and the other developed by dynamic hyperinflation (Pap). With PEEP also considered, a more complete equation of motion can be written:

$$P = Ri\dot{V} + Vi/C + Pex$$

Note, however, only the Pap portion of Pex affects the pressure cost to the patient during unaided or partially assisted breathing. This analysis, although conceptually useful, assumes linear impedance and ignores viscoelasticity, pendelluft inertia, and sundry other pressure losses that may occur in patients with acute illnesses.

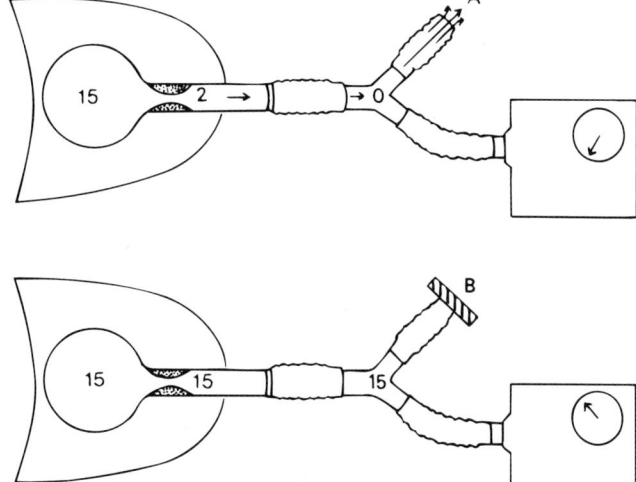

Fig. 10-7. Concept of dynamic hyperinflation and Auto-PEEP. When insufficient time is allowed between inspiratory cycles to permit the lung to deflate to its resting equilibrium volume, alveolar pressure remains positive at end exhalation with respect to that applied at the airway opening, and flow continues throughout the expiratory period (A). This auto-PEEP can be detected by timed occlusion of the expiratory port (B), stopping flow and allowing auto-PEEP to be approximated from the accompanying change in central airway pressure. (From Marini, J. J.: Respiratory Medicine and Intensive Care for the Houseofficer. Baltimore, Williams & Wilkins, 1981, p. 139.)

For a given level of ventilation, the primary means by which the pressure cost of ventilation can be varied is by manipulation of the ventilatory pattern. Whatever the specific components of impedance, the least pressure cost is incurred during constant flow at a small tidal volume and high frequency.[47] Rapid initial flows (as during inflation with constant pressure) require relatively higher levels of alveolar tension. The specific choice of tidal volume and breathing frequency is important; the lower the tidal volume, the lower the elastic pressure cost of each tidal breath. The total pressure-volume product (work) of two breaths, each half as large as their sum, will be considerably less than that of the larger breath (Fig. 10-8). If tidal volume is reduced too far, however, the **effective** component of each tidal breath ventilating the alveolar compartment will fall disproportionately. This occurs as the physiologic dead space fraction, influenced by its relatively fixed "anatomic" (series) component, rises precipitously at very small tidal volumes.[48] Thus, from the standpoint of the energy required to accomplish a given level of alveolar ventilation, an optimal frequency-tidal volume combination exists.

The mechanical work of breathing (Wb) during inspiration is defined as the product of the pressure difference applied across the respiratory system (Pi) and the flow ($\dot{V}$) it produces, integrated over the inspiratory period (ti)[49]:

$$Wb = \int_0^{Ti} Pi\dot{V}dt$$

Expressed differently:

$$Wb = \int_0^{V_T} Pi\, dv$$

These integrals can be graphically assessed as the area enclosed beneath the inspiratory pressure-volume envelope

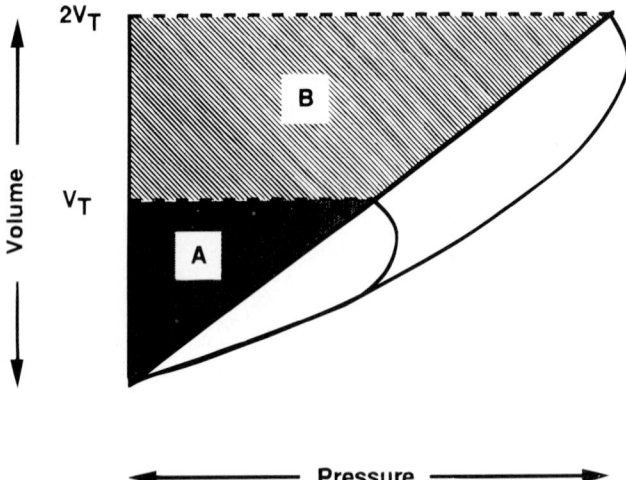

Fig. 10-8. Schematic diagram of the work performed during two breaths of different size in a subject with unchanging impedance to breathing. Two breaths of size V$_T$ are associated with less total work (twice area A) than that of a single breath of size 2V$_T$ (A + B), because of the reduced elastic pressure requirement.

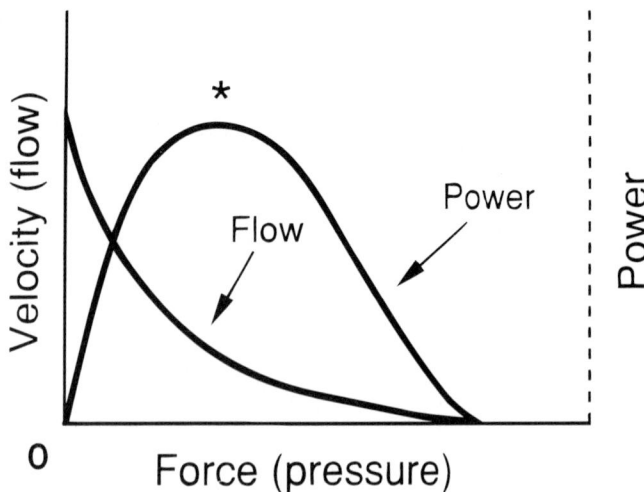

Fig. 10-9. Schematic force-velocity (pressure-flow) relationship for contracting skeletal muscles, such as those that comprise the respiratory system. For a given level of neural stimulation, maximal pressure is developed isometrically (flow = 0). The maximal rate of volume change is developed under completely unloaded conditions (pressure = 0). The pressure flow product, equivalent to work performed per unit time (power), is maximized at some intermediate value (*).

(see Fig. 10-6). **Work** of breathing is not synonymous with **effort** of breathing. For a given impedance condition, however, patient effort tends to parallel the ventilatory workload. The mechanical work accomplished by a given pressure difference is a function of the impedance to movement. No mechanical work is accomplished during isometric efforts, even though the pressure developed and the O$_2$ consumed may be great. The power curve (Fig. 10-9) inscribed across a range of loads and contraction velocities illustrates the fallacy of using work to index effort under conditions of changing afterload to contraction; for this purpose, the pressure-time product is preferable.[50] The directly measurable pressure-time product (PTP) can be defined as the time-weighted integral of the inspiratory pressure (Pi) applied across the lung and airway (Ppl, when assessed during spontaneous breathing), or across the entire respiratory system (Paw, during passive inflation).

Spontaneous Breathing Cycles

The equation of motion summarizes the factors that influence the pressure-time product; therefore, during constant flow:

$$Pi = (V_T/ti)Ri + V_T/2C + Pap$$

$$Pt = (V_TRi) + V_Tti/2C + Papti$$

$$Pt = (V_TRi) + (60z\dot{V}e)/2f^2C + 60zPap/f$$

With all other elements of this equation remaining unchanged, an increased minute ventilation, higher resistance (Ri), lower compliance (C), larger tidal volume (V$_T$), longer inspiratory time fraction (z), lower frequency (f) or greater auto-PEEP (Pap) will each increase the pressure-time product.[41,44,51] When the patient supplies all of the pressure, these are the factors that influence breathing effort. In this context, dynamic hyperinflation deserves special mention. When the respiratory system fails to return to its equilibrium position between tidal cycles, the deflationary pressure that remains presents a threshold load that must be overcome before the inspiratory cycle can begin.[51] This load often adds significantly to the pressure cost of breathing, particularly when inspiratory forces must be generated by a ventilatory pump poised at a mechanically disadvantageous, hyperinflated position (see later in this chapter).

In the clinical setting, the external circuitry can influence the work associated with spontaneous breathing cycles. Early machine circuits added greatly to the ventilatory work of breathing, because inspiratory demand valves were often sluggish, difficult to open, and flow resistive once gas flow was underway.[52] As a general rule, systems that provided continuous flow in the external circuit proved less energy costly, reduced delays, and eliminated opening pressures. Although certain continuous flow circuits are outstandingly efficient,[53] many of the latest generation demand valve circuits are highly responsive and comparable to their continuous flow counterparts.

However efficient an external CPAP circuit may be, the work of inspiring through the endotracheal tube must still be overcome. This single component may account for the major fraction of the patient's inspiratory effort, particularly when minute ventilation is high.[54,55] Tubes left in place for long periods may present resistances significantly higher than those of similar caliber tested in vitro[55] (Fig. 10-10). Because tube resistance relates inversely to the fourth power of tube radius and directly to its length, alter- ations in lumen size caused by secretions, bends or kinks, or impingement of the tube tip against the tracheal mucosa can influence impedance impressively.

Partially Assisted Breathing Cycles

Delineation of the factors that influence patient effort during partially assisted breathing cycles is somewhat more complicated. Here, the equation of motion refers to the entire patient-ventilator system, whereas the component of interest is the patient's alone. During the machine-assisted cycles of **assist-control (AMV)**, the key determinant of the patient's work per breath is the relationship between flow demand and flow delivery.[56-58] Minute ventilation is an obvious influence on ventilatory demand. Factors which influence dyspnea (such as triggering sensitivity and the depth, synchrony, and velocity of the machine cycle) are also crucially important because the machine would easily accomplish the entire work of breathing if the patient could only relax immediately after signalling the need for a breath. The influence of auto-PEEP is noteworthy, because it effectively adds to the pressure threshold that must be overcome to initiate inspiration.[51,57]

The patient's effort during a flow controlled, volume cycled breath can be assessed as the difference in machine work observed during controlled and machine-assisted cycles of identical depth and flow delivery pattern[58] (Fig. 10-11). Because all force generated by the patient originates external to the lungs, the deficit in machine work can be assessed using either the airway or the esophageal pressure, plotted against volume.

It is instructive to compare the patient's work of breathing during the adjacent spontaneous and machine assisted cycles of **synchronized intermittent mandatory ventilation (SIMV)**. Here, the patient's chemical drive to breathe is essentially unchanged from cycle to cycle. Dyspneic subjects fail to alter their breathing effort within the duration of a single inspiration, so that pressure time products computed for adjacent spontaneous and machine-assisted cycles are comparable.[50] The computed external work of breathing, however, is quite different for these same breaths. Surprisingly, the work accomplished during the machine-aided cycle is actually **greater** than that during the spontaneous breath due to the markedly lower effective afterload to muscle contraction.

Pressure support ventilation (PSV) provides another form of partial assistance that deviates significantly from SIMV in several ways. Unlike SIMV, pressure support aids every spontaneous breathing cycle by an amount selected by the clinician.[59] Because the "off-trigger" of pressure support is flow determined, the depth and duration of each breathing cycle are free to vary with the patient's vigor of inspiration. PSV is the only means currently available to help offset the resistance offered by the endotracheal (*ET*) tube. Unless and until central airway pressure is controlled at the carinal end of the ET tube, no CPAP circuit, no matter how perfect, can fulfill this function. For this reason, it is good practice to provide a low level of PSV (3 to 10 cm H$_2$O) to all ventilatory cycles during CPAP or SIMV.[60]

Work of breathing during PSV is computed differently from that during flow controlled, volume cycled ventila-

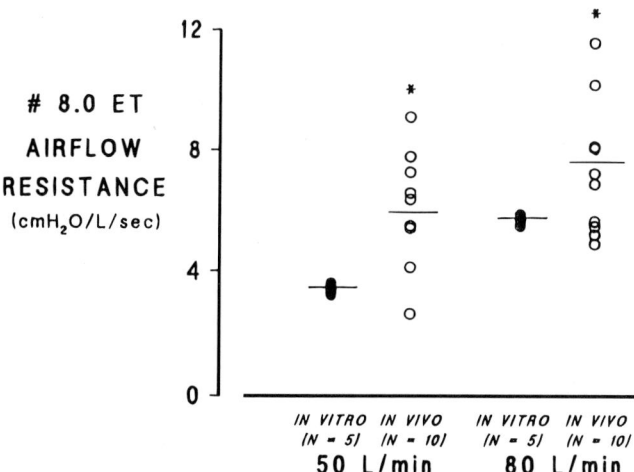

Fig. 10-10. Comparison of the resistance measured through an endotracheal tube of internal diameter 8.0 mm before insertion (in vitro) and after several days of use (in vivo). Certain patients experienced marked increases of tube resistance over that expected, presumably because of secretions, bends, kinks or partial occlusion at the tube tip. (From Wright, P. W., Marini, J. J., and Bernard, G. R.: In vitro versus in vivo comparison of endotracheal tube airflow resistance. Am. Rev. Respir. Dis., *140*:10, 1989.)

tion. Direct calculation of the work of breathing requires placement of an esophageal balloon to estimate intrapleural pressure, the patient's component of the driving force for airflow, and lung expansion. The work of expanding the chest wall must still be estimated independently from its passive inflation characteristics. One simple method for estimating the patient's work during a pressure-supported breathing cycle is to use the modified equation of motion to estimate the total work accomplished by the patient and machine working together, subtracting from this total amount the measured machine component. Ideally, the machine's work contribution (Wm) during pressure-supported inspiration is simply the product of the targeted pressure (PS) and the tidal volume (V_T), assuming that a true square wave of pressure is applied continuously during inspiration:

$$Wm = \int_0^{ti} Pi\dot{V}\, dt = PS \int_0^{ti} \dot{V}\, dt = PS \cdot V_T$$

Although some investigators have suggested that PSV is superior to SIMV in the process of weaning,[59,61] at the present time it has not been convincingly demonstrated that either form of partially assisted ventilation is inherently superior to the other.

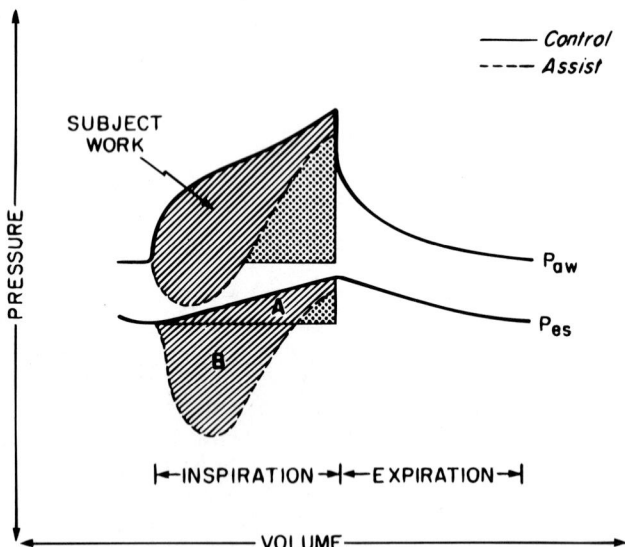

Fig. 10–11. Two methods to estimate the patient's inspiratory work of breathing during flow controlled, volume cycled ventilation. At a constant rate of inspiratory flow and a known tidal volume, subject work can be quantified as the difference in the airway or esophageal pressure-volume areas inscribed during controlled and assisted machine cycles. The principle is to measure the difference in machine work required to accomplish the same overall ventilatory task of moving a constant volume at the same flow rate against an unchanging impedance. Area A refers to the elastic work the subject performs in inflating the chest wall. Area B denotes the work of inflating the lung against the impedance associated with the lungs, airways, and external apparatus. (From Marini, J. J., Smith, T. C., and Lamb, V. J.: External work output and force generation during synchronized intermittent mechanical ventilation: effect of machine assistance on breathing effort. Am. Rev. Respir. Dis., *138*:1169, 1988.)

Table 10–3. Causes of Reduced Ventilatory Drive

Poor nutrition
Chronically elevated breathing workload
Metabolic alkalosis
Sedation/narcotic administration
Sleep deprivation
Hypothyroidism
Central neurologic deficit or injury

Ability to Accomplish the Ventilatory Workload

Ventilatory Drive

Ventilatory drive, the neural signal to the ventilatory apparatus, can be considered to be the integrated result of multiple stimuli (Table 10–3). Ventilatory drive is usually assessed by measuring the output of the ventilatory musculature (gauged by such indices as developed pressure or minute ventilation) in response to altered O_2 saturation and/or $Pa{CO_2}$. Retention of carbon dioxide normally elicits a forceful attempt to restore normocapnia. Sedatives, metabolic alkalosis, poor nutrition, and chronic loading of the ventilatory apparatus (as by airflow obstruction) tend to blunt this chemosensitivity.[62,63] A disproportion between ventilatory drive and ventilatory output gives rise to dyspnea, an important symptom to question in a patient who has experienced acute hypercapnia. (Its absence is virtually diagnostic of blunted ventilatory drive, suggesting a causal role in CO_2 retention.) The chemical drives to breathe begin to revert toward normal within hours after nutrients are given to a semistarved patient (see Chap. 11 and 62.)

Fundamental Properties of Skeletal Muscle Fibers

Three primary characteristics influence the pressure that can be generated during submaximal stimulation:

- The force-frequency relationship
- The force-velocity relationship
- The force-length relationship

The impulse frequency at which the muscle fiber is stimulated by the efferent nerve influences the number of contracting myofibrils and hence the forcefulness of muscular contraction. For a given level of stimulation, the force that can be generated and the velocity of the contraction are inversely related. Thus, the greatest pressure that can be generated at a given volume is isometric pressure, and an unloaded fiber contracts at maximal velocity.[65] The pressure generated at any specific contraction velocity depends on precontractile fiber length, which is an inverse function of chest volume.

Hyperinflation

As already noted, dynamic hyperinflation increases the external work requirement. Acute hyperinflation also seriously compromises the ability of the pump to generate

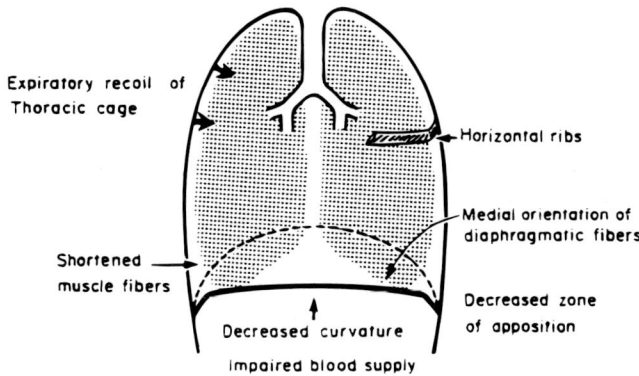

Fig. 10–12. The detrimental effects of acute hyperinflation on respiratory muscle function. Note that several of these disadvantages are attenuated in the long-term setting. (From Marini, J. J.: Ventilatory management of COPD. In Chronic Obstructive Pulmonary Disease. Edited by N. S. Cherniak. Philadelphia, W. B. Saunders, 1991, p. 495.)

pressure and perform work (Fig. 10-12). Apart from reducing the precontractile length of each individual inspiratory muscle fiber, hyperinflation imposes several important mechanical disadvantages on the thoracic pump. Primary among these is a flattening of the diaphragm, a reduction in the effective "zone of apposition" of the diaphragm to the lower rib cage, and a loss of the "bucket handle" motion of the ribs as they turn on their vertical axis.[63-65] With hyperinflation, as during most forms of ventilatory stress or disadvantage, inspiratory power becomes much more dependent on the "accessory" muscles of ventilation, particularly the parasternals, scalenes, and internal intercostals. Such dependence helps to explain the ineffective breathing and O_2 desaturation that occur during the rapid eye movement (REM) phase of sleep in many patients with chronic hyperinflation, as discussed later in this chapter.

The increased work of breathing coupled with the mechanical disadvantages of dynamic hyperinflation make understandable the "panic reaction" experienced by the patient with severe airflow obstruction who is faced with a sudden increase in workload.[65] Any increase in minute ventilation or expiratory resistance will cause the development of auto-PEEP, hyperinflation, and a tendency to unbalance the workload/capability ratio. Furthermore, when dynamic hyperinflation occurs in the setting of positive pressure ventilation, a marked increase in intrathoracic pressure and/or right ventricular afterload may cause a fall in cardiac output and nutritional flow to the exercising muscles.

Fatigue

Fatigue may be defined as the progressive inability to perform a ventilatory task, induced by repetitive effort and reversed by rest. In experimental preparations and in controlled experiments performed by volunteer subjects in a laboratory setting, fatigue can be elicited reproducibly. The ability to generate and sustain pressure is a function of muscle fiber preload and duty cycle. Assuming a normal ti/ttot of 0.3 to 0.5, fatigue tends to develop when the pressure required during each tidal breath exceeds ~40% of the maximal isometric pressure corresponding to that lung volume.[63,66] Higher pressures can be sustained without fatigue when ti/ttot falls to lower values, and lower pressures produce fatigue at longer duty cycles. These relationships are believed to derive from energy delivery/consumption considerations. The product of P/Pmax and ti/ttot expresses the ratio of demand (P $\times$ ti/ttot) to capability (Pmax). Presumably, muscular energy stores cannot be replenished quickly enough between cycles to sustain consistent effort when the "tension-time index" (pressure-time index) is too great.

POST-ICU PHASE OF VENTILATORY FAILURE

Weaning from Mechanical Ventilation

A small but significant percentage of patients receiving mechanical ventilation experience protracted ventilator dependence, a problem associated with physical hazard, disability, and financial cost. Most of these patients have major catabolic illness, profound neuromuscular weakness, or severe cardiopulmonary disease. The need for ventilator assistance often stems from several sources. Psychologic distress, refractory hypoxemia, or cardiovascular problems often develop on resuming spontaneous breathing. The most common reason, however, is an imbalance between ventilatory demand and ability to respond. An effective response requires adequate ventilatory drive and muscular endurance. Adequate drive intensity is seldom the primary problem.[67] Instead, such patients are often weak, malnourished, or deconditioned. Frequently, chest wall instability, impaired coordination, and hyperinflation compromise pump efficiency. Depletion of oxidative enzymes crucial to endurance may be underway within the first 72 hours of total muscle rest, and muscle wasting begins soon thereafter. A considerable percentage of critically ill patients experience forms of drug- or sepsis-related neuromyopathy that were previously unrecognized and are still unexplained.[36,37]

The ventilatory power requirement is jointly determined by the impedance of the respiratory system, and the amount and pattern of ventilation. Rapid, shallow breathing can be an appropriate fatigue-sparing adaptation to weakness or increased breathing workload. Unfortunately, as tidal volume decreases, the deadspace fraction rises and ventilatory efficiency falls. This situation obligates the tachypneic patient either to increase minute ventilation or allow hypercapnia. Whether rapid, shallow breathing proves physiologically adaptive or maladaptive depends on the extent to which ventilatory inefficiency overwhelms the benefit of reduced tidal pressure.

It is always possible to specify some criterion that predicts weaning success or failure in extreme cases, but isolated measures of workload or capability prove disappointing in marginal ones. To judge endurance, any single indicator must reflect both capability and demand. The close interaction between the central control of ventilatory drive and the ventilatory pump is now better appreciated. Well compensated and overtaxed subjects respond differently to ventilatory stress. In response to a potentially exhausting workload, neural outflow may be "down regulated" or modified to avert catastrophic energy depletion.[68] Patients in ventilatory failure may exaggerate the pattern of rapid shallow breathing.

Functional reserve is best assessed empirically during unsupported breathing. At the bedside, the subjective assessment of the breathing trial by an experienced clinician remains the most reliable predictor of weaning success or failure. Tachypnea, paradoxical motion of abdomen or rib cage, respiratory alternans, and vigorous use of accessory ventilatory muscles suggest a load/capability mismatch. These valuable signs, however, are also elicited from normal subjects exposed to moderate breathing workloads, appearing and receding too quickly to be explained by overt fatigue.[69]

Most quantitative indices of functional reserve are technically demanding or require measurements of maximal voluntary effort in uncooperative patients. The proto-inspiratory occlusion pressure (P0.1), however, holds considerable promise; it is not extraordinarily difficult to measure and rises in response to stressful breathing. Although no single value of this drive index sharply distinguishes between compensation and impending fatigue, failure of CO_2 stimulation to augment drive may signal exhausted reserves which allows for better separation.[70]

Irregularity of the breathing rhythm, together with disproportionate changes in respiratory rate or tidal volume are valuable clues to distress, especially when accompanied by tachyarrhythmia or diaphoresis, or when progressive over a 3- to 5-minute period of close observation. Pattern changes tend to stabilize soon after reloading the respiratory system, providing immediate feedback. The frequency to tidal volume ratio quantifies rapid shallow breathing, and during the first minute of machine disconnection appears to provide a simple, yet reliable indicator of weanability.[71]

Although adequate nutrition must be provided to preserve strength and ventilatory drive, overfeeding, lipogenesis, and a high carbohydrate/fat calorie ratio stimulate excessive CO_2 production.[72] The respiratory muscles must not be overtaxed, as recovery from well-established fatigue may require 24 hours or longer. If weaning extends over several days, sufficient nocturnal support should be provided to ensure sleep quality. During REM sleep, the accessory muscles are inhibited, often provoking a crisis of dyspnea or gas exchange in patients dependent on intact diaphragmatic function or full muscle strength.

As already noted, clear superiority of any one weaning mode has not been convincingly demonstrated when each method is appropriately used (Table 10-4). Furthermore, standardized guidelines for the optimal pace of machine withdrawal have not been established. Abrupt removal of machine support works well for most patients with rapidly resolving illness and ample ventilatory reserves. Yet, the hours immediately following abrupt machine withdrawal can be difficult and highly dynamic.[73] Minute ventilation first rises, then falls as pump efficiency or gas exchange improve, fluids redistribute, and metabolic demands subside. Over time, muscles recondition, coordination returns, and drive adjusts to workload. The importance of such adjustments is suggested by the reported success of biofeedback.[74]

A marginal imbalance between capability and demand can often be corrected by a more gradual transition between machine-supported and fully spontaneous breathing. Graded withdrawal of support seems particularly advisable for patients who experience panic reactions, congestive failure, cardiac ischemia, or unusually large breathing workloads when these patients are abruptly disconnected from the ventilator. For these patients, a fine line must be drawn between allowing sufficient adaptation and delaying weaning progress.

Certain aspects of therapy are commonly overlooked. The potential roles of extrapulmonary workloads, impaired cardiovascular function,[75] anemia, fluid or electrolyte imbalance, and endocrine status must be addressed. As a result of attention directed at the resistance and sensitivity of the external breathing circuit, most modern equipment is now quite acceptable for the moderate flows encountered during weaning. In patients with severe airflow obstruction, low levels of PEEP improve the workload, triggering threshold, and dyspnea that accompany dynamic airway compression and auto-PEEP (Fig. 10-13).[76,77] Good arguments can be made to use at least 3 to 5 cm H_2O PEEP in all bedridden, ventilated patients to offset the volume loss associated with recumbent postures.[78] Furthermore, during all spontaneous breathing cycles, sufficient pressure support should be added to overcome endotracheal tube resistance, whatever the mode chosen to supply the ventilatory assistance (SIMV or PSV). To discourage atelectasis during unrelieved shallow breathing, the patient should be as upright and mobile as possible, and periodic deep breaths should be encouraged or provided, e.g., by "high volume" SIMV (e.g., 10 to 12 ml/kg tidal breaths). Although occasional patients express preference,[61] for most it may not matter whether pressure support or well adjusted SIMV (with low level pressure support) provides the machine's power.

There is no general agreement regarding the most appropriate Pa_{CO_2} to target before initiating the weaning process. For patients with ventilatory dysfunction, whether acute or chronic, insistence on maintaining their usual Pa_{CO_2} only increases the breathing workload. Buffer administration may permit "adaptive" hypercapnia.[79] Newer approaches, such as mask-delivered CPAP and noninvasive

Table 10-4. Alternative Weaning Strategies

Primary Source of Machine Assistance			
Pressure Support*		SIMV†	
PSV_{max} →	PSV_5	AMV →	$SIMV_{2/min}$
SIMV	1–2/m	PSV	3–7 cm H_2O
CPAP	3–5 cm H_2O	CPAP	3–5 cm H_2O

* When PSV is chosen, the supporting pressure is tapered from the value giving a tidal volume of 10 ml/kg to ~5 cm H_2O. One to two volume cycles per minute (SIMV, 10 ml/kg) and a small amount of CPAP are supplied to prevent basilar atelectasis as PSV is reduced.
† A similar rationale is followed when SIMV is selected. Here low level PSV is added to overcome endotracheal tube resistance.

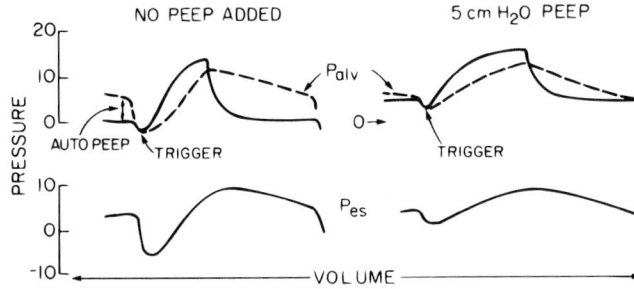

Fig. 10–13. Effect of adding PEEP to the airway of a patient with dynamic airway compression and auto-PEEP during tidal breathing. Auto-PEEP must be counterbalanced by inspiratory muscle activity before central airway pressure can fall sufficiently to trigger the machine cycle. (Auto-PEEP presents a similar threshold load during spontaneous breathing as well.) In many of these flow limited patients, the addition of a small amount of PEEP narrows the difference between end-expiratory alveolar and central airway pressures, thereby improving effective triggering sensitivity and reducing effort, without substantially increasing peak alveolar pressure. (From Marini, J. J.: Ventilatory management of COPD. In Chronic Obstructive Pulmonary Disease. Edited by N. S. Cherniak. Philadelphia, W. B. Saunders, 1991, p. 495.)

intermittent ventilation[80–82] are promising techniques to help the marginal candidate span the postextubation adjustment period.

Adjunctive Ventilatory Support

Occasional patients cannot be successfully weaned from machine support without the institution of some adjunctive form of ventilatory assistance during the postextubation period. In recent years, the option of applying CPAP or noninvasive ventilation has become feasible, providing a potential bridge across the unstable postsupport period.[82] Such techniques may prove helpful especially at night when REM sleep immobilizes the nondiaphragmatic musculature. Indeed, nocturnal nasal ventilation (by nasal mask or other occlusive fitting) appears to be useful over extended periods for selected patients with irreversible neuromuscular disease, sleep apnea, and airflow obstruction.[80,82] Nocturnal support allows many patients to achieve the sleep quality needed to preserve adequate ventilatory drive and muscle strength.

Muscle Training

The place of muscle training in the recovery phase of ventilatory failure and or the peri-extubation period remains highly uncertain at this time. Although most published data support the conceptual value of muscle training, its benefits must still be considered unproven.[83,84] Biofeedback techniques to improve the efficiency of the ventilatory pattern are interesting but clearly experimental adjuncts.

REFERENCES

1. Murray, J. F.: The Normal Lung. 2nd Ed. Philadelphia, W. B. Saunders, 1986, p. 178.
2. Comroe, J. H. Physiology of respiration. Chicago, Yearbook Medical Publishers, 1974, p. 104.
3. Sechzer, P. H., et al.: Effect of CO_2 inhalation on arterial pressure, ECG and plasma catecholamines and 17-OH corticosteroids in normal man. J. Appl. Physiol., 15:454, 1960.
4. Raimondi, A. C., and Raimondi, G. A.: Hypoxemia due to hyperventilation and reduced R value. Chest, 81:391, 1982.
5. Kandel, G., and Aberman, A.: Mixed venous oxygen saturation: its role in the assessment of the critically ill patient. Arch. Intern. Med., 143:1400, 1983.
6. Czer, L. S. C., and Shoemaker, W. C.: Optimal hematocrit value in critically ill patients with postoperative patients. Surg. Gynecol. Obstet., 147:363, 1978.
7. Marini, J. J.: Hemodynamic monitoring using the pulmonary artery catheter. Crit. Care Clin., 2:551, 1986.
8. Coggeshall, J. W., Marini, J. J., and Newman, J. H.: Improved oxygenation after muscle relaxation in the adult respiratory distress syndrome. Arch. Intern. Med., 145:1718, 1985.
9. Field, S., Kelly, S. M., and Macklem, P. T.: The oxygen cost of breathing in patients with cardiorespiratory disease. Am. Rev. Respir. Dis., 126:9, 1982.
10. Viires, N., et al.: Regional blood flow distribution in dog during induced hypotension and low cardiac output: spontaneous breathing versus artificial ventilation. J. Clin. Invest., 72:935, 1983.
11. Pesenti, A.: Target Blood gases during ARDS ventilation management. Intensive Care Med., 16:349, 1990.
12. Marini, J. J.: Controlled Ventilation: targets, hazards and options. In Ventilatory Failure. Edited by J. J. Marini, and C. Roussos, Berlin, Springer-Verlag, 1991, p. 269.
13. Webb, H., and Tierney, D.: Experimental pulmonary edema due to intermittent positive pressure ventilation with high inflation pressures: protection by positive end-expiratory pressure. Am. Rev. Respir. Dis., 110:556, 1974.
14. Dreyfuss, D., Basset, G., Soler, P., and Saumon, G.: Intermittent positive pressure hyperventilation with high inflation pressures produces pulmonary microvascular injury in rats. Am. Rev. Respir. Dis., 132:880, 1985.
15. Maunder, R. J., et al.: Preservation of normal lung regions in the adult respiratory distress syndrome: analysis by computed tomography. JAMA, 255:2463, 1986.
16. Lamy, M., et al.: Pathologic features and mechanics of hypoxemia in adult respiratory distress syndrome. Am. Rev. Respir. Dis., 114:267, 1976.
17. Gattinoni, L., Pesenti, A., and Bombino, M.: Relationships between lung computed tomographic density, gas exchange and PEEP in acute respiratory failure. Anesthesiology, 69:824, 1988.
18. Woodring, J. H.: Pulmonary interstitial emphysema in the adult respiratory distress syndrome. Crit. Care Med., 13:786, 1985.
19. Albelda, S. M., et al.: Ventilator-induced subpleural air cysts: clinical, radiographic, and pathologic significance. Am. Rev. Respir. Dis., 127:360, 1983.
20. Churg, A., Golden, J., Fligiel, S., and Hogg, J. C.: Bronchopulmonary dysplasia in the adult. Am. Rev. Respir. Dis., 127:117, 1983.
21. Marini, J. J., and Culver, B. H.: Systemic air embolism consequent to mechanical ventilation in ARDS. Ann. Intern. Med., 110:699, 1989.
22. Marini, J. J.: Lung mechanics in the adult respiratory distress syndrome. In Clinics in Chest Medicine. Edited by H. P. Wiedemann, M. A. Matthay, and R. A. Matthay, Philadelphia, W. B. Saunders, 1990, p. 673.
23. Pesenti, A., et al.: Mean airway pressure vs positive end-expiratory pressure during mechanical ventilation. Crit. Care Med., 13:34, 1985.

24. Koltan, M., Cattran, C. B., and Kent, G.: Oxygenation during high frequency-ventilation in two models of lung injury. Anesth. Analg., 61:323, 1982.
25. Matamis, D., et al.: Total respiratory pressure volume curves in the adult respiratory distress syndrome. Chest, 86:58, 1984.
26. Kimball, W. R., Leith, D. E., and Robins, A. G.: Dynamic hyperinflation and ventilator dependence in chronic obstructive pulmonary disease. Am. Rev. Respir. Dis., 126:991, 1982.
27. Lynch, J. P., Mhyre, J. G., and Dantzker, D. R.: The influence of cardiac output on intrapulmonary shunt. J. Appl. Physiol., 46:315, 1979.
28. Gurevitch, M. J., Van Dyke, J., Young, E. S., and Jackson, K.: Improved oxygenation and lower peak airway pressure in severe adult respiratory distress syndrome: treatment with inverse ratio ventilation. Chest, 89:211, 1986.
29. Tharatt, R. S., Allen, R. P., and Albertson, T. E.: Pressure controlled inverse ratio ventilation in severe adult respiratory failure. Chest, 94:755, 1988.
30. Kacmarek, R. M., and Hess, D.: Panacea or Auto-PEEP? Respir. Care, 35:945, 1990.
31. Duncan, S. R., Rizk, N. W., and Raffin, T. A.: Inverse ratio ventilation: PEEP in disguise? Chest, 92:390, 1987.
32. Cole, A. G. H., Weller, S. F., and Sykes, M. K.: Inverse ratio ventilation compared with PEEP in adult respiratory failure. Intensive Care Med., 10:227, 1984.
33. Marcy, T. W., and Marini, J. J.: Inverse ratio ventilation in ARDS: rationale and implementation. Chest, 100:494, 1990.
34. Hickling, K. G., Henderson, S. J., and Jackson, R.: Low mortality associated with permissive hypercapnia in severe adult respiratory distress syndrome. Intensive Care Med., 16:372, 1990.
35. Al-Saady, N., and Bennett, E. D.: Decelerating inspiratory flow waveform improves lung mechanics and gas exchange in patients on intermittent positive pressure-ventilation. Intensive Care Med., 11:68, 1985.
36. Zochodne, D. W., et al.: Critical illness polyneuropathy: a complication of sepsis and multiple organ failure. Brain, 110:819, 1987.
37. Douglass, J. A., et al.: Acute myopathy following treatment of severe life-threatening asthma (SLTA). (Abstract.) Am. Rev. Respir. Dis., 141(Suppl.):AA97, 1990.
38. Elliott, C. G.: Pulmonary sequelae in survivors of the adult respiratory distress syndrome. Clin. Chest. Med., 11:789, 1990.
39. Roussos, C., and Macklem, P. T.: The respiratory muscles. N. Engl. J. Med., 307:786, 1982.
40. Sharp, J. T.: The Chest Wall and Respiratory Muscles in Obesity, Pregnancy and Ascites. In The Thorax (Part B). Edited by C. Roussos, and P. T. Macklem. New York, Marcel Dekker, 1985, p. 999.
41. Otis, A. B., Fenn, W. O., and Rahn, H.: Mechanics of breathing in man. J. Appl. Physiol., 2:592, 1950.
42. Cherniack, R. M.: The oxygen consumption and efficiency of the respiratory muscles in health and emphysema. J. Clin. Invest., 38:494, 1959.
43. Bigland, B., and Lippold, O. C. J.: The relation between force, velocity and integrated electrical activity in human muscles. J. Physiol. (Lond.), 123:214, 1954.
44. Otis, A. B.: The work of breathing. Physiol. Rev., 34:449, 1954.
45. Peters, R. M.: The energy cost (work) of breathing. Ann. Thorac. Surg., 7:51, 1969.
46. Moxham, J., et al.: Sternomastoid muscle function and fatigue in man. Clin. Sci. Mol. Med., 59:463, 1980.
47. Hamalainen, R. P., and Viljanen, A. A.: Modeling the respiratory airflow pattern by optimization criteria. Biol. Cybern., 29:143, 1978.
48. Nunn, J. F., and Hill, D. W.: Respiratory dead space and arterial to end-tidal O_2 tension difference in anesthetized man. J. Appl. Physiol., 15:383, 1960.
49. Roussos, C.: Energetics. In The Thorax. Edited by C. Roussos, and P. T. Macklem. New York, Marcel Dekker, 1985, p. 437.
50. Marini, J. J., Smith, T. C., and Lamb, V. J.: External work output and force generation during synchronized intermittent mechanical ventilation: effect of machine assistance on breathing effort. Am. Rev. Respir. Dis., 138:1169, 1988.
51. Smith, T. C., and Marini, J. J.: Impact of PEEP on lung mechanics and work of breathing in severe airflow obstruction: the effect of PEEP on Auto-PEEP. J. Appl. Physiol., 65:1488, 1988.
52. Gibney, R. T. N., Wilson, R. S., and Pontoppidan, H.: Comparisons of work of breathing on high gas flow and demand valve continuous positive airway pressure systems. Chest, 82:692, 1982.
53. Sassoon, C. S. H., Giron, A. E., Ely, E. A., and Light, R. W.: Inspiratory work of breathing on flow-by and demand flow continuous positive airway pressure. Crit. Care Med., 17:1108, 1989.
54. Gottfried, S. B., et al.: Noninvasive determination of respiratory system mechanics during mechanical ventilation for acute respiratory failure. Am. Rev. Respir. Dis., 131:672, 1985.
55. Wright, P. W., Marini, J. J., and Bernard, G. R.: In vitro versus in vivo comparison of endotracheal tube airflow resistance. Am. Rev. Respir. Dis., 140:10, 1989.
56. Marini, J. J., Rodriguez, R. M., and Lamb, V. J.: The inspiratory workload of patient-initiated mechanical ventilation. Am. Rev. Respir. Dis., 134:902, 1986.
57. Fleury, B. D., et al.: Work of breathing in patients with chronic obstructive pulmonary disease in acute respiratory failure. Am. Rev. Respir. Dis., 131:822, 1985.
58. Marini, J. J., Capps, J. S., and Culver, B. H.: The inspiratory work of breathing during assisted mechanical ventilation. Chest, 87(5):612, 1985.
59. MacIntyre, N. R.: Respiratory function during pressure support ventilation. Chest, 89:677, 1986.
60. Marini, J. J.: Strategies to Minimize Breathing Effort during Mechanical Ventilation. Crit. Care Clin., 6:635, 1990.
61. Brochard, L., et al.: Comparison of three techniques of weaning from mechanical ventilation: results of an European multicenter trial. Am. Rev. Respir. Dis., 4:A602, 1991.
62. Weissman, C., et al.: Amino acids and respiration. Ann. Intern. Med., 98:41, 1983.
63. Rochester, D. F., and Arora, N. S.: Respiratory muscle failure. Med. Clin. North. Am., 67:573, 1983.
64. Macklem, P. T.: Hyperinflation. Am. Rev. Respir. Dis., 129:1, 1984.
65. Marini, J. J.: Ventilatory management of COPD. In Chronic Obstructive Pulmonary Disease. Edited by N. S. Cherniack. Philadelphia, W. B. Saunders, 1991, p. 495.
66. Bellemare, F., and Grassino, A.: Effect of pressure and timing of contraction on human diaphragm failure. J. Appl. Physiol., 53:1190, 1982.
67. Murciano, D., et al.: Tracheal occlusion pressure: a simple index to monitor respiratory muscle fatigue during acute respiratory failure in patients with chronic obstructive pulmonary disease. Ann. Intern. Med., 108:800, 1988.
68. Roussos, C., and Moxham, J.: Respiratory muscle fatigue. In The Thorax. Edited by C. Roussos, and P. T. Macklem. New York, Marcel Dekker, 1985, p. 829.
69. Tobin, M. J., et al.: The pattern of breathing during successful and unsuccessful trials of weaning from mechanical ventilation. Am. Rev. Respir. Dis., 134:1111, 1986.

70. Montgomery, A. B., et al.: Prediction of successful ventilator weaning using airway occlusion pressure and hypercapnic challenge. Chest, *4*:496, 1987.
71. Yang, K. L., and Tobin, M. J.: A prospective study of indexes predicting the outcome of trials of weaning from mechanical ventilation. N. Engl. J. Med., *324*:1445, 1991.
72. Rochester, D. F., and Esau, S. A.: Malnutrition and the respiratory system. Chest, *85*:411, 1984.
73. Gilbert, R., Auchincloss, J. H. Jr, Peppi, D., and Ashutosh, K.: The first hours off a respirator. Chest, *65*:152, 1984.
74. Holliday, J. E., and Hyers, T. M.: The reduction of weaning time from mechanical ventilation using tidal volume and relaxation biofeedback. Am. Rev. Respir. Dis., *141*:1214, 1990.
75. LeMaire, F., et al.: Acute left ventricular dysfunction during unsuccessful weaning from mechanical ventilation. Anesthesiology, *69*:171, 1988.
76. Marini, J. J.: Should PEEP be used in airflow obstruction? Am. Rev. Respir. Dis., *140*:1, 1989.
77. Petrof, B. J., et al.: Continuous positive airway pressure reduces work of breathing and dyspnea during weaning from mechanical ventilation in severe chronic obstructive pulmonary disease. Am. Rev. Respir. Dis., *141*:281, 1990.
78. Marini, J. J., et al.: Influence of head-dependent positions on lung volume and oxygen saturation in chronic airflow obstruction. Am. Rev. Respir. Dis., *129*:101, 1984.
79. Darioli, R., and Perret, C.: Mechanical controlled hypoventilation in status asthmaticus. Am. Rev. Respir. Dis., *129*:385, 1984.
80. Gay, P. C., Patel, A. M., Vigianno, R. W., and Hubmayr, R. D.: Nocturnal nasal ventilation for treatment of patients with hypercapnic respiratory failure. Mayo Clin. Proc., *66*:695, 1991.
81. Marini, J. J.: Weaning from mechanical ventilation. N. Engl. J. Med., *324*:1496, 1991.
82. Branthwaite, M. A., Elliott, M. W., and Simonds, A. K.: Ventilatory Failure: innovative Support Techniques. *In* Ventilatory Failure. Edited by J. J. Marini, and C. Roussos. Berlin, Springer-Verlag, 1991, p. 430.
83. Belman, M., and Mittman, C.: Ventilatory muscle training improves exercise capacity in chronic obstructive pulmonary disease patients. Am. Rev. Respir. Dis., *121*:273, 1980.
84. Aldrich, T. K., et al.: Weaning from mechanical ventilation: adjunctive use of inspiratory muscle resistive training. Crit. Care Med., *17*:143, 1989.

Chapter 11

DISORDERS OF CONTROL OF VENTILATION

MELVIN LOPATA

Patients with unexplained chronic or acute on chronic CO_2 retention always present a challenge to the clinician. Sorting out the cause or disease entity is often an unstructured, confusing process and, until recently, therapeutic options were limited and less than efficacious. The goal of this chapter is to put the problem of disorders of respiratory control into perspective for the clinician, to explain the nature and pathophysiology of impaired control of ventilation, and provide a logical and practical scheme for working up such a patient and instituting proper therapy. I will begin by illustrating the scope of the clinical problem by presenting brief vignettes of three actual patients.

Patient 1: A 46-year-old obese male, 40-pack/year smoker, presents with chronic cough, effort dyspnea, and a recent history of increasing daytime somnolence. Admission arterial blood gases are: Pa_{O_2} 52 mm Hg, Pa_{CO_2} 55 mm Hg, pH 7.36. Results of recent pulmonary function tests: FVC 2.4 L, FEV_1 1.4 L.

Patient 2: A 34-year-old female with known progressive, severe kyphoscoliosis presents with increasing dyspnea, peripheral edema, and obtundation. Admission arterial blood gases: Pa_{O_2} 34 mm Hg, Pa_{CO_2} 76 mm Hg, pH 7.22. Results of recent pulmonary function tests: FVC 0.9 L, FEV_1 0.7 L.

Patient 3: A 54-year-old, nonsmoking female presents with fatigue, daytime sleepiness, and peripheral edema. Admission arterial blood gases: Pa_{O_2} 61 mm Hg, Pa_{CO_2} 63 mm Hg, pH 7.33. Results of recent pulmonary function tests: FVC 2.7 L, FEV_1 2.5 L.

The three described patients have quite different primary diseases that share a common result of hypercapnic respiratory failure, a term which can be used interchangeably with alveolar hypoventilation and CO_2 retention. Although the primary pathology in these diseases is different, there is a commonality of pathophysiology. By virtue of the presence of CO_2 retention, these diseases are disorders of respiratory control. Although by different mechanisms or pathways, the many and varied disorders of respiratory control all impact on the respiratory control system and impair the function of the complex regulatory process that normally maintains a narrow range of Pa_{CO_2}.

The three patients presented with alveolar hypoventilation; however, the chronicity and severity of the CO_2 retention was obviously different. Patients 1 and 3 had chronic respiratory failure, whereas patient 2 had acute on chronic failure. Thus, each patient may require a different clinical and therapeutic approach, (i.e., the second patient is likely a candidate for admission to the ICU). In our experience, most patients with hypoventilation syndromes present with chronic manifestations of their disease and fit into the so-called pre-ICU phase and undergo diagnostic studies to identify the primary disease as well as therapeutic evaluations. These patients are all at risk for their disease to exacerbate or progress to the acute or ICU phase, and some patients may initially present with the state of their disease requiring ICU admission. Finally, all (surviving) patients will enter the post-ICU phase where definitive chronic therapy is instituted.

The design of this chapter will be to approach disorders of ventilatory control or hypoventilation syndromes according to the three illness phases that have been emphasized in this book. In the pre-ICU phase, I will discuss differential diagnosis and clinical and laboratory evaluation of the hypoventilating patient aimed at arriving at a disease diagnosis, and at instituting the appropriate therapy. In the ICU phase, I will discuss indications or criteria for admission to the ICU and specific therapeutic modalities available and used to treat these acutely ill patients. Finally, in the post-ICU phase, I will present therapeutic alternatives and recommendations for the long-term management of these usually chronic disease processes.

PRE-ICU PHASE

The number of diseases associated with alveolar hypoventilation is legion (Table 11-1). To understand how a given disease may cause CO_2 retention, however, one must have an understanding of the organization of the respiratory control system which is composed of central and peripheral nervous system, respiratory muscle, and bellows (lung and chest wall) components that serve in concert to control ventilation.[1] Thus, the primary drive to breathe is initiated in the brain stem, transmitted to the spinal cord and the respiratory motor neurons of the peripheral nerves, which carry the impulses to the respiratory muscles whose contraction powers the bellows to effect ventilation (Fig. 11-1). Alveolar ventilation primarily serves to regulate alveolar and consequently arterial Pa_{CO_2}. Various feedback processes, via the peripheral and central chemoreceptors and by way of reflexes generated in the airways, lung parenchyma, and chest wall serve to fine tune the control system such that under varied metabolic, environmental, and even disease states a narrow normal range of Pa_{CO_2} is maintained or the level is decreased, the latter to optimize the Pa_{O_2}.[2] By functionally interrupting the control system anywhere along the control arc, from the central nervous system (CNS) to the bellows, certain disease

DISORDERS OF CONTROL OF VENTILATION

Table 11-1. Causes of Hypoventilation

CENTRAL (CNS)
  Idiopathic (primary)
  CVA, tumor, infection
  Syringobulbia
  Trauma
  Metabolic hypothyroidism, metabolic alkalosis
NEUROMUSCULAR
  Anterior horn cells
    Poliomyelitis
    Amyotrophic lateral sclerosis
    Syringomyelia
  Peripheral nerves
    Polyneuropathy (Gullain-Barré Syndrome)
    Phrenic nerve injury (secondary to cardiac hypothermia)
    Multiple sclerosis
    Postpolio syndrome
  Motor end plate
    Myasthenia gravis
    Eaton-Lambert syndrome
    Botulism
  Muscle
    Dystrophies
    Myopathies
      Hereditary (acid maltase deficiency)
      Inflammatory
      Metabolic (hypophosphatemia)
BELLOWS
  COPD
  Kyphoscoliosis
  Obesity

Table 11-2. Hypoventilation Syndromes Classification

Bellows dysfunction
Neuromuscular disease
Primary (idiopathic) alveolar hypoventilation
Sleep apnea syndrome

which the disease impacts. Table 11-1 shows a list of diseases along these anatomic lines which categorizes the diseases as: central, neuromuscular (divided into anterior motor horn cell, peripheral nerves, motor end-plate, muscle), and bellows. The list is not exhaustive but reflects the more common and well-known disease entities causing or associated with hypoventilation. Certain diagnoses are not easily classified because they may affect more than one component of the control system (e.g., hypothyroidism may impair both central control and respiratory muscle function).[4,5] Sleep apnea, commonly associated with morbid obesity, is an important cause of hypoventilation. Patients with the obesity-hypoventilation syndrome (OHS) in the great majority of instances have sleep apnea such that, in my view, the two diagnoses are interchangeable. OHS also affects the control system at two levels: sleep apnea by causing sleep fragmentation, nocturnal hypoxia, and acidosis over a long period of time may eventually impair central ventilatory control; obesity by its mass loading effect on the respiratory system impairs bellows function.[6] It is probably that both conditions (sleep apnea and obesity), each contributing to a variable degree in a given patient, are necessary for hypoventilation to develop.

When considering the differential diagnosis of a patient with a hypoventilation syndrome, rather than evoke the extensive listing in Table 11-1, I find it convenient to consider the differential in light of a limited but very practical set of categories (Table 11-2). The practicality is in formulating the workup such that the differential is narrowed to the four disease classes that emphasize the common processes that cause hypoventilation, and the order of the listing puts the workup, especially its conceptual sequence, into perspective. In such a sequence, diseases affecting the bellows must first be considered, mainly chronic obstructive pulmonary disease (COPD) because it is the most common disease causing hypoventilation. Once bellows dysfunction as the primary cause is ruled out, the broad category of neuromuscular disease must be considered. Despite the many diseases in this class, a generic approach to the workup can result in the exclusion or inclusion of this category before specific and possibly sophisticated diagnostic methods are used to isolate the particular disease. If neuromuscular disease is ruled out, primary alveolar hypoventilation (PAH) as a diagnosis of exclusion now enters the picture. At this point, however, a sleep study would be done in part to establish or exclude the presence of sleep apnea, namely obstructive sleep apnea. As noted earlier, this diagnostic sequence is largely conceptual; one may have strongly considered sleep apnea earlier than at this point in the workup, but the sequence emphasizes that at some point in the workup, whether sleep apnea is considered early, late, or not at all,

processes may impair the ability of the system to normally regulate ventilation resulting in inappropriately low alveolar ventilation and CO_2 retention.[1] This scenario implies that CO_2 retention is essentially due to a respiratory neuromechanical defect. This statement is not, however, entirely correct because gas exchange abnormalities due to ventilation-perfusion mismatching can impair CO_2 elimination and potentially cause CO_2 retention.[3] In the presence of a normal control system, however, disease-associated hyperventilation should serve to maintain the Pa_{CO_2} in the normal or hypocapnic range. Even with impaired gas exchange, CO_2 retention likely occurs only when some component of the control system is functionally impaired.

In listing the differential diagnoses of alveolar hypoventilation, I find it informative to list the disease processes according to the component of the control system on

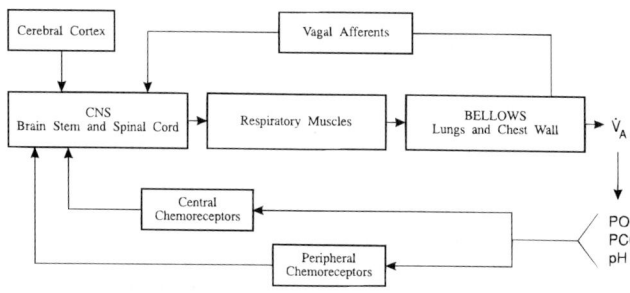

Fig. 11-1. Scheme of the respiratory control system depicting the "closed loop" negative feedback that regulated alveolar ventilation ($\dot{V}_A$). (Courtesy of George Morrison, ACT/PC.)

most, if not all patients with hypoventilation (excluding COPD), should undergo a sleep study. The rationale for this course as well as a detailed discussion of the workup of patients with unexplained CO_2 retention now follows.

The History and Physical Examination

The workup obviously starts with the history. With the disease categories discussed earlier in mind, it is clear that inquiries regarding a past medical history of pulmonary, neurologic, chest wall, and metabolic disease as well as prescription drug usage (i.e., diuretics), must be made. A history of recent open heart surgery (i.e., coronary artery bypass), or a more likely scenario of a difficult to wean postoperative coronary surgery patient, should immediately suggest phrenic nerve injury due to cardiac hypothermia.[7] Careful family history can be important in directing the workup towards genetic neuromuscular diseases.

Symptoms offered by patients with chronic hypoventilation syndromes are often nonspecific or are common to many of the causative diseases. Complaints of fatigability, daytime somnolence, disturbed sleep, and morning headaches can be elicited by most patients, which points to the detrimental effects all of these disease have on sleep. Disabling hypersomnolence coupled with disturbing snoring, especially in an obese patient, certainly suggests sleep apnea, but even in this disease the symptoms may not be classically dramatic.

Specific symptoms such as effort dyspnea, cough with sputum production, especially in a smoker, must direct the workup to investigate the presence and, most importantly, the severity of obstructive lung disease. Patients with neuromuscular disease will variably complain of dyspnea in the upright position but often not to a severe degree, while patients with PAH may not be dyspneic at all.[8,9] An important variant of the complaint of shortness of breath is worsening of dyspnea in the supine position. This symptom, which should be elicited from all these patients, characteristically evokes neuromuscular disease with diaphragmatic paralysis as the causative disease process.[9,10] The reasons for this deduction will be discussed later in this chapter.

In the physical examination, the following abnormalities must be sought: evidence of airway obstruction (wheezing, rhonchi, prolonged expiration), kyphoscoliosis, obesity, muscular weakness, neurologic deficits (sensory and motor), and signs of cor pulmonale and congestive heart failure. The latter cardiac findings are not specific for any disease entity but their presence is evidence of severe sequelae of the disease process. Complimenting supine dyspnea as a symptom of diaphragmatic dysfunction is the physical sign of supine-induced paradoxic chest wall movement such that during the respiratory cycle the rib cage and abdomen do not move synchronously or in and out together, but paradoxically (i.e., during inspiration the rib cage moves outward and the abdomen inward with this pattern reversing during expiration).[10] The explanation of these phenomena will be discussed later in this chapter.

Laboratory Evaluation

The laboratory examination continues the investigative process and hopefully will help narrow the etiologic

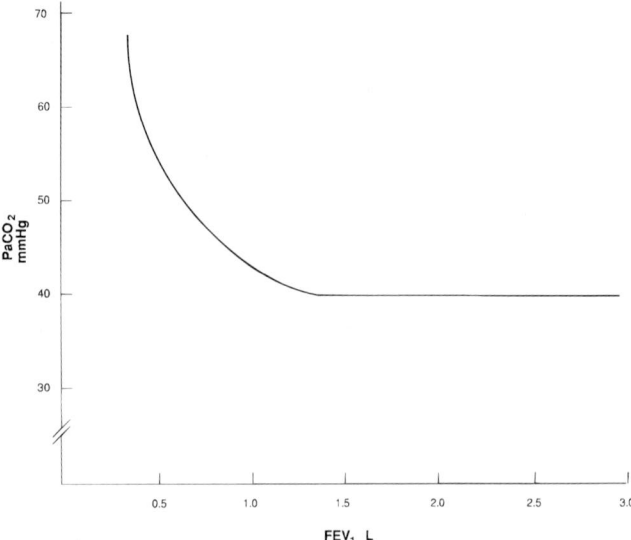

Fig. 11–2. Relationship between airways obstruction (FEV_1) and arterial P_{CO_2} (Pa_{CO_2}) in patients with chronic obstructive pulmonary disease. On average, CO_2 retention does not occur until the FEV_1 is at or below 1.0 L. (Courtesy of ACT/PC.)

choices and result in a definitive diagnosis. To start, basic blood studies should be performed. Serum electrolytes and biochemistry, along with arterial blood gases will enable the identification of metabolic abnormalities that either cause or contribute to hypoventilation such as metabolic alkalosis, hypokalemia, hypophosphatemia, hypomagnesemia, as well as hypothyroidism.[4,5,11–13]

The next step in the workup process involves the pulmonary function laboratory and according to the conceptual framework of Table 11–2, is directed at establishing the presence of Bellows dysfunction and, if so, its causative role in the hypoventilation process. Because COPD is the most common cause of CO_2 retention, the question to be asked is: Does the patient have airways obstruction, and if so, is it severe enough to cause alveolar hypoventilation? In patients with COPD, the level of Pa_{CO_2} is hyperbolically related to the degree of airways obstruction as reflected by the FEV_1 (Fig. 11–2). As per this relationship, Pa_{CO_2} is maintained at eucapnic or hypocapnic levels as the FEV_1 declines with progressive disease until a critical level of obstruction at an FEV_1 or 1 to 1.3 L is reached, after which CO_2 retention tends to occur.[8] Thus, when due to COPD, hypoventilation occurs in the face of severe airways obstruction typically at an FEV_1 of less than 1 L. As such, in the presence of obstructive lung disease, an FEV_1 of greater than 1 to 1.3 L suggests that a process other than COPD is causing or contributing to the CO_2 retention.

Similarly, patients with kyphoscoliosis typically hypoventilate only when a severe degree of chest wall distortion and functional impairment is reached. Thus, most such patients will have severe lateral scoliosis with a Cobb's angle of greater than 120° and a vital capacity of less than 1 L.[14]

Another relatively simple test to assess mechanical limitation is to determine the effects of voluntary hyperventilation on the Pa_{CO_2}. A normal individual, or patients with central and often neuromuscular causes of hypoventilation, will be able to decrease the Pa_{CO_2} more than 20 torr; a patient with bellows dysfunction severe enough to cause hypoventilation will be able to reduce the Pa_{CO_2} no more than 10 torr.[8] Thus, at this point in the workup the next question to be asked is: can patients lower their Pa_{CO_2} with voluntary hyperventilation? A 20 torr decrease in Pa_{CO_2} makes mechanical impairment of the bellows unlikely as a major cause of CO_2 retention. The ability to adequately hyperventilate is consistent with the presence of PAH and OHS, but does not exclude neuromuscular disease.[9]

If the foregoing procedures eliminate bellows dysfunction as a cause of CO_2 retention, then the workup proceeds to include or exclude neuromuscular disease as the causative process. Certainly patients may have diseases that are quite evident or easily diagnosed, especially if the process is diffuse or systemic with neural or muscle group involvement other than that of the respiratory system. But in many diseases the respiratory motor neurons, nerves, or muscles may be the first, the only, or the major components involved, resulting in significant diaphragmatic dysfunction or paralysis.[9] These patients may present with CO_2 retention without obvious neurologic deficits and the effects of diaphragm paralysis may be subtle and overlooked.[9,15]

An approach to the workup of neuromuscular disease is first to demonstrate the presence of a diaphragm paralysis and thereby establish its role in the hypoventilation state. Subsequently (or concurrently), the diagnosis of the specific disease entity must be determined. Respiratory muscle function and to some extent that of the diaphragm can be assessed using the pulmonary function laboratory and radiologic techniques.

There are no specific effects of diaphragm paralysis on pulmonary function tests, but characteristic changes do occur and when present do support or focus on the presence of neuromuscular disease. A 50% or greater decrease of the forced vital capacity (FVC) in the supine position is highly consistent with the presence of bilateral diaphragm weakness or paralysis,[9,15,16] and points to the importance of performing upright and supine spirometry. A nonconcentric restrictive process occurs typically in patients with neuromuscular disease and diaphragm paralysis. As such, the resting lung volume is relatively well preserved, but the inspiratory capacity is markedly impaired, resulting in a normal or slightly reduced functional residual capacity (FRC) and a markedly reduced vital capacity (VC) and total lung capacity (TLC)[17] (Fig. 11-3). Of interest and importance, obesity may result in a nonconcentric restrictive defect that is opposite to that just described because the FRC (and especially the expiratory reserve volume) is decreased, whereas the VC and TLC are relatively well preserved[18] (Fig. 11-3). In kyphoscoliosis the FRC is decreased, mostly due to expiratory reserve volume reduction, and the VC and TLC are markedly impaired resulting in concentric restriction[14] (Fig. 11-3).

The measurement of respiratory pressures developed by maximum isometric contraction of the inspiratory and expiratory muscles is another sensitive way to screen for and document quantitatively the presence of respiratory muscle weakness.[19,20] Mouth pressure can be measured

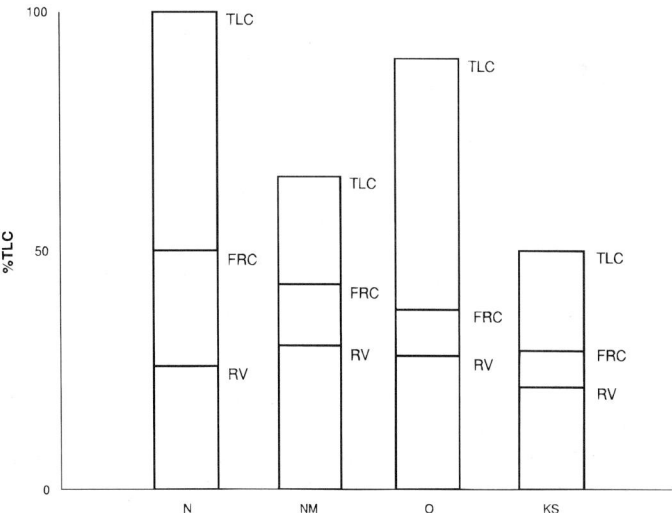

Fig. 11-3. Subdivisions of lung volumes in normal subjects (N) and in patients with neuromuscular disease (NM), obesity (O), and kyphoscoliosis (KS). TLC, Total lung capacity; FRC, functional residual capacity; RV, residual volume; ERV = FRC − RV. (Courtesy of ACT/PC.)

very easily and noninvasively while the patient maximally inspires or expires against a closed airway. The ability to generate maximum mouth pressure is diminished in patients with respiratory muscular dysfunction and both inspiratory and expiratory pressures can be diminished, though not necessarily to an equal degree.[20,21] Similar results are evident when pleural or transdiaphragmatic pressures are recorded.[10,21,22] Impaired pressure generation, especially when patient cooperation and optimal effort is ensured, provides strong support for neuromuscular disease as the culprit in the hypoventilation workup. Normal pressures[19] do not rule out this category of disease, but do make it unlikely.

Fluoroscopy has been the time-honored method used to detect diaphragm dysfunction or paralysis. The lack of diaphragm movement or more specifically, paradoxical, upward movement during a brief inspiratory effort has been regarded as the classic sign of diaphragm paralysis. Unfortunately, this technique, the results of which are often difficult to interpret, can provide misleading, false negative data.[10] This occurs because patients, especially early in the course of their disease, often manifest predominantly inspiratory muscle dysfunction, and the preservation of expiratory abdominal muscle function permits patients to compensate for their diaphragm paralysis. Compensation occurs with the development of a strategy of breathing that utilizes the functioning abdominal muscles to support the action of the nonfunctioning diaphragm.[9,10] This involuntary strategy entails contracting the abdominal muscles during expiration forcing the diaphragm upward or cephalad such that during the subsequent inspiration gravity and passive recoil of the thorax cause the diaphragm to descend and thus effect inspiration. This action of the expiratory muscles promotes and assists inspiration allowing the patient to compensate for the lack of diaphragmatic function. If one were viewing diaphragm movement via fluoroscopy in a patient effecting these maneuvers, the diaphragm would be seen to descend during inspiration, therefore causing the false negative result.[10]

It should be apparent that this successful strategy of breathing depends in large part on gravity and the upright position. When the patient assumes the supine position, neither gravity nor thoracic recoil assists inspiratory movement of the diaphragm and compensation is lost, resulting in the classic symptom of supine dyspnea.

Normally, the rib cage and abdomen move synchronously with respiration, outward with inspiration and inward with expiration. This synchrony occurs because diaphragm contraction results in descent of the diaphragm which increases abdominal pressure that moves the abdominal wall outward. Concurrently, diaphragm action elevates the lower rib cage, moving it outward, and any intercostal recruitment will expand and displace outward the upper rib cage. All these actions cause outward synchrony during inspiration which reverses during expiration.[10] With diaphragm paralysis, the intact inspiratory intercostal and accessory muscles elevate and move the rib cage outward increasing thoracic volume and decreasing intrathoracic pressure pulling the diaphragm cephalad along with the abdominal contents and the abdominal wall moves inward; rib cage and abdomen now move paradoxically.[9,10] As discussed earlier, expiratory recruitment of the abdominal muscles can elicit compensation to prevent such paradoxic movement of the rib cage and abdomen. Indeed, through simple observation or by recording rib cage and abdominal motion with specific sensing devices, one can easily document supine paradoxic movement supporting the diagnosis of diaphragm paralysis.

If these physiologic tests support the presence of neuromuscular disease as the cause of the hypoventilation syndrome then a vigorous neurologic evaluation must ensue. This should include nerve conduction studies and electromyography to detect generalized neurologic involvement and to distinguish between neuropathic and myopathic disease. In the latter case a muscle biopsy will likely be indicated.

If respiratory muscle function is intact and no neurologic deficits are evident (in essence ruling out a neuromuscular etiology), then one is left with the third category of disease, PAH.[16-18] Because no specific test exists for this disease, it essentially becomes a diagnosis of exclusion. Therefore, one can entertain a diagnosis of PAH when chronic hypercapnic respiratory failure occurs in the absence of pulmonary disease, chest wall disease, neuromuscular disease, and obstructive sleep apnea (OSA).

Characteristically, because of the so-called impairment of automatic brain stem respiratory function, there is a diminished or absent ventilatory response to CO_2 and hypoxic stimulation as well as to exercise.[23-25]

At this point even if one is secure in a diagnosis there is one more test that must be part of any workup of hypoventilation and that is a nocturnal sleep study. A sleep study may have already been considered or indicated because of a high suspicion of sleep apnea, yet symptoms of OSA may be subtle or mild, overlap with that of the other diseases, especially PAH, such that OSA may be missed.

Thus, there are two reasons to perform a sleep study on these patients: (1) to determine the presence or absence of OSA, a treatable disease; and (2) to determine the degree of arterial oxygen desaturation and CO_2 elevation during sleep in patients with kyphoscoliosis, neuromuscular disease, and PAH and to assess their response to assisted ventilation.[9,26-28] This latter reason is based on data that clearly show that patients in these categories will demonstrate significant worsening of their hypoxemia, hypercapnia, and acidosis during sleep, especially rapid eye movement (REM) sleep, and this nocturnal deterioration of ventilation and gas exchange creates a vicious cycle that promotes progression of the hypoventilation state and its sequelae (i.e., cor pulmonale and right heart failure).[29] Breaking this cycle with nocturnal ventilatory assist provides a therapeutic modality for these patients which will be discussed later in this chapter.

Nocturnal polysomnography, the monitoring of multiple physiologic parameters during sleep, will detect the presence of sleep disordered breathing which will be different in patients with OSA compared to those in the other disease categories. OSA patients will demonstrate periodic, usually repetitive apneas (cessation of airflow at nose and mouth), during which there is continuing evidence of respiratory muscle activity (i.e. chest wall movement).[30] In patients with kyphoscoliosis, neuromuscular disease, and PAH, there may be irregular breathing, short central apneas, or diminished tidal volume and chest wall excursions, or there may be little overt evidence of disordered breathing, but all are associated with prolonged oxygen desaturation, or worsening of the arterial blood gases, this being especially severe during REM sleep.[29]

Once a diagnosis is secure and the status of sleep disordered breathing is known, the next step would be to consider therapeutic alternatives for the chronic disease state. Before we begin this part of the chapter, I will discuss the management of the ICU phase of these diseases, a phase entered because of acute exacerbation of the usually chronic process.

ICU PHASE

Many of the details involved in treating acute respiratory failure will not be described since they will be covered in other chapters of this book. I focus on criteria for ICU admission and general approaches to treatment.

By definition we are dealing with patients who have chronic hypercapnic respiratory failure; all will have a variable degree of stable CO_2 retention and compensated respiratory acidosis as well as hypoxemia as part of the primary disease. Progression of the disease process, but more likely addition of a complicating secondary process such as infection, can result in acute deterioration of the already compromised respiratory function and worsening of the ventilatory failure and arterial blood gases (ABGs).[31] Aside from obvious clinically emergent situations (i.e., overwhelming infection or sepsis, hemodynamic instability, obtundation, or coma), the ABGs, which must be compared to the patient's baseline gases, are the best guide for assessing acutely ill patients for possible ICU admission. A 20mm Hg or more rise in Pa_{CO_2} associated with a decrease in pH to less than 7.25, especially when associated with signs of CO_2 narcosis clearly relegates the patient to an ICU setting. Absolute levels of $Paco_2$ will range from 65 to 90mm Hg. With these levels of $Paco_2$ the Pao_2 will be severely depressed, usually to values less than 40 to 50mm Hg.[32]

Once in the ICU, treatment will have to be tailored to the patients and will depend on the clinical presentation and the degree of ABG deterioration. Patients with severe acidosis (pH < 7.15), obtundation, or coma, are candidates for intubation and mechanical ventilation. The majority of patients, however, will not present so drastically and could be considered for a more conservative form of management as has been clearly effective in treating patients with COPD in acute exacerbation.[32,33] As long as the acidosis is not life threatening and the patient is hemodynamically stable, treatment must be primarily directed at the severe hypoxemia, otherwise these patients will succumb to hypoxia. Controlled oxygen administration at a low Fio_2, ideally via a Venturi mask (24 to 28% Fio_2) or a nasal cannula (1 to 2 L/min) to achieve and maintain a Po_2 between 50 to 60mm Hg should forestall the fatal effects of severe hypoxemia while therapy can be directed at reversible components of the acute process (i.e., airways obstruction, excessive bronchial secretions, infection, and cardiac failure). This management practice has been found to be effective in patients with COPD and may be successfully used as well for patients with other hypoventilation disorders. The principle of maintaining an appropriate degree of oxygenation while treating reversible conditions allows one to bide time for the patient to survive the acute episode and allow for eventual return to the prior functional level. There are no controlled studies comparing low flow oxygen versus mechanical ventilation and though the broad experience with the conservative approach to therapy is limited to COPD patients, anecdotal experience does support its use in patients who do not have COPD and who do not meet criteria for intubation and mechanical ventilation. The latter therapeutic approach is then relegated to those patients who fail conservative management and demonstrate continued deterioration of the ABGs or clinical state. As with oxygen therapy, mechanical ventilation allows one to gain time to permit the acute process to be reversed.

Intubation may have other beneficial effects on the therapy of patients with acute or chronic respiratory failure. A trial of mechanical ventilation with clear improvement in blood gases and acidosis may improve CNS and/or muscle function resulting in more rapid clinical improvement compared to conservative therapy. In patients with sleep apnea, intubation will essentially reverse obstructive apneas and dramatically improve the patient's condition. In addition, there is the advantage of controlling secretions by tracheal suction and preventing aspiration.

For all patients the decision to intubate and ventilate must be made in light of the known prior state of the chronic condition, the perceived ability to reverse the present acute process, wean the patient from the ventilator, and eventually return to a clinical state acceptable for the patient. This decision involves medical and ethical considerations that are often difficult and not unique to the ICU.

An alternative to low flow oxygen and invasive mechanical ventilation in treating acute exacerbation of hypoventilation disorders is that of "noninvasive" mechanical ventilation. Using a treatment modality that has become common in managing the chronic hypoventilation state (see later in this chapter), it entails ventilating the patient via a tight fitting nasal mask. Found to be efficacious in ventilating the stable chronic hypoventilator, recent experience has shown that this approach can be effective in the acutely ill patient as well.[34-38] The ability to ventilate the patient this way obviously avoids intubation and the morbidity it entails, and may allow one to adequately oxygenate the patient with less concern about worsening the degree of CO_2 retention than with use of low flow oxygen. At present there are no standard criteria for patient selection, contraindications, or methods of noninvasive ventilation, clearly demonstrating the need for extensive clinical studies, especially controlled studies comparing noninvasive ventilation with conventional therapy. However, failing such studies, mechanical ventilation via a nasal mask should be considered as a way to manage acute on chronic respiratory failure in patients with a hypoventilation syndrome.

POST-ICU PHASE

This phase essentially is relegated to long-term therapy of chronic hypoventilation. There are principles of therapy generic to most patients with chronic hypoventilation as well as therapeutic interventions specific to certain diseases. Neurologic diseases that can be specifically treated are myasthenia gravis and debatably, multiple sclerosis, though the latter is rarely associated with respiratory failure. Hypothyroidism is treatable and electrolyte imbalance, whether it be metabolic alkalosis, hypophosphatemia, hypomagnesemia, or hypokalemia, is usually reversible.

Two common diseases associated with alveolar hypoventilation, COPD and sleep apnea, can be singled out for the specific approach to their treatment.

Patients with severe irreversible airways obstruction typically receive an intensive regimen of bronchodilators including inhaled beta agonists and anticholinergics, theophylline, and often steroids. The efficacy of these drugs is variable, but even when there is significant improvement of airways obstruction and symptoms, it is unlikely that respiratory failure will be reversed in patients with COPD. Because these patients also manifest severe hypoxemia, they are invariably candidates for chronic home oxygen therapy. Indeed this is the one therapeutic regimen that can result in improved survival in these patients and should be the mainstay of treatment.[39,40]

More pertinent to the chronic hypercapnic respiratory failure in COPD patients is the consideration of two therapeutic approaches that are at present still investigational: inspiratory muscle training (IMT) and inspiratory muscle rest (IMR). The first is based on the assumption that the functionally impaired inspiratory muscles of these patients can be improved by specific training techniques. Indeed, both muscle strength and endurance can be improved by training directed at these ends. Clinical studies have shown variable results, some demonstrating subjective and objective clinical improvement, others no benefit.[41-46] Until more definitive, randomized studies are performed, including comparisons of IMT to exercise programs, which can also result in similar clinical improvement, IMT cannot be added to the therapeutic armamentarium for COPD.

If one assumes that respiratory failure in COPD is dependent on the development of diaphragmatic fatigue,[47,48] then the use of IMR is a logical extension of this assumption. Unfortunately, no data support the premise that patients with severe COPD develop inspiratory muscle fatigue. It has been shown in patients with COPD that ventilatory support with negative or positive pressure ventilation can unload and "rest" the diaphragm. Certain clinical trials have tested the efficacy of intermittent assisted ventilation in such patients with chronic hypoventilation.[49-53] The studies have generally been nonrandomized and noncontrolled, have had a variable time of ventilator use, and did not necessarily demonstrate that the method of ventilation suppressed spontaneous diaphragm activity. Again, the results have not been uniform, some demonstrating improvement in the clinical status and arterial blood gases of the treated patients, other studies demonstrating no effect. Of importance, the best designed trial thus far carried out with patients randomized to either daytime negative pressure ventilation or sham ventilation, failed to show any benefit of IMR.[54] Therefore, it would seem that current data would not support IMR as an effective form of therapy in hypoventilating patients with COPD. However, recent trials using positive pressure ventilation via a nasal mask have shown promising results.[35,36,38,55] These results coupled with the relative ease and comfort of using this form of ventilatory assist, especially during sleeping hours, should stimulate large and properly designed trials to test this methodology. Because of the relatively high prevalence of this disorder and the great expense of home ventilatory therapy, definitive data confirming the efficacy of IMR is mandatory before it can be accepted as a therapeutic option in these patients.

The association of obesity with cardiorespiratory failure was recognized early in this century and was codified in the medical literature as the pickwickian syndrome.[56] It is now clear that most pickwickians or, stated more appropriately, patients with OHS, have OSA. Hypoventilation, usually associated with cor pulmonale is a serious sequelae of the sleep apnea syndrome, which along with these complications is eminently treatable. Although the therapeutic options for sleep apnea are relatively broad, including surgical (i.e., uvulpalatopharyngoplasty [UPPP], mandibular advancement), pharmacologic, positional, and dietary approaches,[57-61] in the hypoventilating patient with significant morbidity and likely increased mortality,[62] only two forms of therapy should be considered, tracheostomy and nasal continuous positive airway pressure (NCPAP).[63,64] The former will clearly cure obstructive apnea and result in dramatic clinical and blood gas improvement, but the latter therapeutic modality may be just as effective, yet is noninvasive and relatively free of complications and side effects.[63,64] NCPAP, which is administered by means of a high flow air compressor via tight fitting nose mask to achieve pressure levels of 5 to 15 cm H_2O, essentially results in splinting the upper airway and preventing its passive collapse that causes the obstructive apneas.[64] If NCPAP is found to be effective in preventing obstructive apneas and reversing the sleep disruption and oxygen desaturation evident in the baseline polysomnography, and if it is tolerated and accepted by the patient, it is the preferable method of treatment.[65] Failing those criteria, tracheostomy becomes the treatment of choice. Patients treated with NCPAP must be carefully followed up to ensure compliance with therapy.[66] Effective therapy should result in improvement and likely resolution of the CO_2 retention.[67,68] This response along with the expected dramatic clinical improvement is most gratifying and stresses the importance of recognizing and diagnosing this disease so that it can be so treated.

The two diseases just discussed, COPDS and sleep apnea, are both rather prevalent and can coexist in the same patient. This overlap of two highly morbid diseases probably results in additive effects of both disease processes on the sleep-induced blood gas impairment and on daytime respiratory dysfunction as well. The presence of the mechanical and gas exchange abnormalities of airways obstruction in patients with predominantly sleep apnea may well contribute to the development of hypercapnia and pulmonary hypertension in these patients.[69-71] On the other hand, the presence of sleep apnea in patients with chronic airways obstruction may contribute to or independently result in hypercapnia and pulmonary hypertension that may be attributed to COPD because the presence of sleep apnea is overlooked or its importance to the clinical picture is not recognized. Such recognition is critical for proper management because unlike COPD, sleep apnea is treatable and its complications reversible.[72-74] Patients with COPD who have sleep apnea usually demonstrate obesity, daytime somnolence, snoring, etc.[73] One must be especially aware of the COPD patient with CO_2 retention who does not manifest the severe degree of airways obstruction that is characteristically associated with hypercapnia. An FEV_1 of greater than 1 to 1.3 L in such a clinical setting should arouse suspicion of disease in addition to COPD, mainly sleep apnea, and warrants the appropriate workup. The remarkable clinical benefit from treating sleep apnea should not be missed by failing to consider this diagnosis in certain patients with chronic airways obstruction.

Common to most patients with hypoventilation is the risk of experiencing sleep disordered breathing which is associated with nocturnal worsening of the already impaired blood gases. Especially vulnerable during REM sleep, these patients as a rule manifest sleep induced hypoxemia, hypercapnia, and respiratory acidosis.[27,28,75-78] Except for sleep apnea where sleep is associated with repetitive upper airway occlusions, the mechanism of sleep disordered breathing is not understood. Sleep, especially during REM, may result in further central depression of ventilatory drive, or selective inhibition of intercostal/accessory muscle activity.[79-80] Either perturbation can result in worsening hypoventilation and the above noted changes in blood gases as well as sleep disruption and fragmentation. The common daytime symptoms of fatigue and somnolence may be a product of this secondary sleep disorder.

Sleep-induced hypoventilation can be prevented by instituting ventilatory support of the patient during sleep. This support can be accomplished by a number of methods of assisted ventilation, including the rocking bed, negative pressure, and positive pressure ventilation.[81] The rocking bed, a classic but time worn ventilator is rather inefficient and its use has generally been supplanted by newer technology. Negative pressure ventilation (NPV) classically was effected by means of the iron lung, but these days more likely via the cuirass ventilator the pneumowrap (poncho).[81] NPV can be quite effective in ventilating hypoventilating patients, even those with kyphoscoliotic chest wall deformity.[82-86] It is often difficult, however, to capture the patient who tends to breathe around or through the negative pressure cycles. When successful, NPV has one significant drawback: the generated negative airway pressure may result in passive collapse of the upper airway and intermittent upper airway obstruction (i.e., obstructive sleep apnea), with the same consequence to gas exchange and sleep architecture as found in primary sleep apnea.[87] Under these circumstances continued efficacious use of NPV necessitates treatment of sleep apnea, either NCPAP or tracheostomy. This course makes NPV a less than desirable treatment option.

Positive pressure ventilation (PPV) obviates the upper airway problems of NPV. In addition, by utilizing the assist/control mode of a volume cycled ventilator, PPV allows for easier capture of the patient's ventilatory cycle than with NPV. The drawback of PPV has been that its use necessitated a tracheostomy for access to the airway for the ventilator.[88] This problem has been obviated recently by the demonstrated ability to effect PPV via the nose by means of a tight fitting nasal mask.[89,90] Nasally applied positive pressure ventilation (NPPV) is convenient and can be easily effected. It has been shown to inhibit spontaneous respiratory muscle activity in normal subjects and hypoventilation patients so ventilation can be controlled or assisted.[55] Though a relatively new method of providing assisted ventilation, there is accumulating evidence of the short- and long-term efficacy of NPPV and the relatively high rate of patient acceptance and compliance with its use.[91-94] The described side effects of NPPV (e.g., gastric distention, nasal bridge abrasion, and mask leak), have been mild and infrequent.[50,86,89] At the present time NPPV is probably the preferred choice for instituting nocturnal ventilatory assist in these patients.

It must be emphasized that most patients with hypoventilation syndromes, though manifesting chronic respiratory failure, are not ventilator dependent and can sustain adequate ventilatory function during waking hours. It is during nocturnal sleep that ventilatory assistance is required to prevent the disease related deterioration of respiratory control and its sequelae. It is also apparent that the effects of this sleep disordered breathing are causally related to the progression of daytime respiratory failure and the downhill course of the hypoventilation process. Nocturnal support of ventilation, whether by NPV or PPV, can effect marked clinical improvement (i.e., decreased fatigue, somnolence, dyspnea, sleep disruption and improvement of cor pulmonale with resolution of CHF), and most important, improvement of the arterial blood gases, even normalization of the Pa_{CO_2}.[89-94] It is important to emphasize that resolution of alveolar hypoventilation with successful nocturnal ventilation clearly denotes the critical importance of the sleep disorder in the pathophysiology of the disease process. Although the primary disease initiating the hypoventilation state may not be treatable, the sleep disordered breathing can well be controlled and its effects reversed.

Prior to initiating chronic assisted ventilation, the degree of sleep disordered breathing must be determined by baseline nocturnal polysomnography. There are no tested criteria that can be promulgated for instituting nocturnal ventilation, but the presence of O_2 desaturations greater than 6 to 10% or to levels less than 75 to 80% and Pa_{CO_2} increases of more than 10 to 15 mm Hg in patients with chronic hypercapnia certainly warrants therapy. Subsequently, the prevention of documented sleep-induced dysfunction by the chosen form of ventilation must be verified by a second, therapeutic study. Ideally, these trials should be performed with monitoring the arterial Pa_{CO_2} (with an indwelling arterial line), in addition to the usual physiologic parameters. The reason for the ability of nocturnal therapy to effect global improvement of chronic hypoventilation without affecting the primary elements of the disease process is unknown. As in sleep apnea, the effects of the nighttime perturbation on the CNS may result in further impairment of respiratory control, this being prevented and possibly reversed by the use of nocturnal ventilation. One may also speculate that assisted ventilation results in resting the stressed, functionally remaining respiratory muscles so that their overall function is improved.[55] These are interesting ideas and the subject of further investigation.

Nocturnal assisted ventilation must be considered life-long therapy. Patients with nonprogressive disease (i.e., PAH), some neuromuscular disorders and possibly kyphoscoliosis, can do well and remain stable for an indefinite period.[88-94] Patients with progressive neuromuscular disease, or those with a superimposed respiratory infection may be unable to sustain adequate ventilation even during waking hours and require ventilatory support either continuously or for a major part of the day. Noninvasive NPPV can be effective in these patients, but if such daytime ventilatory needs are long term, PPV via a tracheostomy or NPV may be more efficacious than NPPV.[86] The need for chronic, continuous ventilatory support at home or in an institution will depend on the nature of the primary disease and its natural history. The problem of long-term care is discussed in detail in Chapter 24.

EPILOGUE

Patient 1: The patient's hypoventilation had been ascribed to his COPD, but the relatively well-preserved FEV_1 and a subsequently elicited history of daytime somnolence and snoring led to ordering a nocturnal polysomnogram that showed severe obstructive sleep apnea (apnea index of 60 per hour, maximum O_2 desaturation to 40%) that was completely reversed with NCPAP at 10 cm H_2O. After 3 months of nightly NCPAP use his followup ABGs were: Pa_{O_2} 70 mm Hg, Pa_{CO_2} 42 mm Hg, pH 7.42.

Patient 2: The patient was admitted to the MICU. The

chest radiograph showed severe scoliosis with a new right lower lobe infiltrate. She was intubated, ventilated with a volume cycled ventilator, and after 24 hours the Pa_{CO_2} stabilized at 60 mm Hg with a pH of 7.32. After three days of mechanical ventilation and parenteral antibiotics, she was extubated. Her ABGs on room air were: Pa_{CO_2} 48 mm Hg, Pa_{CO_2} 56 mm Hg, pH 7.35. A subsequent nocturnal sleep study, while receiving O_2 at 2 L per minute via nasal cannula, revealed mild hypoventilation and O_2 desaturation in NREM sleep, but periods of marked decrement in tidal volume and chest wall excursions with severe O_2 desaturation to 50% during REM sleep. These episodes of sleep-disordered breathing were essentially prevented by NPPV. Three months after hospital discharge and nightly use of NPPV her ABGs were: Pa_{O_2} 66 mm Hg, Pa_{CO_2} 49 mm Hg, pH 7.38.

Patient 3: Subsequent history revealed a brother who died of "sleep apnea" at age 31 and who had a tracheostomy at the time of his death. The patient had jugular venous distention and clinical evidence of cor pulmonale: right parasternal lift, accentuated pulmonic second heart sound (P2), and a soft right-sided S3 and S4. With voluntary hyperventilation, her Pa_{CO_2} decreased from 63 mm Hg to 38 mm Hg. Ventilatory response to CO_2 rebreathing was markedly blunted. Nocturnal polysomnography showed frequent hypopneas and central apneas (10 to 30 seconds) in NREM and especially REM sleep associated with severe O_2 desaturation (decreasing to less than 50% in REM) worsening hypercapnia (Pa_{CO_2} as high as 85 mm Hg with a pH of 7.19). There were no obstructive apneas. Sleeping with NPV (cuirass) improved the overall hypoventilation but the patient developed frank obstructive apneas. With NPPV, obstructive apneas were avoided while the primary sleep-induced breathing disorder was well controlled (only occasional hypopneas, no apneas, no O_2 desaturation or CO_2 elevation greater than 4% and 5 mm Hg, respectively). Four months after nightly use of NPPV, she no longer had CHF; physical findings of cor pulmonale had receded and her daytime ABGs were: Pa_{O_2} 77 mm Hg, Pa_{CO_2} 46 mm Hg, pH 7.39.

REFERENCES

1. Lopata, M., and Lourenco, R. V.: Evaluation of respiratory control. Clin. Chest Med., 1:33, 1980.
2. Irsigler, G. B., and Severinghaus, J. W.: Clinical problems of ventilatory control. Annu. Rev. Med., 31:1009, 1980.
3. West, J. B.: Causes of carbon dioxide retention in lung disease. N. Engl. J. Med., 284:1232, 1971.
4. Weiner, M., Chausow, A., and Szidon, P.: Reversible respiratory muscle weakness and hypothyroidism. Br. J. Dis. Chest, 80:391, 1986.
5. Zwillich, C. W., et al.: Ventilatory control in myxedema and hypothyroidism. N. Engl. J. Med., 292:662, 1975.
6. Lopata, M., and Onal, E. L.: Mass loading, sleep apnea and the pathogenesis of obesity hypoventilation. Am. Rev. Respir. Dis., 126:640, 1982.
7. Kohorst, W. R., Schonfeld, S. A., and Altman, M.: Bilateral diaphragmatic paralysis following topical cardiac hypothermia. Chest, 85:65, 1984.
8. Rhoads, G. G., and Brody, J. S.: Idiopathic alveolar hypoventilation: clinical spectrum. Ann. Intern. Med., 71:271, 1969.
9. Newsom-Davis, J., Goldman, M., Loh, L., and Casson, M.: Diaphragm function and alveolar hypoventilation. Q. J. Med., 45:87, 1976.
10. Loh, L., Goldman, M., and Newsom-Davis, J.: The assessment of diaphragm function. Medicine, 56:165, 1977.
11. Javaheri, S., and Kazemi, H.: Metabolic alkalosis and hypoventilation in humans. Am. Rev. Resp. Dis., 36:1011, 1987.
12. Newman, J. H., Neff, T. A., and Ziporin, P.: Acute respiratory failure associated with hypophosphatemia. N. Engl. J. Med., 296:1101, 1977.
13. Dhingra, S., Solven, F., Wilson, A., and McCarthy, D. S.: Hypomagnesia and respiratory muscle power. Am. Rev. Respir. Dis., 129:497, 1984.
14. Bergofsky, E.: Respiratory failure disorders of the thoracic cage. Am. Rev. Respir. Dis., 119:643, 1979.
15. Sivak, E. D., et al.: Respiratory insufficiency in adult-onset acid maltase deficiency. South. Med. J., 80:205, 1987.
16. Sivak, E. D., and Streib, E. W.: Management of hypoventilation in motor neuron disease presenting with respiratory insufficiency. Ann. Neurol., 7:188, 1980.
17. Rideau, Y., Jankowski, L. W., and Grellet, J.: Respiratory function in the muscular dystrophies. Muscle Nerve, 4:155, 1981.
18. Ray, C. S., et al.: Effects of obesity on respiratory function. Am. Rev. Respir. Dis., 128:501, 1983.
19. Black, L. F., and Hyatt, R. E.: Maximal respiratory pressures: normal values and relationship to age and sex. Am. Rev. Resp. Dis., 99:696, 1969.
20. Black, L. F., and Hyaff, R. E.: Maximal static respiratory pressures in generalized neuromuscular disease. Am. Rev. Respir. Dis., 103:641, 1971.
21. Demedts, M., Beckers, J., Rochette, F., and Bulcke, J.: Pulmonary function in moderate neuromuscular disease without respiratory complaints. Eur. J. Respir. Dis., 63:62, 1982.
22. Gibson, G. J., Pride, N. B., Newsom-Davis, J., and Loh, L.: Pulmonary mechanics in patients with respiratory muscle weakness. Am. Rev. Respir. Dis., 115:389, 1977.
23. Richter, T., West, J. R., and Fishman, A. P.: The syndrome of alveolar hypoventilation and diminished sensitivity of the respiratory center. N. Engl. J. Med., 256:1165, 1957.
24. Fishman, A. P., Goldring, R. M., Turino, G. M.: General alveolar hypoventilation: a syndrome of respiratory and cardiac failure in patients with normal lungs. Q. J. Med., 35:261, 1966.
25. Mellins, R. B., Balfour, H. H., Turino, G. M., and Winters, R. W.: Failure of automatic control of ventilation (Ondine's Curse). Medicine, 49:487, 1970.
26. Braun, N. M. T., Arora, N. S., and Rochester, D. F.: Respiratory muscle and pulmonary function in polymyositis and other proximal myopathies. Thorax, 38:616, 1983.
27. Mezon, B. L., West, P., Israel, J., and Kryger, M.: Sleep breathing abnormalities in kyphoscoliosis. Am. Rev. Respir. Dis., 122:617, 1982.
28. Guilleminault, C., Kurlame, G., Winkle, R., and Miles, L. E.: Severe kyphoscoliosis, breathing and sleep. Chest, 79:626, 1982.
29. George, C. P. F.: Sleep in neuromuscular diseases. In Principles and Practice of Sleep Medicine. Edited by M. H. Kyger, T. Loth, and W. C. Dement, Philadelphia, W. B. Saunders, 1985, p. 630.
30. Orr, W. C.: Utilization of polysomnography in the assessment of sleep disorders. Med. Clin. North Am., 69:1153, 1985.
31. Grippi, M. A., and Fishman, A. P.: Respiratory failure in structural and neuromuscular disorders involving the chest bellows. In Pulmonary Diseases and Disorders. Edited by A. P. Fishman. New York, McGraw-Hill, 1988, p. 2299.
32. Campbell, E. J. M.: The management of acute respiratory failure in chronic bronchitis and emphysema. Am. Rev. Respir. Dis., 96:626, 1967.

33. Francis, P. B.: Acute respiratory failure in obstructive lung disease. Med. Clin. North Am., *67*:657, 1983.
34. Muir, J. E., et al.: Management of acute respiratory failure (ARF) in elderly patients with nasal intermittent positive pressure ventilation (NIPPV). Am. Rev. Respir. Dis., *141*:A237, 1990.
35. Laier-Groenveld, G., Huttemann, U., and Criee, C. P.: Noninvasive nasal ventilation in acute and chronic ventilatory. Am. Rev. Respir. Dis., *141*:A237, 1990.
36. Waldhorn, R. E., Robinson, R., Murthy, R., and Jennings, C.: Nasal intermittent positive pressure ventilation (NIPPV) with bi-level positive airway pressure (BIPAP) in acute and chronic respiratory failure. Am. Rev. Respir. Dis., *141*:A238, 1990.
37. Brochard, L., et al.: Face mask inspiratory positive airway pressure (IPAP) versus conventional therapy for acute exacerbation of chronic obstructive pulmonary disease (COPD). Am. Rev. Respir. Dis., *141*:A238, 1990.
38. Meduri, G. U., et al.: Noninvasive face mask mechanical ventilation in patients with respiratory failure. Am. Rev. Respir. Dis., *141*:A238, 1990.
39. Nocturnal Oxygen Therapy Trial Group. Continuous or nocturnal oxygen therapy in hypoxemic chronic obstructive lung disease. Ann. Intern. Med., *93*:391, 1980.
40. The Medical Research Council Working Party. Long-term domiciliary oxygen therapy in chronic hypoxic cor pulmonale complicating chronic bronchitis and emphysema. Lancet, *1*:681, 1981.
41. Belman, M. T., and Mittman, C.: Ventilatory muscle training improves exercise capacity in chronic obstructive disease patients. Am. Rev. Respir. Dis., *121*:273, 1980.
42. Pardy, R. L., Remington, R. N., Despas, P. T., and Macklem, P. T.: The effects of inspiratory muscle training on exercise performance in chronic airflow limitation. Am. Rev. Respir. Dis., *123*:426, 1981.
43. Sonne, L., and Davis, J.: Increased exercise performance in patients with severe COPD following inspiratory resistive training. Chest, *81*:436, 1982.
44. Larson, J. L., Kim, M. J., Sharp, J. T., and Larson, D. A.: Inspiratory muscle training with a pressure threshold breathing device in patients with chronic obstructive pulmonary disease. Am. Rev. Respir. Dis., *138*:689, 1988.
45. Chen, H. I., Dukes, R., and Martin, B. J.: Inspiratory muscle training in patients with chronic obstructive pulmonary disease. Am. Rev. Respir. Dis., *131*:251, 1985.
46. Belman, M. T., and Shadmehr, R.: Targeted resistive ventilatory muscle training in chronic obstructive pulmonary disease. J. Appl. Physiol., *65*:2726, 1988.
47. Macklem, P. T., and Roussos, C.: Respiratory muscle fatigue: a cause of respiratory failure. Clin. Sci., *53*:419, 1977.
48. Kongragunta, V. R., Druz, W. S., and Sharp, J. T.: Dyspnea and diaphragmatic fatigue in patients with chronic obstructive pulmonary disease: responses to theophylline. Am. Rev. Respir. Dis., *137*:662, 1988.
49. Braun, N., and Marino, W. D.: Effect of daily intermittent rest of respiratory muscles in patients with severe chronic airflow limitation (abstract). Chest, *85*:59S, 1984.
50. Van Weerden, G. J.: Preliminary results of periodic ambulant ventilatory treatment in patients suffering from severe chronic non-specific respiratory disease. Folia Med. Neerl, *9*:125, 1966.
51. Cropp, A., and DiMarco, A. F.: Effects of intermittent negative pressure ventilation in respiratory muscle function in patients with severe chronic obstructive pulmonary disease. Am. Rev. Respir. Dis., *135*:1056, 1987.
52. Gutierrez, M., et al.: Weekly cuirass ventilation improves blood gasses and inspiratory muscle strength in patients with chronic airflow limitation and hypercarbia. Am. Rev. Respir. Dis., *138*:616, 1988.
53. Zibrak, J. D., et al.: Evaluation of intermittent long-term negative pressure ventilation in patients with severe chronic obstructive pulmonary disease. Am. Rev. Respir. Dis., *138*:1515, 1988.
54. Martin, J. G.: Clinical intervention in chronic respiratory failure. Chest, *97*:105, 1990.
55. Carrey, Z., Gottfried, S. B., and Levy, R. D.: Ventilatory muscle support in respiratory failure with nasal positive pressure ventilation. Chest, *97*:150, 1990.
56. Burwell, C., Rabin, E., Whaley, R., and Bilkman, A.: Extreme obesity associated with alveolar hypoventilation: a Pickwickian syndrome. Am. J. Med., *21*:811, 1956.
57. Fujita, S., Conway, W., Zorick, F., and Roth, T.: Surgical correction of anatomic abnormalities in obstructive sleep apnea syndrome: uvulopalatopharyngoplasty. Otolaryngol. Head Neck Surg., *89*:923, 1981.
58. Powell, N. B., Guilleminault, C., Riley, R. W., and Smith, L.: Mandibular advancement and obstructive sleep apnea syndrome. Bull. Eur. Physiopathol. Respir., *19*:607, 1983.
59. Strohl, K. P., et al.: Progesterone administration and progressive sleep apneas. JAMA, *245*:1230, 1980.
60. Braunell, L. G., et al.: Protriptyline in obstructive sleep apnea. N. Engl. J. Med., *307*:1037, 1982.
61. Smith, P. L., et al.: Weight loss in mildly to moderately obese patients with obstructive sleep apnea. Ann. Intern. Med., *103*:850, 1985.
62. Ke, J., et al.: Mortality and apnea index in obstructive sleep apnea: experience in 385 male patients. Chest, *94*:9, 1988.
63. Guilleminault, C., et al.: Obstructive sleep apnea and tracheostomy: long-term follow-up experience. Arch. Intern. Med., *141*:985, 1981.
64. Sullivan, C. E., Issa, F. G., Berthon-Jones, M., and Eves, L.: Reversal of obstructive sleep apnea by continuous positive airway pressure applied through the nares. Lancet, *1*:862, 1981.
65. Popkin, J., et al.: A one-year randomized trial of nasal CPAP versus protryptyline in the management of obstructive sleep apnea. Sleep, *17*:237, 1988.
66. Grunstein, R. R., Dood, M. J., Costas, L., and Sullivan, C. E.: Home nasal CPAP for sleep apnea—acceptance of home therapy and its usefulness. Aust. N. Z. J. Med., *16*:635, 1986.
67. Rapoport, D. M., Sorkin, B., Garay, S. M., and Goldring, R. M.: Reversal of the "Pickwickian Syndrome" by long-term use of nocturnal nasal airway pressure. N. Engl. J. Med., *307*:931, 1982.
68. Firth, R. W., and Cont, B. R.: Severe obstructive sleep apnea treated with long-term nasal positive airway pressure. Thorax, *40*:45, 1985.
69. Bradley, T. D., et al.: Role of diffuse airway obstruction in the hypercapnia of obstructive sleep apnea. Am. Rev. Respir. Dis., *134*:920, 1986.
70. Bradley, T. D., et al.: Role of daytime hypoxemia in the pathogenesis of right heart failure in the obstructive sleep apnea syndrome. Am. Rev. Respir. Dis., *131*:835, 1985.
71. Leech, J. A., Önal, E., Bahr, P., and Lopata, M.: Determinants of hypercapnia in patients with sleep apnea syndrome. Chest, *92*:807, 1987.
72. Guilleminault, C., Cummiskey, J., and Motta, J.: Chronic obstructive airflow disease and sleep studies. Am. Rev. Respir. Dis., *122*:397, 1980.
73. Flenley, D. C.: Sleep in chronic obstructive lung disease. Clin. Chest. Med., *6*:651, 1985.
74. Fletcher, E. C., Schaaf, J. W., Miller, J., and Fletcher, J. G.: Long-term cardiopulmonary sequelae in patients with sleep

apnea and chronic lung disease. Am. Rev. Respir. Dis., *135:* 525, 1987.
75. Wynne, J. W., et al.: Disordered breathing and oxygen desaturation during sleep in patients with chronic obstructive lung disease (COLD). Am. J. Med., *66:*537, 1979.
76. Arand, D. L., McGinty, D. J., and Littner, M. R.: Respiratory patterns associated with hemoglobin desaturation during sleep in chronic obstructive pulmonary disease. Chest, *80:* 183, 1981.
77. Skatrud, J., et al.: Determinants of hypoventilation during wakefulness and sleep in diaphragmatic paralysis. Am. Rev. Respir. Dis., *121:*587, 1980.
78. Smith, P. E. M., Calverly, P. M. A., and Edwards, R. H. T.: Hypoxemia during sleep in Duchenne muscular dystrophy. Am. Rev. Respir. Dis., *137:*884, 1988.
79. Muller, N. L., et al.: Mechanism of hemoglobin desaturation during REM sleep in normal subjects and in patients with cystic fibrosis. Am. Rev. Respir. Dis., *121:*463, 1980.
80. Johnson, M. W., and Remmers, J. E.: Accessory muscle activity during sleep in chronic obstructive pulmonary disease. J. Appl. Physiol., *57:*1011, 1984.
81. Hill, N. S.: Clinical applications of body ventilators. Chest, *90:*897, 1986.
82. Holtackers, T. R., Loosbrock, L. M., and Gracey, D. R.: The use of the chest cuirass in respiratory failure of neurologic origin. Respir. Care, *27:*271, 1982.
83. Goldstein, R. S., et al.: Reversal of sleep-induced hypoventilation and chronic respiratory failure by nocturnal negative pressure ventilation in patients with restrictive ventilatory impairment. Am. Rev. Respir. Dis., *135:*1049, 1987.
84. Driver, A. G., Blackburn, B. B., Marcuard, S. P., and Austin, E. H.: Bilateral diaphragm paralysis treated with cuirass ventilation. Chest, *136:*1276, 1987.
85. Celli, B. R., Rassulo, J., and Corral, R.: Ventilatory muscle dysfunction in patients with bilateral idiopathic diaphragmatic paralysis: reversal by intermittent external negative pressure ventilation. Am. Rev. Respir. Dis., *136:*1276, 1987.
86. Mohr, C. H., and Hill, N. S.: Long-term follow up of nocturnal ventilatory assistance in patients with respiratory failure due to Duchenne-type muscular dystrophy. Chest, *97:*91, 1990.
87. Glenn, W. W., et al.: Combined central alveolar hypoventilation and upper airway obstruction. Treatment by tracheostomy and diaphragm pacing. Am. J. Med., *64:*50, 1978.
88. Hoeppner, V. H., Cockcroft, D. W., Dosman, J. A., and Cotton, D. J.: Nighttime ventilation improves respiratory failure in secondary kyphoscoliosis. Am. Rev. Respir. Dis., *129:*240, 1984.
89. Kirby, G. R., Mayer, L. S., and Pingleton, S. K.: Nocturnal positive pressure ventilation via nasal mask. Am. Rev. Respir. Dis., *135:*738, 1987.
90. Leger, P., Jennequin, J., Gerard, M., and Robert, D.: Home positive pressure ventilation via nasal mask for patients with neuromuscular weakness or restrictive lung or chest-wall disease. Respir. Care, *34:*73, 1989.
91. Ellis, E. R., Bye, P. T., Bruderer, J. W., and Sullivan, C. E.: Treatment of respiratory failure during sleep in patients with neuromuscular disease: positive-pressure ventilation through a nose mask. Am. Rev. Respir. Dis., *135:*148, 1987.
92. DiMarco, A. F., Connors, A. F., and Altose, M. D.: Management of chronic alveolar hypoventilation with nasal positive pressure breathing. Chest, *92:*952, 1987.
93. Ellis, E. R., et al.: Noninvasive ventilatory support during sleep improves respiratory failure in kyphoscoliosis. Chest, *94:*811, 1988.
94. Bach, J. R., and Alba, A. S.: Management of chronic alveolar hypoventilation by nasal ventilation. Chest, *97:*52, 1990.

SUPPLEMENTAL READINGS

Benhamou, D., et al.: Nasal mask ventilation in acute respiratory failure. Chest, *102:*912, 1992.
Brochard, L., et al.: Reversal of acute exacerbation of chronic obstructive pulmonary disease by inspiratory assistance with a face mask. N. Engl. J. Med., *323:*1523, 1990.
Carney, Z., Gottfried, S. B., and Levy, R. D.: Ventilatory muscle support in respiratory failure with nasal positive pressure ventilation. Chest, *97:*150, 1990.
Chevrolet, J. C., et al.: Nasal positive pressure ventilation in patients with acute respiratory failure. Chest, *100:*775, 1991.
Elliott, M. W., et al.: Domiciliary nocturnal nasal intermittent positive pressure ventilation in COPD: mechanisms underlying changes in arterial blood gas tensions. Eur. Respir. J., *4:*1044, 1991.
Foglio, C., et al.: Acute exacerbations in severe COLD patients. Treatment using positive pressure ventilation by nasal mask. Chest, *101:*1633, 1992.
Gay, P. C., Patel, A. M., Viggiano, R. W., and Hubmayr, R. D.: Nocturnal nasal ventilation for treatment of patients with hypercapneic respiratory failure. Mayo. Clin. Proc., *66:*695, 1991.
Goldstein, R. S.: Hypoventilation: neuromuscular and chest wall disorders. Clin. Chest Med., *13:*507, 1992.
Goldstein, R. S., DeRosie, J. A., Avendano, M. A., and Dolmage, T. E.: Influence of noninvasive positive pressure ventilation on inspiratory muscles. Chest, *99:*408, 1991.
Heckmatt, J. Z., Loh, L., and Dubowitz, V.: Night-time nasal ventilation in neuromuscular disease. Lancet, *10:*579, 1990.
Hill, N. S.: Noninvasive ventilation. Does it work, for whom, and how? Am. Rev. Respir. Dis., *147:*1050, 1993.
Marino, W.: Intermittent volume cycled mechanical ventilation via nasal mask in patients with respiratory failure due to COPD. Chest, *99:*681, 1991.
Meduri, G. U., et al.: Noninvasive face mask mechanical ventilation in patients with acute hypercapneic respiratory failure. Chest, *100:*445, 1991.
Meduri, G. U., Conoscenti, C. C., Menashe, P., and Nair, S.: Noninvasive face mask ventilation in patients with acute respiratory failure. Chest, *95:*865, 1989.
Pennock, B. E., et al.: Pressure support ventilation with a simplified mask in patients with respiratory failure. Chest, *100:* 1371, 1991.
Piper, A. J., et al.: Nocturnal nasal IPPV stabilized patients with cystic fibrosis and hypercapnic respiratory failure. Chest, *102:*846, 1992.
Strump, D. A., et al.: Nocturnal positive-pressure ventilation via nasal mask in patients with severe chronic obstructive pulmonary disease. Am. Rev. Respir. Dis., *144:*1234, 1991.
Strumpf, D. A., Millman, R. P., and Hill, N. S.: The management of chronic hypoventilation. Chest, *98:*474, 1990.
Waldhorn, R. E.: Nocturnal nasal intermittent positive pressure ventilation with bi-level positive airway pressure (BIPAP) in respiratory failure. Chest, *101:*516, 1992.

Chapter 12

MANAGEMENT OF THE UPPER AIRWAY IN THE CRITICALLY ILL PATIENT

MANI S. KAVURU
ISAAC ELIACHAR
EDWARD D. SIVAK

PRE-ICU PHASE

Upper airway obstruction (UAO) is an infrequent cause of admission to the ICU. UAO is a disease with a dramatic presentation, however, with a high risk/benefit ratio. When the characteristic clinical findings are recognized and appropriate and aggressive therapy instituted, the outcome is usually excellent.

Factors that dictate the clinical presentation of UAO include:

- The site of obstruction (upper versus lower, intrathoracic versus extrathoracic)
- Pace of obstruction (acute versus chronic)
- The cause of obstruction
- The underlying physiologic reserve or the preexisting size of the airway

In general, UAO is a more common and serious problem in the pediatric age group than in adults because of several unique anatomic features of the upper airway in children. UAO does occur, however, in adults and therefore familiarity with the differential diagnosis and management strategies of UAO is essential to the intensivist. Figures 12-1 and 12-2 represent the normal anatomic relationship of the larynx and proximal trachea.

Symptoms and Diagnosis

UAO may produce symptoms of dyspnea, cough, wheeze, difficulty clearing secretions, sore throat, and hoarseness.[1] Patients may be febrile, may drool and have difficulty swallowing secretions, may be toxic in appearance, and may have varying degrees of respiratory distress. The hallmark of extrathoracic UAO is stridor which is a harsh, whistling sound that initially occurs on inspiration during hyperventilation and can subsequently progress to involve the entire respiratory cycle. Stridor will result with either mechanical obstruction from edema, inflammation, or mass lesion in the pharynx, larynx, or trachea, or from vocal cord dysfunction. Brief history and a neck examination demonstrating the classic stridor may often be adequate to establish a tentative diagnosis of UAO. In some patients with an atypical presentation or in patients with underlying obstructive parenchymal lung disease, however, physical examination may be misleading.

Pulmonary function tests are useful in the diagnosis of UAO. The forced vital capacity maneuver, graphically displayed as a flow-volume loop, may provide insight into the nature of airway obstruction.[2,3,4] Typically, there is limitation of airflow at high lung volumes, which produces a sharp peak in the flow-volume loop during periods of maximal flow. Miller and Hyatt described characteristic patterns of the loop that help to localize the site of obstruction[4] (Figure 12-3). With UAO the shape of the loop is related to the level of the obstruction (above or below the thoracic inlet) and the net effect of pressures acting on the extrathoracic and intrathoracic airway, including the atmospheric pressure, intraluminal pressure, and intrapleural pressure (Fig. 12-4).[5] The extrathoracic airway tends to collapse with inspiration (tracheal pressure is less than atmospheric pressure); the intrathoracic airway tends to collapse with expiration (a situation where tracheal pressure is less than pleural pressure). This explains why stridor and flow limitation are mainly inspiratory in extrathoracic UAO and expiratory (with wheezes) in intrathoracic UAO. In general, other physiologic parameters such as diffusing capacity, distribution of ventilation, and oxygenation are usually normal in UAO.

Causes of UAO in adults can be broadly classified as:

- Infectious/inflammatory
- Dynamic
- Anatomic or space occupying
- Traumatic

Discussion in this chapter will be limited to infectious, inflammatory, and dynamic disorders of the upper airway. Head and neck tumors are discussed in Chapter 13.

Infectious/Inflammatory

Supraglottitis

Supraglottitis, a more accurate designation than epiglottitis, represents an acute infection of the supraglottic laryngeal and contiguous tissues which can cause life-threatening UAO.[6] For many years, this disorder was viewed exclusively as a pediatric disorder. In the past decade, however, there have been several series which have highlighted the importance of adult supraglottitis.[7-13] The incidence of supraglottitis in adults is unclear, but an 8-year

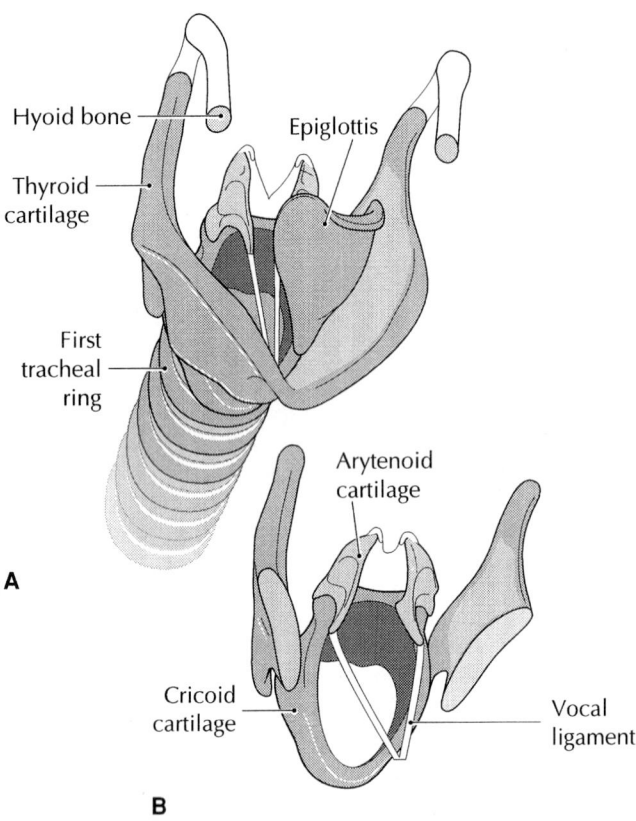
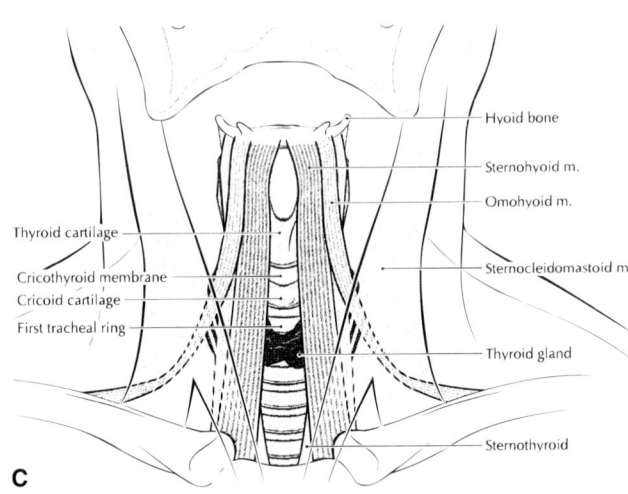

Fig. 12–1. *A*, Schematic illustrating the normal anatomy of the larynx, glottis, and the proximal trachea. *B*, Magnified schematic view of the glottis. *C*, Schematic illustration of the normal anatomy of the anterior aspect of the neck.

study in the state of Rhode Island found 56 cases, for an annual incidence of 9.7 cases per million adults, with an increase during the study period.[9] Similarly, Murrage and colleagues from Western Ontario noted a bimodal age distribution for supraglottitis, with 35% of all patients during a 10-year period being adults.[10] Whether these data represent an actual increase in the incidence of adult supraglottitis or simply an increased recognition remains unclear.

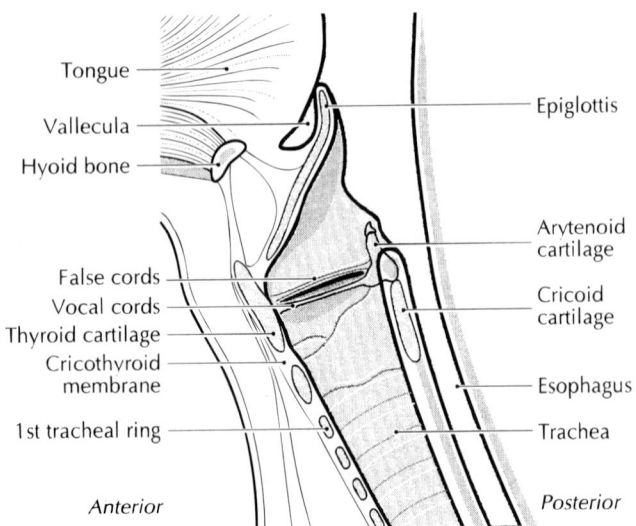

Fig. 12–2. Parasagittal view of the normal larynx and proximal trachea.

Clinical manifestations of adult supraglottitis appear to be less severe than the well-recognized counterpart in children.[10] Children with Haemophilus influenzae supraglottitis have a much more fulminant presentation including fever, dyspnea, drooling, and toxic appearance, with a mean duration of symptoms before presentation of 6 hours.[14] Also, the appearance of the supraglottic tissues on physical examination has a striking "cherry red" swelling.[6] In contrast, adult symptoms may range from sore throat to dysphagia to odynophagia with usual onset over several days. Physical examination commonly shows mild erythema and swelling of the supraglottic structures. In children, supraglottitis is almost always caused by H. influenzae type B, and several reports suggest that the incidence of bacteremia ranges between 79% and 100%.[14] MayoSmith reported a 23% incidence of H. influenzae bacteremia in their adult series consistent with other reports in the literature.[9] Even in adults, H. influenzae remains the most frequently identified pathogen, although the frequency of bacteremia is considerably lower than in children.[10] Throat cultures in both children and adults are not reliable in identifying a causative organism. MayoSmith identified bacteremia as a significant risk factor for more fulminant disease in adults.[10]

Significant controversy remains in the optimal management of adult supraglottitis. The conventional practice in pediatric epiglottitis is a very aggressive approach toward securing a safe and stable airway as soon as a diagnosis of supraglottitis is suspected.[14] If a patient is stable enough, then a plain lateral neck radiograph may be cautiously performed to distinguish supraglottitis from acute viral laryn-

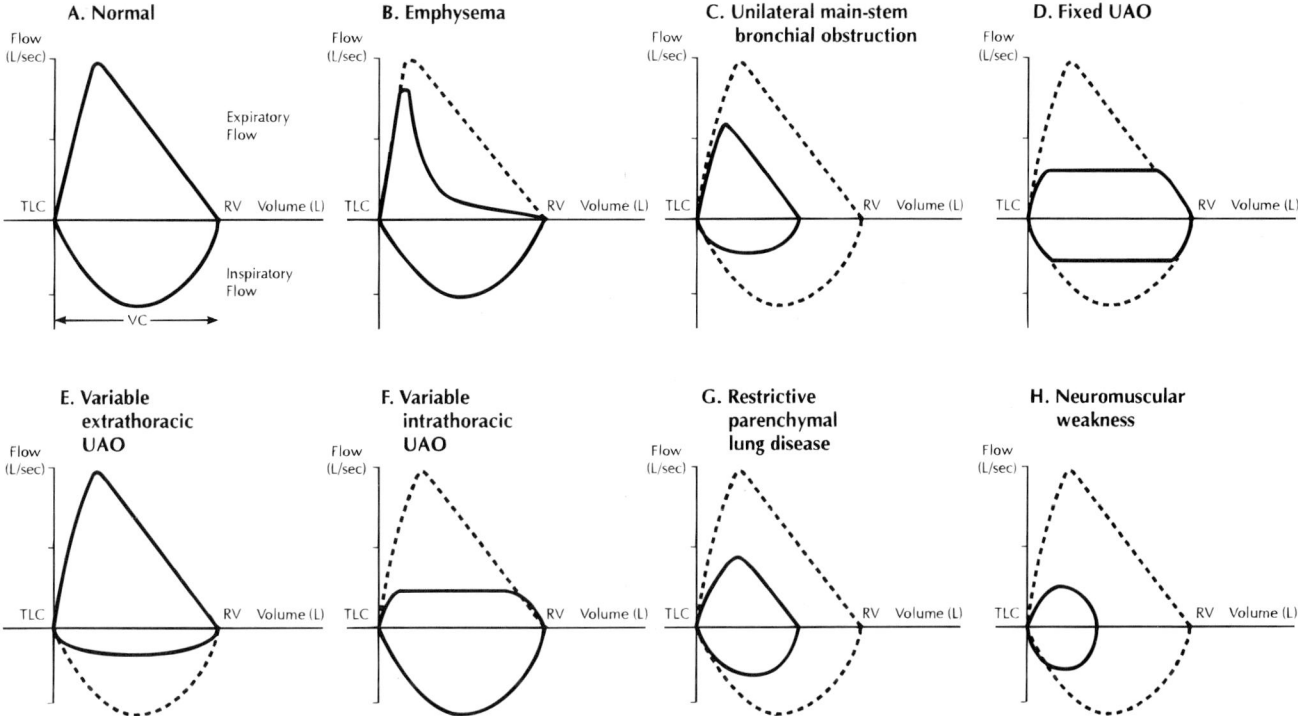

Fig. 12-3. Depicted is a graphic display of the forced vital capacity maneuver as a flow-volume loop. A, Normal loop; B to H, loops from a variety of disorders affecting the flow-volume loop. Flow is displayed on the vertical axis as liters per second, whereas volume is displayed on the horizontal axis as liters. Forced expiration begins at total lung capacity (TLC), and inspiration begins at residual volume (RV). Each loop is composed of an expiratory limb (where flow rates are displayed as a positive value on the graph) and an inspiratory limb (where flow rates are displayed as a negative value). In B: patient with emphysema demonstrates a predominant abnormality in the expiratory limb with a reduction in flow rates at all lung volumes, the dotted line representing the normal. The inspiratory limb is fairly normal. D is an example of a fixed upper airway obstruction (UAO) demonstrating a box-like flattening of both the expiratory and inspiratory limbs. Fixed obstruction anywhere in the upper airway that affects both inspiration and expiration may result in a loop with this configuration. E shows a variable extrathoracic UAO with a flattening of the inspiratory limb of the loop; an example may be bilateral vocal cord paralysis or polyps. F is a variable intrathoracic UAO with predominant flattening of the expiratory limb of the loop; an example is a lesion affecting the mid- or distal trachea such as tracheomalacia. C shows a unilateral main stem bronchial obstruction resulting in a loop with a fairly normal configuration except for a "restricted" appearance with smaller volumes. In G, a loop as seen in restrictive parenchymal lung disease (an example is pulmonary fibrosis) with a reduction in lung volumes and flows. In H, a loop as seen in a patient with neuromuscular weakness, with severe extrathoracic restrictive disease secondary to respiratory muscle weakness. (Modified from O'Reilly, M. J., et al.: Sepsis from sinusitis in nasotracheally intubated patients: a diagnostic dilemma. Am. J. Surg., 147:601, 1984.)

geal tracheitis. Direct laryngoscopy is generally not recommended for fear of precipitating complete airway obstruction. Patients are usually taken immediately to the operating room for laryngoscopy and emergency airway management, usually with nasotracheal intubation.[14] Several studies have shown less morbidity and mortality with nasotracheal intubation than tracheostomy and studies show no long-term sequelae after translaryngeal intubation in an 8-year follow-up. The risk of sudden, total airway obstruction in children is so high that there is a general consensus toward immediate intubation. There is some controversy, however, in adults. Some authors have recommended an artificial airway for all adults suspected of supraglottitis,[7] whereas others have recommended close observation while therapy is being provided.[10] There is clearly a margin of safety in adult patients that is not present in children. It is reasonable for a stable patient to be observed in an intensive care setting where an experienced endoscopist can view the subglottic larynx at any time and airway support can be readily instituted.[6,13] A ventilating rigid bronchoscope used by an experienced endoscopist may provide a safe airway at anytime.

Antibiotic therapy for supraglottitis should target a presumed H. influenzae infection until the results of beta lactamase testing are available. A second generation cephalosporin or a combination of chloramphenicol and ampicillin are equally acceptable. Intravenous therapy can be started in the hospital for several days and therapy can subsequently be continued orally for 10 to 14 days at home. Although steroids have been anecdotally used, there is little objective evidence of the efficacy of steroids in this disease. Mortality in children with supraglottitis has dropped to less than 1% since the use of prophylactic airway intubation. Several reports indicate that the mortality

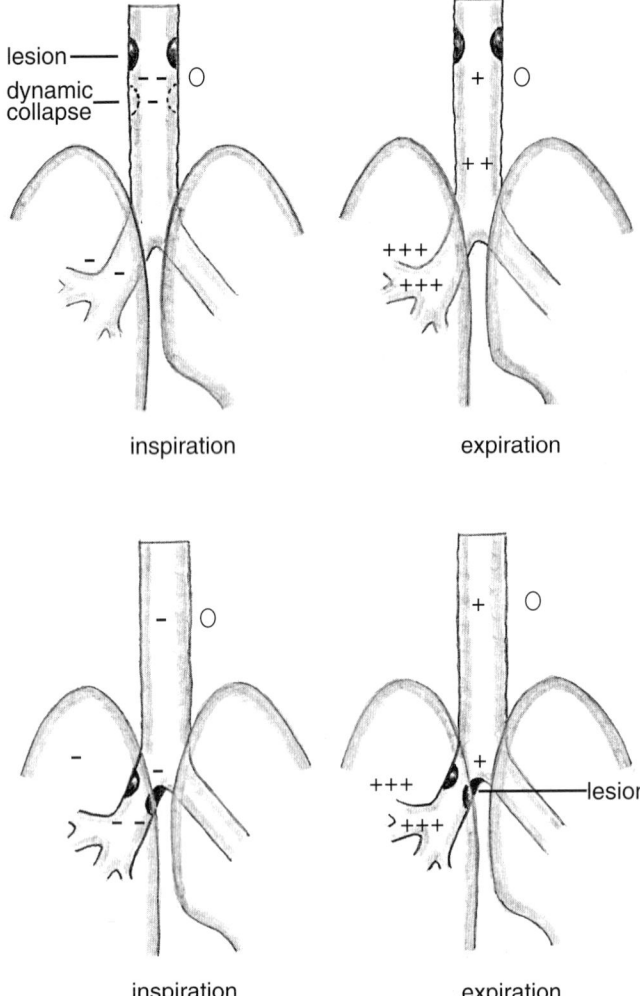

Fig. 12-4. Pressure events during the respiratory cycle with extrathoracic (A) and intrathoracic (B) obstructing lesions. See text for details.

among adults remains 6% and suggest the need for more aggressive airway management in adults.[7]

Ludwig's Angina

Ludwig's angina is a progressive submaxillary cellulitis that involves the neck and floor of the mouth. In a recent review, Moreland described 141 cases of this entity since 1945 and compared the findings to 315 cases from the preantibiotic era.[15] Mean age of patients was 29, and most were previously healthy. Many had evidence of dental disease, however, with a history of lower molar toothache or recent extraction described in 79% of patients. Clinical symptoms including submandibular swelling, elevation of the tongue, dysphagia, and trismus were present in more than 50% of patients. Streptococci and anaerobes were most frequently isolated from soft tissue cultures. Airway obstruction due to edema of the suprahyoid tissues is the most life-threatening problem of Ludwig's angina, but only 2 of the 141 patients described since 1945 died of airway obstruction, probably credited to aggressive airway management over the years. There is no consensus on the timing, need for an artificial airway, or route of intubation of the artificial airway. Similarly, the need for early surgical incision and drainage is controversial, especially in the absence of fluctuance. Computed tomography (CT) scan may be helpful in determining the timing of surgical drainage. Certainly, aggressive early antibiotic therapy targeting streptococci and anaerobes is critical; and perhaps in patients with pharyngitis, including coverage for H. influenzae may be considered as well. There has been a significant drop in mortality rate from 50% in the preantibiotic era to 8.5% since 1945.[15]

Anaphylaxis

Anaphylaxis is a generalized, immediate, and often life-threatening reaction caused by release of bioactive mediators from mast cells and basophils.[16,17] UAO as manifested by hoarseness and stridor is potentially a life-threatening problem that may complicate a subset of patients with anaphylaxis from any cause. In many cases of anaphylaxis, an inciting antigen may be identified such as antibiotics, foreign proteins, immunotherapy, insect stings, or various foods. Common causes of anaphylactoid reactions include contrast media, muscle depolarizing agents, or complement activation secondary to blood products. A recent review of 276 patients with anaphylaxis revealed that cardiovascular collapse occurs in 92% of patients, erythema in 48%, bronchospasm in 29%, angioedema in 24%, along with rash, gastrointestinal symptoms, generalized edema, and pulmonary edema in less than 10%.[17]

Angioedema

Angioedema most frequently involves the periorbital areas, lips, tongue, hands, feet, and genitalia. Patients may have angioedema on the basis of:

- Allergy
- Congenital deficiency of the inhibitor of the first component of complement (hereditary angioedema)
- Idiopathic, no external trigger can be identified

Angioneurotic edema is a rare but important side effect of angiotensin-converting enzyme (ACE) inhibitor.[18-20] It manifests as a well-demarcated swelling of the tongue, lips, and edema of the upper respiratory tract which can result in serious acute respiratory distress, airway obstruction, and death. A recent literature review suggested that angioedema occurs in 0.1% to 0.2% of patients receiving ACE inhibitors.[18] The onset usually occurs within hours or at most 1 week after starting therapy. It reverses within hours after stopping the drug and does not appear to be dose related. Patients with a history of idiopathic angioedema may be at increased risk for developing angioedema from ACE inhibitors.[19] The mechanism for this reaction is speculative but may involve autoantibodies, bradykinin, or complement-system components.[18] Treatment involves expectant airway management, epinephrine, antihistamines, and possibly corticosteroids. Therapy for the underlying cardiovascular disorder should be with an alternative class of antihypertensive agents.

Table 12-1. Comparison of Clinical Features of Hereditary and Allergic/Idiopathic Angioedema

Clinical Features	Hereditary	Allergic or Idiopathic
Duration	lifelong	<1 y
Itching/urticaria	rare	common
UAO	common (50%)	rare
Induced by trauma	common	rare
Abdominal pain	common	rare
Positive family history	common (80%)	rare

Hereditary angioedema accounts for a small fraction of all angioedema and should be included in the differential diagnosis of any patient with unexplained angioedema.[21] A recent study suggested that patients with hereditary angioedema had symptoms for an average of 21 years before their disease was diagnosed.[22] Several clinical clues may favor a diagnosis of hereditary angioedema as opposed to the allergic or idiopathic variety (Table 12-1).[23] First, patients with the hereditary form have a lifelong disorder whereas patients with the other forms have a history of less than 1 year. Second, urticaria and pruritus are usually not features of the hereditary variety. Third, UAO occurs in about 50% of all patients with hereditary angioedema, which is considerably more often than in patients with other forms of the disorder. Fourth, over 50% of the episodes of hereditary angioedema are precipitated by trauma such as dental surgery. Trauma does not appear to be related to the course of other types of angioedema. Fifth, episodes of cramping abdominal pain are perhaps the best single clinical feature that discriminates hereditary angioedema from other kinds of angioedema. If unrecognized, the abdominal pain can be so perplexing that the patients may undergo exploratory laparotomy for this problem. Finally, about 85% of patients with hereditary angioedema have a positive family history.

The clinical syndrome of hereditary angioedema is directly related to an inherited deficiency of C1 inhibitor (C1 INH), which inhibits the activated form of the first component of complement.[22] The absence of control by C1 INH leads to unopposed activation of the C1r and C1s subunits and these patients have free circulating activated C1s in their plasma during attacks of their disease, but not during asymptomatic intervals. The single most reliable screening test for diagnosis is measurement of C4, which is always decreased, even during asymptomatic periods, though the decrease may be more significant during symptomatic periods.[23] C4 is a better screening test than C3 or total hemolytic complement levels. When a subnormal C4 level has been established, it is essential to confirm the diagnosis by performing an assay for C1 INH by either an immunoassay or a functional assay. Family studies have shown that the hereditary angioedema exhibits an autosomal dominant inheritance pattern and children have a 50% chance of inheriting the disease regardless of gender, and generations are not skipped. Management of hereditary angioedema involves three separate issues. First, therapy for an acute attack mainly involves maintenance of airway patency if obstruction is imminent, and the administration of intravenous hydration if the patient has severe vomiting. Second, prophylaxis before surgical trauma with either repletion of C1 INH levels (fresh frozen plasma or occasionally a purified C1 INH) or plasmin inhibitors (aminocaproic acid). Third, in patients with disability due to frequent attacks, suppression or elimination of all symptoms can be achieved by chronic treatment with androgens (Stanozolol or Danazol).

Idiopathic Anaphylaxis

Wiggins described the evaluation and classification of a group of 123 patients with idiopathic anaphylaxis (IA).[24] The episodes in all patients consisted of urticaria or angioedema with concomitant life-threatening manifestations of UAO, bronchospasm, hypotension, or loss of consciousness. In some patients, other associated symptoms included generalized flushing and gastrointestinal symptoms (IA with generalized symptoms). This occurred in 63 of 123 patients with IA. In 43 of 123 patients, IA occurred with life-threatening UAO. The outcome for both groups of patients was felt to be similar with no deaths. Therapy was based on frequency of episodes, with prophylactic therapy by prednisone given for patients with frequent episodes. By definition, there was no identifiable antigen responsible for episodes of IA, and no underlying disease in these patients. Some authors have suggested a mast cell-basophil activation mechanism. Wiggins concluded that IA may represent the most severe form of a spectrum of diseases that includes idiopathic urticaria and angioedema.[24]

Dynamic Vocal Cord Paralysis

Vocal cord paralysis (VCP), either unilateral or bilateral, is an uncommon disorder caused by a variety of diseases which may locally affect the recurrent laryngeal nerve. The functional consequences of unilateral and bilateral VCP differ significantly. The paralyzed cord is usually in a paramedian position. With unilateral VCP, patients develop hoarseness and occasionally symptoms related to aspiration, but UAO is usually absent because the contralateral functional vocal cord is able to abduct away from the midline during inspiration. The left vocal cord is more commonly involved because the left recurrent laryngeal nerve is more vulnerable to injury by its longer, circuitous route in the chest. Conditions including lung cancer with mediastinal adenopathy, left atrial or pulmonary outflow tract enlargement, and aortic aneurysms can compress the nerve and result in left VCP. Unilateral right VCP can occur by right-sided Pancoast tumors or metastases to the right superior mediastinum, by damaging the right recurrent laryngeal nerve.

In bilateral VCP, both cords are adducted in the midline of the airway. During exhalation, the vocal cords passively abduct, being pushed aside by positive airway pressure. Because of the neutral position of the cords in the midline, the voice may be relatively preserved. During inspiration, the flaccid cords adduct acting as one way valves, thereby obstructing the airway. Stridor may develop and result in respiratory failure. Other symptoms may include nocturnal stridor, monotone voice, and conscious suppression of cough and laughter. Bilateral VCP may simulate UAO from a variety of other conditions including laryngotracheal tumors and aspirated foreign bodies.[25]

Parnell and Brandenberg, in a survey of 1,407 patients with VCP reported that the etiology was related to: thyroid surgery (33%), malignant neoplasm (24%), other "mechanical" forces including aortic aneurysm (8%), central nervous system disease (4%), and idiopathic (23%).[26] In a review by Hollinger and colleagues of 389 cases of partial or complete bilateral VCP, 240 cases occurred in adults age 13 or older.[27] The most frequent causes included: 138 of 240 followed thyroidectomy; 52 of 240 were associated with various neurologic disorders including poliomyelitis, Parkinson's disease, strokes, Guillain-Barré syndrome, multiple sclerosis; 16 of 240 were due to malignant neoplasms of the neck and mediastinum; 34 of 240 were due to miscellaneous or idiopathic causes. A Mayo Clinic review of 1088 patients with VCP found that 202 (18%) had bilateral paralysis.[28] In 13 patients (6% of 202), no cause for paralysis was found initially despite thorough examination. During a follow-up period, 4 of the 13 patients had partial or complete return of vocal cord function, usually within 6 months of the onset of upper airway symptoms. Five of the 13 patients required tracheostomy. There have been reports of bilateral VCP and UAO in patients with bilateral cortical stroke,[29] extrapyramidal disorders such as Parkinson's disease,[30] and vocal cord fixation secondary to severe rheumatoid arthritis.[31]

The decision to treat VCP depends on the severity of voice dysfunction and dyspnea, whether the paralysis is unilateral or bilateral, whether the disorder is VCP or fixation, and the underlying cause of the disease. In general, unilateral paralysis is better tolerated than bilateral paralysis. Most patients with bilateral paralysis will require intubation for management of airway obstruction. The airway can then be converted to a tracheostomy for long-term management, and a one-way valve can be attached to the tracheostomy tube to allow exhalation through the normal airway and preserve speech. Rarely, external beam radiation therapy or chemotherapy directed at the mediastinal tumor may return function to one or both cords if the nerve was only compressed, as opposed to disruption by direct neoplastic invasion. However, VCP is more commonly permanent. Several surgical procedures are available to allow removal of the tracheostomy tube. These techniques include laser arytenoidectomy and reinnervation.

Vocal Cord Dysfunction/"Factitious Asthma"

Over the past decade, several reports have described patients with functional vocal cord disorders that mimic attacks of bronchial asthma.[32,33] The typical history involves episodes of wheezing and dyspnea that are refractory to standard therapies for asthma. These individuals may have wheezing that is often loudest over the upper airway, but the wheezing is often transmitted over both lung fields and may be misdiagnosed as bronchial asthma. During episodes of wheezing, the maximal expiratory and inspiratory flow-volume loop is consistent with variable extrathoracic obstruction.[32] The pathophysiology in these individuals, as noted by laryngoscopy, appears to be adduction of the true and false vocal cords throughout the respiratory cycle, including the inspiratory phase. During asymptomatic periods, both the flow-volume loop and the laryngoscopic examination are normal. Interestingly, methacholine provocation testing for bronchial asthma is usually negative. Christopher and colleagues described a variety of personality styles and psychiatric diagnoses in these individuals and suggested that this disorder is a form of conversion reaction.[32] They described a dramatic response to speech therapy and psychotherapy in these patients with factitious vocal cord dysfunction. Tracheostomy may be rarely required.

Treatment

In acute UAO, evaluation and management often have to proceed simultaneously. The management typically involves three phases:

- Initial airway management
- Nonspecific adjunctive measures
- Specific measures to treat the underlying cause of the UAO

Initial Airway Management

The preeminent issue in the pre-ICU phase in patients with acute UAO is to ensure a stable, patent airway. If a conservative approach is elected, patients should be carefully observed and monitored in an intensive care setting where there is expertise for emergent establishment of an artificial airway if needed. If a decision has been made to bypass an UAO, the options include translaryngeal intubation (nasal or oral), ventilating rigid bronchoscopy, cricothyroidotomy, or a tracheostomy. Attempting intubation by direct laryngoscopy or over a fiberoptic bronchoscope can often bypass the obstruction. There is a risk of exacerbating the obstruction by manipulation of the airway, especially in patients with severe obstruction. In children with supraglottitis, most investigators strongly recommend that this should be undertaken in the operating room in cooperation with an experienced surgeon. In adults with UAO it may be reasonable to attempt translaryngeal intubation initially, provided that experienced personnel and equipment are available.

Nonspecific Adjunctive Measures

Several nonspecific adjunctive measures may be used in the acute management of UAO pending a more definitive treatment. Respiratory depressants of all types must be avoided in the setting of UAO. Gas exchange is usually well maintained in patients with UAO, although hypoxemia may occur secondary to ventilation-perfusion mismatching or to alveolar hypoventilation. In general, supplemental oxygen therapy should be used. Inhalation therapy with alpha adrenergic agonists are often used to promote mucosal vasoconstriction and reduce edema. For adults, 1.5 to 2.5 ml of either the racemic mixture (Vaponefrin) or 1% of epinephrine is nebulized in 10 to 15 minutes. The effect is usually short-lived for 1 to 2 hours and a rebound increase in UAO can occur if the underlying process has not been corrected. Although there are many reports to suggest its effectiveness, especially in children with laryngotracheitis, there are no prospective studies in adults with other causes of UAO. Likewise, systemic corticosteroids have been felt to be useful in pediatric viral laryngotracheitis and this practice has often been used in adults with a variety of UAO. Some clinicians have advocated steroids and vasoconstrictive medications to be administered several hours prior to removal of an endotracheal tube in patients with prolonged intubation.

Helium-oxygen mixtures have been widely used in patients with acute UAO. Airway resistance is reduced when a patient with UAO is breathing a He-O$_2$ mixture. Flow in the upper airways is turbulent and resistance depends on gas density. Helium is a gas with a density one seventh that of nitrogen. Therefore, patients with UAO achieve higher flow and have less respiratory distress and stridor while breathing He-O$_2$. Although this therapy is theoretically attractive, several technical requirements must be satisfied prior to use:

- Patients must be able to tolerate a tight fitting mask.
- F$_{IO_2}$ should be less than 0.4.
- The equipment is cumbersome and careful calibration is required.
- Equipment is not always available.

Specific Measures

After the stability of the airway has been addressed and the nonspecific adjunctive measures have been instituted, then long-term specific treatment of the underlying cause of UAO should be addressed for definitive management.[34] This treatment may include antibiotic therapy for an underlying airway infection, drainage of an abscess, removal or resection of a foreign body, airway tumor, or other specific therapy as indicated. Specific treatment of various causes of airway obstruction are listed in Table 12-2.

ICU PHASE: TRACHEAL INTUBATION, INDICATIONS, TECHNIQUES, AND COMPLICATIONS

Access to and control of the upper airway is a preeminent issue that confronts the initial management of critically ill patients. The issues related to tracheal intubation may be addressed by paramedic personnel in the field,[35] emergency room physicians, or by intensivists after semielective transfer to an ICU. The trachea can be intubated by four distinct routes: oral, nasal, laryngeal (via cricothyroid membrane), or tracheal (via tracheotomy). Broadly speaking, access to the trachea can be considered under: (1) acute UAO (specific causes previously discussed in the pre-ICU phase), or (2) a wide variety of medical and surgical disorders requiring control of the airway. A recent consensus conference of the National Association of the Medical Directors of Respiratory Care outlined four indications for tracheal intubation:[36]

- Maintenance of airway patency
- Protection of the airway from aspiration
- Facilitation of secretion clearance

Table 12-2. Specific Treatment for Upper Airway Obstruction

Condition	Treatment
Lugwig's angina	Penicillin or clindamycin
Epiglottitis	First choice: cefuroxime, cefotaxime, ceftazidime, or ceftriaxone, second choice: chloramphenicol: household contacts <4 years of age: rifampin (20 mg/kg/day to maximum 600 mg/day × 4 days)
Peripharyngeal abscess	Surgical drainage, antibiotics (clindamycin, cefoxitin, or penicillin)
Diphtheria	Antitoxin, erythromycin, or penicillin
Angioneurotic edema	Epinephrine SC or IM, antihistamines
Hereditary angioneurotic edema	Androgens (prophylactic), C1 inhibitor
Tracheal stenosis	Bronchoscopic dilation, surgical repair, laser resection
Vocal cord paralysis	Surgery, tracheostomy
Tumors	Endoscopic resection, surgery, radiation, laser resection
Relapsing polychondritis	Steroids, dapsone, immunosuppressants
Papillomatosis	Endoscopic resection

(From Kryger, M. H., and Perez-Padilla, R. J.: Upper airway obstruction. *In* Current Therapy of Respiratory Disease. Edited by R. Cherniak. Philadelphia, B. C. Decker, 1989, p. 25.)

- Making mechanical ventilatory support possible

Translaryngeal Intubation

In patients without a specific upper airway disorder, translaryngeal intubation is by far the most common and first-line mode of airway access in acute care settings. Selecting the specific route of translaryngeal intubation, nasotracheal versus orotracheal, is to some extent a matter of an individual practitioner's expertise and familiarity. Both routes have particular advantages and disadvantages, however, and one may be preferred over the other in certain clinical settings and the critical care physician should be skilled in both approaches. Intubation should be performed by individuals with specific training[37] and there is increasing pressure for institutions to credential personnel on the basis of training, experience, and available backup.

The relative advantages and disadvantages of oral and nasal intubation are summarized in Table 12-3. In general, oral tube insertion is faster, is direct, and is less traumatic. A wider and shorter tube can usually be passed by this route facilitating suctioning, passage of a fiberoptic bronchoscope if needed, and theoretically has the advantage of less tube related air-flow resistance and slightly decreased anatomic dead space. This route avoids nasal and paranasal complications (Table 12-4). Therefore, specific clinical circumstances where oral access may be preferred include the setting of specific nasal pathology, underlying coagulopathy, and in circumstances when the anticipated need for intubation is less than 1 week. The advantages with the nasal route are greater patient comfort in long-term use, improved oral hygiene, and ability to swallow oral secretions. There is also potential for improved communication. Usually, there is better tube anchoring and less chance for inadvertent extubation or occlusion of orotra-

Table 12-3. Comparison of Oral and Nasal Intubation

Orotracheal intubation
    Advantages
- Insertion is faster, easier
- Wider and shorter tube is tolerated
- Avoid nasal complications
- Preferred in presence of coagulopathy

    Disadvantages
- Risk of tube occlusion by biting
- Mouth care is more difficult
- Greater risk of self-extubation

Nasotracheal intubation
    Advantages
- Greater patient comfort, easier mouth care
- Better tube anchoring
- May be performed without muscle relaxants
- Readily performed over fiberoptic bronchoscope

    Disadvantages
- Risk of sinusitis, otitis, epistaxis
- Blind insertion requires spontaneous breathing
- Narrower and longer tube is tolerated

---

cheal tube by biting. Specific clinical circumstances where nasal route may be preferred include: longer term need for translaryngeal intubation in conscious patients, specific oral or maxillofacial surgery or disorders, and in the presence of trismus where there is concern for tetanic biting of the oral tube. The potential disadvantages of nasal intubation include septal trauma, bleeding, necrosis, sinusitis,[38-43] and increased tube-related airway resistance secondary to longer and smaller tube placement.

The technique of tracheal intubation, whether elective, urgent, or emergent should proceed in a methodical fashion with attention to several key steps. Despite the frenzy that often exists, most intubations should be considered semielective and all available help should be used at the bedside with the operator at the head of the bed directing traffic. The initial emphasis is placed on establishing the ABCs of basic life support protocols.[44] Emphasis should be placed on effective oxygenation and ventilation with a self-inflating resuscitation bag with a properly fitting face mask connected to a 100% oxygen source.[45] Once this procedure is accomplished and circulation is stable then the process of intubation can proceed in an orderly fashion. If a patient is conscious, the steps involved in the intubation procedure should be described to the patient.

Table 12-4. Predisposing Conditions and Complications of Nasal Intubation

Predisposing conditions
- Deviated septum
- Turbinate hypertrophy
- Nasal polyposis
- Allergic/vasomotor rhinitis
- Coagulopathy

Complications
- Difficult insertion
- Epistaxis
- Septal trauma and perforation
- Paranasal sinus infection
- Eustachian tube dysfunction
- Otitis media

The pharmacologic preparation of the patient is important and it involves agents that are often used for various indications in the ICU. Options include short-acting barbiturates, benzodiazepines such as midazolam, or narcotic drugs such as morphine or fentanyl. Paralytic drugs are sometimes used in addition to the sedating agents if muscle relaxation is necessary and they should be given only if full ventilatory support is immediately available. A variety of agents including succinylcholine, and nondepolarizing agents such as vecuronium and pancuronium are occasionally used. Emphasis should be placed on topical anesthesia especially for the conscious or semiconscious patient. This can be accomplished with 2 or 4% lidocaine delivered by an atomizer or a tip applicator. Alternatives include 2% tetracaine or 14% benzocaine spray. Vasoconstriction and topical anesthesia must be accomplished in the nose with cocaine or with phenylephrine, together with effective lubrication. Anticholinergic agents are useful to decrease the volume of secretions.

A continuous suction (Yankauer) catheter connected to a wall suction unit should be readily available. Typically, the same catheter is used for both the oral and the nasal routes, in general an 8.5- to 9-mm oral tube is used for men and an 8-mm oral tube for women, and usually a half size less for the nasal route. The tube length can be estimated by placing the tube next to the patient's head and assuming that the carina is at the level of the sternal angle. The aim is to place the tip of the endotracheal tube 4 or 5 cm above the carina. A critical step in successful intubation by either the oral or the nasal route is the appropriate positioning of the patient. The axis of the mouth, pharynx, and larynx need to be aligned in a straight line, and this alignment requires flexion of the neck at the lower cervical vertebrae and extension of the head at the atlanto-occipital joint (Fig. 12-5). This can be accomplished with the patient being placed in a so-called "sniffing position," with several rolled towels under the patient's head (Fig. 12-6). With the patient in the appropriate position and preoxygenated by bag and mask ventilation, oral intubation can proceed with the lips and teeth being opened with the right hand using the crossed finger technique. The laryngoscope is inserted into the mouth held by the nondominant hand, pushing the base of the tongue forward and to the left. A curved MacIntosh blade or a straight Miller blade can be used, the former passed forward until its tip rests in the vallecula and the latter used to lift the epiglottis (Fig. 12-7). Manual pressure on the cricoid cartilage by an assistant may help expose the vocal cords during intubation. A lubricated tube is gently advanced through the glottis under direct visualization.

Nasal intubation procedure may be either performed blind[46] or guided by a laryngoscope together with Magill forceps which grasp and advance the tip of the tracheal tube once it reaches the pharynx (Fig. 12-8). Documenting proper tube position within the trachea is essential and should be initially assessed by physical examination for bilateral equal air entry into the lung fields, and by the absence of gastric dilatation. During blind passage of a nasotracheal tube, audible breath sounds from the tube may signal placement in the proximal trachea rather than

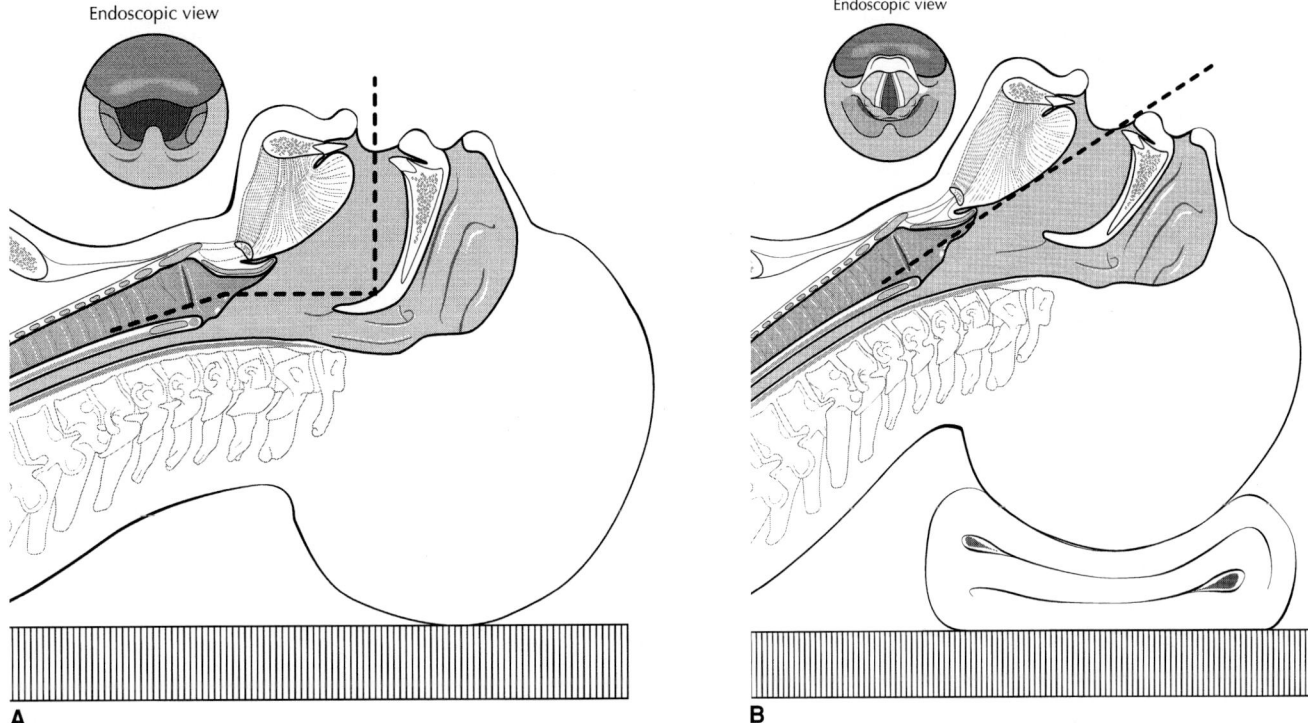

Fig. 12–5. *A,* Supine position demonstrating the axial planes of mouth, pharynx, and trachea. The endoscopic view (inset) only visualizes the posterior pharynx. *B,* Supine position with flexion of the lower portion of the cervical spine and extension of the atlanto-occipital joint. With proper positioning, the mouth, pharynx, and trachea are in proper alignment for directly visualized oral intubation. The endoscopic view (inset) with the head in a "neutral" position clearly shows the glottis and the vocal cords.

the esophagus.[46] The appearance of tracheal secretions into the tube is suggestive of proper placement. A portable chest radiograph is mandatory. Studies suggest that tube repositioning is required in 15% of the patients based on the result of the chest radiograph. Ideal position for a tracheal tube is in the center of the tracheal lumen 4 to 5 cm above the carina.[47] An alternative technique to ensure proper tube position is by fiberoptic tracheobronchoscopy through the endotracheal tube.

The success of intubation is to some extent dependent on the expertise and familiarity of the operator. The inability to intubate a patient is acutely life-threatening and therefore an organized alternative management plan is essential for the difficult intubation (Table 12-5). A difficult intubation has been variously defined as a circumstance when a well-trained individual with at least 12 months of experience fails to intubate the trachea on three successive attempts.[48] In anesthesia practice at teaching hospitals this has been estimated to be in the range of 2 to 4%.[49] Murrin and colleagues summarized the causes of difficult intubation under categories of:[50]

- Anatomic abnormalities
- Congenital airway abnormalities

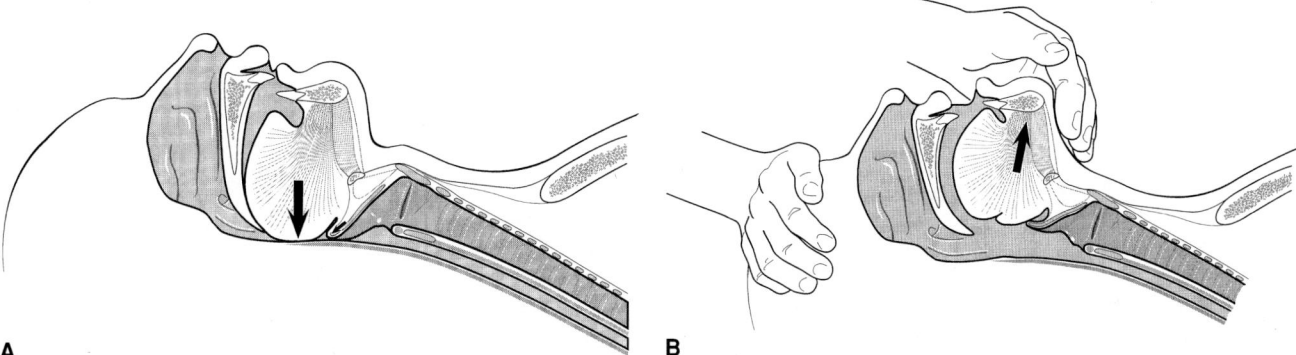

Fig. 12–6. *A,* In the supine, unconscious patient, upper airway obstruction can occur secondary to collapse of the flaccid tongue and epiglottis onto the posterior pharyngeal wall. *B,* This obstruction can be relieved by various maneuvers, as described in the text.

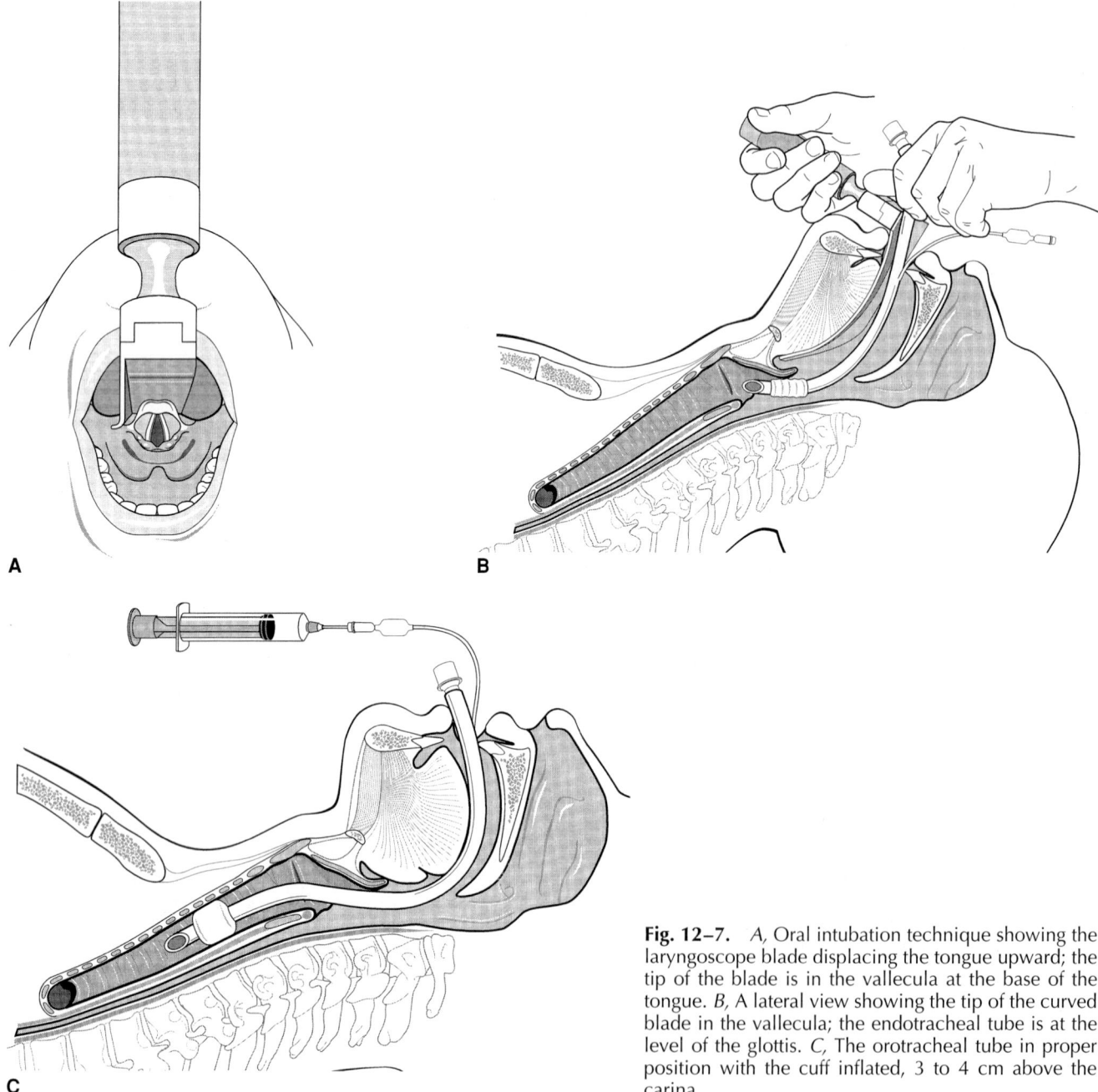

Fig. 12-7. *A,* Oral intubation technique showing the laryngoscope blade displacing the tongue upward; the tip of the blade is in the vallecula at the base of the tongue. *B,* A lateral view showing the tip of the curved blade in the vallecula; the endotracheal tube is at the level of the glottis. *C,* The orotracheal tube in proper position with the cuff inflated, 3 to 4 cm above the carina.

- Head and neck trauma
- Infectious disease
- Neoplastic disease
- Inflammatory rheumatologic disease

In the absence of these specific conditions, common pitfalls in translaryngeal intubation are listed in Table 12-6. The most frequent error is malpositioning of the patient's head and neck. Various techniques and devices are available to assist one in difficult intubations, including various stylets and flexible guide wires.[49-52] In these circumstances, flexible fiberoptic bronchoscopy can be invaluable in visually directing a tube placed over the bronchoscope either via the nasal or the oral route.[53] This procedure does require familiarity and expertise with a flexible fiberoptic laryngoscope or bronchoscope. In general, it is well suited for the conscious patient, preferably in the upright sitting position. The patient should be capable of cooperation under effective topical anesthesia with control of oropharyngeal secretions.

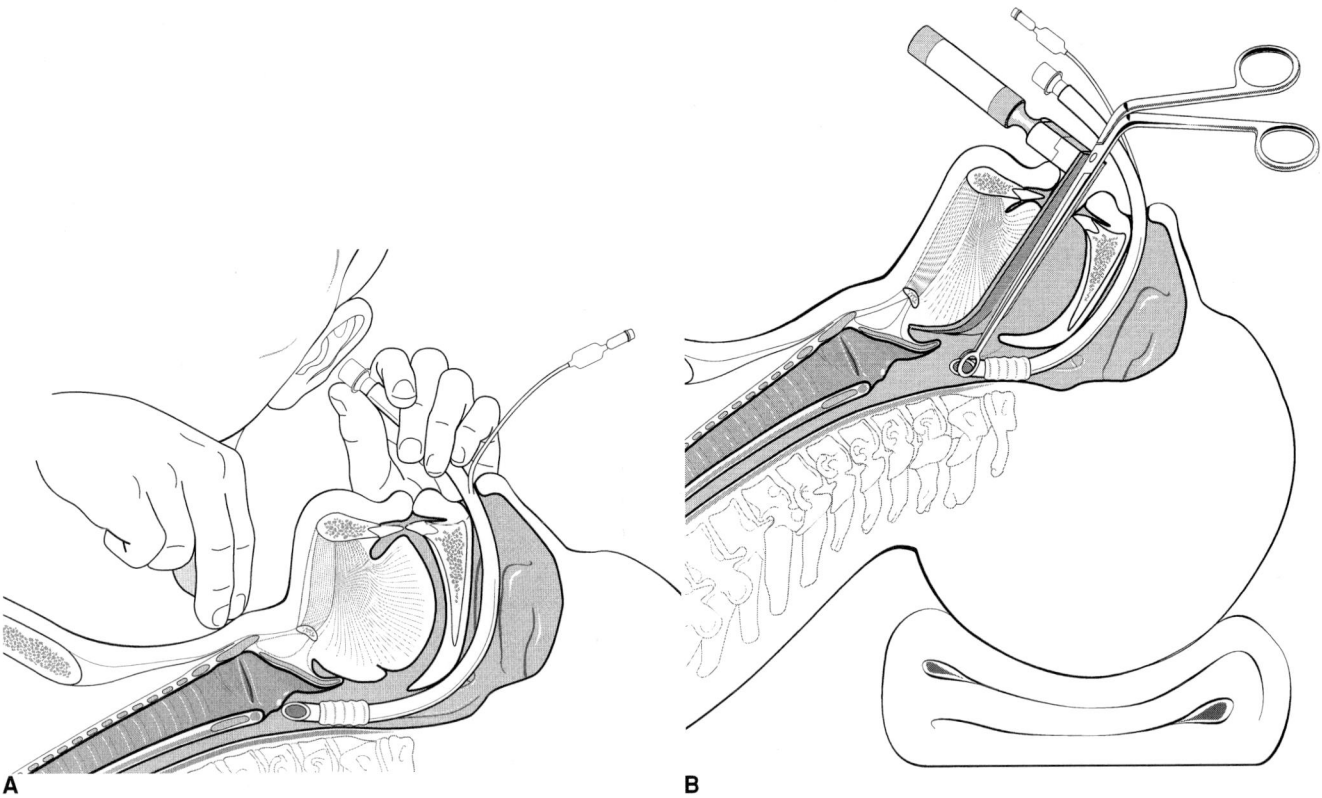

Fig. 12–8. *A*, Technique of "blind" passage of the nasotracheal tube. See text for details. *B*, Technique of nasotracheal intubation under direct visualization by the use of Magill forceps. See text for details.

Tracheotomy

Tracheotomy is considered to be an elective operative procedure preferably performed in the operating room under either local or general anesthesia.[54,55] More recently, this procedure has been adapted as a controlled bedside procedure in the intensive care unit by a skilled and well-equipped surgical team.[56,57] The standard tracheotomy is performed with a 3- to 5-cm vertical or horizontal skin incision entering the trachea at the region of the second or third tracheal ring.[58] The technique involves separation of the strap muscles and elevation or division of the thyroid isthmus with blunt dissection from the trachea. Horizontal incisions between the third and fourth tracheal rings with the creation of a window and removal of a midportion of the third or fourth tracheal ring is often performed. The window is subsequently dilated and a cuffed tracheostomy tube is inserted and sewn to the adjacent skin. Several variations of this conventional tracheotomy technique are occasionally performed.

Cricothyroidotomy is in essence a laryngotomy. This procedure is usually performed as an emergent temporary procedure when an acute translaryngeal intubation is un-

Table 12–5. Plan for Failed Intubation

Position patient head down and on left side, if patient has a full stomach
Oxygenate by positive pressure bagging; use oropharyngeal airway and suction pharynx
Repeated and prolonged attempts at intubation should be avoided
If equipment and expertise are available, consider intubation over a fiberoptic bronchoscope or rigid ventilating bronchoscopy
If foregoing techniques are unsuccessful, proceed to cricothyroidotomy (or large-bore angiocatheterization via cricothyroid membrane)

Table 12–6. Common Pitfalls in Translaryngeal Intubation

Inadequate training, practice, and experience
Failure to assemble essential intubation equipment before starting
Selection of the incorrect route of intubation
Inadequate topical anesthesia, sedation, or muscle relaxation
Failure to use vasoconstrictors before attempted nasal intubation
Failure to preoxygenate and preventilate the patient
Improper positioning and alignment of the head and neck
Using the laryngoscope to pry open the airway and using the teeth as a fulcrum for the laryngoscope
Forcing the tracheal tube forward against tissue resistance
Passing the tracheal tube too far into the trachea after entering the glottis
Prolonged (>30 seconds) or repeated intubation attempts without oxygenation and ventilation
Performing "crash" intubation when bag and mask ventilation would provide time to intubate more slowly and carefully
Equipment malfunction

(From Stauffer, J. L.: Medical management of the airway. Clin. Chest Med., *12*:474, 1991.)

Table 12-7. Complications of Tracheostomy

Early
    Bleeding
    Pneumothorax, pneumomediastinum, subcutaneous emphysema
    Tube displacement
    Aspiration
    Stomal infection
Late
    Bacterial colonization, pneumonia
    Tracheoinominate fistula
    Tracheoesophageal fistula
    Tracheal and laryngeal stenosis
    Swallowing dysfunction

successful or there is complete obstruction of the upper airway and immediate access to the trachea is needed.[59] The cricothyroid membrane is located at 1 cm below the vocal cords just within the subglottic larynx. Most surgeons feel that a cricothyroidotomy should be limited to emergency settings and should be formally converted to a conventional tracheotomy within a few hours after the patient is stable. There are some advocates, however, who recommend cricothyroidotomy for long-term access to the airway as well. This approach is criticized by most otolaryngologists, especially those involved in laryngotracheal reconstruction. A minitracheotomy was developed as a means of access to the airway with a 1 cm stab incision for placement of a narrow endotracheal tube. A variety of percutaneous techniques have been developed to perform either a cricothyroidotomy or a minitracheotomy usually restricted for emergency access.[58-61]

Intraoperative complications of tracheotomy include bleeding, pneumothorax and pneumomediastinum, recurrent laryngeal nerve injury, tracheoesophageal (T-E) fistula, and pulmonary edema.[62-64] Major intraoperative hemorrhage is rare and is usually due to anatomic abnormalities, errors in surgical technique, or coagulopathy. Pneumothorax and pneumomediastinum occur in around 5% of adults and 10% to 17% of children. It occurs more commonly in children because the dome of the pleura often extends superiorly. Accidental laceration through the posterior membranous trachea into the esophagus could result in a T-E fistula. This rare complication can be prevented by attention to surgical detail and if a fistula is created it should be repaired at the time of initial surgery. Untreated T-E fistula could progress to mediastinitis, pneumomediastinum, and empyema, and may be complicated by life-threatening aspiration. Recurrent laryngeal nerve injury during the dissection process would result in either unilateral or bilateral vocal cord paralysis, which would not be noticed in the tracheotomized patient unless a laryngoscopy is performed to view the cords. Of course, this result would become obvious and cause airway problems during or following the decannulation process.

Postoperative complications include hemorrhage, wound infection, subcutaneous emphysema, tube obstruction, or displacement of the tube (Table 12-7).[63] Stock reviewed the comparative incidence of perioperative complications of tracheostomy in recent literature (Table 12-8).[64] Postoperative bleeding occurs in about 5% of tracheostomy patients. It is the most common complication. The bleeding occurs from generalized venous oozing in the surgical site which is felt to be related to postoperative volume expansion and normalization of hemodynamics. More than 10 ml of fresh bleeding 48 hours or longer after the surgery raises concern for erosion of innominate artery. Jones reported that over 50% of life-threatening bleeding episodes through the tracheotomy tube in the 72 hours after the surgery were secondary to innominate artery erosion, and 72% of innominate artery bleeds occur between 1 and 3 weeks postoperatively.[70] The range for this complication to occur, however, is 30 hours to 7 months. The innominate artery is located anterior to the trachea 4 to 8 cm below the cricothyroid cartilage below the level of the jugular notch. The incidence of this life-threatening bleeding has been described to be 0.4% to 4.5% of tracheotomies performed. The pathophysiology of innominate bleeding is felt to be on the basis of a downward erosion of the caudal tip of the tube and excessive cuff overinflation over time.

A tracheotomy that is performed too low (i.e., around the fourth tracheal ring) may predispose innominate artery bleeding. Once this diagnosis is suspected, the focus of management should be to alert the surgical team and mobilize the patient for emergent operative intervention, usually with a sternotomy and ligation of the vessel. Temporizing measures should include hyperinflating the tracheostomy cuff and, perhaps, digital compression of the artery by placing the finger through the tracheostomy stoma with anterior pressure on the retrosternal area. The acute clinical scenario is usually such that ancillary studies such as an angiogram are not feasible.

Another potential major complication in the perioperative period is the accidental displacement of the tube within the first 72 hours. This complication has been reported in up to 7% of various tracheostomy series. In this

Table 12-8. Comparative Incidence of Perioperative Complications of Tracheostomy in Recent Reports

Source	No. of Patients	Displaced Tubes	Moderate Bleeding	Obstruction	Subcutaneous Emphysema	Pneumothorax	Aspiration	Perioperative Morbidity
Chew & Cantrell,[65] 1972	100	7	1	2	0	0	10	11
Dane & King,[66] 1975	40	0	3	2.3	0	5	0	1
Stauffer et al.,[67] 1981	51	0	36	4	9	4	8	20
Stock et al.,[64] 1986	81	0	2.4	0	0	2.4	0	6
Goldstein et al.,[68] 1987	124	1.6	0	0	0	1.6	0	5.6
Astrachan et al.,[69] 1988	52	0	0	0	0	0	0	14

(Adapted from Stock, M. C., et al.: Perioperative complications of elective tracheostomy in critically ill patients. Crit. Care Med., 14:861, 1986.)

Table 12–9. Comparison of Translaryngeal Intubation and Tracheostomy

Translaryngeal intubation
    Advantages
        Ease and speed of access
        Less skill required
        Less expensive, operating room not required
        Fewer complications, lower mortality rate
    Disadvantages
        Patient discomfort
        Interferes with swallowing, speech
        Mouth care is difficult
        Laryngeal complications
Tracheostomy
    Advantages
        Long-term comfort
        Facilitates mouth care, feeding, speech
        Better anchoring, improved mobility, care outside of hospital
        Avoids laryngeal complications
    Disadvantages
        Greater expense, need for general anesthesia
        Risk of perioperative mortality
        Greater risk of tracheal and laryngeal stenosis
        Greater risk of bacterial colonization, aspiration

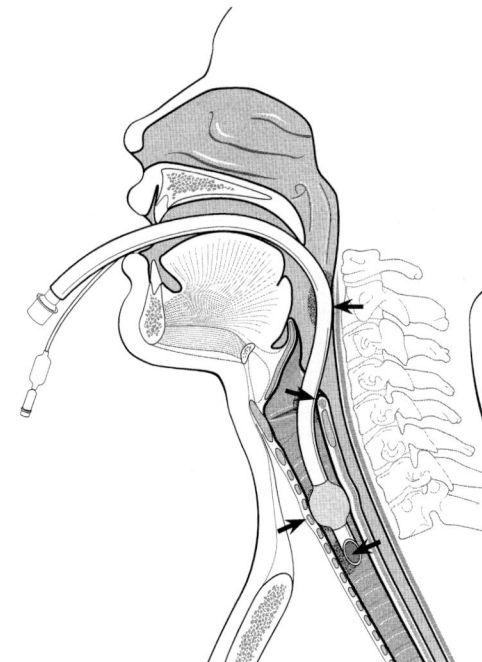

Fig. 12–9. Sagittal view of a translaryngeal endotracheal tube showing the points of mucosal contact between the tube and the airway at the level of the glottis as well as the trachea. See text for details.

situation, stabilization by emergency transstomal or translaryngeal intubation in the absence of UAO is preferred. The tracheotomy tube can be reinserted electively under more controlled conditions. The problem in this immediate postoperative period is that the tracheotomy tube has not developed a secure tract and efforts to reinsert a dislodged tube could lead to misplacement through a false channel in the pretracheal fascia. Some surgeons routinely employ tracheal flaps and traction sutures in a tracheostomy to help exteriorize the trachea, and to facilitate bedside recannulation in the event of such accidental dislodgement.

The relative advantages and disadvantages of translaryngeal intubation and tracheostomy are listed in Table 12–9. Prolonged need for mechanical ventilation and ventilator dependence in a subset of patients with chronic respiratory failure is a fact of current intensive care medicine. The overall approach to rehabilitation in these patients will be discussed elsewhere in this chapter. Airway management in this patient population, the conversion of "short-term" translaryngeal intubation to "longer-term" tracheostomy, and the optimal timing for such a procedure is an area of much confusion, debate, and dogma.[71–74] Theoretical factors that influence the decision include the potential long-term complications to the larynx and trachea of prolonged translaryngeal intubation[75–79] weighed against both the short- and long-term risks of tracheostomy.[65,80]

Translaryngeal intubation is clearly the procedure of choice for acute control of the airway. The main advantages of translaryngeal intubation include the fact that it is easier to perform in any location, can be established very quickly, and it has far fewer immediate complications with lower mortality rate. Concerns with prolonged translaryngeal intubation include potential for chronic laryngeal damage and tracheal cuff stenosis (Table 12–10 and Fig. 12–9), along with inadvertent decannulation with the attendant risks, the potential for bacterial colonization with subsequent aspiration and pneumonia, and issues related to patient comfort, nursing care, and difficulties with speech. Potential benefits of tracheostomy include sparing of direct laryngeal injury, greater patient comfort, and ease of delivering better oral care, increased likelihood of initiating speech, and a more secure airway which may permit transfer and care of the patient outside of the ICU. These benefits must be balanced against the perioperative surgical complications, the risks of stomal and cuff stenosis (Fig. 12–10), of bacterial colonization, and of nosocomial pneumonia, and the overall greater cost of this more invasive procedure.

Numerous clinical and experimental studies have considered the risks and benefits of prolonged translaryngeal intubation versus tracheostomy, especially on laryngeal and tracheal anatomy. Studies comparing airway injury with the duration and route of tracheal intubation are summarized in Table 12–11. Heffner summarized the limitations of study design in the available literature:[72]

Table 12–10. Complications of Translaryngeal Intubation

Direct laryngeal injury
    Posterior commissure stenosis
    Ulceration of the vocal cords
    Cricoarytenoid ankylosis or subluxation
    Epiglottic dysfunction
    Vocal cord, arytenoid fixation
Subglottic
    Subglottic stenosis and granuloma formation
    Cuff-related stenosis
    Tip granuloma, stenosis

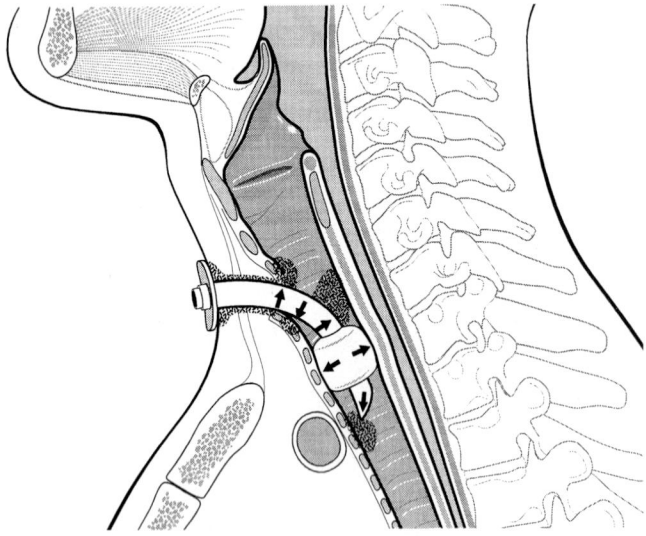

Fig. 12–10. Injuries inflicted on the trachea by the curved tracheostomy tube with several points of contact. The illustration also demonstrates an overinflated cuff.

- Studies have considered patients with diverse underlying conditions.
- Studies have been observational and retrospective.
- Operative technique and perioperative complication rate is variable between studies.

- Studies have used dissimilar anatomic end points with dissimilar clinical significance (i.e., laryngeal dysfunction has a different natural history than tracheal-stenosis).
- Studies have failed to consider the effect of translaryngeal intubation on tracheostomy complications.
- Incomplete long-term follow-up

In general, tracheostomy has more complications than translaryngeal intubation, and the complications tend to be more severe. Heffner described an algorithm on the timing of tracheostomy in patients intubated and mechanically ventilated (Fig. 12-11).

Tracheal Intubation and Nosocomial Pneumonia

Numerous studies have addressed the frequency and seriousness of nosocomial pneumonia and the enhanced risk of mechanical ventilation.[86-91] Multiple complex mechanisms appear to contribute to the risk of pneumonia in critically ill patients who are intubated.[92,93] The common pathway appears to be increased gram negative airway colonization and reduced local defenses.

In a prospective study of over 13,000 general hospitalized patients, Cross and Roup reported a 0.3% incidence of nosocomial pneumonia in patients not intubated or ventilated compared to a rate of 1.3% among those patients with an endotracheal tube on a ventilator.[94] The nosocomial pneumonia rate was 25% in tracheotomized patients

Table 12–11. Studies Comparing Airway Injury with Duration and Route of Tracheal Intubation

Source	# of pts	Age Range (% women)	Study Population	Mean Duration of TLI to Trache	Airway Exam Prior to Trache (Lundholm grade)	% Converted from TLI to Trache	Acute Laryngeal Abnormalities (&)	Symptomatic Laryngeal Damage	Chronic Laryngeal Stenosis (%)	Chronic Tracheal Stenosis (%)	Cuff Site Abnorm (%)	Total F/U Period (mos)	Comments
Dane[66] (1975)	25	43	Flail chest 15, ARDS 6, hypovent 3	4.2	N/A	100%	N/A	0		2/25 (8%)			both required surgery
Stauffer[67] (1981)	150	17–88 (36%)	61% ARF, 16% TLI for OR, 12% did not require vent	5.7	N/A	51/150 (33%)	N/A	1 pt		<50%:14 >50%: 2 (5%)			long term laryngeal or tracheal complications were rare; population was less seriously ill; higher incidence of short term complications
Pecora[81] (1982)	21	N/A	ARF 2 to pneumonia	1.46	N/A	0	N/A		0	0			TLI 727 d in 3 pts
Kastanos[82] (1983)	19	59 (32%)	COPD 10, Asthma 3, ARDS 2, Pneu 4	2–14	N/A	0	N/A	3/19		2/19 (10%)			
Whited[83] (1984)	Group I: 50	N/A	Adult upspec	2–5	45/50 I or II	0	3/50 (6%)		0	0	0	3–6 mths	highest incidence of chronic LTS (required specific therapy) occured in pts with grade II, IV changes prior to back; most with chronic LTS underwent conversion from TLI to trach; TLI >> 10d as unacceptable
	Group II: 100			6–10	16/100 III or IV	16%	3/32 (9%)		5/100 (5%)		0		
	Group III: 50			>>11	18/50 III or IV	32%			6/50 (12%)	6/50 (12%)	N/A		
Raskin[51] (1986)	61	19–93 (44%)	TLI > 3d	12.4		11/61 (18%)	N/A		N/A	N/A			
Elliott[84] (1988)	30	13–62	Survivors of ARDS	18	N	0/3	N/A		3 (All women)	3			all 3 pts required surgical repair
Colice[85] (1989)	54	25–88	VA, 18 COPD, 11 post op, 6 pneu, 19 misc	9.7		11/54 (20%)	mild: 52% mod/severe: 58%	0	0	0	0		

* See text.
ARDS, Adult respiratory distress syndrome; ARF, acute respiratory failure; TLI, translaryngeal intubation; trache, tracheostomy; VA, Veterans Administration Hospital; N/A, not available.

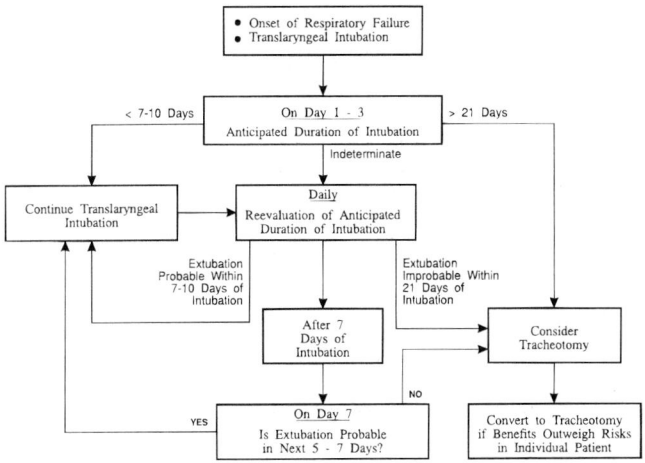

Fig. 12–11. An approach to timing of tracheostomy in intubated patients in the intensive care unit. See text for details. (Redrawn by George Morrison from Heffner, J. E.: Timing of tracheotomy in ventilator-dependent patients. Clin. Chest Med., *12:* 611, 1991.)

and 66% in those patients with combined tracheotomy and mechanical ventilation. Other studies documented a 12 to 38% incidence of nosocomial pneumonia in intubated patients. Numerous studies have documented that longer duration carries a greater risk of pneumonia, with perhaps the first 10 days posing the greatest risk. Lavine and Niederman summarized the direct and indirect effects of artificial airways contributing to the risk of nosocomial pneumonia.[95] Direct effects include:

- Direct access for bacteria to the lower tract
- Impaired local host defenses by blunting the cough reflex and mucociliary escalator
- Failure to fully prevent aspiration around the tube and cuff
- A foreign body reservoir for bacteria

Indirect effects include increased bacterial adherence and colonization of the airways as a result of local airway injury and secretion stasis.

Microaspiration in intubated patients is a common occurrence. The incidence is reported to be lower for the currently used high-volume low-pressure cuffs.[96-98] Bernhard and colleagues reported that cuff pressures of 34 cm H_2O prevented clinical aspiration,[99] whereas Cameron described that cuff inflation was not as effective.[100] Also, the presence of nasogastric tubes has been reported to enhance the risk of aspiration, probably by interfering with swallowing and gastroesophageal sphincter function and by providing a surface for retrograde migration of bacteria. A recent multivariate prospective study by Celis and coworkers, however, did not find that the presence of a nasogastric tube predisposed to pneumonia.[101] The data are not available regarding the relative risk of aspiration comparing laryngotracheal intubation and tracheotomy.

Nutrition

Nutritional support in the ICU will be discussed more extensively later in this book (see Chap. 62). Discussion here will be limited to special challenges unique to patients with an artificial airway. In individuals with a functioning gut, every effort should be made to begin enteric nutrition as soon as the patient has stabilized from acute decompensation (i.e., stable circulation and airway). In patients with translaryngeal intubation, choice is limited to nasoenteric tube feeding. In patients with a tracheotomy, additional options include oral feeding and gastrotomy/jejunostomy feeding.

Nasoenteric route is perhaps most often used in the ICU, due to the ease of placement of the tube by nonphysician care givers and the relative patient comfort by these small-bore tubes. These tubes tend to function best with the lowest incidence of reflux and aspiration when placed in the duodenum. Fluoroscopy may be required to achieve this. The head of the bed should be elevated 30° to 45°, and continuous feedings rather than bolus feedings should be used. It is preferable to use the enteric tubes exclusively for tube feeding, rather than as a multipurpose catheter for medications. The potential limitations of naso-enteric tubes include a 1 to 5% incidence of misplacement in the tracheobronchial tree, with potentially catastrophic consequences including pneumothorax, empyema, and pneumonia.[93] Proper placement of these tubes should be confirmed by either portable radiography or by fluoroscopy, and one should not rely solely on bedside clinical criteria. Indeed, a translaryngeal or tracheotomy tube may predispose misplacement by compressing the upper esophagus by means of the inflated cuff. Many ICU patients are critically ill with various metabolic abnormalities and their gastrointestinal tract may not function optimally (i.e., "low grade" ileus). In such patients, initiating tube feedings is frequently frustrating and is limited by abdominal distention and gastric residuals. Beyond the technical factors associated with starting tube feedings, the overall effectiveness of this form of nutrition on clinical outcome has not been adequately studied.

An important advantage with tracheostomy over translaryngeal intubation is the potential for oral nutrition. Longstanding tracheostomy however, does significantly affect the normal reflexive glottic function by various mechanisms. These tubes compress the esophagus, interfere with deglutition, and prevent the upward movement of the larynx during the swallowing process, and hence jeopardize glottic closure and protection. Before initiating oral nutrition, patients should be carefully evaluated for ability to handle oral secretions, presence of the gag and cough reflexes, and level of consciousness and motivation. Flexible fiberoptic laryngoscopy allows evaluation of vocal cord movement and laryngeal competence. It is appropriate to obtain a formal modified barium swallow by a speech pathologist, often with the benefit of a monitored cine-esophagogram. The patients should be taught to "practice" swallowing. Oral nutrition should be initiated with colored semisoft materials, such as pudding or jello, and slowly advanced. The impact of successful oral nutrition on a chronically ill patient's psychosocial makeup is favorable.

Extubation

When the underlying cause for the critical illness and respiratory failure are resolved, patients are gradually weaned from mechanical ventilation by criteria discussed in other chapters of this book. The decision to extubate a patient, from either translaryngeal intubation or tracheostomy, should be carefully considered and viewed as an independent decision separate from discontinuing mechanical ventilation. The prerequisite criteria needed prior to extubation have not been as well studied as criteria commonly used prior to weaning from mechanical ventilation. In general, there should be stabilization or reversal of the underlying medical or surgical condition which originally required intubation, whether this is COPD exacerbation or ARDS or postoperative nosocomial pneumonia. Patients should have adequate ventilatory reserve and have demonstrated spontaneous breathing (off CPAP and pressure support) for perhaps 24 or 48 hours, monitored by clinical parameters, oxygen saturation, and respiratory mechanics. If UAO was the cause for the intubation, such as infection, laryngospasm, vocal cord paralysis, etc., then this should be fully resolved prior to extubation. Other criteria that are, at least anecdotally, associated with successful extubation include an awake and cooperative patient, presence of an effective and intact cough and gag reflex, and the absence of excessive secretions. The problem of excess secretions frequently delays extubation and is particularly troublesome. There is no accepted definition of "excess secretions," but if a patient is requiring suctioning every one to two hours for a large volume of secretions, it is unlikely that such a patient would tolerate extubation. The reason for such excess secretions should be evaluated. The presence of an infectious process in the lung parenchyma or tracheobronchial tree may be the cause and an empiric trial of antibiotics may be warranted. Also, impaired ability to swallow oral secretions may lead to aspiration past the endotracheal tube and cuff. In some cases, the secretions may be due to the artificial airway producing laryngotracheal inflammation.

During the extubation process patients should be adequately oxygenated and ventilated, be awake and free from sedation, be in a 30° head-elevated position, and preferably receiving nothing by mouth: trachea should be suctioned and the catheter left in place. After the cuff is deflated, the trachea is again suctioned as the tube is being removed. Use of supplemental oxygen and cool bland aerosol is routine after extubation. The patients often complain of mild sore throat and difficulty with hoarseness on initial speech. Mackenzie reported postextubation severe stridor in 6 of 1290 patients (0.5%).[102] Laryngoscopy in these patients indicated laryngeal edema and inflammation to be the primary mechanism of airway obstruction, not laryngospasm. In this series, patients with this complication required an average of 3 reintubations. Conservative measures that are used, and are believed to be anecdotally effective, include aerosolized racemic epinephrine 0.5 cc of 2.25% solution in 3 cc saline, helium-oxygen mixture to decrease airway frictional resistance, and occasionally systemic corticosteroids.[102]

Inadvertent or self-extubation appears to be a relatively common and potentially serious complication in ICUs. Reported incidence ranges from 8.5% by Zwillich (30 of 354),[103] 11% by Coppolo and May (12 of 112),[104] 13% by Stauffer (29 of 226),[67] and 16% by Jayamanne (17 of 104).[105] Coppolo and May were unable to retrospectively identify risk factors for self-extubation.[104] Their study does indicate, however, that 70% of self-extubations occurred in patients who had been intubated for less than 48 hours and 69% occurred on the evening shift (3 to 11 PM). They were unable to ascribe these events to a lapse in nursing coverage. Moreover, sedation and use of restraints were believed to be appropriate. Coppolo did note a trend toward fewer self-extubations in patients who were nasally intubated.

Published reintubation rate after inadvertent extubation ranges from 31%[104] to 53%.[105] The only outcome data are available from Coppolo and May, who described serious complications (i.e., myocardial infarction, arrhythmia) in 4 of 13 self-extubated patients (31%).[104] No deaths occurred. These authors made a further distinction between "deliberate" and "inadvertent" self-extubation and noted only an 11% reintubation rate in the former group. It is not clear from their data how this distinction is made, however.

Postextubation laryngospasm, and indeed any cause of UAO, has been associated with pulmonary edema.[106-109] In a review of adult cases of UAO requiring intubation or tracheostomy, 11% developed pulmonary edema.[108] Willms and Shure reviewed a series of 26 patients with pulmonary edema and UAO and found that the most common cause of UAO was laryngospasm (11 of 26 patients or 42%), with all but 2 cases occurring shortly after extubation.[108] It appears that pulmonary edema usually occurs after relief of UAO. In most cases, recognition of pulmonary edema occurred within minutes of relief of UAO. All cases of laryngospasm-induced pulmonary edema resolved within 36 hours. It is postulated that the principal factor is the generation of a markedly negative intrathoracic pressure due to forceful inspiratory effort against a closed upper airway, resulting in a decrease in interstitial pressure favoring transudation of edema fluid. The UAO creates a more positive pressure during expiration which serves as a form of auto-PEEP to oppose transudation until the obstruction is removed. Recognition of this syndrome of pulmonary edema in the postextubation period is important so that aggressive diagnostic and therapeutic interventions may be avoided. Supportive care with maintenance of oxygenation and the establishment of a patent airway are the mainstays of treatment.

Postextubation airway complications include glottic edema, laryngeal dysfunction, and hoarseness. In general, these are mild and resolve with time. If hoarseness is severe, fiberoptic laryngoscopy should be performed to exclude vocal cord paralysis, which is uncommon. The usual cause for this complication is injury to the cricoarytenoid joint and recurrent laryngeal nerve by the translaryngeal tube itself and usually is not secondary to the tracheostomy surgery. If cord paralysis is noted, and is compensated by a contralateral mobile cord, observation alone for 6 to 12 months is usually adequate. If the larynx is incompetent, translaryngeal injection of Gelfoam temporarily medializes the paralyzed vocal cord for two to three months. For a more permanent problem, Teflon injections or surgical laryngoplasty may be required for vocal cord medialization.

POST-ICU PHASE: SPEECH, DECANNULATION

Discussion of airway management in the initial ICU phase of the illness focused on establishing immediate access to the airway (translaryngeal intubation), and the decision and timing of conversion to a tracheostomy. During the ICU phase, emphasis is usually placed on treating and reversing the underlying problems causing acute respiratory failure and the attendant nosocomial complications. In patients with an artificial airway, either translaryngeal or tracheostomy, there are special challenges with respect to preservation or reestablishment of speech and a normal route of nutrition, which are often neglected or relegated a less important role in the early ICU phase.

The rehabilitation phase actually begins in the ICU. After stabilization of circulation and establishment of an artificial airway, issues of communication and nutrition should be addressed. Issues related to decannulation and management of postextubation complications are addressed in this section.

Communication

Loss of speech is devastating to the conscious, critically ill patient who has an artificial airway. The fear engendered by the life-threatening illness, the isolation and depression that frequently accompany such an experience are aggravated by the frustrating inability of the patient to communicate with family members or medical personnel. Efforts to establish communication with the patient should be made in all ICU patients. Health care givers should actively inform intubated patients, in general terms, of the problems being addressed, the overall progress, and a brief management plan. Involving the patient, and obtaining permission for routine ICU procedures, is essential. Frequently orienting the patient to time, day, location and encouraging visitation by family and friends would help minimize the ICU alienation.

Intubated patients often attempt to express themselves by nonverbal gestures. This form of communication can be facilitated by attempting to lip read and by use of signboards. In alert patients who have the strength and dexterity, writing on paper with a felt-tip pen or on a Magic-Slate board is often effective. Portable electronic keyboards with a display screen or voice synthesizers are available commercially and do represent an option. These devices are not yet used widely, however, because of their relative expense and the manual dexterity needed to use such equipment. Additionally, by the time that the patient has recovered to a point where it is possible to use a medium of communication such as an electronic keyboard, written communication is just as effective.

Production of speech normally requires a power source (lung), amplifier (larynx), and articulators (tongue, lips).[107] Tracheostomy normally bypasses the amplifier by interrupting the airflow across the vocal cords.[110] Various options are available to establish effective, intelligible communication in the patient with a tracheotomy. The likelihood of success with effective speech is favorably dictated by the following factors:

- Low to moderate minute ventilation requirement
- Ability to sustain spontaneous ventilation for even short intervals
- Absence of upper airway pathology
- Absence of copious secretions
- Fairly alert and motivated patient

In stable ventilator dependent individuals, slight deflation of the cuff permits a cuff leak during the machine inspiratory cycle. Patients can be taught to time articulation with the passage of cuff leakage through the vocal cords, resulting in short phrases. The inner cannula of a cuffed fenestrated tracheostomy tube is usually nonfenestrated. When the inner cannula is removed temporarily, a patient may produce speech even with the cuff inflated. In patients who are not ventilator dependent and who do not aspirate, use of cuffless fenestrated tubes results in effective speech while the airway is secured by a tracheostomy (Fig. 12–12).

Specialized devices for speech in patients with a tracheotomy include:

- Pneumatic talking tracheotomy tube
- Tone generator catheter placed in the oropharynx
- Speaking one-way valves
- Electrolarynx

A unique tracheostomy tube is available for patients requiring constant inflation of the cuff (e.g., a CommuniTrach). The single-cuff, double-lumen tube was conceived to provide speech capability while the patient is on the ventilator with the cuff inflated. A special air channel directs controlled airflow from an outside source, other than the ventilator, towards the vocal cords. The patient or an attendant can control the flow of air (usually 1 to 10 L of gas flow per minute) through the glottis, providing patients with the ability to phonate by means of their own larynx. This tube may be effective when properly applied. Patients and staff may require several days of instruction and training. Though this device is claimed to be effective in clearing secretions accumulated above the inflated cuff, its maintenance is time consuming and secretions frequently occlude the special air channel and its parts.

Speaking one-way valves attached to the preferably fenestrated tracheostomy tubes are designed to serve patients who can produce voice when the expired air is directed towards their glottis, yet they depend on the tracheostomy for inhalation. Without these valves, a patient with a tracheostomy can only phonate by occluding the tube with a finger. The built-in valve opens during inhalation and closes during exhalation to direct and force the air through the vocal cords. These valves (examples include: Trach-Talk, Olympic, Passy-Muir, Silicone Membrane Tracheal Cannula Valve, Ball-Valve) are all effective and useful in voice and cough production. A 2-cm H_2O negative inspiratory force is required for the valve to open, and this may contribute slightly to the work of breathing. These valves may become occluded by secretions and therefore must be readily detachable for cleaning.

A fenestrated tracheostomy tube with the inner cannula also fenestrated, or removed, allows the spontaneously breathing patient to occlude the port and speak through the native airway. Limitations of the fenestrated tracheostomy tube include the standard position of the fenestration along the tube's greater curvature. The fenestra are in a

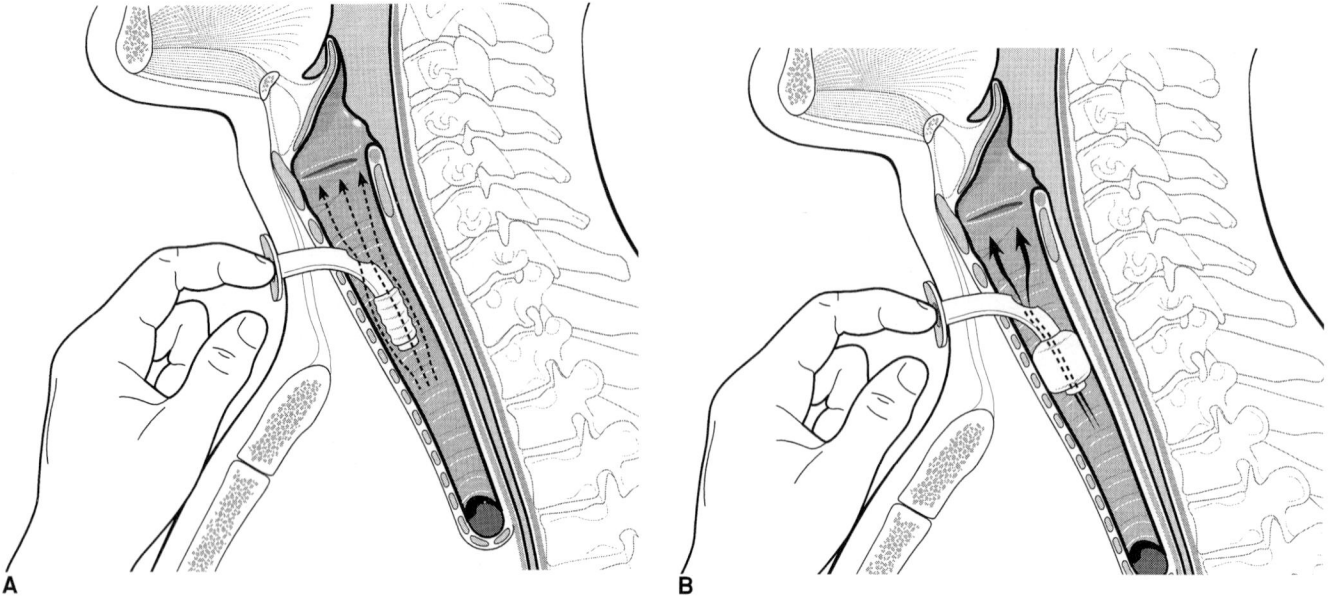

Fig. 12-12. A, Fenestrated tracheostomy tube with the inner cannula removed to allow spontaneous breathing and speech through the native airway. B, Tracheostomy tube with the cuff inflated permits expired gases to flow across the larynx, but air flow is significantly restricted.

fixed location on a tube and, because of individual variation in anatomy, the fenestra may occasionally occlude by abutting against the anterior or posterior tracheal walls. Also, the fenestration may occlude as granulation tissue grows into the orifice. Tube designs that have multiple small fenestrations overcome some of these problems.

Long-Term Tracheostomy

The standard technique for performing a tracheostomy is indicated and applicable in patients who require relatively short term, temporary airway management. Long-term tracheostomies are recommended for patients who will require prolonged or permanent airway control. When tracheostomy is performed in the standard technique, serious damage to the laryngotracheal complex may result if maintained for months or years. In some longstanding standard tracheostomies, progressive erosion of the upper anterior tracheal wall and eventually cricoid arch is observed, often with growth of granulation tissue and secondary subglottic stenosis. The structural changes in the anterior tracheal wall and the larynx occur as a result of pressure, friction, and deformation by the relationship between the curved cannula, the trachea, the larynx, and the upper border of the sternum. Little attention has been paid in the literature to measures to prevent these problems.

Indications for long term tracheostomy include:

- Neuromuscular disorders such as ALS, muscular dystrophy, or multiple sclerosis where a decision for long-term mechanical ventilation has been made
- Severe obstructive sleep apnea
- Bilateral vocal cord paralysis
- Laryngeal or tracheal stenosis or incompetence
- Chronic respiratory failure of any cause where a decision for long-term ventilation has been made

Goals of long-term tracheostomy include providing a direct access to the trachea that is tube free. This would improve the ease of management and patient acceptance. This type of stoma would avoid raw surfaces (minimize pain, infection, and granulation tissue) and avoid stoma contracture or collapse. They are best managed with specially designed Stoma-Stents that may be one-way valved to promote comfort, speech, and a patent airway. The surgical technique primarily involves shortening of the tracheal-cutaneous gap and the establishment of a noncollapsing, circumferential, mucocutaneous junction. Our surgical technique and experience have been published elsewhere.[111-114]

Decannulation

Decannulation from a tracheostomy tube requires essentially the same prerequisite criteria discussed for translaryngeal extubation. Patients should be initially evaluated by cuff deflation, and if they tolerate this for 24 hours, then attempts to manually occlude the tracheostomy should proceed. During this period, the patient should be evaluated for stridor, difficulty with secretions and the presence of respiratory distress. In the absence of any of these difficulties over a few days, and after a decision has been made that the patient no longer requires access to the airway, the tracheostomy tube can simply be removed. The walls of the stoma can be approximated by several sterile strips and dressed with a gauze. The stoma tract typically closes rapidly by second intent over several days. Occasionally, poor wound healing may interfere with spontaneous stomal closure and may require local surgical intervention. In patients with a more tenuous respiratory status, an alternative decannulation strategy is to insert progressively smaller caliber cuffless cannulae over days or weeks prior to complete removal.

A subset of patients need access to the trachea for a longer term basis for several reasons:

- Slow rehabilitation from underlying respiratory failure
- Require nocturnal positive pressure ventilation
- Upper airway pathology

There are numerous devices which maintain patency of the tracheostomy stoma, yet avoid the local complications and increased airway resistance of a bulky tracheostomy tube. These devices are short cylinders designed to fit in the tracheostomy stoma without extending into the tracheal lumen beyond the anterior tracheal wall. Examples of the devices include the Kistner polyvinyl acetate tracheostomy tube, the Olympic tracheostomy button made of hollow Teflon, and the Stoma-Stent made of silicone (Fig. 12-13). There are slight differences between these devices with respect to the need for external ties and the mechanism for sizing and ensuring an optimal fit in a patient's stoma. In general, they are better tolerated than the standard curved tracheostomy tube.

Late Complications of Tracheostomy

Other late complications of a tracheostomy include laryngeal or tracheal stenosis and tracheomalacia. Perhaps the most significant lesions occur at the stomal site by posterior buckling of the anterior suprastomal tracheal wall, along with formation of exophytic granulation tissue. Other lesions include a cuff stenosis lower down the trachea. The stenotic areas are often circumferential and may have a weblike appearance on laryngoscopy. The two stenotic areas between the stomal stenosis and cuff stenosis may be interposed by an area of tracheomalacia that can produce dynamic airway obstruction. In patients who have prolonged translaryngeal intubation, a cuff stenosis can occur in the proximal trachea along with the laryngeal complications discussed earlier in this chapter.

These complications of the trachea may be suspected initially by difficulty with decannulation. However, patients may become symptomatic between 2 weeks and 3 to 6 months after decannulation. Patients may present with difficulty clearing secretions, coughing, wheezing, or insidious dyspnea on exertion. These symptoms are frequently misdiagnosed as asthma, congestive heart failure, or a recurrence of the patient's underlying problem. Proper diagnosis is made by awareness of these complications and a high suspicion, along with appropriate ancillary studies. Occasionally, the tracheal air column on a plain chest radiograph, especially when overpenetrated, may show a focal narrowing suggestive of UAO. Lateral plain neck radiographs, tomograms, and xeroradiography may

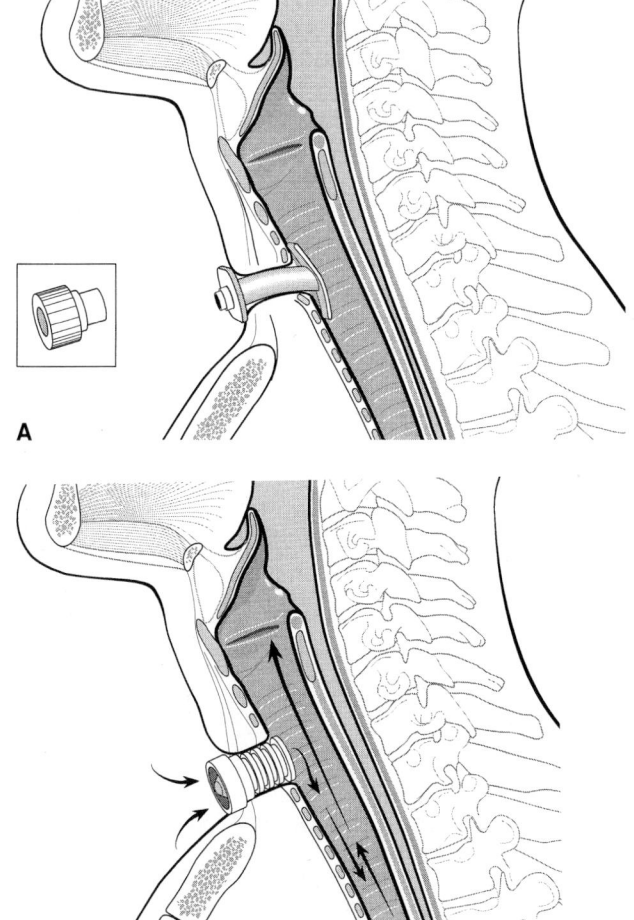

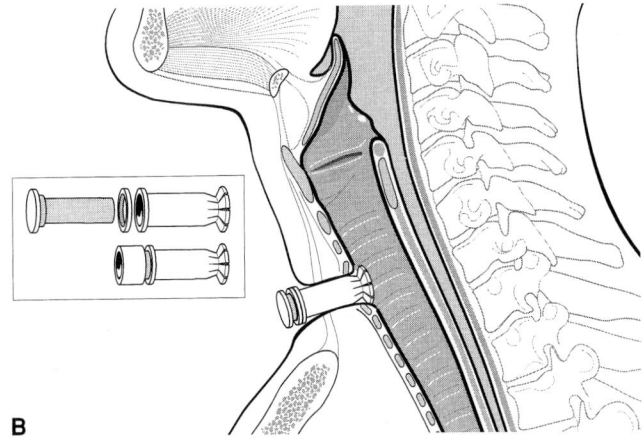

Fig. 12-13. *A,* Sagittal projection of a long-term tracheostomy with the StomaStent in place. *B,* Tracheostomy stoma with the Olympic button in place, with the insert showing the various parts. *C,* Stoma with Kistner button. See text for details.

also aid in a timely diagnosis. CT and MRI scans of the neck are excellent modalities in establishing the diagnosis, and defining the exact location and extent of the lesion. Pulmonary function testing may give clues to the presence of UAO by the configuration of the flow-volume loop and the measured flow rates with several classic patterns as previously discussed. Bronchoscopy represents the gold standard to establish a diagnosis of tracheal-stenosis. This procedure should be cautiously performed because patients with significant stenosis do not tolerate it well. Flexible fiberoptic endoscopy may be readily achieved at the patient's bedside or ambulatory clinic through the nose, mouth, or tracheostomy site to verify the diagnosis of tracheal-stenosis.

Management of Long-term Complications

The management of post-tracheostomy tracheal stenosis and tracheal malacia is controversial. Treatment options include endoscopic surgery followed by placement of a silicone rubber T-tube in the trachea, treatment with laser, rigid bronchoscopic dilatation, a segmental resection of the trachea with end-to-end anastomosis, or when indicated by complex reconstruction of the larynx and trachea. The choice of these approaches is dependent on the severity of the underlying problem, the overall expected prognosis, the likelihood for recurrent mechanical ventilation, and certainly by personal and institutional bias and practice.

A soft, malleable T-tube (Montgomery tube) was developed in the early 1960s and provides a satisfactory solution for some patients. The T-tube is designed to be inserted through an existing stoma and is retained in position in the trachea by virtue of its design, obviating the need for ties or sutures to prevent its expulsion or aspiration. With the T-tube in place, breathing occurs normally through the oral pharynx, the voice is preserved, and no special care of the tube is required. This tube helps to temporarily support the tracheal wall and the lower subglottic larynx. The free upper and lower margins of the T-tubes must extend beyond the stenotic lesions, and they should not be in close proximity to the glottis or to the carina (Fig. 12–14).

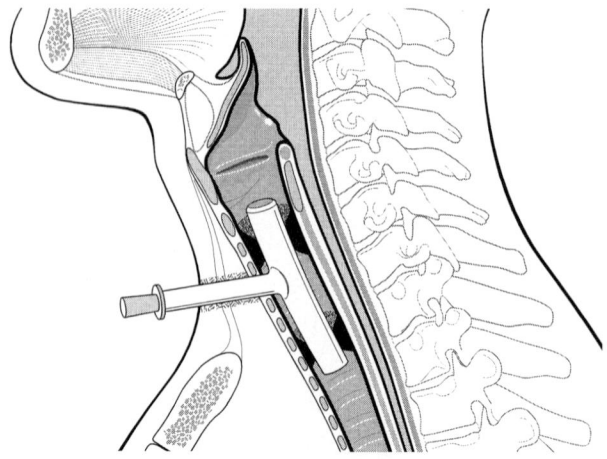

Fig. 12–14. A silicone T-tube above and below the level of the tracheostomy site, stenting stenotic lesions.

In cases where the larynx and in particular the glottis itself must be stented, the T-tube can be extended above the vocal cords at the risk of aspiration. Because T-tubes lack an inner cannula, they are dangerous and difficult to manage, they become occluded by encrusted and inspissated secretions, and they require frequent and continuous ambulatory care. In addition, ambulatory patients who go to local hospital emergency rooms may encounter personnel who are not trained to manage complications associated with the T-tube.

Laser resection with dilatation of the tracheal stenosis may provide symptomatic relief. Several series suggest that recurrent stenosis occurs in a significant majority of such patients within 8 weeks. There is some concern that additional damage to the tracheal mucosa and cartilage can occur with repeated laser therapy.

Surgical revision of the trachea is indicated in a subset of patients with tracheal stenosis.[115] The exact indications have not been well defined. Surgical technique typically involves approach through the neck, sometimes in conjunction with division of the upper portion of the sternum but a full sternotomy is usually unnecessary. A right posterolateral thoracotomy is occasionally used. Once the trachea is mobilized and the diseased segment is excised, an end-to-end circumferential anastomosis with interrupted absorbable sutures is performed. Surgical maneuvers to reduce tension on the suture line are usually employed. Important elements in surgical success include preservation of the tracheal blood supply and recurrent laryngeal nerves, avoidance of tension at the anastomosis, and full resection of the stenotic and inflamed area back to the healthy trachea. Postoperative care requires maintaining neck flexion for approximately seven postoperative days, which is sometimes accomplished by placing a suture from the chin to the manubrium to help maintain this flexion. Typically, a 3- to 4-cm section of the trachea can be removed.

In summary, the management of the upper airway in the critically ill patient crosses the traditional disciplines in medicine. The intensivist functions in a capacity to ensure a stable, patent airway in the initial management of critically ill patients. The issues are complex and disparate enough, however, to warrant frequent consultation with various medical and surgical subspecialties, both for acute issues and for long-term management. Using the format pre-ICU phase, ICU-phase, and post-ICU phase, this chapter attempted to review comprehensively both the common and the uncommon issues related to the management of the upper airway in the critically ill patient. Clearly, many controversies remain in this evolving area.

REFERENCES

1. Proctor, D. F.: State of the art: the upper airways. Am. Rev. Respir. Dis., *115*:315, 1977.
2. Bass, H.: The flow volume loop: normal standards and abnormalities in chronic obstructive pulmonary disease. Chest, *63*:171, 1973.
3. Golish, J. A., Ahmad, M., and Yarnal, J. R.: Practical application of the flow-volume loop. Cleve. Clin. Q., *47*:39, 1980.
4. Miller, R. D., and Hyatt, R. E.: Evaluation of obstructing

lesions of the trachea and larynx by flow-volume loops. Am. Rev. Respir. Dis., *108*:475, 1973.
5. Loughlin, G. M., and Taussig, L. M.: Upper airway obstruction. Semin. Respir. Med., *1*:131, 1979.
6. Baker, A. S., and Eavey, R. D.: Adult supraglottitis (editorial). N. Engl. J. Med., *314*:1185, 1986.
7. Baxter, F. J., and Dunn, G. L.: Acute epiglottitis in adults. Can. J. Anaesth., *35*:428, 1988.
8. Hanallah, R., and Rosales, J. K.: Acute epiglottitis: current management and review. Can. Anaesth. Soc. J. *25*:84, 1978.
9. MayoSmith, M. F., Hirsch, P. J., Wodzinski, S. F., and Schiffman, E. J.: Acute epiglottitis in adults. N. Engl. J. Med., *314*:1133, 1986.
10. Murrage, K. J., Janzen, V. D., and Ruby, R. R.: Epiglottitis: adult and pediatric comparisons. J. Otolaryngol., *17*:194, 1988.
11. Shapiro, J., Kavey, K. D., and Baker, A. S.: Adult supraglottitis: a prospective analysis. JAMA, *259*:563, 1988.
12. Sheikh, K. H., and Mostow, S. R.: Epiglottitis—an increasing problem for adults. West. J. Med., *151*:520, 1989.
13. Shih, L., Hawkins, D. B., and Stanley, R. B.: Acute epiglottitis in adults: a review of 48 cases. Ann. Otol. Rhinol. Laryngol., *97*:527, 1988.
14. Vernon, D., and Sarhaik, A. P.: Acute epiglottitis in children: a conservative approach to diagnosis and management. Crit. Care Med., *14*:23, 1986.
15. Moreland, B. W., Corey, J., and McKenzie, R.: Ludwig's angina: report of a case and review of the literature. Arch. Intern. Med., *148*:461, 1988.
16. Sheffer, A. L.: Anaphylaxis. J. Allergy Clin. Immunol., *75*:227, 1985.
17. Fisher, M. M., and Baldo, B. A.: Acute anaphylactic reactions. Med. J. Aust., *149*:34, 1988.
18. Israili, Z. H., and Hall, W. D.: Cough and angioneurotic edema associated with angiotensin—converting enzyme inhibitor therapy. Ann. Intern. Med. *117*:234, 1992.
19. Jain, M., Armstrong, L., and Hall, J.: Predisposition to and late onset of upper airway obstruction following angiotensin-converting enzyme inhibitor therapy. Chest, *102*:871, 1992.
20. Wood, S. M., and Mann, R. D.: Angio-edema and urticaria associated with angiotensin converting enzyme inhibitors. Br. Med. J., *294*:91, 1987.
21. Frank, M. M., Gelfand, J. A., and Atkinson, J. P.: Hereditary angioedema: the clinical syndrome and its management. Ann. Intern. Med., *84*:580, 1976.
22. Arreaza, E. E., Singh, K., and Grant, J. A.: Hereditary angioedema: clinical and biochemical heterogeneity. Ann. Allergy, *61*:69, 1988.
23. Ruddy, S.: Hereditary angioedema undersuspected, underdiagnosed. Hosp. Pract., *23*:91, 1988.
24. Wiggins, C. A., DyKewicz, M. S., and Patterson, R.: Idiopathic anaphylaxis: classification, evaluation, and treatment of 123 patients. J. Allergy Clin. Immunol., *82*:849, 1988.
25. Cormier, Y., Kashima, H., Summer, W., and Menkes, H.: Upper airways obstruction with bilateral vocal cord paralysis. Chest, *75*:423, 1979.
26. Parnell, F. W., and Brandenburg, J. H.: Vocal cord paralysis: a review of 100 cases. Laryngoscope, *80*:1036, 1970.
27. Holinger, L. D., Holinger, P. C., and Holinger, P. H.: Etiology of bilateral abductor vocal cord paralysis: a review of 389 cases. Ann. Otol., *85*:428, 1976.
28. Neel, H. B., Townsend, G. L., and Devine, K. D.: Bilateral vocal cord paralysis of undetermined etiology. Ann. Otol., *81*:514, 1972.
29. Shaw, G. L.: Airway obstruction due to bilateral vocal cord paralysis as a complication of stroke. South. Med. J., *80*:1432, 1987.
30. Vincken, W. G., et al.: Involvement of upper airway muscles in extrapyramidal disorders: a cause of airflow limitation. N. Engl. J. Med., *311*:438, 1984.
31. Lawry, G. V., et al.: Laryngeal involvement in rheumatoid arthritis. Arthritis Rheum., *28*:873, 1984.
32. Christopher, K. L., et al.: Vocal-cord dysfunction presenting as asthma. N. Engl. J. Med., *308*:1566, 1983.
33. Downing, E. T., Braman, S. S., Fox, M. J., and Carrao, W. M.: Factitious asthma: physiological approach to diagnosis. JAMA, *248*:2878, 1982.
34. Kryger, M. H., and Perez-Padilla, R. J.: Upper airway obstruction. In Current Therapy of Respiratory Disease. Edited by R. Cherniak, Philadelphia, B. C. Decker, 1989, p. 25.
35. Jacobs, L. M., et al.: Endotracheal intubation in the prehospital phase of emergency medical care. JAMA, *250*:2175, 1983.
36. Plummer, A. L., and Gracey, D. R.: Consensus conference on artificial airways in patients receiving mechanical ventilation. Chest, *96*:178, 1989.
37. Orlowski, J. P., Kanoti, G. A., and Mehlman, M. J.: The ethics of using newly dead patients for teaching and practicing intubation techniques. N. Engl. J. Med., *319*:439, 1988.
38. Deutschman, C. S., et al.: Paranasal sinusitis associated with nasotracheal intubation: a frequently unrecognized and treatable source of sepsis. Crit. Care Med., *14*:111, 1986.
39. Fassoulaki, A., and Pamouktsoglov, P.: Prolonged nasotracheal intubation and its association with inflammation of paranasal sinuses. Anesth. Analg., *69*:50, 1989.
40. Guerin, J. M., et al.: Purulent rhinosinusitis is also a cause of sepsis in critically ill patients. (Letter.) Chest, *93*:893, 1988.
41. Inodel, A. R., and Beckman, J. F.: Unexplained fevers in patients with nasotracheal intubation. JAMA, *248*:868, 1982.
42. Kronberg, F. G., and Goodwin, W. J. Jr.: Sinusitis in intensive care unit patients. Laryngoscope, *95*:936, 1985.
43. O'Reilly, M. J., et al.: Sepsis from sinusitis in nasotracheally intubated patients: a diagnostic dilemma. Am. J. Surg. *147*:601, 1984.
44. American Heart Association: Standards and guidelines for cardiopulmonary resuscitation and emergency cardiac care. J.A.M.A., *255*:2841, 1986.
45. Columbine, D. L., and Cohen, N. H.: Airway management of the non-intubated patient. J. Intensive Care Med., *2*:354, 1987.
46. Iserson, K. V.: Blind nasotracheal intubation. Ann. Emerg. Med., *10*:468, 1981.
47. Connardy, P. A., et al.: Alteration of endotracheal tube position: flexion and neck extension of the neck. Crit. Care Med., *4*:8, 1976.
48. Wilson, M. E., et al.: Predicting difficult intubation. Br. J. Anaesth., *61*:211, 1988.
49. Salem, M. R., Mathrubhuttam, M., and Bennett, E. J.: Difficult intubation. N. Engl. J. Med., *295*: 878, 1976.
50. Murrin, K. R.: Intubation procedure and causes of difficult intubation. In Difficulties in tracheal intubation. Edited by I. P. Latto, and M. Rosen. London, Bailliere Tindall, 1985, p. 75.
51. Rashkin, M. C., and Davis, T.: Acute complications of endotracheal intubation. Chest, *89*:165, 1986.
52. Samsoon, G. L. T., and Young, J. R. B.: Difficult tracheal intubation: a retrospective study. Anaesthesia, *42*:487, 1987.
53. Rosenbaum, S. H., et al.: Use of the flexible fiberoptic bron-

choscope to change endotracheal tubes in critically ill patients. Anesthesiology, 54:169, 1981.
54. Heffner, J. E.: Tracheal intubation in mechanically ventilated patients. Clin. Chest Med., 9:23, 1988.
55. Orringer, M. B.: Endotracheal intubation and tracheostomy: indications, techniques, and complications. Surg. Clin. North Am., 60:1447, 1990.
56. Heffner, J. E.: Medical indications for tracheotomy. Chest, 96:186, 1989.
57. Goldstein, S. I., Breda, S. D., and Schneider, K. L.: Surgical complications of bedside tracheostomy in an otolaryngology residency program. Laryngoscope, 97:1407, 1987.
58. Heffner, J. E., Miller, K. S., and Sahn, S. A.: Tracheostomy in the intensive care unit part I: indications, techniques, management. Chest, 90:269, 1986.
59. Esses, B. A., and Jafek, B. W.: Cricothyroidotomy: a decade of experience in Denver. Ann. Otol. Rhinol. Laryngol., 96:519, 1987.
60. Ciaglia, P., Fiorsching, R., and Syniec, C.: Elective percutaneous dilatational tracheostomy: a simple bedside procedure, preliminary report. Chest, 87:715, 1985.
61. Matthews, H. R., and Hopkinson, R. B.: Treatment of sputum retention by minitracheotomy. Br. J. Surg., 71:147, 1984.
62. El-Kihany, S. M.: Complications of tracheostomy. Ear Nose Throat J., 59:59, 1980.
63. Heffner, J. E., Miller, K. S., and Sahn, S. A.: Tracheostomy in the intensive care unit part II: complications. Chest, 96:430, 1986.
64. Stock, C. M., et al.: Respiratory complications of elective tracheostomy in critically ill. Crit. Care Med., 14:861, 1986.
65. Chew, J. Y., and Cantrell, R. W.: Tracheostomy: complications and their management. Arch. Otolaryngol., 96:538, 1972.
66. Dane, T. E. B., et al.: A prospective study of complications after tracheostomy for assisted ventilation. Chest, 67:398, 1975.
67. Stauffer, J. L., Olson, D. E., and Petty, T. L.: Complications and consequences of endotracheal intubation and tracheotomy: a prospective study of 150 critically ill adult patients. Am. J. Med., 70:65, 1981.
68. Goldstein, S. I., Breda, S. D., and Schneider, K. L.: Surgical complications of bedside tracheostomy in an otolaryngology residency program. Laryngoscope, 97:1047, 1987.
69. Astrachan, D. I., Kirchner, J. C., and Goodwin, W. J. Jr.: Prolonged intubation vs. tracheotomy: complications, practical and psychological considerations. Laryngoscope, 98:1165, 1988.
70. Jones, J. W., et al.: Tracheoinominate artery erosion: successful surgical management of a devastating complication. Ann. Surg., 194:184, 1976.
71. Bishop, M. J.: The timing of tracheotomy: an evolving consensus. Chest, 96:712, 1989.
72. Heffner, J. E.: Timing of tracheotomy in ventilator-dependent patients. Clin. Chest Med. 12:611, 1991.
73. Marsh, H. M., Gillespie, D. J., and Baumgartner, A. E.: Timing of tracheostomy in the critically ill patient. Chest, 96:190, 1989.
74. Heffner, J. E.: Timing of tracheostomy in mechanically ventilated patients. Am. Rev. Respir. Dis., 147:768, 1993.
75. Dixon, T. C., et al.: A report of 342 cases of prolonged endotracheal intubation. Med. J. Aust., 2:529, 1968.
76. Dunham, C. N., et al.: Prolonged tracheal intubation in the trauma patient. Trauma, 24:120, 1984.
77. Dubick, M. N., and Wright, B. D.: Comparison of laryngeal pathology following long-term oral and nasal endotracheal intubations. Anesth. Analg., 57:663, 1978.
78. Dobrin, P., and Canfield, T.: Cuffed endotracheal tubes: mucosal pressures and tracheal wall blood flow. Am. J. Surg., 133:562, 1977.
79. Weymuller, E. A., et al.: Quantification of intralaryngeal pressure exerted by endotracheal tubes. Ann. Otol. Rhinol. Laryngol., 92:444, 1983.
80. Sasaki, C. T., Horiuchi, M., and Koss, N.: Tracheostomy-related subglottic stenosis: bacteriologic pathogenesis. Laryngoscope, 89:857, 1979.
81. Pecora, D. V., Seinige, U.: Endotracheal intubation. (Letter.) Chest, 82:130, 1982.
82. Kastanos, N., et al.: Laryngotracheal injury due to ETT. Crit. Care Med., 11:362, 1983.
83. Whited, R. E.: A prospective study of laryngotracheal sequelae in long-term intubation. Laryngoscope, 94:367, 1984.
84. Elliott, C. G., Rasmusson, B. Y., and Crapo, R. O.: Upper airway obstruction following adult respiratory distress syndrome: an analysis of 30 survivors. Chest, 94:526, 1988.
85. Colice, G. L., Stukel, T. A., and Dain, B.: Laryngeal complications of prolonged intubation. Chest, 96:877, 1989.
86. Baigelman, W., et al.: Bacteriologic assessment of the lower respiratory tract in intubated patients. Crit. Care Med., 14:864, 1986.
87. Craven, D. E., and Driks, M. R.: Nosocomial pneumonia in the intubated patient. Semin. Respir. Infect., 2:20, 1987.
88. Craven, D. E., et al.: Risk factors for pneumonia and fatality in patients receiving continuous mechanical ventilation. Am. Rev. Respir. Dis., 133:792, 1986.
89. Fagon, J. Y., et al.: Nosocomial pneumonia in patients receiving continuous mechanical ventilation: prospective analysis of 52 episodes with use of a protected specimen brush and quantitative culture techniques. Am. Rev. Respir. Dis., 139:877, 1989.
90. Fagon, J. Y., et al.: Detection of nosocomial lung infection in ventilated patients: use of a protected specimen brush and quantitative culture techniques in 147 patients. Am. Rev. Respir. Dis., 138:110, 1988.
91. Niederman, M. S., et al.: Pneumonia in the critically ill hospitalized patient. Chest, 97:170, 1990.
92. Palmer, L. B.: Bacterial colonization: pathogenesis and clinical significance. Clin. Chest Med., 8:455, 1987.
93. Pingleton, S. K., Hinthorn, D. R., and Liu, C.: Enteral nutrition in patients receiving mechanical ventilation: multiple sources of tracheal colonization include the stomach. Am. J. Med., 80:827, 1986.
94. Cross, A. S., and Roup, B.: Role of respiratory assistance devices in endemic nosocomial pneumonia. Am. J. Med., 70:681, 1981.
95. Lavine, S. A., and Niederman, M. S.: The impact of tracheal intubation on host defenses and risks for nosocomial pneumonia. Clin. Chest Med., 12:523, 1991.
96. Spray, S. B., Zuidema, G. D., and Cameron, J. L.: Aspiration pneumonia: incidence of aspirations with endotracheal tubes. Am. J. Surg., 131:701, 1976.
97. Burgess, G. E., et al.: Laryngeal competence after tracheal extubation. Anesthesiology, 51:73, 1979.
98. Grillo, H. C., et al.: A low pressure cuff for tracheostomy tubes to minimize tracheal injury. J. Thorac. Cardiovasc. Surg., 62:898, 1971.
99. Berhnhard, W. N., et al.: Adjustment of intracuff pressure to prevent aspiration. Anesthesiology, 50:363, 1979.
100. Cameron, J. L., Reynolds, J., and Zuidema, G. D.: Aspiration in patients with tracheostomies. Surg. Gynecol. Obstet., 136:68, 1973.
101. Celis, R., et al.: Nosocomial pneumonia: a multivariant analysis of risk and prognosis. Chest, 93:318, 1988.

102. MacKenzie, C. F., et al.: Severe stridor after prolonged endotracheal intubation using high volume cuffs. Anesthesiology, *50:*235, 1979.
103. Zwillich, C. W., et al.: Complications of assisted ventilation: a prospective study of 354 consecutive episodes. Am. J. Med., *57:*161, 1974.
104. Coppolo, D. P., and May, J. J.: Self-extubation: a 12-month experience. Chest, *98:*165, 1990.
105. Jayamanne, D., Nadipati, R., and Patel, D.: Self-extubation: a prospective study. Chest, *94:*3S, 1988.
106. Lorch, D. G., and Sahn, S. A.: Post-extubation pulmonary edema following anesthesia induced by upper airway obstruction. Chest, *90:*802, 1986.
107. Godwin, J. E., and Heffner, J. E.: Special critical care considerations in tracheostomy management. Clin. Chest Med., *12:*573, 1991.
108. Willms, D., and Shure, D.: Pulmonary edema due to upper airway obstruction in adults. Chest, *94:*1090, 1988.
109. Tami, T. A., Chu, F., Wildes, T. O., and Kaplan, M.: Pulmonary edema and acute upper airway obstruction. Laryngoscope, *96:*506, 1986.
110. Blom, E. D.: Alternative methods of communication for intubated patients in critical care. Indiana Med., *81:*398, 1988.
111. Eliachar, I., and Oringher, S. F.: Performance and management of long-term tracheostomy. Oper. Tech. Otolaryngol. Head Neck Surg., *1:*56, 1990.
112. Eliachar, I., et al.: Planning and management of long-standing tracheostomy. Otolaryngol. Head Neck Surg., *97:*385, 1987.
113. Eliachar, I., et al.: Permanent tracheostomy. Head Neck Surg., *7:*99, 1984.
114. Eliachar, I., and Papay, F. A.: Laryngotracheal devices. *In* Complications in Head and Neck Surgery. Edited by Y. P. Krespi, and R. H. Ossoff. Philadelphia, W.B. Saunders, 1993, p. 233.
115. Grillo, H. C., and Mathisen, D. J.: Surgical management of tracheal strictures. Surg. Clin. North Am., *68:*511, 1988.

Chapter 13

POSTOPERATIVE MANAGEMENT FOLLOWING HEAD AND NECK SURGERY

PIERRE LAVERTU
MARY LYNN DROUGHTON

Head and neck surgery can be defined as any surgery performed for the treatment of tumors arising between the base of skull superiorly and the chest inferiorly. A variety of lesions are encountered in different sites. The commonly recognized sites are:

- Lip and oral cavity
- Pharynx (naso, oro, and hypopharynx)
- Larynx
- Paranasal sinus
- Salivary gland
- Thyroid gland

The American Cancer Society estimates that there will be approximately 30,500 new cancers of the lip, oral cavity and pharynx diagnosed in the United States in 1990, an incidence of 3% of all cancers. Twelve-thousand laryngeal and 12,000 thyroid cancers will be found, with each group making up about 1% of all cancers.[1] Other sites are much less common. Excluding salivary gland and thyroid sites, the great majority of head and neck cancers arise from the mucosal lining of the upper aerodigestive tract and most are squamous cell carcinomas. With the exception of sinonasal and nasopharyngeal lesions, most squamous cell carcinomas result from chronic tobacco and alcohol use. For example, less than 5% of oral carcinomas are seen in nonusers of tobacco. The male/female ratio varies from 2:1 to 8:1, depending on the site. These tumors can be found in all age groups, but more commonly in patients in their fifth and sixth decades.

In this chapter, the evaluation and treatment of these patients is briefly outlined. More emphasis is placed on the postoperative management in the intensive care setting. All aspects of care including patient positioning, airway management, wound care, nutritional management, communication and medications are addressed. Management and rehabilitation after discharge from the intensive care setting are also discussed.

PRE-ICU PHASE

Squamous cell carcinoma of the head and neck may be treated with different modalities, including:

- Radiation therapy
- Surgery
- Chemotherapy

Without detailing treatment decision, earlier or smaller tumors are treated either with surgery or radiation. For larger or more advanced tumors, surgery and radiation are used in combination. With the combined approach, depending on the preference of the treating team, radiation is given either preoperatively or postoperatively. More recently, research protocols have added aggressive chemotherapy to the treatment of more advanced tumors.[2] When used with curative intent, chemotherapy is always combined with radiation therapy and/or radiation and surgery. The use of chemotherapy as a single modality is reserved for palliation.

Because of previous chronic tobacco and alcohol use, the majority of patients undergoing head and neck surgery have increased risks for cardiac, vascular, and pulmonary abnormalities. Liver dysfunction is also common and may be associated with nutritional and coagulation deficiencies. The tumor may interfere with deglutition and contribute to a catabolic state, with weight loss and diminished resistance to surgical trauma and infection. Prior use of radiation therapy and/or chemotherapy may further compromise the patient's overall medical condition and nutritional status.

Medical condition should be thoroughly evaluated by an appropriate medical colleague and managed to as optimal a level as possible preoperatively, keeping in mind that definitive treatment for the lesion must be begun promptly. Delays in treating larger tumors may make the difference between success and failure. Additionally, even after minor surgery, admission to the ICU may be required because of the patient's medical condition.

Patients with no significant underlying medical condition are admitted to the intensive care postoperatively based on the following criteria:

- Extent of surgery
- Need for monitoring
- Level of nursing care required

Extensive and lengthy surgical procedures often result in increased risks of fluid imbalance, hemorrhage, and airway compromise. Close monitoring by an experienced nursing team is required. Therefore, operations such as neck dissection, mandibulectomy, maxillectomy, pharyngectomy, and laryngectomy may require admission to such a specialized unit.

Patients needing frequent recording of vital signs, urinary output, drainage, airway management, monitoring of flaps, or with arterial and/or central lines should be managed in a unit with a nurse/patient ratio of 1:2, to 1:4.

The volume of head and neck surgery in specialized centers has created the need for a designated ward where these patients can be managed postoperatively. Nurses in such units become subspecialized and capable of managing cases requiring regular intensive care in other centers. Conversely, many hospitals will not have this luxury and, therefore, an integrated care team of ICU personnel and primary surgeon should be provided.

The basic indications for admission to ICU for these patients is the need to monitor:

- Hemodynamics
- Airway
- Wound and flaps

ICU PHASE

Aside from the need to maintain patients hemodynamically stable, admission to an intensive care setting can ensure maintenance of the airway and provide close observation of the surgical wound. Prevention and/or immediate recognition of a wound complication minimizes the risks of major wound breakdown, pharyngocutaneous fistula, or carotid artery blowout, and results in optimal healing and early discharge. During this phase of recovery, the following aspects of care should be emphasized:

- Patient positioning
- Airway management
- Wound management
- Nutritional management
- Speech and swallowing

Patient positioning

In order to minimize venous and arterial pressure in the neck, which increases the risk of swelling and hemorrhage, a 30° to 45° elevation of the head of the bed is recommended. The neck is maintained in a slightly flexed position to minimize tension on suture lines. Further neck flexion or rotation may be necessary to further decrease tension and/or compression:

- On pedicled flaps used in reconstruction
- To end-to-end tracheal anastomosis following segmental tracheal resection
- To patients after total laryngopharyngoesophagectomy in whom the stomach is sutured to the pharynx

Head and neck patients may be promptly mobilized postoperatively. Despite extensive surgery, pain rarely limits early ambulation. The typical patient sits in his chair the following day and is seen ambulating in the hallway two days postoperatively. This situation is probably why deep venous thromboses and subsequent pulmonary emboli are rarely encountered. The risk of these complications is, however, greater in patients suffering from other disease conditions (see Chap. 23).

Airway Management

Maintenance and protection of the airway is of utmost importance in a majority of head and neck surgical patients. Some degree of airway obstruction is often present, either from tumor, edema from radiation therapy, and/or surgery performed in the vicinity. One example might be a patient who undergoes bilateral neck dissections where venous congestion causes laryngeal edema and obstruction. Laryngeal paralysis secondary to involvement of the ipsilateral recurrent laryngeal nerve classically results in a vocal cord in paramedian position which further compromises the airway. Patients who previously had a tracheotomy have a relative tracheal stenosis which could add to the problem. Even a patient with previous radiation and/or surgery to the neck, who is intubated for an unrelated surgical procedure, is at increased risk for laryngeal edema which, even if minimal, may result in obstruction if the airway is already compromised.

The first step in the treatment of impending upper airway obstruction is to recognize the problem. The patient often appears restless, respirations are noisy and difficult, and inspiratory stridor is noted. Blood gases, when obtained, may show some degree of hypoxemia. When the situation is recognized, the patient should immediately be placed in an almost sitting position. With mild obstruction, racemic epinephrine inhalation and systemic steroids such as dexamethasone (Decadron 10 mg IV) are administered. Oxygen with cool mist is also added to the therapy. When the severity of upper airway obstruction is not readily apparent, the adequacy of the airway can be assessed by flexible laryngoscopy. With severe obstruction or when the situation deteriorates, orotracheal intubation or tracheotomy should be considered immediately. The choice between intubation and tracheotomy has to be individualized. Close communication between the anesthesiologist and/or intensivist and the head and neck surgeon is essential to identify the patients at risk for airway obstruction and determine appropriate therapy. In most cases immediate intubation in the intensive care setting is the best approach. A patient who is difficult to intubate and may require a tracheotomy should, when time permits, be brought to the operating room for the procedure. When anatomic reasons or a recent operation on the airway preclude laryngeal intubation, or if intubation is unsuccessful, immediate tracheotomy should be performed. A tracheotomy is also performed when intubation is required for more than 48 hours. The tracheotomized patient, unlike the intubated patient, can be allowed early ambulation and discharge from the intensive care setting.

To prevent emergency airway situations a planned tracheotomy is usually done at the time of surgery. A cuffed tracheotomy tube is used through this temporary tracheostomy (Fig. 13-1). The reasons for a cuffed tube are threefold:

- It permits assisted ventilation in the immediate postoperative period when the patient is late waking up.
- It prevents blood from entering the tracheobronchial tree.

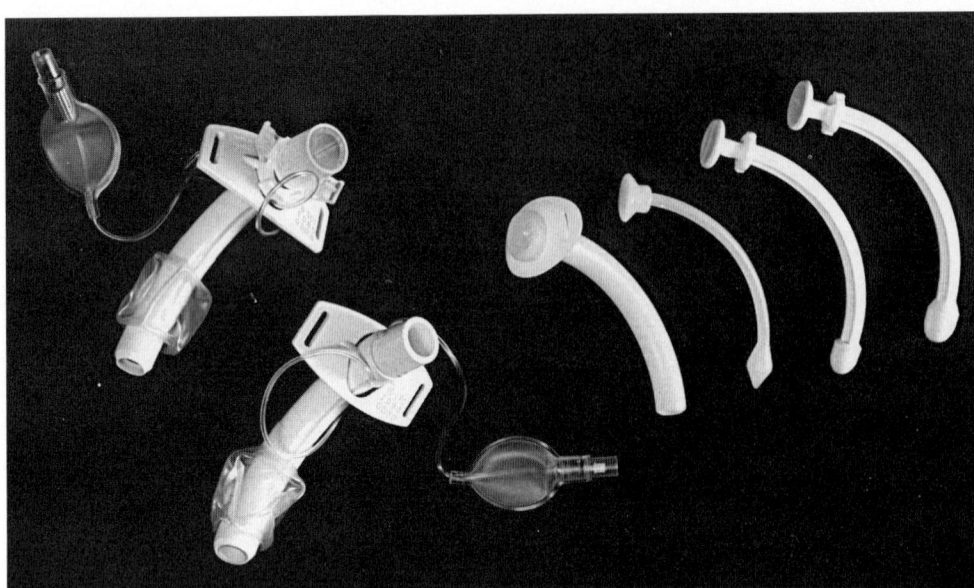

Fig. 13–1. Cuffless (right) and cuffed (left) tracheotomy tubes.

- It prevents bronchial soilage from the patient's pharyngeal and gastric secretions.

The tracheotomy tube is secured with ties fastened around the neck and often sutured to the adjacent skin to prevent accidental dislodgement. If the tube becomes dislodged, the patient should be placed on his back with a roll under his shoulders to provide some extension of the neck (this is the position in which the procedure was performed), the opening in the trachea visualized and the tube reinserted. Blind attempt at reinsertion, especially when the patient's position is incorrect, is likely to result in the creation of a false tract and further compromise the airway.

Inflation of the cuff is maintained until the morning after the surgery, or until patients can handle their own secretions. Thereafter, even with low pressure cuffs, the cuff should be deflated at least every 8 hours to reduce tracheal damage resulting from cuff pressure on the tracheal wall. Routine deflation of the cuff may permit aspiration of the secretions accumulated above the cuff and, therefore, should be followed by thorough tracheobronchial suctioning. Suctioning every 2 to 4 hours is recommended to prevent any buildup of secretions in the tracheobronchial tree or in the tracheotomy tube. When the airway becomes compromised from such a buildup, the patient should be vigorously suctioned. If simply suctioning does not relieve the obstruction, blockage often corresponds to where the suction catheter meets resistance. Tracheotomy tube blockage is first handled by removing and cleaning the inner cannula (present in most commercially available types of tubes). When the tube lacks an inner cannula or it remains blocked after cleaning, the entire tube should be replaced. Obstruction distal to the tracheotomy tube is addressed first by instilling sterile saline to soften and dislodge thickened and dried secretions. This procedure is followed immediately by vigorous suctioning. When this fails, the entire tracheotomy tube is removed and the procedure repeated (the plug may be wider than the diameter of the tube). The next step would be to proceed to a bronchoscopic lavage and aspiration. Prophylactic use of cool mist via T-tube or cervical mask helps prevent this situation. Patients should receive aggressive respiratory therapy including forced inspiration, chest physiotherapy, and, if necessary, aerosol and systemic bronchodilators.

When a cuffed tube is no longer needed, but usually not earlier than three days following the creation of the tracheotomy, a cuffless tracheotomy tube is inserted (Fig. 13-1). This tube has the advantage of being less traumatic to the trachea, interferes less with normal deglutition, and minimizes aspiration. When the tube is temporarily occluded with the patient's finger or for a longer time with a special tracheotomy plug (when the airway is not obstructed), phonation is restored. This situation is a significant psychologic help to these patients. A cuffless tracheotomy tube is kept in place during the process of decannulation. When patients are able to handle and/or expectorate their secretions and have an adequate airway, the tube is plugged for increased periods of time. The size of the tube may also be reduced accordingly. When patients breathe without difficulty with a plugged tube and aspiration is not a problem, the tube may be removed and the tracheotomy allowed to close by secondary intention (often after discharge from the ICU and even from the hospital).

Total Laryngectomy

Patients who undergo total laryngectomy are left with a permanent stoma. The distal cut end of the trachea is sutured circumferentially to an opening in the lower aspect of the skin of the neck. The trachea is therefore completely and permanently separated from the digestive tract (Fig. 13-2). Unless there is wound breakdown resulting in a pharyngocutaneous fistula, oropharyngeal secretions

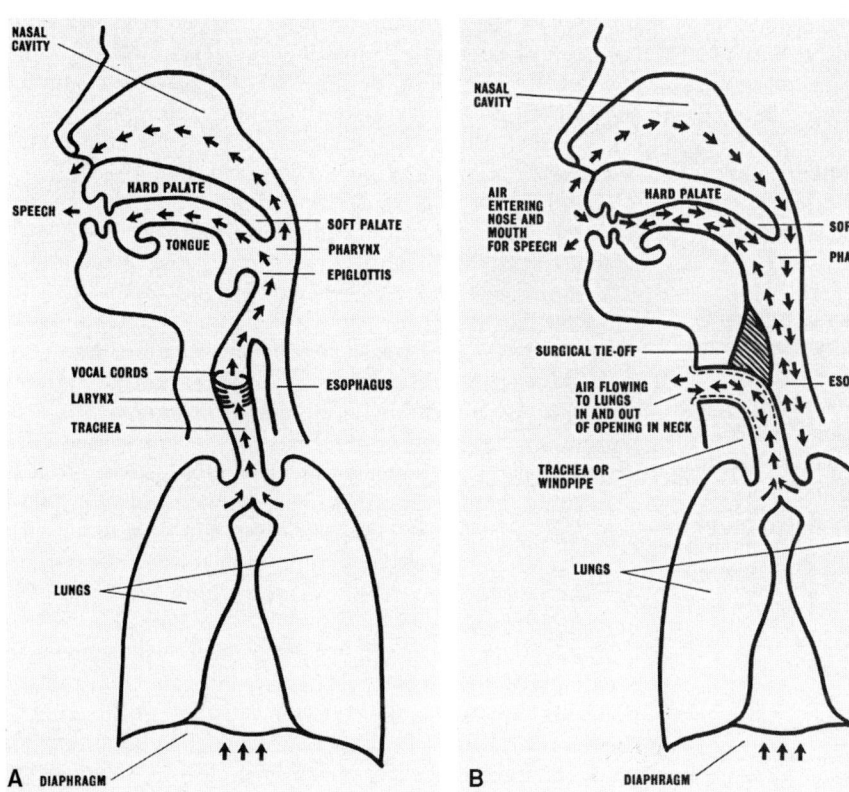

Fig. 13–2. Physiology of the head and neck before (A) and after (B) total laryngectomy. (From the program of the International Association of Laryngectomees, American Cancer Society, 1978.)

cannot be aspirated into the tracheobronchial tree. One other exception is patients who have planned tracheoesophageal fistulas created for voice restoration postlaryngectomy. With this technique, a small hole is created in the superior back wall of the trachea into the pharynoesophagus which can permit some salivary soilage of the tracheobronchial tree. This tract is stented with a catheter or most often with a regular nasogastric tube (size 16 or 18 Fr) and usually aspiration is insignificant.

In the postoperative period after total laryngectomy, the airway is secured with a cuffed tracheotomy tube. As soon as the patient is sufficiently awake and can breathe on his or her own, the tube can be replaced with an uncuffed "laryngectomy" tube or stoma vent (Fig. 13-3). There is no contraindication to leaving the cuffed tracheotomy tube in place longer but the cuff does not need to be inflated. Many patients do not require any tracheotomy tube but it is customary to leave a stoma vent in place until the stoma has matured and there is no risk of stomal stenosis. The period of time before complete maturation and stability of the stomal opening varies from patient to patient but is usually no sooner than one month after surgery or after completion of radiation therapy (when radiation is used postoperatively). A patient rarely requires a permanent tube to prevent stenosis. With a total laryngectomy patient there is no risk of losing the airway if the tracheotomy tube becomes dislodged. If this occurs, there is no danger because the trachea is sutured to the skin and the tracheal lumen is readily visible. The tube is then gently reintroduced and the ties refastened around the neck.

Tracheotomy care of a laryngectomized patient is the same as for the tracheotomized patient and includes regular cleaning of the tube and routine suctioning of the tracheobronchial tree.[3] Adequate humidity is of utmost importance to prevent the formation of plugs from pulmonary secretions. These patients have lost the physiologic capability to humidify inspired air through the nasal and pharyngeal passages and remain at risk for mucous plug formation for a prolonged period and, in some cases, forever. Management of plug formation is described in the section on tracheotomized patients.

Once the immediate postoperative period is over and the patient starts to ambulate, the tracheostoma is covered with a bib to prevent foreign material from entering the airway and also to conceal the opening. Should a cardiopulmonary emergency occur, the airway can be secured through the neck and is easily accessible. Oral intubation will, of course, be useless and should never be attempted (see Fig. 13-2).

Wound Management

Management of the wound is an important aspect in the care of head and neck surgical patients. Unlike abdominal or thoracic surgery, head and neck surgery often requires extensive elevation of skin flaps. Moreover, the wound is often contaminated at the time of surgery because the upper aerodigestive tract must be entered and many surgeries are performed in a radiated field where healing qualities of tissue is less than optimal. The combination of local tissue matters gives rise to a perfect setting for hematoma, wound dehiscence, necrosis, pharyngocutaneous fistula, carotid artery rupture, and other complications. Prevention of such events starts in the intraoperative period and is the responsibility of the surgeon. A well-designed and executed operation with adequate hemostasis, careful pharyngeal closure, good placement of subcutaneous drains, and meticulous skin closure is of utmost importance. Despite all these measures, complications can still occur. They often can be prevented or minimized by careful wound management.

Wound Assessment

Most head and neck surgeons use closed suction drainage for major surgery and leave the surgical site exposed (no dressing), thus facilitating wound assessment. The external suture line, closed with interrupted or running sutures, or, most often, with skin staples, is readily visible. In the immediate postoperative period, the care team should become familiar with the appearance of the wound. Changes from this initial evaluation should result in immediate attention and any corrective measures needed. The skin flaps' viability is assessed by noting color, temperature, capillary refill, and induration. Slight erythema and induration of the skin flaps because of surgical incisions and previous radiation is often noted postoperatively. The incision lines are kept free of crusting and exudates achieved by gentle cleaning with hydrogen peroxide, followed by the application of antibiotic ointment every 8 hours until the wound is sealed (3 to 7 days). Drain exit sites and tracheotomy incisions receive the same care. Slight bleeding from skin edges is often seen in the immediate postoperative period. This bleeding should not be confused with a more diffuse ooze of darker blood seen with a hematoma under tension, where the wound is also massively swollen.

Closed Drainage System Assessment

Optimal healing of the wound depends on adequate apposition of the skin flaps to the underlying tissues (deep muscles of the neck and pharynx). Closed drainage with continuous suction eliminates dead space and prevents accumulation of blood, serum, and other secretions under the skin flaps. Many commercially available drainage systems (Davol, Hemovac, Jackson-Pratt) provide continuous negative pressure of 80 to 120 mm Hg (Fig. 13-4).

Drainage systems must be monitored frequently for function, air leak, type, and amount of drainage. Drain malfunction with loss of negative pressure results in accumulation of material under the skin flap and flap elevation. This situation can result in massive hematoma under tension which requires immediate surgical exploration with control of bleeding and restoration of the drainage system. Even excessive bleeding alone may overcome a properly functioning drainage system and may result in a similar situation. Later, changes are more subtle, resulting in less noticeable flap elevation. If unrecognized, this condition may lead to vascular compromise of the skin flaps with external and/or internal wound breakdown. It also increases the risk of abscess formation which may also result in wound breakdown.

Problems may also result if air continuously seeps into the drainage system and prevents maintenance of negative pressure. Not only is there poor apposition of the flaps to the deep structures, but the wound may be contaminated. Inadequate skin closure, pharyngeal closure, malposition of the drains (too close to the external and/or internal suture line), a tracheotomy site that communicates with the wound, or surgical violation of other structures (paranasal sinuses, eustachian tube), can result in such air leakage, which must be corrected as soon as possible. When the air leak is through the skin suture line the problem can be solved by adding sutures or applying thick antibiotic ointment to the incision. Many leaks cease when a circular pressure dressing is applied to the neck, but care must be taken not to compromise blood supply to reconstruction flaps. If the leak is minimal, high wall suction may allow

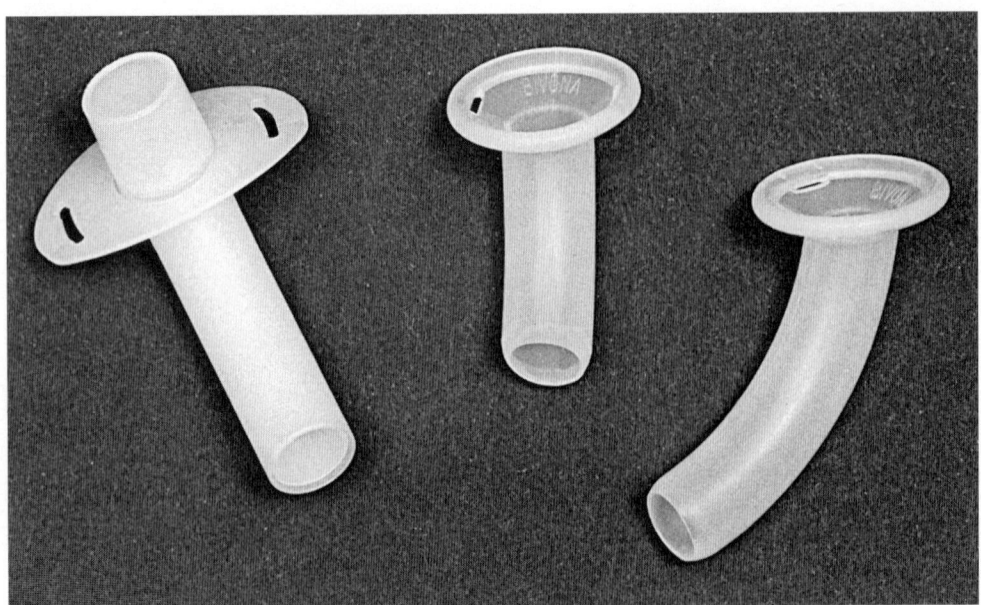

Fig. 13-3. Postlaryngectomy tubes: standard on the right; tube with stoma vents on the left.

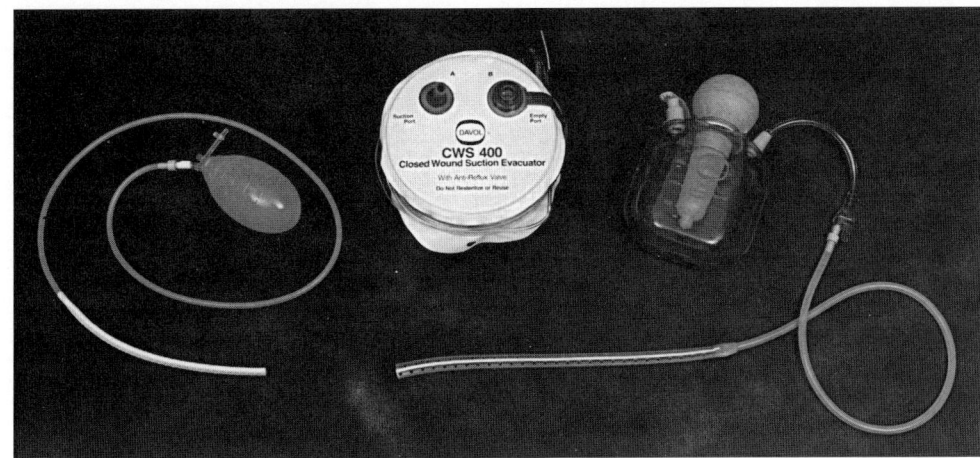

Fig. 13-4. Closed suction drainage systems. (Courtesy of Davol, Inc., Cranston, RI.)

proper tissue apposition and sealing of the air leak. Massive air leak requires removal of the involved drain or even surgical reexploration and closure of the defect and/or proper drain placement.

The type and amount of drainage is monitored and recorded every 8 hours. The amount of drainage for the first few shifts is highly variable and can vary from less than 100 to 300 ml. Volumes of drainage higher than 300 ml/24 hours are not often encountered in the early postoperative period. High volumes can result in drain obstruction and hematoma formation. Initially the drainage is sanguinous to serosanguinous. The drainage progressively decreases from one recording to the next and becomes more serous in nature. Minimal drainage or an abrupt drop in volume suggests a malfunctioning drain and a possible fluid collection under the skin flaps and requires immediate attention. All the drains should be checked for patency either by manually milking them or by increasing the negative pressure to the suspicious drain (syringe, high wall suction). At the same time, the wound is examined for evidence of fluid collection. In the event of a blocked drain and fluid collection undermining the skin flap, surgical drainage is indicated, and the patency of the drainage system should be reestablished.[4] After extensive neck surgery, drains may be removed when drainage is less than 300 ml every 24 hours. If drainage volume does not decrease as expected a pressure dressing may be applied to the neck if a reconstruction flap has not been utilized. Significant opaque serous drainage which turns white with enteral feedings is typical of chyle fistula (see discussion later in this chapter). Purulent and/or granular looking odorous drainage mixed with air points toward probably pharyngocutaneous fistula.

Intraoral Incision Care

The intraoral wound is accessible for assessment and care when a tumor has been removed from the oral cavity.[5] The viability of a flap used to reline the intraoral defect may be assessed directly. A split thickness skin graft is sometimes used intraorally to line the defect. The graft is held in place with a bolster dressing 5 to 7 days after which it is removed at bedside. Surgery in the oral cavity interferes with deglutition and results in pooling of saliva, debris, and unpleasant odors. Therefore, frequent oral hygiene is paramount in caring for these patients.

Intraoral hygiene is the responsibility of the care team in the immediate postoperative period. Secretions are gently suctioned using a soft catheter or a pharyngeal tip suction (Fig. 13-5). Early care of the intraoral suture line is left to the surgical team. Regular inspection and cleaning of contaminated material (e.g., saliva and debris) minimizes the risk of infection and permits early detection of wound dehiscence.

Three or 4 days postoperatively the patient begins active participation in intraoral care. Oral rinses consisting of normal saline, half normal saline and hydrogen peroxide, water with sodium bicarbonate or a combination of saline, peroxide, and Cepacol are prescribed 4 to 5 times a day. Patients are instructed to swish and spit or suction the rinse. Lemon glycerin swabs and full strength commercial mouthwashes should be avoided because they cause excessive drying of the mucous membranes.[6] Commercial mouthwashes have been implicated in the etiology of squamous cell carcinoma of the upper digestive tract[7] and are probably best avoided or diluted.

Later, most patients regain the ability to swallow their own secretions and repeated suctioning is unnecessary. On the other hand, many tend to retain food particles in certain denervated or reconstructed areas of the oral cavity and therefore need to rinse regularly, especially after meals. After the initial healing phase (10 to 15 days), oral hygiene may be supplemented with a Water Pik apparatus and/or manual cleaning.

Split-Thickness Skin Graft

Split-thickness skin grafts are used on occasion to reline mucosal or skin defects in and around the head and neck. They may also be used to reline the harvest site of a free flap. The upper thigh is the usual donor site for such a graft. The donor site may be cared for with either of the following dressings: (1) gauze, or (2) transparent.

A commercial gauze dressing impregnated with antibiotic ointment (Xeroform) is first used to cover the defect. A thick gauze dressing, supplemented with a circumferential dressing around the thigh, is applied. Two days later, all of the dressing that peels away easily is removed leaving the remainder open to air. As the edges of the remaining dressing dry and peel, they are progressively trimmed. Five to 7 days postoperatively patients are instructed to soak the site in the bathtub. This procedure facilitates removal of the remaining gauze from the donor site.[5] Reepithelialization is usually complete in 10 to 14 days.[8,9]

A transparent dressing can also be used (Op site).[8] This dressing covers the wound for 5 to 10 days, during which time reepithelialization occurs. If the dressing leaks serosanguinous fluid, a gentle pressure dressing is applied over the Op site or a new transparent dressing is applied. Any excessive drainage accumulating under the transparent dressing must be drained.[5]

Reconstruction Flaps

Extended surgical resections often require reconstructive tissue from other body sites for wound closure or functional rehabilitation. Losses of skin, mucosa, and soft tissue (e.g., muscle, jawbone) are usually reconstructed using a variety of "flaps." Those used in head and neck reconstruction are either pedicled or free flaps.

Pedicled flaps are harvested from regional tissues and transposed into the surgical defect still attached to their vascular supply (pedicle). The most commonly used pedicled flap in head and neck reconstruction is the pectoralis major myocutaneous flap (Fig. 13-6). An island of skin and subcutaneous tissue is outlined on the chest over the pectoralis major muscle, freed from the surrounding tissue and left attached to the underlying muscle. A strip of muscle is preserved surrounding the vascular pedicle. The flap is then rotated superiorly (most often subcutaneously) and sutured into the defect. The island of skin is easily monitored when used to replace external skin but on occasion only the muscle is harvested for this purpose and a split thickness skin graft is placed over the muscle. The flap is "buried" and is not readily visible when used to reline the mucosal lining of the oral cavity or pharynx. Postoperatively, the affected neck may appear full compared to the opposite side. A subcutaneous bulge over the clavicle corresponds to the area where the cuff of muscle and the vascular pedicle cross it.

It is important to minimize tension and/or pressure on the vascular pedicle. The head is flexed and rotated toward the side where the flap was harvested. Nothing should be tied around the neck: no tracheotomy ties, circumferential neck dressings, gown, nor even the mask used to provide tracheotomized patients with humidity. Any change in the external appearance of the neck and/or drain malfunction should be reported immediately since the tension caused by a hematoma may compromise the vascular supply. When the island of skin is visible, direct observation of skin color (especially changes), capillary refill, and temperature are also noted.

Free flap reconstruction of head and neck defects is now common in major centers. A free flap consists of harvested tissue completely divided from its donor site and anastomosed to recipient vessels close to the defect (microvascular anastomosis). For example, a segment of jejunum may be harvested from the abdomen and transferred to the neck to reconstruct a circumferential defect of the pharynx following total pharyngolaryngectomy. Flaps containing bone and soft tissue (e.g., scapula, iliac

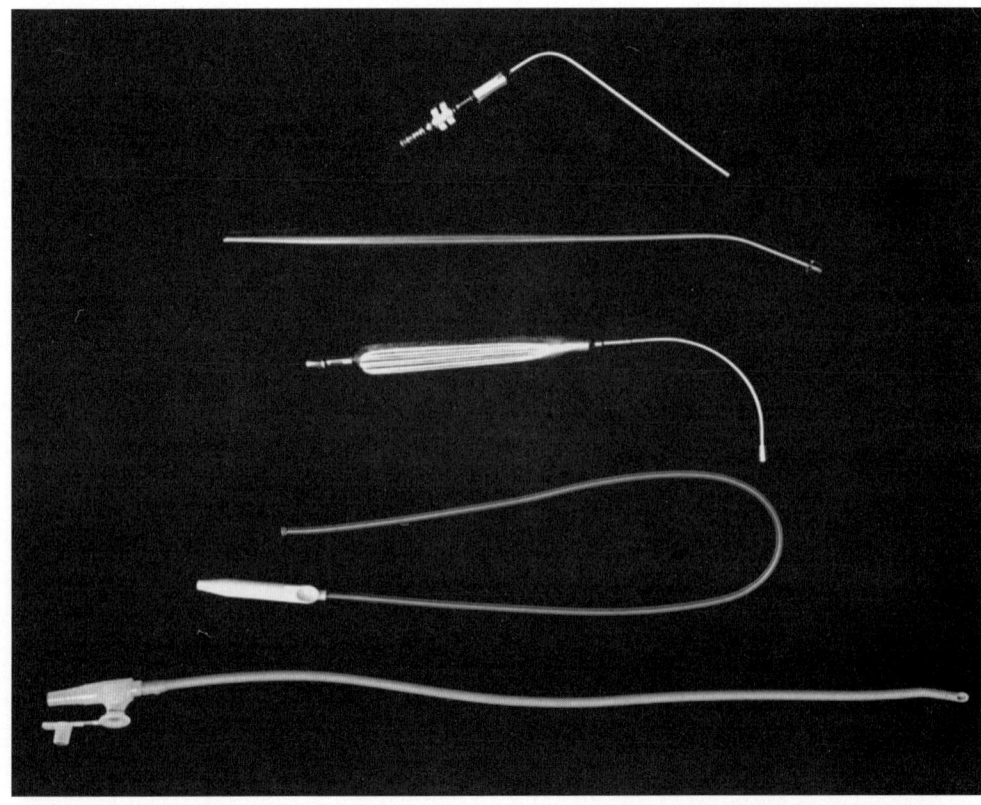

Fig. 13-5. Suction tips and catheters.

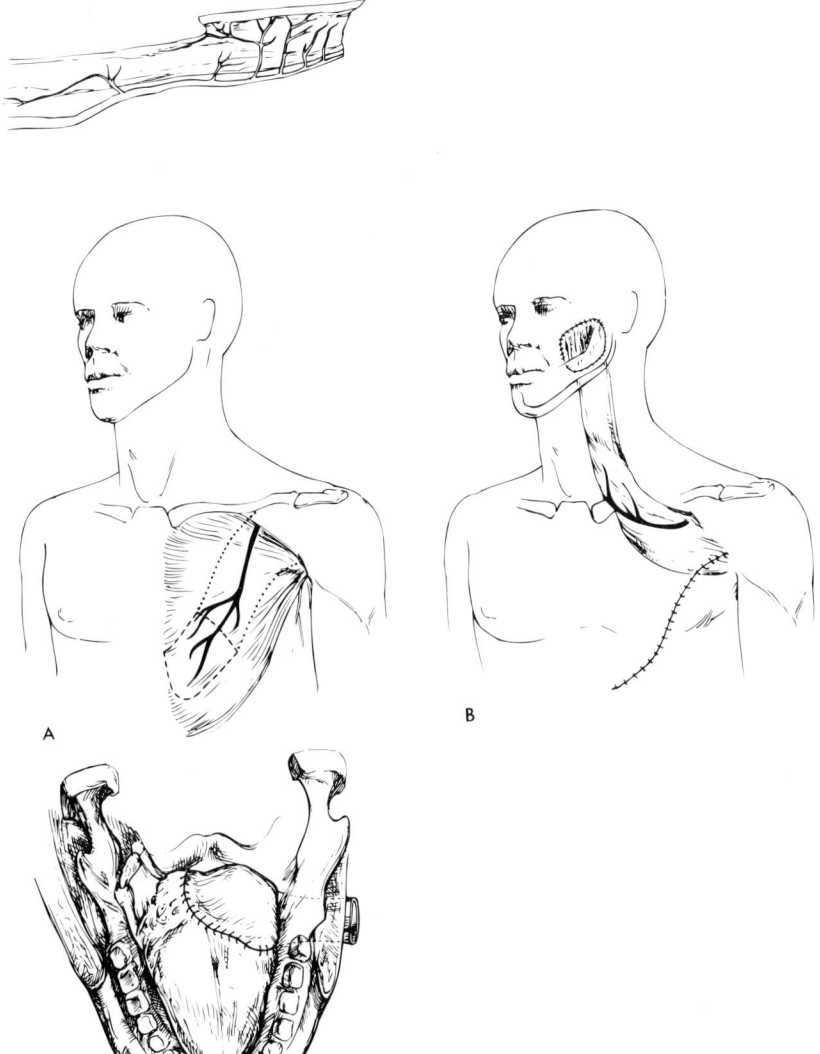

Fig. 13–6. Pectoralis major myocutaneous flap (*A*) used to reconstruct an intraoral defect (*B* and *C*). (From Parsons, J. T., and Million, R. R.: Treatment of tumors of the oropharynx. In Comprehensive Management of Head and Neck Tumors. Edited by S. E. Thawley, W. R. Panje, J. G. Batsakis, and R. D. Lindberg. Philadelphia, W. B. Saunders, 1987, p. 744.)

crest) may be used to reconstruct the mandible after mandibulectomy.

Close postoperative monitoring of these flaps is of utmost importance. Avoiding tension and/or pressure on the vascular pedicle as outlined above for pedicled flaps should be applied to the free flap, as well. In addition, patency for the vascular anastomoses and/or the perfusion of the transferred tissues must be monitored.[10,11] Direct observation of the skin flap is reliable when available; for this reason some surgeons exteriorize a small segment of buried flaps. Doppler is commonly used to confirm patency of the anastomoses. The exact area where the Doppler should be applied is determined by the surgeon at the time of the anastomoses. Hourly assessments are done at least for the first 24 hours. Although currently unavailable, continuous monitoring of distal tissue perfusion would be ideal. Early detection of vascular compromise is important because salvage is possible only for a short period of time prior to the "no-reflow" phenomenon, which is the time when the extent of tissue injury is such that revascularization cannot be successfully established.[11]

Another important consideration in the postoperative care of free flaps is blood viscosity. The hematocrit is usually maintained below 30 and allowed to fall as low as 25 before consideration is given to transfusing the patient. Dextron 40 (Rheomacrodex) can be used at a rate of 25 to 50 ml/hr for 5 days. Low dose aspirin and even heparin are used by some surgeons.

Wound Complications

Postoperative wound complications arise because of fluid collection, injection, and/or vascular disruption. These include:

- Hematoma
- Seroma
- Infection and wound dehiscence
- Chyle fistula
- Carotid artery rupture

Hematoma. Hematoma occurs in 2 to 4% of head and neck surgery cases.[12,13] Acute postoperative hematoma usually happens in the first 12 hours following the procedure. The neck becomes massively enlarged, dark blood is seen seeping through the incision line, drains are occluded, and the patient complains of significant discomfort. When drain patency cannot be reestablished immediately the cerebral vascular supply can be compromised and, in a nontracheotomized patient, the airway is at risk. If necessary, the wound can be opened at the bedside to relieve the tension, discomfort, and/or airway compromise. Immediate arrangements should be made to take the patient to the operating room to verify hemostasis and reestablish the drainage system.[14]

Subacute hematoma is less dramatic and usually presents as a mild to moderate, often localized area of swelling. The surgeon either decides to manage the problem conservatively or surgically, based on the amount of undermining, location, and progression of the hematoma. Flap undermining compromises vascular supply to skin flaps, increases the risks of infection, wound dehiscence, fistula formation, etc. Thus, the surgeon must drain any significant collection.

Seroma. This minor complication occurs infrequently and is noted as a fluid-filled (serous) swelling under the skin flap. Seromas are usually noted 5 to 10 days postoperatively and are managed by sequential sterile needle aspirations,[14] and occasionally supplemented with pressure dressing.

Infection and Wound Dehiscence. Postoperative wound infection is the source of significant morbidity in the head and neck surgical patients. Antibiotic prophylaxis has reduced the incidence of infection to 5 to 25% of cases. Many risk factors for infection have been described by Tabet and Johnson.[15] Preoperative weight loss, diabetes, smoking and drinking, large tumors, previous radiation, and previous tracheotomy are associated with an increased incidence or severity of infection. Intraoperatively, size and location of tumor and the technical ability of the surgical team are mentioned. Postoperative factors include poor nutritional status, inadequate drainage, and dehiscence of the oropharyngeal suture line.[15]

The same authors grade the status of the neck as it relates to infection from 0 to 5:

0: Normal
1: Erythema within 1 cm of suture line
2: 1 to 5 cm erythema
3: Induration and >5 cm erythema
4: Purulent drainage
5: Mucocutaneous fistula[15]

Limited induration and erythema are normally seen around the incision lines for a short period postoperatively (grade 1 to 3). Infection is considered significant and will require attention when:

- Grade 1—purulent drainage, or saliva is noted in the drainage system (usually early: <5 days)
- Grade 2—purulent or salivary collection forms underneath the skin flaps and causes undermining
- Grade 3—pus and/or saliva leaks through a dehiscent skin incision

Most infections are secondary to seepage of saliva through a dehiscent oropharyngeal suture line. Such dehiscence may be noted from postoperatively (due to a technical error) to weeks later (related to poor healing), but most are noted within 3 weeks of surgery.[16] Patients with impending fistula often have low grade temperature.

Management of infection and/or fistula requires adequate drainage of any subcutaneous collection in order to prevent further undermining and loss of tissue. The wound is opened in a dependent portion away from the cervical vessels, if possible. A penrose-type drain or packing (i.e., Nu-gauze) is left in the opening and a dressing is placed around the neck. Depending on the amount of drainage the dressing and packing are changed when soiled, up to three times a day. The fistula site is examined daily to assure adequate drainage and remove necrotic tissue. In most cases healthy granulation tissue forms progressively around the fistula site, the amount of drainage decreases, and the fistula closes spontaneously. Most fistulas heal with this conservative approach. Problem fistulas which do not respond to conservative treatment persist more than 6 weeks, and threaten the integrity of the carotid artery require surgical closure.

Chyle Fistulas. Chyle fistulas are reported in approximately 1 to 2% of all neck dissections.[17,18] Recently Spiro and colleagues reported an incidence of 1.9% in 823 neck dissections.[19] Chyle fistulas occur predominantly in the left neck and are related to injury to the thoracic duct. Chyle contains most of the ingested fat, electrolytes, and white cells, mainly lymphocytes. Anatomy of the thoracic duct is highly variable and sometimes chyle fistulas are seen on the right side. More often such a fistula is detected between the second and fifth postoperative days, usually on resumption of enteral feedings. A chyle fistula presents as a swelling in the lower anterior neck region or as increased drainage or both. The appearance of this drainage changes depending on the fat content because the more drainage will be milky white. A common presentation is flap undermining by semiopaque, gray yellowish coagulum. Chylothorax may also result from a neck dissection in which case shortness of breath or other related symptoms are present and chest radiograph shows a pleural effusion.

Drainage from such a fistula can amount to two to four liters a day. A severe and/or persistent fistula can result in severe metabolic deficit from loss of fluid, electrolytes, and proteins.

Three factors should be considered in the management of a chyle fistula:

- Fluid and electrolytes replacement
- Dietary considerations
- Management of the leakage site

Depending on the severity of the chyle leak, fluid, electrolytes, and proteins can either be provided enterally or parenterally. With smaller chyle leaks, enteral alimentation is maintained, but centered around medium-chain triglycerides. Medium-chain triglycerides are absorbed directly in the portal system and result in a decreased production of chyle. With larger chyle leaks, total parenteral nutrition should be considered.

Conservative management of the fistula site is indicated initially.[19] This program consists of proper drainage and application of a pressure dressing to the area. If after 4 to 5 days there has been no response, or if the volume is greater than 500 to 600 ml per day with no signs of regression, surgical intervention is recommended.[17-19] Localization of the fistula is facilitated by preoperative ingestion of fat (chyle will become white) and the use of the operating microscope. Prolonged conservative management (1 to 2 months) may eventually result in closure of the fistula but at the expense of a lengthy hospital stay. Chylothorax is managed by placing a chest tube to drain the collection and restore adequate pulmonary and circulatory functions. Depending on the amount of drainage, early thoracotomy may be considered.

Carotid Artery Rupture (Blowout). Carotid rupture is the most feared complication of head and neck surgery. This complication is seen most frequently when neck dissection is performed along with entry into a mucosalined viscus. The majority of patients also have had preoperative radiation therapy to the head and neck area. Rupture is usually preceded by wound infection, often secondary to the breakdown of the internal suture line and resulting pharyngocutaneous fistula. The artery is exposed to purulent material and/or air. Then, the adventitia and media are weakened, an aneurysm forms, and eventually the artery ruptures. The incidence of this complication is between 3 to 5% of major head and neck resections.[12,20,21] Many techniques have been described to provide extra protection to the carotid artery in the event of a possible pharyngocutaneous fistula.[21,22] Dermal grafts and/or muscle rotation flaps (e.g., levator scapulae, pectoralis major) are used by many surgeons to provide coverage to the artery, especially when radiation has been used previously, the mucosal lining is violated, or the tissues are believed to be of poor quality. Although this extra barrier should theoretically reduce the incidence of rupture, no studies thus far confirm this assumption and ruptures still occur.

Although rupture can sometimes occur underneath an intact skin suture line with no obvious signs of underlying infection, most often a pharyngocutaneous fistula and exposure of the carotid artery is recognized or suspected before rupture. The surgeon assures adequate drainage to prevent collections under the flaps, further necrosis, and tissue slough. When possible, the fistula is directed away from the carotid vessels. If the fistula does not show signs of prompt healing and the carotid artery is at risk, a reconstruction flap may be used to provide additional protection to the artery and close the fistula.

When artery rupture seems inevitable, elective occlusion either by progressive clamping or by intraarterial balloon occlusion is a good alternative to watchful waiting. Brisk, severe bleeding through the incision line, the mouth and/or tracheotomy, leading to shock with cessation of bleeding is often seen when the artery initially ruptures. The patient should be brought to the operating room immediately, the necrotic segment of the artery excised, and the distal and proximal stumps ligated in healthy tissue.

When a patient is at risk of carotid rupture, special precautions should be instituted. Patients are admitted to an ICU with adequate monitoring. Enteral nutrition (especially oral) is discontinued. Intravenous access lines are installed and the patient is maintained on bed rest. Blood should be available for immediate replacement. When blood may be aspirated into the tracheobronchial tree, a cuffed endotracheal or tracheotomy tube should be available. Immediate, direct manual pressure to the bleeding point is the most effective way to control it. This procedure should be performed by whoever is first in the room after rupture to minimize hypotension, the risk of permanent neurologic sequelae, and/or death. With the bleeding under control, the airway should be secured, IV fluids and blood transfusion instituted and the patient moved to the operating room for further treatment.

Mortality from carotid rupture approaches 30 to 50%. Significant neurologic sequelae of either aphasia and/or contralateral hemiplegia is seen in up to 50% of survivors.[21,23]

Nutritional Management

Malnutrition is a common problem in head and neck cancer patients. Goodwin and Torres estimated that malnutrition occurs in 30 to 50% of such patients.[24] Bassett and Dobie found 60% of their patients with fair to poor nutrition.[25] Malnutrition can be secondary to the patient's nutritional habits, or because of tumor, or pain interfering with deglutition.

Malnourished patients generally suffer more surgical complications such as impaired wound healing, infection, and fistula.[24,26] Therefore, nutritional assessment, planning, and management are essential in this patient population.

Nutritional Assessment

The dietician is an integral part of the head and neck multidisciplinary team. Nutritional status is based on eating habits, weight, height, weight loss, etc. In 1980, Buzby and colleagues developed a prognostic nutritional index (PNI) derived from serum albumin and transferrin, triceps skinfold, and delayed hypersensitivity skin testing.[27] PNI was found to be useful in predicting postoperative complications in head and neck cancer patients.[24,26] Additional methods have also been described to assess nutritional status.[25,28] (see Chap. 62.)

Nutritional management for this patient population may consist of any of the following:

(1) Counseling on oral intake and supplements
(2) Enteral nutrition
(3) Parenteral nutrition

Preoperatively, or during the course of radiation and/or chemotherapy, patients with a fair to good nutritional status are recommended a well-balanced diet high in proteins and calories.

Oral supplements are recommended for patients with slight nutritional deficit who have no more than minimal dysphagia. Lactose free preparations are used because they are better tolerated, especially in patients with lactose intolerance (i.e., diarrhea, bloating and cramping).[29] Lactose products can also increase oral and pharyngeal mucus production. The same type of supplements are recommended postoperatively when swallowing is still somewhat impaired.

Many head and neck cancer patients will need some form of enteral nutrition during the course of treatment. Enteral nutrition offers nutritional and immunologic advantages over isocaloric parenteral nutrition.[30] Therefore, enteral nutrition is preferred over parenteral nutrition in patients with an intact intestinal tract and good tolerance to feedings.

Enteral therapy can be instituted if swallowing is impaired by tumor (pharyngeal stenosis), mandibular excursion (trismus), pain (odynophagia), the patient's reaction to the disease (depression), or by a combination of these factors. In addition, local reaction (mucositis) during radiation therapy and/or chemotherapy may cause or increase patient's dysphagia and necessitate enteral nutrition.

If the digestive tract has been entered during surgery, oral feedings are not permitted for approximately 10 days.

Enteral nutrition may be administered by:

- Nasogastric tube
- Pharyngotomy
- Esophagostomy
- Gastrostomy
- Jejunostomy

Nasogastric Tube

Most head and neck cancer patients require a nasogastric tube, proper management of which cannot be overemphasized. Head and neck patients may have an ileus for 24 to 48 hours, during which time the nasogastric tube is used for decompression. When the digestive tract has not been entered (i.e., neck dissection), and in absence of dysphagia and/or aspiration, the nasogastric tube is discontinued and oral alimentation resumed.

The nasogastric tube has a triple role when the digestive tract has been entered. It is used for nutrition and for medication after the decompression period. Because of the risk of disrupting the internal suture line, the nasogastric tube should not be reinserted if dislodged until sufficient healing has occurred. To prevent accidental dislodgement the nasogastric tube is often sutured to the nasal septum and taped to the nose. When the nasogastric tube becomes dislodged or is accidentally removed in the early postoperative period, despite these measures, the decision to reinsert the tube should be made only by the surgeon who is familiar with the details of surgical resection, reconstruction, and location of the internal suture lines. If the tube cannot be reinserted, the patient is limited to IV fluids or given parenteral nutrition until healing is judged sufficient for oral alimentation.

During nutritional use of the nasogastric tube, tube clogging from medications or blenderized food should be prevented. For this reason, a No. 16 french Silastic tube is preferred over smaller tubes. In a survey of 91 hospitals, 58% reported significant occlusion and mechanical problems when smaller diameter feeding tubes were used.[31] In the event that the nasogastric tube is obstructed, it may be flushed with water or club soda, or even meat tenderizer may be used to unclog it.

A large syringe filled with warm water may be used to flush the tube. Assuming that the tube is not kinked or in an improper position, significant pressure may be applied which usually unclogs the tube. Club soda may also be used to flush the tube and is left for 10 minutes before plunging. Meat tenderizer (1 tsp. of meat tenderizer with 120 ml of warm water) can also be left in the nasogastric tube for 10 minutes before syringing several times.[32] Substances such as cranberry juice, which interacts with commercial feedings, and sugar-based sodas should be avoided because they promote clogging.

Nasogastric tubes are not free of risks. They can be a source of irritation to the nose and throat, they may interfere with deglutition, they can increase pulmonary complications,[33] and they may disrupt the internal suture line. Sofferman and colleagues recently reported cases of postcricoid laryngeal ulceration resulting in cord paralysis secondary to N/G tubes.[34] Therefore, they are recommended for short-term use, usually no longer than 1 month.

Pharyngotomy and Cervical Esophagostomy

These techniques are not as popular today as in the past. In 1989, Williams and Meguid stated that cervical esophagostomy was underused.[33] In the short term (<1 month), these techniques have no advantage over a nasogastric tube, require an operation, and add another risk of complication in the recently operated neck. They are also a source of concern if radiation therapy was or is to be used postoperatively. In the long term, they have been largely supplanted by gastrostomy, especially the percutaneous endoscopic gastrostomy (PEG), which is comfortable for the patient and can be done under topical anesthesia with minimal morbidity. The advantages of the gastrostomy techniques include a tube easily concealed under clothing and less risk of esophageal reflux.

Gastrostomy

Gastrostomy is recommended for long-term enteral nutrition (>1 month). In patients with cancer of the head and neck, it may be used before any treatment if the patient is nutritionally deficient on first evaluation and/or is likely to have further swallowing difficulties during or following treatment.

Gastrostomy tubes may be inserted by open surgery (laparotomy) or by guided PEG. If flexible esophagoscopy is technically possible (the tumor can prevent access into the esophagus), this latter is the procedure of choice. First described in 1980 by Gauderer and colleagues[35] for long-term enteral feeding in the pediatric population, it has gained wide acceptance in head and neck cancer patients.[36] It can be performed under local anesthesia and with minimal complications. It may even be performed at the time of initial panendoscopy evaluation.[33]

The following complications have been described following gastrostomy:

- Gastric content leakage around the tube
- Skin excoriation and granulation
- Pain and tenderness around the tube
- Chronic granulation of the gastrointestinal tract

Table 13-1. Enteral Feeding Administration Protocol

Lactose-free product	½ strength at 50 ml/h × 8 h
	½ strength at 75 ml/h × 8 h
	½ strength at 100 ml/h × 8 h
	Full strength at 75 ml/h × 8 h
	Full strength at 100 ml/h × 8 h
	Bolus 300–400 ml 6/day over 20–30 min

- Gastric or peritoneal hemorrhage
- Gastric erosion and/or perforation
- Abscess, infection, peritonitis
- Accidental removal of tube
- Pyloric obstruction by tube[37]

Nonetheless, these complications are uncommon, and generally the advantages outweigh the disadvantages.

Jejunostomy

This technique is used when the stomach is unavailable (previous surgery), or has been used for pharyngoesophageal reconstruction (gastric pullup). Another indication is severe gastroesophageal reflux. A laparotomy is required to insert a jejunostomy tube. Special nutritional preparations are utilized to maximize absorption and minimize diarrhea. Isotonic enteral formula is delivered by continuous drip method which is best regulated by infusion pump.

Enteral Feeding Administration

Commercially prepared enteral products vary in content (i.e., lactose, lactose free, varying amounts of fiber, carbohydrate, protein, and fat). The product used is determined by patient nutritional status and requirements.

Lactose-free products (e.g., Osmolyte, Isocal) are used most commonly. An example of a feeding administration protocol is shown in Table 13-1. This protocol may be used for all types of enteral feeding tubes, with the exception of the jejunostomy tube.

Prior to administration of bolus enteral feedings, stomach residuals are measured. If the residual is greater than 100 ml the tube feeding is withheld. The patient's upper body is positioned in a sitting or semisitting position during the feeding to minimize aspiration. Daily weight and frequent monitoring of urinary sugar and ketones are also part of the protocol.

Patients may complain of abdominal bloating and distention, nausea, flatus, and/or diarrhea. Increasing the patient's activity and decreasing the infusion rate and/or concentration of enteral formula can minimize these symptoms. When there is no response to these measures, the formula can be changed from hypertonic to isotonic or from isotonic to a blenderized formula. Preparation of blenderized meals in the hospital setting is a major undertaking, mostly because of sanitary regulations. Once the patient is home, however, blenderized food is less of a financial burden, and self-administration of "real" food through the feeding tube may provide a psychologic boost.

Multivitamin supplements are provided. Malnourished alcoholic patients receive thiamine 100 mg daily as well as folic acid 1 mg daily. Other supplements are added as necessary.

Total Parenteral Nutrition

Total parenteral nutrition (TPN) is used for patients with dysfunctional gastrointestinal tracts. This procedure is unusual in head and neck cancer patients.

Medications

Antibiotics

Clean head and neck surgery (thyroidectomy, parotidectomy), in which the aerodigestive tract is not entered, has a rate of infection of around 2% which does not justify antibiotic prophylaxis.[38] Clean contaminated surgery in which a previously uninfected surgical site becomes contaminated at the time of surgery by oropharyngeal secretions, requires antibiotic prophylaxis.[15] Microorganisms found in oropharyngeal secretions are: (1) aerobic gram(+), mainly streptococcus and staphylococcus, and (2) anaerobes, most bacteroides species. Tabet and Johnson conclude that an adequate dosage of either a cefazolin (ANCEF), a third generation cephalosporin, clindamycin, or metronidazole with cefazolin constitutes adequate prophylaxis. They also conclude that medication should be administered intravenously starting 1 or 2 hours preoperatively and maintained for no longer than 24 hours.[15]

Analgesics

Pain severity is subjective and should be assessed based on the patient's perception of the pain. The goal of pain management is pain relief and patient comfort. Patients participate more actively in their care if their pain is well managed.

Pain resulting from head and neck surgery is generally less severe than that of abdominal surgery.[39] In the immediate postoperative period the patient may complain of discomfort from tubes and positioning, but the pain is usually minimal. Sensory innervation to the surgical site is often interrupted at the time of surgery, thus minimizing pain. A skin graft or dermal graft obtained from the leg or a flap harvested from the chest often generates more discomfort than the neck wound. For the first 24 hours or until enteral alimentation is started, pain can be controlled with intravenous codeine (30 mg every 4 to 6 hours). Some patients may benefit from stronger medications such as meperidine, buprenorphine (Buprenex), or morphine. A combination of acetaminophen and codeine is often used orally or enterally as soon as the patient's condition permits. This combination is also used after hospital discharge.

POST-ICU PHASE

The care of patients undergoing head and neck surgery does not stop with hospital discharge. Only a few resume all their former activities. The majority of patients are considered disabled and are unable or unwilling to find gainful employment. Many need the financial help provided through social services.

Speech and Swallowing

Speech and swallowing are two important functions related to the head and neck. Speech involves sound production at the vocal cord level and further modulation of this in the oral cavity producing speech. Fine musculature control of the tongue is required for this last step in speech production. During this process, adequate velopharyngeal control is also necessary (nasality). Swallowing requires the handling of food and secretions in the oral cavity, propulsion of the bolus into the pharynx, and then into the esophagus. During this process, velopharyngeal closure is required to prevent nasal regurgitation. Laryngeal closure prevents aspiration of food and secretions into the airway. These functions are under the control of the neurologic system and require constant interaction of multiple sensory input at the brain stem and cortical levels followed by voluntary and instant reflex motor output.

Tumors of the larynx, pharynx, and oral cavity and their treatment may alter structural competence and affect swallowing and speech. Involvement of cranial nerves IX and X, and to a lesser degree nerves VII and XII, also interferes with speech. The airway must be protected from aspiration during swallowing. Disorders of speech and/or swallowing are best evaluated and treated by a speech pathologist experienced in their treatment. Speech and swallowing evaluation and rehabilitation start when the surgeon deems it appropriate, which could be the day after the surgery if the pharynx has not been entered, to 7 to 10 days when the pharynx has been entered.

Laryngeal Surgery

Hemilaryngectomy

This consists of the removal of one vocal cord anterior to the arytenoid cartilage. Although there is some risk of aspiration initially, normal deglutition usually resumes promptly with minimal instruction.[40,41] When the operation is extended posteriorly to include the arytenoid, however, the risk of aspiration is increased. Rehabilitation includes swallowing exercises to promote adequate laryngeal closure and may occasionally take several months to learn.[42] Voice is altered following hemilaryngectomy but usually improves with short-term speech therapy. When glottic incompetence (breathy voice and/or aspiration), persists for more than 2 to 3 months, surgical revision may be considered.

Supraglottic Laryngectomy

This operation requires the removal of the laryngeal structures above the vocal folds including the false cords and the epiglottis, which have an important role in protection of the airway during swallowing. Their removal will result in some degree of aspiration in all patients. Swallowing must be relearned and patients are taught the "supraglottic swallow." This technique involves swallowing at the end of inspiration, followed by a voluntary cough to clear the airway of any aspirated material. Within 2 to 3 months of the surgical procedure, most patients have resumed oral intake without significant aspiration. When this operation is extended superiorly to include the tongue, laterally to the pharynx, or inferiorly to include the arytenoid, aspiration is likely to be more severe.[43] Voice may also be affected with some changes in pitch, increased breathiness, and hoarseness.

Total Laryngectomy

Total laryngectomy is complete removal of the larynx and permanent separation of swallowing function (pharyngoesophagus) from breathing (trachea) (see Fig. 13-2). Aspiration is not a concern, but patients may experience some changes in chewing and tongue movement and possibly changes in the pharyngoesophageal segment that can result in some degree of dysphagia.[44]

Normal phonation is lost following this procedure. Patients and families are counseled preoperatively regarding alternate methods of communication. In the immediate postoperative period, patients communicate by writing or by using a communication board (Fig. 13-7). Instructions on the use of an artificial larynx are given by the speech pathologist 24 to 48 hours after the surgery (Fig. 13-8). Once healing has occurred, or following postoperative radiation, the patient may learn esophageal speech or have a laryngeal prosthesis placed through a surgically created tracheoesophageal puncture.

Pharyngeal Surgery

Although these patients usually have a normal voice, pharyngeal sensation and peristalsis are hampered resulting in possible aspiration. A diet consisting of liquids or semiliquids is usually recommended. Thicker foods are more difficult to pass through the pharynx because they require greater peristalsis.[40]

Oral Cavity Surgery

Glossectomy, mandibulectomy, and/or palatectomy may affect mouth closure, tongue, and jaw movement. Articulation, chewing, and propulsion of the food bolus into the pharynx may be compromised.[45] Different eating techniques and food of different consistencies are recommended by the speech pathologist. Intraoral prosthesis to lower the palate and permit better apposition to the remaining tongue or to act as an obturator may assist in eating more effectively and in speaking with better intelligibility.

Cranial Nerve Deficits

Loss of sensation and/or motor function of oropharyngolaryngeal structures due to cranial nerve injury may interfere with speech and swallowing. Isolated paralysis of cranial nerves V, VII, IX, X, or XII is usually well tolerated. However, paralysis of multiple nerves and/or surimposed structural defects are likely to result in significant problems. Paralysis of cranial nerves IX, X, XI, and sometimes XII seen in association with base of skull surgery may result in significant problems with swallowing and speech. Besides initial speech pathology techniques, different surgical approaches have been described to solve voice and aspiration problems.[46] Most techniques are effective in improving voice but help with aspiration is less satisfactory.

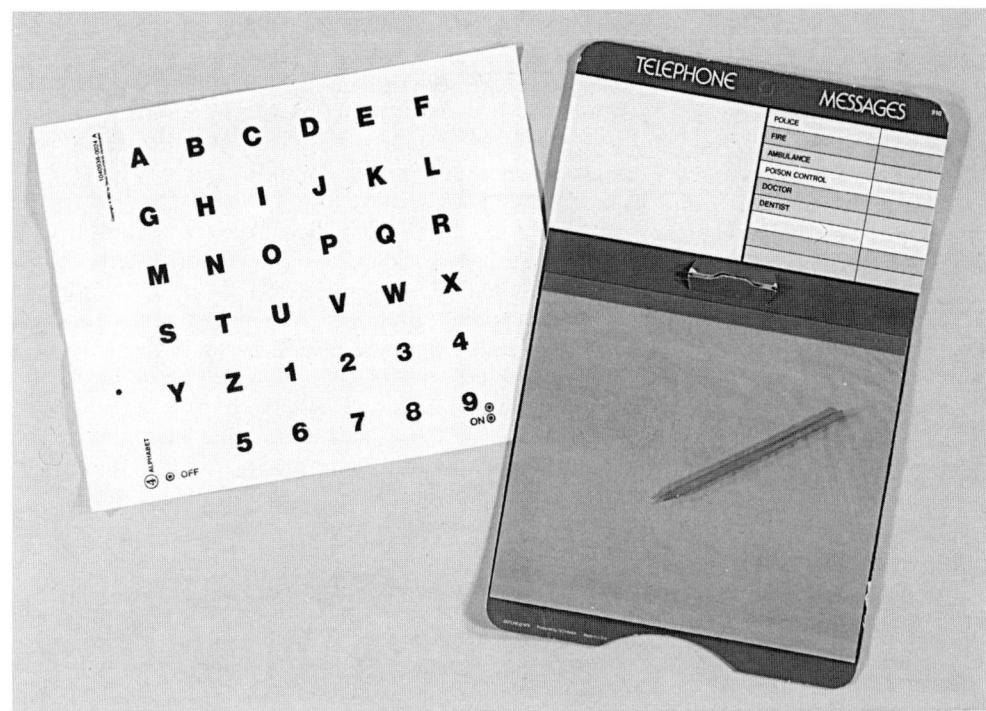

Fig. 13–7. Communication means immediately following tracheotomy or laryngectomy.

Patients who undergo the previously mentioned procedures usually require tracheotomy and placement of a nasogastric tube. Management of the tracheotomy tube and of the nasogastric tube has been reviewed in detail earlier in this chapter. When the patient is incapable of resuming oral alimentation within a reasonable amount of time following his or her surgery, arrangements are made for discharge with these tubes in place. These patients are followed regularly in the outpatient clinic and aggressive speech and swallowing therapy is provided. As the patient's swallowing improves, oral alimentation is resumed and the tubes removed. If dysphagia persists for more than

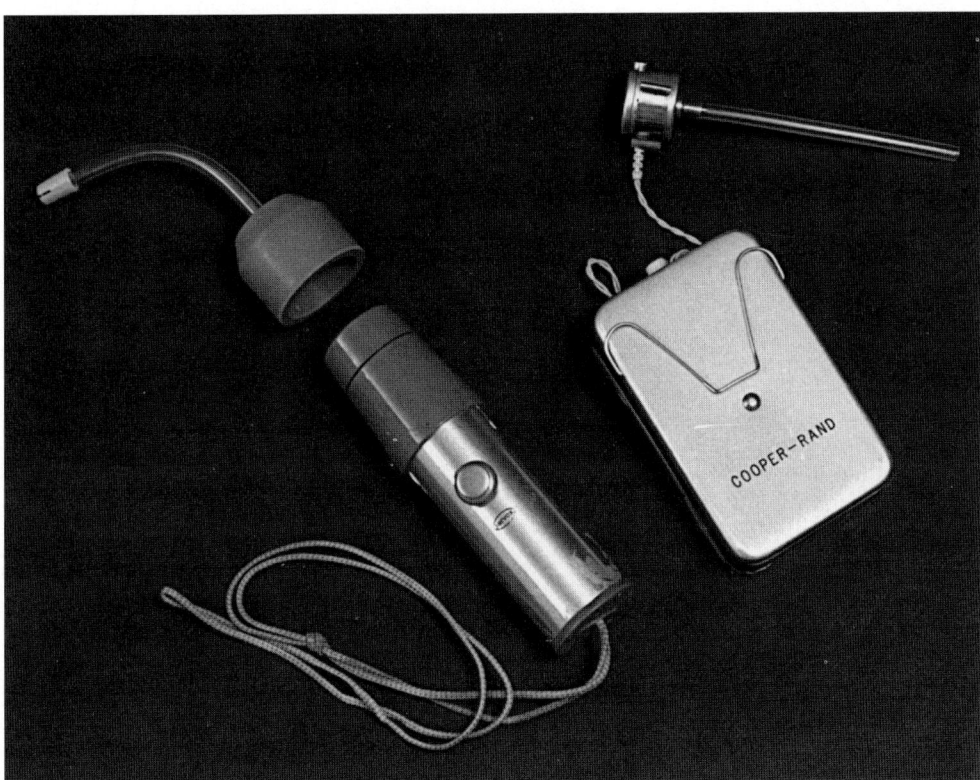

Fig. 13–8. Electronic devices used following laryngectomy. (Cooper Rand Electrolarynx, Luminaud, Inc., Mentor, OH.)

3 to 6 months, revision surgery, permanent tracheotomy, and/or permanent enteral alimentation are considered.

Treatment of cancer of the head and neck often results in significant changes in external appearance and/or function. Cosmesis may be improved in many different ways: revision surgery, makeup, prosthetic devices. Defects and scars may be concealed under adapted closing, wigs, or hats. Swallowing impairments are evaluated by the speech pathologist. When necessary, the diet is modified or different swallowing techniques are recommended. Revision surgery or prosthetic devices may be necessary. When oral alimentation is impossible or insufficient to maintain adequate nutrition, permanent enteral nutrition is instituted. Difficulty with speech can be helped by prosthetic devices, speech techniques, and revision surgery.

Patients who undergo head and neck surgery often complain of neck discomfort and stiffness, which can be secondary to the position of the head (extreme rotation and/or extension) during surgery. Months later, the discomfort and stiffness are secondary to scarring. Shoulder discomfort is a common complaint in patients who undergo neck dissection. Sacrifice or extensive manipulation of the accessory nerve (cranial nerve XI) as it travels in the posterior aspect of the neck results in trapezius muscle weakness. The functions of the trapezius muscle are: (1) rotation of the scapula to raise the shoulder during arm abduction, and (2) drawing of the scapula backward. Complete or partial loss of function results in the "shoulder drop syndrome" where the shoulder droops forward and inferiorly and abduction of the arm is restricted. This situation results in some discomfort around the acromioclavicular joint. Physical therapy is instituted within a week from the time of surgery to maintain the normal range of motion, prevent ankylosis and stiffness, and minimize the patient's discomfort.

Patients with squamous cell carcinoma are at risk of a second primary cancer, not only in the head and neck, but also in the rest of the upper aerodigestive tract, as well as in the urinary tract. The majority of these patients are long-term abusers of tobacco and alcohol. They should be encouraged to change their habits to decrease chances of local recurrence or secondary primary cancer. This recommendation is not an easy task for someone who is already under significant stress from the disease and its treatment as well as loss of employment and income. Depression is common, and psychiatric help may be required.

Patients are followed closely on an outpatient basis. Monthly visits are recommended for the first 6 months and are then spaced out to every 2 to 4 months. After the third year, patients are seen every 6 months up to 5 years, after which they are seen yearly. At each visit, a thorough head and neck examination is performed to detect any recurrence or a new primary tumor. An annual chest radiograph is obtained because the lungs are the most common site of a secondary primary tumor as well as the first site of distant metastasis from a primary tumor of the head and neck. Routine blood tests are not part of regular follow-up, however. Hypothyroidism is seen frequently in patients who have extensive surgery and radiation to the head and neck.[47,48] Therefore, thyroid-stimulating hormone (TSH) levels should be obtained and proper therapy administered when necessary.

Despite aggressive treatment of head and neck cancer lesions, 5-year survival of patients with advanced tumors is well below 50%. These patients not only die of recurrent disease or secondary primary tumors, but also of an array of medical conditions.

In conclusion, head and neck cancer represents only 5% of all cancers. The location of these tumors often renders their treatment difficult. Specialized postoperative care to promote proper healing and minimize complications is mandatory. Important aspects in the care of these patients in the immediate postoperative period have been presented. Close communication between the surgical team and members of the postoperative care team improves the final outcome. A multidisciplinary approach to the care of this patient population is required.

REFERENCES

1. American Cancer Society: Cancer facts and figures, 1990.
2. Al-Sarraf, M.: Head and neck cancer: chemotherapy concepts. Semin. Oncol., 15:70, 1988.
3. Levine, H., and Miller, C.: Tracheotomy Care Manual. 2nd Ed. New York, Thieme, 1988.
4. Johnson, J. T., and Myers, E.: Management of complications of therapeutic intervention. In Cancer of the Head and Neck. 2nd Ed. Edited by E. Myers and J. Suen. New York, Churchill Livingstone, 1989, p. 953.
5. Hannon, L. M.: Cancer of the oral cavity. Semin. Oncol. Nurs., 5:150, 1989.
6. Wilson, D.: Make mouth care a must for your patients. RN, 49:39, 1986.
7. Wheaver, A.: Personal communication, 1988.
8. James, J. H., and Watson, C.: The use of Opsite, a vapor permeable dressing, on skin graft donor sites. Br. J. Plast. Surg., 28:107, 1975.
9. Reid, W.: Free grafts-kin and other tissues. Nurs. Times, 73:1627, 1977.
10. Jones, N. F.: Postoperative monitoring of microsurgical free tissue transfers for head and neck reconstruction. Microsurgery, 9:159, 1988.
11. Urken, M. L., et al.: Free flap design in head and neck reconstruction to achieve an external segment for monitoring. Head Neck Surg., 115:1447, 1989.
12. Gall, A. M., Sessions, D. G., and Ogura, J. H.: Complications following surgery for cancer of the larynx and hypopharynx. Cancer, 39:624, 1977.
13. Johnson, J. T., and Cummings, C. W.: Hematoma after head and neck surgery—a major complication? Otolaryngology, 86:171, 1978.
14. Johnson, J. T., and Myers, E. N.: Management of complication of therapeutic intervention. In Cancer of the Head and Neck, 2nd Ed. Edited by E. Myers and J. Suen. New York, Churchill Livingstone, 1989.
15. Tabet, J. C., and Johnson, J. T.: Wound infection in head and neck surgery: prophylaxis, etiology, and management. J. Otolaryngol., 19:197, 1990.
16. Conley, J. J.: Oropharyngocutaneous fistula. In Complications of Head and Neck surgery. Philadelphia, W. B. Saunders, 1979, p. 92.
17. Conley, J. J.: Operative complications. In Complications of Head and Neck surgery. Philadelphia, W. B. Saunders, 1979, p. 30.
18. Crumley, R. L., and Smith, J. D.: Postoperative chylous fistula prevention and management. Laryngoscope, 86:804, 1976.

19. Spiro, J. D., Spiro, R. H., and Strong, E. W.: The management of chyle fistula. Laryngoscope, *100:*771, 1990.
20. Ketcham, A. S., and Hoye, R. C.: Spontaneous carotid artery hemorrhage after head and neck surgery. Surgery, *110:*649, 1965.
21. Hillerman, B. L., and Kennedy, T. L.: Carotid rupture and tissue coverage. Laryngoscope, *92:*985, 1982.
22. Costantino, P. D., Atiyah, B. A., Mico, A. S., and Sisson, G. A.: The prevention of carotid artery rupture with isobutyl-2 cyanoacrylate. Laryngoscope, *98:*377, 1988.
23. Porto, D. P., Adams, G. L., and Foster, C.: Emergency management of carotid artery rupture. Am. J. Otolaryngol., *7:*213, 1986.
24. Goodwin, W. J., and Torres, J.: The value of prognostic nutritional index in the management of patients with advanced carcinoma of the head and neck. Head Neck Surg, *6:*932, 1984.
25. Bassett, M. R., and Dobie, R. A.: Patterns of nutritional deficiency in head and neck cancer. Otolaryngol. Head Neck Surg., *91:*119, 1982.
26. Hooley, R., et al: Predicting head and neck complications using nutritional assessment: the prognostic nutritional index. Arch. Otolaryngol., *109:*83, 1983.
27. Buzby, G. P., et al: Prognostic nutritional index in gastrointestinal surgery. Am. J. Surg., *139:*160, 1980.
28. Brookes, G. B.: Nutritional status: a prognostic indicator in head and neck cancer. Otolaryngol. Head Neck Surg., *93:* 69, 1985.
29. Stefee, W. P., and Krey, S. H.: Enteral hyperalimentation for patients with head and neck cancer. Otolaryngol. Clin. North Am., *13:*437, 1980.
30. Thompson, J. S., et al: The effect of the route of nutrient delivery on gut structure and diamine oxide levels. JPEN J. Parenter. Enteral Nutr., *11:*28, 1987.
31. Petrosino, B. M., Meravigilia, M., and Becker, H.: Mechanical problems with small diameter enteral feeding tubes. J. Neurosci. Nurs., *19:*276, 1987.
32. Asbeck, C., Imbrosciano, S., Matarese, L. E., and Tyus, F.: Tube Feeding Instruction for Home. Cleveland, Cleveland Clinic Foundation, 1988.
33. Williams, E. F., and Meguid, M. M.: Nutritional concepts and considerations in head and neck surgery. Head Neck Surg, *11:*393, 1989.
34. Sofferman, R. A., Haisch, C. E., Kinchrer, J. A., and Hardin, N. J.: The nasogastric tube syndrome. Laryngoscope, *100:* 962, 1990.
35. Gauderer, M. W. L., Ponsky, J. L., and Izant, R. J.: Gastrostomy without laparotomy: a percutaneous endoscopic technique. J. Pediatr. Surg., *15:*872, 1980.
36. O'Dwyer, T. P., Gullane, P. J., Awerbuch, D., and Chia-Sing, J.: Percutaneous feeding gastrostomy in patients with head and neck tumors: a five-year review. Laryngoscope, *100:*29, 1990.
37. Dudrick, S. J., O'Donnell, J. J., and Weinman-Winkler, S.: Nutritional management of head and neck tumor patients. *In* Comprehensive Management of Head & Neck Tumors. Vol. I. Philadelphia, W. B. Saunders, 1987, p. 14.
38. Johnson, J. T., and Wagner, R. L.: Infection following uncontaminated head and neck surgery. Arch. Otolaryngol. Head Neck Surg., *113:*368, 1987.
39. Schwartz, S. S., and Yuska, C. M.: Common patient issues following surgery for head and neck cancer. Semin. Oncol. Nurs., *5:*191, 1989.
40. Litton, W. B., and Leonard, J. R.: Aspiration after partial laryngectomy: cinefluorographic studies. Laryngoscope, *79:*887, 1969.
41. Logemann, J. A.: Aspiration in head and neck surgical patients. Ann. Otol. Rhinol. Laryngol., *94:*373, 1985.
42. Logemann, J. A.: Speech and swallowing rehabilitation for head and neck tumor patients. *In* Cancer of the Head and Neck. Edited by E. Myers and J. Suen. New York, Churchill Livingstone, 1989, p. 1021.
43. Norris, K. L., Goepfert, H., and Wendt, C. D.: Supraglottic laryngectomy for intermediate-stage cancer: U.T.M.D. Anderson Cancer Center experience with combined therapy. Laryngoscope, *100:*831, 1990.
44. McConnel, F. M.: Analysis of pressure generation and bolus transit during pharyngeal swallowing. Laryngoscope, *98:*71, 1988.
45. Logemann, J. A.: Swallowing and communication rehabilitation. Semin. Oncol. Nurs., *5:*205, 1989.
46. Lavertu, P., and Tucker, H. M.: Neurologic disorders of the larynx. *In* Diseases of the Nose, Throat, Ear, Head and Neck. 14th Ed. Edited by J. J. Ballenger. Philadelphia, Lea & Febiger, 1993.
47. Posner, M. R., et al: Incidence of hypothyroidism following multimodality treatment for advanced squamous cell cancer of the head and neck. Laryngoscope, *94:*451, 1984.
48. Liening, D. A., Duncan, N. O., Blakeslee, D. B., and Smith, D. B.: Hypothyroidism following radiotherapy for head and neck cancer. Otolaryngol. Head Neck Surg., *103:*10, 1990.

SUPPLEMENTAL READINGS

Bailey, C. E., Lucas, C. E., Ledgerwood, A. M., Jacobs, J. R.: A comparison of gastrostomy techniques in patients with advanced head and neck cancer. Arch. Otolaryngol. Head Neck Surg., *118:*124, 1992.

Complications in Head and Neck Surgery, Edited by David W. Eisele, St. Louis, C. V. Mosby, 1993.

Gibson, S. E., Wenig, B. L., and Watkins, J. L.: Complications of percutaneous endoscopic gastrostomy in head and neck cancer patients. Ann. Otol. Rhinol. Laryngol., *101:*46, 1992.

Grandis, J. R., et al.: Postoperative wound infection: a poor prognostic sign for patients with head and neck cancer. Cancer, *70:*2166, 1992.

Johnson, J. T., et al.: Prophylactic antibiotics for head and neck surgery with flap reconstruction. Arch. Otolaryngol. Head Neck Surg., *118:*488, 1992.

Complications in Head and Neck Surgery, Edited by Y. P. Krespi and R. H. Ossoff, Philadelphia, W. B. Saunders, 1993.

Pelczar, B. T., et al.: Identifying high-risk patients before head and neck oncologic surgery. Arch. Otolaryngol. Head Neck Surg., *119:*861, 1993.

Rao, M. K., Reilley, T. E., Schuller, D. E., and Young, D. C.: Analysis of risk factors for postoperative pulmonary complications in head and neck surgery. Laryngoscope, *102:*45, 1992.

Weber, R. S., and Callender, D. L.: Antibiotic prophylaxis in clean-contaminated head and neck oncologic surgery. Ann. Otol. Rhinol. Laryngol., *101:*16, 1992.

Weber, R. S., et al.: Ampicillin-sulbactam vs clindamycin in head and neck oncologic surgery: the need for gram-negative coverage. Arch. Otolaryngol. Head Neck Surg., *118:*1159, 1992.

Chapter 14

BRONCHOSPASTIC DISEASE

DAN J. HENDRICKSON
RICHARD J. MARTIN

Bronchospasm and wheezing can be a component of a variety of disease processes including asthma, chronic obstructive pulmonary disease, pulmonary thromboembolism, and aspiration. This chapter discusses the evaluation and management of patients with reversible obstructive airway disease (i.e., asthma) who have an acute, severe exacerbation.

The prevalence of asthma varies widely in different populations of the world, but has been estimated to affect approximately 3% of the United States population and lead to approximately 459,000 hospitalizations annually.[1] Asthma is undoubtedly a common medical problem necessitating evaluation in the office or emergency room. Although deaths from asthma occur infrequently, they merit our attention and evaluation since many of these deaths may be preventable, and most disturbing is the probable recent rise in asthma mortality. Asthma mortality rates have risen throughout the world and also in the United States since 1977.[2-4] In 1985, 4800 deaths from asthma occurred in the United States, 1.1 deaths from asthma per 100,000 population.[5] This contrasts with the 2400 deaths recorded in 1977, 0.6 deaths from asthma per 100,000 population (Fig. 14-1).

This near doubling of the United States asthma mortality rates over the past decade has occurred despite a wider availability of diagnostic testing, increasing data base on the pathophysiology of the disease, wider availability and spectrum of pharmaceutical agents, more aggressive use of corticosteroids, and other interventions. The cause(s) of the rise in death rates is probably multifactorial, and numerous factors have been offered in explanation.[5-7] Regardless, the challenge to the practicing physician is to identify the asthmatic patient at greatest risk for morbidity and mortality so that appropriate therapy can be promptly delivered.

PRE-ICU PHASE: ASSESSING RISK IN THE BRONCHOSPASTIC PATIENT

History and Physical Examination

The utility of the history and physical examination in assessing the severity of a bronchospastic attack has a long history but its efficacy has come under recent scrutiny. Clearly, patients who can provide only truncated histories secondary to extreme dyspnea are potentially high risk patients. Additionally, the patient's judgment of the severity of his or her symptoms can be an important factor in assessing the risk of an acute exacerbation. Patients may be more able to predict their degree of airflow obstruction than experienced physicians who base their assessment on the physical examination alone.[8] Hence, it is important to listen carefully to the patient's history of symptoms, because this can identify a serious exacerbation of bronchospastic disease. Many patients will also underestimate, however, the severity of their airflow obstruction based on their perceptions alone. This situation has been documented both clinically and experimentally. Hospitalized patients recovering from a severe bronchospastic attack were asymptomatic yet had a mean forced expiratory volume in 1.0 second (FEV_1) of methacholine inhalation studies.[10,11] Hence, symptoms may enable one to identify a severe bronchospastic attack, but they may not accurately reflect the severity of the underlying pathophysiologic process (Fig. 14-2).

Common precipitating factors include medical noncompliance, viral respiratory infections, and exposures to nonspecific bronchial irritants or specific allergens.

The length of symptoms may also help identify the high risk patient. In one detailed and well-planned evaluation of deaths in patients with asthma, most patients had several days of progressive symptoms, and only 11% of the deaths were secondary to a sudden, precipitous onset of symptoms and a rapid downhill course.[12] These unusual patients are probably the victims of anaphylactic reactions from a drug (e.g., aspirin-like drugs). In contrast, the majority of deaths from asthma appear to be associated with a prolonged attack of bronchospasm which has been inadequately assessed and treated.[2,12-14]

The past medical history also helps identify patients at greatest risk from their exacerbations. Retrospective analysis of asthma mortality data has identified the following historical factors as markers of a high risk patient (Table 14-1).[14-17]

- Patient's age: Asthma deaths are rare in the very young and are bimodal in distribution, with peaks in the adolescent/young adult population and the middle aged and elderly populations. In the United States, the most dramatic increase in asthma mortality has occurred in the over 85-year-old population, almost tripling from 1968-1984.[3]
- Race: Nonwhites appear to be at higher risk because the asthma mortality rates for blacks has risen more rapidly than for whites in the United States.[3] It is im-

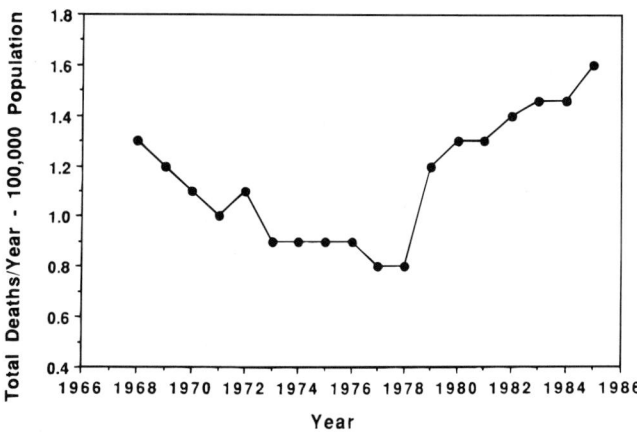

Fig. 14–1. Rising asthma mortality rates in the United States from 1968 to 1984. (From Robin, E. D.: Death from bronchial asthma. Chest, 93:614, 1988.)

Table 14–1. Historical and Physical Examination Findings Characteristic of High Risk Patients*

1. The elderly and young adult populations.
2. Patients who are unwilling or unable to assume responsibility for their care (e.g., rebellious adolescent or psychotic patients).
3. A prior history of severe bronchospastic attacks requiring hospitalization and especially intubation and mechanical ventilation.
4. A gradual, progressive increase in symptomatology despite adequate medication and especially corticosteroids.
5. The patient's judgment that the attack is severe.
6. Sinus tachycardia > 120 beats per minute.
7. Respiratory rates > 30 breaths per minute.
8. Presence of diaphoresis, accessory muscle use, and/or pulsus paradoxus > 15 mm Hg.
9. Underlying major medical disease(s).

* Note that no index correlating numerous variables with risk for admission has proved successful when studied prospectively. These are guidelines and do not substitute for clinical judgment.

possible to discriminate socioeconomic factors versus genetic predisposition as the cause of this increased risk.

- Psychosocial factors: Many young patients who have died of asthma apparently had a behavioral history of rejecting parental and medical supervision, often minimized their symptoms, and were unwilling or unable to accept responsibility for the management of the disease. Older patients who have died of asthma may have had a similar behavioral profile, perhaps complicated by psychiatric disease, alcoholism, or dementia, but most appear to have been at risk secondary to the chronicity, severity, and inadequate management of their disease.
- Prior history of severe attacks: Patients who have a history of prior severe bronchospastic attacks are at higher risk for asthma mortality. Those patients who have been hospitalized for asthma in the past 12 months or required 2 or more outpatient consultations within the last 12 months are at highest risk.
- Prior therapy: Symptoms no longer controlled by previously effective therapy are a marker for increased mortality risk. This is especially true if the patient is having persistent or increased symptoms while taking corticosteroids.

Physical signs associated with acute bronchospasm include tachycardia, tachypnea, diaphoresis, use of accessory respiratory muscles, pulsus paradoxus, wheezing, and hyperinflation. Note that the subjective assessment of the degree of wheezing is an unreliable index of the severity of the underlying airflow obstruction.[18] The average pulse rate of an emergency room (ER) patient with acute bronchospasm is approximately 100 bpm, and the respiratory rate is generally between 25 and 28 breaths per minute.[19] Heart rates greater than 120 bpm and respiratory rates greater than 30 occur in 20 to 25% of these patients. Diaphoresis, accessory muscle use, and pulsus paradoxus are thought to be the physical findings most closely associated with severe bronchospasm, and the latter two findings are present in 30 to 40% of ER patients prior to treatment.[9,19,20] Pulsus paradoxus values greater than 15 mm Hg are found in less than 20% of these patients, which this is generally associated with an FEV_1 of less than 1.0L (< approximately 25% of predicted).[18,21-23]

Although these physical findings may help one to identify the high risk patient, they are not universal. The absence of these findings does not necessarily indicate less severe bronchospasm and airflow obstruction. To be manifest, a pulsus paradoxus requires large negative intrathoracic pressure swings. If the patient is breathing with high frequency and low tidal volumes, these findings may not be present. Patients with an FEV_1 of less than 0.7 L (<20% predicted) who did not manifest a pulsus paradoxus have been reported.[18]

Hence, both the patient and the physician may underestimate the severity of airflow limitation from acute bron-

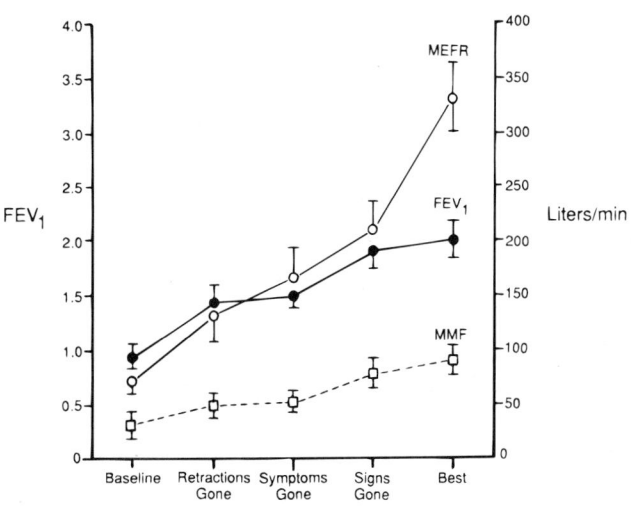

Fig. 14–2. Low correlation between clinical symptoms and flow rates. (From McFadden, E. R., Kiser, R., and DeGroot, W.: Acute bronchial asthma: relations between clinical and physiological manifestations. N. Engl. J. Med., 288:221, 1973.)

chospasm based on historical factors alone. Additionally, the physical examination may fail to identify the high risk bronchospastic patient and is probably not helpful in discriminating the patient who needs admission to the ward versus the ICU (see Table 14-1).

Pulmonary Function and Blood Gases

Because the history and physical examination can be misleading, objective data must be obtained in the assessment process of the patient with acute bronchospasm. The pathophysiology is that of airflow obstruction with resultant gas exchange abnormalities and it is appropriate to quantify this process. The pulmonary function derangements of the usual ER patient have been well documented. The ER patient usually manifests hyperinflation with the residual volume averaging 400% of predicted and the functional residual capacity approximately doubles the predicted value.[9] Lung volume data is rarely obtained, however, secondary to the technical difficulties of performing the diagnostic measurements in the acutely bronchospastic patients. Despite considerable individual variability in the measurement of airflow, the forced expiratory time is prolonged, and the forced vital capacity (FVC) and the FEV_1 are reduced. Generally, the FVC is 50% and the FEV_1 is 30 to 35% of the predicted value in the acutely bronchospastic patient.[9,18,24] The peak expiratory flow rate (PEFR) is often reduced to 135 to 200 L per minute (normal 350 to 550 L per minute).[21,22,25] A small proportion of asthmatic patients will be falsely judged as not significantly improving with bronchodilator therapy if airflow alone is measured. These patients have a decrease in hyperexpansion with no discernible increase in airflow which is, however, a physiologic and clinical improvement. That is, a significant decrement in the abnormally high lung volumes (TLC, FRC, and RV) occurs.

The FEV_1 and the PEFR are the most commonly used airflow measurements in the acute bronchospastic attack and there is considerable data on their use. The absolute FEV_1 value, the percentage of predicted FEV_1, and the improvement following therapy have all been used to discriminate patients who require admission and those who can be successfully managed on an outpatient basis (Table 14-2). A FEV_1 value of less than 1.6 to 2.0 L, a FEV_1 of less than 50 to 60% of predicted, and improvements of less than 400 ml in the FEV_1 following initial therapy have all been promoted as identifying the patients who will require admission to the hospital.[18,26-29] Initial PEFR of less than 20% predicted (approximately 100 L per minute), failure of the PEFR to improve greater than 20% after a single, initial injection of a beta-2-adrenergic agonist, and post-treatment values of less than 60% of the predicted PEFR value (approximately 300 L per minute) have also been used to discriminate the patient requiring hospitalization.[29-31]

Hence, measurement of airflow in acute bronchospasm can help reliably discriminate the mild attack from the more severe physiologic derangements and predict the need for hospitalization. Airflow measurement can also help predict the need for an arterial blood gas (ABG) measurement as there is a rough correlation between airflow obstruction and ABG findings. Most ER patients (70 to 75%) manifest a combination of mild hypoxemia, hypocapnia, and respiratory alkalosis.[28,32,33] The exact values depend on the local elevation and resultant alveolar/arterial oxygen gradient. Most of these patients have mild to moderate bronchospastic attacks. In such cases, the oxyhemoglobin saturation as measured by pulse oximetry is normal or nearly normal.

Most patients with acute bronchospasm with significant hypoxia have marked airflow limitation. At sea level, most patients with PaO_2 less than 60 mm Hg also have an FEV_1 of less than 0.7 to 1.0 L or 25% of predicted.[28,29,32] The relationship between airflow and the $PaCO_2$ is more reliable. Carbon dioxide retention ($PaCO_2 > 42$ mm Hg at sea level) does not occur until the FEV_1 or PEFR drops below 25% of the predicted value.[25,31,32,34] It has been suggested that bronchospastic patients should have an initial airflow measurement, and if the airflow is greater than 25% of predicted (e.g., a $FEV_1 > 1.01$ L or PEFR > 200 L per minute) an ABG can be safely deferred.[25,31] These criteria have not been prospectively tested, however.[35] If there is any question regarding oxygenation and especially ventilation, or if the initial airflow determination places the patient in the severe bronchospastic attack group, an ABG should be obtained.

Hypercapnic patients are clearly at higher risk for requiring intubation and mechanical ventilation. In one large series, approximately 27% of bronchospastic episodes in asthma patients were associated with hypercapnia, but only approximately 8% of hypercapnic episodes required intubation. No patient who presented with a $PaCO_2$ less than 38 mm Hg required intubation.[36] In adults, metabolic acidosis is rare but is associated with severe airflow obstruction and a high risk intubation and mechanical ventilation.[37]

Other Laboratory Tests

The value of other, more routine laboratory evaluations is much less defined. A chest radiograph is commonly obtained in bronchospastic patients who present to the ER although there is little objective data on the utility or indications for this diagnostic evaluation. One study found no significant correlation between the chest film interpreta-

Table 14-2. Suggested Admission Criteria*

1. FEV_1 50–60% of predicted.
   PEFR < 16–20% of predicted.
2. Failure to increase $FEV_1 > 400$ ml despite ER therapy.
   Failure to increase PEFR > 16% despite ER therapy.
   Post-treatment PEFR < 60% of predicted.
3. Moderate or severe hypoxemia (i.e., $PaO_2 < 55$ mm Hg at sea level).
4. Respiratory acidosis and/or carbon dioxide retention ($PaCO_2 > 42$ mm Hg at sea level).
5. Metabolic acidosis.
6. Clinical pneumonia or underlying major medical disease.
7. Presence of barotrauma.
8. Right axis deviation or P pulmonale on electrocardiography.
9. Moderate to severe hypokalemia and theophylline toxicity.

* See also Tables 14-1 and 14-3. These are guidelines only and do not substitute for clinical judgment.

tion and the need for hospitalization.[38] Another study found a small incidence of unsuspected pneumothorax and pneumomediastinum, however, in patients requiring hospital admission.[34] It is probably reasonable to obtain chest radiographs on patients who require admission to the hospital (especially those with a severe episode of bronchospasm) and those with clinical signs and symptoms consistent with a bacterial infection (e.g., fever).

Electrocardiographic abnormalities in patients requiring admission to the hospital are not uncommon. Sinus tachycardia is the most common, but right axis deviation, clockwise rotation, right bundle branch block, P pulmonale, right ventricular hypertrophy (dominant R in V1, dominant S in V5), ventricular ectopic beats, and ST-T wave abnormalities have all been described.[34,39,40] These findings are generally transient and resolve as therapy reverses the airflow obstruction and hypoxia. A rightward axis or P pulmonale may identify a high risk bronchospastic patient as these electrocardiographic findings have correlated with pulsus paradoxus and respiratory acidosis.[40]

These studies have documented that sinus tachycardia is common but appears to be secondary to the disease process rather than the drug therapy. Several studies have shown that as the airflow obstruction is reversed, the tachycardia partially resolves despite the use of beta agonists. Hence marked, persistent sinus tachycardia may indicate a patient at high risk who will require close observation.

The routine laboratory evaluation of the bronchospastic patient is generally of marginal benefit in assessing the severity of the bronchospastic attack. Some of these tests become important, however, in certain populations with complications of the disease and/or the therapy. The white blood cell count is often elevated from the sympathomimetic and/or corticosteroid therapy and will not assist in identifying the patient with a concomitant infection unless a left shift is present. A Gram stain and culture of the sputum in these patients may then be indicated. The serum potassium is often an important laboratory value, especially in the elderly population with their higher prevalence of diuretic drug use, coronary artery disease, and subsequent hypoxia, possible theophylline toxicity, and beta agonist use (which can lead to hypokalemia) can further aggravate a predisposition towards ventricular ectopy, and diligent monitoring of the serum potassium and can then be of major importance. Additionally, the serum theophylline concentration should be measured to aid decisions in regards to the use or discontinuation of this therapy (see later in this chapter).

Special Patient Populations (Table 14–3)

Two populations have been largely ignored in clinical research for which the foregoing criteria may not apply: the pregnant and elderly bronchospastic populations. Asthma during pregnancy is not uncommon and has been reported to have a prevalence of 0.4 to 1.3% in pregnant women, and the effects of pregnancy on bronchospastic disease are variable.[42] Approximately one fourth of asthmatic women have worsening symptoms during pregnancy.[43] Studies predating current standards of corticoste-

Table 14–3. Special Patient Populations with Additional Risk Factors*

PREGNANCY
1. Maternal Pa_{O_2} < 60 mm Hg.
2. Maternal Pa_{CO_2} > 38 mm Hg or pH < 7.35.

ELDERLY
1. Underlying major medical illnesses, especially cardiopulmonary.
2. New onset asthma in this age group, this may be a diagnostic error.
3. Patients with marked dyspnea and a high work of breathing in this age group are at increased risk of ventilatory failure secondary to the lower ventilatory reserve as a function of normal senescence.

* See also Tables 14–1 and 14–2.

roid use suggested increased perinatal and maternal mortality in pregnancies in asthmatic patients, but more recent studies have shown an elimination of maternal mortality with the use of corticosteroids.[44,45] This data suggest that if asthma is well controlled during pregnancy, adverse consequences are minimized.

Regardless, some of these patients will have severe exacerbations requiring admission to the hospital and perhaps the ICU. Several factors are important in assessing the pregnant patient which may alter the criteria for admission and subsequent management. The issues are complex as the physician is simultaneously caring for two patients—the woman and the fetus.

During a normal pregnancy, the tidal volume increases with a subsequent increase in the minute ventilation. This situation results in a compensated respiratory alkalosis with pH ranging from 7.40 to 7.47 and the partial pressure of arterial carbon dioxide ranging from 25 to 32 mm Hg, conditions which optimize fetal respiratory exchange.[42,46] Hence, a Pa_{CO_2} in the normal range may represent impending ventilatory failure in the pregnant asthmatic during an acute exacerbation. It has been suggested that pregnant patients with an arterial pH below 7.35 and/or Pa_{CO_2} above 38 mm Hg should be placed in an ICU.[47] This recommendation stems from the fact that acidosis can impair respiratory exchange to the fetus. Evaluation of oxygenation in the pregnant asthmatic is also altered. Although a Pa_{O_2} slightly below 60 torr at sea level may be well tolerated by the nonpregnant asthmatic, fetal jeopardy is possible secondary to hypoxia with maternal Pa_{O_2} values below 60 mm Hg.[42,43,46,47] Hence, it is clear that ABG analysis assumes a greater importance in the evaluation of the pregnant asthmatic during an acute exacerbation and that the threshold for admission to the hospital and the ICU is lower than in nonpregnant asthmatics.

The elderly population is challenging to assess and treat. This population group has incurred dramatic increases in asthma mortality rates, yet there is a paucity of data directed specifically at bronchospastic disease in the elderly. This is typical of most of the diseases in the above-65 age group who are difficult to study because most will have complicating secondary diagnoses.

Asthma in the elderly is not uncommon; a single epidemiologic study found a prevalence rate of 6.5% in the above-70 population.[48] Important findings were that men were more commonly affected than women with worse underlying pulmonary function, most did not have childhood asthma, nocturnal dyspnea was a common symptom, and it was often difficult to separate patients with chronic bronchitis. Most of these elderly patients, however, continue to have the usual symptoms of cough, wheezing, and dyspnea. Many patients had an underlying fixed airflow limitation with a large reversible component. An important distinguishing characteristic of the elderly asthmatic is that it is uncommon for the disease to present in this population. It has been estimated that only 1% of patients with asthma have the onset of their disease after age 70.[49] Hence, it is critical to entertain the entire differential diagnosis in the wheezing elderly population who often have concomitant disease and risks, especially those with no prior history of bronchospastic disease. The differential diagnosis includes asthma, chronic obstructive pulmonary disease (COPD), upper airway obstruction secondary to laryngospasm or tumor, endobronchial obstruction secondary to foreign body or tumor, acute left ventricular failure, pulmonary thromboembolism, and aspiration which may be chronic, perhaps from upper airway dysfunction.

Perhaps even more caution than usual must be used in the physical examination when assessing the elderly bronchospastic patient.[50] For a given degree of abnormality in the ABG or airflow, the elderly patient may be less tachycardiac and less likely to manifest a pulsus paradoxus. It is more difficult to interpret laboratory results in this population, and both the Pa_{O_2} and airflow (FEV_1) decrease with age. Predicted values have often been extrapolated from younger populations.

Hence, assessing the elderly patient with acute bronchospasm is perhaps more difficult than in younger patients. The clinician should probably have a lower admission threshold in this age group and also a lower threshold for ICU if the patient is deemed a unit candidate. The elderly have a lower physiologic reserve as a function of age, they often have serious underlying medical problems which can be exacerbated by the increased work of breathing and hypoxia that accompanies an acute, severe bronchospastic attack. An elderly patient with only mild bronchospasm may require ICU admission secondary to active coronary ischemia, worsening congestive heart failure, need for continued chronic renal dialysis, or some other severe, underlying medical condition(s). The elderly are also more likely to have complicated medical regimens and are prone to iatrogenic side effects (e.g., hypokalemia as discussed earlier), and may have less social support and transportation access (Table 14-3).

Paradoxic vocal cord motion or vocal cord dysfunction may mimic asthma with potentially harmful results.[51,52] The entity may be more common in females. Some patients have acute upper airway obstruction and have been treated with intubation or tracheostomy. Other patients have a history of intermittent dyspnea and wheezing that generally has failed to respond to standard asthma therapy. When severe, the analysis is generally unremarkable for respiratory failure or hypoxia, but the flow-volume curve may be remarkable for a variable truncation of the inspiratory loop of the flow-volume tracing and perhaps also the expiratory loop. Direct laryngoscopy reveals pyridoxic inspiratory adduction of the true vocal cords. Several maneuvers such as deep inspiration (inspiratory adduction near total lung capacity is normal), panting, phonation, or exercise may be required to demonstrate vocal cord dysfunction. Patients have responded to speech therapy. A point of differential diagnosis is that auscultation of the lungs reveals clear breath sounds while auscultation of the upper airway may reveal inspiratory and expiratory wheezing. Patients appear to be apprehensive and may have audible wheezing noted in the upper airway even without listening with a stethoscope.

In summary, the assessment of the acutely bronchospastic patient begins with the history and physical which unfortunately can be misleading. However, several historical factors delineate patients at higher risk for a given bronchospastic attack. Patients with a history of prior severe bronchospastic attacks requiring hospitalization and especially intubation and patients with recurring or worsening symptoms despite use of corticosteroids demarcate higher risk groups. Additionally, asthmatics who are pregnant or elderly require special consideration as noted earlier. Physical signs that generally signal a severe bronchospastic attack include marked tachycardia above 120 bpm, tachypnea greater than 30 breaths per minute, and pulsus paradoxicus greater than 15 mm Hg. Providing the patient can cooperate with diagnostic testing, airflow rates delineate the subgroup at greatest risk for ventilatory insufficiency and probably hypoxia (FEV_1 or PEFR < 25% of predicted). Electrocardiographic abnormalities may also delineate patients with marked airflow obstruction and increased risk. Most of these criteria have been discerned in the hopes of discriminating those patients who require admission to the hospital and those patients who can be treated and released from the ER. Other than the unusual patient who requires immediate intubation and mechanical ventilation (e.g., severe respiratory acidosis and mental status changes), the determination of which patients should be admitted to the ICU remains an empiric process. There is no prospective data which delineates criteria for intensive care and especially intubation and mechanical ventilation.

Ultimately, one of the key factors in this assessment process is the patient's response to therapy. For example, patients who are otherwise healthy and present with severe airflow limitation and mild to moderate respiratory acidosis (e.g., pH 7.30 to 7.35 and Pa_{CO_2} < 48 torr) but have significant airflow improvement with initial therapy can readily be managed in either the observation unit or on the ward. Patients with moderate airflow limitation who continue to worsen despite several hours of medical therapy may require intensive care therapy, however, as they may soon require intubation if their downhill course continues. Additionally, patients with significant medical codiagnoses such as angina, chronic congestive heart failure, pregnancy, or other problems may merit an ICU admission simply because of the requirements for more frequent attention by the medical staff and closer monitoring and observation.

Hence, each of these decisions must then be approached on an individualized basis reflecting the resources of the institution, the patient's response to therapy, other underlying medical conditions, subjective assessment on whether the patient can sustain the considerable work of breathing until airflow improves from therapy as well as other considerations. It is important to know your institution's ability to monitor these patients, the frequency at which nebulization therapy can be given on the ward by the nursing and respiratory therapy staff, and other therapeutic details. For example, patients who are responding to therapy may warrant several more hours of more frequent therapy in the observation unit of the ER and then admission to the ward rather than admission to the ICU. This procedure may avoid more expensive delivery of care and yet effectively treat the patient's bronchospastic attack.

Several other circumstances worth discussion include the physician's familiarity with the patient and the presence of barotrauma. Patients who are seen for the first time with bronchospasm may be more difficult to assess than patients who are well known to the physician and have a history of multiple attacks which generally respond readily to intensive medical therapy. Additionally, the older the age of presentation with new onset of bronchospasm, the physician should be suspicious of other items in the differential diagnosis as noted previously. Patients with barotrauma on admission are at risk for a precipitous decline and perhaps mortality secondary to tension pneumothorax. If physical examination or radiography demonstrates subcutaneous emphysema, pneumomediastinum, or a small pneumothorax, the patient is at risk for progression and ventilatory embarrassment if he or she continues to have marked bronchospasm. It is appropriate to hospitalize all patients with barotrauma and consider intensive care for patients with a small pneumothorax who are in the midst of a bronchospastic attack as large intrathoracic pressure swings could worsen this situation. If a tube thoracostomy is necessary, caution and close supervision will be required in the use of analgesia in the nonintubated acutely bronchospastic patient.

ICU Phase

Therapy of the bronchospastic attack will have been initiated prior to the patient's arrival to the ICU. Generally, the ICU care will be a continuation of medical therapy unless the patient has complications and/or such severe bronchospasm and airflow limitation that intubation and mechanical ventilation are required. A review of respiratory pharmacology is then germane. The physician has a variety of agents available including beta-2 adrenergic agonists, anticholinergics, methylxanthine derivatives, corticosteroids, and supplemental oxygen.[14,53]

Drug Therapy

Beta agonists are commonly the first line of therapy in the acute situation. This includes subcutaneous epinephrine or terbutaline although tachyphylaxis may limit the use of these agents to the initial hours of therapy. Terbutaline given subcutaneously should be given in high enough doses for a full pharmacologic effect (Table 14-4). Some of these agents should be avoided or used with extreme caution in patients with known coronary artery disease and probably those patients with multiple coronary artery disease risk factors (e.g., an elderly diabetic, hypertensive, smoking male patient).

Table 14-4. Drug Therapy in Acutely Bronchospastic Patients

INJECTABLE BETA AGONISTS

Epinephrine HCL (1:1,000)	0.3-0.5 ml sq q 20 min., repeat 2-4 times
Terbutaline sulfate	0.3-0.5 mg sq q 30 min., repeat 1-2 times

INHALED BETA AGONISTS

Isoetharine	(a) 1% solution for nebulization: 0.5 ml in 3.0 ml NS
	(b) MDI (isoetharine mesylate): 0.34 mg/puff
Terbutaline sulfate	(a) nebulization solution not available
	(b) MDI: 0.20 mg/puff
Metaproterenol sulfate	(a) 5% solution for nebulization: 0.3 ml in 3.0 ml NS
	(b) MDI: 0.65 mg/puff
Albuterol sulfate	(a) 0.083% solution for nebulization, no dilution required
	(b) 0.5% solution for nebulization, 0.5 ml in 3.0 ml NS
	(c) MDI: 90 μg/puff
Pirbuterol acetate	(a) nebulization solution not available
	(b) 0.2 mg/puff

ANTICHOLINERGICS

Atropine sulfate for nebulization: 0.5-1.0 mg in 2-3.0 ml NS
Ipatroprium Br MDI: 18 μg/puff

ISOPROTERENOL INFUSION

Isoproterenol HCl	(a) bolus: 0.2 mg diluted in 10 ml NS, 0.01-0.02 mg (0.5-1.0 ml of the solution)
	(b) infusion: 2 mg in 500 ml D5W (4 μg/ml); titrate up to 5 μg/min (75 ml/h)

METHYLXANTHINES

Aminophylline	(a) load: 6-9 mg/kg of ideal body weight, reduce dose or await serum drug level if prior use
	(b) infusion: 0.4-1.0 mg/kg/hour
Theophylline	(a) load: 5-7.5 mg/kg ideal body weight, reduce dose if necessary
	(b) infusion: 0.4-0.8 mg/kg/hour

The number of inhaled beta agonists has recently increased in the United States. A partial list includes epinephrine, isoproterenol, isoetharine, metaproterenol, terbutaline, albuterol, and pirbuterol (Table 14-4). Some of these agents are not available in both a metered dose inhaler (MDI) delivery system or solution for nebulization. There is no data establishing the superiority of any one of the agents in the ICU population, and the literature is conflicting on ranking beta-2 selectivity after the least beta-selective drugs, epinephrine and isoproterenol.[54] Beta-2 selectivity can be important in patients with other underlying major medical illnesses (e.g., angina), but beta-2 selectivity of these drugs is often lost when used in frequent high doses commonly employed in therapy of the acute bronchospastic attack. Most physicians start treatment with a more beta-2-selective agent such as metaproterenol or albuterol.

Beta adrenoreceptors are distributed primarily in the peripheral airway smooth muscle.[55] Direct human airway innervation has been disputed and the primary stimulation probably is secondary to circulating and locally released catecholamines.[56] The beta adrenoreceptor is coupled to the guanine nucleotide regulatory protein and thus adenylate cyclase. Increases in cyclic adenosine monophosphate and cytoplasmic calcium will produce smooth muscle relaxation. Beta receptor expression also increases in vivo following cortisol stimulation.[57]

The mechanism of delivery (i.e., MDI versus nebulization) and dosing frequency should be individualized based on an assessment of the patient's severity of airflow limitation, gas exchange abnormalities, background of other medical diseases, and the patient's ability to cooperate. Finally, the dosing frequency may be limited by drug side effects (e.g., tremor). Although the drugs can all cause tachycardia, this is generally secondary to the disease process rather than the treatment (as noted generally secondary to the disease process rather than the treatment (as noted earlier). Hence, if tachycardia persists or worsens markedly, it is probably best to reassess the patient's status including gas exchange while continuing the drug therapy. Many physicians treat the severely bronchospastic patient with nebulized drug rather than using a MDI with or without an auxiliary device. The advantages of nebulization include continuous drug delivery during inspiration (inspiratory airflow is often limited during an acute attack) and that some patients have poor hand-breath coordination with the MDI system, particularly when acutely ill. Compressed air or oxygen nebulizer systems deliver aerosol particles of similar size and deposit an equivalent amount of drug within the lung when compared to MDI systems (although a higher dose of the drug is given when compared to MDI systems). A common practice should be to administer 2 to 3 nebulized treatments of the drug in the first hour and then begin tapering the frequency of the treatments dependent on the patient's response to therapy.

Delivery of the drug with a MDI and reservoir bag in multiple doses has been reported to successfully treat severe acute airflow obstruction in mixed asthmatic and COPD populations.[58,59] This delivery mechanism has the advantages of less cost and increased speed than nebulization of a medication. Also, the treatment can be started with equipotent bronchodilation. However, this has not been prospectively studied in the ICU population, and most physicians continue to use the compressed air or oxygen nebulization. Finally, intermittent positive pressure breathing (IPPB) for drug delivery should probably be avoided. This delivery system has no greater efficacy than compressed gas nebulization,[60] and it has been associated with mortality, often secondary to barotrauma.[61] Additionally, some patients may "fight" the delivery of the preset volume, and IPPB may worsen hyperexpansion and worsen the already deranged pulmonary mechanics. An occasional carefully selected patient with marked fatigue may avoid intubation with IPPB if they have a rapid, large bronchodilator response.

Intravenous therapy with sympathomimetics, primarily with isoproterenol in the United States, has been used with varying success and complications.[62,63] The drug has considerable potential toxicity and should probably be reserved for desperate situations involving younger patients (less likely to suffer potentially fatal cardiac toxicity) when prior therapy has failed to reverse critical airflow obstruction. It is prudent to monitor cardiac enzymes when using this drug, and discontinue intravenous therapy as soon as the patient's airflow or peak dynamic airway pressures improve.

Anticholinergic agents used in the therapy of asthma include atropine and ipratropium bromide. There are no clinical trials in the ICU population, but these drugs have been shown to increase bronchodilation in some non-ICU patients when used in combination with other medications.[64] One study of ER asthma patients found increased bronchodilator response when beta agonists and nebulized ipatroprium bromide (currently unavailable for nebulization in the United States at this time) were used as compared to beta agonist inhalation alone. Inhalation of anticholinergics generally avoids the systemic toxicity of intravenous doses, and the drugs have a more delayed onset of action than sympathomimetics.[65] If airflow limitation remains severe or ventilator dynamic airway pressures remain high despite manipulations, then an empiric trial of anticholinergics is certainly reasonable.

Methylxanthines are commonly used in the therapy of asthma and COPD, although the use of these agents has become controversial. Some studies have failed to document any bronchodilation increase provided that beta agonists have been used maximally, and one review of the drug in acute, severe asthma revealed contradictory data.[66,67] In nonacute situations, such as nocturnal asthma, methylxanthines may have considerable benefits.[68,69] The mechanism of action of methylxanthines in bronchospasm remains unclear. Theophylline does inhibit phosphodiesterase which leads to an intracellular increase in cyclic adenosine monophosphate, yet the levels achieved in vivo are inadequate to significantly inhibit the enzyme.[70] Methylxanthines have also been thought to exert their effect via antagonism of adenosine receptors which modulate adrenergic tone. However, the methylxanthine enprofylline has been shown to provide dose dependent bronchodilation in bronchospastic patients despite its lack of adenosine antagonism.[71]

Methylxanthines have a low therapeutic ratio and the toxicity potential is increased in the setting of hypoxia. Nevertheless, many physicians routinely employ these agents in severe bronchospastic attacks with an appropriate loading dose followed by an infusion. The drug may rapidly accumulate in the setting of right heart or ciprofloxacin drug therapy.[70,72] Additionally, patients who smoke or require phenobarbital or phenytoin therapy may have lower than expected theophylline levels as these other drugs cause increased hepatic biotransformation of methylxanthines.[70,73] It is mandatory to follow serum drug levels. Toxicity is reduced to an acceptable level when serum levels of 10 to 20 µg/ml are maintained. If nausea, vomiting, marked tachycardia, tachyarrhythmias, irritability, confusion or other adverse reactions develop, the infusion should be stopped and a serum drug level obtained. The potentially fatal toxic complications of tachyarrhythmias and seizures may occur without a prodromal period of nausea, vomiting, tachycardia, or tremors.

Toxicity usually resolves with discontinuation of the drug alone. Patients with heart rate greater than 120 bpm, multifocal atrial tachycardia, frequent premature ventricular contractions, hypotension, seizures, or coma have severe theophylline toxicity, however.[74] These patients and asymptomatic patients with drug levels of 40 to 60 µg/ml should be urgently treated with repetitive doses of 30 to 60 g of activated charcoal via the oral or nasogastric tube route.[70,75] Cathartics are often used to speed the excretion of the bound drug although severe hypermagnesemia has been reported following the use of magnesium citrate.[76] Sorbitol is then a more logical choice to avoid this iatrogenic complication. Patients who have theophylline levels greater than 60 µg/ml should be considered for charcoal hemoperfusion which will rapidly lower the serum levels, but this is much more effective when instituted prior to the onset of seizures.

Corticosteroids are essential in the therapy of severe, acute bronchospasm. These drugs decrease the cellular airway inflammation invariably present in these patients and other potentially important effects include increasing the sensitivity of the beta receptors.[77] The optimal dose, interval, route of administration, and agent remain unestablished, but data suggests a dose-response relationship with increasing doses of methylprednisolone and the rate of response of the FEV_1.[78] In the acute setting, a common dosing pattern is to use 60 to 125 mg of methylprednisolone intravenously at 6 to 8 hour intervals for 24 to 48 hours and then changing to lower doses or prednisone orally at 40 to 60 mg as the clinical situation allows. Although data suggesting hospitalized, nonventilated patients have an equivalent response in airflow to oral corticosteroids,[79] many physicians choose intravenous therapy in the ICU setting. Note that although the employed doses of corticosteroids are high, it is the length of administration of the drug rather than the total dose that is most closely associated with steroid side effects. Hence, it is inappropriate to withhold the drugs for concern of possible side effects in the setting of severe bronchospasm.

Antibiotics should be used when indicated. Those patients with a fever leukocytosis and "left-shiff," or a radiographic infiltrate should be considered for antibiotic therapy for pneumonia (assuming no other source is found on physical examination and screening labs) based on the usual pathogen in that clinical setting.

Therapeutically, little is altered in the pregnant asthmatic. Beta adrenergic agonists, theophylline, and corticosteroids are generally safe for the patient and are not teratogenic.[42,46] The choice of which beta agonist to employ in the pregnant asthmatic is subject to debate and little controlled trial data is available. Epinephrine has a long clinical history of efficacy and safety, but terbutaline has been safely used as a tocolytic. Hence, it may be a more logical choice secondary to its beta selectivity. Corticosteroids should be used as in any other acutely bronchospastic patient. Ampicillin and erythromycin are thought safe if an infection is present,[80] but tetracycline must be avoided secondary to its well known effects on fetal osseous and dental anlage.

Asthma drug therapy in the elderly is similar to the general population, but many of these patients have coexisting medical diseases with multiple medications that may yield more complications and possible drug interactions. The elderly appear to have a decreased beta receptor sensitivity which may slow the response to beta agonist therapy.[81]

There is some evidence, however, that the elderly population may have a comparatively greater bronchodilator response to anticholinergic agents.[82] No apparent age-related differences exist in the metabolism of methylxanthine derivatives and side effects. Additionally, most elderly asthmatics have severe, chronic diseases with slower response to therapy and less pulmonary reserve. Because of this condition, early use of corticosteroids in this population may be of greater importance. With chronic use, they may be most likely to incur the adverse drug effects such as salt retention, glucose intolerance, hypokalemia, osteopenia, and cataract formation. Regardless, corticosteroids should not be withheld in cases of severe life threatening bronchospasm in the elderly.

Mechanical Ventilation

Despite aggressive and timely pharmacologic intervention, some patients will unfortunately require intubation and mechanical ventilation. Clearly this procedure is a life-saving technologic intervention but it is unfortunately associated with morbidity and mortality. Complications include malfunction of the endotracheal tube, malfunction of the ventilator, alveolar hypoventilation, pneumonia, and barotrauma (pneumomediastinum, pulmonary interstitial emphysema, subcutaneous emphysema, and pneumothorax). The mortality of conventional mechanical ventilation has ranged from 0 to 38% in several series.[83-86] The incidence of pneumothorax and pneumomediastinum on the ventilator in this disease appears to be between 10 to 30% with an approximate 33% mortality.[83-85] Other causes of death are probably not as strongly correlated with asthma alone compared to other ventilator populations. Despite these shortcomings, the majority of patients survive intubation and mechanical ventilation.

Few patients have ventilatory failure and the immediate need for intubation as a presenting condition. Instead, most patients who require intubation continue to worsen or fail to respond to drug therapy over the course of hours. The question of when to intubate the patient is an empiric decision for which there is little data available. It is a difficult decision as the above data suggest that mechanical ventilation has a significant mortality mostly secondary to barotrauma yet asthmatic patients who suffer a respiratory arrest do extremely poor. The clinician must balance the risk of intubation and mechanical ventilation with that of waiting too long with potentially catastrophic results. It is better to conservatively and electively intubate the patient, however, rather than take the aggressive route and risk respiratory arrest. Mechanical ventilation is supportive until the severe airway inflammation, edema, and bronchospasm have resolved with drug therapy. General guidelines for the timing of intubation in the bronchospastic patient include:

- Severe respiratory acidosis with an arterial pH of less than 7.20
- Worsening respiratory acidosis despite adequate therapy
- Mental status changes
- Clinical impression of impending muscular exhaus-

tion, deteriorating hemodynamic status, or active coronary ischemia

Again, each patient and each decision needs to be individualized and these are guidelines. Hypoxemia is generally correctable with supplemental oxygen and is rarely the cause for intubation.

It is paramount to place the largest possible endotracheal tube (preferably 8.0 mm). This allows for less expiratory resistance, lowers peak airway pressures, and reduces the risk of barotrauma.[87,88] Oral intubation is the placement of choice as this can be performed the most expeditiously by a skilled operator, especially when sedatives and paralytics are employed. Sedatives and paralytics are strongly recommended as they increase the speed and safety of this procedure in patients who are highly anxious and potentially combative (with potentially catastrophic results). Although nasotracheal intubation is probably more comfortable to the patient, many, especially younger patients, will respond to therapy within 24 to 48 hours such that they can be extubated. Hence, a quick and effective procedure is more important in this setting rather than the long-term comfort of the nasotracheal tube and oral intubation allows for a larger caliber tube and easier suctioning. Again, sedatives and paralytics during intubation maximizes the safety and efficacy of these important therapeutic goals.

Drugs with theoretical problems for an elective intubation of the bronchospastic patient include succinylcholine and D-tubocurarine which can cause histamine release and may increase the airflow limitation. Pancuronium or vecuronium are probably the paralytic agents of choice.[89] Additionally, morphone may also cause histamine release and benzodiazepines are possibly the preferred sedatives to accompany the use of paralytics.

Introduction of the endotracheal tube may irritate receptors in the airway and worsen bronchospasm, presumably vagally medicated.[90] The physician should be aware of this potentially disastrous complication in the bronchospastic patient which can be treated with inhaled atropine or perhaps 0.4 to 1.0 mg of the drug IM or IV if the situation is critical.

Conventional volume-cycled ventilators are routinely employed to ventilate the severely bronchospastic patient. There is not data establishing the superiority of any ventilator mode in this or any setting, but the assist control or continuous mechanical ventilation mode allows for several important functions. First, it allows for the lower work of breathing and resting of the respiratory musculature.[91,92] Additionally, unless the patient is heavily sedated, they may become anxious and uncomfortable in the intermittent mandatory ventilation (IMV) mode when they self-ventilate between mechanical tidal volumes (unless the set rate closely matches the patient's own intrinsic rate). This mode employs a demand valve with a greater negative inspiratory pressure requirement, and the awake patient may feel that they are not obtaining enough ventilation between the mechanical tidal volumes.[91] In patients who are extremely alkalotic secondary to a rapid respiratory rate in the assist control mode, the IMV mode tends to correct this imbalance. Few data are available regarding the use of IMV with pressure support ventilation in the acute asthmatic patient. Regardless, empiric bedside adjustments are needed at times with trials of sedatives. We prefer the assist control mode to ventilate the asthmatic patient. A tidal volume in the standard range of 10 to 15 ml/kg is recommended, but a smaller tidal volume may be appropriate. Large tidal volumes may yield inordinately high dynamic peak airway pressures and thereby increase the risk of barotrauma. Oxygenation is normally readily achieved in the asthmatic patient requiring mechanical ventilation as the pathophysiology is ventilation/perfusion mismatching rather than shunting.[93]

Besides the mode of ventilation, respiratory rate, fraction of inspired oxygen, and tidal volume, astute clinicians will concern themselves with the peak inspiratory flow and the inspiratory:expiratory ratio. As the pathophysiology is that of expiratory airflow obstruction, it is important to adjust the ventilator to provide the longest possible expiratory phase. This must be balanced, however, with the dynamic peak airway pressures and risk for barotrauma, clearly increased when exceeding levels of 50 cm H_2O.[94] Setting the ventilator with a high respiratory flow rate may allow for a prolonged expiratory phase, but this unfortunately may cause unacceptably high peak airway pressures. The physician must empirically adjust the minute volume, tidal volume, and inspiratory flow rates to provide for acceptable peak airway pressures and gas exchanges. This situation will require periodic reevaluation, and at times is best accomplished in a slightly sedated patient.

Positive end-expiratory pressure (PEEP) is generally employed to improve oxygenation in markedly hypoxic patients (e.g., adult respiratory distress syndrome). PEEP should not routinely be used in the mechanical ventilation of the patient with airflow obstruction because it can potentially increase the hyperexpansion leading to hemodynamic compromise and increase the risk of barotrauma.[95]

An alternative to conventional volume-cycled mechanical ventilation in the acutely bronchospastic patient is controlled mechanical hypoventilation. This method evolved through an appreciation of the significant barotrauma and mortality associated with conventional mechanical ventilation in patients with acute bronchospasm. The strategy employed is to oxygenate the patient with a high fraction of inspired oxygen within paradoxically low mechanical minute volumes in the controlled mechanical ventilation mode. The minute volume (entirely mechanical in this mode) is determined not by the patient's $Paco_2$ or acid/base status, but instead by the peak airway pressure. The $Paco_2$ is allowed to remain high or drift upwards, and if the pH falls too low (e.g., <7.20), a bicarbonate infusion is employed. Hence, if the peak airway pressure exceeds an arbitrary value of 50 cm H_2O, then the tidal volume and/or the peak inspiratory flow rate is lowered. This effectively lowers the mean airway pressure and the barotrauma risk. This mode often requires sedation and paralysis, and patients have undergone mechanical ventilation for days in this state. The limited data available are encouraging, with zero mortality, but these data have not been compared with those for conventional mechanical ventilation in a clinical trial.[96,97] Controlled mechanical hypoventilation should probably be considered in patients who have a deteriorating status despite adequate pharmacologic

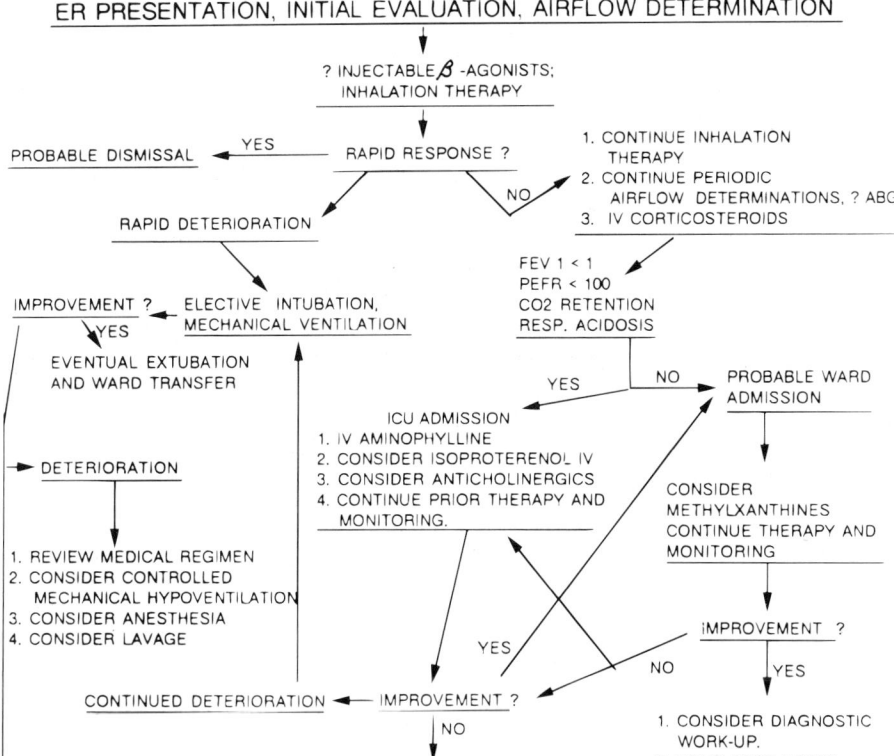

Fig. 14-3. Acute bronchospastic attack algorithm. ABG, arterial blood gas; FEV$_1$, forced expiratory volume in 1 second; PEFR, peak expiratory flow rate; Resp., respiratory.

therapy including sedation during conventional mechanical ventilation, inordinately high peak airway pressures, or already manifest barotrauma. An algorithm for treatment is demonstrated in Figure 14-3.

Heroic Measures

Most patients who are intubated and mechanically ventilated will improve when more of the work of breathing is assumed by the ventilator, and the various medications gradually improve the bronchospasm. Some patients will continue to worsen, however, despite appropriately aggressive medical and mechanical therapy. In such cases, serious consideration should be given to the technique of controlled mechanical hypoventilation and the drug therapy reviewed for omissions of potentially beneficial agents. If the situation continues to deteriorate, it may be appropriate to consider several techniques that are best viewed as desperate and heroic. All described reports have been entirely anecdotal and the exact role remains undefined. Each is associated with a significant potential for morbidity and mortality.

Magnesium infusions have been employed in acute bronchospastic attacks with initial reports documenting increases in airflow rates.[98,99] A single randomized double-blind study has found increased airflow in nonventilated patients who did not double their PEFR following two beta agonist nebulizations. A single dose of magnesium, 1.2 g IV over 20 minutes, produced a significant improvement in PEFR within 20 minutes of infusion. Magnesium infusions are probably contraindicated in patients who are hemodynamically tenuous, have mental status changes, or have severe chronic renal insufficiency or require renal dialysis.

Use of anesthetic agents in the treatment of acute, severe bronchospasm has been described since at least the 1930s. With currently available pharmacotherapeutics, however, fewer patients fail to improve on medical and mechanical therapy and the use of anesthetic agents has markedly decreased. Isolated reports showing utility in the deteriorating patient continue to be reported, however.[100-102] Halothane is often thought to be the anesthetic agent of choice in the asthmatic patient because it is known to be a bronchodilator in both animals and man although the mechanism is unclear.[103] The agent is often given through the ventilator circuitry or through anesthesia machines at concentrations of 0.5 to 3.0%, but the exact dose is titrated to clinical response or limited by the side effects. Halothane is a myocardial depressant and a vasodilator. Hypotension is often the limiting factor in using this agent for these situations. A Swan-Ganz catheter may aid management in these cases, especially in those patients with underlying cardiac disease. Additionally, the drug can increase ventricular irritability, not an insignificant concern in acidotic patients who may have electrolyte abnormalities and have received maximum doses of aminophylline and sympathomimetics. Clearly, the use of halothane requires diligent monitoring of the serum potassium, drug levels, cardiac rhythm, and blood pressure. Diethyl ether at concentrations of 15 to 20% through inhalation has been used successfully in patients refractory to halothane inhalation.[102]

Bronchoalveolar lavage has also been attempted to salvage patients with severe acute bronchospasm. Many of these reports antedated the currently accepted early and aggressive use of corticosteroids as well as several other drugs currently available. A variety of solutions have been employed with mixtures of saline including aminophylline, corticosteroids, and N-acetyl-L-cysteine delivered through a double lumen endotracheal tube, rigid bronchoscopy, or through flexible fiberoptic bronchoscopy.[104-108] The results have been optimistic in the literature, but it is unclear whether this therapy is appropriate within the context of available medical and mechanical therapy. Extracorporeal membrane oxygenation has also been attempted.[108]

Monitoring Response

In the ICU, laboratory tests of particular importance include the serum potassium as the drug therapy may cause hypokalemia as noted earlier. This situation is especially true if the patient is also receiving diuretic therapy. Additionally, it is pertinent to monitor the serum theophylline level in those patients on an infusion.

Obviously, those patients who require mechanical ventilation will also require a periodic ABG until their condition begins to improve, especially if the patient had a respiratory acidosis. If controlled mechanical hypoventilation is utilized, the monitoring of the acid/base status with an ABG is crucial, even more so if the patient requires a bicarbonate infusion. In those cases requiring frequent ABGs (more than 5 to 10 ABG draws in 24 hours), an arterial line is appropriate.

For nonintubated patients, airflow determinations should be continued in the ICU. This procedure will allow objective documentation of the response to therapy. For the intubated patient, improvement is more difficult to assess but is generally noted by lower peak airway pressures, decreasing minute volume, perhaps less hyperexpansion on the chest radiograph, and normalization of the ABG. Many patients have less wheezing on examination but again wheezing is an unreliable index of the severity of airflow limitation in the nonintubated patient.[18] When the patient has been judged to have improved, it is important to consider whether extubation is possible. Criteria have been developed which correlate with successful extubation and include.[14]

- The patient is awake and alert
- Fraction of inspired oxygen of <50%
- Spontaneous minute volume of <10.0 L, able to spontaneously double the minute volume on command
- Spontaneous tidal volume of >5 ml/kg
- Spontaneous vital capacity of >10 to 15 ml/kg
- Negative inspiratory force of ≤20 to 25 cmH$_2$O

These criteria were developed in a heterogenous population of ventilator patients but appear to apply to asthmatics. If the above criteria are met, it is appropriate to proceed to a 15 to 30 minute T-piece trial and check an ABG. If the patient tolerates the T-piece trial with an adequate ABG, then extubation will generally be successful. Patients who are otherwise healthy can often be rapidly extubated following this short trial and rarely are prolonged, repetitive T-piece trials or gradual IMV decrements necessary once a satisfactory response to therapy has occurred.

Once extubated, most physicians maintain the patient in the ICU for another 24 to 48 hours, gradually transferring the patient from IV drugs to the oral route. The question of when to transfer the patient from the ICU is an empiric decision which must be individualized for each patient and each institution. For those patients who were successfully treated without mechanical ventilation, there should be a clear improvement in the airflow (FEV$_1$ or PEFR) prior to transfer to the floor.

POST-ICU

Following ICU discharge and while the patient is recovering from a severe bronchospastic attack, the medical regimen will be adjusted. Obviously, the patient will be changed from IV and probably nebulized routes to oral and MDI therapy. We prefer to first place the patient on oral corticosteroids and methylxanthines and then on MDI beta agonists although there is no data suggesting a logical order of conversion. A medical regimen should be planned which will control the bronchospasm and allow for compliance. One must consider each patient's past history to elucidate possible contributing circumstances such as an atopic history, environmental exposures, exercise history, gastroesophageal reflux, infection, and importantly the nocturnal worsening of asthma in order to intelligently prescribe medications which may control the patient's disease. A review of the etiology of asthma is beyond the scope of this chapter, but these factors need to be considered in order to most effectively control the asthma and prevent another life threatening bronchospastic attack. A peak flowmeter for both the remaining hospitalization and home can demonstrate those patients with marked circadian variation in lung function. Further diagnostic testing for other etiologies would be appropriate at this time or in the outpatient setting after the patient has approached baseline.

In addition to inhaled beta agonists, these patients should be discharged on oral corticosteroids, usually prednisone at 40 to 60 mg per day. Too often a rapid taper is done with the patient returning to the ER with recurrent severe bronchospasm. The rate at which the drug is subsequently tapered is individualized but a slow taper over 2 to 3 weeks should be prescribed. The use of methylxanthines is important in treating asthmatics with nocturnal worsening.[68,69] Cromolyn sodium should also be considered for therapy of moderate to severe, chronic asthma with an allergic or exercise component.

Inhaled corticosteroids are clearly effective in many asthmatic patients. Aggressive use of these agents may allow tapering of oral steroids to a dose with acceptable side effects or even discontinuation of the oral drug. Data suggest that high dose inhalation therapy may be particularly effective in patients with chronic disease.[109] Higher doses are well above that recommended by the manufacturer and the transition period between oral and inhaled steroids which often requires several weeks.

Review of asthma mortality data suggests that patient education and early aggressive institution of therapy may prevent asthma fatality. In perhaps the most detailed evaluation, avoidable factors were identified in the events that led to 82% of the deaths.[12] Few patients fail to respond to adequate therapy. Most of the patients who perish have not received adequate instruction regarding their disease, and many of the patients with life threatening asthma have not received optimal therapy. This situation is often secondary to a lack of appreciation of the severity of the attack. Hence, it is difficult to avoid the conclusion that improved patient and physician education will have a favorable impact on the rising asthma mortality rates. Education of the patient in regards to the disease process, medication, and knowing when to seek medical attention can help prevent hospitalizations and hopefully life threatening attacks. Compliance and education are often overlooked factors which lead to frequent bronchospastic attacks, and the ICU physician may be the first to recognize this important component of the patient's care. Since both the patient and the physician may underestimate the severity of airflow limitation on historical factors alone, patients will benefit from use of a peak flow meter at home. This procedure will give both the patient and the physician an objective measure of the severity of an attack and, one hopes, will lead to earlier and more rational therapeutic decisions.

REFERENCES

1. Evans, R., et al.: National trends in the morbidity and mortality of asthma in the U.S. Chest, *91*:65S, 1987.
2. Benatar, S. R.: Fatal asthma. N. Engl. J. Med., *314*:423, 1986.
3. Sly, R. M.: Increases in deaths from asthma. Ann. Allergy, *53*:20, 1984.
4. Paulozzi, L. S., Coleman, J. J., and Buist, A. S.: A recent increase in asthma mortality in the northwestern United States. Ann. Allergy, *56*:392, 1986.
5. Robin, E. D.: Death from bronchial asthma. Chest, *93*:614, 1988.
6. Evans, R.: Recent observations reflecting increases in mortality from asthma. J. Allergy Clin. Immunol., *80*:377, 1987.
7. Buist, A. S.: Is asthma mortality increasing? Chest, *93*:449, 1988.
8. Shim, C. S., and Williams, M. H.: Evaluation of the severity of asthma: patients versus physicians. Am. J. Med., *68*:11, 1980.
9. McFadden, E. R., Kiser, R., and DeGroot, W.: Acute bronchial asthma: relations between clinical and physiological manifestations. N. Engl. J. Med., *228*:221, 1973.
10. Burdon, J. G. W., et al.: The perception of breathlessness in asthma. Am. Rev. Respir. Dis., *126*:825, 1982.
11. Rubinfield, A. R., and Pain, M. C.: Perception of asthma. Lancet, *2*:882, 1976.
12. British Thoracic Association: Death from asthma in two regions in England. Br. Med. J., *285*:1251, 1982.
13. Stableforth, D.: Death from asthma. Thorax, *38*:801, 1983.
14. Fernandez, E., and Martin, R.: Treatment of acute, severe asthma. Semin. Respir. Med., *8*:227, 1987.
15. Sears, M. R., Rea, H. H., Beaglehole, R., et al.: Asthma mortality in New Zealand: a two-year national study. N. Z. Med. J., *98*:271, 1985.
16. Sutherland, D. C., et al.: Death from asthma in Auckland: circumstances and validation of causes. N. Z. Med. J., *97*:845, 1984.
17. Rea, H. H., et al.: A case control study of deaths from asthma. Thorax, *41*:833, 1986.
18. Kelsen, S. G., et al.: Emergency room assessment and treatment of patients with acute asthma: adequacy of the conventional approach. Am. J. Med., *64*:622, 1986.
19. McFadden, E. R.: Clinical physiologic correlates in asthma. J. Allergy Clin. Immunol., *77*:1, 1986.
20. Knowles, G. K., and Clark, T. J. H.: Pulsus paradoxicus as a valuable sign indicating severity of asthma. Lancet, *2*:1356, 1973.
21. Fischl, M. A., Pitchenir, A., and Gardner, L. B.: An index predicting relapse and need for hospitalization in patients with acute bronchial asthma. N. Engl. J. Med., *305*:783, 1981.
22. Rose, C. C., Murphy, J. G., and Schwartz, J. S.: Performance of an index predicting the response of patients with acute bronchial asthma to intensive emergency department treatment. N. Engl. J. Med., *310*:573, 1984.
23. Rebuck, A. S., and Pengeley, D. L.: Development of pulsus paradoxicus in the presence of airways obstruction. N. Engl. J. Med., *288*:66, 1973.
24. Fanta, C. H., Rossing, T. H., and McFadden, E. R.: Emergency room treatment of asthma. Relationships among therapeutic combinations, severity of obstruction, and time course of response. Am. J. Med., *72*:416, 1982.
25. Martin, T. G., Elenbaas, R. M., and Pingleton, S. H.: Use of peak expiratory flow rates to eliminate unnecessary arterial blood gases in acute asthma. Ann. Emerg. Med., *11*:70, 1982.
26. Nowak, R. M., Gordon, K. R., and Wroblewski, D. A.: Spirometric evaluation of acute bronchial asthma. J. Am. Coll. Emerg. Physicians, *8*:9, 1979.
27. Nowak, R. M., et al.: Comparison of peak expiratory flow and FEV_1 admission criteria for acute bronchial asthma. Ann. Emerg. Med., *11*:64, 1982.
28. McFadden, E. R., and Lyons, H. A.: Arterial blood gas tensions in asthma. N. Engl. J. Med., *278*:1027, 1968.
29. Corre, K. A., and Rothstein, R. J.: Assessing severity of adult asthma and need for hospitalization. Ann. Emerg. Med., *14*:45, 1985.
30. Banner, A. S., Shah, R. S., and Addington, W. W.: Rapid prediction of need for hospitalization in acute asthma. JAMA, *235*:1337, 1976.
31. Nowak, R. M., et al.: Arterial blood gases and pulmonary function testing in acute bronchial asthma. JAMA, *249*:2043, 1983.
32. Rees, H. A., Millar, J. S., and Donald, K. W.: A study of the clinical course and arterial blood gas tensions of patients in status asthmaticus. Q. J. Med., *37*:541, 1968.
33. Miyamoto, T., Mizuno, K., and Furuya, K.: Arterial blood gases in bronchial asthma. J. Allergy Clin. Immunol., *45*:248, 1970.
34. Rebuck, A. S., and Read, J.: Assessment and management of severe asthma. Am. J. Med., *51*:788, 1971.
35. Raffin, T. A.: Indications for arterial blood gas analysis. Ann. Intern. Med., *105*:390, 1986.
36. Mountain, R. D., and Sahn, S. A.: Clinical features and outcome in patients with acute asthma presenting with hypercapnia. Am. Rev. Respir. Dis., *138*:535, 1988.
37. Appel, D., Rubenstein, R., Schrager, K., and Williams, M. H.: Lactic acidosis in severe asthma. Am. J. Med., *75*:580, 1983.
38. Findley, L. J., and Sahn, S. A.: The value of chest roentgenograms in acute asthmatic adults. Chest, *80*:535, 1981.
39. Grossman, J.: The occurrence of arrhythmias in hospitalized asthmatic patients. J. Allergy Clin. Immunol., *57*:310, 1976.
40. Gelb, A. F., et al.: P pulmonale in status asthmaticus. J. Allergy Clin. Immunol., *64*:18, 1979.
41. Lipworth, B. J., McDevitt, D. G., and Struthers, M. D.: Prior

41. (continued) treatment with diuretic augments the hypokalemic and electrocardiographic effects of inhaled albuterol. Am. J. Med., *86*:653, 1989.
42. Greenberger, P. A., and Patterson, R.: Management of asthma during pregnancy. N. Engl. J. Med., *312*:896, 1985.
43. Turner, E. S., Greenberger, P. A., and Patterson, R.: Management of the pregnant asthmatic patient. Ann. Intern. Med., *93*:905, 1980.
44. Greenberger, P. A., and Patterson, R.: Beclomethasone dipropionate for severe asthma during pregnancy. Ann. Intern. Med., *98*:478, 1983.
45. Schatz, M., et al.: Corticosteroid therapy for the pregnant asthmatic patient. JAMA, *233*:804, 1975.
46. Huff, R. W.: Asthma in pregnancy. Med. Clin. North Am., *73*:653, 1989.
47. Hernandez, E., Angell, C. S., and Johnson, J. W. C.: Asthma in pregnancy: current concepts. Obstet. Gynecol., *55*:739, 1980.
48. Burr, M. L., Charles, T. J., Roy, K., and Seaton, A.: Asthma in the elderly: an epidemiological survey. Br. Med. J., *1*: 1041, 1979.
49. Derrick, E. H.: The significance of the age of onset of asthma. Med. J. Aust., *1*:1317, 1971.
50. Peheram, I., Jones, D. A., and Collins, J. V.: Assessment and management of acute asthma in the elderly: a comparison with younger asthmatics. Postgrad. Med. J., *58*:149, 1982.
51. Christopher, K. D., et al.: Vocal cord dysfunction presenting as asthma. N. Engl. J. Med., *308*:1566, 1987.
52. Martin, R. J., et al.: Pyridoxic vocal cord motion in presumed asthmatics. Semin. Respir. Med., *8*:332, 1987.
53. Fitzgerald, J. M., and Hargreave, F. E.: The assessment of acute life-threatening asthma. Chest, *95*:888, 1989.
54. Popa, V.: Beta-adrenergic drugs. Clin. Chest Med., *7*:313, 1986.
55. Carstains, J. R., et al.: Autoradiographic localization of beta-adrenoreceptors in human lung. Eur. J. Pharmacol., *103*: 189, 1984.
56. Zaagsma, J., et al.: Adrenergic control of airway function. Am. Rev. Respir. Dis., *136*:S45, 1987.
57. Brink, C., Ridgway, P. G., and Douglas, J. S.: Modification of airway smooth muscle responses in the guinea pig by hydrocortisone, in vitro and in vivo. J. Pharmacol. Exp. Ther., *203*:1, 1977.
58. Shim, C. S., and Williams, H. M.: Effect of bronchodilator therapy administrated by cannister versus jet nebulizer. J. Allergy Clin. Immunol., *73*:387, 1984.
59. Turner, J. R., et al.: Equivalence of continuous flow nebulizer and metered-dose inhaler with reservoir bag for treatment of acute airflow obstruction. Chest, *93*:476, 1988.
60. Goldberg, I., and Cherniack, R. M.: The effect of nebulized bronchodilator delivered with and without IPPB on ventilatory function in chronic obstructive emphysema. Am. Rev. Respir. Dis., *91*:13, 1965.
61. Karetzky, M. S.: Asthma mortality associated with pneumothorax and intermittent positive-pressure breathing. Lancet, *1*:828, 1975.
62. Klaustermeyer, W. B., DiBernardo, R. L., and Hale, F. C.: Intravenous insoproterenol: rationale for bronchial asthma. J. Allergy Clin. Immunol., *55*:325, 1975.
63. Kurland, G., Williams, J., and Lewiston, N. J.: Fatal myocardial toxicity during continuous infusion intravenous isoproterenol therapy of asthma. J. Allergy Clin. Immunol., *63*: 407, 1979.
64. O'Driscoll, B. R., et al.: Nebulized salbutamol with and without ipratropium bromide in acute airflow obstruction. Lancet, *1*:1418, 1989.
65. Ziment, I., and Au, J. P.: Anticholinergic agents. Clin. Chest Med., *7*:355, 1986.
66. Rossing, T. H., et al.: Emergency therapy of asthma: comparison of the acute effects of parenteral and inhaled sympathomimetics and infused aminophylline. Am. Rev. Respir. Dis., *122*:365, 1980.
67. Littenberg, B.: Aminophylline treatment in severe, acute asthma. JAMA, *259*:1670, 1988.
68. Zwillich, C. W., et al.: Nocturnal asthma therapy, inhaled bilolterol versus sustained-release theophylline. Am. Rev. Respir. Dis., *139*:475, 1989.
69. Martin, R. J., et al.: Circadian variations in theophylline concentrations and the treatment of nocturnal asthma. Am. Rev. Respir. Dis., *139*:475, 1989.
70. Miech, R. P., and Stein, M.: Methylxanthines. Clin. Chest Med., *7*:331, 1986.
71. Lunell, E., et al.: Intravenous enprofylline in asthma patients. Eur. J. Respir. Dis., *65*:28, 1984.
72. Raoof, M. B., et al.: Ciprofloxacin increases serum levels of theophylline. Am. J. Med., *82(Suppl. 4A)*:115, 1987.
73. Marquis, J. F., et al.: Phenytoin-theophylline interaction. N. Engl. J. Med., *307*:1189, 1982.
74. Greenberg, A., et al.: Severe theophylline toxicity: role of conservative measures, antiarrhythmic agents, and charcoal hemoperfusion. Am. J. Med., *76*:854, 1984.
75. Goldberg, M. J., Park, G. D., and Berlinger, W. G.: Treatment of theophylline intoxication. J. Allergy Clin. Immunol., *78*: 811, 1986.
76. Weber, C. A., and Santiago, R. M.: Hypermagnesmia, a potential complication during treatment of theophylline intoxication with oral activated charcoal and magnesium-containing cathartics. Chest, *95*:56, 1989.
77. Ellul-Micallef, R., and Fenech, F. F.: Effect of intravenous prednisolone in asthmatics with diminished adrenergic responsiveness. Lancet, *2*:1269, 1975.
78. Haskell, R. J., Wong, B. M., and Hansen, J. E.: A double-blind, randomized clinical trial of methylprednisolone in status asthmaticus. Arch. Intern. Med., *143*:1324, 1983.
79. Harrison, B. D., et al.: Need for intravenous hydrocortisone in addition to oral prednisolone in patients admitted to hospital with severe asthma without ventilatory failure. Lancet, *8474*:181, 1986.
80. Greenberger, P., and Patterson, R.: Safety of therapy of allergic symptoms during pregnancy. Ann. Intern. Med., *89*:234, 1978.
81. Vestal, R. E., Wood, A. J. J., and Shand, D. G.: Reduced beta-adrenoreceptor sensitivity in the elderly. Clin. Pharmacol. Ther., *26*:181, 1979.
82. Ullah, M. I., Newman, G. B., and Saunders, K. B.: Influence of age on response to ipratroprium and salbutamol in asthma. Thorax, *36*:523, 1981.
83. Scoggins, C. H., Sahn, S. A., and Petty, T. L.: Status asthmaticus, a nine-year experience. JAMA, *238*:1158, 1977.
84. Webb, A. K., Bihon, A. H., and Hanson, G. C.: Severe bronchial asthma requiring ventilation. A review of 20 cases and advice on management. Postgrad. Med. J., *55*:161, 1979.
85. Westerman, D. E., Benatar, S. R., Potgieter, P. D., and Fergoson, A. D.: Identification of the high-risk asthmatic patient: experience with 39 patients undergoing ventilation for status asthmaticus. Am. J. Med., *66*:565, 1979.
86. Luksza, A. R., et al.: Acute severe asthma treated by mechanical ventilation: 10 years' experience from a district general hospital. Thorax, *41*:459, 1986.
87. Habib, M. P.: Physiologic implications of artificial airways. Chest, *96*:180, 1989.
88. Wright, P. E., Marini, J. J., and Bernard, G. R.: In vitro versus

in vivo comparison of endotracheal tube airflow resistance. Am. Rev. Respir. Dis., *140:*10, 1989.
89. Levin, N., and Dillon, J. B.: Status asthmaticus and pancuronium bromide. JAMA, *222:*1265, 1972.
90. Gal, T. J.: Pulmonary mechanics in normal subjects following endotracheal intubation. Anesthesiology, *52:*27, 1980.
91. Christopher, K. L., et al.: Demand and continuous flow intermittent mandatory ventilation systems. Chest, *87:*625, 1985.
92. Marini, J. J., Rodriguez, M., and Lamb, V.: The inspiratory workload of patient initiated mechanical ventilation. Am. Rev. Respir. Dis., *134:*902, 1986.
93. Rodriguez-Roisin, R., et al.: Mechanisms of hypoxemia in patients with status asthmaticus requiring mechanical ventilation. Am. Rev. Respir. Dis., *139:*732, 1989.
94. Haake, R., Schlichtey, R., Ulstad, D. R., and Hehschen, R. R.: Barotrauma: pathophysiology, risk factors and prevention. Chest, *91:*608, 1987.
95. Tuxen, D. V.: Detrimental effects of positive end-expiratory pressure during controlled mechanical ventilation of patients with severe airflow obstruction. Am. Rev. Respir. Dis., *140:*5, 1989.
96. Dariole, E., and Perret, C.: Mechanical controlled hypoventilation in status asthmaticus. Am. Rev. Respir. Dis., *129:*385, 1984.
97. Menitove, S. M., and Goldring, R. M.: Combined ventilator and bicarbonate strategy in the management of status asthmaticus. Am. J. Med., *74:*898, 1983.
98. Okayama, H., et al.: Bronchodilating effect of intravenous magnesium sulfate in bronchial asthma. JAMA, *257:*1076, 1987.
99. Skobeloff, E. M., et al.: Intravenous magnesium sulfate for the treatment of acute asthma in the emergency department. JAMA, *262:*1210, 1989.
100. O'Rourke, P. P., and Crone, R. K.: Halothane in status asthmaticus. Crit. Care Med., *10:*341, 1982.
101. Schwartz, S. H.: Treatment of status asthmaticus with halothane. JAMA, *251:*2688, 1984.
102. Robertson, C. E., Steedman, D., Sinclair, C. J., and Brown, D.: Use of ether in life-threatening acute severe asthma. Lancet, *1:*187, 1985.
103. Snider, S. M., and Papper, E. M.: Anesthesia for the asthmatic patient. Anesthesiology, *22:*886, 1961.
104. Thompson, H. T., Pryor, W. J., and Hill, J.: Bronchial lavage in the treatment of obstructive lung disease. Thorax, *21:*557, 1966.
105. Rogers, R. M., Shuman, J. F., and Zubrow, A. B.: Bronchopulmonary lavage in bronchial asthma. Chest, *63:*62S, 1973.
106. Donaldson, J. C., et al.: Acetylcysteine for life-threatening acute bronchial obstruction. Ann. Intern. Med., *88:*656, 1978.
107. Shridharani, M., and Maxson, T. R.: Pulmonary lavage in a patient in status asthmaticus receiving mechanical ventilation: a case report. Ann. Allergy, *49:*156, 1982.
108. MacDonnell, K. F., Moon, H. S., Thomandram, S. S., and Ahluwalia, M. P.: Extracorporeal membrane oxygenator support in a case of severe status asthmaticus. Ann. Thorac. Surg., *31:*171, 1981.
109. Salmeron, S., et al.: High doses of inhaled corticosteroids in unstable chronic asthma. Am. Rev. Respir. Dis., *140:*167, 1989.

Chapter 15

MANAGEMENT OF CHRONIC OBSTRUCTIVE PULMONARY DISEASE

RICHARD MENZIES
PETER GOLDBERG

Because of the chronic, irreversible, and progressive nature of chronic obstructive pulmonary disease (COPD) most patients admitted to the ICU tend to be near the end stage of their disease. Intubation and institution of mechanical ventilation will significantly prolong survival for some patients, but others will suffer prolonged dependence on mechanical ventilation, with resultant pain and suffering as well as potentially devastating financial burdens for patients and their families. Management decisions in the ICU should be based an understanding of the prognosis and factors affecting the course of COPD, to identify those who will benefit from mechanical ventilation.

This chapter will review the natural history, factors affecting the course, and pharmacologic therapy of patients with COPD. The major causes, pathophysiology and treatment of respiratory failure, and associated hemodynamic changes will be summarized. Options for ventilatory assistance, problems, and solutions in weaning the patients from mechanical ventilation will be reviewed in detail. Finally, for the patients who are successfully discharged from the ICU a number of therapeutic options, in addition to standard pharmacologic therapy, should be considered. These include:

- Smoking cessation
- Rehabilitation
- Oxygen therapy
- Nutrition therapy

Home ventilation may be indicated for a few carefully selected patients who remain dependent on mechanical ventilation, while lung transplantation may be considered for even fewer.

One of the greatest problems in any discussion of COPD is the lack of a precise, universally accepted definition, making it difficult to compare results from different centers, particularly those in different countries. It is generally accepted that this disorder is comprised of several entities. Bronchitis and emphysema are universally included in the definition of COPD, even though both may occur without significant airways obstruction.[1] **Chronic bronchitis** is defined as cough productive of sputum persistent for three months, recurring in at least two consecutive years.[2] **Emphysema** is defined by the pathologic finding of destruction of alveolar septa with cystic enlargement of air spaces.[2] **Asthma** may be considered part of COPD, because it is a chronic disorder with airways obstruction, but usually only if there is a component of irreversible airways obstruction. This has been termed chronic asthmatic bronchitis by Burrows[1] and has a very different clinical course, response to therapy and prognosis.[1] **Bronchiectasis** and **cystic fibrosis** are also usually considered part of COPD.[2]

An excellent definition of COPD was formulated at a recent conference at the National Heart, Lung, and Blood Institute: "COPD may be defined as a process characterized by the presence of chronic bronchitis or emphysema that may lead to the development of airways obstruction. Airways obstruction need not be present at all stages of the process. The airways obstruction may be partially reversible."[3]

In this chapter, respiratory insufficiency will be defined as worsening of dyspnea and gas exchange that requires hospitalization, while respiratory failure will be defined as requirement for mechanical ventilation.

PRE-ICU PHASE

Etiology and Pathogenesis

Normal Changes In Lung Function With Aging

The normal development of the lung in adolescence, and adulthood has been elucidated in several large community based studies in Boston[4] and in Tucson, Arizona.[5] In nonsmoking healthy persons, lung growth continues up to age 25 or even 30. This is followed by a long plateau period which extends to age 35 in men. Thereafter, FEV_1 begins to decline, initially at the rate of 10 to 20 ml per year, which gradually increases to 40 ml per year by age 43[6] and more than 50 ml per year after age 50.[6] Among smokers the onset of lung function decline occurs earlier, without plateau so that lung function begins to decline as early as age 25,[4] and this decline is more rapid at all ages.[7] In community based studies, decline of FEV_1 among smokers exceeded that of nonsmoking age-matched cohorts by only 10 ml per year.[4,6] On the other hand, patients with COPD who continue to smoke have decline in FEV_1 of 80 to 100 ml per year.[8] An important finding first noted by Fletcher,[7] and confirmed by others, is that among those who quit smoking the decline in lung function quickly reverts to the same level as the nonsmoking cohort, as shown in Figure 15-1.

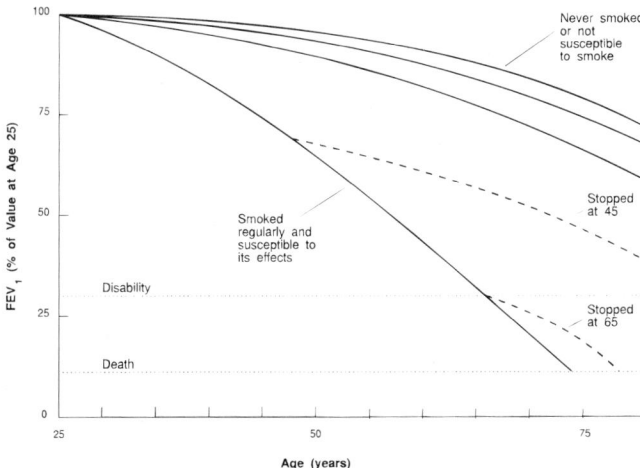

Fig. 15-1. Effect of smoking and smoking cessation on disability and death. (Redrawn courtesy of ACT/PC from Fletcher, C. M., and Peto, R.: The natural history of chronic airflow obstruction. Br. Med. J., 1:1645, 1977.)

Pathogenesis of Smoking-Related COPD

In the early studies of the natural history of COPD conflicting findings arose which gave rise to two opposing theories of the pathogenesis of COPD. In the first theory, among British male railway workers, of whom a high proportion smoked heavily, the development of COPD was almost exclusively related to cigarette smoking.[7] This lead to the "British hypothesis" that the development of COPD was related entirely to smoking and not to asthma.[7] On the other hand, a community based study conducted in the Netherlands, which included males and females and did not exclude asthmatics, found that the presence of an asthmatic tendency was a strong predictor for the development of fixed airways obstruction among those who smoked.[10] It is now accepted that 80 to 90% of COPD cases are attributable to smoking,[9,11] but that an asthmatic tendency will heighten a smoker's risk of developing COPD.[1,12]

It is unknown why only 15% of those who smoke develop COPD. There are four possible explanations for this apparent difference in individual susceptibility to the effects of cigarette smoking. (1) A local lung protease deficiency similar to, but less severe than that of patients with alpha-1 antitrypsin (AAT) deficiency;[1,9,12] (2) those who develop COPD have consumed more cigarette smoke. In support of this dose dependency hypothesis is that lung function is strongly correlated to pack/years of cigarettes smoked.[1] Differences in lung function among those with similar smoking histories may be a result of differences in initial lung function, or that pack/years does not measure actual consumption. Serum or urine cotinine levels, which are accepted as accurate measures of consumption, may be equal among individuals smoking as little as 15 or as much as 40 cigarettes.[13] Further evidence that the development of COPD is dose dependent is the correlation of COPD with other diseases such as lung cancer[14] in which an exposure-response relationship to cigarette smoking has been shown; (3) bronchial hyperreactivity has been detected in 50 to 100% of patients with COPD, although this may be secondary to inflammatory changes, and appears to be of less importance than among patients with asthma. Prospective studies would be needed in order to know the temporal sequence of the development of bronchial reactivity in these patients;[1] and (4) patients who have had childhood respiratory illnesses may be at increased risk for the development of COPD.[1]

The agent in cigarette smoke responsible for the lung injury and the mechanism of injury are unknown. The pathologic events have been described from autopsy and pathologic studies of lungs of smokers.[15,16] The earliest pathologic changes are bronchiolar inflammation without any evidence of airflow obstruction or emphysema.[15] With the development of mild airways obstruction the bronchiolar inflammation is more severe but there is no evidence of emphysema. As the airways obstruction worsens, the bronchiolar inflammation remains severe and there is increasing severity of parenchymal emphysema. Severe airflow obstruction is associated with severe emphysema, at which point patients may die of their disease and come to autopsy.[16] The importance of bronchiolar inflammation and injury has been underestimated in past autopsy series of patients with severe airways obstruction. Whether bronchiolar inflammation and the development of emphysema are pathogenetically related remains unclear, however.[1,3,11]

Other Factors—Personal

In 1964, Errikson described patients with severe emphysema developing at a young age in whom circulating levels AAT were extremely low.[17] Currently, AAT accounts for approximately 1% of all patients with COPD in the United States.[1,3] This is an autosomal recessive genetic defect with a prevalence of approximately 1 in 2000 among North American caucasians. Heterozygotes have lower serum levels of AAT yet have no evidence of increased incidence of COPD. The development of COPD is accelerated by cigarette smoking. Among those who smoke, lung function decline may exceed 150 ml per year and average age of presentation with dyspnea is 40 years among smokers compared to 53 years among nonsmokers.[3] Currently, replacement therapy is available, but is only recommended for those over age 18 with abnormal lung function and AAT levels of less than 11 μmol/L.[18] A weekly infusion of human AAT (prolactin) prepared from pooled human plasma should be given.[18]

Other Factors—Environmental

Passive smoking is associated with increased respiratory symptoms and lower lung function among children whose parents smoke. The effect of the long-term exposure in childhood on respiratory symptoms or lung function among adults is unknown.[1,3]

Air pollution may cause deterioration in lung function in patients with established COPD but the role of air pollution in the pathogenesis of COPD itself is uncertain. Lower socioeconomic status (SES) is associated with increased respiratory symptoms, as well as, lower lung function. It is unclear if this is due to the effects of more frequent childhood respiratory illnesses, to increased exposure to personal and passive smoking or some other adverse effects of poverty on respiratory health.[19]

Occupational exposures have been implicated.[20] In several community based longitudinal surveys, the relationship between nonspecific exposure to dust, heat, and fumes has been associated with increased rates of lung function decline and development of COPD.[6,20] In a study of 550 factory workers resident in Paris who were followed for 12 years, FEV_1 declined by: 42 ml per year in those with no occupational exposure to dust, heat, and fumes; 44 ml per year among those with slight exposure; 53 ml per year among those with moderate to heavy exposure to dust at work; 55 ml per year among those exposed to dust and heat at work; and 60 ml per year among those exposed to dust, heat, and fumes at work.[21] It is significant to note that those who changed to occupations with less exposure subsequently had slower decline of FEV_1.[21]

Epidemiology

Morbidity

In 1985 there were 5,448,000 prevalent cases of COPD in the United States among the population aged over 55.[22] Prevalence is equal in males and females up to age 55, after which there is an increasing male predominance. Prevalence is highest among those aged 65 to 75, of whom 13.6% of males and 11.4% of females have COPD.[22] In 1985 this condition was responsible for 5% of all physician office visits, and 13% of all acute care hospital admissions. Patients with COPD suffer on average 55 days of restricted activity and 28 days of bed disability due to illness each year. Among those aged 55 and over, patients with COPD spend an average of 3.1 days in hospital annually compared to an average of 1.5 days for the entire population of that age.[22]

Mortality

Of all deaths in the United States in 1985; COPD was the direct cause in 3.6% and a contributory cause in 4.3%.[11,22] In total this disorder was the fifth most common cause of death, accounting for 164,650 deaths, over 90% of which occurred among those aged over 55. Eighty-four percent of the deaths among males and 79% among females could be attributed to smoking.[9] It has been estimated that smoking-related COPD was directly responsible for approximately 500,000 potential years of life lost in 1985.[9]

The mortality rate from all causes of COPD in the United States has risen steadily from 1950 until 1985, as seen in Figure 15-2, even after adjustment for revisions in the international classification of diseases.[22] Mortality from chronic bronchitis has apparently declined while deaths due to all COPD have risen. This apparent contradiction is most likely due to changes in diagnostic habits; because bronchitis is viewed as a less serious illness, so it is attributed less often as a cause of death.[22] There has been a similar steady increase in mortality from COPD of all forms in Canada, although the increase among females has been less than in the United States.[23] On the other hand, mortality from COPD among females in Britain has risen rapidly between 1960 and 1985 with little change in the mortality of males in those years.[24]

In summary, COPD is a disease of older men and to an increasing extent, older women. This is most likely related to the different smoking patterns particularly among the older cohorts in which the proportion of female smokers was lower. Despite a significant decrease in the proportion of the population that smokes and an absolute decrease in the number of smokers and tobacco consumption[9] it has been estimated that the prevalence and mortality from COPD will continue to rise particularly among women, for at least another decade.[9,11]

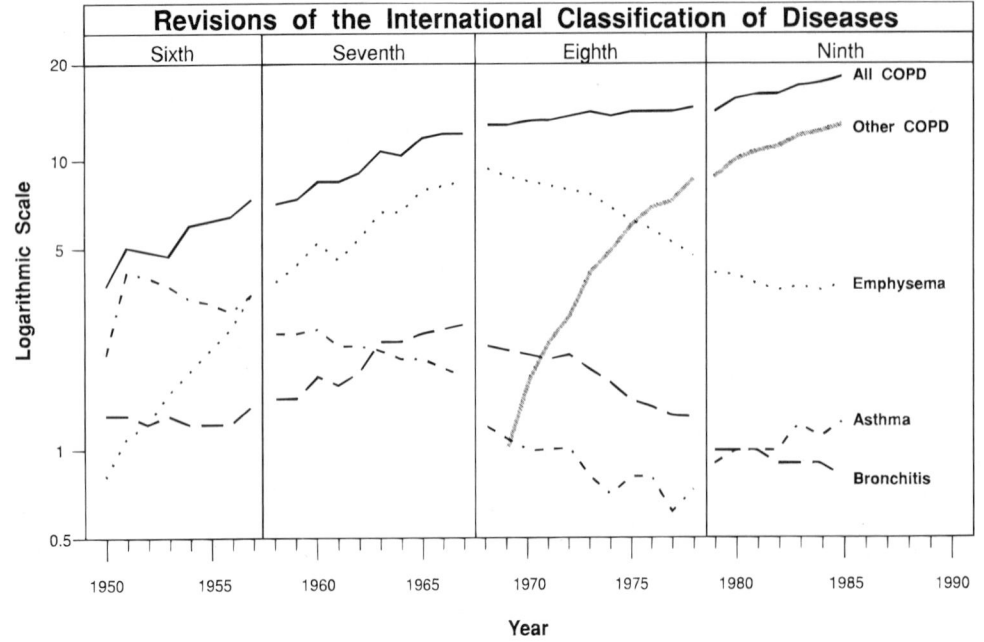

Fig. 15–2. Mortality from COPD and its subcategories standardized to the total United States population in 1940. (Redrawn by George Morrison, ACT/PC from Feinleib, M., et al.: Trends in COPD morbidity and mortality in the United States. Am. Rev. Respir. Dis., *140*:S9, 1989.) (Source: National Vital Statistics Systems, 1950 to 1985).

Table 15-1. Prognosis and Prognostic Factors in COPD Stable Outpatients

Author (year)	No. of Patients	Age (mean)	Males (%)	FEV_1 (L)	Survival 1 yr (%)	2 yr (%)	3 yr (%)	Prognostic Factors Significant	Not Significant
Burrows (1969)	200	59	89	1.0	93	79	66	FEV_1 Resting HR Functional class Edema Alb/Glob ratio Hypercarbia Cor Pulm on ECG	Age Sex
VandenBurgh (1973)	64	54	94	1.0	100	97	93	Bronchodilator response (−) Exercise ABGs Cor Pulm on ECG	Age FEV_1 Pao_2 $Paco_2$ HR rest
Boushy (1973)	663		100		88	82	75	FEV_1 Emphysema on CXR Age $Paco_2$ (+/−)	PAP & PVR Pao_2 RV InspRes
Postma (1979)	129	54	80	0.6	94	88	80	Bronchodilator response $Paco_2$ Functional class Resting HR $FEV_1 <$ 450 ml	Age Sex SES
Traver (1979)	200	59	89	33% Pred.	91	78	66	Age FEV_1 Cor Pulm on ECG Dyspnea Edema	Sex Smoke Alb/Glob ratio

Course and Prognosis

Numerous longitudinal studies of the prognosis and prognostic factors among patients with COPD have been done. Valid comparison of the results of these studies is hampered because of differences in criteria for population selection. For example, mortality is lowest among patients followed from the onset of dyspnea, intermediate among those followed from an episode of acute respiratory insufficiency requiring hospitalization, and very high among patients identified after an episode of acute respiratory failure requiring mechanical ventilation. The course and prognostic factors among patients with COPD have been summarized separately in Tables 15-1 and 15-2 for patients who were selected from the onset of dyspnea, or from an episode of worsening dyspnea requiring hospitalization with or without respiratory failure.

Mitchell followed a cohort of outpatients who presented with dyspnea due to emphysema, among whom mortality over 5 years was 18%.[25] Longitudinal surveys of similar cohorts of patients are summarized in Table 15-1[26-33] and in Figure 15-3.[28,34,35] Three-year survival ranged from 65[26] to 100%[27]. As seen in Table 15-1, some of the differences between studies may be ascribed to differences of age and lung function of the study populations. It appears that survival is no different in the earliest compared to the most recent series. This suggests that despite significant advances in therapy of this disorder in the intervening 20 years the major determinant of prognosis is still the severity of the underlying disease.

As reviewed by Hodgkin,[36] the factors associated with survival are:

- Lung function
- Exercise capacity
- Diffusing capacity (D_{LCO})
- Age
- Pulmonary artery pressure
- Malnutrition
- AAT deficiency
- Lung function decline (longitudinal)

Almost all studies have shown that lung function, particularly postbronchodilator FEV_1, is the most important prognostic factor, as seen in Figure 15-4. In longitudinal surveys, patients with more rapid decline in lung function had worse prognosis. It has been stated that smoking cessation will not improve long-term survival, because mortality in the first 1 to 2 years is higher among those who quit, presumably because sicker patients tended to stop smoking.[37] Postma and colleagues reported that improved survival after cessation of smoking was seen only after 7 years, as seen in Figure 15-5.[8] Arterial hypoxemia contributes to mortality only if supplemental oxygen is not given.[37] Elevated pulmonary artery pressures adversely affected survival only if they did not normalize with administration of supplementary oxygen.[37] Mucus hypersecretion is not related to mortality, although it is related to cigarette smoking and airflow obstruction.[38] The absence of an independent relationship with mortality suggests that mucus hy-

Table 15–2. Prognosis and Prognostic Factors in COPD

A. Patients with acute respiratory failure

Author (year)	No. of Patients	Age (mean)	FEV₁	Males (%)	Init. Episode	Survival 1 yr (%)	Survival 2 yr (%)	Survival 3 yr (%)	Prognostic Factors Significant	Not Significant
Sulumalchantra (1966)	43	62		86	82%	74	58	54	Cor pulmonale on ECG Disability	Age FEV₁ FVC
Martin (1982)	34	61	.99	100	94%	86	72		Right heart failure	

B. Patients requiring mechanical ventilaton

Author (year)	No. of Patients	% Placed on MV	Age (mean)	Males (%)	% Weaned	Survival 1 yr (%)	Survival 2 yr (%)	Survival 3 yr (%)	Prognositic Factors Significant	Not Significant
Bradley (1964)	29	100	57	79		38	14			
Jessen (1967)	111	100	60	93		46	38	38	Degree of disability	Age Cause Cor pulmonale on ECG
Asmundsson (1969)	146	50	61	100	60	44	29	20	Age Anemia Weight loss FEV₁ FVC	
Wesselass (1970)	43	100	50	60	60	40	26	20	FEV₁ FVC Cor pulmonale on ECG	Age
Gillespie (1986)	47	100	68		75	50				
Menzies (1989)	95	100	70	53	74	34			Disability FEV₁ Albumin Dyspnea	Cause Age

persecretion is a separate process that is not of major pathogenetic importance.[1,38]

As seen in Table 15–2, prognosis is worse among patients selected after an episode of acute respiratory insufficiency.[34,39] In two series, 54%[39] and 72%[34] of patients survived 2 years. The prognosis of patients requiring mechanical ventilation for acute respiratory failure (ARF) is even worse.[40–45] Bradley[40] reported 1-year survival of 38% among 30 patients with emphysema who required mechanical ventilation (MV) for ARF between 1961 to 1962. Menzies reported 1-year survival of 34% among 95 patients with COPD who required MV in 1984 to 1987.[45] Petty reported that among patients at Colorado University Hospital who required mechanical ventilation for ARF due to ARDS, mortality in 1969, 1974, 1978, and 1981 was 38%, 44%, 42% and 40%, respectively.[46] From this it would appear that the prognosis of patients with ARF from COPD or ARDS is unchanged over the last 20 to 25 years.

As seen in Table 15–2, prognostic factors among patients with COPD who develop ARF have not been clarified as fully as for stable outpatients. This is because patients with ARF do not have complete premorbid data, or this information is obtained retrospectively. Factors associated with survival are:

- Degree of disability (judged from performance of activities of daily living)
- Lung function
- Serum albumin (or other markers of malnutrition)
- Severity of dyspnea

In two studies,[41,45] the most important prognostic factor was the degree of disability as estimated from patients' performance of activities of daily living, as shown in Table 15–3. The prognosis of patients, based on this classification of disability, has not been validated by prospective studies. This measure can be considered to summarize the severity of the disease, other co-morbid illnesses, and psychologic factors such as the patients' response to their illness.

The course of patients after their initial hospitalization for respiratory insufficiency has been reported in only one study. Gottleib and colleagues[47] followed 30 patients with COPD from the time of their first hospitalization for ARF, during which 19 (63%) required MV. Among the survivors a second episode of ARF occurred after a mean interval of 8 months, and among those still surviving a third episode occurred after a mean of another 4 months. Cumulative mortality after each of these episodes as 30%, 60%, and 67%, respectively. Overall, only one third of patients remained alive one year after their initial hospitalization for respiratory insufficiency.[47]

In summary, the course of patients with COPD is that of variable decline. Prognosis does not appear to be affected by exacerbations per se,[36] but rather those patients that develop acute respiratory failure, particularly if me-

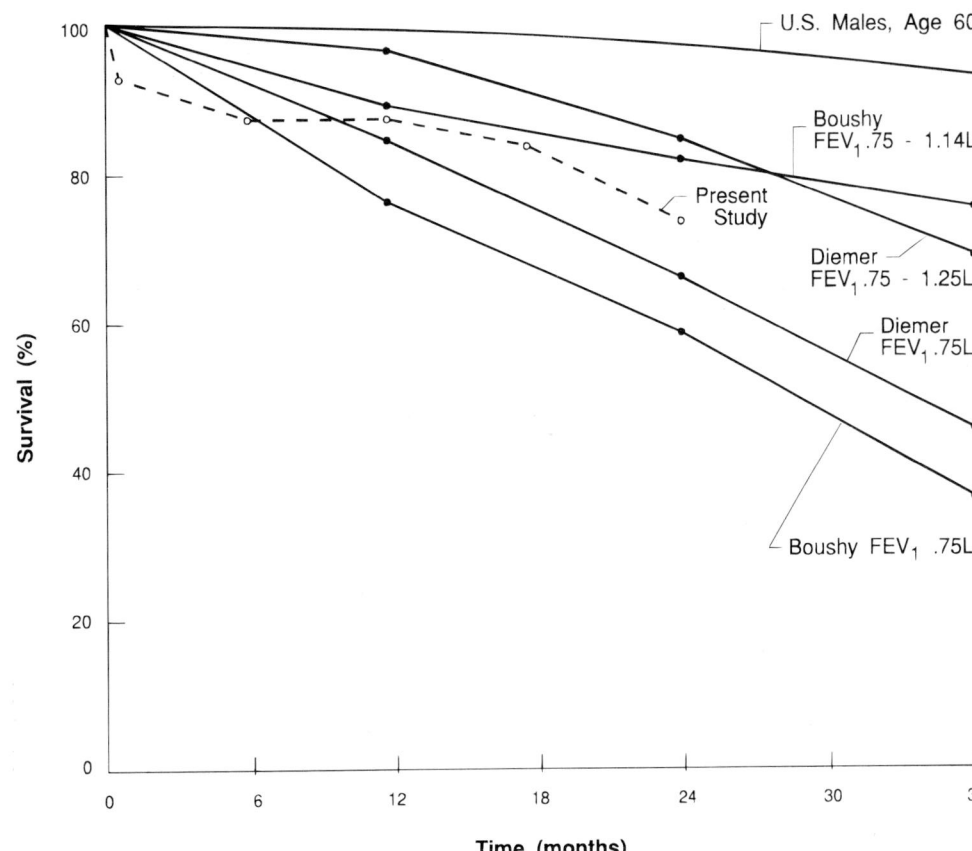

Fig. 15-3. Effect of lung function on mortality among patients with COPD compared to the general population (present study refers to a study of stable outpatients by Martin et al.). (Redrawn courtesy of ACT/PC from Hudson, L. D.: Survival data in patients with acute and chronic lung disease requiring mechanical ventilation. Am. Rev. Respir. Dis., *140*:S19, 1989.)

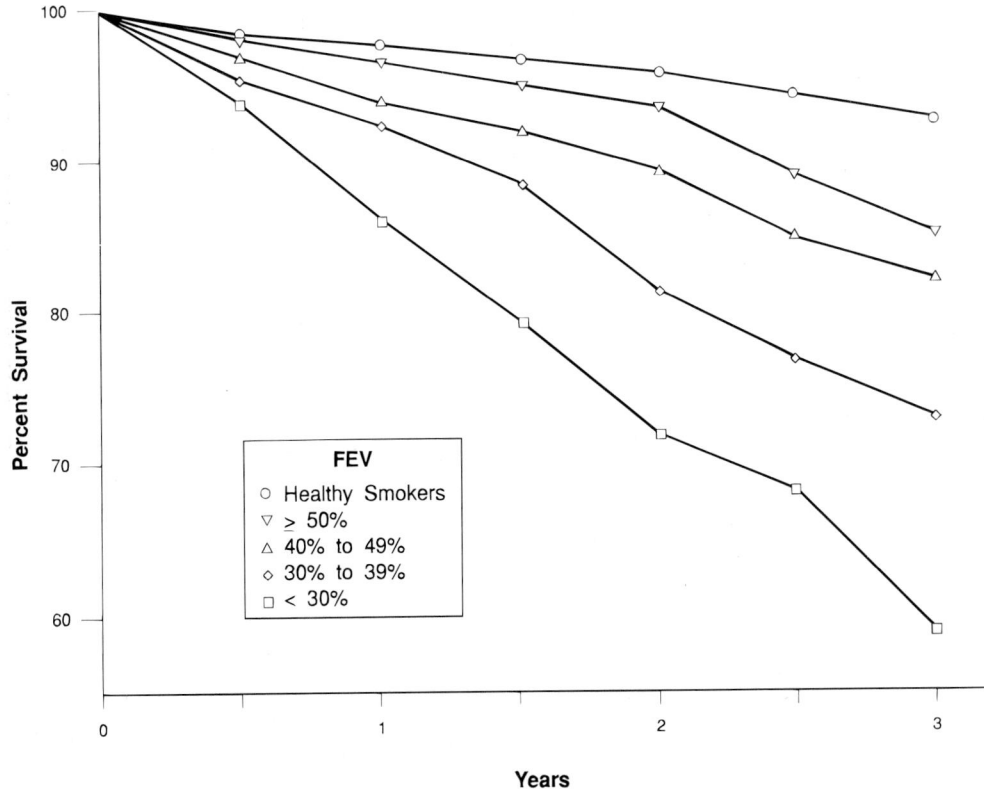

Fig. 15-4. Survival in groups segregated according to baseline postbronchodilator FEV_1. (Redrawn by George Morrison, ACT/PC from Anthonisen, N. R., et al.: Prognosis in chronic obstructive pulmonary disease. Am. Rev. Respir. Dis., *133*:14, 1986.)

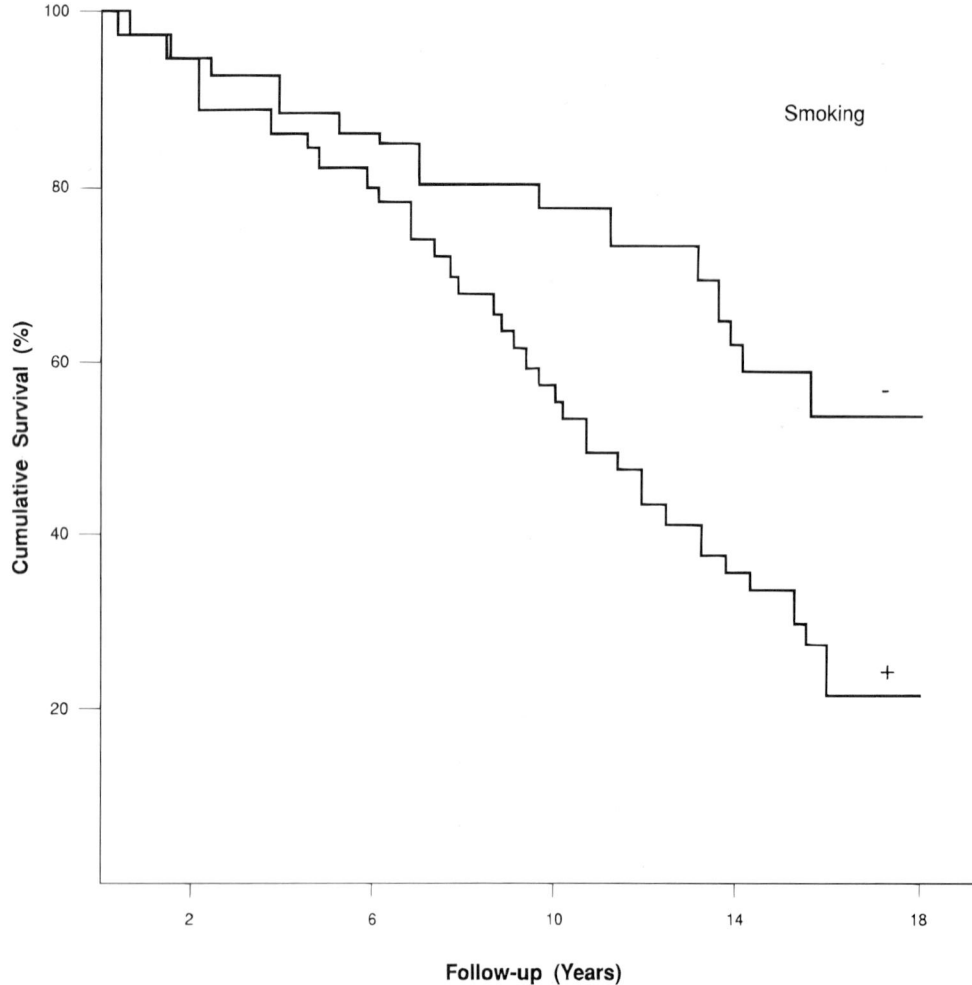

Fig. 15–5. Cumulative survival curves of continuing smokers (+) and ex-smokers (−). (Redrawn by George Morrison, ACT/PC from Postma, D. S., and Sluiter, H. J.: Prognosis of chronic obstructive pulmonary disease: the Dutch experience. Am. Rev. Respir. Dis., 140:S100, 1989.)

chanical ventilation is required, have worse underlying disease. As such they are likely to have recurring episodes of ARF, and mortality on initial and subsequent episodes is extremely high. Prognosis is strongly associated with worse lung function, arterial hypoxemia (unless corrected by supplemental oxygen), pulmonary hypertension, and malnutrition. Degree of disability, estimated from performance of activities of daily living, has been shown to be strongly predictive of outcome in two retrospective studies. Despite advances in pharmacologic therapy and critical care, the prognosis of patients with COPD, with or without episodes of ARF, has not changed significantly over the last 25 years and remains related to the severity of the underlying disease.

Symptoms and Signs

The major symptoms of COPD are dyspnea, cough and sputum production.[2] Patients in whom airflow obstruction develops remain asymptomatic for years although they may note a diminishing exercise tolerance. Dyspnea at rest is usually noted when the FEV_1 declines to less than 1 liter, at the time of an acute exacerbation. Cough is common, particularly among those who smoke. Sputum production is present among those with mucus hypersecretion, and

Table 15–3. Impact of Premorbid Disability on Weaning and One Year Survival (All patients with COPD and ARF requiring MV)

Author (year)	Jessen (1967) No. of patients	% surviving 1 yr	Menzies (1989) No. of patients	% surviving 1 yr	% Weaned from MV
Total	111	38	95	34	72
Fully independent/working	53	62	19	74	95
Able to get out of the house	46	37	22	45	77
Housebound (bed or chair)	12	8	54	22	69

is independent of the presence of airflow obstruction.[38] More severely ill patients may experience orthopnea, but paroxysmal nocturnal dyspnea is uncommon. They may also experience leg edema. Chest pain is not commonly seen. If other problems such as pneumonia, pneumothorax, pulmonary embolus, or congestive heart failure occur, the symptoms will be specific to these illnesses.

The body habitus is usually normal, or of diminished weight. On chest examination there are usually signs of hyperinflation with both diaphragms being lower than normal. The chest is hyperresonant to percussion. The most notable finding on auscultation is reduced air entry in all lung fields with reduced breath sounds. There may be wheezing particularly during episodes of acute worsening of airflow obstruction.

The patients may have signs of right heart failure such as jugular venous distention, hepatojugular reflux, and leg edema. Cardiac examination is usually normal, although heart sounds may be distant and the apical impulse may be felt only in the epigastrium. In severe cor pulmonale, there may be a right ventricular heave and the murmur of tricuspid insufficiency, and a right ventricular S3 gallop may be heard.

Pharmacologic Therapy

The literature on pharmacologic therapy in COPD is voluminous and is only briefly summarized here. For further details, please refer to three excellent reviews.[48-50]

Beta Agonists

Beta agonists form the foundation of bronchodilator therapy for COPD. Almost all patients demonstrate some bronchodilator response, particularly if it is expressed relative to their actual rather than their predicted FEV_1.[48] In a survey of over 1000 consecutive patients with COPD, approximately 20% of patients had a postbronchodilator increase in FEV_1 of more than 10% relative to their predicted FEV_1.[48] This group is traditionally regarded as bronchodilator responsive.[48] As well, beta agonists may have pulmonary vasodilator effects,[51] which in turn may enhance cardiac output.

Onset of action after inhalation is within 15 minutes and lasts 4 to 6 hours.[48,50] Typical initial dose is 2 puffs every 6 hours, but maximal improvement may be achieved only after as many as 8 puffs.[2,50] Because the use of the MDI requires coordination of respiration with hand action, delivery of medication may be worse in patients who are older and more debilitated. Larger droplets impact in the upper airways and may be associated with unwanted oral and upper airways side effects and some systemic absorption. A simple device known as a spacer can eliminate the need for coordinated action, reduce local side effects and systemic absorption, and improve overall delivery to the lungs.[50] Beta agonists can also be given by nebulized aerosol solution. The major advantage of this method of administration is that a dose up to 50 times greater than that of a single puff from a MDI can be given.[48,50]

The earliest beta agonists introduced, epinephrine and isoproterenol, had significant cardiac side effects. With the newer agents, selective beta-2 agonists, salbutamol, fenoterol, and terbutaline, systematic absorption is minimal, and cardiac effects toxicity very rare.[48,50] Tremor after inhalation of these agents is dose dependent and is commonly seen after aerosol administration but may also be seen after frequent use of an MDI. Oral preparations are available but are not recommended because of extremely erratic absorption.[50] Beta agonists may be given parenterally but this is not recommended because cardiac toxicity is significantly increased and there is no evidence of increased therapeutic benefit compared to aerosol administration.[48,50]

Anticholinergics (Ipratropium Bromide)

Interest in the anticholinergic agents has been stimulated by findings within the last 10 years of significant bronchodilator effect of these agents, among patients with asthma and COPD.[52] The exact mechanism of action is unknown but it has been found experimentally that there is increased cholinergic tone in inflamed airways.[50] After inhalation the onset of bronchodilator effect occurs in 1.5 to 2 hours with duration of over 6 hours.[52] This relatively slow onset of action may explain why patients experience no subjective improvement with the use of these agents. Ipratropium has a bronchodilator effect that is additive to that of concurrently administered beta agonists.[52] This effect is not seen if high doses of beta agonists are given prior to the administration of ipratropium.[53] It has recently been suggested that an optimal dose of ipratropium is 8 puffs with the MDI or 0.4 mg in aerosolized solution.[54,55]

Side effects from inhalational therapy are minimal because this is a quaternary ammonium compound which is, not absorbed systemically. Secretions are not dried and mucus clearance is not impaired in contrast to the effects of atropine given as an aerosol.[54] Given orally, less than 30% is absorbed systemically. Side effects are infrequently seen with oral preparations but this is probably because the serum levels achieved are subtherapeutic. When given parenterally, ipratropium causes significant tachycardia and other signs of cholinergic blockade.[50]

Based on the benefits demonstrated experimentally and in clinical trials, it has been suggested that ipratropium should be the initial therapy for patients with COPD.[54] This recommendation is not widely accepted at the present time.

Theophylline

Of current therapies for COPD, theophylline has the longest history of use, but despite this, its present role remains unclear. Bronchodilation begins at serum concentrations of 10 mg/L and increases in direct proportion to serum concentrations up to 20 mg/L.[56] The bronchodilator effect is additive to that of concurrently administered beta agonists, but the effect of theophylline given after the administration of beta agonists and anticholinergic agents has not been measured.[48,50] In a randomized controlled trial of COPD patients with an acute exacerbation given a standard regimen of beta agonists, corticosteroids, and antibiotics, the addition of theophylline was of no benefit.[57] In a second, similar study of COPD patients with acute exacerbations seen in an emergency room, the addition of theophylline to a regimen of beta agonists and oxygen was of no benefit.[58]

Theophylline has other actions which may be of benefit, including pulmonary vascular dilatation which should reduce pulmonary vascular resistance and right ventricular afterload. Right ventricular function is further improved because theophylline independently increases right ventricular contractility.[59] Aubier and colleagues have reported that blood flow to the diaphragm and diaphragmatic contractility was increased after intravenous infusion of theophylline.[60] There are few well-designed clinical trials which demonstrate a consistent benefit among patients with COPD from theophylline. In one randomized double-blind placebo control trial, theophylline administration was associated with significant increases in vital capacity, tidal volume and minute ventilation, although there were no changes in dyspnea, blood gases, or exercise tolerance.[48] In another trial, FEV_1 increased in proportion to increasing doses of theophylline.[56] Despite the inconsistent evidence, theophylline is still considered important in the therapy of patients with COPD.[2]

One of the major problems in the clinical use of this agent is the narrow therapeutic window between serum levels that are effective and those that are toxic. As seen in Figure 15-6, this window is affected by other medications, age and co-morbid illnesses of the patients,[50] so careful monitoring of serum levels is essential. Toxic effects include cardiac toxicity manifested as tachycardia, supraventricular and ventricular arrhythmias, and central nervous system effects manifested initially as increased irritability and insomnolence, although at higher serum levels seizures and coma may occur. The prognosis of theophylline-induced seizures is extremely poor; in one series, however, this complication resulted in 50% mortality.[61] As well, many patients complain of nausea and gastrointestinal upset. This is believed to be CNS related to stimulation in the medulla oblongata, rather than a direct gastrointestinal effect.[50]

Corticosteroids

Corticosteroids are fundamental to reversing the airways obstruction of asthma, but patients with COPD do not have reversible airways obstruction (by definition) and therefore the role of corticosteroids in the therapy of COPD is controversial. The three clinical situations for which steroids may be considered are stable outpatients, acute exacerbations, and acute respiratory failure. The evidence for the use of corticosteroids will be reviewed for these three clinical settings:

Stable Outpatient. Between 1963 and 1986, 13 randomized placebo-controlled double blind trials have been conducted,[62-74] as summarized in Table 15-4. Of these studies, five showed no benefit[64,66,69,73,74] although in one of these[66] only 5 mg of prednisone was given daily for a total of 1 week. In three studies,[65,70,71] improvements were reported as changes in mean values of the entire group treated, with lower $Paco_2$ and increased diffusing

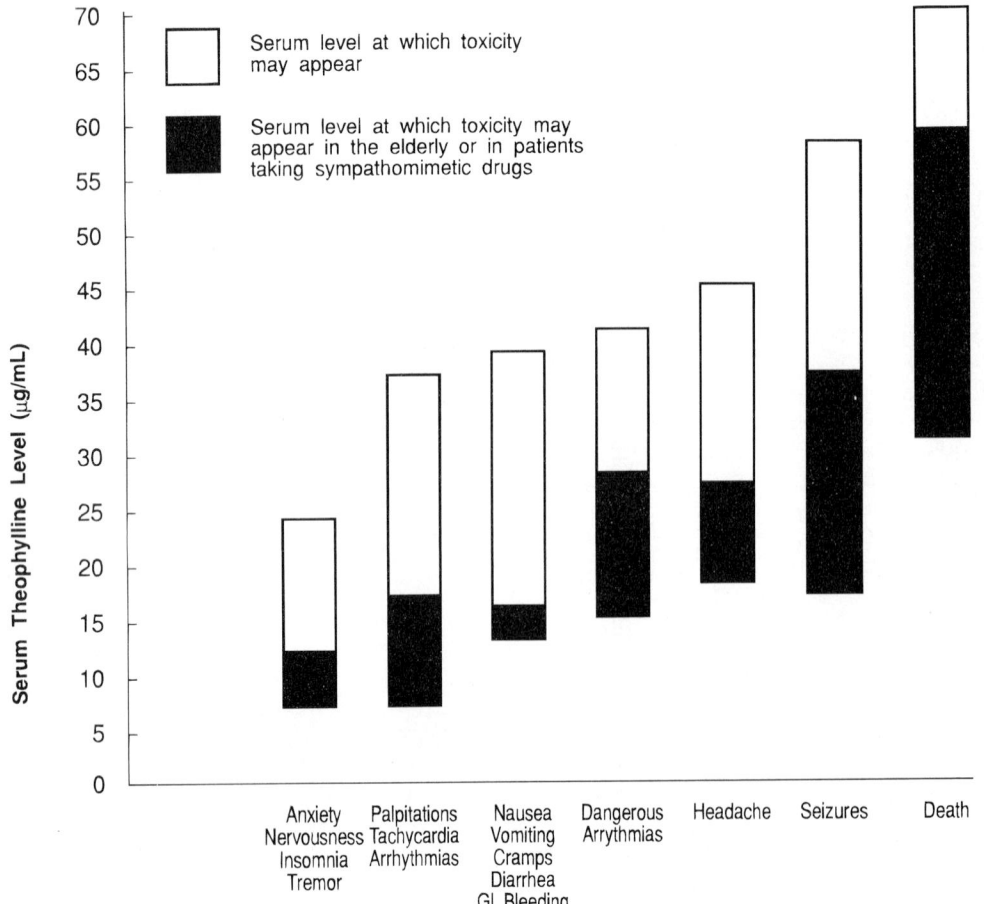

Fig. 15-6. Correlation between serum theophylline levels and major side effects. (Redrawn courtesy of ACT/PC from Ziment, I., and Au, J. P.: Making the best use of aminophylline in the ICU. J. Crit. Illness, *1*:21, 1986.)

Table 15-4. Results of Trials of Corticosteroids in Stable COPD Patients

Author	No. of patients	Study Design	Diagnosis (FEV$_1$)	Doses of CS (Duration)	Benefits of RX
Blair (1984)	44	RCT*	COPD .7	40 mg 1.5 wk	8/29 responders
Strain (1984)	13	Crossover	COPD 1.1	40 mg 2 wk	None
Eliasson (1986)	16	Crossover	COPD 1.2	40 mg 2 wk	1/16 Responders
Beerel (1963)	10	RCT	emphysema <0.6	30 mg 2 wk	2/5 responders 0/5 placebo
Hurford (1963)	39	RCT	bronchitis 0.6–1.8	30 mg 1 wk	4/19 responders 1/20 placebo
Morgan (1964)	7	Crossover	emphysema .7–2.2	45 mg 4 wk	0/7 responders
Beerel (1971)	23	Crossover	emphysema	30 mg 8 wk	↓ mean Paco$_2$ ↑ mean D$_2$co
Evans (1974)	10	Crossover	emphysema .5–1.7	5 mg 1 wk	Worse
Shim (1978)	24	Crossover	asthmatics COPD .75	30 mg 1 wk	7/24 responders (3/7 replaced with MDI)
Mendella (1982)	46	Crossover	COPD 1.03	40 mg 2 wk	8 responders (3/8 replaced with MDI)
O'Reilly (1982)	10	Crossover	COPD .8	20 mg 2 wk	None
Lam (1983)	16	Crossover	COPD .85	40 mg 2 wk	↑ FEV$_1$ ↑ FVC ↑ 14 MD (means)
Mitchell (1984)	43	Crossover	COPD 1.0	40 mg 2 wk	↑ FEV$_1$ ↑ FVC % responders same

* Note—RCT, Randomized Clinical Trial.

capacity in one,[65] increased FEV$_1$, FVC and 12 minute walking distance in the second,[70] and increased FEV$_1$ and FVC in the third.[71] In the remaining five studies, significant improvement was seen in 21 to 40% of those given prednisone.[62,63,67,68,72] Those who responded were more likely to have a significant bronchodilator response[68,72] and in one study response to therapy was associated with sputum or serum eosinophil.[67]

Only about two thirds of steroid responsive patients can be identified from bronchodilator response, however, so it is currently recommended that a trial of steroids be given to all patients with stable COPD.[48-50]

For patients who respond, recommendations for maintenance therapy have not been established. Inhaled steroids have been assessed in 2 studies.[68,75] In the first study, only 4 of 12 who responded to oral corticosteroids could be maintained with inhaled,[68] compared to 3 of 7 responders in the second study.[75]

Although inhaled steroids have far fewer side effects because of their minimal systemic absorption, they cannot be recommended to replace oral corticosteroids without further clinical trials to evaluate their use as maintenance therapy in COPD.

Mild Exacerbations of COPD. The only study of the effectiveness of steroids in this setting was conducted among patients seen in an emergency room among whom FEV$_1$ measured after 12 and 72 hours of treatment with intravenous corticosteroids was no different from that after treatment with placebo. As well, there was no difference in the proportion requiring hospitalization.[76]

Hospitalized Patients with Acute Respiratory Failure. In the often quoted clinical trial 44 patients hospitalized for an acute exacerbation of COPD were randomized to receive 72 hours of intravenous corticosteroids or placebo.[77] Improvement in FEV$_1$ was more rapid and greater among the steroid treated patients. There were no differences in gas exchange and other outcomes were not reported. Based on this one study it is currently recommended that all acute exacerbations of COPD be treated with intravenous corticosteroids.

Complications of corticosteroids are frequent although it has been assumed that complications arising after 1 to 2 weeks of therapy were minimal. Among the 13 randomized clinical trials mentioned earlier, side effects were not reported in 12 studies. In the one study in which side effects are mentioned, 6 out of 23 patients developed serious side effects on corticosteroids compared to none on placebo.[65] None of the clinical trials of corticosteroids published to date have had sufficient numbers of patients in each treatment arm to have adequate power to detect significant differences in the incidence of side effects, which could be done only by combining results from many studies. It is hard to draw firm conclusions except that there are significant excess of complications among steroid treated groups.[49]

Antibiotics

Until 1988, 9 double-blind placebo controlled trials had been reported, none of which showed benefit of antibiotics in exacerbations of COPD.[48,50] These trials were flawed by lack of clearly defined outcomes, and small numbers in each study so that benefits occurring only in subgroups of patients could not be detected. Anthonisen and colleagues conducted a randomized placebo controlled clinical trial among 173 patients with COPD who developed 362 exacerbations during follow-up over 3 to 5 years.[78] During this time, patients who presented with an exacerbation not requiring hospitalization were randomized to receive antibiotics or placebo. The study was strengthened by the design feature that patients randomized to one arm of therapy on their initial exacerbation were assigned to the opposite arm of therapy on a subsequent exacerbation. Of episodes of exacerbation treated with antibiotics, 68% improved and 10% deteriorated, compared to 55% and 19%, respectively, among those episodes managed with placebo. These differences were highly significant for both outcomes. As well, peak flow improved significantly more rapidly among those treated with antibiotics. Analysis within subgroups revealed that those with increased sputum production demonstrated the greatest benefit whereas those who presented primarily with wheeze and dyspnea without significant sputum production had no benefit from antibiotics.[78] Based on the results of this trial, it is currently recommended that among patients with COPD who present with exacerbations not requiring hospitalization associated with increased amount and/or prevalence of sputum should be treated with antibiotics such as tetracycline, ampicillin, or trimethoprim sulfate.[2,48,50] Sputum culture has not been shown to be helpful nor cost effective and is not recommended.[48,50]

Other Therapy

Annual administration of influenza vaccine is recommended because influenza can cause substantial morbidity and mortality among patients with COPD.[2] At the time of an epidemic, amantadine can be given to those who are unvaccinated, although this is effective only for prevention of influenza A. Pneumococcal vaccine is not recommended routinely for patients with COPD because this form of pneumonia is relatively rare among these patients.[2] Vaccines for other bacteria such as Haemophilus influenzae have been used in European trials with beneficial results. These have not been tested in trials in North America and are not currently part of standard practice here.[2]

Mucolytic agents are of no proven benefit. The respiratory stimulant almitrine has been shown to diminish arterial CO_2 and increase arterial O_2, but without improvement in exercise tolerance or mortality.[50] As well, use of almitrine has been associated with weight loss and increased pulmonary artery pressures.[50] Therefore, this agent needs further evaluation before its use can be recommended. Sedatives have been used for patients with severe dyspnea and normal blood gases, but may precipitate acute respiratory failure[50] and should be avoided.

Digoxin has not been demonstrated to be of benefit in right ventricular failure[79] because it may result in increased pulmonary vascular resistance.[80] Both ventricular and supraventricular arrhythmias are commonly seen in patients with right ventricular failure given digoxin.[79,80] Therefore, supraventricular tachycardias should be managed with a calcium channel antagonist while right ventricular failure associated with left ventricular failure should be initially managed with an angiotensin converting enzyme inhibitor.[59] Left ventricular failure remains the only indication for the use of digoxin in patients with right heart failure. Diuretics may be prescribed for symptomatic relief of peripheral edema of patients with right heart failure, but the most important therapy for right heart failure is oxygen, because long-term use of pulmonary vasodilators have not been shown to be of benefit among outpatients.[81]

Considerations Upon Admission to the ICU—Prediction of Outcome

The clinician who is considering institution of MV for COPD patients with ARF must weigh the benefits against the risks of this intervention. Institution of MV for acute respiratory failure in patients with COPD is potentially life saving. There is considerable risk of complications, however, including long-term dependence on mechanical ventilation. The decision to institute MV will depend on the physician's estimates of the patient's longevity, functional status, and quality of life after recovery.[82,83] These estimates may be quite inaccurate,[82,84] however, even among those with considerable experience.[82]

As seen in Table 15-2, one-year survival is only 32 to 45% after an episode of ARF requiring MV among patients with COPD.[40-45] There is a subgroup with prolonged survival,[45] however, and accurate identification of that subgroup would be of great benefit to the clinician. The predictors of survival among patients with COPD and acute respiratory failure are:

- Lung function
- Indicators of malnutrition, such as serum albumin
- The capacity of patients to perform activities of daily living

The last predictor is readily available from information obtained from the patient or the family. More sophisticated tests such as pulmonary artery pressures (see Table 15-2) may be helpful in occasional cases, but are seldom available to the clinician at the time that the decision to institute MV must be made.

Accurate identification of patients who are at high risk to remain dependent on MV would also be of benefit. Using physiologic and clinical measures taken after MV is begun to predict success in weaning will not prevent the high risk patient from becoming dependent on MV. Therefore, prediction of weaning must be based on premorbid factors such as lung function or functional status. Hilberman and colleagues prospectively studied 124 patients undergoing cardiac surgery to determine premorbid factors associated with difficulty weaning in the immediate postoperative period. Severity of dyspnea, lung function, and inspiratory mouth pressure were most strongly associated with difficulty weaning.[85] Menzies and co-workers retrospectively surveyed 95 patients requiring MV for ARF. Failure to be weaned from MV was significantly associated with lower lung function, serum albumin less than 3 g/dl, and severely impaired activities of daily living as seen in Table 15-3. Of 54 patients who were housebound, 37 (67%) were weaned compared to 36 of 41 patients (88%) who regularly got out of their homes.[45] Use of one factor to predict likely outcome may provide a reasonable estimate, but use of two factors should improve the precision.

Although using 4 or 5 factors would improve the accuracy of estimation of likely outcome, it is conceptually and practically impossible.[84] Predictive models developed using logistic regression can provide a mathematical estimate of the likelihood of outcome.[45,82] Such models were formulated by Menzies and colleagues,[45] but have not yet been validated by application in a prospective manner to a different population. Use of the premorbid characteristics such as lung function, evidence of malnutrition, hypercarbia, and the degree of disability can provide a reasonably accurate estimate of outcome. While information derived from these predictive models cannot be relied on absolutely, it would be of use to the clinician, particularly in discussing this difficult decision with patients and their families.

ICU PHASE

Acute Respiratory Insufficiency

Although often in chronic hypercapnic and hypoxemic respiratory failure, individuals with COPD not infrequently require admission to the ICU for assessment and treatment of an acute increase in their level of dyspnea. While the sensation of increased dyspnea is usually accompanied by an increased respiratory rate, the other signs and symptoms characterizing the clinical state will be determined in large part by the etiology of the decompensation, all of which may ultimately lead to respiratory failure and the requirement for mechanical ventilation. Although Table 15-5 suggests several common causes for these acute decompensations, to date, few studies have delineated the frequency with which each presents.

Acute Bronchitis

In their study, Smith and colleagues[86] examined the frequency with which various pathogens are linked etiologically with acute bronchitis—the so-called acute exacerbation—in patients with COPD. Although bacterial pathogens such as H. influenzae and pneumococci have commonly been linked to such acute respiratory infections,[87] these authors failed to confirm such a relationship and were able to document a specific etiologic agent in only 20% of events. Rhinoviruses were the most common pathogen identified. These authors speculated that the etiology of the remaining 40 to 80% of events was due to other viral pathogens such as coronavirus that are difficult to isolate.

Fagon and colleagues[88] have demonstrated using the protected brush technique that up to 50% of episodes of acute exacerbations could not be attributed to bacterial infection. In the remaining 50%, they isolated a variety of pathogens of which haemophilus species, in particular Haemophilus parainfluenzae and Streptococcus pneumoniae, were the most common. They concluded that nearly half the episodes of acute bronchitis in this patient population must be attributable to noninfectious causes or perhaps to nonbacterial infections such as viruses, mycoplasma, and chlamydia.

Hydrostatic Pulmonary Edema

The role that increased lung water plays in worsening the dyspnea in these patients has been the subject of several investigations.[89,90] The most common precipitant of increased lung water, left ventricular dysfunction, has been considered for many years to be associated with chronic pulmonary disease, that dysfunction attributed to decreased arterial oxygen levels, increased amounts of CO_2, and an increased hydrogen ion concentration. Kohama and colleagues[91] found that the degree of left ventricular hypertrophy and fibrosis correlated with that found in the right ventricle suggesting that the same pathologic process affects both ventricles. They attributed these changes to the possible humoral consequences of chronic cor pulmonale such as increased plasma epinephrine levels, chronic hypoxia, arterial acidosis, or hypokalemia secondary to hypoxia induced adrenal stimulation. Although these authors did not examine the cardiac function in their subjects, their findings may in part explain the impairment of left ventricular function as documented in several other studies by systolic-time intervals,[92] two-dimensional echocardiography,[93] and by radionuclide angiography.[94]

Despite these laboratory indices of dysfunction, clinical left-sided failure has been assessed to be quite uncommon in COPD patients. Although Christianson[95] was also able to demonstrate laboratory evidence of abnormal left ventricular function angiographically in 14 of 15 patients with COPD, none of these patients had clinical evidence of left-sided failure, making the clinical import of the abnormal cardiac findings cited earlier unclear.

More important, left ventricular dysfunction has been found, even in the setting of acute COPD decompensation to be uncommon. Steele and colleagues[96] assessed left ventricular ejection fractions in 92 such patients and found that only 20% had ejection fractions of less than 40%, of whom 60% were noted to have evidence of coronary artery disease.

Even in the absence of left ventricular dysfunction, lung water may still be elevated in an acute exacerbation. The

Table 15-5. Causes of Increasing Shortness of Breath in Patients With COPD

Acute bronchitis
Hydrostatic pulmonary edema
Thromboembolic disease
Pneumonia
Pneumothorax
Pharmacologic agents
    Inappropriate uses, e.g., beta blockers
    Poor compliance

Table 15-6. Factors Responsible for Promoting Increased Lung Water in an Acute Exacerbation of COPD

Markedly negative intrapleural pressures
Increased venous return
Increased left ventricular afterload
Decreased left ventricular compliance

---

markedly negative intrapleural pressure (e.g., -80 cm H_2O) generated by the patient may significantly lower the perivascular interstitial fluid pressure, thereby facilitating, by virtue of the Starling forces, the egress of fluid from the alveolar capillaries into the interstitium.[97] Additional factors that enhance this egress of fluid are listed in Table 15-6 and are depicted graphically in Figure 15-7.

Because of the severe pulmonary arterial hypertension that is often a feature of the advanced COPD patient, right-sided cardiac pressures are often found to be elevated. Although unlikely in and of themselves to induce pulmonary edema, these increased pressures may severely limit the clearance of already established pulmonary edema. In a series of animal studies Allen, Laine, and colleagues[98,99] demonstrated that by raising right-sided pressures both cardiogenic and endotoxic-induced increases in lung water could be significantly worsened.

Therefore, while clinically relevant left ventricular failure has been reported to be unusual in the setting of the acute decompensation of COPD, the role of lung water in that worsening has yet to be clearly delineated. Although no consensus exists, several authors[100] have suggested that diuretics may be used in these patients judiciously and in a controlled setting (see later).

Thromboembolic Disease

At postmortem, significant pulmonary thromboembolic disease has been found in up to 50% of individuals with COPD.[101] Although these patients would appear at high risk given the venous stasis that accompanies their elevated right-sided cardiac pressures such a relationship has been difficult to document clinically. Prescott and colleagues[102] found the presence of deep vein thromboses, a suggested marker of pulmonary embolism, in only 2 of 45 patients (4%). They concluded that pulmonary embolism is an unusual cause of decompensation in this patient population. This conclusion, however, may be premature because others have found a poor correlation between the presence of deep vein thromboses and pulmonary emboli.[103] Therefore, when pulmonary embolism is clinically suspected a direct assessment of the pulmonary vascular tree is essential.

Although severely limited in its application in this patient population given the underlying pulmonary vascular pathology, the ventilation-perfusion (V/Q) scan should represent the first step in visualizing the pulmonary vascular tree in the off chance that a completely normal or high probability result is obtained. More realistically, the results of this scan are used in guiding the angiographer to the pulmonary vascular tree which is most highly suspected. This is suggested given the reported mortality in patients with pulmonary arterial hypertension undergoing main pulmonary arterial trunk contrast injections[104] and the recent report[105] in which 67 patients with severe pulmonary hypertension underwent selective angiography without any significant complications or mortality. Such selective injections assume an even greater importance in the COPD patient in whom visualization of small distal vessels are essential.

Pneumonia

As with the other causes of increased dyspnea in this population, neither the incidence of pneumonia nor the etiologic agents responsible have been elucidated. It must be remembered, however, that while these patients often present with the usual clinical and radiologic findings of pneumonia caused by the usual community acquired etiologic agents the long-term use of systemic steroids in this population may firstly inhibit a febrile response and in combination with their frequent hospitalizations may make them at risk for opportunistic infections as has been recently reported.[106]

Pneumothorax

The incidence of pneumothorax precipitating an acute decompensation as been studied. Dines reviewed 22,000 patients at the Mayo Clinic and found that only 57 patients (0.4%) suffered a total of 95 episodes of pneumothorax.[107] These findings suggest that while this diagnosis must always be sought with, for example, inspiratory and expiratory chest radiographs, it is indeed a rare cause of increased shortness of breath in these patients.

Drugs

Although increased breathlessness in this patient population has been clearly linked to the injudicious use of oral beta blockers, such a relationship has not been commonly appreciated to exist between the use of topical beta blockers and increased dyspnea.[108] To that extent, beta-1-selective topical medications should be used in these patients.

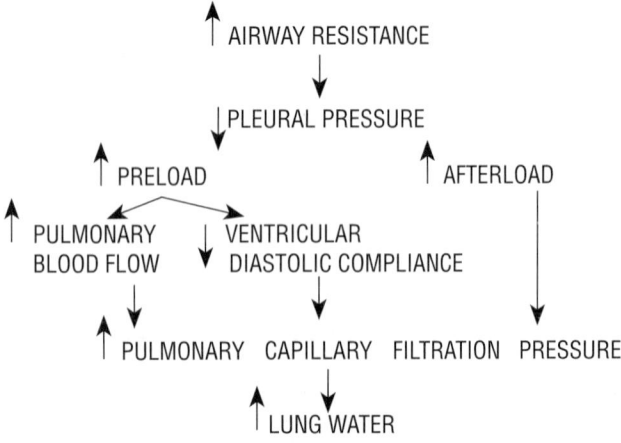

Fig. 15-7. Schematic illustration of factors contributing to increased lung water in COPD exacerbation.

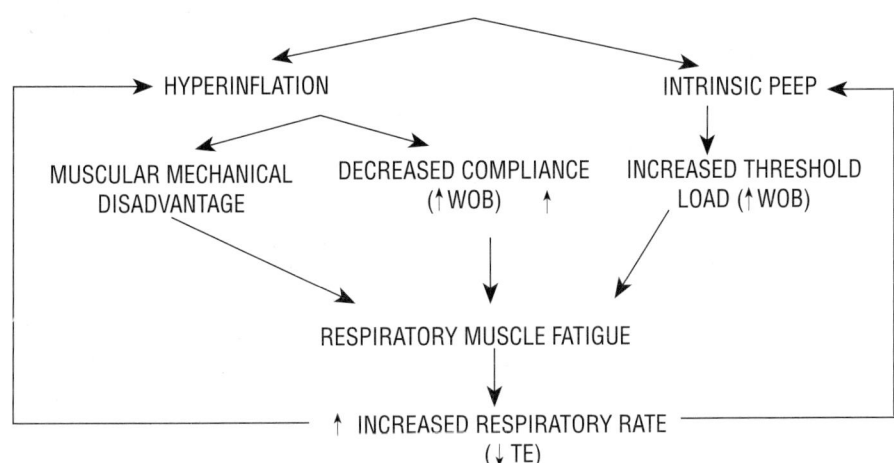

Fig. 15–8. Schematic illustration of the pathophysiology of acute respiratory failure and the link between increased airway resistance and respiratory muscle fatigue. (WOB = Work of breathing; TE = Expiratory Time)

Pathophysiology of Respiratory Failure

As outlined in Figure 15–8, the initiating event, whatever it may be, in an episode of increased dyspnea in the patient with COPD is accompanied by an increase in the work of breathing whether that increase represents an elastic or resistive load. For the purposes of the following discussion it will be assumed that the patient is suffering an episode of acute bronchitis in which airway edema, increased purulent secretions, and increased smooth muscle tone all lead to an increased resistive load. Furthermore, the delayed emptying of gas exchange units results in both hyperinfection and the generation of intrinsic PEEP (PEEPi). These events lead, on the one hand, to the placing of the diaphragm at mechanical disadvantage (shortening of the muscle) while at the same time placing increased elastic, resistive, and threshold loads on those disadvantaged muscles.

Hyperinflation, whatever its genesis, imposes several critical constraints on the respiratory muscles and, in particular, the diaphragm, the principal muscle of inspiration.[109] That muscle, like other skeletal muscles, operates along a length-tension curve that describes a relationship between the resting length of the muscle and the tension it is able to generate for a given degree of stimulation (Fig. 15–9). When hyperinflation and diaphragmatic shortening ensues, the diaphragm, forced downward and to the left (Fig. 15–9), is placed at mechanical disadvantage in that for a given degree of stimulation lesser amounts of tension can be generated.[110,111] Although there is evidence that chronic hyperinflation may lead to diaphragmatic adaptation,[112] it is certainly not an issue in the acute setting.

For the diaphragm to act as an efficient muscle of inspiration it must be capable of converting the tension it is able to develop into pressure; this conversion will be determined by the radius of the muscle as articulated mathematically by the Laplace law (Pressure = 2 × Tension/Radius). When flattened, as occurs in the hyperinflation of COPD, the radius of the diaphragm approaches infinity implying that the diaphragm can no longer effectively convert tension to pressure.[113]

In normal subjects, when the diaphragm contracts, the increased abdominal pressure is transmitted to the thorax via the zone of apposition thereby facilitating rib cage expansion.[114] This zone refers to that region of contiguity between the costal diaphragm and the lateral chest wall. With hyperinflation and diaphragmatic shortening the diaphragm is pulled away from the chest wall thereby diminishing their contact. Finally, at the extremes of hyperinflation, both the intercostal muscles and diaphragm may be actually converted to an expiratory role.[115]

While the inspiratory muscles may be severely compromised the work imposed upon them may be increased several-fold. In the example of acute bronchitis, the implications of an increased resistive load are instinctively appreciated. By virtue of the accompanying hyperinflation,

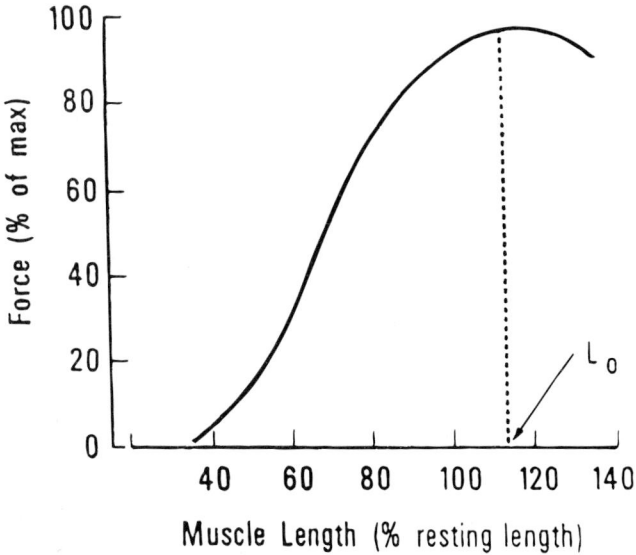

Fig. 15–9. The relationship between muscle length and the percentage of maximal force generated by that muscle. (From Goldberg, P., and Roussos, C.: The assessment of respiratory muscle chronic dysfunction in chronic obstructive lung disease. Med. Clin. North Am., 74:643, 1990.)

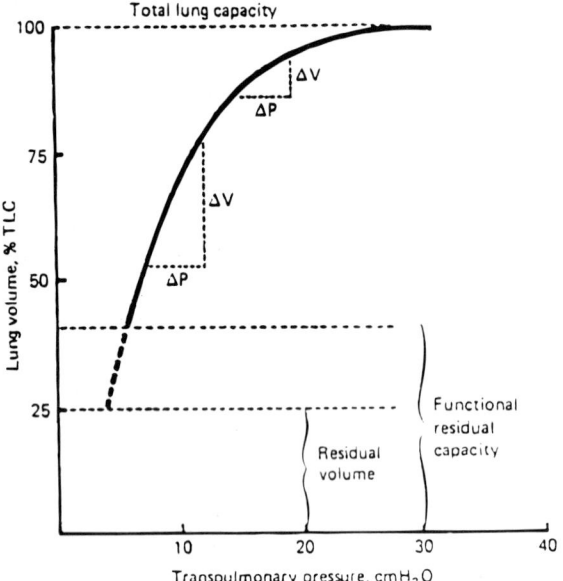

Fig. 15-10. Pressure-volume curve of the lung. The compliance is greater at low lung volumes than at high lung volumes. Therefore, when hyperinflation occurs, as in the setting of an acute exacerbation of COPD, the lung becomes increasingly difficult to inflate, as it sends up to and the right along its compliance curve. This additional elastic load increases the work of breathing in this condition. (From Altose, M.: Pulmonary mechanics. In Pulmonary Diseases and Disorders. 2nd Ed. Edited by A. T. Fishman. New York, McGraw-Hill, 1988, p. 173.)

however, the lung is less compliant, having moved upward and to the right along its compliance curve (Fig. 15-10). This change implies that for a given volume displacement (tidal volume) the individual must generate greater transpulmonary pressures (i.e., must increase the work of breathing).

Over the last several years the concept of PEEPi has received increasing attention by several authors, including Pepe[116] and Rossi and colleagues.[117] In brief, this concept suggests that because of the long time constants (resistance [R] × Compliance [C]) for alveolar emptying implicit in patients with COPD, the respiratory system fails to reach its resting equilibrium at end-expiration such that the elastic recoil of the respiratory system continued to be positive. This implies that before any flow into the lungs is permitted that positive elastic recoil must be first overcome, making PEEPi a threshold load. In ambulatory patients with COPD, Rossi[118] noted an average PEEPi of approximately 2.5 cm H_2O, whereas Murciano and colleagues[119] discovered an average PEEPi of 10 cm H_2O in COPD patients experiencing an exacerbation of their disease.

Respiratory muscle fatigue which has been defined as "a condition in which there is loss in the capacity for developing force and/or velocity by a muscle in response to a load and that is reversible by rest"[120] will occur theoretically whenever energy demands outstrip energy supply.[114] Clearly, the events set in motion during an acute exacerbation of COPD would appear to favor such an eventuality.

It must be cautioned, however, that although inspiratory muscle fatigue can be clearly induced in the laboratory setting[121] its role in hypercapnic respiratory failure has yet to be defined as a clinical entity.[120]

In just such an attempt, Cohen and colleagues[122] correlated the electromyographic (EMG) indices of diaphragmatic fatigue with simultaneously observed clinical signs. They suggested a characteristic sequence of events which are heralded by and follow the onset of EMG-defined fatigue (Table 15-7). The first clinical manifestation is an increase in respiratory rate which is followed by abdominal paradoxic breathing movements (inward abdominal displacement during inspiration) which may or may not be accompanied by respiratory alternans (the variation from breath to breath of rib cage and abdominal contribution to tidal volume). Increasing hypercapnia and worsening respiratory acidosis may accompany the discoordinate respiratory movements but severe acidemia is usually a late manifestation. The onset of bradypnea (a slowing respiratory rate) and decreased minute ventilation appear late in the course of inspiratory muscle fatigue and indicate imminent respiratory arrest.

Although more recent work has called into question the relationship between thoracoabdominal abnormal movements (THAM) and inspiratory muscle fatigue,[123] there appears a consensus that whatever the pathophysiology patients encountering high respiratory loads adopt a breathing pattern characterized by rapid and shallow breaths.[124] Once the patient adopts a pattern of rapid, shallow breathing, the vicious downward cycle outlined in Figure 15-8 is complete. That is, the amount of intrinsic PEEP which must be overcome is dependent not only on the length of the time constants but also on the time within the respiratory cycle available for expiration (Te). With the adoption of a rapid respiratory rate, and a decreasing time available for expiration, the amount of PEEPi will gradually increase, thereby making each successive breath more difficult. As Figure 15-8 suggests, such a pattern of breathing may be pursued to ultimately result in ventilatory failure. Therapy, therefore, must be directed at different points along that pathway thereby interrupting the downward spiral.

Therapeutic Intervention

Pharmacotherapy

As outlined previously, the acute onset of increased dyspnea in a patient with COPD has diverse etiologies and as such therapy must be so tailored. As mentioned earlier, it

Table 15-7. Proposed Clinical Correlates of Inspiratory Muscle Fatigue (in Order of Appearance)

Increased respiratory rate
Thoracoabdominal abnormal movements
    Respiratory alternates
    Paradoxic respiration
Respiratory acidosis
Decreased respiratory rate

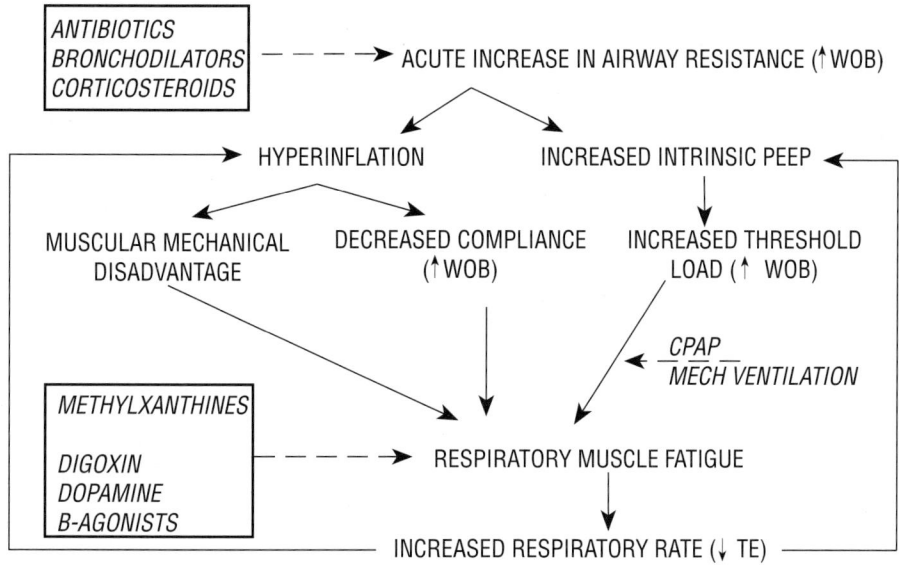

Fig. 15-11. Approach to treatment based on the pathophysiology of respiratory failure.

is assumed for the purposes of this discussion that the worsening dyspnea is secondary to an episode of acute bronchitis. Figure 15-11 outlines schematically where the various therapeutic agents are believed to intervene and inhibit the generation of respiratory muscle fatigue and ventilatory failure.

The proposed mechanisms of action of the individual drugs have been outlined in the pre-ICU section; Table 15-8 lists these agents and suggested dosing schemes.

While the commonly encountered signs and symptoms of theophylline toxicity are listed in Table 15-9 it must be remembered that many of them, notably the onset of multifocal atrial tachycardia, may appear while the theophylline level is still well within the suggested therapeutic range of 10 to 20 μg/ml.[125] Moreover, while the most dreaded potential toxicity—grand mal seizures—has not been associated with drug levels still within the therapeutic range, it has, nevertheless, been associated with only minimal (25 μg/ml) elevations.[61]

While the loading dose is dependent only on its previous (within 24 hours) use and volume of distribution, the maintenance dose range suggested in Table 15-8 is highly dependent on the variables listed in Table 15-10. This latter table describes the host variables and drug interactions that are thought to influence the hepatic metabolism of this drug which have led to wide and unpredictable intersubject variability in serum levels. As such, and because of the narrow toxic to therapeutic ratio of this drug alluded to previously, close monitoring of serum levels are absolutely essential if this agent is to be used. Whereas the maintenance dosing schedule (Table 15-8) should be used as an initial guide, blood levels drawn 6 hours after the initiation of that maintenance dose should be used to determine further therapy.[125]

Whereas the cardiovascular and central nervous system manifestations of theophylline toxicity have been well characterized, the metabolic consequences have not. Kear-

Table 15-8. Suggested Guidelines for Drug Therapy in an Acute Exacerbation of COPD

First Line Therapy
    Beta agonists, e.g., Salbutamol aerosol 2.5-5 mg q 20 minutes or MDI 0.4 mg q 20 minutes to response or to toxicity;
    and/or
    Anticholinergics, e.g., Ipratropium bromide aerosol 500 μg q 4-6 hours or MDI 200 μg q 4-6 hours;
    and
    Corticosteroids, e.g., methylprednisolone 0.5 mg/kg q 6 hours;
    and
    Antibiotics, e.g., Trimethoprim–sulfamethoxazole 160/80 mg bid
    Amoxicillin 0.25 g qid
    Deoxycycline 0.1 g q day

Second Line Therapy
    Theophylline
    Loading Dose: In the absence of theophylline therapy within the preceding 24 hours; 5 mg/kg ideal body weight/30 minutes;
    otherwise
    Maintenance: 2.5 mg/kg ideal body weight/30 minutes; 0.2-0.7 mg/kg/hr (see text for details)

Table 15-9. Adverse Reactions to Theophylline

System	Adverse Effect(s)
Gastrointestinal	Nausea, vomiting, epigastric pain, hematemesis, diarrhea.
Central nervous system	Headaches, irritability, restlessness, insomnia, reflex hyperexcitability, muscle twitching, clonic and tonic generalized convulsions.
Cardiovascular	Palpitations, tachycardia, extrasystoles, flushing, hypotension, circulatory failure.
Respiratory	Tachypnea
Renal	Potentiation of diuresis, albuminuria, increased excretion of renal tubular cells and red blood cells.
Other	Hyperglycemia, syndrome of inappropriate antidiuretic hormone secretion.

(From Miech, R.P., and Stein, M.: Methylxanthines Clin. Chest Med., 7: 331, 1986.)

Table 15-10. Factors Affecting Theophylline Clearance

Increased Theophylline Clearance—Decreased Levels
  Cigarette smoking
  High protein/low carbohydrate diet
  Charcoal broiled diet
  Drugs
    Phenobarbital
    Phenytoin
    Carbamazepine
    Rifampim
Decreased Theophylline Clearance—Increased Levels
  Hepatic cirrhosis
  Cor pulmonale
  Congestive heart failure
  Drugs
    Propranolol
    Allopurinol (> 600 mg/day)
    Erythromycin
    Cimetidine
    Oral contraceptives
    Troleandomycin

(From Seligman, M.: Bronchodilators. In The Pharmacologic Approach to the Critically Ill Patient. Edited by B. Chernow. Baltimore, Williams & Wilkins, 1988, p. 927).

ney and colleagues[42] implicated the beta-adrenergic system in the generation of the hypokalemia, hypophosphatemia, hyperglycemia, metabolic acidosis, and hypotension associated with toxic levels of theophylline in that these effects could be reversed or blunted by beta blockade. Similarly, McPherson and co-workers[127] were able to document an association between hypercalcemia and theophylline—both toxic and therapeutic levels—the latter reversed by propranolol. These two latter studies, while not examining the issue directly, to raise the question of the utility of beta-blockade in the management of theophylline toxicity.

There has been to date no data in this patient population comparing the efficacy of parenteral beta-agonists to aerosol administration. This issue has been addressed in the setting of severe asthma, and while there is no clear consensus on this issue, the majority of reports have documented no additional benefit of intravenously administered beta-agonists when compared to aerosol administration.[128-130] One study has, however, reported such a benefit[131] and another has suggested a potentially additive effect of inhaled and systemic beta-agonists.[132]

The toxicity associated with beta-agonist therapy—tachycardia, tremor, and nervousness—is a function, primarily, of its dose and secondarily, of its mode of administration—systemic administration resulting in more side effects than its aerosolized form.[129,132] Walters and colleagues[133] have reported both a dose-related bronchodilator response and dose-related toxicity demonstrating that while an aerosol dose of 3.0 mg is not as efficacious as 7.5 mg, the side effects associated with the latter dose are quite troublesome. They concluded, however, that the highest tolerated dose of salbutamol should be given.

As with theophylline, salbutamol results in a decrease in serum potassium, the result of its effect on the beta-2-receptor linked to the sodium-potassium ATPase in skeletal muscle.[134] Indeed, a recent study[135] has exploited this relationship by demonstrating the utility of aerosolized salbutamol in the treatment of renal failure associated hyperkalemia. Other potential side effects include hypotension[51]—through unopposed beta-2-agonist-induced vasodilatation—and worsening hypoxemia,[53] the latter attributed to the inhibition of ventilation-perfusion matching mechanisms by the nonspecific pulmonary vasodilatory effects of salbutamol.

Ipratropium bromide, a quaternary amine, has virtually no systemic absorption and as such is nearly completely free of any systemic side effects, most notably on the volume and viscoelastic properties of the mucus, and on pupillary and urinary sphincter function.[54] Despite early concerns, no local ill effects on mucociliary clearance have been demonstrated even when the drug has been administered in large doses and over prolonged periods.[54] Finally, there have been a few reports[136] documenting paradoxic bronchoconstriction to aerosolized ipratropium, a response attributed to the bromine constituent of the drug.

A review of the varied toxicities attributed to high dose corticosteroid therapy is beyond the scope of this chapter. Note, however, should be made of the hyperglycemia and fluid retention commonly induced by these agents and of the less frequently encountered episodes of psychosis, all of which may greatly complicate the care of these patients. High dose steroid therapy, in this patient population, has been associated both with the development of opportunistic infections[106] and inspiratory muscle myopathy,[137] the latter leading to difficulty in weaning from mechanical ventilation. In view of these potential toxicities and given that the study supporting their use in this setting has been challenged as statistically flawed[138] steroids should be used for defined and limited periods, for example, 2 to 3 weeks.

Oxygen Therapy

Given that its administration may lead to the retention of CO_2 in this patient population, oxygen must be administered in a rigorously controlled fashion in the setting of an acute decompensation. While the mechanism of CO_2 retention can no longer be attributed to the diminution of hypoxic drive, the rise in P_{CO_2} in response to the administration of high concentrations of oxygen is no less real. This rise is due mainly to an oxygen-induced increase in the inhomogeneity of V/Q distributions within the lung.[139] In this context the use of controlled amounts of oxygen, for example, by the use of a Venturi mask, is stressed as opposed to the use of low flow uncontrolled oxygen, as for example, by nasal cannulae. Although the former method will deliver, at the most, the preset amount of oxygen, the concentration of the latter is extremely variable and dependent on the patient's inspiratory flow[140] and has the potential for delivering an oxygen concentration of 100%. A reasonable approach, therefore, would be to prescribe the least amount of oxygen able to achieve an arterial P_{O_2} of 60 mm Hg (saturation 90%).

Although care must be exercised when oxygen is administered, the fear of inducing increasing levels of CO_2 should never be used as the premise for withholding adequate amounts of administered oxygen. Paramount to the care of any critically ill patient is the assurance that adequate amounts of oxygen be delivered to the tissues, a goal which demands, in part, that adequate amounts of exogenous oxygen be administered to ensure sufficient hemoglobin saturation. If adequate oxygenation necessitates a dangerous rise in CO_2, then mechanical ventilation may have to be instituted, as discussed later in this chapter.

A major thrust of therapy in the treatment of an acute decompensation of COPD is the reversal of the acute increase in pulmonary arterial hypertension and the support for an acutely stressed and overloaded right ventricle. Although it has been thought that the precipitant for increased pulmonary arterial pressure was the accompanying hypoxemia and acidemia,[141] Degaute and colleagues failed to demonstrate a reversal of this hypertension during the short-term administration of oxygen to a group of patients with acutely decompensated COPD.[142] This unexpected finding appears to challenge the accepted hypothesis that has been advanced to explain the development of pulmonary arterial hypertension and has been further supported by the results of a more long-term study by Morrison and co-workers[143] who examined the effects of 1 month of continuous low flow oxygen on hemodynamics. These authors found that whereas oxygen administration improved right ventricular ejection fraction, cardiac output, and oxygen delivery there was no appreciable change in pulmonary arterial pressure which suggests that the improvement attributed to the oxygen was on the basis of tissue delivery (i.e., oxygen delivery to the myocardium and enhanced myocardial contractility), rather than on a decrease in the afterload to right ventricular ejection. Whatever the mechanism, however, oxygen administration, in a controlled manner as outlined previously, constitutes an appropriate first-line therapeutic approach in this setting.

Diaphragmatic Inotropic Agents

Much has been written about the pharmacologic enhancement of inspiratory, particularly diaphragmatic, contractility in this patient population. Aubier and co-workers,[60] studying normal subjects, were the first to explore the relationship between theophylline and diaphragmatic contractility. Since that time, several studies[144,145] have reported that therapeutic levels of theophylline both increase contractility and prevent and reverse the onset of diaphragmatic fatigue in several populations, including that with COPD. While the mechanism of action has yet to be clearly delineated, transcellular calcium flux has been implicated, a concept supported by the finding[144] that verapamil, a calcium-channel blocking agent reverses the theophylline-induced potentiation of diaphragmatic contractility.

In addition to theophylline, other pharmacologic agents have been investigated as to their effect on diaphragmatic performance. Aubier and colleagues[146] reported that therapeutic levels of digoxin augmented transdiaphragmatic pressure by approximately 20% in a population of COPD patients during acute respiratory failure. These same authors have also reported[147] that the beta agonist terbutaline, while having no effect on the fresh diaphragm, significantly increased its contractility when fatigued, an effect completely abolished by beta-blockade. Finally, the administration of dopamine to a group of COPD patients in acute respiratory failure was shown to enhance diaphragmatic contractility by approximately 30%, the same amount by which blood flow to that muscle had been increased.[148]

Notwithstanding these reports, the clinical utility of theophylline in this population setting has yet to be defined. Previous studies[57] that have examined its role in the acutely decompensated COPD patient have used spirometric indices as the primary end point. To appropriately answer this question, however, it will be necessary, for example, to determine whether the administration of this drug will decrease the need for mechanical ventilation. At this time, its use even within our own institution is controversial.

Ventilatory Support

Continuous Positive Airway Pressure

As noted previously, during the past several years the concept of intrinsic PEEP (PEEPi) and its role in the genesis of acute respiratory failure in this patient population has received increasing attention. Both Simkovitz and colleagues[149] and Smith and Marini[150] have shown that the addition of extrinsic PEEP (PEEPe) to COPD patients with PEEPi did not result in hyperinflation as long as the amount applied extrinsically was less than the amount of PEEPi. Indeed, both these groups have shown that by increasing the amount of external PEEP the amount of PEEPi decreases, the former counterbalancing the latter. The implications of these findings suggested that the administration of extrinsic PEEP through a continuous positive airway pressure (CPAP) circuit would decrease the work of breathing by diminishing the amount of PEEPi. This hypothesis has been tested in two different settings.

Petroff and colleagues[151] examined the effects of CPAP on COPD patients undergoing weaning from mechanical ventilation. They demonstrated that the addition of CPAP resulted in a statistically significant decrease in the work of breathing and in the pressure-time products (the latter a reflection of the metabolic cost of muscle contraction) for both the inspiratory muscles and for the diaphragm.

This same group, therefore, investigated whether CPAP applied noninvasively to a patient experiencing an acute exacerbation of COPD could successfully delay or prevent the need for invasive mechanical ventilation by decreasing the work of breathing thereby permitting adequate time for drug therapy. In a preliminary report, Goldberg and colleagues[152] demonstrated that the application of both 5 and 7.5 cm H_2O of CPAP effected a significant decrease in tidal excursion of esophageal pressure and significantly diminished the pressure-time integral of the inspiratory muscles (the latter a measure of the oxygen cost of muscle metabolism). In addition, application of CPAP tended to improve breathing pattern, maintain minute volume constant, and decrease P_{CO_2}. The clinical implications of this study are clear but whether such a therapeutic approach can ultimately diminish the need for invasive mechanical ventilation must, however, await further studies.

Virtually all COPD patients suffering from worsening dyspnea, except perhaps those patients with pneumothorax, are candidates for CPAP trial. The only absolute contraindication is a decrease in the level of consciousness and the presence of bradypnea (<RR 12/minute). And while not a contraindication, the expectoration of copious amounts of sputum and the need, therefore, for the recurrent removal of the mask will make this therapeutic approach difficult to implement.

Noninvasive Mechanical Ventilation

Several years ago, Ellis and colleagues[153] demonstrated the successful use of noninvasive positive-pressure mechanical ventilation in a group of neuromuscular patients. Since that time several groups have reported a similar experience with the use of cycling nasal or full-face ventilation in the treatment of a COPD exacerbation, in one such study over a period of days.[154]

No clear cut guidelines can be used in deciding whether to initiate CPAP or noninvasive mechanical ventilation. They are interchangeable in many respects. Whereas a depressed level of consciousness and bradypnea are both contraindications to the former, noninvasive ventilation can still be effectively implemented in this setting. Although presently used almost routinely in our ICU, attention must be addressed to the dangers of facial tissue necrosis that may ensue secondary to the high pressure at the mask-skin interface. To this end, the mask is removed every 2 hours for a period of approximately 20 minutes.

Because of the danger of gastric distension and its implications for gastric content aspiration and for worsening thoracic compliance, it is imperative that all patients, regardless of the method of ventilatory support (CPAP, noninvasive and invasive mechanical ventilation) have a nasogastric tube placed for gastric decompression.

As in the case of CPAP, the presence of copious amounts of thick secretions also makes the application of noninvasive mechanical ventilation problematic. It has been our experience that the repeated necessity to remove the mask to allow expectoration and/or the inability of the patient to raise secretions on his or her own has ultimately led us to abandon this approach in favor of intubation and ventilation.

Intubation and Mechanical Ventilation

There is no consensus as to when mechanical ventilation, of whatever form, should be initiated. When it can be applied noninvasively as described previously, the issue becomes less critical. When intubation, with its physical and psychological implications is a prerequisite, however, then this issue assumes an added importance. Most would agree that a depressed level of consciousness with the inability to control the airway constitutes such an indication. Another relative indication, as alluded to earlier, is to permit adequate tracheal toilet when the patient is unable to expectorate secretions adequately.

A more contentious indication is the presence of circulatory shock, whatever the latter's cause. In a provocative study several years ago, Aubier and colleagues[155] demonstrated that the institution of ventilatory support in dogs rendered hypotensive prevented their ventilatory deaths as compared to the respiratory failure and death in all the animals which were permitted to breathe spontaneously. Moreover, blood flow studies performed in those animals demonstrated that the mechanical ventilatory support permitted the redistribution of blood flow away from the inspiratory muscles in favor of other critical organ systems.

Arterial blood gas abnormalities in and of themselves are rarely an indication for mechanical ventilation. As in the non-COPD population the need for adequate oxygenation alone is an unusual indication for mechanical support. Nor is an increased level of CO_2 by itself an indication for mechanical ventilation, certainly not when the blood pH is greater than 7.30. Similarly, the critical level of pH at which mechanical ventilation should be instituted is unclear. In making that decision in the absence of clear guidelines, the clinician must weigh the impact of the adverse effects of the raised CO_2—its effect, for instance on diaphragmatic contractility,[156] and its effect on electrolyte movement—against the costs of an invasive intubation and against the likelihood of a quick resolution of the hypercapnia. Most authorities would probably agree that a respiratory acidosis of pH less than 7.2 without any realistic expectation for a rapid reversal of that trend would justify ventilatory support whatever its mode.

Probably as accurate and certainly a far earlier indicator of the need for the institution of mechanical ventilation, however, is the patient's respiratory mechanics and, in particular, the respiratory rate and tidal volume. Although the role of inspiratory muscle fatigue has yet to be defined as a clinical entity, the study by Cohen and co-workers,[122] referred to previously, described tachypnea as the earliest clinical manifestation of inspiratory muscle fatigue. As discussed in more detail later (see under weaning), several authors[124,157] have pointed to these two variables as accurate predictive indices of weaning failure. Moreover, from a theoretic point of view, if the foregoing schema outlining the pathophysiology of respiratory failure in this patient population is accurate, then the adverse implications of a rapid respiratory rate are immediately apparent. It has therefore become routine at our institutions to seriously consider intubation for those patients with a respiratory rate of greater than 35 per minute regardless of the arterial blood gases; we keep in mind that the earliest arterial blood gas manifestation of inspiratory muscle fatigue may be hypocapnia and respiratory alkalosis.[122]

As noted earlier, the physiologic implication of disordered thoracoabdominal movements is yet to be determined. At the present time, patients with such disordered breathing are observed closely in a constant care area, but in the absence of a pattern of rapid, shallow breathing, these movements, by themselves, are rarely an indication for mechanical support (Table 15-11).

Table 15–11. Indications for Intubation and Mechanical Ventilation

---
Depressed level of consciousness
Circulatory shock
Respiratory rate > 35/min
Respiratory acidosis—pH < 7.2
Copious amounts of tracheobronchial secretions

Maintenance of Hemodynamic Status

Assessment

The primary hemodynamic derangement in COPD is pulmonary arterial hypertension (PAH) and impedance to right ventricular outflow which results from both the anatomic destruction of the pulmonary vascular bed and from alveolar hypoxia-induced reflex vasoconstriction. Indeed, Weitzenblum and colleagues[158] have shown that while there is a tentative relationship between the fall in FEV_1 and the development of pulmonary hypertension there is a much stronger correlation between the latter's development and the onset of hypoxemia and hypercapnia. While there may be quite modest progression of the pulmonary hypertension in the stable COPD patient (approximately 0.56 mm Hg/year) this is in sharp contrast to the marked and sudden increases in pulmonary arterial pressures that occur in the setting of acute respiratory failure.[159] These changes, however, most often abate with the resolution of the acute event.[160]

At the beginning of this century, Bernheim was the first to suggest that the overloaded left ventricle could adversely affect the function of the right ventricle by rightward deviation of the interventricular septum.[161] Since then, a variety of authors have confirmed the interrelationship between the two ventricles; a relationship that is a function of common muscle fibers, a shared deformable interventricular septum, and the pericardium. This concept suggests that as the volume of one ventricle is increased, the resulting increased pressure in that ventricle is transmitted to the other resulting in either an increase in latter's filling pressure, a decrease in the latter's filling volume, or a combination of the two.[161]

In the setting of acute respiratory failure, the right ventricle may acutely distend in its attempt to overcome the marked increase in its afterload.[162] As such, the hemodynamic assessment may reveal not only an elevated right atrial pressure (RA = CVP) but, in addition, an elevated pulmonary capillary wedge pressure (PCWP = "wedge" pressure). In this setting the elevated "wedge" pressure would in no way reflect intrinsically impaired left ventricular function but rather would be reflective of a decreased left ventricular compliance, the latter a result of a right-sided circulatory event. Therapy, therefore, aimed at lowering the high "wedge" pressure would not only be misdirected but may well be deleterious (see later).

Two other considerations, besides left ventricular dysfunction, may explain the finding of an elevated PCWP. Pepe and Marini[116] were the first to draw attention to the concept that intrinsic positive end-expiratory pressure (PEEPi), by increasing end-expiratory intrathoracic and juxtacardiac pressures could effect an increase in the measurement of PCWP. Other authors[119,163] reported that the COPD patient experiencing an acute decompensation may develop up to 22 cm H_2O of PEEPi. Clearly, such high levels of PEEPi may have a significant impact on the measurement of vascular pressures. The extent of that impact depends on the degree to which those airway pressures are transmitted to the juxtacardiac space which is, in turn, dependent on the compliance of the lung and chest wall.

Butler and colleagues[164] have hypothesized that the elevated wedge pressure during exercise in the COPD patient could be attributed to lower lobe gas trapping, hyperinflation, and direct compression of the cardiac fossa; moreover, such an increase in pressure, unlike that associated with PEEPi, would escape detection in the clinical setting because the strictly localized increase in juxtacardiac pressure would not be reflected by an increase in esophageal (pleural) pressure. These authors reported that hyperventilation alone to a rate of 28 +/− 11 breaths per minute, in the absence of exercise, resulted in a rise in the wedge pressure by 2 +/− 3 mm Hg. If it is accepted, as suggested earlier, that the patient with COPD in acute respiratory failure, adopts a pattern of rapid, shallow breathing then, once again, the finding of an elevated PCWP in this setting may reflect disturbed respiratory mechanics rather than an abnormal left ventricle.

The detection of left ventricular dysfunction in this setting can be very challenging. Elevated jugular venous pressures and peripheral edema denote elevated right-sided pressure quite consistent with pulmonary arterial hypertension alone. Moreover, the auscultatory findings of a gallop rhythm may also be a right-sided event. As in non-COPD critically ill patients, the clinical examination is often unhelpful in determining the presence or absence of an elevated wedge pressure. In one study, only 3 of 20 patients were correctly identified as having an elevated wedge pressure on the basis of the clinical examination.[165] Even when correctly identified, the meaning of a raised PCWP can be quite confusing. Therefore, while the finding of a low to normal "wedge" pressure is helpful the recording of an elevated value is not, and may be misleading. In this setting, we have found the echocardiogram, easily performed at the bedside, to be of inordinate help in sorting out these patients. Although challenging to do in the face of marked hyperinflation, this test can give valuable information about ventricular size, septal deviation, adequacy of contractility, and, in the presence of tricuspid insufficiency, an accurate estimate of pulmonary arterial pressures.

The other hemodynamic hallmark of acute decompensation of COPD is the exaggerated swings of pleural pressures—increasingly negative during inspiration and increasingly positive during expiration, the latter due to positive elastic recoil or PEEPi. Mention has already been made concerning the implications of these changes on lung water and increasing the after-load to left ventricular ejection.

Finally, since the concept was first introduced by Danek and colleagues[166] a decade ago, several authors have described supply dependence of oxygen consumption in a variety of disorders. Such a phenomenon has been recently described by Mohsenifar and colleagues[167] who documented oxygen supply dependent oxygen consumption in COPD patients with pulmonary hypertension. This situation suggests that in this patient population as more oxygen is made available to metabolizing tissues more oxygen will be consumed. Whether the clinician should augment such oxygen delivery to very high levels must await further studies.

Therapy

The tendency to increased lung water has led to the use of diuretics in the treatment of the decompensated COPD patient. Not only would the effects of lung water on gas exchange be minimized, but the worsening compliance and airway resistance which may be attributable to that water may be ameliorated. Moreover, the septal shift caused by volume overload of the right ventricle may be lessened thereby enhancing left ventricular function.[168] Although diuretics may be used judiciously in a controlled setting, their potential side effects in this setting must be realized. First, they may induce a metabolic alkalosis that may further depress respiratory drive, but more important, the increased vascular compliance initially and the later decrease in circulating volume result in a decrease in the mean systemic pressure, so critical in ensuring adequate venous return and hence cardiac output, especially in these patients with high right atrial pressures.[169]

When hypotension is present, volume challenges may be tried. Although many of these patients are edematous on presentation a careful fluid challenge is appropriate in an attempt to augment mean systemic pressures and venous return. The clinician must understand that the response to fluid challenge cannot be accurately predicted, however. In a study, Reuse and co-workers[170] were unable to find any correlation between baseline right atrial pressures and increase in stroke volume in response to a fluid challenge. Conversely, in a preliminary communication, Magder and colleagues[171] were successful in predicting the response to fluid loading by the baseline presence or absence of an inspiratory fall in right atrial pressures. In spite of these observations, fluid therapy is not without its risks. Two groups have reported the paradoxic drop in cardiac output in response to fluid loading presumably on the basis of aggravating interventricular independence, leftward shift of the septum, and further compromise of left ventricular integrity.[170,172]

While there appears to be consensus on the usefulness of phlebotomy in enhancing exercise performance in these patients, no such agreement surrounds its use in the acute setting.[168] This therapy is based on the hypothesis that the increased blood viscosity which may characterize many of these polycythemic patients may further increase impedance to right ventricular outflow. When examined in stable COPD patients at rest this therapeutic approach was found to decrease both pulmonary arterial pressure and oxygen delivery but maintain both cardiac output and, more importantly, oxygen consumption constant.[173] For the present, however, until such time as this approach is examined in the unstable decompensated state, phlebotomy should be reserved for the severely polycythemic patient who is resistant to the usual therapeutic approaches.[168]

Vasodilators. As indicated previously, the hemodynamic hallmark of the decompensated COPD patient is pulmonary arterial hypertension. Given the success of vasodilators on the left side of the circulation these drugs have been investigated for their potential role in this condition. These investigations have been made all the more difficult, however, because the desired end points of this therapy are difficult to articulate. Even if they should fail to decrease pulmonary arterial pressure, vasodilators may still be of clinical benefit if they induce a decrease in pulmonary vascular resistance and increases in cardiac output (hence pulmonary pressures remaining constant) and oxygen delivery. In this regard, Brent[174] reported hydralazine to be superior to both nitroprusside and nitroglycerin despite the finding that the latter two effected a decrease in pulmonary artery pressures while hydralazine did not. The increased benefit attributed to hydralazine is its ability to increase right ventricular ejection fraction, cardiac index, and oxygen delivery whereas the other two agents decreased preload, cardiac index, and oxygen delivery.[174]

A variety of other vasodilators have been similarly studied. Agostoni and colleagues[175] demonstrated that while its beneficial effects dissipated over time (8 weeks), the calcium antagonist nifedipine, in substantial doses (180 mg), could induce pulmonary vascular dilatation in the acute setting. Captopril, an angiotensin converting enzyme inhibitor, was found to decrease pulmonary vascular resistance and PAH while increasing cardiac output and oxygen delivery.[176] The vasodilatory prostaglandin E_1 has been noted to improve hemodynamics in the setting of acute respiratory failure.[177]

In addition to their bronchodilator properties, beta agonists have been shown to induce pulmonary vascular vasodilation. In their study, Brent and colleagues[178] demonstrated that terbutaline, a beta-2-selective agonist effected a decrease in pulmonary vascular resistance while enhancing the cardiac index and oxygen delivery.

Regardless of the choice of vasodilator, it would be appropriate to initiate therapy while assessing the patient's hemodynamic status through the use of a right heart catheter both to allow for an accurate evaluation of their efficacy and, as importantly, to monitor their potentially toxic effects. The two major potential toxicities of these agents are systemic hypotension and worsening hypoxemia, the latter probably through the inhibition of the hypoxic vasoconstriction reflex.[168]

Because of the uncertainty relating to therapeutic goals and concern over possible toxicity, Rubin[179] has offered four guidelines to determine whether vasodilator therapy is successful and should be continued (Table 15-12).

Inotropic Agents. A host of inotropic agents have been tried in this setting. Digitalis, although an appropriate choice in the treatment of left ventricular failure, has no role in right-sided dysfunction.[79,80] While digitalis does improve right ventricular contractility, it also increases pulmonary vascular resistance thus offsetting any potential benefit the drug may offer. While the mechanism may still be unclear patients treated with this agent are at greater risk for the development of cardiac arrhythmias, hypoxia

Table 15-12. Guidelines for the Continued Use of Vasodilators

Reduction in pulmonary vascular resistance > 20%
Cardiac output increased or unchanged
Pulmonary arterial pressure decreased or unchanged
Minimal effect on systemic blood pressure

being the most often cited explanation for this occurrence.[80] Furthermore, Sylvester and co-workers[169] have reported that digitalis increases the unstressed volume of the circulation leading to a decrease in the mean systemic pressure, the effective pressure head for venous return to the right side of the heart which in the absence of appropriate and sufficient reflexes will lead to a fall in cardiac output.

Mention was made earlier to the extrapulmonary effects of theophylline and, in particular, of its inotropic properties. Several studies have demonstrated that this drug can enhance biventricular function both by a direct inotropic effect and indirectly, by decreasing pulmonary vascular resistance.[59]

Over the past several years considerable attention has been focused on the therapeutic benefits of the alpha agonist sympathomimetics such as norepinephrine and phenylephrine. Many authors consider ischemia to be the ultimate determinant of right ventricular failure. This hypothesis suggests that as pulmonary arterial pressure increases, the right ventricle, in its attempt to overcome this increased impedance to its outflow, exploits its Frank-Starling relationship such that right ventricular end-diastolic volumes, and hence end-diastolic pressure, increase.

The right ventricular free wall and a portion of the interventricular septum is perfused by the right coronary artery which arises from the aorta. The perfusion of this coronary artery is critically dependent on the difference between mean aortic pressure and mean right ventricular pressure. While mean right ventricular pressure rises in response to right ventricular dilatation, mean aortic pressure may fall as the output from a failing right ventricle decreases. After the compensatory right coronary vasodilation is overwhelmed, myocardial ischemia ensues, leading to a vicious downward cycle marked by increasing mean right ventricular pressures, decreasing mean aortic pressures, and worsening circulatory failure[180] (Fig. 15-12).

The critical role that right coronary arterial perfusion plays in the genesis of right ventricular dysfunction has been the subject of several investigations. Brooks and co-workers[181] have shown that animals subjected to right coronary occlusion were able to withstand a far lower right ventricular afterload than a cohort with a normal coronary circulation, a failure that could be reversed by reperfusion of that coronary artery. In an experimental model of pulmonary embolism, Spotnitz and colleagues[182] successfully reversed right ventricular failure by occluding the descending aorta and thereby increasing right coronary perfusion pressure. Vlahakes[180] demonstrated that right ventricular failure induced by progressive increases in right ventricular afterload was associated with decreased right ventricular coronary artery driving pressure and free wall blood flow and increased concentrations of the metabolic markers of ischemia. All of these changes could be reversed by the infusion of phenylephrine, presumably through the measured augmentation in right coronary arterial perfusion pressure. Finally, several other authors have reported the successful use of norepinephrine in reversing right ventricular failure induced by an increased afterload.[172,183]

An additional benefit of these alpha-agonist agents is their failure to induce a tachycardia given the latter's negative impact on cardiac oxygen consumption. This is in marked contradistinction to such agents such a dopamine which, at dosages sufficient to result in vasoconstriction, will virtually always induce a sinus tachycardia. To this end, norepinephrine can be infused through a central line (this agent must not be administered peripherally because of the risk of extravasation and tissue necrosis) at a starting rate of 4 μg per minute titrated to response. Dopamine in dopaminergic doses is administered concurrently to counteract the renal arterial vasoconstricting effects of the drug.[184] If phenylephrine is selected, it is started centrally, at a dose of 1 μg/kg per minute and titrated to response.

In summary, oxygen is the drug of first choice both to increase oxygenation and right heart function and thereby to increase oxygen delivery. Simultaneously, beta-agonist therapy is initiated primarily as a bronchodilator but also with a view to its positive impact on cardiac output. In that subgroup of patients who are in frank circulatory shock because of right heart failure a modest fluid challenge would be appropriate which, if unsuccessful, should be followed by an alpha agonist such as norepinephrine or phenylephrine. Vasodilators may be used, under central monitoring guidance, in the presence of both elevated right-sided pressures and systemic hyper or normotension.

Nutrition

Whatever the mechanism or mechanisms, a substantial proportion of patients with COPD are underweight, and not uncommonly cachectic. Patients with emphysema (DLCO <60%) are more malnourished than their bronchitic counterparts (DLCO >80%).[185] In their study of malnourished patients without any pulmonary disorder, Arora and Rochester[186] noted that whereas diaphragm muscle mass was reduced in proportion to reduction in body weight, respiratory muscle strength and endurance as assessed by inspiratory and expiratory mouth pressures and a 12-second maximum minute ventilation were diminished out of proportion to the loss in diaphragm area. This suggested

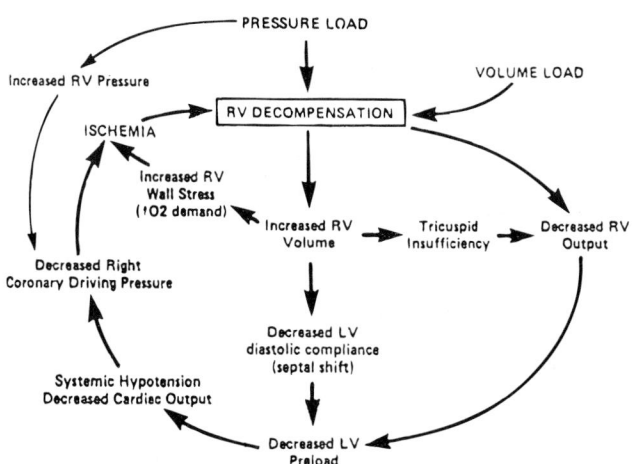

Fig. 15-12. Pathophysiology of acute right ventricular failure: the vicious cycle. (From Weidemann, H., and Mathay, R.: Right ventricular failure. *In* Heart and Lung Interactions in Health and Disease. Edited by S. M. Scharf and S. S. Cassidy. New York, Marcel Dekker, 1989.)

the coexistence of a myopathic process, presumably secondary to the malnutrition.

While it is probable that the mass of the diaphragm is similarly an important determinant of inspiratory muscle strength and endurance in COPD, the effect of COPD on the size of that muscle is unclear. Several authors have reported that diaphragm dimensions are diminished in COPD whereas others have reported muscular hypertrophy, presumably secondary to the chronically increased work of breathing. Rochester and colleagues[187] have suggested that these results may represent two antithetical trends in these patients because the net effect is determined by the amount of weight loss leading to a decreased diaphragm mass on the one hand and hypertrophy on the other hand.

Regardless of the influence of weight loss on diaphragmatic mass and its strength, Rochester and co-workers[188] have reported that in one half the COPD patients they studied inspiratory muscle strength was depressed more than could be accounted for by the length-tension characteristics of the muscle suggesting a superimposed myopathy. In that study, only a minority of these patients was underweight. It is probable, therefore, that while weight loss may contribute to respiratory muscle weakness there are other factors at work such as hypoxemia, hypercapnia, and electrolyte abnormalities that may depress respiratory muscle function.

The role of nutritional repletion on respiratory muscle strength has been studied by several authors. Kelly and colleagues[189] reported that in 59 critically ill patients there was a significant correlation between body cell mass (skeletal muscle) and maximal inspiratory mouth pressures. Of the 29 patients who underwent serial measurements, the 21 patients who increased their body cell mass consequent to parenteral nutrition also increased their mouth pressures while in those eight patients who suffered a fall in body cell mass mouth pressures did not change.

Several groups have studied the impact of nutritional support on weaning from mechanical ventilation. In 42 patients who retrospectively were not felt to have received adequate nutrition, only 48% were weaned successfully in contrast to a 90% weaning success in those 28 patients who had received adequate nutritional replacement.[190] To date, however, there is no study controlled for such variables as underlying respiratory mechanics, severity of illness, age, and sex that has examined this issue in a prospective fashion. Therefore, while there may be mounting evidence that nutritional replacement impacts importantly on the success or failure of weaning this issue is yet to be definitively resolved.

Although much attention has been paid to the impact of malnutrition and its reversal on respiratory muscle function, refeeding has additional implications for the respiratory system. Issues such as the prevention of lung injury and the promotion of lung parenchymal repair have been linked to adequate nutrition as has the production of adequate amounts of surfactant. Additionally, both ventilatory drive in response to hypoxia and hypercapnia have been found to be depressed during hypocaloric diets and enhanced by adequate caloric intake.[185]

If one accepts the premise that nutritional repletion of the COPD patient will improve his or her outcome (a premise which despite a body of suggestive evidence has yet to be proven), then aggressive nutritional support should be initiated. To this end, parameters such as total nonprotein calories per day, total protein per day, and the relative amounts of carbohydrate and lipid have to be established (see Chap. 62.)

Askanazi and co-workers[191] have shown that the administration of total parenteral nutrition composed primarily of carbohydrate significantly increases both CO_2 production and minute ventilation, the latter marked primarily by an increase in tidal volume. This increase in CO_2 production has been explained by an increase in the respiratory quotient (RQ) as the patient switches from using his or her endogenous lipids (RQ = 0.7) in favor of the exogenously supplied carbohydrate (RQ = 1.0). Moreover, if excess calories are administered, the excess carbohydrate is metabolized to lipid (RQ > 1.0). The authors concluded that such nutrition formulas could precipitate hypercapnic respiratory failure in some patients and suggested that lipids be used, in part, as a caloric source.

In a follow-up study,[192] the same authors compared the metabolic effects of a carbohydrate-enriched total parenteral nutrition (TPN) formula with one in which half those calories were in the form of lipid. These authors found that both CO_2 production and minute ventilation increased significantly in the carbohydrate group. Over the last several years, many reports have linked the onset of hypercapnic respiratory failure to high carbohydrate nutritional formulas most often in patients with limited ventilatory reserve, such as in patients with COPD.[193]

There can be little doubt that carbohydrate feeds result in the increased production of CO_2 and the resulting increase in minute ventilation. This finding has been documented even in an ambulatory group of COPD patients.[194] Whether carbohydrate formulas are responsible for failure to wean from mechanical ventilation is as yet unsettled, however. In a preliminary communication, Al-Saady and colleagues have reported that in eight patients with respiratory failure a low carbohydrate-high fat enteral diet was associated with both a lower Pa_{CO_2} when compared to a high carbohydrate-low fat formula and a significant reduction in ventilator days.[195] These latter findings must await further confirmation.

Askanazi and colleagues noted that, in a subgroup of patients who were acutely ill, not only did their CO_2 production increase, but also their oxygen consumptions rose, in addition to the effects on CO_2 production.[192] These findings may have significant implications for the patient with limited cardiovascular reserve unable to respond to those demands.

Although concern has been raised over the metabolic cost of carbohydrate loads, several investigators have described the ill effects of intravenous lipids in both animal and human studies.[196] Greene and colleagues[197] demonstrated that the infusion of 500 ml 10% intralipid over 4 hours resulted in a decrease in diffusion capacity at rest and during submaximal exercise in normal subjects, an effect attributed to intrapulmonary prostaglandin metabolism.[196] Venus and co-workers[198] reported that intralipid administered at clinically appropriate rates worsened the right-to-left shunt in a group of patients with adult respiratory distress syndrome. These findings have led several

Table 15-13. Determinants of Arterial CO_2

Pa_{CO_2}	$\dfrac{V_{CO_2}}{\left(1 - \dfrac{V_D}{V_T}\right) \dot{V}_E}$
V_{CO_2}	CO_2 Production
V_D/V_T	Dead space/tidal volume
$\dot{V}_E$	Minute ventilation

authors to suggest that intralipid should be used very judiciously in patients with underlying lung disease.[199] Their potential toxicity in the population with COPD is unknown.

Weaning from Mechanical Ventilation

Certain practical and theoretical considerations must be considered when weaning a patient from mechanical ventilation. Such issues as adequacy of oxygenation, airway control, tracheal toilet, and hemodynamic stability (the converse of the indications for the institution of mechanical ventilation as listed in Table 15-11) must be assessed. Fundamental to the weaning process is the patient's ability to sustain spontaneous ventilation and effectively eliminate CO_2. A useful framework, therefore, with which to approach the patient is through the articulation of the determinants of arterial CO_2 as listed in Table 15-13. This equation suggests that if one of the determinants of CO_2 is abnormal in the absence of appropriate compensation by the others CO_2 retention will ensue and weaning will fail.

Broadly stated, the weaning process is dominated by the following considerations:

- Requirements for minute ventilation and the efficiency of the process
- Assessment of ventilatory capacity including respiratory drive; and respiratory muscle strength, endurance, and fatigue
- The amount of rest versus exercise
- The mode of ventilation employed during the weaning process
- Assessment of respiratory mechanics

Requirements for Minute Ventilation

Increased CO_2 Production. Under normal circumstances, at rest, CO_2 production is approximately 100 ml/min/m². In the critically ill patient, however, production is often augmented and should be measured at the bedside when weaning from mechanical ventilation becomes problematic. When found to be elevated, a careful search for its possible causes must be undertaken (Table 15-14). Fundamental to this approach is the appreciation that under normal conditions increases in CO_2 production are easily compensated for by an increase in minute ventilation $\dot{V}_E$. In cases of CO_2 retention, the patient will not or cannot adequately increase his or her minute ventilation. Such an inability should not be unexpected in the case of COPD in which severe airflow obstruction places extreme limitations on the patient's maximum minute ventilatory capacity.

Increased Metabolic Rate. Any state that leads to an increase rate of metabolism will result in an increased production of CO_2. It has been estimated that CO_2 production will rise by approximately 14% for each degree rise (Celsius) in temperature above 37°.[200] Furthermore, the hyperventilation that usually accompanies the septic state will further increase that production. These findings have led to the suggestion that patients who are septic or febrile, whatever the cause, should not be weaned from mechanical ventilation.[201]

Increased Muscular Activity. Clearly such factors as agitation and shivering will result in an increased production of CO_2, up to tenfold in some instances.[200] Macklem has reported that resistive breathing is accompanied by a CO_2 production of between 700 to 800 ml per minute,[202] which is of obvious relevance to the patient with COPD.

Substrate Utilization. As noted previously, several investigators have linked high carbohydrate feeding loads with an increase both in CO_2 production and minute ventilation. Therefore, it has been suggested that in those patients in whom weaning failure is linked to an increase in CO_2 production, a trial of a high-lipid and low-carbohydrate diet would be appropriate. Beyond the issues of substrate utilization, nutritional repletion will stress the cardiovascular-respiratory system in other ways. Upon refeeding, the ventilatory drive both to hypoxia and hypercapnia increases as does the metabolic rate;[185] the former will lead to an increase in CO_2 production on the basis of an increased work of breathing while the latter on the basis of increased metabolism.

Increased Dead Space. The measurement of dead space which is normally 33% at rest and 40 to 60% in mechanically ventilated patients is usually expressed as a percentage of tidal volume. This implies that this ratio can be increased either by an absolute increase in dead space or by a fall in tidal volume in the presence of a constant deadspace. Table 15-15 lists the common causes of such an increased ratio which can also be easily measured at the bedside.

Pulmonary embolism is the paradigm of an acute dead space producing disease. Although typically this entity presents with respiratory alkalosis (decreased CO_2) and hypoxemia, it does so because of the patient's ability to com-

Table 15-14. Causes of Increased CO_2 Production

Increased Muscular Activity
  Shivering
  Increased work of breathing
  Agitation
Increased Metabolic Rate
  Fever
  Sepsis
  Injury
  Hyperthyroidism
Substrate Utilization
  High carbohydrate load

Table 15–15. Causes of Increased V_D/V_T

Increased Physiologic Dead Space
    Acute pulmonary embolism
    Hypotension
    Positive pressure ventilation
    Positive end-expiratory pressure
Decreased Tidal Volume
    Pattern or rapid, shallow breathing

pensate for the increase in dead space, the increase in minute ventilation induced by a variety of proposed mechanisms. There have now been several reports in the literature relating the acute onset of hypercapnia as the presenting blood gas abnormality in patients on mechanical ventilation who could not increase their minute ventilation.[203] Therefore, an unexplained increase in physiologic dead space should lead the clinician to investigate the possibility of new pulmonary vascular disease.

Ventilatory Capacity

When the normal minute ventilation of 5 to 7 liters per minute is found to be decreased an anatomic approach to its cause can be useful, as outlined in Table 15–16.

Respiratory center output can be easily measured in the ICU by assessing the P0.1 (the pressure that the patient can generate during the first 100 msec of an occluded breath), a period during which the patient is felt to be consciously unaware of the occlusion.[204] To perform this measurement one need not install any specialized machinery as the first 100 msec of a triggered ventilator breath has been found to correlate with an occlusion-valve measurement.[205] As will be discussed later, a depressed level of respiratory center output is rarely the cause of failure to wean in the COPD population.

Obviously a complete neurologic assessment is critical to eliminating any systemic neurologic illnesses that may preclude an adequate minute ventilation. Such entities as amyotrophic lateral sclerosis, Guillain-Barré, and myasthenia gravis rarely afflict the respiratory axis alone. An entity termed the polyneuropathy of the critically ill has been described that may initially present as the inability to wean from mechanical ventilation.[206] Clinically, this entity may resemble Guillain-Barré but is characterized by different csf and EMG findings.[207]

Respiratory Muscle Fatigue. When the respiratory muscles are no longer able to generate adequate pressure but are anticipated to be able to do so after a period of rest then inspiratory muscle fatigue is said to exist.[120] It has been suggested that inspiratory muscle fatigue will ensue when the rate of energy consumption exceeds the rate of energy supplies.[208] Thus, underlying strength, the imposed work load placed on those muscles, energy supplies, energy stores, and the efficiency of those muscles must be considered when assessing inspiratory muscle fatigue.[208]

One of the fundamental concepts relating to this entity to emerge over the last decade is the notion that the ratio between the pressure needed to generate a tidal volume breath and the maximum inspiratory pressure that the individual is able to generate that is critical in approaching respiratory muscle fatigue. In brief, both Roussos and Macklem[121] and Bellemare and Grassino[209] have described, in the laboratory setting, in both normal subjects and in patients with COPD that the inspiratory muscles fatigue depending on the duration of inspiration and, more fundamentally, on the fraction of the maximum inspiratory pressure analyzed per breath. They found that if the pressure per breath were less than 40% of the maximal pressure, the subject could continue breathing indefinitely; if that fraction were greater than 50% the time to fatigue would depend on the degree by which that percentage was exceeded. It becomes apparent, therefore, why many current bedside measurements of weaning have such poor sensitivity and specificity. The maximal inspiratory force that is commonly measured at the bedside assesses only

Table 15–16. Causes of Alveolar Hypoventilation

Decreased central drive
    Drugs, e.g., sedatives
    Neurologic disease, e.g., encephalitis
    Primary alveolar hypoventilation
    Ondine's curse
Spinal cord disease
    Trauma
    Transverse myelitis
    Tetanus
Motor neuron disease
    Amyotrophic lateral sclerosis
    Poliomyelitis
Neuropathy
    Guillain-Barré syndrome
    Toxic (lead, vincristine, Dilantin, arsenic, alcohol)
Neuromuscular junction defect
    Muscular dystrophy
    Polymyositis
    Metabolic myopathies
    Disuse atrophy
Chest wall and pleural abnormalities
    Kyphoscoliosis
    Obesity
    Flail chest
    Ankylosing spondylitis
    Thoracoplasty
    Fibrothorax
    Abdominal distention
    Diaphragmatic rupture
    Pleural effusion
    Pneumothorax
Lung and airway diseases
    Chronic obstructive airway disease
    Interstitial lung disease
    Pulmonary edema
    Asthma
    Pneumonia
    Respiratory distress syndrome
    Upper airway obstruction
Other causes
    Metabolic alkalosis
    Endocrine disorders
    Sepsis
    Sleep apnea
    Circulatory shock
    Electrolyte abnormality
    Malnutrition

(From Goldberg, P., and Roussos, C.H.: Alveolar hypoventilation and respiratory muscle fatigue. *In* Current Therapy in Critical Care Medicine. Edited by J. Parillo. Philadelphia, B. C. Decker, 1987.)

the patient's normal inspiratory strength, whereas the inspiratory pressure that patient must generate for each breath remains unknown.

The maximal inspiratory force is dependent on a variety of variables that Roussos has delineated. Energy stores (i.e., adequate nutritional status) have been discussed earlier. In addition, electrolyte deficits, in particular potassium, calcium, phosphate, magnesium can all result in diminished muscle strength.[210,211] Energy supplies depend on the delivery of nutrients to the muscles, in particular oxygen, fatty acids, and glucose. In this regard, as indicated earlier, Aubier and co-workers[155] have demonstrated that in animals rendered hypotensive mechanical ventilation significantly prolonged survival when compared to a spontaneously breathing cohort while redistributing blood flow away from respiratory muscles to other organ systems. The implications of this study are that a diminished flow (e.g., cardiac output) and by extension, the delivery of nutrients, resulted in the failure of the respiratory muscles as pressure generators. These findings would suggest that not only is an insufficient delivery of oxygen an adequate reason not to actively pursue weaning, but also suggests that hypotension per se, whatever the cause, constitutes a relative indication for ventilatory support.

The pressure that must be generated per breath is also a function of several variables, the most important of which are the elastic, resistive, and threshold-load forces that must be overcome before an adequate tidal volume can be effected. In the intubated patient, each of these variables can be easily measured and followed sequentially for improvement.[212]

A decrease in the elastic forces may be accomplished, for example, by decreasing lung water through the use of diuretics and by diminishing the degree of hyperinflation by increasing inspiratory flow and through the use of various bronchodilators. Airway resistance can be minimized through the use of bronchodilators, by increasing the size of the endotracheal tube, or even by removing the latter in favor of a tracheostomy. Similarly, the threshold load (PEEPi) may be minimized by decreasing alveolar time constants with the use of bronchodilators and by augmenting inspiratory flow thereby increasing the time available for expiration.

Finally, other factors that may increase the work of breathing include metabolic acidosis and sepsis with their effect on the respiratory center output and any cause of increased metabolic rate with its increased oxygen consumption and CO_2 production.

Rest Versus Exercise

If respiratory muscle fatigue is to be implicated in ventilatory failure then respiratory muscle rest, either partial (use of medications) or complete (mechanical ventilation) is the most important treatment modality available.[213] If complete rest is chosen as the appropriate therapeutic option then rest must be ensured. Common ventilatory modes, such as assist/control, have recently been shown not to necessarily ensure such rest, however, and frequently may demand that the patient perform even more work than that expected in a spontaneously breathing normal subject despite being on ventilatory support.[214,215] In this latter study, the authors reported that the mechanically ventilated patient was placed completely at rest only when inspiratory flow was set at 65 L per minute; sensitivity at -2 cm H_2O; and tidal volume of 12 ml/kg.

Even when on mechanical ventilation, intrinsic PEEP may play an adverse role by significantly increasing the amount of ventilatory work that the patient must perform. The ventilator, even if set to trigger at a sensitivity of -2 cm H_2O, will do so only when the patient is able to lower the pressure at the airway opening 2 cm H_2O below that level of end-expiratory pressure sensed by the machine (i.e., the amount of externally applied PEEP or, in its absence, atmospheric pressure. The patient with COPD, however, before being able to lower the pressure at the airway opening, must first overcome his or her intrinsic PEEP. Therefore, to compensate for this threshold load undelivered by the ventilator, external PEEP, equal to the intrinsic PEEP, should be applied.

Intermittent mandatory ventilation (IMV) has emerged as the most popular instituted mode of ventilation. Although no studies to date have clearly documented the superiority of one ventilatory mode over another, nevertheless certain aspects of the IMV mode must be appreciated. Integral to the internal IMV circuit of all ventilators is a demand valve which the patient must open to gain access to the IMV reservoir. The triggering of such a demand valve requires that work be performed by the patient, work that has been measured by Gibney and colleagues[216] and found to be variable depending on the ventilator but always higher than an external flow-by circuit. Several reports have described patients with limited ventilatory capacities whose failure to wean has been linked to such internal IMV circuits.[217] It is suggested therefore that if the IMV mode is to be instituted, an external circuit, in which there is no demand valve, be employed.

If inspiratory muscle fatigue underlies the development of ventilatory failure then muscle rest, as proposed previously, is fundamental to any treatment regimen.[213] It has also been demonstrated, however, that significant diaphragmatic atrophy results after just 11 days of mechanical ventilation in the normal animal.[218] Atrophy may prolong inspiratory muscle dysfunction and the need for mechanical ventilation. The issue, therefore, is when to "rest" the muscles and when to "exercise" them.

The notion of inspiratory muscle training in the ambulatory COPD population has been the subject of numerous investigations with varying results.[219,220] What appears clear from these studies is that if such training is to be successful then training targeted at the inspiratory muscles must be undertaken. A recent report has described the successful use of such training in promoting weaning from mechanical ventilation.[221]

Because of the uncertainty over whether rest or exercise should be pursued, it is the practice in our institutions to initially rest the patient by minimizing ventilator-associated increases in the work of breathing while interspersing brief periods (approximately 15 minutes every 4 to 6 hours) of spontaneous breathing while gradually increasing those periods of spontaneous breathing over a period of days to weeks. If weaning is still problematic after approximately 2 to 3 weeks despite the optimization of all respiratory and nonrespiratory variables, then a careful analysis of the requirement for rehabilitation should be instituted (See Chapter 24 on Rehabilitation of the Ventilator-Dependent Patient).

Ventilatory Mode

Ultimately, because of the unreliability of weaning parameters, the patient should be allowed to breathe spontaneously, to some degree, under close scrutiny. The ventilation mode used to facilitate this process has also been the subject of controversy. Although a report by Tomlinson and co-workers[222] failed to document any difference between IMV and T-piece, this report primarily studied a postsurgical population containing few patients who were difficult to wean. Moreover, by design, the authors replaced the demand valve in the IMV circuit with a low resistance H valve to circumvent the added burden of work that is inherent in currently available ventilators because of the demand valves.[216]

In their report, Petroff and co-workers[151] examined the use of CPAP as a weaning mode in this patient population. Because of the concerns over the effect that PEEPi may impose on the COPD patient, and given that previous work had demonstrated that external PEEP could counterbalance the PEEPi,[149,150] these investigators compared T-piece trials with those of CPAP. They found that the work of breathing and metabolic cost of the inspiratory muscles were significantly lower on CPAP and that the patients all felt subjectively less dyspneic. As a result, it has become routine in our institutions to wean patients with PEEPi on CPAP circuits.

Brochard and co-workers[223] investigated the use of pressure support ventilation in eight patients in whom previous attempts at weaning from mechanical ventilation had failed. This mode of ventilation allows the patient to control the respiratory rate, tidal volume, and inspiratory time. These authors examined whether this mode of ventilation would allow spontaneous activity of the diaphragm to continue (thereby avoiding muscle atrophy), while preventing the onset of fatigue. The authors defined the optimal level as the lowest amount of support not associated with EMG evidence of diaphragm fatigue. Although the level of such support varied among the different patients, it was nevertheless associated, in all subjects, with the identical amount of ventilatory work—8 to 10 joules per minute. The authors concluded that pressure support ventilation could indeed prevent diaphragm fatigue while allowing for substantial diaphragmatic activity. The invasive techniques employed in this report to determine the level of such support would tend to make such an approach somewhat limited. These authors also noted, however, that the EMG activity of the sternomastoid muscle fell to its lowest value at that optimal level of pressure support. The electrical activity of the sternomastoid muscle was, moreover, associated with the contractile activity of that muscle. The authors suggested, therefore, that the optimal level of pressure support could be determined noninvasively by increasing the amount of that support until contractile activity of the sternomastoid muscle, assessed by palpation, disappears. Although the implications of this report for weaning are clear, the efficacy of pressure support in

Table 15-17. Weaning Criteria: Commonly Used Indices of Respiratory Mechanics

Tidal volume > 5-7 ml/kg
Vital capacity > 10-12 ml/kg
Maximal inspiratory pressure > -20 cm H_2O
Minute ventilation < 10 L/min
Ability to double resting minute ventilation

weaning must remain a subject of speculation until a properly designed study answers that question.

Assessment of Respiratory Mechanics

Several indices of respiratory mechanics have been proposed as guidelines in clinical assessment of when the patient is ready for a trial of spontaneous breathing; the most commonly used ones are listed in Table 15-17. Maximum inspiratory pressure (Pimax) is a global assessment of inspiratory muscle strength which was introduced by Sahn and Lakshminarayan more than a decade ago.[224] In their study, a Pimax of greater (more negative) than -30 cm H_2O was always associated with weaning success whereas those patients unable to generate a pressure greater than -20 cm H_2O were unable to sustain spontaneous ventilation; values between -20 and -30 cm H_2O were not predictive. Since that time, however, several authors have documented the limitations of this measurement. Tahvanainen and co-workers[225] reported that a Pimax of greater than -30 cm H_2O was falsely negative in 100% of patients and falsely positive in 26%. These discrepant findings may be due to the different patient populations studied. The earlier study examined patients ventilated for brief periods of mechanical ventilation. Moreover, from a theoretical point of view, as alluded to previously, Pimax assesses only the muscle's maximal ability to sustain inspiratory pressures. Without a concomitant assessment of the load imposed on that muscle per tidal volume breath one would expect this measurement to have a limited predictive value. Similar limitations have been found with respect to the other commonly employed indices—vital capacity, minute volume, and maximum voluntary ventilation.[226]

In searching for an accurate predictive index of weaning success, several investigators have proposed that an index of respiratory drive, the P0.1 (i.e., the airway pressure generated during the first 100 msec of an occluded breath) be so used. Sassoon and colleagues[227] studied 12 patients with COPD and noted that those patients with a P0.1 of greater than 6 cm H_2O at the beginning of the trial all failed to wean. Those subjects with a P0.1 of less than 6 were all successful. In a different study design, Murciano and co-workers[228] followed 16 patients with COPD who underwent mechanical ventilation for ventilatory failure secondary to airway infection. All patients were ultimately extubated based on bedside assessment:

- Apyrexia
- Diminished tracheal secretions
- Acceptable arterial blood gases
- A maximal inspiratory pressure higher than -20 cm H_2O

Those patients, however, who could ultimately sustain spontaneous ventilation had, over the period of their ventilatory support, a significant decrease in P0.1 to levels (4 cm H_2O) seen in patients with stable COPD. Those patients, however, who failed and required reintubation within 24 to 48 hours had not demonstrated any such decrease. On the other hand, Montgomery[229] failed to demonstrate the positive predictive utility of this index but did report that the ratio of CO_2-stimulated P0.1 to the baseline P0.1 was greater in those patients who weaned successfully as compared to those who failed.

Several investigators have examined a host of other variables to assess their predictive value. These studies have yielded, by and large, contradictory results. Both Swartz and Marino[230] and Pourriat and co-workers[157] reported on the value of measuring transdiaphragmatic pressures (Pdi = gastric pressure [Pga] − esophageal pressure [Peso]), the latter in a group of patients with COPD, during a trial of spontaneous breathing. Swartz and Marino reported that despite a rise in Pco_2 and a failed weaning attempt Pdi rose during the weaning trial suggesting that, at least in these patients, diaphragmatic failure was not the cause of CO_2 retention and weaning failure. On the other hand, Pourriat reported that both Pdi breath and Pdi maximum, when measured early during the weaning period, were significantly lower in the group failing to wean compared to the group who succeeded. Most intriguing was that of the 19 patients who ultimately failed to wean 13 showed a Pdi/Pdimax ratio of greater than 40%, whereas 16 of the 18 patients who could sustain spontaneous respiration showed a ratio of less than 40%, results quite reminiscent of the original findings of Roussos and Macklem.[121]

Although of enormous research potential, the measurement of Pdi is impractical because its use demands an invasive procedure and somewhat sophisticated equipment. The same reservations can be made in relation to the work of breathing calculations advanced by several authors to represent accurate predictors of weaning success.[231-233] Several authors, therefore, have tried to identify the clinical correlates of inspiratory muscle fatigue. As mentioned earlier, Cohen and colleagues[122] documented that a rapid respiratory rate heralded the onset of EMG muscle fatigue and was followed by an ordered sequence of clinical events which are listed in Table 15-7. Such a pattern of rapid shallow breathing has been reported by several authors to predict weaning failure. Tobin and co-workers[124] reported that those patients who, immediately on the discontinuation of mechanical support, adopted a rapid (> 30/min), shallow (tidal volume < 300 ml) breathing pattern ultimately failed. By combining these two indices, Tobin and Yang[235] have reported that a frequency/tidal volume ratio of greater than or equal to 100 breaths per minute per liter was associated with weaning failure in 86% of patients and success in only 10%. In the study cited previously,[157] Pourriat documented the adoption of such a pattern of breathing but not until well into the weaning period, several hours after the development of a declining Pdi and Pdimax and an increasing Pdi/Pdimax. In their longitudinal study referred to previously, Murciano and colleagues[228] reported that in that cohort ultimately able to breathe spontaneously the respiratory frequency decreased significantly when compared to baseline whereas the tidal volume increased substantially; these two parameters did not change in that group requiring further ventilatory support. On the other hand, Swartz and Marino[230] were unable to document any progressive changes in either respiratory rate or tidal volume in the patients who failed their weaning attempts but, it must be noted, all of the patients in this latter study started their weaning trials with high respiratory frequencies and low tidal volumes.

Unlike Cohen and colleagues, Tobin and co-workers[123] were unable to relate abdominal paradox to weaning failure. These authors reported the onset of abnormal ribcage and abdominal motion in both patients who were and who were not successfully weaned from mechanical ventilation. Although the difference in the group mean data was significant, the considerable overlap between the two groups tended to eliminate this clinical sign as a usable predictive index. Moreover, this same group of investigators showed in a companion paper that abnormalities in abdominal and rib cage motion were related not to inspiratory muscle fatigue but primarily to the increase in the imposed respiratory load.[234] Although the former study demonstrates the difficulty in using abnormal thoracoabdominal movements as an accurate predictor of weaning success, the latter study calls into question the entire concept of this physical finding as it relates to inspiratory muscle fatigue.

At the moment there is no single index with which to accurately predict the success or failure of weaning. The limitations of the traditionally used weaning parameters listed in Table 15-17 have been discussed previously. Although requiring further validation, a P0.1 of greater than 6 cm H_2O may preclude successful weaning. In combining ease of measurement and predictive value respiratory rate and tidal volume are two valuable parameters, however. A respiratory rate of greater than 30 per minute should alert the clinician. Such a rapid rate, especially when combined with a tidal volume of less than 300 ml will probably result in an unsuccessful weaning trial.

Finally, in an elegant but preliminary report Yang and Tobin[235] have described a weaning index that attempts to integrate the maximal capacity of the inspiratory muscles with the load imposed on them, a measurement that can be made at the bedside noninvasively. Prior to weaning, dynamic compliance (Cdyn) as described by Marini[212] is measured. A tidal volume (VT) that is anticipated to meet the ventilatory needs of the patient is estimated (e.g., 5 to 7 ml/kg). The pressure, therefore, that the inspiratory muscles will have to generate to produce that predicted spontaneous tidal volume can be calculated by VT/Cdyn. Once Pi-breath (the pressure that must be generated by the inspiratory muscles per breath) is known, its ratio to Pimax can be determined keeping in mind, once again, that a Pdi/Pdimax of greater than 40% has been associated with the development of fatigue.[121] In a modification of this index, Yang reported that they were accurate in predicting successful weaning outcome in nearly 90% of cases.

POST-ICU PHASE
Smoking cessation

In the management of patients with COPD who still smoke, the most important intervention is smoking cessation.[2] The incidence of coronary heart disease is diminished by 50% within 1 year of quitting and returns to normal after 10 years.[11] Incidence of lung cancer diminishes slowly and returns to that of the nonsmoking population after 12 to 15 years.[11] Among patients with COPD, the most immediate benefits are a reduction in cough and sputum which occurs within weeks of quitting.[8] In longitudinal studies, the accelerated lung function decline seen among smokers slows after quitting so that within 1 to 2 years, lung function decline is similar to that of nonsmokers.[7] As was seen in Figure 15–1, this is particularly important among patients with COPD who appear to have increased susceptibility manifested by accelerated lung function decline of 80 to 90 ml per year.[1,7] In a longitudinal community based survey, diffusing capacity (DLco) was significantly lower among healthy smokers compared to nonsmokers, and improved among those that quit smoking, suggesting that smoking is associated with reversible gas exchange abnormalities.[236] In a community based study of patients with COPD, those who stopped smoking had similar mortality for the first 7 to 8 years as those who continued to smoke, after which survival was significantly better among patients who had quit smoking.[8] The absence of survival advantage in the first 7 years has been attributed to the selection bias that sicker patients usually were more likely to stop smoking.[237]

Smoking cessation methods vary; those that are more intensive and costly appear to have the highest long-term success.[238] Advice from physicians may be effective in 5 to 10% of smokers. Self-help programs (such as those offered by the American Lung Association) may be effective in approximately 10% of smokers.[238] On the other hand, more expensive commercially available programs (such as SmokeEnders) may achieve quit rates of 40 to 50% after 1 year. Hypnosis therapy has been shown effective in small trials, but acupuncture has not been shown to be superior to placebo.[239] Nicotine is now recognized to be an addictive substance by the American Foundation of Addiction;[13] therefore pharmacologic therapy such as nicotine-containing gum or transdermal patches should enhance smoking cessation success. Twelve of 13 studies comparing the nicotine-containing gum to placebo demonstrated higher quit rates among those given the gum.[13] In 8 studies where the nicotine gum was compared to other methods of smoking cessation the gum was of equal or superior effectiveness.[13] Among 25 smokers given clonidine, over 25% quit for at least 1 year.[13] Of those who successfully stop smoking, only 30% remain nonsmokers after 1 year.[238] In the MRFIT trials, a high proportion of those who said they had quit or substantially reduced smoking had elevated or urine cotinine levels indicating continued heavy smoking.[240] It was this failure to sustain smoking cessation and inaccuracies in patient histories that accounted for the lower than expected effectiveness of smoking cessation programs in improving health outcomes.[240]

In conclusion, smoking cessation is the most important intervention for a patient with COPD who still smokes. The early benefits are a reduced incidence of coronary heart disease and reduced cough and sputum production. Long-term benefits include slower decline in lung function, substantially reduced incidence of coronary heart disease and lung cancer, and improved survival after an interval of 7 to 8 years.

Rehabilitation in COPD

In 1969, Petty reported that a comprehensive exercise and rehabilitation program for patients with COPD resulted in diminished hospitalization and improved functional status.[241] Since then there has been continued interest in this form of intervention, particularly because of its apparent cost-effectiveness.[242] The components of pulmonary rehabilitation include ventilatory muscle training, exercise training, and psychosocial support.[242,243] The actual benefits of this program are difficult to measure in an unbiased manner, because the intervention cannot be applied in a double-blind fashion. Using historical controls, however, Hodgkin has pointed out that survival appears to be improved.[242]

Ventilatory muscle training is achieved through the maneuver of breathing through a resistive device (inspiratory muscle training) or through the performance of isocapnic voluntary hyperventilation. Almost all investigations of this method have reported improvement in strength and endurance of the ventilatory muscles, without significant change in dyspnea, pulmonary function, or exercise test performance.[243–250] On the other hand, patients who undergo exercise training, either through treadmill, bicycle or walking, have significant improvement in exercise tolerance and endurance.[242,243,251–254] In these studies, patients show a dramatic improvement in the work output, without change in maximal oxygen consumption, implying that the major training effect is to increase muscle efficiency.[251–253]

The cardiovascular adaptation in normal persons after exercise training is increased stroke volume and reduced heart rate at the same levels of exercise. This adaptation is not seen among patients with COPD, because these patients exercise capacity is so limited by ventilation that the cardiac response does not usually reach even 50% of the maximal predicted heart rate.[242]

The improvement seen in exercise capability is often very specific to the training exercise. This specificity was demonstrated in two studies.[251,254] In one study, upper extremity training was performed among 28 patients with COPD who had significantly improved performance of upper extremity exercise without improvement on treadmill exercise test.[254] In the other study, the benefits of walking were compared to those of treadmill exercise. Patients who walked had greater improvement in 6-minute walking distance whereas those who exercised on the treadmill performed better on the treadmill test.[251] The benefit of exercise can be seen after a period of training of as little as 12 days and can be maintained for 3 to 6 months with only minimal continuing exercises.[255] There was considerable concern initially that exercise itself might be dangerous to patients with COPD. Holle reported that among 44 patients with COPD who exercised, 33% desaturated and 20% had evidence of cardiac disease.[251] Moser reported that 31 of 39 patients had arterial desaturation during exercise.[252] Despite this, there are no reports of sudden death or other complications resulting from pulmonary rehabilitation.[243,251]

Psychosocial support has been included in most rehabilitation programs because it is frequently needed by these chronically ill, debilitated patients. Interventions of this kind are more difficult to quantify and their effects difficult to measure. It has been noted that mood and motivation correlate better with exercise endurance than pulmonary function.[256] In a prospective study in which psychologic indices were measured prior to beginning the rehabilitation, patients with a more positive psychologic index were found to have a better response to the rehabilitation program.[256] Anecdotal experience from many rehabilitation programs suggests that only highly motivated patients complete the programs.[241] It is possible that the benefit of rehabilitation is a result of the selection bias that these programs enroll only the most highly motivated patients.

Ventilatory Muscle Rest

When it was recognized that respiratory muscle fatigue was important in the pathogenesis of both chronic and acute respiratory failure, it was hypothesized that the rest of these muscles would improve their function.[257] To test this hypothesis, a randomized placebo controlled trial was conducted[258] on 186 patients with severe COPD. These patients were randomized to receive nocturnal negative pressure ventilation using a cuirass ventilator for 3 months or a sham intervention. Patients underwent pulmonary function and exercise testing at baseline and at monthly intervals. Ventilatory muscle rest (VMR) was confirmed through measurement of transdiaphragmatic pressures and diaphragmatic electromyograms for patients receiving the active arm of therapy. VMR was not associated with significant improvement in any of the outcomes viewed including dyspnea, gas exchange, bicycle exercise endurance, 6-minute walking distance, or lung function. Analysis within subgroups of patients with partially reversible airways obstruction or patients with hypercapnia failed to demonstrate any benefit of this therapy.[258] This study was well designed and conducted and of sufficient size to convincingly demonstrate that, using currently available technology, VMR is of no benefit in patients with severe COPD.

Nutritional Support

The association of malnutrition and emphysema was noted as early as the 19th century and became part of the clinical definition of the typical emphysematous patient ("the pink puffer"). Among patients with COPD, the prevalence of significant malnutrition, defined as weight less than 90% of the ideal body weight, ranges between 30 to 50%,[259,260] and is higher among those with more severe obstructive airways disease.[260] This association is unexplained because the oral intake of malnourished patients with COPD is similar to normal persons of equal weight and to well-nourished patients with COPD of similar lung function.[259] Possible contributory factors are:

- Gastrointestinal disturbances such as peptic ulcers which are more common among COPD patients
- Arterial desaturation after eating a meal seen in a significant minority of patients
- Patients with COPD are hypermetabolic because of the greater metabolic demand of respiratory muscles[259]

It has been hypothesized that weight loss occurs during episodes of acute respiratory failure and hospitalization. After recovery from these episodes, the weight may never fully be recovered.[259]

Malnutrition has been shown to blunt the hypoxic respiratory drive in experimental animals and human volunteers. In autopsy, as well as in animal studies of severe malnutrition, ventilatory muscles are of reduced bulk and weight in proportion to the wasting seen in other muscle groups. Underweight patients with COPD have reduced ventilatory muscle strength and diminished peak exercise performance, as compared to those of normal weight.[261] In the NIH IPPB trial, mortality was related to malnutrition independently of lung function.[237]

Nutrition interventions have been studied in a number of settings. ICU patients receiving TPN have had improvements in inspiratory muscle strength directly proportional to increases in body mass.[262] Intensive feeding programs among hospitalized patients with COPD have resulted in significant weight gain which in turn have resulted in significant increases in hand-grip strength and inspiratory muscle pressures.[259] Lewis and colleagues randomized 21 malnourished outpatients with COPD to receive supplementary feedings or normal diet.[263] Those patients who received supplementary feedings demonstrated no significant improvement in respiratory muscle strength compared to the controls. This study may have been negative because the supplementary feedings were given in an unsupervised manner and these patients reduced their normal dietary intake so that actual caloric intake in the two treatment groups were not significantly different.[263]

In a similar study among 14 malnourished outpatients with COPD, those randomized to receive supplementary feedings for three months had no change in gas exchange or lung function but had significant improvement in inspiratory muscle strength, hand-grip strength, dyspnea scores, and 6-minute walking distance.[264] These improvements were noted one month after initiation of the supplementary feedings. The measurements improved throughout the three month feeding period but all parameters had returned to baseline levels within three months of cessation of supplementary feedings.[264] In a third study, six malnourished patients with COPD received 1000 calories by nasoenteric feeding tube in addition to their regular diet, whereas four matched controls received sham nasoenteric feeding. Lung function did not change, but there was significant improvement in inspiratory muscle strength in the group that received supplementary feeding as compared to the control group.[265]

In summary, malnutrition is common in patients with severe COPD and is associated with diminished respiratory muscle strength. Nutrition interventions such as dietary supplements, nasoenteric feeding or parenteral nutrition, will result in improved inspiratory muscle strength and exercise capability. These benefits are short lived, however, and further study is needed of the feasibility, benefits, and problems associated with long-term nutrition supplementation.

Oxygen Therapy

Current recommendations for oxygen therapy are based on the results of 2 important clinical trials[266,267] which will be reviewed briefly. The first study compared mortality over 5 years among 87 British patients randomized to receive supplementary oxygen for 12 to 15 hours per day or no oxygen.[266] These patients all had severe COPD and cor pulmonale with mean FEV_1 of 0.65 L, Pa_{O_2} of 45 torr and Pa_{CO_2} of 51 torr. After 5 years, 30 of 45 controls (67%) had died, compared to 19 of 42 (47%) of those who received supplemental oxygen. Annual mortality was 12% among oxygen-treated males, compared to 29% among control males. Among oxygen-treated females annual mortality was 4 to 5%, compared to 30% among control females.[266] In the second study, 203 American patients were randomized to continuous oxygen (greater than 19 hours per day) or nocturnal oxygen (12 to 15 hours per day).[267] After follow-up of 12 to 24 months (mean 19 months), annual mortality was 21% among those receiving nocturnal oxygen, compared to 11.9% for those receiving continuous oxygen, or 1.94 times higher among nocturnal compared to continuous oxygen. The subgroup of patients with arterial hypercarbia showed even greater benefit from continuous oxygen therapy. Pulmonary vascular resistance and pulmonary artery pressures were improved only among those receiving continuous oxygen therapy.[267]

The reduction in mortality associated with oxygen therapy in these two studies was so significant that long-term oxygen therapy came into widespread use. Currently, it is recommended if the resting arterial oxygen concentration is less than 55 torr or if it is less than 60 torr and there is evidence of cor pulmonale or polycythemia.[2] Oxygen should be given by nasal catheter at a rate sufficient to increase the arterial oxygen saturation to 91 to 95%. This rate should be increased by 1 liter per minute during sleep or exercise.[2]

Other possible indications for long-term oxygen therapy are sleep or exercise desaturation, both of which are common in patients with COPD. An American Thoracic Society statement recommended that if there was evidence on sleep studies of significant sleep desaturation without obstructive apneas that oxygen should be prescribed.[2] Among patients who showed desaturation with exercise, the ATS recommended that oxygen be prescribed only for those who show significant improvement in exercise tolerance with supplemental oxygen. It was further recommended that the need for supplemental oxygen should be evaluated by performing exercise testing with and without supplemental oxygen in a manner such that the patient was unaware of receiving oxygen.[2]

Home Ventilation

Home ventilation is becoming feasible because of the development of new ventilatory assistance and monitoring technology. At present, it is mainly applicable for patients with neuromuscular disorders in whom there are fewer concomitant medical problems, lung compliance is normal so that ventilation is relatively easy, infections are uncommon, and secretions minimal so that suctioning is infrequently needed. Home ventilation has not been as successful among patients with COPD. This is because they tend to be older, have increased airway resistance making ventilatory assistance more difficult, and have increased secretions requiring frequent suctioning. Oxygen and aerosol therapy may be needed as well. These patients need close medical and nursing supervision because they are not in stable condition, they have an average life expectancy of approximately 6 months, and they frequently require rehospitalization.[47] Because of these problems, home ventilation will be an option for only a few highly selected patients with COPD.

Lung Transplantation

With the advent of cyclosporine, long-term survival following lung transplantation has become a possibility. Initially, lung transplantation was performed as part of heart-lung transplantation for primary pulmonary hypertension. Double lung transplantation without cardiac transplantation was introduced by the Toronto group for patients with interstitial fibrosis. In the last 5 years an increasing number of centers have reported successful lung transplantation for patients with COPD.

Heart-lung transplantations are still the most frequent transplantation operation performed for COPD. Up until 1991, approximately 100 had been reported to the International Lung Transplant Registry. Actuarial survival is 62% for one year.[268] Double lung transplant has been advocated for patients with COPD because it avoids the need for cardiopulmonary bypass,[269] and eliminates the problem of cardiac rejection which can occur independently of lung rejection.[268,270] Up to 1991, 73 patients have received double lung transplantations, of whom 55% were still alive.[268]

Single lung transplantation (SLT) is now considered the procedure of choice for patients with interstitial fibrosis.[268] This was thought to be hazardous in patients with COPD, because the remaining native lung might overinflate, resulting in mediastinal shift and compression of the grafted lung, leading to ventilation perfusion and gas exchange abnormalities. However, since these reports, SLT has been performed successfully among 44 patients with COPD,[271-273] of whom 31 survived more than 6 months. Mediastinal shift towards the grafted lung does occur but without significant ventilation perfusion mismatch or abnormalities of gas exchange.[268]

Problems following lung transplantation are similar among patients with COPD compared to patients with other pulmonary disorders. The major causes of death are infection and rejection. Progressive bronchiolitis obliterans, which appears to be a rejection phenomenon, develops in approximately 20% of patients. This problem can be detected early with transbronchial biopsies, and managed by intensifying immunosuppressant therapy.[270]

Functional outcome of these patients after transplantation is excellent and in all reports recipients no longer require oxygen therapy. Exercise testing performed 3 months[274] and 1 to 2 years[275] after transplantation have shown a dramatic improvement in exercise ability. Gibbons showed that the major exercise limitation among patients with COPD after SLT was deconditioning and peripheral muscle weakness.[271] This limitation was believed to be related to the inactivity prior to transplantation, and the corticosteroid therapy following transplantation.[271]

In conclusion, COPD is a chronic illness manifested by worsening dyspnea due to slowly progressive airways obstruction. Prognosis is closely related to the severity of the underlying airways obstruction, and has changed little over the last 25 years. Acute respiratory insufficiency requiring hospitalization arises in those with severe airways disease. The acute worsening in respiratory status may be due to pneumonia, heart failure, pulmonary embolus or pneumothorax, although in 50% of instances no definite cause is found. These latter, termed acute exacerbations, may result from viral or bacterial bronchitis. Whatever the initiating event, respiratory insufficiency may evolve into respiratory failure with hypoventilation and hypercarbia, worsening gas exchange with hypoxemia, and finally respiratory muscle fatigue. It is usually at this point that the intensive care specialist becomes involved and must decide rapidly whether to institute MV, often with little clinical information and no prior knowledge of the patient. Institution of MV may be life-saving, but for patients with COPD there is a substantial risk of complications, including long-term dependance on MV. Identification of those most likely to benefit from MV, who can be weaned from MV, can be better made with knowledge of the pre-morbid functional status, lung function, and signs of cor pulmonale or malnutrition.

At present, for those who survive their initial ICU admission, management includes pharmacologic and nonpharmacologic therapy, in an effort to avoid subsequent episodes of respiratory failure with attendant high mortality. After discharge from the ICU, management should include pharmacologic therapy, with an oral theophylline preparation, and inhaled beta agonists. Ipratropium appears to be of benefit, while oral corticosteroids are of use in approximately 20% of patients. For those who respond to oral steroids, replacement with inhaled steroids is successful in only one third. Top priority should be given to smoking cessation for patients who are still smoking. Rehabilitation and nutritional supplementation should be offered to all patients, because these programs will hasten recovery after a major illness, will improve exercise tolerance and functional status, and may prevent subsequent hospitalizations. VMR, although theoretically attractive, is not effective, at least using currently available technologies. Home ventilation may be considered for ventilator-dependent patients who are in stable condition, have minimal secretions, have considerable social/family support, and are highly motivated. Finally, unilateral lung transplantation may be considered for those with emphysema who are young, uninfected, and without co-morbid illnesses. Given the dismal prognosis of COPD patients after their first episode of ARF, and the current expansion of lung transplantation, this may become the management of choice for patients with COPD whose disease is so severe as to result in debilitating or life threatening disease.

REFERENCES

1. Burrows, B.: Airways Obstruction Diseases: pathogenetic mechanism and natural histories of the disorders. Med. Clin. North Am., *74*:547, 1990.
2. American Thoracic Society. Standards for the diagnosis and care of patients with chronic obstructive pulmonary disease (COPD) and asthma. Am. Rev. Respir. Dis., *136*:225, 1987.
3. Snider, G. L.: Changes in COPD Occurrence. Chronic Obstructive Pulmonary Disease: a definition and implications of structural determinants of airflow obstruction for epidemiology. Am. Rev. Respir. Dis., *140*:S3, 1989.
4. Tager, I. B., Segal, M. R., Speizer, F. E., and Weiss, S. T.: The Natural History of Forced Expiratory Volumes. Effect of cigarette smoking and respiratory symptoms. Am. Rev. Respir. Dis., *138*:837, 1988.
5. Burrows, B.: Factors Related to Survival. The course and prognosis of different types of chronic airflow limitation in a general Population Sample from Arizona: comparison with the Chicago "COPD" Series. Am. Rev. Respir. Dis., *140*:S92, 1989.
6. Sherrill, D. L., Lebowitz, M. D., and Burrows, B.: Epidemiology of chronic obstructive pulmonary disease. Clin. Chest Med., *11*:375, 1990.
7. Fletcher, C., Peto, R., Tinker, C., and Speizer, F. E.: The natural history of chronic bronchitis and emphysema. London, Oxford University Press, 1976.
8. Postma, D. S., and Sluiter, H. J.: Prognosis of chronic obstructive pulmonary disease: the Dutch experience. Am. Rev. Respir. Dis., *140*:S100, 1989.
9. Davis, R. M., and Novotny, T. E.: Changes in risk factors: the epidemiology of cigarette smoking and its impact on chronic obstructive pulmonary disease. Am. Rev. Respir. Dis., *140*:S82, 1989.
10. Orie, N. G., et al.: The host factor in bronchitis. *In* Bronchitis. Edited by N. G. Orie, and H. J. Sluiter. Assen, Royal Vangorcum, 1961, p. 43.
11. United States Department of Health and Human Services: Chronic Obstructive Lung Disease: The Health Consequences of Smoking. A Report of the Surgeon General. Public Health Service Publication No. 84-50205. Rockville, MD, U.S. Government Printing Office, 1984.
12. Snider, G. L.: Chronic obstructive pulmonary disease: risk factors, pathophysiology and pathogenesis. Ann. Rev. Med., *40*:411, 1989.
13. Benowitz, N. L.: Pharmacologic aspects of cigarette smoking and nicotine addiction. N. Engl. J. Med., *319*:1318, 1988.
14. Tockman, M. S., Anthonisen, N. R., Wright, E. C., and Donithan, M. G.: Airway obstruction and the risk for lung cancer. Ann. Intern. Med., *106*:512, 1987.
15. Nagai, A., West, W. W., Paul, J. L., and Thurlbeck, W. M.: The National Institutes of Health Intermittent Positive-Pressure Breathing Trial: pathology studies. I. Interrelationship between morphologic lesions. Am. Rev. Respir. Dis., *132*:937, 1985.
16. Nagai, A., West, W. W., and Thurlbeck, W. M.: The National Institutes of Health Intermittent Positive-Pressure Breathing Trial: pathology studies. II. Correlation between morphologic findings, clinical findings, and evidence of expiratory airflow obstruction. Am. Rev. Respir. Dis., *132*:946, 1985.
17. Erikson, S.: Pulmonary emphysema and alpha 1-antitrypsin deficiency. Acta. Med. Scand., *175*:197, 1964.
18. American Thoracic Society. Guidelines for the approach to the patient with severe hereditary alpha 1-antitrypsin deficiency. Am. Rev. Respir. Dis., *140*:1494, 1989.

19. Becklake, M. R.: Occupational exposures: evidence for a causal association with chronic obstructive pulmonary disease. Am. Rev. Respir. Dis., *140*:S85, 1989.
20. Steinberg, M., and Becklake, M. R.: Socio-environmental factors and lung function. S. Afr. Med. J., *70*:270, 1986.
21. Kauffman, F., Drouet, D., Lellouch, J., and Brille, D.: Occupational exposure and 12 year spirometric changes among Paris area workers. Br. J. Ind. Med., *39*:221, 1982.
22. Feinleib, M., et al.: Trends in COPD morbidity and mortality in the United States. Am. Rev. Respir. Dis., *140*:S9, 1989.
23. Manfreda, J., Mao, Y., and Litven, W.: Morbidity and mortality from chronic obstructive pulmonary disease. Am. Rev. Respir. Dis., *140*:S19, 1989.
24. Backhouse, A., and Holland, W. W.: Trends in mortality from chronic obstructive airways disease in the United Kingdom. Thorax, *44*:529, 1989.
25. Mitchell, R. S., Webb, W. C., and Filley, G. F.: Chronic obstructive bronchopulmonary disease. III. Factors influencing prognosis. Am. Rev. Respir. Dis., *89*:878, 1964.
26. Burrows, B., and Earle, R. H.: Course and prognosis of chronic obstructive lung disease. N. Engl. J. Med., *280*:397, 1969.
27. Vandenbergh, E., Ziment, I., and van de Woestijne, K. P.: Course and prognosis of patients with advanced chronic obstructive disease: evaluation by means of functional indices. Am. J. Med., *55*:736, 1973.
28. Boushy, S. F., et al.: Prognosis in chronic obstructive pulmonary disease. Am. Rev. Respir. Dis., *108*:1373, 1973.
29. Postma, D.S., et al.: Prognosis in severe chronic obstructive pulmonary disease. Am. Rev. Respir. Dis., *119*:357, 1979.
30. Traver, G. A., Cline, M. G., and Burrows B.: Predictors of mortality in chronic obstructive pulmonary disease: a 15-year follow-up study. ARRD, *119*:895, 1979.
31. Weitzenblum, E., et al.: Prognosis value of pulmonary artery pressure in chronic obstructive pulmonary disease. Thorax, *36*:752, 1981.
32. Kawakami, Y., Kisha, F., Yamamoto, H., and Miyamoto, K.: Relation of oxygen delivery, mixed venous oxygenation, and pulmonary hemodynamics to prognosis in chronic obstructive pulmonary disease. N. Engl. J. Med., *308*:1045, 1983.
33. Kanner, R. E., et al.: Predictors of survival in subjects with chronic airflow limitation. Am. J. Med., *74*:249, 1983.
34. Martin, T. R., Lewis, S. W., and Albert, R. K.: The Prognosis of patients with chronic obstructive pulmonary disease after hospitalization for acute respiratory failure. Chest, *82*:310, 1982.
35. Diener, C. F., and Burrows, B.: Further observations on the course and prognosis of chronic obstructive lung disease. Am. Rev. Respir. Dis., *108*:1373, 1973.
36. Hodgkin, J. E.: Prognosis in chronic obstructive pulmonary disease. Clin. Chest Med., *11*:555, 1990.
37. Anthonisen, N. R.: Prognosis in chronic obstructive pulmonary disease: results from multicenter clinical trials. Am. Rev. Respir. Dis., *140*:S95, 1989.
38. Peto, R., et al.: The Relevance in adults of air-flow obstruction, but not of mucus hypersecretion, to mortality from chronic lung disease: results from 20 years of prospective observation. Am. Rev. Respir. Dis., *128*:491, 1983.
39. Sukumalchantra, Y., Dinikara, P., and Williams, M. H. Jr.: Prognosis of patients with chronic obstructive pulmonary disease after hospitalization for acute ventilatory failure: a three-year follow-up study. ARRD, *93*:215, 1966.
40. Bradley, R. D., Spencer, G. T., and Semple, S. J. G.: Tracheostomy and artificial ventilation in the treatment of acute exacerbations of chronic lung disease. A study in twenty-nine patients. Lancet, *1*:854, 1964.
41. Jessen, O., Kristensen, H. S., and Rasmussen, K.: Tracheostomy and ventilation in chronic lung disease. Lancet, *2*:9, 1967.
42. Asmundsson, T., and Kilburn, K. H.: Survival of acute respiratory failure: a study of 239 episodes. Ann. Intern. Med., *70*:471, 1969.
43. Wessel-Aas T, Vale JR, Hauge HE. Artificial ventilation in chronic pulmonary insufficiency. Indications and prognosis. Scand. J. Respir. Dis., *72(Suppl)*:36, 1979.
44. Gillespie, D. J., Marsh, H. M. M., Divertie, M. B., and Meadows, J. A.: Clinical outcome of respiratory failure in patients requiring prolonged (>24 hours) mechanical ventilation. Chest, *90*:364, 1986.
45. Menzies, R., Gibbons, W., and Goldberg, P.: Determinants of weaning and survival among patients with COPD who require mechanical ventilation for acute respiratory failure. Chest, *95*:398, 1989.
46. Petty, T. L.: Editor's perspective. Semin. Respir. Med., *4*:321, 1983.
47. Gottlieb, L. S., and Balchum, O. J.: Course of chronic obstructive pulmonary disease following first onset of respiratory failure. Chest, *63*:5, 1973.
48. Anthonisen, N. R.: Recent advances in pharmacotherapy: chronic obstructive pulmonary disease. Can. Med. Assoc. J., *138*:503, 1988.
49. Hudson, L. D., and Monti, C. M.: Rationale and use of corticosteroids in chronic obstructive pulmonary disease. Med. Clin. North Am., *74*:661, 1990
50. Ziment, I.: Pharmacologic therapy of obstructive airway disease. Clin. Chest Med., *11*:461, 1990.
51. Wyse, S. D., Gibson, D. G., and Branthwaite, M. D.: Hemodynamic effects of salbutamol in patients needing circulatory support after open-heart surgery. Br. Med. J., *3*:502, 1974.
52. Gross, N. J., and Skorodin, M. S.: Role of the parasympathetic system in airway obstruction due to emphysema. N. Eng. J. Med., *311*:421, 1984.
53. Karpel, J. P., Pesin, J., Greenberg, D., and Gentry, E.: A Comparison of the effects of ipratropium bromite and metaproterenol sulfate in acute exacerbations of chronic obstructive pulmonary disease. Chest, *98*:835, 1990.
54. Gross, N.: Ipratropium bromide. N. Engl. J. Med., *319*:486, 1988.
55. Ward, M. J., Fentem, P. H., Roderick, W. H., and Davies, D.: Ipratropium bromide in acute asthma. Br. Med. J., *282*:598, 1981.
56. Vozeh, S., et al.: Theophylline serum concentration and therapeutic effect in severe acute bronchial obstruction: the optimal use of intravenously administered aminophylline. Am. Rev. Respir. Dis., *125*:181, 1982.
57. Rice, K. L., et al.: Aminophylline for acute exacerbations of chronic obstructive pulmonary disease. Ann. Intern. Med., *107*:305, 1987.
58. Seidenfield, J. J., et al.: Intravenous Aminophylline in the treatment of acute bronchospastic exacerbations of chronic obstructive disease. Ann. Emerg. Med., *13*:284, 1984.
59. Matthey, R. A.: Effects of theophylline on cardiovascular performance in chronic obstructive pulmonary disease. Chest, *88*:1125, 1985.
60. Aubier, M., et al.: Aminophylline Improves Diaphragm Contractility. N. Engl. J. Med., *305*:249, 1981.
61. Zwillich, C. W., et al.: Theophylline-induced seizures in adults: correlation with serum concentrations. Ann. Intern. Med. *82*:784, 1975.
62. Beerel, F., Jick, H., and Tyler, J. M.: A controlled study of the effect of prednisone on air-flow obstruction in severe pulmonary emphysema. N. Engl. J. Med., *268*:226, 1963.

63. Hurford, J. V., Little, G. M., Loudon, W. G.: The use of prednisolone in chronic bronchitis. Br. J. Dis. Chest, 57: 133, 1963.
64. Morgan, W. K. C., and Rusche, E.: A Controlled trial of the effects of steroids in obstructive airway disease. Ann. Intern. Med., 61:284, 1964.
65. Beerel, F. R., and Vance, J. W.: Prednisone treatment for stable pulmonary emphysema. Am. Rev. Respir. Dis., 104: 264, 1971.
66. Evans, J. A., Morrison, I. M., and Saunders, K. B. A controlled trial of prednisone, in low dosage, in patients with chronic airways obstruction. Thorax, 29:401, 1974.
67. Shim, C., Stover, D. E., and Williams, M. H. Jr. Response to corticosteroids in chronic bronchitis. J. Allergy Clin. Immunol., 62:363, 1978.
68. Mendella, L. A., Manfreda, J., Warren, P. W., and Anthonisen, N. R.: Steroid response in stable chronic obstructive pulmonary disease. Ann. Intern. Med., 96:17, 1982.
69. O'Reilly, J. F., Shaylor, J. M., Fromings, K. M., and Harrison, B. D.: The use of the 12 minute walking test in assessing the effect of oral steroid therapy in patients with chronic airways obstruction. Br. J. Dis. Chest, 76:374, 1982.
70. Lam, W. K., So, S. Y., and Yu, D. Y. C.: Response to oral corticosteroids in chronic airflow obstruction. Br. J. Dis. Chest, 77:189, 1983.
71. Mitchell, D. M., et al.: Effects of prednisolone in chronic airflow limitation. Lancet, 1:193, 1984.
72. Blair, G. P., and Light, R. W.: Treatment of chronic obstructive pulmonary disease with corticosteroids: comparison of daily vs alternate-day therapy. Chest, 86:524, 1984.
73. Strain, D. S., Kinasewitz, G. T., Franco, D. P., and Goerge, R. B.: Effects of steroid therapy on exercise performance in patients with irreversible chronic obstructive pulmonary disease. Chest, 88:718, 1985.
74. Eliasson, O., et al.: Corticosteroids in COPD: a clinical trial and reassessment of the literature. Chest, 89:484, 1986.
75. Shim, C. S., and Williams, M. H.: Aerosol beclomethasone in patients with steroid-responsive chronic obstructive pulmonary disease. Am. J. Med., 78:655, 1985.
76. Emerman, C. L., et al. A randomized controlled trial of methylprednisone in the emergency treatment of acute exacerbations of COPD. Chest, 95:663, 1989.
77. Albert, R. K., Martin, T. R., and Lewis, S. W.: Controlled clinical trial of methylprednisolone in patients with chronic bronchitis and acute respiratory insufficiency. Ann. Intern. Med., 92:753, 1980.
78. Anthonisen, N. R., et al.: Antibiotic therapy in exacerbations of chronic obstructive pulmonary disease. Ann. Intern. Med., 106:196, 1987.
79. Mathur, P. N., et al.: Effect of digoxin on right ventricular function in severe chronic airflow obstruction. Ann Intern Med, 95:283, 1981.
80. Mecca, T. E., Elam, J. T., and Caldwell, R. W.: Mechanism of the pulmonary vasoconstrictor action in dogs. J. Cardiovasc. Pharmacol., 7:833, 1985.
81. Dal Nogare, A. R., and Rubin, L. J.: The effects of hydralazine on exercise capacity in pulmonary hypertension secondary to chronic obstructive pulmonary disease. Am. Rev. Respir. Dis., 133:385, 1986
82. Pearlman, R. A., Inui, T. S., and Carter, W. B.: Variability in physician bioethical decision-making: a case study of euthanasia. Ann. Intern. Med., 97:420, 1982.
83. Perkins, H. S., Jonsen, A. R., and Epstein, W. V.: Providers as predictors: using outcome predictions in intensive care. Crit. Care Med., 14:105, 1986.
84. Perkins, H. S.: Using outcome predictions to make treatment decisions. Chest, 91:475, 1987.
85. Hilberman, M., et al.: An analysis of potential physiological predictors of respiratory adequacy following cardiac surgery. J. Thorac. Cardiovasc. Surg., 71:711, 1976.
86. Smith, C. B., Golden, C. A., Kanner, R. E., and Renzetti, A. D.: Association of viral and mycoplasma pneumonia infections with acute respiratory illness in patients with chronic obstructive pulmonary diseases. Am. Rev. Respir. Dis., 121: 225, 1980.
87. Gump, D. W., et al. Role of infection in chronic bronchitis. Am. Rev. Respir. Dis., 113:465, 1976.
88. Fagon, J. Y., et al.: Characterization of distal bronchial microflora during acute exacerbation of chronic bronchitis. Am. Rev. Respir. Dis., 142:1004, 1990.
89. Ng, M. L., Levy, M. N., DeGeest, H., and Zieske, H.: Effects of myocardial hypoxia on left ventricular performance. Am. J. Physiol., 211:43, 1966.
90. Downning, S. E., Talner, N. S., and Gardner, T. H.: Influences of hypoxemia and acidemia on left ventricular function. Am. J. Physiol., 210: 1327, 1966.
91. Kohama, A., et al.: Pathologic involvement of the left ventricle in chronic cor pulmonale. Chest, 98:794, 1990.
92. Hooper, R. G., and Whitecomb, M. E.: Systolic time intervals in chronic obstructive pulmonary disease. Circulation, 50: 1205, 1974.
93. Jardin, F., et al.: Two-dimensional echocardiographic assessment of left ventricular function in chronic obstructive pulmonary disease. Am. Rev. Respir. Dis., 129:135, 1984.
94. Chipps, B. E., et al.: Noninvasive evaluation of ventricular function in cystic fibrosis. J. Pediatr., 95:379, 1979.
95. Christianson, L. C., Shah, A., and Fisher, V. J.: Quantitative left ventricular cineangiography in patients with chronic obstructive pulmonary disease. Am. J. Med., 66:399, 1979.
96. Steele, P., et al.: Left ventricular ejection fraction in severe chronic obstructive airway disease. Am. J. Med., 59:21, 1975.
97. Loyd, J. E., Nolop, K. B., Parker, R. E., and Roselli, R. J.: Effects of inspiratory resistance loading on lung fluid balance in awake sheep. J. Appl. Physiol., 60:198, 1986.
98. Allen, S. J., et al.: Elevation of superior vena caval pressure increases extravascular lung water after endotoxemia. J. Appl. Physiol., 62:1006, 1987.
99. Laine, G. A., et al.: Effect of systemic venous pressure elevation on lymph flow and lung edema formation. J. Appl. Physiol., 61:1643, 1986.
100. Heinemann, H. O.: Right-sided heart failure and the use of diuretics. Am. J. Med., 64:367, 1978.
101. Mitchell, R. S., Silvers, G. W., Dart, G. A., and Petty, T. L.: Am. Rev. Respir. Dis., 97:54, 1968.
102. Prescott, S. M., et al.: Venous Thromboembolism in Decompensated Chronic Obstructive Pulmonary Disease. Am. Rev. Respir. Dis., 123:32, 1981.
103. Hull, R. D., et al.: Pulmonary angiography, ventilation lung scanning, and venography for clinically suspected pulmonary embolism with abnormal perfusion lung scan. Ann. Intern Med., 98:891, 1983.
104. Goodman, P. C.: Pulmonary angiography. Clin. Chest Med., 5:465, 1984.
105. Nicod, P., et al.: Pulmonary angiography in severe chronic pulmonary hypertension. Ann. Intern. Med., 107:565, 1987.
106. Wiest, P. M., et al.: Serious infectious complications of corticosteroid therapy for chronic obstructive pulmonary disease. Chest, 95:1180, 1989.
107. Dines, D. E., Clagett, O. T., and Payne, W. S.: Spontaneous pneumothorax in emphysema. Mayo Clin. Proc., 45:481, 1970.

108. Charan, N. B., and Lakshminarayan, S.: Pulmonary effects of topical timolol. Arch. Intern. Med., 140:843, 1980.
109. Sharp, J. T.: The chest wall and respiratory muscles in airflow limitation. In The Thorax. Part B. Edited by C. Roussos and P. T. Madelem. New York, Marcel Dekker, 1985, p. 1155.
110. Kim, M. J., et al.: Mechanics of the canine diaphragm. J. Appl. Physiol., 41:369, 1976.
111. Braun, N. M. T., Arora, N. S., and Rochester, D. F.: Force-length relationship of the normal human diaphragm. J. Appl. Physiol., 53:405, 1982.
112. Farkas, G. A., and Roussos, C.: Adaptability of the hamster diaphragm to exercise and/or emphysema. J. Appl. Physiol., 53:1263, 1982.
113. Goldberg, P., and Roussos, C.: Assessment of respiratory muscle dysfunction in chronic obstructive lung disease. Med. Clin. North Am., 74:643, 1990.
114. Roussos, C.: Function and fatigue of respiratory muscles. Chest, 88:1245, 1985.
115. Tobin, M. J.: Respiratory muscles in disease. Clin. Chest Med., 9:263, 1988.
116. Pepe, P. E., and Marini, J. J.: Occult positive end-expiratory pressure in mechanically ventilated patients with airflow obstruction: the auto-PEEP effect. Am. Rev. Respir. Dis., 126:166, 1982.
117. Rossi, A., et al.: Measurement of static compliance of the total respiratory system in patients with acute respiratory failure during mechanical ventilation. Am. Rev. Respir. Dis., 131:672, 1985.
118. Dal Vecchio, L., Polese, G., Poggi, R., and Rossi, A.: "Intrinsic" positive end-expiratory pressure in stable patients with chronic obstructive pulmonary disease. Eur. Respir. J., 3: 74, 1990.
119. Murciano, D., et al.: Comparison of esophageal, tracheal, and mouth occlusion pressure in patients with chronic obstructive pulmonary disease during acute respiratory failure. Am. Rev. Respir. Dis., 126:837, 1982.
120. Macklem, P. T.: The importance of defining respiratory muscle fatigue. Am. Rev. Respir. Dis., 142:274, 1990.
121. Roussos, C. S., and Macklem, P. T.: Diaphragmatic fatigue in man. J. Appl. Physiol., 43:189, 1977.
122. Cohen, C. A., et al.: Clinical manifestations of inspiratory muscle fatigue. Am. J. Med., 73:308, 1982.
123. Tobin, M. J., et al.: Konno-Mead analysis of ribcage-abdominal motion during successful and unsuccessful trails of weaning from mechanical ventilation. Am. Rev. Respir. Dis., 135:1320, 1987.
124. Tobin, M. J., et al.: The pattern of breathing during successful and unsuccessful trials of weaning from mechanical ventilation. Am. Rev. Respir. Dis., 134:1111, 1986.
125. Miech, R. P., and Stein, M.: Methylxanthines. Clin. Chest Med., 7:331, 1986.
126. Kearney, T. E., Manoguerra, A. S., Curtis, G. P., and Ziegler, M. G.: Theophylline toxicity and the beta-adrenergic system. Ann. Intern. Med., 102:766, 1985.
127. McPherson, M. L., et al.: Theophylline-induced hypercalcemia. Ann. Intern. Med., 105:52, 1986.
128. Pierce, R. J., et al.: Comparison of intravenous and inhaled terbutaline in the treatment of asthma. Chest, 79:506, 1981.
129. Lawford, P., Jones, B. J. M., and Milledge, S. S.: Comparison of intravenous and nebulized salbutamol in initial treatment of severe asthma. Br. Med. J., 1:84, 1978.
130. Williams, S. J., Winner, S. J., and Clark, T. S. H.: Comparison of inhaled and intravenous terbutaline in acute severe asthma. Thorax, 36:629, 1981.
131. Williams, S., and Seaton, W.: Intravenous or inhaled salbutamol in acute severe asthma. Thorax, 32:555, 1977.
132. Shim, C., and Williams, M. H.: Bronchial response to oral versus aerosol metaproterenol in asthma. Ann. Intern. Med., 93:428, 1980.
133. Walters, E. H., et al.: Optimal dose of salbutamol respiratory solution: comparison of three doses with plasma levels. Thorax, 36:625, 1981.
134. Gelmont, D. M., Balmes, J. R., and Yee, A.: Hypokalemia induced by inhaled bronchodilators. Chest, 94:763, 1988.
135. Allon, M., Dunlay, R., and Copkney, C. H.: Nebulized albuterol for acute hyperkalemia in patients on hemodialysis. Ann. Intern. Med., 110:426, 1989.
136. Patel, K. R., and Tullet, W. M.: Bronchoconstriction in response to ipratropium bromide. Br. Med. J., 286:1318, 1983.
137. Janssens, S., and Decramer, M.: Corticosteroid-induced myopathy and the respiratory muscles. Chest, 95:1160, 1989.
138. Glenny, R. W.: Steroids in COPD: the scripture according to Albert. Chest, 91:289, 1987.
139. Aubier, M., et al.: Effects of the administration of O_2 on ventilation and blood gases in patients with chronic obstructive pulmonary disease during acute respiratory failure. Am. Rev. Respir. Dis., 122:747, 1980.
140. Johanson, W. G., and Peters, J. I.: Respiratory failure: general principles and initial approach. In Textbook of Respiratory Medicine. Edited by J. F. Murray and J. A. Nadel. Philadelphia, W. B. Saunders, 1988, p. 1973.
141. Enson, Y. et al.: The influence of hydrogen ion concentration and hypoxia on the pulmonary circulation. J. Clin. Invest., 43:1146, 1964.
142. Degaute, J. P., et al.: Oxygen delivery in acute exacerbation of chronic obstructive pulmonary disease. Am. Rev. Respir. Dis., 124:26, 1981.
143. Morrison, D. A., Henry, R., and Goldman, S.: Preliminary study of the effects of low flow oxygen on oxygen delivery and right ventricular function in chronic lung disease. Am. Rev. Respir. Dis., 133:390, 1986.
144. Viires, N., et al.: Effects of aminophylline on diaphragmatic fatigue during acute respiratory failure. Am. Rev. Respir. Dis., 129:396, 1984.
145. Murciano, D., Aubier, M., Lecocquic, Y., and Pariente, R.: Effect of theophylline on diaphragmatic strength and fatigue in patients with chronic obstructive pulmonary disease. N. Engl. J. Med., 311:349, 1984.
146. Aubier, M., Murciano, D., Viires, N., and Lebargy, F.: Effects of digoxin on diaphragmatic strength generation in patients with chronic obstructive pulmonary disease during acute respiratory failure. Am. Rev. Respir. Dis., 135:544, 1987.
147. Aubier, M., Viires, N., Murciano, D., and Medrano, G.: Effects and mechanisms of action of terbutaline on diaphragmatic contractility and fatigue. J. Appl. Physiol., 56:922, 1984.
148. Aubier, M., et al.: Dopamine effects on diaphragmatic strength during acute respiratory failure in chronic obstructive pulmonary disease. Ann. Intern. Med., 110:17, 1989.
149. Simkovitz, P., et al.: Interaction between intrinsic and externally applied PEEP during mechanical ventilation. Am. Rev. Respir. Dis., 135:A202, 1987.
150. Smith, T. C., and Marini, J. J.: Impact of PEEP on lung mechanics and work of breathing in severe airflow obstruction. J. Appl. Physiol., 65:1488, 1988.
151. Petroff, B. J., et al.: Continuous positive airway pressure reduces work of breathing and dyspnea during weaning from mechanical ventilation in severe chronic obstructive pulmonary disease. Am. Rev. Respir. Dis., 141:281, 1990.
152. Goldberg, P., Reissmann, H., Ranieri, M., and Gottfried, S.: CPAP reduces inspiratory effort during acute respiratory

failure in chronic obstructive pulmonary disease. Chest, *98:* 76S, 1990.
153. Ellis, E. R., Bye, P. T. P., Bruderer, J. W., and Sullivan, C. E.: Treatment of respiratory failure during sleep in patients with neuromuscular disease. Am. Rev. Respir. Dis., *135:* 148, 1987.
154. Meduri, G. U., Conoscenti, C. C., Menashe, P., and Nair, S.: Noninvasive face mask ventilation in patients with acute respiratory failure. Chest, *95:*865, 1989.
155. Aubier, M., Trippenbach, T., and Roussos, C. H.: Respiratory muscle fatigue during cardiogenic shock. J. Appl. Physiol., *51:*499, 1981.
156. Schnader, J. Y., et al.: Arterial CO_2 partial pressure affects diaphragmatic function. J. Appl. Physiol., *58:*823, 1985.
157. Pourriat, J. L., et al.: Diaphragmatic fatigue and breathing pattern during weaning from mechanical ventilation in COPD patients. Chest, *90:*703, 1986.
158. Weitzenblum, E., et al.: Long-term course of pulmonary arterial pressure in chronic obstructive pulmonary disease. Am. Rev. Respir. Dis., *130:*993, 1984.
159. Abraham, A. S., et al.: Factors contributing to the reversible hypertension of patients with acute respiratory failure studied by serial observations during recovery. Circu. Res. *24:* 51, 1969.
160. Weitzenblum, E., Loiseau, A., Hirth, C., and Mirhom, R.: Course of pulmonary hemodynamics in patients with chronic obstructive lung disease. Chest, *75:*656, 1979.
161. Janicki, J. S., Shroff, S. G., and Weber, K. T.: Ventricular interdependence. *In* Heart-Lung Interactions in Health and Disease. Edited by S. M. Scharf and S. S. Cassidy. New York, Marcel Dekker, 1989.
162. Sibbald, W., Driedger, A. S., Myres, M. L., and Short, A. I. K.: Biventricular function in the adult respiratory distress syndrome. Chest, *84:*126, 1983.
163. Broseghini, C., et al.: Respiratory mechanics during the first day of mechanical ventilation in patients with pulmonary edema and chronic airway obstruction. Am. Rev. Respir. Dis., *138:*355, 1988.
164. Butler, J., et al.: Cause of the raised wedge pressure on exercise in chronic obstructive pulmonary disease. Am. Rev. Respir. Dis., *138:*350, 1988.
165. Kline, L. E., et al.: Noninvasive assessment of left ventricular performance in patients with chronic obstructive pulmonary disease. Chest, *72:*558, 1977.
166. Danek, S. J., Lynch, J. P., Weg, J. G., and Dantzker, D. R.: The dependence of oxygen uptake on oxygen delivery with adult respiratory distress syndrome. Am. Rev. Respir. Dis., *122:*387, 1980.
167. Mohsenifar, Z., Jasper, A. C., and Koerner, S. K.: Relationship between oxygen uptake and oxygen delivery in patients with pulmonary hypertension. Am. Rev. Respir. Dis., *138:*69, 1988.
168. Matthay, R. A., Niederman, M. S., and Wiedemann, H. P.: Cardiovascular-pulmonary interaction in chronic obstructive pulmonary disease with special reference to the pathogenesis and management of cor pulmonale. Med. Clin. North Am., *74:*571, 1990.
169. Sylvester, J. T., Goldberg, H. S., and Permutt, S.: The role of the vasculature in the regulation of cardiac output. Clin Chest Med., *4:*11, 1983.
170. Reuse, C., Vincent, J. L., and Pinsky, M. R.: Measurements of right ventricular volumes during fluid challenge. Chest, *98:*1450, 1990.
171. Magder, S. A., Cheong, T. H., and Georgiadis, G.: Respiratory variations in CVP predict response to fluid challenge. Chest, *98:*118S, 1990.
172. Ghignone, M., Girling, L., and Prewitt, R.: Volume expansion versus norepinephrine in treatment of a low cardiac output complicating an acute increase in right ventricular afterload in dogs. Anesthesiology, *60:*132, 1984.
173. Weisse, A. B., et al.: Hemodynamic effects of staged hematocrit reduction in patients with stable cor pulmonale and severely elevated hematocrit levels. Am. J. Med., *58:*92, 1975.
174. Brent, B. N., et al.: Contrasting acute effects of vasodilators (nitroglycerin, nitroprusside, and hydralazine) on right ventricular performance in patients with chronic obstructive pulmonary disease and pulmonary hypertension: a combined radionuclide-hemodynamic study. Am. J. Cardiol., *51:* 1682, 1983.
175. Agostoni, P., et al.: Nifedipine reduces pulmonary pressure and vascular tone during short- but not long-term treatment of pulmonary hypertension in patients with chronic obstructive pulmonary disease. Am. Rev. Respir. Dis., *139:* 120, 1989.
176. Burke, C. M., et al.: Captopril and domiciliary oxygen in chronic airflow obstruction. Br. Med. J., *290:*1251, 1985.
177. Naeije, R., Melot, C., Mols, P., and Hallemans, R.: Reduction in pulmonary hypertension by prostaglandin E1 in decompensated chronic obstructive pulmonary disease. Am. Rev. Respir. Dis., *125:*1, 1982.
178. Brent, B. N., Berger, H. J., Matthay, R., and Mahler, D.: Physiologic correlates of right ventricular ejection fraction in chronic obstructive pulmonary disease: a combined radionuclide and hemodynamic study. Am. J. Cardiol., *50:*255, 1982.
179. Rubin, L. J.: Cardiovascular effects of vasodilator therapy for pulmonary arterial hypertension. Clin. Chest Med., *4:* 309, 1983.
180. Vlahakes, G. J., Turley, K., and Hoffman, J. I. E.: The pathophysiology of failure in acute right ventricular hypertension: hemodynamic and biochemical correlations. Circulation, *63:*87, 1981.
181. Brooks, H., et al.: Performance of the right ventricle under stress: relation to right coronary flow. J. Clin. Invest., *50:* 2176, 1971.
182. Spotnitz, H. M., Berman, M. A., and Epstein, S. E.: Pathophysiology and experimental treatment of acute pulmonary embolism. Am. Heart J., *82:*511, 1971.
183. Molloy, W. D., et al.: Treatment of shock in a canine model of pulmonary embolism. Am. Rev. Respir. Dis., *130:*870, 1984.
184. Schaer, G. L., Fink, M. P., and Parrillo, J. E.: Norepinephrine alone versus norepinephrine plus low-dose dopamine: enhanced renal blood flow with combination pressor therapy. Crit. Care Med., *13:*492, 1985.
185. Wilson, D. O., Rogers, R. M., and Hoffman, R. M.: Nutrition and chronic lung disease. Am. Rev. Respir. Dis., *132:*1374, 1985.
186. Arora, N. S., and Rochester, D. F.: Respiratory muscle strength and maximal voluntary ventilation in undernourished patients. Am. Rev. Respir. Dis., *126:*5, 1982.
187. Rochester, D. F., Arora, N. S., Braun, N. M. T., and Goldberg, S. K.: The respiratory muscles in chronic obstructive pulmonary disease (COPD). Bull. Eur. Physiopathol. Respir., *15:* 951, 1979.
188. Rochester, D. F., and Braun, N. M. T.: Determinants of maximal inspiratory pressure in chronic obstructive pulmonary disease. Am. Rev. Respir. Dis., *132:*42, 1985.
189. Kelly, S. M., et al.: Inspiratory muscle strength and body composition in patients receiving total parenteral nutrition therapy. Am. Rev. Respir. Dis., *130:*33, 1984.
190. Rochester, D. F: Malnutrition and the respiratory muscles. Clin. Chest Med., *7:*91, 1986.

191. Askanazi, J., et al.: Respiratory changes induced by the large glucose loads of total parenteral nutrition. JAMA, *243:*1444, 1980.
192. Askanazi, J., et al.: Nutrition for the patient with respiratory failure. Anesthesiology, *54:*373, 1981.
193. Covelli, H. D., Black, J. W., Olsen, M. S., and Beekman, J. F.: Respiratory failure precipitated by high carbohydrate loads. Ann. Intern. Med., *95:*579, 1981.
194. Angelillo, V. A., et al.: Effects of low and high carbohydrate feedings in ambulatory patients with chronic obstructive pulmonary disease and chronic hypercapnia. Ann. Intern. Med., *103:*883, 1985.
195. Al-Saady, N., Blackmore, C., and Bennett, E. D.: Low carbohydrate (CHO), high fat, enteral feeding in patients requiring intermittent positive pressure ventilation (IPPV), lowers Paco$_2$, and reduces the period of ventilation. Clin. Nutr., *6(Suppl.):*77, 1987.
196. Skeie, B., et al.: Intravenous fat emulsions and lung function: a review. Crit. Care Med., *16:*183, 1988.
197. Hageman, J. R., and Hunt, C. E. Fat emulsions and lung function in nutrition and respiratory disease. Clin. Chest Med., *7:*69, 1986.
198. Venus, B., et al.: Cardiopulmonary effects of intralipid infusion in critically ill patients. Crit. Care Med., *16:*587, 1988.
199. Maini, B. S.: Nutritional support in the intensive care patient. *In* Intensive Care Medicine. Edited by J. M. Rippe, R. S. Irwin, J. S. Alpert, J. E. Dalen. Little Brown & Co., 1985, p. 762.
200. Roussos, C.: Ventilatory failure and respiratory muscles. *In* The Thorax, Part B. Edited by C. Roussos and P. T. Macklem. New York, Marcel Dekker, 1985, p. 1253.
201. Morganroth, M. L., Morganroth, J. L., Nett, L. M., and Petty, T. L.: Criteria for weaning from prolonged mechanical ventilation. Arch. Intern. Med., *144:*1012, 1984.
202. Macklem, P. T.: Respiratory muscles: the vital pump. Chest, *78:*753, 1980.
203. Padmanabhan, K., and Dhar, S. R.: Irreversible hypercapnia secondary to embolic occlusion of the pulmonary artery. Chest, *86:*927, 1984.
204. Whitelaw, W. A., Derenne, J. P., and Milic-Emili, J.: Occlusion pressure as a measure of respiratory center output in conscious man. Respir. Physiol., *23:*181, 1975.
205. Fernandez, R., et al.: Inspiratory effort and occlusion pressure in triggered mechanical ventilation. Intensive Care Med., *14:*650, 1988.
206. Witt, N. J., et al.: Peripheral nerve function in sepsis and multiple organ failure. Chest, *99:*176, 1991.
207. Bolton, C. F., Gilbert, J. J., Hahn, A. F., and Sibbald, W. J., Polyneuropathy in critically ill patients. J. Neurol. Neurosurg. Psychiatry, *47:*1223, 1984.
208. Roussos, C., Fixley, M., Gross, D., and Macklem, P. T.: Fatigue of inspiratory muscles and their synergistic behaviour. J. Appl. Physiol., *46:*897, 1979.
209. Bellemare, F., and Grassino, A.: Force reserve of the diaphragm in patients with chronic obstructive lung disease. J. Appl. Physiol., *55:*8, 1983.
210. Aubier, M., et al.: Effects of hypophosphatemia on diaphragmatic contractility in patients with acute respiratory failure. N. Engl. J. Med., *313:*420, 1985.
211. Aubier, M., et al.: Effect of hypocalcemia on diaphragmatic strength generation. J. Appl. Physiol., *58:*2054, 1985.
212. Marini, J. J.: Monitoring during mechanical ventilation. Clin. Chest Med., *9:*73, 1988.
213. Grassino, A., and Macklem, P. T.: Respiratory muscle fatigue and ventilatory failure. Ann. Rev. Med., *35:*625, 1984.
214. Marini, J. J., Rodriguez, R. M., and Lamb, V.: The inspiratory workload of patient-initiated mechanical ventilation. Am. Rev. Respir. Dis., *134:*902, 1986.
215. Ward, M. E., et al.: Optimization of respiratory muscle relaxation during mechanical ventilation. Anesthesiology, *69:*29, 1988.
216. Gibney, R. T. N., Wilson, R. S., and Pontoppidan, H.: Comparisons of work of breathing on high gas flow and demand valve continuous positive airway pressure systems. Chest, *82:*692, 1982.
217. Williams, H. M.: IMV and weaning. Chest, *78:*804, 1980.
218. Anzueto, A., et al.: Effect of prolonged mechanical ventilation on diaphragmatic function: a preliminary study of a baboon model. Am. Rev. Respir. Dis., *135:*A201, 1987.
219. Harver, A., Mahler, D. A., and Daubenspeck, A. J.: Targeted inspiratory muscle training improves respiratory muscle function and reduces dyspnea in patients with chronic obstructive pulmonary disease. Ann. Intern. Med., *111:*117, 1989.
220. Pardy, R. L., Reid, W. D., and Belman, M. J.; Respiratory muscle training. Clin. Chest Med., *9:*287, 1988.
221. Aldrich, T. K., et al.: Weaning from mechanical ventilation: adjunctive use of inspiratory muscle resistive training. Crit. Care Med., *17:*143, 1989.
222. Tomlinson, J. R., et al.: A prospective comparison of IMV and T-piece weaning from mechanical ventilation. Chest, *96:*348, 1989.
223. Brochard, L., Harf, A., Lorino, H., and Lemaire, F.: Inspiratory pressure support prevents diaphragmatic fatigue during weaning from mechanical ventilation. Am. Rev. Respir. Dis., *139:*513, 1989.
224. Sahn, S. A., and Lakshminarayan, S.: Bedside criteria for discontinuation of mechanical ventilation. Chest, *63:*1002, 1973.
225. Tahvanainen, J., Salenpera, M., and Nikki, P.: Extubation criteria after weaning from intermittent mandatory ventilation and continuous positive airway pressure. Crit. Care Med., *11:*702, 1983.
226. Tobin, M. J., and Yang, K.: Weaning from mechanical ventilation. Crit. Care Clin. *6:*725, 1990.
227. Sassoon, C. S. H., Te, T. T., Mahutte, C. K., and Light, R.: Airway occlusion pressure: an important indicator for successful weaning in patients with chronic obstructive pulmonary disease. Am. Rev. Respir. Dis., *135:*197, 1987.
228. Murciano, D., et al.: Tracheal occlusion pressure: a simple index to monitor respiratory muscle fatigue during acute respiratory failure in patients with chronic obstructive pulmonary disease. Ann. Intern. Med., *108:*800, 1988.
229. Montgomery, A. B., Holle, R. H. O., and Neagley, R. N.: Prediction of successful ventilatory weaning using airway occlusion pressure and hypercapnic challenge. Chest, *91:*496, 1987.
230. Swartz, M. A., and Marino, P. L.: Diaphragmatic strength during weaning from mechanical ventilation. Chest, *88:*736, 1985.
231. Proctor, H. J., and Woolson, R.: Prediction of respiratory muscle fatigue by measurement of the work of breathing. Surg. Gynecol. Obstet., *136:*367, 1973.
232. Peters, R. M., Hilberman, M., and Hogan, J. S.: Objective indications for respiratory therapy in post-trauma and post-operative patients. Am. J. Surg., *124:*262, 1972.
233. Fiastro, J. F., Habib, M. P., and Shon, B. Y.: Comparison of standard weaning parameters and mechanical work of breathing in mechanically ventilated patients. Chest, *94:*232, 1988.
234. Tobin, M. J., et al.: Does ribcage-abdominal paradox signify respiratory muscle fatigue? J. Appl. Physiol., *62:*851, 1987.
235. Yang, K. L., and Tobin, M. J.: Decision analysis of param-

eters used to predict outcome of a trail of weaning from mechanical ventilation. Am. Rev. Respir. Dis., *139*:A98, 1989.
236. Knudson, R. J., Kaltenborn, W. T., and Burrows, B.: The effects of cigarette smoking and smoking cessation on carbon monoxide diffusing capacity of the lung in asymptomatic subjects. Am. Rev. Respir. Dis., *140*:645, 1989.
237. Anthonisen, N. R., et al.: Prognosis in chronic obstructive pulmonary disease. Am. Rev. Respir. Dis., *133*:14, 1986.
238. Godenick, M. T.: A review of available smoking cessation methods, 1989. MMJ, *38*:277, 1989.
239. Godenick, M. T.: A review of available smoking cessation methods, 1989. Part II. MMJ, *38*:377, 1989.
240. Kuller, L. H., et al.: The epidemiology of pulmonary function and COPD mortality in the Multiple Risk Factor Intervention Trial. Am. Rev. Respir. Dis., *140*:S76, 1989.
241. Petty, T. L., et al.: A comprehensive care program for chronic airway obstruction. Ann. Intern. Med., *70*:1109, 1969.
242. Hodgkin, J. E.: Pulmonary Rehabilitation. Clin. Chest Med., *11*:447, 1990.
243. Belman, M. J.: Exercise in chronic obstructive pulmonary disease. Clin. Chest Med., *7*:585, 1986.
244. Ambrosino, N., Paggiaro, P. L., Roselli, M. G., and Contini, V.: Failure of resistive breathing training to improve pulmonary function tests in patients with chronic obstructive pulmonary disease. Respiration, *45*:455, 1984.
245. Anderson, J. B., and Falk, P.: Clinical experience with inspiratory resistive breathing training. Int. Rehabil. Med., *6*:183, 1984.
246. Chen, H., Dukes, R., and Martin, B. J.: Inspiratory muscle training inpatients with chronic obstructive pulmonary disease. Am. Rev. Respir. Dis., *131*:251, 1985.
247. Goldstein, R., et al.: Applicability of a threshold loading device for inspiratory muscle testing and training in patients with COPD. Chest, *96*:564, 1989.
248. Harver, A., Mahler, D. A., and Daubenspeck, J. A.: Targeted inspiratory muscle training improves respiratory muscle function and reduces dyspnea in patients with chronic obstructive pulmonary disease. Ann. Intern. Med., *111*:117, 1988.
249. Larson, M., and Kim, M. J.: Respiratory muscle training with the incentive spirometer resistive breathing device. Heart Lung, *13*:341, 1984.
250. Levine, S., Weiser, P., and Gillen, J.: Evaluation of a ventilatory muscle endurance training program in the rehabilitation of patients with chronic obstructive pulmonary disease. Am. Rev. Respir. Dis., *133*:400, 1986.
251. Holle, R. H., and Williams, D. V.: Increased muscle efficiency and sustained benefits in an outpatient community hospital-based pulmonary rehabilitation program. Chest, *94*:1161, 1988.
252. Moser, K. M., et al.: Results of a comprehensive rehabilitation program. Arch. Intern. Med., *140*:1596, 1980.
253. Pineda, H., Haas, F., and Axen, K.: Treadmill exercise training in chronic obstructive pulmonary disease. Arch. Phys. Med. Rehabil., *67*:155, 1986.
254. Ries, A. L., Ellis, B., and Hawkins, R. W.: Upper extremity exercise training in chronic obstructive pulmonary disease. Chest, *93*:688, 1988
255. Carter, R., et al.: Exercise conditioning in the rehabilitation of patients with chronic obstructive pulmonary disease. Arch. Phys. Med. Rehabil., *69*:118, 1988.
256. Singh, B. S., Lewin, T.: Predictors of initial and final work capacity in a chronic obstructive airway disease rehabilitation program. Aust. N. Z. J. Psychiatry, *17*:321, 1983.
257. Martin, J. G., and Levy, R. D.: Respiratory muscle rest. Probl. Respir. Care, *3*:534, 1990.
258. Shapiro, S. S., et al.: Effect of negative pressure ventilation in severe chronic obstructive pulmonary disease. Lancet, *340*:1425, 1992.
259. Wilson, D. O., Rogers, R. M., and Openbrier, D.: Nutritional aspects of chronic obstructive pulmonary disease. Clin. Chest Med., *7*:643, 1986.
260. Openbrier, D., et al. Nutritional status and lung function in patients with emphysema and chronic bronchitis. Chest, *83*:17, 1983.
261. Gray-Donald, K., Gibbons, L., Shapiro, S., and Martin, J. G.: Effect of nutritional status on exercise performance in patients with chronic obstructive pulmonary disease. Am. Rev. Respir. Dis., *140*:1544, 1989.
262. Wilson, D. O., et al.: Nutritional intervention in malnourished patients with emphysema. Am. Rev. Respir. Dis., *134*:672, 1986.
263. Lewis, M. I., Belman, M. J., and Dorr-Uyemura, L.: Nutritional supplementation in ambulatory patients with chronic obstructive pulmonary disease. Am. Rev. Respir. Dis., *135*:1062, 1987.
264. Efthimiou, J., Fleming, J., Gomes, C., and Spiro, S. G.: The Effects of supplementary oral nutrition in poorly nourished patients with chronic obstructive pulmonary disease. Am. Rev. Respir. Dis., *137*:1075, 1988
265. Whittaker, J. S., Ryan, C. F., Buckley, P. A., and Road, J. D.: The Effects of refeeding on peripheral and respiratory muscle function in malnourished chronic obstructive pulmonary disease patients. Am. Rev. Respir. Dis., *142*:283, 1990.
266. Medical Research Council Working Party: Long term domiciliary oxygen therapy in chronic hypoxic cor pulmonale complicating chronic bronchitis and emphysema. Lancet, *1*:681, 1981.
267. Nocturnal Oxygen Therapy Trial Group: Continuous or nocturnal oxygen therapy in hypoxemic chronic obstructive lung disease (a clinical trial). Ann. Intern. Med., *93*:391, 1980.
268. Patterson, G. A.: Lung transplantation for chronic obstructive pulmonary disease. Clin. Chest Med., *11*:547, 1990.
269. Cooper, J. D., Patterson, G. A., Grossman, R., and Maurer, J.: Double-lung transplant for advanced chronic obstructive lung disease. Am. Rev. Respir. Dis., *139*:303, 1989.
270. Higenbottam, T., Stewart, S., Penketh, A., and Wallwork, J.: The Diagnosis of lung rejection and opportunistic infection by transbronchial lung biopsy. Transplant. Proc., *19*:3777, 1987.
271. Gibbons, W. J., et al.: Cardiopulmonary exercise responses after single lung transplantation for severe obstructive lung disease. Manuscript submitted for publication.
272. Mal, H., et al.: Case reports: unilateral lung transplantation in end-stage pulmonary emphysema. Am. Rev. Respir. Dis., *140*:797, 1989.
273. Trulock, E. P., et al.: Single lung transplantation for severe chronic obstructive pulmonary disease. Chest, *96*:738, 1989.
274. Frost, A. E., et al.: Exercise tolerance in patients undergoing double lung transplant for end stage pulmonary disease. Am. Rev. Respir. Dis., *137(Suppl)*:377, 1988.
275. Theodore, J.: Cardiopulmonary function at maximum tolerable constant work rate exercise following human heart-lung transplantation. Chest. *92*:433, 1987.

Chapter 16

MECHANICAL VENTILATION

CYRIL M. GRUM

PRE-ICU PHASE

Mechanical Ventilation in Perspective

In order to properly approach the patient at risk for requiring mechanical ventilation, we must first put this intervention in perspective. Although there are isolated reports of human trials dating back as early as the sixteenth century, mechanical ventilation has been used clinically only over the past 40 years.[1] Initially, the ventilation consisted of negative pressure ventilation systems, such as the iron lung and the cuirass, which became widespread during the poliomyelitis epidemic in the 1950s. The advent of positive pressure ventilation to support patients in an ICU setting has become popularized only since physically separate ICUs were developed in the late 1960s and early 1970s. Positive pressure ventilation was used initially to support the patient during surgical anesthesia. With the development of medical ICUs, the role of positive pressure ventilation expanded to include acutely ill patients who needed transient respiratory support. However, the 1970s and 1980s saw an exponential broadening of the spectrum of patients who were placed on mechanical ventilators, sometimes without regard to prognosis or to cost.

The technologic advances of mechanical ventilators have been extensive over the past 20 years. Each succeeding generation of ventilator has greater capability, with an ever wider array of functions and monitoring systems. The design of ventilators has radically changed over the last 10 years due to the use of computer technology and the ability to miniaturize components. These changes have allowed ICU physicians to support ventilation even in patients with the highest order of respiratory embarrassment. Indeed, it is becoming exceedingly rare for patients to die in ICUs due to an inability to provide adequate ventilation.

The current state of mechanical ventilation technology has far outpaced scientific explanation and critical scientific validation. New ventilation features and approaches are introduced and proliferate, long before studies can be done comparing them to more established techniques. New modes generally get accepted due to personal experience, ease of use, and small clinical trials. Because there are many variables relating to ultimate patient outcome, scientific validation of a new facet of mechanical ventilation is exceedingly difficult to achieve. Therefore, many studies use various clinical and physiologic parameters as specific end points rather than patient outcome. In addition, the critical nature of patient illness and the complexity of treatment does not lend itself to prospective, randomized, blinded clinical trials. Most of the mechanical ventilation modes and techniques that are widely accepted today have achieved their status largely due to tincture of time.

Risk Factors for Requiring Mechanical Ventilation

Patients that are at risk for needing mechanical ventilation must be identified early. Often the patient presents to the ICU in fulminant respiratory failure, such as occurs during an arrest situation. Emergency intubation and institution of mechanical ventilation is, however, fraught with anxiety, prone to miscalculations, and suffers an increased rate of complications. Therefore, a goal of critical care practitioners is to educate their professional counterparts to help identify those patients at highest risk for requiring mechanical ventilation. Knowledge and identification of these patients could lead to mechanical ventilation being avoided in some cases, but certainly should allow the institution of mechanical ventilation to be done in an elective and controlled manner whenever possible. Some of the most common causes of respiratory failure are listed in Table 16-1.

Patient symptoms and the physical examination alone are often not early predictors of impending respiratory failure in the setting of acute obstructive lung disease. Sequential pulmonary function testing of people with asthma or chronic obstructive lung disease is critical to predict which patients will progress to frank respiratory failure. In an asthmatic exacerbation, both the patient's subjective assessment or the physician's clinical assessment have been shown to be unreliable in predicting severity of obstruction.[2] Proper monitoring of these patients, in addition to the clinical examination, therefore requires the use of spirometry, measurement of peak expiratory flow, and the use of arterial blood gas analysis. An asthmatic at risk for requiring mechanical ventilation is characterized by an FEV_1 less than 1 L or a peak expiratory flow of less than 200 L per minute.[3] Confusion, disorientation, and fatigue in asthmatic patients are clear signs that mechanical ventilation will be required. In the asthmatic, the response to initial therapy is more important than the initial values of either the arterial blood gas or a spirometric assessment. A severe decline in respiratory function that does not respond to initial therapy signifies a very high risk group of patients that will likely need mechanical ventilation (see Chap. 14).

In chronic obstructive pulmonary disease (COPD), clinical assessment often aids the identification of the patient

Table 16–1. Common Causes of Respiratory Failure

Intrinsic lung disease
  Obstructive lung diseases
    Asthma
    COPD
    Emphysema
  Acute parenchymal disease
    Pneumonia
    Adult respiratory distress syndrome
Depressed ventilatory drive
  Central alveolar hypoventilation
  Drugs, especially narcotics and sedatives
  Central nervous system disease, such as strokes, trauma, hypoxia, or encephalitis
Neuromuscular diseases
  Guillain-Barré syndrome
  Myasthenia gravis
  Poliomyositis
  Muscular dystrophy
  Amyotrophic lateral sclerosis
  Acid maltase deficiency of the adult
Musculoskeletal problems
  Chest trauma
  Spinal deformity; e.g., kyphoscoliosis, thoracoplasty
  Obesity
  Pleural disease, effusion, or pneumothorax
  Diaphragmatic rupture or paralysis
Miscellaneous
  Upper airway obstruction (laryngospasm, foreign body, or epiglottitis)
  Hypothyroidism
  Hyperosmolar ketoacidosis
  Hypomagnesemia
  Hypophosphatemia

at risk for developing acute respiratory failure. Certainly, serial spirometry and arterial blood gases indicate which patients are at highest risk. The chronic presence of symptoms, however, blur the subjective distinction of impending respiratory failure versus an increase in symptomatology. In COPD patients, mental status changes, the presence of right heart failure, the use of accessory muscles of respiration, and diaphoresis are often a helpful adjunct to measurement of pulmonary function. Because infection is a leading cause of respiratory failure in these patients, extra vigilance should be afforded those patients who develop either viral or bacterial upper or lower respiratory tract infections.

Perhaps the most common cause of depressed ventilatory drive is the use of and the overdose of sedative drugs. The acute sedative overdose is easily recognized. Often sedative agents are, however, part of a complex picture leading to respiratory failure. Use of any sedative drugs, in patients with intrinsic lung diseases, in geriatric patients, and in patients on multiple pharmaceutical agents must be done with extreme caution. In these patients, even "normal" doses of sedative agents precipitate respiratory insufficiency.

Sequential monitoring of spirometry, particularly the FEV_1 is critical in patients with neuromuscular diseases. Serial measurements of respiratory muscle function indicate the need for mechanical intervention. In addition to the FEV_1 and FVC, maximum negative inspiratory force is a useful adjunct in predicting when mechanical ventilation will be necessary. A reduction of the FEV_1 or the FVC to less than 40% of predicted or the reduction of the negative inspiratory force to less than 30 cm of water identifies the patient at high risk for needing mechanical ventilation. The course of the patient's disease and the pattern of decline in respiratory function is more important, however, than the absolute values of pulmonary function tests. The more precipitous the decline in respiratory function, the more likely the need for mechanical ventilation. Sequential evaluation of these patients also allows for heightened awareness of complications such as atelectasis, pneumonia, left ventricular dysfunction, and pulmonary embolus, which can easily precipitate acute respiratory failure. The administration of any pharmacologic agents must be carefully reviewed. For example, the use of small doses of sedatives, or the use of aminoglycoside antibiotics (which are weak neuromuscular blocking agents), has been shown to precipitate acute respiratory failure in patients with neuromuscular diseases. Finally, the careful monitoring of patients with progressive and incurable neuromuscular disease (e.g., amyotrophic lateral sclerosis or muscular dystrophy) allows adequate time for discussion with the patient and family as to whether mechanical ventilation is desirable in each particular case. Once these patients are placed on mechanical ventilation, discussion regarding the appropriateness of stopping mechanical ventilation clearly becomes more difficult (see Chap. 82).

Signs and Symptoms of Acute Respiratory Failure

The bedside clinical assessment of respiratory function in patients with chronic diseases, such as COPD or chronic neuromuscular diseases is most useful. In these patients with longstanding severe impairment of pulmonary function tests, clinical judgment appears to be most helpful in making the decision to institute mechanical ventilation. In contrast, patients with acute respiratory compromise (e.g., drug overdose or acute asthma), more reliance needs to be placed on sequential pulmonary function testing and arterial blood gas analysis, as with moderate respiratory impairment the clinical examination can be misleading. Ideally, transfer to the ICU should take place in these patients before overt clinical signs of respiratory failure occur.

Perhaps the best bedside assessment of respiratory failure is an increase in respiratory rate.[4] A respiratory rate greater than 20, and especially greater than 30, is a sensitive physical marker of impending respiratory failure. A slow respiratory rate of less than 8 breaths per minute indicates imminent respiratory fatigue particularly when accompanied by altered mental status. Monitoring respiratory rate above 35 breaths per minute is considered a critical value necessitating urgent intubation and mechanical ventilation.

The major clinical manifestations of impending respiratory failure are presented in Table 16-2. These signs and symptoms are often nonspecific, therefore, clinical impressions must be quickly confirmed by arterial blood gas analysis. Patient anxiety is characteristically manifested by the patient's facial expression. Mental status changes can range from subtle changes in judgment to frank coma. Frequently, the patient is hypertensive. Central or facial cya-

Table 16–2. Clinical Signs and Symptoms of Respiratory Failure

Tachypnea
Dyspnea
Irregular respiratory rate
Shallow respirations
Use of accessory muscles of respiration
Dyscoordination of the abdominal musculature with the thoracic cage
Severe anxiety
Diaphoresis
Alterations in mental status
Central cyanosis (usually a late finding)

---

nosis is a notoriously unreliable sign because it requires the amount of reduced hemoglobin to exceed 5 g. Therefore, the likelihood of a patient to manifest cyanosis is both a function of severe hypoxemia and of total hemoglobin of concentration. Peripheral cyanosis is even less helpful because it may reflect changes in the local circulation. Wheezing, prolonged expiratory time, or absence of breath sounds in a hemithorax may be present in certain situations.

If there is doubt as to the adequacy of ventilation, especially when the patient is semicomatose or hypotensive, immediate measure to restore adequate ventilation must be undertaken before waiting for arterial blood gases. Ventilatory assistance may be given emergently mouth-to-mouth, or preferably by mask and ventilating bag. Although intubation offers many advantages in situations of ventilatory collapse, intubation must be considered a semielective procedure, because ventilation can be maintained quite easily by proper external application of a mask. Ideally, this should be done prior to all intubation attempts to partially compensate for the hypoxia and hypoventilation (see Chaps. 10, 15, and 24).

On a physiologic level, ventilation should be assigned by mechanical means when there is either a failure to maintain adequate alveolar ventilation or when there exists severe gas exchange ineffectiveness. Critical values for considering the institution of mechanical ventilation, depending upon the clinical conditions are listed in Table 16-3.[5,6] The critical value of $Paco_2$ assumes the absence of metabolic acidosis. In the presence of metabolic acidosis, hyperventilation should be seen, and the expected $Paco_2$ can be calculated.[7] Although these guidelines are useful in deciding to initiate mechanical ventilation, trends in these values and clinical judgment should be the final arbitrator of when mechanical ventilation is necessary.

Table 16–3. Clinical Values for Starting Mechanical Ventilation

Respiratory rate	>35 breaths/min
Negative inspiratory force	<−30 mm Hg
Vital capacity	<10 ml/kg
Minute ventilation	<3 L/min
Pao_2 (100% oxygen)	<60 mm Hg
$Paco_2$ (acutely)	>45 mm Hg
A-a O_2 difference (100% oxygen)	>450 mm Hg
pH fall due to hypoventilation	>0.10

A common example of the need to apply clinical judgment occurs in the acute young asthmatic patient who presents with a $Paco_2$ in a "normal" range (e.g., 38 to 40 mm Hg). This value represents an ominous prognostic indicator of impending respiratory failure as it indicates that the patient is unable to ventilate in the face of severe bronchospasm. The physiologic response to asthma is hyperventilation, and failure to do so indicates inadequate respiratory reserve. Similarly, a rapidly progressing severe illness should also predispose the clinician to early institution of mechanical ventilation before physiologic numbers achieve critical values. Specific examples which merit early institution of mechanical ventilation include the:

- Hypotensive patient
- Patient developing septic shock
- Patient with cardiac arrest
- Patient with overwhelming pneumonia
- Patient developing the adult respiratory distress syndrome (ARDS)
- Patient with severe chest trauma to stabilize the chest wall[8-10]
- Patient with fatigued respiratory muscles[11]

There is general consensus that early institution of mechanical ventilation in situations of severe respiratory failure may serve to minimize complications and irreversible injury by at least preserving lung volumes and preventing atelectasis.

Need for Intubation

Although often regarded in tandem, it is necessary to separate the decision to intubate with the decision to initiate mechanical ventilation. Several indications for tracheal intubation do not require initiation of mechanical ventilation. Indications for tracheal intubation include:

- To assist in the clearance of secretions
- To protect the lungs from aspiration
- To preserve patency of the upper airway
- To provide a means for the initiation of mechanical ventilation

The patency of the upper airway must especially be preserved in situations of depressed consciousness, inflammation, trauma, malignancy, and upper airway infection. Sometimes intubation alone can avert imminent respiratory failure in a patient with respiratory distress (e.g., upper airway obstruction) without the need for mechanical ventilation. It is very common, however, to place these people on the ventilator at least for a short period as sedation and rest can be beneficial. Mechanical ventilation must be initiated whenever spontaneous ventilation is inadequate to sustain life. In addition, patients that are critically ill are often intubated to gain control of the patient's airway and ventilation, and as prophylaxis for an impending collapse of other physiologic functions. In situations of increased intracranial pressure, intubation and hyperventilation may temporize neurologic status. Finally, mechanical ventilation is done electively in the operating theater.

Appropriateness of Instituting Mechanical Ventilation

Technology has allowed us to provide mechanical support to a wider spectrum of chronically ill patients with respiratory embarrassment.[12] Often not enough attention is paid to the sociology of instituting mechanical ventilation, however. The critical questions of today's physician and patient generation has become: When is it appropriate to use our technical ability for ventilation? Clearly, this is a question with ethical, quality of life, and financial considerations.[13] An increasing number of physicians and patients believe that, in certain situations, mechanical ventilation provides no advantage in prolonging a meaningful quality of life and its use should be sociologically limited (see Chap. 24). Consensus between the patient and long-term caregiver prior to the critical event is the most rational approach in a chronic illness. In patients who are unable to provide an opinion in advance, discussion with the family is helpful; however, some courts have maintained that family members have no legal status unless the patient has left them specific instructions (e.g., a living will).[14] If the family and the patient can reach a consensus (ideally prior to ICU admission), it is prudent to follow that approach. Asking legal opinion or the court such fundamental questions should be a maneuver of last resort. Court opinions are, in general, never satisfying to the patient, the patient's family, or the physician.

The clear precedent has been set that competent patients have the right to determine their own course. This includes declining mechanical ventilation, even if it means certain death, or persistence of mechanical ventilation even when there is minimal hope for any improvement. A murky area, however, exists in situations where the medical profession believes that mechanical ventilation is a futile maneuver. In this situation, most physicians tend to continue providing mechanical support despite its uselessness. Increasing financial burden and the scant availability of resources may change this common practice, however.

Mechanical ventilation is expensive technology; it adds $1500 per day and more to a patient's already astronomical medical bill. Sociologists, ethicists, and others have questioned whether these resources, often coming from public funds, can be used in other health-related areas for the greater common good. As the acuity of hospitalized patients increases, the limitation in ICU beds promises to be another factor in determining the appropriateness to initiate mechanical ventilation. The availability of noninvasive respiratory care units has taken some pressure off the ICUs, but the relief has been insufficient.[15,16]

Several basis tenets ought to be kept in mind when considering the appropriateness of providing mechanical ventilation to a patient:

- Modern medical practice probably provides mechanical ventilation in far too many cases.
- Despite ethical and legal opinions to the contrary, mechanical ventilation is often viewed as a special form or higher level of therapy by the medical profession

Table 16–4. Alternatives to ICU Admission in Chronic Respiratory Failure

Noninvasive mask ventilation
Negative-pressure ventilation
   Iron lung
   Cuirass
   Poncho
   Pneumobelt
Full-body tilt (i.e., rocking bed)
Diaphragmatic pacing

and the population at large, and therefore, the decision to withdraw this form of treatment becomes emotionally difficult once it has been initiated.
- With advancing technology and the availability of improved pharmacologic agents, the ability to keep the patient alive frequently exceeds all expectations.
- The allocation of ICU beds can be a major logistical problem in many hospitals, and indiscriminate use of mechanical ventilation will continue to strain the physical limits.

Alternatives to ICU Admission

Although acute respiratory failure necessitates intubation and transfer to an ICU setting, some specialized situations of chronic respiratory failure may allow alternatives.[5,17] Most hospitals proscribe that positive pressure ventilation must be done within an ICU setting. Mechanical devices that do not require intubation, however, often can be used on general medical floors (Table 16-4).

These devices have limited applications, but may be a special consideration for people with neuromuscular diseases, old polio, or blunted drive to breathe.[18] These devices are very effective in the proper setting, are less invasive than positive pressure ventilators, and are simple mechanically which makes them suitable for long-term home ventilation. In general, all negative pressure ventilators work best in patients who have normal lung compliance. None of the negative pressure ventilatory devices should be used in patients with severe pulmonary parenchymal disease, or for acute respiratory failure. Patients that have wide fluctuations in their intrinsic lung compliance also are not considered for negative pressure ventilators. Common disadvantages to all negative pressure ventilatory systems include the prohibition for eating and drinking while using a negative assist device because of the increased risk for aspiration. Negative pressure ventilators are clearly contraindicated in patients who have upper airway obstruction. These devices have seen a resurgence in recent times due to social and economic pressures that are increasing the practice of home ventilation in today's medical practice.[19–21]

The pneumobelt compresses abdominal contents resulting from diaphragmatic motion. It is usually used in patients with incomplete spinal cord injury and inspiratory insufficiency. Although incapable of providing total ventilatory assistance, the device will augment respirations when the patient is in a sitting position.[20]

The rocking bed is infrequently used in patients with

chronic respiratory failure who have normal lung compliance and airway resistance. The rocking bed has the obvious limitations of being cumbersome, sometimes causing motion sickness, and clearly making patient care difficult. A minority of carefully selected patients (especially old polio patients), however, prefer the rocking bed to a tracheostomy, or to the often claustrophobic iron lung. In these patients, the rocking bed has been used as a reasonable alternative for many decades.[19]

A final alternative to chronic ventilatory support is diaphragmatic pacing. Diaphragmatic pacing has been primarily used in patients with cervical cord injury or severe alveolar hypoventilation.[22,23] It is most successful in children with quadriplegia. Diaphragmatic pacing has the absolute requirement of intact bilateral phrenic nerves.[24] Although phrenic nerve pacing has been available for 20 years, it has never received widespread acceptance.[25] Major disadvantages include the fact that electrical failure in a patient with total respiratory insufficiency can be disastrous without proper monitoring devices. Despite drawbacks, some patients with quadriplegia still prefer phrenic pacing to conventional positive pressure ventilation.[23]

ICU PHASE

Initial Ventilatory Settings

A simple, but effective method of initiating mechanical ventilation is to use the assist control mode and the 12/12 rule; that is, tidal volume of 12 ml/kg with a back-up rate of 12 breaths/minute (Table 16-5).[6,26] Even though more complex formulas exists, they are often time-consuming and easily forgotten. Although often later switched to other modes, it is important that the initial mode be assist/control because it allows the patient to increase machine-delivered ventilation with a minimum of inspiratory effort. This practice, therefore, allows the patients to set their own minute ventilation based on ventilatory needs. Clinically significant hyperventilation is infrequent in circumstances of acute respiratory failure and can easily be corrected at a later time. The initial use of other modes may, however, cause significant hypoventilation if the patient is unable to supplement machine-delivered ventilation. This may be especially true in the critical phase of illness as the patient's ventilatory requirements may fluctuate drastically. An initial inspired oxygen fraction (FIO_2) of 1.0 is necessary to provide immediate oxygenation in the setting of acute respiratory failure. Often these patients have a high degree of ventilation-perfusion mismatching along with varying degrees of shunt and inadequate cardiac output which make low levels of inspired oxygen inadequate to meet the body's demands. Because the amount of required oxygen is often underestimated, it is wiser to start with an inspired oxygen concentration that may be excessive and gradually decrease the oxygen fraction as able. The widespread availability and use of pulse oximeters in ICUs can allow a rapid reduction in inspired oxygen concentration if it is demonstrated that the patient does not need high oxygen concentrations.

In the setting of acute respiratory failure, initiation of mechanical ventilation should be done with a volume-cycled ventilator.[27] These ventilators, which deliver a preset volume, are used almost exclusively in medical ICUs, because the critically ill patient often has dramatic changes in respiratory compliance or resistance which renders pressure-cycled ventilators inadequate to maintain a set amount of ventilatory support. For this reason, the recently introduced pressure support mode is also not indicated as an initial respiratory mode.

Evaluation of the adequacy of oxygenation and ventilation with the mechanical ventilator must be done with arterial blood gas levels. The first blood gas measurement should be done approximately 10 minutes after initiation of mechanical ventilation. This period is adequate for equilibration of arterial Po_2 in most patients, with the exception of patients with severe obstructive lung disease.[28] The equilibration of carbon dioxide is almost never a clinical problem because of its high solubility properties. Although patients with severe obstructive lung disease may require 25 minutes for stabilization of arterial Po_2, even in this patient group. A subsequent arterial blood gas is usually obtained 30 minutes after initiation of mechanical ventilation. Because of the often hectic nature surrounding the initiation of mechanical ventilation, this early and aggressive approach at obtaining arterial blood gas values is helpful to provide perspective on the clinical situation. In practice, for logistical reasons, the obtaining of an arterial gas inevitably takes longer to obtain than initially planned. In today's ICU, continuous monitoring with finger oximeter compliments the arterial blood gas evaluation. Overdependence on the finger oximeter, however, must be guarded against because it provides no indication of the proper level of ventilation.

Adequacy of oxygenation at the tissue level cannot be reliably determined by methods available in clinical practice. Until methods become clinically applicable, an oxygen tension of 60 mm Hg in the arterial circulation is a reasonable goal since this allows oxygen saturation to remain in the flat portion of the oxygen-hemoglobin dissociation curve, when it is located in its normal position.[30,31] Ventilatory rate is then adjusted so that the $Paco_2$ is between 35 and 40 in most patients. A back-up rate is set at 2 or 3 breaths/minute below what is required to maintain the desired $Paco_2$ to be adjusted to the patient's baseline level, as indicated by the respiratory component of the pH. Often this requires use of lower tidal volumes and lower respiratory rates than that used in other patients. On the other hand, a larger tidal volume and respiratory rate is generally used in the face of metabolic acidosis to provide some respiratory compensation for the acidosis.

An initial flow rate of 40 L per minute allows an inspiratory-to-expiratory ratio of at least 1:3. In patients with very high inspiratory demands, higher flow rates may be re-

Table 16-5. Initial Ventilatory Settings with Assist Control Mode

Ventilator rate	12
Tidal volume	12 ml/kg
Flow rate	40 L/min
Inspiratory:expiratory ratio	1:3
Oxygen	100%

quired in order to decrease inspiratory work in these patients.[32] On the other hand, patients with high mean airway pressures may do better with lower flow rates, which allow lower airway pressures and may potentially reduce barotrauma. Lower mean airway pressures may also assist venous return and permit a higher cardiac output. As the flow rate is decreased, caution must be exercised so that the expiratory time is maintained as much as possible. Clearly, the lowering of mean airway pressure must be balanced against an increasing inspiratory time. The current generation of ventilators which contain microprocessing capabilities also allow inspiratory flow to be given at differing rates over the inspiratory cycle. These various inspiratory patterns may offer some advantage in an individual patient, but their overall benefit has not been established.

Oxygen Administration

After demonstrating adequate Pa_{O_2} or an adequate saturation with pulse oximetry, the F_{IO_2} should be rapidly reduced to maintain a saturation above 90% and a Pa_{O_2} above 60 mm Hg.[30] In patients at risk from ischemic vascular disease, or in situations of severe asthma, the Pa_{O_2} should be maintained at a higher level, especially if this can be done at an F_{IO_2} of less than .5. A Pa_{O_2} of 80 to 100 with a saturation above 95% often provides a small measure of safety in the unstable patient and outweighs the theoretic risk of increased oxygen toxicity. This higher level of oxygen protects the patient from hypoxia during suctioning and from that which may occur with change in position, mucus plugging, or retained secretions. The F_{IO_2} is optimized as rapidly as possible to minimize potential oxygen toxicity to the lung.[33] Deleterious effects of high oxygen concentration include impaired mucociliary clearance, increased epithelial permeability, and impairment of vascular endothelial function.[34,35] In addition, pulmonary edema and pulmonary fibrosis may occur. Although it is known that oxygen toxicity is influenced both by the concentration of inspired oxygen and the duration of exposure, threshold levels cannot reliably be documented. In general, exposure to 40% oxygen for long periods probably causes minimal damage.[36] On the other hand, concentrations above 60% have an exponential likelihood of causing some pulmonary changes. Even oxygen levels of 40 and 50% for 2 days have been shown to increase lung lavage albumin concentration and modulate clearance of substances suggesting that even at these often used levels of inspired oxygen concentration, there may be some increased epithelial permeability.[37] The risk of oxygen toxicity must always be minimized in the ICU, however, the immediate catastrophic effects of tissue ischemia often dictate the F_{IO_2}.

Positive End-Expiratory Pressure (PEEP)

The use of PEEP during mechanical ventilation is a maneuver that maintains intrathoracic pressure persistently above atmospheric pressure during exhalation. This maintains the lung at a higher end-tidal volume. PEEP can be used with many modes of positive pressure mechanical ventilation. It has become popular over the last 25 years, and particularly in the postoperative setting and for treatment of ARDS.[38] PEEP increases the functional residual capacity (FRC) which tends to prevent small airway closure, the magnitude depending on lung compliance.[39] The primary goal of PEEP is to increase the Pa_{O_2} in severe hypoxemia. PEEP has no intrinsic therapeutic value; its usefulness in the ICU is as an alternative to raising the F_{IO_2} in severely hypoxemic patients.[40] PEEP has been shown to improve gas exchange in patients with hypoxemia. PEEP decreases shunting, increases dead space ventilation, and decreases ventilation/perfusion heterogeneity, causing more lung units to have balanced ventilation/perfusion ratios.[41] In addition, it may minimize atelectasis. Therefore, PEEP is generally useful in combating the hypoxemia of both cardiac and noncardiac pulmonary edema.

The optimal amount of PEEP in any given situation should be the least amount necessary to maintain oxygenation and allowing for a reasonable level of F_{IO_2}. The optimum level of PEEP depends on its intended goal. For example, in a patient with a good cardiac output, good peripheral perfusion, and good delivery of oxygen to the tissues, who requires a high F_{IO_2}, PEEP may be increased fairly aggressively in an attempt to decrease the F_{IO_2}. In this situation, the primary goal of administering the PEEP is to lower F_{IO_2}, and it appears the patient's cardiovascular integrity would permit the application of PEEP. On the other hand, a patient in shock and hypoxemia despite 1.00 F_{IO_2} may tolerate only very small amounts of PEEP without precipitating cardiovascular catastrophe. In this situation, calculating the maximal tissue oxygen delivery to guide levels of PEEP is probably appropriate. The measurement of static total lung compliance to determine "best PEEP," is of limited value as lung compliance often does not parallel the desired end point.[42,43] Levels of PEEP above 20 cm H_2O are clinically unwarranted because of the exponential increase in complications and the lack of clinical data demonstrating benefit.

Because PEEP often reduces cardiac output with the consequences of systemic hypotension, monitoring is critical.[44,45] Baseline hemodynamic, compliance, and gas exchange parameters are measured prior to and with each subsequent change of PEEP. PEEP is applied at the smallest pressure to achieve an improvement in oxygenation. If hypoxia precludes reduction of PEEP, often systemic hypotension can be ameliorated by the administration of fluids to expand intravascular volume, the use of inotropic and or vasopressor drugs, or the use of lower body compressive trouser.[46] Rapid cessation of PEEP must be done with caution as it may cause collapse of tenuous alveoli and markedly increased shunt.

The application of positive pressure mechanical ventilation (especially when used in conjunction with PEEP) can have a profound influence on pressures obtained with a pulmonary artery catheter. The division of the lung into three zones based on the relative magnitudes of arterial, venous, and alveolar pressures is a useful concept in understanding distribution of pulmonary blood flow and vascular pressures (Fig. 16-1).[47,48] When alveolar pressure exceeds venous pressure (i.e., zones 1 and 2), the pressures measured by the pulmonary artery catheter will reflect alveolar pressure changes in addition to venous pressure.

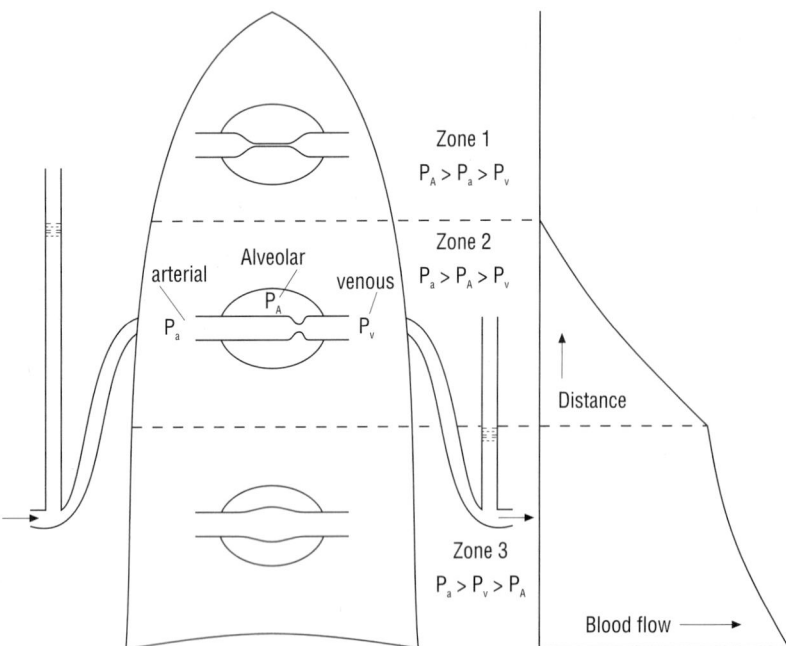

Fig. 16-1. Three-zone model that accounts for the distribution of blood flow in the lung. In zone 1, alveolar pressure exceeds arterial pressure and no flow occurs. In zone 2, arterial pressure exceeds alveolar pressure, but alveolar pressure exceeds venous pressure, and flow is dependent on the arterial-alveolar pressure difference. In zone 3, venous pressure now exceeds alveolar pressure, and flow is determined by the alveolar-venous pressure difference. (From West, J. B., Dollery, C. T., and Naimark, A.: Distribution of blood flow in isolated lungs; relation to vascular and alveolar pressures. J. Appl. Physiol., 19:713, 1964.)

PEEP tends to increase alveolar pressure and, therefore, may increase the amount of lung that is in zone 1 and 2. When the pulmonary catheter is in the upper portions of the lung, the applied alveolar pressure has a large influence on the measured pulmonary artery catheter pressure. This situation can be minimized if the pulmonary artery catheter is located in the dependent portions of the lung (zone 3), where vascular compression by increased alveolar pressure is likely. A cross-table lateral chest roentgenogram is occasionally helpful to document the position of the pulmonary artery catheter in the dependent portion of the lung.[49] Because most patients are supine in the ICU, the tip of the pulmonary artery catheter should be directed posteriorly on the lateral chest roentgenogram.

It must be kept in mind that PEEP is a temporary mechanical maneuver to support oxygenation that has no long-term curative value. PEEP, even if applied early, has no effect on the incidence of ARDS.[50] In addition, PEEP does not change the mortality of ARDS or the complications associated with ARDS. PEEP does not decrease extravascular lung water, and has not been shown to be useful in prophylaxis against atelectasis in a postoperative setting.[38,51,52] PEEP also does not aid the resolution of acute lung injury.[53] The use of PEEP has several drawbacks, the principal one being an increase in the incidence of barotrauma. PEEP also reduces cardiac output as indicated earlier, however, this effect varies depending on the cardiovascular status and intravascular volume. Finally, the routine use of PEEP after coronary bypass surgery may depress myocardial function.[45]

In summary, PEEP is a useful alternative to maintain adequate oxygenation in addition to the F_{IO_2}. The use of PEEP rather than increasing F_{IO_2} depends on the clinical situation. Clearly, indiscriminate use of PEEP is not justified because it has no direct therapeutic effect, and there are significant complications associated with its use especially depression of cardiac output and barotrauma.

Inverse Ratio Ventilation

Inverse ratio ventilation is an experimental mode of ventilation in which the inspiratory phase is prolonged such that it exceeds the expiratory phase, causing a net increase in mean airway pressure. Inspiratory:expiratory ratios (I:E) up to 4:1 have been reported in the clinical setting. Its use has been almost exclusively in the setting of respiratory failure due to acute lung injury (neonatal or adult respiratory distress syndrome).[54] Its major goal is to improve arterial oxygen tension. It has no direct therapeutic value (similar to PEEP), and should be viewed as a maintenance strategy until the hypoxemia resolves. Two forms of inverse ratio ventilation have been described: pressure controlled inverse ratio ventilation (PC-IRV), and volume controlled inverse ratio ventilation (VC-IRV).[55] The vast majority of clinical reports delineate experience with PC-IRV, although there may be some advantages in using the alternative VC-IRV. VC-IRV has the strong advantage of guaranteeing minute ventilation, especially in a patient who has a changing pattern of compliance. With VC-IRV, however, the airway pressures may vary extensively, warranting extreme vigilance. PC-IRV has the advantage of tightly controlling peak airway pressures, but at the expense of a changing tidal volume. Minute ventilation must therefore be monitored closely and adjusted with PC-IRV.

The postulated rationale for using IRV is that it may recruit and stabilize previously closed or partially functioning alveolar units.[55] The short expiratory time prevents the recruited alveoli from falling below their closing volume, therefore, maintaining lung recruitment. The stabilization of pulmonary units is purported to lead to improved gas exchange. Proponents of IRV have suggested that the increase in mean airway pressure with a decrease in peak inspiratory pressure, allows for improved oxygenation while minimizing barotrauma and preserving hemodynamic variables. No controlled clinical trials validate these assumptions, however.

IRV has mainly been advocated as a mode to improve oxygenation in patients with ARDS.[56,57] Mortality in ARDS, however, is generally due to sepsis and/or multiorgan failure. It is, therefore, not surprising that inverse ratio ventilation has not been shown to change ARDS mortality. There have also been no controlled studies to show the benefit of IRV over conventional methods in reducing the morbidity of ARDS. The ineffectiveness of IRV in a substantial number of patients with ARDS has been noted.[54] Although some investigators have found no hemodynamic effect due to IRV when using ratios of 2:1 or less,[58,59] as the I:E ratio increases to 4:1 the risk of hemodynamic compromise becomes significant.[60] Because mean airway pressure appears to be both the major detriment of oxygenation and a key determinant in the development of hemodynamic compromise, it is unlikely in the final analysis that IRV (which increases mean airway pressure) will be able to consistently achieve improved oxygenation without hemodynamic compromise. Limitations that will probably relegate IRV to a minor role in modern ICUs include:

- Its most important benefit (i.e., improving oxygenation) can often be achieved by manipulating conventional respiratory settings.
- In acute lung injury, adequate oxygenation does not appear to be the limiting factor in determining patient mortality.
- IRV ventilation increases the mechanical complexity of ventilation.
- Because it is uncomfortable, IRV usually requires deep sedation and paralysis of the patient.
- IRV requires extremely close monitoring to prevent the development of air trapping, and increasing risks of barotrauma.

Because of the shortened expiratory time, claims of decreased potential for barotrauma are unlikely to be substantiated.

In summary, IRV ventilation has not been validated by clinical studies and must still be considered an unproven method. The major benefit of IRV may be that it has forced the clinician to consider alternative techniques in the attempt to recruit alveoli and to improve oxygenation. Conventional ventilation already offers many options, however, that allow for the implementation of these concepts without the need for new mechanical devices or heavy sedation. Judicious application of PEEP and the delivery of ventilation with sustained inflation time without inverting the I:E ratio is often sufficient even in the most difficult cases of ARDS. If IRV is implemented, the I:E ratios should be limited as ratios of greater than 2:1 have an exponential risk of barotrauma and impairment of hemodynamic parameters with little evidence of any benefit. Careful monitoring is mandatory, especially the monitoring of end-expiratory pressure.

Mechanical Options

The initial response to acute respiratory failure includes intubation, ventilation, and usually the administration of supplemental oxygen. These processes often occur simultaneously, and are accompanied by continual assessment to ensure adequate Po_2 and Pco_2. Once the airway has been secured, and the patient is receiving adequate ventilation and oxygenation, consideration can be given to which ventilation mode will be most beneficial for the patient. Ventilatory requirements can change during the patient's ICU stay, consequently the ventilation mode must be reassessed periodically.

Assist-Control Mode

The assist-control mode of ventilation delivers a physician-determined preset volume of ventilation when the machine is triggered by the patient's inspiratory effort. If the patient is incapable of respiratory efforts a back-up provides for adequate minute ventilation. The frequency of respiration is set by the patient. The assist-control mode is often the mode preferred by the patient. This mode is the initial ventilatory mode of choice in most hospitals, because it allows patients to increase their minute ventilation on demand even if respiratory efforts are diminished.[61] In addition, patients who have sudden increases in their ventilatory needs (e.g., development of the septic syndrome) can easily increase minute ventilation with this mode. Assist-control ventilation is associated with increased work of breathing, compared to continuous mandatory ventilation.[62] Significant exertion of respiratory musculature persists throughout patient-initiated cycles.[63] This effort may prevent disuse atrophy of respiratory muscle, however, it also may perpetuate muscle fatigue in selected patients. Because ventilation can be increased with minimum effort, the assist-control mode can also predispose the patient to hyperventilation if the patient is very agitated or has a central neurologic problem; however, this is a clinical problem only in a minority of cases.

Intermittent Mandatory Ventilation Mode

Although initially intermittent mandatory ventilation (IMV) was advocated as a weaning method,[64] this mode has rapidly become the overwhelming clinical choice despite the lack of scientific evidence showing superiority to the older assist-control mode.[63-67] Clearly IMV is a reasonable and safe option. In a national survey done in 1987, IMV was shown to be the most common mode of ventilation for both maintenance of mechanical ventilation and during weaning from mechanical ventilation.[68] This mode is similar to the assist-control mode in that a preset volume of gas is administered at a set rate to the patient, however, respiratory efforts above the back-up ventilatory rate result in ventilations that are governed by the patient's own efforts. In the assist-control mode, the ventilator delivers a full breath for each patient effort. In contrast, during IMV only a set number of breaths are fully supported. The patient's contribution towards total minute ventilation, therefore, depends on their ability for spontaneous respiratory efforts. Today's generation of ventilators have synchronized the IMV mode so that the machine senses and delivers breaths at the time when the patient makes respiratory efforts. The synchronization was designed to prevent the patient from receiving an excessive tidal volume when a mandatory machine breath is introduced on top of a patient's spontaneous breath.

Postulated advantages of IMV over other modes are in dispute. Initially, it was speculated that the IMV mode is less likely to cause respiratory alkalosis than the assist-control ventilation.[69] Studies have shown, however, that respiratory alkalosis during mechanical ventilation is more likely to be due to patient circumstances rather than the particular mode of ventilation.[70,71] In weaning patients from mechanical ventilation, arguments have been raised claiming both increased and decreased weaning time with the IMV mode.[65-67] Part of the difficulty centers around the fact that patients who are weanable, wean regardless of ventilatory mode. Because of this, it is doubtful that any mode can be shown to be superior in a controlled study. IMV has some intrinsic disadvantages which would not make it the mode of choice in situations of rapid changes in acid/base status. Similarly IMV should be avoided in the patient with respiratory muscle fatigue in whom it is determined that respiratory muscles need to be rested. In these patients, the IMV mode carries the risk of increasing respiratory work if the ventilator is not synchronized properly. Alternatively, IMV is preferred in patients with central hyperventilation.

Pressure Support Ventilation

Pressure support ventilation has recently become widely used in ICUs across the country. Pressure support ventilation is the augmentation of spontaneous ventilation with a preselected inspiratory pressure which is maintained throughout inspiration. Its features include the fact that it is patient initiated and pressure limited, however, it delivers a variable tidal volume and a variable flow. During pressure support ventilation, the patient must initially generate negative inspiratory pressure, at which point the ventilator value opens to maintain a plateau pressure at the preselected level until the patient's inspiratory effort ceases. The patient, therefore, controls the inspiratory time, but the tidal volume varies depending on patient effort and the preset level of pressure. As opposed to continuous positive airway pressure (CPAP), pressure is maintained only during inspiration. Pressure support ventilation is available as an option with the newer ventilators. Pressure support ventilation differs from other modes because it allows the patient to control both the respiratory rate and the inspiratory time. As with IMV and other ventilatory modes, pressure support ventilation has not been rigidly scrutinized. Possible advantages of pressure support include:

- Reduced respiratory muscle work[72,73]
- Improvement in patient-ventilator synchronization and comfort level[74]
- A decreased inspiratory work caused by endotracheal tubes[75]
- Less predisposition to diaphragmatic fatigue[76]

Despite its advantages, pressure support has several drawbacks. If the patient is solely on pressure support, there is no guarantee of a minimum minute ventilation. Clearly pressure support is impedance dependent, and therefore, contraindicated in patients whose lung compliance may change rapidly, especially patients with secretions. Finally, pressure support ventilation may compromise cardiac filling because no negative intrathoracic pressure is generated in this mode.

To initiate pressure support ventilation, the pressure is set initially so that the patient is comfortable with an emphasis on reducing the respiratory rate to around 20. This is accomplished by matching the volume delivered on the initial pressure support setting to the patient's tidal volume before initiation of pressure support. The initial pressure support should not be higher than 25 to 30 cm H_2O. An alternative way to determine the initial pressure support is to set it approximately half the peak inspiratory pressure. Pressure support ventilation is clearly contraindicated as the sole source of ventilation in severely ill patients, especially those with an impaired respiratory drive. In unstable situations, fluctuation of the patient's compliance (e.g., mucus plugging) can cause a precipitous fall in the minute ventilation. On the other hand, in a stable patient who is ready to wean, pressure support ventilation is widely used and may be more comfortable for the patient.[77] It provides adequate ventilation and oxygenation in the stable patient.[78]

High Frequency Ventilation

High frequency ventilation has been used sporadically over the last 20 years in an attempt to provide an alternate mode of ventilation that optimizes ventilation to perfusion matching, with relatively low peak airway and intrathoracic pressures, and that avoids rapid fluctuations in alveolar pressures. The essence of high frequency ventilation is the administration of very low tidal volumes (less than dead space), at a high respiratory frequency.[79,80] The most common types of high frequency are high frequency jet ventilation (HFJV), high frequency oscillation (HFO), and high frequency positive pressure ventilation (HFPPV).[81,82] Comparative volumes and frequencies of these types are shown in Table 16-6. HFJV is probably the high frequency ventilation method of choice in the United States today.[83] A small cannula delivers the gas to the patient at a driving pressure of 15 to 50 psi. The delivered gas can be humidified taking advantage of the pulsatile flow to aerosolize saline as it enters the endotracheal tube. Additional oxygen can be introduced through a side port. HFO employs an oscillating of a piston at very high frequencies. HFO can be used in parallel with conventional ventilation. HFPPV represents an extension of conventional mechanical ventilation to high respiratory rates and low tidal volumes. The

Table 16-6. High Frequency Ventilator Features

Type	Tidal Volumes	Frequency
Jet ventilation (HFJV)	2–5 ml/kg	100–200 breaths/min
Oscillation (HFO)	1–3 ml/kg	300–3000 breaths/min
Positive pressure ventilation (HFPPV)	3–5 ml/kg	60–100 breaths/min

mechanism of gas exchange in the setting of high frequency ventilation is unclear. It is thought that convection and facilitated diffusion are important mechanisms.[82]

Although high frequency ventilation has been used sporadically for a wide range of clinical conditions, evidence for its benefit is sparse.[84] In the adult population, most of the clinical experience has been with the high frequency jet ventilator, especially in the context of ARDS.[85] The decision to use high frequency ventilation is generally made on a case-by-case basis. Despite there being no clear indications for its use, clinical circumstances sometimes demand that it be considered. High frequency ventilation is tried occasionally when respiratory failure is refractory to conventional ventilation. High frequency ventilation in this scenario offers the hope of improved gas exchange at lower airway pressure and with less cardiac depression. Controlled trials comparing HFJV with conventional mechanical ventilation have failed to show a clear cut advantage of HFJV. Clearly there is no difference in overall survival for patients with acute respiratory failure.[86] HFPPV has also been used to ventilate patients undergoing laryngeal or tracheal surgery.[87]

The most accepted ICU use of high frequency ventilation has been in the treatment of refractory bronchopleural fistula that has failed conventional mechanical ventilation.[88] It has been suggested that jet ventilation may lower proximal airway pressure causing a decrease in flow to the bronchopleural fistula. In practical application, however, the HFJV can either increase or decrease air leak through a bronchopleural fistula.[89] Despite this controversy, HFJV may be of clinical value in certain subgroups of patients.[90] Jet ventilation is particularly useful in treatment of bronchopleural fistula under the following conditions:

- Proximal fistulas with normal lung parenchyma
- Adequate oxygenation (patient requiring no more than 50% oxygen)
- Hypercarbia with conventional ventilation
- High peak pressures with large airway leak

In patients with these circumstances, many intensivists believe that HFJV should be considered as the primary mode of ventilation. In other cases of refractory bronchopleural fistula, a trail of jet ventilation seems reasonable, provided that jet ventilation and gas exchange are carefully monitored. Guidelines for initiation of high frequency ventilation appear in Table 16-7. There are several difficulties in managing a patient with HFJV. The primary difficulty of high frequency ventilation is the lack of appropriate monitoring techniques to determine delivered minute ventilation. Certainly, repeated blood gas measurements or transcutaneous P_{CO_2} monitors have their limitations. Furthermore, although airway is monitored during high frequency ventilation, this may not reflect alveolar pressure, which may be higher in some cases. Difficulties with adequate humidification of the air that is delivered through

Table 16–7. Initiation of High Frequency Ventilation

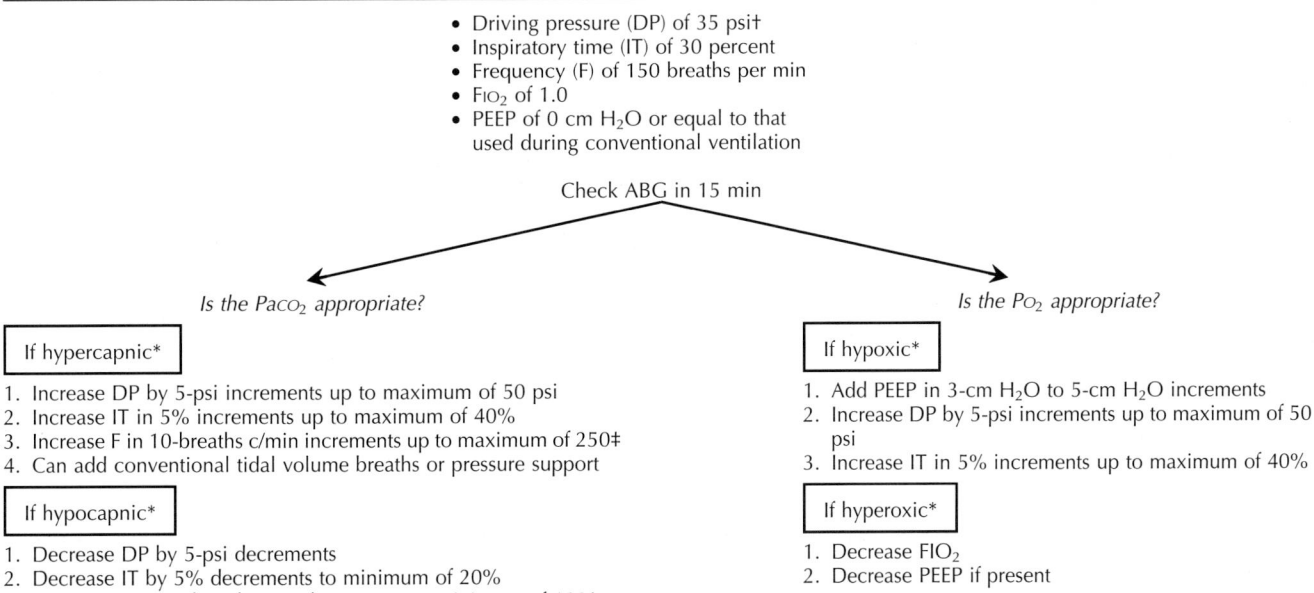

* Careful monitoring of peak, mean, and end-expiratory airway pressures and minute ventilators, as well as oximetry should be performed when any change in ventilatory parameters are made. Only experienced personnel should use HFJV: ABG; Arterial blood gas levels.
† If patient was hypoxic on CMV, then DP should be adjusted as necessary to achieve mean airway pressure (MAP) equal to that present during CMV. If minute ventilation ($\dot{V}E$) under those conditions is not at least equal to that present during CMV, then DP should be further increased until this condition is met prior to obtaining ABG. If patient was hypercapnic on CMV, than DP should be adjusted as necessary to achieve $\dot{V}E$ two times that present during CMV. If MAP exceeds 110% of MAP present during CMV prior to obtaining that $\dot{V}E$, then ABG should be obtained at that point prior to further increasing DP.
‡ In individual patients, changes in rate may have opposite effects.
(From Standiford, T. J., and Morganroth, M. L.: High-frequency ventilation. Chest, 96:1380, 1989.)

the high frequency jet ventilator remains a problem. Finally, tracheal stenosis has been described using HFJV.

Pharmacologic Interventions During Mechanical Ventilation

Sedation is frequently needed for optimal management of the patient during mechanical ventilation. Before sedating medications are used, however, one must document that the agitation or uncomfortableness of the patient is not due to inadequate ventilation and gas exchange, or a mechanical problem with the ventilator. After determination, preferably by arterial blood gases, that ventilation and oxygenation are optimized for the seriousness of the condition, the ventilator should be manipulated in an attempt to synchronize patient-ventilatory interaction. Sensitivity of the threshold valve should be adjusted to the patient does not unduly struggle to receive a tidal volume. Life-threatening complications such as tension pneumothorax or malposition of the endotracheal tube (e.g., right mainstem intubation or a partial extubation) must be excluded. Accumulation of pulmonary secretions is a common problem that can be improved by suctioning. The inspiratory flow rate adjustments will often permit a patient to be on the ventilator more comfortably. Pressure support ventilation seems to be very comfortable for many patients, however, some patients still prefer assist-control ventilation, and other IMV. It is impossible to generalize in these cases, and empiric trials are indicated. After the appropriate adjustments are done, the patient's ventilation and oxygenation must again be assessed.

Sedating and paralyzing agents should be thought of as items of last resort in an attempt to synchronize patient breathing during mechanical ventilation. A sedative agent or narcotic alone often can provide the desired effect without the need of a paralyzing agent. In the acute situation, morphine still appears to be the drug of first choice. It can be given IV 2 to 5 mg and repeated as often as necessary. Its onset of action is very short and often can last a few hours. The prime advantage of morphine is that it can be readily antagonized or neutralized by the administration of naloxone. This is an invaluable safety feature, especially in the hemodynamically unstable patient. All sedating agents have the potential for causing or exacerbating hypotension. No drug has the potential to be as quickly reversed as morphine, however, morphine tends to be a more potent vasodilating agent than some of the other sedatives. Diazepam, 5 mg IV, repeated as often as necessary, has withstood the test of time and is probably the most commonly used sedative drug in ICUs. Its onset of action is rapid and sedation usually lasts 3 hours. The incidence of cardiac depression with diazepam, however, is not trivial, especially when used in combination with other sedating drugs. Lorazepam 1 to 2 mg IV may have less hemodynamic effects and is widely used. Midazolam is a newer generation of sedative drug which has the theoretical advantage of providing some amnesia during its use. It is given intravenously between 2 and 10 mg and has a similar onset and duration of action as diazepam or morphine. It might have less of a propensity to cause hypotension, and may be given as a continuous infusion at 2 to 5 mg per hour.

If ventilator maneuvers and sedative alone are inadequate to make the patient comfortable during mechanical ventilation, then muscle relaxants must be utilized. Pancuronium is a long acting muscle relaxant and clearly the most widely used for prolonged paralysis. A reasonable initial dose is 0.08 mg/kg IV and the patient can then be maintained between 0.02 and 0.06 mg/kg IV. The dose must be titrated for the individual patient as there is always a fluctuation in patient requirements. Pancuronium is popular because it is inexpensive and does not need refrigeration. It is, however, excreted both through the kidney and metabolized in the liver. Therefore, it is metabolized more slowly in patients with failure of these organs. There have been reports of prolonged action of this drug in patients with renal or hepatic failure. In addition to allowing easier ventilator synchronization, benefits of muscle relaxing agents include decreased total body oxygen consumption and decreased cardiac demand. Often the hemodynamic instability may be improved and the patient actually may experience better gas exchange. Because muscle relaxants do not sedate or relieve anxiety, they must always be given in conjunction with a sedative. Morphine or diazepam generally work very well. A newer neuromuscular blocking agent that has become recently available is atracurium. Atracurium is administered in an initial bolus of 0.3 to 0.5 mg/kg and then can be administered by continuous infusion for maintenance of neuromuscular blockage. Although the manufacturer recommends 5 to 9 μg/kg per minute to maintain continuous neuromuscular blockade, occasionally doses higher than this are necessary. The reported rate of hypotension or tachycardia is quite low; however, the drug still needs to withstand the test of time. As with other neuromuscular blocking agents, a sedative agent or narcotic must be administered concomitantly to depress sensorium and reduce anxiety. A unique feature of atracurium is that it breaks down spontaneously in the plasma at body temperature and pH. It has a short half-life, approximately 19 minutes, and is independent of both liver and kidney function for its elimination from the body. There have been reports of its successful use in renal failure because of this property. The spontaneous breakdown and its low level of adverse hemodynamic side effects make this a potentially very useful drug in the ICU.

Monitoring the Patient During Mechanical Ventilation

The patient receiving mechanical ventilation requires frequent (at least once an hour) monitoring and recording of vital signs, the monitoring of the adequacy of gas exchange, and the monitoring of lung and chest wall compliance.[91] Arterial blood gas analysis is the gold standard in assessing the adequacy of blood oxygenation and carbon dioxide elimination. In the acutely ill patient, the placement of an arterial catheter is invaluable for repeated arterial blood gas measurements. This catheter eases the burden of frequent arterial blood pressure monitoring and blood sampling. The benefits of the arterial catheter usually far outweigh the potential complications, especially if the catheter is placed in the radial artery. The presence of an arterial line also facilitates the obtaining of arterial blood gases, which can easily be delayed or done too infrequently if a separate arterial puncture is required to obtain the sample. Arterial blood gases should be viewed as the cornerstone for assessing the adequacy of gas exchange.

Technology has made the continuous monitoring of arterial oxygen saturation easy to accomplish.[92] Transmission oximetry is most commonly performed on digits using a pulse oximeter.[93] When used in conjunction with arterial blood gases and clinical observation of the patient, the use of the finger oximeter can be very helpful. However, caution must be exercised in using oximetry so that the medical staff does not overextend its utility. It is easy for the staff to forget that the oxygen saturation does not reflect the adequacy of ventilation, especially in the face of supplemental oxygen administration. Oximetry is also available on the tip of a pulmonary arterial catheter to continuously monitor the mixed venous oxygen saturation. A reduction in the mixed venous saturation may indicate a decrease in oxygen delivery, but also may indicate increased extraction or decreased peripheral shunting. In the stable patient, a decrease in the mixed venous saturation may alert the medical team to search for potential causes. Although the use of the mixed venous oxygen saturation can be helpful, overreliance on a stable number may not be warranted as unfortunately the mixed venous saturation is influenced by a number of factors. For example, a decreasing oxygen delivery in the presence of increasing peripheral shunting may cause the mixed venous saturation to remain stable despite critical changes in the patient's status. Furthermore, the mixed venous saturation is not sensitive at low oxygen delivery values[94] and may correlate poorly with arterial saturation or oxygen delivery in the postoperative patient.[95]

Ventilator Monitoring

The required pressure necessary to deliver the preset volume should be noted initially. A pressure alarm system is then set approximately 10 cm H_2O above this level. When the initial pressure is exceedingly high (e.g., above 70 cm H_2O) or the patient continues to supersede the alarm mechanisms, mechanical ventilation should be interrupted and the patient should be manually ventilated with a ventilating bag until machine problems or airway obstruction are eliminated as potential causes.

The patient who is maintained on mechanical ventilation not infrequently experiences acute respiratory distress. The cause of this distress can usually be identified by examining peak and static pressures on the ventilator manometer.[26,96] If the respiratory distress comes on suddenly, it is often beneficial to remove the patient from the ventilator during the acute distress and attempt manual ventilation until the problem is identified and corrected. Calculation of the patient's dynamic and static compliance often assists in identifying the cause of acute respiratory distress.[97] Repeated documentation of these values is useful in providing trends in the patient with intrinsic lung disease. Dynamic compliance is obtained by dividing the tidal volume by the peak inspiratory pressure. Dynamic compliance will decrease if there is a reduction in lung or chest wall compliance, or if there is an increase in airways resistance. Static compliances are obtained by dividing

Table 16–8. Common Ventilator Dilemmas

Observed Problem	Investigate
Low static and dynamic compliance (high plateau and peak pressure)	Pulmonary edema, consolidation, atelectasis, mainstem bronchus intubation, tension pneumothorax, chest wall constriction
Low dynamic compliance and normal static compliance (increased difference between peak and static pressure = ↑ resistance)	Bronchospasm Increased secretions Obstructed inspiratory circuit)
Spontaneous positive end-expiratory pressure (Auto-PEEP)	Obstructed expiratory circuit (for example, H_2O in tubing) Insufficient flow rate/expiratory time
Increased respiratory rate	Change in clinical status (for example, desaturation, bronchospasm, secretions, pulmonary embolism, sepsis) Low tidal volume Insufficient flow rate
Low exhaled volumes	Leak from circuit Cuff leak Insufficient delivery/low flow rate Bronchopleural fistula Inaccurate measurement of exhalation
Increased exhaled volumes ("stacking breaths")	Hypersensitivity of demand valve High minute ventilation Insufficient flow rate Low I:E ratio
No spontaneous breaths	Backup rate too high, causing relative respiratory alkalosis Sedation Central nervous system lesion
Temperature/humidity problems	Check temperature and moisture daily at connection to endobronchial tubing

(From Grum, C.M., and Chauncey, J.B.: Conventional mechanical ventilation. Clin. Chest Med., 9:37, 1988.)

tidal volume by the static pressure, which can be obtained by occluding the exhalation port just prior to exhalation. Static compliance is therefore not affected by airway resistance, but is reduced by a decrease in chest wall or lung compliance. A decrease in dynamic compliance without similar decrease in static compliance indicates increased airway resistance (e.g., retained secretions, obstructed tubing, or increased bronchospasm). Symmetric decreases in both static and dynamic compliance would indicate increased resistance due to lung parenchyma or chest wall problems (e.g., tension pneumothorax, right mainstem intubation, pulmonary edema, pneumonia, or atelectasis). Common ventilator problems and reasonable investigative approaches are outlined in Table 16-8.[26] Complications are due in part to the patient's inherent illness which minimizes physiologic reserves, and to the application of an external mechanical device (Table 16-9). Zwillich and co-workers found over 400 complications in a total of 354 episodes of mechanical ventilation.[98] In this large study, right mainstem intubation, endotracheal tube malfunction, and alveolar hypoventilation correlated with increased mortality. These complications were seen in 6 to 10% of these patients. Complications that were not associated

Table 16–9. Complications During Mechanical Ventilation

Hemodynamic instability
Barotrauma
    Pneumothorax
    Subcutaneous emphysema
    Pneumomediastinum
    Pneumoperitoneum
    Bronchopleural fistula
Atelectasis
Gastrointestinal hemorrhage
Pulmonary embolism
Nosocomial pneumonia

---

with increased mortality included pneumonia, pneumothorax, atelectasis, gastric distention, and ventilator malfunction. We suggest that careful attention to the recognition and prevention of these complications may minimize the consequences of patients' morbidity and mortality.[98]

Hemodynamic Instability

Hemodynamic instability is a common event that occurs in mechanically ventilated patients. The causes of hemodynamic instability are usually multifactorial and are often based on preexisting conditions. Mechanical ventilation clearly increases the risk of hemodynamic instability due to the application of the positive pressure superimposed on the presence of underlying critical illness. The major determinant of the hemodynamic effect of mechanical ventilation is the mean airway pressure.[99] The effects of positive pressure ventilation on the cardiovascular system are generally that of depressed cardiac output and a decrease in the systemic blood pressure.[100] This is especially true if PEEP is administered. This effect is not uniform, however, and occasionally left ventricular ejection fraction can increase with the institution of mechanical ventilation especially in patients with overt left ventricular failure. Patients that require mechanical ventilation are frequently older and frequently have smoking-related obstructive lung disease. This population has a high prevalence of coexisting arteriosclerotic heart disease which may limit cardiac reserve. The heart disease may also predispose the patients to arrhythmias which can cause further hemodynamic embarrassment. In acutely ill patients, the likelihood of arrhythmias is frequently increased due to imbalances in electrolytes and acid/base status, hypoxemia, and hypercarbia. Furthermore, pharmacologic therapy aimed at the patient's lung disease or other underlying illness can increase the incidence of arrhythmias. Finally, underlying COPD is a frequent cause of supraventricular arrhythmias. Patients who require prolonged mechanical ventilation are also at very high risk for development of sepsis and multiple organ failure. These latter two conditions frequently lead to severe and often unresponsive hypotension.

Hemodynamic monitoring of patients during mechanical ventilation is critical to assess the cardiovascular system. Perhaps the most neglected monitoring device in ICUs today is the frequent physical examination. Often signs of cardiac failure are appreciated quickly at the bedside and lead to intervention, stabilizing the situation before catastrophic changes occur. At a minimum, a daily chest radiograph is mandatory and can provide valuable information regarding cardiac size, the engorgement of the pulmonary vasculature, and the presence of interstitial or alveolar edema. Continuous monitoring of the patient's heart rate and blood pressure (usually with an arterial line) in the critically ill situation proves to be an invaluable early warning system. The pulmonary artery catheter is a proven tool that aids in diagnosis and treatment of hemodynamic instability in the ICU.[49] Although there exists much controversy regarding its benefits, a pulmonary artery catheter would seem reasonable to use in the mechanically ventilated patient under the following conditions:

- Respiratory failure in association with myocardial dysfunction
- Lack of hemodynamic improvement with fluid challenge and vasopressor therapy
- Decreasing urine output in the face of increasing levels of PEEP
- Pulmonary edema of unclear origin
- Severe hypoxemia refractory to high F_{IO_2}

A sudden onset of hypotension is a frequent emergency in patients on mechanical ventilation. Most common causes of hypotension in patients on mechanical ventilation are shown in Table 16-10. In addition, other conditions such as congestive heart failure, the presence of arrhythmias, or the development of an acute myocardial infarction may complicate the situation. Bradycardia that can occur during suctioning can be minimized by administration of nebulized atropine.[101] Aside from gastrointestinal hemorrhage, other situations of volume loss would include vomiting or diarrhea, and renal losses due to overdiuresis. Occasionally, internal sequestration of fluid (e.g., ascites, or retroperitoneal or intra-abdominal bleeding) can cause hemodynamic instability. Finally, cardiac output can be severely depressed by cardiac tamponade or in the presence of massive pulmonary embolism.

The approach to the patient with sudden hypotension requires a comprehensive assessment of all the causes of hypotension as outlined earlier. The initial physical examination should assess the probability of pneumothorax, of congestive failure, and of gastrointestinal bleeding. A stat ECG and chest radiograph are required. Initial blood work should include an arterial blood gas, hematocrit, white blood cell count with differential, and serum electrolytes.

Table 16–10. Most Common Causes of Hypotension in Patients on Mechanical Ventilation

Hypovolemia (especially in debilitated patients)
Sepsis
Cardiac failure
Gastrointestinal hemorrhage
Pneumothorax
Sedation overdose

Medication given over the last 8 hours should be checked for hypotensive potential. Naloxone may be given empirically, but this is seldom effective unless specifically given as a narcotic antagonist. A nasogastric tube to determine the presence of upper gastrointestinal hemorrhage should be placed if the cause of hypotension is not obvious. Insights into the patient's fluid status can often be obtained by examining the patient's intake and output over the past few days. A pulmonary artery catheter should be inserted without delay if the cause of hypotension is not obvious. An immediate echocardiogram is indicated if the physical examination or the pulmonary artery measurements are suspicious for cardiac tamponade. Rare causes of hypotension include adrenal failure and anaphylactic reaction to administered medication. A final cause of hypotension is severe cerebral anoxia or autonomic insufficiency. If the cause of the patient's hypotension is not discernable after the first hour of assessment, experience shows that sepsis is by far the most likely culprit, and empiric antibiotic coverage is indicated. If the specific cause can be found, treatment should be directed at this cause. Often empiric therapy with vasoactive agents is appropriate. Although there are many agents and many strategies at increasing arterial pressure, dopamine remains a favorite of ICU physicians because it has both alpha- and beta-adrenergic effectiveness. Dopamine is the empiric drug of choice because septic shock is such a frequent cause of hypotension in the mechanically ventilated patient. Initial management of the patient with hemodynamic instability is often reduced to empiric stabilization and meticulous vigilance until the problems are resolved.

Barotrauma

The risk of barotrauma is always present when external positive pressure is applied.[102] The most dangerous manifestation of barotrauma is a pneumothorax. Other manifestations include subcutaneous emphysema, pneumomediastinum, and pneumoperitoneum. Systemic gas embolization is an infrequent, but potentially lethal complication due to barotrauma. The triad of livedo reticularis, cerebral infarction, and myocardial injury is highly suggestive of this syndrome.[103] The risk of barotrauma increased when high peak airways pressures are required, during the application of PEEP, and when the underlying lung disease causes a marked decrease in lung compliance. Chest radiographs ought to be obtained and a physical examination performed whenever the patient develops respiratory distress, especially when manifested by high peak and high plateau pressures. When considering the possibility of a pneumothorax, the chest radiograph must be taken in the upright position, otherwise pneumothorax may loculate anteriorly and be missed on the chest roentgenogram. The presence of an inspiratory lag on the affected side is often a diagnostic clue to the presence of a pneumothorax. Other diagnostic clues include abrupt increase in peak airway pressure, hypotension, decreasing urine output, and deterioration in oxygenation.

A pneumothorax, regardless of the magnitude, necessitates the placement of a chest tube in the opinion of most medical experts. The risk of a tension pneumothorax is too high to allow one to observe even a small pneumothorax. On the other hand, if the patient has clinical signs of tension pneumothorax or exceedingly high peak airway pressures, immediate relief may often be obtained temporarily by the insertion of a 14-gauge catheter in the anterior second intercostal space. A chest tube should be placed thereafter. Initially, the chest tube is applied to suction, but frequently after a day, it can be placed on a waster seal. In the otherwise stable patient in the ICU, an alternative to the chest tube placement, is the insertion of a small intrathoracic catheter known as the Heimlich valve.[104] These catheters permit the escape of air from the pleural space, but do not allow for the collection of fluid. The Heimlich valves are less bulky than chest tubes, and may be more comfortable for the patient. Bronchopleural fistula as a complication of pneumothorax occurs in approximately 2% of mechanically ventilated patients.[105] The persistence of bronchopleural fistula causes significantly increased mortality. In patients with persistent bronchopleural fistula, adequate ventilation can usually be achieved by adjusting the minute ventilation to minimize the lead.[106] HFJV should be considered in refractory cases.[89,90] Although most bronchopleural fistulas close with conservative treatment, bronchoscopy and thoracoscopy have been used to instill an occluding agent.[107] These techniques have not been evaluated critically to prove efficacy.

The risk of barotrauma can be minimized by maintaining a low mean airway pressure,[108] and limiting the peak inspiratory pressure.[109] This is especially crucial in patients who are predisposed to barotrauma (e.g., patients with COPD, necrotizing pneumonia, ARDS, or restrictive lung diseases). Peak inspiratory pressures can be limited by decreasing flow rates and by decreasing tidal volume, at the expense of increasing the respiratory rate. The inspiratory time should be reduced, and PEEP should be avoided or limited to less than 10 cm H_2O. Careful vigilance must be maintained for right mainstem intubation, which is a leading cause of iatrogenic barotrauma in the ICU. Chest wall procedures, such as subclavian cannulation, need to be minimized. Finally, in the very high risk patient, in whom reductions in mean airway pressures are not possible, a chest tube tray should be at the bedside.

Atelectasis

Mechanical ventilation predisposes the lung to the development of atelectasis. The presence of atelectasis leads to ineffective gas exchange by increasing the ventilation/perfusion mismatching, and right to left shunt, with hypoxemia being a common clinical manifestation. The risk of atelectasis increases with higher inspired oxygen concentration due to absorption atelectasis. In certain diseases, such as ARDS, pulmonary surfactant is depleted or destroyed which increases alveolar surface tension and promotes the development of atelectasis. If the atelectasis is segmental or lobar in scope, it can easily be demonstrated on the chest radiograph. The presence of microatelectasis, however, may only be inferred from arterial blood gas measurements showing difficulty in gas exchange. The formation of atelectasis may be minimized by the application

Table 16–11. Factors That Minimize the Formation of Atelectasis

High tidal volumes
Period sigh breaths
PEEP
Aggressive bronchopulmonary hygiene
   Suctioning
   Percussion
   Postural drainage
   Irrigation with normal saline
Rotation of the patient
Use of bronchodilators

---

of several preventative and therapeutic measures (Table 16-11).

Tidal volumes above 10 ml/kg are often efficacious in preventing atelectasis. If lower tidal volumes are used, the application of sigh breaths at twice the normal tidal volume will minimize atelectasis. Pharmacologic therapy may be of benefit, especially with obstructive lung disease or in the presence of excessive secretions. This would include theorphylline, anticholinergic agents, sympathomimetics, and corticosteroids. The sympathomimetics have the advantage of not only causing bronchodilation, but also increasing mucociliary clearance.[110] The use of bronchoscopy as a means of identifying and removing mucous secretions especially in the presence of lobar or segmental atelectasis is controversial.[111] Often suctioning is sufficient, but occasionally bronchoscopy must be used when these conservative measures fail to resolve the atelectasis. The use of a mucolytic agent (i.e., acetylcysteine) to break down the tenacious pulmonary mucous has been used in certain centers. Because of the inherent irritating effect of acetylcysteine and the potential of increasing bronchospasm, however, it cannot be advocated on a routine basis.

Gastrointestinal Hemorrhage

Gastrointestinal hemorrhage related to stress ulceration has been reported to occur in 5 to 30% of mechanically ventilated patients in the absence of prophylaxis.[112,113] Both gastric acid hypersection and the inability to keep gastric mucosal integrity have been implicated as factors involved in this increased incidence of gastrointestinal hemorrhage. Aggressive therapy aimed at increasing the gastric pH or by stabilizing gastric mucosa has been shown to markedly reduce the incidence of gastrointesinal hemorrhage in ICU patients. Gastric pH can be increased by the intensive administration of antacids or by administration of H_2-receptor antagonists. With aggressive antacid therapy the patient must be monitored for diarrhea and hypophosphatemia. H_2-receptor antagonists can cause mental status changes, especially in the elderly.[114] Both intensive antacid regimens and the administration of H_2-receptor antagonists may lead to increasing gastric colonization by gram negative bacteria. This has been shown to increase the incidence of nosocomial pneumonia in ICUs.[115] An alternative approach effective in preventing stress ulcerations is the administration of sucralfate. Sucralfate preserves the integrity of the gastrointestinal mucosa without increasing the gastric pH, and therefore, does not predispose to increase gastric bacterial colonization.[116]

Pulmonary Embolism

Patients on mechanical ventilation are at a substantially increased risk for the development of venous thrombosis and subsequent pulmonary embolism,[113,117] which clearly leads to increased morbidity and mortality in these patients. During mechanical ventilation, factors that predispose to development of venous thrombosis include immobilization, and the frequent presence of edema and cardiac failure which leads to venous stasis. The management of pulmonary embolism in these patients is complicated by the fact that diagnosis is difficult. Physical signs of venous thrombosis are often absent and the chest radiograph and arterial blood gases are of limited value. Because of the frequent presence of underlying lung disease, a ventilation/perfusion scan is rarely useful in these patients. Therefore, pulmonary angiography remains the necessary test to demonstrate the presence of embolization. Pulmonary angiography is probably under used in the ICU patient because of logistical problems in moving the patient to the angiography suite, and because of the concern for complications from angiography. The mortality and morbidity associated with pulmonary embolism, however, clearly exceeds the potential risks of angiography. Prophylactic treatment is mandatory in all patients on mechanical ventilation unless a specific contraindication exists. Subcutaneous heparin at 5000 U every 12 hours remains the preferred choice. Oral warfarin (Coumadin) is an acceptable alternative. If pulmonary emboli are documented by angiography and the patient has contraindication to the institution of anticoagulation therapy, then a Greenfield filter can be placed in the inferior vena cava.

Nosocomial Pneumonia

Nosocomial pneumonia is much more frequent in patients requiring mechanical ventilation, and incidences of 50% and more have been reported in patients that are on respiratory assist devices.[112,113] The risk apparently increases with prolonged mechanical ventilation, as nosocomial pneumonia is not seen in patients that require mechanical ventilation for 24 hours or less.[118] The presence of underlying diseases and the severity of illness are clear factors in increasing the likelihood of nosocomial pneumonia. Other risk factors for nosocomial pneumonia include: an immunocompromised state, the presence of multiorgan failure, and the presence of central nervous system disease. The contribution of contaminated respiratory therapy equipment and medications has been minimized since the recognition of these infection sources, and the introduction of disposable nebulizers with frequent changing of ventilator tubing.[119,120] The incidence of nosocomial pneumonia is particularly high in patients with ARDS. An important mechanism for the development of nosocomial pneumonia appears to be aspiration of oral secretions.[121] The colonization of the gastrointestinal tract with gram negative bacilli is an important reservoir in the development of nosocomial pneumonia. The use of antacids and histamine blockers may potentiate the development of nosocomial pneumonia by increasing the stomach reservoir of gram-negative bacilli in an alkaline environment.[115]

Procedures During Mechanical Ventilation

Tracheostomy

Tracheostomy is often done on the patients who require mechanical ventilation for prolonged periods. Modern endotracheal tubes with large high compliant cuffs have made immediate tracheotomy a procedure of the past. There remains, however, some controversy between prolonged endotracheal intubation versus early tracheostomy. Laryngeal injury and dysfunction is the main complication of prolonged endotracheal intubation that can be avoided by tracheotomy.[122] This complication is rare, however, and cannot be implicated as a rationale for early tracheostomy placement. Tracheotomy placement has its own inherent risks and complications including bleeding, increased bacterial contamination of the upper trachea, injury to adjacent structures, and the potential for a pneumothorax.[123,124] On the other hand, tracheostomy does offer the patient certain advantages.[125] In addition to sparing the patient from direct laryngeal injury, it improves patient comfort and facilitates nursing care in the patient who will have a prolonged period on mechanical ventilation. Placement of the tracheotomy certainly increases patient mobility, permits speech, facilitated oral nourishments, and provides a certain amount of psychologic benefit.[126] The ability to speak may be an important determining factor in the patient's ability to wean. The tracheotomy also decreases the incidence and the crisis of extubation, and should therefore, be considered in a patient who will not tolerate extubation even for short periods. Occasionally, the placement of a tracheotomy facilitates transfer from the ICU setting, as many hospitals preclude the use of an endotracheal tube on a general medical ward. It appears that for periods less than 10 to 21 days, the benefits of tracheostomy are not justified.[127] Most practitioners, therefore, prefer to leave the endotracheal tube in place for at least 2 to 3 weeks before considering a tracheotomy. There are situations, however, in which a tracheotomy tube may be considered during the first week of mechanical ventilation. These would include patients in whom it is obvious that the length of time on a mechanical ventilator will be more than a month (e.g., severe neurologic trauma, Guillain-Barré, and other neuromuscular conditions), and patients who would not tolerate even a brief period of extubation. On the other hand, clinical features that would delay the placement of tracheostomy include an extremely grave prognosis or a decreased level of consciousness where the benefits of tracheostomy may not be appreciated by the patient (see Chaps. 12 and 24 for additional discussion).

Bronchoscopy

Fiberoptic bronchoscopy is a safe and effective procedure for mechanically ventilated patients when they are carefully selected and where proper precautions are taken to prevent potential complications.[128,129] The indications for fiberoptic bronchoscopy during mechanical ventilation include:

- To insert an endotracheal tube
- To evaluate airway damage
- To localize minor bleeding or obstruction
- To perform BAL, brushings, and transbronchial biopsy

In addition, fiberoptic bronchoscopy can be used to document endotracheal position under direct visualization.[130] Relative contraindications to fiberoptic bronchoscopy would include patients with hemodynamic instability, especially those that are dependent on high doses of inotropic agents.[131] Other contraindications are patients who are unable to maintain Pa_{O_2} above 60 despite high levels of F_{IO_2}.[132] Finally, rigid bronchoscopy is preferred in patients with massive hemoptysis.

The procedure of fiberoptic bronchoscopy during mechanical ventilation is tailored to the individual patient with caution to avoid potential complications. The endotracheal tube should be a size 8 or larger to prevent high driving pressures by the ventilator and air trapping.[129,133] The use of the newer bronchoscopes which have narrower diameters certainly facilitates the process. During the procedure, the patient is ventilated with 100% oxygen with continuous monitoring of oxygen saturation by pulse oximetry. The saturation should be above 90 during the procedure. After bronchoscopy, the patient should be supplemented with oxygen for a period determined by the pulse oximeter.[128] An experienced respiratory therapist should be at the controls of the ventilator to react to changes in flow rates and tidal volumes. An elbow adaptor fitted with a rubber diaphragm prevents loss of tidal volume during the procedure. The ECG should be monitored for arrhythmias.

The use of fiberoptic bronchoscopy in the management of secretions and mucus plugging is still debated. Although useful in identifying the presence and location of secretions, evidence that suctioning through the fiberoptic bronchoscope is any more beneficial than percussion and endotracheal catheter suctioning is lacking.[111] Despite repeated attempts in some patients, it is difficult to guide the endotracheal catheter into the left mainstem bronchus to loosen and agitate the secretions, and the fiberoptic bronchoscope may be helpful in this setting. Direct instillation of normal saline in the areas of mucus plugging, may facilitate its removal. Intensive bronchodilators combines with aggressive endotracheal suctioning and chest physiotherapy still remains the standard in controlling mucus secretions.

The complications of fiberoptic bronchoscopy during mechanical ventilation are fortunately few. The patient is always at risk for barotrauma, however, especially to the development of a pneumothorax. Careful monitoring by the respiratory therapist of ventilator pressures and the obtaining of a chest radiograph immediately after the procedure can serve to minimize the consequences of this complication. During a bronchoscopy the use of suction should be used only for brief periods as a decrease in patient tidal volume has been noticed with overuse. The problems of hypoxia and hypercarbia can usually be obviated by careful monitoring and by having the respiratory therapist initiate changes in the ventilator parameters.

Bronchoalveolar Lavage

Bronchoalveolar lavage has now become a common procedure in the ICU. Studies have documented that it is safe and easily done. Its greatest usefulness is in the immunocompromised patient in whom a pulmonary infection is suspected.[134-137] It is especially useful to document Pneumocystis carinii in the AIDS population.[130] Bronchoalveolar lavage has been shown to be an excellent method for diagnosing nonbacterial infections (e.g., fungi and tuberculosis). This procedure, however, is less useful to delineate noninfectious processes and is less useful in immunocompetent patients. Its principal value is that it can be done easily with a minimal amount of complications. Frequently in very sick patients, the use of transbronchial biopsy or open lung biopsy cannot be done. Although the yield may be quite small, generally in these very sick patients diagnostic procedures are limited. Therefore, bronchoalveolar lavage is a reasonable partial step in an attempt to obtain diagnosis.

Transbronchial Biopsy

The ability to safely perform transbronchial biopsy during mechanical ventilation has been described. Transbronchial biopsy in conjunction with bronchial brushing has established diagnosis in 45% of patients reported in a small study.[138] This yield is markedly less than an open lung biopsy, but because transbronchial biopsy has much lower morbidity than the open lung approach, it has been advocated as an initial approach in the critically ill patient with diffuse lung disease. Animal studies have also provided evidence that transbronchial biopsy can be done safely during mechanical ventilation.[139,140] The most serious complication of transbronchial biopsy during mechanical ventilation is clearly that of a pneumothorax. With proper vigilance, a pneumothorax should be readily diagnosed and treated. Hypoxemia and hypercapnia are no more of a problem during transbronchial biopsy than during the performance of fiberoptic bronchoscopy alone, or the performance of bronchoalveolar lavage. Certainly, patients with coagulopathy and patients with severe hemodynamic compromise would not be candidates for transbronchial biopsy. Similarly, patients with severe hypoxia who could not tolerate a transient pneumothorax should not be considered the gold standard in obtaining a diagnosis in critically ill patients. It offers, however, an alternative which may provide some information in the very critically ill patients for whom options are limited.

Open Lung Biopsy

In a patient with acute diffuse lung injury of unknown etiology, an open lung biopsy, if technically possible, is best in determining a diagnosis.[141,142] Certainly, less invasive approaches such as discussed earlier are a useful first step and may prevent the morbidity of an open lung biopsy. Mechanical ventilation is routinely managed in the operating room and is not a contraindication to the performance of an open lung biopsy.[143] Situations where an open lung biopsy is most helpful include the immunosuppressed patient and patients likely to have an infectious process, or a drug reaction.[144-147] On the other hand, open lung biopsy usually does not yield any useful information in an ARDS patient with a typical clinical picture and predisposing factors.[141] An open lung biopsy should not be done if the patient has severe coagulopathy, is hemodynamically unstable, or has difficulty being oxygenated despite an F_{IO_2} of 100% and PEEP. One must bear in mind that the open lung biopsy requires the presence of a general anesthesia and the need for a chest tube postoperatively. The latter may be a formidable management problem in the patient receiving chronic corticosteroids. Technically, the open lung biopsy should involve a new area of disease or an area that is moderately involved, as studies have shown that the severely involved lung is likely to be helpful because of total destruction of lung tissue.[141] In a patient with a diffuse process, one biopsy is sufficient as numerous biopsies do not show different pathologic features.[143]

POST-ICU PHASE

Preparing for Weaning

As a patient is recovering from his or her acute respiratory failure, consideration should be given to prepare the patient for eventual weaning from mechanical ventilation. A systemic organ based review for reversible problems should be done. Cardiovascular attention is focused on correction and stabilization of cardiac output, as subclinical congestive heart failure may be an important factor in weaning failure. Anemia, if severe, should be corrected to provide maximum oxygen carrying capacity. Potential renal impediments to weaning include metabolic acidosis, electrolyte disturbances, and fluid overload. Occasionally acetazolamide may be useful in correcting some of the metabolic alkalosis. It is not uncommon for the patient to gain a significant amount of total body water during the process of mechanical ventilation and treatment of the acute illness, even with meticulous attempts to match intake and output.[142] The serum phosphate, potassium, calcium, and magnesium should be normalized to maximize the strength of the respiratory muscles. Central nervous system depression by sedatives needs to be minimized. Musculoskeletal integrity can be improved by physical therapy and proper nutrition. Pulmonary function can be maximized with aggressive pulmonary suctioning, along with percussion and postural drainage to enhance secretion clearance. Optimization of obstructive lung disease should be done including the administration of theophylline, beta agonists, anticholinergics, and usually corticosteroids. Calories from carbohydrates may need to be limited to prevent excess carbon dioxide production. Finally, the patient's tidal volume may gradually need to be reduced so that the tidal volume given by the mechanical ventilator more closely approximates the volume that the patient can generate. By decreasing the tidal volume, it allows the patient to adjust to the smaller tidal volumes that will occur during spontaneous ventilation.

The process of extubation should be distinguished from the process of weaning. Often patients that can be discontinued from mechanical ventilation need the presence of an endotracheal tube or a tracheotomy tube for the management of copious secretions. Indeed, mucus plugging and inability to clear mucus secretions is one of the most frequent causes for chronic ventilator patients to be returned to the ICU after being discharged. Finally, the endotracheal or tracheotomy tube occasionally needs to be left in place, longer than mechanical ventilation is necessary to prevent massive aspiration, or in the presence of upper airway swelling or mass. (For a more detailed discussion on weaning and rehabilitation, see Chap. 24.)

Prognosis in Mechanically Ventilated Patients

Although mechanical ventilation is often viewed acutely as a lifesaving technique, the prognosis of people that have been on mechanical ventilation for a prolonged period is poor. Ventilatory assistance is a expensive commodity, both in physical and in emotional terms, yet few patients are aware of the usual outcome of this technology. Spicher and Whyte reviewed 250 consecutive patients that had a minimum of 10 days of ventilatory support.[149] Overall survival was only 39% at discharge and survival at 1 year was only 28.6%. Unfortunately, of those patients who survived at discharge, approximately 40% were institutionalized and an additional 33% were confined to their homes. Only 3% of the patients had no deficits, and only 25% of the patients had mild deficits according to a functional scale. Their study also clearly indicated that preadmission function was a heavy influence of survival. These authors also found both age and the cause of respiratory failure to be an important predictor of survival.[143] Patients with postoperative respiratory complications had the best survival rates, while patients with chronic obstructive pulmonary disease had a uniformly poor prognosis. The duration of mechanical ventilation was not related to mortality. Although the study was retrospective, their data do indicate that long-term success in patients who receive prolonged mechanical ventilation is usually poor. Other investigators have shown that patients with certain disease categories have an exceedingly poor prognosis. For example, Schuster and Marion have shown that only 4 of 52 patients who required mechanical ventilation for hematologic malignancy ever left the hospital.[150]

Knaus and colleagues have developed a severity of illness scoring system which has been applied in an attempt to model prognosis for patients on mechanical ventilation.[151] Their system shows that severity of illness, the patient's age, and chronic health status affect the patient's probability of survival. Their model was a good predictor of mortality based on ICU admission values. In addition, scores obtained after 3 days of ICU treatments, demonstrated a 97% accuracy in their estimation of hospital mortality.[152] The recurrent principle in the available literature is that if the respiratory failure does not respond quickly, the prognosis drops rapidly if mechanical ventilation is necessary for more than a week. Factors associated with increased mortality include:

- Age
- Severity of illness
- Severe underlying COPD
- Development of complications during acute respiratory failure (especially nosocomial pneumonia)

The survival data in patients with acute and chronic lung diseases requiring mechanical ventilation have been recently reviewed.[153] The data were segregated into 2 diagnostic entities: COPD and ARDS. Mortality data of patients with COPD and acute respiratory failure were reviewed from 9 studies over 1958 to 1978. In these combined studies, a total of 180 patients with COPD required mechanical ventilation. Eighty-three of these patients, or 46%, died during the acute event. Although the decision to place people on mechanical ventilation varied considerably from study to study, the mortality rate was consistently high. Furthermore, even in patients with COPD who survived the episode of acute respiratory failure, their clinical course is grim. The mean interval between the first and second episode of acute respiratory failure in surviving patients was approximately 8 months. Prognosis for survival decreased for a second or subsequent episode of acute respiratory failure. Prognosis in a particular patient appeared to depend on the degree of underlying lung disease.

Numerous studies have shown that the mortality of patients with ARDS has remained at approximately 60%, unchanged over the last 25 years. Increasing number of organ systems failures, or the presence of sepsis define the highest mortality group. Bartlett and colleagues have shown that in 490 patients the mortality from respiratory failure alone is 40%.[154] The addition of one organ failing increases the mortality to 56%, two organs failing to 73%, three organs failing to 83%, and four organs failing to 100%. One third of the deaths in ARDS are due to the underlying illness, whereas two thirds of the deaths are due to a multiorgan system failure and/or sepsis.[153] These data, in summary, indicate a high baseline mortality in patients with acute respiratory failure secondary to ARDS who require mechanical ventilation. In addition, if sepsis or multiorgan system failure develops, the prognosis becomes negligible.

Failure of Mechanical Ventilation

As indicated by the survival data, the patient will not respond to therapeutic interventions often despite mechanical ventilation. Once it is obvious that the prognosis for functional recovery is extremely slim, difficult decisions regarding the continuation of mechanical ventilation must be addressed. The situation is complicated by the fact that the severity of illness usually leaves the patient incompetent and unable to participate in decisions regarding future care. Ideally, with excellent physician-family rapport, a consensus can be reached regarding the benefits of continuing mechanical ventilation. The decision to withdraw care or limit intervention is often a difficult decision for the physician, for the nursing staff, and for the patient's family. Sometimes setting a time limit for continued interventions is a good psychologic technique to assist in limiting intervention. For example, it can be decided that if no response is seen after another 5 to 7 days of acute intervention, intervention will stop. Occasionally consensus can be reached that ventilation be discontinued. In practice, however, it is much easier simply to limit further intervention and let nature take its course. One technique occasionally useful in this regard is to withhold new drugs and to limit inotropic and ventilator support at the current level. If the patient's condition is stable, ventilatory support and inotropic medication are decreased. Once decreased, the new support level becomes the baseline which is never increased. It is also often helpful if the burden of these decisions is borne mainly by the physicians and the ICU team, with input from the family involved. The medical team taking care of the patient should initiate a rational plan of limiting or withdrawing care and present it to the family. Shorn of this decision-making burden, many families find this approach comfortable to accept. Appropriate dialogue and rapport with the patient's family early often prevent problems as the illness progresses and frequently keep decision making between the physician and the family, avoiding a legal quagmire.

REFERENCES

1. Petty, J.: A historical perspective of mechanical ventilation. Crit. Care Clin., *6*:489 1990.
2. Shim, C., and Williams, M.: Evaluation of the severity of asthma: patients versus physicians. Am. J. Med., *68*:11, 1980.
3. Jederlinic, P., and Irwin, R.: Status asthmaticus. J. Intensive Care Med., *4*:166, 1989.
4. Gravelyn, T., and Weg, J.: Respiratory rate as an indicator of acute dysfunction. JAMA, *244*:1123, 1980.
5. Grum, C. M., and Morganroth, M. L.: Initiating mechanical ventilation. J. Intensive Care Med., *3*:6, 1988.
6. Pontoppidan, H., Geffin, B., and Lowenstein, E.: Acute respiratory failure in the adult. N. Engl. J. Med., *287*:690, 743, 799, 1972.
7. Naris, R., and Emmett, M.: Simple and mixed acid-base disorders: a practical approach. Medicine, *59*:161, 1980.
8. Hopeman, A.: Chest trauma. In Pulmonary emergencies. Edited by S. Sahn Edinburgh, Churchill Livingstone, 1982, p. 328.
9. Nealon, T.: Trauma to the chest. In Pulmonary diseases and disorders. Edited by A. Fisherman. New York, McGraw-Hill, 1980, p. 1567.
10. Trinkle, J. et al.: Management of flail chest without mechanical ventilation. Ann. Thorac. Surg., *19*:355, 1975.
11. Braun, N., et al.: When should respiratory muscles be exercised? Chest, *84*:76, 1983.
12. Rosen, R., and Bone, R.: Financial implications of ventilator care. Crit. Care Clin., *6*:797, 1990.
13. Snider, G. L.: Thirty years of mechanical ventilation. Arch. Intern. Med., *143*:745, 1983.
14. Luce, J.: Withholding and withdrawing life support from the critically ill: how does it work in clinical practice? Respir. Care, *36*:417, 1991.
15. Elpern, E., Silver, M., Rosen, R., and Bone, R.: The noninvasive respiratory care unit. Patterns of use and financial implications. Chest, *99*:205, 1991.
16. Krieger, B., Ershowsky, P., and Spivack, D.: One year's experience with a noninvasively monitored intermediate care unit for pulmonary patients. JAMA, *264*:1143, 1990.
17. Shneerson, J.: Assisted ventilation. 5. Non-invasive and domiciliary ventilation: negative pressure techniques. Thorax, *46*:131, 1991.
18. Levine, S., Levy, S., and Henson, D.: Negative-pressure ventilation. Crit. Care Clin., *6*:505, 1990
19. Donohue, W., et al.: Long-term mechanical ventilation: guidelines for management in the home and at alternative community sites. Chest, *90*:1S, 1986.
20. Kacmarek, R., and Spearman, C.: Equipment used for ventilatory support in the home. Respir. Care, *31*:311, 1986.
21. Wiers, P., et al.: Cuirass respirator treatment of chronic respiratory failure in scoliotic patients. Thorax, *32*:221, 1977.
22. Glenn, W., Holcomb, W., Gee, J., and Rath, R.: Central hypoventilation: long-term ventilatory assistance by radiofrequency electrophrenic respiration. Ann. Surg., *172*:755, 1970.
23. Glenn, W., Hogan, J., and Phelps, M.: Ventilatory support of the quadriplegic patient with respiratory paralysis by diaphragm pacing. Surg. Clin. North A., *60*:1055, 1980.
24. Glenn, W., et al.: Diaphragm pacing radiofrequency transmission in the treatment of chronic ventilatory insufficiency. J. Thorac. Cardiovasc. Surg., *66*:505, 1973.
25. Phrenic nerve pacing in quadriplegia. Lancet, *336*:88, 1990.
26. Grum, C. M., and Chauncey, J. B.: Conventional mechanical ventilation. Clin. Chest Med., *9*:37, 1988.
27. Schuster, D.: A physiologic approach to initiating, maintaining, and withdrawing mechanical ventilatory support during acute respiratory failure. Am. J. Med., *88*:268, 1990.
28. Howe, J., et al.: Return of arterial P_{O_2} values to baseline after supplemental oxygen in patients with cardiac disease. Chest, *67*:256, 1975.
29. Sherter, C., Jabbour, S., Kovnat, D., and Snider, G.: Prolonged rate of decay of arterial P_{O_2} following oxygen breathing in chronic airways obstruction. Chest, *67*:259, 1975.
30. Anthonisen, N.: Hypoxemia and O_2 therapy. Am. Rev. Respir. Dis., *126*:729, 1982.
31. Thomas, H., et al.: The oxyhemoglobin dissociation curve in health and disease. Am. J. Med., *57*:331, 1974.
32. Marini, J., Capps, J., and Culver, B.: The inspiratory work of breathing during assisted mechanical ventilation. Chest, *87*:612, 1985.
33. Bryan, C., and Jenkinson, S.: Oxygen toxicity. Clin. Chest. Med., *9*:141, 1988.
34. Davis, W., Rennard, S., Bitterman, P., and Crystal, R.: Pulmonary oxygen toxicity. Early reversible changes in human alveolar structures induced by hyperoxia. N. Engl. J. Med., *309*:878, 1983.
35. Deneke, S., and Fanburg, B.: Normobaric oxygen toxicity of the lung. N. Engl. J. Med., *303*:76, 1980
36. Lodato, R.: Oxygen toxicity. Crit. Care Clin., *6*:749, 1990.
37. Griffith, D., et al.: Effects of common therapeutic concentrations of oxygen on lung clearance of 99mTc DTPA and bronchoalveolar lavage albumin concentration. Am. Rev. Respir. Dis., *134*:233, 1986.
38. Weisman, I., Rinaldo, J., and Rogers, R.: Positive end-expiratory pressure in adult respiratory failure. N. Engl. J. Med., *307*:1381, 1982.
39. Popovich, J. J.: Mechanical ventilation. Postgrad. Med., *79*:217, 1986.
40. Rounds, S., and Brody, J.: Putting PEEP in perspective. N. Engl. J. Med., *311*:323, 1984.
41. Dantzker, D., et al.: Ventilation-perfusion distributions in the adult respiratory distress syndrome. Am. Rev. Respir. Dis., *120*:1039, 1979.
42. Connors, A., McCaffree, D., and Rogers, R.: The adult respiratory distress syndrome. Dis. Mon., *27*:1, 1981.
43. Suter, P., Fairley, H., and Isenberg, M.: Optimum end-expiratory airway pressure in patients with acute pulmonary failure. N. Engl. J. Med., *292*:284, 1975.
44. Luce, J.: The cardiovascular effects of mechanical ventilation and positive end-expiratory pressure. JAMA, *252*:807, 1984.
45. Tittley, J., et al.: Hemodynamic and myocardial metabolic consequences of PEEP. Chest, *88*:496, 1985.
46. Payen, D., et al.: Lower body positive pressure vs. dopamine during PEEP in humans. J. Appl. Physiol., *58*:77, 1985.

47. West, J., Dollery, C., and Naimark, A.: Distribution of blood flow on isolated lungs; relation to vascular and alveolar pressures. J. Appl. Physiol., 19:713, 1964.
48. Glazier, J., Hughes, J., and Maloney, J.: Measurements of capillary dimensions and blood volume in rapidly frozen lungs. J. Appl. Physiol., 26:65, 1969.
49. Swan, H.: The pulmonary artery catheter. Dis. Mon., 37:475, 1991.
50. Pepe, P., Hudson, K., and Carrico, C.: Early application of positive end-expiratory pressure in patients at risk for the adult respiratory-distress syndrome. N. Engl. J. Med., 311:281, 1984.
51. Good, J., et al.: The routine use of positive end-expiratory pressure after open heart surgery. Chest, 76:397, 1979.
52. Risk, N., and Murray, J.: PEEP and pulmonary edema. Am. J. Med., 72:381, 1982.
53. Luce, J., et al. The effects of expiratory positive pressure on the resolution of oleic acid-induced lung injury in dogs. Am. Rev. Respir. Dis., 125:716, 1982.
54. Sassoon, C. S. H.: Positive pressure ventilation. Alternate modes. Chest, 100:1421, 1991.
55. Mawrcy, T. W., and Marini, J. J.: Inverse ratio ventilation in ARDS. Rationale and implementation. Chest 100: 494, 1991.
56. Tharratt, R. S., Allen, R. P., and Albertson, T. E.: Pressure controlled inverse ratio ventilation in severe adult respiratory failure. Chest, 94:755, 1988.
57. Gurevitch, M. J., Van Dyke, J., Young, E. S., and Jackson, K.: Improved oxygenation and lower peak airway pressure in severe adult respiratory distress syndrome. Treatment with inverse ratio ventilation. Chest, 89:211, 1986.
58. Poelaert, J. I., Vogelaers, D. P., and Colardyn, F. A.: Evaluation of the hemodynamic and respiratory effects of inverse ratio ventilation with a right ventricular ejection fraction catheter. Chest, 99:1444, 1991.
59. Abraham, E., and Yoshihara, G.: Cardiorespiratory effects of pressure controlled inverse ratio ventilation in severe respiratory failure. Chest, 96:1356, 1989.
60. Cole, A. G., Weller, S. F., and Sykes, M. K. Inverse ratio ventilation compared with PEEP in adult respiratory failure. Intensive Care Med., 10:227, 1984.
61. Sassoon, C., Mahutte, C., and Light, R.: Ventilator modes: old and new. Crit. Care Clin., 6:605, 1990.
62. Marini, J., Rodriguez, R., and Lamb, V.: The inspiratory workload of patient-initiated mechanical ventilation. Am. Rev. Respir. Dis., 134:902, 1986.
63. Marini, J.: Strategies to minimize breathing effort during mechanical ventilation. Crit. Care Clin., 6:635, 1990.
64. Downs, J. et al.: Intermittent mandatory ventilation: a new approach to weaning patient from mechanical ventilators. Chest, 64:331, 1973.
65. Luce, J., Pierson, D., and Hudson, L.: Intermittent mandatory ventilation. Chest, 79:678, 1981.
66. Weisman, I., Rinaldo, J., Rogers, R., and Sanders, M.: Intermittent mandatory ventilation. Am. Rev. Respir. Dis., 127:641, 1983.
67. Willatts, S.: Alternative modes of ventilation. Part 1. Disadvantages of controlled mechanical ventilation; intermittent. Intensive Care Med., 11:51, 1985.
68. Venus, B., Smith, R., and Mathru, M.: National survey of methods and criteria used for weaning from mechanical ventilation. Crit. Care Med., 15:530, 1987.
69. Down J., Perkins, H., and Modell, J.: Intermittent mandatory ventilation: an evaluation. Arch. Surg., 109:519, 1974.
70. Culpepper, J., Rinaldo, J., and Rogers, R.: Effect of mechanical ventilator mode on tendency towards respiratory alkalosis. Am. Rev. Respir. Dis. 132:1075, 1985.
71. Hudson, L., Hurlow, R., Craig, K., and Pierson, D.: Does intermittent mandatory ventilation correct respiratory alkalosis in patients receiving assisted mechanical ventilation? Am. Rev. Respir. Dis., 132:1071, 1985.
72. Brochard, L., Pluskwa, F., and Lemaire, F.: Improved efficacy of spontaneous breathing with inspiratory pressure support. Am. Rev. Respir. Dis., 136:411, 1987.
73. Hurst, J. M., Branson, R. D., David, K Jr., and Barrette, R. R.: Cardiopulmonary effects of pressure support ventilation. Arch. Surg., 124:1067, 1989.
74. MacIntyre, N.: Respiratory function during pressure support ventilation. Chest, 89:677, 1986.
75. Fiastro, J. F., Habib, M. P., and Quan, S. F.: Pressure support compensation for inspiratory work due to endotracheal tubes and demand continuous positive airway pressure. Chest, 93:499, 1988
76. Brochard, L., Harf, A., Lorino, H., and Lemaire, F.: Inspiratory pressure support prevents diaphragmatic fatigue during weaning from mechanical ventilation. Am. Rev. Respir. Dis., 139:513, 1989.
77. Prakash, O., and Meij, S.: Cardiopulmonary response to inspiratory pressure support during spontaneous ventilation vs conventional ventilation. Chest, 88:403, 1985.
78. Valentine, D., et al.: Distribution of ventilation and perfusion with different modes of mechanical ventilation. Am. Rev. Respir. Dis., 143:1262, 1991.
79. Gillespie, D.: High frequency ventilation: a new concept in mechanical ventilation. Mayo Clin. Proc., 58:187, 1983.
80. Sykes, D.: High frequency ventilation. Thorax, 40:161, 1985.
81. Gallagher, T., Klain, M., and Carlon, G.: Present status of high frequency ventilation. Crit. Care Med., 10:613, 1982.
82. Standiford, T., and Morganroth, M.: High-frequency ventilation. Chest, 96:1380, 1989.
83. Gallagher, T.: High-frequency ventilation. Med. Clin. North Am., 67:663, 1983.
84. Saari, A., Rossing, T., and Drazen, J.: Physiological bases for new approaches to mechanical ventilation. Annu. Rev. Med., 35:165, 1984.
85. Mal, H., Rouby, J., Benhamou, D., and Viars, P.: High frequency jet ventilation in acute respiratory failure: which ventilator settings? Br. J. Anaesth., 58:18, 1986.
86. Froese, A., and Bryan, A.: High-frequency ventilation. Am. Rev. Respir. Dis., 135:1363, 1987.
87. Shikowitz, M., Abramson, A., and Liberatore, L.: Endolaryngeal jet ventilation: a 10-year review. Laryngoscope, 101:455, 1991.
88. Powner, D., and Grenvik, A.: A ventilatory management of life-threatening bronchopleural fistulae. Crit. Care Med., 9:54, 1981.
89. Bishop, M., Benson, M., Sato, P., and Pierson, D.: Comparison of high frequency ventilation with conventional mechanical ventilation for bronchopleural fistula. Anesth. Analg., 66:833, 1987.
90. Baumann, M., and Sahn, S.: Medical management and therapy of bronchopleural fistula in the mechanically ventilated patient. Chest, 97:721, 1990.
91. Guidelines for standards of care for patients with acute respiratory failure on mechanical ventilatory support. Task Force on Guidelines; Society of Critical Care Medicine. Crit. Care Med., 19:275, 1991.
92. Wiedemann, H., and McCarthy, K.: Noninvasive monitoring of oxygen and carbon dioxide. Clin. Chest Med., 10:239, 1989.
93. Schnapp, L. M., and Cohen, N. H.: Pulse oximetry: uses and abuses. Chest, 98:1244, 1990.
94. Tobin, M.: Respiratory monitoring. JAMA, 264:244, 1990.

95. Marini, J.: Monitoring during mechanical ventilation. Clin. Chest Med., *9:*73, 1988.
96. Wiedemann, H., and Matthay, R.: Cardiovascular-pulmonary monitoring in the intensive care unit. Chest, *85:*537, 656, 1984.
97. Demers, R., Pratter, M., and Irwin, R.: Use of the concept of ventilator compliance in the determination of static total compliance. Respir. Care, *26:*644, 1981.
98. Zwillich, C., et al.: Complications of assisted ventilation. Am. J. Med., *57:*161, 1974.
99. Goertz, A., Heinrich, H., Winter, H., and Deller, A.: Hemodynamic effects of different ventilatory patterns. A prospective clinical trial. Chest, *99:*1166, 1991.
100. Pinsky, M.: The effects of mechanical ventilation on the cardiovascular system. Crit. Care Clin., *6:*663, 1990.
101. Winston, S., Gravelyn, T., and Sitrin, R.: Prevention of bradycardia responses to endotracheal suctioning by prior administration of nebulized atropine. Crit. Care Med., *15:*1009, 1987.
102. Petersen, G., and Horst B.: Incidence of pulmonary barotrauma in a medical ICU. Crit. Care Med., *11:*67, 1983.
103. Marini, J., and Culver, B.: Systemic gas embolism complicating mechanical ventilation in the adult respiratory distress syndrome. Ann. Inter. Med., *110:*669, 1989.
104. Sargent, E., and Turner, A.: Emergency treatment of pneumothorax. Am. J. Roent., *109:*531, 1970
105. Pierson, D., Horton, C., and Bates, P.: Persistent bronchopleural air leak during mechanical ventilation. Chest, *90:*321, 1986.
106. Pierson, D.: Persistent bronchopleural air leak during mechanical ventilation: a review. Respir. Care, *27:*408, 1982.
107. Powner, D., and Bierman, M.: Thoracic and extrathoracic bronchial fistulas. Chest, *100:*480, 1991.
108. Pierson, D.: Complications associated with mechanical ventilation. Crit. Care Clin., *6:*711, 1990.
109. Peevy, K., Hernandez, L., Moise, A., and Parker, J.: Barotrauma and microvascular injury in lungs of nonadult rabbits: effect of ventilation pattern. Crit. Care Med., *18:*634, 1990.
110. Ziment, I.: Theophylline and mucociliary clearance. Chest, *92 (suppl):*38S, 1987.
111. Marini, J., Pierson, D., and Hudson, L.: Acute lobar atelectasis: a prospective comparison of fiberoptic bronchoscopy and respiratory therapy. Am. Rev. Respir. Dis., *119:*971, 1979.
112. Pingleton, S.: Complications of acute respiratory failure. Med. Clin. North Am., *67:*725, 1983.
113. Strieter, R. M., and Lynch, J. P.: Complications in the ventilated patient. Clin. Chest Med., *9:*127, 1988.
114. Dellinger, R.: Pathophysiology, monitoring, and management of the ventilator-dependent patient: considerations for drug therapy, emphasis on stress ulcer prophylaxis. DICP, *24 (suppl 11):*S8, 1990.
115. Craven, D., et al.: Risk factors for pneumonia and fatality in patients receiving continuous mechanical ventilation. Am. Rev. Respir. Dis. *133:*792, 1986.
116. Tryba, M.: Sucralfate versus antacids or H$_2$-antagonists for stress ulcer prophylaxis: a meta-analysis on efficacy and pneumonia rate. Crit. Care Med., *19:*942, 1991.
117. Moser, K., LeMoine, J., Nachtwey, F., and Spragg, R.: Deep venous thrombosis and pulmonary embolism. Frequency in a respiratory intensive care unit. JAMA, *246:*1422, 1981.
118. Cross, A., and Roup, B.: Role of respiratory assistance devices in endemic nosocomial pneumonia. Am. J. Med., *70:*681, 1981.
119. Craven, D. E., et al.: Contamination of mechanical ventilators with tubing changes every 24 or 48 hours. N. Engl. J. Med. *306:*1505, 1982.
120. Craven, D., et al: Contaminated medication nebulizers in mechanical ventilator circuits. Am. J. Med., *77:*834, 1984.
121. Pingleton, S., Hinthorn, D., and Liu, C.: Enteral nutrition in patients receiving mechanical ventilation. Am. J. Med., *80:*827, 1986.
122. Stauffer, J. L., Olson, D. E., and Petty, T. L.: Complications and consequences of endotracheal intubation and tracheotomy. Am. J. Med., *70:*65, 1981.
123. Niederman, M., Ferranti, R., and Zeigler, A.: Respiratory infection complicating long-term tracheostomy: the implication of persistent gram negative tracheobronchial colonization. Chest, *85:*39, 1984.
124. Heffner, J. E., Miller, S., and Sahn, S. A.: Tracheostomy in the intensive care unit. Part 2: complications. Chest, *90:*430, 1986.
125. Heffner, J. E.: Tracheal intubation in mechanically ventilated patients. Clin. Chest Med., *9:*23, 1988.
126. Heffner, J.: Airway management in the critically ill patient. Crit. Care Clin., *6:*533, 1990.
127. Plummer, A. L., and Gracey, D. R.: Consensus conference on artificial airways in patients receiving mechanical ventilation. Chest, *96:*178, 1989.
128. Barrett, C. J.: Flexible fiberoptic bronchoscopy in the critically ill patient. Chest, *73:*746, 1978.
129. Shinnick, J., Johnston, R., and Oslick, T.: Bronchoscopy during mechanical ventilation using the fiberscope. Chest, *65:*613, 1974.
130. O'Brien, D., Curran, J., and Conroy, J.: Fibre-optic assessment of tracheal tube position. A comparison of tracheal tube position as estimated by fibre-optic bronchoscopy and by chest x-ray. Anaesthesia, *40:*73, 1985.
131. Lundgren, R., Haggmark, S., and Reiz, S.: Hemodynamic effects of flexible fiberoptic bronchoscopy performed under topic anesthesia. Chest, *82:*295, 1982.
132. Fulkerson, W.: Current concepts: fiberoptic bronchoscopy. N. Engl. J. Med., *311:*511, 1984.
133. Baier, H., Begin, R. and Sackner, M.: Effect of airway diameter, suction catheters and the bronchofiberscope on airflow in endotracheal and tracheostomy tubes. Heart Lung, *5:*235, 1976.
134. Stover, D., White, D., Romano, P., and Gellene, R.: Diagnosis of pulmonary disease in acquired immune deficiency syndrome. Am. Rev. Respir. Dis., *130:*659, 1984.
135. Stover, D., et al.: Bronchoalveolar lavage in the diagnosis of diffuse pulmonary infiltrates in the immunosuppressed host. Ann. Intern. Med., *101:*1, 1984.
136. Young, J., Hopkins, J., and Cuthbertson, W.: Pulmonary infiltrates in immunocompromised patients: diagnosis by cytological examination of bronchoalveolar lavage fluid. J. Clin. Pathol., *37:*390, 1984.
137. Chauncey, J., Lynch, J., Hyzy, R., and Toews, G.: Invasive techniques in the diagnosis of bacterial pneumonia in the intensive care unit. Semin. Respir. Infect., *5:*215, 1990.
138. Papin, T., Grum, C., and Weg, J.: Transbronchial biopsy during mechanical ventilation. Chest, *89:*168, 1986.
139. Maurer, J., et al.: The risk/yield of invasive diagnostic procedures during PEEP in a canine model of pneumonia. Am. Rev. Diagnostics, *2:*129, 1983.
140. Moser, K., et al.: Sensitivity, specificity, and risk of diagnostic procedures in a canine model of streptococcus pneumoniae pneumonia. Am. Rev. Respir. Dis., *125:*436, 1982.
141. Gaensler, E.: Open and closed lung biopsy. *In* Diagnostic Techniques in Pulmonary Disease. Edited by M. Sackner. New York, Marcel Dekker, 1981, 579.
142. Matthay, R., and Moritz, E.: Invasive procedures for diagnos-

ing pulmonary infection: a critical review. Clin. Chest Med., 2:3, 1981.
143. Hill, J., et al.: Pulmonary pathology in acute respiratory insufficiency: lung biopsy as a diagnostic tool. J. Thorac. Cardiovasc. Surg., 71:64, 1976.
144. Gaensler, E., and Carrington, C.: Open biopsy for chronic diffuse infiltrative lung disease: clinical, roentgenographic, and physiological correlations in 502 patients. Ann. Thorac. Surg., 30:411, 1980.
145. Rossiter, S., et al.: Open lung biopsy in the immunosuppressed patient: is it really beneficial? J. Thorac. Cardiovasc. Surg., 77:338, 1979.
146. Toledo-Pereyra, L., et al.: The benefits of open lung biopsy in patients with previous nondiagnostic transbronchial lung biopsy. Chest, 77:647, 1980.
147. Cheu, H., et al.: Open lung biopsy in the critically ill newborn. Pediatrics, 86:561, 1990.
148. Sladen, A., Laver, M., and Pontoppidan, H.: Pulmonary complications and water retention in prolonged mechanical ventilation. N. Engl. J. Med., 279:448, 1968.
149. Spicher, J., and White, D.: Outcome and function following prolonged mechanical ventilation. Arch. Intern. Med., 147:421, 1987.
150. Schuster, D., and Marion, J.: Precedents for meaningful recovery during treatment in a medical intensive care unit. Outcome in patients with hematologic malignancy. Am. J. Med., 75:402, 1983.
151. Knaus, W., Draper, E., Wagner, D., and Zimmerman, J.: An evaluation of outcome from intensive care in major medical centers. Ann. Intern. Med., 104:410, 1986.
152. Knaus, W.: Prognosis with mechanical ventilation: the influence of disease, severity of disease, age, and chronic health status on survival from an acute illness. Am. Rev. Respir. Dis., 140:S8, 1989.
153. Hudson, L.: Survival data in patients with acute and chronic lung disease requiring mechanical ventilation. Am. Rev. Respir. Dis., 140:S19, 1989.
154. Bartlett, R., et al.: A prospective study of acute hypoxic respiratory failure. Chest, 89:684, 1986.

SUPPLEMENTAL READINGS

Blanch, P. B., Jones, M., Layon, A. J., and Camner, N.: Pressure-preset ventilation. Part 1. Physiologic and mechanical considerations. Chest, 104:590, 1993.

Blanch, P. B., Jones, M., Layon, A. J., and Camner, N.: Pressure-preset ventilation. Part 2. Mechanics and safety. Chest, 104:904, 1993.

Brunet, F., et al.: Extracorporeal carbon dioxide removal and low-frequency positive-pressure ventilation: improvement in arterial oxygenation with reduction of risk of pulmonary barotrauma in patients with adult respiratory distress syndrome. Chest, 104:889, 1993.

Consensus Conference on the Essentials of Mechanical Ventilation. Respir. Care, 37:999, 1992.

East, T. D., et al.: A successful computerized protocol for clinical management of pressure control inverse ratio ventilation in ARDS. Chest, 101:697, 1992.

Leach, C. L., Fuhrman, B. P., Morin, F., and Rath, M. G.: Perfluorocarbon-associated gas exchange (partial liquid ventilation) in respiratory distress syndrome: a prospective, randomized, controlled study. Crit. Care Med., 21:1270, 1993.

Mercat, A., et al.: Cardiorespiratory effects of pressure-controlled ventilation with and without inverse ratio in the adult respiratory distress. Chest, 104:871, 1993.

Munoz, J., et al.: Pressure-controlled ventilation versus controlled mechanical ventilation with decelerating inspiratory flow. Crit. Care Med., 21:1143, 1993.

Ravenscraft, S. A., et al.: Tracheal gas insufflation augments CO_2 clearance during mechanical ventilation. Am. Rev. Respir. Dis., 148:345, 1993.

Slutsky, A. S.: Mechanical ventilation: ACCP Consensus Conference. Chest, 104:1833, 1993.

Stauffer, J. L., et al.: Survival following mechanical ventilation for acute respiratory failure in adult men. Chest, 104:1222, 1993.

Talpers, S. S., Romberger, D. J., Bunce, S. B., and Pingleton, S. K.: Nutritionally associated increased carbon dioxide production: excess total calories vs high proportion of carbohydrate. Chest, 102:551, 1992.

Chapter 17

THE ADULT RESPIRATORY DISTRESS SYNDROME

JOHN W. CHRISTMAN
JEAN E. RINALDO

The concept of the adult respiratory distress syndrome (ARDS) has evolved significantly since the first description appeared in the literature.[1,2] ARDS was originally termed ARDS because it appeared to be similar to the respiratory distress syndrome (RDS) which occurs in premature infants. This term has proven to be a misnomer because the pathology of ARDS and RDS are not similar. RDS results from an absolute deficiency of surfactant due to immature type II pneumocytes whereas the pathophysiology of ARDS involves damage to the epithelial and endothelial cells. In ARDS, type I epithelial cells are damaged and the epithelial cell surface is regenerated with surfactant producing type II pneumocytes.[3,4] The damaged endothelial and epithelial surfaces in ARDS contributes to a loss of the selective barrier properties of the alveolar-capillary membrane. Salt, water, and proteins flood the interstitial and alveolar compartments and disrupt the gas exchange process.

Initially, ARDS appeared to be a serious but potentially reversible disease process limited to the lungs. Advances in supportive technology were spawned and applied to patients with increasing enthusiasm, but without appreciable impact on survival. A notion has arisen that ARDS is a systemic process where the lung pathophysiology is combined with extrapulmonary abnormalities which typically involve the circulatory, digestive, hematopoietic, and metabolic systems. The interactions between these organ systems dominates the clinical manifestations of ARDS, dictate supportive treatments, and appears to predict the outcome.[5-7] The mortality of ARDS is closely associated with the presence of pulmonary and extrapulmonary infections.[6,8] Infection both predisposes to ARDS and is a poor prognostic indicator. This theme of a systemic reaction to an infection or an infectious-like process fits well with our evolving concepts of the network of cellular events which culminate in ARDS. Despite recognition of this syndrome for at least two decades and new ideas regarding the pathogenesis of ARDS, our understanding of it remains incomplete and treatment remains largely supportive and controversial.

In this chapter, we will explore the events which predispose to and alter the outcome from ARDS. We will discuss the current concepts of ARDS, elaborate on the prevailing theories of the pathogenesis of ARDS, and outline the current modes of supportive treatments. We will investigate the predictors of outcome and will discuss the studies which have evaluated the residual pulmonary dysfunction that occurs in those who survive ARDS.

DEFINITION OF ARDS

A syndrome is a group of signs and symptoms that collectively characterize or indicate a particular disease or abnormal condition. ARDS is a clinical constellation of radiologic and physiologic abnormalities that occur following an identifiable cataclysmic occurrence. ARDS has been recognized in all ages and occurs with equal prevalence in both sexes. The definition of ARDS usually includes chest radiographic, arterial blood gas, and pulmonary physiologic criteria. The chest radiograph typically shows diffuse five lobe interstitial and alveolar infiltrates. Arterial blood gas measurements reveal severe arterial hypoxemia despite oxygen administration. The compliance of the lungs is usually decreased[9] and the pulmonary vascular resistance is frequently elevated.[10] The threshold for the diagnosis of ARDS is variable. Most definitions of ARDS have originated for the purpose of clinical investigations and have propagated the idea that ARDS is an "all or none" phenomenon. The validity of this hypothesis has not been tested and the notion that ARDS is a phenomenon that varies in severity is increasing in popularity.[11,12] Rinaldo identified 27 patients over a 3 month period who appeared to have ARDS based on "broad clinical criteria."[12] These clinical criteria included: (1) a recognized predisposition to ARDS; (2) diffuse alveolar infiltrates on the chest radiograph; (3) respiratory failure requiring mechanical ventilation with an F_{IO_2} of greater than 0.4; and (4) the absence of a clinical history of roentgenologic findings of congestive heart failure. Only 7 out of 27 patients actually met published criteria for ARDS and the mortality of this subgroup was 71% (5/7). Seventy-four percent (20/27) of the patients did not meet published criteria for ARDS because they never achieved an alveolar/arterial ratio of less than 0.3 on PEEP, or did not require placement of a pulmonary artery catheter. In this group of patients, the mortality was only 30% (6/20). These observations seem to indicate that ARDS may occur in at least a mild and severe category. Rocker and colleagues studied 50 individuals with a range of severity of respiratory failure and risk factors for ARDS.[11] Twenty-two patients met criteria for ARDS at some point in the study, whereas 28 patients did not develop ARDS. Both populations had a spectrum of respiratory failure which these authors found was related to intravascular and intra-alveo-

Table 17-1. Diagnostic Criteria for ARDS

Appropriate clinical setting (see Table 17-2)
Diffuse radiographic pulmonary infiltrates
$PaO_2 < 60$ mm Hg on a $FIO_2 > 0.4$
Absence of hydrostatic pulmonary edema (PAOP $\leq$ 18 cm)
Lung compliance < 40 ml/cm

Table 17-3. Diseases that Can Mascarade as ARDS

Pulmonary microemboli	Bleomycin lung toxicity
Miliary tuberculosis	Varicella pneumonia
Mycosis fungoides	Neuroleptic malignant syndrome
Blastomycosis	Alveolar cell carcinoma
Histoplasmosis	Legionella pneumonia
Pneumocystis carinii	Idiopathic pulmonary fibrosis

lar neutrophil elastase levels and capillary permeability. This study suggests that a continuum of severity of lung injury exist and that the current threshold for identifying ARDS may fail to identify patients with early or mild disease. The spectrum of ARDS may range from a subclinical process of mild compensated pulmonary dysfunction which is easily treated with oxygen and/or PEEP to severe progressive pulmonary edema with irreversible acute respiratory failure.

Diagnostic Criteria

Although unequivocal diagnostic criteria for ARDS do not exist, the phenomenon is clearly and frequently recognized. A reasonable clinical definition appears in Table 17-1. Clinically, ARDS occurs in the setting of trauma or sepsis, although a great variety of inciting events have been associated with the syndrome. For two decades, case reports and small series have reported increasingly more complex and unusual association between etiologic events and ARDS. Important etiologic events that predispose to ARDS are listed in Table 17-2. In many cases, ARDS occurs as the direct or indirect consequence of an adverse situation or a cataclysmic event. This concept may have implications in terms of pathogenesis. ARDS appears to be initiated by a seminal incident that leads to a uncontrolled cascade of cellular and subcellular events which climax in pulmonary dysfunction. These events can be exacerbated and prolonged by persistent, untreated, or recurrent infections. If an antecedent event cannot be clearly identified, the clinician should strongly consider an alternate diagnosis such as the differential diagnoses listed in Table 17-3. An increasing number of patients who present with unexplained hypoxemic respiratory failure and diffuse infiltrates are found to have Pneumocystis carinii pneumonia associated with the acquired immunodeficiency syndrome (AIDS). Miliary tuberculosis, legionella pneumonia, and hypersensitivity pneumonitis are prominent examples of diseases which can be confused with ARDS. Ashbaugh and Maier have reported 10 patients who presented with an ARDS-like picture underwent open lung biopsy that diagnosed idiopathic pulmonary fibrosis.[13]

ARDS is recognized by a collection of clinical findings which include: diffuse infiltrates by chest radiography, arterial hypoxemia, the absence of hydrostatic pulmonary edema, decreased pulmonary compliance, and increased pulmonary vascular resistance. These criteria are arbitrarily defined and, therefore, each component is intrinsically disputable. The presence of diffuse radiograph pulmonary infiltrates is probably not sensitive enough to identify subtle pulmonary dysfunction since arterial hypoxemia may precede or be out of proportion to the demonstration of pulmonary infiltrates by chest radiography. Conversely, the chest radiograph can lag behind improvements in gas exchange.

The threshold for a diagnostic abnormality in gas exchange is also arbitrary and may require further definition as a more precise definition of ARDS becomes available. Typically, the arterial blood gas measurements show respiratory alkalosis (pH > 7.45) with hypoxemia ($PaO_2 < 50$) that only partially corrects with oxygen administration. An early improvement in arterial hypoxemia in response to treatment with positive end-expiratory pressure (PEEP) is a good prognostic indicator for survival from ARDS.[14]

Study criteria usually exclude patients with cardiogenic pulmonary edema. It is impossible to totally exclude this group of patients from the critical care unit. In fact, there appears to be an association between myocardial infarctions and ARDS.[15] In addition, enthusiastic fluid management in ARDS may inadvertently result in an expanded intravascular volume and superimposed hydrostatic pulmonary edema. Thus, permeability and hydrostatic pulmonary edema may coexist and interact with one another.

PRE-ICU AND PRE-ARDS CONSIDERATIONS

Risk Factors, Host Factors, and Clinical Setting

The incidence of ARDS in a civilian population is unknown but a widely quoted figure of 150,000 cases per year is prevalent in the literature. This incidence has been recently questioned because of new information gathered from the study of ARDS in a sequestered population. In 1989, a careful epidemiologic study of an island population indicated that the incidence of carefully defined ARDS was 1.5 cases per 100,000 persons per year and using more liberal criteria, 3.5 cases per 100,000.[16] If this study can be applied to the population of the United States at large, it suggests a yearly incidence of 36,000 to 84,000 persons per year. These findings are in agreement with the studies of Fowler[17] and Webster[18] who found incidence of ARDS at 5.2 cases per 100,000 and 4.5 cases per 100,000, respec-

Table 17-2. Predisposition to ARDS

Sepsis	Fat embolism
Shock	Aspiration pneumonia
Diabetic ketoacidosis	Infectious pneumonia
Pancreatitis	Myocardial infarction
Thoracic trauma	Near drowning
Head trauma	Drug overdosage
CNS hemorrhage	Amniotic fluid embolism

tively. Baumann and colleagues reported only a 2% incidence of ARDS in a prospective analysis of 11,112 high risk patients who entered the emergency room of a large metropolitan hospital.[19] Even if ARDS is less common than previously believed, the syndrome remains important because of its potential to occur in previously healthy individuals.

Clearly defined events which predispose to ARDS include: near drowning, multiple long bone fractures, hemorrhagic blood loss and multiple emergency transfusion, pulmonary contusions, aspiration of gastric acid, pancreatitis, and gram-negative bacteremia (see Table 17-2).[20] Most studies of predisposing risk factors have focused on the external events which are associated with or result in ARDS. Host factors have not been examined critically in clinical studies. The presence of premorbid malnutrition, diabetes mellitus, chronic obstructive pulmonary disease, chronic liver disease, malignancy, immunodeficiency, organ transplantation, and atherosclerotic coronary artery disease may be among those conditions which adversely effect survival if full blown ARDS should develop.

A liver-lung alliance may be an important feature that determines prognosis of ARDS.[21] The combinations of end-stage liver failure and ARDS have a 100% mortality.[22] ARDS associated with the rejection of a liver allograft has been observed to resolve following hepatic retransplantation.[23] Hepatic dysfunction observed during the first week of ARDS appears to be a major determinant of survival.[24] Taken together, these findings may indicate that the hepatic function is essential for detoxifying pro-inflammatory substances in ARDS.

ICU Phase of ARDS

The clinical findings of ARDS are nonspecific, but of monumental proportions. Altered vital signs and mental status usually herald the onset of ARDS and precipitate transfer to the ICU. Tachypnea is the predominant change in the vital signs, but fever and hypotension may be present depending on the predisposing cause of ARDS. The physical findings of ARDS are remarkable for impressive respiratory distress and auscultation of the chest frequently reveals bilateral crackles. The laboratory evaluation is helpful to identify arterial hypoxemia and to evaluate concurrent disease, such as pancreatitis and sepsis. The chest radiograph excludes other pulmonary causes for respiratory failure, such as pneumothorax, and reveals diffuse alveolar and interstitial infiltrates. The current definition of ARDS requires that all patients develop severe respiratory distress which necessitates tracheal intubation and mechanical ventilation with PEEP.

Pathophysiology of ARDS

A physiologic feature of ARDS is decreased pulmonary compliance which contributes significantly to the altered lung mechanics seen in ARDS.[16] The dynamic compliance of the total thoracic unit is usually measured by dividing the mechanically delivered tidal volume by the peak inspired positive pressure. Values less than 40 ml/cm water pressure are considered abnormal and consistent with the decreased compliance and increased resistance seen in ARDS. Mild pulmonary artery hypertension and elevated pulmonary vascular resistance are also thought to be a universal feature of ARDS.[19] Pulmonary artery pressure is difficult to estimate with noninvasive techniques and must be directly measured using a right heart catheter with a pressure transducer. The indication for right heart catheterization and its contribution to patient management is difficult to objectively determine and has recently been considered controversial.

Pathogenesis of ARDS

The tissue reaction seen in ARDS can be divided into three superimposed components: injury, inflammation, and repair. The injury component consists of damage and death to the microvascular endothelial and type I pulmonary epithelial cells. Lung inflammation appears to precede lung repair and is identified by the presence of granulocytic and mononuclear phagocytes in the lung. The repair component of the histopathology of ARDS involves the proliferation and altered function of endothelial cells, type II pulmonary epithelial cells, and interstitial matrix cells. Any theory of the pathogenesis of ARDS must account for injury, inflammation, and repair and provide for an interaction between the various cell types of the alveolar space. The evolution of concepts concerning the pathogenesis of ARDS has included at least three distinct phases, which we will refer to as the permeability phase, complement-mediated neutrophil activation phase, and the cytokine network phase.

Permeability Phase

With ARDS, the lungs accumulate edema as a result of altered barrier properties of the alveolar-capillary membrane. The variables which are known to determine the flux of fluid across the alveolar-capillary membrane are mathematically defined by Starling's equation:

$$Qf = K(P_{cap} - P_{is}) - K_o(\pi_{cap} - \pi_{is})$$

where K = capillary filtration coefficient, Pcap = hydrostatic pressure in the capillary space, Pis = hydrostatic pressure in the interstitial space, πcap = colloid oncotic pressure in the capillary space, πis = colloid oncotic pressure in the interstitial space, and o = reflection coefficient. Starling's equation relates the intravascular filtration forces (oncotic pressure and hydrostatic pressure) to those of the interstitial compartment. Pulmonary edema is an abnormal accumulation of liquid in the lungs which occurs when the net Starling's force favors the egress of salt and water into the pulmonary interstitial compartment at a rate which exceeds reabsorptive capacity. "Permeability" pulmonary edema is distinguished from "hydrostatic" pulmonary edema. In the case of permeability edema, flux increases because of altered permeability coefficients whereas hydrostatic edema results from an increase in intraluminal filtration pressures. Microvascular permeability has proved extremely difficult to measure in humans but has been shown to be increased by sensitive techniques in ARDS patients.[25,26] Rinaldo and colleagues measured lung microvascular transport properties using indication dilution technology using ^{51}Cr-erythrocytes, ^{125}I-albumin, ^{14}C-urea, and ^{3}H-water as tracers.[26] In this study, the ^{51}Cr-erythrocytes and ^{125}I-albumin were chosen as intravascular reference curves. The tracer ^{14}C-urea was chosen as a barrier-limited marker of the transport properties of the lung microvasculature, and the tracer ^{3}H-water was chosen as a measure of extravascular water. In this study, the mean values of the lung microvascular permeability surface area product for urea (^{14}C-PSu) and the extra-vascular lung water (EVLW) were significantly elevated in 10 ARDS patients compared to 5 control patients. Using identical methodology, Harris and colleagues studied two groups of ARDS patients: those who progressed during the course for the study (N = 23) and those who reversed the criteria for ARDS during the course of the study (N = 16).[25] These investigators reported a significant difference in the ^{14}C-PSu between the two groups even though the usual clinical measurements of lung function was similar. The role of lung edema has not been established as a direct cause of arterial hypoxemia. Brigham and colleagues have shown that lung edema, reflected by ^{3}H-water indicator dilution measurements of EVLW, does not correlate with the degree of arterial hypoxemia in 14 ARDS patients.[27] Thus, abnormalities in the measurements of ^{14}C-PSu and EVLW appear to be sensitive indicators of ARDS, but insufficient data are present in the literature to assess the specificity of these measurements. Currently, permeability pulmonary edema is thought to be a market of lung injury and inflammation.

Complement-Mediated Neutrophil Activation Phase

In the early 1980s, attention turned to activated neutrophils as a probable factor for increased lung microvascular permeability. Complement activation during hemodialysis utilizing cellophane dialysis membranes cause hypoxemia which is associated with the sequestration of neutrophils in the pulmonary vascular compartment. Such predisposers to ARDS, as trauma, pancreatitis, and endotoxemia are associated with complement activation. Complement activation generates phylogisins such as the complement breakdown product, C5a, which can directly activate peripheral blood neutrophils and can serve as a chemotactic agent to direct the movement of neutrophils according to a concentration gradient. In a small but provocative study, Hammerschmidt and associates found that complement activation, measured as neutrophil aggregating activity, was increased in patients with sepsis who developed ARDS.[28] Other investigators have been unable to reproduce the correlation, however.[29-32] Several studies implicate neutrophils as mediators of lung injury in ARDS. Some studies have shown that circulating neutrophils are activated in ARDS patients,[33] and have decreased adherence properties in vitro.[34] Other investigators have observed transient leukopenia associated with development of ARDS which may be due to sequestration in the pulmonary capillary bed.[35] ^{111}Indium-labeled neutrophils have been shown to accumulate in the lungs of ARDS patients.[36] Neutrophil and neutrophil products have been identified in bronchoalveolar lavage (BAL) samples taken from ARDS patients.[37] There is a positive correlation between the increased numbers of lavage neutrophils and abnormalities of gas exchange, lung protein permeability, and neutrophil activation products.[38] A deterioration in gas exchange is associated with resolution of leukopenia in patients who received chemotherapy.[39] These and other bits of data support the complement-mediated neutrophil activation theory.

Yet like all general hypotheses, contradictory findings raise questions regarding the validity of this theory.[40] ARDS has been shown by several different investigators to occur in severely neutropenic hosts.[41-42] In more recent studies, biologic and immunologic assays of complement activation were found to be nonspecifically associated with sepsis and septic shock syndrome and to lack a correlation with progression to ARDS.[29-32] Intrapulmonary neutrophil accumulation and soluble inflammatory mediators have been identified in the BAL fluid of individuals at risk for ARDS, but who do not meet physiologic criteria for the disorder.[43] Whether the presence of neutrophils in the lung is an epiphenomenon, perhaps a marker of lung injury, or a etiologic agent remains controversial. It appears from the available information that although complement activation and neutrophils may contribute to ARDS, they are not essential for the development of the syndrome.

Cytokine Network Phase

Cytokines are "communication proteins" produced by a certain cell type and have an action on the same or different cell type. The production of cytokines by activated lung cells may mediate many of the local and systemic manifestation of ARDS. Activation is a process by which a cell acquires new or additional functional capacities as the result of exposure to external blood or airborne stimuli. Cytokines are small-molecular-weight proteins that act as ligands to specific surface receptors on effector cells.[44] The production of each cytokine is governed by a regulatory mechanism. A particular cytokine may have multiple actions on different effector cells. Each individual cytokine may be counteracted by a cytokine with an opposing action. These principles allow cytokines to interact with one another and may determine the events that lead to the clinical manifestations of ARDS on a tissue level.

Several of the cytokines implicated in the pathogenesis of ARDS, have systemic actions. Serum tumor necrosis factor (TNF) levels have been shown to be increased in experimental gram-negative endotoxemia,[45] and TNF has recently been detected in the bronchopulmonary secretions of five patients with ARDS.[46] Serum TNF levels are increased in patients with septic shock, and patients with detectable levels have a higher incidence and severity of ARDS.[47] When TNF is injected into normal volunteers, it has activated the coagulation cascade.[48] The relationship between circulating TNF and ARDS has not been established, but the implications of this intriguing possibility have been reviewed.[49] A mechanism that relates TNF concentrations to the diffuse endothelial damage thought to occur in ARDS has not been forwarded.

Other cytokines implicated in the pathogenesis of ARDS include the interleukins 1, 2, and 8. Interleukin-1 is a proinflammatory cytokine with a wide range of biologic actions.[50] Interleukin-2 causes diffuse third space and pulmonary permeability edema when infused in cancer patients and causes hemodynamic effects that are indistinguishable from those seen in septic shock.[51] Interleukin-8 (IL-8) is a potent monocyte/macrophage-derived neutrophil chemotactic cytokine. Preliminary studies have implicated an IL-8-like chemoattractant in ARDS.[52]

Potential Role of the Alveolar Macrophage in ARDS

The resident airspace cells consist of capillary endothelial cells, type I and type II pulmonary epithelial cells, fibroblasts, alveolar macrophages (AM), lymphocytes (LYS), polymorphic nuclear leukocytes (PMN), mast cells, and eosinophils (EOS). Among these contenders, the AM has emerged as a potential central figure in the pathogenesis of ARDS by virtue of its ability to release cytokines. The AM, the principal resident phagocyte of the lung, is important in maintaining the homeostatic sterile environment of the lungs. The AM can phagocytize bacteria and foreign particles that reach the airspace. The cell then undergoes a respiratory burst that results in the death of ingested bacteria. Along with this process, the AM can release proteolytic enzymes and potentiate the production of reactant oxygen species. When activated, macrophages release a broad array of cytokines that can potentially interact with other lung cell types. These cytokines include IL-1 and TNF, which may participate in the systemic manifestations of ARDS. Endotoxin-stimulated alveolar macrophages also release IL-8, which is a potent chemoattractant for peripheral blood neutrophils.[53] Recruitment of the neutrophil is a fundamental component of the acute inflammatory response. The secondary role of the neutrophil may be to further contribute to lung injury by releasing proteolytic enzymes and potentiating the production of reactant oxygen species. Alveolar macrophages also release a variety of cytokines, such as transforming growth factor beta (TGF-beta); fibroblast growth factor (FGF), and platelet growth factor (PDGF), which affect the proliferation rates and synthetic capacity of matrix cells. These events, and their possible interactions with a variety of other cell types, are shown schematically in Figure 17–1.

Other cells can also release cytokines which may contribute to ARDS. For example, IL-8 can be released by peripheral blood monocytes, endothelial cells, fibroblasts, epithelial cells, and hepatoma cells.[54] Understanding the regulation of multiple cytokines by a variety of lung cell types may provide insight into the events which culminate into ARDS.

Bronchoalveolar Lavage Markers of ARDS

BAL is a powerful and safe tool which can be used to sample the secretion and nonadherent cells of the alveolar space. BAL has been used to investigate the specific details of the cellular and biochemical aspects of ARDS. BAL has the potential of providing information regarding the injury, inflammation, and repair which characterize ARDS.

Angiotensin-converting enzyme is elevated in the serum and BAL fluid of septic ARDS patients.[55,56] This finding may indicate diffuse endothelial injury, since this enzyme is primarily a component of the endothelial cell surface.

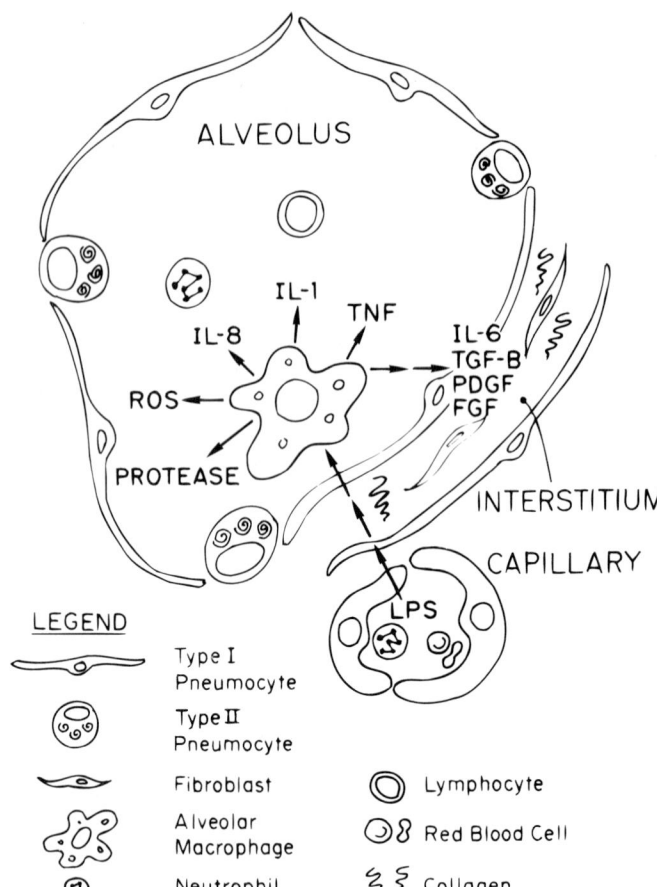

Fig. 17–1. A hypothetic model of ARDS that proposes a central role of the alveolar macrophage as a producer of cytokines, reactive specifics of oxygen, and proteolytic enzymes. The pathways are discussed in the text. LPS, endotoxin; IL-1, interleukin-1; IL-8, interleukin-8; TNF, tumor necrosis factor; ROS, reactive species of oxygen; protease, proteolytic enzymes; IL-6, interleukin-6; TGF-beta; transforming growth factor-beta; PDGE, platelet derived growth factor; and FGF, fibroblast growth factor. The cell types are depicted as icons in the legend at the bottom of the figure. The intravascular, alveolar, and interstitial spaces are labeled as capillary, alveolus, and interstitium.

Alteration in the phospholipid composition of surfactant obtained by BAL in ARDS patients has been thought to indicate altered type II pneumocyte functional capacity.[4] Fibrin depositions in ARDS have been attributed to increases in procoagulant activity which have been measured in the BAL fluid of ARDS patients.[57]

The neutrophil is the predominant cell type recovered by BAL in ARDS. Products of both activated neutrophils and eosinophils have been measured in BAL fluid from ARDS patients.[58] The balance between neutrophil protease and pulmonary antiprotease activates has been measured by BAL[59] although controversy exists regarding the dominant activity. Several investigators have taken different approaches in an attempt to explain the presence of neutrophils in BAL. Parsons and colleagues have characterized a chemotactic agent in the cell-free portion of BAL in 14 of 16 ARDS patients which was not present in 5 control subjects.[52] Although this factor was not completely characterized, it may be identical to the chemotactic cytokine, IL-8. Products of complement activation have been identified in the lower respiratory tract of ARDS patients suggesting that C5a may also contribute to the influx of neutrophils in this disorder.[60] Chemotactic factor inactivator (CFI), an agent in BAL fluid which inactivates C5a, has been shown to be functionally deficient in ARDS patients.[61] Leukotrienes, which may also contribute to the inflammatory phase of ARDS, have been shown to be increased in BAL fluid from ARDS patients, and those at risk for ARDS.[62] Another protein cytokine referred to as enzyme releasing peptide (ERP) has been partially purified and shown to be increased in the BAL fluid of ARDS patients.[63]

Alveolar macrophages from ARDS patients release greater amounts of IL-1 which may play a role in the resolution of acute lung injury.[64] Collagenase activity, which may reflect remodeling of the interstitium of the lung, has been shown to be elevated in 12 of 17 ARDS patients and none of 10 control subjects.[65] Polypeptide growth factors that regulate the proliferation of lung cells have been shown to be produced by alveolar macrophages and circulating monocytes.[66] These polypeptides, which include transforming growth factor-beta (TGF-beta), platelet derived growth factor (PDGF), and fibroblast growth factor (FGF), are capable of stimulating the proliferation and phenotypic expression of lung fibroblast.[67-69] There is an expanding interest in these and other growth factors in the pulmonary fibrosis which may result in the survivors of ARDS. BAL is a technique that will allow recovery of AM where molecular and immunologic probes can be used to identify and implicate these molecules in the pathogenesis of ARDS.

Clinical Finding and Criterion for Admission to a Special Unit

ARDS presents with the insidious onset of dyspnea, tachycardia, and cyanosis which may ultimately progress to hypoxemia respiratory failures. The physical signs of ARDS are nonspecific and consist of altered vital signs, change in consciousness, and early inspiratory bibasilar rates. The central nervous system manifestations of ARDS are associated with hypoxemia and other metabolic derangements attributable to the underlying disorder (see Table 17-2).

ARDS is a devastating illness which usually requires transfer to a special care unit when it is initially recognized. Transfer criteria are nonspecific. Altered mental status, increasing requirement for supplemental oxygen, oliguria, fever and hypotension lead the clinician to transfer a patient to the ICU. Otherwise, obvious clinical circumstances identify the patient at a high risk for developing ARDS and themselves are indications for ICU transfer. The principles of management of ARDS include titrated bedside care, attention to details, and continuous close observation. ARDS is a syndrome which crosses medical and surgical specialties. The techniques of supportive management require both invasive and noninvasive continuous monitoring, and expedient diagnostic and therapeutic interventions (Table 17-4).

Table 17-4. Principles of Supportive Management of ARDS

Airway management
Mechanical ventilation with PEEP
Vital sign monitoring
Salt/water management
Nutritional support
Minimization of invasive monitoring devices
Identification and prompt treatment of infections

Supportive Treatments for ARDS

It is beyond the scope of this chapter to discuss all of the details of the supportive managements of ARDS patients but four areas deserve special attention: mechanical ventilation with PEEP, fluid managements, nutritional intervention, and infection surveillance (Table 17-5).

Mechanical Ventilation with PEEP

A cardinal feature of ARDS is hypoxemia that is refractory to oxygen administration. In ARDS, hypoxemia is usually associated with an increased elastic work of breathing, increased metabolic demands, and an inefficient pattern of carbon dioxide elimination (ventilation). Without intervention, ARDS results in death from asphyxiation. Intervention consists of airway management, ventilatory support, and PEEP. Of these three measures, PEEP was developed specifically for the supportive management of ARDS and is effective in prolonging life and improving survival.[70,71] An early response to PEEP appears to be a good prognostic indicator.[14] PEEP maintains arterial oxygen saturation while minimizing the exposure of lungs to an oxidant stress. PEEP therapy is directed at increasing the functional residual capacity (FRC) of acutely injured lungs which results in improved arterial oxygenation. Although it has been suggested that PEEP may decrease interstitial lung water, the preponderance of clinical evidence suggests that PEEP results in either a significant increase or no change in extravascular lung water.[72] PEEP is thought to improve gas exchange by increasing FRC by both increasing alveolar size and recruiting collapsed alveoli.[72] This process increases the surface area for gas exchange and decreases the physiologic left to right shunting of desaturated mixed venous blood. The result is improved arterial blood oxygenation which allows the clinician to decrease the concentration of inspired oxygen and presumably reduce the probability of oxygen toxicity. In general, the goal of PEEP treatment is to reduce the fraction of inspired oxygen to less than 0.6, while maintaining an arterial blood oxygen saturation of 90%.

Table 17-5. Pharmacologic Studies in ARDS (reference in parentheses)

Ibuprofen (100)	Corticosteroids (92-94)
n-Acetylcyteine (103)	Prostacyclin (106)
Vitamin E (104)	Almitrine (107)
Prostaglandin E$_1$ (95)	Ketoconazole (108)
Exogenous surfactant (105)	

PEEP therapy must be used in the context of a comprehensive approach to improving oxygenation which requires a thorough understanding of the factors which cause worsened oxygenation in mechanically ventilated patients.[73] For example, ARDS causes an elevation in the right-sided cardiovascular pressures which can result in an anatomic right to left shunt through a patient foramen ovale.[74] PEEP would be expected to increase pulmonary vascular resistance and exacerbate this pathophysiologic process. PEEP can have a paradoxic effect of improving gas exchange by reducing oxygen delivery to the periphery. PEEP affects right and left ventricular performance primarily by reducing the return of blood to the left atria.[75] This process leads to a decreased cardiac output and lowers the delivery of oxygen-enriched blood to vital organs. This effect can usually be minimized by judicious use of volume expansion to maintain preload and maximize oxygen delivery to the brain, kidneys, and other vital organs. We support the view that the best PEEP is the minimal amount necessary to reduce the incidence of oxygen toxicity.[76] We consider an F_{IO_2} of 0.6 as an achievable goal in most patients if a Pa_{O_2} value of 60 torr is used as a therapeutic end point. Although the prophylactic use of PEEP has been advocated, a prospective randomized clinical trial did not find evidence of efficacy.[77] The dictum that PEEP "heals" is not supported by objective data, and PEEP should be viewed as a physical method for improving gas exchange while minimizing the use of oxygen enrichment. Guidelines for the rational use of PEEP have recently been reviewed by Petty.[78] Petty recommends the use of PEEP in the range of 5 to 15 cm H_2O when F_{IO_2} greater than 0.4 to 0.5 is required for more than a few hours, but cautions us to titrate the use of PEEP to the degree of measured hypoxemia.[78]

Most ARDS patients can be managed with conventional volume-cycled ventilation. The benefits of high frequency jet ventilation and high frequency oscillation ventilation have not been clearly established in the treatment of ARDS. Inverse ration ventilation appears to improve oxygenation, possibly by inducing an "occult PEEP" effect and progressively recruiting collapsed alveoli.[79,80] Recently, intriguing preliminary data has emerged examining the role of extracorporal carbon dioxide removal (ECCO$_2$R), but none of the available clinical studies has been randomized or has used concurrent control groups. In the early 1970s, a NIH funded multicenter study of extracorporal membrane oxygenation (ECMO) determined that this level of technology was insufficient to reduce the mortality of severe ARDS.[81] The role of ECCO$_2$R in the supportive treatment of ARDS awaits careful peer review.

Fluid Management in ARDS

Many ARDS patients present with unstable hemodynamic parameters. Frequently, they are in shock with an unknown volume status and receive relatively large amounts of intravenous fluids. Intriguing clinical data has emerged that indicates that uncontrolled salt and water weight gain is a poor prognostic indicator and that forced diuresis may improve the outcome from ARDS.[82,83] Simmons and colleagues found that ARDS patients who gained 3 kg or more had a much higher mortality than those who lost weight.[82] Humphrey and associates extended this observation to show in a retrospective analysis that management strategies which cause a 25% reduction in the pulmonary artery obstructing pressure were significantly correlated with survival.[83] One explanation for these observations is that salt and water weight gain is a manifestation of a generalized alteration in microvascular permeability. The initial volume status of a critically ill patient is impossible to predict without objectively determined physiologic parameters. The use of right heart catheterization in ARDS must be judiciously controlled by weighing the relative risks with the potential benefits of measuring right ventricular pressures, pulmonary artery occlusion pressure, cardiac output, and mixed venous oxygen saturation. The risks of right heart catheterization include pneumothorax, perforation of cardiovascular structures, inducing ventricular arrhythmias, and catheter related nosocomial infections. The use of right heart catheterization has not had an appreciable effect on survival from ARDS and a controversial study has shown a negative impact on the survival of myocardial infarction patients.[84]

Nutritional Interventions

Malnutrition in elderly and chronically ill patients is endemic in the United States, particularly in those patients who require hospitalization. This affects some patients who develop ARDS and enter the ICU in a nutritionally depleted state. Virtually all patients with ARDS are catabolic and waste nitrogen according to the degree of muscle proteolysis. TNF, which is also known as a cachectic, may contribute to loss of lean body mass in cachectic patients. The subcutaneous injection of recombinant TNF in humans has been shown to alter plasma amino acid concentrations much like starvation.[85] There is a belief that aggressive nutrition intervention is necessary to maintain muscle mass and respiratory muscle performance. Unfortunately, there have been no carefully performed clinical studies in ARDS patients to prove this hypothesis. We advocate early and aggressive nutrition support in ARDS patients. Nutrition therapy should be closely monitored with nitrogen balance measurements and by serial measurement of visceral protein.[86]

Infection Surveillance

Nosocomial infections are those which are identified in patients following a 72-hour infection-free period of hospitalization. The incidence, location, and microbiology of nosocomial infections in ARDS patients is not entirely clear. Several studies indicate that the lung is the most common cause of serious nosocomial infections in ARDS patients. Montgomery and colleagues reported that pneumonia was evident in 20 of 47 patients who developed sepsis after the onset of ARDS.[5] Seidenfield and associates reported an incidence of nosocomial pneumonia of 53% in 129 patients.[8] A preliminary report by Carlet and colleagues indicates an incidence of nosocomial pneumonia of 34% in 583 patients.[87]

The difficulty in diagnosing nosocomial pneumonia has been highlighted by the study of Andrews and colleagues.[88] They evaluated the clinical diagnosis of pneumonia by autopsy in 30 patients who died of ARDS. Of the 17 patients who had histologic evidence of pneumonia, one third were not thought to be infected per clinical criteria at the time of death. Of 13 patients without histologic pneumonia, one fifth were diagnosed and being treated for pneumonia. In their study, Andrews could not retrospectively distinguish patients without pneumonia from those with pneumonia on the basis of fever, leukocytosis, sputum pathogens, or asymmetric radiographic infiltrates.

The major risk factor for the development of nosocomial pneumonia appears to be violation of the intact airway by endotracheal intubation. Endotracheal intubation and mechanical ventilation are associated with a sevenfold increased incidence of nosocomial pneumonia.[89] Endotracheal intubation disrupts the normal cough reflex and mucociliary escalation of lower respiratory trace secretions. Repeated endotracheal suction and endotracheal intubation may damage and denude the respiratory epithelial surface making it more susceptible to infection.[90] The presence of an endotracheal tube appears to promote introduction of upper airway microbial flora into the lower respiratory tract where the combination of inoculum, pooled secretions, and denuded respiratory epithelial results in nosocomial infections.

The difficulty in identifying pulmonary nosocomial infections in ARDS is legendary. The techniques available, including sputum Gram staining and cultures, are insufficient to either diagnose or exclude pneumonia in the presence of diffuse pulmonary infiltrates. The thoracic CT scan has recently been forwarded as a noninvasive study that may give clinical information regarding the presence of a lung abscess or pleural effusion which are not evident on portable supine anteroposterior chest radiographs. The use of a protected specimen brush and quantitative cultures has been suggested as a cost effective way of diagnosing pulmonary infections in mechanically ventilated patients while avoiding unnecessary treatment with antibiotics.[91]

Other invasive devices, including central venous lines, arterial lines, nasogastric tubes, and foley catheters are all associated with local and systemic infections. ARDS patients are susceptible to endocarditis, septic embolization, sinusitis, erosive esophagitis, prostatitis, and urinary tract infections as a result of using these invasive devices. A management goal in ARDS is to avoid unnecessary invasive devises and to expediently remove those devices when measurements have been consummated.

Treatment with antibiotics should be as specific as possible based on probable site, likely bacterial species, and specific culture information. Broad spectrum antibiotics should be used in those patients with a high probability infection of unknown site and bacterial species. The complications of liberal use of broad-spectrum antibiotics are not trivial and include superinfection with candida species, unnecessary renal and auditory nerve damage, coagulation abnormalities, and antibiotic related diarrhea. We advocate a conservative use of antimicrobials based on the probability of infection, likely site of infection, and confirmation by careful cultures taken prior to antibiotic therapy.

Pharmacologic Treatment of ARDS

The use of high doses of corticosteroids has been forwarded for theoretical reasons as a potential treatment of ARDS. The rationale was that the antiinflammatory effects of steroids might block the acute inflammation which is evident in ARDS and that the risk of drug toxicity was minimal. Several well-designed studies have failed to show a difference between steroid treated and control ARDS patients on the basis of either physiologic manifestations or the outcome of ARDS.[92-94] Thus, no rationale currently exists for the use of corticosteroids in ARDS. A randomized double-blind, multicenter study of prostaglandin E_1 failed to show an enhancement in survival although pharmacologically improved oxygen availability and consumption in ARDS patients was observed.[95]

Recently, the National Institutes of Health (NIH) has funded a multicenter trial of the intravenous nonsteroidal antiinflammatory drug (NSAID), ibuprofen, as a potentially beneficial agent in ARDS. NSAID inhibits cyclo-oxgenase thereby diminishing the synthesis of thromboxane A_2 and prostacyclin.[96] NSAIDs diminish platelet and neutrophil aggregation and leukocyte lysosomal and oxygen radical release.[97-99] Bernard and colleagues have reported preliminary data that rectal ibuprofen resulted in higher blood pressure, lower heart rate, and decreased minute ventilation in 15 patients with sepsis.[100] Despite concerns over the nephrotoxic effect of NSAIDs, no renal dysfunction was noted in this study.

Because endotoxemia is an important cause of ARDS, substantial interest has been applied to developing antibodies to endotoxin for therapeutic purposes. Ziegler and colleagues reported a randomized prospective study of 304 patients with sepsis who were treated with either preimmune serum or a human anticore endotoxin antiserum obtained from healthy men who had been immunized with heat-killed Escherichia coli J5, a mutant that does not synthesize oligosaccharide side chains for its endotoxin.[101] In this study, treatment with J5 antiserum decreased the mortality rate from 38 to 24% in patients with gram-negative infections as a whole and from 76 to 46% in patients with gram-negative septic shock. Preliminary results of a large multicenter trial of monoclonal antibodies to endotoxin in the treatment of sepsis have demonstrated safety but not efficacy.[102] The role of antiendotoxin antibodies is not firmly established at this time and requires additional investigation. Many other agents have been tried in small preliminary studies of ARDS, however (see Table 17-5).

ARDS as a Systemic Illness and Prognostic Indicator

The incidence and outcome of ARDS may be in constant flux. As an example, better supportive measures for immunocompromised patients who developed septic shock may have the undesirable consequence of increasing the incidence of irreversible ARDS in the "survivors" of the septic event. It is conceivable that a shift in patient population has occurred since ARDS was reported two decades ago. A detailed comparison has not been made between contemporary ARDS patients and those of previous decades.

Mortality of patients with ARDS is usually due to extrapulmonary organ system failure. The majority of deaths that occur within 72 hours of onset of ARDS, are because of the underlying disorder, whereas the majority of late deaths are related to infection and multiorgan system failure.[5] Infection is fundamentally related to ARDS as both a predisposing factor and a principal complication. Gram-negative septicemia has emerged as an important hospital acquired complication with a high mortality. Several studies have clearly related gram-negative sepsis to ARDS and have suggested a mortality of this combination approaching 90%.[109,110] The pathogenesis of gram-negative septicemia is mediated by endotoxin in the cell wall of the bacteria. This biologically active agent has the potential to activate alveolar macrophages and other lung cell types and initiate the cellular event that leads to ARDS. Ironically, antibiotics effective against gram-negative organisms may increase the release of endotoxin in the circulation. Blood culture negative infections of unknown premorbid location are particularly poor prognostic indicators.[6] Gram-negative pulmonary infections infrequently invade the blood stream, are difficult to diagnose, and have the worst mortality of all.[8] The overall accuracy of diagnosing pneumonia in the presence of diffuse lung injury is not better than 70%.[88] Gram-negative intra-abdominal infections are more frequently blood culture positive and can often be treated surgically.[111] A theoretically potential endogenous pool of endotoxin exists as the normal bacterial flora of the intact gastrointestinal (GI) tract. Any disease which alters the mucosal integrity of the GI tract could result in the mobilization of this endogenous pool of endotoxin. The combination of circulating endotoxin and complement fragments has been associated in clinical studies to the development of ARDS.[111]

Patients with ARDS who develop multisystem organ failure syndrome (MSOF) have a high mortality.[7] The metabolic abnormalities that exist in ARDS suggest a generalized disorder which is best conceptualized as a diffuse injury to the endothelial cell barrier of many organ systems. The pan-endothelial inflammation and injury affects virtually all organ systems, but the overt manifestations of the disorder are dominated by abnormalities of the circulatory, digestive, hematopoietic, and metabolic systems. Certain investigators have shown a pathologic dependency of oxygen uptake to oxygen delivery in ARDS and sepsis.[112–115] The GI complications of ARDS include GI edema and enteral feeding intolerance.[116] Disseminated intravascular coagulopathy is frequently associated with ARDS and localized abnormalities in coagulation and fibrinolytic pathways have been forwarded as having a role in the pathogenesis of ARDS.[117] Persistent metabolic acidemia and azotemia are poor prognostic variables in ARDS patients.[118]

POST-ICU PHASE–OUTCOME
Pulmonary Sequelae of ARDS

A spectrum of pulmonary impairment may follow an episode of ARDS. This impairment may range from mild asymptomatic abnormalities that require sophisticated laboratory measurements to overt symptomatic disease. ARDS has the capacity to progress to extensive fibrosis in 2 to 4 weeks.[119] There appears to be a difference between the degree of fibrosis which occurs in nonsurvivors versus survivors of ARDS. In an autopsy study, Zapol and colleagues found a two to threefold increase in collagen content of 12 ARDS patients as compared to the control population.[120] Collins and associates confirmed these postmortem observations and suggested that the increased amount of collagen in ARDS patients was related to the use of high levels of PEEP and prolonged exposure to high concentrations of inspired oxygen.[121] Yet, in survivors of ARDS, only mild abnormalities consisting of reductions of pulmonary volumes, decreased carbon monoxide diffusion capacity (D_{LCO}), and a mild increase in the resting alveolar-arterial oxygen pressure gradient occur during the early post-ICU recovery period.[122] Using the American Thoracic Society recommendations for evaluating impairment, Ghio and colleagues reported that 65% of survivors of ARDS had physiologic evidence of impairment more than a year after ARDS, and 30% of these had moderate or severe pulmonary impairment.[123] In other studies of survivors of ARDS, these abnormalities appear to be related to the therapeutic use of oxygen support with an $F_{IO_2} > 0.6$ for more than 24 hours appearing to be a sensitive and specific predictor of an abnormal D_{LCO} a year following ARDS.[124] Surprisingly, increasing levels of PEEP applied from days four through seven of ARDS appear to be associated with better long-term values for total lung capacity.[125] Long-term abnormalities of lung volumes are related to higher pulmonary artery resistance, higher pulmonary artery pressures, higher alveolar-arterial oxygen pressure gradients and a worse radiographic appearance beyond the fourth day of ARDS.[125]

REFERENCES

1. Murray, J. F., Matthay, M. A., Luce, J. M., and Flick, M. R.: An expanded definition of the adult respiratory distress syndrome. Am. Rev. Respir. Dis., *138*:720, 1988.
2. Petty, T. L.: Adult respiratory distress syndrome: refinement of concept and redefinition. Am. Rev. Respir. Dis., *138*:724, 1988.
3. Bachofen, M., and Weibel, E. R.: Alternation of the gas exchange apparatus in adult respiratory insufficiency associated with septicemia. Am. Rev. Respir. Dis., *116*:589, 1977.
4. Hallman, M., et al.: Evidence of lung surfactant abnormality in respiratory failure: study of bronchoalveolar lavage phospholipid, surface activity, phospholipase activity, and plasma myoinositol. J. Clin. Invest., *70*:673, 1982.
5. Montgomery, A. B., Stager, M. A., Carrico, C. J., and Hudson, L. D.: Causes of mortality in patients with the adult respiratory distress syndrome. Am. Rev. Respir. Dis., *132*:485, 1985.
6. Bell, R. C., Coalson, J. J., Smith, J. D., and Johanson, W. G.: Multiple organ system failure and infection in adult respiratory distress syndrome. Ann. Intern. Med., *99*:293, 1983.
7. Dorinsky, P. M., and Gadek, J. E.: Mechanism of multiple nonpulmonary organ failure in adult respiratory distress syndrome. Chest, *96*:885, 1989.
8. Seidenfeld, J. J., et al.: Incidence, site, and outcome of infections in patients with the adult respiratory distress syndrome. Am. Rev. Respir. Dis., *134*:12, 1986.
9. Wright, P. E., and Bernard, G. R.: The role of airflow resistance in patients with the adult respiratory distress syndrome. Am. Rev. Respir. Dis., *139*:1169, 1989.
10. Zapol, W. M., and Snider, M. T.: Pulmonary hypertension

in severe acute respiratory failure. N. Engl. J. Med., *296:* 476, 1977.
11. Rocker, G. M., Wiseman, M. S., Pearson, D., and Shale, D. J.: Diagnostic criteria for adult respiratory distress syndrome: time for reappraisal. Lancet, *8630:*120, 1989.
12. Rinaldo, J. E.: The prognosis of the adult respiratory distress syndrome: inappropriate pessimism? Chest, *90:*470, 1986.
13. Ashbaugh, D. G., and Maier, R. V.: Idiopathic pulmonary fibrosis in adult respiratory distress syndrome. Arch. Surg., *120:*530, 1985.
14. Bone, R. C., et al.: An early test of survival in patients with the adult respiratory distress syndrome: the Pao_2/Fio_2 ratio and its differential response to conventional treatment. Chest, *96:*849, 1989.
15. Keren, A., Klein, J., and Stern, S.: Adult respiratory distress syndrome in the course of acute myocardial infarction. Chest, *77:*161, 1980.
16. Villar, J., and Slutsky, A. S.: The incidence of the adult respiratory distress syndrome. Am. Rev. Respir. Dis., *140:*814, 1989.
17. Fowler, A. A., et al.: Adult respiratory distress syndrome: risk with common predispositions. Ann. Intern. Med., *98:* 593, 1983.
18. Webster, N. R., Cohen, A. T., and Nunn, J. F.: Adult respiratory distress syndrome—How many cases in the UK? Anaesthesia, *43:*923, 1988.
19. Baumann, W. R., et al.: Incidence and mortality of adult respiratory distress syndrome: a prospective analysis from a large metropolitan hospital. Crit. Care Med., *14:*1, 1986.
20. Pepe, P. E., et al.: Clinical predictors of the adult respiratory distress syndrome. Am. J. Surg., *144:*124, 1982.
21. Matuschak, G. M., and Rinaldo, J. E.: Organ interactions in the adult respiratory distress syndrome during sepsis: role of the liver in host defense. Chest, *94:*400, 1988.
22. Matuschak, G. M., et al.: Effect of end-stage liver failure on the incidence and resolution of the adult respiratory distress syndrome. J. Crit. Care, *2:*162, 1987.
23. Matuschak, G. M., and Shaw, B. W.: Adult respiratory distress syndrome associated with acute liver allograft rejection: resolution following hepatic retransplantation. Crit. Care Med., *15:*878, 1987.
24. Schwartz, D. B., Bone, R. C., Balk, R. A., and Szidon, J. P.: Hepatic dysfunction in the adult respiratory distress syndrome. Chest, *95:*871, 1990.
25. Harris, T. R., et al.: Lung microvascular transport properties measured by multiple indicator dilution methods in patients with adult respiratory distress syndrome: a comparison between patients reversing respiratory failure and those failing to reverse. Am. Rev. Respir. Dis., *14:*272, 1990.
26. Rinaldo, J. E., et al.: Assessment of lung injury in the adult respiratory distress syndrome using multiple indicator dilution curves. Am. Rev. Respir. Dis., *133:*1006, 1986.
27. Brigham, K. L., et al.: Correlation of oxygenation with vascular permeability surface area but not with lung water in humans with acute respiratory failure and pulmonary edema. J. Clin. Invest., *72:*339, 1983.
28. Hammerschmidt, D. E., et al.: Association of complement activation and elevated plasma C5a with adult respiratory distress syndrome. Lancet, *1:*947, 1980.
29. Duchateau, J., Haas, M., and Schregen, H.: Complement activation in patients at risk for developing the adult respiratory distress syndrome. Am. Rev. Respir. Dis., *130:*1058, 1984.
30. Parsons, P. E., and Giclas, P. C.: The terminal complement complex (sC5b-9) is not specifically associated with the development of the adult respiratory distress syndrome. Am. Rev. Respir. Dis., *141:*98, 1990.

31. Sprung, C. L., et al.: Complement activation in septic shock patients. Crit. Care Med., *14:*525, 1986.
32. Weinberg, P. F., et al.: Biologically active products of complement and acute lung injury in patients with the sepsis syndrome. Am. Rev. Respir. Dis., *130:*791, 1984.
33. Zimmerman, G. A., Renzetti, A. D., and Hill, H. R.: Functional and metabolic activity of granulocytes from patients with adult respiratory distress syndrome: evidence for activated neutrophils in the pulmonary circulation. Am. Rev. Respir. Dis., *127:*290, 1983.
34. Zimmerman, G. A., Renzetti, A. D., and Hill, H. R.: Granulocyte adherence in pulmonary and systemic arterial blood samples from patients with adult respiratory distress syndrome. Am. Rev. Respir. Dis., *129:*798, 1984.
35. Thommasen, H. V., Russell, J. A., Boyko, W. J., and Hogg, J. C.: Transient leucopenia associated with adult respiratory distress syndrome. Lancet, *14:*809, 1984.
36. Warshawski, F. J., Sibbald, W. J., Driedger, A. A., and Cheung, H.: Abnormal neutrophil-pulmonary interaction in the adult respiratory distress syndrome: qualitative and quantitative assessment of pulmonary neutrophil kinetics in humans with in vivo ^{111}Indiumneutrophil scintigraphy. Am. Rev. Respir. Dis., *133:*797, 1988.
37. Lee, C. T., et al.: Elastolytic activity in pulmonary lavage fluid from patients with adult respiratory distress syndrome. N. Engl. J. Med., *304:*192, 1981.
38. Weiland, J. E., et al.: Lung neutrophils in the adult respiratory distress syndrome: clinical and pathophysiologic significance. Am. Rev. Respir. Dis., *133:*218, 1986.
39. Rinaldo, J. E., and Borovetz, H. S.: Deterioration of oxygenation and abnormal lung microvascular permeability during resolution of leukopenia in patients with diffuse lung injury. Am. Rev. Respir. Dis., *131:*579, 1985.
40. Rinaldo, J. E.: Mediation of adult respiratory distress syndrome by leukocytes: clinical evidence and implication for therapy. Chest, *89:*590, 1986.
41. Ognibene, F. P., et al.: Adult respiratory distress syndrome in patients with severe neutropenia. N. Engl. J. Med., *315:* 547, 1986.
42. Maunder, R. J., et al.: Occurrence of the adult respiratory distress syndrome in neutropenic patients. Am. Rev. Respir. Dis., *133:*313, 1986.
43. Fowler, A. A., et al.: The adult respiratory distress syndrome. Cell populations and soluble mediators in the air spaces of patients at high risk. Am. Rev. Respir. Dis., *136:*1225, 1987.
44. Kelley, J.: Cytokines of the lung. Am. Rev. Respir. Dis., *141:* 765, 1990.
45. Michie, H. R., et al.: Detection of circulating tumor necrosis factor after endotoxin administration. N. Engl. J. Med., *318:* 1481, 1988.
46. Millar, A. B., et al.: Tumor necrosis factor in bronchopulmonary secretions of patients with adult respiratory distress syndrome. Lancet, *2:*712, 1989.
47. Marks, J. D., et al.: Plasma tumor necrosis factor in patients with septic shock: mortality rate, incidence of adult respiratory distress syndrome and effects of methylprednisolone administration. Am. Rev. Respir. Dis., *141:*94, 1990.
48. van der Poll, T., et al.: Activation of coagulation after administration of tumor necrosis factor to normal subjects. N. Engl. J. Med., *322:*1622, 1990.
49. Tracey, K. J., Lowry, S. F., and Cerami, A.: Cachetin/TNF-alpha in septic shock and septic adult respiratory distress syndrome. Am. Rev. Respir. Dis., *138:*1377, 1988.
50. Dinarello, C. A.: Interleukin-1. Rev. Infect. Dis., *6:*51, 1984.
51. Rosenberg, S. A., et al.: A progress report on the treatment of 157 patients with advanced cancer using lymphokine

51. activated killer cells and interleukin-2 or high dose interleukin-2 alone. N. Engl. J. Med., *316*:889, 1987.
52. Parsons, P. E., Fowler, A. A., Hyers, T. M., and Henson, P. M.: Chemotactic activity in bronchoalveolar lavage fluid from patients with adult respiratory distress syndrome. Am. Rev. Respir. Dis., *132*:490, 1985.
53. Sylvester, I., et al.: Secretion of neutrophil attractant/activation protein by lipopolysaccharide-stimulated lung macrophages determined by both enzyme-linked immunosorbent assay and N-terminal sequence analysis. Am. Rev. Respir. Dis., *141*:683, 1990.
54. Baggiolini, M., Walz, A., and Kunkel, S. L.: PMN activating peptide-1/interleukin-8, a novel cytokine that activates PMN. J. Clin. Invest., *84*:1045, 1989.
55. Fourrier, F., et al. Angiotensin-converting enzyme in human adult respiratory distress syndrome. Chest, *83*:593, 1983.
56. Idell, S., et al.: Angiotensin converting enzyme in bronchoalveolar lavage in adult respiratory distress syndrome. Chest, *91*:52, 1987.
57. Idell, S., et al.: Procoagulant activity in bronchoalveolar lavage in adult respiratory distress syndrome. Contribution of tissue factor associated with factor VII. Am. Rev. Respir. Dis., *136*:1466, 1987.
58. Halligren, R., Samuelsson, T., Venge, P., and Modig, J.: Eosinophil activation in the lung is related to lung damage in adult respiratory distress syndrome. Am. Rev. Respir. Dis., *135*:639, 1987.
59. Wewers, M. D., Herzyk, D. J., and Gadek, J. E.: Alveolar fluid neutrophil elastase activity in the adult respiratory distress syndrome is complexed to alpha-2-macroglobulin. J. Clin. Invest., *821*:260, 1988.
60. Robbins, R. A., Russ, W. D., Rasmussen, J. K., and Clayton, M. M.: Activation of the complement system in the adult respiratory distress syndrome. Am. Rev. Respir. Dis., *135*:651, 1987.
61. Robbins, R., et al.: Functional loss of chemotactic factor inactivator in the adult respiratory distress syndrome. Am. Rev. Respir. Dis., *141*:1463, 1990.
62. Stephenson, A. H., et al.: Increased concentration of leukotrienes in bronchoalveolar lavage fluid of patients with adult respiratory distress syndrome or at risk for adult respiratory distress syndrome. Am. Rev. Respir. Dis., *138*:174, 1988.
63. Cohen, A. B., et al.: A peptide from alveolar macrophages that releases neutrophil enzymes into the lungs in patients with the adult respiratory distress syndrome. Am. Rev. Respir. Dis., *137*:1151, 1988.
64. Jacobs, R. F., Tabor, D. R., Burks, A. W., and Campell, G. D.: Elevated interleukin-1 release by human alveolar macrophages during the adult respiratory distress syndrome. Am. Rev. Respir. Dis., *140*:1686, 1989.
65. Christner, P., et al.: Collagenase in the lower respiratory tract of patients with adult respiratory distress syndrome. Am. Rev. Respir. Dis., *131*:690, 1985.
66. King, R. J., Jones, M. B., and Minoo, P.: Regulation of lung cell proliferation by polypeptide growth factors. Lung Cell Mol. Physiol., *1*:L23, 1989.
67. Assoian, R. K., et al.: Expression and secretion of type beta transforming growth factor by activated human macrophages. Proc. Natl. Acad. Sci. USA, *84*:6020, 1987.
68. Shimokado, K. E., et al.: A significant part of macrophage-derived growth factor consists of at least two forms of PDGF. Cell, *43*:277, 1985.
69. Gospodarowicz, D. G., Neufeld, G., and Schweigerer, L.: Fibroblast growth factor as a survival agent. Proc. Natl. Acad. Sci. USA, *73*:4120, 1976.
70. Ashbaugh, D. G., Petty, T. L., Bigelow, D. B., and Harris, T. M.: Continuous positive-pressure breathing (CPPB) in adult respiratory distress syndrome. J. Thoarc. Cardiovas. Surg., *57*:31, 1969.
71. Springer, R. R., and Steven, P. M.: The influence of PEEP on survival of patients in respiratory failure. Am. J. Med., *66*:196, 1979.
72. Shapiro, B. A., Cane, R. D., and Harrison, R. A.: Positive end-expiratory pressure therapy in adults with special reference to acute lung injury: a review of the literature and suggested clinical correlations. Crit. Care Med., *12*:127, 1984.
73. Glauser, F. L., Polatty, R. C., and Sessler, C. N.: Worsening oxygenation in the mechanically ventilated patient: cause, mechanisms, and early detection. Am. Rev. Respir. Dis., *138*:458, 1988.
74. Dewan, N. A., et al.: Persistent hypoxemia due to patent foramen ovale in a patient with adult respiratory distress syndrome. Chest, *89*:611, 1986.
75. Potkin, R. T., Hudson, L. D., Weaver, L. J., and Trobaugh, G.: Effect of positive end-expiratory pressure on right and left ventricular function in patients with the ARDS. Am. Rev. Respir. Dis., *135*:307, 1987.
76. Carroll, G. C., et al.: Minimal positive end-expiratory pressure (PEEP) may be "best PEEP." Chest, *93*:1020, 1988.
77. Pepe, P. E., Hudson, L. A., and Carrico, C. J.: Early application of positive pressure in patients at risk for the adult respiratory distress syndrome. N. Engl. J. Med., *311*:281, 1984.
78. Petty, T. L.: The uses, abuses, and mystique of positive end-expiratory pressure. Am. Rev. Respir. Dis., *138*:475, 1988.
79. Gurevitch, M. J., Van Dyke, J., Young, E. S., and Jackson, K.: Improved oxygenation and lower peak airway pressure in severe adult respiratory distress syndrome: treatment with inverse ration ventilation. Chest, *89*:211, 1986.
80. Tharratt, R. S., Allen, R. P., and Albertson, T. E.: Pressure controlled inverse ratio ventilation in severe adult respiratory distress syndrome. Chest, *94*:755, 1988.
81. Zapol, W. M., et al.: Extracorporal membrane oxygenation in severe acute respiratory failure: a randomized prospective study. J. Am. Med. Assoc., *242*:2193, 1979.
82. Simmons, R. S., et al.: Fluid balance and the adult respiratory distress syndrome. Am. Rev. Respir. Dis., *135*:924, 1987.
83. Humphrey, H., et al.: Improved survival in ARDS patients associated with a resolution in pulmonary capillary wedge pressure. Chest, *97*:1176, 1990.
84. Gore, J. M., et al.: A community-wide assessment of the use of pulmonary artery catheters in patients with acute myocardial infarction. Chest, *92*:721, 1987.
85. Warren, R. S., et al.: The acute metabolic effect of tumor necrosis factor administration in humans. Arch. Surg., *122*:1396, 1987.
86. Pingleton, S. K., and Harmon, G. S.: Nutritional management in acute respiratory failure. J. Am. Med. Assoc., *257*:3094, 1987.
87. Carlet, J., et al.: Infection and ARDS: a complex interaction: a prospective study of 583 patients [abstract]. Am. Rev. Respir. Dis., *139*:A270, 1989.
88. Andrews, C. P., Coalson, J. J., Smith, J. D., and Johanson, W. G.: Diagnosis of nosocomial bacterial pneumonia in acute, diffuse lung injury. Chest, *80*:254, 1981.
89. Celis, R., et al. Nosocomial pneumonia: a multi-variate analysis of risk and prognosis. Chest, *93*:318, 1988.
90. Ramphal, R., et al.: Adherence of *Pseudomonas aeroginosa* to tracheai cells injured by influenza infection or endotracheal intubation. Infect. Immun., *27*:614, 1980.
91. Fagon, J. Y., et al.: Detection of nosocomial lung infections in ventilated patients: use of a protected specimen brush

and quantitative culture techniques in 147 patients. Am. Rev. Respir. Dis., *138:*110, 1988.
92. Bernard, G. R., et al.: High-dose corticosteroids in patients with the adult respiratory distress syndrome. N. Engl. J. Med., *317:*1565, 1987.
93. Luce, J. M., et al.: Ineffectiveness of high-dose methyl prednisolone in preventing parenchymal lung injury and improving mortality in patients with septic shock. Am. Rev. Respir. Dis., *138:*62, 1988.
94. Bone, R. C., et al.: Early methylprednisolone treatment for septic syndrome and the adult respiratory distress syndrome. Chest, *92:*1033, 1987.
95. Bone, R. C., et al.: Randomized double-blind, multicenter study of prostaglandin E₁ in patients with the adult respiratory distress syndrome. Prostaglandin E1 study group. Chest, *96:*114, 1989.
96. Petrak, R. A., Balz, R. A., and Bone, R. C.: Prostaglandins, cyclooxygenase, inhibitors and thromboxane synthetase inhibitors in the pathogenesis of multiple systems organ failures. Crit. Care Clin., *5:*303, 1989.
97. Ogletree, M. L.: Overview of physiological and pathological effects of thromboxane A₂. Fed. Proc., *46:*133, 1987.
98. Simchowitz, L., Mehta, J., and Spilberg, I.: Chemotactic factor-induced generation of superoxide radicals by human neutrophils. Arthritis Rheum., *22:*755, 1979.
99. Spanguolo, P. S., et al.: Thromboxane A₂ mediates augmented polymorphonuclear leukocyte adhesiveness. J. Clin. Invest., *66:*406, 1980.
100. Bernard, G. R., et al.: Effects of a short course of ibuprofen in patients with severe sepsis [abstract]. Am. Rev. Respir. Dis., *137:*A138, 1988.
101. Ziegler, E. J., et al.: Treatment of gram-negative bacteremia and shock with human antiserum to a mutant *Escherichia coli*. N. Engl. J. Med., *307:*1225, 1982.
102. Bernard, G. R., et al.: Multicenter trial of a monoclonal anti-endotoxin antibody in gram negative sepsis [abstract]. Chest, *96:*137S, 1989.
103. Bernard, G. R., et al.: Glutathione repletion by n-acetylcysteine in patients with the ARDS. Am. Rev. Respir. Dis., *139:* 4, 1989.
104. Seeger, W., Ziegler, A., and Wolf, H. R.: Serum alpha-tocopherol levels after high-dose enteral vitamin E administration in patients with acute respiratory failure. Intensive Care Med., *13:*395, 1987.
105. Merritt, T. A., et al.: Exogenous surfactant treatment for neonatal respiratory distress syndrome and their potential role in the adult respiratory distress syndrome. Drugs, *38:* 591, 1989.
106. Rademacher, P., et al.: Prostacyclin for the treatment for pulmonary hypertension in the adult respirator distress syndrome: effects on pulmonary capillary pressure and ventilation-perfusion distributions. Anesthesiology, *72:*238, 1990.
107. Reyes, A., et al.: Effect of almitrine on ventilation-perfusion distribution in adult respiratory distress syndrome. Am. Rev. Respir. Dis., *137:*1062, 1988.
108. Slotman, G. J., Burchard, K. W., D'Arezzo, A., and Gann, D. S.: Ketokonazole prevents acute respiratory failure in critically ill surgical patients. J. Trauma, *28:*648, 1988.
109. Fein, A., et al.: The risk factors, incidence, and prognosis of adult respiratory distress syndrome following septicemia. Chest, *83:*40, 1983.
110. Kaplin, R. L., Sahn, S. A., and Petty, T. L.: Incidence and outcome of the respiratory distress syndrome in gram-negative sepsis. Arch. Intern. Med., *139:*867, 1979.
111. Parsons, P. E., et al.: The association of circulating endotoxin with the development of the adult respiratory distress syndrome. Am. Rev. Respir. Dis., *140:*294, 1989.
112. Dantzker, D. R., et al.: Ventilation-perfusion distribution in the adult respiratory distress syndrome. Am. Rev. Respir. Dis., *120:*1039, 1979.
113. Annat, G., et al.: Oxygen delivery and uptake in the adult respiratory distress syndrome: lack of relationship when measured independently in patients with normal blood lactate concentration. Am. Rev. Respir. Dis., *133:*999, 1986.
114. Dorinsky, P. M., Costello, J. L., and Gadek, J. E.: Relationship of oxygen uptake and oxygen delivery in respiratory failure is not due to the adult respiratory distress syndrome. Chest, *93:*1013, 1988.
115. Russell, J. A., et al.: Oxygen delivery and consumption and ventricular preload are greater in survivors than in nonsurvivors of the adult respiratory distress syndrome. Am. Rev. Respir. Dis. *141:*659, 1990.
116. Brison, R. R., and Pitts, W. M.: Gastrointestinal complications of acute respiratory failure: analogy between adult respiratory distress syndrome, gastrointestinal edema, and enteral feeding intolerance. Crit. Care Med., *17:*841, 1989.
117. Idell, S., et al.: Local abnormalities in coagulation and fibrinolytic pathways predispose to alveolar fibrin deposition in the ARDS. J. Clin. Invest., *84:*695, 1989.
118. Fowler, A. A., et al.: Adult respiratory distress syndrome: prognosis after onset. Am. Rev. Respir. Dis., *132:*472, 1985.
119. Pratt, P. C., et al.: Pulmonary morphology in a multihospital collaborative extracorporal membrane oxygenation project. Am. J. Pathol., *95:*191, 1979.
120. Zapol, W. M., et al.: Pulmonary fibrosis in severe acute respiratory failure. Am. Rev. Respir. Dis., *119:*547, 1979.
121. Collins, J. F., Smith, J. D., Coalson, J. J., and Johanson, W. G.: Variability in lung collagen amounts after prolonged support of acute respiratory failure. Chest, *85:*641, 1984.
122. Yahav, J., Lieberman, P., and Molho, M.: Respiratory function following the adult respiratory distress syndrome. Chest, *74:*247, 1978.
123. Ghio, A. J., et al.: Impairment after adult respiratory distress syndrome. Am. Rev. Respir. Dis., *139:*1158, 1989.
124. Elliott, C. G., et al.: Prediction of pulmonary function abnormalities after adult respiratory distress syndrome. Am. Rev. Respir. Dis., *135:*634, 1987.
125. Peters, J. I., et al.: Clinical determinants of abnormalities in pulmonary function in survivors of the adult respiratory distress syndrome. Am. Rev. Respir. Dis., *139:*1163, 1989.

SUPPLEMENTAL READINGS

Anderson, H. L. III, et al.: Early experience with adult extracorporeal membrane oxygenation in the modern era. Ann. Thorac. Surg., *53:*553, 1992.

Bone, R. C., et al.: Adult respiratory distress syndrome: sequence and importance of development of multiple organ failure. The Prostaglandin E1 Study Group. Chest, *101:*320, 1992.

Chollet-Martin, S., et al.: Subpopulation of hyperresponsive polymorphonuclear neutrophils in patients with adult respiratory distress syndrome. Role of cytokine production. Am. Rev. Respir. Dis., *146:*990, 1992.

High, K. M., et al.: Clinical trials of an intravenous oxygenator in patients with adult respiratory distress syndrome. Anesthesiology, *77:*856, 1992.

Jepsen, S., et al.: Antioxidant treatment with N-acetylcysteine during adult respiratory distress syndrome: a prospective, randomized, placebo-controlled study. Crit. Care Med., *20:* 918, 1992.

Kiiski, R., Takala, J., Kari, A., and Milic-Emili, J.: Effect of tidal volume on gas exchange and oxygen transport in the adult respiratory distress syndrome. Am. Rev. Respir. Dis., *146:* 1131, 1992.

Leff, J. A., et al.: Increased serum catalase activity in septic patients with the adult respiratory distress syndrome. Am. Rev. Respir. Dis., *146:*985, 1992.

Lykens, M. G., Davis, W. B., and Pacht, E. R.: Antioxidant activity of bronchoalveolar lavage fluid in the adult respiratory distress syndrome. Am. J. Physiol., *262:*L169, 1992.

Mitchell, J. P., Schuller, D., Calandrino, F. S., and Schuster, D. P.: Improved outcome based on fluid management in critically ill patients requiring pulmonary artery catheterization. Am. Rev. Respir. Dis., *145:*990, 1992.

Rossaint, R., et al.: Inhaled nitric oxide for the adult respiratory distress syndrome. N. Engl. J. Med., *328:*399, 1993.

Suter, P. M., et al.: High bronchoalveolar levels of tumor necrosis factor and its inhibitors, interleukin-1, interferon, and elastase, in patients with adult respiratory distress syndrome after trauma, shock, or sepsis. Am. Rev. Respir. Dis., *145:*1016, 1992.

Winer-Muram, H. T., Rubin, S. A., Miniati, M., and Ellis, J. V.: Guidelines for reading and interpreting chest radiographs in patients receiving mechanical ventilation. Chest, *102(5 Suppl 1):*565S, 1992.

Chapter 18

ACUTE INHALATION INJURY

EDWARD F. HAPONIK

Respiratory injury caused by inhalation of irritant gases is a major problem of progress,[1-23] Industrialization of our society assures a continuous risk of exposures to varying concentrations of numerous, potentially injurious agents. The possibility of acute massive inhalational exposures following industrial accidents or relating to transport of toxic materials threatens virtually every community. Tragically, numerous mass disasters have underscored the impact of this hazard. Catastrophes such as the 1929 Valley Disaster, 1984 Bhopal casualty, and 1986 Cameroon disaster and conflagrations such as the Cocoanut Grove, Hartford Circus, Dellwood, and Las Vegas Hotel fires stir the imagination because of their horror and unpredictability.[1-11] Lethal exposures also occur on a daily basis on a much smaller scale (Fig. 18-1). The personal and economic tolls of all of these are obvious and have direct implications for critical care physicians.

Just as progress has created this dilemma, it has also provided unprecedented opportunities to intervene for these devastating injuries.[8-21] Enhanced recognition of the hazards of irritant gases, appreciation of the spectrum of respiratory and systemic problems that ensue, and innovative approaches to accurate diagnosis and supportive care of inhalational exposure victims have been major developments.[8-11,21] The acuity, diversity, and multisystemic nature of clinical syndromes encountered after inhalation injury and the roles of new technologies in their acute management mandate central roles for the intensive care physician. Defining these functions and delineating priorities for optimum patient care require thorough understanding of the pathogenesis of inhalation injury, familiarity with the toxins most likely to be encountered, and appreciation of both obvious and insidious clinical presentations of serious injury. The intensivist must possess specific knowledge of those particular hazards that predominate within his or her own community and be familiar with all of the resources immediately available to implement the most efficient, effective responses. Moreover, responsibilities may range from coordinating hospital disaster plans with community-based emergency medicine services personnel, to dealing with the unannounced arrival of mass casualties, to appraising personnel needs and calling in of off-duty staff.

PATHOGENESIS OF ACUTE INHALATION INJURY

Inhalation exposures may cause asphyxiation, systemic toxicity, immunologically mediated responses, or most commonly direct cellular damage.[9-12,16] Generally the irritant gases associated with severe, direct respiratory injury are highly reactive acids or bases. Their inhalation and hydration within the lung leads to oxidation or denaturation of cellular constituents. For many agents, the injurious potential should appear obvious because of the noxious nature of the compound: Interaction of inhaled chlorine with water may result in generation of hypochlorous (HOCl) and hydrochloric acids and other highly reactive compounds; sulfur dioxide may produce local injury by sulfuric and sulfurous acids; inhalation of oxides of nitrogen generates nitrous and nitric acids; and ammonia leads to liquefaction necrosis.

Asphyxiation results from diverse mechanisms:[9,10] reduction of alveolar oxygen tension to critical levels (as by its consumption during the "flash over" phase of a fire when a room bursts into flames), displacement by other gases (as with the high concentrations of methane or carbon dioxide responsible for mining or silo casualties and the massive carbon dioxide release causing the Cameroon disaster), and compromise of tissue delivery and cellular utilization of oxygen (as with cyanide, hydrogen sulfide, or carbon monoxide intoxications). With such displacement of oxygen, asphyxia is said to occur when oxygen concentrations fall below 15%, with unconsciousness followed by death occurring at concentrations below 6 to 8%.[17] Some asphyxiants may also cause direct pulmonary damage, but profound systemic poisoning generally occurs despite relatively well-preserved lung structure and function. In addition, pulmonary absorption of heavy metals such as mercury or of volatile hydrocarbons may lead to severe neurologic sequelae, whereas renal or hepatic failure may follow inhalations of cadmium, arsine, or serine.[11,17] Intravascular hemolysis may be seen with arsenic or may occur as a result of disseminated intravascular coagulation (DIC) complicating shock. Inhalation exposure may trigger complement activation; release an array of humoral mediators; and as after exposures to isocyanates, platinum salts, and anhydrides, result in predominantly immunologically mediated responses.

Primary Mechanisms of Injury

In most instances, irritant gases produce direct cellular damage[9-17,23-30] (Fig. 18-2). The anatomic distribution and severity of respiratory and systemic effects are determined by the concentration of the agent, its physical and chemical properties (especially its water solubility, diffusing characteristics, and reactivity with tissue components), the duration of exposure, and the setting in which it oc-

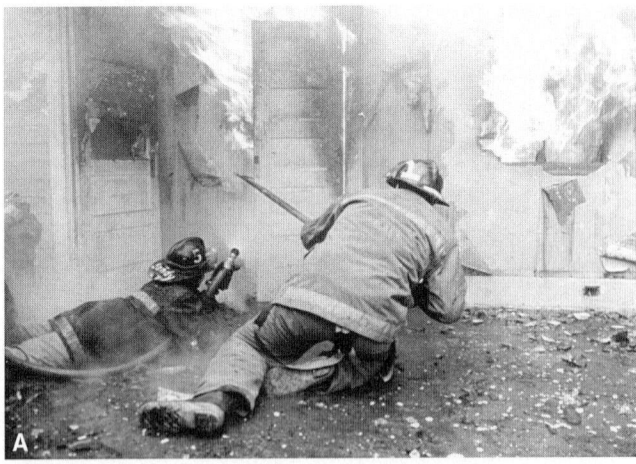
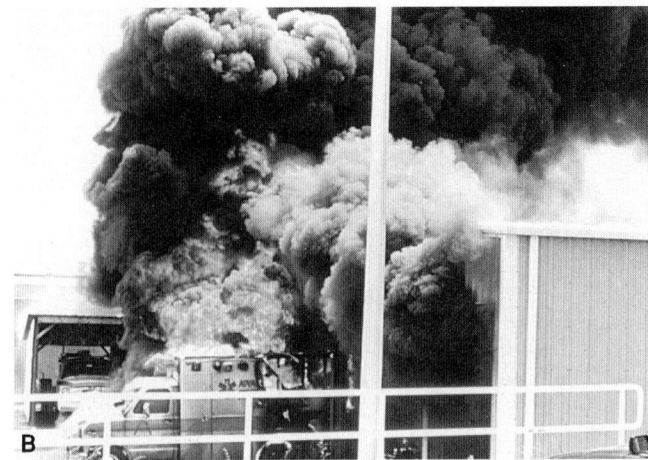

Fig. 18–1. Settings for acute inhalation injury and risks for severe exposure may vary considerably, as seen with this residential fire *(A)* and burning ambulance *(B)*. (Courtesy of Dr. Ralph Leonard.)

curred.[8-12] It has been suggested that adherence of gases or mists to particulates (as with smoke inhalation) may prolong the residence time of a noxious agent within the lung, accentuating possible toxic effects. In one test of this hypothesis, inhalation of an activated carbon "carrier" aerosol did not augment the pulmonary response to sulfur dioxide.[31] Direct mucosal damage by heat is an additional factor important not only during fires, but also in a number of industrial settings of exposure. Because of the effectiveness of the central airways as a heat sink and the protective functions of the glottis, however, true thermal injury to the lung is unusual even in the presence of severe upper airway damage.[32] These natural defenses may be overcome during aspiration of hot liquid,[33] inhalation of steam (with its markedly increased heat-carrying capacity), injuries in hyperoxic environments, and following inhalation of the ignited ether vehicle of the crack form of cocaine,[34] resulting in true pulmonary burns.

The chemical activity and water solubility of inhaled agents require particular emphasis because of direct implications for the extent of acute respiratory exposure.[8-12] Such historical information about the nature of the inhaled agent may provide important early clues to subsequent management needs. Irritants such as ammonia, sulfur dioxide, and hydrogen fluoride are highly water soluble, predisposing to mucous membrane and pharyngeal damage. Aldehydes commonly encountered in smoke (acrolein, acid acetaldehyde, and formaldehyde) also share this characteristic. Nasal and conjunctival irritation may have protective effects by providing an important early warning of expo-

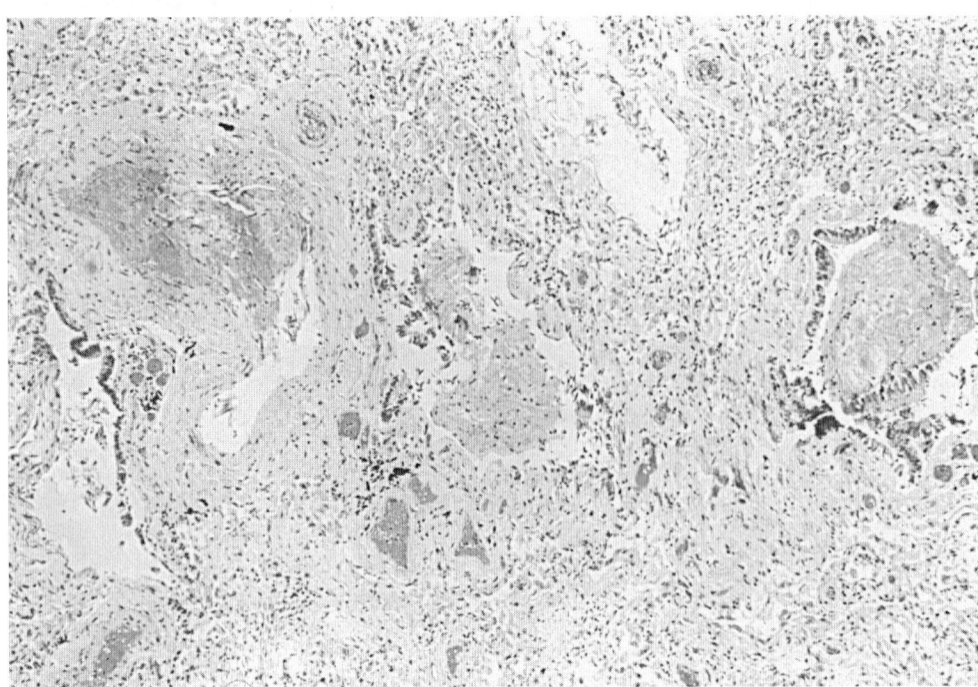

Fig. 18–2. Despite marked variations among inhaled irritant gases and exposures, histologic effects of severe pulmonary injury are generally nonspecific, characterized by cellular filtration, exudation, and edema. These changes and their physiologic effects are generally indistinguishable from acute lung injuries sustained in other settings.

sure and allowing the victim sufficient time to escape. Conversely, these characteristics may contribute to incapacitation and entrapment, as with the acute blinding of a refrigeration worker following an ammonia spill, resulting in more intense exposure with global respiratory injury. In other instances, the noxious odors of irritants (e.g., high levels of hydrogen sulfide) may lead to olfactory fatigue, and increasing, dangerous concentrations may not be recognized.[17] More insidious clinical presentations may follow exposures to gases having lower water solubilities, such as phosgene and oxides of nitrogen. A relative paucity of irritative mucosal and upper airway signs and symptoms may delay recognition of the danger until after severe lower respiratory injury has occurred. Clinical experience suggests that as the concentration of the agent and duration of exposure are increased, so does the likelihood of damage to all levels to the respiratory tract; the impact of differential water solubilities may then become a less important determinant of injury.

Cellular Events

These initial events trigger an acute inflammatory response that appears to be modulated and, in some instances perpetuated, by diverse cytokines, which may amplify the effects of direct chemical damage.[35,36] Observations in well-controlled animal models suggest that similar cascades are activated as seen with other acute lung injuries.[35-51] Varying roles for tumor necrosis factor, interleukins, and products of arachidonate metabolism have been proposed. Lipid peroxidation seems to be a fundamental event that is well documented in animal models of smoke inhalation and cutaneous burns and is under assessment in humans.[37-40] Generation of free radicals after inhalation of sulfur dioxide, ozone, and nitrogen dioxide appears to present a paradigm of events following inhalation injury.[26-28,39-44]

Support for a prominent role of polymorphonuclear leukocytes (PMN) in the pathogenesis of inhalation injury has come from the attenuation of experimental smoke inhalation injury by pretreatment of the animal with nitrogen mustard.[49] Basadre and colleagues showed that leukopenic sheep had less severe elevations of pulmonary artery pressure, pulmonary vascular resistance, and pulmonary lymph flow, better oxygenation, lower levels of plasma-conjugated dienes (indicating less oxygen radical production), and higher lung lymph alpha$_2$-macroglobulin levels (suggesting less consumption of antiprotease) in comparison to nonleukopenic controls.[49] In experimental smoke inhalation, interstitial and airway accumulation of PMN appears to be mediated by alveolar macrophages.[50] The role of alveolar macrophages in modulating these injuries requires further investigation.

Reduced concentrations and activity of pulmonary antiproteases after smoke inhalation injury suggest their consumptive depletion by proteases. Increased interstitial concentrations of beta glucuronidase have been demonstrated following smoke inhalation.[52] Niehaus and co-workers suggested that this inhalation injury could result from direct proteolytic degradation of the microvasculature or from enzymatic activation of reactive oxygen metabolites or eicosanoids.[53]

Differential susceptibilities of airway epithelial cell types to damage by specific irritant gases seem to have major importance, but relatively little is known about this determinant of clinical effects of acute inhalation injury. These factors have been detailed in Loke's superb text.[10] In animal models, ciliated cells are more vulnerable than nonciliated epithelium to nitrogen dioxide, sulfur dioxide, and ozone inhalation.[10,26-28] The common pathway of oxidant-induced damage includes an early increase of pericellular permeability owing to disruption in the strands of tight junctions.[10] Within minutes of cellular damage, increased membrane permeability or inhibition of sodium-calcium exchange leads to a rise of intracellular calcium, an important factor in the control of junctional contacts.[10] A well-controlled model of smoke inhalation injury demonstrated exfoliation of ciliated epithelium to be the earliest pathologic event;[54] subsequently, Lykens et al.[45] has shown desquamated bronchial epithelial cells in the bronchoalveolar lavage (BAL) fluid of smoke inhalation victims within hours of acute exposures.

Variation in susceptibility of alveolar cells to inhalation injury has also been observed, with type I pneumocytes the most sensitive alveolar component.[10,26,30,46,47] Acute ammonia toxicity leads to denudation of the tracheobronchial epithelium, edema of the lamina propria, and marked alveolar edema, with congestion and hemorrhage. Electron microscopy in patients with fatal exposures has shown marked swelling and imbibitional edema of type I alveolar epithelial cells, suggesting that these represent the primary target of acute alveolar wall injury.[10,30] Specific alterations of lung structure caused by inhalation of oxidants have been reviewed by Crapo et al.,[30] and Evans[51] has underscored the sensitivity of type I alveolar epithelial cells and ciliated epithelial cells to these agents. Injuries due to ozone and nitrogen dioxide are characterized primarily by damage and remodeling of the alveolar epithelium and are associated with recruitment of increased numbers of alveolar macrophages.

Several host factors might influence these responses to inhalation injury and include patient age, history of previous exposure, and, later in the course, the presence of superimposed infection. In animals, species differences and varying concentrations of vitamin E and other antioxidants have been related to the degree of damage.[10] In some models, modifying factors, including ambient temperature, humidity, air flow, and the presence of pathogens, have been implicated. Variable host responses related to these factors seem to have clinical relevance, but delineating their precise roles in humans in the acute setting is generally unfeasible.

Major Physiologic Sequelae

The physiologic effects of these acute events are similar to those associated with lung injuries described in other chapters.[8,36] The primary airway site of injury is manifest by increased airway resistance, occurring on the basis of not only an inflamed mucosal surface with anatomic narrowing, but also lumenal obstruction by exudate and sloughed epithelium. Either bronchorrhea or strategically located viscid plugs obstructing central airways may become major management problems. Bronchospasm is another component of this dynamic air flow obstruction, presenting not only during the acute setting, but also as a reactive airways dysfunction syndrome (RADS) that may persist long after the acute injury should have resolved.[55,56] Mucosal inflammation is associated with an increased physiologic dead space (with its deleterious impact on alveolar ventilation) and markedly increased bronchial blood flow.[7]

In several elegant models, increased lung lymph and its protein concentration suggest an increase in alveolar capillary membrane permeability following severe inhalation exposures.[37,38,52,57-60] With increased lung water, thoracic compliance becomes markedly reduced, posing major difficulties in mechanical ventilation of patients with severe permeability edema. Acute inhalation of smoke has been shown to inactivate surfactant, a change accompanied by near-immediate microatelectasis.[60] Not surprisingly these acute changes in airways and alveoli are associated with an increased work of breathing. Varying degrees of ventilation-perfusion mismatch result in hypoxemia.[61] Not only may pulmonary hypertension ensue, but also, depending on the reserve of the individual and nature of the toxic agent, cardiovascular collapse may supervene.

COMMON INHALATION EXPOSURES

Although inhalation injury encompasses acute and chronic exposures to virtually innumerable noxious agents and their combinations, several commonly encountered materials represent the spectrum of clinical sequelae seen after acute massive exposure (Table 18-1).[9-12] Respiratory complications caused by inhaled recreational drugs,[10] including opiates, marijuana, phencyclidine (PCP), cocaine, nitric oxide, toluene, hydrocarbons, and aerosol propellants (fluorocarbons); are not addressed in this chapter. All of these may have direct respiratory toxicities similar to the spectrum described with other agents or predispose to other respiratory injuries (e.g., aspiration, trauma). Also not addressed are the poorly quantifiable, chronic low dose exposures to inhaled gases and mists that are associated with environmental pollution and occupational and home exposures. Moreover, exposures to even low concentrations of many of these agents (e.g., sulfur dioxide, ammonia) may trigger acute exacerbations of chronic obstructive airways disease.

As noted previously, special familiarity with the agents related to local industries or transported through one's own community is particularly important. The most frequently encountered causes of inhalation injury may vary in their propensities to produce either respiratory or systemic injury and in the type of respiratory problems that are most likely to ensue. Even for rarely encountered exposures, however, similar principles of acute evaluation and management apply. Most severe inhalation exposures result from smoke inhalation and industrial accidents, but such irritants have been used purposefully in riot control, chemical warfare, and recreational drug use. Clearly each of these situations has added effects on evaluation and management strategies.

Table 18-1. General Characteristics of Commonly Encountered Toxic Gases, Fumes, and Mists

Agent	Major Mechanism of Injury*	Setting of Exposure
Acrolein	D	Plastic, rubber, textile resin maker
Acrylonitrile	A	Synthetic fiber, acylic resin, rubber maker
Arsine	S	Smelting, refining
Cadmium fume	I,S	Ore smelting, alloying, welding
Carbon dioxide	A	Foundry work, mining
Carbon disulfide	S	Degreasing, electroplating, sulfur processing
Carbon monoxide	A	Foundry work, petroleum refining, mining
Chlorine	D	Bleaching, disinfectant and plastic making
Copper fume	S	Welding
Formaldehyde	I,D	Disinfectant, embalming fluid use, paper and photography industry
Hydrogen chloride	D	Refining, dye making, orlonic chemical synthesis
Hydrogen cyanide	A	Electroplating, fumigant work, steel industry
Hydrogen fluoride	D	Etching, petroleum industry, silk-working
Hydrogen sulfide	A,D	Natural gas making, paper pulp, sewage treatment, tannery work
Magnesium oxide fume	S	Welding, alloy, flare, filament making

D, Direct toxicity; A, asphyxiant; S, systemic; I, immunologic.
(Data from references 9 to 17.)

Carbon Monoxide

The prototypic asphyxiant, carbon monoxide (CO) is the most commonly recognized cause of inhalation injury.[8,9,62-64] This ubiquitous compound is generated in any situation in which incomplete combustion occurs and is the most important cause of early fatalities due to smoke. Foundries, petroleum refining, and mining industries are important occupational settings of major exposures. Although it was believed previously that the sole effects of CO related to compromised tissue oxygenation based on binding of hemoglobin and a leftward shift of the oxyhemoglobin dissociation curve, interference with cellular respiration owing to uncoupling of the cytochrome system has been suggested in animal models. In addition, direct alveolar injury resulting in noncardiogenic pulmonary edema has been implicated occasionally. Central nervous system (CNS) and cardiac dysfunction are hallmarks of severe CO poisoning. The possibility of long-term neurologic residual is well recognized, but its precise frequency and cause are unknown, contributing to major controversies regarding management. Whether this complication can be avoided with general use of hyperbaric oxygen (HBO) therapy is unresolved. As with other asphyxiants, the severity of the patient's symptoms and organ dysfunction also relates to the acuity and duration of exposure and to the patient's preexisting functional reserve.

Cyanide

Exposures to cyanide commonly occur in the steel and electroplating industries.[65-70] Acrylonitrile (vinyl cyanide) is encountered in manufacture of synthetic fibers, rubbers, plastics, and resins. Significant exposure to this cytochrome poison has been noted in up to one fourth of smoke inhalation victims and may occur to some degree in nearly all such patients.

Ammonia

Ammonia is used in diverse occupational settings.[71-76] Large volumes of pressurized ammonia have been released during trailer or railroad crashes or in accidents in the refrigerator, explosive, and fertilizer industries. On a smaller scale, clinically severe exposures may accompany use of household cleaners in enclosed spaces. The high water solubility of this agent leads to prominent upper airway, conjunctival, and nasal symptoms. Blindness owing to corneal burns may preclude escape and lead to lethal respiratory exposures; ammonia is one of the agents associated with global respiratory damage. Resolution of the acute injury has been followed by chronic respiratory dysfunction, in which bronchiolitis, bronchiectasis, and airways hyperreactivity may occur.

Sulfur Dioxide

Sulfur dioxide (SO_2) is another highly water-soluble agent with a wide spectrum of clinical presentations similar to that of ammonia.[9,77-80] A virtually ubiquitous air pollutant generated from combustion of fossil fuels, SO_2 is well recognized as an industrial hazard in paper manufacturing, bleaching, and refrigeration industries. Rhinorrhea, cough, lacrimation, burning throat, odynophagia, dysphasia, headache, nausea, and vomiting all may follow acute exposures and are relatively nonspecific presentations. Long-term physiologic dysfunction (with both restrictive and obstructive ventilatory defects), bronchiolitis, and RADS have occurred. Generation of bisulfite may be an important factor in the acute airway hyperresponsiveness caused by SO_2 inhalation.[10]

Hydrogen Fluoride

Expansion of the semiconductor industries during the past two decades has increased the possibility of accidental exposure to hydrogen fluoride (H_2F).[81-83] This highly water-soluble compound is also used widely in the ceramics and glass etching industries and causes a clinical presentation similar to that of ammonia and SO_2 intoxications. Severe cutaneous burns may also occur, with their severity underestimated at the time of initial injury. Because H_2F binds magnesium and calcium in tissues, clinically important hypomagnesemia and hypocalcemia may develop and must be addressed during acute management.

Chlorine

Use of chlorine as a chemical warfare agent during World War I underscored the lethal potential for this irritant gas. Currently, widespread exposures may accompany use of this agent in water purification, chemical manufacturing, and bleaching processes.[84-88] In addition to these industrial exposures, chlorine intoxication may also occur in the home in relation to swimming pool accidents and the widespread practice of mixing combinations of cleaning agents. Because this reactive gas is intermediate in its water solubility, a delayed onset of severe respiratory injury may occur.

Phosgene

Another chemical warfare agent, phosgene ($COCl_2$) has a lower water solubility than chlorine and may result in a more insidious delayed clinical presentation of parenchymal lung injury.[9,10,89-91] This dense gas is used in the synthesis of dyes and insecticides, is used in the pharmaceutical industry, and is also generated during arc welding and production of isocyanates. Importantly, high concentrations of phosgene evolve with combustion of polyvinyl chloride (PVC), a ubiquitous component of plastic furnishings.

Oxides of Nitrogen

Exposures of nitrogen dioxide (NO_2) and other oxides of nitrogen are important causes of inhalation injury commonly encountered during chemical manufacturing, welding, and fire fighting.[92-102] In addition, N_2O_2 is generated during combustion of aircraft and rocket fuels and the storage of silage. The low water solubility of this heavy, yellow to red-brown gas predisposes to delayed clinical presentations and pulmonary parenchymal damage. Biphasic and triphasic clinical presentations have been recognized. An initial episode of acute, nonspecific respiratory symptoms may be followed by apparent resolution, only to have recurrence of even more severe signs and symptoms. The latter may also clear completely, insidiously lead to long-term sequelae, or progress to fulminant acute respiratory failure. An apparently increased propensity of such exposures to cause bronchiolitis obliterans has provided some justification for acute treatment with corticosteroids, but more information is needed about the benefits of this approach. Exposure of N_2O_2 may also potentiate airway reactivity in asthmatics. Severe exposure to oxides of nitrogen can also result in methemoglobinemia, compromising oxygen delivery.

Hydrogen Sulfide

Hydrogen sulfide (H_2S) exposures are widespread in the waste disposal, natural gas, drilling, and refining industries.[11,103-108] H_2S is not only a mucosal irritant, but also a cytochrome poison. As with other asphyxiants, neurologic dysfunction is a prominent clinical presentation.

Ozone

Ozone is a low-water-solubility gas widely recognized as an air pollutant and generated in high concentrations around ultraviolet light sources, around electrical arcs, and during welding. Exposures have been associated with acute and chronic air flow obstruction and, when severe, pulmonary edema.[9-11,109]

Table 18-2. Common Toxic Products of Incomplete Combustion

Source	Product
Polyvinyl chloride	Hydrogen chloride, chlorine phosgene, carbon monoside
Wool, silk, nylon, polyurethane, melamine resins	Hydrogen cyanide, ammonia, isocyanates
Nitrocellulose film, fabrics	Oxides of nitrogen
Wood, cotton, paper, petroleum products	Acrolein, acetaldehyde, acetic acid, carbon monoxide
Fluorinate resins	Hydrogen fluoride, hydrogen bromide
Sulfur-containing compounds	Sulfur dioxide
Petroleum products	Benzene

(From Haponik, E. F., and Munster, A. M. (Eds.): Respiratory Injury: Smoke Inhalation and Burns. New York, McGraw-Hill, 1990.)

Smoke Inhalation

Exposures to combinations of asphyxiant and irritant gases during fires is perhaps the most common cause of inhalation injury.[1-4,7,8,23,36] Smoke is a product of thermal demutation during pyrolysis (in the presence of low oxygen concentrations, without visible flame) or burning (in higher oxygen environments, with visible flame). The heterogeneous mixture of particulates and gases varies with each fire scenario, hindering efforts to model this injury. Asphyxiants and irritants commonly generated during fires are outlined in Table 18-2 and lead to markedly diverse clinical presentations.[22-25,110,111] Acrolein, an intense airways irritant, has been especially noteworthy during residential fires, whereas PVC polymers from household furnishings make phosgene, hydrogen chloride, and cyanide important exposures. It is suspected that the mixture of agents may cause synergistic respiratory damage, but this speculation is unproved.

Metallic Compounds

Inhalation of the fumes from metals may also lead to acute injuries ranging from life-threatening multisystem organ failure to the relatively benign but annoying course of metal fume fever. The latter acute illness is characterized by systemic symptoms including fever, chills, myalgias, and malaise beginning 4 to 6 hours after exposure.[9,11,112] The presence of a peripheral leukocytosis may suggest an infectious cause. Typically, manifestations decrease in severity as the work week progresses, a tolerance to exposure that should suggest the diagnosis. History of exposure to zinc oxide and other fumes generated during welding or smelting of metals in enclosed spaces, with the lack of respiratory symptoms and roentgenographic abnormalities, may help to differentiate this problem from other, more serious inhalational injuries. Polymer and organic dusts may cause similar febrile, systemic syndromes, also with tolerance to exposure. The latter illnesses may be complicated by interstitial or alveolar radiographic abnormalities.

Metal hydrides are used widely in the semiconductor industry, and inhalations of arsine, phosphine, and diborine are especially important.[9,11,17] Severe exposures to these agents may lead to pulmonary edema and CNS dysfunction. In addition, arsine may cause intravascular hemolysis, with bilirubinemia and hematuria. Exchange transfusion may be required to clear the arsenic-hemoglobin complex, whereas hemodialysis may be necessary to manage associated acute renal failure. In a similar fashion, acute exposure to cadmium oxide during welding or smelting may result in combined respiratory and renal failure.[9] Industrial bronchitis or interstitial pneumonitis may also follow inhalation of manganese, cobalt, nickel carbonyl, vanadium, and mercury, whereas inhalation of platinum-halide complexes or cobalt may result in occupational asthma.[9-11]

Anhydrides and Isocyanates

Exposures to these reactive compounds have well-documented, immunologically mediated respiratory sequelae. Trimellitic anhydride is used in manufacture of epoxy resins and as an anticorrosive and may cause delayed-onset pulmonary hemorrhage.[9-18] Anemia, dyspnea, massive hemoptysis, and severe shock-related hypoxemia all may ensue. Toluene disocyanate (TDI) may be produced in high concentrations from polyurethane foams, fibers, and coatings.[113,114] Although high dose exposure may produce nonspecific, chemically mediated upper respiratory symptoms, most noteworthy is the delayed-onset, immunologically mediated syndrome. Exposures to low concentrations of these agents may result in asthma and rhinitis and follow a prolonged (e.g., 1 to 5 years) symptom-free interval after exposure. Less often encountered is a much more severe syndrome characterized by a combination of constitutional symptoms and delayed-onset respiratory effects mimicking hypersensitivity pneumonitis.

Chemical Warfare Agents

Tragically recognition of the adverse effects of inhaled toxins through their historical application as chemical warfare agents has continued in the current development and use of such weapons. In Urbanetti's comprehensive review of battlefield chemical inhalation injuries, these are classified as choking agents (e.g., phosgene, diphosgene, chlorine, chloropicrin), blood agents (e.g., cyanide), nerve agents (e.g., sarin, sonan, tabun, VX), incapacitants (e.g., BZ), blister agents (e.g., sulfur mustard, nitrogen mustard, Lewisite, phosgene oxime), and organic toxins (e.g., botulinus toxin, staphylococcus enterotoxin B, ricin).[115] Riot control agents (e.g., chloroacetophenone, chlorobenzylidene) generally have less severe effects. As in other circumstances, the possibility of multiple adverse effects of a single exposure must be considered. For example, organophosphates may cause several respiratory problems ranging from bronchospasm, bronchorrhea, and pulmonary edema to hypoventilatory respiratory failure due to respiratory muscle paralysis.

GENERAL CLINICAL PRESENTATIONS

Despite the diversity of causative agents and exposure scenarios, the clinical manifestations of inhalation injury

Table 18–3. Anatomic Classification of Acute Inhalation Injury

Anatomic Level of Injury	Predominant Clinical Presentation	Usual Timing of Onset	Primary Mechanism of Injury	Principal Physiologic Presentation(s)
Systemic/Neurologic	Obtundation	Early	Chemical	Tissue asphyxia
Respiratory				
Conducting airways	Respiratory distress			
Upper		Early	Chemical ± thermal	Airway obstruction ± alveolar hypoventilation
Tracheobronchial		Early	Chemical	Airway obstruction ± alveolar hypoventilation, mild hypoxemia, atelectasis
Parenchymal	Respiratory distress	Delayed	Chemical	Hypoxemic respiratory failure, pulmonary edema

(From Haponik, E. F., and Munster, A. M. (Eds.): Respiratory Injury: Smoke Inhalation and Burns. New York, McGraw-Hill, 1990.)

are relatively limited and nonspecific (Fig. 18–3). These events appear to reflect a stereotypic response of the respiratory system and are markedly similar to those seen with other acute lung injuries. Classification in anatomic and mechanistic terms permits concise description of the nature of injury in an individual patient and should contribute to prompt, systematic delineation of therapeutic priorities. This simple approach is fortunate because in many instances the precise nature of the offending agent or its toxicity may not be apparent to managing clinicians at the time when vigorous supportive treatment must be initiated.

Simple anatomic classification partitions the respiratory and systemic effects of the inhalation exposure[8] (Tables 18–3, and 18–4). For the most part, the latter include numerous end organ toxicities of agents absorbed over the alveolar capillary membrane. Although in some instances these effects are mediated directly by an inhaled toxin, in others they reflect compromised oxygen delivery and parallel events seen with multisystem organ failure in other clinical settings. Because absorption via the respiratory tract is the most significant route of entry for toxic metals, such as lead, mercury, manganese, cadmium, antimony, and cobalt, particular attention toward systemic effects as well as local irritative respiratory problems must be considered after such inhalation exposures. Skornik has reviewed the inhalation toxicity of metals extensively.[116]

Direct respiratory injuries, in turn, can be characterized as those with predominant airway and pulmonary paren-

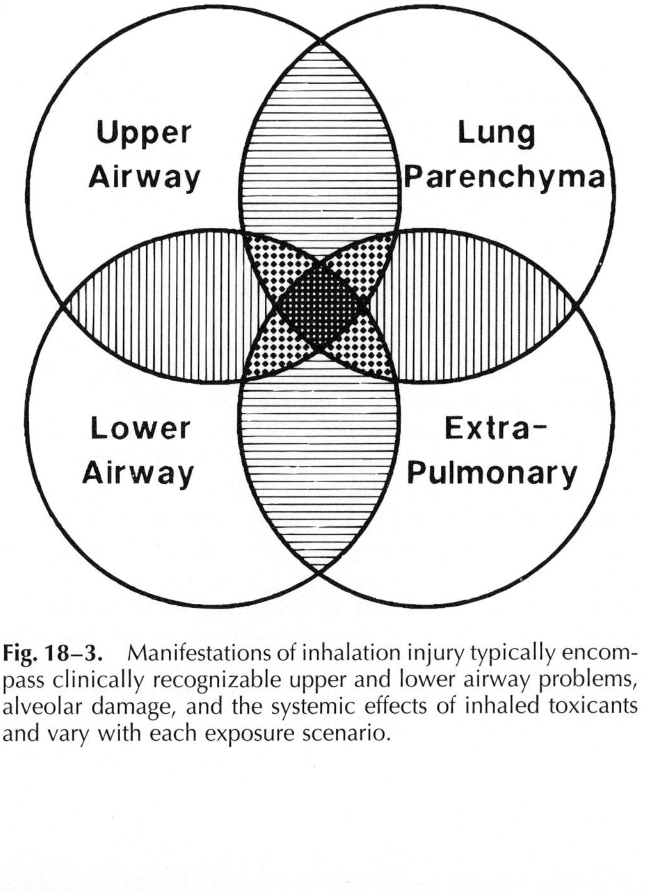

Table 18–4. Major Respiratory Complications of Irritant Gas Inhalation

Inhalation injury*
  Asphyxia
    Hypoxia
    Carbon monoxide, cyanide intoxication
  Direct respiratory injury
    Airway responses
      Upper airway obstruction
      Tracheobronchitis
      Bronchiolitis
      Atelectasis
    Alveolar-capillary membrane injury (permeability pulmonary edema)
Effects of cutaneous burns
  Pulmonary dysfunction
    Chest wall restriction (e.g., circumferential thoracic burns, soft tissue edema)
    Upper airway compression (e.g., circumferential cervical burns)
Combined inhalation with cutaneous burn
Concomitant chest trauma
Nosocomial/iatrogenic problems
  Hydrostatic pulmonary edema (over-resuscitation)
  Pneumonia (aerogenous, hematogenous)
  Sepsis-related permeability edema
  Drug-induced
    Hypoventilation (e.g., morphine)
    Hyperventilation (e.g., topical mafenide)
  Pneumothorax
    Ventilator-induced barotrauma
    Central venous access procedures
  Pulmonary embolism
  Complications of artificial airways
  Aspiration
Exacerbation of preexisting cardiopulmonary disease
  Cardiogenic pulmonary edema
  Chronic obstructive pulmonary disease

(From Haponik, E. F., and Munster, A. M. (Eds.): Respiratory Injury: Smoke Inhalation and Burns. New York, McGraw-Hill, 1990.)

Fig. 18–3. Manifestations of inhalation injury typically encompass clinically recognizable upper and lower airway problems, alveolar damage, and the systemic effects of inhaled toxicants and vary with each exposure scenario.

chymal (visceral) manifestations.[117,118] The former include airway obstruction at supraglottic, glottic, and tracheobronchial levels, whereas the latter focus on alveolar capillary membrane injury with resulting increased permeability. In some instances, there is a predominance of one of these clinical manifestations that surprisingly often parallels recognized physical characteristics of the inhaled gas. After overwhelming exposures (often owing to the patient's entrapment by the physical setting of exposure or incapacitation by neurologic or other trauma), all of these levels are affected. This potential for interaction of multiple sites of respiratory and systemic injury is outlined in Figure 18-3. At the time of earliest presentation and triage, such manifestations of injury must be addressed simultaneously. Their impact on clinical presentations and management priorities is outlined in Table 18-3.

Just as respiratory complications of inhalation injury may be partitioned according to the anatomic level of airway involvement, they also can be characterized by their temporal onset.[8,20] In a sheep model of smoke inhalation, the time course of microvascular injury (assessed with measures of selective sieving of macromolecules and lymph protein flux) varied with the anatomic site of damage. Tracheal protein flux occurred earlier (8 hours after exposure) than that in the lung (24 hours after exposure).[119]

Careful analysis of microvascular permeability through estimates of the reflection and filtration coefficients in an ovine smoke inhalation model demonstrated that lung edema formation is multifactorial, associated with marked elevations of both capillary pressure and permeability. The relative impact of these factors varied with the time after inhalation injury. Whereas increased permeability predominated at 24 hours after injury, accounting for approximately two thirds of increased capillary filtration, at 48 hours after injury, three fourths of the increased capillary filtration was due to increased capillary pressure.[120] The acute elevation of pulmonary microvascular permeability was associated with oxygen-free radical release (reflected by elevated plasma conjugated dienes).

"Early" clinical problems during the first 24 hours after exposure typically include systemic intoxication by asphyxiants, upper airway obstruction, and tracheobronchial obstruction. Although acute pulmonary edema based on not only adult respiratory distress syndrome (ARDS), but also congestive heart failure or iatrogenic volume overload during resuscitative efforts may be an early pulmonary complication of severe exposure to virtually any agent, it more often has a delayed onset during the second or third day. The spectrum of late complications following inhalation injury (e.g., pneumonia, sepsis, pulmonary embolism) is similar to that seen in other hospitalized patients. Inhalation injury victims are especially predisposed to nosocomial infection, which has a particularly high morbidity and mortality.

PREHOSPITAL ASSESSMENT AND MANAGEMENT OF INHALATION INJURY

Acute elevation and management begin at the scene of exposure and require immediate recognition of potentially severe respiratory and systemic injury. Fundamental priorities of these acute resuscitative strategies are establishing the airway, administering oxygen, initiating and maintaining alveolar ventilation, and ensuring circulatory support. As noted elsewhere, these diagnostic efforts must be merged with timely therapy. Among priorities more specific to inhalation exposures, protection of the patient from further injury, airway maintenance, and early administration of antidotes require added emphasis.

Evacuation and Decontamination

The noxious nature of the agents causing injury demands that continued exposure to the agent be interrupted so as to avoid more severe acute and long-term sequelae. Prompt physical removal of the victim from the scene and at least supply of uncontaminated air (as with supplemental oxygen administration) is a key, empiric early maneuver. When significant cutaneous as well as inhalation exposures have occurred, as for example after a "drenching" accident, thorough washing of the patient to limit the extent of cutaneous injury or absorption of the toxin is necessary. As soaked clothing is removed and the patient is washed down, health care personnel should cautiously avoid contamination. In the case of battlefield chemical exposures, topical decontamination using standard powders and solutions is a priority.[10,115] Gentle manipulation of trauma sites or concomitant burns is necessary to avoid exacerbating the injury.

During these efforts, health care professionals and other members of the evacuation team must recognize the possibility of personal injury or incapacitation and take appropriate precautions. These might include use of self-contained breathing apparatus or protective outerwear. Practical applications of this strategy have resulted in effective rescue functions by firefighters (as in the case of smoke inhalation) or soldiers (as during exposures to chemical warfare agents). Failure to take proper safeguards may result in severe injury. For example, exposures to high concentrations of phosgene and other products of PVC pyrolysis may occur during the cleanup, "overhaul" phase after a fire, when some firefighters or rescue personnel may be tempted to discard their protective gear.

Upper Airway Management

Obstruction owing to acute pharyngeal inflammation is the most treatable of the serious early respiratory complications,[21,117] but if unrecognized, it has tragic consequences. Objective endoscopic evaluations have shown that supraglottic rather than glottic edema is the major site of injury. Inflammation of the arytenoid eminences, edema and obliteration of the aryepiglottic folds, and interarytenoid edema are seen characteristically[121,122] (Fig. 18-4). Edematous supraglottic tissue prolapses to occlude the airway, and these changes can be accentuated by rapid administration of resuscitative fluid.[123] In addition, to these direct effects of exposure to irritants, one must consider mechanical obstruction by foreign bodies or traumatic injury.

Early endotracheal intubation is the standard of care for established or impending upper airway obstruction or ina-

ACUTE INHALATION INJURY

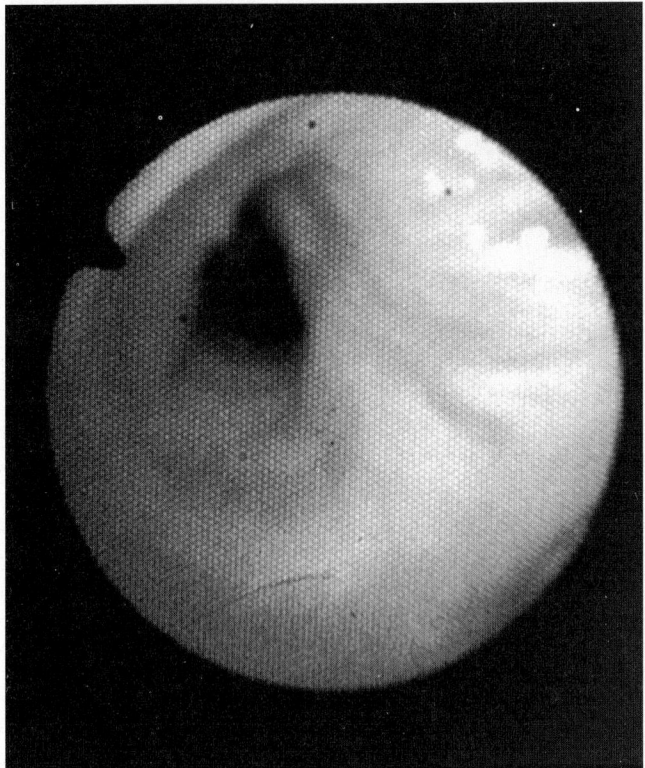

Fig. 18-4. Upper airway edema with obscuration of supraglottic landmarks is an important sign of inhalation injury, and effacement of normal landmarks (e.g., arytenoid eminences) is a significant finding. Clinically important physiologic dysfunction may be present despite an apparently patent glottic lumen, and anatomic obstruction may progress rapidly with intravenous fluid administration.

bility to protect the airway because of neurologic compromise.[124-130] The acute supraglottitis or laryngitis owing to irritant gases (especially those that are highly water soluble), thermal injury, or aspiration of hot liquids creates an emergency akin to acute infectious epiglottis in children. The jeopardized upper airway requires prompt management by a true expert, and there is no margin for error (Fig. 18-5). Tracheotomy and cricothyrotomy are generally reserved for circumstances when an airway otherwise cannot be secured safely. Coexisting facial and cervical burns with massive edema may require these modes of airway support. The adage "when in doubt, intubate" is an appropriate description for the low threshold for endotracheal intubation that must be maintained in patients with inhalation injury because of the possibility of rapid progression to complete airway occlusion.

There is considerable debate about the optimum route for intubation, with no clearly established superiority for one approach.[20,21] The skills and experience of the intubator and the anatomic limitations presented by the individual patient are key determinants. In anticipation of major requirements for suctioning and possible bronchoscopy, as large an orotracheal tube as possible is usually selected. Because fatal hyperkalemia has been associated with succinylcholine during the first 8 to 12 hours after burn injuries,[131,132] nondepolarizing muscle relaxants are advisable for rapid sequence intubation. Once placed, endotracheal tubes must be secured appropriately because of the exceedingly high frequency and risk of self-extubation in this setting. In one report, all patients requiring emergency tracheostomy for lost airways after burns experienced fatal cardiopulmonary arrests.[133]

Administration of Antidotes

Administration of antidotes must begin during field management. Most obvious (and best supported) are the administration of high concentrations of oxygen to patients with CO intoxication and the acute therapy of cyanide poisoning. Oxygen is the most important antidote. Empiric early administration of the highest oxygen concentrations possible is essential in persons exposed to asphyxiants. Despite its theoretic attractiveness, the precise role of HBO is unclear in patients with CO intoxication.[134-137] The controversies surrounding this therapy have been addressed in a consensus conference and medical publications and remain hotly debated. In the presence of neurologic dysfunction or cardiovascular and cerebrovascular disease, HBO is generally advocated; end organ dysfunction (rather than a particular carboxyhemoglobin (COHb) level) is the most appropriate criterion for therapy.[64] The value of HBO in preventing delayed neurologic deficits remains unknown. Practical issues concerning availability of a chamber, transportation, and other acute resuscitative needs must influence patient selection for therapy. In particular, it must be assured that oxygen therapy and other supportive care are not compromised pending HBO. HBO has also been advocated for treatment of patients sustain-

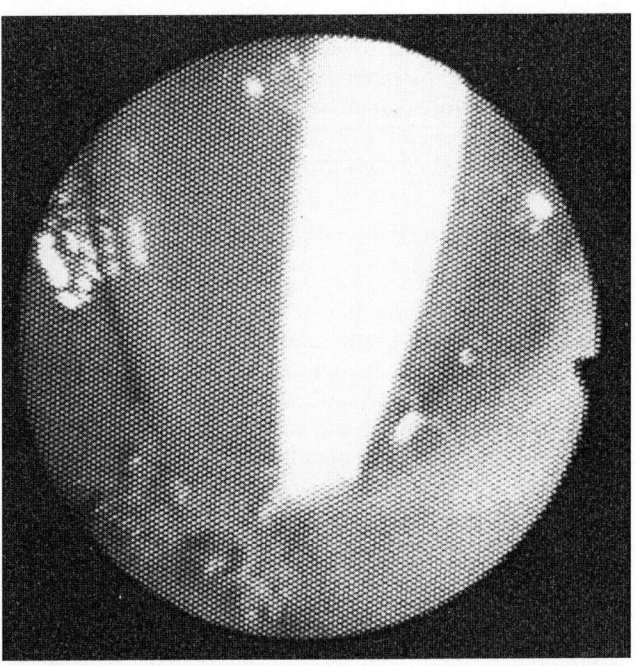

Fig. 18-5. Early, elective endotracheal intubation is essential because of airway compromise by extensive supraglottic edema and copious secretions.

ing other asphyxiant injuries (e.g., as with cyanide or H_2S inhalations),[103] but its role in these settings is even less clear.

As the impact of cyanide intoxication has been appreciated increasingly, empiric administration of antidotes in the field has been considered more often, but firm guidelines for early treatment are not delineated because of potential risk of empiric therapy[67-70] and delays in laboratory confirmation of cyanide intoxication. Neurologic dysfunction in patients at high risk is the primary criterion for therapy. Sequential administration of nitrites and thiosulfate is the standard treatment for cyanide intoxication and is facilitated by use a commercially available kit.[9,11,69] Initially methemoglobinemia is produced through administration of amyl nitrite perles and 3% sodium nitrite, resulting in binding of cyanide to produce cyanomethemoglobin. Systemic hypotension may complicate nitrite administration. Administration of sodium thiosulfate then results in regeneration of methemoglobin with formation of thiocyanate, which is excreted by the kidneys. The roles of other medications, including hydroxycobalamin (generating cyanocobalamin), dicobalt edentate aminophenols, and stroma-free methemoglobin, are under investigation. If benefits of hydroxycobalamin are confirmed, the threshold for empiric safer treatment of residential fire victims would lower considerably.[69]

Nitrites (without thiosulfate) have also been used for treatment of sulfhemoglobinemia associated with H_2S intoxication but are controversial because of concerns about methemoglobinemia generation.[11] Caution in applying these strategies is especially important in children, in whom fatal methemoglobinemia may occur. Methemoglobinemia in turn is treated by administration of methylene blue.[9,11] Calcium administration (as in the subcutaneous injection of calcium gluconate to patients suffering hydrogen fluoride burns) may help to avoid profound hypocalcemia. Pralidoxime (to regenerate cholinesterase) and atropine (to address the respiratory effects of accumulated acetylcholine) are standards in treating organophosphate inhalation.[10,115] Administration of these and other antidotes are detailed elsewhere.

General Risk Appraisal

During the acute evaluation, several characteristics of the inhalation exposure may help to predict a greater likelihood of significant inhalation injury.[8,138] The nature of the toxin (if known), its concentration, and duration of exposure have obvious importance. Exposures in an enclosed space setting, often with the victim's entrapment or incapacitation, increase this possibility. The presence of unconsciousness, restlessness, or other alterations of sensorium should suggest not only hypoxemia, severe aveolar hypoventilation, coexisting head trauma, or circulatory collapse. but also the systemic effects of a variety of neurotoxins.[139] Although transient, self-limited airway irritation is common, any respiratory signs or symptoms must be regarded as a potential marker of severe injury. Cough (including hemoptysis), dyspnea of varying degrees, and chest discomfort (often expressed as "tightness," "congestion," or frank pain) occur frequently. Hoarseness and painful swallowing should be recognized as important markers of pharyngeal inflammation and potential upper airway obstruction. During the initial field evaluation, it generally cannot be predicted whether these nonspecific symptoms will resolve or progress. The absence of either respiratory symptoms or abnormalities on the physical examination does not exclude significant inhalation injury.

Sputum may appear grossly purulent (reflecting intense airway inflammation) in the absence of superimposed infection. Expectoration of carbonaceous secretions by smoke inhalation victims represents only a marker of exposure, without prognostic significance.[6] When cutaneous burns are present, their distribution has special importance. Although the mere presence of facial burns owing to direct exposures to flame or chemicals is an inaccurate predictor of inhalation injury, involvement of the "respiratory area" of the face has correlated with multiple respiratory complications.[140,141] Such burns around the lips and nose are not only associated with an increased likelihood of inhalation injury, but also have major implications for endotracheal intubation. As facial and associated pharyngeal edema progress, eversion of the lips and fixation of the jaw impose grave technical limitations.

Although simple laboratory studies are performed occasionally in the field (e.g., expired CO determinations, peak flow rate measurements), the physical examination provides the primary means of identifying persons with the most severe inhalation injuries. The significance of obvious signs, such as cyanosis, stridor, recruitment of accessory respiratory muscles, tachypnea or apnea, and altered sensorium, must be appreciated. The "cherry red" facies characteristics of CO intoxication, green tongue of vanadium toxicity, and green face and chest of H_2S toxicity are seen infrequently. Soot covering a smoke inhalation victim and burns related to heat or immersions in noxious liquids all may obscure cyanosis. Moreover, hypoperfusion in the most severely injured individuals may further reduce the yield of such "classic" cutaneous signs. In some instances, characteristic odors may identify a particular irritant gas, and victims' clothing may reek of the agents to which they have been exposed. The pungent aromas of H_2S, SO_2, and smoke are widely recognized. The odor of bitter almonds has been associated with cyanide toxicity and that of garlic suggests arsine exposure, but these are seldom appreciated on the breath of exposure victims.

For clinicians evaluating patients at the scene of injury, information from rescue personnel or, as after an industrial accident, the patient's co-workers often provides added insights. The abrupt collapse of an individual after a massive inhalation exposure usually makes the diagnosis obvious. Even in these instances, however, recognition of the breadth of respiratory problems that can develop and the anticipation of the supportive measures most likely to become required may prevent problems later in management. In some circumstances, more chronic low level exposure can cause severe respiratory illness, especially when these events are superimposed on preexisting lung disease (e.g., obstructive airway disease in a long-term smoker). Differentiation of the relative components of the patient's chronic symptoms from those of acute injury in the latter setting can be quite difficult.

Table 18–5. Early Clinical Presentations of Inhalation Injury

Irritant gas exposure, without overt respiratory dysfunction
   No respiratory injury (normal objective tests; e.g., spirometry, peak flow rates)
   Subclinical injury (abnormal objective tests; ? borderline normal tests)
Clinically overt respiratory dysfunction (respiratory symptoms, signs, ± abnormalities of objective tests)
Cardiopulmonary arrest at scene, successful resuscitation
Asphyxiant death at scene of exposure

(Modified from Clark, W. R., and Nieman, G. F.: Smoke inhalation. Burns, 14:473, 1988.)

Triage Issues

Initial triage decisions in victims of inhalation injury are complicated by the possible delayed onset of life-threatening problems. Awareness that a significant lag time may occur, especially following inhaling less water-soluble agents, must lower the clinician's thresholds for hospitalization and objective diagnostic testing. In many instances, evaluating physicians cannot provide patients with reassurances that they seek even after an apparently minor exposure has occurred. Clinical errors in both under-estimating and overestimating the extent of injury occur frequently, accentuating these uncertainties.

Generally, anatomic considerations are merged with key information about the circumstances of exposure, the clinical presentation, and the severity of the respiratory injury documented objectively by diagnostic tests (when available). A gradation of clinical presentations occurs, ranging from exposures without overt adverse effects to death occurring at the scene of the inhalation exposure (Table 18–5). The categories of injury that are frequently encountered clinically can be described further according to the individual characteristics of the inhaled toxin. A practical, "common-sense" approach to triage is suggested in Table 18–6.[11] On arbitrary grounds, exposures of longer dura-

Table 18–6. Action Criteria for Acute Inhalation Exposures and Acute Inhalation Injury

Criteria for Hospitalization
High risk exposures (e.g., CO > 20%)
High risk patients
   Elderly, preexisting disease
     Limited access to care
Symptoms/signs present (respiratory, neurologic, cardiac)
Abnormal physiology
Burns present
Associated injuries
Candidates for Outpatient Observation
Low risk exposures
Low risk patients
   Young, previously well
   Access to follow-up
Symptom/signs absent
Normal physiology
Burns absent/minor
Other injury unlikely

(Modified from Wald, P. H., and Balmes, J. R.: Respiratory effects of short-term, high-intensity toxic inhalations: smoke, gases, and fumes. J. Intensive Care Med., 2:260, 1987.)

Table 18–7. Combined Anatomic/Physiologic Classification of Acute Respiratory Injuries Following Irritant Gas Inhalation Exposures

Grade	Criteria
0	Gas exposure (0_S), cutaneous burns (0_B), or their combination (0_{S+B}), without clinical evidence of respiratory injury
I	Evidence of either isolated asphyxiant exposure (I_{Asph}), upper airway (I_{UA}), lower airway (I_{LA}), or parenchymal ($I_{Parench}$) dysfunction, not meeting criteria for grade II or III.

II	Evidence of combined respiratory injuries (IIa–IIe) but with no individual component meeting criteria for grade III:
	   IIa: Asph & UA
	   IIb: UA + LA
	   IIc: Asph + UA + LA
	   IId: UA + LA + Parench
	   IIe: Asph + UA + LA + Parench

III	Any isolated or combined injury in which one of the following is present:
	   IIIa: COHb ≥ 20%, CN > 1, or any elevation of COHb and/or CN with neurologic dysfunction
	   IIIb: Stridor, physiologic or endoscopic evidence of UAO
	   IIc: Alveolar hypoventilation (Pa_{CO_2} ≥ 45 mm Hg) present
	   IIId: Major shunt-related hypoxemia (Pa_{O_2}/Fi_{O_2} ≤ 250) present

IV	Combined injuries (as in grade II) in which two or more criteria in III are present.
V	Injuries with which respiratory arrest has occurred.

Asph, Asphyxiant; UA, upper airway dysfunction; LA, lower airway dysfunction; parench, parenchymal dysfunction.
(From Haponik, E. F., and Munster, A. M. (Eds.): Respiratory Injury: Smoke Inhalation and Burns. New York, McGraw-Hill, 1990.)

tion, in enclosed spaces, or to "high risk" toxins alone might justify hospitalization even in the absence of obvious respiratory compromise.

Another grading scale outlined in Table 18–7 combines commonly obtained information about the anatomic and physiologic extent of injury and has direct implications for management.[8] For most patients with grade I injury, hospitalization is necessary. In most of these individuals, mere close observation and nonspecific supportive care would be sufficient to ensure that progression to more severe clinical dysfunction does not occur. Usually persons with grade 0 injuries at the time of initial evaluation are managed effectively on an ambulatory basis, so long as appropriate provisions for timely return to medical care are made should the patient deteriorate. Initial emergency evaluation and disposition of the patient must also include appropriate patient and, whenever feasible, family education about potential delayed signs and symptoms related to the exposure, with clearly specified action criteria for return to medical care and documentation of these recommendations.

Such thresholds, focused for the most part on the degree of respiratory injury, must be modified based on other factors, including the likelihood of the agent to cause delayed-onset respiratory sequelae or extrapulmonary dysfunction. Other factors influencing management include physiologic reserve and the added vulnerability conferred by preexisting illnesses and the patient's age. Persons at the extremes of age appear to be especially vulnerable to such injuries, and thresholds for hospitalization must be lowered accordingly. Whether there is an age-related variation in oxidant defenses or predispositions to irritant gas injury is unknown in humans. Importantly, the availability of family, other support systems, and transportation are added practical determinants of triage. As can be seen, "when in doubt, hospitalize" is a conservative but appropriate strategy for this type of unpredictable injury.

In most circumstances, all patients with grades III, IV, and V inhalation injuries will require ICU management. Moreover, depending on the nature of the institution and levels of supportive care available, most patients with grade II injury would benefit from the careful observation offered by the ICU setting. In this instance, planned, graded interventions can be introduced systematically should a patient's status deteriorate. Clinical worsening would be more likely appreciated early rather than "after the crash" and a reactionary management approach thus avoided.

Communication and Documentation

Responding to the demands of acute evaluation and management often limits the quality of records of events at the scene of injury. To whatever extent circumstances permit, however, as detailed a description as possible recording the patient's clinical presentation, objective findings, and circumstances of exposure should be communicated to subsequent caregivers.[142] This task might be especially difficult when dealing with patients sustaining severe injuries or with mass casualties, but such information may be crucial during later phases of management. Too often critical data available from initial field evaluation and management by rescue personnel are lost, and opportunities for modifications of management are compromised. Consequently, retrospective piecing together of events using fragmentary information is done. Even crude maps or diagrams made at the time of rescue (showing, for example, the victims' relative positions with respect to sources of an irritant gas or liquid) may help to estimate the severity of exposure and likelihood of delayed sequelae. On a larger scale (as after the wreck of a trailer or train transporting volatile chemicals), relative risks and varying natures of exposures to communities can often be estimated. Enhanced descriptions of chlorine exposures, for example, have taken into consideration wind conditions and topography of an area; such estimates of the relative concentrations and distributions of the gas have guided plans for evacuation and mobilization of health care resources. In industrial settings in particular, the extent of the hazard may be estimated more precisely with simple, rapidly performed field measurements of ambient toxins and relating these to established National Institute of Occupational Safety and Health guidelines and recognized risks for pulmonary sequelae.

HOSPITAL CONFIRMATION OF THE PRESENCE AND EXTENT OF INHALATION INJURY

As diagnostic and therapeutic interventions initiated in the field are continued in the hospital setting, the presence and severity of respiratory injury can be confirmed with

Table 18–8. Major Considerations in Clinical Diagnosis of Inhalation Injury

Spectrum and time course of respiratory problems
Classic clinical predictors
  Exposure characteristics
    Closed space setting, entrapment
    Unconsciousness
    Known inhaled toxin
  Respiratory signs, symptoms
  Facial, cervical burns
  Carbonaceous sputum or purulent
Objective diagnostic tests
  Measurement of asphyxiants (carboxyhemoglobin, cyanide)
  Arterial blood gases (cooximetry)
  Chest roentgenogram
  Direct airway observation (laryngoscopy or nasopharyngoscopy, bronchoscopy)
  Radionuclide scanning
  Pulmonary function testing (Spirometry, complete flow volume curves)

(From Haponik, E. F., and Munster, A. M. (Eds.): Respiratory Injury: Smoke Inhalation and Burns. New York, McGraw-Hill, 1990.)

other objective information. Importantly basic support should not be interrupted or delayed pending results of this evaluation. There are few published reports about the diagnostic yields of many laboratory tests as they relate to specific noxious gases. Perhaps the most extensive body of data is derived from management of large numbers of patients with smoke inhalation.[8] It seems reasonable to extrapolate major principles derived from this experience to develop strategies for evaluating patients with less complex exposures to individual irritant gases. Because these confirmatory diagnostic tests differ in their availability, yields, positive and negative predictive values, levels of complexity, and requirements for technical support, their appropriateness necessarily varies substantially with institutional resources. The diversity of worthwhile studies provides considerable latitude to the clinician, who must define the algorithms most appropriate for his or her center (Table 18–8).

Measurements of toxins or their metabolites in peripheral blood (e.g., as with co-oximetry), arterial blood gas analysis, imaging procedures (including not only chest roentgenograms, but also radionuclide studies), endoscopic visualization of airway patency and the extent of mucosal injury, and objective measurements of respiratory mechanics have valuable, complementary roles. The relative frequencies of abnormalities found on physical examination and such laboratory tests differ considerably among reporting centers. The nature and severity of the acute exposure, the time elapsed until clinical presentation, and the effects of emergency treatment influence the relative frequencies and significance of abnormalities that are detected. Despite a focus on respiratory injury, seeking evidence of other end organ injury is an important priority of the overall evaluation that should not be minimized. For example, an electrocardiogram is a basic test to assess occult myocardial ischemia owing to compromised oxygen delivery. The broad overview of the patient is particularly important in dealing with the inhaled systemic toxins and in excluding coexisting traumatic injuries.

Hematologic Studies

Even the gross appearance of blood may provide helpful information: A blue or chocolate-brown color should suggest mathemoglobinemia. Evidence of intravascular hemolysis might accompany shock-related DIC but should also suggest exposure to arsenicals. Simple measurement of the complete blood count and differential and serum electrolytes provides basic, albeit nonspecific information. Peripheral leukocytosis should not be surprising in the presence of acute inhalation injury alone and does not necessarily connote infection. Serum electrolytes, with measurement of the anion gap, can assist recognition of lactic acidosis. Although this finding might accompany hypoperfusion in a patient with any type of inhalation exposure, toxicity owing to CO or cyanide should be considered especially. Measurements of serum lactate greater than 10 correlated with cyanide intoxication in victims of residential fires. In patients with known hydrogen fluoride exposure, hypocalcemia should be sought and corrected;[11] alternatively the presence of hypocalcemia should suggest exposure to this toxin. Elevated transaminases and renal dysfunction are especially noteworthy with arsenical inhalations but may accompany shock after any severe exposure. Elevations of serum lactic dehydrogenase have been seen in patients with severe phosgene exposures and may occur with severe inhalation injury in other settings.

Co-oximetry adds an especially important dimension to the acute evaluation. Essential to assessment of CO intoxication, this rapidly performed measurement is also worthwhile in documenting elevations of methemoglobin[143] (in persons exposed to smoke or oxides of nitrogen) and sulfhemoglobin (e.g., as following H_2S or severe SO_2 inhalations). Such measurements enhance recognition of threats to tissue oxygen delivery. Most information about asphyxiants derives from experience with CO intoxication, the most common lethal inhalation injury. Although it must be appreciated that arterial COHb measurements do not have the prognostic import assigned to them in the past, they contribute information when interpreted in the context of the time elapsed since the exposure, and whether or not oxygen was administered properly in the field and during transport to the medical facility. Such measurements might also imply that other toxic exposures have occurred. For example, smoke inhalation victims with high COHb levels are also more likely to have inhaled high concentrations of other dangerous gases; elevated COHb levels have correlated with cyanide determination.[144] The impact of CO and other tissue asphyxiants must also be interpreted within the context of the patient's physiologic reserve and, in particular, the presence of coexisting cardiovascular or cerebrovascular disease.

In the past, much emphasis has been placed on relationships between the severity of symptoms, the likelihood of systemic dysfunction, or chronic residual effects to specific arterial COHb measurements, but such relationships have been shown to be unreliable. Far more important is the demonstration of end organ dysfunction following exposure. In this regard, neuropsychologic testing has been clinically valuable in the acute appraisal for neurologic injury. The limitations of widely performed pulse oximetry in this setting must be appreciated. The presence of high COHb levels contributes to overestimates of hemoglobin oxygen saturation determined by this method, whereas methemoglobin elevations lead to underestimates of oxyhemoglobin.[145] A surprisingly large number of physicians also remain unaware that SaO_2 estimated from arterial blood gas analysis (without co-oximetry) does not take into account asphyxiants. These confounding practical problems must be recognized and communicated to avoid serious management errors.

When major discrepancies exist between the apparent results of co-oximetry and the severity of clinical dysfunction after smoke inhalation (as, for example, in the patient who remains comatose despite normalization of COHb levels), alternative explanations (e.g., such as mixed exposures) should be sought vigorously. In this regard, cyanide measurements have been performed more frequently with recently increased appreciation of the role of this toxin in early deaths owing to residential and aircraft fires. As with COHb determinations, ranges of potentially toxic (> 0.1 mg/dl) or lethal (1 to 3 mg/dl) serum levels can be noted, but the extent of organ dysfunction in the exposed patient is the major indicator of injury. Unfortunately, the time delays for such assays (up to 5 hours), accentuated when laboratory personnel perform them infrequently, may limit their timely use. Profound neurologic dysfunction and otherwise unexplained lactic acidosis are among clinical clues to cyanide intoxication.

Rapid analysis of arterial blood gases is available widely. Emphasis should be placed not only on the absolute values of pH, PaO_2 and $PaCO_2$ (with their obvious, immediate implications for management), but also on the degree of inappropriateness for the clinical situation (e.g., as with "normal" $PaCO_2$ measurements in tachypneic, hyperpneic individuals or "normal" PaO_2 measurements in persons receiving high doses of supplemental oxygen). Combined acid/base disturbances are encountered frequently in these patients, who suffer not only respiratory injury, but also acute systemic collapse. Arterial hypoxemia is a common sequela of the ventilation/perfusion mismatch accompanying lung parenchymal injury, frequently preceding obvious chest roentgenographic abnormalities.[146,147] Facility with recognizing a widened alveolar-arterial oxygen gradient and major physiologic shunt is essential to early identification of patients with established alveolar capillary membrane injury. Importantly, normal oxygenation does not establish that severe inhalation injury has not occurred. The delayed onset of hypoxemia is well documented following smoke inhalation injury or exposures to gases with moderate and low water solubility (e.g., oxides of nitrogen). A decreased or absent alveolar-oxygen gradient has been observed with cyanide poisoning and attributed to inability to use oxygen.[17] In addition to their acute diagnostic role, arterial blood gases are essential to appropriate modifications of oxygen therapy and mechanical ventilation throughout the hospital course.

Because of the frequent roles of alcohol and other drugs in many inhalation exposure scenarios, measurements of these substances are important components of acute evaluation. For example, alcohol intoxication has been implicated in about half of unconscious victims of residential fires and is an important cause of industrial accidents. Analyses of urine for offending toxins, illicit drugs, and their metabolites are another component of the early laboratory evaluation. Such information may be important not only in acute management of the patient, but also in subsequent reconstructions of the nature of the accident. Input from the intensivist is often sought in such inquiries as efforts are made to prevent future recurrences and in medicolegal contexts.

To date, no single laboratory test provides a definitive diagnosis of inhalation injury. Recently, however, several potential markers of pulmonary injury have been identified. Although their clinical usefulness requires further clarification, these may provide added insights about mechanisms of damage. Brizio-Molteni and co-workers found elevated serum and BAL angiotensin-converting enzyme ACE activity in a canine model of smoke inhalation and in burned patients with smoke inhalation injury.[148] Serum ACE levels were significantly higher in patients with smoke inhalation and burns in comparison to individuals with surface burns alone.[148] Serum and BAL ACE levels were highest on the initial day after injury and both fell subsequently. In addition, elevations of serum immunoreactive calcitonin, with preferential release of procalcitonin, have been observed in burn patients with inhalation injury.[149-151] These changes, attributed to injury of pulmonary neuroendocrine cells present in the bronchial epithelium, correlated with mortality and with the severity of inhalation injury, as reflected by the need for mechanical ventilation and the extent of shunt-related hypoxemia.[149]

Radiologic Tests

As with arterial blood gas analyses, a normal chest roentgenogram at the time of initial presentation does not exclude significant inhalation injury. A spectrum of radiographic abnormalities has been identified;[152,153] none of these is specific for particular inhaled toxins. Focal opacities might suggest segmental or major atelectasis or, especially in individuals with depressed sensorium, aspiration of gastric contents. Air trapping with marked hyperinflation may accompany severe bronchospasm; at the other extreme, marked restriction of lung capacity may be radiographically obvious. Diffuse bilateral interstitial and alveolar infiltrates should suggest severe inhalation injury, and roentgenographic patterns may strongly suggest a noncardiogenic (permeability) pulmonary edema. As noted previously, ARDS is a nonspecific manifestation after severe exposures to virtually all irritant gases.

As in other critically ill patients, excluding coexisting lung injury sustained at the scene of exposure (e.g., chest trauma) or as a complication of acute management (e.g., pneumothorax following emergency central line placement) confers an added value to chest roentgenograms. The usefulness of serial studies is well documented. Careful analysis of the pattern of roentgenographic abnormality may help to distinguish cardiogenic from noncardiogenic pulmonary edemas, although uncertainties in this area (and efforts to optimize oxygen delivery) frequently require hemodynamic monitoring for more definitive information. Subtle changes in the chest roentgenogram can have a predictive role. In patients with smoke inhalation injury who require fluid resuscitation for coexisting burns, widening of the mediastinal silhouette of the great vessels, the "vascular pedicle," has accurately predicted volume overload and the subsequent onset of alveolar flooding during the first 3 days of management (Fig. 18–6).[154] Such information can assist decisions regarding earlier modifications of fluid resuscitation. Thus, details gleaned from the clinician's personal review of each chest film is an essential component of not only the initial evaluation, but also continuing care.

Radionuclide lung scans have also had worthwhile applications in patients following smoke inhalation injury,[155-157] and far less often, after other inhalation exposures.[158] Because of the similarities in the effects of irritant gases, such lung scans would be expected to have a role, but no large series are available. Inhomogeneous ventilation owing to mechanical and physiologic air flow obstruction is detected readily. Delayed clearance and focal retention of radionuclide (typically xenon) can be an early diagnostic finding, antedating radiographic changes. The integrity of the alveolar capillary membrane as well as the extent of airway disease can be investigated. Increased epithelial permeability has been suggested by abnormalities of technetium-99m (^{99m}Tc) diethylenetriaminepentaacetic acid (DTPA) lung scans in some patients with smoke inhalation, but the practical roles of such scans in "all corners" with inhalation injury have not yet been defined, and this should be regarded as an investigational tool.[113] The requirements for timely availability of radionuclides, technical staff to perform the study, the acuity of patients' respiratory symptoms, the possibility of false-positive abnormal examinations (for example, owing to preexisting lung disease or superimposed aspiration or lung contusion), and the usefulness of alternative, more readily available diagnostic tests have limited the general application of radionuclide scanning.

In a similar regard, chest computed tomography (CT) has demonstrated parenchymal abnormalities as a result of inhalation injury but has not supplanted more immediately available, less costly chest roentgenograms. In carefully selected patients, however, chest CT may be a worthwhile adjunct in evaluating late sequelae of parenchymal injury (as with thin section scans), central airway complications, or superimposed pleural space problems (e.g., empyema). Abdominal CT or ultrasonography may provide important diagnostic information about subdiaphragmatic origins (e.g., concomitant trauma) of atelectasis or pleural effusions.

Endoscopic Procedures

Direct examination of the airway to assess the presence and extent of mucosal injury has been facilitated by relatively noninvasive endoscopic techniques, and all intensivists who manage patients with acute inhalation injury should be proficient in these procedures. When performed by experienced endoscopists in appropriate circumstances, little morbidity has been associated with them. Considerable clinical experience has established the value and safety of fiberoptic nasopharyngoscopy and bronchos-

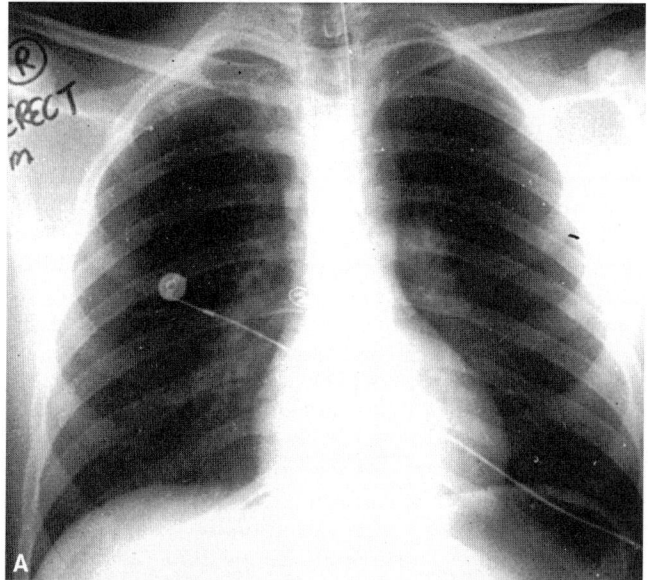
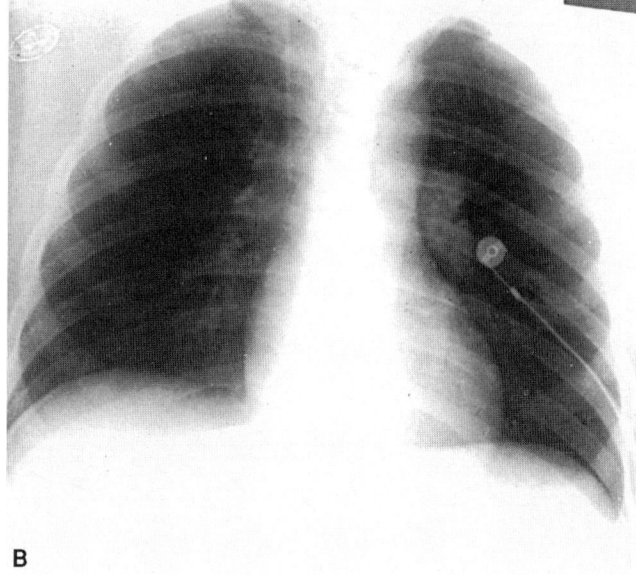
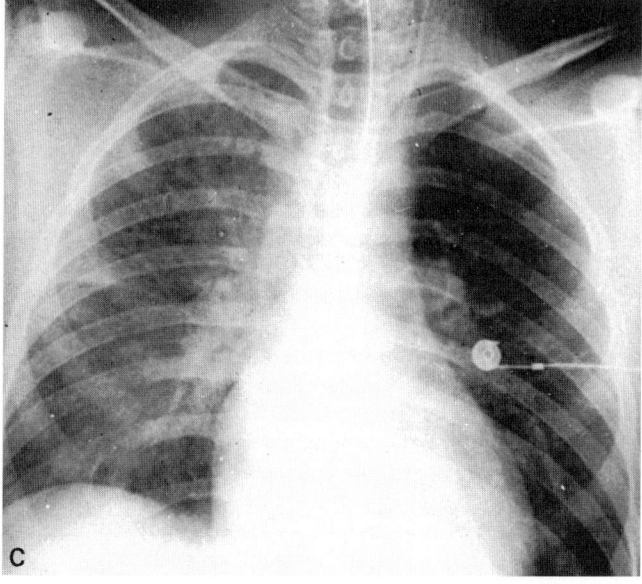

Fig. 18–6. Serial roentgenographic studies provide important diagnostic information. Although this patient with cutaneous burns and smoke inhalation had a normal admission roentgenogram (A), pulmonary edema developed by the third hospital day (C). Widening of the vascular pedicle (B) during the first day of fluid resuscitation indicated increased circulating blood volume, and may antedate frank alveolar flooding. (From Haponik, E. F., et al.: Vascular pedicle widening preceding burn-related pulmonary edema. Chest, 90:649, 1986.)

copy in patients with smoke inhalation.[114,119,121,122,159–161] Although less is written about use of these procedures in other inhalation victims, their potential applications are obvious. Frietag et al. have reported the value of bronchoscopy in acute evaluation of the extent of upper airway injury in victims of mustard gas inhalation.[123,162] In addition, this procedure was helpful in pulmonary toilet and, during subacute and chronic stages of injury, evaluation and management of tracheobronchial stenoses.

Urgent evaluation of the upper airway is especially important because of its immediate implications for decisions about endotracheal intubation. Severe mucosal inflammation, edema, and even ulceration can be seen after inhalation of irritant gases; these changes may be accentuated with coexisting thermal injuries. Especially likely after inhalation of highly water-soluble gases, fulminant upper airway injury can be seen after a severe exposure to virtually any agent. This problem becomes compounded by the presence of upper airway cinders, blistering, and mechanical occlusion by aspirated food or other foreign bodies. Trauma caused by attempts at upper airway management in the field superimposes other anatomic abnormalities readily assessed by this technique.

Experience with patients with smoke inhalation has underscored that the supraglottic mucosa, with its high capacity to swell rapidly with edema fluid, is an especially important site for careful examination.[121,122] Such edematous mucosa prolapses to occlude the airway. Anecdotal experience suggests that the same concerns apply to inhalation victims in other settings. After smoke inhalation, supraglottic damage is generally more severe than infraglottic injury.[8] A completely normal upper airway examination makes severe lower airway damage less likely but, especially in the case of low-solubility gases, does not ensure an uneventful course. The presence of severe upper airway injury should alert the clinician to the increased possibility

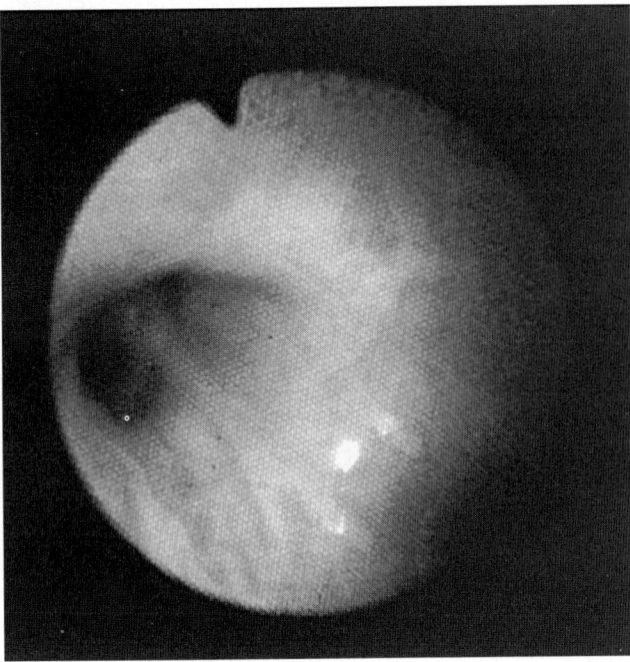

Fig. 18-7. Airway edema and the presence of copious carbonaceous secretions are among the endobronchial manifestations of smoke inhalation injury seen at bronchoscopy, but have only variable relationships with management needs and outcomes.

that tracheobronchial changes will be seen. Tracheobronchial edema, erythema and ulcerations (with or without soot in the presence of smoke inhalation), and extramucosal abnormalities such as copious secretions or blood all may be seen, depending on the degree of inhalation injury (Fig. 18-7).

Bronchoscopic findings have represented the major diagnostic criterion for inhalation injury at some centers, and such objectively documented changes have correlated with increased mortality. Precise gradation of the degree of endobronchial abnormalities or other scoring systems, however, have not consistently predicted the need for mechanical ventilation, the severity of hypoxemia, or prognosis.[160] Thus, it is not established that bronchoscopy must be performed in every patient with inhalation injury. Such examination has little risk for persons already intubated for upper airway obstruction or indications for mechanical ventilation, but it is not clear whether finding endoscopic abnormalities truly adds substantially to management. It should be well appreciated, however, that an obstructed upper airway should not be bypassed solely for purposes of a bronchoscopic assessment of subglottic disease; clearly the airway must be under control first. In this regard, fiberoptic bronchoscopy has had useful applications in assisting difficult intubations in patients with inhalation injury.[163-165] The bronchoscope is used as a stylet over which the endotracheal tube is passed readily, and the acute diagnostic evaluation is merged with timely therapy. Intensivists must be skilled in this technique. At the Baltimore Regional Burn Center, however, we found that therapeutic bronchoscopies were seldom required for either difficult intubations or management of atelectasis.

In selected patients with severe inhalation injuries or major compromise of tracheobronchial clearance, repeated evaluative and therapeutic bronchoscopies may be necessary.[166] Frietag et al. noted that each of their patients required a mean of seven procedures.[162]

Bronchoscopy has also been used to help time extubations in patients with pharyngeal edema, but its value in this application is unclear. In our experience with patients with smoke inhalation, repeat procedures for upper airway assessment provided helpful information contributing to management decisions and were well tolerated by patients. Endoscopic visualization of the endotracheal tube enveloped by swollen mucosa obscuring the glottis suggests that extubation should be deferred, but an apparently patent upper airway and resolving glottic edema does not guarantee safe extubation. Bronchoscopic culture techniques using bronchoalveolar lavage (BAL) or protected catheter brushes have contributed to evaluation of ventilator-associated pneumonia, an important complication of inhalation injury. Philosophies about (and validation of) this procedure vary markedly among centers, and its specific roles in patients with inhalation injury are not established. During later phases of injury, bronchoscopy is useful in evaluation of selected patients for residual tracheobronchial damage (e.g., polyps, subglottic stenosis) causing chronic respiratory limitations.

Fiberoptic bronchoscopy has also had important applications to the investigation of inhalation injury. In numerous animal models, visualization of abnormalities in central airways has provided interesting insights about mechanisms of inhalation injury. BAL has clarified cellular events in more distal airways and lung parenchyma in this setting.[166-168] In one model, the presence of a polymorphonuclear leukocytosis and elevated protein concentrations demonstrated at BAL appeared to be the most sensitive cellular indicator of phosgene inhalation.[10] Initial observations in animals and in humans with smoke inhalation suggest that a polymorphonuclear alveolitis is a component of the early inflammatory events, and its perpetuation appears particularly ominous.[166-168] Lykens and co-workers have shown that such an alveolitis correlated with increased permeability to protein and with clinical outcomes. In addition, desquamation of bronchial epithelial cells can be detected by BAL in patients with smoke inhalation.[45] These changes antedated physiologic and radiologic abnormalities and correlated with worsened prognosis. The diagnostic role of BAL in the routine clinical assessment of patients with injuries due to smoke and other irritant gases requires further clarification. In a carefully standardized ovine model of smoke inhalation, the degree of tracheobronchial hyperemia could be measured objectively with bronchoscopic laser flowmetry and correlated with arterial carboxyhemoglobin levels.[169] Clinical investigations are needed to determine whether this will represent a worthwhile adjunct to bronchoscopic evaluation of humans with inhalation injuries.

Physiologic Measurements

Simple pulmonary function testing with spirometry, peak air flow measurements, and complete flow volume curves appears to provide the most sensitive bedside physiologic indicator of inhalation injury.[8] Such observations should not be surprising in view of the primary mucosal site of injury. In both animal models of inhalation exposure and anecdotal reports in patients, the presence of obstructive or restrictive ventilatory defects has been inferred from timing the duration of each component of the respiratory cycle. Lengthening of expiratory time has been associated with obstructive defects, whereas shortening of both inspiratory and expiratory times has been associated with restriction. A "reflex restriction" of respiration, characterized by rapid shallow breathing, was described by Haldane and co-workers in World War I victims of gas warfare.[10] Obstructive and restrictive ventilatory defects were observed in Bhopal victims who sustained massive exposure to methyl isocyanate, and acute bronchodilator responsiveness was confirmed with such physiologic measurements in some patients.[6] Restrictive and obstructive ventilatory defects are common in smoke inhalation victims.[170] Their severity parallels the clinical course of injury and burn resuscitation. The severity of restriction has correlated with reduced colloid oncotic pressure and fluid administration and may also reflect extrapulmonary factors, such as unyielding chest wall eschars.

Reproducible studies of appropriate quality (sometimes difficult to achieve in this acute situation) often permit demarcation of the relative components of upper and lower airway damage.[121,122,124] In persons with smoke inhalation, the combination of normal spirometry and flow volume curves has an exceedingly high predictive value: Patients with such normal findings are unlikely to require endotracheal intubation for acute upper airway or tracheobronchial injuries.[8] Complete flow volume loops demonstrating patterns of variable or fixed extrathoracic obstruction or reproducible oscillations ("sawtoothing") help to identify patients with upper airway instability noninvasively.[121,122,124] Such abnormalities have correlated with (and often have preceded) endoscopic evidence of evolving, anatomic upper airway obstruction in patients who do not require immediate endotracheal intubations. Serial measurements are quite useful and may guide decisions about management or the need for follow-up bronchoscopy.

These applications, noted for the most part in smoke inhalation victims, should also apply to virtually all patients with irritant gas exposures, but remarkably few data are available. Kamat and co-workers[6] observed similar flow volume curve abnormalities in Bhopal victims: Inspiratory sawtoothing, reduced flow rates at low lung volumes, "doming" of the expiratory loop, and a rectangular configuration to the loop attributed to restrictive ventilatory. Alford and Haponik have identified reduced inspiratory flow rates and loops suggesting variable extrathoracic obstruction after accidental acute SO_2 inhalation.[171] Flow volume curve patterns can help to partition the relative affects of acute inhalation injury on the upper and lower airway, but it must be recognized that because of the effort dependence of peak flow rate measurements and in particular of the inspiratory limb of the loop, assurance of the quality of curves is essential. The severity of illness of patients (who often have depressed sensorium based on neurologic injury or medications) limits the role of such testing after acute inhalation exposures.

More complex monitoring of respiratory mechanics and other parameters might also contribute to early evaluations, but more information is needed. Reduced diffusing capacity has been associated with inhalation injury, but this test is not generally performed in these acutely ill patients. As in individuals with other acute lung injuries in whom increased permeability of the alveolar capillary membrane results in exudation into air spaces, estimates of lung water might provide useful information about the extent of damage.[172,173] Increased thermal volume has correlated with early smoke inhalation injury, and in particular with later onset sepsis-related ARDS, this study has remained an investigative tool.

General Diagnostic Approaches

Strategies incorporating diagnostic tests vary considerably with individual patients' needs and the institutional resources at hand. As in other circumstances, limiting diagnostic investigations to only those that provide sufficient information to guide management decisions (and clearly result in modifications of care) is necessary: Not all studies are indicated for every patient. Basic information derived from co-oximetry, arterial blood gas analyses, the chest roentgenogram, endoscopy, and pulmonary function testing, however; complements that gleaned from the history and physical examination. Pulmonary function tests would appear to have particular usefulness in the triage of large numbers of patients with acute inhalation injury, but the practical application of this strategy has not been documented. For any patient at risk for significant inhalation injury, direct visualization of the upper airway is indicated. Fiberoptic techniques have particular advantage over either the physical examination or the widely performed (and more traumatic) inspection with the laryngoscope. The latter procedure, especially when performed by less experienced individuals, may have great potential for exacerbating upper airway damage. The portability of small fiberoptic endoscopes with compact light sources and simple pulmonary function equipment (e.g., peak flowmeters or spirometers) makes them well suited for the field evaluation of victims in mass disasters, but published information about this strategy is presently unavailable.

Most often, these diagnostic tools are used after the patient's triage to the hospital setting. Generally empiric field management (e.g., intubation of persons with marginal or questionable upper airway status) should not be delayed pending results of hospital-based diagnostic tests. The timely application of these diagnostic procedures imposes considerable demands for an integrated team approach. Advance preparations are essential for dealing with unpredictable, mass casualties so each patient is managed optimally and are especially important for medical centers located in industrial communities, where high intensity, accidental exposures are most likely to occur.

HOSPITAL MANAGEMENT OF INHALATION INJURY

The episodic nature of inhalation injury and the inherent variability of exposures and treatment regimens have con-

Table 18-9. Treatment of Acute Inhalation Injury

Respiratory problem	Therapeutic measure
Asphyxia/systemic toxicity	Oxygenation, antidotes, general support, specific therapy of end organ dysfunction
Airway obstruction	Early, elective endotracheal intubation (rarely, cricothyrotomy or tracheotomy)
Upper airway	Chest physiotherapy (percussion, postural drainage)
Tracheobronchial	Bronchodilators
Mild	(Occasional) therapeutic bronchoscopy
Severe (with hypoventilatory failure)	?Anti-inflammatory agents, mucolytics
Alveolar-capillary membrane injury	
Mild	Supplemental oxygen (e.g., Low F_{IO_2} generally achievable by nasal prongs/mask delivery)
Severe (with hypoxemic respiratory failure)	Oxygenate (High F_{IO_2} ([O_2 via ET tube]) (mechanical ventilation)
	Increase lung volume (CPAP, PEEP)
	? Adjustments of resuscitative fluid volumes, composition, and infusion rates
	?Vasoactive, inotropic drugs
	?Minimize ongoing damage/leak (e.g., experimental use of antioxidants, antiproteases)

founded efforts to define specific therapies directed toward the pathogenesis of respiratory damage. There are numerous anecdotal reports of successfully administered, theoretically attractive innovative treatments to patients with inhalation injuries but little support from controlled investigations. For example, in management of ARDS owing to accidental inhalation of zinc chloride, intravenous and nebulized acetylcysteine were administered in an effort to enhance urinary excretion of zinc, and L-3,4-dehydroproline was given in an effort to arrest pulmonary collagen deposition.[174] For the most part, general supportive approaches validated in other critically ill patients have been applied successfully to victims of inhalation exposures (Table 18-9). Careful neurologic monitoring is essential in all of these patients, but especially after exposure to asphyxiants and other agents with well-recognized neurotoxicty (e.g., hydrocarbons, phosphine, diborane). During the hospital phase, other supportive therapy is administered according to the toxic profile of the agent. For example, hemodialysis and exchange transfusion might be necessary in therapy of arsine intoxication and dialysis used for renal failure in patients with cadmium poisoning.

As in other patients with permeability edemas, philosophies about the optimum approaches to intravenous fluid administration and hemodynamic support continue to evolve and vary considerably among institutions. The relative proportions of crystalloid and colloid vary among resuscitative regimens, with no one combination offering clearly superior outcomes. The hazards of either overresuscitation (with worsened alveolar flooding) or underresuscitation (with failure to meet tissue oxygen needs) are well established.[175-180] Demling and co-workers have reported that oxygen consumption in sheep with small burns becomes oxygen delivery dependent with the addition of smoke inhalation injury.[181] This change occurred despite the absence of hypoxemia or increased lung water and was associated with markedly increased lung lipid peroxidation. Patients with smoke inhalation generally receive approximately 30% more fluid than that predicted based on burn size,[177,178] but limiting fluid to spare the lung may jeopardize perfusion to critical beds.[179,180] Thus, this aspect of management remains highly individualized.

When hypoventilatory respiratory failure complicates inhalation injury, mechanical ventilation using volume ventilators is used as in other circumstances.[8,20,182] Theoretical advantages notwithstanding, the superiority of newer ventilators and ventilatory techniques (e.g., pressure control, inverse ratio modes) in management of patients with inhalation injury has not been proved, nor has it been established that particular strategies result in better outcomes for this population. One investigation in burn patients attributed a lower incidence of pneumonia and higher survival (compared with historical controls) to use of high frequency percussive ventilation,[183] but prospective controlled studies of this issue are not yet available. Neither has the superiority of any one approach to weaning patients from this treatment yet been established; experience with multiple weaning approaches is necessary to design plans optimal for individual patients' needs.

Carefully monitored supplemental oxygen and positive end-expiratory pressure (PEEP) are used as in other settings for management of hypoxemia and has established benefits.[184,185] Despite claims to the contrary,[186] it has not been shown that prophylactic administration of PEEP protects patients with inhalation injury from hypoxemic respiratory failure.

Immediate administration of positive pressure ventilation with PEEP improves survival in sheep with severe smoke inhalation injury and was associated with decreased tracheobronchial cast formation, compared to controls receiving delayed ventilation and PEEP after development of hypoxemia or respiratory distress.[187,188] This therapy did not prevent the development of hypoxia and was associated with increased pleural fluid formation.

In addition to its well-recognized effects on lung volume and recruitment of alveoli, PEEP decreases bronchial blood flow, which, in turn, has been associated with reduced lung edema after smoke inhalation injury. Investigators have speculated that this effect on bronchial hyperemia and airway edema also helps to reduce tracheobronchial cast formation.[189] Follow-up experiments showed that bronchial blood flow was not reduced below normal levels, and focal airway ischemia due to PEEP was unlikely.[190]

The use of venovenous extracorporeal membrane oxygenation (ECMO) has improved survival in sheep with severe smoke inhalation and was associated with reduced peak inspiratory pressure and mechanical ventilator requirements.[191] The role of ECMO in humans with inhalation injury is unknown. The intravascular oxygenator (IVOX) has been used to facilitate gas exchange in animal models of inhalation injury, but it also requires further investigation.

Because mechanical airway clearance is an important priority, chest postural drainage, humidification, and other respiratory care adjuncts are applied as in other settings.[182] Therapeutic bronchoscopy may be required for clearing atelectasis unresponsive to these more conservative measures or when the severity of associated hypoxemia does not allow the time to perform them. There is no present support for therapeutic BAL or intrapulmonary instillation of buffer solutions. The benefits of aerosolized antimicrobials, mucolytics, and expectorants are also undefined, and their use varies with institutional philosophies. Prophylactic antibiotics, widely recommended in the past, are generally not administered because of the hazards of selecting out multidrug-resistant pathogens. The roles of innovative strategies to prevent nosocomial pneumonia have not yet been defined critically in inhalation injury victims.

Despite their widespread administration, there is remarkably little proof of the efficacy of inhaled and systemic bronchodilator therapy in this population. The impact of inhalation injury on central airways, together with anecdotally documented benefits of inhaled anticholinergics (e.g., ipratropium bromide) and beta sympathomimetics, suggests that these agents might be effective, but there is no large published experience documenting this strategy. Inhalation of anticholinergic agent (atropine) and an anti-inflammatory medication (disodium cormoglycate nedocromil) has attenuated the increased airway resistance owing to SO_2 exposure in asthmatics, and the combination of these medications may be especially effective.[10] Whether these observations should be extrapolated to persons with preexisting airways disease and following other acute inhalation injuries requires further study.

The potential value of corticosteroids has represented an especially long-standing, yet unresolved controversy.[192-198] In the presence of cutaneous burns, controlled investigation of persons with smoke inhalation has demonstrated that corticosteroids are associated with an increased mortality and should be avoided.[196] In the absence of burns, however, it is unclear whether a short-term course of therapy would result in improved outcomes. An abbreviated course of corticosteroids might be well tolerated and considered in patients with smoke inhalation alone, but there is no proof of the benefit of this approach. In Las Vegas Hotel fire victims, without burns, outcomes did not differ among steroid-treated and nonsteroid-treated individuals.[197] It has been suggested that steroids might lessen the likelihood of bronchiolitis obliterans, especially that complicating severe exposures to oxides of nitrogen, ammonia, or sulfur dioxide. Interestingly, discontinuation of such treatment has been associated with exacerbations of pulmonary edema owing to oxides of nitrogen; reports of benefits in small series of such patients provide perhaps the strongest arguments for their use. Clearing of severe injuries after inhalation of household cleaners has been attributed to steroids,[198] and anecdotal, memorable reports of good outcomes in individual patients with severe injuries has influenced many clinicians to use an abbreviated course of steroids empirically. At the present time, routine administration of corticosteroids to "all corners" with inhalation injury is not the standard of care but might be considered on an individualized basis (in the absence of major contraindications). There is neither compelling support for nor consensus about this issue, and we have not advocated their general use.

More widely accepted, short-term use of steroids has been reserved for treatment of acute exacerbations of obstructive airways disease triggered by irritant gas exposures or for management of severe bronchospasm unresponsive to bronchodilators. The widely used practice of steroid administration to patients with pharyngeal edema following inhalation injury, especially after failed attempts at endotracheal extubation, is of unknown benefit in this setting. Inhaled corticosteroids might have a role in carefully selected persons who present with very mild initial injuries and may be supported by the efficacy and safety of early anti-inflammatory therapy in the outpatient management of asthmatics. Whether or not airway damage would be helped by such topical therapy in patients who experience severe exposure is an important question. Investigations of these therapeutic issues are needed.

The central role of inflammation in the pathogenesis of inhalation injury has led to considerable interest in other pharmacologic interventions. Encouraging observations of beneficial effects in numerous animal models of inhalation exposures owing to single individual irritant gases have led to proposed roles for antioxidants, free radical scavengers, and other drugs.[199] In some models, pharmacologic administration of antioxidants has had protective effects: Superoxide dismutases, catalase, glutathione, peroxide, glutathione reductases, and allopurinol are of particular interest. Interactions of vitamin E with free radicals or its preferential oxidation by the offending gas (preventing subsequent evolution of lipid peroxides) may influence the course of injury.[10] The role of antioxidant defenses in inhalation injury, particularly in treating patients following such exposures, requires further investigation.

Administration of nebulized dimethysulfoxide (DMSO), a free radical scavenger, has been associated with less severe pulmonary injury, suggesting an important role of oxygen-free radicals in the pulmonary edema due to smoke inhalation.[208] Whether DMSO has a clinical role in patients with inhalation injury has not been established. Experimental smoke inhalation causes increased protease activity in the lung interstitium demonstratable by reductions of antiprotease activity (elastase inhibitory capacity) and immunoreactive alpha$_2$-macroglobulin. Administration of a synthetic antiprotease, gabexate mesilate, has attenuated increased transvascular fluid and protein flux due to smoke and has improved gas exchange.[53]

Heparin has been nebulized into airways in an effort to clear tracheobronchial casts due to smoke.[209] In an ovine model, continuous infusion of heparin reduced cast formation improved oxygenation (with a lower requirement for PEEP) and lessened gravimetrically measured pulmonary edema. The output of thin, yellow, proteinaceous tracheal fluid appeared to increase in animals receiving intravenous heparin. Among many potential mechanisms, it was speculated that heparin may prevent thrombin-mediated microvascular injury, in addition to its more direct effects on airway casts.[209]

Acute smoke inhalation causes deactivation of pulmonary surfactant, but therapeutic administration of exogenous surfactant (Exosurf) in a rabbit model of wood smoke inhalation failed to reduce pulmonary edema, to improve gas exchange or mechanical abnormalities, or to restore surfactant function.[210]

In further evaluation of the sequestration of white cells in the pulmonary circulation, increased attention has been directed toward cytokines and the roles of intercellular adhesion molecules. In one investigation, administration of monoclonal antibody directed toward the CD 18 adhesion complex of PMN failed to ameliorate inhalation injury.[211] Modulation of responses to smoke inhalation by platelet activating factor (PAF) has been suggested by elevated malondialdenhyde levels (in blood and BAL fluid), and increased BAL thromboxane B_2 (TXB_2) levels following smoke inhalation. Administration of a PAF antagonist ameliorated these changes, suggesting that PAF influences inhalational injury by modulating lipid oxygenation.[212] Despite their benefits in individual experiments, the roles of these agents in humans with inhalation injury are unknown.

ACUTE OUTCOMES AND LONG-TERM SEQUELAE

Acute outcomes of inhalation injury vary considerably among reports but show striking parallels to those described with acute respiratory failure of other causes. In addition, the adverse impact of increasing severity of illness reflected in failure of other systems is associated with increased mortality.[213] Because of these relationships, meticulous attention to the details of daily supportive care is essential. The requirement for mechanical ventilatory support for management of inhalation injury in patients with coexisting burns has been associated with extraordinary high mortality.[213,214] The interaction of inhalation injury with superimposed infection has an especially ominous major impact. Smoke inhalation predisposes not only to nosocomial pneumonia, but also has been associated with increased translocation of gut flora and resultant sepsis.[215] In their major review of the experience at Brooke Center, Shirani et al. noted that the presence of inhalation injury increased in burn mortality by 20%, whereas pneumonia independently increased burn mortality by 40%.[216] The combination of these injuries resulted in a 60% increase in deaths. This lethal impact seen in smoke inhalation victims is consistent with classic descriptions of pneumonias superimposed on inhalation injuries caused by chemical warfare.

In experimental models, the severity of inhalation injury has been graded according to the level of mucosal damage. With mild exposures, injury is limited to superficial ciliated epithelium, whereas nonciliated and basal epithelial cells appear spared.[10] After more severe exposures, mature differentiated epithelial cells are damaged as well, but basal cells remain intact. With a yet higher intensity of injury, the entire mucosal layer is affected, exposing the basement membrane. The rapidity of healing relates to the extent of these mucosal changes, ranging from hours to weeks. With more severe damage, the basement membrane becomes disrupted, and protracted time is required for healing. In both animal models and in humans, these direct epithelial effects of irritant gases are accompanied by acute and chronic inflammation with recruitment of fibroblasts resulting in varying degrees of scar.

Table 18-10. Major Sequelae of Inhalation Injury/Management

Subclinical air flow obstruction	Bronchiolitis obliterans
Chronic bronchitis	Pulmonary fibrosis
Tracheal stenosis	Tracheobronchial polyps
Bronchiectasis	Reactive airways distress syndrome
Bronchial stenosis	? Sarcoidosis

Even after massive exposures with development of ARDS, the prognosis of inhalation injury appears to be good, but surprisingly few detailed descriptions of long-term outcomes are available (Table 18-10). Although most patients resolve their acute illnesses with little residual physiologic or functional impairment, a variety of clinical syndromes and varying degrees of residual restrictive or obstructive ventilatory defects may occur.[9-11,217-220] Chronic bronchitis, obstructive and restrictive ventilatory defects, RADS, bronchiectasis, and bronchiolitis obliterans have all been reported after irritant gas injuries.[23] Central airways polyps and tracheal and bronchial stenosis may follow severe exposures. It has been proposed that chronic airway inflammation may lead to bronchial hyperreactivity clinically manifest by RADS.[18] Global respiratory injuries owing to oxides of nitrogen, ammonia and SO_2, and isocyanates appear to have been more often associated with more severe sequelae, but long-term effects could follow any severe exposure. To these problems are added the complications of hospital management (e.g., tracheal damage from endotracheal tubes[221,222] (Fig. 18-8). Although more data are available regarding the effects of chronic, low dose exposures, even single massive inhalations may result in permanently disabling pulmonary disease.

Interestingly, firefighters appear to have an increased risk of dying of nonmalignant respiratory diseases.[223] Recently, the presence of three patients with sarcoidosis among a cohort of firefighters has raised the question of whether smoke inhalation injury, perhaps with superimposed respiratory infection, also predisposes persons to this problem.[224] Elevated serum neopterin levels suggested that firefighters may have an increased risk of T-lymphocyte activation.[224]

PREVENTION OF INHALATION INJURY

Because of the limitations and nonspecificity of most of the treatment for already established inhalation injury and the potential for fatalities and permanent disability even after optimum management, prevention of the exposures that lead to this problem is essential. In patients who have sustained acute inhalation injury, recurrent exposures must generally be avoided because of the unquantitated potential for even more severe respiratory damage. The latter may be especially noteworthy in patients with immunologically mediated injuries, as with trimellitic anhydride

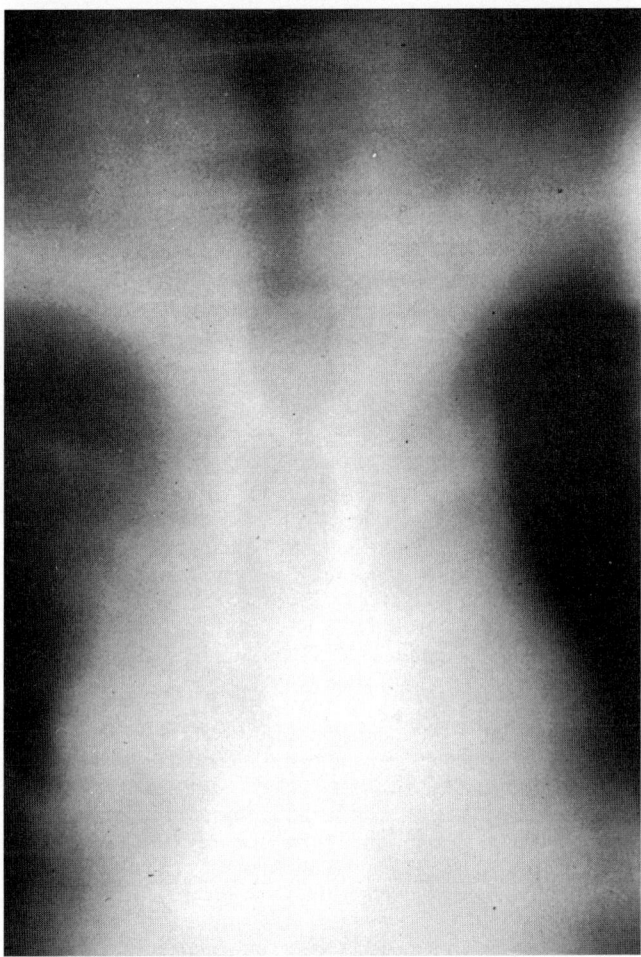

Fig. 18-8. Tracheal stenosis is among the late sequelae of inhalation injury and its management. Prevention of this complication requires particularly close monitoring of the use of endotracheal tubes. (From Colice, G. L., Munster, A., M., and Haponik, E. F.: Tracheal stenosis complicating cutaneous burns: an underestimated problem. Am. Rev. Respir. Dis., *134*:1315, 1986.)

and isocyanates.[18] Do Pico[18] has related such persistent airways hyperresponsiveness to multiple inhalation exposures. Because of uncertainties in those patients who have residual dysfunction after inhalation injury or other coexisting cardiopulmonary disease, avoidance of further exposures is prudent.

Appropriate preventive strategies focus on the ubiquitous risks for inhalation injury and take several forms, including public educational programs, delineation and enforcement of already established industrial safety policies, and design of programs to address newly identified hazards. Such advanced preparation can be exceedingly effective and may range from the routine use of smoke detectors in efforts to avoid the risks of residential fires,[225] appropriate training of farmers about the dangers of entering a silo filled with fresh silage,[95,97,98] education and monitoring of industrial workers' use of protective masks,[9] and homemakers' avoidance of mixtures of bleaches with ammonia-containing and chlorine-containing cleaning compounds, among other considerations.[226-229]

Thus, the responsibilities of the intensive care physician do not end with the expert evaluation and management of inhalation injury victims.[230,231] Levy has addressed these roles of the intensive care physician in the reporting of occupational inhalation hazards and in initiating and promoting preventive measures.[231] Because of his or her central role in the acute assessment and management of patients, the intensive care physician not only has a major function in delineating evaluation and management algorithms, but also must provide input about triage and preventive programs. In the latter role, the time spent as a consultant to industry may provide even greater benefits to large numbers of potential inhalation victims than does the acute care administered to an individual patient after acute exposure. Although time consuming, the importance and potential impact of these educational functions should not be minimized.

In many instances, the exposures leading to serious injuries truly prove to be not only accidental, but also unavoidable. In others, there have been clear breaches of appropriate procedures in dealing with these injurious agents, resulting in avoidable catastrophes. Because of particular knowledge of the nature of the injury and specific details about its effects, the clinician has major roles in investigation of the events surrounding acute inhalations. These activities may have profound social benefits for the community affected by this exposure, as well as for the individual victim of inhalation injury.

REFERENCES

1. Cope, O.: Management of the Cocoanut Grove burns at the Massachusetts General Hospital. Ann. Surg., *117*:801, 1943.
2. Aub, J. C., Pittman, H., and Brues, A. M.: The pulmonary complications: a clinical description. Ann. Surg., *117*:834, 1943.
3. Finland, M., Davidson, C. S., and Levenson, S. M.: Clinical and therapeutic aspects of conflagration injuries to respiratory tract sustained by victims of Cocoanut Grove disaster. Medicine, *25*:215, 1946.
4. Zawacki, B. E., et al.: Smoke, burns, and the natural history of inhalation injury in fire victims: a correlation of experimental and clinical data. Ann. Surg., *185*:100, 1977.
5. Haponik, E. F., and Summer, W. R.: Respiratory complications in burned patients: pathogenesis and spectrum of inhalation injury. J. Crit. Care, *2*:49, 1987.
6. Kamat, S. R., et al.: Early observations on pulmonary changes and clinical morbidity due to the isocyanate gas leak at Bhopal. J. Postgrad. Med., *31*:63, 1985.
7. Clark. W. R., and Nieman, G. F.: Smoke inhalation. Burns, *14*:473, 1988.
8. Haponik, E. F., and Munster, A. M. (eds.): Respiratory Injury: Smoke Inhalation and Burns. New York, McGraw-Hill, 1990.
9. Seaton, H., and Morgan, W. K. C.: Toxic gases and fumes. *In* Occupational Lung Diseases. Edited by W. K. C. Morgan and H. Seaton. Philadelphia, W. B. Saunders, 1975.
10. Loke, J. (Ed.): Pathophysiology and Treatment of Inhalational Injuries. New York, Marcel Dekker, 1988.
11. Wald, P. H., and Balmes, J. R.: Respiratory effects of short-term, high-intensity toxic inhalations: smoke, gases, and fumes. J. Intens. Care Med., *2*:260, 1987.
12. Summer, W., and Haponik, E. F.: Inhalation of irritant gases. Clin. Chest Med., *1*:121, 1987.

13. Ziskind, M. M., Ellithorpe, D. B., and Weill, H.: The relationship of lung disease to air pollutants and noxious gases. *In* Textbook of Pulmonary Disease. Edited by C. L. Baum. Boston, Little, Brown, 1974.
14. Linz, D. H., et al.: Occupational toxic inhalations. Top. Emerg. Med., 7:21, 1985.
15. Schwartz, D. A.: Acute inhalation injury. *In* Occupational Medicine. State Art Rev., 2:297, 1987.
16. Jones, R. N.: Acute and accidental exposures to irritant gases. *In* Pulmonary Diseases and Disorders. Edited by A. P. Fishman. New York, McGraw-Hill, 1980.
17. Kizer, K. W.: Toxic inhalations. Emerg. Med. Clin., 2:649, 1984.
18. do Pico, G. A.: Pulmonary injury from chemicals and gases. Pulm. Clin. Update Am. Coll. Chest Phys., 4:20, 1989.
19. Connor, E. H., DuBois, A. B., and Comroe, J. H., Jr.: Acute chemical injury of the airway and lungs. Experience with six cases. Anesthesiology, 23:538, 1962.
20. Haponik, E. F., and Summer, W. R.: Respiratory complications in burned patients. Diagnosis and management of inhalation injury. J. Crit. Care, 2:121, 1987.
21. Clark, W. F., Bonaventura, M., and Myers, W.: Smoke inhalation and airway management at a regional burn unit. 1974–1983. Part I: Diagnosis and consequences of smoke inhalation. J. Burn Care Rehab., 10:52, 1989.
22. Dressler, D. P.: Laboratory background on smoke inhalation. J. Trauma, 19:913, 1979.
23. Haponik, E. F.: Clinical smoke inhalation: pulmonary effects. Occup. Med., 8:431, 1993.
24. Davies, J. W. L.: Toxic chemicals versus lung tissue—an aspect of inhalation injury revisited. J. Burn Care Rehab., 7:213, 1986.
25. Traber, D. L., Linares, H. A., and Herndon, D. N.: The pathophysiology of inhalation injury—a review. Burns, 14:357, 1988.
26. Man, S. F. P., and Hulbert, W. C.: Airway repair and adaptation to inhalation injury. *In* Pathophysiology and Treatment of Inhalational Injuries. Edited by J. Loke. New York, Marcel Dekker, 1988.
27. Mustafa, M. G., and Tierney, D. F.: Biochemical and metabolic changes in the lung with oxygen, ozone, and nitrogen dioxide toxicity. Am. Rev. Respir. Dis., 118:1061, 1978.
28. Welsh, M. J., Shasky, M., and Husted, R. M.: Oxidants increase paracellular permeability in a cultured epithelial cell line. J. Clin. Invest., 76:1155, 1985.
29. Burns, T. R., Mace, M. L., Greenberg, S. D., and Jachimczyk, J. A.: Ultrastructure of acute ammonia toxicity in the human lung. Am. J. Forensic Med. Pathol., 6:204, 1985.
30. Crapo, J. B., Barry, B. E., Chang, L. Y., and Mercer, R. R.: Alterations in lung structure caused by inhalation of oxidants. J. Toxicol. Environ. Health, 13:301, 1984.
31. Kulle, P. J., et al.: Pulmonary effects of sulfur dioxide and respirable carbon aerosol. Environ. Res., 41:39, 1986.
32. Moritz, A. R., Henriques, F. C., and MacLean, R.: The effects of inhaled heat on the air passages and lungs, an experimental investigation. Am. J. Pathol., 21:311, 1945.
33. Garland, J. S., Rice, T. B., and Kelley, K. J.: Airway burns in an infant following aspiration of microwave-heated tea. Chest, 90:621, 1986.
34. Taylor, R. F., and Bernard, G. R.: Airway complications from free-basing cocaine. Chest, 95:476, 1989.
35. Lykens, M., and Haponik, E. F.: Direct and indirect lung injuries in burned patients. Crit. Care Rep., 2:101, 1990.
36. Kinsella, J.: Smoke inhalation. Burns, 14:269, 1988.
37. Demling, R. H., LaLonde, C., Liu, Y., and Zhu, D.: The lung inflammatory response to thermal injury: relationship between psychologic and histologic changes. Surgery, 106:62, 1989.
38. Loke, J., Paul, E., Virgulto, J. A., and Smith, G. J. W.: Rabbit lung after acute smoke inhalation. Arch. Surg., 119:956, 1984.
39. Till, G. O., et al.: Lipid peroxidation and acute lung injury after thermal trauma to skin. Evidence of a role for hydroxyl radical. Am. J. Pathol., 119:376, 1985.
40. Daryani, R., et al.: Effect of endotoxin and a burn injury on lung and liver lipid peroxidation and catalase activity. J. Trauma, 30:1330, 1990.
41. Till, G. O., et al.: Oxygen radical dependent lung damage following thermal injury of rat skin. J. Trauma, 23:269, 1983.
42. Ward, P. A., Johnson, K. J., and Till, G. O.: Oxygen radicals and microvascular injury of lungs and kidneys. Acta Physiol. Scand., 548:79, 1986.
43. Quinn, D. A., Robinson, D., Jung, W., and Hales, C. A.: Role of sulfidopeptide leukotrienes in synthetic smoke inhalation injury in sheep. Am. J. Phys. Soc., 68:1962, 1990.
44. Youn, Y. K., Lalonde, C., and Demling, R.: Oxidants and the pathophysiology of burn and smoke inhalation injury. Free Radical Biol. Med., 12:409, 1992.
45. Lykens, M. G., Haponik, E. F., Meredith, J. W., and Bass, D. A.: Bronchial epithelial cell damage after inhalation injury: assessment by bronchoalveolar lavage. Chest, 100:12S, 1991.
46. Linares, H. A., Herndon, D. N., and Traber, D. L.: Sequence of morphologic events in experimental smoke inhalation. J. Burn Care Rehab., 10:27, 1989.
47. Herndon, D. H., et al.: The pathophysiology of smoke inhalation in a sheep model. J. Trauma, 24:1044, 1981.
48. Kimura, R., et al.: Increasing duration of smoke exposure induces more severe lung injury in sheep. J. Appl. Physiol., 64:1107, 1988.
49. Basadre, J. O., et al.: The effect of leukocyte depletion on smoke inhalation injury in sheep. Surgery, 104:208, 1988.
50. Stein, M. D., et al.: Production of chemotactic factors and lung cell changes following smoke inhalation in a sheep model. J. Burn Care Rehab., 7:117, 1986.
51. Evans, M. J.: Oxidant gases. Environ. Health Perspect., 55:85, 1984.
52. Traber, D. L., Schlag, G., and Redl Her, L. D.: Pulmonary edema and compliance changes following smoke inhalation. J. Burn Care Rehab., 6:490, 1985.
53. Niehaus, G. D., et al.: Administration of a synthetic antiprotease reduces smoke-induced lung injury. J. Appl. Physiol., 69:694, 1990.
54. Abdi, S., et al.: Inhalation injury to tracheal epithelium in an ovine model of cotton smoke exposure. Am. Rev. Respir. Dis., 142:1436, 1990.
55. Brooks, S. M., Weiss, M. A., and Bernstein, I. L.: Reactive airways dysfunction syndrome (RADS). Chest, 88:375, 1985.
56. Boulet, L. P.: Increases in airway responsiveness following acute exposure to respiratory irritants. Chest, 94:476, 1988.
57. Loke, J., Paul, E., Virgulto, J. A., and Walker-Smith, G. J.: Rabbit lung after acute smoke inhalation. Cellular responses and scanning electron microscopy. Arch. Surg., 119:956, 1984.
58. Haponik, E. F., et al.: Smoke inhalation. Am. Rev. Respir. Dis., 138:1060, 1988.
59. Loke, J., Paul, E., and Virgulto, J.: Smoke exposure chamber and bronchoalveolar lavage as a method for the evaluation of toxicity of pyrolysis and combustion products in laboratory animals. J. Combust. Toxicol., 8:37, 1981.
60. Nieman, G. F., Clark, W. R., Wax, S. D., and Webb, W. R.:

The effect of smoke inhalation on pulmonary surfactant. Ann. Surg., *191:*171, 1980.
61. Robinson, N., et al.: Ventilation and perfusion alterations after smoke inhalation injury. Surgery, *90:*352, 1981.
62. Zikra, B. A., et al.: Smoke and carbon monoxide poisoning in fire victims. J. Trauma, *12:*641, 1972.
63. Strohl, K. P., Feldman, N. T., Saunders, N. A., and O'Connor, N.: Carbon monoxide poisoning in fire victims: a reappraisal of prognosis. J. Trauma, *20:*78, 1980.
64. Stewart, R. D., Stewart, R. S., Stamm, W., and Seelen, R. P.: Rapid estimation of carboxyhemoglobin level in fire fighters. JAMA, *235:*390, 1976.
65. Symington, I. S., et al.: Cyanide exposure in fires. Lancet, *2:*91, 1978.
66. Hall, A. H., and Rumack, B. H.: Clinical toxicology of cyanide. Ann. Emerg. Med., *15:*1067, 1986.
67. Baud, F. J., et al.: Elevated blood cyanide concentrations in victims of smoke inhalation. N. Engl. J. Med., *325:*1761, 1991.
68. Vogel, S. N., Sultan, R. F., and TenEyck, R. P.: Cyanide poisoning. Clin. Toxicol 18:367–383, 1981.
69. Kulig, K.: Cyanide antidotes and fire toxicology. N. Engl. J. Med., *325:*1801, 1991.
70. Berlin, C.: Cyanide poisoning—a challenge. Arch. Intern. Med., *137:*993, 1977.
71. Montague, T. J., and MacNeil, A. R.: Mass ammonia inhalation. Chest, *77:*496, 1980.
72. Levy, D. M., Divertie, M. B., Litzow, T. J., and Henderson, J. W.: Ammonia burns of the face and respiratory tract. JAMA, *190:*873, 1964.
73. Greene, J. B.: A prospective study of pulmonary function abnormality following ammonia burns. Chest, *2:*995, 1987.
74. Walton, M.: Industrial ammonia gassing. Br. J. Ind. Med., *30:*78, 1973.
75. Ward, K., Costello, G. P., and Murray, B.: Acute and long-term pulmonary sequelae of acute ammonia inhalation. Ir. Med. J., *76:*279, 1983.
76. Cloase, L. B., Catlin, F. L., and Cohn, A. M.: Acute and chronic effects of ammonia burns of the respiratory tract. Arch. Otolaryngol., *106:*151, 1980.
77. Woodford, D. M., Coutin, R. E., and Gaensler, E. A.: Obstructive lung disease from acute sulfur dioxide exposure. Respiration, *38:*238, 1979.
78. Charan, N. B., Myers, C. G., Lakshminarayan, M. S., and Spencer, T. M.: Pulmonary injuries associated with acute sulfur dioxide inhalation. Am. Rev. Respir. Dis., *119:*555, 1979.
79. Rom, W. N., et al.: Longitudinal evaluation of pulmonary function in copper smelter workers exposed to sulfur dioxide. Am. Rev. Respir. Dis., *135:*830, 1986.
80. Harkonen, H., Nordman, H., Korhonen, O., and Winblad, I.: Long term effects of exposure to sulfur dioxide. Am. Rev. Respir. Dis., *128:*890, 1983.
81. Braun, J., Stob, H., and Zober, A.: Intoxication following inhalation of hydrogen fluoride. Arch. Toxicol., *56:*50, 1984.
82. Caravat, E. M.: Acute hydrofluric acid exposure. Am. J. Emerg. Med., *6:*143, 1988.
83. Mayer, L., and Guelich, J.: Hydrogen fluoride (HF) inhalation and burns. Arch. Environ. Health, *7:*445, 1963.
84. Jones, R. N., Hughes, J. M., Glindmeyer, H., and Weill, H.: Lung function after acute chlorine exposure. Am. Rev. Respir. Dis., *134:*1190, 1986.
85. Kowitz, T. A., Reba, R. C., Parker, R. T., and Spicer, S. S.: Effects of chlorine gas upon respiratory function. Arch. Environ. Health, *14:*545, 1967.
86. Charan, N. B., Lakshminarayan, S., Myers, G. C., and Smith, D. D.: Effects of accidental chlorine inhalation on pulmonary function. West. J. Med., *143:*333, 1985.
87. Weill, H., George, R., Schwartz, M., Ziskind, M.: Late evaluation of pulmonary function after acute exposure to chlorine gas. Am. Rev. Respir. Dis., *99:*374, 1969.
88. Wood, B. R., Colombo, J. L., and Benson, B. E.: Chlorine inhalation intoxicity from vapors generated by swimming pool chlorinator tablets. Pediatrics, *79:*427, 1987.
89. Diller, W. F., and Zante, R.: A literature review: therapy for phosgene poisoning. Toxicol. Ind. Health, *1:*117, 1985.
90. Wang, Y. T., Lee, L. K., and Poh, S. C.: Phosgene poisoning from a smoke grenade. Eur. J. Respir. Dis., *70:*126, 1987.
91. Everett, E. D., and Overhold, E. L.: Phosgene poisoning. JAMA, *205:*243, 1968.
92. Horvath, E. P., et al.: Nitrogen dioxide-induced pulmonary disease. J. Occup. Med., *20:*103, 1978.
93. Ainslie, G.: Inhalation injuries produced by smoke and nitrogen dioxide. Respir. Med., *87:*169, 1993.
94. Becklake, M. K., Goldman, H. I., Bosman, A., and Freed, C. C.: The long-term effects of exposure to nitrous fumes. Am. Rev. Tuberc., *76:*398, 1967.
95. Lowery, T., and Schuman, L. M.: "Silo-filler's disease"—a syndrome caused by nitrogen dioxide. JAMA, *162:*153, 1956.
96. Robertson, A., Dogson, J., Collings, P., and Seaton, A.: Exposure to oxides of nitrogen: respiratory symptoms and lung function of British coal miners. Br. J. Ind. Med., *41:*214, 1984.
97. Douglas, W. W., Norman, G., Hepper, G., and Colby, T. V.: Silo-filler's disease. Mayo Clin. Proc., *64:*291, 1989.
98. Epler, G. R.: Silo-filler's disease: a new perspective. Mayo Clin. Proc., *64:*368, 1989.
99. Blank, M. L., et al.: Sequential changes in phospholipid composition and synthesis in lungs exposed to nitrogen dioxide. Am. Rev. Respir. Dis., *117:*273, 1978.
100. Guidotti, T. L.: Toxic inhalation of nitrogen dioxide: morphologic and functional changes. Exp. Mol. Pathol., *33:*90, 1980.
101. Ramirez, J., and Dowell, A. R.: Silo filler's disease: nitrogen dioxide induced lung injury—longterm follow-up and review of the literature. Ann. Intern. Med., *74:*569, 1971.
102. Yockey, C. C., Eden, B. M., and Byrd, R. B.: The McConnell missile accident—clinical spectrum of nitrogen dioxide exposure. JAMA, *244:*1221, 1980.
103. Whitcraft, D. D., Bailey, T. D., and Hart, G. B.: Hydrogen sulfide poisoning treated with hyperbaric oxygen. J. Emerg. Med., *3:*23, 1985.
104. Hoidal, C. R., et al.: Hydrogen sulfide poisoning from toxic inhalations of roofing asphalt fumes. Ann. Emerg. Med., *15:*826, 1986.
105. Mack, R. B.: World enough and time—hydrogen sulfide poisoning. N. C. Med. J., *48:*33, 1987.
106. Stine, R. J., Slosberg, B., and Beachman, B. E.: Hydrogen sulfide intoxication—a case report and discussion of treatment. Ann. Intern. Med., *85:*756–758, 1976.
107. Burnett, W. W., King, E. G., Grace, M., and Hall, W. F.: Hydrogen sulfide poisoning: review of five years' experience. Can. Med. Assoc. J., *117:*1277, 1977.
108. Ravizza, A. G., et al.: The treatment of hydrogen sulfide intoxication: hydrogen versus nitrites. Vet. Hum. Toxicol., *24:*241, 1982.
109. Stokinger, H. E.: Ozone toxicology: a review of research and industrial experience. Arch. Environ. Health, *10:*719, 1965.
110. Terrill, J. B., Montgomery, R. R., and Reinhardt, C. F.: Toxic gases from fires. Science, *200:*1343, 1978.

111. Bowes, P. C.: Smoke and toxicity hazards of plastics in fires. Ann. Occup. Hyg., 17:143, 1974.
112. Mueller, E., and Seger, D. L.: Metal fume fever: a review. J. Emerg. Med., 2:271, 1985.
113. Clark, W. F., Grossman, Z. D., Ritter-Hincirik, C., and Warner, F.: Clearance of aerosolized ^{99m}Tc-Diethylenetriamine pent-acetate before and after smoke inhalation. Chest, 94:22, 1988.
114. Moylan, J. A., Adib, K., and Birnbaum, M.: Fiberoptic bronchosocpy following thermal injury. Surg. Gynecol. Obstet., 140:541, 1975.
115. Urbanetti, J. S.: Battlefield chemical inhalation injury. In Pathophysiology and Treatment of Inhalation Injuries. Edited by J. Loke. New York, Marcel Dekker, 1988, p. 281.
116. Skornik, W.: Inhalation toxicity of metal particles and vapors. In Pathophysiology and Treatment of Inhalation Injuries. Edited by J. Loke. New York, Marcel Dekker, 1988.
117. Clark, W. R., Bonaventura, M., and Kellman, R.: Smoke inhalation and airway management at a regional burn unit: 1974 to 1983. II. Airway management. J. Burn Care Rehabil., 11:121, 1990.
118. Isago, T., et al.: Determination of pulmonary microvascular reflection coefficient in sheep in venous occlusion. J. Appl. Physiol., 69:2311, 1990.
119. Barrow, R. E., Morris, S. E., Basadre, J. O., and Herndon, D. N.: Selective permeability changes in the lungs and airways of sheep after toxic smoke inhalation. J. Appl. Physiol., 68:2165, 1990.
120. Isago, T., et al.: Analysis of pulmonary microvascular permeability after smoke inhalation. J. Appl. Physiol., 71:1403, 1991.
121. Haponik, E. F., et al.: Upper airway function in burn patients: correlation of flow volume curves and nasopharyngoscopy. Am. Rev. Respir. Dis., 129:251, 1984.
122. Haponik, E. F., et al.: Acute upper airway injury in burn patients: serial changes of flow-volume curves nasopharyngoscopy. Am. Rev. Respir. Dis., 135:360, 1987.
123. Prakash, U. B. S.: Chemical warfare and bronchoscopy. Chest, 100:1486, 1991.
124. Epstein, B. S., et al.: Comparison of orotracheal intubation with tracheostomy for anesthesia in patients with face and neck burns. Anesth. Analg., 45:352, 1966.
125. Bartlett, R. H., et al.: Acute management of the upper airway in facial burns and smoke inhalation. Arch. Surg., 111:744, 1976.
126. Waymack, J. P., et al.: Acute upper airway obstruction in postburn period. Arch. Surg., 120:104, 1985.
127. Echauser, F. E., Billore, J., Burke, J. F., and Quinby, W. C.: Tracheostomy complicating massive burn injury: a plea for conservatism. Am. J. Surg., 127:418, 1974.
128. Hunt, J. L., Purdue, G. F., and Gumming, T.: Is tracheostomy warranted in the burn patient? Indications and complications. J. Burn Care Rehabil., 7:492, 1986.
129. Haponik, E. F., and Lykens, M. G.: Acute upper airway obstruction in burned patients. Crit. Care Rep., 2:28, 1990.
130. Schwartz, D. E., and Weiner-Kronish, J. P.: Management of the difficult airway. Clin. Chest Med., 12:483, 1991.
131. Tolmie, J. D., Joyce, T. H., and Mitchell, G. D.: Succinylcholine danger in the burned patient. Anesthesiology, 28:467, 1967.
132. Bush, G. H., et al.: Danger of suxamethonium endotracheal intubation in anaesthesia for burns. Br. Med. J., 2:1081, 1962.
133. Jones, W. G., et al.: Tracheostomies in burn patients. Ann. Surg., 209:471, 1989.
134. NHLBI Workshop Summary: Hyperbaric oxygenation therapy. Am. Rev. Respir. Dis., 141:1414, 1989.
135. Gabb, G., and Robin, E. D.: Hyperbaric oxygen. A therapy in search of disease. Chest, 92:1074, 1987.
136. Boutros, A. R., and Hoyt, J. L.: Management of carbon monoxide poisoning in the absence of hyperbaric oxygenation chamber. Crit. Care Med., 4:144, 1976.
137. Raphael, J. C., et al.: Trial of normobaric and hyperbaric oxygen for acute carbon monoxide intoxication. Lancet, 2:414, 1989.
138. Haponik, E. F., and Munster, A. M.: Diagnosis, classification, and impact of inhalation injury. In Respiratory Injury: Smoke Inhalation and Burns. Edited by E. F. Haponik and A. M. Munster. New York, McGraw-Hill, 1990.
139. Phillips, A. W., Tanner, J. W., and Cope, O.: Burn therapy. IV. Respiratory tract damage (an account of the clinical, x-ray and postmortem findings) and the meaning of restlessness. Ann. Surg., 158:799, 1963.
140. Phillips, A. W., and Cope, O.: Burn therapy. III. Beware the facial burn. Ann. Surg., 156:759, 1962.
141. Wroblewski, D. A., and Bower, G. C.: The significance of facial burns in acute smoke inhalation. Crit. Care Med., 7:335, 1979.
142. Leonard, R. B., and Teitelman, U.: Manmade disasters. Crit. Care Clin., 7:293, 1991.
143. Hoffman, R. S., and Sauter, D.: Methemoglobinemia resulting from smoke inhalation. Vet. Hum. Toxicol., 31:168, 1989.
144. Clark, C. J., Campbell, D., and Rein, W. H.: Blood carboxyhaemoglobin and cyanide levels in fire survivors. Lancet, 1:1332, 1981.
145. Barker, S. J., et al.: The effects of carbon monoxide on non-invasive oxygen monitoring. Anesth. Analg., 65:S12, 1986.
146. Luce, E. A., Su, C. T., and Hoopes, J. E.: Alveolar-arterial oxyten gradient in the burn patient. J. Trauma, 16:212, 1976.
147. Hudson, L.: Delayed hypoxemia in smoke inhalation. Clin. Res., 19:191, 1971.
148. Brizio-Molteni, L., et al.: Angiotensin-1-converting enzyme activity as index of pulmonary damage in thermal injury with or without smoke inhalation. Ann. Clin. Lab. Sci., 22:1, 1992.
149. O'Neill, W. J., et al.: Serum calcitonin may be a marker for inhalation injury in burns. J. Burn Care Rehab., 13:605, 1992.
150. Nylen, E. S., et al.: Serum procalcitonin as an index of inhalation injury in burns. Horm. Metab. Res., 24:439, 1992.
151. Becker, K. L., et al.: Hypercalcitonemia in inhalation burn injury: a response of the pulmonary neuroendocrine cell? Anat. Rec., 236:136, 1993.
152. Peitzman, A. B., et al.: Smoke inhalation injury: evaluation of radiographic manifestations and pulmonary dysfunction. J. Trauma, 29:1232, 1989.
153. Teixidor, H. S., Rubin, E., Novick, G. S., and Alonso, D. R.: Smoke inhalation: radiologic manifestations. Radiology, 149:383, 1983.
154. Haponik, E. F., et al.: Vascular pedicle widening preceding burn-related pulmonary edema. Chest, 90:649, 1986.
155. Agee, R. N., et al.: Use of ^{133}xenon in early diagnosis of inhalation injury. J. Trauma, 16:218, 1976.
156. Moylan, J. A., Wilmore, D. W., Moulton, D. E., and Pruit, B. A.: Early diagnosis of inhalation injury using Xenon lung scan. Ann. Surg., 176:477, 1972.
157. Schall, G. L., et al.: Xenon ventilation-perfusion lung scans. The early diagnosis of inhalation injury. JAMA, 140:2442, 1978.
158. Taplin, G. V., Chopra, S., Yanda, R. L., and Elam, D.: Radionuclide lung-imaging procedures in the assessment of injury due to ammonia inhalation. Chest, 698:582, 1976.

159. Clark, C. J., et al.: Respiratory injury in burned patients. The role of flexible bronchoscopy. Anesthesiology, 38:35, 1983.
160. Bingham, H. G., Gallagher, T. J., and Powell, M. D.: Early bronchoscopy as a predictor of ventilatory support for burned patients. J. Trauma, 27:1286, 1987.
161. Hunt, J. L., Agee, R. N., and Pruitt, B. A.: Fiberoptic bronchoscopy in acute inhalation injury. J. Trauma, 27:1286, 1987.
162. Frietag, L., Firusian, N., Stamatis, G., and Greschuchna, D.: The role of bronchoscopy in pulmonary complications due to mustard gas inhalation. Chest, 100:1436, 1991.
163. Schneider, W., Berger, A., Maihnder, P., and Tempak, A.: Diagnostic and therapeutic possibility for fiberoptic bronchoscopy in inhalation injury. Burns, 14:537, 1988.
164. Rogers, S. N., and Benumof, J. L.: New and easy techniques for fiberoptic endoscopy-aided tracheal intubation. Anesthesiology, 59:569, 1983.
165. Lee, K. C., Weedman, D., and Peres, W. J.: Use of fiberoptic bronchoscope to place endotracheal tubes in patients with burned airways: case report. J. Burn Care Rehabil., 7:348, 1986.
166. Clark, C. J., et al.: Role of pulmonary alveolar macrophage activation in acute lung injury after burns and smoke inhalation. Lancet, (2) 872, 1988.
167. Lykens, M. G., Haponik, E. F., Meredith, J. W., and Bass, D. A.: Neutrophil (PMN) sequestration and lung permeability after burn injury: assessment by bronchoalveolar lavage (BAL). Am. Rev. Respir. Dis., 143:A582, 1991.
168. Lykens, M. G., Haponik, E. F., Meredith, S. H., and Bass, D. A.: Survival after acute thermal inhalation injury: clinical and BAL predictors. Am. Rev. Respir. Dis., 145:A417, 1992.
169. Loick, H. M., et al.: Endoscopic laser flowmetry: a valid method for detection and quantitative analysis of inhalation injury. J. Burn Care Rehabil., 12:313, 1991.
170. Whitener, D. R., et al.: Pulmonary function measurement in patients with thermal injury and smoke inhalation. Am. Rev. Respir. Dis., 122:731, 1980.
171. Alford, P. T., and Haponik, E. F.: Clinical and physiologic sequelae of accidental sulfur dioxide inhalation. Unpublished observations, 1993.
172. Tranbaugh, R. F., Lewis, F. R., and Christensen, J. M.: Lung water changes after thermal injury: the effect of crystalloid resuscitation and sepsis. Ann. Surg., 192:479, 1980.
173. Herndon, D. N., et al.: Extravascular lung water changes following smoke inhalation and massive burn injury. Surgery, 102:341, 1987.
174. Hjorts, E., et al.: ARDS after accidental inhalation of zinc chloride smoke. Intensive Care Med., 14:71, 1988.
175. Goodwin, C. W., Dorethy, J., Lam, V., and Pruitt, B. A.: Randomized trial of efficacy of crystalloid and colloid resuscitation on hemodynamic response and lung water following thermal injury. Ann. surg., 197:520, 1983.
176. Clark, W. R., Nieman, G. F., Goyette, D., and Gryzboski, D.: Effects of crystalloid on lung field balance after smoke inhalation. Ann. Surg., 108:56, 1988.
177. Navar, P. D., Affle, J. R., and Warden, G. D.: Effect of inhalation injury on fluid resuscitation requirements after thermal injury. Am. J. Surg., 150:716, 1985.
178. Scheulen, J. J., and Munster, A. M.: The Parkland formula in patients with burns and inhalation injury. J. Trauma, 22:869, 1982.
179. Dries, D. J., and Waxman, K.: Adequate resuscitation of burn patients may not be measured by urine output and vital signs. Crit. Care Med., 19:327, 1991.
180. Waxman, K.: Toward a re-evaluation of burn resuscitation. Crit. Care Med., 17:1077, 1989.
181. Demling, R. H., Knox, J., Youn, Y. K., and Lalonde, C.: Oxygen consumption early postburn becomes oxygen delivery dependent with the addition of smoke inhalation injury. J. Trauma, 32:593, 1992.
182. Haponik, E. F.: Smoke inhalation injury: some priorities for respiratory care professionals. Resp. Care, 37:609, 1992.
183. Cioffi, W. G., et al.: Prophylactic use of high-frequency percussive ventilation in patients with inhalation injury. Ann. Surg., 213:575, 1991.
184. Davies, L. K., Poulton, T. J., and Modell, J. H.: Continuous positive airway pressure is beneficial in the treatment of smoke inhalation. Crit. Care Med., 11:726, 1983.
185. Jin, L. J., Lalonde, C., and Demling, R. H.: Effect of anesthesia and positive pressure ventilation on early postburn hemodynamic instability. J. Trauma, 26:26, 1986.
186. Venus, B., et al.: Prophylactic intubation and continuous positive airway pressure in the management of inhalation injury in burn victims. Crit. Care Med., 9:519, 1981.
187. Herndon, D. N., Adams, T., Traber, L. D., and Traber, D. L.: Inhalation injury and positive pressure ventilation in a sheep model. Circ. Shock, 12:107, 1984.
188. Cox, C. X., et al.: Immediate positive pressure ventilation with positive end-expiratory pressure (PEEP) improves survival in ovine smoke inhalation injury. J. Trauma, 6:821, 1992.
189. Salahadin, A., et al.: Bronchial blood flow reduction with positive end-expiratory pressure after acute lung injury in sheep. Crit. Care Med., 18:1152, 1990.
190. Stothert, J. C., Traber, L., and Traber, D.: Does positive end-expiratory pressure significantly reduce airway blood flow? J. Trauma, 35:437, 1993.
191. Brown, M., et al.: The use of venovenous extracorporeal membrane oxygenation in sheep receiving severe smoke inhalation injury. Burns, 13:34, 1987.
192. Skornik, W. A., and Dressler, D.: The effects of short-term steroid therapy on lung bacterial clearance and survival in animals. Ann. Surg., 179:415, 1974.
193. Dressler, D. P., Skornik, W. A., and Kupersmith, S.: Corticosteroid treatment of experimental smoke inhalation. Ann. Surg., 183:46, 1975.
194. Welch, G. W., et al.: The use of steroids in inhalation injury. Surg. Gynecol. Obstet., 145:539, 1977.
195. Levine, B. A., et al.: Prospective trials of dexamethasone and aerosolized gentamicin in the treatment of inhalation injury in the burned patient. J. Trauma, 18:188, 1978.
196. Moylan, J. A.: Diagnostic technique and steroids. J. Trauma, 19:917, 1979.
197. Robinson, N. B., et al.: Steroid therapy following isolated smoke inhalation injury. J. Trauma, 22:876, 1982.
198. Chester, E. H., Kaimal, P. J., Payne, C. B., Jr., and Kohn, P. M.: Pulmonary injury following exposure to chlorine gas. Possible beneficial effects of steroid treatment. Chest, 72:247, 1977.
199. Stewart, R. J., et al.: Effects of ibuprofen on pulmonary edema in an animal smoke inhalation model. Burns, 16:409, 1990.
200. Kimura, R., et al.: Ibuprofen reduces the lung lymph flow changes associated with inhalation injury. Circ. Shock, 24:183, 1988.
201. Shinozawa, Y., et al.: Ibuprofen prevents synthetic smoke-induced pulmonary edema. Am. Rev. Respir. Dis., 134:1145, 1986.
202. Thomson, P. D., et al.: Superoxide dismutase prevents lipid peroxidation in burned patients. Burns, 16:406, 1990.
203. Desai, M. H., et al.: Reduction of smoke-induced lung injury with dimethysulfoxide and heparin treatment. Surg. Forum, 36:103, 1985.

204. Desai, M. H., et al.: Nebulization treatment of smoke inhalation injury in sheep model with dimethylsulfoxide, heparin combination and Nacetylcysteine. Crit. Care Med., *14:*321, 1986.
205. Ryozo, K., et al.: Treatment of smoke-induced pulmonary injury with nebulized Dimethylsulfoxide. Circ. Shock, *25:*333, 1988.
206. Brown, M., et al.: Dimethylsulfoxide with heparin in the treatment of smoke inhalation injury. J. Burn Care Rehab., *9:*22, 1988.
207. Demling, R., et al.: Fluid resuscitation with deferoxamine prevents systemic burn-induced oxidant injury. J. Trauma, *31:*583, 1991.
208. Kimura, R., et al.: Treatment of smoke-induced pulmonary injury with nebulized dimethylsulfoxide. Circ. Shock, *25:*333, 1988.
209. Cox, C. S., et al.: Heparin improves oxygenation and minimizes barotrauma after severe smoke inhalation in an ovine model. Surg. Gynecol. Obstet., *176:*339, 1988.
210. Feldbaum, D. M., et al.: Exosurf treatment following wood smoke inhalation. Burns, *5:*396, 1993.
211. Guna, S. C., et al.: Is the CD18 adhesion complex of polymorphonuclear leukocytes involved in smoke-induced lung damage? A morphometric study. J. Burn Care Rehab., *14:*503, 1993.
212. Ikeuchi, H., et al. The effects of platelet-activating factor (PAF) and a PAF antagonist (CV-3988) on smoke inhalation injury in an ovine model. J. Trauma, *32:*344, 1992.
213. Marshall, W. G., Jr., and Dimick, A. R.: The natural history of major burns with multiple subsystem failure. J. Trauma, *23:*102, 1983.
214. Thompson, P. B., Herndon, D. N., Traber, D. L., and Abstron, S.: Effect on mortality of inhalation injury. J. Trauma, *26:*163, 1986.
215. Morris, S. E., Navaratram, N., and Herndon, D. N.: A comparison of effects of thermal injury and smoke inhalation on bacterial translocation. J. Trauma, *30:*639, 1990.
216. Shirani, K. Z., Pruitt, B. A., and Mason, A. D.: The influence of inhalation injury and pneumonia on burn mortality. Ann. Surg., *205:*82, 1987.
217. Winternitz, W.: Chronic lesions of the respiratory tract initiated by inhalation of irritant gases. JAMA, *73:*689, 1919.
218. Williams, D. O., Vanecko, R. M., and Glassroth, J.: Endobronchial polyposis following smoke inhalation. Chest, *84:*774, 1983.
219. Perez-Guerra, F., Walsh, R. E., and Sagel, S. S.: Bronchiolitis obliterans and tracheal stenosis: late complications of inhalation burn. JAMA, *218:*1568, 1971.
220. Kass, I., Zamel, N., Dobry, C. A., and Holzer, M.: Bronchiectasis following ammonia burns of the respiratory tract. Chest, *62:*282, 1972.
221. Lund, T., et al.: Upper airway sequelae in burn patients requiring endotracheal intubation or tracheostomy. Ann. Surg., *201:*374, 1985.
222. Colice, G. L., Munster, A. M., and Haponik, E. F.: Tracheal stenosis complicating cutaneous burns: an underestimated problem. Am. Rev. Respir. Dis., *134:*1315, 1986.
223. Rosenstock, L., Demers, P., Heyer, N. J., and Barnhart, S.: Respiratory mortality among firefighters. Br. J. Indust. Med., *47:*462, 1990.
224. Kern, D. G,. Neill, M. A., Wrenn, D. S., and Varone, J. C.: Investigation of a unique time-spaced cluster of sarcoidosis in firefighters. Am. Rev. Respir. Dis., *148:*974, 1993.
225. Council on Scientific Affairs, American Medical Assocation: Preventing death and injury from fires with automatic sprinklers and smoke detectors. JAMA, *257:*1618, 1987.
226. Reisz, G. R., and Gammon, R. S.: Toxic pneumonitis from mixing household cleaners. Chest, *89:*49, 1986.
227. Murphy, D. M. F., Fairman, R. P., Lapp, N. L., and Morgan, W. K. C.: Severe airway disease due to inhalation of fumes from cleansing agents. Chest, *69:*372, 1976.
228. Gapany-Gapanavicius, M., Molho, M., and Tirosh, M.: Chloramine-induced pneumonitis from mixing household cleaning agents. Br. Med. J., *185:*1086, 1985.
229. Zanen, A. L., and Rietveld: Inhalation trauma due to overheating in a microwave oven. Thorax, *48:*300, 1993.
230. Himmelstein, J. S., and Frumkin, H.: The right to know about toxic exposures. Implications for physicians. N. Engl. J. Med., *312:*687, 1985.
231. Levy, B. S.: Acute toxic inhalations: beyond treatment. J. Intensive Care Med., *2:*239, 1987.

Chapter 19

LIFE-THREATENING PULMONARY HEMORRHAGE

JAMES W. LEATHERMAN
CONRAD IBER

There are two fundamentally different ways in which life-threatening pulmonary hemorrhage occurs. First, massive hemoptysis that originates from a focal bleeding source (focal pulmonary hemorrhage [FPH]), may overwhelm the patient's ability to clear the airway, leading to death by drowning in one's own blood. Second, diffuse alveolar hemorrhage (DAH) owing to widespread bleeding from the pulmonary microvasculature can result in extensive areas of blood-filled alveoli, with a clinical and roentgenographic pattern similar to adult respiratory distress syndrome (ARDS). Although FPH and DAH share the common feature of massive bleeding that originates downstream from the larynx, they differ with respect to underlying cause, diagnostic evaluation, and therapeutic approach. Familiarity with these two conditions is important for several reasons. First, respiratory failure in some cases may be prevented by early recognition and treatment of the underlying disorder responsible for lung hemorrhage, before bleeding becomes life-threatening. Second, the diagnostic approach to massive hemoptysis and DAH is different from that used for other causes of acute respiratory failure. Finally, appropriate treatment of life-threatening pulmonary hemorrhage is often rewarded by a better outcome than with other catastrophic pulmonary disorders.

DIFFUSE ALVEOLAR HEMORRHAGE

The term DAH refers to widespread bleeding that originates in the pulmonary microvasculature, resulting in large regions of confluent blood-filled alveoli.[1] Many different disorders have been associated with DAH (Table 19-1). High pulmonary venous pressure, coagulopathies, drugs, leukemia, vascular tumors, bone marrow transplantation, infections, and a variety of airborne or intravascular insults to the pulmonary capillary bed may on occasion result in sufficient bleeding that the clinicopathologic features are essentially those of DAH.[2-18] DAH, however, is most often due to one of several disorders that are believed to have an immunopathogenesis.[19] This chapter focuses primarily on immune DAH, but nonimmune disorders are also discussed in relationship to the diagnostic steps required in the evaluation of a patient who presents with suspected DAH.

The fundamental process involved in DAH, regardless of the underlying cause, is frank bleeding from multiple microvascular sites within the acinar portion of the lung. Because nearly all severe pulmonary insults may give rise to some bleeding into alveoli, DAH is distinguished clinically and pathologically from other more common alveolar filling disorders by the *degree* of hemorrhage. In other alveolar filling disorders (e.g., hydrostatic pulmonary edema, ARDS, pneumonia), frank widespread hemorrhage is unusual and is rarely the predominant cause of alveolar filling. With DAH, there is pure hemorrhage resulting in truly blood-filled alveoli.

Pre-ICU Phase

Clinical and Roentgenographic Features of Diffuse Alveolar Hemorrhage

Although DAH occasionally presents with fulminant respiratory failure, more often there is a preceding period during which the patient is seen in the outpatient clinic or on the hospital ward with one or more of the four cardinal manifestations of DAH:

- Hemoptysis
- Alveolar shadowing on chest radiograph
- Anemia
- Dyspnea with hypoxemia

Hemoptysis is a presenting symptom in many cases of DAH. Although occasionally absent,[20] hemoptysis occurs in the majority of cases of immune DAH. Because bleeding originates distal to the terminal airways, however, extensive DAH may give rise to a relatively small amount of hemoptysis, and massive hemoptysis (> 500 ml/24 hours) is unusual. An equivalent amount of intrapulmonary bleeding typically leads to much less hemoptysis when the bleeding is diffuse than when bleeding arises from the airway or a focal inflammatory parenchymal lesion.

With certain types of DAH, hemoptysis is distinctly uncommon.[10,17,18] For example, hemoptysis is virtually never a feature of DAH related to autologous bone marrow transplantation (BMT).[17] The reason that hemoptysis occurs more often in immune DAH than after autologous BMT may be a matter of case definition. Immune DAH is usually recognized clinically by the triad of hemoptysis, alveolar shadows on x-ray film, and a fall in serum hemoglobin that occurs in the clinical setting of a systemic immunologic disorder (see later). This may result in detection of relatively more severe degrees of intra-alveolar bleeding, with

Table 19–1. Causes of Immune/Idiopathic Diffuse Alveolar Hemorrhage

Antibasement membrane antibody disease
Systemic vasculitides/collagen vascular diseases
    Wegener's granulomatosus
    Nonspecific systemic necrotizing vasculitis, "overlap vasculitis" (includes "microscopic polyarteritis")
    Systemic lupus erythematosus
    Henoch-Schönlein syndrome
    Behçet's disease
    Essential mixed cryoglobulinemia
    Rheumatoid arthritis
    Progressive systemic sclerosis
    Mixed connective tissue disease
Alveolar hemorrhage and glomerulonephritis unrelated to antibasement membrane antibody disease, vasculitis, or collagen vascular disease
    Thrombotic thrombocytopenic purpura
    Membranoproliferative glomerulonephritis
    IgA nephropathy
    Diffuse endocapillary proliferative glomerulonephritis
    Focal proliferative glomerulonephritis
Alveolar hemorrhage due to drugs or chemicals
    D-penicillamine
    Trimellitic anhydride
    Isocyanates
    Nitrofurantoin
Idiopathic pulmonary hemosiderosis

less severe episodes that are unaccompanied by hemoptysis or a fall in hemoglobin going unrecognized. In contrast, DAH in the immunocompromised host and after autologous BMT has been defined by bronchoalveolar lavage (BAL) criteria that may permit detection of less extensive intraalveolar hemorrhage.[15-18] In one series, none of the four patients who had BAL-defined DAH related to autologous BMT had a change in hemoglobin level, despite the uniform presence of dyspnea, hypoxemia, and diffuse consolidation on chest roentgenogram and need for mechanical ventilatory support in two cases.[18] This would indicate that the alveolar filling process could not have been "pure" hemorrhage, as is generally the case with immune DAH.

A variety of roentgenographic patterns may be seen during active DAH.[21] With mild DAH, the chest radiograph may show one or more focal areas of alveolar shadowing, in which case infection may be suspected. It is not uncommon for patients with DAH to receive one or more empiric courses of antibiotics for presumed pneumonia before a correct diagnosis is made. In contrast to pneumonia, DAH does not respect fissures, and thus an exquisitely lobar distribution favors infection. No other single roentgenographic criterion is particularly helpful in differentiating DAH and pneumonia, but serial films may be helpful. The resolution of DAH, either spontaneously or in response to therapy, tends to occur over a few days up to a couple of weeks, depending in part on the extent of alveolar bleeding. This rate of resolution is much faster than would be expected if infection were responsible for the alveolar infiltrates. An even more common radiographic differential diagnosis is DAH versus hydrostatic pulmonary edema or ARDS because DAH is usually bilateral and often symmetric. Central vascular congestion or Kerly B lines suggest that hydrostatic pulmonary edema rather than DAH occurs in the setting of rapidly progressive glomerulonephritis. Again observation of changes on serial films may be useful. Complete clearing over 24 to 48 hours in response to diuresis or dialysis suggests hydrostatic pulmonary edema rather than DAH. In brief, several roentgenograms are of much greater value than single films in differentiating DAH from other disorders.

As is the case with the chest roentgenogram, serial observations of serum hemoglobin are of greater diagnostic utility than individual values. Moderate to severe DAH is associated with a concomitant reduction in serum hemoglobin because of acute blood loss into the lungs. In the appropriate clinical setting (e.g., acute glomerulonephritis), progressive alveolar shadowing on chest film that is accompanied by a significant fall in hemoglobin (usually ≥2 g/dl) is suggestive of DAH, provided that other causes of acute blood loss and hemolysis are excluded. Conversely, a stable hemoglobin in the face of major roentgenographic progression is not consistent with a diagnosis of immune DAH because frank hemorrhage sufficient to cause widespread alveolar shadows would not occur without a change in hemoglobin. Chronic blood loss into the lung may lead to iron deficiency anemia because the hemoglobin-bound iron that enters alveoli is not effectively reused for erythropoiesis.

Dyspnea and hypoxemia occur at some point during the course of DAH in the majority of cases. When DAH is sufficiently severe to cause overt or impending acute respiratory failure, the patient is transferred to the ICU and enters the ICU phase of the disease process (see later).

Diagnostic Approach to Suspected Diffuse Alveolar Hemorrhage

In approaching a patient with suspected DAH, it is helpful to consider the following questions: How convincing is the evidence that frank hemorrhage is indeed the cause of alveolar filling seen on chest film? If the evidence for DAH seems convincing, does the patient have defined risk factors that can lead to frank alveolar bleeding, such as elevated pulmonary venous pressure, coagulopathy, acute leukemia, or prior autologous BMT? Does the clinical setting suggest a multisystem immune disorder?

Defining the Presence of Diffuse Alveolar Hemorrhage. A diagnosis of DAH is usually first considered because of the coexistence of unexplained infiltrates with hemoptysis or anemia. In immune disorders, the full triad of hemoptysis, alveolar infiltrates, and anemia is observed in most cases but is of course not specific for DAH. For instance, a patient could have hemoptysis and infiltrates on chest radiograph owing to a variety of common pulmonary insults and be anemic for a different reason. It is therefore necessary to determine whether the alveolar filling process actually represents frank hemorrhage. As noted earlier, a marked fall in hemoglobin coincident with frank hemoptysis and progressive alveolar infiltrates may be sufficient for a diagnosis of DAH, provided that there is convincing clinicopathologic evidence for one of the underlying immune disorders known to cause DAH, and other more common pulmonary disorders do not appear to be likely. More often, some uncertainty exists about the nature of the alveolar filling process, and additional tests are indicated. The presence of blood-filled alveoli can be diagnosed by BAL,[15-17] by measurement of the diffusing capacity for carbon monoxide (DLCO),[21-24] and by lung biopsy.[1]

BAL in the setting of DAH typically reveals a blood lavage effluent and hemosiderin-laden macrophages. The latter are important because they indicate that bleeding did not occur as a result of the procedure itself. (Nonetheless, rare patients do not for some reason, demonstrate abundant hemosiderin in macrophages, despite otherwise convincing clinicopathologic evidence of DAH.) A study involving DAH in the setting of autologous BMT found that the initial BAL aliquot was often clear but that subsequent aliquots were blood by gross visual inspection.[17] With immune DAH, the bronchoscopic findings are often less subtle. Not only is the lavage effluent generally bloody throughout, but also before lavage the bronchoscopist often sees blood welling up from numerous subsegmental bronchi. In less severe cases of immune DAH, the bronchoscopic findings could be less obvious. It would be difficult, however, to attribute an alveolar filling process to DAH if the BAL in an appropriate area showed neither a bloody effluent nor abundant hemosiderin-laden macrophages. A false-positive lavage may occur if bleeding is induced from scope trauma during the procedure and Prussian-blue positive deposits related to smoking are attributed to prior alveolar bleeding.[25] Travis and colleagues have compared the staining pattern of macrophages in smokers with those due to prior DAH.[1] Smoker's macrophages may contain a finely granular brown pigment that stains positively with Prussian blue but tends to be relatively faint. In contrast, iron pigment from prior DAH is usually coarsely granular and stains strongly positive with Prussian blue.[1] Because of the preceding considerations, bronchoscopy with BAL should be viewed as a useful adjunctive diagnostic tool in evaluating patients with suspected DAH, especially because it also provides for visual inspection of the airway to exclude a focal bleeding source and material for culture and special stains to exclude infection. Reliance on BAL findings as the sole diagnostic criteria for DAH, however, without correlation to the entire clinical picture is not advisable.

A second way to confirm the presence of blood-filled alveoli is by measuring the DLCO. With fresh (<48 hours) bleeding into alveoli, extravascular erythrocytes bind CO, thereby resulting in higher DLCO than would otherwise be expected.[21-24] A DLCO that is 1.3 times the baseline value or greater (or a single value in excess of 130% of predicted) would suggest recent DAH.[24] Values that are two to three times the predicted DLCO can be observed.

Finally, open lung biopsy can be used to confirm the presence of DAH.[1] Although open lung biopsy may occasionally be indicated, especially if the differential diagnosis centers primarily on DAH versus opportunistic infection, the use of careful clinical assessment, DLCO, and bronchoscopy with BAL relegates open lung biopsy to a relatively minor role in the evaluation of suspected DAH. If lung biopsy is undertaken, an open rather than transbronchial approach is recommended. The latter may lead to sampling error, insufficient material to define the presence of capillaritis (see later) and for immunofluorescence, and problems with differentiating preexisting hemorrhage from bleeding caused by the procedure.

Diffuse Alveolar Hemorrhage: Immune or Not Immune? Establishing the presence of DAH does not prove that the patient has an underlying immune disorder. Many nonimmune pulmonary insults can also lead to substantial alveolar bleeding. Furthermore, patients with an underlying immune disorder can bleed into their lungs as a result of intercurrent nonimmune insults. Thus it is imperative that all known causes of DAH be considered and excluded, to the extent possible, before accepting that DAH is immune mediated. Differentiation of DAH from cardiographic pulmonary edema and ARDS as the cause of acute respiratory failure is discussed later (see under ICU Phase). Most other causes of DAH are suspected because of the clinical setting. A special problem, however, is presented by the occurrence of DAH in the setting of acute leukemia or following BMT.[10,15,17,18] DAH can occur with acute leukemia and autologous BMT in the absence of infection.[10,17] Infection must always be excluded, however, (generally by BAL) because of the propensity for these immunocompromised patients to develop angioinvasive infections that could lead to substantial hemorrhage, particularly when coagulation parameters are abnormal.[15] The approach to the immunocompromised patient with pneumonia is discussed elsewhere (see Chap. 22).

Immune Diffuse Alveolar Hemorrhage. The immune disorders that cause DAH are for the most part systemic diseases that typically cause glomerulonephritis but may also involve extrarenal organs.[19,24,26-28] Isolated DAH occurs in idiopathic pulmonary hemosiderosis and occasionally as an early manifestation of antibasement membrane antibody (ABMA) disease, systemic lupus erythematosus (SLE), or systemic necrotizing vasculitis. In the great majority of cases, however, there is evidence of glomerulonephritis, sometimes with extrarenal features of vasculitis, at the time of initial presentation with DAH.[10] A physical examination that detects extrarenal vasculitis (e.g., palpable purpura, mononeuritis multiple) or a urinalysis that suggests glomerulonephritis may provide the initial clue to a diagnosis of immune DAH. The urinalysis is particularly helpful because the great majority of patients with immune-related DAH have microscopic hematuria, and a glomerular origin of bleeding may be indicated by the presence of deformed red blood cells under the microscope.[29]

Diagnosis of Origin of Immune Diffuse Alveolar Hemorrhage. Diagnosis of the specific cause of immune-related DAH is established by renal biopsy and serology (Table 19–2). Immune-related DAH is usually due to ABMA disease, SLE, Wegener's granulomatosis, or a nonspecific systemic necrotizing vasculitis.[19] In ABMA disease, there is no involvement of organs other than the lungs or kidneys.[24] Renal histopathology is variable but there is a characteristic immunofluorescent pattern of intense linear staining of glomerulus for IgG.[30] This linear pattern represents deposition of ABMA along glomerular capillaries and is the hallmark of ABMA-mediated glomerulonephritis. The presence of circulating ABMA is reliably confirmed by radioimmunoassay (RIA) or by enzyme-linked immunosorbent assay (ELISA). Both types of assay for ABMA have sensitivities and specificities exceeding 90%.[31,32] Indirect

Table 19–2. Differential Diagnosis of the Major Causes of Immune/Idiopathic Alveolar Hemorrhage

Disorder	Extrapulmonary Features	Serology	Glomerular Pathology Histopathology	Glomerular Pathology IF/EM	Essential Diagnostic Criteria
ABMA disease	GN >90% Extrarenal disease rare	+ ABMA	Variable-segmental necrosis, crescents common	Linear IgG by IF	+ Serum ABMA Linear IgG in glomeruli
SLE	GN >90% Extrarenal disease common (e.g., arthritis, serositis, purpura, photosensitivity)	+ ANA	Variable-segmental necrosis, crescents in minority	Granular IgG by IF, electron dense deposits by EM	Clinical features, +ANA, immune complexes in glomeruli by IF, EM
WG	GN >90% Extrarenal disease Distinctive—upper airway disease, pulmonary nodules Nonspecific (e.g., arthritis, purpura, mononeuropathy)	+ ANCA	Segmental necrosis, crescents	Negative (granular IF in minority)	Necrotizing granulomatous vasculitis in upper airway or lung biopsy or Pauci-immune necrotizing GN with extensive upper airway disease or cavitary lung nodules
Nonspecific systemic necrotizing vasculitis (microscopic polyarteritis, polyangiitis, overlap syndrome)	GN >90% Extrarenal disease variably present (e.g., arthritis, purpura, mononeuropathy)	± ANCA (usually + if include p-ANCA)	Segmental necrosis, crescents	Negative (granular IF in minority)	Necrotizing, crescentic GN (or pathologic evidence vasculitis elsewhere) and exclude WG to extent possible
Idiopathic pulmonary hemosiderosis	None	None	Normal		Exclusion all other causes

IF, Immunofluorescence; EM, electron microscopy; ABMA, antibasement membrane antibody; SLE, systemic lupus erythematosus; WG, Wegener's granulomatosis; GN, glomerulonephritis; ANA, antinuclear antibody; ANCA, antineutrophil cytoplasmic antibody; p-ANCA, perinuclear ANCA.

immunofluorescence can also be used to detect serum ABMA but is less sensitive than RIA or ELISA. Diagnosis of ABMA disease can be made by lung biopsy if linear deposits of IgG are found along alveolar septa.[1] False-negative results do occur, however, at least with the transbronchial biopsy approach.[33] ABMA disease is easily diagnosed by serology and renal biopsy. Even when the kidneys appear to be uninvolved, renal biopsy may still show linear immunofluorescence.[34] Thus lung biopsy is virtually never required to diagnose ABMA disease.

Unlike ABMA disease, the vasculitides and SLE are multisystem disorders that can affect many organs. Renal biopsy and serology are also useful for diagnosis of these disorders, but the findings are not as specific as for ABMA disease. SLE is diagnosed by a positive antinuclear antibody (ANA) in serum, immune-complex-mediated glomerulonephritis demonstrated by renal histopathology and immunofluorescence, and compatible clinical features. Hypocomplementemia is usually found in active SLE. Renal biopsy findings in Wegener's granulomatosis and nonspecific systemic vasculitis are identical. A segmental necrotizing glomerulonephritis with absent or sparse immune deposits is characteristic of renal vasculitis.[35] In Wegener's granulomatosis, serology usually reveals the presence of antinuclear cytoplasmic antibody (ANCA).[36,37] When both the perinuclear (p-ANCA) and cytoplasmic (c-ANCA) staining patterns are considered positive, most patients with nonspecific systemic necrotizing vasculitis also test positive for serum ANCA.[38] Thus DAH associated with pauci-immune segmental necrotizing glomerulonephritis and a positive serum ANCA could be due to Wegener's granulomatosis or nonspecific systemic vasculitis.

The histopathologic correlate of immune DAH is usually a pulmonary capillaritis, or microangiitis, regardless of whether the responsible disorder is Wegener's granulomatosis or nonspecific systemic vasculitis or SLE.[39-43] Capillaritis also can be detected in cases of ABMA and idiopathic pulmonary hemosiderosis.[1] If the chest roentgenogram shows focal nodules or cavitary lesions in addition to diffuse alveolar infiltrates, biopsy of these focal areas is likely to establish a diagnosis of Wegener's granulomatosis. Otherwise, open lung biopsy of DAH generally reveals fairly nonspecific changes that add little to the diagnostic information provided by the combination of renal biopsy, serology, and clinical examination. Open lung biopsy would be indicated when DAH occurs without extrapulmonary disease or circulating ABMA. If pulmonary capillaritis is detected without vasculitis in larger vessels and without immune deposits by immunofluorescence, a diagnosis of idiopathic pulmonary hemosiderosis may still be appropriate.

Treatment of immune DAH depends on the specific underlying disorder. In brief, combined immunosuppression and plasma exchange is recommended for ABMA disease, whereas corticosteroids plus cyclophosphamide are usually given for SLE, Wegener's granulomatosis, and nonspecific systemic vasculitis.[19,24,35,44-46] Corticosteroids alone are given for idiopathic pulmonary hemosiderosis.[19]

Empiric therapy should be started as pulse methylprednisolone, followed by daily prednisone, as soon as active DAH is diagnosed.[19] In most cases, active DAH ceases within 24 to 72 hours after pulse methylprednisolone is begun.[19] Therapy other than empiric methylprednisolone is added as the underlying disorder is clarified by clinical examination, renal biopsy, and serology. The goals of therapy are to halt further activity of DAH and to treat extrapulmonary disease. The major long-term complication in patients with DAH is renal failure rather than respiratory failure. The outcome for renal failure depends on renal function at presentation and the underlying disorder. In ABMA disease, prognosis is good if the serum creatinine is less than 6 mg/dl and the patient is nonoliguric. Oliguria and a serum creatinine level greater than 6 mg/dl predict little chance for recovery,[47] and therapy should probably be withheld to avoid complications of therapy, unless DAH is active.[48] The prognosis for renal recovery in the vasculitides is also better if renal function is normal or only mildly impaired. Vasculitis-related acute renal failure, however, may reverse with therapy.[49] Thus, in contrast to the case with ABMA disease, therapy should be given form the outset, regardless of the degree of renal impairment, unless renal biopsy reveals an end-stage kidney.

Recommendations regarding therapy of DAH cannot be considered definitive because prospective, controlled trials have not been conducted to evaluate the different types of therapy. Use of methylprednisolone is often followed by cessation of active DAH,[19] but bleeding could in some cases have resolved spontaneously. Because methylprednisolone can be given easily and safely and probably has true benefit, its empiric use for immune DAH is recommended. Empiric use of plasmapheresis is a different matter. Plasmapheresis is safe in experienced hands but is certainly more complex and resource intensive than giving pulse corticosteroids. It would seem appropriate to reserve plasma exchange for cases of DAH caused by ABMA disease. The rationale for its use in this disorder is to remove circulating ABMA quickly while immunosuppressive therapy (prednisone and cyclophosphamide) is given to prevent antibody resynthesis. Certainly one could not quarrel with the use of empiric plasma exchange for immune DAH unrelated to ABMA disease if there is no response to pulse methylprednisolone.

Issues regarding empiric treatment of DAH that presents with respiratory failure and of long-term therapy are discussed in the sections dealing with the ICU and post-ICU phases.

ICU Phase

The ICU phase of DAH is entered when the patient requires admission to the ICU for the purpose of close clinical monitoring of respiratory status or because of the need for mechanical ventilation. The principles of diagnosis and treatment of DAH in the ICU are similar to those described in the pre-ICU phase (see earlier), with a few important differences. In the ICU, the presence of respiratory insufficiency limits the utility of the DLCO for diagnosing DAH. Although bronchoscopy with BAL can generally be easily and safely performed via the endotracheal tube in mechanically ventilated patients, this procedure may not be well tolerated in the nonventilated patient with moderate-to-severe respiratory insufficiency. Indeed, elective intubation may be required to perform bronchoscopy in such patients. Critically ill patients in the ICU usually have Foley catheters and may have an elevated creatinine level owing to a variety of nonimmune insults. Thus, determining whether or not glomerulonephritis is present may be difficult without renal biopsy. The latter may be performed with greater hesitation in the setting of critical illness. These constraints on defining the presence of DAH and its origin, together with the need for urgent therapy when DAH has caused respiratory (and often renal) failure, requires that empiric treatment of severe DAH with respiratory failure be given at a point where the degree of confidence in the correct diagnosis is somewhat less than in the less severely ill patient.

In our experience, the majority of patients with DAH have spent some time in the ICU during their hospital course, and more than one third have required mechanical ventilation.[19] We believe that it is reasonable to adopt a policy of early ICU admission when DAH causes significant impairment in gas exchange. This is because an acute exacerbation of intrapulmonary bleeding in a patient with already compromised gas exchange can quickly lead to frank respiratory failure. Furthermore, patients with DAH are often otherwise healthy and have a good short-term and long-term prognosis even if respiratory failure occurs. Patients who have a respiratory rate greater than 30 breaths per minute require an FiO_2 greater than 0.4 or who have poor respiratory reserve because of preexisting disease should generally be monitored in an ICU. Another less common reason for ICU admission is the presence of massive hemoptysis related to DAH (see focal pulmonary hemorrhage, later).

When previously undiagnosed DAH presents as acute respiratory failure, the differential diagnosis centers on primarily two common causes of widespread diffuse alveolar filling: acute hemorrhagic pulmonary edema owing to elevated pulmonary venous pressure and ARDS. An echocardiogram is helpful for excluding mitral value disease and evaluating the status of left ventricular systolic and diastolic performance by echocardiography. If there is any doubt as to whether the pulmonary venous pressure could be elevated, a pulmonary artery catheter should be inserted to measure the wedge pressure and to help detect intermittent V waves. The need to exclude increased pulmonary venous pressure remains even when there is substantial hemoptysis. In the absence of mitral stenosis, major hemoptysis is an uncommon manifestation of intermittent or sustained elevations of pulmonary venous pressure, but it can occur. We have seen cases of major hemoptysis with DAH, caused solely by left-sided heart disease, which completely abated with appropriate diuretic, vasodilator, or anti-ischemic therapy.

A second major differential diagnostic consideration may be severe DAH versus ARDS. ARDS usually occurs in the setting of sepsis, trauma, gastric aspiration, or another readily identifiable insult. The cause of ARDS, however, is not always apparent, as in the case of primary lung infection or occult aspiration. Thus it may in some cases be difficult to determine whether the patient with combined respiratory and renal failure has ARDS with acute tubular necrosis (ATN) or immune DAH with glomerulonephritis. This is especially true when there is little or no preceding hemoptysis and gross blood is not suctioned from the endotracheal tube. Bronchoscopy with lavage may prove useful in that some estimate of the degree of alveolar bleeding can be made, and cultures and stains for microorganisms can be obtained. If visual inspection of the lower airway reveals gross blood welling up from numerous subsegmental bronchi or a nontraumatic lavage yields gross blood in the effluent and abundant hemosiderin-laden macrophages, DAH is almost certain to be present. The degree of alveolar bleeding in ARDS, however, can be quite variable, and in some cases the lavage effluent may appear serosanguineous. In these cases of ARDS associated with greater degrees of alveolar bleeding, hemosiderin-laden macrophages might also be seen if the onset of lung injury occurred more than a day or two before bronchoscopy. In brief, there are cases in which one simply cannot be sure based on clinical features and bronchoscopy whether respiratory failure is due to DAH or ARDS.

Most patients with DAH have concomitant glomerulonephritis. Because ARDS is associated with ATN but not glomerulonephritis, clarification of the cause of renal insufficiency may be of great value in differentiating DAH and ARDS. Inspection of the urine may be diagnostic of glomerulonephritis if red blood cell casts are readily apparent. As noted earlier, the presence of microscopic hematuria is not particularly helpful because an indwelling Foley catheter is usually present. Deformation in the red cell membrane suggests a glomerular origin of bleeding but is not sufficient for diagnosis. Renal biopsy is strongly recommended because it reliably differentiates glomerulonephritis from ATN and helps clarify the cause of DAH if the former is detected. Nephrologists are often understandably reluctant to perform a renal biopsy in the setting of respiratory failure requiring ventilatory support. Nonetheless, by using the therapeutic paralysis, movement of the kidney can be controlled, and percutaneous biopsy is not contraindicated. An alternative is open renal biopsy. This procedure can be performed under local anesthesia.[50] Open lung biopsy might also be considered to distinguish DAH from the diffuse alveolar damage of ARDS.

If a tissue biopsy specimen cannot be obtained, diagnosis may of necessity be made solely based on serologic studies. If the clinical picture is more suggestive of DAH than ARDS and a strongly positive assay for either ABMA or ANCA is obtained, a presumptive diagnosis can be made and therapy appropriate for ABMA disease or vasculitis may be given. Because most centers do not perform the ABMA (by RIA or ELISA) or the serum ANCA assay, serum must usually be sent out to referral laboratories. To avoid undue delays in receiving the results, the physician must ensure that the laboratory performing the test understands that the patient is critically ill so the sample is not simply batched with other samples and the test performed at a later date. Referral laboratories are generally responsive to such urgent requests, permitting rapid turnaround in receiving test results.

When suspected DAH causes respiratory insufficiency, it is important that empiric therapy with corticosteroids be given before defining the underlying disorder. Indeed it is prudent to give corticosteroids even if the presence of DAH is less certain, as long as it is a strong clinical consideration. Even if the underlying disorder later proved to be ARDS related to sepsis, viral pneumonia, or another cause, it is unlikely that a couple of days of high-dose corticosteroids would significantly worsen the prognosis for recovery.[51] Administration of other immunosuppressive drugs (e.g., cyclophosphamide) or plasmapheresis cannot be recommended, however, unless the evidence for vasculitis or ABMA disease is entirely convincing. Once the underlying immune disorder has been clarified, therapy appropriate for the specific disease process should be given (see pre-ICU phase, earlier).

DAH may in some cases prove to be entirely refractory to therapy and lead to death from intractable respiratory failure. More often, there is initially severe gas exchange impairment that gradually improves once active intrapulmonary bleeding ceases. Unlike ARDS, even severe DAH requiring high levels of inspired oxygen and positive end-expiratory pressure (PEEP) has a favorable outcome.[19] The ventilator management of acute respiratory failure is essentially the same as that used for ARDS (see Chap. 17). In brief, PEEP is indicated to reduce intrapulmonary shunt when an F_{IO_2} greater than 0.5 is required to achieve an arterial oxygen saturation of 90% or greater. If high levels of PEEP (e.g., > 10 cm H_2O) are required, use of a pulmonary artery catheter may be advisable to measure cardiac output and to measure wedge pressure. It is not clear that wedge pressure reduction would benefit gas exchange in DAH, but exacerbation of bleeding owing to high pulmonary venous pressure seems feasible. As in ARDS, inverse ratio ventilation might be tried if hypoxemia is refractory to PEEP.[52]

Respiratory failure from DAH usually necessitates no more than 1 to 2 weeks of mechanical ventilation. In some cases, however, the course is more protracted, as in ARDS. When there is need for prolonged ventilatory support, the risk of nosocomial pneumonia or another intercurrent serious infection increases. A difficult decision regarding continuation of immunosuppressive therapy must be made. In general, nosocomial bacterial infections should not require discontinuation of corticosteroids or cyclophosphamide, unless the latter has resulted in severe neutropenia. Because the chance for recovery from vasculitis-related DAH and glomerulonephritis is good, even when mechanical ventilation and dialysis are required, corticosteroids and cyclophosphamide should be continued whenever possible. ABMA-mediated renal disease that is severe enough to require dialysis seldom reverses.[47] Thus, when a serious infection arises early in the course of therapy for ABMA diseases, it may be reasonable to discontinue treatment if renal function has become seriously impaired, unless DAH is still active.

Mechanically ventilated patients with DAH are often able to be extubated and take food by mouth in less than a week after intubation. There are no data to suggest that patients with DAH are particularly hypermetabolic. Thus it is not inappropriate to delay institution of nutritional support for a few days after intubation to see if recovery will be relatively rapid. Apparent need for ongoing mechanical ventilation beyond 4 to 5 days would be a reasonable indication for beginning nutritional support. Earlier nutritional support would be indicated for preexisting malnutrition, documented hypermetabolism, or presence of persistently febrile course that might be expected to increase energy needs.

Criteria for extubating the patient with DAH are basically the same as those used for other causes of respiratory failure. Acceptable weaning parameters followed by a successful trial of spontaneous ventilation without tachypnea (>30 breaths/min), tachycardia (>120 beats/min), use of accessory muscles of respiration, or need for an F_{IO_2} greater than 0.4 would predict a high likelihood of safe extubation. Patients with respiratory failure owing to DAH, however, should also meet an additional criteria for extubation—no evidence for active bleeding for at least 24 to 48 hours. Inactivity of DAH is evidenced by a stable hemoglobin, improving oxygenation, and lack of fresh blood suctioned through the endotracheal tube.

Post-ICU Phase

Once DAH has improved to the point that respiratory insufficiency is no longer present or an ongoing threat, transfer out of the ICU is appropriate. Therapy begun previously is continued, with tapering of prednisone over a few weeks to an every-other-day dosing schedule. There are no good data on which to base a decision as to how long to treat vasculitis-related DAH and glomerulonephritis. When preservation of renal function is not a goal of therapy because of end-stage disease, it may be reasonable to opt for a shorter course of therapy. In this situation, the primary goal of treatment is to prevent recurrence of DAH. Once pulmonary disease has been quiescent for several weeks, it seems appropriate to withdraw therapy gradually and follow the patient so as to avoid the complications of immunosuppression. The same rationale would apply to patients with idiopathic pulmonary hemosiderosis; i.e., the need for treatment with prednisone beyond a few weeks after the last episode of DAH is uncertain. In the future, use of the serum ANCA to follow therapy of Wegener's granulomatosis and systemic necrotizing vasculitis may prove to be useful, but at present there are insufficient data available to justify basing treatment solely on the ANCA.

For ABMA disease, it is uncertain that treatment needs to be continued much beyond the time that ABMA disappears from serum. Therefore, a relatively short course of treatment (e.g., 2 to 3 months) may be reasonable.[47] As with the vasculitides, however, there are no really good data on which to base such decisions. For patients with ABMA disease, it is especially important to discourage cigarette smoking because smoking was shown in one study to be an important co-factor in the development of DAH.[53]

Outpatient follow-up of patients with immune DAH should include careful attention to respiratory symptoms, hemoglobin, and renal function. When a patient who is receiving immunosuppressive therapy for immune DAH develops new respiratory symptoms and new infiltrates on chest roentgenograms, an infection must be carefully excluded before a flare-up of DAH is diagnosed, even if there has been hemoptysis and a fall in hemoglobin. Flare-ups of DAH during therapy are not common, whereas the patient is at significant risk for opportunistic infection. The roentgenographic distinction of DAH and opportunistic infection is usually difficult. Also, certain types of opportunistic infection, especially invasive aspergillus, can lead to substantial lung hemorrhage.[15] If BAL, with or without transbronchial biopsy, does not clarify the underlying disorder, open biopsy to distinguish capillaritis with DAH from opportunistic infection should be considered. Accurate distinction of infection from an exacerbation of DAH is especially crucial because the latter may be managed with intensification of immunosuppressive therapy.

FOCAL PULMONARY HEMORRHAGE

Most patients with FPH do not have a life-threatening episode of airway hemorrhage. Only 1 to 5% of patients seeking medical care for hemoptysis die as a result of the effects of pulmonary hemorrhage or its treatment.[54-59] The majority of patients with life-threatening hemoptysis present with initially explosive bleeding rather than recurrent minor "sentinel" bleeding.[54] Survival from explosive bleeding may be determined by rate of bleeding, airway clearance, and underlying cardiopulmonary reserve. Intervention in this setting is focused on skilled airway management and rapid institution of specific therapy to prevent further bleeding. Blood and clot must be cleared from the airway, and adequate ventilation and oxygenation should be ensured. Immediate airway examination to localize the bleeding site is requisite to specific therapy. Occasionally isolation of the involved portion of the tracheobronchial tree may be necessary to prevent recurrent episodes of asphyxiation.

Surgical resection of the bleeding focus is clearly the most definitive and permanent solution to life-threatening pulmonary hemorrhage from a focal site, yet patients who survive initial moderate bleeding can often be managed without surgery. Although early retrospective studies showed a high mortality rate associated with medical therapy of hemoptysis of 600 ml/16 to 24 hours,[54,60] the indiscriminate recommendation of surgical resection for all cases of operable FPH has been challenged.[54,56] Surgical management may be particularly suited for operable patients with hemoptysis of greater than 1000 ml/24 hours[56] and with severe hemoptysis from diseases with high recurrence rates, such as tuberculosis or aspergillomas. Surgical resection should be considered only in patients who have had certain localization of the bleeding site.

Depending on the case referral patterns, 30 to 80% of patients with hemoptysis are not operable because of severe underlying cardiopulmonary disease or short life expectancies from co-morbid clinical problems. In these patients, surgical removal of the focus of bleeding may carry unacceptable risks of morbidity and mortality as compared with nonsurgical management. The most specific, effective nonsurgical therapy for focal pulmonary hemorrhage in this setting is bronchial arterial embolization. In 75 to 90% of selected patients, hemoptysis can be initially controlled with this technique.[61-65]

Mortality following life-threatening hemoptysis is determined by not only the tendency for hemoptysis to recur, but also the prognosis of the disease producing the pulmonary bleeding. Patients with lung cancer and leukemia have an understandable poor long-term prognosis after initial management of hemoptysis. Patients who have self-limited hemoptysis from treatable infection, such as bronchitis, pneumonia, lung abscess, or fungal infections, usually have resolution of hemoptysis with eradication of the infection. When bronchial arterial neovascularization accompanies chronic inflammatory conditions, such as aspergilloma or bronchiectasis, significant hemoptysis may be recurrent over many years, unless the abnormal vessels are embolized or the involved tissue is resected.

Pre-ICU Phase

Focal massive bleeding can rapidly lead to respiratory failure, in which case the life-threatening nature of the pulmonary hemorrhage is apparent and issues of airway management, prompt localization of bleeding, and control of the bleeding source are of immediate concern. These areas are discussed under ICU Phase. In many cases, however, substantial hemoptysis occurs without immediate detrimental effects on respiratory function. In the latter instance, an attempt to assess the risk of further bleeding and its likely impact on respiratory function is important. Although any patient who experiences acute hemoptysis of moderate amount is potentially at risk for asphyxial death on recurrence of bleeding, there are certain factors that help to stratify such patients as to relative risk of fatal hemoptysis.

Risk Assessment

Three factors of considerable importance in assessing risk from hemoptysis are:

- Cause of bleeding
- Bleeding rate
- Baseline cardiopulmonary reserve

The risk of asphyxiation may be affected by the cause of focal pulmonary bleeding. Despite the high incidence of bronchitis as a cause of hemoptysis, massive bleeding is uncommon in conditions such as bronchitis that produce only capillary or small vessel injury. The pathology of massive FPH usually involves erosion or disruption of vessels larger than the capillary bed (Table 19-3). Chronic inflammatory conditions, such as lung abscess, tuberculosis, bronchiectasis, cavitary fungal infection, and aspergilloma, cause neovascularization of the bronchial arterial system with erosion of these vessels in the inflammatory focus. Erosive pseudoaneurysms of the pulmonary artery may also occur in this setting. Patients with chronic inflammatory or cavitary lung conditions are at risk for FPH (Table 19-4).

Newly diagnosed tuberculosis was associated with daily hemoptysis of 250 to 1000 ml in 1.3% of patients in one series.[61] Bronchiectasis is a common residua of inactive destructive tuberculosis and may produce serious pulmonary bleeding more frequently than in patients with active tuberculosis. Bronchiectasis may also complicate diverse conditions such as cystic fibrosis,[66] dysmotile cilia syndrome, immunoglobulin deficiencies, allergic bronchopulmonary aspergillosis, and destructive pneumonia and produce life-threatening pulmonary hemorrhage. Massive hemoptysis is disturbingly common in cystic fibrosis.[66-68] In one retrospective review of 728 patients with cystic fibrosis, 5% had hemoptysis totaling 300 ml or more in 24 hours, and 45% of the patients with massive bleeding had recurrent bleeding.[65] In another series, 13 of 19 patients with cystic fibrosis who had initial hemoptysis of greater than 500 ml were dead within 6 months.[69] Eighty-five percent of 111 patients with allergic bronchopulmonary aspergillosis in one study had hemoptysis, although only 4% exceeded bleeding rates of more than 240 ml/day.[70] Eleven percent to 15% of patients with lung abscess have hemoptysis, and approximately 5% have massive hemoptysis.[71] Chronic cavitary histoplasmosis is associated with hemoptysis in up to 22% of patients, although massive bleeding is unusual.[72] Aspergillomas carry perhaps the highest risk of massive hemoptysis compared with other specific diagnoses (Fig. 19-1). Seventy-eight percent of patients with aspergillomas in one series had hemoptysis during long-term observation (8.7 years).[73] The incidence of hemoptysis exceeding 150 ml/24 hours was 25% in this study.

Congenital or acquired arteriovenous communications may produce brisk bleeding but are not uncommon com-

Table 19-3. Vascular Sources of Focal Pulmonary Hemorrhage

Mechanism	Diseases
Localized neovascularization of bronchial artery system	Cavitary infections Bronchiectasis Aspergilloma Lung cancer
Pseudoaneurysm of pulmonary artery	Cavitary infections
Vascular rupture	Trauma Thoracic aortic aneurysm
Dilated communications between bronchial vein and pulmonary vein	Mitral stenosis
Dilated communications between pulmonary artery and vein	Arteriovenous malformation

Table 19-4. Selected Inflammatory Conditions Producing Severe Focal Pulmonary Hemorrhage

Condition	Incidence
Aspergilloma[73,101-105]	5-25%
Cystic fibrosis[66-68]	5-7%
Lung abscess[71]	5%
Allergic bronchopulmonary aspergillosis[70]	4%
Tuberculosis[61]	1%
Cavitary fungal infections	—

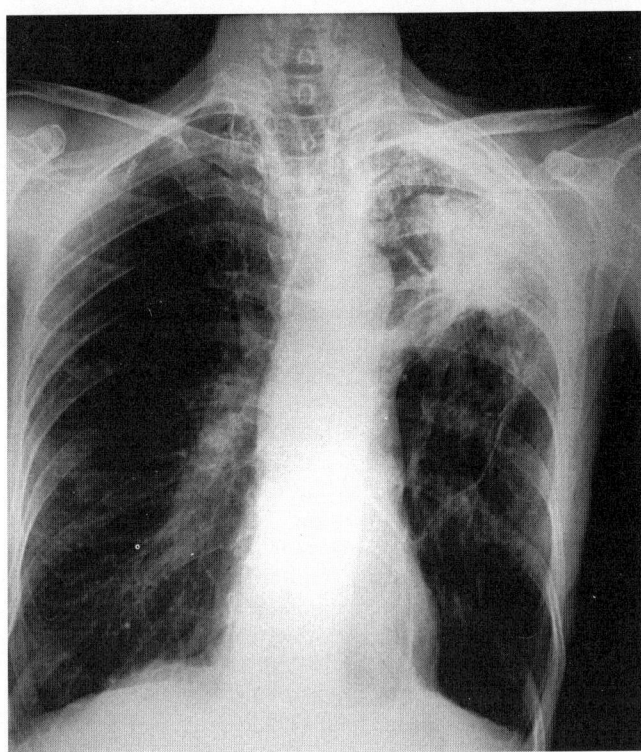

Fig. 19-1. Left upper lobe aspergilloma in a patient with recurrent hemoptysis. The radiographic finding of a "ball in a cavity" is relatively specific for fungus colonization of a preexisting cavity and is a common cause of severe focal pulmonary hemorrhage. Even with focal radiographic findings, bleeding sites should always be confirmed by endoscopic examination or bronchial arteriography before any definitive management is begun.

pared with inflammatory causes for FPH. Congenital vascular anomalies, such as pulmonary arteriovenous malformations and capillary hemangiomatosis, may be unsuspected before onset of hemoptysis. Massive hemoptysis complicating mitral stenosis likely represents bleeding from engorged pulmonary to systemic venous anastomosis (bronchial "varices") and requires immediate reduction in pulmonary venous pressures (often valvular surgery).[3,74] Rupture of an enlarging thoracic aortic aneurysm that has eroded into the pulmonary parenchyma produces bleeding rates that are unparalleled by most other causes of FPH. Also, in contrast to other causes of pulmonary hemorrhage, sudden death may occur as a result of exsanguination rather than asphyxiation. In this condition, hemoptysis may occur simultaneously with bleeding into the pleural space of mediastinum, producing hypovolemic shock that is disproportionate to pulmonary bleeding.

In addition, acquired endobronchial neoplasms may cause serious hemoptysis. Approximately 1% of patients with lung cancer develop massive hemoptysis. More than 80% of these patients have squamous carcinoma, often associated with mainstream tumors of cavitation.[75] Laser therapy and brachytherapy have been associated with hemoptysis in patients with endobronchial lung cancer. More modest hemoptysis is associated with diverse conditions resulting in endobronchial erosion, such as carcinoid tumors, endometriosis,[76] and Kaposi's sarcoma.

In one prospective study, mortality rate with hemoptysis was clearly stratified according to bleeding rate. Mortality was 71% with hemoptysis totaling 600 ml in 4 hours, 45% with 600 ml in 4 to 16 hours, and 5% with 600 ml in 16 to 48 hours.[77] Another retrospective study demonstrated a mortality rate of 58% in patients with hemoptysis of 1000 ml or more in 24 hours compared with a 9% mortality for patients with less than 1000 ml over 24 hours.[56] Measured bleeding rates are understandably only approximations of actual blood volume output into the airway and may be underestimated in patients with significant aspiration of blood. In one study, mortality was higher in patients with focal bleeding who had evidence of aspirations on chest radiographs.[56]

There are theoretical reasons why patients with impaired cardiopulmonary reserve would be expected to be at greater risk for respiratory distress during periods of airway flooding from hemoptysis as compared with more vigorous patients. Patients with severe chronic restrictive or obstructive lung disorders have reduced ventilatory reserve. Resting ventilation is a larger proportion of maximal sustainable ventilatory capacity in this setting as compared with normal subjects. Any further encumbrance on ventilation may reduce sustainable ventilatory capacity below resting ventilatory needs, producing respiratory muscle fatigue. Respiratory muscle fatigue may be accentuated by hypoxia associated with the underlying lung disease. Impairment of effective cough may also interfere with airway clearance. Patients with reduced expiratory flow rates from chronic obstructive pulmonary disease (COPD), or patients with depressed cough reflexes may be at greater risk for aspiration of blood during periods of rapid intrabronchial flooding. Finally, increased work of breathing has been shown to produce ischemia in patients with underlying coronary artery disease.[78] The increased work of breathing associated with airway flooding in massive hemoptysis may be sufficient to provoke ischemia and acute left ventricular failure in susceptible patients. All of these considerations are well-recognized factors that should be reviewed when evaluating the need for ventilatory support of airway clearance in patients with underlying cardiopulmonary disease. Because of the unpredictability of hemoptysis, it is unlikely that prospective studies could be designed to assess risks of ventilatory failure from hemoptysis accurately according to coexisting disease process or severity.

Triage Strategy

The risk of massive airway bleeding and adequacy of cardiopulmonary reserve are probably the best determinants of the need for ICU monitoring and the timing of diagnostic and therapeutic procedures. Although there are no well-verified protocols for management of hemoptysis, strategies can be based on practical considerations, such as rate of bleeding, respiratory compromise, and prior history of massive bleeding. Patients with rapid rates of hemoptysis (estimated volume of $\geq$ 600 ml in the initial 14 to 16 hours or $\geq$ 1000 ml in the first 24 hours) should probably be monitored in the ICU and have immediate bronchoscopy for localization of bleeding site. Patients with sufficient airway flooding from hemoptysis to produce respiratory distress or severe derangements in gas exchange should be monitored in the ICU and have immediate bronchoscopy for the purpose of (1) localization of bleeding site and (2) facilitation of airway clearance. Patients with lower rates of bleeding and adequate cardiopulmonary reserve should probably be hospitalized if they have had prior life-threatening hemoptysis. Finally, the decision to hospitalize patients for definitive management of hemoptysis may not require ICU management. Patients may be admitted electively for chronic small volume hemoptysis for the purposes of lung resection or bronchial arterial embolization.

ICU Phase

The ICU phase of major hemoptysis centers on four essential areas:

- Airway control must be achieved so as to prevent death from asphyxiation.
- Localization of the bleeding source, an essential requisite for both prevention of massive aspiration of blood into nonbleeding areas of the lung and definitive control of the bleeding source, must be accomplished promptly.
- A specific diagnosis should be pursued to determine appropriate management strategy.
- Measures to control the source of bleeding should be applied whenever feasible.

Airway Management

Asphyxia owing to airway flooding is the major cause of early mortality from FPH. Rapid rates of bleeding may overwhelm patients' ability to clear the airway. In contrast to pulmonary bleeding from immune causes, FPH may produce sufficient clot in the airway to result in thrombotic obstruction of the tracheobronchial lumen and ventilatory failure. Alveolar flooding and tracheobronchial obstruction may produce shunt with severe hypoxia that may further impair ventilatory reserve. Underlying cardiopulmonary disease or depressed consciousness may act in concert to impair airway clearance.

Rigid bronchoscopy or intubation with fiberoptic bronchoscopy[79] may be used to provide ventilatory support during removal of large thrombotic obstructions of the endobronchial tree. If ventilation cannot be performed because of impaction of the airways with thrombus, judicious use of intrabronchial streptokinase may facilitate clearance.[80] There is some controversy about the effectiveness of rigid versus fiberoptic bronchoscopy in achieving airway clearance. Over the last 20 years since the dissemination of fiberoptic bronchoscopy techniques, the majority of diagnostic procedures for hemoptysis have been performed with fiberoptic bronchoscopy.[54,56,79]

Fiberoptic bronchoscopy is often the most immediately available method to facilitate timely clearance of the airway in the initial management of a patient with life-threatening bleeding. A 7.5-mm or larger endotracheal tube should be placed to allow adequate ventilation during fiberoptic procedures. The bronchoscope should be passed through an airtight adapter into the airway. High peak airway pressures may be needed to ventilate patients during the procedure. Loss of ventilation may occur as a result of prolonged suctioning, leaking around the bronchoscope adapter, or volume loss in compliant ventilator tubing. Continuous heart rate and oximetry monitoring should be performed during prolonged bronchoscopic procedures in this setting. Monitoring of expired volume and use of noncompliant ventilator tubing or higher tidal volumes may ensure adequate ventilation if airway pressures are increased. Air trapping frequently occurs as a result of high airway resistance in this setting and should be minimized with slow respiratory rates and judicious use of sedation to prevent triggering of the ventilator. Patients frequently require high concentrations of oxygen during prolonged irrigation and suctioning of the tracheobronchial tree.

If the rate of bleeding or volume of thrombotic obstruction prevents adequate clearance with a fiberoptic bronchoscope, rigid bronchoscopy or isolation of the airway may need to be performed. Rapid bleeding from the right tracheobronchial tree can be isolated by endoscopic placement of a left main stem endotracheal tube, which allows clearance and ventilation of the left tracheobronchial tree. Because intubation of the right main stem bronchus may obstruct the right upper lobe orifice, isolation of left tracheobronchial tree in this setting often requires balloon occlusion of the left main stem bronchus and placement of the ventilating endotracheal tube above the main carina.[55] Double lumen tubes are effective in isolating the right and left main stem but are often too small to allow adequate clearance during periods of active bleeding and intrabronchial clot formation. Balloon occlusion of a segmental airway has been used anecdotally to isolate (and presumably tamponade) focal pulmonary bleeding. This technique requires adequate visualization and identification of the segmental source of bleeding—both of these maneuvers are difficult to accomplish in patients with life-threatening bleeding. Topical epinephrine and thrombin have been used to control endoscopically localized bleeding from endobronchial biopsy but may be difficult to perform in patients who have airways flooded with blood.

Localization of Bleeding

In patients with life-threatening focal pulmonary bleeding, localization of bleeding site is prerequisite to elective or emergent local management. Massive bleeding from the nasopharynx that accompanies traumatic aneurysms or coagulopathies is usually easily identified by patient and physician as an upper airway source. Massive nasal bleeding from traumatic pseudoaneurysm may require unilateral carotid ligation. Localization by patients of bleeding sites downstream from the larynx is less precise. Fewer than 10% of patients can correctly identify which lung is the site of intrapulmonary bleeding.[81] Physical examination and chest roentgenogram correctly identify the site of bleeding in 50 to 60% of patients. Chest film findings in aspergilloma (see Fig. 19-1) and bronchiectasis may have relatively high diagnostic specificity but not allow certain localization of bleeding site. Chest films showing middle mediastinal widening or smooth deformity of the aortic profile should raise the suspicion of aortic aneurysm rupture as a cause of hemoptysis. Computed tomography (CT) scans with intravenous contrast material or aortic angiography is requisite to surgical management of thoracic aortic aneurysm rupture and should be performed as soon as possible if this diagnosis is a reasonable consideration. CT scans may also be helpful in patients with suspected lung cancer or bronchiectasis, although localization of bleeding site is understandably poor in bilateral disease. Thin-section and high-resolution CT scans are particularly sensitive in detecting cystic bronchiectasis but are less denotive in detecting cylindrical or varicose bronchiectasis.[82] Occasionally lung cancers located in the hilum or proximal to the mediastinum may be detected by CT scan when not visualized on routine chest roentgenograms. Chest CT scans have not, however, proved sufficiently accurate to be used indiscriminately in localizing the origin of hemoptysis.[83]

Bronchoscopy is the most commonly used method of identifying site of focal pulmonary bleeding. The availability of trained fiberoptic bronchoscopists and its ease of use in spontaneously breathing patients have promoted fiberoptic bronchoscopy as the most common diagnostic tool. Endoscopic examination may uncover relatively specific findings, such as the mucosal friability of hyperemia seen with bronchitis, foreign body, endobronchial tumors, bronchial varices, and Kaposi's sarcoma. The yield of specific diagnostic findings by bronchoscopy increases with the volume of hemoptysis.[84] Even when bronchoscopy does not reveal specific diagnosis, it may allow localization of bleeding site by bronchoscopy in 86 to 93%[81-85] of patients with focal pulmonary bleeding. Although no standard definition of bronchitis has been used in reported series of patients with hemoptysis, the finding of diffuse mucosal friability in a patient with a normal chest roentgenogram is associated with a relatively low risk of life-threatening hemoptysis.[86]

Timing of bronchoscopic procedures may be more relevant to localization of bleeding site than specific diagnostic cause. In one retrospective study of 129 patients with hemoptysis, early (and presumably timely) bronchoscopy localized bleeding in 34%, whereas delayed endoscopy identified bleeding site in only 11%.[87] Although no difference in management occurred as a result of early versus delayed bronchoscopy in this study, it would seem judicious to perform bronchoscopy during active bleeding in all patients who require timely localization of bleeding site to direct emergency surgical or bronchial arteriographic procedures. Bronchoscopy should be performed even if the chest radiograph does not suggest a focal site of bleeding. Smokers over 50 years of age with hemoptysis but a normal chest radiograph have a high probability of having lung cancer.[84]

Preliminary studies suggest that radionuclide imaging may be useful for localizing bleeding in pediatric or other patients who are unable to undergo bronchoscopic examination. Extravascular radiolabeled red blood cells or technetium sulfur colloid may be identified in perhaps 50% of patients with massive hemoptysis and require ongoing blood loss of approximately 6 ml/min for maximum sensitivity.[88,89] In practice, bronchoscopy is superior to radionuclide techniques because of the ease and timeliness of bedside endoscopic examination and the specificity of bronchoscopy in patients with endobronchial disease.

Diagnosis of Specific Causes

Defining the specific cause of focal pulmonary bleeding may help in immediate decisions regarding management of patients with massive pulmonary hemorrhage. Bronchoscopic identification of inoperable stage III non-small-cell lung cancer or small cell carcinoma mitigates against surgical management in almost all cases. The specific yield of bronchoscopic procedures in endobronchially visible neoplasms is approximately 90%. Unfortunately massive bleeding frequently dilutes specimens obtained for cytologic examination, making the yield less optimal.

Many pulmonary infections that produce FPH may be diagnosed by examination and culture of sputum or bronchoscopically obtained material. Identification of a specific infectious agent does not obviate the need for surgical resection or bronchial embolization in patients with uncontrolled bleeding. Similarly, in life-threatening FPH, definite control of bleeding source may need to be accomplished before a specific infectious agent is identified. The suspicion of specific infectious causes should be tempered by the nature of the host, regional disease frequencies (as in legionellosis, histoplasmosis, coccidioidomycosis, and blastomycosis), the nature of the illness (such as putrid sputum in anaerobic lung abscess), and other epidemiologic factors. In special circumstances, a specific infectious cause may be highly suspected by the radiographic appearance. Cavitation of a chronic infiltrate with development of an intracavitary mass following resolution of profound and prolonged (> 3 weeks) leukopenia is nearly pathognomonic of invasive aspergillosis or mucormycosis.[90] Aspergillomas should be suspected as a cause of hemoptysis in patients with preexisting cavities from tuberculosis and cystic sarcoidosis. In other circumstances, morphology of the organism on smear of bronchial secretions or sputum may provide an early specific diagnosis (e.g., blastomycosis, tuberculosis, coccidioidomycosis, nocardia). BAL increases yield to more than 80% in tuberculosis[91] and 50% in invasive opportunistic fungal infections.[92] Serologic tests are diagnostic in the majority of nonimmunocompromised patients with histoplasmosis and coccidioidomycosis, although chronic or disseminated infections in debilitated hosts are less reliably diagnosed by serologic criteria.[93] Histoplasmosis complement fixation tests are positive in 75 to 100% of patients with chronic cavitary histoplasmosis.[94] Titers of 1:32 or greater and a positive immunodiffusion carry a high specificity for active histoplasmosis in the proper clinical setting.

Surgical Repair and Excision

In patients with rapid bleeding rates and an identified unilateral bleeding site, surgical resection provides definitive resolution of bleeding in almost all cases. Surgical repair is the only reliable management for major vascular disruption, such as trauma or rupture of a thoracic aortic aneurysm. Surgical resection of focal pulmonary bleeding sites should be limited to patients whose pulmonary reserve is adequate to undergo resection of the involved lung tissue and should be withheld in most patients who have poor short-term survival from other coexisting medical conditions, such as untreatable metastatic tumor. Thoracotomy may complicate subsequent lung transplantation, making bronchial artery embolization a more attractive management strategy for lung transplant candidates.

Retrospective reviews of long-term survival following surgical resection versus medical therapy in FPH are undoubtedly biased: Patients selected for surgery are likely to have better cardiopulmonary reserve, and deaths occurring abruptly before localization of bleeding site may be ascribed to failure of medical management. Although some studies suggest high mortality (79 to 85%) in medically managed patients and low mortality (< 20%) in surgically managed patients,[77,95] other studies report a low mortality (0 to 25%) in patients managed without surgical resection.[75,76,96,97] Surgical complications may be more common in patients with extensive parenchymal destruction owing to loss of pulmonary reserve and debility. Resection of inflammatory conditions associated with extensive pleural involvement, such as necrotizing aspergillosis, may be complicated by postoperative bronchopleural fistulas or empyema. The role of surgical resection should be determined by weighing the risks of life-threatening bleeding and the surgical risk. Patients with rapid bleeding rates (> 600 ml/4 hours or > 1000 ml/24 hours) with localized unilateral disease and good cardiopulmonary reserve would seem most likely to benefit from surgery. The risk of surgical resection should be gauged by coexisting cardiac disease,[98] severity of air-flow limitation in COPD, and volume of lung resected.[99]

Angiographic Localization and Embolization

Angiography is useful for localization and embolic obstruction of vessels supplying focal areas of pulmonary hemorrhage. Patients who would be expected to have a high operative mortality, poor long-term survival, or bilateral disease are more appropriately treated with angiographic embolization rather than surgical resection. Patients with cystic fibrosis who are candidates for bilateral lung transplantation may be more appropriately treated with angiography rather than surgery.

More than 90% of patients with angiographically identifiable vascular abnormalities have a bronchial arterial (as opposed to pulmonary arterial) source for bleeding.[100] Of these patients, perhaps 75 to 90% have cessation of bleeding after bronchial arterial embolization.[61-65] Rebleeding occurs in approximately 20% of patients who have undergone initially successful embolization.[61] Recurrences are most common in the first 6 months of follow-up and are thought to be related to bilateral disease or progression of local disease as well as technical failures of the procedure. The procedure requires a skilled angiographer and may take several hours for successful identification and embolization of involved vessels. Complications such as spinal artery embolism are rare (< 1%) in large series of patients undergoing this procedure.[62] Erosive pulmonary arterial aneurysms and pulmonary arterial malformations require arteriographic studies of the pulmonary circulation for localization and embolization. When multiple pulmonary arteriovenous malformations occur, angiographic embolization may be more appropriate than multistage surgical procedures.

Post-ICU Phase

In patients who have not had definitive management of a bleeding source in FPH, recurrence of hemoptysis may occur unpredictably after spontaneous cessation of a life-threatening episode. Recurrence rates are lowest for patients who have abnormal or nonlocalizing chest roentgenograms and a bronchoscopic examination demonstrating either normal mucosa or diffuse changes of bronchitis. In one study of 67 patients who met these latter criteria, hemoptysis resolved in 57% of patients before hospital discharge and recurred in only 7.5% of patients.[86]

Patients who have persisting, ineffectively treated inflammatory conditions have relatively frequent recurrences of significant hemoptysis. Surgical management in these patients is often obviated by the presence of bilateral disease, such as bronchiectasis, or by severe underlying pulmonary disease in the setting of unilateral lesions, such as aspergilloma. Control of bleeding with bronchial artery embolization may be a determinant of mortality and frequency of rebleeding in this setting. In one study, 5 of 6 deaths from continued bleeding occurred in 14 patients with unsuccessful bronchial artery embolization, as compared with 1 death from unrelated causes in 50 patients with initially effective bronchial artery embolization.[62]

REFERENCES

1. Travis, W. D., Colby, T. V., Lombard, C., and Carpenter, H. A.: A clinicopathologic study of 22 cases of diffuse pulmonary hemorrhage with lung biopsy confirmation. Am. J. Surg. Pathol., *14:*1112, 1990.
2. Schwartz, E. E., Teplick, J. G., Onesti, G., and Schwartz, A. B.: Pulmonary hemorrhage in renal disease: Goodpasture's syndrome and other causes. Radiology, *122:*39, 1977.
3. Schwartz, R., Myerson, R. M., Lawrence, L. T., and Nichols, W. T.: Mitral stenosis, massive pulmonary hemorrhage, and emergency valve replacement. N. Engl. J. Med., *275:*755, 1966.
4. Finley, T. N., Aronow, A., Cosentino, A. M., and Golde, D. W.: Occult pulmonary hemorrhage in anticoagulated patients. Am. Rev. Respir. Dis., *142:*23, 1975.
5. Robboy, S. J., et al.: Pulmonary hemorrhage syndrome as a manifestation of disseminated intravascular coagulation: analysis of ten cases. Chest, *63:*718, 1973.
6. Godwin, J. E., Harley, R. A., Miller, K. S., and Hefner, J. E.: Cocaine, pulmonary hemorrhage, and hemoptysis. Ann. Intern. Med., *110:*843, 1989.
7. Sternlieb, I., Bennet, B., and Scheinberg, I. W.: D-penicillamine-induced Goodpasture's syndrome in Wilson's disease. Ann. Intern. Med., *82:*673, 1975.
8. Patterson, R., Nugent, K. M., Harris, K. E., and Eberle, M. E.: Immunologic hemorrhagic pneumonia caused by isocyanates. Am. Rev. Respir. Dis., *141:*226, 1990.
9. Bucknall, C. E., Adamson, M. R., and Bauham, S. W.: Nonfatal pulmonary hemorrhage associated with nitrofurantoin. Thorax, *42:*475, 1987.
10. Smith, L. T., and Katzenstein, A. L. A.: Pathogenesis of massive pulmonary hemorrhage in acute leukemia. Arch. Intern. Med., *142:*2149, 1982.

11. Spragg, R. G., et al.: Angiosarcoma of the lung with fatal pulmonary hemorrhage. Am. J. Med., 74:1072, 1983.
12. Carter, E. J., Bradburne, R. M., Jhung, J. E., and Ettensohn, D. B.: Alveolar hemorrhage with epithelioid hemangioendothelioma. Am. Rev. Respir. Dis., 142:700, 1990.
13. Berrigan, T. J., Carsky, E. W., and Heitzman, E. R.: Fat embolism: roentgenographic pathologic correlation in three cases. Am. J. Roentgenol., 96:967, 1967.
14. Wierty, L. M., Gagnon, J. H., and Anthonisen, N. R.: Intrapulmonary hemorrhage with anemia after lymphography. N. Engl. J. Med., 288:1264, 1971.
15. Kahn, F. W., Jones, J. M., and England, D. N.: Diagnosis for pulmonary hemorrhage in the immunocompromised host. Am. Rev. Respir. Dis., 136:155, 1987.
16. Drew, W. L., Finely, T. N., and Golde, D. W.: Diagnostic lavage and occult pulmonary hemorrhage in thrombocytopenic immunocompromised patients. Am. Rev. Respir. Dis., 116:215, 1977.
17. Robbins, R. A., et al.: Diffuse alveolar hemorrhage in autologous bone marrow transplant recipients. Am. J. Med., 87:511, 1989.
18. Chao, N. J., et al.: Corticosteroid therapy for diffuse alveolar hemorrhage in autologous bone marrow transplant recipients. Ann. Intern. Med., 114:145, 1991.
19. Leatherman, J. W., Davies, S. F., and Hoidal, J. R.: Alveolar hemorrhage syndromes: Diffuse microvascular lung hemorrhage in immune and idiopathic disorders. Medicine, 63:343, 1984.
20. Abud-Mendoya, C., Diaz-Jovaneu, E., and Alarcon-Segovia, D.: Fatal pulmonary hemorrhage in systemic lupus erythematosus: occurrence with hemoptysis. J. Rheum., 12:558, 1985.
21. Bowley, N. B., Hughes, J. M. B., and Steiner, R. E.: The chest x-ray in pulmonary capillary hemorrhage: correlation with carbon monoxide uptake. Clin. Radiol., 30:413, 1979.
22. Ewan, P. W., Jones, H. A., Rhodes, G. C., and Hughes, J. M. B.: Detection of intrapulmonary hemorrhage with carbon monoxide uptake. N. Engl. J. Med., 295:1391, 1976.
23. Addleman, M., Logan, A. S., and Grossman, R. F.: Monitoring intrapulmonary hemorrhage in Goodpasture's syndrome. Chest, 87:119, 1985.
24. Rees, A. J.: Pulmonary injury caused by antibasement membrane antibody. Semin. Respir. Med., 5:264, 1984.
25. Kim, C. C., Saleba, K., Baughman, R. P., and Wesseler, T. A.: Iron staining on bronchoalveolar lavage smears for detecting occult pulmonary hemorrhage: it is reliable? [Abstract]. Acta. Cytol., 33:716, 1989.
26. Haworth, S. J., et al.: Pulmonary hemorrhage complicating Wegener's granulomatosis and microscopic polyarteritis. Br. Med. J., 290:1775, 1985.
27. Holdsworth, S., Boyce, N., Thomson, N. M, and Atkins, R. C.: The clinical spectrum of acute glomerulonephritis and lung hemorrhage (Goodpasture's syndrome). Q. J. Med., 216:75, 1985.
28. Eagen, J. W., et al.: Pulmonary hemorrhage in systemic lupus erythematosus. Medicine, 54:545, 1978.
29. Fasset, R. G., Hogan, B. A., and Matthew, T. H.: Detection of glomerular bleeding by phase contrast microscopy. Lancet, 1:1432, 1982.
30. Glassock, R. J.: Goodpasture's syndrome. In Textbook of Nephrology. S. G. Massry and R. J. Glassock. Baltimore, Williams & Wilkins, 1983, p. 108.
31. Wilson, C. B.: Nephritogenic immune responses involving basement membrane and other antigens in or of the glomerulus. In Immune Mechanisms in Renal Disease. Edited by N. Cummings, A. F. Michael, and C. V. Wilson. New York, Plenum Press, 1983, p. 233.
32. Fish, A. J., Kleppel, M., Jeraj, K., and Michael, A. F.: Enzyme immunoassay of antiglomerular basement membrane antibodies. J. Lab. Clin. Med., 105:700, 1985.
33. Johnson, J. P., et al.: Therapy of anti-glomerular basement membrane antibody disease: analysis of prognostic significance of clinical, pathologic and treatment factors. Medicine, 64:219, 1985.
34. Zimmerman, S. W., Varanasi, V. R., and Hoff, B.: Goodpasture's syndrome with normal renal function. Am. J. Med., 66:163, 1979.
35. Balow, J. E.: Renal vasculitis. Kidney Int., 27:954, 1985.
36. VanderWoude, F. J., et al.: Autoantibodies against neutrophils and monocytes: tool for diagnosis and market of disease activity in Wegener's granulomatosis. Lancet, 1:425, 1985.
37. Nolle, B., et al.: Anticytoplasmic autoantibodies: their immunodiagnostic value in Wegener's granulomatosis. Ann. Intern. Med., 111:28, 1989.
38. Falk, R. J., et al., and the Glomerular Disease Collaborative Network: Clinical course of anti-neutrophil cytoplasmic autoantibody, glomerulonephritis, and systemic vasculitis. Ann. Intern. Med., 113:656, 1990.
39. Myers, J. L., and Katzenstein, A. L. A.: Microangiitis in lupus-induced pulmonary hemorrhage. Am. J. Clin. Pathol., 85:552, 1986.
40. Stokes, T. C., et al.: Acute fulminating intrapulmonary hemorrhage in Wegener's granulomatosis. Thorax, 37:315, 1982.
41. Travis, W. D., Carpenter, H. A., and Lie, J. T.: Diffuse pulmonary hemorrhage. An uncommon manifestation of Wegener's granulomatosis. Am. J. Surg. Pathol., 11:702, 1987.
42. Myers, J. L., and Katzenstein, A. L. A.: Wegener's granulomatosis presenting with massive pulmonary hemorrhage and capillaritis. Am. J. Surg. Pathol., 11:895, 1987.
43. Mark, E. J., and Ramirez, J. F.: Pulmonary capillaritis and hemorrhage in patients with systemic vasculitis. Arch. Pathol. Lab. Med., 109:413, 1985.
44. Balow, J. E., et al.: Lupus nephritis. Ann. Intern. Med., 106:79, 1987.
45. Fauci, A. S., Katz, P., Haynes, B. F., and Wolff, S. M.: Cyclophosphamide therapy of severe sytemic necrotizing vasculitis. N. Engl. J. Med., 301:235, 1979.
46. Fauci, A. S., Haynes, B. F., Katz, P., and Wolff, S. M.: Wegener's granulomatosis: Prospective clinical and therapeutic experience with 85 patients over 21 years. Ann. Intern. Med., 98:76, 1983.
47. Peters, D. K., Rees, A. J., Lockwood, C. M., and Pusey, C. D.: Treatment and prognosis of antibasement membrane antibody mediated nephritis. Transplant. Proc., 14:513, 1982.
48. Flores, J. C., et al.: Clinical and immunological evolution of oligoanuric anti-GBM nephritis treated by hemodialysis. Lancet, 1:5, 1985.
49. Hind, C. R. K., et al.: Prognosis after immunosuppression of patients with crescentic nephritis requiring dialysis. Lancet, 1:263, 1983.
50. Chodak, G. W., Gill, W. B., Wald, V., and Spargo, B.: Diagnosis of renal parenchymal diseases by a modified open kidney biopsy technique. Kidney Intern., 24:804, 1983.
51. Bernard, G. R., et al.: High-dose corticosteroids in patients with the adult respiratory distress syndrome. N. Engl. J. Med., 317:1565, 1987.
52. Abraham, E., and Yoshihara, G.: Cardiorespiratory effects of pressure controlled ventilation in severe respiratory failure. Chest, 98:1445, 1990.
53. Donaghy, M., and Rees, A. J.: Cigarette smoking and lung hemorrhage in glomerulonephritis caused by autoanti-

bodies to glomerular basement membrane. Lancet, 2:1390, 1983.
54. Bobrowitz, I. D., Ramakrishna, S., and Shim, Y. S.: Comparison of medical vs. surgical treatment of major hemoptysis. Arch. Intern. Med., 143:1343, 1983.
55. Conlan, A. A., et al.: Massive hemoptysis. J. Thorac. Cardiovasc. Surg., 85:120, 1983.
56. Corey, R., and Hla, K. M.: Major and massive hemoptysis: reassessment of conservative management. Am. J. Med. Sci., 294:301, 1987.
57. Jones, D. K., and Davies, R. J.: Massive hemoptysis. Br. Med. J., 300:889, 1990.
58. Life-threatening hemoptysis [edit.]. Lancet, 1:1354, 1987.
59. Winter, S. M., and Ingbar, D. H.: Massive hemoptysis: pathogenesis and management. J. Intern. Care Med., 3:171, 1988.
60. Israel, R. H., and Poe, R. H.: Hemoptysis. Clin. Chest. Med., 8:197, 1987.
61. Nath, H.: When does bronchial arterial embolization fail to control hemoptysis? [Editorial]. Chest, 97:515, 1990.
62. Uflacker, R., et al.: Bronchial artery embolization in the management of hemoptysis: technical aspects and long-term results. Radiology, 157:637, 1985.
63. Muthuswamy, P. P., et al.: Management of major or massive hemoptysis in acute pulmonary tuberculosis by bronchial arterial embolization. Chest, 92:77, 1987.
64. Remy, J., et al.: Treatment of hemoptysis by embolization of bronchial arteries. Radiology, 122:33, 1977.
65. Rabkin, J. E., Astafjev, V. I., Gothman, L. N., and Grigorjev, Y. C.: Transcatheter embolization in the management of pulmonary hemorrhage. Radiology, 163:361, 1987.
66. Stern, R. V., et al.: Treatment and prognosis of massive hemoptysis in cystic fibrosis. Am. Rev. Respir. Dis., 117:825, 1978.
67. Porter, D. K., VanEvery, M. J., Anthracite, R. F., and Mach, J. W., Jr.: Massive hemoptysis in cystic fibrosis. Arch. Intern. Med., 143:287, 1983.
68. di Sant'Agnese, P. A., and David, P. B.: Cystic fibrosis in adults. Am. J. Med., 66:121, 1979.
69. Holsclaw, D. S., Grand, R. J., and Schwachman: Massive hemoptysis in cystic fibrosis. J. Pediatr., 76:829, 1970.
70. McCarthy, D., and Pedys, J.: Allergic bronchopulmonary aspergillosis. Clinical immunology: clinical features. Clin. Allergy, 2:261, 1971.
71. Thomas, N. W., Wilson, R. F., Puro, H. E., and Arbulu, A.: Life-threatening hemoptysis in primary lung abscess. Ann. Thorc. Surg., 14:347, 1972.
72. Goodwin, R., et al.: Chronic pulmonary histoplasmosis. Medicine, 55:413, 1976.
73. Jewkes, J., Kay, P. H., Paneth, M., and Citron, K.: Pulmonary aspergilloma. Thorax, 38:572, 1983.
74. Scarlat, A., Bodner, G., and Liron, M.: Massive hemoptysis as the presenting symptom in mitral stenosis. Thorax, 41: 413, 1986.
75. Miller, R. R., and McGregor, D. H.: Hemorrhage from carcinoma of the lung. Cancer, 46:200, 1980.
76. Bateman, E. D., and Morrison, S. C.: Catamenial hemoptysis from endobronchial endometriosis—a case report and review of previously reported cases. Respir. Med., 84:157, 1990.
77. Crocco, J. A., et al.: Massive hemoptysis. Arch. Intern. Med., 121:495, 1968.
78. Lemaine, F., et al.: Acute left ventricular dysfunction during unsuccessful weaning from mechanical ventilation. Anesthesiology, 69:171, 1988.
79. Johnston, I. H., and Reisz, G.: Changing spectrum of hemoptysis. Arch. Intern. Med., 149:1666, 1989.
80. Brandstetter, R. D.: The use of a Swan-Ganz catheter and streptokinase in the management of massive hemoptysis. N.Y. J. Med., 90:33, 1990.
81. Pursel, S. E., and Lindskig, G. E.: Hemoptysis: a clinical evaluation of 105 patients examined consecutively on a thoracic surgical service. Am. Rev. Respir. Dis., 84:329, 1961.
82. Muller, N. L., Bergin, C. J., Ostrow, D. N., and Nichols, D. M.: Role of computed tomography in the recognition of bronchiectasis. Am. J. Roentgenol., 143:971, 1984.
83. Haponik, E. F., Britt, E. J., Smith, P. L., and Bleecker, E. R.: Computed chest tomography in the evaluation of hemoptysis. Chest, 91:80, 1987.
84. Poe, R. H., et al.: Utility of fiberoptic bronchoscopy in patients with hemoptysis and a non-localizing chest roentgenogram. Chest, 92:70, 1988.
85. Smiddy, J. F., and Elliott, R. C.: The evaluation of hemoptysis with fiberoptic bronchoscopy. Chest, 64:158, 1973.
86. Adelman, M., Haponik, E. F., Bleecker, E. R., and Britt, J.: Cryptogenic hemoptysis. Am. Intern. Med., 102:829, 1985.
87. Gong, H., and Salvatierra, C.: Clinical efficacy of early and delayed fiberoptic bronchoscopy in patient with hemoptysis. Am. Rev. Respir. Dis., 124:221, 1981.
88. Coel, M. N., and Druger, G.: Radionuclide detection of the site of hemoptysis. Chest, 81:242, 1982.
89. Haponik, E. F., Rothfeld, B., Britt, E. J., and Bleeker, E. R.: Radionuclide localization of massive pulmonary hemorrhage. Chest, 86:208, 1984.
90. Albelda, S. M., et al.: Pulmonary cavitation and massive hemoptysis in invasive pulmonary aspergillosis. Am. Rev. Respir. Dis., 131:115, 1985.
91. de Gracia, J., et al.: Diagnostic value of bronchoalveolar lavage in suspected pulmonary tuberculosis. Chest, 93:329, 1988.
92. Kah, F. W., Jones, J. M., and England, D. M.: The role of bronchoalveolar lavage in the diagnosis of invasive pulmonary aspergillosis. Am. J. Clin. Pathol., 86:518, 1986.
93. Davies, S. F.: Diagnosis of pulmonary fungal infections. Semin. Respir. Infect., 3:162, 1988.
94. Davies, S. F.: Serodiagnosis of histoplasmosis. Semin. Respir. Infect., 1:9, 1986.
95. Garzon, A. A., and Gourin, A.: Surgical management of massive hemoptysis. Ann. Surg., 187:267, 1978.
96. Yang, C. T., and Berger, H.: Conservative management of life-threatening hemoptysis. Mt. Sinai J. Med., 45:329, 1978.
97. Yeoh, C. B., Hubaytar, R. T., Ford, J. M., and Wylie, R. H.: Treatment of massive hemorrhage in pulmonary tuberculosis. J. Thorac. Cardiovasc. Surg., 54:503, 1967.
98. Goldman, L., et al.: Multifactorial index of cardiac risk in noncardiac surgical procedures. N. Engl. J. Med., 297:845, 1977.
99. Miller, J. I., and Hatcher, C. R.: Limited resection of bronchogenic carcinoma in the patient with marked impairment of pulmonary function. Ann. Thorac. Surg., 44:340, 1987.
100. Remy, J., et al.: Massive hemoptysis of pulmonary arterial origin: diagnosis and treatment. Am. J. Roentgenol., 143: 963, 1984.
101. Borkin, M. H., Arena, F. P., Brown, A. E., and Armstrong, D.: Invasive aspergillosis with massive fatal hemoptysis in patient with neoplastic disease. Chest, 78:835, 1980.
102. Karas, A., et al.: Pulmonary aspergillosis: an analysis of 41 patients. Ann. Thorac. Surg., 22:1, 1976.
103. Varkey, B., and Rose, H. D.: Pulmonary aspergilloma: a rational approach to treatment. Am. J. Med., 61:626, 1976.
104. Rafferty, P., Biggs, B., Crompton, G. K., and Grand, I. W.: What happened to patients with aspergilloma? Analysis of 23 cases. Thorax, 38:579, 1983.
105. Butz, R. O., Zvetra, J. R., and Leininger, B. J.: Ten years

experience with mycetomas in patients with tuberculosis. Chest, 87:356, 1985.

SUPPLEMENTAL READINGS

Bigby, T. D., Serota, M. L., Tierney, L. M., and Matthay, M. A.: Clinical spectrum of pulmonary mucormycosis. Chest, 89: 435, 1986.

Charan, N. B., Turk, G. M., and Dhand, R.: The role of bronchial circulation in lung abscess. Am. Rev. Respir. Dis., 131:121, 1985.

Ferris, E. J.: Pulmonary hemorrhage. Chest, 80:710, 1981.

Goldman, J. M.: Hemoptysis: Emergency assessment and management. Emerg. Med. Clin. North Am., 7:325, 1989.

Gourin, A., and Garzon, A. A.: Operative treatment of massive hemoptysis. Ann. Thorac. Surg., 18:52, 1974.

Gutierrez-Rodero, F., and Andres Am Praga, M.: Diffuse pulmonary hemorrhage and crescentic glomerulonephritis. Nephron, 47:156, 1987.

Haponik, E. F., and Chin, R.: Hemoptysis: clinicians' perspectives. Chest, 976:469, 1990.

Heaton, R. W.: Should patients with hemoptysis and a normal chest x-ray be bronchoscoped? Postgrad. Med. J., 63:947, 1987.

Hiebert, C. A.: Balloon catheter control of life-threatening hemoptysis. Chest, 66:308, 1974.

Imgrund, S. P., et al.: Clinical diagnosis of massive hemoptysis using the fiberoptic bronchoscope. Crit. Care. Med., 13:438, 1985.

Karas, A., et al.: Pulmonary aspergillosis: an analysis of 41 patients. Ann. Thorac. Surg., 22:1, 1976.

Katho, O., et al.: Bronchoscopic and angiographic comparison of bronchial arterial lesions in patients with hemoptysis. Chest, 91:486, 1987.

Klasa, R. J., Abboud, R. T., Ballon, H. S., and Grossman, L.: Goodpasture's syndrome: recurrence after a five year remission. Am. J. Med., 84:751, 1988.

Leatherman, J. W.: Immune alveolar hemorrhage. Chest, 91:891, 1987.

Lederle, F. A., Nichol, K. L., and Parenti, C. M.: Bronchoscopy to evaluate hemoptysis in older men with nonsuspicious chest roentgenograms. Chest, 95:1043, 1989.

Magee, G., and Williams, M. H., Jr.: Treatment of massive hemoptysis with intravenous pitressin. Lung, 160;165, 1982.

Middleton, J. R., et al.: Death producing hemoptysis in tuberculosis. Chest, 72:601, 1977.

Nakao, M. A.: The use of a Swan-Ganz catheter and streptokinase in the management of massive hemoptysis. (Editorial.) N.Y. State J. Med., 90:270, 1990.

Olopade, C. O., and Prakash, U. B. S.: Bronchoscopy in the critical care unit. Mayo Clin. Proc., 64:1255, 1989.

Panos, R. J., Barr, L. F., Walsh, T. J., and Silverman, H. J.: Factors associated with fatal hemoptysis in cancer patients. Chest, 94:1008, 1988.

Pape, L. A., et al.: Fatal pulmonary hemorrhage after use of the flow-directed balloon tipped catheter. Ann. Int. Med., 90: 344, 1979.

Patterson, R., Nugent, K. M., Harris, K. E., and Eberle, M. E.: Immunologic hemorrhagic pneumonia caused by isocyanates. Am. Rev. Respir. Dis., 141:226, 1990.

Prager, R. L., Laws, K. H., and Bender. H. W.: Arteriovenous fistula of the lung. Ann. Thorac. Surg., 36:231, 1983.

Remy, J., et al.: Massive hemoptysis of pulmonary arterial origin: diagnosis and treatment. Am. J. Roentgenol., 143:963, 1984.

Research Committee of the British Thoracic and Tuberculosis Association: Aspergilloma and residual tuberculosis cavities—the results of a resurvey. Tubercle, 51:227, 1970.

Rogol, P. R.: Fatal hemoptysis due to lung abscess and pulmoaortic fistula. Chest, 94:441, 1988.

Rubinstein, I., Baum, G. L., Hiss, Y., and Solomon, A.: Hemoptysis as the presenting manifestation of sarcoidosis. (Editorial). Chest, 91:931, 1987.

Scarlat, A., Bodner, G., and Liron, M.: Massive hemoptysis as the presenting symptom in mitral stenosis. Thorax, 41:413, 1986.

Shah, K. B., Rao, T. L. K., Laughlin, S., and El-Etr, A. D.: A review of pulmonary artery catheterization in 6,245 patients. Anesthesiology, 61:271, 1984.

Shapiro, M. J., Albelda, S. M., Mayock, R. L., and McLean, G. K.: Severe hemoptysis associated with pulmonary aspergilloma. Chest, 94:1225, 1988.

Sherman, J. M., et al.: Time course of hemosiderin production and clearance by human pulmonary macrophages. Chest, 86:409, 1984.

Smiddy, J. R., and Elliott, R. C.: The evaluation of hemoptysis with fiberoptic bronchoscopy. Chest, 64;:158, 1973.

Smith, L. T., and Katzenstein, A. L. A.: Pathogenesis of massive pulmonary hemorrhage in acut eleukemia. Arch. Intern. Med., 142:2149, 1982.

Stamatis, G., and Greschuchna, D.: Surgery for pulmonary aspergilloma and pleural aspergillosis. Thorac. Cardiovasc. Surg., 36:356, 1988.

Syabbalo, N. C.: Medical management of hemoptysis. (Editorial). Chest, 96:1441, 1989

Tadavarthy, S. M., et al.: Systemic to pulmonary collaterals in pathological states. Radiology, 144:55, 1982.

Trento, A., Estner, S. M., Griffith, B. P., and Hardesty, R. L.: Massive hemoptysis in patients with cystic fibrosis: three case reports and a protocol for clinical management. Ann. Thorac. Surg., 39:254, 1985

Tsukamoto, R.: Medical bronchial artery embolization. (Editorial). Chest, 93:1316, 1988.

Wedzicha, J. A., and Pearson, M. C.: Management of massive hemoptysis. Respir. Med., 84:9, 1990.

Wollschlager, C., and Kahn, F.: Aspergillomas complicating sarcoidosis: a prospective study in 100 patients. Chest, 86:585, 1984.

Chapter 20

MANAGEMENT OF THE GENERAL THORACIC SURGICAL PATIENT

THOMAS W. RICE
THOMAS L. HIGGINS
THOMAS J. KIRBY

PREOPERATIVE CONSIDERATIONS (RISK PHASE)

Consideration of cardiac and pulmonary reserve is essential for all patients undergoing surgical intervention but particularly critical for those undergoing major noncardiac thoracic operations. Thoracic operations are among the most dangerous and challenging, particularly when adequate oxygen delivery must be maintained in the face of one-lung ventilation. The essential questions to answer for a specific patient include:

- What factors are present that have already reduced physiologic reserve in major organ systems, particularly the heart and lungs?
- What is the planned surgical procedure, and how will surgery and anesthesia affect the patient both acutely and chronically (i.e., how much pulmonary reserve will remain postoperatively, particularly if the resection winds up more extensive than initially planned?
- Can any adverse factors be modified by preoperative, perioperative, or postoperative interventions (i.e., smoking cessation, bronchodilators, mode of ventilation, cardiac support)?
- What surgical, anesthetic, and intensive care factors may have impact on the patient's outcome, and what steps may be taken to identify and limit these factors?

This chapter focuses on addressing these questions by developing a profile for the patient at particular risk for complications following thoracic surgery and then discusses methods of risk modification and therapeutic choices that might further minimize risks.

Preoperative Evaluation

The thoracic surgery patient may be young and healthy but is typically older with concurrent medical problems, possibly debilitated by cancer, and often saddled with significant abnormalities of lung function. Pulmonary abnormalities may have arisen from occupational exposure, tobacco use, or a primary disease process. Thus a careful history is indicated, with particular attention to clues of extrapulmonary system dysfunction. Appropriate exploration of the extent of these problems can then be accomplished, as detailed in Chapter 59. A history of dyspnea may indicate either heart or lung disease, and thus it is helpful to quantitate the degree of effort required to produce dyspnea. Ability to climb stairs is a simple, noninvasive, and inexpensive measure of pulmonary reserve.[1] A history of asthma, wheezing, or allergic airway responses is important, both as a risk factor and to identify patients in whom bronchodilator management will be needed in the intraoperative or postoperative period. Forced vital capacity (FVC) alone is insufficiently sensitive and specific as the sole physiologic predictor of postoperative pulmonary function, and more extensive pulmonary function testing is indicated in the majority of patients.

One approach to the thoracotomy patient, based on a comprehensive review,[2] is to conduct a staged evaluation as follows:

- All patients should have a careful general history and physical examination.
- Arterial blood gas analysis and formal pulmonary function testing are essential when resection of lung tissue is comtemplated.
- Indicators of high risk include Pco_2 determined by greater than 45 mm Hg and abnormal FVC, forced expiratory volume in 1 second (FEV_1), and carbon monoxide diffusion capacity ($DLco_2$) (Table 20-1).

Patients with initially abnormal values should have abnormalities confirmed and then be considered for more sophisticated tests. Those with expected postresection FEV_1 values close to the limits to be described subsequently may also be candidates for further tests. These tests include split perfusion scanning,[3,4] exercise testing with measurement of maximal O_2 consumption,[5,6] and right heart catheterization to determine pulmonary vascular resistance during exercise.[7] The values and implications of each of these tests are described subsequently.

Preoperative pulmonary function testing is of proven benefit in predicting outcome for patients undergoing lung resection and is endorsed for identification of patients at high risk for complications after lung resection[8] (Tables 20-1 and 20-2). Spirometry is simple, reliable, and cost-effective in providing preoperative information. FEV_1, which is affected by inspiratory muscle strength, elastic recoil, and degree of obstructive air trapping, provides a good indicator of the patient's postoperative ability to cough effectively and clear secretions.

Table 20-1. Pulmonary Function Criteria Suggesting High Risk in Resective Surgery

Forced vital capacity <50% of predicted
Forced expiratory volume in 1 sec 50% of forced vital capacity, or <2 L absolute value
Maximal voluntary ventilation <50% of predicted
Residual volume/total lung capacity ratio >50%
Diffusing capacity <50% of predicted

(Adapted from Olsen, G. N., et al.: Pulmonary function evaluation of the lung resection candidate: a prospective study. Am. Rev. Respir. Dis., *111*:379, 1975.)

Simple spirometric criteria of surgical resectability include a minimum preoperative FEV_1 of 1.7 to 2.0 L for pneumonectomy and 1.2 to 1.5 L for lobectomy.[6,9] The decrease in FEV_1 after lung resection for bronchogenic carcinoma is not necessarily a simple proportionate relationship because lesser decreases in FEV_1 than calculated are noted when an obstructed lobar or main stem bronchus is present. Patients with minimal obstructive pathology are more likely to have a greater postoperative decrease in FEV_1 (formula: postoperative FEV_1 = preoperative FEV_1 [1 − % perfusion to resected lung]). A cutoff value for postpneumonectomy FEV_1 of 800 ml is commonly used as a criterion of resectability, although this value has not been tested prospectively, and some studies recommend the cutoff to be 1 L. Another predictor of pulmonary complications following resection surgery is reduction of maximum O_2 consumption during exercise to less than 15 ml/kg/min, which in an initial study that has been shown to be a sensitive predictor.[5] Pulmonary vascular resistance (PVR) values greater than 190 dyne-sec/cm^5 during exercise are associated with poor outcome;[7] preoperative identification of excessive PVR may be useful in identifying those patients at risk for severe postoperative right ventricular dysfunction. Table 20-3 summarizes the results of several major studies and compares the sensitivity and specificity of spirometry, exercise PVR, and combined tests.[2,7,9,11-13]

Lung surgery affects postoperative lung function, and entering the chest cavity, even without resection of tissue, produces substantial changes. Lateral thoracotomy in particular is associated with postoperative pulmonary impairment. Marked decreases occur in FVC, and functional residual capacity (FRC), usually to less than 60% of the preoperative value on the first postoperative day. Subsequent return to baseline can take 14 days or longer. The decline in FRC is especially important because the resulting atelectasis causes physiologic shunting and hypoxemia. Postoperative lung function changes less with median sternotomy than with lateral thoracotomy, partly because the midline incision is less painful, and patients have less splinting and thus less difficulty reexpanding atelectatic segments. For this reason, a median sternotomy incision may be preferred to the more routine lateral thoracotomy in patients with borderline lung function, if there is an option.[14]

Scoring Preoperative Severity of Illness

No scoring system for stratifying preoperative severity of illness in the thoracic surgery patient is currently in widespread use. This hampers efforts at quality assurance and mortality comparisons because so many factors other than operative skill can affect outcome. The widely used American Society of Anesthesiologists (ASA) physical status classification[15] (Table 20-4) provides a rough guideline of anesthetic risk but is not specific for thoracic surgery patients and has been found to suffer from inconsistency in ratings.[16] Determining severity of illness in the thoracic surgery population must take into account both pulmonary and nonpulmonary risk factors that might predispose a patient to postoperative respiratory complications. These factors include not only the respiratory criteria of fitness for surgery, but also age, body habitus, smoking history, disease-related factors (in particular, cardiac and renal function), and factors related to the operation itself (type of surgery, location of incision, and anesthetic technique).

Although such testing guidelines have been outlined for the thoracic surgical population at large, there may be additional benefit in examining other variables in the subset of patients with severe pulmonary compromise. A study of 53 operations in 42 patients with severe chronic obstructive disease suggests that the best predictors of postoperative ventilation requirements were the arterial Po_2 less than 70% of predicted for age and the presence of dyspnea at rest.[17] In patients undergoing elective thoracic or abdominal surgery, the risk of postoperative pneumonia was increased by:

- Low serum albumin concentration on admission
- High ASA physical status classification
- History of smoking
- Longer preoperative stay
- Longer operative procedure
- Thoracic or upper abdominal surgical site[18]

Identification of the patient at risk extends beyond simple prognosis because there is evidence that intervention in the high risk population with cessation of smoking, bronchodilatation, antibiotics, humidification, and aggressive chest physiotherapy may reduce postoperative morbidity and mortality.[19]

Numerous studies implicate advanced age, particularly age greater than 80 years,[20] as a risk factor for adverse postoperative outcome, although questions have been raised about selection bias in reports from large tertiary-care centers.[21] Malnutrition is common in the elderly, and hypoalbuminemia correlates with increased risk of perioperative complications in elderly patients undergoing car-

Table 20-2. Criteria of Operability

Mean pulmonary artery pressure on balloon occlusion and exercise <35 mm Hg
Systemic Pao_2 value on balloon occlusion and exercise >45 mm Hg
Predicted postpneumonectomy FEV_1 value >0.8 L

(Adapted from Olsen, G. N., et al.: Pulmonary function evaluation of the lung resection candidate: a prospective study. Am. Rev. Respir. Dis., *111*:379, 1975.)

Table 20-3. Preoperative Pulmonary Function Evaluations in Patients with Lung Cancer

Study	Year	Study Design and Number of Patients	Tests	Pulmonary Complications Studied	Sensitivity of Test for Outcome	Specificity of Test for Outcome
Keagy et al.[11]	1983	Retrospective, 101	Spirometry	Death	0.08 0.0–0.27	0.89 0.82–0.96
				Any pulmonary complication	0.16 0.0–0.32	0.91 0.84–0.98
Fee et al.[7]	1978	Prospective, 39	Spirometry, ABG	Death	0.20 0.0–0.65	0.77 0.59–0.93
			Exercise PVR at catheterization	Death	1.00 0.09–1.0	0.79 0.64–0.94
Peters et al.[12]	1978	Retrospective, 43	Spirometry	Death	0.50 0.0–1.0	0.49 0.32–0.66
Smith et al.[13]	1984	Prospective, 22	Spirometry, MVV split perfusion	Any pulmonary complication	0.72 0.41–1.00	0.45 0.11–0.79
			Maximal oxygen consumption		0.91 0.7–1.0	0.82 0.55–1.0
Bechard & Wetstein[6]	1987	Prospective, 50	Maximal oxygen consumption	Any pulmonary complication	0.63 0.23–1.0	0.95 0.87–1.00

ABG, Arterial blood gas; PVR, pulmonary vascular resistance; MVV, maximum ventilatory volume. (Adapted from Zibrak, J. D., O'Donnel, C. R., Marton, K.: Indications for pulmonary function testing. Ann. Intern. Med., *112*:763, 1990.)

diac thoracic procedures.[22] Inability to exercise worsens cardiac prognosis in elderly patients undergoing noncardiac surgery.[23] Elderly patients have age-related changes in pulmonary function, including decreased elastic recoil and progressive stiffening of the chest wall, increase in the ratio of FRC to total lung capacity, and diminished vital capacity and FEV_1.[24] The activity of elderly upper airway reflexes is blunted,[25] which may result in impaired clearance of secretions and ability to protect the airway. In one study of 138 patients aged 65 and older, only 13.5% of patients had normal measured hemodynamic, respiratory, and oxygen transport function.[26] Twenty-three percent of this same population were considered unacceptable risks for major surgery. In another study examining only patients over the age of 70 undergoing thoracotomy, hospital mortality was 7.5% and complication rate 17%.[27] A number of studies have examined the additional risk imposed by severe obesity.[28,29] Obesity results in decreases in FRC and expiratory reserve volume (ERV), to the point that ERV may drop below closing volume (CV), resulting in perfused, unventilated segments of lung and a widened (A-a) Po_2 gradient. Obese patients are more likely to cough poorly, retain secretions, and develop basilar atelectasis.[30]

Cigarette smoking is well recognized for its contribution to perioperative morbidity via effects on the cardiovascular system, elevation of carbon monoxide levels, impairment of mucus secretion and clearance, small airway narrowing, immune suppression, and hepatic enzyme induction.[31] Cigarette exposure is conventionally measured in "pack-years" (i.e., the average number of packages of 20 cigarettes smoked per day times the number of years as a smoker). The risk of chronic obstructive pulmonary disease (COPD) and development of malignancy rises with increasing "pack-years" of smoking history. The benefit of smoking cessation before elective surgery is well recognized, although data in coronary artery bypass patients suggest that cessation of smoking within 8 weeks of surgery may actually increase the risk of postoperative pulmonary

Table 20-4. Physical Status Classification of the American Society of Anesthesiologists (ASA)

ASA Class	Patient Characteristics	Example
I	No organic, physiologic, biochemical, or psychiatric disturbance. The pathologic process for which operation is to be performed is localized and does not entail a systemic disturbance	Removal of benign nodule in otherwise healthy individual
II	Mild-to-moderate systemic disturbance caused either by the condition to be treated surgically or by other pathophysiologic processes	Bronchoscopy and mediastinoscopy in patient with diabetes and chronic obstructive pulmonary disease
III	Severe systemic disturbance or disease from whatever cause with the potential for perioperative complications	Lobectomy in patient with angina pectoris
IV	Severe systemic disorders that are already life-threatening, not always correctable by operation	Elective descending thoracic aneurysm repair in patient with congestive heart failure and renal insufficiency
V	Moribund with little chance of survival	Pulmonary embolectomy for saddle embolus
E	Emergency operation—letter "E" is placed beside the numerical classification to indicate increased risk and poorer physical condition associated with emergency procedure	Any emergency procedure, often associated with hemodynamic instability

(From Dripps, R. D., Lamont, A., and Eckenhoff, J. E.: The role of anesthesia in surgical mortality. JAMA, *178*:261, 1961.)

Table 20-5. Classification of Risk of Pulmonary Complications of Thoracic and Abdominal Procedures

Category	Points*
Expiratory spirogram	
Normal (%FVC + %FEV$_1$/FVC >150)	0
%FVC + %FEV$_1$/FVC = 100 − 150	1
%FVC + %FEV$_1$/FVC <100	2
Preoperative FVC <20 ml/kg	3
Postbronchodilator FEV$_1$/FVC <50%	3
Cardiovascular system	
Normal	0
Controlled hypertension, myocardial infarction without sequelae for more than 2 years	0
Dyspnea on exertion, orthopnea, paroxysmal nocturnal dyspnea, dependent edema, congestive heart failure, angina	1
Arterial blood gases	
Acceptable	0
Pa$_{CO_2}$ >50 mm Hg or Pa$_{O_2}$ <60 mm Hg on room air	1
Metabolic pH abnormality >7.50 or <7.30	1
Nervous system	
Normal	0
Confusion, obtundation, agitation, spasticity, discoordination bulbar malfunction	1
Significant muscular weakness	1
Postoperative ambulation	
Expected ambulation (minimum, sitting at bedside) within 36 hours	0
Expected complete bed confinement for at least 36 hours	1

* 0 Points = low risk, 1–2 Points = moderate risk. 3 Points = high risk. (Adapted from Shapiro, B. A., Harrison, R. A., Kacmarek R. M., and Cane, R. D.: Clinical Application of Respiratory Care. 3rd Ed. Chicago, Year Book, 1985.)

Table 20-6. Absolute Contraindications for Lung Transplantation

Active drug and alcohol dependency
Another major organ failure
Psychologically unfit
On prednisone >20 mg/day

complications,[32] possibly owing to a transient increase in sputum volume. Early cessation of smoking (more than 8 weeks before surgery) is one of the conceptually easiest and practically difficult ways to modify risk effectively.

A system for classification of the risk of pulmonary complications following thoracic and abdominal procedures was developed by Shapiro and colleagues[33] (Table 20-5). By applying 0 to 3 points for spirometric valves, cardiovascular history, arterial blood gases, central nervous system, and expected postoperative ambulation, patients can be classified as low risk, moderate risk, or high risk. Low risk patients do not generally require oxygen therapy after recovery room discharge. Moderate risk patients require several days of postoperative observation. The high risk patient often requires postoperative intensive care and significant prophylactic interventions.

Special Considerations Preoperatively in the Lung Transplant Patient

Potential single or double lung transplant recipients must be thoroughly screened by a transplant team before acceptance for transplantation. Tables 20-6 and 20-7 outline our absolute and relative contraindications for lung transplantation. Recipients are obviously in incipient or frank respiratory failure and have many special considerations that must be addressed. These patients are often malnourished and in suboptimal physical condition because respiratory disease severely restricts physical activity. An attempt should be made to correct these problems before transplantation, and in most instances this is possible. Patients can be started on a modest exercise program under the direction of a physical therapist using a pulse oximeter to monitor oxygenation and supplementing inspired oxygen requirements as needed. In consultation with a nutritionist, the patient should be placed on a diet that provides adequate caloric and protein intake while attempting to correct any previously identified nutritional deficiencies. Patients with cystic fibrosis may be seen by an infectious disease consultant to decide on appropriate perioperative antibiotic coverage based on the most recent culture results.

In single lung transplantation, preoperative investigations, including a quantitative ventilation/perfusion scan and a computed tomography (CT) scan of the chest, help to identify the lung with the most compromised function, which in general is selected as the side for transplantation. In double lung transplantation, the lung with the poorer function is transplanted first, allowing in most cases the patient to be supported on the remaining lung without the need for cardiopulmonary bypass during this part of the procedure. Once the first lung has been transplanted, it usually functions adequately to support the patient while the opposite side is being grafted. This bilateral sequential single lung transplantation technique, using a bilateral submammary fourth intercostal space incision and a transverse sternotomy, allows 70 to 80% of patients to be transplanted without using cardiopulmonary bypass, thus avoiding full systemic heparinization in patients who are at significant risk of bleeding because of associated pleural and mediastinal adhesions and fibrosis. The risk of chest wall bleeding is most significant in those with prior empyemas and fibrosis, especially when cystic fibrosis is the underlying diagnosis.

Single lung transplantation in patients with systemic pulmonary hypertension, most often based on primary pulmonary hypertension or Eisenmenger's physiology secondary to a patent ductus arteriosus or an atrial or ventricular septal defect, present a challenging group of patients for any lung transplant program.[34] This group of patients, up

Table 20-7. Relative Contraindications for Lung Transplantation

Ventilator dependent
On prednisone <20 mg/day
Age >60 years
Life expectancy >18 months

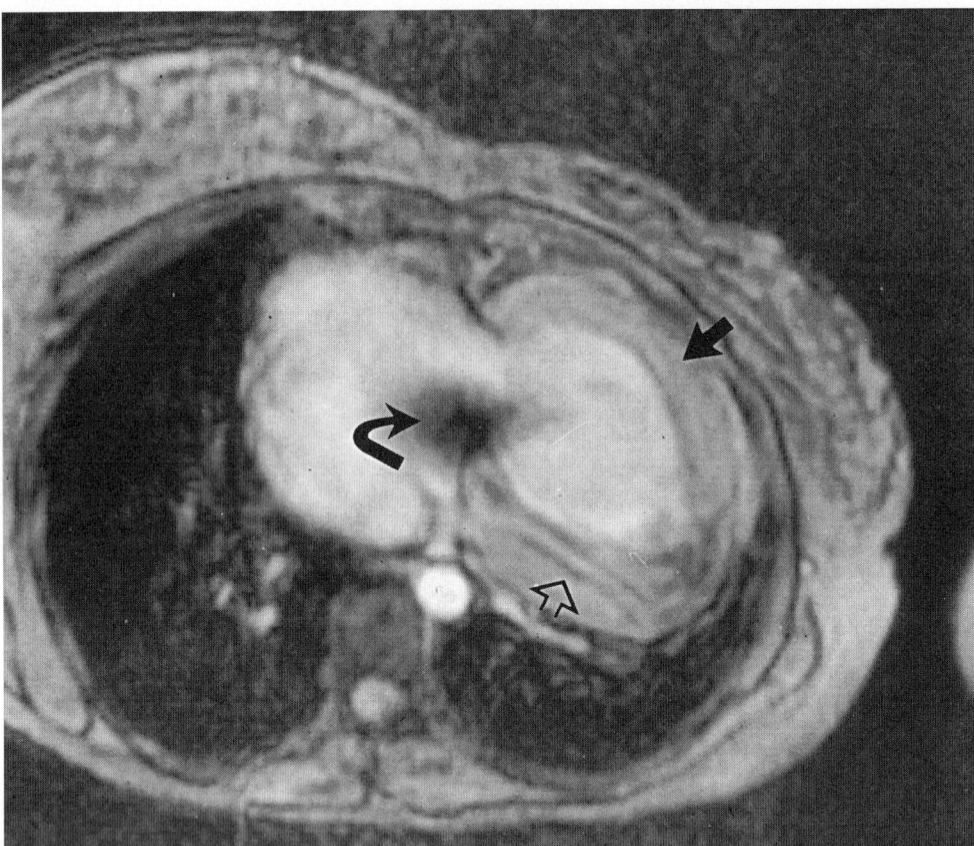

Fig. 20-1. An MRI scan of the chest in a patient with Eisenmenger's syndrome illustrates the dilated hypertrophied right atrium compressing the left ventricle (open arrow). A jet of tricuspid regurgitation is shown by the curved arrow.

until the past 2 years, were the classic candidates for heart-lung transplantation but more recently have been successfully managed with single lung transplantation. This approach has many advantages, including allowing three organs (two lungs, one heart) to be used in three different recipients instead of one heart-lung graft in one recipient. Initially there was concern that the often compromised right ventricular function in these individuals would not recover following single lung transplantation. We have carefully documented right ventricular function preoperatively and postoperatively and have found that magnetic resonance imaging (MRI) is particularly valuable in this area, in addition to documenting accurately the presence and degree of associated tricuspid regurgitation (Fig. 20-1). We have shown full recovery of right ventricular function in patients who preoperatively often had ejection fractions of less than 10%.[35] Clinically if patients are in florid, uncontrolled right ventricular failure (ascites, hepatomegaly, peripheral edema), we believe these are appropriate candidates for heart-lung transplantation.

Our preference is to perform a right single lung transplantation in patients with pulmonary hypertension because it is easier to place the patient on cardiopulmonary bypass through the right chest, cannulating the ascending aorta and right atrium instead of using femoral-femoral bypass where adequate venous return can be a problem. Donor organ supply is always a problem in all organ transplantation but is particularly acute with lung transplantation. Donor criteria (Table 20-8) results in only 15 to 20% of all cardiac donors having lungs that are acceptable for lung transplantation.

Preoperative Outcome Assessment in the Thoracic Surgical Patient

The candidate for thoracic surgery may have both pulmonary and cardiac disease, and consideration should be given to quantifying cardiac risk as well in this population. The risk assessment of Goldman and colleagues[36] tallies clinical findings to predict cardiac risk in noncardiac surgical procedures, although not specifically for thoracic patients. Patients with suspected myocardial compromise should be screened for clinical criteria of cardiac risk (his-

Table 20-8. Lung Donor Criteria*

Age <50 years
<10 pack-year history of smoking
On ventilator <10 days
P_{O_2} >300 mm Hg on F_{IO_2} of 1.00
ABO compatibility
Correct size match
Clear chest radiograph
Bronchoscopy normal
Gram stain and KOH preparation negative for significant pathogens

*Although it is not necessary that all the above criteria be met, donors that fall outside of these criteria are often found to be unsuitable or to increase the risk of graft failure post-transplantation.

tory of angina, myocardial infarction, congestive heart failure, diabetes, or Q wave on electrocardiogram [ECG]).[37] Further workup (thallium imaging after exercise or dipyridamole (Persantine), coronary arteriography) can then be used to assess those at increased risk by clinical criteria. Stepwise discriminant analysis has been used to predict those at risk for postoperative ventilation[17] and pneumonia,[18] but as yet there is no score specifically tailored to predict outcome in the thoracotomy patient.

APACHE-II, a system for ICU severity scoring, has been applied to the evaluation of surgical lung carcinoma patients and found to be useful when coupled with tumor-node-metastasis (TNM) staging. In a retrospective analysis of 59 high risk patients with a mortality of 12.4%, APACHE-II demonstrated sensitivity of 75%, specificity of 95%, and a total correct classification rate of 55.6%. The total mortality ratio (actual deaths/predicted deaths) was 0.94.[38] The reader is referred to Chapter 79 for a more complete discussion of scoring systems and particularly the potential difficulties with using physiologic scoring systems in surgical patients, in whom the degree of physiologic derangement at ICU admission is a function of operative events.

Table 20–9. Staging of Bronchogenic Carcinomas

T: Primary Tumor
- T1 Tumor 3 cm or less in greatest dimension
  Local invasion limited by pulmonary parenchyma
  Without bronchoscopic evidence of invasion proximal to lobar bronchus
- T2 Tumor that has one of the following features:
  More than 3.0 cm in greatest dimension
  Invades the visceral pleura
  Involves the main bronchus, 2 cm or more distal to the carina
  Atelectasis or obstructive pneumonitis that extends to the hilar region but does not involve the entire lung
- T3 Tumor that has one of the following features:
  Any size
  Invades any of the following: chest wall (including superior sulcus tumors), diaphragm, mediastinal pleura, parietal pericardium
  Involves the main bronchus less than 2 cm distal to the carina but without involvement of the carina
  Atelectasis or obstructive pneumonitis of the entire lung
- T4 Tumor that has one of the following features:
  Any size
  Invades any of the following: mediastinum, heart, great vessels, trachea, esophagus, vertebral body
  Involves the carina
  Malignant pleural effusion

N: Regional Lymph Nodes
- N0 No regional lymph node metastasis
- N1 Metastasis to ipsilateral peribronchial and/or ipsilateral hilar lymph nodes, including direct extension
- N2 Metastasis to ipsilateral mediastinal and/or subcarinal lymph node(s)
- N3 Metastasis to contralateral mediastinal or hilar lymph nodes, or scalene or supraclavicular lymph nodes

M: Distant Metastasis
- M0 No distant metastasis
- M1 Distant metastasis

Stage Grouping

Stage	T	N	M
Stage I	T1	N0	M0
	T2	N0	M0
Stage II	T1	N1	M0
	T2	N1	M0
Stage IIIa	T1	N2	M0
	T2	N2	M0
	T3	N0, N1, N2	M0
Stage IIIb	Any T	N3	M0
	T4	Any N	M0
Stage IV	Any T	Any N	M1

Table 20–10. Staging of Esophageal Carcinomas

T: Primary Tumor
- T1 Tumor invades lamina propria or submucosa
- T2 Tumor invades muscularis propria
- T3 Tumor invades periesophageal tissue
- T4 Tumor invades adjacent structures

N: Regional Lymph Nodes
- N0 No regional lymph node metastases
- N1 Regional lymph node metastases

M: Distant Metastasis
- M0 No distant metastasis
- M1 Distant metastasis

Stage Grouping

Stage	T	N	M
Stage I	T1	N0	M0
Stage IIa	T2	N0	M0
	T3	N0	M0
Stage IIb	T1	N1	M0
	T2	N1	M0
Stage III	T3	N1	M0
	T4	Any N	M0
Stage IV	Any T	Any N	M1

Staging

The survival of patients with carcinoma is directly related to the stage of the disease at diagnosis and treatment. Staging systems have been published for the staging of small cell,[39] non-small-cell,[40] and other types of cancer by histologic type.[41,42] These systems are TNM based. To determine the stage of the disease, one must first determine the status of:

- Primary *t*umor (T)
- Regional lymph *n*odes (N)
- Distant site *m*etastases (M)

Subsets of TNM groups are arranged into staging sets with similar prognosis (Tables 20–9 and 20–10).[43-45] The staging of thymomas and mesotheliomas is presently less sophisticated. The stage of a thymoma is determined by the extent of local invasion and whether or not distant metastases exist (Table 20–11).[46] The invasive nature of a thymoma is sometimes best appreciated by the surgeon and

Table 20–11. Staging of Thymomas

Stage I	Macroscopic encapsulation, no microscopic capsular invasion
Stage II	Invasion into the capsule, surrounding fatty tissue, or mediastinal pleura
Stage III	Invasion into neighboring structures (pericardium, great vessels or lung)
Stage IVA	Pleural or pericardial metastases
Stage IVB	Lymphogenous or hematogenous metastases

(From Masaoka, A., Monden, Y., Nakahara, K. and Tanioka, T. Follow-up study of thymomas with special reference to their clinical stages. Cancer, *48*:2485, 1981.)

Table 20-12. Staging of Mesotheliomas

Stage I	Tumor confined to homolateral pleura, lung, and pericardium
Stage II	Tumor invades chest wall or involves mediastinal structures, e.g., esophagus, heart, opposite pleura Lymph node involvement outside the chest
Stage III	Tumor penetrates diaphragm to involve peritoneum directly Lymph node involvement outside the chest
Stage IV	Distant blood-borne metastases

(From Butchart, E. G., Ashcroft, T., Barnsley, W. C., and Holden, M. P.: Pleuropneumonectomy in the management of diffuse malignant mesothelioma of the pleura. Thorax, *31:*15, 1976.)

is generally not predictable by histology or cytology. Mesotheliomas are staged according to the number of mesothelial-lined cavities involved (Table 20-12).[39,47]

OPERATIVE CONSIDERATIONS

Premedication

The amount and type of premedication ordered depend on the patient's general physical status (age, height, weight, preexisting disease), anxiety level, and need for cooperation if multiple invasive lines need to be placed. The choice between long-acting and short-acting agents also depends on whether early extubation is a desired goal. Preoperative opiates can linger to cause postoperative respiratory and neurologic depression at a time when the respiratory system is already compromised because of the operative procedure. Antisialagogues (such as atropine, glycopyrrolate, or scopolamine) can reduce the copious secretions that sometimes occur during upper airway endoscopy and manipulation but cause uncomfortable dryness of the mouth. Typical premedication orders for an adult patient call for diazepam, 5 mg orally, plus scopolamine, 0.4 to 0.6 mg/60 kg body weight, if prophylactic use of a parasympatholytic agent is specifically indicated. Scopolamine can contribute to postoperative confusion, especially in the elderly patient.

Monitoring and Invasive Devices

Minimal monitoring for all procedures performed under anesthesia includes continuous ECG, noninvasive blood pressure determinations at regular intervals, temperature monitoring, and assessment of oxygenation and gas exchange (Table 20-13). Oxygenation is generally assessed by pulse oximetry and gas exchange by end-tidal carbon dioxide determination or mass spectrometry. Use of both pulse oximetry and end-tidal carbon dioxide measurements may obviate the need for frequent blood gas sampling, although at least one arterial blood gas sample may be necessary to determine the gradient between end-tidal CO_2 and arterial CO_2. It is helpful to place the pulse oximeter probe on the lower arm when the patient is placed in the lateral thoracotomy position as a monitor of limb perfusion.

A large-bore peripheral intravenous catheter is indicated for rapid fluid resuscitation. It is also worthwhile to insert a nasogastric tube, not only to prevent intraoperative gastric distention, but also to provide the surgeon with a guide to identifying the esophagus in difficult cases, such as in patients undergoing pulmonary resections following a course of chemotherapy or radiation therapy.

Beyond the basic monitoring set, further monitoring may be indicated based on individual risk/benefit determinations. Most patients undergoing a major thoracic procedure are provided with a bladder (Foley) catheter for assessment of urine output. Continuous intra-arterial blood pressure monitoring is indicated in individuals with significant cardiovascular disease and in addition facilitates sampling arterial blood gas to cross check and augment the noninvasive monitors. Central venous cannulation, although not essential for every case, provides immediate access to the venous circulation during hemodynamic instability and allows more accurate assessment of volume status during long cases or procedures involving significant blood loss. Because volume status may be difficult to determine in the patient with severe pulmonary disease or right heart failure secondary to pulmonary artery hypertension, insertion of a pulmonary arterial line is often helpful. A pulmonary artery catheter can be useful in a pneumonectomy patient with cardiac disease because pulmonary artery pressures may rise significantly and compromise right ventricular function as the pulmonary artery is clamped. Pressure readings, particularly pulmonary capillary wedge pressure, must be carefully interpreted in light of the pulmonary artery catheter tip location relative to the "West" zone of the lung.[48] If the catheter tip is positioned in zone I or II, occlusion pressures reflect alveolar pressure rather than venous pressure (Fig. 20-2)[49] (see Chaps. 76 and 77). Optimally the pulmonary artery catheter tip should terminate in zone III of the nonoperative lung, although such selective placement of the catheter is difficult to accomplish without fluoroscopy. In the patient at risk for compromise during induction and intubation, it is reasonable to place a pulmonary artery catheter before induction, withdrawing it into the right atrium should it interfere with later surgical plans.

Airway Obstruction

Selected patients are prone to airway obstruction on induction of anesthesia: patients with airway compromise

Table 20-13. Intraoperative Monitoring and Devices

Minor Procedures	
Bronchoscopy	Continuous ECG
Mediastinoscopy	Blood pressure
Open lung biopsy	Temperature
	O_2 saturation/pulse oximeter
	Inspired oxygen concentration
	Adequacy of ventilation
	Large-bore peripheral IV
Major Procedures	
Lung resections	Monitoring as for minor procedures plus:
Esophagectomy	Arterial blood pressure line
Bullectomy	Central venous pressure line
	Swan-Ganz line when indicated
	End-tidal CO_2
	Bladder catheter
	Nasogastric tube

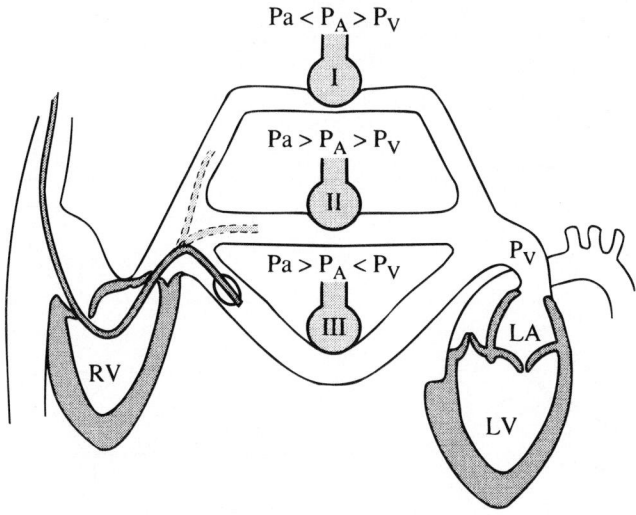

Fig. 20-2. The relationship between wedge pressure measurements and actual filling pressures (Pv) of the left side of the heart is affected by the position of the tip of the pulmonary artery catheter. When the catheter tip is higher than the plane of the left atrium, arterial (Pa) and venous pressures become increasingly lower relative to alveolar pressure (PA). In the top two zones, PA exceeds Pv. Thus a "wedge" pressure will be influenced by alveolar pressures rather than pulmonary venous pressure. The difference may be significant with high levels of PEEP or high mean airway pressures, as with pressure controlled inverse-ratio ventilation. Pv will be accurately estimated only in zone 3 of the lung. Positioning of the catheter can be checked with a portable chest radiograph; however, one cannot easily determine from anteroposterior chest films the vertical position of the catheter when the patient is supine. (From O'Quinn, R., and Marini, J. J.: Pulmonary artery occlusion pressure: clinical physiology, measurement, and interpretation. Am. Rev. Respir. Dis., 128:319, 1983.)

owing to critical airway lesions and pediatric patients with foreign bodies or large anterior mediastinal masses.[50] Factors that predispose for tracheal compression by mediastinal masses include the relaxant effect of general anesthesia on airway structures, supine body position, and elimination of glottic regulation of air flow by endotracheal intubation. In a patient with an anterior mediastinal mass with signs or symptoms of airway compression, cardiac compression, or superior vena caval obstruction, upright and supine flow volume loops are indicated during preoperative workup. When general anesthesia cannot be avoided, special precautions must be taken (Fig. 20-3).[51] Preoperative sedation is sufficiently hazardous enough to be contraindicated in these patients. No anesthetic agents should be given until all monitoring apparatus is in place, and the surgical staff is present and ready to intervene with rigid bronchoscopy or immediate thoracotomy should the airway become completely obstructed.

Choice of Anesthesia

Considerations in the choice of anesthetic technique involve the need to use high inspired oxygen concentrations, particularly during one-lung anesthesia, and the benefit of early extubation, which could be delayed by administration of long-acting intravenous agents, such as opioids. Regional techniques alone (e.g., spinal, epidural) are generally not applicable to operative anesthesia in thoracic procedures because of the difficulty in providing a high enough spinal level to allow surgery without affecting the brain stem or muscles of respiration. Controlled ventilation is also mandatory to sustain respiration during any open-thorax procedure. Epidural anesthesia has been used in conjunction with a general anesthetic,[52] and there is a suggestion that this technique could affect outcome by minimizing the stress response.[53] Other preliminary evidence suggests that the neuroendocrine responses to thoracotomy may not be altered by epidural opiate analgesia.[54] Current anesthetic technique employs either potent inhalational agents (e.g., enflurane, isoflurane) or short-acting intravenous agents (e.g., propofol, ketamine, midazolam) and neuromuscular blocking agents to provide the necessary lack of awareness, muscle relaxation, and control of sympathetic discharge. Intravenous agents coupled with high frequency jet ventilators are useful when the airway may be disrupted.[55] Intravenous opiates are often avoided or used in limited amounts, unless prolonged postoperative ventilation is planned. The usual goal is to have the patient awake, comfortable, and extubated at the end of the procedure, thus avoiding the potential stress on fresh suture lines from positive pressure ventilation and coughing or bucking on the endotracheal tube.

Endobronchial Intubation

Indications for selective endobronchial intubation include protection against airway soilage (hemorrhage or secretions), differential bronchospirometry, or selective ventilation of the lung (Table 20-14). One-lung ventilation allows the surgeon to operate on a quiet, collapsed lung and allows the airway to be maintained during major airway procedures, such as tracheal reconstruction or "sleeve" resection. Various reusable red-rubber and disposable polyvinyl versions of double-lumen tubes are available in odd sizes between 35 and 41 French. The Robertshaw-type tubes are available in left-sided or right-sided configurations. Carlens tubes (left-sided) and White tubes (right-sided) are distinguished by the presence of a carinal hook, which better stabilizes the tube but may complicate insertion. Right-sided tubes are slightly easier to place; however, the bronchial cuff has a tendency to occlude the orifice of the right upper lobe, even when

Table 20-14. Indications for Use of Endobronchial Intubation

Absolute
    To prevent soilage of contralateral lung with pus, blood, or secretions
    To control distribution of ventilation
        Bronchopleural fistula
        Cystic lesions
        Differential lung compliance
    For unilateral bronchopulmonary lavage
    For unilateral lung transplantation
Relative
    Surgical exposure—pneumonectomy and thoracic aneurysm
    Surgical convenience—esophageal resection and lobectomy

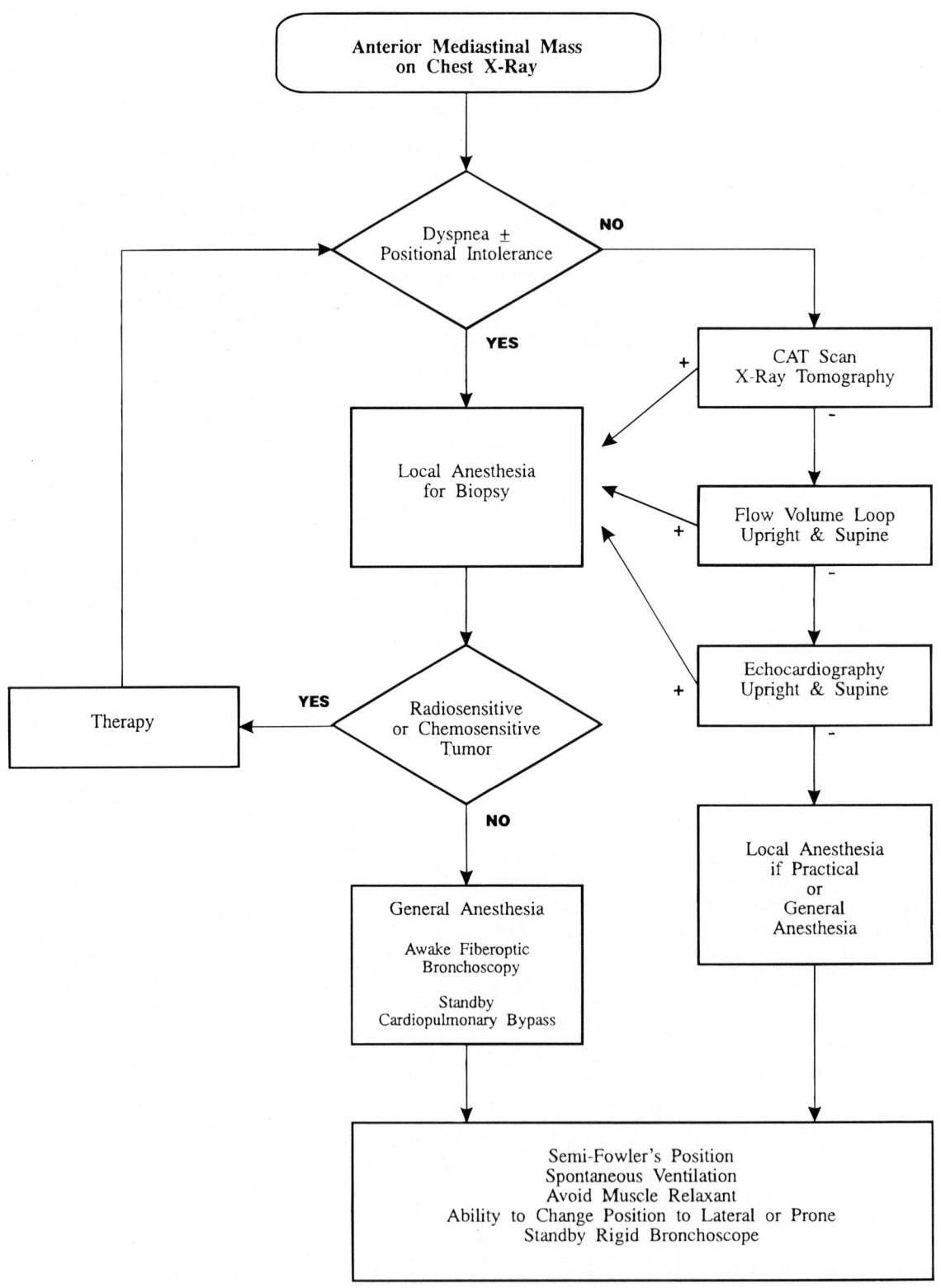

Fig. 20-3. Flow chart describing the preoperative evaluation of the patient with an anterior mediastinal mass + indicates positive finding; − indicates negative workup. Expiratory plateau seen with extrinsic intrathoracic airway. (Redrawn from Neumann, G. G., et al.: The anesthetic management of the patient with an anterior mediastinal mass. Anesthesiology, 60:144, 1984.)

carefully placed. A large Macintosh-type laryngoscope blade is preferred to a Miller (straight) blade to provide more room to manipulate the tube during laryngoscopy. The nonoperative bronchus is often chosen for selective intubation in lobectomies and pneumonectomies, so surgical manipulation does not displace the tube and disrupt lung isolation and to allow resection of the main stem bronchus should that become necessary. When selective endobronchial intubation is impossible (as in pediatric patients, extremely small adults, laryngectomy patients), a bronchial blocker can be placed under fiberoptic guidance to occlude a bronchus selectively (Fig. 20-4).

One-lung ventilation alters the ventilation-perfusion relationship, and the blood passing through the unventilated lung effectively causes a right-to-left shunt and reduces arterial oxygenation. Perfusion of the unventilated lung is reduced by physical collapse of the lung and hypoxic pulmonary vasoconstriction,[56] but it is sometimes necessary briefly to inflate the unventilated lung, to apply positive end-expiratory pressure (PEEP) to the ventilated lung, or to provide a small amount of continuous positive airway pressure (CPAP) to the operative lung using an oxygen flow/meter and PEEP valve (Fig. 20-5). High frequency jet ventilation has been experimentally used to ventilate the operative lung but does not substantially improve ventilation or cardiac function compared with conventional one-lung ventilation.[57] Rarely occlusion of the pulmonary artery to the nonventilated lung is required to eliminate the shunt.

Because the double-lumen endotracheal tube is large with the potential to cause airway trauma and edema, prone to moving if the patient shifts position, and more difficult to suction through, it is generally removed at the end of the operation and replaced by a single-lumen tube if continued mechanical ventilation is required. Specific indications for continued selective endobronchial intubation would include the need to protect against soilage (pus or blood) and provision of different levels of PEEP to lungs of different compliance. Use of pressure-controlled inverse ratio ventilation may also accomplish effective ventilation in noncompliant lung segments, however, by allowing sufficient time for transfilling (Fig. 20-6). The need for differential levels of PEEP frequently occurs in emphysematous patients undergoing single lung transplantation.[58,59] This switch may be accomplished in the operating room or the ICU. A fiberglass resin tube changer or a pediatric fiberoptic bronchoscope are essential tools that should be available because airway edema or bleeding may obscure vision during direct laryngoscopy.

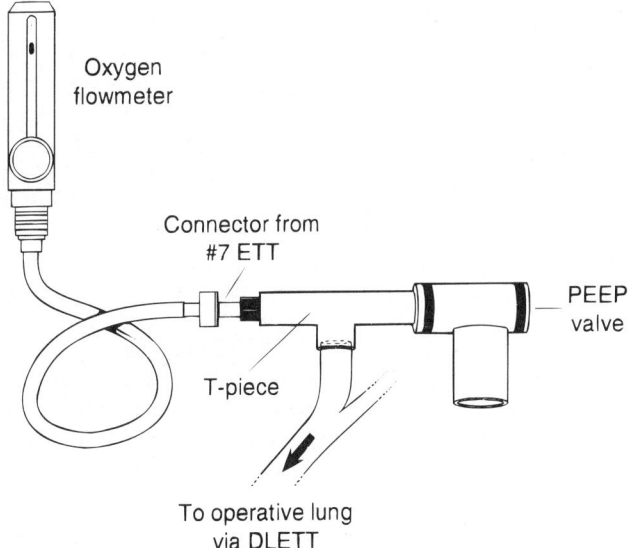

Fig. 20-5. Method for delivering positive end-expiratory pressure (PEEP) to operative lung during one-lung anesthesia via double lumen endotracheal tube (DLETT).

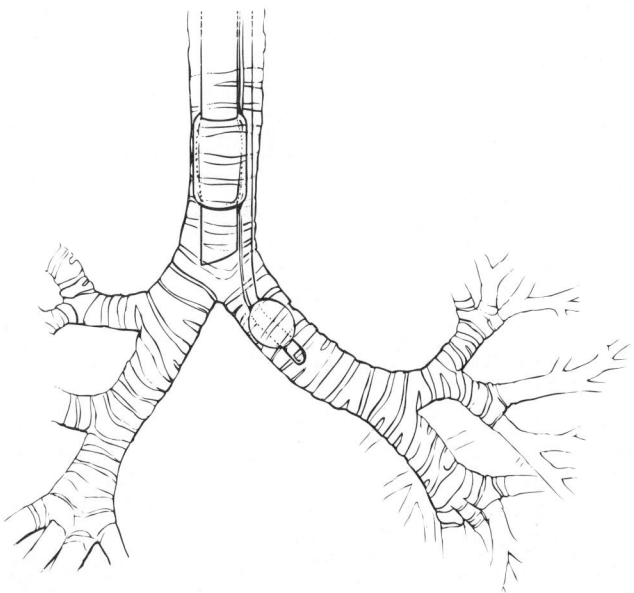

Fig. 20-4. Fogarty embolectomy catheter used as a bronchial blocker.

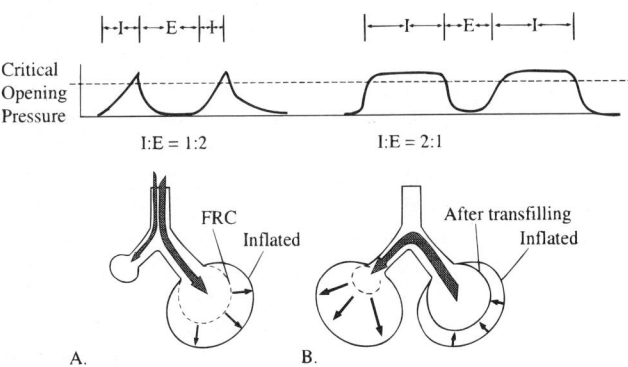

Fig. 20-6. Comparison of conventional (I:E = 1:2) volume ventilation (CVV) with pressure controlled inverse ratio (I:E = 2:1) ventilation (PC-IRV). With CVV, ventilated breath follows the path of least resistance, overinflating normal lung segments but failing to open atelectatic areas because pressure rarely exceeds critical opening pressure. With PC-IRV, pressure remains above the critical opening value for a longer part of the ventilatory cycle, to allow transfilling inflation of closed segments and thus better V/Q matching.

Antibiotic Prophylaxis

The value of antimicrobial prophylaxis in general thoracic surgical procedures is debated.[60] Most authorities recommend antibiotic coverage for the immediate perioperative period only. A first-generation cephalosporin (such as cefazolin sodium) is appropriate; such coverage has a moderately long serum half-life and adequately guards against staphylococcal infection without selecting for resistant gram-negative organisms.[61,62] Our procedure is to give 1 g of cefazolin preoperatively and two doses postoperatively at 8- to 12-hour intervals. Patients with known preoperative infection (empyema, pneumonia, lung abscess, esophageal perforation) or in whom gross intraoperative contamination occurs should be treated with broad-spectrum antibiotics chosen to cover the most likely organisms.

POSTOPERATIVE CONSIDERATIONS

The choice of recovery area following operation depends primarily on the degree of patient illness and the ability of a particular nursing unit to deal with postoperative ventilation or hemodynamic monitoring. At our institution, patients undergoing bronchoscopy, mediastinoscopy, esophageal dilatation, esophagoscopy, gastrostomy, jejunostomy, laryngoscopy, pleuroscopy, or scalene node biopsy are generally recovered in the postanesthesia recovery unit (PACU). Patients undergoing esophagectomy, esophagogastrectomy, and pneumonectomy, because they often require postoperative ventilation or critical monitoring, are normally recovered in the ICU. Patients undergoing lobectomy, segmental or wedge pulmonary resections, hiatal hernia repairs, or Heller myotomy are triaged to either PACU or ICU depending on chronic health condition and length and difficulty of operation. (The ability to perform esophageal myotomy with a thorascope may eventually change this recommendation.) Extubation can often be accomplished in the operating room, but specific considerations (concurrent cardiac illness, inability to protect airway, malnutrition, coexisting lung disease) may mandate continued intubation. Silent aspiration of gastric contents is an important complication following esophagectomy or esophagogastrectomy, and maintenance of endotracheal intubation for 24 hours postoperatively has been shown to decrease the occurrence of pneumonia and the operative mortality rate in this type of patient.[63] Transportation from the operating room to recovery area requires hemodynamic monitoring and provision of supplemental oxygen or mechanical ventilation. Two chest tubes are usually inserted to drain the surgical site at the end of the procedure except with pneumonectomy patients, in whom the standard practice is to avoid a chest tube unless there is the need to monitor the pneumonectomy space postoperatively. Chest tubes should never be clamped during transport because of the dangers of unrecognized bleeding and tension pneumothorax. Immediately on arrival in the PACU or ICU, patients should have a quick but comprehensive examination, including vital signs, auscultation of breath sounds, and visual inspection of monitoring lines and chest tube connections. The chest tubes are

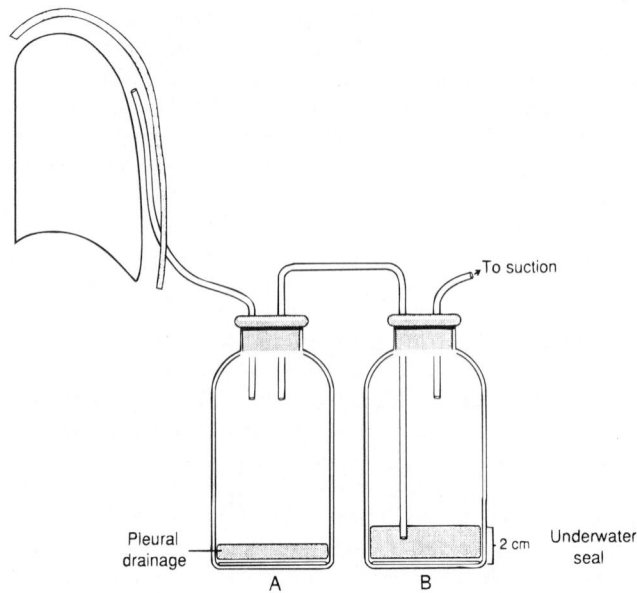

Fig. 20-7. The traditional two-bottle setup to provide underwater seal drainage of the pleural space. Bottle A collects pleural fluid drainage and bottle B provides an underwater seal.

connected to a vacuum regulator to provide -20 cm H_2O of suction except for those tubes in pneumonectomy spaces. A chest radiograph should be ordered immediately for confirmation of endotracheal, nasogastric, and chest tube placement and identification of pneumothorax, mediastinal shift, or significant atelectasis. Patients who have undergone pneumonectomy and have a chest tube in place should have this tube connected to straight drainage with an underwater seal (Fig. 20-7) or to a "balanced" type of pleural drainage (Fig. 20-8). Commercially available units, such as the Thora-klex (Fig. 20-9), provide calibrated drainage chambers, a blow-off chamber for excessive positive pressure, and regulated amounts of negative pressure, similar to that of a three-bottle system. Baseline blood work generally includes a hemoglobin or hematocrit, white cell count, electrolytes, blood urea nitrogen or creatinine, blood glucose in diabetics, arterial blood gases, and clotting studies (prothrombin time, partial thromboplastin time). Minimal monitoring includes intermittent blood pressure determinations to detect hypotension, continuous electrocardiography to detect dysrhythmia, and pulse oximetry to detect arterial desaturation. In selected patients, volume status and cardiopulmonary function may require use of central venous pressure or pulmonary artery catheters.

Although anesthesia is generally terminated in the operating room, a growing body of evidence suggests that complex patients may benefit through ablation of the stress response into the early postoperative period.[64] These patients may be maintained on continuous infusions of morphine, fentanyl, midazolam, or propofol while mechanical ventilation is continued during a period of postoperative instability. (Details on postoperative sedation and pain relief are covered in Chap. 63.)

MANAGEMENT OF THE GENERAL THORACIC SURGICAL PATIENT

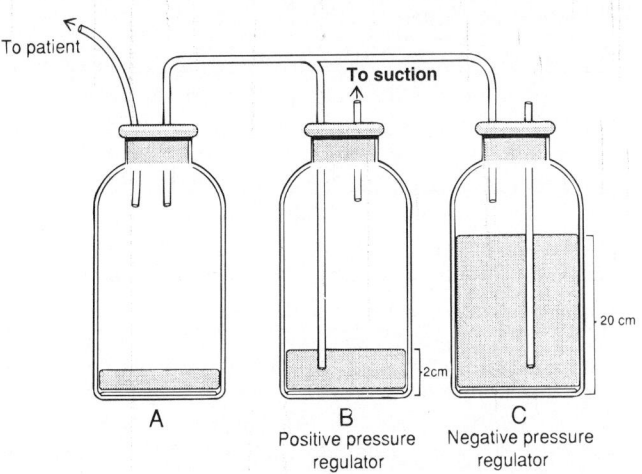

Fig. 20-8. A "balanced" system used in pneumonectomy patients to prevent excessive "swings" in intrapleural pressures. Bottle A is the collection chamber. Bottle B provides 2 cm of underwater seal and allows air to escape when intrapleural pressure exceeds 2 cm H_2O. Bottle C provides a negative pressure valve, allowing air to enter the system if the negative pressure within the chest builds up beyond 20 cm.

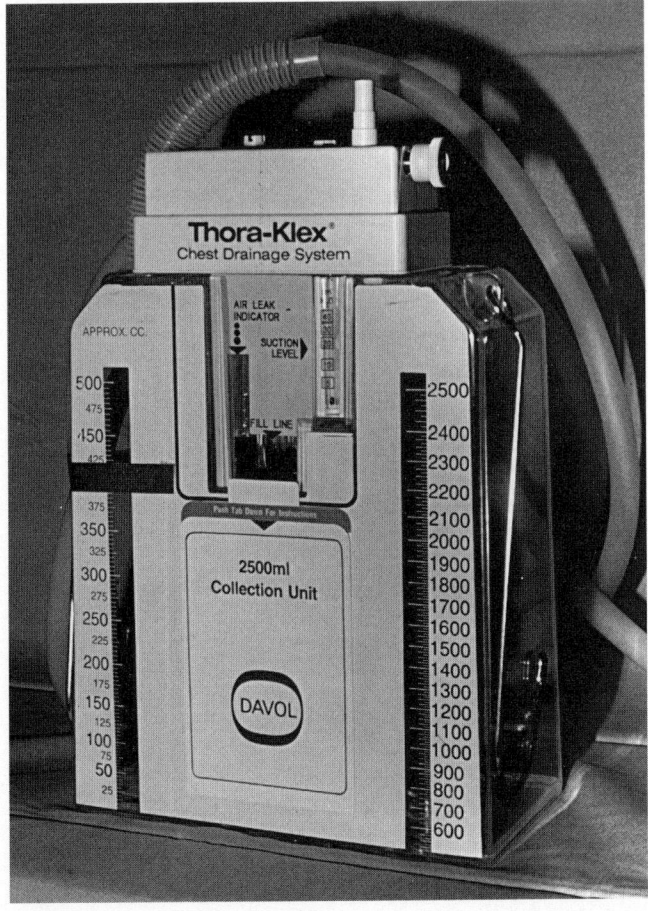

Fig. 20-9. The two- and three-bottle systems (see Figs. 20-7 and 20-8) have been replaced with a simpler one-"bottle" system that combines both underwater seal and collection chambers.

Extubation and Airway Concerns

Patients are extubated when the effects of anesthetic agents (e.g., opiates, neuromuscular blockers) have dissipated and when a suitable level of consciousness and neuromuscular strength has been regained. Measurement of maximal inspiratory pressure (MIP) (previously called negative inspiratory pressure) can be helpful in determining respiratory muscle strength, although the MIP required to maintain ventilation is far less than the muscle strength required to protect the airway.[65] Checking a set of arterial blood gases while on CPAP is another convenient method of assessment for the short-term ventilated patient. Standard accepted criteria for extubation include:

- Awake, cooperative patient
- Good gag reflex (i.e., ability to protect airway)
- Vital capacity of more than 10 ml/kg
- MIP more than 25 cm H_2O
- Respiratory rate less than 25 breaths/min on CPAP
- Adequate oxygenation with an inspired oxygen concentration of less than 0.50

Although many patients do not strictly meet these criteria for extubation, it is usually best to attempt weaning and extubation rather than risk the complications of continued ventilation in this group of patients. Specific indications for prolonged intubation include:

- Poor pulmonary reserve
- Compromised myocardial function, particularly when large fluid shifts are expected
- Severe neurologic impairment
- Continued bleeding with the possibility of reexploration
- Airway compromise

Esophageal surgery patients are at particular risk for reflux and subsequent aspiration and should generally be left intubated overnight to facilitate pain control and allow full recovery of airway reflexes.[66] After extubation, continued nasogastric suction and keeping the head and thorax elevated to 30 degrees or more are also mandatory to prevent aspiration.

Weaning ventilatory support in the patient requiring mechanical ventilation beyond 48 hours requires an individualized approach, covered in detail in Chapter 24. Controversy still exists over the proper timing of tracheostomy; this has been the subject of a consensus conference from the American College of Chest Physicians.[67] Our approach is to proceed with tracheostomy in patients who have required more than 2 weeks of ventilatory support when further support is inevitable, and earlier in patients when secretions or upper airway lesions make it unlikely that extubation will be accomplished in less than 3 weeks' time.

An acceptable alternative to formal tracheostomy is a percutaneous tracheostomy that can be quickly and safely performed at the patient's bedside in the ICU. A number of authors[68-70] have reported on the success of percutaneous tracheostomy in the management of patients requiring long-term ventilatory support, protection of the airway, or for tracheobronchial toilet. Complications with this method (5 to 10%) are less than those reported for standard tracheostomy (up to 33%),[71-73] although follow-up had not been long enough to report on the incidence of subglottic and tracheal stenoses. Although the technique is not suitable for all patients (i.e., difficult anatomy, "bull" neck, severe neck edema), it offers distinct advantages to a formal tracheostomy, including fewer complications and a procedure that can be rapidly performed at the patient's bedside even in emergency conditions.

A "minitracheostomy" kit is now available for percutaneous placement by the Seldinger technique (Fig. 20-10). The minitracheostomy's primary role is to provide access for suctioning in the patient who cannot clear secretions well but who does not need a full-sized tracheostomy for ventilation. Minitracheostomies can be inserted at bedside and appear to have few complications, although aspiration of the device itself has been reported.[74]

Laryngeal and glottic edema may occur, particularly after intubation with a large double-lumen endotracheal tube or with airway manipulation. The presence of serious edema can be determined by first suctioning the posterior pharynx, then deflating the endotracheal tube cuff, occluding the endotracheal tube, and watching for evidence of airway obstruction. Endotracheal intubation may need to be maintained while edema resolves. Racemic epinephrine and corticosteroids are useful adjuncts. If there is any doubt about airway patency, the endotracheal tube should be removed only under direct laryngoscopic or fiberoptic observation, with a percutaneous tracheostomy set immediately at hand to provide airway access should reintubation be impossible because of airway swelling.

Postoperative Fluids

Initial intravenous maintenance fluid administration should be kept to a minimum (50 to 75 ml per hour) in all patients in whom postoperative pulmonary capillary integrity may be a problem. This includes patients in whom there has been significant lung retraction, patients undergoing pulmonary resections, and lung transplant recipients. Misplaced concerns about causing pulmonary edema or adult respiratory distress syndrome (ARDS) should not delay aggressive fluid replacement in hypovolemic patients or those developing circulatory shock. Patients who have had large resections with considerable dissection and mobilization of tissue planes, in whom there is significant potential for third space losses (e.g., esophagectomy, esophagogastrectomy, excision of large mediastinal tumors), require large volumes (typically ≥2 L) of fluid replacement. This fluid is generally spontaneously mobilized beginning on the second to third postoperative day, which may pose a problem if the patient has cardiac or renal compromise. In some cases, continued ICU care with invasive monitoring and aggressive intervention with inotropes and diuretics is necessary. It is probably safer to hydrate and ventilate a patient adequately than to limit fluids and cause hypovolemic hypoperfusion.

Urinary output is recorded hourly, with 0.5 ml/kg/hour considered acceptable. If intravascular fluid volume is required, the usual considerations apply relative to hemodilution and translocation of fluid. Because colloid (albumin, hetastarch, plasma) tends to remain in the intravascular compartment longer than crystalloid, administration of colloid reduces the total amount of volume required by up to 66%. This can be an important consideration in the

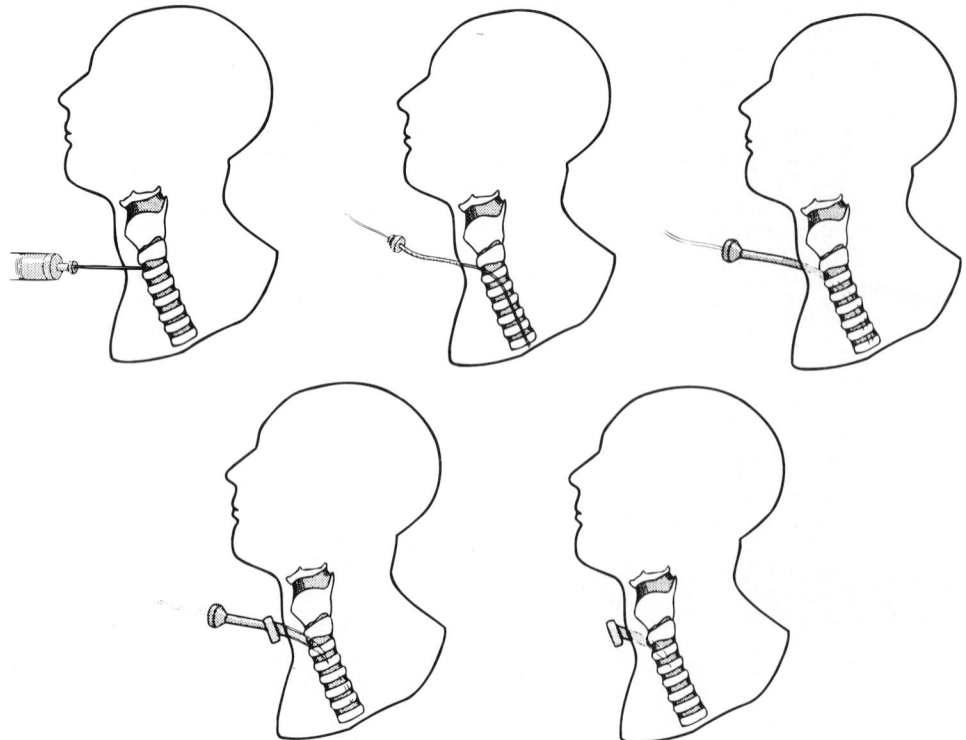

Fig. 20-10. The percutaneous placement of a minitracheostomy.

patient with preexisting cardiac compromise or when pulmonary edema is likely (post-transplant, postpneumonectomy). To maintain oxygen carrying capacity, the patient's hemoglobin should initially be followed at 4- to 6-hour intervals and repleted via transfusion to provide appropriate oxygen delivery: Generally a hematocrit of about 25% in a healthy patient or 30% or greater in those with organ system compromise is acceptable.

Many of the patients who have undergone routine pulmonary resections can begin oral intake within the first 24 hours. Patients who have undergone a pneumonectomy are generally given nothing by mouth for 24 to 48 hours. The mediastinal shift, diaphragmatic elevation, alteration of the esophageal hiatus, and possible damage to the vagus and recurrent laryngeal nerves make aspiration more likely in these patients. Because aspiration is a life-threatening complication (in any patient but particularly in the pneumonectomy patient), it is advisable to ensure an intact swallowing mechanism and adequate gag reflex before the institution of oral intake. Consideration should be given to early institution of parenteral or enteral nutrition in patients with complex clinical problems, particularly those expected to receive nothing by mouth for more than 48 hours, those expected to require long-term ventilation, and those with preoperative cachexia. Patients who suffered from dysphagia preoperatively are often severely malnourished, and parenteral support should be employed until recovery is complete.[75]

Most patients stabilize rapidly and can then be followed with hourly vital signs, followed by progressively longer intervals as indicated by clinical condition. Patients undergoing simple procedures (bronchoscopy, mediastinoscopy) can frequently be discharged to home on the same day, and most patients are discharged from the recovery room or ICU to the postoperative thoracic surgery nursing floor within the first 24 hours.

Hourly output from chest tubes should be recorded and the surgeon notified if drainage is more than 100 ml/hour for more than 4 hours or if more than 200 ml of drainage is recorded in any 1-hour observation period. Expected chest tube drainage in the first 24 hours is 300 to 600 ml, tapering to less than 200 ml by the second day. Daily chest radiographs are obtained while the chest tubes are in place. The level of fluid in the water seal should fluctuate with each respiration (assuming no air leak) and should be checked frequently to assure chest tube patency. Clotted tubes can be cleared in a sterile fashion using a Fogarty catheter. The function of commercially available drainage systems can be confusing to the novice: Tracing the path of air and fluid flow as if it were a conventional system (see Fig. 20–8) helps to avoid confusion between abnormal air leaks and normal bubbling seen in the vacuum chamber. Most patients who have undergone pulmonary resection return with mild-to-moderate air leaks, which become problems in the ICU only if the underlying lung parenchyma does not completely expand to fill the pleural space or if the patient is losing a significant percentage of tidal volume out the chest tubes. In such circumstances, additional pleural drainage may be required or changes in ventilation made that minimize the air leak and optimize ventilation. Frequently leaks occur only above a given inflation pressure, and ventilation techniques, such as smaller volumes at higher rates or pressure-controlled inverse ratio ventilation, can minimize leaking and allow a seal to develop. Once all air leaks have resolved and drainage is minimal (less than 100 ml in 24 hours), chest tubes may be removed during the expiratory phase of ventilation or while the patient performs a Valsalva maneuver.

Ventilator Support

The combination of thoracic surgery and compromised preoperative pulmonary function can necessitate mechanical ventilation for 48 hours or more after a procedure. The immediate goals are to provide sufficient ventilation for prevention of respiratory acidosis and CO_2 retention and sufficient parenchymal inflation to prevent hypoxemia and loss of compliance. In most postoperative patients, a tidal volume of 10 to 12 ml/kg delivered at a rate of 8 to 10 breaths/min with 3 to 5 H_2O PEEP accomplishes these goals. In thoracic surgery patients, reduction of barotrauma becomes an additional consideration, which may require reductions in both total volume and PEEP. Low tidal volumes (6 ml/kg) cause a small but clinically irrelevant decrease in oxygenation and may decrease morbidity,[76] although this has not been evaluated specifically in thoracotomy patients. Normal individuals breathe with an inspiration-to-expiration ratio of 1:2; thus this I:E ratio is normally used as the routine starting point. Longer inspiratory times reduce peak airway pressure, but in patients with significant airway obstruction, this may not allow sufficient time for expiration, resulting in auto-PEEP[77] or stacking of breaths. This can cause hemodynamic compromise because cardiac filling is diminished during the inspiratory phase of positive pressure ventilation.

Intermittent mandatory ventilation is ideal for early postoperative management because the intermittent mandatory ventilation circuit allows patients to breathe spontaneously above the machine rate as they awaken from anesthesia and metabolize residual neuromuscular blockers. The F_{IO_2} in the early postoperative period is generally set at 50 to 60% and then adjusted as clinically appropriate. F_{IO_2} values of 50% or higher have been implicated in the development of oxygen toxicity,[78] and very high inspired oxygen concentrations promote absorption atelectasis because a nonabsorbed gas such as nitrogen acts as a stent to keep FRC above the critical closing volume.

Arterial blood gas determinations are used to assess ventilation, although the combination of pulse oximetry and end-tidal CO_2 monitoring may be helpful in minimizing arterial sampling. The ideal target for oxygen saturation is 92% or higher in white patients and 95% or higher in black patients.[79] End-tidal CO_2 is frequently (30%) incorrect in indicating direction of change with weaning.[80]

A complete discussion of ventilatory modes and application of PEEP can be found in Chap. 16. Controversy still exists as to the optimal level of PEEP in the thoracic surgery patient. Low levels of PEEP (3 to 5 cm) may be helpful in restoring FRC and substituting for the "physiologic PEEP" of the glottis. The occurrence of "auto-PEEP"[77] in the patient with obstructive pulmonary disease should be sought for and treated if it occurs. In the patient with a bronchopleural fistula or a fragile bronchial stump, it is not clear whether low levels of PEEP, with resultant airway closure, are more harmful than higher levels of PEEP, with resultant barotrauma.

High frequency jet ventilation (HFJV) has found a role in the operating room during laryngoscopy, bronchoscopy, microlaryngeal procedures, and airway surgery. Advantages include a quieter operative field, reduced airway pressures, and elimination of competition between the anesthesiologist and surgeon for space within the airway. A study of 65 patients undergoing lobectomy, which randomized patients to conventional ventilation via a double lumen endotracheal tube versus HFJV at a rate of 150 with a driving pressure of 1.4 to 1.7 atm, concluded that the HFJV group had a shorter ICU stay, lower incidence of chest infections, and higher P_{O_2} at 4 and 24 hours and 7 days.[81]

The role of HFJV in the ICU, particularly for management of hypoxemic respiratory failure, is less well defined. A study of patients with ARDS concluded that although HFJV as an adjunct to spontaneous ventilation resulted in lower peak airway pressures than intermittent mandatory ventilation, airway pressures were lower with conventional ventilation than with HFJV in the absence of spontaneous ventilation.[82] One accepted application of this mode of therapy is the ventilation of a patient with a bronchopleural fistula.[83-85] Under ideal circumstances, required ventilation can be attained with HFJV at lower airway pressures than conventional ventilation. The reduction in ventilation pressure minimizes the amount of air passing through the fistula and may promote healing by allowing adjacent tissues to approximate and possibly seal the fistula. In the face of decreased pulmonary compliance, the beneficial effect of HFJV in lowering airway pressure may be lost.[84]

With adequate separation of the right and left lungs using either a double lumen endotracheal tube or a combination bronchial blocker and insufflation catheter, it is possible to ventilate each lung independently.[86] Selected commercially available ventilators (such as the Servo 900-C) can be linked together in a master-slave combination allowing a synchronized respiratory cycle, with independent control of CPAP, tidal volume, and pressure limits for each lung. A single ventilator may also be used to ventilate one lung, while apneic ventilation with a small amount of CPAP is applied to the other lungs.[87] These systems allow the establishment of differential airway pressures. This is beneficial in the setting of bronchopleural fistula or other unilateral lung pathology, in which application of sufficient pressure to ventilate the diseased lung could produce overdistention and poor V/Q matching in the healthy lung. Independent lung ventilation is particularly useful in the unilateral lung transplant patient in whom sufficient PEEP to open the atelectatic transplanted lung leads to auto-PEEP and overinflation of the native lung.[58,59] Proper sizing of the double lumen tube is critical to avoid excessive cuff inflation pressure and subsequent tracheal or bronchial trauma. Disadvantages of this technique include the difficulty of placing and maintaining the double lumen endotracheal tube and the limitations of suctioning and bronchoscopy through the narrower individual lumens of the double lumen endotracheal tube. This technique should be used for the shortest time possible, usually only when the differential level of pressure between the lungs is greater than 10 cm H_2O. Newer ventilation techniques, such as pressure-controlled inverse ratio ventilation (PC-IRV), can sometimes achieve reexpansion of atelectatic segments when substantial inhomogenicity of lung tissue exists (Fig. 20-6).

Respiratory Therapy

Patients presenting for general thoracic procedures often have significant underlying COPD, impairment of mucociliary clearance, excessive secretions, and increased closing volumes, all of which predispose to atelectasis. The respiratory therapist plays an important role in providing intensive care, from simple incentive spirometry through chest physiotherapy (percussion and vibration). Other modalities supporting an uncomplicated recovery include humidified oxygen, adequate hydration, aerosolized bronchodilators, and early identification and treatment of infection of the tracheobronchial tree. Chest physiotherapy should begin when the patient has recovered sufficiently from anesthesia to cooperate. Many patients are able to cough effectively, particularly if provided with adequate analgesia. Mucolytic agents (such as N-acetylcysteine) are helpful in solubilizing thick secretions but may cause a risk of bronchospasm. Oral or nasotracheal suctioning is reserved for selected patients because of discomfort and the possibility of complications (hypoxemia, vagal-mediated bradycardia, or cardiac arrest). The minitracheostomy can occasionally be used for access to the lower airway in patients with thick secretions. Major difficulties with retained secretions, including lobar collapse, can be handled with a combination of vigorous chest physiotherapy and humidified oxygen. Inadequate clearance of secretions occasionally mandates flexible bronchoscopy, which is of greatest benefit in the extubated patient who cannot adequately be suctioned.[88-90] When pulmonary parenchymal involvement is confined to one lung, altering body positioning can improve gas exchange, by changing the relationships between ventilation and perfusion. The lateral decubitus position, with the uninvolved lung down, allows maximal blood flow to ventilated areas during spontaneous ventilation. This relationship may be altered with mechanical breaths and application of PEEP. Specialized beds, such as the Roto Rest kinetic bed, can be set to supine, lateral, or rotating modes to optimize oxygenation.[91]

Appropriate protein and caloric intake is important in the thoracic patient, particularly those debilitated before surgery as a result of their underlying disease process. In pulmonary resection patients unable to start oral intake within 48 hours, consideration should be given to starting total parenteral nutrition. Esophagectomy patients are generally managed with placement of a feeding jejunostomy (J-tube) at operation, so feedings can begin within 12 to 24 hours of surgery. Nutritional support is slowly advanced to full caloric intake (generally 2000 to 2400 kcal every 24 hours of full-strength enteral feeding). Esophagectomy patients who do not have J-tubes should be started on total parenteral nutrition within 24 hours of surgery because recovery of adequate bowel function can often take up to 10 days, and placement of a gastric tube across the anastomosis and feeding via the stomach is undesirable.

Postoperative Analgesia

Options for control of pain are discussed in detail in Chapter 63. Several considerations apply specifically to the thoracic surgery patient. The majority of patients undergoing a lateral thoracotomy require medication for adequate pain relief. This is essential not only for comfort, but also to minimize the splinting and atelectasis that otherwise result. Patients undergoing median sternotomy appear to require substantially lower amounts of postoperative narcotics than those undergoing lateral thoracotomy. This may be due to the nature of the incision, which divides minimal soft tissue, has a secure immobile bony closure, and does not involve retraction of or trauma to any cutaneous nerves. This may also be influenced, however, by the liberal use of narcotic-based anesthesia in most median sternotomy patients undergoing cardiac procedures and the caution with which anesthesiologists administer intraoperative opiates to lateral thoracotomy patients. Systemic pain relief may be accomplished with intravenous or intramuscular opiates, such as morphine and meperidine; however, the potential for respiratory depression exists. The peaks and valleys of intermittent opioid administration can be minimized by the use of a continuous infusion of narcotics, resulting in a lower overall dose and hence less respiratory depression. Patient-controlled analgesia modifies this technique by providing a basal infusion and allows the patient to self-administer predetermined amounts of an analgesic at specified minimal intervals.[92] Newer nonopiate agents, such as the parenteral prostaglandin inhibitor ketorolac,[93] offer a viable alternative to opioids.

Epidural analgesia, using opioids, local anesthetics, or both, is increasingly popular for postoperative pain control. There is some controversy over the contribution of direct effect of opioids at the nerve roots versus systemic absorption and at least one study suggesting that epidural and intravenous infusions may be clinically indistinguishable after lower extremity operations.[94] Randomized, double-blind trials do indicate that lumbar epidural infusions are highly effective compared with systemic morphine in post-thoracotomy patients and that epidural management improves respiratory function.[95] Epidural catheters may be placed at either the lumbar or thoracic level, although locations above the cauda equina require an added degree of operator experience. A single bolus injection of preservative-free morphine provides 6 hours or more of effective analgesia; continuous epidural infusions of opiates with or without local anesthetics can be used for several days when necessary. The major disadvantages to epidural analgesia are the potential for inadvertent entry of the needle or catheter into the subarachnoid space ("wet tap") with subsequent spinal headache, increased risk (albeit negligible) of infection with another skin entry site, neurologic injury including epidural hematomas with compression (extremely rare), urinary retention, pruritus (common), and delayed respiratory depression as the result of circulation of opiates from the epidural space to the brain stem respiratory center. This last complication suggests a need for close monitoring of the patient, although one study suggests that although hypercarbia commonly occurs, life-threatening respiratory depression is sufficiently rare that this technique may be safely used outside the ICU.[96]

Intrathecal administration of morphine has also been used extensively in the thoracotomy population[97,98] and offers the advantage of ease of administration. Similar to epidural administration, intrathecal administration carries the risk of delayed respiratory depression. Typical doses in the thoracotomy patient are 0.25 to 0.5 mg of preservative-free morphine in normal saline given at the L3 or L4 interspace.[98]

Intercostal nerve blocks effectively relieve postoperative pain and muscle spasm. These may be performed intraoperatively before chest closure under direct vision, but this technique provides only limited postoperative analgesia. Percutaneous intercostal block is generally performed in the posterior lateral area at the level of the surgical incision, one interspace below the site (Fig. 20–11). Signifi-

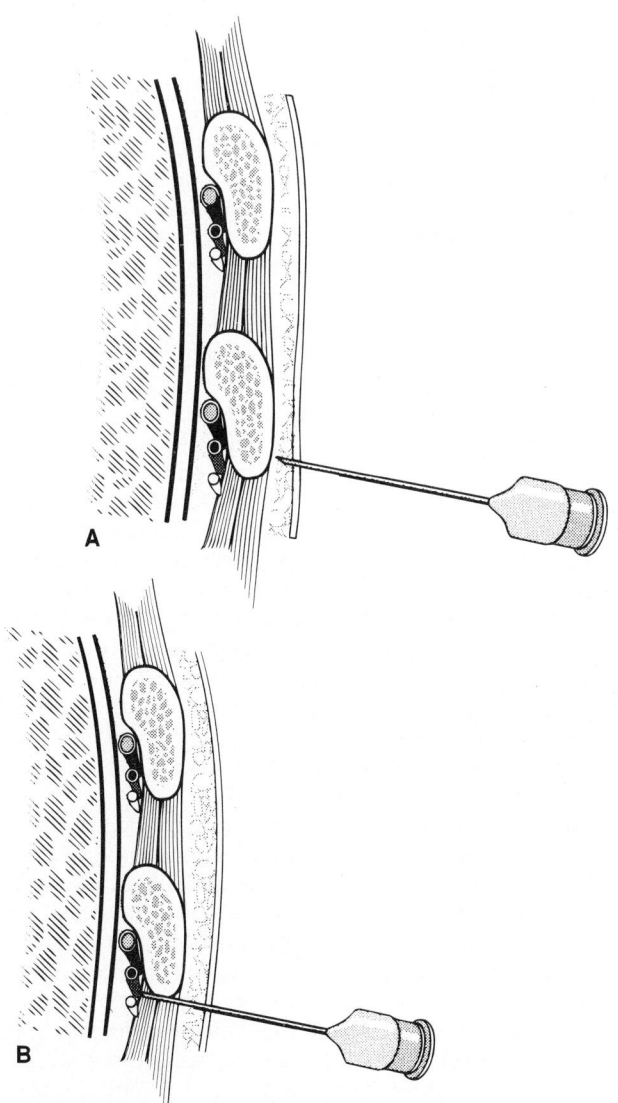

Fig. 20–11. *A,* The intercostal bundle is located by first identifying the inferior border of the adjacent rib. *B,* The needle is then advanced below and deep to the inferior rib border. (From Contemp. Surg., June: front cover, 1992.)

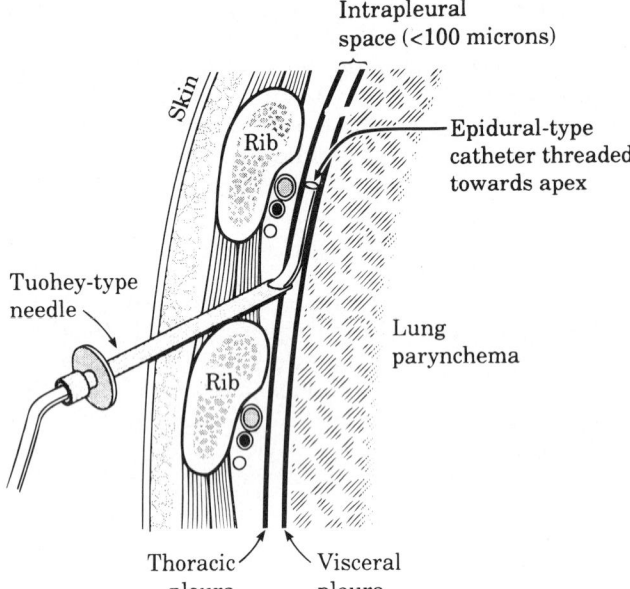

Fig. 20–12. The correct placement of an intrapleural catheter.

cant pain is also present at the chest tube insertion site(s), and these may also be blocked either directly (ring block) or proximally. Intercostal nerve blocks are relatively contraindicated in the postpneumonectomy patient because of the risks of entering or contaminating the empty chest cavity and also because splinting on the side of the pneumonectomy may actually be beneficial in reducing atelectasis in the remaining lung. The block should be performed under sterile conditions, using a 1.5-inch (3.4-cm) 23-gauge needle, using 4 to 5 ml of 0.5% bupivacaine at each site. Appropriate caution should be exercised to prevent pneumothorax, intravascular injection, toxicity from local anesthetic, and "total spinal." The latter complication can occur if the intercostal block is performed too close to the patient's midline, such that local anesthetic is deposited directly into the outpouchings of the subarachnoid space around nerve roots. With a properly performed intercostal block, analgesia generally lasts 6 to 12 hours, and in some patients, a single procedure is all that is required. Contraindications to intercostal block include chest wall resection with loss of appropriate landmarks, infection or tumor at the injection site, and pneumonectomy.

Intrapleural catheters have been used to administer local anesthetics after thoracic, breast, renal, and upper abdominal surgery and in the treatment of multiple rib fractures. A catheter is inserted in the posterior pleural cavity and is threaded toward the apex of the lung (Fig. 20–12), and local anesthetics (commonly bupivacaine or lidocaine) are supplied by intermittent bolus or continuous infusion. Controversy exists about the exact mechanism of pain relief, but it is likely that the anesthetic agents block afferent pain fibers in the thoracic sympathetic chain and also back-diffuse to some extent into intercostal nerve roots at the costovertebral angle[99] to the intercostal nerves as well. A single 20-ml injection of 0.5% bupivacaine with epinephrine can be expected to supply between 3 and 10 hours of pain relief.[100] Complications include pneumothorax, toxicity to the local anesthetic (often in patients with abnormal pleura), and tachyphylaxis to the local anesthetic with time. In one study evaluating blind insertion of catheters in 21 patients subsequently subjected to thoracotomy, correct placement occurred in 11 (52%), holes were noted in the lung surface in 8 (38%), and 3 patients had a pneumothorax.[101] Other reports suggest lower complication rates.[102] Contraindications to interpleural catheters include pleural effusion (which dilutes the local anesthetic), pleural fibrosis, and allergy to local anesthetic. Putative advantages compared with the intercostal block include less tachyphylaxis, fewer injections, and perhaps a longer period of pain relief. Compared with epidural administration of narcotics, interpleural local anesthetics avoid respiratory depression and urinary retention.

Rectal indomethacin (100 mg), administered at 8-hour intervals, has been shown to be safe and effective after thoracotomy and to have an additive effect when used adjunctively with cryoanalgesia.[103]

Specific Postoperative Complications

Complications seen in patients undergoing thoracic surgery are of two types: those that may follow any operation and complications specific to thoracic surgery. Postoperative circulatory problems and dysrhythmias are common but are covered elsewhere in this text. If we consider only the specific complications related to thoracic procedures, it is perhaps easiest to classify these complications into site-specific complications. Table 20–15 lists general and Table 20–16 lists specific complications following thoracic surgery.

Airway Complications

Operations in or about the thoracic cavity many times require prolonged intubation with large endotracheal

Table 20–15. Postoperative Complications following Any Thoracic Procedures

Airway edema/stridor
Arrhythmias (especially atrial fibrillation, multifocal atrial tachycardia)
Arytenoid dislocation
Aspiration of gastric contents
Atelectasis
Bronchospasm
Bronchopleural fistula
Chylothorax
Congestive heart failure
Deep venous thrombosis
Empyema
Hemorrhage
Hemothorax
Infection (superficial, deep)
Lobar collapse
Lobar torsion
Myocardial infarction
Pain and splinting
Pleural effusion
Pneumothorax
Pulmonary embolus
Re-expansion pulmonary edema
Respiratory failure
Retained secretions
Subcutaneous emphysema
Tension pneumothorax

Table 20-16. Complications of Specific Thoracic Procedures

Procedure	Complications
Anterior mediastinotomy (Chamberlain)	Damage to recurrent laryngeal nerve (particularly left)
Bronchoscopy/mediastinoscopy	Bleeding from major vessels if torn, air leak with biopsy of bronchus
Bronchopleural fistula repair	Persistent leak, dehiscence
Bronchopulmonary lavage	Respiratory distress/contralateral spillage
Bullectomy	Tension pneumothorax; air leak
Chest wall reconstruction	Blood loss, altered chest wall compliance, unstable chest, infected prosthetic material
Clagett window	Air leak
Collis Belsey	Gastric leak, splenic injury
Decortication	Blood loss, air leak(s)
Esophageal dilatation	Esophageal perforation, pleural effusion, airway obstruction
Esophagoscopy	Esophageal perforation
Esophagogastrectomy	"Third-spacing" of fluids, anastomotic leak, gastric devascularization, splenic injury, gastric torsion
Heller myotomy	Esophageal tear
Lobectomy	Bronchial leak, lobar collapse, lobar torsion
Mediastinal tumor excision	Airway obstruction with sedation/anesthesia; damage to recurrent laryngeal nerve
Nissen fundoplication	Esophageal obstruction (with tight wrap), splenic injury
Pectus repair	Costrochondritis, unstable sternum
Pleuroscopy	Pharyngeal laceration, air leak
Pneumonectomy	Atrial arrhythmias (atrial fibrillation, MAT), mediastinal shift, cardiac torsion, air embolism, disrupted bronchus
Thoracic aortic aneurysm	Paraplegia, bleeding, aortobronchial fistula, esophageal injury
Thymectomy	In myasthenics, possible weakness and respiratory failure
Lung transplant	Rejection (day 5), reperfusion injury, infection, overdistention of native lung, dehiscence
Tracheal resection	Fixed neck flexion postoperatively; dehiscence, air leak

tubes or double lumen endotracheal tubes, the passage of bronchial blockers, rigid bronchoscopes, or frequent reintubations. All of these procedures can result in trauma or edema of the larynx or trachea. Despite expert technique and the utmost care, airway edema may be seen. Anticipation and prompt recognition are perhaps the most important factors in the management of this problem. On extubation it is prudent to inspect the hypopharynx, supraglottic larynx, and vocal cords. Maneuvers to reduce edema should be promptly administered if significant airway edema is found. Intravenous corticosteroids and racemic epinephrine respiratory treatments are the mainstay of edema reduction. A critical airway may be converted to an adequate airway by the administration of a helium and oxygen mixture.[104] Helium, which replaces the more viscous gas nitrogen, allows maintenance of laminar flow through the critically swollen upper airway. On occasion, prolonged endotracheal intubation or temporary tracheostomy is required to allow resolution of the edema.

Many thoracic surgical operations are carried out about the recurrent laryngeal nerves in the neck of the chest. The recurrent laryngeal nerves originate from the vagus nerves as they enter the chest. The right recurrent laryngeal nerve arises high in the apex of the right chest and loops around the right subclavian artery to travel back to the larynx in the tracheoesophageal groove. The left recurrent laryngeal nerve, which is more susceptible to injury, wraps around the aortic arch in the left chest before it enters the tracheoesophageal groove. The surgeon should be alert to any excessive traction, aggressive dissection about these nerves, or the possible sacrifice of these nerves during surgery along the route of the recurrent laryngeal nerves. Mediastinoscopy, anterior mediastinotomy, left pulmonary resection with subaortic exenteration, and resections of mediastinal tumors are common operations in which the recurrent laryngeal nerve may be damaged. It is expedient to visualize the vocal cords on extubation in these situations because early recognition and treatment minimize the possible complications. The problems may be aggravated by the late realization of the injury because the associated airway and laryngeal edema may allow for adequate coaptation of the vocal cords for the first days postextubation and prevent identification of the problem until after discharge from the ICU. The resultant ineffective cough, aspiration, and potential for airway obstruction (when both nerves have been damaged) may have disastrous effects in the thoracic surgical patient. It is our practice on recognition of the injury to augment the affected vocal cord by injection of Gelfoam or Teflon if it lies in an abducted position and is not mobile. It is best to use an absorbable material such as Gelfoam, which allows a midline shift of this nonfunctioning vocal cord until the neurapraxia resolves. If in the judgment of the surgeon there is permanent damage or division of the recurrent laryngeal nerve, augmentation of the vocal cord with a long-lasting substance such as Teflon may be considered. In the early postoperative period, it is best to perform simple augmentation of the nerve rather than permanent augmentation or extensive laryngeal reconstruction because this may always be performed at a later date and indeed may not be required at all. In many instances, aggressive chest physiotherapy, careful airway management, and temporary alternate means of nutrition and avoidance of oral feeding may eliminate the need for any intervention until recovery of the nerve function has occurred. Arytenoid dislocation, an uncommon cause of postextubation respiratory failure, is characterized by intermittent noisy inspiration and painful swallowing.[105] Treatment consists of surgical reduction, using gentle pressure with a laryngeal spatula, and must be accomplished before the cricoarytenoid joint becomes fibrosed in poor position.

Retained secretions and blood in the airway are frequently seen after thoracic operations. This is especially common if the airway is opened, as it is during a bronchoplastic procedure or closure of the bronchial stump with a suture technique. It is mandatory that before extubation all patients be suctioned through their endotracheal tube. If there has been excessive or bloody secretions in the airway, flexible fiberoptic bronchoscopy with clearance of secretions is wise before extubation. The mechanical airway obstruction secondary to secretions may be aggravated by bronchospasm. Many patients have reactive airways, and their preoperative bronchodilators should be continued in the perioperative and postoperative course. This bronchodilator therapy coupled with good bronchopulmonary hygiene minimizes airway obstruction and bronchospasm.

Closure of the bronchus proximally after resection of the lung or lobe or more distally after wedge resections or segmentectomies must be meticulous to minimize the possibility of a postoperative **bronchopleural fistula.** Most postoperative air leaks, however, are the result of distal fistula between tiny bronchiolus or respiratory units and the pleural cavity. One of the main functions of the chest tube is to evacuate air from these small air leaks and ensure complete expansion of the lung and coaption of the cut surface of the lung to the parietal pleura. with the avoidance of pleural spaces and assurance of complete expansion of the lung, these small air leaks seal. Careful examination of the chest radiograph, repositioning of the chest tubes or insertion of further chest tubes into undrained spaces, adequate suction applied to the pleural cavity, and assurance of full expansion of the lung with vigorous chest physiotherapy and bronchodilator treatments are all necessary to guarantee closure of these small distal fistula.

If there is a substantial persistent air leak from the chest tube, however, or there is incomplete or no expansion of the lung in the pleural cavity, a significant bronchopleural fistula should be suspected. Major proximal airway problems, such as failure of the anastomosis of a bronchoplastic procedure, disruption of a bronchial closure, or retained secretions or foreign bodies, should be excluded early in the postoperative course by bronchoscopy. Bronchopleural fistulas following pulmonary resections occur in three time sequences. In the acute phase, within the first 7 postoperative days, the fistula is usually secondary to a technical problem. In the subacute phase, usually more than 1 week after the operation but usually within the first 6 weeks, the fistula is usually associated with an empyema or local peribronchial abscess. The late occurrence of a bronchopleural fistula, usually more than 6 months after the operation, should lead one to consider recurrent lung carcinoma. The confirmation of a disruption of the bronchial closure usually requires reoperation with correction of the technical problem, drainage of all sepsis, and reinforcement of the closure with an acceptable well-vascularized flap, such as the omentum, the pleuropericardial fat pad, or a muscle flap.

The occurrence of a bronchopleural fistula in the early postoperative course of a patient who has undergone a pneumonectomy is a surgical emergency. The typical presentation of a postpneumonectomy bronchopleural fistula in the acute or subacute setting is the sudden expectoration of copious amounts of pink, frothy sputum. Rather than assume that this is pulmonary edema, a bronchopleural fistula and drainage of the pneumonectomy fluid into the airway should be immediately entertained. The patient should be positioned without delay so the operated or pneumonectomy side is down. This traps the remaining fluid in the pneumonectomy space and protects the patient from drowning in his or her own pleural fluid. When the patient is stabilized, a chest radiograph can be performed, which shows loss of fluid from the pneumonectomy space. Next a chest tube should be placed into the pneumonectomy cavity; remembering that there is significant shift in the mediastinum and diaphragm, the tube should be placed high in the midaxillary line. This should be done in a sterile manner so as not to contaminate the pleural space because there may not be an associated empyema. The fluid should be immediately sent for Gram stain and culture. Bronchoscopy is then performed to determine the security of the closure of the bronchial stump. In the early stages, if the fluid is not contaminated and the bronchial closure has dehisced, reoperation and resection of the necrotic bronchus and repeat closure of the bronchial stump with fortification either by intercostal muscle or similar flaps should be undertaken.

If the bronchopleural fistula is associated with an **empyema,** the complexity of the problem and the postoperative management is intensified. The empyema is initially treated with tube drainage and antibiotic therapy. The bronchopleural fistula may be a source of pulmonary contamination and respiratory failure; if this is the case, intubation and assisted ventilation is necessary. If there is difficulty ventilating, this is the ideal clinical setting for jet ventilation or intubation of the remaining main stem bronchus with either a single lumen tube or double lumen tube and conventional ventilation. Also the fistula may be temporarily occluded with a bronchial blocker to prevent contamination of the remaining lung and to allow adequate contralateral ventilation. Once the patient has been stabilized and if the bronchopleural fistula is of minimal clinical significance, the treatment of the empyema predominates. Eventually drainage of the empyema cavity should be converted from closed tube drainage to open tube drainage. This is done by opening the chest tube to air. A chest film is then taken to determine if the mediastinum is fixed or has shifted and compressed the contralateral remaining lung. Once the stability of the mediastinum has been confirmed, the drainage of the cavity may be permanently converted to open drainage. This is done by performing a rib resection and marsupialization of the pneumonectomy cavity (Clagett window or Eloessor flap). With time, the pneumonectomy cavity shrinks in size, and with dressing changes and irrigation, contamination is minimized. If possible, it is favorable to close the bronchopleural fistula through a clean, noninvolved area. This is generally via a median sternotomy by transpericardial closure of the bronchial stump. At a later date, the Clagett window may be closed in the classic fashion or with muscle or omental flap filling of the space and reinforcement of the bronchial stump closure. If median sternotomy is not available for transpericardial closure of the bronchial stump, muscle flap omental or pleuropericardial fat pad flap closure of the bronchopleural fistula and closure of the Clagett window can be undertaken. If the bronchopleural fistula is the result of the recurrent malignant disease, the chance of closure and resection for cure is highly unlikely, and the patient should be palliated for tube drainage. Radiation therapy may aggravate the bronchopleural fistula.

Vascular Complications

Pulmonary emboli, a serious complication in any patient, have disastrous effects in patients who have recently had a pulmonary resection. Prophylaxis, as undertaken in any operative procedure, should be carried out in patients undergoing thoracic procedures. Subcutaneous heparin and vascular compression stocking should be used in all patients. The placement of prophylactic inferior vena caval filters in patients who cannot be anticoagulated, who have had previous deep venous thrombosis, or who are at an increased risk of pulmonary emboli should be considered. In the postoperative period, pulmonary emboli are sometimes difficult to diagnose because hypoxemia may be due to sepsis, ARDS, or pneumonia. If pulmonary embolism is highly suspected, ventilation perfusion scanning and pulmonary angiography should be done. Treatment, as for all postoperative patients, is anticoagulation or lytic therapy. If these are contraindicated, an inferior vena caval filter should be placed.

Systemic tumor emboli, although uncommon, may be seen after pulmonary resections for primary bronchogenic carcinomas or metastatic sarcomas. These patients present with peripheral systemic emboli with resection. Intraoperatively the surgeon notices a bulky tumor possibly with invasion of the pulmonary vein, and it may be reported that there was difficulty in obtaining an adequate venous resection margin. Arteriography confirms the embolus and its location; however, the nature of the embolus cannot be determined unless an embolectomy is indicated. Therefore a high index of suspicion is required to make the diagnosis of tumor emboli.

Massive postoperative hemorrhage may be a lethal complication in pulmonary resection patients. Early significant shock occurring on transfer of the patient to the recovery room is a life-threatening emergency. It generally requires emergent reoperation and is the result of a slipped tie from the pulmonary artery or more commonly the pulmonary vein. This complication is seen when these major vessels are controlled with a single, simple tie.

Postoperative hemorrhage is more commonly a slower process and is generally the result of small bleeding arteries or veins in the mediastinum or chest wall. Reoperation is required for control of bleeding, but just as important is the evacuation of the hemothorax and prevention of fibrothorax and restrictive lung disease in the future. If exploration is not undertaken but bleeding is controlled, the hemothorax may be evacuated later in the postoperative course, when the patient is more stable, by thoracoscopy.

Pulmonary Parenchymal Complications

Atelectasis is a common complication, perhaps the most common complication after thoracic surgery. Its origin is multifactorial, the result of splinting, hypoventilation, bronchospasm, inadequate cough, retained secretions, absorption atelectasis, and intraoperative trauma to the lung. Atelectasis may be the forerunner of further complications and therefore should not be overlooked. The increased work of breathing and impaired gas exchange, owing to the inherent ventilation-perfusion mismatch, may precipitate respiratory failure in a patient with marginal pulmonary reserve. Retained bronchial secretions and the frequent colonization of the airway in patients with COPD facilitate the progression of atelectasis to postoperative pneumonia. As well, atelectasis is one of the many precipitating causes of postoperative arrhythmias.

Patients with atelectasis may initially be asymptomatic, and the diagnosis is made on chest x-ray findings. With clinically significant atelectasis, however, the patient may present with fever, tachypnea, tachycardia, arrhythmias, hypoxia, or respiratory failure. On physical examination, there may be decreased motion of the involved chest. Percussion and auscultation reveals the signs of a consolidated portion of lung. The chest x-ray film may show patterns of platelike atelectatic collapse, to segmental, lobar, or total atelectasis of the lung. Although the operative side is more frequently involved, contralateral lung and bilateral involvement may be seen.

Prevention of atelectasis is mandatory in all patients undergoing thoracic surgery, and therefore prevention is the mainstay of treatment. Prevention requires careful preoperative assessment and education. Vigorous preoperative preparation with cessation of smoking, chest physiotherapy, bronchodilator therapy, and antibiotics, if required, should be initiated 2 to 3 weeks before the operation. Postoperatively the treatment is directed at expanding the collapsed lung and clearing the airway of retained secretions. Incentive respirometry, chest physiotherapy, inhalation therapy, and bronchoscopy are the principle means of treating atelectasis postoperatively. Identification of high risk patients also helps to minimize this complication; patients with impaired pulmonary function, bronchitis, bronchiectasis, cystic fibrosis, poor pain control, and those undergoing bronchoplastic procedures are at increased risk of this postoperative complication. Along with early identification, early prophylactic measures may be advantageous. Adequate pain relief, aggressive bronchodilator therapy, incentive respirometry, physiotherapy, patient positioning, early ambulation, and appropriate antibiotic administration may minimize the occurrence of atelectasis and pneumonia. Routine bronchoscopy has been shown not to be advantageous; however, its role in established atelectasis is invaluable.[90] The need for repeated bronchoscopy should lead to the percutaneous placement of a minitracheostomy.[70] Expansion of the atelectatic portions of the lung by CPAP or intubation and selective ventilation should not be routinely used but should be reserved for the recalcitrant or perilous case.

Lobar collapse is most commonly seen after right upper lobectomy but may be seen after any thoracic operation. All the factors that foster atelectasis are aggravated by the altered bronchial geometry following right upper lobectomy. The horizontal fissure rises and rotates to lie perpendicularly along the mediastinal pleura. The resultant twisting and kinking of the long and narrow middle lobe bronchus renders it susceptible to occlusion. This complication should prompt early bronchoscopy to rule out torsion and repeated bronchoscopy to remove retained secretions.

Lobar torsion is an uncommon complication that results from the twisting of a mobile piece of pulmonary parenchyma about its hilar structures with resultant bronchial, arterial, and venous occlusion.[106] This occurs most commonly after right upper lobectomy. If the remaining portion of the major fissure between the middle and lower lobes has been completed at surgery or is relatively complete, the middle lobe has no anchoring attachments except the middle lobe bronchus, artery, and vein. This one point fixation and the absence of the upper lobe allow the middle lobe to rotate freely, during the surgery, about its hilum. Lobar torsion may be seen after bilobectomy on the right with torsion of the remaining upper or lower lobe or after lobectomy on the left with torsion of the remaining lobe. Prevention is the key to treating this complication and requires a careful inspection of the pulmonary parenchyma, fissures, and hilum before closure of the thoracotomy incision. This complication can be prevented by fixing mobile portions of pulmonary parenchyma to nearby structure; this provides multiple point fixation and thus averts torsion. This is most commonly practiced after right upper lobectomy, when the middle lobe is fixed to the lower lobe at the fissure by one or two superficial stitches in the visceral pleura and the peripheral pulmonary parenchyma, thereby closing the major fissure. Postoperatively this complication may be recognized early by appreciating the potential for torsion after lobectomy, most notably right upper lobectomy. The patient may be asymptomatic or may present as a patient with atelectasis. On physical examination, there may be the findings of collapse of a portion of the lung. Careful study of the postoperative chest film demonstrates more atelectasis or collapse than expected in the early postoperative period. Later in the course, the film shows complete "white out" of the involved segment or lobe. Early on there may be no abnormalities of gas exchange or biochemistry. As ischemia progresses to infarction, however, all the biochemical signs of tissue necrosis may be seen, and the patient may cough up bloody, purulent, malodorous secretions. Similar chest tube drainage may be found.[106] Early bronchoscopy demonstrates abrupt occlusion of the involved airway; however, it may be possible to pass the bronchoscope distally into the twisted airway. The altered orientation of cartilaginous to membranous airway with a spiral effect may be appreciated. Pulmonary angiography and perfusion scans demonstrate lack of flow to the involved portion of lung; however, these tests are not diagnostic. The differential diagnosis includes atelectasis, pulmonary hematoma, and hemothorax. Once diagnosed, urgent thoracotomy with detorsion is required. Questionably viable tissue should be left, and a second-look thoracotomy may be required. If frozen section review of the tissue or if gross tissue inspection demonstrates necrosis, excision is necessary.

Reexpansion pulmonary edema may occur after rapid removal of a large pleural effusion or after reexpansion of a pneumothorax. It is characterized by unilateral alveolar pulmonary edema, which resolves rapidly.[107]

Postpneumonectomy pulmonary edema is an uncommon complication after pneumonectomy or on occasion lesser pulmonary resections. It is usually seen 24 to 72 hours after operation. The onset is insidious and is heralded by the appearance of a fine interstitial infiltrate on the early postoperative chest film. The patient becomes progressively tachypneic and tachycardic with marked hypoxia, often requiring reintubation and reinstitution of mechanical ventilation. The origin of postpneumonectomy pulmonary edema is multifactorial. It is not the result of increased hydrostatic pressures owing to cardiac failure but due to defects in the membrane permeability with resultant increased lung water. This complication may be avoided by judicious perioperative and postoperative fluid management. Once postpneumonectomy pulmonary edema has been established, reintubation, ventilation, pulmonary artery pressure and cardiac output monitoring, and close attention to fluid balance are required. All causes of ARDS should be excluded.[108] The authors have had anecdotal success with the use of terbutaline for postpneumonectomy pulmonary edema on extension of the concept proposed by Basran et al.[109] that beta-adrenergic agents reduce transmembrane permeability. The mechanism of terbutaline's action in this regard has not been determined.

Respiratory insufficiency may complicate thoracic surgical procedures, especially pulmonary resections. This may be irreversible and due to inadequate pulmonary reserve. The complication may be the result of too aggressive a resection, the consequence of poor assessment preoperatively, and an incorrect estimation of vital capacity and FEV_1 postoperatively or the result of technical problems that required a larger than predicted resection. Once this state has been realized, the patient's pulmonary status should be optimized. If there is failure to wean from the ventilator and to extubate, arrangement must be made for long-term support (see Chap. 24). Presently this complication is not an indication for pulmonary transplantation and therefore should be avoided by careful preoperative evaluation of pulmonary function, realistic preoperative prediction of postoperative pulmonary function, and meticulous surgical technique with the use of parenchymal sparing operations whenever feasible.

Respiratory failure may be reversible, the result of some superimposed treatable complication or the acute reduction in pulmonary function secondary to anesthesia and thoracotomy. Infection, fluid overload, aspiration, pulmonary edema, pulmonary embolus, or pneumothorax in the setting of acute respiratory insufficiency postoperatively should be identified and quickly treated. In this setting, extracorporeal membrane oxygenation has not been shown to improve survival in adults. Not until acute lung injury is treatable and reversible is successful acute support a clinical reality. Regrettably acute lung injury frequently progresses to fibrosis and chronic lung failure.

Pleural Complications

Fluid and air may possibly collect in the pleural space during the postoperative period. Adequate drainage of these areas is necessary and obtained by the correct positioning of a sufficient number of appropriately sized chest tubes. This is best accomplished during the operation, but undrained and possibly loculated collections may require drainage postoperatively. The portable chest radiograph may help in the positioning of these tubes, but often it is difficult to place the tube adequately with only two-dimensional imaging. CT scanning with placement after or during the scan is beneficial. At the bedside, however, loculated fluid collections are best located and drained with surface ultrasound guidance.

A **pneumothorax** after thoracic surgery can be found with or without an air leak. Either situation should prompt the assurance of proper chest tube function. The drainage system should be checked to guarantee it is a closed system with adequate underwater seal. Chest tube patency should next be ascertained. Declotting chest tubes may require vigorous stripping of the tubes or opening the system and using a balloon occlusion (Fogarty) catheter to remove the obstructing material. If the pneumothorax is not associated with an air leak and the previous steps have ensured a properly functioning tube and drainage system, a loculated pneumothorax with no communication with the drainage system or a large bulla are the most likely explanations. A persistent pneumothorax not associated with an air leak or signs of sepsis is generally not a problem. A persistent pneumothorax may require increased suction on the present system or possibly a new chest tube placed in the loculated pneumothorax. The majority resolve with expectant therapy, however, and few become infected.[110] A persistent pneumothorax associated with an air leak means there is an established bronchopleural fistula; diagnosis and management have been discussed previously under airway complications.

Significant **persistent pleural fluid drainage** should prompt thoracentesis for diagnosis. If a hemothorax is found, prompt management as described under vascular complications should be initiated. A transudative pleural effusion should be drained by thoracentesis, but attention should be turned to treatment of the extrathoracic cause. An exudative pleural effusion should lead one to consider an empyema even if cultures of the fluid are negative. The clinical setting and low pH of the fluid may further verify the diagnosis.[111] Empyemas after thoracic surgery should be treated with chest tube drainage. The primary cause of the empyema should be identified and corrected. Once the primary cause has been treated and the space has been drained, every effort should be taken to maintain full expansion of the lung and obliteration of the empyema cavity. Once the pleural space has resolved and the pleural surfaces are fused, the chest tube may be opened to air, cut 2 to 3 inches from its entry site, and treated as a regular drain. It is slowly removed from the chest cavity, ensuring that the chest tube tract closes about the exiting tube. This ensures that no space is allowed to develop and therefore there will be no persistence of the empyema cavity. If, however, the lung does not expand to fill the pleural space, two methods may be undertaken. In either situation, the chest tube should be left for drainage. When the pleural surfaces have fused and the mediastinum is fixed, the chest tube may be opened to the atmosphere to confirm this occurrence. The drainage may then be converted to open drainage (e.g., Clagett window, Eloesser flap). At a later date, decortication and closure of the window may be considered. If the patient is thought to be an adequate candidate for decortication, however, the chest tube may be left as the sole means of drainage, and the patient and cavity are prepared for operation. Six to 8 weeks after the initial drainage of this empyema, the patient may be brought to the operating room for decortication and pleurectomy.

Chylothorax can complicate operations in the chest about the aorta, esophagus, or lung. Any dissection in the posterior mediastinum may result in an injury to the thoracic duct. This should be identified operatively and repaired. The drainage can be quite serous, however, and its true nature, rate, and site of origin may not be easily determined. If there is a suspected injury to the thoracic duct and this injury cannot be found, the supradiaphragmatic ligation of the thoracic duct is an acceptable intraoperative approach, at the time of the original procedure. This is done by mobilizing the tissue between the azygous vein and the aorta posteriorly and continuing the dissection toward the esophagus anteriorly, at or just above the diaphragm. This is the most constant position of the thoracic duct in the chest. This tissue, which contains the thoracic duct, is then ligated. If the damage to the thoracic duct is not noted preoperatively but postoperatively, the physician is challenged with the management of high output fistula. Volumes of 1 to 3 L per day are common. Because there is a high concentration of lymphocytes and protein, there may be significant losses of these and other elements. The diagnosis should be confirmed by analysis of the fluid, which has a high protein content, a large proportion of lymphocytes, and most notably an elevated concentration of chylomicrons. A contrast lymphangiogram or nuclear lymphangiogram using ^{99m}technetium antimony colloid may be used to confirm the diagnosis but more importantly locate the site of injury.[112] Initially the management consists of placing the thoracic duct at rest and complete drainage of the pleural space ensuring full expansion of the lung. The pleural space is managed with chest tube drainage. The thoracic duct flow can be kept to a minimum by giving the patient nothing by mouth. Nutrition may then be supplemented by either intravenous hyperalimentation or feedings through gastrointestinal tract using medium-chain triglyceride formulas. If after 1 week there is not resolution of the chylothorax, thoracotomy with ligation of the thoracic duct is indicated. Care should be taken to ensure that the thoracic duct is the site of injury. Lymphatic leakage after mobilization of the internal mammary artery or extensive mediastinal lymphadenectomy has been known to cause a significant lymphatic leak, simulating a chylothorax. Confirmation of the diagnosis and site of leakage is paramount before surgery. Therapy may then be directed at the site of injury or the thoracic duct proximal to the site of injury. Intraoperative identification of the site of injury may be aided by the preoperative ingestion of cream or similar fatty food. Pleuroperitoneal shunting is an option in the management of recalcitrant chylothorax.[113]

Chest Wall Complications

Infection of thoracic incisions is uncommon. The use of prophylactic antibiotics intraoperatively and in the early postoperative course has further decreased the incidence, and the routine use of an antibiotic with good coverage of Staphylococcus aureus is recommended. There is an increased incidence, however, of thoracic wound infections during operations in which there is a septic complication or if the gastrointestinal tract is opened. These procedures commonly include operations for empyema, lung abscess, mediastinitis, or perforated esophagus. Posterior lateral thoracotomies are sometimes complicated by a subscapular abscess. This is particularly true if large tissue planes are opened during the formation of the incision. This abscess is uncommon and may be difficult to diagnose early in its formation. CT scanning may be helpful in confirming and locating these abscesses.

Infections of the costal cartilage and costal arch present a most difficult management problem. Once the perichondrium is disturbed, the underlying cartilage is rendered ischemic. If infected, the cartilage acts as a foreign body and the infection will not be controlled until the dead cartilage is excised. As well, the infection has been reported to spread across the cartilaginous xiphoid process to involve contralateral costal cartilage. To deal with this problem, wide excision of the infected, avascular cartilage must be undertaken. Sometimes this necessitates excision of a costal arch and xiphoid process. Generally these wounds are left opened to granulate in, a process that may take weeks. Because they are generally located inferiorly and anteriorly, there may be a significant flail component of the chest wall.

Subcutaneous emphysema is the result of tracking of air into the subcutaneous space and dissecting along the path of least resistance. The driving pressure is that of positive pressure ventilation, if the patient is intubated and mechanically ventilated or the positive pressure generated on expiration or coughing. Although alarming, subcutaneous emphysema does not generally adversely affect the patient's outcome. The treatment consists of the placement of a properly functioning chest tube into the pleural space; the tube should be placed to suction drainage. Rarely massive emphysema in a nonintubated patient compromises the airway and requires urgent intubation or tracheostomy for control of the upper airway. The patient with subcutaneous emphysema should be assured that this temporary problem will resolve. If the air tracks to the upper eyelids and closes them, causing inability to see, the air can be released by carefully puncturing the upper eyelid with a no. 25 gauge needle after sterile preparation.

Bullectomy

Bullectomy for bullous emphysema is an uncommon operation because chronic obstructive pulmonary disease is a diffuse process, and the entire lung is usually involved. In selected patients, however, in whom large compressive bullae are present, resection of these bullae allows expansion of relatively normal compressed lung with marked clinical improvement. The major cause of postoperative morbidity is nonexpansion or delayed expansion of the remaining lung, resulting in persistent air leak, pneumonia, or empyema. Preoperative preparation is crucial in these patients. Attention to secure closure of the base of a bulla during the operation minimizes air leaks and postoperative spaces. Patient selection is the most important factor in avoiding postoperative respiratory insufficiency.

Mediastinal Complications

Patients with **myasthenia gravis** may undergo therapeutic thymectomy, based on observed clinical improvement with sustained lowering of thymic hormone activity.[114] These patients were once routinely ventilated for a day or more postoperatively, but in our experience, the majority may be safely extubated on the table or shortly after arrival in the ICU if neuromuscular blockade is monitored and adequately reversed. In a series of 92 patients, only eight (8.7%) required prolonged mechanical ventilation, ranging in duration from 15 hours to 3 days.[115] The need for postoperative mechanical ventilation can be predicted by four key factors:[116]

- Duration of myasthenia gravis greater than 6 years
- History of chronic respiratory disease not related to myasthenia
- Pyridostigmine dose greater than 750 mg/day
- Preoperative vital capacity less than 2.9 L

Patients with severe myasthenia gravis treated with preoperative plasma exchange require less mechanical ventilation and have a shorter ICU length of stay.[117]

Cardiac Dysrhythmias

Cardiac dysrhythmias constitute a major, life-threatening complication of thoracic procedures. Rhythms that are seemingly benign in other settings (e.g., atrial fibrillation, supraventricular tachycardia) assume greater prognostic significance in the post-thoracotomy patient. One assessment of 236 patients undergoing pneumonectomy with normal sinus rhythm preoperatively demonstrated a 22% incidence of dysrhythmias in the perioperative period.[118] Of the total, 64% had atrial fibrillation, 23% had supraventricular tachycardia, and 13% had atrial flutter. Twelve of 53 patients with tachydysrhythmias had increased levels of creatinine phosphokinase (CPK) associated with an elevated MB fraction, and 25% of these died within 30 days of operation, a significant difference from the mortality rate (7%) without dysrhythmias. Patients who underwent intrapericardial dissection or who developed postoperative interstitial or perihilar pulmonary edema had the highest incidence of dysrhythmias. These findings suggest that careful attention to heart rate and fluid balance might be beneficial in reducing the morbidity and mortality from cardiac events. Prophylactic administration of digoxin has been associated with a lower 30-day mortality rate (4 versus 14%) in a retrospective analysis of 125 thoracotomy patients,[119] but controlled, prospective information is lacking.

Multifocal atrial tachycardia is common in elderly patients and those with pulmonary disease, although the mechanism is not clearly established.[120] Multifocal atrial tachycardia is occasionally seen in the postoperative thoracic surgery patient, although less commonly than other supraventricular tachycardias. Drugs such as beta-agonists and aminophylline exacerbate multifocal atrial tachycardia at therapeutic levels, and this dysrhythmia often resolves with discontinuing or decreasing the dose of these agents.

Esophageal Complications

The major complication after esophageal surgery is leakage of esophageal contents from the site of esophageal surgery, a myotomy, hiatal hernia repair, excision site of a foregut cyst, or from an esophagogastric or esophagocolic anastomosis. In a study of 138 patients undergoing gastric interposition following transhiatal esophagectomy, the leak rate was 10.9%, with aspiration occurring in 4.3% and gastric perforation in 1.5%.[121] The authors suggest that with a high incidence of suspicion for perforation (evidenced by postoperative fever), use of water-soluble contrast media is preferable to extravasation of barium.

Early esophageal perforation should be managed with thoracotomy, secure closure, reinforcement of the closure with a pedicle wrap, drainage, and defunctioning of the esophagus. This defunctioning may be as simple as a nasogastric tube or as complex as an esophagostomy and gastrostomy. After prolonged leakage from an esophageal perforation and soilage of the pleural space and mediastinum, the possibility of repair is less likely. If the repair is undertaken, it must be protected by a gastrostomy and some means of draining the esophagus, either tube or formal esophagoscopy.

On occasion with a late perforation or a perforation associated with distal pathology that will not allow healing of any closure of the perforation, resection should be contemplated. Reconstruction is undertaken if the reconstruction can be done in a sterile field. Otherwise, the esophagus should be defunctioned with an end cervical esophagostomy and a tube gastrostomy. With this resection and defunctioning, a substernal colon interposition may be used at a later date without entering the posterior mediastinum.

Anastomotic leaks should be confirmed by radiographic means. The tissue should be examined by endoscopy to ensure viability. If there is a small leak with a viable anastomosis, it should be drained locally. The patient should be given nothing by mouth and supported nutritionally. If the anastomosis is widely disturbed because of technical problems or necrotic owing to ischemia, take-down of the anastomosis and defunctioning of the gastrointestinal tract are required.

Manipulation of the esophagus generates release of all three isoenzymes of CPK, limiting the use of CPK for diagnosis of perioperative myocardial infarction. The small serum CPK-MB bands generated by esophageal manipulation can be differentiated from those seen in acute myocardial infarction and infarction confirmed by simultaneous analysis of serum lactate dehydrogenase (LDH) isoenzymes.[122]

Complications following Lung Transplantation

Lung transplant recipients are prone to the usual postoperative complications after major thoracic surgery that have been reviewed here and in previous chapters. We discuss specific complications inherent to patients in the ICU setting after single or double lung transplantation that can make these patients difficult management problems in the postoperative period.

Considerations after Lung Transplantation

First 48 Hours. Lung transplant recipients can present formidable management problems both in immediate and late postoperative periods. Patients may initially be in unstable condition and thus may return to the ICU fully monitored with arterial and venous lines. Once adequate urine output has been established, full immunosuppression is started with cyclosporine (3 to 5 mg/kg/intravenously), azathioprine (2 mg/kg/intravenously), and corticosteroids (methylprednisolone, 125 mg intravenously every 8 hours for 48 hours, then prednisone, 0.5 mg/kg). We believe that the adverse effects of steroids on bronchial healing have been exaggerated, and we have demonstrated in a dog model of lung transplantation that it is possible to give immunosuppressive doses of steroids in the perioperative period and not increase the risk of bronchial dehiscence.[123] Clinically, with more than 40 bronchial anastomoses at risk, we have only a single patient who has required stenting for a recalcitrant bronchial stenosis and no instances of bronchial dehiscence despite the immediate use of steroids.

Many patients are extremely hemodynamically unstable on returning to the ICU and often require significant inotropic support. One or both transplanted lungs often develop **"reperfusion" pulmonary edema** (Figs. 20-13 and 20-14), resulting in problems with oxygenation and increasing pulmonary artery pressures that further aggravate the situation. The chest radiograph in Figure 20-13A was taken immediately postoperatively after a double lung transplantation. The left lung was implanted first and was subsequently exposed to the entire cardiac output while the right pulmonary artery was clamped and the right allograft implanted. When the right pulmonary artery clamp was released, the right lung did not develop the pulmonary edema seen on the left side. The chest radiograph in Figure 20-13B was obtained 4 days later, showing resolution of the pulmonary edema. The same problem with reperfusion edema can be seen following single lung transplantation in the setting of pulmonary hypertension. Figure 20-14 shows massive edema 24 hours after left lung transplantation in a patient with Eisenmenger's syndrome and systemic pulmonary artery pressures before transplantation. Here again, the entire cardiac output is directed toward the donor lung because of the high vascular resistance present in the native lung. This finding is in some ways analogous to high flow pulmonary edema, but is compounded by the ischemic injury that occurs to the vascular endothelium and subsequent increased endothelial permeability. Measures in the ICU that can be used to counter this complication include controlling fluid intake, keeping the patient "dry," diuretics, PEEP, and positioning the patient with the transplanted lung up. Although various centers have reported survival rates of between 50 and 60% in this setting, Cooper in St. Louis has successfully performed single lung transplantation in 17 or 18 patients with pulmonary hypertension (personal communication). In an attempt to circumvent the problem of reperfusion edema with a single lung transplantation, some transplant centers are exploring the appropriateness of double lung transplantation in this setting.

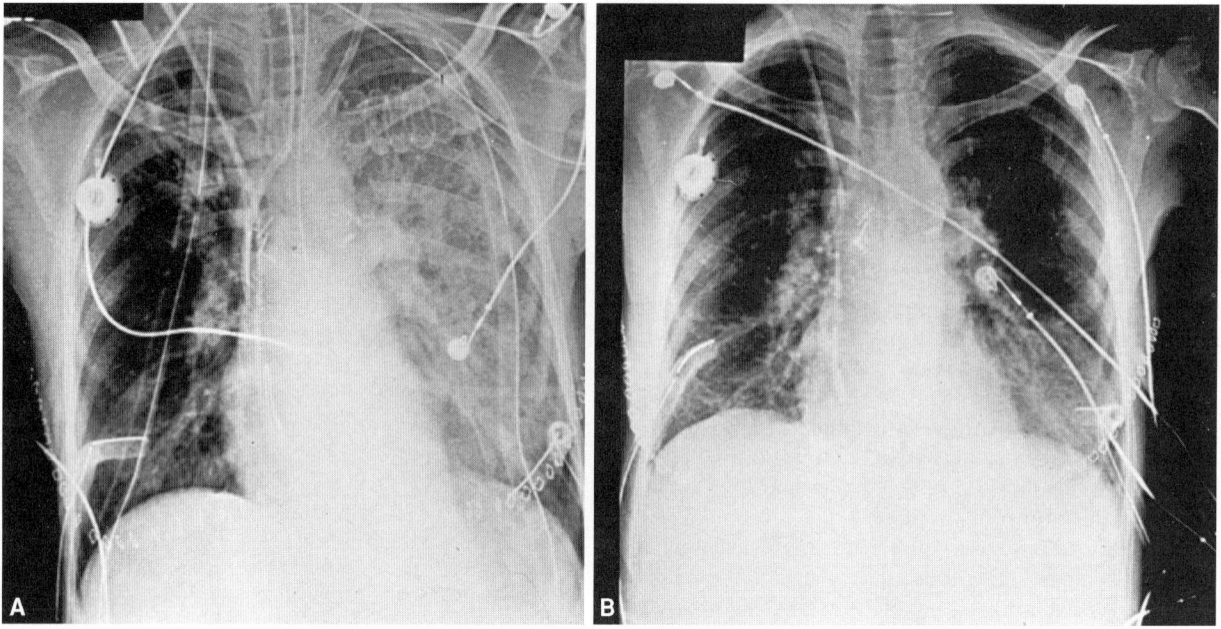

Fig. 20–13. *A*, The chest radiograph is from a double lung transplant recipient immediately postoperatively. Marked "reperfusion" edema is present in the left lung. *B*, Five days later, this edema cleared.

Another major problem in the immediate postoperative period is the development of hyperexpansion of the native lung and compression of the allograft in patients that have had a single lung transplantation for emphysema.[124] This is a result of the highly compliant native lung accepting most of the ventilation compared with the relatively low compliance in the transplanted lung. In most cases, hyperexpansion is not seen, and it is difficult to predict which recipients are at risk to develop this complication. It is our belief, however, that patients with bullous-type emphy-

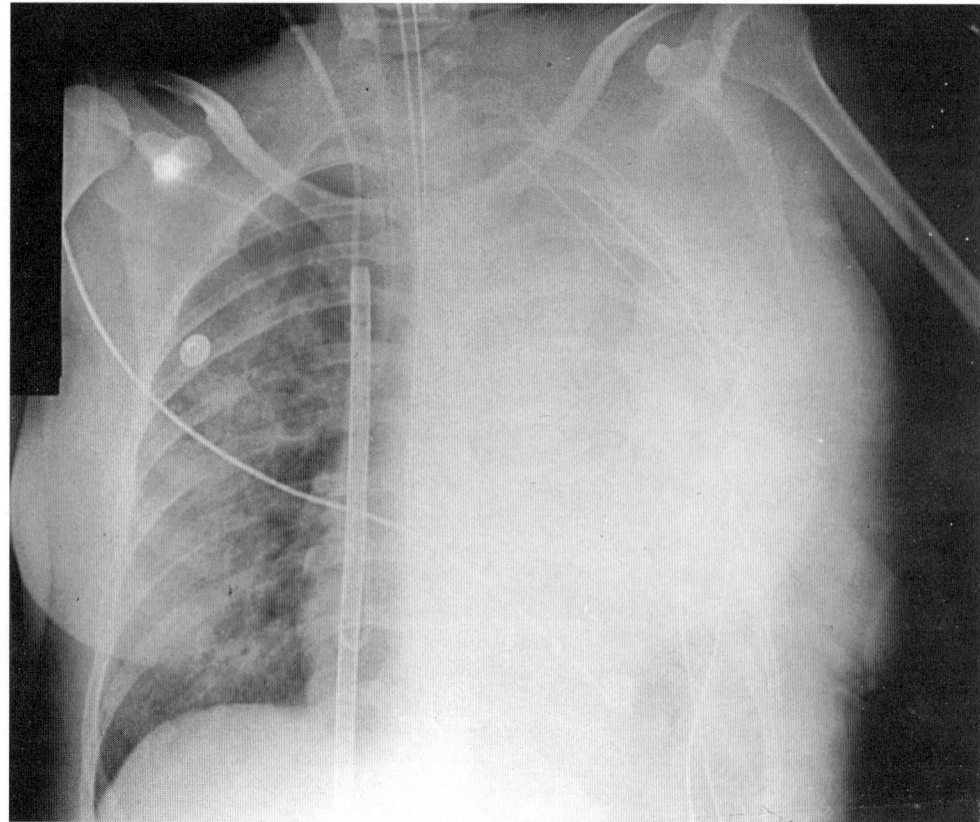

Fig. 20–14. Postoperative chest radiograph in a left single lung transplant recipient with Eisenmenger's syndrome. Massive edema is present in the left lung. An ECMO cannula can be seen lying in the vena cava. This was necessary to support gas exchange in this setting.

sema represent the highest risk group and should be considered for double lung transplantation to avoid this problem. Although unusual, this complication is best dealt with a double lumen tube and selective ventilation of each lung until the patient has sufficiently recovered to be extubated.

Uncomplicated lung transplant recipients are able to be extubated within the first 48 hours. We are not advocates of extubation in the immediate postoperative period because we have seen too many patients require reintubation if this is attempted. Before extubation, an epidural catheter is placed for pain control. Soon after extubation, the patient may be slowly advanced to a regular diet and the immunosuppression switched to oral medication (cyclosporine, 5 to 10 mg/kg; azathioprine, 1 to 2 mg/kg; and prednisone, 1 mg/kg). Patients with uneventful postoperative courses are usually able to be discharged from the ICU in 7 to 10 days and from the hospital in 3 to 4 weeks.

48 Hours to 2 Weeks. The major problem with lung transplants during this time period is the differentiation of infection from rejection.[125] The clinical (dyspnea, malaise, fever), radiologic (perihilar infiltrate, pleural effusion), and laboratory findings (hypoxia, elevated white blood count) are similar, making differentiation on this basis difficult. Transbronchial biopsy is probably the most specific investigation that can be performed to demonstrate rejection, but it should be done under fluoroscopy, which is often not available in the ICU setting. As well, transbronchial biopsy lacks overall accuracy because of sampling error, and the similar histologic changes can be seen in rejection and certain infections (i.e., cytomegalovirus, pneumocystis).

Our preferred management algorithm in recipients in whom the question of rejection versus infection arises is to perform a bronchoscopy, BAL, and, if possible, a transbronchial biopsy. BAL and brushings have been shown to be accurate at detecting infection, so if the Gram stain on these specimens is negative along with a negative cytomegalovirus cell spin, we treat the patient for rejection. Our standard regimen for acute rejection is a course of methylprednisolone, 500 mg intravenously daily, for 3 days. If rejection is the diagnosis, a dramatic improvement in the patient's clinical course and oxygenation should occur within 12 to 24 hours. One caveat that should always be borne in mind is that a patient may be suffering from a combination of rejection and infection and therefore need to be treated for both. Recalcitrant rejection is treated with the murine monoclonal antibody OK$_3$ or antilymophocyte globulin.

Bronchial dehiscence used to be one of the major causes of postoperative mortality in lung transplant recipients but today is seen in only 5 to 8% of cases and in most instances can be handled conservatively. Before extubation, which usually occurs within 72 hours in an uncomplicated transplant, we use bronchoscopy to assess airway healing. Patients in whom there is concern over airway healing undergo bronchoscopy in the future on a regular basis to assess airway healing. Mucosal sluffing is not uncommon and is of little consequence but does represent ischemic damage to the airway and thus may portend poor anastomotic healing. Partial dehiscences are the rule, and most heal in time without further intervention. Occasionally bronchomalacia or stenosis develops in the area of concern requiring repeated dilatation and in some cases the insertion of a Silastic bronchial stent. Complete bronchial dehiscence is a rare complication today. It requires either reoperation and resuturing of the anastomosis, or in the presence of complete distal airway ischemia/necrosis, retransplantation is necessary.

REHABILITATION/POST-ICU CARE

Discharge Considerations for the General Thoracic Surgery Patient

Wound dressings are changed at 48 hours and then as required. Most patients can be discharged from the ICU within 24 hours if they are sent to a nursing unit familiar with management of thoracic patients and accompanying chest tubes and if sufficient respiratory support personnel are available for monitoring and chest physiotherapy. Readmissions within 48 hours are used as a quality improvement statistic, and readmissions should constitute less than 3% of all discharges from the unit. The major reason for readmission is respiratory decompensation, owing to fluid overload, aspiration, or failure to cough and breathe well enough to prevent atelectasis and retained secretions. Good pain management with epidural or intravenous patient-controlled analgesia[92] helps avoid splinting and inadequate respiratory effort.

Respiratory Therapy after Transfer to the Nursing Floor

All thoracic surgery patients should be followed by the respiratory therapy team for the first several days after transfer from the ICU. Atelectasis is a continuing threat and can be avoided by insisting that the patient properly use the incentive spirometer at hourly intervals while awake. Patients unable to cooperate fully with incentive spirometry can often be managed with intermittent positive-pressure breathing treatments. Bronchodilators and mucolytics are added as needed. More intensive intervention, in the form of percussion, postural drainage, and nasotracheal suctioning, may be needed when secretions are thick or atelectasis is persistent. Follow-up care should include periodic chest radiographs and at least daily physical examination by the primary care physicians. Arterial blood gases and intermittent oxygen saturation measurements using a portable pulse oximeter are helpful adjuncts.

Because of the high incidence of swallowing difficulties after esophageal surgery or prolonged intubation, it is wise to evaluate ability to swallow carefully before allowing oral intake. Consideration should be given to maintaining nothing by mouth status in neurologically impaired patients and those with documented swallowing difficulty. The patient with compromised cardiac or renal function is prone to accumulation of excess fluid and eventual congestive heart failure. Daily weights and balancing of intake and output can point to the need for diuretic or cardiotonic therapy before respiratory distress develops.

Psychologic Support

Meeting the psychologic needs of the thoracic surgery patient begins in the ICU. When so much attention is given to the physical injuries of these acutely ill patients, it is common to overlook their psychologic injuries. Because the majority of the patients undergoing thoracic surgery have a malignancy, their major acute need is dealing with the diagnosis and its implications. Psychiatric consultations may be helpful in this setting.

REFERENCES

1. Bolton, J. W., et al.: Stair climbing as an indicator of pulmonary function. Chest, 92:783, 1987.
2. Zibrak, J. D., O'Donnel, C. R., and Marton, K.: Indications for pulmonary function testing. Ann. Intern. Med., 112:763, 1990.
3. Olsen, G. N., Block, A. F., and Tobias, J. A.: Prediction of postpneumonectomy pulmonary function using quantitative macroaggregate lung scanning. Chest, 66:1, 1974.
4. Olsen, G. N., et al.: Pulmonary function evaluation of the lung resection candidate: a prospective study. Am. Rev. Respir. Dis., 111:379, 1975.
5. Smith, T. P., et al.: Exercise capacity as a predictor of postthoracotomy morbidity. Am. Rev. Respir. Dis., 129:730, 1984.
6. Bechard, D., and Wetstein, L.: Assessment of exercise oxygen consumption as preoperative criterion for lung resection. Ann. Thorac. Surg., 44:344, 1987.
7. Fee, J. H., et al.: Role of pulmonary vascular resistance measurements in preoperative evaluation of candidates for pulmonary resection. J. Thorac. Cardiovasc. Surg., 75:519, 1978.
8. American College of Physicians: Preoperative pulmonary function testing. Ann. Intern. Med., 112:793, 1990.
9. Neuhaus, H., and Chemiak, N. S.: A bronchospirometric method estimating the effect of pneumonectomy on the maximum breathing capacity. J. Thorac. Cardiovasc. Surg., 55:144, 1968.
10. Boushy, S. F., Billig, D. M., North, J. B., and Helgason, A. H.: Clinical course related to preoperative and postoperative pulmonary function in patients with bronchogenic carcinoma. Chest, 59:383, 1971.
11. Keagy, B. A., et al.: Correlation of preoperative pulmonary function testing with clinical course in patients after pneumonectomy. Ann. Thorac. Surg., 36:253, 1983.
12. Peters, R. M., Clausen, J. L., and Tisi, G. M.: Extending resectability for carcinoma of the lung in patients with impaired pulmonary function. Ann. Thorac. Surg., 73:316, 1978.
13. Smith, T. P., et al.: Exercise capacity as a predictor of postthoracotomy morbidity. Am. Rev. Respir. Dis., 129:730, 1984.
14. Falor, W. H., and Traylor, R.: Extended indications for the median sternotomy incision. Am. Surg., 48:582, 1982.
15. Dripps, R. D., Lamont, A., and Eckenhoff, J. E.: The role of anesthesia in surgical mortality. JAMA, 178:261, 1961.
16. Owens, W. D., Felts, J. A., and Spitznagel, E. L.: ASA physical status classifications. Anesthesiology, 49:239, 1978.
17. Nunn, J. F., Miledge, S., Chen, D., and Dore, C.: Respiratory criteria of fitness for surgery and anesthesia. Anaesthesia, 43:543, 1988.
18. Garibaldi, R. A., et al.: Risk factors for postoperative pneumonia. JAMA, 70:677, 1981.
19. Stein, M., and Cassara, E. L.: Preoperative pulmonary evaluation and therapy for surgery patients. JAMA, 211:787, 1970.
20. Djokovic, J. L., and Hedley-Whyte, J.: Prediction of outcome of surgery and anesthesia in patients over 80. JAMA, 242:2301, 1979.
21. Warner, M. A., et al.: Effects of referral bias on surgical outcomes: A population-based study of surgical patients 90 years of age or older. Mayo Clin. Proc., 65:1185, 1990.
22. Rick, M. W., et al.: Increased complications and prolonged hospital stay in elderly cardiac surgical patients with low serum albumin. Am. J. Cardiol., 63:714, 1989.
23. Gerson, M. C., et al.: Cardiac prognosis in noncardiac geriatric surgery. Ann. Intern. Med., 103:832, 1985.
24. Wahba, W. M.: influence of aging on lung function—clinical significance of changes from age twenty. Anesth. Analg., 62:764, 1983.
25. Pontoppidan, H., and Beecher, H. K.: Progressive loss of protective reflexes in the airway with the advance of age. JAMA, 174:2209, 1960.
26. DelGuercio, L. R. M., and Cohn, J. D.: Monitoring operative risk in the elderly. JAMA, 243:1350, 1980.
27. Ebner, H., Sudkamp, N., Wex, P., and Dragojevic, D.: Selection and preoperative treatment of over-seventy-year-old patients undergoing thoracotomy. Thorac. Cardiac. Surg., 33:268, 1985.
28. Latimer, G., et al.: Ventilatory patterns and pulmonary complications after upper abdominal determined by preoperative and postoperative computerized spirometry and blood gas analysis. Am. J. Surg., 122:622, 1971.
29. Putman, H., Jenicek, J. A., Cellan, C. A., and Wilson, R. D.: Anesthesia in the morbidly obese. South. Med. J., 67:1411, 1974.
30. Laver, M. B., and Bendixen, H. H.: Atelectasis in the surgical patient: recent conceptual advances. Prog. Surg., 5:1, 1966.
31. Pearce, A. C., and Jones, R. M.: Smoking and anesthesia: preoperative abstinence and perioperative morbidity. Anesthesiology, 61:576, 1984.
32. Warner, M. A., et al.: Role of preoperative cessation of smoking and other factors in postoperative pulmonary complications: a blinded prospective study of coronary artery bypass patients. Mayo Clin. Proc., 64:609, 1989.
33. Shapiro, B. A., Harrison, R. A., Kacmarek, R. M., and Cane, R. D.: Clinical Application of Respiratory Care. 3rd Ed. Chicago, Year Book, 1985.
34. Levine, S. M., et al.: Single lung transplantation for primary pulmonary hypertension. Chest, 98:1107, 1990.
35. Kirby, T. J.: Single lung transplantation and pulmonary hypertension. Transplant. Sci., 2:15, 1992.
36. Goldman, L., et al.: Multifactorial index of cardiac risk in noncardiac surgical procedures. N. Engl. J. Med., 297:845, 1977.
37. Eagle, K. A., et al.: Dipyridamole-thallium scanning in patients undergoing vascular surgery. JAMA, 257:2185, 1987.
38. Gianguiliani, G., et al.: APACHE II in surgical lung carcinoma patients. Chest, 98:627, 1990.
39. Abrams, J., Doyle, A., and Aisner, J.: Staging, prognostic factors, and special considerations in small cell lung cancer. Semin. Oncol., 15:261, 1988.
40. Little, A. G., and Stitik, F. P.: Clinical staging of patients with non-small cell lung cancer. Chest, 97:1431, 1990.
41. Yoshimura, K.: A clinical statistical study of lung cancer patients in Japan with special reference to the staging system of TNM classification: a report from the Japan Joint Committee of Lung Cancer Associated with the TNM System of Clinical Classification (UICC). Radiat. Med., 1:186, 1983.
42. Yoshimura, K.: A clinical statistical analysis of 4,931 lung cancer cases in Japan according to histological type—field study results—a report from the Japanese Joint Committee of Lung Cancer Associated with the TNM System of Clinical Classification (UICC). Radiat. Med., 2:237, 1984.
43. Mountain, C. F.: A new international staging system for lung cancer. Chest, 89:2255, 1986.

44. American Joint Committee on Cancer: Manual for Staging of Cancer. Philadelphia, J. B. Lippincott, 1988, p. 63.
45. Little, A. G., and Stitik, F. P.: Clinical staging of patients with non-small cell lung cancer. Chest, 97:1431, 1990.
46. Masaoka, A., Monden, Y., Nakahara, K., and Tanioka, T.: Follow-up study of thymomas with special reference to their clinical stages. Cancer, 48:2485, 1981.
47. Butchart, E. G., et al.: Pleuropneumonectomy in the management of diffuse malignant mesothelioma of the pleura. Thorax, 31:15, 1976.
48. West, J. B.: Respiratory Physiology—The Essentials. Baltimore, Williams & Wilkins, 1974, p. 44.
49. O'Quinn, R., and Marini, J. J.: Pulmonary artery occlusion pressure: clinical physiology, measurement, and interpretation. Am. Rev. Respir. Dis., 128:319, 1983.
50. Prakash, U. B. S., Abel, M. D., and Hubmayr, R. D.: Mediastinal mass and tracheal obstruction during general anesthesia. Mayo Clin. Proc., 63:1004, 1988.
51. Neuman, G. G., et al.: The anesthetic management of the patient with an anterior mediastinal mass. Anesthesiology, 60:144, 1984.
52. Temeck, B. K., Schafer, P. W., Pary, W. Y., and Harmon, J. W.: Epidural anesthesia in patients undergoing thoracic surgery. Arch. Surg., 124:415, 1989.
53. Yeager, M. P., Glass, D. D., and Neff, R. K.: Epidural anesthesia and analgesia in high-risk surgical patients. Anesthesiology, 66:729, 1987.
54. Wasnick, J., Hurford, W., Gelb, C., and Chernow, B.: Epidural opiate analgesia does not alter the neuro-endocrine response to thoracotomy. Anesth. Analg., 70:S1, 1990.
55. McCarthy, G., Coppel, D. L., Gibbons, R., and Cosgrove, J.: High frequency jet ventilation for bilateral bullectomy. Anaesthesia, 42:411, 1987.
56. Bergman, N. A.: Hypoxic pulmonary vasoconstriction. Semin. Anesth., 6:188, 1987.
57. Jenkins, J., Cameron, E. W. J., Milne, A. C., and Hunter, R. M.: One lung anaesthesia. Anaesthesia, 42:938, 1987.
58. Smiley, R. M., Navedo, A. T., Kirby, T., and Schuloman, L. L.: Postoperative independent lung ventilation in a single-lung transplant recipient. Anesthesiology, 74:1144, 1991.
59. Popple, C., et al.: Unilateral auto-PEEP in the recipient of a single lung transplant. Chest, 103:297, 1993.
60. Abramowicz, M.: Antimicrobial prophylaxis in surgery. Med. Lett., 31:806, 1989.
61. Skinner, D.: Recent advances in the management of thoracic surgical infections. Ann. Thorac. Surg., 31:191, 1981.
62. Ilves, R., Cooper, J. D., Todd, T. R. T., and Pearson, F.: Prospective, randomized double blind study using prophylactic cephalothin for major elective general thoracic operations. J. Thorac. Cardiovasc. Surg., 81:813, 1981.
63. DeHaven, C. B., Hurst, J. M., and Branson, R. D.: Evaluation of two different extubation criteria: attributes contributing to success. Crit. Care Med., 14:92, 1986.
64. Mangano, D. T., Brownder, W. S., and Hollenberg, M.: Association in perioperative myocardial ischemia with cardiac morbidity and mortality in men undergoing noncardiac surgery. N. Engl. J. Med., 323:1781, 1990.
65. Pavlin, E. G., Holle, R. G., and Schoene, R. B.: Recovery of airway protection compared with ventilation in humans after paralysis with curare. Anesthesiology, 70:381, 1989.
66. Kawasaki, K., Ogawa, Y., Kido, Y, and Mori, T.: An important role of silent aspiration of gastric contents as a cause of pulmonary complications following surgery for esophageal cancer. Jpn. J. Surg., 17:455, 1987.
67. Plummer, A. L., and Gracey, D. R.: Consensus conference on artificial airways in patients receiving mechanical ventilation. Chest, 96:178, 1989.
68. Hazard, P. B., et al.: Bedside percutaneous tracheostomy: experience with 55 elective procedures. Ann. Thorac. Surg., 46:63, 1988.
69. Schachner, A., et al.: Rapid percutaneous tracheostomy. Chest, 98:1266, 1990.
70. Matthews, H. P., Fischer, B. J., Smith, B. E., and Hoopkinson, R. B.: Minitracheostomy: a new delivery system for jet ventilation. J. Thorac. Cardiovasc. Surg., 92:673, 1986.
71. Stauffer, J. L., Olson, D. E., and Petty, T. L.: Complications and consequences of endotracheal intubation and tracheostomy: a prospective study of 150 critically ill adult patients. Am. J. Med., 70:65, 1981.
72. Heffner, J. E., Miller, K. S., Sahn, S. A.: Tracheostomy in the intensive care unit: II. complications. Chest, 90:430, 1987.
73. Hazard, P., Jones, C., and Benitone, J.: Comparative clinical trial of standard operative tracheostomy with percutaneous tracheostomy. Crit. Care Med., 19:1018, 1991.
74. Charnley, R. M., and Verma, R.: Inhalation of a minitracheotomy tube. Int. Care Med., 12:108, 1986.
75. Stizmann, J. V.: Nutritional support of the dysphagic patient: methods, risks, and complications of therapy. Jpn. J. Parenter. Enteral Nutr., 14:60, 1990.
76. Lee, P. C., Helsmoortel, C. M., Cohn, S. M., and Fink, M. P.: Are low tidal volumes safe? Chest, 97:430, 1990.
77. Pepe, P. E., and Marini, J. J.: Occult positive end-expiratory pressure in mechanically ventilated patients with airflow obstruction. Am. Rev. Respir. Dis., 126:166, 1982.
78. Register, S. D., Downs, J. B., Stock, M. C., and Kirby, R. T.: Is 50% oxygen harmful? Crit. Care Med., 15:598, 1977.
79. Jubran, A., and Tobin, M. J.: Reliability of pulse oximetry in titrating supplemental oxygen therapy in ventilator-dependent patients. Chest, 97:1420, 1990.
80. Dess, D., et al.: An evaluation of the usefulness of end-tidal Pco_2 to aid weaning from mechanical ventilation following cardiac surgery. Respir. Care, 36:837, 1991.
81. Nevin, M., Van Besouw, J. P., Williams, C. W., and Pepper, J. R.: A comparative study of conventional versus high-frequency jet ventilation with relation to the incidence of postoperative morbidity in thoracic surgery. Ann. Thorac. Surg., 44:625, 1987.
82. Holzapfel, L., et al.: Comparison of high-frequency jet ventilation to conventional ventilation in adults with respiratory distress syndrome. Intern. Care Med., 13:100, 1987.
83. Klain, M., and Keszler, H.: High-frequency jet ventilation. Surg. Clin. North Am., 65:917, 1985.
84. Baumann, M. H., and Sahn, S. A.: Medical management and therapy of bronchopleural fistulas in the mechanically ventilated patient. Chest, 97:721, 1990.
85. Stadiford, T. J., and Morganroth, M. L.: High frequency ventilation. Chest, 96:1380, 1989.
86. Carlon, G. C., et al.: Criteria for selective positive end-expiratory pressure and independent synchronized ventilation of each lung. Chest, 74:501, 1978.
87. Banner, M. J., and Gallagher, T. J.: Respiratory failure in the adult: ventilatory support. In Mechanical Ventilation. Edited by R. R. Kirby, R. A. Smith, and D. A. Desautels. New York, Churchill Livingstone, 1985, p. 209.
88. Ovassapian, A., and Dykes, M. H. M.: The role of fiberoptic endoscopy in airway management. Semin. Anesth., 6:93, 1987.
89. Tsao, T. C. Y., et al.: Treatment for collapsed lung in critically ill patients. Chest, 97:435, 1990.
90. Marini, J. J., Pierson, D. J., and Hudson, L. D.: Acute lobar atelectasis: a prospective comparison of fiberoptic bronchoscopy and respiratory therapy. Am. Rev. Respir. Dis., 119:971, 1979.
91. Nelson, L. D., and Anderson, H. B.: Physiologic effects of

steep positioning in the surgical intensive care unit. Arch. Surg., *124*:352, 1989.
92. White, P. F.: Patient-controlled analgesia: a new approach to the management of postoperative pain. Semin. Anesth., *3*:255, 1985.
93. Yee, J. P., Koshiver, J. E., Allbon, C., and Brown, C. R.: Comparison of intramuscular ketorolac tromethamine and morphine sulfate for analgesia of pain after major surgery. Pharmacotherapy, *6*:253, 1986.
94. Loper, K. A., et al.: Epidural and intravenous fentanyl infusions are clinical equivalent after knee surgery. Anesth. Analg., *70*:72, 1990.
95. Shulman, M., et al.: Postthoracotomy pain and pulmonary function following epidural and systemic morphine. Anesthesiology, *61*:569, 1984.
96. Busch, E. H., and Stedman, P. M.: Epidural morphine for postoperative pain on medical-surgical wards—a clinical review. Anesthesiology, *67*:101, 1987.
97. Gray, J. R., et al.: Intrathecal morphine for post-thoracotomy pain. Anesth. Analg., *65*:873, 1986.
98. Nordberg, G., Hedner, T., Mellstrand, T., and Dahlstrom, B.: Pharmacokinetic aspects of intrathecal morphine analgesia. Anesthesiology, *60*:448, 1984.
99. Camporesi, E. L.: Intrapleural analgesia: a new technique. J. Cardiothorac. Anesth., *3*:137, 1989.
100. Reiestad, F., and Stromskag, K. E.: Interpleural catheter in the management of postoperative pain—a preliminary report. Reg. Anesth., *11*:89, 1986.
101. Symreng, T., et al.: Intrapleural bupivacaine—technical considerations and intraoperative use. J. Cardiothorac. Anesth., *3*:139, 1989.
102. Covino, B. G.: Interpleural regional analgesia. Anesth. Analg., *67*:427, 1988.
103. Keenan, D. J. M., Cave, K., Langdon, L., and Lea, R. E.: Comparative trial of rectal indomethacin and cryoanalgesia for control of early postthoracotomy pain. Br. Med. J., *287*:1335, 1983.
104. Skrinskas, G. J., Hyland, R. H., and Hutcheon, M. A.: Using helium-oxygen mixtures in the management of acute upper airway obstruction. Can. Med. Assoc. J., *128*:555, 1983.
105. Castella, X., Gilabert, J., and Perez, C.: Arytenoid dislocation after tracheal intubation: an unusual cause of acute respiratory failure? Anesthesiology, *74*:613, 1991.
106. Mulin, M. J., et al.: Pulmonary lobar gangrene complicating lobectomy. Ann. Surg., *175*:62, 1972.
107. Hymphreys, R. L., and Berne, A. S.: Rapid re-expansion of pneumothorax: a cause of unilateral pulmonary edema. Radiology, *96*:509, 1970.
108. Deschamps, C., Pairolero, P. C., Allen, M. S., and Trastek, V. F.: Postpneumonectomy pulmonary edema. Chest Surg. Clin. North Am., *2*:785, 1992.
109. Basran, G. S., et al.: Beta-2-adrenoceptor agonists as inhibitors of lung vascular permeability to radiolabelled transferrin in adult respiratory distress syndrome in man. Eur. J. Nucl. Med., *12*:381, 1986.
110. Kirsh, M. M., et al.: Complications of pulmonary resection. Ann. Thorac. Surg., *20*:62, 1975.
111. Potts, D. E., Levin, D. C., and Sahn, S. A.: Pleural fluid pH in parapneumonic effusions. Chest, *70*:3, 1976.
112. Rice, T. W., Kirsh, J. C., Schacter, I. B., and Goldberg, M.: simultaneous occurrence of chylothorax and subarachnoid pleural fistula after thoracotomy. Can. J. Surg., *30*:256, 1987.
113. Milsom, J. W., et al.: Chylothorax: an assessment of current surgical management. J. Thorac. Cardiovasc. Surg., *89*:221, 1985.
114. Twomey, J. J., et al.: Myasthenia gravis, thymectomy and serum thymic hormone activity. Am. J. Med., *66*:639, 1979.
115. Eisenkraft, J. B., et al.: Predicting the need for postoperative mechanical ventilation in myasthenia gravis. Anesthesiology, *65*:79, 1986.
116. Leventhal, R., Orkin, F. K., and Hirsch, R. A.: Prediction of the need for postoperative ventilation in myasthenia gravis. Anesthesiology, *53*:26, 1980.
117. D'Empaire, G., Hoaglin, D. C., Perlo, V. P., and Pontoppidan, H.: Effect of prethymectomy plasma exchange on postoperative respiratory function in myasthenia gravis. J. Thorac. Cardiovasc. Surg., *89*:592, 1985.
118. Krowka, M. J., et al.: Cardiac dysrhythmia following pneumonectomy: clinical correlates and prognostic significance. Chest, *91*:490, 1987.
119. Shields, T. W., and Ujiki, G. T.: Digitalization for prevention of arrhythmias following pulmonary surgery. Surg. Gynecol. Obstet., *126*:743, 1968.
120. Kastor, J. A.: Multifocal atrial tachycardia. N. Engl. J. Med., *322*:1713, 1990.
121. Agha, E. P., Orringer, M. B., and Amendola, M. A.: Gastric interposition following transhiatal esophagectomy: radiographic evaluation. Gastrointest. Radiol., *10*:17, 1985.
122. Graeber, G. M., et al.: Serum creatine kinase and lactate dehydrogenase isoenzyme levels in patients after major esophageal surgery, esophageal dilation, and acute myocardial infarction. Ann. Thorac. Surg., *43*:279, 1987.
123. Auteri, J. S., et al.: Normal bronchial healing without bronchial wrapping in canine lung transplantation. Ann. Thorac. Surg., *53*:80, 1992.
124. Smiley, R. M., Navedo, A. T., Kirby, T. J., and Schulman, L.: Postoperative independent lung ventilation in a single lung transplant recipient. Anesthesiology, *74*:1144, 1991.
125. Kirby, T. J.: Diagnosis and management of acute and chronic lung rejection. Semin. Cardiovasc. Surg., *4*:126, 1992.

Chapter 21

PNEUMONIA IN THE NONCOMPROMISED HOST

DAVID L. LONGWORTH

Community-acquired pneumonia and nosocomial pneumonia remain major clinical problems and cause significant morbidity and mortality. About 3 million cases of pneumonia occur annually in the United States, of which approximately 300,000 cases are nosocomial in origin.[1,2] Pneumonia was the leading cause of infection-related mortality in the United States in 1986 through 1988 and the sixth most common cause of death overall.[3] Pneumonia accounts for 500,000 hospital admissions per year with an estimated annual cost of 1.5 billion dollars.[4]

Fortunately, most cases of community-acquired pneumonia can be successfully managed in the outpatient setting with excellent clinical outcome. In more seriously ill patients requiring hospitalization, the mortality of community-acquired pneumonia has been 5 to 15% and up to 30% in the elderly.[5-11] The disease may be fatal in up to 50% of individuals requiring admission to the ICU for community-acquired pneumonia.[12]

In contrast to community-acquired pneumonia, nosocomial pneumonia, by definition, is acquired within the hospital and is therefore not present or incubating at the time of hospitalization. Many cases arise in patients who are already hospitalized in an ICU or recovery room setting. The mortality of nosocomial pneumonia has approached 55% and has been as high as 70% with selected pathogens, such as Pseudomonas aeruginosa.[13-15]

To reduce the significant morbidity and mortality associated with nosocomial pneumonia and selected cases of community-acquired pneumonia, prompt diagnosis and appropriate therapy are essential. Moreover, the early recognition and appropriate triage to the ICU of patients with more severe disease is crucial. This chapter reviews the clinical manifestations, epidemiology, microbiology, diagnosis, and therapy of community-acquired and nosocomial pneumonia. Emphasis is placed on the timely identification of patients who may benefit from ICU support. The discussion is confined to immunocompetent patients. A discussion of pneumonia in the immunocompromised host follows in Chapter 22.

PRE-ICU PHASE

There is an obligatory pre-ICU phase for patients with community-acquired pneumonia, even if it is brief and confined to the emergency room or admitting physician's office. Patients present with an illness, the diagnosis of pneumonia is suspected, and a decision is made to admit the patient to the hospital. In selected individuals, the gravity of illness necessitates transfer to the ICU, either at presentation or later in the hospital course. The approach to the patient with community-acquired pneumonia in the pre-ICU phase necessitates careful consideration of the microbiology, epidemiology, and clinical manifestations of pneumonia together with an assessment of the severity of the illness. In most patients, diagnostic evaluation and initial therapy are initiated before transfer to the ICU. By contrast, patients with nosocomial pneumonia represent a mixed population of hospitalized patients. Many are already in the ICU for other medical or surgical problems and require ongoing ICU support. For those individuals not in the ICU, a decision must also be made regarding whether the gravity of illness necessitates ICU admission. For both populations, however, a knowledge of the microbiology, epidemiology, clinical manifestations, and optimal therapy of nosocomial pneumonia are essential. For purposes of clarity of discussion, the microbiology, epidemiology, and clinical manifestations of nosocomial pneumonia are discussed under the pre-ICU phase, along with those of community-acquired pneumonia.

Microbiology and Epidemiology

Successful treatment of patients with pneumonia requires the selection and prompt administration of appropriate antimicrobial chemotherapy. Unfortunately, empiric therapy must often be started in the absence of a definitive microbiologic diagnosis. Knowledge of the most common causes of community-acquired pneumonia and nosocomial pneumonia is therefore essential in selecting an antibiotic regimen.

Data from 15 series describing the microbial etiology of community-acquired pneumonia in the past decade are summarized in Table 21-1.[1,6-11,16-23] These data must be interpreted with caution because some studies did not rigorously look for viral infections, Mycoplasma pneumoniae, Chlamydia pneumoniae (TWAR), or legionellosis. Aspiration pneumonia was also not included in the tabulation of several series. Nevertheless, it is evident that Streptococcus pneumoniae remains the most common etiologic agent in most studies over the past decade. Also of note is the significant percentage of cases in most studies in which no microbiologic diagnosis was established.

The prevalence of legionellosis varies from one geographic area to another, which likely accounts for the variability in incidence of legionnaires' disease in the respective studies. Legionnaires' disease usually occurs in late summer or early autumn. Sporadic cases occur with higher frequency in alcoholics; in males; and in patients with un-

Table 21-1. Etiology of Community-Acquired Pneumonia,* 1980–1990

Series	No. of Patients	Percent Pneumococcus	Percent Legionella	Percent Mycoplasma	Percent Viral	Percent S. aureus	Percent H. influenzae	Percent Gram-negative Bacilli	Percent Aspiration	Percent Other	Percent No Diagnosis
Elbright, 1980[23]	106	36	—	—	—	3	1	10	—	3	47
White, 1981[22]	210	12	2	14	15	4	2	2	—	4	52
MacFarlane, 1982[21]	127	76	15	2	9	2	3	1	—	6	2
Klimek, 1983[1]	204	36	14	—	—	8	15	22	4		
McNabb, 1984[20]	80	50	1	—	6	4	6	1	—	3	36
Marrie, 1985[11]	138	9	1	17	3	9	3	15	18	17	44
Berntsson, 1985[19]	127	54	1	14	18	1	5	—	—	4	21
Holmberg, 1987[9]	147	47	3	5	11	1	10	—	—	5	30
Marrie, 1987[17]	301	9	4	3	16	5	6	2	11	20	37
British Thoracic Society, 1987[8]	453	34	2	18	7	1	6	1	—	7	33
Aubertin, 1987[18]	274	25	21	17	5	4	7	6	1	6	49
Levy, 1988[10]	116	26	4	4	4	3	12	7	3	14	35
Ausina, 1988[7]	207	39	6	17	4	1	1	3	—	9	20
Lim, 1989[6]	106	42	3	8	18	3	9	8	—	8	23
Fang, 1990[16]	349	15	7	2	—	3	11	6		9	

* In some instances, percentages total >100% owing to mixed infections in some patients.

derlying malignancy, diabetes mellitus, renal failure, and chronic obstructive pulmonary disease.[24] Additional predisposing factors include occupational exposure as a construction worker or residence near excavation sites.[25]

Haemophilus influenzae is a common cause of community-acquired pneumonia in patients with chronic obstructive pulmonary disease and accounts for 1 to 15% of cases in different series.[26] M. pneumoniae has produced up to 18% of cases of community-acquired pneumonia over the past decade. Epidemics occur every 4 to 8 years, more commonly in summer and fall.[27] Mycoplasma disease should be suspected in young adults and adolescents with pneumonia, especially in institutional settings such as dormitories or military barracks. Staphylococcus aureus is an infrequent cause of community-acquired pneumonia, accounting for 1 to 8% of cases over the past decade. It should be considered in intravenous drug users with tricuspid valve bacterial endocarditis or in patients with recent influenza.

Aspiration pneumonia may be encountered in elderly or debilitated patients and is often polymicrobial with mouth aerobes and anaerobes. Enteric gram-negative bacilli are unusual causes of community-acquired pneumonia in healthy immunocompetent individuals. Residents of nursing homes or chronic care facilities who become colonized with enteric gram-negative rods in their oropharynx, however, may develop necrotizing gram-negative pneumonia following aspiration.[28]

Branhamella catarrhalis and C. pneumoniae (TWAR) are more recently recognized pathogens that may produce community-acquired pneumonia.[17,29,30] In one study from Nova Scotia, C. pneumoniae (TWAR) accounted for 6% of cases of community-acquired pneumonia, and epidemics have been reported in military conscripts in Scandinavia.[17,31] Additional unusual causes of community-acquired pneumonia include Coxiella burnetti (Q fever), Chlamydia psittaci (psittacosis), Histoplasma capsulatum, Blastomyces dermatitidis, and Mycobacterium tuberculosis. In one study from France, M. tuberculosis accounted for 10% of cases of community-acquired pneumonia.[10]

Viral pneumonia has accounted for up to 18% of cases of community-acquired pneumonia in series reported over the past 10 years. Common pathogens in adults include influenza A, influenza B, and adenovirus. In children, respiratory syncytial virus and parainfluenza viruses are common etiologic agents. Although viral pneumonia is often considered a benign disease, one study that examined patients with community-acquired pneumonia requiring admission to the ICU found that viral pathogens accounted for 18% of cases in which an etiologic diagnosis was established.[32]

The microbiology of nosocomial pneumonia is different from that of community-acquired pneumonia. Gram-negative bacilli account for the majority of these infections. Although precise prevalence figures may vary from one institution to another, data from the National Nosocomial Infections Study are consistent with the experience in many hospitals.[33] In that study, the responsible pathogens, in descending order of prevalence, included:

- Pseudomonas aeruginosa (15.9%)
- Staphylococcus aureus (12.9%)
- Klebsiella species (11.6%)
- Enterobacter species (9.4%)
- Serratia species (5.8%)
- Proteus species (4.2%)

The striking difference in the microbiology of nosocomial pneumonia compared with community-acquired pneumonia is partly attributable to differences in pathogenesis. Community-acquired pneumonia most often arises from inhalation of aerosolized infectious agents or, less commonly, aspiration. Clinically significant infection may develop when the inoculum is sizable, the offending agent is virulent, or intrinsic defects in pulmonary host defense are present. The pathogenesis of nosocomial pneumonia is more complex. Aspiration and microorganisms colonizing the oropharynx is the most common mechanism, but bacteremic spread of remote infection to the lung can occasionally produce nosocomial pneumonia.

The propensity for gram-negative bacilli to produce nosocomial pneumonia is likely attributable to the fact that these organisms rapidly and commonly colonize the oropharynx and upper airway mucosa in hospitalized patients, especially those who were intubated, critically ill, azotemic, or have received recent antibiotic therapy.[28,34,35] Acid neutralization in the stomach with antacids or H_2 blockers also permits colonization of the upper gastrointestinal tract with gram-negative bacilli.[36,37] Retrograde spread of these organisms to the oropharynx and upper airway may predispose to the development of nosocomial pneumonia as well. The ability of gram-negative bacilli to colonize oropharyngeal and gastrointestinal mucosa in such individuals is attributable to a combination of factors, including the presence of foreign bodies, such as nasogastric or endotracheal tubes; defects in local host defense; and organism-specific virulence factors. The glycoprotein fibronectin, which is normally present on the surface of oropharyngeal epithelial cells, is an important component of mucosal host immunity. Fibronectin inhibits the binding of gram-negative bacilli to these cells and preferentially mediates the attachment of certain gram-positive organisms, such as streptococci and staphylococci.[38] In hospitalized and critically ill patients, mucosal fibronectin may be digested by increased levels of salivary proteases, thereby predisposing to colonization of the oropharyngeal epithelium with gram-negative bacilli.[39,40] Bacterial virulence factors, such as pili on the surface of certain gram-negative bacilli, may also be important in mediating the adherence of certain organisms to the oropharyngeal epithelium.[38,41]

B. catarrhalis and H. influenzae are less common causes of nosocomial pneumonia, although they are occasionally encountered in patients with chronic obstructive lung disease. Nosocomial legionellosis varies considerably in incidence from one institution to another. Although uncommon in many hospitals, nosocomial legionnaires' disease has accounted for up to 29% of nosocomial pneumonias in some centers.[42] Respiratory syncytial virus may be a common nosocomial pathogen in the pediatric ICU. Outbreaks with this organism usually occur in the winter or early spring, paralleling the seasonal occurrence of this infection in the community. Influenza A is an unusual cause of nosocomial pneumonia in adults and also occurs in the winter.

It is apparent that the microbiology of nosocomial pneumonia may differ from one institution to another. Legionellosis is a problem in some places and is rare in others. Although gram-negative bacilli are the most common culprits, variability from one institution to another with regard to specific microorganisms and their antibiotic susceptibilities must be anticipated. A knowledge of the most common institutional causes of nosocomial pneumonia, together with the antibiotic susceptibility profile of these organisms, is therefore essential for the practicing intensivist. Ongoing infection control surveillance for outbreaks of pneumonia due to specific pathogens is necessary for the timely diagnosis and appropriate therapy of patients with hospital-acquired lower respiratory tract infection.

Clinical Manifestations

The clinical features of patients with community-acquired pneumonia may provide a clue to the microbiologic diagnosis, which may permit a more rational selection of empiric antibiotic therapy. Community-acquired pneumonia has traditionally been divided into the syndromes of atypical pneumonia and typical bacterial pneumonia, although the differential diagnostic value of this classification scheme has been questioned.[16] The major features of these two clinical syndromes are summarized in Table 21-2.

Patients with atypical pneumonia tend to be children, adolescents, or young adults, although this syndrome can occur in older individuals. Patients usually present with the subacute onset of fever, a dry cough, prominent headache, and constitutional symptoms. Cough is frequently a minor complaint at the onset but predominates with time. Leukocytosis is uncommon, and chest radiographs often disclose patchy infiltrates, frequently involving the lower lobes. The most common pathogens responsible for producing the atypical pneumonia syndrome include:

- M. pneumoniae
- Legionella species
- Various viruses

Of these, legionnaires' disease is most likely to produce an illness of sufficient severity to warrant admission to an ICU. Less common causes of the atypical pneumonia syndrome include:

- Chlamydia pneumoniae (TWAR)
- Chlamydia psittaci
- Coxiella burnetii
- Mycobacterium tuberculosis
- Fungi such as Coccidioides immitis and Histoplasma capsulatum

Patients with "typical bacterial pneumonia" usually present with the sudden onset of fever and shaking chills, pleuritic chest pain, and a prominent productive cough.

Table 21-2. Distinguishing Features of "Typical" Bacterial Pneumonia and "Atypical" Pneumonia

	Atypical Pneumonia	Typical Pneumonia
Usual Host	Child, adolescent or young adult	Middle-aged or elderly
Onset	Gradual over several days	Sudden
Respiratory Complaints	Cough less prominent, dry at onset, may be productive over time Pleurisy uncommon	Productive cough often prominent Pleurisy common
Constitutional Symptoms	May overshadow respiratory complaints initially	Less prominent
Leukocytosis	WBC <10,000 in 80%	Common
Radiographic Features	Patchy infiltrates frequently involving lower lobes	Lobar consolidation or bronchopneumonia
Common Pathogens	Mycoplasma pneumoniae, Legionella species, Chlamydia pneumoniae, Viruses	Streptococcus pneumoniae, Haemophilus influenzae

This syndrome is more commonly encountered in middle-aged or elderly adults. Leukocytosis is common, and the chest radiograph usually discloses lobar consolidation or bronchopneumonia. S. pneumoniae is the most common culprit, but H. influenzae, legionella species, S. aureus, and gram-negative bacilli may also produce this syndrome, as can aspiration pneumonia.

A careful history should be taken in every patient presenting with community-acquired pneumonia with regard to circumstances of onset, residence, recent travel, occupation, animal contact, or exposure to similarly ill patients. Such information may suggest the presence of unusual pathogens. For example, an exposure to ill parrots, cockatiels, turkeys, or canaries might suggest the diagnosis of psittacosis. Similarly, a history of occupational or casual contact with cattle, sheep, or goats might suggest the diagnosis of Q fever. An outbreak of Q fever occurred following exposure to a parturient cat.[43] Recent travel to the southwestern United States would necessitate consideration of coccidioidomycosis.

The season and circumstances of onset are also important. Pneumonia presenting in the peak of influenza season in the winter should alert one to the possibility of primary influenza pneumonia or secondary bacterial pneumonia with S. aureus or pneumococcus. Community-acquired pneumonia in a young person in an institutional setting, such as school dormitory or military barracks, should suggest C. pneumoniae (TWAR) or M. pneumoniae. Patients residing in or traveling to the Mississippi or Ohio River valleys may present with primary pneumonia caused by H. capsulatum. Residents of nursing homes or other chronic care facilities who have impaired gag reflexes are predisposed to aspiration pneumonia with aerobic and anaerobic mouth flora, enteric gram-negative bacilli, S. aureus, S. pneumoniae, and H. influenzae.

Risk factors for infection with the human immunodeficiency virus (HIV) should be sought in every patient presenting with community-acquired pneumonia, especially in young and middle-aged individuals. A history of male homosexuality, hemophilia, sexual promiscuity, or intravenous drug abuse should prompt more serious consideration of HIV-related infections. The incidence of pneumococcal pneumonia and H. influenzae pneumonia appears to be increased with intravenous drug users with HIV infection.[44] Pneumocystis carinii pneumonia (PCP), pulmonary tuberculosis, and cryptococcal pneumonia must also be considered in patients with potential HIV infection. The clinical presentation of PCP in patients with AIDS is highly variable. Patients usually present with a subacute, indolent illness with nonproductive cough and mild dyspnea on exertion.[45] Occasionally, however, in patients with previously undiagnosed HIV infection, PCP may present as an acute, fulminant illness characterized by high fever, dry cough, dyspnea, and significant hypoxemia. The chest radiograph usually discloses patchy or diffuse interstitial infiltrates but may be normal in mild cases of PCP. Unusual radiographic findings of pulmonary pneumocystosis include pneumatoceles, nodules, cavities, pneumothoraces, and pleural effusions.[46] These are being recognized with increasing frequency, especially in HIV-infected patients receiving aerosolized pentamidine prophylaxis.

Certain findings on physical examination may provide useful clues to the diagnosis in patients with community-acquired pneumonia. In the absence of underlying heart disease or therapy with beta-blockers, the presence of relative bradycardia should suggest M. pneumoniae, legionellosis, or pneumonia with C. psittaci or C. pneumoniae (TWAR). Splenectomized or asplenic patients are predisposed to overwhelming infections with encapsulated organisms such as S. pneumoniae or H. influenzae.[47] Bullous myringitis has been associated with M. pneumoniae, although this has been disputed.[48,49] Stigmata of intravenous drug abuse in a patient with pneumonia should suggest the presence of right-sided bacterial endocarditis and septic pulmonary emboli owing to S. aureus or gram-negative bacilli such as P. aeruginosa. PCP in association with underlying HIV infection should also be considered in such individuals. The presence of new-onset splenomegaly in a patient with pneumonia should suggest the diagnoses of psittacosis or Q fever. In patients with risk factors for HIV infection, the presence of oral thrush or hairy leukoplakia, Kaposi's sarcoma, or diffuse lymphadenopathy should suggest underlying infection with HIV.

The clinical manifestations of pneumonia in the elderly deserve special comment because they may be much more subtle than in younger individuals.[50,51] Fever, malaise, or confusion may be the only clinical clues. Cough may sometimes be absent. In patients with bacteremic pneumococcal pneumonia, rigors and pleuritic chest pain were less common in the elderly in one study.[50] The diagnosis of pneumonia should be considered in elderly patients with unexplained fever or altered mental status.

The recognition of nosocomial pneumonia is often much more difficult than community-acquired pneumonia. In some patients, the classic findings of fever, productive cough, purulent sputum, and leukocytosis may be present. Elderly patients who aspirate while residing on the nursing floor may simply develop dyspnea, confusion, or fever. The diagnosis may be equally difficult in patients hospitalized in the ICU who may develop fever and leukocytosis for other reasons. In such individuals, important clinical clues in the diagnoses of nosocomial pneumonia include a rising fever, worsening hemodynamic instability, increasing leukocytosis, a new or progressive infiltrate on chest radiography, and an increasing amount and purulence of the sputum. In patients with underlying congestive heart failure or adult respiratory distress syndrome, the distinction between tracheobronchitis and nosocomial pneumonia may be especially difficult.

Diagnosis of Community-Acquired Pneumonia

A clinical diagnosis of pneumonia is supported by the finding of a pulmonary infiltrate on a chest radiograph. Although the configuration of the infiltrate seldom permits a precise causative diagnosis, several features may sometimes be helpful in predicting the likely pathogens.[10] Lobar consolidation, cavitation, and the presence of a large pleural effusion are all suggestive of a bacterial etiology. Pneumococcal pneumonia may present with lobar consolidation or bronchopneumonia. M. pneumoniae pneumonia commonly produces patchy infiltrates in the lower lobes.

Legionella pneumonia may appear similar radiographically to M. pneumoniae pneumonia at the onset but often is lobar and frequently progresses to involve several additional lobes. Small thin-walled areas of cavitation, termed pneumatoceles, are typical of staphylococcal pneumonia but may be seen with other gram-negative bacilli and rarely with H. influenzae. Extensive cavitation is characteristic of certain gram-negative pathogens, such as P. aeruginosa, but may also develop in patients with anaerobic pneumonia following aspiration. Diffuse interstitial pulmonary infiltrates should suggest a viral cause, mycoplasma, or PCP. Aspiration pneumonia usually involves the posterior segments of the upper lobes or the superior or basilar segments of the lower lobes, depending on whether the patient is recumbent or upright at the time of aspiration.

The initial diagnostic evaluation should begin with a Gram stain examination of an adequate sputum specimen. If necessary, a specimen should be induced by inhalation of nebulized hypertonic saline. An adequate specimen is defined as one that contains fewer than 10 epithelial cells and more than 25 white blood cells per low-powered microscopic field.[52] The presence of pulmonary alveolar macrophages suggests that the specimen has originated in the lower respiratory tract; however, such specimens may nevertheless be contaminated with oropharyngeal flora if more than 10 epithelial cells are present per low-powered field. One study demonstrated that the finding of many polymorphonuclear leukocytes and a predominant organism on sputum Gram stain has a high predictive value for selecting an appropriate antibiotic regimen in patients with bacteremic community-acquired pneumonia.[53] The sensitivity and specificity of identifying pneumococci on a sputum Gram stain, which appear as gram-positive diplococci, have been shown to be 62 and 85%.[54] A predominance of other organisms on sputum Gram stain may also be helpful in suggesting a specific diagnosis. Staphylococci appear as gram-positive cocci in grapelike clusters. The presence of gram-negative coccobacilli would suggest H. influenzae or B. catarrhalis as the responsible pathogen. A sputum specimen containing many polymorphonuclear leukocytes, few squamous epithelial cells, and a mixed population of gram-positive and gram-negative cocci and bacilli might suggest a mixed aerobic and anaerobic process, as sometimes occurs following aspiration.

Examination of expectorated sputum may sometimes be helpful in patients with suspected PCP and acquired immunodeficiency syndrome (AIDS). Sputum specimens stained with Giemsa, Gomori, methenamine silver, or methylene blue may disclose the organism in up to 80% of patients with AIDS and PCP.[55] Patients with suspected tuberculosis should have sputum examined for acid-fast bacilli.

Specimens of blood should be obtained for culture before the initiation of antibiotic therapy in patients with community-acquired pneumonia. If a significant pleural effusion is present, diagnostic thoracentesis should be performed because this may provide a microbiologic diagnosis and disclose the presence of empyema, which would necessitate tube thoracostomy. A sputum specimen should be obtained for routine bacterial culture, although the value of this has been disputed.[56] Special cultures for legionella and mycobacteria should be performed when clinically indicated.

Newer diagnostic techniques have been developed that may facilitate a more rapid microbiologic diagnosis in some patients with community-acquired pneumonia. Direct fluorescent antibody staining of sputum or a lower respiratory tract specimen for legionella species is about 25 to 70% sensitive and 95% specific in patients with suspected legionella pneumonia.[24,57] Fluorescein-labeled monoclonal antibodies and DNA probes have been used to detect P. carinii, legionella species, and several viruses in upper respiratory tract secretions. These are not yet widely available for P. carinii, but a DNA probe for legionella species has been marketed. A test to detect Legionella pneumophila serogroup 1 antigen in urine has also been developed and is 75 to 90% sensitive and extremely specific. Acute and convalescent serum specimens should be collected in patients in whom M. pneumoniae, legionella species, C. psittaci, and C. pneumoniae (TWAR) are suspected because diagnostic confirmation may require the demonstration of seroconversion.

Some patients may be unable to provide sputum specimens for Gram stain and appropriate cultures. Depending on the severity of the illness, further diagnostic evaluation may be necessary. An otherwise healthy young adult with community-acquired pneumonia and a mild illness may be empirically treated for M. pneumoniae pneumonia with erythromycin. If the patient has risk factors for infection with HIV or is critically ill, lower respiratory tract specimens should be obtained by fiberoptic bronchoscopy or transtracheal aspiration. Transtracheal aspiration should be performed only by those experienced with the procedure. Few data exist regarding the sensitivity of transtracheal aspiration in patients with AIDS and suspected PCP. Bronchoscopy is the procedure of choice in such patients if they are unable to produce sputum for initial examination. Studies have examined the diagnostic sensitivity and specificity of protected specimen brush and quantitative bronchoalveolar lavage (BAL) cultures in the diagnosis of pneumonia. These are discussed in the section dealing with the diagnosis of nosocomial pneumonia in the ICU phase. Open lung biopsy is rarely necessary in patients with community-acquired pneumonia and should be reserved for critically ill patients who are failing broad-spectrum therapy and in whom bronchoscopy has not provided a microbiologic diagnosis.

Assessing Need for Hospitalization and Transfer to the ICU

A crucial decision in the management of patients with community-acquired pneumonia in whether hospitalization is indicated. Most studies examining outcome in patients with community-acquired pneumonia have focused on predictors of mortality in hospitalized patients.[8,21,58,59] Factors portending an increased risk of death have included:

- Advanced age
- Significant underlying disease
- Respiratory rate > 30 at admission
- Diastolic blood pressure ≤ 60 mm Hg at admission

For pneumococcal pneumonia, numerous studies have defined certain factors that increase the risk of mortality, which include

- Advanced age
- Leukopenia at presentation
- Multiple lobe involvement
- Alcoholism
- Significant underlying disease, such as diabetes mellitus, malignancy, or chronic lung and heart disease[51,60-62]

In patients with suspected pneumococcal pneumonia in whom these factors are present, hospitalization should be considered.

For many patients, the microbiologic diagnosis is uncertain at the time admission is contemplated. In such individuals, indications for hospitalization have been defined using a modified version of Appropriateness, Evaluation, Protocol (AEP), which is a validated tool used by quality assurance and utilization review organizations.[4,63] These indications for hospitalization include:

- Vital sign abnormality defined as heart rate >140/min, respiratory rate >30/min, or systolic blood pressure <90 mm Hg
- Hypoxemia defined as Po_2 <60 mm Hg on a room air blood gas analysis
- A significant hematologic, electrolyte, or metabolic laboratory abnormality that is new
- Evidence of metastatic infection, including meningitis, endocarditis, empyema, or septic arthritis
- A concomitant acute medical illness requiring hospitalization, such as myocardial infarction

Patients with such abnormalities should be hospitalized. Unfortunately many patients do not possess any of these factors, and the decision regarding hospitalization may therefore not be clear-cut. A prospective, observational study examined outcome in such patients, which included mortality as well as a complicated course.[4] Five predisposing risk factors for a complicated course were identified in patients who did not have an AEP-defined indication for hospitalization. These risk factors for adverse outcome included:

- Age >65 years
- Temperature >38°C at presentation
- Premorbid illness (diabetes mellitus, renal insufficiency, congestive heart failure, or hospitalization within the prior year)
- Immunosuppression with systemic corticosteroids or cancer chemotherapy
- High risk bacterial cause (staphylococcal, gram-negative bacilli, postobstructive pneumonia, or aspiration pneumonia)[4]

In this study, patients with more than one of these risk factors would have benefited from hospitalization. Patients who are poorly compliant or in whom the home situation is suboptimal should also probably be hospitalized for initial therapy.

Table 21-3. Factors at Presentation in Patients with Community-Acquired Pneumonia Predicting the Ultimate Need for ICU Admission

Bronchopneumonia or lobar pneumonia involving >2 lobes
Respiratory rate >30/min
PaO_2 <8 kPa
Clinical signs or hemodynamic parameters suggesting sepsis
Confusion
Renal insufficiency
Abnormal liver function studies and/or low serum albumin

(Data from References 32 and 64.)

In a more seriously ill patient, ICU support may be necessary. The utility, however, of intensive care management in altering the outcome of certain types of community-acquired pneumonia, such as bacteremic pneumococcal pneumonia, has been questioned. One study demonstrated a mortality of 76% in patients with bacteremic pneumococcal pneumonia admitted to the ICU.[62] The mortality rate was 80% in those requiring mechanical ventilation and 93% in patients who required vasopressor support. These mortalities are comparable to those reported 19 years earlier by Austrian and Gold,[59] leading the authors to conclude that improvements in ICU management have not altered the mortality of bacteremic pneumococcal pneumonia.

Clearly, some patients may present with serious, far advanced illness that cannot be reversed by even the most aggressive antimicrobial chemotherapy and supportive care. Nevertheless, the challenge remains to identify patients early in their illness who have predictors of adverse outcome and who might benefit from aggressive intensive care management. Several retrospective studies have begun to analyze factors in patients with community-acquired pneumonia that influence the need for ICU admission.[32,64] Factors present at the time of presentation that predict the need for ultimate ICU admission are summarized in Table 21-3. Although these factors predicted the need for ICU support in these studies, it has not been demonstrated that early admission to the ICU has a favorable impact on outcome in such patients. Nevertheless, the presence of these clinical or laboratory abnormalities in patients who are hospitalized for community-acquired pneumonia should prompt consideration of early transfer to the ICU.

Many patients who develop nosocomial pneumonia are already hospitalized in the ICU. In such individuals, the issue of transfer to the ICU is moot. Selected patients, however, develop nosocomial pneumonia outside the ICU. In such individuals, a decision must be made regarding whether ICU support is required. A prospective study assessed risk factors associated with mortality in a cohort of 118 non-neutropenic patients who developed nosocomial pneumonia.[65] Factors associated with an increased risk of fatal outcome included:

- Age >60 years
- Bilateral infiltrates
- Development of respiratory failure
- Presence of an ultimately or rapidly fatal underlying illness

In addition, certain high risk nosocomial pathogens increased the risk of fatal outcome, including P. aeruginosa, Enterobacteriaceae, acinetobacter species, Streptococcus faecalis, S. aureus, candida species, and aspergillus species. Although it is not clear that ICU support alters outcome in patients with these risk factors, such care should probably be considered in critically ill patients with one or more of these factors who develop nosocomial pneumonia.

ICU PHASE

In patients with community-acquired pneumonia, the ICU phase of the illness focuses on the initial selection or continuation of empiric antibiotic therapy; the optimization of the antimicrobial regimen based on microbiologic data; necessary supportive ventilatory, hemodynamic, and nutritional care; and the prevention, rapid identification, and appropriate management of complications. The aforementioned issues are also important in patients with nosocomial pneumonia. In addition, because many patients develop nosocomial lower respiratory tract infection while hospitalized in the ICU for other reasons, the diagnosis of pneumonia is also frequently an issue during the ICU phase of these patients' illnesses.

Therapy of Community-Acquired Pneumonia

The selection of empiric antibiotic therapy in patients with community-acquired pneumonia is dictated by the severity of illness and the certainty of the microbiologic diagnosis. Treatment recommendations for the common causes of community-acquired pneumonia are summarized in Table 21-4. Patients with a compatible history, chest radiograph, and sputum Gram stain for pneumococcal pneumonia may be treated with penicillin G, 600,000 units intravenously every 12 hours. In patients with pneumococcal meningitis, empyema, septic arthritis, or endocarditis, high dose intravenous therapy with 20 million units of penicillin G per day in divided doses should be used. The penicillin-allergic patient with uncomplicated pneumonia may be treated with erythromycin. A third-generation cephalosporin or chloramphenicol should be used in penicillin-allergic patients with pneumococcal meningitis. Septic arthritis or endocarditis in such patients may be treated with vancomycin or a third-generation cephalosporin. In some regions of the world, penicillin-resistant pneumococci are prevalent.[66,67] This is fortunately rare in the United States at this time. Vancomycin is the drug of choice for patients with suspected penicillin-resistant pneumococcal infection.[66]

Erythromycin is the preferred treatment for patients with suspected M. pneumoniae pneumonia. Empiric therapy with erythromycin has the additional advantage of providing excellent coverage against S. pneumoniae and legionella species. Patients with suspected C. pneumoniae (TWAR) should receive doxycycline because erythromycin appears to be less effective.[29] C. pneumoniae (TWAR) pneumonia is usually a relatively mild disease and rarely necessitates admission to the ICU.

Empiric therapy in patients with suspected H. influenzae pneumonia should be dictated by the local prevalence of beta-lactamase-producing strains of H. influenzae. In areas where these strains are uncommon, ampicillin is an appropriate empiric choice. In some parts of the United States, more than 25% of strains of H. influenzae produce beta-lactamases. In such areas, a third-generation cephalosporin is an appropriate choice and preferable to second-generation drugs, such as cephamandole. Of the third-generation cephalosporins, ceftriaxone, ceftizoxime, and cefotaxime have comparable in vitro activity against H. influenzae but differ in pharmacokinetics and, at times, cost. Any of these drugs would be appropriate empiric choices in patients with suspected H. influenzae pneumonia in areas where beta-lactamase-producing strains are common.

Community-acquired staphylococcal pneumonia may be treated with a penicillinase-resistant penicillin, such as oxacillin or nafcillin, or a first-generation cephalosporin. Vancomycin is an acceptable alternative in the penicillin-allergic patient. Fortunately methicillin-resistant S. aureus is uncommon in the community but may be encountered in intravenous drug abusers or residents of nursing homes or long-term care facilities who develop S. aureus pneumonia. In such individuals, empiric therapy with vancomycin is appropriate pending the antibiotic susceptibilities of the isolate.

Erythromycin is the drug of choice for patients with suspected legionellosis at parenteral doses of 2 to 4 g per

Table 21-4. Treatment Recommendations for Community-Acquired Pneumonia Requiring Parenteral Therapy*

Pathogen	Recommended Regimen	Alternative Regimen
Mycoplasma pneumoniae	Erythromycin 500 mg IV q6h	Doxycycline 100 mg IV q12h
Legionella species	Erythromycin 1 g IV q6h	Doxycycline 100 mg IV q12h + rifampin 600 mg po qd
Chlamydia pneumoniae	Doxycycline 100 mg IV q12h	
Streptococcus pneumoniae	Penicillin G 600,000 U IV q12h	Erythromycin 500 mg IV q6h
Haemophilus influenzae	Third-generation cephalosporin (e.g., ceftizoxime, cefotaxime, ceftriaxone)	Trimethoprim-sulfamethoxazole 5 mg/kg IV q12h
Staphylococcus aureus	Oxacillin or nafcillin 2 g IV q4h (vancomycin if MRSA suspected)	Vancomycin 1 g IV q12h
Aspiration		
Community acquired	Clindamycin 600 mg IV q6h	Penicillin G 2 MU IV q4H
Nursing home acquired	Penicillin G 2 MU IV q4h or clindamycin 600 mg IV q6h + third-generation cephalosporin or aminoglycoside	Ticarcillin-clavulanate 3.1 g IV q6h

* For adults with normal liver and kidney function.
MRSA, Methicillin-resistant S. aureus.

day. Seriously ill patients with suspected legionnaires' disease should receive erythromycin, 1 g intravenously every 6 hours. Some individuals develop tinnitus or hearing loss on this dose of erythromycin, which is fortunately reversible with dosage reduction or discontinuation of the medication. Rifampin may be added to the regimen in critically ill patients, although no data clearly demonstrate improved outcome with two-drug therapy. Alternative agents for the treatment of legionnaires' disease include doxycycline or tetracycline. Studies comparing the efficacy of erythromycin versus doxycycline or tetracycline have unfortunately not been performed.

Patients with community-acquired aspiration pneumonia may be treated with parenteral penicillin or clindamycin. Residents of nursing homes or long-term care facilities and recently hospitalized patients may be colonized in their oropharynx with gram-negative bacilli. Aspiration pneumonia in such patients should be treated with an antibiotic regimen with activity against these organisms as well as mouth aerobes and anaerobes. An appropriate regimen would include penicillin or clindamycin plus a third-generation cephalosporin or aminoglycoside. A third-generation cephalosporin is probably preferable to an aminoglycoside, given the poor penetration of aminoglycosides into pulmonary parenchyma and respiratory secretions. These regimens cover S. pneumoniae, mouth anaerobes, and most enteric gram-negative bacilli. H. influenzae is also covered if a third-generation cephalosporin is used. Single-agent therapy with ticarcillin-clavulanic acid would be an acceptable alternative.

Patients with PCP in the setting of AIDS may be treated with either trimethoprim-sulfamethoxazole or pentamidine. Most studies have suggested that these drugs are equally effective, although a randomized prospective trial demonstrated improved survival in trimethoprim-sulfamethoxazole recipients compared with patients who receive pentamidine.[68] Parenteral therapy is indicated in patients with moderate or severe disease at a dose of 15 to 20 mg/kg/day in two divided doses. Oral therapy, which is appropriate in patients with mild PCP, should not be used for patients with disease of sufficient severity to warrant ICU admission. Pentamidine should be administered at a dose of 4 mg/kg/day by slow intravenous infusion. Both medications are unfortunately complicated by frequent side effects. Trimethoprim-sulfamethoxazole may produce adverse effects in up to 50% of AIDS patients, including fever, rash, leukopenia, or hepatitis.[69] Significant side effects associated with pentamidine include intractable hypoglycemia, renal failure, hyperglycemia, hypotension, fever, and leukopenia.[70] Corticosteroids have been demonstrated to improve outcome in patients with moderate or severe PCP and should be used in most patients requiring admission to the ICU.[71]

The selection of empiric antibiotic therapy is most difficult in seriously ill patients with community-acquired pneumonia in whom the microbial cause is uncertain. Such patients require broad-spectrum antibiotic therapy pending a microbiologic diagnosis. A regimen consisting of erythromycin and a third-generation cephalosporin provides excellent coverage against S. pneumoniae, legionella species, H. influenzae, and M. pneumoniae. The third-generation cephalosporins ceftriaxone, cefotaxime, and ceftizoxime provide good coverage against many enteric gram-negative bacilli except for P. aeruginosa. This organism rarely produces community-acquired pneumonia except in patients with underlying cystic fibrosis. In such individuals, an antipseudomonal penicillin or third-generation cephalosporin, such as ceftazidime, should be used together with an aminoglycoside. If staphylococcal pneumonia is a differential diagnostic concern, a semisynthetic penicillin or vancomycin should be added to the regimen, pending results of cultures. Newer antibiotics, such as imipenem-cilastatin and ciprofloxacin, seldom have a role in the treatment of community-acquired pneumonia. Imipenem-cilastatin is expensive and has an extremely broad spectrum of antimicrobial activity, which is usually unnecessary in such patients. Although some studies have shown ciprofloxacin to be efficacious in the treatment of community-acquired pneumonia, its in vitro activity against S. pneumoniae and anaerobic mouth flora is relatively poor.[72,73]

Although broad-spectrum antibiotic therapy is warranted in severely ill patients with community-acquired pneumonia, the antibiotic regimen should be modified based on culture results from specimens of lower respiratory tract secretions, blood, and pleural fluid. If a microbiologic diagnosis is established based on these cultures, the optimal regimen for the identified microorganism should be used. Ideally, the spectrum of the antimicrobial regimen should be narrowed so as to prevent the emergence of resistant strains and bacterial colonization and superinfection with nosocomial pathogens.

Diagnosis of Nosocomial Pneumonia

Despite advances, the accurate diagnosis of nosocomial pneumonia remains a problem. Clinical manifestations are insensitive and nonspecific in patients with nosocomial pneumonia. Fever, leukocytosis, hypoxemia, and pulmonary infiltrates may all develop in hospitalized patients for reasons unrelated to pneumonia. In patients with underlying congestive heart failure or adult respiratory distress syndrome, the presence of purulent respiratory secretions may be indicative of either tracheobronchitis or pneumonia. The clinical distinction between these two entities in such individuals is difficult. Elderly or immunosuppressed patients may not develop the characteristic clinical manifestations of pneumonia but may simply present with respiratory distress or confusion. Clearly, a high index of suspicion is necessary in hospitalized patients at risk for the development of nosocomial pneumonia.

The difficulty in diagnosis of nosocomial pneumonia was highlighted in a study in which the clinical impression was compared with autopsy findings in patients with suspected nosocomial pneumonia or adult respiratory distress syndrome.[74] Postmortem findings were discordant with the clinical impression in 29% of patients in this study. Despite the most careful diagnostic evaluation, some patients receive empiric therapy for suspected pneumonia when it is absent, whereas others do not receive appropriate therapy when pneumonia is nevertheless present.

The initial diagnostic evaluation should include a Gram

stain examination of a lower respiratory tract specimen. Specimens obtained via endotracheal suctioning may be contaminated with upper respiratory tract secretions and are often unreliable. The presence of pulmonary alveolar macrophages and elastin fibers corroborate the lower respiratory tract origin of a specimen but do not exclude confounding upper respiratory contamination. The presence of elastin fibers was a specific finding in patients with nosocomial pneumonia in one study but had a sensitivity of only 52%.[75]

Additional techniques may sometimes be useful in obtaining adequate specimens of lower respiratory tract secretions in patients with suspected nosocomial pneumonia. Transtracheal aspiration may be used in selected cases by physicians experienced with the procedure but is not appropriate in intubated patients. Percutaneous transthoracic thin needle aspiration is specific but relatively insensitive in diagnosing nosocomial pneumonia because of the small sample size. In addition, patients receiving positive pressure ventilation are at risk of developing pneumothorax with this procedure.

Fiberoptic bronchoscopy using the protected specimen brush to obtain samples of lower respiratory tract secretions has received a great deal of attention. In one study in ventilated patients with suspected nosocomial pneumonia, the sensitivity of this technique was 100% in identifying patients with nosocomial pneumonia when organisms were isolated in concentrations greater than 10^3 cfu/ml.[76] The specificity of the techniques was 87% in patients who had not received prior antibiotic therapy but fell to 42% in patients who had received prior antimicrobials. Preliminary studies examining the utility of quantitative cultures of BAL fluid in intubated baboons with nosocomial pneumonia were promising.[77] A follow-up study in humans, however, comparing the performance of BAL and the protected specimen brush in correctly identifying patients with suspected nosocomial bacterial pneumonia demonstrated that quantitative BAL cultures failed to discriminate between patients with and without pneumonia.[78] In this study, quantitative cultures of material obtained using the protected specimen brush had a sensitivity and specificity of 100% when a cut-off of greater than 10^3 cfu/ml was used.[78] The quantification of cells containing intracellular bacteria recovered by BAL was also helpful in distinguishing patients with pneumonia from those who were not infected. The presence of intracellular organisms in more than 25% of recovered cells had a sensitivity and specificity of 100% in patients with pneumonia.[78] Quantitative BAL cultures, total and differential cell counts in BAL, and quantification of extracellular organisms in BAL were less helpful in distinguishing patients with and without pneumonia. Several studies have examined the diagnostic utility of the antibody-coded bacteria test in patients with suspected pneumonia. Winterbauer et al.[79] examined this technique on specimens obtained at bronchoscopy in nonintubated patients with pneumonia and found a sensitivity of 73% and a specificity of 98%. A pilot study in intubated patients found that this technique had a sensitivity of 48% and a specificity of 100% in correctly identifying patients with pneumonia.[80] Unfortunately this technique is not available in most hospitals and remains investigational.

Although controversy remains regarding the optimal diagnostic method for patients with suspected nosocomial pneumonia, seriously ill patients should undergo fiberoptic bronchoscopy with quantitative culture of specimens obtained using the protected specimen brush. Unfortunately quantitative cultures and antibiotic susceptibilities of recovered isolates are seldom available within 24 hours of the procedure. Although quantification of cells containing intracellular organisms may aid in the discrimination between patients with and without pneumonia, empiric antibiotic therapy usually must be administered in the absence of definitive microbiologic data.

Therapy of Nosocomial Pneumonia

The definitive antibiotic therapy of nosocomial pneumonia is dictated by the identity and antibiotic susceptibility profile of microorganisms cultured from appropriate lower respiratory tract specimens. Unfortunately, such results are seldom available at the time empiric antimicrobial therapy is initiated. The selection of empiric antibiotics in patients with nosocomial pneumonia is governed by several considerations. These include:

- Prevalence of specific nosocomial pathogens within the institutions
- Antibiotic susceptibility profile of these pathogens
- Circumstances of onset of pneumonia in the patient
- Presence or absence of prior antibiotic therapy
- Severity of illness
- Results of recent sputum cultures
- Specific host considerations

Gram stain results of appropriately obtained lower respiratory tract specimens may aid in the selection of empiric antibiotic therapy as well.

General treatment recommendations for common pathogens producing nosocomial pneumonia are outlined in Table 21–5. These recommendations must be individu-

Table 21–5. Treatment Recommendations for Common Causes of Nosocomial Pneumonia*

Pathogen	Recommended Regimen
Staphylococcus aureus	
Methicillin sensitive	Oxacillin or nafcillin 2 g IV q4h
Methicillin resistant	Vancomycin 1 g IV q12h
In-hospital aspiration	Clindamycin 600 mg IV q6h + third-generation cephalosporin
	or
	Ticarcillin-clavulanate 3.1 g IV q6h
Legionella species	Erythromycin 1 g IV q6h
Gram-negative bacilli	
Escherichia coli	Cefazolin 2 g IV q8h
Klebsiella	±
pneumoniae	Aminoglycoside†
Pseudomonas aeruginosa	Ceftazidime or ureidopenicillin + aminoglycoside
Serratia species	Third-generation cephalosporin
Enterobacter species	(cefotaxime, ceftizoxime or ceftriaxone) + aminoglycoside

* Therapy must be individualized depending on antimicrobial susceptibilities of institutional isolates. Dosages assume normal renal and hepatic function in the adult.
† Add aminoglycoside in the critically ill patient.

alized in any given institution based on antibiotic susceptibility profiles of common isolates. Patients with nosocomial aspiration pneumonia generally have polymicrobial infections, which include mouth anaerobic bacteria and gram-negative enteric bacteria, and should receive a regimen with activity against these microorganisms. Appropriate antimicrobial combinations include clindamycin or penicillin plus an aminoglycoside or third-generation cephalosporin. Aminoglycosides tend to penetrate poorly into pulmonary parenchyma and respiratory tract secretions, owing in part to the low pH in these sites. For this reason, a third-generation cephalosporin is often preferable to an aminoglycoside for gram-negative enteric coverage in this setting. Some mouth anaerobic bacteria may be resistant to penicillin, and clindamycin may be preferable. Metronidazole should not be used because facultative mouth anaerobes may also be resistant to this antibiotic. Monotherapy with ticarcillin-clavulanate or imipenem-cilastatin may be appropriate in certain patients because these antibiotics provide broad coverage against anaerobic bacteria and many gram-negative bacilli. The antimicrobial spectrum of imipenem is extremely broad and sometimes unwarranted in patients with nosocomial aspiration pneumonia, unless prior sputum cultures have demonstrated resistant gram-negative bacilli.

Patients with serious nosocomial gram-negative pneumonia should receive a third-generation cephalosporin or ureidopenicillin, together with an aminoglycoside. If P. aeruginosa is suspected, the third-generation cephalosporin ceftazidime is an appropriate choice, as is a ureidopenicillin, such as piperacillin, ticarcillin, or mezlocillin. Antibiotic susceptibilities of P. aeruginosa may vary from one institution to another, and empiric therapy for suspected pseudomonas pneumonia should be dictated by local institutional experience.

Monotherapy for gram-negative nosocomial pneumonia with a third-generation cephalosporin or carbapenem, such as imipenem-cilastatin, has received considerable attention in the literature. Although outcome has been comparable to two-drug therapy in some studies, emerging resistance has often been a problem with monotherapy. The rationale for two-drug therapy has been to provide antimicrobial synergy and to minimize the likelihood of emerging resistance. Two-drug therapy is generally indicated in patients with more serious gram-negative pathogens, including P. aeruginosa, Serratia marcescens, and selected enterobacter species. Monotherapy may be appropriate in patients with gram-negative pneumonias caused by Escherichia coli, proteus species, or Klebsiella pneumoniae, but two-drug therapy should be considered in critically ill patients.

Patients with suspected staphylococcal nosocomial pneumonia should receive vancomycin, pending antibiotic susceptibilities of the isolate. In institutions where methicillin-resistant S. aureus is uncommon, a semisynthetic penicillin, such as oxacillin or nafcillin, may be used empirically pending microbiologic information. If legionellosis is a problem within an institution, empiric therapy in patients with suspected nosocomial pneumonia may require the addition of erythromycin pending more microbiologic information. In many institutions, however, legionellosis is extremely uncommon, and empiric therapy with erythromycin may not be indicated.

If prior surveillance cultures of sputum are available in patients with suspected nosocomial pneumonia, the presence of specific pathogens may provide a clue as to the diagnosis and help to guide empiric antibiotic therapy.

Because of the significant morbidity and mortality associated with nosocomial pneumonia, new strategies for the treatment of these infections have been actively investigated. Several approaches have been used. A prospective randomized study examined the utility of systemic antibiotics together with the direct installation of the aminoglycoside sisomicin into the respiratory tract via the endotracheal or tracheostomy tube.[81] Patients receiving sisomicin into the respiratory tract fared better than patients who did not receive this therapy and had a similar incidence of bacterial superinfection with resistant microorganisms. Because of the narrow therapeutic ratio for aminoglycosides in serum and the poor penetration of these agents into pulmonary parenchyma and sputum, alternative strategies have been developed to optimize delivery of these agents to the infected lung. These have included computer-assisted dosing as well as the use of unconventionally high aminoglycoside doses to achieve high serum levels. One study suggested that patients with serious gram-negative nosocomial pneumonia fared better if peak aminoglycoside levels exceeded 6 µg/ml of gentamicin or tobramycin or 24 µg/ml of amikacin.[82]

In addition to antibiotic therapy, considerable interest has developed in immunotherapy for patients with gram-negative pneumonia. Pseudomonas hyperimmune globulin is presently under study in patients with P. aeruginosa pneumonia. The monoclonal antibody HA1A against bacterial endotoxin was demonstrated to be effective in selected patients with gram-negative septicemia.[83] Its specific utility in gram-negative pneumonia remains to be defined. Studies with monoclonal antibody against tumor necrosis factor are ongoing to assess its efficacy in patients with the sepsis syndrome and pneumonia.

Management of Complications

Patients with community-acquired and nosocomial pneumonia may develop numerous complications in the ICU. Failure to respond to the empiric antibiotic regimen should prompt several considerations. These include the selection of an inappropriate regimen, the presence of a metastatic focus of infection, or complicating empyema or lung abscess. Patients with a pleural effusion should undergo diagnostic thoracentesis because this may disclose the presence of empyema, which would necessitate tube thoracostomy for definitive therapy. Empyema fluid is usually exudative and characterized by a pH of less than 7.2, lactate dehydrogenase of greater than 600 mg/dl, and a glucose level less than 40 mg/dl.[84] The presence of large numbers of microorganisms on Gram's stain examination of pleural fluid is also suggestive of empyema. A feculent odor often accompanies anaerobic empyema. Although bacteria are frequently visualized on Gram's stain examination of empyema fluid, this is not invariably the case. If Gram's stain is negative and empyema is nevertheless suspected, pleural fluid should be tested for bacterial antigen using latex agglutination or countercurrent immunoelectrophoresis for bacterial antigen. In patients with suspected legionellosis or tuberculous empyema, specific stains of pleural fluid for these organisms may corroborate the diagnosis.

Appropriate drainage of pleural empyema remains the treatment of choice and usually requires tube thoracostomy. This approach is successful in about two-thirds of patients.[85] Tubes are left in place until drainage is less than 50 ml/day, at which point they are removed. If significant pleural adhesions exist, tubes are sometimes cut and gradually withdrawn over several weeks.

Patients who fail tube thoracostomy or who have large loculated empyemas with thick fluid may require surgical intervention with rib resection and external drainage. Decortication may ultimately be required in those with a thick pleural peel and restrictive pulmonary disease. This is generally delayed for at least 1 month after the initial infection. Chronic pleural empyema is often not amenable to tube thoracostomy and may require open window thoracostomy.

Some patients may respond initially to antibiotic therapy, only to develop recurrent fever several days into therapy. In such patients, the differential diagnosis for recurrent fever is broad and includes:

- Drug fever
- Deep venous thrombosis
- New nosocomial infections such as line sepsis
- Nosocomial urinary tract infection
- Nosocomial sinusitis
- Infected sacral decubitus ulcer
- New nosocomial pneumonia
- Antibiotic-associated colitis

Generally a specific clue is identifiable in most patients, either based on physical examination or after routine laboratory and radiographic studies. Patients experiencing recurrent fever should have specimens for culture obtained of blood, urine, and sputum. If diarrhea is present, stool should be tested for Clostridium difficile. If intravenous lines have been in place for several days, these should be removed and the catheter tips cultured using the method of Maki.[86] Intravenous lines should ideally be changed to a new site if they have been in place for more than 72 hours and should not be rewired. If chest radiography discloses a new pulmonary infiltrate, additional specimens of lower respiratory tract secretions should be obtained for Gram's stain and culture.

In patients in whom no source of new infection is evident, occult sources of fever and infections should be pursued. Nosocomial sinusitis is common in patients with indwelling nasogastric or nasoendotracheal tubes and may simply present with fever or leukocytosis. Patients in the ICU are frequently sedated or unresponsive and therefore unable to provide complaints referable to the sinuses. In such individuals, a sector computed tomography scan of the sinuses may be invaluable in establishing the diagnosis. Other common causes of unexplained fever in the absence of localizing signs or symptoms include drug fever, deep venous thrombosis, and neuroleptic malignant syndrome, a frequently forgotten cause of fever in the ICU in patients receiving neuroleptics.

Additional complications may sometimes occur in patients with community-acquired pneumonia and nosocomial pneumonia. These include adult respiratory distress syndrome, restrictive lung disease secondary to a residual pleural peel in those with inadequately drained pleural empyema, and the postinfectious variant of bronchiolitis obliterans organizing pneumonia (BOOP), an uncommon complication generally seen in children following viral or mycoplasma infection or as a chronic sequela of unresolved tuberculosis or bacterial pneumonia.[88,89] BOOP is characterized histopathologically by intraluminal inflammation and fibrosis of distal air spaces with inflammatory cells, connective tissue, and fibroblast proliferation involving alveoli and terminal bronchioles.[90] Patients usually present with persistent dyspnea and may exhibit solitary, multiple patchy, or diffuse infiltrates on chest radiographs. Diagnosis generally requires transbronchial or open lung biopsy. In the idiopathic variant of BOOP, corticosteroids appear to be beneficial. Their utility in postinfectious BOOP is unclear.

Disseminated intravascular coagulation is also an occasional complication in such patients with community-acquired and nosocomial pneumonia. More complete discussions of these various complications are beyond the scope of this chapter and are reviewed elsewhere.

Criteria for Discharge from the ICU

Patients with community-acquired pneumonia who are admitted to the ICU require hemodynamic or ventilatory support (or both). Hospitalization in the ICU is necessary until these problems are resolved. Selected patients with chronic respiratory failure may be managed in units on regular nursing floors capable of caring for patients on ventilators; most patients, however, should be hospitalized in the ICU until extubation is accomplished and oxygenation by face mask or nasal cannula is acceptable. Hemodynamic instability and clinical signs of sepsis should also be resolved before transfer to the regular nursing unit. Other complications, including disseminated intravascular coagulation and new nosocomial infections, should be adequately controlled before contemplating transfer out of the ICU.

In patients with nosocomial pneumonia, the same considerations apply with regard to the duration of ICU hospitalization. In addition, other complicating illnesses requiring ICU support must be successfully treated before contemplating discharge to the regular nursing floor.

POST-ICU PHASE

The post-ICU phase in patients with nosocomial and community-acquired pneumonia focuses on the administration of an appropriate course of parenteral antibiotic therapy, management of complications, rehabilitation, and late diagnostic procedures to confirm the microbiologic diagnosis.

The duration of antimicrobial therapy in patients with community-acquired pneumonia must be individualized depending on the circumstances of the patient. Patients with uncomplicated pneumococcal pneumonia often may be successfully treated with 5 to 7 days of parenteral penicillin G, followed by a course of oral penicillin to complete 10 to 14 days of total therapy. Oral therapy may be completed in the outpatient setting. Patients with complicated pneumococcal pneumonia with metastatic infection, such as meningitis, generally require 10 to 14 days of parenteral high dose penicillin G therapy in the hospital. Patients with H. influenzae pneumonia should receive 10 to 14 days of parenteral therapy. Individuals with legionnaires' disease should receive a 3-week course of therapy, of which 10 to 14 days should be parenteral erythromycin. Shorter courses of therapy have been associated with a higher rate of relapse. Community-acquired staphylococcal and gram-negative pneumonia generally require 2 to 4 weeks of parenteral therapy, depending on the clinical course. Patients with complicating empyema may require longer courses of therapy, up to 4 weeks.

The duration of antimicrobial therapy in patients with nosocomial pneumonia is empiric and must be individualized as well, depending on the clinical course of the patient. Patients with in-hospital aspiration pneumonia generally require 10 to 14 days of antibiotic therapy. Patients with nosocomial gram-negative or staphylococcal pneumonia may require 3 to 4 weeks of antibiotic therapy. The clinical response as evidenced by defervescence, resolution of leukocytosis, and improvement in the pulmonary infiltrates on chest radiography should be followed to assist in the determination of the appropriate duration of antibiotic therapy. Well-designed prospective studies have not been reported to define the optimal duration of therapy in patients with nosocomial pneumonia, and this remains a matter of clinical judgment. Patients with complicating pleural empyema, secondary to either community-acquired or nosocomial pneumonia, generally require at least 3 to 4 weeks of parenteral antibiotic therapy for this complication.

In selected patients, the microbiologic diagnosis may remain uncertain, despite the best attempts to culture appropriate specimens. If legionnaires' disease, C. pneumoniae pneumonia, M. pneumoniae pneumonia, psittacosis, or Q fever are differential diagnostic considerations, appropriate convalescent serum specimens should be obtained in 4 to 6 weeks to test for a fourfold rise in antibody titer to these respective pathogens. This may permit a retrospective diagnosis of the cause of pneumonia in selected patients with community-acquired pneumonia or nosocomial legionellosis.

The management of pulmonary complications, such as pleural empyema or lung abscess, may be continued in the post-ICU phase of the hospitalization. Patients who have required tube thoracostomy for management of pleural empyema should have the tubes placed to water seal and ultimately removed if a bronchopleural fistula is present. In patients with extensive pleural adhesions, tubes may ultimately be advanced and withdrawn over several weeks, but this may often be accomplished in the outpatient setting. Selected patients with lung abscess may complete their course of parenteral antibiotic therapy through a home intravenous antibiotic program if this is available and appropriate support systems exist in the home setting. Patients considered for such programs should be medically stable, compliant, and have adequate nursing and family support.

Finally, the post-ICU phase should focus on pulmonary and general medical rehabilitation through appropriate physical therapy and nutritional support. These aspects of patient care are discussed elsewhere in this book.

REFERENCES

1. Klimek, J. J., et al.: Community-acquired bacterial pneumonia requiring admission to hospital. Am. J. Infect. Control, *11:* 79, 1983.
2. Gross, P. A.: Epidemiology of hospital-acquired pneumonia. Semin. Respir. Infect., *2:*2, 1987.
3. Centers for Disease Control: M. M. W. R., *38:*117, 1989.
4. Fine, M. J., Smith, D. N., and Singer, D. E.: Hospitalization decision in patients with community-acquired pneumonia: a prospective cohort study. Am. J. Med., *89:*713, 1990.
5. Wollschlager, C. M., Khan, F. A., and Khan, A.: Utility of radiography and clinical features in the diagnosis of community-acquired pneumonia. Clin. Chest. Med., *8:*393, 1987.
6. Lim, I., et al.: A prospective hospital study of the aetiology of community-acquired pneumonia. Med. J. Aust., *151:*87, 1989.
7. Ausina, V., et al.: Prospective study on the etiology of community-acquired pneumonia in children and adults in Spain. Eur. J. Clin. Microbiol. Infect. Dis., *7:*343, 1988.
8. British Thoracic Society: Community-acquired pneumonia in adults in British Hospital in 1982–1983: a survey of aetiology, mortality, prognostic factors and outcome. Q. J. Med., *62:* 195, 1987.
9. Holmberg, H.: Aetiology of community-acquired pneumonia in hospital treated patients. Scand. J. Infect. Dis., *19:*491, 1987.
10. Levy, M., et al.: Community-acquired pneumonia: importance of initial noninvasive bacteriologic and radiographic investigations. Chest, *92:*43, 1988.
11. Marrie, T. J., et al.: Community-acquired pneumonia requiring hospitalization: is it different in the elderly? J. Am. Geriatr. Soc., *33:*671, 1985.
12. Woodhead, M. A., et al.: Aetiology and outcome of severe community-acquired pneumonia. J. Infect., *10:*204, 1985.
13. Gross, P. A., et al.: Deaths from nosocomial infections: experience in a university hospital and a community hospital. Am. J. Med. *68:*219, 1980.
14. Craven, D. E., et al.: Risk factors for pneumonia and fatality in patients receiving continuous mechanical ventilation. Am. Rev. Respir. Dis., *133:*792, 1986.
15. Stevens, R. M., et al.: Pneumonia in an intensive care unit. Arch. Intern. Med., *134:*106, 1974.
16. Fang, G. D., et al.: New and emerging etiologies for community-acquired pneumonia with implications for therapy: a prospective multicenter study of 359 cases. Medicine, *69:* 307, 1990.
17. Marrie, T. J., et al.: Pneumonia associated with the TWAR strain of Chlamydia. Ann. Intern. Med., *106:*507, 1987.
18. Aubertin, J., et al.: Prevalence of legionellosis among adults: a study of community-acquired pneumonia in France. Infection, *15:*328, 1987.
19. Berntsson, E., et al.: Etiology of community-acquired pneumonia in patients requiring hospitalization. Eur. J. Clin. Microbiol., *4:*268, 1985.
20. McNabb, W. R., Shanson, D. C., Williams, T. D., and Lant, A. F.: Adult community-acquired pneumonia in central London. J. R. Soc. Med., *77:*550, 1984.

21. MacFarlane, J. T., Fince, R. G., Ward, M. J., and Macrae, A. D.: Hospital study of adult community-acquired pneumonia. Lancet, 2:255, 1982.
22. White, R. J., et al.: Causes of pneumonia presenting to a district general hospital. Thorax, 36:566, 1981.
23. Elbright, K. R., and Rytel, M. W.: Bacterial pneumonia in the elderly. J. Am. Geriatr. Soc., 28:220, 1980.
24. Esposito, A. L., and Gantz, N.: Legionnaires' disease: the distance traveled since Philadelphia. Pediatr. Infect. Dis. J., 5:163, 1986.
25. Storch, G., et al.: Sporadic community-acquired Legionnaires' disease in the United States: a case control study. Ann. Intern. Med., 90:596, 1979.
26. Garibaldi, R. A.: Epidemiology of community-acquired respiratory tract infections. Am. J. Med., 78:32, 1985.
27. Foy, H. M., et al.: Long-term epidemiology of infections with Mycoplasma pneumonia. J. Infect. Dis., 139:681, 1979.
28. Valenti, W. M., Trudell, R. G., and Bentley, D. W.: Factors predisposing to oropharyngeal colonization with gram-negative bacilli in the aged. N. Engl. J. Med., 298:1108, 1978.
29. Grayston, J. T., et al.: A new Chlamydia psittacti strain, TWAR, isolated in acute respiratory tract infections. N. Engl. J. Med., 315:161, 1986.
30. Nicotra, B., et al.: Branhamella catarrhalis as a lower respiratory tract pathogen in patients with chronic lung disease. Arch. Intern. Med., 146:890, 1986.
31. Grayston, J. T., et al.: Countrywide epidemics of Chlamydia pneumoniae, strain TWAR, in Scandinavia, 1981–1983. J. Infect. Dis., 159:1111, 1989.
32. Ortqvist, A., Sterner, G., and Nilsson, J. A.: Severe community-acquired pneumonia: factors influencing the need of intensive care treatment and prognosis. Scand. J. Infect. Dis., 17:377, 1985.
33. Centers for Disease Control: National Nosocomial Infections Study Report. Annual Summary 1984. M. M. W. R., 35:1755, 1986.
34. Johanson, W. G., Pierce, A. K., Sandor, J., and Thomas, G. D.: Nosocomial respiratory infections with gram-negative bacilli: the significance of colonization of the respiratory tract. Ann. Intern. Med., 77:701, 1972.
35. Louria, D. B., and Kaminski, T.: The effects of four antimicrobial regimens on sputum superinfection in hospitalization patients. Am. Rev. Resp. Dis., 85:649, 1962.
36. Driks, M. R., et al.: Nosocomial pneumonia in intubated patients given sucralfate as compared with antacids or histamine type 2 blockers. N. Engl. J. Med., 25:1562, 1982.
37. DuMoulin, G. C., et al.: Aspiration of gastric bacteria in antacid-treated patients: a frequent cause of postoperative colonization of the airway. Lancet, 1:242, 1982.
38. Woods, D. E.: Role of fibronectin in the pathogenesis of gram-negative bacillary pneumonia. Rev. Infect. Dis., 9:S386, 1987.
39. Woods, D. E., et al.: Role of adherence in the pathogenesis of Pseudomonas aeruginosa lung infection in cystic fibrosis patients. Infect. Immun., 30:694, 1980.
40. Woods, D. E., et al.: Role of salivary protease activity in adherence of gram-negative bacilli to mammalian buccal epithelial cells in vivo. J. Clin. Invest., 68:1435, 1981.
41. Woods, D. E., et al.: Role of pili in adherence of Pseudomonas aeruginosa to mammalian buccal epithelial cells. Infect. Immun., 29:1146, 1980.
42. Yu, V., et al.: Legionnaires disease: new clinical perspectives from a prospective pneumonia study. Am. J. Med., 73:357, 1982.
43. Langley, J. M., et al.: Poker players' pneumonia. An urban outbreak of Q fever following exposure to a parturient cat. N. Engl. J. Med., 319:354, 1988.
44. Selwyn, P. A., et al.: Increased incidence of bacterial pneumonia in HIV-infected intravenous drug abusers without AIDS. AIDS, 2:267, 1988.
45. Kovacs, J. A., et al.: Pneumocystis carinii pneumonia: a comparison between patients with acquired immunodeficiency syndrome and patients with other immunodeficiencies. Ann. Intern. Med., 100:663, 1984.
46. Edelstein, H., and McCabe, R. E.: Atypical presentations of Pneumocystis carinii pneumonia in patients requiring inhaled pentamidine prophylaxis. Chest, 98:1366, 1990.
47. Bisno, A. L.: Hyposplenism and overwhelming pneumococcal infection: a reappraisal. A. J. Med. Sci., 262:101, 1971.
48. Murray, H. W., et al.: The protean manifestations of Mycoplasma pneumoniae infections in adults. Am. J. Med., 58:229, 1975.
49. Roberts, D. B.: The etiology of bullous myringitis and the role of mycoplasmas in ear disease: a review. Pediatrics, 65:761, 1980.
50. Verghese, A., and Berk, S. L.: Bacterial pneumonia in the elderly. Medicine, 62:271, 1983.
51. Esposito, A. L.: Community-acquired bacteremic pneumococcal pneumonia: effect of age on manifestations and outcome. Arch. Intern. Med., 144:945, 1984.
52. Murray, P. R., and Washington, J. A.: Microscopic and bacteriologic analysis of expectorated sputum. Mayo Clin. Proc., 50:339, 1975.
53. Gleckman, R., et al.: Sputum gram stain assessment in community-acquired bacteremic pneumonia. J. Clin. Microbiol., 26:846, 1988.
54. Rein, M. F., et al.: Accuracy of the Gram's stain in identifying pneumococci in sputum. JAMA, 239:2671, 1978.
55. Hopewell, P. C.: Pneumocystis carinii pneumonia: diagnosis. J. Infect. Dis., 157:1115, 1988.
56. Barrett-Connor, E.: The non-value of sputum culture in the diagnosis of pneumococcal pneumonia. Am. Rev. Respir. Dis., 103:845, 1971.
57. Finegold, S. M.: Legionnaires disease—still with us. N. Engl. J. Med., 318:571, 1988.
58. Daley, J., et al.: Predicting hospital-associated mortality for Medicare patients: a method for patients with stroke, pneumonia, myocardial infarction, and congestive heart failure. JAMA, 260:3617, 1988.
59. Austrian, R., and Gold, J.: Pneumococcal bacteremia with especial reference to bacteremic pneumococcal pneumonia. Ann. Intern. Med., 60:759, 1964.
60. Perlino, C. A., and Runland, D.: Alcoholism, leucopenia, and pneumococcal sepsis. Am. Rev. Respir. Dis., 132:757, 1985.
61. Chomet, B., and Gach, B. W.: Lobar pneumonia and alcoholism: an analysis of thirty-seven cases. Am. J. Med. Sci., 253:300, 1967.
62. Hook, E. W., Horton, C. A., and Schaberg, D. R.: Failure of intensive care unit support to influence mortality from pneumococcal bacteremia. JAMA, 249:1055, 1983.
63. Gertman, P., and Pestuccia, J.: The evaluation protocol: a technique for assessing unnecessary days of hospital care. Med. Care, 19:855, 1981.
64. Van Eeden, S. F., Coetzee, A. R., and Joubert, J. R.: Community-acquired pneumonia—factors influencing intensive care admission. S. Afr. Med. J., 73:77, 1988.
65. Celis, R., et al.: Nosocomial pneumonia. A multivariate analysis of risk and prognosis. Chest, 93:318, 1988.
66. Penicillin resistant pneumococci [edit.]. Lancet, 1:1142, 1988.
67. Feldman, C., et al.: Community-acquired pneumonia due to penicillin-resistant pneumococci. N. Engl. J. Med., 313:615, 1985.
68. Sattler, F., et al.: Trimethoprim-sulfamethoxazole compared

with pentamidine for treatment of Pneumocystis carinii pneumonia in the acquired immunodeficiency syndrome. Ann. Intern. Med., *109:*280, 1988.
69. Gordin, F. R., et al.: Adverse reactions to trimethoprim-sulfamethoxazole in patients with the acquired immunodeficiency syndrome. Ann. Intern. Med., *100:*495, 1984.
70. Waskin, H., et al.: Risk factors for hypoglycemia associated with pentamidine therapy for Pneumocystis pneumonia. JAMA, *260:*345, 1988.
71. Masur, H., et al.: Consensus statement on the use of corticosteroids as adjunctive therapy for Pneumocystic pneumonia in the acquired immunodeficiency syndrome. N. Engl. J. Med., *323:*1500, 1990.
72. Khan, F., and Basir, R.: Sequential intravenous-oral administration of ciprofloxacin vs. ceftazidime in serious bacterial respiratory tract infections. Chest, *96:*528, 1989.
73. Chow, J. W., and Yu, V. L.: Antibiotic studies in pneumonia: pitfalls in interpretation and suggested solutions [edit.]. Chest, *96:*453, 1989.
74. Andrews, C. P., et al.: Diagnosis of nosocomial bacterial pneumonia in acute, diffuse lung injury. Chest, *80:*254, 1981.
75. Salata, R. A., et al.: Diagnosis of nosocomial pneumonia in intubated, intensive care unit patients. Am. Rev. Respir. Dis., *135:*426, 1987.
76. Chastre, J., et al.: Prospective evaluation of the protected specimen brush for the diagnosis of pulmonary infections in ventilated patients. Am. Rev. Respir. Dis., *130:*924, 1984.
77. Johanson, W. G., et al.: Bacteriologic diagnosis of nosocomial pneumonia following prolonged mechanical ventilation. Am. Rev. Respir., *137:*259, 1988.
78. Chastre, J., et al.: Diagnosis of nosocomial bacterial pneumonia in intubated patients undergoing ventilation: comparison of the usefulness of bronchoalveolar lavage and the specimen brush. Am. J. Med., *85:*499, 1988.
79. Winterbauer, R. H., et al.: The use of quantitative cultures and antibody coating of bacteria to diagnose bacterial pneumonia by fiberoptic bronchoscopy. Am. Rev. Respir. Dis., *128:*98, 1983.
80. Wunderlink, R. G., et al.: The diagnostic utility of the antibody-coated bacteria test in intubated patients. Chest, *99:*84, 1991.
81. Klastersky, J., et al.: Endotracheal-administered antibiotics for gram-negative bronchopneumonia. Chest, *75:*586, 1979.
82. Moore, R. D., Smith, C. R., and Lietman, P. S.: Association of aminoglycoside plasma levels with therapeutic outcome in gram-negative pneumonia. Am. J. Med., *77:*657, 1984.
83. Ziegler, E. J., et al.: Treatment of gram-negative bacteremia and septic shock with HA-1A human monoclonal antibody against endotoxin. N. Engl. J. Med., *324:*429, 1991.
84. Light, R. W.: Parapneumonic effusions and infections of the pleural space. *In* Pleural Diseases. Edited by R. W. Light. Philadelphia, Lea & Febiger, 1983, p. 101.
85. Lemmer, J. H., Botham, M. J., and Orringer, M. D.: Modern management of adult thoracic empyema. J. Thorac. Cardiovasc. Surg., *90:*849, 1985.
86. Maki, D. G., Weise, C. E., and Sarafin, H. W.: A semiquantitative culture method for identifying intravenous catheter-related infection. N. Engl. J. Med., *296:*1305, 1977.
87. Guze, B. H., and Baxter, L. R.: Neuropleptic malignant syndrome. N. Engl. J. Med., *313:*163, 1985.
88. Epler, G. R., and Colby, T. V.: The spectrum of bronchiolitis obliterans. Chest, *83:*161, 1983.
89. Sulavik, S. B.: The concept of "organizing pneumonia." Chest, *96:*967, 1989.
90. Cordier, J. F., Loire, R., and Brune, J.: Idiopathic bronchiolitis obliterans organizing pneumonia: definition of characteristic clinical profiles in a series of 16 patients. Chest, *96:*999, 1989.

Chapter 22

PNEUMONIA IN THE COMPROMISED HOST

LIONEL A. MANDELL
COLEMAN ROTSTEIN

A compromised host can be thought of as someone whose defense mechanisms have been impaired, ablated, or bypassed either temporarily or permanently. As a result, repeated, often serious infections may occur. Of all the infections from which such patients are at risk, pneumonia is the most common as well as the most frequently fatal, with mortality rates that can exceed 50%.

To deal with such infections, the physician must first have an understanding of normal defense mechanisms and how they can be impaired in relation to both the patient in general and the lungs in particular. In an attempt to provide the reader with some of the requisite information, this chapter is structured so as to deal first with general aspects of host defenses and then to focus in on defense mechanisms of the lung, pathogenesis of pneumonia, and issues related to the diagnosis and management of this condition.

DEFENSE MECHANISMS

A wide array of defenses exist to protect us from infection. These vary from simple mechanical processes, such as flushing and peristalsis, to more sophisticated processes involving complex mediators. The defense mechanisms can be categorized simply as first-line and second-line defenses. The first-line defenses are innate and rather nonspecific in terms of their role, whereas the second-line defenses are more specific in their role and in their response to challenge by microbial pathogens (Table 22-1). In addition to the defenses outlined in Table 22-1, two other processes deserve mention: the normal microbial flora of humans and the acute phase response.

The healthy individual is normally colonized by microorganisms that form part of the so-called normal commensal flora.[1] The presence of a normal resident flora helps to prevent infection in a variety of ways. They compete for available nutrients and receptors and play an important role in maintaining the relatively high levels of expression of the class II histocompatibility molecule on monocytes, so important for antigen presentation to the T cells. The role of the normal flora and of colonization of the oropharynx by pathogenic organisms is now increasingly recognized as a factor in the development of pneumonia. This is discussed in greater detail later.

The acute-phase response is a cytokine-mediated, non-antigen-specific reaction to challenge by an infecting pathogen. The extent and degree of the response depend on the severity of infection. The response itself is composed of a number of changes, including elevated temperature (fever), increased number and immaturity of circulating neutrophils, and reduction in serum iron and zinc levels as well as increased production of substances such as complement components, insulin, and glucagon.[2]

In addition to understanding defenses, we must also realize the large number of ways in which these various defenses can be impaired or bypassed, thereby predisposing patients to infection.

PREDISPOSING CONDITIONS TO INFECTION

This can be approached by dividing patients into those with non-neoplastic or neoplastic conditions.

Non-Neoplastic Conditions

Non-neoplastic conditions can be generally classified as:

- Bypassing mechanical barriers
- Splenectomy
- Malnutrition
- Diabetes mellitus
- Rheumatic diseases
- Uremia
- Alcoholism
- Drugs and radiation
- Infection

Bypassing Mechanical Barriers. The skin provides the major barrier mechanism against infection. Most bacteria are incapable of penetrating the stratified epithelium, and skin surface organisms are shed when the keratinized cells desquamate. An antibacterial effect is also provided by the lipids excreted by sebaceous glands and by the acid pH of the skin surface.[3] Breaches of the skin barrier that occur in parenteral drug abusers and burn patients may have serious sequelae in terms of infection.

Splenectomy. The spleen is a site of antibody production and removal of circulating opsonized organisms.[4] The increased susceptibility to infection seen in splenectomized patients may also be due to the lack of the enzyme tuftsin endocarboxypeptidase, which is involved in the activation of phagocytes by the tetrapeptide tuftsin.[5]

Malnutrition. Patients with severe protein-calorie malnutrition suffer losses in the integrity of surface defenses

Table 22-1. Selected Host Defense Mechanisms

Factors	First-line—Innate Immunity (Nonspecific)	Second-line—Adaptive Immunity (Specific)
Surface and mechanical	Skin Cough reflex Ciliary motion Flushing action (e.g., urine)	Immunoglobulins (e.g., immunoglobulin A)
Humoral	Complement Lysozyme Fibronectin Cytokines	Antibodies (e.g., immunoglobulins M and G)

Cellular	Phagocytes
	  Neutrophils
	  Monocytes
	  Eosinophils
	Natural killer cells
		Cell-mediated immunity

such as the skin and mucous membranes. This is compounded by reduced levels of immunoglobulin A in the gut, which allow bacteria colonizing the colon to enter the systemic circulation.[6] One may also find defective opsonization resulting from low complement levels, impaired cell-mediated immunity and neutrophil chemotaxis, and impaired phagocytic activity in cells of the fixed tissue monocyte macrophage type.[7,8]

Diabetes Mellitus. Phagocytic function and microbicidal activity of granulocytes are reduced in diabetic patients.[9] In addition to this, barrier defenses of these patients are bypassed with insulin injections or as a result of intravascular lines or urinary catheters inserted during hospitalization. Diabetic neuropathy and associated vascular disease may also lead to disruption of the skin surface.

Rheumatic Diseases. Two rheumatic diseases have been extensively investigated with regard to changes in host defense mechanisms. These are systemic lupus erythematosus (SLE) and rheumatoid arthritis. In cases of active SLE, neutropenia secondary to antigranulocyte antibodies may develop, and chemotaxis may be impaired as a result of defective generation of chemotactic factors as well as the appearance of chemotactic inhibitors in serum.[10,11] An inhibitor of phagocytosis and neutrophil degranulation has also been reported, as has impaired cell-mediated immunity.[12]

In patients with active rheumatoid arthritis, a substance in synovial fluid has been shown to impair neutrophil phagocytosis, and impaired chemotaxis and monocyte microbicidal function have also been reported.[13,14]

Uremia. Both quantitative and qualitative problems with neutrophils have been found in patients with renal failure. The former are due to decreased granulocyte reserves in the bone marrow, and qualitative defects, such as impaired chemotaxis, are probably due to defective generation of chemotactic factors.[15] Uremic patients have also been found to have impaired cell-mediated immunity and impaired antibody responses to primary immunization.[16]

Alcoholism. Alcoholics are at increased risk of pneumonia for two reasons. One is the gross aspiration that may occur when the level of consciousness is reduced and the cough reflex is impaired. The other is the silent aspiration of oropharyngeal organisms that occurs during sleep. Alcoholics are more likely to have oropharyngeal colonization by gram-negative bacilli, and they also have impaired microbicidal clearance by pulmonary alveolar macrophages.[17] Defects in complement activity, granulocyte response to bacterial infection, and cell-mediated immunity have also been noted in alcoholics.[18]

Drugs and Radiation. It is neither possible nor practical to try to cover all types of drugs that may affect host defenses, so only certain broad classes of agents are touched on. Steroids cause transient lymphopenia and monocytopenia with more selective effects on the T-cell subpopulations. Functional defects have also been described, including altered microbicidal activity of neutrophils and monocytes and impaired cell-mediated immunity.[19] Cytotoxic agents such as methotrexate and cyclophosphamide induce neutropenia and lymphocytopenia with resultant impairment of defenses associated with neutrophils, monocytes, and B and T cells.

Radiation affects cells with rapid renewal rates, such as the gastrointestinal epithelium, with the result that gut organisms may gain access to the systemic circulation. Radiation can also destroy the pool of mitotic cells resulting in granulocytopenia.

Infection. Organisms themselves have mechanisms that allow them to bypass or inhibit the defense mechanisms of humans. In addition to this, infection with certain pathogens can itself lead to suppression of host defenses. Cell-mediated immunity may be impaired following infection by viruses such as the human immunodeficiency virus (HIV), cytomegalovirus, and Epstein-Barr virus.

Infection is the major cause of morbidity and mortality in patients with neoplastic disease, particularly those suffering from hematologic malignancies. As well as being a complication of both the neoplastic disease itself and the treatment of the disease, infection may also complicate staging procedures in such malignancies as Hodgkin's disease.

Neoplastic Conditions

Neoplastic conditions that predispose the host to infection can be classified as:

- Bypassing mechanical barriers
- Granulocytopenia
- Cell-mediated and humoral immunosuppression
- Obstruction of natural passages
- Chemotherapy
- Broad-spectrum antibiotics

Bypassing Mechanical Barriers. Use of intravascular access lines, such as the Hickman or Broviac catheter, has been associated with an increased incidence of infections owing to Staphylococcus epidermidis and JK diphtheroids. The infections may be local or on occasion may result in sepsis.[20]

Granulocytopenia. Of all the factors predisposing to infection in cancer patients, this is the most important by far. The risk of infection is related not only to the severity of neutropenia, but also to its duration. A marked increase in the incidence of infection is seen in patients with granulocyte levels less than 500/mm^3. Patients with neutrophil counts below 100/mm^3 for prolonged periods of time are at great risk from infection, including some that can be rapidly fatal, such as gram-negative rod sepsis.[21]

The neutrophil issue may be a qualitative as well as a quantitative one. For example, in patients with acute myelogenous leukemia, cells that appear to be morphologically mature may in fact have impaired bactericidal and fungicidal activity.[22]

Cell-Mediated and Humoral Immunosuppression. Problems with cell-mediated and humoral immunity may be seen in disease states in which T-cell and B-cell function are impaired (for example, hematologic malignancies, Hodgkin's disease, and multiple myeloma). A balance between the helper T and cytotoxid/suppressor T cells is necessary for T-cell function to proceed normally. In HIV infection, the infecting virus selectively destroys helper T cells, whereas in Hodgkin's disease, there is an excess of suppressor T cells.[23]

Humoral immunity is disturbed when either insufficient or abnormal immunoglobulin is produced. In chronic lymphocytic leukemia, a progressive decrease in normal immunoglobulin and antibody response occurs. In plasma cell dyscrasias, there may be excessive amounts of homogeneous immunoglobulin molecules or fragments produced with a progressive decrease in antibody response.[24]

Obstruction of Natural Passages. Partial or complete obstruction of passages, such as the bronchi, ureters, or biliary tree, may result in infection owing to overgrowth of microorganisms. The urinary tract may become blocked in cases of prostatic, ovarian, or renal carcinoma, whereas branches of the bronchial tree may become occluded in carcinoma of the lung, resulting in postobstructive pneumonia. Obstruction of the biliary tree secondary to neoplastic disease can lead to acute cholangitis.

Chemotherapy. Some of the drugs used to treat malignant disease are themselves myelosuppressive and immunosuppressive. Their use often results in granulocytopenia and mucositis with its attendant infectious complications.

Broad-Spectrum Antibiotics. Although the use of broad-spectrum antibiotics is often necessary in the management of cancer patients, their use, especially if prolonged, may result in alterations of the normal microbial flora of the patients. Colonization and occasionally superinfection with resistant bacteria or fungi may then result.

PRE-ICU PHASE—THE RISK FOR PNEUMONIA

Pneumonia is the leading cause of death from nosocomial infection in the United States, and in the cancer population specifically, mortality rates for patients with pneumonia far exceed mortality rates from infection at other sites.[25] In leukemia and lymphoma patients, pneumonia is particularly serious. In acute leukemia patients in relapse, episodes of pneumonia have been documented once every 60 days of patient risk, and in lymphoma patients undergoing chemotherapy, the lung is the most common site of serious infection and death from infection.[26,27]

The previous section dealt with host defenses in general and how they may become impaired. In this section, we deal specifically with pulmonary defenses, how these defenses are breached, and the pathogenetic mechanisms involved in pneumonia.

Pulmonary Defense Mechanisms

The lung has a formidable and effective array of defenses to protect itself against invasion from pathogens. These may be classified in a number of ways, although a functional classification is probably best, e.g., resident or surveillance mechanisms versus augmenting mechanisms. One can also use an anatomic approach, although this essentially simply indicates the type of functional defense used at a particular point in the respiratory tree. For example, from the oropharynx to the level of the respiratory bronchioles, mechanical methods of clearance predominate, whereas beyond the respiratory bronchioles to the alveoli, cellular and humoral defense mechanisms predominate. A detailed description of pulmonary defense mechanisms is beyond the scope of this chapter, and the interested reader is referred elsewhere.[28,29]

The resident or surveillance mechanisms referred to previously are primarily mechanical or anatomic and are operative from the point of air entry to the respiratory bronchioles. Beyond this point, mechanical defenses are essentially ineffective, and resident or surveillance mechanisms that rely on immunoglobulin and phagocytic cells take over. In response to invasion by potential pathogens, the augmenting mechanisms are recruited, and these include the generation of an inflammatory response and an immune response. These defenses, along with defects and potential infections resulting from such defects, are given in Table 22-2.

The balance between health and disease can at times be a precarious one. In the case of pulmonary infection, the occurrence of disease depends not only on the integrity of host defenses, but also on the type of microbial challenge. A particularly virulent organism or a large inoculum of a less virulent pathogen may overwhelm even normal defenses. Once defense mechanisms are impaired, infection even by usually nonpathogenic organisms may occur.

The resident or surveillance mechanisms listed in Table 22-2 are nonspecific in their action as opposed to the augmenting mechanisms, which are quite specific. The humidification and aerodynamic filtration system provided by the upper airways and tracheobronchial tree along with mucociliary clearance and coughing aid in the trapping and expulsion of particles and pathogens. If pathogens manage to elude or bypass the physical or mechanical defenses and reach the terminal airways and alveoli, another aspect of the lung defenses becomes important.

These are shown in Figure 22-1 and include proteins such as complement and immunoglobulins, the phospholipid surfactant and phagocytes such as alveolar macrophages, and polymorphonuclear neutrophils (PMNs). Interaction among complement, immunoglobulins, and an infecting organism may result in activation of the alternate complement pathway with generation of chemotactic factors and may also help to opsonize the pathogen, thereby aiding both attachment and ingestion by phagocytic cells, such as the alveolar macrophage.[28,30]

Table 22–2. Lung Host Defenses to Airway Challenge

Host Defenses	Defect	Potential Infection Problem
Surveillance mechanisms		
Ciliated and squamous epithelium in naso-propharynx	Poor nutrition	Colonization with pathogenic gram-negative bacteria
Conducting airways		
Mechanical barriers (larynx) and airway angulation	Bypassing barriers with an endotracheal tube or tracheostomy	Aspiration, direct entry of microorganisms into airway
Mucociliary clearance	Structural defects in cilia	Stagnant secretions, bronchiectasis
Cough	Depressed cough reflex	Poor removal of secretions
Bronchoconstriction	Hyperactive airways, intrinsic asthma	Aspergillus, use of corticosteroids
Local immunoglobulin coating—secretory IgA	IgA deficiency'	Sinopulmonary infections
	Functional deficiency from breakdown by bacterial IgA$_1$ proteases	Abnormal colonization with certain bacteria (bronchitis)
Alveolar milieu		
Other immunoglobulin classes (opsonic IgG)	Acquired hypogammaglobulinemia, IgG$_4$, IgG$_2$ deficiency	Pneumonia with encapsulated bacteria
Iron-containing proteins (transferrin, lactoferrin)	Iron deficiency	May not inhibit certain bacteria (Pseudomonas, E. coli)
Alternate complement pathway activation	C$_3$ and C$_5$ deficiency	Trouble with infection but not life-threatening
Surfactant	Decreased synthesis, acute lung injury	Loss of opsonization activity
Alveolar macrophages	Subtle effects from immunosuppression, cannot kill intracellular microbes	Propensity for P. carinii and legionella sp. infections; poor inactivation of mycobacterium
Polymorphonuclear granulocytes	Absent because of immunosuppression; intrinsic defect in motility or lack of chemotactic stimulus	Poor inflammatory response, propensity for gram-negative bacillary infection and fungus (aspergillus)
Augmenting mechanisms		
Initiation of immune responses (humoral antibody and cellular)	Not described except as part of deficiency syndrome	Inadequate S-IgA or IgG antibody (?viral or mycoplasma infection and with encapsulated bacteria)
Generation of an inflammatory response (influx of polymorphonuclear granulocytes, eosinophils, lymphocytes, and fluid components)	Generally reflects status and supply of PMNs	Same as for PMNs; C$_5$ deficiency might decrease inflammatory response

PmNs, Polymorphonuclear neutrophils.
(From Reynolds, H. Y.: Normal and defective respiratory host defenses. *In* Respiratory Infections: Diagnosis and Management. 2nd ed. Edited by J. E. Pennington. New York, Raven Press, 1989.)

The pulmonary alveolar macrophage has a dual role both as a phagocyte/scavenger cell and as a cell with an effector role in the immune response. As a phagocyte, the macrophage serves as an integral part of the first-line or surveillance defense mechanisms of the lung. This is in contrast to the PMN, which does not normally reside in the alveoli in significant numbers and must be recruited from the adjacent intravascular compartment as part of the inflammatory response. As an immune effector cell, the alveolar macrophage is capable of processing antigens and presenting them to T helper cells and of releasing a large number of mediators that help to modulate both the inflammatory and the immune responses triggered by an infection that is not contained by the surveillance mechanisms alone.[31]

That the macrophage has such a dual role is critical. Although the cell can ingest and kill many commonly encountered bacterial pathogens, a number of organisms are able to survive within the macrophage, and their elimination depends on cell-mediated immune mechanisms. Some examples of these are Listeria monocytogenes, Legionella pneumophila, Pneumocystis carinii, cytomegalovirus, and mycobacteria.[29]

In normal lungs, PMNs constitute less than 1 to 2% of alveolar cells, and they normally reside in the interstitial areas of the lung and in adjacent capillaries.[29] Their recruitment into the alveoli depends on the generation of chemoattractants, which are necessary for the directed migration of PMNs into the alveoli.

By means of C3b and Fc receptors on their surface, PMNs are able to recognize and ingest opsonized organisms, and killing them takes place by both oxygen-dependent and oxygen-independent systems within the PMN.[33] As a result of the generation and release of toxic oxygen radicals as well as some of the enzymes normally contained within the PMN, host lung tissue may also be damaged. In more severe cases, interactions among inflammatory cells, vasoactive mediators, cytokines, and reactive oxygen radicals may lead to the development of the adult respiratory distress syndrome.

In compromised patients, particularly those with hematologic malignancies, quantitative defects of neutrophils are commonly seen following myelosuppressive therapy. The reduction in the peripheral white blood cell count and marginated pool means that the source of PMNs from which these cells are recruited into the lung is reduced. The relationship is not quite as clear, however, for the pulmonary alveolar macrophage. These cells have a substantially longer life span than the PMN, and it was found

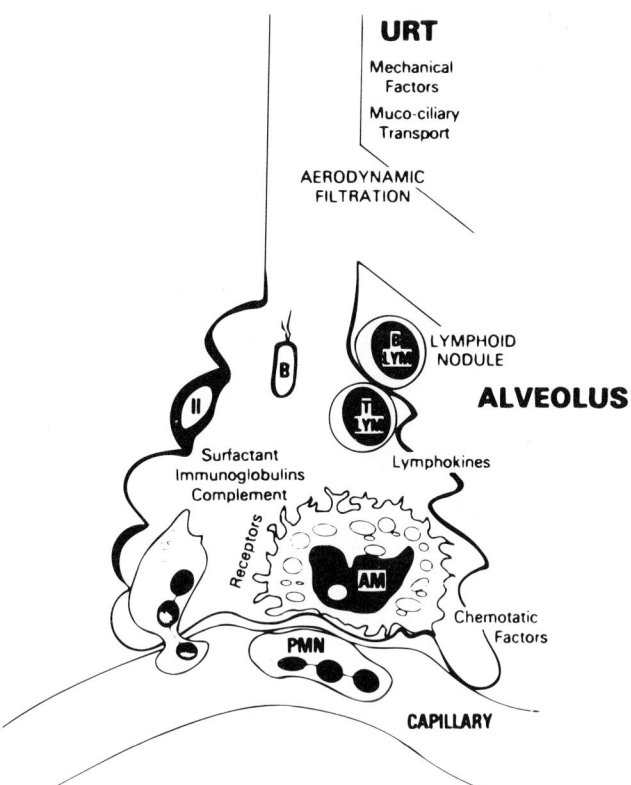

Fig. 22-1. Factors responsible for clearance of bacteria (B) inhaled into the lungs are different in the upper airway (URT) and in the lower respiratory tract, here represented by enlargement of an alveolus. A bacterium of critical size, which escapes mechanical removal from the URT and is deposited in an alveolus, may encounter surfactant and/or immunoglobulins (antibodies) and complement proteins that condition it for phagocytosis by a resident alveolar macrophage (AM). Antibody with specific opsonizing potential could facilitate attachment of the bacterium to the AM surface membrane through specialized cell receptors. A complement (C3) might augment such attachment. At least two alternate mechanisms could be activated to enhance killing and clearance of the microbe. First, the AM can liberate chemotactic factors that attract nearby polymorphonuclear phagocytes (PMNs), marginated in a lung capillary adjacent to the alveolus, and thus initiate an inflammatory response. Second, the bacterium may trigger immune lymphocytes (T-lym) to release effector substances (lymphokines) that may activate or stimulate AM phagocytic activity. (From Reynolds, H. Y.: Normal and defective respiratory host defenses. In Respiratory Infections: Diagnosis and Management. 2nd Ed. Edited by J. E. Pennington. New York, Raven Press, 1989.)

that in patients undergoing treatment for monocytic leukemia, the induced monocytopenia was not reflected in the number of alveolar macrophages found on lung lavage.[34]

Pathogenesis of Pneumonia

Having briefly reviewed the defense mechanisms of the lung, we can now go on to a consideration of how pneumonia occurs, particularly in the compromised host. In the section dealing with general defense mechanisms of the body, we discussed how pneumonia might develop in patients with a solid tumor and impaired clearance of a lung segment. Other defects in host defenses can predispose the patient to infection by a particular pathogen (Table 22-3).

One of the main questions to consider in the pathogenesis of pneumonia is how the various organisms gain access to the lower respiratory tract. Generally organisms reach this site by one of three routes:

- Inhalation
- Aspiration
- Hematogenous spread

The importance of each of these varies depend on the pathogen.

For bacterial pneumonia, particularly if due to gram-negative bacilli, aspiration into the tracheobronchial tree of organisms colonizing the oropharynx appears to be the most important route.[35,36] With fungal infections, however, other mechanisms predominate. Opportunistic fungal pathogens that typically cause pneumonia in patients with impaired defenses are aspergillus, the phycomycetes (mucor, rhizopus, absidia), candida species, and Torulopsis glabrata. Aspergillus species are molds, and their aerosolized conidia are inhaled into the lung where, in granulocytopenic patients in particular, they may cause active disease.[37] Candida is more likely to reach the lung via the hematogenous route, usually in the setting of an immunocompromised patient with disseminated candida infection.[26,37] Pneumonia caused by such diverse agents as Mycobacterium tuberculosis, P. carinii, and viruses such as herpes simplex is usually the result of reactivation of a latent infection.[38,39] Extrapulmonary lesions associated with pulmonary infection in the immunocompromised host are listed in Table 22-4.

Once the organisms have reached the lower respiratory tract, whether or not they are effectively cleared depends on their virulence, the inoculum size, and the extent of suppression of the host defenses.

Oropharyngeal Colonization

Oropharyngeal colonization by gram-negative bacilli is relatively uncommon in healthy persons. Once individuals become ill, however, the situation changes, and gram-negative colonization occurs quite rapidly.[40] In a study of the relationship of such colonization to nosocomial pneumonia, the investigators found that the indicators of severity of illness associated with colonization were:

- Respiratory tract disease
- Tracheal intubation
- Coma
- Hypotension
- Acidosis
- Azotemia
- Marked leukocytosis or leukopenia[35]

This study also examined the relationship between oropharyngeal colonization by gram-negative bacilli and nosocomial pneumonia. Of 213 patients admitted to a medical ICU, 95 became colonized, and nosocomial infection de-

Table 22-3. Infectious Agents Seen in Association with Specific Immune Lesions

Immune Lesion*	Conditions Associated	Predisposed to Infections With
Antibody formation (B lymphocytes or regulation thereof)	Primary and acquired humoral deficiency Lymphoproliferative disease (especially myeloma) AIDS (especially new antigens) Corticosteroids, immunosuppressive agents	Bacteria: highly encapsulated Streptococcus pneumonia Haemophilus influenzae Neisseria meningitidis Pyogenic: S. aureus, streptococci, P. carinii
Cellular-mediated/ T-lymphocyte-regulated	Lymphoma Uremia (chronic) AIDS Corticosteroids, immunosuppressive agents Radiation therapy	Viruses: cytomegalovirus, herpes simplex, varicella zoster Parasites: P. carinii, T. gondii, amebae, S. stercoralis Fungi: C. neoformans, candida, H. capsulatum, C. immitis, B. dermatitidis Bacteria: legionella, N. asteroides, salmonella, L. monocytogenes Mycobacteria: tuberculosis and avium complex
Granulocyte/phagocyte defects	Granulocytopenia Splenectomy Splenic dysfunctions (alcoholism, sickle cell, myeloproliferative, lymphoma) Myeloproliferative disease Corticosteroids Hemolysis	Encapsulated (above) Gram-negative: E. coli, klebsiella, pseudomonas, S. aureus, mycobacteria, salmonella Fungi: cryptococcus, aspergillus, candida, torulopsis, mucor species
Serum complement	Primary Alcoholism/malnutrition	Encapsulated bacteria

* Few lesions are specific enough to exclude any pathogen group.
(From Fishman, J. A.: Diagnostic approach to pneumonia in the immunocompromised host. Semin. Respir. Infect., 1:133, 1986.)

veloped in 22 (23%). Pneumonia developed in only 4 of 118 noncolonized patients, however (3.3%).[35]

The increased colonization by gram-negative bacilli is likely related to impairment of pharyngeal clearance mechanisms and to increase adherence of gram-negative bacilli to epithelial cells. In healthy individuals, mucosal cells are coated with cell surface fibronectin, which prevents attachment of gram-negative bacilli to receptors on the underlying cells.[41] Loss of cell surface fibronectin and increased adherence by gram-negative bacilli have been demonstrated in patients before colonization by these organisms.[42] The loss of the fibronectin has been attributed to increased salivary protease activity; one source for this protease appears to be PMNs in airway secretions.[43] Although a true cause-and-effect relationship between oropharyngeal colonization and pneumonia has not yet been proved, the association is a strong one.

One of the main questions to consider as well is, what are the potential sources of organisms that colonize the oropharynx? These sources can be exogenous as well as endogenous, with the latter referring primarily to the gastrointestinal tract.

Normally the acid pH of the stomach is hostile to most bacteria. If gastric pH increases, however, as can occur with the use of antacids and histamine type 2 (H_2 blockers), there is a substantial increase in gastric colonization

Table 22-4. Extrapulmonary Infectious Lesions Associated with Pulmonary Infection in the Immunocompromised Host

Site	Lesions	Major Organism(s)
Skin	Ecthyma gangrenosum (vasculitis with bacteremia) Also: cellulitis, abscesses, infected ulcers, "shingles", lymphangitis	Bacteria: P. aeruginosa, aeromonas, other gram-negative bacteria Also: nocardia, vibrios, mycobacteria, neisseria Fungi: cryptococcus, aspergillus, blastomyces, coccidioides, trichosporan, zygomycetes Viral: varicella zoster, herpes simplex, measles
Upper respiratory	Peritonsillar abscess, Ludwig's angina, epiglottitis, sinusitis, otitis	Bacteria: streptococci (especially group A, beta-hemolytic), staphylococci, oral anaerobes, pseudomonas, H. influenzae
Eye	Retinitis, conjunctivitis	Fungi: zygomycetes, aspergillus, candida, mucor agents Viral: cytomegalovirus Parasites: toxoplasma
CNS	Abscess Meningoencephalitis Cavernous sinus thrombosis Spinal abscess	Bacteria: streptococci (especially pneumoniae, alpha-hemolytic), staphylococcus, pseudomonas, mycobacteria, nocardia, neisseria Fungi: cryptococcus, aspergillus, coccidioides Viruses: varicella zoster, herpes simplex, HTLV-III/LAV Parasites: toxoplasma, strongyloides
Gastrointestinal tract	Colitis Ingestion	Bacteria: L. monocytogenes Parasites: E. histolytica, Strongyloides (with gram-negative), paragonimus

(From Fishman, J. A.: Diagnostic approach to pneumonia in the immunocompromised host. Semin. Respir. Infect., 1:133, 1986.)

by gram-negative rods.[44,45] Based on data from several studies, it appears that gastric colonization with gram-negative bacilli precedes oropharyngeal colonization with these organisms. The stomach may act as a reservoir for bacteria, which subsequently colonize the oropharynx and are then aspirated into the tracheobronchial tree.[44,46,47]

The correlation between gastric colonization with gram-negative bacilli and the incidence of pneumonia in ICU patients was carefully studied by Driks et al.[48] They examined incidence rates of nosocomial pneumonia in mechanically ventilated patients given sucralfate or antacids or H_2 blockers. Patients in the sucralfate group had a higher proportion of gastric aspirates with pH less than 4.0 and a significantly lower number of gram-negative bacilli in culture specimens than did patients in the antacid/H_2 antagonist group. Pneumonia occurred in 11.5% of the sucralfate group and in 23.3% of the antacid/H_2 blocker group. Mortality rates in the two groups were 29.5 and 46.4%. The results of this study suggest that elevation of gastric pH increases the risk of nosocomial pneumonia in ventilated patients by promoting gastric colonization with gram-negative bacilli.

Diagnosis

As in any medical or surgical condition, the diagnosis of pneumonia is made by weighing the evidence obtained from a carefully taken history, a carefully done physical examination, and appropriate laboratory tests and procedures. This is particularly true of the immunocompromised host in whom the diagnosis of pneumonia is being considered. Despite the large number of diagnostic possibilities in such patients, an organized and methodical approach can help to narrow the alternatives.

History

When confronted with a compromised patient with a chest infiltrate, one of the first things the clinician must sort out is whether in fact it is pneumonia. In other words, is an infectious or a noninfectious process responsible for the pulmonary findings? The clinician must also bear in mind the fact that more than one disease process may coexist in the same patient at any one time. For example, a febrile neutropenic leukemic patient who is undergoing remission induction chemotherapy may be short of breath and have a pulmonary infiltrate because of a gram-negative bacillary pneumonia or a pulmonary hemorrhage that is complicating the patient's severe thrombocytopenia. Some of the infectious and noninfectious causes of pulmonary infiltrates in compromised hosts are given in Table 22–3.

As indicated in Table 22–3, certain defects in host defense are typically associated with certain pathogens. The issue is more complicated than the table implies, however, because patients may well have more than one defect at a time. For example, patients with Hodgkin's disease typically have impaired cell-mediated immune function. While undergoing remission induction therapy, however, they can be made severely neutropenic. During this time, they are at risk from pathogens that are normally handled by cell-mediated immune mechanisms as well as pathogens handled by neutrophils. In attempting to sort through the various possibilities, it is important to consider the following:

1. Does the patient have any previous infections that might be reactivated by the current state of immunosuppression? These include mycobacterial infections as well as certain endemic systemic fungal infections, such as histoplasmosis and coccidioidomycosis.
2. Is the pneumonia community acquired or hospital acquired? A community-acquired pneumonia in a patient whose underlying disease was relatively quiescent may be due to such commonplace organisms as Streptococcus pneumoniae or the influenza virus if it is known to be present in the community. As reported by Rubin and Greene,[49] in their experience the single most common bacterial infection in the cancer patient and renal transplant patient is S. pneumoniae, and other than cytomegalovirus, influenza is the most common viral infection in the renal transplant patient.
3. What is the time course of the illness? This information may be particularly helpful in attempting to determine the nature of the causative pathogen. Lung infections in immunocompromised patients can be broadly categorized according to their rate of progression as acute, subacute, and insidious or chronic.

Infections with an acute onset usually occur over a 24-hour period or less and are typically bacterial, although P. carinii can also be dramatic in its onset. Subacute infections that develop over a period of several days are suggestive of organisms such as aspergillus or mucormycosis or viral infections such as cytomegalovirus. A more insidious progression suggests other fungal infections, nocardia, and tuberculosis.[49,50]

Another factor that must be kept in mind in dealing with pneumonia, particularly in granulocytopenic patients, is that because the inflammatory response is blunted, the typical features that one associates with lung infection may be minimal or absent. For example, even with a gram-negative rod pneumonia, there may be little or no purulent sputum production, and if there is pleural involvement, there may be little, if any, accompanying chest pain. Even radiologic findings may be diminished or absent. In one report, up to 58% of cancer patients with severe granulocytopenia who died were found to have had clinically unrecognized pneumonia.[51]

Physical Examination

Although it can occasionally be unrevealing, the physical examination is nevertheless an important, integral part of the diagnostic assessment of the patient. As mentioned previously, findings, particularly in the severely granulocytopenic patient, may be minimal, but the physician must nevertheless diligently search for any clues. The physical examination is probably best considered under the following headings: thoracic and extrathoracic.

Thoracic Examination. Despite the lack of a productive cough, and with few findings on percussion or auscultation of the chest, the finding of an increased respiratory rate and especially the use of accessory muscles of respiration may help to point to a pulmonary focus of infection.

The presence of a pleural friction rub in the patient with suspected pneumonia normally suggests that the infectious process has involved the pleural surfaces and that a pleuritis has developed. In granulocytopenic patients, such a finding takes on special significance. Certain pathogens, such as aspergillus, are capable of invading along blood vessels and causing thrombosis and pulmonary infarction. If this occurs in a peripheral area of the lung, a clinical presentation resembling acute pulmonary embolism and pulmonary infarction may be seen.[52]

Extrathoracic Examination. Occasionally the pathogen causing pneumonia also causes infection in other body sites or is associated with certain extrathoracic manifestations, which might suggest a particular organism. Some examples of these are ecthyma gangrenosum in the setting of pseudomonas sepsis and fundoscopic findings of choroidal lesions in patients with disseminated candida infection. Table 22-4 provides a list of various extrapulmonary lesions that have been associated with pulmonary infection in the immunocompromised patient.

Laboratory Tests and Procedures

In addition to the information gained from the history and physical examination, the physician also has a number of laboratory tests and procedures at his or her disposal that can be used to pinpoint the diagnosis further. These can be categorized in a number of ways, but the simplest is to divide them into noninvasive and invasive tests.

Noninvasive Tests. Noninvasive tests include:

- X-ray and ultrasound studies
- Immunologic tests
- Microbiologic tests

X-ray and Ultrasound Studies. X-ray studies include routine posterioanterior and lateral as well as portable chest films, apical lordotic films, and tomograms. The computed tomography (CT) scan may also be used to detect early cavity formation and to differentiate pleural from parenchymal disease. Ultrasound studies are usually used to define the size and extent of a pleural effusion, particularly when one is considering a drainage procedure. Certainly the most frequently used test, however, is the routine chest film.

We have all learned from experience, however, that the x-ray appearance is not pathognomonic of a particular disease process and that with the possible exception of radiation pneumonitis, which follows the boundaries set by radiation fields rather than any known anatomic boundaries, one cannot make a definitive diagnosis based on the x-ray appearance. The radiographic pattern, however, may help in narrowing the diagnostic possibilities, particularly when assessed in the context of information gleaned from the history and physical examination.

Radiographic patterns generally fall into three main groups: nodular or cavitary, diffuse, and focal or consolidative. Some of the infectious and noninfectious conditions associated with these three patterns are given in Table 22-5.

Immunologic Tests. These include skin and serologic tests. Skin tests have little role to play in the diagnosis of pulmonary infection in the compromised host. For example, in a patient with suspected tuberculosis who has received intensive myelosuppressive therapy for lymphoma or leukemia, the tuberculosis and control skin tests (e.g., mumps, candida, streptokinase streptodornase) may well be negative even in a patient with active infection simply as a result of the extensive immunosuppression secondary to the chemotherapy.

As well, serologic diagnosis is not usually of great help in the compromised host, particularly in a patient with a rapidly advancing pulmonary infection. There is a problem not only with the sensitivity and specificity of many of the tests, especially those for viral and fungal infection, but also the severely immunosuppressed patient may not be able to mount an effective antibody response to a particular pathogen, thereby resulting in a false-negative test.

Microbiologic Tests. These tests refer to stains and cultures of expectorated sputum samples and blood cultures.

Table 22–5. Radiographic Appearance of Pulmonary Infiltrates in Immunocompromised Patients

Nodular or Cavitary	Diffuse	Focal or Consolidative
Infectious		
Bacteria (e.g. staphylococcus, pseudomonas)	Viral	Bacteria (including legionnaires')
Legionella	Pneumocystis	Tuberculosis
Nocardia	Candida	Nocardia
Cryptococcus	Aspergillus	Aspergillus
Aspergillus	Cryptococcus	Mucormycosis
		Cryptococcus
		Viral
Noninfectious		
Neoplasm	Pulmonary edema	Neoplasm
Septic emboli	Pulmonary hemorrhage	Pulmonary hemorrhage
Pulmonary hemorrhage	Radiation pneumonitis	
	Lymphocytic carcinomatosis	
	Leukemic involvement	
	Drug-induced	
	Nonspecific interstitial pneumonitis	

Technically the latter is an invasive procedure, but we have taken some license and included it among the noninvasive tests. The most frequently done stains are the Gram and acid-fast stains. The usefulness of sputum culture and Gram stain in particular has been the subject of considerable debate. Nevertheless, these are simple, relatively inexpensive procedures that should be carried out. Samples should be screened to rule out sputum that is inappropriate for culture because of excessive oropharyngeal contamination. The specimens should be examined under low power and are considered appropriate for culture if there are less than 10 squamous epithelial cells or more than 25 PMNs per low power field.[53] Obviously this may be difficult in a patient who is neutropenic.

It is always helpful when dealing with immunocompromised patients in whom pneumonia is suspected to discuss the patient with the microbiologist. By alerting the laboratory regarding the possible pathogens, specialized stains or culture media for certain opportunistic organisms can be used. A detailed discussion of the various stains and culture techniques is beyond the scope of this chapter. The interested reader is referred to the June 1988 issue of *Seminars in Respiratory Infections*.[54] The entire issue is devoted to the diagnosis of pneumonia and provides an in-depth review of invasive and noninvasive techniques useful for the diagnosis of pneumonia.

Invasive Tests. Invasive tests include:

- Needle aspiration
- Bronchoscopy
- Thorascopy
- Open lung biopsy

Noninvasive tests, such as chest film, sputum Gram stain, and cultures of blood and sputum, are the main ones used for the diagnosis of most cases of nosocomial pneumonia that do not involve immunosuppressed patients. The compromised host, however, is more difficult to deal with because of the increased number of noninfectious as well as infectious causes that must be considered. Although information obtained from the history, physical examination, and noninvasive tests may certainly help to narrow the diagnostic possibilities, they unfortunately often do not provide a specific diagnosis, and the clinician must decide whether to resort to empiric therapy or to use invasive procedures in the quest for a specific diagnosis. In a study of 80 immunosuppressed patients with diffuse pulmonary infiltrates, the use of noninvasive tests resulted in a specific diagnosis in only 10% of patients.[55]

There are two key questions that relate to the use of invasive techniques. The first is, when does one use such tests? The second question follows from the first: Having decided that an invasive procedure is necessary, which of the many that are available does one use?

When to Use Invasive Procedures. Generally, one should consider an invasive test to establish a specific diagnosis if there is a high likelihood of finding a pathogen, the treatment of which is associated with considerable adverse events. Rather than listing when one should consider using invasive procedures, it may be easier simply to consider situations in which they definitely should not be used. Generally invasive procedures should not be used if the test is unlikely to yield information that will change therapy and if the risks of the procedure are too great. An example of the former is the patient with recently diagnosed acute myelogenous leukemia undergoing remission induction therapy who develops a focal infiltrate on chest film and who is febrile and neutropenic as well. In such patients, the likely pathogen is bacterial and not necessarily opportunistic. Such a patient would routinely be started on empiric therapy with antibacterial agents. In most centers, such a patient would be followed closely, and an invasive procedure would not routinely be done initially. An example of a patient with an unacceptably high risk is one with an uncorrectable bleeding diathesis or a patient whose pulmonary function is so impaired the patient could not tolerate either the procedure itself or any adverse sequelae that might complicate the procedure.

Which Invasive Procedure to Use. Having decided that an invasive procedure is necessary, the next step is to decide which one is best. In making this decision, the clinician must consider the patient's underlying disease and any associated illnesses, the nature of the pulmonary infiltrate on x-ray film, and its rate of progression. A number of invasive procedures exist, each with its own particular advantages and disadvantages. They include the following:

- Needle aspirations—transtracheal and transthoracic
- Bronchoscopy-related procedures—plugged telescoping catheter, brush, bronchial washings, transbronchial needle aspiration, transbronchial biopsy, and bronchoalveolar lavage
- Thoracoscopy—guided biopsy
- Open lung biopsy

Transtracheal needle aspiration was originally developed to allow cultures to be obtained without the risk of contamination by oropharyngeal organisms. Its main advantage is its low false-negative rate, but it has a high false-positive rate of 21%.[56] Because of the risk of potentially serious complications, it is no longer used in most centers.

Needle aspiration using the transthoracic approach has shown some promise as a diagnostic tool. By using a fine gauge needle (18 G to 25 G), the complication rates seen with the Vim-Silverman and Cope needles and Trephine drill are avoided. Transthoracic needle aspirations should be considered for focal lesions, such as discrete nodules or cavities, especially if peripherally located.[49] Using an ultrathin 24- to 25-gauge needle in patients with infectious/inflammatory disease, sensitivity and specificity rates of 83% and 100% have been reported.[57] In a study of needle aspiration in immunocompromised patients who had undergone previous diagnostic tests that had been unrewarding, the yield with the transthoracic approach was 73%.[58] The procedure is less useful, however, for the diagnosis of diffuse lung disease.

A distinct drawback to the procedure before the use of ultrathin needles was the complication rate. In one review, the incidences of pneumothorax and hemoptysis were 20 to 30% and 3 to 10%.[59] In contrast with these rates, the complications in Zavala and Schoebl's study[57] in which ultrathin needles were used were minimal.

The development of the fiberoptic bronchoscope has led to a number of procedures that can be used in the diagnosis of pneumonia. The plugged telescoping catheter brush was developed as a way of avoiding the inevitable contamination that occurs as the bronchoscope traverses the oropharyngeal area. When used with quantitative culture techniques ($>10^3$ cfu/ml), pulmonary pathogens can usually be distinguished from colonizing organisms.[60] In a study evaluating fiberoptic bronchoscopy in immunocompromised patients, the plugged catheter provided the same information as transbronchial biopsy in patients with nonfungal pneumonia.[61] Bronchial washings and transbronchial needle aspiration offer no advantages over the protected catheter technique.[62,63]

In immunocompromised patients with a diffuse infiltrative process on chest film, the physician has a choice between two types of invasive procedures. The less invasive approach is fiberoptic bronchoscopy plus bronchoalveolar lavage or transbronchial biopsy, and the more invasive one is open lung biopsy. If it is not absolutely imperative to make a definitive diagnosis immediately, the usual approach is to proceed first with bronchoscopy.

Transbronchial biopsy offers a means of actually sampling pieces of lung parenchyma, whereas bronchoalveolar lavage offers the physician the opportunity to sample up to 1 million alveoli. In one review, the yield with transbronchial biopsy in immunocompromised patients ranged from a low of 26% to a high of 68%.[64] By combining transbronchial biopsy with bronchoalveolar lavage, however, the yield can be increased. A study in acquired immunodeficiency syndrome (AIDS) patients showed sensitivities of 50% with transbronchial biopsy and 73% with bronchoalveolar lavage, but when the two were combined, a diagnostic yield of 85% was obtained.[65] In cases of nonspecific interstitial pneumonitis, samples obtained by transbronchial biopsy may be particularly difficult to interpret. In such cases, transbronchial biopsy may have to be followed by open lung biopsy.

The major disadvantages of transbronchial biopsy are the risks of bleeding and pneumothorax, and the procedure is in fact contraindicated in patients with uncontrolled bleeding diatheses and severe hypoxemia. Bronchoalveolar lavage is considerably safer. In fact, in immunocompromised patients in whom transbronchial biopsy is considered too risky, bronchoalveolar lavage alone may be done, particularly for the diagnosis of diffuse pulmonary infiltrates.

The gold standard, however, for the diagnosis of pulmonary infection is still open lung biopsy. This invasive approach is recommended under the following circumstances:

- When patients are hypoxemic despite supplemental oxygen
- When the pulmonary infiltrates are advancing rapidly and a definitive diagnosis is required
- When the patient is unable to cooperate for fiberoptic bronchoscopy

In a review of six published studies of open lung biopsy in immunosuppressed patients, specific diagnoses were found in 55 to 90% of cases, and in a study from the Mayo Clinic, the figure was 81%.[64,66] The procedure is used most frequently in non-AIDS patients who are immunosuppressed, for example, bone marrow transplant recipients who develop a pulmonary infiltrate. The open lung biopsy allows a direct look at the involved lung tissue and also enables the surgeon to control hemostasis. The procedure is generally well tolerated, with pneumothorax being the most frequent complication (approximately 8% incidence). Bleeding complications occur in less than 1% of cases.[64]

The major question that must be asked regarding open lung biopsy is this: Despite its high diagnostic yield, does the information provided substantially alter patient treatment and, most importantly, patient survival? In a retrospective analysis of 64 immunosuppressed patients who had undergone open lung biopsy, the information obtained from the procedure resulted in a change in treatment for 45 of the patients. Only nine of the patients, however, clearly had a beneficial response as a result.[67] A prospective study also addressed this issue. In one arm of the trial, patients were randomized to open lung biopsy, while patients in the other study arm received empiric therapy with trimethoprim-sulfamethoxazole plus erythromycin. If there was no clinical improvement after 4 days of treatment, patients then underwent open lung biopsy.[68] With survival rates as the end point, no significant differences between the two groups were noted.

The final procedure that deserves brief mention is the thoracoscopy-guided biopsy. In one small series in which the procedure was evaluated, a diagnostic yield of 99% was reported, and complication rates were low.[69] More studies, however, are needed to assess the utility of this technique.

It must be stressed that the decisions to proceed with an invasive test and which test to use must be made on an individual basis. The various factors outlined in this section as well as the patient's ultimate prognosis from his or her underlying disease must all be taken into account.

Treatment of Pneumonia

The initiation of therapy to halt the pathophysiologic processes occurring in pneumonia is of paramount importance in the compromised host. As stated previously, mortality can exceed 50% in this patient group. Therapy centers around maintaining adequate ventilatory status, while eradicating the respiratory pathogens. This is accomplished initially with oxygen therapy, antimicrobial agents, and the provision of hemodynamic stability. In an effort to maintain adequate ventilation, the clinician must often decide if admission to the ICU is necessary. In particular, the subsequent decision to provide mechanical ventilatory support for a compromised host may be an onerous one. Subgroups of patients with leukemia, lymphoma, and solid tumors exist within the compromised host population who have a uniformly grim prognosis with little chance of a meaningful recovery, thus making the decision to use mechanical ventilation much more difficult.

Owing to the variety of infectious and noninfectious causes of pulmonary infiltrates in compromised hosts and

Table 22-6. Empiric Therapy for Pneumonia: Antimicrobial Therapy

Host Defect	Focal Infiltrate	Diffuse Infiltrates
Granulocytopenia	Antipseudomonal beta-lactam + aminoglycoside or monotherapy. Add in: amphotericin B if no response by 5–7 days. Then TMP-SMX + erythromycin if still no response by 8 days	Antipseudomonal beta-lactam + aminoglycoside or monotherapy + TMP-SMX + erythromycin. Add in: amphotericin B by 3 days
Granulocytopenia + T-cell defect	Antipseudomonal beta-lactam + aminoglycoside or monotherapy + erythromycin. Add in: amphotericin B by 5–7 days	Antipseudomonal beta-lactam + aminoglycoside or monotherapy + TMP-SMX + erythromycin. Add in: amphotericin B by 3 days ? ganciclovir
T-cell defect	TMP-SMX + erythromycin	TMP-SMX + erythromycin
B-cell defect	Third-generation cephalosporin + erythromycin or cefuroxime + aminoglycoside + erythromycin	Third-generation cephalosporin + erythromycin or cefuroxime + aminoglycoside + erythromycin
Solid tumors (no particular host defect)	Cefuroxime + aminoglycoside or clindamycin + aminoglycoside	Cefuroxime + aminoglycoside + erythromycin or third-generation cephalosporin + erythromycin

TMP-SMX, Trimethoprim-sulfamethoxazole.

the wide spectrum of disease severity observed, the clinician is often faced with diverse therapeutic intervention strategies. With lack of evidence to the contrary, one must always assume that the compromised host with cancer and pulmonary infiltrates is infected until proved otherwise. Therefore therapeutic strategies for the treatment of pulmonary infiltrates focus on antimicrobial therapy. Such therapy may be prescribed empirically (i.e., the exact cause of the pulmonary infiltrate is unknown) or specifically for a known pathogen. The empiric antimicrobial therapy used is predicated on the host's underlying immune defect as outlined in Table 22-6.

Granulocytopenic Hosts

Granulocytes are the most important defense against infection. Granulocytopenia, if present, is the overriding host defense defect predisposing patients with cancer to infection. Because bacteria followed by fungi are the main pathogens encountered in granulocytopenic patients, the incidence and severity of these infections are inversely proportional to the absolute neutrophil count and the duration of granulocytopenia.[70]

In the initial febrile episode of a granulocytopenic patient with a lobar or focal pneumonia, the causative pathogens are usually gram-negative bacilli (Enterobacteriaceae and Pseudomonas aeruginosa), Staphylococcus aureus, and less commonly the opportunistic fungi candida and aspergillus.[71,72] Because gram-negative bacilli aspirated from the upper airways and oropharynx account for a significant portion of the infectious mortality, empiric therapy with broad-spectrum antibiotics active against gram-negative bacilli is a universally accepted principle[73] (see Table 22-6). In choosing the initial empiric antibiotic regimen, one should consider the type, incidence, and antibiotic susceptibilities of the indigenous bacterial isolates usually found in granulocytopenic patients. Other issues also to be considered include penicillin allergy, renal or hepatic dysfunction, and the coadministration of nephrotoxic drugs such as cisplatin. The recommended therapeutic intravenous options are:

- A combination of an aminoglycoside with an antipseudomonal beta-lactam antibiotic

- A combination of two broad-spectrum antipseudomonal beta-lactam antibiotics
- Monotherapy with a single broad-spectrum antipseudomonal beta-lactam antibiotic
- Vancomycin in combination with a broad-spectrum antipseudomonal beta-lactam antibiotic with or without an aminoglycoside[73]

There are potential drawbacks to each of the aforementioned regimens. Aminoglycoside-containing combination regimens are associated with the development of nephrotoxicity and ototoxicity. Double beta-lactam regimens are safe but costly, and the possibility of antagonism of some combinations with certain bacterial infections remains. Finally, definitive data on the efficacy of monotherapy for pneumonia is currently not available. As a result, the specific composition of the empiric regimen remains controversial.

A number of studies have confirmed that response rates for pneumonias in granulocytopenic patients are worse than for other types of infection.[74] Although broad-spectrum synergistic combinations have been demonstrated to be beneficial for patients with rapidly fatal disease and shock,[75] monotherapy for pneumonia with a potent broad-spectrum beta-lactam antibiotic may be equally efficacious. Moreover, the main factor responsible for a favorable response in granulocytopenic patients with pneumonia is neutrophil recovery rather than the empiric regimen used. Monotherapy with ceftazidime, cefoperazone, or imipenem/cilastatin may not suffice for P. aeruginosa pneumonia in a granulocytopenic patient, in whom combination therapy is preferred. For pneumonia caused by known resistant pathogens, therapy should be adjusted accordingly.

Fungal pathogens account for a small proportion of focal pulmonary infiltrates occurring early in the course of granulocytopenia. In one study, only 13% of focal pneumonias were caused by fungi (aspergillus and candida).[72] These infections are usually observed after the first week of profound granulocytopenia. The scenario of persisting fever and granulocytopenia in a patient with leukemia and pulmonary infiltrates unresponsive to 5 to 7 days of antibacterial therapy mandates the empiric initiation of amphotericin B at a dosage of 0.6 to 1 mg/kg/day.[73] In addition, the appearance of a new, localized pulmonary infiltrate and fever in a persistently granulocytopenic individual on antibiotics is likely to be a fungal pneumonia and necessitates the prompt administration of empiric amphotericin B. If the fungal pathogen is known, amphotericin B would still be the choice for susceptible organisms. Pneumonias caused by aspergillus are often relatively more resistant to amphotericin B and require dosages of 1 mg/kg/day. The imidazole antifungals, miconazole and ketoconazole, have produced poor results in granulocytopenic patients with fungal pneumonia.[76] The impact of the new triazoles, such as fluconazole and itraconazole, has yet to be ascertained.

Opportunistic pathogens, such as resistant gram-negative or gram-positive bacteria, Mycoplasma pneumoniae, or Nocardia asteroides, may on rare occasions produce an initial focal pulmonary infiltrate in a granulocytopenic patient. These pneumonias are refractory to the initial empiric antibacterial regimen. When assessed at 48 to 72 hours, the patient remains febrile and clinically unwell. If the pathogen is known, therapy should be directed appropriately. If the organisms are unknown, however, empiric therapy is used. The empiric approach here would once again include the use of amphotericin B. If the clinical picture does not improve within 72 hours of the initiation of amphotericin B, however, one may decide to alter the empiric antibacterial regimen or perform an invasive diagnostic procedure, such as bronchoscopy with bronchoalveolar lavage. The latter consideration would be advisable only if the risk-to-benefit ratio was sufficiently low. Faced with the high risk of complications in granulocytopenic patients, empirically switching to another broad-spectrum antibacterial regimen and adding trimethoprim-sulfamethoxazole (10 to 20 mg/kg/day in four divided doses) plus erythromycin (1 g every 6 hours intravenously) is preferred.

Diffuse pneumonitis in a granulocytopenic patient demands a different therapeutic approach than that outlined for a localized pneumonia. Diffuse disease is more commonly caused by opportunistic pathogens, such as aspergillus, candida, P. carinii, cytomegalovirus, and legionella, or noninfectious processes, such as adult respiratory distress syndrome (ARDS),[77] leukemia, hemorrhage,[72] or nonspecific pneumonitis.[78] In the absence of a known pathogen, empiric therapy for a febrile granulocytopenic patient with diffuse pneumonia should consist of broad-spectrum antibiotic coverage for gram-negative rods as discussed previously, plus trimethoprim-sulfamethoxazole (20 mg/kg/day in four divided doses) with erythromycin (1 g every 6 hours intravenously).[79] Failure to improve on this regimen in 3 days should again prompt a clinician to administer amphotericin B. In situations in which granulocytopenia is combined with an underlying T-cell defect, as in Hodgkin's disease, empiric ganciclovir may also be warranted.

If the diagnostic procedures discussed earlier result in a clearly identifiable pathogen responsible for the diffuse pulmonary infiltrates, therapy can be tailored to the specific pathogen. Nevertheless, broad-spectrum antibiotics are still advocated owing to the presence of granulocytopenia. Erythromycin is used for legionella, mycoplasma, and chlamydia, whereas trimethoprim-sulfamethoxazole is used for P. carinii pneumonia. As discussed previously, amphotericin B remains the gold standard for microbiologically documented fungal pneumonia.

Cell-Mediated Host Defects

For cell-mediated defects in immunocompromised hosts, e.g., those with Hodgkin's lymphoma, therapy for focal pulmonary infiltrates may also be empiric or tailored to a specific pathogen. A reasonable empiric regimen for focal disease is trimethoprim-sulfamethoxazole plus erythromycin.[79] Initially it is unnecessary to augment this regimen with other antibiotics because trimethoprim-sulfamethoxazole provides adequate coverage for S. aureus and many aerobic gram-negative rods with the exception of P. aeruginosa. Moreover, antibiotic treatment can subsequently be easily tailored to a specific pathogen.

Diffuse pulmonary infiltrates in this patient group pose a more difficult therapeutic challenge. The differential diagnosis is extensive and includes both infectious and noninfectious causes. Studies have shown the P. carinii, viruses, mycoplasma, or legionella may represent the most likely infectious causes.[80,81] Here, too, empiric therapy with trimethoprim-sulfamethoxazole and erythromycin has been found to be successful.[78] Early efforts to establish a definitive diagnosis of viral origin, such as cytomegalovirus or tuberculosis, are certainly worthwhile owing to the availability of ganciclovir and antituberculous medication and allow one to avoid drugs with potential adverse effects.

B-Cell Host Defects

B-cell dysfunction, such as is seen in multiple myeloma, classically is complicated by pulmonary infections owing to encapsulated organisms, such as pneumococci, Haemophilus influenzae, and S. aureus. This pattern has changed, however, with an increasing incidence of gram-negative pneumonias.[82] Therefore empiric therapy for both focal and diffuse infiltrates in such individuals must also take these latter pathogens into account. One must also be wary of atypical pathogens, such as legionella or mycoplasma. Possible empiric regimens include a broad-spectrum third-generation cephalosporin plus erythromycin or cefazolin or cefuroxime with an aminoglycoside plus erythromycin. It is noteworthy that more successful outcomes in gram-negative pneumonias are achieved when adequate peak serum aminoglycoside levels are achieved.[83] If a specific pathogen is identified, antibiotic therapy can be modified accordingly.

Solid Tumors

Pneumonias constitute the majority of infections in patients with certain types of solid tumors. Those with head and neck and lung cancers are particularly susceptible.[84,85] For patients with head and neck cancers, therapy should be directed against anaerobes as well as gram-positive cocci and gram-negative rods. Empiric regimens, such as clindamycin with an aminoglycoside, metronidazole with a broad-spectrum third-generation cephalosporin, imipenem-cilastatin, or ticarcillin-clavulanic acid, are reasonable. In patients with lung cancer, gram-positive cocci and gram-negative bacilli are the most common pathogens. Therefore cefazolin or cefuroxime plus an aminoglycoside or a broad-spectrum third-generation cephalosporin are appropriate. Erythromycin should be added if diffuse pulmonary infiltrates are present. Once more, if the cause for the pulmonary infiltrate has been determined, therapy may be modified accordingly.

Although we currently possess potent antimicrobial agents, the mortality rates for pneumonia in immunocompromised patients remains high. Future directions to reduce the high mortalities for pneumonia point to the use of immune modulating agents. A human monoclonal IgM antibody, HA-1A, has been demonstrated to reduce mortality rates in patients with gram-negative bacteremia and septic shock,[86] but unfortunately it has been withdrawn from investigation. This antibody has some activity against tumor necrosis factor, which plays a role in the pathogenesis of ARDS.[87] Inhibitors of platelet activating factor, reactive oxygen metabolites, neutrophil proteases, and interleukin-8 used as a cocktail may also prove beneficial in gram-negative pneumonia and ARDS[88] in the future.

ICU ADMISSION

One of the key decisions to be made by a clinician in the management of the cancer patient with pneumonia is whether admission to the ICU is required. Criteria for admission may include:

- Hemodynamic instability
- Respiratory failure requiring mechanical ventilation
- An FIO_2 >0.40 to maintain a PaO_2 >70 mm Hg
- Severe electrolyte abnormalities requiring close monitoring
- Continuing hemorrhage

Because of often severe underlying systemic illness (cancer), clinicians may consider withholding life-support measures. Mechanical ventilatory support is a particularly vexing problem in patients afflicted with cancer and having a limited life expectancy. One may have to balance the use of life-sustaining supportive action, such as mechanical ventilation, versus prolongation of the dying process at the cost of unnecessary suffering and loss of dignity for the patient. Moreover, the cost-to-benefit ratio for such patients cannot be ignored in the present era of spiraling medical costs. Caring for some patients may be 100 times more expensive than caring for others, at a time when resources are limited.[89] Clinicians must also be cognizant of the fact that once mechanical ventilation has been instituted, withdrawal of this supportive action may produce considerable stress and anguish for both health care personnel and relatives.[90] These decisions are difficult under the duress of patient physical decompensation.

A review of the literature demonstrates that cancer patients have a grim prognosis when admitted to the ICU with respiratory problems. Turnbull and coworkers[91] and Snow and colleagues[92] reviewed respiratory failure among cancer patients in the ICU setting and noted mortality rates of 22.3 and 26%. Both studies commented that the mortality rates were comparable with historical rates of other patient groups. Hauser et al.,[93] however, in a case-control analysis found a higher fatality rate among patients with cancer (55%) than those without cancer (17%).[93] Moreover, patients with cancer and respiratory failure (75%) or respiratory failure due to ARDS (86%) had the highest mortality rates. It is evident that granulocytopenic patients with leukemia and lymphoma who develop acute respiratory failure owing to an infectious cause and require mechanical ventilation have a uniformly grave prognosis.[94] Poor survival rates have also been observed for nonsurgical lung cancer patients with respiratory failure.[95] Those patients with cancer without respiratory failure have mortality rates comparable to those patients without cancer (25 versus 17%).[93] Patients admitted to the ICU for intensive monitoring or for antineoplastic chemotherapy fare well.[96]

The critical care physician therefore faces a formidable challenge in assessing a cancer patient for admission to the ICU. Clearly, patients with malignant disease who have exhausted all therapeutic options and are destined to die within a short time are low priorities for an ICU admission, whereas patients sustaining complications of an initial course of aggressive antineoplastic chemotherapy that are theoretically reversible and for whom hope for remission exists are almost always candidates for admission.[89] For patients who lie between the two extremes, the use of the acute physiology assessment and chronic health evaluation (APACHE II)[97] may be helpful in making a decision about ICU admission. Although no "magical" APACHE II score may ever be determined for withholding necessary life support or denying cancer patients access to the ICU, an elevated score may provide evidence for making an educated decision about the prognosis of cancer patients with respiratory failure. In addition, such information may be used to convey an accurate prognosis to the patient's family members so a rational decision about care measures can be made in this crisis situation. Cancer patients are nevertheless entitled to ICU care and the life-supportive measures offered in this unit just as other types of patients are, if there is a reasonable expectation of recovery.

ICU PHASE ("SUPPORTIVE PHASE")

Infection Control

With the initiation of antimicrobial therapy, admission to the ICU, and stabilization of the patient's status, the "risk phase" of pneumonia in the cancer patient blends into the next phase of clinical management—the ICU or "support" phase. The support phase revolves around supportive care measures and monitoring of the patient, including hemodynamic, respiratory, laboratory, nutritional, and neurologic monitoring. These issues are not addressed here because they are dealt with elsewhere. An often forgotten aspect of supportive care for cancer patients in the ICU, however, is infection control measures.

Infection control measures have a direct impact on the care of cancer patients in the ICU. Microorganisms may be acquired from the ICU environment or health care personnel.[98] Often multiply-resistant organisms are indigenous to the ICU, and these organisms colonize cancer patients. These colonizers may later be implicated as the pathogens responsible for bacteremia and pneumonia, particularly in granulocytopenic patients.[99] As a result, the basic infection control tenet to be followed by health care personnel in caring for cancer patients is excellent handwashing technique.[100] Handwashing reduces the interpersonal transmission of organisms. Gloves are useful adjuncts for personnel with open skin lesions or dermatitis. Other techniques, such as reverse isolation, are of little benefit.[101]

When caring for granulocytopenic patients who have been treated in a high efficiency particulate arresting (HEPA) filtered environment, an ICU should have facilities to maintain such a protective environment. HEPA filtration has been demonstrated to reduce the incidence of infectious complications[102] and invasive aspergillosis[103] in granulocytopenic individuals.

At times, other specific infection control measures must be adopted for cancer patients in the ICU. Specific respiratory precautions used by health care personnel, including the donning of masks and sometimes gowns, are required for patients with tuberculous pneumonia. Infections caused by methicillin-resistant S. aureus mandate the use of contact isolation, although some institutions have adopted strict isolation procedures involving hats, masks, gowns, and gloves.

Another important infection control principle regarding cancer patients in the ICU setting is the avoidance of any unnecessary devices. Contaminated devices and solutions used with these devices are potential sources of nosocomial pathogens. Devices that circumvent host defenses or facilitate the entry of bacteria or fungi into normally sterile areas are of particular concern. Such problems are magnified in granulocytopenic patients owing to their lack of cellular defenses. Nasogastric tubes and enteral feeding, resuscitation bags, Foley catheters, and endotracheal tubes may all increase the risk of infection.[104] Although such devices may be necessary initially, they should be removed as quickly as possible to reduce the risks of nosocomial infection in the ICU setting.

Clinical Re-Evaluation During Support Phase

With the initiation of antimicrobial therapy, admission to the ICU, and establishment of appropriate monitoring, the patient may stabilize. During the following 72 hours, the patient is closely evaluated for signs of response to pneumonia therapy. Some of the results of bacterial, fungal, and viral studies become known by the end of this time period and provide new data to facilitate therapeutic decisions. Antimicrobial therapy may then be tailored based on clinical information about the specific pathogen(s) causing pneumonia. Often refinements are made to the regimen with the deletion or addition of antimicrobial agents. If improvement continues, antimicrobial therapy is maintained for at least 10 to 14 days in most instances of bacterial infection. Treatment for P. carinii and viral pneumonias is also approximately 14 days in cancer patients, whereas therapy for fungal pneumonias is usually considerably longer. As improvement accelerates, the patient's course moves into the rehabilitative phase.

Improvement in the patient's condition is not guaranteed. Deterioration in the patient's clinical status at the 72-hour mark after ICU admission may occur. Faced with this situation, ICU physicians must decide on a course of action. If further information from cultures is not forthcoming,[105] the physician has three alternatives: Continue the current treatment and watch the patient deteriorate; seek further clinical information, i.e., proceed to an invasive diagnostic procedure; or prescribe additional empiric therapy. The first alternative may be chosen if a decision not to pursue further aggressive therapy has been made. This may be a reasonable decision if a patient has been admitted to the ICU as a medical emergency, and it has become evident or been requested that heroic measures should not be pursued.

Choosing between the latter two alternatives may prove difficult in cancer patients. At times, an empiric approach is advisable if coagulopathy, refractory thrombocytopenia, or profound respiratory compromise make the risk of an invasive procedure too great, and the results are unlikely to change the final outcome. In other situations, such as diffuse pulmonary infiltrates, both alternatives may be options. Yet the use of an invasive diagnostic procedure must be carefully weighed.

One may consider an escalating approach to the invasive diagnostic procedures recognizing that bronchoscopy with bronchoalveolar lavage may yield clinically significant information but is less invasive than open lung biopsy. If therapy was begun empirically, bronchoscopy with bronchoalveolar lavage should be considered. Similarly if bronchoscopy with bronchoalveolar lavage had initially failed to provide an answer, escalation to bronchoscopy with transbronchial biopsy and finally open lung biopsy may be warranted. Often, however, a clinician does not have the luxury of enough time for this escalating approach and merely opts for the gold standard, which is open lung biopsy. The risk of the morbidity of an open lung biopsy for pulmonary infiltrates, which may be of infectious or noninfectious origin, should be counterbalanced by the benefit of establishing a definitive diagnosis. Clearly the deciding factor is whether open lung biopsy will affect the patient's outcome.

The literature on the use of open lung biopsy in cancer patients is hampered by the lumping together of different subsets of patients. If one focuses on the experience of patients with acute leukemia and granulocytopenia, open lung biopsy was of little help in directing medical therapy or influencing clinical outcome.[106,107] Among nongranulocytopenic patients, survival was greater (83 versus 67%) and complications fewer in a randomized trial comparing empiric therapy with open lung biopsy.[107] In the subset of patients who did not improve after 4 days of empiric treatment, open lung biopsy established a diagnosis in 75%. Nevertheless, no change in therapy was made because patients were already receiving appropriate therapy before the open lung biopsy. As a result, it appears that open lung biopsy will establish a diagnosis but not have a major impact in altering therapy. Using empiric therapy for patients may be preferred.[68,107] Particularly in granulocytopenic cancer patients with focal or diffuse infiltrates, one is far less likely to use an invasive procedure that has a narrow margin of safety and will not have an impact on therapy.

Table 22–7. Summary of Prophylaxis

	Acute Nonlymphocytic Leukemia	Acute Lymphocytic Leukemia, Lymphoma	Solid Tumors
Antibacterial	Ciprofloxacin*	TMP-SMX†	Ciprofloxacin
Antifungal	Fluconazole‡	Fluconazole	Fluconazole
Antiviral—herpes simplex	Acyclovir§	Acyclovir	Acyclovir

* Ciprofloxacin, 500 mg b.i.d. po.
† TMP-SMX (trimethoprim-sulfamethoxazole), 160/400 mg b.i.d. po.
‡ Fluconazole, 400 mg once daily.
§ Acyclovir, 400 mg b.i.d.

Superinfection

Although cancer patients benefit from close monitoring with invasive devices in the ICU setting, this care is not without risk. Superinfections in the ICU are common, serious complications. Superinfections may be acquired in the ICU secondary to the use of invasive devices, such as central venous catheters, arterial catheters, indwelling bladder catheters, or endotracheal tubes, or they may be endogenous in nature, for example, a fungal superinfection in a granulocytopenic patient. Whatever the origin, such infections can prove devastating in the cancer patient recovering from a pneumonia. Not only may these infections prolong ICU stay, but superinfections have a negative impact on the probability of final recovery.

The most recent National Nosocomial Infections Surveillance System information regarding nosocomial infections in the ICU found that P. aeruginosa, S. aureus, coagulase-negative staphylococci, enterococci, Enterobacteriaceae, and Candida albicans were the most common pathogen.[108] ICU physicians must be mindful of the spectrum of pathogens and be cognizant of multiply-resistant organisms indigenous to their ICUs. For example, central-catheter-related sepsis due to methicillin-resistant, coagulase-negative staphylococci has become the scourge of many ICUs.

Physicians must be particularly vigilant about pulmonary superinfections in cancer patients with pneumonia. Should this occur, both the diagnostic and therapeutic decision-making processes must once again be undertaken. Mortality is greatly increased in such situations.[108]

POST-ICU, REHABILITATIVE PHASE

With resolution of pneumonia and the weaning of the patient from life support systems, consideration is given to the patient's discharge from the ICU. Although antimicrobial therapy may be continued, the patient has passed the "crisis" stage. With discharge from the ICU, the patient's potential risks diminish, and the rehabilitative phase commences.

Decisions about the duration of antimicrobial therapy are finalized during this phase. As mentioned previously, antimicrobial therapy for pneumonia in a cancer patient may extend from 10 days to several months depending on the origin of the infectious process. Although therapy must be given via the parenteral route during the risk and support phases, efforts to switch to oral therapy are appropriate during the rehabilitative phase. In addition, increasing mobilization of the patient and an exercise physiotherapy program are warranted. The mobilization process may be slow, particularly for the individual with diffuse pulmonary infiltrates in whom residual fibrosis remains. Patients should be counseled regarding their expected rate of recovery and final performance status.

Because the patient's underlying malignancy may remain, and thus the possibility of further infections may loom in the future, it is prudent for physicians to educate their patients about their future potential susceptibility to infection. Avoidance of large crowds or exposure to friends or family members with infections is advisable. As well, prophylactic antimicrobial agents are useful should there be exposure to subsequent antineoplastic chemotherapy.[110] A scheme of prophylactic antimicrobials based on underlying malignancy is provided in Table 22–7.

Pneumonia places the compromised cancer patient at great risk of developing life-threatening respiratory and hemodynamic compromise. The most likely causative agents of pneumonia are predicted on the host's underlying immunologic deficiency. Diagnostic and therapeutic decisions may be difficult in oncology patients because clinicians must carefully weigh the risk-to-benefit ratio of each decision for the patient. At times, invasive procedures, such as bronchoscopy or open lung biopsy, are warranted, whereas in other situations, empiric therapy or no therapy at all is appropriate. Cancer patients are entitled to admission to the ICU based on the probability that there is an expectation of recovery from the acute illness and a reasonable duration of life and some quality of life after discharge from the hospital. Adherence to good infection control practices may optimize the ICU phase of supportive care and prevent superinfections. Management of pneumonia in cancer patients in the ICU calls for a collaborative approach owing to the high mortality associated with this clinical entity. The rehabilitative phase may be prolonged in these patients owing to their underlying disease state. In the future, it is hoped that we will continue to make advances in the management of pneumonias in cancer patients.

REFERENCES

1. Mackowiak, P. A.: The normal microbial flora. N. Engl. J. Med., *307*:83, 1982.
2. Dinarello, C. A.: Interleuklin-1 and the pathogenesis of the acute-phase response. N. Engl. J. Med., *311*:1413, 1984.
3. Reichert, U., Saint Leger, D., and Schaeffer, H.: Skin surface chemistry and microbial infection. Semin. Dermatol., *1*:91, 1982.
4. Schumacher, M. J.: Serum immunoglobulin and transferrin

levels after childhood splenectomy. Arch. Dis. Child., 45: 114, 1970.
5. Naijar, V. A., and Fridkin, M.: Antineoplastic, immunogenic and other effects of tetrapeptide tuftsin: a natural macrophage activator. Ann. N. Y. Acad. Sci., 419:1, 1983.
6. Phillips, I., and Wharton, B.: Acute bacterial infection in kwashiorkor and marasmus. Br. Med. J., 1:407, 1968.
7. Edelman, R., Suskind, R., Olson, R. E., and Sirisinka, S.: Mechanisms of defective delayed cutaneous hypersensitivity in children with protein-calorie malnutrition. Lancet, 1: 506, 1973.
8. Deo, M. G., Bhan, I., and Ramalingaswami, V.: Influence of dietary protein on phagocytic activity of the reticuloendothelial cells. J. Pathol., 109:215, 1973.
9. Tan, J. S., Anderson, J. L., Watanakunakorn, C., and Phair, J. P.: Neutrophil dysfunction in diabetes mellitus. J. Lab. Clin. Med., 85:26, 1975.
10. Clark, R. A., Kimball, H. R., and Decker, J. L.: Neutrophil chemotaxis in systemic lupus erythematosus. Ann. Rheum. Dis., 33:167, 1974.
11. Perez, H. D., Lipton, M., and Goldstein, I. M.: A specific inhibitor of complement (C5) derived chemotactic activity in serum from patients with systemic lupus erythematosus. Clin. Res., 26:519A, 1978.
12. Zurier, R. B.: Reduction of phagocytosis and lysosomal enzyme release from human leucocytes by serum from patients with lupus erythematosus. Arthritis Rheum., 19:73, 1976.
13. Mowat, A. G., and Baum, J.: Chemotaxis of polymorphonuclear leukocytes from patients with rheumatoid arthritis. J. Clin. Invest., 59:2541, 1971.
14. BarEli, M., Ehrenfeld, M., Litvin, Y., and Gallily, R.: Monocyte function in rheumatoid arthritis. Scand. J. Rheumatol., 9:17, 1980.
15. Salant, D. J., et al.: Depressed neutrophil chemotaxis in patients with chronic renal failure and after renal transplantation. J. Lab. Clin. Med., 88:536, 1976.
16. Boulton-Jones, J. M., Vick, R., Cameron, J. S., and Black, P. J.: Immune response in uremia. Clin. Nephrol., 1:351, 1973.
17. Laurenzi, G. A., and Guarneri, J. J.: Effects of bacteria and viruses on ciliated epithelium. A study of the mechanisms of pulmonary resistance to infection: the relationship of bacterial clearance to ciliary and alveolar macrophage function. Am. Rev. Respir. Dis., 93:134, 1966.
18. Brayton, R. G., Stokes, P. E., Schwartz, M. S., and Louria, D. B.: Effect of alcohol and various diseases on leukocyte mobilization phagocytosis and intracellular bacterial killing. N. Engl. J. Med., 282:123, 1970.
19. Fauci, A. S.: Mechanism of the immunosuppressive and anti-inflammatory effects of glucocorticosteroids. J. Immunopharmacol., 1:1, 1967.
20. Karp, J. E., et al.: Empiric use of vancomycin during prolonged treatment-induced granulocytopenia. Am. J. Med., 81:237, 1986.
21. Schimpff, S. C.: Therapy of infection in patients with granulocytopenia. Med. Clin. North Am., 61:1101, 1978.
22. Cline, M. J.: A test of individual phagocyte function in a mixed population of leukocytes. Identifications of a neutrophil abnormality in acute myelocytic leukemia. J. Lab. Clin. Med., 81:311, 1973.
23. Engleman, E. J., et al.: Autologous mixed lymphocyte reaction in patients with Hodgkin's disease. J. Clin. Invest., 66: 149, 1980.
24. Owens, A. H.: The malignant lymphomas. In The Principles and Practice of Medicine. 22nd Ed. Edited by A. McHarvey, et al. East Norwalk, Appleton & Lange, 1988.
25. Singer, C., Kaplan, M. H., and Armstrong, D.: Bacteremia and fungemia complicating neoplastic disease. Am. J. Med., 62:731, 1977.
26. Sickles, E. A., Youong, V. M., Greene, W. H., and Wiernik, P. H.: Pneumonia in acute leukemia. Ann. Intern. Med., 79: 528, 1973.
27. Bishop, J. F., Schimpff, S. C., Diggs, C. H., and Wiernik, P. H.: Infections during intensive chemotherapy for non-Hodgkin's lymphoma. Ann. Intern. Med., 95:549, 1981.
28. Toews, G. B.: Determinants of bacterial clearance from the lower respiratory tract. Semin. Respir. Infect., 1:68, 1986.
29. Reynolds, H. Y.: Normal and defective respiratory host defenses. In Respiratory Infections: Diagnosis and Management. 2nd Ed. Edited by J. E. Pennington. New York, Raven Press, 1989.
30. Reynolds, H. Y., et al.: Receptors for immunoglobulin and complement on human alveolar macrophages. J. Immunol., 114:1813, 1975.
31. Nathan, C. F., Murray, H. W., and Cohn, Z. A.: The macrophage as an effector cell. N. Engl. J. Med., 303:622, 1980.
32. Perlo, S., Jalowayski, A. A., Durand, C. M., and West, J. B.: Distribution of red and white blood cells in alveolar walls. J. Appl. Physiol., 38:117, 1975.
33. Lehrer, R. I., et al.: Neutrophils and host defense. Ann. Intern. Med., 109:127, 1988.
34. Golde, D. W., Finley, T. N., and Cline, M. J.: The pulmonary macrophage in acute leukemia. N. Engl. J. Med., 290:875, 1974.
35. Johanson, W. G., Jr., Pierce, A. K., Sanford, J. P., and Thomas, G. D.: Nosocomial respiratory infections with gram-negative bacilli. Ann. Intern. Med., 77:701, 1972.
36. Pennington, J. E.: Nosocomial respiratory infection. In Principles and Practice of Infectious Diseases. 3rd Ed. Edited by G. L. Mandell, R. G. Douglas, Jr., and J. E. Bennett. New York, Churchill Livingstone, 1990.
37. Pennington, J. E.: Opportunistic fungal pneumonias. In Respiratory Infections: Diagnosis and Management. 2nd Ed. Edited by J. E. Pennington. New York, Raven Press, 1989.
38. Young, L. S.: Pneumocystis carinii. In Respiratory Infections: Diagnosis and Management. 2nd Ed. Edited by J. E. Pennington. New York, Raven Press, 1989.
39. Ramsey, P. G., et al.: Herpes simplex virus pneumonia: clinical, virologic and pathologic features in 20 patients. Ann. Intern. Med., 97:813, 1982.
40. Johanson, W. G., Pierce, A. K., and Sanford, J. P.: Changing pharyngeal bacterial flora of hospitalized patients: emergence of gram negative bacilli. N. Engl. J. Med., 281:1137, 1969.
41. Woods, D. E., Straus, D. C., Johanson, W. G., Jr., and Bass, J. A.: Role of fibronectin in the prevention of adherence of Pseudomonas aeruginosa to buccal cells. J. Infect. Dis., 143: 784, 1981.
42. Woods, D. E., Straus, D. C., Johanson, W. G., Jr., and Bass, J. A.: The role of salivary protease activity in adherence of gram negative bacilli to mammalian buccal epithelial cells in vivo. J. Clin. Invest., 68:1435, 1981.
43. Dal Nogare, A. R., Toews, G. B., and Pierce, A. K.: Increased salivary elastase precedes gram-negative bacillary colonization in post-operative patients. Am. Rev. Respir. Dis., 135: 671, 1987.
44. du Moulin, G. C., Paterson, D. G., Hedley-Whyte, J., and Lisbon, A.: Aspiration of gastric bacteria in antacid-treated patients: a frequent cause of postoperative colonization of the airway. Lancet, 1:242, 1982.
45. Snepar, R., et al.: Effect of cimetidine and antacid on gastric microbial flora. Infect. Immunol., 36:518, 1982.
46. Goularte, T. A., Lichtenberg, D. A., and Craven, D. E.: Gastric colonization in patients receiving antacids and mechani-

46. cal ventilation: A mechanism for pharyngeal colonization. Am. J. Infect. Control, 14:88, 1986.
47. Daschner, F., et al.: Stress ulcer prophylaxis and ventilation pneumonia: prevention by antibacterial cytoprotective agents? Infect. Control Hosp. Epidemiol., 9:59, 1988.
48. Driks, M. R., et al.: Nosocomial pneumonia in intubated patients given sucralfate as compared with antacids or histamine type 2 blockers. N. Engl. J. Med., 317:1376, 1987.
49. Rubin, R. H., and Greene, R.: Etiology and management of the compromised patient with fever and pulmonary infiltrates. In Clinical Approach to Infection in the Compromised Host. 2nd Ed. Edited by R. H. Rubin and L. S. Young. New York, Plenum Medical Book Company, 1988.
50. Fanta, C. H., and Pennington, J. E.: Pneumonia in the immunocompromised host. In Respiratory Infections: Diagnosis & Management. 2nd Ed. Edited by J. E. Pennington. New York, Raven Press, 1989.
51. Bodey, G. P., Buckley, M., Sathe, Y. S., and Freireich, E. J.: Quantitative relationships between circulating leukocytes and infection in patients with acute leukemia. Ann. Intern. Med., 64:328, 1966.
52. Sinclair, A. J., Rosoff, A. H., and Coltman, C. A.: Recognition and successful management in pulmonary aspergillosis in leukemia. Cancer, 42:2019, 1978.
53. Murray, P. R., and Washington, J. A., III: Microscopic and bacteriologic analysis of expectorated sputum. Mayo Clin. Proc., 50:339, 1975.
54. Gerding, D. N. (ed.): Diagnosis of pneumonia. Semin. Respir. Infect., 3, 1988.
55. Singer, C., et al.: Diffuse pulmonary infiltrates in immunosuppressive patients: prospective study of 80 cases. Am. J. Med., 66:110, 1979.
56. Bartlett, J. G.: Diagnostic accuracy of transtracheal aspiration bacteriologic studies. Am. Rev. Respir. Dis., 115:777, 1977.
57. Zavala, D. C., and Schoebl, J. E.: Ultrathin needle aspiration of the lung in infectious and malignant disease. Am. Rev. Respir. Dis., 123:125, 1981.
58. Castellino, R. A., and Blank, N.: Etiologic diagnosis of focal pulmonary infections in immunocompromised patients by fluoroscopically guided percutaneous needle aspiration. Radiology, 132:563, 1979.
59. Bartlett, J. G.: Invasive diagnostic techniques in pulmonary infections. In Respiratory Infections: Diagnosis and Management. 2nd Ed. Edited by J. E. Pennington. New York, Raven Press, 1989.
60. Pollock, H. M., et al.: Diagnosis of bacterial pulmonary infections with quantitative protected catheter cultures obtained during bronchoscopy. J. Clin. Microbiol., 17:255, 1983.
61. Williams, D., et al.: The role of fiberoptic bronchoscopy in the evaluation of immunocompromised hosts with diffuse pulmonary infiltrates. Am. Rev. Respir. Dis., 131:880, 1985.
62. Bartlett, J. G., et al.: Should fiberoptic bronchoscopy aspirates be cultured? Am. Rev. Respir. Dis., 114:73, 1976.
63. Lorch, D. G., et al.: Protected transbronchial needle aspiration and protected specimen brush in the diagnosis of pneumonia. Am. Rev. Respir. Dis., 136:565, 1987.
64. Matthay, R. A., and Moritz, E. D.: Invasive procedures for diagnosing pulmonary infection. A critical review. Clin. Chest Med., 2:3, 1981.
65. McKenna, R. J., Jr., Campbell, A., McMurtrey, J. J., and Mountain, C. F.: Diagnosis for interstitial lung disease in patients with acquired immunodeficiency syndrome (AIDS): A prospective comparison of bronchial washings, alveolar lavage, transbronchial lung biopsy and open lung biopsy. Am. Thorac. Surg., 41:318, 1986.
66. Cockerill, F. R., et al.: Open lung biopsy in immunocompromised patients. Arch. Intern. Med., 145:1398, 1985.
67. Hiatt, J. R., Gong, H., Mulder, D. G., and Ramming, K. P.: The value of open lung biopsy in the immunosuppressed patient. Surgery, 92:285, 1982.
68. Potter, D., et al.: Prospective randomized study of open lung biopsy versus empirical antibiotic therapy for acute pneumonitis in nonneutropenic cancer patients. Am. Thorac. Surg., 40:422, 1985.
69. Dijkman, J. H., et al.: Transpleural lung biopsy by the thoracoscopic route in patients with diffuse interstitial pulmonary disease. Chest, 82:76, 1982.
70. Bodey, G. P., Buckley, M., Sathe, Y. S., and Freireich, E. J.: Quantitative relationships between circulated leukocytes and infections in patients with acute leukemia. Ann. Intern. Med., 64:329, 1966.
71. Pennington, J. E., and Feldman, N. T.: Pulmonary infiltrates and fever in patients with hematologic malignancy: assessment of transbronchial biopsy. Am. J. Med., 62:581, 1977.
72. Tenholder, M. F., and Hooper, R. G.: Pulmonary infiltrates in leukemia. Chest, 78:469, 1980.
73. Hughes, W. T., et al.: Guidelines for the use of antimicrobial agents in neutropenic patients with unexplained fever. J. Infect. Dis., 161:381, 1990.
74. Bodey, G. P., et al.: Beta-lactam regimens for the febrile neutropenic patient. Cancer, 65:9, 1990.
75. Anderson, E. T., Young, L. S., and Hewitt, W. L.: Antimicrobial synergism in the therapy of gram-negative rod bacteremia. Chemotherapy, 24:45, 1978.
76. Fainstein, V., et al.: Amphotericin B or ketoconazole therapy of fungal infections in neutropenic cancer patients. Antimicrob. Agents Chemother., 31:11, 1987.
77. Ognibene, F. P., et al.: Adult respiratory distress syndrome in patients with severe neutropenia. N. Engl. J. Med., 315:547, 1986.
78. Browne, M. J., et al.: A randomized trial of open lung biopsy versus empiric antimicrobial therapy in cancer patients with diffuse pulmonary infiltrates. J. Clin. Oncol., 8:222, 1990.
79. Masur, H., Shelhammer, J., and Parillo, J. E.: The management of pneumonias in immuncompromised patients. JAMA, 253:1769, 1985.
80. Singer, C., et al.: Diffuse pulmonary infiltrates in immunosuppressed patients: Prospective study of 80 cases. Am. J. Med., 66:110, 1979.
81. Brown, M. J., et al.: Excess prevalence of pneumocystis carinii pneumonia in patients treated for lymphoma with combination chemotherapy. Ann. Intern. Med., 103:338, 1986.
82. Shaikh, B. S., Lombard, R. M., Appelbaum, P. C., and Bentz, M. S.: Changing patterns of infections in patients with multiple myeloma. Oncology, 39:78, 1982.
83. Moore, R. D., Smith, C. R., and Lietman, P. S.: Association of aminoglycoside plasma levels with therapeutic outcome in gram-negative pneumonia. Am. J. Med., 77:657, 1984.
84. Hussain, M., et al.: The role of infection in the morbidity and mortality of patients with head and neck cancer undergoing multimodality therapy. Cancer, 66:593, 1991.
85. Perlin, E., et al.: The impact of pulmonary infections on the survival of lung cancer patients. Cancer, 66:593, 1990.
86. Ziegler, E. J., et al.: Treatment of gram-negative bacteremia and septic shock with HA-1A human monoclonal antibody against endotoxin: A randomized, double-blind, placebo-controlled trial. N. Engl. J. Med., 324:429, 1991.
87. Marks, J. D., Marks, C. B., and Luce, J. M.: Plasma tumor necrosis factor in patients with septic shock. Am. Rev. Respir. Dis., 141:94, 1990.

88. Streiter, R. M., et al.: Host responses in mediating sepsis and adult respiratory distress syndrome. Semin. Respir. Infect., 5:233, 1990.
89. Carlon, G. C.: Admitting cancer patients to the intensive care unit. Crit. Care Clin., 4:183, 1988.
90. Youngner, S. J., et al.: Resolving problems at the intensive care unit/oncology unit interface. Perspect. Biol. Med., 31:299, 1988.
91. Turnbull, A., Goldiner, P., Silverman, D., and Howland, W.: The role of an intensive care unit in a cancer center: An analysis of 1,035 critically ill patients treated for life threatening complications. Cancer, 37:82, 1976.
92. Snow, R. M., Miller, W. C., Rice, D. L., and Ali, K.: Respiratory failure in cancer patients. JAMA, 241:2039, 1979.
93. Hauser, M. J., Tabak, J., and Baier, H.: Survival of patients with cancer in a medical critical care unit. Arch. Intern. Med., 142:527, 1982.
94. Schuster, D. P., and Marion, J. M.: Precedents for meaningful recovery during treatment in a medical intensive care unit: outcome in patients with hematologic malignancy. Am. J. Med., 75:402, 1983.
95. Ewer, M. S., et al.: Outcome of lung cancer patients requiring mechanical ventilation for pulmonary failure. JAMA, 256:3364, 1986.
96. Sculier, J. P., et al.: Role of intensive care unit in a medical oncology department. Eur. J. Clin. Oncol., 24:513, 1988.
97. Knaus, W. A., Draper, E. A., Wagner, D. P., and Zimmerman, J. E.: APACHE II: a severity of disease classification system for acutely ill patients. Crit. Care Med., 6:685, 1985.
98. Maki, D. G.: Control of colonization and transmission of pathogenic bacteria in the hospital. Ann. Intern. Med., 89:777, 1978.
99. Bodey, G. P.: Antibiotics in patients with neutropenia. Arch. Intern. Med., 144:1845, 1984.
100. Steere, A. C., and Mallison, G. F.: Handwashing practices for prevention of nosocomial infections. Ann. Intern. Med., 83:683, 1975.
101. Nauseef, W. M., and Maki, D. G.: A study of the value of simple protective isolation in patients with granulocytopenia. N. Engl. J. Med., 304:448, 1981.
102. Buckner, C. D., et al.: Protective environment for marrow transplant recipients: A prospective study. Ann. Intern. Med., 304:448, 1981.
103. Rhame, F. S., et al.: Extrinsic risk factors for pneumonia in the patient at high risk of infection. Am. J. Med., 76:42, 1984.
104. Craven, D. E., Barber, T. W., Steger, K. A., and Montecalvo, M. A.: Nosocomial pneumonia in the 1990s: update of epidemiology and risk factors. Semin. Respir. Infect., 5:157, 1990.
105. Bustamante, C. I., and Wade, J. C.: Treatment of interstitial pneumonia in cancer patients: is empiric antibiotic therapy the answer. J. Clin. Oncol., 8:200, 1990.
106. McCabe, R. E., Brooks, R. G., Mark, J. B. D., and Remington, J. S.: Open lung biopsy in patients with acute leukemia. Am. J. Med., 78:609, 1985.
107. Browne, M. J., et al.: A randomized trial of open lung biopsy versus empiric antimicrobial therapy in cancer patients with diffuse pulmonary infiltrates. J. Clin. Oncol., 8:222, 1990.
108. Horan, T., et al.: Pathogens causing nosocomial infections: preliminary data from the National Nosocomial Infections Surveillance System. Antimicrob. Newslett., 5:65, 1988.
109. Craven, D. E., et al.: Nosocomial infection and fatality in medical and surgical intensive care unit patients. Arch. Intern. Med., 148:1161, 1988.
110. Bodey, G. P.: Antimicrobial prophylaxis for infection in neutropenic patients in current clinical topics in infectious diseases. Edited by J. S. Remington and M. N. Swartz. New York, McGraw-Hill, 1988.

Chapter 23

PULMONARY EMBOLISM: PREVENTION, DIAGNOSIS, AND MANAGEMENT IN THE CRITICALLY ILL

GARY E. RASKOB
J. DEAN SANDHAM
RUSSELL D. HULL

The management of venous thromboembolism in the critically ill is a challenging problem. Diagnosis may be difficult because definitive tests such as pulmonary angiography and venography may be contraindicated or impractical, and lung scanning and noninvasive tests for venous thrombosis have some practical limitations in the critically ill. Patients in the intensive care unit (ICU) may be at high risk of bleeding with anticoagulant or thrombolytic therapy because of their underlying disorder (e.g., recent surgery or trauma, gastrointestinal bleeding, etc.) or the presence of invasive lines. This chapter addresses two main themes:

- The diagnosis and management of patients who present with clinically suspected life-threatening pulmonary embolism
- The prevention, diagnosis, and management of venous thrombosis and pulmonary embolism in patients who are hemodynamically stable, but who require the ICU for management of their primary illness

The chapter is organized into three sections. In the first section, on the pre-ICU phase, the natural history and clinical course, risk factors, and prevention of venous thromboembolism are reviewed. In the second section, on the ICU phase, the management of patients with clinically suspected pulmonary embolism or venous thrombosis is discussed, and the initial treatment of patients with established venous thromboembolism is described. In the third section, on the post-ICU phase, the long-term treatment of patients with venous thromboembolism is reviewed.

In making specific recommendations, the strength of the evidence from clinical trials is considered. To qualify the strength of the evidence supporting a recommendation, we used the "Levels of Evidence" approach adopted by the American College of Chest Physicians for the consensus conference on antithrombotic therapy.[1] The definitions of levels I to V evidence are shown in Table 23-1. A firm recommendation is made when it is supported by the findings of adequately designed and executed clinical trials (level I evidence). It is recognized, however, that the ICU physician may often be forced to make clinical decisions in the absence of definitive data (level I evidence). When definitive data from clinical trials are unavailable, possible options will be discussed, and the level of evidence supporting these options will be specified.

PRE-ICU PHASE

Pulmonary embolism is a leading cause of death in hospitals and is responsible for 100,000 or more deaths each year in the United States.[2] Many such deaths occur in terminally ill patients, but a significant proportion occur in patients who otherwise would have survived to lead a normal life (e.g., patients undergoing elective major orthopedic surgery). Most patients who die from pulmonary embolism succumb abruptly or within two hours after the acute event,[3] before therapy can be initiated or take effect. Prevention is the key to reducing death and morbidity from venous thromboembolism. This applies both to patients outside the ICU and also to patients in the ICU who are at high risk for venous thromboembolism because of their primary medical or surgical illness.

Natural History and Clinical Course of Venous Thromboembolism

Venous thrombosis of the leg may occur in the superficial veins, the deep veins of the calf (calf vein thrombosis), or the popliteal or more proximal deep veins (proximal vein thrombosis). Superficial thrombophlebitis may occur with or without associated deep vein thrombosis; in the absence of associated deep vein thrombosis, it is usually benign and self-limiting. Deep vein thrombosis which remains confined to the calf veins is associated with a low risk (<1%) of clinically important pulmonary embolism.[4-8] Untreated, however, 20 to 30% of calf vein thrombi extend into the proximal deep veins.[4,9]

Proximal vein thrombosis is a serious and potentially lethal disorder. Untreated proximal vein thrombosis is associated with a 10% risk of fatal pulmonary embolism, and a high risk (20 to 50%) of recurrent venous thromboembolic events.[10,11] The fatality rate of 10% for untreated proximal vein thrombosis is based on the following:

- Studies showing that pulmonary embolism occurs in 50% or more of patients with proximal vein thrombosis[4,5,12]

Table 23-1. Levels of Clinical Evidence

Level	Study Design Features
I*	Large randomized trials with definite results (low chance of alpha or beta error)
II	Small randomized trials with uncertain results (moderate to high alpha or beta error)
III	Nonrandomized Concurrent controls
IV	Nonrandomized Historical controls
V	No controls Case series

* For studies evaluating the accuracy of diagnostic tests, the requirements for level I are: prospective, consecutive patients, broad-spectrum of patients, independent gold-standard, blinded interpretation of test, and gold-standard.
(Adapted from Sackett, D. L.: Rules of evidence and clinical recommendations on the use of antithrombotic agents. Chest, 95(Suppl.):25, 1989.)

- A mortality rate of 25% for untreated pulmonary embolism[13]
- Studies in patients undergoing total hip replacement that document a strong association between proximal vein thrombosis and fatal pulmonary embolism.[14-17] In the absence of prophylaxis, 20 to 30% of such patients develop proximal vein thrombosis and 2 to 3% die from pulmonary embolism.[14-17]

Pulmonary embolism originates from thrombi in the deep veins of the leg in 90% or more of patients. Most clinically important pulmonary emboli arise from thrombi in the proximal deep veins of the leg.[18-23] The clinical significance of pulmonary embolism depends on the size of the embolus and the cardiorespiratory reserve of the patient. Other less common sources of pulmonary embolism include the axillary veins, deep pelvic veins, renal veins, inferior vena cava, and right heart. Central venous catheters are commonly used in ICU patients and may be a source of pulmonary embolism.

Risk Factors and Classification of Risk

Clinical risk factors for venous thromboembolism include:

- Advanced age
- Previous venous thromboembolism
- Surgery or trauma
- Prolonged immobility or paralysis
- Malignancy
- Congestive cardiac failure
- Oral contraceptive use
- Pregnancy

Certain surgical procedures, including orthopedic surgery to the lower limbs, and extensive pelvic or abdominal surgery for advanced malignant disease, are associated with a particularly high risk of postoperative venous thromboembolism. Inherited abnormalities which predispose to venous thromboembolism include deficiencies of antithrombin III, protein C, protein S, or heparin cofactor II, and dysfribrinogenemia. Other conditions that may be associated with venous thromboembolism include abnormalities of the fibrinolytic system, polycythemia vera, and systemic lupus erythematosus.

In general, patients can be classified as low, moderate, or high risk for developing venous thromboembolism, as summarized in Table 23-2. In the absence of prophylaxis, the frequency of fatal pulmonary embolism ranges from 0.1 to 0.8% in patients undergoing general abdominal or thoracic surgery,[24] from 2 to 3% in patients undergoing elective hip or knee replacement,[17] and from 4 to 7% in patients undergoing surgery for fractured hip.[25] In medical patients, such as those with myocardial infarction or stroke, venous thrombosis occurs in 20 to 30% in the absence of prophylaxis.[26,27]

Prevention of Venous Thromboembolism

Two approaches can be taken to prevent fatal pulmonary embolism: (1) **primary prophylaxis** using drugs or physical methods that are effective for preventing deep vein thrombosis and pulmonary embolism; and (2) **secondary prevention** by the early detection and treatment of subclinical venous thrombosis by screening patients postoperatively with objective tests that are sensitive for venous thrombosis.

Primary prophylaxis is the preferred approach in most patients. Effective and safe primary prophylaxis is now

Table 23-2. Risk Categories for Postoperative Venous Thromboembolism

Risk Category	Calf Vein Thrombosis	Proximal Vein Thrombosis	Fatal Pulmonary Embolism
High Risk 1. general surgery in patients >40 yr with a recent history of DVT or PE 2. extensive pelvic or abdominal surgery for malignant disease 3. major orthopedic surgery of lower limbs	40–80%	10–30%	1–5%
Moderate Risk* 1. general surgery in patients >40 yr lasting 30 min or more.	10–40%	2–10%	0.1–0.8%
Low Risk 1. uncomplicated surgery in patients <40 yr with no additional risk factors 2. minor surgery (i.e., less than 30 min) in patients >40 yr with no additional risk factors	<10%	<1%	<0.01%

* The risk is increased by advanced age, malignancy, prolonged immobility, cardiac failure, and a past history of venous thromboembolism.

available for most patients. Secondary prevention by screening (case-finding) is a costly approach for averting pulmonary embolism because of the hospital and treatment costs incurred in treating patients who develop deep vein thrombosis.[28,29] Screening should never replace primary prophylaxis. Screening is reserved for patients in whom effective primary prophylaxis is contraindicated or unavailable. Screening may also be used to supplement primary prophylaxis in very high risk patients (for example, patients with a history of venous thromboembolism who must undergo surgery).

The forms of primary prophylaxis that have been evaluated clinically include anticoagulant drugs (such as heparin or warfarin sodium), antiplatelet agents (e.g., aspirin), and physical methods such as intermittent pneumatic leg compression. Heparin and oral anticoagulants prevent thrombosis by inhibiting blood coagulation. Heparin markedly accelerates the inhibition by antithrombin III of the activated coagulation factors XII, XI, IX, X, and thrombin. Because the biochemical reactions of blood coagulation are amplified by each successive step in the coagulation cascade, much lower doses of heparin are required to inhibit the initiation of blood coagulation and prevent thrombus formation that are required for the treatment of established thrombosis.[10,11,24] Oral anticoagulants inhibit the synthesis of functionally active vitamin-K dependent coagulation factors II, VII, IX, and X. Antiplatelet drugs such as aspirin inhibit the interaction between platelets and the damaged vessel wall; however, clinical trials (level 1) indicate that antiplatelet drugs have a limited role, if any, in preventing venous thromboembolism. Intermittent compression prevents venous thrombosis by enhancing blood flow in the deep veins of the leg, thereby preventing venous stasis. It also enhances blood fibrinolytic activity, which may contribute to its antithrombotic properties.

Table 23-3. Recommended Prophylactic Approaches for the Alternative Risk Categories and Surgical Groups

Risk Category	Recommended Approaches
Low Risk	Graduated compression stockings
Moderate Risk	
General abdominal or thoracic surgery*	Low dose heparin (q12h or q8h) Intermittent compression Low molecular weight heparin
Neurosurgery	Intermittent compression
Urologic surgery	Intermittent compression
Medical patients	Low dose heparin Intermittent compression
High Risk	
General abdominal or thoracic surgery	Oral anticoagulants Adjusted-dose heparin Low dose heparin (q8h) ± intermittent compression Low molecular weight heparin
Elective hip surgery	Oral anticoagulants Low molecular weight heparin
Fractured hip	Oral anticoagulants Dextran
Major knee surgery	Intermittent compression

*In patients with a high risk of bleeding, intermittent pneumatic compression is the prophylaxis of choice.

The choice of primary prophylaxis depends on the patient's risk category and the surgical procedure. The recommended prophylactic approaches for the alternative risk categories and surgical groups are summarized in Table 23-3 (all recommended approaches are supported by level I evidence).

In high risk medical patients, either low dose heparin (5000 U subcutaneously q 8h or q 12h), or intermittent leg compression can be used. Intermittent compression is preferred in patients at high risk of bleeding (e.g., recent stroke). In patients with acute transmural myocardial infarction, low dose heparin is effective for preventing venous thromboembolism,[26] but is not effective for preventing left ventricular mural thrombosis[30] and systemic embolism. A practical heparin regimen that is effective for preventing mural thrombosis[30] and also protects against venous thromboembolism is 12,500 units subcutaneously every 12 hours (level I).

In patients with very recent proximal vein thrombosis who require urgent surgery, insertion of a vena caval filter (Greenfield filter) may be considered to prevent massive pulmonary embolism during surgery or in the early postoperative period while treatment is interrupted.

ICU PHASE: DIAGNOSIS AND MANAGEMENT OF VENOUS THROMBOEMBOLISM IN THE CRITICALLY ILL

General Considerations

The clinical diagnosis of pulmonary embolism is highly nonspecific because none of the symptoms or signs of pulmonary embolism is unique, and each may be caused by a variety of cardiorespiratory disorders. More than half of all patients with clinically suspected pulmonary embolism do not have this diagnosis confirmed by objective testing.[21,22,31,32] Objective testing is required to establish or exclude the presence of pulmonary embolism.

The ICU physician is frequently asked to assess patients who are hemodynamically unstable and have varying degrees of respiratory compromise, in whom pulmonary embolism is part of the differential diagnosis. These patients represent emergency situations and require immediate physiologic support and initiation of therapy while the provisional diagnosis of pulmonary embolism is quickly confirmed or excluded.

The ICU physician may also be confronted with patients who are hemodynamically stable, but who require ICU for other reasons, the clinical course is complicated by suspected pulmonary embolism. In this latter group, the diagnostic process can usually be carried out according to a protocol which includes lung scanning, objective testing for venous thrombosis, and pulmonary angiography, together with a clinical assessment of the patient's cardiorespiratory reserve.

Pulmonary embolism may present clinically as one of several syndromes as summarized in Table 23-4. These syndromes may overlap considerably but for practical clinical purposes, they can be grouped into two categories:

- Syndromes that include clinical findings of an unstable circulation, and are usually associated with massive pulmonary embolism, but may also result from sub-

Table 23-4. Clinical Syndromes Associated with Pulmonary Embolism

Syndrome	Symptoms
Circulatory arrest	Hypotension, asystole
Persistently unstable circulation	Hypotension, syncope, end organ dysfunction-oliguria, lactic acidosis, CNS dysfunction
Transciently unstable circulation	Right heart failure, severe dyspnea, tachypnea
Pulmonary infarction (ischemic pneumonitis or incomplete infarction)	Pleuritic chest pain, cough, hemoptysis, pleural effusion and pulmonary infiltrates
Transient dyspnea and tachypnea	Absence of clinical findings
Nonspecific clinical features	Unexplained arrhythmias, resistant cardiac failure, wheezing, fever

massive embolism in patients with poor cardiac reserve because of underlying disorders such as severe congestive cardiac failure
- Syndromes that do not include clinical findings of hemodynamic instability

The management of patients with clinically suspected pulmonary embolism is outlined later in this chapter according to whether the patient is hemodynamically stable or unstable at the time of presentation. First, a brief consideration of the ancillary test findings (chest radiograph, electrocardiogram (ECG), etc.) is provided.

Serum enzymes (LDH, SGOT) and bilirubin, and arterial blood gases, are insensitive and nonspecific for pulmonary embolism.[31,33,34] These tests should not be used for diagnostic purposes in patients with suspected pulmonary embolism. A normal arterial Po_2 (> 80 mm Hg) does not exclude pulmonary embolism.[31,33,34] In the UPET study, a Po_2 greater than 80 mm Hg was found in 12% of 167 patients with pulmonary embolism by pulmonary angiography, including some patients with massive pulmonary embolism.[31,34]

The ECG is frequently normal in patients with suspected pulmonary embolism. The classic ECG findings associated with pulmonary embolism (right axis shift, $S_1Q_3T_3$ pattern) are uncommon and nonspecific.[33] The ECG is most useful for differentiating between pulmonary embolism and myocardial infarction.

The chest radiograph abnormalities associated with pulmonary embolism are nonspecific and occur in many other pulmonary disorders. These abnormalities include the presence of an infiltrate or consolidation, elevated hemidiaphragm, pleural effusion(s), atelectasis, prominent pulmonary arteries, an enlarged right or left ventricle, and focal oligemia (Westermark sign). Patients with pulmonary embolism may have a normal chest radiograph at presentation.[31,33-35] The chest radiograph is helpful for demonstrating other causes of chest symptoms (e.g., pneumothorax), and is important for interpreting the lung scan findings.

Hemodynamically Unstable Patients

Autopsy studies indicate that less than one third of patients who die with clinically important pulmonary embolism have this diagnosis established antemortem (including those patients in whom pulmonary embolism is judged to be the immediate cause of death).[36] Pulmonary embolism should be part of the differential diagnosis each time the ICU physician is asked to assess a hemodynamically unstable patient (and especially if the patient is in the moderate or high risk category for venous thromboembolism, see Table 23-2).

Most patients who die from pulmonary embolism succumb abruptly or within 2 hours of the acute event.[3] In patients who survive for more than 2 hours, the prognosis with standard anticoagulant therapy is very good. Circulatory failure is the major factor that leads to death from pulmonary embolism. The immediate objectives in the hemodynamically unstable patient with suspected pulmonary embolism are:

- To stabilize the circulation and restore the hemodynamics towards normal
- To provide adequate anticoagulant therapy to prevent thrombotic extension of the existing embolus and/or recurrent pulmonary embolism

Initial Physiologic Support

The initial physiologic support includes appropriate measures to ensure adequate ventilation and oxygenation, and measures to stabilize the circulation and restore normal hemodynamics. The decision regarding the optimum route of oxygenation and ventilation remains a clinical judgment based on the usual indications for supplemental oxygen by nasal prongs, nonbreathing mask, or intubation and ventilation.

Currently, no data are available from clinical trials on the impact of intubation and ventilation on circulatory function in patients with massive pulmonary embolism, or the optimum ventilator technique in such patients. One study in an experimental animal model of massive pulmonary embolism suggests that high frequency jet ventilation is more effective than intermittent positive pressure ventilation, but the clinical relevance of these findings remains uncertain.[37]

Shock which occurs secondary to pulmonary embolism is the result of extensive pulmonary vascular obstruction, resulting in high pulmonary artery pressures, increased right ventricular afterload, and right ventricular failure.[38,39] The management of patients with shock secondary to massive pulmonary embolism has been based on case reports and extrapolation of data from experimental animal studies.[38-41] The traditional therapy has been to use volume expansion to increase mean systemic pressure and to increase cardiac output.[38] However, in a canine model of massive pulmonary embolism with shock, Molloy and colleagues demonstrated that norepinephrine is more effective than either volume expansion or isoproterenol for acute resuscitation and short-term maintenance of hemodynamic stability.[40] The improvement in ventricular function with norepinephrine may be due to a direct increase in contractility and/or an increased contractility secondary to improved right ventricular perfusion.[39,40]

Recent data in experimental animals and also from patients with massive pulmonary embolism provide potentially important information about the hemodynamic response to pulmonary embolism.[39-43] These data suggest that massive pulmonary embolism is associated with both right ventricular failure, and also inadequate left ventricular function due to poor diastolic filling. The latter is particularly true if right sided pressures are high which results in expansion of the right atrium and right ventricle with pericardial constraint and septal shift.[42,43] Consequently, there is an impairment of left ventricular filling and decreased cardiac output with reduced systemic flow. These physiologic data suggest that the traditional therapeutic approach of volume loading is inappropriate, and support two alternative approaches:

- Reducing right ventricular preload (for example, using nitroglycerin or a phlebotomy)
- Therapy using a drug with both inotropic and systemic vasoconstrictor effects such as norepinephrine (Levophed), which increases systemic pressures and helps to restore normal septal position

The foregoing physiologic data are based on studies in experimental animals, and the relevance to the clinical management of massive pulmonary embolism is uncertain. Nevertheless, the use of measures to decrease right ventricular preload, and agents with inotropic and systemic vasoconstrictor effects may be considered in selected patients. In patients with moderately depressed cardiac output, who are not hypotensive, the use of inotropic therapy and/or a pulmonary vasodilator may be sufficient.

The role of hemodynamic monitoring using the pulmonary artery (Swan-Ganz) catheter is currently uncertain. The role of hemodynamic monitoring remains uncertain because the benefits and risks have not been adequately evaluated by randomized clinical trials in patients with suspected pulmonary embolism. Advocates of invasive monitoring suggest that it aids in the initial assessment of the patient's physiologic status, and allows serial hemodynamic measurements to assess the impact of specific treatments. On the other hand, opponents of hemodynamic monitoring point out that inflation of the catheter balloon may be deleterious in patients who already have severe pulmonary vascular obstruction, and that placement of the catheter may dislodge thromboemboli present in the right heart or main pulmonary arteries (leading to further embolic obstruction). At present, it is not possible to make specific recommendations on the use of invasive hemodynamic monitoring because of a lack of data from clinical trials. Furthermore, placement of the catheter through internal jugular or subclavian veins may predispose patients to excessive site bleeding if thrombolytic therapy is used.

Specific Therapy and Clinical Course

Anticoagulant therapy is commenced with a 5000-U intravenous bolus of heparin, followed by a continuous intravenous heparin infusion of 40,000 U per 24 hours. This relatively high initial infusion dose is chosen to ensure an adequate anticoagulant response (activated partial thromboplastin time 1.5 or more times control). Patients with pulmonary embolism may have higher heparin dose requirements than patients with venous thrombosis,[44] particularly those patients with massive pulmonary embolism. Thus, in the setting of the hemodynamically unstable patient who may have massive pulmonary embolism, the clinician should not be timid about using relatively high doses of heparin to ensure that adequate therapy is obtained immediately. Further practical details of intravenous heparin therapy are discussed under the heading "Practical Protocol For Continuous Intravenous Heparin Therapy." After initial physiologic support and anticoagulant therapy is provided, the early clinical course can be described, for practical purposes, as falling into one of three categories:

- Rapid stabilization after a brief period of physiologic support. These patients show normalization of blood pressure, adequate gas exchange with or without supplemental oxygen (by mask or nasal prongs), and adequate tissue perfusion as indicated by normal central nervous system (CNS) function, adequate urine output, and the absence of lactic acidosis.
- Those who remain unstable and require continued physiologic support. These patients may require the use of vasopressors and/or inotropic agents to maintain adequate blood pressure, or intubation and ventilation to maintain adequate arteriolar oxygenation and CO_2 excretion. With this physiologic support, however, these patients show evidence of adequate tissue perfusion indicated by satisfactory CNS function, urine output, and the absence of lactic acidosis.
- Those who remain unstable and continue to deteriorate clinically. These are patients who despite the use of vasopressors and inotropic agents, remain hemodynamically unstable with tachycardia, hypotension, and/or arrhythmias, and who require intubation and ventilation with a high F_{IO_2} to maintain adequate oxygenation. Despite this physiologic support, these patients continue to deteriorate as evidenced by altered CNS function, inadequate urine output and the development of lactic acidosis.

In the first group of patients discussed, the prognosis with standard anticoagulant therapy is excellent. In these patients, the diagnostic process should be carried out to confirm or refute the diagnosis of venous thromboembolism. The protocol is the same as for the hemodynamically stable patient (outlined later).

In the second group of patients, there is an urgent need to confirm (or refute) the diagnosis of pulmonary embolism; if pulmonary embolism is confirmed, thrombolytic therapy should be considered. The diagnosis can be established rapidly by proceeding directly to pulmonary angiography without first performing lung scanning. If pulmonary embolism is confirmed, then thrombolytic therapy is indicated in the absence of absolute contraindications. Thrombolytic therapy with streptokinase, urokinase, or tissue plasminogen activator has been shown by randomized trials (level I) to be more effective than heparin alone for inducing rapid resolution of recent pulmonary embolism.[31,45,46] To date, however, no clinical trial has established that the use of thrombolytic therapy is associated with a reduction in mortality from pulmonary embolism compared to intravenous heparin therapy alone. Thrombolytic therapy has been shown, however, to result in significant improvements in the hemodynamics,[31,45,46] and has the potential to be lifesaving in those patients with massive pulmonary embolism, or submassive pulmonary embolism on a background of severe cardiopulmonary disease. The practical details of thrombolytic therapy are outlined under the heading "Protocol for Thrombolytic Therapy."

Patients in the third group outlined previously have a poor prognosis. The ICU physician must decide whether to add thrombolytic therapy or to consider surgical embolectomy. Unfortunately, no data from clinical trials are available to guide this decision. The decision to use pulmonary embolectomy depends on the resources available in the hospital. If the expertise and facilities are available to perform pulmonary embolectomy, and the surgical team can be mobilized quickly, then the procedure should be considered. If the patient would require transfer to another hospital, however, or if surgery is delayed beyond a brief period, then thrombolytic therapy is preferred to pulmonary embolectomy because the available data indicate that patients who survive for 2 hours or more have a good prognosis with heparin and/or thrombolytic therapy.

Hemodynamically Stable Patients

These patients are evaluated according to a protocol which includes ventilation-perfusion lung scanning, objective tests for deep vein thrombosis, pulmonary angiography, and clinical assessment of the patient's cardiorespiratory reserve.

Lung Scanning

Perfusion lung scanning has a pivotal role. A normal perfusion scan excludes clinically important pulmonary embolism (Fig. 23-1).[32,47,48] it is possible that the perfusion scan may be normal in the presence of a saddle embolus which does not obstruct the main pulmonary outflow tract, but such patients are rare.

A recent prospective study evaluated the alternative diagnoses in 515 consecutive patients with clinically suspected pulmonary embolism and normal perfusion lung scans.[47] With knowledge of normal findings by perfusion lung scanning, an alternative diagnosis was established in 71% of patients. A wide variety of alternative diagnoses were found (Table 23-5). In a considerable proportion (29%) of patients, however, the cause of symptoms remained uncertain.[47]

An abnormal perfusion scan is nonspecific,[21,22,32] and may be caused by conditions that produce either abnormal chest radiograph findings (such as pneumonia, atelectasis pleural effusion, or pulmonary edema), or a regional reduction in ventilation (such as chronic obstructive lung disease, acute asthma, bronchial mucous plugs, and bronchitis), which are frequently associated with normal chest radiograph findings.

Ventilation imaging was introduced into clinical practice to improve the specificity of an abnormal perfusion scan by differentiating embolic occlusion of the pulmonary vasculature from perfusion defects occurring secondary to a primary disorder of ventilation (e.g., chronic obstructive pulmonary disease, asthma, emphysema, etc.).[49-52] The concept, however, that perfusion defects which ventilate normally (ventilation-perfusion mismatch) are due to pul-

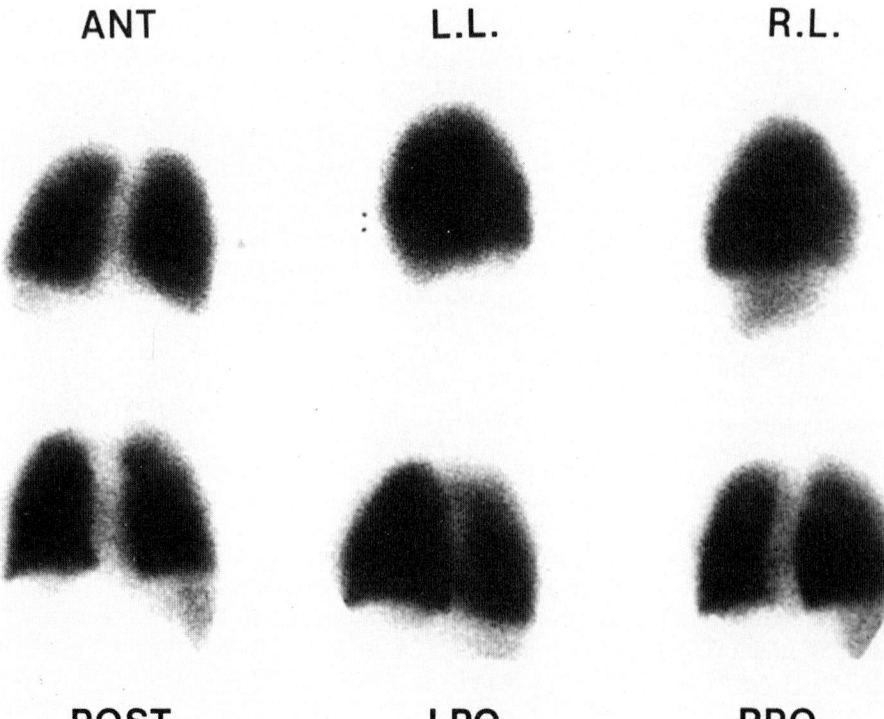

Fig. 23-1. A normal six-view perfusion lung scan (^{99m} technetium MAA). ANT, Anterior; POST, posterior; L.L., left lateral; R.L., right lateral; LPO, left posterior oblique; RPO, right posterior oblique.

Table 23-5. Alternative Diagnoses in 515 Consecutive Patients with Suspected Pulmonary Embolism and Normal Perfusion Scans

Diagnosis	No. of Patients (%) (n = 515)
Musculoskeletal disorder	133 (26%)
Other specific conditions involving chest wall*	34 (7%)
Cardiac disorder†	85 (16%)
Pleuritis	
viral	26 (5%)
due to other documented condition‡	11 (2%)
Pneumonia	22 (4%)
Esophagitis	14 (3%)
Asthma	8 (1%)
Chronic obstructive pulmonary disease	7 (1%)
Carcinoma of lung	4 (1%)
Miscellaneous§	23 (4%)
Unknown	148 (29%)

* Including injury, costochondritis, pathologic rib fracture, rheumatoid arthritis, disc space infection, and herpes zoster.
† Including myocardial infarction or ischemia, and congestive cardiac failure, percarditis, and tachyarrhythmias.
‡ Including systemic lupus erythematosus, and rheumatoid arthritis.
§ Including tuberculosis, sarcoidosis, bronchiectasis, pulmonary fibrosis, lymphoma, thoracic outlet syndrome, post-transfusion reaction, cholecystitis, peptic ulcer, and perforated viscus.
(From Hull, R. D., Rashob, G. E., Coates, G., and Panju, A. A.: Clinical validity of a normal perfusion scan in patients with suspected pulmonary embolism. Chest, 97:23, 1990.)

monary embolism, whereas matching ventilation-perfusion abnormalities are due to other disorders, has been shown to be incorrect by recent prospective clinical trials (Level I-diagnostic studies).[21,22,32]

Between 1976 and 1980, attempts were made to improve the predictive value of ventilation-perfusion lung scanning by classifying the perfusion defects according to size and number, and the presence of matched or mismatched ventilation defects.[50-52] The classic criteria developed by Biello[51] and by McNeil[52] are the basis for the widely used concept of high, intermediate, and low probability lung scan patterns (Table 23-6). The classic high probability and low probability lung scan patterns are shown in Figures 23-2 and 23-3, respectively. The data supporting the use of these probability patterns were derived from retrospective studies or nonconsecutive patient series.[50-53]

More recently, two large prospective studies[21,22,32] have assessed the value of ventilation-perfusion scanning in patients with suspected pulmonary embolism. The findings of these level I diagnostic studies are consistent. The data support the concept of "high probability" lung scan patterns; 86 to 88% of such patients had pulmonary embolism by angiography.[22,32] The data indicate the concept of "low probability" ventilation-perfusion scan patterns is incorrect, however; 12 to 40% of patients with lung scan patterns considered "low probability" had pulmonary embolism.[22,32] Further, in two prospective studies in which objective testing for venous thrombosis was performed routinely in all patients, proximal vein thrombosis (the precursor of pulmonary embolism) was detected in 8 to 25% of patients with "low probability" scan patterns.[22,23] Most of these proximal vein thrombi were clinically silent. These findings have important implications for patient management because inadequately treated proximal vein thrombosis is associated with a high risk (20 to 50%) of recurrent venous thromboembolism.[10,11]

The conclusions from recent prospective studies[21,22,32] are as follows: Ventilation lung scanning is only helpful in patients with large perfusion defects (> 75% of a lung segment) and then only if a large ventilation-perfusion mismatch is found (high probability scan). Combining the clinician's pretest estimate of the probability of pulmonary embolism with the lung scan findings is helpful only in a minority of patients.[22,32] Further investigations are required in most patients who have high abnormal ventilation-perfusion scan patterns that are "high probability" for pulmonary embolism. These patterns, which have traditionally been regarded as either "low probability" or intermediate probability for pulmonary embolism, include matching ventilation-perfusion defects, moderate or small subsegmental defects with ventilation mismatch, or perfusion defects that correspond to an area of increased density on the chest radiograph (indeterminate perfusion scan).

The additional investigations for patients who do not have high probability lung scans include pulmonary angiography and objective testing for venous thrombosis. The

Table 23-6. Classic Criteria for the High, Intermediate, and Low Probability Lung Scan Categories

Lung Scan Probability Category	Criteria Biello[51]	McNeil[52]
High	Large* perfusion defect(s) with ventilation mismatch	Segmental or larger perfusion defect(s) with ventilation mismatch
Intermediate	1. Moderate perfusion defect(s) with ventilation mismatch 2. Perfusion defect(s) corresponding to area of chest x-ray abnormality	1. Perfusion defect(s) corresponding to area of chest x-ray abnormality
Low	1. Perfusion defects (any size) with ventilation match 2. Small perfusion defect(s) with ventilation mismatch	1. Perfusion defects (any size) with ventilation match 2. Subsegmental perfusion defect(s) with ventilation mismatch

* Large (> 75% of a lung segment); moderate (25% to 75% of a lung segment), small (25% of a lung segment).

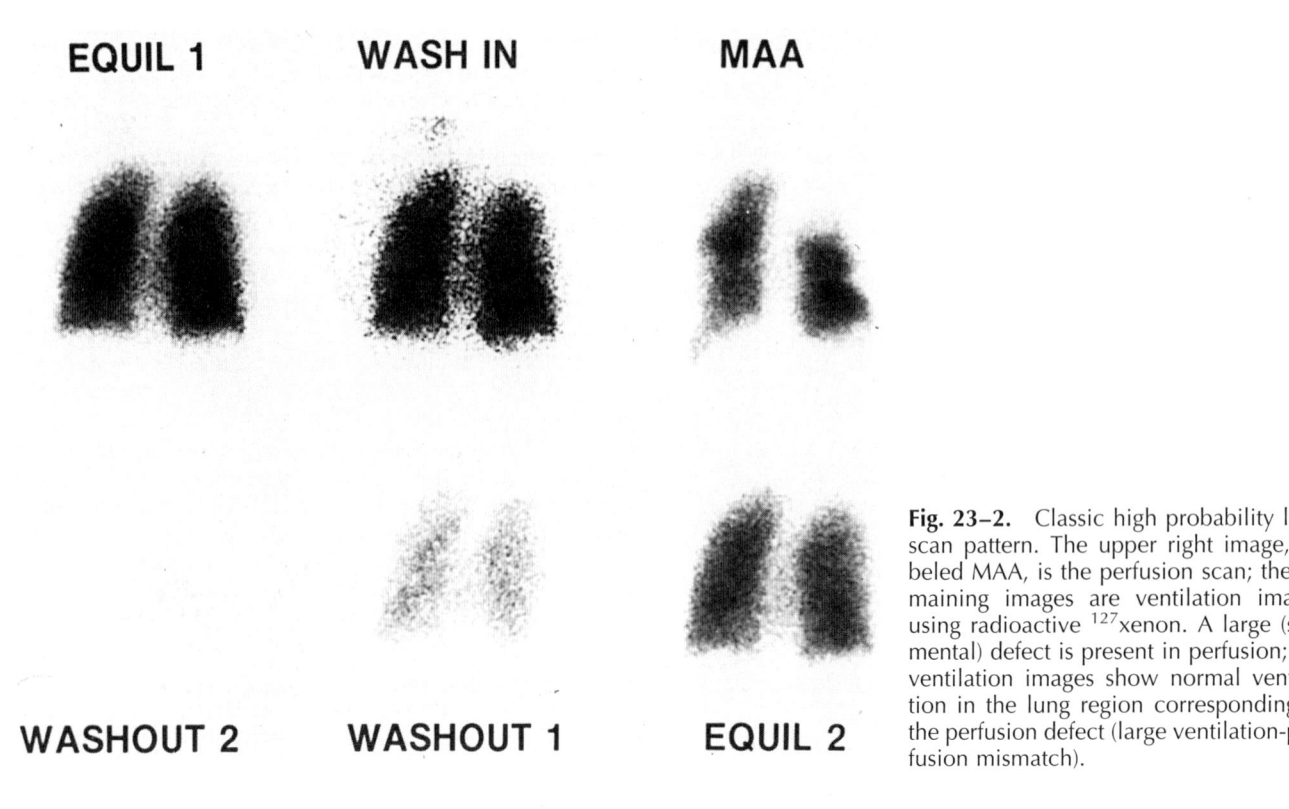

Fig. 23-2. Classic high probability lung scan pattern. The upper right image, labeled MAA, is the perfusion scan; the remaining images are ventilation images using radioactive ^{127}xenon. A large (segmental) defect is present in perfusion; the ventilation images show normal ventilation in the lung region corresponding to the perfusion defect (large ventilation-perfusion mismatch).

morbidity associated with pulmonary angiography and venography is substantially less than the morbidity from unnecessary anticoagulant therapy, and these invasive tests should be used when other approaches are unavailable or inconclusive. Furthermore, no morbidity is associated with the noninvasive tests for venous thrombosis such as impedance plethysmography or B-mode venous ultrasound, which provide clinically useful information in many patients (see the section of this chapter on the Role of objective testing for venous thrombosis).

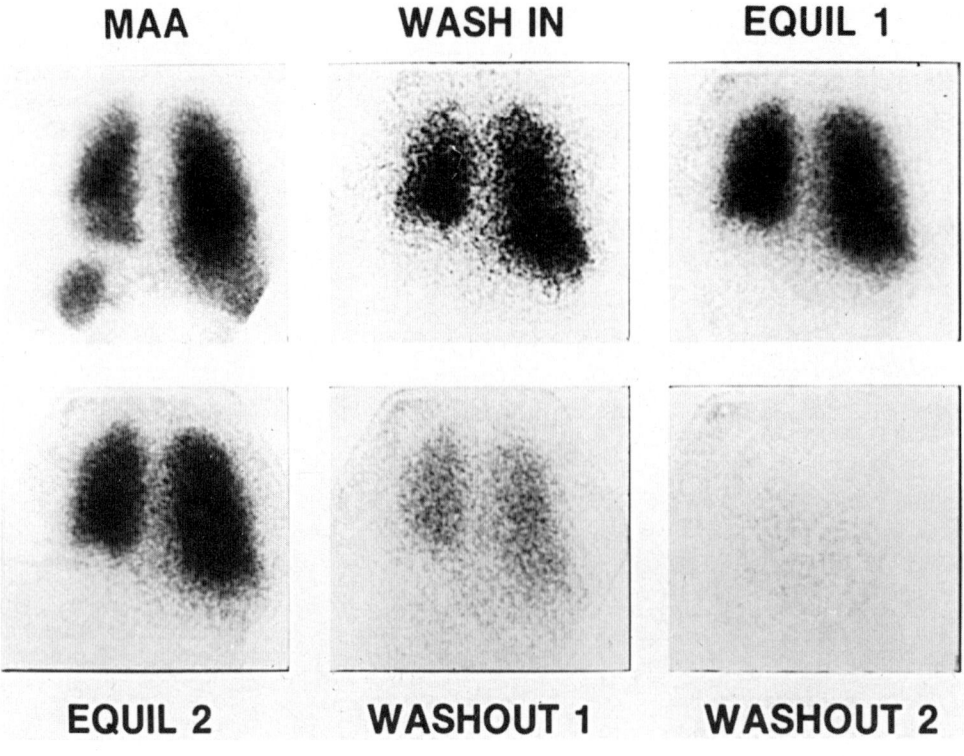

Fig. 23-3. Classic "low probability" lung scan pattern. The upper left image, labeled MAA, is the perfusion scan (posterior view); the remaining images are ventilation images using radioactive ^{127}xenon. A perfusion defect is present in the left lower lobe; the ventilation images show that ventilation is absent in this area (ventilation-perfusion match).

Pulmonary Angiography

Pulmonary angiography is the accepted diagnostic reference standard for pulmonary embolism.[54-55] A diagnosis of pulmonary embolism is established if there is either an intraluminal filling defect or abrupt termination (cut-off) of a vessel greater than 2.5 mm in diameter which is constant on all films.[55] Other abnormalities, such as oligemia, vessel pruning, and loss of filling of small vessels, are nonspecific and occur in a variety of conditions, including pneumonia, atelectasis, bronchiectasis, emphysema, and pulmonary carcinoma.

In recent years, the diagnostic resolution of pulmonary angiography has been markedly improved, and the risk to the patient decreased by using selective catheterization with repeated injections of small volumes of dye. Selective pulmonary angiography is a safe technique in the absence of severe chronic pulmonary hypertension or severe cardiac or respiratory decompensation.[56] Clinically significant complications including tachyarrhythmias, endocardial or myocardial injury, cardiac perforation, cardiac arrest, and hypersensitivity reactions to contrast medium occur in up to 3 to 4% of patients undergoing pulmonary angiography.[21,22,35,54,56] Pulmonary angiography should not be performed in patients with a history of allergy to radiopaque dye.

The clinical validity of a negative pulmonary angiogram in patients with suspected pulmonary embolism has been tested by long-term follow-up in four studies.[32,35,53,57] These studies report a 1 to 3% frequency of objectively confirmed pulmonary embolism on follow-up in patients with negative angiograms.

A practical limitation of pulmonary angiography is that many patients in the ICU may be too ill to undergo the procedure. In addition, the findings may be inconclusive due to inadequate visualization of the pulmonary vasculature in 2 to up to 15% of patients.[21,22,32,54]

Role of Objective Testing for Venous Thrombosis

Postmortem and surgical studies[18-20] and recent prospective clinical trials[21,22] have shown that the majority of patients with pulmonary embolism have associated deep vein thrombosis of the legs. Deep vein thrombosis by venography is present in 70% of patients with pulmonary embolism by pulmonary angiography.[21] Most of these patients do not have symptoms or signs of venous thrombosis at the time of presentation.

Objective testing for venous thrombosis has practical value in the diagnosis of patients with suspected pulmonary embolism. In most patients, the treatment of deep vein thrombosis and pulmonary embolism is the same. The finding of deep vein thrombosis by objective testing is an indication for treatment,[9-11] and avoids the need for pulmonary angiography. The noninvasive tests such as impedance plethysmography or B-mode venous ultrasound have the advantages that they are easily performed at the bedside and are readily repeatable (see the discussion of noninvasive testing for venous thrombosis for further details).

If therapy is started on the basis of documented deep vein thrombosis, the patient's respiratory status should be closely monitored to detect disorders such as pneumonia, that may be present but not evident at the time of presentation. The objective confirmation of venous thrombosis does not necessarily establish a diagnosis of pulmonary embolism because venous thrombosis may have occurred in association with another primary respiratory illness, which placed the patient at high risk for venous thromboembolism. If respiratory symptoms persist and the cause remains uncertain, pulmonary angiography will distinguish between pulmonary embolism and other respiratory problems.

A negative result by objective testing for venous thrombosis cannot be used to exclude pulmonary embolism. A negative venogram occurs in 30% of patients with angiographically documented pulmonary embolism.[21] There are two possible explanations for this finding. First, pulmonary embolism may have originated from a source other than the deep veins of the legs, such as the right heart, axillary veins, deep pelvic veins, renal veins, or inferior vena cava. Alternately, the emboli originated from thrombosis in the deep veins of the legs, but all or most of the thrombus embolized, leaving no residual thrombosis detectable at the time of presentation. Recent data[23] support the latter explanation.

At present, pulmonary angiography is required to confirm or exclude pulmonary embolism in patients with non-high probability lung scan patterns and negative findings by objective testing for venous thrombosis. Pulmonary angiography may be impractical, unavailable, or of limited access, however. An alternative in patients who do not have severely limited cardiac or respiratory reserve (defined in the section of this chapter on practical diagnostic approach) is to perform serial objective testing for proximal vein thrombosis. This approach is based on the following concepts:

- In most patients, recurrent pulmonary embolism comes from proximal vein thrombosis, and clinically important pulmonary embolism is unlikely in the absence of proximal vein thrombosis.
- Isolated pelvic vein thrombosis or calf vein thrombosis is not associated with clinically important pulmonary embolism provided they do not extend into the proximal venous segment.
- Thrombotic extension of submassive pulmonary embolism is not an important cause of morbidity in patients with adequate cardiorespiratory reserve.

These concepts are supported by the findings of a recent prospective study.[23,58] The findings suggest that serial objective testing for proximal vein thrombosis is effective for separating patients with non-high probability lung scans who have adequate cardiorespiratory reserve into two groups: (1) patients with proximal vein thrombosis in whom treatment is indicated[10,11]; and (2) those negative by serial testing, who have a good prognosis without anticoagulant therapy. Only 12 of 627 patients (1.9%, 95% confidence limits 0.8 to 3.0%) negative by serial testing for proximal vein thrombosis had venous thromboembolism on long-term follow-up, compared with 4 of 586 patients (0.7%) with normal perfusion scans, and 8 of 145 patients (5.5%) with high probability scans who received anticoagulant therapy.[23] The prognosis in patients negative by serial testing for proximal vein thrombosis is similar to the 2% rate of pulmonary embolism on follow-up in patients with negative pulmonary angiograms.[32,35,53,57] If the findings of this study are confirmed, then serial objective testing for proximal vein thrombosis will provide a practical noninvasive alternative to pulmonary angiography in patients with non-high probability lung scans and adequate cardiorespiratory reserve (see the following section for details).

Practical Diagnostic Approach

A practical algorithm for the management of clinically suspected pulmonary embolism is shown in Figure 23-4. The findings of a normal perfusion lung scan exclude clinically important pulmonary embolism. Conversely, therapy can usually be commenced without further investigation in patients with one or more large (> 75% of a lung segment) perfusion defects with ventilation mismatch (high probability scan), and in patients with non-high probability lung scan patterns in whom deep vein thrombosis is detected by objective testing.

Pulmonary angiography is indicated in patients with abnormal non-high probability lung scan patterns who are negative by objective testing for venous thrombosis at presentation. If the patient has adequate cardiorespiratory reserve, serial objective testing for proximal vein thrombosis can be used instead of pulmonary angiography.

The cardiorespiratory reserve is defined as adequate if **none** of the following are present:

- Pulmonary edema
- Right ventricular failure
- Hypotension (systolic < 90 mm Hg)
- Syncope
- Acute tachyarrhythmias
- Respiratory insufficiency shown by severely abnormal spirometry (FEV_1 < 1.0 or VC < 1.5) or blood gas measurements (Po_2 < 50 mm Hg or Pco_2 > 45 mm Hg on room air)

Objective testing for proximal vein thrombosis should be repeated 4 to 5 times over the 14 days following presentation (for example, the day after presentation and then on the third, fifth to seventh, tenth, and 14th day).[23] Anticoagulant therapy can be safely withheld if the results by serial testing remain negative.[23]

Serial testing for proximal vein thrombosis can also be used in patients with temporary inadequate reserve, in whom the reserve improves to adequate within 10 days. In these patients, intravenous heparin is given during the period of inadequate cardiorespiratory reserve. When adequate cardiorespiratory reserve is achieved (as defined previously), heparin therapy is withdrawn, and the patient is followed with serial testing for the next 14 days.

A considerable proportion of patients in the ICU may have persistent inadequate cardiorespiratory reserve (for 10 days or more). In these patients, the strategy of repeated testing for proximal vein thrombosis is not recommended to avoid the risk of serious morbidity or death from pulmonary emboli already present, and responsible in part for the inadequate cardiorespiratory reserve. These patients are usually readily identified at the time of presentation with suspected pulmonary embolism because of clinically overt underlying cardiorespiratory disorders such as severe chronic obstructive pulmonary disease or severe congestive cardiac failure. If pulmonary angiography is contraindicated or impractical, then it may be prudent to err on the side of treatment rather than risk death from pulmonary embolism in these patients.

Diagnosis of Venous Thrombosis

Clinical Features and Differential Diagnosis

The clinical features of venous thrombosis include leg pain, tenderness or swelling, a palpable cord (i.e., a thrombosed vessel that is easily palpable as an obvious cord), discoloration, distension and prominence of the superficial veins, and cyanosis. The clinical diagnosis of venous thrombosis is highly nonspecific, and in more than 50% of symptomatic patients, venous thrombosis is not confirmed by objective testing.[6-8,59-63] Objective testing is mandatory in order to confirm or exclude a diagnosis of venous thrombosis. It should be emphasized that patients with relatively minor symptoms and signs may have extensive deep vein thrombosis, whereas patients with florid leg pain and swelling, suggesting extensive deep vein thrombosis, frequently are negative by objective testing.

The differential diagnosis in patients with suspected ve-

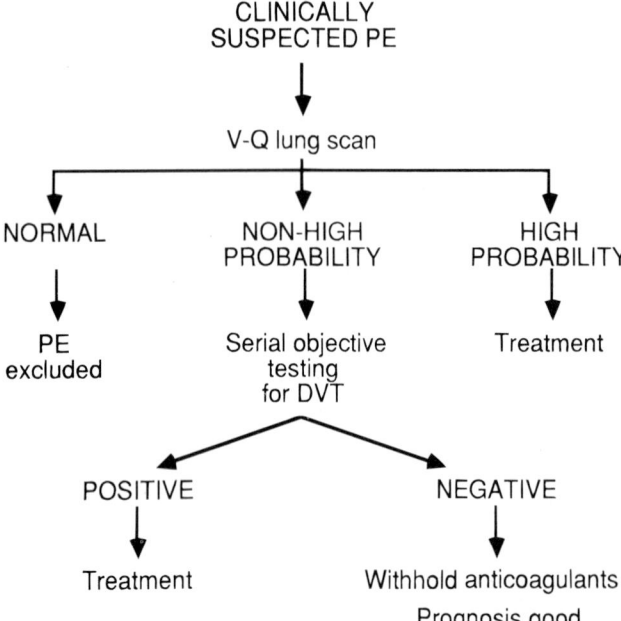

Fig. 23-4. Practical diagnostic approach for clinically suspected pulmonary embolism (PE) in the hemodynamically stable patient. Serial objective testing for proximal vein thrombosis can be used instead of pulmonary angiography in patients who do not have high probability lung scan patterns and who have adequate cardiorespiratory reserve (see text for details). Pulmonary angiography is indicated for patients who do not have high probability lung scans and who have persistent inadequate cardiorespiratory reserve. V-Q, Ventilation-perfusion; DVT, deep vein thrombosis.

nous thrombosis includes the following:[64] muscle strain (usually associated with unaccustomed exercise), muscle tear, direct twisting injury to the leg, vasomotor changes in a paralyzed leg, venous reflux, lymphangitis, lymphatic obstruction, Baker's cyst, cellulitis, internal derangement of the knee, hematoma, and the postphlebitic syndrome. An alternate diagnosis is frequently not evident at the time of presentation, and without objective testing, it is impossible to exclude venous thrombosis. The cause of symptoms can often be determined by careful follow-up once a diagnosis of venous thrombosis has been excluded by objective testing. In 25% of patients with negative venograms, however, the cause of pain, tenderness, and swelling remains uncertain even after careful follow-up.[64]

Venography

Venography is the accepted reference standard for the diagnosis of venous thrombosis.[64,65] It is an invasive procedure which produces significant foot and calf pain in some patients. The high ionic contrast media may produce superficial phlebitis and even deep vein thrombosis in 1 to 2% of patients who have normal venograms.[64] Other less common complications of venography include hypersensitivity reactions to the radiopaque medium, and local skin and tissue necrosis due to extravasation of dye at the site of injection.

Recent studies have demonstrated that the risk of nephrotoxicity in patients with diabetes mellitus, renal insufficiency or both, is low with both low-ionic and high-ionic contrast media.[66,67] Exclusion of very high risk patients and careful attention to hydration and to technical details can eliminate most serious adverse reactions including renal insufficiency. It is prudent to avoid venography in patients with a history of allergy to radiographic dyes.

Noninvasive Testing for Venous Thrombosis

Numerous noninvasive techniques for diagnosing venous thrombosis have been developed including:

- ^{125}I-fibrinogen leg scanning
- Impedance plethysmography
- Doppler ultrasonography
- B-mode venous ultrasound imaging
- Duplex scanning (B-mode imaging combined with Doppler ultrasound)
- Strain gauge plethysmography
- Thermography
- Radioisotope venography

The most extensively evaluated approaches are impedance plethysmography (with or without the addition of leg scanning), Doppler ultrasonography, and venous imaging using real-time B-mode ultrasound. Only three approaches, however, have been evaluated by prospective clinical trials incorporating long-term follow-up to determine the safety of withholding therapy in patients with negative findings by noninvasive testing. These approaches are combined impedance plethysmography and ^{125}I-fibrinogen leg scanning,[61] serial impedance plethysmography,[6-8,63] and serial B-mode venous ultrasound imaging.[68] Because ultrasound imaging technology has been widely disseminated to many hospitals, venous imaging using real-time ultrasound is the real contender among the noninvasive tests in the 1990s. Impedance plethysmography is a low cost technology that continues to play an important role in centers in which this test is available.

Impedance plethysmography is highly sensitive and specific for proximal vein thrombosis in symptomatic patients,[6-8,21,59-61,69] but fails to detect most calf vein thrombi. This potential limitation is overcome for practical clinical purposes, either by adding ^{125}I-fibrinogen leg scanning (which is highly sensitive to calf vein thrombosis) to impedance plethysmography,[61] or by performing serial impedance plethysmography.[6-8,69] The combined approach of impedance plethysmography and leg scanning can replace venography in most patients with clinically suspected venous thrombosis.[61] The combined approach has been replaced, however, by serial impedance plethysmography as the preferred approach.[6-8,63] ^{125}I-fibrinogen leg scanning is now of historical interest only, because of concern about the potential transmission of HIV infection from donor fibrinogen.

The use of serial impedance plethysmography is based on the concept, now confirmed by clinical observation,[6-8,63] that calf vein thrombi are only clinically important when extension into the proximal veins occurs, at which point, detection with impedance plethysmography have been evaluated by prospective clinical trials[6-8,63] in patients with suspected venous thrombosis. Based on the data provided by these studies, the following conclusions can be made: (1) a positive result by impedance plethysmography is highly predictive of acute proximal vein thrombosis (positive predictive value greater than 90%); and (2) it is safe to withhold therapy in patients with clinically suspected deep vein thrombosis who remain negative by serial impedance plethysmography over 10 to 14 days.

Occlusive impedance plethysmography is performed with the patient supine and the lower limb elevated 20 to 30°, the knee flexed 10 to 20°, and the ankle 8 to 15 cm higher than the knee. A pneumatic cuff 15 cm in width is applied to the midthigh and inflated to 45 cm H_2O, thereby occluding venous return. After a predetermined period, the cuff is rapidly deflated, and the changes in electrical resistance (impedance) resulting from alterations in blood volume distal to the cuff are detected by circumferential calf electrodes and recorded on an ECG paper strip. These changes in impedance during cuff inflation and deflation are measured, and both the total rise (venous filling) during cuff inflation and the fall occurring in the first 3 seconds of deflation (venous emptying) are plotted on a two-way impedance plethysmography graph.[59] The graph includes a "discriminant line" that was developed by discriminant function analysis to provide optimal separation of results into normal and abnormal for proximal vein thrombosis.[59]

The accuracy of impedance plethysmography is critically dependent on the degree of venous filling during cuff occlusion.[60] Venous filling is frequently suboptimal after only 45 seconds of cuff occlusion (as was originally recommended), and this may compromise the accuracy of the test. Venous filling is improved by two maneuvers: (1) prolonging the period of cuff occlusion from 45 seconds to

2 minutes; and (2) performing repeated sequential testing. These maneuvers increase both venous filling and the sensitivity and specificity of the test.[60] As venous filling is increased, there is a corresponding increase in venous emptying in normal legs but not in legs with proximal vein thrombosis, so the regression lines relating venous filling and emptying for normal and abnormal legs diverge. Thus, increased venous filling increases the separation between normal and abnormal impedance plethysmography results and enhances the accuracy of the test.[60]

Impedance plethysmography does not distinguish between thrombotic and nonthrombotic obstruction to venous outflow. Therefore, falsely positive results may occur if the patient is positioned incorrectly or is inadequately relaxed with constriction of veins by contracting leg muscles, if the vein is compressed by an extra vascular mass, or if venous outflow is impaired by raised central venous pressure or by positive pressure ventilation. Reduced arterial inflow to the limb due to severe obstructive arterial disease may also produce a falsely positive result.

The availability of high resolution real-time ultrasound probes has led to the application of ultrasound imaging for the diagnosis of deep vein thrombosis.[62,68,70] The term "Duplex" ultrasound refers to the technique in which real-time ultrasound imaging is combined with doppler ultrasound.[70] The concept is that real-time imaging provides direct visualization of the major deep veins whereas the doppler component is used to assess venous flow. Recent technologic advances enable the doppler signal from moving blood to be converted into a color-flow doppler or color imaging. Venous imaging using real-time B-mode ultrasound is a promising technique for evaluating patients with clinically suspected deep vein thrombosis.[62,68,70] A recent prospective study has shown that the single criterion of vein compressibility is highly sensitive and specific for proximal vein thrombosis in symptomatic patients (sensitivity and specificity 100% and 99% respectively).[62] Other criteria such as echogenicity or change in venous diameter during a Valsalva maneuver are less useful. The visualization of an echogenic band is highly sensitive for proximal vein thrombosis, but nonspecific (specificity 50%).[62] The percent change in venous diameter during a Valsalva maneuver is both insensitive (sensitivity 55%) and relatively nonspecific (specificity 67%).[62]

Real-time B-mode venous ultrasound is insensitive for isolated calf vein thrombosis.[70] Therefore, serial testing is required to detect patients who develop proximal extension. A recent randomized clinical trial (level I)[68] indicates that serial testing with B-mode venous ultrasound is as effective as impedance plethysmography, and confirms the safety of withholding anticoagulant therapy in symptomatic outpatients who remain negative on repeated testing with either approach. B-mode venous ultrasound may fail to detect isolated iliac vein thrombi.[62,70,71] This is a practical clinical limitation in patient groups in whom isolated iliac vein thrombosis is not uncommon (such as the pregnant patient).[63,72] Color flow imaging or other future technologic advances may improve the ability of B-mode venous imaging to detect isolated iliac vein thrombi and calf vein thrombi; clinical trials are awaited with interest.

B-mode venous imaging has a practical advantage in specificity over impedance plethysmography in selected ICU patients, such as those with raised central venous pressure (e.g., patients with congestive cardiac failure, in whom impedance plethysmography may be falsely positive). In addition, venous imaging may identify patients with extrinsic venous compression (e.g., due to Baker's cyst), which can lead to false-positive impedance plethysmography results.

If noninvasive tests for the diagnosis of venous thrombosis are not available or inconclusive, then ascending venography should be performed to objectively confirm or exclude venous thrombosis.

Practical Diagnostic Approach

A practical diagnostic approach for clinically suspected deep vein thrombosis is illustrated in Figure 23–5. If impedance plethysmography or B-mode venous imaging is positive in the absence of clinical conditions known to produce false-positive results, a diagnosis of venous thrombosis is established. A positive result by impedance plethysmography in the presence of conditions known to produce false-positive findings (e.g., congestive cardiac failure) should be confirmed by venography. If the result

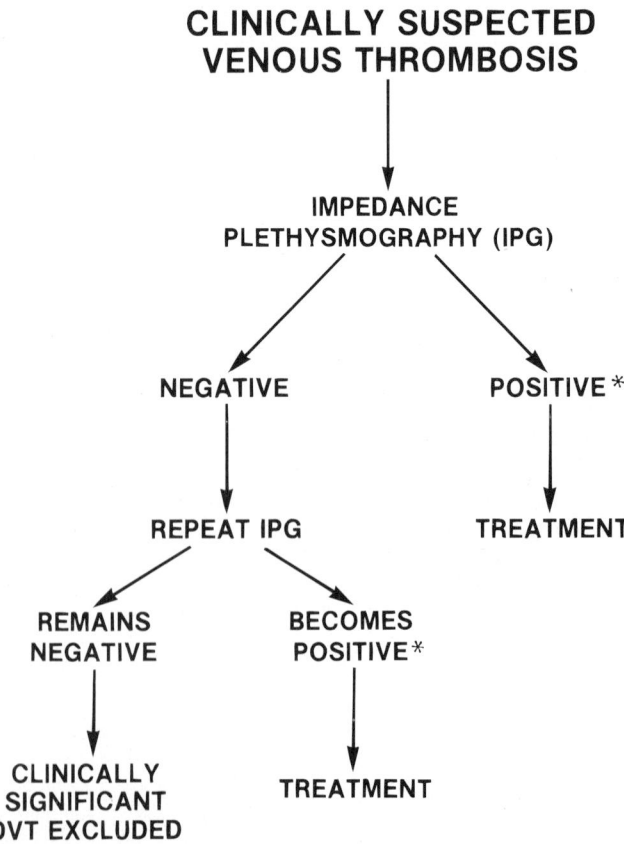

Fig. 23–5. Practical diagnostic approach for clinically suspected deep vein thrombosis. The asterisk indicates that if patients have clinical conditions that may produce a false-positive IPG result, venography should be performed. B-mode venous ultrasound imaging can be used in place of IPG.

Table 23-7. Contraindications to Anticoagulant Therapy

Absolute Contraindications
    Subarachnoid or cerebral hemorrhage
    Serious active bleeding (postoperative, spontaneous, or associated with trauma)
    Recent brain, eye, or spinal cord surgery
    Malignant hypertension
Relative Contraindications
    Active gastrointestinal hemorrhage
    Hemorrhagic diathesis
    Recent stroke
    Recent major surgery
    Severe hypertension
    Bacterial endocarditis
    Severe renal failure
    Severe hepatic failure

of the initial impedance plethysmography or B-mode ultrasound evaluation is negative, therapy is withheld and the test is repeated on several occasions over the 10 to 14 days following presentation.[6-8,63,68] If the results of serial impedance plethysmography remain negative over 10 to 14 days, clinically important venous thrombosis is excluded, and therapy can be safely withheld.[6-8,63,68]

Initial Treatment of Venous Thromboembolism

The therapeutic options in patients with established venous thromboembolism include:

- Anticoagulant therapy
- Thrombolytic therapy
- Vena caval filter (Greenfield filter)

The absolute and relative contraindications to anticoagulant therapy and thrombolytic therapy are listed in Tables 23-7 and 23-8, respectively. Inferior vena caval interruption, using a transvenously inserted filter (the Greenfield filter), is the management of choice for preventing pulmonary embolism in patients in whom anticoagulant therapy is absolutely contraindicated, and in the rare patient in whom anticoagulant therapy is ineffective. If relative contraindications to anticoagulant therapy exist, the patient should be treated with either carefully controlled continuous intravenous heparin, maintaining the anticoagulant effect near the lower limit of the therapeutic range, or with inferior vena caval interruption.

Anticoagulant Therapy

Intravenous heparin is the initial treatment of choice for most patients with acute proximal vein thrombosis or pulmonary embolism.[11,13,73] Low dose subcutaneous heparin (e.g., 5000 U every 8 hours), although effective for preventing venous thrombosis in surgical patients, is not effective for preventing recurrent venous thromboembolism in patients with established proximal vein thrombosis.[10] The difference in the dose of heparin required for the prevention and treatment of proximal vein thrombosis is probably due to the biochemical amplification that occurs with each successive step in the blood coagulation pathway. Consequently, much lower doses of heparin are required to prevent the formation of venous thrombi than are required to prevent the extension of recurrence of established thrombosis.

Intravenous heparin administered in doses which prolong the activated partial thromboplastin time (APTT) to 1.5 to 2 times control is effective and is associated with a low frequency (5%) of recurrent venous thromboembolism.[11,74] The findings of a randomized trial comparing intermittent subcutaneous heparin with continuous intravenous heparin strongly suggest a relationship between the intensity of anticoagulant response and the effectiveness of heparin therapy for proximal vein thrombosis.[11] In the subcutaneous heparin group, 36 to 57 patients (63%), had an APTT response < 1.5 times control during the initial 24 hours or more, compared with 17 of 58 patients (29% receiving continuous intravenous heparin ($p < 0.001$). The frequency of symptomatic recurrent venous thromboembolism confirmed by objective testing was 19% in the subcutaneous group (11 of 57 patients), compared with only 5% (3 of 58 patients) given continuous intravenous heparin ($p = 0.024$). All but one of the recurrences occurred in patients with an inadequate initial anticoagulant response (APTT < 1.5 times control). Recurrent venous thromboembolism was virtually eliminated in patients whose response to initial heparin therapy was above the lower limit of the therapeutic range set before the study began (APTT > 1.5 times control).[11] Thus, the episodes of recurrent venous thromboembolism were associated with, and likely the result of, an inadequate anticoagulant response. These results strongly suggest that an adequate initial anticoagulant response is required to prevent recurrent venous thromboembolism, and support the practice of monitoring heparin therapy with the APTT to ensure that an adequate response is obtained. The importance of adequate initial heparin treatment is also supported by the findings of a randomized trial comparing intravenous hepa-

Table 23-8. Contraindications to Thrombolytic Therapy

Absolute Contraindications
    Active internal bleeding
    Recent (within 2 months) cerebrovascular accident or other active intracranial processes
Relative Major Contraindications
    Recent (< 10 days) major surgery
    Recent obstetric delivery
    Recent organ biopsy
    Recent previous puncture of noncompressible vessels
    Recent serious gastrointestinal bleeding
    Recent serious trauma
    Severe hypertension (systolic > 200 mm Hg, diastolic > 110 mm Hg)
Relative Minor Contraindications
    Recent minor trauma including CPR
    High likelihood of left heart thrombus (e.g., mitral stenosis with atrial fibrillation)
    Bacterial endocarditis
    Diabetic hemorrhagic retinopathy
    Pregnancy
    Age > 75 years

rin with oral anticoagulants alone for the initial treatment of proximal vein thrombosis.[73]

It has been common clinical practice to continue intravenous heparin for 10 days, with oral anticoagulant therapy added on day 5 to 10 and continued long term. Recent clinical trials[75,76] indicate that the length of initial heparin treatment can be reduced to 5 days, without loss of effectiveness or safety, if oral anticoagulants are commenced on the first day. In patients at extremely high risk of bleeding, however, such as those who have just had surgery, those with multiple invasive lines, or those who have conditions that predispose them to major bleeding, it would be prudent to delay oral anticoagulant treatment, because the effect of heparin can be reversed almost instantly, but it may take six to eight hours to reverse the effect of oral anticoagulants. Heparin is discontinued on the fifth day following the initiation of oral anticoagulant therapy, provided the prothrombin time is prolonged above the lower limit of the therapeutic range (International Normalized Ratio ≥ 2.0).

Bleeding is the most common side effect of heparin, and occurs in 5 to 12% of patients during initial continuous intravenous heparin therapy.[11,74,76] The risk of bleeding is greater with intermittent intravenous heparin than for continuous intravenous heparin.[74,77,78]

A recent clinical trial (level 1)[76] provides new information about the relation between risk factors for bleeding, heparin dose, and the frequency of major bleeding complications. Before commencing heparin, patients were classified according to the presence or absence of one or more of the following risk factors for bleeding:

- Surgery within the previous 14 days
- A history of peptic ulcer disease, or of bleeding into the gastrointestinal or genitourinary tract
- Disorders or conditions predisposing the patient to bleeding (for example, multiple invasive lines)
- Thrombotic stroke within the previous 14 days
- Thrombocytopenia (platelet count $< 150 \times 10^9$/L)

If none of the foregoing risk factors were present (low risk), the initial heparin infusion dose was 40,000 U per 24 hours. Patients with one or more risk factors (high risk) were commenced at an infusion dose of 30,000 U per 24 hours. Major bleeding complications occurred in 12 of 111 (11%) high risk patients, compared with only 1 of 88 (1%) low risk patients (p = 0.007), even though the low risk patients were commenced on a higher initial heparin dose.[76] Six of the 13 patients suffered major bleeding, while the APTT was within the prescribed therapeutic range. Many patients without bleeding complications had APTT values more than 2.5 times control during the course of therapy. The findings suggest that the risk of bleeding is determined mainly by the presence or absence of predisposing factors, rather than the heparin dose or APTT response. In the absence of readily identifiable clinical risk factors (outlined previously), the risk of major bleeding complications is low (1%) even when these patients receive relatively high initial heparin infusion doses (40,000 U per 24 hours).[76]

Thrombocytopenia is now a well-recognized complication of heparin treatment. It usually has its onset 7 to 10 days after the initiation of therapy, but may occur earlier. Arterial thromboembolism is a rare but potentially devastating complication that occurs together with thrombocytopenia. The diagnosis of heparin-associated thrombocytopenia. The diagnosis of heparin-associated thrombocytopenia is made by excluding other causes of thrombocytopenia. This may be particularly difficult in ICU patients who may be septic or who may have received a number of different drugs that can cause thrombocytopenia. Heparin should be discontinued in all cases because it is impossible to predict which patients may develop thrombotic complications.

Other less common side effects of heparin include hypersensitivity to heparin, alopecia, a bluish discoloration of the toes associated with a burning sensation, and acquired hyperaldosteronism.

Protocol for Initial Continuous Intravenous Heparin Therapy. The following practical protocol has been developed based on the findings of clinical trials.[11,76,79] Heparin is given as an initial intravenous bolus of 5000 U, followed by a maintenance dose of 30,000 to 40,000 U per 24 hours (1250 to 1660 U/hour) by continuous intravenous infusion. If risk factors for bleeding are absent (as outlined previously)[76] then the initial infusion dose of 40,000 U per 24 hours should be used; if one or more risk factors for bleeding are present, the infusion dose of 30,000 U per 24 hours is used. Sufficient heparin should be given to maintain the APTT above 1.5 times the control value. A practical protocol for intravenous heparin therapy is described in Tables 23-9 and 23-10. Once the patient's anticoagulant (APTT) response and heparin dose requirements are stabilized, the APTT is measured daily for the duration of therapy.

Low Molecular Weight Heparin. Heparin in use clinically is a mixture of polysaccharide molecules ranging in

Table 23-9. Intravenous Heparin Protocol for Patients With Venous Thromboembolism

Initial intravenous heparin bolus: 5000 U
Continuous intravenous heparin infusion: commence at 42 ml/hr of 20,000 U (1680 U/hr) in 500 ml of diluent (a 24-hr heparin dose of 40,320 U), except in the following patients, in whom the heparin infusion is commenced at a rate of 31 ml/hr (1240 U/hr) (i.e., a 24-hr dose of 29,760 U):
  Patients who have undergone surgery within the previous 2 weeks
  Patients with a previous history of peptic ulcer disease, gastrointestinal bleeding or genitourinary bleeding
  Patients with recent stroke (i.e., thrombotic stroke within previous 2 weeks)
  Patients with a platelet count $< 150 \times 10^9$/L
  Patients with miscellaneous reasons for a high risk of bleeding (e.g., invasive line, hepatic failure, etc.)
APTT is performed in all patients thus:
  4 hours after commencing heparin, the heparin dose is adjusted
  4-6 hours after implementing the first dosage adjustment
  The APTT is then performed for the first 24 hours of therapy
  Thereafter, the APTT is performed once daily, unless the patient is subtherapeutic, in which case, the APTT should be repeated 4 hours after increasing the heparin dose

(From Hull, R., et al.: Optimal therapeutic level of heparin therapy in patients with venous thrombosis. Arch. Intern. Med., *152*:1589, 1992.)

Table 23–10. Intravenous Heparin Dose-Titration Nomogram Using the APTT for Patients with Venous Thromboembolism*

APTT (sec)	IV Infusion Rate Change (ml/hr)	Dose/Change (U/24 hr)	Additional Action
≤ 45	+6	+5,760	Repeat APTT in 4–6 hr
46–54	+3	+2,880	Repeat APTT in 4–6 hr
55–85	0	0	None†
86–110	−3	−2,880	Stop heparin for 1 hour Repeat APTT 4–6 hours after restarting heparin
> 110	−6	−5,760	Stop heparin for 1 hour Repeat APTT 4–6 hours after restarting heparin

* Using Actin-FS thromboplastin APTT reagent (Dade). Heparin concentration 20,000 U in 500 ml = 40 U/ml.
† During the first 24 hours, repeat APTT in 4 to 6 hours. Thereafter, the APTT is done once daily, unless subtherapeutic.
(From Hull, R., et al. Optimal therapeutic level of heparin therapy in patients with venous thrombosis. Arch. Intern. Med., *152*:1589, 1992.)

molecular weight from 5000 to 30,000 daltons, with a mean of 15,000 daltons. In recent years, low molecular weight fractions of heparin have been prepared with a mean molecular weight of 4000 to 5000 daltons.[80,81] Pharmacokinetic studies performed in the early and mid-1980s documented some potentially useful properties of low molecular weight heparin. These properties are:

- Very high bioavailability (90% or more) after subcutaneous injection
- A long half-life compared with unfractionated heparin
- A high correlation between body weight and the anticoagulant response to a given dose of low molecular weight heparin

The pharmacokinetic studies demonstrated that low molecular weight heparin administered as a single daily subcutaneous injection in a fixed dose (units per kilogram) could achieve a sustained anticoagulant effect throughout the 24-hour period, without the need for laboratory monitoring and dose adjustment. Two randomized clinical trials have evaluated the clinical outcomes of recurrent venous thromboembolism, bleeding, and death in patients with proximal vein thrombosis who were treated initially with either unfractionated intravenous heparin or subcutaneous low molecular weight heparin.[80,81] These clinical trials evaluated two different low molecular weight heparin fractions: Logiparin[80] and Fraxiparine.[81]

In the trial evaluating Logiparin, Hull and colleagues found that 15 (6.9%) of 219 patients who received intravenous unfractionated heparin had new episodes of symptomatic venous thromboembolism confirmed by objective testing, compared with only 6 (2.8%) of 213 patients who received Logiparin. This result represented a risk reduction of 59% in the incidence of recurrent venous thromboembolism, which did not quite achieve statistical significance (p = 0.07). Time to event analysis, however, demonstrated a significant difference in the frequency of recurrent venous thromboembolic events (p = 0.049).

Major bleeding associated with initial therapy occurred in 11 patients (5.5%) receiving intravenous heparin, compared with only 1 patient (0.5%) receiving low molecular weight heparin (a statistically significant risk reduction of 91%). Importantly, treatment with low molecular weight heparin was also associated with a 51% risk reduction in total mortality; 21 patients (9.6%) given intravenous heparin died, compared with 10 patients (4.7%) receiving low molecular weight heparin (p < 0.05).[80]

Similar reductions in the risk of recurrent venous thromboembolism, major bleeding, and mortality were reported in the study by Prandoni and colleagues evaluating Fraxiparine.[81] This trial had a smaller sample size however, and the observed differences in outcome did not achieve statistical significance (level II).

These two studies indicate that low molecular weight heparin is at least as effective and safe as intravenous unfractionated heparin for the initial treatment of patients with proximal vein thrombosis. At present, it remains uncertain whether the findings associated with one preparation of low molecular weight heparin can be extended to a different preparation. Therefore, each low molecular weight heparin fraction will have to be evaluated by randomized clinical trials before being introduced into clinical practice. The results of these initial trials evaluating clinical outcome are impressive and support the expanded evaluation of low molecular weight heparin in the treatment of acute venous thromboembolism.

Thrombolytic Therapy

Thrombolytic therapy with streptokinase, urokinase, or tissue plasminogen activator (rt-PA) is more effective than heparin alone for inducing rapid resolution of recent pulmonary embolism[31,45,46] or venous thrombosis.[82-86] The clinical role of thrombolytic therapy has not been completely resolved, however. Thrombolytic therapy is indicated for the management of patients with life-threatening massive pulmonary embolism. Thrombolytic therapy should also be considered in patients with pulmonary embolism and coexisting severe primary cardiac or pulmonary disease, in whom even a small embolus may be life-threatening.

The role of the thrombolytic therapy in patients with venous thrombosis is less certain. Thrombolytic therapy may benefit selected patients with acute massive venous thrombosis, such as those with phlegmasia cerulea dolens and impending venous gangrene. Such patients, however, comprise less than 1% of all patients with symptomatic venous thrombosis. In most patients with acute deep vein thrombosis, the role of thrombolytic therapy remains controversial.

The use of thrombolytic therapy in patients with venous thrombosis is based on the premise that early thrombolysis will minimize or prevent venous valvular damage and prevent the postphlebitic syndrome. This pathophysiologic concept remains an unresolved question. Unfortunately, because venous valvular damage may occur early in the formation of venous thrombosis, it may not necessarily be restored by thrombolysis. Although thrombolytic therapy is more effective than heparin alone for inducing complete lysis of recent deep vein thrombosis, it is currently uncertain if this improved lysis is associated with a decreased frequency of the postphlebitic syndrome. This issue can only be resolved by adequately designed and executed randomized clinical trials that measure clinical outcome (the postphlebitic syndrome). At present, the effectiveness of thrombolytic therapy for preventing the postphlebitic syndrome remains uncertain.[82]

Bleeding is a more frequent complication of thrombolytic therapy with streptokinase than with heparin treatment alone.[82] The risk of major bleeding with streptokinase treatment in patients with venous thrombosis is increased approximately two to three times compared to that with intravenous heparin.[82] Intracranial hemorrhage occurs in 1% of patients treated with thrombolytic therapy using streptokinase—about twice as frequently as with intravenous heparin.[87] The risk of hemorrhage during thrombolytic therapy with streptokinase or urokinase increases with the length of infusion; a short course of therapy (12 to 24 hours) lessens the risk of bleeding, but in patients with venous thrombosis, treatment may have to be continued for as long as 72 hours to achieve complete lysis. Initial randomized trials of rt-PA infusions in patients with venous thrombosis have reported bleeding rates of 7 to 30%.[84-86] The optimal regimen of rt-PA is currently uncertain; further trials are required to determine if rt-PA should be given as a continuous infusion or as a bolus injection.

The risk of bleeding with thrombolytic therapy can be minimized, but not completely avoided, by careful selection of patients. The following guidelines are recommended for patient selection for thrombolytic therapy:[87] (1) the presence of an appropriate clinical indication including an objectively documented diagnosis and evidence that the venous thromboembolic event is of recent origin (less than 7 days); and (2) careful evaluation of contraindications (see Table 23–8). If pulmonary angiography is used to confirm a diagnosis of pulmonary embolism, the angiography catheter should be inserted into an arm vein, where hemostatis is easier to achieve than the femoral vein. In addition, attention should be given to avoiding (if possible) the use of central venous lines and arterial lines in patients with suspected pulmonary embolism and hemodynamic instability who may be candidates for thrombolytic therapy.

There are practical limitations to the routine use of thrombolytic therapy in patients with deep vein thrombosis. The guidelines outlined previously are stringent in order to enhance effectiveness and minimize the risk of bleeding, but this also significantly reduces the number of patients who are eligible for thrombolytic therapy. Clinical trials[6-8] in patients with symptomatic venous thrombosis indicate that many have symptoms for more than 7 days, which makes them unsuitable for thrombolytic therapy by the suggested guidelines.[84,86]

In view of the documented increased risk of bleeding, and the lack of definitive evidence of improved long-term benefit, the routine use of thrombolytic therapy in patients with venous thrombosis is not recommended. Further clinical trials may modify these recommendations but, at present, anticoagulant therapy remains the treatment of choice for most patients with acute proximal vein thrombosis.

Protocol for Thrombolytic Therapy. Before initiating thrombolytic therapy, a baseline hemoglobin, hematocrit, and platelet count should be obtained, as well as a prothrombin time, partial thromboplastin time, and thrombin clotting time. To minimize the risk of bleeding, invasive arterial procedures should be avoided and venipuncture should be kept to an absolute minimum. If arterial blood samples are required, blood should be taken from the radial artery and local compression maintained for at least 20 minutes.

The most extensively evaluated thrombolytic agents are streptokinase, urokinase, and tissue plasminogen activator (t-PA). Streptokinase, a product of hemolytic streptococci, is antigenic in humans and stimulates the production of neutralizing antibodies. Streptokinase complexes with plasminogen to form a plasminogen-streptokinase complex, which then acts on uncomplexed plasminogen to produce plasmin. Urokinase is a naturally occurring activator of plasminogen produced by renal parenchymal cells and is present in human urine. Urokinase is a nonantigenic in humans. Tissue plasminogen activator is a naturally occurring protein produced by endothelial cells which catalyzes the conversion of plasminogen to plasmin. Other thrombolytic agents which have been less extensively evaluated in venous thromboembolic disease are acylated plasminogen-streptokinase activator complex (APSAC), and recombinant single chain urokinase plasminogen activator (rscu-PA).

Streptokinase. Streptokinase therapy is initiated with a loading dose of 250,000 U administered intravenously over 30 minutes, followed by a maintenance dose of 100,000 U by continuous intravenous infusion.[31,82,83,87] Larger loading doses may be indicated in patients with life-threatening massive pulmonary embolism in order to ensure that the patients streptokinase antibodies have been neutralized and thus to ensure an adequate lytic effect.

The systemic effect of streptokinase can be determined by monitoring the thrombin clotting time or euglobulin lysis time, but there is currently no evidence that monitoring with these tests predicts clinical efficacy or reduces bleeding complications. The thrombin clotting time should be performed approximately 2 hours after the loading dose is given, at which time it should be prolonged to four to five times the control value. A lesser degree of prolongation suggests that the patient's streptokinase antibodies have not been adequately neutralized and is an indication for streptokinase-resistance test and adjustment of the dose accordingly.

Once a thrombolytic state is established, the thrombin clotting time should be repeated at four hour intervals. If the thrombin clotting time remains two to five times the control value, no change in dose is required. A thrombin time that is less than twice the control value indicates an excess of plasminogen-streptokinase complex relative to uncomplexed plasminogen, and the dose should be decreased by 25 to 50%. A thrombin clotting time in excess of five times the control value indicates a lack of streptokinase-plasminogen complex relative to uncomplexed plasminogen, and the maintenance dose should be increased to approximately 200,000 U per hour to increase the rate of complex with free plasminogen.

Urokinase. The recommended dose of urokinase for patients with pulmonary embolism is a loading dose of 4400 IU per kilogram body weight given intravenously over 10 minutes, followed by a maintenance dose of 4400 IU per kilogram per hour by continuous intravenous infusion.[31]

A short course of therapy (12 to 24 hours) with streptokinase or urokinase lessens the risk of bleeding and is preferred in patients with pulmonary embolism. In patients with venous thrombosis, patients may have to be continued for as long as 72 hours to achieve complete lysis.

Recombinant Tissue Plasminogen Activator (rt-PA). The optimal regimen of rt-PA in patients with venous thromboembolism remains uncertain. In one randomized trial, rt-PA given by continuous intravenous infusion in a dose of 50 mg per hour for 2 hours was more effective than urokinase in producing clot lysis at 2 hours (by repeat angiography) and for improving the hemodynamics.[46] The rt-PA and urokinase regimens achieved similar improvements in lung scan reperfusion at 24 hours.[46]

The efficacy of rt-PA administered as a single bolus dose has been evaluated by a randomized trial in patients with pulmonary embolism.[88] The rationale for this study was the finding in experimental animals that rt-PA produces continued thrombolysis after it is cleared from the circulation, and the thrombolysis is both increased and accelerated, and bleeding reduced, when rt-PA is administered over a short period. A bolus dose of rt-PA (0.6 mg/kg over two minutes) produced a greater than 50% resolution in perfusion lung scan defects at 24 hours in 11 of 32 patients (34%), compared with three of 25 patients (12%) who received heparin alienate (P — 0.026).[88] By seven days, the lung scan resolution was similar in the rt-PA and intravenous heparin groups. Importantly, this randomized trial did not evaluate the early (2-hour) thrombolytic effect or hemodynamic response. Therefore, based on the available data, if rt-PA is used for patients with massive pulmonary embolism, the continuous infusion regimen should be used (50 mg per hour for 2 hours) (level 1).[46] Further randomized clinical trials are required to determine if rt-PA should be given by continuous infusion or bolus injection.

After thromboembolic therapy is discontinued, it should be followed by full dose intravenous heparin therapy and then long-term anticoagulant therapy to prevent recurrent venous thromboembolism.[10,11]

POST-ICU PHASE: LONG-TERM TREATMENT OF VENOUS THROMBOEMBOLISM

Failure to follow the initial course of intravenous heparin with adequate long-term therapy exposes patients with proximal vein thrombosis to a high risk (40 to 50%) of recurrent venous thromboembolism; this risk is markedly reduced to 2% by adequate long-term anticoagulant therapy.[10] Oral warfarin sodium is the preferred long-term approach in most patients.[89] Adjusted dose subcutaneous heparin is an effective and safe alternative to warfarin sodium;[90] it is the long-term regimen of choice in pregnant patients, and in patients returning to geographically remote areas which lack the facilities for anticoagulant monitoring (in whom the dose is adjusted during the first few days of long-term therapy and then fixed).

Long-term anticoagulant therapy for venous thromboembolism can now be given with a low risk of bleeding (< 5%). Either less intense oral warfarin sodium (INR 2.0 to 3.0)[91] or adjusted dose subcutaneous heparin[90] are effective for preventing recurrent venous thromboembolism while markedly reducing the risk of bleeding associated with the more intense warfarin therapy traditionally used in North America (INR 3.0 to 4.5).

Long-term anticoagulant therapy is continued for three months in patients with their first episode of proximal vein thrombosis or pulmonary embolism. A longer course of therapy is indicated in patients with recurrent venous thromboembolism, and in patients in whom there is a continuing risk factor for venous thromboembolism. In patients with recurrent venous thrombosis, therapy should probably be continued for at least one year because stopping anticoagulant therapy at three months is associated with a 20% frequency of recurrent venous thromboembolism during the following year and a 4% risk of fatal pulmonary embolism.[92] In patients with a continuing risk factor that is potentially reversible (e.g., fractured hip), anticoagulant therapy should be continued until the risk factor is reversed. Anticoagulant therapy should be continued indefinitely in patients with an irreversible risk factor (e.g., antithrombin III deficiency or protein C deficiency).

Special Issues in Venous Thromboembolism

Management of Calf Vein Thrombosis

The optimal management of patients with isolated calf vein thrombosis has not been completely resolved. Venous thrombosis that remains confined to the deep calf veins is associated with a low risk of clinically important pulmonary embolism,[4-8] but 20% of calf vein thrombi extend into the proximal venous segment.[4-9] An alternative to anticoagulant treatment in patients with calf vein thrombosis is to monitor for proximal extension using serial impedance plethysmography or B-mode venous ultrasound (which is insensitive for calf vein thrombosis but highly sensitive for proximal vein thrombosis). This approach is supported by the findings of prospective clinical trials[6-8,63,68] in patients with clinically suspected venous thrombosis (level 1). These trials indicate that anticoagulant therapy can be safely withheld if the results of impedance plethysmography remain negative on repeated testing over 10 to 14 days.[6-8,63,68] Thus, surveillance with serial impedance plethysmography or B-mode venous ultrasound can be used to separate the 20% of patients with calf vein thrombosis who develop proximal extension (and require treatment), from the remaining 80% who do not extend, in whom the risks of anticoagulant therapy may outweigh the benefits. If these tests are unavailable to monitor for extension, then patients with calf vein thrombosis should be treated initially with heparin therapy followed by adequate long-term anticoagulant therapy.[9]

Axillary Vein Thrombosis

The most common cause of axillary vein thrombosis is indwelling catheters. This fact makes axillary vein thrombosis an important issue for the ICU physician because of the common use of catheters in ICU patients. Wherever possible, measures should be taken to prevent catheter-induced thrombosis. A practical regimen that may be effective in patients with central venous catheters is a fixed low dose (2 mg per day) of warfarin sodium (level 3).[93] Other less common causes of axillary vein thrombosis include an anatomic abnormality of the thoracic inlet that compresses the axillary vein, or unusually strenuous arm exercise involving marked adduction of the arm (so-called "stress thrombosis").

The clinical features of axillary or subclavian vein thrombosis include swelling of the entire arm, pain, tenderness, and the development of venous collaterals around the shoulder. Axillary vein thrombosis may be complicated by pulmonary embolism. Patients with axillary vein thrombosis may suffer recurrent episodes and may develop marked postphlebitic symptoms.

Of the noninvasive tests, B-mode venous ultrasound is best suited for application to upper extremity. The role of venous ultrasound imaging or other noninvasive tests in the diagnosis of upper extremity thrombosis is currently uncertain, however. Therefore, venography is indicated to confirm or refute a clinical diagnosis of axillary vein thrombosis.

The optimal management of patients with confirmed axillary vein thrombosis remains uncertain; the issue has not been addressed by randomized clinical trials. At present, a reasonable approach would be to treat these patients like patients with deep vein thrombosis of the leg, using full dose continuous intravenous heparin for 5 to 10 days followed by oral anticoagulant for 6 weeks to 3 months. Alternately, thrombolytic therapies may be considered if the thrombus is of recent origin and there are no contraindications (which is usually not the case in patients in the ICU). The objective of thrombolytic therapy is to minimize postphlebitic symptoms, but its effectiveness for this purpose remains uncertain. In patients with suppurative thrombophlebitis in whom surgical drainage and ligation is not feasible, case reports document successful therapy with combined anticoagulants and antibiotics.[94]

Suspected Pulmonary Embolism During Pregnancy

Although the absolute incidence of venous thromboembolism during pregnancy is low, pulmonary embolism among the leading causes of maternal mortality.[95] The pregnant patient with clinically suspected pulmonary embolism poses major diagnostic and therapeutic challenges.

If the patient is hemodynamically stable at the time of presentation, then the management is as outlined previously for "the hemodynamically stable patient." The dose of radioisotope for perfusion lung scanning can be reduced to minimize fetal exposure. If pulmonary angiography is required, appropriate measures should be taken to shield the fetus from radiation exposure. A prospective study (level 1) in pregnant patients with clinically suspected deep vein thrombosis indicates that if serial testing with impedance plethysmography remains negative, anticoagulant therapy can be safely withheld.[63] These data, together with previous data in patients with clinically suspected pulmonary embolism,[23] suggest that serial testing for proximal vein thrombosis with impedance plethysmography may be a useful alternative to pulmonary angiography in patients with nonhigh probability lung scan findings who have adequate cardiorespiratory reserve. B-mode venous ultrasound is useful if positive results are found (using the criteria of vein compressibility), but because this test may fail to detect isolated iliac vein thrombi[70,71] (which is not uncommon in pregnant patients),[63,72] the safety of withholding therapy in pregnant patients with negative findings by B-mode ultrasound remains uncertain.

The pregnant patient with suspected massive pulmonary embolism who is hemodynamically unstable is a more difficult problem. In general, the principles outlined in our discussion of the hemodynamically unstable patient apply. Although pregnancy is listed as a contraindication to thrombolytic therapy, this may be the only option in patients with life-threatening pulmonary embolism if facilities and expertise for immediate embolectomy are unavailable. There have been case reports of pulmonary embolectomy performed successfully during pregnancy with both maternal and fetal survival.[96-98] The appropriate management in pregnant patients with suspected massive pulmonary embolism remains a clinical judgment in the individual case, which depends on the available facilities and expertise, as well as an appropriate weighing of both maternal and fetal welfare.

REFERENCES

1. Sackett, D. L.: Rules of evidence and clinical recommendations on the use of antithrombotic agents. Chest, *95(Suppl.)*: 2S, 1989.
2. Dalen, J. E., and Alpert, J. S.: Natural history of pulmonary embolism. Prog. Cardiovasc. Dis., *17*:249, 1975.
3. Donaldson, G. A., Williams, C., Scanell, J., and Shaw, R. S.: A reappraisal of the application of the Trendelenburg operation to massive fatal embolism. N. Engl. J. Med., *268*:171, 1963.
4. Kakkar, V. V., et al.: Natural history of post-operative deep-vein thrombosis. Lancet, *2*:230, 1969.
5. Moser, K. M., and LeMoine, J. R.: Is embolic risk conditioned by location of deep venous thrombosis? Ann. Intern. Med., *94*:439, 1981.
6. Hull, R. D., et al.: Diagnostic efficacy of impedance plethysmography of clinically suspected deep-vein thrombosis: a randomized trial. Ann. Intern. Med., *102*:21, 1985.
7. Huisman, M. V., Buller, H. E., Ten Cate, J. W., and Vreeken, J.: Serial impedance plethysmography for suspected deep venous thrombosis in outpatients. The Amsterdam General Practitioner Study. N. Engl. J. Med., *314*:823, 1986.
8. Huisman, M. V., et al.: Management of clinically suspected acute venous thrombosis in outpatients with serial impedance plethysmography in a community hospital setting. Arch. Intern. Med., *149*:511, 1989.
9. Lagerstedt, C. I., et al.: Need for long-term anticoagulant treatment in symptomatic calf vein thrombosis. Lancet, *2*: 515, 1985.
10. Hull, R. D., et al.: Warfarin sodium versus low-dose heparin in the long-term treatment of venous thrombosis. N. Engl. J. Med., *301*:855, 1979.

11. Hull, R. D., et al.: Continuous intravenous heparin compared with intermittent subcutaneous heparin in the initial treatment of proximal-vein thrombosis. N. Engl. J. Med., 315:1109, 1986.
12. Huisman, M. V., et al.: Unexpected high prevalence of silent pulmonary embolism in patients with deep venous thrombosis. Chest, 95:498, 1989.
13. Barritt, D. W., and Jordan, S. C.: Anticoagulant drugs in the treatment of pulmonary embolism. A controlled trial. Lancet, 1:1309, 1960.
14. Stamatakis, J., et al.: Femoral vein thrombosis and total hip replacement. Br. Med. J., 2:223, 1977.
15. Harris, W. H., et al. Aspirin prophylaxis of venous thromboembolism after total hip replacement. N. Engl. J. Med., 297:1246, 1977.
16. Nillius, A. S., and Nylander, G: Deep-vein thrombosis after hip replacement: a clinical and phlebographic study. Br. J. Surg., 66:324, 1979.
17. Coventry, M. B., Nolan, D. R., and Beckenbaugh, R. D.: Delayed prophylactic anticoagulation: a study of results and complications in 2,012 total hip arthroplasties. J. Bone Joint Surg., 55-A:1487, 1973.
18. Sevitt, S., and Gallagher, N.: Venous thrombosis and pulmonary embolism. A clinicopathological study in injured and burned patients. Br. J. Surg., 48:475, 1961.
19. Havig, G. O.: Source of pulmonary emboli. Acta Chir. Scand., 478(Suppl.):42, 1977.
20. Mavor, G. E., and Galloway, J. M. D.: The iliofemoral venous segment as a source of pulmonary emboli. Lancet, 1:871, 1967.
21. Hull, R. D., et al.: Pulmonary angiography, ventilation lung scanning and venography for clinically suspected pulmonary embolism with abnormal perfusion lung scan. Ann. Intern. Med., 98:891, 1983.
22. Hull, R. D., et al.: Diagnostic value of ventilation-perfusion lung scanning in patients with suspected pulmonary embolism. Chest, 88:819, 1985.
23. Hull, R. D., et al.: A new non-invasive management strategy for patients with suspected pulmonary embolism. Arch. Intern. Med., 149:2549, 1989.
24. International Multicentre Trial. Prevention of fatal post-operative pulmonary embolism by low doses of heparin. Lancet, 2:45, 1975.
25. Sevitt, S., and Gallager, N. G.: Prevention of venous thrombosis and pulmonary embolism in injured patients. A trial of anticoagulant prophylaxis with phenidine in middle-aged and elderly patients with fractured necks of femur. Lancet, 2:981, 1959.
26. Warlow, C., et al.: A double-blind trial of low doses of subcutaneous heparin in the prevention of deep-vein thrombosis after myocardial infarction. Lancet, 2:934, 1973.
27. Turpie, A. G., et al.: A randomized double-blind trial of ORG 10172 low molecular weight heparinoid in the prevention of deep-vein thrombosis in thrombotic stroke. Lancet, 1:523, 1987.
28. Salzman, E. W., and Davies, G. C.: Prophylaxis of venous thromboembolism: Analysis of cost-effectiveness. Ann. Surg., 191:207, 1980.
29. Hull, R. D., Hirsh, J., Sackett, D. L., and Stoddart, G.: Cost effectiveness of primary and secondary prevention of fatal pulmonary embolism in high-risk surgical patients. Can. Med. Assoc. J., 127:990, 1982.
30. Turpie, A. G., et al.: Comparison of high-dose with low-dose subcutaneous heparin to prevent left ventricular mural thrombosis in patients with acute transmural anterior myocardial infarction. N. Engl. J. Med., 320:352, 1989.
31. Urokinase Pulmonary Embolism Trial: a National Co-operative Study. Circulation (Suppl. II):1, 1973.
32. PIOPED Investigators. Value of the ventilation/perfusion scan in acute pulmonary embolism. Results of the Prospective Investigation of Pulmonary Embolism Diagnosis (PIOPED). JAMA, 263:2753, 1990.
33. Szucs, M. M., et al.: Diagnostic sensitivity of laboratory findings in acute pulmonary embolism. Ann. Intern. Med., 74:161, 1971.
34. Bell, W. R., Simon, T. L., and DeMets, D. L.: The clinical features of submassive and massive pulmonary emboli. Am. J. Med., 62:355, 1977.
35. Hull, R. D., et al.: Pulmonary embolism in outpatients with pleuritis chest pain. Arch. Intern. Med., 148:838, 1988.
36. Dismuke, S. E., and Wagner, E. H.: Pulmonary embolism as a cause of death. The changing mortality in hospitalized patients. JAMA, 255:2039, 1986.
37. Murray, I. V., Mikail, M. S., Banner, M. J., and Modell, J. H.: Pulmonary embolism: high-frequency jet ventilation offers advantages over conventional mechanical ventilation. Crit. Care Med., 15:114, 1987.
38. Vlahakes, G. J., Turley, K., and Hoffman, J. I. E.: The pathophysiology of failure in acute right ventricular hypertension: hemodynamic and biochemical correlations. Circulation, 63:87, 1981.
39. Ducas, J., and Prewitt, R. M.: Pathophysiology and therapy of right ventricular dysfunction due to pulmonary embolism. Cardiovasc. Clin., 17:191, 1987.
40. Molloy, W. D., et al.: Treatment of shock in a canine model of pulmonary embolism. Am. Rev. Respir. Dis., 130:870, 1984.
41. Duca, J., Girling, L., Shick, U., and Prewitt, R. M.: Pulmonary vascular effects of hydralazine in a canine preparation of pulmonary thromboembolism. Circulation, 73:1050, 1986.
42. Belenkie, I., Dani, R., Smith, E. R., and Tyberg, J. V.: Ventricular interaction during experimental acute pulmonary embolism. Circulation, 78:761, 1988.
43. Jardin, F., et al.: Quantitative two-dimensional echocardiography in massive pulmonary embolism: emphasis on ventricular interdependence and leftward displacement. J. Am. Coll. Cardiol., 10:1201, 1987.
44. Hirsh, J., et al.: Heparin kinetics in venous thrombosis and pulmonary embolism. Circulation, 53:691, 1976.
45. Goldhaber, S. Z., et al.: Acute pulmonary embolism treated with tissue plasminogen activator. Lancet, 2:886, 1986.
46. Goldhaber, S. Z., et al.: Randomized controlled trial of recombinant tissue plasminogen activator versus urokinase in the treatment of acute pulmonary embolism. Lancet, 2:293, 1988.
47. Hull, R. D., Raskob, G. E., Coates, G., and Panju, A. A.: Clinical validity of a normal perfusion scan in patients with suspected pulmonary embolism. Chest, 97:23, 1990.
48. Kipper, M. S., Moser, K. M., Kortman, K. E., and Ashburn, W. L.: Long-term follow-up of patients with suspected pulmonary embolism and a normal lung scan. Chest, 82:411, 1982.
49. Denardo, G., et al. The ventilatory lung scan in the diagnosis of pulmonary embolism. N. Engl. J. Med., 282:1334, 1974.
50. Alderson, P. O., Rujanavech, N., Secker-Walker, R. H., and McKnight, R. C.: The role of ^{133}Xe ventilation studies in the scintigraphic detection of pulmonary embolism. Radiology, 120:633, 1976.
51. Biello, D. R., Mattar, A. G., McKnight, R. C., and Siegel, B. A.: Ventilation-perfusion studies in suspected pulmonary embolism. AJR, 133:1033, 1979.
52. McNeil, B. J.: Ventilation-perfusion studies and the diagnosis of pulmonary embolism: concise communication. J. Nucl. Med., 21:319, 1980.
53. Cheely, R., et al.: The role of non-invasive tests versus pulmo-

nary angiography in the diagnosis of pulmonary embolism. Am. J. Med., 70:17, 1981.
54. Dalen, J. E., et al.: Pulmonary angiography in acute pulmonary embolism. Indications, techniques, and results in 367 patients. Am. Heart J., 81:175, 1971.
55. Bookstein, J. J., and Silver, T. M.: The angiographic differential diagnosis of acute pulmonary embolism. Radiology, 110:25, 1974.
56. Mills, S. R., et al.: The incidence etiologies, and avoidance of complications of pulmonary angiography in a large series. Radiology, 136:295, 1980.
57. Novelline, R. A., et al.: The clinical course of patients with suspected pulmonary embolism and a negative pulmonary arteriogram. Radiology, 126:561, 1978.
58. Hull, R., et al.: A noninvasive strategy for the treatment of patients with suspected pulmonary embolism. Arch. Intern. Med., 154:289, 1994.
59. Hull, R. D., et al. Impedance plethysmography using the occlusive cuff technique in the diagnosis of venous thrombosis. Circulation, 53:696, 1976.
60. Hull, R. D., et al.: Impedance plethysmography: the relationship between venous filling and sensitivity and specificity for proximal-vein thrombosis. Circulation, 58:898, 1978.
61. Hull, R. D., et al.: Replacement of venography in suspected venous thrombosis by impedance plethysmograph and ^{125}I-fibrinogen leg scanning: a less invasive approach. Ann. Intern. Med., 94:12, 1981.
62. Lensing, A. W., et al.: Detection of deep-vein thrombosis by real-time B-mode ultrasonography. N. Engl. J. Med., 320:342, 1989.
63. Hull, R. D., Raskob, G. E., and Carter, C. J.: Serial impedance plethysmography in pregnant patients with clinically suspected deep-vein thrombosis. Clinical validity of negative findings. Ann. Intern. Med., 112:663, 1990.
64. Hull, R. D., et al.: Clinical validity of a negative venogram in patients with clinically suspected venous thrombosis. Circulation, 64:622, 1981.
65. Rabinov, K., and Paulin, S.: Roentgen diagnosis of venous thrombosis in the leg. Arch. Surg., 104:134, 1972.
66. Parfrey, P. S., et al.: Contrast material-induced renal failure in patients with diabetes mellitus, renal insufficiency, or both: a prospective controlled study. N. Engl. J. Med., 320:143, 1989.
67. Schwab, S. J., et al.: Contrast nephrotoxicity: a randomized controlled trial of a nonionic and an ionic radiographic contrast agent. N. Engl. J. Med., 320:1459, 1989.
68. Heijboer, H., et al.: A comparison of real-time compression ultrasonography with impedance plethysmography for the diagnosis of deep-vein thrombosis in symptomatic outpatients. N. Engl. J. Med., 329:1365, 1993.
69. Wheeler, H. B., and Anderson, F. A. Jr.: Can noninvasive tests be used as the basis for treatment of deep-vein thrombosis? In Noninvasive Diagnostic Techniques in Vascular Disease. 3rd Ed. Edited by E. F. Bernstein. St. Louis, C. V. Mosby Co., 1985, p. 805.
70. White, R. H., McGahan, J. P., Daschbach, M. M., and Hartling, R. P.: Diagnosis of deep-vein thrombosis using Duplex ultrasound. Ann. Intern. Med., 111:297, 1989.
71. Gocke, J. E., and Harlan, J.: Detection of deep-vein thrombosis by B-mode ultrasonography (letter). N. Engl. J. Med., 321:613, 1989.
72. Bergqvist, A., Bergqvist, D., and Hallbrook, T.: Deep-vein thrombosis during pregnancy. A prospective study. Acta Obstet. Gynecol. Scand., 62:443, 1983.
73. Brandjes, D. P. M., et al.: Acenocoumarol and heparin compared with acenocoumarol alone in the initial treatment of proximal-vein thrombosis. N. Engl. J. Med., 327:1485, 1992.
74. Salzman, E. W., Deykin, D., Shapiro, R. M., and Rosenberg, R.: Management of heparin therapy: controlled prospective trial. N. Engl. J. Med., 292:1046, 1975.
75. Gallus, A., et al.: Safety and efficacy of warfarin started early after submassive venous thrombosis or pulmonary embolism. Lancet, 2:1293, 1986.
76. Hull, R. D., et al.: Heparin for 5 days as compared with 10 days in the initial treatment of proximal venous thrombosis. N. Engl. J. Med., 322:1260, 1990.
77. Glazier, R. L., and Crowell, E. B.: Randomized prospective trial of continuous versus intermittent heparin therapy. JAMA, 236:1365, 1976.
78. Wilson, J. R., and Lampman, J.: Heparin therapy: a randomized prospective study. Am. Heart J., 97:155, 1979.
79. Hull, R. D., et al.: Optimal therapeutic level of heparin therapy in patients with venous thrombosis. Arch. Intern. Med., 152:1589, 1992.
80. Hull, R. D., et al.: Subcutaneous low molecular weight heparin compared with continuous intravenous heparin in the treatment of proximal-vein thrombosis. N. Engl. J. Med., 326:975, 1992.
81. Prandoni, P., et al.: Comparison of subcutaneous low-molecular-weight heparin with intravenous standard heparin in proximal deep-vein thrombosis. Lancet, 339:441, 1992.
82. Goldhaber, S. Z., Buring, J. E., Lipnick, R. J., and Hennekens, C. H.: Pooled analyses of randomized trials of streptokinase and heparin in phlebographically documented acute deep-venous thrombosis. Am. J. Med., 75:393, 1984.
83. Rogers, L. Q., and Lutcher, C. L.: Streptokinase therapy for deep vein thrombosis: a comprehensive review of the English literature. Am. J. Med., 88:389, 1990.
84. Turpie, A. G. G., et al.: Tissue plasminogen activator (rt-PA) vs heparin in deep-vein thrombosis. Results of a randomized trial. Chest, 97(Suppl):172S, 1990.
85. Goldhaber, S. Z., et al.: Randomized control trial of tissue plasminogen activator in proximal deep venous thrombosis. Am. J. Med., 88:235, 1990.
86. Verhaeghe, R., Besse, P., Bounameaux, H., and Marbet, G. A.: Multicenter pilot study of the efficacy and safety of systemic rt-PA administration in the treatment of deep-vein thrombosis of the lower extremities and/or pelvis. Thromb. Res., 55:5, 1989.
87. Thrombolytic therapy in thrombosis. A National Institutes of Health Consensus Development Conference. Ann. Intern. Med., 93:141, 1980.
88. Levine, M., et al.: A randomized trial of a single bolus dosage regimen of recombinant tissue plasminogen activator in patients with acute pulmonary embolism. Chest, 98:1473, 1990.
89. Hull, R. D., Raskob, G., Hirsh, J., and Sackett, D. L.: A cost-effectiveness analysis of alternative approaches for long-term treatment of proximal venous thrombosis. JAMA, 252:235, 1984.
90. Hull, R. D., et al. Adjusted subctuaneous heparin versus warfarin sodium in the long-term treatment of venous thrombosis. N. Engl. J. Med., 306:189, 1982.
91. Hull, R. D., et al.: Different intensities of oral anticoagulant therapy in the treatment of proximal-vein thrombosis. N. Engl. J. Med., 307:1676, 1982.
92. Hull, R. D., et al.: The diagnosis of acute recurrent deep-vein thrombosis: a diagnostic challenge. Circulation, 67:901, 1983.
93. Bern, M. M., et al.: Prophylaxis against central vein thrombosis with low dose warfarin. Surgery, 99:216, 1986.
94. Verghese, A., Widrich, W. C., and Arbeit, R. D.: Central venous septic thrombophlebitis—the role of medical therapy. Medicine, 64:394, 1985.

95. Kaunitz, A. M., et al.: Causes of maternal mortality in the United States. Obstet. Gynecol., 65:605, 1985.
96. Richards, S. R., Burrows, H., and O'Shaughnessy, R.: Intrapartum pulmonary embolus: a case report. J. Reprod. Med., 30: 64, 1985.
97. Blegrad, S., Lund, O., Nielsen, T. T., and Guldholt, I.: Emergency embolectomy in a patient with massive pulmonary embolism during second trimester pregnancy. Acta Obstet. Gynecol. Scand., 68:267, 1989.
98. Splinter, W. M., Dwane, P. D., Wigle, R. D., and McGrath, M. J.: Anaesthetic management of emergency Caesarean section followed by pulmonary embolectomy. Can. J. Anaesth., 36: 689, 1989.

ns is a condition in which the capacity of a rested muscle to generate force is impaired."[14]

Chapter 24

REHABILITATION OF THE VENTILATOR-DEPENDENT PATIENT

EDWARD D. SIVAK

The technology of mechanical ventilation has evolved along two pathways—maintenance of respiration through anesthesia, and surgery and maintenance of respiration through critical illness.[1] As surgical techniques improve and new treatments for medical illnesses develop, increasing numbers of patients will receive the benefits of mechanical ventilation. By the same token, the risk of patients requiring longer periods of ventilatory support and the possibility of permanent ventilator dependency will also increase. Some patients may benefit from prolonged ventilation whereas others will live a life of maintenance and custodial care because of an inability to sustain spontaneous ventilation.[2] Under these circumstances, ventilator dependency, weaning from mechanical ventilation, and rehabilitation rather than weaning from mechanical ventilation have become true societal issues.[3-6]

In discussing these issues, ventilator dependency will be defined as the requirement for mechanical ventilation beyond the limits of critical illness or acute events associated with acute respiratory failure. The interpretation of this description is the requirement for mechanical ventilation beyond 24 to 48 hours for surgical patients, for patients who have sustained and recovered from a cardiac arrest, or from the clinical conditions summarized in Table 24-1.

For some patients, especially those with neuromuscular disease or chest wall restriction, predisposition to ventilator dependency may occur when the work of spontaneous ventilation exceeds their ability to maintain spontaneous ventilation. In this setting, the development or redevelopment of the signs, symptoms, and laboratory findings of respiratory insufficiency as summarized in Table 24-2 takes place. The clinical conditions that dictate this dependency serve as impediments to sustained spontaneous ventilation and must be controlled or reversed before the patient can be free of the ventilator.[10-13]

The physiologic basis for ventilator dependency, regardless of the cause, is respiratory muscle fatigue and/or weakness and less frequently, loss of the drive to breathe. These concepts were recently defined by the "Respiratory Muscle Fatigue Workshop Group" sponsored by the Division of Lung Diseases (Structure and Function Branch), National Heart, Lung, and Blood Institute, and National Institutes of Health as follows, "Muscle fatigue is a condition in which there is a loss in the capacity for developing force and velocity of a muscle, resulting from muscle activity under load and which is reversible by rest. Muscle weakness is a condition in which the capacity of a rested muscle to generate force is impaired."[14]

The implications of these definitions applied to the ventilator-dependent patient are best understood in light of the work of Roussos and Macklem[15] and Bellemare and Grassino.[16] Each group demonstrated in both normal individuals and in patients with chronic obstructive pulmonary disorder (COPD) that the proportion of effort at spontaneous ventilation in relation to maximum ability to generate respiratory muscle contraction force (**strength**) for ventilation would determine the degree to which the individual could sustain spontaneous ventilation (**endurance**). If the force for spontaneous ventilation was less than 40% of the maximum force that could be generated, the effort could continue indefinitely.[16] If the effort exceeds this ratio, however, fatigue is likely to ensue. Thus, the factors that reduce the maximum force or the ability to sustain the maximum force will predispose the ventilator patient to muscle fatigue and weakness and further dependency (see Chapter 15 for further discussion in addition to the following section).

In addition to factors that affect the strength and endurance of the respiratory muscles, there are also clinical conditions which affect the function of the drive to breathe—the pacemaker or the respiratory pump. Alteration in the drive to breathe will produce inefficient ventilation which ultimately culminates in respiratory insufficiency and failure. The management of these conditions is reviewed in Chapter 11.

PRE-ICU PHASE OF ILLNESS

Clinical Considerations in the Implementation of Mechanical Ventilation

The decision to institute mechanical ventilation should always carry some certainty that the result will be a patient who can be weaned from the ventilator. Thus, the decision making should be based upon prior knowledge of the patient's physiologic condition and the speculation of his or her future physiologic condition (see Table 24-1). Table 24-1 summarizes three basic physiologic causes, along with clinical conditions for mechanical ventilation:

- Alteration in the drive to breathe
- Alteration in respiratory muscle function
- Alteration in the process of oxygenation

Table 24-1. Annotated Classification of Causes of Respiratory Failure or Insufficiency

Alteration in the drive to breathe
   *Cerebral vascular accident—brain stem, lower pons
   Pharmacological suppression—drug overdose, over sedation, post-anesthesia states
   Respiratory alkalosis
   Myxedema
   *Postpolio states—previous bulbar involvement
   *Idiopathic alveolar hypoventilation
Alteration in respiratory muscle function
   Neuromuscular disease (Progressive deterioration in muscle strength)
     *Guillain-Barré syndrome
     *Muscular dystrophy
     *Amyotrophic lateral sclerosis
     *Acid maltase deficiency of the adult
     Myasthenia gravis
     States of malnourishment
     *Cervical spine injury
   Chest wall restriction (Perpetuation of respiratory muscle fatigue)
     *Kyphoscoliosis
     *Old thoracoplasty
     Pneumonectomy
     Pleuritis—collagen vascular disease
   Chronic obstructive lung disease (inefficiency of the respiratory muscles—altered mechanical advantage)
   Hypokalemia, hypophosphatemia, hypomagnesemia
   *Diaphragmatic paralysis following surgery
Disruption in the process of oxygenation
   Pneumonia
   Pulmonary edema
   Acute bronchospasm

* Conditions more likely to be associated with long term requirements for mechanical ventilation beyond the ICU and/or hospitalization.

Practically speaking, requirements for mechanical ventilation are due to some combination of these three problems.[17]

The weaning and rehabilitation of the ventilator-dependent patient necessitates that the underlying clinical conditions responsible for respiratory failure must be preferably reversed totally or minimally in part before weaning from mechanical ventilation will be possible. Clinically, it is best to consider this process a "mirror image" exercise in which the events leading to respiratory failure are totally controlled and reversed in the opposite sequence of their occurrence.[10,18] The simple principle of accounting last in first out (LIFO), applies quite well. The clinician should also be mindful that certain clinical categories (e.g., muscular dystrophy, amyotrophic lateral sclerosis) may necessitate long-term commitment to mechanical ventilation beyond hospitalization or intermittent nighttime use of mechanical ventilation (e.g., kyphoscoliosis, diaphragmatic paralysis following heart surgery).[19-21] Obviously, the clinical conditions responsible for the respiratory failure may not be reversible. Thus, circumstances in the pre-ICU phase of illness may define the strategy required for ventilator management in the ICU and post-ICU phase of illness.

Elective Use of Mechanical Ventilation

There are few risks for ventilator dependency involved in the elective use of mechanical ventilation. This application is almost exclusively used for elective surgery and the postanesthesia recovery period. The preoperative assessment, including cardiac and pulmonary status, is done with the expectation of reducing the risks of postoperative morbidity (see Chap. 59). Conversely, there are preexisting conditions which might prolong the postoperative course including:

- **Preexisting neuromuscular disease**
  (Amyotrophic lateral sclerosis, muscular dystrophy, myasthenia gravis, old polio, polymyositis, adult onset acid maltase deficiency, cervical cord injury)
- **Restrictive chest wall disease**
  [Kyphoscoliosis, thoracoplasty, postpneumonectomy (remote)]
- **Chronic obstructive lung disease**
  (Emphysema, asthma)

To minimize the risk of prolonged ventilation, optimization or stabilization of underlying disease processes preoperatively is imperative.

Neuromuscular Disease

In this group, the risk of postoperative ventilator dependency following elective surgery is greater because of inherent underlying weakness of the respiratory muscles. Therefore, the clinician should be mindful that the following conditions increase the risk of postoperative ventilator dependency:

- Orthopnea and disturbed sleep (suggestive of diaphragmatic weakness or paralysis)
- Difficulty clearing secretions
- Dysarthria (suggestive of bulbar dysfunction)
- Inability to perform personal care during the recovery process (indicative of the overall functional status of the patient)

Objectively, the findings of decreased lung volumes (vital capacity less than 40 to 50% predicted), basilar atelec-

Table 24-2. Clinical Indicators of Risk of Ventilator Dependency in Patients with Altered Drive to Breathe, Neuromuscular, or Restrictive Chest Wall Disease

Clinical symptoms[7-9]
   Generalized fatigue
   Orthopnea
   Hypersomnolence or disturbed sleep
   Morning headache
   Decreased exercise tolerance
Physical findings
   Generalized debilitation from muscle weakness
   Ineffective cough to clear secretions
   Chronic aspiration due to bulbar dysfunction
   Paradoxic motion of the abdomen on inspiration
   Edema in the lower extremities
   Cor pulmonale
Laboratory findings
   Vital capacity less than 50% of predicted (in association with diaphragmatic dysfunction)
   Basilar atelectasis on chest radiograph
   Resting P_{CO_2} > 50 mm Hg
   Resting hypoxemia on room air (P_{O_2} < 55 mm Hg)

tasis on chest radiograph, arterial carbon dioxide elevation of 50 mm Hg or more and obvious inspiratory abdominal paradox in the supine position (diaphragmatic weakness/paralysis) are clinical indicators for risk of postoperative ventilator dependency. Conversely, a preoperative vital capacity greater than 40% of predicted, the absence of orthopnea, normal motion of the diaphragm when supine, normal arterial carbon dioxide tension, and sufficient strength to sit upright are reasonable indicators that the postoperative risk of ventilator dependency is minimal.

Special consideration should be given to the patient with myasthenia gravis who will undergo thymectomy. Similar adherence to the recommendations listed above is essential. In addition, when anticholinesterase therapy is required, a period of disease stability of one to two months reduces postoperative risks. The preoperative administration of a regularly scheduled dose of anticholinesterase medication is recommended.[22,23] Similar stability is also suggested if plasmapheresis is used or has been recently instituted in appropriate cases (see Chap. 8).

Restrictive Chest Wall Disease. There are few guidelines in minimizing risks for ventilator dependency following elective surgery in patients with restrictive chest wall disease. Generally, the presence of symptoms listed in Table 24-2 should alert the clinician to potential postoperative problems. In the absence of these symptoms, the clinician can usually recommend surgery with postoperative vigilance being the same as for any normal patient.

Chronic Obstructive Lung Disease. The increased risks of postoperative ventilator dependence are discussed in Chapters 15 and 59. The issues of weaning in this particular group of patients are also discussed in Chapter 15.

Nonelective Application of Mechanical Ventilation

In contrast to the elective use of mechanical ventilation, the lifesaving application of mechanical ventilation in the face of respiratory failure in a patient with previously compromised respiratory reserve carries a higher risk for ventilator dependency. The clinical circumstances which require this emergent use of mechanical ventilation are listed in Table 24-3. The tendency to "try mechanical ventilation for a few days" should be avoided if possible. The principal question is whether the application of the ventilator carries the potential for reversal of the underlying conditions leading to respiratory failure. If neither of these expectations can be achieved, one must ask if the patient and his family will be able to adapt to a life of ventilator dependency if it occurs?

A large body of literature and clinical experience suggests that a life of total or partial ventilator dependency is possible and desirable in some patients.[2,5,19,24-27] Practically speaking, this type of intervention may facilitate rehabilitation in some patients with neuromuscular disease (usually in association with diaphragmatic paralysis), and chest wall restriction. Having weighed these issues prior to intubation, the clinician should be able to proceed with some certainty about the outcome of mechanical ventilation in this population (see the following discussion).

Noninvasive Methods of Assisted Ventilation

In light of the foregoing discussion, it is important to consider the application of noninvasive methods of assisted ventilation before a patient deteriorates to the point where the emergency use of mechanical ventilation is required because of respiratory failure (Table 24-3). The earliest application of this logic was determined many years ago in patients who recovered from acute poliomyelitis developed respiratory muscle weakness which could not be completely reversed. Assisted ventilation during a part of a 24 hour period (nighttime) with either negative pressure (iron lung) or with altered body position (rocking bed) proved successful in preventing respiratory failure.[28] This logic has been further extended to patients with neuromuscular diseases (e.g., amyotrophic lateral sclerosis, muscular dystrophy and the adult form of acid maltase deficiency) and chest wall restriction (e.g., kyphoscoliosis and thoracoplasty).[2,28-30,32] In addition, application of mask or nasal ventilation has been recently demonstrated to reverse clinical symptoms in some of these same patients.[33-36] Table 24-4 summarizes the clinical circumstances of three patients with amyotrophic lateral sclerosis and diaphragmatic paralysis assisted with BiPAP(R) (Respironics, Murraysville, PA) ventilation.[37,38] Similar application of assisted ventilation with negative pressure ventilation has been reported in patients with chronic respiratory insufficiency due to chronic obstructive lung disease.[39]

Although not explicitly stated in medical literature, the logic of the application of assisted ventilation to prevent respiratory failure in patients with respiratory muscle weakness or fatigue is to rest the inspiratory muscles completely. This situation essentially means that the assisted respiratory rate and tidal volume must provide sufficient minute ventilation to suppress all activity of the respiratory muscles (i.e., controlled ventilation). This application normalizes the arterial carbon dioxide tension and may be associated with a respiratory alkalosis (pH 7.45 to 7.50) when receiving assisted ventilation. Most important is the necessity to recognize the clinical events and patient types which dictate a trial of noninvasive mechanical ventilation before respiratory failure ensues (Tables 24-1 and 24-2) (see Chap. 11). The ultimate benefits of this type of therapeutic intervention may be demonstrated in the form of improved exercise tolerance, reversal of the clinical signs listed in Table 24-2 and a reduction in the resting arterial carbon dioxide.[19]

Table 24-3. Indications for the Emergency Use of Mechanical Ventilation

---
Altered mental status
Inability to control airway secretions
Progressive hypercarbia with pH < 7.20
Worsening oxygenation
Tachypnea beyond 35 respirations per minute in association with the foregoing items
Metabolic acidosis with the advent of shallow breathing, abdominal paradoxic motion on inspiration
Sudden loss of respiratory effort
Cardiac arrest

Table 24-4. Clinical Application of BiPAP(R) to Patients with Amyotrophic Lateral Sclerosis

Age	Gender	Vital Capacity (Sitting)	Vital Capacity (Supine)	BiPAP Setting	Clinical Findings
66	M	37% Predicted	25% Predicted	*IPAP 10 cm *EPAP 4 cm Rate 15 30% IPAP	Fatigue Hypersomnolence Disturbed sleep
		45% Predicted (2 months after BiPAP started)	26% Predicted	Same Settings	Symptoms reversed
51	M	34% Predicted (pH 7.37, P_{CO_2} 51, P_{O_2} 75)		IPAP 12 cm EPAP 4 cm Rate 17, 40% IPAP	Fatigue Hypersomnolence Disturbed sleep
		28% Predicted (2 months after BiPAP started) (pH 7.38, P_{CO_2} 45, P_{O_2} 79)		Same settings	Symptoms reversed
52	F	46% Predicted (pH 7.41, P_{CO_2} 48, P_{O_2} 83)	18% Predicted	IPAP 12 cm EPAP 4 cm Rate 20, 40% IPAP	Orthopnea Disturbed sleep

* IPAP, Inspiratory positive airway pressure; EPAP, Expiratory positive airway pressure; %IPAP, percent of respiratory cycle spent in inspiration. Both patients placed in timed mode of ventilation.[35]

Decision to Institute Mechanical Ventilation

In the pre-ICU phase of illness, situations in which the respiratory status is compromised will necessitate transfer of a patient to the ICU for further monitoring and institution of mechanical ventilation (Table 24-3). The principal concern is, "If mechanical ventilation is instituted, will it be possible to wean the patient following reversal of the acute events?" No guidelines exist to facilitate the decision-making process, but the questions outlined in Table 24-5 may be of some assistance.

The final question is, "Does the clinician think that the patient will fall into a custodial or rehabilitative category?" A custodial care patient will require the constant presence of a caregiver. There is no potential for rehabilitation based on permanence of the clinical conditions causing ventilator dependency. A rehabilitative patient will require only minimal assistance, if any, from a caregiver. The latter patient will be able to perform all activities of daily living without assistance. Under these circumstances, the goals of mechanical ventilation that are summarized in Table 24-6 should be considered in the pre-ICU phase of illness by all clinicians, particularly outside of the ICU.[13,18] Careful and timely consultation with the critical care specialist is essential to long-term management and should be ideally undertaken prior to acute decompensation. It is certainly appropriate to withhold mechanical ventilation if a patient and his or her physician feel that the quality of life will not improve with the institution of mechanical ventilation, or if the quality of life will be less desirable in the eyes of the patient (see Chap. 82). Additionally, if the underlying disease process is chronic and debilitating and cannot be reversed, the clinician should be prepared to deal with ventilator dependency beyond the ICU.

ICU-PHASE OF ILLNESS: REVERSAL OF IMPEDIMENTS TO THE REHABILITATION PROCESS

Magnitude of Ventilator Dependency

One of the most stressful ICU resource constraints is the requirement of critically ill patients to receive mechanical ventilation. Numerous publications have suggested that reimbursement for such care is insufficient for available resources.[3,4,6,40-42] For the ICU caregiver, a different perspective is appreciated. Essentially, long-term ventilator patients eliminate ICU beds from use. For example, in 1988, there were 501 patient admissions to the medical

Table 24-5. Questions to Raise Prior to the Institution of Mechanical Ventilation

Is the deterioration in respiratory status acute in a previously healthy individual? If so, proceed with mechanical ventilation.
Is the acute deterioration due to an event or disease process that will also serve as an impediment to any recovery? If so, long-term care might be expected.
Is there a chronic underlying disease which has slowly deteriorated to the point where rehabilitation is required? If so, the risk of ventilator dependency is increased.
Is the chronic underlying disease an impediment to rehabilitation? If so, there is higher risk of permanent ventilator dependency.
If the answers to these questions are unclear, does the prior experience of the clinician dictate that it is reasonable to offer mechanical ventilation in the hope of reversing the acute or chronic disease processes? If so, clinical experience may facilitate recommendations for or against mechanical ventilation.

Table 24-6. The Goals of Mechanical Ventilation (Based on patient care classification)

Goals of custodial care
  Patient comfort and discharge from the ICU
  Continued patient comfort in the home or extended care facility
  Patient and family acceptance of the finality of requirements for mechanical ventilation
  Adequate care to guarantee the patient's maximum physical comfort
  Emotional stabilization of patient and family
Goals of rehabilitative care
  Involvement of patient in activities of daily living
  Increasing independence from mechanical ventilation
    For a part of the day
    For the daytime hours
    Completely
  Complete mobility outside of the home
  Return to previous employment of activities of daily living

(Adapted from Sivak, E. D., et al.: Home care ventilation: the Cleveland Clinic experience from 1977 to 1985. Respir. Care, *31*:294, 1986.)

Table 24-7. Hospital Outcome of Mechanical Ventilation

Author	Year Reported	Patient #	Average Age	Major Associated Conditions	Average Duration of Ventilation (days)	Hospital Mortality
Nunn[44]	1979	100	NA	Cardiac failure, postoperative states following cardiac arrest	NA	53%
Snow[45]	1979	180	50.4	Malignancies of blood/reticuloendothelial solid tumors	NA	74%
Davis[46]	1980	100	66.7	Cardiopulmonary disorders, postoperative states	8.9	56%
Sivak[18]	1980	15	59.7	COPD, neuromuscular disease	29.4	13%
Fedullo[47]	1980	94*	70+	Disorders of respiratory or cardiovascular system, following cardiac arrest	NA	35%
Schmidt[48]	1983	137	55.1	ARDS, COPD postoperative state	14.7	64%
Morganroth[13]	1984	11	46	COPD, postoperative state	53	30%
McLean[49]	1985	54*	75+	Noncardiac surgery	6.2	46.3%
Witek[50]	1985	100	68 s / 66 ns	COPD, postoperative state, following cardiac arrest	1.6 s / 3.0 ns	50%
Ewer[51]	1986	46	58	Nonsurgical lung carcinoma	NA	85%
Gillespie[52]	1986	327	62.2 s	Acute lung injury. Multisystem organ failure, previous lung disease	11.8	33.9%
Papadakis[53]	1987	78	64.7	Pneumonia, COPD, sepsis, following cardiac arrest	8.4	76%
Spicher[54]	1987	250	59.6	COPD, pneumonia, postoperative states	31	60.8%
Peters[55]	1988	116	58.2 s	Hematologic malignancy	24.7 s	82%
Swinburne[56]	1988	1538		Pulmonary edema, ARDS, COPD, neuromuscular disease, following cardiac arrest		41.4%
Menzes[57]	1989	95	69.6	COPD	20	22%
Sivak[43]	1991	218	59	Hematologic malignancies, postoperative states, GI bleeding, pulmonary edema	10.5	56%

* Partial series; s, Survivor; ns, nonsurvivor.

ICU of the Cleveland Clinic Hospital. Two hundred eighteen or 44% of admissions required mechanical ventilation and consumed 72% of patient days. Of these 218 patients, 26 consumed more than one half of patient days spent on mechanical ventilation.[43] Additionally, the hospital mortality for the 218 admissions was 56%. Table 24-7 lists other series which demonstrate that the long-term outcome of mechanical ventilation has been associated with a high mortality. Practically speaking, the necessity to identify the potential ventilator-dependent patient as early as possible is essential to the management of any ICU. This identification should lead to early institution of therapy to maximize rehabilitation potential or realize limits of therapeutic intervention. Conversely, if appropriate, only supportive care without mechanical ventilation outside of the ICU can be undertaken.

Patient Management Theme for Weaning and Rehabilitation

If the acute event responsible for deterioration of the respiratory status is reversed, patients may be rapidly weaned from mechanical ventilation. Indeed, if the criteria defined by Sahn and colleagues are met, a short period of spontaneous ventilation (i.e., one to two hours) may be followed by immediate extubation.[58] These criteria are summarized in Table 24-8. A careful observation for the signs of respiratory muscle fatigue must be made during this period (Table 24-9).[59] If a pattern of fatigue is observed, a logic other than repeated attempts at weaning before reversing impediments to the process of weaning must be employed. At this point, a coordinated long-term plan for mechanical ventilation must be outlined.

Ideally, in order to successfully wean a ventilator-dependent patient, the following conditions should be met:

- An awake cooperative patient
- Patient is able to breathe spontaneously without dyspnea
- Requires no active infusions of vasoactive drugs
- Is able to take in nutrition enterally
- Is free of life support systems

Table 24-8. Minimal Acceptable Criteria for the Discontinuation of Mechanical Ventilation After Acute Respiratory Failure

Parameter	Acceptable Level
Minute ventilation	< or = 10 L
Respiratory rate	< or = 25/min
Vital capacity	> or = 10–15 ml/kg
Maximum inspiratory pressure	< or = −25 cmH$_2$O

(Adapted from Sahn, S. A., and Laksnminarayan, S.: Bedside criteria for discontinuation of mechanical ventilation. Chest, 63:1002, 1973.)

Table 24-9. Clinical Signs of Respiratory Muscle Fatigue

Respiratory rate > 30 per minute
Abdominal paradoxic motion
Respiratory alternans
Hypercarbia
Decreased inspiratory forces
Bradypnea
Decreased ventilation-acidosis

(Adapted from Cohen, C. A., et al.: Clinical manifestations of respiratory muscle fatigue. Am. J. Med., 73:308, 1982.)

Table 24-10. Altered Functions as Impediments to Rehabilitation

Critical Success Factor	Causes of Altered Function	Impediment to Rehabilitation
Central nervous system	Confusion, disorientation, cerebrovascular accident, fever, hyperglycemia, hypernatremia, hypomagnesemia, hypophosphatemia, azotemia, medications, ICU psychosis	Patients who are not alert and cooperative cannot participate in the rehabilitation process
Cardiovascular system	Postoperative myocardial infarction, cardiac tamponade; preexisting deficiency in myocardial function; arrhythmias due to hypokalemia, hypomagnesemia, or hypoxemia	Poor perfusion of the respiratory muscle fatigue and failure
Respiratory system	Dysfunction of the upper airway because of glottic incompetence, paralysis of the vocal cords, formation of granuloma, or tracheomalacia; poor function of the pulmonary parenchyma due to pneumonia, excess secretions, atelectasis, bronchospasm, large pleural effusion, and fatigue of respiratory muscles from malnutrition or diaphragmatic paralysis	Recurrent aspiration will cause persistent hypoxemia and atelectasis, and predispose to pneumonia; hypoxemia and its causes will cause increased work of breathing and predispose the patient to respiratory failure
Gastrointestinal system	Postoperative ileus because of medications, pancreatitis, cholecystitis, or recurrent hypotension; fever may be due to cholecystitis, ischemic bowel, perforated ulcers, or diverticulitis	Persistent abdominal distention and fever will constantly increase the work of breathing and predispose to respiratory failure
Renal system	Decreased cardiac output, toxic antibiotics, recurrent hypotension; previously existing renal vascular disease	Debilitation, alterations in fluid balance, and nutritional support will predispose to respiratory failure

(From Sivak, E. D., and Krawtz, S. M.: Critical success factors in weaning the ventilator dependent patient after heart surgery. In Anesthesia and the Heart Patient. Edited by F. G. Estafanous. Boston, Butterworths, 1989, p. 307.)

The last two items on the list can be interpreted loosely since parenteral nutrition and dialysis may facilitate the weaning process. Then, before consideration of weaning, one should identify any impediments to achieving these goals (Table 24-10).

Critical Success Factors in Weaning

As mentioned previously, certain conditions should exist before one considers attempts at weaning. Morganroth and colleagues elaborately defined these conditions in an **adverse factor score**.[13] Conditions which serve as impediments to weaning were weighted and scored. Additionally, these authors included physiologic assessment in the form of a **ventilator score** (see Chapter 79 for further discussion). These two scores summarize best the approach that one should take in weaning the ventilator-dependent patient [i.e., elimination of adverse factors (Impediments) to weaning and optimization of physiologic status].

Before attempting to optimize physiologic status, goals of mechanical ventilation should always be considered first. In short, one uses a technology to support a patient until he is awake and cooperative; able to support spontaneous ventilation without dyspnea or chest pain; to consume an adequate amount of nutrition without extraordinary means; and not rely on mechanical devices to survive. These goals essentially mean that the following organ systems must function adequately with sufficient reserve:

- Central nervous system
- Respiratory system
- Cardiovascular system
- Gastrointestinal system
- Renal system

If one employees a checklist approach in the review of these systems, impediments to adequate function of these systems are easily identified. Simultaneously, the impediments to rehabilitation and weaning are identified. Table 24-10 summarizes this approach. Before weaning occurs, the clinician must first eliminate any impediments to the rehabilitation process. Otherwise, there will always be a potential for respiratory failure and ventilator dependency. Although seemingly simplistic, this approach has not varied much in the last 20 years.[10,18,60]

Common Impediments to the Process of Weaning

In addition to eliminating the impediments listed in Table 24-10, a concise protocol which will allow for periods of work of breathing interspersed with periods of rest during the weaning process is equally important. There are also requirements for further rehabilitation of patients who are often extremely debilitated from critical illness and prolonged bed rest. These patients may often require periods of sedation during periods of hemodynamic and respiratory instability for days or weeks. This process will necessitate gradually increasing orientation to reality through the early phases of rehabilitation. The surrounding environment may seem foreign as consciousness is regained. Table 24-11 suggests steps through which a pa-

Table 24-11. The Evolution of Reorientation for the Long-Term Ventilator-Dependent Patient Following Prolonged Detachment From Reality

Eyes open; observation of environment
Communication through gestures
Communication by attempting to speak
Communication by writing. (Writing ability may be variable, depending on education and the frequency with which the patient used this method to communicate before the critical illness.)

(Adapted from Sivak, E. D., and Krawtz, S. M.: Critical success factors in weaning the ventilator dependent patient after heart surgery. In Anesthesia and the Heart Patient. Edited by F. G. Estafanous. Boston, Butterworths, 1989, p. 307.)

Table 24-12. Graded Sequence of Physical Activity to Follow During Rehabilitation and Weaning from Mechanical Ventilation

Passive range of motion of extremities
Active range of motion of extremities
Sit in bed with support (reclining chair)
Active sitting in straight back chair
Sit on the edge of the bed; begin to bear weight and stand with pivot into the bedside chair
Walk with assistance and sit in a wheelchair for transportation to the department of physical therapy (Spontaneous ventilation for at least 2 hours)
Walk with minimal assistance
Rehabilitation to the point where the ventilator is unnecessary

(Adapted from Sivak, E. D., and Krawtz, S. M.: Critical success factors in weaning the ventilator dependent patient after heart surgery. In Anesthesia and the Heart Patient. Edited by F. G. Estafanous. Boston, Butterworths, 1989, p. 307.)

tient will evolve in reorientation. The caregiver should carefully reorient the patient to time, place, and person often. In addition, appropriate establishment of rapport with the patient and identification of primary caregivers should take place as the patient becomes more aware of his or her environment. As this awareness evolves and the rehabilitation process is started, a program of gradually increasing activity can be instituted (Table 24-12). The process of increasing activity and increasing time off of the ventilator should evolve in parallel, if possible, as if to use the ventilator as a "crutch" to facilitate the rehabilitation process. The rehabilitation process should also be a multidisciplinary approach and include the physical therapists, occupational therapists, speech pathologists, dieticians, and, if necessary, psychiatrists.

Special Considerations

As the patient proceeds through the rehabilitation process, there are additional problems which should be appropriately managed. These include:

- The sedative-hypnotic abstinence syndrome
- Restoration and maintenance of nutrition status
- Maintenance of patient and family interest in the rehabilitation process
- The timing of tracheostomy tube placement
- Management of problems of glottic dysfunction and the upper airway
- Special considerations for the patient with diaphragmatic dysfunction, neuromuscular disease, and restrictive chest wall disease

The **sedative-hypnotic abstinence syndrome** refers to a set of clinical circumstances that occur within 24 hours of discontinuance of narcotics or benzodiazopenes. Tremors, weakness, insomnia, and restlessness may develop. Fluctuation in blood pressure may compound management difficulties. More severe manifestations include myoclonic muscular contractions and hallucinosis.[61] This problem is likely to occur when the major effects of infection, azotemia, hepatic insufficiency and electrolyte imbalance have subsided and the clinician wishes to proceed with weaning. The reader should refer to Chapter 2 for methods of minimizing the likelihood of this syndrome developing. The starting point in any weaning process is an awake, cooperative patient.

Restoration of adequate nutrition status is essential to the rehabilitation process. In the face of poor nutrition status, the risks of perpetuation of ventilator dependency have been well documented.[62-68] Practically speaking, the clinician should not plan sustained attempts at weaning until visceral protein stores are reasonable (serum albumin, 3.0 g/dl and serum transferrin > 150 mg/dl). In addition to caloric intake, the caregiver should also be aware that diaphragmatic weakness has been reported in association with hypomagnesemia[69] and with hypophosphatemia.[70] For appropriate prescription of replacement and maintenance of nutrition, the reader is referred to Chapter 62.

The long drawn out course of critical illness requires the necessity to **maintain the interest of the patient's family members or friends.** As the patient proceeds through the rehabilitation process, efforts must be made to avoid depression and maintain interest in working toward ICU discharge and hospital discharge. It is important for the patient and family members to have psychologic stress minimized and to focus on long-term goals (see Chap. 73). By the same token, all efforts should be made to involve these individuals in the slow process of rehabilitation. Schedules of visitation, physical and occupational therapy and so forth, should be made so as to give the patients events to look forward to each day. Communication among caregivers, patients and their families, and friends should be mandated and facilitated.

Bergbom-Engbert and Haljamae found that 47% of 158 patients experienced anxiety and/or fear during the process of mechanical ventilation. The principle reason was the inability to talk or communicate. These investigators noted that these factors also contributed to an inability of these patients to sleep.[77] In addition to problems of anxiety and fear contributing to the sleep-wakefulness pattern, the clinician should also heed the observations of Chen and Tang.[72] They found that sleep loss impairs inspiratory muscle endurance. These factors suggest that quiet, safe environments which emphasize rehabilitation rather than critical illness are best for weaning the long-term patient (see the section on Post-ICU management for further discussion).

The timing of the placement of tracheostomy has always been a perplexing problem for clinicians. The principle reason for this problem is the lack of specific indices to predict the duration of mechanical ventilation. The minimization of damage to the upper airway and patient comfort remain the principle benefits of tracheostomy. Marsh and colleagues succinctly suggested that the major determining factor for proceeding with tracheostomy should be the time needed for continued intubation and the anticipation that the underlying illness would extend to the point where tracheostomy would be needed.[73] Practically speaking, if intubation is expected beyond 7 to 10 days, tracheostomy should be planned if the process has already exceeded 10 to 14 days. The only deterrents to this rule

Table 24-13. Potential Problems of the Upper Airway in the Long-Term Ventilator-Dependent Patient

Posterior commissure stenosis
Ulceration of the vocal cords
Cricoarytenoid ankylosis
Epiglottic dysfunction
Subglottic stenosis and granuloma formation
Inward buckling of anterior cartilaginous skeleton of the larynx (above tracheostomy stoma)
Chronic aspiration of oral secretions due to failure of patient to sense presence of secretions

(From Sivak, E. D.: Management of ventilator dependency following heart surgery. Semin. Thorac. Cardiovasc. Surg., 3:53, 1991.)

would be anticipation of death or imminent recovery and easy extubation.[73]

The **problems of glottic and upper airway dysfunction** are particularly perplexing as one proceeds through the rehabilitation process. Some of the problems encountered are summarized in Table 24-13. For the patient who has been extubated with no previous requirement for tracheostomy, such dysfunction can be associated with symptoms of hoarseness, a "breathiness" to the voice, and respiratory insufficiency due to aspiration of the oropharyngeal secretions. Repeated episodes of hypoxemia, respiratory distress, and possible respiratory failure suggest that there are problems with the glottis and/or upper airway. For the patient who has a tracheostomy in place, the clinical scenario is one of repeated necessity to suction the trachea with a return of clear-to-whitish secretions. Indeed, a nurse or therapist may suction secretions from the trachea and not 15 to 30 minutes later, the clinician will examine the patient and inquire why the patient's trachea has not been kept free of secretions. Another clinical clue is the presence of secretions constantly draining from the tracheostomy stoma. The stoma dressing is usually saturated with these secretions. The long-term management of the problems summarized in Table 24-13 is discussed in Chapter 12. In these situations, rehabilitation of the function of the upper airway must take place before the patient can be totally free of the potential to redevelop respiratory failure.

For the patient who has **diaphragmatic dysfunction** associated with ventilator dependency, the clinician is usually faced with the difficulty of making the diagnosis as well as formulating long-range plans for rehabilitation and weaning. This problem has been associated with local hypothermia during heart surgery, closed chest trauma, subclavian and internal jugular venipuncture, and thoracic surgical procedures.[74-79] The clinical symptoms are usually those of alveolar hypoventilation as listed in Table 24-2. These symptoms apply to all patients regardless of the cause. The diagnostic dilemma occurs when the critical illness associated with infection, hemodynamic instability, or a complicated postoperative course masks the presence of the problem. In these latter situations, the clinical course is characterized by patient restlessness, arrhythmias, repeated extubations and intubations, recurrent pneumonia, confusion, and apprehension due to fear of falling asleep and not awakening. The key to the clinical diagnosis should be the presence of orthopnea and the observation of inward paradoxic motion of the abdomen when the patient is breathing in the supine position.[7] Because dysfunction of the diaphragm muscle produces symptoms when both hemidiaphragms are involved, it is usually unnecessary to document dysfunction if only one hemidiaphragm is suspected as being dysfunctional.

Electrophysiologic confirmation of dysfunction is considered to be the method of choice for diagnosis.[80] Such methods require a trained electromyographer, however, and may not be available at all institutions. Measurement of transdiaphragmatic pressure is another acceptable method for diagnosis.[8] Similar to electrophysiologic confirmation, the placement of esophageal and gastric balloons for measurement requires some skill and may be uncomfortable for the critically ill or ventilator-dependent patient. A third technique often used to confirm unilateral diaphragmatic paralysis is fluoroscopy. This test is not valid for the patient who has bilateral dysfunction because inspiratory effort may cause downward motion if the tidal volume is large enough or else no motion is seen whatsoever.[7,8]

Practically speaking, the best approach is to assume that a patient has diaphragm dysfunction until proven otherwise. The weaning protocol remains the same regardless of whether or not dysfunction exists. As a process of rehabilitation ensues, it will be possible to measure sitting and supine vital capacity. A greater than 50% decrease in vital capacity (VC) when the patient assumes the supine position should be sufficient to diagnosis diaphragmatic dysfunction. Caution should be used, however, in the interpretation of this measurement in the extremely debilitated patient. The VC may be so small that there is no difference in either position. In this situation, I allow a patient 24 to 48 hours of complete ventilator support and then observe for supine paradoxic motion of the abdomen during spontaneous ventilation. Therapeutic intervention during the rehabilitation process should be directed toward minimizing the symptoms of orthopnea and disturbed sleep. Periods of spontaneous ventilation should be conducted with the patient in the upright position only. Attempts to wean with the patient in bed will only perpetuate apprehension. Ventilation should be completely supported during the hours of rest and sleep for the purpose of completely resting the assessory muscles of respiration. Because the diaphragm is the principal muscle of respiration during REM sleep, the patient is unlikely able to enter into deep sleep without the support of ventilation.[81]

The initial weaning protocol should be directed at complete weaning during the daytime hours and complete support of ventilation during the night. There is usually some requirement for nighttime ventilation following ICU discharge (see the section on Post-ICU Phase later in this chapter).[20,21] Similar logic is applied to patients with neuromuscular disease and chest wall restriction.[15-17]

Physiologic Considerations

The themes for consideration in weaning are similar to those for instituting mechanical ventilation. The first is the **control of ventilation.** The spectrum of patients with alteration in the control of ventilation is covered extensively in Chapter 11. The second is the **strength and en-**

Table 24-14. Causes of Hypoxemia and Clinical Intervention

Cause	Intervention
Hypoventilation	Assisted ventilation
Ventilation/Perfusion mismatch	Add supplemental oxygen
Shunt	Add PEEP
Diffusion impairment	Enhancement of surface area for gas exchange-diuresis
Decreased inspired oxygen	Not applicable in ICU
Decreased cardiac output	Inotropic and pressor agents

durance of the respiratory muscles. The third is the **function status of the lung parenchyma** (the process of oxygenation), itself. In keeping with the "mirror image"[10,18] concept of weaning, one must work backward through these three considerations. Oxygenation, the respiratory muscles, and finally the drive to breathe must be assessed. The common categories of causes of hypoxemia and the clinical response to these categories are listed in Table 24-14. In the weaning process, step six is eliminated first, with the logic of reversing the most recently applied intervention first. One would not expect to begin the weaning process if a patient was dependent on vasopressors or inotropic agents to maintain hemodynamic status. Since problems of decreased inspired oxygen and diffusion do not apply to this setting, one should next consider the minimum requirements for adequate oxygenation before further weaning. With respect to the process of oxygenation, an inspired oxygen concentration of 40% with acceptable oxygen saturation and no more than 5 cm end-expiratory pressure is an acceptable threshold to consider further weaning. The figure of 40% appears numerous times in the literature without substantiation.[10,18,60,82] It can be further translated as follows: (PA-a)o_2 with 100% oxygen at < 350 mm Hg; Pao_2/Fio_2 > 200 mm Hg; QsQ_T < 20%). Its recurrent appearance over the years, however, suggests that there may be at least some consensus and therefore, it represents an acceptable starting point to consider further weaning. Once these criteria are met, one should further consider the ability of the patient to sustain spontaneous ventilation. It is assumed that the previously listed impediments to further weaning have been minimized at this point (see Table 24-10).

Following the point where oxygenation is acceptable, there is considerable controversy about further weaning from mechanical ventilation. On one hand, there has been a generation of attempts to define an acceptable index which predicts the ability of a patient to continue to breathe without support. These attempts are based on various physiologic measurements which will be summarized below. On the other hand, there have been numerous explanations that these measurements will be dependent on the physiologic reserve of the patient and that such factors as hemodynamic status, nutrition status, infectious status, mental status, and overall strength should be addressed before attempts at weaning are made.[83] In reality, both approaches are correct, but neither in and of itself. Controversy exists for a number of reasons including:

- Lack of definition of terms of weaning (Rapid versus gradual)
- The method employed to wean a patient (Intermittent mandatory ventilation, "T-piece," pressure support, continuous positive airway pressure (CPAP)
- Resistance in the airway and ventilator circuit
- The existence of impediments to weaning when the weaning process is attempted or quantitated
- The necessity for many patients to be rehabilitated before weaning can be completed

The physiologic parameters that have been used in the weaning process are summarized in Table 24-15, which groups them according to measurement of the following categories:

- Strength
- Endurance
- Combined indices

Strength

The parameters of VC and maximum inspiratory pressure (Pimax) are used to define respiratory muscle strength or force of contraction. Their limitation is the inability to determine the capacity to sustain the periodic or repetitive force of contraction for spontaneous ventilation over time.

Table 24-15. Parameters Used to Predict Acceptability of Weaning

Assessment	Measurement	Normal	Acceptable	Reference
Strength	Vital capacity (VC)	65–75 ml/kg	10–15 ml/kg	Sahn[58,84] Milbern[85]
Endurance	Maximum inspiratory pressure (Pimax)	115 ± 27 cm H$_2$O	−30 cm H$_2$O	Tahvanainen[86]
	Maximum voluntary ventilation (MVV)	50–250 L/min	<10 L/min with voluntary doubling	Tahvanainen[86] Sahn[58]
	Airway occlusion pressure (P 0.1)	<2 cm H$_2$O	>6 cm H$_2$O predicts failure	Sassoon[87]
	Respiratory pattern	>25 breaths/min and VT 300 ml		Tobin[88]
	Work of breathing	0.45–.65 J/L	<.70 J/L	Taylor[89]
	Pressure time index (PTI)		<0.15	Tobin[83]
Combined indices	Compliance, rate, oxygenation and pressure (CROP)		≥13	Yang[90,91]
	Weaning index (WI)	<4	>4	Jabour[92]

When measured at the beginning and end of periods of spontaneous ventilation, they may, however, serve to indicate the effect of sustained work of breathing on the overall endurance of the respiratory muscles. Practically speaking, a significant decline in these parameters at the end of a specified period of spontaneous ventilation suggests the limits of a patient's ability to breathe spontaneously without fatigue.

Endurance

When measuring the strength of the respiratory muscles during the weaning process, a correlation with an estimation of endurance or the patient's ability to sustain spontaneous ventilation should be made. The minute ventilation to maximum minute ventilation ratio, electromyographic power spectrum, mouth occlusion pressure, breathing pattern and pressure time index have been proposed as estimates of endurance of the respiratory muscles. As in the case of strength measurements, these measurements must be compared to maximum values. The determination of minute ventilation to maximum voluntary minute ventilation (VE/MVV) is difficult in the ventilator-dependent patient because of the degree of cooperation required for measurement of maximum voluntary minute ventilation. An alternative of this measurement is the ability of the patient to be able to voluntarily increase minute ventilation by more than two times the resting minute ventilation. This measurement may indicate that a patient is able to sustain spontaneous ventilation indefinitely.[84]

Measurement of the electromyographic (EMG) signals from the diaphragm with an esophageal electrode reveals both high and low frequency discharges. A reduction in the ratio of high to low frequency discharge suggests that the respiratory muscles are fatiguing from the work of breathing.[93] This measurement, referred to as the power spectrum, is not practical to measure at the bedside because of the requirement for placement of an esophageal electrode.

Although not extensively studied, Sasson and colleagues used mouth occlusion pressure (P 0.1) to estimate the ability to sustain spontaneous ventilation after abrupt discontinuation from mechanical ventilation. A value > 6 cm H_2O predicted inability to continue spontaneous ventilation.[94] Montgomery and colleagues used the addition of hypercapnic challenge in the ventilator-dependent patient and found that lack of an increase in P 0.1 suggests inability to wean.[95] As in the case of the power spectrum, this measurement is not always practical at the bedside.

The studies by Cohen and colleagues suggest that as the diaphragm fatigues, the assessory or chest wall muscles continue to support ventilation, diaphragmatic contraction markedly decreases, and thus paradoxic motion of the abdomen is seen.[59] Figure 24-2 illustrates this sequence, which is also outlined in Table 24-9. Tobin, however, has suggested that this pattern may not be entirely suggestive of respiratory muscle fatigue.[83] More important is the relationship of the contribution of the inspiratory effort from both chest wall and abdominal muscles. In the face of a fatiguing work load, there is initially asynchronous motion of rib cage (i.e., abdominal motion with the abdominal motion following the rib cage motion in inspiration). Following the development of this pattern, abdominal paradox is seen.[83] These observations can be translated into clinically simplified terms by the observation of respiratory rate and tidal volume. A respiratory frequency above 25 and a tidal volume of less than 300 ml may suggest that weaning trials may be unsuccessful.[83,96,97]

Numerous investigators have demonstrated that the inspiratory work in proportion to the patient's maximum respiratory muscle strength will determine the limits of a patient's ability to sustain spontaneous ventilation.[14-17] Figure 24-1 illustrates this concept.[98] On the abscissa, the ratio of the force of diaphragmatic contraction on spontaneous ventilation to maximum force of contraction is shown (Pdi/Pdi max). As the ratio increases, the patient is likely to have less reserve if greater force is necessary to maintain spontaneous ventilation. On the ordinate, the ratio of the inspiratory time to the total duty cycle (T_I/T_{TOT})

(duty cycle = inspiratory time + expiratory time)

If the time spent in inspiration increases, the overall inspiratory time each minute required for ventilation is increased. This situation represents an increased requirement for force of contraction over each minute. Normally, resting spontaneous ventilation is far to the left (Fig. 24-1). Increased work of breathing as manifested by increased time for inspiration and/or decreased force reserve of the respiratory muscles will predispose the patient to limited

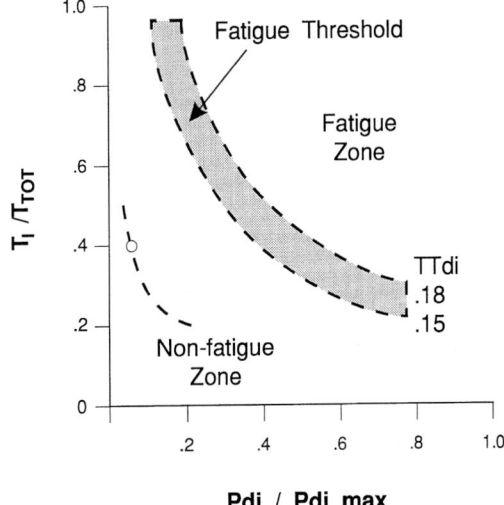

Fig. 24-1. T_I/T_{TOT} is the relationship between inspiratory time and cycle duration. Pdi/Pdimax is the mean transdiaphragmatic pressure expressed as a percentage of maximal Pdi. The solid circle is the pattern of breathing held during resting breathing. Fatigue threshold: Breathing patterns falling in this zone can be sustained for 45 minutes or longer. TTdi: Product of pdi/Pdimax × T_I/T_{TOT}. Fatiguing patterns: Breathing sustained with any pattern falling in this area result in respiratory muscle failure in less than 1 hour. (Redrawn by George Morrison, ACT/PC, from Grassino, A., and Mackleim, P. T.: Respiratory muscle fatigue and ventilatory failure. Annu. Rev. Med., 35:625, 1984.)

periods of spontaneous ventilation. As this increased work of breathing continues, the respiratory pattern is likely to follow the sequence listed in Table 24-9. The consequences are illustrated in Figure 24-2. In this figure, an additional measurement of diaphragmatic fatigue is illustrated by a shift in the power spectrum measured by electromyography (esophageal electrode measuring signals from the costal portion of the diaphragm). As fatigue ensues, there is a reduction in the ratio of high frequency discharge to low frequency discharge. These discharges are from contractions of muscle fibers Chap. 10).[99]

The product of (Pdi/Pdi max) and (TI/TTOT) is referred to as the pressure-time index (PTI). Field and colleagues have determined there there is an inverse correlation between this index and diaphragmatic endurance in normal subjects.[100] Additionally, Tobin and colleagues have demonstrated that a PTI of < 0.15 predicts successful weaning.[88] The logic of this measurement is fairly straightforward. The less force exerted over time during spontaneous ventilation, the less likely that respiratory muscle fatigue will ensue. Despite the ease of measurement, however, the accuracy of this measurement as a predictor of a successful weaning trial remains to be established.

Combined Indices

To this point, the entire discussion on weaning has emphasized the interdependency of clinical conditions that are associated with increased work of breathing relative to physiologic strength and endurance. Because of the

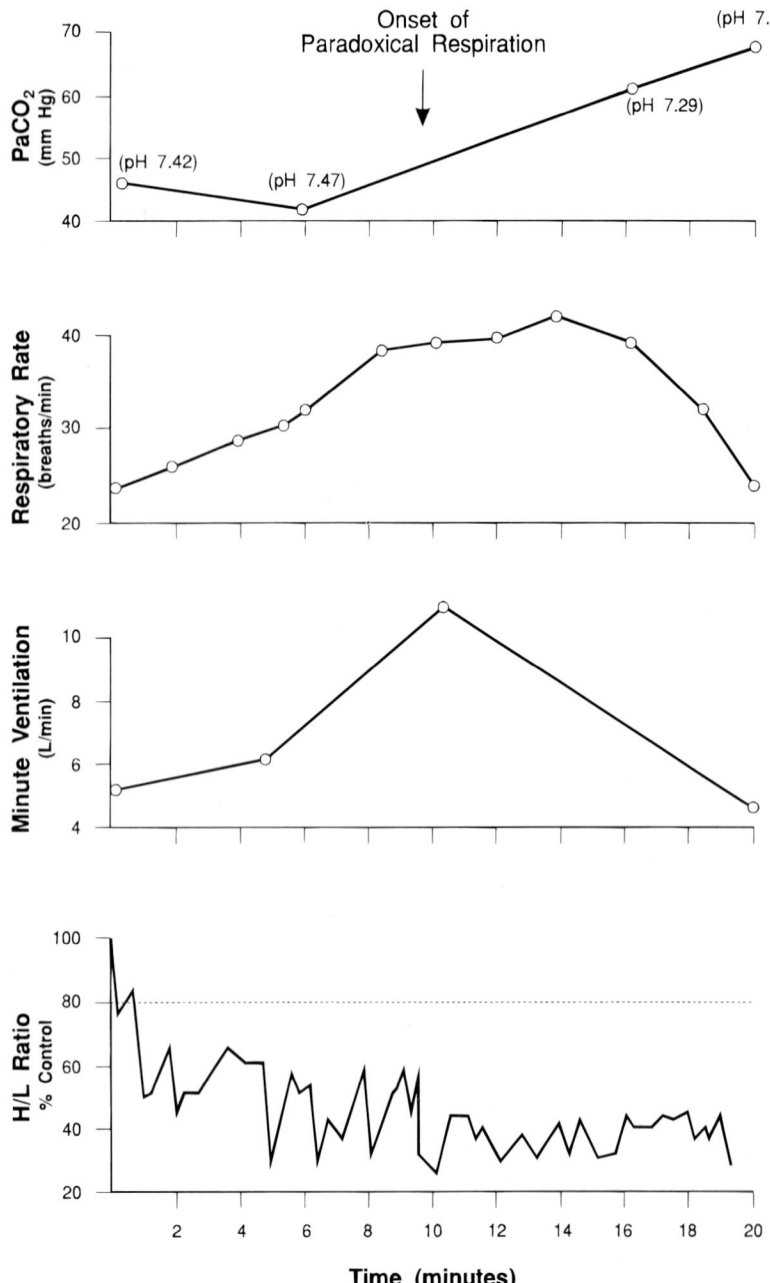

Fig. 24-2. Sequence of changes in $Paco_2$, respiratory rate, minute ventilation, and high/low (H/L) ratio of the diaphragm in a patient being weaned from mechanical ventilation during a 20-minute attempt at discontinuation. The initial change was the fall in high/low ratio, followed by a progressive increase in respiratory rate. The $Paco_2$ initially fell, and the patient became alkalemic. Paradoxic abdominal displacements were not noted until after a substantial increase in respiratory rate and minute ventilation. Hypercapnia and respiratory acidosis did not develop until after abdominal paradox and alternation between rib cage and abdominal breaths were noted. Just before artificial ventilation was reinstituted, there was a sharp fall in respiratory frequency and minute ventilation. (Redrawn by George Morrison, ACT/PC, from Cohen, C. A., et al.: Clinical manifestations of inspiratory muscle fatigue. Am. J. Med., 73:308, 1982.)

complexity of the clinical conditions, no single measurement has been shown to predict successful weaning trials. Two combined indices, the CPOP index and the Weaning Index, have been proposed, however. The CROP index (compliance, rate, oxygenation, and pressure) is as follows:

$$CROP = (Cdyn \times Pimax \times (Pa_{O_2}/PA_{O_2}))/R$$

where:

$Cdyn$ = Dynamic compliance
$Pimax$ = Maximum inspiratory pressure
R = Rate

Using this index, Wang and Tobin found that patients with high values for this index had an 87% chance of successful weaning compared to 55% for minute ventilation of 10L or less, and 61% for Pimax of more negative than −30 cm H_2O.[90] This index is expressed in units of ml/breath/per minute. A value of ≥ 13 is the threshold that predicted successful weaning outcome.[91] The logic of this index suggests that the better the compliance and greater the strength in association with adequate oxygen and lower respiratory rate, the more likely that spontaneous ventilation could continue indefinitely.

In a more extensive study, these same investigators found that the ratio of respiratory rate to tidal volume (f/VT ratio) was slightly more accurate than the CROP index in predicting success in weaning.[91]

The Weaning Index evaluates the relationship between ventilation required to maintain arterial carbon dioxide and the endurance of the respiratory muscles based on the PTI, since both influence the work of breathing.[92] It is expressed as follows:

$$WI = PTI \times V_{E40}/V_{Tsb}$$

where:

WI = Weaning Index
PTI = Pbreath/NIP $\times$ T_I/T_{TOT}
Pbreath = Peak airway pressure − PEEP $\times$ V_{TSB}/V_{TMV}
V_{TSB} = Spontaneous tidal volume
V_{TMV} = Ventilator tidal volume
T_I = Inspiratory time
T_{TOT} = Total respiratory cycle time
V_{E40} = minute ventilation required to achieve Pa_{CO_2} of 40 mm Hg
V_{E40} = (fmv $\times$ V_{TMV}/BW $\times$ Pa_{CO_2}mv/40
fmv = respiratory rate in control or assist mode
V_{TMV} = ventilator tidal volume in control or assist mode
BW = body weight
Pa_{CO_2}mv = Pa_{CO_2} during mechanical ventilation

Although the variables in this index make it seem complex, the logic seems straightforward. The probability of successful weaning is proportional to the mechanics of lungs and chest wall; respiratory muscle strength and endurance and the adequacy of gas exchange quantitated by ventilatory efficiency in relationship to size of tidal volume.[92] Using the index, Jabour and colleagues found a positive predictive value to detect failure to wean of 96% and a negative predictive value (predicting success of 95% in its application to 46 weaning trials) of 38 patients.[92] These findings were qualified by the finding that the age of the patients (55 +/− 18 yr) and a better level of consciousness than other published weaning series may have been responsible for the high degree of predictability.[92] The value of this index is expressed as a number per minute with a value of 4 or greater predicting success and less than 4 predicting failure.

Both indices take into account the proportion of work required for spontaneous ventilation compared to an assessment of the maximum work possible under conditions imposed by respiratory mechanics and gas exchange. The CROP index additionally takes into account an additional variable of respiratory rate. A dissimilarity in the indices is the use of the ratio of arterial to alveolar oxygen tension (Pa_{O_2}/PA_{O_2}) in the CROP index and the minute ventilation required to achieve an arterial Pa_{CO_2} of 40 mm Hg in the WI. Table 24-16 provides additional insight into the relationship of the predictive powers of these indices to other conventional parameters.[91]

Clinical Protocol for Weaning

Figure 24-3 illustrates an algorithm for rehabilitation of the ventilator-dependent patient. The first step in the protocol is to identify the impediments to weaning as listed in Table 24-10. During this step, the clinician should develop the discipline of creating a checklist of the common impediments, to search for them, and then eliminate them as soon as possible. One would then determine the adequacy of the lung parenchyma.

If the requirements for supplemental oxygen are 40% or less with no more than 5 cm of end-expiratory pressure, one can proceed with further weaning from mechanical ventilation. This process is done by selecting an appropriate mode of ventilation from the following list:

- Spontaneous ventilation (with or without CPAP)
- Intermittent mandatory ventilation
- Pressure support ventilation

Regardless of the mode, the clinician should be watchful for signs of respiratory muscle fatigue. If the pattern of respiratory muscle fatigue listed in Table 24-9 develops, full rest of the respiratory muscles with ventilatory support is essential. It should also be kept in mind that the "assist" mode of ventilation can be associated with significant work of breathing.[101,102] Therefore, to ensure a period of rest for the respiratory muscles, the clinician should select sufficient machine ventilation to suppress the function of the respiratory muscles.

If one begins weaning with short periods of sponta-

Table 24-16. Effect of Mechanical Ventilation (<8 days or ≥8 days) on the Accuracy of Indices in Predicting Weaning Outcome*

Index	Sensitivity <8 Days	Sensitivity ≥8 Days	Specificity <8 Days	Specificity ≥8 Days	Positive Predictive Value <8 Days	Positive Predictive Value ≥8 Days	Negative Predictive Value <8 Days	Negative Predictive Value ≥8 Days
Minute ventilation	0.79	0.75	0.75	0.08	0.65	0.35	0.40	0.33
Respiratory frequency	0.89	1.00	0.31	0.42	0.69	0.53	0.63	1.00
Tidal volume	1.00	0.88	0.50	0.58	0.78	0.58	1.00	0.88
Tidal volume/patient's weight	0.96	0.88	0.38	0.42	0.73	0.50	0.86	0.83
Maximal inspiratory pressure	1.00	1.00	0.00	0.25	0.64	0.47	1.00	1.00
Dynamic compliance	0.75	0.63	0.69	0.25	0.81	0.36	0.61	0.50
Static compliance	0.82	0.50	0.56	0.08	0.787	0.27	0.64	0.20
Pa_{O_2}/PA_{O_2} ratio	0.79	0.88	0.38	0.17	0.69	0.41	0.50	0.67
Frequency/tidal volume ratio	1.00	0.88	0.63	0.67	0.82	0.64	1.00	0.89
CROP index	0.82	0.75	0.56	0.58	0.77	0.55	0.64	0.78

* Values shown were derived from the complete prospective-validation data set of 64 patients; among whom 44 patients (28 who were successfully weaned and 16 who had weaning failure) required <8 days of mechanical ventilation, and 20 patients (8 who were successfully weaned and 12 who had weaning failure) required ≥8 days of mechanical ventilation. (From Yang, K. L., and Tobin, M. L.: A prospective study of indices predicting the outcome of trials of weaning from mechanical ventilation. N. Engl. J. Med., *321*:1445, 1991.)

neous ventilation, aside from the requirements for oxygenation previously listed, the spontaneous tidal volume should be at least 2 to 3 times the anatomic deadspace (1 ml/pound of body weight), and the respiratory rate less than 30 to 35 breaths per minute. There are times when such attempts will be associated with significant dyspnea and tachycardia. The respiratory rate may exceed 35 breaths per minute. From this point onward, regardless of whether spontaneous unassisted ventilation or else pressure support ventilation is employed, the parameters of minute ventilation, maximum inspiratory force, and respiratory rate should be measured both at the beginning and at the end of each period of ventilation. Ventilation should be stopped if respiratory rate exceeds 30 to 35 per minute or if impediments reoccur (Table 24-10). The clinician may wish to use the CROP or WI but these indices require calculations and may not replace the clinical rule that a rapid respiratory rate may be the earliest sign of a predispostion to respiratory muscle fatigue.[59,91,103,104]

If pressure support ventilation is employed, it is my policy to increase time on pressure support alone until the patient has reached 2 hours on this mode of ventilation. The initial level of pressure support selected is the minimal pressure to maintain spontaneous respiratory rate at < 30 per minute. If respiratory rate remains less than 30 and if vital capacity and inspiratory forces remain similar at the end of the trial period as at the beginning, the pressure support is decreased by 2 cm for two hour increments until down to 0 cm. Once at 0 cm, the time of spontaneous ventilation is increased keeping within the guidelines of respiratory rate of less than 30 and VC and inspiratory forces remaining unchanged or improved from beginning of the trial to the end.

The sequence of longer and longer periods of spontaneous ventilation interspersed with periods of rest is supported by the investigations of Fiastro and colleagues.[103] In a small series of 17 patients, 6 were considered to require prolonged ventilation. The best predictor of weaning was work of breathing rather than various spontaneous ventilatory parameters. It is reasonable to conclude that the best way to ensure the ability to perform more work is with periods of rest in between work. Similarly, strength and conditioning are improved with periods of gradually increasing amounts of work—in the case of weaning, longer periods of spontaneous ventilation. Figure 24-4 illustrates the difference between those patients who were rapidly weaned (less work required per minute to breathe) and those who required longer periods of mechanical ventilation (increased work per minute and per liter of minute ventilation). Tobin further interpreted these results by suggesting that simple clinical parameters of spontaneous respiratory rate may be a reasonable indicator of work of breathing.[104] He noted that in Fiastro's patients the initial respiratory rate per minute of the ventilator-dependent patients was higher (32.4 +/− 3.6, SE) than those patients who weaned rapidly (18.5 +/− 1.5 SE). Further support to the importance of the work of breathing as an important factor in weaning is demonstrated in a small series of 8 patients reported by Shikora and colleagues.[105] These investigators expressed work of breathing as the difference in oxygen consumption on and off of mechanical ventilation. For 5 to 8 patients whose oxygen consumption during spontaneous ventilation was less than 15% of resting oxygen consumption, weaning was accomplished in less than 2 weeks. Of the 12 patients who exceeded 15%, none were weaned.[105]

The clinician should also be mindful that endotracheal tubes provide resistance to the work of breathing. Figure 24-5 illustrates the contribution to the work of breathing by variously sized endotracheal tubes.[106] With increasing levels of pressure support, the additional work of breathing created by the endotracheal tube is reduced. These findings suggest that it is reasonable to reduce added work of breathing with supplemental pressure support as shown. The reader is encouraged to review Chapters 10 and 15 for additional discussion about work of breathing and the contributions which ventilator circuits and modes of ventilation add to this work.

Aside from the mode of ventilation and resistance in the endotracheal-respiratory circuit, the consequences of

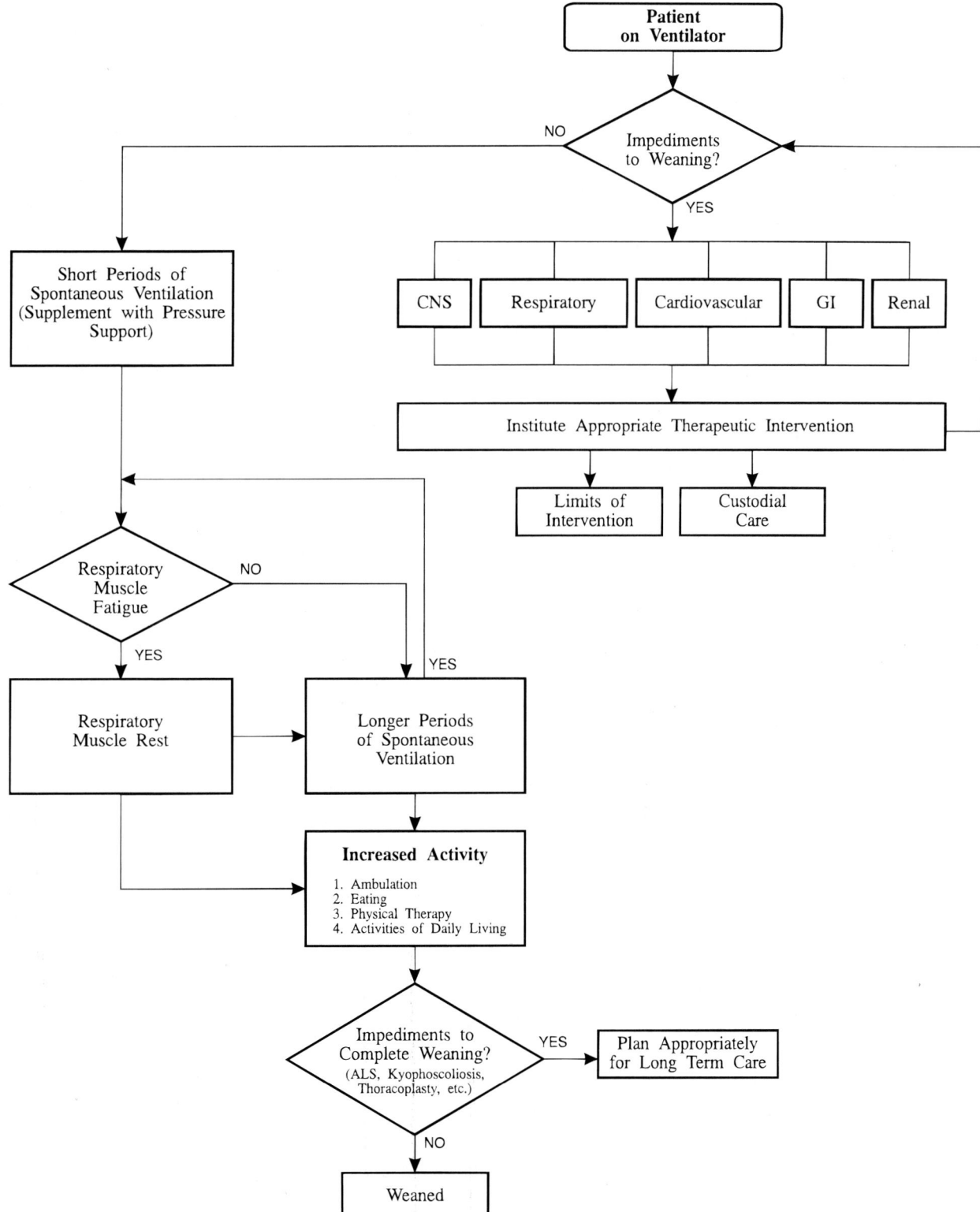

Fig. 24-3. An algorithm for weaning from mechanical ventilation begins with the question of whether any impediments to the weaning process exist. If none exist, then the process proceeds through signs of respiratory muscle fatigue. Otherwise, the impediments should be corrected carefully before weaning takes place. As the weaning process ensues, further emphasis is placed on rehabilitation with increasing activity to the point of complete or partial weaning. (Prepared by George Morrison, ACT/PC.)

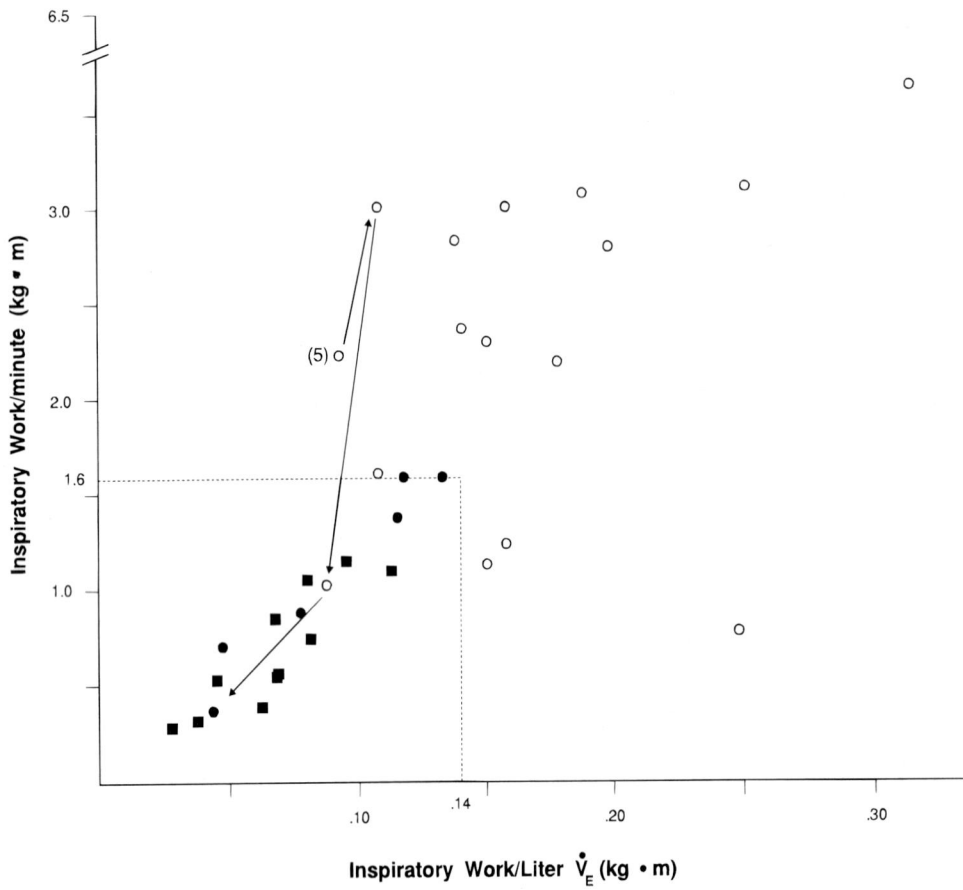

Fig. 24-4. Inspiratory work per minute (WI/min) versus inspiratory work per liter (WI/L) in all studies of patients in group 1 (solid boxes) and group 2 (solid circles) represent the final studies during successful weaning; open circles represent all other studies. The WI/min ≤ 1.60 and WI/L ≤ 0.14 kg/m were both necessary prior to extubation. Serial studies are plotted (arrows) for case 5 in group 2 from study entry until successful extubation. The first two studies were recorded during ventilator dependence (requiring constant assist control and intermittent mandatory ventilation, respectively); the next to last study (open circle) occurred during successful weaning (45-minute T-piece trials), and a decrease in both measures of WI reflected this change. (Redrawn by George Morrison, ACT/PC, from Fiastro, J. F., et al.: Comparison of standard weaning parameters and the mechanical work of breathing in mechanically ventilated patients. Chest, 94:232, 1988.

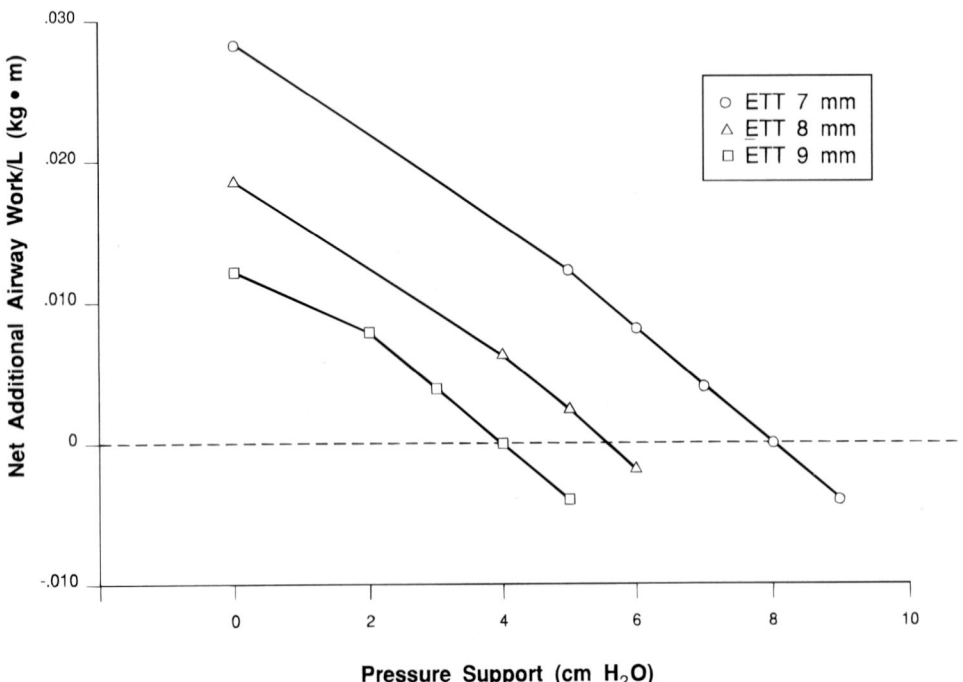

Fig. 24-5. Net additional work by mechanical respiratory system (positive Waw) resulting from an endotracheal tube (ETT) and ventilator circuit with increasing pressure support for 9-, 8-, and 7-mm endotracheal tubes at a respiratory rate of 20 per minute and VT of 0.5 L. (Redrawn by George Morrison, ACT/PC, from Fiastro, J. F. Habib, M. P., Quan, S. F.: Pressure support compensation for inspiratory work due to endotracheal tubes and demand continuous positive airway pressure. Chest, 93:499, 1988.

dynamic hyperinflation should also be considered during the weaning process. Dynamic hyperinflation, also known as auto-PEEP (intrinsic positive end-expiratory pressure, occult PEEP), occurs when the expiratory time is insufficient for establishment of resting equilibrium between inspiratory/expiratory cycles. Under the circumstances, alveolar pressure exceeds airway pressure and thus there is the added necessity of overcoming increased alveolar pressure for inspiration to take place.[107-109] The clinical consequences of this phenomenon include barotrauma (i.e., increased work of breathing and hypertension.[92] The increased work of breathing should be minimized during the weaning process. Sasson and colleagues have demonstrated that the application of CPAP, or pressure support ventilation, were associated with decreased pressure time product and decreased auto-PEEP during the weaning process.[110] Attempts to measure and reduce auto-PEEP during the early phases of weaning should be made to reduce the work of breathing. Under such circumstances, the addition of CPAP or pressure support should result in decreased respiratory rate. Please refer to Chapter 10 for further discussion of these points.

The principal logic of clinical protocols in weaning is outlined in Figure 24-6 in which a hypothetic patient's respiratory course is shown in relation to work of breathing. In this illustration, the respiratory rate begins to increase with the development of pneumonia, as does minute ventilation. As the Po_2 falls, the inspired oxygen concentration is increased. With continued infection, the work of breathing begins to affect the strength of the respiratory muscles. The maximum force of contraction of the respiratory muscles is reduced over time (Pdimax) whereas the proportion of diaphragmatic force for inspiratory effort to Pdimax increases. The proportion of inspiratory time over each minute increases (more contraction of the respiratory muscles each minute as opposed to the baseline state). The patient is placed on mechanical ventilation until the primary disease reverses itself with treatment. During the recovery process, the patient develops a perforated duodenal ulcer, the cycle repeats itself, and after appropriate intervention the process of weaning is repeated. Eventually, the patient recovers from surgery and nutrition depletion. Weaning and rehabilitation begin at a time when overall strength is reduced, manifested by decreased Pdimax and increased PTI. Periods of spontaneous ventilation are characterized by high TI/TTOT and high Pdi/Pdimax. The respiratory rate is increased, minute ventilation is high, and requirements for supplemental oxygen are also increased. With improvement in strength TI/TTOT decreases, Pdi/Pdimax decreases and overall, the amount of strength and endurance of the respiratory muscles increases.

Preparation for ICU Discharge

Many patients who receive ventilator support in an ICU reach a point where discharge is feasible. From some, the efforts have been unsuccessful and represent the limits of therapeutic intervention. Some patients represent a component of ICU mortality because of underlying illness. There are others who may still represent the limits of therapeutic intervention and remain ventilator dependent.

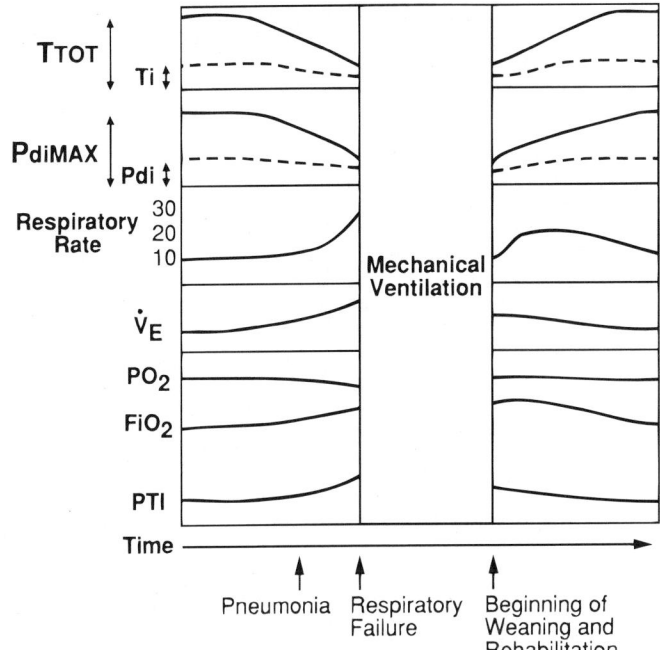

Fig. 24-6. Physiologic considerations in weaning should take into account the ratio of requirements for spontaneous ventilation to total possible function for maximum voluntary ventilation. In the text, reference is made to a patient who develops pneumonia. Note that the inspiratory time (TI) in relation to total respiratory cycle time (TT) increases as does the ratio of diaphragmatic contraction pressure (Pdi) to maximum possible pressure (Pdimax). These changes signify diminished endurance of the respiratory muscles. Continued respiratory distress is indicated by an increasing respiratory rate and minute ventilation ($\dot{V}E$), falling oxygen level with increased FIO_2, and increased tension time index (PTI). These trends are reversed following treatment of pneumonia and progression of the weaning and rehabilitation process (see text).

These latter individuals may require further assisted ventilation in a step-down unit or beyond hospitalization in the home care setting. Proper classification of these two groups is necessary to define the amount of ventilator care necessary beyond the ICU. For patients who are to receive only custodial care, it is important to determine if home care will be possible. For patients who can be rehabilitated with the assistance of mechanical ventilation, proper equipment selection, caregiver selection, patient education and discharge planning are necessary. Most importantly, at sometime during the course of the ICU stay, careful consideration should be given to the long-term care categories outlined in Table 24-1.

Table 24-17 lists criteria to be considered prior to discharging a patient who will receive long-term ventilator care outside of the ICU.

POST-ICU PHASE

Rehabilitation and Long-Term Use of Mechanical Ventilation

The major issues following ICU discharge for patients who have received mechanical ventilation or require long-term ventilation include:

Table 24-17. ICU Discharge Criteria

Hemodynamic stability for at least 1 week
No need for infusion of vasoactive medication
Inspired oxygen concentration of no more than 45%, with more than 5 cm end-expiratory pressure
Tracheostomy in place for at least 1 week
"Do not resuscitate" order for patients with terminal illness
Classification in custodial or rehabilitation care group prior to ICU discharge

(Adapted from Cordasco, E. M., Sivak, E. D., and Perez-Trepichio, A.: Demographics of long term ventilator dependent patients outside the intensive care unit. Cleve. Clin. J. Med., 58:505, 1991.)

- Continued rehabilitation
- Anticipation and prevention of complications which necessitate readmission to the intensive care unit
- Decannulation of the tracheostomy stoma
- Management of complications of long-term tracheostomy and long-term intubation
- Requirements for long-term mechanical ventilation beyond hospital discharge

Following discharge from the ICU, continued rehabilitation will guarantee hospital discharge if the underlying medical conditions have improved. Emphasis should be placed on maintaining nutrition status, monitoring for signs of infection, and increasing physical activity. While in the ICU, most long-term patients undergo a period when they depend completely on caregivers and therefore, some transition is required. The patient's family members should be brought into the rehabilitation process to maintain the focus on the purpose of the care plan (i.e., hospital discharge). This joint effort also will allow patient and family members to adjust to becoming more independent.

Techniques of decannulation of the tracheostomy stoma are outlined in Chapter 12. This process is usually uneventful, but on occasion is associated with numerous complications which require rehabilitation in themselves. The rehabilitation effort often necessitates retraining the patient to swallow and to eliminate oral secretions which accumulate in the posterior pharynx. There may also be requirements to use a prosthetic device to facilitate communication which necessitates instruction for optimum use. These services should be provided by a trained speech pathologist, as outlined in Chapter 12.

While adherence to the prior philosophy of rehabilitation and weaning technique will often result in success, one should be mindful that hospital mortality for patients who require mechanical ventilation beyond the usual course of illness remains high (see Table 24-7 for further discussion). In addition, the financial consequences often exceed the payment schedules provided for these patients particularly for patients who have complex or multiple medical illnesses.[112] Lastly, the requirement for care of these patients strains the resources of ICUs to the point that more bed spaces are required for continued care of critically ill patients. These facts underscore the necessity for options beyond the ICU to provide the continued care of the ventilator-dependent patient.

Noninvasive Respiratory ICU

In the early 1980s there was considerable emphasis on home care for the ventilator-dependent patient. This option, however, may not be available to all patients because of financial, sociologic, or psychologic constraints. Since home care represented the extreme of long-term care, it became obvious that intermediate care options would be required in hospitals.[113] Bone and colleagues have developed the concept of the noninvasive respiratory care unit as a less costly option for the patient receiving long-term mechanical ventilation.[113] They have further suggested that the non-ICU areas have benefits beyond financial issues. The benefits may include reduced complications from invasive studies and improved patient environment with less background noise and increased time for family visitation.[113]

Elpern and colleagues have suggested a "model" for the noninvasive respiratory care unit. This concept is based on reduced staffing (one third to one fifth nursing equivalents per patient as opposed to one to one half in the ICU), noninvasive monitoring, microprocessor based ventilators, noninvasive expiratory gas monitoring but no facilities for invasive arterial or pulmonary artery catheters. In addition, there is emphasis on strategy for long-term weaning.[114] The two major admission criteria to this noninvasive respiratory care unit are: requirement for specialized respiratory monitoring and/or support and hemodynamic stability.[114]

Cordasco and colleagues have suggested a model for care of selected long-term patients on conventional nursing units. This program emphasizes a patient care team with increased education in respiratory care for the caregivers. Specific ICU discharge criteria are summarized in Table 24-17.[114] Additional criteria for this ICU alternative for ventilator care have been outlined for patients following cardiac surgery.[12] These criteria emphasize that patients are awake and cooperative, ambulatory with moderate assistance, and able to be free of requirements for mechanical ventilation long enough to tolerate 45 minutes of physical therapy.[12]

There is little information available on the types of patients who can be managed in the non-ICU environment. In a population of 136 patients reported by Elpern and colleagues, the average age was 60.6 years with a range between 16 and 87.[114] Cordasco and colleagues reported an average age of 57 years for custodial patients and 60 years for rehabilitative patients.[111] Table 24-18 summarizes the diversity of the patient population in this latter study.

The outcome of the care delivered in the non-ICU setting will always be a function of the severity and reversibility of the condition which precipitates respiratory failure. Elpern and colleagues reported a 53% hospital mortality for 136 patients.[114] Cordasco and associates reported a hospital mortality of 25% for 99 patients reflecting discharge of some ventilator patients to home and nursing homes.[111] The populations were most likely dissimilar and the higher mortality figure reflects the differences in patient acuity. In Cordasco's patients, 50% required either full or partial mechanical ventilation at the time of hospital discharge.[111]

Table 24–18. Clinical Diagnoses Expected to Require Long-Term Mechanical Ventilation

Custodial conditions
    Amyotrophic lateral sclerosis
    Muscular dystrophy
    Chronic obstructive pulmonary disease (COPD)
    Parkinsonism
    Multiple sclerosis (rare)
    Spinal cord injury
Rehabilitative conditions
    Kyphoscoliosis
    Thoracoplasty
    Diaphragmatic paralysis
    Primary alveolar hypoventilation
    COPD

(Adapted from Cordasco, E. M., Sivak, E. D., and Perez-Trepichio, A.: Demographics of long term ventilator dependent patients outside the intensive care unit. Cleve. Clin. J. Med., *58*:505, 1991.)

Patient Selection for Long-Term Ventilatory Support

As outlined in the pre-ICU phase of this discussion, certain clinical conditions are likely to result in a long-term requirement for mechanical ventilation to achieve some degree of rehabilitation. Practically speaking, they include neuromuscular diseases, disorders of the drive to breathe (see Chap. 11), and patients with restriction of the chest wall. For the critical care practitioner, patients who require long-term mechanical ventilation (beyond 30 days) should be identified according to necessity of either custodial or rehabilitative care (see Table 24–6). Table 24–19 lists reports that summarize experience with long-term patients in the home care setting. The principal point to be extracted from these experiences is that the clinician should not always expect to wean certain patients completely and that valuable ICU resources should not be expended on such efforts.

In this context, the question of which patients qualify for long-term ventilation should be addressed. This question can be easily answered by returning to the pre-ICU phase of illness. Patients with designated diagnoses as outlined in Table 24–1 are likely to require long-term ventilation if the clinical history is one of progressive loss of exercise tolerance associated with the signs and symptoms of alveolar hypoventilation. Patients are unlikely to have detailed laboratory studies which define an end point that predicts freedom from ventilatory support and the requirement to begin rehabilitation assisted with mechanical ventilation.[120] The principal consideration to emphasize is that the decision to commit to long-term ventilation for rehabilitation is usually based on clinical judgment.

With this knowledge, appropriate care plans should be outlined in anticipation of hospital discharge. The most important factor in the consideration of home care ventilation is identification of the primary caregiver. In the case of patients in the rehabilitation care category, it is preferable that this individual be the patient himself. Although not always expected, independence is the goal of rehabilitative care.[2] For a patient in the custodial care category, the nature of their underlying diseases makes independence impossible. Experience with patients with amyotrophic lateral sclerosis best summarizes the nature of long-term custodial care.[30] In a small series of 6 patients with this disease, Sivak and colleagues concluded that home care was not suited for every patient.[30] The ideal candidate was one who had previously established coping skills to deal with adverse circumstances. Preexisting conflicts for patient and family members were often merged with stress and anxiety from the primary illness. If patients received some initial benefit from mechanical ventilation, the impact of the deteriorating physical condition was delayed until patients could no longer ambulate. Finally, the success of home care could not be guaranteed by any individual or group of caregivers. It is the responsibility of the patient and his or her family to make home care ventilation a successful venture.[30]

It is advisable that the contraindications to home care ventilation be carefully reviewed with the patient care team before such plans are discussed with the patient and his family. Basic contraindications include:

- Lack of a primary patient caregiver
- Inappropriate family situation
- Lack of economic resources for equipment
- Altered mental status
- Terminal disease state such as end stage cardiac disease or carcinoma

Once a patient is deemed suitable for home care, an appropriate protocol should be followed to properly educate the patient and his or her family in the use of equipment and patient care plans for home care.[115]

Equipment Selection for Home Care

As equally important as patient selection and caregiver identification, appropriate selection of equipment is neces-

Table 24–19. Supplemental Reference List—Home Care Reference

Author	Year	Restrictive Lung Disease Patients	COPD Patients	No Using Positive Pressure Ventilations	Years of Follow-Up
Make[116]	1986	23	15	29	1–4
Sivak[2]	1986	33	2	25	0.2–17
Robert[117]	1983	162	60	222	1–25
Fischer[24]	1982	15	14	29	0.1–5.5
Splaingard[25]	1983	47	0	47	1 day–11 years
Kopacz[118]	1984	14	4	18	0.1–3.6
Indihar[119]	1984	12	2	14	0.1–2.1

(Adapted from Make, B. J., and Gilmartin, M. E.: Rehabilitation and home care for ventilator assisted individuals. Clin. Chest Med., *7*:679, 1986.)

sary to facilitate the care process. In the event of requirements for long-term positive pressure ventilation, the use of small portable ventilations should be employed in the hospital setting prior to discharge. This procedure will allow the patient to adjust to the flow patterns of the smaller ventilators and to be trained in the use of equipment suitable for the home care setting.[121] For the most part, small portable machines which are classified as volume cycled ventilators are ideally suitable for home care.

The patient-ventilator interface must be accomplished with the sole purpose of providing rest to the respiratory muscles during the hours of rest and during sleep. For the patient with neuromuscular disease and/or with diaphragmatic paralysis, complete control of the process of ventilation should be accomplished by overriding the patient's spontaneous respiratory efforts. This process is accomplished by selecting an appropriate tidal volume and respiratory effort to maintain a mild respiratory alkalosis (i.e., pH 7.45 to 7.50). Of particular importance for the patient with diaphragmatic paralysis is the necessity to prevent hypoxemia during REM sleep.[81,122] This will help facilitate the sleep process for these patients since the diaphragm is the principal muscle of respiration during REM sleep. Restful sleep is usually not possible without some support to allow the patient to fall into this level of sleep. For the patient with idiopathic alveolar hypoventilation, it is important to prevent hypoxemia and hypercarbia during sleep to prevent development of long standing pulmonary hypertension and cor pulmonale. This problem can usually be avoided with suitable nighttime ventilation.

In most cases, positive pressure ventilation via tracheostomy will be required for long-term rehabilitation following critical illness. In order to facilitate the beginning of the weaning process, a tracheostomy should be placed if there is the anticipation of long-term requirements for mechanical ventilation. It is important for those patients who might require long-term ventilation beyond hospitalization to receive a type of tracheostomy which will not be susceptible to fibrosis and destruction of the anterior tracheal wall. The placement of appropriate tracheostomy type should be discussed with the surgeon performing the procedure according to the guidelines outlined in Chapter 12.

For patients with blunted drive to breathe or diaphragmatic paralysis, the use of a rocking bed may be sufficient to accomplish ventilation during the hours of sleep or rest. This device has also been employed for patients with old polio, diaphragmatic dysfunction after cardiac surgery, diaphragmatic dysfunction in neuromuscular diseases such as acid maltase deficiency and primary alveolar hypoventilation. Physiologically, the most important requirement for use of the rocking bed is compliance of the lung and chest wall. If compliance is reduced because of chest wall stiffness or retention of secretions, adequate ventilation and patient interface with the motion of the bed is unlikely. Although no specific studies are available, certain inferences are available on the use of the rocking bed. Goldstein and colleagues were unable to lower carbon dioxide levels using rocking beds in a group of seven patients with nonobstructive ventilatory impairment with an average VC of 43% of predicted.[123] This observation suggests that patients with vital capacity at or below this level may not receive adequate therapeutic benefit for rocking bed assisted ventilation. It is possible that patients may proceed through the rehabilitation process and eventually achieve suitable VC but still require conventional positive pressure ventilation to facilitate the process (see Chap. 25 on Respiratory Therapy).

There are various negative pressure devices available for facilitation of ventilation which have been employed in patients with old polio,[28] chronic obstructive lung disease,[38] and other neuromuscular diseases. This technology is best used in the pre-ICU phase of illnesses and applied earlier in the development or respiratory insufficiency before respiratory failure takes place.

The use of noninvasive face or nasal mask ventilation should also be considered for long-term care in appropriately selected patients. As discussed in the pre-ICU phase of illness, this method of ventilation is best applied prior to the onset of respiratory failure.

Home Going Prescription

The home going prescription should be made with the premise that the patient and family members together are self sufficient with respect to respiratory care on discharge from the hospital. Proper selection of the home care supplier should be made with the provision that 24 hour coverage by trained respiratory therapists is always available. Patient and family members should be thoroughly trained in tracheostomy care, tube changes, and management of the ventilator and ventilatory circuits. This training also includes proper cleaning of equipment and basic trouble shooting for circuit and ventilator malfunction.

For the patient in the custodial care category, a second ventilator should be available in the home if 24 hour ventilatory support is required. Additionally, public utilities, police and fire authorities must be notified of the patient's presence in the home so that special consideration can be provided in the event of emergencies. For the patient in the rehabilitative category, carefully designed protocols for increasing levels of physical activities should be established. If the patient can only be weaned to nighttime ventilation, proper emphasis on requirements for continued ventilator use should be made. For the patient with diaphragmatic paralysis, kyphoscoliosis or thoracoplasty, the care plan should be continued use of the ventilator. It should be emphasized that the patient should not independently attempt to wean completely. Otherwise, these efforts will only predispose to repeated respiratory failure. Table 24-20 outlines typical home care assessments according to the goals of care.

In summary, the assessment of the ventilator-dependent patient should always begin with a definition of the long-term goals of patient care. Careful definition of the impediments to weaning should be outlined and followed by classification of the patient into custodial or rehabilitative care categories. For the patient with no identified impediments prior to ICU admission, the prognosis for complete weaning may be good. For the patient with preexisting neuromuscular disease, restrictive chest wall disease or altered

Table 24–20. Assessments According to Types of Care

Rehabilitative Care	Custodial Care
1st month	1st month
(a) Documentation of the level of physiologic and psychologic function	(a) Tracheostomy change every 3 weeks
(b) Examination of tracheostomy stoma; auscultation of the lungs and heart; examination of the lower extremities for edema	(b) Gastrostomy or jejunostomy tube change monthly
(c) Vital capacity; negative inspiratory force stability of arterial blood gases should be established before discharge	(c) Examination of tracheostomy stoma; vital signs, physical examination of chest, abdomen, skin
(d) Ventilator circuit check; review of patient's use and maintenance of equipment	(d) Ventilator circuit check; equipment use and maintenance by primary caregiver
	(e) Observe patient and family members for signs of anger, fear, depression, anxiety, or resentment
	(f) Oximetry
2nd month	2nd month
a–d above	a–f above
3rd month	3rd month
a–d above	a–f above
6th month	6th month
a–d above	a–f above
12th month	12th month
a and b above	a–f above. Complete history and physical examination by physician
Thereafter	Thereafter
Influenza vaccine may be given each year as appropriate. Items a–d every 6 months for one year and then annually	Assessments a–f above every 3 months and yearly examinations

(From Sivak, E. D., and Steinel, J. A.: Ventilatory management of the home care patients. *In* Current Respiratory Care Techniques and Therapy. Edited by R. M. Kacmarek and J. K. Stoller. Toronto, B. C. Decker, 1988, p. 250.)

drive to breathe, long-term ventilator support beyond hospitalization may be indicated.

As the clinician proceeds with weaning of the appropriately selected patient, the impediments to weaning such as infection, malnutrition, debilitation and so forth must be eliminated. Throughout the weaning process, careful emphasis should be placed on increasing the strength and endurance of the respiratory muscles. As the process continues, the clinician must minimize the risks for the development of respiratory muscle fatigue. As strength and endurance improve, the patient can be withdrawn completely from the ventilator. As such, the ventilator should be viewed as a "crutch" to facilitate rehabilitation. The use of this crutch is both an art and a science.[125] With respect to weaning, it is still evident that the true scientist may actually be an accomplished artist in his or her own right.

REFERENCES

1. Snider, G. L.: Historical perspective on mechanical ventilation: from simple life support system to ethical dilemma. Am. Rev. Respir. Dis., *140*:S2, 1989.
2. Sivak, E. D. et al.: Home care ventilation: the Cleveland Clinic experience from 1977 to 1985. Respir. Care, *31*:294, 1986.
3. Douglas, P. S., Rosen, R. L., Butler, R. W., and Bone, R. C.: DRG payment for long-term ventilator patients. Implications and recommendations. Chest, *92*:413, 1987.
4. Gracey, D. R. et al.: Financial implications of prolonged ventilator care of medicare patients under the prospective payment system. A multicenter study. Chest, *91*:424, 1987.
5. Goldberg, A.I.: Life-sustaining Technology and the Elderly. Prolonged mechanical ventilation factors influencing the treatment decision. Chest, *94*:1277, 1988.
6. Wagner, D. P.: Economics of prolonged mechanical ventilation. Am. Rev. Respir. Dis. *140*:S14, 1989.
7. Newsom-Davis, J., Goldman, M., Loh, L., and Casson, M.: Diaphragm function and alveolar hypoventilation. Q. J. M., *177*:87, 1976.
8. Loh, L., Goldman, M., and Newsom, D. J.: The assessment of diaphragm function. Medicine, *56*:165, 1977.
9. Bergofsky, E. H.: Respiratory failure in disorders of the thoracic cage. Am. Rev. Respir. Dis., *119*:643, 1979.
10. Hall, J. B., and Wood, L. D. H.: Liberation of the patient from mechanical ventilation. JAMA, *257*:1621, 1987.
11. Sivak, E. D., and Kratz, S. M.: Critical success factors in weaning the ventilator dependent patient after heart surgery. *In* Anesthesia and the Heart Patient. Edited by F. G. Estafanous. Boston, Butterworths, 1989, p. 307.
12. Sivak, E. D.: Management of ventilator dependency following heart surgery. Semin. Thorac. Cardiovasco. Surg., *3*:53, 1991.
13. Morganroth, M. L., et al.: Criteria for weaning from prolonged mechanical ventilation. Arch. Intern. Med., *144*:1012, 1984.
14. Respiratory Muscle Fatigue. Report of the respiratory muscle fatigue workshop group. Am. Rev. Respir. Dis., *142*:474, 1990.
15. Roussos, C. S., and Macklem, P. T.: Diaphragmatic fatigue in man. J. Apply. Physiol.: Respirat. Environ. Exercise Physiol, *43*:189, 1977.
16. Bellemare, F., and Grassino, A.: Force reserve of the diaphragm in patients with chronic obstructive pulmonary disease. J. Appl. Physiol.: Respirat. Environ. Exercise Physiol., *55*:8, 1983.
17. Roussos, C., and Macklem, P. T.: The respiratory muscles. N. Engl. J Med. *307*:786, 1982.
18. Sivak, E. D.: Prolonged mechanical ventilation. An approach to weaning. Cleve. Clin. Q., *47*:89, 1980.
19. Garay, S. M., Turino, G. M., and Goldring, R. M.: Sustained reversal of chronic hypercapnea in patients with alveolar hypoventilation syndromes. Long-term maintenance with noninvasive nocturnal mechanical ventilation. Am. J. Med., *70*:269, 1981.
20. Sivak, E. D., et al.: Long-term management of diaphragmatic paralysis complicating prosthatic valve replacement. Crit. Care Med., *11*:438, 1983.

21. Abd, A. G., et al.: Diaphragmatic dysfunction after open heart surgery: treatment with a rocking bed. Ann. Intern. Med., *111*:881, 1989.
22. Sivak, E. D., Mehta, A. Hanson, M., and Cosgrove, D. M.: Post operative ventilatory dependence following thymectomy for myasthenia gravis. Cleve. Clin. Q., *51*:585, 1984.
23. Graham, T. R., Pearson, D. T., and Holden, M. P.: Letter. Re: Post operative ventilatory dependency following thymectomy for myasthenia gravis. Cleve. Clin. Q., *53*:115, 1986.
24. Fisher, D. A., and Prentice, W. S.: Feasibility of home care for certain respiratory-dependent restrictive or obstructive lung disease patients. Chest, *82*:739, 1982.
25. Splaingard, M. L., et al.: Home positive-pressure ventilation. Twenty years' experience. Chest, *84*:376, 1983.
26. Make, B., et al.: Rehabilitation of ventilator-dependent subjects with lung diseases. The concept and initial experience. Chest, *86*:358, 1984.
27. Home Care in the 1990's. Council on Scientific Affairs. JAMA, *263*:1241, 1990.
28. Affeldt, J. E., Bower, A. G., Dail, C. W., and Arata, N. N.: Prognosis for respiratory recovery in severe poliomyelitis. Arch. Phys. Med. Rehabil., *38*:16, 1957.
29. Curran, F. J.: Night ventilation by body respirators for patients in chronic respiratory failure due to late stage Duchenne muscular dystrophy. Arch. Phys. Med. Rehabil., *62*:270, 1981.
30. Sivak, E. D., Gipson, W. T., and Hanson, M. R.: Long-term management of respiratory failure in amyotrophic lateral sclerosis. Ann. Neurol., *12*:18, 1982.
31. Sivak, E. D., Ahmad, M., Hanson, M. R., and Mitsumoto, H.: Respiratory insufficiency in adult-onset acid maltase deficiency. South. Med. J., *80*:205, 1987.
32. Hoeppner, V. H., Cockcroft, D. W., Dosman, J. A., and Cotton, D. J.: Nighttime ventilation improves respiratory failure in secondary kyphoscoliosis. Am. Rev. Respir. Dis., *129*:240, 1984.
33. Ellis, E. R., Bye, P. T. P., Bruderer, J. W., and Sullivan, C. E.: Treatment of respiratory failure during sleep in patients with neuromuscular disease. Positive-pressure ventilation through a nose mask. Am. Rev. Respir. Dis., *135*:148, 1987.
34. Kerby, G. R., Mayer, L. S., and Pingleton, S. K.: Nocturnal positive pressure ventilation via nasal mask. Am. Rev. Respir. Dis., *135*:738, 1987.
35. Leger, P., Jennequin, J., Gerard, M., and Robert, D.: Home positive pressure ventilation via nasal mask for patients with neuromuscular weakness or restrictive lung or chest-wall disease. Respir. Care, *34*:73, 1989.
36. Strumpf, D. A., et al.: An evaluation of the Respironics BiPAP Bi-Level CPAP device for delivery of assisted ventilation. Respir. Care, *35*:415, 1990.
37. Brochard, L., et al.: Reversal of acute exacerbations of chronic obstructive lung disease by inspiratory assistance with a face mask. N. Engl. J. Med., *323*:1523, 1990.
38. Marino, W.: Intermittent volume cycled mechanical ventilation via nasal mask in patients with respiratory failure due to COPD. Chest, *99*:681, 1991.
39. Cropp, A., and DiMarco, A. F.: Effects of intermittent negative pressure ventilation on respiratory muscle function in patients with severe chronic obstructive pulmonary disease. Am. Rev. Respir. Dis., *135*:1056, 1987.
40. Munoz, E., et al.: DRG prospective, "All Payor Systems," Financial risk, and hospital cost in pulmonary medicine Non CC stratified DRGs. Chest, *94*:855, 1988.
41. Munoz, E., et al.: Healthcare financing policy for hospitalized pulmonary medicine patients. Chest, *95*:174, 1989.
42. Elpern, E. H., et al.: Long-term outcomes for elderly survivors of prolonged ventilator assistance. Chest, *96*:1120, 1989.
43. Sivak, E. D., and Perez Trepichio, A.: Quality assessment in the intensive care unit: continued evolution of a data model. Qual. Assur. Util. Rev., *7*:42, 1992.
44. Nunn, J. F., Milledge, J. S., and Singaraya, J.: Survival of patients ventilated in an intensive therapy unit. Br. Med. J., *1*:1525, 1979.
45. Snow, R. M., et al.: Respiratory failure in cancer patients. JAMA, *1*:2039, 1979.
46. Davis, H., Lefrak, S. S., Miller, D., and Malt, S.: Prolonged mechanically assisted ventilation. JAMA, *243*:43, 1980.
47. Fedullo, A. J., and Swinburne, A. J.: Relationship of patient age to cost and survival in a medical ICU. Crit. Care Med., *11*:155, 1983.
48. Schmidt, D., et al.: Prolonged mechanical ventilation for respiratory failure: a cost benefit analysis. Crit. Care Med., *11*:407, 1983.
49. McLean, R. F., et al.: Outcome of respiratory intensive care for the elderly. Crit. Care Med., *13*:625, 1985.
50. Witek, T. J., et al.: Mechanically assisted ventilation in a community hospital. Arch. Intern. Med., *145*:235, 1985.
51. Ewer, M. S., et al.: Outcome of lung cancer patients requiring mechanical ventilation of pulmonary failure. JAMA, *256*:2264, 1986.
52. Gillespie, D. J., Marsh, H. M., and Divertie, M. B.: Clinical outcome of respiratory failure in patients requiring prolonged (> 24 hours) mechanical ventilation. Chest, *90*:364, 1986.
53. Papadakis, M. A., and Browner, W. S.: Prognosis of noncardiac medical patients receiving mechanical ventilation in a veterans hospital. Am. J. Med., *83*:687, 1987.
54. Spicher, J. E., and White, D. P.: Outcome and function following prolonged mechanical ventilation. Arch. Intern. Med., *147*:421, 1987.
55. Peters, S. G., Meadows, J. A., and Gracey, D. R.: Outcome of respiratory failure in hematologic malignancy. Chest, *1*:99, 1988.
56. Swinburne, A. J., Fedullo, A. J., and Shayne, D. S.: Mechanical ventilation: analysis of increasing use and patient survival. J. Inten. Care Med., *3*:315, 1988.
57. Menzies, R., Gibbons, W., and Goldberg, P.: Determinants of weaning and survival among patients with COPD who require mechanical ventilation of acute respiratory failure. Chest, *95*:398, 1989.
58. Sahn, S. A., and Lakshnminarayan, S.: Bedside criteria for discontinuation of mechanical ventilation. Chest, *63*:1002, 1973.
59. Cohen, C. A., et al.: Clinical manifestations of inspiratory muscle fatigue. Am. J. Med., *73*:308, 1982.
60. Hodgkin, J. E., Bowser, M. A., and Burton, G. G.: Respiratory weaning. Crit. Care Med., *2*:96, 1974.
61. Khantzian, E. J., and McKenna, G. J.: Acute toxic and withdrawal reactions associated with drug use and abuse. Ann. Intern. Med., *90*:361, 1979.
62. Rich, M. W., et al.: Increased complications and prolonged hospital stay in elderly cardiac surgical patients with low serum albumin. Am. J. Cardiol., *63*:714, 1989.
63. Wilson, D. O., Bogers, R. M., and Hoffman, R. M.: Nutrition and chronic obstructive lung disease. Am. Rev. Respir. Dis., *132*:1347, 1986.
64. Apelgren, K. N., et al.: Comparison of nutritional undues and outcome in critical ill patients. Crit. Care Med., *10*:305, 1982.
65. Pingleton, S. K., and Harmon, G. S.: Nutritional management of acute respiratory failure. JAMA, *257*:3094, 1987.

66. DeValut, G. A.: Nutritional support of the critically ill: writing the TPN prescription. J. Crit. Illness, 4:54, 1989.
67. Askanazi, J.: Nutrition for the patient with respiratory failure: glucose vs. fat. Anesthesiology, 54:373, 1981.
68. Doekel, R. C., et al.: Clinical semistarvation. Depression of hypoxic ventilatory response. N. Engl. J. Med., 295:358, 1976.
69. Fiaccadori, E., et al.: Muscle and serum magnesium in pulmonary intensive care unit patients. Crit. Care Med., 16:751, 1988.
70. Aubier, M., et al.: Effect of hypophosphatemia on diaphragmatic contractility in patients with acute respiratory failure. N. Engl. J. Med., 313:420, 1985.
71. Bergbom-Engbert, I., and Haljamae, H.: Assessment of patients' experience of discomforts during respiratory failure. Crit. Care Med., 17:1068, 1989.
72. Chen, H., and Tang, Y.: Sleep loss impairs inspiratory muscle endurance. Am. Rev. Respir. Dis., 140:907, 1989.
73. Marsh, H. M., Gillespie, D. J., and Baumgartner, A. E.: Timing of tracheostomy in the critically ill patient. Chest, 96:190, 1989.
74. Benjamin, J. L., et al.: Left lower lobe atelectasis and consolidation following cardiac surgery: the effect of tropical cooling on the phrenic nerve. Radiology, 142:11, 1982.
75. Chandler, K. W., et al.: Bilateral diaphragmatic paralysis complicating local cardiac hypothermia during open heart surgery. Am. J. Med., 77:243, 1984.
76. Baraka, A., et al.: Post operative paralysis of phrenic and recurrent laryngeal nerves. Anesthesiology, 55:78, 1981.
77. Mickell, J. J., et al.: Clinical implications of postoperative unilateral phrenic nerve paralysis. J. Thorac. Cardiovasc. Surg., 76:297, 1978.
78. Vest, J. V., Perlira, M., and Senior, R. M.: Phrenic injury associated with venipuncture of the internal jugular vein. Chest, 78:777, 1980.
79. Wheeler, W. E., et al.: Etiology and prevention of topical cardiac hypothermia-induced phrenic nerve injury and left lower lobe atelectasis during cardiac surgery. Chest, 88:680, 1985.
80. Moorthy, S. S., et al.: Electrophysiologic evaluation of phrenic nerves in severe respiratory insufficiency requiring mechanical ventilation. Chest, 88:211, 1985.
81. Skatrud, J., et al.: Determinants of hypoventilation during wakefulness and sleep in diaphragmatic paralysis. Am. Rev. Respir. Dis., 121:587, 1989.
82. Hudson, L. D.: Ventilator management. In Care of the trauma patient. 2nd Ed. Edited by B. T. Shires. New York, McGraw-Hill, 1979, p. 487.
83. Tobin, M. J.: Which respiratory parameters can predict successful weaning? J. Crit. Illness, 5:819, 1990.
84. Sahn, S. A., Lakshminarayan, S., and Petty, T. L.: Weaning from mechanical ventilation. JAMA, 235:2208, 1976.
85. Milbern, S. M., et al.: Evaluation of criteria for discontinuing mechanical ventilation support. Arch. Surg., 113:1441, 1978.
86. Tahvanainen, J., Salempera, M., and Nikki, P.: Extubation criteria after weaning from intermittent mandatory ventilatory and continuous positive airway pressure. Crit. Care Med., 11:703, 1983.
87. Sasson, C. S. H., et al.: Airway occlusion pressure: an important indicator for successful weaning in patients with chronic obstructive pulmonary disease. Am. Rev. Respir. Dis., 135:107, 1987.
88. Tobin, M. J., et al.: The pattern of breathing during successful and unsuccessful trials of weaning from mechanical ventilation. Am. Rev. Respir. Dis., 134:1111, 1986.
89. Taylor, R. F., et al.: "Bedside estimation of respiratory drive during machine assisted ventilation." Am. Rev. Respir. Dis., 135:A51, 1987.
90. Yang, K. L., and Tobin, M. J.: Decision analysis of parameters used to predict outcome of a trial of weaning from mechanical ventilation. Am. Rev. Respir. Dis., 137:A98, 1989.
91. Yang, K. L., Tobin, M. J.: A prospective study of indexes predicting the outcome of trials of weaning from mechanical ventilation. N. Engl. J. Med., 321:1445, 1991.
92. Jabour, E. R., Rabil, D. M., Truwitt, J. D., and Rochester, D. F.: Evaluation of a new weaning index, based on gas exchange, tidal volume and effort. Am. Rev. Respir. Dis., 141:A517, 1990.
93. Gross, D., Grassino, A., Ross, W. R. D., and Macklem, P. T.: Electromyogram pattern of diaphragmatic fatigue. J. Appl. Physiol., 46:1, 1979.
94. Sasson, C. S. H., Te, T. T., Mahutte, C. K., and Light, R. W.: Airway occlusion pressure. An important indicator for successful weaning in patients with chronic obstructive pulmonary disease. Am. Rev. Respir. Dis., 135:107, 1987.
95. Montgomery, A. B., et al.: Prediction of successful ventilator weaning using airway occlusion pressure and hypercapnic challenge. Chest, 91:496, 1987.
96. Tobin, M. J., et al.: Konno-Mead analysis of ribcage-abdominal motion during successful and unsuccessful trials of weaning from mechanical ventilation. Am. Rev. Respir. Dis., 135:1320, 1987.
97. Tobin, M. J., et al.: Does ribcage abdominal paradox signify respiratory muscle fatigue? J. Appl. Physiol., 63:851, 1987.
98. Grassino, A., and Macklem, P. T.: Respiratory muscle fatigue and ventilatory failure. Annu. Rev. Med., 35:625, 1984.
99. Marini, J. J.: Lung mechanics determination at the bedside: instrumentation and clinical application. Respir. Care, 35:669, 1990.
100. Field, S., Sanci, S., and Grassino, A.: Respiratory muscle oxygen consumption estimated by the diaphragm pressure-time index. J. Appl. Physiol., 57:44, 1984.
101. Flick, G. R., Bellamy, P. E., and Simmons, D. H.: Diaphragmatic contraction during assisted mechanical ventilation. Chest, 96:130, 1989.
102. Marini, J. J., Rodriguez, R. M., and Lamb, V.: The inspiratory workload of patient-initiated mechanical ventilation. Am. Rev. Respir. Dis., 134:902, 1986.
103. Fiastro, J. F., et al.: Comparison of standard weaning parameters and the mechanical work of breathing in mechanically ventilated patients. Chest, 94:232, 1988.
104. Tobin, M. J.: Predicting weaning outcome (editorial). Chest, 94:227, 1988.
105. Shikora, S. A., et al.: Work of breathing: reliable predictor of weaning and extubation. Crit. Care Med., 18:157, 1990.
106. Fiastro, J. F., Habib, M. P., and Quan, S. F.: Pressure support compensation for inspiratory work due to endotracheal tubes and demand continuous positive airway pressure. Chest, 93:499, 1988.
107. Pepe, P. E., and Marini, J. J.: Occult positive end-expiratory pressure in mechanically ventilated patients with airflow obstruction. Am. Rev. Respir. Dis., 136:880, 1987.
108. Rossi, A., et al.: Measurement of static compliance of the total respiratory system in patients with acute respiratory failure during mechanical ventilation: the effect of intrinsic positive end-expiratory pressure. Am. Rev. Respir. Dis., 131:672, 1985.
109. Hoffman, B. A., Ershowsky, P., and Krieger, B. P.: Determination of auto-PEEP during spontaneous and controlled ventilation by monitoring changes in end-expiratory thoracic gas volume. Chest, 96:613, 1989.
110. Sasson, C. S. H., et al.: Pressure-time product during contin-

uous positive airway pressure, pressure support ventilatory and T-piece during weaning from mechanical ventilation. Am. Rev. Respir. Dis., *143:*469, 1991.
111. Cordasco, E. M., Sivak, E. D., and Perez-Trepichio, A.: Demographics of long term ventilator dependent patients outside the intensive care unit. Cleve. Clin. J. Med., *58:*505, 1991.
112. Spivack, D.: The high cost of acute health care: a review of escalating costs and limitations of such exposure in intensive care units. Am. Rev. Respir. Dis., *136:*1007, 1987.
113. Bone, R. C., and Balk, R. A.: Non-invasive respiratory care unit. Chest, *93:*390, 1988.
114. Elpern, E. H., Silver, M. R., Rosen, R. L., and Bone, R. C.: The non-invasive respiratory care unit. Patterns of use and financial implications. Chest, *99:*205, 1991.
115. Make, B. J., and Gilmartin, M. E.: Rehabilitation and home care for ventilator assisted individuals. Clin. Chest Med., *7:*679, 1986.
116. Make, B. J.: Long-term management of ventilator-assisted individuals: the Boston experience. Respir. Care, *31:*303, 1986.
117. Robert, D., et al.: Domicilliary mechanical ventilation by tracheostomy for chronic respiratory failure. Rev. Fr. Mal. Respir., *11:*923, 1983.
118. Kopacz, M. A., and Moriarty-Wright, R.: Multidisciplinary approach for the patient on a home ventilator. Heart Lung, *13:*255, 1984.
119. Indihar, F. J., and Walkner, N. E.: Experience with a prolonged respiratory care unit revisited. Chest, *86:*616, 1984.
120. Sivak, E. D., Cordasco, E. M., Gipson, W. T., and Stelmak, K.: Clinical considerations in the implementation of home care ventilation: observations in 24 patients. Cleve. Clin. Q., *50:*219, 1983.
121. Kacmarek, R. M., and Spearman, C. B.: Equipment used for ventilatory support in the home. Respir. Care, *31:*311, 1986.
122. Barlow, P. B., et al.: Idiopathic hypoventilation syndrome: importance of preventing nocturnal hypoxemia and hypercarbia. Am. Rev. Respir. Dis., *121:*141, 1980.
123. Goldstein, R. S., et al.: Assisted ventilation in respiratory failure by negative pressure ventilation and by rocking bed. Chest, *92:* 470, 1987.
124. Sivak, E. D., and Steinel, J. A.: Ventilatory management of the home care patient. *In* Current Respiratory Care Techniques and Therapy. Edited by R. M. Kacmarek and J. K. Stoller. Toronto, B. C. Decker, 1988, p. 250.
125. Milic-Emili, J.: Is weaning an art or a science. Am. Rev. Respir. Dis., *134:*1107, 1986.

Chapter 25

UTILIZATION OF RESPIRATORY CARE SERVICES AND RELATED TECHNOLOGY IN THE HIGH RISK PATIENT

JOHN J. KOMARA, JR.
LUCY KESTER
DENNIS K. GILES

Currently, our health care system is under tremendous pressure to reduce costs. Respiratory therapy services, once embraced by hospital administrators as "revenue generators," are now commonly viewed as "cost centers" secondary to the labor intensive nature of the service, changing reimbursement strategies, and the spiraling costs of new technology. This has forced many institutions to reduce personnel and focus on improving methods for the delivery of respiratory care services. As health care resources become limited, it is necessary to define and establish a scientific basis for the delivery of appropriate respiratory care. Many orders for common respiratory therapy modalities are generated by personnel who have had minimal education and training regarding their efficacy.[1-3] In an era of limited health care resources and a prospective payment reimbursement system, the importance of minimizing unnecessary and inappropriate procedures cannot be over emphasized.

Studies have demonstrated a significant reduction in inappropriate respiratory therapy procedures when respiratory care practitioners become involved in patient assessments and evaluations. In 1988, Shapiro and associates[4] reported a 61% decrease in non-ICU bronchial hygiene therapy (BHT) after implementing a formal evaluation system. Estimated cost savings exceeded $250,000 after one year with no reported increase in morbidity or mortality. Other investigators have demonstrated that the development and implementation of medical necessity guidelines, criteria-based evaluation systems, and clinical practice protocols have yielded similar results in regards to reducing procedures such as arterial blood gases (ABGs), oxygen therapy, aerosol therapy, and bronchial hygiene therapy without negatively affecting patient outcomes.[5-10] Overuse and misallocation of respiratory therapy procedures appears to increase costs to both the consumer and provider of health care.

By reducing the volume of therapy that has questionable benefit, resources can be redirected toward the high acuity, high risk patient. Such a philosophy will hopefully improve the quality of care as well as the efficiency of our health care system. Carefully designed studies are needed to identify those procedures and techniques which are most likely to provide maximal benefit to the patient. A comprehensive listing of the respiratory care services available in the care of the high risk patient are summarized in Table 25-1.

We firmly believe that consultation with practitioners highly knowledgeable in the field of respiratory care will result in an appropriate care plan without overuse of health care resources and technology. With this theme in mind, in this chapter we will explore the role of respiratory therapy modalities and related technology in the monitoring, treatment and management of the high risk patient. In addition, we will attempt to define the scope of services available for patient care in the pre-ICU phase of illness through ICU, and into rehabilitation and discharge. The clinical application of many procedures and techniques apply to each phase of illness, however the manner, frequency, and intensity with which they are applied may vary with each area or stage of hospitalization.

RESPIRATORY CARE SERVICES IN THE PRE-ICU PHASE OF ILLNESS

The objective of respiratory care in the pre-ICU phase of illness is to identify the high risk patient and to prevent or minimize the incidence of pulmonary complications. This objective may be accomplished by various screening techniques, comprehensive patient assessments, and the implementation of clinically indicated therapeutic procedures.

The following characteristics, if present, predispose the patient to an increased likelihood for the development of complications that may lead to increased morbidity, mortality, or length of hospitalization. The presence of multiple risk factors presents an even greater challenge regarding patient management issues. These patient risk factors include:

- Smoking history
- Advanced age (>60)
- Obesity
- Poor or inadequate nutrition status
- Chronic obstructive pulmonary disease (COPD) and asthma
- Neuromuscular disease
- Congestive heart failure or cor pulmonale
- Type and location of surgical procedure

Table 25-1. Scope of Respiratory Therapy Services Provided to the High Risk Patient

Arterial blood gas analysis and sampling
Aerosolized bronchodilator therapy
Metered dose inhaler therapy
Bedside pulmonary function testing
Bronchopulmonary hygiene therapy
CPAP therapy—PEP therapy
Oxygen therapy—aerosol therapy
Incentive spirometry—IPPB therapy
Pulse oximetry—CO_2 monitoring
Mechanical ventilation and weaning
Airway management
Patient evaluation and assessment
Pulmonary rehabilitation and education
Transport of the high risk patient

Patient Assessment and Evaluation

Patient assessment and application of the correct therapeutic modality has been a long standing controversial issue particularly regarding pre- and postoperative respiratory care. Several factors may be responsible for the general lack of consensus among health care providers regarding this topic. First, in order to clearly demonstrate the efficacy of one modality or care plan as compared to another, large scale and carefully designed studies need to be conducted. This is certainly not an easy task to perform considering health care's diverse patient populations and high acuity levels. Secondly, the complex medical-legal and economic climate in which we provide health care urges practitioners to establish "safety margins" by ordering procedures with only marginal or questionable benefit. Finally, education of health care workers has been less than adequate regarding such issues as indications, expected benefits, resource allocation, and associated costs.

A recent study conducted at the University of Virginia Medical Center[7] demonstrated the effects of practitioner-physician interaction in regards to the appropriateness of respiratory care modalities. After 6 months, inappropriate orders decreased from 48 to 11% resulting in improved allocation of limited resources. Other anticipated benefits from such a "consultation" approach include enhanced employee job satisfaction, improved education of physician and nursing personnel, and more efficient use of health care resources.

Torrington and co-workers[11] developed a perioperative program for respiratory care which included patient assessments for the purpose of identifying the high risk patient. Expected benefits included improved patient care to those in need and cost savings to those low risk patients who would not likely benefit from therapy.

An example of a simple bedside risk assessment form can be seen in Figure 25-1. This particular system uses a scale from 1 to 5, where 1 equates to the most severely ill (high risk) patient and 5 to the low risk patient. This particular risk assessment and protocol system incorporates eight specific criteria in order to classify "severity of illness" including:

- Pulmonary history
- Medical/surgical history
- Auscultation findings
- Cough and sputum evaluation
- Mental status
- Respiratory pattern
- Level of mobility
- Chest x-ray studies

Once classified, this system can be used to determine the nature and type of care plan, frequency of therapy, and in times of staffing shortages, which patients can be seen on a less frequent basis without subjecting them to unnecessary risk. The following is summary of how such a process would operate if a practitioner driven protocol or "consultation" service were available to the ordering physician.

- Chart review for medical/surgical history, laboratory data, etc.
- Patient assessment and observation
- Perform bedside spirometry, pulse oximetry or ABG if warranted
- Based on clinical and laboratory findings, initiate care plan according to medically approved clinical practice guidelines
- Notify and discuss with physician therapeutic plan and alternatives
- Perform periodic assessment and reevaluation as necessary

Consideration in the Monitoring and Detection of Respiratory Insufficiency

Bedside Spirometry

Recent advances in microprocessor technology has lead to the development of portable hand-held spirometers designed primarily for bedside measurements of pulmonary function. Table 25-2 lists the various parameters that can be obtained with these devices. Although not intended to replace referrals to the inpatient pulmonary function laboratory, these instruments offer the clinician a valuable tool in the diagnosis and management of patients with impaired ventilatory function, diaphragmatic fatigue, and respiratory muscle weakness. Specific factors contributing to pulmonary dysfunction are listed in Table 25-1.

Fig. 25-1. Patient assessment forms can assist in the identification and categorization of the high risk patient. Such forms are based on the patient's medical history, observed symptoms, and clinical findings. From such classifications as illustrated in this form used at our institution therapeutic respiratory care plans can be developed. Triage 1 indicates a high "severity of illness" and high risk, and conversely, triage 5 indicates minimal risk for development of pulmonary complications. (CCF, Cleveland Clinic Foundation.) (Courtesy of the Cleveland Clinic Foundation, Cleveland, OH.)

RESPIRATORY CARE AND RELATED TECHNOLOGY

CCF RESPIRATORY THERAPY EVALUATION

DATE _____

TIME _____

DIAGNOSIS _____ AGE _____

RESPIRATORY THERAPIST _____

ADDRESSOGRAPH

CHART ASSESSMENT

Points	0	x	1	x	2	x	3	x	4	x	POINTS
Pulmonary History	(-)History (-)Smoking		Smoking History < 1 pk a day		Smoking History > 1 pk a day		Pulmonary Disease		Severe or chronic with exacerbation		
Surgical	No Surgery		General Surgery		Lower Abdominal		Thoracic or Upper Abdominal		Thoracic with Pulmonary Disease		
Chest Xray	Clear or not indicated		Chronic radiographic changes		Infiltrate or Atelectasis or Pleural effusions		Infiltrates in more than one lobe		Infiltrate + Atelectasis +/or Pleural effusion		

DATE: LAB TEST: _____ WBC_____ Hb_____ PLTS_____

DATE: _____ Ph _____ HCO3 _____ PaCO2 _____ PaO2 _____ Sat / FiO2 _____

PULMONARY FUNCTION TEST:
FEV1 _____ FEF25-75 _____
FVC _____ PEAK FLOW _____

VITAL SIGNS: TEMP _____ ANTIPYRETIC THERAPY YES ___ NO ___
HR _____ BP _____ RR _____

PATIENT ASSESSMENT

	0	x	1	x	2	x	3	x	4	x	POINTS
Respiratory Pattern	Regular Pattern RR 12-20		Increased RR 20-25		Dyspnea on Exertion Irregular Pattern		Use of Accessory Muscles, Prolonged Expiration, or Decreased VC *		Severe Dyspnea, Use of Accessory Muscles, RR > 30		
MENTAL STATUS	Alert Oriented Cooperative		Disoriented Follows Commands		Obtunded Uncooperative		Obtunded		Comatose		
BREATH SOUNDS	Clear to Auscultation		Decreased Unilaterally		Decreased Bilaterally		Crackles in Bases		Wheezing or rhonchi		
COUGH	Strong Spontaneous Non-Productive		Strong Productive		Weak Non-productive		Weak Productive		No Spontaneous cough or may require suctioning		
LEVEL OF ACTIVITY	Ambulatory		Ambulatory with Assistance		Non-Ambulatory		Paraplegic		Quadraplegic		

* VC < or = minimal predicted (males: 50 + (2.4 x inches > 60 inches)
(female: 45 + (2.4 x inches > 60 inches)
multiply above ideal body wt. x 15 for minimum VC

Total Points _____

TRIAGE 1 > 20	TRIAGE 2 (16-20)	TRIAGE 3 (11-15)	TRIAGE 4 (6-10)	TRIAGE 5 (0-5)

Triage #

Table 25-2. Bedside Pulmonary Function Testing Parameters

Forced Vital Capacity (FVC)
Forced Expiratory Volume (FEV_1)
FEV_1/FVC Ratio
Peak Expiratory Flowrate (PEF)
Forced Expiratory Flow 25-75% (FEV_{25-75})
Maximum Voluntary Ventilation (MVV)
   Respiratory Rate (RR)
Tidal Volume (V_T)*
Minute Volume (MV)*
Maximum Voluntary Ventilation (MVV)*
Negative Inspiratory Force (NIF)*

*Extubation parameters—Respiradyne II Plus (Sherwood Medical)

The American Association for Respiratory Care (AARC) published guidelines and recommendations concerning the appropriate use and testing methods for spirometry.[12] These standards were designed for use in a number of areas including the inpatient pulmonary function laboratory, bedside testing, public screening, and the outpatient office or clinic setting. The AARC guidelines recommend that spirometry be used in the following manner:

- Preoperative assessment of lung function
- Occupation and or environment exposure assessment
- Monitoring the severity and progression of existing disease
- Monitoring the effects of therapeutics (i.e., pharmacologic agents)
- Screening for the detection of pulmonary dysfunction

Preoperative Assessment

Quantitative assessment of ventilatory function is of particular benefit in identifying the high risk patient. Early diagnosis of the patient at risk and subsequent implementation of an appropriate preoperative and postoperative respiratory care regimen has been associated with a reduction in pulmonary complications.[3,11,13-16] It is well recognized that postoperative complications are a major cause of morbidity and mortality. Under certain circumstances, however, laboratory measurements of pulmonary function may be both unavailable and/or impractical. For example, consider the "after hours" or weekend hospital admission patient who requires same or next day surgery. With the availability of portable bedside spirometry, pulmonary function testing can now be performed in a nonlaboratory environment using instrumentation that complies with the 1987 ATS Standards for spirometry (see Chap. 59).

Bedside Screening Devices

The Puritan-Bennett corporation currently manufactures and markets a device that complies with these updated standards—the PB 100 Portable Spirometer (Fig. 25-2). This particular device incorporates the use of disposable pneumotachs which effectively minimizes the potential risk of cross-infection in addition to providing a graphic representation of flow-volume and/or volume-time displays.

Sherwood Medical (St. Louis, MO) also markets a small portable pulmonary function/ventilation monitor—the Respiradyne II Plus—designed for bedside measurements of pulmonary function including parameters designated by the manufacturer as "extubation parameters" (Fig. 25-3). The Respiradyne II Plus is a battery operated self-calibrating device that also incorporates a microprocessor and solid-state pressure transducer. The disposable flow sensors possess a rather unique nonwoven fabric filter design. Unlike the PB 100 spirometer, this particular unit can be used to obtain measurements of pulmonary mechanics (see Table 25-2) on intubated patients with use of a specially designed disposable adapter.

A cooperative and well motivated subject is necessary in order to provide for a reliable and accurate assessment of pulmonary function. Therefore, it is strongly recommended that personnel performing these tests be well educated and trained in the various aspects of testing. Inadequately or poorly trained technicians have been shown to increase the likelihood of invalid or inaccurate test results.[12,18-20]

Pulmonary Function Assessment in COPD and Asthma

Both of these diseases are characterized by variable degrees of airflow obstruction.[18,94-96] Quantitative assessment of ventilatory function may provide valuable objective information considering that patient perception of symptoms and/or exacerbation may be inaccurate. The monitoring of peak expiratory flow rates (PEFR) appear to be gaining in popularity particularly in the management of asthma. Despite concerns regarding their accuracy, reliability and sensitivity,[19] measurements of PEFR are performed in the home, office, emergency room, and inpatient setting. Beasley and colleagues[21] recommend immediate medical attention for an observed PEFR less than 150 to 200 L per minute. PEFR monitoring in both the morning and evening may prove useful in detecting circadian (day/night) fluctuations in pulmonary function.[18] One must recognize that this test is highly effort dependent, however, and that suboptimal efforts will result in invalid and potentially misleading data.[19]

Peak flow devices are relatively inexpensive and simple to operate. Devices currently available for home monitoring include the Assess Peak Flow meter, shown in Figure 25-4 (HealthScan, Cedar Grove, NJ), the mini-Wright peak flow meter (Clement Clarke, Columbus, OH) and the Vitalograph (Vitalograph, Lenexa, KS).

Measurements of PEFR are often performed in hospitalized patients with more sophisticated devices than those previously discussed in this section. In this setting, the monitoring of FVC, FEV_1 and FEF_{25-75} may yield a more accurate and sensitive indication of airflow obstruction and subsequent response to therapy. It remains unclear whether the monitoring of PEFR can affect morbidity, mortality, or hospital admissions. Yet, many experts in the field

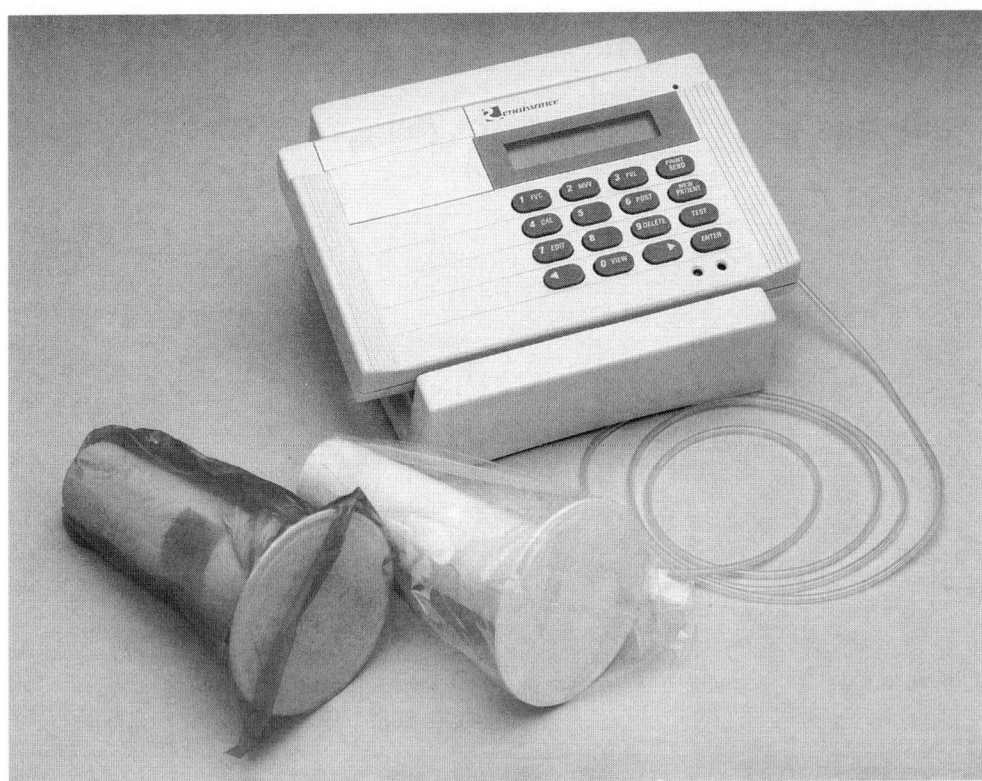

Fig. 25-2. The PB 100 hand-held spirometer provides a graphic representation of flow volume and/or volume time at the bedside. Disposable pneumotachs minimize the potential risk of cross-infection. (Courtesy of Puritan-Bennett Corp., Carlsbad, CA.)

firmly believe that peak flow monitoring is superior to subjective self-assessments of symptoms in the home setting.[18,20]

In addition to the monitoring of PEFR, the use of bedside spirometry is often used to assess the effectiveness of bronchodilator and steroid therapy in patients diagnosed with asthma and COPD. In many circumstances, the periodic assessment of pulmonary mechanics including measurements of maximal inspiratory pressures may also be of value in the management of patients diagnosed with neuromuscular disease. The results of serial measurements are of particular value when observed over a period. Early recognition of impending respiratory failure may avert the need for admission to the ICU or a prolonged hospital stay.

Pulse Oximetry Technology

First introduced commercially in the mid-1970s, pulse oximetry technology has rapidly gained acceptance and popularity in adult, pediatric, and neonatal patients. By 1988, the number of manufacturers of pulse oximetry technology had risen to more than 30. Figures 25-5 and 25-6 are current examples of pulse oximeter units available commercially in both the United States and abroad. Because pulse oximetry is widely used in a multitude of clinical settings, we consider it an important issue to explore. This explosion into clinical practice has prompted the AARC to recently publish a comprehensive set of guidelines for its use including indications, device limitations, and appropriate documentation procedures.[12] Table 25-3 summarizes the charting and documentation necessary to increase the validity and clinical significance of the measurement.

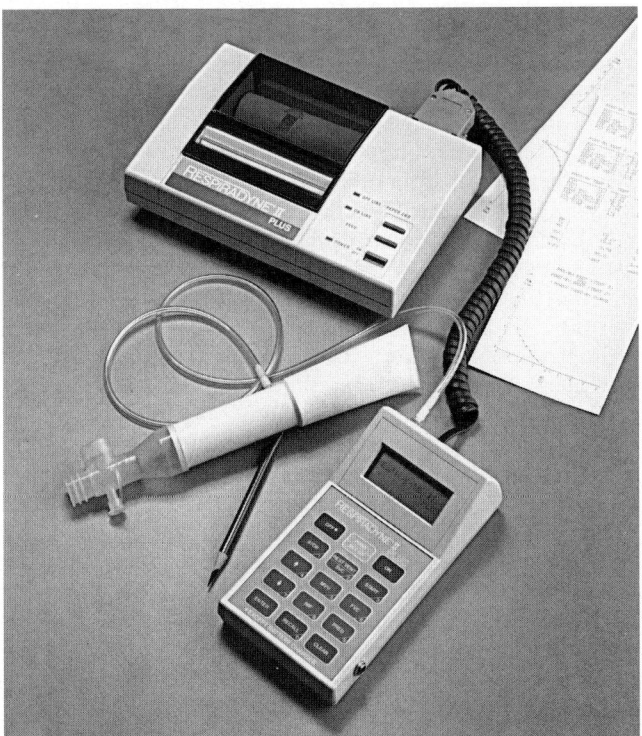

Fig. 25-3. The Respiradyne II Plus, another version of a bedside spirometer, has the additional utility of measurement of pulmonary mechanics (see Table 25-2) in intubated patients when a specially designed disposable adapter is applied. (Courtesy of Sherwood Medical Co., Watertown, NY.)

466 THE HIGH RISK PATIENT: MANAGEMENT OF THE CRITICALLY ILL

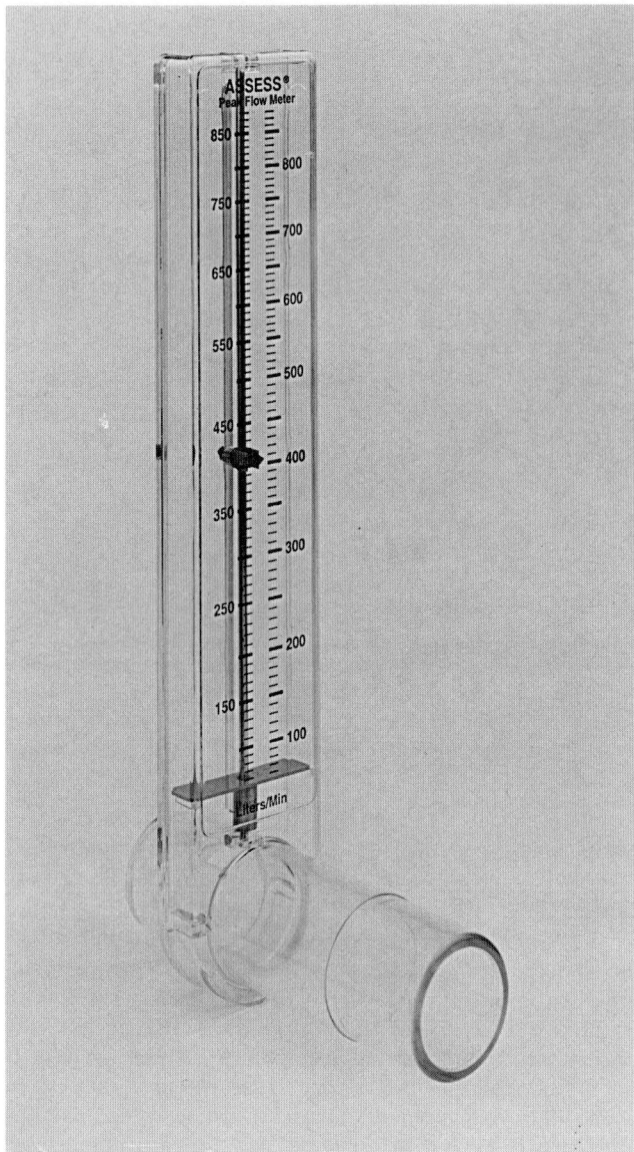

Fig. 25–4. Peak flow meters have been developed for outpatient management and assessment of asthmatic patients. In the hospital, they provide an inexpensive method of monitoring the effect of therapeutic intervention in patients who are receiving treatment for bronchospasm compromising respiratory function. The Assess Peak Flow Meter is shown. (Courtesy of HealthScan Products, Cedar Grove, NJ.)

Table 25–3. Charting and Documentation of Pulse Oximetry

Appropriate date, time, and patient activity level
Pulse oximeter readings of SpO_2 and heart rate
FiO_2 and/or oxygen flow including device
Probe site and type
Pulse oximeter model
Results of simultaneous ABG results if appropriate
Stability and reproducibility of reading
Clinical assessment of patient
Correlation of ECG/palpitation heart rate with oximetry heart rate

---

Technical Considerations. Pulse oximetry technology incorporates the use of two light-emitting diodes (LEDs) of specific wavelengths. Infrared light (920 nm) and red light (660 nm) are emitted by these diodes and subsequently transverse the arterial vascular bed. Directly opposite these diodes is a photodetector that measures the intensity of the transmitted light (Fig. 25–7). Oxygenated and deoxygenated hemoglobin possess uniquely different light absorption characteristics. Therefore, based on the differences of light received by the photodetector, the pulse oximeter unit is able to compute the hemoglobin oxygen saturation or more commonly referred to as "SpO_2."[22] Disposable sensors are available for a wide range of application including adult, pediatric, and neonatal monitoring. These sensors are designed and calibrated for use in a particular site and must be applied according to manufacturer recommendations. A detailed discussion of the technical aspects of pulse oximetry including the principles of optical plethysmography and spectrophotometry can be found in Chapter 77.

Several manufacturers have developed an alternative sensor for temple or forehead application. This method may be of particular benefit in conditions of peripheral vasoconstriction, patient movement, and during exercise and stress testing. The particular design of this sensor also incorporates both LEDs and a photodetector. In contrast to conventional transmissive technology, however, these particular sensor positions are aligned differently (Fig. 25–8).

Clinical Application and Considerations. The ability of pulse oximetry to provide the clinician with a noninvasive method for the detection of arterial desaturation has caused this technology to be recognized as a standard monitoring device intraoperative and postoperative in the postanesthesia care unit (PACU). Preliminary evidence suggests that intraoperative hypoxia related morbidity and mortality has been reduced as a result of pulse oximetry monitoring.[23-24] It remains unclear, however, whether the use of this technology will result in similar success in other settings. In fact, Bowton and colleagues[25] reported their alarming findings regarding the use of continuous pulse oximetry monitoring of general medical-surgical patients in a large tertiary care university based hospital. Despite the presence of desaturation in 30 of 40 patients to a SpO_2 value of less than 90% and in 23 patients to less than 85%, these events resulted in changes in respiratory care orders in 20% and 26% of the patients, respectively. In addition, documentation of these desaturation events occurred in only 33% of the nursing notes, and in 7% of the physician notes.

Of great concern is the perception that pulse oximetry technology is an inexpensive monitoring tool. Patient costs are estimated to range from $17 to $48 for each measurement or "spot check." In fact, the cost of one disposable digit sensor to the institution is in excess of $20 depending on the manufacturer. Continuous oximetry monitoring charges are estimated to range from $48 to more than $153 for a 24-hour period. To say that this technology is inexpensive, at least as far as the patient is concerned, is certainly inaccurate.

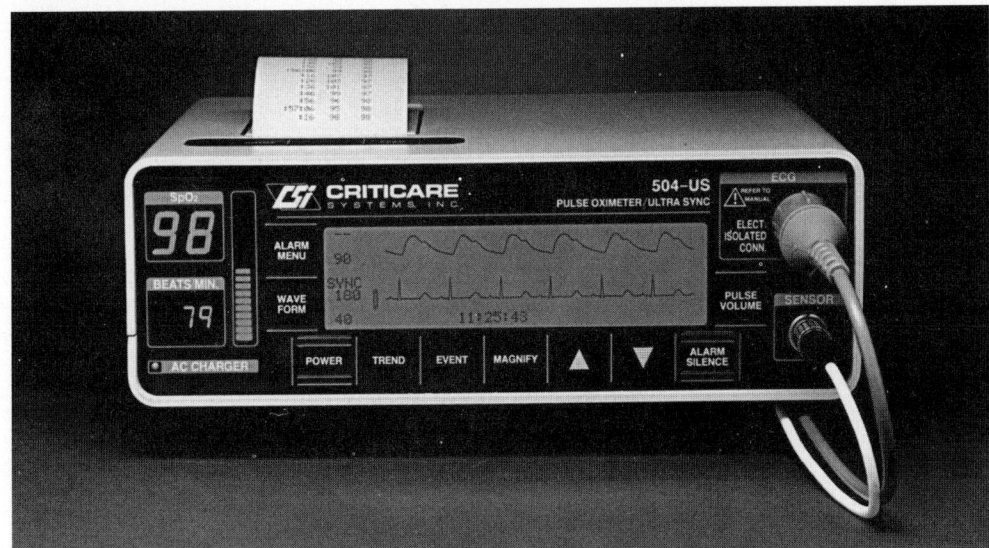

Fig. 25-5. An example of a current pulse oximeter is shown. Note that an electrocardiographic trace as well as the pulse plethysmograph can be viewed on the LCD. The digital readout is also provided to assist the caregiver monitoring these parameters. (Courtesy of Criticare Systems, Waukesha, WI.)

Often in routine clinical practice, measurements are ordered and subsequently performed on a "want to know" versus a "need to know" basis.[25,26] For example, it is not uncommon for an order to be generated for a "stat" pulse oximeter measurement based on a clinical assessment of confusion, lethargy, or some other nonspecific finding. Certainly, mental status changes may be the result of arterial hypoxemia. What is the likelihood that this event will occur, however, without either clinical changes including dyspnea, tachypnea, tachycardia, or other symptoms? How sensitive is a one time "spot check" in assessing the presence and/or absence of arterial desaturation? Despite extensive research and technologic improvements regarding both pulse oximetry design and software, these and many other questions need to be explored before the "fifth vital sign" becomes a routine standard of practice in all hospitalized patients. Educational efforts regarding the indications, limitations, accuracy, and associated costs should be directed at all health care personnel responsible for its use in the management of the high risk patient.[26,27] A more detailed discussion on the clinical application and limitations of pulse oximetry monitoring will follow in the ICU phase of illness section.

Therapeutic Strategies in the Prevention and Treatment of Atelectasis

Atelectasis is a relatively common finding in the postoperative patient population that results from changes in pulmonary function as a consequence of anesthesia, pain-management, and impaired mucociliary clearance.[28] These pulmonary changes include a reduction in:

- tidal volume (V_T)
- vital capacity (VC)
- functional residual capacity (FRC)

In the following discussion, we will briefly examine the various "hyperinflation" techniques available for treatment and prevention of atelectasis.

Incentive Spirometry

Introduced by Barlett[17] in 1973, incentive spirometry (also referred to as sustained maximal inspiration) is one of the most common, inexpensive, and simple hyperinflation maneuvers used in clinical practice today.[14] In 1985, O'Donohue[14] reported that incentive spirometry (IS) was pre-

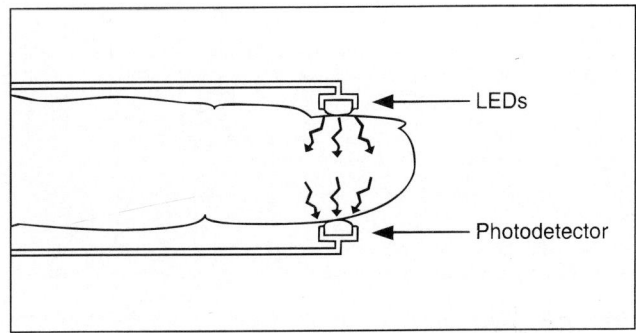

Fig. 25-6. The Nellcor N-200 pulse oximeter unit is shown. Note that the display contains only digital readouts of the oxygen saturation measured by oximetry and the pulse rate. (Courtesy of Nellcor, Haywood, CA.)

Fig. 25-7. Components of the transmission digit sensor used in pulse oximetry. (Courtesy of Nellcor, Haywood, CA.)

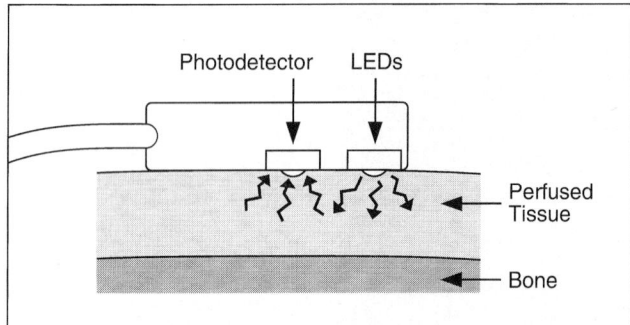

Fig. 25-8. Components of the reflectance forehead sensor used in pulse oximetry. (Courtesy of Nellcor, Haywood, CA.)

scribed for the treatment of postoperative atelectasis in 95% of United States hospitals. Most spirometers incorporate a floating ball or bellows system within the device (Fig. 25-9). In particular, this maneuver is intended to mimic the natural sigh mechanism. In most instances, this can be accomplished by encouraging the patient to inhale at a predetermined flow while sustaining inspiration for a minimum of 2 to 3 seconds. This procedure is then repeated 10 to 15 times per hour during waking hours. The purpose of the incentive spirometer is to provide feedback to the patient by displaying estimated volumes while encouraging and reinforcing maximal effort without incurring fatigue. In order to be effective, patients should be able to generate at least their predicted minimal VC (15 ml/kg of ideal body weight). In addition to achieving adequate inspiratory volumes, it appears patients may achieve better oxygenation if they are able to sustain the inspiratory hold for at least three seconds.[29] Based on the findings of Lederer and co-workers,[30] frequent patient reinforcement may also improve the efficacy of IS therapy. In contrast, other investigators[31] have reported that incentive spirometry therapy is of no therapeutic value in low risk patients fol-

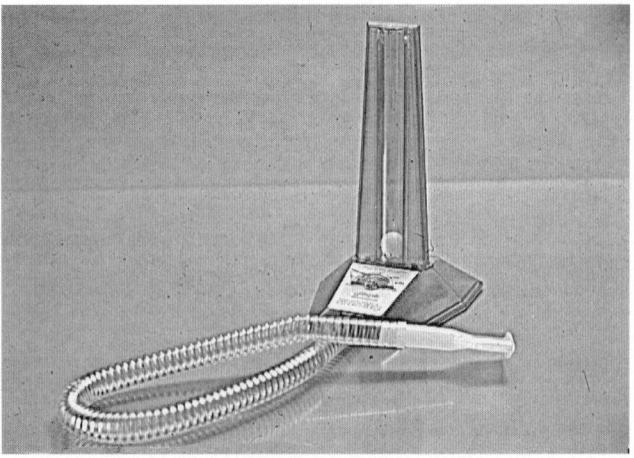

Fig. 25-9. An example of a floating ball-type incentive spirometer is shown. Resistance to inspiration can be varied depending on the strength and clinical condition of the patient. (Courtesy of Intertech Resources, Lincolnshire, IL.)

lowing elective cholecystectomy. A summary of recommended indications[12] for the use of incentive spirometry includes:

- Postoperative respiratory care particularly following thoracic and upper abdominal surgery
- Treatment of suspected or diagnosed atelectasis
- Following surgery in the high risk patient (i.e., COPD and neuromuscular disease)
- Restrictive lung disease

In circumstances where patients are unable to generate their predicted minimal vital capacity and have evidence of persistent atelectasis, alternative therapy may be considered. Intermittent positive airway pressure (IPPB), mask continuous positive airway pressure (Mask CPAP), and positive expiratory pressure (PEP) are examples of positive pressure hyperinflation techniques that are designed to increase both inspiratory volumes and FRC.

Intermittent Positive Pressure Breathing

Early enthusiasm for the use of IPPB therapy in the 1970s as a postoperative modality for the prevention of atelectasis has waned. Despite widespread use, little scientific evidence could be found to substantiate its theoretical benefit.[32] In fact, Iverson,[15] Sands,[33] and Van de Water[16] all reported significant complication rates despite the postoperative use of IPPB therapy. Despite these findings, evidence does support the therapeutic trial of IPPB in the treatment of clinically diagnosed atelectasis and certain neuromuscular diseases.[34] In addition, IPPB therapy may be appropriate for patients with poor inspiratory volumes who have a predisposition for the development of atelectasis. Exhaled tidal volumes must be monitored to ensure delivery of a therapeutic inspiratory volume.

Continuous Positive Airway Pressure (CPAP) and Positive Expiratory Pressure (PEP)

The application of CPAP therapy has been demonstrated to increase FRC in spontaneous breathing patients by mask.[35] Linder and co-workers[36] reported greater improvement in VC and FRC as compared to standard incentive spirometry. These findings have been confirmed by several recent investigations and have spawned recent interest in its application in the postoperative non-ICU setting.[37] CPAP therapy requires a continuous flow of gas and either a preset or adjustable valve. F_{IO_2} can be regulated by using either a high flow generator (Fig. 25-10) or an air/oxygen blending device to appropriate level. Both the level of CPAP and F_{IO_2} can be titrated according to the patient's response, measured by pulse oximetry or ABG.

Although similar in nature, PEP therapy does not require an inspiratory gas source. With this technique, the patient actively inspires through a one-way valve and then exhales through a preset or adjustable pressure valve. The fact that PEP therapy does not necessitate a continuous flow of gas makes this particular therapy attractive, secondary to its ease of operation and simple design (Fig. 25-11). There exists some evidence, however, that PEP may be associated with an increased work of breathing as compared

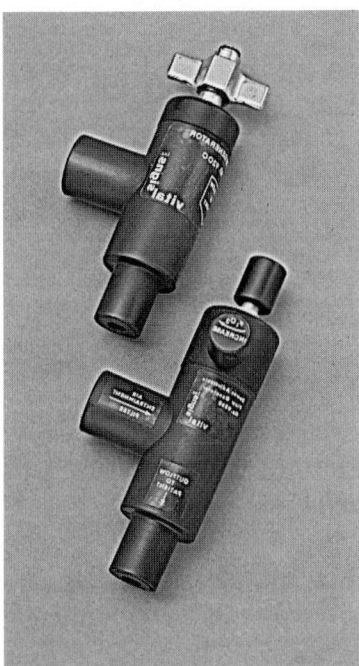

Fig. 25–10. Flow generators may be used for administering CPAP therapy. The top device has variable flow rate adjustment and the bottom has an F_{IO_2} adjustment. (Courtesy of Vital Signs, Totowa, NJ.)

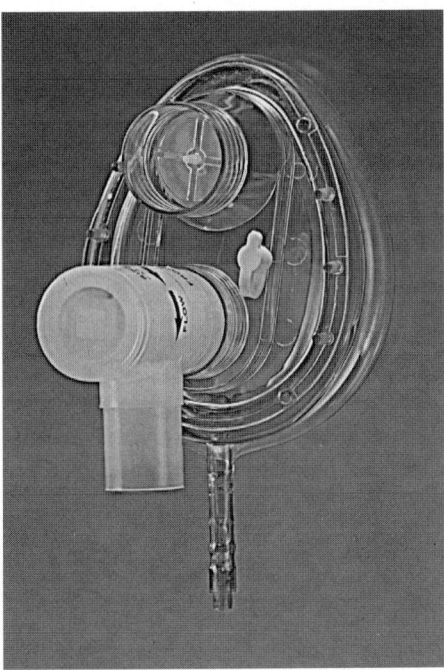

Fig. 25–11. A face mask and PEEP valve (lower end of mask) for application of positive expiratory pressure (PEP) is shown. Inspiration is through the flutter valve at the top portion of the mask. The seal can be adjusted with the instillation of air through the small valve on the lower portion of the mask. (Courtesy of Vital Signs, Totowa, NJ.)

Table 25–4. Indications for Oxygen Therapy (Inpatient)

Documented hypoxemia
  In adults, children, and infants older than 28 days:
    PaO_2 <60 torr or an SaO_2 <90% breathing room air and/or SaO_2 below desirable range for specific clinical situation.
  In neonates:
    PaO_2 <50 torr and/or SaO_2 <88% or capillary oxygen tension <40 torr.
An acute situation in which hypoxemia is suspected. Documentation of hypoxemia is required within an appropriate period of time following initiation of therapy.
Severe trauma.
Acute myocardial infarction.
Short-term therapy (e.g., postanesthesia recovery)

(From AARC clinical practice guidelines. Respir. Care, *36*:1402, 1991.)

to continuous flow CPAP therapy. Despite this limitation, Rickstein and co-workers[37] reported the superiority of PEP and CPAP as compared to deep breathing exercises (incentive spirometry) in 43 patients undergoing upper abdominal surgery with regards to alveolar-arterial oxygen difference ([A-a] O_2 diff), stabilization of lung volumes, and incidence of atelectasis.

Under investigation is the hypothesis that PEP therapy can aid in secretion clearance by mechanical bronchodilation of the airways.[38] In theory, retained secretions can be more easily expectorated as a result of both increased lung volumes and expiratory flow rates. It remains to be seen whether these initial claims can be validated in carefully designed clinical trials.

Oxygen Therapy and Oxygen Therapy Delivery Devices

Oxygen Therapy

The need for supplemental oxygen administration must be carefully substantiated by clinical indicators and or laboratory measurements according to the current AARC guidelines for oxygen therapy listed[12] in Table 25–4. Although there is no absolute contraindication for oxygen when an indication is present, there are several precautions that should be taken when prescribing this drug. These specific precautions and safety considerations are outlined in Table 25–5.

Oxygen Therapy Delivery Systems

For the purpose of this discussion, the delivery of oxygen can be basically divided into two distinct categories, high flow systems (HFS) and low flow systems (LFS). High flow oxygen systems can provide 100% of the patient's inspiratory flow demands (Fig. 25–12). In contrast, low flow oxygen systems provide only partial supplementation of the patient's inspiratory flow and volume requirements. HFSs are generally recommended when the patient requires moderate to high F_{IO_2} (>45%). Tachypnic patients with high inspiratory flow rates and/or high minute volumes normally benefit from oxygen therapy when administered by these systems as compared to low flow devices.

There are several types of oxygen delivery devices that can technically be classified as high flow systems. Jet mix-

Table 25–5. Associated Hazards and Possible Complications of Oxygen Therapy

With a PaO_2 >60 torr, ventilatory depression may occur in spontaneously breathing patients with an elevated $PaCO_2$ value.
With an FIO_2 >50%, absorption atelectasis, oxygen toxicity, and/or depression of ciliary and/or leukocytic function may occur.
In newborns:
  In premature infants: PaO_2 of >80 torr should be avoided because of the possibility of retinopathy of prematurity.
  Increased PaO_2 can contribute to closure or constriction of the ductus arteriosus—a possible concern in infants with ductus-dependent heart lesions.
Supplemental oxygen should be administered with caution in patients suffering from paraquat poisoning and patients receiving bleomycin.
During laser bronchoscopy, minimal levels of supplemental oxygen should be used to avoid intratracheal ignition.
Fire hazard is increased in the presence of elevated oxygen concentrations.
Bacterial contamination associated with certain neublization and humidification systems is a possible hazard.

(From AARC clinical practice guidelines. Respir. Care, 36:1402, 1991.)

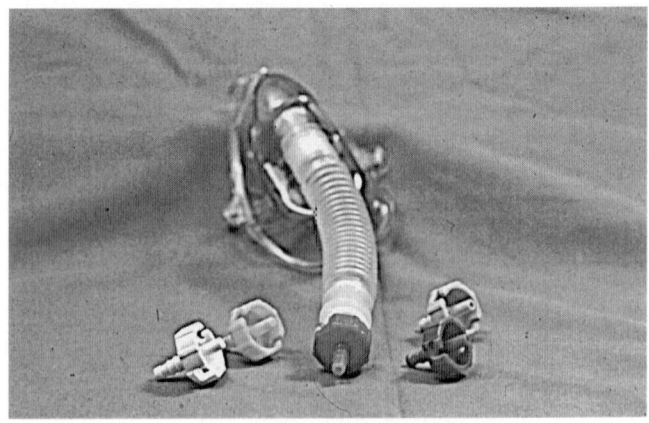

Fig. 25–13. A jet mixing "air entrainment" mask is shown. Various oxygen concentrations can be obtained using one of the various adapters. Concentrations of 24%, 28%, 31%, 35%, 40%, and 50% are typically available. Because of limitations of flow rates, concentrations above 50% are available. (Variable concentration mask, courtesy of Baxter HealthCare Corp., Valencia, CA.)

ing "air entrainment" masks are available for use with or without supplemental aerosol administration (Fig. 25–13). These particular devices rely on Bernoulli's principle for the mixing of 100% oxygen (source gas from 50 PSI outlet) and room air (FIO_2 of 21%) to provide a selected oxygen concentration. Oxygen concentrations normally available with this style mask are 24%, 28%, 31%, 35%, 40%, and 50%. Because these devices are unable to provide high flow rates when FIO_2 settings are above 50%, most manufacturers limit the devices to this 50% concentration setting.

Flow Generating Devices

Another device that incorporates the Bernoulli principle is the Downs flow generator (Vital Signs, Inc.). This partic-

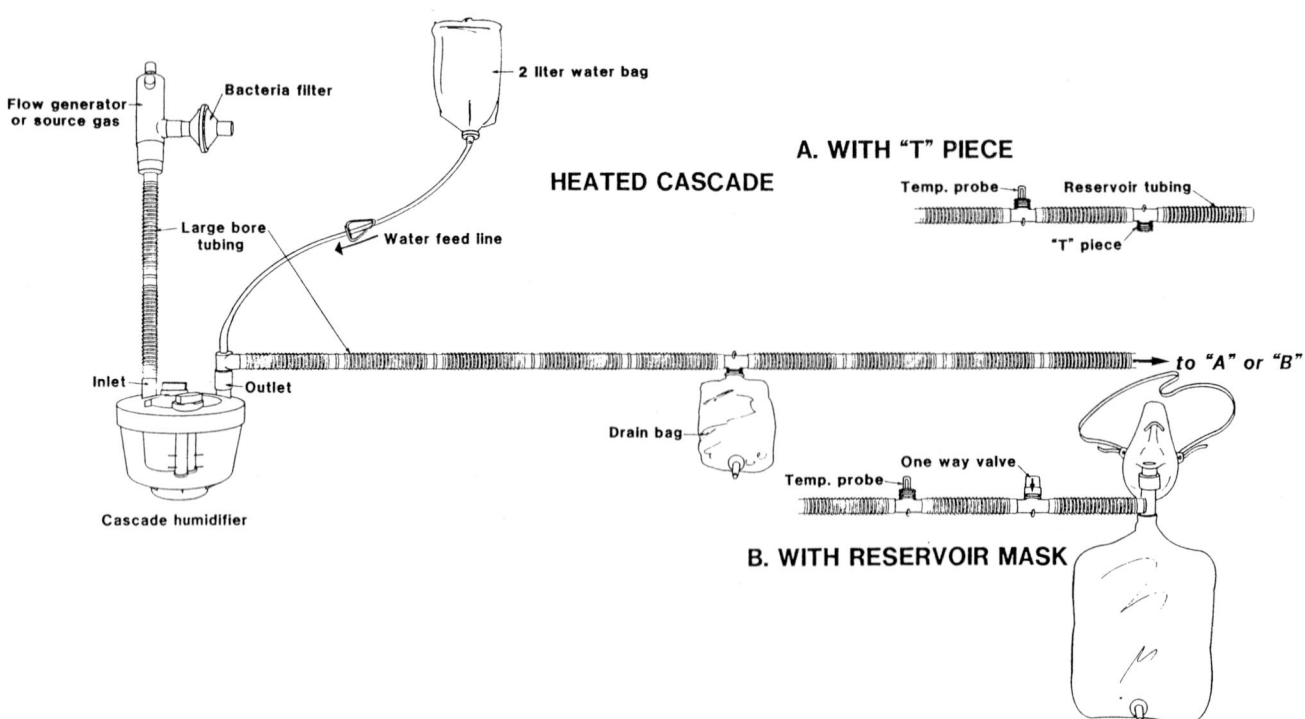

Fig. 25–12. A high flow oxygen delivery system is illustrated. A demonstrates the circuitry for connection to a standard 15-mm outer diameter airway in an intubated patient. B demonstrates the connection to a reservoir mask. Both circuits are connected to a common delivery system that provides oxygen and humidification.

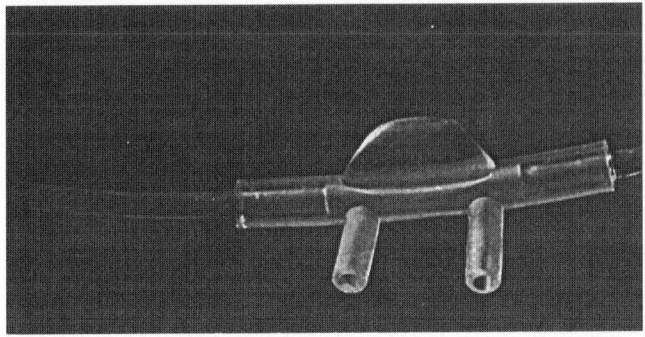

Fig. 25–14. The nasal cannula is the most common low flow oxygen delivery appliance. Continuous oxygen up to a concentration of approximately 40% at a flow of 6 L per minute is possible. Flows in excess of 6 L are not appropriate because the high flow may generate sufficient pressure to dissect along tissue plains and cause subcutaneous emphysema.

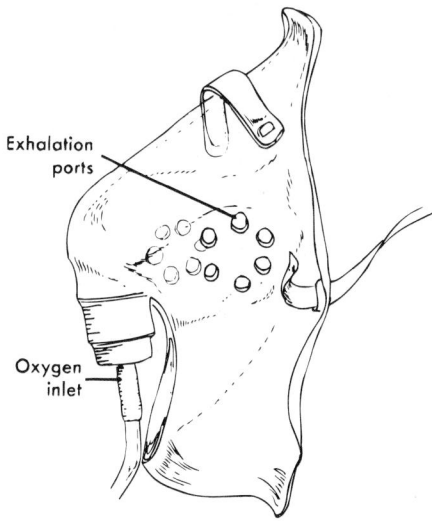

Fig. 25–15. The "simple" oxygen mask is capable of delivering 35 to 50% oxygen at flow rates between 5 and 10 L. The reservoir size of the mask necessitates that flow rates be at least 5 L per minute.

ular flow device connects to a 50 PSI oxygen outlet and is capable of providing flows in excess of 100 LPM regardless of the F_{IO_2} setting. This system can be used to supply oxygen therapy via mask or to patients with artificial airways. A major advantage of the flow generator is that it only requires one 50 PSI gas source for its operation.

An alternative to the Downs flow generator in providing high inspiratory flow rates and high inspired oxygen concentrations can be accomplished by blending air and oxygen. This mixing of air and oxygen requires the use of an oxygen controller, or more commonly referred to as an air/oxygen "blender." With this device, the F_{IO_2} and flow rate can be regulated accurately. Although reliable, set-up is far more difficult and requires two 50 PSI (air and O_2) gas sources.

Low Flow Oxygen Delivery Systems

These oxygen delivery devices are classified as such because they meet only a portion of the patient's inspiratory flow requirements. Mixing of oxygen with tidal breathing often results in the delivery of an unpredictable and varying F_{IO_2}, particularly when variations in breathing patterns occur. These are formulas available that assist the practitioner in estimating F_{IO_2} concentrations under certain conditions. These are often of limited value in clinical practice, however. Despite this limitation, low flow oxygen administration is commonly prescribed in both the inpatient and home settings. In most circumstances, low flow oxygen is titrated by adjustments in LPM according to clinical response and direct measurements of Pa_{O_2} and Sp_{O_2}. Therefore, knowledge of the exact concentration of inspired oxygen is not of primary importance.

Nasal Oxygen. The nasal cannula is probably the most common method of low flow oxygen delivery in patients with acute and chronic conditions requiring oxygen administration (Fig. 25-14). This simple, lightweight device is well tolerated by the patient and provides continuous, uninterrupted oxygen administration during ambulation, meals, nursing care, etc. It is capable of providing an estimated F_{IO_2} of approximately 40% at flow rates of 6 L per minute. In certain circumstances, the clinician may need to determine the estimated F_{IO_2} delivered by this device with various flow rates. Each liter per minute of oxygen flow corresponds to an increase in F_{IO_2} of 4%. Changes in respiratory frequency, tidal volume, and/or peak inspiratory flow rates will alter these estimates, however. The routine humidification of this device is probably not warranted when using flow rates of 4 L per minute or less.

Mask Oxygen. Often referred to as a "simple" mask, this device is capable of delivering 35 to 50% oxygen at flow rates of 5 to 10 L per minute (Fig. 25-15). Because this particular mask has a reservoir of 100 to 200 ml (depending on mask size), it is necessary to maintain a flow rate of at least 5 L per minute to prevent rebreathing of exhaled gases. This particular type of device is not well tolerated by most patients who require oxygen therapy for extended periods. In certain circumstances, interruption of oxygen therapy during meals, nursing care, etc., may be undesirable. Therefore, current use is limited primarily to short-term oxygen therapy.

Partial Rebreathing Mask and Nonrebreathing Mask. Both types of masks are similar in design with one exception. The nonrebreather mask incorporates the use of a one-way valve located between the reservoir bag and face mask (Fig. 25-16 right). In contrast, the partial rebreathing mask allows for a portion of the patient's exhaled gas (anatomic dead space) to inflate the reservoir bag with the remaining tidal breath exhaled through the side ports of the mask (Fig. 25-16 left). If adequate inspiratory flow rates are used, both masks can achieve inspired oxygen concentrations in excess of 60%.

Considerations in the Use of Aerosol Therapy

Aerosol administration is one of the cornerstones of respiratory therapy. Aerosolization of pharmacologic agents is one of the fastest methods of achieving a clinical re-

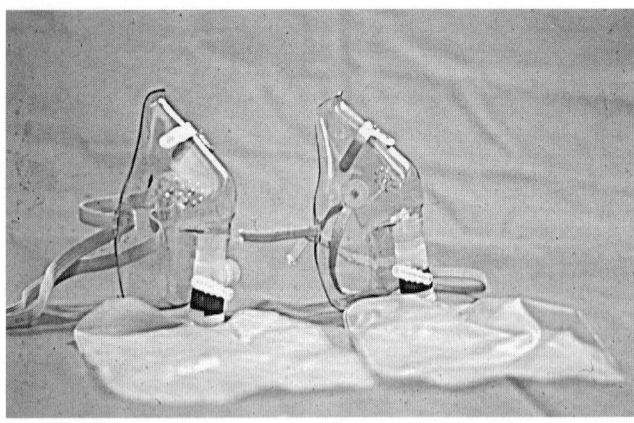

Fig. 25–16. The partial rebreathing mask (left) and the nonrebreathing mask (right) are similar in design, except that the nonrebreather mask incorporates a one-way valve located between the reservoir bag and the face mask. The one-way valve permits the bag to fill with oxygen, as opposed to the partial rebreather mask, which permits the reservoir to fill with a portion of the patient's exhaled tidal volume. Both masks are capable of delivering in excess of 60% oxygen if inspiratory flow rates are sufficiently high.

sponse, second only to intravenous administration.[3,8,18] By direct application of the drug to its intended site of action, the patient can avoid many of the associated systemic side effects. A complete listing of the indications and side effects of pharmacologic agents administered by aerosol or MDI can be found in Table 25-6. These drugs may be administered by either small volume nebulizer (SVN) and/or metered dose inhalers (MDI) (Figs. 25-17 and 25-18). Several classifications of drugs have been developed over the years for use in treating respiratory disorders and disease. These drugs can be divided into seven specific categories:

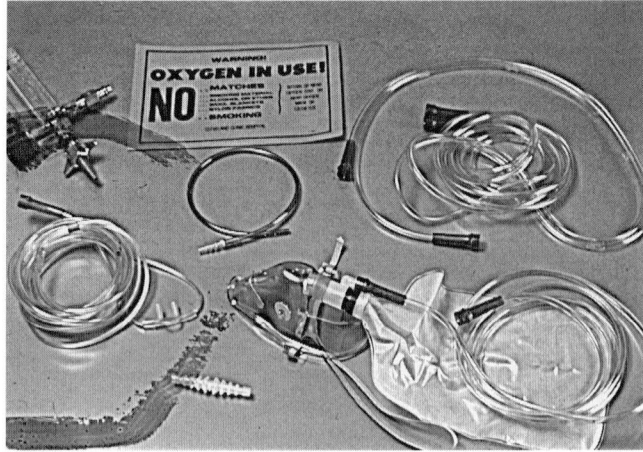

Fig. 25–17. A small volume medication nebulizer is shown. Such devices are portable and suitable for home use. (Courtesy of De Vilbiss, Somerset, PA.)

- Bland aerosols
- Mucolytics
- Beta-adrenergic agents
- Anticholinergics
- Anti-inflammatory agents
- Antimicrobial agents
- Antiviral agents

Recommended dosages for both adult and pediatric use are listed in Table 25-7.

Bland Aerosols

Little scientific evidence exists that substantiates the routine use of bland aerosols (i.e., water and saline) in the treatment of pulmonary disease.[3,39] Some reports, how-

Table 25–6. Indications for and Side Effects of Commonly Used Drugs in Respiratory Care

Drug Classification	Examples	Indications for Use in Respiratory Care	Side Effects
Beta-adrenergic agents	Albuterol, metaproterenol	Treatment of bronchospasm Increase in mucociliary escalation	Palpitations, tachycardia, restlessness, anxiety, tension, tremor, and dizziness
Anticholinergic agents	Ipratroprium bromide, atropine sulfate	Usually used in combination with inhaled beta-adrenergics for the treatment of bronchospasm	In aerosol preparations, drying of the mouth is the most common side effect; however in higher doses one may see reduced secretions, inhibition of sweating, dizziness, fatigue, sedation, and decreased heart rate
Anti-inflammatory drugs			
Steroids	Beclomethasone dipropionate, triamcinolone acetonide	Allergic asthma to prevent or suppress the inflammatory response	In aerosol preparations: upper airway fungal infections, hoarseness, coughing, dry mouth
Cromolyn sodium	Cromolyn sodium	Prophylactic maintenance for asthma	Local irritation, bronchospasm, maculopapular epistaxis, urticaria, cough, congestion, sneezing
Antimicrobial drugs			
Antibacterial	Pentamidine isethionate	Used for the treatment and prophylaxis of Pneumocystis carinii pneumonia	Local irritation
Antiviral	Virazole	Used in the treatment of respiratory syncytial virus	Conjunctivitis, suppression of immunity

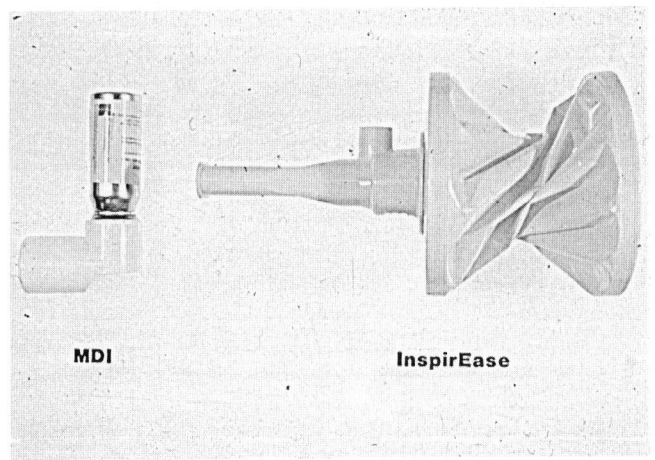

Fig. 25–18. Two types of metered dose inhalers (MDI) are illustrated. The canister (left) may not deliver a proper dose of medication if the patient does not inhale slowly. Medication may impact against the posterior pharynx and may not be delivered to the airways. In contrast, the reservoir type (right) provides an atmosphere of medication for inhalation.

ever, have shown bland aerosols to cause a slight increase in mucociliary clearance in normal subjects as well as patients with chronic bronchitis.[40] It may be of therapeutic benefit to administer a trial of bland aerosol therapy prior to postural drainage and chest clapping in patients known to have tenacious secretions (i.e., cystic fibrosis and bronchiectasis) and/or suspected evidence of peripheral mucous plugs. Bland aerosol therapy has also been advocated for use in sputum inductions.[3] Bigby and colleagues[41] reported good success in the use of a hypertonic saline solution (3%) for identifying the organism responsible for PCP pneumonia. Therapy is normally given over 15 to 20 minutes under the close observation of the practitioner.

Mucolytic Agents

Several aerosolized mucolytics have been tested and commercially marketed for the treatment of liquifying retained secretions. Most reports have failed to demonstrate any therapeutic value in the routine treatment of COPD, however.[42] More favorable results have been reported in the breakdown and subsequent removal of mucous plugs.[3] The most notable and widely used mucolytic is N-acetylcysteine. This sulfhydryl compound breaks disulfide bonds

Table 25–7. Pharmacologic Agents Used in Respiratory Care

Drug	Available Form for Use in Respiratory Care	Standard Adult Dosage	Standard Pediatric Dosage
Beta Agonists			
Albuterol	0.5% Solution for nebulization	0.5 ml of a 0.5% solution q4–6h, diluted with 2–3 ml of saline	0.1–0.15 mg/kg of a 0.5% solution in 2 ml of saline q4–6h, maximum 5.0 mg
	Metered dose inhaler 0.90 mg/puff	2 puffs q4–6h	2 puffs q4–6h
Metaproterenol	5% Solution for nebulization	0.3 ml of 5% solution q4–6h diluted with 2–3 ml of saline	0.25–0.50 mg/kg of a 5% solution in 2 ml of saline q4–6h, maximum 15.0 mg
	Metered dose inhaler 0.65 mg/puff	2 puffs q4–6h	
Isoetharine	1% Solution for nebulization	0.5 ml of a 1% solution q4h diluted with 2–3 ml of saline	Generally not used in pediatrics
	Metered dose inhaler 0.34 mg/puff	2 puffs q4h	
Terbutaline	Metered dose inhaler 0.20 mg/puff	2 puffs q4h	2 puffs q4h
Pirbuterol	Metered dose inhaler 0.2 mg/puff	2 puffs q4h	2 puffs q4h
Bitolterol	Metered dose inhaler 0.37 mg/puff	2 puffs q8h	2 puffs q8h
Anticholinergics			
Ipratropium bromide	Metered dose inhaler 0.018 mg/puff	2 puffs q4h	2 puffs q4h
Atropine sulfate	Not approved by FDA for aerosolization	0.025 mg/kg q3–4h diluted with 2–3 ml of saline	0.05 mg/kg tid to qid diluted with 2–3 ml of saline
Anti-inflammatory drugs			
Cromolyn sodium	Metered dose inhaler 1 mg/puff	2 puffs bid to qid	2 puffs bid to qid
	Dry powder inhaler 20 mg/capsule	1 capsule bid to qid	1 capsule bid to qid
	Nebulizer solution 20 mg/ampule	1 ampule bid to qid	1 ampule bid to qid
Beclomethasone dipropionate	Metered dose inhaler 0.050 mg/puff	2 puffs tid to qid	2 to 4 puffs bid to qid
Triamcinolone acetonide	Metered dose inhaler 0.10 mg/puff	2 puffs tid to qid	2 to 4 puffs bid to qid
Antimicrobial drugs			
Pentamidine isethionate	Dried powder for reconstitution with sterile water	60–300 mg/treatment	60–300 mg/treatment
Virazole	Dried powder for reconstitution with sterile water	Generally not used in adults	300 ml of a 20 mg/ml solution nebulized for 12 to 18 h per day, licensed for use with the SPAG-2 system only

in mucoproteins and mucopolysaccharides in vitro. Available in 10 and 20% solution form, it is normally given by either SVN or by direct administration into the artificial airway. Mucolytics have been reported to have an irritative effect on the airways and may precipitate the onset of bronchospasm, particularly in patients with hyperreactive airways.[42] Therefore, it is recommended that bronchodilator therapy be given prior to its administration. Ziment[43] recommends a 2 to 5 ml of a 10% solution or 1 to 5 ml of a 20% solution as often as required based on clinical observations and severity of mucous plugging.

Beta-Adrenergic Agents

Aerosolized beta agonists have replaced the common practice of subcutaneous preparations and intravenous theophylline as the first line treatment of bronchospastic disorders.[18,44] This choice is most likely due to its effectiveness, quick response in producing the desired clinical effect, and beta$_2$ specificity. Several of the more commonly prescribed beta agonists used in the United States include albuterol (Proventil, Ventolin), metaproterenol (Alupent/Metaprel), and isoetharine (Bronkosol). Isoproterenol still remains commercially available, but is rarely used secondary to its known cardiovascular side effects. The previously mentioned drugs are available in solution form for aerosolization and as metered dose inhalers. Certain beta agonists are currently available in MDI form only. These include: bitolterol (Tornalate), pirbuterol (Maxair), and terbutaline (Brethine, Bricanyl). Despite pharmaceutical recommendations, the prescribed frequency of beta agonists largely depends on institutional guidelines, physician preference, and severity of airflow obstruction. Of interest is the recommendations for beta-agonist therapy found in the 1991 report: *Executive Summary: Guidelines for the Diagnosis and Management of Asthma.*[44] In this report, adults who present with clinical symptoms of acute airflow obstruction and who have no underlying cardiovascular disease may receive beta-agonist therapy as frequently as every 20 to 30 minutes. In pediatric cases, nebulized albuterol was reported to be safe when administered as frequently as every 20 minutes. In cases of persistent severe airflow obstruction, albuterol may be administered continuously if necessary.

Anticholinergics

This particular drug classification is used primarily in the treatment of airflow obstruction in patients diagnosed with asthma and COPD. Anticholinergics have been reported to have a synergistic effect when used in conjunction with beta agonists for the treatment of chronic airflow obstruction.[45] Examples include ipratropium bromide (Atrovent) and atropine sulfate. Technically, atropine is not an FDA approved drug for aerosol therapy. On occasion, however, it is prescribed in situations were MDI administration of Atrovent is not feasible. If given in aerosol form, the patient should be closely monitored for potential side effects (see Table 25-7). Ziment[43] recommends using .025 mg/kg of a 1% solution. At this present time, atrovent is available only in MDI form.

Anti-inflammatory Agents

The use of anti-inflammatory agents including corticosteroids and cromolyn sodium have been the center of much discussion regarding the treatment of airflow obstruction, particularly in the case of asthma.[18-44] Research has identified the presence of a significant inflammatory component in patients with reactive airways disease.[44] Therefore, it seems logical that patients with airway inflammation will derive clinical benefit from inhaled corticosteroids (Azmacort and Vanceril) in addition to beta-agonist therapy.

Cromolyn sodium (Intal) is thought to stabilize mast cells found in the lung. It is commercially available in solution form (2 ml/20 mg) or via MDI. By preventing the release of chemical mediators including histamine and serotonin that lead to inflammation and edema, the consequences of airflow obstruction can be minimized or avoided. Neither cromolyn sodium nor corticosteroids are of clinical benefit in treating acute airflow obstruction. In most instances, it requires 6 to 9 hours for steroids to reduce airway edema. Stabilization of mast cells may require several days of therapy to be of clinical significance.[45]

Antimicrobials

Initially described by Baroch in 1942, the use of aerosolized antimicrobials entered medical practice with interest and enthusiasm. During the 1950s, many studies were conducted to determine if this particular method of delivery offered any therapeutic advantages. Despite extensive research, little evidence could be found to recommend this method of administration in the treatment of bacterial pulmonary infections, except for patients with chronic conditions as seen in cystic fibrosis. Aerosolized antimicrobials are irritating to the mucosal surface of the lung and have been known to cause reactive bronchoconstriction.[45]

During the 1980s, an increase in the number of patients diagnosed with Pneumocystis carinii pneumonia (PCP) due to the acquired immunodeficiency syndrome (AIDS) led to a rekindling of interest in aerosolized antimicrobial agents. In 1986, it was reported that aerosolized pentamidine was found to be effective in preventing PCP in rodents that were immunosuppressed.[46] Subsequent studies in human patient populations were found to be favorable and eventually led to FDA approval for the prophylactic treatment of PCP.[47] Pentamidine, a relatively toxic preparation, is now commonly used in the treatment of this parasitic lung infection. Dosages range from 60 mg for maintenance schedules to 300 to 600 mg for acute infections. Several manufacturers of medication nebulizers have added an expiratory filter to limit the practitioners' exposure to aerosolized pentamadine (Fig. 25-19). Aerosolized pentamidine has been shown to be as effective as intravenous administration without the occurrence of systemic side effects.[46,47] In addition, many patients were reported to develop an intolerance to pentamidine when given via intramuscular injection.[46]

Antiviral Agents

The use of antiviral drugs in aerosol form is currently limited to ribavirin. This synthetic nucleoside analogue re-

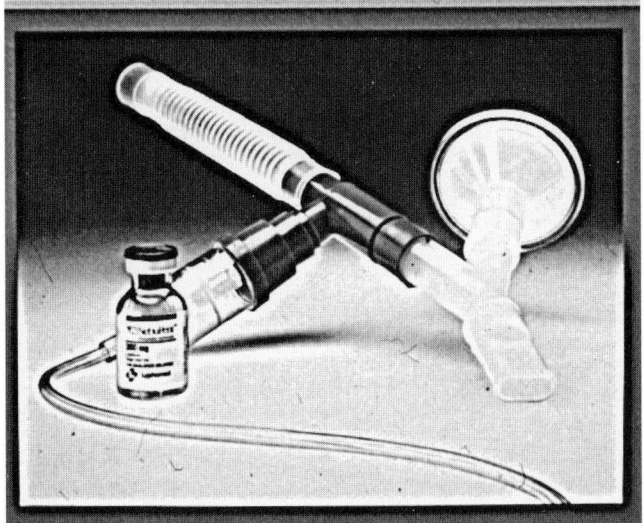

Fig. 25–19. The environmental exposure to pentamidine carries potential risks. In an effort to reduce the exposure of health care workers to aerosolized pentamidine, certain manufacturers have developed medication delivery devices with expiratory filters. This specific type of device generates aerosols with a mass median aerodynamic diameter of approximately 0.90 μg. (Respirgard-II Nebulizer System, courtesy of Marquest Medical Products, Englewood, CO.)

lated to guanosine is used primarily in the treatment of the respiratory syncytial virus (RSV). It is licensed to be administered in aerosol form with a specially designed small particle aerosol generator (SPAG) unit (Fig. 25-20). This particular device produces 95% of its particles with a mean mass diameter of less than 5 μg. Most often, this nebulizer is connected to an infant hood or tent. If used with mechanical ventilation, special precautions must be taken to ensure that the endotracheal tube and/or ventilator circuitry does not become occluded with the precipitated drug.

Bronchopulmonary Hygiene Therapy

Bronchopulmonary hygiene therapy (Bph) consists of a series of therapeutic maneuvers that are specifically designed to enhance secretion clearance thereby decreasing the likelihood of pulmonary complications such as atelectasis, pneumonia, and arterial hypoxemia. These maneuvers may be employed individually or in conjunction with other respiratory therapy modalities which include the following:

- Cough and deep breathing exercises
- Chest percussion and vibration
- Postural drainage techniques

Cough and Deep Breathing Exercises

Cough and deep breathing exercises should be considered standard care for all nonambulatory patients, postoperative patients, and patients with chronic pulmonary disease. When instructing the patient on the proper breathing technique, emphasis should be placed on a slow inspiratory phase with a slight breath hold followed by a vigorous cough. Adequate inspiratory volumes and expiratory flow rates must be achieved in order to mobilize pulmonary secretions.

Chest Percussion and Vibration

Percussion and vibration maneuvers are externally applied manipulations of the chest wall that use kinetic energy to enhance secretion mobilization. Chest percussion is normally performed by tapping the chest wall over specific lung segments in a rhythmic manner while the practitioner's hands are in a "cupped" position. Mechanical devices for chest physiotherapy may be substituted for manual percussion if fatigue or other factors reduce the effectiveness of the practitioner. Chest vibrations are normally applied during the expiratory phase of breathing resulting in a tremorous action which in theory, is transmitted through the lung parenchyma and into the airways.

Postural Drainage Therapy (PDT)

PDT is normally performed by positioning of the patient in such a manner that gravity will assist in mobilizing pulmonary secretions. Each pulmonary segment has a specific position that will allow for secretion clearance under certain conditions. This primarily depends on the anatomic position of the larger airways (or bronchi), secretion volume, and secretion consistency. In theory, pulmonary secretions will migrate into the carina from peripheral bronchi where they can be removed by cough or suctioning. Several of these positions are illustrated in Figure 25-21.

The scientific basis for bronchial hygiene therapy (i.e., postural drainage, chest percussion, and vibration) is

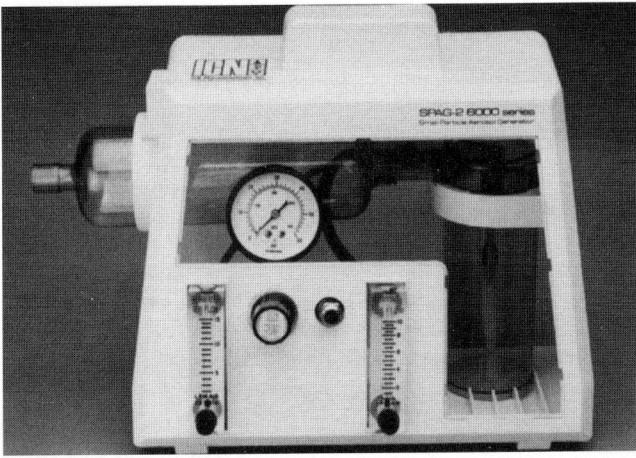

Fig. 25–20. Due to the recent availability of antiviral drugs in aerosol form, specially designed small particle aerosol generators (SPAG) have been designed. The SPAG-2 r produces 95% of its particles at a mean mass diameter of less than 5 μg. Caution during use is necessary to prevent artificial airways and ventilator circuits from becoming occluded with precipitated drug. (Courtesy of ICN Pharmaceuticals, Costa Mesa, CA.)

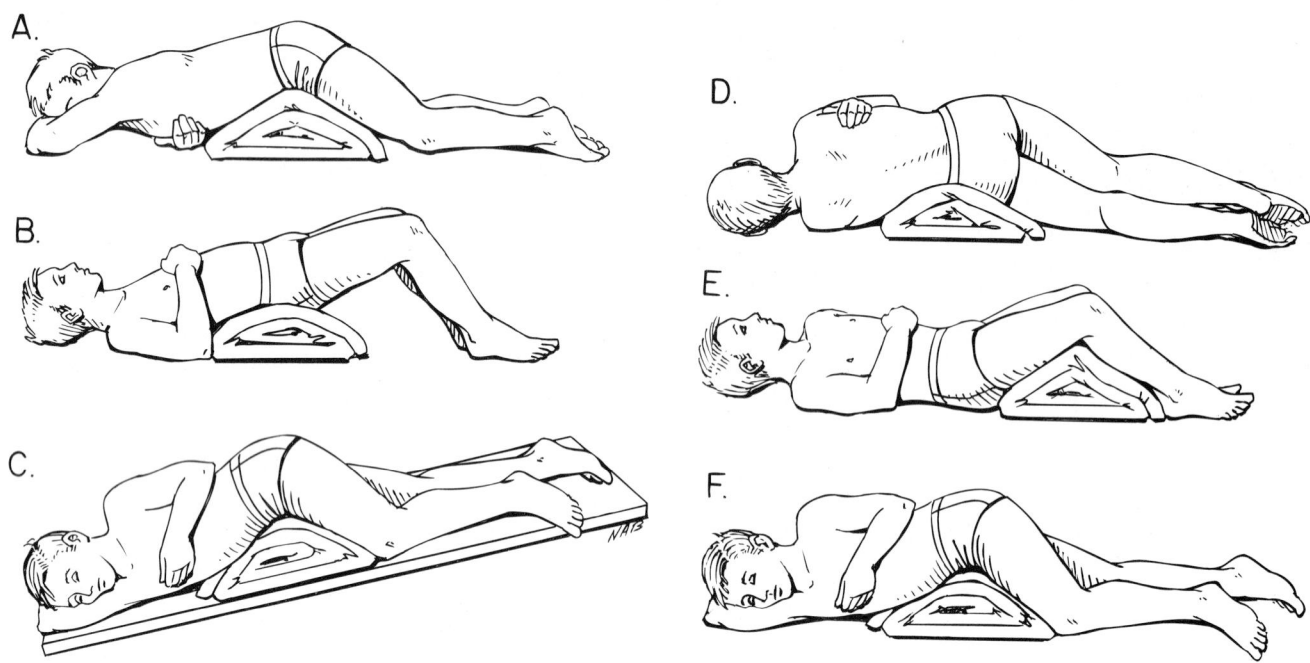

Fig. 25-21. Postural drainage positions are illustrated. *A,* The prone position with a pillow under the lower abdomen is utilized for drainage of the lower lobes. Percussion, if indicated, is done over the lower ribs. *B,* Lying on the back with a pillow under the hips allows for drainage of the anterior portion of the chest. Percussion is done over the lower ribs. *C,* Lying on the right side with a pillow under the lower abdomen allows for drainage of the left lower lobe. Percussion is done over the lower ribs. *D,* Lying on the left side with a pillow under the lower abdomen allows for drainage of the right lower lobe. Percussion is done over the lower ribs. *E,* Lying on the back, slightly turned to one side with a pillow under the knee, allows for drainage of the anterior basal segment of the lower lobe. Percussion is done over the lower ribs. *F,* Lying on the right side with the feet higher than the head and with a pillow between hip bone and bottom ribs allows for drainage of the lingular segment. Percussion is done over the left nipple area.

somewhat controversial.[3,4,6,48-53] The relative lack of standardized studies and control groups has clouded the issue regarding their clinical indications and expected benefits. Despite this fact, it appears that under certain circumstances these maneuvers are of clear therapeutic benefit.[3,12] Figure 25-22 illustrates the use of a symptom-based flow chart which may be used to determine the need for Bph maneuvers. In a published report by Eid and colleagues,[54] these maneuvers were found to be of particular benefit in the following conditions: atelectasis secondary to mucous plugging, after extubation of the newborn, cystic fibrosis, chronic bronchitis, and bronchiectasis. In contrast, little evidence of therapeutic benefit could be determined in cases of viral bronchiolitis, pneumonia, and in the management of low risk postoperative patients.[12] In fact, Torrington and associates found that chest physiotherapy was of no therapeutic value in the prevention of postoperative complications following upper abdominal surgery. Additional findings included increased patient discomfort and increased hospital costs.[55] A comprehensive listing of both the relative and absolute contraindications associated with Bph therapy can be found in Table 25-8.

An intuitive look at the conditions and disease processes where bronchopulmonary hygiene techniques have been found to be of clinical benefit leads us to a more general conclusion regarding their use. It seems quite apparent that these techniques are of therapeutic value in patients who produce moderate to large volumes of sputum.[3,49,50]

With the exception of cough and deep breathing exercises, the use of Bph techniques may actually lead in certain circumstances to the development of pulmonary complications including atelectasis and arterial hypoxemia.[50,51,53] This subject is discussed in further detail in the sections of this chapter on ICU phase of illness and post-ICU recovery.

RESPIRATORY CARE SERVICES IN THE ICU PHASE OF ILLNESS

In most circumstances, patients are admitted to the intensive care setting for closer monitoring and observation, specialized nursing care, and more intensive therapeutic interventions than available on regular nursing units. Patients who require the services of the respiratory care practitioner (RCP) in the ICU are those admitted with a primary or secondary diagnosis of respiratory insufficiency and/or impending respiratory failure. In addition, early recognition and identification of the high risk patient in the ICU setting may ultimately prevent respiratory failure from occurring if an appropriate care plan is implemented. If respiratory failure does occur, efforts should be directed toward reversal of the underlying cause when possible. As both cost concerns and resource constraints become more of an issue prevalent in the ICU, our attention and efforts must be directed towards improving patient outcomes without overusing health care resources. This goal can be accomplished by prompt implementation of appropriate

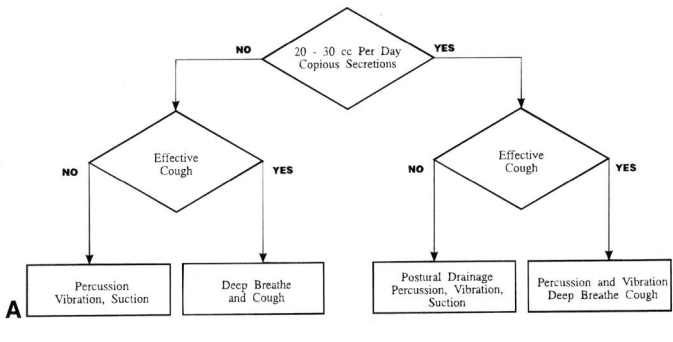

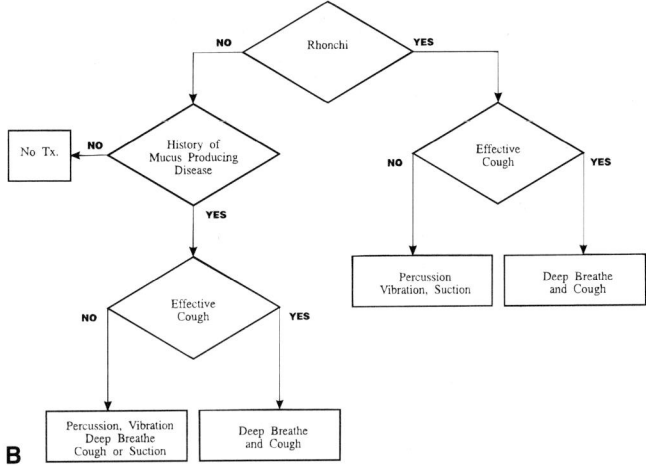

Fig. 25-22. An algorithm used at the Cleveland Clinic Foundation for determining the appropriateness of bronchopulmonary hygiene therapy. *A,* The definition of a productive cough depends on the amount of secretions produced. *B,* The key point of treatment for nonproductive cough depends on a history of mucus-producing disease. (From Stoller, J. K., et al.: Physician-ordered respiratory care vs physician-ordered use of a respiratory therapy consult service: early experience at the Cleveland Clinic Foundation. Respir. Care, *38:*1143, 1993.)

respiratory care plans that would guide the application of various monitoring techniques and therapeutic interventions. In the following section, we closely examine the role of respiratory care modalities and related technology in the management, monitoring, and treatment of high risk critically ill patients.

Monitoring techniques for those patients with clinical signs and symptoms of respiratory insufficiency and/or impending respiratory failure may include the following:

- ABG analysis and hemoximetry
- Hemodynamic monitoring
- Assessment of respiratory mechanics
- Pulse oximetry monitoring
- Capnography

Therapeutic modalities which may be used in the treatment and management of the ICU patient with respiratory dysfunction include interventions that are primarily intended to reduce the work of breathing (WOB), while improving carbon dioxide (CO_2) elimination and arterial oxygenation (Pao_2). These include:

- Oxygen therapy (high and low flow)
- Aerosol/humidity therapy
- Aerosolized pharmacologic agents
- Bronchopulmonary hygiene techniques
- Incentive spirometry
- IPPB
- CPAP
- Mechanical ventilation

To provide consistency and continuity of care for the critically ill patient, it is essential that individualized care plans be constructed including goal-oriented therapeutic objectives. Ideally, these care plans would include:

- The type of monitoring required by the patient, including monitoring criteria
- The appropriate oxygen device or ventilatory support parameters
- Airway care techniques and considerations
- Therapeutic respiratory therapy modalities including type and frequency
- Weaning strategies
- ICU discharge plans

The development of an appropriate respiratory care plan involves a thorough and comprehensive assessment of the patient for indications of each planned intervention. In addition, the clinician must also consider the potential side effects of each modality in terms of the risk/benefit ratio for each patient. Failure to do this may result in the delivery of inappropriate therapy while also subjecting the patient to unnecessary risks. Recent studies suggest that when RCPs evaluate patients for respiratory care modalities following established ICU clinical guidelines and protocols, the number of unnecessary and inappropriate therapies decrease.[5,7,9,54] Often, this results in substantial cost savings to the institution, the patient, and third-party payors. Therefore, the use of RCPs as evaluators for establishing and implementing respiratory care plans may promote better allocation of ICU resources. Table 25-9 summarizes the steps taken and rationale for periodic assessments, observation, and monitoring of the critically ill.

Table 25-8. Relative and Absolute Contraindications for Bph Maneuvers

Bph Maneuver	Relative Contraindication	Absolute Contraindication
All positioning	Intracranial pressure > 20 mm Hg Recent spinal surgery/injury Active hemoptysis Empyema Bronchopleural fistula Pulmonary edema associated with CHF Large pleural effusions Pulmonary embolism Aged, confused, or anxious patients who do not tolerate positioning Rib fractures with or without flail chest Surgical wound or healing tissue	Head and neck injury until stable Hemorrhage with hemodynamic instability
Trendelenburg	Intracranial pressure > 20 mm Hg Patients in whom increased intracranial pressure is to be avoided Uncontrolled hypertension Distended abdomen Esophageal surgery Recent gross hemoptysis related to recent lung carcinoma treated surgically or with radiation Uncontrolled airway at risk for aspiration (tube feeding or recent meal)	
Reverse Trendelenburg	Hypotension or vasoactive medications	
Percussion/vibration	Subcutaneous emphysema Recent epidural spinal infusion or spinal anesthesia Recent skin grafts, or flaps on the thorax Burns, open wounds, and skin infections of the thorax Recently placed transvenous pacemaker or subcutaneous pacemaker (particularly if mechanical devices are to be used) Suspected pulmonary tuberculosis Lung contusion Bronchospasm Osteomyelitis of the ribs Osteoporosis Coagulopathy Complaint of chest-wall pain	

(From AARC clinical practice guidelines. Respir. Care, 36:1402, 1991.)

Monitoring Respiratory Insufficiency

Peripheral Artery Catheterization

As a general rule, peripheral arterial catheters are primarily inserted in the hemodynamically unstable patient for the purpose of continuous monitoring of arterial blood pressure while at the same time providing vascular access for ABGs, hemoximetry, and other laboratory values. For new admissions to the ICU, a principal concern would be to establish the appropriateness of arterial catheterization for blood pressure monitoring. If warranted, routine sampling of arterial blood for analysis could be performed as well. If catheter placement is not indicated for blood pressure monitoring, does the frequency of projected blood sampling or the lack of suitable puncture sites justify the insertion of an arterial line? Recent literature supports the practice of peripheral artery catheter insertion by personnel who are not physicians but have had specialized education and training.[56-58]

When performing arterial cannulation, the radial artery is normally considered the primary site of choice because of its ease of access and the normal presence of adequate collateral circulation via the ulnar artery.[56-58] The existence of adequate collateral circulation minimizes the complications that may occur from thrombus formation or inadequate perfusion. If radial artery cannulation cannot be performed, consideration should be given to other sites including the brachial, femoral, and dorsalis pedal arteries. Femoral artery cannulation may be used when hypotension or other factors preclude the use of other sites. The proximity of the femoral vein and nerve, the potential for hemorrhage and the relative difficulty in care of this site makes it the least desirable, however.[59-61]

Peripheral artery catheterization is certainly not without risk. The occurrence of infection and distal ischemia appear to be the most commonly reported complication.[58-67] Fortunately, with careful attention to both catheter placement and subsequent care of the site, the incidence of these complications can be minimized.[65,66] Several other potential hazards have been associated with indwelling peripheral catheters including:

- Thrombus formation
- Retrograde embolus secondary to prolonged line flush

Table 25-9. Patient Evaluation and Assessment

Perform periodic patient assessments based on acuity level
Identify therapeutic objectives based on clinical findings
Implement goal-oriented patient care plan and evaluate response
Modify care plan in response to acuity or clinical changes

- Impaired circulation distal to catheter site
- Iatrogenic anemia

Smoller and Kruskall[68] reported significant blood loss (mean 944 ml) secondary to diagnostic phlebotomy in a study of 100 patients admitted to a tertiary care institution. These amounts did not include whole blood that was discarded during the sampling procedure or arterial line flushing. Considering the current critical shortage of available blood supplies, it is hoped these findings will prompt close and careful examination of current practices regarding blood sampling techniques and procedures to minimize unnecessary blood loss to the ICU patient.

Some controversy exists regarding the frequency of catheter removal and reinsertion. Based on the findings by Norwood and colleagues,[65] catheter changes are performed every 4 days if an alternative site is readily accessible. In the event an alternative site is unavailable, however, the catheter may remain in place for a longer period if close observation and meticulous care of the site is provided. Conversely, Thomas and associates[59] failed to demonstrate a correlation between duration and occurrence of infection and therefore do not believe that the practice of catheter reinsertion every 4 days is warranted. Rather than attempt to establish routine policies regarding this issue, it would seem prudent to consider each patient individually as to risk of infection, availability of alternative sites, ease of insertion, and projected duration of catheter placement.

ABGs and Hemoximetry

Information obtained from ABG analysis is essential in documenting the necessity for the administration of supplemental oxygen as well as aiding the practitioner in the selection of the appropriate concentration of oxygen. (Devices for the delivery of oxygen therapy, including CPAP, and their specific concentration capabilities have previously been described in the pre-ICU phase.) If arterial hypoxemia is present, it is important to explore the potential causes of this condition as other therapeutic interventions may be indicated in order to treat the underlying pathophysiology. In addition to identifying metabolic disturbances that would affect acid/base balance (i.e., acidemia and alkalemia), monitoring ABGs is useful for assessing the process of oxygenation (comparing the Pa_{O_2} to F_{IO_2} ratio), and the efficiency of ventilation (comparing Pa_{CO_2} to respiratory rate and minute ventilation).

The routine sampling of arterial blood for blood gas analysis is a common occurrence in the ICU setting, particularly in those patients who have indwelling arterial lines. Concerns regarding the "routine" sampling of arterial blood despite the absence of clinical indicators prompted investigation of this practice.[5,69] Thorson and colleagues[69] studied 29 clinically stable patients in the ICU for variation in arterial pH, Pa_{O_2} and Pa_{CO_2} values. Significant variability occurred in Pa_{O_2} values without the need for therapeutic intervention. This situation suggests that transient fluctuations of arterial Pa_{O_2} do occur in the seriously ill, but are often unaccompanied by significant clinical changes. Using Pa_{O_2} values as a sole criterion for clinical decision making may lead to unnecessary changes in patient management. Durbin and co-workers[5] reported an average reduction of 1.85 blood gas samples per patient day after the education of housestaff, nurses, and RCPs regarding the indications and appropriateness of ABG sampling. Significant cost reductions were noted in terms of supplies, personnel, and laboratory costs. Since this report, many institutions have incorporated the surveillance of arterial blood sampling into their quality assurance monitoring programs.

Advances in technology have lead to the development of specialized indwelling catheters that possess the capability to monitor arterial pH, Pa_{CO_2}, and Pa_{O_2} values continuously.[70] Whether these catheters will gain acceptance once introduced and made available on a widespread commercial basis is unclear. The potential advantages of continuous monitoring in unstable patients certainly warrants serious consideration for their use in selected cases, however.

The presence of dysfunctional hemoglobins may impair oxygen transport and produce erroneous pulse oximetry readings. To identify and quantitate carboxyhemoglobin (COHb) and methemoglobin (metHb) accurately, hemoximetry should be considered if abnormally high levels of these species are suspected.

Other methods that aid the practitioner in the monitoring of patients at risk for developing respiratory failure and/or respiratory insufficiency include bedside spirometry, continuous or intermittent pulse oximetry, and capnography.

Hemodynamic Monitoring

Hemodynamic monitoring is a useful tool in assessing the effects of mechanical ventilation and PEEP on cardiac output and oxygen transport. Impairment of oxygen transport occurs in a variety of serious clinical conditions including sepsis, pulmonary edema, myocardial infarction, pulmonary emboli, and ARDS. Serial measurements of cardiac output, intrapulmonary shunt fraction (Q_S/Q_T), arteriovenous oxygen difference (A-V D_{O_2}), and venous oxygen concentration may be helpful in management of mechanically ventilated patients. The accuracy and validity of these parameters in patients with sepsis and ARDS have been questioned. Noninvasive monitoring of patients receiving mechanical ventilation and PEEP therapy appears to be gaining popularity with the development of pulse oximetry and end-tidal CO_2 monitoring devices. Nevertheless, many clinicians continue to insert Swan-Ganz catheters for the assessment of pulmonary artery pressure (PAP), pulmonary capillary wedge pressure (PCWP) and cardiac output in the hemodynamically unstable patient. Careful monitoring of these parameters is particularly useful if high levels of PEEP (> 10 cm H_2O) are anticipated for the treatment of refractory hypoxemia.[73-76]

Bedside Spirometry

Serial measurements of tidal volume, vital capacity, expiratory flow rates, respiratory rate, and negative inspiratory force can provide valuable information when evaluating ventilatory function. Monitoring trends in respiratory mechanics may indicate the need to alter patient management or possibly to support ventilation. One must understand, however, that the accuracy and validity of such measurements depends largely on the level of effort, coordination, and cooperation displayed by the patient. Despite this limitation, serious consideration should be given to the potential development of respiratory insufficiency if the patient meets two or more of the following criteria:

- Tidal volume < 7 ml/kg ideal body weight
- Vital capacity < 15 ml/kg ideal body weight
- Respiratory rare > 30 breaths per minute
- Negative inspiratory force (NIF) < 20 cm H_2O
- Peak expiratory flow rate (PEFR) < 150 LPM
- Forced expiratory volume/forced vital capacity ratio (FEV_1) of < 75%

The various types of bedside spirometry devices have previously been described in the pre-ICU section of this chapter. In addition to these portable spirometers, there currently exists noninvasive continuous monitoring systems (respiratory inductive plethysmography) that can document respiratory rate, apneas, and hypopneas.[77] These systems use belts placed around the abdomen and chest which electronically sense deflection signals from the patient. In turn, these signals are transformed into visual patterns and recorded. As with all direct measuring systems, the limitations and accuracy of the device must be fully understood before its data can be considered useful clinical information.

Pulse Oximetry Technology

Since its commercial availability in the 1970s, pulse oximetry technology has rapidly gained popularity as a noninvasive monitoring tool in a wide variety of clinical environments including the operating room, PACU, and the ICU. This technology provides the clinician with an estimate of arterial oxyhemoglobin saturation (SaO_2) by incorporating specific wavelengths of light through a capillary bed to determine the oxyhemoglobin saturation (SpO_2).[22,23] Unfortunately, pulse oximetry technology possesses certain inherent limitations. Reports of both false-negative results and false-positive results in hypoxemia, normoxemia, and hyperoxemia may lead to incorrect management decisions.[12,25-27,78,80] Table 25-10 summarizes the various factors and conditions that may affect the accuracy and performance of pulse oximetry technology.

The use of continuous pulse oximetry in the ICU is indicated for those patients who exhibit, or who are at risk for developing arterial oxyhemoglobin desaturation. Jurban and colleagues[79] reported that of 25 hospital ICUs

Table 25–10. Factors and Conditions Affecting the Accuracy of Pulse Oximetry

Dysfunctional hemoglobins (COHb) and (metHb)
Severe anemia and fetal hemoglobin
Ambient light interference (infrared and fluorescent)
Hypoperfusion conditions and venous pulsation
Venous pulsation
Skin pigmentation
Motion artifact
Intravascular dyes (indocyanine, indigo carmine, and methylene blue)
Arterial saturations < 85%
Peripheral edema at the sensor site
Optical shunting
Optical cross-talk (placement of two sensors in close proximity)
Nail polish (particularly green, black, blue, and reddish brown)

Table 25–11. Indications for Pulse Oximetry Monitoring of the High Risk Patient

FIO_2/PEEP titration	Intraoperative period
Endotracheal intubation	Postoperative period
Bronchoscopy	Asymmetric pulmonary disease
Endoscopic procedures	Hemodynamic instability
Central line insertion	Refractory hypoxemia
Transport	Hemodialysis
Diagnostic procedures outside the ICU	

surveyed, 88% used pulse oximetry during FIO_2 titration of patients requiring mechanical ventilation. Despite this high use of pulse oximetry, ABGs were performed frequently in order to verify adequate arterial oxygenation. The survey also reported a lack of consensus regarding the appropriate SpO_2 criterion for FIO_2 titration with responses ranging from 85 to 95%.

Careful consideration of the possible use of pulse oximetry monitoring should also be given to the patient who requires therapeutic and diagnostic interventions that may affect arterial oxygenation (Table 25-11). It is essential, however, that before the clinician can use pulse oximetry with a high degree of confidence, that a positive correlation should be established between arterial saturation (SaO_2) and the pulse oximeter measurement (SpO_2). This correlation must be reevaluated periodically as changes occur in the patient's clinical status. In most circumstances, hemoglobin saturation values are calculated from ABG values and are therefore affected by several factors including pH, body temperature, PaO_2, and 2,3-DPG levels.

Pulse oximetry accuracy and reliability is often adversely affected in the ICU patient, particularly in the presence of hypovolemia, hypotension, vasoconstrictor infusions, and hypothermia.[12,26,27,80,81] Clayton and co-workers[80] recently evaluated the performance of 20 pulse oximeters in 120 patients with poor peripheral perfusion who had undergone cardiopulmonary bypass with hypothermia. Their comparative study demonstrated significant variability regarding pulse oximeter performance under conditions of poor perfusion. Only 2 oximeter units consistently fell within 4% of the 95% confidence limits as referenced to the co-oximeter reading. Therefore, careful consideration and evaluation must be made when making decisions regarding the purchase of pulse oximeter units.

Capnography

Noninvasive monitoring of end-tidal CO_2 ($ETCO_2$) provides for rapid real-time assessment of ventilation. End-tidal CO_2 monitoring often incorporates a numerical display and corresponding wave form. The characteristics of a normal capnogram are displayed in Figure 25-23. As with all monitoring techniques, for $ETCO_2$ monitoring to be successful, its use must receive cooperation from all members of the critical care team.[81] The inconsistent and sporadic recording of values offer little if any clinical benefit. Continuing inservice programs which include recognition and interpretation of waveform abnormalities are quite beneficial.

Under normal circumstances, a 2- to 6-mm Hg difference or gradient exists between arterial $PaCO_2$ and the $ETCO_2$

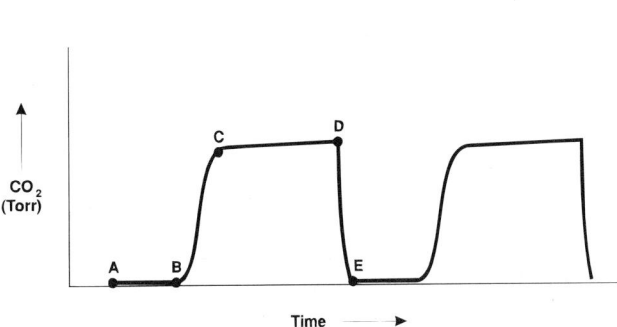

Fig. 25–23. A normal capnogram is illustrated. The various components of the waveform represent different events during exhalation. A is the beginning of expiration; B to C is the expiratory upstroke or ascending limb (CO_2 increases as alveolar gas appears); C to D is the alveolar plateau; D is the end-tidal (peak expired concentration); D to E is the inspiratory downstroke or descending limb (non-CO_2 gas begins to replace alveolar gas). (See Chap. 78 for further description of the abnormal capnograph.) (Waveform from Criticare Systems, Waukesha, WI.)

value.[82–84] During anesthesia and/or mechanical ventilation, this gradient may be expected to increase to approximately 5 to 10 mm Hg. Once the clinician has determined a stable $Paco_2$-$ETco_2$ gradient, then end-tidal monitoring may be used to estimate arterial carbon dioxide levels. One must consider that clinical conditions such as hypovolemia, hypotension, and pulmonary embolism may alter this relationship.[85–88] Therefore, periodic measurements of $Paco_2$ and $ETco_2$ are necessary to assess the effect of cardiorespiratory function on this gradient correctly. End-tidal monitoring may be of particular benefit during weaning trials in the hemodynamically stable patient and in the detection of equipment malfunction or disconnect.[88,89] Unfortunately, most software designs limit the range of end-tidal monitoring to a maximum value of 99 mm Hg. This limitation may be of particular concern in the pediatric patient population. It remains uncertain, however, if $ETco_2$ monitoring will become a standard of practice in the monitoring of the high risk patient. As with all monitoring technique, one must carefully consider the potential benefit versus the additional cost and operational expense associated with this technology (see Chap. 77).

Before discussing the more common therapeutic modalities used in the treatment of the ICU patient, it is important to recognize that technology should not be considered a replacement for the well trained and highly skilled observer at the bedside. Rather, technology should be used to assist the practitioner in quantitating or qualifying what they believe to be occurring based on their clinical observations and physical assessment.

Common Respiratory Therapy Modalities Used in the Treatment of the Critically Ill

Aerosol and Humidity Therapy

If the presence of copious or thick secretions is observed or suspected, then specific techniques to facilitate secretion mobilization should be implemented. Controversy exists as to the efficacy of the use of bland aerosols for thinning retained secretions.[3,12,45] This issue was discussed in the pre-ICU phase of this chapter. In the ICU, however, where frequent assessment of the patient occurs, a bland aerosol (either continuously or as a 20- to 30-minute treatment before bph therapy) may be given a therapeutic trial. If after careful observation and assessment, it appears that secretions are less tenacious and more easily expectorated or evacuated by tracheal suctioning, then it seems reasonable to continue therapy. Proper documentation for improvement in secretion mobilization sufficient to warrant the continuation of therapy would include the approximate volume of secretions expectorated or suctioned along with a description of its consistency and color.

Patients with artificial airways whose anatomic heating and humidification structures have been bypassed and that demonstrate the presence of secretions should have heated humidity administered to their airway.[90] Failure to provide adequate water content to the airway may result in obstruction of the tube or severe mucous plugging of the peripheral airways. Scientific evidence indicates that prolonged periods of inadequate hydration may lead to malfunction of the mucociliary transport mechanisms.[3,12,45]

Humidity, in the form of molecular water vapor, is not associated with causing an increase in airway resistance (Raw) as are aerosols. In addition, certain humidification devices are less likely to transmit bacteria than aerosol generators.[12] Caution must be exercised, however, to prevent contamination when using high flow systems with either heated humidifiers or aerosol generators when connected to patients with an artificial airway. There currently exists a lack of definitive studies documenting infection and contamination risks associated with respiratory therapy equipment in the ICU patient population. Therefore, it is recommended that each ICU establish infection control procedures including surveillance measures to ensure that the frequency of equipment changes is sufficient to prevent nosocomial infection.[12,90,91]

If conventional humidity and bland aerosol therapy prove ineffective in mobilizing retained secretions, then consideration should be given to a therapeutic trial of a mucolytic agent such as N-acetylcysteine. This particular agent can be directly instilled into the artificial airway or given via aerosol, even though little scientific evidence exists to substantiate the efficacy of these particular methods of administration.[42,92,93] As in the case of bland aerosols, a short trial of aerosolized mucolytic therapy may be warranted followed by a careful assessment and evaluation of the patient's response to therapy. A more detailed analysis of mucolytic therapy will follow in the discussion of the post-ICU management of patients diagnosed with chronic obstructive lung disease.

Bronchopulmonary Hygiene Therapy

In addition to liquifying secretions, it may be beneficial to employ bronchopulmonary hygiene techniques to aid in their mobilization and subsequent removal. These techniques include postural drainage, chest percussion, vibration, and deep breathing exercises. The indications, contraindications, and hazards associated with these techniques have been previously described in the pre-ICU phase. The primary indications for the application of these procedures in the ICU patient include the presence of copious secretions in excess of 25 to 30 ml per day, those with an ineffective cough, and those with a history of a secretion producing disease such as cystic fibrosis, bronchiectasis, and chronic bronchitis.[12] The effectiveness of such techniques should be well documented by recording sputum production, the effect on breath sounds, pulmonary function, gas exchange, and overall increase or decrease in symptoms. It is recommended that postural drainage with or without percussion and vibration not be performed on critically ill patients without proper indications and reasonable expectation of benefit. Placing these patients in the Trendelenburg position can cause ventilation to perfusion (V/Q) mismatching resulting in hypoxemia, hypercapnia, and acute increases in intracranial pressure (ICP).[51-53] Connors and associates[53] reported a significant drop in arterial Pao_2 values following postural drainage (PDT) and chest percussion in 22 nonsurgical patients with a variety of pulmonary disorders who produced little or no sputum. This observation of post-therapy arterial desaturation has also been reported by other investigators.[51] Therefore, the decision to use PDT in the ICU should be based on a careful analysis of the potential risk or benefit to the patient.

Therapeutic Bronchoscopy

If airway patency and secretion clearance cannot be achieved by noninvasive methods, then nasotracheal suctioning or therapeutic bronchoscopy may be considered. Care must be taken to provide adequate oxygenation and ventilation during these procedures to avoid hypoxemia, cardiac arrhythmias, or atelectasis. Therapeutic bronchoscopy for secretion removal of foreign body obstruction can also be accomplished safely in the ICU setting where close monitoring and emergency support systems are readily available should complications arise. Patients who require mechanical ventilation can also undergo a diagnostic or therapeutic bronchoscopy if necessary. During the procedure, the Fio_2 should be increased to 100% and if large tidal volume losses are observed, appropriate alterations in inspiratory flow settings and minute ventilation should be made.

Aerosolized Pharmacologic Agents

Many patients admitted to the ICU require the administration of various pharmacologic agents including beta-adrenergic agents, anticholinergics, mucolytics, and anti-inflammatory agents. The indications, dosages, and potential side effects of these particular drug classifications were previously outlined in the pre-ICU phase discussion on aerosol therapy. In addition, the clinical application of these agents will be further discussed in the post-ICU phase regarding the management of COPD.

Of particular relevance to the ICU phase of illness, is the increasing popularity and use of MDIs for the mechanically ventilated patient population. Significant reductions in costs, both in terms of personnel and supplies, have been reported when nebulized bronchodilators have been substituted by MDI therapy in nonintubated hospitalized patients.[8] These findings have spawned recent investigation to determine if MDI therapy may be considered a viable alternative to conventional SVM therapy in intubated, mechanically ventilated patients with clinical evidence of reversible airways obstruction. For example, Gay and colleagues[94] reported equivalent responses to albuterol for both methods of delivery (3 puffs 270 μg versus 2.5 mg nebulized) in a series of 18 ventilator-dependent patients. Despite these preliminary findings, the appropriate dosage and optimal delivery method for the administration of MDI therapy in mechanically ventilated patients remains the subject of much discussion and controversy.

It also remains unclear whether anticholinergics (Atrovent) and anti-inflammatory drugs (Azmacort, Aerobid) can also be effectively administered via MDI in this setting. In the meantime, continued clinical investigation and research are needed in order to determine the appropriate dosage (i.e., number of puffs) and other variables including ventilatory settings, placement of the MDI, and time of actuation of the device with regards to the inspiratory and expiratory cycle.[95]

Of equal interest and importance is the use of SVN in the delivery of therapeutic aerosols to the mechanically ventilated patient. The most commonly used technique in clinical practice at this time appears to be continuous nebulization with placement of the nebulizer proximal to the endotracheal tube.[96] Despite its routine use, several potential problems have been observed with SVNs in this patient population and are summarized in Table 25-12. A report by Hughes and Saez[96] described the effect of nebulizer position and mode (continuous versus intermittent) on the quantity of aerosol theoretically delivered to an intubated patient. Placement of the nebulizer at the ventilator circuit manifold with operation only during inspiration resulted in the greatest delivery of aerosol. Conversely, the lowest quantity of aerosol was delivered during continuous operation with the nebulizer proximal to the endotracheal tube. One may assume that placement of the SVN at the manifold (distal to the patient) allowed for the inspiratory tubing to act as a reservoir for holding the aerosol in suspension. During delivery of the ventilator breath, the suspended aerosol is administered through the endotracheal tube and into the airways. This procedure was of course only a hypothetic model but certainly warrants further clinical investigation.

Mechanical ventilation of the patient with persistent and significant airflow obstruction poses a serious challenge to the clinician. Elevation of peak airway pressures, air trapping, hyperinflation, and the development of "intrinsic PEEP" are serious consequences of severe airflow obstruction. If this condition worsens or is irreversible, the development of tension pneumothorax, pulmonary barotrauma, or cardiovascular compromise may result in impaired oxygen transport. It is hoped that additional re-

Table 25–12. Potential Problems Associated With SVN in the Mechanically Ventilated Patient

Potential source of bacterial contamination
Potential source of unrecognized leak with resultant loss of tidal volume (VT)
Increases in VT and peak airway pressure during therapy
Potential interference with ventilator sensitivity to patient inspiratory effort

search on this subject will provide further insight into the effective use of therapeutic aerosols via both MDI and SVN in the treatment of airflow obstruction in this patient population.

Techniques for the Prevention and Treatment of Atelectasis

When persistent atelectasis is caused by pleural effusions, spontaneous pneumothorax, elevated diaphragms or other contributing factors, attempts should be made to treat the underlying conditions along with implementing therapy to reexpand the affected area of the lung. If aggressive incentive spirometry and bronchopulmonary hygiene techniques prove unsuccessful, then one should consider alternative forms of therapy.

IPPB has limited application in the prevention and treatment of pulmonary complications.[3,12] One should consider a therapeutic trial for the patient with persistent atelectasis, however, when conventional methods have failed. This situation is particularly true for those patients who have poor inspiratory volumes (less than 75% of their predicted minimal vital capacity), secondary to diaphragmatic dysfunction, respiratory muscle fatigue, or pulmonary disease. For proper administration, IPPB therapy should be volume oriented rather than pressure oriented. Exhaled volumes should be measured and reach at least 75% of the patient's predicted minimal vital capacity to be of therapeutic benefit.

Another therapeutic option for the treatment and prevention of atelectasis is CPAP. CPAP may be administered as a series of treatments by mask or be delivered continuously by mask, endotracheal tube, or tracheostomy tube (Fig. 25-24). The therapeutic benefit of this form of therapy is achieved primarily by its ability to increase intrapulmonary pressures thereby increasing FRC.[36] The indications, contraindications, and complications associated with CPAP therapy are listed in Table 25-13. Currently, the majority of CPAP therapy is administered in the ICU setting. As patient acuity continues to increase in the acute care hospital and as the availability of ICU beds becomes limited, however, it appears likely that CPAP therapy will be encountered more frequently on routine nursing floors.

Table 25-13. Continuous Positive Airway Pressure (CPAP)

Indications
   Prevention and treatment of alveolar collapse (atelectasis)
   Interstitial pulmonary edema
   Refractory hypoxemia
   Obstructive sleep apnea
Contraindications
   Acute respiratory failure
   Bullous disease
   Untreated pneumothorax
   Hemodynamic instability
Hazards
   Increase in the work of breathing
   Pulmonary hyperinflation
      (increase deadspace to tidal volume ratio)
                    OR
      (increase in intrapulmonary shunt fraction)
   Pulmonary barotrauma
   Cardiovascular compromise
   Aspiration of gastric contents (Mask CPAP therapy)

Respiratory Therapy Techniques in the Management of the Critically Ill

Airway Management

Complications associated with endotracheal intubation and tracheostomy have been well documented and reported in several excellent reviews on the subject.[97-100] A summary of many of these complications appears in Table 25-14. Potential complications associated with artificial airways may be avoided or minimized by early recognition and detection. For example, in situations where persistent coughing and "fighting the ventilator" occur and the presence of unexplained high ventilating pressures are noted, the following possibilities should be explored:

- Airway obstruction by blood, mucous, or foreign material
- Endobronchial intubation
- Kinked or inappropriately positioned airway
- Esophageal intubation
- Cuff overinflation and herniation
- Ventilator malfunction

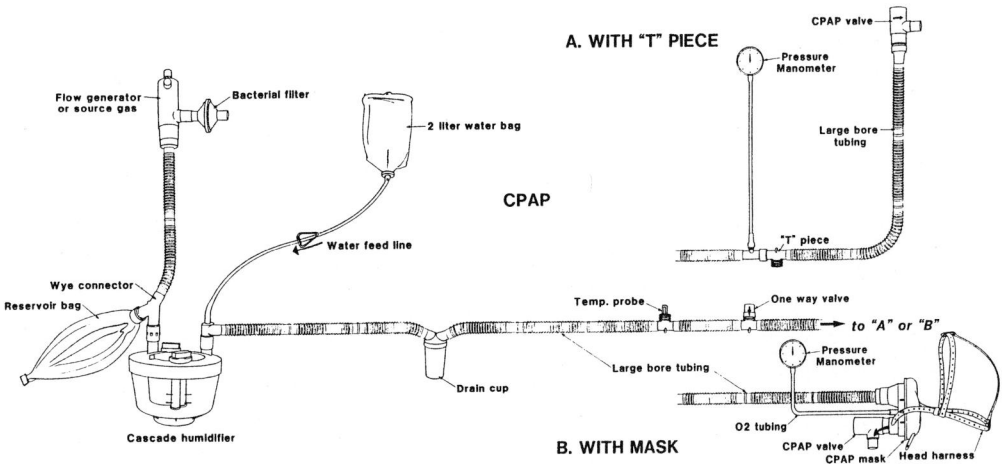

Fig. 25-24. CPAP may be administered as a series of treatments by mask or continuously by mask, endotracheal tube, or tracheostomy tube. A high flow CPCP system for connection to a standard 15-mm outer diameter airway and a mask (B) are illustrated.

Table 25-14. Complications of Tracheal Intubation

Intubation Procedure	While Intubated	Post Intubation
Epistaxis	Erosion or rupture of the trachea	Sore throat, dysphagia
Tooth trauma	Subcutaneous emphysema	Paresis or paralysis of vocal cords or tongue
Retropharyngeal, hypopharyngeal perforation	Pneumothorax	Ulceration of lips, mouth, pharynx, larynx
Subcutaneous mediastinal emphysema	Tracheal bleeding	Laryngitis, sinusitis
Laceration of pharynx or larynx	Aspiration	Laryngitis, edema granulomas, or polyps
Arytenoid dislocation	Respiratory tract infection	Laryngeotracheal membranes, webs
Aspiration	Laryngeal edema, necrosis	Tracheal stenosis
Esophageal intubation	Tracheal dilation	Tracheomalacia
Bronchial intubation	Tracheoesophageal fistula	
Laryngeal spasm		
Cardiac arrhythmias		
Arterial hypotension		

Of critical importance in the management of the high risk patient is the monitoring of intracuff pressures. Despite the widespread use of low-pressure "soft" cuffed endotracheal and tracheostomy tubes, tracheal injury still persists.[97-101] Often, this complication is the result of cuff overinflation. The practice of intermittent cuff deflation for other than clearing retained secretions at the cuff site appears not to affect the incidence or severity of tracheal wall injury. Significant increases in both intracuff and tracheal wall pressures have been observed in low pressure "soft" cuffed airways after minimal increases in cuff volume of 1 to 2 ml beyond the minimal occluding volume (MOV).[98,101] Therefore, the routine monitoring of MOV and documentation of intracuff pressure appears warranted when using cuffed airways. The anatomic complications associated with excessive intracuff pressures (> 20 mm Hg) are summarized in Figure 25-25. In addition to excessive cuff pressure, impaired oxygen transport and nutrition deficiencies may further aggravate tracheal wall injury in the severely ill patient.[98-101]

Compared to high pressure "hard" cuffs, low pressure type airways have been shown to exert substantially less tracheal wall pressure when properly used.[98-101] Table 25-15 lists commonly used tracheostomy tubes that are currently available with a low pressure cuff design. Meticulous care should be taken to ensure that the lowest intracuff pressure and volume are maintained at all times. In addition to monitoring these two parameters, particular attention should be given to the oxygen and ventilatory tubing apparatus attached to the airway. Excessive motion and torque created by poorly positioned equipment may further promote tracheal and stomal injury including the potential for accidental extubation and decannulation.

Tracheobronchial aspiration, when indicated by the presence of retained secretions, should be performed under sterile conditions in an attempt to minimize the potential for infection. Care must be taken to avoid unnecessary aspiration procedures as repeated passage of the catheter into the airway may cause injury to the respiratory epithelium. Proper hyperinflation and oxygenation during the procedure can reduce the potential complications associated with tracheobronchial suctioning including hypoxemia, atelectasis, and cardiac arrhythmias.[100-103] In addition, the use of inappropriately high aspiration pressures and poorly designed catheters may also contribute to tracheal injury.[101,103]

Endotracheal Intubation

In emergency situations, when it is imperative that an endotracheal tube be immediately inserted, the oral route

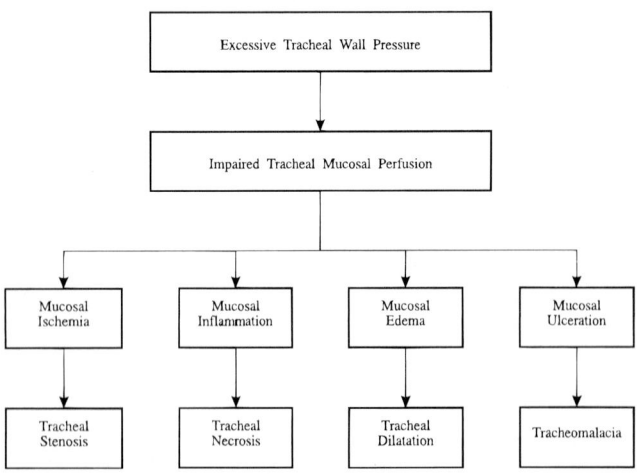

Fig. 25-25. The anatomic complications of excessive cuff pressure begin with abnormally high tracheal wall pressures. When tracheal wall pressure exceeds mucosal capillary perfusion pressure, mucosal ischemia, inflammation, edema, and ulceration result. Delayed consequences include tracheal necrosis and dilatation and the more severe problems of tracheal stenosis and tracheomalacia. (Adapted from references 98 and 100.)

Table 25-15. Low Pressure Design Cuffed Tracheostomy Tubes

Type of Tube	Use	Type of Cuff
Shiley	Mechanical ventilation	High volume
	Maintain a patent airway	Low pressure
Fenestrated Shiley	Facilitate speech	High volume
	Mechanical ventilation	Low pressure
Lantz	Mechanical ventilation	High volume Pressure regulated
Bivona	Prolonged ventilation	Foam cuff
	Prevent aspiration	Self-fill
Rusch	Adjustable length and cuff position	High volume Low pressure

is preferred in most instances. In more controlled non-emergent conditions, passage of the airway through the nares may be a more suitable alternative. Nasal tubes are considered more stable than oral tubes and are believed to cause less trauma to the vocal cords due to reduced movement of the airway.[98] Depending on the configuration of the patient's nasal anatomy, however, passage of an acceptable diameter tube via this route may be difficult. Recent literature on the subject of endotracheal intubation contains several reports which clearly demonstrate that specially trained nonphysician personnel (i.e., nursing and respiratory care practitioners) can also perform this procedure with a high degree of skill and manual dexterity.[104-107]

Under most circumstances, the internal diameter (ID) of a nasal airway will be approximately half to one size smaller than the oral route. In general, the largest size airway that can safely be inserted should be used to minimize airway resistance and maximize access to retained secretions. The use of small diameter tubes may significantly increase both RAW and ventilating pressures.[108,109] This condition can impose an increase in WOB for patients in spontaneous modes or during weaning trials.[109,110,114,115]

Mechanical Ventilation

Current advances in medical technology offer the clinician a wide variety of highly sophisticated, complex and expensive mechanical ventilators.[111] Most modern critical care units use volume cycled or volume controlled microprocessor ventilators which provide for accurate and consistent volume delivery. In addition, these "newer generation" mechanical ventilators (Fig. 25-26) offer a wide range of modes, computer-interfaced monitoring capabilities, and clinical data collection. In lower acuity institutions where the availability and choice of ventilators may be limited, however, alternatives to expensive microprocessor technology may be considered without adversely affecting patient outcomes. In instances when respiratory failure is a result of central nervous system dysfunction, drug overdose, or other conditions not affecting pulmonary compliance, patients may be effectively ventilated with a less sophisticated volume or a pressure cycled ventilator. It remains unclear if the "newer generation" technology will improve patient outcomes or reduce morbidity and mortality in patients with acute respiratory failure. The issue of "technology in search of application" continues to be the subject of much discussion and debate.[109,111]

The multiplicity and complexity of these newer modes and features plus the rapidity with which they are modified mandates continuing inservice education for all personnel responsible for their operation.[111] Respiratory care practitioners can be invaluable not only in the initiation and monitoring of these modes and features, but also in the education of new and existing staff as to their appropriate use, complications, and hazards. In the following section, we will provide a brief technical description and discussion of the more common modes of ventilation currently available.

Modes of Mechanical Ventilation

Control. In this mode of ventilation, inspiration is initiated automatically at a rate predetermined by the clinician

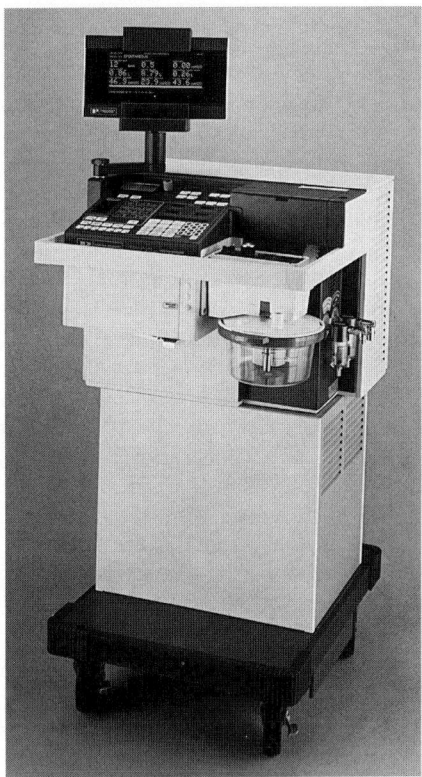

Fig. 25-26. Newer generation mechanical ventilators offer various modes of ventilation and computer-interfaced monitoring capabilities for data collections because microprocessors control their mechanical operations. The Puritan-Bennett 7200 Series Microprocessor Ventilator is shown. (Courtesy of Puritan-Bennett Corp., Carlsbad, CA.)

which results in the delivery of a specific minute ventilation regardless of patient effort. This situation may be very anxiety producing for those patients who are awake, alert, and/or capable of spontaneous breathing. In order to reduce patient anxiety and minimize the potential for poorly synchronized ventilation, these patients should be sedated and carefully monitored. Perhaps a better option would be to select the assist/control or SIMV mode with an appropriate level of sedation if necessary. In fact, several of the newer generation ventilators have eliminated the control mode entirely.

Assist. This particular mode of ventilation delivers a predetermined tidal volume (volume ventilators) in response to the inspiratory effort of the patient. In the event the patient becomes apneic or is unable to initiate inspiration, however, ventilation will cease. For obvious reasons, this mode is outdated and is unavailable on current mechanical ventilators.

Assist/Control. In assist/control ventilation, inspiration can be initiated by either a spontaneous breath or in case of apnea, automatically at a rate determined by the clinician. This particular mode invites the potential for producing hypocapnia and respiratory alkalosis should the patient develop tachypnea in response to pain, anxiety, fever, etc. If tachypnea persists and the patient demonstrates evidence of bronchospasm, the clinician must be alerted to the possible development of pulmonary hyperinflation, intrinsic PEEP, and/or cardiovascular compromise. Assist/control ventilation may be considered, however, in clinical situations for temporary correction of metabolic acidosis and in the management of acute respiratory failure. Crucial to the success of this mode of ventilation is the appropriate setting of inspiratory flowrate. Failure to provide adequate inspiratory flows may significantly increase the patient's WOB.[112] Active inspiration by the patient has been observed throughout the entire inspiratory phase of ventilation in situations where inappropriate flow rates have been provided. In addition, several investigators have reported clinically significant differences in the amount of patient effort (sensitivity) required to initiate inspiration in the assist/control mode.[109,113] This situation may further impose an additional load on the WOB which in the critically ill patient can be of serious consequence.[112,114,115] Therefore, careful consideration should be given regarding the purchase and subsequent use of mechanical ventilators for all patient populations.

IMV/SIMV. Intermittent mandatory ventilation (IMV) allows for unassisted spontaneous breathing in conjunction with mandatory positive pressure breaths determined at a rate selected by the clinician. Table 25-16 summarizes the putative advantages and potential disadvantages associated with this mode of ventilation. Synchronized IMV is essentially the same as IMV, however with SIMV, the ventilator "pauses" before each breath for a brief period to allow the patient the opportunity to initiate the positive pressure breath. If a spontaneous breath is not sensed by the ventilator, a mandatory positive pressure breath is subsequently delivered. SIMV may avoid the "stacking" of spontaneous and mechanically supported breaths that have been reported to occur in the time-cycled IMV mode of ventilation. Although investigators have reported a statistical increase in both mean and peak airway pressure with IMV as compared to SIMV, this difference is rarely of clinical significance.[109] Conversely, reports by Christopher, Gibney, and Kacmarek revealed significant increases in the WOB with various SIMV systems that could be of particular importance in the critically ill or difficult to wean patient.[114,115]

All of the newer generation microprocessor ventilators now incorporate the SIMV mode despite previous concerns of its efficacy, WOB requirements and additional expense.[111] The introduction of more sophisticated technology and improvements in circuit design have resolved several of the early issues concerning the WOB making SIMV one of the more popular modes of ventilation.[110]

Either IMV or SIMV may be used for weaning by gradual reduction of mandatory breaths over time, depending on patient tolerance of independent spontaneous ventilation. In addition to weaning, either mode can be employed as a method of ventilation in the management of patients diagnosed with acute respiratory failure (ARF).

Pressure Control. In this mode of ventilation, the maximum pressure used to deliver a breath is preset on the ventilator along with inspiratory time and flow rate. This preset pressure will not be exceeded during the inspiratory phase, however, it does not end inspiration. Rather, the inspiratory time setting will determine the point at which inspiration is terminated. In this case, tidal volume delivery will be the function of pressure, time and flow rate and may vary from breath to breath depending on resistance and compliance changes. Pressure control may allow for ventilation of patients with decreased lung compliance without the use of exceedingly high peak pressures. Mean airway pressures may or may not be lower, as compared to conventional volume controlled ventilation depending on individual patient characteristics.

Mandatory Minute Ventilation. MMV is a mode employed for weaning patients from the ventilator. It allows for a preset minute volume to be established that will be accomplished in part by the ventilator and in part by the patient. If at any time, patient contribution falls below what is necessary to maintain the preset minute volume, the ventilator will make up the additional volume required by either increasing the rate or the volume delivered. The mechanism by which this is accomplished varies from ventilator to ventilator. Caution must be exercised if the patient develops tachypnea in addition to low spontaneous volumes in this mode. Under these circumstances, the preset minute ventilation may be achieved, but with a higher deadspace to total volume ratio and increase in the WOB.

Continuous Positive Airway Pressure. CPAP as named on most current generation ventilators is a misnomer in that when this mode is employed, it allows for independent spontaneous breathing only. Depending on the type of ventilator used, the patient may breathe either through a demand valve or receive a continuous flow of gas with or without a predetermined positive pressure level as selected by the clinician. This mode may be used during the weaning process, or may be used to improve oxygenation in patients that exhibit ventilation perfusion abnormalities resulting in hypoxemia and/or atelectasis. In this latter instance, when it is evident that the patient will not require ventilatory support, consideration should be given to a less expensive means of providing CPAP (i.e., a continuous high flow system).

Features of Mechanical Ventilators

Multiple Flow Patterns

The flow patterns available on current commercially available ventilators include:

Table 25-16. Advantages and Disadvantages of IMV/SIMV Ventilation

Advantages
 Decreased need for sedation
 Lower mean airway pressure
 Prevention of atrophy of ventilatory muscles
 Reduction of cardiovascular compromise
 Avoidance of respiratory alkalosis
Disadvantages
 Increased risk of hypercapnia
 Increased work of breathing
 Respiratory muscle fatigue
 Prolonged weaning times

Table 25–17. Effect of Inspiratory Flow Patterns on Airway Pressures Inspiratory Time and Inspiratory:Expiratory Ratio

Flow Pattern	Peak Airway Pressure	Mean Airway Pressure	Inspiratory Time	I:E Ratio
Accelerating	↑	↓	↓	↓
Constant (square wave)	↑	↓	↓	↓
Decelerating	↓	↑	↑	↑
Sinusoidal	↓	↑	↑	↑

- Square wave flow patterns
- Decelerating flow patterns
- Accelerating flow patterns
- Sinusoidal flow patterns

Preliminary studies have failed to demonstrate that flow distribution is influenced by alterations in inspiratory flow patterns.[117] Evidence indicates that peak airway pressure and inspiratory time may indeed, however, be affected by variation in flow patterns. The theoretical effect of various inspiratory flow patterns on these parameters is listed in Table 25–17. The flow pattern chosen will depend on how it alters these parameters and how these alterations influence the patient's ventilation (i.e., gas exchange, airway pressures, etc.). Unfortunately, little clinical evidence exists to support the use of one flow pattern over another. Rather, choice of inspiratory flow pattern appears to be based on clinician preference and anecdotal observations.

Pressure Support

Pressure support refers to the addition of a preset amount of pressure to the inspiratory phase of a spontaneous breath. Depending on the ventilator being used, this pressure will be ended by either a decrease in flow rate or by time. Low levels of pressure support (5 to 10 cm H_2O) may be used to decrease the work of breathing by overcoming the resistance of the endotracheal tube and/or ventilator circuitry.[108-115] Higher levels of pressure support (> 10 cm H_2O) may be used to augment the patient's tidal volume. The use of pressure support may be advantageous for patients who are difficult to wean.[113-115] Care must be taken not to misinterpret the tidal volumes accomplished with the aid of pressure support levels greater than 10 cm H_2O as equivalent to the mechanics of spontaneous breathing.

Continuous Flow (Flow-By)

Continuous flow provides a constant supply of gas to the ventilator circuit from which the patient may breathe spontaneously. Patients with weak respiratory muscles may fatigue easily when breathing with demand systems that do not respond quickly or easily enough to minimize the WOB. Continuous flow may facilitate weaning in these types of patients.[109,110,116] The subject of weaning and its associated problems have been discussed in previous chapters.

Inverse I:E Ratio Ventilation

Inverse I:E ratio (inspiratory time exceeds expiratory time) ventilation may be considered in critically ill patients exhibiting refractory hypoxemia. Controversy exists as to the exact mechanism responsible for increases in arterial Pao_2 that have been reported after application of inverse I:E ratio ventilation. Many clinicians contribute improvements in gas exchange to the development of "auto-PEEP" or intrinsic PEEP.[73-75,111] With inverse ratio ventilation, the relatively short expiratory time does not allow for complete exhalation to occur, therefore gas is "trapped" in the alveoli creating a PEEP effect. This additional PEEP and subsequent increase in FRC is what most observers believe to be responsible for increases in Pao_2 during application of this mode. The potential hemodynamic consequences (i.e., arterial hypotension and impaired cardiac output) associated with this increase in mean airway pressure mandates close attention and monitoring, however. In addition, reports of pulmonary barotrauma, including pneumothorax, have been reported with the use of inverse ratio ventilation.[117] Procedures are available that allow the clinician to quantitate intrinsic PEEP levels but vary depending on the ventilatory circuit design and manufacturer. The Siemens 300 ventilator allows for measurements of auto-PEEP by a simple manipulation of one dial (Fig. 25–27).

Respiratory Mechanics

Several of the new generation microprocessor ventilators possess the capability of measuring respiratory mechanics including VC, negative inspiratory force (NIF), RAW, and pulmonary compliance (dynamic and static). The accuracy and reproducibility of certain parameters, particularly the NIF, have been questioned, however, by several investigators.[111] Measurements of pulmonary mechanics using the technology associated with the mechanical ventilator may eliminate the need for additional equipment and supplies. Further study is needed, however, to determine the accuracy and validity of pulmonary me-

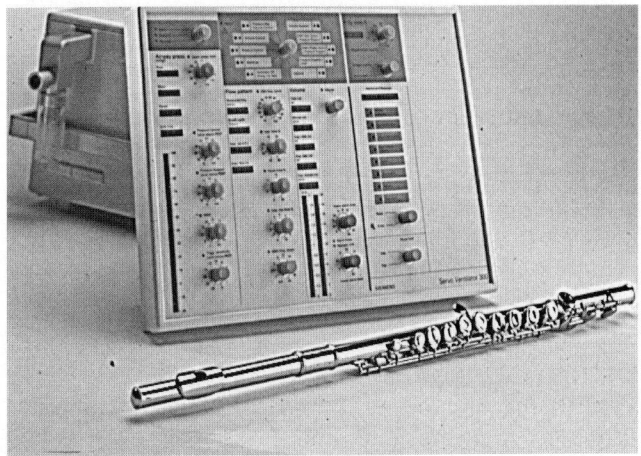

Fig. 25–27. The Siemens 300 ventilator allows for measurements of "auto-PEEP" by the simple manipulation of one dial. (Courtesy of Siemens Medical Systems, Danvers, MA.)

chanic measurements when performed under these circumstances.

Ventilator Graphics and Waveforms

Graphic display of ventilator wave forms depicting airway pressure, volume, and flow may be helpful in assessing the influence of changes in ventilator settings and the detection of intrinsic PEEP (auto-PEEP). Often, these observations are of more benefit in regards to teaching theory than aiding the practitioner in clinical decisions. When well understood, however, these wave forms may be of assistance to the clinician when ventilating difficult patients.

Graphic representation of ventilator waveforms plot patterns of flow, airway pressure, and volume over time. In situations where expiratory time is insufficient to allow for complete exhalation of inspiratory volumes, analysis of ventilator waveforms may aid the clinician in detecting such conditions. For example, in this scenario peak airway pressure increases and expiratory pressure will fail to return to baseline. The clinician will also notice continued expiratory flow until the next ventilator breath occurs. Finally, a discrepancy will occur between inspired and exhaled tidal volumes.

In situations where inspiratory flow rates are inadequate to meet patient inspiratory flow demands, the WOB normally increases placing a further burden on oxygen delivery and CO_2 elimination. The clinicians may notice a decrease or fluctuation in the airway pressure despite relatively constant measurements of flow.

In instances where the clinician has the ability to manipulate continuous flow (PB-7200 Volume Ventilator), ventilator waveforms may be helpful in determining the appropriate level of continuous flow for each patient. Flow should be adjusted to allow for a minimal fluctuations in inspiratory pressure without increasing resistance to exhalation or expiratory pressure.

Therapeutic response to bronchodilator therapy may also be determined by observation of waveforms and airway pressures. Reversal of airflow obstruction will result in a decrease in peak airway pressures along with an improvement in expiratory flow patterns. If airflow obstruction resulted in significant air trapping, the clinician will note a return to baseline of both expiratory flow and airway pressure. Examples of various waveform patterns are depicted in Figure 25-28.

Transport of the Critically Ill

It is often necessary to transport a critically ill patient from the ICU to another area of the hospital for therapeutic and/or diagnostic testing. Some of these procedures include:

- CAT scanning
- MRI scanning
- Angiograms
- Nuclear medicine techniques
- Radiation therapy

Although several studies demonstrate the relative safety of transports outside of the ICU environment,[118,119] it is only with extreme caution and with adequate preparation that these transports be undertaken. The likelihood that critical incidents occur undetected during transport is a distinct possibility considering the high acuity level of many of these patients.[120-122] If mechanical ventilation is required during transport, it is essential that practitioners skilled in airway management accompany the patient. Careful monitoring and observation of the patient's cardiorespiratory status as well as equipment must be maintained at all times.

Concerns exist as to the adequacy of manual ventilation as compared to mechanical ventilation via a transport ventilator.[120] Weg and Haas[118] reported that manual ventilation was found to be as consistent and reliable as a portable ventilator and with less expense. Based on these findings, manual ventilation by skilled practitioners appears to be sufficient in most circumstances. If the institution has several ICUs that require frequent transports of the critically ill, however, the expense of providing a specialized transport ventilator may be justified.

The use of a mechanical ventilator during a diagnostic or therapeutic procedure is often advisable particularly when the procedure requires an extensive amount of time (longer than 20 to 30 minutes), or if hazardous conditions are present that may adversely affect the health of the transport team. At this time, ventilators are available that may be used during magnetic resonance imaging (MRI) procedures and would eliminate human exposure to magnetic fields (Fig. 25-29).

Continuous pulse oximetry is a valuable noninvasive monitoring tool that can be used during transport of the high risk patient. It is particularly helpful for those patients that require high oxygen concentrations and/or PEEP to maintain adequate oxygenation. Sudden and precipitous decreases in SpO_2 can alert the attending personnel to equipment failure as well as to changes in the patient's clinical condition. Several institutions have described the assembly of specialized transport carts for use in the transport of the high risk patient. These carts are fitted with oxygen, a portable ventilator, pulse oximeter, and suction equipment. The frequency of transports conducted may influence the decision whether it is of sufficient benefit to assemble such equipment.

Finally, the time, expense, and possible complications of transporting critically ill patients for diagnostic tests and treatment dictates that procedures be ordered only when indicated and when the information obtained will affect the management of the patient.[122]

Weaning and Extubation

Weaning

When it has been determined that the patient is ready to begin the weaning process, it is important to establish a weaning plan including criteria for the discontinuation of weaning (failure criterion) as well as criteria for continuation of the weaning trials. The particular method of weaning chosen normally depends on institution or clinician preference. Little scientific evidence exists that clearly demonstrates the superiority of one technique over another. Various techniques that may be employed in the weaning of the ventilator-dependent patient include:

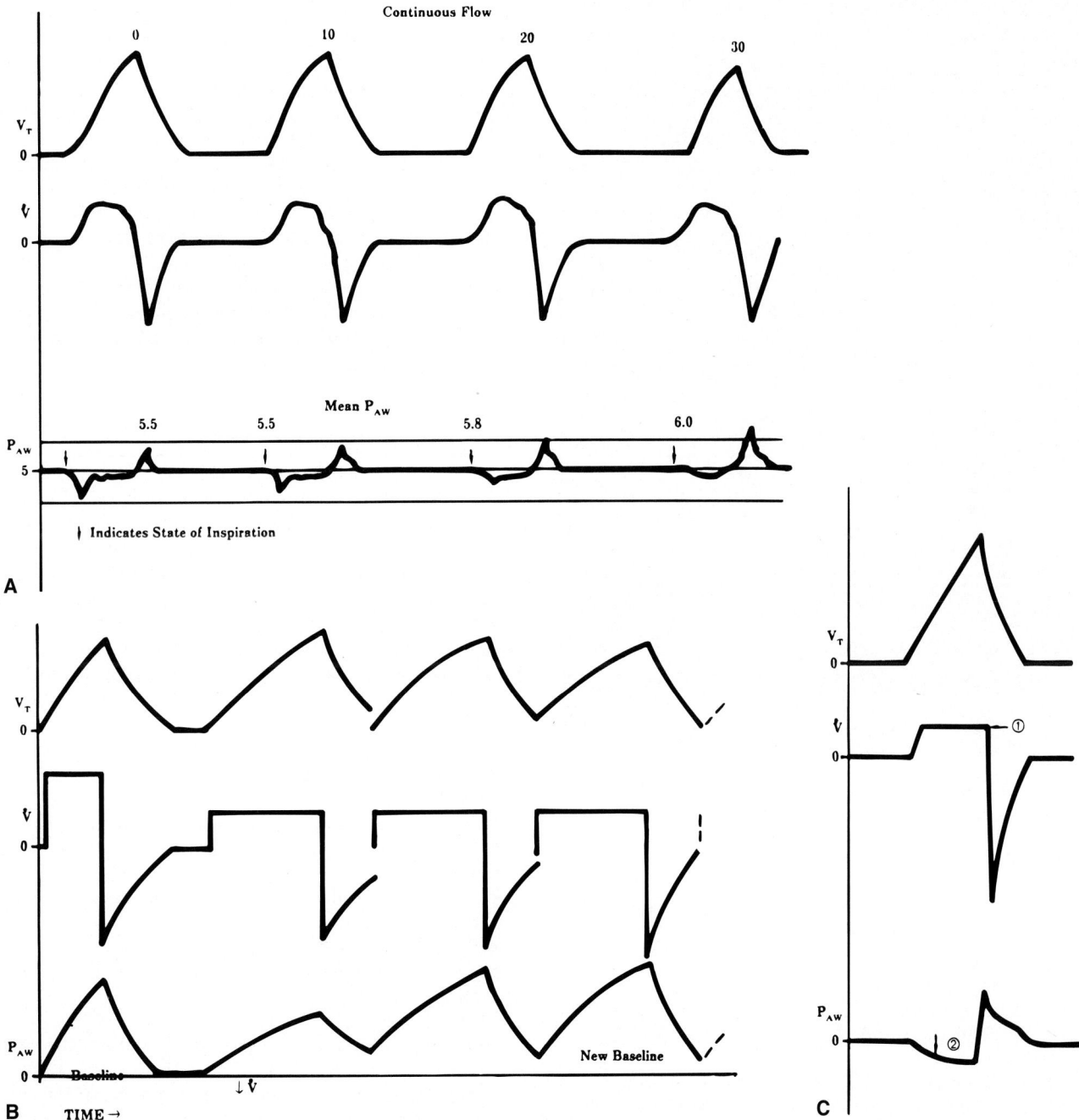

Fig. 25-28. A, The effect of continuous flow on the work of breathing is illustrated. The four wave forms represent increase from 0 to 30 L per minute (top). The upward deflection on the middle wave form pattern represents inhalation with a downward deflection in the mean airway denoting a decreasing airway pressure (Paw). The downward deflection in the middle wave form represents expiration. Note as continuous flow increases, the mean airway pressure increases, and the peak expiratory airway pressure (point of maximum expiratory flow on middle wave forms) increases. This represents increased work of breathing most likely from increased resistance to exhalation caused by an excessively high continuous flow setting. B, The effect of air trapping on pressure and flow curves is illustrated. Note on the bottom wave form that the airway pressure fails to return to the previous level with the establishment of a new baseline. The middle wave form representing inspiration (upward inflection) and expiration (downward deflection) demonstrates that expiratory volumes do not equal inspiratory volumes. C, A pressure-flow wave form depicting the patient's inspiratory flow demands exceeding the ventilator present inspiratory flow is illustrated. Point 1 represents the beginning of expiration. The top wave form represents increasing volume of inspired air. Point 2 shows a decrease in airway pressure during the inspiratory phase of a ventilator-assisted breath representing an increased demand for inspiratory flow beyond values present on the ventilator.

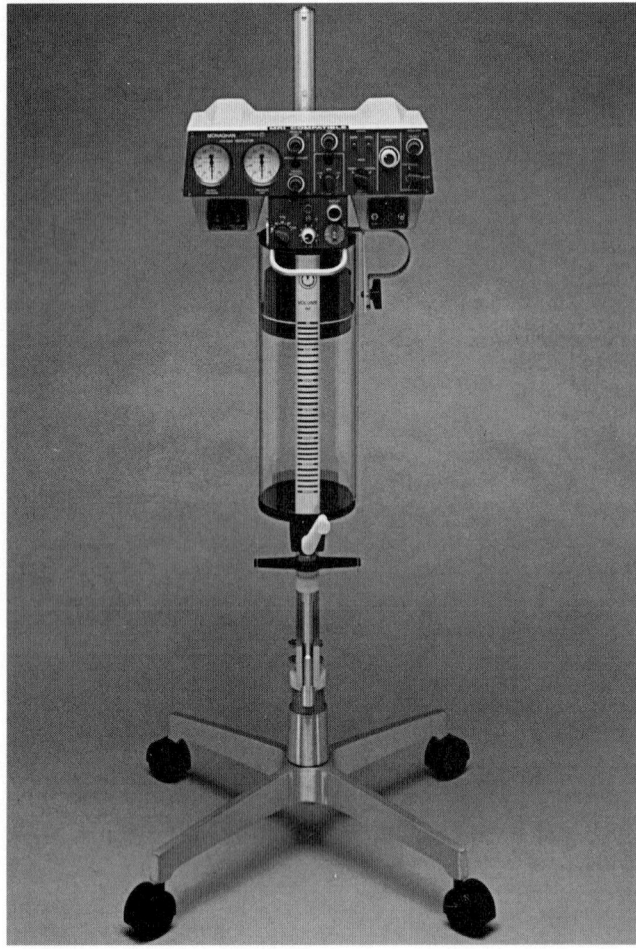

Fig. 25-29. The Monaghan 225/SIMV Volume Ventilator can be used to support ventilation during diagnostic imaging with magnetic resonance. (Courtesy of Monaghan Medical Corp., Plattsburgh, NY.)

- SIMV/IMV
- "T" piece trials
- Pressure Support
- Continuous Flow
- Combinations of the above

Patients known to have poor respiratory muscle function and limited ventilatory reserve pose the greatest challenge to the ICU staff. The development of respiratory muscle fatigue is most often characterized by tachypnea, paradoxic abdominal breathing, and respiratory alternans.[123,124] In cases where these conditions occur, the use with ventilators equipped with pressure support and/or continuous flow may be of particular benefit. Continuous flow from either a "T" piece or through a microprocessor controlled ventilator substantially reduces work of breathing requirements as compared to demand valve systems.[116] The application of pressure support can not only compensate for resistance in the ventilator circuitry and artificial airway, but can also augment tidal volume until such time as the patient is capable of adequate spontaneous ventilation.[113,114]

Emotional support from the ICU staff is imperative to the success of weaning, especially for those who are difficult to wean and must undergo repeated trials. These patients in particular require constant reassurance and encouragement.

Vigilant monitoring and close observation of the patient is vital to the success of weaning difficult patients. The use of continuous pulse oximetry and/or end-tidal CO_2 monitoring may prove helpful in providing noninvasive real-time measurements of ventilatory function. Bedside spirometry performed before, during, and after weaning trials can provide additional information regarding ventilatory mechanics. Close attention to vital signs will help to ensure that the patient is not unduly stressed which, if undetected for even short periods, may contribute to respiratory muscle fatigue and myocardial ischemia further delaying the weaning process.

Extubation

Extubation of the high risk patient should not be attempted unless qualified personnel are immediately available should complications arise and reintubation be necessary. Prior to the actual extubation procedure, equipment should be assembled to provide the appropriate postextubation FIO_2. In most circumstances, a large volume aerosol generator and aerosol mask are used during the postextubation period (normally 2 to 4 hours). These particular devices provide adequate inspiratory flow rates and humidity. The following list summarizes the extubation procedure:

- Place patient in sitting position
- Suction the airway
- Suction the oropharynx
- Insert suction catheter in airway
- Deflate endotracheal tube cuff while simultaneously applying suction
- Remove tube during end inspiration; suction the oropharynx
- Provide appropriate FIO_2 and humidity
- Monitor for signs or symptoms of respiratory muscle fatigue

Following extubation, the patient should be closely observed for the development of postextubation stridor, laryngospasm, and respiratory insufficiency. If stridor develops, aerosolized racemic epinephrine may be administered via SVN.

Preparation for Discharge from the ICU

In preparation for discharge of the patient to a regular nursing floor, the equipment necessary to support the patient's respiratory care (e.g., oxygen, CPAP, humidity, ventilator, etc.) should be appropriate for the non-ICU environment. In addition, patients who have had an extended ICU stay will need emotional preparation and support to prepare them for the change in environment. Advanced notification should be given regarding the transport and subsequent arrival of the patient to the nursing unit. A complete set of respiratory care transfer orders including oxygen concentration, aerosolized medications, Bph, and monitoring devices should be completed to ensure continuity and consistency of care. Finally, a complete report on the patient's medical condition and care plan should be discussed with the appropriate staff including expectations of the post-ICU recovery phase.

RESPIRATORY THERAPY SERVICES IN THE POST-ICU PHASE OF ILLNESS

The decision to discharge patients from the ICU environment is based on the assumption that the patient will no longer benefit from traditional ICU services and specialized nursing care. As cost constraints in the ICU become more prevalent, however, it appears likely that alternative "non-ICU" settings such as the development of noninvasive respiratory care units as described by Elpern and associates[125] will be developed to care for the severely ill. With the development of these noninvasive nursing units, the demand for respiratory therapy services will undoubtedly increase. Once exclusively performed in the traditional ICU setting, ventilatory management and weaning procedures are becoming more common in the general nursing units as well. As patient acuity continues to increase in the non-ICU setting, the need for well trained and highly skilled respiratory care practitioners becomes of utmost importance.

The health care practitioner will encounter a wide variety of patients discharged from the ICU setting. Often, these patients were initially admitted to the ICU because of the need for intensive monitoring of their cardiopulmonary system, regardless of the diagnosis. Therefore, we feel it is not necessarily the patient's post-ICU discharge diagnosis that determines the need for respiratory care, but rather his or her severity of illness, clinical presentation, and profile of risk factors. This philosophy will, one hopes, encourage personnel to carefully assess each patient discharged from the ICU. The primary goal of respiratory care in the post-ICU patient is to prevent the development of pulmonary complications and to restore the patient's pulmonary status to a functional level. It is recognized, however, that certain patients will be discharged from the critical care environment with a poor prognosis and little likelihood for recovery. In this situation, provisions should be made for the delivery of supportive care or rehabilitation if determined feasible by the primary physician.[126]

Failure to identify the high risk patient and implement an appropriate care plan may lead to increased morbidity, mortality, and length of hospitalization including possible readmission to the intensive care setting. The major characteristics of the high-risk post-ICU patient include:

- History of pulmonary disease/pulmonary dysfunction
- Recent upper abdominal and thoracic surgery
- Presence of an artificial airway
- Impaired immune system
- Nutrition deficiencies
- Morbid obesity
- Altered mental status
- Ventilator dependency
- Smoking history
- Neuromuscular disease
- Immobility (debilitation)

Goals of Management

The intent of respiratory care in the post-ICU recovery phase is to reduce both the incidence and severity of pulmonary complications that may occur secondary to changes in pulmonary function, mucociliary clearance, and gas exchange. These complications often include but are not limited to atelectasis, bronchospasm and mucosal edema, hypoxemia, hypoventilation, and pneumonia.[11,13,14,16,17,40] The frequency and severity of these complications can be minimized by identifying the high risk patient (see "Risk assessment form" discussed in the Pre-ICU section) and implementing an appropriate respiratory care plan which includes careful monitoring and observation of the patient. The respiratory care practitioner should be alert for clinical signs and symptoms associated with respiratory impairment (see Table 25–18). Early recognition and treatment may prevent the development of more serious complications which may ultimately prevent an extended hospital stay or readmission to the intensive care setting.

Chronic Obstructive Pulmonary Disease

Patients discharged from the ICU environment with a history of COPD are at an increased risk for developing pulmonary complications. In cases where these patients have experienced an acute episode of respiratory failure, the likelihood of further and more frequent exacerbations increases. Depending on the severity of their illness, these patients often present with some degree of bronchospasm, arterial desaturation with or without hypercarbia, and impaired mucociliary clearance.

Therapeutic Aerosol Therapy in COPD

The use of aerosolized beta agonists via SVNs or MDIs have shown to improve FVC, $FEF_{25-75\%}$, FEV_1, peak flow rates (PEFR) and mucociliary transport.[3,8,9,18] It appears as though beta agonists are gaining popularity in the United States and are being considered as the drug of choice for the treatment of bronchospastic disorders.[18,21,44] This classification of drug has a fairly rapid onset of action (5 to 15

Table 25–18. Clinical Signs and Symptoms of Respiratory Impairment

Dyspnea and/or tachypnea
Confusion or mental status changes
Increased use of accessory muscles
Productive cough/purulent sputum
Presence of wheezing/rhonchi/rales
Diminished or absent breathsounds
Fever with or without cough
Changes in vital signs
Chest pain (pleuritic)
Cyanosis

minutes) when given by aerosol.[21,44,45] In most circumstances, the side effects associated with the administration of beta-adrenergic agents are reversible by either decreasing the dosage or frequency of therapy. When they do occur, it is often not severe and usually manifests itself in the form of tachycardia, tremors, nausea, and nervousness.[9,44]

Recently, anticholinergics have been available in the United States in the form of a MDI. Ipratropium bromide (Atrovent) is thought to have its greatest effect on the central airways as opposed to the beta agonists. Clinical onset of action varies from 30 to 60 minutes and has been associated with a significant decrease in side effects as compared to aerosolized atropine.[45]

In addition to the anticholinergics, the administration of aerosolized corticosteroids appears to demonstrate a therapeutic benefit in these patients by improving airflow obstruction caused by inflammation and edema.[43-45] The three most commonly used corticosteroids available in MDIs include: beclomethasone (Vanceril), triamcinolone (Azmacort), and flunisolide (Aerobid).

The reduction of systemic side effects observed with inhaled corticosteroids is promising for those patients with significant airway obstruction who require maintenance doses of steroids. Side effects associated with inhaled corticosteroids include throat discomfort, hoarseness, and oropharyngeal colonization with candida.[43-45] These side effects may be minimized by instructing patients to rinse their mouths vigorously after each treatment.

Supplemental Oxygen Therapy in COPD

The most common cause of arterial hypoxemia in the COPD patient is ventilation-perfusion (V/Q) mismatching. Hypoxemia leads to pulmonary vasoconstriction and subsequent pulmonary hypertension. In addition, secondary polycythemia may develop as a compensatory mechanism in an attempt to increase the oxygen carrying capacity of the blood. Clinical evidence has clearly demonstrated that the administration of supplemental oxygen therapy can minimize these physiologic effects and improve exercise tolerance, survival, and the quality of life in patients with severe hypoxemia.[127-131] Based on the results of two well publicized clinical trials, (NIH) Nocturnal Oxygen Therapy Trial[129] and the (MRC) British Medical Research Council multicenter trial,[127] continuous oxygen therapy is recommended for those patients who demonstrate an arterial Pa_{O_2} of 55 mm Hg or less. If the patient exhibits evidence of right heart failure and/or polycythemia, it is advised that oxygen therapy be instituted if the arterial Pa_{O_2} is less than 60 mm Hg.[128,132]

Current literature supports the assumption that patients with COPD may experience significant arterial desaturation during exercise and sleep.[131-133] Therefore, the use of awake, resting Pa_{O_2} measurements in order to determine the need for low flow oxygen therapy should not be considered the sole indicator. Table 25-19 summarizes current medicare guidelines for reimbursement of oxygen therapy in the home setting.

Oxygen Delivery Devices

Hypoxemia in these patients can normally be treated by the administration of supplemental low-flow oxygen using a nasal cannula. This type of device is well tolerated by the patient and offers a reasonably comfortable and lightweight method for oxygen delivery during ambulation and exercise. The routine use of humidifiers is not warranted in these patients when receiving flows of 4 LPM or less. In situations where significant ventilation perfusion mismatching occurs, high-flow moderate concentration masks are available. Regardless of the type of system used, careful titration of supplemental oxygen should be performed in order to assess the patient's response to therapy as measured by ABG or pulse oximetry.

Transtracheal oxygen therapy may be considered an alternative to conventional low-flow therapy in patients requiring long-term oxygen therapy. Complications resulting from continuous low-flow oxygen administration have been reported and may affect patient tolerance.[134] In cases of poor patient tolerance or hypoxemia refractory to nasal oxygen administration, transtracheal oxygen therapy may be considered as a therapeutic alternative in the administration of long-term continuous oxygen. Unfortunately, several complications have been reported with transtracheal administration including bronchospasm, infection, bleeding, and paroxysmal coughing episodes.[134] Careful consideration should also be given to catheter care as the side ports have a tendency to become obstructed with secretions. Therefore, it is highly recommended that patients and caregivers be well educated and trained regarding catheter care and cleaning procedures before hospital discharge.

Outpatient Oxygen Therapy

Three distinct types of oxygen delivery systems are routinely used in the outpatient setting: compressed gas cylinders (CGC), oxygen concentrators (OC), and liquid oxygen (LOX) systems. Each has certain advantages and disadvantages regarding issues of economics, ease of ambulation, and concentration and/or flow rate capabilities. Table

Table 25-19. Medicare Guidelines for Reimbursement of Home Oxygen Therapy

A diagnosis of chronic lung disease including COPD, IPF, bronchiectasis, cystic fibrosis, or carcinoma
ABSOLUTE CRITERIA
  Arterial Pa_{O_2} value of less than or equal to 55 mm Hg (measured on room air)
  Arterial oxygen saturation of less than or equal to 88% measured by pulse/ear oximetry (measured on room air)
ALTERNATIVE CRITERIA
  Arterial Pa_{O_2} value of less than or equal to 59 mm Hg (measured on room air) **AND** documentation of "end-organ" dysfunction as characterized by one of the following:
    Hematocrit greater than 56%
    ECG P-wave greater than 3 mm in leads II, III, or aVf
    Dependent edema
    Evidence of cor pulmonale and/or pulmonary hypertension
    Cognitive impairment

(From Golish, J., and Meden, G.: The Physiologic Basis for Long-Term Oxygen Therapy: Home Respiratory Care. Norwalk, CT, Appleton & Lange, 1988, p. 3.)

Table 25-20. Prescription for Outpatient Oxygen Therapy

Diagnosis including evidence of "end-organ" dysfunction if appropriate
Diagnostic evidence of hypoxemia
Oxygen flow rate and/or oxygen concentration
Initial duration of need
Frequency of use (i.e., number of hours)

25-20 summarizes the information that is necessary for prescription of home oxygen therapy. Careful consideration and planning must be given prior to discharge in order to determine the appropriate system for outpatient use.

Pulse Oximetry Technology in COPD

Noninvasive measurements of arterial saturation using pulse oximetry technology have gained popularity in clinical medicine and are currently considered as an acceptable form of documentation by both medicare and HCFA for reimbursement of home oxygen therapy.[133,135,136] At this time, a room air SpO_2 measurement of 88% or less qualifies the patient for home reimbursement.

The accuracy of using SpO_2 measurements to determine the need for oxygen therapy has been questioned. Carlin and co-workers[136] reported that in their study of 55 patients, 80% had observed SpO_2 measurements of greater than 85% despite arterial PaO_2 values of less than 55 torr. These findings are similar to those described by Golish and McCarthy[137] in which simultaneous measurements of SpO_2, SaO_2 and blood oximetry were performed on 287 patients. In their patient population, only 7 of 16 individuals (44%) demonstrated an SpO_2 value of 85% or less despite arterial PaO_2 values of 55 torr or less. As a result of these clinical findings, medicare has raised its criterion for oxygen therapy reimbursement from 85 to 88%.

At the present time it remains unclear if measurements of SpO_2 are definitive and sensitive enough to accurately assess the presence and degree of arterial hypoxemia. The consequences of replacing or substituting traditional measurements of arterial PaO_2 with pulse oximetry technology may result in the inappropriate prescription for oxygen therapy based on current standards.[136] This opinion has been expressed by others.[133,137] Further research is needed to determine if pulse oximetry can replace or be considered the equivalent to direct measurements of arterial PaO_2 values in determining the need for supplemental oxygen therapy in patients with COPD during rest, sleep, or exercise.

Airway Management in COPD: Therapeutic Alternatives

Therapeutic strategies aimed at enhancing secretion clearance and improving the distribution of ventilation play an important role in the post-ICU phase of the patient recovering from an acute exacerbation of COPD. Failure to establish and implement an appropriate care plan designed to improve secretion mobilization and decrease airflow obstruction may subsequently lead to secretion retention, atelectasis, pneumonia, and respiratory insufficiency thereby further prolonging hospitalization. Therefore, the goal of respiratory therapy in the post-ICU phase should be directed towards the delivery of techniques aimed at improving both airway patency and measures of pulmonary function as well as decreasing the symptoms associated with the disease. In the following section, we will closely examine the role of these techniques in the airway management and subsequent rehabilitation of the patient with COPD.

Bronchopulmonary Hygiene Therapy (Bph). Controversy still exists regarding the efficacy of certain Bph techniques including percussion, vibration, and postural drainage in the treatment and prevention of pulmonary complications secondary to secretion retention. A review of the medical literature involving this subject reveals both conflicting and inconclusive results.[49-53] Three controlled long-term studies on the effects of postural drainage and chest percussion in hospitalized patients with pneumonia and chronic bronchitis failed to demonstrate improvement in pulmonary function, gas exchange, or secretion clearance.[49,50,54,138] Conversely, Cochrane and co-workers[139] reported significant improvement in FEV_1 and specific airways conductance following Bph therapy in patients who produced > 30 ml of sputum daily. Improvement in both expiratory flow rates and secretion clearance have also been reported following Bph therapy in patients diagnosed with chronic bronchitis and cystic fibrosis having significant daily sputum production.[54] It appears as though the routine use of Bph therapy including chest percussion, vibration, and postural drainage is not warranted in all patients with a diagnosis of COPD. The effect of these procedures on secretion clearance and pulmonary function is often highly variable and difficult to objectively assess in the clinical setting. Essentially, each patient should then act as their own control. Therapeutic trials of Bph therapy should be given to those patients who demonstrate impaired secretion clearance as evidenced by adventitious breath sounds, x-ray abnormalities, or deteriorating pulmonary function. Bph therapy may be of particular benefit to those patients who produce relatively large quantities of sputum. If little or no benefit is achieved after a therapeutic trial, serious consideration should be given to either discontinue or modify therapy. The continuation of these time consuming procedures in the absence of clinical benefit may lead to increased hospital costs and waste valuable practitioner time and effort.

Aerosol Therapy. In addition to Bph techniques, mucolytic agents and the administration of bland aerosols have also been used in an effort to improve secretion clearance in patients with COPD. The specific techniques and equipment used for administration have been discussed in the pre-ICU section. Despite the widespread use of these agents, many clinicians firmly believe that systemic hydration offers the most effective therapeutic option regarding mucolysis.[39,42] At the present time, few controlled or clinical studies exist that substantiate the role of bland aerosol therapy in secretion mobilization. It does appear, however, that solutions of saline (particularly hypertonic), are better tolerated and assist in stimulating the cough reflex. The use of high density nebulizers such as ultrasonic units are not well tolerated by the majority of patients and have been associated with an increase in airway resistance. Consequently, their popularity has diminished in recent years. In conclusion, our clinical experience has shown the same variability regarding patient response and potential benefit with bland aerosol therapy as with Bph therapy. Therefore, we recommend the same philosophy of carefully performed therapeutic trials on a case-by-case basis.

Mucolytic Agents. The administration of aerosolized mucolytic agents such as N-acetylcysteine is intended to reduce the viscosity of mucous thereby improving mucociliary transport. There currently exists a lack of clinical evidence, however, to substantiate the efficacy of this therapy. In fact, reports of bronchial irritation and bronchospasm have minimized the popularity and routine clinical use of these aerosolized agents.[42,92,93] (The recommended dosage of mucolytics has been previously stated in the pre-ICU phase discussion on aerosols.) Fortunately, this has not been the case regarding the administration of oral preparations. Published studies demonstrated that oral mucolytic therapy reduced both the incidence and severity of acute exacerbations in patients with chronic bronchitis.[92,93] The results of The National Mucolytic Study as described by Petty,[42] revealed similar findings with the administration of 60 mg of iodinated glycerol given four times daily. If the clinician believes a therapeutic trial of aerosolized mucolytic therapy is warranted, then it is highly recommended that the mucolytic be administered in conjunction with a beta agonist such as albuterol sulfate (Proventil). Mucolytic agents may play an important role in the management of secretion clearance in certain patients with chronic bronchitis. It remains unclear, however, if aerosolized N-acetylcysteine offers any therapeutic benefit based on current observations.[42,92,93]

CONSIDERATIONS IN THE PREVENTION AND TREATMENT OF POSTOPERATIVE PULMONARY COMPLICATIONS

Patients transferred from the PACU, OR, or surgical ICU require careful monitoring in their postoperative recovery phase. Pulmonary complications have been reported to be directly responsible for increased morbidity and mortality, particularly in patients who have undergone upper abdominal and thoracic surgery.[11,14,28,32,35] The incidence of postoperative atelectasis in these patients has been reported to exceed 50%.[14,15,31] Postoperative pulmonary complications may manifest themselves in a variety of ways including:

- Bronchospasm
- Secretion retention (secondary to mucociliary depression)
- Hypoventilation and reduced lung volumes
- Pulmonary atelectasis
- Hypoxemia (ventilation/perfusion mismatch)
- Pneumonia and infection

As discussed in the pre-ICU section of this chapter, early identification of the high risk patient and implementation of an appropriate respiratory care plan can often prevent or minimize the incidence of postsurgical pulmonary complications. This situation is of particular importance during the first 72 hours of postoperative recovery when lung volumes (FRC, VT, and VC) are reduced secondary to the effects of anesthesia, pain, and postoperative analgesia.[13,17,28,35,36] After major upper abdominal surgery, a patient's VC can decline by as much as 60 to 75%.[3,11,28] In addition, significantly high complication rates have been reported in thoracotomy patients who undergo resection of lung tissue. Perioperative respiratory care has been shown to significantly decrease both the incidence and severity of pulmonary complications.[11,13] The inappropriate or over zealous use of respiratory care procedures, however, has also been associated with increased hospital costs.[4,5,7,10] Therefore, extreme care must be undertaken when developing care plans in order to ensure an appropriate cost-benefit ratio. An example of a symptom-based algorithm used to determine the appropriateness of various hyperinflation techniques that may be used during postoperative care is illustrated in Figure 25-30. The scientific basis for respiratory care modalities in the prevention and treatment of postoperative pulmonary complications has been reviewed previously.

MALNUTRITION AND ITS CONSEQUENCES ON PULMONARY FUNCTION

Malnutrition is a systemic disorder that affects virtually all organ systems. Although nutrition support can correct many of the deficiencies in respiratory function, the respiratory care practitioner may be called on to optimize lung function until such time as the nutrition status of the patient returns to normal. This condition may occur in either the pre-ICU, ICU, or post-ICU phase of illness. Poor or inadequate nutrition may play a significant role in the development or exacerbation of respiratory dysfunction. This fact may be of critical importance in those patients with sepsis, preexisting pulmonary disease, or the long-term ventilator-dependent patient. The consequences of malnutrition on pulmonary function can manifest itself in three distinct areas including respiratory muscle function, control of ventilation, and lung (organ) function.

Malnutrition leads to a reduction in minute ventilation (Ve), inspiratory flow rates, and maximal voluntary ventilation (MVV). Additional findings include a decrease in diaphragmatic muscle mass which often results in a reduction in both inspiratory and expiratory pressures.[140,141]

Alterations in the control of ventilation have also been reported in the nutritionally deficient patient. These include a reduction in the sigh frequency, blunting of the hypoxic drive, and, in certain patients, a decrease in the ventilatory response to hypercapnia.[140,141]

The effects of malnutrition are evident in the lung itself. Compared to healthy individuals, surfactant levels have been found to be abnormal. This condition increases the likelihood for the development of atelectasis and intrapulmonary shunting. Secondly, a reduction in parenchymal elasticity is thought to contribute to the development of emphysematous changes. Finally, malnutrition has been associated with a depressed immune response, thereby increasing the risk for the occurrence of pulmonary infection and pneumonia.

These specific changes in pulmonary mechanics and

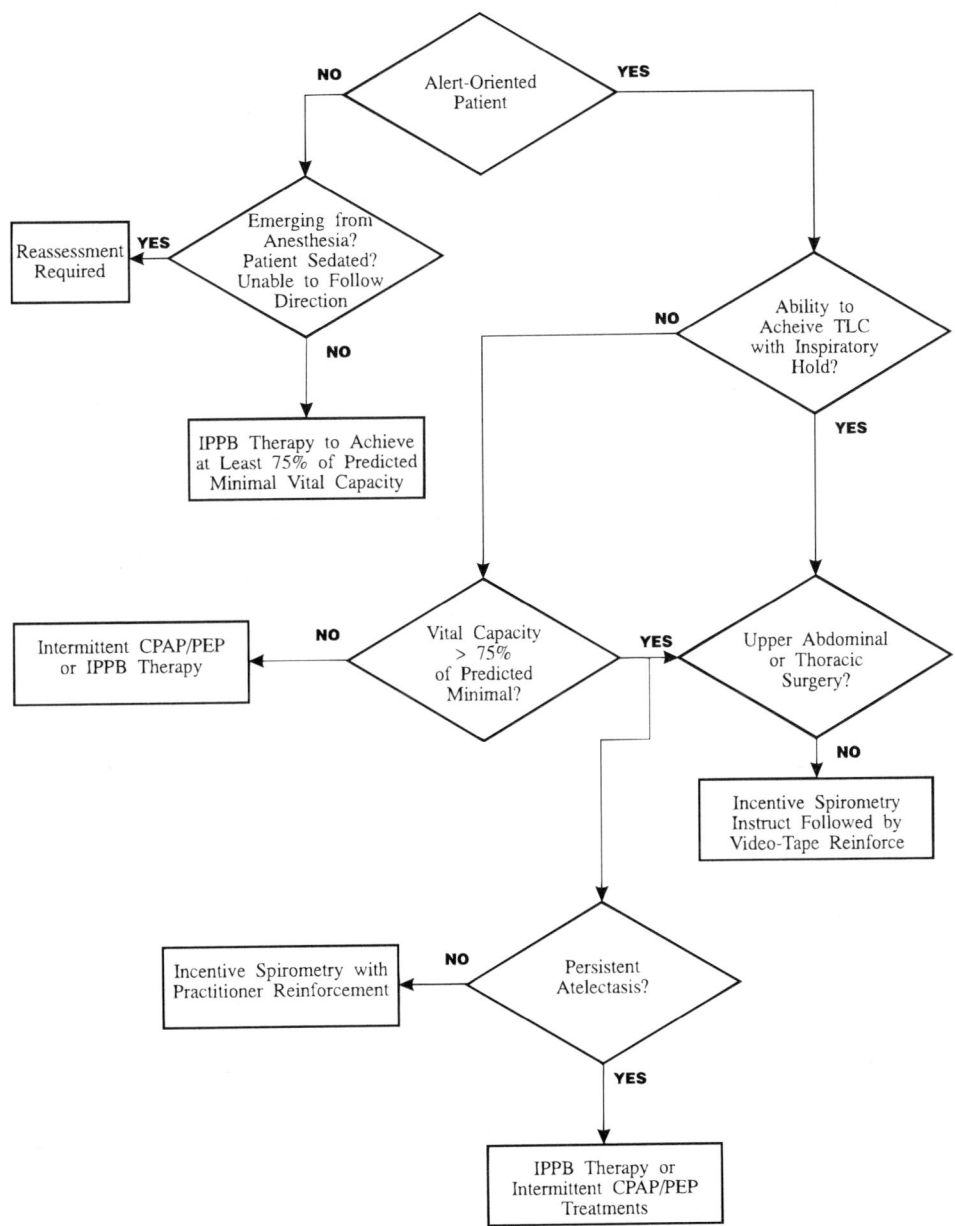

Fig. 25-30. A respiratory care plan for hyperinflation therapy is shown in this algorithm. This therapy is indicated to prevent atelectasis, to promote alveolar expansion, and to treat suspected or documented atelectasis. (From Stoller, J. K., et al.: Physician-ordered respiratory case vs physician-ordered use of a respiratory therapy consult service: early experience at the Cleveland Clinic Foundation. Respir. Care, 38:1143, 1993.)

pulmonary function (see Table 25-21) may lead to an ineffective cough, secretion retention, atelectasis, and hypoxemia. Therefore, an appropriate respiratory care plan should be implemented (see the discussion in this chapter on patient risk-assessment form, pre-ICU phase), including respiratory care modalities aimed specifically at treatment of the previously mentioned findings. These might include:

- Hyperinflation techniques (atelectasis)
- Bph therapy (secretion mobilization)
- Oxygen therapy (hypoxemia)

OBESITY AND THE HIGH RISK PATIENT

Regardless of the primary admitting diagnosis to the ICU, the obese patient possess a particular challenge in

Table 25-21. Effects of Malnutrition on Pulmonary Function

Respiratory muscle function
   Reduction in minute ventilation and maximal voluntary ventilation
   Decrease in diaphragmatic muscle mass
   Reduced inspiratory and expiratory airway pressures
Control of ventilation
   Reduction in the sigh frequency
   Blunting of the hypoxic drive
   Decrease in the ventilatory response to hypercapnia
Lung pathophysiology and function
   Reduction in surfactant production
   Depressed immune response
   Occurrence of emphysematous changes
   Reduction in pulmonary elasticity
---

the post-ICU recovery phase. Defined as a body mass exceeding 20% of predicted body weight, obesity has been associated with an increased incidence of arterial hypertension, coronary atherosclerosis, diabetes mellitus, and pulmonary dysfunction.[142]

Pulmonary function testing normally reveals a restrictive ventilatory defect characterized by a reduction in MVV, FRC, and VC.[13,143] In addition, patients weighing more than 100 kg commonly exhibit clinical signs and symptoms of arterial hypoxemia and hypercapnia. This obesity-hypoventilation syndrome is thought to be associated with a defective ventilatory response to CO_2 and not to body weight alone.[144]

Obesity reduces chest wall compliance and subsequently leads to an increase in the WOB and poor gas distribution.[142-144] This situation often manifests itself in the form of hypoxemia and atelectasis. In most circumstances, the use of low flow oxygen therapy and hyperinflation techniques (incentive spirometry, IPPB, and CPAP/PEP therapy) may prove beneficial in alleviating or improving these symptoms until weight reduction can be achieved.

THERAPEUTIC METHODS IN THE TREATMENT OF OSA: NASAL CPAP

In recent years, nasal CPAP therapy has been employed as a nonsurgical therapeutic alternative for the treatment of obstructive sleep apnea (OSA).[144-146] The application of positive airway pressure during sleep may minimize the incidence and severity of hypoxemic and hypercapnic nocturnal episodes associated with this condition. Internal "pneumatic splinting" of the hypopharyngeal area and increases in FRC are most likely responsible for these improvements noted in gas exchange.[145] Sanders[146] reported a reduction in the frequency of both obstructive and mixed apneas in 18 patients diagnosed with OSA after the application of nasal CPAP. This reduction in apneic episodes occurred in both rapid eye movement (REM) and non-REM stages of sleep.

Not all patients are able to tolerate this particular form of therapy. When presented with the surgical alternative, however, most appear willing to cooperate in a clinical trial. Recent improvements in CPAP unit design allow for the gradual increase of positive pressure to preset levels over time. Response to therapy is quite variable and requires careful titration of airway pressure (and FIO_2 if necessary) in order to achieve optimal results. This process can be most effectively accomplished during polysomnography testing.[77]

Although nasal CPAP can be provided by the use of compressed gas sources, new innovations in technology have lead to the development of a commercially available microprocessor-based servofeedback unit—Tranquility Plus, Healthdyne Technologies, Marietta, GA (Fig. 25-31). This particular unit is portable, relatively lightweight, and simple to operate. The Tranquility Plus allows for the consistent delivery of patient airway pressures despite variations in inspiratory flow rates. In addition, this model is able to compensate for minor leaks in the patient system as well as other variables including altitude, atmospheric pressure, and ambient temperature. In theory, these features may

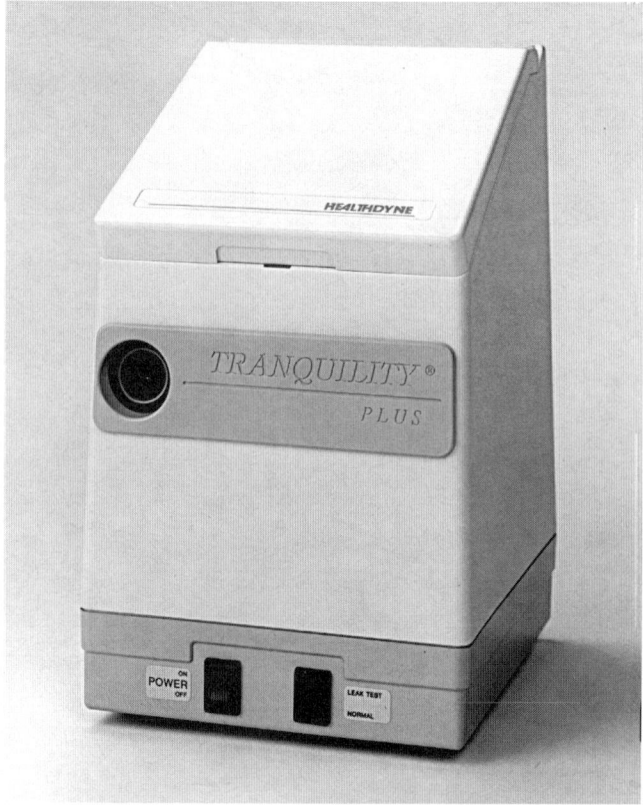

Fig. 25-31. The Healthdyne Tranquility Plus (Model 7100) Nasal CPAP unit allows for consistent delivery of patient airway pressures despite variations in inspiratory flow rates. (Courtesy of Healthdyne Technologies, Marietta, GA.)

increase the likelihood of a successful clinical trial of CPAP therapy as a result of enhanced patient comfort and improved patient compliance. Home maintenance essentially consists of periodic filter and circuit cleaning. The blower unit is connected to a nasal mask or pillows by use of a 22 mm diameter corrugated tubing. Careful consideration should be given when determining the appropriate size and style mask. Many "CPAP trial failures" can be attributed to poor mask fit or inadequate preparation of the patient. Complications of nasal abrasions, nasal irritation, rhinitis, and patient discomfort have been reported.[146,154]

Additional features now available on selected nasal CPAP units allow for incremental increases of airway pressure over a specified period that is predetermined by the clinician. Referred to as "Ramp Time," patient airway pressures can be gradually increased in user-selected intervals between 5 to 30 minutes. Control of this parameter may be of particular value during initial CPAP trials, or in individuals who experience difficulty adjusting to CPAP flow and pressure when attempting to sleep.

CARE OF THE VENTILATOR-DEPENDENT PATIENT IN THE NON-ICU SETTING

As the number of patients who are dependent on a ventilator on a long-term basis continues to increase, alternative sites for the delivery of care have been established in order to preserve ICU resources and reduce health care costs.[147-150] Several investigators have reported the ability to provide care at lower costs to ventilatory-dependent patients in the "noninvasive" ventilator ward without affecting morbidity or mortality. Elpern and associates[125] reported substantial cost savings of greater than $1000 per ventilator day without negatively affecting patient outcomes. In addition, Cordasco and Sivak[150] described their experience during an 8-year period with 99 long-term ventilator-dependent patients who were discharged to the regular nursing floors for either custodial or rehabilitative care. Reduction in overall costs of care and improved use of existing personnel were noted. Despite these preliminary findings, comparison of the efficacy between geographically consolidated ventilator units ("the noninvasive respiratory care unit") versus discharge to a nonspecialized nursing unit ("the dispersal strategy") has yet to be determined. This topic has been the subject of editorials and discussion.[151,152] Nevertheless, both "internal" and "external" pressures concerning resource and cost constraints continue to provide the impetus for prompt ICU discharge into either of these environments depending on the institution and/or availability of the noninvasive ventilator wards.[125,147-152]

Based on the goals outlined in the ICU discharge summary, patients can normally be classified according to their severity of illness and likelihood for recovery. In most circumstances, long-term ventilator-dependent patients can be classified as candidates for either custodial or rehabilitative care. Table 25-22 lists specific diseases and conditions that may necessitate the need for long-term mechanical ventilation.

Patients discharged from the acute care setting should meet specific transfer criterion or "medical readiness" guidelines in order to prevent the transport of clinically unstable patients (see Table 25-23). Premature discharge of patients out of the ICU environment should be avoided if at all possible. Respiratory care in the post-ICU recovery phase of illness must be tailored according to individual patient needs. Custodial patients with little likelihood for recovery or hospital discharge may require only basic nursing care, routine airway care, and simple maintenance of the ventilatory support system. This may include observation and documentation of ventilator operation as well as equipment changes based on departmental guidelines. In contrast, patients who are actively being weaned or who are involved in rehabilitation with a good prognosis for hospital discharge may require more intensive levels of care including aggressive respiratory care, noninvasive monitoring, and, if necessary, transport to other areas of the hospital for therapeutic or diagnostic procedures. If transport is required, then extreme care and caution must be taken to ensure the safety of the patient while away from the nursing unit.[118-122] In order to reduce the risk of a "critical incident," only personnel who are familiar with the patient, equipment, and monitors should be responsible for the transport. In addition, the patient must also be constantly reassured in order to prevent unnecessary stress, anxiety, and apprehension.

Table 25-22. Diseases and Conditions That May Require the Need for Long-Term Mechanical Ventilation

Diaphragmatic defects
Chest wall abnormalities
   Kyphoscoliosis
Neuromuscular disorders
   Central nervous system disorders
   Pheripheral nerve conditions
   Spinal cord injury and disease
Anterior horn cell (lower motor neuron)
   Amyotrophic lateral sclerosis
   Wernig-Hoffman syndrome
   Poliomyelitis
Peripheral nerve disorders
Pulmonary dysfunction
   Chronic bronchitis and emphysema
   Interstital lung disease
   Cystic fibrosis and bronchiectasis
   Adult respiratory distress syndrome
   Bronchopulmonary dysplasia

Table 25-23. ICU Discharge Criteria for Long-Term Ventilator-Dependent Patients

Absence of significant cardiac arrhythmias
Hemodynamically stable
Absence of acute infection
Stable metabolic status
Absence of sustained or prolonged dyspnea and tachypnea
FIO_2 requirements less than 50%
PEEP requirements less than 5 cm H_2O
Presence of a stable airway (tracheostomy preferred)
Clearly defined cardiopulmonary resuscitation guidelines

Technical Aspects of Non-ICU Mechanical Ventilation

Recent advances in microprocessor technology have allowed for the development and manufacture of mechanical ventilators that are versatile, offer a wide range of ventilator modes, and are relatively easy to operate. As a result, multiple ventilator options including safety features and alarm systems are far more sophisticated than those available in the past. Although far more expensive than portable ventilators such as the LP-10 Volume Ventilator (Aequitron Medical, Inc.), these newer generation models offer distinct clinical and safety advantages in certain circumstances. These advantages are of particular importance during weaning trials if pressure support of flow-by is required. Despite this fact, the exclusive use of microprocessor technology is probably not warranted in a variety of clinical scenarios, particularly in the custodial care of the unweanable patient. Therefore, the decision to employ a specific type of mechanical ventilator should be made on an individual basis by the clinician after a thorough analysis of the patient's status and ventilatory requirements.

Secondary alarm systems and back-up electrical power for all ventilators and monitoring systems should be available at all times. In addition, careful consideration must be given to the location and physical surroundings of the non-ICU nursing unit. Ideally, the unit should be designed and constructed in such a manner that direct observation of the patient can be accomplished by the medical staff at all times. If private rooms are present, then one may consider telemetry or some type of central monitoring station including the use of noninvasive respiratory monitoring. Despite preliminary reports of success and cost savings, it remains unclear whether care of the long-term ventilatory-dependent patient in the non-ICU setting offers a safe, viable option to traditional ICU management.[151]

Discharge Planning for the Long-term Ventilator-Dependent Patient

One must recognize the eventual need for discharge of the clinically stable ventilator-dependent patient from the acute hospital setting to either an extended care facility or to the home. In large health care institutions, discharge planning is normally performed by a multidisciplinary team including a physician, social worker, nurse, respiratory care practitioner, dietitian, occupational therapist, physical therapist, durable medical equipment (DME) company, and other health care professionals. It is possible to provide this service with fewer health care practitioners, however, if the members involved in discharge planning possess the necessary skills and training in the evaluation, assessment, and rehabilitation of home care patients. A thorough analysis of the patient and home environment is necessary to determine the feasibility of providing ventilatory support in this setting. Before discharge, the patient, family members, and caregivers should be thoroughly trained in all aspects of care related to the individual needs of the patient. In the event that the provision of home ventilation is determined unrealistic, then alternative arrangements can be made for extended care outside the acute care hospital.

The transition from the acute care setting to the home should be made as smooth as possible for the patient and family members. One can easily understand the apprehension, fear, and overwhelming anxiety of leaving the relative security of hospital care. Many of these fears can be minimized or avoided, however, by constant reassurance and adequate preparation of all those involved. In contrast, the premature discharge of a home care candidate combined with inadequate instruction of the family members and caregivers can truly be an exercise in futility.

THERAPEUTIC ALTERNATIVES TO CONVENTIONAL NOCTURNAL VENTILATION: BiPAP

Nocturnal intermittent positive airway pressure ventilation (IPPV) via nasal mask has been used successfully in the treatment of chronic hypoventilation in patients diagnosed with kyphoscoliosis and neuromuscular disease. In most circumstances, this is accomplished by using a conventional ventilator similar to those required by ventilator-dependent patients. This success has spawned recent interest in the development of an alternative device for the provision of nocturnal ventilation. BiPAP, or bilevel nasal continuous positive airway pressure, may provide a relatively inexpensive and simple alternative to conventional nocturnal ventilation in selected patients.[152]

The BiPAP device provides for a timed (user determined) or assisted cyclical delivery of positive airway pressure during both the inspiratory and expiratory phases of breathing. IPAP (inspiratory positive airway pressure) and EPAP (expiratory positive airway pressure) can be adjusted by the clinical based on patient compliance and desired ABG values. Strumpf and co-workers[153] reported the successful conversion from nasal IPPV to BiPAP in three patients diagnosed with kyphoscoliosis, muscular dystrophy and postpoliomyelitis syndrome. BiPAP may be considered for selected patients who require only intermittent or nocturnal ventilatory support. Because the device is pressure limited, it should be used with extreme caution in conditions presenting with increased airway resistance or poor lung compliance.

Sanders[154] recently reported the successful use of BiPAP therapy in the treatment of OSA. By allowing for independent adjustment of both inspiratory and expiratory airway pressures, OSA-related symptoms were minimized but at a lower mean airway pressure as compared to traditional nasal CPAP therapy. In theory, this result may allow for improved patient compliance as well as minimizing the risk for cardiovascular compromise.

More clinical studies are needed to determine the efficacy of BiPAP in these and other patient populations. In the meantime, BiPAP should only be employed in selected patients under close supervision and guidance by the medical staff.

PULMONARY REHABILITATION

The intent of pulmonary rehabilitation is to stabilize or slow the progression of the physiologic and psychologic consequences and manifestations of chronic pulmonary disease.[159] The ultimate goal is to return the patient to his or her highest functional level. Realistically, the achievement of this goal will depend on their degree of pulmonary impairment, motivational aspects of the patient and caregivers, and their willingness to comply with therapeutic regimens. The specific components of pulmonary rehabilitation include:

- Education, nutrition, smoking cessation, and immunization
- Occupational therapy, vocational rehabilitation, psychosocial rehabilitation, exercise conditioning
- Oxygen administration, bronchopulmonary hygiene, breathing exercises
- Aerosolized medications: bronchodilators, mucolytics, steroids, anticholinergics and cromolyn sodium
- Nonaerosolized medications: diuretics, antimicrobials, antifungals, expectorants and psychotherapy agents
- Home mechanical ventilation and noninvasive ventilatory techniques (BiPAP)

Most experts agree that pulmonary rehabilitation programs are effective.[155-158] There appears to be a consensus opinion, however, that measurements of airflow and gas exchange are not enhanced by rehabilitation if these variables are optimized prior to discharge. Nevertheless, Holden and co-workers[157] reported that individuals enrolled in their program demonstrated an improvement in walking capacity and functional status as measured by a modified dyspnea index. In addition, a reduction in respiratory symptoms and hospital admissions have been reported by other investigators.[155,156]

Specific respiratory care techniques and procedures used in pulmonary rehabilitation including medical necessity guidelines for oxygen administration have been previously discussed in this section. Technologic advances in ambulatory oxygen (i.e., portable liquid systems) have been directly responsible for improving patient compliance with therapy. This situation in turn has resulted in an improved quality of life and a return to meaningful employment for many individuals with chronic pulmonary disease.

Chronic pulmonary disease affects millions of individuals in the United States alone. The projected costs of health care, lost wages, and reduced productivity as a result of pulmonary disease are estimated in the billions of dollars.[159] As health care costs continue to soar, it is hoped that rehabilitation efforts can assist individuals in returning to the daily activities of life (i.e., family life and employment), thereby reducing their dependence on inpatient and outpatient medical care. By achieving the goals of self-dependence and self-reliance, pulmonary rehabilitation efforts will truly have been successful for not only health care providers but also for society as a whole.

CONTINUOUS QUALITY IMPROVEMENT (CQI): MONITORING THE PROVISION OF RESPIRATORY CARE SERVICES

The tremendous changes that have occurred in the health care environment over the past decade make it both desirable and necessary to conduct ongoing assessments in order to ensure the quality, appropriateness, and efficacy of health care as a whole. By establishing specific clinical indicators such as criteria for performance, respiratory therapy services can be monitored for both appropriateness and effectiveness. We hope that this process will result in improved allocation of health care resources and technology.[160] Figure 25–32 illustrates the concepts of CQI depicted in a flow diagram format. The overall focus and intent of CQI lies not in identifying the "bad apple," but rather in enhancing job design and providing a sense of clear direction and purpose for the providers of health care services.

The Joint Committee on Accreditation of Healthcare Organizations (JCAHO) mandates that quality improvement monitors be conducted for many aspects of hospital care. Several models for the monitoring of respiratory care services have been described in recent literature.[160] Specifically, these programs have focused on the monitoring and subsequent reporting of:

- Clinical indicators and criteria
- Adherence to performance guidelines and protocols
- Timeliness issues
- The frequency and intensity of adverse events
- Adherence to charting and documentation standards

To assist those responsible for the delivery of respiratory care services, the AARC has recently published a compre-

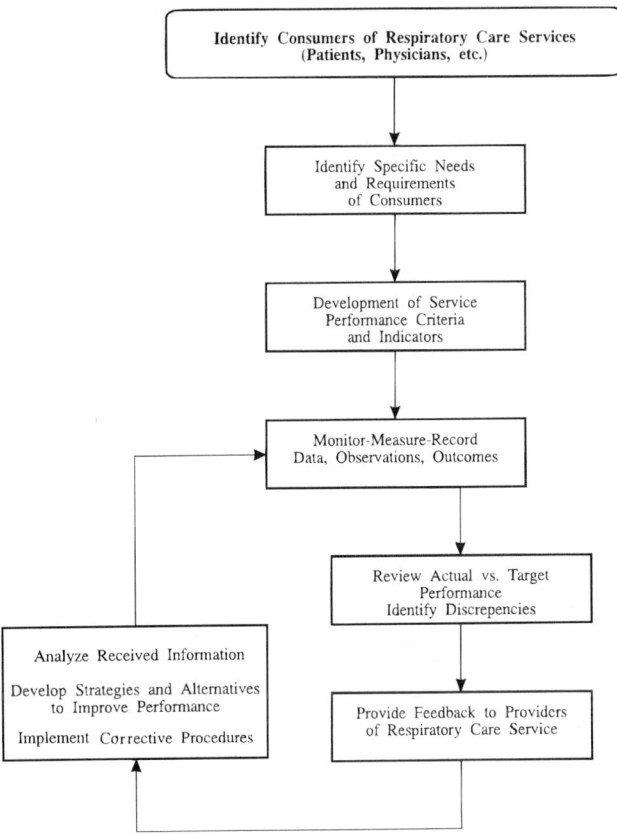

Fig. 25–32. An algorithm for continuous quality improvement (CQI) relating to the provision of respiratory care services is illustrated. The starting point is the identification of consumers of respiratory care services. The principal "fuel" for the entire process is the information derived from monitoring of patient care. (Adapted from Maxwell, C. I.: Design and implementation of the quality improvement process of a community teaching hospital. Am. J. Med. Qual., *8*:87, 1993.)

hensive set of clinical practice guidelines[12,90] for the following practices:

- In-hospital oxygen therapy
- Outpatient oxygen therapy
- Incentive spirometry
- Postural drainage techniques
- Spirometry
- Pulse oximetry technology
- Bronchial provocation testing
- Exercise testing for hypoxemia and/or desaturation
- ABG sampling
- Nasotracheal suctioning
- Aerosol delivery device selection
- Patient-ventilator system checks

Included in these comprehensive guidelines are recommendations for the indications, contraindications, monitoring, and assessment of each modality.

Undoubtedly, both "internal and external" pressures to reduce operating expenses will continue to play a major role in the daily operation of respiratory care services.[148,149] Despite this fact, purchasers of disposable respiratory care equipment should be made aware that quality, reliability, and durability must not be sacrificed in an attempt to reduce expenditures. Equipment failures attributed to poor design, structure, or faulty manufacturing have been reported.[161,162] Therefore, a careful and thorough evaluation of disposable equipment should be performed before being released into the clinical setting. This evaluation is of particular importance when new items are being introduced for the first time. Health care providers must not rely solely on the claims made by the manufacturers of these products.

A continuous quality improvement monitoring program should be designed that requires the examination of clinical procedures on a routine basis. Often, these procedures are categorized based on the potential risk to the patient. Examples of "high risk" procedures might include tracheostomy tube changes, arterial punctures, initiation of mechanical ventilation, and arterial catheterization. Procedures that are performed on a frequent basis but subject the patient to a lower level of risk may include aerosol therapy, spirometry, low flow oxygen therapy, and postural drainage techniques. In addition to clinical procedures, attention must also be directed toward equipment maintenance and sterilization procedures, safety inspections, and collaboration efforts with other health care disciplines.

Information obtained from CQI monitoring can be analyzed and compared against designated standards and criteria. If deficiencies are noted, then appropriate measures can be undertaken including efforts directed at staff education if deemed necessary. A comprehensive on-going program provides valuable information regarding the appropriateness and efficacy of respiratory care services being delivered. To be successful, however, the entire health care team must be committed to the appropriate use of resources. The ultimate goal is to ensure the safe and cost-efficient administration of health care resources directed at improving patient outcomes and quality of life.

REFERENCES

1. Pierson, D. J.: Respiratory care as a science. Respir. Care, 33:27, 1988.
2. Walton, J. R., and Baker, J. P.: Routine Respiratory Therapy (editorial). Respir. Care, 28:1113, 1983.
3. Conference on The Scientific Basis of In-Hospital Respiratory Therapy. Am. Rev. Respir. Dis., 122(Suppl.):1, 1980.
4. Shapiro, B. A., Cane, R. D., Peterson, J., and Weber, D.: Authoritative medical direction can assure cost-beneficial bronchial hygiene therapy. Chest, 93:1038, 1988.
5. Browning, J. A., Kaiser, D. L., and Durbin, C. G.: The effect of guidelines on the appropriate use of arterial blood gas analysis in the intensive care unit. Respir. Care, 34:269, 1989.
6. Walton, J. R., Shapiro, B. A., and Harrison, C. H.: Review of a bronchial hygiene evaluation program. Respir. Care, 28:174, 1983.
7. Hart, S. K., Dubbs, W., Gil, A., and Myers-Judy, M.: The effects of therapist evaluation of orders and interaction with physicians on the appropriateness of respiratory care. Respir. Care, 34:185, 1989.
8. Bowton, D. L., Goldsmith, W. M., and Haponik, E. F.: Substitution of metered-dose inhalers for hand-held nebulizers. Chest, 101:305, 1992.
9. Smoker, J. M., et al.: A protocol to assess and administer aerosol bronchodilator therapy. Respir. Care, 31:780, 1986.
10. Brougher, L. I., Blackwelder, A. K., Grossman, G. D., and Staton, G. W.: Effectiveness of medical necessity guidelines in reducing cost of oxygen therapy. Chest, 90:646, 1986.
11. Torrington, K. G., and Henderson, C. J.: Perioperative respiratory therapy. Chest, 93:946, 1988.
12. AARC Clinical Practice Guidelines. Respir. Care, 36(12):1402, 1991.
13. Scuderi, J., and Olsen, G. N.: Respiratory therapy in the management of postoperative complications. Respir. Care, 34:281, 1989.
14. O'Donohue, W. J., Jr.: National survey of the usage of lung expansion modalities for the prevention and treatment of postoperative atelectasis following abdominal and thoracic surgery. Chest, 87:76, 1985.
15. Iverson, L. I., Ecker, R. R., Fox, H. E., and May, I. A.: A comparative study of IPPB, the incentive spirometer, and blow bottles: the prevention of atelectasis following cardiac surgery. Ann. Thorac. Surg., 25:197, 1978.
16. Van De Water, J., et al.: Prevention of postoperative pulmonary complications. Surg. Gynecol. Obstet., 135:779, 1972.
17. Bartlett, R. H., Brennan, M. L., Gazzaniga, A. B., and Nanson, E. L.: Studies on the pathogenesis and prevention of postoperative pulmonary complications. Surg. Gynecol. Obstet., 137:925, 1973.
18. Williams, M. H.: Evaluation of Asthma. Chest, 76:3, 1979.
19. Van As, A.: The accuracy of peak expiratory flow meters (editorial). Chest, 82:263, 1982.
20. Williams, M. H.: The pulmonary function laboratory—who needs it? (Editorial.) Chest, 89:769, 1986.
21. Beasly, K., Cushley, R., and Holgate, S. T.: A self-management plan in the treatment of asthma. Thorax, 44:200, 1989.
22. Chapman, K. R., Liu, L. W., Watson, R. M., and Rebuck, A. S.: Range of accuracy of two wavelength oximetry. Chest, 89:540, 1986.
23. Harris, K.: Noninvasive monitoring of gas exchange. Respir. Care, 32:544, 1987.
24. Mihm, F. G., and Halperin, B. D.: Noninvasive detection of profound arterial desaturations using a pulse oximetry device. Anesthesiology, 62:85, 1985.
25. Bowton, D. L., Scuderi, P. E., Harris, L., and Haponik, E. F.: Pulse oximetry monitoring outside the intensive care unit: progress or problem? Ann. Inter. Med., 115:450, 1991.
26. Ries, A. L.: Oximetry: know thy limit. (Editorial.) Chest, 91:316, 1987.
27. Schnapp, L. M., and Cohen, N. H.: Pulse oximetry: uses and abuses. Chest, 98:1244, 1990.
28. Demers, R. R., and Saklad, S.: The etiology, pathophysiology, and treatment of atelectasis. Respir. Care, 21:234, 1976.
29. Ward, R. J., Danziger, J. J., Allen, G. D., and Bowes, J.: An evaluation of postoperative respiratory care maneuvers. Surg. Gynecol. Obstet., 137:1, 1973.
30. Lederer, D. H., Van de Water, J. M., and Indeck, R. B.: Which deep breathing device should the postoperative patient use? Chest, 77:610, 1980.
31. Schwieger, I., et al.: Absence of benefit of incentive spirometry in low risk patients undergoing elective cholecystectomy. Chest, 89:5, 1986.
32. Celli, B. R., Rodriguez, K. S., and Snider, G. L.: A controlled trial of intermittent positive pressure breathing, incentive spirometry, and deep breathing exercises in preventing

33. Sands, J. H.: A controlled study using routine intermittent positive pressure breathing in the postsurgical patient. Chest, 40:128, 1961.
34. Respiratory Care Committee of the American Thoracic Society: Guidelines for the use of intermittent positive pressure breathing (IPPB). Respir. Care, 25:365, 1980.
35. George, R. B.: Intermittent CPAP to prevent atelectasis in postoperative patients. (Editorial.) Respir. Care, 28:71, 1983.
36. Linder, K. H., Lotz, P., and Ahnefeld, F. W.: Continuous positive airway pressure effect on functional residual capacity, vital capacity and its subdivisions. Chest, 92:66, 1987.
37. Rickstein, S. E., et al.: Effects of periodic positive airway pressure by mask on postoperative pulmonary function. Chest, 89:774, 1986.
38. Christensen, E. F., Nedergaard, T., and Dahl, R.: Long-term treatment of chronic bronchitis with positive expiratory pressure mask and chest physiotherapy. Chest, 97:645, 1990.
39. Wanner, A.: The role of mucus in chronic obstructive pulmonary disease. Chest, 97:11S, 1990.
40. Gamsu, G., et al.: Postoperative impairment of mucous transport in the lung. Am. Rev. Respir. Dis., 114:673, 1976.
41. Bigby, T. D., et al.: The usefulness of induced sputum in the diagnosis of Pneumocystis carinii pneumonia in patients with the acquired immuno-deficiency syndrome. Am. Rev. Respir. Dis., 133:515, 1986.
42. Petty, T. L.: The National Mucolytic Study. Chest, 97:75, 1990.
43. Ziment, I.: Respiratory Pharmacology and Therapeutics. Philadelphia, W. B. Saunders, 1978.
44. National Heart, Lung and Blood Institute: National Asthma Education Program Expert Panel Report. Guidelines for the diagnosis and management of asthma. Allergy Clin. Immunol., 88:425, 1991.
45. Lourenco, R. V., and Cotromanes, E.: Clinical aerosols. Arch. Intern. Med., 142:2299, 1982.
46. Montgomery, A. B., et al.: Selective delivery of pentamidine to the lung by aerosol. Am. Rev. Respir. Dis., 137:477, 1988.
47. Camus, F., et al.: Pulmonary tolerance of prophylactic aerosolized pentamidine in human immunodeficiency virus-infected patients. Chest, 99:609, 1991.
48. Rochester, D. F., and Goldberg, S. K.: Techniques of respiratory physical therapy. Am. Rev. Respir. Dis., 122:133, 1980.
49. Van Der Schans, C. P., Piers, D. A., and Postma, D. S.: Effect of manual percussion on tracheobronchial clearance in patients with chronic airflow obstruction and excessive tracheobronchial secretion. Thorax, 41:448, 1986.
50. Mohsenifar, Z., Rosenberg, N., Goldberg, H. S., and Koermer, S. K.: Mechanical vibration and conventional chest physiotherapy in outpatients with stable chronic obstructive lung disease. Chest, 87:483, 1985.
51. Tyler, M. L.: Complications of positioning and chest physiotherapy. Respir. Care, 27:458, 1982.
52. Mackenzie, C. F., et al.: Cardiorespiratory function before and after chest physiotherapy in mechanically ventilated patients with post-traumatic respiratory failure. Crit. Care Med., 13:483, 1985.
53. Connors, A. F., Hammon, W. E., Martin, R. J., and Rogers, R. M.: Chest physical therapy: the immediate effects on oxygenation in acutely ill patients. Chest, 78:559, 1980.
54. Eid, N. E., Buchheit, J., Neuling, M., and Phelps, H.: Chest Physiotherapy in Review. Respir. Care, 36:270, 1991.
55. Torrington, K. G., Sorenson, D. E., and Sherwood, L.: Postoperative chest percussion with postural drainage in obese patients following gastric stapling. Chest, 86:891, 1984.
56. Lamb, J.: Intra-arterial monitoring. Nursing, Nov.:65, 1977.
57. Bartlett, R. H., and Munster, A. M.: An improved technique for prolonged arterial cannulation. N. Engl. J. Med., 279:92, 1968.
58. Gauer, P. K., and Downs, J. B.: Complications of arterial catheterization. Respir. Care, 27:435, 1982.
59. Thomas, F., et al.: The risk of infection related to radial vs femoral sites for arterial catheterization. Crit. Care Med., 11:807, 1983.
60. Band, J. D., and Maki, D. G.: Infections caused by arterial catheters used for hemodynamic monitoring. Am. J. Med., 67:735, 1979.
61. Morris, T., and Bouhoutsos, J.: The dangers of femoral artery puncture and catheterization. Am. Heart J., 89:260, 1975.
62. Chang, C., et al.: Air embolism and the radial arterial line. Crit. Care Med., 16:141, 1988.
63. Singh, S., et al.: Catheter colonization and bacteremia with pulmonary and arterial catheters. Crit. Care Med., 10:736, 1982.
64. Lowenstein, E., Little, J. W., and Lo, H. H.: Prevention of cerebral embolization from flushing radial-artery cannulas. N. Engl. J. Med., 283:1414, 1971.
65. Norwood, S. H., et al.: Prospective study of catheter-related infection during prolonged arterial catheterization. Crit. Care Med., 16:836, 1988.
66. Eyer, S., et al.: Catheter-related sepsis: prospective, randomized study of three methods of long-term catheter maintenance. Crit. Care Med., 18:1073, 1990.
67. Gauer, P. K., and Downs, J. B.: Complications of arterial catheterization. Respir. Care, 27:435, 1982.
68. Smoller, B. R., and Kruskall, M. S.: Phlebotomy for diagnostic laboratory tests in adults: patterns of use and effect on transfusion requirements. N. Engl. J. Med., 314:1233, 1986.
69. Thorson, S. H., et al.: Variability of arterial blood gas values in stable patients in the ICU. Chest, 84:14, 1983.
70. Shapiro, B. A., and Cane, R. D.: Blood gas monitoring: yesterday, today and tomorrow. Crit. Care Med., 17:573, 1989.
71. Heard, S. O.: Is capnography useful in the intensive care unit? J. Intens. Care Med., 5:199, 1990.
72. Szaflarski, N. L., and Cohen, N. H.: Use of pulse oximetry in critically ill adults. Heart Lung, 18:444, 1989.
73. Popovich, J., Jr.: PEEP: maximizing the benefits without hampering the heart. J. Respir. Dis., 7:33, 1986.
74. Bone, R. C.: Complications of mechanical ventilation and positive end-expiratory pressure. Respir. Care, 27:402, 1982.
75. Shapiro, B. A., Cane, R. D., and Harrison, R. A.: Positive end-expiratory pressure in acute lung injury. Chest, 83:558, 1983.
76. Hubmayr, R. D., Abel, M. D., and Rehder, K.: Physiologic approach to mechanical ventilation. Crit. Care Med., 18:103, 1990.
77. Tobin, M. J.: Noninvasive evaluation of respiratory movement. In Noninvasive respiratory monitoring. Edited by M. L. Nochomovitz and N. S. Cherniak. New York, Churchill Livingstone, 1986.
78. Nickerson, B. G., Sarkisian, C., and Tremper, K.: Bias and precision of pulse oximeters and arterial oximeters. Chest, 93:515, 1988.
79. Jurban, A., and Tobin, M. J.: Reliability of pulse oximetry in titrating supplemental oxygen therapy in ventilator dependent patients. Chest, 97:1420, 1990.
80. Clayton, D. G., et al.: A comparison of the performance of 20 pulse oximeters under conditions of poor perfusion. Anaesthesia, 46:3, 1991.

81. Morley, T. F.: Capnography in the intensive care unit. J. Intens. Care Med., 5:209, 1990.
82. Yakulis, R., et al.: Mass spectrometry monitoring of respiratory variables in an intensive care unit. Respir. Care, 23:671, 1978.
83. Osborn, J. J.: Use of end-tidal P_{CO_2} in monitoring. Practical Cardiol., 8:85, 1982.
84. Carlon, G., et al.: Capnography in mechanically ventilated patients. Crit. Care Med., 16:550, 1988.
85. Lepilin, M. G., Vasilyev, A. V., Bildinov, O. A., and Rostovtseva, N. A.: Endtidal carbon dioxide as a noninvasive monitor of circulatory status during cardiopulmonary resuscitation: a preliminary clinical study. Crit. Care Med., 15:100, 1987.
86. Murray, I. P., et al.: Titration of PEEP by the arterial minus end-tidal carbon dioxide gradient. Chest, 85:100, 1984.
87. Healey, C. J., Fedullo, A. J., Swinburne, A. J., and Wahl, G. W.: Comparison of noninvasive measurements of carbon dioxide tension during withdrawal from mechanical ventilation. Crit. Care Med., 15:764, 1987.
88. Hess, D.: Capnometry and capnography: technical aspects, physiologic aspects and clinical applications. Respir. Care, 6:557, 1990.
89. Weingarten, M.: Respiratory monitoring of carbon dioxide and oxygen: a ten year perspective. J. Clin. Monit., 3:217, 1990.
90. AARC clinical practice guidelines. Respir. Care, 37:882, 1992.
91. Guidelines for standards of care of patients with acute respiratory failure on mechanical ventilator support. Crit. Care Med., 19(11):275, 1991.
92. Parr, G. D., and Huitson, A.: Oral fabrol (oral N-acetylcysteine) in chronic bronchitis. Br. J. Dis. Chest, 81:341, 1987.
93. Rasmussen, J. B., and Glennow, C.: Reduction in days of illness after long-term treatment with N-acetylcysteine controlled-release tablets in patients with chronic bronchitis. Eur. Resp. J., 1:351, 1988.
94. Gay, P. C., et al.: Metered dose inhalers for bronchodilator delivery in intubated, mechanically ventilated patients. Chest, 99:66, 1991.
95. Hess, D.: How should bronchodilators be administered to patients on ventilators? Respir. Care, 36:377, 1991.
96. Hughes, J. M., and Saez, J.: Effects of nebulizer mode and position in a mechanical ventilator circuit on dose efficiency. Respir. Care, 32:1131, 1987.
97. Zwillich, C. W., et al.: Complications of assisted ventilation: a prospective study of 354 consecutive episodes. Am. J. Med., 57:161, 1974.
98. Stauffer, J. L., and Silvestri, R. C.: Complications of endotracheal intubation, tracheostomy, and artificial airways. Respir. Care, 27:417, 1982.
99. Bishop, M. J.: Mechanisms of laryngotracheal injury following prolonged tracheal intubation. Chest, 96:185, 1989.
100. Stauffer, J. L., Olson, D. E., and Petty, T. L.: Complications and consequences of endotracheal intubation and tracheotomy. Am. J. Med., 70:65, 1981.
101. Off, D., Braun, S. R., Tompkins, B., and Bush, G.: Efficacy of the minimal leak technique of cuff inflation in maintaining proper intracuff pressures for patients with cuffed artificial airways. Respir. Care, 35:1280, 1990.
102. Preusser, B. A., et al.: Effects of two methods of preoxygenation on mean arterial pressure, cardiac output, peak airway pressure, and postsuctioning hypoxemia. Heart Lung, 17:290, 1988.
103. Barnes, C. A., and Kirchhoff, K. T.: Minimizing hypoxemia due to endotracheal suctioning: a review of the literature. Heart Lung, 15:164, 1986.
104. Downs, J. B.: Who should intubate? (Editorial.) Respir. Care, 26:331, 1981.
105. McLaughlin, J. A., and Scott, W.: Training and evaluation of respiratory therapists in emergency intubation. Respir. Care, 26:333, 1981.
106. Conley, J. M., and Smith, D. J.: Emergency endotracheal intubation by respiratory care personnel in a community hospital. Respir. Care, 26:336, 1981.
107. Tenny, D., Sneider, R., and Jacobson, J.: Emergency endotracheal intubation by respiratory care practitioners. Respir. Ther., Nov/Dec:67, 1985.
108. Fiastro, J. F., Habib, M. P., and Quan, S. F.: Pressure support compensation for inspiratory work due to endotracheal tubes and demand continuous positive airway pressure. Chest, 93:499, 1988.
109. Shapiro, B. A.: When is the work of breathing clinically significant? (Editorial.) Crit. Care Med., 18:681, 1990.
110. Christopher, K. L., et al.: Demand and continuous flow intermittent mandatory ventilation systems. Chest, 87:625, 1985.
111. Chatburn, R. L.: A new system for understanding mechanical ventilators. Respir. Care, 36:1123, 1991.
112. Kanak, R., Fahey, P. J., and Vanderwarf, C.: Oxygen cost of breathing. Chest, 87:126, 1985.
113. Brochard, L., Pluskwa, F., and Lemaire, F.: Improved efficacy of spontaneous breathing with inspiratory pressure support. Am. Rev. Respir. Dis., 136:411, 1987.
114. Kacmarek, R. M.: The role of pressure support ventilation in reducing work of breathing. Respir. Care, 33:99, 1988.
115. Brochard, L., Harf, A., Lorino, H., and Lemaire, F.: Inspiratory pressure support prevents diaphragmatic fatigue during weaning from mechanical ventilation. Am. Rev. Respir. Dis., 139:513, 1989.
116. Gibney, R. T. N., Wilson, R. S., and Pontoppidan, H.: Comparison of work of breathing on high gas flow and demand valve continuous pressure airway systems. Chest, 82:692, 1982.
117. Cane, R. D., and Shapiro, B. A.: Mechanical ventilatory support. JAMA, 254:87, 1985.
118. Weg, J. G., and Haas, C. F.: Safe intrahospital transport of critically ill ventilatory-dependent patients. Chest, 96:631, 1989.
119. Vincent, J. L., Dufaye, P., and Kahn, R. J.: A complete system for transportation of critically ill patients with acute respiratory failure. Acute Care, 10:33, 1984.
120. Smith, I., Fleming, S., and Cernaianu, A.: Mishaps during transport from the intensive care unit. Crit. Care Med., 18:278, 1990.
121. Insel, J., et al.: Cardiovascular changes during transport of critically ill and postoperative patients. Crit. Care Med., 14:539, 1986.
122. Indeck, M., Peterson, S., Smith, J., and Brotman, S.: Risk, cost and benefit of transporting ICU patients for special studies. J. Trauma, 28:1020, 1988.
123. Viale, J. P., et al.: Additional inspiratory work in intubated patients breathing with continuous positive airway pressure systems. Anesthesiology, 63:536, 1985.
124. Marini, J. J.: The role of the inspiratory circuit in the work of breathing during mechanical ventilation. Respir. Care, 32:419, 1987.
125. Elpern, E. H., et al.: The noninvasive respiratory care unit—patterns of use and financial implications. Chest, 99:205, 1991.
126. Elpern, E. H., et al.: Long-term outcomes for elderly survivors of prolonged ventilator assistance. Chest, 96:1120, 1989.
127. Conference on Home Oxygen Therapy: Problems in pre-

scribing and supply oxygen for Medicare patients. Am. Rev. Respir. Dis., *134*:340, 1986.
128. Report of the Medical Research Council Working Party: long-term domiciliary oxygen therapy in chronic cor pulmonale complicating bronchitis and emphysema. Lancet, *1*:681, 1981.
129. Nocturnal Oxygen Therapy Trial Group. Continuous and nocturnal oxygen therapy in hypoxemic chronic obstructive lung disease: a clinical trial. Ann. Intern. Med., *93*:391, 1980.
130. Neff, T. A., and Petty, T. L.: Long-term continuous oxygen therapy in chronic airway obstruction: mortality in relation to cor pulmonale, hypoxemia and hypercapnia. Ann. Intern. Med., *72*:621, 1970.
131. Weitzenblum, E., et al.: Long-term oxygen therapy can reverse the progression of pulmonary hypertension in patients with chronic obstructive pulmonary disease. Am. Rev. Respir. Dis., *131*:493, 1985.
132. New problems in supply, reimbursement and certification of medical necessity for long-term oxygen therapy: consensus conference report. Respir. Care, *35*:990, 1990.
133. Escourrou, J. L., Delaperche, M. F., and Visseaux, A.: Reliability of pulse oximetry during exercise in pulmonary patients. Chest, *97*:635, 1990.
134. Adamo, J. P., et al.: The Cleveland Clinic's initial experience with transtracheal oxygen therapy. Respir. Care, *35*:153, 1990.
135. Nelson, C. M., et al.: Clinical use of pulse oximetry to determine oxygen prescriptions for patients with hypoxemia. Respir. Care, *31*:673, 1986.
136. Carlin, B. W., Clausen, J. L., and Ries, A. L.: The use of cutaneous oximetry in the prescription of long term oxygen therapy. Chest, *94*:239, 1988.
137. Golish, J., and McCarthy, K.: Limitations of pulse oximetry in detecting hypoxemia. (Abstract.) Chest, *94(Suppl.)*:50, 1988.
138. Newton, D., and Stephenson, A.: Effect of physiotherapy on pulmonary function. Lancet, *2*:228, 1978.
139. Cochrane, G. M., Webber, B. A., and Clarke, S. W.: Effects of sputum on pulmonary function. Br. Med. J., *2*:1181, 1977.
140. Askanazi, J., et al.: Nutrition and the Respiratory System. Crit. Care Med., *10*:163, 1982.
141. Branson, R. D., and Hurst, J. M.: Nutrition and respiratory function: food for thought. Respir. Care, *33*:89, 1988.
142. Pasuika, P. S., Bistrain, B. R., Benotti, P. N., and Blackburn, G. L.: The risks of surgery in obese patients. Ann. Intern. Med., *104*:540, 1986.
143. Bedell, G. N., Wilson, W. R., and Seebohm, P. M.: Pulmonary function in obese persons. J. Clin. Invest., *37*:1059, 1958.
144. Mishoe, S. C.: The diagnosis and treatment of sleep apnea syndrome. Respir. Care, *32*:183, 1987.
145. Strohl, K. P., and Redline, S.: Nasal CPAP therapy, upper airway muscle activation, and obstructive sleep apnea. Am. Rev. Respir. Dis., *134*:555, 1986.
146. Sanders, M. H.: Nasal CPAP effect on patterns of sleep apnea. Chest, *86*:839, 1984.
147. Bone, R. C., and Balk, R. A.: Noninvasive respiratory care unit. Chest, *93*:390, 1988.
148. Douglass, P. S., Rosen, R. L., Butler, P. W., and Bone, R. C.: DRG payment for long-term ventilator patients. Chest, *91*:413, 1987.
149. Gracey, D. R., et al.: Financial implications of prolonged ventilator care of medicare patients under the prospective payment system. Chest, *91*:424, 1987.
150. Cordasco, E. M., Jr., Sivak, E. D., and Perez-Trepichio, A.: Demographics of long term ventilator-dependent patients outside the intensive care unit. Cleve. Clin. J. Med., *58*:505, 1991.
151. Stoller, J.: Caring for the hospitalized ventilator-dependent patient outside the ICU: united and stand, or divided and fall? Cleve. Clin. J. Med., *58*:537, 1991.
152. Nochomovitz, M., Montenegro, H., Parran, S., and Daly, B.: Placement alternatives for ventilator-dependent patients outside the intensive care unit. Respir. Care, *36*:199, 1991.
153. Strumpf, D. A., et al.: An evaluation of the Respironics bipap bi-level CPAP device for delivery of assisted ventilation. Respir. Care, *35*:415, 1990.
154. Sanders, M. H., and Kern, N.: Obstructive sleep apnea treated by independently adjusted inspiratory and expiratory positive airway pressures via nasal mask. Chest, *98*:317, 1990.
155. Fishman, D. B., and Petty, T. L.: Physical, symptomatic, and psychological improvement in patients receiving comprehensive care for chronic airway obstruction. J. Chronic Dis., *24*:775, 1971.
156. Sonne, L. J., and Davis, J. A.: Increased exercise performance in patients with severe COPD following inspiratory resistive training. Chest, *4*:436, 1981.
157. Belmon, M. J., and Mittan, C.: Ventilatory muscle training improves exercise capacity in chronic obstructive pulmonary disease patients. Am. Rev. Respir. Dis., *121*:273, 1980.
158. Holden, D., et al.: The impact of a rehabilitation program on functional status of patients with chronic lung disease. Respir. Care, *35*:332, 1990.
159. Hodgkin, J. E.: Home care and pulmonary rehabilitation. *In* Current Respiratory Care. Edited by R. M. Kacmarek and J. K. Stoller. Philadelphia, B. C. Decker, 1988, p. 216.
160. Hastings, D.: The AARC's model quality assurance plan. ARRC Times, *12*:25, 1988.
161. Hess, D., Horney, D., and Snyder, T.: Medication-delivery performance of eight small-volume, handheld nebulizers: effects of diluent volume, gas flowrate, and nebulizer model. Respir. Care, *34*:717, 1989.
162. Alvine, G. F., Rodgers, P., Fitzsimmons, K. M., and Ahrens, R. C.: Disposable jet nebulizers. Chest, *101*:316, 1992.

Section Three

THE CARDIOVASCULAR SYSTEM

Chapter 26

DETERMINANTS OF CARDIAC FUNCTION

PHILIP F. BINKLEY

Accurate recognition and measurement of determinants of cardiac function are essential for the appropriate diagnosis and therapeutic management of the critically ill patient. Accurate recognition of abnormalities of cardiac performance is necessary to determine the cause of overall systemic hemodynamic decompensation. Similarly, precise definition of the nature of cardiac dysfunction is essential, given that varying cardiovascular disease states may require diametrically opposed modalities of therapy in the face of similar manifestations of systemic hemodynamic decompensation.

This chapter outlines the primary determinants of cardiac performance in a manner related to the clinical syndromes that are most likely to influence these determinants. Specifically, following an initial discussion of such variables, an outline of the clinically relevant disease states that most closely influence these variables is provided. These disease states constitute the predisposing conditions that may ultimately lead to the necessity for an intensive care admission or dictate further intervention for the ICU patient. In the ICU phase of illness, hemodynamic focus on specific techniques that are applicable to the serial evaluation of determinants of cardiac performance guarantees optimum patient management. Emphasis is placed on those parameters that are most suitable for the sequential evaluation of the patient, as is necessary in critical care management. Both standard methods of evaluation as well as newer techniques currently under development are discussed, because the latter may ultimately play a significant role in further patient management strategies. Finally, the utility of these various techniques for the evaluation of the patient following discharge from the ICU is reviewed. Thus, it may be seen that appropriate recognition of the determinants of ventricular performance and their influence by disease states may lead to an intelligent selection of diagnostic techniques for the evaluation of the patient and the assessment of the progress of therapeutic intervention.

PRINCIPAL DETERMINANTS OF CARDIAC PERFORMANCE

The essential determinants of cardiac performance as they are recognized today were perhaps initially most clearly outlined by the work of E. H. Starling.[1] Although many of Starling's concepts were based on the fundamental work of numerous investigators who preceded him, his demonstration of these principles and his proposal of a unified concept of the factors governing ventricular performance constitute a major foundation in the understanding of cardiovascular performance. Although, as discussed later in this chapter, these concepts have been modified in many respects, they still provide the essential paradigm for the major variables that must be examined in any assessment of ventricular performance.

Starling's work involved an elaborate model of the heart as it was linked to the native circulation.[1] In this model, however, the return of blood from the venous system to the heart, as well as the resistance against which the heart was forced to contract, could be modified. Through variation of venous return, or the resistance of the systemic circulation, Starling and his co-workers noted that the performance of the ventricle could be significantly altered. Thus arose the concepts of **preload** and **afterload**, which will be discussed in greater detail.

The third major element determining cardiac performance was implied by Starling in his analysis of the energetics of the ventricle in this model of the circulation. Specifically, it is the **intrinsic contractility,** or what has been termed the inotropy of the ventricle.[2,3] The inotropic state of the ventricle is defined as the innate ability of the myocardial muscle to perform contractile work. It is a quality distinct from the preload and afterload states of the ventricle. As will be seen, it is often extremely difficult to distinguish whether changes in ventricular performance arise from changes in preload or afterload or are in fact due to some change in inotropic state of the ventricle. Such a distinction, however, may be essential in both the diagnosis of a variety of disease states and the assessment of various therapeutic interventions.

Preload: The Initial Conditions of Myocardial Contraction

The preload of the ventricle may be considered to comprise the initial conditions that exist before the onset of active muscle contraction.[2-9] These initial conditions play a major role in determining the manner in which the ventricle will perform as it encounters the load imposed during the subsequent contraction. Classically, the preload of the ventricle determines the initial fiber length of the myocardial muscle, which in turn determines the overlap of actin myosin filaments in the individual myocyte.[3,4] This concept was proposed by Starling in his original experiments, although he had no knowledge of the ultrastructure of the myocardium. However, his observations regarding the energetics of the intact heart under different preload conditions and the augmented performance of myocardial fi-

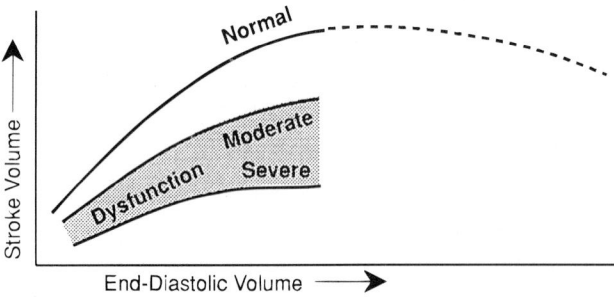

Fig. 26-1. Relation of end-diastolic pressure or volume (preload) to ventricular function. In the normal ventricle, increasing preload leads to a progressive augmentation of ventricular function. After an optimal preload has been attained, a plateau in ventricular performance is noted. With further increases in preload, a decrease in ventricular performance or the so-called descending limb of the Starling curve is observed (dashed line—see text). The curve relating ventricular function and preload becomes progressively depressed with increasingly severe ventricular dysfunction. (Adapted from Binkley, P. F., and Boudoulas, H.: Measurement of myocardial inotropy. In Cardiotonic Drugs: A Clinical Survey. Edited by C. V. Leier. New York, Marcel Dekker, 1986, p. 5.)

bers with increasing ventricular volumes led him to conclude that there was some favorable effect on the contractile elements of the myocytes with increasing muscle fiber length. As he stated,

> So we must conclude that the governor mechanism, in virtue of which the heart is able to do more or less work, according to the amount of blood which has to be sent on and the resistance to the flow presented by the arterial pressure, must be situated in the walls of the heart itself and presumably in the muscle fibers of which these are composed.[1]

These observations and subsequent detailed analysis of the ultrastructure of the myocardium have led to the now familiar concept of actin-myosin filament overlap.[2-4] Simplistically, as the individual myocyte is tretched, the overlap of actin and myosin filaments increases. During active muscle contraction, the actin-myosin filaments form cross bridges in the presence of free calcium, which results in shortening of the myocyte and the myocardial muscle. Thus, an increase in the overlap of these filaments leads to enhanced myocardial contractility and augmented performance of the intact ventricle.

This effect is displayed in the classic curve relating ventricular performance to its degree of filling during relaxation or diastole (Fig. 26-1). If some index of ventricular performance, such as stroke volume, is plotted on the vertical axis and ventricular volume is plotted on the horizontal axis, it is seen that there is a steady increase in ventricular performance with increased diastolic filling of the ventricle. This occurs until a point at which a plateau is reached in the curve, after which, ventricular performance does not improve further. According to Starling's original theory, if ventricular filling continues past this plateau phase, ventricular function will in fact decline.[1] In terms of the relationship between actin and myosin filaments, this would represent a decrease in the number of actin-myosin filaments that overlap as the individual myocytes are stretched to an even greater length. Much controversy still exists regarding this so-called "descending limb of the Starling curve." As discussed later in this chapter, in the clinical setting, this phenomenon may relate more importantly to the relationship between preload and afterload conditions encountered by the ventricle in the intact circulation rather than to a disadvantageous relationship between the actin and myosin filaments.[8] Furthermore, it is important to note that the true preload of the ventricle is the volume rather than the pressure encountered at the end of ventricular diastolic filling. Because the optimization of muscle length at the end of ventricular filling augments the subsequent ventricular contraction, it stands to reason that volume, which depends on the muscle length, is the most accurate measure of ventricular preload. In certain disease states, listed later, the ventricular volume at the end of diastole may be associated with a much higher diastolic pressure than is seen in a normal ventricle. The true preload of both ventricles, however, may be the same. This becomes important in the clinical setting, because many of the techniques used to monitor the critically ill patient rely on estimates of end-diastolic pressure rather than volume and thus may lead to misperceptions regarding the preload status of the ventricle.

The dependence of the ventricle on preload in determining its contractile performance emphasizes the importance of venous return as an integral variable determining ventricular function.[8,10,11] In the context of current models of ventricular performance, the heart in fact functions as a demand pump. This was indeed the concept proposed by Starling, who believed that ever increasing venous return would be accompanied by ventricular dilatation and enhanced contractility, thus continuing to circulate the augmented venous return. The importance of venous return has been reexamined and reemphasized in more recent studies, such as those by Guyton and others.[8,10,11] The cardiac output of the normal ventricle is in fact determined by the volume of systemic venous return. As has been demonstrated in animal models, vasodilating influences that fail to augment venous return or in fact decrease venous return are accompanied by significant decreases in performance of the normal ventricle.[11] In contrast, as ventricular failure develops, myocardial performance becomes more dependent on afterload, and preload becomes relatively fixed (see following discussion). In this case vasodilating influences may beneficially affect ventricular performance because augmented forward stroke volume is accompanied by either little change or in fact an increase in venous return. Thus, in the construct of the Starling model, the heart functions much like a demand pump in its normal state. It has the capacity to eject the volume of blood that is returned to it by the systemic venous circulation. In the absence of an adequate return in the normally functioning ventricle, severe decreases in cardiac output may result.

Disease States Influencing Preload Conditions

The preceding discussion clearly points out the integral role that preload conditions play in determining cardiac

Table 26–1. Abnormal Preload States

Impaired relaxation of the ventricle
  Systemic hypertension
  Aortic outflow obstruction
    Valvular, subvalvular and supravalvular aortic stenosis
  Hypertrophic cardiomyopathy
  Myocardial ischemia
  Hyperkalemia
Impaired ventricular filling
  Pericardial disease
    Constrictive pericarditis
    Pericardial tamponade
  Valvular inflow obstruction
    Mitral stenosis
    Tricuspid stenosis
  Obstruction of venous return
    Superior vena cava syndrome
    PEEP
  Infiltrative disease of the myocardium
    Amyloidosis
  Hypovolemia
Elevated preload states
  Ventricular dilatation
    Dilated cardiomyopathy
    Ischemic cardiomyopathy
    Myocarditis
  Regurgitant valvular lesions
    Mitral regurgitation
    Tricuspid regurgitation
    Aortic insufficiency

PEEP, positive end-expiratory pressure.

performance. A variety of cardiovascular states exert their major pathophysiologic influence through derangements in ventricular preload (end-diastolic volume). As an example, recent studies have indicated that as many as 40% of patients presenting to the emergency room with symptoms of congestive heart failure are noted to have abnormalities in ventricular filling rather than in ventricular contraction or ejection.[12] As noted in Table 26-1, disease states that influence preload conditions may be segregated into three broad categories. The first category comprises those diseases in which normal ventricular volumes at the end of diastole may be obtained only with abnormally high ventricular pressures. As noted previously, the actual preload of the ventricle is the end-diastolic volume. Thus, these disease states may obtain normal preload only through abnormally high ventricular filling pressures. Classic among these groups of disorders are diseases associated with abnormal hypertrophy of the ventricular muscle such as that encountered in long-standing essential hypertension, valvular obstructive disease such as aortic stenosis, and that class of primary muscle diseases or cardiomyopathies characterized by hypertrophy of the ventricular muscle (the hypertrophic cardiomyopathies).[13–16] In addition, myocardial ischemia may also significantly impair relaxation of ventricular muscle, resulting in abnormally high pressures during ventricular diastole.[17]

The next major classification of diseases affecting preload of the ventricle comprises those that impair ventricular filling.[13,18,19] Classic among these is pericardial constriction.[18] Fibrosis and scarring of the pericardium limit adequate filling of the ventricle, thus preventing an adequate level of preload, which may ultimately impair ventricular performance. To a degree, this phenomenon is also observed in pericardial tamponade, in which tense pericardial effusions impair ventricular filling. Mimicking much of the physiology of pericardial constriction are the infiltrative cardiomyopathies, which lead to myocardial restriction, such as amyloid infiltration of the myocardium.[16] Conditions such as amyloid infiltration of the myocardium may lead to so-called myocardial restriction, which again impairs ventricular diastolic filling in much the same way as pericardial constriction. Finally, ventricular filling may be disturbed by disease states extrinsic to the heart itself. Conditions such as pericardial constriction or hypovolemia are associated with a reduction of venous return to the ventricle and lead to a limitation of adequate ventricular preload and as a result diminish ventricular performance.[20]

The third major classification includes disease states in which abnormally high levels of ventricular preload are required to maintain normal ventricular performance. In particular, this includes disease states leading to dilatation and failure of the left ventricle. As a compensatory response to impaired ventricular systolic performance—which may arise from myocardial infarction, primary muscle diseases such as idiopathic dilated cardiomyopathy or myocarditis, or long-standing regurgitant valvular lesions such as aortic or mitral insufficiency—the left ventricle dilates, thus augmenting ventricular systolic function by the Starling mechanism. In these states, an elevated left ventricular diastolic pressure is often required to maintain an adequate level of preload required for a compensatory increase in ventricular systolic function.[15] This is of importance clinically in that patients with ventricular failure of any cause may require a significantly higher end-diastolic pressure than normal ventricles to maintain normal function. As a consequence, lowering ventricular diastolic pressures to levels in the normal range will prevent the compensatory increase in ventricular function that arises as a result of the Starling mechanism and may in fact lead to a deterioration in ventricular performance.

It is thus seen that the variation of ventricular preload may profoundly influence ventricular performance in a variety of disease states. An awareness of the preload characteristics of a given cardiovascular disease and the manner in which variations in preload may in fact compensate for abnormal ventricular function is essential in the management of the critically ill patient.

Afterload: The Resistance to Ventricular Ejection

The second major element determining ventricular performance consists of the load encountered by the ventricle as it initiates active contraction.[2,4–7,21–28] This load, termed afterload, is analogous to the force encountered by an isolated muscle strip as it begins to contract.[21–23] The classic example demonstrating this concept consists of a muscle strip that is attached to a lever from which is suspended a certain amount of weight. The weight, which the muscle strip must lift as it contracts, constitutes the afterload. This concept was incorporated in the intact ventricular model of Starling in the form of a variable resistance that could be imposed in the systemic circulation.[1] Thus, the force against which the intact ventricle must contract constitutes its afterload. As discussed later, the determination of which parameters most precisely describe afterload in the intact circulation remains somewhat controversial.

The relationship between afterload and ventricular function may again be classically defined in the experiments of Starling. As noted in Figure 26-2, if some index of ventricular performance is plotted on the vertical axis (e.g., shortening of an isolated muscle or stroke volume of the intact ventricle) and afterload is plotted on the horizontal axis, one sees an almost exponential decline in ventricular performance with increasing afterload. With increasing levels of afterload, a point is ultimately reached at which the muscle strip can no longer contract or the ventricle can no longer eject volume. This point is defined as an isovolumetric contraction of the ventricle (isometric contraction in the isolated muscle strip) in which the ventricular afterload is equal to the force that the contracting ventricular muscle can generate.

The magnitude of afterload that the actively contracting ventricle can sustain is related to the intrinsic contractility of the ventricle.[23-28] A normal ventricle can sustain relatively high levels of afterload before ventricular performance declines. Thus, fairly marked elevations in systolic pressure are required before a normally functioning ventricle will fail. In the setting of ventricular failure, however, relatively small elevations in ventricular afterload may lead to marked reductions in ventricular performance (Fig. 26-3). In fact, the magnitude of afterload that a ventricle can sustain is one of the more recent indices of myocardial contractility, as discussed later in this chapter.

The accurate definition of afterload in the intact circulation varies from fairly simplistic concepts relating systolic pressure to ventricular performance to more sophisticated models that incorporate wall tension and wall stress. In simple terms, the afterload may be regarded as the pressure encountered by the ventricle during its contraction. This is probably accurate when comparing two ventricles

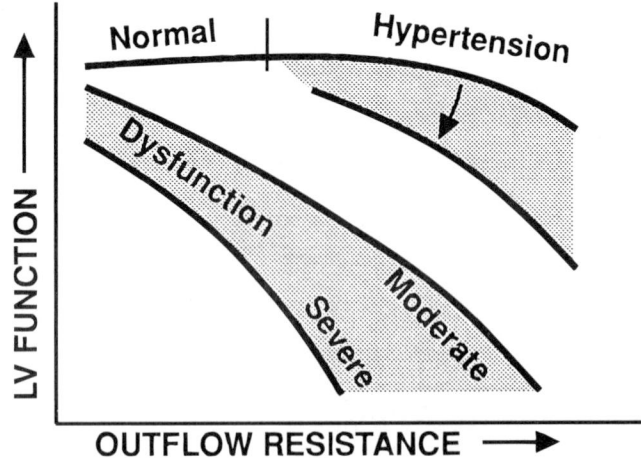

Fig. 26-3. Sensitivity of normal and failing ventricles to ventricular afterload. The normal ventricle can continue to function at a normal level until very high levels of afterload are encountered. In disease states such as hypertension or with abnormal systolic function of the ventricle, increasing sensitivity to elevated afterload is noted. Levels of afterload that do not impair function of the normal ventricle may lead to significant reductions in ventricular performance in these disease states. (Adapted from Binkley, P. F., and Boudoulas, H.: Measurement of myocardial inotropy. In Cardiotonic Drugs: A Clinical Survey. Edited by C. V. Leier. New York, Marcel Dekker, 1986, p. 5.)

that are equal in terms of all other factors. The basic law of LaPlace, however, more accurately indicates that the total load on the ventricle is directly related to the diameter of the ventricular chamber and the thickness of the ventricular wall.[2,5-7] This thus defines the wall stress on the ventricle, which may be thought of as the force per unit cross-sectional area of the ventricle. Therefore, ventricles of different diameters that encounter the same amount of systolic pressure in fact differ in the amount of stress they sustain during contraction. Similarly, ventricles of the same diameter but differing myocardial thickness will also differ in the amount of stress they sustain, despite equivalent systolic pressures. The ventricle having greater wall thickness will distribute the forces encountered during contraction over a greater amount of muscle mass and thus sustain a lesser degree of stress. This in fact accounts for the compensatory mechanism of ventricular hypertrophy that evolves in a state of chronic ventricular pressure overload, thus allowing a normalization of ventricular wall stress.[13] It can be seen that measurements of ventricular wall stress in fact are more accurate determinants of ventricular afterload than measurement of pressure alone. However, if serial measurements of ventricular function are performed in the same ventricule when dimension or thickness of the ventricle is not likely to change, a more simple measurement such as systolic ventricular pressure may adequately reflect afterload because other determinants of afterload are not changing.

Afterload of the ventricle varies with time throughout ventricular systole. The initial pressure and volume encountered by the ventricle at the onset of ejection differ from that encountered at the midpoint of ejection and at

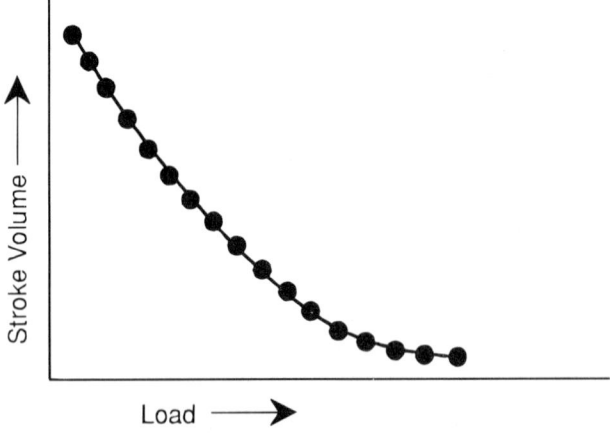

Fig. 26-2. Relation of afterload and velocity of shortening of the myocardium. With increasing afterload, there is decreasing velocity of shortening. With extreme levels of afterload, there is no shortening of muscle and an isometric contraction occurs.

Table 26-2. Abnormal Afterload States

Valvular disease
 Aortic outflow obstruction (see Table 26-1)
Systemic hypertension
 Essential hypertension
 Renovascular hypertension
 Pheochromocytoma
 Coarctation

the end of systole. Ventricular wall stress varies throughout the course of ventricular ejection. Therefore, afterload itself is a variable parameter throughout ventricular ejection.[29] Selection of a particular point in the cycle of ventricular ejection that is reflective of ventricular afterload and is related to ventricular contractility therefore is an important consideration when deriving various parameters of ventricular performance. The pressure or stress at end systole is often chosen as an index of afterload in various parameters of ventricular contractility because, for theoretic reasons, it more purely reflects afterload and depends less on patterns of ventricular ejection and variations in ventricular contractility that may occur as a result of preload conditions. These factors will be discussed in more detail when serial measures of ventricular performance are considered.

A variety of disease states are characterized by either long-standing elevations in afterload, which ultimately contribute to ventricular failure, or inappropriate elevations in afterload given the reduced performance of the ventricle.[13,15,30] As indicated in Table 26-2, among the most common disease states leading to chronic elevations in afterload are lesions obstructing ventricular outflow such as valvular aortic stenosis or the less common subvalvular and supravalvular aortic stenoses. Second, the chronic elevation in afterload posed by long-standing systemic hypertension will similarly impair ventricular systolic performance and ultimately lead to ventricular failure. Finally, in any state in which ventricular systolic performance is impaired, such as primary cardiomyopathy or ventricular dysfunction that is due to ischemic disease, the afterload imposed by the systemic circulation may be inappropriately matched for the level of ventricular performance.[16] As noted previously, a dilated ventricle will sustain a larger degree of stress, according to the law of LaPlace, for any given level of blood pressure because it is functioning with a greater than normal diameter throughout its ejection phase. Thus, in such a failing ventricle, even a normal systemic blood pressure may represent an elevated afterload.

The level of afterload is an important determinant in both short-term and long-term ventricular performance. Aberrations in afterload conditions may ultimately lead to significant impairment of ventricular performance in a variety of disease states. Thus, in addition to a recognition of the preload conditions of the ventricle, accurate description of the afterload state of the ventricle is essential in delineating the pathophysiology of the individual patient as well as guiding appropriate therapy for that patient.

Inotropy: Intrinsic Contractility of the Ventricle

The third major determinant of ventricular performance is the intrinsic contractility of the myocardium independent of the influence of preload and afterload conditions. This property of the ventricle, known as inotropy, is determined by the biochemical factors that govern the contraction of the individual myocytes.[1-9,31-33]

The inotropic state of the ventricle is in essence related to the availability of intracellular calcium and the subsequent influence of calcium on actin-myosin coupling.[31-33] Thus, interventions that tend to increase inotropy are in general those that by a variety of mechanisms enhance the availability of intracellular calcium. Examples are the catecholemines such as dobutamine and dopamine, which increase the formation of cyclic adenosine monophosphate (AMP), which then promotes the phosphorylation of a number of membrane transport proteins, which increase intracellular calcium concentration. Similarly, a newer class of agents termed the phosphodiesterase inhibitors such as amrinone or milrinone increases the concentration of cyclic AMP by inhibiting the breakdown of this compound, thus again augmenting membrane transport protein phosphorylation.[34]

In the truest sense, inotropy is independent of the loading conditions of the ventricle. This may be illustrated again in the isolated muscle strip, as shown in Figure 26-4. If tension of the contracting muscle is measured on the Y axis and a range of afterloads is plotted on the X axis, a baseline curve relating afterload and tension development may be generated. If this muscle strip is now exposed to catecholamine stimulation, the entire curve relating tension and afterload will be shifted upward, indicating an increased contractile state of the muscle. Thus, under these new conditions, with the same level of afterload, a greater degree of tension is developed with active muscle contraction. The improved performance of the muscle may be ascribed purely to an increase in intrinsic contractility or inotropy of the muscle rather than to any change in loading conditions.

In the clinical setting, it may be difficult to segregate

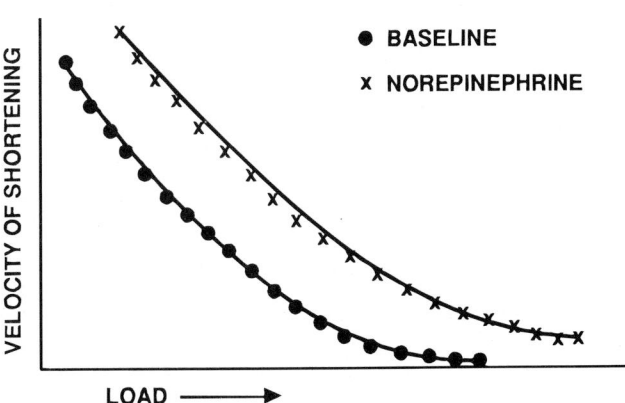

Fig. 26-4. Relation of afterload to shortening velocity of ventricular muscle with varying degrees of inotropy. With the positive inotropic stimulation of norepinephrine, the curve relating performance of the muscle to afterload is shifted up, indicating enhanced contractility. (Adapted from Binkley, P. F., and Boudoulas, H.: Measurement of myocardial inotropy. In Cardiotonic Drugs: A Clinical Survey. Edited by C. V. Leier. New York, Marcel Dekker, 1986, p. 5.)

Table 26-3. Changes in Inotropic State

Ischemic heart disease
Cardiomyopathy
    Idiopathic
    Toxic
    Metabolic
Myocarditis

---

changes in intrinsic contractility of the muscle from changes in ventricular performance that result from alterations in loading conditions.[35,36] Nevertheless, such distinctions may be of great importance in diagnosing the cause of ventricular failure and in planning the appropriate strategy for the treatment of such failure. Ideally, one would wish to have an index of ventricular contractility that segregates loading conditions from the inotropic state of the ventricle. Recently, a variety of parameters of ventricular performance have been proposed that appear to be relatively insensitive to loading conditions and conversely are influenced only by the contractile state of the ventricle. A number of these are summarized in the subsequent sections of this chapter. Although many such parameters have been proposed, and a few appear to attain the goal of accurately distinguishing inotropy from loading conditions, none are perfect, and in many situations, the question as to whether changes in ventricular performance may be ascribed to loading conditions or to the intrinsic contractility of the myocardium remains unanswered.

The disease states that may primarily affect inotropy are summarized in Table 26-3.[2-7] Myocardial ischemia, either in the form of threatened myocardial infarction or completed myocardial infarction, may reduce the capacity of the myocardium to contract in a normal fashion, in essence, reducing the inotropic state of the ventricle. The various cardiomyopathies are characterized by an intrinsic abnormality in the contractility of the myocardium.[16] This arises either in the idiopathic cardiomyopathies or in those that appear to be due to toxic or metabolic factors such as alcoholic cardiomyopathy. Similarly, viral myocarditis is associated with a profound reduction in the intrinsic contractility of the ventricle leading to, in many cases, irreversible ventricular failure.

These three major fractors—preload, afterload, and contractility—are the primary determinants of ventricular performance. Although clearly delineated for the purposes of this discussion, all three factors may be simultaneously affected by a given disease process, thus exerting their separate influences on ventricular performance. A classic example is the patient with acute myocardial ischemia who simultaneously has diminished contractility of the myocardium with elevated preload that is due to diastolic abnormalities of the ventricle and potentially elevated afterload that is due to reflex increases in systemic vascular resistance. In such cases, determining which is the primary influence on ventricular performance and which are secondary or reflex changes may be critical in the successful management of the patient.

Fallacy of the Descending Limb of the Starling Curve

As noted previously, the original Starling model described a plateau in the relation between preload and ventricular performance, which was followed by a descending limb in which further increases in preload resulted in a reduction in ventricular performance. This was ultimately ascribed to a reduction in the overlap between actin and myosin filaments as the muscle fibers are stretched beyond an optimal length. Recent evidence has suggested that, although a so-called descending limb of the Starling curve may exist in the clinical setting, this may be due to a different mechanism than originally proposed by Starling.[36-38] Observations in animal models have indicated that with increasing preload a limit is reached in the mid-wall sarcomere length of the myocardium that does not supersede the optimal overlap between actin and myosin filaments.[38] Therefore, some factor other than "overstretch" of the sarcomere is responsible for the descending limb of the Starling curve. In most cases, clinically, this situation appears to represent what has been termed afterload mismatch with limited preload reserve.[8-11] As ventricular failure develops, there is progressive dilatation of the ventricle with augmentation of ventricular preload to enhance cardiac contractility by the Starling mechanism. A point is reached at which no further preload augmentation may occur, either as a result of the geometric limitations of ventricular dilatation or the limits of the availability of venous return to augment ventricular preload. At this point, no further preload is available to augment ventricular contractility, and any increase in ventricular afterload will result in a decline in ventricular performance. The result is an apparent descending limb of the Starling curve. This situation defines afterload mismatch with limited preload reserve. In very severe cases of ventricular dysfunction, this situation may exist even in the resting state. The importance in the recognition of this phenomenon lies in the realization that, in such settings, afterload reduction rather than preload reduction may have a profound and beneficial influence on ventricular performance. In fact, this mechanism provides much of the basis for afterload reduction therapy in severe ventricular failure.

RIGHT VENTRICULAR FUNCTION

Because of technical limitations, information regarding the determinants of right ventricular performance has lagged behind that available for the left ventricle. With recent advances in a variety of noninvasive imaging modalities, however, an increasing amount of information is now available regarding the performance of the right ventricle. Furthermore, right ventricular performance has been found to be a major determinant in overall circulatory function.[39-45] As an example, right ventricular infarction may be a devastating complication of ischemic heart disease, and dysfunction of the right ventricle may contribute to the symptoms of congestive heart failure in the dilated cardiomyopathies.

Until the development of techniques such as radionuclide ventriculography (described in greater detail later in this chapter), which permit accurate in vivo assessment of right ventricular volumes and contractility, clinical examination of the determinants of right ventricular function were limited.[40-48] Given, however, that many of the isolated heart models employed by Starling and his contemporaries to describe the influence of loading conditions on ventricular performance in fact isolated the right rather than the left ventricle for examination, it is perhaps not surprising that modern in-vivo studies have demonstrated that the right ventricle obeys the principles of afterload, preload, and inotropy discussed previously for the left ventricle.[1] Curves relating right ventricular pressure and volumes have been generated that demonstrate preload and afterload sensitivity of the right ventricle similar to that observed for the left ventricle. In this case, preload is determined by the systemic venous return, and ventricular afterload is the pressure and resistance imposed by the pulmonary circulation. With the various techniques now available for examination of right ventricular volumes, the clinical importance of afterload and preload in governing right ventricular performance is increasingly apparent.

For example, recent investigations have shown that right ventricular ejection fraction and stroke volume may be significantly reduced by the application of positive end-expiratory pressure (PEEP) during assisted ventilation.[49,50] The increased pulmonary pressures attendant to this form of ventilation resulted in elevated pulmonary artery pressures, which in fact represent elevated right ventricular afterload, which may diminish right ventricular function. The degree to which right ventricular function is impaired by PEEP depends on the baseline right ventricular function. Otherwise normal right ventricles, however, may be capable of sustaining PEEP with little change in stroke volume, whereas abnormal right ventricles may show marked decline in stroke volume with PEEP. Therefore, the right ventricle exhibits a sensitivity to afterload much like that of the left ventricle, and this sensitivity increases with diminished intrinsic contractility of the right ventricle in a fashion analogous to that seen in the left ventricle. In fact, this sensitivity may be greater in the right than left ventricle, given the differences in structure of these two chambers. The relatively thin-walled and less muscular right ventricle is structured so that it possesses a relatively large surface/volume ratio.[51] It is thus "designed" simplistically as a "volume pump" rather than a "pressure pump." The muscular left ventricle in contrast can sustain much higher pressures and functions more as the latter type of pump. The importance of these differences in the two ventricles in defining the in vivo determinants of ventricle performance is an object of further clinical investigation.

Although the function of the right or left ventricle is often examined and described as if each ventricle were isolated, the two ventricles in fact interact in such a way that the functional state of one ventricle may have a significant influence on the performance of the other. This phenomenon of ventricular interdependence has been described in both experimental models and the clinical setting.[51] Berheim originally demonstrated that changes in left ventricular volume appeared to result in compression of the right ventricle and consequent systemic venous congestion.[51] More recent investigations have shown that changes in the filling volume of one ventricle may lead to marked changes in the diastolic pressure volume relations of the other ventricle as well as to significant changes in systolic function of that ventricle.[51] Further investigations have shown that large portions of the right ventricular free wall may be transected or damaged with preservation of systolic function of the right ventricle, implying that left ventricular contraction may in some way assist right ventricular systolic function.[51]

The mechanisms accounting for this ventricular interdependence remain incompletely defined. The simple fact that the two ventricles are connected in series accounts for a portion of this interaction so that both forward flow from the right to left ventricle and increased diastolic pressures transmitted from the left to the right ventricle may be important variables connecting ventricular performance. Even more important is the role of the interventricular septum in mediating ventricular interdependence. Several investigations have demonstrated that volume or pressure overload of one ventricle may lead to a geometric distortion of the interventricular septum, which then results in significant changes in systolic and diastolic performance of the other ventricle.[51] In addition, the pericardium appears to play a role in governing the interaction of ventricular performance. Although ventricular interdependence may be demonstrated in the absence of pericardial constraint, the presence of an intact pericardium appears to magnify the interdependence of ventricular performance.

In the clinical setting, the phenomenon of ventricular interdependence may be observed in both normal physiologic responses as well as disease states. The recognized decrease in left ventricular stroke volume that occurs with inspiration may in part result from diminished left ventricular diastolic function and diastolic filling, which may be ascribed to the influence of the increase in right ventricular volume as systemic venous return is augmented. This mechanism appears to play a role in the setting of mechanical ventilation with positive end-expiratory ventilation, in which it has been found that significant changes in left ventricular geometry and diastolic function result apparently from the influence of the increased right ventricular pressure that accompanies this mode of ventilation (see preceding discussion).[49,50] A variety of investigations have demonstrated that disease states resulting in right ventricular volume overload—such as atrial septal defect, tricuspid regurgitation, and pulmonary insufficiency—may ultimately be accompanied by reduction of left ventricular systolic performance that is due to the phenomenon of ventricular interdependence. As noted, left ventricular systolic function appears to assist in right ventricular contraction, as evidenced by the fact that right ventricular performance may be preserved despite destruction of significant portions of the right ventricular free wall. By analogy, hemodynamically significant right ventricular infarction does not appear to occur in either experimental models or in the clinical setting in the absence of ischemic damage to a portion of the left ventricle and in particular the left interventricular septum.

Conflicting data exist regarding changes in left ventricular function in the setting of right ventricular dysfunction that may accompany chronic obstructive pulmonary disease (cor pulmonale). Evidence suggests that left ventricular function as measured by pressure/volume curves becomes abnormal as right ventricular failure develops in the setting of chronic lung disease but is not seen if the lung disease is associated with preservation of right ventricular function. These observations are consistent with investigations that report that there is no clear association between left ventricular dysfunction and the degree of hypoxia or hypercapnea in this setting. Other investigators have reported the development of left ventricular hypertrophy in the setting of cor pulmonale even if left ventricular systolic function is preserved, suggesting that right ventricular pressure overload is in some way a stimulus for left ventricular hypertrophy. The failure to find consistent reports of left ventricular dysfunction in the setting of cor pulmonale may in part be ascribed to the variability in the parameters of ventricular function that have been employed, and this important clinical problem continues to warrant further investigation. In general, ventricular interdependence is an important phenomenon to consider when assessing the overall circulatory performance of the critically ill patient and illustrates the importance of carefully investigating the functional state of both ventricles.

The interaction of these determinants of cardiac function governs the ultimate state of ventricular function (Fig. 26-5). To a degree, augmented preload will improve ventricular performance until the plateau of the Starling curve is attained. Increased afterload may reduce the stroke volume of the ventricle, and reduced afterload may improve ventricular performance. The magnitude of the changes in ventricular performance that result from variations in preload and afterload is governed by the innate contractility of the ventricle or its inotropic state. Thus, an increase in contractility of the failing ventricle may move its function curve toward normal and reduce its sensitivity to afterload. Conversely, because a ventricle having decreased contractility is characterized by a relatively flat curve relating preload and afterload (see Fig. 26-1), a reduction in preload under these conditions may lead to no or small reductions in cardiac output as compared to the normal ventricle. Therefore, a summation of preload and afterload conditions and the contractile state of the myocardium will determine the net functional status of the ventricle. A summary of normal right- and left-sided measures of af-

Table 26-4. Normal Values for Right and Left Ventricular Preload and Afterload Conditions

	Right (Pulmonary Circulation)	Left (Systemic Circulation)
Atrial	Mean, 0–8 mm Hg	Mean, 1–10 mm Hg
Ventricle	Systolic, 15–30 mm Hg	Systolic, 100–140 mm Hg
	End-diastolic, 0–8 mm Hg	End-diastolic, 3–12 mm Hg
Arterial	Systolic, 15–30 mm Hg	Systolic, 100–140 mm Hg
	Diastolic, 3–12 mm Hg	Diastolic, 60–90 mm Hg
	Mean, 9–16 mm Hg	Mean, 70–105 mm Hg
Resistance	20–120 dynes/sec/cm^5	770–1500 dynes/sec/cm^5

Pulmonary resistance
$$= \frac{(\text{mean pulmonary artery pressure} - \text{mean left atrial pressure})}{\text{cardiac output}} \times 80$$

Systemic resistance
$$= \frac{(\text{mean systemic pressure} - \text{mean right atrial pressure})}{\text{cardiac output}} \times 80$$

terload and preload as well as expected ranges of cardiac outputs is shown in Table 26-4.

SERIAL EVALUATION OF VENTRICULAR PERFORMANCE: EVALUATION IN THE ICU SETTING

Recognizing the variables discussed in the previous section, ventricular performance may be measured with a perspective on the various factors by which it is determined using a variety of techniques available in the intensive care setting. A brief description of the most frequently used methodologies for the serial bedside assessment of ventricular performance in the critically ill patient follows. Principally, these are the techniques of radionuclide ventriculography, two-dimensional echocardiography, Doppler echocardiography, and noninvasive pulse wave recordings. Following a general description of the nature of these techniques, their application for the serial bedside assessment of ventricular systolic and diastolic performance is discussed. The potential ways in which these noninvasive

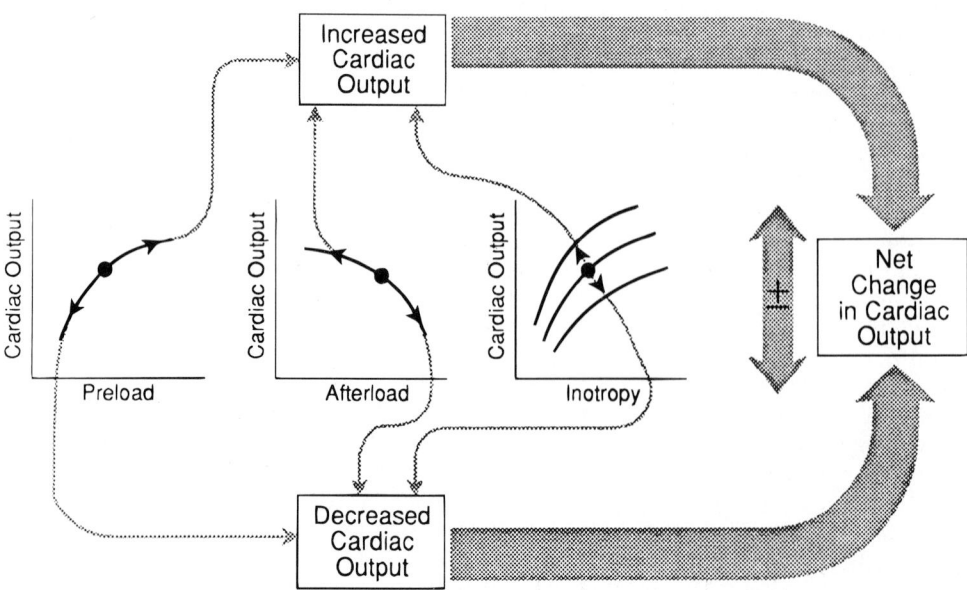

Fig. 26-5. The three major determinants of ventricular performance interact to determine the resultant cardiac output. Increasing preload and inotropic state augment cardiac output whereas increases in afterload may lead to significant decreases in cardiac output especially if myocardial inotropic state is initially depressed.

Noninvasive Techniques

Radionuclide Ventriculography

The technique of radionuclide ventriculography provides a moving image of the right and left ventricles throughout the cardiac cycle[52,53] (Figs. 26-6 and 26-7). As such, it provides an excellent opportunity to globally visualize ventricular systolic function and, as described subsequently, to quantify ventricular systolic and diastolic performance.

This technique entails the labeling of the patient's red blood cells with a radioactive material that allows visualization of the blood cells as they accumulate in the ventricles.[52,53] By filtering out background radiation, a clear and distinct image of the right and left ventricles may be obtained. Specifically, the patient's red blood cells are labeled with technetium, which is injected intravenously.[52-54] Before the injection of technetium, stannous pyrophosphate is administered, which acts as a reducing agent and enhances the intracellular accumulation of technetium. The labeled red blood cells are allowed to circulate throughout the blood, after which time images are acquired with a gamma camera. Because the radioactive label is confined to the red blood cell pool, the image acquired by the gamma camera as it is positioned over the chest comprises the right and left ventricles as well as the atria.

The nuclear camera can be interfaced with a computer, which allows processing of the image in such a way that a moving picture of the ventricle is produced. Simplistically, the patient's electrocardiogram (ECG) is detected by the computer, which then may divide the time between ventricular contractions into a predetermined number of intervals. Commonly, the interval between R waves of the ECG is divided into 20 segments. The computer may then acquire an image for each of these intervals for each of the cardiac cycles for which an image is obtained. Therefore, if the R-to-R interval is divided into 20 time intervals, 20 pictures of the ventricle in different phases of ventricular contraction are acquired for each R-to-R interval. As image acquisition continues, further images for each of these 20 intervals are assigned for each contraction of the ventricle. At the end of image acquisition, each of these 20 images may then be reconstructed to provide the moving picture of the ventricle throughout ventricular contraction. The longer the image acquisition, the more radioactivity in each of the 20 frames that compose the moving image of the heart. As a result, the better the definition of the picture of the ventricle and there is more confidence in the accuracy of the ventricular image.

The radionuclide ventriculogram is therefore similar to

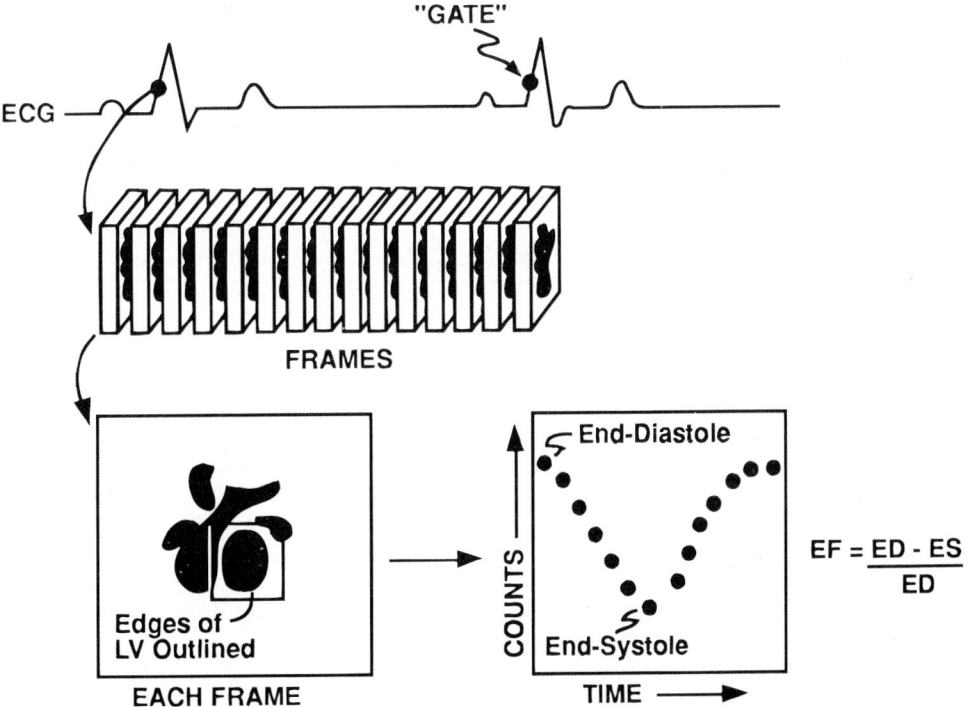

Fig. 26-6. Schematic representation of the acquisition of a gated radionuclide ventriculogram. Images of the ventricle are taken as consecutive frames and are timed in relation to the R wave of the electrocardiogram. The outline of the ventricle in each frame is detected, and the number of counts in the ventricle in each frame is plotted to form the time activity curve of the ventricle (bottom right). This curve in essence represents the filling curve of the ventricle over time. The ejection fraction may be determined by subtracting the end-diastolic counts (ED) and end-systolic counts (ES) and dividing by the end-diastolic counts. (Adapted with permission from Bashore, T. M., and Shaffer, P. B.: Nuclear cardiology. *In* Diagnostic Procedures in Cardiology: A Clinician's Guide. Edited by J. V. Warren and R. P. Lewis. Chicago, Year Book, 1985, p. 143.)

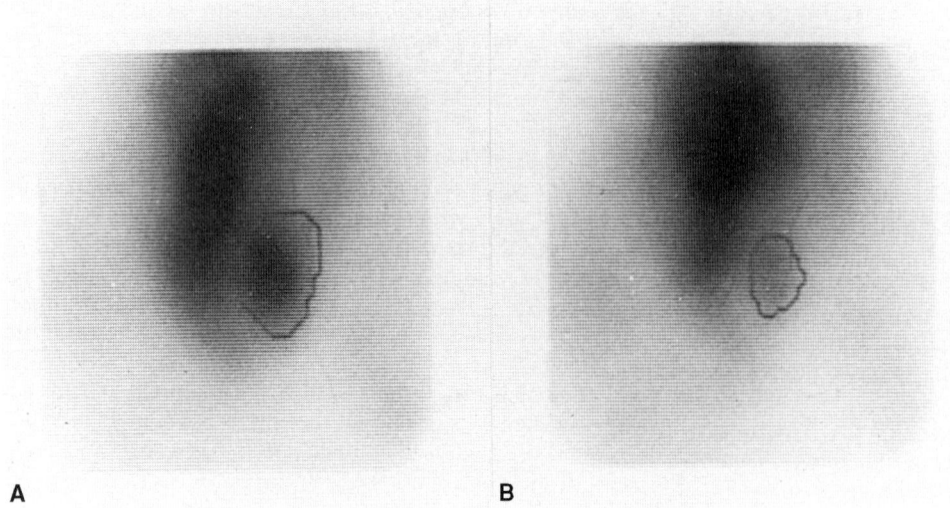

Fig. 26–7. Radionuclide ventriculogram with ventricles at end-diastole (A) and end-systole (B). The left ventricle is outlined, and the right ventricle lies to the left of the outline in this projection.

a motion picture of the heart composed of a given number of frames that are played back in a continuous loop (see Fig. 26-6). These images may be acquired using a portable nuclear camera as well as a portable computer at the bedside in the intensive care setting. Furthermore, because of the half-life of technetium, a number of images of the ventricle may be obtained in a serial fashion over a period of 4 to 5 hours after the initial injection of technetium.

As noted, one major advantage of this system is that it provides images of the right as well as the left ventricle (see Fig. 27-7). However, because in most of the views obtained, the right ventricle is overlapped by the left ventricle, a complete picture of the right ventricle may be lacking. Therefore, to provide better visualization of the right ventricle, a so-called "first-pass" radionuclide ventriculogram may be obtained.[40-45] Using this technique, the initial bolus of radiolabeled blood is followed through the heart, and images are acquired before the radioactive label equilibrates in the blood pool. In this way, images of the right ventricle alone may be acquired before radiolabeled cells have entered the left ventricle. This image may itself be processed to provide a moving image of the right ventricle and thus provide measures of right ventricular performance in an isolated fashion. Typically, a first-pass radionuclide ventriculogram is obtained, followed by the so-called equilibrium study, which comprises images of both the right and left ventricles.

A further approach to the assessment of right ventricular function uses an adaptation of the thermodilution technique for cardiac output determination to derive measures of the right ventricular ejection fraction. The technique requires a thermistor, which possesses a rapid response time, permitting the identification of the diastolic plateaus in the temperature curve that are due to the virtual absence of forward flow during this phase of the cardiac cycle.[49,50] The successive changes in temperature between diastolic plateaus will be related to the stroke volume of each contraction, and thus the relative change in temperature from one diastolic plateau to the next may be used to calculate the right ventricular ejection fraction. This method permits serial determination of the right ventricular ejection fraction over relatively short periods of time; this is not possible using nuclear angiographic techniques, which are limited to one or two injections of labeled blood cells for any given 24-hour period. Although, as suggested previously, no true gold standard currently exists as to the measurement of right ventricular function, a reasonably good correlation has been noted between the right ventricular ejection fractions measured by nuclear angiography and those determined by the thermodilution method. Furthermore, significant changes in right ventricular function that accompany interventions, such as positive end-expiratory ventilation, appear to be detectable by this method. However, agreement between these techniques is not uniformly reported under all conditions. For example, heart transplant recipients may have a marked divergence in ejection fraction measured by these two techniques, and this discrepancy may in part be due to the high incidence of tricuspid regurgitation in these patients.[55] Further investigation is required to define the strengths and limitations of this promising technique.

Radionuclide ventriculography may also be used to provide data regarding end-diastolic and end-systolic volumes of the ventricles, which may subsequently be useful in determining ventricular size and the nature of the ventricular preload. If a blood sample is obtained when the images are acquired, the number of radioactive counts per unit volume of blood may be determined. Using this value, the total number of counts over the ventricle may be obtained and used to extrapolate the volume of blood in the ventricles.[52-54] A noninvasive measure of ventricular volumes is provided. In addition, with measurement of the ejection fraction and the simultaneous determination of stroke volume by the thermodilution method, ventricular volumes may also be estimated from the radionuclide ventriculogram.

This technique provides high resolution pictures of the right and left ventricles, which are then amenable to the derivation of a number of the parameters of ventricular performance discussed later in this chapter. These advantages are offset by the expense of the study as well as the size of the equipment required to perform this evaluation.

However, in settings that require detailed information regarding the nature of ventricular function, the disadvantages are relatively minor. Second, radionuclide ventriculography does not encounter the problems with image acquisition that are occasionally noted with transthoracic echocardiography, discussed later. Therefore, in situations in which image quality is inadequate to evaluate ventricular performance with echocardiography, the radionuclide ventriculogram will often provide the necessary information.

Two-Dimensional and Doppler Echocardiography

The second major imaging modality that is readily applied to the serial evaluation of the critically ill patient is the technique of ultrasonic imaging of the ventricle (echocardiography). This technique relies on the transmission of ultrasound via a transducer placed on the chest wall.[56,57] The ultrasound waves that are reflected by the cardiac structures are reconstructed to form an image of the right and left ventricles, the atria, and the valvular structures of the heart. The two-dimensional images may be obtained in a variety of imaging planes, and many of the views are relatively easily interpreted with a basic knowledge of cross-sectional anatomy, as shown Figure 26-8. Images are displayed in a real-time format so that the ventricles can be observed to contract on a beat by beat basis. These images may also be videotaped to allow further study and analysis at a later time.

From the two-dimensional images of the heart, ventricular volumes may be estimated by a variety of techniques that are either present in on-board software installed in the echocardiographic unit or in a variety of available viewing stations in which the videotaped images are played back.[56,57] In any of these methods, the ventricular outline may be traced to provide an estimate of ventricular volumes and size by a variety of geometric models of the ventricle. As discussed later, these methods allow the derivation of many parameters of ventricular performance. In addition to the two-dimensional images, a single slice through the ventricle may be obtained, creating an image known as the M-mode echocardiogram, as shown in Figure 26-9. This image represents a single section of the two-dimensional image plane over time, and although it does not provide the capacity to measure volumes, dimensions of the left ventricle in a single axis may be measured, and these may be used to derive further indexes of ventricular performance.

In addition to the information provided regarding ventricular performance, the echocardiogram allows a visual inspection of the mobility and function of the cardiac valves. It is an excellent tool to rapidly identify the valvular lesions that may contribute to abnormal afterload and preload states. This type of information is not available using nuclear angiographic techniques.

Coupled with two-dimensional echocardiography, Doppler echocardiography provides important information regarding blood flow through the cardiac chambers.[58-60] This technique relies on the changes in velocity of transmitted ultrasound, which results from blood flow either toward or away from the ultrasound beam. By the Doppler principle, blood flowing toward the ultrasound beam will return with an increased frequency, which then may be interpreted in terms of direction and velocity of blood flow based on the change in the frequency.[58] Simi-

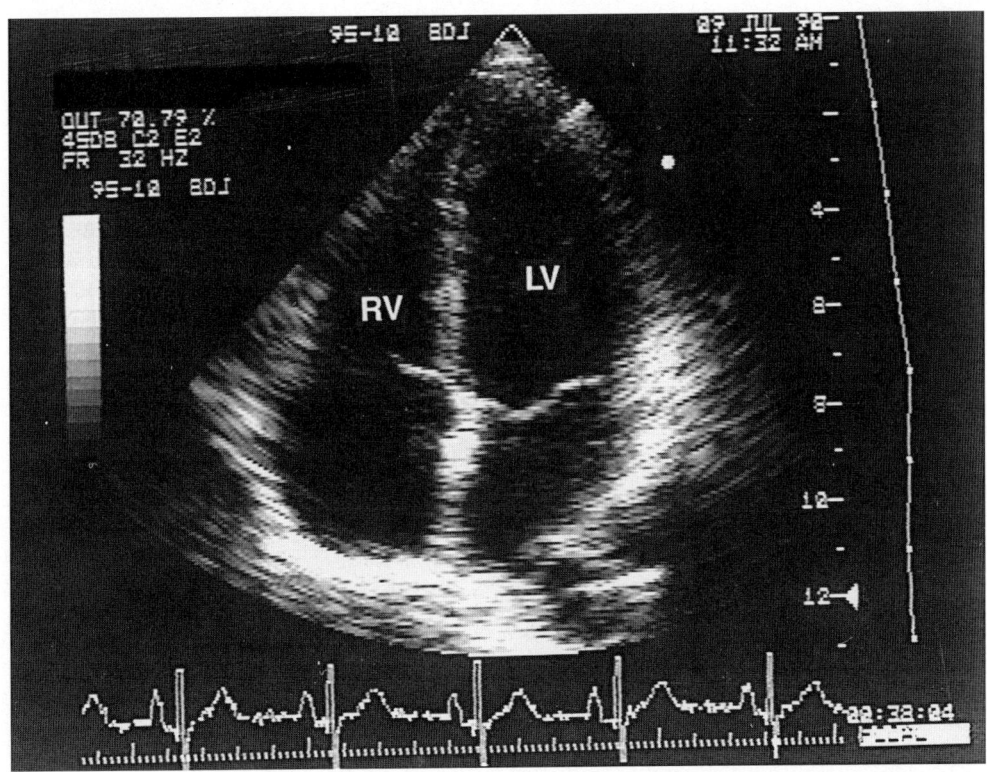

Fig. 26-8. Two-dimensional echocardiogram. The left ventricle (LV) and right ventricle (RV) appear at the top of the image in this view. The respective atria lie below the ventricles. This projection, known as the apical four-chamber view, is typically used for two-dimensional assessment of ventricular function.

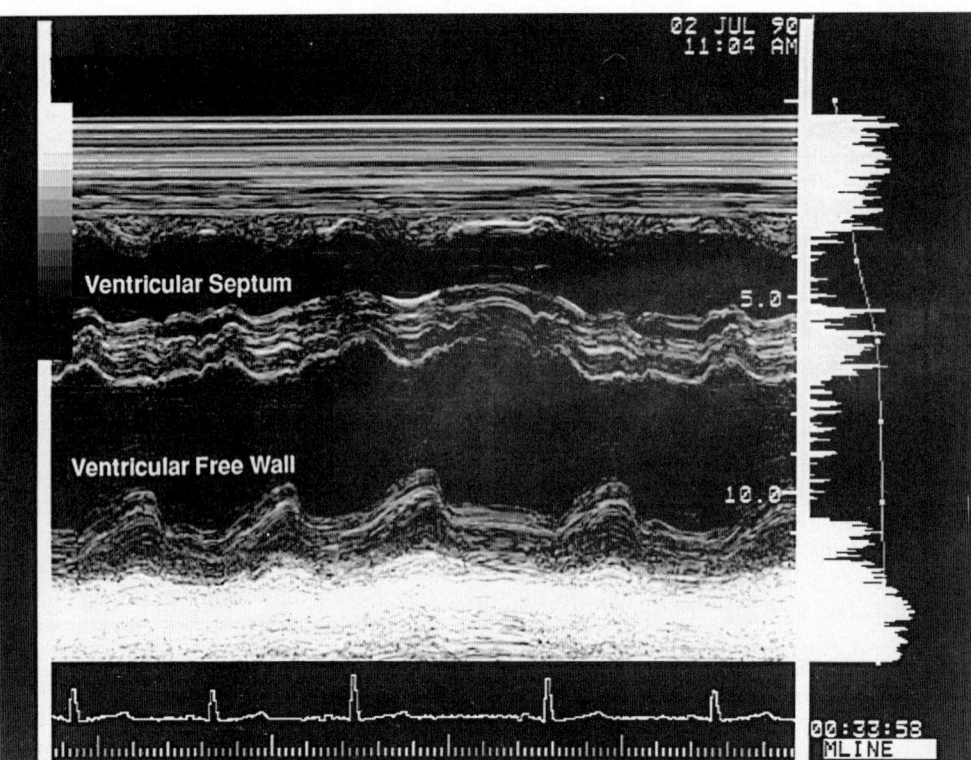

Fig. 26–9. M-mode echocardiogram of left ventricular chamber. The ventricular septum and free wall are noted and are seen to move toward each other in ventricular systole. One-dimensional measurements of ventricular chamber size may be obtained from the M-mode echocardiogram and can be used to derive a variety of parameters of ventricular performance.

larly, blood flowing away from the ultrasound beam will cause the ultrasound to return at a reduced frequency, which then may also be interpreted in terms of direction and velocity. Doppler ultrasound has a variety of applications but perhaps is most importantly summarized as follows: (1) the degree of valvular stenosis and valvular regurgitation may be accurately estimated and quantified using this technique; two-dimensional echocardiography alone may imply valvular lesions based on the structure and motion of the valves but does not provide quantitative information to the extent that Doppler echocardiography may provide; (2) estimates of systolic and diastolic function of the ventricle may be derived through an analysis of the characteristics of the blood flow velocity profiles.[58–60] These are discussed in greater detail later.

Two-dimensional and Doppler echocardiography provide a powerful bedside tool for the serial evaluation of ventricular and valvular function. The Doppler echocardiographic units are easily transportable and ideally suited for the evaluation of the critically ill patient. Furthermore, serial evaluations may be readily performed without the introduction of a radioactive material such as is used for radionuclide ventriculography. Limitations may exist in the adequacy of image quality, given that not all patients have adequate windows for echocardiographic evaluation. In particular, patients maintained on mechanical ventilatory support may be prone to this limitation as a result of hyperinflation of the lungs, which may obscure an adequate echocardiographic view of the heart. Nevertheless, these limitations are seen in a relatively limited number of patients, and this technique is useful in a variety of situations to evaluate ventricular performance.

Indirect Pulse Recordings

Although not commonly used clinically, occasionally, indirect recordings of arterial pulses such as the carotid pulse or the left ventricular apical impulse may be of use in a variety of the parameters of ventricular contractility, which are reviewed later.[61] In particular, the indirect carotid pulse tracing may be useful to measure the left ventricular ejection time. The apex cardiogram is used to assess parameters such as electrical mechanical coupling time, which is necessary for the timing of some diastolic events.

These recordings are generally obtained using an air-filled pressure manometer system with application of a funnel-type device to either the carotid pulse or the apical impulse.[61] The pressure manometer is in essence the same type of manometer that can be used to measure fluid-filled catheter invasive pressure recordings. The noninvasive pressure waveform is then amplified and displayed on a graphic screen or paper printout and used to measure timing intervals.

These pulse recordings and timing intervals maintain a somewhat limited use in the clinical setting but in particular cases may be valuable in the derivation of specific parameters of ventricular function. In certain situations, parameters such as the left ventricular ejection time may alternatively be measured using echocardiographic techniques.

Measurement of Systolic Function

The clinical value in recognizing determinants of ventricular performance lies in the capability of the clinician

Table 26–5. Some Measures of Ventricular Systolic Function (All Values for Left Ventricle Except Where Noted)

Parameter	Formula	Normal Values
Ejection fraction	(EDV − ESV)/EDV × 100	Left ventricle ≥50% Right ventricle ≥45%
Percent fractional shortening	(EDD − ESD)/EDD × 100	34–44%
Mean rate of circumferential fiber shortening (Vcf)	(EDD − ESD)/(EDD × ET)	1.02–1.94 circumferences/sec
Mean P/T	(Dias P − PCWP (mean))/PEP	>1000 mm Hg/sec
Cardiac index	Cardiac output (L/min)/Body surface area (meters^2)	2.5–4.2 L/min/m^2
Stroke volume	Cardiac output (L)/heart rate (beats/min) × 1000 ml/L	65–80 ml/beat
Stroke volume index	Stroke volume (ml/beat)/body surface area (m^2)	30–65 ml/beat/m^2
Left ventricular stroke index	SVI × mean aortic pressure × .0136	30–110 g − m/m^2
Right ventricular stroke index	SVI × mean PA pressure × .0136	4–14 g − m/m^2

EDV, End-diastolic volume; ESV, end-systolic volume; EDD, echocardiographic end-diastolic dimension; ESD, echocardiographic end-systolic dimension; ET, ejection time of the ventricle determined from echo or indirect pulse recordings; Dias P, systemic diastolic pressure; PA, pulmonary artery; PCWP, pulmonary capillary wedge pressure; PEP, preejection period of the left ventricle determined from pulse recordings or echocardiograph; SVI, stroke volume index; .0136 is a conversion factor from mm Hg-cm^{-3} to grams-meters.
(Summarized from references 2, 5, 7, and 10)

to ascertain the cause of altered states of ventricular function and to subsequently treat the underlying abnormalities that lead to reduced ventricular function. This requires reliable measures of ventricular systolic function that can be readily obtained and followed in a serial fashion.

A variety of parameters have been advocated as measures of systolic function of the ventricle (Table 26-5). The chief discriminating factor among these different indexes is how completely they may segregate the determinants of ventricular performance described at the beginning of this chapter. Of all of these parameters, that which continues to be the most reliable and frequently used by the clinician is the **ejection fraction.** This is simply defined as the percentage of the end-diastolic volume ejected by the ventricle in a given contraction. It is calculated as the difference between the end-diastolic and end-systolic volume divided by the end-diastolic volume of the left or right ventricle and is expressed as a percentage.[28,62,63] The major advantages of this parameter are that it is simple to calculate by a variety of techniques, is reproducible, and provides a general measure of ventricular performance that can be assessed in a serial fashion. The major deficiencies are that it is extremely sensitive to changes in both preload and afterload and is influenced by the inotropic state of the ventricle. Therefore, changes in the ejection fraction may be noted throughout a course of therapy or the progression of cardiovascular disease, which may be ascribed to any one or a number of the determinants of ventricular performance that cannot be clearly delineated by this measurement. The simplicity and reproducibility of this measure, however, continue to make it among the most clinically useful parameters of ventricular systolic performance.

The ejection fraction may be readily calculated from the **radionuclide ventriculogram.**[52,53] Because the count rate of radioactivity in any frame of the ventricular image is directly related to the volume of blood in the ventricle, the ejection fraction may be simply calculated as the difference between radioactive count rates at end-diastole and end-systole divided by the count rate at end-diastole expressed as a percentage. It can be seen that geometric considerations are not required for the measurement of the ejection fraction using radionuclide ventriculography. This is a major advantage of this technique, because it circumvents the inaccuracies introduced in geometric models of ventricular shape, which are often inadequate in disease states.[63] For example, ischemic heart disease is often characterized by regional abnormalities of ventricular contraction that result in irregular configurations of the ventricle that are not easily fit by geometric models. Furthermore, because of these considerations, the radionuclide ventriculography is ideal for measurement of right ventricular ejection fractions, given that the shape of the right ventricle is not readily fit by geometric models used to determine left ventricular volumes and ejection fraction.

The ejection fraction may also be derived from the two-dimensional echocardiogram.[56,57] In this case, visualization of the left ventricle in the two-dimensional image allows a tracing of the ventricle at end-diastole and end-systole with a calculation of the area of the ventricle at both times in the cardiac cycle. From this area determination, a volume estimation may be made using any of a number of geometric models of the ventricle. A commonly used formula is the so-called prolate ellipse model, which assumes an elliptic shape of the ventricular chamber and employs measures of the major and minor axis of the ventricle.[63] The ejection fraction is then calculated from the estimated volume. This technique is appealing in that it is easily performed at the bedside and is easily reproduced. The major disadvantage is that the two-dimensional echocardiogram is a segmental study and may use planes of the left ventricle, which are not truly representative of global ventricular performance. Second, the accuracy of right ventricular ejection fraction measurement by two-dimensional echocardiographic techniques remains uncertain. Preliminary investigations suggest that with the appropriate geometric models, this technique may accurately assess the right ventricular ejection fraction; however, further investigation is required to confirm this.[56,57] Regardless of a numeric value, this technique at least provides a subjective assessment of the adequacy of right ventricular systolic performance.[64,65]

A related parameter derived from the M-mode echocardiogram is the so-called percent fractional shortening of the minor axis of the left ventricle.[56,57] This is not a true volume determination of ejection fraction but is derived from measurement of the short axis of the left ventricle. From the M-mode echocardiogram, the short axis of the left ventricle is measured at end-diastole and end-systole. The percentage of fractional shortening is then determined as the difference between end-diastolic and end-systolic minor axis divided by the end-diastolic dimension. This value is also expressed as a percentage, and in most laboratories the lower limit of normal is 26%. This value again does not provide a true volume measurement and may be misleading if the plane of examination is not representative of the true ventricular performance. It is, however, a simple measurement and one that is easily reproduced and continues to have utility in the clinical setting.

As noted, the ejection fraction is not truly independent of afterload or preload conditions of the ventricle. One effort to arrive at a parameter that is somewhat less sensitive to loading conditions is the determination of the velocity of circumferential fiber shortening.[25,57,66-68] This parameter extrapolates the velocity of shortening of an individual muscle fiber to the velocity of contraction of a segment of the left ventricle. In the clinical setting, it is simply derived from measurement of the percent fractional shortening of the ventricle, as described previously, divided by the ejection time of the ventricle. Therefore, it simply measures the extent of contraction of the left ventricle along with rapidity at which this contraction occurs. The left ventricular ejection time can be measured from an indirect recording of the carotid pulse. In this case, the ejection time is the interval from the rapid upstroke of the carotid pulse to the dichrotic notch.[61,69-71] Alternatively, the ejection time can be measured from the M-mode echocardiogram of the aortic valve by measuring the time of the opening of the aortic valve to the time of the closing of the valve.[56,57] This parameter is therefore relatively easily obtained, and the on-board software of many echocardiographic units currently incorporates this measure in routine analysis. Although this measure of ventricular performance is somewhat less sensitive to loading conditions than the simple ejection fraction, it remains sensitive to afterload conditions and, to a degree, preload states.

A variety of parameters of ventricular performance that are theoretically independent of preload and incorporate afterload have been proposed and are based on very intricate measures of ventricular performance in experimental animal models and isolated heart preparations.[35,72-79] Specifically, these are based on the relationship between end-systolic pressure and end-systolic volume over a range of afterloads. Simplistically, the greater the inotropic state of the ventricle, the smaller its end-systolic volume for a given end-systolic pressure. Therefore, if the end-systolic volume of the ventricle is measured over a range of end-systolic pressures, a line may be drawn through these various points, and the slope of that line will be directly related to the contractility of the ventricle (Fig. 26–10). Under physiologic conditions, this relationship is truly linear and is relatively independent of preload. Because it incorporates afterload in its determination, the slope of the line is in essence a pure measure of the inotropic state of the ventricle independent of the loading conditions.

Obviously, such a detailed assessment of the ventricular

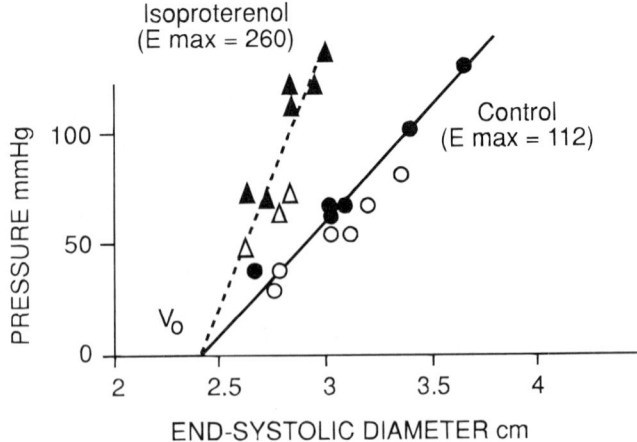

Fig. 26–10. The relation between ventricular end-systolic pressure (vertical axis) and end-systolic volume (horizontal axis) under states of normal and enhanced inotropic state because of norepinephrine infusion. With increased contractility, there is an increase in the slope at the line relating end-systolic pressure and volume. (From Sagawa, K., Suga, H., Shoukas, A. A., and Bakalar, K. M.: End-systolic pressure-volume ratio: a new index of ventricular contractility. Am. J. Cardiol., *40*:748, 1977).

performance is rarely, if ever, possible in the clinical setting. Therefore, a number of simplified parameters based on these more sophisticated measurements have been proposed.[80-88] These have included the simple ratio of the end-systolic pressure to measured end-systolic dimension or volume of the ventricle. In this case, end-systolic pressure may be estimated from the noninvasively measured carotid pulse tracing.[81,84-86,89] By scaling the carotid pulse tracing to measured systemic pressure, the pressure at the dichrotic notch may be estimated and used as the end-systolic pressure. The end-systolic dimension or volume may be obtained from the echocardiogram or from the simultaneously obtained radionuclide ventriculogram.[90]

Other parameters have included measurement of end-systolic stress rather than simple end-systolic pressure. These parameters may be obtained by measurement of the thickness of ventricular wall by the echocardiogram, and when they are used with the estimated end-systolic pressure, end-systolic stress may be derived.[91] The load dependence of the velocity of circumferential fiber shortening may be eliminated in part by an adaptation of this technique. The ratio of the velocity of circumferential fiber shortening to the end-systolic stress has been proposed as a further index of contractility that is independent of loading conditions.[88] Preliminary studies have suggested that this indeed may be a relatively load-independent parameter of the ventricular contractile state. A related parameter is the percent fractional shortening to the end-systolic pressure or stress.[80] Recent comparative studies have suggested that this may be the most sensitive indicator of diminished contractility when compared to other related parameters.[92]

In addition to measures using end-systolic pressure, it has been proposed that peak systolic pressure may be coupled with end-systolic dimension or volume as a similar load-independent measure of ventricular contractility.[90,93,94] In this way, simple measures of systolic blood pressure may be coupled with nuclear or echocardiographically derived end-systolic dimensions or volumes, thus further simplifying the derivation of these indices. Although for theoretical reasons, peak systolic pressure may not be as accurate as the use of end-systolic pressure, it may further simplify the derivation of these indexes and allow their application in the clinical setting.

These measures are relatively easy to obtain and can be performed in a serial fashion. They provide the advantage of segregating, to a degree, the loading conditions that may influence ventricular performance and the intrinsic contractile state of the ventricle.[94,95] Their limitations are that although they are based on elegant measurements of ventricular contractility, their simplifications sacrifice to a degree true load independence of these measures.[94] Nevertheless, this may be a reasonable compromise in the clinical setting to permit application of the principles that define these indexes. Further investigation in the clinical setting will determine the future utility and accuracy of these parameters.

In addition to the preceding methods, Doppler echocardiographic techniques have been advocated as one possible noninvasive modality for the assessment of systolic ventricular performance.[58,96-98] In particular, characteristics of the aortic flow velocity profile appear to be related to systolic function of the ventricle. The time required for the attainment of peak aortic flow velocity, or the so-called acceleration time, and of the peak aortic velocity itself has been found to be related to ventricular systolic function.[96-98] These indexes are based on more formal experimental measurements of aortic flow velocity, which again appear to be related to ventricular systolic function. They are relatively easy to derive with the standard Doppler echocardiographic examination. These indexes however, are not strictly independent of loading conditions and again can be influenced by afterload conditions. Further clinical investigation is required to more carefully establish their utility as bedside measures of ventricular systolic function.

In addition, the Doppler echocardiographic examination may provide information regarding the cause of systolic dysfunction of the ventricle. In particular, Doppler echocardiographic examination of the aortic flow velocity provides information regarding the pressure gradient across the aortic valve and thus may allow determination of whether or not critical valvular obstruction exists and thus constitutes a cause of ventricular systolic failure.[99]

These noninvasive measurements of ventricular performance may be coupled with pressure and flow data obtained invasively to derive further parameters of ventricular dysfunction.[100-105] Among these is an adaptation of the measurement of the peak rise in developed left ventricular pressure, or what has been termed the peak dP/dT of the ventricle.[106] By this technique, the developed pressure of the ventricle is determined by taking the difference between the diastolic systemic blood pressure and the mean capillary wedge pressure. This pressure is divided by some measure of the time over which the pressure is generated, thus providing an index that incorporates the speed as well as magnitude of pressure developed by the ventricle in the earliest stages of systole. A complete description of the manner in which these intervals is obtained is beyond the scope of this chapter. However, such timing of events can be obtained by noninvasive pulse recordings and recordings of the apex cardiogram. (The interested reader is referred to the reference list at the end of the chapter.[106]) This index of contractility is termed the mean dP/dT and again is a relatively load-insensitive parameter of ventricular contractility. Thus, it offers advantages over measurements such as the ejection fraction in selected settings. A variety of parameters using the cardiac output and stroke volume, which may be derived by the thermodilution technique using a Swan-Ganz catheter, have been proposed.[2] Simply measuring the stroke volume or the cardiac output alone does not in and of itself provide accurate information regarding ventricular systolic function.[8,62,107] However, various derivatives of these measures that incorporate the afterload encountered by the ventricle may give some indication of ventricular contractile performance. For example, left ventricular stroke work, which is calculated as the stroke volume multiplied by the mean left ventricular systolic pressure, is a commonly used index of ventricular performance.[108,109] This may be expressed as a rate of work performed per minute by multiplying the stroke work by the heart rate.[67] An analagous measurement is the stroke power, which is the stroke work divided by the left ventricular ejection time.[2,67] These measurements incorporate afterload conditions and thus provide some normalization of ventricular systolic function for afterload conditions. Although not true measures of contractility, they are reasonable and easily reproducible measurements of ventricular systolic performance if invasive bedside hemodynamic monitoring is performed.

A wide array of parameters is available for the bedside serial assessment of ventricular systolic performance. The parameters chosen are governed by the availability of the techniques that may be used to assess ventricular performance and by the specific diagnostic or therapeutic question that must be addressed. Because many of these parameters are further investigated in the clinical setting, their utility as well as their limitations will be further defined.

Assessment of Diastolic Function

Fewer measurements of parameters for the clinical assessment of the diastolic function of the ventricle are available than those for systolic function. In part, this is due to the complex nature of relaxation of the ventricle and consequently the diverse array of factors that must be measured to define ventricular relaxation.[110,111] The parameters used in a clinical setting are in essence simplifications of the pressure and volume measurements that are made with very sophisticated high fidelity measurement systems used in the research laboratory. As with parameters of systolic function of the ventricle, both nuclear angiographic and Doppler echocardiographic techniques may be employed to assess diastolic function at the bedside.

Nuclear angiographic techniques to assess diastolic function are derived from a measurement of the number of counts in each frame of the nuclear angiogram throughout the cardiac cycle.[112,113] As shown in Figure 26-6, when the number of counts per frame is plotted against time from the R wave of the ECG, a curve that in essence represents the volume curve of the ventricle throughout the cardiac cycle is created. The initial decrease in counts corresponds to the contraction of the ventricle as radiolabeled blood is ejected from the ventricle. A subsequent increase in counts represents the filling phase of the ventricle. The most rapid rate of filling of the ventricle may be determined from this curve and is termed the peak filling rate of the ventricle. This constitutes the principal clinically useful parameter of diastolic function that may be derived from radionuclide ventriculography. The second parameter is the time from the R wave to this peak filling rate. The time to peak filling rate itself is also a parameter of diastolic function of the ventricle but is somewhat less sensitive to diastolic function, given that the time resolution of the image acquisition used in most clinical settings is not sufficient for the detection of small changes of the peak filling rate. An increase in the peak filling rate of the ventricle and a decrease in the time to peak filling indicate improvement in diastolic function. Various clinical studies have demonstrated that these techniques may detect significant changes in diastolic function of the ventricle over time.[113]

Nuclear ventriculography techniques have the advantage of allowing an assessment of diastolic function along with the more routine measurement of systolic function. The technique is limited by factors such as the previously noted time resolution and theoretical considerations as to whether or not the values are normalized for ventricular volumes. Because the clinical assessment of diastolic function remains a relatively new area, many laboratories may not have established normal values for these various parameters. The utility of this technique in the clinical setting continues to be tested and evaluated.

Doppler echocardiographic techniques possess perhaps the greatest potential for the accurate evaluation of diastolic performance in the clinical setting.[114-116] Doppler parameters of diastolic function are derived largely from measurement of the flow velocities across the mitral valve during ventricular filling.[115] These flow velocities are in general related to the changes in pressure gradient between the left atrium and left ventricle. Among the most useful parameters is the time course of decrease in blood flow velocity across the mitral valve after the initial rapid filling velocity,[114-116] as demonstrated in Figure 26-11. A prolonged decrease in the initial rapid inflow velocity is suggestive of a decrease in diastolic function of the ventricle. In essence, impairment of ventricular relaxation will be associated with a longer period of time when the ventricle may fill and thus a longer time when the flow velocity will decline to a baseline value. A second index of diastolic performance is seen in the relative magnitude of the filling velocity that is due to early rapid filling and the flow velocity associated with atrial contraction. As shown in Figure 26-12, the velocity of blood flow across the mitral valve is composed of the early rapid filling velocity and a second peak in velocity, which is due to atrial contraction. Normally, the early filling peak is higher than atrial filling velocity. In conditions in which relaxation of the ventricle is impaired, however, the atrial filling velocity may exceed the early rapid filling velocity (see Fig. 26-11). This is a second major indicator of diastolic dysfunction of the ventricle.[58]

These changes, which are reflected by the Doppler echocardiogram, are those that result from impaired filling of the ventricle resulting from muscle hypertrophy or ventricular failure. The Doppler echocardiogram, however, may also provide evidence of other disease states that impair ventricular filling such as constrictive pericarditis.[58] Unlike impaired relaxation that is due to ventricular hypertrophy, constrictive pericarditis impairs later diastolic filling of the ventricle. Thus, the only time when filling can occur is in the very early portions of diastole. As a result, the mitral velocity flow profile is characterized by a very high peak velocity in early filling (greater than 1 m per second) and a very rapid falloff in this velocity. This thus contrasts with the pattern noted in ventricular hypertrophy or other states primarily involving the cardiac muscle in which the flow velocity decline is greatly prolonged. Thus, the Doppler echocardiogram is a highly sensitive tool in distinguishing these two very different entities that impair ventricular filling by different mechanisms. This, of course, may be imperative in determining the therapeutic strategy for a given patient.

In addition, the two-dimensional echocardiographic examination provides the opportunity to detect structural abnormalities that may contribute to impaired ventricular filling. As an example, the two-dimensional echocardiogram may display the abnormal pericardial thickening that characterizes constrictive pericarditis. Mitral valve stenosis, which also impairs ventricular filling, may also be readily recognized by this examination. The severity of stenotic lesions may be further characterized by the Doppler echocardiographic examination as well. Therefore, two-dimensional echocardiography combined with Doppler echocardiography is a powerful tool in both describing diastolic performance of the ventricle and delineating various causes of diastolic dysfunction.

In addition to these noninvasive techniques, invasive information obtained in the critical care setting may be coupled with this noninvasive information. In particular, the left ventricular end-diastolic pressure may be estimated from the pulmonary capillary wedge pressure obtained with a Swan-Ganz catheter. This information may be coupled with end-diastolic volumes or dimensions derived by either nuclear ventriculography or echocardiographic techniques to describe the relationship between end-diastolic pressure and end-diastolic volume or stress, as shown in Figure 26-13.[110,111] If these data are available over a range of pulmonary capillary wedge pressures, a curve describing the relationship between end-diastolic pressure and volume may be created, which, in essence, defines the diastolic function curve of the ventricle. A very steep curve indicates impaired diastolic filling, and various points along this curve can be followed in a serial fashion to assess changes in diastolic performance.

FOLLOW-UP OF THE CRITICALLY ILL PATIENT

The previously described noninvasive techniques used to assess ventricular performance are readily applicable

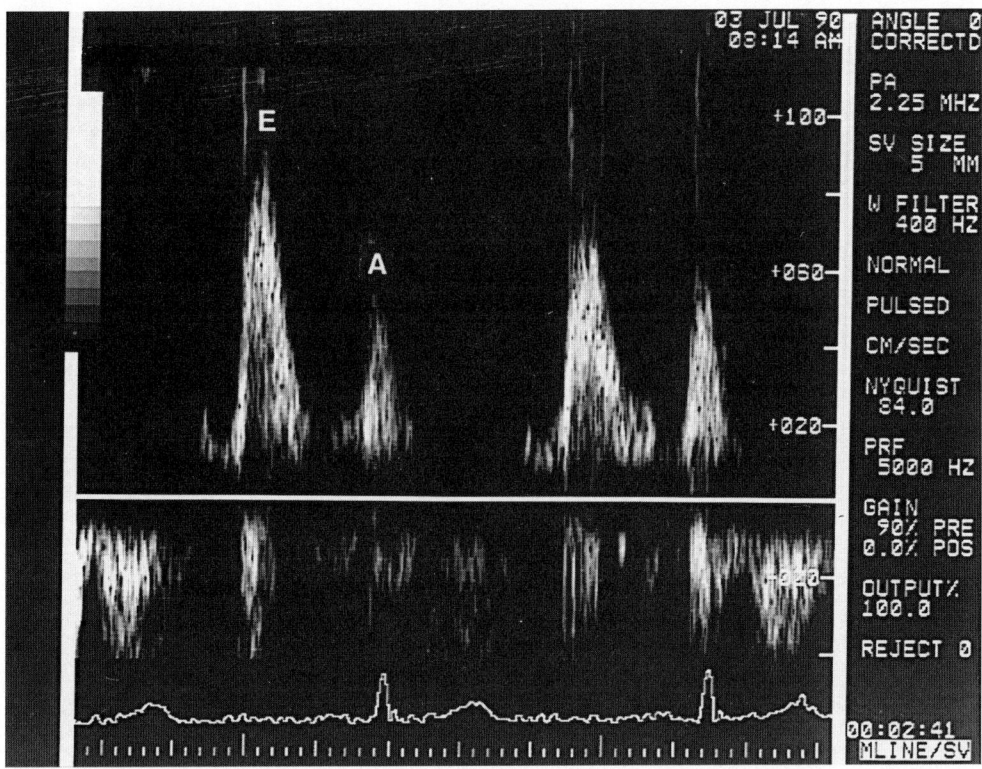

Fig. 26–11. Doppler echocardiogram of blood flow velocity across the mitral valve in a normal subject. An early filling peak of velocity is noted at the beginning of diastole (E wave). A second, smaller velocity peak is noted at the time of atrial contraction (A wave). Normally, the E velocity peak is greater than the A peak.

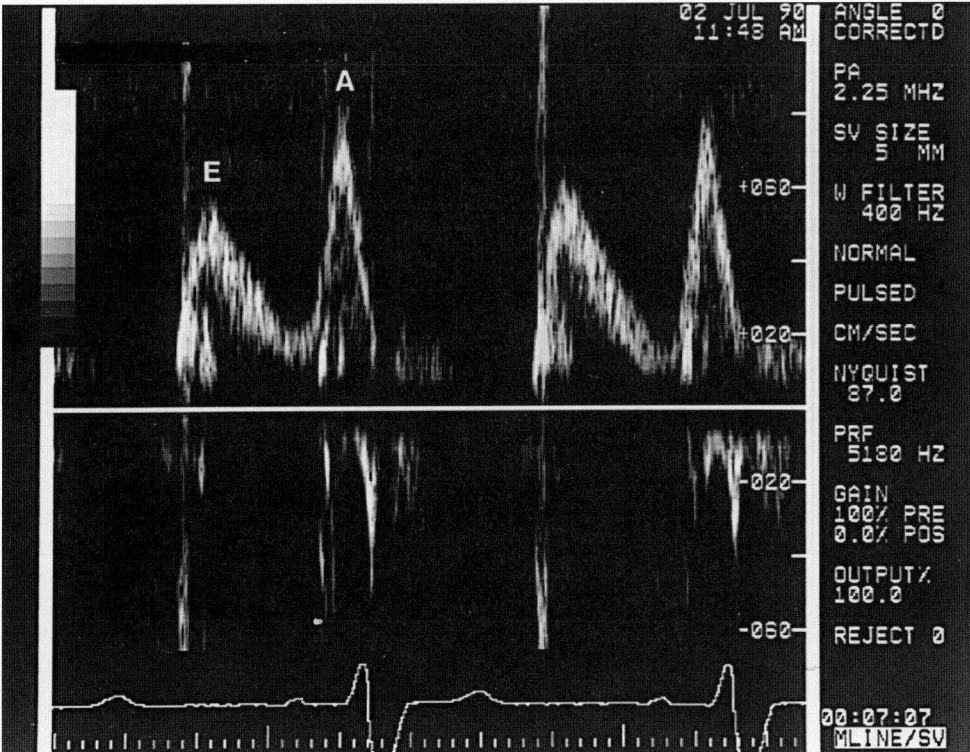

Fig. 26–12. Doppler flow velocity across mitral valve in a patient with hypertension. In contrast to the normal subject noted in Figure 26–10, the A wave velocity is greater than the early diastolic E wave. This suggests abnormal diastolic function of the ventricle with impaired early relaxation resulting in a greater contribution of active atrial filling of the ventricle.

to the patient following critical care management (Table 26-6). In particular, radionuclide ventriculography as well as echocardiographic examination are easily performed in a serial fashion to allow subsequent assessment of the status of ventricular systolic and diastolic function. These data are important in terms of (1) assessing right and left ventricular performance in the absence of influencing factors that were required in the intensive care setting but have

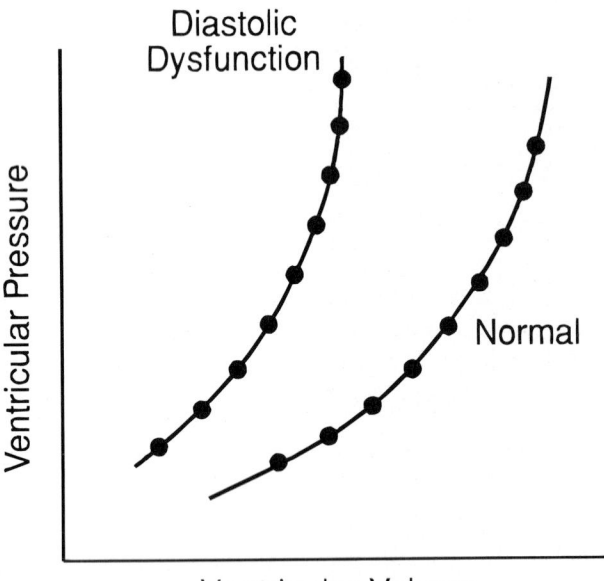

Fig. 26-13. Plotting diastolic ventricular volumes (such as those which may be derived from echocardiography or radionuclide ventriculography) against ventricular diastolic pressures (such as those obtained from pulmonary capillary wedge pressures) provides a measure of the diastolic function to the left ventricle. As shown, with the development of diastolic dysfunction, an upward shift in this curve will result, indicating that higher pressures are required to attain a given ventricular diastolic volume.

been withdrawn (such as assisted ventilation); (2) the assessment of regional wall motion abnormalities, which may be diagnostic of an event such as a myocardial infarction; (3) assessment of residual left and right ventricular function following an ischemic insult such as a myocardial infarction; and (4) assessment of the severity of valvular lesions detected in the intensive care setting and their impact on ventricular performance.

As noted in the preceding discussion, a variety of supportive interventions employed in the intensive care setting may have profound influence on both right and left ventricular performance. Mechanical ventilation may directly influence right ventricular performance and indirectly alter left ventricular performance through the phenomenon of ventricular interdependence. Vasopressor agents required for hemodynamic support may directly augment ventricular contractility through positive inotropic effects or may alter ventricular performance through changes in ventricular preload and afterload. Therefore, assessment of ventricular performance following discharge from the ICU permits an assessment of ventricular function in the absence of these factors that may obscure the true contractile state of the ventricles.

Such an assessment of ventricular performance provides crucial diagnostic and prognostic information, which may govern the further evaluation and management of the patient. Segmental abnormalities in ventricular contraction, which are detectable using either radionuclide ventriculography or echocardiography, may be diagnostic of a myocardial infarction. Thus, this assessment may provide confirmatory evidence of an ischemic cause for ventricular dysfunction, which may have been suspected in the critical care setting. Furthermore, the degree to which ventricular function is impaired is perhaps the most important determinant of mortality in a patient who has suffered a myocardial infarction. The mortality of the postmyocardial infarction patient may therefore be stratified, based on the extent to which ventricular contractile function is decreased as measured by the ejection fraction. Finally, both the status of ventricular function and the degree of valvular dysfunction in patients with valvular stenosis or regurgita-

Table 26-6. Diagnostic Tests for Representative Diseases Influencing Systolic and Diastolic Function

Disease State	Test	Finding
Diastolic dysfunction		
Impaired relaxation (e.g., hypertension, in some cases of ischemic heart disease)	Doppler echocardiogram	Accentuated atrial filling velocity
Reduced compliance (pericardial constriction, myocardial restriction)	Doppler echocardiogram	Abnormal high early filling velocity, rapid deceleration of early filling
Systolic dysfunction		
Myocardial infarction	Rest RNA echocardiogram	Segmental wall motion abnormality, may be diffuse reduction of function with reduced EF
	Stress RNA or echocardiogram	May be no change if no coronary disease outside region of infarction
	Rest thallium	Filling defect in image of ventricle
	Stress thallium	No change in defect or "fixed defect" if no ischemia in region of or remote from region of infarction
Coronary artery stenosis	Stress RNA or echocardiogram	New wall motion abnormality with stress; may have fall in EF
	Stress thallium	Defect in image immediately following stress, which is not present following recovery or "reversible defect"
Idiopathic myopathy or viral myocarditis	Rest RNA or echocardiogram	Diffuse reduction in ventricular function and EF; may in some cases have segmental abnormalities
	Stress RNA or echocardiogram	May be no change in EF; occasionally, segmental abnormalities with stress

EF, Ejection fraction; RNA, radionuclide angiography.

tion may be assessed following recovery from acute hemodynamic decompensation.

In addition to the measurement of right and left ventricular dysfunction, which may be obtained by either radionuclide ventriculography or echocardiography, the severity of valvular stenosis and regurgitation may be determined through Doppler echocardiography. This information may be critical in determining the need for valve replacement or repair and may direct possible invasive evaluation of valvular dysfunction using cardiac catheterization. The degree of ventricular impairment may dictate whether valvular lesions are amenable to surgical intervention. For example, decreased left ventricular function in a patient with mitral or aortic insufficiency may indicate that such a patient is at high risk for perioperative ventricular failure following valve replacement and may thus not be a candidate for such a surgical approach.

Doppler echocardiographic techniques for the assessment of diastolic dysfunction, as discussed previously, may provide an assessment of the efficacy of therapy instituted in the intensive care setting such as pharmacologic interventions designed to treat hypertension and attendant diastolic dysfunction. As can be seen, careful determination of the nature of ventricular function is essential in determining further management strategies following the intensive care phase of the patient's care.

In addition to the determination of resting ventricular performance, stress-induced changes in ventricular function provide data that further direct patient evaluation and management. Radionuclide ventriculography performed during exercise, usually supine bicycle ergometry, may be diagnostic of significant coronary artery disease. A fall in ejection fraction and/or a decrease in contractility of a distinct segment of the myocardium during exercise suggests significant coronary artery disease, which may require definitive diagnosis and coronary angiography. Similar abnormalities in global and regional myocardial function may be detected using exercise stress echocardiography in which images of the ventricle are obtained at baseline and immediately following either bicycle or treadmill exercise. As well as providing information regarding the development of left ventricular ischemia, both of these techniques may provide information about right ventricular function at rest and with stress, which may reveal the presence of right ventricular infarction, right ventricular ischemia, or right ventricular dysfunction, which results from pressure or volume overload. Thus, right and left ventricular contractile reserve may be assessed by stress testing with imaging and can provide important diagnostic clues as to the cause of abnormalities in right and left ventricular systolic dysfunction.

It is important to recognize that not all resting or stress-induced changes in global or segmental ventricular performance may necessarily be ascribed to ischemic disease. Global abnormalities in resting ventricular function in which the entire ventricle is found to be decreased in its systolic function may be ascribed to cardiomyopathies, myocarditis, or severe long-standing mitral regurgitation, aortic insufficiency, or aortic stenosis in addition to global ischemia or diffuse myocardial damage following an extensive or multiple myocardial infarctions. As noted earlier in this chapter, extreme elevations in ventricular afterload as imposed by systemic hypertension may be associated with resting left ventricular dysfunction, and the greater the compromise in intrinsic contractility of the ventricle, the greater the sensitivity to such increases in afterload (see Fig. 26-3). In addition to ischemic insults, resting right ventricular performance may similarly be abnormal as a result of involvement with cardiomyopathies; myocarditis; tricuspid regurgitation; volume overload that is due to right-to-left shunting of blood, as is found in atrial or interventricular septal defects; and right ventricular pressure overload that is due to elevated pulmonary artery pressures. Resting and stress-induced segmental abnormalities in myocardial function in which only a portion of the ventricle demonstrates decreased contractility may also be secondary to factors other than ischemia. Myocarditis has been shown to be associated with only regional abnormalities of ventricular performance rather than diffuse contraction abnormalities. Valvular regurgitation may be associated with rest or stress-induced changes in segmental ventricular performance that are due to uneven stress imposed by the volume overload which result from the regurgitation. In particular, the ventricular apex appears to be prone to these segmental abnormalities because the thickness of the myocardium is at a minimum at this point and thus sustains the greatest stress. Apical contraction abnormalities of the left ventricle therefore may be seen in patients with systemic hypertension either at rest or when undergoing stress in the absence of significant coronary artery disease. This phenomenon may also be seen in patients with diffusely dilated ventricles, such as in the case of dilated cardiomyopathy, in which ventricular wall stress is increased as a result of the marked increase in the radius of the ventricular chamber.

As can be seen, resting or stress-induced abnormalities in global or segmental ventricular performance may have multiple different causes and are not specific for abnormalities in coronary artery blood flow or coronary artery disease. A noninvasive test that reflects the status of coronary blood flow therefore is useful in further defining the cause of ventricular dysfunction. Thallium imaging of the myocardium provides a noninvasive technique that addresses this need. Thallium is taken up and metabolized by the myocardium in a manner similar to potassium.[52] Therefore, regions of the myocardium that are normally perfused will take up thallium that is labeled with radioactive iodine. Imaging of the ventricle with a gamma camera will create a picture in which normally perfused portions of the myocardium are darkly shaded, and regions with either reduced or absent perfusion will appear to be lightly shaded or completely transparent. Therefore, in the absence of coronary artery disease, an image of the left ventricular wall and interventricular septum results. A defect in this image or region of decreased density in the ventricular walls indicates decreased blood flow in that region (Fig. 26-14). Such a defect in a resting image implies either a region of myocardial infarction or resting ischemia.

The resting thallium image thus may be used to confirm the diagnosis of a myocardial infarction. When coupled with exercise stress testing, thallium imaging may be used to delineate areas of ischemia that correspond to signifi-

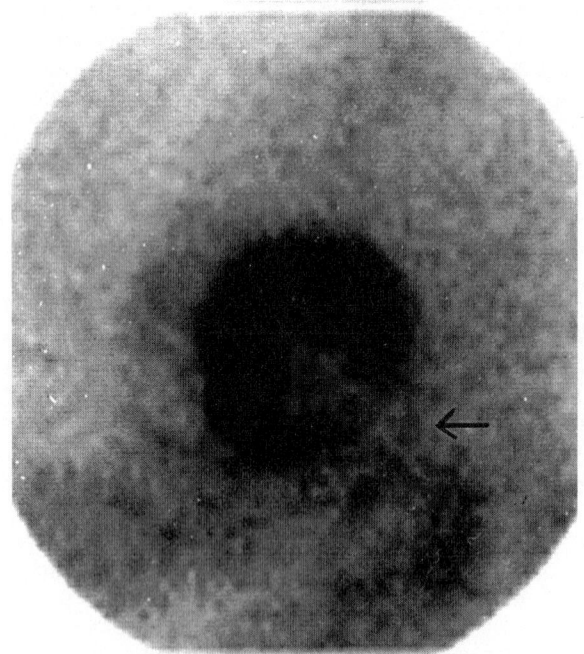

Fig. 26–14. A thallium image of the ventricle demonstrating a region of myocardial infarction. A lightly shaded region (arrow) surrounded by the darkly shaded normal myocardium represents a region of absent myocardial perfusion and consequent infarcted myocardium.

cant stenosis of coronary arteries. Typically, the patient undergoes exercise stress testing using either a treadmill or bicycle ergometer. At the peak of stress, radiolabeled thallium is injected intravenously and thus circulates to normally perfused segments of the myocardium. Images of the heart are obtained immediately after the patient stops exercise so that abnormally perfused segments of the ventricle may be detected. These will appear as regions of the ventricle that are less densely shaded than the remainder of the normal myocardium. Further images of the ventricle are obtained 2 to 3 hours after the patient has completed exercise. Areas of the myocardium that have had decreased blood flow during stress but normal perfusion at rest will now take up circulating thallium and will appear as a shaded region of the myocardium of density equal to the remainder of the ventricle. Such a pattern, known as a reversible defect in the thallium image, indicates a significant stenosis of a coronary artery; a less than normal amount of thallium is taken up by the myocardium supplied by that vessel during exercise, and a normal amount of thallium is in this region following recovery from exercise, which is due to normal myocardial perfusion under resting conditions. This pattern implies viable myocardium that is not adequately perfused during periods of increased oxygen demand and contrasts with the pattern observed in an area of infarcted myocardium, in which density of the region of the myocardial infarction is decreased both immediately following stress and during recovery. Such a pattern is known as a fixed thallium defect and is due to the absence of blood flow and viable myocardium both at rest and during stress. As can be seen, thallium imaging can provide important diagnostic information regarding the presence of coronary artery disease and is complementary to techniques that assess regional and global ventricular function but only indirectly infer the presence of significant coronary artery stenosis.

A significant number of patients may not be able to perform exercise stress testing. Stress imposed by various pharmacologic interventions therefore has been used, and increasing experience with these techniques is proving that they offer a valuable alternative to exercise testing. Agents such as dipyridamole or adenosine, which promote vasodilatation in normal coronaries but fail to augment flow in regions of coronary stenosis, have been used in conjunction with thallium perfusion imaging to elicit reversible thallium defects similar to those observed with traditional exercise stress testing. Infusion of dobutamine to promote enhanced myocardial oxygen demand has been used during echocardiographic imaging of the ventricles to detect the appearance of segmental wall motion abnormalities, which imply ischemia in the region of the wall motion abnormality. The use of such pharmacologic stress tests thus allows the diagnostic power of the various available imaging techniques to be applied to patients who cannot participate in exercise stress testing.

In addition to providing insight into the possible cause of abnormal ventricular function, evaluation of stress-induced changes in ventricular performance may direct further invasive evaluation of ventricular function and coronary anatomy and may point to the need for further therapeutic intervention. A patient who has suffered a myocardial infarction and who during stress testing is found to develop an exercise-induced segmental wall motion abnormality or reversible thallium defect in a region distinct from the myocardial infarction is at increased risk for further ischemic injury. Such "ischemia at a distance" from the region of prior infarction identifies a patient who would benefit from precise definition of coronary anatomy by coronary angiography and who will possibly require some form of revascularization of the region of "jeopardized myocardium." Therefore, patients who have suffered a myocardial infarction frequently undergo limited exercise stress testing (with a less than maximal heart rate as the end point of stress) before discharge from the hospital to further stratify the patient's risk for further ischemic events and identify the potential need for invasive evaluation.

Recognition of the basic elements governing ventricular performance allows appropriate selection of an ever increasing number of techniques available for the assessment of ventricular performance. Further advances in still newer technology not discussed in this chapter, such as rapid computed tomography imaging of the myocardium and magnetic resonance imaging, promise to provide yet more diverse and detailed information regarding ventricular performance. These techniques as well as the more conventional methods described here continue to evolve in their role in the therapeutic and diagnostic management of the patient and will further assist the clinician in the management of the critically ill patient.

REFERENCES

1. Chapman, C. B., and Mitchell, J. H.: Starling on the Heart. London, Dawson of Pall Mall, 1965, p. 119.
2. Binkley, P. F., and Boudoulas, H.: Measurement of myocardial inotropy. *In* Cardiotonic Drugs: A Clinical Survey. Edited by C. V Leier. New York, Marcel Dekker, 1986, p. 5.
3. Katz, A. M.: Energetics of muscle: energy utilization (work and heat). *In* Physiology of the Heart. New York, Raven Press, 1977, p. 73.
4. Mason, D. T., Spann, J. F., Jr., Zelis, R., and Amsterdam, E. A.: Alterations of hemodynamics and myocardial mechanics in patients with congestive heart failure: pathophysiologic mechanisms and assessment of cardiac function and ventricular contractility. Prog. Cardiovasc. Dis., *12:*507, 1970.
5. Rushmer, R. F.: Functional anatomy of cardiac contraction. *In* Organ Physiology: Structure and Function of the Cardiovascular System. Philadelphia, W. B. Saunders, 1972, p. 33.
6. Braunwald, E., Sonnenblick, E. H., and Ross, J., Jr.: Contraction of the normal heart. *In* Heart Disease: A Textbook of Cardiovascular Medicine. Edited by E. Braunwald. Philadelphia, W. B. Saunders, 1984, p. 409.
7. Schland, R. C., Sonnenblick, E. H., and Gorlin, R.: Normal physiology of the cardiovascular system. *In* The Heart. Edited by J. Willis Hurst, et al. New York, McGraw-Hill, 1982, p. 75.
8. Ross, J., Jr.: Cardiac function and myocardial contractility: a perspective. J. Am. Coll. Cardiol. *1:*52, 1983.
9. Katz, A. M.: Contractile proteins. *In* Physiology of the Heart. New York, Raven Press, 1977, p. 89.
10. Guyton, A. S., Jones, C. E., and Coleman, T. G.: Circulatory Physiology: Cardiac Output and its Regulation. 2nd Ed. Philadelphia, W. B. Saunders, 1973.
11. Pouleur, H., Covell, J. W., and Ross, J., Jr.: Effects of nitroprusside on venous return and central blood volume in the presence and absence of acute heart failure. Circulation, *61:*328, 1980.
12. Dougherty, A. H. et al.: Congestive heart failure with normal systolic function. Am. J. Cardiol., *54:*778, 1984.
13. Frohlich, E. D.: Left ventricular hypertrophy, cardiac diseases and hypertension: recent experiences. J. Am. Coll. Cardiol., *14:*1587, 1989.
14. Spirito, P., and Maron, B. J.: Relation between extent of left ventricular hypertrophy and diastolic filling abnormalities in hypertrophic cardiomyopathy. J. Am. Coll. Cardiol., *15:*37:808, 1990.
15. Rahimtoola, S. H.: Perspective on valvular heart disease: an update. J. Am. Coll. Cardiol., *14:*1, 1989.
16. Unverferth, D. V. (Ed.): Dilated Cardiomyopathy. Mount Kisco, NY, Futura Publishing, 1985.
17. Parter, J. D., Ledwich, M. B., and West, R. O.: Reversible cardiac failure during angina pectoris. Circulation, *39:*745, 1969.
18. Shabeti, R.: The pericardium: an essay on some recent developments. Am. J. Cardiol., *42:*1036, 1978.
19. Cameron, J., Oesterle, S. N., Baldwin, J. C., and Hancock, E. W.: The etiologic spectrum of constrictive pericarditis. Am. Heart J., *113:*354, 1987.
20. Perez, C. A., Presant, C. A., and Amburg, A. L.: Management of superior vena cava syndrome. Service Oncol., *5:*123, 1978.
21. Fry, D. L., Griffs, D. M., and Greenfield, F. C.: Myocardial mechanics: tension-velocity-length relationships in heart muscle. Circ. Res., *14:*73, 1964.
22. Downing, S. E., and Sonnenblick, E. H.: Cardiac muscle mechanics and ventricular performance: force and time parameters. Am. J. Physiol., *207:*705, 1964.
23. Sonnenblick, E. H.: Force-velocity relations in mammalian heart muscle. Am. J. Physiol., *202:*931, 1962.
24. Lundin, G.: Mechanical properties of cardiac muscle. Acta Physiol. Scand., *20:*7, 1944.
25. Ross, J., Jr.: Assessment of cardiac function and myocardial contractility. *In* The Heart. 5th Ed. Edited by J. Willis Hurst. Atlanta, McGraw-Hill, 1982, p. 310.
26. Boudoulas, H. et al.: Effect of afterload on left ventricular performance in experimental animals. Comparison of the pre-ejection period and other indices of left ventricular contractility. J. Med., *13:*373, 1982.
27. Reeves, T. J. et al.: The hemodynamic determinants of the rate of change in pressure in the left ventricle during isometric contraction. Am. Heart. J., *60:*745, 1960.
28. Parker, J. O., and Case, R. B.: Normal left ventricular function. Circulation, *60:*4, 1979.
29. Holt, J. P.: Regulation of the degree of emptying of the left ventricle and effects of epinephrine and heart rate on the ratio. Circ. Res., *32:*314, 1973.
30. Grossman, W., Jones, D., and McLaurein, L. P.: Wall stress and patterns of hypertrophy. J. Clin. Invest., *56:*36, 1975.
31. Adelstein, R. S., Pato, M. D., and Conti, M. A.: The role of phosphorylation in regulating contractile proteins. *In* Advances in Cyclic Nucleotide Research. Vol. 14. Edited by J. E. Dumond, P. Greengard, and G. A. Robinson. New York, Raven Press, 1981, p. 361.
32. Tsein, R. W.: Cyclic AMP and contractile activity of the heart. *In* Advances in Nucleotide Research. Vol. 8. Edited by P. Greengard and G. A. Robinson. New York, Raven, Press, 1977, p. 363.
33. Katz, A. M., Jada, M., and Kirchberber, M. A.: Control of calcium transport in the myocardium by the cyclic-AMP-protein kinase system. *In* Advances in Cyclic Nucleotide Research. Vol. 5. Edited by G. I. Drummond, P. Greengard, and G. K. Robinson. New York, Raven Press, 1975, p. 453.
34. Kukovetz, W. R., Poch, G., and Wurm, A.: Quantitative relations between cyclic AMP and contraction as affected by stimulators of adenylate cyclase and inhibitors of phosphodiesterase. *In* Advances in Cyclic Nucleotide Research. Vol. 1. Edited by G. I. Drummond, P. Greengard, and G. K. Robinson. New York, Raven Press, 1975, p. 395.
35. Sagawa, K.: Editorial. The end-systolic pressure-volume relation of the ventricle: definition, modifications, and clinical use. Circulation, *63:*1223, 1981.
36. Katz, A. M.: The descending limb of the Starling curve and the failing heart. (Editorial.) Circulation, *32:*871, 1965.
37. Monroe, R. G. et al: Left ventricular performance at high end-diastolic pressures in isolated, perfused dog hearts. Circ. Res., *26:*85, 1970.
38. Grimm, A. F., Lin, H. L., and Grimm, B. R.: Left ventricular free wall and intraventricular pressure-sarcomere length distribution. Am. J. Physiol., *239:*H101, 1980.
39. Baker, B. J. et al.: Relation of right ventricular ejection fraction to exercise capacity in chronic left ventricular failure. Am. J. Cardiol., *54:*596, 1984.
40. Maddahi, J. et al.: Right ventricular ejection fraction during exercise in normal subjects and in coronary artery disease patients: assessment by multiple-gated equilibrium scintigraphy. Circulation, *62:*133, 1980.
41. Maddahi, J. et al.: A new technique for assessing right ventricular ejection fraction using rapid multiple-gated equilibrium cardiac blood pool scintigraphy. Circulation, *60:*581, 1979.
42. Morrison, D. A., Turgeon, J., and Ovitt, T.: Right ventricular ejection fraction measurement: contract ventriculography versus gated blood pool and gated first-pass radionuclide methods. Am. J. Cardiol., *54:*651, 1984.

43. Xue, Q. F. et al.: Can right ventricular performance be assessed by equilibrium radionuclide ventriculography? Thorax, *38:*486, 1983.
44. Morrison, D. et al.: An improved method of right ventricular gated equilibrium blood pool radionuclide ventriculography. Chest, *82:*607, 1982.
45. Holman, B. L., Wynne, J., Zielonka, J. S., and Idoine, J. D.: A simplified technique for measuring right ventricular ejection fraction using the equilibrium radionuclide angiocardiogram and the slant-hole collimator. Radiology, *138:*429, 1981.
46. Konstam, M. A. et al.: Comparison of left and right ventricular end-diastolic pressure-volume relations in congestive heart failure. J. Am. Coll. Cardiol., *5:*1326, 1985.
47. Konstam, M. A. et al.: Vasodilator effects on RV function in congestive heart failure and pulmonary hypertension: end-systolic pressure-volume relations. Am. J. Cardiol., *54:*132, 1984.
48. Yamaguchi, S. et al.: Effect of left ventricular volume on right ventricular end-systolic pressure-volume relation. Circ. Res., *65:*623, 1989.
49. Martin, C. et al.: Right ventricular function during positive end-expiratory pressure. Chest, *92:*999, 1987.
50. Schulman, D. S. et al.: Effect of positive end-expiratory pressure on right ventricular performance. Am. J. Med., *84:*57, 1988.
51. Bove, A. A., and Santamore, W. P.: Ventricular interdependence. Prog. Cardiovasc. Dis., *23:*365, 1981.
52. Bashore, T. M., and Shaffer, P. B.: Nuclear cardiology. *In* Diagnostic Procedures in Cardiology: A Clinician's Guide. Edited by J. V. Warren and R. P. Lewis. Chicago, Year Book, 1985, p. 143.
53. Boucher, C. A.: Assessment of Left Ventricular Function in Noninvasive Cardiac Imaging. Edited by J. Morgenroth, A. Parisi, and G. M. Pohost. Chicago Year Book Medical Publishers, 1983, p. 71.
54. Kato, M.: In vivo labelling of red blood cells with stannous phydorylideneaminates. J. Nucl. Med., *20:*1071, 1979.
55. Starling, R. C., Hammer, D. F., Wooding-Scott, M., and Binkley, P. F.: A comparison of thermodilution versus radionuclide assessment of ejection fraction in cardiac transplant recipients. Clin. Res., *38:*886A, 1990.
56. Feigenbaum, H.: Echocardiographic evaluation of cardiac chambers. *In* Echocardiography. Philadelphia, Lea & Febiger, 1981, p. 119.
57. Popp, R. L.: Echocardiographic assessment of cardiac disease. *In* Reviews of Contemporary Laboratory Methods. Edited by A. M. Weissler. Dallas, American Heart Association, 1980, p. 197.
58. Hattle, L., and Angelsen, B.: Doppler Ultrasound in Cardiology. Philadelphia, Lea & Febiger, 1985.
59. Nishimura, R. A. et al.: Doppler echocardiography: theory, instrumentation, technique and application. Mayo Clin. Proc., *60:*321, 1985.
60. Huntsman, L. L. et al: Noninvasive Doppler determination of cardiac output in man: clinical validation. Circulation, *67:*593, 1983.
61. Tavel, M. E.: Clinical Phonocardiography and External Pulse Recording. Chicago, Year Book Medical Publishers, 1978.
62. Ventricular Function from Cardiac Catheterization Data to Hemodynamic Parameters. Philadelphia, F. A. Davis, 1972, p. 157.
63. Dodge, H. T., Sandler, H., Baxley, W. A., and Hawley, R. R.: Usefulness and limitations of radiographic methods for determining left ventricular volume. Am. J. Cardiol., *18:*10, 1966.
64. Bommer, W. et al.: Determination of right atrial and right ventricular size by two-dimensional echocardiography. Circulation, *60:*91, 1979.
65. Vitolo, E. et al.: Two-dimensional echocardiographic evaluation of right ventricular ejection fraction: comparison between three different methods. Acta Cardiol., *43:*469, 1988.
66. Hirschleifer, J., Crawford, M., O'Rourke, R. A., and Karliner, J. S.: Influence of acute alterations in heart rate and systemic arterial pressure on echocardiographic measures of left ventricular performance in normal human subjects. Circulation, *52:*895, 1975.
67. Slutsky, R. et al.: Assessment of right ventricular function at rest and during exercise in patients with coronary heart disease: a new approach using equilibrium radionuclide angiography. Am. J. Cardiol., *45:*63, 1980.
68. Quinonis, M. A., Gaasoh, W. H., and Alexander, J. K.: Echocardiographic assessment of left ventricular function: with special emphasis to normalized velocities. Circulation, *50:*42, 1974.
69. Weissler, A. M., and Garrand, C. L., Jr.: Systolic time intervals in cardiac disease. Mod. Concepts Cardiovasc. Dis., *40:*1, 1971.
70. Boudoulas, H. et al.: Assessment of ventricular function by combined noninvasive measures: factors accounting for methodologic disparities. Int. J. Cardiol., *2:*493, 1982.
71. Aronow, W. S.: Isovolumic contraction and left ventricular ejection time. Am. J. Cardiol., *26:*238, 1970.
72. Bunnel, I. L., Grant, C., and Green, D. G.: Left ventricular function derived from the pressure-volume diagram. Am. J. Med., *39:*881, 1965.
73. Grossman, W. et al.: Contractile state of the left ventricle in man as evaluated from end-systolic pressure-volume relations. Circulation, *56:*845, 1977.
74. Mehmel, H. C. et al.: The linearity of the end-systolic pressure-volume relationship in man and its sensitivity for assessment of left ventricular function. Circulation, *63:*1216, 1981.
75. Suga, H., and Sagawa, K.: Instantaneous pressure-volume relationships and their ratio in the excised, supported canine left ventricle. Circ. Res., *35:*117, 1974.
76. Mahler, F., Covell, J. W., and Ross, J., Jr.: systolic pressure-diameter relations in the normal conscious dog. Cardiovasc. Res., *9:*447, 1975.
77. Weisfeldt, M. L. et al.: E-max as a new contractility index in man. (Abstract). Circulation, *54(Suppl. 2):*114, 1976.
78. Sagawa, K., Suga, H., Shoukas, A. A., and Bakalar, K. M.: End-systolic pressure-volume ratio: a new index of ventricular contractility. Am. J. Cardiol., *40:*748, 1977.
79. Suga, H., Sagawa, K., and Shoukas, A. A.: Load independence of the instantaneous pressure-volume ratio of the canine left ventricle and effects of epinephrine and heart rate on the ratio. Circ. Res., *32:*314, 1973.
80. Borow, K. M., Green, L. H., Grossman, W., and Braunwald, E.: Left ventricular end-systolic stress-shortening and stress-length relations in humans: normal values and sensitivity to inotropic state. Am. J. Cardiol., *50:*1301, 1982.
81. Borow, K. M. et al.: Left ventricular end-systolic pressure dimension relation in patients with thalassemia major: a new noninvasive method of assessing contractile state. Circulation, *66:*980, 1982.
82. Brodie, B. R., McLaurin, L. P., and Grossman, W.: Combined hemodynamic-ultrasound method for studying left ventricular wall stress: comparison with angiography. Am. J. Cardiol., *37:*864, 1976.
83. Marsh, J. D. et al.: Left ventricular end-systolic pressure-dimension and stress-length relations in normal human subjects. Am. J. Cardiol., *44:*1311, 1979.
84. Borow, J. M., Newmann, A., and Wynne, J.: Sensitivity of

end-systolic pressure-dimension and pressure-volume relations to the inotropic state in humans. Circulation, 65:988, 1982.
85. Binkley, P. F., Lewe, R. F., Unverferth, D. V., and Leier, C. V.: Preservation of the end-systolic pressure/end-systolic dimension relations following pindolol in congestive heart failure. Am. Heart J., 115:1245, 1988.
86. Binkley, P. F., Lewe, R. F., Unverferth, D. V., and Leier, C. V.: Late systolic indices of ventricular function: noninvasive derivation in congestive heart failure. Am. Heart J., 116:1276, 1988.
87. Brodie, B. R., McLaurin, L. P., and Grossman, W.: Combined hemodynamic-ultrasound method for studying left ventricular wall stress: comparison with angiography. Am. J. Cardiol., 37:864, 1976.
88. Colan, S. D., Borow, K. M., and Neuman, A.: Left ventricular end-systolic wall stress velocity of fiber shortening relation: a load-independent index of myocardial contractility. J. Am. Col. Cardiol., 4:715, 1984.
89. Stefadourous, M. A., Dougherty, M. J., Grossman, W., and Craige, E.: Determination of systemic vascular resistance by a noninvasive technique. Circulation, 47:101, 1973.
90. Aroney, C. N. et al.: Linearity of the left ventricular end-systolic pressure-volume relation in patients with severe heart failure. J. Am. Coll. Cardiol., 14:127, 1989.
91. Takahaski, M., Sasayama, S., Kawai, C., and Kotoura, H.: Contractile performance of the hypertrophied ventricle in patients with systemic hypertension. Circulation, 62:116, 1980.
92. Roman, M. J., Devereux, R. B., and Cody, R. M.: Ability of left ventricular stress-shortening relations, end-systolic stress/volume ratio and indirect indexes to detect severe contractile failure in ischemic or idiopathic dilated cardiomyopathy. Am. J. Cardiol., 64:1338, 1989.
93. Dehmer, G. T. et al.: Exercise-induced alterations in left ventricular volumes and the pressure-volume relationship. Circulation, 63:1008, 1981.
94. Carabello, B. A., and Spann, J. F.: The uses and limitations of end-systolic indexes of left ventricular function. Circulation, 69:1064, 1984.
95. Carabello, B. A., Nolan, S. P., and McGuire, L. B.: Assessment of preoperative left ventricular function in patients with mitral regurgitation: value of the end-systolic wall stress-end-systolic volume ratio. Circulation, 64:1212, 1981.
96. Gardin, J. M.: Doppler measurements of aortic blood flow velocity and acceleration: load-independent indexes of left ventricular performance? Am. J. Cardiol., 64:935, 1989.
97. Bedotto, J. B., Eichhorn, E. J., and Grayburn, P. A.: Effects of left ventricular preload and afterload on ascending aortic blood velocity and acceleration in coronary artery simultaneous high fidelity left atrial and ventricular pressures in idiopathic dilated cardiomyopathy. Am. J. Cardiol., 64:1173, 1989.
98. Isaaz, K. et al.: A new Doppler method of assessing left ventricular ejection force in chronic congestive heart failure. Am. J. Cardiol., 64:81, 1989.
99. Stamm, R. B., and Martin, R. P.: Quantification of pressure gradients across stenotic valves by Doppler ultrasound. J. Am. Coll. Cardiol., 2:707, 1983.
100. Landry, A. B., Jr., and Goodyer, A. V. N.: Rate of rise of left ventricular pressure: indirect measurement and physiologic significance. Am. J. Cardiol., 15:660, 1965.
101. Gleason, W. L., and Braunwald, E.: Studies on the first derivative of the ventricular pressure pulse in man. J. Clin. Invest., 41:80, 1962.
102. Mason, D. T., Braunwald, E., Ross, J., Jr., and Morrow, A. G.: Diagnostic valve of the first and second derivatives of the arterial pressure pulse in aortic valve disease and hypertrophic subaortic stenosis. Circulation, 30:90, 1964.
103. Wallace, A. G., Skinner, N. S., Jr., and Mitchell, J. H.: Hemodynamic determinants of the maximal rate of rise of left ventricular pressure. Am. J. Physiol., 30:205, 1963.
104. Mason, D. T.: Usefulness and limitations of the rate of rise of intraventricular pressure (dp/dt) in the evaluation of myocardial contractility in man. Am. J. Cardiol., 23:516, 1969.
105. Mason, E. H. et al.: Assessment of myocardial contractility in man: relationship between the rate of pressure rise and developed pressure throughout isometric left ventricular contraction. Circulation, 36(Suppl. 2):183, 1967.
106. Diamond, G. et al.: Mean electromechanical P/t. Am. J. Cardiol., 46:291, 1972.
107. Rushmer, R. F.: The cardiac output. In Organ Physiology: Structure and Function of the Cardiovascular System. Boston, W. B. Saunders, 1972, p. 70.
108. Snell, R. E., and Luchsinger, P. C.: Determination of the external work and power of left ventricle in intact man. Am. Heart J., 69:529, 1965.
109. Topham, W. S.: Comparison of methods for calculation of left ventricular stroke work. J. Appl. Physiol., 27:767, 1969.
110. Gilbert, J. C., and Glantz, S. A.: Determinants of left ventricular filling and of the diastolic pressure-volume relation. Circ. Res., 64:827, 1989.
111. Lew, W. Y. W.: Evaluation of left ventricular diastolic function. Circulation, 79:1393, 1989.
112. Magorien, D. J. et al.: Assessment of left ventricular pressure-volume relations using gated radionuclide angiography, echocardiography, and micromanometer pressure recordings. Circulation, 67:844, 1983.
113. Binkley, P. F., Shaffer, P. B., Ryan, J. M., and Leier, C. V.: Augmentation of diastolic function with phosphodiesterase inhibition in congestive heart failure. J. Lab. Clin. Med., 114:266, 1989.
114. Rokey, R. et al.: Determination of parameters of left ventricular diastolic filling with pulsed Doppler echocardiography comparison with cineangiography. Circulation, 7:543, 1985.
115. Appleton, C. P., Hatle, L. K., and Popp, R. L.: Relation of transmitral flow velocity to left ventricular diastolic function. J. Am. Coll. Cardiol., 12:426, 1988.
116. David, D. et al.: Comparison of Doppler indexes of left ventricular diastolic function with simultaneous high fidelity left atrial and ventricular pressures in idiopathic dilated cardiomyopathy. Am. J. Cardiol., 64:1173, 1989.

Chapter 27

COMMON DISORDERS OF CARDIAC RHYTHM AND CONDUCTION IN THE CRITICALLY ILL PATIENT

BRUCE L. WILKOFF
STEPHEN L. MOORE

Accurate recognition of disturbances of cardiac conduction is essential for appropriate diagnosis and therapeutic management of critically ill patients. Improved techniques of intracardiac recording and stimulation have identified mechanisms underlying the pathophysiology of many common arrhythmias and provides a rational basis for their diagnosis and treatment.[1-6] Some arrhythmias are benign and may not warrant intervention, whereas others are disabling and life-threatening and should be treated aggressively. Appropriate therapy should be determined by the following:

- The pathophysiology of the arrhythmia
- The natural history of the disorder
- The efficacy of treatment

This chapter analyzes conduction disturbances in the critically ill patient in three phases: pre-ICU phase (risk phase), ICU (support phase), and post-ICU phase (rehabilitation phase).

PRE-ICU PHASE (RISK PHASE)

The general approach to accurate diagnosis and appropriate therapy of conduction disturbances in the critically ill patient requires careful analysis of the patient's history, physical examination, electrocardiogram (ECG), as well as an understanding of the nature of these rhythm disturbances and available therapeutic modalities. When possible, one should adhere to this approach in evaluating patients with rhythm disturbances.

Two physiologic mechanisms account for most ectopic arrhythmias: reentry and enhanced automaticity.[7-11] Reentry is precipitated by a variety of alterations in refractoriness, impulse formation, and conduction velocity[9] (Fig. 27-1). The therapy is aimed at interruption of the reentrant circuit by changing one of the three conditions from reentry—an obstruction, slow conduction, and unidirectional block—that divides the conducted impulses. Enhanced automaticity leads to repetitive firing from a single focus within the heart.[10] Therapy is aimed at reducing the stimulus to or response from spontaneous depolarizations within the action potential. In many cases the cause of a cardiac arrhythmia, regardless of its mechanism, cannot be determined. The cause is then generally assigned to any associated cardiac disease. Common causes of arrhythmias that are sometimes overlooked include the following:

- Extracardiac disorders (i.e., thyrotoxicosis)
- Electrolyte abnormalities (hyperkalemia or hypokalemia and acid/base disorders)
- Hypotension, hypoxia, and hypercapnia that are due to poor ventilation (chronic obstructive lung disease or after pulmonary surgery)
- Adverse effects of drugs such as digitalis, quinidine, propranolol, aminophylline, and beta-adrenergic agonists[1,2,6,7,8,12]

On reviewing a patient's history, frequently, the physician will examine the patient after the arrhythmia has terminated. If the arrhythmia was not documented by ECG or rhythm strip, the history may give clues to the diagnosis. It is important to determine the circumstances that preceded the arrhythmia: exercise, stress, emotion, caffeine intake, angina, hypoxia, ethanol intake, or metabolic abnormality. If possible, the patient must be thoroughly interrogated by asking such questions as the following:

Is this the first episode?
How often do the episodes occur?
Are they paroxysmal?
How long do they last?
Are you aware of the heart beat?
Is it fast or slow?
Is it regular or irregular?
Did it cause palpitations?
Dizziness?
Presyncope or syncope?
Did you check your pulse?
Did you note any sensation of flushing, choking, or throbbing in the neck before losing consciousness?
How was the arrhythmia terminated?

The answer to these questions may aid in the diagnosis of the arrhythmia as well as underlying cause. Symptoms or a history of any disease that may directly or indirectly influence the cardiovascular system should be listed. The pa-

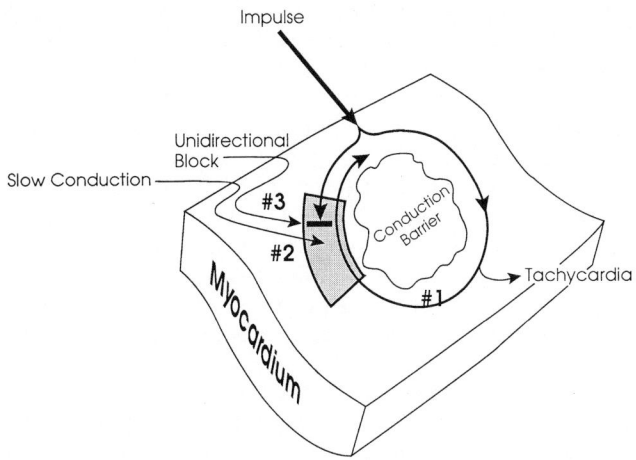

Fig. 27-1. For reentry to cause a sustained arrhythmia, three conditions must be maintained: #1, an anatomic or functional obstruction; #2, slow conduction; and #3, unidirectional block around. These conditions are frequently met in the area of a scar from a myocardial infarction.

tient's medications should be carefully reviewed. For all patients, it is imperative to determine whether there is any serious underlying heart disease because treatment must be directed not only at the arrhythmia but at the cause.

Physical examination should include taking blood pressure and both apical and peripheral pulses. When evaluating an arrhythmia, three particularly helpful parts of the cardiovascular examination include: intensity of the first heart sound, splitting of the second heart sound, and jugular venous pulse. All of these should be observed closely for patterns of atrial activity and atrioventricular synchrony.[13]

The **first heart sound** (S_1) corresponds to the closure of the atrioventricular (AV) valves with the more intense mitral valve closure sound preceding the softer tricuspid valve closure sound. Intensity of S_1 depends primarily on the position of the valve at the onset of ventricular systole as well as the rate of rise of pressure distension in the ventricle.[14] Rheumatic scarring or other diseases may affect the mobility of the valvular leaflets and thus the intensity of S_1. If ventricular systole occurs after a short PR interval, when the valves are still widely open, S_1 will be loud as the valves snap back.[13] With marked prolongation of the PR interval, as occurs in the first-degree AV block, the valves have time to float back to their closed position before the onset of ventricular systole, resulting in a soft S_1.[13] If the PR interval is constantly changing—as occurs in complete heart block, Mobitz type-II AV block, and junctional or ventricular tachycardia with AV dissociation—the intensity of S_1 will vary.[13] Other arrhythmias with varying times of activation between the atrium and ventricles include atrial fibrillation, atrial flutter with varying block, and atrial tachycardia with varying block. Premature ventricular beats may also cause variation of S_1 intensity. Because the ability to appreciate how loud or soft S_1 is may depend on habitus and the presence of associated lung disease or pulmonary edema, the most useful part of this examination is to listen for variation and intensity.[13,14]

The **second heart sound** (S_2) corresponds to the closure of the semilunar valves, with aortic valve closure preceding pulmonary valve closure. Splitting of these two sounds corresponds to the slight asynchrony between ventricles as a result of slight increased filling of the right ventricle during inspiration.[14] Slow activation of the right ventricle because of right bundle branch block or a pressure volume overload of the right ventricle may accentuate the delay between the aortic and pulmonary closure, with a wider split S_2. If the right ventricle is activated before the left ventricle, as in patients with an artificial pacemaker or in patients with left bundle branch block, splitting of the second heart sound will be paradoxic, with the pulmonary component preceding the aortic component.[13]

Examination of the **jugular venous pulse** allows evaluation of the mechanical activity of the right atrium. Examination of the jugular venous pulse is the best bedside method for detection of right-sided congestive heart failure and is reliable in most patients.[13] Normal right atrial systole causes an A wave with relaxation starting the X descent. As isovolumic right ventricular contraction displaces the tricuspid valve upward, the X descent is interrupted by the C wave. As the right atrium fills during right ventricular contraction, the V wave is seen. After right ventricular systole and opening of the tricuspid valve, the V wave collapses with the Y descent. Hemodynamic alterations, such as tricuspid stenosis, pulmonary stenosis, and pulmonary hypertension will all transmit high pressures to the atrium, resulting in a giant A wave. Cannon A waves result from atrial contraction against a closed tricuspid valve and may be seen with AV dissociation. If there is retrograde conduction to the atrium with junctional or ventricular tachycardia, cannon A waves will be frequent. Commonly, cannon A waves are seen with ventricular premature beats, ventricular pacing, and complete heart block. In atrial flutter, flutter waves may be seen in the jugular pulse occurring at a rapid rate and corresponding to the flutter waves seen on an ECG. In any case, examination of the jugular pulse is very difficult and impossible to interpret correctly if not performed with adequate lighting and proper position. Misinterpretation of carotid pulsations must be avoided. Jugular venous pulsations are most useful for detecting AV dissociation and identifying atrial flutter.[13,14]

Certain cardiac maneuvers use vagal stimulation to produce slowing or termination of arrhythmias and provide an additional modality for diagnosing cardiac arrhythmias.[13] Many patients with paroxysmal tachycardias may volunteer the fact that they themselves have discovered methods to terminate their arrhythmias. Many of these are variations of the Valsalva maneuver or other ways to increase vagal tone. The arrhythmia that most commonly terminates with vagal stimulation, such as Valsalva's maneuver, is paroxysmal AV nodal tachycardia. This termination is usually abrupt. Sinus tachycardia may slow during vagal stimulation, while ventricular tachycardia will show no response. In patients with atrial flutter or atrial tachycardia with block, vagal stimulation increases the amount of block but does not terminate the arrhythmia. This maneuver helps to establish the diagnosis as the flutter or P waves become more apparent on the ECG. With atrial fibrillation, Valsalva's maneuver may slow the ventricular response, but it returns to the prior rate after the maneuver is completed.[15] In some reciprocating tachycardias, vagal stimulation may also terminate the arrhythmia or may have no effect.

Carotid sinus massage should be performed as a diagnostic aid only after auscultation to exclude carotid bruits has been undertaken.[13,16] Initially, pressure is gently applied to make certain that the patient does not have a hypersensitive carotid sinus. Pressure may be applied with a massaging action for no longer than 4 to 5 seconds while simultaneously accessing the response of the arrhythmia, usually with electrocardiographic monitoring. Stimulation may have to be repeated five or six times before abrupt conversion of arrhythmia has been accomplished. The most likely rhythm to terminate with sinus massage is an AV nodal tachycardia.[13,16] Sinus tachycardia and atrial fibrillation may temporarily have a slower ventricular response. Atrial flutter and atrial tachycardia with block may have a higher degree of block. Ventricular tachycardia will not respond.

Laboratory studies should also be obtained for all patients before admission to the ICU. Electrolytes (including potassium, calcium, and magnesium), arterial blood gases, antiarrhythmic drug levels, and thyroid function should be measured. A chest radiograph should be employed as a basic method in evaluating a patient with cardiac arrhythmia. The surface ECG is an indispensable tool for proper diagnosis and treatment of arrhythmias.[1,17] Inability to differentiate between atrial depolarizations coinciding with ventricular depolarizations or repolarizations indicates the need for other procedures to assist in the diagnosis. These procedures include vagal stimuli, carotid sinus massage, Valsalva's maneuver, and obtaining an atrial electrogram (EGM).[17,18] Long rhythm strips with evaluation of multiple leads may aid in diagnosing various arrhythmias in question. Leads AVF and V_1 are generally most valuable in identifying atrial activity. Recording the rhythm strip at 50 mm per second may help discriminate P waves. When P waves are not apparent with the standard 12-lead ECG, exploring electrodes on the chest may allow distinction in certain cases. Bipolar exploring leads (Lewis leads) may accentuate atrial activity, using lead I with the left arm electrode placed posteriorly or over the left ventricular apex and the right arm electrode used to explore the precordium.[1,13] The two electrodes are moved to different positions on the chest, and lead I is monitored for the appearance of P waves. If they appear, further manipulation may increase their size. If successful, this technique may aid in the diagnosis of supraventricular arrhythmias.

The atrial EGM is a recording of the electrical activity of the heart from electrodes in direct contact with or in close proximity to the atria, thus enabling a differentiation of atrial from ventricular activity. There are three ways to obtain an atrial EGM: (1) placement of an esophageal electrode; (2) placement of a transvenous temporary pacing electrode; or (3) temporary epicardial electrodes placed at the time of cardiac surgery.[18-20] Many modern pacemakers have atrial and ventricular EGM capabilities (Fig. 27-2).

Esophageal electrodes may be necessary to identify atrial activity.[18] Placement of an electrode in the esophagus behind the heart may permit the recording of P waves because of the proximity to the atria. Optimal atrial recordings are obtained 40 to 50 cm from the nares. Special esophageal electrodes are available. When the electrode is in position and the ECG is being recorded, the electrode may be withdrawn to maximize the atrial EGM and minimize the ventricular EGM. Identification of atrial activity is facilitated if surface ECG and intracardiac leads can be monitored simultaneously. A-wave activity is generally of short duration, in synchrony with P waves on the surface ECG and frequently not during the surface QRS. If an esophageal lead is not available, one can be made by passing a temporary pacemaker wire through a nasogastric tube. The electrode tip of the pacemaker wire should not be extended beyond the terminal part of the tube when it is passed into the esophagus. The nasogastric tube should be passed to approximately 50 cm, and the proximal end of the pacing wire should be attached to an exploring electrode. The pacemaker wire should then be extruded from the distal end of the nasogastric tube, and a search should be made for electrical activity. Having the patient hold a midinspiration breath reduces respiratory motion. Permanent transvenous pacemaker leads can be used without a nasogastric tube. Placement is facilitated with the use of a pacemaker electrode stylet that has been stiffened in a freezer for 15 minutes.

Endocardial atrial ECGs can be obtained if other methods are inadequate. Direct recording from inside the atrium is the most accurate way to record atrial activity but has the disadvantage of being invasive.[19] This procedure should be done under sterile conditions, with an electrically isolated ECG machine or special amplifier. It requires insertion of a temporary pacing electrode into a peripheral or central vein with advancement to the right atrium. If insertion is not performed under fluoroscopy, the electrode should be connected to the ECG and constantly monitored for the appearance of a large atrial deflection. Connection of the electrode to the V lead of the ECG will provide a unipolar tracing. Bipolar EGMs can be accomplished by connecting the two electrodes on the temporary lead to the right and left arm electrodes of the ECG mode with alligator clips while monitoring standard lead I. Sometimes the electrode can be used to terminate the arrhythmia by overdrive pacing.[21] Extreme care must be taken to avoid displacement of the temporary electrode into the ventricle during rapid pacing of the atrium.

Atrial recordings may also be obtained in patients immediately following open heart surgery, when atrial and ventricular pacing electrodes have been placed.[19-21] These epicardial electrodes, which exit through the chest wall, are easily applied at the time of surgery and easily removed before a patient's discharge. They provide a safety factor for the patient if bradycardia pacing is required and diagnostic ease if an arrhythmia develops. Unipolar or bipolar EGMs can be obtained. The unipolar EGM is a recording of the difference of electrical potential between the atria and the skin. It provides information about both ventricular and atrial activity and permits assessment of the relationship of activation. The bipolar atrial EGM is a recording of the difference between the two atrial electrodes, thus demonstrating atrial activity with little or no ventricular activation deflection. The bipolar EGM is preferred when

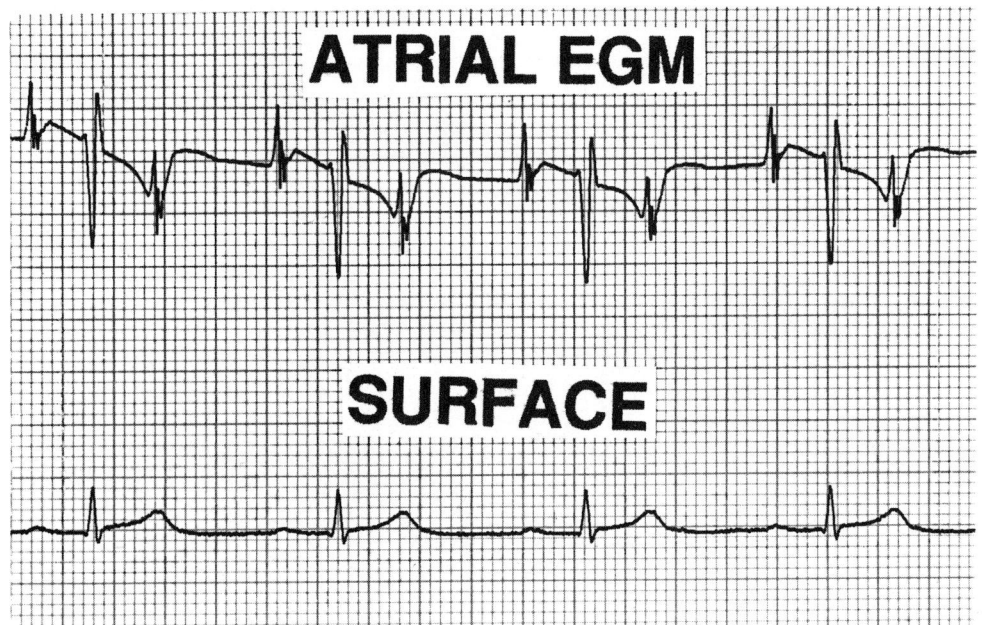

Fig. 27-2. An atrial electrogram (EGM) records the electrical activity from a localized portion of the atrial myocardium. This study uniquely demonstrates the depolarization of the atria as distinct from the ventricles. The surface ECG shows QRS complexes at a rate of 70 beats per minute, but the atrial electrogram shows complexes simultaneous with the surface ECG and additional deflections on either side of the QRS occurring at 140 beats per minute. This electrogram demonstrates 2:1 AV conduction of an atrial tachycardia. This is an example of atrial tachycardia with block secondary to digitalis toxicity.

an atrial EGM is done simultaneously with a surface ECG or ECG to permit clear identification of atrial activation; when the rhythm diagnosis is unclear from the surface ECG record; when the rhythm is rapid or irregular; or when there is difficulty in differentiating the P wave from the QRS complex[20] (Fig. 27-3). Once a diagnosis has been made, overdrive pacing may be performed through the same electrodes when appropriate.[21]

In summary, several types of patients are more likely to end up in the ICU than others, but there are many exceptions. Histories of significant syncope, palpitations, cardiac arrest, ischemia, myocardial infarction, or chronic lung disease all suggest that an arrhythmia may complicate future care. Times of instability such as hypoxemia, ischemia, or hypokalemia and hypomagnesemia related to diuretic use are also frequent precursors to arrhythmias requiring ICU therapy. Unfortunately, more people die suddenly from sustained ventricular tachycardia or fibrillation, frequently without the identification of previous heart disease, than die of cancer each year. Whether or not the pre-ICU risk

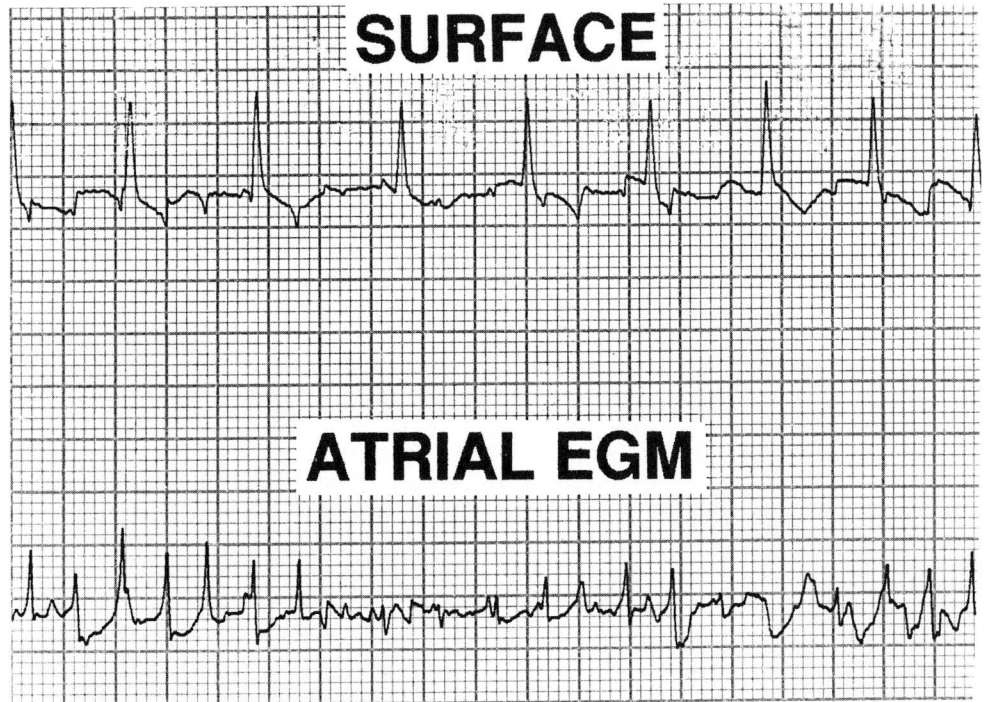

Fig. 27-3. In atrial fibrillation, the fibrillation waves of the chaotically depolarizing atrium are much more clearly seen on the atrial electrogram than on the surface ECG. The surface ECG suggests that the rhythm might be atrial flutter, but the atrial electrogram shows that the electrograms continuously change in shape and rate. Atrial flutter can be terminated by pacing, but atrial fibrillation is not responsive to pacing.

is identified, the clinician must use all the clues available to make the diagnosis of the arrhythmia in the pre-ICU phase. First and foremost, it must be determined if the patient is hemodynamically compromised and whether an arrhythmia is responsible. Next, review of the ECG with attention to rate, regularity, QRS axis, width and morphology, AV dissociation, and P waves may lead to the diagnosis. The history and physical examination provide further evidence. Finally, response to cardiac maneuvers and drugs and the use of specialized electrode techniques may confirm the diagnosis. Although none of these steps alone may be diagnostic, together, they should allow narrowing the differential diagnosis to one or two possibilities. The symptoms of an arrhythmia may not be apparent at the onset. In arrhythmias of longer duration, there may be progressive deterioration of cardiac function, with impaired perfusion of vital organs from decreased cardiac output. The patient may then develop symptoms resulting from inadequate perfusion of the brain, heart, kidneys, skin, and extremities. That the patient tolerates the arrhythmia at the outset does not guarantee that circulatory embarrassment will not develop with time. If the rhythm is determined to jeopardize the patient by resulting in hemodynamic compromise, he should be moved to the ICU for further monitoring, evaluation, and treatment.

ICU PHASE (SUPPORT PHASE)

Before treating the patient with cardiac arrhythmias, it is important to consider reversible precipitating factors that might be corrected. Hypoxia can induce arrhythmias, and acidosis lowers the threshold for ventricular fibrillation.[12] It is not commonly appreciated, however, that alkalosis is even more likely than acidosis to produce ventricular arrhythmias. Establishment of a physiologic partial pressure of oxygen (Po_2), partial pressure of carbon dioxide (Pco_2), and pH can be of major therapeutic benefit in most ICU patients. Hypokalemia predisposes to ventricular arrhythmias and must be suspected in any patient who is taking diuretics. The correction of hypokalemia is of prime importance in the treatment of arrhythmias caused by digitalis toxicity.[22] Hypomagnesemia, which is associated with diuretic use and hypercalcemia, may also provoke digitalis-induced arrhythmias.[23]

Cardiac arrhythmias are common in patients with respiratory failure from chronic obstructive pulmonary disease (COPD) but because such arrhythmias may derive from coexisting arrhythmogenic conditions, or from the use of beta adrenergics in these patients, quantifying their frequency has been difficult. Incalzi and colleagues have studied ventricular arrhythmias in the absence of confounding factors in men with respiratory failure and found that depressed left ventricular diastolic performance seems to predict ventricular arrhythmias in these patients.[24] Decompensated respiratory failure was defined as a worsening of dyspnea in the last week (with or without bronchopulmonary infection) coupled with a partial pressure of oxygen in arterial blood (Pao_2) of less than 70 mm Hg that decreased more than 10% over the last control measure. Appropriate therapy was administered, and stabilized respiration was obtained when blood gas levels were close to each patient's "compensated" base for greater than or equal to 5 days. Incalzi et al. hypothesized that hypoxia may affect left ventricular performance and, thus, increase the risk of ventricular premature contractions and respiratory failure in patients with COPD.[24] Such left ventricular function may be attributed to silent ischemia or left ventricular dependence on an overloaded right ventricle. In other COPD patients, sinus tachycardia, supraventricular ectopic beats, and premature ventricular beats are common among patients with theophylline toxicity; however, sustained or supraventricular tachyarrhythmias that require antiarrhythmic therapy are uncommon.[25]

Myocardial ischemia is commonly associated with ventricular arrhythmias. About 60% of patients with ischemic disease die suddenly, presumably as a result of ventricular fibrillation.[1,2] Appropriate treatment of myocardial ischemia with nitrates, beta blockers, and calcium channel blockers may alleviate arrhythmias in these patients. Enlargement of a failing left ventricle stretches individual myocardial cells and thereby enhances automaticity.[14] Reduction of left ventricular volume by the administration of digitalis, diuretics, or vasodilators helps control arrhythmias that are precipitated by this mechanism.

Increased sympathetic activity, whether the result of anxiety, exercise, exogenous catecholamines, acute myocardial infarction, or congestive heart failure can lead to ectopic, atrial, or ventricular beats.[26] Part of the antiarrhythmic action of propranolol is probably related to its beta-blocking capabilities, although the drug also suppresses arrhythmias by a direct quinidine-like effect.[27] Exercise-induced ventricular tachycardia can be controlled with beta blockers and verapamil.[28,29] Reflex tachycardia may also be due to acute beta-blocker withdrawal. Vagal tone may protect against ventricular fibrillation in an acutely ischemic myocardium. Atropine can sometimes induce ventricular tachycardia in ischemic myocardium, not only by precipitating excessive sinus tachycardia, which intensifies the ischemia, but also by its vagolytic action.[26,30] This must be considered in the ICU because some patients with COPD are given atropine-like medications for treatment of their lung disease. Clinically, this phenomenon is more likely to occur when high doses (greater than 1 mg intravenously) are used but is rare when lower doses (0.5 to 0.75 mg intravenously) are given to treat bradyarrhythmias in acute myocardial infarction.

Bradycardia itself can lead to ventricular arrhythmias by causing a temporal dispersion of refractory periods among the Purkinje fibers. Appropriate treatment with atropine or cardiac pacing to increase the heart rate may be essential in the management of these patients with bradycardia. Overdrive pacing at a rate of 90 to 110 beats per minute may also be effective in abolishing persistent ectopic tachyarrhythmias in patients with normal resting heart rates.[20,31]

Prolongation of the QT interval results in a dispersion of refractory periods among ventricular Purkinje fibers, creating an electrical gradient between adjacent cells, and is associated with ventricular tachycardia and ventricular fibrillation.[32] Torsades de pointes is a polymorphic ventricular tachycardia that is characterized by alternating electrical polarity and is typically seen in patients with prolonged QT intervals. A prolonged QT interval may be congenital or acquired.[33] The congenital form is sometimes associated with congenital deafness. Acquired causes of prolonged QT intervals include hypokalemia, hypomagnesemia, and the use of certain antiarrhythmic drugs, such as quinidine, disopyramide, or amiodarone, and tricyclic antidepressant medications such as amitriptylene. Management of acquired forms of prolonged QT interval syndrome is directed at the removal of the causative agent and the administration of certain antiarrhythmic drugs, such as phenytoin, propranolol, or bretylium. Intravenous magnesium sulfate has also been proven to be very effective for torsades de pointes.[23] Overdrive ventricular pacing, which reduces dispersion of refractory periods, is very effective. Isoproterenol can be given to increase the heart rate and to shorten the QT interval, but this drug may be dangerous in patients with ischemic heart disease.

It is beyond the scope of this chapter to describe in detail the differentiation and treatment of all the arrhythmias; therefore, the remainder of this section will deal with recognition and management of specific arrhythmias, the use of several antiarrhythmic medications, techniques of cardioversion, and general principles of cardiac pacing. Once the diagnosis has been established, additional therapy should be directed at the correction of underlying abnormalities such as hypoxia, acid/base or electrolyte imbalance, hypotension, anxiety, and heart failure. This alone may terminate the arrhythmia and may be necessary if other therapeutic modalities are to be effective. Throughout the remaining text of this chapter, antiarrhythmic medications have been classified according to the Vaughn Williams classification (Table 27-1). Type I medications have their primary action in blocking sodium chemicals, while beta blockers are classified as type II, and calcium blockers are designated type IV antiarrhythmics. Type III medications prolong repolarization by various means and are typified by the action of amiodarone. Table 27-1 also describes the subclassifications of these medications.

Supraventricular Arrhythmias

Sinus tachycardia is defined as a sinus rhythm with a heart rate faster than 100 beats per minute.[1] Sinus tachycardia is a normal response to a stress not a pathologic rhythm. It is imperative to determine and direct therapy at the underlying cause. Attempts to slow the heart rate may be detrimental because the sinus tachycardia may be a physiologic response to maintain adequate cardiac output and tissue oxygenation. Causes of sympathetic stimulation to be excluded include anemia, hemorrhage, hypoxia, hyperthyroidism, fever, hypovolemia, myocardial ischemia, congestive heart failure, and vasopressor therapy with inadequate volume replacement. Drugs such as sympathomimetic amines and other adrenergic agonists, atropine, alcohol, and caffeine can also cause sinus tachycardia. When the rate of the tachycardia ranges between 150 and 180 beats per minute, however, other diagnoses should be entertained.

Treatment of sinus tachycardia itself is rarely required because it is frequently necessary to maintain cardiac output. Primary therapy corrects the underlying abnormality. When antiarrhythmic therapy is needed, propranolol, 10 to 40 mg orally every 6 hours or 1-mg intravenous aliquots with a total intravenous dose not to exceed 0.15 mg/kg acutely, is generally effective. Digoxin is usually not helpful unless heart failure is present.

Atrial premature complexes (APCs) occur in patients of all ages but frequently reflect underlying heart disease. They are exacerbated by myocardial ischemia, pericardial inflammation, drugs, disturbances in acid/base or electrolyte balance, and pulmonary disease. Emotional stress, the use of caffeine, tobacco, or alcohol may also increase the frequency of APCs. APCs are characterized by a P wave, which may have an abnormal configuration, and are followed by a normal QRS complex. Late coupled APCs may be conducted normally, but early coupled APCs are frequently associated with a prolonged PR interval or a widened QRS complex.[1,2] Very early APCs may block in the AV node or His bundle and result in a pause simulating a sinus pause or exit block. APCs usually reset the sinus node, thus resulting in a premature P- to sinus P-wave interval similar to the sinus P-to-P interval.[34] Asymptomatic patients without evidence for sustained atrial tachycardia require no specific therapy acutely, other than elimination of the underlying or precipitating factors. Symptomatic APCs may be suppressed with Vaughn Williams class Ia drugs such as quinidine, procainamide, or disopyramide (see Table 27-1).[35] Patients with a history of atrial fibrillation or

Table 27-1. Vaughn Williams Classification of Antiarrhythmic Medication*

Type I (action by blocking sodium channels)
  IA: Quinidine, procainamide, disopyramide
  IB: Lidocaine, phenytoin, tocainide, mexiletine
  IC: Flecainide, encainide, indecainide, lorcainide, propafenone
Type II (beta blockers)
  Cardioselectives
    Acebutolol
    Atenolol
    Esmolol
    Metoprolol
  Noncardioselective
    Labetalol
    Nadolol
    Oxprenolol
    Pindolol
    Propranolol
    Sotalol
    Timolol
Type III (prolong repolarization)
  Amiodarone
  Bretylium
  Sotalol
Type IV (calcium blockers)
  Calcium antagonists
  Verapamil
  Diltiazem
  Nifedipine

* The Vaughn Williams classification divides antiarrhythmic medications into categories according to their mechanism of action. Type I are sodium-channel blockers, type II are beta blockers, type III prolong repolarization, and type IV are calcium-channel blockers.
(Adapted from Vaughn Williams, E. M.: Classification of anti-arrhythmic drugs. In Symposium on Cardiac Arrhythmias. Edited by E. Sandoe, E. Flensted-Jensen, and K. H. Olesen. Sodertalje, Sweden, A. B. Astra, 1970, p. 449.)

flutter with a rapid ventricular response should not receive these drugs without concomitant therapy with AV nodal depressant drugs: digoxin, propranolol, or verapamil (to control the ventricular response). Patients with APCs initiating recurrent supraventricular tachycardia resistant to therapy with AV nodal depressant drugs should be treated with quinidine, procainamide, or disopyramide. These drugs can be used as single agents if there is no history of atrial fibrillation or flutter. Patients with no structural heart disease can also be treated with Vaughn Williams class Ic drugs such as flecainide, encainide, or propafenone. These drugs must not be used if there is evidence of a recent or remote myocardial infarction as recently demonstrated in the Cardiac Arrhythmia Suppression Trial (CAST) study.[36]

Atrial fibrillation is probably one of the most frequent arrhythmias that the internist is asked to evaluate. The three main causes of atrial fibrillation are lone atrial fibrillation, without disease of the heart or other organs; atrial fibrillation secondary to underlying heart disease; and atrial fibrillation related to systemic problems such as hypoxia, hypothyroidism, electrolyte imbalance, hypotension, or administration of sympathomimetic amines such as aminophylline. It is important to examine the patient for the precipitating factor and consider this in the treatment. Discreet atrial activity is not present on the ECG, and the ventricular response is usually, in the absence of complete heart block, an irregularly irregular rhythm (Fig. 27-4). The rate is between 160 and 200 beats per minute unless blunted with medications. Carotid sinus massage may slow the ventricular rates transiently but generally does not restore sinus rhythm. Atrial fibrillation with a regular ventricular response should always raise the suspicion of digoxin toxicity because it may be indicative of a junctional pacemaker and AV dissociation.[22] A slow ventricular response of less than 120 beats per minute in an untreated patient implies underlying disease of the AV conduction system.

Atrial flutter is not as common as atrial fibrillation but is more often associated with underlying heart disease. Atrial flutter is a more organized rhythm than atrial fibrillation and generally has a constant atrial rate of 240 to 350 beats per minute (Fig. 27-5). Unless modified by type Ia antiarrhythmics, which may slow the rate to 200 beats per minute, the ventricular rate varies with the degree of AV block, which is usually 2:1 in untreated patients. Although 1:1 conduction is rare, it may occur, especially in patients with preexcitation syndromes or those receiving class Ia antiarrhythmic agents in the absence of AV nodal depressants. Waldo et al. have classified atrial flutter in two categories, based on atrial rate and response to atrial pacing.[19] Type I atrial flutter has a slower atrial rate and can be interrupted by overdrive pacing, whereas type II atrial flutter is resistant to pacing and requires aggressive treatment with drugs to slow the ventricular response. The important clinical point to remember is that atrial flutter must be considered in the differential diagnosis of any tachycardia, even if classic flutter waves are not evident. This diagnosis can be made with the aid of vagal maneuvers, Lewis leads, esophageal electrodes, and intra-atrial or direct atrial recordings.

Paroxysmal supraventricular tachycardia may occur in patients of all ages, with or without underlying heart disease. When one hears the phrase paroxysmal supraventricular tachycardia, one immediately thinks of paroxysmal atrial tachycardia or AV nodal reentrant tachycardia, which is in fact the most common (60%) but not the only variety.[34] Today, paroxysmal supraventricular tachycardia is a general term referring to a number of arrhythmias with different electrophysiologic mechanisms. Supraventricular tachycardia is most often due to reentry, generally within the AV node or involving an accessory pathway, although sinus node reentry, intra-atrial entry, and supraventricular tachycardia that are due to enhanced

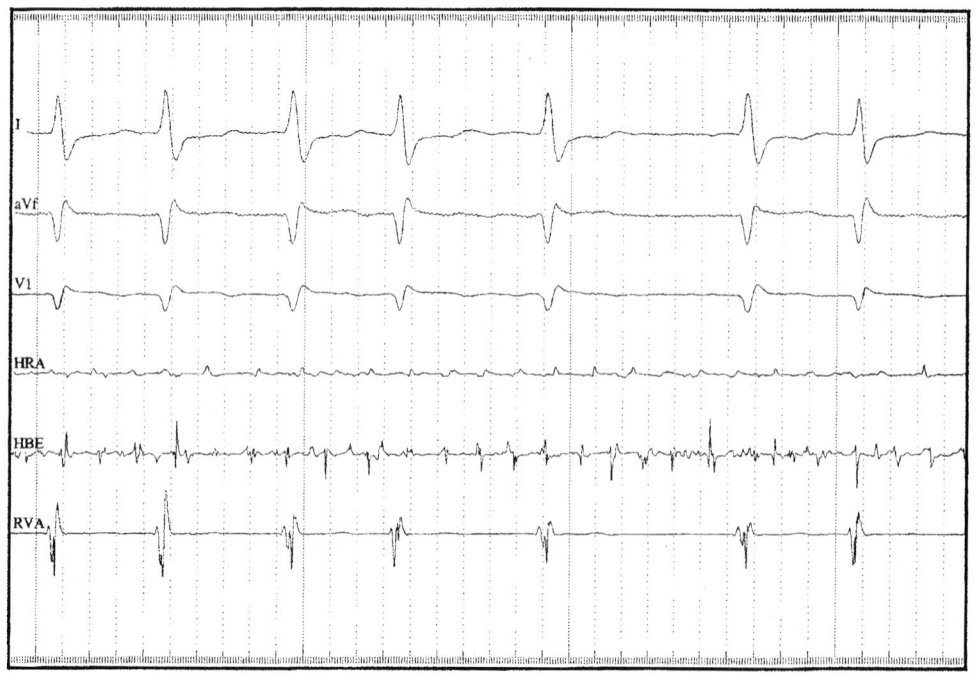

Fig. 27-4. Atrial fibrillation. Three surface ECG leads (I, aVF, and V₁) demonstrate a narrow QRS with a grossly irregular RR interval (380 to 760 milliseconds). On the intracardiac leads (high right atrium—HRA; His bundle electrogram—HBE), rapid and discrete atrial electrograms are of variable amplitude, morphology, and rate. On the right ventricular apex (RVA) electrogram, the deflections demonstrate the same information obtained from the surface leads. Notice the lack of atrial information recorded on the surface leads.

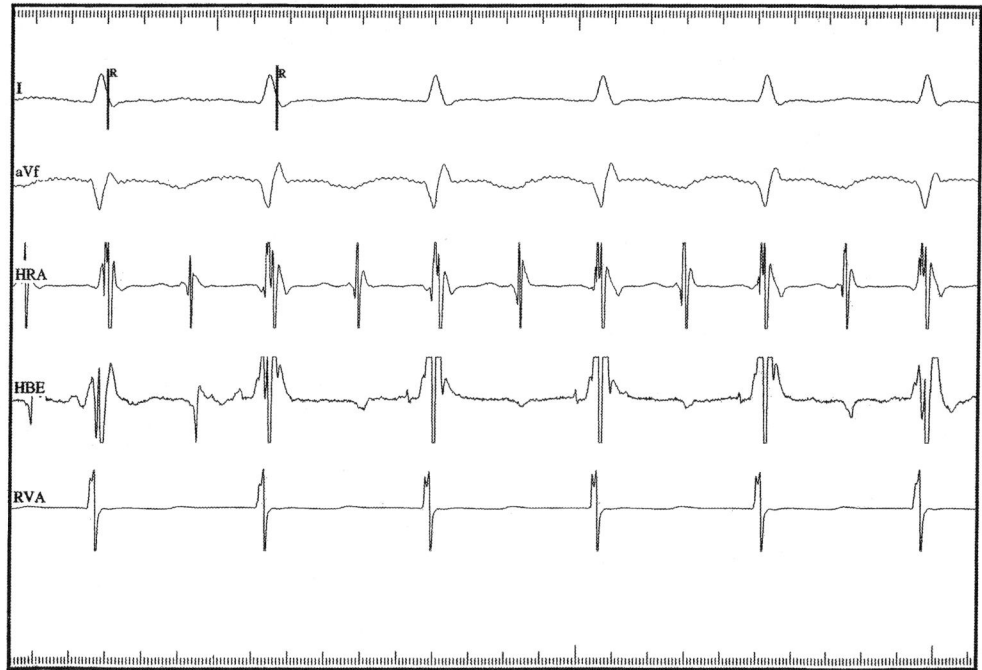

Fig. 27-5. Atrial flutter. Two surface ECG leads (I and aVF) demonstrate a rapid and regular normal QRS rhythm with a rate of 130 bpm (460 milliseconds). P waves are difficult to discern, but the intracardiac signals (high right atrium—HRA; His bundle electrogram—HBE; right ventricular apex—RVA) reveal the remainder of the information. The RVA shows only the ventricular (V) deflections, and these are useful for timing the signals on the HRA and HBE. The HRA shows a regular deflection at 260 bpm (230 milliseconds) that represents the atrial flutter depolarizations. The HBE has poor atrial (A) deflections, but large V deflections that are preceded by sharp and small His bundle electrograms. The His to V time is 40 milliseconds. Thus, there are two A deflections on the HRA for every His and V pair on the HBE. Therefore, the rhythm is atrial flutter with 2:1 atrial to ventricular conduction.

automaticity may also occur. The response to therapy depends on the mechanism of the tachycardia. The rate of these arrhythmias range from 150 to 250 beats per minute. The QRS complex is generally normal, but QRS aberration can occur.

Atrioventricular nodal reentry is the most common cause of supraventricular tachycardia, occurring in approximately 60% of cases.[34] (Fig. 27-6). The reentrant circuit is localized to the AV node and is due to longitudinal dissociation of the AV node into functionally distinct pathways (Fig. 27-7). During supraventricular tachycardia, antegrade conduction occurs over one pathway and retrograde conduction over the other, thus resulting in near simultaneous atrial and ventricular activation. As a result, retrograde P waves are buried within the QRS complexes and are not visible on the surface ECG or appear immediately after the QRS complex. Atrioventricular nodal reentry cannot exist in the presence of AV nodal block but can persist if AV block is intra- or infra-His.[34]

Accessory bypass tract tachycardias including Wolff-Parkinson-White syndrome are the second most common form of supraventricular tachycardia and account for approximately 25% of cases.[34] The reentrant circuit involves the atrial muscle, AV node, His-Purkinje system, ventricular muscle, and an accessory pathway.[34,37] This tachycardia requires two AV pathways, one of which is usually the AV node. The accessory pathways may be manifest or concealed. Manifest accessory pathways conduct quickly antegrade during sinus rhythm, producing a characteristic delta wave on the ECG, thus reflecting ventricular preexcitation[37] (Fig. 27-8). Concealed accessory pathways conduct only retrograde, and ventricular preexcitation is not present during sinus rhythm.[37] Orthodromic supraventricular tachycardia occurs with manifest or concealed accessory pathways and is the most common type.[34] During orthodromic supraventricular tachycardia, the antegrade conduction occurs through the AV node to the ventricles and returns retrograde by the accessory pathway to excite the atria, thus resulting in a P wave that immediately follows the QRS complex (Fig. 27-9). In most patients with orthodromic supraventricular tachycardia, the accessory pathway is left-sided.[34] During supraventricular tachycardia, the atrial activation proceeds left to right, and the P wave is generally negative in lead I. The ventricular activation is normal, so the QRS complex appears normal unless aberration occurs over a bundle branch.[34,37] Antidromic supraventricular tachycardia is rare and can occur only in manifest accessory pathways. The resulting P wave immediately follows the QRS complex but may be difficult to detect because of the repolarization abnormality. During antidromic supraventricular tachycardia, the ventricle is exclusively activated by the accessory pathway; therefore, the delta wave and wide QRS resemble ventricular tachycardia.

Sinus node reentry is a rare cause of supraventricular tachycardia.[34,37] The reentrant circuit is localized to the sinus node; therefore, during supraventricular tachycardia,

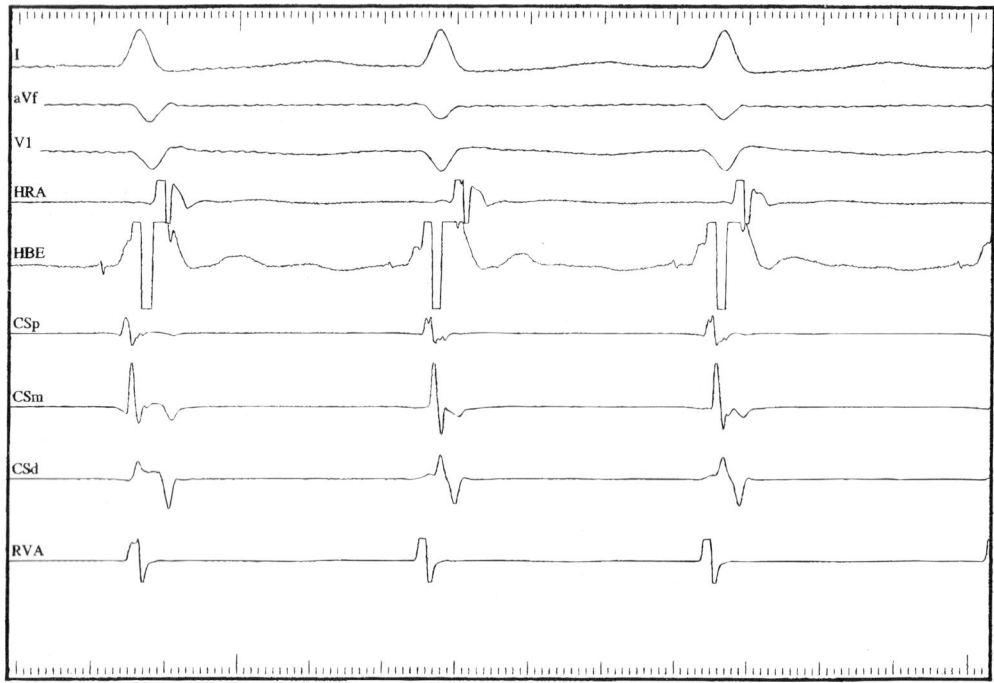

Fig. 27-6. Atrioventricular node reciprocating tachycardia. Three surface ECG leads (I, aVF, and V_1) demonstrate a narrow QRS rhythm at a rate of 150 bpm (RR = 400 milliseconds). Because this is a narrow QRS rhythm with no clear P waves, we need to look at the intracardiac electrograms to figure out what relationship the atrial depolarizations have to the ventricular depolarizations. The electrograms are listed in anatomic order from the high right atrium (HRA) to the His bundle electrogram (HBE) to the proximal, mid-, and distal coronary sinus (CSp, CSm, CSd), and finally the right ventricular apex (RVA) electrograms. The earliest electrogram is the His deflection seen on the HBE followed by a wide combined AV electrogram. The timing of the atrial deflections progress in sequence from the crux of the heart outward; CSp to CSm to CSd to HRA. Notice that the RVA electrogram occurs almost simultaneously with the atrial depolarizations seen on the coronary sinus electrograms. Thus, P waves cannot be distinguished from the QRS deflections on the surface ECG leads on most AV nodal reentry tachycardias.

the P-wave morphology is identical to that during normal sinus rhythm. The AV node is not part of the reentrant circuit, and the PR interval or presence of AV block depends on intrinsic properties of the AV node. Other forms of supraventricular tachycardia include intra-atrial reentrant (5%) and automatic atrial foci (5%)[34,37] (Fig. 27-10). In intra-atrial reentry, the P wave precedes the QRS, thus indicating an antegrade atrial activation sequence. During automatic atrial foci reentry, the P-wave morphology depends on the location of the ectopic pacemaker.

Multifocal atrial tachycardia usually occurs in patients with severe pulmonary disease or severe heart failure in the context of acute respiratory insufficiency. Multiple causative or exacerbating factors may be noted, such as digoxin intoxication, theophylline administration, postoperative state, electrolyte or metabolic imbalance, pulmonary edema, septicemia, hypoxia, and hypercarbia. Three or more different ectopic P-wave morphologies characterize multifocal atrial tachycardia on the ECG.[1,2] There is a variable PR interval with an atrial rate of 100 to 200 beats per minute. Nonconductive P waves in an isoelectric baseline are common. A chaotic atrial mechanism has the same morphologic characteristics and differs only in that the atrial rate is less than 100 beats per minute. Therapy should be again be directed at the underlying causes with particular attention to the patient's pulmonary status.

Therapeutic Intervention for Supraventricular Tachycardia

The therapy of supraventricular tachycardia combines the use of intravenous medications, overdrive pacing, and cardioversion. These therapies are summarized in Table 27-2. Remember that the acute therapy for supraventricular tachycardia in a patient who has angina or is hemodynamically compromised should include prompt termination of the supraventricular tachycardia by immediate cardioversion. Vagal maneuvers may also terminate some supraventricular tachycardias by increasing the parasympathetic tone while inhibiting sympathetic outflow. Carotid sinus massage is the preferred method of enhancing the vagal tone.[37] Verapamil is the drug of choice for terminating AV nodal reentrant tachycardia.[38] The dose is generally 5 to 10 mg intravenously administered over 2 to 3 minutes. This should be used cautiously in older patients and is contraindicated in patients with hypotension or AV block of high degree. Adenosine, given in 6- or 12-mg aliquots is quickly gaining acceptance in terminating any supraventricular tachycardia involving the AV node. Patients, if not intubated, who have a history of asthma are contraindicated for adenosine administration. Beta-adrenergic antagonists are also effective in terminating reentrant supraventricular tachycardias involving the sinus and AV

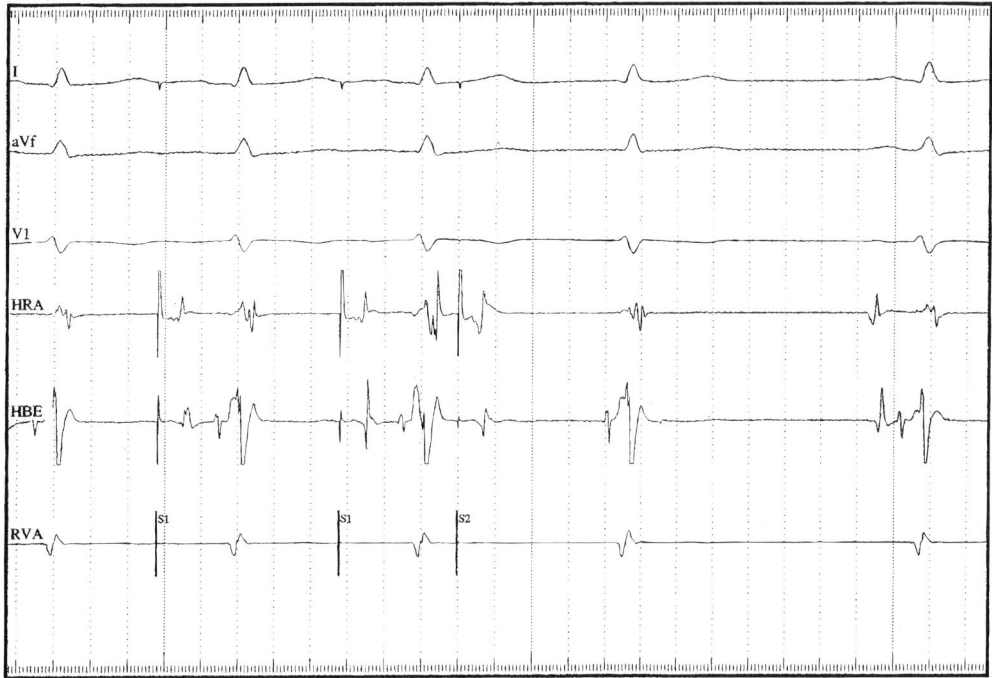

Fig. 27-7. Dual AV node pathways. Three surface ECG leads (I, aVF, and V_1) demonstrate an atrial paced rhythm with conduction to ventricles. Lead I shows atrial capture as evidenced by distinct P waves after the first and second pacing artifacts and a change in the T-wave morphology of the third QRS for the third pacing artifact. The last beat is a nonpaced or intrinsic beat. The first and second artifacts are labeled on the right ventricular apex (RVA) electrogram as S_1, and the third pacing artifact is labeled S_2. The S_1–S_1 interval is 500 milliseconds, and the S_1–S_2 (premature) interval is 320 milliseconds. The pacing artifacts are seen on all three intracardiac electrograms (high right atrium—HRA: His bundle electrogram—HBE; right ventricular apex—RVA) and line up with the signal on the surface lead I. The HRA electrogram has deflections that represent the pacing artifact, the atrial (A) and ventricular (V) events. The A deflection follows S_1 by 70 milliseconds, and the V deflection follows the A by 170 milliseconds. After S_2, the A follows by 70 milliseconds and the V follows the A by 400 milliseconds. Examination of the HBE proves that the prolongation of AV conduction occurred in the AV node instead of the His-Purkinje system. The HBE shows, in order, the S_1, the A, the His (H), and the V. The AH interval is 90 milliseconds, and the HV interval is 40 milliseconds. After S_2, the AH interval is 330 milliseconds, and the HV interval is 40 milliseconds. This represents a jump in the AH interval if, when a slightly less premature (S_1–S_2 interval = 340 milliseconds) produced an AH interval of less than or equal to 280 milliseconds. In actuality, the AH interval was 120 milliseconds, which means a 320 − 120 = 200-millisecond jump in the AH interval when S_1 to S_2 interval was reduced only by 20 milliseconds. This was observed on tracings not included in this chapter. The RVA electrogram shows the stimuli and the V deflections and adds little to the interpretation of the situation.

nodes.[37] Propranolol or esmolol are good agents to treat patients with supraventricular tachycardia. The dose of propranolol is 0.15 mg/kg given intravenously in 1-mg aliquots per minute. Esmolol is a beta-1-selective antagonist that is less likely to induce bronchospasm. Over a 1-minute period, a loading dose of 500 μg/kg is given followed by 4-minute maintenance infusion of 50 μg/kg per minute. If an adequate response is not observed, the same loading dose may be repeated, and the maintenance infusion can be increased to 100 μg/kg per minute. when the desired response is obtained, the loading dose can be omitted and the maintenance increment reduced. Blood pressure, heart rate, and respiratory function should be monitored closely when giving these agents. Digoxin can also be given as an initial dose of 0.5 to 0.75 mg intravenously or orally followed by aliquots of 0.25 mg every 4 hours as needed. Quinidine and procainamide in conventional dosages may be helpful in patients with intra-atrial reentry and to a lesser extent in patients with AV node reentrant or automatic atrial tachycardias. Either elective cardioversion or rapid atrial pacing may be required if the foregoing medications prove unsuccessful. Reentrant forms of supraventricular tachycardia are almost always responsive, but automatic supraventricular tachycardia generally is not. It should always be remembered that patients with Wolff-Parkinson-White syndrome with atrial fibrillation and a rapid ventricular response are at great risk of ventricular fibrillation; therefore, such patients should be treated acutely with immediate cardioversion.[39,40] Atrial fibrillation with a moderate ventricular response can be treated with procainamide, quinidine, or disopyramide to block conduction through the accessory pathway. Digoxin and verapamil may enhance conduction and should not be used as single agents in patients with Wolff-Parkinson-White syndrome unless prior electrophysiologic study has demonstrated their safety.[40]

The history is important in all patients with **atrial fibrillation** because cardioversion should not be attempted if the process is chronic and the patient's blood has not been anticoagulated. If an underlying systemic disorder, such

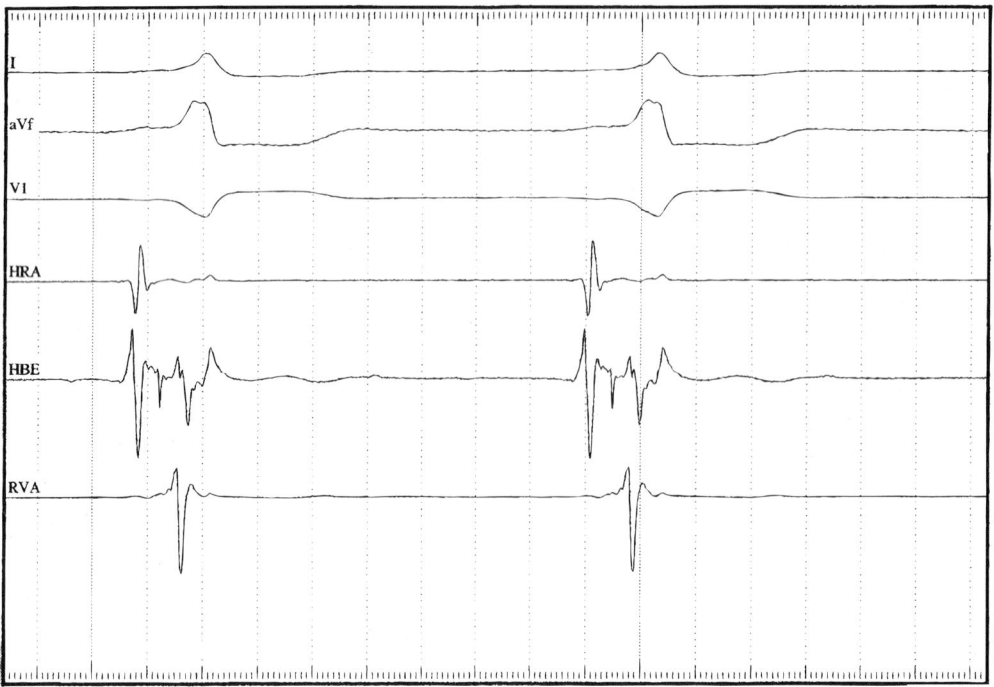

Fig. 27-8. Wolff-Parkinson-White (WPW) Syndrome. Three surface ECG leads (I, aVF, and V₁) demonstrate slurring of the early segment of the QRS complex. There is poor definition of the end of the P wave and the start of the QRS which is characteristic of WPW preexcitation. Three intracardiac leads represent the high right atrium (HRA), His bundle electrogram (HBE), and right ventricular apex (RVA) electrograms. The atrial electrogram interval and the ventricular electrogram interval are each 830 milliseconds. This represents a rate of 60,000/830 = 72 bpm. The HBE demonstrates the atrial, His bundle, and ventricular electrogram. The atrial to His (HV) interval is 70 milliseconds, and the His to ventricle (HV) interval is 30 milliseconds. Normally, HV intervals are 35 to 55 milliseconds, and this shorter interval is consistent with preexcitation of the ventricles through the accessory connection (not the His bundle).

as thyrotoxicosis or hypoxia has not been corrected, the chances of maintaining a regular sinus rhythm are diminished. Control of the ventricular response in atrial fibrillation is the first goal of treatment. Immediate cardioversion should be carried out in patients with hemodynamic compromise or angina. If the patient is hemodynamically stable, digoxin, propranolol, or verapamil may be given intravenously or orally to slow the ventricular response. Maintenance dosages of digoxin, verapamil, or propranolol should control the ventricular response to 70 to 90 beats per minute at rest. Combining these medications is frequently beneficial. Serum digoxin levels considered toxic in other circumstances may be necessary to control the ventricular response. Careful attention should be given to the serum potassium level when large dosages of digoxin are used. The decision to attempt to maintain normal sinus rhythm should be made on the basis of left atrial size, the duration of the arrhythmia, and the necessity to reestablish sinus rhythm, knowing that atrial systole contributes approximately 10 to 15% of the cardiac output. Elective restoration to sinus rhythm can be attempted medically by the administration of type Ia or type Ic antiarrhythmics and amiodarone. Procainamide, disopyramide, or quinidine for 2 days restores this sinus rhythm in approximately 30% of patients.[37] These agents also reduce the energy requirement for direct current (DC) cardioversion. The ventricular response should be controlled before the administration of type Ia agents.

There are several indications for anticoagulation in patients with atrial fibrillation.[41] If elective cardioversion will be performed, the patient should receive a 3-week course of oral anticoagulation before cardioversion and for 2 to 3 weeks afterward. Patients undergoing urgent cardioversion, especially those with a history of embolism or evidence of mitral valve disease, should receive heparin therapy before cardioversion and continued anticoagulation for 2 to 3 weeks thereafter unless there is a strong contraindication. Oral anticoagulation is advised for patients with concomitant mitral valve disease, left ventricular dysfunction, or cardiomyopathy. It should also be considered for patients older than 60 years, because the risk of stroke is greater in this population. Cardioversion should not be delayed for anticoagulation in an emergency.

Once the diagnosis of **atrial flutter** is established, one of three main options of therapy may be selected, depending on the individual patient: electrical cardioversion, drug therapy, or overdrive pacing. The same considerations regarding anticoagulation of patients with atrial fibrillation is applicable with atrial flutter. Atrial flutter can be chronic and in some cases well tolerated, but restoration of normal sinus rhythm with efficient atrial contraction and improved cardiac output is desired.

If the patient is hemodynamically compromised, or has angina, cardioversion should be performed immediately. If the patient is hemodynamically stable, digoxin, verapamil, and propranolol may be used alone or in combination to

COMMON DISORDERS OF CARDIAC RHYTHM AND CONDUCTION

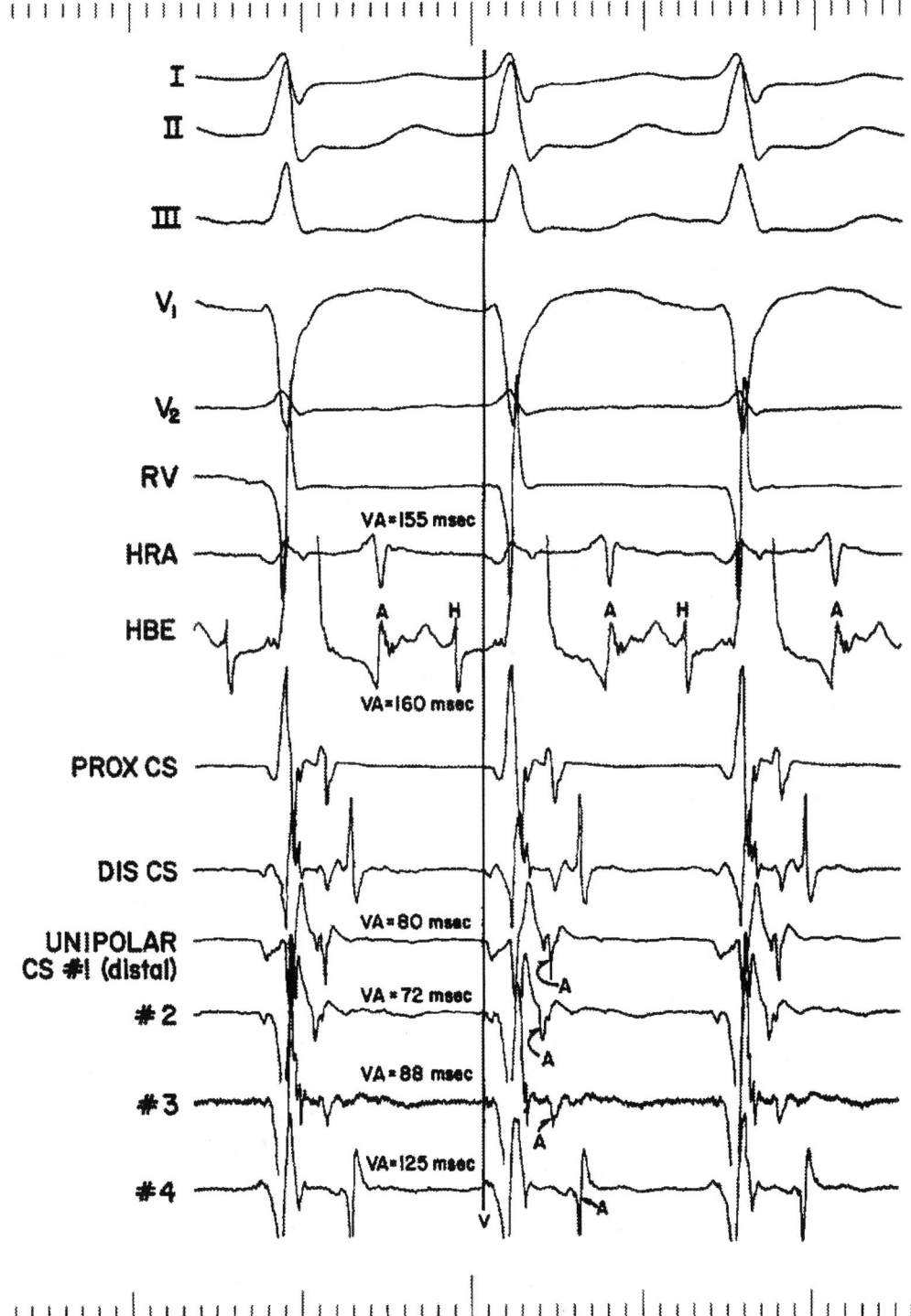

Fig. 27–9. Wolff-Parkinson-White tachycardia. Five surface ECG leads (I, II, III, V_1, and V_2) record a narrow QRS tachycardia. The QRS is normal, and atrial activity is difficult to discern. The other signals are intracardiac electrograms (right ventricular—RV; high right atrial—HRA; His bundle electrogram—HBE; proximal and distal coronary sinus—PROX CS and DIS CS; and four special unipolar coronary sinus electrograms—UNIPOLAR CS #1 (distal), #2, #3, and #4). All signals show the ventricular activation simultaneous with the surface QRS. The time to atrial activation is recorded at different times after the ventricular signal according to the location of the electrodes. This represents the spread of atrial activation from the bypass tract first seen in the UNIPOLAR CS #2 and then seen on #1, #3, and last on #4. The PROX CS also appears "early," but the HRA, HBE, and DIS CS are all "late." Thus, the tachycardia circuit proceeds from atrium, through the His bundle (see H on HBE), to the ventricle, and then up a bypass tract that is located near CS #2 (left side of heart). Once the atrium is reactivated, the process continues in a circular fashion.

control the ventricular response. Pharmacologic cardioversion can be used in atrial flutter patients who are hemodynamically stable. These agents should not be used until ventricular response has been controlled. If atrial flutter is refractory to medical management, electrical cardioversion is the therapy of choice. In the majority of patients, cardioversion from atrial fibrillation to normal sinus rhythm succeeds at low energy (less than 50 joules) and atrial flutter may be converted with even lower discharges (less than 10 joules). Overdrive pacing, using rapid atrial pacing, is a relatively easy way to convert atrial flutter to sinus rhythm. It has the advantage of avoiding electrical cardioversion and/or acute drug therapy. It is useful when there is concern about cardioversion in patients who have received large amounts of digoxin. It has the disadvantage of requiring an electrode in the atrium, but once the electrode is in position, the entire procedure is usually accomplished in less than 5 minutes.

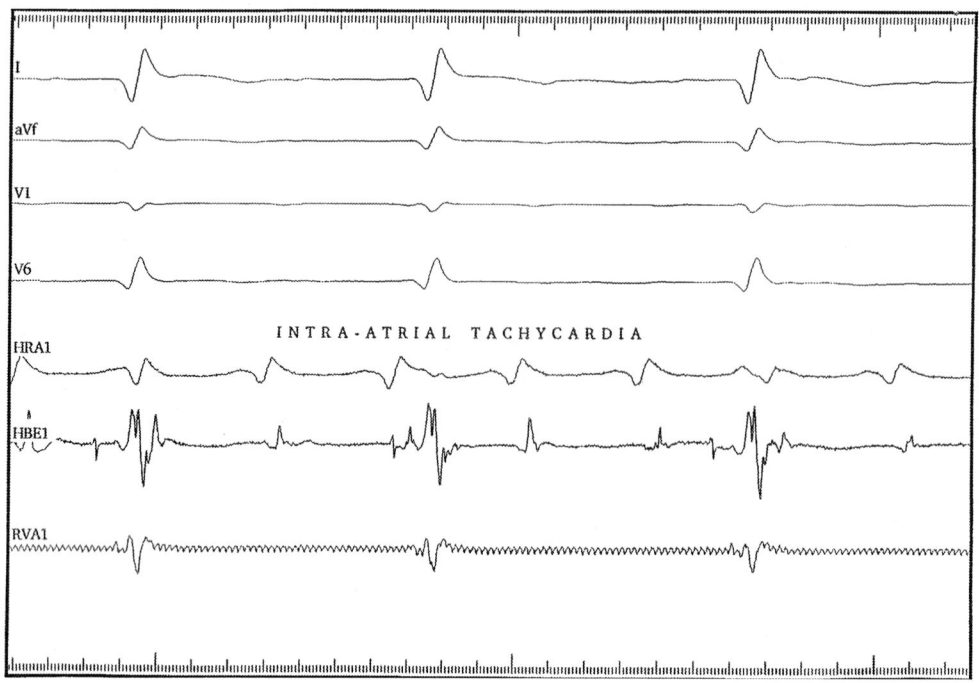

Fig. 27–10. Intraatrial tachycardia. Four surface ECG leads (I, aVF, V_1 and V_6) demonstrate a relatively slow ventricular rhythm with an RR interval of 850 milliseconds (71 bpm). The high right atrial lead (HRA_1) demonstrates a rapid and regular rhythm with an AA interval of 340 milliseconds (176 bpm). The His bundle electrogram (HBE_1) shows three large deflections coincident in timing with the surface QRSs. Eighty-five milliseconds before these ventricular deflections is a distinct deflection representing the His bundle activation. The remainder of the deflections on the HBE_1 represent local atrial activity with a ratio of 2 or 3 atrial deflections for every His and ventricular depolarization recorded. The right ventricular apex (RVA_1) electrogram confirms the surface QRS complexes. Also recorded is 60-cycle electrical noise on RVA_1.

Because **multifocal atrial tachycardia** is usually related to lung disease, the use of bronchodilators, and/or hypoxemia, administration of oxygen to the acutely hypoxic patient may be beneficial. Attempts must be made to optimize the ventilatory status. Digoxin is rarely beneficial and may be harmful. Propranolol may reduce the ventricular response, but the majority of these patients cannot tolerate beta blockade because of the potential bronchospastic effects. Verapamil or quinidine in maintenance dosages may be effective but should never be the primary treatment until the underlying causes have been corrected.

Ventricular Arrhythmias

Premature ventricular depolarizations (PVDs) are due to intraventricular reentry or disturbances in automaticity and occur in normal subjects as well as patients with heart disease.[1,2] PVDs may be exacerbated by electrolyte imbalance, acid/base imbalance, hypoxia, thyrotoxicosis, and a variety of medications. Digoxin, thiocyanide, tricyclate, antidepressants, and antiarrhythmic agents may increase or decrease the frequency of PVDs. In the absence of heart disease, PVDs are generally not associated with an increased risk of sudden death.[42] They are associated with a poorer prognosis in the presence of coronary artery disease, cardiomyopathy, and possibly mitral valve prolapse. PVDs are noted as premature QRS complexes, which are generally bizarre in morphology and greater than 120 milliseconds in duration on the ECG. The T wave is generally large and opposite in direction to the major QRS deflection. The QRS is not preceded by a premature P wave. Differentiation of a PVD from a supraventricular beat conducted with aberrant conduction is not always possible; however, the presence of a compensatory pause, fusion beats, and initial QRS forces different in direction from normal sinus beats favors ventricular origin.

The differentiation of ventricular tachycardia from supraventricular tachycardia with aberrant conduction is often difficult in patients with a QRS duration of 120 milliseconds or more. Wellens and co-workers found that the following changes favored a ventricular origin:[43]

- QRS duration exceeding 140 milliseconds
- Left axis deviation
- Atrioventricular dissociation
- Capture of fusion beats
- Monophasic (R or biphasic) qR, QR, or RS (complexes in V_1)
- A qR or a QS complex in lead V_6

The diagnosis of a supraventricular origin was favored by the following:[43]

- A triphasic QRS complex, especially if there was initial negativity in leads I and V_6
- Ventricular rates exceeding 170 beats per minute
- QRS duration greater than 120 milliseconds but less than or equal to 140 milliseconds
- The presence of preexcitation syndrome

Table 27-2. Therapy of Supraventricular Rhythms*

Sinus Tachycardia
Treat the underlying cause (anemia, hypoxia, shock, etc.)
Propranolol   10–40 mg PO q6h
                1 mg IV bolus (total dose <0.15 mg/kg)
Digoxin   0.5–0.75 mg IV load
(If CHF   0.25 mg/day
present)   Do not use as single agent in WPW unless proven safe by EPS

Atrial Premature Complex
Treat the underlying cause
Class Ia medication   For subjects with symptoms or SVT resistant to treatment with AV nodal-depressant drugs
Class Ic medication   Only if no structural heart disease

Paroxysmal Supraventricular Tachycardia
Vagal stimuli   Valsalva's maneuver, carotid sinus massage
Adenosine   6- to 12-mg aliquots IV
Verapamil   5–10 mg IV
                Do not use as single agent in WPW unless proven safe by EPS
Propranolol   0.15 mg/kg IV in 1-mg aliquots/min
Esmolol   500 mg/kg IV bolus 50 mg/kg/min maintenance and titrate heart rate
Class Ia medication   See Table 27-3 for dosing
Overdrive pacing   All reentrant SVT (not for atrial fibrillation)
Cardioversion   For hemodynamic compromise or medically refractory

Atrial Fibrillation
Treatment of underlying cause (hypoxia, thyrotoxicosis, etc.)
Vagal stimuli   Valsalva's maneuver, carotid sinus massage
Digoxin   0.5–0.75 mg IV load: 0.25–0.375 mg/day
              Do not use as single agent in WPW unless proven safe by EPS
Verapamil   5–10 mg IV
                Do not use as single agent in WPW unless proven safe by EPS
Propranolol   0.15 mg/kg IV in 1-mg aliquots/min
Class Ia medication   For subjects with symptoms or SVT resistant to treatment with AV nodal depressant drugs
Class Ic meds   Only if no structural heart disease
Amiodarone   Must use loading doses; see Table 27-3
Cardioversion   For hemodynamic compromise or medically refractory

* The treatment of supraventricular arrhythmias is outlined in Table 27-2. The treatment depends on the mechanism, but any rhythm associated with significant hemodynamic compromise requires cardioversion. AV, atrioventricular; CHF, congestive heart failure; EPS, electrophysiologic study; IV, intravenous; SVT, supraventricular tachycardia; WPW, Wolf-Parkinson-White syndrome.

With wide QRS complexes, the diagnosis of ventricular tachycardia can also be made on the basis of the following criteria:

- The QRS complexes during the tachycardia are 120 milliseconds or greater in duration and totally different from the complexes during supraventricular rhythm.
- Atrioventricular dissociation or ventricular atrial block is present.
- Intermittent fusion and normal capture beats occur.
- Atrial pacing to rates in excess of the tachycardia does not produce aberration.
- No His bundle potential precedes ventricular activation during the tachycardia during electrophysiologic testing.[1,2,43]

The prompt treatment of **sustained ventricular tachycardia** is essential. If the rhythm is nonsustained without symptoms or consists of frequent PVDs, however, the need for treatment is less clear.[44] Symptoms must clearly be related to a tachycardia for treatment to be effective. Vague fatigue or vertigo is not suggestive of tachycardia. Syncope, presyncope, rapid regular palpitations, or sudden dyspnea with palpitations, however, are characteristic of these arrhythmias. No study has conclusively demonstrated improved survival if asymptomatic nonsustained ventricular tachycardia is treated with antiarrhythmic drugs. Almost all antiarrhythmic drugs have arrhythmogenic potential and may exacerbate asymptomatic nonsustained ventricular tachycardia into a sustained symptomatic ventricular tachycardia or ventricular fibrillation in up to 15% of patients.

Initial attempts to assess the risk of PVDs led Lown and Wolff to propose a grading system for ventricular ectopy, which was modified by the addition of grades IA and IB (Table 27-3).[45] Recently, quantitative subscripts were added. Complex and frequent ectopy has been associated with an increased risk of sudden death, whereas low grade ectopy has a benign prognosis. Objections to the Lown classification include the fact that a patient is characterized by the highest grade, although characteristics of lower grades may also be present. One must be cautious in this grading system, because it does not take into account the underlying heart disease. The individual with asymptomatic ventricular tachycardia and coronary artery disease may have a different prognosis than one with asymptomatic ventricular tachycardia and mitral valve prolapse. Thus, it is important to know the underlying anatomic substrate. Despite various criticisms, the Lown classification system is an important tool in managing arrhythmias. Suppression of high grades of ventricular ectopy with antiarrhythmic therapy in symptomatic patients who are survivors of sudden cardiac death is associated with improved survival. Suppression is defined with the use of multiple Holter monitors and exercise tests.[44] With all variables in consideration, it is imperative to evaluate each patient carefully and to know which studies are indicated for each particular problem. The degree of further evaluation de-

Table 27-3. Lown Classification*

Grade 0	No VPBs
Grade 1A	<30 VPBs/hr and <1/min
Grade 1B	<30 VPBs/hr and occasionally >1 VPB/min
Grade 2	Frequent VPBs >30/hr
Grade 3	Multiform VPBs
Grade 4A	Repetitive VPBs, couplets
Grade 4B	Repetitive VPBs, runs of VT (3 or more repetitive VPBs)
Grade 5	Early R-on-T VPBs

* The Lown classification classifies a patient's arrhythmia as the highest class of ventricular ectopy seen during all monitoring, regardless of frequency of the arrhythmia. In the setting of coronary artery disease and left ventricular dysfunction, arrhythmias of grade 3 and above are associated with a significantly reduced prognosis.
VPB, ventricular premature beat; VT, ventricular tachycardia.
(Adapted from Lown, B., and Wolf, M.: Approach to sudden death from coronary heart disease circulation, *44*:130, 1971.)

pends on the complexity of ventricular ectopy and the degree of symptoms.

The issue of treating patients with asymptomatic PVDs to reduce the risk of sudden cardiac death remains problematic. Decisions to treat patients with asymptomatic PVDs should be made only after considering the risk/benefit ratio of administering antiarrhythmic agents to asymptomatic patients. One should realize that approximately 30 to 40% of patients receiving antiarrhythmic medications develop adverse reactions that necessitate the termination of these agents.[46] Antiarrhythmic agents have also been shown to aggravate ventricular arrhythmias in 10 to 15% of patients.[46] Because PVDs in the absence of organic heart disease are not generally associated with an increased risk of sudden death, most cardiologists do not recommend specific treatment unless patients are symptomatic.[46] PVDs in the presence of organic heart disease may be more ominous, but no definitive data demonstrate that their suppression reduces the risk of sudden cardiac death or that empiric treatment reduces the incidence of sudden cardiac death. Acute suppression of PVDs is best achieved after correcting all possible underlying causes such as hypoxia, electrolyte, and acid/base abnormalities and heart failure. The acute suppression is best achieved using intravenous lidocaine or procainamide (Table 27-4). Chronic suppression of PVDs may occur with the use of class I agents. Beta-adrenergic antagonists and calcium channel antagonists are rarely effective. Amiodarone should be reserved for sustained ventricular tachyarrhythmias that fail to respond to conventional agents.

Ventricular tachycardia occurs most often in the setting of the following:

- Ischemic heart disease
- Cardiomyopathy
- Prolonged QT syndromes
- Mitral valve prolapse
- Drug toxicities
- Metabolic disorders

Ventricular tachycardia may be either nonsustained or sustained (Fig. 27-11). The rate is generally 140 to 220 beats per minute, regular, and the QRS duration is greater than 120 milliseconds. Atrioventricular dissociation is usually present on the surface ECG and can be checked by an atrial EGM to distinguish ventricular tachycardia from supraventricular tachycardia with aberrancy (Fig. 27-12). Criteria mentioned in the preceding section should also be employed. If ventricular tachycardia is associated with severe hemodynamic compromise, immediate defibrillation is indicated with concomitant lidocaine therapy. If the rate is rapid with less severe hemodynamic compromise, cardioversion with synchronized discharge and concomitant lidocaine or procainamide therapy are indicated. If ventricular tachycardia is not accompanied by hemodynamic compromise, the institution of antiarrhythmic agents may terminate the arrhythmia, but if the ventricular tachycardia does not respond promptly, cardioversion should be performed. Lidocaine infusion at 1 to 4 mg per

Table 27-4. Therapy of Ventricular Rhythms*

Premature Ventricular Depolarizations	
Usually no therapy	
Nonsustained Ventricular Tachycardia	
Usually no therapy	
Sustained Ventricular Tachycardia	
Cardioversion	1–360 joules
Overdrive pacing	10–20% faster than tachycardia rate
Lidocaine	1–2 mg/kg IV followed by 20–40 µg/kg/min infusion
Quinidine	200–600 mg PO q 6–8 h
Procainamide	10–15 mg/kg IV (½ hour) then 1–4 mg/min
	250–1500 mg PO q6h for sustained release preparation
Disopyramide	150–300 mg PO q6–12 h
Phenytoin	50–100 mg/5 min IV up to 1 g, then 200–400 mg/day
Tocainide	400–600 mg PO q8h
Mexiletine	150–300 mg PO q6–8h
Flecainide	50–200 mg PO q12h
Propafenone	150–300 mg PO q8h
Moricizine	200–300 mg PO q8h
Bretylium	5–10 mg/kg IV for 10–30 minutes, then 1–4 mg/min
Amiodarone	1200–1800 mg PO daily for 5 days, then 400–600 mg PO daily
Torsades de Pointes	
Correct hypokalemia, hypomagnesemia	
Remove the inciting antiarrhythmic (Type Ia is common but not exclusive culprit)	
Overdrive pacing	
Isuprel	1–4 mg/min to increase sinus rate 10–20%
Ventricular Fibrillation	
Cardioversion	
Correct ischemia	
Antiarrhythmics as per ventricular tachycardia therapy	

* Choosing among the many options requires the assessment of hemodynamic compromise, frequency, or recurrence and associated medical conditions.

minute should be started after an initial bolus of 1 mg/kg and a second intravenous bolus of 0.5 mg/kg. As a second drug of choice, procainamide infusion of 2 to 4 mg per minute should be started after a loading dose of 10 to 15 mg/kg. For ventricular tachycardia that is resistant to other therapies, bretylium may be given with caution because of its hypotensive effects.[47] Initially, 5 to 10 mg/kg should be given in a 1:4 solution with D5W by infusion over 8 to 10 minutes. The antiventricular tachycardia effects of bretylium are delayed several hours. In ventricular fibrillation, however, bretylium can sometimes cause reversion of the arrhythmia with or without defibrillation.

In recent years, amiodarone therapy has become more popular for treatment of refractory ventricular tachycardia, but usage in the acute setting is limited by its long half-life (30 to 45 days). In refractory ventricular tachycardia, an oral loading dose is instituted at dosages between 1000

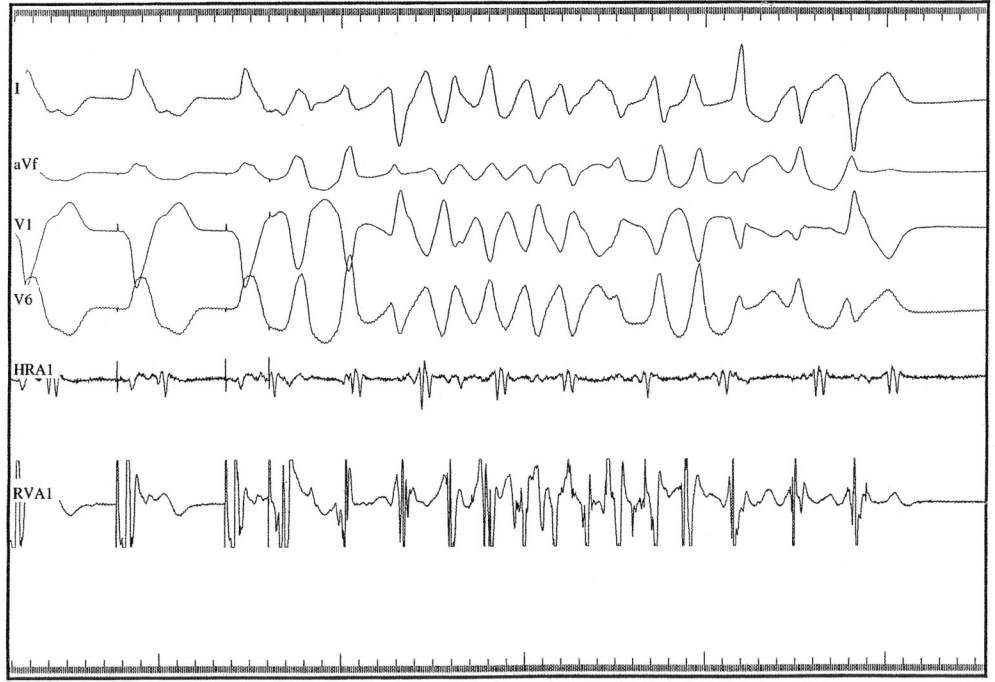

Fig. 27-11. Nonsustained polymorphic ventricular tachycardia. Four surface ECG leads (I, aVF, V_1, and V_6) demonstrate the induction of a rapid, irregular, and self-terminating tachycardia by programmed electrical stimulation (EPS study). The first three beats are of a similar morphology and are spaced at 600 milliseconds (100 bpm). Preceding each beat is a sharp but small deflection, which is the pacing artifact. There is one additional pacing artifact 240 milliseconds after the third paced beat pacing artifact. This represents the premature stimulus and initiates the arrhythmia. The tachycardia lasts 13 beats and has a calculated (2800 divided by 13) average cycle length of 215 milliseconds (60,000/215 = 279 bpm). The high right atrial (HRA_1) lead shows (best noted on the first full paced complex) the pacing artifacts, followed by ventricular electrograms that are then followed by the atrial electrograms. This produces a diagnosis of retrograde (VA) conduction at an interval of 230 milliseconds. After the premature ventricular paced beat, the atrial deflections occur at a regular and comparatively slow rate of 158 bpm (380 milliseconds). Notice the relatively irregular and rapid electrograms on the right ventricular apex (RVA_1) electrogram. Notice that 230 milliseconds after the last two ventricular (RVA_1) beats are atrial electrograms (HRA_1). This represents VA conduction at the same interval that was observed during the ventricular paced beats described previously.

mg to 1800 mg daily for 5 days. After 4 to 8 weeks, maintenance dosing should be adjusted to 200 to 400 mg per day. With more patients on amiodarone therapy today, clinicians should be aware of several complications. Patients who have received amiodarone may be at risk of developing atropine-resistant bradycardia associated with decreased peripheral resistance and contractility.[48] Inotropic agents produce little effect on heart rate or peripheral vascular resistance in these patients. There is also a higher incidence of respiratory complications necessitating possible longer intubation or ICU stay in patients who are receiving chronic amiodarone therapy.[49]

Overdrive ventricular pacing can also be used to terminate drug-refractory ventricular tachycardia. This method of termination should be performed only by experienced personnel because it requires invasive techniques, such as the insertion of a temporary pacing lead into the right ventricular apex.[20]

Bradyarrhythmias

Treatment of arrhythmias in the ICU phase would not be complete without describing briefly the uses of temporary pacemakers. The major indication for cardiac pacing is treatment of bradyarrhythmias. The optimal hemodynamic response to cardiac pacing is achieved when AV synchrony is preserved. In normal patients, a reduction of cardiac output in the order of 10 to 15% may be observed with loss of atrial synchrony, and this effect may be more pronounced in patients with noncompliant ventricles and high diastolic filling pressures.[20] In most patients, however, the cardiac output depends more on the heart rate. Dual-chamber pacing with atrial sensing provides AV synchrony and prevents the development of pacemaker syndrome, which is reported in 5 to 10% of patients with ventricular demand (VVI) pacemakers alone (Table 27-5).[50] Pacemaker syndrome is characterized by retrograde atrial activation, cannon A waves, vasodilatation, and hypotension. Atrial EGMs can be obtained from many permanent and all temporary atrial pacing catheters. These can be used to diagnose cardiac arrhythmias. Classic usage is to differentiate between a supraventricular tachycardia with wide QRS complex at a rate of 150 beats per minute and a 1:1 AV relationship, and a ventricular tachycardia of 150 beats per minute with a wide QRS complex and AV dissociation[52] (Fig. 27-13).

THE HIGH RISK PATIENT: MANAGEMENT OF THE CRITICALLY ILL

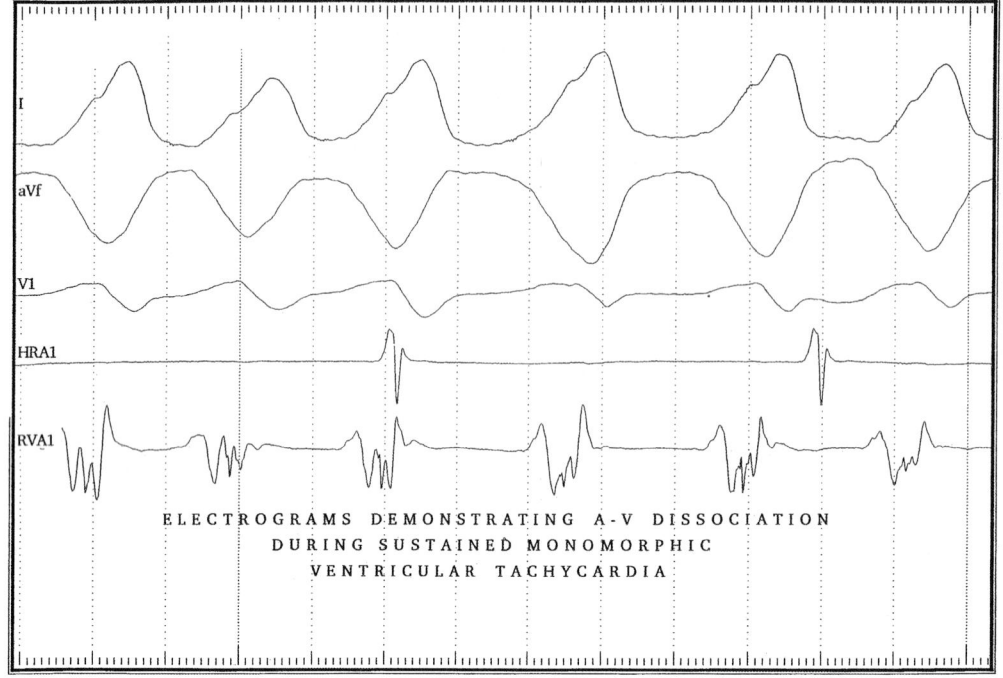

Fig. 27–12. Sustained rapid monomorphic ventricular tachycardia. Three surface ECG leads (I, aVF, and V_1) demonstrate a wide QRS tachycardia. Because little to no evidence of atrial depolarization exists on these leads, it will be necessary to use the atrial electrogram (HRA) to confirm the atrial rate. The RR interval is inconsistent and varies between 195 and 260 milliseconds (230 and 308 bpm). The QRS duration varies in duration between 150 and 180 milliseconds. Because of the variation in QRS duration and RR intervals, some people might consider this rhythm polymorphic ventricular tachycardia. Others, because of the rapid rate, might consider this rhythm ventricular flutter. Most likely this rhythm would behave as monomorphic ventricular tachycardia in that it is likely pacing and low energy cardioversion shock convertible to a normal rhythm. The most important characteristic of the tracing is demonstrated by the high right atrial (HRA_1) and right ventricular apex (RVA_1) electrograms. Notice how easy it is to see that the atrial interval (AA = 580 milliseconds) is dissociated from the ventricular interval (VV = 195 to 260 milliseconds). A wide QRS tachycardia with AV dissociation is virtually always ventricular tachycardia.

Indications for temporary pacing in bradyarrhythmias include the following (Figs. 27-14 to 27-17):

- Symptomatic second- or third-degree heart block from a transient drug intoxication or electrolyte imbalance
- Complete heart block
- Mobitz II or bifascicular block in the setting of acute myocardial infarction
- Symptomatic sinus bradycardia
- Atrial fibrillation with a slow ventricular response

These bradycardias may necessitate temporary pacing until the temporary situation resolves or a permanent pacemaker can be inserted.[20,50]

Indications for permanent pacing and bradyarrhythmias generally include the following:

Table 27–5. The NASPE/BPEG Generic (NBG) Pacemaker Code*

		Position (Category)		
I	II	III	IV	V
Chamber(s) paced	Chamber(s) sensed	Response to sensing	Programmability, rate modulation	Antitachyarrhythmia function(s)
0 = None	0 = None	0 = None	0 = None	
A = Atrium	A = Atrium	T = Triggered	P = Simple programmable	0 = None
V = Ventricle	V = Ventricle	I = Inhibited	M = Multiprogrammable	P = Pacing (antitachycardia)
D = Dual (A + V)	D = Dual (A + V)	D = Dual (T + I)	C = Communicating	S = Shock
			R = Rate modulation	D = Dual (P + S)

* The NASPE/BPEG generic, or NBG, code describes pacemaker function according to the chambers of the heart that paced or sensed. Although not completely descriptive of pacemaker function, it provides a good overall sense of what is expected from the pacemaker. NASPE, North American Society for Pacing and Electrophysiology; BPEG, British Pacing and Electrophysiology Group
(From Bernstein, A. D., et al.: The NASPE/BPEG generic pacemaker code for antibradyarrhythmia and adaptive-rate pacing and antitachyarrhythmia devices. PACE, *10*:794, 1987.)

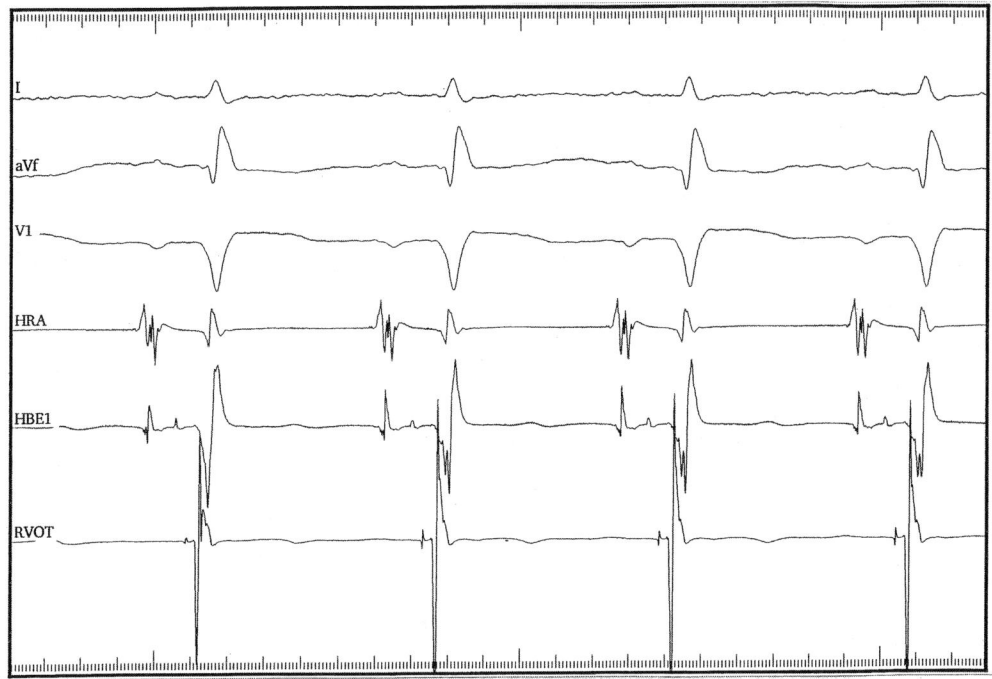

Fig. 27-13. Normal sinus rhythm. Three surface ECG leads (leads I, aVF, and V$_1$) demonstrate normal P, QRS, and T waves. The three additional intracardiac electrograms (high right atrium—HRA, His bundle electrogram—HBE$_1$, right ventricular outflow tract—RVOT) demonstrate the characteristics of normal conduction and rhythm. The HRA shows the atrial deflection under the P waves and a slightly smaller ventricular deflection under the QRS complex. Similarly, the HBE$_1$ shows the atrial (A) and ventricular (V) deflections, but a third discrete deflection in between the A and V represents the activation of the His bundle. The A to His time, which represents the conduction time through the AV node, is 70 milliseconds, and the His to V time, which represents the conduction time from the His bundle to the ventricles, is 60 milliseconds. On the RVOT electrogram a large deflection representing the ventricular activation is preceded by a small deflection. This deflection represents the right bundle branch activation 30 milliseconds before the ventricular activation. The right bundle potential looks a lot like the His bundle deflection, except His to ventricular activation times are always more than 35 milliseconds.

- Congenital complete heart block associated with symptoms
- Bradycardia or failure to increase heart rate with exercise
- Symptomatic second- or third-degree AV block
- Second- or third-degree intra-His or infra-His block
- Bifascicular block that progressed to complete heart block in the setting of acute myocardial infarction and symptomatic sinus bradycardia.[50]

Indications for temporary pacing in the setting of tachyarrhythmias include atrial flutter, AV nodal reentry, and supraventricular tachycardia using accessory bypass tracts. These can generally be terminated by rapid atrial pacing. Atrial fibrillation, type II atrial flutter, and sinus tachycardia are not terminated by atrial pacing.[50] When atrial flutter or reentry supraventricular tachycardia occurs frequently, the pacing electrodes can be left positioned into the right atrium for multiple use. This is better than DC cardioversion because it avoids skin and skeletal muscle trauma and minimizes the discomfort to the patient. Sustained ventricular tachycardia can often be repetitively terminated by rapid ventricular pacing, which provides a bridge until a successful drug regimen can be instituted. Again, it is of great importance that cardiac pacing during ventricular tachycardia is performed only by experienced physicians because the pacing may cause degeneration of the rhythm to ventricular fibrillation. In patients with bradycardia-dependent ventricular tachycardia or with ventricular tachycardia/ventricular fibrillation complicating intrinsic or drug-induced QT prolongation, pacing at rates faster than the intrinsic sinus rate frequently prevents spontaneous recurrence. This temporary increase in heart rate usually decreases the dispersion of refractoriness in the ventricular myocardium, thus abolishing the conditions necessary for reentrant arrhythmias.[52]

Patients who manifest recurrent sustained ventricular arrhythmias should be considered for invasive electrophysiologic studies (EPSs). Such a study is designed to establish the drug therapy most apt to obviate the arrhythmia. If such therapy cannot be advised, mapping and excision of the ectopic focus and/or implantation of an automatic implantable cardioverter defibrillator (ICD) can be performed.

Figures 27-4 to 27-17 demonstrate many of the rhythms described in the text. Each description includes the EGM labels, the EGM characteristics, and the thought process appropriate to the rhythm interpretation. The tracings are recorded at different paper speeds. The time lines across the top and bottom of the tracings have larger and

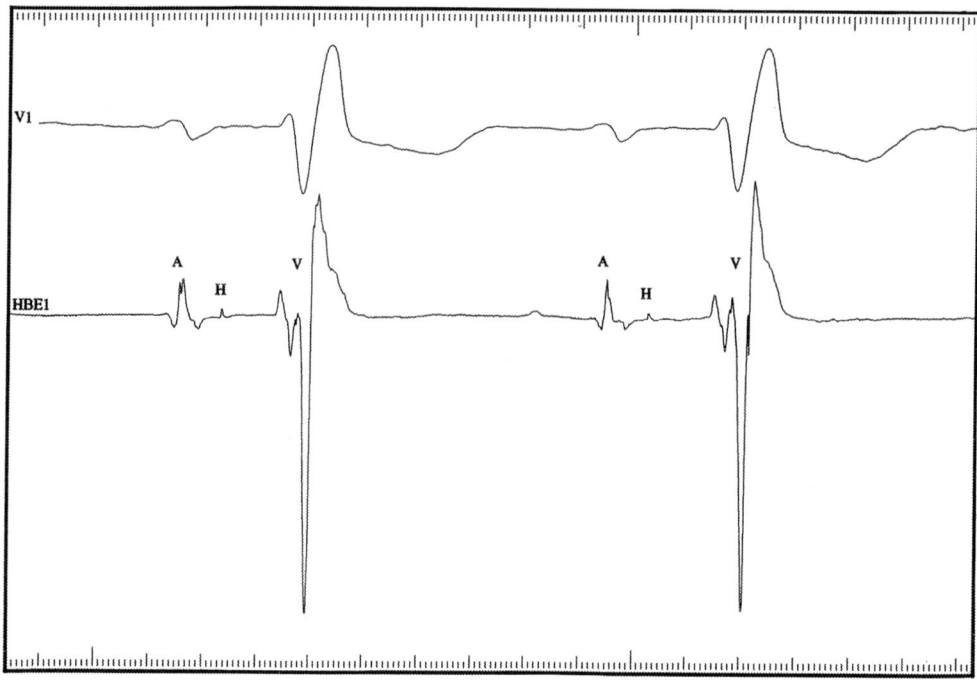

Fig. 27–14. First-degree AV block—normal sinus rhythm. Surface ECG lead V₁ is recorded. Apparent are the P, right bundle branch block QRS (140-millisecond duration), and T waves. The PR interval of 260 milliseconds demonstrates first-degree AV block. The His bundle tracing (HBE₁) comes from a catheter positioned near the crux of the heart. Labeled are the atrial (A), His (H), and ventricular (V) deflections. The atrial to His or AH interval and the His to ventricular or HV intervals are both 100 milliseconds. Because normal HV conduction intervals are between 35 and 55 milliseconds, the prolongation of the PR interval is related to His-Purkinje system disease. By surface electrocardiographic criteria, the first-degree AV block and right bundle branch block with or without a left anterior fascicular block suggested His-Purkinje disease, but these criteria alone are frequently misleading. The decision for pacing is a clinical decision based on symptoms, but these data would be useful in a patient whose symptoms are difficult to interpret.

smaller markings. The time between two of the larger markers is 100 milliseconds, and the time between the smaller markings is 10 milliseconds. Because the paper speed changes, the distance that represents 100 or 10 milliseconds changes from tracing to tracing. Intervals important to the interpretation of the tracing are recorded in the figure legends. To confirm the interval measurements, one should use calipers fixed to the interval of interest and then compare the interval to the time lines on the same tracing.

POST-ICU PHASE (REHABILITATION PHASE)

The primary question one asks when an arrhythmic patient is discharged from the ICU is whether the arrhythmia is likely to recur or whether it was due to a transient and nonrecurrent precipitating factor. One must also ask if the patient requires further evaluation by invasive procedures such as cardiac catheterization or EPSs or if noninvasive testing is sufficient. If the patient left the ICU receiving antiarrhythmic therapy, is this patient at a greater risk of sudden cardiac death than if he was not treated? Last, is this drug therapy sufficient, or should additional measures such as antiarrhythmia surgery, antitachycardia pacemakers, or ICDs be considered? Most of these decisions should be based on the arrhythmia mechanism, the frequency of the occurrence, and their underlying heart disease and symptoms. Most patients with infrequent episodes in the ICU that are not associated with disabling symptoms usually require only correction of the underlying causes without progression to long-term therapy. On the other hand, patients with frequent episodes or episodes associated with disabling symptoms should be treated chronically if they persist after all electrolyte or acid/base imbalances are corrected. EPSs using percutaneous endocardial catheter electrodes to record intracardiac EGMs and programmed electrical stimuli to evaluate complex supraventricular and ventricular arrhythmias may be necessary. The primary uses of EPS follow:

- Identify the mechanism of a tachycardia
- Select an effective antiarrhythmic regimen
- Localize the anatomic substrate of an arrhythmia in preparation for possible surgical intervention
- Evaluate conduction abnormalities for permanent pacemaker implantation[34]

These studies are especially accurate in identifying the mechanisms of supraventricular tachycardia. An EPS induces supraventricular tachycardia in 90 to 95% of patients with clinical episodes of AV nodal reentrant tachycardia

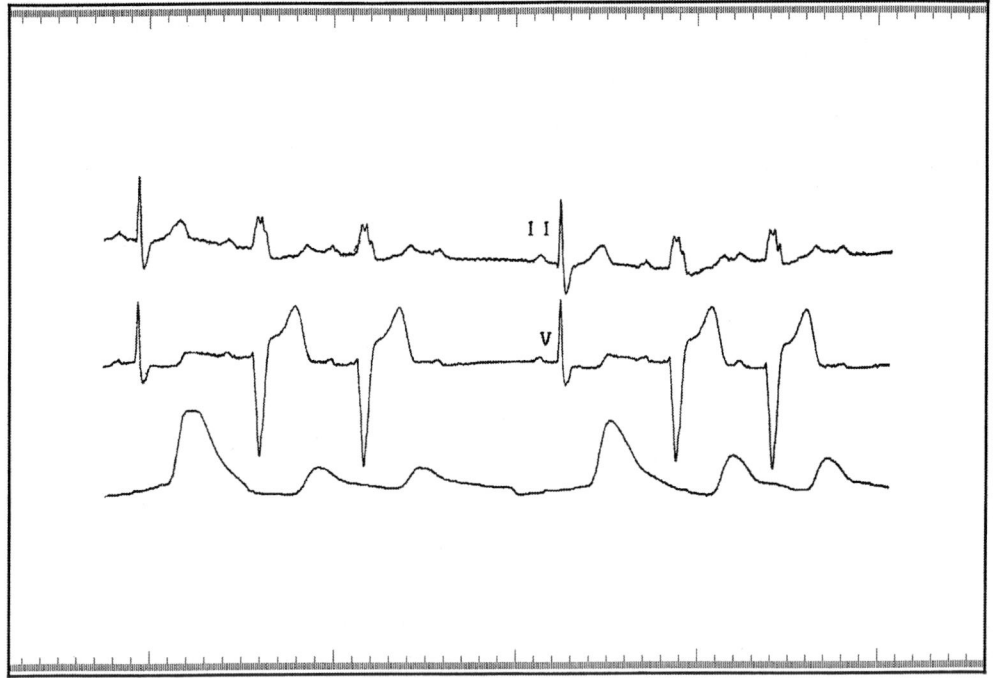

Fig. 27–15. Second-degree heart block (Mobitz II). Two surface ECG leads (II and V) demonstrate a regular atrial rate with conduction to the ventricular chambers on all but two (fourth and eighth) beats. Grouped beating is evident, with an abnormal prolongation of the QRS in four of the QRS complexes (2, 3, 5, and 6). The PR interval does not gradually prolong before failing to conduct to the ventricles. The wide QRS complexes exhibit a left bundle branch configuration. Thus, the left bundle is blocked on the second, third, and fourth complexes of the group, and the right bundle is blocked only on the fourth beat. This represents Mobitz II, second-degree AV block. If there were His bundle recordings, these would likely demonstrate prolonged His to ventricle times and an atrial and His deflection without a ventricular deflection on the blocked beat. Also of note is the third tracing representing the arterial blood pressure. Note that the altered ventricular depolarization on the left bundle beats produces a poor hemodynamic response.

or Wolff-Parkinson-White syndrome and induces sustained ventricular tachycardia or ventricular fibrillation in 75% of survivors of sudden cardiac death and in 95% of patients with sustained monomorphic ventricular tachycardia.[39] Whether an EPS identifies patients with nonsustained ventricular tachycardia at risk of sudden death is still rather controversial. In patients treated with an antiarrhythmic agent that prevented induction of sustained ventricular tachycardia previously induced by EPS, a recurrence rate of 10% can be expected in the first 2 years of therapy compared with a recurrence rate of approximately 50% in patients treated with an agent that failed to prevent induction of ventricular tachycardia.[43]

Patients with a permanent pacemaker should have regular follow-up. Follow-up should include at least two visits during the first year and thereafter at least yearly. The ECG should be repeated if symptoms occur, to determine the pacing rate of the pacemaker in the presence of possible competitive arrhythmias. Sophisticated monitoring techniques are currently available and can be used over telephone lines to supplement other observations. Pacemaker function can also be checked via telephone transmission every 3 months, then increased to monthly as the projected end of battery life approaches. Antibiotic prophylaxis should probably be used for dental and operative procedures in patients with permanent pacemaker implantation and definitely for all patients with an ICD. Patients with permanent pacemakers should be followed for the following possible complications:

- Battery depletion
- Electrode fracture
- Electrode dislodgment
- Infection
- Perforation of the myocardium
- Myopotential sensing or stimulation causing muscle twitching
- Pacemaker-mediated tachycardia and pacemaker syndrome

As clinicians, we should always be aware that any cardiac arrhythmia can occur at any time. The main emphasis is to control risk factors that increase the likelihood of clinical coronary events, especially hypertension, hyperlipidemia, diabetes, and electrolyte and acid/base imbalances.

In summary, accurate recognition of disturbances of cardiac conduction is essential for the appropriate diagnosis and therapeutic management of critically ill patients. Some arrhythmias are benign and may not warrant intervention, whereas others are disabling and life-threatening and should be treated aggressively. We have attempted to analyze common conduction disturbances in the critically ill patient through the risk phase, support phase, and rehabili-

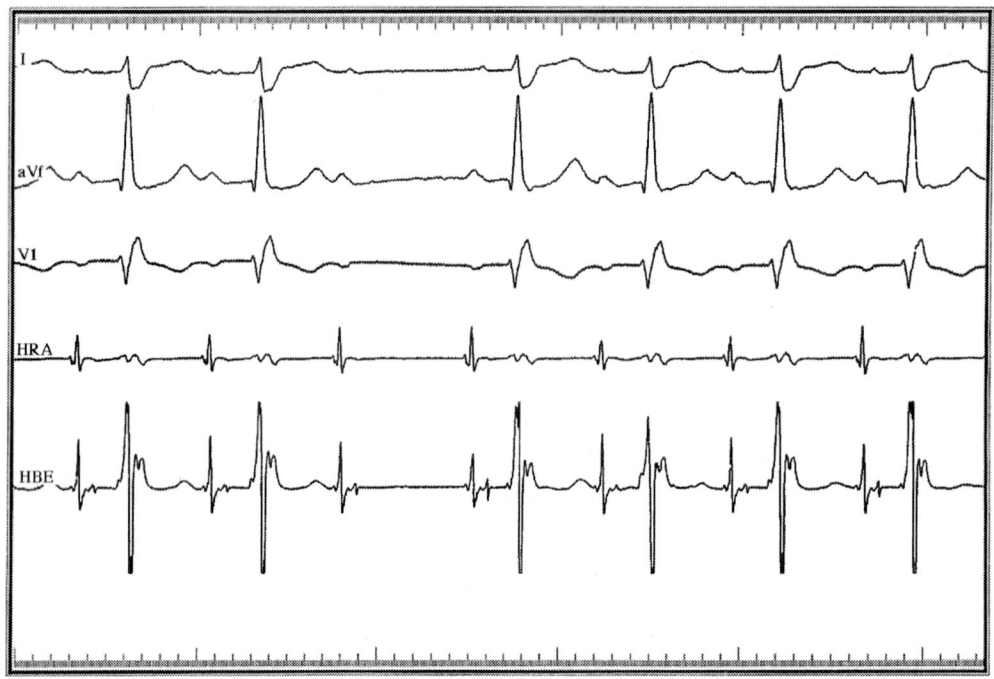

Fig. 27-16. Second-degree AV block (Mobitz II). Three surface ECG leads (I, aVF, and V$_1$) demonstrate a regular atrial rate with conduction to the ventricular chambers on all but the third beat. The QRS complex is in a right bundle branch block configuration. The PR interval does not gradually prolong before failing to conduct to the ventricles. This represents Mobitz II, second-degree AV block. The two additional leads (high right atrium—HRA$_1$; His bundle electrogram—HBE) demonstrate the anatomic sight of the AV block. The HRA$_1$ shows an atrial deflection simultaneous with the surface ECG P waves and smaller ventricular depolarizations during the QRS complexes. The HBE also shows the atrial and ventricular depolarizations, but also demonstrates (100 milliseconds after each atrial deflection) a small His bundle activation. After the third His, there is no ventricular activation. This represents AV block resulting from failure of conduction below the level of the His bundle. There is conduction through the left bundle and none through the right bundle causing a right bundle branch block configuration. On the blocked beats, the left bundle also fails to conduct.

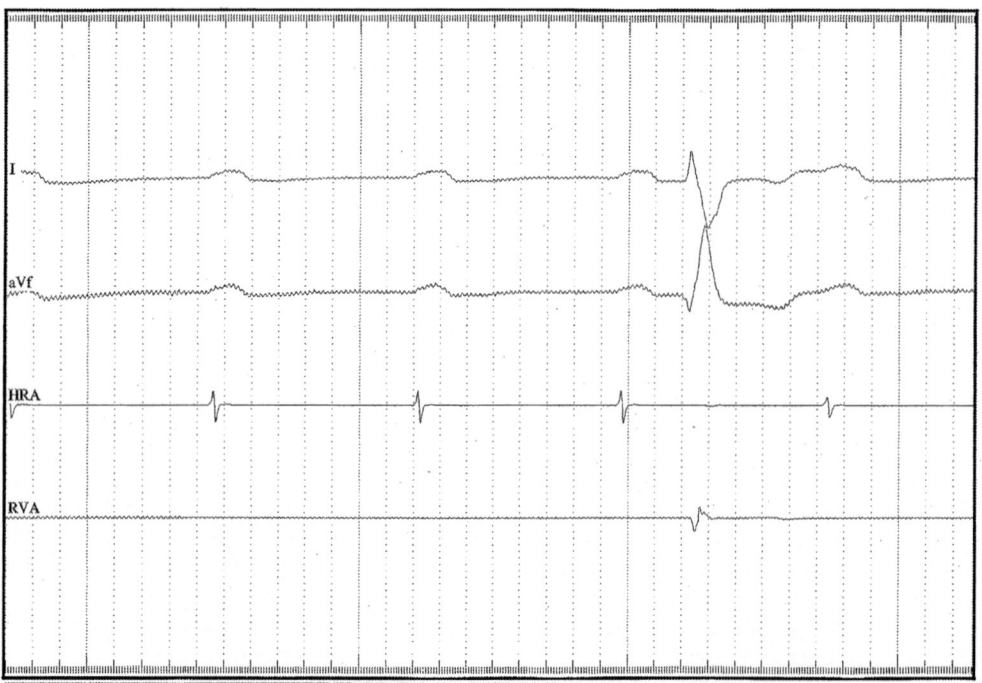

Fig. 27-17. Complete (third-degree AV) heart block. Two surface ECG leads (I and aVF) demonstrate five P waves and one QRS complex. The QRS duration is 160 milliseconds and the atrial rate is 79 bpm (760 milliseconds). The high right atrium (HRA) electrogram confirms the atrial activity and a recording of the single ventricular depolarization is evident on the right ventricular apex (RVA) electrogram.

tation phase of the ICU. Awareness that disturbances of cardiac rhythm and conduction can be responsible for some of the most frequent and potentially serious ICU complications must be employed. Potential causes and precipitating factors must be recognized and corrected. Appropriate therapy must be determined by the pathophysiology of the arrhythmia, the natural history of the disorder, the efficacy of its treatment, and prevention of recurrence.

REFERENCES

1. Chung, E. K.: Principles of Cardiac Arrhythmias. 2nd Ed. Baltimore, Williams & Wilkins, 1977.
2. Cranefield, P. F., Wit, A. L., and Hoffman, B. F.: Genesis of cardiac arrhythmias. Circulation, 47:190, 1973.
3. Horowitz, L. N., Josephson, M. E., and Harken, A. H.: Epicardial and endocardial activation during sustained ventricular tachycardia in man. Circulation, 61:1227, 1980.
4. Myerburg, R. J.: Electrocardiographic analysis of cardiac arrhythmias. Hosp. Pract., 15:51, 1980.
5. Wellens, H. J. J.: Value and limitations of programmed electrical stimulation of the heart in the study and treatment of tachycardias. Circulation, 57:845, 1978.
6. Wellens, H. J. J., Durrer, D. R., and Lie, K. I.: Observations on mechanisms of ventricular tachycardia in man. Circulation, 54:237, 1976.
7. Rosen, M. R., Hoffman, B. F., and Wit, A. L.: Electrophysiology and pharmacology of cardiac arrhythmias. 5. Cardiac antiarrhythmic effects of lidocaine. Am. Heart J., 89:526, 1975.
8. Schamroth, L.: The pathogenesis and mechanism of ventricular arrhythmias. In Progress in Cardiology. Edited by P. N. Yu and J. R. Goodwin, Phiadelphia, Lea & Febiger, 1974, p. 75.
9. Spurrell, R. A. J.: Reciprocation: a mechanism for tachycardias. Am. Heart J., 91:409, 1976.
10. Vera, Z., and Mason, D. T.: Reentry versus automaticity: role in tachyarrhythmia genesis and antiarrhythmic therapy. Am. Heart J., 101:329, 1981.
11. Wellens, H. J. J.: Pathophysiology of ventricular tachycardia in man. Arch. Intern. Med., 135:473, 1975.
12. Ayres, S. M., and Grace, W. J.: Inappropriate ventilation and hypoxemia as causes of cardiac arrhythmias. Am. J. Med., 46:495, 1969.
13. Harvey, W. P., and Ronan, J. A., Jr.: Bedside diagnosis of arrhythmias. Prog. Cardiovasc. Dis., 8:419, 1966.
14. Sinno, M. Z., and Gunnar, R. M.: Hemodynamic consequences of cardiac dysrhythmias. Med. Clin. North Am., 60:69, 1976.
15. Lee, W. K.: Clinical approoch to atrial fibrillation. Cardiovasc. Rev. Rep., 6:958, 1986.
16. Lown, B., and Levine, S. A.: The carotid sinus: clinical value of its stimulation. Circulation, 23:766, 1961.
17. Katz, L. N., and Pick, A.: Clinical Electrocardiography. Part 1: The Arrhythmias. Philadelphia, Lea & Febiger, 1956.
18. Gallagher, J. J. et al.: Esophageal pacing: a diagnostic and therapeutic tool. Circulation, 65:336, 1982.
19. Waldo, A. L. et al.: The use of temporary placed epicardial atrial wire electrodes for the diagnosis and treatment of cardiac arrhythmias following open heart surgery. J. Thorac. Cardiovasc. Surg., 76:500, 1978.
20. Moore, S. L., and Wilkoff, B. L.: Rhythm disturbances after cardiac surgery. Semin. Thorac. Cardiovasc. Surg., 3:24, 1991.
21. Waldo, A. L., and MacLean, W. A. H.: Diagnosis and treatment of cardiac arrhythmias following open heart surgery. In Emphasis on the Use of Atrial and Ventricular Epicardial Wire Electrodes. Mt. Kisco, NY, Futura, 1980.
22. Fisch, C., and Knoebel, S. B.: Digitalis cardiotoxicity. J. Am. Coll. Cardiol., 5:91A, 1985.
23. Keren, A., and Tzivoni, D.: Magnesium therapy in ventricular arrhythmias. PACE, 13:937, 1990.
24. Incalzi, R. A. et al.: Cardiac arrhythmias and left ventricular function in respiratory failure from chronic obstructive pulmonary disease. Chest, 97:1092, 1990.
25. Myerburg, R. J. et al.: Clinical, electrophysiologic and hemodynamic profile of patients resuscitated from prehospital cardiac arrest. Am. J. Med., 68:568, 1980.
26. Malliani, A., Schwartz, P. J., and Zanchetti, A.: Neural mechanisms in life-threatening arrhythmias. Am. Heart J., 100:705, 1980.
27. Stephenson, L. W. et al.: Propranolol for prevention of postoperative cardiac arrhythmias: a randomized study. Ann. Thorac. Surg., 29:113, 1980.
28. Wu, D., Kou, H. C., and Hung, J. S.: Exercise triggered paroxysmal ventricular tachycardia. Ann. Intern. Med., 95:410, 1981.
29. Palileo, E. V. et al.: Exercise provocable right ventricular outflow tract tachycardia. Am. Heart J., 104:185, 1982.
30. Schweitzer, P., and Mark, H.: The effect of atropine on cardiac arrhythmias and conduction. Am. Heart J., 100:119, 1980.
31. Barold, S. S.: Therapeutic uses of cardiac pacing in tachyarrhythmias. In His Bundle Electrocardiography and Clinical Electrophysiology. Edited by O. S. Narula. Philadelphia, F. A. Davis, 1975, p. 407.
32. Bhandari, A. K. et al.: Electrophysiologic testing in patients with the long QT syndrome. Circulation, 71:63, 1985.
33. Vlay, S. C. et al.: Documented sudden cardiac death in prolonged QT syndrome. Arch. Intern. Med., 144:833, 1984.
34. Josephson, M. E., and Seides, S. F.: Clinical Cardiac Electrophysiology Techniques and Interpretations. Philadelphia, Lea & Febiger, 1979.
35. Vaughn Williams, E. M.: Classification of antiarrhythmic drugs. In Symposium on Cardiac Arrhythmias. Edited by E. Sandoe, E. Flensted-Jensen, and K. H. Olesen. Sodertalje, Sweden, A. B. Astra, 1970, p. 449.
36. Cardiac Arrhythmia Suppression Trial (CAST) Investigators: Preliminary report: effect of encainide and flecainide on mortality in a randomized trial of arrhythmia suppression after myocardial infarction. N. Engl. J. Med., 322:406, 1989.
37. Khein, G. J., Yee, R., and Leitch, J. W.: Pharmacological management of supraventricular tachycardia. PACE, 13:1516, 1990.
38. Gray, R. J. et al.: role of intravenous verapamil in supraventricular tachyarrhythmias after open-heart surgery. Am. Heart J., 104:799, 1982.
39. Cox, J. L., and Ferguson, T. B., Jr.: Surgery for Wolff-Parkinson-White syndrome: the endocardial approach. Semin. Thorac. Cardiovasc. Surg., 1:34, 1989.
40. Rinne, C. et al.: Relation between clinical presentation and induced arrhythmias in the Wolff-Parkinson-White syndrome. Am. J. Cardiol. 60:576, 1987.
41. Mancini, G. B. J., and Goldberger, A. L.: Cardioversion of atrial fibrillation: consideration of embolization, anticoagulation, prophylactic pacemaker and long-term success. Am. Heart J., 104:617, 1982.
42. Prystowsky, E. N.: Antiarrhythmic therapy for asymptomatic ventricular arrhythmias. Am. J. Cardiol., 61:102A, 1988.
43. Wellens, H. J. J., Fritz, W. H. M., and Lie, K. I.: The value of electrocardiogram in the differential diagnosis of tachycardia with a widened QRS complex. Am. J. Med., 64:27, 1978.

44. Prystowsky, E. N., Katz, A., and Knilaus, T. K.: Ventricular arrhythmias: risk stratification and approach to therapy after the cardiac arrhythmia suppression trial (CAST). PACE, *13:* 1480, 1990.
45. Lown, B., and Wolf, M.: Approach to sudden death from coronary heart disease. Circulation, *44:*130, 1971.
46. Siddoway, L. A.: Selectivity appropriate first-line antiarrhythmic agents: comparative pharmacological profiles. PACE, *13:* 1488, 1990.
47. Meisseubuttel, R. H., and Bigger, J. T. J.: Bretylium tosylate, a newly available antiarrhythmic drug for ventricular arrhythmias. Ann. Intern. Med., *91:*229, 1979.
48. Gallagher, J. D. et al.: Amiodarone-induced complications during coronary artery surgery. Anesthesiology, *55:*186, 1989.
49. Tuzcu, E. M. et al.: Cardiopulmonary effects of chronic amiodarone therapy in the early postoperative course of cardiac surgery patients. Cleve. Clin. J. Med., *54:*491, 1987.
50. Furman, S., Hayes, D. L., and Holmes, D. R.: A practice of cardiac pacing. Mt. Kisco, NY, Futura Publishing, 1989, p. 209.
51. Waldo, A. L. et al.: Temporary cardiac pacing: applications and techniques in the treatment of cardiac arrhythmias. Cardiovasc. Dis. *23:*451, 1981.
52. Bernstein, A. D. et al.: The NASPE/BPEG generic pacemaker code for antibradyarrhythmia and adaptive-rate pacing and antitachyarrhythmia devices. PACE, *10:*794, 1987.

SUPPLEMENTAL READINGS

Craddock, L. et al.: Resuscitation from prolonged cardiac arrest with high-dose intravenous magnesium sulfate. J. Emerg. Med., *9:*469, 1991.

DiMarco, J. P.: Electrophysiology of adenosine. J. Cardiovasc. Electrophysiol., *1:*340, 1990.

Donovan, K. D., Dobb, G. S., and Lee, K. Y.: Hemodynamic benefit of maintaining atrioventricular synchrony during cardiac pacing in critically ill patients. Crit. Care Med., *19:*320, 1991.

Fish, F. A., Prakash, C., and Roden, D. M.: Suppression of repolarization related arrhythmias in vitro and vivo by low-dose potassium channel activators. Circulation, *82:*1362, 1990.

Garratt, C. et al.: Comparison of adenosine and verapamil for termination of paroxysmal junction tachycardia. Am. J. Cardiol., *64:*1310, 1989.

Goldberger, J., Kruse, J., Ehlert, F. A., and Kadisk, A. K.: Temporary transvenous pacemaker placement: what criteria constitute an adequate pacing site. (Editorial) Am. Heart J., *126:*488, 1993.

Greer, G. S., Wilkinson, W. E., McCarthy, E. A., and Pritchett, E. L.: Random and nonrandom behavior of symptomatic paroxysmal atrial fibrillation. Am. J. Cardiol., *64:*339, 1989.

Grubb, B. P., Temesy-Armos, P., Hahn, H., and Elliott, L.: The use of external, noninvasive pacing for the termination of ventricular tachycardia in the emergency department setting. Ann. Emerg. Med., *21:*174, 1992.

Hedhes, J. R. et al.: Pro-hospital transcutaneous cardiac pacing for symptomatic bradycardia. PACE, *14:*1473, 1991.

Huycke, E. C. et al.: Intravenous diltiazem for termination of reentrant supraventricular tachycardia. J. Am. Coll. Cardiol., *13:* 538, 1989.

Jackman, W. M. et al.: The long QT syndromes: a critical review, new clinical observation and unifying hypothesis. Prog. Cardiovasc. Dis., *31:*115, 1988.

Mohabir, R., Clusin, W. T., and Lee, H. C.: Intracellar calcium alternans and the genesis of ischemic ventricular fibrillation. *In* Cardiac Electrophysiology From Cell to Bedside. Edited by D. P. Zipes and J. Jalife. Philadelphia, W. B. Saunders, 1990, p. 448.

Muller, G. I., Ulmer, H. E., and Bauer, J. A.: complications of chest thump for termination of supraventricular tachycardia in children. Eur. J. Pediatr., *151:*12, 1992.

Roden, D. M.: Usefulness of sotalol for life-threatening ventricular arrhythmias. Am. J. Cardiol., *72:*51A, 1993.

Schuger, C. D. et al.: The excitable gap in AV nodal reentrant tachycardia. Circulation, *80:*324, 1989.

Shander, D.: Serial chest thumps for the treatment of ventricular tachycardia in patients with coronary heart disease. Clin. Cardiol., *15:*A28, 1992.

Stanton, M. S.: Arrhythmias involving accessory pathway and management. ACC Curr. J. Rev., *2:*62, 1993.

Tzivoni, D. et al.: Treatment of torsades de pointes with magnesium sulfate. Circulation, *77:*392, 1988.

von Planta, M., and Chamberlain, D.: Drug treatment of arrhythmias during cardiopulmonary resuscitation. Resuscitation, *24:* 227, 1992.

White, R. D.: Pre-hospital recognition of multifocal atrial tachycardia. Ann. Emerg. Med., *21:*753, 1992.

Zipes, D. P.: Specific arrhythmia: diagnosis and treatment. *In* Heart Disease. A Textbook of Cardiovascular Medicine. Edited by E. Braunwald. Philadelphia, W. B. Saunders, 1992, p. 692.

Chapter 28

CARDIOPULMONARY RESUSCITATION

JAMES P. ORLOWSKI

Since its inception in the early 1960s, modern cardiopulmonary resuscitation (CPR), consisting of mouth-to-mouth, or expired air, ventilation, external defibrillation, and external cardiac compression, has gone through several stages (Fig. 28-1). During the 1960s, a period of initial skepticism was followed by scientific and medical acceptance. In the 1970s we witnessed a zeal for widespread acceptance of dogma and an appeal for mass public education and application of the techniques.[1] In the 1970s and 1980s, the dogma was questioned and a scientific basis for what was being taught was considered necessary.[2,3] This led to improvements and limitations to CPR based on scientific studies and the testing of hypotheses. In the 1990s we will see continued refinements and restrictions placed on the techniques we call CPR.[4] We hope that methods of resuscitating the brain will be discovered, which will improve the outcome of resuscitation, because the brain is the organ most sensitive and most irreparably harmed by interruptions in oxygenation, ventilation, and perfusion. CPCR, or cardiopulmonary-cerebral resuscitation, will be the culmination of a major research thrust in the field of reanimation.

The techniques of modern CPR were developed over centuries, although the synthesis of the various techniques into a defined and unified approach to the victim of cardiopulmonary arrest did not occur until the early 1960s. Some of the early attempts were crude, barbaric, or humorous by modern standards and were based on assumptions of a need to restore warmth and to physically stimulate the body of the victim.

Expired air ventilation, or mouth-to-mouth resuscitation, was recorded in the Bible (2 Kings 4:34-35), when the prophet Elisha successfully resuscitated a child, and was widely and successfully used in the eighteenth century to resuscitate newborns, near-drowned persons, and victims overcome by smoke or fumes.[5] A reservoir bag and mask for manual ventilation was even developed during this time. Unfortunately, preposterous stories of successful resuscitations after days or weeks of submersion or death were not uncommon during these times, and these exaggerated reports detracted from the veracity and credibility of legitimate reports and studies. It was not until the late 1950s[6] that studies proved that mouth-to-mouth ventilation was clearly superior to the postural-manual methods such as Shafer's back-pressure technique, and the Nielsen back-pressure, arm-lift method.[7,8]

External cardiac massage was first reported to be successful in resuscitating cats in 1878 by Boehm, and in humans by Franz Koenig in 1882.[9] In 1892, Maas modified Koenig's technique, closely simulating modern techniques, and successfully resuscitated two children.[10] In 1904, Crile[11] successfully used external compression and epinephrine to resuscitate a patient undergoing thyroidectomy with ether anesthesia, and in 1906 Crile reported on the experimental success of external compression to maintain circulation in dogs.[12] Almost in parallel were the developments of internal or direct cardiac massage. Moritz Schiff reported success in animals in 1874, and in 1906, Greene reported 40 attempts at direct cardiac massage in humans with a 22% complete recovery rate.[4,9,10]

Defibrillation of the heart was also being perfected during the same period. Prevost and Battelli in 1899 had thoroughly studied the effects of electrical defibrillation on the heart in mammals,[4,9] followed by Carl Wigers's work in the 1930s. In 1947, Claude Beck successfully defibrillated a human heart with an internal defibrillator,[13] and in 1956, Zoll successfully performed external defibrillation on a human victim of ventricular fibrillation.[14] In 1957, Kouwenhoven reported on a portable alternating current (AC) external defibrillator.[15]

The birth of modern CPR occurred with the serendipitous and concurrent developments of all three modalities—expired air ventilation, external cardiac massage, and defibrillation—coming together at about the same time with human successes around 1960. Kouwenhoven, Jude, and Knickerbocker described closed chest cardiac massage in 1960;[16] Gordon et al.[8] and Safar[7] described mouth-to-mouth ventilation in 1958; and Zoll et al. in 1956[14] and Kouwenhoven et al. in 1957[15] described external defibrillation.

GENERAL PRINCIPLES OF CARDIOPULMONARY RESUSCITATION

Cardiopulmonary resuscitation refers to those measures used to restore ventilation and circulation in victims in whom these functions have been interrupted. Effective CPR requires a knowledge of anatomy and physiology as well as a knowledge of the drug dosages, which are calculated on the basis of body weight.[16]

Airway

Airway obstruction, or anoxia, is almost always present and is occasionally the precipitating event in cardiopulmonary arrest. The initial priority in CPR is the establishment of an adequate airway. The sedated, poisoned, or uncon-

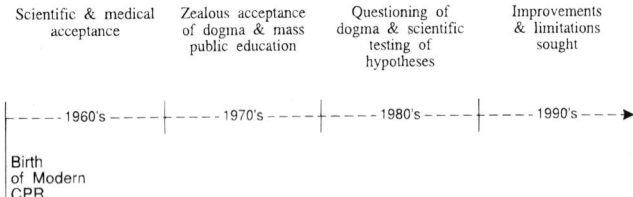

Fig. 28-1. Growth of modern CPR. (Courtesy, George Morrison, CD, Inc.)

scious victim may have airway compromise simply from positional narrowing of the airway. Proper positioning of the head and pulling of the mandible forward may entirely relieve the airway obstruction and permit the victim to breathe unlabored. The neck should not be excessively hyperextended, because marked hyperextension may collapse the trachea. After the airway has been established, it should be cleared of any obstructing or potentially obstructing material by suctioning the posterior oropharynx if possible before commencing breathing. Mouth-to-mouth or bag and mask ventilation provides time to await the arrival of an experienced individual. Considerable damage can be produced by unskilled attempts at intubation, so that experienced individuals may then have difficulty intubating the patient. Intubation should be reserved for the individual most skilled an adept in performing the procedure.

In the emergency situation, one frequently must decide on the size of the endotracheal tube to use. A quick and easy formula is that the size in millimeters of the internal diameter of the endotracheal tube is calculated by adding 16 to the patient's age in years, then dividing that sum by four. One then takes one size larger and one size smaller by 0.5 mm and has all three tubes prepared and ready at the time of intubation. Adult-sized tubes are 7.5, 8.0, and 8.5 mm. The appropriate size tube is then identified by direct laryngoscopy. Another quick method of estimating the size of the endotracheal tube is that the diameter of the trachea is approximately equal to the width of the patient's fifth finger.

Ventilation

The adult requires a ventilation rate of 12 breaths per minute, while the young adolescent or older child should have a ventilatory rate of 16 breaths per minute. Oxygen should be provided to the hypoxic patient at the earliest possible time and in the highest concentrations possible without concern in the emergency situation for the risks of oxygen toxicity. The effectiveness and adequacy of oxygen delivery and ventilation should be assessed by sampling of arterial blood gases.

Circulation

The establishment of an adequate airway and ventilation may be all that is required to resuscitate many patients. Bradycardia and hypotension that are due to hypoventilation will frequently be corrected with adequate delivery of oxygen. Once an adequate airway and ventilation have been established, the next priority in cardiopulmonary resuscitation is the assessment or establishment of adequate circulation. The best places to check for a pulse are the carotid, brachial, and femoral artery regions. If a good pulse is palpable and circulation appears to be good in terms of color of the extremities, circulation is probably adequate. The adequacy of circulation can then be checked by measurement of blood pressure and arterial blood gases. If a pulse cannot be found in the brachial, femoral, or carotid areas, external cardiac massage should be instituted.[17] Precordial chest thumps may be employed in witnessed and documented ventricular fibrillation. Cardiac compression should be about 50% of cycle time. This is achieved by maintaining a distinct pause at maximal compression.[18] The adequacy of external cardiac massage can be assessed by the following:

- The color and perfusion of the extremities
- The adequacy of palpable pulses (especially the brachial and femoral pulses)
- Blood pressure measurements
- Assessment of the arterial blood gases for metabolic acidosis

There is some controversy as to how external chest compression (ECC) results in the movement of blood through the heart and vascular system. One school of thought maintains that ECC results in direct cardiac compression (thus, the term external cardiac massage) between the sternum and the vertebral column, with propulsion of blood in a manner similar to direct internal cardiac massage. Another school of thought maintains that ECC works because of fluctuations in intrathoracic pressure and that the heart functions only as a passive conduit.

Support for the importance of fluctuations in intrathoracic pressure came from observations on cough CPR. In cough CPR, if a patient developing ventricular fibrillation begins to cough repetitively at a rate of 40 to 60 times per minute, they can often maintain consciousness for 1 to 2 minutes, permitting time for defibrillation.[19] Studies demonstrated that the rise and fall of intrathoracic pressure with each cough propelled blood and maintained a degree of circulation.[20] Other clinical evidence supporting the importance of fluctuations in intrathoracic pressure was the difficulty in resuscitating patients with flail chest,[21] despite the fact that a flail chest should not interfere with direct cardiac compression but would reduce intrathoracic pressure fluctuations. A number of experimental studies have documented the importance of intrathoracic pressure changes in the perfusion that results from ECC.[22]

Factors supporting the importance of direct cardiac compression of external cardiac massage included the difficulty of resuscitating patients with barrel chest from chronic obstructive pulmonary disease (COPD), bilateral pneumothoraces, or kyphoscoliosis where the heart does not lie between the sternum and vertebral column.[23] In each of these cases, changes in intrathoracic pressure occurred or were even accentuated, and yet successful CPR was unlikely. Experimental studies have also shown that the cardiac valves function during ECC,[24] suggesting that the heart is being compressed, and studies in dogs have confirmed direct cardiac compression with ECC.[25]

The most recent data suggest a compromise between the two schools. Apparently, early in cardiac arrest and ECC, direct cardiac compression occurs, with cardiac valves functioning and blood propelled by both cardiac massage and changes in intrathoracic pressure.[26] This observation nicely explains why the success rate for CPR rapidly declines after about 5 to 10 minutes of ECC.

ECCs consists of serial, rhythmic applications of pressure over the lower one third of the sternum. The heel of one hand of the rescuer is placed on the victim's sternum so that the long axis of the heel of the hand is directly over the long axis of the sternum, and the other hand of the rescuer is placed on top of this hand with fingers either interlaced or extended. The elbows are locked with the arms straight and extended, and the shoulders of the rescuer are positioned directly over the rescuer's hands so that the compression thrust is straight down on the sternum. The sternum is then compressed 1.5 to 2 inches rhythmically, with complete release between each compression, at a rate of about 100 compressions per minute. Properly performed, ECC should produce systolic blood pressure peaks of greater than 100 mm Hg.

One of the most common causes of difficulty with CPR is the attendant anxiety and excitement. Resuscitation invariably occurs in a tense and dramatic setting, and even the most experienced individual will have increased epinephrine. It is sometimes worthwhile to sacrifice a few seconds to collect one's thoughts for a rational approach. Another common problem is physical overcrowding. A resuscitation effort typically attracts a crowd of people, the majority of whom are simple onlookers. The resuscitation team leader should clear the scene of all extraneous individuals. Good record keeping is an integral part of CPR, and an individual member of the team should be assigned to the function of recording and timing all procedures and the administration of drugs and their dosages.

PRIMARY RESUSCITATION DRUGS

CPR demands familiarity with many drugs, their proper dosages, and their effects (Tables 28-1 and 28-2). Drug dosages in CPR should be based on body weight. The dosages in the following sections are all listed as dose per kilogram of body weight. Thus, epinephrine (1:10,000) is dosed at 0.1 ml/kg or 0.01 mg/kg, and the standard adult dose is 5 ml or 0.5 mg. It would be more appropriate to base adult doses on weight also. A 40-kg woman requires a significantly different dose than a muscular 100-kg male. The following drugs are most commonly employed during resuscitation.

Oxygen

Oxygen is not usually thought of as a drug, but because of its key role in cardiopulmonary resuscitation, it will be discussed as a primary resuscitation drug. Haldane put the problem in proper perspective many years ago when he stated, "Oxygen lack not only stops the motor, but also wrecks the machinery."[13] Many factors in cardiac arrest contribute to severe hypoxia. The amount of oxygen delivered to the tissues depends on the amount of oxygen carried by the blood (oxygen content) and the ability of the heart to deliver the oxygen and blood to the tissues (cardiac output). Oxygen content, in turn, depends on inspired oxygen concentration, transfer of oxygen to the blood, and the amount of hemoglobin in the blood. Expired air ventilation (mouth-to-mouth resuscitation) provides about 16 to 17% oxygen (F_{IO_2}), and under ideal circumstances of resuscitation) no more than 80 torr of alveolar oxygen tension can be obtained. The cardiac output is usually low (25 to 30% of normal), even when CPR is being done properly, and therefore mixed venous blood is severely desaturated and acidotic.[27] Such desaturated blood passing across right-to-left shunts contaminates arterial blood and further lowers the oxygen tension. Intrapulmonary right-to-left shunting and ventilation-perfusion abnormalities intensify the magnitude of arterial hypoxemia. With so many factors contributing to low arterial oxygen tension, it is readily apparent why supplemental oxygen should be added to the treatment regimen as soon as possible. Oxygen should be administered in the presence of suspected hypoxemia of any cause and obviously in all cases of cardiopulmonary arrest.[28] Oxygen should be delivered in the highest concentration available without a concern for possible risk of oxygen toxicity, which is not a hazard in the immediate period of acute resuscitation and should not preclude the use of 100% oxygen.[13] A pink color of the mucous membranes is a good indicator of satisfactory ventilation and oxygenation. Cardiac dysrhythmias that often accompany hypoxemia will frequently revert to normal sinus rhythms when adequate oxygenation is provided.[29]

Epinephrine

Epinephrine (Adrenalin) is an endogenous catecholamine that stimulates beta-adrenergic receptors and alpha-adrenergic receptors. Its usefulness in cardiac arrest situations has been substantiated over many years of clinical experience. Recent studies have reaffirmed the fact that the chief mode of action of epinephrine in asystole is its alpha-adrenergic effect with vasoconstriction and improvement of coronary perfusion. The beta-adrenergic effects can be blocked, and epinephrine will still successfully resuscitate the asystolic heart, but if the alpha-adrenergic actions are blocked, epinephrine is unsuccessful in resuscitation. During CPR, epinephrine has been shown to achieve the following:

- Elevate perfusion pressure generated during cardiac compression.
- Improve myocardial contractility.
- Stimulate spontaneous contraction.
- Increase myocardial tone.

These events may convert fine ventricular fibrillation to coarse ventricular fibrillation, which is more susceptible to termination by electrical countershock. The dosage of epinephrine is 0.1 ml/kg of a 1:10,000 solution or 0.01 mg/kg of body weight. The central venous route is the preferred route of administration during resuscitation. It

Table 28-1. First-Line and Second Line Resuscitation Drugs

Drugs	Route	Dose	Note	Usual Adult Dose
Oxygen	ET	0.50–1.00 F_{IO_2}	Give highest doses possible; never withhold in emergencies because of concern for toxicity	0.50–1.0
Epinephrine	IV ET	0.1 ml/kg of 1:10,000	Use 1:1000 for high dose; avoid intracardiac injection	5 ml (0.5 mg)
Sodium bicarbonate	IV	1.0 ml/kg (0.9 mEq/kg)	Give one dose only; repeat doses after pH and base deficit determination	50 mEq
Calcium chloride (27% Ca^{++})	IV	20–50 mg/kg (0.2–0.5 ml/kg) (max. 2.0 g/dose)	Preferred form of Ca^{++}; push slowly; use extreme caution in digitalized patients	1.0 g
Atropine	IV ET	0.01 mg/kg	Use for treatment of sinus bradycardia accompanied by severe hypotension	0.5–1.0 mg
Lidocaine	IV ET	0.5–1.0 mg/kg	Use for ventricular tachycardia or ventricular fibrillation; should be followed by continuous infusion if premature ventricular contractions or ventricular tachycardia recurs	50 mg
Bretylium	IV	5 mg/kg; increase by 5 mg/kg to max., 30 mg/kg	Use for refractory ventricular contractions or ventricular fibrillation, especially when lidocaine fails	5–10 mg/kg
Adenosine	IV	0.1–0.2 mg/kg (max. 12/mg)	Rapid IV bolus	6–12 mg
Magnesium sulfate	IV	20–50 mg/kg	Dilute in D-5-W and administer over 1–2 minutes; treatment of choice for torsades de pointes	1–2 g

ET, Endotracheal; IV = intravenous.

may be necessary to repeat this dose at 5-minute intervals because of its short duration of action. This drug may be administered by a peripheral intravenous route or intraosseous route if a central intravenous line is not readily available. If there is a delay in establishing an intravenous route, or if because of severe hypoperfusion (shock) an intravenous route cannot be readily established, epinephrine can be instilled directly into the tracheobronchial tree via an endotracheal tube. Absorption from this site is rapid and has a direct action on the heart. When administered down an endotracheal tube, the epinephrine should be 10 times the intravenous dose (1:1000) and should be diluted to a total volume of 5 to 10 ml with sterile water, injected down the endotracheal tube, then bag ventilated into the periphery. If one thinks about this route of administration teleologically,[30] it makes good sense, because the epinephrine will cross the alveolar capillary membrane, then pass to the left side of the heart, which is an excellent site of action for the epinephrine. The risks of intracardiac administration of epinephrine are numerous and include interruption of cardiac compression and ventilation, cardiac tamponade, coronary artery laceration, myocardial necrosis, and pneumothorax.[31] Epinephrine should not be added directly to a bicarbonate infusion, because catecholamines may be partially inactivated by an alkaline solution.

Table 28-2. Emergency Drugs Given by Continuous Infusion

Drugs	Dose	Indications
Dopamine	Low dose: 1–7 μg/kg/min Moderate dose: 7–20 μg/kg/min High dose: >20–30 μg/kg/min	Increase renal blood flow Increase cardiac output Systemic vasoconstriction
Dobutamine	0.5–20 μg/kg/min	Cardiogenic shock
Isoproterenol	Starting dose 0.02 μg/kg/min; rarely need to exceed 0.5 μg/kg/min	Status asthmaticus; diminished cardiac contractility or bradycardia
Epinephrine	Starting dose 0.02–0.05 μg/kg/min; most patients respond to doses less than 0.2 mg/kg/min; doses >0.5 μg/kg/min may cause excessive vasoconstriction	Augmentation of cardiac output and support of blood pressure in shock after restoration of intravascular volume
Norepinephrine (Levophed)	0.02–0.1 μg/kg/min	Peripheral vascular collapse without significant peripheral vasoconstriction
Nitroprusside	Dosage range: 0.5–8.0 μg/kg/min Average dose is 3 μg/kg/min	Immediate reduction of blood pressure in hypertensive crisis; afterload reduction
Lidocaine	No CHF: 36–88 μg/kg/min Mild CHF: 12–35 μg/kg/min Moderate-to-severe CHF: 5–12 μg/kg/min	Management of acute ventricular arrhythmias
Aminophylline	6 mg/kg over 15 min as loading dose, followed by 1 mg/kg/hr by continuous infusion	Bronchospasm
Insulin	0.1 to 0.2 U/kg/hr	Diabetic ketoacidosis; hyperglycemia

CHF, Congestive heart failure.

Lidocaine

Lidocaine was originally developed as a local anesthetic but has subsequently been shown to have many beneficial cardiac effects, including the following:

- Reduction of the automaticity and the ectopic pacemakers of the ventricles
- Termination of reentrant ventricular tachycardias
- Increase of the fibrillation threshold, especially in the ischemic myocardium[32]

In therapeutic doses, lidocaine has negligible effects on the atrial muscle fibers, myocardial contractility, cardiac output, or atrioventricular conduction times. Lidocaine is metabolized in the liver, and the serum blood levels reflect not only the dose given but hepatic metabolism as well. In the presence of liver dysfunction, such as in congestive heart failure or hepatitis, lidocaine must be given in reduced doses to avoid tax blood levels.[33] Lidocaine toxicity can result in the following adverse effects:

- Depression of myocardial contractility
- Depressed cardiac output
- Ventricular ectopy
- Slowing of the atrioventricular and ventricular conduction with resultant heart block and asystole

The early central nervous system symptoms of toxicity that may precede cardiovascular abnormalities in non-CPC situations include nausea, vomiting, lethargy, disorientation, coma, and seizures.

Lidocaine is effective in controlling several forms of ventricular ectopic activity, in which treatment should be instituted promptly:

- Frequent ventricular premature beats (greater than six per minute)
- Close-coupled premature ventricular contractions (R on T phenomenon)
- Multifocal premature ventricular contractions
- Short bursts of ventricular tachycardia or premature ventricular contractions (salvos)
- Ventricular tachycardia and fibrillation

Ventricular premature beats, ventricular tachycardia, or ventricular fibrillation may be secondary to severe persistent metabolic acidosis, metabolic alkalosis, hypoxemia, or electrolyte disturbances, and these problems should be corrected first. Lidocaine is usually given in an initial intravenous bolus of 1 mg/kg of body weight; because of the short half-life of lidocaine, a continuous low dose infusion should be started simultaneously if a continued antiarrhythmic effect is necessary (Table 28-2).

SECONDARY RESUSCITATION DRUGS

(See Table 28-1).

Sodium Bicarbonate

Cardiopulmonary arrest results in both respiratory and metabolic acidosis. Poor perfusion results in the generation of lactic acid and the development of metabolic acidosis, and ventilatory failure leads to carbon dioxide retention and respiratory acidosis. Prompt and efficient ventilation of the lungs is essential for the elimination of carbon dioxide as well as for oxygenation.

Persistent ventilatory insufficiency has been shown to be an important contributor to the genesis of refractory acidosis during cardiopulmonary arrest.[28] Effective ventilation with the generation of a mild-to-moderate respiratory alkalosis can counteract a substantial amount of metabolic acidosis by normalizing the pH. Sodium bicarbonate is indicated for clinically and hemodynamically significant metabolic acidosis, especially in the setting of lactic acidosis secondary to cardiopulmonary arrest. A low arterial pH that is due to respiratory acidosis should be treated by improving the patient's ventilation, and hyperventilation can be used to correct some of the components of metabolic acidosis. Administration of sodium bicarbonate results in a simple acid/base reaction in which the bicarbonate ion combines with the hydrogen ion in the blood and thereby elevates the blood pH:

$$(HCO_3 + H^+ \to H_2CO_3 \to CO_2 + H_2O)$$

Carbon dioxide is generated during this reaction which again emphasizes the need for adequate alveolar ventilation during resuscitation.

The excessive and indiscriminate use of sodium bicarbonate is accompanied by many dangers and should be avoided. The excessive use of sodium bicarbonate may lead to metabolic alkalosis,[34] hypernatremia,[35] and hyperosmolar states, which have been implicated in intracranial hemorrhage in infants.[36] Severe hyperosmolar states during resuscitation have been documented and patients with cardiac and renal disease may not be able to tolerate the sodium load. The precipitous correction of acidosis systemically with sodium bicarbonate may result in worsening of intracerebral acidosis with further depression of the central nervous system.[37] Many of the other primary resuscitation drugs, particularly the catecholamines and calcium, are inactivated in alkaline solutions, and the intravenous lines must be cleared of sodium bicarbonate before these drugs are administered. The dose of sodium bicarbonate varies and should be determined by measurements of arterial pH when feasible. In a situation of unwitnessed cardiopulmonary arrest, the recommended dose is 1 mEq/kg of body weight as a one-time dose. Any subsequent doses are calculated on the basis of measured pH and base-deficit determinations from arterial blood gas samples, as follows:

$$NaHCO_3(mEq) = \frac{HCO_3 \text{deficit}(mEq/l) \times \text{bodyweight}(kg)}{8}$$

Calcium

The calcium ion has long been known to increase myocardial contractile force.[38] Calcium ions may also enhance ventricular excitability and increase conduction velocities through the ventricular muscle. Calcium may be useful in cases of profound cardiovascular collapse with an orderly electrical rhythm but an ineffective mechanical ejection of the blood (electromechanical dissociation) or pulseless non-perfusing rhythm and in some instances of ventricular standstill. Precautions in the use of calcium include the speed of administration and its use in digitalized patients. Rapid administration of calcium salts, if the heart is beating, may produce severe sinus bradycardia or sustained contraction of myocardial muscle with ventricular standstill. Calcium must also be used very cautiously in patients who have received digitalis, because some clinical studies suggest that calcium potentiates digitalis-related dysrhythmias and may result in asystole that is unresponsive to all measures.[38] The dosage of calcium chloride is 20 to 50 mg/kg (with a maximum of 1 g per dose). This should be given as a slow intravenous infusion with continual monitoring of cardiac rate and rhythm.

Atropine

Atropine is the competitive antagonist of acetylcholine and is described as a parasympatholytic drug. It reduces vagal tone with resultant increase in the rate of sinoatrial node discharge and an increase in the conduction through the atrioventricular node. In addition to these peripheral effects, atropine has a central effect and at low doses stimulates the medullary vagal nuclei, which may result in a decreased heart rate with slowing of atrioventricular conduction (a paradoxic central effect). Atropine is indicated for hemodynamically significant bradycardia; that is, bradycardia associated with hypotension or ventricular ectopy. Atropine may also be useful in the temporary treatment of second- and third-degree heart block and slow idioventricular rates. It is important to remember that both atrial and ventricular tachyarrhthmias may be precipitated by atropine,[39] and in insufficient doses, atropine may cause a paradoxic bradycardia secondary to its central actions. The dosage of atropine is 0.01 mg/kg of body weight, with a minimum dose of 0.10 mg and a maximum dose of 2 mg.

Bretylium

Bretylium is useful for parenteral treatment of life-threatening ventricular tachycardia or fibrillation refractory to other therapy. Most studies have indicated that bretylium can stabilize rhythm in about one half of patients with resistant ventricular fibrillation or recurrent tachycardia that does not respond to lidocaine.[40] The mechanism of the antiarrhythmic action of bretylium has not yet been fully defined, but it is believed that at least part of its antiarrhythmic action derives from its effect on sympathetic function. Bretylium was originally developed as an antihypertensive agent, and it can produce hypotension that is due to sympathetic blockade. The recommended intravenous dose of bretylium is 5 mg/kg of body weight, with increases by 5 mg/kg of body weight increments to a maximum of 30 mg/kg.

Amiodarone

The treatment of life-threatening ventricular arrhythmias remains a therapeutic problem. A promising new treatment is intravenous amiodarone. A recent report suggests that intravenous amiodarone may be rapidly effective in terminating ventricular tachycardia or ventricular fibrillation refractory to other antiarrhythmic drugs.[41] Intravenous amiodarone was administered to 14 patients during prolonged in-hospital resuscitation from refractory cardiac arrest caused by ventricular tachycardia or ventricular fibrillation. Resuscitation had been ongoing for at least 30 minutes before amiodarone was administered, and none of the patients was in a perfusing rhythm at the time amiodarone was given. Eleven (79%) of the 14 patients survived their prolonged cardiac arrest after being given intravenous amiodarone.

Adenosine is the drug of choice for paroxysmal supraventricular tachycardia.[4] It is an endogenous purine nucleoside that depresses AV node and sinus node activity. The half-life of adenosine is less than 5 seconds. Transient periods of sinus bradycardia and ventricular ectopy are common after termination of SVT with adenosine. Because of adenosine's short half-life, PSVT may recur (in 50 to 60%) and can be treated with either additional doses of adenosine or a calcium-channel blocker. Adenosine produces little harm in patients with ventricular tachycardia and converts many cases of wide QRS-complex tachycardia.

Magnesium is the treatment of choice for patients with torsades de pointes.[4] Magnesium deficiency is associated with cardiac arrhythmias and even sudden cardiac death. Hypomagnesemia can cause refractory ventricular fibrillation, and magnesium replacement is indicated in refractory or recurrent ventricular fibrillation and ventricular tachycardia.

Other Drugs

Naloxone (Narcan) is used to reverse the respiratory depression of opiate poisonings, and physostigmine (Antilirium) is valuable for reversing the central nervous system depression in other poisonings, including an overdosage of diazepam (Valium). Flumazenil (Romazicon) is a specific antagonist for benzodiazepene overdosage. Morphine is used for relief of pain and is also effective in reducing preload in congestive heart failure. Diazepam, phenytoin, and phenobarbital are employed for the treatment of epileptic seizures. Although diazepam is probably the best initial choice drug for treating status epilepticus, it is short acting, and to prevent further seizures, the patient should be started on phenytoin and/or phenobarbital. Diazoxide (Hyperstat) is used for the treatment of hypertensive crises and must be given intravenously as rapidly as possible. Mannitol is used for treating intracranial hypertension and cerebral edema in the emergency situation, then dexamethasone (Decadron) is used for a more prolonged and sustained treatment of intracranial hypertension. Furosemide is a potent loop diuretic and is used for treating overhydration states and pulmonary and cerebral edema. Digoxin is a cardiac drug that is used for treating congestive heart failure and is a valuable antiarrhythmic for the treatment of paroxysmal atrial tachycardia. Propranolol (Inderal) is a beta-blockade agent that is used for treating sympathetic overactivity. Chapter 27 discusses the use of digoxin, propranolol, and other antiarrhythmics in detail.

For hypovolemic shock states (hypoperfusion), 10 to 15 ml/kg of Ringer's lactate, 5% albumin (Albumisol) or type-specific or O-negative whole blood may be used. The dose of 25% albumin is 1 g/kg of body weight.

Glucose

It is important to remember that even 5% glucose solution can produce hyperglycemia if given rapidly enough. One ampule (50 ml) of 50% glucose solution (D50) is indicated in suspected hypoglycemia pending determination of blood glucose concentrations.

Dopamine

Dopamine is a chemical precursor of epinephrine, which occurs naturally in humans and has dopaminergic, alpha-adrenergic, and beta-adrenergic receptor-stimulating actions, depending on the dosage employed (Table 28-2). It differs from epinephrine, norepinephrine, and isoproterenol in that it dilates renal, mesenteric, coronary, and cerebral blood vessels in dosages that may not increase heart rate or blood pressure (1 to 7 μg/kg per minute).[42] At low doses, the primary effect of dopamine is to increase renal and coronary artery blood flow with either a slight decrease or no change in peripheral vascular resistance secondary to beta-adrenergic vascular dilatation. Low doses of dopamine in congestive heart failure may decrease peripheral vascular resistance sufficiently to raise cardiac output and unload strain on the heart.[43] At moderate doses, more beta stimulation results in an increase in myocardial contractility, heart rate, and stroke volume, with a resultant increase in cardiac output. Total peripheral vascular resistance may increase, which, coupled with the increased cardiac output, results in increased blood pressure. Renal blood flow at moderate doses probably continues to increase.[42] At high doses of dopamine, there is an increase in alpha-adrenergic stimulation, resulting in a decrease in renal blood flow and marked increase in peripheral vasoconstriction. Stroke volume, myocardial contractility, and cardiac output increase, but heart rate may level off secondary to improved cardiac hemodynamics and improved perfusion pressure.[44] The indications for the use of dopamine include the following:

- Improvement in tissue perfusion in septic states (the mechanism of action is said to be a reduction in peripheral arteriovenous shunting with a consequent improvement in capillary perfusion)[45]
- Augmentation of cardiac output in other shock states after correction of hypovolemia
- Augmentation of renal blood flow and perhaps cardiac output in chronic or acute congestive heart failure

The toxicity from dopamine is minimal at reasonable doses. Tachycardia and tachyarrhythmias may occur, and an excessive hypertensive response can result if blood pressure is not closely monitored. Excessive diuresis can also occur. Alkaline solutions, including solutions containing calcium, inactivate dopamine. Dopamine may be safely given into a peripheral vein, provided that the intravenous site and surrounding skin are closely observed for cyanosis, pallor, and coolness.

Dobutamine

Dobutamine is a synthetic catecholamine derived from chemical manipulation of isoproterenol, which is indicated for short-term treatment of cardiac decompensation that is due to refractory heart failure (Table 28-2).[46] Dobutamine increases myocardial contractility with minimal peripheral vasoconstriction.[47]

Dobutamine increase myocardial contractility by direct action on myocardial beta$_1$-adrenergic receptors. Beta-adrenergic blocking agents may make the drug ineffective. Unlike isoproterenol, dobutamine only occasionally causes tachycardia and, unlike norepinephrine, produces little vasoconstriction at usual therapeutic doses. Dobutamine does not dilate renal and mesenteric vessels as dopamine does, but renal and mesenteric blood flow may increase as a consequence of improved cardiac output. The adverse effects of dobutamine include hypertension, arrhythmias (usually premature ventricular contractions), nausea, vomiting, and headache. Dobutamine is contraindicated in idiopathic hypertrophic subaortic stenosis because it can increase the obstruction to cardiac outflow.

Positive inotropic effects from dobutamine can occur at doses as low as 0.5 μg/kg per minute, but the usual dosage range is 2.5 to 10 μg/kg per minute. Doses above 20 μg/kg per minute should be used with special caution because they are more likely to cause tachycardia and arrhythmias. Dobutamine is recommended for the treatment of shock only when the shock is caused by inadequate cardiac contractility. Many clinicians continue to prefer dopamine because of its effect on renal circulation and longer experience with its use. For a more detailed discussion of dobutamine and other inotropic drugs, the reader is referred to Chapter 65.

Isoproterenol

Isoproterenol may be used for states of diminished cardiac contractility unresponsive to digoxin and dopamine and may be indicated for bradycardias not responsive to vagal blockade with atropine. Isoproterenol is contraindicated in ischemic heart disease, including aortic stenosis. It is important to remember that isoproterenol is used diagnostically in the cardiac catheterization laboratory to provoke obstruction in idiopathic hypertrophic subaortic stenosis. Isoproterenol is a synthetic sympathomimetic drug with almost pure beta-adrenergic receptor stimulation. The effects of isoproterenol on the cardiovascular system include increases in heart rate, myocardial contractility and tone, automaticity, myocardial oxygen consumption, and venous return to the heart.[48] Isoproterenol causes peripheral arterial dilatation, particularly in skeletal muscle; if the patient is hypovolemic or dehydrated, there is an increased risk of hypotension with an infusion of isoproterenol.[43] Because isoproterenol is a powerful positive inotropic agent, a rising cardiac output frequently compensates for the decreased peripheral resistance, and blood pressure will not fall with infusion of isoproterenol if the patient is normovolemic. The starting dosage of isoproterenol should not exceed 0.2 μg/kg per minute, and the maximum dose required rarely exceeds 0.50 μg/kg per minute. Tachycardia associated with the use of an infusion of isoproterenol is often striking and results from a combination of direct cardiac stimulation and decreased peripheral resistance. Cardiac arrhythmias are especially likely if hypoxemia, acidosis (pH less than 7.20), or hypovolemia is present. Cardiac tachyarrhythmias are also likely to occur in the setting of digitalis toxicity or preexisting tachyarrhythmias. The duration of action of isoproterenol is very short, so arrhythmias can often be terminated simply by stopping the infusion. One should have lidocaine and a defibrillator available, however, in case problems occur.

Epinephrine

Epinephrine as a continuous low dose infusion is indicated for the augmentation of cardiac output and the support of blood pressure in any shock state after the restoration of intravascular volume (Table 28-2).[43] In low doses, epinephrine decreases peripheral vascular resistance while greatly increasing cardiac output, and it raises the systolic blood pressure while widening the pulse pressure.[48] Renal blood flow is either decreased or unchanged, and epinephrine may be combined with dopamine or with sodium nitroprusside to maintain renal blood flow. The starting dose for a continuous low dose infusion of epinephrine is 0.02 to 0.05 µg/kg per minute. Most patients respond to doses of less than 0.20 µg/kg per minute, and doses exceeding 0.50 µg/kg per minute will frequently result in excessive peripheral vasoconstriction and poor peripheral perfusion. The toxicities associated with the use of epinephrine as a continuous low dose infusion include the following:

- Tachycardia
- Tachyarrhythmias
- Peripheral vasoconstriction that can lead to gangrene, especially if epinephrine is being infused into a peripheral intravenous line
- Hyperglycemia
- Glycosuria
- Pupillary dilatation

An infusion of epinephrine may be turned off for the 2 to 3 minutes necessary to read central venous pressure without loss of effect.

Norepinephrine

Norepinephrine (Levophed) is a naturally occurring catecholamine. The indications for its use are systemic vascular collapse manifested by hypotension and the absence of peripheral vasoconstriction. Norepinephrine is a potent peripheral vasoconstrictor (alpha-receptor-stimulating agent) that generally results in elevation of blood pressure. Norepinephrine produces marked peripheral vasoconstriction with resultant decreases in renal, mesenteric, hepatic, cerebral, and skeletal muscle blood flow.[43] Coronary blood flow is usually increased as a result of both direct coronary artery vasodilatation and the increase in blood pressure. Norepinephrine produces a slightly more rapid blood pressure response than other catecholamines, including dopamine. The initial starting dose for an infusion of norepinephrine should be 0.02 to 0.10 µg/kg per minute titrated to the patient's clinical response. With the clinical usefulness of dopamine having been established over a wide range of doses, the use of norepinephrine has diminished, but it still remains a useful drug, especially if additional alpha-adrenergic stimulation is desired. Norepinephrine may be continued for hours to days but should be tapered with close monitoring of blood pressure. Abrupt cessation of therapy may result in acute severe hypotension. When hypovolemia is present, extreme degrees of vasoconstriction may occur and result in a critical decrease in organ blood flow, even with a "normal" blood pressure is recognizable clinically. Ischemic necrosis and sloughing of superficial tissues may result if extravasation of norepinephrine is allowed to occur at the site of injection.

Nitroprusside

Nitroprusside is a potent, rapid-acting antihypertensive. Its effect is the result of peripheral vasodilatation as a consequence of direct action on blood vessels. Its effect is almost immediate and ends when the intravenous infusion is stopped. Nitroprusside is indicated for the immediate reduction of blood pressure in hypertensive crises and for the relief of afterload strain on the heart in syndromes of congestive heart failure characterized by low cardiac output and high systemic vascular resistance. The dosages of nitroprusside employed range from 0.5 to 8.0 µ/kg per minute, with the average dose for optimum response being approximately 3.0 µg/kg per minute. The end product of the metabolism of nitroprusside is thiocyanate, and blood levels of thiocyanate should be monitored in any patient receiving high doses or prolonged therapy with nitroprusside and in any patient with renal insufficiency. Thiocyanate levels must not be allowed to exceed 10 mg/dl, and a blood cyanide level of 0.34 mg/dl is toxic. Vitamins B_{12} and A have been reported to reduce the formation of cyanide. Nitroprusside can be dissolved only in 5% dextrose in water and must be protected from light. The solution should be used only for 4 hours, and if any colored reaction products form in the solution, the infusion should be replaced.

Lidocaine

Lidocaine was discussed previously in the section entitled "Primary Resuscitation Drugs." The therapeutic range of lidocaine levels in plasma is 2.4 to 6.0 µg/ml. The monitoring of lidocaine plasma levels will help in the clinical management of patients and will also reduce the incidence of toxicity.

DEFIBRILLATION

Defibrillation produces a simultaneous depolarization of a critical mass of myocardial cells, after which a spontaneous beat may resume if the myocardium is oxygenated and is not acidotic. When a victim is found to be without a pulse, early defibrillation is the standard of care in the adult. If ventricular fibrillation is demonstrated by electrocardiograph (ECG), defibrillation should be attempted as soon as possible. The electrode paddles should be placed so that one is to the right of the sternum at the level of the second rib and the other is in the left mid-clavicular line at the xiphoid level. The dosage for defibrillation is an initial dose of 2 to 3 watt seconds (joules) per kilogram of body weight. If this is unsuccessful, the energy dose is then doubled.[49] If the higher dose does not effectively defibrillate the heart, attention should be directed to the acid/base status and oxygenation before the dosage is further increased. It is well-known that electrical stimulation potentiates the effect of digoxin. The use of the usual levels of electrical shock in the presence of bound digoxin in the myocardium may cause irreversible cardiac arrest. It is therefore recommended that if a patient is known to be receiving digoxin at the time of fibrillation, the amount of energy delivered to such a patient should be a low dose. If defibrillation is not successful, the energy should be slowly and cautiously increased.

RECENT ADVANCES AND RESEARCH DEVELOPMENTS LIKELY TO AFFECT CPR

Certain recent discoveries and research developments are being applied to CPR and adopted as standards or guidelines for CPR.[4] These include the following:

- High dose epinephrine[50]
- Higher compression rate[51,52]
- Higher compression force ECC[52,53]
- End-tidal carbon dioxide (P_{ETCO_2})[54-57] monitoring during CPR
- The intraosseous route as an alternative when intravenous access cannot be achieved[58,59]
- A return to open-chest cardiac massage in selected circumstances[60]

High dose epinephrine is an experimental pharmacologic alteration of the present standards and guidelines that potentially will benefit some victims of cardiac arrest. It is based on the observation that some patients who fail to respond to the standard dose of epinephrine will respond to much higher doses, apparently without adverse effects.[50] Doses as high as 10 times the recommended dose have been shown to result in improved systolic and diastolic arterial blood pressures, in a near-linear dose-response fashion. Similar results have been demonstrated with the intratracheal administration of epinephrine. The recommended dose of epinephrine for endotracheal administration has been the same as the intravenous dose, and yet certain authors have reported on the failure of the standard dose by the endotracheal route as compared to the intravenous route.[61,62] In fact, the endotracheal route of administration of epinephrine has been characterized as unreliable compared to other alternatives to intravenous administration such as the intraosseous route. One study suggested that the endotracheal dose needed to be 10 times as large to achieve the same success rate as the intravenous route.[63]

Other alterations of the standard techniques of CPR that have received recent attention include increasing the rate and/or force of compression in external cardiac massage.[51-53] Increasing compression rates over a range from 60 to 150 per minute results in a continuous improvement in cardiac output and mean aortic pressure, whereas total coronary blood flow optimizes at a manual compression rate between 100 and 120.[51,52] Some of the improvements seen with increased rates of compression may reflect a greater proportion of the duty cycle being occupied by the compression. At rates of 60 compressions per minute, compression accounts for less than 20% of the duty cycle, whereas at rates of 150, the compression accounts for about 50% of the duty cycle. Studies have also shown that increasing the compression force from 20 to 140 pounds steadily increases systolic blood pressure, although diastolic blood pressure remains unchanged.[52,53]

(P_{ETCO_2}) monitoring is gaining increasing acceptance as a noninvasive method of monitoring the effectiveness of ECC and as an early predictor of the return of spontaneous circulation (ROSC).[54-57] P_{ETCO_2} depends on ventilation, perfusion, and carbon dioxide production. Perfusion depends on both cardiac output and lung perfusion. If ventilation is kept constant, P_{ETCO_2} will reflect perfusion and has been used during CPR as a noninvasive means of monitoring cardiac output. During cardiopulmonary arrest, P_{ETCO_2} drops to zero and increases slightly during ECC. With the ROSC, P_{ETCO_2} elevates very rapidly, and even exceeds normal values, reflecting a washout of carbon dioxide from the tissues. It then returns to normal, assuming normal pulmonary and cardiac function.

Recent studies have demonstrated that the intraosseous route is superior to the only other approved alternative to intravenous access, the endotracheal route. Not only is the intraosseous route equivalent to the central venous route in drug effectiveness, but any medication or fluid that can be administered by the intravenous route can be administered by the intraosseous route.[58,59] Whereas the endotracheal route of administration is restricted to only a few drugs such as succinylcholine, atropine, lidocaine, isoproterenol, naloxone and epinephrine (mnemonic "SALINE"), all resuscitation drugs, fluids and blood products can be administered by the intraosseous route. Studies also suggest that the endotracheal route is less reliable than the intravenous or intraosseous route for the most critical of resuscitation drugs, epinephrine.[61-63] Another potential advantage of the intraosseous route as an alternative to the intravenous route is that laboratory studies may be obtainable from the bone marrow, permitting diagnostic studies to be obtained in an emergency.[58]

Intraosseous techniques are being taught to prehospital, as well as emergency room personnel, as an important emergency alternative to intravenous access when establishment of intravenous access is either impossible or will be critically delayed. The intraosseous infusion technique consists of inserting a bone marrow aspirate needle into the marrow of the distal femur, proximal tibia, or medial or lateral malleoli, and then infusing colloids, blood or crystalloids, or administering resuscitation drugs.

The rejuvenation of the technique of open-chest cardiac massage is based on experimental and clinical studies demonstrating that open-chest cardiac massage is superior to closed chest or external cardiac compression in both organ perfusion and the number of patients successfully resuscitated.[60] Because external cardiac compression is safer and effective, what needs to be decided is when to proceed to open-chest cardiac massage in terms of indications and timing. It is likely that there will be a window of time when it becomes clear that closed chest cardiac compression will not be effective and when moving to open-chest cardiac massage will still be effective in restoring cardiac activity without producing an unacceptable increase in neurologic deficits. At the present time, the indications for open-chest cardiac massage are penetrating or crushed chest trauma, cardiac arrest when the chest has already been surgically opened, and thoracic or cardiac abnormalities that make closed chest ECC impossible or ineffective.[60] Because open-chest cardiac massage is not a technique that can be employed by laypersons or most health-care personnel, its use is much more restricted. Nevertheless, its superiority to closed chest cardiac compression should be kept in mind in the hospital setting when confronted with "a heart too good to die" that is not responding to external cardiac massage.

Research breakthroughs were incorporated into the 1986[12] and 1992[4] standards and guidelines for CPR, once human studies confirmed their utility and benefit. These changes included a reduced role for sodium bicarbonate[64,65] and calcium[66-68] as resuscitation drugs, an optional position for external cardiac compression in infants and children,[69] and early defibrillation in the field[70] as well as the hospital. Other changes, such as teaching only one-rescuer CPR to the public, and teaching only one maneuver for the obstructed airway, were adopted to simplify the learning process.[3] The most important of the already adopted changes was the more restricted use of sodium bicarbonate to counteract metabolic acidosis. Studies had demonstrated that the indiscriminate use of sodium bicarbonate worsened hemodynamics, increased acidosis on the venous side of the circulation, and did not improve outcome. Excessive use of sodium bicarbonate resulted in metabolic alkalosis with its concomitant problems. Although sodium bicarbonate still has a role in counteracting severe metabolic acidosis, the first steps should be adequate ventilation, oxygenation, and perfusion and the use of moderate hyperventilation to reverse respiratory acidosis and counteract some of the metabolic acidosis before resorting to treatment with sodium bicarbonate.[64,65,71]

Another important change has been the move to early defibrillation as the standard of care for both prehospital and in-hospital cardiac arrest. Early defibrillation is important because the most frequent initial rhythm in sudden cardiac arrest is ventricular fibrillation, which is most effectively treated by electrical defibrillation.[72-74] The probability of successful defibrillation diminishes rapidly with time, with ventricular fibrillation deteriorating to asystole within minutes. Although basic CPR can sustain a victim for a short time, it cannot directly restore an organized cardiac rhythm.

The reasons for reducing the use of calcium chloride were based largely on experimental evidence that calcium accumulation results in cell necrosis and the potential beneficial effects of calcium-channel blockers in ameliorating cerebral and myocardial damage after anoxia and ischemia.[66-68] Now that the results of the clinical trials on the calcium-channel blocker, lidoflazine, are in, and it has not been shown to be beneficial,[75] the risk that calcium would counteract the potential beneficial effects of the calcium-channel blockers may be less important. Calcium chloride is clearly a potent inotropic agent and still has an important role in treating ionized hypocalcemia.[76,77]

Another change in the "Standards and Guidelines for Cardiopulmonary Resuscitation (CPR) and Emergency Cardiac Care (ECC)," recommended by the American Heart Association in 1986 and 1992 was the sternal landmark position for external cardiac compression in infants and young children.[3,4] Previously, the location of the heart in the thorax of infants and young children was assumed to be more cephalad than in adults, based on postmortem studies and a presumed increase of abdominal visceral injuries in children.[1,2] Recent radiologic and physiologic studies in infants and children have demonstrated that the heart lies under the lower third of the sternum in infants and children, just as it does in adults, and that ECC over the lower third of the sternum produces better arterial pressures and stroke volumes.[69]

The advent of external pacemakers now makes it possible to electrically pace the heart without the need for internal wires.[78,79] External pacing is being tried in the field and is being used increasingly in the emergency department by code teams in the hospital and in ICUs. It is effective in some cases of complete heart block, hemodynamically significant bradycardia, and some bradyarrhythmias. Early studies suggest that external pacemakers do not improve the outcome of prehospital arrests with asystole or electromechanical dissociation (EMD).[78,79] Whether any of these changes in CPR techniques will improve survival and will be acceptable in terms of risks versus benefits remains to be seen.

COMPLICATIONS OF CPR

Since the study by Adelson of the anatomic changes in the heart resulting from open-chest cardiac massage,[80] it has been recognized that risks are involved in our attempts to benefit the victim by resuscitation (Table 28-3). Adelson emphasized that the cardiac injuries produced by direct cardiac compression were a function of technique and skill more than duration.[80] He described gross laceration of the heart in six cases (10%).[80] He also showed that prolonged successful massage of more than 1 hour's duration could be carried out without producing significant cardiac damage.[80]

Recent studies of closed chest external cardiac massage have characterized a number of potential complications from the procedure.[81,82] Rib and sternal fractures occur in 20 to 30% of cases, and anterior mediastinal hemorrhage in about 20%. Pulmonary bone marrow and fat emboli have been reported in 10% to as high as 80% of victims. Abdominal visceral complications have been noted in 30% with a 3% incidence of liver injury or rupture and a less than 1% incidence of splenic or gastric rupture. Pulmonary contusion or rupture also occurs in less than 1% of cases. Life-threatening complications, such as heart and great vessel injury, occur in less than 0.5% of cases.[8,82]

Cerebral edema and consumptive coagulopathy (DIC) are to be expected in patients who have been successfully resuscitated from a prolonged anoxic-ischemic insult. Ce-

Table 28-3. Complications of Cardiopulmonary Resuscitation

Rib fractures
Sternal fracture
Anterior mediastinal hemorrhage
Pulmonary bone marrow emboli
Fat emboli
Cardiac contusion
Cardiac tamponade
Pulmonary contusion
Pneumothorax
Hemothorax
Pneumomediastinum
Hepatic contusion or rupture
Splenic rupture
Gastric rupture
Cardiac rupture
Aortic dissection or tear
Rupture of great vessels
Anoxic-ischemic encephalopathy
Myocardial ischemia or infarction
Intracranial hypertension
Disseminated intravascular coagulation
Acute tubular necrosis—acute vasomotor nephropathy
Acute respiratory distress syndrome
Shock liver
Bowel ischemia
Postresuscitation pulmonary edema
Adrenal insufficiency
Costochondritis
Postresuscitation psychologic sequelae
Organic brain syndrome
Diabetes insipidus

rebral edema can be controlled by hyperventilation to a partial pressure of carbon dioxide in arterial blood (Pa_{CO_2}) of 30 ± 2 mm Hg, and mannitol if signs of increased intracranial pressure (ICP) persist. Monitoring of ICP is probably not indicated except in unusual circumstances, because studies have suggested that monitoring does not alter outcome. DIC should be treated by replacement of required components. Other organ systems can also be injured by the anoxia-ischemia, including the kidneys, liver, lungs, gastrointestinal tract, and heart. Support of the organ systems may be indicated in select cases, although, obviously, the greater the number of organ systems injured or failing, the worse the prognosis. Post-CPR pulmonary edema has recently been described as a common occurrence.[83] Costochondritis can be a morbid complication in survivors of CPR.[84]

PRE-ICU PHASE

The pre-ICU phase of CPR can be conveniently separated into two subphases: prehospital and intrahospital. The emergency department serves as a transition zone between these two subphases.

A number of studies have looked at prehospital or out-of-hospital cardiac arrest and the factors that influence survival.[85-90] Certain factors influence both the ability to successfully resuscitate, as well as eventual outcome as measured by discharge from the hospital alive. These include age of the victim,[91-93] underlying disease,[85-90] presenting cardiac rhythm,[85-90] early bystander CPR,[94-97] time to advanced cardiac life support,[98] early defibrillation,[85-90] and time to ROSC.[85-90] Overall, approximately one third of out-of-hospital cardiac arrest victims will be admitted to the hospital alive, and only about half of those successfully resuscitated will be discharged from the hospital alive.[85-90] Of the survivors, the majority will have no significant neurologic dysfunction.[85-90]

Time from collapse to receiving definitive care has an obvious effect on outcomes, with victims receiving early CPR, early defibrillation, and early advanced cardiac life support (ACLS) (generally defined as less than 8 to 10 minutes) having better rates of resuscitation and survival to hospital discharge. Initial cardiac rhythm also plays a critical role, with ventricular fibrillation and ventricular tachycardia having much better prognoses than asystole, pulseless idioventricular rhythm, electromechanical dissociation, or bradyarrhythmias (Table 28-4). The better outcome of ventricular fibrillation and ventricular tachycardia is also supporting evidence for early defibrillation in the field and the use of the automatic external defibrillator in prehospital CPR. Age is no longer considered an independent factor in deciding to resuscitate cardiac arrest victims outside of the hospital. Age alone does not separate those patients who will do well from those who will not. Likewise, even though elderly patients are more likely to die following hospitalization, their hospital stay is not longer, they do not have more residual neurologic impairment, and their survival following hospital discharge is similar to that seen in younger patients.

The most important factors in the prehospital environment influencing successful resuscitation and good outcome are early recognition of the signs and symptoms of acute myocardial infarction and other emergencies requiring immediate intervention, rapid and early access of the emergency medical system (EMS), using a 9-1-1 system preferably before cardiopulmonary arrest, layperson CPR training, early defibrillation, and quick response of paramedic units and advanced life support teams.[85-90,98] A recent study demonstrated that CPR instruction given by telephone to laypersons during an emergency not only can increase the rate of bystander CPR but also improves the quality of CPR performed by persons with prior CPR training.[99] This dispatcher-delivered telephone CPR instruction can alleviate anxiety and refresh skills of previously trained laypersons in an emergency, as well as possibly instruct and guide the untrained on the spot.[99]

One of the ethical dilemmas involving CPR in the pre-

Table 28-4. Initial Cardiac Arrest Rhythm and Outcome[73,78,82,84,87]

Rhythm	Number (%)	Admitted (%)	Discharged (%)
Ventricular fibrillation	1238 (58)	620 (50)	385 (31)
Ventricular tachycardia	50 (2)	36 (72)	23 (46)
Asystole	576 (27)	52 (9)	11 (2)
Idioventricular	162 (8)	27 (17)	5 (3)
Other or unknown	125 (6)	46 (37)	19 (15)
Total	2151	781 (36)	443 (21)

hospital environment is the management of patients who are DNR (do not resuscitate) or should be. These may include not only patients living or being cared for at home but also patients in nursing homes or chronic care facilities. EMS personnel are specifically trained and oriented to attempt to resuscitate persons and save lives. They are not legally empowered to withhold resuscitation efforts except in cases of obvious long-standing death or decapitation.[1-3] The best solution to the dilemma created by DNR patients outside of the hospital environment is not to call the EMS. A call to EMS is interpreted as a request for emergency intervention, and the EMS personnel are required to attempt resuscitation. There is no time to assess the appropriateness and legitimacy of a verbal or written DNR order or request at the scene. Movements are underway to establish mechanisms for DNR orders to exist outside the hospital, which would be recognized by EMS personnel. Home-care hospice programs are working with the EMS to develop medically and legally sound documents and mechanisms that will permit DNR orders to be established and respected on patients who choose to die at home (see Chap. 82).

EMERGENCY DEPARTMENT CPR

One dilemma is the termination of futile CPR in the field.[100] Some EMS systems are experimenting with physician-monitored decision making using paramedics at the scene. Patients are usually either resuscitated at the scene with ROSC before transport, or they are declared dead at the scene with the decision to cease CPR made by the base-station physician in concert with the paramedics at the scene. Protocols are being developed that factor in variables such as presenting rhythm, witnessed or unwitnessed collapse, bystander CPR, time from collapse to ACLS, age, and response to ACLS in the field—all of help decide which victims should be transported and which declared dead at the scene.

Once the patient arrives at the hospital, and treatment is assumed by the emergency department team, new factors enter into the survival equation. Patients who have had ROSC before arrival at the hospital have a better chance of long-term survival than patients who are still in cardiopulmonary arrest (CPA) on admission to the emergency department. Both "downtime," or time from CPA until CPR is commenced, as well as time to ROSC, are inversely correlated with long-term survival. The latter, measured as time from initiation of CPR until ROSC, is usually more precisely known than the former.[85-90]

The factors that influence outcome of CPR include the following:

- Age
- Underlying diseases
- Hypothermia
- Cause of arrest
- Presenting rhythm

Fewer than 10% of patients who present to the hospital with CPA will survive to hospital discharge. One study that directly examined the question found that of 240 consecutive patients presenting to the emergency department after failed prehospital ACLS, 13% were successfully resuscitated in emergency department, but only 1.7% survived to hospital discharge.[101] Fifty percent of the survivors had good neurologic outcomes, and 50% had severe neurologic deficits and were discharged to nursing homes. The 2 patients with good outcomes had undergone cardiac arrest shortly before arrival in the emergency department. These authors characterized in-hospital resuscitation after unsuccessful prehospital ACLS as an "exercise in futility."[101]

Arrival at the emergency department permits the institution of more advanced diagnostic and therapeutic resuscitation techniques including placement of arterial and central venous catheters, endotracheal intubation of victims receiving mouth-to-mouth or bag and mask ventilation or replacements of an esophageal-obturator airway (EOA) with an endotracheal tube, and potentially important diagnostic techniques such as radiographs and laboratory studies. Intra-arterial access is best achieved by cutdown either of the radial, brachial, or femoral arteries. Central venous access can be achieved by either cutdown or the percutaneous approach. Percutaneous approach sites include jugular veins, subclavian veins, femoral veins, auxiliary or brachialcephalic veins.[102] Venous cutdown sites are usually the femoral or antecubital areas. During CPR, the more peripheral or distal sites are usually easier and do not require interruption of external cardiac massage. In the more controlled environment of the emergency department, other diagnostic and therapeutic modalities such as arterial and mixed-venous blood gas monitoring, P_{ETCO_2} monitoring, radiographic and laboratory studies, pericardiocentesis, volume resuscitation, or evacuation of a tension pneumothorax can be employed.

Nevertheless, the prognosis remains poor for victims who are still in CPA on presentation to the emergency department, and most victims will not profit from the more sophisticated diagnostic and therapeutic modalities available in the hospital. A few authors have attempted to generate guidelines for discontinuing prehospital CPR in the emergency department.[103] These authors have suggested that CPR be terminated in the emergency department when victims have failed to respond with ROSC to adequate ACLS, including intubation, defibrillation, IV medications, and external cardiac massage in the field, and present to the emergency department in asystole or severe bradyarrhythmias.[103] Likewise, victims who have failed to respond to ACLS for more than 45 minutes (both prehospital and emergency department times combined) and who have no intrinsic cardiac activity cannot be resuscitated by current standard techniques, and CPR may be discontinued. These guidelines are always qualified by the proviso that victims of hypothermia cannot be pronounced dead until their core body temperature has been raised to 35 to 36°C.

Patients brought to the emergency department with ventricular fibrillation or ventricular tachycardia should receive vigorous resuscitation attempts, especially if the patient has received only external cardiac massage without the benefit of defibrillation. Similarly, victims with a witnessed cardiac arrest who have received immediate CPR but not ACLS may benefit from emergency department resuscitation efforts, even if they have a severe bradyarrhythmia.

Unfortunately, as in all of medicine, there are exceptions to the rules or guidelines, and patients who defy all the odds will still survive.[104] The bell-shaped curve is not necessarily our friend and does not always work to our benefit.

Patients who are successfully resuscitated from prehospital or emergency department CPA are almost always admitted to the ICU. Another important source of ICU admissions is the patient who has a cardiac arrest in the hospital. Survival following an attempt at CPR in the hospital has not changed appreciably over the past 25 years. Only 10 to 20% of patients who receive CPR in hospital survive to discharge from the hospital, and 20 to 25% of these survivors will die within 6 months of discharge.[105-107] These figures are even more discouraging when one realizes that attempts at CPR are made on only a third of patients who die in the hospital.

In one large study of CPR in the hospital, no patients with sepsis, pneumonia, or metastatic cancer preceding their CPA survived to hospital discharge,[105] and no patient in whom resuscitation took longer than 30 minutes survived to be discharged.[105] In most studies of CPA in the hospital, the overwhelmingly important factor influencing survival is the patient's underlying disease or diseases.[105,107] In particular, patients with severe congestive heart failure (New York Heart Association class III or IV), end-stage renal disease, metastatic cancer, or acquired immune deficiency syndrome (AIDS) have the poorest prognosis following CPA (Fig. 28-2).

Outcome studies of CPA with CPR in the hospital reveal that 25 to 50% of victims cannot be resuscitated (Fig. 28-3). Of the victims successfully resuscitated, approximately 25% die within 24 to 48 hours of their initial CPA (Fig. 28-3). Only 10 to 20% of patients undergoing CPR in the hospital survive to hospital discharge (Fig. 28-3).

CPR of in-hospital CPA victims does not differ substantially from CPR of CPA victims in the emergency department. The cause of the arrests may differ, however. The emergency department sees more trauma-associated and primary cardiac arrests, whereas the hospital-based population has a greater prevalence of underlying diseases, more respiratory-associated arrests, some of which are due to oversedation or overmedication, and a greater incidence of iatrogenic complication-associated CPA.

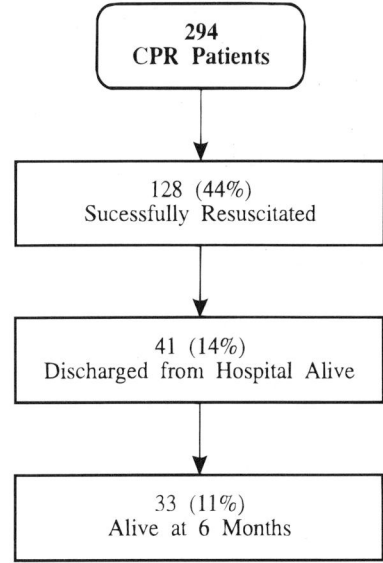

Fig. 28-3. Results of in-hospital CPR as reported by Bedell et al. with follow-up to 6 months. (Redrawn from Bedell, S. E., Delbanco, T. L., Cook, E. F., and Epstein, F. H.: Survival after cardiopulmonary resuscitation in the hospitals. N. Engl. J. Med., 309:569, 1983.)

A special area of concern consists of intraoperative and anesthesia-associated cardiac arrests.[108] The incidence of cardiac arrests that are due solely to anesthesia is estimated at approximately 2.0/10,000 anesthetics given, with a resultant mortality of about 1.0/10,000 anesthetics. When deaths in which anesthesia is considered a contributory factor are included, the incidence increases to approximately 6.0/10,000. Of interest, the pediatric age group has a threefold higher risk than adults, and emergency patients experience an anesthetic-associated cardiac arrest rate six times that of elective patients. Even more important, half of the cardiac arrests are the result of inadequate pulmonary ventilation, and one third are caused by anesthetic overdose. Specific errors in anesthetic management can be identified in about three fourths of cases, whereas hemodynamic instability in very ill patients is associated with about one fourth of anesthetic-associated cardiac arrests. Progressive bradycardia almost invariably preceded a cardiac arrest caused by anesthesia, occurring in 265 of 270 patients in one series.[108] The ACLS management of cardiac arrest in the operating room does not differ substantially from CPR in other areas of the hospital, except that confirming placement of the endotracheal tube should receive a high priority, and moving to open-chest cardiac massage may occur sooner or more often than in other areas of the hospital.

ICU PHASE

The ICU is a unique environment for CPA and CPR for a number of reasons, not the least of which is that a primary role of the ICU is to prevent CPA. Therefore, when

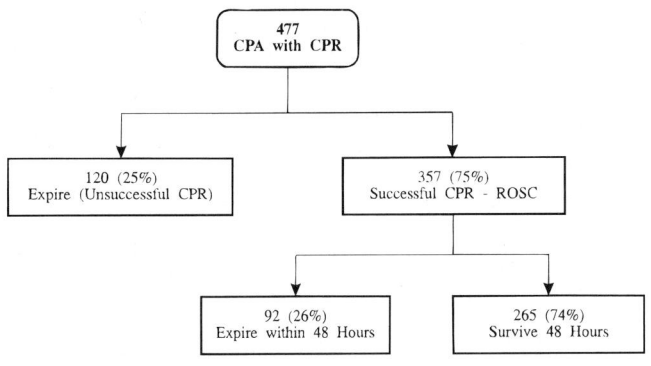

Fig. 28-2. Results of in-hospital CPR at the Cleveland Clinic in 1989. (Drawing Courtesy of George Morrison, CD, Inc.)

a CPA occurs in the ICU, it is often a manifestation of a rapid or slow downhill progression in a critically ill patient and portends a grave prognosis. Many patients gain admission to the ICU because of a CPA or impending CPA. As such, they are at increased risk for CPA in the ICU. Except in the rare case of a malignant arrhythmia occurring in association with myocardial disease, the occurrence of a CPA in the ICU usually signifies a deterioration despite the optimum monitoring and therapy characteristic of the ICU.

We can, therefore, separate patients who undergo cardiac arrest in the ICU into two groups. In the first group, the arrest is unexpected and unanticipated, and the chances of a good outcome including restoration of neurologic function are high, and therefore, an aggressive approach including CPR is justified. In the second group, arrest is an anticipated progression of their acute disease despite maximal support or is a not unexpected consequence of their underlying disease processes; therefore, CPR is probably not justified, because it is either highly unlikely to be successful, or the outcome is likely to be poor in terms of neurologic or vital organ function. CPR can be justified in the patients who do not fit neatly into one of these categories, on the basis that, when in doubt, one should err on the side of life. The management of patients who are DNR is discussed in Chapter 82.

CPR in the ICU has certain advantages over CPR in other areas of the hospital. The patients are being continually monitored, and so downtimes are both known and short, which equates with a greater chance of successful CPR. Catheters are frequently already in place such as arterial lines, central venous pressure lines, or pulmonary artery catheters, permitting not only more rapid institution of ACLS but also more effective monitoring of the success of therapies. Arterial and central venous pressures can be monitored during CPR, giving a precise picture of the adequacy of external cardiac massage and ACLS in terms of systolic, diastolic, and mean arterial pressures, as well as coronary perfusion pressure.[109] Arterial and mixed venous blood gases can be monitored during CPR,[110,111] and prearrest variables are often known. P$_{ET}$CO$_2$ monitoring during CPR may also be available. Many patients will already be intubated; for those who are not, establishing an artificial airway and providing the maximum fraction of inspired oxygen (F$_{IO_2}$) and adequate ventilation should be more rapid than in other areas of the hospital. Access to equipment, specialized techniques, and personnel should also be more facile in the ICU. Because many of the patients in the ICU will be intubated and receiving mechanical ventilation before their CPA, their acid/base status tends to differ. Initial arterial blood gases of patients who undergo cardiac arrest in the emergency department or hospital floors tend to be more acidotic (pH < 7.15) and hypercarbic (Paco$_2$ > 50) than those of patients who undergo cardiac arrest in the ICU (mean pH 7.28, mean Paco$_2$ 40 mm Hg).[99] These acid/base abnormalities have a bearing on the ability to resuscitate and the outcome of resuscitation. Nevertheless, if a patient undergoes cardiac arrest in the ICU despite careful monitoring and support, it often portends a grave prognosis, especially if resuscitation requires multiple doses of drugs and more than a few minutes of CPR. Additionally, if the CPA occurs unexpectedly, the circumstances should be carefully analyzed for deviation from accepted standards of care.

POST-ICU PHASE

The two aspects of the post-ICU phase discussed in this section are CPA in the post-CPR, or post-ICU phase, and postresuscitation care of the CPA victim who is successfully resuscitated, beyond support of vital organ functions.

CPR in the post-ICU phase does not differ significantly from hospital-based CPR in the pre-ICU phase. Except in the case of a drug-induced CPA—for example, hypokalemia secondary to amphotericin-B or diuretics—where specific treatment directed at the electrolyte abnormality may be required, the CPR is based on ACLS protocols. Other causes of iatrogenic CPA in the post-ICU phase may include respiratory failure secondary to narcotics, accumulation of secretions, electrolyte disturbances, fluid imbalances from excessive losses or disproportionate replacement, and unusual or rare complications such as pericardial tamponade from atrial erosion by a central venous catheter. As a general rule of thumb, a patient who sustains another CPA after successful CPR and discharge from the ICU has a poor prognosis, unless the CPA is secondary to an easily reversible iatrogenic complication or arrhythmia.

Patients with irreversible disease states such as New York Heart Association class III or IV congestive heart failure, end-stage pulmonary disease, metastatic cancer, end-stage organ failure, or AIDS who have survived to ICU discharge after organ failure or CPR are likely to profit from CPR in the post-ICU phase. DNR status should be discussed with the patient or family in the case of an incompetent patient, as soon as possible, to avoid the institution of futile therapy.

Survivors of CPR with good outcome may be faced with psychologic sequelae, some of which have profound implications. Nightmares, mild organic brain syndrome, and denial have all been described in survivors of resuscitation and may be misinterpreted by others.[112]

In conclusion, approximately 20% of patients in whom CPR is attempted leave the hospital alive, and most are as functional as they were before the cardiac arrest. Recovery is better if the event is unexpected (e.g., adverse drug reaction) is easily reversible, occurs early in myocardial infarction, or occurs in a critical care unit. The long-term survival of resuscitated patients probably reflects their underlying disease. About 75% of successfully resuscitated patients who survive to hospital discharge live 1 year, and about 50% live 3 years.[105,107] CPR can and does save lives, and it is critically important that ICU personnel maintain their CPR skills.

REFERENCES

1. Standards for cardiopulmonary resuscitation (CPR) and emergency cardiac care (ECC). JAMA, *227(Suppl)*:833, 1974.
2. Standards and guidelines for cardiopulmonary resuscitation (CPR) and emergency cardiac care (ECC). JAMA, *244*:453, 1980.
3. Standards and guidelines for cardiopulmonary resuscitation

(CPR) and emergency cardiac care (ECC). JAMA, *255:*2905, 1986.
4. Guidelines for cardiopulmonary resuscitation and emergency cardiac care. JAMA, *268:*2171, 1992.
5. Hermreck, A. S.: The history of cardiopulmonary resuscitation. Am. J. Surg., *156:*430, 1988.
6. Liss, H. P.: A history of resuscitation. Ann. Emerg. Med., *15:*65, 1986.
7. Safar, P.: Ventilatory efficacy of mouth-to-mouth artifical respiration. Airway obstruction during manual and mouth-to-mouth artificial respiration. JAMA, *167:*335, 1958.
8. Gordon, A. S. et al.: Mouth-to-mouth versus manual artificial respiration for children and adults. JAMA, *167:*320, 1958.
9. Pearson, J. W.: Historical and Experimental Approaches to Modern Resuscitation. Springfield, IL, Charles C. Thomas, 1965, p. 1.
10. Morris, N.: The history of cardiac resuscitation. *In* Cardiac Arrest and Resuscitation. Edited by H. E. Stephenson. St. Louis, C. V. Mosby, 1958, p. 15.
11. Crile, G. W.: The resuscitation of the apparently dead and a demonstration of the pneumatic rubber suit as a means of controlling the blood pressure. Trans. South Surg. Gynecol. Assoc., *15:*362, 1904.
12. Crile, G., and Dolley, D. H.: An experimental research into the resuscitation of dogs killed by anesthesia and asphyxia. J. Exp. Med., *8:*713, 1906.
13. Meyer, J. A.: Claude Beck and cardiac resuscitation. Ann. Thorac. Surg., *45:*103, 1988.
14. Zoll, P. M. et al.: Treatment of unexpected cardiac arrest by external electric stimulation of the heart. N. Engl. J. Med., *254:*541, 1956.
15. Kouwenhoven, W. B. et al.: Closed chest defibrillation of the heart. Surgery, *42:*550, 1957.
16. Kouwenhoven, W. B. et al.: Closed chest cardiac massage. JAMA, *173:*1064, 1960.
17. Todres, I. D., and Rogers, M. C.: Methods of external cardiac massage in the newborn infant. J. Pediatr. *86:*781, 1975.
18. Taylor, G. J. et al.: Importance of prolonged compression during cardiopulmonary resuscitation in man. N. Engl. J. Med., *296:*1515, 1977.
19. Criley, J. M., Blaufuss, A. N., and Kissel, G. L.: Cough induced cardiac compression. JAMA, *236:*1246, 1976.
20. Niemann, J. T. et al.: Cough CPR: documentation of systemic perfusion in man and an experimental model. Crit. Care Med., *8:*141, 1980.
21. Rudikoff, M. T. et al.: Mechanisms of blood flow during cardiopulmonary resuscitation. Circulation, *61:*345, 1980.
22. Chandra, M., Guerci, A., and Weisfeldt, M. L.: Contrasts between intrathoracic pressures during chest compression and cardiac massage. Crit. Care Med., *9:*789, 1981.
23. Orlowski, J. P.: Mechanisms of blood flow during CPR. Circulation, *62:*1141, 1980.
24. Deshmukh, H. G. et al.: Echocardiographic observations during cardiopulmonary resuscitation: a preliminary report. Crit. Care Med., *13:*904, 1985.
25. Babbs, C., Weaver, J. C., Ralston, S., and Geddes, L.: Cardiac, thoracic, and abdominal pump mechanisms in cardiopulmonary resuscitation. Am. J. Emerg. Med., *2:*299, 1984.
26. Deshmukh, H. G. et al.: Mechanisms of blood flow generated by precordial compression during CPR 1. Studies on closed chest precordial compression. Chest, *95:*1092, 1989.
27. Goldberg, A. H.: Cardiopulmonary arrest. N. Engl. J. Med., *290:*381, 1974.
28. Fillmore, S. J., Shapiro, M., and Phillip, T.: Serial blood gas studies during cardiopulmonary resuscitation. Ann. Intern. Med., *72:*465, 1970.
29. Ayres, N. et al.: Inappropriate ventilation and hypoxemia as causes of cardiac arrhythmias. The control of arrhythmias without antiarrhythmic drugs. Am. J. Med., *46:*495, 1969.
30. Robert, J. R., Greenberg, M. I., and Baskin, S. I.: Endotracheal epinephrine in cardiorespiratory collapse. J. Am. Coll. Emerg. Phys., *8:*515, 1979.
31. Schecter, D. C.: Transthoracic epinephrine injection in heart resuscitation is dangerous. JAMA, *234:*1184, 1975.
32. Collinsworth, K. A., Kalman, S. M., and Harrison, D. C.: The clinical pharmacology of lidocaine as an antiarrhythmic drug. Circulation, *50:*1217, 1974.
33. Thompson, P. D. et al.: Lidocaine pharmacokinetics in advanced heart failure, liver disease, and renal failure in humans. Ann. Intern. Med., *78:*499, 1973.
34. Bishop, R. L., and Weisfeldt, M. L.: Sodium bicarbonate administration during cardiac arrest. Effect on arterial pH, PCO_2, and osmolality. JAMA, *235:*506, 1976.
35. Worthley, L. I. G.: Sodium bicarbonate in cardiac arrest. Lancet, *2:*903, 1976.
36. Eidelman, A. L., and Hobbs, J. F.: Bicarbonate therapy revisited. A study in therapeutic revisionism. Am. J. Dis. Child., *132:*847, 1978.
37. Posner, J. B., and Plum, F.: Spinal-fluid PH and neurologic symptoms in systemic acidosis. N. Engl. J. Med., *277:*605, 1967.
38. Chidsey, C. A.: Calcium metabolism in the normal and failing heart. Hosp. Pract, *8:*65, 1972.
39. Massumi, R. A. et al.: Ventricular fibrillation and tachycardia after intravenous atropine for treatment of bradycardias. N. Engl. J. Med., *287:*336, 1972.
40. Holder, D. A. et al.: Experience with bretylium tosylate by a hospital cardiac arrest team. Circulation, *55:*541, 1977.
41. Williams, M. L. et al.: Intravenous amiodarone during prolonged resuscitation from cardiac arrest. Ann. Intern. Med., *110:*839, 1989.
42. Schoeppe, W.: Effects of dopamine on kidney function. Proc. R. Soc. Med., *70(Suppl.):*36, 1977.
43. Goldberg, L. I.: Recent advances in the pharmacology of catecholamines. Intensive Care Med., *3:*233, 1977.
44. Thompson, W. L.: Dopamine in the management of shock. Proc. R. Soc. Med., *70(Suppl.):*25, 1977.
45. Goldberg, L. I.: Dopamine—clinical uses of an endogenous catecholamine. N. Engl. J. Med., *291:*707, 1974.
46. Tuttle, R. R., and Mills, J.: Dobutamine: development of a new catecholamine to selectively increase cardiac contractility. Circ. Res., *36:*185, 1975.
47. Akhtar, N. et al.: Hemodynamic effect of dobutamine in patients with severe heart failure. Am. J. Cardiol., *36:*202, 1975.
48. Tarazi, R. C.: Sympathomimetic agents in the treatment of shock. Ann. Intern. Med., *81:*364, 1974.
49. Tacker, W. A. et al.: Energy dosage for human trans-chest electrical ventricular defibrillation. N. Engl. J. Med., *290:*214, 1974.
50. Gonzalez, E. R. et al.: Dose-dependent vasopressor response to epinephrine during CPR in human beings. Ann. Emerg. Med., *18:*920, 1989.
51. Maier, G. W. et al.: The influence of manual chest compression rate on hemodynamic support during cardiac arrest: high-impulse cardiopulmonary resuscitation. Circulation, *74(Suppl.):*IV-51, 1986.
52. Maier, G. W. et al.: The physiology of external cardiac massage; high-impulse cardiopulmonary resuscitation. Circulation, *70:*86, 1984.
53. Ornato, J. P. et al.: The effect of applied chest compression force on systemic arterial pressure and end-tidal carbon

dioxide concentration during CPR in human beings. Ann. Emerg. Med., *18:*732, 1989.
54. Garnett, A. R., Ornato, J. P., Gonzalez, E. R., and Johnson, E. B.: End-tidal carbon dioxide monitoring during cardiopulmonary resuscitation. JAMA, *257:*512, 1987.
55. Gudipathi, C. V. et al.: Expired carbon dioxide: a noninvasive monitor of cardiopulmonary resuscitation. Circulation, *77:*234, 1988.
56. Sanders, A. B. et al.: End-tidal carbon dioxide monitoring during cardiopulmonary resuscitation. JAMA, *262:*1347, 1989.
57. Falk, J. L., Rackow, E. C., and Weil, M. H.: End-tidal carbon dioxide concentration during cardiopulmonary resuscitation: a prognostic indicator for survival. N. Engl. J. Med., *318:*607, 1988.
58. Orlowski, J. P., Porembka, D. T., Gallagher, J. M., and VanLente, R.: The bone marrow as a source of laboratory studies. Ann. Emerg. Med., *18:*1348, 1989.
59. Orlowski, J. P. et al.: Comparison study of intraosseous, central intravenous, and peripheral intravenous infusions of emergency drugs. Am. J. Dis. Child., *144:*112, 1990.
60. Bircher, N., and Safar, P.: Open-chest CPR: an old method whose time has returned. Am. J. Emerg. Med., *2:*568, 1989.
61. Quinton, P. N., O'Byrne, G., and Airkenhead, A. R.: Comparison of endotracheal and peripheral intravenous adrenaline in cardiac arrest: Is the endotracheal route reliable? Lancet, *1:*828, 1987.
62. Orlowski, J. P., Gallagher, J. M., and Porembka, D. T.: Endotracheal epinephrine is unreliable. Resuscitation, *19:*103, 1990.
63. Ralstom, S. H., et al.: Endotracheal versus intravenous epinephrine during electromechanical dissociation with CPR in dogs. Ann. Emerg. Med., *14:*1044, 1985.
64. Graf, H., Leach, W., and Arieff, A.: Evidence for a detrimental effect of bicarbonate therapy in hypoxic lactic acidosis. Science, *227:*754, 1985.
65. Graf, H., and Arieff, A. L.: The use of sodium bicarbonate in the therapy of organic acidosis. Intensive Care Med., *12:*285, 1986.
66. Thompson, B. M. et al.: Calcium: limited indications, some danger. Circulation, *74(Suppl.):*IV-90, 1986.
67. Steuven, H. A. et al.: Lack of effectiveness of calcium chloride in refractory asystole. Ann. Emerg. Med., *14:*630, 1985.
68. Weaver, W. D.: Calcium-channel blockers and advanced cardiac life support. Circulation, *74(Suppl.):*IV-94, 1986.
69. Orlowski, J. P.: Optimum position for external cardiac compression in infants and young children. Ann. Emerg. Med., *15:*667, 1986.
70. Weaver, W. D. et al.: Improved neurologic recovery and survival after early defibrillation. Circulation, *69:*943, 1984.
71. Jaffe, A. S.: Cardiovascular pharmacology I. Circulation, *74(Suppl.):*IV-70, 1986.
72. Eisenberg, M. S. et al.: Treatment of out-of-hospital cardiac arrests with rapid defibrillation by emergency medical technicians. N. Engl. J. Med., *302:*1379, 1980.
73. Stults, K. R. et al.: Prehospital defibrillation performed by emergency medical technicians in rural communities. N. Engl. J. Med., *310:*219, 1984.
74. Eisenberg, M. S. et al.: Treatment of ventricular fibrillation: emergency medical technician defibrillation and paramedic services. JAMA, *251:*1723, 1984.
75. Abramson, N. S.: Effect of calcium entry blocker (lidoflazine) administration on comatose survivors of clinical cardiac arrest. Crit. Care Med., *17:*S132, 1989.
76. Paraskos, J. A.: Cardiovascular pharmacology III: atropine, calcium, calcium blockers, and beta blockers. Circulation, *74(Suppl. IV):*IV-86, 1986.
77. Urban, P., Scheidegger, D., Buchmann, B., and Barth, D.: Cardiac arrest and blood ionized calcium levels. Ann. Intern. Med., *109:*110, 1988.
78. Barthell, E. et al.: Prehospital external cardiac pacing: a prospective, controlled clinical trial. Ann. Emerg. Med., *17:*1221, 1988.
79. Weaver, W. D. et al.: Use of the automatic external defibrillator in the management of out-of-hospital cardiac arrest. N. Engl J. Med., *319:*661, 1988.
80. Adelson, L.: A clinicopathologic study of the anatomic changes in the heart resulting from cardiac massage. Surg. Gynecol. Obstet., *104:*513, 1957.
81. Bedell, A. E., and Fulton, E. J.: Unexpected findings and complications at autopsy after cardiopulmonary resuscitation (CPR). Arch Intern. Med., *146:*1725, 1986.
82. Krischer, J. P., Fine, E. G., David, J. H., and Nagel, E. L.: Complications of cardiac resuscitation. Chest, *92:*287, 1987.
83. Dohli, S.: Postcardiopulmonary resuscitation pulmonary edema. Crit. Care Med., *2:*434, 1983.
84. Samet, J. H., Flinn, M. S., Balady, G., and Skinner, M.: Costochondritis: a morbid complication in a survivor of cardiopulmonary resuscitation. Am. J. Med., *83:*362, 1987.
85. Roackswold, G. et al.: Follow-up of 514 consecutive patients with cardiopulmonary arrest outside the hospital. J. Am. Coll. Emerg. Physicians, *8:*216, 1979.
86. Einarsson, O., Jakobsson, F., and Sigurdsson, G.: Advanced cardiac life support in the prehospital setting: the Reykjavik experience. J. Intern. Med., *225:*129, 1989.
87. Cummins, R. O., and Eisenberg, M. S.: Prehospital cardiopulmonary resuscitation. JAMA, *253:*2408, 1985.
88. Roth, R., Stewart, R. D., Rogers, K., and Cannon, G. M.: Out-of-hospital cardiac arrest: factors associated with survival. Ann. Emerg. Med., *13:*237, 1984.
89. Myerburg, R. J. et al.: Survivors of prehospital cardiac arrest. JAMA, *247:*1485, 1982.
90. Edgren, E., Kelsey, S., Sutton, K., and Safar, P.: The presenting ECG pattern in survivors of cardiac arrest and its relation to the subsequent long-term survival. Acta Anaesthesiol. Scand., *33:*265, 1989.
91. Tresch, D. D., Thakur, F., Hoffman, R. G., and Brooks, H. L.: Comparison of resuscitation of out-of-hospital cardiac arrest in persons younger and older than 70 years of age. Am. J. Cardiol. *61:*1120, 1988.
92. Tresch, D. D. et al.: Should the elderly be resuscitated following out-of-hospital cardiac arrest? Am. J. Med., *86:*145, 1989.
93. Hazzard, W. R.: Should the elderly be resuscitated following out-of-hospital cardiac arrest? Why not? Am. J. Med., *86:*143, 1989.
94. Sanders, A. B. et al.: Neurologic benefits from the use of early cardiopulmonary resuscitation. Ann. Emerg. Med., *16:*142, 1987.
95. Troiano, P. et al.: The effect of bystander CPR on neurologic outcome in survivors of prehospital cardiac arrests. Resuscitation, *17:*91, 1989.
96. Ritter, G. et al.: The effect of bystander CPR on survival of out-of-hospital cardiac arrest victims. Am. Heart J., *110:*932, 1985.
97. Stueven, H. et al.: Bystander/first responder CPR: ten years experience in a paramedic system. Ann. Emerg. Med., *15:*707, 1986.
98. Eisenberg, M. S. et al.: Management of out-of-hospital cardiac arrest. JAMA, *243:*1049, 1980.
99. Kellerman, A. L., Hackman, B. B., and Somes, G.: Dispatcher-assisted cardiopulmonary resuscitation validation of efficacy. Circulation, *80:*1232, 1989.

100. Frank, M.: Should we terminate futile resuscitations in the field? Can we afford not to? Ann. Emerg. Med., *18:*594, 1989.
101. Kellerman, A. L., Staves, D. R., and Hackman, B. B.: In-hospital resuscitation following unsuccessful prehospital advanced cardiac life support: "heroic efforts" or an exercise in futility? Ann. Emerg. Med., *17:*589, 1988.
102. Dronen, S., Thompson, B., Nowak, R., and Tomlanovich, M.: Subclavian vein catheterization during cardiopulmonary resuscitation. JAMA, *247:*3227, 1982.
103. Smith, J. P., and Bodai, B. I.: Guidelines for discontinuing prehospital CPR in the emergency department—a review. Ann. Emerg. Med., *14:*1093, 1985.
104. Langdon, R. W., Swiecegood, W. R., and Schwartz, D. A.: Thrombolytic therapy of massive pulmonary embolism during prolonged cardiac arrest using recombinant tissue-type plasminogen activator. Ann. Emerg. Med., *18:*678, 1989.
105. Bedell, S. E., Delbanco, T. L., Cook, E. F., and Epstein, F. H.: Survival after cardiopulmonary resuscitation in the hospital. N. Engl. J. Med., *309:*569, 1983.
106. Hershey, C. O., and Fisher, L.: Why outcome of cardiopulmonary resuscitation in general wards is poor. Lancet, *1:*31, 1982.
107. Burns, R., Graney, M. J., and Nichols, L. O.: Prediction of in-hospital cardiopulmonary arrest outcome. Arch. Intern. Med., *149:*1318, 1989.
108. Keenan, R. L., and Boyan, C. P.: Cardiac arrest due to anesthesia. JAMA, *253:*2373, 1985.
109. Paradis, N. A. et al.: Coronary perfusion pressure and the return of spontaneous circulation in human cardiopulmonary resuscitation. JAMA, *263:*1106, 1990.
110. Weil, M. H. et al.: Difference in acid-base state between venous and arterial blood during cardiopulmonary resuscitation. N. Engl. J. Med., *315:*153, 1986.
111. Chazan, J. A., and McKay, D. B.: Acid-base abnormalities in cardiopulmonary arrest: varying patterns in different locations in the hospital. N. Engl. J. Med., *320:*597, 1989.
112. Druss, R. G., and Kornfeld, D. S.: The survivors of cardiac arrest: a psychiatric study. JAMA, *201:*291, 1967.

SUPPLEMENTAL READINGS

Berg, R. A., et al.: Bystander cardiopulmonary resuscitation: is ventilation necessary? Part 1. Circulation, *88:*1907, 1993.
Bonnin, M. J., et al.: Distinct criteria for termination of resuscitation in the out-of-hospital setting. JAMA, *270:*1457, 1993.
Brown, C. G., et al.: A comparison of standard-dose and high-dose epinephrine in cardiac arrest outside the hospital. N. Engl. J. Med. *327:*1051, 1992.
Callaham, M., et al.: A randomized clinical trial of high-dose epinephrine and norepinephrine vs. standard dose epinephrine in prehospital cardiac arrest. JAMA, *268:*2667, 1992.
Cohen, T. J., et al.: Active compression-decompression: a new method of cardiopulmonary resuscitation. JAMA, *267:*2916, 1992.
Kellerman, A. L., Hackman, B. B., and Somes, G.: Predicting the outcome of unsuccessful prehospital advanced cardiac life support. JAMA, *270:*1433, 1993.
Levine, R. L.: Prospective evidence of a circadian rhythm for out-of-hospital cardiac arrests. JAMA *267:*2935, 1992.
Proceedings of the Methodology in Cardiac Arrest Research Symposium. Ann. Emerg. Med., *22:*1, 1993.
Sack, J. B., Kesselbrenner, M. B., and Bregman, D.: Survival from in-hospital cardiac arrest with interposed abdominal counterpulsation during cardiopulmonary resuscitation. JAMA, *267:*379, 1992.
Schneider, A. P., Nelson, D. J., and Brown, D. D.: In-hospital cardiopulmonary resuscitation: a 30-year review. J. Am. Board Fam. Pract., *6:*91, 1993.
Steill, I. G., et al.: High-dose epinephrine in adult cardiac arrest. N. Engl. J. Med., *327:*1045, 1992.
Tang, W., et al.: Augmented efficacy of external CPR by intermittent occlusion of the ascending aorta. Part 1. Circulation, *88:*1916, 1993.
Tucker, K. J., et al.: Active compression-decompression resuscitation: analysis of transmittal flow and left ventricular volume by tranesophageal echocardiography in humans. J. Am. Coll. Cardio., *22:*1485, 1993.
Tunstall-Pedoe, H., et al.: Survey of 3765 cardiopulmonary resuscitations in British hospitals (the BRESUS study): methods and overall results. B. Med. J., *304:*1347, 1992.

Chapter 29

ACUTE MYOCARDIAL INFARCTION

PAUL N. CASALE
BENJAMIN ROBALINO

Each year, approximately 1.2 million people in the United States suffer an acute myocardial infarction. Of these people, over 500,000 will not survive the acute event, the majority of whom die before reaching the hospital.[1,2] Most of these deaths that occur within the first hour of symptoms are due to ventricular fibrillation.[3]

Contributing to the prehospital mortality is the delay between the onset of the patient's symptoms and the time intensive care therapy is initiated. There are many factors contributing to this delay including the interval between the onset of symptoms and the time the patient decides to seek medical attention, transportation to the hospital, triage procedures in the emergency room, and admitting.[4,5]

In this chapter, we will discuss the patient who presents with myocardial ischemia or infarction, focusing on the important considerations for admission to the ICU and indications for invasive monitoring. Short-term interventional therapy and rehabilitation after myocardial infarction will also be reviewed.

PRE-ICU CONSIDERATIONS

The clinical presentation is of vital importance in evaluating the patient prior to admission to the ICU. Despite many recent technologic advances in cardiology, the patient's history remains of substantial value in establishing a diagnosis. A complaint of chest discomfort can be elicited in 20 to 60% of patients with acute myocardial infarction.[6,7] The pain is variable in intensity, but usually severe in most patients, and sometimes intolerable. It lasts for at least 30 minutes and often persists for several hours. Patients will describe the pain as a retrosternal heavy squeezing or choking pain which may radiate down the left arm or up into the neck and jaw. The pain may be burning or stabbing in quality and at times may begin in the epigastrium or radiate to the shoulders or interscapular area.

Instead of presenting with chest discomfort, some patients, particularly the elderly, have symptoms of congestive heart failure or profound weakness associated with diaphoresis and nausea and vomiting, which may cause the acute infarction to be unrecognized. The nausea and vomiting are thought to be due to activation of a vagal reflex and occur more frequently in association with inferior myocardial infarction. Occasionally, the patient may complain of diarrhea during an acute myocardial infarction. The clinical picture may be confused with that of acute cholecystitis, gastritis, or peptic ulcer disease, particularly if the pain is epigastric in location and associated with nausea and vomiting.

There is no precipitating factor for most patients with acute myocardial infarction. Some studies have reported an increased number of myocardial infarctions occurring soon after severe physical activity.[8-10] Other factors include respiratory infections, hypoxemia, hypoglycemia, serum sickness, allergy, and administration of ergot preparations. Emotional stress may also initiate an acute myocardial infarction.[11] Surgical procedures associated with hypotension or severe blood loss can also precipitate a myocardial infarction. A study of patients undergoing elective coronary artery bypass surgery found that perioperative ischemia occurs commonly and was an independent risk factor for postoperative myocardial infarction.[12] There is evidence from the Multicenter Investigation of Limitation of Infarct Size (MILIS) study which suggests that there is an increased risk of myocardial infarction in the morning with a peak incidence at about 9:00 A.M.[13] The early morning hours are also associated with elevation in plasma catecholamines and increases in platelet aggregability. It is possible that the early morning increase in vasospastic and prothrombotic factors are clinically relevant to the onset of acute myocardial infarction.

Physical Examination

The general appearance of patients with an acute myocardial infarction is one of anxiety and distress. They are often restless and unable to find a comfortable position. They may be clutching their chest (Levine's sign). If congestive heart failure is present, the patient may have cold perspiration and may be sitting on the side of the bed markedly dyspneic, with a feeling of suffocation. If the patient is in cardiogenic shock, the skin is cool and clammy with mottling over the extremities and cyanosis of the lips and nailbeds.

The vital signs are also important indicators of a patient's clinical status. The heart rate is commonly rapid and regular initially and slows as the patient's pain and anxiety are relieved. Marked bradycardia may occur, particularly with inferior myocardial infarction. Although most patients are normotensive during the early phase of acute myocardial infarction, some patients will exhibit a hypertensive response presumably due to an adrenergic discharge secondary to pain and agitation. This hypertension often resolves with sedation and relief of chest pain. Many previously hypertensive patients will become normotensive following an acute myocardial infarction, but will subsequently regain their elevated blood pressure 3 to 6 months after infarction. Hypotension occurs in patients with very large infarcts, and in those in cardiogenic shock. Hypotension can also be seen as a manifestation of excessive vagal tone, particularly in inferior myocardial infarction or when the latter is complicated by right ventricular infarction.

Low grade fever can be seen with acute myocardial infarction. It usually develops within 24 to 48 hours after the infarction and is thought to be a nonspecific response to tissue necrosis. The respiratory rate may be elevated in some patients soon after the onset of acute myocardial infarction, secondary to pain and anxiety or to left ventricular failure.

The jugular venous pulse is a reflection of right heart pressures and is usually not elevated in patients with acute myocardial infarction. Distended neck veins are noted in the presence of right ventricular infarction or cardiogenic shock. The carotid arterial pulse is an indirect measure of left ventricular stroke volume. A weak pulse suggests a reduced stroke volume, whereas a sharp upstroke suggests severe mitral insufficiency or ruptured ventricular septum with a left-to-right shunt.[14] Palpation of the precordium may reveal a prominent pulsation at the left parasternal border. This condition is usually present in large anterior wall infarctions.

Auscultation of the heart may reveal a variable first heart sound that occurs in the presence of heart block. Paradoxic splitting of the second heart sound may occur with marked left ventricular dysfunction or left bundle branch block. A fourth heart sound secondary to reduced left ventricular compliance is almost always present. It is commonly heard in patients with chronic ischemic heart disease as well as in older patients. As a result, it is of no diagnostic value.

A third heart sound caused by rapid inflow of blood during early diastole is associated with large infarctions and reflects severe left ventricular dysfunction. The in-hospital mortality of patients with acute myocardial infarction who have a third heart sound is significantly higher.[15] Third and fourth heart sounds are best heard at the apex when they arise in the left ventricle. A right ventricle gallop may be present in patients with right ventricular infarction and are heard best along the left sternal border.

Systolic murmurs are commonly heard and are usually due to mitral regurgitation caused by papillary muscle dysfunction. This condition is more common in inferior or lateral infarctions. A loud, apical holosystolic murmur may represent a ruptured interventricular septum or severe mitral regurgitation due to papillary muscle infarction or rupture.

Pericardial friction rubs are heard in 7 to 20% of all patients, especially those with transmural infarctions.[16,17] They are usually transient and most commonly noted on the second or third day after the acute myocardial infarction.[17]

Laboratory Examination

Although serum enzyme levels are important for establishing the diagnosis of acute myocardial infarction, they

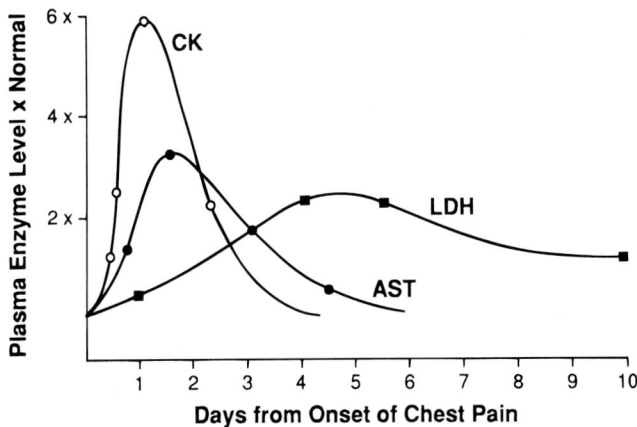

Fig. 29–1. Plasma levels of creatine kinase (CK), aspartate aminotransferase (AST), and lactic dehydrogenase (LDH) of typical patient with acute myocardial infarction.

are of little value in the pre-ICU phase. The standard enzymes for the laboratory diagnosis of myocardial infarction are serum creatinine kinase (CK), aspartate aminotransferase (AST; formerly termed SGOT), and lactic dehydrogenase (LDH) (Fig. 29-1). Serum CK is the most useful because it begins to rise within the first few hours of a myocardial infarction, peaks at 24 hours, and returns to normal in 3 to 4 days. CK can be falsely elevated in patients with muscle disease or trauma, intramuscular injection, alcohol intoxication, and vigorous exercise.[18]

Three isoenzymes of CK (MM, MB, and BB) have been identified by electrophoresis. The MM isoenzyme is present in skeletal muscle and the BB isoenzyme is present in the brain and kidney. The MB isoenzyme is present almost exclusively in the heart; elevated levels of MB isoenzyme are a highly specific indicator of myocardial infarction.[19-22] A radioimmunoassay has recently been developed to measure MB isoenzyme which has increased the sensitivity and specificity of the test.[21]

Serum AST begins to increase 8 to 12 hours after the onset of a myocardial infarction, peaks at 18 to 36 hours, and returns to normal in 3 to 4 days. The high incidence of false positive elevations of this enzyme makes it less useful in diagnosing acute myocardial infarction. Serum LDH levels begin to rise 24 to 48 hours, peak at 3 to 6 days, and return to normal in 8 to 14 days after infarction. Five isoenzymes of LDH are known, and the heart contains primarily LDH_1. Increases in serum LDH and in the ratio of LDH_1 to total LDH occur in more than 95% of patients with acute myocardial infarction,[16,22] and an LDH_1/LDH_2 ratio greater than 1.0 is highly sensitive and specific for the diagnosis of acute myocardial infarction.[19]

Serum enzyme levels are particularly helpful in diagnosing acute myocardial infarction when the electrocardiographic changes are difficult to assess. Examples include patients with left bundle branch block, ventricular pacing, or left ventricular hypertrophy with strain on the electrocardiogram.

In most patients with acute myocardial infarction, the electrocardiogram will document some change when com-

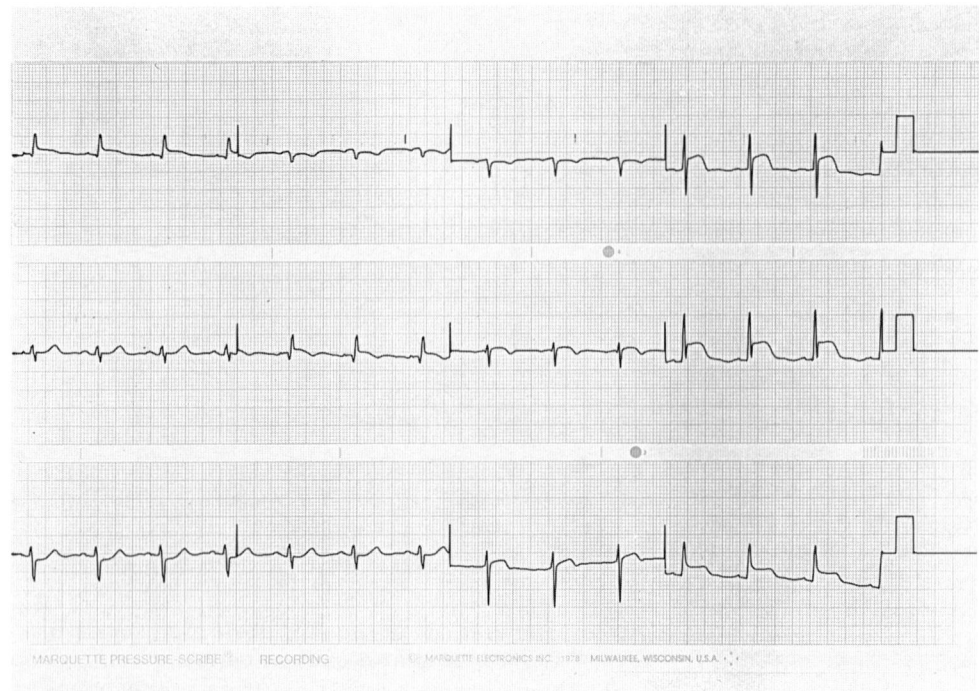

Fig. 29-2. Electrocardiogram in a patient with an acute anterior myocardial infarction demonstrating characteristic ST-segment and T-wave elevation in the precordial and lateral leads with reciprocal ST-segment depression in the inferior leads. There is already loss of R wave in the precordial and lateral leads.

paring serial recordings. The usefulness of the electrocardiogram is limited by the presence of intraventricular conduction disturbances (specifically LBBB), the presence of old myocardial infarction, and electrolyte imbalance.

The initial electrocardiographic change in Q-wave infarction is ST-segment elevation (Fig. 29-2). The T waves are often peaked and then become inverted with time. The most specific electrocardiographic change of acute myocardial infarction is the development of a new Q-wave. There is general agreement on electrocardiographic criteria for localizing an infarction of the anterior or inferior wall, but criteria for localization of a posterior or lateral wall infarction is more controversial.[25]

Right ventricular infarction is seen in up to 43% of patients with inferior infarction.[26] The most sensitive and specific electrocardiographic findings are the presence of ST-segment elevation of at least 1.0 mm and patterns of necrosis (QS or QR) in right precordial leads, especially V_3R and V_4R.[27] The diagnosis of non-Q-wave myocardial infarction by the electrocardiogram is nonspecific. Common changes include ST-segment depression or inversion of T waves. The diagnosis of non-Q-wave infarction depends more on clinical findings and serum enzyme changes than on the electrocardiogram.

The chest roentgenogram may provide important noninvasive information in regards to left ventricular function in the patient with acute myocardial infarction. If the initial chest film shows cardiac enlargement, this suggests preexisting myocardial disease. Serial chest films may show gradual enlargement of the heart as a result of left ventricular dilatation. Characteristic changes of the pulmonary vasculature could be seen if left ventricular failure is present. The degree of congestive heart failure and the size of the left ventricle on the initial chest film are independent predictors of increased mortality in patients with acute myocardial infarction.[28]

General Considerations

The development of mobile coronary care units has been important in decreasing mortality for acute myocardial infarction because most deaths occur within the first hours of the onset of symptoms, usually the result of ventricular arrhythmias.[29] These mobile units, which are equipped with personnel trained in the recognition and early treatment of acute myocardial infarction, have successfully reduced mortality during transportation of the patient to the hospital.[30-32] This reduction has been accomplished primarily through the rapid recognition and treatment of ventricular fibrillation by emergency medical technicians who perform cardiopulmonary resuscitation (CPR), administer lidocaine and DC countershock.

When the patient arrives in the emergency room, alleviation of chest pain is of prime importance because it will also reduce anxiety and diminish sympathetic nervous system activity. Intravenous morphine sulfate should be administered, initially 4 to 10 mg and then dosages of 2 to 4 mg repeated as needed. Benzodiazepines may also be beneficial in relieving anxiety which persists after chest pain has resolved.

In general, patients with acute myocardial infarction should receive oxygen therapy because they often develop hypoxemia.[33] The hypoxemia is usually a result of ventilation-perfusion mismatch[34] from left ventricular dysfunction, but may also be due to pneumonia or intrinsic pulmonary disease. Mild hypoxemia can be generally treated with 2 to 4 L per minute of oxygen by mask or nasal prongs for 24 to 48 hours.

Reperfusion for Acute Myocardial Infarction

Thrombolytic Therapy

Extensive data support the theory that early reperfusion of an occluded coronary artery decreases infarct size and reduces mortality from myocardial infarction.[35-40] Since it has been shown that coronary thrombosis is almost always present in acute myocardial infarction,[41] much interest has been directed toward the use of thrombolytic agents. Intravenous thrombolytic therapy has become the treatment of choice in patients who present early in the course of acute myocardial infarction. Clinical data suggest that mortality is decreased if thrombolytic therapy is administered within the first 6 hours and may be beneficial if given as late as 24 hours after the onset of symptoms.[42-46]

Several thrombolytic agents have been used for the treatment of acute myocardial infarction. They can be classified by the relative selectivity of the agent for fibrin. The fibrin nonselective agents include streptokinase, urokinase, and anisoylated plasminogen streptokinase activator complex (APSAC). These agents activate both circulating and fibrin-bound plasminogen. In contrast, tissue-type plasminogen activator (t-PA) and single-chain urokinase plasminogen activator (scu-PA) binds actively to fibrin clot but only poorly to circulating plasminogen. The t-PA-fibrin complex has a very high affinity to bind and convert plasminogen to plasmin at the local clot site; thus, it is a relatively fibrin selective agent. Figure 29-3 is a schematic representation of the different methods of action of the thrombolytic agents.

The results of large investigations of the use of thrombolytic therapy for acute myocardial infarction are summarized in Table 29-1, and are discussed in more detail in recent publications.[47,48] Data from the GISSI and ISIS-II trials conclusively demonstrate a reduction of short-term mortality of 20-30%.[35,44] The ISAM study showed a small but significant improvement in left ventricular ejection fraction, regional ejection fraction, and decreased CK-estimated infarct size at three weeks post infarction.[42] All three trials used streptokinase as the thrombolytic agent. The European Cooperative Study Group and the ASSET Trials compared intravenous t-PA to placebo and showed a borderline (5.1%, $p = 0.06$) and a significant reduction (25%, $p = 0.001$), respectively, in short-term mortality in rt-PA treated patients. APSAC was the thrombolytic agent used in the AIMS Trial and also showed a significant (47%) reduction in overall mortality. Recent studies have shown that APSAC and streptokinase are equally effective, with a trend to higher early patency and easier administration for APSAC.[49-51]

After showing a decrease in mortality with the use of intravenous thrombolytic therapy for acute myocardial infarction, research has been directed toward comparing the various thrombolytic agents. Early randomized angiographic[52,53] trials that compared recombinant tissue plasminogen activator (rt-PA) with streptokinase showed that at 90 minutes, t-PA has a higher rate of successful reperfusion than streptokinase[54,55] with less systemic fibrinolytic state. However, rt-PA was not associated with fewer hemorrhagic complications. These trials were not large enough to detect a significant mortality difference and they did not take into account late reperfusion rates.

Three large randomized studies directly compared rt-PA with streptokinase in the early treatment of acute myocardial infarction. GISSI-2 randomized 12,490 patients to treatment with either streptokinase or rt-PA, using combined estimates of absence of death plus severe left ventricular damage as their major end point and found no difference between the 2 agents.[54] The International Study Group 55 also conclude that both agents were equally effective in a trial involving 20,891 patients which used in-hospital mortality as its major end point.

GUSTO (Global Utilization of Streptokinase and Tissue Plasminogen Activator for Occluded Coronary Arteries) is the most recent trial and the first to find that accelerated t-PA provided a survival benefit over streptokinase.[56] The study randomized 41,021 patients to 4 different thrombolytic strategies: streptokinase and subcutaneous heparin; streptokinase and intravenous heparin; accelerated t-PA; and intravenous heparin or a combination of streptokinase with t-PA and intravenous heparin. The mortality rate at 30 days after myocardial interaction was 6.3% for the accelerated t-PA, group as compared to 7.2% for the group receiving streptokinase and subcutaneous heparin, 7.4% for the streptokinase and intravenous heparin group, and 7.0% for the patients receiving the combination of both throm-

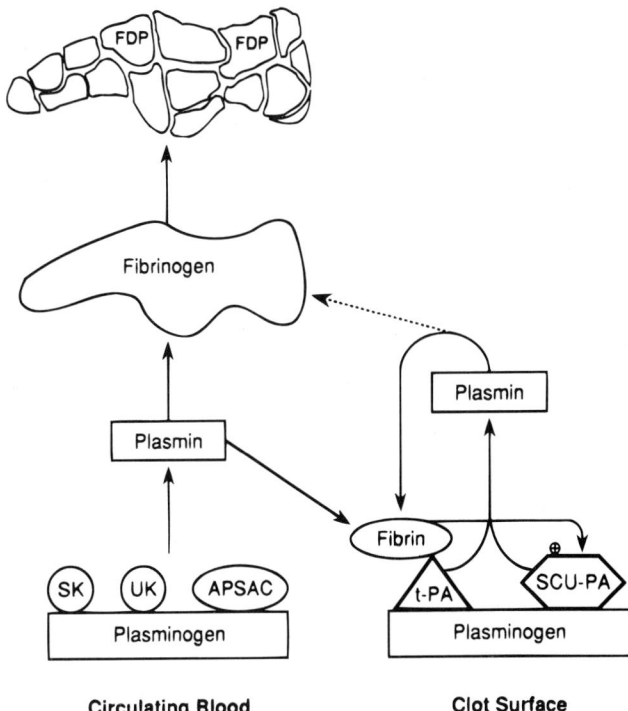

Fig. 29-3. Schematic representation of the action of fibrinolytic enzymes. Streptokinase (SK) and urokinase (UK) and acylated plasminogen streptokinase activator complex (APSAC) work predominantly on circulation plasminogen; tissue-type plasminogen activator (t-PA) and single-chain urokinase plasminogen activator (scu-PA) are relatively clot selective. (From Topol, E. J.: Clinical use of streptokinase and urokinase therapy for acute myocardial infarction. Heart Lung, 16:760, 1987.)

Table 29–1. Large Controlled Randomized Trials of Intravenous Thrombolytic Therapy in Acute Myocardial Infarction

Study	Patients	Agent	Dose	Follow-up (days)	Mortality Treatment %	Mortality Control %	p
GISSI	11,806	SK	1.5 million U	21	10.7	13.0	0.0002
ISAM	1,741	SK	1.5 million U	21	6.3	7.1	NS
AIMS	1,004	APSAC	30 U	30	6.4	12.2	0.0016
ISIS-2	17,187	SK	1.5 million U	35	12.0	9.2	<0.00001
		SK/ASA	1.5 million U/162.5 mg	"	8.0	13.2	<0.0001
		ASA	162.5 mg	"	11.8	23.0	<0.00001
ASSET	5,011	rt-PA	100 mg	30	7.2	9.8	0.0011
ECSG	721	rt-PA	100 mg	14	5.7	62.8	0.06

AIMS, APSAC Intervention Mortality Study; ASA, aspirin; ASSET, anglo-scandinavian study of early thrombolysis; GISSI, grupo italiano per lo studio della streptochinasi nell'infarcto myocardico; ISAM, intravenous streptokinase in acute myocardial infarction; ISIS-2, second international study of infarct survival; SK, streptokinase.

bolytic agents. The rate of hemorrhagic stroke was higher in the accelerated t-PA group (p = 0.03). However, the combined end point of death or disabling stroke was significantly lower in the accelerated t-PA group than in the streptokinase groups (6.9% versus 7.8%; p = 0.06). This study also provided strong evidence that earlier patency of the infarct-related artery was directly related to lower mortality following acute myocardial infarction.

Consensus exists on use of thrombolysis in patients with the following qualifications:

- Age less than 75 years old
- Chest pain suggestive of acute myocardial infarction of less than 6 hours' duration
- At least 1 mm ST segment elevation of two or more contiguous ECG leads[48]

There are some important controversies, however, in the use of thrombolytic agents in some subsets of patients with acute myocardial infarction,[47] and the elderly. The ISIS-II study reported beneficial effects for patients treated up to 24 hours after the onset of symptoms, whereas the GISSI trial revealed that only patients treated during the first 6 hours of infarction had favorable results. In experimental animals, late reperfusion, although not capable of salvaging myocardium, reduces subsequent left ventricular dilation and limits wall thinning and aneurysm formation.[57] The hypothesis of the favorable effects of a patient infarct-related vessel late in the course of acute myocardial infarction requires further research. Both the GISSI and ISIS-II trials failed to show benefit for the use of thrombolytic therapy in patients with ST segment depression as their only electrocardiographic abnormality, and therefore, it is not recommended on patients with unstable angina.

Although patients with an inferior myocardial infarction have a lower overall in-hospital mortality than those with anterior infarction, those with associated right ventricular involvement and/or ST segment depression in precordial leads V_1 to V_4, have a poorer prognosis.[58] Conflicting results were noted between the GISSI trial, which did not show a beneficial effect on mortality in patients with inferior infarction, and the ISIS-II trial which showed a benefit. Results of multiple other smaller randomized and nonrandomized studies, however, seem to justify the use of thrombolytic therapy in patients seen early (less than 2 to 3 hours) in the course of inferior infarction, particularly when accompanied by precordial ST segment depression.[47]

Of the previously cited large trials of thrombolysis in acute myocardial infarction, only GISSI and ISIS-II involved a significant number of patients older than 70 to 75 years because of the fear of bleeding complications in the elderly. The high risk nature of this group of patients is also supported by the fact that almost 50% of all in-hospital deaths from acute myocardial infarction occurred in patients older than 75 years.[59] Beneficial effects with increasing age were reported in these two trials as well as in the GUSTO trial. Therefore, thrombolytic therapy in the elderly should be considered after careful screening for potential bleeding risk.[48]

Absolute contraindications to the use of thrombolytic therapy include:

- Active internal bleeding
- Suspected aortic dissection
- Prolonged or traumatic cardiopulmonary resuscitation
- Recent head trauma or known intracranial neoplasm
- Recent surgery
- Diabetic proliferative retinopathy
- Pregnancy
- History of hemorrhagic stroke[53]

It is estimated that serious side effects from the use of streptokinase are rare, with approximately 3 bleeds requiring transfusion and 3 to 5 cerebral hemorrhages per 1000 treated patients.[44,56] Intracranial hemorrhage with rt-PA at the current recommended dose of 100 mg occurs in 5 to 7 patients per 1000 treated.[56,60] Because most bleeding complications occur at site of vessel puncture, these should be minimized in these patients.

Although some of the post-thrombolysis adjunctive therapy remains empiric, current recommendations include the use of: (1) intravenous heparin (maintaining activated partial thromboplastin time between 1.5 to 2 times control) for several days, beginning at the time of infusion of the thrombolytic agent or immediately after completion of thrombolytic therapy; (2) 160 mg of aspirin daily beginning immediately; (3) intravenous or topical nitroglycerin for 24 to 48 hours; and (4) early intravenous beta blockers, followed by oral administration if indicated (see the section of this chapter on the ICU phase). Angiotensin-converting enzyme inhibitors have been shown to decrease mortality following acute myocardial infarction and should be given to appropriately selected patients.

Percutaneous Transluminal Coronary Angioplasty

Immediately Following Successful Thrombolytic Therapy. The role of immediate coronary angioplasty following thrombolytic therapy has been evaluated by three large trials which are summarized in Table 29-2. Early reperfusion will occur in up to 75% of patients given an intravenous thrombolytic agent.[61] The rationale for performing percutaneous transluminal angioplasty (PTCA) after successful thrombolysis is to obtain a more complete reperfusion in those patients with a residual high grade stenosis in the infarct related artery. The three trials previously mentioned (Table 29-2), however, show that PTCA in this situation not only does not decrease mortality, nor increase global left ventricular ejection fraction (as compared to those patients receiving thrombolysis alone) but is associated with a higher risk of complications, including bleeding and the need for emergency coronary bypass surgery.

Patients Who Fail Thrombolytic Therapy and Have Evidence of Persistent Ischemia, ("Rescue PTCA"). PTCA is indicated in this setting, especially in the patient with post infarction angina associated with ECG changes or in the presence of ventricular tachyarrhythmias refractory to antiarrhythmic therapy.[46] Patients who underwent rescue PTCA in the TAMI-I and TIMI-IIA Trials still had high hospital mortality and reocclusion rates, with no improvement in in-hospital mortality or left ventricular ejection fraction.[61-63] The patients who are more likely to benefit from this treatment strategy are those with a large area of myocardium at risk; however, these patients are difficult to identify by noninvasive methods. Further data are needed to better define the role of rescue PTCA in acute myocardial infarction.

Patient with Contraindications to Thrombolytic Therapy ("Direct or Primary PTCA"). As many as 30 to 40% of patients experiencing an acute myocardial infarction have contraindications to the use of thrombolytic agents[45] and they may be candidates for direct PTCA, when presenting to a hospital with catheterization and angioplasty facilities less than 6 hours from the onset of symptoms. They represent a minority of patients, since only a small percentage of hospitals in the United States have these facilities. Success rates for direct PTCA range from 83 to 95%, acute reocclusion rates from 0 to 14%, and in-hospital mortality from 6.3 to 9.3%.[64-70] The most recent study, PAMI (Primary Angioplasty in Myocardial Infarction) randomized patients within 12 hours of the onset of acute myocardial infarction to either direct angioplasty or to intravenous t-PA.[71] The in-hospital reinfarction rate or mortality rate for the PTCA group was lower than for the t-PA group (5.1% versus 12.0; p = 0.02). At 6 months, reinfarction or death had occurred in 16.8% of patients treated with t-PA, compared to 8.5% treated with PTCA (p = 0.02). Because of these results, there is growing interest in the use of direct PTCA for the treatment of acute myocardial infarction.

Cardiogenic Shock. This represents a special situation in which PTCA has definite potentially favorable effects. This situation will be discussed later under hemodynamic alterations.

Coronary Artery Bypass Surgery

Emergency coronary artery bypass surgery has been evaluated in patients with evolving acute myocardial infarction of less than 6 hours' duration[72-76] and has showed to improve survival and left ventricular function. At present, the indications for emergency or urgent coronary artery bypass surgery include:

- Failed coronary angioplasty with persistent pain or hemodynamic instability
- Post infarction angina with left main or triple-vessel coronary disease or coronary anatomy not suitable for PTCA

Of particular importance are those patients with distant ischemia, suggesting compromise of an artery different

Table 29-2. Randomized Trials of Immediate Coronary Angioplasty Following Thrombolytic Therapy

| | | | | \multicolumn{10}{c}{In-Hospital Events} |
| | | | | Mortality (%) | | Major Bleeding (%) | | CABG (%) | | Reocclusion (%) | | LVEF (%) | |
Study	Patients	Agent	Dose	I-PTCA	D-PTCA	I-PTCA	D-PTCA	I-PTCA	D-PTCA	I-PTCA	D-PTCA	I-PTCA	D-PTCA
TAMI-I	386	rt-PA	150 mg	4	1	21	14	7	2	11	13	53	56
TIMI-IIA	389	rt-PA	100–150 mg	7.2	5.7	20	7**	6.7	1.5*	7	4	50.3	49.0
ECSG	367	rt-PA	100 mg	7	3	10	4	2	0	17	18	51	51

CABG, coronary artery bypass surgery; D (I)-PTCA, deferred (immediate) percutaneous transluminal angioplasty; ECSG, european cooperative study group; LVEF, left ventricular ejection fraction; TAMI, thrombolysis and angioplasty in myocardial infarction; TIMI, thrombolysis in myocardial infarction.
* p = 0.02
** p < 0.001

from that causing the acute myocardial infarction.[77] Coronary artery bypass surgery should also be considered in patients undergoing surgical repair of mechanical complications from myocardial infarction (see later) and with cardiogenic shock when anatomy is unsuitable for angioplasty.

Patients who undergo emergency coronary artery revascularization surgery for failed PTCA usually have a low mortality rate of about 3%.[78,79] They have a higher incidence of myocardial infarction, however, and other complications such as postoperative bleeding, respiratory failure, and sternal problems,[78,79] especially if they entered the operating room with evidence of persistent myocardial ischemia or hemodynamic instability. Therefore, stabilization of these patients with measures such as intra-aortic balloon pumping or perfusion coronary catheters should be attempted provided that there is not a major delay in their transportation to the operating room. Further considerations for pre-ICU care of these patients is presented in Chapter 30.

ICU PHASE

The development of the coronary care unit has contributed to the decrease in mortality for acute myocardial infarction primarily through rapid recognition and treatment of life-threatening arrhythmias. Over the past several years, the focus in the treatment of acute myocardial infarction has been on management prior to admission to the coronary ICU with methods to limit infarct size. The ICU continues to be an important part of the management of the patient with acute myocardial infarction, not only for arrhythmia monitoring, but also for hemodynamic monitoring and pharmacologic intervention.

Pharmacologic Therapy

Beta Blockers

By lowering heart rate and blood pressure, the benefits of beta-blocker therapy in acute myocardial infarction include decreasing myocardial oxygen demand and increasing perfusion of the subendocardium. During the first hours of infarction, the main objectives of beta-blocker therapy are to limit infarct size and decrease mortality.

Short-term randomized trials using intravenous, followed by oral, beta blockers, without thrombolytics, started in the first hours of infarction demonstrate a 15% reduction in 7-day mortality and reinfarction rate.[80,81] The largest of these trials[82-84] are summarized in Table 29-3. Beneficial effects are also seen when beta blockers are given concomitantly with thrombolytic agents. The effects of beta blockers on reduction of infarct size are more difficult to demonstrate, because they depend on the method; however, there seems to be a small favorable effect.[81] It is estimated that treatment of approximately 200 patients with acute myocardial infarction with early beta-blocker therapy would lead to the prevention of one reinfarction during the first 7 days after the acute event.[83] Agents with intrinsic sympathomimetic activity such as pindolol and acebutolol should be avoided because of their potential to increase myocardial oxygen demand.

Early intravenous beta-blocker therapy is indicated in patients with:

- Persistent or recurrent evidence of ischemia
- Supraventricular arrhythmias (such as atrial fibrillation) with a rapid ventricular response
- Reflex tachycardia
- Systolic hypertension

Contraindications to beta-blocker therapy include:

- Moderate to severe left ventricular dysfunction
- Severe bradycardia
- Hypotension
- Advanced atrioventricular block
- Severe chronic obstructive pulmonary disease

The greatest benefit from beta blockers occurs in patients considered to be at high risk for complications as demonstrated by the MIAMI trial.[82] High risk patients in this investigation include:

- Age greater than 60
- Abnormal electrocardiogram
- History of previous myocardial infarction
- Hypertension
- Angina pectoris
- Congestive heart failure
- Diabetes
- Short- or long-term treatment with diuretics or digitalis

Nitrates

Because nitrates produce coronary vasodilatation, increase collateral blood flow, and decrease left ventricular preload, they can be of substantial benefit in the initial management of most patients with acute myocardial infarction. This favorable pharmacologic profile has to be

Table 29–3. Beta-Blocker Therapy in the Early Phases of Acute Myocardial Infarction: Results of Randomized Trials

Study	No. Patients	Thrombolysis	MI duration	Agent	Treatment (%)	Control (%)	p
MIAMI	5,778	−	24 h	Metoprolol	4.3	4.9	NS
ISIS-1	16,027	−	12 h	Atenolol	3.9	4.6	<0.04
TIMI-IIB	1,390	+	4 h	Metoprolol			
Meta-analysis	>27,000	−	−	Varied	3.7	4.3	<0.02

Table 29-4. Intravenous Nitroglycerin for Acute Myocardial Infarction

Study	No. Patients	MI Duration	Cardiac Mortality Treatment (%)	Cardiac Mortality Control (%)	p
Yusuf, et al.	>2000	<24 h	13.3	20.5	<0.01
Judgett, et al.	310	<12 h	14.0	26.0	<0.025

weighed against the potential of nitrates to produce hypotension, reflex tachycardia, and coronary steal syndrome,[85] or aggravation of hypoxemia by ventilation-perfusion mismatch, however.

Table 29-4 outlines the results of investigations of intravenous nitroglycerin[85-89] for acute myocardial infarction. Early studies showed a decrease in mortality and infarct size with the use of this agent; however, the more recent trials (GISSI-3 and ISIS-4) randomized patients to intravenous or oral nitroglycerin or placebo and found no difference in mortality.[90] Patients with congestive heart failure or pulmonary edema derive the greatest benefit from intravenous nitroglycerin therapy.[91] Greater benefit seems to occur when the infusion is started early.

Calcium-Channel Blockers

Diltiazem, nifedipine, and verapamil are the most widely used calcium antagonists in clinical practice. All three decrease blood pressure by lowering peripheral vascular resistance. Diltiazem and verapamil reduce myocardial contractility, and can therefore reduce myocardial oxygen demand. If reflex sympathetic stimulation is prevented, nifedipine has a similar myocardial depressant effect.[92] Diltiazem and verapamil also depress atrioventricular conduction.

Several large studies on the use of calcium antagonists in acute myocardial infarction[93-99] have been completed and the results recently reviewed.[100-106] In brief, despite their favorable hemodynamic and electrophysiologic profile, the routine use of these agents is not associated with decreased mortality,[101] even when started in the early phases of infarction with concomitant thrombolytic therapy.[102] Diltiazem decreases rates of early reinfarction and recurrent ischemic events in patients with non-Q wave infarction, however.[93]

In general, the use of calcium antagonists should be limited to subsets of patients with infarction that present with complications that warrant their use such as:

- Recurrent ischemia
- Systolic hypertension
- Atrial arrhythmias with rapid ventricular response

Calcium-channel blockers are contraindicated if there is concomitant left dysfunction in the early phase of acute myocardial infarction.

Angiotensin-Converting Enzyme Inhibitors

Much interest has recently been shown in inhibition of infarct expansion with the use of angiotensin-converting enzyme (ACE) inhibitors. In the ISIS-4 study, over 50,000 patients with acute myocardial infarction were randomized to receive either oral captopril or placebo, and in the GISSI-3 study, patients were randomized to oral lisinopril or placebo. Both studies found lower mortality rates in the patients treated with ACE inhibitors.[103]

Arrhythmia Monitoring

Ventricular arrhythmias, the occurrence of premature ventricular beats (VPBs), is almost a universal phenomenon in acute myocardial infarction most commonly in the first 48 hours. The presence of frequent VPBs (greater than 5 per minute), closely coupled VPBs ("R on T") multiform VPBs, or short bursts of three of more VPBs in succession were originally considered warning arrhythmias. Current practice is to administer a lidocaine infusion (1 to 3 mg per minute) in patients with acute myocardial infarction demonstrating high grade ventricular ectopic activity. To prevent lidocaine toxicity, this drug should be administered at a reduced dose in:

- Patients older than 70 years
- Congestive heart failure
- Hepatic dysfunction
- Severe renal failure
- Preexisting neurologic dysfunction

Accelerated idioventricular rhythm occurs in 8 to 20% of patients with infarctions and often after successful reperfusion. It is defined as a ventricular rhythm at a rate between 60 and 100 beats per minute. This rhythm usually does not cause hemodynamic instability and is treated only when symptomatic or if associated with rapid ventricular tachycardia. It can be treated by accelerating the sinus rate with atropine or atrial pacing. If the underlying sinus rate is greater than 60 beats per minute, then the ventricular focus can be suppressed with lidocaine.

Ventricular tachycardia occurs in 10 to 40% of cases of acute myocardial infarction[104] and is defined as 3 or more consecutive VPBs at a rate greater than 120 beats per minute. If the patient is hemodynamically stable in this rhythm, then intravenous lidocaine or procainamide can be used initially, but if medications are ineffective or the patient becomes hemodynamically compromised, then one should proceed to electrical cardioversion.

Ventricular tachycardia during the first 24 hours is usually transient and benign. Late ventricular tachycardia is more frequent with transmural infarctions and left ventricular dysfunction, and is associated with a hospital mortality rate of 40 to 50%.[105] The presence of significant ventricular ectopic activity at the time of hospital discharge is a predictor of increased mortality independent of left ventricular function.[106]

Ventricular fibrillation occurs in two forms during acute myocardial infarction. The primary form occurs within the first 24 to 48 hours, and is more common in younger patients and those with first infarctions and no history of high grade arrhythmias. The secondary form is usually a terminal event associated with progressive left ventricular failure and occurs late (1 to 6 weeks) in the course of infarction. Immediate electrical countershock is the treatment of ventricular fibrillation.

The prognostic implication of primary ventricular fibrillation is controversial. The MILIS (multicenter investigation of the limitation of infarct size)[107] study showed that it has no adverse effect in patients without left ventricular failure. A more recent investigation demonstrated an association between primary ventricular fibrillation and increased risk of in-hospital death, however.[108]

Supraventricular Arrhythmias

Sinus bradycardia is a common arrhythmia early in acute myocardial infarction which is usually transient and requires no specific treatment. It is three times more frequent in inferior infarction than anterior infarction. The bradycardia may be secondary to an increase in vagotonia or due to ischemic damage of the sinus node. Sinus bradycardia will most often resolve without treatment. If the sinus rate is slow and associated with hypotension, low cardiac output, or frequent ventricular escape beats, atropine sulfate should be administered (0.3 to 0.6 mg every 3 to 10 minutes up to 2 mg) in an attempt to increase the heart rate and normalize blood pressure.[109,110] If the sinus bradycardia is associated with hypotension and is unresponsive to atropine, then a temporary pacemaker may be needed. Sinus tachycardia (sinus rhythm with a heart rate of greater than 100 bpm) is seen frequently in acute myocardial infarction. Underlying causes of sinus tachycardia include fever, anxiety, hypokalemia, pericarditis, and increased sympathetic stimulation. The most common cause is left ventricular failure. If there is no evidence of left ventricular failure, beta-blocking agents are useful for lowering heart rate and decreasing myocardial oxygen demand.

Atrial fibrillation is seen in up to 15% of patients with acute myocardial infarction and atrial flutter in 2 to 4% of patients. Although these arrhythmias are seen in the presence of post-MI pericarditis, they are most commonly due to left ventricular failure with secondary increases in left atrial pressure.

The ventricular response to the presence of atrial fibrillation is usually fast (greater than 120 bpm) and may result in hemodynamic compromise. Therefore, controlling the ventricular rate is the main focus of treatment and digoxin is the agent used most commonly. If digoxin is insufficient, small doses of intravenous propranolol or verapamil may be used to control the heart rate. If hemodynamic compromise or chest pain is present, one should proceed directly to electrical cardioversion.

Conduction Disturbances

Ischemia of the atrioventricular (AV) node may occur with inferior infarction and may be manifested by AV block. Second-degree block is usually Mobitz type I (Wenckebach) and third-degree block is often preceded by first-degree or second-degree AV block. The escape rhythm in third-degree AV block is usually a junctional escape with a heart rate of 40 to 60 beats per minute and is a narrow complex unless a coexistent bundle branch block is present. The prognosis of AV block in patients with inferior infarction is similar to the overall prognosis for patients with inferior infarction. A temporary pacemaker is required when the slow heart rate is associated with significant chest pain or hemodynamic compromise.

When complete AV block occurs in anterior infarction, it is usually due to extensive infarction with involvement of the bundle of His or all three fascicles of the bundle branch system. Complete AV block is usually preceded by bifascicular block (LBBB, RBBB, and LAHB or alternating RBBB and LBBB). The escape rhythm arises from the ventricle, the rate is slow (20 to 40 bpm) and the QRS complex is wide. Second-degree AV block in the setting of anterior infarction is often Mobitz type II.

Temporary pacing is warranted in patients with anterior myocardial infarction who have symptomatic bradycardia unresponsive to atropine or in patients with new onset of bifascicular or trifascicular block. The AV conduction disturbance almost always resolves during the hospitalization, whereas, intraventricular conduction defects often persist. Because the incidence of sudden death during the first 6 weeks post-MI is higher in this group they should be monitored in the hospital for a longer period of time.[111-113]

The role of permanent pacemaker therapy in acute myocardial infarction is controversial.[114] There is no clear evidence that permanent pacing improves survival. A patient with persistent complete AV block or persistent bifascicular or trifascicular block in the setting of prior complete AV block should be considered for a permanent pacemaker.

Left Ventricular Failure and Cardiogenic Shock

Acute myocardial infarction is often accompanied by some degree of left ventricular failure which usually resolves within the first 48 hours. This resolution may be attributed to recovery of the "stunned" myocardium associated with myocardial infarction.

The Killip classification divides patients into four groups on the basis of clinical signs of left ventricular failure (Table 29-5).[115] Patients with mild left ventricular failure (Killip's class II) can usually be successfully treated with intravenous diuretic therapy. Vasodilator drugs are also useful in treating left ventricular failure. Nitroglycerin is a vasodila-

Table 29–5. Killip Classification of Patients with Acute Myocardial Infarction (MI)

Class	Clinical Definition	Patients with MI Admitted to CCU in this Category (%)	Approximate Mortality (%)
I	No clinical signs of heart failure	30–40	8
II	Rales over ≤50% of lungs and S₃ gallop	30–50	30
III	Rales over ≤50% of lungs, often pulmonary edema	5–10	44
IV	Cardiogenic shock	10	80–100

(From Killip, T., and Kimball, J. T.: Treatment of myocardial infarction in a coronary care unit: a two year experience with 250 patients. Am. J. Cardiol. 20:457, 1967.)

tor with predominant effect on the venous side of the circulation. Because it also dilates epicardial coronary arteries, it is the most useful vasodilator when myocardial ischemia is present. Nitroprusside is another effective vasodilator, but it may cause a "coronary steal," which will preferentially increase coronary flow in nonstenotic areas. Nitroprusside is a balanced vasodilator with similar effects on arterial and venous systems and is very useful in rapidly controlling severe hypertension.[116] A radial artery line and pulmonary artery catheter may be needed to optimize titration of these intravenous agents.

If the left ventricular failure is severe or associated with hypotension, positive inotropic agents such as dopamine and dobutamine should be added.[117] Amrinone, which is an agent with both vasodilating and inotropic properties, can also be used, however hypotension may limit the utility of amrinone and dobutamine. In this situation, combination therapy with dopamine is often effective.

Cardiogenic shock may occur when the infarction involves more than 40% of the left ventricular myocardium. This condition is characterized by severe hypotension, elevated pulmonary capillary wedge pressure, low cardiac output, oliguria, and peripheral vasoconstriction. The mortality associated with cardiogenic shock is more than 80%[108] if treated with medical therapy alone. Hypoxemia should be corrected with administration of oxygen and intubation if necessary. There may be benefits to mechanical ventilation even in the absence of hypoxemia or hypercarbia because the work of breathing can consume up to 20% of cardiac output.[118] Systemic arterial pressure should be maintained with the use of norepinephrine and an intra-aortic balloon pump should be used to increase coronary perfusion and decrease systemic afterload. Consideration should be given to proceeding to the cardiac catheterization laboratory because evidence indicates improved survival in patients with cardiogenic shock who undergo coronary bypass surgery within 12 hours of the onset of symptoms,[119] or who undergo acute PTCA of the infarct-related artery.[120]

Patients with cardiogenic shock should be evaluated for the presence of mechanical complications of acute myocardial infarction such as mitral regurgitation, ventricular free wall or septal rupture. These mechanical complications usually occur 3 to 6 days after infarction and can have a spectrum of clinical presentations ranging from immediate death to a slower progression to shock. One autopsy study involving 1746 patients dying of an acute myocardial infarction, revealed that as many as one third of cardiac ruptures may be subacute which provides time for diagnosis and surgery.[121] Rupture of the free ventricular wall occurs 7 times more often in the left ventricle than in the right, commonly in the area of terminal distribution of the left anterior descending artery. It is usually associated with a large transmural infarction, and is more common in elderly patients, those with long-standing hypertension, females, and anterior infarctions. The usual presentation is that of sudden right heart failure with shock often leading to electromechanical dissociation. Most patients with free wall rupture die within minutes; however, immediate pericardiocentesis, as well as two-dimensional echocardiography when the patient's presentation allows performance of this study will confirm the diagnosis. Removal of pericardial fluid can hopefully stabilize the patient temporarily for transportation to the operating room for repair and myocardial revascularization surgery.

Rupture of the interventricular septum also occurs in transmural infarctions, especially of anterior and anterolateral locations, although it can also be seen in inferior infarctions. Almost all patients have severe multivessel coronary artery disease. The diagnosis is suggested by a new harsh holosystolic murmur at the left lower sternal border and can be confirmed with a pulmonary arterial balloon flotation catheter to document a left-to-right shunt by oximetric measurements. Similar clinical findings (new holosystolic murmur with progressive heart failure) can be seen with papillary muscle rupture. An echocardiogram with Doppler studies (Fig. 29-4) can confirm the diagnosis and help to differentiate it from rupture of the interventricular septum. An intra-aortic balloon pump may be required in patients with ruptured interventricular septum or mitral regurgitation, and prompt surgery is often necessary. Occasionally, a patient may stabilize without pharmacologic and intra-aortic balloon pump support. In such situations, surgery should be delayed for 2 to 4 weeks to allow for complete myocardial healing.[122]

Another important consideration is the presence of a right ventricular infarction which is an entity that occurs almost exclusively as a complication of inferoposterior left ventricular infarction.[123,124] Although some patients with right ventricular infarction can be asymptomatic, other patients can develop the classic clinical and hemodynamic syndrome of predominant right ventricular failure[125] characterized by elevated right heart pressures that exceed left heart pressures, distended neck veins, heart block, and hypotension responding to plasma volume expansion. In the presence of a right ventricular infarction, even patients in shock do not have the ominous prognosis associated with shock due to left ventricular failure, if diagnosed early and treated appropriately.

The goals of therapy in right ventricular infarction are to correct hypotension by rapid administration of intravenous fluids and to avoid preload reducing agents, such as nitroglycerin and diuretics, which may exacerbate the systemic hypoperfusion present in these patients.[126] If left ventricular filling pressure is 18 to 20 mm Hg and the patient remains hypotensive, he or she should be treated with intra-aortic balloon pump counterpulsation and vasopressor agents such as dopamine and dobutamine.[127,128] A rapid improvement in the hemodynamic manifestations of right ventricular infarction has been described in a patient treated successfully with coronary angioplasty.[129]

POST-ICU COURSE

Transfer From the ICU

Most complications from an acute myocardial infarction occur in the first 48 to 72 hours. Therefore, if a patient remains free of chest pain, hemodynamically stable, and without malignant arrhythmias during this period, he or she can be transferred to a regular hospital bed. In patients who have been stabilized after experiencing complications such as congestive heart failure or late ventricular

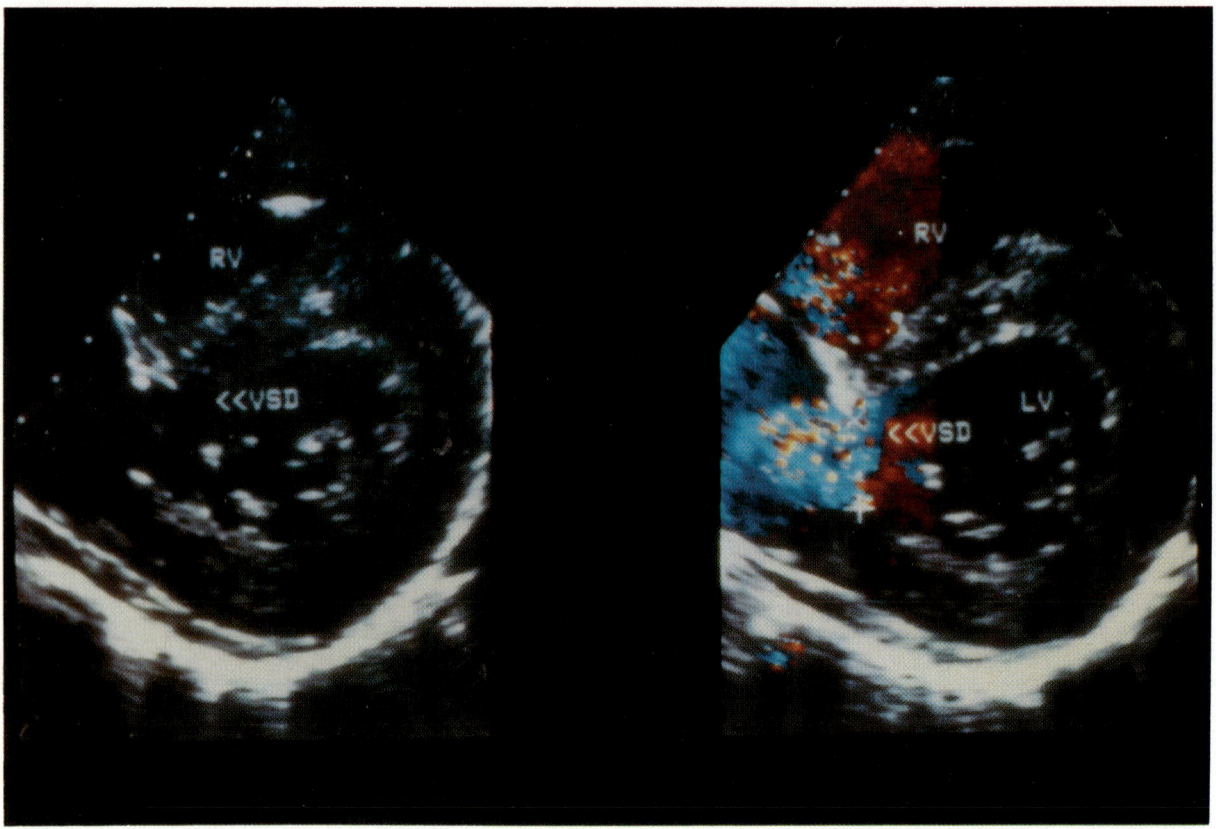

Fig. 29–4. Two-dimensional echocardiogram with color Doppler revealing a ruptured interventricular septum with flow from the left ventricle to the right ventricle.

arrhythmias, transfer to a monitored step-down unit may be more appropriate.

In patients with an uncomplicated post infarction course, out-of-bed activities (e.g., sitting in a bedside chair or short walks to the bathroom) can be started usually on the third or fourth day. Activities should be increased gradually so that the patient is fully ambulatory seven to ten days after infarction which is the time when the patient can be discharged home. Pooled data from 8 trials involving almost 900 patients indicate that an early discharge (7 to 14 days after admission) shows no unfavorable effect on mortality or morbidity.[130] In patients experiencing complications, their clinical conditions should be stable for several days before discharge.

Secondary Prevention of Myocardial Infarction

Risk stratification after myocardial infarction has become increasingly sophisticated as well as clinically useful.[131] Information about a particular patient's long-term prognosis becomes available throughout his hospitalization. The factors associated with increased risk of recurrent cardiac events after myocardial infarction are listed in Table 29–6.

Patients with congestive heart failure (Killip class III or IV), hypotension, recurrent ischemia, late malignant arrhythmias, or suspicion of mechanical complications from infarction, are candidates for cardiac catherization without further noninvasive evaluation. Approximately 60 to 80% of survivors of a first myocardial infarction will lack these high risk indicators during the first weeks of their infarction however, and will require additional testing.[132,133]

In predischarge exercise testing at 6 to 10 days following infarction, a symptom limited submaximal test (end point of 5 METS (metabolic equivalents) or 70% of the maximal predicted heart rate for age) should be used.[133] Results that indicate a high risk of subsequent cardiac events are:

- \>1-mm ST segment depression during exercise
- Low exercise capacity (<4 METS)
- Inability to achieve a peak systolic blood pressure >110 mm Hg or to increase systolic pressure by 10 mm Hg[134]

Patients with one or more of these findings should be considered for early cardiac catherization. If none of these are present, the patient can be discharged and return 4 to 8 weeks later for a repeat symptom limited maximal stress test. The test will help to identify patients at risk for recurrent events and to assess a patient's ability to return to work or to perform strenuous activities. An alternate cost-effective approach in regards to post infarction exercise testing is to perform only one maximal stress test 3 weeks after infarction. This has shown to be safe and of good prognostic value.[135,136] Exercise[201] thallium scintigraphy

Table 29-6. Factors Associated With Increased Mortality After Acute Myocardial Infarction

1. Congestive heart failure (clinical, hemodynamic, or radiographic)
2. Left ventricular ejection fraction less than 0.40
3. Large infarct size (estimated by enzymes, ^{99m}technetium radionuclide scan, electrocardiographic QRS mapping, or echocardiographic techniques)
4. New bundle branch block (any type, including fascicular blocks)
5. Mobitz II second or third-degree heart block
6. Anterior infarction
7. Reinfarction or infarct extension
8. Ventricular fibrillation or ventricular tachycardia
9. Ventricular premature beats (especially if frequent or complex)
10. Supraventricular arrhythmias (other than sinus bradycardia)
11. Abnormal signal-averaged electrocardiogram
12. Inducible sustained monomorphic ventricular tachycardia during electrophysiologic study
13. Postinfarction angina
14. Inability to perform exercise testing
15. Angina pectoris, ST-segment elevation or depression, abnormal blood pressure response, or ventricular ectopy induced by exercise testing
16. Diabetes mellitus
17. Hypertension or loss of preexisting hypertension
18. Age greater than 70 years
19. Female gender

is recommended whenever baseline abnormalities of the electrocardiogram compromise its interpretation. If there is doubt about the interpretation of the thallium exercise stress test, exercise ventriculography by radionuclide scanning or exercise echocardiography can increase the test sensitivity by identifying exercise induced wall motion abnormalities.

Because left ventricular dysfunction is a major predictor of short- and long-term prognosis following acute myocardial infarction, an accurate measurement of left ventricular ejection fraction will identify patients at higher risk. This determination can be done by rest radionuclide ventriculography, echocardiography, or at the time of cardiac catheterization. Higher 1-year mortality rates are seen when left ventricular ejection fractions are below 40%.[137-140] More recently, a cut-off level of 45% was suggested as being more accurate.[141]

If a patient demonstrates electrical instability (such as frequent or complex premature ventricular beats) after the first 48 hours of infarction, a 24-hour Holter monitor should be performed. Patients with 10 or more premature ventricular contractions an hour have a 2-year mortality rate of greater than 20%.[142] Although significant ventricular arrhythmias are associated with left ventricular dysfunction, several large studies have demonstrated them to be an independent risk factor for sudden death.[138,143-145] If runs of ventricular tachycardia are seen, further electrophysiologic testing may be indicated. Sustained ventricular tachycardia and ventricular fibrillation require aggressive management to decrease the incidence of recurrent arrhythmias and sudden death. The goal of therapy for symptomatic, nonsustained ventricular arrhythmias is to alleviate symptoms, usually through the use of long-term antiarrhythmic therapy. The most frequently used agents are procainamide and quinidine.[146] The appropriate management of patients with asymptomatic ventricular arrhythmias remains controversial despite their association with increased risk of sudden death due to the lack of large trials demonstrating the efficacy of antiarrhythmic therapy in this clinical setting.

Beta Blockers

Secondary prevention trials involving thousands of patients[147-149] have demonstrated that long-term beta-blocker therapy initiated in the first few days of infarction and continued for at least 2 years, improved survival and decreased reinfarction rate. The absolute reduction in 2-year mortality achieved by beta blockers in patients without contraindications for their use appears to be 2 to 3%. Favorable effects are observed with both cardioselective and nonselective beta blockers and, as with the acute phases of myocardial infarction, agents with intrinsic sympathomimetic activity should be avoided. No studies address the question of long-term beta-blocker therapy after successful revascularization following myocardial infarction. The benefit of beta-blocker therapy in low risk patients whose 1-year mortality is greater than 2% is more difficult to assess.

Anticoagulants and Antiplatelet Agents

The incidence of deep venous thrombosis of the lower extremities in patients with acute myocardial infarction is 7 to 38% which is as high as that seen in postsurgical patients. The incidence is higher in the presence of massive infarction with heart failure or cardiogenic shock, prolonged immobilization, and in patients older than 70 years. Low dose heparin, 5000 U subcutaneously every 12 hours, started in the first 12 to 18 hours of infarction and continued for 10 days, has decreased the incidence of venous thrombosis in 3 randomized trials from 23 to 4%,[150] and is therefore recommended in all patients with acute myocardial infarction when full anticoagulation is not indicated for other reasons.

Left ventricular mural thrombus occurs in 20% of patients with acute myocardial infarction, in 40% of anterior infarction, and in approximately 60% of large anterior infarctions. Approximately one out of ten patients with a mural thrombus will have a clinically evident systemic embolization.[151] Most of these embolic events occur in the first 3 months after infarction, with the majority occurring in the first 10 days. Therefore, it is recommended that patients with large anterior infarctions be treated immediately with high dose subcutaneous (e.g., 12,500 units every 12 hours) or intravenous heparin to prolong the activated partial thromboplastin time from 1.5 to 2 times control. This treatment should be followed by oral warfarin, adjusting its dose to obtain a prothrombin time control for at least 3 months.

Reocclusion following thrombolytic therapy is reported to occur in 5 to 15% of patients.[152,153] To prevent reocclusion, 160 to 325 mg of aspirin should be started in the emergency room and intravenous heparin should be started immediately with the thrombolytic agent to maintain an activated partial thromboplastin time at 1.5 to 2 times control for 24 to 72 hours.

The ISIS-2 trial demonstrated that aspirin alone reduced

5 week cardiac deaths by 23%, and nonfatal reinfarction by 49%. Furthermore, pooled analysis of 10 large trials in the long-term use of aspirin for secondary prevention of recurrent myocardial infarction and death,[154] indicated that aspirin produces a significant reduction in mortality and reinfarction of 15 and 31%, respectively.

In brief, subcutaneous low dose heparin is recommended for all patients with acute myocardial infarction not receiving thrombolytics. In the presence of a large anterior infarction, full heparinization is indicated and should be followed by oral warfarin for at least 3 months. Finally, in all patients without contraindications, long-term therapy with aspirin is indicated after acute infarction.

Alteration of Coronary Risk Factors

The secondary prevention trials have demonstrated that a 10% reduction in cholesterol can reduce the rate of nonfatal reinfarction by 12%.[155] Because of this fact, any pharmacologic therapy aimed at secondary prevention of myocardial infarction should be coupled with vigorous attempts to lower cholesterol in patients with hypercholesterolemia. To obtain maximum benefits, modification of other coronary risk factors, including smoking cessation and control of hypertension are also necessary. A recently published prospective, randomized, controlled trial has demonstrated that comprehensive life style changes (i.e., low fat vegetarian diet, smoking cessation, stress management training, and moderate exercise) may regress coronary atherosclerosis after only 1 year without the use of lipid-lowering drugs.[156]

REFERENCES

1. Kannel, W. R., Barry, P., and Dawber, T.: Immediate mortality in coronary heart disease. Framingham Study. Proc 4th World Congress Cardio IVB 176, 1963.
2. McNealy, R. H., and Pemberton, J.: Duration of last attack in 998 fatal cases of coronary artery disease and its relation to possible cardiac resuscitation. Br. Heart J., 3:139, 1968.
3. Pantridge, J. F., Webb, S. W., Adgey, A. A. J., and Geddes, J. S.: The first hour after the onset of acute myocardial infarction. In Progress in Cardiology. Edited by P. N. Yu and J. F. Goodman. Philadelphia, Lea & Febiger, 1974.
4. Moss, A. J., Wynar, B., and Goldstein, S.: Delay in hospitalization during the acute coronary period. Am. J. Cardiol., 24:659, 1969.
5. Simon, A. B., Feinleib, M., and Thompson, H. K., Jr.: Components of delay in the prehospital phase of acute myocardial infarction. Am. J. Cardiol., 30:476, 1972.
6. Norris, N. M.: Myocardial Infarction. Edinburgh, Churchill Livingstone, 1982.
7. Alonzo, A. M., Simon, A. B., and Feinleib, M.: Prodromata of myocardial infarction and sudden death. Circulation, 52:1056, 1975.
8. Smith, C., Sauls, H. C., and Ballew, J.: Coronary occlusion: a clinical study of 100 patients. Ann. Intern. Med., 17:681, 1942.
9. French, A. J., and Dock, W.: Fatal coronary arteriosclerosis in young soldiers. JAMA, 124:1233, 1944.
10. Fitzhugh, G., and Hamilton, B. E.: Coronary occlusion and fatal angina pectoris. Study of the immediate causes and their prevention. JAMA, 100:475, 1933.
11. Jenkins, C. D.: Recent evidence supporting psychologic and social risk factors for coronary disease. N. Engl. J. Med., 294:987, 1976.
12. Slogoff, S., and Keats, A. S.: Does perioperative myocardial ischemia lead to postoperative myocardial infarction. Anesthesiology, 62:107, 1985.
13. Muller, J. E., et al.: Circadian variation in the frequency of onset of acute myocardial infarction. N. Engl. J. Med., 313:1315, 1985.
14. Pasternak, R. C., et al.: Acute myocardial infarction. In Heart Disease: A Textbook of Cardiovascular Medicine. 3rd Ed. Edited by E. Braunwald. Philadelphia, W. B. Saunders, 1988.
15. Riley, C., Russell, R. O., and Rackley, C. E.: Left ventricular gallop sound and acute myocardial infarction. Am. Heart J., 86:598, 1973.
16. Sawaya, J. I., Mujais, S. K., and Armenian, H. K.: Early diagnosis of pericarditis in acute myocardial infarction. Am. Heart J., 100:144, 1980.
17. Krainin, F. M., Flessas, A. P., and Spodick, D. H.: Infarction-associated pericarditis. Rarity of diagnostic electrocardiogram. N. Engl. J. Med., 311:1211, 1984.
18. Sobel, B. E., and Shell, W. E.: Serum enzyme determinations in the diagnosis and assessment of myocardial infarction. Circulation, 45:471, 1972.
19. Lee, T. H., and Goldman, L.: Serum enzyme assays in the diagnosis of acute myocardial infarction. Ann. Intern. Med., 105:221, 1986.
20. Roberts, R., Gowda, K. S., Ludbrook, P. A., and Sobel, B. A.: Specificity of elevated serum MB creatine phosphokinase activity in the diagnosis of acute myocardial infarction. Am. J. Cardiol., 36:433, 1975.
21. Roberts, R., and Sobel, B. E.: Creatine kinase isoenzymes in the assessment of heart disease. Am. Heart J., 95:521, 1978.
22. Lott, J. A., and Stang, J. M.: Serum enzymes and isoenzymes in the diagnosis and differential diagnosis of myocardial ischemia and necrosis. Clin. Chem., 26:1241, 1980.
23. Roberts, R., Sobel, B. E., and Parker, C. W.: Radioimmunoassay for creatine kinase isoenzymes. Science, 194:855, 1976.
24. Weidner, N.: Laboratory diagnosis of acute myocardial infarct. Usefulness of determination of lactate dehydrogenase LDH-1 level and the ratio of LDH-1 to total LDH. Arch. Pathol. Lab. Med., 106:375, 1982.
25. Cooksey, J. D., Dunn, M., and Massie, E. (Eds.): Clinical Vectorcardiography and Electrocardiograph. 2nd Ed. Chicago, Year Book, 1977.
26. Braat, S. H., et al.: Value of electrocardiography in diagnosing right ventricular involvement in patients with acute inferior wall myocardial infarction. Br. Heart J., 49:368, 1983.
27. Robalino, B. D., Whitlow, P. L., Underwood, D. A., and Salcedo, E. E.: Electrocardiographic manifestations of right ventricular infarction. Am. Heart J., 118:138, 1989.
28. Brattler, A., et al. The initial chest x-ray in acute myocardial infarction. Prediction of early and late mortality and survival. Circulation, 61:1004, 1980.
29. Bigger, J. T., et al.: Ventricular arrhythmias in ischemic heart disease. Mechanism, prevalence, significance, and management. Prog. Cardiovasc. Dis., 19:255, 1977.
30. Crampton, R. S., et al.: Reduction of prehospital ambulance and community coronary death rates by the community-wide emergency cardiac care system. Am. J. Med., 58:151, 1975.
31. Cobb, L. A., et al.: Resuscitation from out of hospital ventricular fibrillation: 4 years' follow-up. Circulation, 51(Suppl. III):223, 1975.
32. Lewis, R. P., et al.: Reduction of mortality from prehospital myocardial infarction by prudent patient activation of mobile cardiac care system. Am. Heart J., 103:123, 1982.
33. Maroko, P. R., Radvany, P., Braunwald, E., and Hale, S. L.:

Reduction of infarct size by oxygen inhalation following acute coronary occlusion. Circulation, 52:360, 1975.
34. Fillmore, S. J., Shapiro, M., and Killip, T.: Arterial oxygen tension in acute myocardial infarction. Serial analysis of clinical state and blood gas changes. Am. Heart J., 79:620, 1970.
35. Gruppo Italiano Per Lo Studio Della Streptochinasi Nell'Infarcto Miocardico (GISSI): Effectiveness of intravenous thrombolytic therapy in acute myocardial infarction. Lancet, 1:397, 1986.
36. Koren, G., et al.: Prevention of myocardial damage in acute myocardial ischemia by early treatment with intravenous streptokinase. N. Engl. J. Med., 312:1384, 1985.
37. Mathey, D. G., et al.: Nonsurgical coronary artery recanalization in acute transmural myocardial infarction. Circulation, 63:489, 1981.
38. Serruys, P. W., et al.: Coronary recanalization in acute myocardial infarction. Immediate results and potential risks. Eur. Heart J., 3:404, 1982.
39. Serruys, P. W., et al.: Preservation of global and regional left ventricular function after early thrombolysis in acute myocardial infarction. J. Am. Coll. Cardiol., 7:729, 1986.
40. Simoons, M. L., et al.: Early thrombolysis in acute myocardial infarction: limitation of infarct size and improved survival. J. Am. Coll. Cardiol., 7:717, 1986.
41. DeWood, M. A., et al.: Prevalence of total coronary occlusion during the early hours of transmural myocardial infarction. N. Engl. J. Med., 303:897, 1980.
42. ISAM Study Group: A prospective trial of intravenous streptokinase in acute myocardial infarction (ISAM). N. Engl. J. Med., 314:1465, 1986.
43. AIMS Trial Study Group: Effect of intravenous APSAC on mortality after acute myocardial infarction: preliminary report on a placebo-controlled clinical trial. Lancet, 1:545, 1988.
44. ISIS-2 (Second International Study of Infarct Survival) Collaborative Group: Randomized trial of intravenous streptokinase, oral aspirin, both, or neither among 17,187 cases of suspected acute myocardial infarction. ISIS-2. Lancet, 2:349, 1988.
45. Wilcox, R. G., et al.: The ASSET Study Group: trial of tissue plasminogen activator for mortality reduction in acute myocardial infarction: Anglo-Scandinavian Study of Early Thrombolysis (ASSET). Lancet, 2:525, 1988.
46. Van de Werf, F., Arnold, A. E. R., and the European Cooperative Study Group for recombinant tissue-type plasminogen activator (rt-PA). Intravenous rt-PA and size of infarct, left ventricular function and survival in acute myocardial infarction. Br. Med. J., 297:1374, 1988.
47. Becker, R. C., and Alpert, J. S.: Current management of acute myocardial infarction. Curr. Probl. Cardiol., 14:507, 1989.
48. Gunnar, R. M., et al.: Guidelines for the early management of patients with acute myocardial infarction: a report of the American College of Cardiology/American Heart Association Task Force on assessment of diagnostic and therapeutic cardiovascular procedures (Subcommittee to develop guidelines for the early management of patients with acute myocardial infarction). J. Am. Coll. Cardiol., 16:249, 1990.
49. Hogg, K. J., et al.: Comparative effects of antistreplase and streptokinase on coronary artery patency in acute myocardial infarction. (abstract.) Circulation, 80(Suppl. II):II-419, 1989.
50. Pacouret, G., Charbonnier, B., and Trousseau, C. H. U.: Multicentre European randomized trial of anistreplase versus streptokinase in acute myocardial infarction. (abstract.) Circulation, 80(Suppl. II):II-420, 1989.
51. Anderson, J. L., et al.: Comparison of intravenous anistreplase (APSAC) and streptokinase in acute myocardial infarction: interim report of a randomized, double-blind patency study. (abstract.) Circulation, 80(Suppl. II):II-420, 1989.
52. TIMI Study Group: The thrombolysis in myocardial infarction trial: phase I findings. N. Engl. J. Med., 312:932, 1985.
53. European Cooperative Study Group for Recombinant Tissue-Type Plasminogen Activator: Randomized trial of intravenous recombinant tissue-type plasminogen activator versus intravenous streptokinase in acute myocardial infarction. Lancet, 1:842, 1985.
54. GISSI-2: A factorial randomized trial of alteplase versus streptokinase and heparin versus no heparin among 12,490 patients with acute myocardial infarction. Lancet, 2:65, 1990.
55. International Study Group: In-hospital mortality and clinical course of 20,891 patients with suspected acute myocardial infarction randomized between alteplase and streptokinase with or without heparin. Lancet, 2:71, 1990.
56. The GUSTO Investigators: An international randomized trial comparing four thrombolytic strategies for acute myocardial infarction. N. Engl. J. Med., 329:673, 1993.
57. Hochman, J. S., and Choo, H.: Limitation of myocardial infarction expansion by reperfusion independent of myocardial salvage. Circulation, 75:299, 1987.
58. Bates, E.: Reperfusion therapy in inferior myocardial infarction. J. Am. Coll. Cardiol., 12:44A, 1988.
59. Roig, E., et al.: In-hospital mortality rates from acute myocardial infarction by race in U.S. hospitals: findings from the National Hospital Discharge Survey. Circulation, 76:280, 1987.
60. Califf, R. M., et al.: Hemorrhage complications associated with the use of intravenous tissue plasminogen activator in treatment of acute myocardial infarction. Am. J. Med., 85:353, 1988.
61. Topol, E. J., et al.: A randomized trial of immediate versus delayed elective angioplasty after intravenous tissue plasminogen activator in treatment of acute myocardial infarction. N. Engl. J. Med., 317:581, 1987.
62. Simoons, M. L., et al. Thrombolysis with tissue plasminogen activator in acute myocardial infarction: no additional benefit from immediate percutaneous transluminal angioplasty. Lancet, 1:197, 1988.
63. TIMI Research Group: Immediate vs delayed catheterization and angioplasty following thrombolytic therapy for acute myocardial infarction. JAMA, 260:2849, 1988.
64. Hartzler, G. O., et al.: Percutaneous transluminal coronary angioplasty with and without thrombolytic therapy for treatment of acute myocardial infarction. Am. Heart J., 106:965, 1983.
65. Pepine, C. J., et al.: Percutaneous transluminal coronary angioplasty in acute myocardial infarction. Am. Heart J., 107:820, 1984.
66. O'Neill, W., et al.: A prospective randomized clinical trial of intracoronary streptokinase versus coronary angioplasty therapy of acute myocardial infarction. N. Engl. J. Med., 314:813, 1986.
67. Kimura, T., Nosaka, H., Ueno, K., and Nobuyoshi, N.: Role of coronary angioplasty in acute myocardial infarction. Circulation, 74(Suppl. II):II-22, 1986.
68. Rothbaum, D. A., et al.: Emergency percutaneous transluminal angioplasty in acute myocardial infarction: a 3-year experience. J. Am. Coll. Cardiol., 10:264, 1987.
69. Marco, J., et al.: Emergency percutaneous transluminal angioplasty without thrombolysis as initial therapy in acute myocardial infarction. Int. J. Cardiol., 15:55, 1987.
70. Topol, E. J.: Direct or Sequential PTCA in Acute Coronary

Intervention. Edited by E. J. Topol. New York, Alan R Liss, 1988.
71. Grmes, C. L., et al.: A comparison of immediate angioplasty with thrombolytic therapy for acute myocardial infarction. N. Engl. J. Med., 328:673, 1993.
72. DeWood, M. A., et al.: Medical and surgical management of myocardial infarction. Am. J. Cardiol., 44:1356, 1979.
73. Berg, R., et al.: Immediate coronary artery bypass for acute evolving myocardial infarction. J. Thorac. Cardiovasc. Surg., 81:493, 1981.
74. Phillips, S. J., et al.: Reperfusion protocol and results in 738 patients with evolving myocardial infarction. Ann. Thorac. Surg., 41:119, 1986.
75. Flameng, W., Sergeant, P., Van Haecke, J., and Suy, R.: Emergency coronary bypass grafting for evolving myocardial infarction: effects on infarct size and left ventricular function. J. Thorac. Cardiovasc. Surg., 94:124, 1987.
76. Koshal, A., et al.: Urgent surgical reperfusion in acute evolving myocardial infarction: a randomized controlled study. Circulation, 74(Suppl. I):I-171, 1988.
77. Cohn, L. H.: Surgical treatment of acute myocardial infarction. Chest, 93(Suppl. I):135, 1988.
78. Reul, G. J., et al.: Coronary artery bypass for unsuccessful percutaneous transluminal angioplasty. J. Thorac. Cardiovasc. Surg., 88:685, 1984.
79. Golding, A. R., et al.: Early results of emergency surgery after coronary angioplasty. Circulation, 74(Suppl. II):II-26, 1986.
80. Furberg, C. D., and Byington, R. P.: Beta-adrenergic blockers in patients with acute myocardial infarction. Cardiovasc. Clin., 20:235, 1989.
81. Yusuf, S., et al.: Beta blockage during and after myocardial infarction: an overview of the randomized trials. Prog. Cardiovasc. Dis., 27:335, 1985.
82. MIAMI Trial Research Group: Metoprolol in Acute Myocardial Infarction (MIAMI). Am. J. Cardiol., 56:IG, 1985.
83. ISIS-1 (First International Study of Infarct Survival) Collaborative Group: Randomized trial of intravenous atenolol among 16,027 cases of suspected acute myocardial infarction: ISIS-1. Lancet, 2:57, 1986.
84. TIMI Study Group: Comparison of invasive and conservative strategies after treatment with intravenous tissue plasminogen activator in acute myocardial infarction: results of the Thrombolysis in Myocardial Infarction (TIMI) Phase II trial. N. Engl. J. Med., 320:618, 1989.
85. Yusuf, S.: Interventions that potentially limit myocardial infarct size: overview of clinical trials. Am. J. Cardiol., 60:11A, 1987.
86. Stockman, M. D., Verrier, R. L., and Lown, B.: Effect of nitroglycerin on vulnerability of ventricular fibrillation during myocardial ischemia and reperfusion. Am. J. Cardiol., 43:237, 1979.
87. Bussman, W. D., Passek, D., Seidel, W., and Kaltenbach, M.: Reduction of CK and CK-MB indexes of infarct size by intravenous nitroglycerin. Circulation, 63:615, 1981.
88. Judgutt, B. I., and Warnica, J. W.: Intravenous nitroglycerin therapy to limit myocardial infarct size, expansion and complications: effect of timing dosage and infarct location. Circulation, 78:906, 1988.
89. Yusuf, S., Collins, R., MacMahon, S., and Peto, R.: Effect of intravenous nitrates on mortality in acute myocardial infarction: an overview of the randomized trials. Lancet, 1:1088, 1988.
90. ISIS Collaborative Group: ISIS-4: randomized study of oral isosorbide mononitrate in over 50,000 patients with suspected acute myocardial infarction. Circulation, 88(Suppl. I):I-394, 1993.
91. Gunnar, R., et al.: Task Force IV: pharmacologic interventions. Am. J. Cardiol., 50:393, 1982.
92. Fleckenstein, A.: History of calcium antagonists. Circ. Res., 52(Suppl. I):I-3, 1983.
93. Multicenter Diltiazem Postinfarction Trial Research Group: The effect of diltiazem on mortality and reinfarction after myocardial infarction. N. Engl. J. Med., 319:385, 1988.
94. Gibson, R. S., et al.: Diltiazem and reinfarction in patients with non-Q wave myocardial infarction: results of a double-blind, randomized, multicenter trial. N. Engl. J. Med., 315:423, 1986.
95. Muller, J. E., et al.: Nifedipine therapy for patients with threatened and acute myocardial infarction: a randomized, double-blind, placebo-controlled comparison. Circulation, 69:740, 1984.
96. Norwegian Study Group: Nifedipine in acute myocardial infarction: no influence on infarct size. Circulation, 68(Suppl. III):III-22, 1983.
97. Neufeld, H. N.: Calcium antagonists in secondary prevention after acute myocardial infarction: the Secondary Prevention Reinfarct Nifedipine Trial (SPRINT). Eur. Heart J., 7:51, 1986.
98. Wilcox, R. G., et al.: Trial of early nifedipine treatment in patients with suspected myocardial infarction (the Trent Study). Br. Heart. J., 55:506, 1986.
99. Danish Study Group: Verapamil and acute myocardial infarction. Eur. Heart J., 5:516, 1984.
100. Roberts, R.: Recognition, diagnosis, and prognosis of early reinfarction: the role of calcium-channel blockers. Circulation, 75(Suppl. V):V-139, 1987.
101. Skolnick, A. E., and Frishman, W. H.: Calcium channel blockers in myocardial infarction. Arch. Intern. Med., 149:1669, 1989.
102. Erbel, R., et al.: Combination of calcium channel blocker and thrombolytic therapy in acute myocardial infarction. Br. Heart J., 115:529, 1988.
103. ISIS Collaborative Group: ISIS-4: randomized study of oral captopril in over 50,000 patients with suspected acute myocardial infarction. Circulation, 88(Suppl. I):I-394, 1993.
104. Pasternak, R. C., et al.: Acute myocardial infarction. In Heart Disease: A Textbook of Cardiovascular Medicine. 3rd Ed. Edited by E. Brawnwald. Philadelphia, W. B. Saunders, 1988.
105. Meltzer, L. E., and Cohen, H. E.: The incidence of arrhythmias associated with acute myocardial infarction. In Textbook of Coronary Care. Edited by L. E. Meltzer and A. J. Dunning. Philadelphia, Charles Press, 1977.
106. Bigger, J. R., Weld, R. M., and Rolnitzky, L. M.: Prevalence, characteristics and significance of ventricular tachycardia (three or more complexes) detected with ambulatory electrocardiographic recording in the late hospital phase of acute myocardial infarction. Am. J. Cardiol., 48:815, 1981.
107. Toffler, G. H., et al.: Prognosis after myocardial infarction complicated by ventricular fibrillation. Circulation, 74:II-304, 1986.
108. Volpi, A., et al.: In-hospital prognosis of patients with acute myocardial infarction complicated by primary ventricular fibrillation. N. Engl. J. Med., 318:19, 1988.
109. Chadda, K. D., Lichstein, E., Gupta, P. K., and Choy, R.: Bradycardia-hypotension syndrome in acute myocardial infarction: reappraisal of the overdrive effects of atropine. Am. J. Med., 59:158, 1975.
110. Warren, J. V., and Lewis, R. P.: Beneficial effects of atropine in the prehospital phase of coronary care. Am. J. Cardiol., 37:68, 1976.
111. Zoll, P. M., et al.: External noninvasive temporary cardiac pacing clinic trials. Circulation, 71:937, 1985.

112. Topol, E. J., et al.: Hemodynamic benefit of atrial pacing in right ventricular myocardial infarction. Ann. Intern. Med., *96:*594, 1982.
113. Love, J. C., Haffajee, C. I., Gore, J. M., and Alpert, J. S.: Reversibility of hypotension and shock by atrial or atrioventricular sequential pacing in patients with right ventricular infarction. Am. Heart J., *108:*5, 1984.
114. Frye, R. L., et al.: Guidelines for permanent cardiac pacemaker implantation: a report of the Task Force on Assessment of Diagnostic and Therapeutic Cardiovascular Procedures (Subcommittee on pacemaker implantation). J. Am. Coll. Cardiol., *4:*434, 1984.
115. Killip, T., and Kimball, J. R.: Treatment of myocardial infarction in a coronary care unit. A two-year with 250 patients. Am. J. Cardiol., *20:*457, 1967.
116. Franciosa, J. S., et al.: Improved left ventricular function during nitroprusside infusion in acute myocardial infarction. Lancet, *1:*650, 1972.
117. Gillespie, T. A., Ambos, H. D., Sobel, B. E., and Roberts, R.: Effects of dobutamine in patients with acute myocardial infarction. Am. J. Cardiol., *39:*588, 1977.
118. Aubier, M., Trippenbach, T., and Roussos, C.: Respiratory muscle fatigue during cardiogenic shock. J. Appl. Physiol., *51:*499, 1981.
119. Dewood, M. A., et al.: Medical and surgical management of myocardial infarction. Am. J. Cardiol., *44:*1356, 1979.
120. Lee, L., et al.: Percutaneous transluminal angioplasty improves survival in acute myocardial infarction complicated by cardiogenic shock. Circulation, *78:*1345, 1988.
121. Dellborg, M., Held, P., Swedberg, K., and Vedin, A.: Rupture of the myocardium: occurrence and risk factors. Br. Heart J., *54:*11, 1985.
122. Dagget, W. M., et al.: Improved results of surgical management of postinfarction ventricular rupture. Ann. Surg., *196:*269, 1982.
123. Isner, J. M., and Roberts, W. C.: Right ventricular infarction complication left ventricular infarction secondary to coronary heart disease. Am. J. Cardiol., *42:*885, 1978.
124. Ratliff, N. B., and Hackel, D. B.: Combined right and left ventricular infarction: pathogenesis and clinicopathologic correlation. Am. J. Cardiol., *45:*217, 1980.
125. Cohn, J. N., Guiha, N. H., Breder, M. I., and Limas, C. J.: Right ventricular infarction. Clinical and hemodynamic features. Am. J. Cardiol., *33:*209, 1974.
126. Isner, J. M.: Right ventricular myocardial infarction. JAMA, *259:*712, 1988.
127. Dell'Italia, L. J., and Starling, M. R.: Right ventricular infarction: an important clinical entity. Curr. Probl. Cardiol., *9:*1, 1984.
128. Dell'Italia, L. J., et al.: Comparative effects of volume loading, dobutamine, and nitroprusside in patients with predominant right ventricular infarction. Circulation, *72:*1327, 1985.
129. Moreyra, A. E., Suh, C., Porway, M. N., and Kostis, J. B.: Rapid hemodynamic improvement in right ventricular infarction after coronary angioplasty. Chest, *94:*198, 1988.
130. Pryor, D. B., et al.: Early discharge after acute myocardial infarction. Ann. Intern. Med., *99:*528, 1983.
131. Hessen, S. E., and Brest, A. N.: Risk profiling the patient after acute myocardial infarction. Cardiovasc. Clin., *20:*283, 1989.
132. DeBusk, R. F., et al.: Identification and treatment of low-risk patients after acute myocardial infarction and coronary artery bypass graft surgery. N. Engl. J. Med., *314:*161, 1986.
133. American College of Cardiology/American Heart Association: Guidelines for exercise testing: a report of the American College of Cardiology/American Heart Association Task Force on Assessment of Diagnostic and Therapeutic Cardiovascular Procedures (Subcommittee on Exercise Testing). J. Am. Coll. Cardiol., *8:*725, 1986.
134. DeBusk, R. F.: Specialized testing after recent acute myocardial infarction. Ann. Intern. Med., *110:*470, 1989.
135. DeBusk, R. F., and Haskell, W.: Symptom-limited vs heart-rate-limited exercise testing soon after myocardial infarction. Circulation, *61:*738, 1990.
136. DeBusk, R. F., and Dennis, C. A.: "Submaximal" predischarge exercise testing after acute myocardial infarction: who needs it? Am. J. Cardiol., *55:*498, 1985.
137. The Multicenter Postinfarction Research Group. Risk stratification and survival after myocardial infarction. N. Engl. J. Med., *309:*331, 1983.
138. Mukharji, J., et al.: Risk factors for sudden death after acute myocardial infarction: two year follow-up. Am. J. Cardiol., *54:*31, 1984.
139. Taylor, G. J., et al.: Predictors of clinical course, coronary anatomy and left ventricular function after recovery from acute myocardial infarction. Circulation, *62:*960, 1980.
140. Norris, R. M., et al.: Prognosis after recovery from first acute myocardial infarction: determinants of reinfarction and sudden death. Am. J. Cardiol., *53:*408, 1984.
141. Ahnve, S., et al.: Limitations and advantages of the ejection fraction for defining high risk after acute myocardial infarction. Am. J. Cardiol., *58:*872, 1986.
142. Bigger, J. R., et al., for the Multicenter Postinfarction Research Group. The relationships among ventricular arrhythmias, left ventricular dysfunction, and mortality in the two years after myocardial infarction. Circulation, *69:*250, 1984.
143. Rapaport, E., and Remedios, P.: The high-risk patient after recovery from myocardial infarction: recognition and management. J. Am. Coll. Cardiol., *1:*391, 1983.
144. Bigger, J. T., Fleiss, J. L., Rolnitzky, L. M., for the Multicenter Postinfarction Research Group. Prevalence, characteristics and significance of ventricular tachycardia detected by 24-hour electrocardiographic recording in the late phase of acute myocardial infarction. Am. J. Cardiol., *58:*1157, 1986.
145. Kostis, J. B., et al., for the BHAT Study Group. Prognostic significance of ventricular ectopic activity in survivors of acute myocardial infarction. J. Am. Coll. Cardiol., *10:*231, 1987.
146. Curtis, A. B., and Mansour, M.: New approaches to management of arrhythmias after myocardial infarction. Cardiovasc. Clin., *20:*259, 1989.
147. Yusuf, S., et al.: Beta blockage during and after myocardial infarction: an overview of the randomized trials. Prog. Cardiovasc. Dis., *27:*335, 1985.
148. Beta-Blocker Heart Attack Research Group: A randomized trial of propranolol in patients with acute myocardial infarction. I. Mortality results. JAMA, *247:*1707, 1982.
149. Norwegian Multicenter Study Group: Timolol-induced reduction in mortality and reinfarction in patients surviving acute myocardial infarction. N. Engl. J. Med., *304:*801, 1981.
150. Chesbro, J. H., and Fuster, V.: Antithrombotic therapy for acute myocardial infarction: mechanisms and prevention of deep venous left ventricular and coronary artery thromboembolism. Circulation, *74(Suppl. III):*III-1, 1986.
151. Meltzer, R. S., Visser, C. A., and Fuster, V.: Intracardiac thrombi and systemic embolization. Ann. Intern. Med., *104:*689, 1986.
152. Guerci, A. D., et al.: A randomized trial of intravenous tissue plasminogen activator for acute myocardial infarction with subsequent randomization to elective angiography. N. Engl. J. Med., *317:*1613, 1987.
153. Fuster, V., Stein, B., Badimon, L., and Chesbro, J. H.: Anti-

thrombolytic therapy after myocardial reperfusion in acute myocardial infarction. J. Am. Coll. Cardiol., *12(Suppl. A):* 78A, 1988.
154. Acheson, J., et al.: Secondary prevention of vascular disease by prolonged antiplatelet treatment: antiplatelet trialists; collaboration. Br. Med. J., *296:*320, 1988.
155. Rossouw, J. E., Lewis, B., and Rifkind, B. M.: The value of lowering cholesterol after myocardial infarction. N. Engl. J. Med., *323:*1112, 1990.
156. Ornish, D., et al.: Can lifestyle changes reverse coronary heart disease? The lifestyle heart trial. Lancet, *336:*129, 1990.

Chapter 30

SURGICAL INTERVENTION IN MYOCARDIAL ISCHEMIA AND INFARCTION

THOMAS L. HIGGINS
INDERJIT S. GILL
FLOYD D. LOOP

PRE-ICU PHASE

Profile of the Candidate for Myocardial Revascularization

Despite widespread awareness of the risk factors for developing coronary artery disease and improved options for therapy, over 500,000 deaths still occur each year in the United States from myocardial infarction.[1] Over 5 million people suffer from symptomatic coronary artery disease with presentations ranging from stable angina, to myocardial infarction, to sudden cardiac death. Many of these patients are candidates for myocardial revascularization on an elective or emergent basis.

Angina is the subjective sensation associated with myocardial ischemia, brought on by an imbalance between myocardial oxygen supply and demand. Stable angina is the term used to describe precordial discomfort brought about by a known activity whereas unstable angina is used to describe a symptom complex of worsening severity more serious than stable angina pectoris but short of frank myocardial infarction. The Veterans Administration study[2] defines the term "chronic stable angina," by the clinical characteristics of Table 30-1, and the criteria for inclusion into the National Cooperative Study for Unstable Angina[3] are listed in Table 30-2. Strict criteria suitable for study groups are not necessarily representative of the clinical status of most patients. In the Veterans Administration study[2] only 1464 of the 3659 patients originally screened fulfilled the criteria for chronic stable angina. Even the term "chronic stable angina" may be misleading, as symptom stability is not necessarily related to patient stability. The risk of sudden death is better related to coronary anatomy and left ventricular function than anginal symptoms. Natural history data from the Framingham study shows that if angina patients are taken as a group, 30% will die within 8 years of the onset of angina and 44% of these deaths will be sudden.[4]

Myocardial infarction, defined as sudden irreversible damage of the myocardium, results from an acute imbalance between oxygen supply and demand, usually as a result of sudden occlusion of a coronary artery. Prevention of myocardial infarction by medical, surgical, or nonsurgical percutaneous intervention is the mainstay of treatment for the patient at risk. This chapter will concentrate on the perioperative care of patients selected for surgical therapy.

Surgical intervention for myocardial ischemia and its manifestations has evolved both to alleviate the symptoms and to reduce the risk of myocardial damage and death from coronary artery disease. Coronary artery bypass grafting for coronary artery disease was first performed in 1967 by Favalaro.[5] The development of such modalities as thrombolysis, angioplasty, stents, and atherectomy devices has changed the profile of the surgical patient. Primary myocardial revascularization procedures, especially for single-vessel disease, are now less common,[6] whereas the incidence of repeat operation has steadily increased to over 20% in some centers.[7] Thus, compared to a decade ago, patients currently presenting for surgery are often older with more extensive coronary disease and more numerous concurrent medical problems with a higher rate of reoperation (Fig. 30-1).

Indications for Surgery in Stable Angina

The principal objectives of coronary revascularization are relief of angina and prolongation of survival. Secondary end points are the reduction of other late cardiac events and restoration of a more normal life style, including return to work when applicable.

Indications for elective coronary bypass grafting with stable angina are constantly changing as new alternatives emerge, but commonly accepted indications in the early 1990s include:

- Disabling life style restricting symptoms despite optimal medical therapy
- Left main disease (greater than 50% narrowing)
- Proximal high grade stenosis (greater than 70%) in two or three vessels associated with angina and/or ischemia
- Proximal stenosis (greater with 70%) of the left anterior descending artery, supplying a large area of the anterior wall

The concept of "myocardial jeopardy," which is defined as the perceived assessment of the relationship between proximal lesions and retained wall motion, is the most important determinant of coronary artery surgery referral as assessed by referral patterns in a Coronary Artery Surgery Study (CASS) report involving 15 sites.[8]

Table 30–1. Criteria for Chronic Stable Angina
History of stable angina pectoris for at least 6 months
Established medical therapy program for at least 3 months
ECG abnormalities of old infarction, abnormal T waves or ST segments or a positive stress test

Table 30–2. Clinical Criteria of Unstable Angina
Pain
Angina pectoris of new onset
Changing pattern of angina pectoris
Coronary care unit admission-suspected impending infarction
ECG changes associated with angina
New q waves: no enzyme changes in 24 hours
No myocardial infarction within 3 months
Age <71 years

Indications for Surgery in Acute Myocardial Ischemia

Treatment strategies for acute myocardial ischemia, once limited to nitrates, bedrest, sedation, and observation in a coronary care unit, have also grown over the last two decades. Options now include thrombolysis, emergency surgical revascularization, and emergency angioplasty.

Emergency surgical revascularization for unstable angina was first reported by Hill and associates in 1971.[9] Outcome reports from surgical revascularization in this setting have been conflicting and comparisons are limited by differences in patient characteristics.[9] Nonetheless, survival continues to improve[10,11] as experience with grafting techniques has grown, aided by the application of mechanical support (notably the intra-aortic balloon pump),[12] improved methods of myocardial protection, better anesthetic management, and improved pharmacotherapy.

The current indications for surgical intervention in acute myocardial ischemia are:[13]

- Unstable angina and multivessel coronary artery disease with or without hemodynamic instability
- Postinfarction angina, resistant to medical therapy, and with coronary artery anatomy unsuited to percutaneous transluminal coronary angioplasty (PTCA)
- Failed PTCA/thrombolysis in acute myocardial infarction (less than 6 hours' duration)
- Cardiogenic shock with multivessel coronary artery disease
- Myocardial infarction with or without cardiogenic shock associated with the following mechanical defects:
  Rupture of the ventricular septum
  Rupture of the papillary muscle of the mitral valve
  Rupture of the free wall of the left ventricle
- Semi urgent cardiac transplantation with or without a mechanical "bridge" in young patients (less than 55 years old) with a massive acute myocardial infarction.

An "urgent" operation is defined as one performed within 24 hours of an event and an "emergency" operation is one performed as soon as the patient can be brought to the operating room.

As a primary mode of therapy, emergency surgery has several potential advantages beyond abolishing the obstruction responsible for the acute event. For example, other significantly obstructed vessels can be bypassed thereby ensuring more complete revascularization. Putting the patient on cardiopulmonary bypass and decompressing the ventricle is the most effective way of optimizing reperfusion and reducing cardiac work. The use of blood cardioplegia,[14] the addition of substrates such as glutamate, aspartate[15] to the cardioplegia, and use of oxygen free radical scavengers like allopurinol and superoxide dismutase[16] in modifying reperfusion injury have all been proposed to be beneficial.

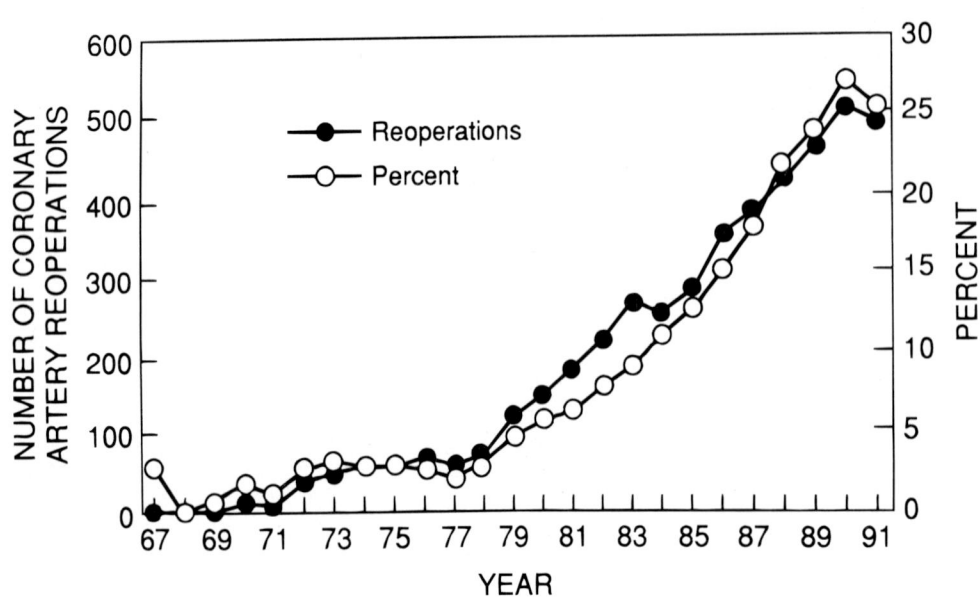

Fig. 30–1. Reoperation rate for isolated coronary artery surgery at the Cleveland Clinic from 1967 to 1991.

The most extensive experience with emergency coronary bypass in acute evolving myocardial infarction is reported from Spokane, Washington.[17,18] This nonrandomized study involved 387 patients with myocardial infarction managed surgically or medically with comparable baseline variables such as age, gender, infarct location, number of diseased vessels, and Killip classification. The in-hospital mortality rate was 5.8% in the surgical group, and 11.5% in the medical group (p < 0.07). Long-term mortalities were 27 and 41%, respectively (p < 0.0007) at 10 to 13 years; however, these data were collected in 1979 before many of the current medical therapies such as thrombolysis were available.

Conflicting surgical results and the introduction of beta blockers to treat unstable angina prompted a variety of preoperative randomized trials to compare urgent coronary bypass surgery with medical therapy. Several studies[19,21] suggest that mortality rates for surgical and medical patients are similar. These studies demonstrated that initial medical management of patients with unstable angina followed later by elective revascularization is safe. This strategy has resulted in markedly improved surgical results. Cohn had an operative mortality of 1.8% in patients who could be controlled medically versus 5.5% in those needing urgent surgery.[22] Similarly, the Stanford group reports an operative mortality of 12%, and an 8% infarction rate in emergency operations, but only 1% mortality and 3% perioperative infarction rate in delayed elective surgery.[23]

Thus, initial medical stabilization, with urgent bypass reserved only for patients with continued refractory ischemia, is now standard protocol for unstable angina in many centers.

For acute evolving infarction, a combination of initial thrombolysis followed by PTCA or appropriately timed bypass may yield the best results.[24] Immediate thrombolytic therapy is the most rational means of establishing early reperfusion, particularly because many patients present to centers were cardiac surgery is not performed.

Approximately 20% of cases need emergency surgical revascularization after failed thrombolytic therapy.[25] Skinner and colleagues report a hospital mortality of 17% in such cases. "Rescue" PTCA in such patients may be indicated and has been examined in a small number of trials. In the TAMI-I trial, 86 such patients had an in-hospital mortality of 10.4%.[26]

Identification of Risk Factors

Identifying risk factors is important not only to facilitate outcome comparison, but also for directing interventions in patients at high risk for complications. Several large studies, using the technique of multivariate analysis, have identified the risk factors in both primary[27-29] and coronary reoperation.[30,31] Other studies have concentrated on individual risk factors or identifying quality of care problems, but the factors most often cited are remarkably consistent (Table 30-3). Patients of advanced age are at higher risk for both mortality and postoperative complications, whether "elderly" is considered over age 65,[32] age 70,[33] or age 80.[34,35] Females appear to be at higher risk than males,[28,35] although this may be primarily due to smaller body and coronary vessel size in females, rather than gender itself.[36] The integrity of the cardiovascular system is also important as concurrent valvular disease,[37] ventricular

Table 30-3. Variables Predicting Operative Mortality

Source (Reference) Era n	CASS (27) 1975-1978 6,176	Montreal Heart (60) 1980 500	Cleveland Clinic (29) 1970-1982 24,672	Newark Beth Israel (61) 1982-1987 3,500	NY State (62) 1989 7,596	Veterans Administration (211) 1987 10,634	Cleveland Clinic (46) 1986-1990 9,212	New England (63) 1987-1989 3,055
Emergency	+	+	+	+	+	+	+	+
Renal dysfunction				+	+	+	+	+
Advanced age	+	+	+	+	+	+	+	+
Poor left ventricular function or congestive heart failure	+	+	+	+	+	+	+	+
Mitral valve disease	+			+	+	+	+	3
Aortic valve disease				+	+		+	3
Other operation	+			+	+	+		3
Left main coronary artery disease	+		+		+			
Left ventricular aneurysm	+			+				0
Female gender	+		+	+	+	1	2	+
Low body weight							+	+
Obesity		+		+				
Prior heart operation		+		+	+	+	+	+
Chronic obstructive pneumonary disease						+	+	+
Peripheral vascular disease						+	+	+
Cerebrovascular disease						+	+	
Diabetes				+	++	+	+	
Other systemic process		+		+			+	

1. VA Study: Females were only 0.8% of the population undergoing coronary artery bypass grafting.
2. Female gender assumes importance in absence of body weight.
3. Study excluded patients undergoing valve or other surgery.

aneurysms,[38] and left ventricular dysfunction[39] have all been shown to increase mortality risk. Some studies implicate coronary anatomy (left main equivalent, multivessel disease) as risk factors, but these risks have been minimized in more recent studies,[29] perhaps due to greater attention to management of operative hypotension, tachycardia, and ischemia.[40-42]

Emergency surgery is a highly significant risk factor. Patients undergoing emergency procedures for treatment of acute coronary insufficiency uncontrolled by medical therapy, ischemic acute valvular dysfunction, unstable hemodynamics, and complications of coronary angiography or percutaneous transluminal angioplasty often have minimal time to be adequately prepared or fully monitored. For example, PTCA in a patient with dissecting left anterior descending artery it is more important to get on bypass quickly than to spend time inserting a pulmonary artery catheter. These patients may present in heart failure, cardiogenic shock, or during resuscitation from a cardiac arrest. Those in cardiogenic shock have the worst prognosis, but emergency surgery after failure of angioplasty also carries a significant risk of postoperative morbidity and mortality.[43,44]

Reoperation (meaning second or higher definitive operation as opposed to immediate postoperative reentry to control bleeding) carries an increased risk of death in most studies[30,31] both because of the generally worse cardiovascular status of these patients, and the potential for surgical technical difficulties. Patients undergoing reoperation frequently have more severe and/or diffuse coronary artery disease, and adequate myocardial protection and/or complete revascularization may not be achieved.[31] Reentry of the chest can be complicated by massive bleeding due to injury of a previous graft of a major vessel. Dissection of adhesions increases the incidence of both intra- and postoperative bleeding. Manipulation of the heart during dissection causes hemodynamic instabilities, and can precipitate arrhythmias and ischemia. Postoperatively, reoperation patients require more vasoactive drug support, and have prolonged ventilation time and intensive care duration.[45] The incidence of perioperative myocardial infarction and surgical complications with reoperation may not be significantly greater, however.[30] Increased experience with reoperations may also be narrowing the morbidity and mortality gap between first time and reoperation patients.[31]

The presence of **extracardiac vascular disease** is a marker for systemic atherosclerosis, and preliminary evidence suggests that patients with a history of carotid disease, or who have undergone prior vascular surgical procedures are at higher risk for postoperative morbidity.[46] Patients with end-stage renal disease have increased risk[47,48] and our experience suggests that even moderate preoperative elevation of serum creatinine is a marker for postoperative events with increased risk demonstrable at values above 1.6 mg %.[46]

Chronic obstructive airway disease is a risk factor for prolonged postoperative ventilation even in nonthoracic operations, and acquires increased significance with lung resection or compromise of the bellows function of the lung.[49] The combination of midexpiratory flow (MMEF 50 to 75) and maximum expiratory pressures is reported to predict the need for prolonged postoperative ventilatory support in adult cardiac patients,[50] however these measurements may not be obtained routinely in all patients. Nonpulmonary factors increasing the risk of respiratory complications following cardiac surgery include congestive heart failure at the time of operation, emergency procedure, reoperation, elevated preoperative creatinine, aortic stenosis, prior vascular surgery, mitral insufficiency, and advanced age.[51] **Smoking cessation,** while advisable, must occur at least 8 weeks before operation to effect substantial improvement.[52] Since recovery of pulmonary function may take 7 days or longer,[53] chronic obstructive pulmonary disease (COPD) may contribute to increased morbidity by prolonging time on mechanical ventilation with attendant risk of superinfection.

Diabetes mellitus is not universally found to be a multivariate risk factor for mortality[27,29] possibly because of the high association of diabetes with other important risks such as left ventricular dysfunction and renal failure. Diabetics are more likely to have cardiovascular lability and subclinical left ventricular abnormalities.[54,55] Diabetes, however, is associated with increased morbidity following coronary artery bypass surgery.[46,51]

Factors known to increase the risk for developing coronary artery disease (i.e., history of smoking, high serum cholesterol level, high triglyceride levels, hypertension), are not necessarily independent risk factors for postoperative mortality following coronary artery surgery, either because of high prevalence in this population, or because these risks are dwarfed in multivariate analysis by the other more important risk factors.

Quantifying Risk by Scoring Systems

Several studies suggest methods by which risks can be quantified. Conventional indices, such as the ASA Physical Status Classification[56] and the Goldman multifactorial index of cardiac risk[57] do not apply to cardiac surgery patients. The New York Heart Association classification grades severity of heart disease on the basis of functional status, but has limited reproducibility and correlates poorly with actual functional ability by treadmill testing.[58] APACHE-II,[59] which scores on the basis of physiologic derangement, is difficult to apply to patients following open heart surgery because many of its variables (e.g., temperature, mean arterial pressure, heart rate, respiratory rate, arterial pH, hematocrit, serum electrolytes, level of consciousness) are deliberately manipulated by the operating room team. Four studies to date have developed either logistic regression equations or simplified scoring systems for cardiac surgical patients.[40,60-63] Factors considered for scoring are compared in Table 30-3. A system that has been prospectively validated at a cross-section of institutions would have applications in adjusting severity of illness for reporting mortality statistics, preoperative patient counseling, quality assurance, and directing special interventions in high risk patients (i.e., renal dopamine infusion, retrograde cardioplegia). Such a study is currently underway, using the system developed at the Cleveland Clinic,[46] which correlates both expected mortality and

Table 30-4. Clinical Severity Scoring System

Preoperative Factors	Score
Emergency case	6
Serum creatinine (mg/dl):	
≥ 1.6 and ≤ 1.8	1
≥ 1.9	4
Severe LV dysfunction	3
Redo operation	3
Mitral valve insufficiency	3
Age (years):	
≥ 65 and ≤ 74	1
≥ 75	2
Prior vascular surgery	2
Chronic obstructive pulmonary disease	2
Anemia (Hct $\leq 34\%$)	2
Aortic stenosis	1
Weight (≤ 65 kg)	1
Diabetes	1
Cerebrovascular disease	1

morbidity with preoperative total score (Table 30-4 and Fig. 30-2).

Peripheral Vascular and Renal Disease

History of claudication or advanced peripheral vascular disease precludes harvesting of veins from the lower extremities since delayed healing and other complications are likely especially in the diabetic patient. The discovery of a carotid bruit, history of a TIA, or cerebrovascular accident mandates a more extensive work-up.[64] Special precautions that may need to be taken at the time of surgery include:

- Simultaneous carotid revascularization[65]
- Maintenance of a higher perfusion pressure on cardiopulmonary bypass (>100 mm Mg (mean) or within 20 mm Hg of preoperative value)

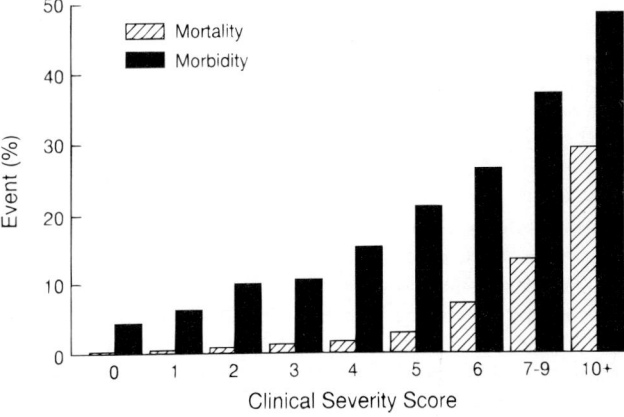

Fig. 30-2. Relationship between preoperative severity score and perioperative morbidity and mortality. Scores are determined by adding the factors in Table 30-4. (From Higgins, T. L., et al.: Stratification of morbidity and mortality outcome by preoperative risk factors in coronary artery bypass patients. JAMA, *267*:2344, 1992.)

- The use of single cross-clamping technique for the construction of the proximal anastomosis to prevent atheroembolism
- The use of intraoperative steroids and barbiturates is controversial[66-68]

Patients with elevated preoperative serum creatinine (>1.6 mg %) are thought to be at risk for postoperative renal failure.[69] While conclusive evidence is lacking, reports suggest a benefit from prophylactic dopamine at renal vasodilating levels (0.5 to 2.0 μg/kg per minute).[70] congestive heart failure is optimized by the use of digitalis, diuretics, and salt and fluid restriction. High risk patients may not have been eating well and can be nutritionally depleted and in need of preoperative enteral or parenteral nutrition. Patients on prolonged bedrest likely benefit from prophylactic subcutaneous heparin (5000 IU every 12 hours) to prevent pulmonary embolism.

Ventricular Dysfunction as a Risk Factor

Ventricular dysfunction has an adverse effect on survival. Ejection fraction (EF), which is calculated from difference between end-systolic and end-diastolic volumes of the ventricle is the most commonly used index of ventricular function and is one of the most important predictors of survival.[71-73]

In a study of 462 patients undergoing between 1981 to 1985, the 5-year survival of patients with an EF of less than 30% was 63.1% versus 77.3% for those patients with a preoperative EF between 30 to 50% (P = 0.0001).[74] Patients with an EF less than 15% and cardiogenic shock are doubtful surgical candidates.[75] Patients with poor ventricular function but suitable coronary anatomy can be offered surgery as an option, however. A major uncertainty when deciding operability based on ejection fraction is its inability to differentiate irreversible fibrosis from viable but depressed myocardium which will recover when revascularized. More sensitive tests such as measurement of dynamic ejection fraction after exercise and scintigraphic[74] studies which provide information about global and regional wall motion are attractive, especially because they are noninvasive.

Mechanical Support Devices and Risk Reduction

Ventricular dysfunction is such an important risk factor because the resulting low cardiac output state compromises all organ system function. Attention has turned to reducing this risk by improving preoperative ventricular dysfunction via mechanical methods. The intra-aortic balloon pump (IABP), which is the time tested method of mechanical circulatory support, increases the cardiac index by about 0.7 L per minute.[76] It increases diastolic perfusion and thus increases coronary blood flow, reduces afterload, thereby reducing myocardial oxygen demand.

IABP placement is achieved using a 40-ml balloon in adults inserted via the femoral artery either percutaneously or by the cut-down technique. The tip of the balloon lies in the descending thoracic aorta, and the balloon is timed to inflate with the R wave of the ECG. When properly timed, the balloon inflates at the dicrotic notch of the arterial wave, (which coincides with onset of diastole) and augments the diastolic pressure in the aorta thus increasing coronary blood flow. The balloon deflates in systole, emptying the ascending aorta and thus reducing the afterload. Current indications for balloon counterpulsation are noted in Table 30-5.

Since the introduction of percutaneous insertion, the incidence of balloon-related complications has decreased to less than 6% for all morbidity and a 2% incidence of vascular injury. These risks are slightly higher in women.

Contraindications for IABP insertion are:

- Aortic regurgitation
- Thoracic and abdominal aneurysm/dissection
- Previous aortofemoral grafts
- Severe atherosclerotic disease of the femoroiliac system

The prophylactic use of IABP in unstable angina is often a decision based on experience and available resources, which is often controversial. Gold reported 85% success in relieving ischemic pain unresponsive to medical therapy with a 3% hospital mortality.[77] Similarly, Weintraub found that preoperative insertion of the IABP in 60 patients for refractory angina relieved symptoms in 95% with a 1.7%[78] mortality and 5% perioperative infarction rate. Although IABP insertion has not been proven to reduce perioperative risk, it is effective in relieving anginal pain.

Ventricular Assist Devices (VAD)

Despite advances in surgical technique, advances in cardiothoracic anesthesia, and myocardial preservation, approximately 4% of patients after cardiac surgery have profound ventricular failure.[79] With appropriate adjustments in preload, manipulation of pharmacotherapy, and the use of the intra-aortic balloon pump, 70% of these patients can be eventually weaned off cardiopulmonary bypass.[80]

In addition, it has been estimated that 10 to 15% of patients with acute myocardial infarction in cardiogenic shock may be candidates for some form of ventricular assist,[81] to provide temporary support to allow the "stunned" but viable myocardium to recover, or as a "bridge" to transplantation.[82] Little has been written about preoperative use of VADs, although studies are now underway to examine the impact of VADs on outcome in patients awaiting heart transplantation.

The two major types of VADs are:

Pulsatile devices: Pierce Donachy (Thoratec Laboratory, Berkeley, California), HeartMate® (Thermedics Inc., Woburn, Massachusetts), Novacor (Novacor Medical Inc., Oakland, California). These are costly and not readily available, unless an institution is part of a clinical trial.

Nonpulsatile or continuous flow devices: Biomedicus (Biomedicus, Eden Prairie, Minnesota) centrifugal pump. These are less expensive and more readily available. At our hospital, 57 patients were supported postcardiotomy with the Biomedicus centrifugal pump, either with univentricular or biventricular support from 1984 to 1987 and 28 (49%) were weaned and 13 (23%) were long-term survivors.[83]

General criteria for selecting patients for mechanical support are:

- Age less than 55 years (this limit is not absolute and experience is growing with use in elderly patients)
- Patients who have had technically successful cardiac surgery but develop a cardiac index of less than 1.8 L/min/m^2, left atrial pressure less than 25 mm Hg, systolic blood pressure greater than 90 mm Hg, unresponsive to maximal inotropic vasoactive and intra-aortic balloon pump support
- Acute cardiogenic shock, postmyocardial infarction, or a potentially reversible cause of cardiac failure (e.g., digitalis toxicity)

The role of ventricular device support in the septic patient has not been fully explored. Although sepsis is generally a contraindication to device insertion, there might be a role for temporary support while clearing myocardial depressant factor(s) from the circulation.

The main contraindications to using assist devices are:

- Metastatic carcinoma or other untreatable, preterminal illness
- Severe or fixed pulmonary hypertension (pulmonary vascular resistance greater than 6 Wood units or mean pulmonary artery pressure more than 50% of systemic pressure)
- Severe peripheral vascular or cerebral vascular disease
- Active infection

Bleeding is the most common complication because of the need to maintain at least partial anticoagulation with some devices.[83] Other complications include stroke due to clot formation, embolization, and infection at sites of anastomoses or drive lines. Experimental devices soon to be available will reduce the infection risk by inductively coupling energy to the pump across intact skin.

The **Nimbus Hemopump** (Johnson & Johnson International System Co., Rancho Cordova, CA) is a recent addition to the group of mechanical devices.[84] This small axial flow pump is mechanically similar to an Archimedes screw and capable of generating flows up to 3.8 L per minute. The inflow cannula of the hemopump is positioned across the aortic valve and pumps blood directly from the left ventricle into the proximal ascending aorta. The first version of this miniature pump is 7 mm in diameter and 16 mm long, and is normally positioned under fluoroscopy. Successful positioning by echo Doppler, however, has been accomplished in the operating room.

Currently, it is inserted by the cutdown technique, but a smaller 14-F version for percutaneous insertion is under development, which may make the device directly competitive with IABP use. It cannot provide total assist because flow through the Hemopump (generally around 3 L) is only a fraction of total needs. Since flow assistance is inversely related to afterload, hemodynamic manipulation (afterload reduction) is usually needed to optmize flow with this device. To date, the Hemopump has provided significant support in patients with cardiogenic shock, and in selected patients has offered improved survival (30-day overall survival of 32% in patients with refractory cardiogenic shock.[85] At this writing, however, the Nimbus pump has been withdrawn pending further modifications.

Centrifugal pumps, such as the disposable Biomedicus centrifugal pump (Biomedicus Inc., Eden Prairie, MN) are in common use, both for temporary support in the patient who cannot be weaned from cardiopulmonary bypass, and as a bridge to transplant. The Biomedicus device can be used for left ventricular assistance (L-VAD), for right ventricular assistance (R-VAD) or, with two devices simultaneously, to support both circulations (Bi-VAD). It is possible to add oxygenators to the VAD circuit to provide extracorporeal membrane oxygenation (ECMO), and also common to add a dialysis filter to allow continuous hemofiltration. Bleeding is the most frequent complication associated with VAD usage. The major cause of death associated with use of the device is failure of the heart ventricle to recover, but sepsis and stroke are also important.[86] The most recent advance in ventricular support is the HeartMate implantable pump. This device, which operates on the pusher-plate principle, is currently in experimental use for bridging to transplant. The version in common use operates via compressed air, coupled into the patient via a pneumatic drive line from an external console mounted on a wheeled cart. The next version of the device will operate using an electrical power source, coupled through intact skin to a belt worn around the patient's waist. An internal battery will supply sufficient backup power to allow removal of the belt pack when showering or dressing. Published data are minimal because of limited experience, but initial observations suggest that the device not only functions as well or better than previous ventricular assist devices, but that the mobility provided facilitates substantial cardiac rehabilitation and improves the patient's comfort.

The use of various forms of mechanical assist devices has resulted in survival in only 40 to 50% of patients. The combined registry under the auspices of the International Society for Heart Transplantation as of December 1985 had 451 patients entered. Fifty percent of these patients were weaned off the circulatory support and only 24% were discharged home.[86]

Experience at our institution from 1979 through 1992 with 105 patients yielded similar results with centrifugal devices. Since 1992, survival with heparin-coated extracorporeal membrane oxygenation (ECMO) has been over 45%, and survival with the HeartMate device has been over 75% (P. McCarthy, personal communication, 1993).

In summary, elective bypass surgery is one accepted treatment in selected patients with stable angina. The great majority of patients with unstable anginal syndromes can be controlled at least temporarily by medical management. Supportive therapy (i.e., bed rest, sedation, vasodilation, inotropic agents, beta-adrenergic blockers, and calcium-channel antagonists) provide the physician with a formidable armamentarium to stabilize a patient in whom surgery must be delayed. Approximately 10% of anginal patients will be resistant to medical measures, and will continue to have pain. The addition of IABP will further stabilize a majority of these patients, allowing surgery to be carried out on an elective basis (Table 30-5). The HeartMate and other assist devices appear promising, although few data on preoperative use have been published.

Table 30–5. Indications for Intra-aortic Balloon Counterpulsation

Preoperative
   Angina or ECG changes, refractory to optimal medical therapy
   Severe pain or ischemia ECG changes in a patient with left main stenosis and/or marked severe left ventricular dysfunction
   Hemodynamic instability as a result of failed PTCA
   Postinfarction ischemic pain, with hemodynamic instability
   Mechanical complications of MI-VSD myocardial dysfunction, acute mitral regurgitation
Operative
   Inability to wean off cardiopulmonary bypass despite maximal inotropic support. At our institute, 76% of balloon insertions fall into this or the following category.
Postoperative
   Low cardiac output states unresponsive to standard pharmacologic therapy
   Postoperative myocardial infarction and refractory dysrhythmias

OPERATIVE/ICU PHASE

Preoperative Considerations

Detailed patient information is necessary for planning the operation and postoperative care. Drugs altering platelet function (specifically aspirin) should be stopped 7 days before surgery to allow for physiologic recovery of platelet function. In emergency situations when cessation of these drugs is impossible, platelet transfusions should be anticipated and available. Heparin infusion in patients is often stopped 4 to 6 hours prior to surgery, although some centers continue the heparin infusion up to induction of anesthesia if the patient has ongoing ischemia. Nitrates, beta-blockers and calcium-channel blockers are continued right up to the time of surgery to reduce the risk of rebound angina and hypertension. Long-acting insulin in diabetics is generally administered at half the usual dose on the morning of surgery and blood glucose levels carefully followed perioperatively. All other medications generally should be held. Cefazolin or cefamandole have traditionally been used prophylactically against wound infections because they offer adequate coverage against the most common pathogens such as coagulase positive staphylococcus. The use of cefamandole and cefazolin is gradually being supplemented by newer agents such as cefuroxime which are more cost-effective primarily because of longer half-life and less frequent dosing.[87] In penicillin/cephalosporin-allergic patients, vancomycin is commonly given as 1 g every 12 hours for four doses.

Intraoperative Care

Major risks result from tachycardia and hypotension, so the anesthetic technique must be chosen to avoid extreme hemodynamic changes. Hypotension diminishes coronary perfusion and hypertension increases myocardial oxygen demand. Tachycardia has been shown to influence postoperative ischemic changes.[88] Arrhythmias should be anticipated and avoided by careful attention to oxygenation, electrolyte levels, and sufficient premedication (for example, 0.1 mg/kg morphine sulfate IM or 5 to 10 mg diazepam orally) to relieve patient anxiety and modify the stress response. The stress response to intubation can be ameliorated with opioids and adrenergic blocking agents.[89]

Routine monitoring involves radial or brachial artery cannulation, central venous pressure (CVP) catheter, and an indwelling bladder catheter for urine output. The use of pulmonary artery catheterization is hotly debated,[90-93] but favored by many clinicians in such high risk cases as unstable angina, repeat operation, concurrent valve surgery, or poor preoperative left ventricular function. Temperature is monitored at two sites (core and shell) using thermistors built into pulmonary artery catheters, bladder catheters, or nasopharyngeal probes. Vascular access is achieved before anesthetic induction, but placement of these devices can be accomplished once the patient is asleep. The anesthetic plan should consider the lack of stimulation between intubation and skin preparation and again between skin preparation and incision and adjust accordingly to avoid hypotensive episodes.

In the unlikely event of cardiac arrest prior to median sternotomy, the patient should be immediately heparinized, and closed chest massage carried out while the femoral artery and vein are cannulated to allow initiation of cardiopulmonary bypass. The patient should be systematically cooled (28°C or lower) to reduce oxygen demand, and median sternotomy expeditiously carried out.

Operative Technique

Technical details of the operation are beyond the scope of this text, but certain points are relevant for optimal perioperative care. With advances in myocardial protection (hyperkalemic crystalloid cardioplegia or cold blood cardioplegia), myocardial preservation is far better than a decade ago and has resulted in improved postoperative function. The effects of cardioplegia are most apparent in higher risk patients.[94] The use of retrograde coronary sinus cardioplegia may further improve protection.[95]

Operative strategy is designed to first revascularize the area in jeopardy. Distal anastomosis are carried out to the vessels affected and then cardioplegia is infused down the vein grafts to optimize myocardial protection. The proximal anastomoses may be carried out under one aortic cross-clamp to reduce embolic events with multiple clamping and unclamping. A recent autopsy study emphasizes that postoperative complications are related to atheroembolism from the ascending aorta, with atheroembolic events occurring in 37% of patients with severe atherosclerosis of the aorta versus 2% of those without significant ascending aorta disease.[96] The hazards of atherosclerotic debris from the ascending aorta are thus minimized by avoiding the need to partially cross-clamp the aorta for proximal anastomosis. In patients with advanced peripheral atherosclerotic disease, evidence of such emboli can be spotted in more than 10%.[97]

The incidence of perioperative mortality in first-time elective bypass with normal left ventricular function is less than 1%.[29,46] Poor left ventricular function, preoperative congestive heart failure or renal failure, emergent operation, simultaneous valve procedure, advanced age, cerebral or peripheral vascular disease, COPD, and incomplete revascularization increase the risk and thus the index of suspicion for postoperative vents. Long pump runs and the need for inotropic support following cardiopulmonary bypass (CPB) also predict worse outcome.

Operative mortality for emergencies such as unstable angina, failed angioplasty, and failed thrombolysis runs closer to 3 to 6%.[11] Operative mortality for unstable angina and established infarction is similar,[98] however, cardiogenic shock, ruptured ventricular septum, ruptured papillary muscle, and rupture of the free wall of the left ventricle are catastrophic events associated with operative mortality of 30 to 60%, a figure that has remained constant for the last 10 years.[99] As the mechanical problems associated with these conditions should have been completely corrected postoperatively, the reasons for higher mortality

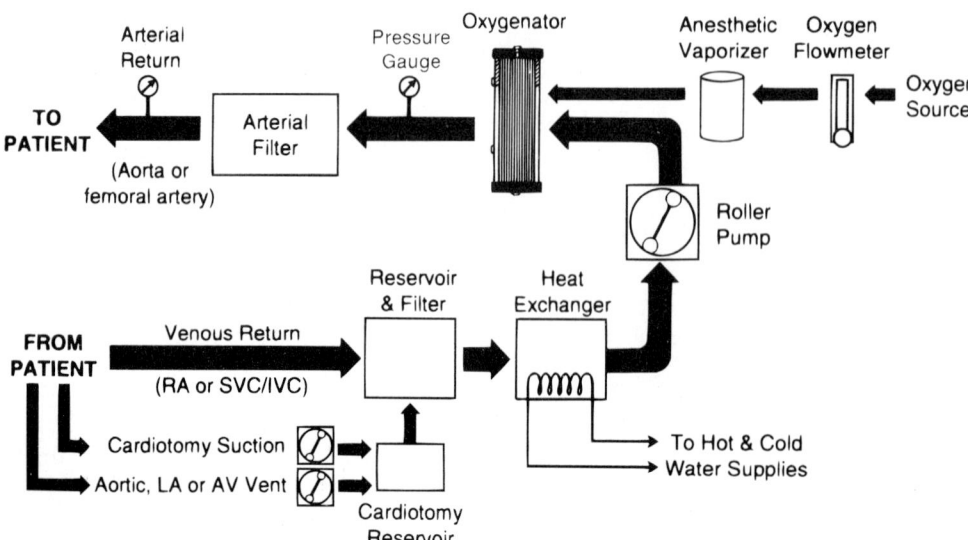

Fig. 30-3. Simplified diagram of a cardiopulmonary bypass circuit using a membrane oxygenator. The thick arrows outline the course of circulation during bypass. Auxilliary roller pumps maintain suction and venting. (For a detailed discussion of cardiopulmonary bypass equipment, the reader is referred to Hessel, E. A.: Cardiopulmonary bypass equipment and circulatory assist devices. *In* Cardiac Anesthesia: Principles and Clinical Practice. Edited by F. G. Estafanous, P. G. Barash, and J. G. Reves. Philadelphia, J. B. Lippincott, 1994, p. 241.)

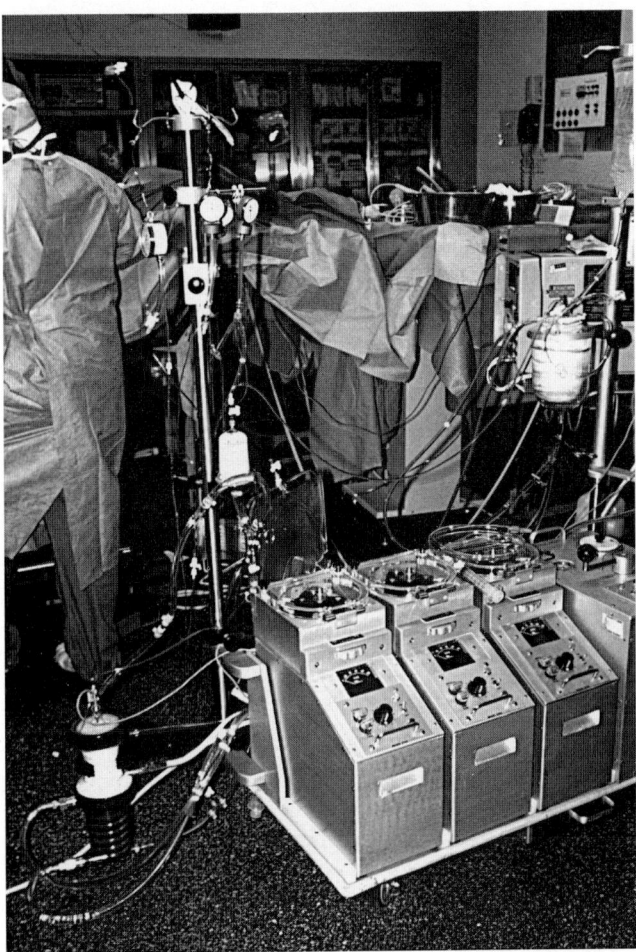

Fig. 30-4. Cardiopulmonary bypass pump, set up for a pediatric case, using a small membrane oxygenator and heat exchanger, visible in the lower left corner. Three identical roller pumps, for circulation, venting, and cardiotomy suction, form the bulk of the unit. A fourth pump is sometimes used for circulating cardioplegia solution. The gauge on each pump monitors the pump flow, which is controlled by the black knob in the center of the panel. The cylindric device above the main roller pump is the arterial filter; pressure manometers are mounted on the same pole. Above and to the left of the right-hand roller pump are the venous return reservoir and filter. Connections between the components of the bypass pump are outlined in Figure 30-3. The actual physical location of these devices may vary by perfusionist preference. Not visible in this picture are the oxygen flowmeter and anesthetic vaporizer, temperature monitoring apparatus, and the connections between the heart exchanger and water supplies.

are still unclear, but may lie in the domain of ineffective myocardial preservation, reperfusion injury, or both.

Pathophysiology of Cardiopulmonary Bypass (CPB)

Most patients undergoing CPB and hypothermia experience a typical pattern of physiologic changes, an understanding of which is essential to their postoperative management. A typical cardiopulmonary bypass circuit is shown in Figure 30-3, and how it is deployed in the operating room is shown in Figure 30-4. Cardiopulmonary bypass is conducted under full anticoagulation, typically 300 to 400 U/kg of heparin, titrated as needed with additional doses to produce to an activated clotting time (ACT) of 400 seconds or more. Venous blood drains into a reservoir that is often in a combined system with the oxygenator and heat exchanger in a single disposable unit. Following oxygenation and ventilation (CO_2 elimination) in the oxygenator, blood passes through a roller pump and filter to be returned to the patient's aorta or femoral artery. The process of CPB produces certain hormonal changes, including elevation of norepinephrine and epinephrine,[100] and increased secretion of antidiuretic hormone (ADH). Serum complement is activated which increases vascular permeability through kinin activation.[101] These factors, and the use of crystalloid prime for the CPB pump are associated with a marked increase in total body water and increased interstitial edema. Hence, these patients need minimal maintenance fluid requirement, with little or no sodium. This excess fluid is rapidly mobilized by otherwise healthy patients, but in those patients with moderate or poor ventricular dysfunction, it may not be redistributed until the second and third postoperative day, and require diuretic therapy.[102]

Hemodilution and hypothermia affect the coagulation factors and platelet function. Peripheral vasoconstriction accompanies hypothermia, and as the patient rewarms in the ICU, vasodilation may lead to hypovolemia and hypotension. This process reaches its peak 3 to 6 months after surgery. Calcium is often used at separation from CPB to improve contractility. Calcium administration has been associated with pancreatic injury after bypass, however.[103]

Postoperative Care

Coordination of care of the postoperative patient involves interaction between the cardiothoracic surgeon, ICU physicians and nurses, the cardiologist, the anesthesiologist and the internist or primary care physician. A good operating room team gleans valuable information from observation of the patient in the operating room and can pass on valuable data to the clinicians involved in postoperative management. For example, optimal filling pressure by vascular monitoring can be correlated with direct visualization of the heart while the chest is still open, bearing in mind that ventricular compliance changes during recovery from CPB.

Complications in the postoperative period can be divided into early concerns (e.g., temperature instability, hemodynamics, ventilatory support, recovery from anesthesia, ischemia, bleeding) and late ICU concerns (Table 30-6). The occurrence of complications is influenced by preoperative clinical condition[46] and also by intraoperative events and postoperative management.

Early ICU Concerns

The most immediate goal following operation is the smooth and uneventful transfer of the patient from operating room to ICU. Physiologic changes and mishaps associated with transport include hypertension and hypoten-

Table 30-6. Postoperative ICU Concerns

Early ICU Concerns
    Temperature instability
    Hemodynamics
    Ventilatory support
    Recovery from anesthesia
    Ischemia
    Bleeding
Late ICU Concerns
    Neurologic injury
    Infection
    Gastrointestinal bleeding/ischemia
    Failure to wean/prolonged mechanical ventilation
    Renal failure
    Multisystem organ failure

sion, arrhythmias, major bleeding, decreased oxygen saturation, and loss of airway continuity. It has been suggested that these adverse events can be minimized by continuous monitoring, maintenance of near-normal cardiac filling pressures, preservation of normothermia, and attention to detail.[104] It may be difficult however, to maintain the same intensity of monitoring during transport as in the operating room or ICU. Electronic and mechanical devices that allow continuous monitoring without the need to reconnect cables and recalibrate transducers simplify patient transfer.[105] Ideally, the postoperative unit should be physically contiguous to the operating room to avoid lengthy hallway passages or elevator rides. When this arrangement is impossible, more expensive alternatives such as dedicated elevators or hiring additional transport personnel must be considered. An organized method of transport must be developed that accounts for the multiple devices attached to the typical cardiac surgical patient: chest tubes, pacemakers, endotracheal tubes, bladder catheters, multiple infusion pumps, and occasionally intra-aortic balloon pumps or ventricular assist devices. At our institution, a system has evolved using racks for infusion pumps that can be lowered from a support arm in the operating room onto the patient's bed, and then resuspended from a support arm in the ICU. This system allows rapid and safe transfer not only from OR to ICU, but in the reverse direction should short-term reexploration be required.[105,106]

In the early postoperative period, continuous monitoring of temperature, heart rate, mean arterial blood pressure, central venous pressure, or pulmonary artery pressure, hourly intake/output, and chest tube drainage is carried out and charted by the ICU nurses. Standardized orders can include limits to prompt notification of the responsible physician. Chest radiograph, 12-lead ECG, hematocrit, serum electrolytes, and blood gases and cardiac enzymes are obtained on arrival. The position of the intra-aortic balloon, if present, is ascertained by chest radiograph. The tip should be in the the second intercostal space, just distal to the origin of the subclavian artery. Other common radiographic findings include malposition of endotracheal and chest tubes and presence of pneumothoraces.

The time course of **recovery from anesthesia** varies with the anesthetic regimen used, amounts given, and the age and physiologic reserve of the patient. High dose opioids such as fentanyl and sufentanil are most commonly employed in conjunction with neuromuscular blocking agents, and often a sedative-hypnotic such as midazolam. Typically, sufficient anesthetic is given to keep the patient asleep well into the postoperative period with the expectation of overnight ventilation. Care must be taken to ensure that the patient does not awaken while still neuromuscularly blocked, which may precipitate hypertension and tachycardia. The tradition of overnight ventilation and a 2-day ICU stay is increasingly challenged in this era of cost containment, and some clinicians feel that early extubation is preferable to late extubation.[107] Earlier awakening and extubation can be achieved with a variety of techniques, including infusions of opioids, benzodiazepines, or propofol. Preliminary evidence suggests an advantage to continuing low dose anesthesia into the postoperative period in order to minimize the stress response, thus reducing the incidence of ST-segment changes by ECG.[108] As the most marked increases in oxygen consumption and carbon dioxide production occur during the first 6 postoperative hours,[109] it may be logical to plan continued stress control via anesthetic infusion during this period, and allow emergence to begin thereafter. Perioperative ischemic episodes are most common in these same few hours of hypermetabolism.[110]

Shivering occurs commonly during rewarming following CPB, and may be accomplished by acute respiratory acidosis if the patient is unable to compensate for increased minute ventilation needs as a result of residual opioids or neuromuscular blocking agents. Calculated minute ventilation based on normal temperature will be excessive when the patient is cold, but can become deficient as rewarming occurs. Respiratory alkalosis will worsen hypokalemia and ventricular irritability, and respiratory acidosis will compromise catecholamine function. Continuous end-tidal CO_2 monitoring may be helpful in determining if ventilatory support is adequate.[111,112]

Hypothermia (below 35°C) may necessitate warming blankets and overhead heating lights. This is most important in unstable patients who cannot withstand sternal closure, and are more prone to lose heat by convection and radiation to the surroundings. Heat loss due to shivering may raise oxygen consumption substantially and interfere with mechanical ventilation.[111] Shivering responds to meperidine[113,114] and radiant heat.[115] In severe cases, shivering may need to be controlled with sedation and neuromuscular blockade.

The most common problem in patients after cardiac surgery is **arterial hypertension,** mediated by afferent impulses from the heart and vasoconstriction due to hypothermia, and occurring in 20 to 40% of adult patients.[116] This situation has important clinical implications in suture line disruption and increased myocardial oxygen demand. This is usually managed by sodium nitroprusside infusion to maintain a mean arterial pressure between 80 to 90 mm Hg. Closed-loop systems incorporating feedback from mean arterial pressure to control nitroprusside infusion have been described[117] and are commercially available. Other approaches to treatment of postoperative hypotension include use of labetalol and esmolol infusions[118] and calcium-channel blockers.[119] Other causes of hypertension such as hypoxia, hypercarbia, shivering, pain, anxiety, and bladder distention should be kept in mind and treated as appropriate.

Hemodynamic management is centered around maintaining a cardiac index of greater than 2.1 L/min/m² with adequate perfusion pressure (MAP around 80) and adequate urine output (greater than 0.5 ml/kg per minute) bearing in mind that regional problems with perfusion can exist even with a globally "normal" cardiac output. If the hemodynamic parameters and clinical evaluation indicate a failing myocardium, a sequential plan to optimize the determinants of cardiac output is made, such as heart rate, preload, afterload, and contractility.

Heart rate is best maintained between 80 to 100 beats per minute for maximal efficacy. Atrial or AV sequential pacing may be needed for bradycardia. For tachyarrhythmias, slowing the heart rate with judicious use of digoxin, verapamil,[120] adenosine,[121,122] beta-blockers[123] or altering inotropic support should be considered.

Preload is optimized by infusion of fluids to maintain a left ventricular filling pressure of 12 to 14 mm Hg for a normal ventricle. For a stiff ventricle, a filling pressure of 18 to 20 mm Hg or even higher may be necessary. Correlation with operating room experience or direct comparison via transesophageal echo are useful guides to the proper filling pressures.

After the preload is optimized, the next step is to reduce afterload to improve stroke volume. Nitroprusside is the drug commonly used, started as an infusion of 0.3 to 0.5 μg/kg/min and occasionally titrated to 5.0 μg/kg per minutes. If the low cardiac output state continues, inotropic agents to improve myocardial contractility are indicated.

The first line drugs are dopamine or dobutamine depending on whether concurrent vasoconstriction or vasodilatation will be advantageous. Either can be started at 3 to 5 μg/kg per minute to a maximum of 15 to 20 μg/kg per minute. The major differences between the two drugs occur at higher doses where dopamine in more likely to cause tachycardia and increased SVR as alpha-adrenergic effects begin to predominate. In contrast, high doses of dobutamine are more likely to lower vascular resistance in both the pulmonary and systemic beds. If these agents do not provide the desired response, epinephrine can be started at an initial infusion of 2 to 4 μg/min. Isoproterenol may be chosen if its chronotropic and pulmonary vasodilatory action are needed, especially in patients with pulmonary hypertension. Amrinone or milrinone phosphodiesterase inhibitors may be used as an adjunct to the catecholamines or as a first-line agent when inotropy and vasodilatation are desired.

If the patient has low mean blood pressure, but a high cardiac output, and low systemic vascular resistance, norepinephrine (Levophed) can be started small doses (2 to 4 μg per minute) to improve blood pressure and coronary and renal perfusion pressures. The reader is referenced to a more complete discussion of inotropes and vasopressors found in Chapter 65.

Ventricular Arrhythmia. Pulmonary vital capacity (PVC) (>6 per minute) is significant and should be treated; after excluding hypoxia, acidosis, alkalosis, hypokalemia, and digitalis toxicity. Potassium and magnesium deficiency may be marked following diuresis from a pump priming solution containing mannitol. Overdrive pacing (i.e., by pacing the ventricle at a rate faster than the intrinsic rhythm) will often suppress the ectopic foci. If not, lidocaine or procainamide infusion are started (see Chap. 27).

Supraventricular Arrhythmia. Disordered rhythms such as rapid atrial fibrillation and supraventricular tachycardia can be controlled with verapamil,[120] adenosine,[121,122] short-acting beta-blockers such as esmolol,[123] and occasionally digoxin. Synchronized electrical cardioversion using an external discharge of 50 to 200 joules is indicated in patients who are hemodynamically compromised by their arrhythmia. In the awake patient, such cardioversion must be preceded by sedation (etomidate, midazolam, or propofol are good choices—see Chapter 63 for a more complete discussion of hemodynamic effects of these agents).

Recent publications have highlighted the high incidence (32% following CABG, 64% following combined CABG and mitral valve replacement) and substantial morbidity associated with postoperative atrial arrhythmias.[124,125] Cox has classified patients into three groups: the 5% in whom atrial fibrillation will develop after any type of major operation, including cardiac procedures; the 30% of patients in whom postcardiac operation atrial fibrillation will develop if no prophylaxis is employed; and the remaining 65% in whom atrial fibrillation is unlikely to develop. The first two groups are thought to have nonuniform dispersion of refractoriness in their atria, a condition only identifiable by detailed electrophysiologic study.[125] Multivariate clinical predictors of the risk of postoperative atrial arrhythmias have, however, been identified and include advanced age, female gender, preoperative digoxin therapy, peripheral vascular disease, COPD, and a history of smoking.[124] Because of the high association between atrial arrhythmias and postoperative stroke, ventricular dysrrhythmias, need for permanent pacer placement, and increased length of stay,[124] it may be reasonable to consider pharmacologic prophylaxis in these patients. Optimal prophylactic therapy has yet to be defined; however, beta-adrenergic blockers, alone or combined with digoxin[126] and magnesium sulfate,[127,128] have been shown to be of benefit.

Myocardial Infarction. Perioperative myocardial infarction is recognized by new ECG changes and cardiac enzyme elevation (creatinine kinase MB fraction greater than 8%, aspartate aminotransferase greater than 80 U/dL). Using these criteria, typical rates of myocardial infarction are 3 to 6%. No combination of enzyme activity changes can completely discriminate patients with perioperative myocardial infarction from those without. Creatinine kinase MB exhibits the best diagnostic association with the presence of histologically proven infarction, however.[129] Reinfusion of shed mediastinal and chest tube drainage can complicate enzyme diagnosis of infarction because autotransfusion produces elevations of creatinine kinase, aspartate aminotransferase, and lactic dehydrogenases.[130] The pattern of enzyme rise is significant: myoglobin levels that increase rapidly and peak at 3 hours after reperfusion are expected, but a rise in myoglobin that continues for 24 hours and exhibits a delayed peak is associated with significant myocardial injury.[131]

Acute Tamponade/Bleeding. Approximately 3 to 14% of the patients undergoing cardiac surgery develop excessive bleeding or hemodynamic instability secondary to tamponade and need to undergo surgical reexploration.[132] Sudden cessation of drainage from the chest tubes with rising filling pressures and failing blood pressure suggests acute tamponade. Surface or transesophageal echocardiography, if immediately available, can be helpful in confirming the diagnosis, but the decision is usually made on clinical grounds. Classic signs of tamponade in the medical setting (i.e., pulsus paradoxus, equalization of pressures) may be absent in surgical tamponade because the pericardium is usually left open. Isolated tamponade involving a single chamber may occur and findings may be obscured by concurrent left ventricular dysfunction.[133]

Sometimes the patient deteriorates suddenly in the postoperative unit and needs an emergency sternal reopening to relieve tamponade and control the site of bleeding. A sterile chest set with a sternal retractor and wire cutters thus should be always kept ready and within easy reach in the postoperative unit. Exploration in the operating room is indicated for persistent bleeding: in excess of 350 ml in the first hour; 250 ml in the second hour or greater than 150 ml per hour thereafter.[134] Mediastinal blood can be retransfused from a cardiotomy reservoir to reduce blood use (Fig. 30-5).[135] The use of desmopressin (DDAVP, 1-Desamino-8-D-arginine vasopressin)[136] and aprotinin[137] has been investigated and remains controversial, because the risk of thrombotic events in the heart or elsewhere may exceed the benefits of lower blood loss.[138] At present, such measures are generally reserved for higher risk patients such as those undergoing reoperations. DDAVP may be particularly beneficial in a subset of patients with abnormal platelet fibrinogen function identified by a thromboelastogram with low maximal amplitude.[139] Available evidence suggests that increased positive end-expiratory pressure does not affect mediastinal blood loss in this setting.[140]

Respiratory Management. Certain respiratory system changes are seen following cardiac surgery, including up to 40% decrease in vital capacity, total lung capacity, inspiratory capacity, and functional residual capacity. Significant changes are seen even 2 weeks postoperatively but appear to resolve after several months. The severity of postoperative pulmonary edema is proportionate to time on bypass.[141] Atelectasis which results in increased work of breathing occurs in up to 90% of patients and occurs whether or not prophylactic positive end-expiratory pressure is used.[142] Pain and splinting cause the patient to limit lung expansion, and limit the ability to cough and clear secretions. Respiratory management goals and interventions are outlined in Table 30-7.

Routine postoperative ventilation is normally initiated at a tidal volume of 10 to 12 ml/kg, respiratory rate of 8 to 10 breaths per minute, inspired oxygen percentage of 60%, and 5 to 10 ml of positive end-expiratory pressure (PEEP) unless experience in the operating room dictates otherwise. Increased levels of PEEP will decrease cardiac output, so volume loading must be used to maintain transmural filling pressures.[143,144] The effects of PEEP are most marked in the presence of abnormal right ventricular

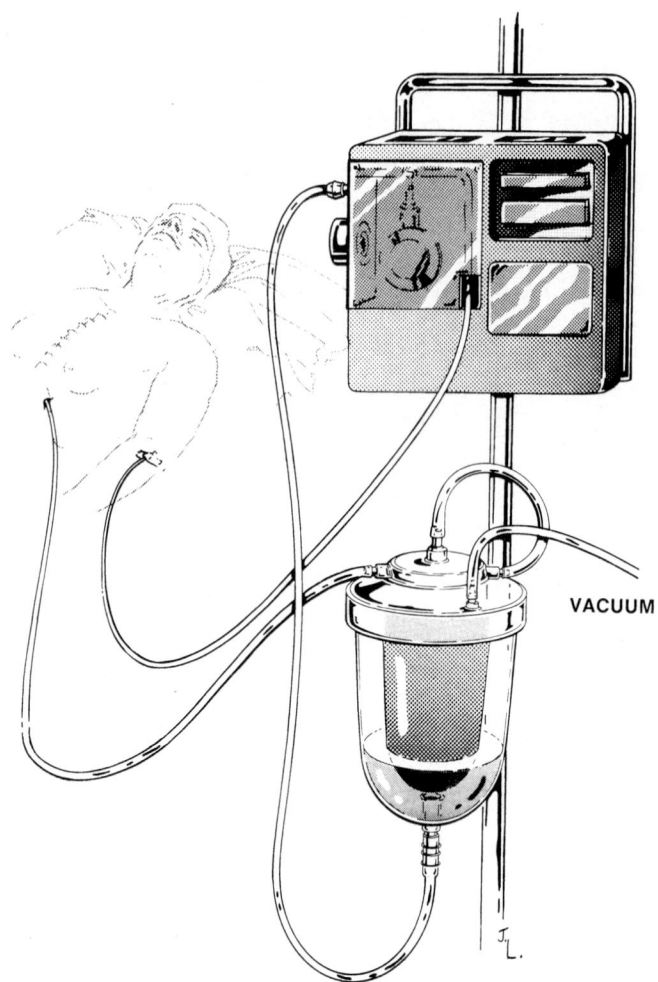

Fig. 30-5. Blood collected in the cardiotomy reservoir is reinfused using a standard infusion pump. The amount of blood collected and transfused and output is tallied hourly. No additional anticoagulation is needed; the cardiotomy filter removes clot and cell debris. Autotransfusion is usually discontinued after 12 hours, or earlier if there is minimal chest tube drainage, fever, or suspected contamination of the system. (From Cosgrove, D. M., Amiot, D. M., and Meserko, J. J.: An improved technique for autotransfusion of shed mediastinal blood. Ann. Thorac. Surg., 40:519, 1985.)

function, particularly if the right coronary artery is stenotic.[145] Because prophylactic application of PEEP neither protects against the development of ARDS[146] nor reduces the amount of mediastinal bleeding,[140] there does not appear to be any advantage in using higher levels. One report, however, concludes that PEEP less than 10 cm H_2O is ineffective to reopen atelectatic lung units.[147]

PEEP supplied by the ventilator is not the only source of end-expiratory pressure. In patients with airflow obstruction, occult positive end-expiratory pressure (Auto-PEEP)[148] may be substantial and dramatically affect hemodynamics. Auto-PEEP can be detected by occlusion of the expiratory port at the end of exhalation, and can be managed with bronchodilators and/or lengthening expiratory time to allow full exhalation to occur.

Table 30-7. Respiratory Management

	Early	Late
Goals:	Complete O_2 saturation of hemoglobin Normocardia Minimization of hemodynamic effects	Extubation with adequate reserve Restoration of FRC
Assessment:	ABGs Cardiac output and filling pressure CXR	Tidal volume, rate on CPAP Vital capacity and MIP ABGs, CXR, Fluid balance Chest tube output
Interventions:	Changes in rate and tidal volume Positive end-expiratory pressure (PEEP) Sedation and neuromuscular blockade Pressure control ventilation	Reversal of narcotics and relaxants Control of secretions Upright position Incentive spirometry

ABG, Arterial blood gases; FRC, functional residual capacity; CXR, chest radiograph; MIP, maximal respiratory pressure.

Endotracheal tube and line placement are confirmed and pneumothorax or atelectasis requiring therapy ruled out with a portable chest radiograph. Arterial blood gases are drawn 30 minutes after the initiation of ventilation and following any adjustments to the ventilator. Since the patient is likely to be hypothermic when their first blood gasp is drawn, mild respiratory alkalosis due to overventilation should be expected and left untreated. As the patient warms, Pco_2 will rise and the alkalosis will resolve without further ventilator changes. Intermittent mandatory ventilation (IMV) is most commonly used for the routine postoperative patient because it allows early spontaneous breathing, and reduces dead space ventilation as compared to control mode ventilation.[149] Control mode ventilation which is useful in the hemodynamically unstable patient and whenever immediate weaning is otherwise contraindicated, may require addition of sedation and neuromuscular blockade.

Extubation time is dictated by certain factors:

- Overall hemodynamic stability
- Respiratory reserve
- Metabolism/redistribution of opioids
- Dissipation of neuromuscular blockade
- Temperature control/rewarming
- Renal function/ability to mobilize fluid loading
- Probability of return to OR for bleeding/tamponade

As previously noted,[107] earlier extubation is gaining adherents, particularly because newer anesthetic agents and techniques make it possible to provide stress control without the need for overnight mechanical ventilation. Aside from efficiency of a shorter ICU stay, earlier extubation allows the patient to cough more effectively[150] and improves preload to both ventricles, thus improving cardiac output.[151] Cited advantages of early endotracheal extubation include improved cardiac performance, decreased length of ICU stay, diminished medication requirements, reduction in morbidity, and improved patient comfort.[152-158] Criteria for extubation are listed in Table 30-8.

Fluid shifts occur during the transition from mechanical to spontaneous ventilation, and may be marked in patients with preoperative congestive heart failure, renal dysfunction, significant mitral valvular lesions, and ventricular dysfunction. Acute left ventricular dysfunction can be precipitated during weaning from mechanical ventilation,[159] and resolution of this problem often requires aggressive diuresis or hemofiltration[160] coupled with inotropic support. Nonrespiratory factors are the strongest determinants of need for prolonged mechanical ventilation, and the presence of congestive heart failure at the time of the operation, an emergency procedure, reoperation, poor preoperative renal function, COPD requiring medication, significant valvular heart disease, diffuse vascular disease, and advanced age should alert the clinician to a possible difficult wean.[161] Sternotomy with internal thoracic artery (ITA) harvesting is accompanied by greater impairment in pulmonary function than when saphenous vein grafts are used alone.[162]

Positioning of the Patient in the Early Postoperative Period. An intriguing study of 277 patients (of whom 102 were from a cardiothoracic ICU) requiring more than 24 hours of mechanical ventilation suggests that supine head positioning during the first 24 hours is a major risk factor for ventilator-associated pneumonia.[163] Other important risk factors for pneumonia were organ system failure, age greater than 60 years, and prior administration of antibiotics. This study raises some interesting questions about perioperative management in the cardiac surgical patient, who may require the Trendelenburg position for blood pressure management. Further study is necessary to determine if supine head position could be avoided by positioning the patient in a "beach-chair" position (head of bed up at 30°, knees bent), more careful attention to fluid balance, and earlier use of vasopressors. In patients who are unavoidably supine, consideration might be given to prophylaxis with an antibiotic regimen[164] or immunoglobulin.[165] Such prophylaxis might best be delivered before a patient who is identified preoperatively to be at risk of postoperative mechanical ventilation[51] or hemodynamic instability arrives in the ICU.

Late ICU Concerns

Prolonged Mechanical Ventilation. Mechanical ventilation for longer than 72 hours is required in about 5% of patients after open heart surgery, with expected variations depending on the type of operation and operative priority. Risk factors for respiratory complications that result in a need for prolonged ventilatory support are given in Table 30-9.[161] Selective digestive decontamination regimens, consisting of application of antibiotic paste to the buccal mucosa and a slurry down the gastric tube, may decrease the incidence of nosocomial pneumonia in this population.[164,166] Prophylaxis for stress ulceration of the gastric mucosa is also indicated in ventilator-dependent patients to reduce the risk of gastric bleeding.

Table 30–8. Extubation Criteria

Neurologic	Awake and cooperative, able to cough and protect airway
	Neuromuscular blockade fully reversed
Cardiac	Stable; not on IABP, index >2 L/min/m²
	MAP >70; no serious arrhythmias
Respiratory	Acceptable CXR, ABGs (pH ≥7.35)
	MIP < −25; Vt >5 ml/kg, Vc >10 ml/kg
	Comfortable on CPAP or T-piece with spontaneous rate ≤24
	Minimal secretions
Renal	Diuresing well; not markedly overloaded
	Urine output >0.5 ml/kg/min
Hematologic	Chest tube drainage <50 ml/hr
Temperature	Fully rewarmed

ABGs, Arterial blood gases; CPAP, continuous positive airway pressure; CXR, chest radiograph; IABP, intra-aortic balloon pump; MAP, mean arterial pressure; MIP, maximal respiratory pressure.

Limiting factors in weaning a patient from mechanical support include renal failure, sepsis, neurologic dysfunction, and unstable hemodynamics. Acute left ventricular dysfunction may be precipitated by the shift from mechanical to spontaneous ventilation in the patient with concurrent pulmonary and cardiac decompensation.[159] Careful attention to fluid balance with aggressive diuresis to optimize cardiac preload and afterload is an important part of therapy. In patients with normal renal function, furosemide or other loop diuretics are effective in reducing total body fluid overload.[167] When renal function is inadequate, considerable success has been achieved using continuous ultrafiltration techniques to remove excess fluid.[160] The catabolic state during prolonged recovery, particularly if sepsis is a component will cause the patient to lose protein mass and cause comparison of postoperative to preoperative weight to be unreliable. It is not unusual for a patient to require diuresis or ultrafiltration to several kilograms **below** their preoperative weight before weaning is successful. Further details on techniques of long-term mechanical support and weaning techniques can be found in Chapter 24.

Table 30–9. Risk Factors for Respiratory Complications After Cardiac Surgery

Factor	Coefficient	S.E.	Odds Ratio	(95% C.I.)
Current CHF	0.788	0.161	2.20	(1.60–3.01)
Emergency case	0.644	0.183	1.90	(1.33–2.72)
Reoperation	0.467	0.087	1.59	(1.34–1.89)
Preop serum Cr ≥1.9	0.447	0.176	1.56	(1.11–2.20)
COPD on medication	0.418	0.107	1.52	(1.23–1.87)
Aortic stenosis	0.366	0.155	1.44	(1.06–1.95)
Prior vascular surgery	0.289	0.110	1.34	(1.08–1.67)
Mitral insufficiency	0.282	0.127	1.32	(1.03–1.70)
Age/decade	0.154	0.043	1.17	(1.07–1.27)

All significant to p < 0.01 except mitral insufficiency, p = 0.027; constant = 2.646; CHF, congestive heart failure; COPD, chronic obstructive pulmonary disease.

The phrenic nerve is at risk for damage or transsection during cardiac procedures, particularly those involving reoperation where pericardial fibrosis increases the difficulty of identifying and protecting nearby nerve fibers. The incidence of diaphragmatic paralysis has not been well characterized. In our experience, transient diaphragmatic dysfunction occurs in about 4% of patients, and bilateral diphragmatic paralysis requiring prolonged ventilatory support occurs in less than 0.1% of patients. Diaphragmatic dysfunction should be suspected when a patient fails to wean from mechanical ventilation or has significant orthopnea, and can be clinically detected by paradoxic movement of the diaphragm during inspiration. This finding can be objectively documented with a fluoroscopic "sniff" test, and if a marked decrease in vital capacity and tidal volume occurs when the patient is moved from a seated to a supine position. Efforts to protect the myocardium with an ice slurry during CPB can cause cold injury to the phrenic nerve,[168] and, although this generally resolves within a few days, full recovery may require up to 2 years.[169] Factors that will contribute to diaphragmatic weakness include sepsis, hypocalcemia,[170] and hypophoshatemia.[171] Therapeutic interventions of reported value include dopamine,[172] aminophylline,[173] and rarely diaphragmatic pacing. Long-term management of diaphragmatic paralysis is simplified by performing a tracheotomy, which facilitates spontaneous daytime ventilation, but allows easy connection of a ventilator for support during sleep. Home ventilation[174] and/or use of a rocking bed[169] are options for the patient who fails to recover.

Oliguric or Anuric Renal Failure. This complication occurs in 1 to 4% post open heart surgery patients, and lesser degrees of renal dysfunction, marked by a rise in serum creatinine occur in 2 to 30%.[175,176] The incidence of postoperative renal complications rises progressively with preoperative serum creatinine values greater than 1.6 mg/dl,[69] low cardiac output at the end of CPB, advanced age, preoperative cardiac failure, need for postoperative circulatory support, blood transfusions, and prolonged time on CPB.[177]

Urine output must be monitored throughout the perioperative period. Dopamine has shown to produce functional improvement in the setting of new onset oliguria following CPB[178] and although the role of prophylactic dopamine has not been well studied, many clinicians advocate the use of "renal" dose dopamine (0.5 to 2 μg/kg per minute) in high risk patients. Dopamine also has been shown to reduce renal vascular resistance during alpha-adrenergic drug therapy,[179] leading to the practice of adding dopamine when norepinephrine must be used. Potassium levels must be monitored carefully during dopamine infusion, as post-CABG patients given dopamine are prone to develop hypokalemia and arrhythmias.[180]

Postoperative renal failure usually presents as one of three well-defined patterns.[181] Abbreviated acute renal failure occurs after an isolated insult, results in a peak in serum creatinine around the fourth postoperative day, and generally has a favorable prognosis if no other events occur. The second pattern is similar to the first, except that the acute insult is accompanied by prolonged circulatory failure. This pattern runs a longer course, with recovery typically occurring in the second or third week after injury, in tandem with improvements in cardiac output. The final pattern begins like the second, but recovery is complicated by a second insult such as sepsis, massive gastrointestinal bleeding, or myocardial infarction. Permanent failure may result from this pattern, and other coexisting organ failure is common. Since fluid overload with renal failure may precipitate respiratory and cardiac failure, there has been a trend toward early application of continuous arteriovenous hemofiltration (CAVH) and related techniques to remove excess fluid.[160]

Neurologic Complications. Such complications following open heart surgery include focal cerebral lesions resulting in hemiparesis and aphasia, severe global encephalopathy, peripheral nerve injury, diaphragmatic injury, and neuropsychiatric changes.[181-184] Prospective studies using sophisticated testing identify early subtle postoperative complications in over 60%.[181] The majority of these will resolve by six months follow-up, and the residual findings are often of little functional importance. Major disability occurs in just over 1%, and is almost always identified early in the postoperative period.[182,183] ICU care of these patients is generally concerned with maintaining reasonable mean arterial (and hence CNS) perfusion pressure, and ensuring continued protection of the airway, as aspiration is a major risk. Seizures are occasionally seen in association with focal neurologic deficits, and as preterminal events, and generally respond to usual measures. Physical therapy and occupational therapy should be started in the ICU once the patient has stabilized to prevent disuse atrophy and strictures and to expedite earlier discharge.

Figure 30-6 outlines an approach to the management of the patient who fails to awaken. All sedatives, narcotics, and muscle relaxants should be withheld, and peripheral neuromuscular function assessed using a nerve stimulator.

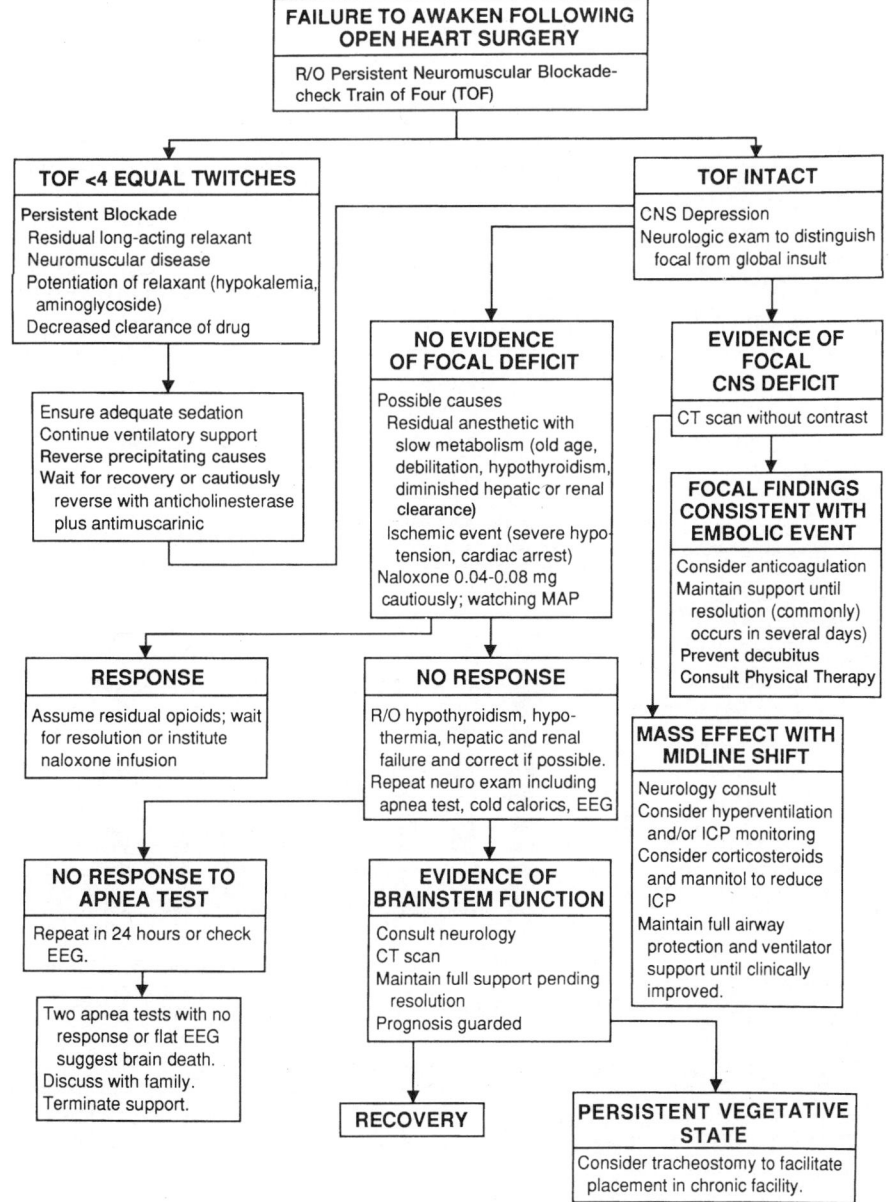

Fig. 30-6. Failure to awaken after open heart surgery. Persistent neuromuscular blockade is surprisingly common and must be ruled out in any patient who does not awaken after open heart surgery. Once this has been ruled out, a careful neurologic examination should be made to search for evidence of a focal central nervous system deficit, which can further be evaluated with computed tomographic scanning. Many focal lesions are of embolic origin, and the prognosis for recovery is good. Persistent coma without evidence of a focal deficit is more worrisome. Aside from the situation in which barbiturate loading has been used for cerebral protection, it is unusual to see a patient fail to metabolize operative anesthetics by the end of 24 hours. If naloxone is used, it should be cautiously titrated in doses of 40 to 80 μg, watching for tachycardia and hypertension. Lack of response to a naloxone challenge requires further workup, and neurologic consultation is well advised at this point. (From Higgins, T. L.: Postoperative complications and intensive care. *In* Cardiac Anesthesia: Principles and Clinical Practice. Edited by F. G. Estafanous, J. G. Reeves, and P. G. Barash. Philadelphia, J. B. Lippincott, 1994, p. 373.)

CT scanning is accomplished to rule out structural problems or cerebral edema prior to lumbar puncture. Electroencephalography is sometimes indicated to assess brain electrical activity and to rule out seizures. Usually, little can be done once a focal or global neurologic injury is identified; prevention of these injuries by avoiding emboli during aortic cannulation[96] and maintaining adequate CNS oxygenation may prove to be the preferred approach.

Transient postoperative delirium occurs in about 7% of patients and resolves in almost all patients by the sixth postoperative day.[184] Initial management of agitation consists of reassurance and orientation of the patient, and control of pain and anxiety. If the patient remains agitated, haloperidol is often useful.[185] (See Chapter 63.)

Mediastinitis, Sternal Dehiscence, or Both. These are serious complications of coronary revascularization, with an incidence of about 1%, but a mortality rate of 13%.[186] Predisposing factors for wound complications after open heart surgery include diabetes, low cardiac output, use of bilateral internal mammary artery grafts, and reoperation for control of bleeding. Mediastinal infection is often manifest as failure to wean, unexplained fever, and an unstable sternum. Confirmation of infection may be difficult, because radionuclide bone scans "light up" during normal healing. Surgical exploration and draining of the wound may be necessary to obtain adequate material for culture. Management of mediastinitis requires selective antibiotic therapy, debridement, irrigation, drainage, and reclosure. In cases of severe sternal necrosis, early debridement and plastic surgical reconstruction using omental and/or myocutaneous flaps are recommended.

Gastrointestinal Complications. Gastrointestinal disorders requiring intervention occur in only 1 to 3% of patients, but are associated with substantial mortality.[187,188] Upper gastrointestinal bleeding from ulceration is the most common complication. Pancreatitis, intestinal ischemia, perforation, or bleeding elsewhere in the gastrointestinal tract are most common in the critically ill patient with developing multisystem failure. Mesenteric ischemia can occur as a result of low perfusion or embolization of atheroma from large vessel manipulation. The incidence of gastrointestinal bleeding can be minimized with antacid therapy, histamine blocker, or barrier protection agents such as sulcralfate. Enteral rather than parenteral nutritional support also appears to better protect the gastric mucosa.[189] Monitoring of intraluminal gastric pH may identify patients at risk for developing multisystem organ failure secondary to poor gut mucosal blood flow.

Jaundice occurs in approximately 20% of patients post CPB and is usually associated with multiple valve replacement, higher transfusion requirements, and longer times on CPB.[190] Acute pancreatitis following cardiac surgery carries a poor prognosis, especially in the setting of multisystem organ failure. Evidence of pancreatitis is found in 25% of autopsied patients dying after open heart surgery.[191] Transient elevation of amylase occurs unrelated to pancreatic injury, making hyperamylasemia less valuable as a diagnostic test, unless it is combined with a serum lipase assay.

POST-ICU PHASE

After uncomplicated open heart surgery, many patients can be sent on the first postoperative day from the ICU to a "stepdown" unit equipped with ECG monitoring on the first postoperative day. Some correlation exists between preoperative severity and average ICU length of stay (Fig. 30–7). At our institution, 55% of the patients remain in the ICU for less than 24 hours and 79% for less than 48 hours.[45] Our criteria for discharge from the ICU are:

- Stable hemodynamics with no inotropic drug support except low dose dopamine or dobutamine
- No arrhythmias other than chronic atrial fibrillation
- Resolution of ongoing ischemia perioperative infarct diagnosed by ECG evidence or elevated cardiac enzymes (CPK MB >80% or ASAT (SGOT) >80)
- Neurologically alert and intact
- Coughing well and able to clear secretions
- Able to maintain adequate oxygenation (PO_2 >60 mm Hg) and elimination of CO_2 on <4 L of oxygen by nasal cannula.
- No evidence of bleeding (chest tube drainage <50 m per hour)
- Adequate renal, hepatic and gastrointestinal function (creatinine and bilirubin within 1 mg/dl of baseline)
- No clinical evidence of infection

Special attention is paid to arrhythmias, congestive heart failure, and respiratory and wound complications. Approximately 4% of the patients need readmission to the ICU, primarily for arrhythmias, congestive failure or respiratory distress[45,186] (Fig. 30–8).

Respiratory therapists should routinely follow patients for the first 3 or 4 postoperative days and encourage deep breathing exercises, provide incentive spirometry, and when needed, chest physiotherapy. We find it helpful to have the ICU staff around on these patients after ICU discharge and thus avert respiratory readmission via timely

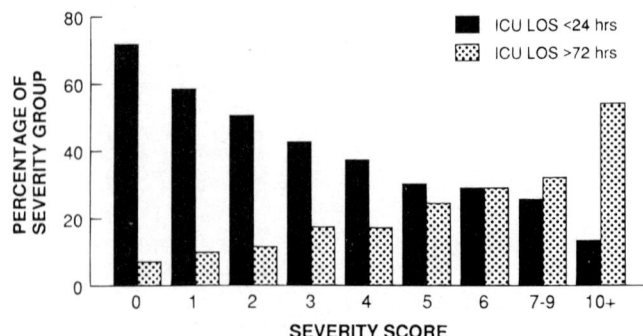

Fig. 30–7. Intensive care length of stay as a function of preoperative severity score. Over 70% of patients with no risk factors are discharged on the first postoperative day. More than half of the patients at highest risk, however, require an ICU stay of 72 hours or longer. (From Higgins, T. L.: Postoperative complications and intensive care. In Cardiac Anesthesia: Principles and Clinical Practice. Edited by F. G. Estafanous, J. H. Reeves, and P. G. Bavash. Philadelphia, J. B. Lippincott, 1994, p. 373.)

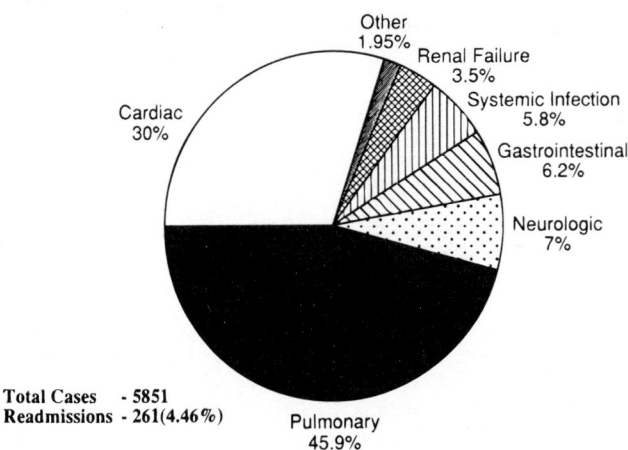

Fig. 30-8. Primary reasons for readmission to the ICU after open heart surgery. (From Higgins, T. L.: Postoperative complications and intensive care. In Cardiac Anesthesia: Principles and Clinical Practice. Edited by F. G. Estafanous, J. G. Reeves, and P. G. Barash. Philadelphia, J. B. Lippincott, 1994, p. 373.)

interventions on the regular nursing floor. Ambulation and a graded exercise program are begun early postoperatively to reduce the likelihood of phlebitis (and consequent pulmonary embolism) and to minimize and reverse atelectasis. If ambulation is not possible, prophylactic heparin (5000 subcutaneously every 12 hours) is considered. A positive attitude emphasizing rehabilitation and discouraging cardiac invalidism is maintained with the help of nursing, respiratory therapy, and rehabilitation specialists. Patients with uncomplicated courses can be discharged home on the fifth or sixth postoperative day. Temporary pacing wires and sutures are removed before hospital discharge. Special attention is paid to catheterization and balloon insertion sites to exclude late pseudoaneurysm formation.

Before discharge, a pamphlet of instructions containing a diagram of the surgical procedure, recommended activities, diet, medications, dates for return appointments and emergency telephone numbers is given to the patient. In larger centers with significant out-of-town referrals, many patients will return to the care of local physicians for all but a simple follow-up visit to the surgical center. Optimal transfer of information should include a dictated summary mailed or faxed to the referring physician in advance of the patient's first postoperative visit.

All patients should be followed for recurrent angina or other symptoms of myocardial dysfunction. Periodic exercise testing and coronary angiograms should be repeated if there is suspicion of graft stenosis or occlusion. Graft occlusion before 6 months is usually due to a technical problem, but after this progression of the disease process is the most common cause.

Delayed Complications

Delayed postoperative pericardial effusion is seen in about 6% of patients, and delayed cardiac tamponade develops in about 1%.[192] On follow-up, the only symptoms may be unexplained dyspnea and lethargy. Clinical examination may reveal pulsus paradoxus, faint heart sounds, hepatomegaly or ascites, and the diagnosis confirmed by an echocardiogram. If the effusion is serosanguineous, pericardiocentesis and treatment with aspirin or indomethacin should suffice. Rarely, evacuation of a hematoma by sternotomy may be indicated.

Pleural effusions usually result from congestive heart failure. They may also result from liquidification of mediastinal hematomas. These may warrant drainage, depending on the patient's symptoms.

Following saphenous vein harvesting, approximately 1% of patients[193] have leg wound complications that delay hospital discharge. There should be minimal undermining of skin edges, careful hemostasis and proper closure in layers, and judicious use of electrocautery at the time of wound closure following harvesting. This is not necessarily the task to assign to the least experienced team member, particularly in patients at higher risk, such as diabetics.

Serum hepatitis is a complication of multiple blood transfusions and becomes manifest about a month after surgery.[194] Hemodilution and blood conservation techniques have greatly reduced the risk of hepatitis by minimizing transfusion requirements.

Long-Term Preventive Goals

Patients following coronary artery bypass for myocardial ischemia remain at an increased risk for subsequent cardiac events including reinfarction, congestive heart failure, and sudden cardiac death. Therefore, measures aimed at preventing these events and enhancing the regression of the primary pathology (coronary atherosclerosis) must be instituted following surgery.

Coronary Atherosclerosis. Epidemiologic evidence strongly supports the relationship between serum cholesterol[195] and coronary heart disease (CHD). Clinical evidence also suggests that lowering of total and LDL cholesterol decreases the incidence of CHD.[196] There is approximately 2% risk reduction for each 1% reduction in serum cholesterol, and it is greatest in patients at highest risk.[197] In the Cholesterol Lowering Atherosclerosis Study (CLAS), the progression of atherosclerosis within both native arteries and bypass grafts was significantly reduced in patients receiving niacin and colestipol 16.2% versus 2% on diet alone.[198]

Smoking Cessation. The detrimental effects of smoking on reinfarction and survival have been extensively and conclusively documented.[199,200] A recent CASS study group confirmed the benefit of smoking cessation in patients with known CHD and, in addition, determined that this could be extended to older patients treated medically or surgically.[201]

Beta-Blockers. In an extensive review of the randomized trials, Yusuf and associates estimated that beta-blocker therapy could reduce long-term mortality and nonfatal infarctions by 22 and 27%, respectively.[202] A variety of beta-blockers with cardioselectivity and membrane stabilizing effects are available, and currently, in patients following acute myocardial infarction, oral beta-blockers are recommended for a minimum of 6 years if no contraindications to their use exist.[203]

Aspirin inactivates platelet cyclo-oxygenase, a potent

platelet aggregating substance, and given the role of platelet thrombi in the pathogenesis of acute coronary thrombosis, randomized trials have been devoted to the role of aspirin in preventing secondary cardiac events and graft patency.[204,205] When direct comparisons are made, low dose aspirin (≤300 mg per day) is as effective as any combination regimen of aspirin and antiplatelet agents and is currently recommended.

Other Measures

The roles of behavior modification, weight loss, and use of other agents such as angiotensin-converting enzyme inhibitors have not been specifically studied in the post-CABG population. Although men with a so-called "type A" behavior pattern have a higher incidence of new coronary heart disease,[206] more recent evidence suggests that of those surviving a coronary event, the long-term mortality rate of those with type A behavior is actually lower than those with type B behavior.[207] More work is needed to determine whether it is truly the type A behavior pattern or how one reacts to stress that determines risk, and furthermore, how this applies to post-CABG patients. Women with intra-abdominal fat deposition are at greater cardiovascular risk than those with obesity alone,[208] but again, the benefit of weight loss following successful CABG surgery remains to be studied. Finally, angiotensin-converting enzyme inhibitors such as enalapril appear to have a beneficial effect on mortality and hospitalizations in patients with chronic heart failure and poor left ventricular function,[209] but data specifically for postrevascularization patients are lacking.

In summary, the perioperative care of the cardiac surgical patient involves a team approach with constant communication between surgeons, anesthesiologists, intensive care physicians, nurses, respiratory therapists, and allied health professionals. Because of the myriad details that require attention, delegation of responsibility is paramount. The attending physician's awareness can be increased by encouraging input from all clinicians involved in the patient's care. At our institution, risk reduction begins with the preoperative visit, at which time the patient's severity score[46] is calculated. This risk estimate is then disseminated to all involved in the care of the patient, helping to focus increased attention on the higher risk individual. Those patients with severity scores greater than 6 will have additional interventions, such as selective digestive decontamination protocol[164,166] or avoidance of the head-down position,[163] to reduce risk.

A recent report suggests that the risk of sepsis after cardiac surgery is reduced when high risk patients are treated with immunoglobulins.[210] We have recently demonstrated that anterograde-retrograde blood cardioplegia improves outcome in high risk patients.[165] In the future, considerable emphasis will be placed on tailoring interventions to those most likely to be of benefit based on preoperative risk assessment.

Of necessity, this chapter has only identified areas of risk in the cardiac surgical patient. Full discussion of therapeutic interventions, specifically with regard to treatment of low output states, therapy of rhythm disturbances, and management of complications found in a wide variety of critically ill patients, can be found elsewhere in this book.

REFERENCES

1. National Center for Health Statistics: Monthly Vital Stat. Rep., 36:13, 1988
2. Murphy, M. L., et al.: Treatment of chronic stable angina: a preliminary report of survival data of the Randomized Veterans Administration Cooperative Study. N. Engl. J. Med., 297:621, 1977.
3. National Cooperative Study Group: Unstable angina pectoris: National Cooperative Study Group to compare medical and surgical therapy: response of protocol of patient population. Am. J. Cardiol., 37:896, 1976.
4. Kanel, W. B., and Feinlab, M.: Natural history of angina pectoris in the Framingham Study. Am. J. Cardiol., 39:154, 1972.
5. Favaloro, R. G.: Saphenous vein graft replacement of severe segmental coronary artery occlusion; operative technique. Ann. Thorac. Surg., 5:334, 1968.
6. Naunheim, K. S., et al.: The changing profile of the patient undergoing coronary artery bypass surgery. J. Am. Coll. Cardiol., 11:494, 1988.
7. Loop, F. D.: Thoracic and cardiovascular disease. The old order changeth. Cleve. Clin. J. Med., 55:15, 1988.
8. Alderman, E. L., et al.: Determinants of coronary surgery in a consecutive patient series from geographically dispensed medical centers: the Coronary Artery Surgery Study. Circulation, 66:6, 1982.
9. Hill, J. D., et al.: Emergency aortocoronary bypass for impending or extending myocardial infarction. Circulation, 43:105, 1971.
10. Keon, W. J.: Urgent surgical therapy for unstable angina. In Unstable Angina, Recognition and Management. Edited by A. G. Adelman and B. S. Goldman. Littleton, PSG Publishing Company, 1981.
11. Golding, L. A., et al.: Emergency revascularization for unstable angina. Circulation, 58:1163, 1978.
12. Langou, R. A., et al.: Surgical approach for patients with unstable angina pectoris. Role of the response to initial medical therapy and intra-aortic balloon pumping in perioperative complications after aortocoronary bypass grafting. Am. J. Cardiol., 42:629, 1978.
13. Cohn, L. M.: Surgical treatment of acute myocardial infarction. Chest, 93:135, 1988.
14. Buckberg, G. D.: A proposed "solution" to the cardioplegic controversy. J. Thorac. Cardiovasc. Surg., 77:803, 1979.
15. Rosencranz, E., et al.: Warm induction of cardioplegia with glutamate-enriched blood in coronary patients with cardiogenic shock who are dependent on inotropic drugs and intra-aortic balloon support. J. Thorac. Cardiovasc. Surg., 86:507, 1983.
16. Stewart, J. R., et al.: Inhibition of surgically induced ischemia/reperfusion injury by oxygen free radical scavengers. J. Thorac. Cardiovac. Surg., 86:262, 1983.
17. De Wood, M. A., et al.: Medical and surgical management of early Q-wave myocardial infarction. I. Effects of surgical reperfusion survival and functional class at 10 years or more of follow-up. J. Am. Coll. Cardiol., 14:65, 1989.
18. De Wood, M. A., et al.: Medical and surgical management of early Q-wave myocardial infarction. II. Effects on mortality and global and regional left ventricular function at 10 or more years of follow-up. J. Am. Coll. Cardiol., 14:78, 1989.
19. Unstable pectoris: National Cooperative Study Group to

Compare Surgical and Medical Therapy. Am. J. Cardiol., *42:* 839, 1978.
20. Pugh, B., et al.: Unstable angina pectoris: a randomized study of patients treated medically and surgically. Am. J. Cardiol., *41:*1291, 1978.
21. Brown, C. A., et al. Prospective study of medical and urgent surgical therapy in randomizable patients with unstable angina pectoris: results of in-hospital and chronic mortality and morbidity. Am. Heart J., *102:*959, 1981.
22. Cohn, L. H., et al.: Changing indications for the surgical treatment of unstable angina. Arch. Surg., *113:*1312, 1978.
23. Miller, D. C., et al.: Discriminant analysis of the changing risks of coronary artery operations: 1971–1979. J. Thorac. Cardiovasc. Surg., *85:*197, 1983.
24. Krebber, H. J., et al.: Management of evolving myocardial infarction by intracoronary thrombolysis and subsequent aorta-coronary bypass. J. Thorac. Cardiovasc. Surg., *83:*186, 1982.
25. Skinner, J. R., Phillips, S. J., Zeff, R. H., and Kongtahworn, C.: Immediate coronary bypass following failed streptokinase infusion in evolving myocardial infarction. J. Thorac. Cardiovasc. Surg., *87:*567, 1984.
26. Topol, E. J., et al.: A randomized trial of immediate versus delayed elective angioplasty after intravenous tissue plasminogen activator in acute myocardial infarction. N. Engl. J. Med., *317:*581, 1987.
27. Kennedy, J. W., et al.: Multivariate discriminant analysis of the clinical and angiographic predictors of operative mortality from the Collaborative Study in Coronary Artery Surgery (CASS). J. Thorac. Cardiovasc. Surg., *80:*876, 1980.
28. Fisher, L. D., Kennedy, J. W., and Davis, K. B.: Association of sex, physical size, and operative mortality after coronary artery bypass in the coronary artery surgery studies (CASS). J. Thorac. Cardiovasc. Surg., *84:*334, 1982.
29. Cosgrove, D. M., et al.: Primary myocardial revascularization. Trends in surgical mortality. J. Thorac. Cardiovasc. Surg., *88:*673, 1984.
30. Foster, E. D., et al.: Comparison of operative mortality and morbidity for initial and repeat coronary artery bypass grafting: the coronary artery surgery study (CASS) registry experience. Ann. Thorac. Surg., *38:*563, 1984.
31. Lytle, B. W., et al.: Fifteen hundred coronary reoperations. Results and determinants of early and late survival. J. Thorac. Cardiovasc. Surg., *93:*847, 1987.
32. Loop, F. D., et al.: Coronary artery bypass graft surgery in the elderly. Indications and outcome. Cleve. Clin. J. Med., *55:*23, 1988.
33. Pelletier, L. C., Castonguay, Y. R., and Chaitman, B. R.: Open-heart surgery in elderly patients. Can. Med. Assoc. J., *128:*409, 1983.
34. Edmunds, L. H., et al.: Open-heart surgery in octogenarians. N. Engl. J. Med., *319:*131, 1988.
35. Loop, F. D., et al.: Coronary artery surgery in women compared with men: analyses of risks and long-term results. J. Am. Coll. Cardiol., *1:*383, 1983.
36. Gibson, C. F., and Loop, F. D.: How different are CABG results in women and men? Cardiovasc. Med., *86:*53, 1986.
37. Lytle, B. W.: Combined surgery for valve and coronary artery disease. Cleve. Clin. J. Med., *55:*79, 1988.
38. Cosgrove, D. M., et al.: Determinants of long-term survival after ventricular aneurysmectomy. Ann. Thorac. Surg., *26:* 357, 1978.
39. Goenen, M., et al.: Preoperative left ventricular dysfunction and operative risks in coronary bypass surgery. Chest, *92:* 804, 1987.
40. Rao, T. L. K., Jacobs, K. H., and El-Etr, A. A.: Reinfarction following anesthesia in patients with myocardial infarction. Anesthesiology, *59:*499, 1983.
41. Knight, A. A., et al.: Perioperative myocardial ischemia: importance of the preoperative ischemic pattern. Anesthesiology, *68:*681, 1988.
42. Mangano, D. T.: Perioperative cardiac morbidity. Anesthesiology, *72:*153, 1990.
43. Parsonnet, V., et al.: Emergency operation after failed angioplasty. J. Thorac. Cardiovasc. Surg., *96:*198, 1988.
44. Golding, L. A. R., et al.: Early results of emergency surgery after coronary angioplasty. Circulation, *74:*26, 1986.
45. Higgins, T. L.: Postoperative care of the cardiac surgery patient. Problems in Anesthesia, *3:*211, 1989.
46. Higgins, T. L., et al.: Stratification of morbidity and mortality outcome by preoperative risk factors in coronary artery bypass patients. JAMA, *267:*2344, 1992.
47. Peper, W. A., et al.: Mortality and results after cardiac surgery in patients with end-stage renal disease. Cleve. Clin. J. Med., *55:*63, 1988.
48. Deutsch, E., et al.: Coronary artery bypass chronic hemodialysis. A case-control study. Ann. Intern. Med., *110:*369, 1989.
49. Tisi, G. M.: State of the art. Preoperative evaluation of pulmonary function. Validity, indications, and benefits. Am. Rev. Respir. Dis., *119:*293, 1979.
50. Peters, R. M., Brimm, J. E., and Utley, J. R.: Predicting the need for prolonged ventilatory support in adult cardiac patients. J. Thorac. Cardiovasc. Surg., *77:*175, 1979.
51. Higgins, T. L., et al.: Risk factors for respiratory complications after cardiac surgery. Anesthesiology, *75:*A258, 1991.
52. Warner, M. A., et al.: Role of preoperative cessation of smoking and other factors in postoperative pulmonary complications: a blinded prospective study of coronary artery bypass patients. Mayo Clin. Proc., *64:*609, 1989.
53. Craig, D. B.: Postoperative recovery of pulmonary function. Anesth. Analg., *60:*46, 1981.
54. Arvan, S., et al.: Subclinical left ventricular abnormalities in young diabetics. Chest, *93:*1031, 1988.
55. Burgos, L. G., et al.: Increased intraoperative cardiovascular morbidity in diabetics with autonomic neuropathy. Anesthesiology, *70:*591, 1989.
56. Owens, W. D., Felts, J. A., and Spitznagel, E. L., Jr.: ASA physical status classifications: a study of consistency of ratings. Anesthesiology, *49:*239, 1978.
57. Goldman, L., et al.: Multifactorial index of cardiac risk in noncardiac surgical procedures. N. Engl. J. Med., *297:*845, 1977.
58. Goldman, L., Hashimoto, B., Cook, E. F., and Loscalzo, A.: Comparative reproducibility and validity of systems for assessing cardiovascular functional class: advantages of a new specific activity scale. Circulation, *64:*1227, 1981.
59. Knaus, W. A., et al.: APACHE II: a severity of disease classification system. Crit. Care Med., *13:*818, 1985.
60. Paiement, B., et al.: A simple classification of the risk in cardiac surgery. Can. Anaesth Soc. J., *30:*61, 1983.
61. Parsonnet, V., Dean, D., and Bernstein, A. D.: A method of uniform stratification of risk for evaluating the results of surgery in acquired adult heart disease. Circulation, *79(Suppl. I):*I-3, 1989.
62. Hannan, E. L., et al.: Adult open heart surgery in New York state. JAMA, *264:*2768, 1990.
63. O'Connor, G. T., et al.: A regional prospective study of in-hospital mortality associated with coronary artery bypass grafting. N. Engl. J. Med., *266:*803, 1991.
64. Reed, G. L. III, Singer, D. E., Picard, E. H., and DeSanctis, R. W.: Stroke following coronary-artery bypass surgery. N. Engl. J. Med., *319:*1246, 1988.
65. Cosgrove, D. M., Hertzer, N. R., and Loop, F. D.: Surgical

management of synchronous carotid and coronary artery disease. J. Vasc. Surg., *3*:690, 1985.
66. Jastremski, M., et al.: Glucocorticoid treatment does not improve neurological recovery following cardiac arrest. JAMA, *262*:3427, 1989.
67. Wynands, J. E.: Barbiturates should be used for brain protection during open heart surgery. J. Cardiothorac. Anesth., *2*:385, 1988.
68. Stevenson, R. L., and Rogers, M. C.: Con: barbiturates for brain protection during cardiopulmonary bypass: fact or fantasy? J. Cardiothorac. Anesth., *2*:390, 1988.
69. Higgins, T. L., Paganini, E. P., Noor, F. A., and Blum, J.: Elevated preoperative creatinine: importance as a risk factor for morbidity and mortality after coronary artery bypass surgery (CABG). Abstr. Soc. Cardiovasc. Anesthesiol., *12*:120, 1990.
70. Davis, R. F., et al.: Acute oliguria after cardiopulmonary bypass: renal functional improvement with low-dose dopamine infusion. Crit. Care Med., *10*:852, 1982.
71. Tyras, D. H., et al.: Global left ventricular impairment and myocardial revascularization: determinants of survival. Ann. Thorac. Surg., *37*:37, 1984.
72. Goenen, M., et al.: Preoperative left ventricular dysfunction and operative risks in coronary bypass surgery. Chest, *92*:804, 1987.
73. Sergeant, P., Flameng, W., Lesaffre, E., and Suy, R.: The value of ejection fraction as a predictor of early and late survival following aortocoronary bypass surgery in patients with moderate to severe depression of the left ventricular function. Thorac. Cardiovasc. Surg., *35*:87, 1987.
74. Gill, I. S., et al.: Left ventricular dysfunction in coronary bypass: prediction of survival. Circulation, *86*:1, 1992.
75. Spencer, F. C.: A critique of emergency and urgent operations for complications of coronary artery disease. Circulation, *74*:1160, 1989.
76. Maccioli, G. A., Lucas, W. J., and Norfleet, E. A.: The Intraaortic balloon pump: a review. J. Cardiothorac. Anesth., *2*:365, 1988.
77. Gold, H. G., et al.: Refractory angina pectoris: follow-up after intraaortic balloon pumping and surgery. Circulation, *54*:41, 1976.
78. Weintraub, R. M., et al.: Medically refractory unstable angina pectoris. I. Long-term follow-up of patients undergoing intra-aortic balloon counterpulsation and operation. Am. J. Cardiol., *43*:877, 1979.
79. McEnany, M. T., et al.: Clinical experience with intraaortic balloon pump support in 728 patients. Circulation, *58*:122, 1978.
80. Pae, W. E., Jr., et al.: Long-term results of ventricular assist pumping in postcardiotomy cardiogenic shock. J. Thorac. Cardiovasc Surg., *93*:434, 1987.
81. Pennock, J. L., et al.: Survival and complications following ventricular assist pumping for cardiogenic shock. Ann. Surg., *198*:469, 1983.
82. Farrar, D. J., Hill, D. J., Gray, L. A., and Pennington, D. Q.: Prosthetic ventricles as a bridge to cardiac transplantation. N. Engl. J. Med., *318*:333, 1988.
83. Golding, L. A. R., Stewart, R. W., and Loop, F. D.: Ventricular assist devices in clinical practice. *In* Assisted Circulation. Edited by F. Unger. New York, Springer-Verlag, 1989, p. 160.
84. Wampler, R. K., et al.: Treatment of cardiogenic shock with the hemopump left ventricular assist device. Ann. Thorac. Surg., *52*:505, 1991.
85. Frazier, O. H., et al.: Clinical experience with hemopump. Trans. Am. Soc. Artif. Int. Organs, *35*:604, 1989.
86. Golding, L. A. R.: Postcardiotomy mechanical support. Semin. Thorac. and Cardiovasc. Surg., *3*:29, 1991.
87. Gentry, L. O., Zeluff, B. J., and Cooley, D. A.: Antibiotic prophylaxis in open-heart surgery: a comparison of cefamandole, cefuroxime, and cefazolin. Ann. Thorac. Surg., *46*:167, 1988.
88. Slogoff, S., and Keats, A. S.: Does perioperative myocardial ischemia lead to postoperative myocardial infarction? Anesthesiology, *62*:107, 1985.
89. Higgins, T. L., and Estafanous, F. G.: Labetalol: time, experience, and adrenergic blockade. J. Clin. Anesth., *1*:161, 1989.
90. Weintraub, A. C., and Barash, P. G.: A pulmonary artery catheter is indicated in all patients for coronary artery surgery. J. Cardiothorac. Anesth., *1*:358, 1987.
91. Bashein, G., and Ivey, T. D.: Con: a pulmonary artery catheter is not indicated for all coronary artery surgery. J. Cardiothorac. Anesth., *1*:362, 1987.
92. Mangano, D. T.: Monitoring pulmonary arterial pressure in coronary-artery disease. Anesthesiology, *53*:364, 1980.
93. Lowenstein, E., and Teplick, R.: To (PA) Catheterize or Not to (PA) Catheterize—That is the Question. Anesthesiology, *53*:361, 1980.
94. Loop, F. D., et al.: Myocardial protection during cardiac operations. Decreased morbidity and lower cost with blood cardioplegia and coronary sinus perfusion. J. Thorac. Cardiovasc. Surg., *104*:608, 1992.
95. Diehl, J. T., et al.: Efficacy of Retrograde coronary sinus cardioplegia in patients undergoing myocardial revascularization. A prospective randomized trial. Am. Thorac. Surg., *45*:595, 1988.
96. Blauth, C. I., et al.: Atheroembolism from the ascending aorta. J. Thorac. Cardiovasc. Surg., *103*:1104, 1992.
97. Gardner, T. J., et al.: Stroke following artery bypass grafting. A ten year study. Am. Thorac. Surg., *40*:574, 1986.
98. Barner, H. B., Lea, J. W. IV, Naumein, K. S., and Stoney, W. S. Jr: Emergency coronary bypass not associated with preoperative cardiogenic shock in failed angioplasty, after thrombolysis and for acute infarction. Circulation, *79(Suppl. I)*:I-152, 1989.
99. Hooshang, B.: Emergency cardiac procedures in patients in cardiogenic shock due to complications of coronary artery disease. Circulation, *79*:1137, 1989.
100. Swain, J. A.: Endocrine responses to cardiopulmonary bypass. *In* Pathophysiology and Techniques of Cardiopulmonary Bypass. Vol. I. Edited by J. R. Utley. Baltimore, Williams & Wilkins, 1982, p. 24.
101. Parker, D. J., et al.: Changes in serum complement and immunoglobulins following cardiopulmonary bypass. Surgery *71*:824, 1972.
102. Utley, J. R., and Stephens, D. B.: Fluid balance during cardiopulmonary bypass. *In* Pathophysiology and Techniques of Cardiopulmonary Bypass. Vol. 2. Edited by J. R. Utley. Baltimore, Williams & Wilkins, 1983, p. 23.
103. Fernandez-del Castillo, C., et al.: Risk factors for pancreatic cellular injury after cardiopulmonary bypass. N. Engl. J. Med., *325*:382, 1991.
104. Edlin, S.: Physiological changes during transport of the critically ill. Int. Care World., *6*:131, 1989.
105. Petre, J. H., Bazaral, M. G., and Estafanous, F. G.: Patient transport: an organized method with direct clinical benefits. Biomed. Instrument. Technol., March/April, 1989.
106. Bazaral, M. G., Petre, J., Cosgrove, D., and Estafanous, F. G.: Operating room design at The Cleveland Clinic Foundation. Cleve. Clin. J. Med., May/June, 1988.
107. Higgins, T. L.: Early endotracheal extubation is preferable

108. Mangano, D. T., et al.: Postoperative myocardial ischemia. Anesthesiology, 76:342, 1992.
109. Chiara, O., et al.: Hypermetabolic response after hypothermic cardiopulmonary bypass. Crit. Care Med., 15:995, 1987.
110. Knight, A. A., et al.: Perioperative Myocardial Ischemia: importance of the preoperative ischemic pattern. Anesthesiology, 68:681, 1988.
111. Sladen, R. N., Renaghan, D., Ashton, J. P., and Wyner, J.: Effect of shivering on mechanical ventilation after cardiac surgery. Anesthesiology, 63:A140, 1985.
112. Sladen, R. N.: Temperature changes and ventilation after hypothermic cardiopulmonary bypass. Anesth. Analg., 62:283, 1983.
113. Burks, L. C., Aisner, J., Fortner, C. L., and Wiernik, P. H.: Meperidine for the treatment of shaking chills and fever. Arch. Intern. Med., 140:483, 1980.
114. Saunders, P. R., Banish, P., Lipton, J. M., and Giesecke, A. H.: Localized regulated radiant heat vs meperidine in the control of postanesthetic shivering. Anesthesiology, 77:3A, 1989.
115. Sharkey, A., Lipton, J. M., Murphy, M. T., and Giesecke, A. H.: Inhibition of postanesthetic shivering with radiant heat. 66:249, 1987.
116. Estafanous, F. G., and Tarazi, R. C.: Systemic arterial hypertension associated with cardiac surgery. Am. J. Cardiol., 46:685, 1980.
117. Bednarski, P., et al. Use of a computerized closed-loop sodium nitroprusside titration system for antihypertensive treatment after heart surgery. Crit. Care Med., 18:1061, 1990.
118. Chauvin, M., Deriaz, H., and Viars, P.: Continuous I.V. infusion of Labetalol for postoperative hypertension. Br. J. Anaesth., 59:1250, 1987.
119. Mullen, J. C., et al.: Postoperative hypertension: a comparison of dilitiazem, nifedipine, and nitroprusside. J. Thorac. Cardiovasc. Surg., 96:122, 1988.
120. Barnett, J. C., and Touchon, R. C.: Short-term control of supraventricular tachycardia with verapamil infusion and calcium pretreatment. Chest, 97:1106, 1990.
121. Vidt, D. G., and Bakst, A. W.: Adenosine: a new drug for acute termination of supraventricular tachycardia. Cleve. Clinic J. Med., 57:383, 1990.
122. Rankin, A. C., and McGovern, B. A.: Adenosine or verapamil for the acute treatment of supraventricular tachycardia? Ann. Intern. Med., 114:513, 1991.
123. Gray, R. J., et al.: Esmolol: a new ultrashort-acting beta-adrenergic blocking agent for rapid control of heart rate in postoperative supraventricular tachyarrhythmias. J. Am. Coll. Cardiol., 5:1451, 1985.
124. Creswell, L. L., Schuessler, R. B., Rosenbloom, M., and Cox, J. L.: Hazards of postoperative atrial arrhythmias. Ann. Thorac. Surg., 56:539, 1993.
125. Cox, J. L.: A perspective of postoperative and atrial fibrillation in cardiac operations. Ann. Thorac. Surg., 56:405, 1993.
126. Kowey, P. R., Taylor, J. E., Rials, S. J., and Marinchak, R. A.: Meta-analysis of the effectiveness of prophylactic drug therapy in preventing supraventricular arrhythmia early after coronary artery bypass grafting. Circulation, 69:963, 1992.
127. Fanning, W. J., et al.: Prophylaxis of atrial fibrillation with magnesium sulfate after coronary artery bypass grafting. Ann. Thorac. Surg., 52:529, 1991.
128. England, M. R., Gordon, G., Salem, M., and Chenow, B.: Magnesium administration and dysrrhythmias after cardiac surgery: a placebo-controlled, double-blind, randomized trial. JAMA, 268:2395, 1992.
129. VanLente, F., et al.: The predictive value of serum enzymes for perioperative myocardial infarction after cardiac operations. An autopsy study. J. Thorac. Cardiovasc. Surg., 98:704, 1989.
130. Wahl, G. W., Feins, R. H., Alfieres, G., and Bixby, K.: Reinfusion of shed blood after coronary operation causes elevation of cardiac enzyme levels. Ann. Thorac. Surg., 53:625, 1992.
131. Kinoshita, K., Tsuruhara, Y., and Tokunaga, K.: Delayed time to peak serum myoglobin level as an indicator of cardiac dysfunction following open heart surgery. Chest, 99:1398, 1991.
132. Czer, L. S. C.: Mediastinal bleeding after cardiac surgery: etiologies, diagnostic considerations, and blood conservation methods. J. Cardiothorac. Anesth., 3:760, 1989.
133. Hoit, B. D., Gabel, M., and Fowler, N. O.: Cardiac tamponade in left ventricular dysfunction. Circulation, 82:1370, 1990.
134. Michelson, E. L., Torosian, M., Morganroth, J., and MacVaugh, H. III: Early recognition of surgically correctable causes of excessive mediastinal bleeding after coronary artery bypass graft surgery. Am. J. Surg., 139:313, 1980.
135. Cosgrove, D. M., Amiot, D. M., and Meserko, J. J.: An improved technique for autotransfusion of shed mediastinal blood. Ann. Thorac. Surg., 40:519, 1985.
136. Hackmann, T., et al. A trial of desmopression (1-Desamino-8-D-argine Vasopressin) to reduce blood loss in uncomplicated cardiac surgery. N. Engl. J. Med., 321:1437, 1989.
137. Royston, D., Bidsturp, B. P., Taylor K. M., and Sapsford, R. N.: Effect of aprotinin on need for blood transfusion after repeat open-heart surgery. Lancet, 2:1289, 1987.
138. Cosgrove, D. M., et al. Aprotinin therapy for reoperative myocardial revascularization: a placebo-controlled study. Ann. Thorac. Surg., 54:1031, 1992.
139. Mongan, P. D., and Hosking, M. P.: The role of desmopressin acetate in patients undergoing coronary artery bypass surgery. A controlled clinical trial with thrombolastographic risk stratification. Anesthesiology, 77:38, 1992.
140. Zurick, A. M., et al.: Failure of postive end-expiratory pressure to decrease postoperative bleeding after cardiac surgery. Ann. Thorac. Surg., 6:608, 1982.
141. Braun, S. R., Brinbaum, M. L., and Chopra, P. S.: Pre- and postoperative pulmonary function abnormalities in coronary artery revascularization surgery. Chest, 73:316, 1978.
142. Ratliff, N. B., et al. Pulmonary injury secondary to extracorporeal circulation. J. Thorac. Cardiovasc. Surg., 65:425, 1973.
143. Good, J. T., Jr et al.: The routine use of positive end-expiratory pressure after open heart surgery. Chest, 76:397, 1979.
144. Guyton, R. A., et al.: The influence of positive-end expiratory pressure on intrapericardial pressure and cardiac function after coronary artery bypass surgery. J. Cardiothorac. Anesth., 1:98, 1987.
145. Boldt, J., et al. Influence of PEEP Ventilation immediately after cardiopulmonary bypass on right ventricular function. Chest, 94:566, 1988.
146. Pepe, P. E., Hudson, L. D., and Carrico, C. J.: Early application of positive end-expiratory pressure in patients at risk for the adult respiratory-distress syndrome. N. Engl. J. Med., 311:281, 1984.
147. Valta, P., Takala, J., Elissa, T., and Milic-Emili, J.: Effects of PEEP on respiratory mechanics after open heart surgery. Chest, 102:227, 1992.
148. Pepe, P. E., and Marini, J. J.: Occult positive end-expiratory

pressure in mechanically ventilated patients with airflow obstruction. Am. Rev. Respir. Dis., *126:*166, 1982.
149. Wolff, G., Brunner, J. X., Ing., D. E., and Gradel, E.: Gas exchange during mechanical ventilation and spontaneous breathing: intermittent mandatory ventilation after open heart surgery. Chest, *90:*11, 1986.
150. Gal, T. H.: Effects of endotracheal intubation on normal cough performance. Anesthesiology, *53:*324, 1980.
151. Dantzker, D. R., et al.: Gas exchange alterations associated with weaning from mechanical ventilation following coronary artery bypass grafting. Chest, *82:*674, 1982.
152. Foster, G. H., et al.: Early extubation after coronary artery bypass: brief report. Crit. Care Med., *11:*603, 1983.
153. Lichtenthal, P. R., Wade, I. D., Niemyski, P. R., and Shapiro, B. A.: Respiratory management after cardiac surgery with inhalation anesthesia. Crit. Care Med., *11:*603, 1983.
154. Klineberg, P. L., Geer, R. T., Hirsh, R. A., and Aukburg, S. J.: Early extubation after coronary artery bypass graft surgery. Crit. Care Med., *5:*272, 1977.
155. Shackford, S. R., Virgilio, R. W., and Peters, R. M.: Early extubation versus prophylactic ventilation in the high risk patient: a comparison of postoperative management in the prevention of respiratory complications. Anesth. Analg., *60:*76, 1981.
156. Gall, S. A., et al.: Beneficial effects of endotracheal extubation on ventricular performance. J. Thorac. Cardiovasc. Surg., *95:*819, 1988.
157. Prakash, O., et al.: Criteria for early extubation after intracardiac sugery in adults. Anesth Analg., *56:*703, 1977.
158. Quasha, A. L., et al.: Postoperative respiratory care: a controlled trial of early and late extubation following coronary-artery bypass grafting. Anesthesiology, *52:*135, 1980.
159. Lemaire, F., et al.: Acute left ventricular dysfunction during unsuccessful weaning from mechanical ventilation. Anesthesiology, *69:*171, 1988.
160. Coraim, F. J., Coraim, H. P., Ebermann, R., and Stellwag, F. M.: Acute respiratory failure after cardiac surgery: clinical experience with the application of continuous arteriovenous hemofiltration. Crit. Care Med., *14:*714, 1986.
161. Higgins, T. L., et al. Risk factors for respiratory complications after cardiac surgery. Anesthesiology, *75:*3A, 1991.
162. Berrizbeitia, L. D., et al.: Effect of sternotomy and coronary bypass surgery on postoperative pulmonary mechanics. Chest, *96:*873, 1989.
163. Kollef, M. H.: Ventilator-associated pneumonia: a multivariate analysis. JAMA, *270:*1965, 1993.
164. Ledingham, E. M. C. A., et al.: Triple regimen of selective decontamination of the digestive tract, systemic cefotaxime, and microbiological surveillance for prevention of acquired infection in intensive care. Lancet, *1:*785, 1988.
165. Loop, F. D., et al.: Myocardial protection during cardiac operations: decreased morbidity and lower cost with blood cardioplegia and coronary sinus perfusion. J. Thorac. Cardiovasc. Surg., *140:*608, 1992.
166. Brun-Bruisson, C., et al.: Intestinal decontamination for control of noscomial multiresistant gram-negative bacilli. Ann. Intern. Med., *110:*873, 1989.
167. Sivak, E. D., et al.: Effects of fuoresemide versus isolated ultrafiltration on extravascular lung water in oleic acid-induced pulmonary edema. Crit. Care Med., *14:*48, 1986.
168. Wilcox, P., et al.: Phrenic nerve function and its relationship to atelectasis after coronary artery bypass surgery. Chest, *93:*693, 1988.
169. Abd, A. G., et al.: Diaphragmatic dysfunction after open heart surgery: treatment with a rocking bed. Ann. Intern. Med., *111:*881, 1989.
170. Aubier, M., et al.: Effects of hypocalcemia on diaphragmatic strength generation. J. Appl. Physiol., *58:*2054, 1985.
171. Aubier, M., et al.: Effect of hypophosphatemia on diaphragmatic contractility in patients with acute respiratory failure. N. Engl. J. Med., *313:*420, 1985.
172. Aubier, M., et al.: Dopamine effects on diaphragmatic strength during acute respiratory failure in chronic obstructive pulmonary disease. Ann. Intern. Med., *110:*17, 1989.
173. Aubier, M., et al.: Aminophylline improves diaphragmatic contractility. N. Engl. J. Med., *305:*249, 1981.
174. Sivak, E. D., Razavi, M., Groves, L. K., and Loop, F. D.: Long-term management of diaphragmatic paralysis complicating prosthetic valve replacement. Crit. Care Med., *11:*438, 1983.
175. Bhat, J. G., Bluck, M. C., Lowenstein, J., and Baldwin, D. S.: Renal failure after open heart surgery. Ann. Intern. Med., *84:*677, 1976.
176. Hilberman, M., et al. Acute renal failure following cardiac surgery. J. Thorac. Cardiovasc. Surg., *77:*880, 1979.
177. Koning, H. M., Koning, A. J., and Leusink, J. A.: Serious acute renal failure following open heart surgery. J. Thorac. Cardiovasc. Surg., *33:*283, 1985.
178. Davis. R. F., et al.: Acute oliguria after cardiopulmonary bypass: renal functional improvement with low-dose dopamine infusion. Crit. Care Med., *10:*852, 1982.
179. Schaer, G. L., Mitchell, P. F., and Parrillo, J. E.: Norepinephrine alone versus norepinephrine plus low-dose dopamine: enhanced renal blood flow with combination pressor therapy. Crit. Care Med., *10:*852, 1982.
180. Smith, M., and Treasure, T.: The effect of dopamine on plasma potassium in man. Clin. Intern. Care, *2:*71, 1991.
181. Myers, B. D., and Moran, S. M.: Hemodynamically mediated acute renal failure. N. Engl. J. Med., *314:*97, 1987.
182. Shaw, P. J., et al.: Neurological complications of coronary artery bypass graft surgery: six month follow-up study. Br. Med. J., *293:*165, 1986.
183. Bojar, R. M., et al.: Neurological complications of coronary revascularization. Ann. Thorac. Surg., *36:*427, 1983.
184. Calabrese, J. R., et al.: Incidence of postoperative delirium following myocardial revascularization. Cleve. Clin. J. Med., *54:*29, 1987.
185. Coyle, J. P.: Sedation, pain relief, and neuromuscular blockade in the postoperative cardiac surgical patient. Semin. Thorac. Cardiovasc. Surg., *3:*102, 1991.
186. Mahfood, S. S., Higgins, T. L., and Loop, F. D.: Management of complications related to coronary artery bypass surgery. *In* Management of Complications Related to Coronary Artery Bypass Surgery. Edited by J. A. Waldhausen and M. B. Orringer. St. Louis, Mosby-Year Book, 1991, p. 265.
187. Krasna, M. J., et al.: Gastrointestinal complications after cardiac surgery. Surgery, *104:*733, 1988.
188. Hanks, J. B., et al.: Gastrointestinal complications after cardiopulmonary bypass. Surgery, *92:*394, 1982.
189. Ephgrave, K. S., Kleinman-Wexler, R. L., and Adar, C. G.: Enteral nutrients prevent stress ulceration and increase intragastric volume. Crit. Care Med., *18:*621, 1990.
190. Sanderson, R. G., Ellison, J. H., Benson, J. A., and Starr, A.: Jaundice following open-heart surgery. Ann. Surg., *165:*217, 1967.
191. Haas, G. S., Warshaw, A. L., Daggert, W. M., and Aretz, H. T.: Acute pancreatitis after cardiopulmonary bypass. Am. J. Surg., *149:*508, 1985.
192. Borkon, A. M., et al.: Diagnosis and management of postoperative pericardial effusions and late cardiac tamponade following open-heart surgery. Ann. Thorac. Surg., *31:*512, 1981.
193. DeLaria, G. A., et al.: Leg wound complications associated

with coronary revascularization. J. Thorac. Cardiovasc. Surg., 81:403, 1981.
194. Rulinson, R. M., Holland, P., Schmidt, P. J., and Morrow, A. G.: Serum hepatitis after open heart complications. J. Thorac. Cardiovasc. Surg., 50:575, 1965.
195. Lipid research clinics program: The lipid research clinics coronary primary prevention trial results II. The relationship of reduction in incidence of coronary heart disease to cholesterol lowering. JAMA, 251:365, 1984.
196. Frick, M. H., et al.: Helsinki Heart Study: primary-prevention trial with gemfibrozil in middle-aged men with dyslipidemia. Safety of treatment, changes in risk factors, and incidence of coronary artery disease. N. Engl. J. Med., 317:1237, 1987.
197. Kannel, W. B., et al.: Overall and coronary heart disease mortality rates in relation to major risk factors in 325,348 men screened for the MRFIT. Multiple Risk Factor Intervention Trial. Am. Heart J., 112:825, 1986.
198. Blankenhorn, D. H., et al.: Beneficial effects of combined colestipol-niacin therapy on coronary atherosclerosis and coronary venous bypass grafts. JAMA 257:3233, 1987.
199. Vietstra, R. E., et al.: Effect of cigarette smoking on survival of patients with angiographically documented coronary artery disease. Report from the CASS registry. JAMA, 255:1023, 1986.
200. Mulcahy, R.: Influence of cigarette smoking on morbidity and mortality for myocardial infarction. Br. Heart J., 49:410, 1983.
201. Hermanson, B., Omenn, G. S., Kornmal, R. A., and Gersh, B. J.: Beneficial six-year outcome of smoking cessation in older men and women with coronary artery disease. Results from the CASS registry. N. Engl. J. Med., 319:1365, 1988.
202. Yusuf, S., et al.: Beta-blockade during and after myocardial infarction. An overview of the randomized trials. Prog. Cardiovasc. Dis., 27:335, 1985.
203. Goldman, L., et al.: Costs and effectiveness of routine therapy with long term B-adrenergic antagonists after acute myocardial infarction. N. Engl. J. Med., 319:152, 1988.
204. Chesboro, J. M., et al.: Effect of dipyridamole and aspirin on late venous graft patency after coronary bypass operation. N. Engl. J. Med., 310:209, 1989.
205. Secondary prevention of vascular disease by prolonged antiplatelet treatment. Antiplatelet Trialists' Collaboration. Br. Med. J. Clin. Res., 296:320, 1988.
206. Jenkins, C. D. Roseman, R. H., and Zyzanski, S. J.: Prediction of clinical coronary heart disease by a test for the coronary-prone behavior pattern. N. Engl. J. Med., 290:1271, 1974.
207. Ragland, D. R., and Brand, R. J.: Type A behavior and mortality from coronary heart disease. N. Engl. J. Med., 318:65, 1988.
208. Peiris, A. N., et al.: Adiposity, fat distribution, and cardiovascular risk. Ann. Intern. Med., 110:867, 1989.
209. The SOLVD Investigators: Effect of enalapril on survival in patients with reduced left ventricular ejection fractions and congestive heart failure. N. Engl. J. Med., 325:293, 1991.
210. Pilz, G., et al.: Early sepsis treatment with immunoglobulins after cardiac surgery in score identified high-risk patients. Chest, 105:76, 1994.
211. Hammermeister, K. E., Burchfiel, C., Johnson, R., and Grover, F. L.: Identification of patients at greatest risk for developing major complications at cardiac surgery. Circulation, 82:IV-380, 1990.

Chapter 31

NONISCHEMIC ALTERATION OF MYOCARDIAL FUNCTION

RICHARD C. BECKER
STEPHEN J. VOYCE

Normal myocardial function is dependent on a complex interaction of events beginning at the cellular level of individual myocytes and ranging to include physiologic restraint at the level of the pericardium. Acknowledging the fact that normal cellular perfusion is a prerequisite for maintaining the structural and functional integrity of all living tissues, an appreciation that myocardial function may be altered independently of abnormalities in perfusion is of critical importance.

Nonischemic alteration of myocardial function considers a broad range of cardiac disorders, including:

- Pericardial disease
  Pericardial effusion
  Pericardial effusion with cardiac tamponade
  Constrictive pericarditis
- Restrictive cardiomyopathy
- Dilated cardiomyopathy
- Hypertrophic cardiomyopathy
- High output heart failure
- Cardiac trauma
- Sepsis-related myocardial dysfunction

PERICARDIAL DISEASE

Anatomy and Physiology

The pericardium encloses the heart and great vessels. It consists of a fibroserous sac with an inner layer (visceral pericardium) and an outer layer (parietal pericardium) which adheres to the vertebral column posteriorly, sternum and costal cartilages anteriorly, diaphragm inferiorly and reflects to the great vessels superiorly (Fig. 31-1). A small physiologic effusion commonly exists (approximately 15 to 30 ml), with constituents similar to those of normal serum.

The pericardium has been a source of curiosity, experimental investigation, and enigmatic concern for centuries. Although some have suggested that the pericardium is a relatively unimportant anatomic structure, it has become increasingly evident that it has numerous physiologic roles:

- *Ligamentous*
  Limits cardiac displacement through attachment to adjacent structures
- *Membranous*
  Reduces external friction from cardiac motion
  Provides a barrier to inflammatory processes originating in contiguous structures
  Provides a buttressing effect for thin-walled myocardial structures (e.g., atria, right ventricle)
- *Mechanical*
  Limits excessive dilation (constraint)
  Prevents or minimizes mitral and tricuspid regurgitation
  Maintains cardiac output in response to venous inflow
  Maintains normal ventricular compliance

Pericardial Effusion

A pericardial effusion is a collection of fluid within the pericardial space which most commonly results from an inflammatory process involving the pericardium (Table 31-1). In addition, however, a broad range of both local and systemic disorders have been associated with the development of a pericardial effusion (Table 31-2).

The **total** pericardial volume consists of the volume within the cardiac chambers **plus** the pericardial fluid volume. The curve relating the total pericardial volume to the pericardial pressure is extremely steep, suggesting that the reserve volume of the pericardium is small (Fig. 31-2). The flat, early portion of the curve is important and reflects normal adaptive changes in cardiac volume associated with respiration and upright posture. The steep portion of the curve reflects the ability of the pericardium to prevent acute dilation, yet at the same time to be responsible for the physiology observed in cardiac tamponade. In this portion of the curve, small changes in pericardial volume cause a marked increase in pericardial pressure.

The development of increased intrapericardial pressure depends on three distinct components:

- The absolute volume of fluid within the pericardial space
- The rate of fluid accumulation
- The ability of the pericardium to stretch (compliance, distensibility)

When fluid accumulates **slowly,** the pericardial space may accommodate one or two liters without a significant change in intrapericardial pressure; however, the normal pericardium will not usually allow more than 100 to 200

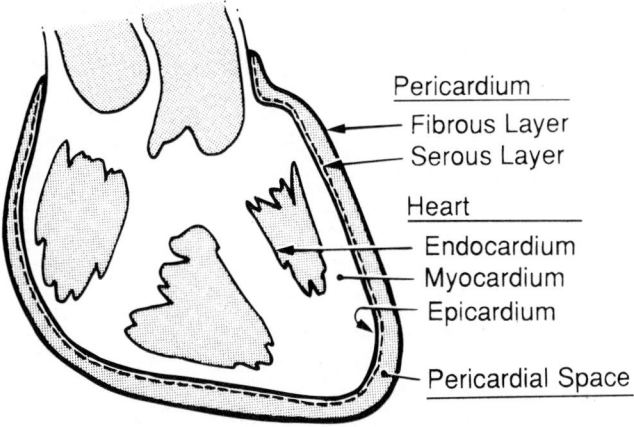

Fig. 31–1. The pericardium including fibrous and serous layers. The pericardial space is shown.

ml of fluid to accumulate **rapidly** without a sharp increase in pressure. In contrast, a thickened, noncompliant pericardium will generate a high pressure with as little as 50 ml of fluid, particularly if accumulation is rapid. An elevation of intrapericardial pressure to levels approaching those generated within the ventricles during diastole impairs filling, and, as a result, decreases total stroke volume and cardiac output. This physiologic condition is referred to as Cardiac tamponade.

Pre-ICU Phase

The **clinical signs and symptoms** in patients with pericardial effusions vary widely and may at times merely reflect the underlying disorder responsible for the effusion rather than the effusion itself. At other times, however, profound hemodynamic abnormalities may predominate with systemic hypotension, cardiogenic shock, or sudden cardiac death.

Previously, pericardial inflammation (acute pericarditis) is the most common cause of a pericardial effusion. The symptoms of acute pericarditis consist typically of sharp and persistent substernal chest pain that is sudden in onset, rapidly progressive, and frequently exacerbated by movement, coughing, swallowing, deep inspiration, or lying supine. The pain may be lessened by sitting upright and leaning forward. Radiation of pain to the left trapezius ridge is considered classic for acute pericarditis; however, the pain may occasionally radiate down the arms thereby simulating acute myocardial infarction. Large pericardial effusions, such as those seen among patients with chronic renal failure, are usually associated with nonspecific precordial discomfort. In addition, large effusions, through direct compression of adjacent mediastinal structures, may cause symptoms including hoarseness (recurrent laryngeal nerve), coughing (bronchi), dyspnea and tachypnea (trachea), or dysphagia (esophagus).

The amount of pericardial fluid by itself does not determine the need for admission to the ICU. Patients with moderate to large pericardial effusions of a chronic nature may be hemodynamically stable, whereas patients with small to moderate effusions developing acutely may deteriorate rapidly. In general, a pericardial effusion associated with either a new or worsening hemodynamic profile warrants an ICU evaluation.

In situations characterized by a sudden increase in pericardial fluid, the patient typically appears cool and clammy with diaphoresis, is tachycardic, and has mottled extremi-

Table 31–1. Causes of Acute Pericarditis

Idiopathic
Infectious
  Viral
  Bacterial
  Mycotic
  Rickettsial
  Parasitic
  Spirochetal
  Mycoplasma
Metabolic
  Uremia (acute, chronic)
  Myxedema
  Gout
  Cholesterol
Collagen Vascular/Immune
  Systemic lupus erythematosus
  Scleroderma
  Rheumatoid arthritis
  Sjögren's Syndrome
  Wegener's granulomatosis
  Serum sickness
  Rheumatic fever
  Inflammatory bowel disease
  Polymyositis (dermatomyositis)
Disorders of Contiguous Structures
  Myocardial infarction (acute)
  Myocardial infarction (chronic; Dressler's syndrome)
  Pneumonia
  Pulmonary embolism
  Aortic dissection
  Endocarditis
Neoplastic
  Primary
  Secondary (metastatic)
Traumatic
Miscellaneous
  Fat embolism
  Fabry's disease
  Pancreatitis (acute)
  Sarcoidosis

Table 31–2. Causes of Pericardial Effusion

Idiopathic causes
Infections
Neoplasia
Connective tissue disease
Uremia
Trauma
Cardiac rupture
Aortic dissection
Aortic aneurysm rupture
Postpericardiotomy
Hypothyroidism
Postirradiation

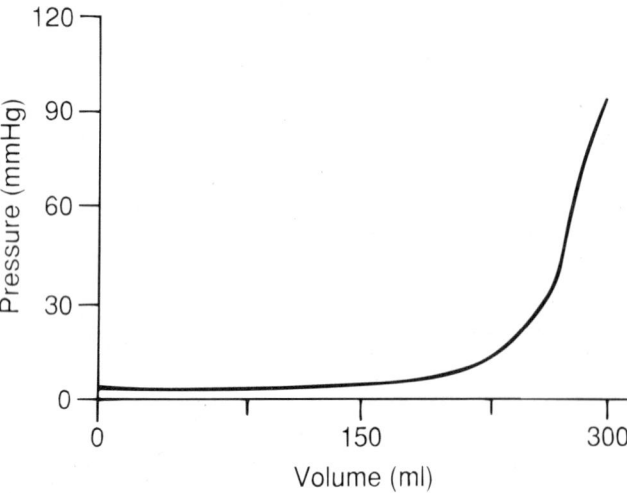

Fig. 31–2. The pericardial pressure-volume curve. Pericardial pressure remains low up to a critical volume at which time a sharp and progressive increase in pressure occurs with accumulation of additional volume.

ties (shock state). In subacute conditions, the systemic blood pressure is low-normal or low with a narrow pulse pressure and an inspiratory decline in systolic blood pressure greater than 10 mm Hg (pulsus paradoxus). Oliguria may be one of the earliest signs of hemodynamic compromise. The heart sounds may be distant and compression of the left lower lung field may produce a focal area of decreased breath sounds (Ewart's signs). Moderate jugular venous distension may also be appreciated.

ICU Phase

Diagnostic Evaluation. *Electrocardiogram (ECG).* The ECG accompanying a pericardial effusion may be normal, have nonspecific ST-T wave abnormalities, or reveal findings that reflect an underlying myocardial or pericardial process such as acute myocardial infarction or pericarditis.[1] With moderate to large effusions, QRS and T-wave amplitudes may be diminished, whereas P-wave amplitude is typically preserved. Electrical alternans may occur and is characterized by alternating contours of P, QRS, ST, T and, occasionally, U waves. Electrical alternans may involve any or all of the ECG components; however, QRS alternans is the most common. Although electrical alternans is a relatively sensitive finding, it is not specific for pericardial effusion, being seen in patients with congestive heart failure, cardiac trauma, hypertensive heart disease, myocarditis, hypocalcemia, drug intoxication, and following partial or complete pneumonectomy.

Chest Radiograph. The size and configuration of the cardiac silhouette depends on the compliance of the pericardium and rate of fluid accumulation. With large subacute or chronic effusions, the heart typically appears enlarged and globular. A change in size and configuration when compared with a previous chest radiograph may be informative. In general, enlargement of the cardiac silhouette does not occur until at least 250 ml of fluid has accumulated in the pericardial space. Enlargement of the cardiac silhouette from a pericardial effusion may, at times, be difficult to distinguish from cardiomegaly; in the former, however, the pericardial sac is distended to the level of the main pulmonary artery or above, and therefore, the hilar vessels may be obscured. In contrast, cardiomegaly rarely obscures the hilar vessels. In addition, when cardiomegaly and congestive heart failure coexist, pulmonary congestion is seen, which is an uncommon finding with pericardial effusion.

CT/MRI. Computed tomography (CT) and magnetic resonance imaging (MRI) may be used to visualize a pericardial effusion. At the present time, however, they are relatively time consuming, costly, and incapable of providing information beyond that of echocardiography. An exception may be in patients with malignant effusions resulting from metastic disease originating in the lungs or other contiguous structures. In this situation, evaluation of both areas may be undertaken concomitantly.

Echocardiography. The noninvasive diagnostic method of choice in the detection and evaluation of patients with either a suspected or established pericardial effusion is the two-dimensional echocardiogram. Although the M-mode echocardiogram is capable of identifying an effusion as an echo-free space between either the chest wall and the right ventricular free wall (Fig. 31–3) or the posterior left ventricular wall and the pericardium, the two-dimensional echocardiogram provides information regarding surrounding structures, ventricular size and performance, the presence of pericardial masses, and the hemodynamic effects of the effusion as well. Two-dimensional echocardiography can also visualize loculated pericardial effusions and reduces the likelihood of "false-positive" results that may occur with M-mode studies in the setting of an enlarged left atrium, ascites, or a descending aortic aneurysm.[2-4]

With small pericardial effusions, an anterior echo-free space is seen and may at times be difficult to distinguish from epicardial fat. Moderate to large effusions typically produce both an anterior and posterior echo-free space (Fig. 31–4), although frequently the fluid is not evenly distributed.

Cardiac motion may be affected by the presence of pericardial fluid. During most of the cardiac cycle, the anterior and posterior myocardial walls appear to move in similar directions ("the swinging heart"). Pseudoprolapse of the mitral and tricuspid valves may also be seen. Doppler ultrasound evaluation may reveal an inspiratory increase in superior vena cava blood flow velocity.

There are a number of echocardiographic findings that support a diagnosis of cardiac tamponade. Diastolic collapse of the right ventricular free wall or right atrium may be seen with effusions causing hemodynamic compromise; the duration of collapse correlating with the hemodynamic severity (Figs. 31–5 and 31–6). Right atrial collapse appears to be a more sensitive finding for tamponade than right ventricular collapse. The latter is more specific, however.[5,6] Diastolic flow velocity within the

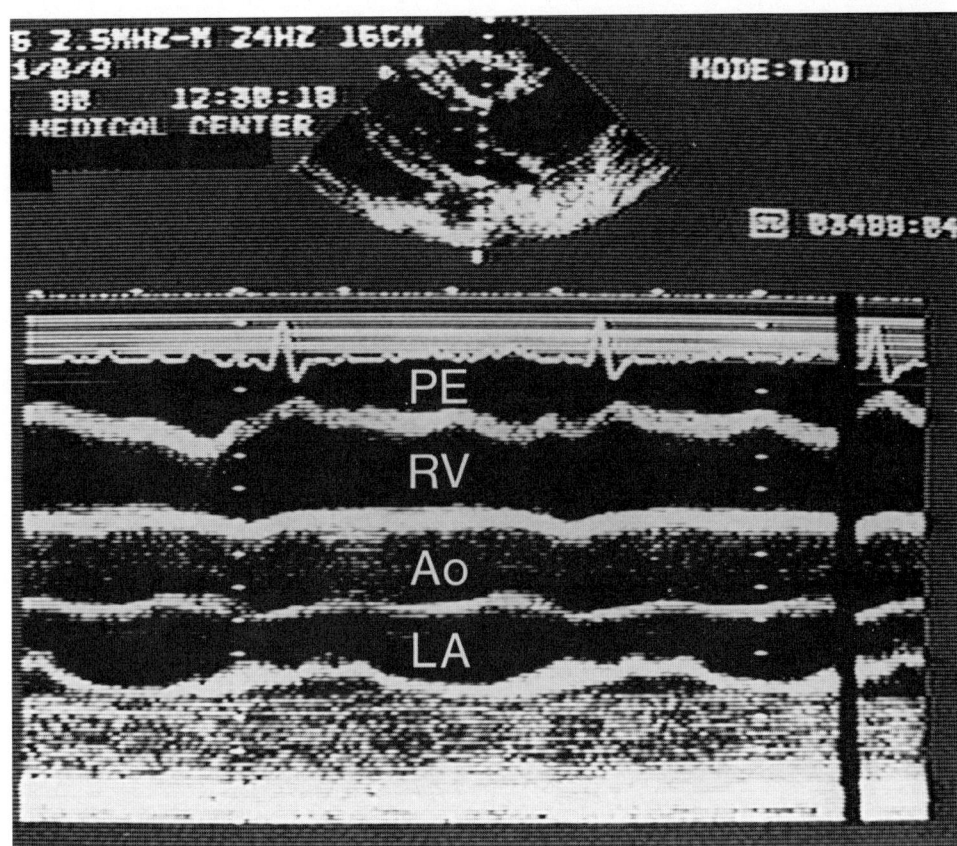

Fig. 31-3. M-mode echocardiogram of a patient with a moderate-sized pericardial effusion. An echo-free space is visualized between the chest wall and the right ventricular free wall. PE, Pericardial effusion; RV, right ventricle; Ao, aorta; LA, left atrium.

superior vena cava is typically reduced or absent during expiration as a result of increased intrapericardial pressure.

Hemodynamic Features. Pulmonary artery catheterization provides confirmatory evidence of tamponade physiology and quantitates the degree of hemodynamic compromise. When used in conjunction with pericardiocentesis, hemodynamic monitoring allows documentation of improvement following pericardial fluid removal, and also provides a way to diagnose coexisting ab-

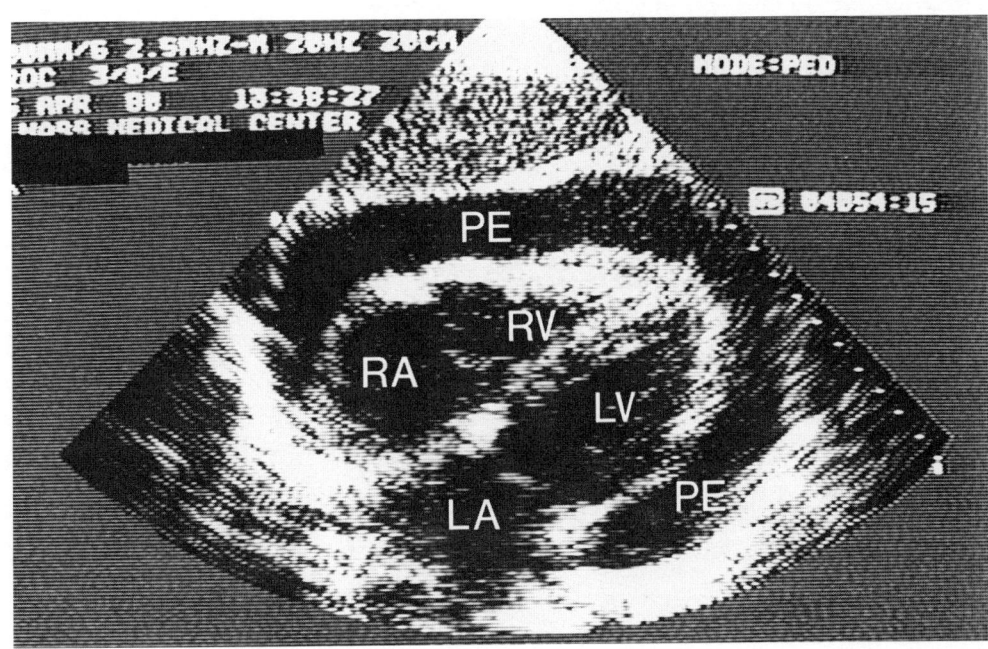

Fig. 31-4. Two-dimensional echocardiogram (subcostal view) of a patient with a moderate to large pericardial effusion. The pericardial effusion (PE) encircles the heart. RV, Right ventricle; RA, right atrium; LV, left ventricle; LA, left atrium.

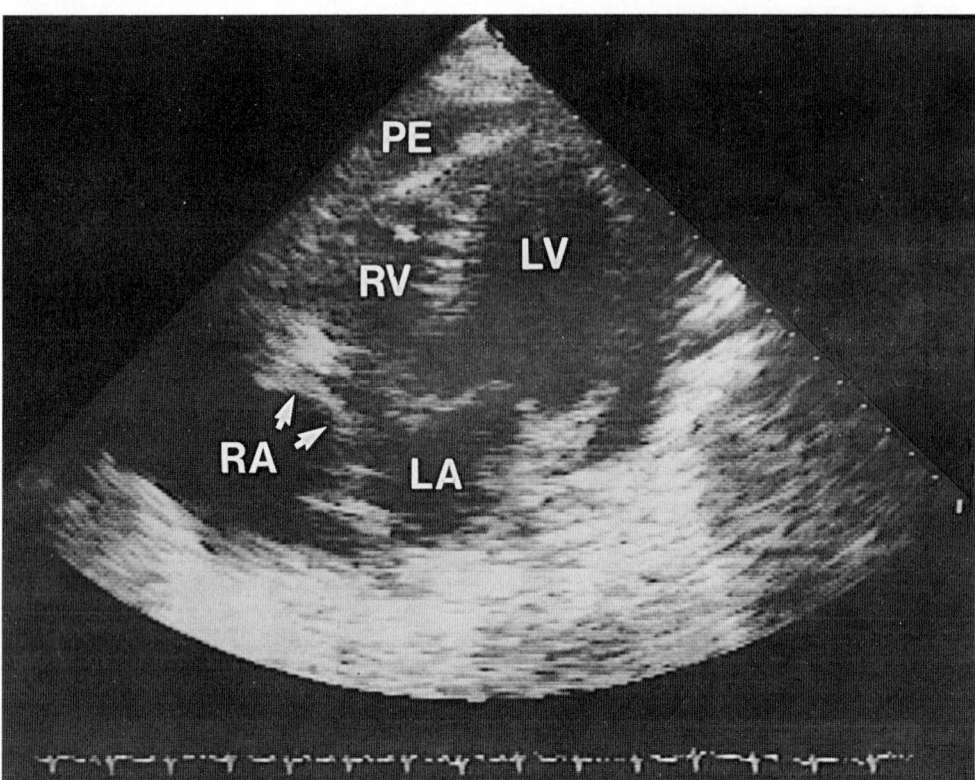

Fig. 31–5. Two-dimensional echocardiogram (apical four chamber view) showing diastolic collapse of the right atrium (arrows) in a patient with a pericardial effusion (PE) causing cardiac tamponade. RV, Right ventricle; RA, right atrium; LV, left ventricle; LA, left atrium.

normalities such as left ventricular dysfunction and effusive-constrictive pericarditis.

Tamponade physiology is characterized by an elevation in right atrial pressure with a prominent X descendent and a diminished or absent Y descent (Fig. 31-7 and Table 31-3).

The X descent reflects a combination of atrial relaxation and downward displacement of the tricuspid valve during right ventricular systole. In contrast, the Y descent is caused by the rapid inflow of blood into the right ventricle during diastole. When right atrial and intrapericardial pressures are obtained simultaneously, they are virtually identi-

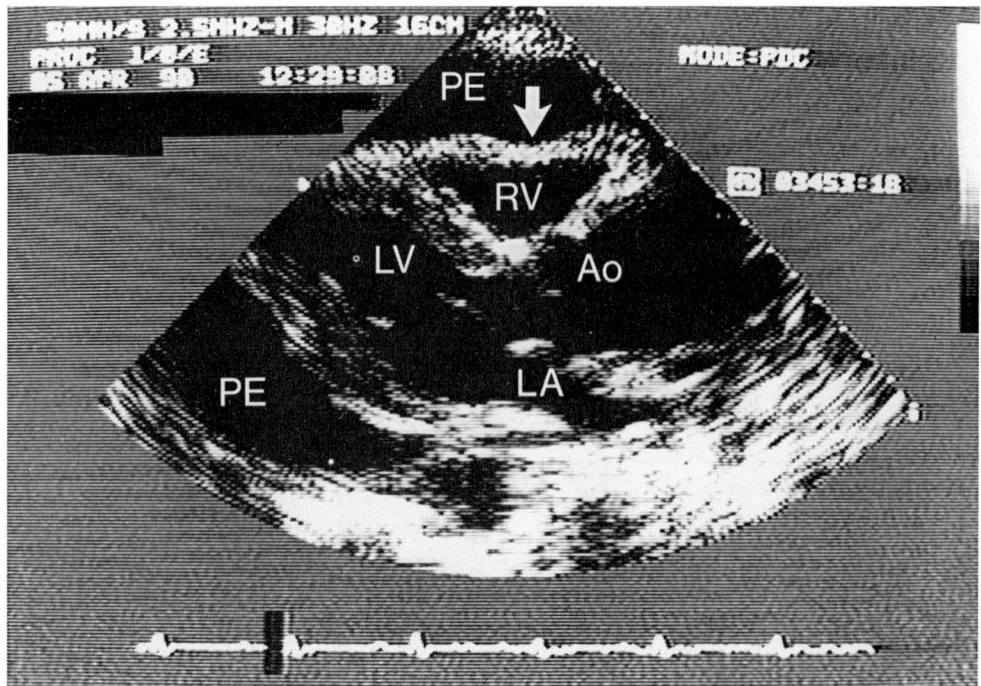

Fig. 31–6. Two-dimensional echocardiogram (parasternal long axis view) showing diastolic collapse of the right ventricle (arrow). PE, Pericardial effusion; RV, right ventricle; LV, left ventricle; LA, left atrium; Ao, aorta.

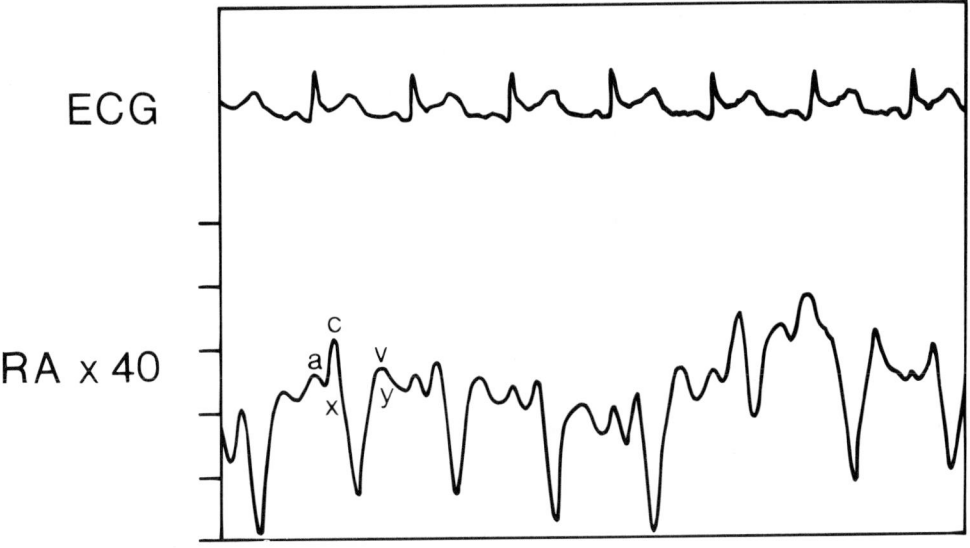

Fig. 31-7. Right atrial (RA) pressure tracing (40 mm Hg scale) of a patient with cardiac tamponade; note the prominent X descent and diminished Y descent (see text for discussion.)

cal (if they are not, the diagnosis of tamponade should be questioned). Right ventricular diastolic and pulmonary wedge pressures may exceed right atrial, right ventricular diastolic, and intrapericardial pressures. In cardiac tamponade, the right ventricular and pulmonary artery systolic pressures reflect the pressure generated by the right ventricle plus the intrapericardial pressure; therefore, they are mild to moderately elevated.

Removal of pericardial fluid results in:

- A lowering of intrapericardial, right atrial, right ventricular, and to a lesser degree pulmonary wedge pressure
- Reappearance of the Y descent in the right atrial pressure tracing
- An improvement in cardiac output
- An increase in systemic blood pressure

Given the steep pressure-volume curve of the pericardial space (see Fig. 31-2), removal of seemingly small amounts of fluid (50 to 100 ml) may result in striking hemodynamic changes.

Differential Diagnosis

- Right ventricular infarction
- Constrictive pericarditis (including constrictive-effusive pericarditis)
- Massive pulmonary embolism with cor pulmonale
- Tension pneumopericardium

Treatment. The presence of a pericardial effusion, in and of itself, may not warrant definitive treatment, particularly if hemodynamic embarrassment is not present and the underlying cause has been ascertained. A diagnostic pericardiocentesis may, however, be of vital importance in situations where the effusion is the result of a systemic disorder or malignant disease. In the setting of cardiac tamponade, a therapeutic pericardiocentesis may be lifesaving (Fig. 31-8). Additionally, care must be exercised to avoid confusion with a diagnosis of congestive heart failure. Above all, narcotics, diuretics, and vasodilators must be avoided because they cause a decrease of venous return (preload), which could cause a fatal fall in cardiac output. In addition to the avoidance of pharmacologic agents that decrease venous return, the clinician should direct therapy to maintain venous return with administration of fluids and, if necessary, vasopressor agents (such as dopamine or norepinephrine).

Pericardiocentesis is performed typically with the patient supine and the thorax elevated to a 30° angle to enhance anterior and inferior pooling of pericardial fluid. The sternal and subxyphoid regions are shaved, cleaned, and prepped. The skin and subcutaneous tissues are then anes-

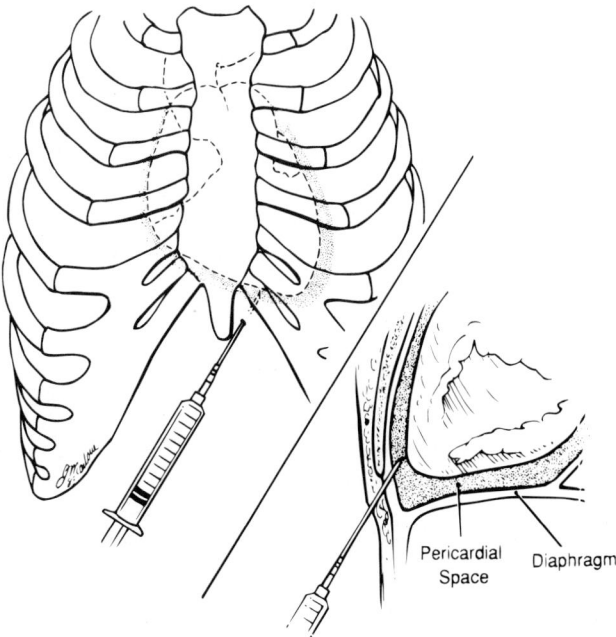

Fig. 31-8. Schematic representation of a pericardiocentesis: a needle is placed below the xiphoid process and slowly advanced into the pericardial space (see text for discussion).

thetized with 1% lidocaine and a small incision is made with a No. 11 blade 0.5 to 2.5 cm below and to the left of the xyphoid process. A long, 16- to 18-gauge needle attached to a hand-held syringe is then advanced (at a 15° posterior tilt) slowly toward either the right or the left shoulder with ECG guidance or, when feasible, echocardiographic guidance. Care should be taken to aspirate continuously while the needle is being advanced; a flash-back of fluid into the syringe will confirm entry into the pericardial space. A floppy guidewire may then be inserted through the needle over which a multiple side hole, soft catheter may be placed to facilitate pericardial drainage. Following the collection of adequate fluid for diagnostic studies or hemodynamic improvement, the catheter should then be sutured securely to the skin and attached via a three-way stopcock to a closed-drainage system. In general, the catheter should not be left in the pericardial space for more than 48 to 72 hours to avoid infection.

Patients undergoing pericardiocentesis should be observed in the ICU for at least 72 hours. Potential complications include:

- Coronary artery laceration
- Myocardial perforation
- Supraventricular arrhythmias
- Ventricular arrhythmias
- Pneumothorax
- Hepatic laceration

Reaccumulation of fluid is usually preceded by a progressive reduction in urine output.

Surgical pericardiectomy or pericardiotomy is preferred over blind pericardiocentesis in patients with traumatic tamponade, leaking aortic or ventricular aneurysms, and with purulent effusions.

Mild to moderate-sized pericardial effusions of idiopathic, viral, and immune-mediated origins may be treated effectively with nonsteroidal anti-inflammatory agents if hemodynamic compromise is not a problem. On occasion, an improvement will not be observed or a recurrent effusion will develop; a short course of corticosteroids may then be required. When corticosteroids are used, care must be taken to taper the dose as rapidly as possible to avoid chronic recurrences and steroid dependency.

Post-ICU Phase

Patients with uncomplicated pericardial effusions rarely require close monitoring following discharge from the ICU. For patients with effusions of unknown origin, diagnostic efforts should continue as needed. Patients experiencing hemodynamic compromise or those requiring emergent pericardiocentesis should be observed closely for evidence of fluid reaccumulation, preferably in a step-down unit or on a monitored floor. Serial echocardiograms may be useful in this regard. Long-term follow-up is determined primarily by the underlying cause.

Constrictive Pericarditis

Constrictive pericarditis is a disorder of the pericardium which is characterized by increased thickness, obliteration of the pericardial space, and impaired diastolic filling of the heart. Although constrictive pericarditis most commonly

Table 31-3. Clinical Manifestations of Cardiac Tamponade

Systemic hypotension
Narrow pulse pressure
Pallor
Dyspnea, orthopnea
Jugular venous distension
Pulsus paradoxus
Distant heart sounds
Shock state

follows acute idiopathic or viral pericarditis, a broad range of causes have been recognized (Table 31-4).

Following an initial episode of acute pericarditis, the early inflammatory phase gives way to a subacute phase characterized by cellular organization, fibrin deposition and resorption of pericardial fluid. In some patients, a chronic phase subsequently develops during which fibrous scarring, calcium deposition, and thickening of the pericardium occurs; if this process is extensive, complete obliteration of the pericardial space may ensue.

Pre-ICU Phase

Clinically, pericardial constriction is typically a chronic process. Therefore, the evolution of its symptoms tends to be gradual. Rarely, however, the symptoms progress rapidly, particularly in effusive-constrictive processes. In general, patients with constrictive pericarditis complain of fatigue, weight loss, generalized weakness, dyspnea on exertion, abdominal distension, and peripheral swelling. Physical examination frequently reveals a chronically ill-appearing individual with generalized muscle wasting and cachexia. The jugular veins are usually distended with a further increase during inspiration (Kussmaul's sign). The systemic blood pressure may be low or normal and pulsus paradoxus may be present. If it is greater than 15 mm Hg, however, a concomitant pericardial effusion should be suspected. The liver may be distended and tender and, not uncommonly, ascites and peripheral edema (reminis-

Table 31-4. Causes of Constrictive Pericarditis

Idiopathic causes
Infections
   Viral
   Fungal
   Tuberculous
   Parasitic
Neoplasia
   Primary
   Secondary (metastatic)
Trauma
Postpericardiotomy
Collagen Vascular Disease
   Systemic lupus erythematosus
   Rheumatoid arthritis
   Scleroderma
Irradiation
Chronic Renal Failure
Rheumatic Heart Disease

cent of severe right-sided congestive heart failure or chronic liver disease) are observed.

In its earliest phase, constrictive pericarditis may not be accompanied by significant clinical manifestations. In later stages of development, or when accompanied by a moderate to large pericardial effusion (effusive-constrictive pericarditis), hemodynamic embarrassment is not uncommon, however. Therefore, the decision underlying ICU admission should rest on the overall clinical status (hemodynamic status) of the patient.

ICU Phase

Diagnostic Evaluation. *ECG Features.* These features of constrictive pericarditis are typically nonspecific, although decreased QRS voltage and generalized T-wave inversions may be seen. On occasion, conduction abnormalities and infarct patterns (Q-waves) occur, reflecting extension of the fibrocalcific process to the myocardium and rarely, compression of one or more coronary arteries.[7]

Chest Radiograph. The cardiac silhouette may be normal in size and configuration; enlargement frequently suggests the presence of a concomitant pericardial effusion. More than 50% of patients have a right pleural effusion. Abnormal left-heart filling pressures may result in prominent hilar vessels, Kerlye B lines, and vascular redistribution. Although intrapericardial calcification supports the diagnosis of pericardial constriction, it is present in fewer than 50% of patients and, moreover, is not a specific finding.

MRI. An MRI may provide useful information regarding the pericardium A pericardial thickness of greater than 4.0 mm is supportive, but not diagnostic, of constrictive pericarditis.[8]

Echocardiography. The two-dimensional echocardiogram can provide useful information, particularly in attempts to exclude processes that may mimic constrictive pericarditis such as restrictive cardiomyopathy and chronic cor pulmonale. In patients with constrictive pericarditis, a number of echocardiographic findings have been described including mid-diastolic flattening of the posterior left-ventricular wall, paradoxic ventricular septal motion, early diastolic atrial or ventricular septal notching, and respiratory variations in both left ventricular isovolumic relaxation time and mitral inflow.[9–11]

Hemodynamic Features. A thickened, noncompliant pericardium impairs diastolic filling of all cardiac chambers equally. Therefore, diastolic pressures are elevated and "equalized" in the right atrium, right ventricle, left atrium, and left ventricle.

Ventricular pressure tracings reveal a characteristic dip and plateau in diastole or "square root sign," whereas tracings within the right atrium show equal A and V waves with an accentuated Y descent (Fig. 31-9). This is in contrast to the sharp X descent seen in tamponade (see Fig. 31-7). (The positive presystolic A wave is produced by right atrial contraction, whereas the late systolic V wave reflects an increase in blood volume within the right atrium during ventricular systole when the tricuspid valve is closed. The X descent is due to a combination of atrial relaxation and the downward displacement of the tricuspid valve during right ventricular systole. Following the V wave is a negative descending limb, the Y descent, caused by the rapid inflow of blood into the right ventricle.) The pulmonary arterial systolic pressure is normal or mildly elevated with a narrow pulse pressure (similar to that seen with cardiac tamponade, but unlike myocardial restriction which typically causes an elevation in pulmonary arterial systolic pressure to greater than 50 mm Hg). The cardiac index is usually low normal or mildly decreased.

Differential Diagnosis. The differential diagnosis includes the following:

- Restrictive cardiomyopathy (Tables 31-5 and 31-6)
- Superior vena cava syndrome
- Chronic liver disease
- Chronic/subacute renal failure
- Chronic cor pulmonale

Treatment. In the majority of cases, constrictive pericarditis is a subacute or chronic process that requires confirmatory diagnostic procedures rather than emergency therapeutic intervention. On rare occasions, however, an effusive-constrictive process may cause rapidly evolving hemodynamic embarrassment which dictates urgent or emergent pericardial drainage (see earlier discussion on cardiac tamponade-pericardiocentesis).

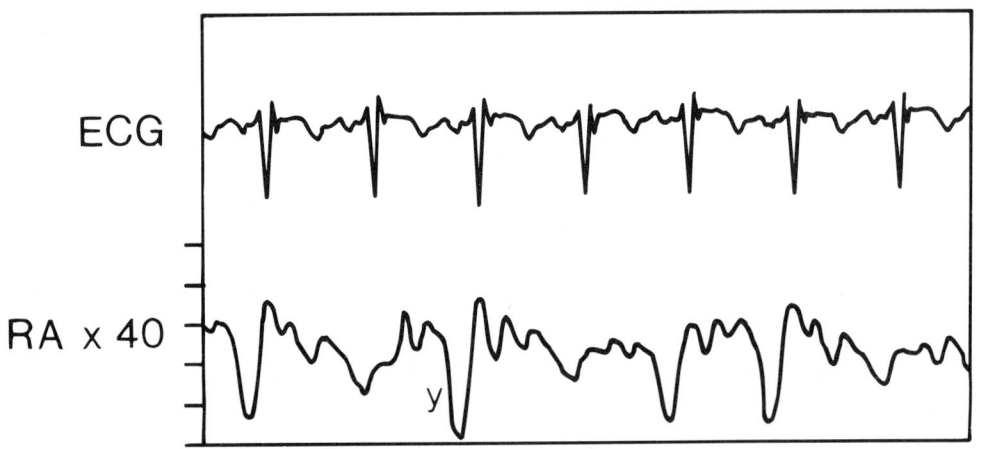

Fig. 31-9. Right atrial (RA) pressure tracing (40 mm Hg scale) of a patient with constrictive pericarditis; note the prominent Y descent (see text for discussion).

Table 31-5. Differentiating Pericardial Constriction from Myocardial Restriction

Study	Constriction	Restriction
Chest radiograph	Calcification	none
Echocardiogram	Thickened pericardium; no mitral or tricuspid insufficiency (MR, TR)	Thickened, granular walls, MR, TR
MRI	Thickened pericardium	none
Hemodynamic features	Equalization of diastolic pressures; classic "square root" sign in RV tracing	LVEDP > RVEDP by 5–10 mm Hg slow, continuous rise in pressure during mid-diastole
Ventricular filling	Rapid through first half of diastole	Rapid very early in diastole, then slows
Endomyocardial biopsy	none	May provide diagnosis

Constrictive pericarditis accompanied by systemic hypotension creates an interesting therapeutic dilemma. Although patients appear markedly fluid overloaded, vigorous diuresis will result in a reduction in venous return (preload) and a further decrease in cardiac output and blood pressure. Vasodilators are also contraindicated. Adequate preload is of critical importance and despite the external appearance of fluid overload intravenous volume expansion with either crystalloid or colloid solutions may be required to maintain systemic blood pressure and vital organ perfusion. Vasopressors may occasionally be required as well.

The definitive therapeutic procedure for constrictive pericarditis is surgical pericardiectomy. The most common surgical approach is a median sternotomy with cardiopulmonary bypass which allows mobilization of the heart and complete pericardial resection.

Table 31-6. Causes of Restrictive Cardiomyopathy

Amyloidosis*
Hemochromatosis
Fabry's disease
Becker's disease
Whipple's disease
Endomyocardial fibrosis
Loeffler's disease
Carcinoid heart disease
Gaucher's disease
Neoplastic infiltration
Pseudoxanthoma elasticum
Endocardial fibroelastosis
Sarcoidosis

* Cardiac amyloidosis may occur as an isolated entity, or as myocardial involvement in a systemic disorder. In either condition, protein-polysaccharide complexes are deposited diffusely leading to a wide variety of cardiovascular manifestations.

Post-ICU Phase

In many patients with constrictive pericarditis, immediate hemodynamic and symptomatic improvement is achieved following surgery. In others, however, improvement may be less pronounced requiring weeks or even months. In the latter situation, certain possibilities should be considered, including:

- Incomplete pericardiectomy
- Concomitant myocardial fibrosis/calcification
- Restrictive cardiomyopathy

DILATED CARDIOMYOPATHY

Dilated cardiomyopathy is a disorder of the myocardium that typically affects each heart chamber causing progressive dilation and, ultimately, congestive heart failure. Although a major impairment in systolic function predominates, abnormalities in diastolic function are invariably present as well.

In most cases, dilated cardiomyopathy follows a viral infection or is of idiopathic origin; however, many potential causes must be considered (Table 31-7). Marked four-chamber enlargement is usually present, the ventricles typically show greater involvement than the atria. Histologic findings include interstitial and perivascular fibrosis, myocardial cell degeneration, and patchy areas of necrosis. Cellular infiltrates may be seen, being more prominent with active myocarditis.[12]

Pre-ICU Phase

In a majority of patients, symptoms develop gradually over weeks or months. With acute myocarditis, however, rapid evolution is common. The symptoms of dilated cardiomyopathy reflect a compromised cardiac output which causes fatigue, generalized weakness, dyspnea on exertion, orthopnea, and paroxysmal nocturnal dyspnea. Prominent findings obtained on physical examination include a low or low-normal systemic blood pressure, an elevated heart rate, jugular venous distension, and pulmonary rales. Evaluation of the precordium may reveal a left and/or right ventricular heave. Although an S4 gallop may precede the development of heart failure, an S3 is the rule once overt heart failure is present. A summation gallop (S3-S4) may be appreciated, particularly in the presence of heart rates exceeding 100 beats per minute. Murmurs of mitral and tricuspid insufficiency are not uncommon and reflect ventricular dilation and distortion of supporting structures within the subvalvular apparati. Late physical findings include hepatomegaly, ascites, and peripheral edema from right ventricular failure.

A thorough physical examination may also reveal important clues to underlying systemic disorders associated with the development of dilated cardiomyopathy[6] (as listed in Table 31-7).

The clinician is likely to admit the patient with cardiomyopathy for therapeutic intervention with inotropic agents or for stabilization before heart transplantation.

Table 31-7. Causes of Dilated Cardiomyopathy

Idiopathic causes
Familial "X linked" disease
Collagen vascular disease
    Systemic lupus erythematosus
    Rheumatoid arthritis
    Dermatomyositis
Infections
    Coxsackie virus A, B
    Echovirus
    Arbovirus
    Toxoplasma gondii
    Trypanosoma cruzi
    Vericella
    Influenza
    Lyme disease
    Cryptococcus
    Neoformans
    Cytomegalovirus
    Mumps
    Psittacosis
    Candida albicans
    Trichinella spiralis
    Schistosoma mansoni
    Leptospira
    Human immunodeficiency virus
Nutritional deficiencies
    Thiamine deficiency
    Vitamin C deficiency
    Selenium deficiency
    Carnitine deficiency
Toxicity
    Ethanol
    Cobalt
    Doxorubicin (Adriamycin)
    Emetine
    Lithium
    Chloroquine
    Bleomycin
    Lead
    Phenothiazines
    Mercury
    Catecholamines
    Reserpine
    Insect bites
    Carbon monoxide
Endocrine disease
    Acromegaly
    Thyrotoxicosis
    Myxedema
    Cushing's disease
    Diabetes mellitus
    Pheochromocytoma
Miscellaneous conditions
    Postpartum status
    Obesity
    Sulfonamides
    Transplant rejection
    Thrombotic thrombocytopenic purpura
    Muscular dystrophies

ICU Phase

Diagnostic Evaluation

ECG Features. Poor ventricular performance necessitates an increased heart rate to maintain cardiac output and vital organ perfusion. Sinus tachycardia, therefore, is the most common ECG finding among patients with dilated cardiomyopathy. A broad spectrum of atrial and ventricular tachyarrhythmias have also been observed (not infrequently adding to hemodynamic and clinical deterioration). In the early stages of the disease process, diffuse nonspecific ST-segment and T-wave changes are common, as is increased QRS voltage resulting from ventricular dilation and increased myocardial mass. In later stages, however, decreased QRS voltage frequently exists which reflects a critical loss in functional myocardium.

Chest Radiograph. The left ventricle frequently appears dilated and generalized cardiomegaly is often present. Signs of pulmonary venous hypertension, including hilar prominence, vascular redistribution, interstitial and alveolar edema, and pleural effusions are typically seen in patients with progressive ventricular dysfunction.

Echocardiogram. Two-dimensional echocardiography provides helpful information regarding the extent of cardiac chamber dilation and functional impairment. In addition, it plays an important role in excluding conditions such as primary valvular heart disease, pericardial effusions with tamponade, and coronary artery disease—specifically, myocardial infarction with focal wall motion abnormalities. In general, the echocardiogram reveals four-chamber dilation with a global reduction in systolic wall thickening. The end-diastolic and end-systolic dimensions are increased significantly (Fig. 31-11). Variable degrees of mitral and tricuspid insufficiency may be appreciated on Doppler examination.

Hemodynamic Features

Early hemodynamic assessment may be vital in patients with dilated cardiomyopathy manifesting systemic hypotension and congestive heart failure. In addition to providing diagnostic information, hemodynamic monitoring can be used to assess treatment response as well. Patients with dilated cardiomyopathy have elevated right- and left-heart pressures. Although the pathologic process is diffuse, the left ventricle is frequently the most severely affected. The pulmonary wedge pressure is, therefore, elevated to a greater degree than right atrial and right ventricular diastolic mean pressures. Typically, the cardiac output and index are moderately to severely reduced with an accompanying elevation in systemic vascular resistance.

Endomyocardial Biopsy

Although it was believed originally that routine endomyocardial biopsy would provide pathogenetic information allowing for specific treatment of patients with dilated cardiomyopathy, this has not been the case.[13] Even in the setting of acute myocarditis, endomyocardial biopsy may not provide important information except in patients with progressive clinical deterioration[13,14] (Fig. 31-10). A biopsy may be helpful, however, when attempting to identify myocardial disorders for which a specific treatment has been identified (Table 31-8).

Treatment

Because a majority of dilated cardiomyopathies are of idiopathic origin, the initial treatment is usually supportive

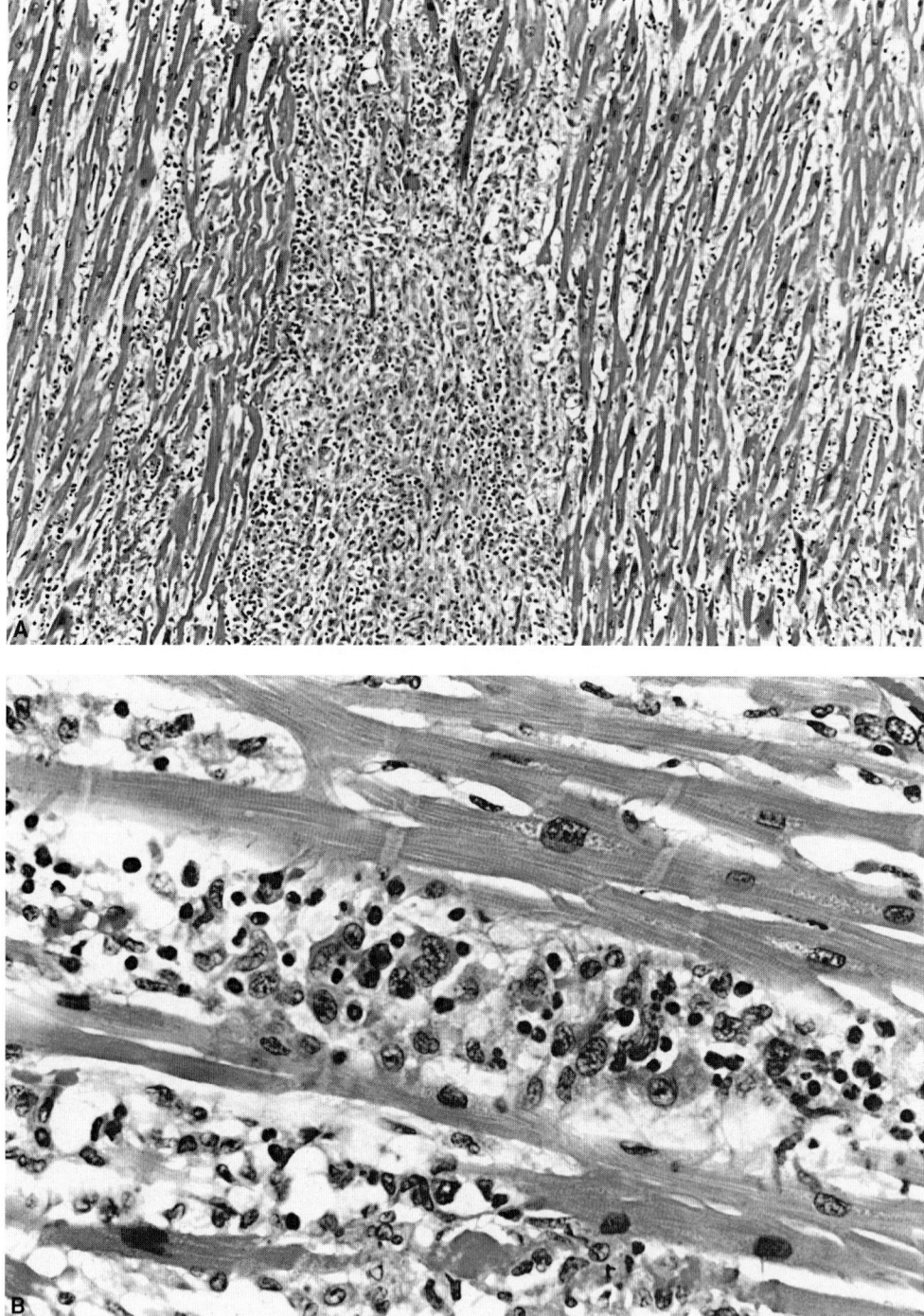

Fig. 31-10. Endomyocardial biopsy specimen from a 24-year-old patient with congestive heart failure; *A*, Foci of inflammatory cells infiltrate the myocardium (mag. 25×); *B*, Higher magnification shows that the cells are mononuclear (100×).

in nature. Arterial Po_2 should be maintained using endotracheal intubation and mechanical ventilation if clinically indicated. An intravenous inotropic agent such as dobutamine, amrinone, or milrinone should be used to increase cardiac output. Although dopamine in low doses may improve renal blood flow and urine output, larger doses may increase systemic vascular resistance and pulmonary wedge pressure thereby neutralizing its overall benefits.[15]

Afterload reduction with intravenous nitroprusside may increase cardiac output and should be titrated to maintain a mean arterial pressure of approximately 80 mm Hg. Antiarrhythmic agents, DC-cardioversion, and overdrive pacing should be used as indicated to treat hemodynamically significant cardiac arrhythmias. The end point of pharmacologic intervention is improvement in systemic blood pressure, oxygenation, and urine output.

Patients with severe hemodynamic compromise in whom supportive measures are unsuccessful may be candidates for cardiac transplantation. Once candidacy has been established, insertion of a ventricular assist device may be required to achieve hemodynamic stability while awaiting transplantation.

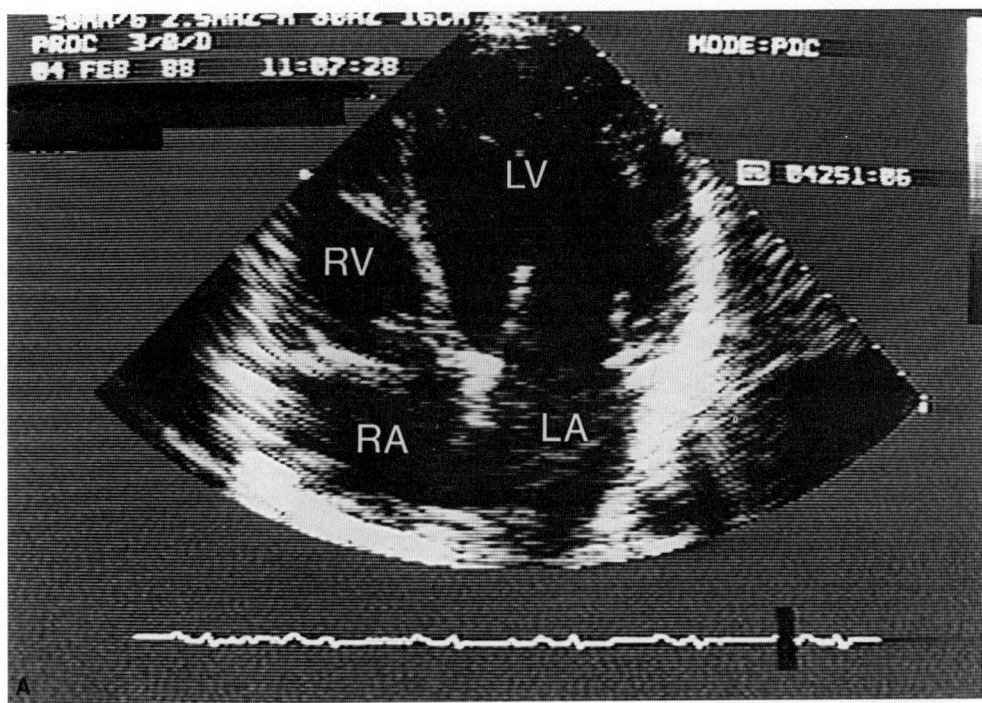
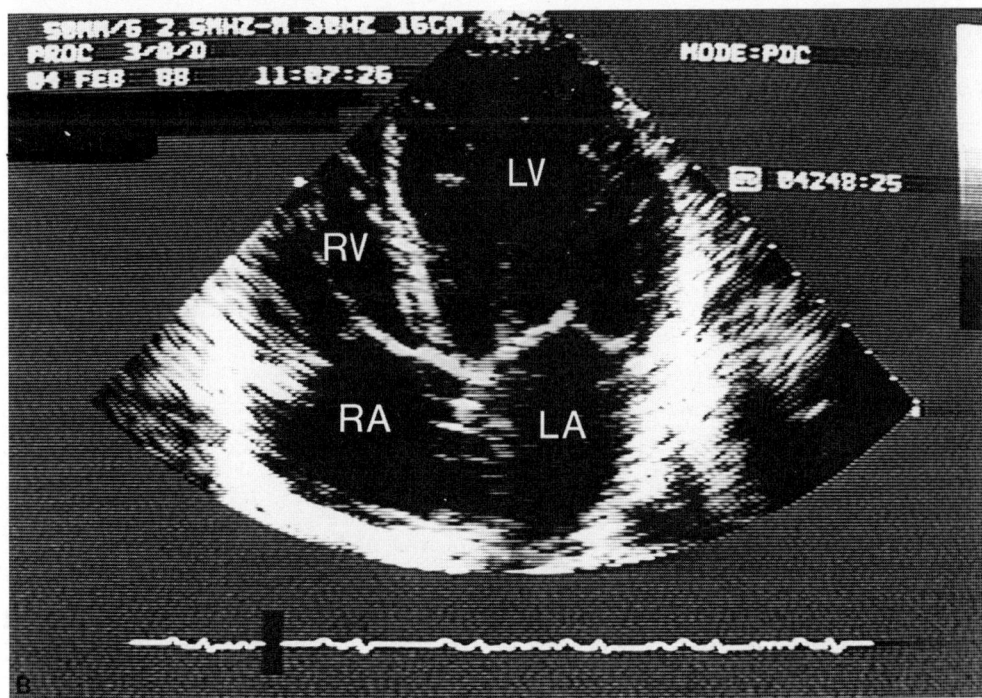

Fig. 31-11. Two-dimensional echocardiogram (apical four-chamber view) of the patient described in Figure 31-10. *A*, Ventricular diastole: there is marked four chamber dilation. *B*, Ventricular systole: the end-systolic cavity dimensions are essentially unchanged reflecting a profound decrease in myocardial contractility. RV, Right ventricle; RA, right atrium; LV, left ventricle; LA, left atrium.

Table 31-8. Identification by Endomyocardial Biopsy of Treatable Disorders

Giant cell myocarditis
Hypereosinophic "Loeffler's" cardiomyopathy[99]
Anthracycline cardiomyopathy (incipient)
Cardiac hemochromocytosis
Lyme carditis[100]
Carnitine deficiency[101]
Cardiac sarcoidosis[102]

Post-ICU Phase

Patients with dilated cardiomyopathy, in general, represent a high risk population with a guarded long-term prognosis. Although some patients can be stabilized initially, most experience recurrent episodes of congestive heart failure and, indeed, a 5-year mortality rate of greater than 50% can be expected.[16] Treatment in most patients includes digitalis in combination with either a direct vasodilator such as hydralazine[17] or an angiotensin-converting enzyme (ACE) inhibitor (e.g., enalapril).[18] The doses must be tailored individually as determined primarily by the systemic blood pressure and overall renal function. In general, we recommend that an ACE inhibitor at low doses be introduced while the patient is in the ICU, titrating slowly thereafter while carefully following urine output, daily weight, blood urea nitrogen (BUN) and creatinine levels, as well as daily heart and lung examinations.

Diuretics are also a mainstay of long-term therapy, however, caution must be exercised to avoid a reduction in preload and subsequent worsening of ventricular function. Patients in whom excessive diuresis has occurred commonly complain of worsening fatigue and general malaise, both manifestations of a low cardiac output. Long-term warfarin therapy is also recommended given the high risk of mural thrombus formation and thromboembolic events in these patients.

Patients with histologic evidence of myocarditis may benefit from prednisone therapy,[19] however, a long-term benefit has not been documented. Ongoing clinical trials will assess the potential benefit of cyclosporine and prednisone in patients with myocarditis.

Cardiac transplantation represents the most effective treatment among patients with dilated cardiomyopathy and refractory congestive heart failure. In carefully selected patients, cardiac transplantation can improve survival.[20,21]

Patients with dilated cardiomyopathy and chronic low output congestive heart failure may benefit from intermittent (48 hour) or continuous intravenous infusions of dobutamine.[23-28] Outpatient administration should be instituted with caution, however, as prospective, controlled trials have not established its overall safety and efficacy.[29,30]

HYPERTROPHIC CARDIOMYOPATHY

Hypertrophic cardiomyopathy, also referred to as idiopathic hypertrophic subaortic stenosis (IHSS) and hypertrophic obstructive cardiomyopathy (HOC), occurs sporadically, or more commonly, as an inherited autosomal dominant disorder. It is characterized by pronounced myocardial hypertrophy involving the interventricular septum of a nondilated left ventricle.[31]

A marked increase in left ventricular mass, with disproportionate involvement of the interventricular septum, develops at the expense of the left ventricular cavity; as a result, left ventricular filling is compromised. In many cases, the ratio of the septal to left ventricular free wall thickness exceeds 1.3 to 1 (normal 1:1); however, concentric left ventricular hypertrophy, particularly in older patients, or hypertrophy localized to the ventricular apex may also occur. Long-standing hypertrophic cardiomyopathy may also progress to a state of left ventricular dilation and end-stage heart disease.

In hypertrophic cardiomyopathy, a dynamic pressure gradient occurs within the left ventricular outflow tract during systole. Although the mechanism(s) are still being explored, progressive obstruction of an already narrowed outflow tract as a result of systolic anterior motion (SAM) of the mitral valve may be directly involved. Whether a primary or secondary phenomena, the volume of blood actually limited by the dynamic outflow obstruction during systole is relatively small.

In many patients with hypertrophic cardiomyopathy, including those with nonobstructive forms of the disease, diastolic dysfunction is a prominent feature. There is evidence that abnormalities in ventricular relaxation, distensibility (compliance), and diastolic filling exist, most likely as a result of increased ventricular mass, interstitial fibrosis, cellular disorganization, and myocardial ischemia.[32,33]

Pre-ICU Phase

Clinically, patients with hypertrophic cardiomyopathy frequently experience symptoms by the second or third decades of life. In some cases, however, symptoms may not appear until the sixth or seventh decades.[34,35] The most common symptom is dyspnea on exertion, however, the clinical presentation varies widely and may include fatigue, palpitations, angina, syncope, and sudden death. In patients experiencing angina, differentiation from coronary heart disease may be difficult. In addition, some patients with hypertrophic cardiomyopathy have recurrent episodes of congestive heart failure.

The major findings on physical examination include lateral displacement of the point of maximum impulse (PMI), a prominent fourth heart sound, a mid-systolic murmur, and brisk carotid upstrokes. The murmur of hypertrophic cardiomyopathy is typically a harsh, crescendo-decrescendo systolic murmur heard best between the apex and left-lower sternal border. Maneuvers that decrease afterload such as the inhalation of amyl nitrate or decrease preload (e.g., Valsalva maneuver), will commonly increase the outflow gradient, and as a result, augment the systolic murmur. A separate holosystolic murmur heard best at the apex and radiating to the axillae may represent concomitant mitral insufficiency. The carotid upstrokes are brisk initially. They frequently decline during mid to late systole, however, with the development of ventricular outflow obstruction (Bisferiens pulse).

Patients with hypertrophic cardiomyopathy requiring ICU admission commonly fall into one of three distinct categories:

- Progressive angina pectoris
- Congestive heart failure
- Potentially life-threatening tachyarrhythmias

In many instances, the diagnosis of hypertrophic cardiomyopathy has previously been established, whereas in others subsequent evaluation of one or more of the previously mentioned clinical abnormalities will uncover the underlying problem.

ICU Phase

Diagnostic Evaluation

ECG Features. A normal ECG is a rare finding among patients with hypertrophic cardiomyopathy. Most commonly, ST-T wave abnormalities, increased QRS voltage and signs of left ventricular hypertrophy are present. Deeply inverted T waves in the precordial leads may be seen, particularly in the apical variant of hypertrophic cardiomyopathy. Prominent Q waves may appear in the infe-

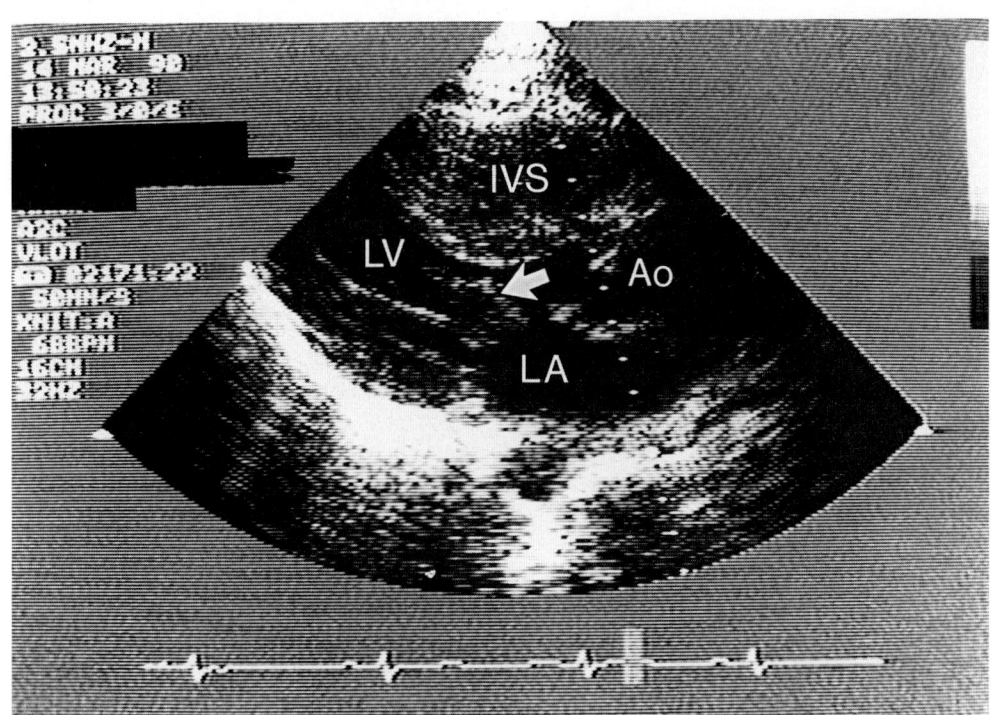

Fig. 31-12. Two-dimensional echocardiogram (parasternal long axis view) in a patient with familial hypertrophic cardiomyopathy. The intraventricular septum (IVS) is markedly thickened. Systolic anterior motion of the mitral valve (arrow) is also seen. LV, Left ventricle; LA, left atrium; Ao, aorta.

rior and lateral leads reflecting abnormal depolarization of myopathic cells in the interventricular septum or possibly increased right ventricular mass. Uncommonly, Q waves may represent an abnormality in myocardial perfusion sufficient to cause a myocardial infarction. A wide variety of supraventricular and ventricular arrhythmias can be seen.

Chest Radiograph. The radiograph findings can vary from a normal study to one demonstrating marked left ventricular prominence. Left atrial enlargement with straightening of the left heart border is common. Patients with congestive heart failure develop hilar prominence, interstitial edema, alveolar edema, and vascular redistribution.

Echocardiography. The two-dimensional echocardiogram is the noninvasive diagnostic method of choice in evaluating patients with hypertrophic cardiomyopathy. The cardinal feature is left ventricular hypertrophy with a maximal septal dimension being observed midway between the base and apex of the heart. The thickened septum is commonly greater than 15 mm in width. The ventricular cavity is small with complete or near-complete obliteration during systole (Fig. 31-12). The narrowed left ventricular outflow tract is formed by the intraventricular septum anteriorly and the anterior leaflet of the mitral valve posteriorly. As mentioned previously, the mechanism(s) underlying the dynamic outflow tract obstruction in hypertrophic cardiomyopathy are being investigated and may relate either to a "venturi effect" or malpositioning of the papillary muscle-mitral valve apparatus.[36]

Pulsed doppler findings include the identification of a "step-up" in flow velocity within the left ventricular outflow tract (Fig. 31-13). Reduced early diastolic filling velocity (E wave) and an increased velocity of atrial contraction (A wave) are considered supportive of diastolic dysfunction, as is a prolonged isovolumic relaxation time. Mitral insufficiency of varying severity may also be seen.

Asymmetric hypertrophy of the interventricular septum is an echocardiographic finding which is not specific for hypertrophic cardiomyopathy; it may be seen in patients with hypertensive heart disease, infiltrating tumors, Pompe's disease, Fabry's disease, acromegaly, Turner's syndrome, and hyperthyroidism as well.

In the ICU setting, serial echocardiograms may be clinically useful in assessing the therapeutic response to therapies aimed at increasing ventricular relaxation and decreasing left ventricular outflow obstruction.

Hemodynamic Features

With the exception of cases in which the hypertrophic process involves the right ventricle, or when long-standing pulmonary venous hypertension exists, the right atrial, right ventricular, and pulmonary artery pressures are frequently normal. The most dramatic feature of hypertrophic cardiomyopathy is the systolic intraventricular pressure gradient which exists between the body of the left ventricle and the ventricular outflow tract. The aortic waveform has a typical spike in the early ejection phase followed by a dip in pressure and a dome-shaped wave form prior to the dicrotic notch. The "spike and dome" configuration is most evident following a ventricular extrasystolic contraction or the Valsalva maneuver; the arterial pulse pressure may also paradoxically narrow "Brockenbrough-Braunwald sign" (Fig. 31-14).

Treatment

The preload-dependency of the hypertrophic left ventricle demands adequate diastolic filling time and atrioventricular synchrony. Thus, a supraventricular tachyarrhythmia such as atrial fibrillation with a rapid ventricular response may have profound hemodynamic consequen-

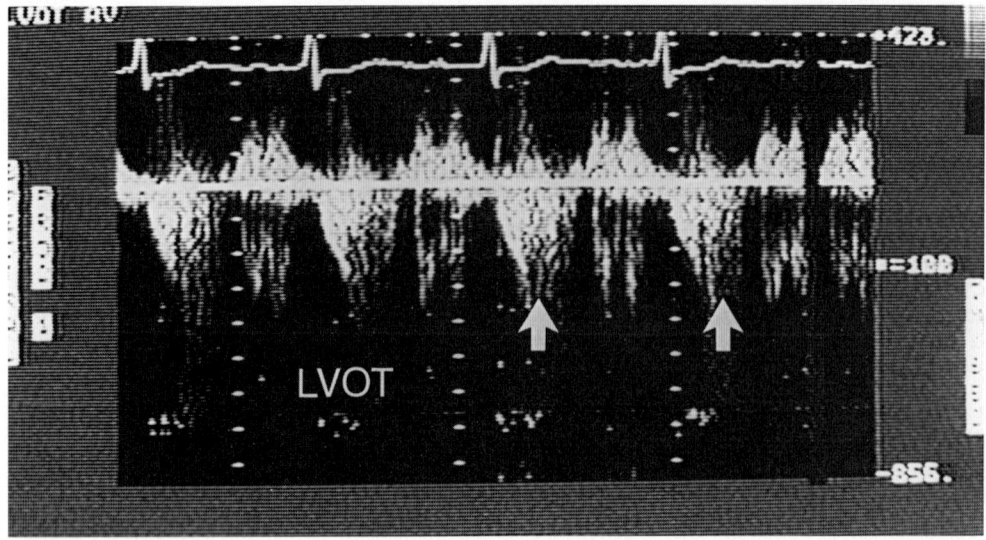

Fig. 31–13. Pulsed-doppler echocardiogram of the left ventricular outflow tract (LVOT) showing high-velocity flow (arrow) in a characteristic "dagger" configuration.

ces. Although rate control with digitalis, verapamil, diltiazem, adenosine, or a beta blocker may provide hemodynamic improvement, many patients require immediate DC cardioversion. Patients with ventricular tachycardia complicated by systemic hypotension, angina pectoris, or congestive heart failure also require emergent synchronized DC cardioversion. Patients with high degree AV block frequently experience hemodynamic improvement with dual-chamber pacing (Table 31–9).

Congestive heart failure, although at times a manifestation of end-stage hypertrophic cardiomyopathy with ventricular dilation and systolic dysfunction, is more commonly the result of diastolic dysfunction. Treatment considerations must, therefore, be tailored specifically to the diastolic properties of the heart. As mentioned previously, tachyarrhythmias and AV conduction abnormalities must be treated promptly to maintain diastolic filling. As with other forms of congestive heart failure, adequate arterial oxygenation is critical and early endotracheal intubation and mechanical ventilation should be considered as clinically indicated in patients whose respiratory status is also compromised. Inotropic agents are ineffective in diastolic dysfunction and, in fact, may cause progressive hemodynamic deterioration. Intra-aortic balloon counterpulsation and afterload reduction are also ineffective. Diuresis will frequently result in symptomatic improvement. Excessive diuresis may decrease preload and cardiac output, however. Therefore, we recommend that patients with hypertrophic cardiomyopathy requiring ICU admission undergo pulmonary artery catheterization and bedside two-dimensional echocardiography with doppler examination to aid in clarifying hemodynamic status and response to subsequent treatment. These diagnostic modalities are also vital in assessing the hemodynamic response to intravenous volume expansion in patients with hypovolemia, in whom the clinical interpretation of intravascular volume status and cardiac output is often difficult.

At present, attempts to improve diastolic relaxation with either intravenous beta blockers or calcium-channel antagonists form the mainstay of treatment.[37,38] Verapamil and diltiazem can be given as intravenous infusions,[39] and serial bedside echocardiograms can be performed to document a reduction in outflow-tract velocity (gradient) and an improvement in diastolic filling. The intravenous beta-

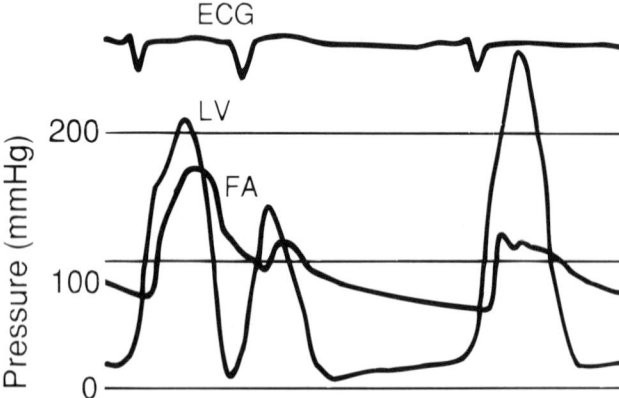

Fig. 31–14. Pressure tracings (200 mm Hg scale) taken concomitantly from the femoral artery (FA) and left ventricle (LV) in a patient with hypertrophic cardiomyopathy. Under baseline conditions, the LV pressure exceeds the FA pressure by approximately 20 mm Hg. Following a ventricular extrasystole, however, there is a marked increase in LV pressure and a decrease in FA pressure (see text for discussion).

Table 31–9. Indications for DC Cardioversion in Patients with Hypertrophic Cardiomyopathy and Supraventricular Tachyarrhythmias*

Systemic hypotension
Refractory angina pectoris
Congestive heart failure
   New onset
   Progressive/worsening

* Ventricular rate control may be attempted initially by pharmacologic means (see text).

adrenergic blocker esmolol may also improve ventricular diastolic function. Most important, the clinician must distinguish between hypovolemic states that worsen outflow obstruction and fluid overload states that worsen diastolic function.

Post-ICU Phase

Following discharge from the ICU, an emphasis should be placed on providing therapy which controls patient symptoms and identifies those individuals at risk for sudden cardiac death.

Long-term therapy with oral beta blockers has been shown to reduce angina, dyspnea, lightheadedness, and syncope; large doses may be required (e.g., propranolol, 640 mg per day), however, to maintain clinical improvement. Calcium-channel blockers (e.g., verapamil, 420 mg per day) may also provide clinical benefits and may, at times, be used in combination with beta blockers. Patients must be observed carefully for bradyarrhythmias and conduction disturbances when high-dose monotherapy or combination therapy is used.

Disopyramide and amiodarone may be used in patients unresponsive to beta blockers or calcium-channel antagonists or in patients with concomitant supraventricular or ventricular tachyarrhythmias. Daily diuretic therapy may be useful. As mentioned previously, excessive diuresis should be avoided however.

Patients with progressive or recurrent symptoms unresponsive to medical therapy may be candidates for surgery. First performed in 1958, surgical therapy, including either septal myectomy, myotomy or mitral valve replacement, is designed to relieve the dynamic outflow tract obstruction.[40] Although many patients experience a clinical improvement after surgery, the operative mortality averages 5 to 8%, symptoms may recur and patient survival may not differ significantly from patients treated medically.

The overall annual mortality rate among patients with hypertrophic cardiomyopathy approaches 2 to 4%.[41] The majority of deaths are sudden and may be either hemodynamic or arrhythmic in origin. Patients with a family history of sudden death or syncope are known to be at increased risk, as are patients with nonsustained ventricular tachycardia as determined by holter monitoring.[42] An abnormal signal-averaged electrocardiogram may also identify high risk patients.

Patients with documented ventricular tachycardia may experience an improved long-term survival with amiodarone therapy.[43] Antiarrhythmic therapy or surgical intervention (cardioverter-defibrillation) cannot be recommended routinely for all patients, however.

HIGH OUTPUT HEART FAILURE

Cardiac output may be defined as the quantity of blood leaving the heart required to perfuse peripheral tissues and vital organs; under normal conditions approximately 6 to 7 L per minute are delivered. A normal increase in cardiac output occurs with exercise and other conditions that increase metabolic demand. A sustained increase in cardiac output, however, particularly when metabolic demands are not increased, is abnormal and may lead to cardiac decompensation.

Table 31-10. High Output Heart Failure

Anemia (blood loss, hemolysis, bone marrow failure)
Hyperthyroidism
Systemic arteriovenous fistulas
   Congenital including Rendu-Osler-Weber disease
   Acquired (traumatic, aortic aneurysm rupture, surgical, neoplastic)
Beriberi heart disease
Paget's disease
Fibrous dysplasia (Albright's syndrome)
Pregnancy
Multiple myeloma
Carcinoid syndrome
Hepatic disease
Hyperkinetic heart syndrome
Hyperviscosity syndrome

In high output states, the peripheral vascular resistance (afterload) is reduced and the venous return (preload) is increased. A marked increase in preload increases both left ventricular end-diastolic volume and pressure. A marked increase in left ventricular end-diastolic pressure may cause congestive heart failure even in the presence of normal myocardial contractility. With time, volume-overload (eccentric) hypertrophy may ensue thereby causing a subsequent rise in end-diastolic pressure and an increase in the propensity for overt heart failure. In addition, an end-stage manifestation of long-standing eccentric hypertrophy is chamber dilation and systolic dysfunction. Some forms of high output heart failure may be associated with a direct impairment of myocardial metabolism (e.g., athyrotoxicosis, beriberi), whereas others may impair myocardial function indirectly (e.g., tissue hypoxemia from long-standing anemia).

Overall, the ability of the heart to compensate for the demands of a high output state depends on the rate of development and the presence or absence of underlying heart disease; rapidly developing high output states and increased metabolic demands on an already compromised myocardium typically lead to a more severe and progressive decompensation (Table 31-10).[44-46]

Pre-ICU Phase

Patients with high output heart failure exhibit clinical findings similar to other forms of congestive heart failure which include fatigue, dyspnea on exertion, and paroxysmal nocturnal dyspnea. A broad range of symptoms reflecting the presence of an underlying disease state may also be encountered. The physical findings of high output heart failure include tachypnea, tachycardia, bounding peripheral pulses, and a widened pulse pressure. "Pistol-shot" sounds may be appreciated over the femoral arteries (Duroziez's sign) and subungual capillary pulsations (Quincke's pulse) are not uncommon. A grade I-III/VI midsystolic flow murmur can frequently be heard along the left sternal border and, at times, a diastolic murmur, reflecting a marked increase in blood flow across the mitral valve may also be appreciated. A systolic murmur suggestive of a pericardial friction rub has been reported in patients with high output states; the "Means-Lerman scratch" is thought to be caused by rubbing of the pleural and pericardial surfaces. In most instances, the heart sounds are accentuated and the PMI is hyperdynamic. On rare occasions, however, the findings of a hyperdynamic circulation are entirely absent. In this setting, concomitant myocardial disease should be suspected.

The physical findings associated with a systemic arteriovenous fistula are determined by the location of the shunt. Typically, the overlying skin is warm and a continuous machinery murmur with an accompanying thrill is appreciated. A slowing of the heart rate with manual compression of the fistula (Branham's sign) is strongly suggestive of hemodynamic significance. Rarely, arteriovenous fistula may become infected (endarteritis).

In classic beriberi, heart failure is accompanied by findings of generalized malnutrition, vitamin deficiencies, peripheral edema, and a generalized sensorimotor peripheral neuropathy.

ICU admission should be considered strongly for patients when high-cardiac output states are accompanied by signs and symptoms of progressive cardiac decompensation. In addition, patients with previously diagnosed high cardiac output states and noncardiac conditions (e.g., infection) that may increase metabolic demands leading to hemodynamic deterioration should be considered for ICU admission as well.

ICU Phase

Diagnostic Evaluation

ECG Features. Sinus tachycardia is present in most patients, frequently exceeding 110 beats per minute, and may be as high as 200 beats per minute. A variety of supraventricular arrhythmias may also occur, particularly with thyrotoxicosis, which is associated with a 5 to 10% incidence of atrial fibrillation. Diffuse, nonspecific ST-T-wave changes are frequently seen. In patients with underlying coronary artery disease, ischemic changes can occur and, on occasion, changes consistent with acute myocardial infarction are encountered. Both abnormalities are a reflection of excessive myocardial oxygen demand.

Chest Radiograph. Although the heart size may be normal, it is more commonly increased in size. Patients with cardiac decompensation will manifest typical findings of pulmonary congestion.

Echocardiography. Increased wall motion and a hyperdynamic contractile pattern are observed on two-dimensional echocardiography, unless an underlying coronary arterial or a primary myocardial disease is present in which case focal wall motion abnormalities or global hypokinesis may be present, respectively. Compensatory hypertrophy (eccentric) may be seen and, on occasion, four chamber dilation is present, suggesting either end-stage decompensation or a concomitant dilated cardiomyopathy[47] (e.g., alcoholic cardiomyopathy and beriberi).

Hemodynamic Features

The cardiac output may be as high as 12 L per minute. However, a gradual decrease occurs with progressive decompensation. Patients with underlying myocardial disease may have a normal cardiac output originally, however, with progressive decompensation cardiac output decreases.

The mixed venous O_2 saturation is typically low; therefore, the a-vO_2 difference is increased, and if maximum extraction reserve is used, the mixed venous O_2 saturation may approach a physiologic low of 35%. The pulmonary arterial and capillary wedge pressures are both increased to a moderate degree.

Treatment

Cardiac involvement in high output states is typically a secondary phenomenon, therefore, treatment of the underlying disorder is of considerable importance. Cardiac stabilization may be achieved initially with systemic blood pressure support, oxygen supplementation, and intravenous diuretics. Inotropic agents and peripheral vasodilator are of limited value in high output heart failure, with the exception of end-stage decompensation or concomitant myocardial disease.

Patients with profound anemia complicated by high output heart failure require blood replacement. It must be given slowly (1 to 2 U per 6 to 12 hours), however, to avoid sudden expansion of an already expanded blood volume. In patients with hemolytic or megaloblastic anemias, supplementation with folate or vitamin B_{12} should also be provided.

In hyperthyroid states, care must be taken to address the endocrine abnormality early in the course of treatment. Although beta blockers may be used to control ventricular response with rapid atrial fibrillation, myocardial suppression preceding a reduction in systemic metabolic demands may precipitate congestive heart failure.

Patients with beriberi heart disease have been shown to respond to digitalis, diuretics, and thiamine supplementation. If thiamine is given prior to initiating diuretic therapy, however, systemic vascular resistance may increase and in the setting of volume expansion can precipitate low output congestive heart failure. Arteriovenous fistulae complicated by high output heart failure require prompt surgical ligation.

Post-ICU Phase

Patients with high output heart failure require close follow-up after discharge from the ICU. In most cases, initial cardiac stabilization can be achieved. Correction of the underlying disorder, with the exception of surgically correctable arteriovenous fistulas, frequently requires time, however. During that time, patients may be susceptible to recurrent episodes of heart failure requiring repeated ICU admissions. In general, if the underlying disease state can be corrected, the long-term prognosis is favorable.

Diuretic therapy may be necessary in certain patients to control intravascular volume status while investigation of the underlying disorder is in progress. Long-term beta-blocker therapy is useful in patients with the hyperkinetic heart syndrome.

TRAUMATIC MYOCARDIAL DYSFUNCTION

High speed motor vehicle accidents and escalating civilian violence have increased the frequency and severity of traumatic cardiac injuries. Furthermore, improved prehospital management and rapid transportation to regional trauma centers make it likely that an increasing number of patients with cardiac trauma will be encountered in the future. Typically, traumatic myocardial injuries have been categorized as either penetrating or nonpenetrating (blunt), depending on the underlying mechanism of injury. Penetrating and nonpenetrating cardiac trauma differ significantly in their presentation, method of diagnosis, treatment and follow-up evaluation; they will, therefore, be discussed separately.

Penetrating Cardiac Traumas

The thoracic cage offers little protection from penetrating trauma and, as a result, only 20 to 40% of patients with penetrating cardiac injuries are alive on hospital arrival.[48-50] Penetrating injuries occurring in the civilian population result mainly from stab and gunshot wounds.[51] The mortality resulting from stab wounds is somewhat less than that associated with projectiles, but the number of gunshot wounds in the United States has been increasing steadily.[48] Although the overall survival from penetrating cardiac trauma is improving, gunshot injuries, particularly shotgun wounds, still portend a poor prognosis.[52,53]

Penetrating cardiac trauma should be suspected in patients with wounds in the "danger zone" which includes the precordium, epigastrium, and superior mediastinum.[54] The frequency of injury to a particular cardiac chamber relates directly to the surface area exposed to the anterior chest wall; the right ventricle subtends 55% of the anterior surface of the heart while the left ventricle covers approximately 20%.[48,50,51,53] In a collective review of 1802 patients suffering penetrating cardiac trauma, Karrel and co-workers[55] found right ventricular involvement in 42% and left ventricular injury in 33%; the right atrium (15%), left atrium (6%), and intrapericardial great vessels (3%) were less frequently involved.

Pre-ICU Phase

The clinical manifestations of penetrating cardiac trauma are a composite of the primary and secondary consequences of this injury including:

- Cardiac tamponade
- Chamber communication(s)
- Valvular disruption
- Coronary artery laceration
- Myocardial damage
- Severe hemorrhage

The relative roles of cardiac tamponade and hemorrhage depend on the size and location of the injury, as well as the state of the pericardium.[50] If the pericardial wound is sealed by thrombus or adjacent fat, blood from the injured cardiac chamber is trapped within the pericardial space and, as a result, cardiac tamponade develops. In patients suffering stab wounds, the pericardium frequently seals and, consequently, approximately 90% of these patients present with cardiac tamponade.[51,52] As little as 60 to 100 ml of blood accumulating acutely in a noncompliant pericardial sac may result in clinical tamponade. (The pathophysiology of tamponade is discussed in detail elsewhere in this chapter.) Gunshot wounds result frequently in significant tissue destruction and large pericardial defects. Hemorrhage, in the presence of an open pericardium will, therefore, dominate the clinical picture. In addition, coronary artery injury, myocardial injury, valvular disruption, and chamber communications can also occur; these complications will be discussed separately.

As mentioned previously, 60 to 80% of patients with penetrating cardiac injuries die before they arrive at the hospital; therefore, rapid transportation to a treatment facility is of utmost importance. Cardiac injury should be suspected immediately in a hypotensive patient suffering a penetrating wound of the chest, neck, or epigastrium. As in all trauma cases, treatment must begin with a rapid assessment and control of the "ABCs" of resuscitation; after maintaining an airway, assuring ventilation and establishing intravenous access via large bore peripheral catheters, a central venous catheter should be placed. Arterial and central venous pressures should be monitored. Routine chest roentgenograms are of little value in diagnosing acute cardiac tamponade or in defining the extent of myocardial injury; they will, however, aid in establishing the presence of a concurrent pneumothorax, hemothorax, or pneumopericardium. Evacuation of the pleural space by chest tube insertion may improve ventilation and oxygenation and enable a more accurate assessment of central venous pressure.[51] A rapid infusion of 2 to 4 L of intravenous fluid is frequently necessary to achieve hemodynamic stability. Subsequent emergency management is determined by the patient's overall hemodynamic status (Fig. 31-15). The definitive treatment of penetrating cardiac wounds accompanied by hemodynamic instability is cardiorrhaphy.

The respective role(s) of emergent pericardiocentesis, a limited pericardial window, and emergency room thoracotomy are outside the scope of this chapter; the reader is referred to recent reviews of these specific topics.[48,50,51,53,55]

Coronary artery injuries, fistulas, intracardiac shunts, valvular damage, retained foreign bodies, and pericarditis may complicate penetrating cardiac trauma in up to 50% of cases.[53] Coronary artery injuries have been reported in 4 to 12% of patients with penetrating trauma and are usually diagnosed intraoperatively.[48] Damage to distal coronary arteries, if less than 1.0 mm in diameter, may be treated with ligation. Damage to larger coronary vessels should be repaired or bypassed during the initial surgery, however.[56]

Coronary-cameral and coronary-venous fistulas may develop after penetrating injuries. Patients with these complications may present with either angina pectoris or congestive heart failure. Coronary angiography, contrast echocardiography, and CT scanning have been employed as a means of diagnosis; operative repair of these lesions is recommended. In contrast, penetrating valvular and in-

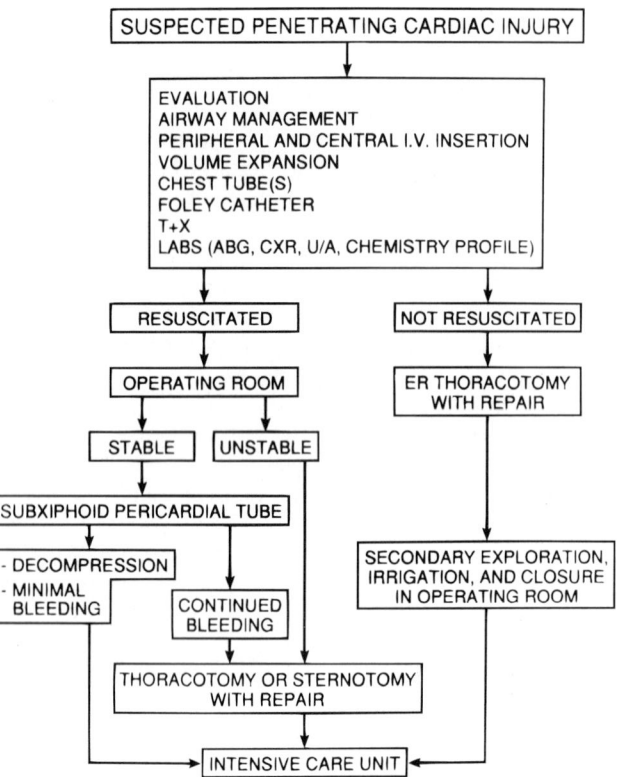

Fig. 31–15. Algorithm for pre-ICU evaluation and treatment of patients with suspected penetrating cardiac injury. ABG, Arterial blood gas; CXR, chest x-ray; U/A, urinalysis; T&X, blood type and crossmatch; IV, intravenous. (Adapted from Chitwood, W. R., and Austin, E. H.: Cardiac Trauma: penetrating and blunt. In Trauma Surgery. Edited by J. A. Moylan. Philadelphia, J. B. Lippincott, 1988.)

terventricular septal injuries may not require acute operative repair if the patient is hemodynamically stable.[56]

In general, patients with penetrating chest injuries should be stabilized initially with intravenous volume expansion and vasopressor agents as needed. Prompt consultation with the cardiovascular surgery team is of vital importance.

ICU Phase

Patients surviving an operation will require intensive medical support in the postoperative period. Physicians caring for these patients must be aware of specific complications and potential late sequelae among survivors of penetrating cardiac trauma. All patients require careful monitoring of their cardiac rhythm, hemodynamic status, urine output, blood counts, and metabolic parameters. Serial assessment of the neurologic status is also recommended since air or solid-particle emboli, systemic hypotension, coexisting head trauma, and preinjury drug or alcohol intoxication may cause neurologic abnormalities. Mattox and associates[57] recommend that survivors of penetrating cardiac trauma be followed with serial physical examination, ECGs, and cardiac enzyme determinations. Patients with clinical symptoms or abnormal physical findings should undergo further investigation (Fig. 31-16).

Significant intracardiac shunts are usually heralded by the development of either:

- A new murmur
- A palpable thrill
- Refractory congestive heart failure

Pulmonary artery catheterization with oximetric studies, two-dimensional Doppler color-flow echocardiography[58] and formal cardiac catheterization may each provide diagnostic information in these settings. Stable patients with large intracardiac shunts (pulmonary to systemic flow ratio of greater than 1.5:1) should undergo elective surgery in 4 to 6 weeks. The timing of surgery in symptomatic patients should be dictated by the patient's overall clinical status. Other causes of refractory congestive heart failure, such as valvular damage or ventricular aneurysm formation, can frequently be diagnosed by echocardiographic techniques. Cardiac catheterization may be used to assess the hemodynamic significance of these lesions as well as the timing of operative repair.

Retained foreign bodies (i.e., bullets, shrapnel) are not uncommon after surgical repair of a penetrating cardiac injury. Intramyocardial foreign bodies may rarely embolize, serve as a nidus for infection, erode into adjacent structures, or cause "cardiac neurosis." Despite these potential complications, however, many clinicians feel that ventricular intramyocardial foreign bodies can be removed on an elective basis.[59]

Post-traumatic pericarditis, typically appearing four to six weeks after the initial event, is heralded by chest pain, fever, and a pericardial friction rub. The etiology of pericarditis appears to be similar to that following elective surgery (i.e., postpericardiotomy syndrome) and usually responds to anti-inflammatory agents. The physician should be

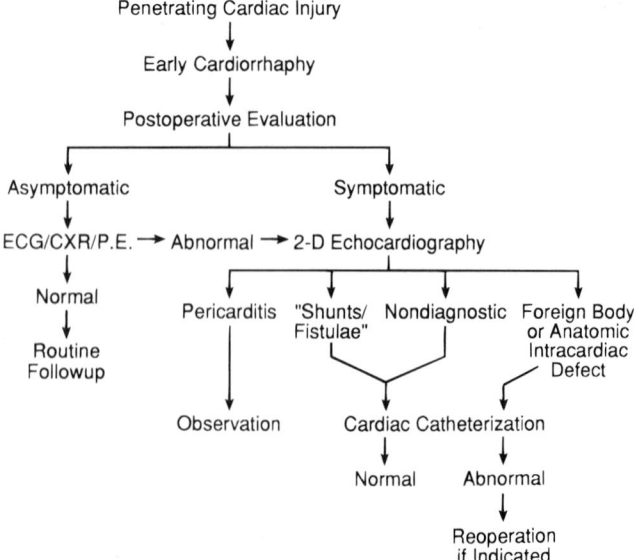

Fig. 31–16. Recommended decision schema for post-cardiorrhaphy patients. ECG, Electrocardiogram; P. E., physical examination. (Adapted from Mattox, K. L., et al.: Cardiac evaluation following heart injury. J. Trauma, 25:758, 1985.)

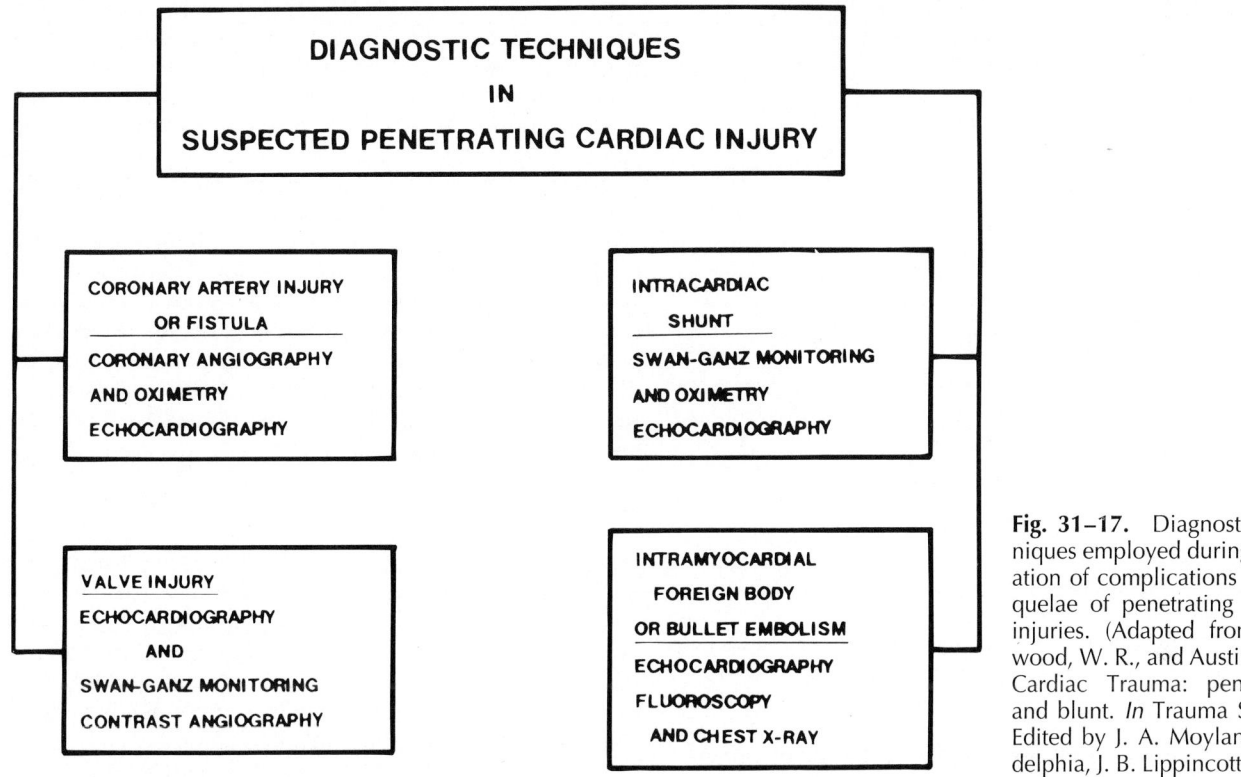

Fig. 31-17. Diagnostic techniques employed during evaluation of complications and sequelae of penetrating cardiac injuries. (Adapted from Chitwood, W. R., and Austin, E. H.: Cardiac Trauma: penetrating and blunt. In Trauma Surgery. Edited by J. A. Moylan. Philadelphia, J. B. Lippincott, 1988.)

aware, however, that post-traumatic pericardial effusions can cause cardiac tamponade or become suppurative. The diagnostic techniques recommended in the evaluation of patients with penetrating cardiac trauma are outlined in Figure 31-17.

Post-ICU Phase

Following clinical stabilization in the ICU, most patients can be transferred to a general medical or surgical floor. The clinician must keep in mind, however, that intracardiac shunts may persist and intramyocardial foreign bodies may embolize relatively late in the patient's course. In the report by Mattox,[57] the mean hospital stay for cardiac trauma patients with suspected complications was 11.3 days; considerably longer than for patients without complications. Asymptomatic patients with documented left-to-right cardiac shunts must have repeat echocardiography within three months of discharge and every 3 to 6 months thereafter until a complete resolution is confirmed or surgical correction is deemed necessary.

Nonpenetrating Cardiac Trauma

Motor vehicle accidents account for approximately 2,000,000 injuries and 55,000 fatalities annually in the United States. The incidence of associated cardiac trauma varies from 16% in autopsy series to 76% in clinical series. Data from the University of California, San Diego suggests that "clinically significant" myocardial injury (life-threatening cardiac complication or death) occurs in approximately 5 to 15% of patients with severe nonpenetrating chest trauma.[60] It must be appreciated, however, that non-penetrating cardiac injuries are the most common unsuspected visceral injury likely to cause death among accident victims.

The mechanisms underlying nonpenetrating cardiac trauma include:

- Rapid deceleration or acceleration
- Direct trauma
- Abrupt increases in intrathoracic or intra-abdominal pressure
- Compression of the heart between the sternum and the thoracic spine[53]

Blunt chest injury occurs most commonly when the driver of a high-speed motor vehicle impacts the steering wheel. Blunt cardiac trauma has also been reported, however, in cases of rapid deceleration from velocities of less than 20 miles per hour.

The spectrum of nonpenetrating cardiac injury ranges from a mild cardiac contusion to overt myocardial necrosis and rupture. Damage to the cardiac valves and supporting structures, coronary arteries, and pericardium may also occur as well. A list of nonpenetrating cardiac injuries is provided in Table 31-11.

Myocardial contusion is usually defined as a blunt cardiac injury which causes identifiable histopathologic changes within the myocardium. The area of contusion resembles a myocardial infarction, although the zone of injury is more sharply defined in the former. Subepicardial, subendocardial, or intramyocardial hemorrhage can also be seen along with myocardial cell necrosis and leukocyte infiltration (Fig. 31-18). The overall clinical significance

Table 31-11. Cardiac Lesions in Nonpenetrating Cardiac Trauma

Myocardial injury
  Wall motion abnormality
  Aneurysm formation
  Free wall rupture
  Ventricular septal rupture
  Myocardial laceration
Rhythm or conduction disturbances
  Atrial arrhythmias
  Ventricular arrhythmias
  First-, second-, or third-degree heart block
Valvular injury
  Cusp or leaflet tear
  Papillary muscle injury
Coronary artery injury
  Laceration
  Thrombosis
  Fistula
Pericardial injury
  Rupture or laceration
  Hemopericardium
  Pericarditis with effusion
  Constrictive pericarditis (late)

(From Symbas, P. N.: Traumatic heart disease. Curr. Probl. Cardiol., 7:3, 1982.)

of cardiac contusion relates directly to the development of complications, which may include:[61]

- Arrhythmias
- Valvular dysfunction
- Septal rupture
- Thromboembolic events
- Congestive heart failure
- Ventricular aneurysm formation
- Constrictive pericarditis

Pre-ICU Phase

Cardiac injury should be suspected in all patients who have sustained significant blunt chest trauma. Clinically relevant myocardial injury is most frequently associated with severe thoracic trauma, but has been reported in cases without evidence of significant external chest injury. Snow and colleagues[62] found that 73% of patients with pathologically confirmed myocardial damage had externally evident chest trauma. Of these, 60% had additional thoracic injuries detected by either physical examination or chest radiograph. Nonpenetrating myocardial injury, as mentioned previously, is most commonly the result of a direct blow to the chest from a steering wheel. Falls and various sports-related injuries have been reported as well, however. The right ventricle is the chamber most commonly injured because of its vulnerable position immediately beneath the sternum. In an autopsy series, Parmley and co-workers[63] defined the frequency and sites of nonpenetrating cardiac injury (Table 31-12).

Patients with nonpenetrating cardiac trauma complicated by myocardial rupture typically present to the hospital in extremis. Cardiac rupture is caused either by (1) direct transmission of increased intrathoracic pressure to the cardiac chambers during a vulnerable time in the cardiac cycle; or (2) rapid deceleration of the heart which rotates anteriorly away from the fixed great vessels.[64] Patients with myocardial rupture also have an incidence of aortic rupture that approaches 20%.[63] Patients with myocardial rupture, if they are to survive, require emergency surgery.

In less severe cases of nonpenetrating chest trauma, the decision for ICU admission is based on the history of injury, associated noncardiac injuries and, perhaps most importantly, a high index of clinical suspicion. There are no classic signs or symptoms of blunt myocardial trauma, although some patients may complain of an angina-like chest pain (which typically is not responsive to nitroglycerin). The cardiovascular examination may be normal or reveal signs of acute valvular dysfunction, congestive heart failure, or cardiac tamponade.

ICU Phase

Diagnostic Evaluation. Currently, the greatest area of controversy concerning nonpenetrating cardiac injuries relates to the criteria used for diagnosing cardiac contusion. The diagnostic tests used most often include electrocardiography, serum cardiac isoenzyme determinations, two-dimensional echocardiography, radionuclide ventriculography (RVG) and radionuclide scanning.

ECG Features. The ECG is the most widely used noninvasive test for detecting myocardial injury. It is readily available and should be obtained in all patients with suspected nonpenetrating cardiac trauma. In a review of the literature, Berk[65] noted that 63% of patients with blunt chest trauma exhibited abnormal ECGs; ST and T wave changes were the most common abnormalities. A summary of ECG abnormality observed in nonpenetrating cardiac trauma appears in Table 31-13.

The most common rhythm disturbance following cardiac trauma is sinus tachycardia; however, associated volume depletion from hemorrhage, pain, anxiety, and heightened sympathetic tone make this finding nonspecific. Premature ventricular and atrial contractions may be seen, as may transient conduction abnormalities. It must be appreciated, however, that the surface ECG is neither a sensitive nor a specific marker of myocardial injury. The sensitivity is limited by the predominance of the left ventricle in determining electrical events, frequently masking irregularities of the more commonly involved right ventricle. The ECG may also be interpreted falsely as positive in the presence of preexisting heart disease or when hypoxemia, concomitant pulmonary contusion, electrolyte alterations, and acid-base imbalances exist.

Creatine Phosphokinase Determinations. Measurement of creatine phosphokinase (CK) and its cardiac isoenzyme (CK-MB) have been extrapolated from use in acute myocardial infarction. As with acute myocardial infarction, trauma may damage cellular membranes allowing release of CK-MB into the systemic circulation; serum levels usually peak within 24 hours after myocardial cell damage and return to baseline by 72 hours. The CK-MB fraction should be determined on hospital admission and every 6 to 8 years thereafter for a minimum of 24 hours and preferably until a steady decline in serum levels has been observed.

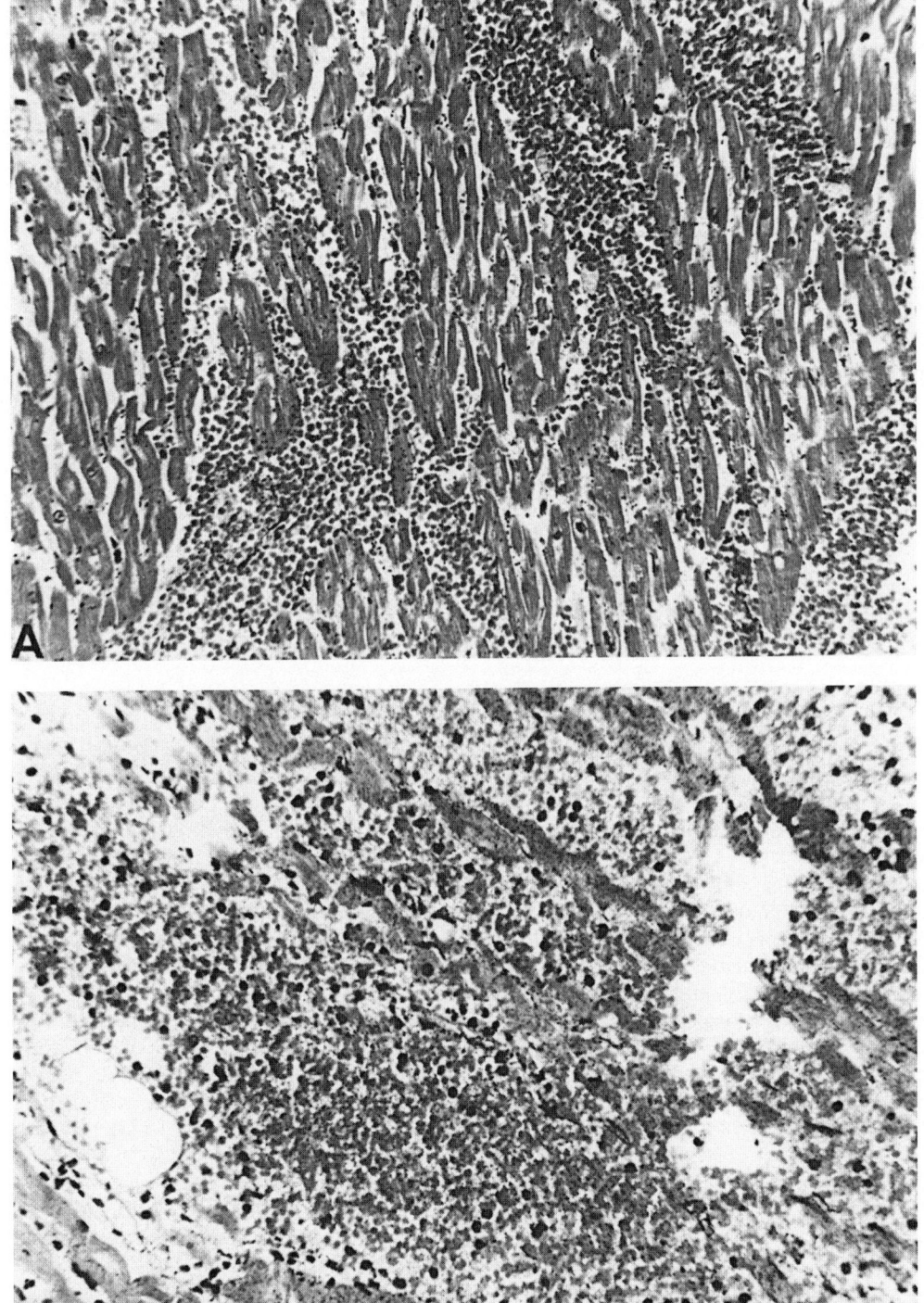

Fig. 31–18. Photomicrographs of myocardial contusion (hematoxylin-eosin, ×176.5). A, Intramyocardial hemorrhage edema, fragmentation and loss of transverse striation of myocardial fibers. B, polymorphonuclear leukocyte infiltration is demonstrated. (From Symbas, P. N.: Traumatic heart disease. Curr. Probl. Cardiol., 7:21, 1982.)

The CK-MB fraction may be elevated in certain noncardiac conditions. For example, crush injuries with total CK values of greater than 20,000 IU/L may cause an elevation in the CK-MB fraction.

The overall sensitivity of CK-MB in diagnosing traumatic myocardial injury has also been questioned. Two separate studies have demonstrated abnormal cardiac wall motion by two-dimensional echocardiograph[66] and RVG[67] respectively without an associated elevation of the serum CK-MB; these findings may represent "myocardial concussion" (myocardial dysfunction without structural myocardial cell damage). A second hypothesis, however, has been proposed by Ingwall[68] who demonstrated negligible CK-MB activity in the muscle of normal ventricles (i.e., young patients without coronary artery disease or pressure overload hypertrophy). Many young, previously healthy pa-

Table 31-12. Cardiac Complications Found in 546 Autopsy Cases of Nonpenetrating Heart Trauma

Type and/or Site of Injury	Number of Cases (Cardiac Only)	Cases (Including Patients with Thoracic Aorta Rupture)	Total Cases
Rupture (cardiac)	273	80	353
Right ventricle	56	10	66
Left ventricle	46	13	59
Right atrium	35	6	41
Left atrium	24	2	26
Interventricular septum	25 (20)*	5 (4)*	30
Interatrial septum	18 (10)*	7 (3)*	25
Multiple chamber ruptures	69	37	106
Myocardial contusion/laceration	105	24	129
Pericardial laceration	18	18	36
Hemopericardium	13	12	25
Valvular laceration/rupture	1 (2)†	0 (4)†	1
Aortic	1 (1)†	0 (2)†	1
Pulmonary	0 (4)†	0	0
Tricuspid	0 (8)†	0	0
Mitral	0 (1)†	0 (1)†	0
Mitral and tricuspid	0 (1)†	1 (1)†	0
Coronary artery laceration/rupture	0 (7)†	1 (2)†	1
Papillary muscle laceration/rupture	1 (23)†	0	1
Total	411	135	546

* Associated with other sites of cardiac rupture.
† Combined with cardiac rupture or other injury.
(From: Parmley, C. F., et al.: Nonpenetrating traumatic injury of the heart. Circulation, *18*:371, 1958. By permission of the American Heart Association, Inc.)

tients with blunt myocardial injury may, therefore, have negligible elevations of serum CK-MB. Despite these potential shortcomings, it is recommended that serial CK-MB measurements be obtained in all patients with nonpenetrating cardiac trauma.

Radionuclide Scanning. Radionuclide scanning with ^{99m}technetium pyrophosphate was applied initially to diagnosing acute myocardial infarction;[69] however, more recently it has been used in the evaluation of traumatic myocardial injury. Although the results of initial animal studies were promising, subsequent clinical investigations have been disappointing.[70] The overall poor sensitivity of ^{99m}technetium pyrophosphate scanning in post-traumatic myocardial dysfunction may be explained by the following: (1) transmural myocardial injury, an uncommon occurrence in blunt trauma, is more likely to cause a positive scan because a large tissue mass is needed to bind a detectable quantity of tracer; and (2) it is technically difficult to separate the thin-walled right ventricle from the overlying sternum and ribs which also accumulate ^{99m}technetium.[69,71,72] Considering these limitations, ^{99m}technetium pyrophosphate scanning cannot be recommended routinely in the diagnostic evaluation of patients with nonpenetrating myocardial injury.

Radionuclide Ventriculography (RVG). Although RVG is somewhat less sensitive for right ventricular as compared with left ventricular abnormalities,[71] it has shown promise in the clinical evaluation of patients with cardiac trauma. Harley and associates[73] studied 74 patients with blunt chest trauma and detected a 74% incidence of abnormal left ventricular wall motion. They concluded that RVG was more sensitive than either electrocardiography or serum CK-MB determinations in diagnosing myocardial trauma. There are some potential limitations of RVG which include its expense, complexity, and lack of widescale availability as a bedside diagnostic technique.[53]

Antimyosin Scanning. The radionuclide labeled FAB fragment of murine antibody to myosin, antimyosin, has been used to detect, localize and quantitate myocardial necrosis in experimental and clinical myocardial infarction,[74] myocarditis,[75] and cardiac allograft rejection.[76] When myocyte necrosis occurs, plasma membrane integrity is lost and, as a result, antimyosin is able to diffuse into the intracellular compartment where it binds to myosin. Radionuclide labeling of antimyosin with ^{111}indium or ^{99m}technetium allows gamma camera imaging.

Because myocardial cell damage may occur following

Table 31-13. Electrocardiographic Findings in 240 Patients with Nonpenetrating Cardiac Trauma

Finding	Percentage of Patients (%)
Patients with abnormal ECG (%)	63
ST-segment or T-wave abnormalities	35
Bundle branch block (total)	10
RBBB	9
LBBB	1
Atrioventricular nodal block	3
Atrial fibrillation	4
Myocardial infarction pattern	2
Sinus bradycardia	2
Ventricular tachycardia	1

RBBB, Right bundle branch block; LBBB, left bundle branch block.
(From Berk, W. A.: Electrocardiographic findings in nonpenetrating chest trauma: a review. J. Emerg. Med., *5*:209; 1987.)

blunt cardiac trauma, the use of antimyosin scanning to localize areas of heart injury is theoretically possible. At our institution, 17 patients with suspected myocardial injury following blunt chest trauma underwent [111]indium antimyosin scanning, two-dimensional echocardiography, serial ECG analysis, and serum CK-MB determinations. Antimyosin scanning demonstrated focal uptake in only one patient; of interest and clinical relevance, this was the only patient shown to have a focal wall-motion abnormality by two-dimensional echocardiography. Electrocardiographic changes and CK-MB, however, did not correlate with antimyosin scan evidence of myocardial injury (Hendel; personal communication). Although theoretically attractive, antimyosin scanning for the detection of nonpenetrating myocardial injury requires further clinical study.

Echocardiography. Two-dimensional echocardiography provides a portable, noninvasive means to rapidly assess the myocardium and pericardial space. The advent of Doppler and color-flow techniques has also increased the sensitivity and specificity for detecting valvular damage and intracardiac shunts. Patients with regional wall motion abnormalities, chamber dilation, pericardial effusions, intramyocardial hemotomas, and mural thrombi can readily be identified.[77]

The sensitivity and specificity of two-dimensional echocardiography in the setting of nonpenetrating cardiac trauma has been investigated. Frazee and colleagues[78] found that 40% of patients with chest trauma and an elevation in serum CK-MB demonstrated echocardiographic abnormalities. In addition, 39% of patients with documented echocardiographic abnormalities experienced cardiac arrhythmias compared with 3% of patients with normal echocardiograms. Reid and colleagues[79] reported that technically adequate two-dimensional echocardiograms could be obtained in 87% of patients with suspected cardiac trauma; in their series 23% of all patients demonstrated specific abnormalities. In contrast, Fabian and associates[80] observed only three abnormal echocardiograms among 21 patients diagnosed as having "myocardial contusion" by either an abnormal ECG or an elevated serum CK-MB concentration.

Hemodynamic Features. Pulmonary artery catheterization may be useful in patients with profound systemic hypotension unresponsive to fluid administration, patients with an abnormal two-dimensional echocardiogram requiring noncardiac surgery, or as a diagnostic aid in patients with new cardiac murmurs. Cardiac catheterization may be used to quantitate intracardiac shunting, assess the severity of valvular regurgitation, diagnose coronary artery injuries, and define the hemodynamic significance of traumatic ventricular aneurysms.

Using the information provided, a diagnostic algorithm for patients with nonpenetrating cardiac trauma may be formulated (Fig. 31–19).

Treatment. The treatment of traumatic myocardial dysfunction is primarily supportive. Rest, cardiac monitoring, supplemental oxygen, a daily 12-lead ECG and serial CK-MB determinations are recommended. The use of prophylactic antiarrhythmic therapy has not been proven in clinical trials. Symptomatic arrhythmias, however, should be treated promptly. Additional diagnostic testing should be

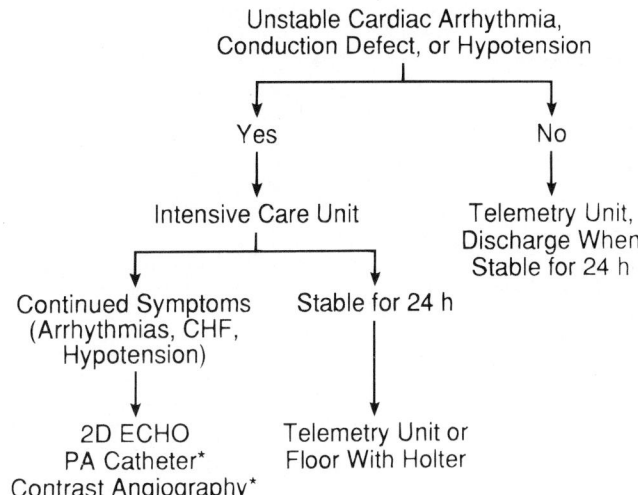

Fig. 31–19. Algorithm for management of patients with nonpenetrating trauma. h, hours; PA, pulmonary artery; 2-D Echo, two-dimensional echocardiography. PA catheterization and contrast angiography should be performed as clinically indicated. (Adapted from Miller, F. B., et al.: Myocardial contusion: when can the diagnosis be eliminated? Arch. Surg., *124*:807, 1989.)

performed as indicated by the patient's overall cardiovascular status (Fig. 31–20).

In patients with blunt cardiac injury, the degree of depression in cardiac output correlates directly with the amount of myocardial damage. Low cardiac output states, however, may also be caused by hypovolemia, cardiac tamponade, ventricular septal rupture, or valvular dysfunction. Echocardiography, pulmonary artery catheterization, or contrast angiography may be used to confirm these diagnoses. Intravenous fluid administration, inotropic support, afterload reduction and, occasionally, intra-aortic balloon counterpulsation[81] may be required to stabilize the patient's hemodynamic status.

Cardiac wall motion abnormalities stemming from blunt cardiac trauma frequently resolve within a few days, typically without sequela. Rarely, however, myocardial contusion heals with excessive scar formation resulting in ventricular aneurysm formation. This usually occurs with transmural left ventricular injury, although it has also been reported following traumatic occlusion of the left anterior descending coronary artery as well.[53] Complications of traumatic left ventricular aneurysms include congestive heart failure, atrial or ventricular arrhythmias, thromboembolic events and, rarely, myocardial rupture. If a ventricular aneurysm is suspected by chest radiograph or two-dimensional echocardiography, cardiac catheterization, and contrast angiography should be performed. Most clinicians recommend elective resection of traumatic ventricular aneurysms.

Post-ICU Phase

Few data are available on which to base recommendations for rehabilitation and follow-up care in patients suffering nonpenetrating myocardial trauma. Overall, how-

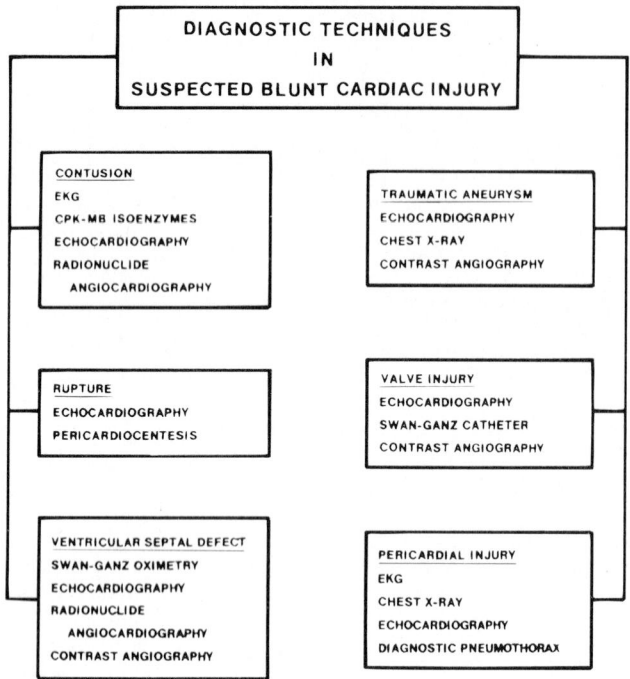

Fig. 31-20. Diagnostic procedures recommended in the evaluation of suspected complications and sequelae of blunt cardiac injury. See text for further discussion. EKG, Electrocardiogram; CPK-MB, creatine phosphokinase-MB fraction. (Adapted from Chitwood, W. R., and Austin, E. H.: Cardiac Trauma: penetrating and blunt. In Trauma Surgery. Edited by J. A. Moylan. Philadelphia, J. B. Lippincott, 1988.)

ever, the prognosis for patients with an uncomplicated cardiac injury is good. Ventricular wall motion abnormalities seen by two-dimensional echocardiography or RVG typically resolve within seven to 10 days, although it occasionally takes up to 10 weeks for complete resolution.[73] Patients with associated complications may require additional diagnostic testing or continued observation while awaiting definitive surgical repair.

Follow-up visits should take place 6 and 12 weeks after hospital discharge and include a complete physical examination and a 12-lead ECG. Patients with an abnormal two-dimensional echocardiogram during hospitalization should undergo a repeat study within 6 weeks of discharge. Patients with minimal valvular damage or small intracardiac shunts should undergo serial two-dimensional echocardiograms until complete resolution or stabilization is confirmed. Long-term guidelines for outpatient follow-up have not been established, however, we recommend that patients with injuries requiring surgical intervention be seen at 6-month intervals for the first 2 years and yearly thereafter. Patients with confirmed myocardial contusion in whom ventricular function is not initially compromised or rapidly returns to normal usually do not require long-term follow-up care.

SEPSIS-RELATED MYOCARDIAL DYSFUNCTION

Sepsis may be defined as a clinical syndrome resulting from the presence of microorganisms or their toxins in the systemic circulation. It is a frequent medical problem in modern ICUs.[82] Many studies of sepsis in humans have focused on gram-negative bacillary infections. Indeed, it has been estimated that 1% of all patients admitted to academic, tertiary care facilities will develop gram-negative bacteremia during their hospitalization.[83] Therefore, up to 300,000 cases of gram-negative bacteremia resulting in 100,000 deaths (assuming a 33% mortality rate) are expected to occur annually in the United States. For patients with documented gram-negative bacteremia complicated by septic shock the mortality rate, even in experienced medical centers, exceeds 50%.[83,84]

Although sepsis and septic shock are most commonly associated with infections caused by gram-negative aerobic bacteria, a wide variety of agents including gram-positive, viral, fungal, mycobacterial, rickettsial, and protozoal micro-organisms may each result in clinical syndromes closely simulating those seen in gram-negative septic shock.[82,84,85]

The physiologic alterations and clinical consequences of sepsis are exceedingly complex and frequently referred to as "the septic syndrome," which includes a wide spectrum of clinical presentations; patients demonstrating signs of infection (e.g., fever) without hemodynamic abnormalities are at one end of the spectrum, while those with hypotension and multisystem failure (septic shock) are at the opposite end. Although the criteria used to diagnose septic shock vary, the following signs and symptoms are commonly included:

- Hypotension; systolic blood pressure less than 90 mm Hg or a mean arterial pressure less than 60 mm Hg
- Hyperthermia (core temperature greater than 38°C) or hypothermia (core temperature less than 35°C)
- Impaired organ perfusion
- Metabolic abnormalities
- Multiorgan failure

The pathogenetic mechanisms causing septic shock are complex (Fig. 31-21), and associated with serious abnormalities in multiple organ systems. (The topic of septic shock is reviewed elsewhere in this text.) This section addresses sepsis-related derangements in the cardiovascular system that include (1) a decrease in systemic vascular resistance; and (2) altered myocardial performance.

The pathogenesis of myocardial depression in septic shock remains ill-defined, however, two basis mechanisms have been proposed:[86]

- Ischemia due to either decreased or maldistributed coronary blood flow
- Circulating myocardial depressant factors

Using thermodilution coronary sinus catheters to measure coronary blood flow, Cunnion and colleagues[87] demonstrated preserved myocardial blood flow in patients with sepsis. Interestingly, a narrowed difference in oxygen content between arterial and coronary sinus blood was noted, which may reflect rapid flow through dilated capillaries (a pattern of arteriovenous shunting similar to that

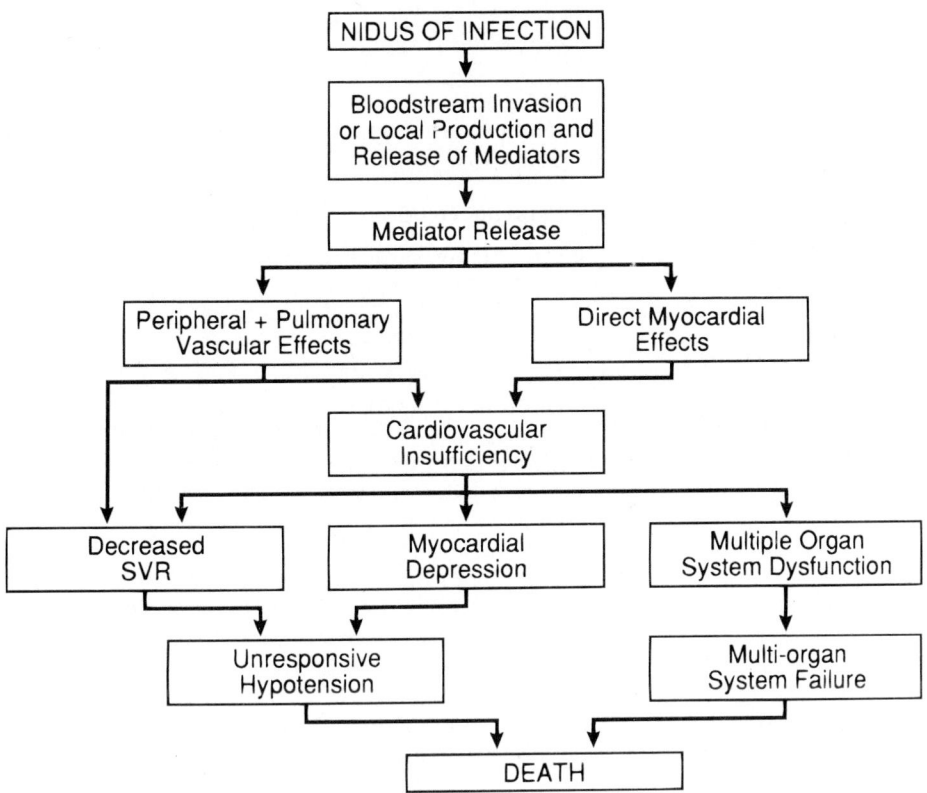

Fig. 31-21. Pathogenesis of human septic shock resulting in patient death. SVR, Systemic vascular resistance. See text for discussion. (Adapted from Cunnion, R. E., and Parrillo, J. E.: Myocardial dysfunction in sepsis: recent insights. Chest, 95:941, 1989.)

seen in the peripheral circulation). These findings have been corroborated by Dhainault and co-workers.[88]

The isolation of circulating myocardial depressant substance(s) (MDS) is an area of intense investigation. Using an in vitro preparation of spontaneously beating rat myocytes, Parrillo and colleagues[89] demonstrated that serum from septic patients with myocardial dysfunction caused a decrease in both the extent and velocity of myocyte contraction. A depression of cellular contraction did not occur with serum from normal volunteers, critically ill nonseptic patients or patients with organ heart disease. Interestingly, the degree of in vitro myocyte depression correlated with the extent of in vivo depression of left ventricular ejection fraction. Of further interest, following recovery from septic shock the serum of these patients no longer induced depression of myocyte contractility.

Certain substances have been identified which possess myocardial depressant activity including endotoxin, interleukins, and tumor necrosis factor (TNF). Endotoxin, a lipopolysaccharide contained within the outerwall of gram-negative bacteria, triggers the release of a number of potent mediators; therefore, it is unclear whether endotoxin itself causes myocardial depression or if myocardial depression is due to the release of one or more mediators which directly affect myocardial performance.[86,90]

The lymphokine, interleukin-2, was found in early clinical trials investigating its antitumor activity to produce marked hemodynamic alterations. In fact, interleukin-2 produced cardiovascular alterations similar to those observed in septic shock.[91] It has not been shown, however, to produce direct depression of in vitro rat myocyte activity.[91]

Tumor necrosis factor is a monokine released from macrophages in response to endotoxin. It appears to be an important mediator of a variety of physiologic processes including neutrophil activation, neutrophil adhesion to endothelial cells, hemostasis, and induction of other mediators of endotoxic shock.[92] Nathanson and colleagues[93] demonstrated in a canine model that intravenous TNF provoked the same hemodynamic effects as endotoxin. TNF has also been shown to directly depress contractility of rat myocytes in vitro.[94] Moreover, mice treated with a polyclonal antibody directed against TNF are resistant to the lethal effects of endotoxin.[95]

Pre-ICU Phase

In 1951, Waisbern reported what is generally accepted as the first description of the septic syndrome: "one group appeared hot, dry and flushed. The pulses were full and bounding." A second group appeared "cold, clammy and lethargic."[96] More recently, the septic syndrome has been divided into three distinct phases[97,98] (Table 31-14). The

Table 31-14. Hemodynamic Findings In Sepsis

	Preshock	Early Shock	Late Shock
Blood pressure	→↓	↓	↓↓
Systemic vascular resistance	↓	↓↓	↓→↑*
Cardiac index	↑↑	↑	↑→↓*
Volume responsive	++	+	−

* See text for details.
(From Harris, R. L., et al.: Manifestations of sepsis. Arch. Intern. Med., 147:1897, 1987.)

preshock phase, also referred to as the hyperdynamic or "warm" phase, is characterized by a normal blood pressure, decreased systemic vascular resistance, and an increased cardiac index. In the early-shock phase, the systemic vascular resistance decreases further with an attendant drop in blood pressure, however, the cardiac index remains elevated. If aggressive therapy is not instituted, the late-shock phase soon develops. Historically, the terminal phase of sepsis was frequently considered to be accompanied by a low cardiac index, normal to high systemic vascular resistance and profound systemic hypotension. Although a progressive decrease in cardiac index is certainly one mechanism responsible for the progressive clinical deterioration seen in overt septic shock, a majority of patients dying from sepsis do not exhibit this hemodynamic profile.

ICU Phase

Diagnostic Evaluation

As outlined previously, significant derangements in myocardial function can occur with sepsis,[83-86] and moreover, can have a profound impact on patient outcome. Primary depression of myocardial function, as assessed by echocardiography and radionuclide ventriculography contributes directly to approximately one third of all patient deaths due to sepsis.[99,100] In general, the myocardial abnormalities observed in sepsis include:

- Depression of left and right ventricular ejection fractions
- Ventricular dilation
- Decreased systolic function
- Abnormal diastolic function

The abnormalities can be manifest at any time between the first and fourth days and typically resolve 7 to 10 days later in surviving patients.[101-104]

Hemodynamic Features

Initially, the myocardial abnormalities may be subtle. In patients with a normal intravascular volume status, the cardiac output may be normal or slightly increased. In the presence of marked peripheral vasodilation, however, a normal or slightly elevated cardiac output may be inadequate to meet the body's overall metabolic demands. It has been suggested that cardiac outputs of greater than 10 L per minute may be required to maintain systemic blood pressure and ensure adequate organ perfusion.[86]

An early study by Weisel and colleagues[105] plotted stroke volume and left ventricular stroke work versus an increasing pulmonary artery wedge pressure in patients with sepsis. A higher ventricular stroke work index was noted among survivors when compared with nonsurvivors. Although certain design flaws may have been present, this study has served as a springboard for further investigation. In a study of 20 patients with sepsis, Parker and colleagues,[101] using bedside radionuclide ventriculography, noted an increase in left ventricular end-diastolic volume index (EDVI) and a decreased ejection fraction in some patients following volume infusion. These patients (largely survivors) developed left ventricular dilation and an elevation in pulmonary artery wedge pressure; however, an increase in stroke work was not observed which

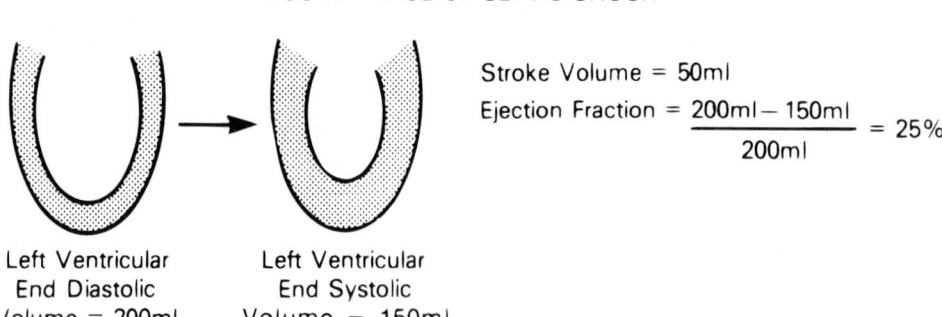

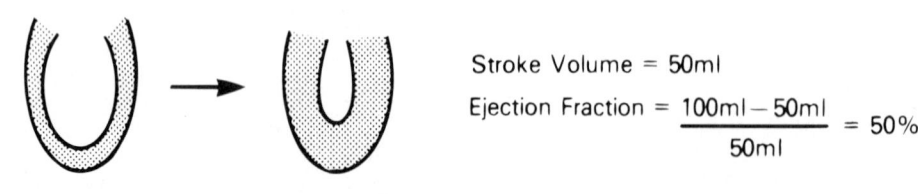

Fig. 31-22. Schematic diagram of cardiac performance changes during the acute and recovery phases of septic shock. An increased end-diastolic volume (EDV) and decreased ejection fraction (EF) occur during the acute phase. EDV and EF return to normal during the recovery phase. See text for discussion. (From Parker, M. M., et al.: Profound but reversible myocardial depression in patients with septic shock. Ann. Intern. Med., 100: 483, 1984.)

suggests an abnormality in ventricular contractility (Fig. 31-22). A second group of patients did not develop ventricular dilation despite volume loading sufficient to cause an increase in pulmonary artery wedge pressure. Although nonsurvivors failed to demonstrate a consistent hemodynamic pattern, these results suggested that left ventricular dilation was an important compensatory mechanism in the setting of sepsis.[83,85,106] A similar compensatory pattern of increased end-diastolic volume and decreased ejection fraction has been observed by other investigators[104,105] using RVG and echocardiography respectively.

Treatment

Patients demonstrating myocardial depression (dysfunction) with a low cardiac output in the setting of markedly increased metabolic demands may respond to an inotropic agent such as dobutamine.[82] Vasopressors including levophed may be required in cases of marked systemic hypotension. Many patients will have already received intravenous fluids and been placed on dopamine in an attempt to maintain systemic blood pressure.

Post-ICU Phase

In general, patients recovering from sepsis who are well enough to leave the ICU can be observed on a regular medical or surgical floor. Some patients may require additional intravenous antibiotics to complete a full treatment course (the duration of which will be determined by the underlying site of involvement and responsible organism). Patients, particularly immunocompromised hosts, must be observed for superinfections caused by resistant bacterial organisms and fungi. Progressive renal insufficiency can also complicate a prolonged antibiotic course when potentially nephrotoxic agents are used; avoidance of this complication requires close monitoring of serum antibiotic levels and meticulous attention to dosing. Risk factors for subsequent infections should be identified and corrected if possible.

Sepsis-related myocardial dysfunction to date has not been shown to cause persistent abnormalities. Myocardial function returns to normal in surviving patients with no prior history of myocardial dysfunction. Follow-up studies are, therefore, not routinely indicated. Indeed, acute, yet transient, abnormalities without residual cardiac dysfunction lend further support to a circulating depressing substance as the underlying etiology for this clinically important phenomenon.

REFERENCES

1. Soffer, A.: Electrocardiographic abnormalities in acute, convalescent and recurrent stages of idiopathic pericarditis. Am. Heart J., *60*:729, 1960.
2. Krozon, I., Cohen, M. L., and Winer, H. E.: Cardiac tamponade by loculated pericardial hematoma: limitations of M-mode echocardiography. J. Am. Coll. Cardiol., *1*:915, 1983.
3. Chen, C. C., Ciang, B. N., and Yeung, S. Y.: Pseudoposterior pericardial effusion due to a large left atrium. Am. Heart J., *108*:1044, 1984.
4. D'Cruz, I. A.: Echocardiographic simulation of a pericardial effusion by ascites. Chest, *85*:93, 1984.
5. Kronzon, I., Cohen, M. L., and Winer, H. E.: Diastolic atrial compression: a sensitive echocardiographic sign of cardiac tamponade. J. Am. Coll. Cardiol., *2*:770, 1983.
6. Williams, G. J., and Partridge, J. B.: Right ventricular diastolic collapse: an echocardiographic sign of tamponade. Br. Heart J., *49*:292, 1983.
7. Levine, H. D.: Myocardial fibrosis in constrictive pericarditis: electrocardiographic and pathologic observations. Circulation, *48*:1268, 1973.
8. Sechtem, V., Tscholakoff, D., and Higgins, C. B.: Magnetic resonance imaging of the pericardium. Am. J. Radiol., *146*:245, 1986.
9. Lewis, B. S.: Real-time two-dimensional echocardiography in constrictive pericarditis. Am. J. Cardiol., *49*:1789, 1982.
10. Agatston, A. S., Rao, A., Price, R. J., and Kinney, E. L.: Diagnosis of constrictive pericarditis by pulsed doppler echocardiography. Am. J. Cardiol., *54*:929, 1984.
11. Hatle, L. K., Appleton, C. P., and Popp, R. L.: Differentiation of constrictive pericarditis and restrictive cardiomyopathy by doppler echocardiography. Circulation, *79*:357, 1989.
12. Bortone, A. S., et al.: Functional and structural abnormalities in patients with dilated cardiomyopathy. J. Am. Coll. Cardiol., *14*:613, 1989.
13. Mason, J. W., and O'Connell, J. B.: Clinical merit of endomyocardial biopsy. Circulation, *79*:971, 1989.
14. Dec, G. W., Fallon, J. T., Southern, J. F., and Palacios, I.: "Borderline" myocarditis: an indication for repeat endomyocardial biopsy. J. Am. Coll. Cardiol., *15*:283, 1990.
15. Leier, C. V., et al.: Comparative systemic and regional hemodynamic effects of dopamine and dobutamine in patients with cardiomyopathic heart failure. Circulation, *58*:466, 1978.
16. McKee, P. A., et al.: The natural history of congestive heart failure: the Framingham study. N. Engl. J. Med., *314*:1547, 1986.
17. Cohn, J. N., et al.: Effect of vasodilator therapy on mortality in chronic congestive heart failure: results of a Veterans Administration cooperative study. N. Engl. J. Med., *314*:1547, 1986.
18. The Consensus Trial Study Group: Effects of enalapril on mortality in severe congestive heart failure: results of the cooperative North Scandinavian Enalapril Survival Study (CONSENSUS). N. Engl. J. Med., *316*:1429, 1987.
19. Parrillo J. E., et al.: A prospective, randomized, controlled trial of prednisone for dilated cardiomyopathy. N. Engl. J. Med., *221*:1061, 1989.
20. Goodwin, J. F.: Cardiac transplantation. Circulation, *74*:913, 1986.
21. Fragomeni, L. S., and Kaye, M. P.: The registry of the International Society for Heart Transplantation: fifth official report 1988. J. Heart Transplant, *7*:249, 1988.
23. Leier, C. V., and Unverferth, D. V.: Diagnosis and treatment. Drugs five years later. Dobutamine. Ann. Intern. Med., *99*:490, 1983.
24. Liang, C. S., et al.: Sustained improvement of cardiac function in patients with congestive heart failure after short-term infusion of dobutamine. Circulation, *69*:113, 1984.
25. Loeb, H. S., Bredakis, J., and Gunnar, R. M.: Superiority of dobutamine over dopamine for augmentation of cardiac output in patients with chronic low output cardiac failure. Circulation, *55*:375, 1977.
26. Leier, C. V., Webel, J., and Bush, C. A.: The cardiovascular effects of continuous infusion of dobutamine in patients with severe cardiac failure. Circulation, *56*:468, 1977.
27. Berkowitz, C., et al.: Comparative responses to dobutamine and nitroprusside in patients with chronic low output cardiac failure. Circulation, *56*:918, 1977.

28. Miller, L. W., Merkel, E. J., and Herrmann, V.: Outpatient dobutamine for end-stage congestive heart failure. Crit. Care Med., 18:S30, 1990.
29. Krell, M. J., et al.: Intermittent, ambulatory dobutamine infusions in patients with severe congestive heart failure. Am. Heart J., 112:787, 1986.
30. Applefeld, M. M., et al.: Outpatient dobutamine and dopamine infusions in the management of chronic heart failure: clinical experience in 21 patients. Am. Heart J., 114:589, 1987.
31. Wigle, D. E.: Hypertrophic cardiomyopathy: a 1987 viewpoint. Circulation, 75:311, 1987.
32. Gaasch, W. H., Levine, H. J., Quinones, M. A., and Alexander, J. K.: Left ventricular compliance: mechanisms and clinical implications. Am. J. Cardiol., 38:645, 1976.
33. Sanderson, J. E., Gibson, D. G., Brown, D. J., and Goodwin, J. F.: Left ventricular filling in hypertrophic cardiomyopathy: an angiographic study. Br. Heart J., 39:661, 1977.
34. Lewis, J. F., Maron, B. J.: Elderly patients with hypertrophic cardiomyopathy: a subject with distinct left ventricular morphology and progressive clinical course late in life. J. Am. Coll. Cardiol., 13:36, 1989.
35. Shenoy, M. M., et al.: Hypertrophic cardiomyopathy in the elderly: a frequently misdiagnosed disease. Arch. Intern. Med., 146:658, 1986.
36. Jiang, L., Levine, R. A., King, M. E., and Weyman, A. E.: An integrated mechanism for systolic anterior motion of the mitral valve in hypertrophic cardiomyopathy based on echocardiographic observations. Am. Heart J., 113:633, 1987.
37. Cody, R. J., et al.: Exercise hemodynamics and oxygen delivery in human hypertension: response to verapamil. Hypertension, 8:3, 1986.
38. Rising, D. R., et al.: Veramapil therapy: a new approach to the pharmacologic treatment of hypertrophic cardiomyopathy. I. Hemodynamic effects. Circulation, 60:1201, 1979.
39. Reiter, M. J., et al.: Pharmacokinetics of verapamil: experience with a sustained intravenous infusion regimen. Am. J. Cardiol., 50:716, 1982.
40. Cannon, R. O., et al.: Effect of surgical reduction of left ventricular outflow obstruction on hemodynamics, coronary flow and myocardial metabolism in hypertrophic cardiomyopathy. Circulation, 79:766, 1989.
41. McKenna, W. J., and Goodwin, J. F.: The natural history of hypertrophic cardiomyopathy. Curr. Probl. Cardiol., 6:5, 1981.
42. Nienaber, C. A., et al.: Syncope in hypertrophic cardiomyopathy: multivariate analysis of prognostic determinants. J. Am. Coll. Cardiol., 15:948, 1990.
43. McKenna, W. J., Oakley, C. M., Krikler, D. M., and Goodwin, J. F.: Improved survival with amiodarone in patients with hypertrophic cardiomyopathy and ventricular tachycardia. Br. Heart J., 53:412, 1985.
44. McBride, W., Jackman, J. D., Gammon, R. S., and Willerson, J. T.: High-output cardiac failure in patients with multiple myeloma. N. Engl. J. Med., 319:1651, 1988.
45. Merillon, R. C., et al.: Left ventricular function and hyperthroidism. B. Heart J., 46:137, 1982.
46. Fowler, N. O., and Holmes, J. C.: Blood viscosity and cardiac output in acute experimental anemia. J. Appl. Physiol., 39:453, 1975.
47. Carson, P.: Alcoholic cardiac beriberi. Br. Med. J., 284:1817, 1982.
48. Symbas, P. N.: Trauma to the Heart and Great Vessels. New York, Grune & Stratton, 1978.
49. Kulshrestha, P., et al.: Cardiac injuries—a clinical and autopsy profile. J. Trauma, 30:203, 1990.
50. Symbas, P. N.: Traumatic heart disease. Curr. Probl. Cardiol., 7:3, 1982.
51. Ivatury, R. R., and Rohman, M.: The injured heart. Surg. Clin. North Am., 369:93, 1989.
52. Ivatury, R. R., et al.: Penetrating cardiac injuries: 20-year experience. Ann. Surg., 53:310, 1987.
53. Chitwood, W. R., and Austin, E. H.: Cardiac trauma: penetrating and blunt. In Trauma Surgery. Edited by J. A. Moylan. Philadelphia, J. B. Lippincott, 1988.
54. Mattox, K. L.: Emergency Department Thoracotomy. J. Am. Coll. Emerg. Physicians, 7:12, 1978.
55. Karrel, R., Schaffer, M. A., and Franszek, J. B.: Emergency diagnosis, resuscitation and treatment of acute penetrating cardiac trauma. Ann. Emerg. Med., 11:504, 1982.
56. Casale, A. S., and Borkon, A. M.: Penetrating cardiac trauma. Trauma Quarterly 4:34, 1988.
57. Mattox, K. L., et al.: Cardiac evaluation following heart injury. J. Trauma, 25:758, 1985.
58. Clyne, C. A., et al.: Traumatic intracardiac communication: detection by color flow mapping. J. Am. Soc. Echocardiogr., 2:342, 1989.
59. Symbas, P. H., and Harlaftis, N.: Bullet emboli in the pulmonary and systemic arteries. Ann. Surg., 185:318, 1977.
60. Shackford, S. R.: Blunt Chest Trauma: the Intensivist's Perspective. J. Intens. Care. Med., 1:125, 1986.
61. Symbas, P. N.: Cardiac trauma. Am. Heart J., 92:387, 1976.
62. Snow, N., Richardson, J. D., and Flint, L. M.: Myocardial contusion: implications for patients with multiple traumatic injuries. Surgery, 92:744, 1982.
63. Parmley, L. F., Manion, W. C., and Mattingly, T. W.: Nonpenetrating traumatic injury of the heart. Circulation, 18:371, 1958.
64. Harmon, P. K., and Trinkle, J. K.: Injury to the Heart. In Trauma. Edited by E. E. Moore and K. L. Mattox. Norwalk, CT, Appleton-Century-Crofts, 1986.
65. Berk, W. A.: ECG findings in nonpenetrating chest trauma: a review. J. Emerg. Med., 5:209, 1987.
66. Helling, T. S., et al.: A prospective evaluation of 68 patients suffering blunt chest trauma for evidence of cardiac injury. J. Trauma, 29:961, 1989.
67. Keller, K. D., and Shatney, C. H.: Creatine phosphokinase-MB assays in patients with suspected myocardial contusion: diagnostic test or test of diagnosis? J. Trauma, 28:58, 1988.
68. Ingwall, J. S., et al.: The creatine kinase system in normal and diseased human myocardium. N. Engl. J. Med., 313:1050, 1985.
69. Tenzer, M. L.: The spectrum of myocardial contusion: a review. J. Trauma, 25:620, 1985.
70. Potkin, R. T., et al.: Evaluation of noninvasive tests of cardiac damage in suspected cardiac contusion. Circulation, 66:627, 1982.
71. Kudsk, K. A., et al.: Myocardial contusion: diagnosis and management. Contemp. Surg., 35:11, 1989.
72. Soutter, D. I., and Rodriguez, A.: Cardiac contusion: diagnosis and management. Trauma Q., 4:16, 1988.
73. Harley, D. P., et al.: Traumatic myocardial dysfunction. J. Thorac. Cardiovasc. Surg., 3:386, 1984.
74. Khaw, B. A., et al.: Acute myocardial infarction imaging with indium-111 labeled monoclonal antimyosin FAB. J. Nucl. Med., 28:1671, 1987.
75. Yasuda, T., et al.: Indium-111 monoclonal antimyosin antibody imaging in the diagnosis of acute myocarditis. Circulation, 76:306, 1987.
76. Frist, W., et al.: Noninvasive detection of human cardiac transplant rejection with indium-111 antimyosin (FAB) imaging. Circulation, 76(Suppl. V):V-81, 1987.

77. Markiewicz, W., et al.: Echocardiographic evaluation after blunt trauma of the chest. Int. J. Cardiol., 8:269, 1985.
78. Frazee, R. C., et al.: Objective evaluation of blunt cardiac trauma. J. Trauma, 26:510, 1986.
79. Reid, C. L., et al.: Chest trauma: evaluation by two-dimensional echocardiography. Am. Heart J., 113:971, 1987.
80. Fabian, T. C., et al.: Myocardial contusion in blunt trauma: clinical characteristics, means of diagnosis and implications for patient management. J. Trauma, 28:50, 1988.
81. Orlando, R., and Drezner, A. D.: Intra-aortic balloon counterpulsation in blunt cardiac injury. J. Trauma, 23:424, 1983.
82. Luce, J. M.: Pathogenesis and management of septic shock. Chest, 91:883, 1987.
83. Parker, M. M., and Parrillo, J. E.: Septic Shock: hemodynamics and pathogenesis. JAMA, 250:3324, 1983.
84. Parrillo, J. E.: Septic shock in humans: clinical evaluation, pathogenesis and therapeutic approach. In Society of Critical Care Medicine, Textbook of Critical Care. Edited by W. H. Shoemaker, et al. Philadelphia, W. B. Saunders, 1988.
85. Parillo, J. E., et al.: Septic shock in humans. Advances in the understanding of pathogenesis, cardiovascular dysfunction and therapy. Ann. Intern. Med., 113: 227, 1990.
86. Cunnion, R. E., and Parrillo, J. E.: Myocardial dysfunction in sepsis: recent insights. Chest, 95:941, 1989.
87. Cunnion, R. E., et al. The coronary circulation in human septic shock. Circulation, 73:637, 1986.
88. Dhainault, J. F., et al.: Coronary hemodynamics and myocardial metabolism of lactate free fatty acids, glucose and ketones in patients with septic shock. Circulation, 75:533, 1987.
89. Parrillo, J. E., et al.: A circulating myocardial depressant substance in humans with septic shock. J. Clin. Invest., 76: 1539, 1985.
90. Nathanson, C., et al.: Role of endotoxemia in cardiovascular dysfunction and mortality: E. Coli and S. Aureus challenges in a canine model of human septic shock. J. Clin. Invest., 83:243, 1989.
91. Ognibene, F. P., et al.: Interleukin-2 administration causes reversible hemodynamic changes and left ventricular dysfunction which are similar to those seen in septic shock. Chest, 94:750, 1988.
92. Beuther, B., and Cerami, A. L.: Cachectin: more than a tumor necrosis factor. N. Engl. J. Med., 316:379, 1987.
93. Nathanson, C., et al.: Endotoxin and tumor necrosis factor challenges in dogs simulate the cardiovascular profile of human septic shock. J. Exp. Med., 169:823, 1989.
94. Hollenberg, S. M., et al.: Tumor necrosis factor depresses myocardial cell function: results using an in vitro assay of myocyte performance. (Abstract.) Clin. Res., 37:538A, 1989.
95. Buetler, B., Milsaik, I. W., and Cerami, A. L.: Passive immunization against cachectin/tumor necrosis factor protects mice from the lethal effects of endotoxin. Science, 229: 869, 1985.
96. Waisbren, B. A.: Bacteremia due to gram-negative bacilli other than salmonella. Arch. Intern. Med., 88:467, 1951.
97. Balk, R. A., and Bone, R. C.: The septic syndrome: definitions and clinical implications. Crit. Care Clin., 5:1, 1989.
98. Harris, R. L., et al.: Manifestations of sepsis. Arch. Intern. Med., 147:1895, 1987.
99. Parker, M. M., et al.: Serial hemodynamic patterns in survivors and nonsurvivors of septic shock in humans. Crit. Care Med., 12:311, 1984.
100. Parker, M. M., et al.: Serial hemodynamic patterns in survivors and nonsurvivors of septic shock in humans. Clin. Res., 31:671A, 1983.
101. Parker, M. M., et al.: Profound but reversible myocardial depression in patients with septic shock. Ann. Intern. Med., 100:483, 1984.
102. Oginbene, F. P., et al.: Depressed left ventricular performance: response to volume infusion in patients with sepsis and septic shock. Chest, 93:903, 1988.
103. Abel, F. L.: Myocardial function in sepsis and endotoxin shock. Am. J. Physiol., 257:R1265, 1989.
104. Elhodt, A. G., et al.: Left ventricular performance in septic shock: reversible segmental and global abnormalities. Am. Heart J., 110:402, 1985.
105. Weisel, R. D., et al.: Myocardial dysfunction during sepsis. Am. J. Surg., 133:512, 1977.
106. Parrillo, J. E.: Cardiovascular dysfunction in septic shock: new insights into a deadly disease. Int. J. Cardiol., 7:314, 1985.
107. Ozier, Y., et al.: Two-dimensional echocardiographic demonstration of acute myocardial depression in septic shock. Crit. Care Med., 12:596, 1984.
108. Kim, C. H., et al.: Steroid-responsive eosinophilic myocarditis: diagnosis by endomyocardial biopsy. Am. J. Cardiol., 53:1472, 1984.
109. Reznick, J. W., et al.: Lyme carditis. Am. J. Med., 81:923, 1986.
110. Ino, T., et al.: Cardiac manifestations in disorders of fat and carnitine metabolism in infancy. J. Am. Coll. Cardiol., 11: 1301, 1988.
111. Lorell, B., Alderman, E. L., and Mason, J. W.: Cardiac sarcoidosis: diagnosis with endomyocardial biopsy and treatment with corticosteroids. Am. J. Cardiol., 42:143, 1978.

Chapter 32

INTENSIVE CARE ASPECTS OF CARDIAC TRANSPLANTATION

ROBERT W. STEWART

Prior to the first human-to-human cardiac transplant, performed in Capetown, South Africa by Dr. Christian Barnard in 1967,[1] nearly a half-century of experimental studies on cardiac transplantation had taken place. These preliminary studies demonstrated the ability of the acutely denervated heart to function adequately after transplantation and also established the operative techniques that are still in use today.

By 1969, over a hundred cardiac transplants had been performed worldwide, with few long-term survivors. Over the next decade, most institutions stopped performing cardiac transplants. A notable exception to this was Stanford Medical Center, where the group led by Dr. Norman Shumway continued an active clinical and investigative effort in transplantation. Shumway's contributions included a process of recipient evaluation, which concentrated mainly on contraindications to transplantation and the diagnosis of rejection by transvenous endomyocardial biopsy.

With the clinical introduction of cyclosporine in 1983, interest in cardiac transplantation resumed, and in 1992 nearly 200 centers in the United States performed a total of 2000 transplants. This number represented a plateau reached in 1990 because of the limited number of donor hearts available. The need, however, continues to exceed the supply of donor hearts. Conservative estimates place the number of patients in the United States who could benefit from cardiac transplantation at 15,000 annually.

CANDIDATES FOR CARDIAC TRANSPLANTATION

Indications

To be considered for cardiac transplantation, a patient must have end-stage heart disease that is progressive and will be fatal within 6 months. Patients considered for transplantation are New York Heart Association Functional class IV; an exception is made in the case of patients with severe progressive cardiac disease who are not yet class IV but who have experienced cardiac arrest. Implicit in the indications for cardiac transplantation is the lack of any alternate form of therapy, either medical or surgical. Cardiac transplantation is reserved for those individuals for whom no therapeutic alternative exists.

Contraindications

Absolute contraindications (Table 32-1) to cardiac transplantation are similar to the contraindications established by other solid organ transplant endeavors. These include active infection (including HIV-positive patients),[2] untreated malignant disease, substance addiction, a history of noncompliance,[3] a strong history of psychologic or social maladjustment, advanced and untreatable peripheral vascular disease, or irreversible end-organ failure, specifically hepatic or renal. Although combined liver and heart transplants, as well as combined kidney and heart transplants, have been performed successfully, liver or kidney failure remains a contraindication to cardiac transplantation.

Certain contraindications are unique to cardiac transplantation (Table 32-1). Irreversible pulmonary vascular disease causes right ventricular failure in the donor heart. Pulmonary vascular disease can result from long-standing left ventricular dysfunction of any origin. Pulmonary embolism resulting in pulmonary infarction prior to transplantation is frequently followed by pneumonitis. Finally, cardiac amyloidosis should be considered a contraindication to transplantation because of the probability of recurrence in the transplanted heart, even though short-term success has been reported.[4]

Evolving contraindications to cardiac transplantation (Table 32-1) include older age or insulin-dependent diabetes.[5] Although originally denied cardiac transplantation, patients between ages 50 to 60 years are now being transplanted with good long-term survival.[6] Our practice is to accept any recipient up to 60 years of age and selectively consider patients up to 65 years of age. Similarly, insulin-dependent diabetics are selectively considered for cardiac transplantation when no evidence of retinopathy, nephropathy, or neuropathy is present.

Evaluation

Patients awaiting transplantation undergo extensive laboratory evaluation (Table 32-2). Some of this testing, such as that for the presence of human immunodeficiency virus (HIV), will directly affect the patients' candidacy for transplantation. Other tests, such as that for antibodies to herpes simplex virus or cytomegalovirus, will be used to direct post-transplantation care.

The potential transplant candidate and his or her family are evaluated at a personal level in order to determine their level of comprehension of transplantation, to uncover any history of noncompliance or drug dependence, and to identify the support people who will help the transplant patient during both the waiting period and also after transplantation. The financial realities of transplantation are discussed at this time. Personnel involved in the evaluation

Table 32-1. Contraindications to Cardiac Transplantation

Obvious
    Irreversible hepatic or renal disease
    Symptomatic peripheral vascular disease
    Cachexia (severe)
    Absence of adequate social support
    Active infection
    Chronic lung disease
    Psychiatric disturbance
    Social instability
    Medical noncompliance
    Recent peptic ulcer disease or diverticulitis
Unique for Cardiac Transplantation
    Severe pulmonary vascular disease
    Recent pulmonary infarction
    Cardiac amyloidosis
Evolving
    Age >65 years
    Diabetes mellitus without either neuropathy, nephropathy, and retinopathy

Table 32-2. Laboratory Evaluation Prior to Cardiac Transplantation

Blood type and screen for preformed antibodies
Tissue typing and screen for preformed anti-HLA antibodies
Viral screen
    Human immunodeficiency virus
    Hepatitis A, B, and C
    Cytomegalovirus
    Herpes simplex
    Epstein-Barr
Miscellaneous screen
    Toxoplasmosis
    Histoplasmosis
    Coccidioidomycosis

Table 32-3. Cardiac Disorders Treated by Transplantation

Cardiomyopathies
    Primary
        Familial (muscular dystrophy)
        Hypertrophic
        Restrictive (endomyocardial fibreolastosis)
    Secondary
        Inflammatory (postviral and idiopathic dilated)
        Toxic (doxorubicin)
        Radiation-induced
        Ischemic
Valvular heart disease
Congenital heart disease
Trauma
Tumors

include a social worker, a nurse, the transplant coordinator, a cardiologist, and a bioethicist. These individuals then convene formally when the evaluation is completed. At that time, the cardiologist presents the history of the present illness together with the pertinent findings and the group makes a recommendation concerning the medical advisability of transplantation. Special family and personal situations are presented by the social worker and bioethicist. Although the transplant surgeons are a part of the committee, their input is usually not a determining factor in recipient evaluation.

Ideally, a potential recipient does not undergo any invasive procedure during the evaluation unless the person is likely to be accepted for cardiac transplantation on the basis of the evaluation provided by the social worker. A right heart catheterization allows the determination of pulmonary vascular resistance (PVR = (PA mean-wedge)/cardiac output). When the PVR is less than or equal to 2.5 U, no further evaluation is needed. When the PVR is greater than 2.5 U, an attempt is made to determine the responsiveness of the pulmonary vasculature. Sodium nitroprusside is infused intravenously until either systemic hypotension occurs or until the PVR is less than or equal to 2.5 U. Patients with PVR greater than 5.0 U on nitroprusside are not considered for heart transplantation. Transpulmonary gradients may be more useful, however, than measurements of pulmonary vascular resistance.[7] Endomyocardial biopsies are necessary in any patient in whom amyloid heart disease is suspected.

Part of the evaluation process is to confirm the presence of severe cardiac disease. All patients undergo surface two-dimensional echocardiograms, and most patients with ischemic heart disease undergo coronary cineangiography. Additional testing includes a metabolic study to measure oxygen consumption, dental examination, sinus radiographs to exclude sinusitis, a multigated angiogram to determine ejection fraction, and a barium enema to evaluate diverticular disease in patients older than 55 years of age. Pulmonary function testing[8,9] and vascular laboratory evaluation are reserved for situations where the severity of lung or peripheral vascular disease is not apparent clinically, but may be severe enough to preclude transplantation. Pneumovax vaccine is administered to all patients awaiting cardiac transplantation.[10]

Although most patients who undergo cardiac transplantation have an original diagnosis of either ischemic heart disease or dilated cardiomyopathy, other diseases are also amenable to transplantation (Table 32-3). Ischemic heart disease and dilated cardiomyopathy account for about 40% of patients requiring transplantation. Ventricular failure resulting from valvular heart disease is seen in 15% of recipients and congenital, and miscellaneous diseases are present in 5%.[11-13] Many patients with either valvular heart disease or congenital heart disease are not candidates for cardiac transplantation because they have irreversible pulmonary vascular disease. Approximately 80% of cardiac transplant recipients are male. The median age of a transplant recipient is 40 years. In 1992, 40% of our 68 transplant patients had undergone previous cardiac surgery.

PRETRANSPLANT PERIOD

Before Donor Identification

About half the potential heart transplant recipients remain at home while awaiting the identification of a donor. Some of these patients depend on intravenous inotropes, most commonly dobutamine, which can be administered at home through an indwelling central line.[14] The decision to hospitalize a patient awaiting transplantation is usually prompted by the patient's inability to maintain fluid balance without the use of intravenous diuretics or because of end-organ dysfunction secondary to low cardiac output. Most hospitalized patients can be managed in a regular nursing unit. Indications for admitting a patient to the ICU include the need for ventilatory support, mechanical circulatory support, or invasive monitoring to titrate continuous intravenous afterload reduction with an agent such as sodium nitroprusside.

The medical management of the patient awaiting transplantation is different from the management of heart failure in nontransplant candidates. Potential transplant candidates can survive their end-stage heart disease if they live long enough to undergo transplantation and if nothing occurs during the waiting period to increase the risk of transplantation. Therefore, the patient awaiting cardiac transplantation should be supported by whatever means are available and every caution should be exercised to ensure that when a donor is identified the recipient will be ready and recovery will be uncomplicated.

Mechanical support of the circulation is indicated when end-organ dysfunction occurs despite maximal medical therapy including angiotensin-converting enzyme inhibitors, inotropes, and intravenous diuretics. No numeric indices are available to dictate when mechanical support is needed; some patients with long-standing heart failure demonstrate stable end-organ dysfunction with cardiac indexes as low as 1.4 L/min/m^2. Most patients, however, display progressive deterioration with indexes less than 1.8 L/min/m^2. Similarly, a systolic blood pressure of less than 80 mm Hg or a pulmonary artery wedge pressure in excess of 30 mm Hg may be tolerated by some patients. Lethargy progressing to unresponsiveness or progressive azotemia are the two most common indications to proceed with mechanical circulatory support. A percutaneously inserted intra-aortic balloon pump is still considered the first choice for mechanical circulatory support. Most transplant candidates who require an intra-aortic balloon pump do so only temporarily. After several days of augmentation, cardiac performance frequently improves, perhaps as a result of more optimal intravascular volume, which is facilitated by the diuretic response obtained with better hemodynamics. Intra-aortic balloon pumps usually increase the cardiac index by 15 to 20%.

When the condition of a transplant candidate deteriorates despite the use of an intra-aortic balloon pump, a left ventricular assist device is indicated.[15] Of the currently available appliances, our experience has been limited to the centrifugal pump, which is external, and the HeartMate implantable left ventricular assist device.[16] This latter appliance has shown fewer complications than the centrifugal pump and is currently our device of choice as a bridge to transplant. Currently, the HeartMate is approved only for patients accepted for cardiac transplantation; it requires a sternotomy and cardiopulmonary bypass for insertion, and, once in place, is not removed. The device is relatively bulky and does not fit in the abdomen of patients who have a body surface area of less than 1.6 m^2.

Care of patients with ventricular assist devices depends on the device. With the centrifugal left ventricular assist device, the most common complications include bleeding in the early phase because of the necessity for heparin-based anticoagulation, inadequate flows because of either right ventricular failure or inadequate intravascular volume, and poor drainage because of positional variability in the left-sided drainage catheter. Late complications are generally thromboembolic, either from the pump or from the native heart. The advantage of the centrifugal pump based left ventricular assist device is that if the heart recovers, the device can be removed.

Complications with the HeartMate have been few,[17] although a true comparison is not possible because of different selection criteria. The HeartMate has been reported to work even with ventricular fibrillation, where adequate pulmonary flow could be obtained without effective right ventricular contraction. A major advantage of the HeartMate system is that the patient can be fully ambulatory with the device in place.

A final form of circulatory support is extracorporeal membrane oxygenation using percutaneous cannulas and heparin-bonded surfaces. Although temporary and probably useful for less than 96 hours, support can be achieved without sternotomy, insertion can be quickly achieved, and support of both ventricles and the lungs can be provided. Complications are generally related to the percutaneously placed femoral cannulas, which can interfere with the circulation to the lower extremity.

Several considerations are worthy of mention in the hospitalized patient during a pretransplant ICU stay. A patient who has undergone cardiac arrest and who has been resuscitated, but who has not awakened, should not undergo cardiac transplantation. A patient who has postarrest encephalopathy that is improving probably should remain on the active list. Improvement in this case may be hastened by the normal perfusion provided by the new heart. An infection in a patient awaiting cardiac transplantation can remove that patient from the waiting list at the time when a donor heart becomes available. Therefore, invasive monitoring (e.g., pulmonary artery catheters, Foley catheters, and arterial lines) should be kept to a minimum. Red cell transfusions should be screened for cytomegalovirus antibodies, and the potential recipient should not be sensitized to HLA antigens by exposure to transfusions containing leukocytes. Most transplant candidates who are sedentary should be prophylactically anticoagulated with warfarin (Coumadin). Both systemic and pulmonary emboli are common during the waiting period.

Arrhythmias should be aggressively treated. Despite early concerns that patients with end-stage heart disease would not tolerate the implantation of an automatic implantable cardioverter-defibrillator, the procedure is well tolerated and does not importantly complicate subsequent transplantation. Therefore, the automatic implantable cardioverter-defibrillator should be considered for patients awaiting cardiac transplantation when antiarrhythmic therapy has failed. Similarly, amiodarone is not contraindicated in potential cardiac transplant recipients. Earlier reports of pulmonary dysfunction and poor donor heart function secondary to amiodarone have not been substantiated.

After Donor Identification

Matching

Matching a donor with a recipient begins when a potential donor is identified. Pertinent data concerning the donor such as age, weight, gender, blood group, and the location of the donor, is submitted to the computer system at the United Network for Organ Sharing (UNOS) in Richmond, Virginia. Hearts are used locally when possible. Potential recipients are grouped according to blood group and weight and, within each of these groups, priority is assigned according to medical urgency and the length of time the patient has been waiting. Although it is possible to use hearts from O blood group donors universally, the practice unfairly prejudices against potential O blood group recipients and may adversely affect outcome in non-O recipients.[18] To address this inequity, identical blood group matches are awarded extra points.

Matching on the basis of weight is influenced both by the donor's gender and the recipient's pulmonary vascular resistance. Ideally, a donor heart weighs approximately what a normal heart would weigh for the given recipient. Female donors tend to have smaller hearts than equally sized males. This discrepancy becomes most marked for females weighing more than 80 kg, in whom heart weight does not continue to increase with body size. Using a heart from an 80-kg woman in a 100-kg man, therefore, may predispose the recipient to inadequate cardiac performance. A better method would be to match hearts on the basis of either cardiac dimensions or lean body mass. In general, hearts from donors weighing 70 to 130% of the recipient are acceptable.

Recipients with elevated pulmonary vascular resistance should receive larger hearts, a process referred to as "oversizing."[19] The rationale for this practice is that the increased right ventricular afterload resulting from pulmonary vascular disease will be better tolerated by a larger right ventricle.

Some recipients have preformed antibodies against HLA antigens.[20] When these antibodies react with more than 10% of lymphocytes in a representative panel, a pretransplant lymphocyte cross-match should be performed. This process requires lymphocyte-rich blood or lymph nodes from the donor. The test is performed at the transplant institution, requires 4 hours for completion, and the results must be available before donor heart procurement can begin.

Recipient

When a potential donor is identified, the recipient is brought to the ICU for blood work, monitoring, and drug administration. Between 2 and 6 U of blood are typed and cross-matched, depending on whether the patient has had previous cardiac surgery. The blood should be cytomegalovirus free and leukocyte poor. If the patient has been taking warfarin, 4 U of fresh-frozen plasma are requested. Additional laboratory work includes a complete blood count, electrolytes, creatinine, and a prothrombin time and partial thromboplastin time. A large-bore triple-lumen central venous line and an arterial line are inserted. A chest radiograph is obtained to confirm line placement and also to evaluate the lung fields for evidence of infection or pulmonary infarction.

If the patient has been receiving warfarin, 10 mg of vitamin K is administered intravenously. Azathioprine (2 mg/kg) is given intravenously and, if an automatic implantable defibrillator-cardioverter is in place, it is programmed to an inactive mode. The recipient is transported to the operating room based on an estimate of when induction should take place, so the recipient is ready to begin cardiopulmonary bypass when the donor heart arrives in the operating room.

Donor

Heart donors are a subpopulation of multiple organ donors (Table 32-4). Currently, about 40% of all donors are suitable for cardiac procurement. The basic criteria for organ donation include documented brain death, no malignant disease except brain tumors, permission from next of kin, age less than 65 years, and a known cause of death. Additionally, donors have been screened for evidence of infection from HIV, hepatitis B, and syphilis. Donors are accepted by some centers when the antibody to the hepatitis B core antigen is positive, but no additional evidence of active hepatitis is present. A history of recent intravenous drug abuse or other life styles that would put the donor at high risk for carrying the HIV are considered adequate justification for not proceeding with organ retrieval. Some centers in the United States accept organ donation in the presence of positive laboratory tests for hepatitis C. The early follow-up of this limited clinical experience to date has been encouraging.

Additional infection screening influences subsequent patient surveillance and antimicrobial therapy of the recipient, but it does not preclude organ harvesting. In this category are tests for cytomegalovirus, herpes simplex, and Toxoplasma gondii.

Cardiac donors represent a select group of the entire population of donors. Until about 1989, cardiac procurement was limited to female donors less than 40 years of age and male donors less than 35. This policy has changed and currently donors up to age 60 years are considered.[21-23] Ideally, these older donors should undergo coronary cineangiography, but unfortunately many hospitals are not equipped to provide this service. Hemodynamic instability that requires high dose inotropic support or pro-

Table 32-4. Criteria for Cardiac Donation

Documented brain death
Known cause of death
Permission
No unwitnessed cardiac arrest
No history of illicit drug use
No active infection (e.g., HIV, hepatitis B, ? hepatitis C)
Negative Venereal Disease Research Laboratory (VDRL) test
No prolonged cardiopulmonary resuscitation
No history of malignant disease (except skin cancer or brain tumors)
Normal cardiac function
Age <65 years

longed cardiopulmonary resuscitation should be viewed as a relative contraindication to harvesting the heart.

Although intravenous drug abuse is considered an absolute contraindication for organ procurement, other forms of drug abuse are not. An exception, however, applies to the heart and cocaine. Cocaine, by any route of administration, has both short- and long-term adverse effects on the heart. On a short-term basis, cocaine depletes the heart of catecholamines. More important, however, are the long-term effects of cocaine: premature coronary atherosclerosis, cardiomyopathies, and eosinophilic myocarditis. For these reasons, cocaine abuse is considered a contraindication for cardiac transplantation.

Although an ECG and myocardial enzyme determination are a routine part of the evaluation of the potential cardiac donor, their results are both nonsensitive and nonspecific. Important abnormalities of the ST segments are common in the brain dead and seem to have little physiologic significance. A two-dimensional surface echocardiogram is the single most useful test currently available. An element of caution is necessary, however, because of the inability of two-dimensional echocardiography to show the right ventricle adequately. When myocardial contusion is suspected, the best method of appraisal will generally be direct visual assessment in the operating room after sternotomy.

Management of the brain dead potential organ donor is aided by an understanding of the physiology of brain death.[24] Although a variety of injuries, including blunt head trauma, penetrating head injuries, and subarachnoid hemorrhage can result in brain death, the final result of these injuries is always brain stem herniation. Brain stem herniation has a reproducible effect which initially is a neuroendocrine stress response followed by endocrine collapse. This latter change is the result of the loss of hypothalamic-pituitary function and concomitant loss of adrenal and thyroid function. In addition to the loss of vasopressin with the resultant obvious diabetes insipidus, there is also a loss of circulating epinephrine, norepinephrine, dopamine, triiodothyronine, and thyroxine. The disappearance of these hormones is more gradual than that of vasopressin and the clinical effect not as readily apparent, but equally important. The observation made repeatedly in the past was that brain death is inexorably followed by somatic death. Only recently, however, has an explanation been forthcoming to explain this link. The loss of the adrenal hormones results in hemodynamic collapse and somatic death. It has been demonstrated, however, that this link can be broken and prolonged somatic viability is possible following brain death when hormonal replacement is provided. A final result of the brain stem herniation is loss of autoregulation of temperature. Brain dead patients are routinely hypothermic and can rapidly assume the temperature of their surroundings.

In addition to the physiologic effects of brain death, the potential organ donor routinely has been subjected to fluid restriction and diuretic administration in an effort to limit cerebral edema. Management of the potential organ donor involves simultaneous assessment and resuscitation. All potential donors require at least two large bore IVs, one of which can be used to monitor central venous pressure. A Foley catheter, an arterial line, an ECG monitor, and a means of monitoring core temperature are mandatory. A pulmonary artery catheter is indicated when the hemodynamics are unstable. The initial assessment of the donor evaluates the adequacy of the cardiac performance. Adequate perfusion is evidenced by easily palpable pedal pulses and warm extremities. Blood pressure does not always reflect the adequacy of the cardiac output, since hypotension, because of the loss of central nervous system controlled vasomotor tone, may be associated with a greater than normal cardiac output. The causes for a low cardiac output include inadequate preload, an elevated afterload, and/or poor myocardial contractility. Occasionally, more than one of these factors may be responsible. Unlike nonbrain dead patients where urine output and heart rate are related to cardiac output, these findings are affected in the brain dead patient by the lack of central nervous system function and are consequently insensitive.

An inadequate preload is the most common cause for a low cardiac output in the brain dead and is a result of both diabetes insipidus and fluid restriction.[25] Resuscitation involves both preventing the continuing inappropriate polyuria and fluid replacement. Vasopressin, 0.5 U per hour, as a continuous intravenous infusion is preferable to bolus administration and can be titrated to achieve a urine output of 100 ml per hour. The type of fluid administered should be determined by the serum electrolytes, which should be reassessed every 2 hours until organ procurement is completed. Most donors are initially severely hypernatremic and the initial choice of fluid is 5% dextrose in water. Because several liters of fluid may be required, the risk of producing hyperglycemia is real. Treatment of blood glucose levels that are in excess of 250 mg is advisable and best achieved with the continuous intravenous administration of insulin. The response of the central venous pressure to fluid administration is a useful guideline to assist in determining the rate of administration.

Some donors have unacceptably low hematocrits during fluid resuscitation. Transfusion therapy in this setting is indicated to maintain a hematocrit near 30%. These blood products should be cytomegalovirus free and leukocyte poor.

Poor myocardial performance can result from either right or left ventricular dysfunction which may be a result of preexisting cardiac disease, myocardial injury accompanying the brain injury, or the loss of the hypothalamic-pituitary-adrenal axis. Myocardial contusion may be missed on the two-dimensional echocardiogram because the injury frequently affects only the right ventricle. Right ventricular myocardial contusion may result in a low cardiac output, elevated central venous pressure, and a normal appearing left ventricle with echocardiography. The diagnosis is generally presumptive. Cardiac procurement does not proceed when a myocardial contusion is strongly suspected.

Myocardial failure because of endocrine collapse is probably the final common pathway for somatic death in the brain dead. Although inotropes are almost routine in managing organ donors, standard practice does not currently reflect scientific knowledge. Currently, inadequate cardiac output is treated with dopamine, and not infrequently doses of 15 to 20 μ/kg per minute are used. A more rational approach, supported by data from clinical investigations, is the use of epinephrine, up to 0.5 μ/kg per minute. The advantage of epinephrine, in addition to increasing the cardiac output, is that it helps to normalize the blood pressure.

Another form of endocrine depletion that has a potential deleterious effect on cardiac function is thyroid dysfunction. Most interest in this area has been from groups involved with cardiac transplantation.[26] Thyroid replacement, using 200 μg of triiodothyronine, has been associated with improved myocardial function and has facilitated the weaning of inotropes. Adverse effects have not been reported.

Most donors are hypotensive with mean arterial blood pressures of less than 70 mm Hg, even when the cardiac output is normal. Although dopamine in high doses helps to maintain the blood pressure, it does so at the expense and risk of depleting the myocardial presynaptic junction of norepinephrine. An occasional donor is hypertensive and should be treated with sodium nitroprusside to optimize pressure. Fluids, inspired gases, and the surroundings should also be warmed. The donor's temperature requires continuous monitoring. Atrial arrhythmias frequently occur when the core temperature falls below 32°C.

In addition to iatrogenically produced hyperglycemia, other metabolic abnormalities are common. Phosphate, calcium, and magnesium levels should be checked and corrected when depletion is established.

Most potential donors have abnormal coagulation profiles. Prolonged administration of parenteral antibiotics without adequate vitamin K administration is a possible mechanism. A moderate hyperfibrinolysis is seen in most patients with head injuries, perhaps most commonly with penetrating head trauma. Full-blown disseminated intravascular coagulation, however, is usual and also is most common in patients with penetrating head injuries. These individuals have clinical evidence of bleeding disorders with prolonged bleeding from puncture sites. Their laboratory evaluation reveals prolonged partial thromboplastin times, elevated prothrombin times, depleted fibrinogen levels, and elevated levels of D-dimers. End-organ dysfunction, notably renal dysfunction, can occur as a result of fibrin deposition. Organ procurement in this setting is contraindicated.

OPERATIVE PHASE

Timing

Heart transplantation involves two teams working in parallel. An ideal result occurs when the donor team arrives at the transplant center with the donor heart at the time that preparation for instituting cardiopulmonary bypass in the recipient has been completed. This obviates unnecessary ischemic time for the donor heart and minimizes anesthesia time and the duration of cardiopulmonary bypass for the recipient. Frequent communication between the two teams is necessary. The donor team should notify the transplant center at the following time points:

- On arrival at the donor institution
- After performing the sternotomy and inspecting the heart
- 20 minutes before heparin is administered
- On leaving the transplant institution

At each of these points, a time estimate is made concerning the interval until the next call. Forty-five minutes are allotted for the time from induction to cannulation in a first-time operation and 1 hour and 45 minutes for reoperations.

Donor

Donor organ procurement involves several teams of surgeons, frequently from different institutions convening at an unfamiliar hospital. Generally, these teams have not worked together before. This fact coupled with the possibility that what may be optimal for one team can be deleterious for the other team produces a situation that is best described as anxious. The local transplant coordinator and the local anesthesiologist are by necessity placed in the middle of this situation.

The donor operating room is warmed to 70°F (21°C) and a heating blanket placed on the table. The donor is positioned with the arms at the sides. Monitoring includes an ECG, an upper extremity arterial line, two upper extremity large-bore catheters (one used for measuring central venous pressure and one for fluid replacement), a thermistor (not a bladder probe), and a Foley catheter. The availability of 4 U of red cells that are cytomegalovirus free and leukocyte poor should be confirmed. The hematocrit is maintained at 25% during procurement. Cefuroxime, 1.5 G, is given IV.

It is the responsibility of each team to check on the following matters:

- That brain death has been documented
- That consent has been obtained for the organ they are harvesting
- That the blood type has been unequivocally established

An anesthesiologist is vital to organ procurement. The donor is ventilated with 100% oxygen, and muscle relaxants are administered. Spinal reflexes are intact in donors, and both muscle activity and hypertension can occur during surgical manipulation.

Because a median sternotomy incision facilitates the exposure needed for the dissection of the intra-abdominal organs, especially the liver, this incision is made at the same time the abdominal incision is made. The pericardium, however, is left intact until the cardiac team is ready to inspect the heart.

Inspection of the heart is both visual and manual. In cases of blunt trauma, the absence of both hematomas of the chest wall and bloody pericardial fluid is indirect evidence against important myocardial contusion. The contractility of the heart is evaluated visually, with the assessment primarily limited to the left ventricle. Congenital abnormalities are excluded at this time, most notably abnormalities of systemic or pulmonary venous return. Palpation is performed to ascertain the presence of thrills and to determine any coronary artery calcification.

Dissection of the heart requires only 5 minutes, and because the manipulation involved with dissection can produce atrial fibrillation, this is postponed until the intra-abdominal organs are completely prepared for removal. Dissection involves placing two ties around the superior vena cava where it crosses the right pulmonary artery and freeing the posterior attachments of the inferior vena cava. A pursestring suture is placed in the ascending aorta at the level that it will eventually be transected and the cardioplegia catheter inserted. Heparin (30,000 U) is given IV. The catheters for perfusion of the abdominal organs are inserted. As soon as the perfusion of the abdominal organs begins the heart is prepared for removal.

Removal of the heart consists of isolation, perfusion, decompression, external cooling, and excision. Isolation involves ligating the superior vena cava, opening the right pleural space to the level of the inferior vena cava, then incising the juncture of the right atrium with the inferior vena cava at a level that leaves adequate tissue on the inferior vena cava for hepatic transplantation. The pleura is opened to allow free drainage of blood from the inferior vena cava, which will preclude venous congestion of the intra-abdominal organs. It will take the heart only a few beats to evacuate any retained blood; the evacuation is assisted by asking the anesthesiologist to manually inflate, or valsalva, the lungs. After this, the donor is disconnected from the ventilator and the aortic cross-clamp applied. Cold (4 to 10°C) crystalloid cardioplegia, 20 ml/kg, is then infused at a rate that achieves an aortic root pressure of 88 mm Hg. The pressure is estimated by palpation. The heart is decompressed by incising the intrapericardial portion of the right superior pulmonary vein. The pericardium is then filled with ice cold saline.

Excision commences after the completion of the infusion of cardioplegia. The superior vena cava is divided above the ligatures and the incision previously made in the inferior vena cava is completed. The aortic cross-clamp is removed and the aorta divided at the level of the pulmonary bifurcation. The apex of the heart is then retracted and the pulmonary veins and the pulmonary arteries are transected flush with the pericardium. The heart is then retracted downward and the reflections of the transverse sinus into the great vessels are incised. It is possible at this point to enter the esophagus. Moreover, if a pulmonary artery catheter or a right atrial line has been placed, it should be retracted before the superior vena cava is ligated.

Preservation during transportation involves cold storage. The heart is sealed with plastic bags containing a small amount of saline, placed in turn within a sealed container, which is placed in an ice chest containing bags of ice. The use of free ice within the ice chest results in excessive cooling. An ideal transport temperature is probably 12 to 14°C.[27] Despite these precautions, most donor hearts are not normal at implantation[28] probably because of ischemic time[29] and injury before removal.

Recipient
Drugs and Anesthesia

Anesthesia for cardiac transplantation involves a combination of inhalation and intravenous agents. After induction, 1.5 g of cefuroxime are administered intravenously and a baseline activated clotting time is obtained. Heparin is administered to obtain an activated clotting time of 480 seconds; initially, 300 U/kg of heparin are given. Additional doses are given to maintain the activated clotting time at 480 seconds. Methylprednisolone, 500 mg, is given intravenously with the initiation of bypass. Protamine, 1 to 3 mg/kg, is given after discontinuation of bypass.

Induction, Preparation, and Cannulation

The recipient arrives in the operating room with arterial and venous lines in place and is not induced until the donor team inspects the heart. After induction and endotracheal intubation, a Foley catheter with a thermal probe is inserted and the recipient prepped from chin to ankles.

A median sternotomy incision is made, and pursestring sutures are placed for high aortic cannulation and for two caval cannulas. The heart is not manipulated to avoid possible embolization. A final aortic pursestring suture is placed for antegrade infusion of cardioplegia.

The technique discussed next is limited to orthotopic transplantation; heterotopic transplantation is reviewed by Desruennes.[30]

Cardiopulmonary Bypass, Cardiectomy, and Implantation

Cardiopulmonary bypass is instituted with the perfusate at 28°C. If the patient has been on warfarin, 2 U of fresh frozen plasma are added to the crystalloid prime. If the hematocrit during bypass is less than 25%, then cytomegalovirus-free leukocyte-poor red cells are transfused, unless the reservoir volume is adequate to allow hemoconcentration. Blood conservation involves reinfusing all of the heparinized blood at the end of cardiopulmonary bypass in addition to washing and transfusing any blood retrieved by the noncardiotomy suction during the procedure. Flows are maintained at 2.5 L/min/m^2 during bypass, and the mean arterial pressure is kept at or above 80 mm Hg.

After the heart has been arrested, the recipient is prepared for orthotopic cardiac transplantation. The right atrium is opened 2 cm from the atrioventricular groove and the intra-atrial septum incised between the medial edge of the fossa ovalis and the tricuspid valve. Working on the left side, incisions are made at the junction of the base of the atrial appendage with the left superior pulmonary vein. These openings are then connected, dividing the atria along their inferior and lateral portions. The aorta and then the pulmonary artery are transected, both at the level of the commissures. This exposes the roof of the left atrium and permits the final division of the atria. The heart is removed from the field and the fossa ovalis inspected for a patent foramen ovale, which is closed. Finally, the aorta is separated from the pulmonary artery up to the pericardial reflection. A final check is made for thrombi in the atrial remnants.

Preparation of the donor heart begins with opening the right atrium at its right lateral wall inferiorly. The fossa is inspected for a patent foramen ovale, and any fibrinous material remaining in the heart from indwelling venous catheters is removed. The tie on the superior vena cava is inspected and the heart turned over. The left atrium is prepared by cutting out the central portion, the limits of this incision being the orifices of the pulmonary veins. The mitral valve is inspected and the heart again rotated. The aorta is freed from the pulmonary artery and the aortic valve inspected. The pulmonary bifurcation is freed from the root of the left atrium with electrocautery and an incision is made opposite the main trunk of the pulmonary artery, connecting the right and left pulmonary arteries. A cuff of pulmonary artery is then fashioned at the level of the pulmonary bifurcation. The length of the aorta above the aortic commissures should be equal to the length of the pulmonary artery above its commissures.

Implantation begins at the most lateral aspect of the left atrium with the donor heart held outside the pericardium. The suture line continues inferiorly, sewing from donor to recipient. The heart is lowered into place with exposure facilitated by the assistant placing two fingers inside the donor left atrium. Suturing continues to the junction of the right and left atria. The other end of the suture is then used, working counterclockwise, and any discrepancies between the perimeters of the two atria are adjusted at this point. The right atrial anastomosis is made next, beginning in the mid portion of the atrial septum where this suture line will overlap the left atrial suture line when the recipient right atrial perimeter exceeds that of the donor, the inferior and occasionally superior portions of the right atrium are plicated, essentially lengthening the inferior and superior vena cava. This produces less distortion of the donor right atrium and tricuspid valve and ideally less tricuspid regurgitation. The medial portion of the right atrial anastomosis is left unfinished, to be closed after the great vessels are anastomosed.

The pulmonary artery anastomosis is performed next. Torsion of the donor pulmonary artery will result in right ventricular outflow obstruction. This situation is avoided by carefully aligning the anterior aspect of the recipient and donor vessel. This anastomosis is done in a single layer but in four quadrants, with the suture being tied in continuity after completing each quadrant. This approach has proved useful because of the possibility of constricting the pulmonary artery. The aortic anastomosis is constructed in two layers working from the outside and creating an entirely everting anastomosis. This result is possible because the final length of the aorta is greater than normal.

The aorta is unclamped and the chambers de-aired. The amount of air remaining in the pulmonary vasculature seems greater than with most cardiac operations and extra time should be spent ensuring complete de-airing.

An alternate technique which is gaining in popularity involves end-to-end anastomosis for both venae cavae. The benefits of this technique are unproven but potentially include less right atrial distortion and therefore less tricuspid regurgitation. Modifications of the recipient cardiectomy are required, and include transection of both venae cavae at their atrial juncture and transecting the left atrium circumferentially just above the pulmonary veins. Preparation of the donor is different because no right atriotomy is made, and the tie on the superior vena cava is removed. Implantation again begins with the left atrial anastomosis. The caval anastomosis can be performed once the cross-clamp is removed, and therefore this technique does not increase the ischemic time.

Myocardial Preservation

During cardiac transplantation, the recipient's heart is arrested with antegrade cold blood cardioplegia. This makes removal easier, because the heart is arrested, and also preserves viability for investigative studies performed by our research colleagues. The donor heart is protected with cold low flow continuous retrograde cardioplegia. A pursestring suture is placed around the coronary sinus and the catheter secured into place. Blood cardioplegia at 4° to 8°C is infused continuously in proportion to heart weight. In general, the flow rates are 100 ml per minute and perfusion pressure about 30 mm Hg. A warm reperfusion is used for the final 3 minutes of cross clamping, with the temperature at 37°C, the pressure no higher than 50 mm Hg, and the flow 200 to 300 ml per minute.

Weaning from Cardiopulmonary Bypass

Monitoring consists of a left atrial line, a pulmonary artery thermistor inserted directly into the pulmonary artery, and four pacing wires: two atrial and two ventricular. Pulmonary artery pressure monitoring is not routine, but is indicated when either the pulmonary vascular resistance is elevated preoperatively, or right ventricular dysfunction occurs after implantation. Weaning the transplant patient from cardiopulmonary bypass is no different than with other cardiac surgical cases:

- The temperature should be 37°C
- The hematocrit should be kept above 25%
- Any bleeding should be controlled
- Potassium, magnesium, calcium, and glucose levels should be brought to normal

Although the newly transplanted heart is anatomically free of disease, its function is generally compromised because of the condition of the donor, the effects of the operation, and the abnormal milieu of the recipient. An optimal situation exists when the cardiac index is equal to or greater than 2.5 L/min/m^2, the left atrial and right atrial pressures are less than 16 mm Hg, and the mean arterial blood pressure is 90 mm Hg.

When the cardiac performance is suboptimal, the transplant patient, like any patient recovering from cardiac surgery, should be assessed systemically and interventions directed toward optimizing preload, afterload, rate, and rhythm.

An optimum preload is achieved when the highest pressure, either right atrial or left atrial is 16 mm Hg. Higher pressures achieve little beneficial effect in increasing stroke volume. Normally, the right atrial pressure is 1 to 2 mm Hg less than the left atrial pressure. An indication that the "limiting ventricle" is the right ventricle occurs when the right atrial pressure exceeds that of the left. An ideal afterload exists when the mean arterial pressure is 90 mm Hg. Pressures lower than this may be inadequate to provide coronary perfusion. Pressures above 90 mm Hg impose an unnecessary burden on the left ventricle.

Norepinephrine and sodium nitroprusside are the drugs of choice for controlling hypotension and hypertension, respectively. When hypotension persists despite 0.1 μg/kg per minute of norepinephrine, then the hematocrit should be increased to 40%.

In regard to rhythm, both inspecting the underlying rhythm and pacing the heart are facilitated by the presence of temporary epicardial pacing wires. An optimal heart rate is 100 to 120, which is faster than generally acceptable for nontransplant cardiac surgery patients. Maintenance of sinus rhythm will assist in optimizing cardiac output; even if the underlying rhythm is an accelerated junctional rhythm, overdrive atrial pacing will improve the cardiac performance. Atrial and ventricular arrhythmias should be treated in the same manner as for the nontransplant cardiac patients.[31-33]

Perhaps the key point in caring for the newly transplanted heart is the realization that right ventricular dysfunction occurs commonly.[34] Indications of isolated right ventricular dysfunction are limited and include an elevated right atrial pressure in the presence of a low left atrial pressure. Echocardiography is helpful in establishing the diagnosis, but frequently empiric therapy is begun without confirming the diagnosis. Therapy is aided by a pulmonary artery catheter that permits monitoring of right ventricular afterload. Right ventricular dysfunction can be primary, secondary, or a combination of both. Primary dysfunction results from donor trauma or poor preservation. Secondary dysfunction results from pulmonary vascular disease or a stenosis of the pulmonary anastomosis.[35] If the latter is suspected, a continuous recording of pulmonary artery pressures should be made during pulmonary artery catheter withdrawal. Therapy for both primary and secondary right ventricular dysfunction includes lowering right ventricular afterload and optimizing right ventricular contractility. Isoproterenol, amrinone, prostaglandin E_1, sodium nitroprusside and nitroglycerin can be used individually or in combination to lower pulmonary vascular resistance. When systemic hypotension occurs, norepinephrine should be infused directly into the systemic arterial circulation either via a left atrial line or into the end of an intra-aortic balloon pump. In this latter regard, an intra-aortic balloon pump is useful in isolated right ventricular dysfunction. The reasons are that it helps to support the systemic perfusion pressure, it lowers left atrial pressure and, in so doing, reduces total pulmonary vascular resistance, it provides a port for infusing pressors, and it assists in myocardial perfusion.

When these measures fail, a right ventricular assist device can be used. The risk of embolization is less with right ventricular assist devices as compared to left ventricular assist devices. Therefore, anticoagulation after insertion can be reduced, keeping the activated clotting time between 160 and 180 seconds.

The choice of inotrope is surprisingly empiric. Isoproterenol, 0.1 μg/kg per minute, and amrinone 10 μg/kg loading dose followed by 5 to 15 μg/kg per minute infusion, are believed to be particularly beneficial for right ventricular dysfunction. Isoproterenol, however, frequently produces an unacceptable degree of atrial tachycardia. Amrinone seems a less potent inotrope and can produce platelet related bleeding problems, both immediately and after prolonged exposure. The dosage of prostacyclin varies and ranges from 0.5 to 5.0 mg/kg per minute.[35]

Dobutamine, 10 μg/kg per minute, epinephrine, 0.1 μg/kg per minute, and dopamine, 10 μg/kg per minute, have all been successfully employed in treating ventricular dysfunction following transplantation. Failure to achieve an adequate inotropic response to one agent should not be viewed negatively; other inotropes may elicit the desired response.

Although the cause of ventricular dysfunction early after transplantation is usually unclear, especially in the absence of isolated right ventricular dysfunction, and is usually treated empirically, one clinical scenario should not be overlooked. Hyperacute rejection, which is mediated primarily by antibodies, can produce early graft dysfunction. It is most likely to occur in patients with preformed antibodies but is not restricted to this group. Retransplantation for this problem is the treatment of choice. Bridging the patient to retransplantation requires extracorporeal membrane oxygenator.

When volume administration, pacing, and afterload optimization fail to achieve a cardiac index of 2.5 L/min/m, then inotropes are initiated. When the transplant patient cannot be weaned from cardiopulmonary bypass using routine inotropes, reappraisal of the situation is indicated. Generally, it is preferable to reinstitute full cardiopulmonary bypass at this point, discontinue all inotropic agents, request an intraoperative echocardiogram, raise the hematocrit to 30%, and inspect the pulmonary artery anastomosis for torsion or constriction. The echocardiogram is useful in distinguishing between isolated right ventricular dysfunction and biventricular global failure: this differentiation affects therapy. Most transplant patients have echocardiographic evidence of tricuspid regurgitation which is not clinically important. A pulmonary artery catheter can be inserted at this time to determine any residual pulmonary hypertension.

Global biventricular failure can be the result of hyperacute rejection, but is more likely the result of poor myocardial preservation. Biventricular support can be achieved with percutaneously placed femoral venous and arterial lines and extracorporeal membrane oxygenator support. Anticoagulation is unnecessary when the entire circuit is heparin bonded. With this form of support, both ventricles can recover, inotropes can be discontinued, and the chest closed.

POSTOPERATIVE ICU PHASE

Early Phase

The early phase of convalescence in the ICU encompasses the period from the operation until the patient is free from inotropic support and extubated. Generally, this process has been accomplished by postoperative day 4. The needs of the heart recipient are best met in the setting of the cardiac surgical ICU. The utility of reverse isolation has never been proven.[37] Cardiac transplant patients at the Cleveland Clinic Foundation are cared for in one of two laminar air flow rooms in the cardiac surgery ICU. The chief advantage of this may lie in protecting the recipient from aspergillosis during periods of renovation and construction. Although the nursing personnel caring for the transplant patient should be familiar with the immunosuppressant agents used, they should recognize that the cardiac transplant patient is best cared for using the same procedures and guidelines as for cardiac surgical patients who have not undergone cardiac transplantation.

Cardiac Considerations

The measures detailed in the section of this chapter on weaning from cardiopulmonary bypass are followed in the ICU. The assessment of the adequacy of the cardiac performance includes measured cardiac indexes and also clinical assessment. An adequate cardiac index correlates closely with the presence of warm extremities, easily palpable pedal pulses, and good urine flow.

When a discrepancy exists between the measured cardiac index and the clinical assessment of cardiac function, determining the oxygen saturation of a specimen of mixed venous blood is useful. Saturations above 75% support the belief that the cardiac index is adequate.

The pericardial silhouette on the chest radiograph is usually unchanged from the preoperative radiograph. The large space within the pericardial cavity is only partly filled by the small donor heart and fills with blood in the first few hours after transplantation. A large cardiac silhouette, therefore, is neither unexpected nor evidence of cardiac tamponade. Excluding tamponade in the transplant patient is best done in the operating room with reexploration. The utility of the chest radiograph or of echocardiography is minimal in either proving or excluding the existence of cardiac tamponade. Postoperative pericardial effusions are seen in 5 to 10% of transplant patients, and their importance remains obscure.[38]

Pulmonary Considerations

Most transplant recipients require mechanical ventilatory support for 24 to 48 hours. Although pulmonary function studies are usually abnormal in the pretransplant patient with end-stage heart disease, the most common causes for prolonged ventilation following cardiac transplantation are hemodynamic instability or general debility.

Renal Considerations

Renal dysfunction, as evidenced by an increasing serum creatinine, occurs more commonly in the cardiac transplant recipient than in other patients following cardiac surgery. Presumably, this is the result of the cumulative effect of pretransplant low cardiac output and the deleterious effects of cardiopulmonary bypass. For this reason, cyclosporine, a known nephrotoxin, is not administered until renal function has normalized.

Diuretics are usually necessary following transplant, especially in individuals who received large doses of diuretics prior to transplantation. Low doses of dopamine, 2 to 3 µg/kg per minute, are used routinely.

If urine output decreases once cyclosporine treatment is initiated, the cyclosporine is discontinued for several hours and renal function is allowed to return to normal before restarting the cyclosporine, which is then given at half the original dose. Nifedipine, 10 mg sublingually, has been effective in maintaining urine flow (and presumably renal function) in patients who become oliguric in response to cyclosporine. A note of caution is needed, however, because nifedipine causes hypotension.

Central Nervous System Considerations

Seizures occur more commonly in transplant recipients than in other cardiac patients. Cerebral overperfusion can result in seizures. This situation occurs when the cardiac index is above 4.0 L/min/m^2. The seizures are generally preceded by headache. Prophylactic or therapeutic reduction in the cardiac index can be achieved by administering 0.5 mg dose of intravenous propranolol. Hypomagnesemia from cyclosporine-induced magnesium wasting also causes seizures and can be prevented by monitoring the serum magnesium level. Although cyclosporine can also cause seizures, it is uncommon in cardiac patients and seizures are usually observed only with excessive blood levels.[39]

Coagulation

Bleeding following cardiac transplantation is more excessive than following nontransplant open heart surgery. The reasons for this have not been rigorously studied. Possible contributing factors, however, include the preoperative administration of warfarin (Coumadin), the presence of hepatic congestion, and the response of the ill patient to cardiopulmonary bypass. Additionally, because of the disparity between the capacity of the pericardium, which has been stretched, and the relatively small size of the new heart, retained intrapericardial blood is common. This condition can contribute to systemic fibrinolysis and bleeding.

The conventional rules regarding reentry to control bleeding also apply to the transplant patient. When bleeding persists but reentry is not indicated, replacement therapy is initiated. The first level of treatment is to administer 12 U of cytomegalovirus-free platelets. The administration of fresh frozen plasma is beneficial when the prothrombin time is elevated. When the partial thromboplastin time is elevated, consideration should be given to administering 25 to 50 mg of protamine to treat heparin rebound. When the fibrinogen level is less than 100 mg or when the prothrombin time or partial thromboplastin times are elevated more than 1.5 times the upper limit of normal, 20 to 40 U of cryoprecipitate are administered.

Fibrinolysis is common after open heart surgery and can be monitored by measuring for the presence of D-dimers. Epsilon amino caproic acid is administered when excessive bleeding is accompanied by fibrinolysis. The loading dose is 10 g followed by 1 g per hour for 10 hours.

Gastrointestinal Considerations

No specific problems of the digestive tract are commonly observed in patients convalescing from cardiac transplantation. Ileus and constipation occur frequently and can be easily monitored with routine x-ray examination. Elevations of the serum amylase occur in some patients who do not have clinical evidence of pancreatitis and who have an uncomplicated recovery without specific therapy. Pancreatitis does occur after cardiac transplantation, however; both corticosteroids and azathioprine have been implicated as causative factors. Therapy includes decompressing the stomach, stopping the azathioprine, and limiting corticosteroids.

Peptic ulcer disease with bleeding or perforation has occurred less frequently in our experience. Although antacids may be beneficial in preventing peptic ulceration, the alteration in gastric flora precludes their use. Sucralfate (Carafate), 1 g every 12 hours, has become the standard prophylaxis for gastric ulceration.

Metabolic Considerations

The usual guidelines for maintaining serum potassium levels at 4.2 mEq/L also apply to the cardiac transplant patient. Magnesium wasting from preoperative diuretics and postoperative cyclosporine requires monitoring and replacement. Ionized calcium levels should be normalized. With the improved oxygen delivery resulting from a normalized cardiac output, the serum phosphate levels fall, a manifestation of nutritional repletion. Sodium or potassium phosphate should be administered either intravenously or orally for several days.

The effects of corticosteroids or exogenous epinephrine are hyperglycemia, even in the previously nondiabetic recipient.[40] Continuous intravenous insulin is preferable to subcutaneous or intravenous boluses of insulin.

Rejection Prophylaxis, Monitoring, and Therapy

Intravenous cyclosporine is begun after renal function has had time to recover following cardiac implantation. Usually, 24 hours are required before this can be ensured. The beginning infusion is 1.0 mg/kg given continuously intravenously over 24 hours.[41] The infusion is stopped if the urine output decreases despite diuretics and nifedipine. Blood levels are monitored daily, targeting for a level of 330 ng/ml using high-pressure liquid chromatography (HPLC) measurements. The method of determining blood levels of cyclosporine is important; the levels reported for HPLC need to be converted for techniques that use radioimmunoassay.[42] Conversion to the oral form of cyclosporine awaits the return of adequate gastrointestinal function. A rule of thumb for conversion of doses from intravenous to oral cyclosporine is 3:1; a patient requiring 2 mg/kg per day of intravenous cyclosporine to maintain a blood level of 330 ng/ml requires 6 mg/kg per day of oral cyclosporine to achieve a trough level of 250 ng/ml. Oral cyclosporine is given twice daily.

Monitoring cyclosporine levels is expensive. Plotting the area under the curve for all patients is unnecessary. Patients who rapidly absorb cyclosporine develop signs of renal toxicity despite low trough levels; monitoring hourly levels enables one to identify this subgroup. Cyclosporine should be given at shortened intervals and smaller doses in these patients.

Certain medications interfere with cyclosporine metabolism (Table 32-5). Education of the patient should begin in the ICU regarding the importance of not taking new medications without full knowledge of their interactions with cyclosporine.

Although cyclosporine produces some adverse reactions, including neurologic dysfunction,[43] renal dysfunction is the most serious (Table 32-6). Some degree of renal impairment occurs in all patients receiving cyclosporine, but the effect is most marked early, and although progression does occur, most patients can continue to take cyclosporine indefinitely.[44-46] Patients who are unable to receive cyclosporine by postoperative day 4 are given muromonab-CD3, a monoclonal antibody to the T3 antigen of the T lymphocyte. The dosage is 5 mg/kg daily IV for 14 days. Azathioprine should be withheld. Corticosteroids should be given in reduced dosage (e.g., 0.2 mg/kg), and should be given as a premedication 30 minutes before the muromonab-CD3 is given. Additional premedication with diphenhydramine (Benadryl), 25 mg, is advised. A first-dose response is seen following the initial exposure to muromonab-CD3 and is manifested by hypotension, chills, pyrexia, and dyspnea.[47] In a volume-overloaded patient, respiratory distress may ensue and may require reintubation. The first-dose response is mediated by cytokine release.

Muromonab-CD3 can elicit host antibodies, which reduces its effectiveness, especially with repeated courses of therapy. Additional complications include cytomegaloviral infections and lymphoproliferative disorders (Table 32-7).[48]

Azathioprine is given daily in a dose of 2 mg/kg. The IV route is preferred until gastrointestinal function resumes. The oral and intravenous dosages are identical. Azathioprine should be withheld when the polymorphonuclear white blood cell count is less than 3000/mm³. Daily moni-

Table 32-5. Cyclosporine Drug Interactions

Drugs that Increase Cyclosporine Levels	Drugs that Decrease Cyclosporine Levels
Bromocriptine	Carbamazepine
Danazol	Phenobarbital
Erythromycin	Phenytoin
Fluconazole	Rifampin
Ketoconazole	Sulfamethoxazole/trimethoprim
Metoclopramide	
Verapamil	

Table 32-6. Adverse Effects of Cyclosporine

Hypertension
Renal toxicity
Liver injury
Hypertrichosis
Tremors
Gingival hyperplasia
Paresthesia
Seizures
Infection
Hyperuricemia

Table 32-7. Adverse Effects of Muromonab-CD3

Infection (especially CMV)
Neoplasia
Headaches
Pulmonary edema
Fever/chills
Nausea
Vomiting
Diarrhea
Hypotension

Table 32-9. Adverse Effects of Corticosteroids

Infection
Cushingoid appearance
Fluid retention
Hunger
Diabetes mellitus
Delayed healing
Cataracts/glaucoma
Osteoporosis
Psychosis
Hypotension
Hypokalemia
Atherosclerosis

toring of the white blood cell count is useful until it has stabilized. Complications of azathioprine use are few (Table 32-8).[49]

Corticosteroids are given in the form of intravenous methylprednisolone, 125 mg every 8 hours for 3 doses then 0.3 mg/kg once daily. Conversion to oral prednisone, 0.3 mg/kg begins after gastrointestinal function has been restored. Complications are well known and protean (Table 32-9).

Rejection monitoring relies exclusively on transvenous biopsy of the right ventricular endomyocardium. The first biopsy is performed on postoperative day 5. Subsequent biopsies are performed one week later unless the first biopsy revealed rejection. In that setting, a repeat biopsy is performed 4 days later. Endomyocardial biopsies are performed with fluoroscopic control in the catheterization laboratory, generally via the right internal jugular vein. The biopsies are interpreted by special immunohistologic staining and light microscopy. A preliminary report from frozen section is available within several hours.

Complications of endomyocardial biopsy are rare.[50] Because the site of the biopsy is the septum and not the free right ventricular wall, perforation is uncommon. Coronary artery to right ventricular fistulas can occur,[51] but their natural history seems benign.

The severity of the rejection process is assessed by the pathologist.[52] The intensity of the rejection, in turn, determines the intensity of the therapy. Mild rejection requires no treatment. For accelerating rejection, the recipient receives 50 mg of methylprednisolone IV daily for 3 days. For moderate rejection, the dose is 100 mg, and for severe rejection, 200 mg. The duration of therapy is always 3 days, followed by a repeat of the biopsy. When severe rejection is accompanied by either hemodynamic instability or evidence of important polymorphonuclear myocardial infiltrate, the patient receives 250 mg of methylprednisolone every 6 hours for 12 doses. Once the 3-day course of therapy has been completed, the original dose of corticosteroid is resumed. Tapering of corticosteroids does not seem necessary.[53]

Steroid resistant rejection is defined as three episodes of severe rejection[54] treated with methylprednisolone. Therapy of steroid resistant rejection uses muromonab-CD3.[55] The administration and cautions are the same as for the use of muromonab-CD3 when cyclosporine is contraindicated. In addition to stopping the corticosteroids and azathioprine, the cyclosporine is reduced. Generally, the cyclosporine will be given continuously, keeping the level at 100 ng/ml.

During severe rejection the coronary circulation is compromised,[56] and myocardial blood flow can become inadequate. Augmented perfusion pressure is needed during this phase and an intra-aortic balloon pump may be helpful. Nitroglycerin, although not proved effective, should be considered. When the rejection process includes complement deposition,[57] heparin should be added to the regimen.

Other techniques for determining rejection have not proved useful.[58] What is required is a screening test with perfect negative accuracy. If a test existed that reliably predicted the absence of rejection, then biopsies could be performed only when the test was positive, even if its positive predictive value were limited. Although some tests have demonstrated a strong correlation with the results of endomyocardial biopsy, none have shown the negative accuracy to serve as a screening tool.

Infection Prophylaxis

Although the procedure is controversial, all cardiac transplant patients at the Cleveland Clinic Foundation receive routine ganciclovir prophylaxis for cytomegalovirus infections. The drug is begun on postoperative day 4, giving 5 mg/kg twice a day intravenously for 2 weeks, then 6 mg/kg daily Monday through Friday for 2 weeks (10 doses). Adverse reactions include azotemia and leukopenia; when these occur the drug is temporarily discontinued. Acyclovir 800 mg 4 times daily for 2 months is begun when the ganciclovir is finished.

Other prophylactic antibiotics include cefuroxime, 1.5 g IV every 12 hours for 4 days, and clotrimazole troches 4 times daily.

Table 32-8. Adverse Effects of Azathioprine

Infection
Nausea/vomiting
Pancreatitis
Liver injury
Leukopenia

Late Phase

After postoperative day 4, the patient is generally extubated, free of inotropic support, and beginning to take oral medications. Care during this interval is less intense. The patient remains in the ICU, generally because of a lack of strength. The most profoundly weak patients are those with preoperative cardiac cachexia. The main interventions during this time are directed at optimizing the cyclosporine dose and treating the hypertension that results from cyclosporine.

Hypertension

Most cardiac transplant recipients require treatment for systemic hypertension.[59-62] The origin of the hypertension is probably multifactorial and may include preoperative hypertension, postoperative volume expansion, and the hypertensive response to cyclosporine. Therapy is empiric and is not guided by measurements of renin or angiotensin II. Therapy is not markedly different than for essential hypertension.

Diuretics, generally loop diuretics, are the first drug of choice. Generally, diuretics alone are not adequate and hydralazine is added. When a third agent is needed, the angiotension-converting enzyme inhibitor enalapril seems preferable to captopril because of captopril's propensity to produce neutropenia. Enalapril can produce a troubling chronic cough, however.

POST ICU PHASE

Hospitalized Patients

Criteria for hospital discharge include a stable immunosuppressive regimen, a biopsy that on two successive occasions has shown no more than improving moderate rejection, and the patient's ability to manage both medication and activities of daily living. Continued intravenous ganciclovir may be given in the home setting with the assistance of visiting nurses.

Discharged Patients

Noncardiac Surgical Procedures

Cardiac transplant recipients seem to be at increased risk of requiring either general surgical operations, such as cholecystectomy,[63-65] or vascular procedures, such as abdominal aortic aneurysmectomy. The denervated transplanted heart tolerates such procedures adequately. No solid information exists that a "steroid prep" is necessary. The policy we have adopted is to continue corticosteroids but to ensure their delivery by giving the maintenance dose intravenously. Azathioprine is similarly given intravenously in a dose identical to maintenance. Cyclosporine is given continuously intravenously, using a 3:1 conversion from total oral daily dose to IV, attempting to achieve a blood level of 200 ng/ml measured by HPLC. All new medications, especially antibiotics, should be screened for interaction with cyclosporine.

Transfused blood should be both lymphocyte poor and screened for cytomegalovirus. Only blood that tests negative for cytomegalovirus should be used, regardless of the recipient's status concerning previous exposure to, or infection with, cytomegalovirus.

Cardiac Surgical Procedures

A similar management protocol should be followed for cardiac procedures. Although such interventions are unusual, occasionally the transplant recipient requires a second open heart procedure for myocardial revascularization, valvular heart surgery, or retransplantation. In the last situation, the immunosuppressive protocol is identical to that used for the initial cardiac transplantation. For procedures other than cardiac retransplantation, management is the same as described for noncardiac operations.

Graft Arteriosclerosis of the Transplanted Heart

Both the transplanted kidney and the transplanted heart are subject to vascular lesions. The terminology describing this process in the heart has been varied, reflecting the underlying uncertainties concerning pathology and etiology. We prefer the term "graft arteriosclerosis" of the heart in preference to "graft atherosclerosis," "allograft coronary disease," or "chronic rejection." These latter terms imply an understanding of etiology and pathology that is unproved. The incidence of this process is alarmingly high.[66] By the fourth year after cardiac transplantation, 30 to 40% of patients have demonstrable graft arteriosclerosis.

Our understanding of the pathology of graft arteriosclerosis has been derived from specimens obtained either at the time of autopsy or at the time of cardiac retransplantation. The hallmark is a diffuse process that involves the entire length of the coronary artery.[67,68] The lesions are intimal and proliferative and can be distinguished from coronary artery atherosclerosis, which can also be seen in transplanted hearts, and which was either present at the time of cardiac transplantation or develops afterward.

The etiology of graft arteriosclerosis is presumably multivariate,[69] but it seems to be related to a chronic process of rejection resulting in repeated injury to the graft,[70] presumably at the level of the endothelium. Therefore, it is not surprising that graft arteriosclerosis is more common in patients with repeated rejection episodes and possibly in those with mismatches for the HLA-DR antigen.[71,72] The occurrence of cytomegaloviral infection in the recipient has been identified as an important risk factor for developing graft arteriosclerosis.[73,74] A possible explanation for this association is again at the level of the endothelium, with viral invasion producing endothelial damage. Finally, hypercholesterolemia and obesity[75] have been identified as incremental risk factors and should be treated.[76]

Most patients with graft arteriosclerosis are asymptomatic. Although angina pectoris has been documented in transplant recipients, it is uncommon because of denervation. As with coronary atherosclerosis, patients with graft arteriosclerosis may present with a short-term occlusive event or, more commonly, with findings of global ventricular dysfunction. Stress testing has not been widely used in cardiac transplant recipients because of the policy of routine annual coronary cineangiography.

Coronary cineangiography lacks sensitivity for the diagnosis of graft arteriosclerosis[77] because the lesion is not focal but diffuse and concentric. Appreciation of the disease process relies on comparison between studies done at intervals. Loss of luminal diameter and loss of small arterial branches are the mainstays of diagnosis.

Treatment for graft arteriosclerosis remains inadequate. Direct revascularization using either percutaneous transluminal angioplasty or surgery is not generally possible for true graft arteriosclerosis because of its diffuse nature.[78] Retransplantation remains the only proven therapy and is indicated when evidence of myocardial dysfunction becomes prominent.

Malignant Disease

Non-Hodgkins lymphomas occur in the transplant recipient at a rate greatly exceeding that in the general population.[79,80] The conventional dogma is that these lymphomas represent the result of Epstein-Barr virus infection[81] resulting in a B-cell lymphoproliferative disorder beginning as a polyclonal gammopathy, which, as it progresses to a true B-cell lymphoma, assumes a mononuclear character. Risk factors include intense immunosuppression, especially with muromonab-CD3, or repeated rejection episodes. Involvement may be extranodal, especially in the brain or the gastrointestinal tract, or nodal. The diagnosis is confirmed by biopsy.

Therapy for lymphoproliferation depends on whether the process has evolved from infection to malignancy. Both stages should be treated with antiviral therapy, acyclovir or ganciclovir. Reduction of immunosuppression also seems prudent. Resectional therapy for gastrointestinal B-cell lymphoma has been successful. Radiation therapy or chemotherapy is also indicated for the malignant form of the disease. Success has been limited, however, and mortality currently approaches 100%.

The second most common malignant lesion in the cardiac transplant recipient is skin cancer, which is treated with standard therapy.

Infections

Fortunately, the incidence of infection after cardiac transplantation has decreased.[82] In the first month following transplantation, infections are virtually limited to the urinary tract, the lungs, the circulation, and the wound. The organisms responsible for these infections are the hospital pathogens that exist institutionally, and therapy is the same as with other patients.[83,84]

Between 1 and 6 months following cardiac transplantation, cytomegalovirus,[85] herpes simplex,[85] and Epstein-Barr virus constitute the major sources of infection. CMV-specific immunoglobulin, in addition to either ganciclovir or foscarnet is recommended for cytomegaloviral infection. Acyclovir is recommended for herpes simplex and Epstein-Barr viral infections.

Late infectious complications are primarily limited to the lungs, and pathogens include Pneumocystis carinii, legionella species, aspergillus, Norcardia asteroides, and mycobacteria.[86] With the exception of aspergillus infections, specific therapy is highly successful.

Toxoplasma gondii transmitted with the donor heart[87] can produce a delayed, frequently fatal, infection, including myocarditis. This diagnosis is based on endomyocardial biopsy. Therapy includes pyrimethamine and sulfadiazine and is highly successful.

REFERENCES

1. Barnard, C. N.: A human cardiac transplant: an interim report of a successful operation performed at Groote Schour Hospital, Capetown. S. Afr. Med. J., 41:1271, 1967.
2. Tzakis, A. G., et al.: Transplantation in HIV + patients. Transplantation, 49:354, 1990.
3. Schweizer, R. T., et al.: Noncompliance in organ transplant recipients. Transplantation, 49:374, 1990.
4. Hosenpud, J. D., et al.: Successful intermediate-term outcome for patients with cardiac amyloidosis undergoing heart transplantation: results of a multicenter survey. J. Heart Transplant., 9:346, 1990.
5. Ladowski, J. S., et al.: Heart transplantation in diabetic recipients. Transplantation, 49:303, 1990.
6. Defraigne, J. O., et al.: Cardiac transplantation beyond 55 years of age. Transplant. Int., 3:59, 1990.
7. Erickson, K. W., et al.: Influence of preoperative transpulmonary gradient on late mortality after orthotopic heart transplantation. J. Heart Transplant., 9:526, 1990.
8. Hosenpud, J. D., Stilbolt, T. A., Atwal, K., and Shelley, D.: Abnormal pulmonary function specifically related to congestive heart failure: comparison of patients before and after cardiac transplantation. Am. J. Med., 88:493, 1990.
9. Bussieres, L. M., et al.: Relationship between preoperative pulmonary status and outcome after heart transplantation. J. Heart Transplant., 9:124, 1990.
10. Amber, I. J., Gilbert, E. M., Schiffman, G., and Jacobson, J. A.: Increased risk of pneumococcal infections in cardiac transplant recipients. Transplantation, 49:122, 1990.
11. DiSesa, V. J., Sloss, L. J., and Cohn, L. H.: Heart transplantation for intractable prosthetic valve endocarditis. J. Heart Transplant., 9:142, 1990.
12. Merchut, M. P., Zdonczyk, D., and Gujrati, M.: Cardiac transplantation in female Emery-Dreifuss muscular dystrophy. J. Neurol., 237:316, 1990.
13. Aravot, D. J., et al.: Primary cardiac tumors—is there a place for cardiac transplantation? Eur. J. Cardiothorac. Surg., 3: 521, 1989.
14. Collins, J. A., Skidmore, M. A., Melvin, D. B., and Engel, P. J.: Home intravenous dobutamine therapy in patients awaiting heart transplantation. J. Heart Transplant., 9:205, 1990.
15. Ott, R. A., Mills, T. C., Eugene, J., and Gazzaniga, A. B.: Clinical choices for circulatory assist devices. ASAIO Trans., 36: 792, 1990.
16. Parnis, S. M., et al.: Anatomic considerations for abdominally placed permanent left ventricular assist devices. ASAIO Trans., 35:728, 1989.
17. McGee, M. G., Parnis, S. M., Nakatani, T., Myers, T., Dasse, K., Hare, W. D., Duncan, J. M., Poirier, V. L., Frazier, O. H.: Extended clinical support with an implantable left ventricular assist device. ASAIO Trans., 35:614, 1989.
18. Nakatani, T., Aida, H., Frazier, O. H., and Macris, M. P.: Effect of ABO blood type on survival heart transplant patients treated with cyclosporine. J. Heart Transplant., 8:27, 1989.
19. Hosenpud, J. D., et al.: Relation between recipient: donor body size match and hemodynamics three months after heart transplantation. J. Heart Transplant., 8:241, 1989.
20. Braun, W. E.: Laboratory and clinical management of the highly sensitized organ transplant recipient. Hum. Immunol., 26:245, 1989.
21. Mulvagh, S. L., et al.: The older cardiac transplant donor.

Relation to graft function and recipient survival longer than 6 years. Circulation, 80:III-126, 1989.
22. Alexander, J. W., and Vaughn, W. K.: The use of "marginal" donors for organ transplantation. The influence of donor age on outcome. Transplantation, 51:135, 1991.
23. Sweeney, M. S., et al.: Extension of donor criteria in cardiac transplantation: surgical risk versus supply-side economics [see comments]. Ann. Thorac. Surg., 50:7, 1990.
24. Frist, W. H., and Fanning, W. J.: Donor management and matching. Cardiol. Clin., 8:55, 1990.
25. Ghosh, S., et al.: Management of donors for heart and heart-lung transplantation. Anaesthesia, 45:672, 1990.
26. Novitzy, D., et al.: Improved cardiac allograft function following triiodothyronine therapy to both donor and recipient. Transplantation, 49:311, 1990.
27. Hendry, P. J., et al.: Are temperatures attained by donor hearts during transport too cold? J. Thorac. Cardiovasc. Surg., 98:517, 1989.
28. Darracott-Cankovic, S., et al.: Effect of donor heart damage on survival after transplantation. Eur. J. Cardiothorac. Surg., 3:525, 1989.
29. Pickering, J. G., and Boughner, D. R.: Fibrosis in the transplanted heart and its relation to donor ischemic time. Assessment with polarized light microscopy and digital image analysis. Circulation, 81:949, 1990.
30. Desruennes, M., et al.: Heterotopic heart transplantation: current status in 1988. J. Heart Transplant., 8:479, 1989.
31. Little, R. E., et al.: Arrhythmias after orthotopic cardiac transplantation. Prevalence and determinants during initial hospitalization and late follow-up. Circulation, 80:III-140, 1989.
32. Miyamoto, Y., et al.: Bradyarrhythmia after heart transplantation. Incidence, time course, and outcome. Circulation, 82(Suppl 5):IV313, 1990.
33. Midei, M. G., et al.: Is atrial activation beneficial in heart transplant recipients. J. Am. Coll. Cardiol., 16:1201, 1990.
34. Fridl, P., Horak, J., Fabian, J., and Kocandrle, V.: Right ventricle in patient after orthotopic heart transplantation. Cor Vasa, 32:206, 1990.
35. Dreyfus, G., Jebara, V. A., Couetil, J. P., and Carpentier, A.: Kinking of the pulmonary artery: a treatable cause of acute right ventricular failure after heart transplantation. J. Heart Transplant., 9:575, 1990.
36. Pascual, J. M., et al.: Prostacyclin in the management of pulmonary hypertension after heart transplantation. J. Heart Transplant., 9:644, 1990.
37. Walsh, T. R., et al.: The value of protective isolation procedures in cardiac allograft recipients. Ann. Thorac. Surg., 47:539, 1989.
38. Valantine, H. A., et al.: Increasing pericardial effusion in cardiac transplant recipients. Circulation, 79:603, 1989.
39. Andrews, B. T., et al.: Neurologic complications of cardiac transplantation. West. J. Med., 153:146, 1990.
40. Ladowski, J. S., et al.: Posttransplantation diabetes mellitus in heart transplant recipients. J. Heart Transplant., 8:181, 1989.
41. Macris, M. P., et al.: Improved immunosuppression for heart transplant patients using intravenous doses of cyclosporine. Transplantation, 47:311, 1989.
42. Zucchelli, G. C., et al.: Evaluation and comparison of radioimmunoassay methods using monoclonal or polyclonal antibodies for the assay of cyclosporine in blood samples. Int. J. Tissue React., 11:315, 1989.
43. Vazquez de Prada J. A., et al.: Cyclosporine neurotoxocity in heart transplantation. J. Heart Transplant., 9:581, 1990.
44. Bantle, J. P., et al.: Long-term effects of cyclosporine on renal function in organ transplant recipients. J. Lab. Clin. Med., 115:233, 1990.
45. Greenberg, A., et al.: Cyclcosporine nephrotoxicity in cardiac allograft patients—a seven-year follow-up. Transplantation, 50:589, 1990.
46. Stein, K. L., Ladowski, J., Kormos, R., and Armitage, J.: The cardiopulmonary response to OKT3 in orthotopic cardiac transplant recipients. Chest, 95:817, 1989.
47. Hosenpud, J. D., et al.: OKT3-induced hypotension in heart allograft recipients treated for steroid-resistant rejection. J. Heart Transplant., 8:159, 1989.
48. Swinnen, L. J., et al.: Increased incidence of lymphoproliferative disorder after immunosuppression with the monoclonal antibody OKT3 in cardiac transplant recipients [see comments]. N. Engl. J. Med., 323:1723, 1990.
49. Perini, G. P., Bonadiman, C., Fraccaroli, G. P., and Vantini, I.: Azathioprine-related cholestatic jaundice in heart transplant patients. J. Heart Transplant., 9:577, 1990.
50. Anastasiou-Nama, M. I., et al.: Relative efficiency and risk of endomyocardial biopsy: comparisons in heart transplant and nontransplant patients. Cathet. Cardiovasc. Diagn., 18:7, 1989.
51. Sutsch, G., Heywood, T., et al.: Coronary artery-right ventricular fistula in a heart transplant patient. J. Heart Transplant., 9:32, 1990.
52. Suit, P. F., et al.: Comparison of whole-blood cyclosporine levels and the frequency of endomyocardial lymphocytic infiltrates (the Quilty lesion) in cardiac transplantation. Transplantation, 48:618, 1989.
53. Wahlers, T., et al.: Treatment of rejection after heart transplantation: what dosage of pulsed steroids is necessary? J. Heart Transplant., 9:568, 1990.
54. Miller, L. W.: Treatment of cardiac allograft rejection with intravenous corticosteroids. J. Heart Transplant., 9:283, 1990.
55. O'Connell, J. B., et al.: Efficacy of OKT3 retreatment for refractory cardiac allograft rejection. Transplantation, 47:788, 1989.
56. Nitenberg, A., et al.: Recovery of a normal coronary vascular reserve after rejection therapy in acute human cardiac allograft rejection. Circulation, 81:1312, 1990.
57. Hammond, E. H., et al.: Vascular (humoral) rejection in heart transplantation: pathologic observations and clinical implications. J. Heart Transplant., 8:430, 1989.
58. Mooney, M. L., et al.: A prospective study of the clinical utility of lymphocyte monitoring in the cardiac transplant recipient. Transplantation, 50:951, 1990.
59. Shapiro, A. P., Rutan, G. H., Thompson, M. E., and Nigalye, R. L.: Hypertension following orthotopic cardiac transplantation. Cardiovasc. Clin., 20:179, 1990.
60. Olivari, M. T., Antolick, A., and Ring, W. S.: Arterial hypertension in heart transplant recipients treated with triple-drug immunosuppressive therapy. J. Heart Transplant., 8:34, 1989.
61. Scherrer, U., et al.: Cyclosporine-induced sympathetic activation and hypertension after heart transplantation [see comments]. N. Engl. J. Med., 323:693, 1990.
62. Farge, D., et al.: Effect of systemic hypertension on renal function and left ventricular hypertrophy in heart transplant recipients [see comments]. J. Am. Coll. Cardiol., 15:1095, 1990.
63. Spes, C. H., et al.: Increased incidence of cholelithiasis in heart transplant recipients receiving cyclosporine therapy. J. Heart Transplant., 9:404, 1990.
64. Parascandola, S. A., Wisman, C. B., Burg, J. E., and Davis, P. K.: Extracardiac surgical complications in heart transplant recipients. J. Heart Transplant., 8:400, 1989.
65. Kirklin, J. K., et al.: Gastrointestinal complications after car-

diac transplantation. Potential benefit of early diagnoses and prompt surgical intervention. Ann. Surg., 211:538, 1990.
66. Eich, D. M., et al.: Accelerated coronary atherosclerosis in cardiac transplantation. Cardiovasc. Clin., 20:199, 1990.
67. Kaufman, C. L., et al.: Propagation of infiltrating lymphocytes and graft coronary disease in cardiac transplant recipients. Hum. Immunol., 28:228, 1990.
68. Gao, S. Z., et al.: Progressive coronary luminal narrowing after cardiac transplantation. Circulation, 82(Suppl 5): IV269, 1990.
69. Radovancevic, B., et al.: Risk factors for development of accelerated coronary artery disease in cardiac transplant recipients. Eur. J. Cardiothorac. Surg., 4:309, 1990.
70. Schutz, A., et al.: The influence of rejection episodes on the development of coronary artery disease after heart transplantation. Eur. J. Cardiothorac. Surg., 4:300, 1990.
71. Petrossian, G. A., et al.: Relation between survival and development of coronary artery disease and anti-HLA antibodies after cardiac transplantation. Circulation, 80:III122, 1989.
72. Ratkovec, R. M., et al.: Influence of corticosteroid-free maintenance immunosuppression on allograft coronary artery disease after cardiac transplantation. J. Thorac. Cardiovasc. Surg., 100:6, 1990.
73. Grattan, M. T., et al.: Cytomegalovirus infection is associated with cardiac allograft rejection and atherosclerosis. JAMA, 261:3561, 1989.
74. Loebe, M., et al.: Role of cytomegalovirus infection in the development of coronary artery disease in the transplanted heart. J. Heart Transplant., 9:707, 1990.
75. Winters, G. L., et al.: Posttransplant obesity and hyperlipidemia: major predictors of severity of coronary arteriopathy in failed human heart allografts. J. Heart Transplant., 9:364, 1990.
76. Kobashigawa, J. A., et al.: Low-dose lovastatin safely lowers cholesterol after cardiac transplantation. Circulation, 82(Suppl. IV):IV-281, 1990.
77. Smart, F. W., et al.: Insensitivity of noninvasive tests to detect coronary artery vasculopathy after heart transplant. Am. J. Cardiol., 67:243, 1991.
78. Copeland, J. G., Butman, S. M., and Sethi, G.: Successful coronary artery bypass grafting for high-risk left main coronary artery atherosclerosis after cardiac transplantation. Ann. Thorac. Surg., 49:106, 1990.
79. Couetil, J. P., McGoldrick, J. P., Wallwork. J., and English, T. A.: Malignant tumors after heart transplantation. J. Heart Transplant., 9:622, 1990.
80. Wilkinson, A. H., et al.: Increased frequency of posttransplant lymphomas in patients treated with cyclosporine, azathioprine, and prednisone. Transplantation, 47:293, 1989.
81. Hanto, D. W., et al.: Confirmation of the heterogeneity of posttransplant Epstein-Barr virus-associated B cell proliferations by immunoglobulin gene rearrangement analyses. Transplantation, 47:458, 1989.
82. Gorensek, M. J., et al.: Decreased infections in cardiac transplant recipients on cyclosporine with reduced corticosteroid use. Cleve. Clin. J. Med., 56:690, 1989.
83. Grossi, P., et al.: Three-year experience with human cytomegalovirus infections in heart transplant recipients. J. Heart Transplant., 9:712, 1990.
84. Boland, G. J., et al.: Early detection of active cytomegalovirus (CMV) infection after heart and kidney transplantation by testing for immediate early antigenemia and influence of cellular immunity on the occurrence of CMV infection. J. Clin. Microbiol., 28:2069, 1990.
85. Goodman, J. L.: Possible transmission of herpes simplex virus by organ transplantation. Transplantation, 47:609, 1989.
86. Novick, R. J., et al.: Nontuberculous mycobacterial infections in heart transplant recipients: a seventeen-year experience. J. Heart Transplant., 9:357, 1990.

Chapter 33

ACUTE VALVULAR REGURGITATION

JOSEPH F. PIETROLUNGO
WILLIAM WITCIK
ALLAN L. KLEIN

ACUTE MITRAL REGURGITATION

Mitral regurgitation (MR) is defined as acute when the severity of the regurgitation develops at such a rate and degree that the ability of the left ventricle to adapt to the increased preload is overwhelmed. Accordingly acute pulmonary edema ensues with its attendant manifestations. MR is by far the most common problem resulting in acute mitral valvular dysfunction and subsequent hemodynamic instability. Rarely a patient with severe mitral inflow obstruction (e.g., stenosis or myxoma) may develop a sustained increase in heart rate (usually atrial fibrillation) or other intercurrent illness that increases the transmitral valvular gradient, causing severe dyspnea.[1,2] The ubiquitous availability of Doppler echocardiography, however, and heightened awareness of these diseases have for the most part eliminated presentations of this type. Acute MR remains a frequent cause of hemodynamic instability requiring admission to an ICU. After a brief discussion of chronic MR to serve as a background for contrast of these two entities, the remainder of the discussion focuses on the various aspects of acute MR, its workup, and its management.

Chronic MR is a distinctly different entity from acute MR. The slow increase in regurgitant volume, usually over many years, results in a gradual elevation in left ventricular end-diastolic volume. Eccentric left ventricular hypertrophy thus ensues as a compensatory response to the elevated left ventricular wall tension and stress imposed by the larger left ventricular end-diastolic volumes. Maintenance of effective forward stroke volume by the larger left ventricular volume that accommodates the regurgitant fraction is primarily responsible for the well-tolerated nature of this disease. Because forward stroke volume is maintained, left ventricular filling pressures and therefore left atrial and pulmonary wedge pressures remain relatively normal over a long period of time. Thus patients tend to have different and less severe symptoms than with acute MR.

Acute MR is generally not well tolerated. Onset of symptoms is rapid, and if not readily recognized and treated, MR may result in death. Prompt identification of this disease with initiation of treatment can be life-saving.

Pre-ICU Phase

The pre-ICU management of acute valvular insufficiency revolves around identifying the cause of the presenting symptom(s) (typically dyspnea and orthopnea) and initial stabilization of vital signs. Presentation varies somewhat with the underlying cause of acute MR, as discussed subsequently, but generally involves the rather sudden, severe onset of dyspnea, orthopnea, and tachypnea. Patients presenting with acute MR owing to myocardial ischemia or infarction tend to be older with risk factors for atherosclerotic coronary artery disease. They may describe symptoms consistent with angina or infarction, but the severity of dyspnea associated with these tends to be far greater than that seen with myocardial ischemia in the absence of MR. Often this occurs 2 to 7 days into the recovery period of a myocardial infarction when myocardial necrosis is at its peak.

Acute MR owing to rupture of a chordae tendineae in a patient with myxomatous valve disease usually occurs in a younger population with less co-morbid disease. The event is dramatic and sudden. Patients can usually relate exactly what they were doing at the exact time of chordal rupture and onset of dyspnea. Their overall good health provides these patients with an improved cardiac reserve; thus they tend to tolerate the hemodynamic derangement better, unless chordal rupture is extensive.

Although the pre-ICU phase of acute MR centers primarily on a search for the underlying cause, initial (and at times empiric) treatment measures are important because these patients tend to be quite ill. Therapy starts with maintaining airway support and providing adequate arterial oxygenation in an organized, escalating fashion. Circulatory support centers on the maintenance of adequate blood pressure by medical and if necessary mechanical means. Once the patient is stable, a thorough, organized search for the cause may ensue.

Cause

Acute MR may result from damage to any part of the mitral valve apparatus. This includes the left atrium, annulus, leaflets, chordae tendineae, papillary muscle, and adjacent left ventricular wall. The integrity as well as the spatial relationship of these structures must remain intact for normal valvular function. One approach to understanding the various causes of acute MR is to categorize them with respect to the diseased mitral valvular anatomy (Table 33-1).

Mitral Valve Leaflets. The incidence of rheumatic heart disease as a cause of acute MR remains largely un-

Table 33–1. Common Causes of Acute Mitral Regurgitation

Disorders of the Mitral Valve Leaflet
    Infective endocarditis
    Postmitral valvuloplasty
    Penetrating and nonpenetrating trauma
    HLA-B_{27} disorders (anklyosing spondylitis)
    Myxomatous degeneration
Disorders of the Mitral Annulus
    Connective tissue diseases
Disorders of the Chordae Tendineae
    Rupture with or without underlying myxomatous degeneration of the valve
    Infective endocarditis
    Trauma
    Connective tissue diseases
    Pregnancy
Disorders of the Papillary Muscles
    Coronary artery disease
        Ischemia of the papillary muscle and ventricular wall
        Infarction and rupture of part or all of the papillary muscle
    Other
        Infective endocarditis and myocardial abscess formation
        Left ventricular dilatation
        Trauma
        Infiltrative cardiomyopathies (amyloidosis, sarcoidosis)
Prosthetic valve dysfunction
    Infective endocarditis
    Dehiscence and strut fracture
    Rupture of a bioprosthetic valve
    Failure or tearing of the leaflet structures

(Modified from Harrington, R. A., and Rippe, J. M.: Acute mitral regurgitation. In Intensive Care Medicine. Edited by J. M. Rippe, et al. Boston, Little, Brown & Company, 1991.)

known, and reports in the literature vary with respect to frequency of occurrence.[3,4] Chronic MR caused by this entity is certainly much more common. When acute MR occurs owing to rheumatic heart disease, it is usually in the setting of acute rheumatic fever or infective endocarditis. In rheumatic fever, a combination of prolapse of the anterior leaflet, elongation of the chordae, and dilatation of the annulus results in regurgitation.[5] Endocarditis, which is much more common, may affect any aspect of the mitral valvular apparatus but is usually associated with inflammation-induced damage to the leaflets or chordae tendineae rupture.[6] Perforation of the leaflets may occur as a result of the infectious process. In patients with aortic insufficiency, repetitive impact of the jet on the anterior mitral leaflet may cause perforation and severe MR. Additionally vegetations may interfere with leaflet coaptation and cause regurgitation.[7] Mitral valve prolapse owing to myxomatous degeneration is a common cause of mitral regurgitation[8] (Fig. 33-1). Abnormalities in the leaflets may occur, but chordae abnormalities and annular deformation account for most of the pathology in this lesion. Rheumatic diseases, such as systemic lupus erythematosus[9] and ankylosing spondylitis,[10] may cause severe fibrosis and scarring of the leaflets precipitating acute MR. Left atrial myxoma[11] may interrupt normal leaflet mobility, and tearing of the leaflets has been reported after mitral valvuloplasty.[12] Penetrating and non-penetrating[13] trauma to the chest is another cause of valve leaflet dysfunction and subsequent MR (Fig. 33-2).

Chordae Tendineae. Chordal rupture is an important and frequent cause of acute MR. It may be spontaneous

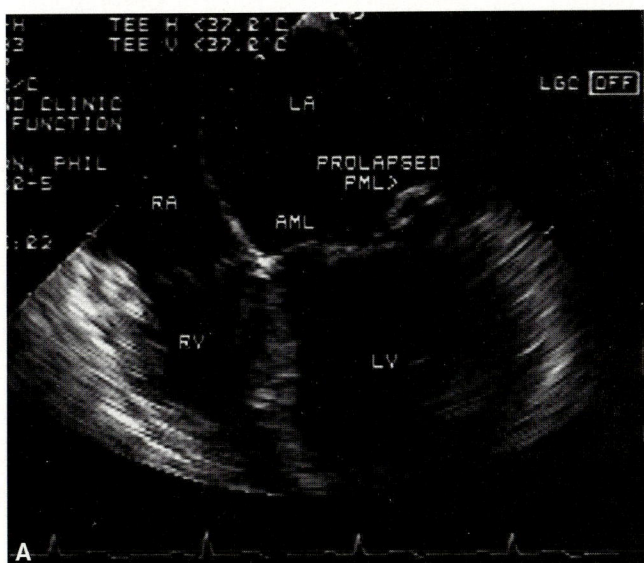 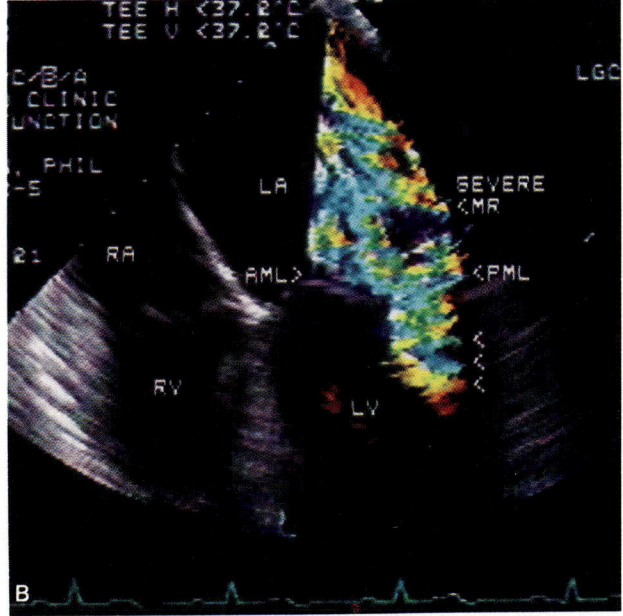

Fig. 33–1. *A*, Transesophageal echocardiogram in the transverse, four-chamber view of a myxomatous mitral valve with severe posterior leaflet prolapse. *B*, Color flow mapping of same image demonstrating severe mitral regurgitation directed anteriorly. Arrowheads depict pre-acceleration (flow convergence) on the ventricular side of the valve, further suggesting the presence of severe mitral regurgitation (see section on echocardiography for description). MR, Mitral regurgitation; RA, right atrium; LA, left atrium; RV, right ventricle; LV, left ventricle; AML, anterior mitral leaflet; PML, posterior mitral leaflet.

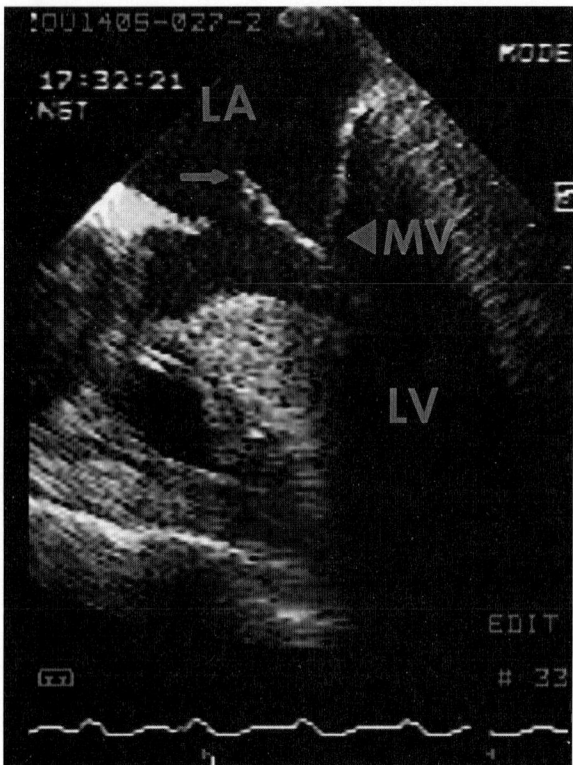

Fig. 33–2. Transesophageal echocardiogram in the transverse, four-chamber view of a patient with severe acute mitral regurgitation owing to a deceleration chest injury sustained in a motor vehicle accident. Traumatic rupture of the base of the anterior mitral valve leaflet is denoted by the arrow. LA, Left atrium; LV, left ventricle; MV, coaptation point for the leaflets of the mitral valve. (Courtesy of Dr. Gerald Cohen.)

and is usually associated with some underlying cardiac abnormality.[14] Frequently this abnormality is myxomatous degeneration with or without associated mitral valve prolapse[15] (Fig. 33–3). It commonly occurs as a consequence of infective endocarditis,[16] Marfan syndrome,[17] and trauma.[18] There have also been rare reports of its association with rheumatic fever,[19] systemic lupus erythematosus,[10] and pregnancy.[20] Recently Wei-Xi et al.[21] reported five patients with hypertrophic obstructive cardiomyopathy and acute MR owing to rupture of the chordae tendineae. The posterior leaflet was found to be more frequently involved presumably as a result of its perpendicular position relative to systolic flow and thus greater shear stress.[21] Given the relative prevalence of this disease, a heightened awareness of the potential for ruptures may help characterize more accurately the pathophysiologic process responsible for the MR frequently associated with this entity.

Papillary Muscles. Ischemia predominates as the major cause of papillary muscle dysfunction and consequently acute MR. These structures are particularly vulnerable to diminished blood flow because they are subserved by the distal branches of the coronary arteries. The posteromedial papillary muscle usually has a single blood supply originating from the posterior descending branch of the dominant coronary artery (usually right coronary artery), and thus it is more prone to ischemia. The anterolateral papillary muscle has the advantage of a dual circulation emanating from the left anterior descending and circumflex arteries. The enriched circulation serves to insulate this papillary muscle from ischemic dysfunction.[22]

Ischemia may be transient or prolonged resulting in variable degrees of papillary muscle dysfunction and MR. Transient dysfunction may result in acute MR during periods of angina or silent ischemia. At times this may be severe enough to promote hemodynamic embarrassment.[23]

Papillary muscle infarction is a consequence of prolonged ischemia. When this occurs, chronic MR is often the result. Infarction of the head(s) of the papillary muscle may result in partial or complete rupture. Rupture of one of the heads of the papillary muscle may be hemodynamically tolerated for a short period usually dependent on intensive medical management. Complete rupture of the main muscle trunk, however, is associated with torrential MR and usually results in rapid circulatory collapse.[24,25]

In addition to ischemia, numerous other causes of papillary muscle dysfunction resulting in acute MR have been reported albeit less frequently. These include left ventricular dilatation owing to cardiomyopathy or left ventricular aneurysm formation, infiltrative diseases of the myocardium (e.g., amyloidosis, sarcoidosis, granulomatous diseases), and trauma.[26-28]

Prosthetic Valve Dysfunction. Failure of a mitral valve prosthesis is an important cause of acute MR and should be readily considered in patients presenting with acute pulmonary edema and an antecedent history of mitral valve surgery. Table 33-1 lists many of the problems seen with prosthetic mitral valves. Two are of particular importance and account for a significant proportion of the associated morbidity and mortality.

Endocarditis is one of the most serious and common complications. An overall incidence of 2 to 4% is reported at most centers.[29] Endocarditis is characterized as early (less than 60 days from valve implantation) and late (more than 60 days from valve implantation).[30] Staphylococcus (particularly S. epidermidis) is the commonest organism found in the early group and is isolated in more than 30% of the late infections as well. Streptococcus viridans accounts for 30% of the late infections and is the commonest pathogen in this group.[31,32] Acute MR may result from destruction of one or more components of the valve apparatus. Large vegetations may disrupt normal coaptation and result in severe MR.

Valvular degeneration is commonly seen with previously replaced mitral valves. Although largely a cause of chronic MR, acute presentations do occur. Bioprostheses develop cusp tears, perforation, and flail or immobile as a consequence of wear and tear. These valves typically exhibit regurgitation, which is valvular in nature, that is, within the sewing ring. Frequently there are calcium deposits, thrombi, and fibrosis adherent to the valve structure. Mechanical valves may fail acutely as well. Although they are more resilient than their bioprosthetic counterparts, degeneration of the metallo-tissue interface may occur over time and produce regurgitant lesions that are perivalvular in location (Fig. 33–4). Silastic discs may lodge

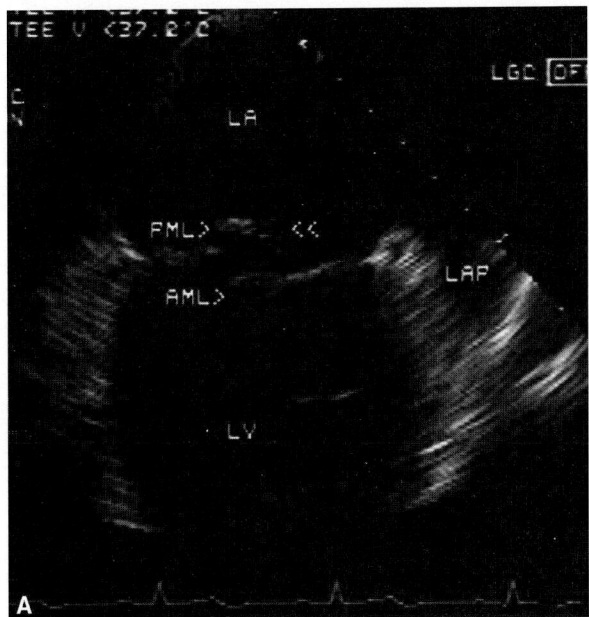 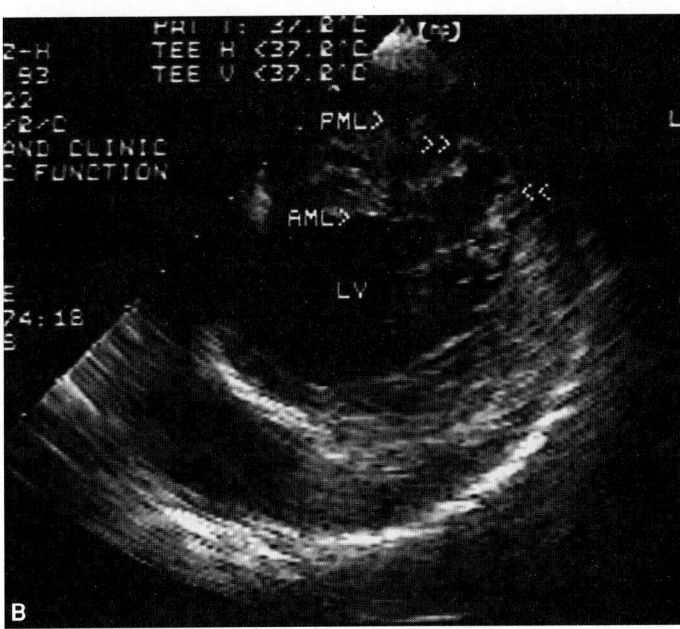

Fig. 33-3. *A*, Transesophageal echocardiogram in the transverse, two-chamber view of a patient with mitral valve prolapse owing to myxomatous degeneration. Flail chordae tendineae are delineated by arrowheads. Severe mitral regurgitation was present. *B*, Transesophageal echocardiogram of same patient in the transverse short axis view of the mitral valve. Arrowheads denote severe prolapse of the posterior mitral leaflet. Flail chordal structures are also seen. PML, Posterior mitral leaflet; AML, anterior mitral leaflet; LV, left ventricle; LA, left atrium; LAP, left atrial appendage. (Courtesy of Dr. Gerald Cohen.)

in the open position or fracture and embolize.[33,34] Reports of strut fracture with the Bjork-Shiley valve have noted.[35] Given the popularity and wide use of this valve, screening for this problem has begun.

Pathophysiology

The clinical sequelae that follow the development of acute MR are due to rapid emptying of left ventricle regurgitant stroke volume into the low resistance, low afterload left atrium. The amount of retrograde flow is proportional to the size of the regurgitant orifice and the pressure gradient between the two chambers. Almost 50% of the left ventricular volume may regurgitate into the left atrium before aortic valve opening.[36] Factors affecting the regurgitant volume are dynamic. Therefore any increase in venous return (preload), resistance to left ventricular emptying (afterload), or size of the regurgitant orifice (left ventricular dilation) results in an increased regurgitant fraction. In patients with acute MR and a noncalcified malleable valvular apparatus, interventions that reduce the cross-sectional area of the mitral annulus generally result in a reduced regurgitant fraction. Thus in these patients, treatment with positive inotropic agents, diuretics, and vasodilators enhance forward cardiac output and improve symptoms.[37,38]

In acute MR, the left ventricular end-diastolic volume is increased and end-systolic volume decreased. The regurgitant fraction that is discharged into the left atrium, together with the pulmonary venous return, is delivered to the left ventricle during the next diastolic interval and is added to the remaining end-systolic volume. This results in increased left ventricular preload. Left ventricular stroke volume is increased owing to the mechanism of Frank-Starling and serves to help maintain an effective forward stroke volume despite the MR. Fortunately myocardial oxygen demand is not significantly elevated with acute MR. The increased velocity of myocardial fiber shortening that results is not as important a determinant of myocardial oxygen demand as are heart rate, contractility, and wall tension, which are less affected.[39] A lower late ventricular systolic pressure and radius result in reduced wall tension. In contrast to chronic MR, however, the pericardium in these patients is tight and noncompliant. The left ventricle operates on the steep portion of the pressure-volume curve, and as such, a sudden increase in left ventricular volume results in a marked rise in left ventricular end-diastolic pressure. The sudden increase in left ventricular volume within a restricting pericardium closely simulates the diastolic filling abnormalities seen in constrictive pericarditis.[40] If the ventricle is unable to expand and accommodate this increased load, stroke volume eventually falls. As MR persists and left ventricular end-diastolic volumes continue to rise, forward cardiac output declines.

The hemodynamic and clinical findings associated with acute MR largely depend on left atrial compliance. Acute MR usually occurs in the setting of normal or reduced atrial compliance. The chamber size remains virtually unchanged, but transmission of the markedly increased left atrial pressure (reflected primarily as a large V wave) back through the pulmonary circuit results in an increased impedance to right ventricular emptying. Pulmonary hypertension and subsequently pulmonary edema often result.[41,42] In addition, right ventricular failure may ensue. This is seen in cases of acute MR due to ruptured chordae tendineae from any cause, papillary muscle dysfunction

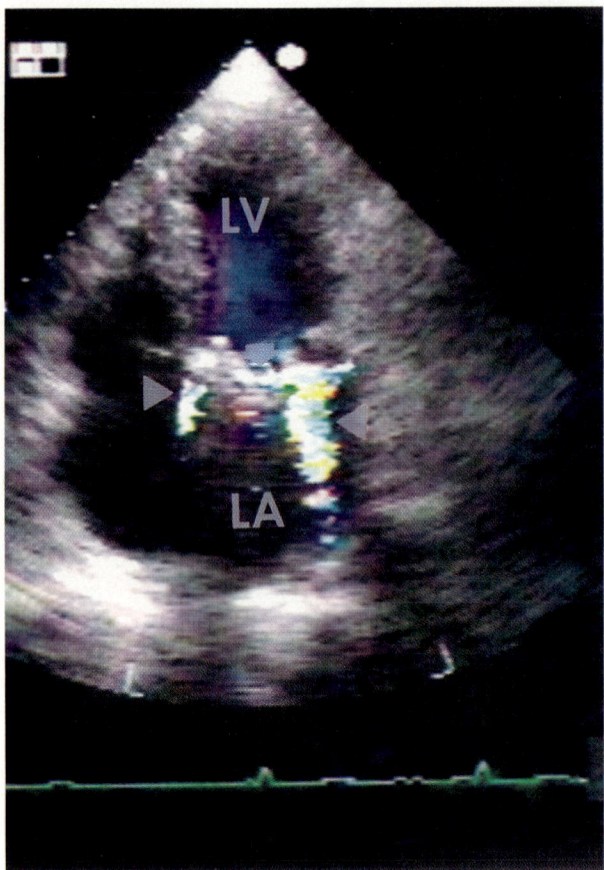

Fig. 33–4. Transthoracic echocardiogram in the apical, four-chamber view of a patient with deterioration of mechanical valve resulting in mitral regurgitation. The arrowheads depict two separate jets of perivalvular mitral regurgitation typical of mechanical valve failure. LA, Left atrium; LV, left ventricle.

due to ischemia or infarction, and mitral leaflet disruption usually due to endocarditis.[43]

MR associated with acute myocardial infarction is a well-recognized phenomenon. The pathogenesis, however, remains incompletely understood.[44] Severe MR owing to papillary muscle infarction and rupture is a well-recognized entity,[45] but there have been several mechanisms proposed to explain the production of MR owing to papillary muscle dysfunction. The first describes an ischemia-induced decreased systolic shortening of the papillary muscle resulting in inadequate tethering of the chordae tendineae. Elongation of the papillary muscle as a result of this causes leaflet prolapse into the left atrium during ventricular contraction.[46] Support for this hypothesis has been put forth in both clinical[47] and experimental studies.[48,49] A second mechanism proposes that infarction of the left ventricular wall near the base of the papillary muscle creates a localized dyssynergy resulting in incomplete closure of the mitral leaflets.[50] Hypokinesia and scarring of the ventricular segment overlying the papillary muscle leads to retraction of the mitral leaflets toward the apex, resulting in insufficient leaflet coaptation.[51] This theory as well has been supported by both experimental[52] and clinical observations.[53,54]

Clincal Characteristics

Presentation. The clinical manifestations of acute MR depend on the underlying cause, degree of regurgitation, and overall left ventricular function. The most prominent symptoms are usually respiratory and due to the sudden increase in left atrial and pulmonary artery pressure. Patients may complain of varying degrees of dyspnea ranging in severity from mild discomfort to frank respiratory failure requiring intubation for severe pulmonary edema.[55] Right ventricular failure owing to abrupt elevation of pulmonary artery pressures may be present. In these cases, increased jugular venous pressure, hepatomegaly, and peripheral edema may be seen. Symptoms related to the underlying illness should be sought as clues to the diagnosis. Although acute MR owing to ruptured chordae tendineae frequently occurs in patients with myxomatous degeneration, physical evidence of connective tissue abnormalities may not be present. When they are obvious, as in Marfan or Ehlers-Danlos syndrome, suspicion for acute MR should remain high. Those presenting with a history of the mitral valve prolapse syndrome are at increased risk and require a heightened awareness of the disease as well.[56] Endocarditis is a frequent cause of acute MR owing to multiple mechanisms as previously noted. Fevere, splenomegaly, and peripheral embolic manifestations may suggest the diagnosis, particularly in the setting of a prosthetic mitral valve, but are frequently absent.[57] Recent antecedent chest trauma, either blunt or penetrating, is an obvious cause. The former occurs owing to a sudden deceleration producing shear on the intrathoracic structures. The latter is often associated with other cardiovascular injuries, such as hemopericardium and pericardial tamponade.[58]

Patients with MR in the setting of myocardial ischemia or infarction constitute an important category. With ischemia, acute MR is usually episodic and due to transient papillary muscle dysfunction. Patients may describe severe dyspnea during their anginal episodes that resolves either partially or completely as the chest pain abates.[59] When acute MR occurs with infarction, the clinical sequelae depend on the extent of myocardial necrosis and papillary muscle damage. Partial rupture of one of the papillary muscle heads often produces severe but hemodynamically tolerated MR if the left ventricular function remains adequate. The infarcts in these patients tend not to involve large amounts of myocardium owing to a predominance of single-vessel or double-vessel coronary artery disease.[60] A small but strategically placed infarct, however, may produce partial or complete rupture of a papillary muscle; the latter is associated with torrential MR and the development of overwhelming pulmonary edema and cardiogenic shock. This usually occurs 2 to 7 days after an acute myocardial infarction and is associated with a poor prognosis. Eighty-three percent die within the first 24 hours, and 80% of the remaining patients die within 2 weeks.[61]

Physical Examination. Table 33–2 lists some of the more common physical findings that may be associated with acute MR. Patients may be hemodynamically stable and able to give a clear history or may present in cardiogenic shock and require intubation. On palpation, the cardiac impulse is accentuated and may be slightly displaced

Table 33–2. Physical Findings in Acute Mitral Regurgitation

Evidence of Underlying Disorder
    Abnormal body habitus suggestive of connective tissue disorder
        Marfan syndrome
        Ehlers-Danlos syndrome
    Systemic manifestations of endovascular infection
        Fever
        Peripheral stigmata of endocarditis (Roth's spots, Osler's nodes, Janeway lesions, petechiae)
        Splenomegaly
    Evidence of penetrating or nonpenetrating chest trauma
    Evidence of previous valve surgery (median sternotomy scar)
Cardiovascular Findings
    Palpation
        PMI vigorous and displaced slightly to the left
        Palpable S_4 may be present
        Thrill
    Auscultation
        P_2 delayed and increased in intensity
        S_1 decreased or completely masked by the murmur
        S_3 may be present. Right-sided S_3 may be present if RV failure prominent
        S_4 usually present. Right-sided S_4 may be present if RV failure prominent
        Holosystolic regurgitant murmur. May radiate widely and mimic aortic stenosis. Usually loud but may be inaudible
        Short early diastolic murmur may be present owing to large volume of blood returned in diastole
    Carotid upstrokes
        Sharp, brief, and small volume
    Jugular vein
        Elevated, especially with RV failure
        Prominent A wave and CV wave if tricuspid regurgitation present

PMI, Point of maximal impulse; RV, right ventricular.

to the left.[62] There is often a palpable early filling wave at the apex. Auscultatory findings differ significantly from chronic MR. S_1 is normal unless associated with a separate problem (e.g., prosthetic valve). S_2 may be widely split owing to early closure of the aortic valve. P_2 is increased in intensity owing to the frequent presence of severe pulmonary hypertension and may be delayed. An S_3 and S_4 are frequently audible. Although a systolic murmur is usually present with both acute and chronic MR, the qualitative aspects of each differ significantly. Acute MR is accompanied by an early systolic murmur or a holosystolic murmur that is decrescendo, diminishing if not ending before the second heart sound. The physiologic mechanism responsible for this early systolic decrescendo murmur is regurgitation into a normal-sized nondistensible left atrium. A steep rise in left atrial V wave approaches left ventricular pressure at end diastole. A late systolic decline in left ventricular pressure predisposes to this phenomenon.[63] The murmur also tends to be lower in pitch and softer than that of chronic MR. The pattern of radiation depends on which leaflet is dysfunctional. The posterior leaflet is more commonly involved and produces an anteriorly directed jet. This has impact on the atrial septum and aortic root producing a murmur that is loudest at the left sternal border radiating to the aortic space and carotids, at times causing confusion with murmur of aortic stenosis.[64] Involvement of the anterior leaflet generates a posteriorly directed jet that strikes the posterior wall. This murmur is transmitted through the vertebral column and is heard in a wide variety of places, including the axilla, back, and top of the head.[65] In the presence of right ventricular decompensation, the murmurs of tricuspid and pulmonary insufficiency may be heard. It is important to realize that when due to ischemia, the murmur of severe MR may be atypical in character[66] and not readily appreciated. This is commonly the case with papillary muscle rupture[67] and has been confirmed in a cohort study of the Thrombolysis in Acute Myocardial Infarction (TIMI) population. These investigators found that 50% of patients with moderately severe to severe MR admitted within 7 hours of an acute myocardial infarction had a physical examination that did not point to the presence of MR.[68] Moreover, if the pitch is high as with prosthetic valve dysfunction, the regurgitant orifice large, or left ventricular function impaired, the murmur may be quite soft or inaudible.

Laboratory Evaluation

Electrocardiography. In acute MR, the electrocardiogram may contribute valuable information and aid in establishing the diagnosis (Table 33–3). Sinus tachycardia may be present but is nonspecific. Occasionally a right ventricular strain pattern is seen owing to sudden and severe right ventricular pressure overload. Evidence of acute or resolving myocardial infarction or ischemia may be present and is of particular help, providing a clue to the underlying problem.

Radiologic Studies. The chest film in acute MR usually reveals a normal or mildly dilated cardiac silhouette in the presence of interstitial or alveolar edema[69] when no preexisting cardiac disease is present. Together with the aforementioned findings, the presence of a mechanical valve in the mitral position should enhance one's suspicion for the presence of acute MR.

Echocardiography. Transthoracic (TTE) and transesophageal (TEE) Doppler echocardiography with color flow mapping is by far the most useful noninvasive modality available for the quantification and evaluation of acute MR. In the acute setting, the use of both techniques applied in a logical sequence may be required to make the correct diagnosis. TTE should be one of the first studies obtained because this modality is readily available and is usually able accurately to semiquantitate the amount of regurgitation, evaluate cardiac chamber size and function, and gain important insight into the underlying cause. TEE may be needed, however, if images are suboptimal for the many technical reasons discussed next.

Doppler echocardiography has been useful in the noninvasive assessment of the hemodynamics of MR, including estimation of mean left atrial pressure, dp/dt, and the time constant of relaxation.[69a,69b]

The ability to discriminate between acute MR and ventricular septal defect in the setting of myocardial ischemia and infarction is of primary importance. Hemodynamic measurements may be imprecise and require the placement of catheters, which may delay the diagnosis. Rapid transthoracic imaging can usually descriminate between these two entities reliably with little delay.

Flail mitral valve leaflet owing to a ruptured chordae

Table 33-3. Laboratory Findings in Acute Mitral Regurgitation

Electrocardiography
   Sinus tachycardia
   Nonspecific ST-T wave changes
   Left atrial abnormality
   Myocardial ischemia or injury pattern (usually inferior and/or posterior distribution)
Radiography
   Normal or slightly enlarged cardiac silhouette
   Pulmonary venous hypertension (interstitial or alveolar pulmonary edema)
   Prosthetic mitral valve
Echocardiography
   Hemodynamics
      Right atrial pressure (IVC diameter)
      Right ventricular systolic pressure
      Pulmonary artery diastolic pressure
      Left atrial pressure
      dp/dt as a measure of LV contractility
   Native valve disease. TEE more thoroughly evaluates valvular and subvalvular apparatus
      Flail leaflet
      Ruptured chordae
      Vegetation(s)
      Myxomatous valvular degeneration
      Segmental wall motion abnormalities due to myocardial ischemia or infarction
      Color and/or Doppler evidence of MR
   Prosthetic mitral valve (TEE imaging better than surface echo due to lack of shielding)
      Dehiscence
      Valve leaflet failure
      Ruptured bioprosthetic valve
      Vegetation(s), ring abscess
      Color and/or Doppler evidence of MR
   Newer Techniques
      Regurgitant Fraction by quantitative Doppler
      Effective regurgitant orifice area
      Left atrial appendage evaluated for thrombus. TEE only
Cardiac Catheterization
   Hemodynamics (right heart)
      Giant C-V waves in pulmonary wedge position
      Pulmonary hypertension
      No oxygen saturation step-up
      Evidence of right heart failure may be present
   Left heart catheterization and angiography
      Angiographic assessment of MR
      Assessment of left ventricular function
      Degree of associated coronary artery disease
      Identification of cardiac anomalies (MVP, anomalous coronary arteries)

MR, mitral regurgitation; LVOT, left ventricular outflow tract; VSD, ventriculoseptal defect; TEE, Transesophageal echocardiography; MVP, mitral valve prolapse.
(Modified from Harrington, R. A., Rippe, M. J.: Acute mitral regurgitation. *In* Intensive Care Medicine. 2nd Ed. Edited by J. M. Rippe, et al. Boston, Little, Brown & Company, 1991.)

---

may well be seen with its characteristic high frequency motion and associated findings, such as leaflet thickening from myxomatous degeneration and prolapse[70] (see Figs. 33-1 and 33-2). Evidence of papillary muscle dysfunction with resultant MR owing to myocardial ischemia or infarction can be obtained by using several echocardiographic modalities. M-mode measurements may be used to assess the wall motion of corresponding myocardial segments. Doppler and color flow images readily identify the presence of MR. Doppler echocardiography and color flow imaging also provide an excellent modality for the determination of the mechanism of MR.[71] With flail or prolapsed leaflets, regurgitant jet orientation (as depicted by color flow mapping) is opposite in direction to the involved leaflet. Thus anterior leaflet prolapse produces a posteriorly directed jet and vice versa (Fig. 33-5). Symmetric disease of both leaflets may result in a centrally directed jet. When rheumatic fibrosis predominates, however, the relatively normal anterior leaflet more often fails to coapt with the fibrosed immobile posterior leaflet resulting in a posteriorly directed jet. Thus in restricted leaflet motion and asymmetric involvement, the jet is directed toward the affected leaflet. The ability to classify the mechanism of mitral regurgitation accurately by echocardiography is useful for both immediate medical and eventual surgical therapy.

Morphologic confirmation of the presence of infective endocarditis can often be obtained using echocardiography. When the study is technically optimal, vegetations as small as 2 to 3 mm may be visualized.[72] Currently, vegetations can be documented by TTE in more than 50% of patients with endocarditis and in some studies as high as 80%.[73]

Prosthetic mitral valve dysfunction in the past has limited the accurate assessment of MR by transthoracic echocardiography owing to shielding from the prosthesis. Using TTE, however, the visualization of preacceleration on the ventricular side of the mitral valve during systole is suggestive of significant MR despite the lack of visualization owing to acoustic shadowing.[74] With the advent of transesophageal imaging probes, clear, accurate information regarding prosthetic mitral valve morphology and function can be readily obtained when TTE is nondiagnostic.[75] In addition, this new modality gives much more detailed information on the various components of the mitral valvular apparatus and should be readily used to aid in the decision-making process, particularly when surface images are suboptimal.[76]

Florid, severe MR is generally easily identified with Doppler echocardiography. At times, however, differentiation of moderate from severe MR may be difficult if shielding or unfavorable body habitus is present. In these situations, TEE is useful. Furthermore, the onset of acute MR is generally accompanied by severe pulmonary edema, which degrades the image quality of TTE. TEE circumvents this problem and produces superior images. In these patients, not only are the images superior to surface echo, but also evaluation of the pulmonary venous flows provides further insight into the severity of MR. A decreased systolic-to-diastolic flow ratio and reversed systolic flow reflect the increasing amplitude of the v wave and the decreasing left atrial pressure a/v ratio seen on the pulmonary wedge or left atrial pressure tracing in patients with severe MR[77] (Fig. 33-6). Recent work has attempted to quantify the degree of MR using the methods of proximal flow convergence and quantitative Doppler.[77]

Cine Magnetic Resonance Imaging. A relatively new technique, cine magnetic resonance imaging (MRI) with ultrafast imaging is based on changing signal characteristics associated with blood flow. Cine MRI is capable of

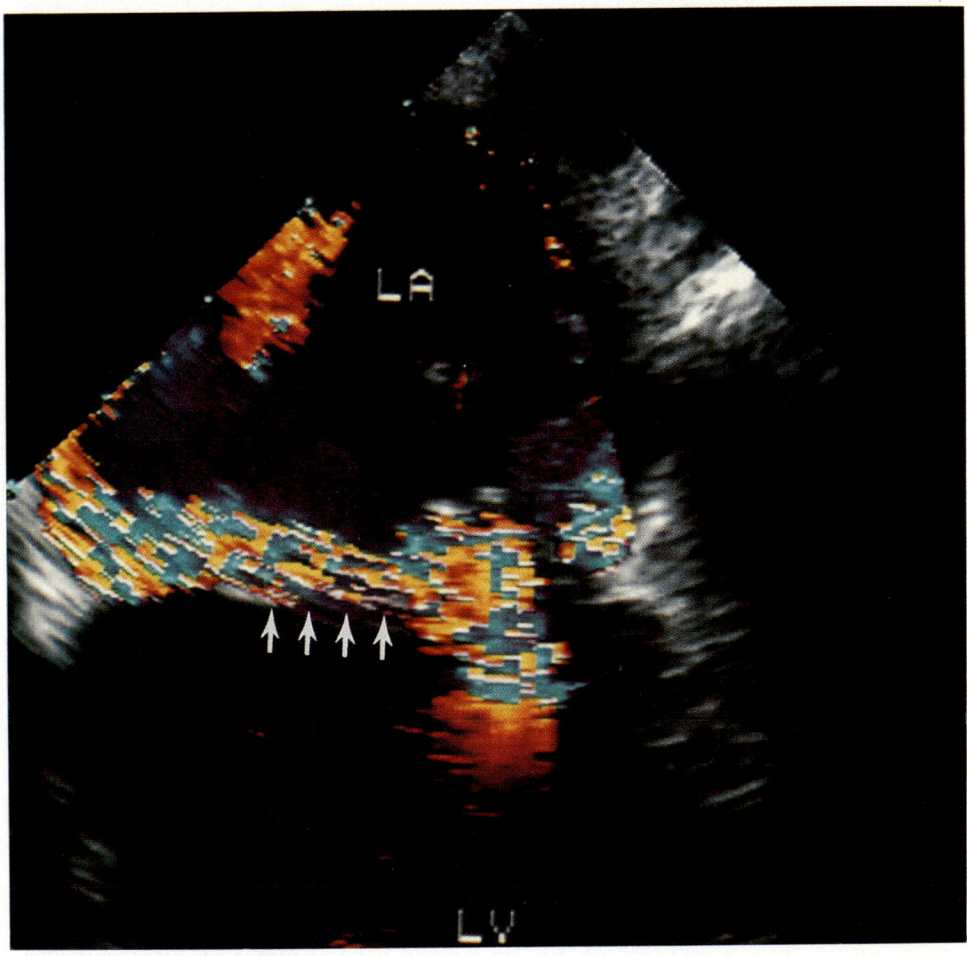

Fig. 33–5. Transesophageal echocardiogram in the transverse view demonstrating eccentric, anteriorly directed jet of mitral regurgitation (arrows) owing to posterior mitral leaflet prolapse. LA, Left atrium; LV, left ventricle.

demonstrating the regurgitant jet as signal dropout, which correlates well with the regurgitation seen with color Doppler echocardiography and angiography.[78,79] The high velocity, turbulent retrograde flow through the incompetent mitral valve is represented by a signal void jet proximal to the closed valve within the otherwise signal enhanced recipient chamber.[80] Based on detection of a jet, MR is identified with a high degree of sensitivity and specificity, with all cases of significant MR having been detected.[81] The limitations of this modality relate to the logistic aspects of the care and transport of severely symptomatic, often unstable patients to the MRI suite.

Cardiac Catheterization. Although much of the important information regarding diagnosis and cause may be readily obtained through the use of echocardiography as previously noted, information obtained at cardiac catheterization may make an important contribution as well as provide continuous hemodynamic measurements used to gauge the effects of treatment. At present, no other modality is capable of visualizing the coronary anatomy in detail, which is indispensable when acute MR accompanies myocardial ischemia or infarction.

Hemodynamics. Doppler echocardiographic assessment of hemodynamics has supplanted hemodynamic assessment by cardiac catheterization.[69b] However, right heart catheterization can usually be performed safely and easily from the bedside using a balloon-tipped, flow-directed catheter. Occasionally severe pulmonary hypertension prohibits easy advancement to the pulmonary artery, and fluoroscopic support is needed. Pulmonary artery and wedge pressures are markedly elevated. There is usually a large systolic regurgitant v wave present on the pulmonary wedge tracing. Although large v waves may be seen in patients with mitral stenosis, ventricular septal defects, mitral prosthesis, and impaired left ventricular function, its present is suggestive of acute MR.[82] Occasionally a systolic left atrial pressure wave is reflected back through the pulmonary capillary circuit to the pulmonary artery and is seen as a large systolic wave located after the dicrotic notch on the pulmonary artery pressure recording. On these tracings, peak pulmonary artery pressures are greater than right ventricular pressures, but this peak occurs in diastole serving as a clue to the mechanism.[43] Pulmonary artery systolic and right ventricular systolic pressures remain equal. This finding is unique to acute MR. The left ventricular end-diastolic pressure is elevated occasionally with a dip and plateau configuration (due to acute volume

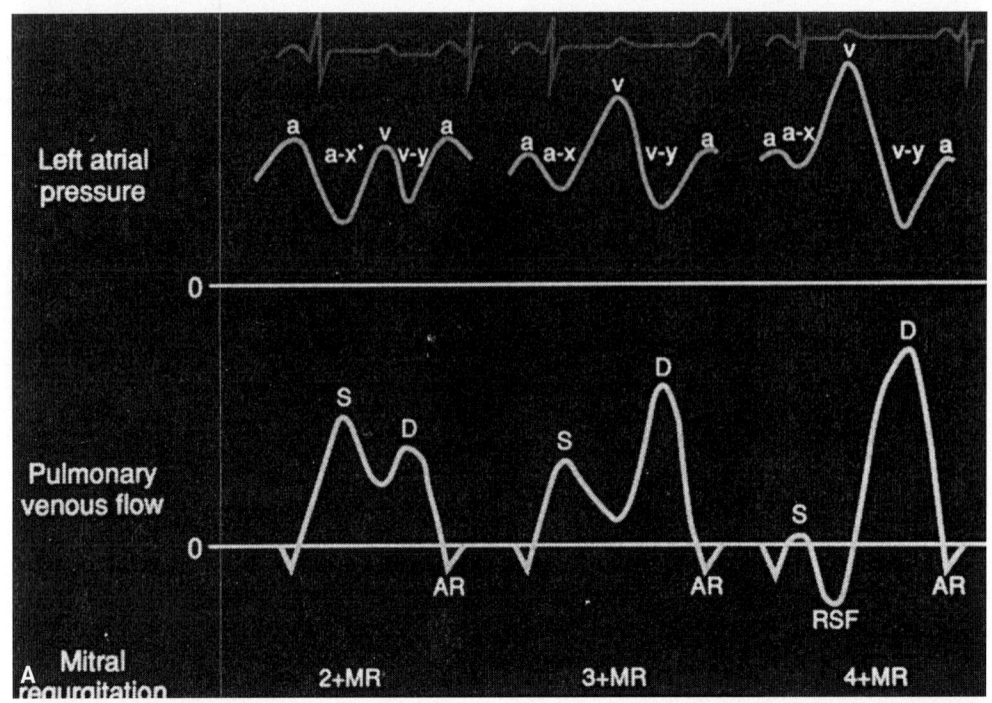
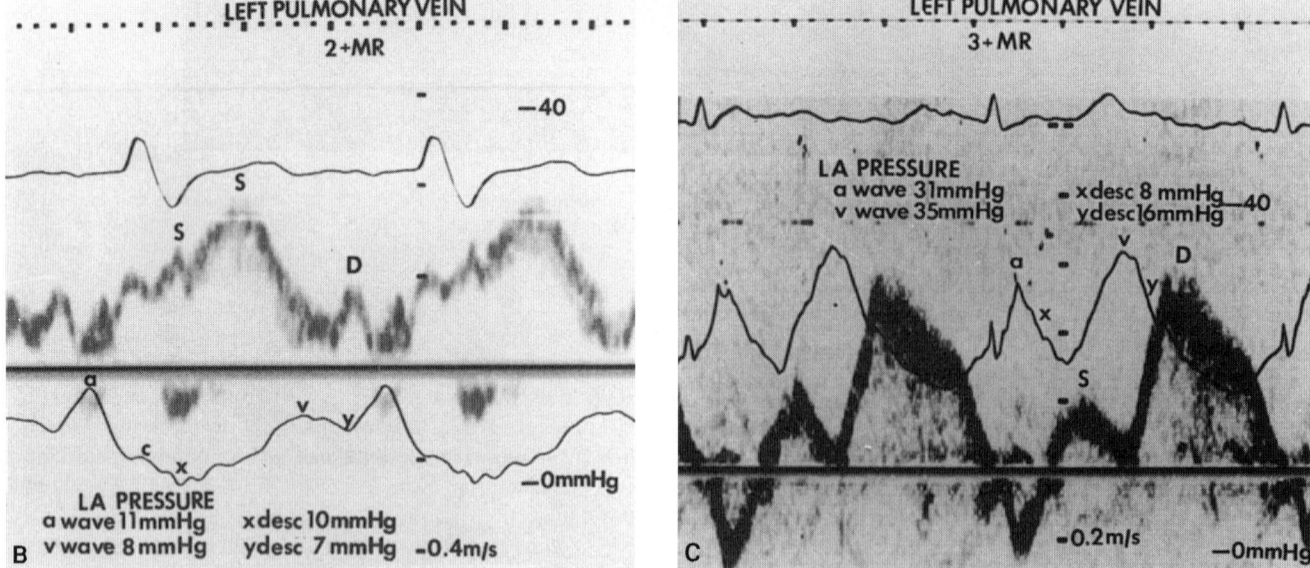

Fig. 33-6. Pulmonary venous flow morphology with increasing severity of mitral regurgitation (MR). *A,* Schematic representation of left atrial pressure tracing plotted against worsening degrees of MR. Normal pulmonary venous inflow consists of an S wave (which correlates to the x-decent on left atrial tracing) and smaller D wave (which correlates to the y-decent on left atrial pressure tracing) (S:D ratio <1.0). This is similar to that seen with mild (2+) MR. As MR increases, however, progressive blunting of the S wave occurs with increase in the D wave velocity. Eventually reversed forward systolic flow (RSF) occurs when severe MR is present. These changes correlate with a blunted a wave (decreased a-x' decent) and increased v wave (increased y-decent) in the left atrial tracing. *B,* Doppler characterization of pulmonary venous inflow obtained by transesophageal echocardiography and plotted against left atrial pressure curve in patient with mild MR. Tracing is similar to that seen in patients without MR. Note that the correlation between Doppler derived and measured pressures are quite good. *C,* Typical Doppler pattern of pulmonary venous flow obtained by transesophageal echocardiography in a patient with moderately severe (3+) MR. Small S wave and large D wave correspond to changes in left atrial tracing as previously noted. These findings can be helpful in accurately classifying severity of MR when color flow mapping is limited (i.e., in the presence of shielding owing to prosthetic mitral valve).

overload of the left ventricle) similar to that seen in constrictive pericarditis as previously described.

In adition to pressure measurements, right heart catheterization enables one to perform a complete saturation run to help exclude ventricular septal defect, which is a major differential diagnosis in the setting of myocardial infarction. An oxygen step-up of greater than 1 vol% between the right atrium and right ventricle is considered by some authors indicative of a hemodynamically significant left-to-right shunt.[83] Often, echocardiography is useful in assessing the presence of a ventricular septal defect.[83a]

Angiography. Contrast left ventricular angiography performed in the right anterior oblique projection provides a well-recognized method of evaluating left ventricular function and quantifying MR.[84] The left ventricle usually contracts vigorously, and the degree of MR as it opacifies the left atrium can be graded. Mild (1+) MR is present when the left atrium clears with each new beat, and there is never full left atrial opacification. Moderate (2+) MR is present when the left atrium does not clear with each new beat. The left atrium is fairly, but completely (faintly) opacified. In moderately severe (3+) MR, the left atrium is completely opacified and to the same degree level as the left ventricle. Severe (4+) MR is denoted by complete opacification of the left atrium after the first beat. This opacification intensifies with each beat, and reflux into the pulmonary veins can be seen. Wall motion abnormalities associated with myocardial ischemia or infarction are characterized as well. One must carefully weigh the information obtained from this study, however, with the risks associated with contrast administration in an often unstable patient when this information can usually be obtained by echocardiography.

ICU Phase

Once the patient has presented, is stabilized, and has a working differential diagnosis that is actively being evaluated with the above-mentioned techniques, rapid triage to an ICU is imperative for optimal management.

The care of a patient with acute MR requires a high index of suspicion for prompt diagnosis, hemodynamic stabilization, and consideration for early surgical intervention to repair any mechanical abnormalities. Management in an ICU setting is fundamental to the management of these patients. In addition, awareness of and specific treatment for the underlying cause is important in tailoring proper management. The sequence of therapeutic interventions depends primarily on the underlying cause and hemodynamic status of the patient. Once a diagnosis is strongly suspected or confirmed, the therapeutic approach to a patient with acute MR starts with a general assessment of clinical status. Attention to optimal oxygenation, ventilation, and hemodynamic stability is mandatory in all patients as previously noted. Adequate arterial oxygenation should be provided with the use of supplemental oxygen and endotracheal intubation as needed. Ventilation may be satisfactory at first, but fatigue often ensues owing to a marked increase in the work of breathing (from pulmonary edema), and mechanical support may be required. Blood pressure may be well maintained, but if cardiogenic shock is present, urgent use of pressors and intra-aortic balloon placement are necessary.

In general, medical management is limited to hemodynamic support until definitive surgery can be performed. There have been several reports of nonsurgical therapy directed specifically toward the underlying disorder, resulting in hemodynamic stabilization and lessening of the regurgitant volume. A notable example of this is acute MR secondary to papillary muscle dysfunction in the setting of ischemia or acute myocardial infarction. Although several studies have reported mixed results, interventions directed toward improving flow in the obstructed coronary artery with the early administration of a thrombolytic agent or percutaneous myocardial revascularization may reduce the amount of MR and improve myocardial salvage;[85-87] unfortunately this is not usually the case. A study by Tcheng and coworkers,[88] found that neither thrombolytic therapy nor percutaneous transluminal angioplasty reliably reversed valvular incompetence. Patients in this study with residual MR at 1 year had a significantly higher mortality rate independent of left ventricular function.[88]

Medical Management. Initiation of proper medical therapy requires constant hemodynamic monitoring to assess the severity of MR and gauge the response to therapeutic intervention. A pulmonary artery monitoring catheter should be inserted at the bedside or using fluoroscopic guidance whenever the clinical situation allows. By no means, however, should this delay the initiation of medical, mechanical, or surgical therapies once the diagnosis is obtained. Continuous arterial pressure measurements are optimal and should be obtained with the placement of an intra-arterial pressure catheter. The preferred site is radial artery, unless the placement of an intra-aortic balloon counterpulsation device is anticipated, which has arterial pressure recording capabilities. Once reliable hemodynamic measurements can be obtained, medication may be more effectively added and titrated to the desired effect. Table 33-4 lists the commonly used medications and their dosages.

The cornerstones of medical therapy for acute MR include decreasing impedance to left ventricular emptying and relief of pulmonary congestion. This is accomplished through preload and afterload reduction and increasing inotropic competence. The beneficial effects of medical therapy are realized by a reduction in pulmonary capillary wedge pressure, pulmonary artery pressure, and improved effective cardiac output. Pulmonary congestion is managed with the usual medications, including diuretics, supplemental oxygen, and morphine sulfate. The drug of choice for afterload reduction in our institution is sodium nitroprusside. It has a rapid onset of action and a short half-life and is easily titratable.[89] The arterial dilating effects of sodium nitroprusside improve forward cardiac output, and because it has beneficial (albeit weaker) venodilating properties that decrease left ventricular end-diastolic volume and thus pressure, it reduces the size of the regurgitant orifice.[90,91] As a cautionary note, sodium nitroprusside is rapidly converted into cyanide and then further metabolized in the liver to thiocyanate. Thiocyanate is renally excreted, and with normal renal function, toxicity does not tend to be a problem. When renal impairment is present,

Table 33-4. Commonly Used Vasodilators in Acute Mitral Regurgitation

Drug	Principal Action	Dosage	Route(s) of Administration	Comments	Major Side Effects
Combination Agents					
Sodium nitroprusside	Vasodilation of arterial and venous smooth muscle	0.25–1.0 μg/kg/min. Titrate up until desired effect obtained	Intravenous only. Onset immediate and effect stops when drug is turned off	Drug of choice in acute MR. Use cautiously when hypotension present	Thiocyanate intoxication (see text). Keep serum levels ≤5–10 mg/dl
Prazosin	Alpha₁-blocker with effects on arterial and venous capacitance	2–5 mg q 6–8 h	Oral only. Effects last 6 hours	Not a first-line drug. Use if subacute or long-term maintenance required	Postural hypotension; "first dose" effect; tachyphylaxis
ACE Inhibitors					
Captopril	Angiotension converting enzyme inhibition. Arterial and venous dilatation	6.25 mg q 6–8 h initially, titrate to 50 mg q 8 h as tolerated	Oral only	Not a first-line drug. Caution with impaired renal function	Cough and hypotension. Rash, dysgeusia, proteinuria, and neutropenia rare
Enalapril	Similar to captopril	2.5–10 mg q 12 h	Oral only	Similar to captopril	Similar to captopril
Enalaprilate	Similar to captopril	0.625–1.25 mg q 8 h	Intravenous only	Experience in acute MR limited. Effects similar to nitroprusside	Similar to captopril
Hydralazine	Arterial smooth muscle vasodilatation	25–50 mg p.o. q 6 h to start. Titrate to 200 mg/d IV 0.3 mg/kg; 10–40 mg IV q 6–8 h	Intravenous. Switch to oral if patient stabilizes and requires more long-term therapy	Good second-line drug if nitroprusside poorly tolerated. Use with nitrates for maximal benefit	Tachycardia, lupus-like syndrome, headache, and nasal congestion
Nifedipine	Calcium entry blocker. Major effect is arterial vasodilatation	10–40 mg q 6–8 h	Oral or sublingual	Not a first-line drug. Use for semiacute and long-term management	Edema and hypotension. Negative inotropic effects offset by peripheral vasodilation and reflex tachycardia
Preload Reducing Agents					
Nitroglycerine	Major effects on venous capacitance vessels	10–200 μg/min IV; ointment 1–3 in. q 3–4 h; sublingual 2.5–15 mg q 2–4 h	Intravenous. Topical ointment and oral better in long-term management	Not ideal for use as a single agent. Works well with pure vasodilators such as hydralazine	Hypotension, headaches, postural symptoms

(Adapted from Kron, J. and Bristow, J. D.: The use of vasodilators in acute and chronic valvular regurgitation. *In* Cardiology. Edited by Parmley, W. W., and Chatterjee, K. Philadelphia, J. B. Lippincott, 1991.)

however, close monitoring of the patients and serum thiocyanate levels is indicated. Thiocyanate intoxication appears at serum levels of 5 to 10 mg/dl and manifests with a variety of symptoms, including nausea, headache, seizure, mental status changes, rash, and rarely respiratory arrest.[89] Many of these manifestations are seen in critically ill patients in the absence of thiocyanate toxicity, and thus we recommend routine measurement of thiocyanate levels with the use of sodium nitroprusside in the presence of impaired renal function.

Pure vasodilating agents, such as intravenous hydralazine, may also be used. A reduction in impedance to left ventricular emptying occurs with lessening of the MR. The magnitude of effect, however, is less than that seen with sodium nitroprusside. Owing to the lack of venodilation with this agent, preload remains relatively unaffected, and thus regurgitant orifice in not lessened.[92] Success with alternative agents, such as angiotensin converting enzyme (ACE) inhibitors, peripheral alpha blocker (prazocin), and calcium channel antagonists (nifedipine), has been reported.[93] With the exception of sodium enalaprilate, however, these medications have the disadvantage of requiring oral or sublingual administration and are not readily titratable. Thus they are best left for use in more stable patients or when surgery is to be delayed.

Preload reduction is accomplished mainly with the use of diuretics (particularly loop diuretics) and intravenous nitroglycerin. These require the concomitant administration of vasodilating agents for optimal benefit. The latter may not be necessary if sodium nitroprusside is used owing to its venodilating properties. The addition of nitroglycerin to hydralazine makes for an effective combination and second-line therapy when there is evidence of thiocyanate toxicity or sodium nitroprusside intolerance.

Inotropic support is a useful adjunct when there is evidence of left ventricle failure and systemic hypotension.

Clinically this is typically seen when systolic blood pressure is less than 90 to 100 mm Hg and cardiac index is less than 2.2 L/min/m². In these situations, systemic vascular resistance is usually elevated in an effort to maintain blood pressure. The exclusive use of vasodilators in these patients may cause rapid deterioration unless cardiac contractility is maintained. Inotropic support is provided with dopamine, dobutamine, and amrinone. Dopamine and dobutamine are synthetic amines that act as beta₂-agonists. The former has dopaminergic and alpha-adrenergic effects as well, depending on the dose. Dopamine may be more useful in the setting of profound hypotension because it is a potent vasopressor when used in higher doses. The vasopressor action of dopamine comes at the expense of increased systemic vascular resistance, which worsens MR. Dobutamine is the preferred agent in acute MR because it is a positive inotrope and pure beta₂-agonist. This results in an increased force of contraction and vasodilatation that reduces regurgitant volume and increases effective cardiac output. Digitalis glycosides play a limited role in the management of severely ill patients with acute MR. They may be potentially useful in the treatment of atrial arrhythmias that develop as a sequela of increased left atrial pressure. Although these arrhythmias can prove refractory to most forms of therapy, digitalis preparations may be worth trying. Accordingly the slow onset of action and narrow therapeutic index of these agents dramatically limit their utility in acute MR.

Amrinone, a phosphodiesterase inhibitor, is also an inotropic agent with peripheral vasodilatory capabilities. It is used in a similar manner to dobutamine. Thrombocytopenia is the major side effect and requires serial measurement of platelet counts.

The use of vasopressors in acute MR owing to ischemic syndromes constitutes an altogether separate entity. In these patients, enhanced contractile force may increase myocardial oxygen consumption and worsen ischemia. Vasopressors should be used judiciously in these situations. These patients are best managed with pure afterload reduction and anti-ischemic and antithrombotic medications as well as intra-aortic balloon counterpulsation. Expeditious arrest of myocardial injury with myocardial revascularization is the principal therapy.

Mechanical Support. Percutaneous intra-aortic balloon counterpulsation (IABP) is generally reserved for patients in whom medical management alone is either inadequate or produces intolerable systemic hypotension. This form of afterload reduction most effectively reduces impedance to left ventricular ejection and augments coronary blood flow. Forward cardiac output is enhanced and pulmonary wedge pressure may be markedly reduced. Although it is of considerable importance for severe acute MR in general, IABP placement may be particularly useful in ischemic MR. It provides additional hemodynamic support during cardiac catheterization and improves tolerance of the procedure.[94]

Placement of an IABP requires insertion of a large catheter usually in the femoral artery. Because of this, frequent rotation of the site (usually every 3 to 5 days), careful assessment of limb viability, and evaluation for infection is required.

It is important to emphasize that the acuity of illness dictates the sequence of therapies and rapidity with which they are executed. Patients presenting in cardiogenic shock require rapid diagnostic assessment as previously outlined, intra-aortic balloon pump insertion, intravenous preload and afterload reduction, and rapid triage for surgical intervention. Often multiple therapies and interventions are performed simultaneously to obtain rapid diagnostic information and stabilization. Patients who are less ill may be successfully managed medically for a period of time while a diagnostic and therapeutic evaluation is performed.

Surgical Management. Surgical therapy is generally considered the treatment of choice for acute MR, focusing on reduction of regurgitation, coronary revascularization, and additional cardiac repair (abscess drainage, other valve surgery, and repair of chest trauma) as needed. In ischemic MR, the need and urgency of definitive surgical intervention may be reduced if successful thrombolytic therapy or percutaneous revascularization can be achieved. Patients with ischemic mitral valve dysfunction should have prompt surgical intervention. First successfully treated surgically by replacement of the mitral valve in 1965 by Austin and associates,[95] the incidence of this syndrome remains relatively low with only 22 surgical cases reported in a 10-year series from the Mayo Clinic.[96] In a similar series from Emory University, only 14 cases were described.[97] Nevertheless, significant morbidity and mortality are associated with its occurrence. Operative mortality has been reported to be 27% with a 7-year survival of 64% for patients discharged from the initial hospitalization. In this patient population, no survival advantage was found for delaying surgical intervention beyond 7 days after myocardial infarction, and thus these patients should be considered for surgery early after the diagnosis is established.[96]

Mitral valve replacement and repair constitute the major forms of surgical therapy directed at reversing the regurgitant pathology. The former is an excellent treatment for valvular incompetence and has been well validated. Owing to the contribution of papillary muscle-annular continuity to overall left ventricular function,[98] efforts to preserve the papillary muscles and chordal attachments are generally undertaken in both ischemic[99] and nonischemic[100] causes of acute MR. Mitral valve repair has gained wide appeal. Owing to a reduced perioperative morbidity, low operative mortality,[101] improved long-term survival, and low incidence of thromboembolic events,[102] it is now considered the operation of choice for most forms of acute MR. A variety of techniques and procedures for the repair have been advocated, but those pioneered by Carpentier (quadrangular resection, chordal shortening, chordal transfer, and ring annuloplasty) seem to have emerged as the most widely used reconstructive method for nearly all mitral valve pathology.[103] Figure 33-1 shows features of a typical myxomatous mitral valve with prolapse and severe MR before repair. Figure 33-7 illustrates features of the same mitral valve after quadrangular resection of the posterior mitral leaflet and repair of flail chordal structures. Color flow mapping reveals no significant MR, and all native structures have been retained. This is the procedure of choice for most forms of acute MR (see later) and should

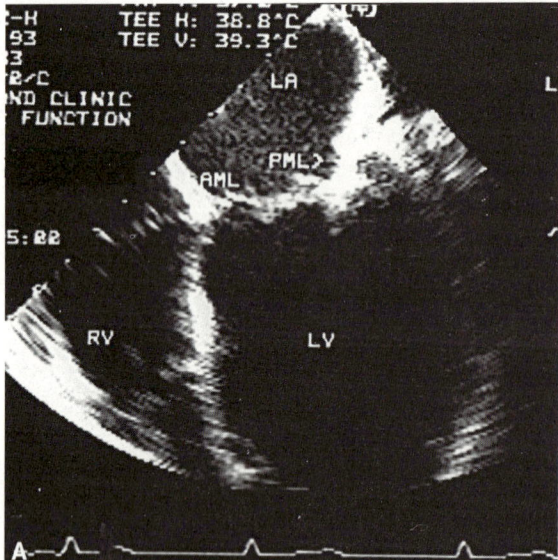 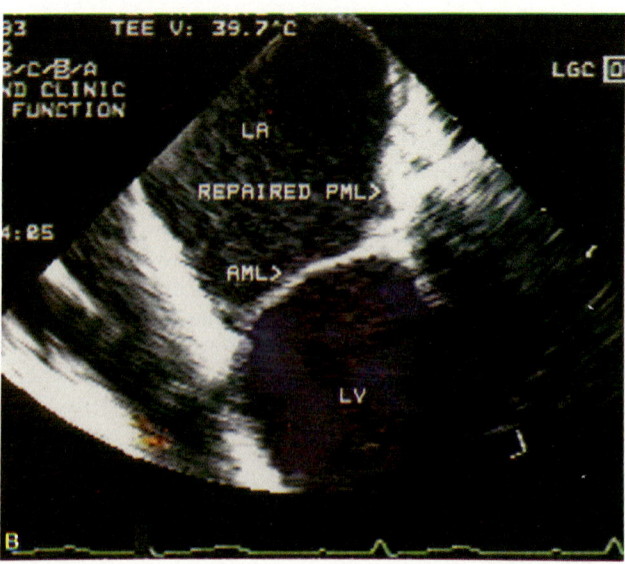

Figure 33-7. A, Intraoperative transesophageal echocardiogram in the transverse, four-chamber view of a myxomatous mitral valve with posterior leaflet prolapse after mitral valve repair. B, Same image in systole shows no evidence of mitral regurgitation using color flow mapping. LA, Left atrium; LV, left ventricle; RV, right ventricle; AML, anterior mitral leaflet; PML, posterior mitral leaflet. (Courtesy of Dr. Gerald Cohen.)

be attempted by all surgeons proficient in its use, unless there is severe calcification of the leaflets or subvalvular apparatus preventing performance of a satisfactory repair.

In acute MR caused by myocardial infarction, the main surgical therapy has remained mitral valve replacement,[104] although investigators at our institution[105] have advocated mitral valve repair for papillary muscle rupture owing to myocardial infarction. This technique, although theoretically preferable, is limited by the quality of the tissue at the insertion site of the papillary muscle. Often the ventricular tissue is necrotic and friable limiting the quality and durability of the repair. Because of this, some authorities continue to recommend mitral valve replacement.[106]

Although controversy exists, most authorities recommend proceeding with coronary angiography whenever possible before valve surgery.[107-110] Although some of the sickest patients are unable to tolerate this additional intervention, through the use of medical therapies and intraaortic balloon counterpulsation, adequate hemodynamic support is achieved so the majority may safely undergo the study. Perioperative and long-term mortality is clearly higher in patients not given the benefit of coronary artery bypass surgery in the setting of ischemic MR.[96]

Mitral valve repair has previously been considered contraindicated in patients with acute mitral valvular endocarditis owing to the chance of reinfection. Dreyfus et al.,[111] however, found a low (2.5%) perioperative and late mortality rate. They believe that early surgical intervention avoids extension of the infectious process, preserves the subvalvular apparatus thus improving left ventricular function, and provides tissues that are more resistant to infection than prosthetic material. Endocarditis did not recur, and long-term valvular integrity was maintained. Thus, extension of this technique to endocarditis infection seems warranted.

Intraoperative assessment of the surgical repair is of paramount importance to ensure a satisfactory outcome. Often this is accomplished through saline filling of the arrested left ventricle. Intraoperative echocardiography with TEE or epicardial imaging, however, has largely supplanted this as the technique of choice owing to its dynamic and versatile nature.[112,113] TEE has been advocated as an improved method of intraoperative assessment.[114] This method is superior to epicardial imaging because it does not obstruct the surgical field and obviates the problems of acoustic interference so frequently encountered with mechanical mitral valves.[115]

The outcome of surgical intervention depends on many factors including:

- Age of the patient
- Severity of the MR
- Left ventricular function
- Underlying cause of the regurgitation
- Extent of co-morbid illness (coronary artery disease, renal impairment)
- Presence of cardiogenic shock
- Urgency of the surgery[116-118]

Although presurgical medical stabilization of the patient with acute MR is important, it should not significantly delay surgical intervention. In patients with acute MR owing to myocardial infarction, it has previously been advocated to attempt medical stabilization of the patient for at least 6 to 8 weeks before performing surgery to allow time for the myocardium to heal.[119,120] This delay reportedly lowers operative mortality rates from 30 to 35% to 15 to 25%.[121] This strategy, however, may select out for those patients with better left ventricular function and less severe MR who can survive the waiting period. In addition, studies that have evaluated this waiting period reveal that although survival of patients who live to undergo surgical repair is improved, approximately half of the patients stabilized on medical management die suddenly while awaiting operation.[122] Other studies of early surgical intervention have had excellent results, with survival perioperatively approaching 100% and 1-year follow-up survival of 90%.[123,124] Thus we recommend early surgical intervention for acute MR in whom thrombolytic therapy or percutaneous revascularization yields suboptimal results.

The decision to continue with surgical repair in an extremely ill patient is a complex and difficult one. Whenever possible, detailed information on left ventricular function, extent of coronary artery disease, and co-morbid illnesses, such as renal impairment, should be ascertained. Patients with severe MR and significant impairment of left ventricular function may do poorly after valve replacement or repair.[125,126] In these patients, the relative merits of complex interventions, including potential for recovery of stunned or hibernating myocardium in the setting of coronary artery disease require careful thought before embarking on an expensive, potentially unhelpful therapeutic course.

Post-ICU Phase

The post-ICU phase is concerned with postoperative convalescence and rehabilitation. Follow-ups of the surgical procedure, progression to oral medication, patient education, and physical rehabilitation are the main components. In addition, medical management of the rare patient not undergoing surgical intervention changes necessitates close follow-up.

Patients recovering from valve surgery require close cardiac follow-up during the first few postoperative weeks to months. Patients may develop any complication associated with open cardiac surgery in the first few days or weeks after operation. In addition to early postoperative hemorrhage, acute myocardial infarction, cerebral hemorrhage or pulmonary embolus, renal failure, infection, and hepatitis are important possible complications. The laboratory and hemodynamic markers of these problems require close attention. Once stable, serial echocardiograms are required to assess function of the prosthetic valve or integrity of a valve repair. We recommend at least one postoperative echocardiogram usually prior to discharge with the patient in stable condition to be used as a baseline study. This is usually followed by a 6-week postoperative evaluation with serial echocardiograms performed every 6 months to 1 year thereafter as needed.

Anticoagulation. Anticoagulation is often a routine part of postoperative care. Patients receiving a mechanical valve require lifelong anticoagulation. Heparin may be started initially with transition to warfarin preparations, but if the patient has been stable and no further interventions are planned, warfarin may be started directly on approximately postoperative day 3 or 4. Therapeutic anticoagulation is followed with the use of International Normalized Ratio (INR) and prothrombin times (PT). The former is a test that corrects for the different index of sensitivity (ISI) of tissue thromboplastins used in various laboratories in North America to perform PTs. Reporting level of anticoagulation in INR units is more reproducible and applicable between different laboratories. Adequate levels of anticoagulation for patients with tissue valves is an INR of 2.0 to 3.0 corresponding roughly to a PT of 1.6 to 1.8 times control value when tissue thromboplastin ISI is 1.8 to 2.8. An INR of 2.5 to 3.5 (PT 1.5 to 2.0 when thromboplastin ISI similar to those noted previously are used) is desirable when a mechanical valve is present.[127] An INR greater than 3.5 (PT ≥2.0 times control) is associated with an increased risk of bleeding without further reduction in incidence of thromboembolic events.[128] At recommended doses, the incidence of anticoagulant associated bleeding is reported to be approximately 1.0 to 1.5% per year, with a 2 to 4% risk of thromboembolism.[129]

Patients undergoing mitral valve repair with the placement of an annular ring may or may not be given oral anticoagulation for 6 to 12 weeks following surgery depending on the type of ring and preferences of the surgical team. Thereafter they can be safely discontinued. The method of anticoagulation is similar to that used with mechanical valves, although the intensity is somewhat less. Numerous studies have confirmed the safety of valve repair with a reported 94% and 96% freedom from thromboembolism and anticoagulant associated hemorrhage at 15 years.[130,131]

Endocarditis Prophylaxis. Antibiotic prophylaxis for the prevention of endocarditis is recommended for all patients after having undergone mitral valve replacement or repair, particularly if the latter involved placement of a supporting mitral annular ring. Patients with prosthetic mitral valves constitute the group at greatest risk, with an overall incidence of 2 to 4%.[29] Prosthetic valve endocarditis occurring within 2 months of surgery carries a high mortality rate of 63 to 88%,[132,133] whereas late onset has a lower mortality rate (25 to 45%).[134] Early reoperation when necessary can be life-saving. Patients are counseled on signs and symptoms of endocarditis and the high risk procedures requiring prior antibiotic prophylaxis. In addition, all are given a wallet-sized pamphlet containing the most recent American Heart Association guidelines.

Management of Underlying Disorder. Close follow-up and treatment of the underlying disorder predisposing to acute MR are important because many of the diseases (most notably the connective tissue disorders) are progressive. Patients with myxomatous disease and particularly Marfan syndrome require close follow-up for aortic valve regurgitation, aortic aneurysm, and aortic dissection. Continuing myxomatous degeneration may involve the repaired or other heart valves producing recurrent regurgitation. Atherosclerotic coronary artery disease requires management on multiple fronts. Attention to lipids, prevention of recurrent ischemia, and use of afterload reducing agents (ACE inhibitors) when significant residual left ventricular dysfunction exists are required in appropriate patients. As noted previously, one report has suggested that residual MR after myocardial infarction is an independant risk factor for mortality 1 year after the event. Thus every effort should be made in these patients to ensure complete revascularization and maintenance of valvular competency. Rheumatic fever may necessitate long-term suppressive therapy with antibiotics. Systemic lupus erythematosus is a systemic disorder that may require lifelong medical therapy and close follow-up. These and other disorders that predispose to recurrent valvular incompetence require attention and treatment in the post-ICU, pre-discharge phase.

ACUTE AORTIC REGURGITATION

Strategies for management of the patient with acute aortic valvular insufficiency parallel those for acute MR. Focus on initial stabilization of vital signs, maintenance of adequate arterial oxygenation, and elucidation of the underlying cause are the primary goals. Presentation is similar with respiratory complaints predominating. Symptoms of severe dyspnea and orthopnea are common and may be accompanied by hemodynamic embarrassment. As with acute MR, prompt recognition and treatment of these symptoms may be life-saving.

Pre-ICU Phase

Aortic regurgitation is the retrograde flow of blood from the aorta to the left ventricle during diastole through an incompetent aortic valve. When aortic regurgitation occurs acutely, the left ventricle is of normal size and cannot accommodate the increased volume of blood.[135] The patient with acute aortic regurgitation may be mildly symptomatic to extremely ill, depending on the acuity and severity of the process. The clinical presentation and physical findings of acute aortic regurgitation are typically much different than those of chronic aortic regurgitation. The patient with acute aortic regurgitation requires prompt diagnosis, aggressive ICU management, treatment of underlying causes, and surgical intervention.

Cause

Acute aortic regurgitation may result from damage to any part of the aortic apparatus. This may result from damage to the cusps, loss of commissural support, aortic root dilatation, or prosthetic valve dysfunction. The following description classifies aortic regurgitation according to the diseased component (Table 33-5).

Cusp Abnormality. The most common cause of acute aortic regurgitation is infective endocarditis.[136,137] Infective endocarditis causes aortic regurgitation through perforation of the aortic cusp. Large, mobile vegetations may be seen on the valve leaflets (Fig. 33-8). This often occurs on a functionally normal valve. Although a congenitally bicuspid valve is more often associated with aortic stenosis, aortic regurgitation may be associated with a bicuspid valve, with or without endocarditis.[138,139] Aortic regurgitation on a bicuspid valve without endocarditis involves reduction in the area of the cusps. Sudden, severe aortic regurgitation is the most frequent cause of death in infective endocarditis.[140] The congenitally bicuspid valve is the most frequent congenital cardiac malformation, with an incidence of 2%.[141] If there is no previously recognized murmur or suspicion of anomaly, antibiotic prophylaxis is not routinely used, and the patient's risk of developing endocarditis is much higher. Other cardiac complications of endocarditis include atrioventricular conduction disturbance (first-degree heart block, Wenckebach, transient or complete atrioventricular block), involvement of the left ventricle wall with sequelae varying from abscess cavity, pericardial friction rub to perforation with tamponade, left-to-right shunts owing to aortic to right atrial or right ventricular fistula, perforation of ventricular septum, periprosthetic valvular regurgitation, and MR caused by extension to the anterior mitral leaflet.

Acute aortic regurgitation secondary to cusp abnormality may be associated with blunt or penetrating trauma to the chest,[142,143] spontaneous rupture of myxomatous leaflets,[144] and rupture of leaflet fenestrations.[145]

Other cusp abnormalities involve reduction in the area of the cusps and include causes such as rheumatic disease, rheumatoid disease, and ankylosing spondylitis.

Loss of Commissural Support. The next most common cause of acute aortic regurgitation is dissection of the ascending aorta with proximal extension to the aortic cusp with loss of commissural support (Fig. 33-9). This is associated with hypertension and may result in leakage of blood into the pericardium and pericardial tamponade. Sudden sagging of an apparently normal cusp, Fallot-type ventricular septal defect, trauma, and syphilis can also cause aortic regurgitation through loss of commissural support. Severe aortic regurgitation may rarely follow balloon

Table 33-5. Common Causes and Mechanisms of Aortic Regurgitation

Cusp abnormality	Bacterial endocarditis
Perforation	Rheumatic disease
Reduction in area	Rheumatoid disease
	Ankylosing spondylitis
	Trauma
	Biscuspid valve
	Rupture of fenestrations
Loss of commissural support	Dissection of the aorta
	Fallot-type VSD
	Trauma
	Syphilis
	Sudden sagging of an apparently normal cusp
Aortic root dilatation	Annuloaortic ectasia
	Cystic medionecrosis of the aorta (isolated or with Marfans syndrome)
	Osteogenesis imperfecta
	Syphilitic aortitis
	Ankylosing spondylitis
	Behçet's syndrome
	Psoriatic arthritis
	Ulcerative colitis
	Relapsing polychondritis
	Reiter's syndrome
	Giant cell arteritis
	Hypertension
	Ehlers-Danlos syndrome
	Pseudoxanthoma elasticum
	Familial
	Idiopathic
Prosthetic valve dysfunction	Infective endocarditis
	Rupture
	Strut fracture

(Modified from Braunwald, E.: Valvular Heart Disease. *In* Heart Disease—A Textbook of Cardiovascular Medicine. Edited by E. Braunwald. Philadelphia, W.B. Saunders, 1988.)

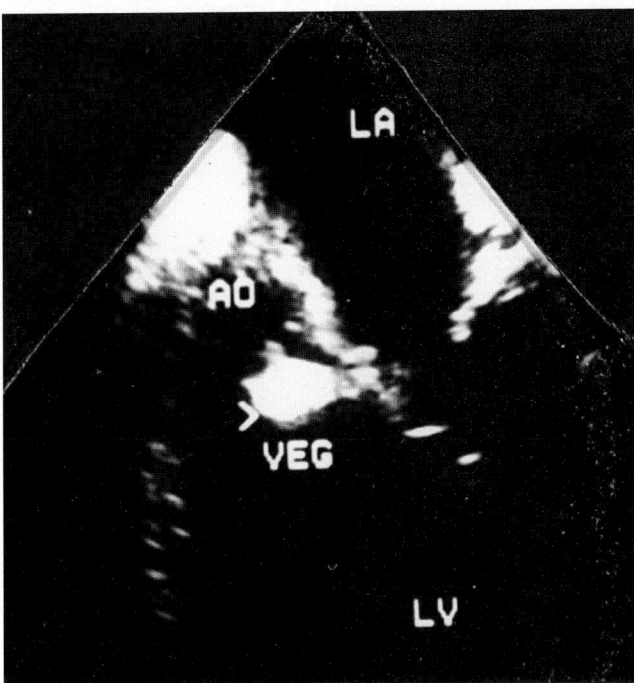

Figure 33-8. Transesophageal echocardiogram showing infective endocarditis with large vegetation on aortic valve and abscess cavity between aortic valve and left atrium. Color Doppler imaging shows two jets of aortic regurgitation, one centrally and one anteriorly. There is also fistulous communication between the abscess cavity and the left atrium, demonstrated by color Doppler. LA, Left atrium; AO, aorta; VEG, vegetation; LV, left ventricle.

aortic valvuloplasty for aortic stenosis, also through loss of commissural support.[146-148]

Aortic Root Dilatation. Acute, severe aortic regurgitation may occur secondary to dilatation of the aortic root, which occurs by a variety of causes, including hypertension, annuloaortic ectasia, cystic medionecrosis of the aorta, and syphilitic aortitis. Acute severe aortic regurgitation has been reported with systemic lupus erythematosus, ankylosing spondylitis, polychondritis,[149] Whipple's disease, and Behçet's syndrome,[150] through dilatation of the aortic root.

Prosthetic Valve Dysfunction. Acute aortic regurgitation may occur postoperatively in patients with aortic prostheses with periprosthetic leakage, rupture of leaflets, strut fracture, or endocarditis of a tissue graft.

Pathophysiology

Because left ventricular volume increases abruptly, there is no opportunity for the left ventricle to compensate through the mechanisms of dilatation and hypertrophy, which occur during chronic aortic regurgitation. Left ventricular end-diastolic pressure rises, total stroke volume rises slightly, forward stroke volume declines, and left ventricular contractility may decline because the left ventricular volume is beyond the peak of the Frank-Starling curve. Left ventricular end-diastolic pressure greatly increases[151] and can equal the aortic diastolic pressure, which is termed diastasis. This equalization may limit the amount of aortic regurgitation and maintain forward stroke volume. Premature opening of the aortic valve in late diastole may occur.[152] Because the aortic diastolic pressure cannot decrease below the left ventricular end-diastolic pressure, pulse pressure shows little increase, in contrast to chronic aortic regurgitation. Because stroke volume cannot increase significantly, cardiac output can increase only through an increase in heart rate. Tachycardia is a common finding in acute aortic regurgitation. As the left ventricular diastolic pressure rises above left atrial pressure in early diastole, diastolic MR ensues as a result of premature mitral valve closure.[153-155] This premature closure of the mitral valve protects the left atrium and pulmonary venous bed against elevations in pressure.[156] Pulmonary edema may develop despite these processes, with transmission of elevated pressures to the right side of the heart.

Clinical Manifestations

Patients with acute aortic regurgitation may develop dyspnea, weakness, and hypotension. Congestive heart failure is common. A known history of bicuspid aortic valve, rheumatic fever, trauma, or previous valve surgery may be a clue to the diagnosis. There may be tachycardia, vasoconstriction, and cyanosis present on physical examination. Manifestations of the underlying disease, such as fever, chest or back pain, and embolic phenomenon, are often present and point toward the diagnosis (Table 33-6).

The peripheral signs of increased pulse pressure seen in chronic aortic regurgitation are not typically seen in acute aortic regurgitation. These include head bobbing with each heartbeat (de Musset's sign),[157] abrupt rise and fall in pulses (water-hammer or Corrigan's pulse), booming systolic and diastolic sounds heard over the femoral artery (Traube's sign), systolic pulsation of the uvula (Muller's sign), and a systolic murmur heard over the femoral artery when it is compressed proximally and a diastolic murmur when it is compressed distally (Duroziez's sign). Capillary pulsations or Quincke's sign may be seen in the lips or fingertips. Popliteal cuff systolic pressure exceeding brachial cuff pressure by more than 60 mm Hg is referred to as Hill's sign. Patients with acute AI usually have normal pulse pressures and, thus, these findings are absent.

Auscultation

In chronic severe aortic regurgitation, there is usually a soft S_1 because of premature closure of the mitral valve, prolongation of the P-R interval, soft or absent A_2, and obscuring of P_2 by the early diastolic murmur.[158] S_2 may be single or absent or be narrowly or paradoxically split. Abrupt distention of the aorta by the large stroke volume may cause a systolic ejection sound. An S_3 may be present and may be useful as an indicator for cardiac catheterization in severe chronic aortic regurgitation.[159]

The diastolic murmur of aortic regurgitation usually begins immediately after A_2 or aortic valve closure and is high pitched, decrescendo in character. It is heard best with the diaphragm of the stethoscope with the patient sitting up and leaning forward, with the breath held in deep expiration. The severity of the aortic regurgitation

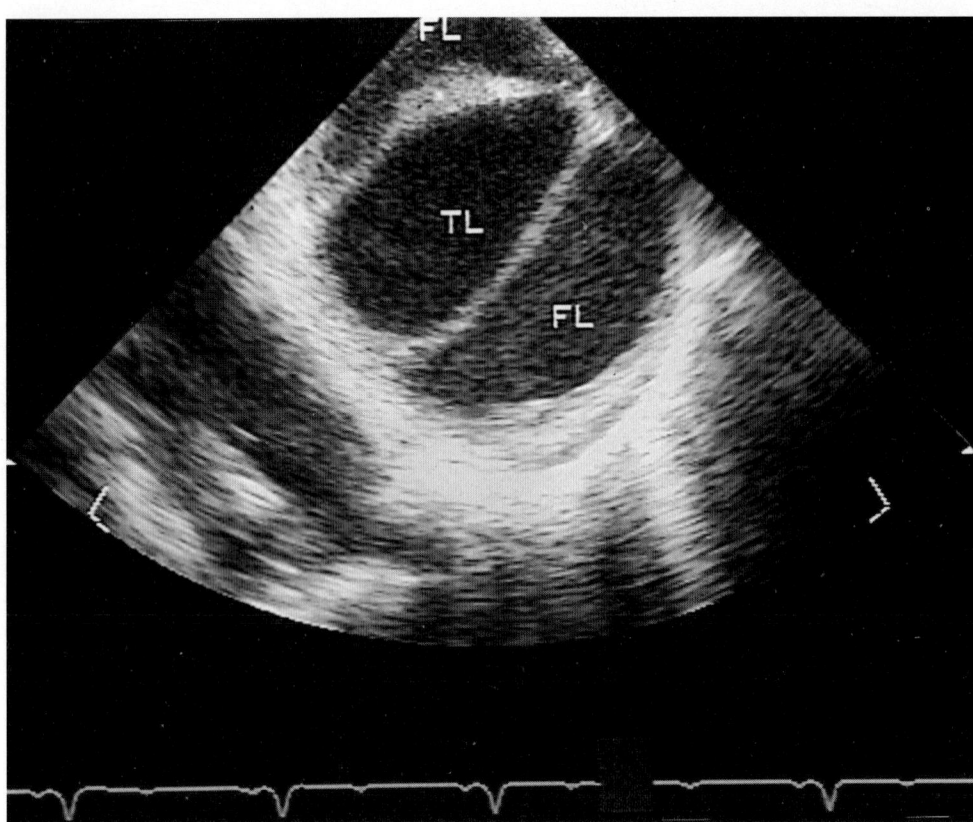

Fig. 33–9. Basal short axis view of ascending aorta by transesophageal echocardiography, showing aortic dissection with true lumen (TL) and false lumen (FL).

correlates best with the duration rather than the intensity of the murmur. The murmur may be early diastolic and high pitched in mild aortic regurgitation or rough and holodiastolic in moderate or severe aortic regurgitation. There may be a musical quality to the murmur in the presence of a torn aortic cusp. As heart failure worsens, S_2 may no longer be split and may show reverse splitting. In severe aortic regurgitation, there may be equilibration of left ventricular and aortic diastolic pressures, in late diastole, eliminating the murmur in late diastole. The Austin Flint murmur, a mid-diastolic and late diastolic apical rumble, is common in severe aortic regurgitation. Traditionally it has been thought to be caused by rapid antegrade flow across a narrowed mitral orifice, secondary to the rapidly rising left ventricular diastolic pressure. It may be similar to the rumble of mitral stenosis. An opening snap and loud S_1 may point toward mitral stenosis, whereas the absence of these support the Austin Flint murmur. The Austin Flint murmur may begin and end earlier as left ventricular end-diastolic pressure rises. Landzberg et al.[160] studied 24 patients with moderate or severe aortic regurgitation, who also had Austin Flint murmurs. The presence of an Austin Flint murmur correlated best with the volume of signal loss associated with the aortic regurgitation jet on cine MRI and the extent of contact of this signal loss with the left ventricular endocardium. They concluded that the Austin Flint murmur is caused by the aortic regurgitation jet abutting the left ventricular endocardium, resulting in the generation of a low pitched diastolic rumbling. A short midsystolic murmur secondary to the increased ejection rate and stroke volume may be heard. It may be transmitted to the carotids but is usually higher pitched than the murmur of aortic stenosis. The murmurs of aortic regurgitation vary concordantly with changes in systemic blood pressure.

In acute aortic regurgitation, the left ventricular impulse

Table 33–6. Physical Findings in Acute Aortic Regurgitation

Evidence of Underlying Disorder
   Systemic manifestations of endovascular infection
     Fever
     Splenomegaly
     Evidence of embolic phenomenon (Roth's spots, Osler's nodes, petechiae)
   Evidence of trauma
   Evidence of previous surgery
   Symptoms of aortic dissection—chest or back pain, decreased peripheral pulses
Cardiovascular Findings
   Nonspecific findings—dyspnea, weakness, hypotension, cyanosis
   Congestive heart failure
     Pulmonary congestion
     Jugular venous distention
     Peripheral edema
   Palpation—usually normal apical impulse
   Auscultation
     Tachycardia
     Soft-to-absent first heart sound
     Soft-to-absent A_2, normal-to-increased P_2
     S_3 common, S_4 absent
     Grade 3 or less systolic murmur—abrupt distention of aorta
     Short, medium-pitched decrescendo aortic regurgitant murmur
     Mid-diastolic rumble, Austin Flint murmur

is usually normal. With premature closure of the mitral valve, S_1 may be soft or absent. Diastolic MR may occur because of premature closure of the mitral valve. The diastolic murmur of acute aortic regurgitation is lower pitched and shorter than that of chronic aortic regurgitation. This occurs owing to a reduced pressure gradient across the aortic valve as elevation of the left ventricular end-diastolic pressure ensues. If the Austin Flint murmur is present, it is brief and ends when left ventricular pressure exceeds left atrial pressure in diastole. Evidence of pulmonary hypertension with an accentuated P_2, along with an S_3 and S_4, may be present. The signs of congestive heart failure, including jugular venous distention, tachycardia, hypotension, and cyanosis, may be present as well.

Laboratory Findings

Electrocardiogram. In acute aortic regurgitation, sinus tachycardia is usually present (Table 33-7). There may be nonspecific ST or T wave changes. Left ventricular hypertrophy is not usually present because there has not been sufficient time for hypertrophy to occur. In chronic aortic regurgitation, left ventricular hypertrophy and left axis deviation may be seen. There may be Q waves present in 1, AVL, and leads V3-V6. There may be nonspecific ST and T wave changes and intraventricular conduction delay, which are usually a sign of severe disease.

Chest Radiography. In acute aortic regurgitation, there may be little cardiac enlargement. Pulmonary venous hypertension and vascular congestion may often be seen and pulmonary artery prominence consistent with pulmonary hypertension identified. There may be calcification and dilatation of the ascending aorta associated with the underlying disease process.

In chronic aortic regurgitation, there is marked enlargement of the cardiac size on chest film usually in a leftward and inferior direction. There may be calcification of the aortic valve if there is combined aortic stenosis and aortic regurgitation. Enlargement of the ascending aorta may be seen with dissection and underlying connective tissue disorders.

Echocardiography. Two-dimensional transthoracic and transesophageal echocardiography and Doppler techniques have emerged as the main imaging methods for aortic regurgitation. Echocardiography is useful in defining the anatomy of the aortic valve and aortic root as well as assessing left ventricular size and function. Numerous abnormalities have been reported in the literature as suggestive of aortic regurgitation and include high frequency diastolic flutter of the anterior mitral valve leaflet or the interventricular septum on M-mode echocardiography, although it is neither sensitive nor specific. It is caused by the high frequency jet of blood regurgitating from the aortic valve. Premature closure and delayed opening of the mitral valve,[161,162] narrowing of the mitral valve orifice, and diastolic opening of the aortic valve[163] with equilibration of the left ventricular and aortic pressures in diastole may all be seen. The E-F slope is reduced, left ventricular end-diastolic dimension is normal or mildly elevated, and fractional shortening is usually normal. Two-dimensional echocardiography is useful in assessing the aortic root and the aortic valve for causes of aortic regurgitation: Thickening of cusps, aortic valve prolapse, flail leaflet, bicuspid valve, aortic dissection, and endocarditis may all be identified with echocardiography. Serial studies may be performed to assess left ventricular function and to determine the optimal timing for surgery.

Doppler echocardiography is superior to two-dimensional echocardiography in assessing aortic regurgitation. It is the most sensitive and accurate noninvasive indicator of aortic regurgitation. Certain methods, including pulsed wave, continuous wave, and color flow mapping and quantitative Doppler[163a] can be used to assess aortic regurgitation. The aortic regurgitation jet is high velocity because of the large pressure difference between the aorta and the left ventricle, although it has a lower velocity than the MR jet. The flow is turbulent because it is passing through a relatively small orifice. In pulsed wave Doppler, the jet generally extends above and below the baseline, and because it exceeds the Nyquist limits for forward and reverse flow, aliasing occurs. The views used to visualize the aortic valve are the apical five chamber and long axis and para-

Table 33-7. Laboratory Evaluation of Acute Aortic Regurgitation

Electrocardiography
  Sinus tachycardia
  Nonspecific ST-T wave changes
Chest Radiography
  Normal to moderately increased left ventricular size
  Pulmonary venous pattern redistributed to upper lobes
  Calcification of aorta
  Pulmonary artery prominence in pulmonary hypertension
Echocardiography
  Hemodynamics
    Right atrial pressure (IVC diameter)
    Right ventricular systolic pressure
    Pulmonary artery diastolic pressure
    Left atrial pressure
  Aortic disease
    Dissection of aorta
    Aortic bicuspid valve
    Calcification
    Flail leaflet
    Vegetation in endocarditis
    Left ventricular size and function
    Color and/or Doppler evidence of AR
  Prosthetic aortic valve (TEE more thoroughly evaluates prostheses due to shielding present on TTE)
    Dehiscence
    Periprosthetic leakage
    Strut fracture
    Endocarditis/vegetation, peforation of leaflets
    Rupture of leaflet
  Newer techniques
    Regurgitant fraction by quantitative Doppler
    Effective regurgitant orifice area
Cardiac Catheterization
  Hemodynamics
    Increased pulmonary capillary wedge pressure
    Pulmonary hypertension sometimes present
    Low or normal cardiac output
  Left heart catheterization and angiography
    Angiographic assessment of aortic regurgitation
    Assessment of left ventricular function
    Degree of associated coronary artery disease
    Identification of cardiac anomalies (number of cusps)

sternal long and short axis views. Pulsed wave Doppler is nearly 100% sensitive and specific in detecting aortic regurgitation and should be performed immediately if the diagnosis is suspected.[164,165] Using pulsed wave Doppler, a technique called flow mapping can be used to assess the amount of aortic regurgitation present. Pulsed Doppler sampling can be done at various sites in the left ventricular outflow tract and left ventricle to determine the amount of aortic regurgitation present. Aortic regurgitation is graded as follows:

- Grade 1 (mild): The jet is detected just below the level of the aortic valve.
- Grade 2 (moderate): The flow disturbance extends up to the level of the tips of the mitral valve leaflet in diastole.
- Grade 3 (severe): The jet is detected below the tips of the mitral valve leaflets.

This grading correlates reasonably well with angiography,[166] although it is only semiquantitative. There are limitations to this technique because it requires a high degree of expertise and is time-consuming. Pulsed wave Doppler techniques have been supplanted by flow mapping.[163a]

Continuous wave Doppler shows diastolic flow in the left ventricular outflow tract and its velocity (V) at various times throughout the cardiac cycle. Aliasing does not occur, and the tracing is above the baseline from the apical view. Using continuous Doppler, left ventricular end-diastolic pressure can be estimated by the following formula:

$$LVEDP = AoEDP - P$$

where $P = 4V^2$ (modified Bernoulli equation); V = velocity of aortic regurgitation jet at end diastole obtained by continuous Doppler; and AoEDP = diastolic pressure obtained with the blood pressure cuff.

The slope of the spectral tracing in aortic regurgitation reflects the speed with which the aortic diastolic pressure equalizes with the left ventricular diastolic pressure[167,168] (Fig. 33-10). In severe aortic regurgitation, the left ventricular diastolic pressure is high, and equalization of pressure occurs rapidly. In mild aortic regurgitation, the left ventricular diastolic pressure is lower, and equilibration takes longer. Studies have shown a correlation between the deceleration slope of the spectral tracing and the amount of aortic regurgitation. A deceleration slope of greater than 2 m per second separated individuals with moderate and severe aortic regurgitation from those with mild. A deceleration slope of 3 m per second correlates with severe (3+ to 4+) when compared with aortic regurgitation using angiography. Pressure half-time of the deceleration slope is also used in assessing aortic regurgitation. The time taken for the peak instantaneous pressure between the left ventricle and aorta to drop by half is measured. The shorter the pressure half-time, the more severe the aortic regurgitation. In one study,[169] a value of 400 m per second distinguished between mild (1+ to 2+) and severe (3+ to 4+) aortic regurgitation. A valve less than 250 msec is associated with severe aortic regurgitation.[163a] Owing to deformity of the valve, eccentricity of the jet, and respira-

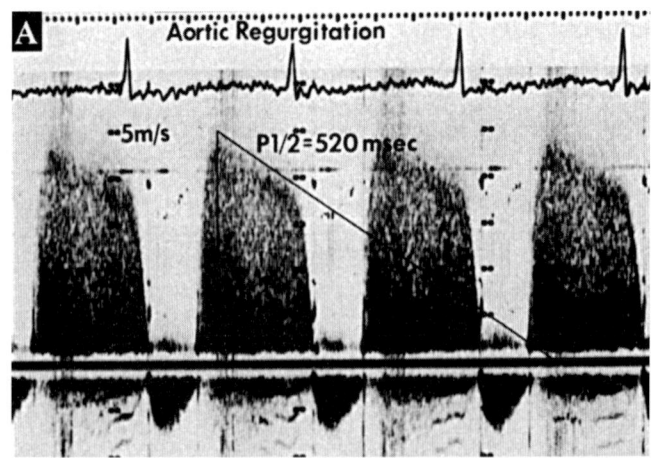

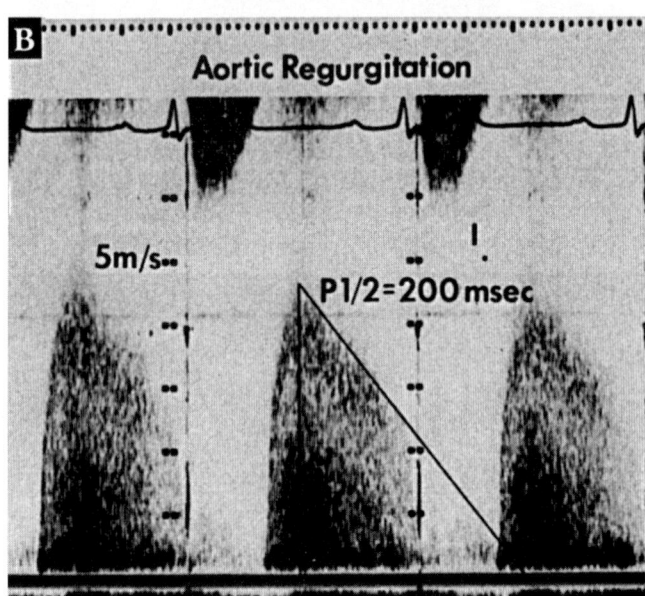

Fig. 33-10. Continuous wave Doppler recording of flow at aortic valve level. A, Signal recording in patient with mild aortic regurgitation, showing mildly decreased half-time index (P1/2) of 520 msec. B, Severe aortic regurgitation with decreased P1/2 of 200 msec. (From Klein, A. L., Davison, M. B., Vonk, G., and Tajik, A. J.: Doppler echocardiographic assessment of aortic regurgitation: uses and limitations. Cleve. Clin. J. Med., 59:365, 1992.)

tory movement, however, there may be difficulty in obtaining adequate spectral signals throughout diastole in some patients with aortic regurgitation.

In addition, the finding of flow reversal in the abdominal aorta is valuable in identifying severe aortic regurgitation (Fig. 33-11). Normally there is only minimal retrograde flow in the aorta. In mild aortic regurgitation, there may be significant retrograde flow, in early diastole only. In patients with severe aortic regurgitation, there is holodiastolic retrograde flow.

Color flow mapping is highly sensitive and specific for aortic regurgitation.[170] Aortic regurgitation is seen as a mosaic colored signal emanating from the aortic valve and extending into the left ventricular outflow tract during

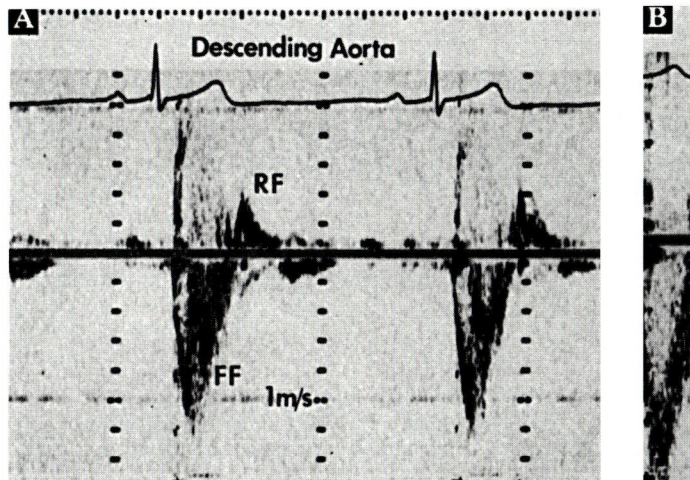
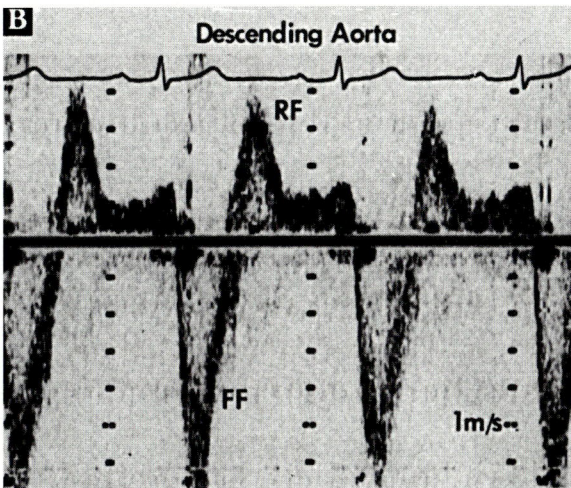

Fig. 33–11. Pulsed wave Doppler recordings. A, Proximal descending aorta in patient with mild aortic regurgitation, showing small and early retrograde diastolic flow compared with forward flow. B, Pulsed wave Doppler in the proximal descending aorta in patient with severe aortic regurgitation, showing retrograde flow to be increased and holodiastolic. (From Klein, A. L., Davison, M. B., Vonk, G., and Tajik, A. J. Doppler echocardiographic assessment of aortic regurgitation: uses and limitations. Cleve. Clin. J. Med., 59:365, 1992.)

diastole (Fig. 33–12). It has been shown that the width of the jet at the aortic valve correlated well with the angiographic assessment of the amount of aortic regurgitation.[171] Reports have shown that the ratio of the aortic regurgitation jet at the level of the aortic valve to the height of the left ventricular outflow tract at the same level correlated with the angiographic grading system better than the area of the regurgitant jet or the depth to which the jet extends into the left ventricle (r = 0.79). A ratio of 1 to 24% predicted an angiographic grade of 1+; 24 to 46% correlated with an angiographic grade of 2+; 47 to 64% correlated with an angiographic grade of 3+; and greater than 64% correlated with an angiographic grade of 4+. The correlation of jet length to angiographic grade of severity was poor. Color M-mode may be useful to help clarify incongruous findings. Color Doppler is useful in assess-

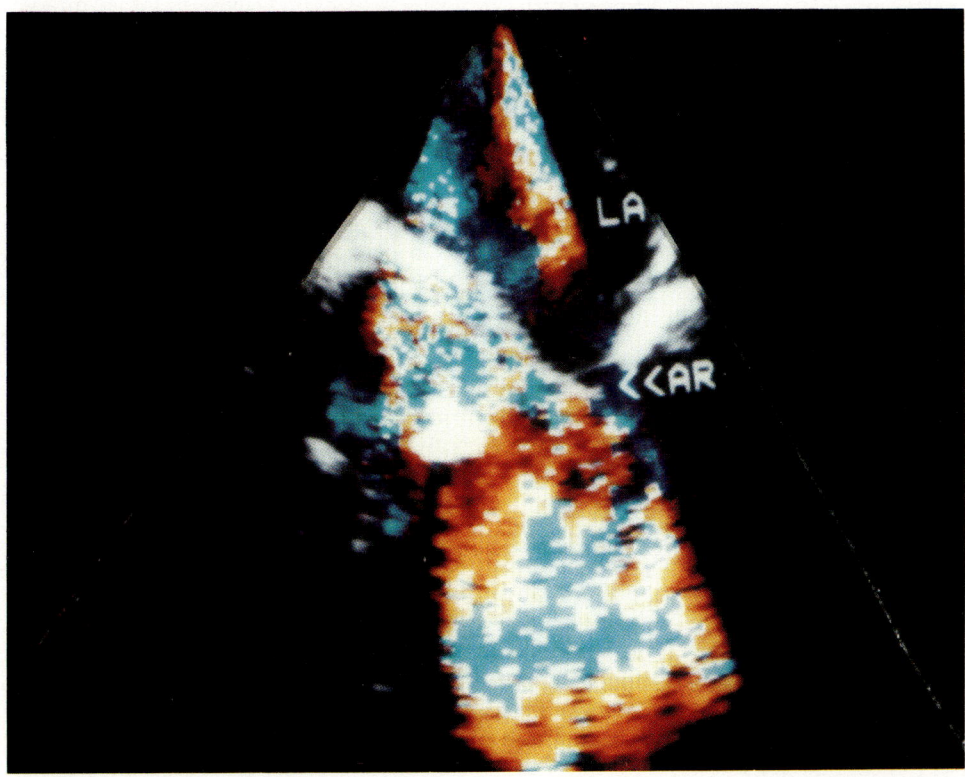

Fig. 33–12. Mosaic colored jet in left ventricular outflow trace representing aortic regurgitation by color flow Doppler by transesophageal echocardiography. LA, Left atrium; AR, aortic regurgitation.

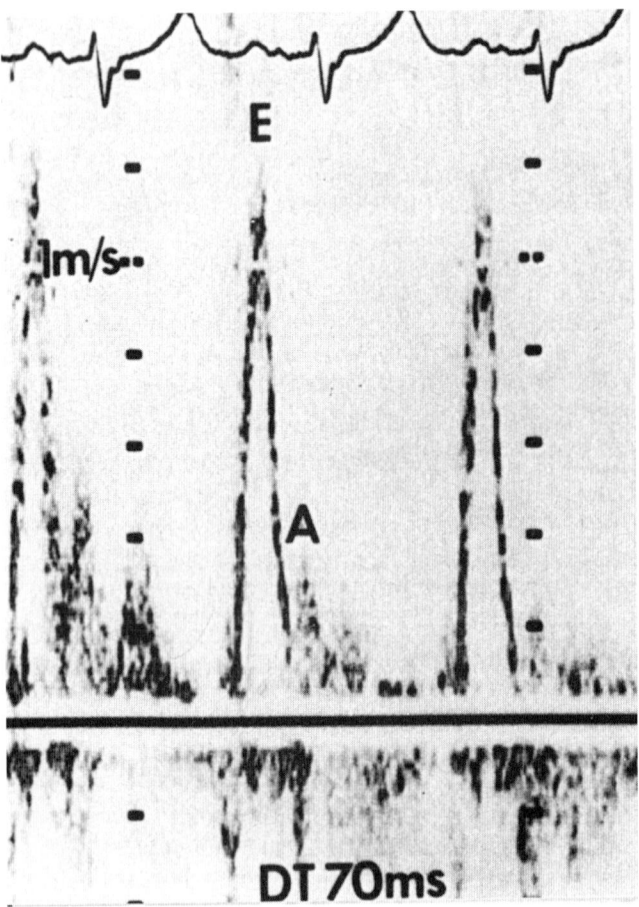

Fig. 33–13. Pulsed wave Doppler recording of the left ventricular inflow in a patient with severe aortic regurgitation. There is an increased E (early) velocity versus A (atrial contraction) velocity, an increased E/A ratio of 4.0, and short deceleration time of E wave filling (70 msec), showing "restrictive physiology." (From Klein, A. L., Davison, M. B., Vonk, G., and Tajik, A. J.: Doppler echocardiographic assessment of aortic regurgitation: uses and limitations. Cleve. Clin. J. Med., 59:365, 1992.)

ing for the presence of retrograde flow in the descending aorta. The color beam also helps guide the cursor for continuous wave Doppler studies. Color easily identifies diastolic mitral regurgitation, which is often present in acute aortic regurgitation. Recently, quantitative Doppler techniques with pulsed-wave Doppler have been used to assess regurgitant volumes and regurgitant fractions in aortic regurgitation.[171a]

Oh et al.[172] noted that in symptomatic severe aortic regurgitation, the Doppler mitral inflow velocity pattern is characteristic, with increased early filling wave velocity (E), increased early-to-late filling wave ratio (E/A), and decreased deceleration time of the E wave (Fig. 33-13). This pattern was more sensitive than premature closure of the mitral valve for detecting hemodynamically significant aortic regurgitation. Presently color flow Doppler mapping, however, is the technique of choice for assessing aortic regurgitation noninvasively.

Assessment of Prosthetic Valves. Valvular regurgitation can be seen on TTE using pulsed wave, continuous wave, and color Doppler echocardiographic techniques. Alam et al.[173] examined 183 clinically normal and 58 dysfunctional valves and found regurgitant flow by pulsed wave Doppler in 92% of the abnormal prostheses. Regurgitation was also found in 10% of the aortic tissue valves. Most normal functioning prosthetic valves and tissue valves have mild intrinsic insufficiency, which can be detected by pulsed wave Doppler. TTE images may be of poor quality when prosthetic valves are present. The beam may have difficulty in penetrating past the sewing ring, valve struts, and occluders present in most mechanical devices. This is termed flow masking and can cause aortic insufficiency to be underestimated or undetected. Doppler echocardiography can be used to assess gradients across prosthetic valves and calculate effective orifice areas using the continuity equation.[173a]

Color flow mapping can also be useful in assessing for aortic regurgitation in prosthetic devices. Kapur et al.[174] studied a series of patients with 126 prostheses, 74 with regurgitation by angiography. Complete agreement was found between color flow Doppler and angiographic grade in 90% of 40 mitral prostheses and 74% of 34 aortic prostheses, using a 1+ to 3+ scale. There were a variety of tissue and mechanical devices. The color Doppler was able to differentiate perivalvular from valvular leakage in 94% of mitral and 81% of aortic valves, and these data were confirmed at surgery.

Underestimation by color Doppler, however, may occur because of flow masking as well as eccentricity of the jet. In two studies,[175,176] color flow mapping underestimated the degree of regurgitation in prosthetic valves.

TEE has emerged as a safe, reliable tool in clinical practice. It can evaluate prosthetic valves more accurately owing to less acoustic interference and attenuation artifact. In nine patients with severe prosthetic regurgitation, transthoracic color flow correctly classified three, whereas transesophageal studies were graded correctly in all nine cases.[177] TEE has proved to be invaluable in grading prosthetic aortic regurgitation and should be readily used whenever possible in the evaluation of this entity. TEE has emerged as the "gold standard" in the detection of aortic dissection, compared with CT scanning, MRI, or angiography.[177a]

TEE has proved to be useful in assessing the heart in infective endocarditis. Karalis et al.[178] studied 55 patients with aortic valve endocarditis, 24 of whom had involvement of subaortic structures. These complications included four with abscess in the mitral-aortic intervalvular fibrosa, four with mitral-aortic intervalvular fibrosa aneurysm, seven with perforation of the mitral-aortic intervalvular fibrosa with communication into the left atrium, two with aneurysm of the anterior mitral leaflet, and seven with perforation of the anterior mitral leaflet. These findings were noted by TEE and confirmed by surgery in 20 and by necropsy in 2 patients. TTE noted these complications in 5 of 24 patients and noted eccentric MR-type jets, which suggested the possibility of these unusual subaortic complications, in 8 more patients, for a total of 13 of 24 patients (54%). This study suggests that subaortic complications are more common than previously thought in aortic valve endocarditis, that patients with aortic valve endocarditis and eccentric jets of MR on TTE should undergo TEE to exclude subaortic complications, that recognition of these complications is of value in the treatment of these patients, and that these complications may be responsible for congestive heart failure and unexplained hemodynamic compromise in some patients with aortic valve endocarditis.

Cardiac Catheterization. Right heart catheterization in aortic regurgitation may show an elevated pulmonary artery wedge pressure, pulmonary hypertension, and low or normal cardiac output. Many of these findings can be obtained using Doppler techniques.[69b] Left heart catheterization is indicated in patients with suspected coronary disease and in adults older than 40 years of age, regardless of presence or lack of anginal symptoms.[179] In a study of patients going to aortic valve surgery,[180] patients with electrocardiographic evidence of coronary artery disease had at least one vessel involvement 84% of the time and three vessel or left main trunk involvement 36% of the time. Sixty-four percent of the patients with no evidence of preoperative coronary artery disease had at least one vessel involvement, and 29% had three vessel or left main trunk involvement. The authors concluded that preoperative cardiac catheterization reduced the risk of cardiac complications in aortic surgery.

Cardiac catheterization can document aortic regurgitation and its severity; evaluate left ventricular function; and identify abnormalities in the aorta, mitral valve, and coronary anatomy. Qualitative assessment of aortic regurgitation, however, is subjective.[181] In 1+ aortic regurgitation, a small amount of contrast material enters the left ventricle in diastole, is essentially cleared with each beat, and never fills the ventricular chamber. In 2+ aortic regurgitation, faint opacification of the entire chamber occurs, and with moderately severe (3+) aortic regurgitation, the entire chamber is opacified and equal in density with the ascending aorta. Severe (4+) aortic regurgitation is marked by complete dense opacification of the left ventricular chamber on the first beat, and the left ventricle can appear more densely opacified than the aorta. The aortic valves can be assessed as well with regard to mobility, calcification, and number of cusps. Involvement of the ascending aorta (extent and type of dissection) is evaluated as well. The aortogram is done in the left anterior oblique projection to separate the ascending aorta, arch, and descending aorta.

Radionuclide Imaging. Radionuclide imaging can be used to assess ejection fraction and stroke volume of the left and right ventricles, both at rest and with exercise. By determining regurgitant fraction and left ventricle/right ventricle stroke volume ratio, it can yield an accurate assessment of aortic regurgitation.[182] Resting ejection fraction and volume measurements using radionuclide angiography appear to be useful in determining the need for aortic valve replacement in patients with few or no symptoms.[183] A decline in exercise ejection fraction suggests myocardial impairment. Serial exercise radionuclide testing can be used to detect and follow early left ventricular dysfunction.

MRI is the newest noninvasive method to evaluate aortic regurgitation. MRI is able to measure accurately cardiac dimensions,[184,185] ejection fraction, volumes,[186] and left ventricular mass[187,188] and may help in assessing optimal timing for surgery.[189,190] MRI is able to image the aortic regurgitation directly by several methods.[191] It can assess the degree of aortic regurgitation by comparing right and left ventricular stroke volumes and computing a regurgitant volume. The amount of aortic regurgitation is estimated by the difference in stroke volumes.[192,193] Phase velocity mapping may be an alternative technique for assessing the degree of aortic regurgitation.[194] MRI is excellent for assessment of aortic disease, which is often present in aortic valve disease and is important to define before surgery. MRI is particularly useful in assessing aortic dissection with respect to the proximal and distal extent of dissection, communications between lumina, involvement of arch vessels, and presence or absence of thrombus.[195] A number of the above techniques may be used to verify the extent of the aortic regurgitation and the level of left ventricular dysfunction.

ICU Phase

Once the patient has presented, is stabilized, and has a working differential diagnosis that is actively being evaluated with the above-mentioned techniques, rapid triage to an ICU is imperative for optimal care. Prompt, aggressive management of acute aortic regurgitation is needed in the ICU setting because these patients may be very sick and die without aggressive management. Initial measures should focus on obtaining hemodynamic stability and ensuring adequate tissue oxygenation. The latter may include endotracheal intubation for respiratory failure secondary to severe pulmonary edema. Because of the possible left ventricular dysfunction, ventricular arrhythmias may be present and require aggressive treatment, usually with lidocaine as a first-line medication. The patient should be on telemetry. Hemodynamic monitoring with a Swan-Ganz catheter is important in assessing filling pressures, pulmonary artery pressures, and cardiac output. Prompt surgical consultation should be sought because surgical repair will be required at some point in the management. Prompt diagnosis and determination of cause are extremely important because the underlying predisposing condition usually requires additional intervention.

While waiting for surgery, medical stabilization of the patient is important. Vasodilator drugs, such as nitroprusside, are the most effective drugs for patients with aortic regurgitation. Nitroprusside is both a venodilator and arterial dilator, although the latter effect predominates. Its venodilating properties can help increase peripheral pooling of blood and decrease venous return of blood to the heart and thus help to relieve pulmonary congestion. Dilatation of the arterial vessels reduces afterload and can significantly decrease the amount of aortic regurgitation. It must be given intravenously, has a rapid onset of action, and has a short half-life, so its hemodynamic effects can quickly be reversed should untoward effects, such as systemic hypotension, ensue. The dose of the drug is titrated against the reduction in wedge pressure. It can be initiated at 15 to 25 mg per minute and increased by 5 to 10 mg per minute until the wedge pressure is less than 15 mm Hg. Side effects include tremulousness, respiratory distress, nausea, vomiting, seizures, hypothyroidism, methemoglobinemia, lactic acidosis, vitamin B_{12} deficiency, and decreased platelet function. Nitroprusside is metabolized to thiocyanate in the liver, and toxic levels of this substance may develop if the drug is given for several days, especially in patients with renal failure.

Loop diuretics, such as furosemide and bumetanide, may be useful in relieving signs and symptoms of pulmonary congestion but do not affect the amount of aortic regurgitation present. Inotropic drugs, such as dobutamine, may be of some value in aortic regurgitation, although myocardial contractility may already be elevated secondary to increased myocardial stretch and elevated circulating levels of catecholamines. Vasopressor agents are contraindicated because an increase in systemic vascular resistance would increase the amount of aortic regurgitation. Intravenous nitroglycerin may be useful as a venodilator in patients with ongoing angina and evidence of ischemia. Intra-aortic balloon counterpulsation is contraindicated because balloon inflation during diastole would increase the amount of aortic regurgitation. In patients with endocarditis as the underlying cause of aortic regurgitation, prompt treatment with broad-spectrum antibiotics should be initiated.

In patients with chronic aortic regurgitation, who are hemodynamically decompensated, surgery is the treatment of choice. If a patient is not a surgical candidate, long-term therapy with a vasodilator, such as an ACE inhibitor, nifedipine, or hydralazine, along with a diuretic and possibly digoxin would be useful. In patients with severe aortic regurgitation, who are not surgical candidates, the long-term prognosis is poor.

Surgical Management

Aortic valve replacement with a biologic or prosthetic valve, along with replacement of the ascending aorta and repair of any other defects when indicated, is the definitive treatment of aortic regurgitation. The choice between a biologic and a mechanical valve is based on a number of variables. The mechanical valve has a better durability and a longer half-life but is prone to thrombus formation and embolization, requiring long-term treatment with warfarin. The biologic valve has a much smaller risk of thromboemboli complication but is much less durable.

In patients with active endocarditis and severe aortic regurgitation, the trend is moving toward earlier surgical intervention. Surgical mortality in several reports[196-199] ranges from 8 to 20%, with increased mortality in patients with severe preoperative left ventricular dysfunction, multiorgan system failure, staphylococcal septicemia, fungal infection, elevated blood urea nitrogen and creatinine, and annular abscess. The prognosis for prosthetic endocarditis was worse in several series,[200-202] with mortality ranging from 7 to 33%. These data supported an aggressive early approach to surgery. In patients with prosthetic valve endocarditis, postoperative complications occurred at an increased rate compared with patients who had surgery for native valve endocarditis.

The primary indications for surgery in patients with aortic regurgitation secondary to endocarditis are:

- Congestive heart failure[203-205]
- Multiple systemic emboli[206,207]
- Fungal endocarditis
- Uncontrolled infection
- Left-to-right cardiac shunt[208]
- Conduction disturbance

The question of which valve, bioprosthetic or mechanical, to use in endocarditis is an important one. The bioprosthetic valve is more resistant to infection early on but less resistant late in the postoperative course.[209] The best results have been obtained with an aortic homograft. This valve has the lowest incidence of postoperative infection because there is no cloth or metal to interact with infected tissue.

In patients with aortic regurgitation secondary to aortic dissection, the earliest surgical intervention is recommended.[210,211] Ascending aortic dissection has a poor natural history without surgical intervention. The mortality rate at 24 hours is 21%; at 48 hours, 37%; at 2 weeks, 74%; and at 3 months, 90%. Operative mortality ranges from 8 to 30%, depending on the series.[212-217] Stroke and renal failure were the major determinants of postoperative outcome.[218]

With aortic dissection, the goal is to reconstruct the insufficient aortic valve and resuspend it on the aortic graft. If the valve cannot be reconstructed or if the patient has Marfan syndrome, a composite graft-valve conduit must be used, and the coronary arteries must be reimplanted into the graft.

In patients with blunt or sharp trauma to the chest, the aortic valve can frequently be injured. Aortic valve replacement is usually necessary in traumatic aortic regurgitation.[219,220] Repair with a pericardial patch may occasionally be done.[221]

A rare cause of severe aortic regurgitation is percutaneous balloon valvuloplasty for severe aortic stenosis. These may improve spontaneously or may require surgical repair.

Other procedures, including coronary artery bypass grafting, abscess drainage, and repair of any other chest trauma, may also be necessary at the time of surgery.

Aortic valvuloplasty or aortic valve repair is becoming an increasingly popular procedure for aortic regurgitation. It maintains the normal valvular architecture and does not require long-term anticoagulation. Carpentier[222] described a series of 95 patients with severe aortic regurgitation who underwent repair from 1971 through 1982. Hospital mortality was 3.3%. Reoperation was necessary 13% of the time for significant residual regurgitation. There was moderate residual aortic regurgitation in 15% not requiring surgery. Repair was possible in about 80% of congenital malformations of the aortic valve but in only about 5% of those with rheumatic aortic regurgitation. Al Fagin et al.[223] described a series of 20 patients with severe rheumatic aortic regurgitation. Repair was done with the use of individually tailored bovine pericardial extensions to the native cusps. There was marked reduction or total correction of the aortic regurgitation over a mean follow-up of 7.5 months. Duran et al.[224] described a series of 107 patients who had

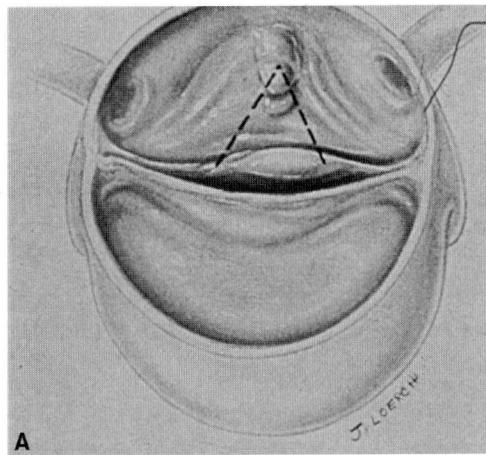

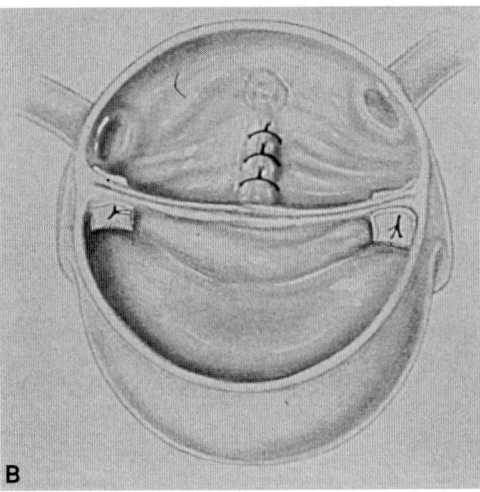

Fig. 33-14. Diagrammatic representation of aortic valve repair for aortic regurgitation. A, When aortic insufficiency results from degenerative disease or valve anomalies, a triangular resection is first made in the free edge of the elongated valve cusp to reduce cusp length to normal. B, The defect is then closed, and sutures are placed at the commissures to reduce annular size and increase cusp coaptation.

aortic valve repair from July 1988 through July 1990. Eighty-four percent were rheumatic; 69 had repair with annular and leaflet plasties, and 38 had cusp extensions with glutaraldehyde-treated pericardium. Death occurred in 1.8%; 4.7% were anticoagulated. There were four reoperations for aortic valve dysfunction. Cusp extension appeared to have a better result than repair. Cosgrove et al.[225] described a series of 28 patients who underwent aortic valvuloplasty for aortic regurgitation caused by leaflet prolapse (Fig. 33-14). The procedure consisted of triangular resection of the free edge of the prolapsing leaflet, annular plication at the commissure, and resection of a raphe when present in bicuspid valves. Seventy-five percent had bicuspid valves in this series. There was a decrease in aortic regurgitation from grade. Death occurred in one patient secondary to intraoperative stroke. One patient required reoperation for recurrent aortic regurgitation caused by partial suture line dehiscence. In 15 patients with late echocardiograms, there was no progression of aortic regurgitation. Intraoperative TEE and epicardial echocardiography are being used increasingly during the repair procedure to look for persistent regurgitation. Progress is being made in aortic valve repair, although it is still in the evolving stage and has limited application at the present time.

Post-ICU Phase

Postoperative Recovery and Evaluation

The immediate postoperative care of the patient with an aortic valve repair or replacement consists of fluid management, hemodynamic monitoring, ventilator management, and treatment of arrhythmias. Patients recovering from valve surgery require close cardiac follow-up, particularly in the early weeks to months. Patients may develop any complication associated with open cardiac surgery in the first few days or weeks after operation. Besides early postoperative hemorrhage, acute Q wave or non-Q wave myocardial infarction, cerebral hemorrhage or embolus, renal failure, infection, and hepatitis are important possible complications. The laboratory and hemodynamic markers of these problems require close attention. Once stable, serial echocardiograms are required to assess function of the prosthetic valve or integrity of a repair. We recommend at least one postoperative echocardiogram with the patient in stable condition, either before hospital discharge or at 6-week follow-up to be used as a baseline study. This is usually followed by evaluation with echocardiogram every 6 months to 1 year thereafter as needed.

Anticoagulation

Anticoagulation is a routine part of the postoperative care. Patients receiving a mechanical valve require lifelong anticoagulation. Heparin may be started initially with transition to warfarin preparations. If the patient has been stable and no further interventions are planned, the latter may be started directly on approximately postoperative day 3 or 4. Therapeutic anticoagulation is achieved with prothrombin times 1.6 to 1.9 times control value and INR of 2.5 to 3.5.[126] A prothrombin time greater than 2.0 times control is associated with an increased risk of bleeding without further reduction in incidence of thromboembolic events.[128] At recommended doses, the incidence of anticoagulant-associated bleeding is reported to be approximately 1.0 to 1.5% per year with a 2 to 4% risk of thromboembolism.[129]

Endocarditis Prophylaxis

Patients with infective endocarditis require a full course of antibiotic treatment and confirmation of infection-free status. Thereafter endocarditis antibiotic prophylaxis is recommended for all patients after having undergone aortic valve replacement and probably repair. Patients with prosthetic aortic valves constitute the group at greatest risk, with an overall incidence of 2 to 4%. Prosthetic valve endocarditis occurring within 2 months of surgery carries a high mortality rate of 63 to 88%,[132,133] whereas late onset has a lower mortality rate of 25 to 45%.[134] Early reoperation when necessary can be lifesaving. Patients are counseled on signs and symptoms of endovascular infection and the high risk procedures requiring prior antibiotic administration. In addition, all are given a wallet-sized pamphlet containing the most recent American Medical Association guidelines.

Management of the Underlying Disorder

Close follow-up and treatment of the underlying disorder predisposing toward acute aortic regurgitation are important because many of the diseases (most notably the connective tissue disorders) are progressive. Patients with Marfan syndrome require close follow-up for aortic valve regurgitation, aortic aneurysm, and aortic dissection. Primary myxomatous degeneration may involve other cardiac valves producing recurrent regurgitation. Rheumatic fever may necessitate long-term suppressive therapy with antibiotics. Systemic lupus erythematosus is a systemic disorder that may require lifelong medical therapy and close follow-up. These and other disorders that predispose to recurrent valvular incompetence require attention and treatment in the post-ICU, predischarge phase.

REFERENCES

1. Dalen, J. E.: Mitral stenosis. *In* Valvular Heart Disease. 2nd ed. Edited by J. E. Dalen and J. S. Alpert. Boston, Little, Brown & Company, 1987.
2. Selzer, A.: Effects of atrial fibrillation upon circulation in patients with mitral stenosis. Am. Heart J., 59:518, 1960.
3. Selzer, A.: Nonrheumatic mitral regurgitation. Mod. Concepts Cardiovasc. Dis., 48:168, 1979.
4. Sanders, C. A., Scannell, J. A., and Harthorne, J. W.: Severe mitral regurgitation secondary to ruptured chordae tendinae. Circulation, 47:248, 1965.
5. Marcus, R. H., et al.: Functional anatomy of severe mitral regurgitation in active rheumatic carditis. Am. J. Cardiol., 63:577, 1989.
6. Oliveiria, D. B. G., Dawkins, K. D., Kay, P. H., and Paneth, M.: Chordal rupture. I. Aetiology and natural history. Br. Heart J., 50:312, 1983.
7. Roberts, W. C., Dangel, J. C., and Bulkley, B. H.: Nonrheumatic valvular cardiac disease: A clinicopathologic survey of 27 different conditions causing valvular dysfunction. *In* Cardiovascular Clinics. Valvular Heart Disease. Edited by W. Likoff. Philadelphia, F. A. Davis, 1973.
8. Tresch, D. D., et al.: Mitral valve prolapse requiring surgery: Clinical and pathological study. Am. J. Med., 78:245, 1985.
9. Paget, S. A., et al.: Mitral valve disease of systemic lupus erythematosus. A cause of severe congestive heart failure reversed by mitral valve replacement. Am. J. Med., 59:134, 1975.
10. Stewart, S. R., Robbins, D. L., and Castles, J. J.: Acute fulminant aortic and mitral insufficiency in ankylosing spondylitis. N. Engl. J. Med., 229:1448, 1967.
11. Penny, J. L., et al.: Calcified left atrial myxoma simulating mitral insufficiency. Circulation, 36:417, 1967.
12. Abascal, V. M., et al.: Mitral regurgitation after percutaneous mitral valvuloplasty in adults: Evaluation of pulsed Doppler echocardiography. J. Am. Coll. Cardiol., 11:257, 1988.
13. McLaughlin, J. S., Cowley, R. A., and Smith, G.: Mitral valve disease from blunt trauma. J. Thorac. Cardiovasc. Surg., 48:261, 1974.
14. Selzer, A., and Katayama, F.: Mitral regurgitation: clinical patterns, pathophysiology, and natural history. Medicine, 51:343, 1972.
15. Hickey, A. J., Wilcken, D. E. L., Wright, J. S., and Warren, B. A.: Primary (spontaneous) chordal rupture: relation to myxomatous valve disease and mitral valve prolapse. J. Am. Coll. Cardiol., 5:1341, 1985.
16. Roberts, W. C., Dangel, J. C., and Bulkley, B. H.: Nonrheumatic valvular cardiac disease: a clinicopathologic survey of 27 different conditions causing valvular dysfunciton. *In* Cardiovascular Clinics. Valvular Heart Disease. Edited by W. Likoff. Philadelphia, F. A. Davis, 1973.
17. Simpson, J. W., Nora, J. J., and McNamara, D. G.: Marfan's syndrome and mitral valve disease. Acute surgical emergencies. Am. Heart J., 77:96, 1969.
18. Parmlley, W. C., Mattingly, T. W., and Manim, L. F.: Penetrating wounds of the heart and aorta. Circulation, 17:953, 1958.
19. Hwang, W. S., and Lam, K. L.: Rupture of the chordae tendineae during acute rheumatic carditis. Br. Heart J., 30:429, 1968.
20. Daves, R. K., and Paneth, M.: Acute mitral regurgitation in pregnancy due to ruptured chordae. Br. Heart J., 34:541, 1972.
21. Wei-Xi, Z., et al.: Mitral regurgitation due to ruptured chorde tenineae in patients with hypertrophic obstructive cardiomyopathy. J. Am. Coll. Cardiol., 20:242, 1992.
22. Estes, E. H., Jr., et al.: The anatomy and blood supply of the papillary muscles of the left ventricle. Am. Heart J., 71:356, 1966.
23. Rankin, J. S., et al.: Ischemic mitral regurgitation. Circulation, 97(Suppl. I):I-116, 1989.
24. Wei, J. Y., Hutchins, G. M., and Bulkley, B. H.: Papillary muscle rupture in fatal acute myocardial infarction. A potentially treatable form of cardiogenic shock. Ann. Intern. Med., 90:149, 1979.
25. Roberts, W. C., and Cohen, L. S.: Left ventricular papillary muscles: description of normal and a survey of conditions causing them to be abnormal. Circulation, 46:138, 1972.
26. Kremkkau, E. L., Gilbertson, P. R., and Bristow, I. D.: Acquired nonrheumatic mitral regurgitation: clinical management with emphasis on evaluation of myocardial performance. Prog. Cardiovasc. Dis., 15:414, 1973.
27. Zoneraich, S., et al.: Myocardial sarcoidosis presenting as acute mitral insufficiency. Chest, 66:452, 1974.
28. Jolly, D. T.: Traumatic rupture of a papillary muscle of the mitral valve due to blunt thoracic trauma. Can. Fam. Phys., 29:1960, 1983.
29. Baumgartner, W. A., et al.: Surgical treatment of prosthetic valve endocarditis. Ann. Thorac. Surg., 35:87, 1983.
30. Dismukes, W. E.: Prosthetic valve endocarditis: factors influencing outcome and recommendations for therapy. *In* Treatment of Endocarditis. Edited by A. Bismo. New York, Grune & Stratton, 1981.
31. Dougherty, S. H., and Simmons, R. L.: Infections in implanted prosthetic devices: prosthetic valve endocarditis. Curr. Probl. Surg., 19:269, 1982.
32. Jones, E. L., Schwarzmann, S. W., Check, W. A., and Hatcher, C. R.: Complications from cardiac prostheses infections, thrombosis, and emboli associated with intracardiac prostheses. *In* Sabiston's Surgery of the Chest. Edited by D. C. Sabiston and F. C. Spencer. Philadelphia, W. B. Saunders, 1983.
33. Samaan, H. A.: Acute massive mitral regurgitation resulting from disc valve replacement of the mitral valve. J. Cardiovasc. Surg., 36:77, 1966.
34. Carlson, C. J., et al.: Mitral regurgitation due to intermittent prosthetic valvular dysfunction. Chest, 71:90, 1977.

35. Ericcsson, A., et al.: Strut fracture with Bjork-Shiley 70 degrees convexo-concave valve. An international multi-institutional follow-up study. Eur. J. Cardiothorac. Surg., 6:339, 1992.
36. Eckberg, D. L., et al.: Mechanics of left ventricular contraction in chronic severe mitral regurgitation. Circulation, 47:1252, 1973.
37. Braunwald, E., Welch, G. H., Jr., and Sarnoff, S. J.: Hemodynamic effects of quantitatively varied experimental mitral regurgitation. Circ. Res., 5:539, 1957.
38. Braunwald, E., and Turi, Z. G.: Pathophysiology of mitral valve disease. In Ionescu's Mitral Valve Disease. Diagnosis and Treatment. Edited by M. I. Ionescu and L. H. Cohn. London, Butterworths, 1985, p. 3.
39. Braunwald, E.: Control of myocardial oxygen consumption. Physiologic and clinical considerations. Am. J. Cardiol., 27:416, 1971.
40. Cheitlin, M. D., and Ardehali, A.: Acute valvular regurgitation. In Cardiology. Edited by W. W. Parmley and K. Chatterjee. Philadelphia, J. B. Lippincott, 1991.
41. Grose, R., Strain, J., and Cohen, M. V.: Pulmonary arterial V waves in mitral regurgitation. Clinical and experimental observations. Circulation, 69:214, 1984.
42. Braunwald, E., and Awe, W. C.: The syndrome of severe mitral regurgitation with normal left atrial pressure. Circulation, 27:29, 1963.
43. Roberts, W. C., Braunwald, E., and Morrow, A. G.: Acute severe mitral regurgitation secondary to ruptured chordae tendineae. Clinical, hemodynamic, and pathologic considerations. Circulation, 33:58, 1966.
44. Heikklia, J.: Mitral incompetence complicating acute myocardial infarction. Br. Heart J., 29:162, 1967.
45. Brand, E. R., Berge, K. G., and Brown, A. L.: Papillary muscles in myocardial infarction. Circulation, 68:183, 1967.
46. Cheng, T. O.: Some new observations on the syndrome of papillary muscle dysfunction. Am. J. Med., 47:924, 1969.
47. Burch, G. E., De Pasquale, N. P., and Phillips, J. H.: The clinical manifestations of papillary dysfunction. Arch. Intern. Med., 12:158, 1963.
48. Tei, C., et al.: Mitral valve prolapse in short-term experimental coronary occlusion: a possible mechanism of ischemic mitral regurgitation. Circulation, 68:183, 1983.
49. Hirakawa, S., et al.: In situ measurement of the papillary muscle dynamics in the dog left ventricle. Am. J. Physiol., 233:H384, 1977.
50. Godley, R. W., et al.: Incomplete mitral leaflet closure in patients with papillary muscle dysfunction. Circulation, 441:174, 1981.
51. Kono, T., et al.: Mechanism of functional mitral regurgitation during acute myocardial ischemia. J. Am. Coll. Cardiol., 19:1101, 1992.
52. Miller, G. E., Cohn, K. E., Kerth, W. J., and Selzer, A.: Experimental papillary muscle infarction. J. Thorac. Cardiovasc. Surg., 56:611, 1968.
53. Ogawa, S., Hubbard, F. E., Mardelli, T. J., and Dreifus, L. S.: Cross-sectional echocardiographic spectrum of papillary muscle dysfunction. Am. Heart J., 97:312, 1979.
54. Kinney, E. L., and Frangi, M. J.: Value of two-dimensional echocardiographic detection of incomplete mitral leaflet closure. Am. Heart J., 109:87, 1985.
55. Becker, E., and Anderson, R. H.: Mitral insufficiency complicating acute miocardial infarction. Eur. J. Cardiol., 2:351, 1975.
56. Rippe, J. M., et al.: Primary myxomatous degeneration of cardiac valves: a clinical, pathological, hemodynamic, and echocardiographic profile. Br. Heart J., 44:621, 1980.
57. Jaffe, A. S., Geltman, E. M., and Rodel, G. E.: Mitral valve prolapse: a consistent manifestation of type IV Ehlers-Danlos syndrome: the pathogenic role of abnormal production of type III collagen. Circulation, 64:121, 1981.
58. Gaffney, F. A., et al.: Abnormal cardiovascular regulation in the mitral valve prolapse syndrome. Am. J. Cardiol., 52:316, 1983.
59. Venkatesh, A., et al.: Mitrazl valve prolapse in anxiety neurosis (panic disorder). Am. Heart J., 100:302, 1983.
60. Nishimura, R. A., et al.: Papillary muscle rupture complicating acute myocardial infarction. Analysis of 17 patients. Am. J. Cardiol., 51:373, 1983.
61. Sanders, R. J., Neubeurger, K. T., and Ravin, B. H.: Rupture of papillary muscles: occurrence of rupture of the posterior muscle in posterior myocardial infarction. Dis. Chest., 31:316, 1957.
62. Reichek, N., Shelburne, J. D., and Perloff, J. R.: Clinical aspects of rheumatic valve disease. Prog. Cardiovasc. Dis., 15:491, 1973.
63. Perloff, J. K.: Physical Examination of the Heart and Circulation. 2nd Ed. Philadelphia, W. B. Saunders, 1990.
64. Antman, E. M., Angoff, G. H., and Sloss, J. J.: Demonstration of the mechanism by which mitral regurgitation mimics aortic stenosis. Am. J. Cardiol., 42:1044, 1978.
65. Merendins, K. A., and Hessel, E. A.: The murmur on the top of the head in acquired mitral insufficiency. JAMA, 199:392, 1967.
66. Phillips, J. H., Burch, G. E., De Pasquale, N. P.: The syndrome of papillary muscle dysfunction. Ann. Intern. Med., 59:508, 1963.
67. Luther, R. R., and Meyers, S. N.: Acute mitral insufficiency secondary to ruptured chordae tendineae. Arch. Intern. Med., 134:568, 1974.
68. Lehmann, K. G., Francis, C. K., Dodge, H. T., and TIMI Study Group: Mitral regurgitation in early myocardial infarction. Incidence, clinical detection, and prognostic implications. Ann. Intern. Med., 117:10, 1992.
69. Raphael, M. J., Steiner, R. E., and Raftery, E. D.: Acute mitral incompetence. Clin. Radiol., 18:126, 1967.
69a. Kuecherer, H. F., et al.: Estimation of mean left atrial pressure from transesophageal pulse Doppler echocardiography of pulmonary venous blood flow. Circulation, 82:1127, 1990.
69b. Nishimura, R. A., and Tasik, A. J.: Quantitative hemodynamics by Doppler echocardiography: a noninvasive alternative to cardiac catheterization. Prog. Cardiovasc. Dis., 36:309, 1994.
70. Mintz, G. S., et al.: Two-dimensional echocardiographic recognition of a ruptured chordae tendineae. Circulation, 57:598, 1978.
71. Stewart, W. J., et al.: Evaluation of mitral leaflet motion by echocardiography and jet direction by Doppler color flow mapping to determine the mechanism of mitral regurgitation. J. Am. Coll. Cardiol., 20:1353, 1992.
72. Gilbert, B. W., et al.: Two-dimensional echocardiographic assessment of vegetative endocarditis. Circulation, 55:346, 1977.
73. Martin, R. P., et al.: Clinical utility of two-dimensional echocardiography in infective endocarditis. Am. J. Cardiol., 43:738, 1979.
74. Cohen, G. I., et al.: A comparison of flow convergence with other transthoracic echocardiographic indexes of prosthetic mitral regurgitation. J. Am. Soc. Echocardiogr., 5:620, 1992.
75. Khandheria, B. K., et al.: Value and limitations of transesophageal echocardiography in assessment of mitral valve prostheses. Circulation, 83:1956, 1991.
76. Seward, J. B., et al.: Transesophageal echocardiography:

77. Klein, A. L., et al.: Effects of mitral regurgitation on pulmonary venous flow and left atrial pressure: an intraoperative transesophageal echocardiographic study. J. Am. Coll. Cardiol., *20:*1345, 1992.
78. Sechtem, V., et al.: Mitral or aortic regurgitation: quantification of regurgitant volumes with cine MR imaging. Radiology, *167:*425, 1988.
79. Utz, J. A., et al.: Valvular regurgitation: dynamic cine MR imaging. Radiology, *168:*91, 1988.
80. Mitchell, L., et al.: Diagnosis and assessment of mitral and aortic valve disease by cine-flow MRI. Magn. Reson. Med., *12:*181, 1988.
81. Nishimura, T., Yamada, N., Itoh, A., and Kunio, M.: Cine MR imaging in mitral regurgitation: comparison with color Doppler flow imaging. AJR Am. J. Roentgenol., *153:*721, 1989.
82. Schwinger, M., Cohen, M., and Fuster, V.: Usefulness of onset of the pulmonary wedge V wave in predicting mitral regurgitation. Am. J. Cardiol., *62:*646, 1988.
83. Meister, S. G., and Helfant, R. H.: Rapid bedside differentiation of ruptured interventricular septum from acute mitral insufficiency. N. Engl. J. Med., *287:*1024, 1972.
83a. Chandraratna, P. A. N., et al.: Echocardiographic observations in ventricular septal rupture. Circulation, *51:*506, 1975.
84. Grossman, W.: Cardiac catheterization, angiography and intervention. *In* Profiles in Valvular Heart Disease. 4th Ed. Edited by W. Grossman and D. S. Baim. Philadelphia, Lea & Febiger, 1991, p. 557.
85. Heuser, R. R., et al.: Coronary angioplasty for acute mitral regurgitation due to acute myocardial infarction. Ann. Intern. Med., *107:*852, 1987.
86. Kusiak, V., and Brest, A. N.: Acute mitral regurgitation: pathophysiology and management. *In* Cardiovascular Clinics. Valvular Heart Disease: Comprehensive Evaluation and Management. Edited by W. S. Frankyl and A.N. Brest. Philadelphia, F. A. Davis, 1986.
87. Hickey, M. St. J., et al.: Current prognosis of ischemic mitral regurgitation: implications for future management. Circulation, *78(Suppl. I):*I-51, 1988.
88. Tcheng, J. E., et al.: Outcome of patients sustaining acute ischemic mitral regurgitation during myocardial infarction. Ann. Intern. Med., *117:*18, 1992.
89. Palmer, R. F., and Lasseter, K. C.: Sodium nitroprusside. N. Engl. J. Med., *292:*294, 1975.
90. Yoran, C., et al.: Mechanism of reduction of mitral regurgitation with vasodilation therapy. Am. J. Cardiol., *43:*773, 1979.
91. Chatterjee, K., and Parmley, W. W.: The role of vasodilator therapy in heart failure. Progr. Cardiovas. Dis., *19:*301, 1977.
92. Greenburg, R. H., Massie, B. M., and Braindodge, B. H.: Beneficial effects of hydralazine in severe mitral regurgitation. Circulation, *58:*673, 1978.
93. Kyron, J., and Bristow, J. D.: The use of vasodilator agents in acute and chronic valvular regurgitation. *In* Cardiology. Edited by W. W. Parmley and K. Chatterjee. Philadelphia, J. B. Lippincott, 1991.
94. Kusiak, V., and Goldberg, S.: Percutaneous intraaortic balloon counterpulsation. Cardiovasc. Clin., *15:*281, 1985.
95. Austin, W. G., et al.: Ruptured papillary muscle: report of a case with successful mitral valve replacement. Circulation, *32:*597, 1965.
96. Kishon, K., et al.: Mitral valve operation in postinfarction rupture of a papillary muscle: immediate results and long-term follow-up of 22 patients. Mayo Clin. Proc., *67:*1023, 1992.
97. Clemments, S. D., et al.: Ruptured papillary muscle, a complication of myocardial infarction: clinical presentation, diagnosis, and treatment. Clin. Cardiol., *8:*93, 1985.
98. Pitarys, C. J., III, Forman, M. B., Panayiotou, H., and Hansen, D. E.: Long term effects of excision of the mitral apparatus on global and regional left ventricular functions in humans. J. Am. Coll. Cardiol., *15:*557, 1990.
99. David, T. E., and Ho, W. C.: The effect of preservation of chordae tendineae on mitral valve replacement for postinfarction mitral regurgitation. Circulation, *74(Suppl. I):*I-116, 1986.
100. Cohn, L. H., et al.: Mitral valve repair for myxomatous degeneration and prolapse of the mitral valve. J. Cardiovasc. Surg., *98:*987, 1989.
101. Kay, J. H., et al.: Mitral valve repair for significant mitral insufficiency. Am. Heart J., *96:*253, 1986.
102. Perier, P., et al.: Comparative evaluation of mitral valve repairs and replacements with Starr Bjork, and porcine valve prostheses. Circulation, *70(Suppl.):*I-187, 1984.
103. Carpentier, A., et al.: Reconstructive surgery of mitral valve incompetence: ten-year appraisal. J. Thorac. Cardiovasc. Surg., *79:*338, 1980.
104. Loisance, D. Y., Deleuze, M. L., and Cachera, J. P.: Are there indications for reconstructive surgery in severe mitral regurgitation after acute myocardial infarction. Eur. J. Cardiothorac. Surg., *4:*394, 1990.
105. Henderson, W. G., et al.: Mitral valve repair for ischemic mitral insufficiency. Ann. Thorac. Surg., *52:*1246, 1991.
106. Cohen, L. H.: Surgical treatment of postinfarction rupture of a papillary muscle [edit.]. Mayo Clin. Proc., *67:*1109, 1992.
107. Radiford, M. J. et al.: Survival following mitral valve replacement for mitral regurgitation due to coronary artery disease. Circulation, *74(Suppl. I):*I-139, 1979.
108. Kay, G. L., et al.: Mitral valve repair for mitral regurgitation secondary to coronary artery disease. Circulation, *74(Suppl. I):*I-188, 1986.
109. Miller, D. C., et al.: Impact of simultaneous myocardial revascularization on operative risk, functional risk, and survival following mitral valve replacement. Surgery, *84:*848, 1978.
110. Killen, D. A., et al.: Surgical treatment of papillary muscle rupture. Ann. Thorac. Surg., *35:*243, 1983.
111. Dreyfus, G., et al.: Valve repair in acute endocarditis. Ann. Thorac. Surg., *49:*706, 1990.
112. Czer, L. S. C., et al.: Intraoperative evaluation of mitral regurgitation by Doppler color flow mapping. Circulation, *76(Suppl. III):*III-108, 1987.
113. Kenny, J., et al.: Doppler echocardiographic evaluation of ring mitral valvuloplasty for pure mitral regurgitation. Am. J. Cardiol., *59:*341, 1987.
114. Reichert, S. L. A., et al.: Intraoperative transesophageal color-coded Doppler echocardiography for the evaluation of residual regurgitation after mitral valve repair. J. Thorac. Cardiovasc. Surg., *100:*756, 1990.
115. Kleinman, J. P., et al.: A quantitative comparison of transesophageal and epicardial color Doppler echocardiography in the intraoperative assessment of mitral regurgitation. Am. J. Cardiol., *64:*1168, 1989.
116. Weldon, C. S., et al.: Clinical recognition and surgical management of acute disruption of the mitral valve. Ann. Surg., *175:*1000, 1972.
117. Cohn, L. H.: Surgical treatment of valvular heart disease. Am. J. Surg., *67:*349, 1974.
118. Salomon, N. W., et al.: Patient-related factors as predictors

119. Merin, G., et al.: Surgery for mitral valve incompetence after myocardial infarction. Am. J. Cardiol., *32*:322, 1973.
120. Mary, D. A., Pakrashi, B. C., and Ionescu, M. I.: Papillary muscle rupture following myocardial infarction. Successful treatment by resection of the akinetic left ventricular area, mitral valve replacement, and aorta to coronary artery bypass graft. Thorax, *28*:390, 1973.
121. Kouchoukos, N. T.: Surgical treatment of acute complications of myocardial infarction. Cardiovasc. Clin., *11*:141, 1981.
122. Bolooki, H.: Emergency cardiac procedures in patients in cardiogenic shock due to complications of coronary artery disease. Circulation, *79(Suppl. I)*:I-137, 1989.
123. Nishimura, R. A., Schaff, H. V., and Gersh, B. J.: Early repair of mechanical complications after acute myocardial infarction. JAMA, *256*:47, 1986.
124. Montoya, A., et al.: Early repair of ventricular septal rupture after myocardial infarction. Am. J. Cardiol., *45*:345, 1980.
125. Rankin, J. S., et al.: Current management of mitral valve incompetence associated with coronary artery disease. J. Cardiovasc. Surg., *4*:25, 1989.
126. Rahimtoola, S. H.: Lessons learned about the determinants of the results of heart surgery. Circulation, *78*:1503, 1988.
127. Hirsh, J. H., Dalen, J. E., and Poller, L.: Oral anticoagulants. Mechanism of action, clinical effectiveness, and optimal therapeutic range. Chest, *102(Suppl.)*:312S, 1992.
128. Rahimtoola, S. H.: Perspectives on valvular heart disease: update II. *In* An Era in Cardiovascular Medicine. Edited by S. B. Knoebel and S. Dack. New York, Elsevier, 1991, p. 45.
129. Bloomfield, P., et al.: A prospective evauation of the Bjork-Shilely, Hancock, and Carpentier-Edwards heart valve prosthesis. Circulation, *73*:12, 1986.
130. Deloche, A., et al.: Valve repair with Carpentier techniques. The second decade. J. Thorac. Cardiovasc. Surg., *99*:990, 1990.
131. Cosgrove, D. M., and Stewart, W. J.: Mitral valvuloplasty. Curr. Probl. Cardiol., *19*:7, 1989.
132. Arnett, E. N., and Roberts, W. C.: Prosthetic valve endocarditis. Am. J. Cardiol., *38*:281, 1976.
133. Wilson, W. R., et al.: Prosthetic valve endocarditis. Ann. Intern. Med., *7*:751, 1975.
134. Child, J. A., Darrell, J. H., Rhys, D. N., and Davies-Dawson, L.: Mixed infective endocarditis in a heroin addict. J. Med. Microbiol., *2*:293, 1969.
135. Dervan, J., and Goldberg, S.: Acute aortic regurgitation: pathophysiology and management. Cardiovasc. Clin., *16*:281, 1986.
136. Morganroth, J., Perloff, J. K., Zeldis, S. M., and Dunkman, W. B.: Acute severe aortic regurgitation—pathophysiology, clinical recognition, and management. Ann. Intern. Med., *87*:223, 1977.
137. Braunwald, E.: Aortic regurgitation. *In* Heart Disease: A Textbook of Cardiovascular Medicine. 4th Ed. Edited by E. Braunwald. Philadelphia, W. B. Saunders, 1992, p. 1043.
138. Stewart, W. J., et al.: Prevalence of aortic valve prolapse with bicuspid aortic valve and its relation to aortic regurgitation: a cross-sectional echocardiographic study. Am. J. Cardiol., *54*:1277, 1984.
139. Roberts, W. C., et al.: Congenitally bicuspid aortic valve causing severe, pure aortic regurgitation without superimposed infective endocarditis. Am. J. Cardiol., *47*:206, 1981.
140. Braniff, B. A., Shumway, N. E., and Harrison, D. C.: Valve replacement in active bacterial endocarditis. N. Engl. J. Med., *276*:1464, 1967.
141. Roberts, W. C.: The congenitally bicuspid aortic valve—a study of 85 autopsy cases. Am. J. Cardiol., *26*:72, 1970.
142. German, D. S., Shapiro, M. J., and Willman, V. L.: Acute aortic valvular incompetence following blunt thoracic deceleration injury: case report. J. Trauma, *30*:1411, 1990.
143. Levine, R. J., Roberts, W. C., and Morrow, A. G.: Traumatic aortic regurgitation. Am. J. Cardiol., *10*:752, 1962.
144. O'Brien, K. P., Hitchcock, G. C., Barratt-Boyes, B. G., and Lowe, J. B.: Spontaneous aortic cusp rupture associated with valvular myxomatous transformation. Circulation, *37*:273, 1968.
145. Marcus, F. I., Ronan, J., Misanik, L. F., and Ewy, G. A.: Aortic insufficiency secondary to spontaneous rupture of a fenestrated leaflet. Am. Heart. J., *66*:675, 1963.
146. Sadaniantz, A., Malhotra, R., and Korr, K. S.: Transient acute severe aortic regurgitation complicating balloon aortic valvuloplasty. Cath. Cardiovasc. Diagn., *17*:186, 1989.
147. Seifert, P. E., and Auer, J. E.: Surgical repair of annular disruption following percutaneous balloon aortic valvuloplasty. Ann. Thorac. Surg., *46*:242, 1988.
148. Alexopoulos, D., and Sherman, W.: Unusual hemodynamic presentation of acute aortic regurgitation following percutaneous balloon valvuloplasty. Am. Heart J., *116*:1622, 1988.
149. Bowness, P., et al.: Complete heart block and severe aortic incompetence in relapsing polychondritis: clinicopathologic findings. Arthritis Rheum., *34*:9, 1991.
150. Comess, K. A., Zibelli, L. R., Gordon, D., and Fredrickson, S. R.: Acute, severe, aortic regurgitation in Behçet's syndrome. Ann. Intern. Med., *99*:639, 1983.
151. Mann, T., McLaurin, L., Grossman, W., and Craige, E.: Assessing the hemodynamic severity of acute aortic regurgitation due to infective endocarditis. N. Engl. J. Med., *293*:108, 1975.
152. Page, A., and Layton, C.: Premature opening of aortic valve in severe aortic regurgitation. Br. Heart J., *37*:1101, 1975.
153. Meyer, T., et al.: Echocardiographic and hemodynamic correlates of diastolic opening of aortic valve in severe aortic regurgitation. Am. J. Cardiol., *59*:1144, 1987.
154. Downes, T. R., et al.: Diastolic mitral regurgitation in acute but not chronic aortic regurgitation: implications regarding the mechanism of mitral closure. Am. Heart J., *117*:1106, 1989.
155. Vanden bossche, J., and Englert, M.: Doppler color flow mapping demonstration of diastolic mitral regurgitation in severe acute aortic regurgitation. Am. Heart J., *114*:889, 1987.
156. Welch, G. H., Braunwald, E., Sarnoff, S. J.: Hemodynamic effects of quantitatively varied experimental aortic regurgitation. Circ. Res., *5*:546, 1957.
157. Sapira, J. D.: Quincke, de Musset, Duroziez, and Hill: some aortic regurgitations. S. Med. J., *74*:459, 1981.
158. Fowler, N. O.: Diagnosis of Heart Disease. New York, Springer-Verlag, 1991.
159. Abdulla, A. M., Frank, M. J., Erdin, R. A., and Canedo, M. I.: Clinical significance and hemodynamic correlates of the third heart sound gallop in aortic regurgitation—a guide to optimal timing of cardiac catheterization. Circulation, *64*:464, 1981.
160. Landzberg, J. S., et al.: Etiology of the Austin Flint Murmur. J. Am. Coll. Cardiol., *20*:408, 1992.
161. Pridie, R. B., Benham, R., and Oakley, C. M.: Echocardiography of the mitral valve in aortic valve disease. Br. Heart J., *33*:296, 1971.
162. Botvinick, E. H., Schiller, N. B., Wickramasekaran, R., and Klausner, S. C.: Echocardiographic demonstration of early

mitral valve closure in severe aortic insufficiency, its clinical implications. Circulation, 51:836, 1975.
163. Tajik, A. J., and Giuliani, E. R.: Diastolic opening of aortic valve—an echographic observation. Mayo Clin. Proc., 52:112, 1977.
163a. Klein, A. L., et al.: Doppler echocardiographic assessment of aortic regurgitation: uses and limitations. Cleve. Clin. J. Med., 59:365, 1992.
164. Esper, R. J.: Detection of mild aortic regurgitation by range-gated pulsed doppler echocardiography. Am. J. Cardiol., 50:1036, 1982.
165. Richards, K. L., Cannon, S. R., Crawford, M. H., and Sorensen, S. G.: Noninvasive diagnosis of aortic and mitral valve disease with pulsed-doppler spectral analysis. Am. J. Cardiol., 51:1122, 1983.
166. Ciobanu, M., et al.: Pulsed Doppler echocardiography in the diagnosis and estimation of severity of aortic insufficiency. Am. J. Cardiol., 49:339, 1982.
167. Kandath, D., and Nanda, N. C.: Assessment of aortic regurgitation by noninvasive techniques. Curr. Probl. Cardiol., 15:45, 1990.
168. Labovitz, A. J., et al.: Quantitative evaluation of aortic insufficiency by continuous wave doppler echocardiography. J. Am. Coll. Cardiol., 8:1341, 1986.
169. Teague, S. M., et al.: Quantification of aortic regurgitation utilizing continuous wave doppler ultrasound. J. Am. Coll. Cardiol., 8:592, 1986.
170. Perry, A. J., et al.: Evaluation of aortic insufficiency by doppler color flow mapping. J. Am. Coll. Cardiol., 9:952, 1987.
171. Switzer, D. F., et al.: Calibration of color doppler flow mapping during extreme hemodynamic conditions in vitro: a foundation for a reliable quantitative grading system for aortic incompetence. Circulation, 75:837, 1987.
171a. Enriquez-Sarano, M, et al.: Quantitative Doppler assessment of valvular regurgitation. Circulation, 87:841, 1993.
172. Oh, J. K., et al.: Characteristic doppler echocardiographic pattern of mitral inflow velocity in severe aortic regurgitation. J. Am. Coll. Cardiol., 14:1712, 1989.
173. Alam, M., et al.: Doppler and echocardiographic features of normal and dysfunctioning bioprosthetic valves. J. Am. Coll. Cardiol., 10:851, 1987.
173a. Chafizadeh, E. R., and Zoghbi, W. A.: Doppler echocardiographic assessment of the St. Jude medical prosthetic in the aortic position using the continuity equation. Circulation, 83:213, 1991.
174. Kapur, K. K., et al.: Doppler color flow mapping in the evaluation of prosthetic mitral and aortic valve function. J. Am. Coll. Cardiol., 13:1561, 1989.
175. Alam, M., et al.: Color flow Doppler evaluation of St. Jude medical prosthetic valves. Am. J. Cardiol., 64:1387, 1989.
176. Alam, M., et al.: Color flow Doppler evaluation of cardiac bioprosthetic valves. Am. J. Cardiol., 64:1389, 1989.
177. Nellessen, U., et al.: Transesophageal two-dimensional echocardiography and color doppler flow velocity mapping in the evaluation of cardiac valve prostheses. Circulation, 78:848, 1988.
177a. Nienaber, C. A., et al.: The diagnosis of thoracic aortic dissection by noninvasive imaging procedures. N. Engl. J. Med., 328:1, 1993.
178. Karalis, D. G., et al.: Transesophageal echocardiographic recognition of subaortic complications in aortic valve endocarditis—clinical and surgical implications. Circulation, 86:353, 1992.
179. Rackley, C. E., Wallace, R. B., Edwards, J. E., and Katz, N. M.: Aortic regurgitation. In The Heart. 7th Ed. Edited by J. W. Hurst, et al. New York, McGraw-Hill, 1990, p. 805.
180. Orecchia, P. M., et al.: Coronary artery disease in aortic surgery. Ann. Vasc. Surg., 2:28, 1988.
181. Grossman, W.: Profiles in valvular heart disease. In Cardiac Catheterization, Angiography and Intervention. 4th Ed. Edited by W. Grossman and D. S. Baim. Philadelphia, Lea & Febiger, 1991, p. 574.
182. Manyari, D. E., Nolewajka, A. J., and Kostuk, W. J.: Quantitative assessment of aortic valvular insufficiency by radionuclide angiography. Chest, 81:170, 1982.
183. Boucher, C. A., Miller, D. D., and Hutter, A. M.: Rest versus exercise ejection fraction and the decision to perform valve replacement in aortic regurgitation. Am. J. Noninvas. Cardiol., 2:19, 1988.
184. Byrd, B. F., Schiller, N. B., Botvinick, E. H., and Higgins, C. B.: Normal cardiac dimensions by magnetic resonance imaging. Am. J. Cardiol., 55:1440, 1985.
185. Friedman, B. J., Waters, J., Kwan, O. L., and DeMaria, A. N.: Comparison of magnetic resonance imaging and echocardiography in determination of cardiac dimensions in normal subjects. J. Am. Coll. Cardiol., 5:1368, 1985.
186. Rehr, R. B., Malloy, C. R., Filipchuk, N. G., and Peshock, R. M.: Left ventricular volumes measured by MR imaging. Radiology, 156:717, 1985.
187. Florentine, M. S., et al.: Measurement of left ventricular mass in vivo using gated nuclear magnetic resonance imaging. J. Am. Coll. Cardiol., 8:107, 1986.
188. Keller, A. M., et al.: In vivo measurement of myocardial mass using nuclear resonance magnetic imaging. J. Am. Coll. Cardiol., 8:113, 1986.
189. Borow, K. M., et al.: End-systolic volume as a predictor of postoperative left ventricular performance in volume overload from valvular regurgitation. Am. J. Med., 68:655, 1980.
190. Kawachi, K., et al.: Relations of preoperative hemodynamics and coronary blood flow to improved left ventricular function after valve replacement for aortic regurgitation. J. Am. Coll. Cardiol., 11:925, 1988.
191. Cranney, G. B., Lotan, C. S., and Pohost, G. M.: Evaluation of aortic regurgitation by nuclear magnetic resonance imaging. Curr. Probl. Cardiol., 15:87, 1990.
192. Underwood, S. R., Firmin, D. N., and Mohiaddin, R. H.: Cine magnetic resonance imaging of vascular heart disease. San Antonio, TX, Society of Magnetic Resonance in Medicine, Abstract No. 723, 1987.
193. Sechtem, U., et al.: Mitral or aortic regurgitation: quantification of regurgitant volumes with cine MR imaging. Radiology, 167:425, 1988.
194. Firmin, D. N., et al.: In vivo validation of MR velocity imaging. J. Comp. Assist. Tomogr., 11:751, 1987.
195. Cranney, G. B., et al.: Diagnosis of thoracic aortic dissection using nuclear magnetic resonance imaging—comparison with other imaging modalities. Aust. N. Z. J. Med., 18:362, 1988.
196. Kay, P. H., et al.: The results of surgery for active endocarditis of the native aortic valve. J. Cardiovasc. Surg., 25:321, 1984.
197. Cukingnan, R. A., Carey, J. S., Wittig, J. H., and Cimochowski, G. E.: Early valve replacement in active infective endocarditis. J. Thorac. Cardiovasc. Surg., 85:163, 1983.
198. Mammana, R. B., et al.: Valve replacement for left-sided endocarditis in drug addicts. Ann. Thorac. Surg., 35:436, 1983.
199. Perry, L. S., et al.: Operative approach to endocarditis. Am. Heart J., 108:561, 1984.
200. Lewis, B. S., et al.: Cardiac operation during active infective endocarditis. J. Thorac. Cardiovasc. Surg., 84:579, 1982.
201. Baumgartner, W. A., et al.: Surgical treatment of prosthetic valve endocarditis. Ann. Thorac. Surg., 35:87, 1983.

202. Raychaudhury, T., Cameron, E. W. J., and Walbaum, P. R.: Surgical management of prosthetic valve endocarditis. J. Thorac. Cardiovasc. Surg., 86:112, 1983.
203. D'Agustino, R. S., Miller, D. C., and Stinson, E.: Valve replacement in patients with native valve endocarditis: what really determines operative outcome? Ann. Thorac. Surg., 40:429, 1985.
204. Frankl, W. S.: The special problems of the patient with valvular prosthesis. Cardiovasc. Clin., 10:415, 1986.
205. Miller, C.: Predictors of outcome in patients with prosthetic valve endocarditis (PVE) and potential advantage of homograft aortic root replacement for prosthetic ascending aortic valve-graft infections. J. Card. Surg., 5:53, 1990.
206. Alsip, S. G., Blackstone, E. H., and Kirklin, J. W.: Indications for cardiac surgery in patients with active infective endocarditis. Am. J. Med., 78:138, 1985.
207. Oikawa, J. H., and Kaye, D.: Endocarditis: epidemiology, pathophysiology, management and prophylaxis. Cardiovasc. Clin., 6:335, 1986.
208. Cohn, L. H., and Birjiniuk, V.: Therapy of acute aortic regurgitation. Cardiol. Clin., 9:339, 1991.
209. Ross, D.: Allograft root replacement for prosthetic endocarditis. J. Card. Surg., 5:56, 1990.
210. Walsh, R. A., and O'Rourke, R. A.: The diagnosis and management of acute left-sided valvular regurgitation. Curr. Probl. Cardiol., 4:5, 1979.
211. Koster, J. K., Cohn, L. H., Mee, R. B. B., and Collins, J. J.: Late results of operation for acute aortic dissection producing aortic insufficiency. Ann. Thorac. Surg., 26:461, 1978.
212. Bachet, J., et al.: Replacement of the transverse aortic arch during emergency operations for type A acute aortic dissection. J. Thorac. Cardiovasc. Surg., 96:878, 1988.
213. Eagle, K. A., and DeSanctis, R. W.: Aortic dissection. Curr. Probl. Cardiol., 4:230, 1989.
214. Ergin, M. A., Galla, J. D., Lansman, S., and Griepp, R. B.: Acute dissection of the aorta—current surgical treatment. Surg. Clin. North Am., 65:721, 1985.
215. Inberg, M. V., Niinikoski, J., Savunen, T., and Vanttinen, E.: Total repair of annulo-aortic ectasia with composite graft and reimplantation of coronary ostia: a consecutive series of 41 patients. World J. Surg., 9:493, 1985.
216. Miller, D. C., et al.: Operative treatment of aortic dissections. J. Thorac. Cardiovasc. Surg., 78:365, 1979.
217. Wheat, M. W.: Acute dissecting aneurysms of the aorta: diagnosis and treatment—1979. Am. Heart. J., 99:373, 1980.
218. Haverich, A., et al.: Acute and chronic aortic dissections—determinants of long-term outcome for operative survivors. Circulation, 72:II22, 1985.
219. Morritt G. N., Taylor, N. C., and Miller, H. C.: Traumatic aortic regurgitation. J. R. Coll. Surg., 24:87, 1979.
220. Kimbler, R. W., Stokes, J. P., and Barnhorst, D. A.: The surgical treatment of traumatic rupture of the aortic valve: report of a case after blunt chest trauma. J. Trauma, 17:168, 1977.
221. Ovil, Y., Wahi, R., Liu, P., and Goldman, B.: Aortic valvuloplasty for traumatic aortic insufficiency: a 2-year follow-up. Ann. Thorac. Surg., 49:143, 1990.
222. Carpentier, A.: Cardiac valve surgery—the "French correction." Ann. Thorac. Cardiovasc. Surg., 86:323, 1989.
223. Al Fagin, M. R., Al Kasab, S. M., and Ashmeg, A.: Aortic valve repair using bovine pericardium for cusp extension. J. Thorac. Cardiovasc. Surg., 96:760, 1988.
224. Duran, C., Kumar, N., Gometza, B., and Al Halees, Z.: Indications and limitations of aortic valve reconstruction. Ann. Thorac. Surg., 52:447, 1991.
225. Cosgrove, D. M., et al.: Valvuloplasty for aortic insufficiency. J. Thorac. Cardiovasc. Surg., 102:571, 1991.

Chapter 34

MANAGEMENT OF A HYPERTENSIVE EMERGENCY

ROBERT J. CODY

Despite an era when hypertension is at least partially treated by a number of classes of antihypertensive agents, patients with hypertensive emergencies continue to present in the emergency room or medical ward setting requiring consideration for an ICU admission. The occurrence of hypertensive emergencies is sufficient to suggest a separate diagnostic category,[1] which facilitates expeditious care and triage. A hypertensive emergency is not a specific disease; rather it represents the occurrence of a diastolic blood pressure greater than 120 mm Hg and one or more symptoms or an associated medical problem, summated as a morbid or premorbid clinical picture. The most commonly accepted hypertensive emergencies are summarized in Table 34-1. With currently available therapies, it is unusual to be placed in a situation in which corrective management of blood pressure cannot be instituted in an expeditious fashion. By the time that a patient is evaluated as a candidate for ICU admission, however, reduction of blood pressure may not be as important or threatening as the associated medical or surgical disorder. Clinical management of a hypertensive emergency requires equal attention to blood pressure reduction and the associated medical problems. A considerable number of review articles have addressed the issue of hypertensive emergencies, and several are cited herein.[2-8] This chapter focuses on the issue of management related to the ICU:

- Initial evaluation and management with a decision regarding requirement for admission to the ICU
- Management, stabilization, and improvement in the ICU
- Discharge from the ICU where long-term blood pressure management, diagnostic workup and treatment of associated problems are established.

This chapter summarizes these three major management stages as greater than 70% of patients with the diagnosis of "hypertensive emergency" continue to require ICU admission.[2]

PRE-ICU PHASE

Circumstances of a Hypertensive Emergency

A full discussion of the pathophysiology of hypertension is outside the scope of this chapter. Furthermore, the exact mechanisms by which a patient with relatively stable hypertension proceeds to develop an unstable picture consistent with a hypertensive emergency remains to be more fully established. Several factors predispose to the diagnosis of hypertensive emergency (Table 34-2). The first issue is the type of hypertension that can result in a hypertensive emergency. Virtually any form of hypertension can produce a hypertensive emergency. It should be noted that "essential" or idiopathic hypertension, by its ranking as the most common form of hypertension, is the most likely cause. The exact factors that trigger a hypertensive emergency or crisis in one patient with essential hypertension as opposed to other patients with essential hypertension remain unknown. Whether this is a superimposition of a form of vasculitis, recent accelerated hypertension, or long-standing poor control of blood pressure has not been defined. Another form of hypertension that may predispose to a hypertensive emergency or crisis is renovascular hypertension. This may also be the result of an associated vasculitis, at least within the kidney, that is aggravated by the hypersecretion of renin. Other factors are listed in Table 34-2. The second issue is the occurrence of an accelerated, severe medical problem that occurs in the setting of poorly controlled hypertension. An example would be the presence of a myocardial infarction or a transient ischemic attack coinciding with poorly controlled hypertension. Under these circumstances, the severity or urgency of the associated medical problem not only intensifies the hypertension, but also confers the diagnosis of hypertensive emergency, thereby intensifying consideration for admission to an ICU. The third issue is the clinical prodrome leading to the diagnosis of hypertensive emergency. One can identify two patients whose hypertensive course, degree of inadequate therapeutic control, and absolute blood pressure are virtually identical. The clinical prodrome, however, may differentiate how each patient is handled. For instance, if one patient is virtually asymptomatic at the time of presentation, such a patient may be treated in the emergency room or on a regular medical unit. The second patient, however, may have associated clinical symptoms or findings, such as left ventricular dysfunction, either systolic or diastolic; obvious neurologic obtundation; or visual impairment, that necessitate more urgent blood pressure management. Many authors attempt to distinguish a hypertensive "emergency" from a hypertensive "urgency." The clinical characteristics that permit this differentiation may vary from patient to patient and may change within minutes. Furthermore, there is no therapeutic end point associated with this differentiation, and the antihypertensive therapies are virtually identical. A final paradoxic twist to this terminology is the fact that the true "urgency" of treat-

Table 34-1. Situations Typically Considered to Be Hypertensive Emergencies When Associated with a Diastolic Pressure Greater Than 120 mm Hg

Neurologic
   Intracranial hemorrhage
     Subarachnoid
     Charcot-Bouchard aneurysm
     Parenchymal
   Cerebral hemisphere infarct
     Completed
     In progress
     Impending (transient ischemic attack)
   Lacunar infarct
   Encephalopathy
   Seizure activity
Cardiac/vascular
   Myocardial infarction or active angina
   Congestive heart failure
   Post coronary artery bypass surgery
   Aortic dissection
   Aortic aneurysm
   Active vasculitis, secondary to connective tissue disorders
Renal
   Acute renal failure
   Glomerulonephritis
   Post renal transplant
Endocrine crises
   Hypothyroidism
   Hyperthyroidism
   Pheochromocytoma
Malignant-phase hypertension
Eclampsia
Severe hypertension associated with
   Postoperative bleeding or instability
   Major vascular or cranial surgical procedures
   Severe burns
   Head trauma
   Preeclampsia

ment is associated with the hypertensive emergency group, rather than patients with asymptomatic elevations of diastolic pressure. For these reasons, "hypertensive urgencies" are not discussed in this chapter. What in fact transpires in many patients is an increasing scale of severity. To have hypertension as a disease process is an obvious factor for cardiac cerebral, vascular, renal, and ophthalmic disease. When the functions of these end organs become altered, additional risk is appreciated, and these end organ changes become disease processes of their own importance. Finally, if the clinical prodrome that develops as a result of the aforementioned disorders implies that major disruption of health status is close at hand, a third order of magnitude of the problem is seen.

Initial Data Acquisition

Features of the initial data acquisition are summarized in Table 34-2. The history provides important clues regarding the origin of hypertension, the duration of hypertension, the difficulty with which hypertension was previously controlled, and the likely outcome of therapy in the ensuing 48 hours. One can attempt to develop some idea regarding the most likely cause of the acceleration of hypertension based on the features that present in the history of the hypertension. These diagnostic considerations are exemplified by the following profiles. If the hypertension occurs in an individual with a positive family history for hypertension, particularly in a middle-aged black individual, one can be reasonably assured that at least part of the hypertensive problem is due to familial or essential hypertension. The absence of a strong family history raises the possibility of recently acquired hypertension, such as renovascular hypertension. This differential is further clarified by identifying the likely duration of hypertension. Long-standing hypertension (more than 5 years) would be an unusual course for renovascular hypertension. Conversely, a middle-aged individual with documented hypertension of only 6 months' duration is atypical for familial essential hypertension, unless the patient is a poor historian or is unaware of his or her previous family history. Additional factors suggesting long-standing hypertension include a previous history of cigarette smoking, diabetes, abnormal lipid profile, or known renal impairment. These factors not only influence the course of hypertension, but also the choice of therapy. Information regarding previous therapy can provide important insights. For instance, if the patient had been previously managed with large doses of an angiotensin-converting enzyme (ACE) inhibitor, yet blood pressure control was never adequately achieved, this would not necessarily exclude a diagnosis of renovascular hypertension but would certainly put this diagnosis somewhat lower on the list. The previously used drug regimens provide information regarding the best general class of therapeutic agent to initiate for the individual. Con-

Table 34-2. Clinical Features of a Hypertensive Emergency

Predisposition to Hypertensive Emergency
   Type of hypertension
     Essential hypertension
     Renovascular hypertension
     Pheochromocytoma
     Hyper- or hypothyroidism
     Acute glomerulonephritis
     Primary aldosteronism
     Coarctation of the aorta
     Hypertension associated with connective tissue disease/vasculitis
   Accelerated medical problem with associated severe hypertension, such as
     Transient ischemic attack
     Myocardial infarction
   Clinical prodrome
     Stable versus unstable presentation
Initial Data Acquisition
   Past medical history
     Family history of hypertension
     Duration of hypertension
     Adequacy of previous blood pressure control
     Associated disorders, such as diabetes
   Major focus of physical examination
     Neurologic findings
     Fundus
     Cardiac
     Vascular
   Laboratory screen
     Electrocardiogram
     Chest film
     Blood sample for electrolytes, blood urea nitrogen, creatinine
     Spot urine for glucose, protein, occult blood, sediment

tinuing along with this same example, if a patient was previously unresponsive to large doses of an ACE inhibitor plus a diuretic, one might consider low renin essential hypertension and would be more predisposed to consider a calcium channel antagonist or a central sympatholytic. Pheochromocytoma is a relatively rare form of hypertension but is one that can present with striking features consistent with the diagnosis of a hypertensive emergency. Perhaps the most important historical factor in these patients is the recent onset of "spells." When asked for further detail, patients often relay a history of dizziness, palpitations, fluttering in the chest, and other nondescriptive circulatory findings. These spells tend to be intermittent and may be associated with headache, tachycardia, and flushing. The occurrence of this profile should lead the physician at least to consider the possibility of a pheochromocytoma. If the patient has no idea of previous medical therapy, this would raise concerns regarding lack of compliance with medication in the past. This may be an issue of true treatment noncompliance or may simply reflect an inadequate understanding on the patient's part as to the importance of therapy. It is also important to solicit the history of previous medical follow-up. If a patient appears to have been reasonably well followed by a physician or nurse practitioner in both the immediate and the remote past, the presentation of a hypertensive emergency raises concerns that accelerated hypertension may be a difficult management problem. Additional important information can be obtained from the history. This includes the time course in change of blood pressure control and associated symptoms. If the patient can provide a reasonable history of gradual increase in blood pressure over the course of several months, this suggests a form of hypertensive emergency resulting from inadequate therapeutic control but at the same time suggests that well-directed therapy over the next 24 to 96 hours will likely achieve blood pressure control. If the patient can provide a reasonable history that blood pressure was well controlled until just days or weeks before presentation, however, this raises concerns regarding malignant phase of hypertension. If the patient is obtunded or unconscious at the time of presentation or cannot provide adequate history, probing into the previous history of the patient by discussing the aforementioned issues with family and friends should at least provide the name of a physician or nurse practitioner who has managed the patient in the recent past. With the wide recognition of the risks of hypertension and the wide range of treatment methods currently available to the practitioner, it is becoming increasingly unlikely to encounter a patient who has not been under the care of a physician in the recent past. A phone call to the practitioner at the time of admission or within the first 12 hours of admission to the hospital or consideration for transfer to the ICU is clearly warranted. This may prevent subsequent unnecessary testing or prolonged admission to the ICU.

Following the history, a brief but directed physical examination is important. The focus of the examination is neurologic and cardiovascular. The extent of the neurologic evaluation depends on the presentation. If the patient is asymptomatic or relatively asymptomatic, the neurologic examination can be limited. If the patient is obtunded, has obvious visual or motor impairment, or manifests confusion or memory loss, however, a more detailed examination is necessary. It may actually be necessary to move to diagnostic neurologic testing rapidly if the examination demonstrates significant neurologic impairment. The funduscopic examination provides important information regarding the severity of hypertension (atrioventricular nicking, spasm/tortuosity), duration of hypertension (hemorrhages and especially exudates) and the diagnosis of malignant-phase hypertension, which is based on the presence of papilledema. Repeated attempts to examine the fundi should be made (by several individuals, if necessary) to document the presence or absence of abnormalities. The cardiovascular examination involves the heart and all accessible blood vessels. This provides an assessment of the extent of vascular impairment that has resulted from hypertension. The cardiac examination provides a quick assessment of left ventricular enlargement or impairment resulting from hypertension, corroborating the duration of hypertension and the likelihood of interventional requirements for left ventricular failure or infarction in the setting of the hypertensive emergency. The vascular examination is often overlooked but provides an excellent window to the duration of hypertension, associated disease, the potential risk of subsequent cerebrovascular events, and the origin of hypertension. The vascular examination can start at the level of the chest and work to the periphery. The likelihood of dilatation or distention of the proximal aorta should be rapidly assessed in consideration of a diagnosis of aortic aneurysm dissection. This, of course, would be supported or refuted by the quality of peripheral pulses. Examination of the carotid arteries for a bruit is important to establish the presence or absence of carotid artery stenosis, particularly in the presence of neurologic findings or a diminished unilateral pulse. It should be specified that the absence of a carotid bruit, particularly in the presence of a diminished carotid pulse, does not exclude the possibility of carotid artery stenosis. In fact, the tightest carotid stenosis may often be associated with the absence of a bruit and a diminished carotid pulse.

The retinal arteries are a literal window of the vascular system (Table 34-3). Narrowing of the arteries, particularly the presence of focal spasm, provides important information regarding the severity of the vascular reaction to the increase in blood pressure. The temporal arteries should also be palpated on examination, despite the fact that coexistent vasculitis or temporal arteritis is relatively infrequent. The abdominal aorta should also be examined in great detail. Widening of the abdominal aorta or dis-

Table 34-3. Retinal Changes in Patients with Hypertension

Grade	
I	Decreased vessel caliber or sclerosis of retinal arteries
II	Generalized and localized narrowing of arteries with exaggerated arterial reflex; arteriovenous nicking
III	Hemorrhages and exudates, superimposed on sclerotic and spastic arterioles
IV	Papilledema

placement to the right or left suggests at least the existence of significant atherosclerosis. This diagnosis is strengthened by the presence of a pulsatile abdominal aorta; however, the latter may frequently be observed in thin elderly subjects whose blood pressure is markedly elevated. Perhaps more compelling is the presence of an abdominal bruit. At least this indicates the presence of atherosclerosis involving the aorta and provides the first clue to the possibility of renovascular disease. The abdominal aorta is a sensitive but not specific marker for renovascular disease. If the patient can be examined in the seated position, it is important to examine the paraspinal areas of the back at the level of the lower rib cage. The presence of a unilateral or bilateral bruit in the lumbar regions is a specific marker for renovascular disease. Finally, the peripheral vessels should be examined for evidence of diminished pulses. This is important in terms of excluding the diagnosis of aortic dissection and identifying the presence or absence of peripheral vascular disease, which may influence therapy and suggests the need to evaluate for coexistent disease, such as diabetes. Following completion of these important aspects of the examination that pertain to the hypertensive emergency, a brief but careful general physical examination should be completed.

As with any other emergency that suggests the need for admission to an ICU, the hypertensive emergency does not permit adequate time for collection of a large laboratory base. An electrocardiogram provides information regarding rhythm abnormalities, such as atrial fibrillation, that are commonly associated with hypertension. It also provides information regarding the presence or absence of myocardial ischemia or infarction, left atrial and ventricular enlargement, and electrolyte abnormalities. The chest film also provides information regarding the presence or absence of cardiac enlargement, current or impending left ventricle failure, and coexistent pulmonary disease. A screening blood sample should include serum electrolytes, serum creatinine, and blood urea nitrogen (BUN). Electrolyte abnormalities, such as hyponatremia and hypokalemia, may provide additional information regarding concurrent therapy, such as diuretics, and also help identify central risks in the ensuing 24 hours. Perhaps the most vulnerable major organ system at risk from hypertension is the kidney. It is difficult to obtain any information regarding kidney status from history or physical examination. Thus the screening laboratory data are the best window to the kidney. The BUN and serum creatinine are a quick way of obtaining information regarding renal function. A screening urinalysis for the presence of proteinuria or hematuria suggests at least passive involvement of the kidney in the hypertensive emergency. Examination of the urine sediment can provide evidence for disorders such as acute tubular necrosis or acute glomerular nephritis.

Organization

The current approach to management presumes that the patient in question is already in the hospital or is assumed to require hospital admission. The issue then becomes a question as to whether the patient requires an ICU bed or regular hospital bed. The factors influencing this decision

Table 34–4. Circumstances that Support Admission to an ICU for Treatment of Hypertensive Emergency

Need for parenteral antihypertensive therapy
Inadequate response of severe hypertension to initial urgent therapy
Associated clinical status
    Neurologic impairment
        Fixed neurologic deficit
        Fluctuating neurologic status
        Somnulence/lethargy
        Memory impairment
        Seizure activity
    Eclampsia and many cases of preeclampsia
    Unstable cardiac status
        Congestive heart failure/pulmonary edema
        Active angina
        Myocardial infarction
    Unstable renal status
        Active macroscopic hematuria
        Oliguria/anuria with renal insufficiency
Active bleeding from an associated medical problem or recent surgery
Insufficient nursing or medical staff on the regular medical unit to monitor frequent pressure recordings and adjust therapy (particularly on the night shift)

are outlined in Table 34-4. It should be emphasized that the presence of extremely high blood pressure levels (e.g., 180/120) does not of itself mandate ICU admission. Such pressure does mandate therapy. A patient who presents with high pressure but has not had symptoms or signs of coexistent disease or a worrisome clinical prodrome can likely be admitted directly to a regular hospital bed. It should again be emphasized that treatment should be initiated promptly. This includes treatment at the time of the initial evaluation and immediately on admission as part of the admitting orders. In view of the rapidly acting, highly effective antihypertensive regimens that exist, blood pressure reduction in such an individual should be achieved within a matter of 1 to 3 hours. Patients who have malignant-phase hypertension, evidence of a true hypertensive emergency, significant coexistent disease together with hypertension, or a worrisome clinical picture are best treated in the ICU even if this is only overnight. Other factors prompting admission to the ICU include need for intravenous therapy, management of coexistent disease, logistical issues such as time of day, and physician/nurse availability, and the need to follow neurologic status.

Three hypertensive emergencies that require particular attention are malignant-phase hypertension, preeclampsia/eclampsia, and pheochromocytoma. The expression "malignant hypertension" is often used inappropriately to signify any case of severe hypertension. Malignant phase or malignant hypertension, however, is a distinct clinical entity that stands apart from any of the several serious presentations of accelerated hypertension or hypertensive emergency. It is distinct in terms of the pathophysiology, the urgency of treatment, the potential for an adverse outcome, and the potential mortality. "Malignant" is not a synonym for accelerated hypertension, hypertensive crisis, or hypertensive emergency. It is a discrete constellation of findings (Table 34-5). The diagnosis of malignant-phase hypertension requires the presence of papilledema on funduscopic examination. Malignant-phase hyperten-

Table 34-5. Characteristics of Malignant-Phase Hypertension

Blood pressure
  Usually greater than 200/130
  Usually associated with a recent accelerated course, regardless of previous control
  Underlying cause is virtually any form of hypertension (although primary hyperaldosteronism and coarctation of the aorta rarely provoke the malignant phase)
Fluctuating signs and symptoms
  Neurologic
    Lethargy
    Visual changes
    Disorientation/memory deficit
  Secondary manifestations of target organ response, such as a cerebrovascular accident or myocardial infarction
Neuroretinopathy (papilledema)
Renal insufficiency, with rapid progression to renal destruction

sion is associated with arteriolar fibrinoid necrosis, which is a marker for the vasculitis aspect of this disorder occurring within target organs, particularly the retina, brain, and kidney. It is apparent that accurate diagnosis of papilledema and characterization of fibrinoid lesions may be obscured in many patients.[1] Clinically this disorder is characterized by a rapid increase in blood pressure over a few days, superimposed on one of the other forms of hypertension. Virtually any form of hypertension can be the substitute of malignant-phase hypertension, although malignant phase is unusual in primary hypersecretion of aldosterone or coarctation of the aorta. Malignant-phase hypertension can proceed to rapid destruction of renal function in a matter of a few days. Unfortunately this process sometimes occurs despite adequate blood pressure reduction. Malignant-phase hypertension is almost always associated with activation of renin system activity, even when the underlying hypertension is "essential." Therefore ACE inhibitors are often effective initial therapy for these patients, but typically two or three drugs are required to achieve satisfactory blood pressure control.

Hypertension during pregnancy may have many expressions (Table 34-6), ranging from transient hypertension to eclampsia that requires emergency delivery of the fetus. Detailed reviews of this topic can be found elsewhere.[9-11] The differentiation of preeclampsia from eclampsia is the presence of seizures in the latter group. Obviously this is another fine line of differentiation because the preeclampsia patient can become an eclampsia patient in a matter of minutes with the onset of seizures. Therefore depending on the assessment of all clinical factors, many patients with preeclampsia may warrant additional monitoring in an ICU, if only overnight, until blood pressure is controlled. Special care must be taken in the choice of therapy in pregnancy. Particular attention is given to factors that do not suppress cardiac output, do not disrupt the uterine-placental interface, and do not adversely affect the fetus in terms of teratogenicity, growth, or neurologic and cardiac function. Therefore, therapy continues to center on traditional therapy with agents such as hydralazine and alpha-methyldopa.[10,11] Newer agents appear to be minimally effective (e.g., ACE inhibitors) or may produce considerable relaxation of uterine contractility (e.g., calcium channel antagonists).[11] In the most urgent situations, data would suggest a role for nitroprusside,[12] although this remains controversial, and labetalol appears promising.[10,11] Therapy of chronic hypertension during pregnancy may require a somewhat different spectrum of antihypertensive therapy.[10]

Pheochromocytoma is an uncommon form of hypertension. It is a disorder that usually appears in the exclusionary diagnostic considerations of the physician who encounters recently uncontrolled hypertension. Unfortunately the diagnosis requires plasma or urine catecholamine determinations that may take several days to return to the patient's chart. A high index of suspension for this diagnosis would be raised by the recent onset of hypertension in someone who describes spells, such as palpations, headache, or blurred vision, as previously mentioned. If the patient or the patient's family offers unsolicited evidence for such spells in the recent history and the hypertension is indeed episodic, one might consider going directly to a computed tomography (CT) scan of the abdomen looking for an adrenal tumor. This does not imply, however, that a CT scan should be a screening test in patients with recent onset of hypertension. In fact, this would be an approach that should be used only by experienced physicians who have some sense of certainty that this is a likely diagnosis.

Outcome of the Pre-ICU Phase

Completion of the evaluation for a hypertensive emergency in the pre-ICU phase should accomplish several goals. These include estimation of the severity of the crisis, a grasp of the previous history, diagnosis and planning for the associated medical problems, and, most important, plans for treatment. It is difficult to treat all of the factors associated with the hypertensive emergency simultaneously. Blood pressure reduction is obviously important. One would obviously not neglect, however, the treatment of a coexistent seizure, myocardial infarction, or congestive heart failure at the time of initiating antihypertensive therapy. Furthermore, one would not wish to lower blood pressure precipitously in the setting of an unstable coexistent medical problem, which might further compound the clinical picture, such as adversely lowering blood pressure in the setting of myocardial infarction, thereby permitting

Table 34-6. Hypertension in Pregnancy versus Hypertensive Emergency in Pregnancy

Spectrum of hypertension in pregnancy
  Transient hypertension (stress, volume retention)
  Preexisting chronic hypertension
  Chronic hypertension/superimposed preeclampsia
  Preeclampsia
  Eclampsia
Preeclampsia—may constitute a hypertensive emergency
  Elevated blood pressure
  Generalized edema formation
  Proteinuria
  Occasionally coagulation/liver function abnormalities
Eclampsia—is a hypertensive emergency
  All features of preeclampsia plus seizure activity

extension of the infarct. Conversely, the urgency to treat associated heart failure or a seizure as well as triage to the ICU may become so paramount that the patient's severe hypertension may go untreated for a considerable period or may even be completely overlooked. There is a risk that antihypertensive therapy may not be instituted for 1 to 2 hours, depending on the time required for transferring the patient to the ICU. Therefore blood pressure reduction should be initiated after an initial expeditious evaluation and before admission to the ICU.

The list of potential medications for the management of hypertensive emergencies can be extensive (Table 34-7). Before choosing therapy, it is important to address the question: How quickly and to what level must I lower blood pressure? There is a tendency in clinical practice to immediately (within minutes) lower blood pressure to normotensive levels. In actuality this may be totally inappropriate, and more experienced physicians now shy away from this approach, particularly with the current wide choice of antihypertensive agents. The speed with which blood pressure is lowered depends on the overall clinical picture. If a patient has been free of symptoms in the previous 2 to 3 days and is currently free of symptoms, blood pressure can be reduced with oral medications in the course of the ensuing few hours and may not require intensive care therapy or an extensive workup. The patient with active seizures or acute pulmonary edema would certainly benefit from a rapid reduction of blood pressure to a diastolic range of 90 to 100 mm Hg. A patient with stroke in progress (particularly if severe carotid disease is present) or a patient with an acute myocardial infarction may be better served by a more gradual reduction of blood pressure over the ensuing 1 to 4 hours, rather than radical swings of blood pressure within a few minutes. In such patients, rapid reduction of diastolic blood pressure to a range of 70 to 80 mm Hg for instance from a baseline of greater than 120 mm Hg may induce considerable ischemia. The decision must also be made as to whether this patient would be stabilized with oral medications or whether parenteral therapy will be required over the next 48 hours.

For the treatment of hypertensive emergencies, diuretics are used primarily as an adjunct to other agents. Their major benefit is to induce natriuresis and reduction of volume overload. Therefore the most effective use of diuretics is in patients with congestive heart failure or renal failure when these clinical situations are a part of the hypertensive emergency. It should be remembered that thiazide-type diuretics are less effective in patients whose serum creatinine level is greater than 2.0.

Traditionally, the central sympatholytic/ganglionic blocking agents were the first antihypertensive agents that proved effective for the treatment of hypertensive emergencies. They consisted primarily of reserpine and guanethidine. These drugs are now less used because of their tendency to induce somnolence, which may obscure an associated or impending neurologic event. Alpha-methyldopa remains an effective agent for antihypertensive emergencies in view of its potential for combined parenteral and oral administration. Furthermore, it has a well-established profile and utilization so many physicians remain comfortable with its use. Clonidine is now used with greater frequency in hypertensive emergencies.[22-25] Over the last decade, its favorable effects in hypertensive emergencies have been documented, and for the most part it appears to be well tolerated and safe. Furthermore, comparative studies now exist between alpha-methyldopa and clonidine in the treatment of hypertension of pregnancy,[11] which therefore improves its profile as a potential drug for hypertensive emergencies associated with pregnancy. Both alpha-methyldopa and clonidine, however, may also induce neurologic changes that may obscure the clinical status of the patient. Trimethaphan is a potent antihypertensive agent that can cause profound reduction of blood pressure well below normotensive ranges. Its use for hypertensive emergencies has decreased with the availability of newer agents. In certain situations, however, particularly aortic dissection and other surgical situations in which there is a risk of bleeding in the perioperative stage, this drug is still used.

Drugs that block the autonomic nervous system have traditionally been used for the treatment of hypertensive emergencies. Beta-adrenergic blockade has long been a standard approach to antihypertensive therapy. It is particularly useful in patients with ongoing coronary ischemia or myocardial infarction in the setting of a hypertensive emergency. Utilization is enhanced by the option of parenteral and oral routes of administration. It should be remembered, however, that blood pressure reduction with beta-adrenergic blockers occurs in the time frame of one to several hours rather than minutes. Its negative inotropic and chronotropic effects, however, occur within a shorter time frame. The clinical expression of alpha-adrenergic blockade is primarily vasodilation. Thus, drugs such as prazosin and terazosin have been used in hypertension primarily for their vasodilating properties. Labetalol has gained particular attention as a compound that combines both alpha-adrenergic and beta-adrenergic blockage. Its favorable profile in hypertensive emergencies is well documented,[26-34] and it has been used with reasonable success and safety in the treatment of hypertension during pregnancy.[10,11] It is also desirable because of its multiple routes of administration. Therapy can be initiated with intravenous bolus or intravenous steady-state infusion. This can be followed with oral administration. Although purely speculative, the fact that labetalol has combined alpha-blocking and beta-blocking properties may be fundamental to its favorable effects in hypertensive emergencies, compared with a drug that has only alpha-blocking or beta-blocking properties.

Direct-acting vasodilators have long been favored in the treatment of hypertensive emergencies.[35] Sodium nitroprusside is a potent vasodilator, and its steady-state infusion characteristics permit for precise titration of blood pressure control. It is generally well tolerated, particularly when infusion rates are less than 48 hours in duration, thereby avoiding cumulative toxicity. Diazoxide is a means of parenteral blood pressure reduction, particularly in the emergency room. As soon as intravenous access has been established, diazoxide can be given by the "mini-bolus" technique, thereby avoiding the excessive hypotension noted when a large intravenous bolus of 300 mg was rec-

Table 34–7. Therapy for Hypertensive Emergencies, According to the Phase of Management

Drug/Drug Class*	Dose†	Route	Comment
Pre-ICU Phase‡			
Diuretics (typically loop agents)	See individual drugs	Intravenous	Acutely, used primarily to achieve volume depletion, such as in treatment of pulmonary edema; diuretics are not usually effective as acute antihypertensive agents.
Sympatholytics§			
Central/ganglionic blockade.			
Reserpine	0.25–5.0 mg	Intravenous	Current primary use is the treatment of aortic dissection; may depress the sensorium
Trimethaphan	1–10 mg/min	Intravenous	Can cause profound hypotension in a dose-dependent fashion; favored when very low pressure required: neurosurgery, aortic dissection; requires arterial pressure catheter
Guanethidine	10–25 mg	Oral	Less favored at the current time, in view of newer alternative agents; still useful for aortic dissection; potential limitation of oral administration
Alpha-methyldopa	250–500 mg over 30 min	Intravenous	Long-standing well-known drug for the treatment of hypertension; a major concern would be drug-induced CNS changes, obscuring the clinical status
Clonidine	0.2 mg; repeat 0.1 mg 1 hour later	Oral	Limited by oral administration and potential CNS changes
Phentolamine	2–20 mg bolus; infusion of 0.2–5 mg/min	Intravenous	Primary use is pheochromocytoma; arterial pressure catheter is preferable
Phenoxybenzamine	1 mg/kg bolus	Intravenous	Primary use is pheochromocytoma
Beta-blockade			
Selective/nonselective	See individual drugs	Intravenous	Antihypertensive effect may lag behind autonomic effect; negative inotropic effect; nonselectives produce bronchoconstriction
Labetalol (combined alpha/beta)	10 mg; repeat 40 mg q 10–15 min ×2	Intravenous	May have a negative inotropic effect similar to beta-blockade; this is often less apparent, owing to the vasodilator properties of alpha-blockade
Vasodilators			
Sodium nitroprusside	0.5–10 µg/kg/min	Intravenous	Requires arterial pressure catheter; photosensitive; probably the best parenteral therapy for most patients
Diazoxide	Repeated 50–100 mg "mini-bolus"	Intravenous	Can give up to the full 300 mg dose; monitor the rate and magnitude of blood pressure reduction
Hydralazine	10–50 mg	Intravenous	Give 10-mg bolus, which can be repeated at 20–30 min intervals to a total dose of 50 mg; can be associated with appreciable reflex tachycardia
Minoxidil	5–40 mg	Oral	May require 1–2 hours for major antihypertensive effect; in view of its potency, it can nonetheless be considered
Nitroglycerin preparations	See individual drugs	Sublingual; topical; intravenous	These agents are not necessarily potent antihypertensive agents; they can be particularly effective when the hypertensive emergency is associated with angina, myocardial infarction, or heart failure
ACE inhibitors			
Enalaprilat	0.5–5 mg	Intravenous	Start with smallest dose, and repeat/increase as necessary
Captopril	6.25–25 mg	Oral	Considered here because of rapid onset of action
Calcium channel antagonists‖			
Verapamil	0.15 mg/kg followed by infusion of 1–2 mg/min	Intravenous	The need for an arterial line is lessened, if only the bolus is given: without continuous infusion, however, the duration of antihypertensive effect may only be approximately 30 min; can produce negative inotropic effects
Dihydropyridines			
Nifedipine	10 mg	Oral; sublingual	Oral onset of action is prompt in most people; the sublingual route has been popularized but can produce hypotension-related adverse effects; can produce negative inotropic effects

(continued)

Table 34-7. Therapy for Hypertensive Emergencies, According to the Phase of Management—*(Continued)*

Drug/Drug Class*	Dose†	Route	Comment
ICU Phase			
Diuretics			
"Loop" type diuretics Thiazide-type diuretics Potassium-sparing diuretics	See individual agents	Intravenous; oral	The ICU phase would be a good opportunity for the transition to oral agents; in addition to volume depletion, the chronic antihypertensive effects can be initiated at this time
Sympatholytics			
Central/ganglionic blockade			
Reserpine	0.25–5.0 mg	Intravenous	Current primary use is the treatment of aortic dissection; may depress the sensorium
Trimethaphan	1–10 mg/min	Intravenous	Can cause profound hypotension in a dose-dependent fashion; favored when very low pressure required: neurosurgery, aortic dissection; requires arterial pressure catheter
Guanethidine	10–25 mg q.d.	Oral	Potent therapy when indicated; CNS symptoms may limit efficacy
Guanabenz	4–16 mg q 12 h	Oral	Properties generally similar to guanethidine; limitations associated with side effects
Alpha-methyldopa	250–500 mg over 30 min (IV) 250–1000 mg q 6 h (p.o.)	Intravenous Oral	Long-standing well-known drug for the treatment of hypertension; a major concern would be drug-induced CNS changes, obscuring the clinical status
Chonidine	0.1–0.3 mg q 12 h	Oral	Limited by oral administration and potential CNS changes
Phentolamine	5–20 mg bolus; infusion of 0.2–5 mg/min	Intravenous	Primary use is pheochromocytoma; arterial pressure catheter is preferable
Phenoxybenzamine	1 mg/kg bolus	Intravenous	Primary use is pheochromocytoma
Alpha-blockade			
Prazosin	1–5 mg q 8–12 h	Oral	Effective vasodilator in hypertension; good evidence for tachyphylaxis in the congestive heart failure population
Terazosin	1–10 mg q 12–24 h	Oral	Second-generation compound, with longer half-life than prazosin
Doxazosin	1–8 mg q 24 h	Oral	New compound; some unique features; needs postmarketing evaluation
Beta-blockade			
Selective/nonselective	See individual drugs	Intravenous; oral	Antihypertensive effect may lag behind autonomic effect; negative inotropic effect; nonselectives produce bronchoconstriction
Labetalol (combined alpha/beta)	20 mg; repeat 40 mg ×2 (IV) 100–400 mg q 12 h (oral)	Intravenous Oral	May have a negative inotropic effect similar to beta-blockade; this is often less apparent, due to the vasodilator properties of alpha-blockade
Vasodilators			
Sodium nitroprusside	0.5–10 µg/kg/min	Intravenous	Requires arterial pressure catheter; photosensitive
Diazoxide	Repeated 50–100 mg "mini-bolus"	Intravenous	Can give up to the full 300-mg dose; monitor the rate and magnitude of blood pressure reduction
Hydralazine	10–50 mg 50–200 mg q 8–12 h	Intravenous Oral	Intravenous characteristics as above; oral therapy may also be associated with considerable reflex tachycardia, which may be problematic in disorders such as coronary ischemia
Minoxidil	5–40 mg q 12–24 h	Oral	May require 1 hour until its effect is apparent; in view of its potency, it can be considered nonetheless
Nitroglycerin preparations	See individual drugs	Sublingual; topical; intravenous	These agens are not necessarily potent antihypertensive agents; they can be particularly effective when the hypertensive emergency is associated with angina, myocardial infarction, or heart failure
ACE inhibitors			
Captopril	6.25–100 mg q 8–12 h	Oral	Dosage of ACE inhibitors reflects most likely range of utilization; lowest effective dosage should be sought initially; although there is concern for adverse renal effects, most patients other than those with bilateral or severe renal artery stenosis should tolerate therapy with these agents
Enalapril	2.5–20 mg q 12–24 h	Oral	
Lisinopril	10–40 mg q 24 h	Oral	
Calcium-channel antagonists			
Verapamil	80–160 mg q 8 h	Oral	All drugs in this class are effective vasodilators; the extent to which individual compounds have negative inotropic properties is variable
Dihydropyridines	See individual drugs	Oral	
Diltiazem	60–120 mg q 6 h	Oral	

(continued)

Table 34-7. Therapy for Hypertensive Emergencies, According to the Phase of Management—*(Continued)*

Drug/Drug Class*	Dose†	Route	Comment
Post-ICU Phase¶			
Diuretics			
"Loop" type diuretics	See individual agents	Intravenous; oral	Use in the post-ICU phase is for volume depletion and the chronic antihypertensive effect; the latter may take 2–3 weeks for maximal response
Thiazide-type diuretics			
Potassium-sparing diuretics			
Sympatholytics			
Central/ganglionic blockade			
Guanethidine	10–25 mg q.d.	Oral	Potent therapy when indicated; side effects such as orthostatic hypotension, impotence, and CNS symptoms may limit efficacy
Guanabenz	4–16 mg q 12 h	Oral	Properties generally similar to guanethidine; limitations associated with side effects
Alpha-methyldopa	250–1000 mg q 6 h	Oral	Less adverse symptoms than the guanethidine-like agents, especially at lower doses; same cautions apply nonetheless
Clonidine	0.1–0.3 mg q 12 h	Oral	Limited by oral administration and potential CNS changes
Alpha-blockade			
Prazosin	1–5 mg q 8–12 h	Oral	Effective vasodilator in hypertension; good evidence for tachyphylaxis in the CHF population
Terazosin	1–10 mg q 12–24 h	Oral	Second-generation compound, with longer half-life than prazosin
Doxazosin	1–8 mg q 24 h	Oral	New compound; some unique features; needs postmarketing evaluation
Beta blockade	See individual drugs	Oral	Antihypertensive efficacy typically would be more apparent at this stage of therapy; any issues regarding adverse effects should have been resolved at this stage
Labetalol (combined alpha/beta)	100–400 mg q 12 h	Oral	May have a negative inotropic effect similar to beta-blockade; this is often less apparent, owing to the vasodilator properties of alpha-blockade
Vasodilators			
Hydralazine	50–200 mg q 8–12 h	Oral	Oral therapy may also be associated with considerable reflex tachycardia, which may be problematic in disorders such as coronary ischemia
Minoxidil	5–40 mg q 12–24 h	Oral	Potent antihypertensive response to oral therapy; secondary fluid retention is common
Nitroglycerin preparations	See individual drugs	Sublingual; topical; intravenous	These agents are not necessarily potent antihypertensive agents; they can be particularly effective when the hypertensive emergency is associated with angina, myocardial infarction, or heart failure
ACE inhibitors			Dosage of ACE inhibitors reflects most likely range of use; lowest effective dosage should be sought initially; although there is concern for adverse renal effects, most patients other than those with bilateral or severe renal artery stenosis should tolerate therapy with these agents
Captopril	6.25–100 mg q 8–12 h	Oral	
Enalapril	2.5–20 mg q 12–24 h	Oral	
Lisinopril	10–40 mg q 24 h	Oral	
Calcium-channel antagonists			All drugs in this class are effective vasodilators; the extent to which individual compounds have negative inotropic properties is variable
Verapamil	80–160 mg q 8 h	Oral	
Dihydropyridines	See individual drugs	Oral	
Diltiazem	60–120 mg q 6 h	Oral	

* This is not intended as an exhaustive list but a list of therapeutic agents that can be used for the three stages of ICU patient management. Also, see references 13–21.
† Based on dosage to control more severe hypertension.
‡ All compounds listed in this subsection are notable for rapid onset of action, usually by an intravenous route.
§ All drugs in this class have the potential limitation of central nervous system (CNS) adverse side effects that could obscure the clinical status of the patient.
|| Long-acting preparations are not covered; effective approaches to use of this class in hypertensive emergencies are given.
¶ There are many forms of therapy; these are representative of typical agents.
ACE, Angiotensin-converting enzyme.

ommended. It is preferably given in a bolus of 50 mg, which can be repeated at 5- to 10-minute intervals until blood pressure is controlled. Minoxidil has been used for more than a decade, and it is characterized as a potent vasodilator. With direct-acting vasodilating agents, there is a tendency for excessive fluid retention in many patients, but this is less important during initial management. Hydralazine remains a favored vasodilator in the treatment of hypertensive emergencies. It may be given by a parenteral or oral route, and the parenteral administration includes intramuscular administration. The latter may not be desirable and can cause erratic blood pressure responses. Nonetheless, this approach can be used in the absence of intravenous access. It is particularly favored when vasodilation is a desired end point in therapy, such as with coexistent pulmonary edema or congestive heart failure. Furthermore, hydralazine has a well-established track record for the treatment of hypertensive emergencies of pregnancy[10,11] and remains a drug of choice under those conditions. Nitroglycerin compounds are frequently used for hypertensive emergencies, particularly in the absence of intravenous access or when prompt reduction of blood pressure is necessary. As an antihypertensive agent, however, nitroglycerin does not have the potency of other compounds. In the presence of coronary ischemia, myocardial infarction, or congestive heart failure, it is a desirable approach to therapy.[21] The ACE inhibitors are a somewhat newer, yet potent class of antihypertensive agents.

In addition to oral therapy, parenteral therapy has been used for hypertensive emergencies. There are now reports with sublingual administration of captopril that are encouraging.[36,37] More specifically, enalaprilat, the active metabolite of enalapril, can be given intravenously.[38] Substantial reductions of blood pressure can be observed within 15 minutes with as little as 1 mg intravenously. The ACE inhibitors are likely to be most effective when the renin system is activated. Thus, in patients with renovascular hypertension or malignant-phase hypertension, the blood pressure response is substantial. In contrast, these agents may be less effective when the hypertensive emergency is characterized by marked fluid overload or in hypertensive emergencies associated with pregnancy.[10] It is sometimes difficult to achieve the kind of dose-response relationship with an ACE inhibitor that one observes with other vasodilators. There may be more of a tendency for "all-or-none" response with this class of agents. Nonetheless, these agents are potent vasodilators that can block the endocrine effects of circulating angiotensin II as well as the secretion of aldosterone. They are of particular benefit in hypertensive emergencies associated with congestive heart failure.

The calcium channel antagonists are potent vasodilators, and much has been written regarding their utilization for the treatment of hypertensive emergencies in the last decade.[39-53] Of the three prototypic classes of calcium channel antagonists, the dihydropyridines appear to be the most frequently used. It should be noted, however, that verapamil can be safely administered by intravenous route and in the absence of known congestive heart failure may not produce clinically relevant negative inotropic effects.[51] Nifedipine is the prototypic dihydropyridine that was developed for oral administration, and other more creative approaches have been used.[56] Several reports have indicated that rapid, effective blood pressure reduction can be obtained by sublingual administration of nifedipine.[20,54-56] Although this has proved safe in many patients, it should be noted that there is the potential for deleterious effects by this route of administration. Rapid reduction of blood pressure from markedly elevated levels to normal within 5 to 10 minutes may not be desirable in many hypertensive emergencies, such as stroke in progress or myocardial infarction. The onset of action of oral nifedipine can be within 15 to 30 minutes, with peak effect at 45 to 90 minutes, thus providing reasonable blood pressure control in a sufficient time frame. Newer dihydropyridines, such as nicardipine, are available in a soluble preparation, so intravenous administration as a bolus or steady-state infusion can produce an effective reduction without adverse cardiac effects in blood pressure.[52]

The considerations listed here are necessary before admission to the ICU. Therapeutic intervention should be executed in a rapid fashion, however, so triage can be expedited. By the time the patient is mobilized for the ICU, there should be a reasonable estimate of a background of hypertension, the likelihood of successful treatment, the delineation of coexistent or concomitant medical illness, inclusion or exclusion of the diagnosis of malignant-phase hypertension, and an estimate of the duration of stay required in the ICU. Most importantly, by the time of admission to the ICU, blood pressure reduction should have been accomplished. Examples of therapy oriented to specific disease processes are given in Table 34-8. This table is not meant to be all inclusive. The purpose, however, is to point out that certain disease processes associated with a hypertensive emergency may require specific forms of therapy. These specific applications are either a drug class

Table 34-8. Examples of Antihypertensive Therapy for Specific Clinical Problems (pending ICU admission)

Clinical Problem	Drug Class
Congestive heart failure	Diuretics Ace inhibitors Direct vasodilators
Myocardial ischemia/infarction	Nitrates Beta-adrenergic blockade Calcium channel antagonists
Aortic dissection	Central sympatholytics Beta-adrenergic blockade
Encephalopathy	Direct vasodilators Calcium channel antagonists
Stroke in progress	Calcium channel antagonists Direct vasodilators ACE inhibitors
Malignant-phase hypertension	ACE inhibitors Calcium channel antagonists Direct vasodilators Central sympatholytics Diuretics
Eclampsia	Hydralazine Alpha-methyldopa Labetalol
Renal failure/glomerulnephritis	Diuretics Direct vasodilators

ACE, Angiotensin converting enzyme.

that is known to have particular favorable effects for this disease or a class that would likely have minimal adverse effects, under the conditions of instability associated with a particular disorder.

ICU PHASE

Circumstances of Management

Blood pressure reduction at the time of ICU admission provides a temporal buffer to stabilize associated medical conditions. It should be reiterated that it is not mandatory for blood pressure to be "normal" at this stage (i.e., 130/80); diastolic pressures of 90 to 100 mm Hg are acceptable in most patients. In most situations, blood pressure in the 150 to 160/90 to 100 range prevents secondary deterioration owing to hypertensive or hypotensive ranges and also provides a time envelope to stabilize associated medical problems. At this stage, the management of the patient should follow the general concepts outlined in Tables 34-7 and 34-8. First, a decision should be made regarding the most likely antihypertensive regimen for the ensuing 24 to 48 hours. As previously noted, it is not mandatory that antihypertensive therapy be given by the parenteral route. Parenteral therapy, however, is necessary if the patient is obtunded, blood pressure is difficult to stabilize in the range stated previously, or concomitant medical illnesses are sufficiently complicated such that the most simple, easily regulated form of antihypertensive therapy should be instituted. A simple rule of therapeutic intervention is to use the simplest, safest therapy to achieve the treatment in point. For the patient in the ICU, placement of an arterial catheter is a relatively direct approach. Second, attention should then be maximized in the direction of the associated problem that has constituted the basis of the diagnosis of hypertensive emergency. Several of these disorders may be relatively easy to stabilize and may in fact stabilize simply as a result of blood pressure control. The frequency and severity of seizure disorders, the symptoms and findings of congestive heart failure, and neuroretinopathic changes are examples of disorders that may stabilize quickly. A cerebrovascular accident, myocardial infarction, or aortic dissection may require further intensive evaluation and therapy. In many patients, the associated medical problem actually becomes the primary management issue over the ensuing days when blood pressure has been controlled. (See Chaps. 5, 29, and 35.)

Data

With stabilization of the patient, additional data are obtained. Follow-up discussions with the patient's family or primary medical care staff permit subtle adjustment of therapy initiated in the ICU. Fluctuations in clinical status should be minimized by monitoring the key features of the physical examination. A neurologic examination, including intermittent assessment of the patient's cognitive status, is particularly important. It would not be unusual to see considerable swings in the neurologic status of a patient with a hypertensive emergency, particularly if such features as confusion, visual impairment, and lethargy were present at the time of admission. If neurologic findings are nonexistent or minimal at the time of admission but subsequently progress in the ICU, neurology consultation, including cranial imaging, should be obtained. The funduscopic examination should also be repeated in the ICU. Hemorrhages and exudates are not likely to show considerable short-term change. Arteriolar spasm, however, should demonstrate resolution as blood pressure is lowered. If papilledema was present at the time of admission as part of a malignant-phase diagnosis, it is unlikely that this will demonstrate rapid improvement. The findings on cardiac examination depend on the associated cardiovascular pathophysiology at the time of admission. If congestive heart failure was a feature, resolution of a gallop rhythm and pulmonary rates should occur. Fluctuation in systolic murmurs would be typical and could change in either direction. The same applies to flow characteristics in the peripheral arteries and the intensity of a bruit that may have been detected at the time of initial evaluation.

Coexistence of aortic dissection may be more difficult to identify and to exclude than aortic aneurysm. A limited aortic dissection may be well masked on examination and screening radiologic evaluation, so more detailed studies may be necessary if this diagnosis is suspected. These issues are covered in greater detail in Chapter 35. A more detailed laboratory database should be acquired at this stage of management. The extent of such studies depends on the nature of coexistent disease, the ease of blood pressure control, and the clinical status of the patient. In situations in which blood pressure has been promptly controlled and the ICU admission is in the range of 24 hours, much of the workup can be deferred to the post-ICU hospital stay on the regular medical unit. Particular attention should be given to the electrolyte status of the patient, which may fluctuate depending on the therapy chosen. At this point, renal function should also be monitored more closely and in a serial fashion. More detailed 24-hour urine collections should be initiated for quantitating catecholamine, aldosterone, and protein excretion as well as glucose and creatinine clearance. In uncontrolled accelerated hypertension, it would not be unusual to observe proteinuria exceeding 1 g in 24 hours, although the protein content is primarily albumin. The magnitude of proteinuria typically resolves as hypertension is controlled. Special laboratory procedures depend primarily on the presentation of the concomitant illness (Table 34-9). The need for such studies and the extent of their utilization depend on consultation with one or more subspecialty groups and consideration of the patient's overall status.

Outcome

After blood pressure stabilization and the identification and management of coexistent processes, a decision must be reached regarding transfer from the ICU to a regular medical or surgical unit (Table 34-10). Within 12 to 24 hours of ICU admission and in the absence of mitigating factors such as obtundation, antihypertensive therapy should have been switched to an oral regimen in sufficient dosage to control blood pressure (see Table 34-7). If the patient's clinical status remains complicated, obviously this patient should remain in the ICU and will likely require

Table 34–9. Management of a Hypertensive Emergency During the ICU Admission

Blood pressure management
  Establish level of pressure reduction desired
  Maintain pressure within desired range
  Initiate transition from parenteral to oral drug regimens, if appropriate
Additional data acquisition
  History
    Follow-up discussions with family and primary medical team
  Physical examination
    Particular focus on neurologic and vascular changes
  Routine laboratory data
    Follow-up chest film and electrocardiogram
    24-hour urine collection for catecholamines, aldosterone, glucose, protein, creatinine
  Special laboratory data
    CT scan or MRI of the head, if warranted by neurologic deficits
    CT or transesophageal echocardiogram if aortic dissection is suspected
    Cardiac catheterization for unstable angina/early infarct, if appropriate
    CT of the abdomen if pheochromocytoma is suspected
Treatment of associated disorders
  Depending on circumstances, this may be of equal of greater importance than reduction of blood pressure

CT, Computed tomography, MRI, magnetic resonance imaging.

continued parenteral medication. Otherwise, it would be reasonable to consider discharge to a regular medical unit, where further treatment and subsequent diagnostic evaluation of hypertension can now be distinguished from any associated medical problems. Each of these latter associated problems should receive their own diagnostic and therapeutic management. This may require more than one team of medical specialists. As in any other complex ICU patient, however, a primary physician responsible for the integrated care of the patient should be identified.

Table 34–10. Factors to Consider When Transfer From the ICU is Contemplated

Stabilization of blood pressure and secondary associated medical problems
Identification of the primary/coordinating physician
Blood pressure management (see Table 34–7)
  Assurance of blood pressure has been stabilized on a rational oral drug regimen
  Maintenance of therapy within known efficacy guidelines
  Use of an effective drug combination
Further diagnostic studies
  Renal studies, which may include
    Renal vein renins
    Renal blood flow and functional studies
    Digital subtraction angiography
    Renal angiogram
  Cardiac evaluation if appropriate
    Exercise testing with/without imaging
    Echocardiogram
    Catheterization
  Neurologic evaluation
    Angiography
    Computed tomography scan
    Positron-emission tomography scan
    Magnetic resonance imaging scan
    Other specialized studies as clinically indicated

As with any form of therapy, antihypertensive therapy can be associated with complications. Based on the nature of drug administration in the ICU and the obvious instability of the patient in the hypertensive emergency, the complication most likely reflects a change in pressure or perfusion that is undesirable. This in fact would be more common than a direct adverse effect of the drug itself. The latter would be more typical once therapy had been instituted for a considerable amount of time. Complications include evidence of target organ ischemia resulting from excessive hypertension and the provocation of sudden relative hypotension. This includes myocardial infarction or a deepening of the extent of a cerebral stroke. Additional neurologic findings could also occur. These include confusion and stupor as well as other mental status changes. Seizures could also occur in a patient who was admitted with neurologic instability. Renal dysfunction may also occur as either a direct effect of the drug or rapid reduction of blood pressure. One complication that is a direct pharmacologic effect typically occurring in the ICU setting is the occurrence of cyanide toxicity resulting from the administration of nitroprusside.

POST-ICU PHASE

Considerations for Therapy and Management

For the purposes of clarity, it is assumed that any associated medical problems are managed as outlined elsewhere in this text. In terms of hypertensive management, it may be best to consider circumstances, data, and outcome in an integrated fashion at this point because the patient's clinical status should be stabilized with the patient advanced to recovery status by the time of discharge from the ICU. Treatment of hypertension at this point would not be unlike many other patients with hypertension (see Table 34–7) with two exceptions. First, it is unlikely that monotherapy will be sufficient for blood pressure control in these patients. Currently both the pharmaceutical and the medical communities are advocating the use of monotherapy, particularly when an agent can be administered once or twice daily. Although this is desirable, evidence that adequate therapeutic end point therapy can be achieved in the majority of hypertensive patients remains inconclusive. Furthermore, in any individual who has experienced a hypertensive emergency, it is not reasonable to cut therapeutic corners. In most patients who have experienced a hypertensive emergency, it is advisable and desirable to use a combination of therapies that are administered with sufficient daily frequency to accommodate the known pharmacology of each of the agents. As health care professionals, we are all confronted with advertising that would suggest that a drug can safely and effectively reduce blood pressure when given only once or twice a day, when the pharmacokinetics of that compound would suggest that it must be administered three or four times a day. Monotherapy may have a role in mild forms of hypertension. This is not germane, however, to the patient with the recent hypertensive emergency. For instance, calcium channel antagonists must be given three or four times a day to be truly effective on a 24-hour basis. Some of the newer long-acting preparations of these compounds, however, may be effective on a once-daily or twice-daily basis. The control of blood pressure in a patient with a recent hypertensive emergency may require administration of as many as 6 to 12 pills a day, but this seems to be a small price to pay for clinical and blood pressure stability.

Second, the patient who has experienced a hypertensive emergency and who was fortunate enough to be stabilized and discharged is different than the patient with "garden variety" hypertension. Frequent initial visits and persistent long-term follow-up in relatively short intervals should be the rule. Particular attention should be given to renal function and cardiac status during long-term follow-up. If a major neurologic event caused the hypertensive emergency, the appropriate rehabilitation and steps to minimize a recurrence should be initiated. Attention to and management of other complicating factors, such as elevated cholesterol level or diabetes, should be initiated and maintained within rigid treatment guidelines.

Renal function may show considerable variation during the early phases of blood pressure control, and it is not unusual to see an increase of serum creatinine and BUN during early therapeutic interventions. The mechanisms for this response are numerous but should not discourage blood pressure reduction. The intrarenal circulatory response to accelerated hypertension is complex, and renal autoregulatory responses occur regardless of changes in the general systemic circulation. Acute and subacute blood pressure reduction to the range of 150/90 is not sufficient to induce renal hypoperfusion except perhaps in the situation of severe bilateral renal artery stenosis. Therefore an increase of serum creatinine or BUN should not be misconstrued as an excessive reduction of blood pressure. In most cases, moderate renal abnormalities typically resolve at some point 1 to 2 weeks after adequate blood pressure control. Rapidly progressing renal insufficiency, however, can be observed in two situations: severe renal artery stenosis and malignant-phase hypertension. In the absence of papilledema and other clinical features suggesting malignant-phase hypertension, the occurrence of rapidly progressing renal insufficiency should focus attention on the possibility of renal artery stenosis. This diagnosis would be further strengthened if marked reduction of blood pressure and accelerated renal insufficiency occurred during therapy with an ACE inhibitor. If papilledema and the other clinical hallmarks of phase hypertension were present at the time of initial evaluation, progressive renal insufficiency unfortunately follows a relentless course often regardless of the adequacy of blood pressure control.

A final word should be mentioned regarding malignant-phase hypertension. It would not be unusual by this stage of therapeutic follow-up for a patient with malignant-phase hypertension to have developed irreversible renal failure requiring dialysis. This remains one of the tragic gaps in our understanding of hypertension. Such patients may continue to require multiple pharmacologic agents for blood pressure control. Blood pressure control, however, is more manageable once dialysis has been initiated.

In summary, when therapy is initiated in an expeditious fashion, management of most hypertensive emergencies can be achieved by early stages of the ICU phase of hospitalization. Unfortunately, some of the sequelae of hypertensive emergencies, such as a cerebral infarct or chronic renal failure, may never resolve. To minimize the latter clinical outcomes, the presence of marked elevation of blood pressure in the setting of a seemingly more important clinical problem must be identified and treated. In one study of hypertensive emergencies,[2] 93% of the patients were previously diagnosed as having hypertension, and 83% were aware of their diagnosis. Therefore, it is unlikely that the occurrence of hypertensive emergencies will abate despite newer treatment methods.

REFERENCES

1. Hickler, R. B.: Hypertensive emergency: a useful diagnostic category. Am. J. Public Health, 78:623, 1988.
2. Bennett, N. M., and Shea, S.: Hypertensive emergency: case criteria, sociodemographic profile and previous care of 100 cases. Am. J. Public Health, 78:636, 1988.
3. Burris, J. F.: Hypertensive emergencies. Am. Fam. Physician, 32:97, 1985.
4. Burris, J. F., and Freis, E. D.: Hypertensive emergencies. Cardiovasc. Clin., 16:164, 1986.
5. Feldstein, J. S.: Hypertensive emergencies. Prim. Care, 13:109, 1986.
6. Ferguson, R. K., and Vlasses, P. H.: Hypertensive emergencies and urgencies. JAMA, 255:1607, 1986.
7. Houston, M.: Hypertensive emergencies and urgencies: pathophysiology and clinical aspects. Am. Heart J., 111:205, 1986.
8. Cody, R. J.: Hypertensive emergencies and aortic dissection. In Current Therapy in Critical Care Medicine. Edited by J. E. Parrillo. Toronto, B. C. Decker, Inc., 1990.
9. Nissen, J. C.: Treatment of hypertensive emergencies of pregnancy. Clin. Pharm., 1:334, 1982.
10. Barron, W. M., Murphy, M. B., and Lindheimer, M. D.: Management of hypertension during pregnancy. In Hypertension. Edited by J. H. Laragh and B. M. Brenner. New York, Raven Press, 1989, p. 1809.
11. Silver, H. M.: Acute hypertensive crisis in pregnancy. Med. Clin. North Am., 73:623, 1989.
12. Stempel, J. E., O'Grady, J. P., Morton, M. J., and Johnson, K. A.: Use of sodium nitroprusside in complications of gestational hypertension. Obstet. Gynecol., 60:533, 1982.
13. Vidt, G. D., and Gifford, R. W., Jr.: A compendium for the treatment of hypertensive emergencies. Cleve. Clin. Q., 51:421, 1984.
14. Masotti, G., et al.: Treatment of hypertensive emergencies: classic and newer approaches. J. Cardiovasc. Pharmacol., 8:46, 1986.
15. Vidt, D. G.: Current concepts in treatment of hypertensive emergencies. Am. Heart J., 111:220, 1986.
16. Bertel, O., Marx, B. E., and Conen, D.: Effects of antihypertensive treatment on cerebral perfusion. Am. J. Med., 82:29, 1987.
17. Garcia, J. Y., Jr., and Vidt, D. G.: Current management of hypertensive emergencies. Drugs, 34:263, 1987.
19. Stumpf, J. L.: Drug therapy of hypertensive crises. Clin. Pharm., 7:582, 1988.
20. Opie, L. H.: Treatment of severe hypertension. In New Therapeutic Strategies in Hypertension. Vol. 3. Edited by N. M. Kaplan, B. M. Brenner, and J. H. Laragh. New York, Raven Press, 1989, p. 183.
21. Cody, R. J.: Treatment of hypertension in patients with cardiovascular disorders. In New Therapeutic Strategies in Hypertension. Vol. 3. Edited by N. M. Kaplan, B. M. Brenner, and J. H. Laragh. New York, Raven Press, 1989, p. 199.

22. Perez Acuna, F., et al.: Acute hypotensive action of clonidine after intravenous infusion in hypertensive emergencies. Eur. J. Clin. Pharmacol., 25:151, 1983.
23. Masotti, G., et al.: Changes in cardiac function after effective of hypertensive emergencies with i.v. clonidine. Eur. Heart J., 5:1036, 1984.
24. Karachalios, G. N.: Hypertensive emergencies treated with oral clonidine. Eur. J. Clin. Pharmacol., 31:227, 1986.
25. Houston, M. C.: Treatment of hypertensive emergencies and urgencies with oral clonidine loading and titration. A review. Arch. Intern. Med., 146:586, 1986.
26. MacCarthy, E. P., and Bloomfield, S. S.: Labetalol: A review of its pharmacology, pharmacokinetics, clinical uses and adverse effects. Pharmacotherapy, 3:193, 1983.
27. Wallin, J. D., and O'Neill, W. M., Jr.: Labetalol. Current research and therapeutic status. Arch. Intern. Med., 143:485, 1983.
28. Wilson, D. J., et al.: Intravenous labetalol in the treatment of severe hypertension and hypertensive emergencies. Am. J. Med., 75:95, 1983.
29. Cressman, M. D., et al.: Intravenous labetalol in the management of severe hypertension and hypertensive emergencies. Am. Heart J., 107:980, 1984.
30. Louis, W. J., McNeil, J. J., and Drummer, O. H.: Pharmacology of combined alpha-beta-blockade. Drugs, 28:16, 1984.
31. Kanto, J. H.: Current status of labetalol, the first alpha- and beta-blocking agent. Int. J. Clin. Pharmacol. Ther. Toxicol., 23:617, 1985.
32. Lebel, M., Langlois, S., Belleau, L. J., and Grose, J. H.: Labetalol infusion in hypertensive emergencies. Clin. Pharmacol. Ther., 37:615, 1985.
33. Ngole, P. M.: Intravenous labetalol in the management of resistant hypertensive emergency. Drug. Intell. Clin. Pharm., 21:512, 1987.
34. Cosentino, F., et al.: The safety of cumulative doses of labetalol in perioperative hypertension. Cleve. Clin. J. Med., 56:371, 1989.
35. Osterziel, K. J., and Julius, S.: Vasodilators in the treatment of hypertension. Compr. Ther., 8:43, 1982.
36. Polonia, J. J., et al.: Influence of sublingual captopril on plasma catecholamine levels during hypertensive emergencies and cold immersion. Am. J. Med., 84:148, 1988.
37. Ceyhan, B., et al.: Comparison of sublingual captopril and sublingual nifedipine in hypertensive emergencies. Jpn. J. Pharmacol., 52:189, 1990.
38. Strauss, R., Gavras, I., Vlahakos, D., and Gavras, H.: Enalaprilat in hypertensive emergencies. J. Clin. Pharmacol., 26:39, 1986.
39. Chia, B. L., Ee, B., Tan, A., and Choo, M.: The immediate hypotensive effect of oral nifedipine. Curr. Med. Res. Opin., 8:139, 1982.
40. Conen, D., Bertel, O., and Dubach, U. C.: An oral calcium antagonist for treatment of hypertensive emergencies. J. Cardiovasc. Pharmacol., 4:378, 1982.
41. Bertel, O., et al.: Nifedipine in hypertensive emergencies. Br. Med. J., 286:19, 1983.
42. McHardy, K. C., and Hutcheon, A. W.: Nifedipine in hypertensive emergencies [letter]. Br. Med. J., 286:648, 1983.
43. Frishman, W. H., et al.: Calcium entry blockers for the treatment of severe hypertension and hypertensive crisis. Am. J. Med., 77:35, 1984.
44. Klein, W. W.: Treatment of hypertension with calcium channel blockers: European data. Am. J. Med., 77:143, 1984.
45. Bertel, O., and Conen, L. D.: Treatment of hypertensive emergencies with the calcium channel blocker nifedipine. Am. J. Med., 79:31, 1985.
46. Sluiter, H. E., Huysmans, F. T., Thien, T. A., and Koene, R. A.: Hemodynamic effects of intravenous felodipine in normotensive and hypertensive subjects. Drugs, 29:144, 1985.
47. Frishman, W. H.: Calcium-channel blockers for hypertensive emergencies. J. Clin. Hypertens., 2:55S, 1986.
48. Houston, M. C.: Treatment of hypertensive urgencies and emergencies with nifedipine. Am. Heart J., 111:963, 1986.
49. Opie, L. H., and Jennings, A. A.: Role of calcium channel blockade in chronic hypertension following successful management of hypertensive emergency. Am. J. Med., 81:35, 1986.
50. Bauer, J. H., and Reams, G. P.: The role of calcium entry blockers in hypertensive emergencies. Circulation, 75:2, 1987.
51. Cody, R. J.: The hemodynamics of calcium channel antagonists in hypertension: vascular and myocardial responses. Circulation, 75(Suppl. II):II-75, 1987.
52. Ryman, K. S., Kubo, S. H., Shaknovich, A., and Cody, R. J.: Influence of baseline hemodynamic states and sympathetic activity on the response to nicardipine, a new dihydropyridine in patients with hypertension or chronic congestive heart failure. Clin. Pharmacol. Ther., 41:483, 1987.
53. Schillinger, D.: Nifedipine in hypertensive emergencies: a prospective study. J. Emerg. Med., 5:463, 1987.
54. Ellrodt, A. G., Ault, M. J., Riedinger, M. S., and Murata, G. H.: Efficacy and safety of sublingual nifedipine in hypertensive emergencies. Am. J. Med., 79:19, 1985.
55. Abraham, G., Shukkur, A., Van Der Muelen, J., and Johny, K. V.: Sublingual nifedipine—a safe and simple therapy for hypertensive emergencies. Br. J. Clin. Pract., 40:478, 1986.
56. Kurosawa, S., et al.: Rectal administration of nifedipine: hemodynamic effects and pharmacokinetics in hypertensives. J. Int. Med. Res., 15:121, 1987.

Chapter 35

THORACIC AORTIC DISSECTIONS AND ANEURYSMS

BRUCE W. LYTLE

AORTIC DISSECTION

Aortic dissection is a potentially lethal condition characterized by a longitudinal separation within the media of the aortic wall. The separation is initiated by a transverse tear (the entry point) through the intima and part of the media, and the longitudinal separation (the false channel or false lumen) is subjected to aortic pressure (Fig. 35-1). Aortic dissection is the most common catastrophe involving the thoracic aorta, and its incidence approaches that of ruptured abdominal aortic aneurysms. The National Center for Health Statistics lists hospital discharge diagnoses for 1987 as follows:

- Dissection, 7000
- Thoracic aneurysms, 3000
- Abdominal aneurysm (nonruptured), 40,000
- Abdominal aneurysm (ruptured), 9000

The major predisposing factor for the occurrence of aortic dissection is systemic hypertension. At least two thirds of patients with dissections have a history of hypertension. Other conditions that have been associated with aortic dissection include bicuspid aortic valve, coarctation of the aorta, cystic medial necrosis, and connective tissue disorders such as Marfan syndrome and Ehlers-Danlos syndrome. Dissection has also been reported in association with pregnancy (usually in the third trimester) and secondary to trauma.[1-6] Dissections are more common in males compared with females, with a ratio of 3:1. Although aortic dissection is most common in the sixth and seventh decades of life, it may occur in any age group. Aortic atherosclerosis by itself probably is not a factor predisposing the patient to a dissection, and, in fact, Roberts[1] has pointed out that the medial scarring that is characteristic of atherosclerosis may serve to limit dissections. Aortic dissection does occur in patients with atherosclerosis, but it is probably related to systemic hypertension, a condition prevalent in patients with atherosclerosis.[1]

Dissections may also occur during or after cardiac surgery. Dissections that occur during cardiac surgery may be secondary to procedures on the ascending aorta, such as aortotomy, the proximal anastomoses associated with coronary bypass grafting, or simply clamping of the aorta. Cardiopulmonary bypass alone and, in particular, the altered flow patterns associated with femoral cannulation and retrograde perfusion may also initiate a dissection.[7] Aortic dissection has also been reported after cardiac catheterization.[6]

Anatomy and Pathophysiology

The pathoanatomic features of aortic dissections explain many of their clinical manifestations, complications, and the rationale behind their treatment. A review by Roberts[1] contains a particularly lucid description of the anatomic features of dissections.

In approximately two thirds of cases of aortic dissection, the intimal tear (entry point) occurs in the ascending aorta, 2 to 3 cm distal to the aortic valve and 1 to 2 cm distal to the coronary orifices (Table 35-1). In about 25% of patients, the entry point is located in the descending aorta, usually just distal to the left subclavian artery. In 10% of patients, the entry point is in the aortic arch. A small number of cases have been reported in which an intimal lesion could not be identified and the dissection consisted solely of an intramural hematoma.

Once an entry point is present, propagation of the false channel is produced by systemic blood pressure and the impulse of left ventricular ejection (dP/dt), which force arterial blood into the false channel. Distal progression of the dissection can occur extremely rapidly, and the entire distal aorta may become dissected virtually instantaneously.

Dissections may also extend in a retrograde direction, and in the majority of cases in which the entry point is in the ascending aorta, some retrograde dissection to the level of the coronary arteries and aortic sinuses does occur. For dissections that originate distal to the ascending aorta, significant retrograde dissection seems to be less common, but the ascending aorta can become dissected retrograde from an entry point in the descending aorta.

Dissections do not inevitably progress the length of the aorta. When a dissection is limited in its longitudinal extent, the false lumen may be largely filled with thrombus, the dissection consisting of an intramural hematoma that has a communication with the true lumen via the entry-point tear.

Anatomic sequelae of dissections include rupture, branch vessel occlusion, and disruption of the aortic valve. Rupture may occur either externally through the adventitia or back into the aortic true lumen (reentry). The entry point of a dissection extends through to the outer half of the media, which means that the outer wall of the false channel is thinner than the inner wall. External rupture therefore appears to be more common than re-entry.

The most common location for the entry point of a dissection is on the greater curvature of the aorta. Therefore

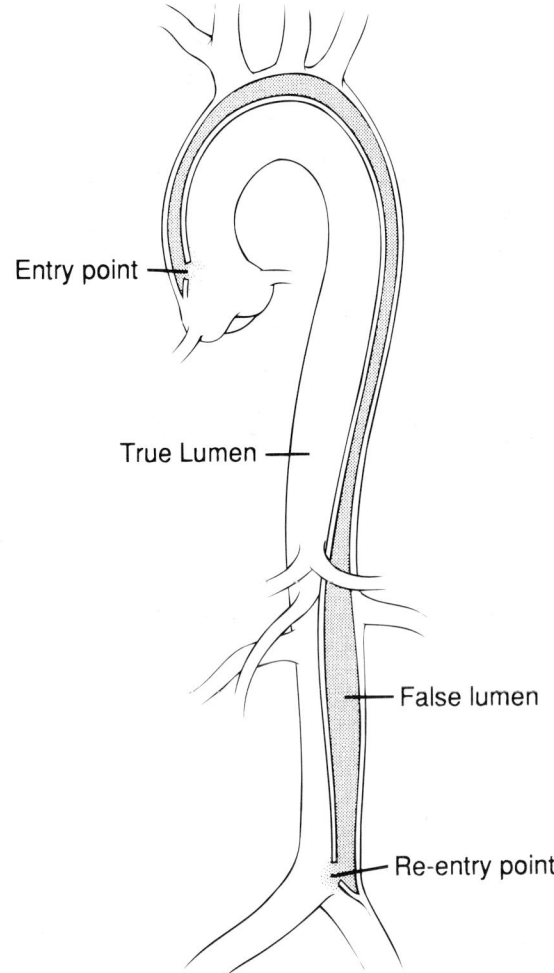

Fig. 35-1. Schematic diagram of aortic dissection. The most common entry point is in the ascending aorta. The false lumen extends distally in the aorta for a variable distance. One of the anatomic sequelae of an aortic dissection is rupture back into the true lumen or "reentry."

in the case of ascending dissections, the right lateral wall of the aorta usually contains the entry point. As dissections progress distally, the false lumen extends down the left side of the descending thoracic aorta in the majority of cases. The most common sites of rupture of ascending aortic dissections are into the pericardial sac and into the pleural space (left more commonly than right). Rupture may occur immediately on the initiation of the dissection or be delayed. In addition to the force of arterial pressure

Table 35-1. Location of Entry Point (Intimal Tear) of Aortic Dissections

Location	Frequency of Occurrence
Ascending aorta	60–70%
Descending aorta	20–30%
Aortic arch	10%
No intimal lesion identified	Rare

within the false lumen, necrosis of the wall of the aorta may contribute to delayed rupture. Some leakage of blood into the pericardium or pleural space without frank rupture is often noted at the time of operation for ascending aortic dissections. This may result from blood infiltrated through the thin external wall of the false channel by arterial pressure or by subadventitial infiltration of blood through the epicardium to mediastinal tissues. It is common to identify hematomas in the periaortic tissues at operation. Dissection of blood into cardiac structures may rarely cause compression of the right atrium or pulmonary artery. Dissections with the entry point in the descending thoracic aorta most commonly rupture into the left pleural space. Less common sites of ruptures of either ascending or descending aortic dissections are into the mediastinum, retroperitoneum, or adherent structures of the gastrointestinal tract.

The frequency of rupture back into the aortic true lumen, or reentry, varies according to whether necropsy or surgical series are examined. In the necropsy series of Hirst and coworkers,[8] about 15% of subjects were found to have reentry sites, with the most common locations being the iliac arteries and the abdominal aorta. The likelihood of reentry appears to be more common in surgical series because those patients have survived long enough to undergo operation. Reentry clearly predisposes to at least short-term survival, and the frequency with which reentry occurs can now be examined with computed tomography (CT) and magnetic resonance imaging (MRI). These imaging techniques have shown that persistence of the distal false lumen after surgery (as a result of flow through the reentry site) is common.[9,10]

Disruption or occlusion of peripheral arterial branches is also common. The intimal connection of a branch vessel may be sheared off completely, at which time the vessel may be adequately supplied by blood flow through the false channel. This event may have no clinical sequelae. If intimal disruption at the branch vessel does not occur, however, the arterial pressure in the false channel may compress the origin of the tributary vessel, causing stenosis or occlusion. Ascending dissections usually begin on the right lateral aspect of the aorta; approximately one half of the circumference of the aorta is involved; and if they progress distally, they tend to follow the greater curvature. Therefore the arch vessels may be jeopardized, and the left renal artery is involved in dissections more often than the right renal artery. Dissections may follow a spiral course, however, or the entire circumference of the aorta may be dissected. Therefore any branch of the aorta can be involved in a dissection. Stenosis of the true lumen of the aorta can be caused by intussusception of the intima or pressure within the false channel.

Aortic valve insufficiency is caused by retrograde dissection of the aorta to the level of the aortic sinuses, a process that destabilizes aortic valve commissures and causes prolapse of one or more of the aortic valve leaflets into the left ventricle during diastole. The commissures that join the noncoronary cusp to the left and right coronary cusps are most commonly involved.

Classification of Dissections

A variety of classification systems have been proposed for dissections. In DeBakey's original system, type I referred to a dissection originating in the ascending aorta and extending beyond the ascending aorta, whereas type II designated a dissection limited to the ascending aorta. Dissections originating in the descending aorta are termed type III. In the system of Daily et al. (Stanford classification), the site of entry point of the dissection is disregarded. If the ascending aorta is dissected, whether or not the entry point is in the ascending aorta, it is called type A. All others are designated as type B. Other authors have called DeBakey types I and II "proximal dissections" and type III "distal dissections." Typing of dissections is important because the treatment plan is different for dissections involving the ascending aorta compared with those involving only the descending aorta.

Another important distinction is the degree of acuity of the dissection. Because approximately 75% of deaths from untreated dissections occur within 2 weeks of onset, dissections recognized within that time span are called acute and others are termed chronic.

Pre-ICU Phase

Clinical Syndromes and Natural History

Because of the lethal nature of aortic dissections, it is an important diagnosis to make, and the physician must maintain a high index of suspicion for dissections in all cases of chest and back pain, acute arterial occlusion, and acute aortic insufficiency (Table 35-2). Pain initiates the clinical syndrome in almost all patients with aortic dissection. In the majority of patients, it is severe and sudden, reaching its greatest intensity immediately. A clue to the diagnosis often lies in the patient's own description of a "ripping, tearing pain." The pain may be migratory, and its changing position may mimic the progress of the dissection. For example, a sudden "tearing" substernal pain progressing to the neck or jaw and then to the back is characteristic of a dissection beginning in the ascending aorta and extending to the descending aorta. Although severe pain is the most common presentation, the pain of aortic dissection can be mild, and painless dissection may occur, although it is not common. In an era in which thrombolytic therapy is often part of the treatment of acute myocardial infarction, it is important to distinguish the pain syndrome of aortic dissection from that caused by myocardial ischemia or infarction. The pain of myocardial infarction often has a crescendo pattern to it, may be described as "squeezing" or likened to pressure, and when migratory usually involves the arms. It is obviously important to avoid giving thrombolytic agents to patients with a dissection.

Aortic dissection is a diagnosis that must be strongly considered for any patient who presents with a syndrome characteristic of acute arterial occlusion. In a literature review of 967 cases of aortic dissection by Sarris and Miller,[11] they noted that 25% of those patients demonstrated some peripheral vascular complications at the time of presentation, including pulse loss, stroke or paraplegia, and renal or visceral ischemia. In addition, dissections may cause myocardial ischemia or infarction by producing stenosis or occlusion of coronary arteries.

Acute left ventricular failure is a clinical syndrome that can be caused by dissection through the production of acute aortic insufficiency, cardiac tamponade owing to intrapericardial rupture, or coronary stenosis or occlusion. Sudden collapse, with either temporary or persistent shock, is also a situation in which dissection must be considered. Less common presentations of acute dissections include pericarditis and findings referable to a space-occupying lesion, such as superior vena cava syndrome, Horner's syndrome, vocal cord paralysis, and a pulsatile substernal mass.

The likelihood of death from a untreated dissection starts out high and remains high for at least 2 weeks.[1,4,6,8] Data from the series of Hirst and coworkers[8] indicate that death occurs at a rate of approximately 1% per hour for the first 48 hours. Within the first 2 weeks, the mortality rises to 75%. The implication of these observations is that there is a particularly high risk within the first 2 days, and this situation should probably be termed "hyperacute dissection." Expeditious diagnosis and treatment are obviously of prime importance. In many patients, however, death is delayed for at least a few hours, leaving a window of opportunity for the diagnosis and treatment of an aortic dissection. A minority of patients survive the acute episode with an unrecognized and untreated dissection and may come to medical attention months to years later. Aortic insufficiency and expansion of the false channel to produce a space-occupying lesion are the most common syndromes of presentation for these truly chronic dissections.

Diagnosis of Acute Dissections

Because rapidity in establishing treatment is important for the salvage of patients with acute aortic dissection, a presumptive diagnosis needs to be established and treatment instituted while a definitive diagnosis is being pursued. The presumptive diagnosis of an acute dissection is best established by history and physical examination. Any patient with a characteristic pain syndrome, acute aortic insufficiency, or an acute pulse loss should be considered to have an acute dissection until proved otherwise. The younger the patient, the more likely these syndromes are due to a dissection. Stroke in the older age group has sev-

Table 35-2. Clinical Syndromes Caused by Acute Aortic Dissection

Pain
Acute arterial occlusions
    Myocardial infarction
    Stroke
    Paraplegia
    Bowel infarction
    Renal failure
    Limb ischemia
    Pulse loss
Acute aortic insufficiency
Cardiac tamponade
Collapse
Superior vena caval syndrome

eral more common causes than aortic dissection, but the diagnosis of dissection must be at least considered.

For patients with suspected dissections, physical examination may reveal aortic insufficiency, and the presence and strength of pulses need to be carefully documented. Pulse deficits are important clues to the presence of a dissection, and pulses may change as the dissection progresses. Although patients may be clammy and vasoconstricted, the blood pressure is often elevated owing to preexisting hypertension, anxiety, or aortic or renal artery stenosis.

Routine diagnostic maneuvers, such as plain chest x-ray film, electrocardiogram (ECG) and laboratory studies such as complete blood count and electrolyte levels, usually provide only suggestive information. On plain chest film, a change in the size or configuration of the aorta or a left pleural effusion may point in the direction of a dissection. There are no diagnostic ECG changes associated with dissection, although signs of myocardial ischemia may suggest that the patient's chest pain is not due to dissection. It is important to remember, however, that a proximal dissection may cause myocardial ischemia.

Indications for ICU Admission

Regardless of the age of the patient or severity of symptoms, ICU admission is mandatory when there is a suspicion of aortic dissection. Beyond suspicion, other indications for admission include:

- Preoperative monitoring with documented dissections
- Control of hypertension
- Evaluation of myocardial ischemia
- Acute pulse loss
- Acute aortic insufficiency

ICU Phase

Definitive Diagnosis

The management of the ICU phase of a patient with suspected dissection should focus on:

- Treatment with antihypertensive and anti-impulse therapies
- Definitive diagnosis of the presence and location of a dissection
- Surgical therapy for patients with an indication for operation

For patients with a suspected aortic dissection, the diagnostic questions that need to be answered in order of importance are as follows:

- Has a dissection occurred?
- Is the ascending aorta dissected?
- Where is the entry point?
- Is there significant coronary atherosclerosis present?
- Is there aortic insufficiency?
- Is cardiac tamponade present?
- What is the size of the false lumen?

The imaging techniques that are available for the evaluation of patients with suspected aortic dissection include echocardiography, contrast aortography, CT scanning, and nuclear MRI. We are in a period of changing technology and are witnessing a shift away from contrast angiography and CT scanning and toward echocardiography and MRI for the evaluation of aortic dissection.

Echocardiography has the distinct and unique advantage that it can be performed at the bedside for a critically ill patient. Conventional transthoracic echocardiography detects ascending aortic dissection in approximately 80% of cases but has been less accurate in examining the descending aorta. The addition of transesophageal echocardiography techniques allows the echocardiographer to examine the aortic arch and descending aorta with more precision, and the further addition of Doppler color-flow mapping techniques enables important information to be obtained regarding blood flow in the true and false lumina and identification of the entry point of dissections. Studies have documented a high degree of sensitivity and specificity in the determination of whether or not the ascending aorta is dissected, and Hashimoto and associates[12] were able to document consistently the location of the entry point in a small series of patients with dissections. Furthermore, echocardiography can reliably examine the aortic valve and establish whether or not a pericardial effusion and cardiac tamponade are present. If an ascending aortic dissection is not identified by echocardiography, however, that does not exclude the diagnosis. In particular, the presence of a limited dissection within the ascending aorta (type II), a situation in which thrombus may limit free flow in the false lumen, can be difficult to document with echocardiography. Other disadvantages of echocardiography are its dependence on the skill and experience of the echocardiographer, a lack of information regarding intrinsic coronary atherosclerosis, and the need for esophageal intubation with a transesophageal probe.[13]

The advantages of CT scanning are that it is available in most institutions, it is noninvasive, and it has a high degree of sensitivity and specificity in the identification of the false lumen of the dissection. Accuracy rates of typing dissections with CT scan according to whether or not the ascending aorta is involved have been reported in excess of 90%.[14] False-positive and false-negative results, however, have been reported, and the overall sensitivity of CT scanning is probably only slightly greater than that of angiography. Furthermore, information concerning the coronary arteries and the aortic valve is unavailable with CT scanning. Clinical disadvantages of CT scanning in the acute setting include the dye load that must be given to the patient and the need to transport the patient to the radiology department for the examination.

From an imaging standpoint, ECG-gated MRI appears to be the most accurate way to establish the presence and extent of an aortic dissection.[15] MRI is able to display differences in the velocity of blood flow that enhances the separation of the true and false lumina of the dissection from each other and from surrounding structures. Furthermore, imaging in multiple planes is possible, enabling the definition of the proximal and distal extent of the dissection as well as more accurate sizing of the true and false lumina. Based on static spin-echo (dark blood) MRI, a sensitivity for the diagnosis of dissection was noted to be more than 95% at the 90% specificity level.[16] Cine-MRI (bright blood) techniques have added to this. The only significant imaging blind spots for MRI are inconsistency in establishing the precise location of the entry point and inability to detect intrinsic coronary atherosclerosis.

The major disadvantages of MRI are practical: the need to transport the patient to the radiology suite and to place the patient in the magnetic scanner. In hemodynamically unstable patients who are receiving medications through infusion pumps, MRI scanning is technically difficult, and its current application for the diagnosis of acute dissection is limited by these considerations. MRI is the best imaging technique that is currently available for stable patients and has supplanted CT scanning in the follow-up of patients after surgery.

In the past, contrast aortography has been the single most useful examination for the diagnosis of acute aortic dissection, and even today many patients undergo some type of angiographic study. Angiography can define the location of the entry point of the dissection, is the only way to know whether or not coronary atherosclerosis is present, and can be helpful in identifying the origins of distal aortic branches. Aortography, however, has a rate of failure to identify dissections that may approach 20%. Other disadvantages of angiography include the time taken for study in an acute situation and the dye load that is given to a patient who may have some compromise of renal function. For patients with acute dissections, the identification of the origin of the distal aortic branches (whether they are supplied by the true or false lumen) is not critical. First, it may take a prolonged, detailed angiographic study to answer those questions, often not in the patient's interest in the acute situation. Second, the initial operation performed in these situations is the same regardless of which lumen supplies the distal branches with blood flow.

Our current approach to obtaining a definitive diagnosis for the patient with the presumptive diagnosis of acute aortic dissection, as listed in Figure 35-2. Echocardiography is often the most rapidly and easily obtainable study, and that is usually our initial maneuver. If echocardiography clearly defines the presence of an ascending aortic dissection, if the patient is less than 40 years of age and has no history of angina, and if the clinical syndrome has occurred less than 24 hours before (hyperacute dissection), or if the patient is at all unstable, we consider the echocardiographic information sufficient to proceed with urgent operation. For patients over 40 years of age with a dissection documented by echocardiography, we proceed with cine angiography, if the patient is stable, to locate any intrinsic coronary atherosclerosis and to attempt to define the entry site precisely. If echocardiography fails to document the presence of a suspected dissection, we proceed with angiography. If these examinations fail to document the presence of dissection, we next perform a MRI examination if the patient is stable or CT scan if the patient is unstable and on life support.

The type of imaging technique that is used most effectively varies among institutions and even within institutions depending on the time of day. The physician investigating a patient with suspected acute aortic dissection must remember that the patient has an ongoing risk of death, and the order in which imaging techniques are preferred is influenced by time considerations. Patients with chronic aortic dissections are almost always stable enough to undergo detailed angiographic studies, although MRI techniques can often provide the necessary information.

Treatment

The objective of the medical treatment of an acute aortic dissection is to lower the systemic blood pressure to normal levels and to lower the velocity with which blood is ejected into the aorta (dP/dt)—anti-impulse therapy. Whether or not surgery is contemplated, initial medical treatment is appropriate for all patients with a presumed or definitive diagnosis of aortic dissection who are not in a state of hemodynamic compromise.

The initial medical treatment of patients with an acute aortic dissection should be undertaken with parenteral medication, in an ICU with precise hemodynamic monitoring, including an indwelling arterial pressure catheter, a central venous pressure catheter for administration of medications, and preferably a Swan-Ganz catheter to monitor pulmonary artery pressure and cardiac output. Heart rate, urine output, systemic blood pressure, and cardiac filling pressures are continuously monitored, and cardiac output is intermittently determined.

The pharmacologic therapy of acute aortic dissection is relatively standardized (Table 35-3).[17] Sodium nitroprusside is a vasodilator that acts directly on arterial and venous smooth muscle and is used to lower systemic blood pressure acutely. Nitroprusside has immediate effect, has a short half-life, and is given by infusion pump at an initial rate of 0.25 to 1 μg/kg/min. The levels that are given are then titrated according to the systemic blood pressure to achieve a systolic pressure of 100 to 110 mm Hg. By itself, administration of sodium nitroprusside can result in an increase in ejection velocity (dP/dt) and tachycardia, both undesirable effects. Therefore concomitant use of beta-adrenergic blockade is required. Other complications of the use of large doses (> 3 μg/kg/min) of sodium nitroprusside include cyanide or thiocyanate toxicity and methemoglobinemia. The cardial sign of cyanide toxicity is metabolic acidosis, and those of thiocyanate toxicity are hyperreflexia, confusion, and convulsion. If treatment is continued for more than 24 hours, even 0.5 to 1.0 μg/kg/min may produce toxicity, particularly in patients with renal insufficiency.

Beta-adrenergic blockade, "anti-impulse" therapy, should be used even in the presence of a normal mean arterial blood pressure. In the short term, the choices of pharmacologic agents include propranolol, esmolol, and labetalol. Esmolol has an advantage of a shorter half-life.[18] The most salient side effect of beta blockade is bronchospasm. This problem usually does not occur unless the patient has a history of bronchospasm, asthma, or chronic obstructive pulmonary disease.

Trimethaphan is a short-acting ganglionic blocking

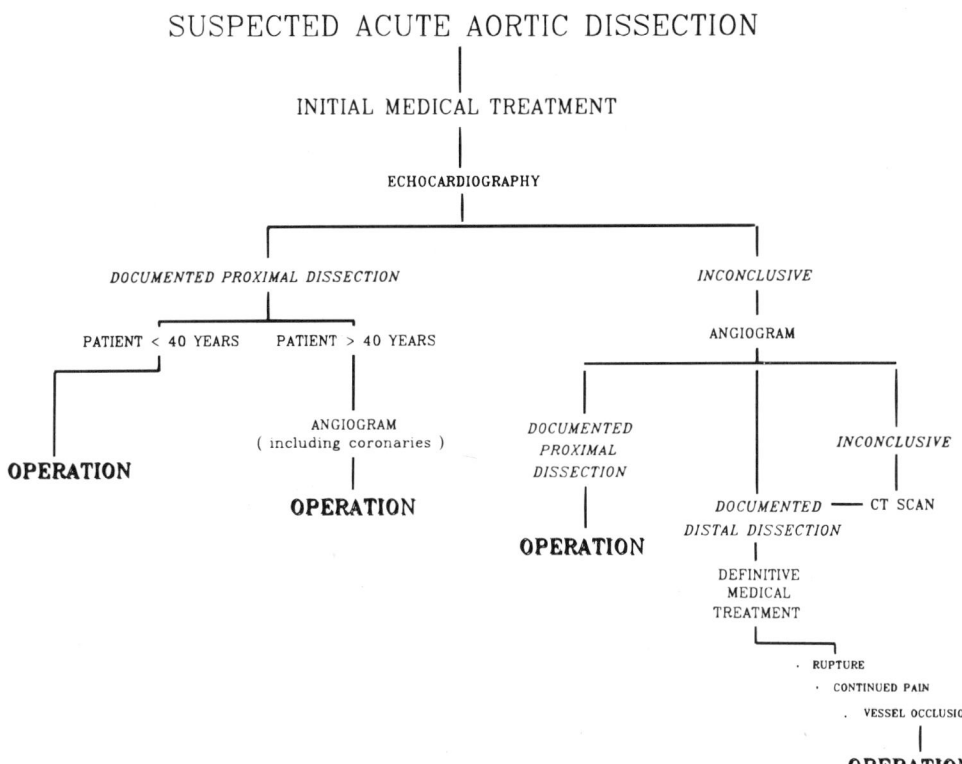

Fig. 35–2. Decision tree for the diagnosis and treatment of acute aortic dissection.

agent that can be used instead of nitroprusside, and in theory it is a superior agent for the treatment of dissection because one of its effects is to provide sympathetic blockade. Most ICU teams, however, are more familiar with the use of nitroprusside. Furthermore, trimethaphan may produce ileus and urinary retention, and tachyphylaxis develops rapidly, often within 24 to 48 hours. Therefore, trimethaphan is a secondary choice and is used in situations in which toxicity to nitroprusside or beta-adrenergic blockade develops or is threatened.

If the long-range plan is to treat the dissection with pharmacologic therapy, an oral treatment program must be instituted. This is most common in the treatment of dissections involving only the descending aorta. We usually delay institution of oral therapy for at least 3 days after the dissection has occurred. First, oral medication may not be well absorbed in the acute setting, and second, we prefer to wait for a few days to see whether or not complications that will indicate surgery develop.

Definitive Therapy of Ascending Aortic Dissections

Virtually all investigators agree that the definitive treatment of acute ascending aortic dissection should be surgical.[3,4,6,19,20] Medical treatment alone has resulted in an in-hospital mortality of at least 75% for patients with acute ascending aortic dissection, whereas the mortality of surgically treated patients should be around 10% even when patients with established complications, such as stroke and renal failure, are included. Dissections that arise in the aortic arch are less frequent, and operation carries with it a higher risk. We recommend surgery for arch dissections if the aortic diameter exceeds 5 cm.

Surgery for ascending aortic dissection is undertaken through a median sternotomy with the aid of cardiopulmonary bypass. After systemic heparinization, arterial cannulation is accomplished through the femoral artery, and venous cannulation is usually accomplished through the right atrium. If evidence of cardiac tamponade is present,

Table 35–3. Pharmacologic Management of Aortic Dissection

| | | Clinical Effect | | |
Agent	Preparation an Dosage	Blood Pressure	Ejection Velocity	Half-Life
Sodium nitroprusside (vasodilator)	50–100 mg in 500 ml D$_5$W IV at initial dose of 25–50 μg/min	↓	↑	Minutes
Trimethaphan (ganglionic blockade)	500 μg/500 ml D$_5$W IV at initial dose of 1 mg/min	↓	—	Minutes
Propranolol (beta blockade)	0.5–1 mg IV followed by 0.5–1 IV every 5 min until heart rate <70 min	↓	↓	3 hours
Esmolol (beta blockade)	5 g/500 ml D$_5$W or NS 500 μg/kg loading dose over 1 min Maintenance at 50–300 μg/kg/min (repeat loading dose may be necesary)	↓	↓	9 min
Labetalol (alpha and beta blockade)	200 mg/200 ml D$_5$W or NS 2 mg/min; titrate to effect	↓	↓	5.5 hours

venous cannulation may be accomplished through the femoral vein so it is possible to establish cardiopulmonary bypass before opening the pericardium. Once the pericardium is opened, a second venous cannula may be placed in the right atrium to provide complete venous drainage. Because many patients with an ascending aortic dissection also have aortic insufficiency, we decompress the left ventricle with a cannula placed through the right superior pulmonary vein, across the mitral valve, and into the left ventricle. Once cardiopulmonary bypass is established, the body temperature is cooled to a nasopharyngeal and bladder temperature of 18°C, a process that usually takes 40 to 45 minutes. If severe aortic insufficiency is not present, the aorta is not clamped, but circulatory arrest is instituted once the 18°C temperature is achieved. If aortic insufficiency begins to distend the left ventricle, the aorta is clamped proximal to the site where the distal anastomosis will be constructed, and the aorta is opened. Blood cardioplegia is used to protect the myocardium during the time the circulation to the coronary arteries is interrupted. The goals of operation for an acute ascending aortic dissection are to:

- Eliminate the entry point to the dissection
- Prevent antegrade blood flow into the false lumina
- Establish a competent aortic valve

The most secure way to accomplish these goals is usually to excise the ascending aorta (which contains the entry point) and to replace the ascending aorta with a Dacron graft.

The distal anastomosis of the graft to the aorta is constructed distal to the extent of the intimal tear. In most cases, this means that this anastomosis is made proximal to the innominate artery, but in a few cases, the intimal tear spirals into the aortic arch, and the anastomosis must be constructed either in the arch of the aorta or distal to the arch. Although the aorta containing the intimal tear is entirely resected, in many cases (type I dissection), the false lumen extends distal to the point of anastomosis. Therefore the false channel must be obliterated in the construction of the distal anastomosis. This is accomplished by "sandwiching" the layers of the aorta back together by placing one layer of Teflon felt on the adventitial surface, one layer on the intimal surface, and a third layer within the false channel, then sewing the Dacron graft to the reconstructed aorta (Fig. 35-3). The Teflon felt is used to distribute tension evenly and to prevent tearing of the fragile tissues. Some authors have reported the successful use of an intraluminal shunt for the construction of the distal anastomosis, a technique we have rarely used.[21] Placement of an aortic cross clamp distal to the distal anastomosis can fracture the intima and allow antegrade flow into the false channel. To avoid placing a clamp on an area of dissection that is not going to be resected, circulatory arrest is used in the construction of the distal anastomosis. Circulatory arrest also allows the surgeon to visualize the anatomy precisely and to construct this anastomosis under ideal circumstances. Once the distal anastomosis is constructed, a clamp can be placed on the graft, flow reestablished via cardiopulmonary bypass, and systemic rewarming started.

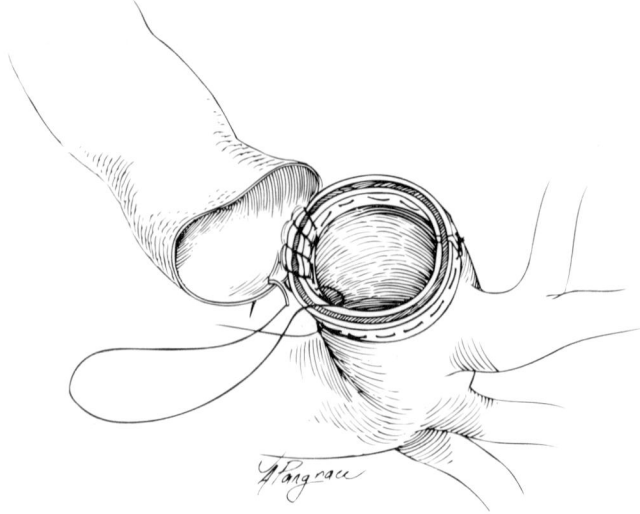

Fig. 35-3. In performing the distal aortic anastomosis for patients with dissections in situations in which the false channel extends further than the point of anastomosis, we reconstruct the layers of the aorta using three layers of Teflon felt, then sew the graft to this reconstructed aorta.

The type of operation performed in the aortic root is governed by the pathology of the aortic sinuses and the aortic valve. In most cases, the aortic valve and aortic sinuses are intrinsically normal, and the intimal tear is distal to the coronary orifices. In this situation, the aortic layers are reconstructed using Teflon felt, and the commissural attachments of the aortic valve are resuspended (Fig. 35-4), thus sparing the aortic valve (see Fig. 35-5C). If the aortic valve is intrinsically abnormal with stenosis or insufficiency but the sinuses are normal, the aortic valve is replaced, and a supracoronary graft is placed (see Fig. 35-5B). If the sinuses are intrinsically abnormal, as is often the case for patients with Marfan syndrome, the entire aortic root is replaced with a composite graft technique (Fig. 35-5A). Once both anastomoses are completed, the clamp on the graft is removed, and the heart is reperfused. When the patient is rewarmed to 36°C and effective myocardial contractions have returned, the patient is weaned off cardiopulmonary bypass. Protamine is used to reverse the heparin effect.

In the past, bleeding after operation for an acute aortic dissection has been of concern, but a number of technical advances have helped surgeons avoid these problems. The combination of "sewability" and low porosity of woven Dacron grafts has been an advance, and before insertion, the graft is baked in an autoclave with 5% albumin to ensure impermeability to blood. The use of Teflon felt in the construction of anastomoses has decreased needle hole bleeding from the friable tissues, and the use of circulatory arrest has increased the precision with which surgeons can construct the distal anastomosis. Finally, the use of blood component therapy, platelets, and fresh frozen plasma has helped to counteract the detrimental effects

THORACIC AORTIC DISSECTIONS AND ANEURYSMS

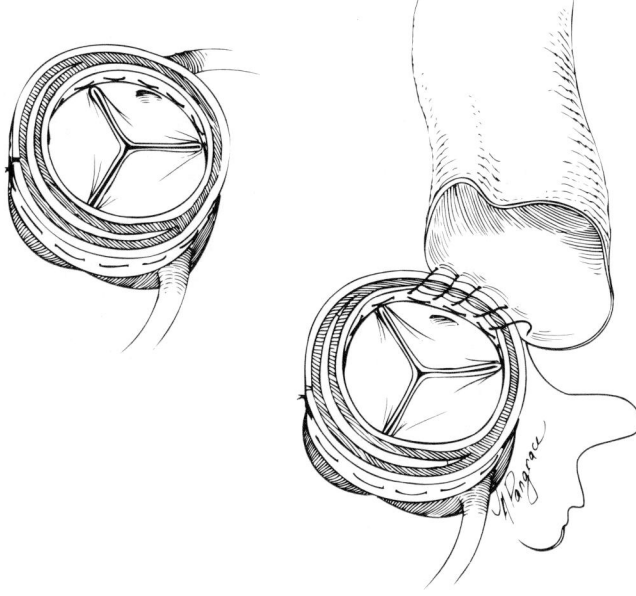

Fig. 35-4. For patients with ascending aortic dissections, a normal aortic valve, and normal aortic sinuses, the aortic valve commissures are resuspended with suture backed with Teflon felt, and the proximal anastomosis is then constructed to the reconstructed aortic root.

that cardiopulmonary bypass and deep hypothermia have on platelet function and the coagulation system.

Postoperative Management of Patients After Operations for Ascending Aortic Dissection

Control of postoperative hypertension is a critical aspect of postoperative care. It is important to remember that some patients have a residual false lumen present in the aorta distal to the location of the graft (Fig. 35-6), and if there was a distal reentry site, there is flow into the false lumen from that reentry site. For control of postoperative hypertension in the ICU, we use the same pharmacologic agents, sodium nitroprusside and beta-blockade, that are used in the preoperative period.

Hemodynamic management is similar to that used after most open heart operations. Systemic arterial pressure, pulmonary artery pressure, heart rate, urine output, and chest tube output are continuously monitored, and cardiac output is intermittently determined by thermodilution techniques using a pulmonary artery catheter. Routine postoperative chest films and ECGs are obtained.

Close attention must be paid to the coagulation system. Platelet count, prothrombin time, and activated partial thromboplastin time are determined on arrival in the ICU, and abnormalities are treated with component therapy.

When the high pressure antegrade flow is removed from the false lumen by operation, pulses that were deficient by the dissection commonly improve. Pulse assessment is important in the postoperative period. It is important to remember that even if pulses have returned, it is possible that end organs may have suffered ischemic damage between the time the dissection occurred and the time the operation effected reperfusion of those organs. For example, in one case, we noted bowel necrosis that did not become clinically evident until 3 days after operation for a dissection. At exploratory laparotomy, the pulses in the distribution of the superior mesenteric artery were normal, but the small bowel was necrotic, presumably because of transient ischemia that occurred before operation. If pulses that were missing preoperatively do not return after operation and if limb or end-organ ischemia is present, local operations for revascularization must be considered. If an effective operation to resect the ascending aorta and to prevent antegrade flow into the false lumen has been carried out, however, persistent organ ischemia is extremely uncommon.

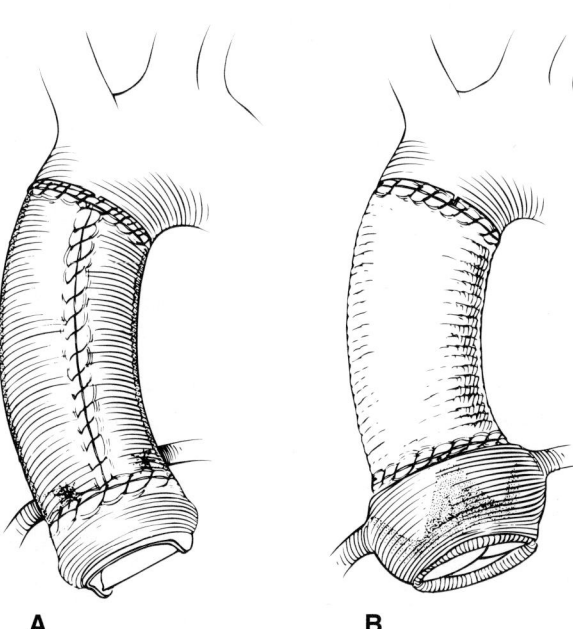
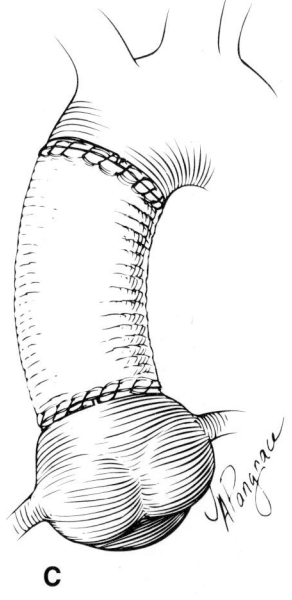

Fig. 35-5. *A*, If the aortic valve and sinuses are abnormal, a composite graft (Dacron tube graft continuous with a prosthetic valve) is used to replace the aortic root, and the coronary arteries are implanted into the graft. *B*, If the aortic valve is abnormal and the aortic sinuses are normal, the aortic valve is replaced, and the aortic graft is sewn above the coronary arteries. *C*, If the aortic valve and sinuses are normal, the graft is sewn above the coronary arteries, and the aortic valve is resuspended (see Fig. 35-4).

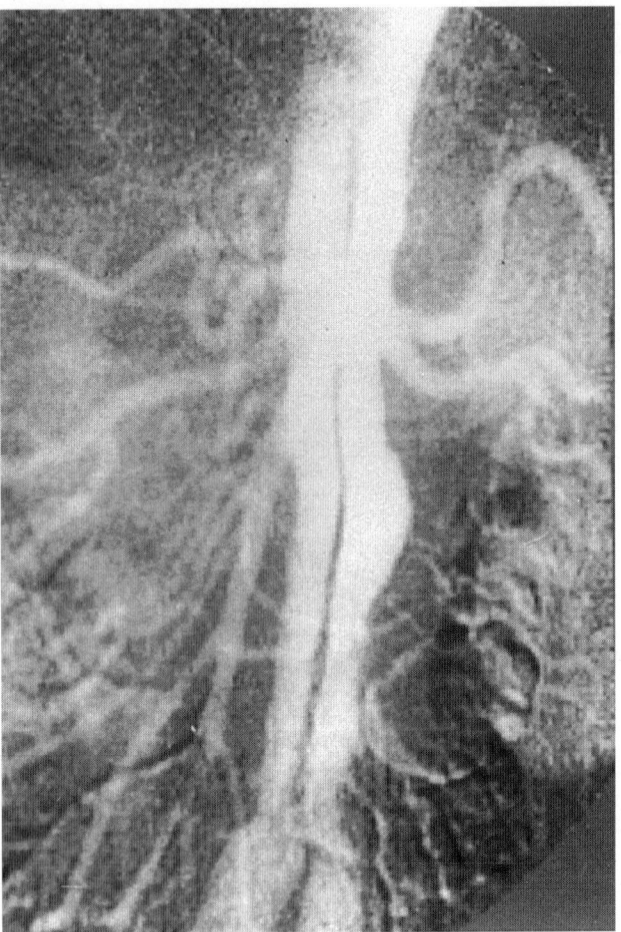

Fig. 35-6. Angiogram showing residual false channel in the abdominal aorta distal to the repair of the dissection.

We do not believe that preoperative neurologic or renal deficits are a contraindication to operation for acute dissection. Such preoperative deficits are rarely immediately corrected by operation, but with tenacious and effective postoperative care, these deficits may resolve.

If things go well in the postoperative period, it may be possible to discharge the patient from the ICU within a day or two. For this to occur, the pharmacologic, antihypertensive, and anti-impulse therapy must be shifted from an intravenous to an oral program.

The in-hospital mortality rates of operations for ascending aortic dissection are related to the acuity of the dissection, the extent of the operation, and the experience of the surgical team.[3,20,22,23] We reviewed the in-hospital mortality rates for patients undergoing resection of the ascending aorta for dissections from 1978 to 1987 and found that patients having surgery for acute dissections had approximately twice the mortality (21%) of patients who underwent operation for chronic dissections (11%).[22] Crawford and associates[23] have noted similar mortality rates of 23% and 11% for acute and chronic dissections. Furthermore, we found that the need to resect the aortic arch doubled the mortality rate. The presence of intrinsic coronary artery disease that required bypass grafting quadrupled the mortality. Finally, when we compared the mortality rate in the first 5 years of the study (1978 to 1983), with that in the second 4 years of the period under review (1984 to 1987), the mortality rate dropped from 23% to 13%.[22]

Surgery for Descending Aortic Dissections

Operations for descending aortic dissections are done through a left thoracotomy. Often the operation can be performed without cardiopulmonary bypass. If there is room distal to the left subclavian artery, the aorta is clamped at that point. At times, however, hematoma in the periaortic tissues or the size of the false lumen of the dissection may obscure the aorta distal to the subclavian, and the proximal aortic cross-clamp must be placed between the left carotid and the left subclavian artery.

When the lung is adherent to the aorta, it may signify that a localized rupture has been contained by the lung and mediastinal structures. In this situation, it may be difficult to gain control of the proximal aorta and may be safest to use cardiopulmonary bypass. Deep hypothermia and circulatory arrest enables the operation to be performed without aortic clamping.

The proximal anastomosis is performed to aorta that is not dissected, usually just distal to the subclavian artery. In the construction of the distal anastomosis, the layers of the aorta are sewn back together, and the graft is sewn to the reconstructed aorta, as has been described in the section on ascending aortic dissections.

Postoperative Care of Patients with Descending Aortic Dissections

In addition to bleeding, specific postoperative complications related to operations for descending aortic dissections often relate to respiratory function. The lateral thoracotomy used for operation on the descending aorta compromises respiratory function more than a median sternotomy does, and some trauma to the lung on the side of the operation may occur, particularly if the patient receives heparin during the procedure and intraparenchymal bleeding occurs in the lung. Furthermore, the left recurrent laryngeal nerve curves around the ligamentum arteriosum and runs in an area where it may be injured by the procedure, causing left vocal cord paralysis that may be temporary or permanent. Patients with vocal cord paralysis may have difficulty coughing after operation, and persistent attention to pulmonary toilet is needed. Pain and splinting are greater with lateral thoracotomy than with median sternotomy, and methods of pain relief such as intercostal block and epidural infusion improve the patient's comfort and pulmonary function.

Late survival after operation for descending aortic dissection was 64% at 5 and 34% at 10 postoperative years in the series reported by Crawford and associates[23] and 90% and 65% as reported by Haverich and colleagues.[26] Late complications related to aortic pathology are common. In Crawford's series, 19% of late deaths were clearly due to ruptured aneurysms, and Haverich et al. reported that aortic reoperation occurred in 13% of patients by 5 and 23% by 10 postoperative years. Late surveillance of patients after successful operation for descending aortic dissections is critical.

Post-ICU Phase

Late Follow-Up for Patients with Ascending Aortic Dissections

After surgery for an ascending aortic dissection, patients should be followed for possible late complications involving the residual aorta (either dissected or not dissected), the aortic graft, aortic valve, and hypertension. Patients who have had an aortic dissection should remain on antihypertensive and anti-impulse therapy for life.

Patients with a residual false channel and nonresected aorta need to have periodic imaging of the aorta to detect late aneurysm formation. The best way to accomplish this is with MRI, the first examination being done within 3 months of operation to provide a baseline and then yearly after that.

If the aortic valve has been resuspended, periodic (yearly) echo Doppler studies are the best way to document the continued competence of the valve. If the aortic valve has been replaced with a mechanical prosthesis, anticoagulation with warfarin for life is indicated. Patients with a prosthetic aortic valve or a prosthetic aortic graft need antibiotic prophylaxis if they have future procedures (particularly dental procedures) that might produce bacteremia.

The late survival rate after ascending aorta operations for dissection is 70 to 75% at 5 postoperative years. The most common causes of late death are cardiac, but 21% of late deaths in the Crawford series were due to rupture of aneurysms, indicating the need for persistent surveillance of these patients.

Treatment of Descending Aortic Dissections

There is no uniform agreement on the optimal treatment for acute distal (type III) aortic dissections, but currently the weight of evidence supports medical therapy for uncomplicated distal dissections. In 1965, Wheat and colleagues[24] reported the treatment of 6 consecutive patients with anti-impulse and antihypertensive pharmacologic therapy with early survival for all patients. This was during a period when the operative mortality for type III dissections was at least 20% even at centers experienced with aortic surgery. Miller and co-workers[20] from Stanford University reported a lower operative mortality of 13% and advocated surgery as the treatment of choice. Glower and associates[25] reported a combined series of patients with acute or chronic type III dissections from Duke and Stanford Universities and found no difference in early or late mortality for patients with uncomplicated dissections when they compared medical and surgical therapy. The 30-day mortality of all acute-care patients treated medically was 18% (10/56) compared with 33% (11/33) for those who had surgery. Seven of the 11 surgical deaths, however, occurred in patients operated on because of rupture. In "good risk" patients without complications of dissections, the mortality was 16% (3/19) with medical treatment and 9% (1/11) with surgery. Five of the 56 acute-care patients initially treated medically subsequently required surgery for rupture or expansion of the false channel. Our current approach is to treat most patients with acute type III dissections medically and reserve operation for the treatment of patients with specific complications of type III dissections. Specific indications for the surgical treatment of acute type III dissections are rupture, pulse loss, progression of the dissection while on medical therapy, continued pain (indicating progression), and dilation of the false channel while on medical treatment.

When definitive medical treatment is planned, it is necessary to switch from intravenous agents to oral agents. All patients receive antiadrenergic agents, and if possible, we prefer to use antenolol and nadolol because they need to be taken only once a day. Any oral beta-blocker, however, can be used. If antiadrenergic agents alone do not control the blood pressure, we add an angiotensin-converting enzyme inhibitor, such as lisinopril, 5 to 40 mg orally once a day.

In addition to death, the most significant complication of operation for resection of the descending thoracic aorta is paraplegia. The reasons for this complication are probably multiple, but the major one is spinal cord ischemia because of interruption of the blood supply to the cord from the intercostal branches of the aorta. The incidence of paraplegia is related to the length of the aorta that needs to be replaced. In large series of operations for dissections reported by Crawford et al.,[23] the incidence of paraplegia ranged from 7% for thoracic aortic replacement to 40% when extensive thoracoabdominal replacement was necessary. Acuity also influenced the rate of paraplegia because patients with acute dissections had twice the incidence of that complication than those with chronic dissections.

THORACIC ANEURYSMS

Thoracic aneurysms are localized dilatations of the aorta that may consist of all layers of aorta (true aneurysms) or the aortic adventitia (false aneurysms).

False Aneurysms

False aneurysms of the thoracic aorta are almost always caused by trauma, usually a deceleration-type injury. Deceleration trauma can exert a shearing force on the aorta, resulting in a tear of the intima and media. This injury usually occurs just distal to the ligamentum arteriosum, probably because the descending aorta is fixed posteriorly to the vertebrae, whereas the aortic arch is more mobile. The most common result of this injury is full-thickness rupture and almost immediate death from exsanguination. In some patients, however, the adventitia is strong enough to contain the rupture, and a false aneurysm is the result.

Clinical Situation and Diagnosis

Aortic traumatic rupture contained by the aortic adventitia (false aneurysm) must be suspected in any patient who has suffered a severe deceleration injury. Because most patients with thoracic aortic injuries have also suffered injuries to the bony thoracic structures or pulmonary contusions, plain chest films may be difficult to interpret. Mediastinal widening or a left pleural effusion, however, may be evident on x-ray film and should raise the question of an aortic injury. Mediastinal hematomas that are not the result of aortic rupture may also occur and can complicate the diagnostic process.

In the acute situation, the definitive diagnosis of aortic rupture is usually established by contrast thoracic aortography. The reliability of less invasive techniques, such as echocardiography, CT scanning, and MRI, in the identification of acute aortic rupture has not yet been established. Because these patients often have intra-abdominal, pelvic, cranial, or long-bone injuries, the timing of arteriography is often determined by the need for the diagnosis and treatment of these other injuries.

Once the diagnosis of an acute traumatic rupture of the thoracic aorta is made, the usual procedure is operation to repair the disruption. Again, the timing of operation may be influenced by the need to deal with associated injuries. Operation is undertaken through a left thoracotomy. The aorta is clamped proximal and distal to the injury. If the transection is partial, simple repair of the aorta may be possible, but at times replacement of the entire aorta with a graft is needed.

Controversy still exists as to the best way to protect the lower body (and, in particular, the spinal cord) during clamping of the proximal descending aorta. The options include simple aortic cross-clamping, use of a heparin-bonded shunt from the proximal to the distal aorta, centrifugal pumps that may require submaximal amounts of systemic heparin, and cardiopulmonary bypass, which requires full heparinization. Because of the frequency of associated injuries in these patients, it is often desirable to avoid systemic heparinization. A study of operations for traumatic aortic rupture by Katz and colleagues[27] demonstrated that when simple aortic cross-clamping was used, the likelihood of paraplegia increased when the cross-clamp time exceeded 30 minutes. At present, heparin-bonded shunts that do not require systemic heparinization and centrifugal pumps that do not require full heparinization are probably the most commonly used methods for minimizing spinal cord ischemia during operations for aortic rupture (Fig. 35-7).[28]

True Aneurysms of the Thoracic Aorta

True aneurysms of the thoracic aorta may involve any portion of the aorta, although they are least common in the region of the aortic arch. Atherosclerosis is the most common pathologic cause of aneurysms in the descending thoracic aorta. These aneurysms may be fusiform or saccular. In the ascending aorta, most aneurysms are associated with cystic medial necrosis. Saccular aneurysms are not common in the ascending aorta, where their form is usually fusiform or annuloaortic ectasia, a situation in which the entire aortic root, including the aortic valve, is involved in the aneurysmal process. The majority of patients with thoracic aneurysms have a history of hypertension.

Clinical Presentations of Ascending Aortic Aneurysms

The majority of ascending aortic aneurysms are associated with aortic valve insufficiency, and this valve lesion

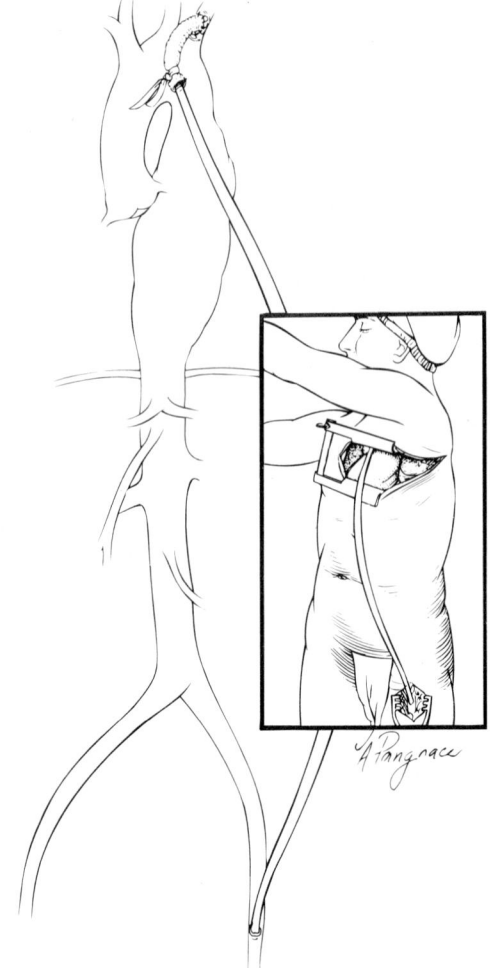

Fig. 35–7. Diagram showing the use of heparin-bonded shunt from the left subclavian artery to the left femoral artery. The shunt maintains flow to the lower part of the body during aortic cross-clamping.

often dominates the clinical presentation by causing dyspnea. An abnormal chest film is another common reason these patients are evaluated. The natural history of ascending aortic aneurysms is not as accurately understood as the history of infrarenal aneurysms is, but data reported by Joyce and associates[29] indicate that when thoracic aneurysms reach 6 cm in diameter, the risk of rupture increases. There is general consensus that 6-cm aneurysm of the ascending aorta should be treated surgically. Moreover, dissection can occur in patients with aneurysms of the ascending aorta and is a common cause of death for these patients.

MRI is the most effective way to image ascending aortic aneurysms because this technique does not require a large dye load and allows imaging of the entire aorta. This second consideration is important because concomitant aneurysms of the descending or abdominal aorta may be present. Cardiac catheterization is indicated to evaluate the aortic and mitral valves for insufficiency and to identify any coronary artery disease that may be present. Echo Doppler studies are also helpful for evaluation of valve function.

Most patients with ascending aortic aneurysms who do not have dissections are evaluated electively, and detailed studies are almost always possible.

Young adults with ascending aortic aneurysms commonly have cystic medial necrosis with or without other stigmata of Marfan syndrome. In Marfan patients, we often recommend operations if the aorta is more than 5 cm in diameter because waiting a year or two before the 6-cm stage is reached is not really worth the risk that a dissection will supervene.

Ascending aortic annuloaortic ectasia is usually treated surgically by composite graft replacement of the aortic root and ascending aorta, as described in the section on ascending aortic dissection. Older patients sometimes have a normal segment of aorta just distal to the aortic valve that contains the coronary orifices, and this situation can often be treated with valve replacement and a supracoronary graft.

Elective operations for ascending aortic aneurysms are quite safe with an overall in-hospital risk of less than 5% even in elderly patients. Postoperative care of these patients is similar to that for routine cardiac surgery, and the most important part is usually attention to postoperative hypertension, both in the hospital setting and after discharge.

Descending Thoracic and Thoracoabdominal Aneurysms

True aneurysms of the descending thoracic or thoracoabdominal aorta are primarily a disease of the elderly. Approximately half of the patients coming to medical attention are asymptomatic, and of those with symptoms, the most common complaint is chest or back pain.[30-33] Symptoms referable to a space-occupying lesion, such as dysphagia owing to esophageal compression, wheezing or hoarseness owing to recurrent pharyngeal nerve involvement, tracheal deviation, and superior vena cava syndrome, may also occur.

The natural history of thoracic and thoracoabdominal aneurysms treated conservatively is not favorable. In Joyce's series, 38% of patients with aneurysms greater than 6 cm in diameter survived 5 years. Bickerstaff and associates[34] calculated a 19% 5-year survival for patients with aneurysms not caused by dissection, in which 50% of the patients died because of rupture of the aneurysm. A series of patients with thoracoabdominal aneurysms followed without surgery showed that only 24% of patients survived 2 years, with half of those deaths also due to aneurysm rupture.[30] There is general agreement that operations should be considered for aneurysms larger than 6 cm in diameter or twice the size of the proximal aorta. Because of the large number of patients who have thoracic aneurysms, however, who also have concomitant cardiovascular or pulmonary disease, careful preoperative evaluation is in order. We recommend preoperative coronary angiography for all patients who are being evaluated for elective resection of a thoracic or thoracoabdominal aneurysm. Sixteen percent of patients in Joyce's series had angina or previous myocardial infarction. In a surgical series of patients with thoracoabdominal aneurysms, 16% had angiographically documented coronary artery disease. Not only does coronary artery disease contribute to perioperative morbidity and mortality, but also late death after successful operation for thoracic aneurysm is often related to coronary artery disease. If coronary angiography documents significant left main stenosis, triple vessel disease, or double-vessel disease involving the anterior descending coronary artery, we recommend elective bypass surgery before elective operation for the thoracic aneurysm. If the patient has single-vessel disease with a large amount of myocardium at risk, we sometimes proceed with bypass surgery or percutaneous transluminal coronary angiography.

Preoperative evaluation of pulmonary function is also important because at least a quarter of patients with thoracic aneurysms also have chronic obstructive pulmonary disease. A lateral thoracotomy, which is used for resection of thoracic or thoracoabdominal aneurysms, induces more postoperative respiratory dysfunction than a median sternotomy does. Retention of carbon dioxide predicts a difficult postoperative course, as does forced first-second vital capacity of less than 1.25 L.

Preoperative renal dysfunction is also evaluated, and in Crawford's series of thoracoabdominal aneurysm patients, 14% had chronic renal insufficiency (creatinine greater than 2 mg/dl).

Operation for thoracic or thoracoabdominal aneurysm is performed through a left thoracotomy or a thoracoabdominal incision, which divides the costal margin, divides the diaphragm, and reflects the abdominal viscera anteriorly. As with other operations on the descending thoracic aorta, paraplegia is a major concern and is related to the length of the aorta that needs to be resected. For patients with atherosclerotic thoracoabdominal aneurysms involving the entire descending thoracic aorta, the incidence of paraplegia is 10% if the upper abdominal aorta is involved and 28% if the entire aorta needs to be replaced. Patients with aneurysms caused by dissection have had a higher risk of paraplegia than those with nondissections. For aneurysms limited to the thoracic aorta, the risk is much lower, 5 to 10%. Unfortunately, despite the use of multiple techniques for trying to decrease the incidence of paraplegia, this problem is far from solved.

The postoperative management of patients with thoracic or thoracoabdominal aneurysm resection starts with respiratory management. We usually continue mechanical ventilation for at least 24 hours after surgery. Once the patient is awake and communicative, we gradually decrease intermittent mandatory ventilation rate while maintaining a moderate degree of positive and excretory pressure to prevent small airway collapse. Postoperative pain and possible recurrent laryngeal paresis or paralysis may make coughing difficult after extubation, and careful attention to pulmonary toilet is important. Positive end-expiratory pressure can be maintained by a mask, and nasotracheal suctioning can be used. Renal dysfunction of mild degree is often seen after surgery for thoracoabdominal aneurysms, and approximately 5% of patients need dialysis during the postoperative course. If patients have preoperative renal dysfunction, the likelihood of dialysis postoperatively is 15 to 20%. We routinely maintain patients on postoperative levels of dopamine (2 to 3 mg/kg) but increase renal blood flow.

Attention to postoperative nutrition is also important. Particularly when patients have undergone resection of thoracoabdominal aneurysms, there is often a postoperative ileus present that may be evident for up to a week. Nutrition is maintained by intravenous hyperalimentation in these patients.

REFERENCES

1. Roberts W. C.: Aortic dissection: anatomy, consequences and causes. Am. Heart J. *101*:195, 1981.
2. Larson, E. W., and Edwards, W. D.: Risk factors for aortic dissection: a necropsy study of 161 cases. Am. J. Cardiol., *53*:849, 1984.
3. Crawford, E. S.: The diagnosis and management of aortic dissection. J.A.M.A. *264*:2537, 1990.
4. DeSanctis, R. W., Doroghazi, R. M., Austen, W. G., and Buckley, M. J.: Aortic dissection. N. Engl. J. Med., *317*:1060, 1987.
5. Doroghazi, R. M., et al.: Long-term survival of patients with treated aortic dissection. J. Am. Coll. Cardiol., *3*:1026, 1984.
6. Cohn, L. H.: *In* Surgery of the Chest. 5th ed. Edited by D. C. Sabiston, Jr., and F. C. Spencer. Philadelphia, W. B. Saunders, 1990, p. 1182.
7. Murphy, D. A., et al.: Recognition and management of ascending aortic dissection complicating cardiac surgical operations. J. Thorac. Cardiovasc. Surg., *85*:247, 1983.
8. Hirst, A. E., Jr., Johns, U. J., Jr., and Kime, S. W., Jr.: Dissecting aneurysms of the aorta: a review of 505 cases. Medicine, *37*:217, 1958.
9. Dicesare, E., et al.: Post-surgical follow up with MR imaging of aortic dissections. Radiology, *173*:105, 1989.
10. White, R. D., Ullyot, D. J., and Higgins, C. B.: MR imaging of the aorta after surgery for aortic dissection. Am. J. Roentgenol., *150*:87, 1988.
11. Sarris, G. E., and Miller, D. C.: Peripheral vascular manifestations of acute aortic dissection. *In* Vascular Surgery. 3rd ed. Edited by R. B. Rutherford. Philadelphia, W. B. Saunders, 1989, p. 842.
12. Hashimoto, S., et al.: Assessment of transesophageal doppler echography in dissecting aortic aneurysm. J. Am. Coll. Cardiol., *14*:1253, 1989.
13. Wilbers, C. R. H., Cariol, C. L., and Hullica, M. A.: Optimal diagnostic imaging of aortic dissection. Texas Heart J. *12*:231, 1990.
14. White, R. D., et al.: Noninvasive evaluation of suspected thoracic aortic disease by contrast enhanced computed tomography. Am. J. Cardiol., *57*:282, 1986.
15. White, R. D., and Higgins, C. B.: Magnetic resonance imaging of thoracic vascular disease. J. Thorac. Imag., *4*:34, 1989.
16. Kersting-Sommerhoff, B. A., et al.: Aortic dissection: sensitivity of MR imaging. Radiology, *166*:651, 1988.
17. Doroghazi, R. M., Slater, E. E., and DeSanctis, R. W.: Medical therapy for aortic dissections. J. Cardiovasc. Med., *6*:187, 1981.
18. Turlaputy, P., et al.: Esmolol: a titratable short-acting intervenous beta blocker for acute critical care settings. Am. Heart J., *114*:866, 1987.
19. Appelbaum, A., Karp, R. B., and Kirklin, J. W.: Ascending vs. descending aortic dissections. Ann. Surg., *183*:296, 1976.
20. Miller, D. C., et al.: Operative treatment of aortic dissections. Experience with 125 patients over a 16-year period. J. Thorac. Cardiovasc. Surg., *78*:365, 1979.
21. Berger, R. L., Romero, L., Chaudhry, A. G., and Dobnik, D. B.: Graft replacement of the thoracic aorta with a sutureless technique. Ann. Thorac. Surg., *35*:231, 1983.
22. Lytle, B. W., Mahfood, S. S., Cosgrove, D. M., and Loop, F. D.: Replacement of the ascending aorta. J. Thorac. Cardiovasc. Surg., *99*:651, 1990.
23. Crawford, E. S., et al.: Aortic dissection and dissecting aortic aneurysms. Ann. Surg. *208*:254, 1988.
24. Wheat, M. W., Palmer, R. G., Bartley, T. D., and Seelman, R. C.: Treatment of dissecting aneurysms of the aorta without surgery. J. Thorac. Cardiovasc. Surg., *50*:364, 1965.
25. Glower, D. D., et al.: Comparison of medical and surgical therapy for uncomplicated descending aortic aneurysm. Circulation, *82*:IV-39, 1990.
26. Haverich, A., et al.: Acute and chronic aortic dissections—determinants of long-term outcome for operative survivors. Circulation, *72(Suppl. II)*:II-22, 1985.
27. Katz, N. M., Blackstone, E. N., Kirklin, J. W., and Karp, R. B.: Incremental risk factors for spinal cord injury following operating for acute aortic transection. J. Thorac. Cardiovasc. Surg., *81*:669, 1981.
28. Verdant, A., et al.: Surgery of the descending thoracic aorta: spinal cord protection with the Gott shunt. Ann. Thorac. Surg., *46*:147, 1988.
29. Joyce, J. W., Fairbainn, J. F. II, Kincaid, O. W., and Juergens, J. L.: Aneurysms of the thoracic aorta: a clinical study with special deference to prognosis. Circulation, *29*:176, 1964.
30. Crawford, E. S., and DeNatale, R. W.: Thoracoabdominal aortic aneurysm: observations regarding the natural course of the disease. J. Vasc. Surg. *3*:578, 1986.
31. Crawford, E. S., et al.: Thoracoabdominal aneurysms: preoperative and intraoperative factors determining immediate and long-term results of operating in 605 patients. J. Vasc. Surg. *3*:389, 1986.
32. Moreno-Cabral, C., et al.: Degenerative and atherosclerotic aneurysms of the thoracic aorta. J. Thorac. Cardiovasc. Surg. *88*:1020, 1984.
33. Pressler, V., and McNamara, J. J.: Aneurysm of the thoracic aorta: review of 260 cases. J. Thorac. Cardiovasc. Surg. *89*:50, 1985.
34. Bickerstaff, L. K., et al.: Thoracic aortic aneurysms: a population-based study. Surgery, *92*:1103, 1982.

# Chapter 36

POSTOPERATIVE CARE OF THE VASCULAR SURGERY PATIENT

ERIC D. MORSE
JAMES W. HOLCROFT

Surgical correction of vascular disease of the abdominal aorta and of its immediate and distal branches frequently requires postoperative critical care. These corrections are directed at aneurysmal disease of the abdominal aorta and atherosclerotic aortoiliac occlusive disease, which frequently require major vascular procedures, such as aortic aneurysmectomy and aortobifemoral bypass, respectively. Postoperatively these patients must be monitored in an ICU. In addition, patients with peripheral arterial occlusive disease of the lower extremities often require infrainguinal bypass procedures to restore adequate distal circulation. Depending on their medical problems, such as cardiac and pulmonary disease, they may also require ICU monitoring postoperatively. Finally, acute arterial occlusion secondary to thrombosis or embolism may necessitate critical care. In this chapter, we discuss important preoperative considerations as well as postoperative intensive care of the vascular surgery patient.

Risk factors for the development of atherosclerosis have been well established and include:[1]

- Elevated blood lipids
- Hypertension
- Diabetes mellitus
- Cigarette smoking

Therefore, control of serum cholesterol and triglycerides, medial therapy for hypertension, tight control of blood glucose, and cessation of cigarette smoking slow the progression of atherosclerotic occlusive disease.[2] Exercise, either by stimulating the development of collateral circulation or by improving metabolic capacity of muscle tissue, may improve the symptoms of atherosclerotic occlusive disease. Hemorheologic agents, most notably pentoxifylline, may improve the symptoms of atherosclerotic occlusive disease.[3] This drug inhibits erythrocyte phosphodiesterase and causes increased phosphorylation of erythrocyte membrane proteins. Through these actions, pentoxifylline produces improved blood flow and oxygen delivery to ischemic areas by improving blood flow in the microcirculation as a result of increased erythrocyte deformability, associated with a minor reduction in blood viscosity. Vasodilators have been tried but have not been found to be effective in the treatment of occlusive disease.[3]

For progressive vascular disease that is unresponsive to medical therapy, there are three general indications for surgery for atherosclerotic occlusive disease. These are:

- Intermittent claudication
- Ischemic rest pain
- Threatened limb loss

The last two are generally accepted as absolute indications for surgery. Intermittent claudication as an indication for surgery is much more controversial. Many vascular surgeons recommend nonoperative measures, such as cessation of cigarette smoking and implementing an exercise program. With these measures, as many as 80% of patients may achieve stability or improvement in their claudication.[4] Only when claudication progresses to a point that it is so disabling that it impinges on the patient's lifestyle should it be considered an indication for surgery. The indications for surgery on abdominal aortic aneurysms (as opposed to occlusive disease) are more urgent. These include:[5]

- Rapid expansion (greater than 0.5 cm increase in diameter in a 3-month period)
- A diameter of 6 cm or greater and development of symptoms (back or abdominal pain)
- Distal arterial embolization from the aortic aneurysm
- Rupture

PRE-ICU PHASE

Postoperative complications after major vascular procedures are inevitable in some patients with severe systemic atherosclerosis. Risk factors that influence postoperative morbidity and mortality include advanced age, diabetes mellitus, hypertension, coronary artery disease, chronic obstructive pulmonary disease, and impaired renal function. Even though these risk factors are heavily concentrated among patients with abdominal aortic aneurysms and aortoiliac occlusive disease, current mortality rates for elective aortic replacement range from 2 to 5%.[6-8] Specific preoperative risk factors that significantly influence postoperative mortality include age greater than 60 years, suspected coronary artery disease, serum creatinine level greater than 2.0 mg/dl, complementary renal artery revascularization, and aneurysm rupture.[6] Further associated risks include intraoperative blood loss along with postoperative myocardial infarction, renal failure, and pulmonary insufficiency.[6]

When assessing risks, the age of the patient must be

Table 36-1. Factors Influencing Postoperative Morbidity and Mortality

Preoperative Risk Factors	Intraoperative/ Postoperative Risk Factors	Postoperative Complications
Advanced age	Blood loss	Stroke
Diabetes mellitus	Myocardial infarction	Congestive heart failure
Hypertension		Retroperitoneal bleeding
Coronary artery disease	Renal failure	Wound infection
Chronic obstructive pulmonary disease	Pulmonary insufficiency	Graft infection
		Renal failure
Impaired renal function		Pulmonary insufficiency
		Myocardial infarction
		Pulmonary embolism
		Colon ischemia

kept in mind because postoperative complications occur with greater frequency with increasing age of the patients. Postoperative morbidity rates range from 20 to 50%. Such complications include stroke, congestive heart failure, retroperitoneal bleeding, wound or prosthetic graft infection, acute renal failure, pulmonary insufficiency, myocardial infarction, pulmonary embolism, and colon ischemia (Table 36-1).

Angiography

Most vascular surgery patients undergo angiography preoperatively. In addition, other patients in the ICU may develop problems that need to be evaluated by angiography. Some of these problems include cardiac ischemia, pulmonary embolism, and acute arterial occlusion from thrombosis or embolism. Studies such as coronary, pulmonary, and aortic angiography with distal runoff need to be performed in these patients. Therefore, knowledge of the complications of angiography is necessary for any physician caring for these patients. These include:

- Acute renal dysfunction
- Reaction to iodinated contrast material
- Hematoma
- Hemorrhage
- Arterial occlusion
- Pseudoaneurysm
- Arteriovenous fistula

The complication rate for angiography ranges from 2 to 4%.[9,10] The mortality rate ranges from 0.03 to 0.06%.[9,10] Angiography is performed via one of three routes: transfemoral, translumbar, or transaxillary. Of these three, the transfemoral route is associated with the lowest overall complication rate.[9]

Acute renal dysfunction and acute renal failure are significant complications of angiography. The incidence of acute renal dysfunction ranges from 0 to 12%, and the incidence of acute renal failure is 0 to 2%.[11,12] Risk factors for the development of postangiographic acute renal dysfunction include diabetes mellitus, acute systemic illness, advanced age, pre-existing renal disease, dehydration, and infusion of large amounts of contrast material.[9,11] Therefore adequate preprocedure and postprocedure hydration and judicious use of angiographic contrast material are important in preventing the occurrence of this complication. Urine output and serum creatinine should be monitored for at least 24 hours after angiography to detect the development of renal dysfunction. When contrast-induced renal dysfunction does occur, most episodes resolve within 7 days.[13]

The incidence of untoward reactions to iodinated contrast material ranges from 4 to 9%.[14] These reactions range from a mild allergic reaction with urticaria to frank anaphylactic reactions with laryngeal edema, airway obstruction, and cardiovascular collapse. The mortality rate from these reactions is 0.002 to 0.009%.[14]

Complications may also occur at the arterial puncture site. The most common complication is a hematoma. Other complications include hemorrhage, arterial obstruction or embolization, pseudoaneurysm formation, or creation of an arteriovenous fistula. Careful postangiography observation for these problems is mandatory for 8 to 12 hours after procedures.

Cardiovascular Considerations

Atherosclerotic heart disease is the leading cause of death in the postoperative period.[7,8,38,39] In fact, postoperative myocardial infarction accounts for 50 to 80% of the postoperative deaths in several studies.[6,7,40,41] Because of the prevalence of atherosclerotic coronary artery disease among patients with peripheral atherosclerotic vascular disease, a thorough cardiac evaluation should be done preoperatively. This evaluation should include a routine cardiac history and a 12-lead electrocardiogram (ECG). Any patient with clinical evidence of cardiac disease (i.e., previous myocardial infarction or angina pectoris by history or Q-waves or ST-T-wave changes on the ECG) should have a complete cardiac assessment. Clinical evidence of atherosclerotic coronary disease is present in 40 to 60% of patients in need of major vascular procedures.[6,41,42] These patients should undergo radionuclide angiography or exercise tolerance testing to determine if coronary artery disease is present. If the results of these tests are abnormal, coronary angiography should be performed to determine if surgically correctable coronary artery disease is present. Coronary revascularization should be done before elective vascular procedures in patients with symptomatic coronary artery disease. Postoperative morbidity and mortality are significantly reduced when coronary revascularization precedes the elective vascular procedure.[6,42-46]

Preoperatively, all patients scheduled to undergo reconstruction of the abdominal aorta should undergo a formal bowel preparation with antibiotics. Such a preparation empties the small and large bowel and facilitates performance of the operative procedure. It also decreases the risk of ischemic colitis.

Neurologic Considerations

The morbidity and mortality associated with postoperative cerebrovascular accidents can be severe. The incidence of postoperative cerebrovascular accidents is approximately 1 to 5% after vascular procedures.[57,59] All patients should be evaluated for cerebrovascular disease preoperatively. Each patient should be questioned for symptoms of cerebrovascular disease and examined for cervical bruits. If symptoms of cerebrovascular disease are present or if a cervical bruit is found on physical examination, a duplex scan of the carotid arteries with Doppler flow analysis should be performed. If stenosis of the internal carotid artery is 80% or greater by these noninvasive methods, a carotid arteriogram should be obtained. If the arteriogram confirms the stenosis or if a badly ulcerated plaque is found, a carotid endarterectomy should be performed before the elective vascular procedure. Otherwise, the vascular procedure can be performed without carotid endarterectomy. There is no direct relationship between an asymptomatic bruit, severity of carotid artery disease, and incidence of preoperative cerebrovascular accident.[57]

ICU PHASE

Intraoperative Considerations

The principal intraoperative concern that has direct bearing on the postoperative course is the effect of the procedure on hemodynamic status. Cross-clamping and unclamping of the aorta during surgery causes significant hemodynamic changes in the cardiovascular system.[15] Aortic cross-clamping suddenly increases the systemic vascular resistance, placing a heavy burden on an often compromised heart, resulting in a decrease in cardiac output, and mean blood pressure frequently falls because of sequestration and pooling of blood in the lower extremities with release of vasodepressor substances, accumulation of metabolic byproducts, and washout acidosis (Fig. 36-1).[16-20] Under these circumstances, two different hemodynamic alterations are frequently seen.[15] On the one hand, a combination of decreased cardiac output and decreased pulmonary arterial wedge pressure can occur because of hypovolemia secondary to inadequate volume loading and because of vasodepressor substances released from ischemic lower extremities. On the other hand, a combination of decreased cardiac output and increased pulmonary arterial wedge pressure can occur because of impaired myocardial function.

The stress of these hemodynamic changes in patients with underlying myocardial disease may contribute to intraoperative and postoperative complications. In fact,

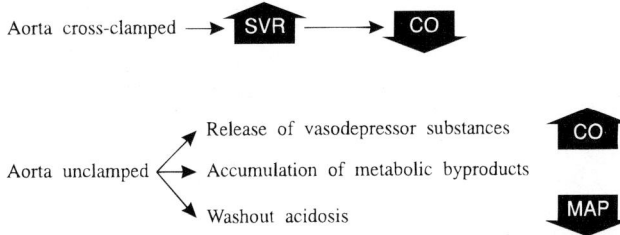

Fig. 36-1. Hemodynamic changes in the cardiovascular system as a result of cross-clamping and unclamping of the aorta. (Courtesy of George Morrison, CD, Inc.)

Table 36-2. Invasive Monitoring of Various Cardiopulmonary Parameters

Monitor	Assessment	Potential Problem
Arterial catheter	Arterial blood gas	Hypoxemia/hypercarbia
	Arterial pressure	Hypotension/hypertension
Central venous line	Central venous pressure	Volume status
Swan-Ganz catheter	Left-heart filling pressures	Volume status
	Vascular resistance	Congestive heart failure
	Cardiac output	Elevated/reduced systemic vascular resistance
		Cardiac dysfunction
Palpation of pedal pulses	Peripheral circulation	Poor perfusion
		Graft thrombosis
		Arterial embolism
Pulse oximeter	Oxygen saturation	Hypoxemia
Foley catheter	Urine output	Renal perfusion

myocardial infarction and congestive heart failure are the leading causes of death following major vascular surgery.[21] Therefore, prevention of hypotension and extremities during aortic clamping, are released with unclamping of the aorta.[16-20] These substances induce hemodynamic changes that may persist in the recovery room as well as in the first few hours in the ICU. In patients undergoing repair of aortic aneurysms who lack collateral circulation, a greater degree of lower extremity ischemia may occur with aortic cross-clamping as compared with patients who undergo surgery for occlusive disease. Therefore, hemodynamic changes are more severe in patients undergoing aortic aneurysm repair.

Intraoperatively, patients undergoing repair of abdominal aortic aneurysms should be anticoagulated with heparin during the time when their aortas are cross-clamped. Patients with aortoiliac occlusive disease do not always require anticoagulation. Straight-forward procedures to bypass occlusive segments that can be done in less than half an hour do not require anticoagulation. More complicated procedures, however, and procedures that take longer than this time do require anticoagulation. For abdominal aortic aneurysm repair, heparin, at a dose of 10,000 U, should be used for anticoagulation. For aortoiliac occlusive disease, the dose of heparin for anticoagulation can be 5 to 15 U/kg. After the initial heparin bolus, if the patient continues to have clot formations, anticoagulation is suboptimal, and additional heparin should be given. On completion of the vascular procedure, protamine, at a dose of 1 mg/100 U of heparin given, should be given to reverse the effects of heparin.

Postoperative Monitoring in the ICU

Postoperatively, invasive monitoring of various cardiopulmonary parameters is often necessary (Table 36-2). Frequently, these monitoring devices are placed either preoperatively or intraoperatively. If patients develop complications postoperatively, however, additional monitoring may be necessary.

All patients should have an arterial catheter for measurements of systemic arterial pressure and blood gases.[23] This allows frequent or continuous assessment of oxygenation and efficiency of ventilation. Frequent monitoring of the systemic arterial pressure allows for early detection of hypotension secondary to sudden hemorrhage from the suture line of the graft, gradual hemorrhage from other sources, or myocardial dysfunction. Hypertension is also detected early. Finally, an arterial catheter aids in the titration of vasodilators used to control hypertension.

Each patient should have a central venous catheter in place. In the case of sudden hemorrhage, crystalloid solutions or blood can be given rapidly to restore intravascular volume; if necessary, vasoactive drugs or cardiotonic agents can be given via this catheter; and, finally, central venous pressure or right atrial pressure can be measured to aid in the assessment of right-sided heart function. It should be remembered, however, that central venous pressure is not a reliable predictor of left ventricular filling pressure.[21,23,24]

For more detailed assessment, a pulmonary arterial catheter (Swan-Ganz catheter) is indicated for any patient with a severe cardiopulmonary derangement.[23] If myocardial function is compromised by myocardial failure or myocardial infarction, this catheter can provide crucial information on the efficacy of pharmacologic support. A Swan-Ganz catheter is also indicated for patients with good cardiopulmonary function who are undergoing major vascular procedures associated with large volume requirements and fluid shifts (complicated aortic procedures, aneurysmal or occlusive disease). Patients with severe cardiac disease and dysfunction should have a pulmonary arterial catheter placed the evening before their elective vascular procedure. Preoperative placement allows accurate assessment of myocardial performance, improvement of myocardial performance, and determination of optimum cardiac parameters (filling pressures, vascular resistances, and contractility), which should be maintained in the postoperative period.

The distal circulation should be monitored closely in the ICU. Palpation of the dorsalis pedis and posterior tibial arteries should be done immediately postoperatively (ideally in the operating room on completion of the procedure) to determine baseline pulses. These pulses should be followed closely postoperatively. Loss of pedal pulses may indicate poor distal perfusion secondary to myocardial dysfunction, graft thrombosis, or distal arterial embolism of debris or thrombus from the aorta. Early detection of these limits morbidity, as discussed subsequently.

The pulmonary status of each patient should be followed for signs of altered oxygenation or ineffective ventilation. Patients with minimal or no pulmonary disease are usually extubated in the operating room or recovery room. Their respiratory rate and level of consciousness are observed for alterations that might indicate pulmonary insufficiency (i.e., elevated respiratory rate > 25 breaths/min or decline in mental status). Should either of these alterations occur, an arterial blood gas value should be obtained to assess adequate oxygenation (Po_2 > 70 mm Hg) and ventilation (Pco_2 < 45 mm Hg). Patients with moderate pulmonary dysfunction and higher risk patients should remain intubated and mechanically ventilated until postoperative day 1. This way pulmonary function is well controlled, and additional support, if needed, can be quickly and easily given. Practically speaking, if there is any degree of anaerobic metabolism during the time of aortic cross clamping, it will be manifested by metabolic acidosis (from lactate production) in the postoperative period. The clinician should be mindful that this can create a burden of increased minute ventilation postoperatively. The benefits of early extubation should be carefully weighed against continued mechanical ventilation to reduce the work of breathing. If there are no complications or deterioration in the postoperative course, the patient can be extubated in the morning. Patients with severe pulmonary disease and prior risk patients should remain intubated and supported with mechanical ventilation until they are stable.

Intubated patients should have their pulmonary function followed closely. Arterial blood gases should be obtained routinely every 4 to 6 hours to ensure adequate oxygenation and ventilation. Acute changes and unstable patients may require more frequent blood gas monitoring. Pulse oximeters have proved extremely useful for continuous monitoring of arterial oxygen saturation in ICU patients.[23] They are noninvasive, are easy to use, and require minimal calibration. The sites used for measurement are the fingertip or the earlobe; however, this technique can be used only in patients who have good perfusion.[23]

Each patient's renal status should be monitored because it reflects adequacy of renal perfusion. A Foley catheter is placed preoperatively before all major vascular procedures. Urine output should be followed and kept greater than 0.5 ml·kg^{-1}·hour^{-1}. Serum creatinine levels should be checked at lease once daily. Should urine output decline or serum creatinine rise, the cause of these disturbances should be determined and aggressively treated. Common causes of these disturbances are discussed later.

Once a patient's postoperative course has stabilized, less invasive monitoring may be appropriate. Invasive lines should be removed as soon as they are no longer needed to make therapeutic decisions. Arterial lines can be removed once blood pressure has stabilized, patients have been extubated for 24 to 48 hours, and there is no need to monitor blood pressure or blood gases frequently. Central venous lines should be removed when there is no longer a threat of sudden hemorrhage, and there is no need of a central line for nutritional support. Pulmonary artery catheters should be removed as soon as hemodynamic function is stable. These catheters should be removed within 72 hours because the risk of infection increases after this time. Foley catheters should be left in place for 5 to 7 days because retroperitoneal dissection of the aorta frequently disrupts nerves to the bladder, resulting in urinary retention and distention of the bladder, which further exacerbates the contractile dysfunction of the bladder. When a Foley catheter is in place, the bladder should be catheterized every 6 to 8 hours if the patient is unable to void.

Maintenance of less intensive monitoring depends on the experience of the clinician and the clinical course of the patient. An experienced clinician may be comfortable with certain less intensive interventions in a situation for which a less experienced clinician might use invasive monitoring. If the patient's recovery deviates from the expected course or if an intervention fails to produce the desired therapeutic effect, more intensive monitoring is frequently necessary.[23]

Just as each of the major organ systems needs close monitoring in the ICU, each organ system may need additional support. Patients with atherosclerotic vascular disease frequently have dysfunction of other organ systems or medical problems that predispose to other organ system dysfunction. In fact, in one study, associated diseases were present in 75% of the patients undergoing major vascular procedures.[7] Each organ system may require little support or maximum support depending on its degree of dysfunction. The physician must be aware of every medical problem and treat each problem aggressively to prevent complications in the vascular surgery patient.

Patients with atherosclerotic peripheral vascular disease frequently have some degree of atherosclerotic coronary artery disease. The coexistence of coronary artery occlusive disease and peripheral arterial disease has been reported to range from 15 to 55%.[25] Coronary artery disease causes some degree of myocardial dysfunction. When myocardial dysfunction becomes severe enough to warrant cardiovascular support, treatment should proceed in an efficient, orderly fashion. Optimization of the hemodynamic status should be accomplished in the following order:[26]

- Identification and correction of hemodynamically significant arrhythmias
- Optimization of filling pressures (preload)
- Reduction of elevated vascular resistances (afterload)
- Augmentation of poor contractility (inotropy)
- Reduction of excessive myocardial oxygen consumption

Identification and Correction of Arrhythmias

Arrhythmias with ventricular rates of less than 60 beats per minute or more than the maximum aerobic rate should be treated.[26] The maximum aerobic rate is calculated as three fourths of the patient's maximum heart rate, which generally equals 220 minus the patient's age in years. Correction of ventricular rate in a patient with a ventricular arrhythmia (described in Chap. 27) usually achieves hemodynamic stability. If correction of the arrhythmia fails to resolve myocardial dysfunction, however, another abnormality must be contributing to the dysfunction. A Swan-Ganz catheter should be inserted to distinguish myocardial dysfunction caused by:

- Suboptimal ventricular filling pressures
- Elevated vascular resistances
- Inadequate myocardial contractility

Optimization of Filling Pressures

Following treatment of arrhythmias, the next therapeutic maneuver is to optimize ventricular end-diastolic volumes.[26] These volumes are usually adequately approximated by right atrial pressures (through the proximal port of the catheter) and pulmonary arterial wedge pressures. It should be remembered, however, that intracavitary atrial filling pressures do not always reliably reflect ventricular end-diastolic volumes. The goal of therapy should be to maximize the cardiac index while minimizing filling pressures—the greater the index, the greater the amount of oxygen delivered to the tissues, and the lower the filling pressures, the less the peripheral and pulmonary edema. The optimum ventricular end-diastolic volumes are determined by monitoring the response of the heart to alterations in filling pressures. The end-diastolic volume can either be increased—by infusing 10 ml/kg of a balanced salt solution—or decreased—by administering furosemide (40 mg initially) to prompt a diuresis. A fluid bolus should be given if filling pressures are 15 mm Hg or less, and furosemide should be given if filling pressures are greater than 20 mm Hg. Cardiac indices should be measured before and after manipulation of the end-diastolic volumes. A myocardial performance curve can be constructed by plotting cardiac index against pulmonary arterial wedge pressure. In addition, by optimizing cardiac index, patients are kept hyperdynamic. Under these circumstances, there is increased likelihood that the graft will remain patent and not thrombose.

Reduction of Elevated Vascular Resistances

If the ventricular rate and filling pressures are adequately adjusted but the cardiac index remains low, elevated systemic or pulmonary vascular resistances, if present, should be reduced.[26] If the heart rate is slow, isoproterenol at an initial dosage of 0.1 $\mu g \cdot kg^{-1} \cdot min^{-1}$ should be used. Isoproterenol dilates the peripheral vasculature and eases ventricular emptying while increasing the cardiac index by increasing contractility and heart rate. The agent's chronotropic activities, however, limit its usefulness in patients whose heart rate approaches the maximum aerobic rate limit. An irritable myocardium is another contraindication because of the agent's arrhythmogenic potential.[27,28]

If the filling pressures are normal or elevated, nitroglycerin, at an initial dosage of 25 μg per minute, should be used. Nitroglycerin usually dilates the systemic resistance vessels effectively and dilates the venules and small veins as well. At times, however, the agent fails to dilate the resistance vessels at all. Thus, as the drug is being titrated, the systemic vascular resistance should be calculated and followed.

If filling pressures are low to normal, sodium nitroprusside at an initial dosage of 0.5 $\mu g \cdot kg^{-1} \cdot min^{-1}$, should be used for peripheral vasodilation. This agent exerts its effect on resistance as well as capacitance vessels. It can usually be used only for a few days because it is metabolized into thiocyanate and cyanide. These metabolites can reach toxic concentrations and result in anaerobic metabolism. Therefore, patients on sodium nitroprusside infusions should have serum lactate levels measured frequently; if therapy continues for more than 2 days, thiocyanate levels should also be measured periodically.[26,27]

Augmentation of Poor Contractility

If myocardial dysfunction persists after optimization of heart rate, end-diastolic volumes, and vascular resistances, attention should be directed toward contractility.[26] Many inotropic agents are available, but dopamine, at an initial dosage of 2 $\mu g \cdot kg^{-1} \cdot min^{-1}$, and dobutamine, at an initial dosage of 5 $\mu g \cdot kg^{-1} min^{-1}$, are usually the agents of choice in surgical ICU patients. Dopamine may dilate the renal arterioles more than dobutamine, but it is more likely to produce a sinus tachycardia. Dobutamine seems to dilate the systemic arterioles more than dopamine; it is the better agent to use when systemic resistance is high. The goal of administration of any inotropic agent is the same as that of all other interventions previously mentioned: to maximize cardiac index while minimizing filling pressures. The overall volume status should be analyzed when using either of these agents. A wedge pressure of 15 mm Hg or greater with dopamine usage, especially in the face of decreased perfusion to the extremities, could suggest either inadequate intravascular volume or poor myocardial function. In this situation, a normal cardiac index usually means a constricted peripheral vascular bed from volume depletion. An elevated pulmonary arterial wedge pressure in the face of a less than normal cardiac output suggests that dobutamine therapy may be beneficial. If the mean blood pressure is less than 80 mm Hg, nitroprusside may produce hypotension. Conversely, dobutamine therapy results in improved cardiac output and reduced pulmonary arterial wedge pressure.

Reduction of Excessive Myocardial Oxygen Consumption

In some patients with myocardial dysfunction caused by myocardial ischemia, the heart continues to pump at rates approaching the maximal aerobic rate. In these patients, myocardial oxygen consumption should be decreased by slowing the heart rate with a beta-blocker.[26] Myocardial oxygen consumption should also be decreased in any patient who demonstrates symptoms or electrocardiographic signs of myocardial ischemia. Esmolol, at an initial dosage of 50 $\mu g \cdot kg^{-1} \cdot min^{-1}$, with gradual increases as needed, is the best agent in this situation. It is the shortest acting of all the beta blockers. It reduces myocardial oxygen consumption by decreasing contractility and heart rate. The reduction in contractility should be monitored closely because most surgical patients need supranormal cardiac indices to maximize microcirculatory flow and to optimize conditions for wound healing.

Once the cardiovascular status has stabilized and the patient is improving clinically, pharmacologic support should be weaned slowly with periodic assessment of hemodynamic function. Once all pharmacologic support has been discontinued and the patient remains stable, cardiovascular monitoring devices can be discontinued as previously mentioned.

Postoperative fluid therapy should be directed at maintaining adequate urine output (> 0.5 ml·kg^{-1}·hour^{-1}) and adequate distal perfusion. In patients with moderate-to-severe cardiac disease, a Swan-Ganz catheter should be used to guide fluid therapy to optimize filling pressures and maximize cardiac index. The cardiac status should be kept hyperdynamic to help keep the prosthetic graft open.

Usual fluid therapy requirements are a balanced salt solution at 100 to 150 ml per hour. Certain preoperative and intraoperative factors may alter postoperative fluid requirements. Patients who have undergone angiography the day before surgery can become hypovolemic because of an osmotic diuresis induced by the angiographic dye. Patients are given nothing by mouth the night before their surgery. A mechanical bowel preparation can also cause some degree of hypovolemia. This hypovolemia should be corrected with preoperative intravenous fluids to negate any adverse effects. These factors must be kept in mind when determining postoperative fluid orders. Intraoperatively, the length of aortic cross-clamp time, the extent of collateral circulation, and the amount of blood loss should be considered in determining postoperative fluid therapy. The longer the aortic cross-clamp time, the greater the degree of lower extremity ischemia, which results in a greater amount of vasodepressor substances being released into the systemic circulation.[16-20] In addition, patients with aneurysmal disease of the aorta as compared with occlusive disease often have less developed distal collateral circulation, which results in a greater degree of ischemia when the aorta is cross-clamped. The fluid requirements to treat these distributions are much greater. With large intraoperative blood losses, patients should receive blood transfusions to a hematocrit of 30 to replace any severe hemoglobin deficit. In addition, fluid therapy should be adjusted to ensure adequate distal organ perfusion. With adequate perfusion, lower concentrations of hemoglobin are better tolerated. Finally, cardiac, pulmonary, and renal complications are minimized when fluid therapy is adjusted to maintain good organ perfusion.[29]

Vascular surgery patients often have other coexisting medical problems. Each of these problems should be treated as described elsewhere in this text. Some of the more common medical problems, however, and their treatment are mentioned here.

Because of a high incidence of smoking, patients with atherosclerotic occlusive disease frequently have some degree of pulmonary disease, such as chronic obstructive pulmonary disease. Maintenance of adequate arterial oxygen tension is a vital part of postoperative care.[23] The goals of pulmonary support include the maintenance of adequate arterial P_{O_2} at a level that provides an oxygen saturation of hemoglobin of at least 90% at the lowest possible fractional concentration of oxygen in inspired gas (F_{IO_2}), preferably less than 50%.[23] Other goals are prevention and treatment of atelectasis, pulmonary toilet, and prevention of pneumonia.[23] Commonly used indications for assisted ventilation include:[23]

- P_{O_2} of less than 60 mm Hg when F_{IO_2} is greater than 50%
- Arterial P_{CO_2} greater than 50 mm Hg with pH less than 7.3
- Tachypnea with respiratory rate greater than 35 breaths per minute
- Signs of impeding respiratory failure, such as tachypnea, hypertension, sweating, and anxiety

As previously mentioned, patients with minimal or no pulmonary disease are usually extubated in the operating room or recovery room. Patients with moderate pulmonary disease and patients with other coexisting medical problems that make them at higher risk for postoperative complications should probably remain intubated overnight and extubated the following morning. Patients with severe pulmonary disease and poor risk patients should remain intubated and supported with mechanical ventilation until the physician caring for the patient is assured that pulmonary function is stable, and there is a low likelihood of postoperative complications that might worsen pulmonary function (see Chaps. 15 & 59).

Vascular surgery patients often have essential hypertension. An elevated blood pressure in the postoperative period, however, should not be automatically attributed to hypertension. Other causes, such as hypoxia, pain, and fluid overload, should be considered. Only after other causes of an elevated blood pressure have been ruled out should hypertension be attributed to preoperative essential hypertension and antihypertensive medication given. Our choice of antihypertensive medication for patients in the ICU is sodium nitroprusside. This agent has a fast time of onset of action, has a short duration of action, and can be titrated to the desired effect on blood pressure. Dosages and side effects of this agent have been previously mentioned. Sublingual nifedipine at a dose of 10 to 20 mg every 4 hours is also useful in reducing an elevated blood pressure.

The incidence of diabetes mellitus among patients undergoing major vascular surgery can be as high as 50%. Postoperatively blood glucose should be followed closely, every 4 to 6 hours, depending on the degree of hyperglycemia. Regular insulin should be given intravenously on a sliding scale basis. The goal of insulin therapy should not be tight control in the early postoperative period. Blood glucose levels in the range of 220 to 250 are adequate. If the renal threshold for glucose is low, however, additional insulin should be given to lower the glucose concentration and prevent an osmotic diuresis.

Hypothermia may occur in the early postoperative period after major vascular procedures. The common causes for hypothermia are infusion of large quantities of cold blood products and complicated abdominal aortic procedures in which the abdomen remains opened for a prolonged time. There are many adverse effects of hypothermia. Hypothermia induces cardiac dysfunction and a resultant decrease in cardiac index. Cardiac arrhythmias are common. Many enzymes that are important for metabolism function optimally at 37°C. With hypothermia, these enzymes function much less efficiently. Hypothermia also impairs the clotting system, which can become a major problem in the postoperative patient. Adverse effects of hypothermia include decreased ability to form stable clots, decreased production of blood clotting factors, and platelet dysfunction.[30,31] Finally, with declining temperature, the hemoglobin dissociation curve shifts to the left, which decreases peripheral oxygen unloading. This shift may be undesirable in the postoperative patient with high metabolic demands and tissue oxygen requirements.

Treatment of hypothermia should proceed expeditiously. All intravenous fluids should be warmed before infusion. All cold blood products should be infused through level I blood warmers. If patients are intubated and being mechanically ventilated, the temperature of inhaled air should be increased to 41°C. Heating pads and warm blankets can be placed on the patient but are not as effective as the first three measures.

Patients should be mobilized as soon as possible in the postoperative period. On postoperative day 1, patients should be encouraged to get out of bed and sit in a chair. Even intubated patients should be assisted out of bed and placed in a chair at least twice daily. Patients must also be encouraged to ambulate as much as possible. Mobilization improves pulmonary function by having patients take deep breaths, which reverses or prevents atelectasis, allows quicker return of gastrointestinal function, and decreases the risk of deep venous thrombolism. A disadvantage might be that sitting in a chair may kink grafts or compromise wound healing in the groin region. The advantages, however, definitely outweigh these concerns in poor risk patients.

Systemic anticoagulation may be indicated in selected patients undergoing vascular procedures. One indication for anticoagulation intraoperatively and postoperatively is to prevent arterial or graft thrombosis. The other indication for anticoagulation is for prophylaxis against deep venous thrombosis and pulmonary embolism. Heparin, on a rare occasion, can be continued postoperatively in patients who have undergone distal arterial reconstruction and who continue to have lower extremity ischemia. More often, dextran, a carbohydrate polymer, is used for postoperative anticoagulation. The antithrombotic properties of dextran are attributed to decreased blood viscosity, reduced platelet interaction with the damaged vessel wall, and an increased susceptibility for fibrin clots formed in the presence of dextran to undergo fibrinolysis.[32] Dextran, which is normally administered as a 6% solution with an average molecular weight of 70,000, is given as a continuous infusion of 500 ml daily for 3 days postoperatively. The indications for dextran are:

- To retain patency of distal reconstitutions to the lower extremities
- All polytetrafluoroethylene bypasses, small femoropopliteal bypasses, and femorodistal lower extremity bypasses
- Aortobifemoral bypasses with reduced outflow owing to small or diseased distal vessels

Occasionally warfarin (Coumadin) is used for postoperative anticoagulation in patients undergoing polytetrafluoroethylene femoropopliteal bypasses. The dose should be adjusted to increase the INR (international normalized ratio) to 2.0.

Anticoagulation is also indicated postoperatively in patients who have a moderate or high risk of developing a deep venous thrombosis or pulmonary embolism. The risk of venous thromboembolism is increased in patients with:[32]

- Primary hypercoagulable states (e.g., antithrombin III deficiency, protein C + S deficiencies)
- Age greater than 40
- Malignant disease
- Anticipated prolonged bed rest postoperatively
- Obesity
- Recent history of venous thromboembolism

Reducing the incidence of venous thromboembolism reduces the morbidity and mortality of venous thromboembolism. The disadvantage of anticoagulation, however, is the risk of postoperative hemorrhage. We advocate two methods of prophylaxis: continuous intravenous infusion of low dose heparin and intermittent pneumatic leg compression. Continuous low dose heparin should be given at a rate to increase the partial thromboplastin time by 5 to 10 seconds. This dosage is usually 500 to 1000 U per hour, and no loading dose is given. Intermittent pneumatic leg compression prevents venous thrombosis by enhancing blood flow in the deep veins of the legs and thus preventing venostasis. It also increases blood fibrinolytic activity. This device, however, should not be used in patients with ischemic lower extremities.

Antibiotic prophylaxis is an important consideration in patients undergoing vascular bypass procedures with prosthetic grafts. We recommend that cefazolin, a first-generation cephalosporin with gram-positive and gram-negative coverage, be given intravenously just before surgery and continued postoperatively for 24 hours. The value of a short perioperative course of prophylactic antibiotics has been clearly demonstrated in two prospective, randomized clinical trials.[33,34] These two studies showed that perioperative antibiotics continued for 24 hours postoperatively decreased the incidence of wound infection as well as graft infection. Some vascular surgeons, however, may recommend continuation of postoperative antibiotics until all indwelling catheters (i.e., central lines, Swan-Ganz catheters, and Foley catheters) are removed because of the potential for bacteremia and subsequent graft infection. Although prolonged antibiotic administration offers the theoretic advantage of protection against infection of the graft by a transient bacteremia in the postoperative period, only in a small percentage of cases has a transient bacteremia been documented to be the source of a graft infection.[34,35] In addition, prolonged antibiotic administration increases the risk of emergence of resistant organisms. Currently there is no evidence available to prove the theory that continuation of systemic antibiotics over several days in the postoperative period reduces the risk of subsequent graft infection.

Other medications used in the postoperative period include analgesics and antiplatelet drugs. Adequate analgesia is necessary to optimize pulmonary function by allowing patients to cough and deep breathe and use the incentive spirometer. Adequate analgesia also allows patients to be mobilized out of bed. We prefer an intravenous narcotic for initial postoperative analgesia. Morphine sulfate, as a dose of 2 to 10 mg, can be given hourly to obtain adequate analgesia. Two significant side effects of intravenous narcotics are arterial hypotension secondary to venodilation and respiratory depression. If intravenous narcotics fail to provide adequate analgesia, epidural anesthesia or patient-controlled analgesia may be used. Epidural anesthesia is accomplished by sterile placement of a catheter into the epidural space and infusion of morphine (Duramorph) or fentanyl either intermittently or continuously. Anticoagulation, however, is a contraindication to epidural catheter placement. Patient-controlled analgesia allows a patient to administer his or her own analgesic therapy. Various parameters can be adjusted to prevent narcotic overdose: dose of narcotic, frequency of administration time interval between doses, and maximum dose per time period. Frequently patients obtain better pain control when they are allowed to administer their own analgesia via this PCA device. Finally, when patients begin oral intake, they are started on oral pain medications. We prefer acetaminophen with codeine or acetaminophen with hydrocodone. Other oral pain medication may be used as per each physician's personal preference.

Commonly used antiplatelet drugs are aspirin and dipyridamole. We recommend giving aspirin, 325 mg daily, once patients tolerate a regular diet but do not use dipyridamole. The latter drug offers no added benefit over aspirin alone.

Patients with aneurysmal disease generally do not do as well postoperatively as patients with aortoiliac occlusive disease. Patients with aneurysmal disease of the aorta are more likely to be obese than patients with occlusive disease. Patients with aneurysms of the aorta have little, if any, preexisting collateral circulation as compared with patients with aortoiliac occlusive disease; therefore aneurysm patients develop a greater amount of lower extremity ischemia following aortic cross-clamping. In addition, psychologic factors may also play a role in the postoperative course. Aneurysm patients are usually asymptomatic before elective repair and therefore experience no improvement in symptoms postoperatively. In contrast, patients with occlusive disease are usually incapacitated with pain preoperatively. Most of them notice an improvement in their circulation early in the postoperative course, sometimes even in the recovery room. This perceived relief of symptoms in the early postoperative period can be a major booster for patient morale.

Postoperative Complications (Table 36-3)

Pulmonary Complications

The main pulmonary complications after major vascular reconstruction are atelectasis, pneumonia, and pulmonary insufficiency. Atelectasis typically occurs 12 to 36 hours postoperatively and is the most common cause of an elevated temperature in the early postoperative period. Pneumonia may occur at any time in the postoperative period. Its incidence is increased with prolonged endotracheal intubation. Pulmonary insufficiency, consisting of hypoxemia owing to atelectasis or retained secretions and hypoventilation from analgesia, may also occur at any time in the postoperative period. Risk of pulmonary insufficiency is affected by the degree of pulmonary dysfunction preoperatively and by the number and severity of nonpulmonary postoperative complications. The main preoperative risk factors for developing pulmonary complications are cigarette smoking and chronic obstructive pulmonary disease. As many as 80% of vascular patients have a significant history of tobacco use, and as many as 20% have sufficient pulmonary dysfunction to warrant the diagnosis of chronic obstructive pulmonary disease.[6]

Patients undergoing any type of upper abdominal surgery may develop changes in lung function and are at increased risk to develop atelectasis.[36] These changes occur

Table 36-3. Postoperative Complications

Organ System	Complication	Time of Occurrence
Pulmonary	Atelectasis	12–36 hours
	Pneumonia	48 hours
	Pulmonary insufficiency	24 hours
	Pleural effusion	48–72 hours
Cardiovascular	Cardiac ischemia	12–24 hours +
	Myocardial infarction	0–72 hours
	Cardiac arrhythmias	0–48 hours
	Congestive heart failure	48–96 hours
	Retroperitoneal hemorrhage	0–24 hours
	Lower extremity ischemia	0–24 hours
	Venous thrombosis	5–7 days
	Pulmonary embolism	7–10 days
	Obligatory edema	24–48 hours
Gastrointestinal	Ileus	0–96 hours
	Colon ischemia	0–72 hours
Renal	Oliguria	0–48 hours
	Acute renal failure	24–48 hours
Metabolic	Hypokalemia	Any time
	Hyperglycemia	Any time
Neurologic	Cerebrovascular accident	24–48 hours +
	Ischemic spinal cord damage	0–12 hours
Hematologic	Anemia	0–72 hours
	Consumptive coagulopathy	12–72 hours
	Disseminated intravascular coagulation	12–72 hours
Infectious	Urinary tract infection	3–7 days
	Graft infection	Days–months
	Graft-enteric fistula	Days–months
	Graft-enteric erosion	Days–months
	Central line sepsis	3–7 days

because of reduced diaphragm activity. Postoperatively there is a shift from predominantly abdominal to rib cage breathing. This shift results in a significant reduction in tidal volume. In addition, long abdominal incisions are frequently used in major vascular procedures, making it painful to breathe, which further reduces tidal volume. Chest x-ray films frequently demonstrate patchy atelectasis. Therefore the reduction in diaphragm function after upper abdominal surgery can be important in the development of atelectasis, reduced vital capacity, and hypoxemia postoperatively.[36]

Atelectasis should be treated promptly in the postoperative period because it may predispose patients to pulmonary dysfunction and pneumonia. Patients should be encouraged to get out of bed, at least to sit in a chair. After ICU discharge, patients should ambulate at least three times daily. They should be instructed on how to cough and deep breathe as well as how to use the incentive spirometer. Aggressive pulmonary toilet reverses atelectasis and minimizes pulmonary complications postoperatively.

Postoperative pneumonia is one of the most common causes of death in the vascular patient.[37] Risk factors for the development of postoperative pneumonia include:[37]

- Colonization of the upper respiratory tract with virulent gram-negative organisms
- Atelectasis secondary to decreased tidal volume
- Gross or subclinical aspiration

To minimize the risk of postoperative pneumonia, certain concepts must be kept in mind. Pulmonary function should be maximized by demanding preoperative cessation of smoking, cough and deep breathing techniques, and aggressive pulmonary toilet. Ideally this should be initiated at least 1 week before surgery but for practical reasons is often instituted 24 to 48 hours before surgery. The duration of preoperative prophylactic antibiotics should be limited to 24 hours to decrease the risk of colonization of the upper respiratory tract with resistant organisms. Finally, gastrointestinal motility may not return postoperatively for many days. A nasogastric tube should be placed to treat the postoperative ileus. Oral feedings should be withheld until 36 to 48 hours after extubation. These measures decrease the risk of aspiration.

The diagnosis of pneumonia should be considered with any of the following signs or symptoms:

- Elevated white blood cell count
- Purulent sputum
- Appearance of an infiltrate on chest film
- Need to increase the Fio_2 or ventilatory support to maintain adequate oxygenation
- Any systemic signs of sepsis, such as an elevated temperature, increased fluid requirements, or glucose intolerance.

Once the diagnosis of pneumonia has been established, therapy should be instituted at once. Secretions should be mobilized by coughing, nasotracheal suctioning, or endotracheal suctioning if the patient is intubated. Appropriate cultures should be sent to the laboratory, and empiric antibiotic therapy should be initiated. The treatment of pneumonia is discussed in greater detail in Chapter 21.

The pulmonary status of each patient should be followed closely. If pulmonary insufficiency develops, patients should be intubated and supported with mechanical ventilation to ensure adequate oxygenation. Full ventilatory support should be maintained until the cause of the pulmonary insufficiency is determined and treated. Ventilatory support is described in detail in Chapter 16.

Postoperatively, patients may develop pleural effusions after major vascular procedures. Pleural effusions may result from large fluid shifts that occur during these procedures; they may also result from dissection of the upper abdominal aorta, near the diaphragmatic crura. In general, thoracentesis or tube thoracostomy should not be performed because of the risk of infection or pneumothorax. Large pleural effusions that compromise pulmonary function, however, should be drained.

Cardiovascular Complications

In patients who are at high risk to develop postoperative myocardial infarction or congestive heart failure, myocardial performance curves should be determined preoperatively. This preoperative assessment allows determination of the optimal filling pressure of the left ventricle, which can then be used as a guide to accurate volume replacement and appropriate drug therapy in the postoperative period. Using this approach, major cardiovascular complications can be drastically reduced.[21] One study reported only one operative death in a series of 110 patients undergoing abdominal aortic aneurysm resection whose pulmonary artery wedge pressures were maintained in the normal range.[47]

Postoperative retroperitoneal hemorrhage can be a serious, life-threatening complication. Risk factors for retroperitoneal hemorrhage include:

- Inadequate reversal of operative anticoagulation
- Technical error involving the aortic anastomosis
- Aortic-graft anastomotic rupture secondary to arterial hypertension.

To prevent mortality, prompt recognition and treatment of this complication must occur. The hematocrit should be followed periodically in all patients in the early postoperative period; patients who are hemodynamically unstable should have their hematocrit checked more frequently, every 2 to 4 hours, to rule out retroperitoneal hemorrhage. Coagulation studies (prothrombin and partial thromboplastin time and platelet count) should be checked postoperatively, and if coagulation abnormalities exist, these should be corrected. Arterial hypertension should be treated aggressively to prevent anastomotic rupture. If retroperitoneal hemorrhage is suspected, prompt operative re-exploration should be undertaken. A combination of hemodynamic instability and falling hematocrit is indicative of hemorrhage and warrants re-exploration.

Leg ischemia after major vascular procedures may occur immediately postoperatively in the recovery room or early in the postoperative period. Factors implicated in causing distal ischemia include:[48]

- Distal embolization of thrombus and debris
- Technical error resulting in stenosis or obstruction of the reconstruction
- Graft occlusion caused by postoperative hypotension
- Decreased distal blood flow via collateral circulation because of disruption of collaterals at the time of exposure of the abdominal aorta

Distal embolization of thrombus and debris is much less common than in the past.[7] The reason is that earlier many proximal aortic anastomoses were made end to side in patients with partial distal aortic obstruction. Distal embolization of thrombi and debris arising in the partially obstructed aorta and iliac arteries occurred at the time of operation. With the more common use of aortic transection and end-to-end proximal aortic anastomosis, embolization occurs much less frequently. Embolization of thrombus and debris, however, is still the most common cause of postoperative leg ischemia.[48] This complication must be recognized promptly to prevent tissue loss and the need for lower extremity amputation. If a patient loses dorsalis pedis and posterior tibial pulses postoperatively and develops lower extremity ischemia, the patient should be immediately anticoagulated with heparin. The patient should then be taken back to the operating room to undergo an on-table femoral arteriogram and Fogarty embolectomy to restore distal circulation.

Venous thrombosis may occur after major vascular procedures. Acute onset of lower extremity pain and swelling should raise suspicion regarding the possibility of deep venous thrombosis. Patients should be empirically anticoagulated with heparin. A bolus of 5000 to 10,000 U of heparin is given initially followed by a constant infusion of 1000 to 2000 U per hour. This rate is adjusted to keep the partial thromboplastin time 2.5 to 3.0 times normal and to alleviate symptoms. The diagnosis can be confirmed with any of several noninvasive tests (impedance plethysmography, Doppler ultrasound) or with a venogram. Once the patient is able to eat, warfarin should be started. Once the dose of warfarin has been adjusted to raise the prothrombin time to 1.25 to 1.50 times normal, the heparin can be discontinued. Warfarin should then be continued for 6 months postoperatively.

Pulmonary embolism should be suspected in any postoperative patient who develops the acute onset of tachypnea, dyspnea, pleuritic chest pain, or decrease in arterial P_{O_2}. To confirm the diagnosis, a pulmonary arteriogram should be obtained. Treatment consists of a bolus of heparin, 500 U, followed by a continuous intravenous infusion of 1250 to 1660 U per hour. Anticoagulation should be continued for 7 to 10 days. A complete description of the diagnosis and treatment of pulmonary embolism can be found in Chapter 23.

Obligatory edema of the lower extremities often develops after revascularization procedures. The physiology of this occurrence is described in Chapter 23. There is no recommended treatment because this eventually resolves with time.

Gastrointestinal Complications

Postoperative paralytic ileus occurs commonly after major vascular procedures involving the abdominal aorta. The retroperitoneal dissection that exposes the abdominal aorta frequently disrupts autonomic nerves supplying the bowel. In addition, the small bowel is frequently eviscerated and placed in a bowel bag at the time of surgery for better exposure of the aorta. The resulting angulation of the small bowel mesentery obstructs the lymphatics and veins, causing small bowel wall edema. Treatment consists of placing a nasogastric tube at the time of surgery. The nasogastric tube may be removed when bowel function returns, usually on postoperative days 3 to 5.

Ischemia of the colon after aortic reconstructive procedures is an occult, yet often lethal, complication. The incidence of ischemic colitis varies from 2 to 10%.[49-53] Among patients undergoing repair of ruptured aortic aneurysms, however, the incidence may be as high as 60%.[51] The overall mortality rate for patients with colon ischemia is approximately 50% but approaches 90% if the ischemia is a transmural process.[49,53-55]

Several risk factors that arise as a result of surgery have been identified that probably affect the development of ischemic colitis postoperatively.[50,55] These include:

- Vascular anatomy of the colon with congenital variation
- Operative sacrifice of the inferior mesenteric artery of its collateral circulation

- Emboli to the inferior mesenteric artery
- Associated low flow states, such as hemorrhagic shock and congestive heart failure

Because most causes of colon ischemia involve the sigmoid colon, ligation of the inferior mesenteric artery and inadequate collateral circulation are probably the most important factors leading to the development of ischemic colitis.

Early diagnosis of ischemic colitis requires a high index of suspicion. Patients may complain of left lower quadrant abdominal or generalized abdominal pain. On physical examination, left lower quadrant tenderness with or without peritoneal signs and abdominal distention may be present. Hypotension, fever, tachycardia, positive fluid balance, diarrhea (which may or may not be bloody), leukocytosis, and acidosis may also be present. This clinical picture may be easily confused with pseudomembranous enterocolitis. Sigmoidoscopic examination is the best way to evaluate the sigmoid colon mucosa to make the diagnosis. This often reveals a cyanotic, friable mucosa with multiple ulcerations. Treatment consists of segmental resection of the ischemic colon with proximal colostomy.

Renal Complications

Acute renal failure can occur postoperatively after major vascular procedures in approximately 5% of patients with normal preoperative renal function.[6] If patients have abnormal renal function (serum creatinine > 2.0 mg/dl) before surgery, however, their chance of postoperative renal failure is approximately 30%.[6] In addition, acute renal failure that develops postoperatively is further associated with high morbidity and mortality rates.[56]

Urine output should be maintained at a rate greater than 0.5 ml·kg^{-1}·hour^{-1}. If urine output declines below this rate, a fluid bolus should be given if hypovolemia is suspected. If fluid challenges fail to improve urine output or if myocardial dysfunction is suspected, a Swan-Ganz catheter, if not already in place, should be placed to measure the various cardiac indices. Cardiac index should be maximized to ensure good renal perfusion. Serum creatinine should be checked daily. A rise in serum creatinine to a level 1.0 mg/dl greater than baseline deserves further investigation (see Chaps. 39 and 40). The common causes of postoperative renal insufficiency include:[56]

- Hypovolemia
- Myocardial dysfunction with poor renal perfusion
- Exacerbation of preexisting renal disease
- Ischemic renal injury secondary to suprarenal clamping of the aorta
- Intraoperative hypotension
- Postoperative hypotension
- Angiographic dye-induced renal injury
- Use of potentially nephrotoxic drugs
- Atherosclerotic renal artery disease

Most often renal failure after aortic surgery is caused by the additive effects of multiple insults that progressively decrease renal reserve.[56]

Metabolic Complications

Hypokalemia may occur postoperatively after major vascular procedures. There are four factors responsible for its occurrence. In response to the stress of surgery, renin and vasopressin are released. Through the renin-angiotensinogen-angiotensin I-angiotensin II pathway, aldosterone is released from the adrenal gland. Aldosterone stimulates tubular reabsorption of sodium and increases renal excretion of potassium. Vasopressin, besides being a vasopressor, potentiates reabsorption of water by the kidneys. This dilutional effect lowers serum potassium. During major vascular procedures, large volumes of crystalloid solutions are often given intraoperatively as well as postoperatively. These solutions are frequently normal saline and Ringer's lactate and contain either no potassium or only small amounts of potassium. Their administration adds to the dilutional effect. Finally, after aortic cross clamping, there is some degree of ischemia to the lower extremities. Because of a lack of adequate distal perfusion, intracellular metabolism becomes anaerobic, and an intracellular acidosis ensues. Hydrogen ion is released from the cells, and concomitantly potassium ions are taken up, thus lowering the serum potassium concentration. The serum potassium concentration should be followed closely in the early postoperative period. Therapy consists of adequate potassium replacement.

Many patients with vascular disease also have diabetes mellitus. Serum glucose concentrations should be frequently monitored and kept under control. The management of the diabetic patient is described in Chapter 56.

Nutritional support in the form of total parenteral nutrition is indicated postoperatively in certain circumstances. Patients with severe infections, such as aortic prosthetic graft infection, require maximal nutritional support because of the high metabolic demands induced by sepsis. Patients who cannot receive enteral feedings and patients with a prolonged postoperative ileus deserve total parenteral nutrition. Examples are patients who undergo repair of aortoduodenal erosions or fistulas and patients with mesentery vascular disease. A complete description of nutritional support is given in Chapter 62.

Neurologic Complications

Ischemic spinal cord damage after temporary clamping of the abdominal aorta has been well deserved by Szilagyi.[60,61] This complication almost always presents as paraplegia or paraparesis. The incidence of ischemic spinal cord damage is 0.25% for all operations for aortic aneurysms. The incidence of damage to the spinal cord is 10 times higher for treatment of ruptured aneurysms.

The cause of ischemic spinal cord damage is probably related to an anatomic abnormality of the blood supply of the spinal cord. The blood supply of the entire cord between T10 and L4 depends on two radicular arterial branches, the most important of which is the great radicular artery or the artery of Adamkiewicz. The usual point of origin of this artery is between the eleventh thoracic and the first lumbar vertebrae, but it may be as low as the second and third lumbar vertebrae. When it is in a normal position, it cannot be harmed by even the highest infradiaphragmatically placed clamp. When it is in an anomalous lower position, however, it may be interrupted even if the occluding clamp is in an infrarenal position. Although the main cause of spinal cord ischemia is inadvertent interruption of blood flow through an anomalous great radicular artery, other contributing factors include concomitant hypotension, pre-existing atherosclerosis, and embolization.

In terms of prognosis, when sensory and motor loss is incomplete, partial or nearly total recovery is more likely. If sensory and motor loss is complete, however, recovery is unlikely, and treatment is limited to supportive and rehabilitative measures.

Hematologic Complications

Postoperatively patients may have some degree of anemia, which relates to the amount of intraoperative blood loss and intraoperative blood replacement. Patients without significant cardiac or pulmonary disease can tolerate hematocrit as low as 25%. Patients with coronary artery disease, chronic obstructive pulmonary disease, or a likelihood of postoperative hemorrhage, however, should be transfused as necessary to maintain a hematocrit of 30 to 35%.[26] This hematocrit ensures adequate oxygen delivery on a cellular level, assuming there is no significant cardiac dysfunction. To minimize the need for banked blood transfusion with its inherent risk of hepatitis and acquired immunodeficiency syndrome (AIDS), patients who are to undergo an elective procedure can contribute and store their own blood preoperatively in an autologous self-directed blood donation program. Vascular procedures also lend themselves well to intraoperative autotransfusion techniques. The process of collection and retransfusion of autologous blood, however, decreases the half-life of these red blood cells. Therefore patients may develop an anemia and require transfusion later in the postoperative period.

Patients may develop a consumptive coagulopathy or frank disseminated intravascular coagulation secondary to large intraoperative blood losses and multiple transfusions. This complication can be severe enough to be lethal.[62] Early recognition is necessary to limit the severity of the coagulopathy and to minimize the number of blood transfusions. Signs of disseminated intravascular coagulation include:

- Blood in endotracheal secretions
- Bleeding from intravenous sites or arterial catheters
- Hematuria
- Various abnormal laboratory tests, such as prolonged prothrombin and partial thromboplastin times, hypofibrinogenemia, markedly positive fibrin split products, and fibrin monomers and thrombocytopenia

Treatment consists of correcting hypothermia if this is present and replacing clotting factors with fresh frozen plasma and platelet transfusions.

Infectious Complications

Vascular surgery is associated with relatively low infection rates but differs from many other surgical procedures in that the morbidity and mortality of infection can be extremely high. In the case of aortic prosthetic graft infections, loss of life or limb occurs frequently. Therefore all patients should receive a short course (24 hours) of prophylactic antibiotics to minimize the risk of infection.

Two of the most common postoperative infections are pneumonia and urinary tract infections. Chronic obstructive pulmonary disease and prolonged postoperative intubation and mechanical ventilation are predisposing factors for postoperative pneumonia. Postoperative pneumonia has been previously discussed. Predisposing factors for urinary tract infections are prolonged indwelling Foley catheterization and prostatism. Significant benign prostatic hypertrophy is estimated to occur in about 20% of men over 50 years of age.[63] Therefore, to minimize the incidence of postoperative urinary tract infections, Foley catheters should be removed as soon as possible. In addition, patients with significant prostatism should have transurethral resection of the prostate before their elective vascular procedure.[64] This prevents the risk of bacteremic seeding of the prosthetic graft from bacteremia induced by transurethral resection of the prostate if the resection is delayed until after prosthetic graft placement. Also, by performing transurethral resection of the prostate first, the risk of postoperative urinary retention is reduced, indwelling Foley catheters can be removed sooner, and the risk of postoperative urinary tract infection is reduced.

Prosthetic vascular graft infections are a relatively uncommon complication of peripheral vascular surgery. This complication, however, is always serious and often leads to loss of life or limb. The incidence of graft infection is approximately 1.5 to 6%.[35,65-67] Mortality ranges from 33 to 75%.[35,65-68] Mortality is highest for proximal aortic graft infection and lowest for distal infections. Conversely, the amputation rate is highest for distal infections.

The time interval between operation and clinical appearance of graft infection varies from a few days to greater than 5 years.[35,65] Szilagyi and coworkers,[35] however found that in 65% of cases, graft infection was detected in the immediate postoperative period.

There are several sources of infection that are responsible for the development of graft contamination. Inguinal skin and subsequent wound infections are responsible for the majority of graft infections.[35] Factors important in the development of groin wound infections include:

- Use of prosthetic material
- Prolonged operative time
- Presence of ischemic tissues
- Transection of infected groin lymphatics
- Diabetes
- Obesity[34,35]
- Contamination by enteric effluent
- Bacteria in perioaortic or aneurysmal tissues
- Unrecognized mycotic aneurysms
- Contamination from bacteremia or intra-abdominal sepsis[69]

Late causes of intra-abdominal graft infections include graft-enteric fistulas, graft-enteric erosions, late bacteremia, and contiguous spread of intra-abdominal infections.[69] Bacteremic seeding of a prosthetic graft has been reported only anecdotally.[35,65,66]

The diagnosis of graft infection is usually straightforward with peripheral infections but may be exceedingly difficult with intra-abdominal graft infections. Signs and symptoms of graft infections include:

- Discharge of pus from surgical wounds
- Development of anastomotic pseudoaneurysms
- Exteriorization of the graft
- Formation of sinus tracts
- Graft thrombosis
- Local hemorrhage
- Systemic sepsis
- Septic emboli[65,66,69]

Gallium scanning or indium-labeled white blood cell scans may localize ill-defined sepsis to a prosthetic graft. An abdominal computed tomography (CT) scan may have findings, such as retroperitoneal gas bubbles or perigraft fluid collections, that are consistent with graft infections.

Management of prosthetic graft infections consists of excision of the infected graft, lower extremity revascularization using an extra-anatomic bypass graft as described by Blaisdell and colleagues,[70] and broad-spectrum or culture specific antibiotic therapy. We believe that when possible, the extra-anatomic bypass graft should be placed before removal of the infected prosthetic graft.[71] If the infected graft is removed before placement of the extra-anatomic bypass graft, both the incidence of lower extremity ischemia and overall morbidity increase significantly.[71]

Graft-enteric fistula is a relatively uncommon complication, occurring in less than 1% of major vascular procedures involving the abdominal aorta.[35] The majority of fistulas are aortoduodenal, but aortojejunal and aortoileal fistulas do occur. Onset of symptoms is usually seen 2 to 8 years postoperatively, but some fistulas have occurred as early as 2 days.[72-74]

The most characteristic presentation of graft-enteric fistula is a triad of abdominal pain, gastrointestinal hemorrhage, and a pulsatile abdominal mass. Patients may experience a ''herald'' hemorrhage before a second, massive uncontrollable hemorrhage and exsanguination.[71-73] After a ''herald'' bleeding episode, upper gastrointestinal endoscopy should be performed promptly in an attempt to see the graft or fistula as well as to rule out other causes of upper gastrointestinal bleeding. Gallium scans, indium-labeled white blood cell scans, and abdominal CT scans may also be useful in making the correct diagnosis.[75] Angiography may show either a pseudoaneurysm or a small amount of extravasation of contrast material at the aortic suture line representing the fistula. If the cause of an upper gastrointestinal hemorrhage cannot be identified in a patient with an abdominal prosthetic graft, the patient should undergo immediate abdominal exploration to rule out the presence of a graft-enteric fistula. Management consists of extra-anatomic bypass, removal of the prosthetic graft, repair of the enteric defect and intravenous antibiotic therapy.

Graft-enteric erosion is a much less frequent complication than graft-enteric fistulas. In fact, there are only 38 cases documented in the literature.[75] The average interval between graft placement and development of a graft-enteric erosion is 2 to 3 years; however, some have occurred as early as in the immediate postoperative period, whereas some have occurred more than 13 years after operation.[75] The majority of graft-enteric erosions occur between the aorta and the third or fourth portions of the duodenum. Erosions into the ileum, jejunum, sigmoid colon, and stomach have also been reported.[75-77] Graft-enteric erosions result from adherence of the bowel to the graft, formation of dense adhesions, and then mechanical erosion of the bowel by the pulsatile graft.

Symptoms of graft-enteric erosions include fever, malaise, sepsis, gastrointestinal hemorrhage, anemia, abdominal pain, nausea, and vomiting.[75] The diagnosis is usually made with barium studies and endoscopy. Management is similar to that of graft-enteric fistulas and consists of extra-anatomic bypass, removal of the prosthetic graft, closure of the enteric defect, and intravenous antibiotic therapy.

The last infectious complication to be discussed is central line sepsis. Because many vascular patients require invasive monitoring postoperatively, the threat of central line sepsis is a definite concern. Central line sepsis may initiate bacteremia from which a prosthetic graft may become infected. Although there are only anecdotal exports of hematogenous seeding of prosthetic grafts,[35,65,66] should this complication occur, it would have serious life-threatening or limb-threatening consequences. Central lines should be removed as soon as possible in patients in whom a prosthesis has been inserted.

POST-ICU PHASE

Once the patient's postoperative course has stabilized and there is no longer a need to monitor intensively, the patient can be transferred to the regular ward. All invasive monitoring devices are removed before transfer. The patient should be examined closely to identify any potential postoperative problems that have been previously mentioned.

After transfer to a regular ward, each organ system should be evaluated daily. Aggressive pulmonary toilet should be continued with instructing the patient to cough and deep breathe as well as continuing incentive spirometry hourly while awake. An arterial blood gas value should be obtained intermittently as long as oxygen therapy is required and until a Pco_2 of 45 mm Hg or less is obtained. The patient must be encouraged to get out of bed often. This not only helps reverse atelectasis, but also decreases the risk of deep venous thrombosis and facilitates resolution of postoperative ileus. Once any ileus has resolved, sips of clear liquids are started. If sips are well tolerated, the volume of clear liquids is increased followed by advancement to a regular diet.

The fluid status is followed daily by having the nurses record the inputs and outputs accurately. Ideally a patient should be in negative fluid balance with output being greater than input. If a patient is continually in positive fluid balance, the cause must be determined. Causes for a positive fluid balance include high intake (unnecessary intravenous fluids, excessive oral intake) and low output (intravascular volume depletion secondary to sepsis or inadequate volume replacement, renal insufficiency, congestive heart failure, inaccurate output reading). Once the cause has been determined, the specific treatment can be initiated. Patients who are receiving intravenous fluid therapy or intravenous hyperalimentation should have their electrolytes checked at least daily. Diabetic patients should have their serum glucose measured every 6 hours by a finger-stick method. Daily NPH and regular insulin therapy should be started once a regular diet is begun and well tolerated. Finally, if a patient is anemic, oral iron therapy should be instituted.

Once a patient is able to function independently and tolerate a diet well and there are no specific postoperative concerns, the patient can be discharged home. The patient should be instructed on use of medications, bathing, and other symptomatic care that requires medical attention.

REFERENCES

1. Kannel, W. G., et al.: Optimal resources for primary prevention of atherosclerotic disease: atherosclerotic study group. Circulation, 70:157A, 1984.
2. Ekroth, R., et al.: Physical training of patients with intermittent claudication: indications, methods and results. Surgery, 84:640, 1978.
3. Taylor, L. M., and Porter, J. M.: Drug treatment of claudication: vasodilators, hemorrheologic agents and antiseritonin drugs. J. Vasc. Surg., 3:374, 1986.
4. Imparto, A. M., Kim, G. E., Davidson, T., and Crowley, J. G.: Intermittent claudication: its natural course: Surgery, 78:795, 1975.
5. Bernstein, E. F., and Chan, E. L.: Abdominal aortic aneurysm in high-risk patients. Outcome of selective management based on size and expansion rate. Ann. Surg., 200:255, 1984.
6. Diehl, J. T., Cali, R. F., Hertzer, N. R., and Beven, E. G.: Complications of abdominal aortic reconstruction. An analysis of perioperative risk factors in 557 patients. Ann. Surg., 197:49, 1983.
7. Crawford, E. S., et al.: Aortoiliac occlusive disease: factors influencing survival and function following reconstructive operation over a 25-year period. Surgery, 90:1055, 1981.
8. Crawford, E. S., et al.: Infrarenal abdominal aortic aneurysm. Factors influencing survival after operation performed over a 25-year period. Ann. Surg., 193:699, 1981.
9. Hessel, J. J., Adams, D. F., and Abrams, H. L.: Complications of angiography. Diagn. Radiol., 138:273, 1981.
10. Lang, E. K.: A survey of the complications of percutaneous retrograde arteriography: Seldinger technic. Radiology, 81:257, 1963.
11. Gomes, A. S., et al.: Acute renal dysfunction after major arteriography. Am. J. Roentgenol. 145:1249, 1985.
12. Swartz, R. D., Rubin, J. E., Leeming, B. W., and Silva, P.: Renal failure following major angiography. Am. J. Med., 65:31, 1978.
13. Port, F. K., Wagoner, R. D., and Fulton, R. E.: Acute renal failure after angiography. Am. J. Roentgenol. 121:544, 1974.
14. Erffmeyer, J. E., Siegle, R. L., and Lieberman, P.: Anaphylactoid reactions to radiocontrast material. J. Allergy Clin. Immunol., 75:401, 1985.
15. Grindlinger, G. A., et al.: Volume loading and vasodilators in abdominal aortic aneurysmectomy. Am. J. Surg., 139:48, 1980.
16. Rittenhous, E. A., et al.: The role of prostaglandin E in the hemodynamic response to aortic clamping and declamping. Surgery, 80:137, 1976.
17. Baue, A. E., and McClerkin, W. W.: A study of shock: acidosis and the declamping phenomenon. Ann. Surg., 161:41, 1965.
18. Brant, B., Armstrong, R. P., and Vetto, R. M.: Vasodepressor factor in declamp shock production. Surgery, 67:650, 1970.
19. Selby, D. M., Haddy, F. J., and Campbell, G. S.: Vasodilator material in ischemic tissues. Surg. Forum, 15:232, 1964.
20. Malette, W. G., Armstrong, R. G., and Criscuolo, D.: A second mechanism in hypotension following release of abdominal aortic clamps. Surg. Forum, 14:292, 1963.
21. Bush, H. L., et al.: Assessment of myocardial performance and optimal volume loading during elective aortic aneurysm resection. Arch. Surg., 112:1301, 1977.
22. Chattergee, K., et al.: Hemodynamic and metabolic responses to vasodilator therapy in acute myocardial infarction. Circulation, 48:1181, 1973.
23. Abrams, J. H., Cerra, F., and Holcroft, J. W.: Cardiopulmonary monitoring. In Care of the Surgical Patient; 1 Critical Care. Edited by D. W. Wilmore, et al. New York, Scientific American, 1989, p. 1.
24. Samii, K., Conseiller, C., and Viars, P.: Central venous pressure and pulmonary wedge pressure. Arch. Surg., 111:1122, 1976.
25. Tomatis, L. A., Fierens, E. E., and Vergrugge, G. P.: Evaluation of surgical risk in peripheral vascular disease by coronary arteriography: a series of 100 cases. Surgery, 71:429, 1972.
26. Holcroft, J. W.: Shock. In Care of the Surgical Patient; 1 Critical Care. Edited by D. W. Wilmore, et al. New York, Scientific American, 1989.
27. Rice, C. L.: Pharmacologic support of the failing heart. In Care of the Surgical Patient; 1 Critical Care. Edited by D. W. Wilmore, et al. New York, Scientific American, 1989.
28. Reves, J. G.: Vasoactive drugs and when to use them. In Manual of Cardiac Anesthesia. Edited by S. J. Thomas. New York, Churchill Livingstone, 1984, p. 43.
29. Cohn, L. H., et al.: Fluid requirements and shifts after reconstruction of the aorta. Am. J. Surg., 120:182, 1970.
30. Rutledge, R., Sheldon, G. F., and Collins, M. L.: Massive transfusion. Crit. Care Clin., 2:791, 1986.
31. Valeri, C. R., et al.: Hypothermia-induced reversible platelet dysfunction. Ann. Surg., 205:175, 1987.
32. Hull, R. D., Raskob, G. E., and Hirsh, J.: Prophylaxis of venous thromboembolism. Chest, 89(Suppl.):374, 1986.
33. Kaiser, A. B., et al.: Antibiotic prophylaxis in vascular surgery. Ann. Surg., 188:283, 1978.
34. Pitt, H. A., et al.: Prophylactic antibiotics in vascular surgery. Ann. Surg., 192:356, 1980.
35. Szilagy, D. E., et al.: Infection in arterial reconstruction with synthetic grafts. Ann. Surg., 176:321, 1972.
36. Ford, G. T., et al.: Diaphragm function after upper abdominal surgery in humans. Am. Rev. Respir. Dis., 127:431, 1983.
37. Martin, L. F., Asher, E. F., Casey, J. M., and Fry, D. E.: Postoperative pneumonia. Arch. Surg., 119:379, 1984.
38. Szilagyi, D. E., et al.: Contribution of abdominal aortic aneurysmectomy to prolongation of life. Ann. Surg., 164:678, 1966.
39. Szilagyi, D. E., et al.: A 30-year survey of the reconstructive surgical treatment of aortoiliac occlusive disease. J. Vasc. Surg., 3:421, 1986.
40. Martinez, B. D., Hertzer, N. R., and Beven, E. G.: Influence of distal arterial occlusive disease on prognosis following aortobifemoral bypass. Surgery, 88:795, 1980.
41. Brown, O. W., et al.: Abdominal aortic aneurysm and coronary artery disease. Arch. Surg., 116:1484, 1981.
42. Hertzer, N. R., et al.: Coronary artery disease in peripheral vascular patients: a classification of 1000 coronary angiograms and results of surgical management. Ann. Surg., 199:223, 1984.

43. Mahar, L. J., et al.: Perioperative myocardial infarction in patients with coronary artery disease with and without aortocoronary artery bypass grafts. J. Thorac. Cardiovasc. Surg., 76:533, 1978.
44. Crawford, E. S., et al.: Operative risk in patients with previous coronary bypass. Ann. Thorac. Surg., 26:215, 1978.
45. Edwards, W. H., Mulherin, J. L., and Walker, W. E.: Vascular reconstructive surgery following myocardial revascularization. Ann. Surg., 187:653, 1978.
46. McCollum, C. H., Garcia-Rinaldi, R., Graham, J. H., and DeBakey, M. E.: Myocardial revascularization prior to subsequent major surgery in patients with coronary artery disease. Surgery, 81:302, 1977.
47. Whittemore, A. D., et al.: Aortic aneurysm repair: reduced operative mortality associated with maintenance of optimal cardiac performance. Ann. Surg., 192:414, 1980.
48. Tchirkow, G., and Beven, E. G.: Leg ischemia following surgery for abdominal aortic aneurysm. Ann. Surg., 188:166, 1978.
49. Ottinger, L. W., et al.: Left colon ischemia complicating aortoiliac reconstruction. Arch. Surg., 105:841, 1972.
50. Smith, R. F., and Szilagyi, D. E.: Ischemia of the colon as a complication in the surgery of the abdominal aorta. Arch. Surg., 80:806, 1960.
51. Hagihara, P. F., Ernst, C. B., and Griffen, W. O., Jr.: Incidence of ischemic colitis following abdominal aortic reconstruction. Surg. Gynecol. Obstet., 149:571, 1979.
52. Ernst, C. B., et al.: Ischemia colitis incidence following abdominal aortic reconstruction: a prospective study. Surgery, 80:417, 1976.
53. Johnson, W. C., and Nabseth, D. C.: Visceral infarction following aortic surgery. Ann. Surg., 180:312, 1974.
54. Young, J. R., et al.: Intestinal ischemia necrosis following abdominal aortic surgery. Surg. Gynecol. Obstet., 115:615, 1962.
55. Bandyk, D. F., Florence, M. G., and Johansen, K. H.: Colon ischemia accompanying ruptured abdominal aortic aneurysm. J. Surg. Res., 30:297, 1981.
56. Bush, H. L.: Renal failure following abdominal aortic reconstruction. Surgery, 93:107, 1983.
57. Turnipseed, W. D., Berkoff, H. A., and Belzer, F. O.: Postoperative stroke in cardiac and peripheral vascular disease. Ann. Surg., 192:365, 1980.
58. Evans, W. E., and Cooperman, M.: The significance of asymptomatic unilateral carotid bruits in preoperative patients. Surgery, 83:521, 1978.
59. Treiman, R. L., Foran, R. F., Shore, E. H., and Levin, P. M.: Carotid bruit significance in patients undergoing an abdominal aortic operation. Arch. Surg., 106:803, 1973.
60. Szilagyi, D. E.: Spinal cord ischemia in surgical procedures with temporary clamping of the abdominal aorta. Surgery, 93:110, 1983.
61. Szilagyi, D. E., Hageman, J. M., Smith, R. F., and Elliott, J. P.: Spinal cord damage in surgery of the abdominal aorta. Surgery, 83:38, 1978.
62. Dean, R. H., Keyser, J. E. III, and Dupont, W. D.: Aortic and renal vascular disease: factors affecting the value of combined procedures. Ann. Surg., 200:336, 1984.
63. Badenoch, A. W.: Diseases of the prostate gland and obstruction of the bladder neck. In Manual of Urology. Edited by A. W. Badenoch. London, William Heineman Medical Books, 1974, p. 469.
64. Morgan, R. J., and Abbott, W. M.: Safe management of patients with simultaneously occurring prostatism and abdominal aortic aneurysm. Am. J. Surg., 143:319, 1982.
65. Goldstone, J., and Moore, W. S.: Infection in vascular prosthesis. Am. J. Surg., 128:225, 1974.
66. Liekweg, W. G., and Greenfield, L. J.: Vascular prosthetic infections: collected experience and results of treatment. Surgery, 81:335, 1977.
67. Yashar, J. J., Weyman, A. K., Burnard, R. J., and Yashar, J.: Survival and limb salvage in patients with infected arterial prostheses. Am. J. Surg., 135:499, 1978.
68. Lindenaur, S. M., Fry, W. S., Schaub, G., and Wild, D.: The use of antibiotics in the prevention of vascular graft infections. Surgery, 62:487, 1967.
69. Bunt, T. J.: Synthetic vascular graft infections. I. Graft infections. Surgery, 93:733, 1983.
70. Blaisdell, F. W., DeMattei, G. A., and Gauder, P. J.: Extraperitoneal aorta to femoral bypass graft as replacement for an infected aortic bifurcation prosthesis. Am. J. Surg., 102:583, 1961.
71. Trout, H. H. III, Kozloff, L., and Giordano, J. M.: Priority of revascularization in patients with graft enteric fistulas, infected arteries or infected arterial prostheses. Ann. Surg., 199:669, 1984.
72. Busuttil, R. W., Rees, W. R., Baker, J. D., and Wilson, S. E.: Pathogenesis of aortoduodenal fistula: experimental and clinical correlates. Surgery, 85:1, 1979.
73. Kleinman, L. H., Towne, J. B., and Berhard, V. M.: A diagnostic and therapeutic approach to aortoenteric fistulas: clinical experience with 20 patients. Surgery, 86:868, 1979.
74. Garrett, H. E., Beall, A. C., Jordan, G. L., and DeBakey, M. E.: Surgical considerations of massive gastrointestinal tract hemorrhage caused by aortoduodenal fistula. Am. J. Surg., 105:6, 1963.
75. Bunt, T. J.: Synthetic vascular graft infections. II. Graft-enteric erosions and graft-enteric fistulas. Surgery, 94:1, 1983.
76. Mannick, J. A., and Nabseth, D. C.: Axillofemoral bypass grafts: a safe alternative to aortoiliac reconstruction. N. Engl. J. Med., 278:461, 1968.
77. Youmans, C. R., and Derrick, J. R.: Gastrointestinal erosion after prosthetic arterial reconstructive surgery. Am. J. Surg., 114:711, 1967.

Chapter 37

POSTOPERATIVE HYPERTENSION

ROBERT M. SAVAGE
FAWZY G. ESTAFANOUS
THOMAS L. HIGGINS

Hypertension is a phenomenon commonly encountered in the perioperative setting. At one time, a postoperative rise in blood pressure was considered to be a favorable indication of clinical improvement. Later, postoperative hypertension (POH) became recognized as a significant contributor to the patient's morbidity and evidence of an underlying physiologic alteration in the patient's condition.[1-7] In 1901, Harvey Cushing first described POH in patients with intracranial hypertension resulting from brain stem herniation.[8] Reports of POH in the setting of perinatal eclampsia soon followed. In the late 1940s, POH was determined to be a significant contributor to mortality following thoracic aortic coarctation resection.[9] In 1953, Sealy reported an overall incidence of "paradoxic" hypertension of 50% following resection of aortic coarctation.[10]

As use of the postoperative recovery unit increased, POH was found to be a relatively common clinical entity. In 1973, Estafanous Tarazi and associates noted a 35 to 50% incidence of POH in patients undergoing myocardial revascularization and a 5 to 10% incidence of POH in those undergoing heart valve replacement.[11] In a 1975 study involving more than 1500 patients, Gal et al. reported a 3% incidence of hypertension in patients following noncardiac surgery.[4] Seltzer et al. reported a 6% incidence of hypertension in patients following noncardiac surgery.[12] Seltzer, however, defined POH as a blood pressure increase of more than 20% over preoperative levels or greater than 140/90 mm Hg;[6] whereas Gal defined it as pressure greater than 190/100 mm Hg.[6]

Since then, multiple reports have been made of POH in a variety of clinical settings with a multitude of different therapeutic approaches, including more recently the automated administration of sodium nitroprusside by a feedback control mechanism.[13-16] The importance of intraoperative and postoperative hypertension as a risk factor for significant perioperative cardiac morbidity has been demonstrated by both Gal[4] and Seltzer.[12] In view of the documented association of prolonged POH or hypertensive crises with the significant postoperative complications of myocardial ischemia, congestive heart failure, cerebrovascular events, and postoperative bleeding, an understanding of the principles and management of POH is crucial for anyone involved in the critical care of the surgical patients in the period immediately following surgery.

This review focuses on the causes of POH and the pathophysiology related to acute and chronic hypertension. Additionally, we will examine in depth the specific causes of POH with particular emphasis on the mechanisms and hemodynamic changes associated with each cause. This will be followed by an overview of the clinical evaluation and therapeutic approach to the surgical patient with POH.

DEFINITION OF POSTOPERATIVE HYPERTENSION

A rise in the patient's blood pressure above normal baseline values does not necessarily constitute POH. The term **POH** is restricted to a rise in the patient's blood pressure that places the patient at significant risks for hypertensive complications. In normotensive patients (i.e., blood pressure less than 140/90 mm Hg), a postoperative blood pressure higher than 160/95 mm Hg is clinically significant. In hypertensive patients, a postoperative rise of 20% or more in either systolic or diastolic pressure is clinically significant.[3,5]

PATHOPHYSIOLOGY OF HYPERTENSION

The circulatory system has highly sophisticated mechanisms for maintaining a mean arterial pressure in the normal range of 90 to 110 mm Hg. These control mechanisms (Table 37-1) act to maintain the blood pressure in survivable ranges as well as to return blood volume to normal levels for hemodynamic homeostasis. The mechanisms for regulating blood pressure may be thought of as either short-term, intermediate, or long-term. Immediate control of blood pressure occurs within seconds of a change in mean arterial pressure outside the normal parameters. These rapidly acting control mechanisms include the baroreceptor feedback mechanism, the chemoreceptor feedback mechanism, and the central nervous system ischemic responses. Intermediate-term mechanisms that become active after 30 minutes to several hours include stress relaxation changes in the vasculature, the renin-angiotensin control mechanism, and capillary fluid shifts into or out of the circulation for the readjustment of blood volume. The long-term regulation of arterial blood pressure compensates for the inability of the short- and intermediate-term mechanisms to actively control arterial pressure after a few

Table 37–1. Blood Pressure Adaptation and Control Mechanisms

Adaptation	Onset	Peak Effect	Duration	Feedback
Short term				
Baroreceptor	<15 sec	30 seconds	2–4 days	Pressure
Chemoreceptor	<15 sec	60 seconds	Prolonged	Po_2, Pco_2, pH
Central nervous system ischemic	<15 sec	Minutes	Prolonged	Ischemia
Intermediate				
Stress relaxation	30 sec	Days	Prolonged	Pressure
Capillary fluid shift	8 min	Days	Prolonged	Pressure
Renin-angiotensin	2 min	45 minutes	Prolonged	Pressure
Long term				
Blood volume	5–120 min	Days	Prolonged	Renal

Pco_2, partial pressure of carbon dioxide; Po_2, partial pressure of oxygen.

days because of adaptations that diminish their responsiveness. Long-term mechanisms are involved mainly with the control of blood volume via the kidney by the renin-angiotensin system and the hormone aldosterone, which is secreted by the adrenal cortex.[17,18]

Short-Term Blood Pressure Regulation

The moment-by-moment control of blood pressure is regulated by the central nervous system via the baroreceptor and chemoreceptor feedback mechanisms as well as the central nervous system ischemic responses. Baroreceptors or pressor receptors are located in the walls of the large arteries of the thoracic and neck region, most notably in the internal carotid artery above the bifurcation in the carotid sinus and in the walls of the thoracic aortic arch (Fig. 37–1). These receptors have "spray-type" nerve endings that are stimulated when stretched. As the blood pressure increases above a normal range, there is an increased inhibition of the medullary vasoconstrictive center and an enhancement of the vagal tone that results in peripheral vasodilatation, diminished heart rate, and diminished force of myocardial contraction.

The carotid sinus and aortic baroreceptors have different responses according to the mean arterial pressure. The carotid baroreceptor response is carried via the nerve of Hering to the glossopharyngeal nerve and ultimately to the medullary center. The aortic baroreceptor response reaches the medullary center via nerve fibers that travel along with the vagus nerve. The carotid sinus baroreceptor responds between a mean arterial pressure range of 60 to 180 mm Hg, whereas the aortic baroreceptor response starts at 90 mm Hg. These overlapping response ranges result in an extremely rapid response to transient changes in pressure, as noted by respiratory variation in heart rate response. With rapid changes in blood pressure, the impulse transmission to the medullary center results in a more rapid compensation and buffering of any acute blood pressure changes. The baroreceptor response adapts to persistent pressure changes over a 24- to 48-hour period such that if the blood pressure is consistently elevated for 48 hours, there is a gradual decrease in afferent nerve transmission to baseline levels during the next 24 to 48 hours. This adaptive response prevents the baroreceptor reflex from functioning as a buffer control mechanism beyond a few days.[19] In patients with atherosclerosis of the carotid sinus vasculature, there is an enhanced transmission of impulses to the medullary center with a resultant overactive response to minimal baroreceptor stimulation. This syndrome, called **carotid sinus hypersensitivity,** is frequently seen in elderly patients.[20]

The chemoreceptors are chemosensitive cells located in the carotid bodies (at the bifurcation of the internal and external carotid arteries) and the aortic bodies. These chemoreceptors are richly supplied with nutrient arteries. When the blood pressure is diminished to a level where the blood flow to the chemoreceptors is reduced, the diminished oxygen supply to the chemoreceptors is detected, as is the accumulation of excess carbon dioxide and hydrogen ions.[21] This results in an enhanced transmission of signals that pass with the baroreceptors through the nerve of Hering and the vagus nerve to the medullary center. Unlike the baroreceptor response that is active in the normal range, the chemoreceptor mechanisms do not respond until the mean arterial pressure falls below 80 mm Hg. With this reduction in blood pressure, there is an increase in nerve transmission to the medullary system. In addition, if the partial pressure of oxygen in arterial blood (Pao_2) falls below normal or the carbon dioxide or hydrogen ion concentration rises above normal, there is a similar increase in nerve transmission to the medullary center resulting in a sympathetic excitation and vagal inhibition that ultimately causes an increase in the blood pressure.[17,18]

In addition to the baroreceptors and chemoreceptors of the carotid artery and aortic arch, low pressure stretch receptors are located in the arterial and pulmonary arteries. With stimulation of these receptors secondary to increased venous return, there is a reflex vasodilatation at the arteriolar level of the peripheral and renal circulation. This increases the peripheral capillary pressure and fluid filtration into the interstitial tissue along with the glomerular filtration rate and fluid filtration into the renal tubules. The increase in arterial size causes further stretching of the sinoatrial node, which may increase the heart rate by 15% via the Bainbridge reflex.[22]

Most blood pressure control by the nervous system is achieved by the baroreceptors, chemoreceptors, and low pressure arterial receptor reflexes. When blood flow to the medullary vasomotor center is diminished to a critical level, however, resulting in ischemia of the vasomotor neurons, a dramatic enhancement of overall sympathetic effer-

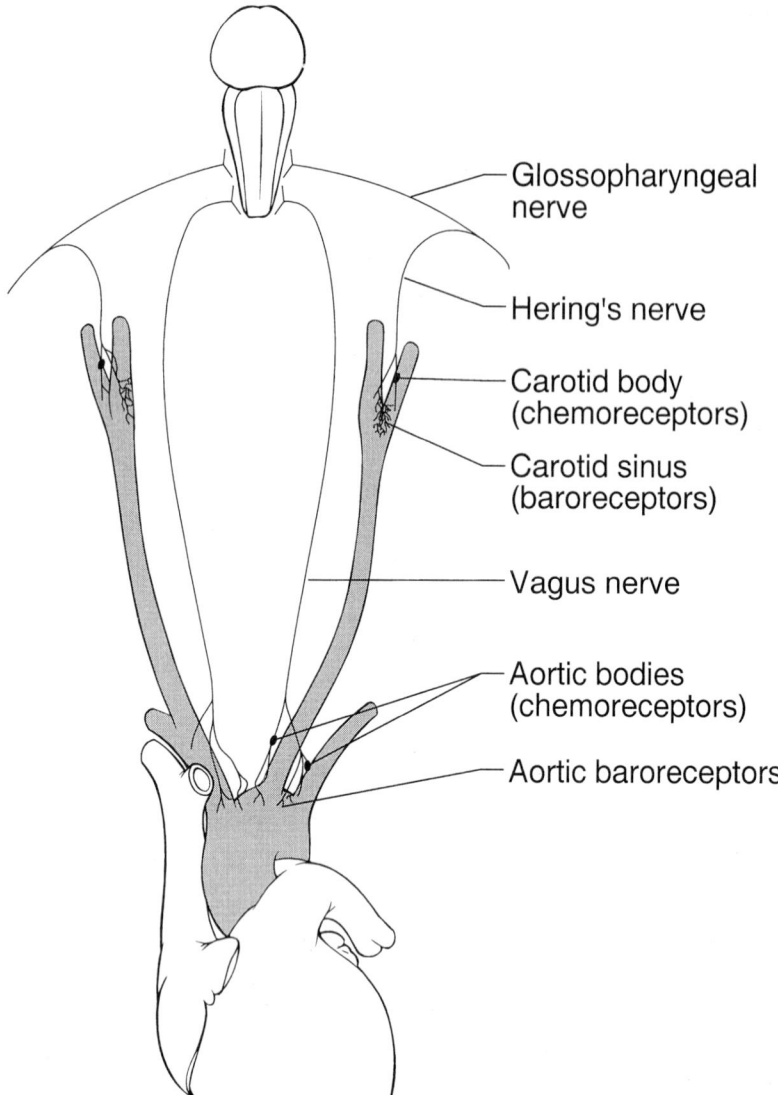

Fig. 37-1. Pressor chemoreceptor location and afferent nerves associated with immediate blood pressure regulation. (Courtesy of the Cleveland Clinic Foundation, Cleveland, OH.)

ent tone occurs, which increases the mean arterial pressure potentially to greater than 200 mm Hg with profound sympathetic nervous system vasoconstriction as well as increased heart rate and force of ventricular contractility. This ischemic response begins at mean arterial pressures below 50 mm Hg and is greatest at 15 to 20 mm Hg. Obviously, such a system operates to prevent decrease blood flow to the brain. With acute increases in blood pressure, the diminished transmission of impulses from the baroreceptors decreases sympathetic activity and enhances vagal tone triggered by the medullary center.[23]

Intermediate-Term Blood Pressure Regulation

Hormonal mechanisms also help regulate mean arterial pressure. Acute drops in blood pressure stimulate the adrenal medulla to release norepinephrine, which increases the heart rate, ventricle contraction force, and vasoconstriction of the venous and arteriolar bed. Because norepinephrine has a circulation half-life of 1 to 3 minutes, it is relatively short-lived, absent hypotension continued. Kidneys have the capacity to maintain a normal glomerular filtration rate and renal blood flow between a mean arterial pressure of 70 and 160 mm Hg. When the mean arterial pressure is acutely increased, the glomerular filtration rate and renal and glomerular blood flow are maintained at a relatively constant level by the tubuloglomerular feedback mechanism with afferent arteriolar vasoconstriction. An acute drop in blood pressure is noted by the juxtaglomerular apparatus (Fig. 37-2), leading to afferent arteriolar vasodilatation and efferent arteriolar vasoconstriction secondary to increased renin release (Fig. 37-3). Persistent low mean arterial pressure maintains the renin release leading to increased levels of angiotensin with eventual vasoconstriction of the afferent arterioles and decreased glomerular blood flows. Arteriolar vasoconstriction conserves as much intravascular volume as possible by preventing glomerular filtration. As displayed in Figure 37-3, renin is secreted from the juxtaglomerular cells of the kidney in response to decreases in pressure in the renal artery, di-

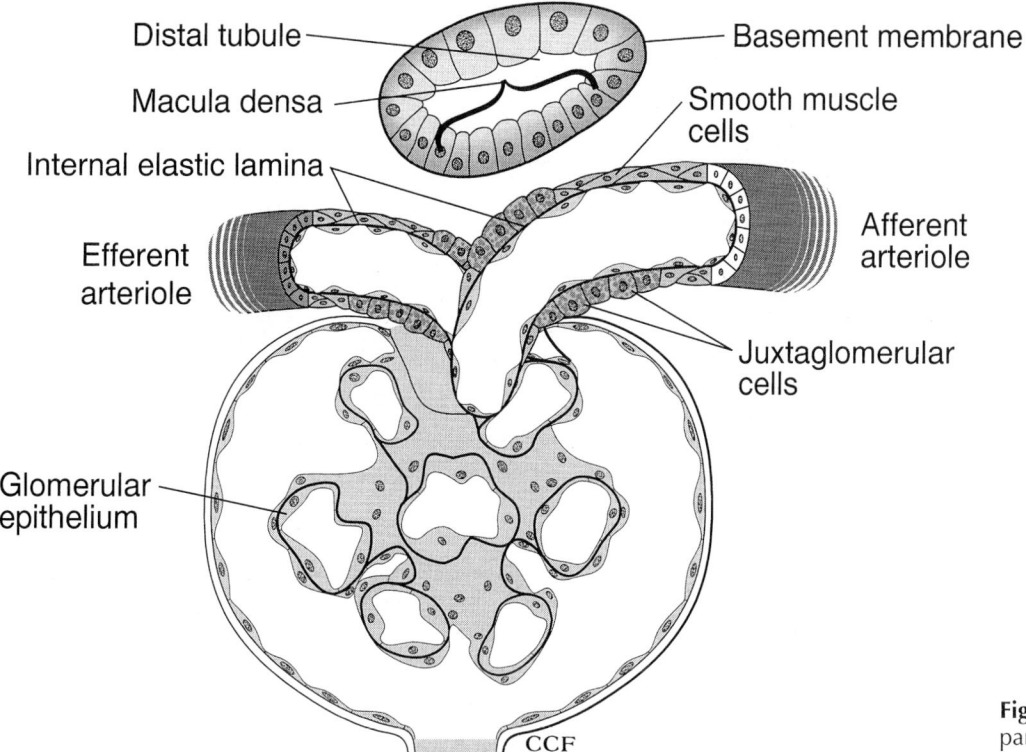

Fig. 37-2. Juxtaglomerular apparatus. (Courtesy of the Cleveland Clinic Foundation, Cleveland, OH.)

minished sodium delivery to the macula densa, and increased sympathetic tone. Renin cleaves its substrate, angiotensinogen, resulting in angiotensin I, which is rapidly converted to angiotensin II by the angiotensin-converting enzyme (ACE) which is found in the lung, kidney, adrenal cortex, and vascular endothelium of the heart. Angiotensin itself is one of the most potent known vasopressor substances and serves to stimulate aldosterone secretion by the adrenal cortex as well as the parasympathetic response.[24]

When the blood pressure falls below 50 mm Hg, the hypothalamus secretes the hormone vasopressin, a direct vasoconstrictor. Vasopressin also plays a role in the long-term control of blood volume via its effect of increasing the reabsorption of water in the distal tubules of the kidney.[25] Further short-term regulation of the blood pressure occurs

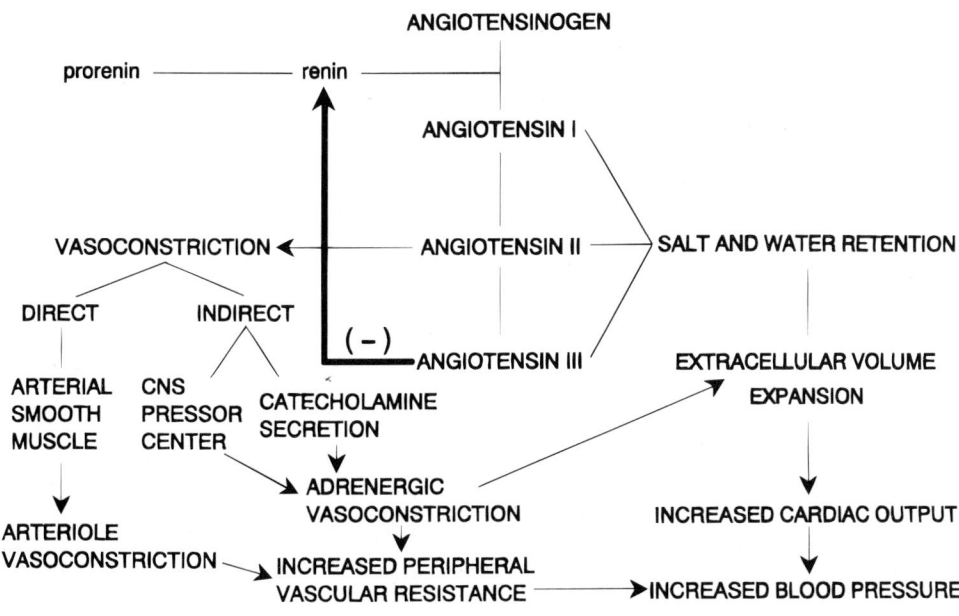

Fig. 37-3. Renin-angiotensin blood pressure effect. CNS, Central nervous system. (Adapted from Miranda, J.V.: Anesth. Analg., 72:667, 1991.)

through capillary fluid shift and the stress relaxation response of the vasculature. As blood pressure increases, there is an increase in transudation of fluid into the tissue interstitium caused by an increase in hydrostatic pressure in the capillary bed. This diminishes the overall venous return and reduces the mean arterial pressure. In addition, the vasculature can accommodate larger amounts of blood when the mean arterial pressure is elevated and smaller amounts of blood when the pressure is reduced. After an acute elevation of pressure caused by an increase in blood volume, the blood pressure will gradually return to normal as a result of increases in the venous capacity caused by this stress relaxation response.[26]

Long-Term Blood Pressure Regulation

The long-term regulation of mean arterial pressure occurs as the capability of short-term regulatory mechanisms diminishes. As elevated blood pressure persists, the kidney increases its capacity for excreting both water and salt, which diminishes blood volume and lowers the mean arterial pressure. As the mean arterial pressure decreases, the renal output of both salt and water decreases, resulting in a gradual normalization of the intervascular volume and mean arterial pressure.[17,18]

In the long-term regulation of mean arterial pressure, physiologic changes associated with hypertension have a profound impact on the cardiovascular, central nervous, and renal systems. The myocardium responds to acute changes in blood pressure (i.e., an increase in the systemic afterload) by gradual increases in the left ventricular end diastolic volume with increasing cardiac work load. This increase in left ventricular end diastolic volume is caused by gradual decreases in stroke volume secondary to the increase in afterload. The increase in stroke volume is matched by an increase in coronary blood flow resulting from an increase of coronary perfusion pressure and from a coronary autoregulation response to the production of local metabolites and vasodilatation of the coronary capillary bed (Fig. 37–4). The normal ventricle responds to acute elevations of afterload by increasing the overall force of contraction.

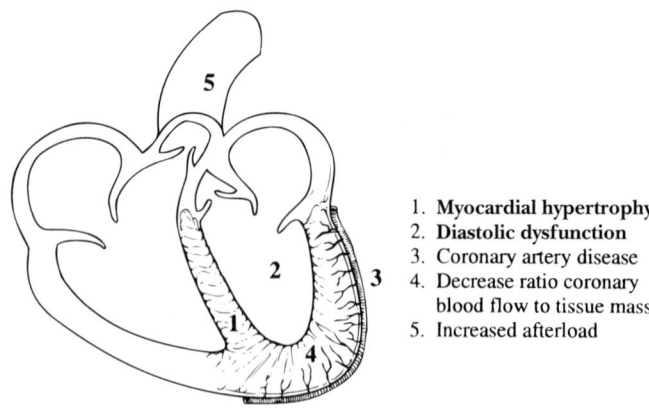

Fig. 37–5. Factors affecting myocardial oxygen supply and demand in chronic hypertension.

With the persistence of increased afterload or output impedance, there is an increase in cardiac mass or hypertrophy. Figure 37–5 demonstrates the effects of hypertension on the myocardial oxygen consumption. Myocardial hypertrophy increases the oxygen demand secondary to the increase in overall muscle mass of the myocardium. In addition, the increase in left ventricular end pressure diminishes compliance or left ventricular distensibility (Fig. 37–6). This diminished compliance is commonly referred to as the diastolic dysfunction of left ventricular hypertrophy. Initially, left ventrical systolic function is not affected; however, reduced ventricular compliance results in a decreased sarcomere recruitment for a given left ventricular end diastolic pressure. The increased myocardial wall mass exerts an extrinsic force on the penetrating coronary vessels, thereby increasing the total coronary vascular resistance and impeding endocardial blood flow.[27]

Another response to persistent blood pressure elevation is arteriolar myogenic hyperplasia of the coronary capillary bed. The coronary capillary bed is autoregulated by local arteriolar responses to metabolic substrates such as lactate or adenosine in addition to tissue oxygen and carbon dioxide levels.[28] When hyperplasia of the muscular layer of the

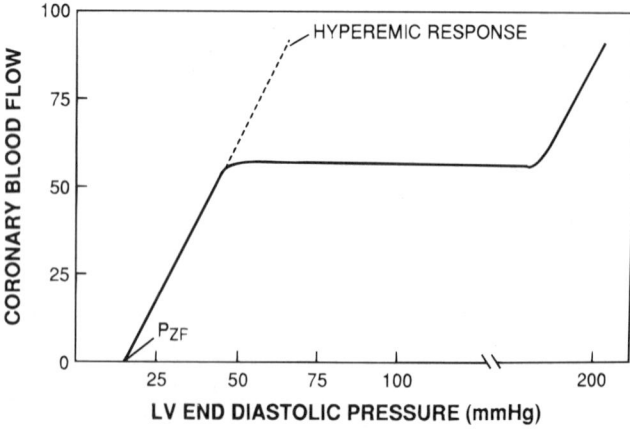

Fig. 37–4. Autoregulation of coronary blood flow. LV, Left ventricular; P$_{ZF}$, pressure at zero coronary blood flow. (Adapted from Miranda, J. V.: Anesth. Analg., 72:667, 1991)

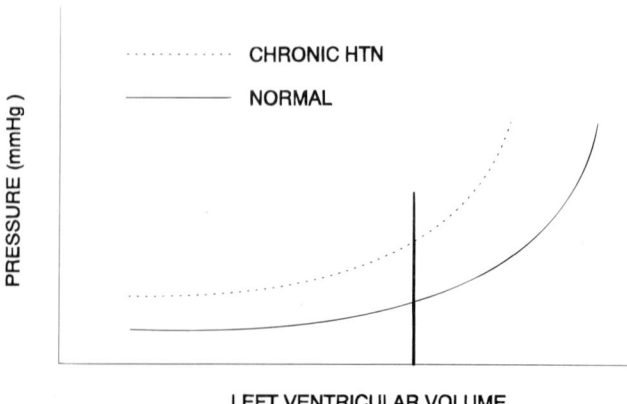

Fig. 37–6. Changes seen in left ventricular compliance (pressure-volume relationship) with chronic hypertension (HTN).

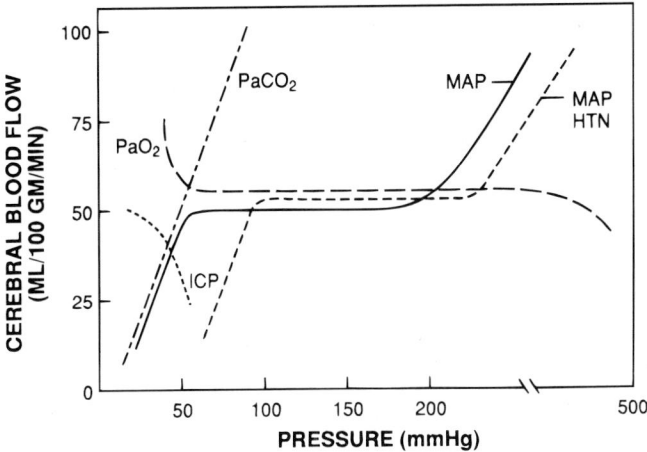

Fig. 37-7. Cerebral blood flow autoregulation in normal circumstances and in chronic hypertension (HTN). ICP, Intracranial pressure; MAP, mean arterial pressure.

vessel wall occurs, autoregulation cannot reduce arteriolar resistance.[29] With the increased oxygen demands caused by the myocardial hypertrophy and increased work load of the myocardium secondary to the increased afterload, this impaired autoregulation cannot provide adequate oxygen supply.[30] Coronary atherosclerosis and chronic hypertension further exacerbate this imbalance of myocardial oxygen supply and demand.

Normally, cerebral blood flow is maintained at a constant flow to the various capillary beds via an autoregulatory mechanism.[31,32] This autoregulatory mechanism (Fig. 37-7) maintains blood flow to the central nervous system vascular capillary beds at 50 ml/100 g of tissue between a mean arterial pressure of 50 mm Hg and 150 mm Hg.[31] With chronic hypertension, this autoregulatory curve is shifted to the right. In the hypertensive patient, the lower limit of autoregulation is at a mean arterial pressure of 85 to 150 mm Hg versus 50 to 70 mm Hg seen in the normal patient.[31] In chronic hypertension, arteriolar or vascular hypertrophy enables the hypertensive patient to tolerate higher mean arterial pressure changes.[33] Arterial or muscular hypertrophy, however, diminishes the ability of the cerebral vascular bed to vasodilate when the mean arterial pressure goes below the lower limit of autoregulation.[34-36] With chronic hypertension, blood pressure below the lower limit of autoregulation results in a blood flow inadequate to maintain cerebral metabolism, which can cause irreversible ischemic damage to the central nervous system.[37-39] The clinical consequences of an upward shift in the autoregulatory curve in patients with chronic hypertension include symptoms of global ischemia if the mean arterial pressure is reduced too rapidly to levels that would otherwise be tolerated by normotensive patients.[40] Morphologic changes in the arterioles of patients with chronic hypertension include hypertrophy of the smooth muscle and elastic fibers of the arterials with eventual fibrous replacement, which narrows the smaller vessels and dilates the larger. In the cerebral circulation, this causes a microaneurysm called Charcot-Bouchard aneurysm.[41,42] In patients with chronic hypertension, as previously discussed, the autoregulatory curve shifts to the right. Though this may be reversed with chronic antihypertensive therapy, extreme caution must be taken in these patients against aggressively lowering the blood pressure. In the setting of increased sympathetic tone, the cerebral blood flow autoregulatory curve shifts to the right acutely because of the resulting constriction of the large cerebral inflow vessels that reduce downstream pressure, thus provoking local autoregulatory vasodilatation. The effect is that the cerebral circulation can withstand higher pressures but at the expense of compromised autoregulatory blood flow at lower pressures. Alpha and ganglionic blockers prevent this acute shift in the autoregulatory and preserve blood flow at lower pressures.

The kidney's mechanisms for maintaining consistent levels of renal blood flow contribute to the mechanisms of renal pathology in the setting of chronic hypertension. As the mean arterial pressure increases and the blood flow becomes too great for the renovascular bed, regulatory afferent vasoconstrictive mechanisms maintain the renal blood flow and glomerular filtration rate at normal to near normal levels. With chronic elevations of mean arterial pressure, hypertrophy of the afferent arteriolar musculature occurs with an impairment of the autoregulatory mechanisms. In a manner similar to that seen in the cerebral circulation, the glomerular blood flow may be reduced if the blood pressure is rapidly reduced or decreased to a "normal" level after this arteriolar muscular hypertrophy has occurred. This may cause glomerular or tubular ischemia and eventually impair overall renal function.[43]

CAUSES OF POSTOPERATIVE HYPERTENSION

Every surgical patient has the potential of developing POH. Table 37-2 lists the most common causes of POH. As patients emerge from anesthesia, their level of "nociceptive" stimulation such as pain, bladder distention, hypothermia with shivering, and prolonged intolerance of endotracheal intubation increases.[44] Surgical patients may experience respiratory difficulties related to airway obstruction or prolonged sedation and neuromuscular blockade that can cause hypercapnia, hypoxemia, or acidosis, which may further accentuate the sympathetic tone.[1,2,4,5] Other common factors associated with POH include hypervolemia, hypovolemia, and preoperative hypertension.

Commonly, POH occurs in response to increased sympathetic nervous system activity that results in both $alpha_1$-

Table 37-2. General Causes of Postoperative Hypertension

1. Pain
2. Anxiety
3. Shivering
4. Hypoxemia
5. Hypercarbia
6. Acidosis
7. Hypervolemia
8. Hypovolemia
9. Intubation
10. Full bladder
11. Previous hypertension

mediated vasoconstriction with increased vascular resistance and venous return as well as beta$_1$-receptor-mediated increases in the heart rate. Usually, this enhanced sympathetic nervous system activity is in response to pain, anxiety, urinary bladder distention, persistent endotracheal intubation, or hypothermia. When the residual anesthesia is inadequate to completely inhibit the "nocioceptive" stimuli, there is a enhanced activity of the hypothalamic-hypophysial adrenal axis and the renin-angiotensin system.[44] Postoperative hypertension may also be associated with decreased parasympathetic activity associated with either parasympatholytic agents or certain muscle relaxants such as pancuronium and gallamine.

Hypoxemia, hypercarbia, or acidosis may result in a reflex increase in sympathetic nervous system activity via the carotid body chemoreceptors. This causes a progressive increase in the patient's heart rate and blood pressure. Unless the metabolic aberrations are reversed, the vasomotor center will eventually fail, resulting in profound sympathetic nervous system hyperactivity. Mechanisms associated with hypercarbia or hypoxemia are commonly related to inadequate postoperative ventilation. Factors that may cause postoperative ventilatory depression include delayed emergence from anesthesia (including residual narcosis) and residual neuromuscular blockade either from a relative overdose or a compounding factor such as hypothermia that may exacerbate the neuromuscular blockade.

Hypervolemia is relatively common during the first 12 to 24 hours after surgery. It is related to intraoperative fluid administration and the increased secretion of the antidiuretic hormone as part of the surgical stress response. The increased fluid volume increases the heart rate as well as the force of contractility via the Bainbridge reflex. Though this may be associated with increased production of the atrial naturetic factor, the ensuing naturesis does not occur rapidly enough to compensate for the increased cardiac output resulting from the venous return.

The presence of hypovolemia may enhance the baroreceptor response as well as the central nervous system adaptive mechanisms that increase sympathetic nervous system activity.[45] This response may be further accentuated by increased chemoreceptor activity triggered by elevations of carbon dioxide and hydrogen ion content that are due to inadequate tissue perfusion and interference with local cellular metabolisms.[45,46] Though the hypovolemia may initially cause a hypertensive response, a continued inadequate volume status would eventually result in hemodynamic instability and hypotension.

The normal response to a lowered body temperature is intense shivering to increase the overall metabolic rate and produce more body heat. This increased metabolic rate increases the demand for oxygen delivery to the tissues, which enhances sympathetic nervous system activity resulting in increased cardiac output. The associated vasoconstriction that accompanies hypothermia elevates the blood pressure by increasing the systemic vascular resistance.

Preoperative hypertension has been linked with POH.[47] This may occur in patients with either recognized or unrecognized hypertension (Table 37-3). With chronic hypertension, there is a relative contraction of the intravascular space with subsequent greater lability of the blood pressure in response to administration of anesthesia and emergence. In addition, the chronic physiologic changes associated with hypertension, such as vascular arteriolar muscular hypertrophy and myocardial hypertrophy, increase sensitivity to sympathetic nervous system stimulation and vasopressor responsiveness.

Myocardial ischemia is included with the more common causes of POH to serve as a reminder of the disastrous consequences that can occur if it is not recognized. Mangano noted that POH is often associated with myocardial ischemia.[48,49] Myocardial ischemia has also been associated with an overall enhancement of sympathetic nervous system tone as well as the level of circulating catecholamines and serotonin in numerous studies.[50-52] Elevated levels of circulating catecholamines are associated with serious arrhythmias, which are presumably due to catecholamine effects on both the slope of phase 4 depolarization and the resting membrane potential. The hypertension associated with extensive myocardial infarction is also associated with this sympathetic response and contributes to significant ventricular dysfunction by increasing afterload.[53] It is not surprising that the extent of myocardial damage, cardiogenic shock, and mortality have been closely correlated with these levels.[53]

Postoperative hypertension also may be associated with the type of surgical procedure (Table 37-4), particularly vascular procedures or those affecting the organs controlling blood pressure homeostasis. Postoperative hyperten-

Table 37-3. Medically Related Causes of Postoperative Hypertension

1. Essential hypertension
2. Renal disease
   Acute or chronic renal failure
   Renovascular hypertension
3. Endocrine-related disorders
   Hypoglycemia
   Hyperthyroidism
   Pheochromocytoma (diagnosed or latent)
   Catecholamine-secreting tumors
   Hyperparathyroidism
   Acromegaly
   Myxedema
   Cushing's syndrome
   Carcinoid syndrome
   Renin-secreting tumors
4. Myocardial ischemia/infarction
5. Medication related
   Rebound: clonidine, beta blockers
   Monoamine oxidase inhibitors
   Tricyclic antidepressants
6. Miscellaneous
   Obesity
   Advanced age
   Pregnancy (preeclampsia or eclampsia)
   Oral contraceptives
   Alcohol or narcotic withdrawal
   Polyarteritis nodosa
   Hypercalcemia
   Increased intracranial pressure

Table 37-4. Surgical and Anesthetic Causes of Postoperative Hypertension

Surgical Causes	Anesthetic Causes

1. Cardiac surgery
   Myocardial revascularization
   Valve repair or replacement
   Heart transplantation
2. Vascular surgery
   Aortic aneurysm resection
   Aortic coarctation
   Carotid endarterectomy
3. Neurosurgical procedures
   Neurovascular procedures
   Increased intracranial pressure
   Autonomic hyperreflexia
4. Abdominal surgery
   Endocrine tumors
   Liver transplantation
   Renal surgery and transplantation
   Urologic surgery
5. Obstetric surgery
   Eclampsia
   Preeclampsia
   Hypertension of pregnancy
6. Radical neck dissection
	1. Intravenous agents
	   Opioids (meperidine)
	   Ketamine
	   Neuroleptic agents
	   Opioid antagonists
	2. Decreasing levels of inhalation agents
	   Halothane
	   Enflurane
	3. Regional anesthesia
	   Systemic absorption of epinephrine
	   Tourniquet pain
	4. Anesthetic emergence
	5. Endotracheal intubation
	6. Induced hypotension rebound
	7. Discontinuation of medication
	   Beta-blocker therapy
	   Clonidine
	8. Residual intraoperative medications
	   Vasopressor effect
	   Anticholinergics
	9. Preoperative medications
	   Monoamine oxidase inhibitors
	   Tricyclic antidepressants
	   Illicit drugs
	   Nonprescription drugs

sion has been shown to occur in up to 50% of patients undergoing cardiac surgery or major peripheral vascular surgery.[11] In addition, POH is commonly associated with patients having an endocrine tumor resection. Other surgeries associated with POH include neurosurgical procedures involving an increase in intracranial pressure, organ transplants, and neck surgery with the potential for carotid sinus denervation. Some anesthetic techniques and agents are also associated with hypertension in the postoperative setting (see Table 37-4). Ketamine hydrochloride use has commonly been associated with perioperative hypertension, as has the use of opioids in patients who have been taking monoamine oxidase inhibitors or tricyclic antidepressants.[54,55]

Surgically Related Causes of Postoperative Hypertension

Myocardial Revascularization

Hypertension has been reported in 35 to 50% of patients undergoing myocardial revascularization, although the prophylactic use of sodium nitroprusside and other antihypertensive agents may mask this incidence.[3,11,56-59] The higher hypertension incidence in patients after myocardial revascularization than valvular heart surgery is thought to be related to the instability of blood pressure control in patients with ischemic heart disease.[60] The rise of blood pressure has been associated with elevated catecholamine levels as well as diminished baroreceptor sensitivity and frequent hypovolemia.[59] Studies suggest that enhanced activity of the renin-angiotensin system is responsible.[61] Weinstein et al., found no difference in plasma renin activity, angiotensin II levels, or aldosterone levels between normotensive and hypertensive patients undergoing myocardial revascularization, despite elevated norepinephrine levels.[62] The blood pressure elevation occurs shortly after the completion of surgery and may last for 8 to 14 hours.[56] Such elevations have not been found to be related to the presence of preoperative hypertension, use of preoperative medications, distribution of specific vascular lesions, use of saphenous vein versus internal mammary artery grafts, anesthetic techniques, or the extent of hypothermia or hypervolemia.[56]

The most common hemodynamic characteristic of hypertension following myocardial revascularization has been reported to be an elevation of the patient's systemic vascular resistance along with an associated increase in heart rate and elevation of the rate of left ventricular pressure rise with little change in cardiac output.[58-59] It should be noted, however, that this particular study was carried out in patients undergoing myocardial revascularization with normal or mildly impaired left ventricular function. Because the baroreceptor pathways may be interrupted during dissection around the aorta, the inhibitory impulses to the vasomotor centers may be diminished or abolished.[59] This hemodynamic pattern is consistent with a sympathetic overdrive with the attending chronotropic cardiac and peripheral vascular pressor reflexes. This may account for the normalization of pressures seen with the ablation of afferent sympathetic impulses by the stellate ganglion block.[63] Another suggestion is that the cardiogenic hypertensive chemoreflex, resulting from interruption of chemoreceptors between the aorta and pulmonary artery, causes the release of serotonin.[50]

Valvular Heart Surgery

Hypertension occurs in up to 12% of patients following aortic valve replacement and 6% following mitral valve replacement.[11,58] The potential causes include an increase in the afferent sympathetic pressor response associated with the myocardial revascularization surgery and the improvements in hemodynamic function commonly seen after valve replacement. The higher incidence of POH following aortic valve replacement is thought to be caused by the pronounced myocardial hypertrophy, with relative preservation of function, in patients with aortic valve disease. The incidence of POH in patients undergoing mitral valve surgery varies according to the underlying disease. In patients with mitral disease related to underlying ischemic heart disease, the presence of significant ventricular dysfunction in association with papillary muscle dysfunction or mitral valve incompetency secondary to annular dilatation may blunt the potential for POH. In patients with rheumatic mitral stenosis, successful valve replacement in the setting of preserved ventricular function would result in a hyperdynamic heart in the setting of an elevated systemic vascular resistance associated with the postoperative increase in circulating catecholamines. Thus, the mechanism of hypertension following valvular heart surgery not only includes elevated systemic vascular resistance but also may include hyperdynamic cardiac function. The incidence of POH in this heterogenous population depends on the residual ventricular function of the patients. Dehring et al. reported both systemic and pulmonary hypertension in association with valvular heart surgery.[60]

Cardiac Transplantation

Postoperative hypertension following orthotopic cardiac transplantation has been reported in 20 to 90% of patients.[64-66] In these patients, POH appears to be multifactorial in nature. To a great extent, the high incidence of POH was related to the underlying compensatory mechanisms prevalent in patients who are candidates for cardiac transplantation, most specifically high systemic levels of circulating catecholamines. Most patients undergoing cardiac transplantation had been in a low output state during their preoperative clinical course. The marked elevation in systemic vascular resistance persists after implantation of the "new" heart and may persist up to 1 year after the transplant.[67]

Other factors related to POH in these patients include the presence of a denervated heart, a tendency to be volume overexpanded, and the associated effects of immunosuppressant agents. The characteristic feature of the denervated transplanted heart is its lack of sympathetic or parasympathetic innervation. Consequently, it is not subject to normal intrinsic baroceptor control operating through the cardioaccelatory and cardioinhibitory reflexes of the sympathetic and vagal pathways. Thus, elevated blood pressures produce no inhibitory cardiac response. These patients also have an elevated level of circulating catecholamines to which the "new heart" has not been exposed. Hyperdynamic responses immediately following implantation are not unusual and may cause profound hypertension, given the relatively fixed nature of the elevated systemic vascular resistance and a hyperdynamic, denervated heart that is unresponsive to the inhibitory neural reflexes.

Immunosuppressive agents commonly administered following heart transplantation include both corticosteroids and cyclosporine. Corticosteroids have a direct effect on the arteriolar sensitivity to catecholamines and enhance retention of sodium by the kidney.[68] Scherrer et al. demonstrated that cyclosporine administration is associated with sympathetic neural activation, which becomes further accentuated in the presence of the denervated transplanted heart.[66] Borrow et al. demonstrated an increased chronotropic responsiveness of the transplanted heart as well as reduced responsiveness to alpha$_1$-agonist.[67] The latter implies a relatively fixed systemic elevation of systemic vascular resistance in the face of a heart with increased responsiveness to adrenergic stimulation. Although these patients do not have elevated renin levels, persistent hypertension has been related to reductions in the glomerular filtration rate associated with chronic cyclosporine therapy.[65] These results occur when vascular glomerular damage elevates levels of plasma renin and angiotensin.

Aortic Aneurysm Resection

Hertzer and Beven and co-workers reported POH in approximately 50% of patients undergoing resection of abdominal aortic aneurysms or aortofemoral bypass.[69] With aortic manipulation, it is thought that denervation of the aortic pressor receptors results in less afferent transmission to the medullary center, which is interpreted centrally as profound hypotension. This causes an immediate increase of sympathetic tone. As a result, there is a diminished cardiac inhibitory response in the face of profound hypertension. In addition, underlying renal vascular disease or renal ischemia secondary to aortic cross-clamping further contributes to the development of POH.

Carotid Endarterectomy

Hypertension following carotid endarterectomy has been reported in 37 to 55% of patients.[70,71] Causes implicated include preoperative hypertension, carotid sinus denervation, and massive cerebral edema related to a postoperative neurologic stroke.[70-73] Also, dissection of the area surrounding the carotid bulb can cause denervation of the baroreceptors in this area. With the attendant decrease of inhibitory impulses to the vasomotor centers, there is an increase in sympathetic activity resulting in an elevated systemic vascular resistance, increased heart rate, and increased contractile state of the myocardium.[73] The application of local anesthetic to the carotid bulb area also mimics denervation with diminished inhibitory impulses to vasomotor center, resulting in enhanced systemic sympathetic vascular tone. Consequently, it has been recommended that physicians discontinue the surgical practice of applying local anesthesia in the carotid bulb area.

Hypertension usually occurs within the first 2 hours following carotid endarterectomy, and it may last up to 9 hours.[72,73] The hemodynamic characteristics include elevated systemic vascular resistance, tachycardia, and hyperdynamic cardiac function. The hypertensive episodes are commonly associated with cerebral vascular events in addition to localized bleeding, hematoma formation, and airway obstruction.[72] They also have been associated with cerebral ischemia related to inadequate collateral blood flow that occurs with carotid cross-clamping.[74] Because of the close association of hypertension and neurologic sequelae, hypertension must be managed aggressively but without inducing hypotension.[72,75]

Resection of Thoracic Aortic Coarctation

Paradoxic hypertension following thoracic aortic coarctation has been recognized since the 1940s.[10] Approximately 50% of the patients who undergo thoracic aortic coarctation develop hypertension.[76-78] A recent review of this hypertension outlined two types of responses.[78] The first occurs within 24 hours. It lasts for just a few hours, is benign, and responds readily to treatment. It has been attributed to a "high set" of the carotid baroreceptors caused by chronic central hypertension and a gradual decline of the afferent impulses traveling from the carotid baroreceptors to the central nervous system.

The second type of hypertensive response occurs 24 to 48 hours postoperatively. From 12 to 26% of the patients suffer delayed POH after thoracic aortic coarctation resection.[77] This type of hypertension is associated with severe acute abdominal pain caused by small bowel necrosis related to severe arteritis of mesenteric vessels originating below the coarctation. Following coarctation resection, the pressure proximal to the coarctation is greatly reduced. When the baroreceptors with a "high set" detect this reduced pressure, the inhibitory impulses to the vasomotor centers are reduced, causing a marked increase of sympathetic activity and circulating catecholamines. Both norepinephrine and angiotensin concentrations remain elevated for 72 to 96 hours postoperative.[77] The overall result is an intense vasoconstriction and vasospasm of the mesenteric vascular bed with diminished blood flow to the small bowel. Aggressive treatment with beta blockers and vasodilators is needed to prevent mesenteric ischemia associated with such hypertensive episodes, and blood pressure must be closely monitored until the patient is hemodynamically stable.[76] In 1988, Behl et al. suggested that perioperative hypertension persisted only in those surgical patients older than 6 years.[79] Common hemodynamic mechanisms in these patients include profound elevations of systemic vascular resistance secondary to the elevated levels of catecholamines caused by the "high set" of the baroreceptors in response to the chronic upper body hypertension with diminished renal blood flow.[76,77]

Neurovascular Surgery

Hypertension following neurovascular procedures has been associated with potentially lethal postoperative complications such as intercranial bleeding, intercranial hypertension, and permanent neurologic deficit.[80-85] Because of this association of perioperative morbidity with intercranial aneurysm hemorrhaging, POH must be controlled. Previously, hypotension was induced to reduce the incidence of intraoperative aneurysmal bleeding; however, such intraoperative hypotension has been clinically associated with vasospasm of the cerebral vessels.[82] The evolution of neurosurgical techniques that permit the transient clipping of vessels proximal to the aneurysm has reduced the rebound hypertension following discontinuation of the hypotensive agents.[86] Causes of hypertension following neurovascular procedures include increased sympathetic stimulation with anesthetic emergence associated with an elevated systemic vascular resistance, heart rate, and contractility of the myocardium. Rebound hypertension following discontinuation of hypotensive agents such as nitroprusside is associated with a marked elevation of the systemic vascular resistance that has been related to elevated plasma renin activity.[86]

Increased Intracranial Pressure

In 1901, Cushing described a reflex consisting of hypertension, bradycardia, and respiratory irregularities in association with head trauma and increased intracranial pressure.[8] There is a direct transmission of the intracranial pressure to the cerebral spinal fluid, which, when elevated above mean arterial pressures, compresses the cerebral arteries, perfusing the vasomotor center in the pons. This results in a reflex sympathetic response that causes intense peripheral vasoconstriction with resulting hypertension.[85] Through the baroreceptor-mediated response, this profound hypertension reflex results in an accompanying bradycardia.[84] This combination of physiologic events is commonly referred to as the Cushing reflex. In addition to space-occupying lesions, other causes of increased intracranial pressure include intracranial bleeding, cerebral edema, hypercapnia, and hypoxemia. Because of the potential for permanent neurologic damage, immediate treatment is indicated.[81] Management is directed at the underlying mechanism responsible for the intracranial hypertension and may warrant immediate surgical intervention. In addition, intracerebral pressure may be gradually lowered by reducing cerebral blood flow by inducing an osmotic diuresis with mannitol, managing hypercapnia via hyperventilation, and administering pharmacologic agents that reduce blood pressure without causing an associated vasodilation. Initially, mannitol may increase intracranial pressure as a result of its effect on volume expansion. Pretreatment with furosemide may prevent this effect. The hypertensive response to increased intracranial pressure may be a protective adaptation that maintains cerebral blood flow in this setting. Consequently, treatment of the patient's hypertension is of secondary importance when the cause of the patient's intracranial hypertension may be severely life-threatening. Treatment may be cautiously initiated after a definitive treatment plan has been established. Those agents include trimethaphan camsylate and urapidil. Urapidil is an antihypertensive agent that blocks postsynaptic alpha$_1$ receptors without increasing cerebral blood flow, thus making it an appropriate drug for treating hypertensive emergencies in neurosurgical patients.

Autonomic Hyperreflexia

Quadraplegic or paraplegic patients with spinal cord injuries above the inhibitory splanchnic outflow level (T4 to T7) have a potential for acute sympathetic hyperactivity in response to stimuli below the level of the transection.[87-89] This generalized sympathetic activity results from reflex stimulation of the sympathetic neurons in the anterolateral column of the spinal cord below the transection level without the inhibitory modulation that comes from the higher centers in the central nervous system. This disorder occurs in 65 to 85% of quadraplegic and high level paraplegic patients, often in response to bladder catheterization or orthopedic procedures such as debridement of pressure sores, osteotomies, or arthrectomies.[89] The responses may be prevented by general anesthesia or regional anesthesia in addition to the local anesthetic infiltration at the surgical site or dense regional block.

Hypertension in these patients is related to profound increases in systemic vascular resistance resulting from the sympathetically mediated vasoconstriction. Autonomic hyperreflexia is commonly associated with a reflex bradycardia mediated by the baroreceptor reflex. In addition, there may be a second reflex arc involving skeletal muscles that produces intense muscle spasm. Treatment of the hypertensive response in autonomic hyperreflexia is directed at reversing elevated systemic vascular resistance with sodium nitroprusside or ganglionic blocking agents such as trimethaphan.[87,89]

Resection of Endocrine-Secreting Tumors

Pheochromocytomas.
Pheochromocytomas are the most common of the catecholamine-secreting tumors. They originate from neural crest chromaffin tissue. In approximately 90% of the patients, pheochromocytomas arise from the adrenal medulla. Of these tumors, 85 to 90% are solitary, with a reported incidence of multiple tumors in 10 to 25% of patients; the contralateral adrenal is the most frequent site. Up to 10% of these tumors may have extrarenal sites or may be malignant.[90]

Hypertension associated with these tumors may be silent or paradoxic in nature in up to 40% of patients.[91] The episodic or silent nature of these tumors may lead to a significant number of patients with undiscovered tumors undergoing surgical procedures unrelated to their tumors. Postoperative hypertension may be the initial clinical presentation of these tumors.[92,93] If hypertension occurs after pheochromocytoma removal, it indicates that either there are tumors remaining that have not been completely removed or the patient has other catecholamine-secreting tumors.[93]

One of the hallmark clinical features of patients with these tumors is their relative volume contraction. This often manifests itself as hypotension following induction or at the time of anesthetic emergence. Initially, hypovolemia may present as hypertension because of the compensatory baroreceptor sympathetic response. In these circumstances, management is directed toward volume resuscitation.[45,46]

It is common for patients with these tumors to have a glucose intolerance requiring intravenous insulin administration preoperatively. After the tumors are removed, the need for insulin is no longer necessary, and its discontinuation must not be overlooked if a continuous infusion has been used. Although infrequent, hypoglycemia may initially manifest itself as POH before hemodynamic instability, which is due to the increased sympathetic outpouring. In patients who are anesthetized and beta blocked, however, there are few clinical signs of hypoglycemia.

Hypotension is common following pheochromocytoma resection because of the removal of the continuous source of catecholamines in the presence of the adrenergic blockade necessary in the cautious preoperative preparation of these patients. Such hypotension may necessitate the administration of fluids to expand the intravascular volume as well as vasopressor agents. Postoperatively, these patients may exhibit an exaggerated response to vasopressor agents. If the patients received inadequate alpha-blocking agents preoperatively, this exaggerated response will become readily apparent.

The stress of surgery or anesthesia commonly stimulates the release of catecholamines into the circulation.[93] Postoperative hypertension resulting from a pheochromocytoma is caused by an increase in circulating levels of both epinephrine and norepinephrine. Consequently, severe ventricular dysrhythmias in addition to pronounced hypertension may be found in these patients. The hemodynamic mechanism of hypertension in these patients is related to the pronounced elevation in systemic vascular resistance and hyperdynamic myocardial function including tachycardia and accentuated contractility. Management is best directed at prevention with preoperative prophylactic alpha-adrenergic blockade using prazosin hydrochloride (up to 1 mg orally, three times daily) or phenoxebenzamine hydrochloride (starting at 30 mg per day up to 200 mg orally per day) while expanding the patient's intravascular volume. If the patient continues to have an elevated heart rate, beta blockers may be added. Caution is indicated when using beta-blocker therapy in patients with catecholamine-secreting tumors. If alpha-blockade therapy is inadequate or discontinued, beta-receptor blockade may result in a profound hypertensive response, which is due to their peripheral blocking properties. Postoperative hypertension is best managed by lowering the systemic vascular resistance with vasodilators in conjunction with the use of alpha and beta blockers.[90] During the preparation phase, once the patient has been adequately alpha-blocked, beta-blockers may be added to avoid unopposed alpha-mediated vasoconstriction. Postoperative hypertension is thus managed with titrated intravenous infusions of nitroprusside or phentolamine mesylate, although labetalol hydrochloride offers a reasonable alternative. Other catecholamine-secreting tumors, such as the glomus jugulare and ciliary and aortic tumors, are also associated with pronounced hypertensive responses following surgical or anesthetic stress.

Carcinoid Tumors.
Carcinoid tumors most commonly originate from the gastrointestinal system, frequently, the appendix. Some carcinoid tumors secrete certain vasoactive amines, such as serotonin, histamine, and kinin substances. These substances are secreted into the circulation and are inactivated in the liver. When these tumors metastasize to the liver, the syndrome associated with these tumors may become clinically apparent.[94] These symptoms include flushing, enhanced gastrointestinal motility, bronchospasm, and the cardiac presentation of carcinoid. In addition, these substances may cause systemic vasoconstriction and paroxysmal hypertension.[95] In addition to the conventional vasodilators, such as nitroprusside or hydralazine hydrochloride, ketanserin has been advocated as a useful agent because of its serotonin s_2-receptor antagonist properties.[95] Steroids and antihistamines are also used in the treatment of the carcinoid syndrome.

Carotid Body Tumors.
These tumors are known to be nonchromaffin-reacting paraganglioma that arise from chemoreceptors. Normal carotid bodies contain neurosecretory cells capable of secreting physiologically active catecholamines. Though few carotid body or glomus jugulare tumors are reported to cause POH, some patients with these tumors have episodic blood pressure elevations.[74] The same surveillance should be applied for these patients as for patients with pheochromocytomas who are undergoing surgery.

Thyrotoxicosis or Thyroid Storm.
In patient's with undiscovered hyperthyroidism or in whom preoperative preparation of their thyroid condition is inadequate, the stress of surgery may contribute to the release of high levels of T_4 hormone from the thyroid gland into the circulation. There is a fine distinction clinically and on the basis of laboratory evaluation between thyrotoxicosis and thyroid storm. Thyroid storm is often associated with elevated lev-

els of the T_4 hormone in comparison to the more frequent elevations of T_3 seen in thyrotoxicosis.[96] Clinically, the patients with thyroid storm present in the perioperative setting with the signs of increased sympathetic tone and the peripheral effects of the thyroid hormone. These patients are most commonly febrile, hypertensive, tachycardic, agitated, and confused. Depending on the patient's cardiovascular status, the increased oxygen demands placed on the heart may precipitate high output failure or uncover underlying ischemic heart disease, resulting in the acute onset of congestive heart failure. Preoperatively, these patients may have demonstrated few clinical signs of hyperthyroidism or they may have the classic presentation of Grave's disease with toxic goiter (nodular or nonnodular) and the associated ophthalmopathology.[97,98] Hemodynamic instability or collapse will shortly ensue unless immediate and appropriate treatment is initiated. Such treatment includes the management of the patient's hyperthermia, the administration of beta-adrenergic blockers (propranolol or esmolol) and inhibitors of the synthesis and release of thyroid hormones (prophylthiouracil, methimazole, and sodium iodide). In severe circumstances, active removal of the thyroid hormone from the circulation is indicated. Such techniques include plasmaphoresis or peritoneal dialysis.[98,99]

Surgery of the Extremities

Arterial hypertension has been associated with the use of a pneumatic tourniquet during surgery on legs and arms. In a review of 699 patients who had a pneumatic tourniquet inflated for at least an hour, there was a 30% increase in arterial pressure in 67% of those patients who had general anesthesia.[100] The highest incidences of "tourniquet hypertension" were associated with lower extremity surgery, old age, long operations, and regional anesthesia. Tourniquet-associated hypertension resolved in most patients within 1 hour postoperatively. The hemodynamic mechanism for hypertension was thought to be related to an increase in pain during anesthetic emergence causing enhanced sympathetic activity and increased systemic vascular resistance. Because of the self-limiting nature of this problem, symptomatic relief of pain is generally sufficient.

Obstetric Surgery

Eclampsia and preeclampsia are degrees of a hypertensive disorder that occurs in approximately 10% of all late pregnancies and causes up to 20% of all maternal deaths.[101] These disorders are thought to be related to an immunologic reaction to the fetal tissue, resulting in placental vasculitis and subsequent ischemia. This ischemia increases angiotensin activity through a release of uterine renin. In addition, there is the release of placental tissue thromboplastin with subsequent glomerular deposition resulting in proteinuria. There is also thought to be an imbalance of prostacyclin and thromboxane production by the placenta, resulting in diminished uteral-placental blood flow and increased platelet aggregation.[102] Complications from this syndrome include convulsions, cerebral hemorrhaging, and death. Fortunately, the hypertensive response associated with this clinical entity usually abates postpartum. There may be, however, persistent postpartum hypertension related to increased sensitivity to either endogenous or exogenous oxytocin or use of vasopressor agents. With elevated levels of renin and angiotensin, a pronounced increase in systemic vascular resistance occurs. Postoperative treatment is directed at reducing systemic vascular resistance with vasodilators and maintaining adequate intervascular volume.[102] Central nervous system hyperactivity becomes manifest after the use of intravenous magnesium sulfate. Oxytocin should be used sparingly, if at all, in the postpartum period to avoid prolonging the hypertension.

Renal Surgery

Acute renal ischemia commonly results from the occlusion of renal arteries during major vascular surgery or following renal transplantation. The lack of blood flow and resulting ischemia of the juxtaglomerular apparatus increases renin secretion and subsequent conversion of angiotensin I to angiotensin II. The primary hemodynamic consequences of this humorally mediated hypertension is marked elevation in the systemic vascular resistance. If myocardial function is normal, there is little hemodynamic effect on myocardial function; however, if there is significant myocardial dysfunction and or coronary artery disease, the increase in systemic afterload may be life-threatening.

Between dialysis treatments, patients with chronic renal failure or those who are anephric are hypervolemic because of their inability to handle normal sodium and water excretion. These patients frequently have an exaggerated response to vasopressor therapy or volume replacement which is due to the chronically elevated renin levels and enhanced vascular responsiveness. These patients' hypertension can be managed with vasodilators or ACE inhibitors. Preoperative hemodialysis records may provide an indication of the patient's optimal volume status. Hemodialysis is effective in patients with volume-sensitive hypertension.

Hypertension following renal transplantation has been associated with stenosis of the renal artery anastomosis, rejection reactions, immunosuppressive therapy, and excessive renin release by the diseased kidneys.[103,104] Improvements in organ preservation methods and surgical techniques have reduced the incidence of hypertension following transplantation.[105] Immunosuppressive therapy with steroids increases the arteriolar-systemic vascular resistance to endogenous catecholamines along with excess renin released from the diseased kidneys. Cyclosporine also has been associated with an increase of sympathetic discharge, which may further exacerbate POH.[104-107] The mechanisms of hypertension following renal transplantation depend on the underlying causes; however, treatment with ACE inhibitors and vasodilators has been advocated.[108]

Urologic Surgery

Special considerations apply to paraplegic and quadriplegic patients undergoing urologic procedures.[109] One to 3 weeks following acute spinal cord injury, autonomic hyperreflexia may develop, as a result of disrupted integration between the spinal and sympathetic pathways. Uncontrolled sympathetic discharge, occurring in response to stimuli such as distention of the bladder, can cause severe hypertension. With higher spinal cord lesions, there is a more unmodulated vasculature that can uncontrollably constrict, and less innervated vasculature left to compensate. This syndrome is most common with cervical and high thoracic lesions, particularly with transverse lesions above T7. Hypertensive reactions can be prevented in the operating room by deep general or regional anesthesia, but there is the possibility of a reaction in the early postoperative period should bladder distention or manipulation occur as the anesthetic is eliminated. Manifestations of autonomic hyperreflexia include not only severe hypertension, but also bradycardia, ventricular arrhythmias, and cardiac arrest resulting from intact vagal reflexes in the face of hypertension. The syndrome of autonomic hyperreflexia generally subsides some weeks after the acute injury, but may occur at any time, even years later.[109]

Liver Transplantation

Systemic arterial hypertension following liver transplantation has been reported in up to 75% of patients.[110] Hypertension in these patients is thought to be related to the administration of immunosuppressive agents, similar to heart and kidney transplant patients. In addition to the increased sympathetic activity and enhanced vascular responsiveness to catecholamines caused by the immunosuppressive agents, cyclosporine is thought to interact with the intercellular metabolism of the calcium ion with the enhancement of vascular tone.[110] Diaz and colleagues have suggested that verapamil or angiotensin offers the most effective control of hypertension in patients receiving liver transplants.[110] Other antihypertensive agents used in this patient population include vasodilators such as hydralazine and nitroprusside.

Radical Neck Dissection

Postoperative hypertension following carotid artery manipulation and subsequent carotid sinus stimulation is a well-recognized complication of radical neck dissection. In 1987, McGuirt et al. reported a 9.6% incidence of POH, by their definition greater than 200/100 mm Hg.[111] Following surgery of the head and neck, hypertension may predispose patients to hemorrhage and hematoma formation within a confined vital area, which may result in airway compromise. Hypertension associated with head and neck surgery peaks at 2½ hours postoperatively. The underlying mechanisms of postoperative hypertension in these patients are most likely related to denervation of the carotid sinus.[112] Systemic hypertension is caused by a combination of increased circulating catecholamines, altered baroreceptor function, and imbalance of the renin-angiotensin hormonal system. In a prospective, randomized double-blind trial, nicardipine hydrochloride was shown to be an effective treatment for POH associated with head and neck surgery. Hypertension was controlled in 83% of patients treated with nicardipine and in 86% of placebo failures subsequently treated with nicardipine. Given the association of sympathetically mediated hypertension and imbalances of the renin-angiotensin-aldosterone system, other effective therapeutic agents include adrenergic blockers, direct vasodilators, and ACE inhibitors.

Medication-Related Postoperative Hypertension

Anesthetic Related

Ketamine is an arylcyclohexylamine used in anesthesia and is chemically related to phencyclidine ("angel dust"). Postoperative hypertension following ketamine administration is attributed to its sympathetic autonomic nervous system-stimulating effect as well as its ability to inhibit the uptake of catecholamines by postganglionic neurons. Such activity elevates systemic vascular resistance and increases the heart rate. In addition, some evidence suggests that ketamine depresses the gamma-amino butyric acid (GABA)-inhibitory neurotransmittors. Ketamine causes cerebral vessel vasodilatation, potentially resulting in intracranial hypertension in certain circumstances. In addition, it causes a dose-dependent increase in heart rate and blood pressure with little change in peripheral vascular resistance. Ketamine is a coronary vasodilator despite its effects on the peripheral circulation. In patients with long-standing congestive heart failure, ketamine may have myocardial depressant effects that are due to the patient's catecholamine-depleted condition.[113] Postoperatively, ketamine's central sympathomimetic effect may continue and be manifest as hypertension related to an increased heart rate, myocardial contractility, and unchanged peripheral vascular resistance.[114]

Vasodilating effects of inhalation agents may necessitate expansion of the intravascular volume, causing a relative hypervolemia following anesthetic emergence. As previously discussed, in the setting of enhanced sympathetic tone experienced during emergence, this relative hypervolemia may be the underlying factor leading to the patient's hypertension. In patients with elevated intracranial pressure, the potential for increased cerebral blood flow exists with all inhalation agents; however, this may be prevented to some extent by hyperventilation. In addition, as suggested by Miller et al., insufficient inhibition of stimuli by inhalation anesthetics may lead to the activation of central hormonal and peripherally activated renin-angiotensin systems.[115] Spinal or epidural anesthetic techniques have been shown to prevent the activation of the renin-angiotensin-aldosterone system.

Neuroleptics, such as droperidol or direct dopamine$_1$-receptor blockers, may block dopamine-mediated peripheral vasodilatation in the setting of sympathetic stimulation, vasopressor administration, or a catecholamine-secreting tumor. This may result in an unopposed vasoconstriction and subsequent paradoxic hypertensive response. Profound hypertension following neuroleptic anesthetic agent administration includes direct vasodilatory effects of dopamine$_1$-receptor blockades.

Medication Withdrawal

Clonidine hydrochloride is a common antihypertensive agent used to decrease the systemic vascular resistance and heart rate without interfering with the normal cardiovascular response to exercise. Acute withdrawal, manifest by hypertension, is quite common in patients who abruptly discontinue treatment regimens of more than 1.2 mg of clonidine per day.[116] This hypertensive response starts within 18 hours and may last up to 3 days unless appropriate therapy, such as transcutaneous clonidine, is reinstituted. On discontinuation of this drug, withdrawal syndrome occurs approximately 18 hours from the last dose. This is associated with pronounced hypertension, tachycardia, and tremulousness. In 1973, Hanson et al. described the acute postoperative clonidine syndrome and its clinical manifestations.[116] Management of the withdrawal syndrome includes the administration of quinidine after institution of emergent antihypertensive medication such as labetalol and/or peripheral vasodilators.[117]

Narcotic withdrawal may be a result of either a patient's declining chronic blood level or the administration of narcotic antagonist such as naloxone in patients using opioids chronically. Symptoms of narcotic withdrawal include diaphoresis, hypertension, restlessness, mydriasis, and central nervous system excitability. Use of opioid agonist-antagonists, such as pentazocine or nalbuphine, may also precipitate narcotic withdrawal.[118,119]

Similar to opioid withdrawal, alcohol or sedative withdrawal may occur as a result of either a decreased chronic level of use or the abrupt withdrawal from these substances as may occur in the perioperative setting. Postoperative symptoms of withdrawal from these agents include central nervous system excitation, diaphoresis, autonomic hyperactivity with associated hypertension, and tachycardia. Though presentation may be confounded by anesthetic emergence, the importance of a history of alcohol or sedative use is apparent. Treatment with beta blockers can reduce the profound sympathetic stimulation associated with the withdrawal syndrome.

Postoperative hypertension has also been associated with rebound following nitroprusside therapy. In 1979, Khamhatta et al. reported a series of 12 patients who received hypotensive anesthesia during the intraoperative surgical resection of cerebral aneurysms.[120] The researchers used nitroprusside to induce hypotension with a mean arterial pressure decrease of 49 mm Hg. Associated with this decrease was an elevation of renin activity four times that of the baseline level. Mean arterial pressure was elevated from a preoperative value of 85 mm Hg to a postoperative value of 112 mm Hg within 30 minutes after discontinuation of the sodium nitroprusside administration. Researchers postulated that the rebound hypertension was due to the longer half-life of renin following discontinuation of sodium nitroprusside.[120]

Abrupt discontinuation of beta blockers preoperatively has been associated with pronounced rebound tachycardia and hypertension.[121] Such rebound episodes may be associated with the development of myocardial ischemia, given the particular patient population commonly receiving these medications.

Drug Interactions

Monamine oxidase inhibitors are used as antidepressant agents because of their ability to block the oxidative deamination of catecholamine to vanillylmandelic acid. Inhibition of monoamine oxidase causes an accumulation of norepinephrine, dopamine, epinephrine, and 5-hydroxytryptamine (5-HT) in sympathetic tissues. Use of indirect-acting sympathomimetic agents, such as ephedrine, or the narcotic meperidine has been associated with exaggerated hypertensive responses secondary to the triggered release of the catecholamines that have accumulated in the nerve terminals.[122] Postoperative hypertension in patients who have been taking monamine oxidase inhibitors may indicate this drug interaction. Commonly, antihypertensive medications may be discontinued preoperatively. With long-term beta-blockade therapy, there is an upregulation of the beta-receptor concentration such that minimal sympathetic stimulation or elevation of circulating catecholamine may result in profound elevations of blood pressure and heart rate. Such withdrawal is managed by reinstituting the beta-blocker therapy.

MANAGEMENT OF PATIENTS WITH POSTOPERATIVE HYPERTENSION

When presented with a patient who has POH, the management goals must remain in the forefront during the clinical assessment, diagnosis, and treatment (Fig. 37–8). These goals include the reversal of any life-threatening condition, prevention of complications commonly associated with POH, expeditious treatment of POH with the avoidance of side effects, and eventual discharge from the critical care setting without the necessity for readmission.

The complications associated with POH (Table 37–5) most frequently involve either surgical bleeding or cardiac complications such as acute ventricular failure, myocardial ischemia or infarction, and acute aortic dissection. Less frequent, yet catastrophic in their nature, are neurologic complications including intracerebral hemorrhage, hypertensive encephalopathy, and cerebral vasospasm. In obstetric patients diagnosed with preeclampsia preoperatively, the inability to control blood pressure postoperatively may lead to eclampsia with seizure activity despite the patient having delivered. Patients with prolonged POH also may develop acute renal insufficiency. Most POH

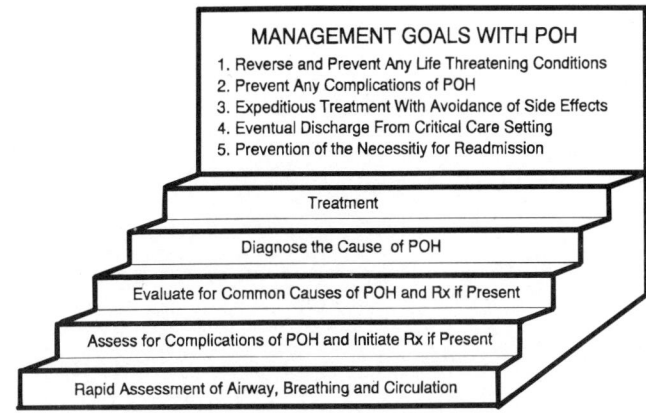

Fig. 37–8. Step-by-step approach to managing postoperative hypertension (POH).

Table 37-5. Complications of Postoperative Hypertension

1. Surgical bleeding
2. Cardiac complications
   Myocardial ischemia
   Left ventricular failure
   Aortic dissection
3. Neurologic complications
   Intracerebral hemorrhage
   Hypertensive encephalopathy
   Cerebral vasospasm
4. Acute renal insufficiency
5. Eclampsia

of a patient's respiratory insufficiency or hemodynamic instability. During the initial assessment, however, whenever such a life-threatening condition is uncovered, control of the patient's airway and ventilation is the highest priority. Urgent treatment cannot await a definitive diagnosis of the underlying cause of the patient's POH in these circumstances. Following the initial management of the patient's respiration, a rapid assessment of the patient's hemodynamic status is performed, including intravascular volume status, myocardial function, and afterload. Any abnormalities revealed as part of this initial evaluation are managed accordingly.

If the cardiorespiratory function is satisfactory, a search for potential complications of POH is undertaken. Any evidence of surgical bleeding or myocardial or neurologic compromise requires immediate treatment to safely lower the patient's blood pressure. If no complications are found that necessitate urgent treatment, the patient's evaluation proceeds with an evaluation of the common causes of POH. A history of hypertension is of great importance in view of the potential for rebound hypertension from many of the patient's antihypertensive drug therapies (e.g., clonidine, beta blockers). As Table 37-3 illustrates, many medical causes may predispose individuals to either POH or the rapid progression to complications of POH.

is related to underlying ventilatory abnormalities and pain.[4] However, despite the sophisticated diagnostic studies and clinical acumen available to diagnose the underlying causes of POH, in up to 17% of patients, no definitive diagnosis is established.[4]

Until proven otherwise, POH must be thought of as a sign of significant underlying aberration in a patient's cardiorespiratory status. As outlined in the management algorithm (Fig. 37-9), when a patient has POH, a rapid assessment of the patient's airway, air exchange, and circulatory status is imperative. In addition to the patient's vital signs, laboratory data including the patient's arterial blood gas and analysis, electrocardiogram, hematocrit, and chest radiograph may be of great assistance in defining the cause

Pain may be managed by intravenous opioids or by regional anesthetic techniques, such as thoracic or lumbar epidurals in patients who have thoracic or abdominal surgi-

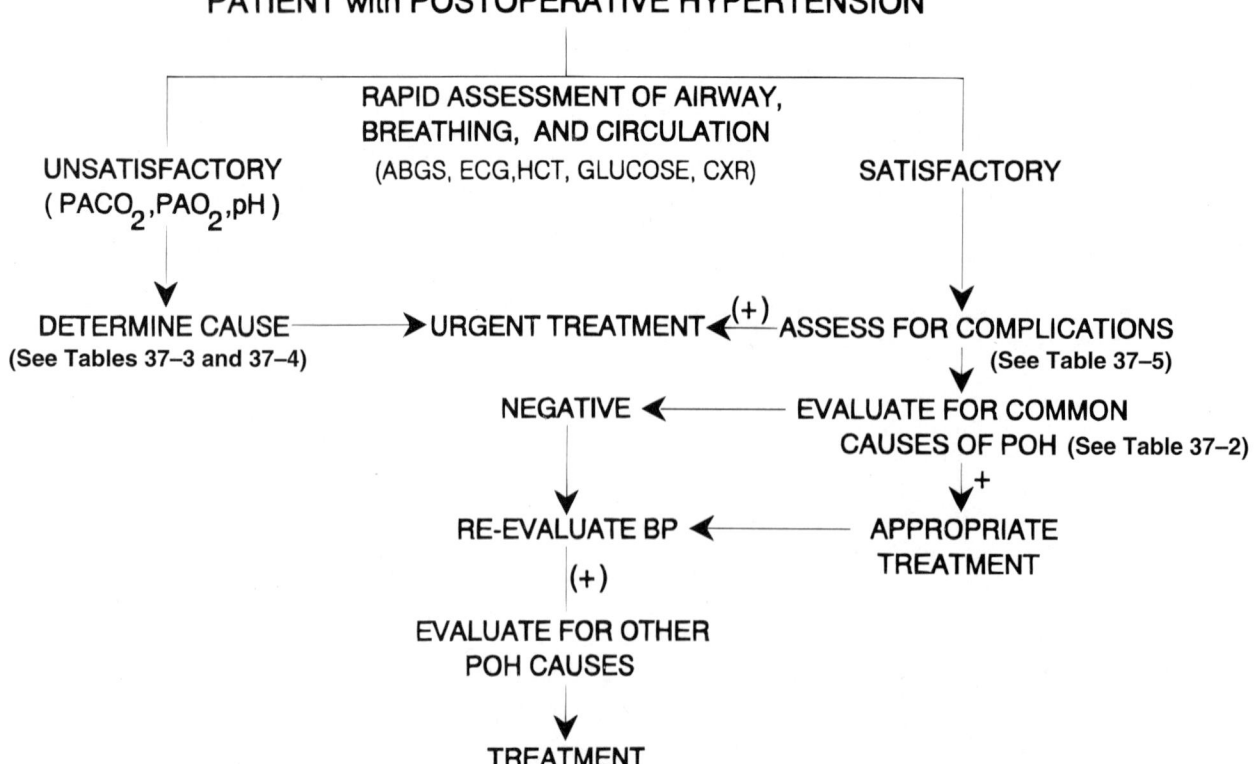

Fig. 37-9. Algorithm for management of postoperative hypertension (POH). ABGS, Arterial blood gases; BP, blood pressure; CXR, chest radiograph; ECG, electrocardiogram; HCT, hematocrit; HTN, hypertension; MAO, monoamine oxidase; $PACO_2$ and PAO_2, partial pressure of carbon dioxide and oxygen, respectively, in arterial blood.

Table 37-6. Specific Treatments for Postoperative Hypertension (See Table 37-8 for dosages.)

Surgical Causes	Treatment	Contraindicated
Cardiac surgery		
Myocardial revascularization	Nitroprusside, nitroglycerin, calcium antagonists, esmolol (if no CHF), nifedipine, nicardipine, labetalol, enalaprilat	Hydralazine, diazoxide, phentolamine; with IHSS or tight aortic stenosis, avoid agents that reduce preload or BP
Valve repair or replacement		
Heart transplantation		
Vascular surgery		
Aortic aneurysm resection	Nitroprusside, esmolol, labetalol	Hydralazine, diazoxide, phentolamine (potential for angina by increasing cardiac oxygen demands)
Aortic coarctation	Nitroprusside, esmolol, labetalol	
Carotid endarterectomy	Labetalol, NTG, esmolol, nitroprusside	
Neurosurgical procedures		
Neurovascular procedures	Nitroprusside or trimethaphan	Methyldopa, clonidine, esmolol, hydralazine, phentolamine, diazoxide
Increased intracranial pressure	Treat underlying cause; urapadil, trimethaphan	
Autonomic hyperreflexia	Nitroprusside or trimethaphan, epidural anesthesia	
Abdominal surgery		
Pheochromocytoma	Phentolamine or nitroprusside then esmolol	Beta blockers alone, methyldopa, droperidol
Carcinoid	Ketanserin	
Liver transplantation	ACE inhibitors, hydralazine, nitroprusside (CNS toxicity)	
Renal surgery and transplantation	Nitroprusside, enalaprilat, labetalol	
Obstetric surgery		
Eclampsia/preeclampsia (always check up-to-date recommendations)	Magnesium sulfate, methyldopa, nifedipine	Diuretics, trimethaphan, beta blockers, nitroprusside (fetal CNS toxicity potential), enalaprilat, nimodipine (relative)
Miscellaneous		
Thyroid storm	Iodine, PTU, beta blockers	
Radical neck dissection	Nitroprusside, enalaprilat, nicardipine, labetalol	

ACE, angiotensin-converting enzyme; BP, blood pressure; CHF, congestive heart failure; CNS, central nervous system; IHSS, idiopathic hypertrophic subaortic stenosis; PTU, propothiouracil; NTG, nitroglycerin.

---

cal incisions. Emergence delirium is a common clinical phenomenon associated with POH. In these patients, repeated reassurances by nurses, other medical team members or family members may avoid the need to administer sedatives or anxiolytics, which could depress respiration and worsen the patient's POH. In addition, hypertension associated with endotracheal intubation is quite common during emergence. If the patient's respiratory or neurologic status assessment is insufficient to warrant extubation, 100 mg of lidocaine may be administered either down the endotracheal tube or as a slow intravenous bolus. This will often permit the patient to better tolerate the endotracheal tube.

Hypoglycemia in the postoperative setting is a silent killer. In the patient who is beta blocked and anesthetized or emerging from anesthesia, there are few clinical signs of hypoglycemia. Unfortunately, establishing the diagnosis of hypoglycemia in this setting is particularly difficult and often associated only with a prolonged failure to awake. A high index of suspicion is warranted in all patients who are diabetic or are receiving hypoglycemic agents.

Despite satisfactory initial ventilatory assessment, one must keep in mind that the postoperative period is a highly dynamic situation and necessitates repeated assessment of the patient's cardiorespiratory status. Arterial blood gases may demonstrate hypercapnia, hypoxemia, or acidosis despite the initial presence of acceptable arterial blood gas values.

If no general causes of postoperative hypertension are identified, the patient's blood pressure is reevaluated. If it has decreased or normalized, no further treatment or in-depth evaluation is warranted. If the hypertension persists, however, the subsequent evaluation consists of a more detailed and comprehensive review of the patient's medical history and is supplemented with information from the patient's family. A thorough physical examination is undertaken, and appropriate laboratory studies are obtained. Treatment may be simultaneously initiated because of the association of postoperative complications with prolonged POH. Treatment should be directed at the underlying causes of POH (Table 37-6) as well as its fundamental mechanisms (Table 37-7).

The concept that blood pressure is the product of the cardiac output and systemic vascular resistance lends itself to a fundamental understanding of the nature of elevations

Table 37-7. Mechanisms of Postoperative Hypertension

Neural (reflex mediated)
  Increased intracranial pressure
  Autonomic hyperreflexia
  Baroreceptor reset/denervation
    Aortic coarctation
    Carotid endarterectomy
    Aortic aneurysm resection
Multifactorial
  Heart transplantation
  Liver transplantation
  Renal transplantation
Humoral
  Endocrine tumors or disorders
  Eclampsia
  Catecholamine-secreting tumors
  Hyperthyroidism
Mechanical
  Myocardial revascularization
  Cardiac valve repair or replacement

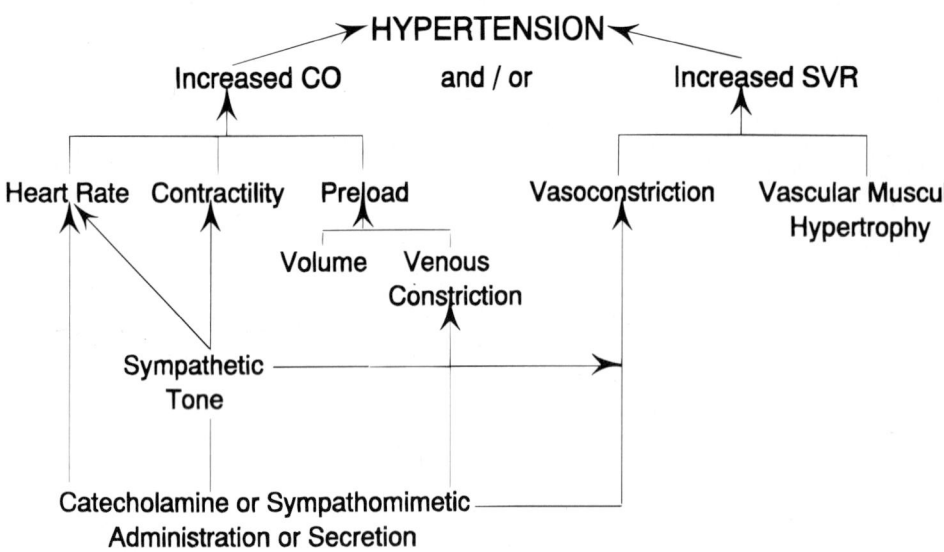

Fig. 37-10. Postoperative hypertension has multiple related and unrelated causes. The final common pathway of hypertension ultimately results, however, from either an increased cardiac output or an increased systemic vascular resistance. CO, Cardiac output; SVR, systemic vascular resistance.

in blood pressure postoperatively (Fig. 37-10). Hypertension results from either an increase in the cardiac output or the systemic vascular resistance or both. Increased heart rate and contractility are commonly associated with enhancement of sympathetic tone or increased circulating catecholamines or sympathomimetic drug administration. In addition, such increases in overall vascular tone increase the circulating blood volume, which further amplifies the potential for hypertension. The peripheral vasoconstrictive response to sympathetic tone may be transient or more prolonged, which may result in vascular muscular hypertrophy. Despite the many diverse causes and mechanisms of POH, the final common pathway ultimately results from an increase in either cardiac output or systemic vascular resistance.

Mechanisms of POH may be classified neural (reflex mediated), humorally mediated, or multifactorial (see Table 37-7). Neural mechanisms leading to POH include increased intracranial pressure and autonomic hyperreflexia as well as those associated with baroreceptor threshold resetting or denervation. Among the factors linked to hypertension following cardiac surgery are a diminished sensitivity of the aortic and carotid baroreceptors, which elicits a profound sympathetic response with increases in sympathetic tone as well as circulating catecholamines. The most common feature of neural-mediated mechanisms of POH is a marked increase in overall sympathetic tone. Consequently, stellate ganglia blockade may be used successfully to manage patients with this type of POH.[63]

Other mechanisms of POH include those associated with release of various humoral substances by endocrine or endocrine-related tissues. This category includes those patients with diagnosed or latent pheochromocytomas and those with other catecholamine-secreting tumors or endocrine disorders. Optimal management of these patients is directed at the specific endocrine-related disorder. The third category is multifactorial, reflecting the diverse nature of some circumstance of POH such as those found following heart or liver transplantation procedures. The hypertension related to orthotopic heart transplant has a number of associated causes. Included among these are the immunosuppressive agents (corticosteroids and cyclosporine), the presence of a denervated heart, the tendency for relative hypervolemia, and baroreceptor denervation as well as the reports of elevated renin levels postoperatively in the patients. These patients are managed with nitroprusside to reduce systemic vascular resistance brought about by an elevation in circulating catecholamines as well as beta-blocker therapy to control the hyperdynamic cardiac state.

The critical care team has a diverse collection of pharmacologic agents from which to choose in managing POH (Table 37-8). The urgency for lowering blood pressure is directed by the degree of elevation of the patient's blood pressure compared to preoperative levels as well as the presence of severe life-threatening complications related to POH. Consequently, when the patient's blood pressure must be lowered rapidly, fast-acting intravenous agents that address the underlying mechanism of hypertension are the drugs of choice. Once again it must be emphasized that in the setting of chronic hypertension, aggressive lowering of the blood pressure may cause profound cerebral ischemia and/or infarction in addition to diminished perfusion of the renal, gastrointestinal, hepatic, and myocardial perfusion beds. Aggressive lowering to "normal" blood pressure values may cause irreversible end organ damage.

If urgent treatment is not indicated, the administration of sublingual, buccal, or oral medications may be considered or even clinically warranted. Such circumstance would include the presence of POH related to myocardial ischemia following myocardial revascularization with an internal thoracic artery that would warrant sublingual administration of the calcium channel blocker nifedipine, or the presence of rebound hypertension related to discontinuation of a patient's clonidine that warrants resumption of the drug.

The antihypertensive medications used to treat POH may be broken down into a number of pharmacologic

Table 37–8. Antihypertensive Medications Used in the Management of Postoperative Hypertension

Mechanism of Action	Drug	Dosage	Onset	Duration of Action	Indications	Contraindications	Side Effects	Comments
Vascular smooth muscle relaxation	Sodium nitroprusside	IV: 0.5–10 µg/kg/min	Immediate	Minutes	Postoperative hypertension Hypertensive crisis	Pregnancy	Hypotension, nausea, and cyanide toxicity (increased renal and hepatic insufficiency)	Invasive pressure monitoring recommended
	Hydralazine	IV: 5–10 mg bolus	15–30 min	2–4 hr	Postoperative hypertension	Severe coronary disease, lupus, aortic stenosis IHSS, hemoglobinpathies	Fluid retention, lupus like rash, headache	Tolerance may develop
	Nitroglycerin	IV: 5–100 µg/min	1–2 min	3–5 min	Myocardial ischemia or infarction postoperative hypertension		Bradycardia, tachycardia, methemoglobinemia, flushing, vomiting, headache	
	Diazoxide	IV: 50–100 mg q5–10min, up to 600 mg IV: 30 mg/min	1–5 min	6–12 hr	Postoperative hypertension	Diabetes, hyperuricemia, CHF	Hypotension, tachycardia, fluid retention, myocardial ischemia, aortic dissection, hyperglycemia, nausea, vomiting, heart failure	May require beta blocker
	Nitric Oxide	Inhaled 15–30 ppm	Immediate	Seconds	Experimental			
Autonomic ganglia blockers	Trimethaphan	IV: 1–5 mg/min	2–5 min	4–12 hr	Postoperative hypertension	Coronary artery disease, prostatism, cerebrovascular insufficiency, diabetes mellitus, glaucoma	Ileus, urinary retention, hypotension, blurred vision, dry mouth, angina	Invasive pressure monitoring recommended
Alpha blockers	Phentolamine	IV: 5–20 mg q10min	Immediate	2–10 min	Pheochromocytoma	Coronary artery disease	Tachycardia, vomiting, angina, hypotension, miosis, dry mouth	
Combined alpha and beta blocker	Labetalol	IV: 10–80 mg q10min IV: 2 mg/min	5–10 min	2–12 hr	Mild to moderate postoperative hypertension	Heart block, asthma, bradycardia, heart failure, hypertension secondary to decreased cardiac output	Hypotension, heart failure, heart block, dizziness, nausea, phlebitis, bronchospasm, cardiac arrest if given with verapamil	Increases digoxin level, prolongs neuromuscular blockade of succinylcholine
Beta blocker	Esmolol	IV: titrated load of 500 µg/kg over 1–2 min and infusion of 50–300 µg/kg/min	<5 min	10–20 min	Coronary artery disease without left ventricle dysfunction, aortic dissection without heart failure, postoperative hypertension related to increased sympathetic tone, hyperthyroidism	Asthma, heart block, sinus bradycardia, heart failure, cardiogenic shock, pregnancy	Heart failure, bronchospasm, heart block, hypotension, phlebitis, dizziness, urinary retention	Elevates digoxin level, prolongs duration neuromuscular blockade with succinylcholine, risk of fatal cardiac arrest if used in conjunction with verapamil
Calcium antagonists	Nifedipine	SL: 10–20 mg q15min	5–10 min	30–60 min	Myocardial ischemia or infarction	Heart block, intravenous beta blockers without pacer backup	Headache, tachycardia, flushing, dizziness, hypotension, phlebitis	
	Nicardipine	IV: 5–15 mg/hr	1–5 min	3–6 hr	Myocardial ischemia or infarction	Severe aortic stenosis, hypersensitivity	Hypotension, tachycardia, nausea, minimal myocardial depression	
	Nimodipine	PO: 60 mg q4hr	1–2 hr	4–6 hr	Subarachnoid hemorrhage	Pregnancy, hepatic impairment	Edema, hypotension, headache, ileus, nausea, abnormal liver function	Administer through NG tube
Centrally acting	Clonidine	IV: 0.1–0.2 mg	30 min–1 hr	6–8 hr	Rebound hypertension following discontinuation of clonidine	Heart block, bradycardia, sick sinus syndrome	Drowsiness, sedation, dry mouth	Reduce dose in elderly, preexisting cerebrovascular or cardiovascular disease: rebound phenomena; treat overdose tolazoline
	Methyldopa	IV:250–500 mg q6hr	2–3 hr	2–12 hr	Postoperative hypertension	Pheochromocytoma, hepatic disease, MAO inhibitors	Drowsiness, hypotension, fever, positive Coombs' test, chronic hepatitis, lupus-like syndrome	
Converting enzyme inhibitors	Enalaprilat	IV: titrated 0.625–1.25 mg q6–8h	10–15 min	6–24 hr	Hypertension related to renal artery stenosis	Pregnancy, renal failure, bilateral renal artery stenosis	Cough and angioedema, fever, urticaria hypotension, pancytopenia	

CHF, congestive heart failure; IHSS, idiopathic hypertrophic subaortic stenosis; MAO, monoamine oxidase; NG, nasogastric.

groupings depending on their mechanism of action (see Table 37-8). These categories include the following:

- Vascular smooth muscle relaxers (e.g., sodium nitroprusside)
- Autonomic ganglia blockers (e.g, trimethaphan)
- Alpha blockers (e.g., phentolamine)
- Combined alpha and beta blockers (e.g., labetalol)
- Selective beta blockers (e.g., esmolol)
- Calcium antagonists (e.g., nicardipine)
- Central-acting antihypertensive medications (methyldopa or clonidine)
- Converting enzyme inhibitors (enalaprilat)

The agent recommended for treatment of specific causes of POH are listed in Table 37-6.

Vascular Smooth Muscle Relaxers

Sodium Nitroprusside

Nitroprusside is a direct-acting vasodilator that acts on the arterioles and venules by decreasing the overall tone of the vascular smooth muscle. This agent reduces the afterload primarily as well as the preload to a lesser extent. Nitroprusside is a light-sensitive medication and is immediate in onset with a duration of action of 3 to 5 minutes. It is initiated in a dose of 0.25 to 1 μ/kg per minute and may be titrated upward to 10 μ/kg/min. Nitroprusside is broken down into cyanide. Consequently, the infusion dose should not exceed 10 μ/kg per minute for extended periods or a total dose of 3 mg/kg per 24 hours. The nitroso-molecule of nitroprusside is rapidly metabolized when ferrous iron reacts with its sulfide group in red cells and tissues. The cyanogen molecule (half-life of 7 days) produced by this reaction is converted by the liver enzyme rhodanase to ferrocyanate, which is excreted by the kidneys. Cyanide inhibits mitochondrial cytochrome oxidase oxygen transport. The accumulated cyanogen molecule may result in metabolic acidosis, an increase mixed venous partial pressure of oxygen (P_{O_2}) or a reduced arteriovenous oxygen ($A V_{O_2}$) difference. The treatment of nitroprusside toxicity includes the initial administration of thiosulfate (150 mg/kg) to provide sulfate donors for conversion of cyanide to thiocyanate.[123] This is followed by amyl nitrate (inhaled) or sodium nitrate (5 mg/kg intravenously), which provide nitrate ions that convert the hemoglobin to methemoglobin, which binds the cyanide molecule. Hydroxycobalamin subsequently converts cyanide to cyanocobalamin. In addition, there have been previous reports of patients with acute myocardial infarction developing worsening of ST-segment elevation during sodium nitroprusside infusion.[124] Reversal of ST-segment changes were seen with nitroglycerin. The potential of a coronary steal phenomenon has been reported to result from sodium nitroprusside vasodilatation in nonischemic zones with reduction of perfusion pressure in the ischemic zone.[124] The noncardiac effects of sodium nitroprusside include increased renal blood flow that is due to increased cardiac output with measurable increases in urine flow, cation excretions, and an increased filtration fraction. Reduced pulmonary artery pressure and pulmonary vascular resistance may reduce regional blood flow to the lung, worsening of the ventilation-perfusion (VQ) ratio, and may cause arterial hypoxemia that is due to dead space ventilation.

Hydralazine

Hydralazine is a direct-acting vasodilator with an onset of action of 15 to 30 minutes (following a 5- to 10-mg bolus) and a duration of action of 2 to 4 hours. Hydralazine is specifically indicated in patients with POH. It is relatively contraindicated in patients with severe coronary disease, because of its potential for reflex tachycardia and potential for precipitating angina. In addition, hydralazine has been reported to cause a lupus-like rash and consequently is contraindicated in patients with systemic lupus. Other side effects related to hydralazine include fluid retention and headache. Patients also may develop tolerance.

Diazoxide

Diazoxide is chemically similar to the thiazides and is a direct-acting vasodilator with rapid onset (1 to 5 minutes) after an intravenous administration (either as a bolus of 50 to 100 mg every 5 to 10 minutes or at a constant infusion of 30 mg per minute). Its duration of action varies from 6 to 12 hours. Because of its relatively rapid action, diazoxide is indicated in the management of POH. Its side effects are numerous, however. Included among these are its association with hyperglycemia, reflex tachycardia that may precipitate angina, and an increase in the sheer force of ventricular ejection that may extend an aortic dissection. Consequently, diazoxide is contraindicated in patients with diabetes, severe coronary disease, hyperuricemia, aortic dissection, or severe congestive heart failure. Diazoxide use may necessitate the addition of a beta blocker to control the resulting reflex tachycardia.

Nitroglycerin

Nitroglycerin is a vasodilator that acts via relaxation of smooth muscles in the venules and arterioles by release of a nitrite ion. It is a functional antagonist of norepinephrine and acetylcholine. Reduction of venous return is a major cause of decreased blood pressure with nitroglycerin. Aside from hypotension, few serious side effects are associated with nitroglycerin. Included among these, however, are headache associated with meningeal vessel dilatation, and a propensity for producing methemoglobinemia. Nitroglycerin has been shown to oxidize hemoglobin to methemoglobin. Nitroglycerin has been reported to have a vasodilatory effect on the internal thoracic artery and on saphenous vein grafts.[125]

Autonomic Ganglia Blockers

Trimethaphan

Trimethaphan (Arfonad) is a ganglionic blocker administered in a continuous infusion of 0.1 to 1 mg per minute. Because of its rapid onset of action (2 to 5 minutes), trimethaphan is indicated in the management of postoperative hyperthermia. It is reported that this medication does not produce a reflex tachycardia; however, it has been associated with urinary retention, hypotension, dry mouth, blurred vision, and gastrointestinal ileus.[126] Consequently, this medication is contraindicated in patients with prostatism, cerebrovascular insufficiency, and glaucoma. Because of its rapid onset of action, arterial pressure monitoring is indicated in these patients. Histamine release is quite common with this medication and consequently should be avoided in patients with pheochromocytomas or those taking monamine oxidase inhibitors.

Alpha Blockers

Phentolamine

Phentolamine is a direct $alpha_1$- and $alpha_2$-blocking agent with immediate onset of action and a duration of 2 to 10 minutes. It is administered in an intravenous dose of 5 to 20 mg per 10-minute period and it is specifically indicated in patients with pheochromocytomas. Because it blocks the $alpha_1$ receptors peripherally and the $alpha_2$ receptors centrally, cardic stimulatory effects are noted. These effects result from both a reflex tachycardia that is due to the peripheral dilatation as well as the enhanced norepinephrine release from neural tissues. It also should be kept in mind that, in patients with pheochromocytomas in whom both alpha and beta blockers are going to be used, alpha blockade must be established before beta blockade. Otherwise, unopposed beta blockade may result in a profound hypertensive response that is due to the unopposed peripheral alpha stimulation. Side effects of phentolamine include profound tachycardia with the potential for precipitating angina in patients with severe coronary disease. Other side effects include miosis and a dry mouth.

Urapadil

Urapadil produces vasodilatation by blockade of the postsynaptic $alpha_1$ receptors. In addition, it may cause modest degrees of $beta_1$ blockade with intrinsic sympathomimetic activity. Because of its lack of $alpha_2$ effects centrally, it does not enhance the neural release of norepinephrine. This agent has been used primarily in many European countries in the management of perioperative hypertension. Treatment with this drug has not been reported to be associated with increased intracranial pressure, and consequently it has great potential for managing POH in the neurosurgical patient most frequently encountered during emergence. The initial dose is reported to be 0.6 mg/kg.[127,128]

Combined Alpha and Beta Blockers

Labetalol

Labetalol (Normodyne) is an $alpha_1$- and nonselective beta-adrenergic antagonist that is relatively safe in patients with chronic obstructive pulmonary disease (COPD). It has an effective beta/alpha potency ratio of 7:1. Consequently, it has an immediate peripheral effect in lowering the systemic vascular resistance without the significant reflex tachycardia seen with the alpha-blocking agents and smooth muscle vasodilators. Because of the enhanced sympathetic tone as well as increased levels of circulating catecholamines in the postoperative period, labetalol is ideal for management of hypertension in this setting. Labetalol is administered in a dose of 5 mg and may be doubled to a maximum dose of 80 mg per 10-minute period. It may also be administered as an infusion of 0.5 to 2 mg per minute. After an intravenous injection of labetalol, its full effect appears within 5 to 10 minutes.[129] Because of its beta-blocking properties, labetalol is relatively contraindicated in patients with congestive heart failure, and it should be avoided in patients prone to bronchospastic disease.[130] In addition, in patients with pheochromocytomas, paradoxic response has occurred because of its relatively greater beta-blocking potential. Labetalol may also block the tachycardia associated with hypoglycemia and therefore should be avoided in patients receiving intravenous insulin or who have received oral hypoglycemic agents preoperatively.[131] Side effects of labetalol include bradycardia, heart block, anaphylaxis, hypotension, and dizziness. It has also been associated with tremors in patients receiving tricyclic antidepressants.

Beta Blockers

Because of the potential for underlying left ventricular failure in patients with POH, the longer acting beta-blocking agents are relatively contraindicated, which is due to their prolonged duration of action and potential for adversely impacting ventricular function.

Esmolol

Esmolol (Brevibloc) is a short-acting cardioselective beta blocker. It has an onset of action in 3 to 5 minutes with a duration of action of 10 to 20 minutes. It has a beta-elimination half-life of 9 minutes, and it is metabolized by red blood cell esterase. It has a dose-related hypotension in 20 to 50% of patients.[132,133] The initial loading dose of esmolol is 500 μ/kg per minute followed by continuous infusion of 50 mg/kg per minute for 4 minutes. This dose is then doubled, following a repeat bolus over subsequent similar periods up to an infusion rate of 300 μ/kg per minute. Despite its relative $beta_1$ selectivity, esmolol is relatively contraindicated in patients with asthma, diabetes, heart block, sinus bradycardia, heart failure, and pregnancy. It may potentiate bronchospasm and has been shown to cross the placental barrier. Esmolol has been demonstrated to elevate digoxin levels and also prolongs the neuromuscular blockade in patients who have been administered succinylcholine. Used in conjunction with verapamil, it has been associated with fatal cardiac arrest. At this time is not approved by the Food and Drug Administration (FDA) for the treatment of perioperative hypertension; however, numerous studies have reported its efficacy in such treatment of intraoperative tachycardia and/or hypertension.[134-136] Reeves et al. demonstrated its safe and efficacious use in patients following open heart surgery.[137] Esmolol has no reported antihypertensive effects in the absence of tachycardia or high catecholamine activity. It has mild antihypertensive activity in patients during surgery, with its response depending directly on the patient's degree of surgical stress. Newsome et al. demonstrated that it has a beta$_1$ attenuation of the hemodynamic responses in coronary artery bypass surgery.[138] The use of esmolol to treat hypertensive crisis is generally not recommended. Like all beta-blocking agents, it reduces systolic blood pressure by decreasing cardiac output. In severe hypertensive episodes where the blood pressure may result from a high systemic vascular resistance, a decrease in cardiac output may significantly compromise perfusion of vital organs. This danger is somewhat offset because of the very short half-life of esmolol, and should myocardial dysfunction result, the medication infusion may be discontinued. Gray et al., in treating postcardiac surgery hypertension, found that esmolol was particularly well suited for the control of moderate POH when hypertension was associated with a hyperdynamic state.[139] This would include those patients who are having a reflex tachycardia that is due to baroreceptor receptor denervation or a resetting of the baroreceptor response.

Gibson et al. reported on the safety of esmolol administration in patients emerging from general anesthesia following neurovascular or intracranial surgery.[140] It was found that esmolol reversed an increase in systolic blood pressure within 1 to 3 minutes of infusion initiation; however, adverse effects occurred in 6 to 21 patients. Two patients experienced mild-to-moderate hypertension, and one patient developed a nodal rhythm and required modification of the dosage. Because of its 9-minute elimination half-life, esmolol can be down-titrated rapidly. This titratability allows more precise degree of beta blockade in comparison to the longer acting nonselective beta blockers.

Calcium Antagonist

Nifedipine

Nifedipine is a calcium-channel blocker that acts as a potent vasodilator and afterload reducer. Potentially, it may cause reflex tachycardia and is useful in patients with concurrent ischemia. When used as a single sublingual doses of 10 to 20 mg, it has been reported to be effective in the management of POH.[141-143] Mullen et al. reported on the use of nifedipine following elective cardiac surgery. Despite mild depression of myocardial performance, it was an effective and safe agent in managing POH.[143] Relative contraindications to nifedipine include hypersensitivity to nifedipine as well as severe congestive heart failure, tight aortic stenosis, and renal insufficiency.[144] Nifedipine should be used only in extreme circumstances in pregnant patients because it has reported teratogenic effects in laboratory animals and does enter maternal breast milk. Side effects include hypotension, tachycardia, syncope, platelet dysfunction, hepatotoxicity, and headache. In patients receiving digoxin, nifedipine increases serum digoxin levels.

Nicardipine

Nicardipine (Cardene) is a short-acting calcium antagonist that is indicated in the treatment of POH. The initial rate of infusion is 5 mg per hour of a 0.1-mg/ml solution increased by 2.5 mg per hour up to a maximum dose of 15 mg per hour. It has an onset of action of 1 to 5 minutes and a duration of action of 3 to 6 hours.[112] Because of its coronary vasodilatory effect, nicardipine is specifically indicated in a setting of postoperative myocardial ischemia or infarction. it has the potential side effects of hypertension, tachycardia, nausea, and minimal myocardial depression. It is contraindicated in patients with tight aortic stenosis and with hypersensitivity reactions.[145,146] In previous studies by David et al., nicardipine was found to be as effective as sodium nitroprusside following coronary bypass surgery. it was noted that it did achieve a therapeutic response sooner than nitroprusside and required less frequent dosage adjustment during the maintenance therapy with fewer episodes of severe hypotension in comparison to nitroprusside.[147] Benammar et al. reported on the use of nicardipine in the management of POH.[148] Of the patients who received nicardipine, 94% had a therapeutic response compared to 12% of the placebo group. The mean onset in those treated with nicardipine was 11.5 minutes with a mean infusion rate of 12.8 mg per hour. A few patients required discontinuation of the drug because of adverse side effects which included hypotension, polyuria, tachycardia, and ST-segment depression. The most frequent adverse effect was hypotension (4.5%) and tachycardia (2.7%).

Nimodipine

Nimodipine is a calcium antagonist that has been used in patients with subarachnoid hemorrhages for prevention of cerebrovasospasm and subsequent neurologic deficits. It is administered orally or via the nasogastric tube in a dose of 60 mg every 4 hours (21 consecutive days) with an onset of action in 1 to 2 hours and a duration of action of 4 to 6 hours. It is contraindicated in pregnancy and nursing mothers. Because of a low incidence of hepatic dysfunction, it is contraindicated in hepatic impairment. Potential side effects of nimodipine include hypotension, edema, headache, ileus, and abnormal liver function tests.

Centrally Acting Antihypertensive Agents

Clonidine

Clonidine is a centrally acting alpha$_2$-receptor agonist that reduces the release of norepinephrine from nerve endings both centrally and peripherally. In addition it modulates tonic and reflex blood pressure control, resulting in a diminished sympathetic outflow as well as an increase of vagally induced reflex bradycardia.[149,150] This results in both a diminished heart rate as well as blood pressure. This drug is particularly indicated in circumstances of clonidine rebound where it has been discontinued preoperatively. It is administered in a dose of 0.1 to 0.2 mg intravenously and may be also administered orally via a nasogastric tube (0.1 mg to 0.3 mg twice daily) or by patch (3.5 cm^2 or 0.1 mg per day) administration. The intravenous form has an onset of action in 30 minutes to 1 hour with a duration of action of 6 to 8 hours. Clonidine is contraindicated in patients with bradycardia, sick sinus syndrome, or heart block and has been associated with drowsiness, sedation, and dry mouth. Of particular note is the need to reduce the dose in elderly patients and in patients with preexisting cerebral or cardiovascular disease, which is due to the bradycardiac response and potential for drowsiness and sedation.

Methyldopa

Methyldopa is a centrally acting antihypertensive medication that is useful in the treatment of POH when administered in a dose of 250 to 500 mg every 6 hours. In this dose, it has an onset of action to 2 to 3 hours with a duration of action of 2 to 12 hours. It is contraindicated in patients with pheochromocytoma, active hepatic disease, liver disorders associated with prior dysfunction, and those receiving monamine oxidase inhibitors. It has side effects of drowsiness, hypotension, positive Coombs' test, chronic hepatitis and a lupus-like syndrome that abates when it is discontinued.

Angiotensin-Converting Enzyme Inhibitors

These agents act by preventing the conversion of angiotensin I to angiotensin II, which is a potent vasoconstrictor (see Fig. 37-3).

Enalaprilat

Enalaprilat is a newer generation ACE inhibitor, which, unlike captopril, has less likelihood of producing leukopenia. It is administered as a titrated dose of 0.625 to 1.25 mg every 6 hours, having an onset of action in 10 to 15 minutes and a duration of action of 6 to 24 hours. It is indicated in the management of hypertension when oral therapy is impractical and in particular when the hypertension is related to unilateral renal artery stenosis. It is contraindicated in pregnancy, with a history of angioedema related to ACE inhibitors, and in renal failure due to bilateral renal artery stenosis. It is associated with side effects of cough and angioedema as well as hypotension. Surgery has been associated with elevated plasma renin levels. In particular, cardiac surgery has been reported to activate the renin-angiotensin system with separate reports of both elevated renin[151] as well as angiotensin II levels after bypass.[152] There have been conflicting reports, however, that demonstrated no significant elevations of renin following open heart surgery.[153] Nonetheless, enalaprilat has been reported by Mirenda et al. to provide a more favorable profile than nitroprusside despite no demonstrable evidence of elevated plasma renin activity, suggesting that the mechanism for blood pressure control involves something more than the renin-angiotensin system.[153]

In summary, the purpose of this discussion regarding POH has been to review the underlying physiologic adaptations that control and regulate blood pressure. In addition, the causes of POH and their underlying pathophysiologic mechanisms have been examined. One key theme throughout this discussion has been the understanding that POH may potentially serve as a sign representing a significant underlying aberration of the patient's cardiorespiratory homeostasis. Given the potential life-threatening nature, it is imperative that the overall management of POH include a thorough assessment of respiration and circulatory hemodynamics as well as the evaluation of potential complications of POH. When the presence of life-threatening conditions or complications are excluded, a more thorough evaluation of the patient to ascertain the cause of POH can be undertaken. Given the dynamic nature of the postoperative period, it is incumbent on the members of the medical team to reevaluate the patient's vital functions. Despite the number and diversity of the pharmacologic agents available for the management of POH, the most appropriate and efficacious treatment regimen is directed by the clinical degree of urgency as well as the underlying mechanism of the patient's hypertension.

REFERENCES

1. Heuser, D., Heinz, G., and Fretschner, R.: Acute blood pressure increase during the perioperative period. Am. J. Cardiol., 63:26C, 1989.
2. Fremes, S. E. et al.: Effects of postoperative hypertension and its treatment. J. Thorac. Cardiovasc. Surg., 86:47, 1983.
3. Estafanous, F. G. et al.: Arterial hypertension in immediate postoperative period after valve replacement. Br. Heart J., 40:718, 1978.
4. Gal, T. J., and Cooperman, L. H.: Hypertension in the immediate postoperative period. Br. J. Anesth., 47:70, 1975.
5. Estafanous, F. G.: Hypertension in the surgical patient: management of the blood pressure and anesthesia. Cleve. Clin. J. Med., 56:385, 1989.
6. Seltzer, J. L. et al.: Hypertension in the perioperative period. NY State J. Med., 80:29, 1980.
7. Seltzer, J. L.: Etiology and prevention of perioperative hypertension. Surg. Rounds, 10:50, 1987.
8. Cushing, H.: Concerning a definite regulatory mechanism of the vasomotor center which controls blood pressure during cerebral compression. Bull. Johns Hopkins Hosp., 12:290, 1901.
9. Crafoord, C., and Nylin, G.: Congenital coarctation of the aorta and its surgical treatment. J. Thorac. Cardiovasc. Surg., 14:347, 1945.
10. Sealy, W. C.: Indications for surgical treatment of coarctation of the aorta. Surg. Gynecol. Obstet., 97:301, 1953.
11. Estafanous, F. G., Tarazi, R. C., Vilojen, J. F., and Tawil, M. Y.: Systemic hypertension following myocardial revascularization. Am. Heart J., 85:732, 1973.
12. Seltzer, J. L., Gerson, J. I., and Grogono, A. W.: Hypertension in the perioperative period. NY State J. Med., 80:29, 1980.
13. Cosgrove, D. M. et al.: Automated control of post-operative hypertension: a prospective randomized multicenter study. Ann. Thorac. Surg., 47:678, 1989.
14. Pomer, S., Elert, O., and Sutter, P.: Effects of the automated management of hypertension after open heart surgery. J. Clin. Pharmacol. Ther. Tox., 22:207, 1984.
15. Gijsman, H., Westeenskow, D. R., and Christopher, M. A.: Evaluation in dogs of a sodium nitroprusside closed-loop delivery device for hypotensive anesthesia. Anesth. Analg., 70:S126, 1990.
16. Bednarski, D. et al.: Use of computerized closed-loop sodium nitroprusside titration system for antihypertensive treatment after open heart surgery. Crit. Care Med., 18:1061, 1990.
17. Guyton, A. C.: Nervous regulation of the circulation and rapid control of arterial pressure and dominant role of the kidneys in long term regulation of the arterial pressure and

in hypertension: the integrated system for pressure control. *In* Textbook of Medical Physiology. Edited by A. C. Guyton. Philadelphia, W. B. Saunders, 1991.
18. Malliani, A.: Cardiovascular sympathetic afferent fibers. Rev. Physiol. Biochem. Pharmacol., *94*:10, 1982.
19. Kreiger, E. M.: Time course of baroreceptor resetting in acute hypertension. Am. J. Physiol., *8*:486, 1970.
20. Huang, S. K. et al.: Carotid sinus hypersensitivity in patients with unexplained syncope: clinical, electrophysiologic, and long term follow-up observations. Am. Heart J., *116*:989, 1988.
21. Mancia, G., Lorenz, R. R., and Shepherd, J. T.: Reflex control of circulation by heart and lungs. Int. Rev. Physiol., *9*:111, 1976.
22. Prather, J. W. et al.: Effect of blood volume, mean circulatory pressure and stress relaxation on cardiac output. Am. J. Physiol., *216*:467, 1969.
23. Mark, A. L., and Mancia, G.: Cardiopulmonary baroreflexes in humans. *In* Handbook of Physiology. Vol. 3. Edited by J. T. Shepherd and F. M. Abboud. Bethesda, Md, American Physiological Society, 1983, p. 397.
24. Oparil, S., and Haber, E.: The renin-angiotensin system (first of two parts). N. Engl. J. Med., *291*:389, 1974.
25. Cowey, A. W. et al.: Vasopressin: Cellular and Integrative Functions. New York, Raven Press, 1988.
26. Brenner, B. M., and Laragh, J. H.: Advances in Atrial Peptide Research. American Society of Hypertension Symposium Series. Vol. 2. New York, Raven Press, 1988.
27. Kaplan, N. M.: Systemic hypertension. *In* Heart Disease: A textbook of Cardiovascular Medicine. 4th Ed. Edited by E. Braunwald. Philadelphia, W. B. Saunders, 1992, p. 870.
28. Bellamy, R. F.: Diastolic coronary pressure-flow relation in the dog. Circ. Res., *43*:92, 1978.
29. Kocke, F. J.: Coronary blood flow in man. Prog. Cardiovasc. Dis., *19*:117, 1976.
30. Bern, R. M., and Rubio, R.: Coronary circulation. *In* Handbook of Physiology. Vol. 1. Edited by R. M. Bern et al. New York, Oxford University Press, 1979, p. 873.
31. Strandgaard, S.: Autoregulation of cerebral blood flow in hypertensive patients. The modifying influence of prolonged antihypertensive treatment on the tolerance to acute drug induce hypotension. Circulation, *53*:720, 1976.
32. Strandgaard, S.: Autoregulation of cerebral circulation with hypertension. Acta Neurol. Scand., Suppl. *66*:1, 1978.
33. Paulson, O. B., Walderman, G., Schmidt, J. F., and Strandgaard, S.: Cerebral circulation under normal and pathologic conditions. Am. J. Cardiol. *63*:2C, 1989.
34. Single, A., Bedi, V.: Trans-paraplegia following sudden lowering of blood pressure. J. Indian Med. Assoc., *82*:214, 1984.
35. Fitch, W., Mackenzie, E. T., and Harpe, A. N.: Effect of decreasing arterial blood pressure on cerebral blood flow in the baboon. Circ. Res., *37*:550, 1975.
36. Sadishuma, S. et al.: Cerebral autoregulation in young spontaneously hypertensive rats. Effect of sympathetic denervation. Hypertension, *7*:392, 1985.
37. Olsen, J., Skin hoy, E., and Lassen, N.: Autoregulation of cerebral blood flow in severe arterial hypertension. Br. Med. J., *1*:507, 1973.
38. Strandgaard, S. et al.: Studies on the cerebral circulation of the baboon in acutely induced hypertension. Stroke, *7*:287, 1976.
39. Barry, D. I.: Influence of antihypertensive drugs on cerebral blood flow. Am. J. Cardiol., *63*:14C, 1989.
40. Mchedlishvili, G.: Physiological mechanisms controlling cerebral blood flow. Stroke, *11*:240, 1980.
41. Russell, R. W. R.: Observations on intracerebral aneurysms. Brain, *96*:425, 1963.
42. Graham, D. I.: Morphologic changes during hypertension. Am. J. Cardiol., *63*:6C, 1989.
43. Gothberg, G. et al.: Apparent and true vascular resistance to flow in SHR and NCR kidneys as related to pre/post glomerular resistance ratio. Acta Physiol. Scand., *105*:282, 1979.
44. Miller, E. et al.: Hemodynamic response to halothane and enflurane in spontaneous-hypertensive rats. Anesth. Analg., *64*:136, 1985.
45. Cohn, J. N.: Paroxysmal hypertension and hypervolemia. N. Engl. J. Med., *275*:643, 1966.
46. Fouad, F. M. et al.: Idiopathic hypovolemia. Ann. Intern. Med., *104*:298, 1986.
47. Prys-Roberts, C.: Anesthesia and hypertension. Br. J. Anesth., *56*:711, 1984.
48. Mangano, D. T. et al.: Postoperative myocardial ischemia, therapeutic trials using intensive analgesia following surgery. Anesthesiology, *76*:342, 1992.
49. Mangano, D. T.: Perioperative cardiac morbidity. Anesthesiology, *72*:153, 1990.
50. James, T. N.: A cardiogenic hypertensive reflex. Anesth. Analg., *69*:633, 1989.
51. Cerenvzynski, L.: Humoral and metabolic reaction by acute myocardial infarction. Arch. Res., *48*:767, 1981.
52. Uple, L. H.: Metabolism of free fatty acids glucose and catecholamine in acute myocardial infarction. Relation to myocardial ischemia and infarct size. Am. J. Cardiol., *36*:938, 1975.
53. Karlsberg, R. P., Guyer, P. E., and Roberts, R.: Serial plasma catecholamine response early in the course of clinical acute myocardial infarction: relation to infarct extent and mortality. Am. Heart J., *102*:24, 1981.
54. Gaines, G. Y., and Rees, D. I.: Electroconvulsive therapy and anesthetic considerations. Anesth. Analg., *65*:1345, 1986.
55. Stoelting, R. K.: Drugs used in treatment of psychiatric disease. *In* Pharmacology and Physiology in Anesthetic Practice. Edited by R. K. Stoelting. Philadelphia, J. B. Lippincott, 1987, p. 347.
56. Estafanous, F. G. et al.: Pattern of hemodynamic alterations during coronary artery operations. J. Thorac. Cardiovasc. Surg., *87*:175, 1984.
57. Fouad, F. M., Estafanous, F. G., and Tarazi, R. C.: Hemodynamics of postmyocardial revascularization hypertension. Am. J. Cardiol., *41*:564, 1981.
58. Estafanous, F. G., and Tarazi, R. C.: Systemic arterial hypertension associated with cardiac surgery. Am. J. Cardiol., *46*:685, 1980.
59. Fouad, F. M. et al.: Possible role of cardioaortic reflexes in postcoronary bypass hypertension. Am. J. Cardiol., *44*:866, 1979.
60. Dehring, D.: Ketanserin in the treatment of pulmonary hypertension after valvular surgery: comparison with sodium nitroprusside. Crit. Care Med., *18*:119, 1990.
61. Taylor, K. M. et al.: Hypertension and renin-angiotensin system following open heart surgery. J. Thorac. Cardiovasc. Surg., *78*:840, 1977.
62. Weinstein, G. S. et al.: The renin angiotensin system is not responsible for hypertension following coronary artery bypass grafting. Ann. Thorac. Surg., *43*:74, 1987.
63. Tarazi, R. C., Estafanous, F. G., and Fouad, F. M.: Unilateral stellate block in the treatment of hypertension after coronary bypass surgery. Am. J. Cardiol., *42*:1013, 1978.
64. Olivari, M. T., Antiolick, A., and Ring, S.: Arterial hypertension in heart transplant recipients treated with triple drug

immunosuppressive therapy. J. Heart Transplant, 8:34, 1989.
65. Rottenbourg, J. et al.: Renal function and blood pressure in heart transplant recipients treated with cyclosporin. J. Heart Transplant., 4:404, 1985.
66. Scherrer, U. et al: Cyclosporin-induced sympathetic activation after heart transplantation. N. Engl. J. Med., 323:693, 1990.
67. Borrow, K. M. et al.: Cardiac and peripheral vascular responses to adrenoceper stimulation and blockade after cardiac transplantation. J. Am. Coll. Cardiol., 14:1229, 1989.
68. Farge, D. et al.: Effect of systemic hypertension on renal function and left ventricular hypertrophy in heart transplant recipients. J. Am. Coll. Cardiol., 15:1095, 1990.
69. Hertzer, N. et al.: Coronary artery disease in peripheral vascular patient. A classification of 1000 coronary angiograms and results of surgical management. Ann. Surg., 199:223, 1984.
70. Gelb, A., and Herrick, I.: Preoperative hypertension does predict post carotid endarterectomy hypertension. Am. J. Neurol. Sci., 17:95, 1990.
71. Skydell, J. et al.: Incidence and mechanism of post carotid endarterectomy hypertension. Arch. Surg., 122:1153, 1987.
72. Archie, J.: The relationship of early hypertension following carotid endarterectomy to intraoperative cerebral ischemia. J. Thorac. Cardiovasc. Anesth., 2:108, 1988.
73. Englund, R., and Dean, R.: Blood pressure aberrations associated with carotid endarterectomy. Ann. Vasc. Surg., 1:304, 1986.
74. Vincent, R. et al.: Esmolol as an adjunct in the treatment of systemic hypertension after operative repair of vascularization of the aorta. Am. J. Cardiol., 65:941, 1990.
75. Towne, J. B., and Bernard, V. M.: The relationship of postoperative hypertension to complications following carotid endarterectomy. Surgery, 80:575, 1980.
76. Leehem, F. et al.: Postoperative hypertension after repair of coarctation of the aorta in children: protective effect of propanolol. Am. Heart. J., 113:1164, 1987.
77. Sealy, W.: Hypertension after repair of the aorta: a review. Ann. Thorac. Surg., 50:323, 1990.
78. Choy, M. et al.: Paradoxical hypertension after repair of the aorta in children: angioplasty versus surgical repair. Circulation, 76:1186, 1987.
79. Behl, P., Sante, P., and Blesovsky, A.: Isolated coarctation of the aorta: surgical treatment and late results. J. Cardiovasc. Surg., 29:509, 1988.
80. Bojar, R., Weimer, B., and Cleveland, R.: Intravenous labetalol for the control of hypertension following repair of the aorta. Clin. Cardiol., 11:639, 1988.
81. Aken, H. V., Cottrell, J. E., Anger, C., and Puchstein, C.: Treatment of intraoperative hypertensive emergencies in patients with intracranial disease. Am. J. Cardiol., 63:43C, 1989.
82. Franklin, S., Sowers, J., and Butzdorf, V.: Relationship between arterial blood pressure and plasma norepinephrine levels in a patient with neurologic hypertension. Am. J. Med., 1:1105, 1986.
83. Plets, C.: Arterial hypertension in neurosurgical emergencies. Am. J. Cardiol., 63:40C, 1989.
84. Jones, J. V.: Differentiation and investigation of primary versus secondary hypertension (Cushing reflex). Am. J. Cardiol., 63:10C, 1989.
85. Simard, J., and Bellefleur, M.: Systemic arterial hypertension in head trauma. Am. J. Cardiol., 3:32C, 1989.
86. Cottrell, J. E. et al.: Rebound hypertension after sodium nitroprusside induced hypertension. Clin. Pharmacol. Ther., 27:32, 1980.
87. Schonwald, G., Fish, K. J., and Perkaash, I.: Cardiovascular complications during anesthesia in chronic spinal cord injured patients. Anesthesiology, 55:550, 1981.
88. Snow, J. C. et al.: Autonomic hyper reflex during cyptoscopy in patients with high spinal cord injuries. Paraplegia, 15:327, 1978.
89. Abin, M. S. et al.: Anesthesia for spinal cord injury. Probl. Anesth., 4:138, 1990.
90. Bravo, E. L., and Gifford, R. W. Jr.: Pheochromocytoma: diagnosis, localization, and management. N. Engl. J. Med., 311:1298, 1984.
91. Cryer, P. E.: Diseases of the sympathochromaffin system. In Endocrinology and Metabolism. 2nd Ed. Edited by P. Felig et al. New York, McGraw-Hill, 1987, p. 651.
92. Samaan, N. A., Hickey, R. C., and Shutts, P. E.: Diagnosis, localization, and management of pheochromocytomas. Pitfalls and follow-up in 41 patients. Cancer, 62:2451, 1988.
93. Roizen, M. F. et al.: A prospective randomized trial of four anesthetic techniques for resection of pheochromocytoma. Anesthesiology, 57:A43, 1981.
94. Kvols, L. K.: Metastatic carcinoid tumors and the carcinoid syndrome. Am. J. Med., 81:49, 1986.
95. Buckley, F. P.: Anesthesia and obesity and gastrointestinal disorders. In Clinical Anesthesia. 2nd Ed. Edited by P. G. Barash, B. F. Cullen, and R. K. Stoelting. Philadelphia, J. B. Lippincott, 1992, p. 1169.
96. Stehling, L. C.: Anesthetic management of the patient with hyperthyroidism. Anesthesiology, 41:585, 1974.
97. Maheswaran, R., and Beeves, D.: Clinical findings in parathyroid hypertension. J. Hypertens., 7:S190, 1989.
98. Bennett, M. H., and Wainwright, A. P.: Acute thyroid crisis on induction of anesthesia. Anaesthesia, 44:28, 1989.
99. Lombardi, A., Chiovato, L., and Braverman, L. E.: Thyroid storm. In Intensive Care Medicine. Edited by J. M. Rippe, R. S. Irwin, J. S. Alpert, and M. P. Fink. Boston, Little, Brown, 1991, p. 976.
100. Vaill, H., Rosenberg, H., Kytta, J., and Neuman, M.: Arterial hypertension associated with the use of a tourniquet. Acta Anesth., 31:279, 1987.
101. Assche, F., Spitz, B., and Vansteelant, L.: Severe systemic hypertension during pregnancy. Am. J. Cardiol., 63:22C, 1989.
102. Dildy, G., and Cotton, D.: Management of severe preeclampsia and eclampsia. Crit. Care Clin., 7:829, 1991.
103. Strandgaard, S., and Hansen, V.: The ischemic factor in hypertension after renal transplantation. Acta Med. Scand., 714:49, 1986.
104. Stanek, B. et al.: Renin-angiotensin-aldosterone system and vasopressor in cyclosporine treated renal allograft recipients. Clin. Nephrol., 8:186, 1987.
105. Guidi, E.: Hypertension and the kidney; lessons learned from transplantation. J. Clin. Hypertens., 3:227, 1987.
106. Baum, W.: Long-term complications of renal transplantation. (Clinical conference.) Kidney, 37:1363, 1990.
107. Murrsran, A., and Mourad, G.: Is renal transplantation useful in the understanding of the pathogenesis of hypertension? Adv. Nepherol., 19:53, 1990.
108. Stanek, B. et al.: Renin-angiotensin aldosterone system and vasopressin in cyclosporine treated renal allograft recipients. Clin. Nephrol., 8:186, 1987.
109. Higgins, T. L.: Anesthesia for Urologic Surgery. In Clinical Anesthesia Procedures of the Massachusetts General Hospital. 3rd Ed. Edited by L. L. Firestone, P. W. Lebowitz, and C. E. Cooke. Boston, Little, Brown, 1988, p. 431.
110. Diaz, M. et al.: Systemic arterial hypertension in the immediate postoperative period of liver transplant. Transplantation, 21:3547, 1989.

111. McGuirt, W., and May, J.: Postoperative hypertension associated with radical neck dissection. Arch. Otolaryngol. Head Neck Surg., *113*:1098, 1987.
112. Halpern, N. et al.: Nicardipine infusion for postoperative hypertension after surgery of the head and neck. Crit. Care Med., *18*:950, 1990.
113. Tweed, W. A. et al.: Circulatory responses to ketamine anesthesia. Anesthesiology, *37*:613, 1972.
114. Wieber, J. et al.: Pharmacokinetics of ketamine in man. Br. J. Anaesth., *53*:27, 1975.
115. Miller, E. D. et al.: Hormonal and hemodynamic response to halothane and enflurance in spontaneously hypertensive rats. Anesth. Analg., *64*:136, 1985.
116. Hanson, L. et al.: Blood pressure crisis following withdrawal of clonidine. Am. Heart J., *85*:605, 1973.
117. Vans-der-Geest, S. et al.: Clonidine withdrawal syndrome in a patient with heart failure. Crit. Care Med., *13*:444, 1985.
118. Jaffe, J. H., and Martin, W. R.: Opioid analgesics and antagonists. *In* The Pharmacological Basis of Therapeutics. 7th Ed. Edited by A. G. Gilman, L. S. Goodman, T. W. Rall, and F. Murad. 1991, p. 531.
119. Wax, P. M., and Delaney, K. A.: Withdrawal. *In* Intensive Care Medicine. Edited by J. M. Rippe, R. S. Irwin, J. S. Alpert, and M. P. Fink. Boston, Little, Brown, 1991.
120. Khamhatta, H., Store, J., and Kam, E.: Hypertension during anesthesia on discontinuation of sudden nitroprusside induced hypotension. Anesthesiology, *54*:127, 1979.
121. Miller, R. R.: Propranolol withdrawal rebound phenomenon: exacerbation of coronary events after abrupt cessation of antianginal therapy. N. Engl. J. Med., *293*:416, 1975.
122. Stack, C. et al.: Monamine oxidase inhibitors and anaesthesia. Br. J. Anaesthesia, *60*:222, 1988.
123. Cole, P.: The safe use of sodium nitroprusside. Anesthesia, *33*:473, 1978.
124. Mann, T. et al.: Effect of nitroprusside on regional myocardial blood flow in coronary artery disease: results in 25 patients and comparison with nitroglycerine. Circulation, *57*:732, 1978.
125. Jett, G. K. et al.: Vasoactive drug effects on blood flow in internal mammary and saphenous vein grafts. J. Thorac. Cardiovasc. Surg., *94*:2, 1987.
126. Taylor, P.: Ganglionic stimulating and blocking drugs. *In* The Pharmacological Basis of Therapeutics. 7th Ed. Edited by A. G. Gilman, L. S. Goodman, T. W. Rall, and F. Murad. New York, Macmillan, 1991, p. 215.
127. Puchstein, C. H. et al.: Urapadil in der perioperativen Phase. Anaesthesist, *33*:224, 1984.
128. VanAken, H. et al.: Anti hypertensive treatment with urapadil does not increase ICP in patients. Crit. Care Med., *12*:106, 1987.
129. Orlowski, J. P. et al.: The hemodynamic effects of intravenous labetalol for postoperative hypertension. Cleve. Clin. J. Med., *56*:30:1989.
130. Leslie, J. B. et al.: Intravenous labetalol for treatment of postoperative hypertension. Anesthesiology, *67*:413, 1987.
131. Cruise, C. et al.: Intravenous labetalol versus sodium nitroprusside for treatment of hypertension post coronary bypass surgery. Anesthesiology, *71*:835, 1989.
132. Reynolds, R., Gorczynslir, R., and Guon, C.: Pharmacology and pharmacokinetics of esmolol. J. Clin. Pharmacol., *26*:A3, 1986.
133. Turlapaty, P. et al.: Esmolol: a titratable short acting intravenous beta blocker for acute critical care settings. Am. Heart J., *114*:866, 1987.
134. Cucchiara, R. F. et al.: Evaluation of esmolol in controlling increases in heart rate and blood control pressure during endotracheal intubation in patients undergoing carotid endarterectomy. Anesthesiology, *65*:528, 1986.
135. Vincent, R. et al.: Esmolol as an adjunct in the treatment of systemic hypertension after operative repair of vascularization of the aorta. Am. J. Cardiol., *65*:941, 1990.
136. Sung, R. et al.: Clinical experience with esmolol, a short acting beta-adrenergic blocker on cardiac arrhythmias and myocardial ischemia. J. Clin. Pharmacol., *26*:A15, 1986.
137. Reeves, J. G. et al.: Esmolol for treatment of intraoperative tachycardia in hypertension of patients having cardiac operations. Bolus loading technique. J. Thorac. Cardiovasc. Surg., *100*:221, 1990.
138. Newsome, L., Roth, J., Hug, C., and Najel, D.: Esmolol altered hemodynamics response during fentanyl-pancuronium anesthesia bypass surgery. Anesth. Analg., *65*:451, 1986.
139. Gray, R. J., Bateman, T. M., and Czer, L. S. C.: Comparison of esmolol and nitroprusside for acute postcardiac surgical hypertension. Am. J. Cardiol., *59*:887, 1987.
140. Gibson, B. E. et al.: Esmolol for the control of hypertension following neurologic surgery. Anesth. Analg., *67*:S71, 1986.
141. Alder, A. G. et al.: Management of perioperative hypertension using sublingual nifedipine: experience in elderly patients undergoing eye surgery. Arch. Intern. Med., *146*:1927, 1986.
142. Ceyber, B. et al.: Comparison of sublingual captopril and sublingual nifedipine in hypertensive emergencies. Jpn. J. Pharmacol., *52*:189, 1990.
143. Mullen, J. C. et al.: Postoperative hypertension: a comparison of diltiazem, nifedipine, and nitroprusside. J. Thorac. Cardiovasc. Surg., *96*:122, 1988.
144. Adler, A. G., Lealy, J., and Cressman, M. D.: Management of perioperative hypertension using sublingual nifedipine. Arch. Intern. Med., *146*:1927, 1986.
145. Kaplan, J.: Clinical considerations for the use of intravenous nicardipine in the treatment of postoperative hypertension. Am. Heart J., *119*:443, 1990.
146. Venkata, C. et al.: Nicardipine and propranolol in the treatment of hypertension: similar antihypertensive but dissimilar hemodynamic actions. Am. Heart J., *119*:463, 1990.
147. David, D. et al.: Comparison of nicardipine and sodium nitroprusside in the treatment of paroxysmal hypertension following aortocoronary bypass surgery. Chest, *99*:393, 1991.
148. Benammar, M. S. et al.: Nicardipine vs. trinitrene for treatment of postoperative hypertension: effects on hemodynamics and left ventricular function. Anesthesiology, *67*:A139, 1987.
149. Ghigrione, M., Calvillo, O., and Quintin, L.: Anesthesia and hypertension: the effect of clonidine on perioperative hemodynamics and isoflurane requirements. Anesthesiology, *67*:3, 1987.
150. Flacke, J. W. et al.: Reduced narcotic requirement by clonidine with improved hemodynamic and adrenergic stability in patients undergoing coronary artery bypass surgery. Anesthesiology, *67*:11, 1987.
151. Roberts, A. J. et al.: Systemic hypertension associated with coronary artery bypass surgery. J. Thorac. Cardiovasc. Surg., *74*:846, 1977.
152. Weinstein, G. et al.: The renin angiotensin system is not responsible for hypertension following coronary artery bypass grafting. Ann. Thorac. Surg., *43*:74, 1987.
153. Miranda, J. V. et al.: Use of intravenous enalaprilat for hypertension following myocardial revascularization. Anesth. Analg., *72*:667, 1991.

Section Four

THE RENAL SYSTEM

Chapter 38

ACID/BASE AND ELECTROLYTE DISORDERS

JAY B. WISH
CAROLYN P. CACHO

NORMAL ACID/BASE METABOLISM

The normal organism is in a continuous state of acid flux. Body cells metabolize nutrients to generate approximately 1 mEq/kg body weight or 60 to 70 mEq of mineral acid per day. Most of these mineral acids consist of sulfates, which are derived from sulfur-containing amino acids in the diet and phosphates, which are abundant in most foodstuffs. The concentration of free hydrogen ion in body fluids is approximately 40×10^{-9} Eq/L; it is obvious that even a slight accumulation of the 60 to 70×10^{-3} Eq of hydrogen ion produced daily would be rapidly fatal. Therefore, endogenously produced acid must be immediately buffered so that free hydrogen ion does not accumulate in body fluids. At the physiologic pH of approximately 7.40, endogenously produced hydrogen ion is immediately buffered by circulating bicarbonate, generating carbon dioxide and water. The kidneys' role in acid/base balance is to excrete the mineral anion associated with the endogenously produced acid and to regenerate the 60 to 70 mEq of bicarbonate consumed daily in buffering the endogenous acid load. The latter function occurs primarily in the distal tubule, where a hydrogen ion is secreted in exchange for a reabsorbed sodium ion, under the influence of aldosterone. The secreted hydrogen ion is then buffered in the urine by weak acids present in the glomerular filtrate and by ammonia, which is generated by the renal tubular cells. This secretion of hydrogen ion into the urine is coupled with regeneration of the bicarbonate ion, which is returned to the extracellular fluid. An individual in acid/base balance will have a net acid excretion of 60 to 70 mEq per day and will regenerate the 60 to 70 mEq of bicarbonate consumed in the initial buffering of acid to maintain a stable plasma bicarbonate concentration.

The proximal renal tubule also defends extracellular bicarbonate concentration by rejecting filtered bicarbonate in excess of 25 to 28 mEq/L, so that, under normal circumstances, bicarbonate cannot accumulate to abnormally high levels in the plasma. The threshold for bicarbonate rejection by the proximal tubule can be modulated by a variety of factors, however, including the following:

- Partial pressure of carbon dioxide in arterial blood ($Paco_2$)
- Extracellular potassium concentration
- Effective extracellular fluid volume
- Mineralocorticoid activity

Metabolic acidosis results when endogenous production of acid exceeds the ability of the kidney to excrete the acid and regenerate bicarbonate, or when there is a loss of extracellular bicarbonate through a renal or extrarenal route. Metabolic alkalosis results when excessive administration or generation of bicarbonate by the distal renal tubule is coupled with a stimulus to the proximal renal tubule to reabsorb the excess bicarbonate, maintaining an abnormally high plasma bicarbonate concentration.

IDENTIFICATION OF ACID/BASE DISORDERS

Compensatory Responses

Whenever an abnormality in acid/base metabolism occurs, the organism attempts to compensate for that abnormality in order to bring pH or hydrogen ion concentration back toward normal. The Henderson-Hasselbalch equation predicts that the hydrogen ion concentration of a solution will be determined by the ratio of the proteinated and unproteinated species of any buffer pair in that solution. The Henderson equation, a simplified variation on this theme, uses the most important buffer pair in physiologic solutions, bicarbonate and carbonic acid, and predicts that hydrogen ion concentration (acidity) will be a function of the ratio of the partial pressure of carbon dioxide (Pco_2) (which is proportional to carbonic acid concentration) and the bicarbonate concentration.

$$H^+ = 24 \times \frac{Pco_2}{Hco_3^-}$$

This very simple equation predicts that hydrogen ion concentration, or acidity, will increase if either the Pco_2 rises (respiratory acidosis) or the bicarbonate concentration falls (metabolic acidosis). Conversely, hydrogen ion concentration will fall (alkalosis) if either the Pco_2 falls (respiratory) or the bicarbonate concentration rises (metabolic). An abnormality in pH secondary to a metabolic disorder is immediately sensed by the lungs, and respiratory compensation occurs to change Pco_2 in the same direction as the change in bicarbonate. Thus, in response to a metabolic acidosis (decreased bicarbonate), hyperventilation will normally occur to drive Pco_2 down and return pH toward normal. Conversely, in a metabolic alkalosis (increased bicarbonate), respiratory drive will decrease, resulting in hypoventilation and a rise in Pco_2 to drive pH back toward normal. Because the hypoventilatory response to metabolic alkalosis is limited by the development of hypoxemia, the rise in P_{CO_2} in response to metabolic alkalosis tends not to be as great as the fall in P_{CO_2} in response to a comparable degree of metabolic acidosis.

As noted in the preceding discussion, reabsorption of bicarbonate by the proximal tubule is modulated by P_{CO_2}. In the setting of respiratory acidosis, with an increase in P_{CO_2}, the reabsorption of bicarbonate by the proximal renal tubule will be accelerated, increasing plasma bicarbonate concentration and offsetting the degree of acidosis. Conversely, in the setting of respiratory alkalosis, the proximal tubule will reject more filtered bicarbonate, decreasing plasma bicarbonate concentration and offsetting the degree of alkalosis. Unlike the respiratory compensation to metabolic acid/base disorders, the renal compensation takes 2 to 3 days to exert its full effect. Respiratory acid/base disorders of shorter duration are generally termed acute; respiratory acid/base disorders in which full renal compensation has occurred are generally termed chronic.

In critically ill patients, it is not uncommon for more than one acid/base disorder to coexist at the same time. It is obvious that the blood can have only one pH even though a number of acid/base disorders may change that pH to different degrees or in different directions. An acidemia is defined as a plasma pH of less than 7.36; an alkalemia is defined as a plasma pH of more than 7.44. This is to be differentiated from acidosis and alkalosis, respectively, which are disorders that tend to perturb plasma pH but whose effect may be modulated by the coexistence of other acid/base disorders. For example, it is possible to have a normal plasma pH in the setting of a metabolic acidosis and respiratory alkalosis that offset each other. It is therefore important to understand the fundamental rules for the interpretation of pH, P_{CO_2}, and bicarbonate values so that the exact nature of all acid/base disorders that might be present can be identified (Table 38-1).

The first step in the interpretation of arterial blood gases is to determine whether an acidemia or alkalemia is present, as defined previously (Table 38-2). If an acidemia is present (pH less than 7.36), then the next step is to assess the P_{CO_2}. If the P_{CO_2} is increased (more than 40 mm Hg), then a respiratory acidosis is definitely present. If the P_{CO_2} is normal or low in the presence of an acidemia, then a metabolic acidosis is definitely present. If a metabolic acidosis is present, then the next step is to determine whether the change in P_{CO_2} is appropriate for the degree of acidosis. Experimental studies have indicated that appropriate respiratory compensation for a simple metabolic acidosis would lead to a 1.0- to 1.3-mm Hg in P_{CO_2} for every 1.0-mEq fall in bicarbonate from normal. Another formula predicts that the expected acid/base for a simple metabolic acidosis should be 1.5 times the bicarbonate concentration $+ 8 \pm 2$ mm Hg. A P_{CO_2} in excess of this predicted value indicates that a respiratory acidosis coexists with the metabolic acidosis; a P_{CO_2} less than this value indicates that a respiratory alkalosis coexists with the metabolic acidosis.

For example, if a patient with diabetic ketoacidosis presents with a serum bicarbonate of 10 mEq/L, then the appropriate respiratory compensation would be for his P_{CO_2} to fall approximately 1.3 times the fall in the bicarbonate from normal. If we assume a normal serum bicarbonate to be 25 mEq/L, the fall in bicarbonate is 15 mEq/L, and the expected P_{CO_2} is $40 - (1.3 \times 15) = 21$ mm Hg. Using the alternate formula, the predicted P_{CO_2} is $(1.5 \times 10) + 8 \pm 2 = 21$ to 25 mm Hg. If the patient's P_{CO_2} fell to only 30 mm Hg in this setting, this represents incomplete compensation, and a diagnosis of coexisting respiratory acidosis could be made. Note the dramatic effect of incomplete respiratory compensation on the blood pH of a patient with metabolic acidosis and a serum bicarbonate of 10 mEq/L. At the predicted P_{CO_2} of 21 mm Hg, the resulting blood pH is 7.27. At a P_{CO_2} of 30 mm Hg, the resulting pH is 7.10, a life-threatening situation.

Table 38-1. Simple Acid/Base Disorders

Disorder	pH	H⁺	P_{CO_2}	HCO_3^-	Primary Problem	Secondary Response
Metabolic acidosis	↓*	↑	↓	↓↓	↓↓HCO_3^-	↓P_{CO_2} $\Delta P_{CO_2} = 1.0 - 1.3 \times \Delta HCO_3^-$ or expected $P_{CO_2} = 1.5 \times HCO_3^- + 8 \pm 2$
Metabolic alkalosis	↑	↓	↑	↑↑	↑↑HCO_3^-	↑P_{CO_2} $\Delta P_{CO_2} = 0.5 - 1.0 \times \Delta HCO_3^-$ or expected $P_{CO_2} = 0.7 \times HCO_3^- + 20 \pm 1.5$
Respiratory acidosis						
Acute	↓↓	↑↑	↑↑	↑	↑↑P_{CO_2}	↑HCO_3^- $\Delta pH = 0.007 \times \Delta P_{CO_2}$ $\Delta HCO_3^- = 0.1 \times \Delta P_{CO_2}$ HCO_3^- does not exceed 30–32 mEq/L
Chronic	↓	↑	↑↑	↑↑	↑↑P_{CO_2}	↑↑HCO_3^- $\Delta pH = 0.003 \times \Delta P_{CO_2}$ $\Delta HCO_3^- = 0.4 \times \Delta P_{CO_2}$
Respiratory alkalosis						
Acute	↑↑	↓↓	↓↓	↓	↓↓P_{CO_2}	↓HCO_3^- $\Delta pH = 0.007 \times \Delta P_{CO_2}$ $\Delta HCO_3^- = 0.25 \times \Delta P_{CO_2}$ HCO_3^- generally ≥ 18 mEq/L
Chronic	↑	↑	↓↓	↓↓	↓↓P_{CO_2}	↓↓HCO_3^- $\Delta pH = 0.001 - 0.002 \times \Delta P_{CO_2}$ HCO_3^- generally ≥ 15 mEq/L

*Upward and downward arrows reflect the relative magnitude of change.

Table 38–2. Identification of Acid/Base Disorders

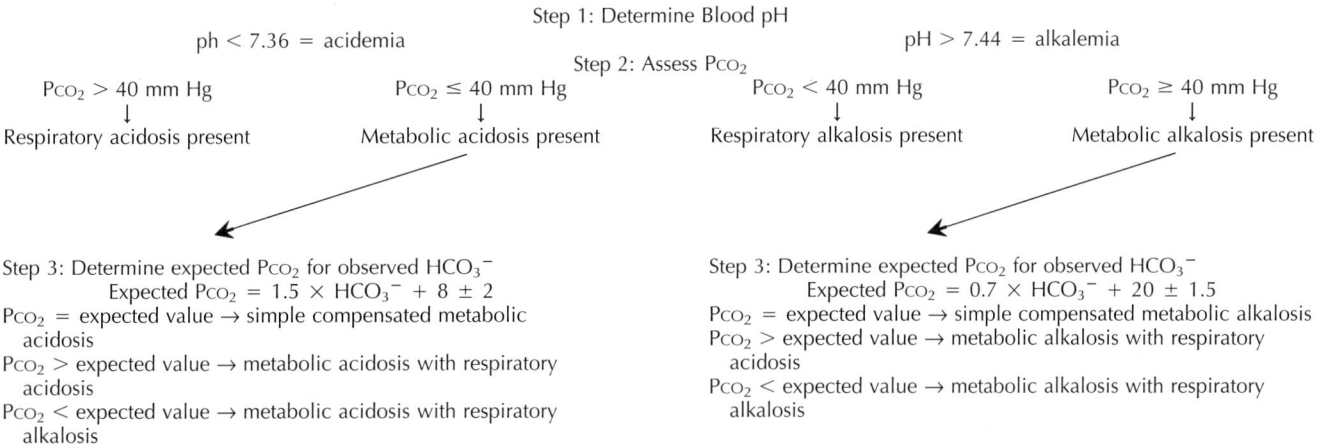

A similar set of rules can be defined for patients whose blood pH is greater than 7.44 (alkalemia). A low P_{CO_2} in this setting indicates that a respiratory alkalosis is definitely present. A normal or high P_{CO_2} in this setting indicates that a metabolic alkalosis is definitely present. Experimental studies have demonstrated that in a simple metabolic alkalosis, P_{CO_2} should fall 0.5 to 1.0 mm Hg for every 1.0-mEq fall in bicarbonate concentration from normal, or that the predicted P_{CO_2} should be equal to 0.7 times the bicarbonate $+ 20 \pm 1.5$ mm Hg. A P_{CO_2} in excess of this predicted value indicates that a respiratory acidosis coexists with the metabolic alkalosis; a P_{CO_2} less than this predicted value indicates that a respiratory alkalosis coexists with the metabolic alkalosis.[1]

For example, if a patient with protracted vomiting presents with a serum bicarbonate of 40 mEq/L, then the appropriate respiratory compensation is for his P_{CO_2} to rise approximately 0.7 times for normal. If we again assume a normal serum bicarbonate to be 25 mEq/L, then the rise in bicarbonate is 15 mEq/L and the expected P_{CO_2} is $40 + (0.7 \times 15) = 50$ mm Hg. Using the alternate formula, the predicted P_{CO_2} is $(0.7 \times 40) + 20 \pm 1.5 = 47 - 50$ mm Hg. An observed P_{CO_2} out of this range indicates the coexistence of a respiratory acidosis (if greater than 50 mm Hg) or alkalosis (if less than 47 mm Hg).

METABOLIC ACIDOSIS

Pre-ICU Phase

An understanding of the basic concepts of acid/base metabolism should allow the physician to predict under which circumstances hydrogen ion will accumulate in the extracellular fluid and a metabolic acidosis will occur. Most simply, situations include the following:

- Acid production in excess of the kidneys' ability to excrete the acid and regenerate bicarbonate
- Decreased ability of the decreased kidney to excrete acid and regenerate bicarbonate
- Loss of bicarbonate from the extracellular fluid either through the kidneys or the gastrointestinal tract

Excessive production of metabolic acids may occur as the result of abnormal cellular metabolism, as in the case of lactic acidosis and ketoacidosis, or may be the result of metabolism of an ingested toxin such as ethylene glycol, methyl alcohol, or salicylate to an acid end product. Decreased renal acid excretion may occur in the setting of a normal or abnormal glomerular filtration rate. Obviously, the patient with decreased nephron mass will have a decreased number of functioning tubules to secrete hydrogen ion and urinary ammonia buffer, limiting acid excretion and regeneration of bicarbonate. Because of the decreased glomerular filtration rate, anions associated with endogenously produced acid will accumulate in the extracellular fluid. A subset of patients may have decreased renal acid excretion leading to the development of a metabolic acidosis in the absence of an abnormal glomerular filtration rate. Because this is primarily a renal tubular defect, it is termed **renal tubular acidosis** and may occur in a variety of settings. Finally, depletion of the extracellular bicarbonate buffer pool, either through gastrointestinal losses with bicarbonate-rich diarrhea or renal losses that are due to the failure of the proximal tubule to reabsorb filtered bicarbonate, will compromise the organism's ability to buffer endogenously produced acid and lead to net acid accumulation within the body.

Risk Factors for the Development of Metabolic Acidosis

Because it is clear that the accumulation of acid in the extracellular fluid is a function of the balance between acid production and acid excretion, any patient with decreased renal function will be at higher risk for developing metabolic acidosis. The normal kidney can adapt to increased acid generation by substantially increasing urinary ammonia production to provide a vehicle for increased net acid excretion. The diseased kidney cannot compensate in like fashion, and this may be further compounded by incomplete proximal tubular absorption of filtered bicarbonate. The result is that even modest increases in endogenous acid production can lead to profound decreases in plasma pH and the development of severe metabolic acidosis in the uremic patient. This is part of the rationale for the institution of low protein diets in such individuals, as the lower protein content limits the load of sulfur-containing amino acids and the generation of sulfuric acid. Because renal hydrogen ion excretion occurs in the distal tubule in exchange for the absorption of sodium, it is essential that adequate sodium be delivered to the distal tubule for net acid excretion to occur. States of volume depletion, by causing increased reabsorption of sodium in the proximal portions of the nephron, may limit delivery of sodium to distal hydrogen exchange sites and may reduce net acid excretion, compounding the acidosis. Therefore, as a rule, patients with, or at risk for, metabolic acidosis should be well hydrated so that adequate amounts of sodium can be delivered to the distal nephron to promote acid excretion.

The reabsorption of filtered sodium in exchange for secreted hydrogen ion in the distal nephron is under the influence of mineralocorticoid. In a variety of situations, mineralocorticoid activity may be decreased, compromising renal acid excretion and promoting the development of metabolic acidosis. The simplest case is primary adrenal insufficiency, in which decreased mineralocorticoid production may be associated with a mild chronic metabolic acidosis. In such individuals, the inability to substantially increase net acid excretion may lead to life-threatening degrees of acidosis if acid production is increased even modestly. A more common syndrome leading to metabolic acidosis out of proportion to the degree of renal insufficiency is hyporeninemic hyperaldosteronism, also known as type 4 renal tubular acidosis, in which the combination of low renin generation by the kidneys, an insensitivity of adrenal mineralocorticoid production to hyperkalemia, and an insensitivity of the renal tubule to the effects of mineralocorticoid all conspire to decrease renal sodium-hydrogen exchange, decrease net acid secretion, and lead to the generation of a chronic metabolic acidosis. Such individuals are also at risk for developing life-threatening degrees of acidemia should acid production increase to even a modest degree.

ICU Phase

Differential Diagnosis of Metabolic Acidosis

When a patient in the ICU develops a metabolic acidosis, the first priority is to determine the cause of the acidosis. Obviously, the medical history is of paramount importance, and in many cases, the cause of the metabolic acidosis can be ascertained on the basis of the history alone. In cases for which the medical history is not sufficient, a variety of laboratory tools have proved extremely useful in the differential diagnosis of metabolic acidosis. The most well-known is the serum anion gap[2] (Table 38-3). The negatively charged anions and positively charged cations in the plasma must be equal for electroneutrality. If one examines only the major cation (sodium) and the two major anions (chloride and bicarbonate) in the plasma, the difference between the sodium concentration and the sum of the chloride and bicarbonate concentrations is normally 10 to 14 mEq/L. If may be somewhat lower if newer multichannel biochemical analyzers are used.[3] This represents unmeasured anions including negatively charged proteins, phosphates, and other weak acids. In the setting of metabolic acidosis, this "anion gap" will increase if the bicarbonate consumed in the buffering of excess acid is quantitatively replaced by the unmeasured anion accompanying that acid. Most forms of metabolic acidosis encountered in the ICU are accompanied by an increase in the anion gap and include lactic acidosis, diabetic ketoacidosis, advanced renal failure, and the acidosis resulting from intoxication with salicylates, methanol, and ethylene glycol. The greater the increase in the anion gap, the more likely the cause of the organic acidosis will be confirmed with further biochemical tests.[4] If the anion gap is greater than 30 mEq/L, the cause can be demonstrated in almost all cases and is usually due to ethylene glycol or methanol intoxication or lactic acidosis (see Table 38-3).

A patient with metabolic acidosis may have a normal anion gap if the consumed or lost bicarbonate is quantitatively replaced by chloride, so that the sum of chloride and bicarbonate concentrations will be a constant, and the difference of this sum from the sodium concentration will be normal. The loss of sodium and bicarbonate from the extracellular fluid, either through diarrhea or proximal renal tubular acidosis, produces a state of volume depletion that accelerates sodium and chloride reabsorption by the proximal tubule, such that the plasma chloride concentration increases to match the fall in plasma bicarbonate concentration. The administration of acid with chloride anion also leads to the development of metabolic acidosis with a normal anion gap, because the administered chloride quantitatively replaces bicarbonate in the plasma. This situation can be encountered in the setting of hydrochloric acid ingestion, hydrochloric acid or arginine hydrochloride administration for the treatment of metabolic alkalosis or in patients with ureterosigmoidostomy. Patients with mild degrees of chronic renal insufficiency may also have a proximal tubular bicarbonate wasting defect leading to the development of a hyperchloremic or normal anion gap metabolic acidosis (see Table 38-3).

A number of renal function studies can be useful in the differential diagnosis of metabolic acidosis (Table 38-4). The blood urea nitrogen (BUN) and serum creatinine, as markers of glomerular filtration rate, provide an index as to the ability of the kidneys to excrete even normal quantities of metabolic acid. Urine studies may also be useful in the differential diagnosis of metabolic acidosis with a normal anion gap. If the metabolic acidosis is due to bicarbonate loss from diarrhea, then the normal kidney should compensate by increasing net acid excretion and bicarbonate regeneration. This will be reflected by an acid urine pH (5 or less) and increased amounts of ammonium in the urine. Although it is not customary to measure urinary ammonium directly, its concentration can be inferred from the "urinary anion gap."[5] As with the serum, the total number of anions and cations in the urine must be equal to maintain electroneutrality. The ions that are easiest to measure in the urine are sodium, potassium, and chloride. If there are large amounts of ammonium in the urine (excreted as ammonium chloride), the chloride concentration will exceed the sum of the sodium and potassium concentrations, leading to a negative urinary anion gap. In the

Table 38-3. Causes of Metabolic Acidosis

Normal Anion Gap	Increased Anion Gap
Loss of Bicarbonate	Overproduction of Organic Acids
Gastrointestinal	Lactic Acidosis
Diarrhea	Post grand mal seizure
Pancreatic or biliary drainage	Sepsis
Renal	Reperfusion of extremities following revascularization procedures
Proximal renal tubular acidosis (type 2)	Ketoacidosis
Recovery phase of diabetic ketoacidosis	Diabetic
Post chronic hypocapnia	Alcoholic
Mild–moderate renal failure	Toxin ingestions
Chloride-containing acid administration	Salicylates
Hyperalimentation with HCl-containing amino acid solutions	Methanol
Overshoot treatment of metabolic alkalosis with HCl	Ethylene glycol
Ureterosigmoidostomy (absorption of NH_4Cl from urine by sigmoid)	Paraldehyde (rare)
Impaired renal acid excretion	Toluene (rare)
Distal renal tubular acidosis (type 1)	Advanced renal failure
Mineralocorticoid deficiency or resistance	
Mild–moderate renal failure	

patient with a normal anion gap metabolic acidosis secondary to renal tubular acidosis, there is an inability to acidify the urine and a defect in renal ammonium excretion. This leads to an inappropriately high urine pH (6 or greater) in the setting of systemic acidemia as well as a decrease in urinary ammonium concentration manifested as a positive urinary anion gap in which the sum of urinary sodium and potassium concentrations exceeds the urinary chloride concentration.

In the patient with metabolic acidosis in whom lactic acidosis or ketoacidosis is suspected, serum lactate and ketone levels can be measured directly, confirming these causes for the acidosis. For those patients in whom no cause for the metabolic acidosis with increased anion gap can be ascertained and in whom blood ketone and lactate levels are normal, a toxic ingestion of ethylene glycol, methanol, or salicylates should be suspected. The medical history would be most helpful in this setting but may be unobtainable if the patient is comatose. A toxic screen should be sent, but unfortunately, the results may not be available for many hours. A more rapid clue to the possibility of a toxin ingestion would be the elevation of the serum osmolal gap. Under normal circumstances, plasma osmolality is primarily determined by the sum of the contributions of anions, cations, glucose, and urea. A rough calculation of plasma osmolality follows:

$$\text{Osmolality} = 2\,[Na^+] + \frac{\text{glucose (mg/dl)}}{18} + \frac{\text{BUN (mg/dl)}}{2.8}$$

If the plasma osmolality determined by the hospital laboratory exceeds the estimated plasma osmolality by more than 10 mOsm/L, then an unidentified osmotically active substance is present in the plasma. To exert a significant effect on plasma osmolality, such a molecule would have to be of small molecular weight. Metabolic acidoses associated with the greatest increase in the osmolal gap are those associated with methanol or ethylene glycol intoxication.[6]

Table 38-4. Use of the "Gaps" in the Differential Diagnosis of Metabolic Acidosis

Gap	Formula	Interpretation
Serum AG	$AG = Na^+ - [Cl^- + HCO_3^-]$ Normal = 10 – 14 mEq/L	An elevated AG generally implies the presence of metabolic acidosis, but an AG < 20 can be observed in other acid/base disorders A metabolic acidosis with an elevated AG is due to overproduction of organic acids, consumption of certain toxins or advanced renal failure A metabolic acidosis with a normal AG is due to bicarbonate loss or administration of Cl^- containing acid The normal range for AG decreased by 2.5 mEq/L for every 1 g/dl fall in serum albumin concentration
Urinary anion gap	$UAG = [UNa^+\ UK^+] - UCl^-$	In the setting of a metabolic acidosis with normal AG, a negative UAG implies normal urinary acidification response to extrarenal HCO_3^- loss or HCl administration; a positive UAG suggests impaired urinary calcification as in distal renal tubular acidosis
Osmolal gap	$Osm = 2[Na] + \dfrac{\text{glu (mg/dl)}}{18} - \dfrac{\text{BUN (mg/dl)}}{18}$ Osmolality as determined by laboratory should not exceed calculated osmolality by > 10 mOsm/kg	Elevated osmolal gap (actual osmolality) in the setting of metabolic acidosis with increased anion gap suggests intoxication with low molecular weight substance such as methanol or ethylene glycol

AG, anion gap; BUN, blood urea nitrogen; UAG, urinary anion gap.

An increased osmolal gap may also be seen in alcoholic ketoacidosis and lactic acidosis.[7]

Signs and Symptoms of Metabolic Acidosis

Although hypotension may lead to the generation of metabolic acidosis as a result of decreased tissue perfusion, severe acidosis may also produce hypotension through depression of myocardial contractility and arterial vasodilatation. In mild-to-moderate acidemia, hypotension is not a common consequence, because high levels of circulating catecholamines will usually antagonize these cardiovascular effects. When blood pH falls below 7.15, however, the effects of the acidemia may predominate, and hypotension results.

The normal respiratory compensation for a metabolic acidosis is to increase minute ventilation, driving down P_{CO_2}, and returning plasma pH toward normal. As a rule, these ventilatory changes are accomplished through an increase in tidal volume rather than through an increase in respiratory rate, resulting in the classic Kussmaul respirations. Severe degrees of metabolic acidosis may exert central nervous system (CNS) effects, including mental status changes, nausea, and vomiting. Coexisting illness may also lead to neurologic sequelae, making the contribution of the acidemia per se on CNS function difficulty to quantify. In most patients with severe acidemia, however, correction of blood pH toward normal does lead to an improvement in cardiovascular and CNS function, even if this occurs before the underlying disease is reversed. As a result, bicarbonate therapy continues to assume a central role in the treatment of a variety of the metabolic acidoses.

Treatment of Metabolic Acidosis

Because the chemical change that defines a metabolic acidosis is a decrease in plasma bicarbonate concentration, bicarbonate therapy for this disorder has great empiric appeal. Indeed, many patients with moderate-to-severe metabolic acidosis will benefit from bicarbonate therapy, because a rise in blood pH to around 7.20 may lead to an improvement in cardiovascular stability and CNS function. As with any other therapeutic intervention, the risks of bicarbonate therapy must be weighed against the benefits. The risks of bicarbonate therapy include fluid overload and hypernatremia associated with the accompanying sodium cation, depression of respiratory drive leading to hypercapnia, and overshoot alkalosis. There are reports that, in certain settings, bicarbonate therapy may actually exacerbate metabolic acidosis by increasing carbon dioxide generation and suppressing ventilation.[8] Because carbon dioxide diffuses much more rapidly in and out of the cerebrospinal fluid than does bicarbonate, a decrease in ventilation may lead to the worsening of cerebrospinal fluid acidosis and greater neurologic sequelae. Finally, some studies have suggested that, in selected settings, bicarbonate therapy may actually increase lactate production, compounding intracellular acidosis and further compromising cellular enzymatic and transport processes.[9]

Therefore, if bicarbonate therapy is considered, the goal should not be to correct the acidemia but merely to stabilize the cardiovascular and neurologic sequelae of the de-

Table 38–5. Bicarbonate Therapy for Metabolic Acidosis

General Guidelines
1. Bicarbonate therapy should be reserved for patients with severe metabolic acidosis, characterized by hemodynamic instability, blood pH < 7.15, and/or serum HCO_3^- < 12.
2. Bicarbonate therapy is most beneficial in patients with metabolic acidosis that is due to bicarbonate loss from the body (e.g., severe diarrhea). It is generally not indicated if accumulated bicarbonate precursor (e.g., ketoacids) can be metabolized to generate bicarbonate once the underlying metabolic is corrected. Bicarbonate therapy may be detrimental in certain forms of lactic acidosis.
3. Goal of bicarbonate therapy is not to normalize serum bicarbonate but to improve hemodynamic and central nervous system function in severe acidemia. Bicarbonate dose should be calculated to increase serum bicarbonate to 15 mEq/L or blood pH to 7.15, no higher.
4. Ongoing generation of acid may require frequent monitoring of response to bicarbonate administration and adjustment of dosage accordingly.

Dosage Calculation
Use as volume of distribution of bicarbonate (V):
  $0.5 \times$ body weight if serum HCO_3^- > 10 mEq/L
  $0.75 \times$ body weight if serum HCO_3^- > 5 to 10 mEq/L
  $1.0 \times$ body weight if serum HCO_3^- < 5 mEq/L
Bicarbonate dose: Body weight (kg) $\times$ V $\times$ (15 − initial serum HCO_3^- concentration).
Administration: 50% of calculated bicarbonate dose immediately by intravenous bolus, remainder over next 6–12 hr by intravenous infusion.

creased blood pH (Table 38-5). The calculation of bicarbonate dose is generally made on the basis of that required to raise plasma bicarbonate concentration to 15 mEq/L. To make this calculation, one multiplies the difference between 15 and the patient's plasma bicarbonate concentration by the distribution volume of bicarbonate. In normal individuals, the bicarbonate distribution space is approximately 50% of lean body weight, and this also applies to acidemia patients with a plasma bicarbonate level of greater than 10. In more severe degrees of acidosis, nonbicarbonate buffers assume an increased role in consuming excess hydrogen ion, and these must be back-buffered by administration alkali before plasma bicarbonate concentration will rise. As a result, the bicarbonate distribution space increases in more severe degrees of acidemia to approximately 75% of lean body weight in individuals whose plasma bicarbonate concentration is 5 to 10 mEq/L and to 100% of lean body weight in individuals whose plasma bicarbonate concentration is less than 5 mEq/L.[10]

As a example, if a 70-kg patient presents with a metabolic acidosis and a plasma bicarbonate concentration of 8 mEq/L, the quantity of bicarbonate required to raise plasma bicarbonate concentration to 15 mEq/L will equal $(15 − 8) \times (0.75 \times 70) = 367.5$ mEq. Approximately half of the calculated bicarbonate deficit is generally given immediately by intravenous bolus, with the remaining deficit administered over the next 6 to 12 hours by infusion. An approximately isotonic solution of sodium bicarbonate can be created by adding three ampules (50 mEq each) of sodium bicarbonate to 1 L of 5% dextrose and water. In the example noted previously, the patient might receive three ampules of sodium bicarbonate intravenously immediately, followed by infusions of sodium bicarbonate in

D5W at 200 ml per hour for 8 hours, to provide a total of 390 mEq of bicarbonate.

Because the process that generated the metabolic acidosis does not necessarily terminate once bicarbonate therapy is initiated, it is important to continuously monitor patients with metabolic acidosis throughout the course of bicarbonate therapy. Continued production of metabolic acid will partially neutralize administered bicarbonate, so that the desired change in plasma bicarbonate concentration and blood pH may not be achieved with the originally calculated dose. Frequent modifications of bicarbonate dosing may be necessary to achieve the desired effect. It is recommended that arterial blood gas and electrolyte determinations be repeated every 1 to 2 hours during the initial phases of management so that appropriate modifications of bicarbonate as well as other electrolyte therapy can be made as needed.

Treatment of Specific Diseases Causing Metabolic Acidosis

Acidosis Associated with Renal Disease. The renal acidoses may be associated with normal or abnormal glomerular filtration rate. Patients with severely impaired glomerular filtration rate and a substantial reduction in renal mass develop metabolic acidosis primarily on the basis of decreased renal ammoniagenesis and net acid excretion, which lags behind daily acid production. If untreated, this may result in a profound acidosis, usually accompanied by an increase in the serum anion gap. Bicarbonate therapy poses an additional risk in this setting, because the compromised kidney may not effectively excrete the sodium load, and pulmonary edema may result. Therefore, bicarbonate therapy, if considered, should be conservative, using only that which is necessary to stabilize cardiovascular and CNS function. Large doses of loop diuretics may be useful to promote sodium excretion in this setting and minimize the risk for extracellular fluid volume overload. Because patients with renal disease may also have a defect in renal potassium excretion, metabolic acidosis may further compound the tendency toward hyperkalemia, and the treatment of the metabolic acidosis with bicarbonate therapy may lead to a favorable reduction in serum potassium concentration. On the other hand, many patients with advanced renal disease have hypocalcemia, and the acidemia protects against tetany by producing a higher proportion of ionized to bound calcium in the serum. The correction of the acidemia may precipitate tetany in this setting and should be accompanied by calcium administration, if appropriate.

Patients with uremic acidosis or who are oliguric, severely azotemic, volume overloaded or who have other electrolyte disorders will probably require dialysis to correct the acidosis. Typical dialysis solutions contain 35 mEq/L of bicarbonate or bicarbonate precursor (lactate or acetate) and provide a favorable gradient for the diffusion of bicarbonate into the extracellular fluid during the treatment.

Renal diseases leading to metabolic acidosis in the absence of abnormal glomerular filtration rate are due to tubular disorders and have been termed **renal tubular acidoses**. The **distal tubular variety (type 1)** is due to the inability to establish a high hydrogen ion concentration gradient between the urine and the plasma, resulting in a failure of urinary acidification (urine pH greater than 6) and net acid excretion that lag behind daily acid production. As a result, there is cumulative retention of acid, which progressively titrates bicarbonate and nonbicarbonate buffers, leading to a variety of metabolic abnormalities including acidosis, demineralization of bone, nephrocalcinosis, and progressive renal failure. Because of the inability to secrete adequate quantities of hydrogen ion in exchange for reabsorbed sodium in the distal tubule, sodium-potassium exchange is favored, renal potassium excretion is accelerated, and severe hypokalemia often results. Rapid correction of the acidemia may shift extracellular potassium back into cells, further compounding the hypokalemia and precipitating skeletal muscle paralysis or rhabdomyolysis. In these patients, therefore, it is important to at least partially correct the cumulative potassium deficit before attempting to correct the acidemia. Once the electrolyte abnormalities are corrected, these patients require chronic alkali therapy to buffer the daily hydrogen ion production that exceeds net acid excretion. An acute self-limited form of distal renal tubular acidosis may be seen in association with certain drugs, most notably amphotericin B.

A proximal tubular defect of bicarbonate reabsorption may lead to the partial depletion of the extracellular buffer pool and has been termed **type 2 renal tubular acidosis.** Because distal tubular acidification mechanisms are intact, however, these individuals generally achieve a steady state of acid/base balance, once plasma bicarbonate concentration falls to a level wherein the filtered load of bicarbonate equals the capacity of the compromised tubules to reabsorb it. Therefore, these individuals generally do not develop the long-term metabolic consequences of bone demineralization, nephrocalcinosis, and progressive renal failure of type 1 renal tubular acidosis, and their hypokalemia tends to be much more modest. Such patients generally achieve a steady-state plasma bicarbonate concentration in the 15- to 20-mEq/L range and, with appropriate respiratory compensation, their plasma pH is generally greater than 7.30. As a result, bicarbonate therapy is generally not indicated and is ineffective, because administered bicarbonate will be rapidly dumped by the proximal tubules and lost in the urine. Type 2 renal tubular acidosis may be seen in association with the administration of carbonic anhydrase inhibitors, streptozotocin, and in the setting of multiple myeloma.

A hyperkalemic form of renal tubular acidosis may be seen in association with certain forms of mild-to-moderate chronic renal insufficiency, especially chronic interstitial renal disease and diabetic nephropathy. In these individuals, the hyperkalemia tends to be much more problematic than the acidosis. The use of diuretics to promote potassium excretion may lead to an increase in hydrogen ion excretion and bicarbonate regeneration, ameliorating the acidosis. In selected cases, the administration of a sympathetic mineralocorticoid, 9-fludrocortisone, to stimulate sodium cation exchange in the distal tubule will correct the hyperkalemia, but a mild chronic acidemia usually persists.

Bicarbonate Loss. The most common cause of extrarenal bicarbonate loss is diarrhea. Patients with prolonged diarrhea that is due to cholera, other enterotoxic bacteria, and, more recently, patients with acquired immune deficiency syndrome (AIDS) may develop substantial bicarbonate as well as other fluid and electrolyte deficits. Renal bicarbonate generation cannot keep up with gastrointestinal bicarbonate losses, and a progressive, life-threatening acidemia may result. In most of these patients, however, volume depletion is the most critical issue at the time of presentation, and intravenous volume replacement is the primary goal of initial therapy. The constituents of that replacement are determined by the nature and severity of electrolyte disorders present on admission as well as by analysis of the diarrheal fluid for electrolyte content. If bicarbonate depletion is severe and life-threatening, a "normal" bicarbonate solution, made by adding 3 ampules of bicarbonate to 1 L of 5% dextrose in water with potassium added, provides the most rapid fluid and bicarbonate replacement. Restoration of adequate circulating volume will improve renal perfusion, allowing the kidneys to more effectively regenerate bicarbonate so that complete bicarbonate replacement is generally not required. Again, the goal of therapy should be to treat the acidosis sufficiently to raise levels of bicarbonate to approximately 15 mEq/L and, assuming the diarrhea is controlled, allow the kidneys to do the rest. In patients with intractable diarrhea, chronic bicarbonate supplementation may be required.

Metabolic Acidosis that is Due to Intoxication. Salicylate, methanol, and ethylene glycol intoxication may lead to profound, life-threatening metabolic acidosis, and bicarbonate therapy is generally recommended in this setting. The metabolic acidosis associated with salicylate intoxication is due to both the accumulation of acetylsalicylic acid and its metabolites as well as the lactic acidosis derived from the uncoupling of oxidative phosphorylation at the mitochondrial level. Aside from providing sufficient bicarbonate to improve the acidemia and correct cardiovascular instability, the treatment of choice is to promote salicylate excretion through the generation of an alkaline diuresis or the institution of hemodialysis. If hemodialysis is used, the relatively high bicarbonate concentration of the dialysate will also improve the acidemia. The metabolic acidosis associated with methanol and ethylene glycol ingestions is partially due to the accumulation of acid metabolites of these compounds. Ethylene glycol intoxication may also lead to acute renal failure through deposition of calcium oxalate crystals throughout the kidneys, leading to a failure of urinary acid excretion and a compounding of the acidosis. Methanol intoxication may also be accompanied by the development of lactic acidosis. The treatment of choice for these intoxications is prompt hemodialysis to remove the toxins and their metabolites from the extracellular fluid as rapidly as possible. The provision of a dialysate with high bicarbonate concentration will generally prove sufficient to treat the acidosis, so additional intravenous bicarbonate therapy is generally not warranted.

Ketoacidosis. The two major forms of ketoacidosis are diabetic ketoacidosis and alcoholic ketoacidosis. In diabetic ketoacidosis, it is important to recognize that the plasma glucose concentration does not necessarily correlate with the degree of acidemia.[11] In fact, it is typical that ketoacid production continues for many hours after glycemic control has been achieved with insulin administration, so that the goal of insulin therapy in this setting should not be the achievement of a normal glucose concentration but should be the achievement of a normal plasma bicarbonate concentration, reflecting a resolution of the ketoacidosis. Patients with diabetic ketoacidosis typically present with a variety of fluid and electrolyte disorders. The sustained osmotic diuresis from hyperglycemia that often precedes the development of ketoacidosis leads to a substantial depletion of body electrolytes, particularly potassium, magnesium, and phosphorus. Substantial, life-threatening reductions in extracellular fluid volume result not only from the osmotic diuresis but also from the excessive renal excretion of sodium along with ketoanions. The primary goals of the initial therapy of the patient with diabetic ketoacidosis should be restoration of adequate extracellular fluid volume, repletion of body potassium stores, and correction of hyperglycemia and ketone generation with insulin therapy. The administration of bicarbonate is generally not necessary in patients with diabetic ketoacidosis, because provision of insulin will lead to adequate endogenous generation of bicarbonate as ketoacids are metabolized by the liver. Because, however, some ketoacids will invariably be lost in the urine before the initiation of therapy, insulin will not generally lead to the prompt normalization of serum bicarbonate, and several days may be required before renal generation of "new" bicarbonate leads to a normalization of plasma bicarbonate levels. Following the administration of adequate insulin, the metabolic acidosis may change from one with an elevated anion gap (reflecting accumulated ketoanions) to one with a normal anion gap, reflecting the ketone (bicarbonate precursor) loss in the urine.[12]

If bicarbonate therapy is considered in the setting of diabetic ketoacidosis, it should be reserved for those patients who present with severe acidemia and circulatory instability, in whom the goal of therapy is to promptly raise plasma pH to around 7.15.[13] Patients with underlying renal disease may have trouble recovering from the non-anion gap metabolic acidosis that may be seen during the recovery phase of diabetic ketoacidosis, because renal bicarbonate regeneration may be compromised. Such patients may benefit from a short term of oral bicarbonate supplements. Serum creatinine concentration may be falsely elevated in the presence of ketoacidosis because acetoacetic acid is a noncreatinine chromogen that is measured as creatinine in the standard colorimetric assay. Therefore, the fall in serum creatinine that occurs following fluid resuscitation and insulin therapy in diabetic ketoacidosis is due not only to improved renal perfusion but also to the elimination of the false assay.

Patients with diabetic ketoacidosis, as noted, may have substantial potassium depletion, and correction of the acidemia may lead to profound hypokalemia as hydrogen ions shift into cells. Therefore, potassium replacement should accompany any alkali therapy. It is also recommended, because of coexisting phosphate depletion, that at least one third of the potassium be administered as the phosphate salt.

Alcoholic ketoacidosis is generally seen in chronic alcoholic patients with poor carbohydrate intake, often with superimposed vomiting. The resulting dehydration leads to impaired renal clearance of prestarvation ketosis and the generation of a metabolic acidosis with an increased anion gap. Because of the increase in reduced nicotinamide adenine dinucleotide (NADH) generation by the liver from the oxidation of ethanol, beta-hydroxybutyrate tends to be the predominant ketoacid produced in this setting. The standard nitroprusside assay for serum ketones detects only acetoacetate and may be negative or only weakly positive in patients with alcoholic ketoacidosis. Therefore, the clinical setting is an essential component in the diagnosis of alcoholic ketoacidosis because these patients may have negligible serum alcohol levels.

The treatment of alcoholic ketoacidosis is restoration of adequate circulating volume with sodium chloride and provision of adequate carbohydrate substrate with glucose. The intravenous administration of a solution containing 5% dextrose and 0.9% sodium chloride is generally adequate, and bicarbonate supplementation is unnecessary.

Lactic Acidosis. Lactic acidosis is the most common cause of metabolic acidosis in the critically ill patient but also the most poorly understood. It tends to be associated with catastrophic illness and, not surprisingly, carries a high mortality. It is estimated that approximately 60 to 70% of all patients with lactic acidosis will not survive their hospitalization and, if the lactic acidosis results from refractory hypotension, mortality approaches 100%.[14]

Because of the catastrophic illness that accompany lactic acidosis, the contribution of the acidemia per se to cardiovascular instability or mental status changes can be difficult to determine. As a result, the role of bicarbonate therapy in this setting remains controversial, and no clear clinical studies demonstrate that the administration of bicarbonate in patients with lactic acidosis improves mortality. It is clear that patients who develop lactic acidosis survive only if the underlying disease that causes the lactic acidosis is reversed. In some patients, these underlying factors are easier to identify than others, and this provides that basis for the classification of lactic acidosis into types A and B. **Type A lactic acidosis** is associated with decreased delivery of oxygen to the tissues, either as a result of hypoxemia or hypotension. Patients with ongoing sepsis may have shunting of blood flow away from the capillaries, leading to tissue hypoxemia in the absence of overt hypotension, and also fall into the type A lactic acidosis group. **Type B lactic acidosis** is due to abnormalities of cellular metabolism, frequently associated with an uncoupling of oxidative phosphorylation. This may be seen in the setting of disseminated malignancy or certain toxins, including cyanide, phenformin, and salicylates. The prognosis of lactic acidosis depends on the reversal of the underlying illness. If the underlying illness cannot be identified or corrected, as is more often the case in type B lactic acidosis, then the prognosis tends to be extremely grave.

The role of bicarbonate therapy in patients with lactic acidosis has become a point of considerable controversy in the literature. However, the arguments can be distilled into a simple issue: is the bicarbonate therapy more helpful than harmful? In a 1986 editorial, Stacpoole[15] argued against the routine use of bicarbonate therapy in patients with lactic acidosis. He emphasized the failure of any scientific study to demonstrate a relationship between the amount of bicarbonate administered to patients with lactic acidosis and the eventual outcome. He also cited experimental studies that bicarbonate administration results in the paradoxic acidification of the spinal fluid, increases carbon dioxide production, and may increase lactic acid production, all resulting in a potential exacerbation rather than amelioration of the acidosis. In a 1987 rebuttal article, however, Narins and Cohen[16] addressed each of these arguments one by one and concluded that the evidence regarding the dangers of indiscriminate use of alkali therapy in lactic acidosis was not convincing and was outweighed by the potential benefits in terms of cardiovascular stability.

It is clear that no consensus exists regarding the role of bicarbonate therapy in the treatment of lactic acidosis. If the underlying disease cannot be identified and/or reversed, the prognosis remains poor with or without bicarbonate therapy. The major role of bicarbonate therapy in this setting is to improve cardiovascular performance, which may, at least theoretically, enhance tissue oxygen delivery and decrease lactate production. The dose and rate of bicarbonate administration should be chosen to bring plasma pH up to approximately 7.20, minimizing fluid overload and hypernatremia.

Some of the arguments leveled against bicarbonate therapy in lactic acidosis have been addressed with alternate alkalizing agents. These include sodium carbonate (Na_2CO_3) and dichloroacetate (DCA). Carbicarb is an equimolar solution of sodium bicarbonate and sodium carbonate that has the theoretical advantage of generating less carbon dioxide than bicarbonate alone, leading to less of a superimposed respiratory acidosis in patients with compromised ventilatory function. When sodium bicarbonate neutralizes a hydrogen ion, carbon dioxide and H_2O are generated. When sodium carbonate neutralizes a hydrogen ion, sodium bicarbonate is generated. Carbicarb has not yet been released by the Food and Drug Administration, and the clinical experience with this drug is limited, although preliminary results are encouraging.[17]

Dichloroacetate stimulates pyruvate dehydrogenase (PDH), thereby diverting pyruvate toward mitochondrial oxidation and decreasing lactate production. Although this concept is appealing and has proved beneficial in experimental animals, the results of DCA therapy in patients with lactic acidosis have been mixed.[18]

Post-ICU Phase

Most patients who develop metabolic acidosis in the critical care setting will not require chronic therapy for acidosis once their underlying disease has been corrected and their acidosis reversed. If the patient has recovered sufficiently from his acute illness for transfer to a non-ICU setting, the recurrence of metabolic acidosis will generally be a function of recurrence or exacerbation of the underlying illness. Measures to keep the underlying illness under control, such as appropriate insulin therapy for diabetics, maintenance of adequate tissue perfusion to prevent lactic acidosis, avoidance of toxins, and measures to maximize renal perfusion, should all minimize the recurrence of metabolic acidosis. Two forms of chronic metabolic acidosis, however, may require ongoing bicarbonate therapy. These have been alluded to in the previous section and include the renal acidosis and chronic diarrhea.

Renal Acidosis

Once the presenting acidosis has been corrected, patients with metabolic acidosis secondary to chronic renal insufficiency or distal renal tubular acidosis may require ongoing bicarbonate therapy. The daily bicarbonate dose required to maintain a steady-state plasma bicarbonate concentration can be determined by estimating the daily endogenous acid production (approximately 1 mEq/kg body weight) and subtracting the daily net acid excretion (urinary ammonium plus urinary titratable acid minus urinary bicarbonate). Even if daily net acid excretion is 0, the maximum daily supplement that would be required to maintain a stable plasma bicarbonate concentration would be 1 mEq/kg body weight, or 60 to 70 mEq per day in the average individual. Each 650-mg sodium bicarbonate tablet contains approximately 8 mEq of bicarbonate, so that no patient with a renal acidosis should require more than about eight sodium bicarbonate tablets per day to maintain a stable plasma bicarbonate concentration. Most patients will actually require less, because they will have some net acid excretion. The major concern in patients with renal insufficiency is the sodium load that accompanies bicarbonate administration and that often will require a higher dose of loop diuretic to promote urinary sodium excretion. Patients with chronic renal insufficiency and the hyperkalemic form of renal tubular acidosis (type 4) may also benefit from chronic administration of synthetic mineralocorticoid (9-fludrocortisone) in doses generally higher than that required for adrenal replacement therapy in patients with Addison's disease, because patients with renal disease often have some resistance to the effects of mineralocorticoid. 9-Fludrocortisone (Florinef) doses of 0.5 to 1.0 mg per day are often required in patients with type 4 renal tubular acidosis to control hyperkalemia. Because of the sodium retention induced by the mineralocorticoid, again, higher doses of loop diuretic may be required in these individuals.

Chronic Diarrhea

Patients with chronic refractory diarrhea may have ongoing bicarbonate requirements, which can be substantial. An increasing number of patients with AIDS and cryptosporidium or other opportunistic diarrheas fall into this category. The coexistence of volume depletion or intrinsic renal disease may further compromise the kidneys' ability to regenerate bicarbonate in this setting, underscoring the role of adequate sodium and fluid replacement to maximize sodium delivery to the distal nephron where it can be exchanged for hydrogen and bicarbonate regenerated to replace diarrheal losses. Liquid stool can be measured for electrolyte content, and an appropriate prescription can be determined to replace those electrolytes either orally or intravenously. Because these patients may also have substantial potassium losses in the diarrheal fluid, care must be taken to adequately replace potassium as well as bicarbonate, so the alkalinization of the plasma does not compound the hypokalemia by producing a shift of potassium into cells.

METABOLIC ALKALOSIS

Pre-ICU Phase

Metabolic alkalosis is the most common acid/base disorder among hospitalized patients, accounting for 51% of acid/base disturbances in one study.[19] The diagnosis of a metabolic alkalosis is made on the basis of an elevated blood pH (greater than 7.44) in the presence of a normal or high Pco_2. In a simple metabolic alkalosis, the pH will be elevated and the plasma bicarbonate will also be greater than normal (25 to 28 mEq/L). Especially in the critically ill patient, however, metabolic alkalosis often coexists with other acid/base abnormalities, particularly metabolic acidosis. If a metabolic alkalosis coexists with a metabolic acidosis with an increased anion gap, the resulting pH may be low, normal or high, depending on which disorder predominates. An important clue to the presence of a metabolic alkalosis in this setting is the degree to which the serum anion gap is elevated above normal, because once the metabolic acidosis is corrected, the anions will be metabolized back to bicarbonate. Therefore, the theoretical serum bicarbonate concentration, if the metabolic acidosis were not present, equals the patient's actual serum bicarbonate concentration plus the increase in the anion gap over normal. If this sum exceeds 28 mEq/L, then a metabolic alkalosis is present.

As an example, a patient with diabetic ketoacidosis and vomiting might have an anion gap of 25 mEq/L and a plasma bicarbonate concentration of 20 mEq/L. The theoretical bicarbonate concentration would equal the increase in the anion gap over normal (25 − 12 = 13) plus the actual bicarbonate concentration (20 mEq/L) equals 33 mEq/L, demonstrating the presence of a "hidden" metabolic alkalosis.

Mechanisms of Metabolic Alkalosis

The development of metabolic alkalosis requires two phases: generation and maintenance. Often, the factors involved in each of these two are different, and successful treatment of metabolic alkalosis requires that the factors related to both phases be corrected. In simplest terms, metabolic alkalosis represents an excess of alkali in the extracellular fluid. This can be due to the following:

- Alkali administration
- Loss of acid from the extracellular fluid leaving alkali behind
- Loss of a fluid with a higher chloride/bicarbonate ratio than that of the plasma

The last example, which is often termed a contraction alkalosis, results from the fact that the total extracellular fluid bicarbonate remains relatively constant, while the fluid in which that bicarbonate is dissolved decreases, resulting in a relative increase in bicarbonate concentration. The loss of extracellular fluid in which the electrolytes are identical to that of plasma, such as in the case of hemorrhage, will not result in a contraction alkalosis and, more often, results in metabolic acidosis if shock supervenes. Diuretics induce the elaboration of a relatively chloride-rich urine and, although "contraction" may be one of the mechanisms by which these agents induce metabolic alkalosis, many other factors are clearly involved.

The second phase in the development of a metabolic alkalosis is the maintenance phase. The kidney normally defends against an abnormal rise in plasma bicarbonate concentration by limiting reabsorption of filtered bicarbonate in the proximal tubule, so that excess bicarbonate is rapidly excreted. As a result, the administration of alkali, in the absence of any other factors that affect renal bicarbonate handling, will rarely result in the generation of a metabolic alkalosis, because the administered alkali will be rapidly excreted in the urine. A variety of factors, however, may lead to augmented bicarbonate reabsorption by the proximal tubule and include the following:

- Volume contraction
- Hypokalemia
- Increased mineralocorticoid activity
- Hypercapnia

In the setting of hypovolemia, the proximal tubule will attempt to reabsorb as much filtered sodium as possible with available filtered chloride. Once the filtered chloride is exhausted through reabsorption, however, the proximal tubule continues to attempt to reabsorb sodium and will do so with the other available anion, bicarbonate. The net effect is that the organism will defend extracellular fluid volume at the expense of acid/base balance, resulting in the maintenance of a higher than normal plasma bicarbonate concentration and a metabolic alkalosis. The majority of cases of metabolic alkalosis encountered in the critical care setting are related to some form of chloride depletion, usually accompanied by volume contraction. This is often compounded by the development of hypokalemia resulting from urinary potassium wasting as the kidney attempts to conserve sodium in the distal tubule through sodium-potassium exchange. Stimulation of the renin-angiotensin-aldosterone axis through volume depletion further augments the urinary potassium losses and can also lead to additional bicarbonate reabsorption in the distal tubule through sodium-hydrogen exchange. The net effect is that even though only one factor, such as vomiting, may have led to the generation of metabolic alkalosis, a number of factors may be involved in the maintenance of metabolic alkalosis, and all these factors must be addressed before the metabolic alkalosis can be corrected.[20,21]

Consequences of Metabolic Alkalosis

As noted previously, metabolic alkalosis often occurs in the setting of other fluid and electrolyte disorders, and therefore, the consequences of the metabolic alkalosis per se on organ function may be difficult to assess. Severe metabolic alkalosis may lead to increased ventricular ectopic activity, but because these cases almost invariably have coexisting hypokalemia, the contribution of the metabolic alkalosis is unclear. Severe metabolic alkalosis may also lead to encephalopathic changes, but again, coexisting hypoxemia resulting from compensatory hypoventilation may also play a role. Alkalemia decreases free calcium concentration by increasing calcium-protein binding, leading to an increased risk of tetany and seizures. In the patient with hepatic disease, alkalemia shifts ammonium equilibrium to the uncharged ammonia form, which more easily penetrates the blood-brain barrier and may compound hepatic encephalopathy. Of course, the underlying disease associated with metabolic alkalosis may also lead to significant organ dysfunction. The development of severe metabolic alkalosis in the critically ill patient is an ominous prognostic sign because of the grave nature of the underlying illnesses involved, and mortality approaches 40% once serum pH rises above 7.55.

Risk Factors for the Development of Metabolic Alkalosis

The most common scenarios leading to the development of metabolic alkalosis in the ICU patient follow (Table 38-6):

- Prolonged vomiting
- Nasogastric suction
- Use of diuretics
- Alkali administration
- Correction of hypercapnia in a patient with chronic respiratory acidosis

Vomiting/Nasogastric Suction. The loss of gastric fluid, which is rich in hydrochloric acid, leads to the development of metabolic alkalosis through several mechanisms. Most simply, the loss of hydrogen ion leaves bicarbonate behind in the extracellular fluid, raising plasma bicarbonate concentration as this bicarbonate is no longer neutralized by the absorption of gastric juice by the intestine. This alone, however, does not lead to the development of metabolic alkalosis, because the normal kidney excretes the excess bicarbonate. The key to the maintenance of the metabolic alkalosis in this setting is the chloride and volume depletion. Volume depletion stimulates the kidney to reabsorb filtered sodium, and because less chloride is available in the proximal tubule to be reabsorbed along with the sodium, bicarbonate reabsorption increases to maintain electroneutrality. The hypokalemia that often accompanies vomiting or nasogastric suction is not due to potassium loss through the vomitus but rather to increased renal potassium excretion, as sodium-potassium exchange is accelerated in the distal tubule. The hypokalemia further accelerates bicarbonate reabsorption in the proximal tubule as well as hydrogen secretion in the distal tubule, leading to the elaboration of an acid urine despite the systemic alkalosis. This has often been termed the "paradoxical aciduria" of metabolic alkalosis. As might be expected, because the kidney attempts to reabsorb so-

Table 38-6. Causes of Metabolic Alkalosis

Cause	Mechanism	Urine Chloride	Treatment
Chloride responsive			
Vomiting, nasogastric suction	Loss of HCl from body, leaving HCO_3^- behind; increased renal absorption of HCO_3^- that is due to volume depletion	Zero or near zero	Provision of Cl^-, restoration of ECV
Diuretic therapy	Cl^- loss in urine, ECV depletion, increased renal HCO_3^- generation, hypokalemia, hypomagnesemia	High during diuretic use; zero or near zero following diuretic use	Provision of Cl^- as NaCl and KCl; restoration of ECV
Posthypercapnia	Renal excretion of acid and generation of HCO_3^- during respiratory acidosis	Zero or near zero	Provision of Cl^-
Chloride resistant			
Minaralocorticoid excess (Cushing's syndrome, hyperaldosteronism, exogenous steroids, renal artery stenosis)	Direct stimulation of Na^+-H^+ and Na^+-K^+ exchange in distal nephron; increased generation of HCO_3^- in distal nephron; increased reabsorption of HCO_3^- in proximal nephron that is due to hypokalemia	High (> 15 mEq/L)	Correction of underlying disorder, spironolactone, K^+ replacement
Bartter's syndrome	Proximal Cl^- reabsorption defect in kidney leading to increased Na^+-H^+ and Na^+-K^+ exchange in distal nephron	High (> 15 mEq/L)	K^+ replacement, nonsteroidal anti-inflammatory drugs, ? ECV expansion
Excessive alkali administration	Usually requires presence of some renal insufficiency; may be due to massive blood transfusions (citrate), hyperalimentation solutions or milk-alkali syndrome	High (> 15 mEq/L)	Cessation of all alkali administration
Severe potassium depletion (K^+ < 2 mEq/L)	Impairment of renal Cl^- reabsorption, leading to increased Na^+-H^+ exchange and generation of HCO_3^-	High (> 15 mEq/L)	K^+ repletion

ECV, extracellular volume.

dium with as much chloride as is available, urinary chloride will be extremely low in the setting of metabolic alkalosis that is due to vomiting or nasogastric suction, and this can often be an important clue to the cause.

Diuretics. Use of diuretics is perhaps the most common cause of metabolic alkalosis in the hospitalized patient. Diuretics promote the development of the metabolic alkalosis through several mechanisms:

The extracellular volume depletion that results from a successful diuresis stimulates the renin-angiotensin-aldosterone axis. Sodium, which may previously have been reabsorbed in the proximal portions of the nephron, is now delivered to the distal tubule, where increased aldosterone activity promotes sodium-hydrogen exchange, leading to the increased generation of bicarbonate, which is returned to the extracellular fluid.

The relatively chloride-rich urine leads to a chloride-depleted state so that the kidney attempts to reabsorb sodium in the proximal tubule with the alternate available anion, bicarbonate, leading to an increase in plasma bicarbonate concentration.

Increased sodium delivery and increased aldosterone activity in the distal tubule lead to increased sodium-potassium exchange and potassium excretion. The resulting hypokalemia increases bicarbonate reabsorption in the proximal tubule and sodium-hydrogen exchange in the distal tubule, resulting in the further generation of bicarbonate, which is delivered to the extracellular fluid.

Diuretic-induced magnesium losses further impair renal potassium conservation, compounding hypokalemia, and further promoting bicarbonate generation and retention by the kidney. Diuretic-induced magnesium depletion is often not appreciated, and magnesium deficits must be repaired before the kidney can adequately conserve potassium and metabolic alkalosis can be corrected in this setting.

Alkali Administration. Alkali administration generally does not result in the development of metabolic alkalosis unless the kidneys' ability to excrete that alkali is impaired. Such an impairment may be physiologic or pathologic. Physiologic examples include the administration of alkali in the setting of volume depletion, in which the kidney chooses to retain the sodium with the bicarbonate anion provided, or hypokalemia, in which accelerated renal sodium-hydrogen exchange allows for reabsorption of additional filtered bicarbonate. Renal insufficiency will also lead to an impaired ability to excrete an alkali load because fewer functioning nephrons are available to excrete the alkali. The most common sources of exogenous alkali in hospitalized patients are intravenous fluids including Ringer's lactate, parenteral nutrition (which contains lactate or acetate), and the citrate that is contained in whole blood as an anticoagulant.[22] Patients receiving large quantities of these fluids in the setting of volume depletion or renal insufficiency often develop a transient metabolic alkalosis, but this will generally impair itself if adequate chloride is administered to replace the retained bicarbonate.

Chronic Hypercapnia. Patients with chronic hypercapnia will develop a compensated respiratory acidosis with an elevated plasma bicarbonate concentration. If these patients experience a sudden improvement in their ventilation, most commonly following intubation, then the elevated plasma bicarbonate will persist following normalization of the P_{CO_2}, and a metabolic alkalosis will result.

Mineralocorticoid Excess. States of mineralocorticoid excess, either primary or secondary, are associated with metabolic alkalosis (see Table 38-6). In primary hyperaldosteronism, enhanced reabsorption of sodium in the distal nephron in exchange for potassium and hydrogen leads to intravascular volume expansion and the development of a hypokalemic metabolic alkalosis. Increased extracellular fluid volume suppresses sodium-chloride reabsorption in the proximal tubule, so that urinary chloride excretion is enhanced. On the other hand, these individuals continue to waste potassium in the urine despite decreasing serum potassium concentrations; the hypokalemia, along with increased bicarbonate generation through sodium-hydrogen exchange, maintains the metabolic alkalosis. Secondary hyperaldosteronism is associated with states of effective intravascular volume depletion, such as congestive heart failure, cirrhosis with ascites, and nephrotic syndrome. In these individuals, decreased effective renal perfusion leads to stimulation of the renin-angiotensin-aldosterone axis. However, because proximal tubular reabsorption of sodium is enhanced in these individuals, relatively little sodium is delivered to the distal tubule to be exchanged for hydrogen or potassium ion, and therefore, metabolic alkalosis generally does not occur unless these patients are treated with a diuretic. Diuretic therapy suppresses proximal sodium reabsorption, delivering more sodium to the distal nephron, where high aldosterone activity promotes sodium reabsorption in exchange for potassium and hydrogen excretion, resulting in a hypokalemic metabolic alkalosis.

ICU Phase

Evaluation of the Patient With Metabolic Alkalosis

The initial steps in the evaluation of the patient with metabolic alkalosis are obviously directed at identifying those factors that may have precipitated the alkalosis as well as determining the patient's volume status. A thorough history and review of the hospital record should be performed to identify factors such as vomiting, nasogastric suction, the administration of diuretics or alkali, other extracellular fluid losses that may have led to depletion of chloride, potassium or magnesium, and changes in the patient's ventilatory status. A thorough physical examination should be performed to identify signs of extracellular fluid volume depletion including postural changes in pulse or blood pressure, dry skin and mucous membranes, and decreased skin turgor. New-onset or difficult to control hypertension may be a sign of mineralocorticoid excess. The presence of edema or a history of an edematous condition such as congestive heart failure, cirrhosis with ascites, or nephrotic syndrome may be associated with secondary hyperaldosteronism. Secondary hyperaldosteronism may also be associated with renal artery stenosis, the signs of which may include an abdominal bruit and accelerated hypertension.

The initial laboratory evaluation of the patient with metabolic alkalosis should be directed at differentiating the chloride-responsive from the chloride-resistant forms of the syndrome (see Table 38-6). The chloride-responsive forms, including diuretic therapy, vomiting, nasogastric suction, posthypercapnia, and other high chloride extracellular fluid losses, will be associated with a low urinary chloride concentration, generally less than 15 mEq/L. The chloride-resistant forms of metabolic alkalosis, including the hypermineralocorticoid states, severe magnesium and potassium deficiency, Bartter's syndrome, and massive alkali administration in the setting of renal disease will be associated with a high urinary chloride concentration, generally greater than 15 mEq/L. If the patient with chloride depletion that is due to diuretic therapy is evaluated for urinary chloride while receiving diuretics, of course, a high urinary chloride concentration may be found, which might be deceptive. Therefore, urinary chloride determinations should be performed only after the patient has been withdrawn from diuretic therapy for at least 24 hours.

The measurement of other electrolyte concentrations may also be helpful in the differential diagnosis as well as the treatment of patients with metabolic alkalosis. Although serum potassium concentration is generally low in patients with metabolic alkalosis, the presence of an extremely low serum potassium concentration (less than 2 mEq/L) is suggestive of primary hyperaldosteronism or prolonged diuretic therapy. A complete set of electrolytes and arterial blood gases should be drawn so that coexisting acid/base disorders can be identified. Recall that in patients with metabolic acidosis and an elevated anion gap, the increase in the anion gap over normal should be added to the plasma bicarbonate concentration to determine the "theoretic" bicarbonate concentration and identify a "hidden" metabolic alkalosis. The serum magnesium level should be determined to rule out hypomagnesemia as a cause of or contributing factor to the alkalosis and hypokalemia.

Treatment of Metabolic Alkalosis

Several strategies are appropriate for the treatment of all forms of metabolic alkalosis. As noted previously, the initial evaluation is directed at determining whether the alkalosis falls into the chloride-responsive or chloride-resistant category. In any event, associated fluid and electrolyte disturbances should be identified and treated simultaneously with the treatment of the metabolic alkalosis. All forms of metabolic alkalosis have both a generation and maintenance phase. The underlying factors relating to the generation of metabolic alkalosis must be identified and reversed. However, unless the factors contributing to the maintenance of the metabolic alkalosis are also identified and corrected, the metabolic alkalosis will persist. The most common factors contributing to the maintenance of metabolic alkalosis are extracellular volume depletion and hypokalemia. Even after the initiating event, such as diuretic therapy or nasogastric suction, has been terminated, unless accumulated fluid and potassium deficits are repaired, the metabolic alkalosis will not be reversed.

Chloride-Responsive Metabolic Alkalosis. Obviously, the mainstay in the treatment of the chloride-responsive forms of metabolic alkalosis is chloride. If the patient has signs of extracellular volume depletion, then much of this chloride can be administered as a saline solution, to address both the volume and chloride deficit. Potassium chloride will address the hypokalemia as well as the chloride deficit. If the patient with a chloride-responsive metabolic alkalosis has neither extracellular fluid volume depletion nor hypokalemia, then consideration should be given to administering the chloride as hydrochloric acid.

The volume of sodium chloride to be administered to a patient with metabolic alkalosis and decreased extracellular fluid volume can be estimated by calculating the chloride deficit. One subtracts the patient's serum chloride concentration from a target value of 100 mEq/L, then multiplies this value by the volume of distribution of chloride, which is approximately 27% of body weight. As an example, if a 70-kg patient has a serum chloride concentration of 80 mEq/L, then the chloride deficit would be equal to the following:

$$(100 - 80) \times 0.27 \times 70 \text{ kg} = 370 \text{ mEq}$$

This deficit would be corrected by the infusion of 2.4 L of 0.9% sodium chloride (normal saline), each liter of which contains 154 mEq of chloride. This volume of saline is generally administered over the first 24 hours, with additional fluids administered as necessary to replace ongoing losses.

Potassium therapy is also essential in the treatment of metabolic alkalosis because administered chloride cannot be retained as long as substantial potassium deficits persist. The calculation of potassium replacement is discussed more fully in the section on hypokalemia but, as a rule, patients with hypokalemic metabolic alkalosis generally require the addition of 40 mEq of potassium chloride to each liter of intravenous normal saline administered. Additional potassium supplements may be required in the setting of profound hypokalemia. Magnesium supplementation, also as the chloride salt, is indicated in patients with hypomagnesemia as administered potassium cannot be retained in a setting of severe magnesium deficits.

The treatment of chloride-responsive metabolic alkalosis in the edematous patient is somewhat more challenging. In this setting, large infusions of saline would provide replacement chloride but would compound the edema. Furthermore, because the sodium-retaining state is a function of decreased effective renal perfusion and not true volume depletion, administered chloride is less likely to suppress renal sodium bicarbonate reabsorption and correct the metabolic alkalosis. In patients with severe metabolic alkalosis and edema, one also cannot administer the required chloride as the potassium salt, because this would pose a risk for hyperkalemia because of the large amounts of potassium required. The administration of hydrochloric acid may be the only option to repair the chloride deficit and to provide hydrogen ion to neutralize excess extracellular bicarbonate.[23] As a rule, a 0.1% normal hydrochloric acid solution (100 mEq/L hydrogen ion) is preferred because it approximates the acid content of the stomach and is reasonably well tolerated when administered through a central vein. Hydrochloric acid cannot be administered through a peripheral vein because of its tendency to cause sclerosis. Because of its potential toxicity, hydrochloric acid is generally reserved for patients with severe metabolic alkalosis (pH greater than 7.50) and the dose administered is generally that required to improve the systemic consequences of the alkalosis but not to completely correct the alkalosis. In estimating the dose of hydrochloric acid to be administered, a target bicarbonate concentration of 35 mEq/L is generally chosen. If a 70-kg person presents with a serum bicarbonate concentration of 45 mEq/L, the the required hydrochloric acid dose would be equal to 45 minus 35 mEq/L times volume distribution of bicarbonate, which is 50% of the body weight. In this individual, the required hydrochloric acid dose would equal the following:

$$10 \times 0.5 \times 70 = 350 \text{ mEq/L}$$

This would equal 3.5 L of a 0.1% normal hydrochloric acid solution, which is administered over at least 24 hours.

Because of the sclerosing property of a pure hydrochloric acid solution, the use of a buffered hydrochloric acid solution such as ammonium chloride or arginine hydrochloride has been proposed. These solutions, however, may be contraindicated in selected patients. Ammonium chloride should not be used in patients with liver disease, because it will increase blood ammonia levels and contribute to hepatic encephalopathy. The administration of arginine hydrochloride has been associated with the development of life-threatening hyperkalemia in patients with renal insufficiency.[24] Some evidence indicates that hydrochloric acid can be administered safely through a peripheral vein when infused along with a fat emulsion.[25]

In patients with metabolic alkalosis, attempts should be made to minimize administration of additional alkali. The buffer content of intravenous hyperalimentation solutions should be reduced. Patients with chloride-responsive metabolic alkalosis and volume overload may actually benefit from the administration of loop diuretics and intravenous replacement of urinary volume with normal saline. Although it may appear paradoxic to treat a chloride-responsive alkalosis with additional diuretics, the resulting urine will generally have a chloride concentration of less than 150 mEq/L and, therefore, replacement with normal saline will result in net chloride administration. Patients with metabolic alkalosis, volume overload, and renal failure who are refractory to diuretics may require some form of dialytic therapy to correct the metabolic alkalosis. Peritoneal dialysis solutions typically contain 40 mEq/L of lactate as the bicarbonate precursor and are, therefore, relatively ineffective in correcting metabolic alkalosis. The solutions used in hemodialysis generally contain 35 mEq/L of bicarbonate (or acetate as the bicarbonate precursor) and may provide a gradient for the removal of bicarbonate in patients with severe metabolic alkalosis and a serum bicarbonate concentration of more than 40 mEq/L. If hemodialysis is unavailable or the patient is hemodynamically unstable, continuous arteriovenous hemofiltration (CAVH) will remove large quantities of extracellular fluid while allowing for the infusion of chloride-containing solutions to raise plasma chloride concentration and correct the metabolic alkalosis. If fluid overload is present, the rate of administration of replacement fluids is less than that of the ultrafiltration, leading to a net reduction of extracellular fluid volume.

When continuous nasogastric suction or vomiting contributes to the persistence of metabolic alkalosis, the use of an intravenous H_2 blocker such as ranitidine will suppress gastric acid secretion and reduce further hydrogen ion loss.[26] Such an agent will only be effective if gastric drainage is, in fact, acidic, which can be confirmed by determining the pH of the gastric fluid. The dose of the H_2 blocker should be titrated to maintain gastric fluid pH above 5. The use of H_2 blockers will not correct the metabolic alkalosis that has already developed; the prophylactic use of H_2 blockers to prevent the development of metabolic alkalosis should be considered in patients who may require prolonged nasogastric suction.

Carbonic anhydrase inhibitors such as acetazolamide (250 to 500 mg, three to four times daily) inhibit bicarbonate reabsorption in the proximal tubule and lead to increased excretion of bicarbonate and sodium in the urine. They may be helpful in the treatment of metabolic alkalosis in the setting of increased extracellular fluid volume. It is still necessary to correct the underlying problem, however, and the carbonic anhydrase inhibitors may be associated with increased urinary potassium loss and decreased extracellular fluid volume, which may tend to compound the alkalosis. Therefore, the use of the carbonic anhydrase inhibitors should be considered a temporizing measure only, until the underlying problem can be corrected.

Chloride-Resistant Metabolic Alkalosis. Patients with chloride-resistant metabolic alkalosis do not have a chloride deficit and typically have a urinary chloride concentration of greater than 15 mEq/L. As a result, they do not respond to chloride-containing solutions and, because extracellular fluid volume is normal, administered chloride is rapidly excreted in the urine. Because the primary defect is generally an increase in mineralocorticoid activity, saline administration may actually worsen the hypokalemia by enhancing sodium presentation to the distal nephron where it is exchanged for excreted potassium.

In patients with hypokalemic metabolic alkalosis, hypertension, and a urinary chloride concentration of greater than 15 mEq/L, a diagnosis of hyperaldosteronism should be considered. If this is due to an adrenal adenoma, removal of the adenoma is curative. If the lesion is nonresectable, then the treatment is to block the action of the aldosterone with an antagonist such as spironolactone or amiloride. Because the associated hypokalemia maintains the alkalosis by enhancing bicarbonate reabsorption in the proximal renal tubule, potassium replacement is necessary in these individuals to correct the alkalosis.

Bartter's syndrome is a relatively rare disorder that produces a chloride-resistant metabolic alkalosis. Enhanced renal prostaglandin activity appears to be a contributing factor in this syndrome, and use of nonsteroidal anti-inflammatory agents, particularly indomethacin, has proved useful in correcting the alkalosis. Potassium supplementation is also required to repair the associated potassium deficit. Bartter's syndrome may be difficult to distinguish from surreptitious diuretic abuse and forced vomiting. The former may be identified by performing a diuretic assay on the patient's urine. Patients with prolonged surreptitious vomiting may become sufficiently hypokalemic that they convert to a chloride-resistant metabolic alkalosis and may have high urinary chloride concentrations. In such cases, the only clue to the vomiting may be the demonstration of an acid pH in the patient's oropharynx.

Post-ICU Phase

Because a majority of the causes of metabolic alkalosis in the hospitalized patient are related to iatrogenic factors such as administration of diuretics, nasogastric suction, and alkali, follow-up treatment of these patients should be directed at avoiding these interventions or taking steps to minimize the recurrence of metabolic alkalosis in patients at risk. As a rule, patients most prone to the development of metabolic alkalosis are those with renal insufficiency or volume depletion in whom the ability of the kidneys to adapt to hydrogen ion loss or alkali administration is compromised. In those patients at greatest risk or in whom prolonged alkalosis-inducing interventions are contemplated, steps should be taken to minimize the development of metabolic alkalosis by addressing the perturbations in electrolyte balance before they occur. For example, in patients requiring prolonged nasogastric suction, adequate replacement fluids, sodium, potassium, and chloride should be administered before hypokalemia or alkalosis develops, and the use of H_2 antagonists should be considered if the pH of the gastric aspirate is less than 5. For patients requiring substantial or prolonged diuretic therapy, consider the concomitant use of a potassium-sparing diuretic such as spironolactone, amiloride, or triamterene, especially if the patient has an underlying condition leading to stimulation of the renin-angiotensin-aldosterone axis, such as congestive heart failure, nephrotic syndrome, or cirrhosis with ascites. In the diuretic-treated patient, be sure to repair potassium deficits with supplemental potassium before potassium depletion itself begins to contribute to the alkalosis. In patients receiving intravenous hyperalimentation, especially in the presence of renal insufficiency, frequent monitoring of electrolytes is vital. Daily adjustments in the hyperalimentation formula may be necessary to repair potassium and magnesium deficits as well as to provide the proper balance of chloride and alkali to correct an acid/base disorder.

DISTURBANCES OF PLASMA OSMOLALITY

Hyponatremia and hypernatremia are disorders of plasma osmolality in which excessive renal water retention or excess water excretion, respectively, occurs. Despite great variations in daily dietary salt and water intake, the extracellular fluid (ECF) volume and plasma osmolality are kept remarkably constant by a complex regulatory system. A fall in plasma osmolality, of which the chief component is the serum sodium concentration, is detected by osmoreceptors in the anterior hypothalamus, which then suppresses antidiuretic hormone (ADH) release. Conversely, increases in plasma osmolality result in increased ADH secretion as well as stimulation of the thirst center in the hypothalamus. ADH, also known as arginine vasopressin, is a polypeptide released from the pituitary gland, which exerts its effects on the renal cortical and medullary collecting tubules. Without ADH, these tubules are unable to reabsorb water and a dilute urine results. When plasma osmolality rises, the collecting tubule under the influence of ADH becomes permeable to water, an antidiuresis or water retention results, and the plasma osmolality can return to normal without any change in the total body sodium. Antidiuretic hormone is also released in response to such nonosmotic stimuli as volume depletion, cardiac failure, adrenal insufficiency, pain, and emotional stress. The ADH response to volume depletion is mediated by the left atrial and carotid baroreceptors and is less sensitive than the osmotic response. In addition, when ECF volume falls, decreased left ventricular filling pressure and mean arterial pressure are detected by the baroreceptors, and the renin-angiotensin system is activated. This stimulates aldosterone release, and the actions of these hormones on the kidney result in sodium retention.

Hyponatremia

Pre-ICU Phase

Hyponatremia is the most common electrolyte disturbance seen in the critically ill patient (Table 38-7). In true hyponatremia, the serum sodium is below 135 mEq/L, and a hypo-osmolar state exists. In pseudohyponatremia, the serum sodium concentration is below 135 mEq/L, but the plasma osmolality is either high, as in hyperglycemia, or normal, as in hyperlipidemia or glycine toxicity.[27] The severity of the illness and urgency with which this problem must be addressed depend on the depth of the sodium level, the age of the patient, and most importantly, the rate at which the hyponatremia developed. Acute hyponatremia develops in less than 48 hours, whereas the chronic form develops over a longer period. Hyponatremia is a disorder of water, not of sodium balance. A low serum sodium concentration can occur when total body sodium is low, normal, or even high. In hyponatremia, there is always a decrease in the proportion of salt to water. In **hypovolemic hyponatremia,** there is loss of salt and water with a greater loss of salt. The losses may be renal or extrarenal, and if these losses are replaced by free water, the hyponatremia worsens.

A typical patient with an extrarenal hypovolemic hyponatremia repeatedly vomits over several days and ingests only a "tea and toast" diet. Renal hypovolemic hyponatremia is not uncommonly seen in the elderly white female who several weeks before her presentation was started on thiazide diuretic therapy. It is unclear why this population is so susceptible to this side effect of diuretic therapy, but the hyponatremia is due to the unique combination of effects caused by the thiazides.[28] In addition to potassium wasting and volume depletion, each of which can cause renal water retention, the thiazides, by their action on the distal tubule, cause salt wasting without the urinary dilution seen with the loop diuretics. The patient continues to drink water, diluting the extracellular sodium which remains, resulting in hyponatremia.

Hypervolemic hyponatremia occurs when there is an excess of both total body water and total body salt with a greater excess of water. Clinically, this is seen in the edematous states: nephrotic syndrome, cirrhosis, congestive heart failure, or renal failure.[29,30] A typical example is the patient with decompensated heart failure who presents with a serum sodium of 125 mEq/L. In this patient, cardiac output is so low that the kidneys "see" effective intravascular depletion and reabsorb more of the filtered load of salt and water in the proximal tubule, with decreased delivery of filtrate to the loop of Henle, where urinary dilution occurs. If free water is ingested in excess of the reduced urinary diluting capacity, it will be retained, and hyponatremia results.

Euvolemic hyponatremia is so named because the patient appears clinically euvolemic. The total body salt content is normal or slightly reduced, but there is an excess of total body water. This is usually due to the syndrome of inappropriate ADH (SIADH) production[31] (Table 38-8). A typical patient with euvolemic hyponatremia has SIADH that is due to a pulmonary or cerebral lesion of infectious or malignant origin. Drugs may also cause a euvolemic

Table 38–7. Hyponatremia: Clinical Settings

Disorder	Clinical Presentation	Differential Diagnosis	Laboratory Findings	Treatment
Pseudohyponatremia	Diabetic, obese	Hypertriglyceridemia Hyperglycemia	Posm, normal ↑Posm, ↓U_{Na}, ↑Uosm True serum sodium = measured serum sodium + 1.6 mEq/100 mg/dl of blood glucose > 180 mg/dl	Treat the underlying conditions
Hypovolemic hyponatremia	Volume depletion, nausea and vomiting, decreased oral salt intake, continued water intake	GI losses Skin losses Renal losses Secondary to diuretic use	↑Posm, ↓U_{Na}, ↑Uosm (↑U_{Na} if diuretic was recently taken)	Normal saline infusion
Hypervolemic hyponatremia	Edema	Congestive heart failure Cirrhosis Nephrotic syndrome	↓Posm, ↓U_{Na}, ↑Uosm	1. Fluid restriction 2. For serum Na < 120 mEq/L, give hypertonic saline
Euvolemic hyponatremia	Appears euvolemic	SIADH Hypothyroidism Hypoadrenalism	↓Posm, ↓U_{Na}, Uosm inappropriately high	1. Fluid restriction 2. Furosemide 40–80 mg qd 3. Demeclocycline 300–600 mg bid

GI, gastrointestinal; Posm, plasma osmolality; SIADH, syndrome of inappropriate antidiuretic hormone; U_{Na}, urine sodium; Uosm, urine osmolality.

Table 38–8. Causes of SIADH

Increased hypothalamic production of ADH
  Neurologic disorders
    Infection
    Inflammation
    Vascular disease
    Malignant disease
  Drugs
    Cyclophosphamide
    Carbamazepine
    Vincristine, vinblastine
    Monoamine oxidase inhibitors
  Pulmonary disease
    Pneumonia
    Tuberculosis
  Postoperative
  Idiopathic
  Psychosis
Ectopic ADH production
  Carcinoma
    Oat cell of lung
    Bronchogenic
    Pancreatic
  Pulmonary tuberculosis
Increased sensitivity to ADH
  Drugs
    Chlorpropamide
    Carbamazepine
    Cyclophosphamide
    Tolbutamide
  Psychosis

ADH, antidiuretic hormone; SIADH, syndrome of inappropriate antidiuretic hormone.

hyponatremia in several ways. Chlorpropamide acts to potentiate the effect of ADH on the distal tubule, whereas cyclophosphamide and carbamazepine cause both an increase in hypothalamic ADH production and an increase in tubular sensitivity to ADH. The hypothyroid or hypoadrenal patient may also present with hyponatremia that is due to excess ADH production. In hypothyroidism, the reason for excess ADH production is not well understood but is thought to be related to the decreased cardiac output and glomerular filtration rate that occur in this condition. The cause of excess ADH production in hypoadrenalism is controversial but appears to be related both to the negative sodium balance caused by mineralocorticoid deficiency and the inability to completely suppress ADH secretion, which occurs with glucocorticoid deficiency.[32]

Symptoms and Signs. The symptoms and signs of hyponatremia vary with the underlying cause, severity, and rate of development of the hyponatremia. At any reduced serum sodium level, the presentation is more dramatic if the hyponatremia develops over a short period. Symptoms include lethargy, disorientation, muscle cramps, nausea, and vomiting (which can also be a cause of hyponatremia), as well as agitation and encephalopathy. On physical examination, the patient may have altered mental status, depressed deep tendon reflexes, hypothermia, Cheyne-Strokes respirations, and depending on the cause of the hyponatremia, the patient may be edematous, dehydrated, or may appear euvolemic.

Laboratory Diagnosis. In addition to the history and physical examination, several laboratory and radiologic studies are useful in the diagnosis of hyponatremia (see Table 38-7). The serum sodium and plasma osmolality are determined to confirm the presence of hyponatremia and a true hypo-osmolar state. If the plasma osmolality is high, then pseudohyponatremia secondary to hyperglycemia should be ruled out. In hyperglycemia, the serum sodium is expected to decrease by 1.6 mEq/L for every 100 mg of glucose above 180 mg/dl. When the plasma osmolality is normal, hyperlipidemia or hyperproteinemia should be suspected, and serum triglyceride and total protein levels obtained. Next, the urine osmolality should be measured to determine whether the urine is maximally and appropriately dilute. A urine osmolality greater than 100 mOsm/kg suggests impaired renal water excretion. The urine sodium differentiates between intravascular volume depletion and the euvolemic states. Urine sodium is less than 15 mEq/L in volume depletion and the edematous states and greater than 20 mEq/L in euvolemic causes of hyponatremia.

Because SIADH is a diagnosis of exclusion that cannot be made in the presence of renal, thyroid or adrenal dysfunction, tests to rule out renal failure, hypothyroidism, and adrenal insufficiency as well as a urine drug screen, if indicated, should be obtained before making the diagnosis of SIADH (see Table 38-8).

ICU Phase

When does a hyponatremic patient require management in the ICU? Clearly, the patient with altered mental status and a serum sodium below 115 mEq/L should be admitted to the ICU until a diagnosis has been established and therapy instituted. In other situations, the decision is less clear and should be based on whether the patient needs ICU-level nursing care or frequent laboratory monitoring. In general, patients with neurologic signs and symptoms, those who are treated with hypertonic saline infusion, and those who require blood work more frequently than every 4 hours should be admitted to the ICU, although this should be left to the judgment of the physician and may vary with the facilities available at individual institutions (Table 38-9).

Much has been written about the management of hyponatremia in recent years, and the controversy revolves around the optimal rate of correction.[33-35] Evidence shows that, under certain conditions, rapid correction or normalization of the serum sodium may lead to central pontine myelinolysis (CPM), a neurologic syndrome that is characterized by paraparesis, dysarthria, dysphagia, coma, and possibly death. It is believed that this rare syndrome is caused by a rapid rise in plasma osmolality, which results in axonal shrinkage and cerebral demyelination. Patients most at risk for development of this syndrome are those who have had an episode of hypoxia or anoxia before the development and treatment of hyponatremia. Malnutrition, which may be seen in alcoholics and burn victims, an increase in serum sodium levels by more than 25 mEq/L during the first 48 hours of treatment, previous liver or central nervous system disease, advanced age, diuretic use, and female gender are also risk factors for the development of CPM. The most important consideration in the management of hyponatremia is the rate of development of the

Table 38-9. Sodium Replacement for Hyponatremia

General Guidelines
1. Patients with mild chronic hyponatremia that is due to one of the edematous states or SIADH may not need saline and often benefit from some combination of fluid restriction, diuretic therapy, or ADH inhibition.
2. Saline administration should be reserved for those patients who develop severe hyponatremia over a short period of time, those with serum sodium <115 mEq/L or those who have developed neurologic signs or symptoms.
3. Saline administration should not raise the serum sodium by more than 1–2 mEq/L/hr in acute hyponatremia or by 0.5–1.0 mEq/L/hr in chronic hyponatremia.
4. The rate of saline administration should be re-evaluated every 12 hours with the aid of frequent serum sodium measurements.

Dosage Calculation
Total Na deficit = 0.6 × lean body weight × (desired serum Na − measured sodium Na)
  0.9% saline = 155 mEq/L Na   Use when patient needs salt and water
  3.0% saline = 513 mEq/L Na   Use when patient needs salt alone

Example
What is the volume and rate of 0.9% or 3.0% saline that should be administered to a 70-kg patient to raise the serum sodium from 110 mEq/L to 116 mEq/L (0.5 mEq/L/hr) over 12 hr?
Na deficit = 0.6 × 70 kg (116 − 110) mEq/L = 252 mEq

$$\text{Volume 0.9\% saline} = \frac{252 \text{ mEq}}{155 \text{ mEq/L}} = 1625 \text{ ml}$$

$$\text{Rate 0.9\% saline} = \frac{1625 \text{ ml}}{12 \text{ hr}} = 135 \text{ ml/hr}$$

$$\text{Volume 3.0\% saline} = \frac{252 \text{ mEq}}{513 \text{ mEq/L}} = 491 \text{ ml}$$

$$\text{Rate 3.0\% saline} = \frac{491 \text{ ml}}{12 \text{ hr}} = 41 \text{ ml/hr}$$

ADH, antidiuretic hormone; SIADH, syndrome of inappropriate antidiuretic hormone.

---

hyponatremia, and the initial goal of therapy should be to raise serum sodium just enough to reverse the symptoms or to reach 120 mEq/L. If the hyponatremia is acute, then rapid correction, at a rate of 1 to 2 mEq/L per hour, in the first 24 hours is appropriate. In chronic hyponatremia, however, a slower rate of correction, 0.5 to 1 mEq/L per hour, is safer.

The next consideration is the underlying condition, particularly the volume and cardiac status of the patient. The hypovolemic hyponatremic patient requires salt and water and, therefore, is the easiest to manage. Such patients are treated with normal saline at a rate calculated to raise the serum sodium by no more than 2 mEq/L per hour in the acute situation or 1 mEq/L per hour in chronic hyponatremia. If the patient has congestive heart failure, then the rate may be lowered or small doses of furosemide given after several hours of volume repletion.

The hypervolemic hyponatremic patient is much more difficult to manage. If the hyponatremia is mild, chronic, and the patient is asymptomatic as in congestive heart failure, a trial of water restriction alone is reasonable. This is often unsuccessful because these patients may have excess thirst driven by their effective intravascular depletion. If the hyponatremia is severe, acute, or the patient is symptomatic as in decompensated cirrhosis, then cautious administration of hypertonic saline should be instituted. The reason for using hypertonic (3.0%) rather than normal (0.9%) saline is that the greater water content of the latter would compound the already volume-overloaded condition of these patients. The volume of hypertonic saline to be given is calculated to increase the serum sodium approximately 1 mEq/L per hour in acute cases and 0.5 mEq/L per hour in chronic cases. Patients who are at risk for pulmonary congestion can be given small doses of furosemide as well.

The euvolemic hyponatremic patient is usually less thirsty as a result of the mildly volume expanded state and can often be managed with fluid restriction alone. For patients with severe (less than 115 mEq/L) or symptomatic hyponatremia, a small amount of hypertonic saline calculated to raise the serum sodium to 120 mEq/L at 0.5 to 1.0 mEq/L per hour may be added. Patients in whom water restriction alone is insufficient to maintain a normal or near-normal serum sodium should be started on furosemide or demeclocycline. Furosemide 40 to 80 mg once daily and a liberal salt diet will lead to urinary dilution and net free water loss while demeclocycline, 300 to 600 mg twice daily, will interfere with ADH action on the distal tubule and, thereby, cause free water losses.[36,37]

In addition to therapy aimed at raising the serum sodium level, there should be frequent monitoring of the intake and output, serum and urine sodium determinations, and serial neurologic examinations as well as therapy specifically directed at correcting the underlying condition. Once the symptoms of hyponatremia have resolved, the serum sodium is above 120 mEq/L, the underlying condition has either resolved or stabilized, and there is no longer any indication for ICU-level nursing care, the patient may be transferred to a regular medical floor.

Post-ICU Phase

Following discharge from the ICU, serum sodium levels should be obtained daily until the level has returned to normal and the patient no longer requires intravenous sodium replacement. The patient with an irreversible underlying condition such as chronic SIADH or cirrhosis with ascites should continue to be water restricted. If this alone does not control the hyponatremia, then demeclocycline or furosemide should also be continued. In patients with hypervolemic hyponatremia, it is frequently not possible to raise their serum sodium levels above 130 mEq/L even with water restriction. Because they are usually asymptomatic at this level, such patients need no further therapy aimed at raising the serum sodium. An effort should be made, however, to avoid large amounts of hypotonic fluids or diuretics in these individuals.

Hypernatremia

Pre-ICU Phase

Hypernatremia is not as common as hyponatremia but is also a disorder of plasma osmolality.[38] In hypernatremia, the serum sodium is above 150 mEq/L and the plasma osmolality is high. The severity of the resulting symptoms depends on the rate of development of the hypernatremia; acute hypernatremia develops in less than 48 hours while chronic hypernatremia develops more slowly. There is always an increase in the proportion of salt to water, although total body sodium and water may be high or low. Because the thirst mechanism is a very effective defense against hypernatremia, only patients with altered thirst that is due to a hypothalamic lesion or patients who are unable to obtain water to satisfy their thirst, the very young, old, or sick will develop hypernatremia.[39]

In hypovolemic hypernatremia, there is a loss of both salt and water with a greater loss of water. These losses may be renal or nonrenal. A typical patient with renal hypovolemic hypernatremia may have central diabetes insipidus (CDI) that is due to a malignancy involving the hypothalamus or nephrogenic diabetes insipidus (NDI) that is due to lithium toxicity.[40] The typical patient with extrarenal hypovolemic hypernatremia is the burn victim whose enormous hypotonic insensible losses have been replaced with isotonic saline.

Hypervolemic hypernatremia occurs much less frequently than does hypovolemic hypernatremia and is usually iatrogenic. There is an excess of both salt and water with a greater excess of salt that is due to the administration of too much hypertonic saline or sodium bicarbonate especially in a patient who cannot excrete the salt and water load.

Symptoms and Signs. The hypernatremic patient frequently has preexisting mental status changes, and therefore, the signs and symptoms of hypernatremia may be missed. Although acute hypernatremia may present in a more dramatic fashion with seizures and coma, the patient with chronic hypernatremia may simply become more lethargic, weak, or irritable. On physical examination, the patient may be edematous or dehydrated depending on the underlying cause of the hypernatremia.

Laboratory Diagnosis. The history and physical examination are often not helpful in establishing a diagnosis in hypernatremia. In addition to the serum sodium and plasma osmolality to confirm the presence of a true hyperosmolar state, the most useful diagnostic test is the urine osmolality (Table 38-10). If the urine osmolality is greater than 800 mOsm/kg, this is an indication that ADH is being secreted and that the kidneys can elaborate a concentrated urine. In this situation, diagnostic considerations include severe dehydration, hypodipsia, or sodium overload. Urine

Table 38–10. Laboratory Findings in Hypernatremia

Uosm	Diagnostic Possibilities	Effect of Exogenous ADH
> 800 mOsm/Kg	Dehydration Hypodipsia Sodium overload	No need to give ADH
300–800 mOsm/kg	Partial CDI Partial NDI Osmotic diuresis	Increase in Uosm; decrease in Posm No change Slight increase in Uosm; decrease in Posm
< 300 mOsm/kg	CDI NDI	Increase in Uosm; decrease in Posm No change

ADH, antidiuretic hormone; CDI, central diabetes insipidus; NDI, nephrogenic diabetes insipidus; Uosm, urine osmolality; Posm, Plasma Osmolality.

osmolality between 300 and 800 mOsm/kg suggests a partial CDI, NDI, or the presence of a solute diuresis that is due to hyperglycemia, saline infusion, or the administration of high osmolality enteral tube feeds. If a solute or osmotic diuresis is suspected, then the urine concentration of sodium, urea, and glucose should be determined. Patients with a urine osmolality less than 300 mOsm/kg and hypernatremia are undergoing a water diuresis that is due to either lack of endogenous ADH secretion or resistance to ADH by the renal distal tubule. These patients, as well as patients with a urine osmolality between 300 and 800 mOsm/kg who are suspected of a partial central or nephrogenic diabetes insipidus should be transferred to the ICU and undergo the water-restriction test, which is described later in this chapter. A computed tomography (CT) scan of the head should also be obtained if a hypothalamic lesion is suspected.

ICU Phase

Diagnostic Considerations. It is not necessary to admit every hypernatremic patient to the ICU. Although there are no absolute criteria for admission, hypernatremic patients with severe mental status changes, serum sodium levels above 165 mEq/L, or whose underlying diagnosis is unknown should be managed in the ICU. Patients who require intensive nursing care or frequent laboratory determinations should also be admitted to ICU until their condition has stabilized. In patients suspected of diabetes insipidus, a water-restriction test should be performed. The patient is weighed and a baseline plasma and urine osmolality are obtained. The patient is then completely fluid restricted and the urine volume, urine osmolality, and body weight are measured hourly. The plasma osmolality and serum sodium are measured every 4 hours, and the test continues until

- Plasma osmolality reaches 300 mOsm/kg
- Urine osmolality stops rising
- Patient has lost 3% of his body weight

The patient is then given 5 units of aqueous vasopressin subcutaneously, and the hourly measurements are continued. Patients with normal hypothalamic and renal function

Table 38–11. Fluid Replacement in Hypernatremia

General Guidelines
1. Volume-expanded patient should be given a loop diuretic and the fluid losses replaced orally with water or intravenously with 5% dextrose in water.
2. Hypovolemic patient should first be given enough isotonic saline to correct the hypovolemia. The serum sodium should then be repeated and the water deficit calculated. The rate of water replacements should not decrease the serum sodium by more than 1–2 mEq/L/hr in acute hypernatremia or 0.5 mEq/L/hr in chronic hypernatremia.

Dosage Calculations

Body water deficit = desired total body water (TBW) − measured TBW

$$= \frac{\text{measured [Na]}}{\text{desired [Na]}} (0.6 \times \text{body weight}) - (0.6 \times \text{body weight})$$

$$= 0.6 \times \text{body weight} \left(\frac{\text{measured [Na]}}{\text{desired [Na]}} - 1 \right)$$

Example
What is the volume and rate of fluid administration for a 70-kg patient with a serum sodium of 165 mEq/L if the hypernatremia is acute?
Goal = to reduce serum sodium to normal (145 mEq/L)

$$\text{Volume body weight deficit} = 0.6 \times 70 \text{ kg} \left(\frac{165 \text{ mEq/L}}{145 \text{ mEq/L}} - 1 \right) = 5.79 \text{ L}$$

$$\text{Rate} \frac{5790 \text{ ml}}{24 \text{ hr}} = 241 \text{ ml/hr}$$

---

will respond to water restriction with a rise in the plasma osmolality, which then stimulates ADH release. The antidiuresis that follows is measured clinically as decreased urine volume and a rise in the urine osmolality. In diabetes insipidus, water restriction does not lead to a fall in urine volume or a rise in the urine osmolality, and the plasma osmolality continues to rise. The administration of exogenous ADH differentiates CDI from NDI. In CDI, all of these abnormalities are corrected following ADH administration because the renal response to ADH is normal. In NDI, however, ADH administration has no effect on the urine volume, urine osmolality, or plasma osmolality.

Treatment. The primary consideration in the treatment of hypernatremia is the rate at which the hypernatremia developed (Table 38–11). Acute hypernatremia can be corrected at a rate of 1 to 2 mEq/L per hour, while chronic hypernatremia should be corrected more slowly to prevent the development of CPM. The second consideration is the type of fluid with which to replace the salt and water losses. Patients with hypovolemic hypernatremia should first be hydrated with isotonic saline and then given hypotonic fluids to complete the normalization of their serum sodium. If hypotonic solutions are used to hydrate the patient, the serum sodium may fall too rapidly, and the patient's neurologic status may deteriorate. Patients who are volume-expanded should be given a diuretic, and the fluid loss should be replaced with water orally or dextrose in water intravenously. Patients with CDI and altered thirst whose hourly urine volume exceeds 150 ml should be started on desmopressin acetate (dDAVP), a 2 amino substitute of arginine vasopressin. The starting dose of 5 μg given intranasally should be titrated to reduce the hourly urine output below 100 ml. Patients on dDAVP are at risk for the development of hyponatremia and should not be given hypotonic fluids. The serum sodium should be checked frequently until it stabilizes.

Once the underlying condition has been managed and the hypernatremia has been corrected or is no longer symptomatic, the patient may be discharged from the ICU for continued treatment and monitoring on a regular hospital floor.

Post-ICU Phase

Once the patient has been transferred to the hospital floor, the serum sodium and plasma and urine osmolality tests should be repeated to ensure that they are normal, and treatment for the underlying condition should continue. Alternative therapies for patients with partial CDI include the use of chlorpropamide or carbamazepine, both drugs that potentiate the effect of ADH on the renal tubule. For patients with NDI, therapy is frequently unnecessary as long as the patient has normal thirst and ready access to water. Those patients who remain hypernatremic or are markedly polyuric can be maintained on a low sodium, low protein diet and given a thiazide diuretic. This seemingly paradoxical combination leads to volume contraction, increasing salt and water reabsorption in the proximal renal tubule. The amount of water delivered to the distal tubule is therefore decreased, and free water losses are diminished. Nonsteroidal anti-inflammatory drugs such as indomethacin are also useful in the treatment of NDI. These drugs increase the urine osmolality through inhibition of renal prostaglandins even in the absence of ADH and are fairly well tolerated when taken with meals. Amiloride, a potassium-sparing diuretic, is specifically indicated in the treatment of lithium-induced NDI because it blocks the sodium channels through which lithium enters the collecting tubule cells.[41]

DISORDERS OF POTASSIUM BALANCE

Potassium is the primary intracellular cation through its continuous translocation from the ECF to the intracellular fluid (ICF) by Na-K-ATPase, which is located in the cell membrane. As a result, only 2% of total body potassium is in the ECF. Because it is the ratio of the ICF/ECF potassium concentration that directly affects neuromuscular excitability, small increments in the plasma potassium level cause a decrease in the resting membrane potential and increase membrane excitability. The extracellular potassium concentration must be tightly regulated and is maintained through transcellular shifts of potassium and the excretion of ingested potassium by the kidney. The effect of an acute potassium load, whether endogenous or exogenous, on the extracellular potassium concentration can be mitigated by the movement of potassium from the ECF to the ICF under the influence of three hormones: epinephrine, insulin, and aldosterone.[42] Epinephrine, by increasing Na-K-ATPase activity, promotes potassium uptake, particularly in muscle cells. Insulin also increases Na-K-ATPase activity and, thereby, increases potassium uptake in liver, muscle, and other tissues. Aldosterone is the major hormone that controls the renal handling of potassium and also has been shown to increase cellular uptake of potassium. Changes in blood pH also result in transcellular shifts of potassium. In general, acidosis causes potassium to move out of cells while alkalosis is associated with movement of potassium into cells. However, the amount by which the serum potassium increases or decreases depends on the cause of the underlying acid/base disorder.

With the exception of a small amount of potassium excreted in the stool and the sweat, most of the dietary potassium as well as potassium released during cell breakdown is excreted by the kidneys. Potassium is freely filtered at the glomerulus, and after reabsorption in the proximal convoluted tubule and the thick ascending loop of Henle, approximately 10% of the filtered load is delivered to the distal tubule. This filtrate then passes through the distal convoluted tubule to the cortical collecting tubule, where potassium is secreted into the lumen if dietary potassium intake is normal or high. If dietary potassium intake is low, the filtrate remains unchanged. Although the final adjustment in the potassium concentration of the urine occurs in the medullary collecting tubule where potassium is absorbed, it is the amount of secretion that takes place in the cortical collecting tubule that controls net potassium excretion and potassium balance. Several factors affect potassium secretion by the cortical collecting tubule. First, increased serum potassium levels directly stimulate Na-K-ATPase activity in the cortical collecting tubules, and this results in increased potassium secretion. Second, aldosterone, which is produced and released in response to high plasma potassium levels, also stimulates Na-K-ATPase activity and increases the permeability of the luminal membrane to potassium. Third, increased fluid delivery to the cortical collecting tubule increases potassium secretion. This mechanism is helpful in preventing changes in potassium balance when abnormalities in sodium balance have caused changes in aldosterone production. For example, in congestive heart failure, aldosterone production is stimulated though the renin-angiotensin system and will result in hypokalemia through increased potassium secretion if this is not balanced by decreased potassium secretion that is due to decreased fluid delivery to the distal tubule.

Hypokalemia

Pre-ICU Phase

Differential Diagnosis. Hypokalemia is defined as a serum potassium less than 3.5 mEq/L and can develop in three ways:

- Extremely low dietary intake
- Shift of serum potassium into the cells leading to low extracellular potassium concentration with normal total body potassium
- Excessive gastrointestinal or urinary potassium losses

Because the kidney has the capacity to excrete as little as 10 mEq of potassium per day, hypokalemia solely on the basis of decreased dietary intake is uncommon. This type of hypokalemia may occur in patients who have received multiple transfusions with frozen red blood cells that are potassium poor. Eating some types of clay, a pica common in the southeastern United States, may bind potassium in the gastrointestinal tract and can result in hypokalemia.

A typical example of hypokalemia secondary to transcellular shifts occurs in patients with hypokalemic periodic paralysis.[43] In this dramatic condition, there is a sudden shift of potassium into the cells, with profound hypokalemia, and muscular paralysis, which can be life-threatening. The episodes are precipitated by glucose and insulin, adrenocorticotropic hormone (ACTH), mineralocorticoids, high carbohydrate meals, and vigorous exercise. The episode may last 6 to 48 hours if untreated. Acute respiratory or metabolic alkalosis can also result in mild hypokalemia, which is due to movement of potassium into the cell. Total body potassium is normal, and the decrease in serum potassium is clinically insignificant unless the patient is receiving digitalis. Digitalis toxicity is increased by both alkalemia as well as by hypokalemia.

Hypokalemia secondary to gastrointestinal losses is typically seen in patients with diarrhea that is due to a villous adenoma or chronic laxative abuse because the intestinal fluid is rich in potassium. In contrast, the hypokalemia that occurs with vomiting is more complex. Gastric fluid does contain 5 to 10 mEq/L of potassium; however, removal of this small amount of potassium during vomiting or nasogastric suction does not account for the hypokalemia that develops. In this case, the removal of gastric hydrochloric acid generates a chloride deficiency alkalosis and volume-depleted state, which results in renal sodium retention. Sodium resorption by the renal tubules in exchange for secreted potassium results in renal potassium losses and the development of hypokalemia.

Hypokalemia that is due to urinary losses of potassium can be classified on the basis of the accompanying acid/base disorder. Hypokalemia and normal acid/base equilibrium is commonly seen with the magnesium deficiency that may develop with intestinal malabsorption, chronic alcoholism, hyperparathyroidism, and aminoglycoside therapy.[44] The mechanism by which magnesium depletion causes hypokalemia is unclear but may be due to enhanced aldosterone secretion. It is important to recognize this entity because the hypokalemia is refractory to potassium therapy unless the hypomagnesemia has first been corrected. Osmotic diuretics such as mannitol and uncontrolled diabetes mellitus without the development of an acidosis may also lead to hypokalemia with normal acid/base status.

Hypokalemia may occur with a coexisting metabolic acidosis. The prototypical example is the distal renal tubular acidosis, which is associated with amphotericin B therapy. This type of hypokalemia can also occur in patients with proximal renal tubular acidosis.

Hypokalemia that occurs in patients with diabetic ketoacidosis (DKA) is more complex. In DKA, the patient loses potassium in the urine during the osmotic diuresis that occurs with hyperglycemia. The serum potassium, however, is usually normal on presentation because the insulin deficiency, hyperosmolarity, and acidosis combine to cause a shift of potassium out of the cells. Insulin therapy then causes movement of potassium into the cell due to both a direct membrane effect and the correction of the acidosis, resulting in hypokalemia.

Finally, urinary losses of potassium can occur in the setting of a metabolic alkalosis. The most common example of this type of hypokalemia is diuretic therapy. The loop and thiazide diuretics cause hypokalemia through several mechanisms. First, they cause ECF volume contraction, which, through stimulation of the renin-angiotensin system, results in secondary hyperaldosteronism. Second, the delivery of filtrate to the distal tubule is increased and, as noted previously, this increases potassium secretion. Finally, the alkalosis itself causes a shift of potassium from the ECF to the ICF as well as increased renal potassium secretion. Patients with mineralocorticoid excess that is due to primary aldosteronism or Cushing's syndrome also have excessive urinary losses of potassium. These patients are usually hypertensive and can be distinguished from patients with hypokalemia secondary to diuretics or vomiting by the resistance of the former to correction with rehydration and chloride replacement.

Symptoms and Signs. Patients with serum potassium levels above 3.0 mEq/L are usually asymptomatic unless they are receiving digitalis or are alkalemic. Potassium levels below 3.0 mEq/L are most commonly associated with skeletal or smooth muscle weakness, which may manifest itself as an intestinal ileus or may be so severe as to cause rhabdomyolysis. Chronic hypokalemia is associated with increased blood pressure, mild glucose intolerance, and several renal abnormalities including decreased ability to maximally concentrate the urine, increased renal excretion of ammonium leading to a decrease in the urine pH, and the development of a tubulointerstitial disease with a characteristic histologic picture. With the exception of the tubulointerstitial disease, these abnormalities can be reversed with potassium repletion. As noted previously, in the setting of mineralocorticoid excess, the patient is usually hypertensive; however, other causes of hypokalemia are associated with a normal or slightly low blood pressure. The electrocardiographic changes seen in hypokalemia are characteristic and correlate roughly with the severity of the hypokalemia. They are due to a delay in ventricular repolarization, which results in ST-segment depression, flattening or inversion of the T wave, a prominent U wave, and a prolongation of the QU interval. A number of cardiac arrhythmias including premature atrial and ventricular beats, sinus bradycardia, junctional tachycardia, and even ventricular tachycardia have been associated with hypokalemia and are more common with concomitant digitalis therapy.

Laboratory Diagnosis. The initial laboratory evaluation of hypokalemia includes the serum and urine electrolytes with calculation of the serum anion gap. In most instances the cause of the hypokalemia is clear from the history and physical examination; however, when the patient cannot give a history, is surreptitiously ingesting laxatives or diuretics, or denies vomiting, the physician must rely on the laboratory examination to reveal the diagnosis. The first step in the differential diagnosis of hypokalemia is to determine whether the potassium losses are renal or extrarenal. The urine potassium is the most useful test in this regard because the normal kidney should conserve potassium if potassium losses are extrarenal, resulting in a urine potassium of less than 20 mEq/L. The urine potassium is greater than 20 mEq/L if the hypokalemia is due to renal potassium wasting. The next step is to determine the acid/base status of the patient and to classify the hypokalemia according to the model in Table 38–12. In the setting of metabolic alkalosis, the urine chloride should be measured to separate a chloride-resistant from a chloride-sensitive alkalosis. Hypertensive patients with a high urine chloride (off diuretics) should have plasma renin and aldosterone levels measured. The serum magnesium level should be checked in patients resistant to potassium replacement therapy, and a serum creatinine level should be measured to evaluate baseline renal function. Patients suspected of laxative abuse should have the stool tested for phenolphthalein.

ICU Phase

Patients with mild-to-moderate hypokalemia do not require confinement to the ICU. Hyperkalemic patients who should be admitted to the ICU include the following:

- Those with a serum potassium less than 2 mEq/L
- Patients receiving digitalis therapy
- Those who have concurrent moderate-to-severe alkalosis

Patients who require electrocardiographic monitoring and those with severe muscle weakness should also be admitted to ICU.

In addition to correcting the underlying cause of hypokalemia, treatment consists of replacing the potassium deficit. Calculating the potassium deficit, however, can be difficult because the total body potassium does not correlate well with the serum potassium level. If the hypokalemia has been caused by a shift of potassium into the cells in the absence of any urinary or gastrointestinal potassium loss, then the patient need only be given enough potassium to prevent the cardiac consequences of hypokalemia. Once the underlying cause of the transcellular shift has been corrected, serum potassium levels will return to normal. If the hypokalemia is due to potassium losses from the body, then the rule of thumb is that a serum potassium of 3.0 mEq/L represents a 200- to 400-mEq deficit, and a serum potassium of 2.0 mEq/L represents a 400- to 800-mEq deficit.

Table 38–12. Differential Diagnosis of Hypokalemia

Step 1: Determine if potassium losses are renal or extrarenal by measuring the urinary potassium concentration (UK^+).
Step 2: Determine the acid/base status.
Step 3: If the patient has a metabolic alkalosis, then measure the urinary chloride (UCl^-).

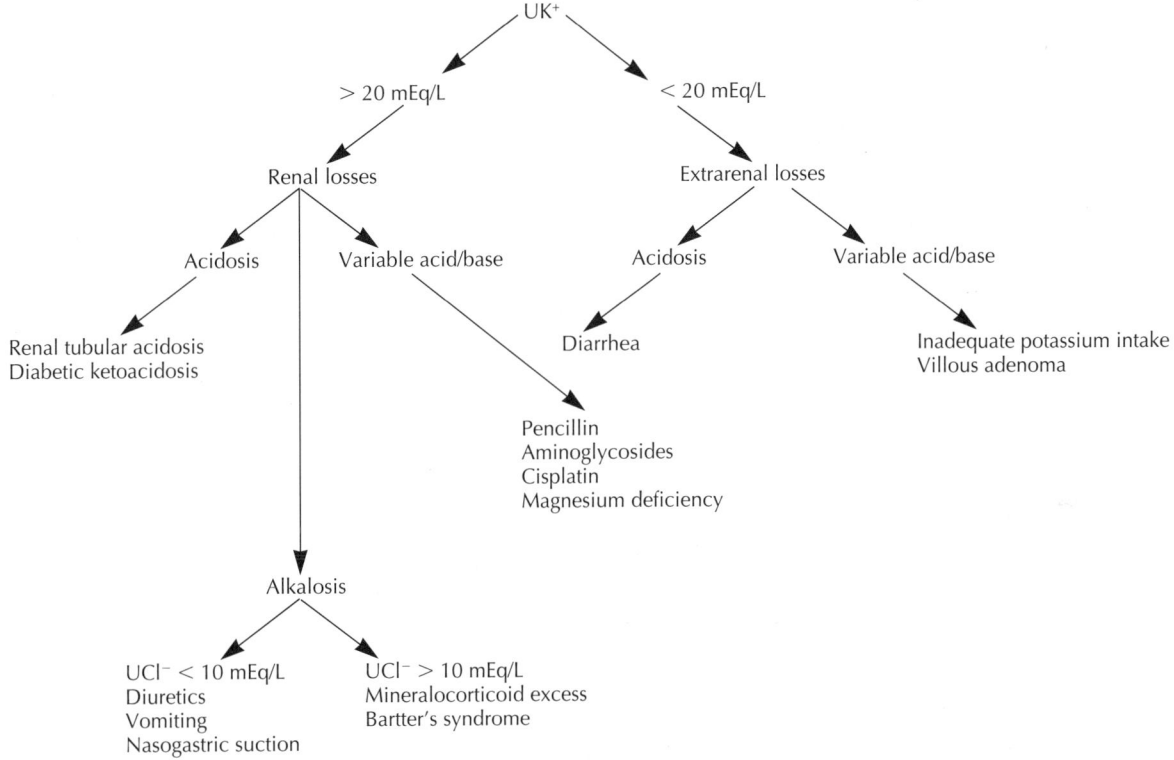

Oral replacement of potassium is preferable to intravenous replacement because larger doses can be given, and there is less danger of hyperkalemia and its consequences. Although many oral potassium preparations have an unpleasant taste, they have few serious side effects. Potassium is available as the chloride, bicarbonate, phosphate, and gluconate salt; however, the chloride salt is generally preferred except when a metabolic acidosis co-exists with the hypokalemia. This is because the chloride helps to correct any concurrent alkalosis and because the chloride is mostly restricted to the extracellular space. Administered phosphate and bicarbonate, however, are partially distributed into the intracellular compartment so that the serum potassium does not rise to the same degree as when an equimolar dose of KCl is given. Oral KCl is available in slow-release tablet, capsule, liquid, and crystalline forms. In chronic mild (K^+ less than 3.0 mEq/L) hypokalemia such as is commonly seen with diuretic use, KCl 40 to 80 mEq per day is sufficient to replace potassium losses. This dose of oral KCl is associated with a transient 1.0 to 1.5 mEq/L rise in serum potassium and, therefore, is an appropriate initial dose when the hypokalemia is more severe. The serum chemistries are followed, and the dose is repeated every 3 to 4 hours as necessary. In very severe symptomatic hypokalemia, an oral dose of up to 160 mEq can be given and will cause a brief 2.5 to 3.5 mEq/L rise in the serum potassium. Extreme caution should be exercised when potassium is given to patients with renal failure because they are unable to excrete potassium and may rapidly develop severe hyperkalemia with potassium replacement. Additional caution is in order when high doses of potassium supplement are given in bolus fashion via feeding tube. The sclerosing properties of the solutions may cause ulcers, edema, and obstruction of the gastrointestinal tract if the tube is located in the duodenum or lower.

Intravenous potassium replacement must be administered to patients without a functioning gastrointestinal tract. Intravenous potassium is more difficult to administer than oral potassium replacement for several reasons. First, intravenous potassium should not be administered in a concentration greater than 60 mEq/L. Thus, it is necessary to give the patient a large fluid volume. For example, a patient with a serum potassium of 3.0 mEq/L would require between 3.3 and 6.6 L of fluid to replace the 200 to 400 mEq potassium deficit. Second, the rate of intravenous potassium administration should not exceed 20 mEq per hour except in the presence of life-threatening arrhythmia. Third, it is preferable to give the potassium in saline instead of dextrose solution because the latter infusion stimulates insulin release, which, in turn, causes potassium to shift into cells, potentially worsening the hypokalemia.

The patient with severe acidosis and hypokalemia presents a difficult management problem. It should be noted that administration of alkali will cause a shift in potassium into the cell and worsen the hypokalemia. Therefore, potassium replacement therapy should be concurrent with the correction of the acidosis. Patients with KDA frequently have a concurrent hypophosphatemia and should have a portion of their potassium deficit replaced as potassium phosphate.

Once the serum potassium is above 3.0 mEq/L and the urine potassium has begun to rise, signalling potassium repletion, there is no further need for cardiac monitoring, and the patient can be safely transferred out of the ICU. If the patient is receiving digitalis, however, he should remain in the ICU until the serum potassium is greater than 3.5 mEq/L.

Post-ICU Phase

After discharge from the ICU, a serum potassium level should be obtained to ensure that it has remained normal. No further follow-up is necessary if the underlying cause has been corrected. Patients receiving diuretics should be reassessed several weeks after potassium supplementation has been initiated or adjusted to ensure that the serum potassium remains normal. Once it has been ascertained that the potassium is normal, there is no need to continue repeating the serum potassium unless the patient's condition changes. In some settings such as mineralocorticoid excess, the potassium loss is ongoing, and it may be difficult to maintain a normal serum potassium level with supplements alone. In this case, the addition of a potassium-sparing diuretic such as spironolactone is useful in controlling both the potassium loss and the hypertension. Patients with hyperaldosteronism should have repeat serum potassium determination every 2 to 3 weeks.

Hyperkalemia

Pre-ICU Phase

Differential Diagnosis. Hyperkalemia does not often occur in normal individuals but is the most life-threatening of all electrolyte disturbances. Mild hyperkalemia is defined as a serum potassium of 5.0 to 6.0 mEq/L, and severe hyperkalemia is defined as a serum potassium greater than 6.0 mEq/L. Because the normal kidney has the capacity to excrete large potassium loads, hyperkalemia that is due to increased intake is uncommon unless renal function is impaired. A typical example is the patient with moderate renal insufficiency who has hypertension and develops hyperkalemia after using a salt substitute in an effort to decrease sodium intake.

Pseudohyperkalemia, transcellular shifts, and decreased renal excretion of potassium are other causes of hyperkalemia. Pseudohyperkalemia is the term used to describe an artifactual hyperkalemia that is due to the movement of potassium out of blood cells after the blood has been drawn. The three causes of this phenomenon are hemolysis, leukocytosis, and thrombocytosis. In hemolysis, mechanical trauma caused by repeated fist clenching or a tight tourniquet ruptures the red cells, spilling their contents, including potassium, and is detected in the lab because the released hemoglobin tints the serum red. During the clotting process, a small amount of potassium is re-

Table 38–13. Drug-Induced Hyperkalemia

Increased intake
   High dose penicillin
Redistribution across the cell membrane
   Digitalis excess
   Insulin deficiency
   Beta blockers
   Succinylcholine
Decreased urinary excretion
   Potassium-sparing diuretics
   Angiotensin-converting enzyme inhibitors
   Nonsteroidal anti-inflammatory drugs
   Cyclosporine
   Heparin

leased from the white cells and platelets and is insignificant when the numbers of these cells are normal. However, a patient with leukemia and a white blood cell count of greater than 100,000/mm^3, or a patient with thrombocytosis and a platelet count of greater than 1,000,000 may be reported to have a serum potassium level greater than 6.0 mEq/L. Pseudohyperkalemia should be suspected if the electrocardiograph (ECG) and renal function are normal. An unclotted specimen should be sent in a heparinized tube for a plasma potassium, which, if normal, confirms the pseudohyperkalemia.

The most common causes of hyperkalemia secondary to transcellular shifts are insulin deficiency and metabolic acidosis. As an example, the patient with diabetic ketoacidosis may present with an elevated or high-normal serum potassium despite decreased total body potassium as a consequence of insulin deficiency and the hyperosmolar environment. The acidosis contributes less to this increase because the organic acidoses are less likely than mineral acidoses to cause hyperkalemia, in part, because the former anions can move into the cell, thus diminishing potassium movement out of the cell. Beta-adrenergic blockers, which block beta$_2$-adrenergic-mediated cellular potassium uptake, and digitalis, which impairs the functioning of the Na-K-ATPase pump, are also causes of hyperkalemia secondary to transcellular shifts that occur especially in patients with impaired renal excretion of potassium (Table 38–13).

Decreased renal potassium excretion is the most common cause of hyperkalemia. Renal failure, renal tubular dysfunction, and mineralocorticoid deficiency of adrenal, renal, or drug origin all result in decreased renal excretion of potassium. This type of hyperkalemia is most typically seen in patients with end-stage renal disease. Unless a patient has a specific condition that impairs distal tubular potassium excretion, the ability to excrete a normal dietary load of potassium is fairly well preserved until the patient becomes oliguric. It is not uncommon, however, for end-stage renal disease patients to become severely hyperkalemic, which is due to dietary indiscretion or missed dialysis treatments. Secondary hypoaldosteronism is also a common cause of hyperkalemia in the setting of renal insufficiency. A typical example is the patient with diabetic- or sickle cell disease-associated hyporeninemic hypoaldosteronism.[45] These patients often have elevated serum potassium and mild-to-moderately impaired renal function. Hyperkalemia out of proportion to the severity of the renal impairment is also seen with nonsteroidal anti-inflammatory drug use and in patients with renal insufficiency secondary to tubulointerstitial disease.[45] Drug-induced hyperkalemia occurs in several ways (see Table 38-13). An example is the patient with renal impairment and a normal serum potassium who develops hyperkalemia in the hospital after receiving "prophylactic low-dose heparin." Heparin, by its direct action on the adrenal gland, decreases aldosterone secretion within 4 to 7 days after the start of therapy.

Symptoms and Signs. The signs and symptoms of hyperkalemia are few. Muscle weakness, which at first may be isolated to the lower extremities, occurs with severe hyperkalemia, but patients with serum potassium levels below 6.5 mEq/L are frequently asymptomatic. It is the potential for the development of life-threatening cardiac arrhythmias, however, that is of most concern. Hyperkalemia leads to a progression of electrocardiographic changes that start with narrowed and peaked T waves and shortening of the QT interval. This is followed by a widening of the QRS complex and prolongation of the PR interval. With the disappearance of the P wave, the T wave and QRS complex converge into the sine wave, which heralds ventricular fibrillation and cardiac standstill. Although the manner in which the ECG changes progress is predictable, the time course and the serum potassium level at which these changes will be manifested is unpredictable. Therefore, the demonstration of narrowed peaked T waves demands therapeutic action.

Laboratory Diagnosis. In addition to the history (which should include questions regarding the use of potassium-sparing diuretics and salt substitutes) and physical examination, the initial workup of hyperkalemia should include the serum and plasma potassium. If the plasma potassium is normal, then the white cell count and platelet count should be obtained to determine the cause of the pseudohyperkalemia. In addition, the blood urea nitrogen (BUN), blood glucose, creatinine, bicarbonate levels, and arterial blood gas should be obtained. When hypoaldosteronism is suspected, serum aldosterone, cortisol, and plasma renin activity should be determined.

ICU Phase

Patients with serum potassium levels greater than 6.0 mEq/L should be admitted to the ICU for cardiac monitoring. End-stage renal disease patients without ECG changes are an exception if they can be dialyzed urgently. Patients with digitalis toxicity should also be placed in the ICU even if the serum potassium is less than 6.0 mEq/L because these patients are particularly at risk for life-threatening cardiac arrhythmias.

The treatment of hyperkalemia can be seen as a four-step process. First, because the most dangerous consequence of hyperkalemia is the potential for the development of cardiac arrhythmias, the myocardium should be protected (Table 38-14). Elevated potassium levels cause a decrease in the resting potential, thereby increasing membrane excitability, and this can be counteracted by increasing the plasma calcium and, thereby, decreasing the threshold potential. This returns membrane excitability to normal. In severe hyperkalemia with ECG changes, 10 ml of a 10% solution of calcium gluconate administered intravenously over 2 to 5 minutes is almost immediately cardioprotective and lasts 30 to 60 minutes. The patient should be on a cardiac monitor when the drug is administered,

Table 38-14. Treatment of Hyperkalemia

Agent	Dose	Mechanism	Onset	Duration	Limitation
Calcium gluconate	10-30 ml 10% solution over 3-4 min	Stabilization of cell membranes	Few minutes	<1 hr	Hypercalcemia
Hypertonic sodium	50-100 mEq NaHCO$_3^-$ to 1 L of isotonic NaCL; infuse at 250 ml/hr	Stabilization of cell membranes	<1 hr	Few hours	Na$^+$ and volume load, alkalemia
Sodium bicarbonate	1-2 ampules (50 mEq each) IV over 5-10 min	Uptake of K$^+$ into cells	<1 hr	Few hours	Na$^+$ and volume load, alkalemia
Glucose ± regular insulin	50 ml of 50% glucose solution rapidly IV (±10 U reg. insulin) followed by 500 ml of 10% glucose solution IV over 30-60 min (±10 U reg. insulin per 100 g infused glucose)	Uptake of K$^+$ into cells	<1 hr	Few hours	Hyperglycemia, hypoglycemia, volume load
Potent diuretics	Furosemide 40 mg IV, higher if renal insufficiency present	Urinary K$^+$ excretion through GI tract	<1 hr	Few hours	Ineffective in advanced renal insufficiency; volume depletion
Kayexalate and sorbitol	Oral: 20-50 g sodium polystyrene sulfonate with 100 ml 20% sorbitol Enema: 50-100 g sodium polystyrene sulfonate with 50-100 ml 70% sorbitol	K$^+$ excretion through GI tract	Few hours	Few hours	Na$^+$ and volume load
Dialysis	Peritoneal dialysis or hemodialysis	Removal of K$^+$ from body	Few minutes after start	Few hours after end	Risks and complications of dialysis

and the dose can be repeated after 5 to 10 minutes if the ECG changes have not reversed. Because calcium can worsen digitalis toxicity, care should be taken in suspected cases of digitalis overdose to infuse the calcium more slowly.

Second, steps should be taken to promote potassium entry into the cells. This can be effected with the administration of sodium bicarbonate and glucose or glucose and insulin. One ampule of $NaHCO_3$ administered intravenously has an onset of action within 15 minutes, lasts for several hours, and is particularly useful in patients who are acidemic. The administration of $NaHCO_3$, however, is limited by the large sodium load that may precipitate congestive heart failure in susceptible individuals. Patients with hypocalcemia, as in the setting of chronic renal failure, may experience seizures and tetany as the blood pH rises with bicarbonate administration. This can be prevented if calcium is given before the bicarbonate. The administration of 1 ampule of 50% dextrose alone in a nondiabetic may stimulate an insulin response large enough to correct the hyperkalemia, but in diabetic and acutely ill patients, 10 units of regular insulin should be given intravenously with the dextrose to ensure an adequate response. The effect is noted within 30 minutes and also lasts several hours.

Third, in patients with elevated total body potassium, potassium can be removed through the administration of a cation-exchange resin or either hemo- or peritoneal dialysis. Sodium polystyrene sulfonate (Kayexalate), given orally in a dose of 15 to 30 g and mixed in 50 to 100 ml of sorbitol to prevent constipation, removes about 1 mEq $K+/g$, and has an onset of action of 4 to 6 hours. Therefore, it should be given as soon as possible after the diagnosis of hyperkalemia is made. The dose can be repeated as many as four to six times per day until the serum potassium is normal. The major concern with this drug is sodium overload because, for every 1 mEq of potassium removed, 1 mEq of sodium is released. Dialysis is the therapy of last resort in patients with severe hyperkalemia. Hemodialysis removes potassium more efficiently and with more precision than does peritoneal dialysis and is, therefore, the dialysis therapy of choice in acute renal failure. Continuous peritoneal dialysis, however, is better for maintaining eukalemia in patients with end-stage renal failure and a high dietary intake of potassium. Finally, in patients with impaired renal potassium excretion, urinary potassium losses can be increased with a loop diuretic or, if the patient is neither hypertensive nor edematous, with fludrocortisone, a synthetic mineralocorticoid.[46]

Once the serum potassium is below 5.5 mEq/L and the patient is clinically stable, ECG monitoring can be discontinued and the patient transferred from the ICU if the underlying cause of the hyperkalemia has resolved or been stabilized.

Post-ICU Phase

Once the patient has been discharged from the ICU, a serum potassium level should be obtained to ensure that a life-threatening hyperkalemia has not recurred. Further follow-up and treatment depends on the underlying cause of the hyperkalemia. Hypertensive patients on potassium-sparing diuretics can be managed with a thiazide or loop diuretic or another first-line antihypertensive agent. Other patients with drug-induced hyperkalemia do not require any specific follow-up or therapy; however, the patient should be advised not to take the offending drug again and to report the drug reaction to any new physicians involved in his care. Patients with hyporeninemic hypoaldosteronism and chronic renal failure should be instructed to adhere to a low potassium diet. If the patient is also hypertensive, a thiazide or loop diuretic may be useful in the management of the hyperkalemia. Patients who are not hypertensive may benefit from the chronic administration of fludrocortisone. Finally, sodium polystyrene sulfonate can be used chronically, although its use is limited by the diarrhea it causes. Dialysis patients should be reminded to avoid potassium-rich foods, and the potassium concentration of the dialysis bath should be lowered.

REFERENCES

1. Narins, R. A., and Emmett, M.: Simple and mixed acid-base disorders: a practical approach. Medicine, 59:161, 1980.
2. Gabow, P. A.: Disorders associated with an altered anion gap. Kidney Int., 27:472, 1985.
3. Winter, S.D. et al.: The fall of the serum anion gap. Arch. Intern. Med., 150:311, 1990.
4. Gabow, P. A. et al.: Diagnostic importance of an increased anion gap. N. Engl. J. Med., 303:854, 1980.
5. Battle, D. C. et al.: The use of the urinary anion gap in the diagnosis of hyperchloremic metabolic acidosis. N. Engl. J. Med., 318:594, 1988.
6. Jacobsen, D. et al.: Anion and osmolal gaps in the diagnosis of methanol and thylene glycol poisoning. Acta Med. Scand., 212:17, 1982.
7. Schelling, J. R. et al.: Increased osmolal gap in alcoholic ketoacidosis and lactic acidosis. Ann. Intern. Med., 113:580, 1990.
8. Cooper, D. J. et al.: Bicarbonate does not improve hemodynamics in critically ill patients who have lactic acidosis. Ann. Intern. Med., 112:492, 1990.
9. Ritter, J. M., Doktor, H. S., and Benjamin, N.: Paradoxical effect of bicarbonate on cytoplasmic pH. Lancet, 335:1243, 1990.
10. Garella, S., Dana C., and Chazan, J.: Severity of metabolic acidosis as a determinant of bicarbonate requirements. N. Engl. J. Med., 289:121, 1973.
11. Brandt, K. R., and Miles, J. M.: Relationship between the severity of hyperglycemia and metabolic acidosis in diabetic ketoacidosis. Mayo Clin. Proc., 63:1071, 1988.
12. Oh, M. S. et al.: Hyperchloremic acidosis during the recovery phase of diabetic ketoacidosis. Ann. Intern. Med., 89:925, 1978.
13. Morris, L. R., Murphy, M. B., and Kitabchi, A. E.: Bicarbonate therapy in severe diabetic ketoacidosis. Ann. Intern. Med., 105:836, 1986.
14. Madias, N. E.: Lactic acidosis. Kidney Int., 29:752, 1986.
15. Stacpoole, P. W.: Lactic acidosis: the case against bicarbonate therapy. Ann. Intern. Med., 105:276, 1986.
16. Narins, R. G., and Cohen, J. J.: Bicarbonate therapy for organic acidosis: the case for its continued use. Ann. Intern. Med., 106:615, 1987.
17. Sun, J. H. et al.: Carbicarb: an effective substitute for $NaHCO_3$ for the treatment of acidosis. Surgery, 102:835, 1987.

18. Stacpoole, P. W. et al.: Dichloroacetate in the treatment of lactic acidosis. Ann. Intern. Med., *108*:58, 1988.
19. Hodgkin, J. E., Soeprono, F. F., and Chan, D. M.: Incidence of metabolic alkalosis in hospitalized patients. Crit. Care Med., *8*:725, 1980.
20. Rimmer, J. M., and Gennari, F. J.: Metabolic alkalosis. J. Inten. Care Med., *78*:482, 1985.
21. Harrington, J. T.: Metabolic alkalosis. Kidney Int., *26*:88, 1984.
22. Driscoll, D. F., Bistrain, B. R., and Jenkins, R. L.: Development of metabolic alkalosis after massive transfusion during orthotopic liver transplantation. Crit. Care Med., *15*:905, 1987.
23. Williams, D. B., and Lyons, J. H.: Treatment of severe metabolic alkalosis with intravenous infusion of hydrochloric acid. Surg. Gynecol. Obstet., *150*:315, 1980.
24. Bushinsky, D. A., and Gennari, F. J.: Life-threatening hyperkalemia induced by argenine. Ann. Intern. Med., *89*:632, 1978.
25. Knutsen, O. H.: New method for administration of hydrochloric acid in metabolic alkalosis. Lancet, *1*:953, 1983.
26. Vaziri, N. D. et al.: Prevention of metabolic alkalosis induced by gastric fluid loss using H_2 receptor antagonist. Gen. Pharmacol., *16*:141, 1985.
27. Sunderrajan, S. et al.: Posttransurethral prostatic resection hyponatremic syndrome: case report and review of the literature. Am. J. Kidney Dis., *4*:80, 1984.
28. Friedman, E., Shadel, M., Halkin, H., and Farfel, Z.: Thiazide-induced hyponatremia. Reproducibility by single dose challenge and an analysis of pathogenesis. Ann. Intern. Med., *110*:24, 1989.
29. Mettauer, B. et al.: Sodium and water excretion abnormalities in congestive heart failure. Ann. Intern. Med., *105*:161, 1988.
30. Schrier, R. W.: Pathogenesis of sodium and water retention in high-output and low-output cardiac failure, nephrotic syndrome, cirrhosis, and pregnancy. N. Engl. J. Med., *319*:1065, 1988.
31. Nolph, K. D., and Schrier, R. W.: Sodium, potassium, and water metabolism in the syndrome of inappropriate hormone secretion. Am. J. Med., *49*:534, 1970.
32. Linas, S. L. et al.: Evidence for vasopressin dependent and independent mechanisms in the impaired water excretion of glucocorticoid deficiency. Kidney Int., *18*:58, 1980.
33. Ayus, J. C., Krothapalli, R. K., and Areff, A. I.: Treatment of symptomatic hyponatremia and its relation to brain damage. N. Engl. J. Med., *317*:1190, 1987.
34. Sterns, R. H.: Severe symptomatic hyponatremia: treatment and outcome. A study of 64 cases. Ann. Intern. Med., *107*:656, 1987.
35. Berl, T.: Treating hyponatremia: what is the controversy all about? (Editorial.) Ann. Intern. Med., *113*:417, 1990.
36. Decaux, G., Waterlot, Y., Genette, F., and Mockel, J.: Treatment of the syndrome of inappropriate secretion of antidiuretic hormone with furosemide. N. Engl. J. Med., *304*:329, 1981.
37. Cox, M. M., Guzzo, J., Morrison, G., and Singer, I.: Demeclocycline and therapy of hyponatremia. Ann. Intern. Med., *86*:113, 1977.
38. Berl, T., Anderson, R. J., McDonald, K. M., and Schrier, R. W.: Clinical disorders of water metabolism. Kidney Int., *10*:117, 1976.
39. Snyder, N. A., Fiegal, D. W., and Arieff, A. I.: Hypernatremia in elderly patients. A heterogenous, morbid, and iatrogenic entity. Ann. Intern. Med., *107*:309, 1987.
40. Boton, R., Gaviria, M., and Battle, D. C.: Prevalence, pathogenesis, and treatment of renal dysfunction associated with chronic lithium therapy. Am. K. Kidney Dis., *10*:329, 1987.
41. Battle, D. C. et al.: Amelioration of polyuria by amiloride in patients receiving long-term lithium therapy. N. Engl. J. Med., *312*:408, 1985.
42. Brown, R. S.: Extrarenal potassium homeostasis. Kidney Int., *30*:116, 1986.
43. Johns, R. J.: Hypokalemic periodic paralysis. Johns Hopkins Med. J., *143*:148, 1978.
44. Solomon, R.: The relationship between disorders of K^+ and Mg^{+2} homeostasis. Semin. Nephrol., *7*:253, 1987.
45. DeFronzo, R. A.: Hyperkalemia and hyperreninemic hypoaldosteronism. Kidney Int., *17*:118, 1980.
46. Sebastian, A. S. et al.: Amelioration of metabolic acidosis with fludrocortisone therapy in hyporeninemic hypoaldosteronism. N. Engl. J. Med., *297*:576, 1977.

SUPPLEMENTAL READINGS

Metabolic Acidosis

Arieff, A.: Indications for use of bicarbonate in patients with metabolic acidosis. Br. J. Anaesth., *67*:165, 1991.

Halperin, M. L., Vasuvattakul, S., and Bayoumi, A.: A modified classification of metabolic acidosis: a pathophysiologic approach. Nephron, *60*:129, 1992.

Mecher, C., et al.: Unaccounted for anion in metabolic acidosis during severe sepsis in humans. Crit. Care Med., *19*:705, 1991.

Metabolic Alkalosis

Brimioulle, S., and Kahn, R. J.: Effects of metabolic alkalosis on pulmonary gas exchange. Am. Rev. Respir. Dis., *141*:1185, 1990.

Koch, S. M., and Taylor, R. W.: Chloride ion in intensive care medicine. Crit. Care Med., *20*:227, 1992.

Marik, D. E., et al.: Acetazolamide in the treatment of metabolic alkalosis in critically ill patients. Heart Lung, *20*:455, 1991.

Hyponatremia

Arief, A.: Management of hyponatremia. Br. Med. J., *307*:305, 1993.

Harris, C. P., Townsend, J. J., and Baringer, J. R.: Symptomatic hyponatremia: can myelinosis be prevented by treatment? J. Neurol. Neurosurg. Psychiatry., *56*:626, 1993.

Kamel, K. S., and Bear, R. A.: Treatment of hyponatremia: a quantitative analysis. Am. J. Kidney Dis., *21*:439, 1993.

Sterns, R. H.: Severe hyponatremia: the case for conservative management. Crit. Care Med., *20*:534, 1992.

Hypernatremia

Allerton, J. P., and Strom, J. A.: Hypernatremia due to repeated doses of charcoal-sorbitol. Am. J. Kidney Dis., *17*:581, 1991.

Oh, M. S., and Carroll, H. J.: Disorder of sodium metabolism: hypernatremia and hyponatremia. Crit. Care Med., *20*:94, 1992.

Vin-Christian, K., and Arieff, A. I.: Diabetes insipidus, massive polyuria, and hypernatremia leading to permanent brain damage. Am. J. Med., *94*:341, 1993.

Hypokalemia

Kruse, J. A., and Carlson, R. W.: Rapid correction of hypokalemia using concentrated intravenous chloride infusions. Arch. Intern. Med., *3*:529, 1990.

Minella, R. A., and Schulman, D. S.: Fatal verapamil toxicity and hypokalemia. Am. Heart J., *121*:1810, 1991.

Perazella, M. A., et al.: Renal failure and severe hypokalemia asso-

ciated with acute myelomonocytic leukemia. Am. J. Kidney Dis., *22:*462, 1993.
Singhal, P. C., et al.: Hypokalemia and rhabdomyolysis. Miner. Electrolyte Metabol., *17:*335, 1991.

Hyperkalemia

Ljutic, D., and Rumboldt, Z.: Should glucose be administered before, with, or after insulin, in the management of hyperkalemia? Renal Fail., *15:*73, 1993.

Michelis, M. F.: Hyperkalemia in the elderly. Am. J. Kidney Dis., *16:*296, 1990.
Schaller, M. D., Fischer, A. P., and Perret, C. H.: Hyperkalemia: a prognostic factor during acute severe hypothermia. JAMA, *264:*1842, 1990.
Velazquez, H., et al.: Renal mechanisms of trimethoprim-induced hyperkalemia. Ann. Intern. Med., *119:*296, 1993.
Wrenn, K. D., Slovis, C. M., and Slovis, B. S.: The ability of physicians to predict hyperkalemia from the ECG. Ann. Emerg. Med., *20:*1229, 1991.

Chapter 39

ACUTE RENAL FAILURE IN THE INTENSIVE CARE SETTING: PREVENTION, DIAGNOSIS, TREATMENT, AND FOLLOW-UP

EMIL P. PAGANINI

The presence of renal dysfunction in the ICU is a common occurrence, especially in the older and more complex patient currently admitted to these units. The underlying renal disease that frequently exists in this same population adds to the predisposition of further renal compromise when these patients are exposed to levels of injury that might not have as far-reaching consequences in patients with "normal" baseline function. Because the unadjusted mortality of patients with acute renal failure has not changed greatly over the past several decades, there is a sense of frustration among care givers. Certainly, the tools developed over this same time frame have allowed for improved care, yet the outcome for this disease has not changed.

Perhaps the answer lies in the type of patient. There has, indeed, been a more complicated patient with an increasing number and level of co-morbid states, which may contribute to a negative outcome.[1-5] If one were to accurately review the case-mix data associated with acute renal failure, one would conclude that it is the patient with multiorgan failure who has the high mortality while the patient with "pure" renal failure has an excellent outcome opportunity. It is thus of importance to identify those conditions that would contribute to patient morbidity if associated with renal failure. Prevention maneuvers aimed at reducing the incidence of renal dysfunction could be focused on this group. Thus, the very patients who would have the greatest difficulty with the addition of renal failure would be the ones who would have the greatest benefit from its prevention.

Once the patient has entered the ICU, the diagnostic and therapeutic approaches to these patients must be focused. It would serve no purpose to treat one aspect of a patient's condition without regard to the effects of such treatment on other systems. Frequently, there also needs to be a trade-off among systems, such as the classic difference between the need for volume in the recovering renal patient and the negative effect of this same volume in the patient being weaned from the ventilator. The type of renal support offered, the differing antibiotic regimen, and the long-term plans for the patient all need to be considered in the formula for renal care.

Finally, the post-ICU period is an often neglected but nonetheless important period for decision and planning. Early patient evaluation to establish an effective renal support plan must be instituted immediately. This will allow for patient referral to appropriate services and result in a smooth flow from an acute phase to perhaps a chronic phase of renal support. Family discussions regarding extended renal support can be initiated, especially if the family members were already part of an organized discussion before patient admission. Also, prolonged renal recovery periods in the elderly may require continued dialytic support at an outpatient facility.

PRE-ICU PHASE: PROTECTIVE INTERVENTIONS

Controversy regarding the use of protective measures and the ultimate outcome of patients subjected to known renal insults continues to give rise to a variety of treatment schedules. Several reports reviewed patient demographics and attempted to identify those patients who would be at higher risk of developing acute renal failure.[6-13] The resulting lists of premorbid states have differed slightly but have generally agreed on several basic conditions (Table 39-1). Certainly, those patients who have a prior history of acute renal failure or those with preexisting chronic renal disease (serum creatinine levels greater than 2 mg/dl) will have a higher risk of renal dysfunction. Co-morbid conditions such as severe peripheral vascular disease, proteinuria, diabetes (type I and II), or moderately severe congestive heart failure are also grouped along with the elderly (greater than 75 years old) as patients at higher renal risk.

In a retrospective look at 5051 patients who underwent open heart surgical procedures at the Cleveland Clinic, Higgins et al.[14] found that using a simplified clinical scoring system developed for preoperative risk assessment proved beneficial in predicting postoperative morbidity and mortality in a subsequent 2-year prospective application of the model (Fig. 39-1). In a similar study, preexisting renal dysfunction was shown to be associated with a higher incidence of morbidity and mortality than had been previously suspected (Fig. 39-1). Case mix adjustment of patient outcomes as well as the use of various discriminate scoring systems are becoming the basis for outcome analysis in both hospitalized and/or disease-specific outpatient care.[15-17] Renal function has played a central role in the analysis of al the severity scoring used in the evaluation of intensive care patients. It thus seems appropriate that the selection of these same patients for preventive measures before a known potential renal insult may be an uncomplicated way to reduce renal morbidity.

Table 39-1. Patient Conditions that Predispose to Acute Tubular Necrosis

Chronic renal failure (creatinine > 2.5 mg/dl)
Diabetes mellitus (with proteinuria)
Proteinuria (esp. light chain and paraproteinuria)
History of allergy (dye/drug)
Chronic liver failure (bilirubin > 3)
Chronic congestive heart failure (ejection fraction < 20%)
Old age (> 75 years)
Peripheral vascular disease (atherosclerosis obliterans, renal artery stenosis)

Fluid Therapy and Balance

The most simple prevention is adequate hydration. Several scoring systems have listed volume depletion as the single most frequent factor fostering acute renal compromise. Patients frequently must refrain from eating or drinking before dye studies or surgery. Patients with an osmotic diuresis from diabetes, however, or those who have lost distal tubular concentrating ability because of chronic renal disease may not be able to conserve water and thus easily develop intravascular depletion. Patients who have received diuretics either as part of their usual therapeutic regimen or in conjunction with other "preventive" maneuvers are also prone to depletion if fluid is not replaced. Preserving the glomerular filtration rate (GFR) is the goal of maintaining effective renal perfusion. Although a certain amount of renal regulation is sustained by local hormonal and vasoactive peptide interaction, patients with moderately severe renal failure may already be using this system to maintain GFR. A reduction in renal blood flow might fall outside the ability of the disease kidney to adequately compensate and result in a GFR reduction. Any disturbance in this system among patients with chronic renal dysfunction would have significant negative effects on the renal regulatory forces. Thus, the use of nonsteroidal anti-inflammatory drug (NSAID) therapy in patients with renal compromise or the addition of medications that may potentiate their actions should be avoided, especially during the period of potential renal insult from a procedure or toxin.[18]

Severe renal artery stenosis, usually in association with peripheral vascular disease, places the kidney at risk from minor variations in systemic blood pressure. Medications that have an effect on prostaglandin synthesis or angiotensin activity would also interfere with renal regulation and thus predispose the patient to the development of renal compromise. Optimizing the relative intravascular volume would go far in avoiding renal blood flow abnormalities.

Administered fluid type and rate must be adjusted to the individual patients' need and circumstance. Just as each fluid type lost will represent a loss from a specific area, so too the addition of volume will be reflected by the areas where the administered fluid usually distributes. The addition of normal saline, for example, will be reflected by an expansion of the extracellular space, while using hypotonic fluid will augment total body water to the extent of the free-water percentage in the delivered solution (Fig. 39-2).

If the object of fluid delivery is the maintenance of an effective intravascular volume, then either appropriate colloid delivery or isotonic or hypertonic crystalloid should be the therapy of choice. There is no place for hypotonic fluid replacement being used in the treatment of intravascular volume deficits other than in conditions that require water rather than salt delivery (hypernatremia, diabetes insipidus, hyperthermia with dermal/respiratory losses). The use of osmotically active substances such as mannitol or albumin, especially in the hypoalbuminemic patient, may expand intravascular volume without expansion of total body fluid. This latter approach is most effective in conditions of excess extravascular total body water, about which it is theorized that one can osmotically mobilize the excessive extravascular volume into the vascular compartment for presentation to the kidneys.[19]

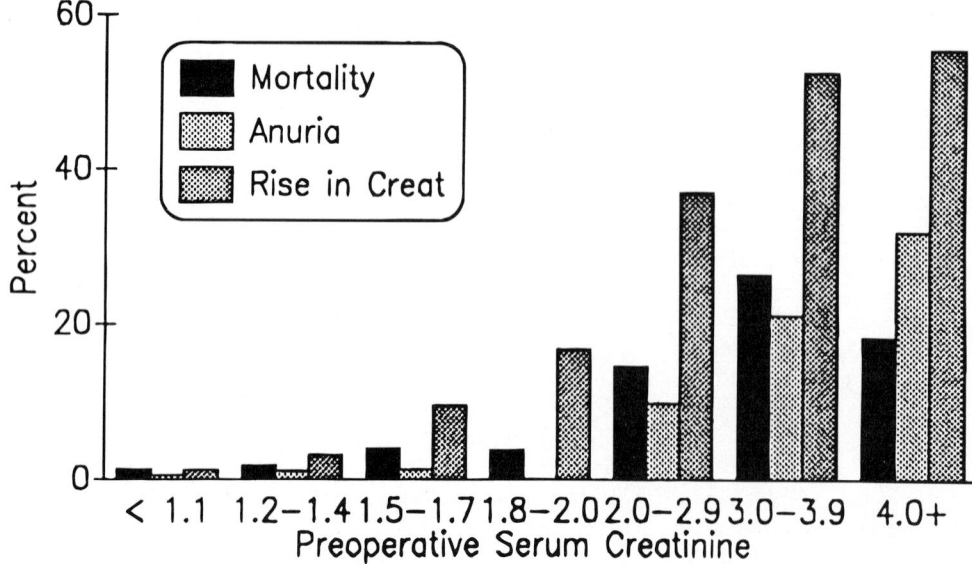

Fig. 39-1. Predictive nature of preoperative serum creatinine levels: morbidity and mortality by preoperative serum creatinine levels. Preoperative serum creatinine (mg/dl) and percentage of occurrence of mortality, anuria, and rise in serum creatinine levels.

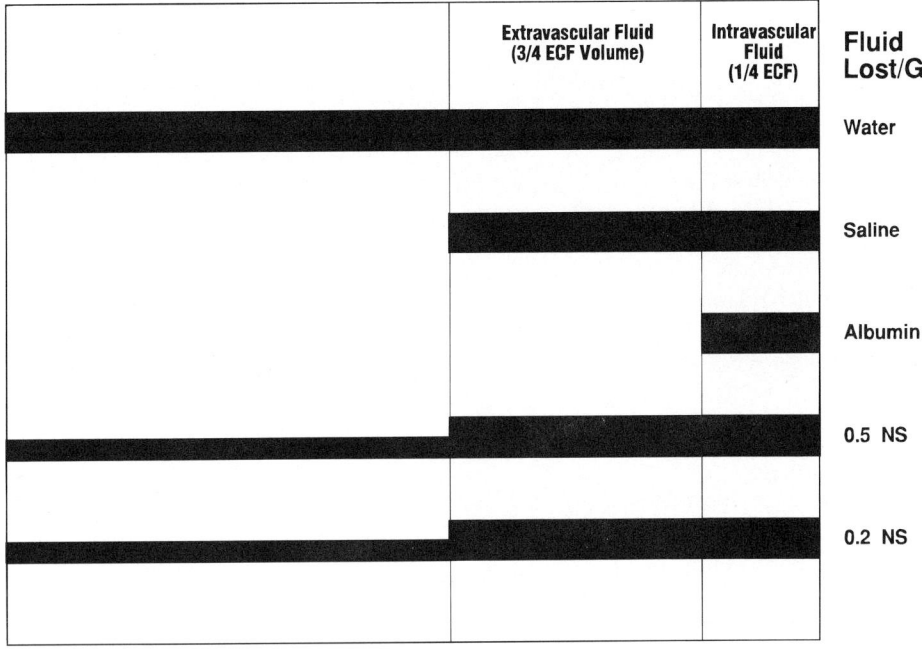

Fig. 39–2. Fluid Distribution when various fluid types are given or lost. The chart shows water added to or lost from all compartments; saline added to or lost from extracellular space; and albumin confined to addition or loss from the vascular compartment. 0.5% Normal saline distributed half its volume across all compartments and half across only the extracellular space; 0.2% normal saline distributed 80% of its volume across all compartments, and 20% of its volume across the extracellular space. (Drawn courtesy of George Morrison, CD, Inc.)

During protective fluid loading, the rate of delivery depends on the following:

- The type of fluid used
- The co-morbid conditions limiting volume expansion
- Residual renal function

Renal failure patients with associated nephrotic syndrome or patients with liver failure and ascites, for example, may benefit from slow albumin infusions combined with normal saline,[20] while patients with diabetes and only marginal reduction of baseline renal function could easily tolerate rapid infusions of saline. Protective fluid therapy should be started at least 12 hours before the potential insult (dye load or surgery) because this time delay will allow for a responsive diuresis and thus establish a euvolemic rather than a hypervolemic state. During the differential evaluation of pre- versus acute renal failure, fluid is typically infused at a rapid rate, and the renal response is observed. Prevention therapy, however, is best done with a more consistent and slower rate of infusion over longer periods of time.

Drug Adjustment and Addition

The approach to patients with the intent of reducing the incidence of acute renal failure (ARF) may require the adjustment of medication, the addition of other drugs, or merely the avoidance of certain situations or therapies that have been shown to be associated with renal dysfunction. The most rewarding results seem to be associated with the adjustment of medications to the patient's renal condition.

Antibiotic dosing frequently needs to be adjusted in renal failure. Not only the parent compound but also the metabolites may be toxic. Indeed, the metabolic products of many drug compounds have a longer half-life than the parent compound, so drug dosage adjustment should also be regulated according to a combination of these various levels. If no alteration is made in drug delivery, renal failure resulting from direct toxicity may result. Whereas acute allergic nephritis rarely is seen with the cephalosporin antibiotics, it occurs more frequently with some penicillins. The tetracyclines tend to potentiate acidosis, raise the blood urea nitrogen (BUN) levels and increase catabolism, whereas amphotericin is commonly associated with nephrotoxicity, renal tubular acidosis, hypokalemia, and nephrogenic diabetes insipidus. Maneuvers such as alkalization of the urine, adequate volume delivery, and avoidance of various combinations will help in minimizing the renal toxic effect.[21]

The classic example and perhaps the most frequently encountered antibiotic-related renal toxicity occurs with the use of aminoglycosides. Although early studies reported a relationship between trough drug levels and serum creatinine, Bennet et al.[22] showed no strong correlation between serum drug levels and nephrotoxicity. Thought to be the effect of the accumulated dose of the aminoglycoside, this renal failure was reported in subsequent studies to have resolved despite continuation of the drug.[23]

Within a class, some drugs are noted to be less toxic than others.[24] The reduced incidence of renal failure with the use of tobramycin over gentamycin is thought to be due to the number of cationic amino groups exhibited by each compound. The higher the number, the more the drug will be concentrated within the proximal tubule cells via its association with the negatively charged phospholipids of the cells' brush borders.[25] Subsequent studies have

Table 39-2. Drugs to Avoid or Use With Caution

Angiotensin-converting enzyme inhibitors (esp. in renal artery stenosis)
Nonsteroidal anti-inflammatory drugs (esp. with chronic renal failure)
Antibiotics (second series) aminoglycosides
  Penicillin associated with allergic nephritis
  Prolonged use of amphotericin

Table 39-3. Protective Drugs and Mechanisms of Protection

Intravascular volume
  Effect on renal plasma flow
  Effect on GFR
  Effect on tubular flow
Mannitol diuresis
  Effect on GFR
  Effect on tubular flow/pressure
Loop diuretic
  Effect on tubular flow
  Effect on cell metabolism
"Renal dose" dopamine
  Effect on plasma flow
  Effect on mesangial cell
Calcium channel blockade
  Effect on plasma flow
  Effect on membrane stability
Oxygen free-radical scavenger
  Effect on cellular enzymes
  Effect on membrane integrity

GFR, glomerular filtration rate.

not, however, confirmed the difference in renal dysfunction. The association of aminogycosides with cephalothin was thought to be associated with an increased incidence of renal failure; however, this has not been universally accepted, and there does not seem to be a similar relationship with other cephalosporins.

Avoiding certain medications in particular disease states will also help in prevention of renal injury (Table 39-2). Certainly, the use of angiotensin-converting enzyme (ACE) inhibition in the face of renal artery stenosis should be avoided. NSAIDs make up another class of medication that patients with chronic renal failure should avoid. Both classes of drugs have been found to adversely affect the kidney's ability to adjust to hemodynamic changes by eliminating or altering the local action of A-II or prostaglandins on the vascular responsiveness of the afferent and efferent glomerular arterioles.

Radiologic and imaging procedures have also been associated with a variable incidence of acute renal failure. Post-contrast renal failure is noted to be more prevalent among diabetics and patients with preexisting renal failure,[26] and the use of nonionic contrast has been considered to offer some protection when compared to the ionic contrast.[27] Schwab et al.[28] have not, however, been able to substantiate this finding. Limiting the contrast dose has been shown to reduce the frequency of nephrotoxicity (less than 125 ml), and Cigarroa et al.[29] have advocated dye limitation in predisposed patients according to the formula

$$\text{contrast limit} = \frac{5 \text{ ml dye/Kg body wt (limit 300 ml)}}{\text{serum creatinine (mg/dl)}}$$

The addition of certain types of drugs seems to have a beneficial effect in protecting the kidney from renal injury (Table 39-3). Calcium blockade prevents the influx of calcium into the injured cell both by membrane-stabilizing effects as well as by direct action on the cell mitochondria.[30-33] The addition of both a loop diuretic and/or an osmotic diuretic to stabilize the cell membrane, promote a brisk diuresis, and thus mechanically "flush" the tubules has also been advocated.[34] Loop diuretics also reduce cellular metabolism by paralyzing the Na-K-adenosine triphosphatase (ATPase) transport system, thereby reducing the metabolic demand of the tubular cell, which may be protective in ischemic states. These effects have all been seen to be variably effective in laboratory animal studies. Free oxygen radical scavengers have been found to be an effective protective agent during the reflow phenomenon of postischemic injury,[35] whereas the so-called "renal-dose" infusion of dopamine either alone or in combination with a loop diuretic has been said to be protective.[36,37] This latter effect is thought to be the result of enhanced renal cortical blood flow and relaxation of the glomerular mesangial cells, thus promoting a change in the K_f of the glomerular basement membrane that is due to structural change. More recently, preservation of intestinal blood flow and thus avoidance of gut ischemia and endotoxin influx associated with vasoactive amine production has been postulated as dopamine's major influence.

With the possible exception of mannitol and calcium-blockade, there have been no well-designed studies in humans that have shown any protective benefit from any of the other drug regimens. Animal and bench research data are more persuasive but may be the result of the controlled atmosphere in which these investigations have been conducted. Of note, in neither laboratory nor clinical trials has any major toxicity from the use of these various drug schema been demonstrated.

Translating this mix of data from the laboratory to the clinics has resulted in the formulation of a "hyperfiltration cocktail" as our generic renal protective maneuver (Table 39-4). High risk patients are usually started with hydration (0.45 to 0.9 N saline) at rates that will promote intravascular repletion and diuresis. Calcium channel blockade

Table 39-4. Renal Hyperfiltration Protective Therapy

Agent	Method
Fluids	0.45–0.9 normal saline (Rate Adjusted to GFR)
Ca^{++} blockade	Nifedipine, 5–10 mg, HS and AM (if not already receiving therapy)
	Or diltiazem, 15–30 mg, HS and AM (if not already receiving therapy)
Diuretics	Lasix (Bumex), 40–100 mg IV, "on call" (may repeat during and after insult as needed q3–4h)
	Mannitol, 25–50 g IV, "on call" (may repeat during and after insult as needed q3–4h)
O^2 Scavenger	Allopurinol 150–300 mg (12 h before insult)
Vascular activity	Dopamine 1.5 μg/kg/min "on call" (continued for 24 h after insult, then slowly taper × 12 h)

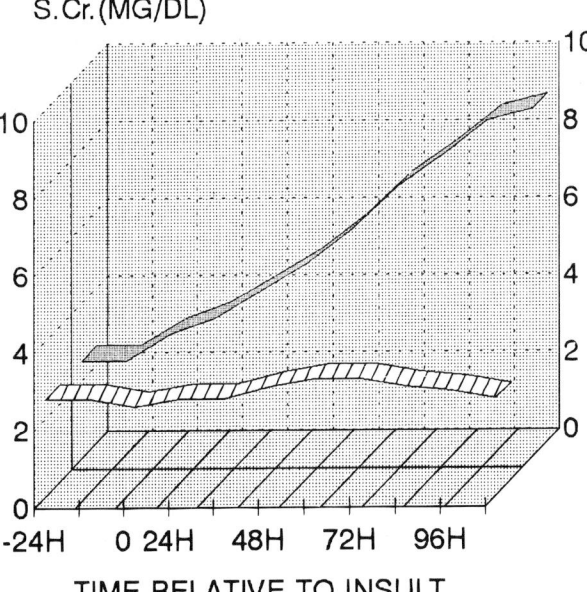
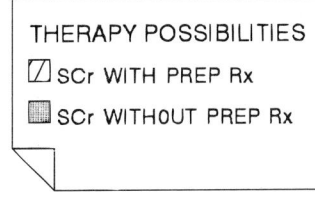

Fig. 39–3. Renal hyperfiltration theory: theoretical response to the "hyperfiltration cocktail." Given the same level of renal dysfunction before insult, the kidneys that had the protection of the "hyperfiltration cocktail" (see text) seem to maintain function while the unprotected kidneys demonstrate a rise in serum creatinine (SCr) levels.

should be started the day before the potential injury (surgery, dye, etc.) is contemplated. On call to the operating room or the radiology suite, an infusion of dopamine (1.5 µg/kg dry weight per minute) is begun, and the patient is also given intravenous mannitol (25 to 50 g) and furosemide (40 to 120 mg), as well as continuing the original fluid infusion. This may necessitate placing a indwelling or condom catheter for urine collection, which is not a problem for patients going to the operating room but is not usually done for radiologic interventions. With instances of expected severe renal ischemia, the addition of allopurinol (100 to 300 mg) to the preoperative regimen would be appropriate. Drug and fluid infusions are continued during the intervention and through the subsequent 12- to 24-hour period with close monitoring of renal function, pulmonary function, and electrolyte balance.

The immediate serum creatinine is usually stable or slightly decreased, reflecting either the expanded volume status of the patient or an induced increase in GFR, a so-called "induced hyperfiltration state." Gradual removal of this therapy is usually accompanied by a slight increase in the serum levels of creatinine and urea which return to baseline over the next 2 to 3 days (Fig. 39-3). If the laboratory pattern shows a persistent decrease in renal function, it has generally been delayed beyond the immediate postinjury time frame, thus allowing for easier patient management.

This approach has its origin in laboratory-based animal investigations of the cause of acute ischemic renal failure. If renal insult can be anticipated, then it indeed seems reasonable to protect the patients most at risk. This approach should not, however, be considered standard practice for all patients, given the expense and associated potential risks. On the other hand, the use of this protocol in patients thought to be a high risk is justified if acute renal failure can be avoided and the related morbidity and expenses eliminated.

ICU PHASE: DIAGNOSIS AND OUTCOME MODIFICATION

Diagnosis

Although the ICU patient frequently has acute renal failure as part of a multisystem dysfunction, the cause of renal failure is discovered following the same rigid analysis one would apply to all patients with single-system renal dysfunction. Classically, the history and physical exam will allow one to categorize the condition as follows:

- Prerenal: congestive heart failure (CHF), hypoalbuminemia, renal bruit, physical and hemodynamic findings consistent with volume depletion, weight changes
- Postrenal: recent abdominal surgery, distended bladder in a diabetic, an enlarged prostate in an elderly male
- Intrinsic: exposure to toxins or drugs, signs of vasculitis, severe hemodynamic instability, septic syndrome, intraoperative catastrophe

Urine volume can be used as an aid in the classification of acute renal disorders but should not be the only factor considered in the categorization of the disease type. Whereas anuria (less than 100 ml per day) is frequent with total obstruction, it can also be present with cortical necrosis, vascular occlusion, severe acute glomerular disease, and acute tubular necrosis (ATN) (especially after open heart surgery). Oliguria (100 to 400 ml per day) is the most frequent presentation of intrinsic renal disease but can also be seen with partial obstruction as well as with prerenal conditions; nonoliguria (more than 400 ml per day) may be seen in prerenal conditions if diuretics have been used but is more frequently seen with intrinsic renal disease and partial or postobstructive states. Fluctuating anuria and polyuria is the hallmark of obstruction, and this diagnosis should be aggressively pursued.

A complete urine analysis should be undertaken in all patients presenting with renal dysfunction. Simple testing and microscopic investigation will have the highest yield at the lowest cost and can often help in making the definitive diagnosis. Generally, the **specific gravity** of the urine produced is not very reliable in differentiating prerenal from renal disease. Specific gravity, which measures the size and density rather than the number of particles in the urine, is easily influenced by such things as contrast dye, dextran, carbenicillin, and mannitol. Indeed, this false elevation (greater than 1.030) could help in establishing the cause in dye-induced renal failure. The specific gravity in prerenal failure is often greater than 1.020, whereas intrinsic disease results in a specific gravity of 1.010. Urine osmolality measures the number of particles in the urine and is classified as hypotonic, isotonic, or hypertonic when compared to the tonicity of serum (285 to 290 mOsm). Prerenal conditions usually have a higher urine osmolality (more than 500 mOsm), and renal conditions will have a lower value (less than 350 mOsm). Although a significant crossover exists, urine/plasma osmolality ratios (U/P osm) may well distinguish prerenal (more than 1.3) from renal (less than 1.0) dysfunction.

Dipstix testing for protein, hemoglobin, ketone, and glucose will aid in framing possible causes. A disparate small amount of protein measured by standard albumin-sensitive calorimetric testing when compared to a large precipitate during sulfosalicylic acid (SSA) testing of the same urine sample points toward Bence-Jones protein states. A large amount of protein (2 to 3 + dipstix) can be seen with CHF, NSAID administration, or acute/chronic glomerular diseases. A positive **hemoglobin test,** accompanied by a negative microscopic examination for red blood cells in a red urine is highly suggestive of myoglobin, whereas glucosuria in a nondiabetic patient may point toward toxin-induced proximal tubular damage. **Urine pH** may be quite alkaline as a result of obstruction-impaired acidification, which would lead to a hyperchloremic acidosis. Careful testing, however, will show impaired acidification in all forms of renal dysfunction.

Electrolyte determination in the urine will often be helpful in distinguishing prerenal from renal dysfunction. When this value is coupled with creatinine determinations of both urine and serum, one can derive either the fractional excretion of sodium or the renal failure index (Table 39–5). The urine/plasma creatinine ratio has less specificity but may be of enormous value when evaluating the recovery of renal function with a patient being supported on continuous renal replacement therapies.

The appearance rates of **BUN** and of **serum creatinine** can help in establishing not only the severity of renal failure but also the overall state of catabolism in a patient with renal failure. The BUN is indeed influenced by protein intake, gastrointestinal bleeding, liver disease, use of medications such as tetracycline or steroids, and fever or sepsis. A total loss of renal function in a patient who is highly catabolic will be accompanied by rise in the BUN of greater than 40 mg/dl per day (galloping azotemia). Given the normal production of 18 to 20 mg/kg per day of creatinine in the male and 12 to 16 mg/kg per day in the female, a rise of greater than 2 mg/dl per day speaks for total renal shutdown. A higher appearance rate is usually seen in conditions of greater muscle breakdown such as rhabdomyolysis.

The urine microscopic examination frequently holds the key to the definitive diagnosis of the renal condition. Whereas prerenal states usually are accompanied by a bland microscopic examination, postrenal causes may be accompanied by crystals such as uric acid (footballs), triple phosphate (coffin lids), calcium oxalate (envelopes), or clots and papillae. Intrinsic renal states are seen with pigmented (dirty brown) casts and/or sheets of renal tubular epithelial cells (ATN), red blood cell casts and/or oval fat bodies (glomerular), and eosinophiluria (interstitial nephritis, atheroembolic disease).

Review of the available hemodynamic data may further aid in establishing the cause of the renal failure. Certainly, the correlation of physical signs and symptoms to the degree of hydration will help in establishing a prerenal picture. Often, central monitoring data will be necessary because the combination of several states may mask the underlying condition of the patient. Administering a fluid challenge to patients will often help in the differentiation of prerenal from intrinsic renal disease, but the blind use of diuretic therapy will not clarify the diagnosis and may actually worsen the overall renal status. Once a diagnosis has been established, the judicious use of loop diuretics, either in repeated doses or as a continuous infusion, may help in the conversion from oliguria to a nonoliguric state.

The relatively simplistic view of renal dysfunction being primarily the consequence of aberrant hemodynamic factors may account for a large portion of renal failure. The not-uncommon occurrence, however, of renal dysfunction without identified hemodynamic alterations may, indeed, have its basis in factors that only now are coming to light.

Radiologic studies may be helpful in establishing a possible cause. Plain films of the abdomen can establish both renal presence and size and may also demonstrate the pres-

Table 39–5. Differential Diagnosis of Prerenal Azotemia Versus Acute Tubular Necrosis

Entity	Prerenal	ATN
Serum creatinine	> 4 rarely	> 4 often
BUN/creatinine	< 20	10–15
Urinary Na	< 20	> 40
Urinary Osm	> 500	< 350
U/P creatinine	> 40	< 20
U/P urea	> 8	< 3
FeNa $\frac{U/P\ sodium}{U/P\ creatinine} \times 100$	< 1%	< 1%
Renal failure index $\frac{Urinary\ Na}{U/P\ creatinine}$	< 1	> 1
Urinary sediment	Scant, hyaline fine granular casts	Renal tubular epithelial cells, muddy casts

ATN, acute tubular necrosis: BUN, blood urea nitrogen; U/P, urine/plasma; FeNa, fractional excretion of sodium.
(From Paganini, E.P., and Bosworth, C.R.: Acute renal failure after open heart surgery: newer concepts and current therapy. Semin. Thorac. Cardiovasc. Surg., 3:63, 1992.)

ence of radiopaque stones. Renal ultrasound has replaced the intravenous pyelogram in the evaluation of obstructive uropathy, while the use of abdominal computed tomography (CT) scanning techniques with dye can further locate pathology and may avoid the use of angiography or venography for the diagnosis of cortical necrosis. Radionuclide scanning techniques have been helpful in the evaluation of renal artery disease, but bilateral disease may not be as easily identified with these techniques. Therefore, one needs to rely on various digital subtraction angiographic techniques to definitively diagnose arterial occlusive disease.

The use of renal biopsy in confirming the cause of the renal dysfunction is an infrequently exploited tool reserved for the patient with no obvious cause of intrinsic renal failure or in patients who require therapy with a drug that may be causing an allergic interstitial nephritis. Treatable systemic diseases may also be diagnosed with this approach. It is of interest that the frequency of unsuspected underlying disease states other than pure ATN has been found to be as high as 40% in some series when the preceding criteria for biopsy are followed.[38]

Cause and Presentation

The clinical presentation of renal dysfunction has been found to follow three general patterns when serum creatinine levels are tracked over time[39,40] (Fig. 39-4). Pattern A reflects a distinct insult with rapid drop in glomerular filtration rate (GFR) and rise in serum creatinine, while patterns B and C reflect a longer duration of continued renal insult and thus a slower but nonetheless steady decline in function. This distinction is useful in the clinical evaluation of patients, because pattern A has the best prognosis, especially when nonoliguric, whereas pattern C has the worst.

Apart from the obvious hemodynamic changes noted during the peri-insult time frame of most acute renal failure, vasoactive intestinal polypeptide (VIP), thromboxane A_2, and endothelin are also emerging as strong players in the renal failure associated with sepsis and have been touted as having some role in the development of multiorgan failure in the patient with "septic syndrome." Furthermore, an increasing body of evidence (Table 39-6) points to the active role of vasoactive polypeptides and cytokines such as tumor necrosis factor (TNF), the leukotrienes, human lymphotoxin (HLT), and endothelin as the basis for additional renal dysfunction.[41-48] This cascade is said to be induced by the back-diffusion of endotoxin produced by normal gut flora and allowed to enter the blood stream through ischemic or damaged intestinal mucosa. This will in turn stimulate macrophage mRNA transcription and translation of TNF. Acting synergistically with interleukin-1, TNF can activate the endothelial cell, pathologically leading to microvascular injury by its enhanced coagulant and inflammatory activity. Endothelin has been noted to be a potent vasoconstrictor, with a 10-fold increased responsiveness of the renal vasculature when compared to coronary, bronchial, and femoral vessels. Thus, organ dysfunction may indeed be the result of immunologic overresponsiveness, initiated by endotoxins and mediated through TNF, finally inducing polymorphonuclear leukocytes (PMNs) to release oxygen radicals and lysosomal enzymes.

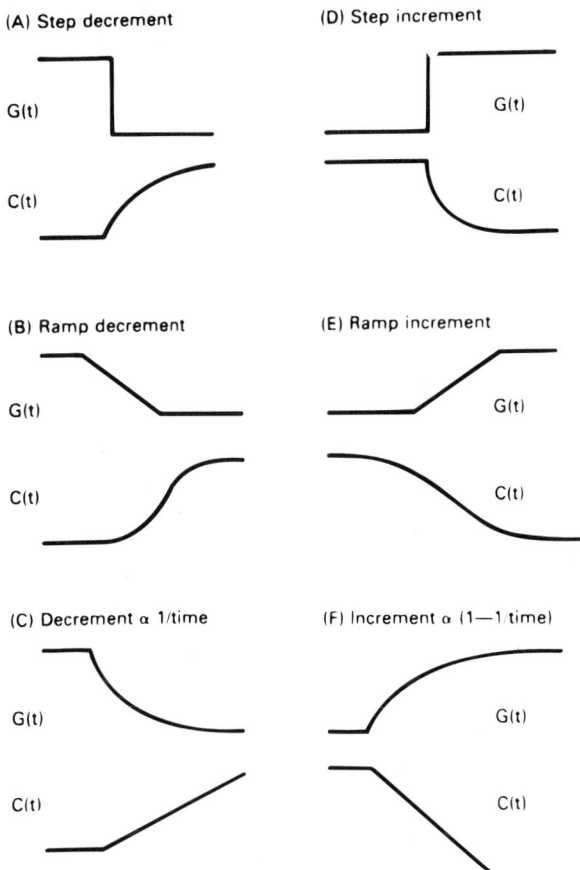

Fig. 39-4. A to C, Patterns of acute renal failure. D to F, Patterns of renal recovery. Where G(t) is the change of glomerular filtration rate over time, and C(t) is the change in serum creatinine levels over time. (Reprinted with permission from Moran, S. M., and Myers, B. D.: Course of acute renal failure studied by a model of creatinine kinetics. Kidney Int., 27:928, 1985.)

Administering endotoxin to animals or normal human volunteers results initially in a hemodynamic state that is indistinguishable from that of sepsis. Continued infusions in animals have lead to hyperdynamic flow states, diffuse intravascular coagulation disorders, and liver and renal failure. In some studies, the outcome of septic shock may correlate with the plasma levels of endotoxin.[49-52]

Inadequate perfusion will injure the intestinal mucosa and increase its permeability and thus the absorption of endotoxin. Other causes of ischemia such as bleeding, sustained systemic hypotension, surgical vascular clamping, or cardiopulmonary bypass may contribute to the decrease in gut mucosal integrity. Other vasoactive polypeptides and neuropeptides that may have potential renal effects include parathormone (PTH), atrial natriuretic factor (ANF), arginine vasopressin (AVP), and angiotensin II.

Early intervention may either attenuate or avoid the immunologic sequelae noted in the preceding scenario. The use of either medical intervention (Tables 39-7 and 39-8) or plasma perfusion over polymyxin B bound to polysty-

Table 39-6. Active Substances in the Development of Multiple Organ Dysfunction

Substance	Chemistry	Source	Stimulus	Synergism	Action
TNF	Polypeptide 51–54 kD	Monocyte Macrophage	ET Others	IL-1	Cell biology Inflammation
IL-1	Polypeptide 17.5 kD	Monocyte Macrophage Endothelial cell PMN	ET TNF IL-1 Others	TNF	Hemostasis Vascular tone Cachexia Tumor
HL	Glycoprotein 60–70 kD	Lymphocyte	TNF IL-1 Others	?	Cytotoxicity

TNF, tumor necrosis factor; IL-1, interleukin 1; HL, human lymphotoxin; ET, endotoxin; PMN, polymorphonuclear leukocyte. (From Paganini, E.P., and Bosworth, C.R.: Acute renal failure after open heart surgery: newer concepts and current therapy. Semin. Thorac. Cardiovasc. Surg., 3:63, 1992.)

Table 39-7. Therapeutic Advances

Drug	Action	Effect
Lipid X	Competitive with lipid A Reduces synthesis of TNF	TNF ↓
Antibodies to ET/lipid A	Inactivates ET/lipid A	TNF ↓
Dexamethasone	Suppresses both ET-stimulated transcription and translation of TNF genetic code	TNF ↓
Oxypentifylline	Suppresses the synthesis of TNF	TNF ↓
Antibodies to TNF	Inactivates TNF	TNF ↓
Allopurinol	Xanthine oxidase inhibitor	Superoxides ↓
DMSO	Hydroxyl radical scavenger	Hydroxyl radicals ↓
PGE$_1$	Smooth vascular muscle Platelets	Vasodilatation inhibits platelet aggregation
Methylprednisone	Phospholipase inhibitor	Eicosanoids =
NSAIDs	TxA$_2$ and PGI$_2$ synthesis inhibitor	TxA$_2$ ↓ PGI$_2$ ↓
TSI	TxA$_2$ synthesis inhibitor	TxA$_2$ ↓
DEC	Lipo-oxygenase inhibitor	LT ↓
FPL 55712	Competitive with LT	LT ↓
Aprotinin	Kallikrein inhibitor	Bradykinin ↓
Ketanserin	Serotonin antagonist	Pulmonary artery pressure ↓

ET, endotoxin; TNF, tumor necrosis factor; NSAID, nonsteroidal anti-inflammatory drug; TxA, thromboxane A$_2$; PGI$_2$, prostacyclin; TSI, thromboxane A$_2$ synthesis inhibitors; LT, leukotriene antagonist; DEC, diethylcarbamazine; FPL 55712, LT antagonist; DMSO, dimethyl sulfoxide.

Table 39-8. Medical Therapy in Early Acute Renal Failure

Substance	Description	Effect	Complications
Fluid	Crystalloid Colloid	Expand fluid; increase intravascular volume, balance electrolytes, convert oliguric to nonoliguric	Water excess, electrolyte imbalance, intravascular overload, pulmonary and cardiac dysfunction
Diuretic	Loop-bolus drip Loop and vasopressor Combo "nephron bomb" Osmotic	Maintains tubular fluid flow: decreases cellular metabolism, stabilizes membrane, converts oliguric to nonoliguric	Intestinal ischemia intravascular depletion, other oxygen oxicity (i.e., ototoxocity, hepatotoxicity)
Drug Trials	NaHCO$_3$	Alkaline urine, control acidosis	Hyponatremia, alkalemia, volume excess
	Dopamine	Maintain GFR: normalizes RBF	Tachyarrhythmias, hypertension
	CA^{++} blockade	Stabilizes membrane: prevents mitochondrial damage	Hypotension, tachyphylaxis
	Epidermal growth factor (r-Hu-EGF)	Promotes hastened cell development and growth	Under study
	Atrial natriuretic peptide		Under study

GFR, glomerular filtration; RBF, renal blood flow.

rene fibers has been shown to either alter the cytokine response to a stimulus or eliminate the stimulus altogether.[53]

TREATMENT VARIANTS AND CONCOMITANT THERAPIES

Medical Approach to Therapy

Managing a patient with established renal failure is limited to the balance of appropriate fluids and medications. With the widespread use of hyperalimentation and the need for drug delivery, frequently, the renal patient will be exposed to a significant fluid challenge. The classic attempt to limit intake has become impossible because both the delivery of medication and the use of invasive monitoring require the administration of a substantial amount of volume. Fluid excess was thought to be bothersome only if it remained intravascular; however, recent evidence has demonstrated the association of volume excess with increased mortality and morbidity in postoperative patients.[54] Thus, aggressive measures must be undertaken to ensure the restriction of unnecessary volume as well as the aggressive removal of excess.

Attempts to convert oliguria to nonoliguria must be done early in the course of renal failure, as close to the insult as possible.[55] As noted previously, pretreatment of patients who are at higher risk for developing renal dysfunction from a known potential insult is the best approach. Obviously, this is not always possible, and the best alternative is to begin drug manipulation as soon as there is evidence of renal decline. Once assured of an effective intravascular volume, one can initiate combination therapy with dopamine and a loop diuretic, or the combined use of loop, osmotic, and proximal/distal tubular diuretics (the so-called "nephron bomb") can aid in the conversion to or maintenance of a nonoliguric status.[56]

Fluid restriction is required in patients with oliguria. This is frequently at odds with the patient's nutritional needs, especially in patients who are highly catabolic. The traditional approach to patients with renal failure has been to restrict both their volume and their nitrogen load, while attempting to deliver adequate calories. More recent studies have pointed to the improved outcome in patients who were treated with both adequate calories and protein.[57-64] Thus, the higher urea appearance rate that accompanies the infusion of increased amounts of hyperalimentation can be counterbalanced by a more aggressive dialytic approach.

Required attention to volume has made the delivery of adequate nutrition to the acutely ill patient with renal failure difficult at best. The fluid restrictions imposed partly by the adverse hemodynamic consequences of volume removal with intermittent dialytic therapy, partly by the need for daily intervention to avoid fulminant fluid-overloaded states, and ultimately by the catabolic state generated by dialysis itself have resulted in the underdelivery of nutrients. This state of starvation has contributed to the high morbidity and mortality rates commonly associated with acute renal failure patients. Bartlett et al.[65] noted that the increased mortality in patients with multiorgan failure seemed to parallel their calorie deficit, and correcting this deficit was accompanied by an improved survival. Asbach et al.[66] noted a decrease in protein catabolism when calories were increased in renal failure patients, and others[61-65] noted an improved renal recovery rate in this same population.

Unfortunately, no recent prospective controlled studies attest to the claim that total parenteral nutrition is crucially linked to patient survival in the intensive care setting. While Abel et al.[57] did indeed find a correlation between glucose intake and outcome in severely ill patients, others have not been able to discern any difference in survival when various forms of amino acid solutions are used as total parenteral nutrition (TPN). In fact, a recent study found continued loss of protein and no increase in body mass in eight critically ill patients receiving aggressive TPN.[67] Restrictions in volume and urea load, however, may have limited the delivered protein. Thus, with the addition of continuous dialytic therapy, this restriction can be lifted with the potential of improving outcome once adequate nutrition is delivered.

Chima et al.[68] estimated the individual protein needs of patients undergoing continuous arteriovenous hemofiltration (CAVH) in the ICU using standard formulas. Correlating these projections with the actually measured needs of the patients, they found the calculated estimates of 1.5 ± 0.25 g protein/kg body weight seemed to match the delivered protein of 1.4 ± 0.5 g via TPN. Although these measures were successful in predicting the protein needs of the group, when individualized these measures did not seem to correlate well with daily protein catabolic rates (1.8 ± 0.75 g/kg). These investigators were able, however, to achieve a positive protein balance in several of their patients. This was only possible because of the fluid removal capacity of the CAVH therapy.

The validity of delivery of unrestricted protein and calories to patients with acute renal failure needs to be thoroughly studied. This practice is promoting the use of therapies that will help in the removal of volume, and if no reduction in mortality or morbidity can be demonstrated, perhaps we are opening patients to unnecessary risks.

Recent work with various growth factors or hormonal manipulations has shown promise in reducing the time of renal shutdown and hastening renal recovery. Atrial natriuretic peptide[69-71] (ANP) has demonstrated the ability to promote a diuresis and natriuresis, to suppress the renin-angiotensin axis, and to increase the GFR in normal kidneys, probably through its effect both on the afferent (where it dilates) and efferent (where it constricts) renal arterioles. Animal studies have also demonstrated a renal preservation effect in both the ischemic and toxic renal failure model. Administration of the hormone even days after the insult may also result in improved renal function and histology.[72] Early prospective human studies are about to be undertaken to investigate the role of ANP in the clinical treatment of acute renal failure.

Genetically engineered epidermal growth factor (EGF), along with transforming growth factor alpha, have been shown to have a direct effect on renal proximal tubular cell growth and proliferation, thus hastening the development of the regenerating tubular cells and reducing the postischemic (or post-toxic) recovery phase in animals with induced ATN.[73] Animal data have also shown the possible beneficial effect of early recombinant human erythropoietin delivery on the rate of renal recovery in rats subjected to cisplatin-induced acute renal failure. Whether these therapies will be effective in patients with multisystem dysfunction and whether shortened recovery time will change the ultimate outcome of this population still need to be studied.

Evidence is also mounting that the choice of dialysis membranes may have an important influence on renal tubular cell recovery.[74,75] Long thought to be merely the result of hemodynamic insults continually induced by the hypotension that frequently accompanies the dialytic process, delayed recovery in patients supported by dialysis was considered a necessary trade-off of the dialytic support process.[76] Animal studies have demonstrated a negative effect of repeated exposure of blood to certain types of dialysis membranes. For example, exposure to cuprophane-based dialytic membranes induces an immunologic cascade, which will ultimately delay renal tubular cell recovery. This phenomenon is not seen with the more biocompatible noncuprophane plastic membranes.[74]

The importance of specific therapeutic approaches rendered to patients with renal failure has thus become more relevant to the ultimate recovery of function. Close attention to the use of various drug types and adherence to the clinical models for drug therapy alteration in patients with renal dysfunction will also be important steps that can be taken by the ICU care giver.

Mechanical Support

There has been a considerable difference of various investigators in the meaning of terms used to describe the techniques used. **Hemofiltration** has been used for ultrafiltration techniques,[77] combined diffusion and convection techniques,[78] and true convective transfer exchanges.[79] "Dialysis" has been used in the description of both convective and diffusive maneuvers,[80] whereas "ultrafiltration" has been described as the removal of fluid associated with hemofiltration or as the description of water loss during the various procedures. Establishing definitions with meaning and adhering to the terminology strictly will allow comparison of data and specific techniques in a particular clinical situation.

The term **ultrafiltration** should refer to the loss of fluid. The type of fluid loss will ultimately depend on the manner in which the volume is removed. For example, if fluid is lost with the use of pure convective forces, either during isolated ultrafiltration or during hemofiltration (see following discussion), then the type of ultrafiltrate is consistent with plasma water. If the loss occurs in conjunction with the diffusive forces of dialysis, the fluid type may differ, depending on the solute concentration of the dialysate. **Hemofiltration** is the removal of plasma water and the replacement of that loss or percentage of the loss with fluid constituted to effect a change in either the acid/base status, electrolyte status, or the concentration of a particular substance such as urea or creatinine. It is principally

Table 39–9. Practical Definitions of Dialytic Therapy Delivered to Patients with Acute Renal Failure

Hemodialysis
A diffusion-based mode of blood cleaning wherein ultrafiltration is limited to the removal of excessive body water. The aim is uremic control as well as fluid and electrolyte balance. It can be intermittent (HD), continuous arteriovenous (CAVHD), or continuous pump-assisted venovenous (CVVHD).

Hemofiltration
A convective mode of blood cleaning wherein large fluid exchanges account for virtually all solute removal. The aim is uremic control as well as fluid and electrolyte balance. It can be intermittent (HF), continuous arteriovenous (CAVH), or continuous pump-assisted venovenous (CVVH).

Ultrafiltration
The removal of plasma water as well as small molecular weight substances (electrolytes, urea) in an attempt at fluid balance. It can be intermittent (IUF) or continuous (SCUF).

thought of as a convective technique. In effect, this process is a plasma water exchange, rather than a volume depletion maneuver.

Hemodialysis is a diffusive exchange of substances across a semipermeable membrane. The kinetics of these elements across the dialysis membranes are classified into two major movement forces: (1) blood flow dependent for the smaller molecular weight substances and (2) membrane dependent for the larger substances. Thus, movement will be affected by both the dialysate and blood flow rates as well as the effective permeability (pore size) of the membrane (Table 39–9).

All techniques can be either intermittent or continuous. Intermittent therapy is offered for a variable period of time (usually less than 5 hours) and is interrupted by periods of nontherapy. Continuous therapy, as the name implies, is offered for the full day of therapy. Thus, the continuous methods may be less efficient for a given period of time of comparison yet offer the same total transfer because the low efficiency is compensated by the long therapy periods.

Access to the blood supply for the particular therapy should also be described in its definition. When using both arterial and venous access, the term **arteriovenous** should be applied to the therapy name. If the venous system alone is used as a blood source, then the term **venovenous** should be used. Venovenous access requires a blood pump to generate blood flow for therapy. Therefore, terms such as "pumpless" or "pump assisted" are implied in the terms describing blood access. Table 39–9 summarizes the definitions and terms that will be used in this discussion, whereas Figures 39–5 to 39–7 picture the various extracorporeal continuous therapies as usually practiced. A complete discussion of the technology behind the various types of therapy is beyond the scope of this review. The reader is referred to several recent texts[81,82] or review articles[83-91] dealing with dialytic therapies.

Therapy Selection and Patient Outcome

It is now well established that the separation of ultrafiltration form diffusion is accompanied by improved patient hemodynamic stability. Silverstein et al.[92] described the use of isolated ultrafiltration in patients with fluid overload, and Neff et al.[93] as well as Shaldon et al.[94] applied the continuous circuit to chronic patients for fluid control with reasonably good results.

The stability of hemofiltration over hemodialysis was originally thought to be due to the slower nature of the solute clearances with hemofiltration. Chen,[95] Paganini et al.,[96] and Chaignon et al.[97] described the active role of the venous side of the circulation as the foundation of this improved hemodynamic stability, and virtually all who reviewed the area of continuous therapies noted that patient selection was predominantly made on the basis of hemodynamic status.[98] Patients with acute renal failure who were labeled "hemodialysis resistant" because of severe hypotensive responses to attempted therapy session were found to be quite tolerant of both CAVH and continuous arteriovenous hemodialysis (CAVHD).[99]

The ability, therefore, to deliver dialysis to patients who normally would have been denied it because of physical conditions framed the patient type for the early experiences with CAVH and slow continuous ultrafiltration (SCUF). In this focused population, any treatment success was applauded, and greater expectations were placed on the therapy than perhaps was clinically evident. Although some described the utility of the techniques as "nephrologist toys" or promoting "bad medicine" because it allowed the patient to receive more fluid instead of restricting the fluid intake, others lauded the attributes of increased nutritional support and reported improved survival rates in various subgroups of patients when compared to historical controls or other studies of similar patient types.[60-63]

Control of azotemia is illustrated in Figure 39-8. The average level of BUN and serum creatinine in our ICU acute renal failure patient population over the past years (1989 to 1991; 320 patients) demonstrates the effectiveness of therapy selection in allowing increased nutritional intake and in controlling the resultant urea generation. Ultimate mortality has not, however, been shown to have been affected by therapy choice. When one compares the out-

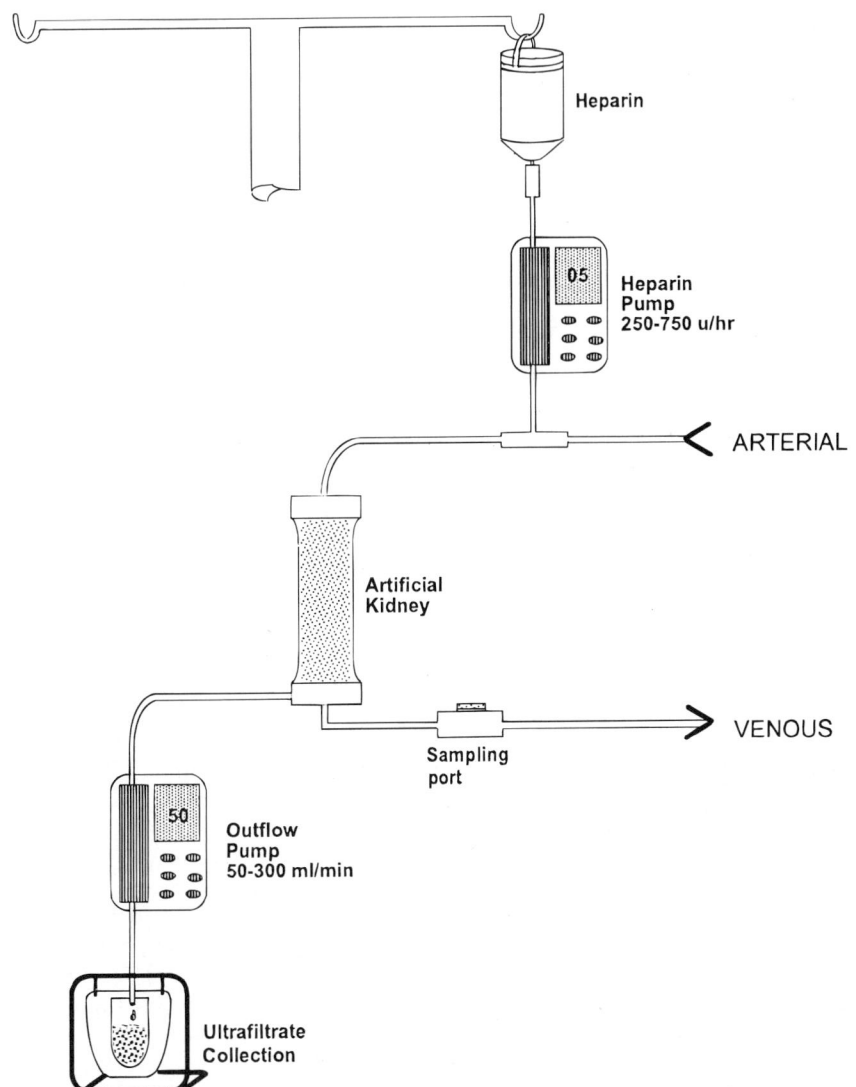

Fig. 39-5. Circuitry for slow continuous ultrafiltration. (From Bosworth, C.: SCVF/CAVH/CAVHD: critical differences. Crit. Care Nurs. Q., *14*:45, 1992.)

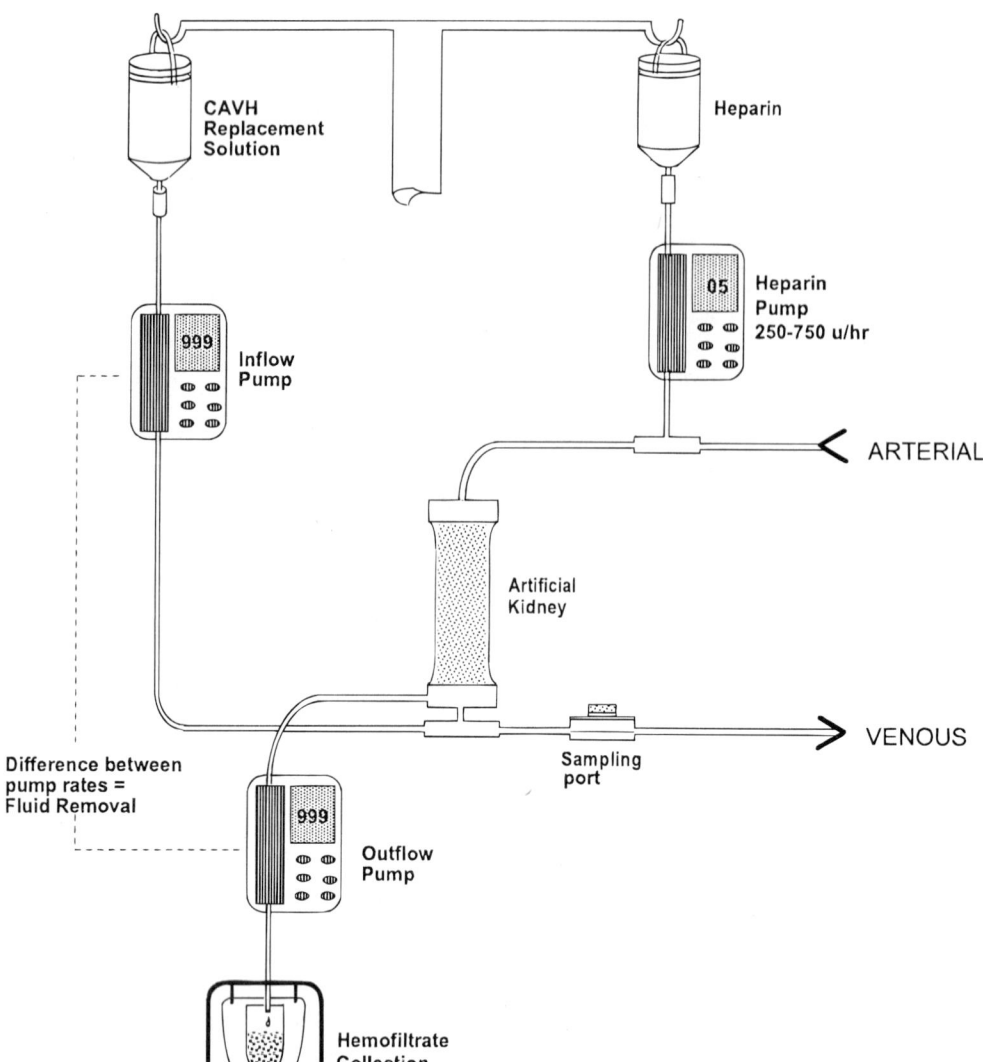

Fig. 39-6. Circuitry for continuous arteriovenous hemofiltration (CAVH). (From Bosworth, C.: SCVF/CAVH/CAVHD: critical differences. Crit. Care Nurs. Q., *14*:45, 1992.)

come of similarly classified patients, survival ranges from a low of 19% in multiorgan failure[100] to an average 24% in patients with similar APACHE II scores.[101-103]

Our survival rates are somewhat higher (32%), but comparison is meaningless unless done as a prospective randomized study. The effectiveness of continuous methodology to provide therapy to the hemodynamically unstable patients has made the randomization of this patient type to intermittent therapy difficult. Recent reviews,[104-106] however, have pointed to the more advanced systems available for the intermittent user that may increase patient stability during therapy. Problems with the differences in access and the inability to control the blood flow accurately in the arteriovenous therapies also make comparative studies difficult. Current therapy using a venovenous approach can be examined as a true therapy comparison,[107] perhaps offering advantages to the arteriovenous approach (Fig. 39-9). The complexity of the currently available venovenous technology and the resistance of many ICU staff to manage these systems make the therapy difficult to establish. The advantage of the arteriovenous therapies is avoidance of this technology literacy requirement, which makes acceptance much easier (Table 39-10).

The decision for applying the appropriate form of therapy to the appropriate group of patients still remains a subjective and difficult process. The admission criteria for varying ICUs differ, and the general patient type may indeed differ, depending on the co-morbid history of these varying patient populations.

In a retrospective analysis of the experience at the Cleveland Clinic since the early 1980s, an average of 80 to 100 patients with acute renal dysfunction were seen in the ICUs each year. Sixty to seventy five percent of these patients received some form of extracorporeal therapeutic intervention. The usual type of therapy delivered was classified as intermittent alone (43%), continuous alone (29.7%) or a combined therapeutic approach (27.3%). Whereas 75% of the acute renal failure was secondary to surgical intervention, 29.5% of the group was seen after open heart surgery, and 58% of the patients with acute renal failure had an initial serum creatinine greater than 1.4 mg/dl on admission to the hospital.

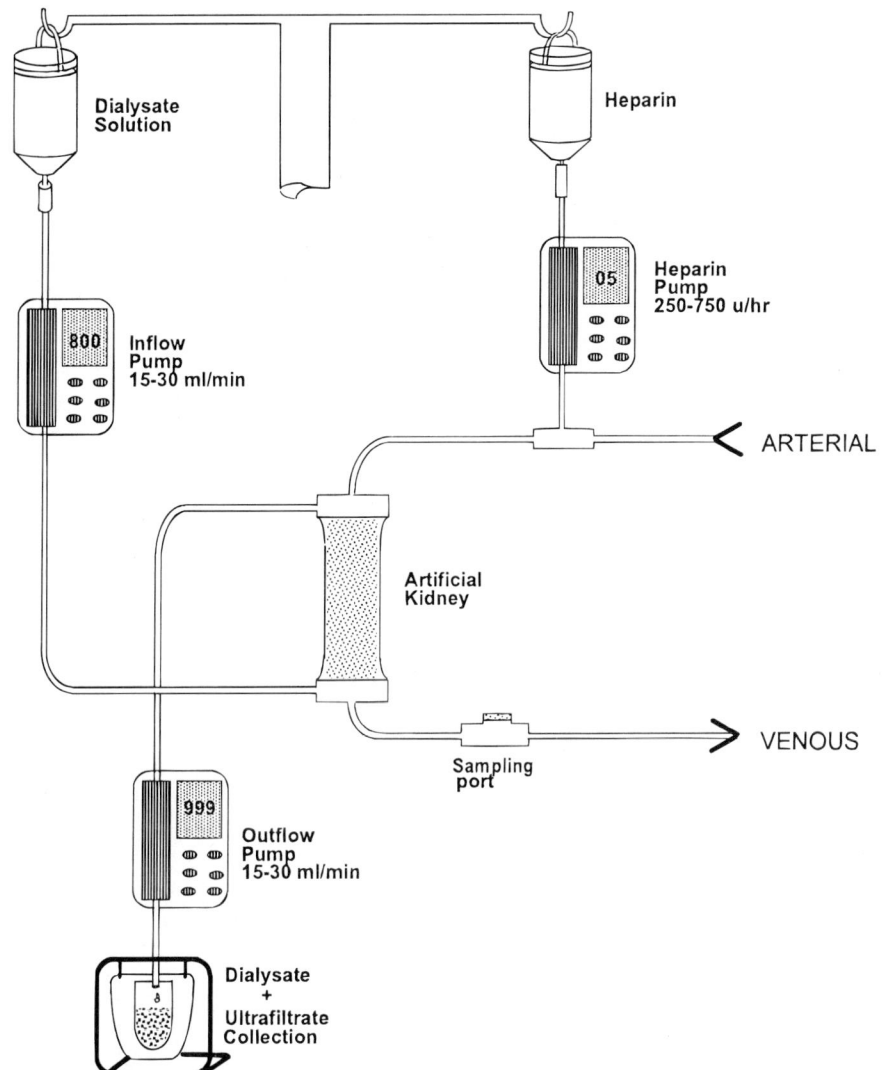

Fig. 39-7. Circuitry for continuous arteriovenous hemodialysis. (From Bosworth, C.: SCVF/CAVH/CAVHD: critical differences. Crit. Care Nurs. Q., *14*:45, 1992.)

Patients were classified with the APACHE II scoring system, calculating their scores on admission to the ICU (A_1) and at the time of the renal consult (A_2). The differences in the APACHE scores were calculated as an A_2/A_1 ratio. In the continuous group, this ratio was noted to be greater than 1, indicating a worsening of the overall physiologic and clinical condition of these patients, whereas the intermittent group showed an improving score during their ICU stay, resulting in a ratio of less than 1. The presence of multiorgan failure, defined as the presence of three or more organ dysfunctions, was also more frequently encountered in the continuous (92%) and the combined (80%) groups, again pointing to the more severely impaired physiologic state of these patients.

Those systems most frequently associated with mortality in the patients with acute renal failure was pulmonary failure (100%), hyperbilirubinemia (74.4%), and hypotension (systolic pressures less than 90 mm Hg) (70%). Thus the continuous therapies should be considered in multisystem failure patients who have low mean arterial pressures. Patients who have the potential for hemodynamic instability if subjected to intermittent hemodialysis techniques and receiving large volume intakes despite established oliguria are another group who might benefit from continuous therapies. Those patients who demonstrate a poor response to diuretic interventions and who are expected to require extracorporeal therapy for longer than 3 days are a third group who might profit from continuous renal replacement, unless a combined approach is envisioned from the beginning. Figure 39-10 describes these variables.

There are, however, subgroups of patients who most likely would not benefit from continuous therapies. The elderly with advanced and severe atherosclerotic vascular disease may not be candidates for arteriovenous access but may require a venovenous approach. This is also true of the patient who has had extensive arterial bypass surgery, because the grafts are prone to infection or bleeding. Severely catabolic patients may generate more urea than hemofiltration techniques can handle, even with the use of venovenous access and the pumped system. Thus, these patients benefit from the more efficient diffusive hemodia-

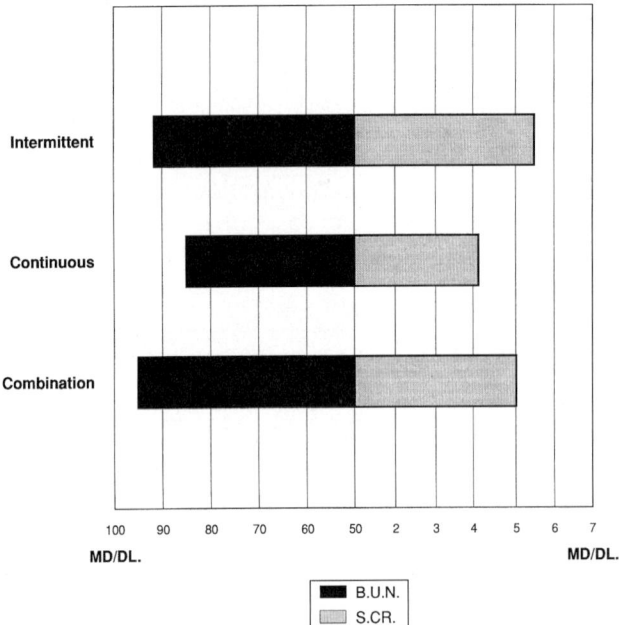

Table 39-10. Comparison of Continuous Venovenous Therapy With Intermittent Therapy

	Continuous Venovenous	Intermittent
Hemodynamic stability	Stable	Unstable
Fluid removal	Slow, gentle, complete	Rapid, harsh, incomplete
Dialysis efficiency	Low efficiency, long time	High efficiency, short time
Anticoagulation	Frequently necessary	0 Heparin possible
Patient mobilization	Possible	Possible
Specialty personnel	Perhaps	Definitely
Drug dosing/delivery	Easier	Difficult
Volume restriction	Minimal	Significant
Physician work	Significant	Moderate
Cost (technical)	Moderate	Significant

Fig. 39-8. Comparison of steady-state blood urea nitrogen (BUN) and serum creatinine (S.CR.) in three general approaches to renal support. Inter, intermittent hemodialysis; cont, continuous forms of renal support therapy; combo, combination of continuous and intermittent therapy. (Drawn courtesy of George Morrison, CD, Inc.)

lytic techniques for urea removal. Ambulatory patients, or those who are scheduled to leave the ICU, are also not prime candidates for femoral arterial access and might be better served with a subclavian or jugular venovenous access. The hemodynamically stable patient, who is not in need of large fluid intakes and can be easily handled by intermittent approaches is another class of patients for whom continuous therapy is questionable. It is possible, however, that this latter group may show an improvement in the overall outcome if they demonstrate periods of notable hemodynamic instability that frequently accompany the intermittent methods of dialysis. It has been theorized that these hypotensive insults delivered to the kidney during dialysis are responsible for prolonging the length of acute renal failure.

Some patients benefit from a combination of intermittent and continuous therapies. The advantages of both techniques are obtained, with the stability of the continuous support seen during the ultrafiltration process[108,109] and then the efficiency of the diffusive forces during the intermittent hemodialysis period of therapy. Thus, the pa-

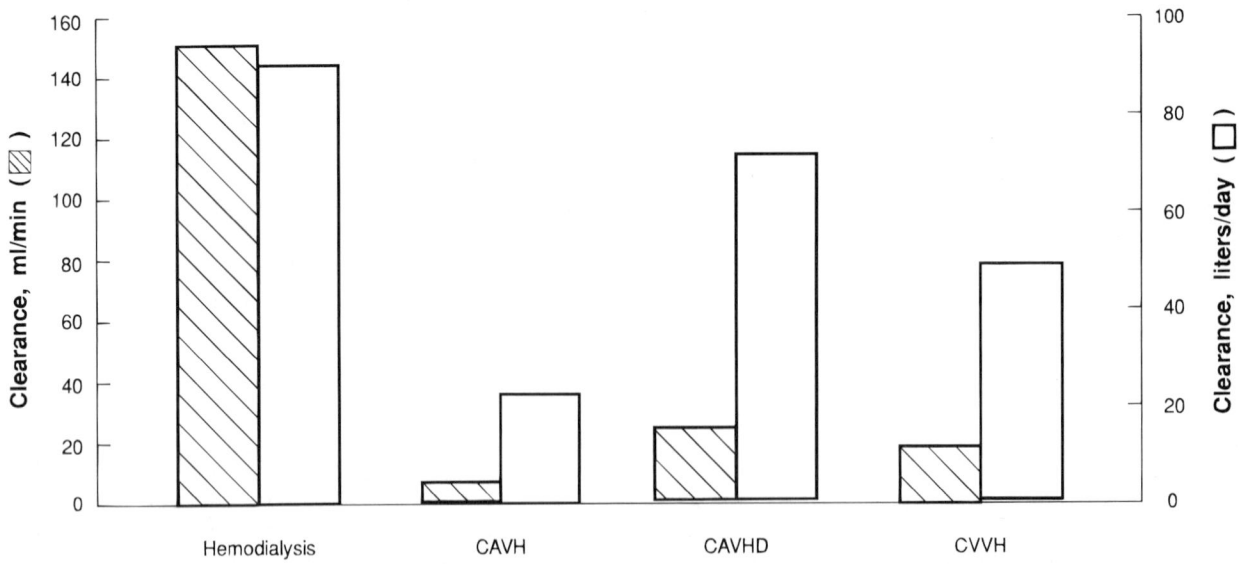

Fig. 39-9. Comparison of the efficiency of various forms of dialytic intervention. Results for continuous arteriovenous hemofiltration (CAVH), continuous arteriovenous hemodialysis (CAVHD), and continuous venovenous hemofiltration (CVVH) are averaged. Daily clearance for hemodialysis was calculated for a daily 4-hour treatment. (Redrawn courtesy of George Morrison, CD, Inc., from Kierdorf, H.: Continuous versus intermittent treatment: clinical results in acute renal failure. Contin. Hemofil. Contrib. Nephrol., 93: 1, 1991.)

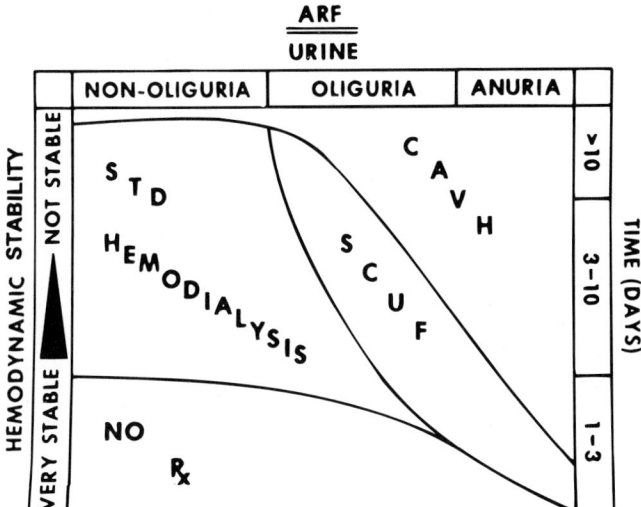

Fig. 39-10. Suggested guideline for use of different therapies in acute renal failure (ARF) supported in various patient types. Urine, spontaneous urine output; time, projected time of renal dysfunction based on insult; CAVH, continuous arteriovenous hemofiltration; SCUF, slow continuous ultrafiltration; Std, standard intermittent; NO Rx = no dialytic intervention needed.

tients still receive the volume obliged by their therapy and are not subject to fluid overload or the instability induced by its removal during the infrequent intermittent procedure.

POST-ICU FOLLOW-UP OF ACUTE RENAL FAILURE

Renal Support

The selection of renal support techniques is much more limited in patients who are discharged from the intensive care setting. Usually supported with intermittent hemodialysis, some patients who had been supported with peritoneal dialysis could continue this method of support. The extracorporeal continuous techniques are not appropriate for the non-ICU setting and should not be continued outside of that setting. Dialytic support is continued until renal function returns. Although this may seem self-evident, the planning for this support must begin as these patients near their discharge from the ICU.

The most important aspect of any hemodialytic support system is the access used for entry to the blood supply. Some authors have advocated the use of femoral catheter placement for each dialysis session,[110] while others have relied on indwelling subclavian or jugular cannulae.[111] With the former, there is a significant increase in both patient and physician inconvenience. With prolonged dialytic support, cannulation becomes both more painful and tedious, frequently resulting in local infections, hematoma formations, and potentially, vascular damage.

The convenience of the indwelling double-lumen catheters has allowed hemodialysis personnel ready access and avoided multiple-vessel puncturing. Prolonged use of the catheter without loss of function has also been reported. Recent data, however, seem to point toward the indwelling catheters as the source of subsequent venous stenosis, especially if left in place for long periods of time. This stenosis will reduce the flow of blood through the subclavian vein and ultimately compromise any future upper extremity arteriovenous access placed on that side for chronic hemodialysis support. Infection and malfunction are the more frequent sequelae of long-term usage of these cannulae and may result in a higher patient morbidity. In a recent report on delivery of acute dialysis, Paganini et al.[112] identified the access catheter as the most frequent cause for poor dialysis delivery in the patient with acute renal failure.

Although predicting the duration of renal compromise may not be accurate, the cause and premorbid patient conditions should be considered when attempting an estimate of renal return. If there is no evidence of increased renal function after 6 weeks, then the likelihood of return diminishes, especially in the elderly with prior renal dysfunction. It is precisely this patient type who should be started on a chronic dialysis support system and be given a surgically constructed arterial access for that support. This will allow the patient to be discharged from the hospital sooner and ensure appropriate follow-up. Return of renal function has been described as late as 4 months from the insult, although this is indeed a rare occurrence.

Long-term care can be facilitated by deciding to "save" an arm for eventual fistula placement early in the course of renal support. This requires that the arm be spared any intravenous lines, blood drawing, or monitors. Blood pressure determinations should also be avoided in this limb. Although this does pose a problem during the ICU stay, it carries the advantage of having a readily available arm for construction of an eventual dialysis fistula.

Resurgence of renal function has been described as being stepwise in increased urine production and frequently accompanied by significant intravascular depletion. With close ICU attention to the acute renal failure patient's volume status, and the availability of continuous therapies that have helped to keep patients closer to their "dry weights," a brisk diuretic phase may not be present. Indeed, although there may be a modest return of urine output, a more dramatic decline in laboratory parameters for a given volume of urine is most frequently noted. Any increase in urine production should be considered a positive sign and should be accompanied by fluid replacement in an effort to ensure intravascular euvolemia. The use of loop diuretics at this stage may also help ascertain returning renal function, especially if an increase in urine production accompanies the diuretic challenge and was not present earlier. Continued diuretic usage will not, however, hasten the recovery phase; it may actually promote depletion and higher metabolic demand by the recovering tubular cells and thus should be avoided.

Resolution of renal dysfunction is often slow, especially in the older patient. Patients who have underlying chronic renal failure may never return to their premorbid renal baseline but, rather, may establish a new lower level of renal function. During this period of resolution, the kidney is quite susceptible to new insults. The higher energy requirements of the regenerating tubules are especially sensitive to ischemia and prerenal factors. Aggressive control of systemic blood pressure or tight glucose control is best reserved for later periods of hospitalization. Resolving function also requires the adjustment of medication doses, continued assessment of support requirements, and planned outpatient follow-up of renal function. The prospect of total return of renal function in patients who have no complicating conditions is excellent.

FUTURE PROSPECTS

Nonrenal Applications of Extracorporeal Therapy

Considerable interest has recently been given to the patient with multiorgan dysfunction (MOD). Although the renal system is frequently involved, other system failures have also been associated with sepsis. Several theories have pointed to the production of cellular mediators that seem to be active in the progression of this syndrome, with the resultant multiorgan involvement.[113-117] One area of particular interest is the progression to the adult respiratory distress syndrome (ARDS) from a variety of causes and the continued high mortality that is associated with this syndrome.[118,119]

Application of continuous techniques to septic MOD patients was accompanied by improved patient outcome in at least one retrospective study,[120] and several descriptive reviews,[121-123] but has not yet been the subject of a controlled prospective design. The ARDS protocol that we have been following,[124,125] however, seems to fulfill this design requirement for the use of CAVH in other organ failures. The pathophysiology of ARDS seems to involve increased vasoactive peptide release and decreased pulmonary clearance of these substances. There have also been several reports[127,128] of many of the same mediators involved in the alteration of renal blood flow or GFR without differences in the usual hemodynamics with which these changes are usually associated. Several investigators[127-129] have also described the presence of various "substances" that have been associated with the depression of myocardial function in association with the septic syndrome.

It would therefore seem reasonable that if these substances could be removed, perhaps the progressive nature of these syndromes might be altered. Some preliminary data have been noted by Coraim and associates[126] in patients with severe heart failure following open heart surgery and resistant to removal from the bypass pump. These patients were able to be removed only after they underwent hemofiltration for the removal of a vague peptide, as yet not clearly identified. Lefer[127] and Parillo et al.[128] postulated the presence of a myocardial depressant in sepsis, and Gomez et al.[129] noted the reversal of this depression when hemofiltration was applied to dogs with sepsis. Hanasawa et al.[130] showed that the elimination of endotoxin from the circulation of dogs with septic shock by means of polymyxin B-immobilized fibers enhanced survival, and Levine et al.[131] noted the presence of TNF in the sera of patients with severe heart failure. Rimondini[132] evaluated CAVH in the treatment of these patients and found limited success, while Golper et al.[133] and McDonald and Mehta[134] anticipated the importance of TNF elimination and have begun to evaluate removal rates using CAVH.

To establish the utility of CAVH in this class of patients, we have been collecting and analyzing ultrafiltrate from patients with severe heart failure. After having obtained several extracts from this fluid, we have added these to a Langendorf heart preparation for evaluation of myocardial depression. A depression of activity has been associated with the ultrafiltrate obtained from patients with heart failure and from patients with renal failure, but not from normal control subjects. Thus, the presence of a substance seems to be evident. Whether this substance is specific for cardiac depression or merely the cardiac activity of another element remains to be established. Nonetheless, we have incorporated the use of CAVH support in several patients with severe heart failure awaiting transplant as well as in patients who have required the use of ventricular assist devices. The cardiac outcome has remained positive in both groups, but a true comparison to patients not given this support has not been undertaken.

Patients with ARDS have also been subject to therapy with CAVH[123] in a prospective and randomized manner in an effort to evaluate the utility of this therapy beyond the fluid removal parameters noted by several investigators.[125] Preliminary results seem to point toward an improved survival in those patients who received CAVH as part of their treatment protocol despite an apparent trend toward improved hemodynamic parameters in the control group. The possibility of using this technology for the protection of organs is indeed exciting.

Work by Tze et al.[135] in the development of bioartificial hybrid organs—where the substructure for cellular growth is a membrane device—may lead the way to a truly innovative artificial kidney that is self-contained and effective in controlling the state of uremia. Once the current system can lose its thrombogenicity, it may be implanted to function as a true continuous device in much the same way that the intravenous oxygenator has been developed.[136] While the glomerular function of filtration can easily be replicated, the tubular function of selective reabsorption/elimination is much more difficult to emulate.

REFERENCES

1. Horn S. D. et al.: Interhospital differences in severity of illness. (Abstract.) N. Engl. J. Med., *313*:20, 1985.
2. Munoz, E. et al.: Diagnosis-related groups, costs, and outcome for patients in the intensive care unit. Heart Lung, *18*:627, 1989.
3. Bekes, E., Fleming, S., and Scott, W. E.: Reimbursement for intensive care services under diagnosis-related groups. Crit. Care Med., *16*:478, 1988.
4. Douglass, P. S., Rosen R. L., Butler, P. W., and Bone, R. L.: DRG payment for long-term ventilator patients. Chest, *91*: 413, 1987.
5. Mayer-Oakes, S. A., Oye, R. K., Leake, B., and Brook. R.H.: The early effect of Medicare's prospective payment system on the use of medical intensive care services in three community hospitals. JAMA, *260*:3146, 1988.
6. McMurray, S. D. et al.: Prevailing patterns and predictor variables in patients with acute tubular necrosis. (Abstract.) Arch. Intern. Med., *138(6)*:950, 1978.
7. Oliveira, D. B., and Winearls, C. G.: Acute renal failure in the elderly can have a good prognosis. (Abstract.) Age Aging, *13*:304, 1984.
8. Rodgers, H., Staniland, J. R., Lipkin, G. W., and Turney, J.

H.: Acute renal failure: a study of elderly patients. (Abstract.) Age Aging, 19:36, 1990.
9. Rasmussen, H. H., Pitt, E. A., Ibels, L. S., and McNeil, D. R.: Prediction of outcome in acute renal failure by discriminant analysis of clinical variables. (Abstract.) Arch. Intern. Med., 145:2015, 1985.
10. Coggins, C. H.: Prediction of outcome in acute renal failure. (Abstract.) Am. J. Nephrol., 7:8, 1987.
11. Shusterman, N. et al.: Risk factors and outcome of hospital-acquired acute renal failure. Clinical epidemiologic study. (Abstract.) Am. J. Med., 83:65, 1987.
12. Cochran, S. T., Wong, W. S., and Roe, D. J.: Predicting angiography-induced acute renal function impairment: clinical risk model. (Abstract.) Am. J. Roentgenol., 141:1027, 1983.
13. Wei, S. S., Lee, G. S., Woo, K. T., and Lim, C. H.: Acute renal failure prognostic induces in hospital inpatients referred for haemodialysis. (Abstract.) Ann. Acad. Med., 20:331, 1991.
14. Higgins, T. L. et al.: Stratification of morbidity and mortality outcome by pre-operative risk factors in coronary artery bypass patients. JAMA, 267:2334, 1992.
15. Schaefer, J. H. et al.: Outcome prediction of acute renal failure in medical intensive care. (Abstract.) Intens. Care Med., 17:19, 1991.
16. Groeneveld, A. B. et al.: Acute renal failure in the medical intensive care unit; predisposing, complicating factors and outcome. (Abstract.) Nephron, 59(4):602, 1991.
17. Maher, E. R. et al.: Prognosis of critically-ill patients with acute renal failure: APACHE II score and other predictive factors. (Abstract.) Q. J. Med., 72:857, 1989.
18. Kiil, F.: The mechanism of renal autoregulation. Sci. J. Clin. Lab. Invest., 41:521, 1981.
19. Baylis, C. et al.: Dynamics of glomerular nitrafiltration effects of plasma protein concentration. Am. J. Physiol., 232:F58, 1977.
20. Vaamonde, C. A.: Selected renal and electrolyte abnormalities in liver disease. (Letter.) AKF Nephrol., 9:13, 1992.
21. Cronin, R. E.: Drug therapy in the management of acute renal failure. (Abstract.) Am. J. Med. Sci., 292:112, 1986.
22. Bennett, W. M., et al.: The influence of dosage regimen on experimental gentamicin nephrotoxicity: dissociation of peak serum levels from renal failure. J. Infect. Dis., 140:576, 1979.
23. Trollfors, B. J.: Gentamicin nephrotoxicity. Antimicrob. Chemo. Ther., 12:285, 1983.
24. Meyers, R. D.: Risk factors and comparisons of clinical nephrotoxicity of aminoglycosides. Am. J. Med., 80:119, 1986.
25. Humes, M. D., Weinberg, J. M., and Knauss, T. C.: Clinical and pathophysiologic aspects of aminoglycoside nephrotoxicity. Am. J. Kidney Dis., 2:5, 1982.
26. Parfrey, P. S. et al.: Contrast material-induced renal failure in patients with diabetes mellitus, renal insufficiency, or both. N. Engl. J. Med., 320:143, 1989.
27. Davidson, C. F. et al.: Cardiovascular and renal toxicity of a nonionic radiographic contrast agent after cardiac catheterization: a prospective trial. Ann. Intern. Med., 110:119, 1989.
28. Schwab, S. J. et al.: Contrast nephrotoxicity: a randomized control trial of a non-ionic and an ionic radiocontrast agent. N. Engl. J. Med., 320:149, 1989.
29. Cigarroa, R. G. et al.: Dosing of contrast material to prevent contrast nephropathy in patients with renal disease. Am. J. Med., 86:649, 1986.
30. Schrier, R. W., and Burke, T. J.: Role of calcium-channel blockers in preventing acute and chronic renal injury. (Abstract.) J. Cardiovasc. Pharmacol., 18(Suppl. 6):S38, 1991.
31. Frei, U. et al.: Calcium channel blockers for kidney protection. (Abstract.) J. Cardiovasc. Pharmacol., 16(Suppl. 6):S11, 1990.
32. Lontzenhiser, R., Epstein, M., and Horton, C.: Inhibition by dilitazem of pressure-induced afferent vasoconstriction in the isolated perfused rat kidney. Am. J. Cardiol., 59:72A, 1987.
33. Loutzenhiser, R., and Epstein, M.: Modification of the renal hemodynamic response to vasoconstrictors by calcium antagonists. (Abstract.) Am. J. Nephrol., 7:6, 1987.
34. Heyman, S. N., Brezis, M., Greenfeld, Z., and Rosen, S.: Protective role of furosemide and saline in radiocontrast-induced acute renal failure in the rat. (Abstract.) Am. J. Kidney Dis., 14:377, 1989.
35. Kaufman, R. P., Jr. et al.: Inhibiton of thromboxane (Tx) synthesis by free radical scavengers. (Abstract.) J. Trauma, 28:458, 1988.
36. Graziani, G. et al.: Dopamine and furosemide in oliguric acute renal failure. Nephron, 37:39, 1984.
37. Lindner, A.: Synergism of dopamine and furosemide in diuretic-resistant, oliguric acute renal failure. Nephron, 33:121, 1983.
38. Sraer, J. D.: Renal biopsy in acute renal failure. Kidney Int., 8:60, 1975.
39. Moran, S. M., and Myers, B. D.: Course of acute renal failure studied by a model of creatinine kinetics. Kidney Int., 27:928, 1985.
40. Myers, B. D., and Moran, S. M.: Hemodynamically mediated acute renal failure. N. Engl. J. Med., 314:97, 1986.
41. Unwin, R. J., Ganz, M. D., and Sterzel, R. B.: Brain-gut peptides, renal function and cell growth. Kidney Int., 37:1031, 1990.
42. Rosa, R. M., Silva, P., Stoff, J. S., and Epstein, F. H.: Effect of vasoactive intestinal peptide on isolated perfused rat kidney. Am. J. Physiol., 249:E494, 1985.
43. Goetz, K. L. et al.: Cardiovascular, renal and endocrine responses to intravenous endothelin in conscious dogs. Am. J. Physiol., 255:R1064, 1988.
44. King, A. J., Brenner, B. M., and Anderson, S.: Endothelin: a potent renal and systemic vasoconstrictor peptide. Am. J. Physiol., 256:F1051, 1989.
45. Firth, J. D., Raine, A. E. G., Ratcliff, P. J., and Ledingham, J. G. G.: Endothelin: an important factor in acute renal failure. Lancet, 2:1179, 1988.
46. Lopez-Farre, A., Montanes, I., Millas, I., and Lopez-Novoda, J. M.: Effect of endothelin on renal function in rats. Eur. J. Pharamcol., 163:187, 1989.
47. Beutler, B., and Cerami, A.: The endogenous mediator of endotoxic shock. Clin. Res., 35:192, 1987.
48. Fischer, D. B., and Badr, K. R.: Managing renal involvement in sepsis: current concepts and future directions. J. Crit. Ill., 7:1446, 1992.
49. Remick, D. G., Kinkel, R. D., Larrick, J. W., and Kinkel, S. L.: Acute in vivo effects of human recombinant tumor necrosis factor. Lab. Inves., 56:583, 1987.
50. Sibbald, W. J.: Circulatory responses to the sepsis syndrome. Prog. Clin. Biol. Res., 308:1075, 1989.
51. Dofferhoff, A. S. M. et al.: Patterns of cytokines, plasma endotoxin, and acute phase proteins during the treatment of severe sepsis in humans. Progr. Clin. Biol. Res., 367:43, 1991.
52. Cumming, A. D., Kline, R., and Linton, A. L.: Association between renal and sympathetic responses to nonhypotensive systemic sepsis. Crit. Care Med., 16:1132, 1988.
53. Cheadle, W. G. et al.: Endotoxin filtration and immune stimulation improve survival from gram-negative sepsis. (Abstract.) Surgery, 110:785, 1991.

54. Lowell, J. A. et al.: Postoperative fluid overload: not a benign problem. Crit. Care Med., *18*:728, 1990.
55. Anderson, R. J., and Schrier, R. W.: Acute tubular necrosis. *In* Diseases of the Kidney. Edited by R. W. Schrier and C. W. Gottschalk. Boston, Little, Brown, 1988, p. 1413.
56. Levinsky, N. G., Bernard, D. B., and Johnson, P. A.: Enhancement of recovery of acute renal failure: effect of mannnitol and diuretics. *In* Acute Renal Failure. Edited by B. Brenner and J. H. Stein. New York, Churchill Livingstone, 1980, p. 163.
57. Abel, R. M., Abbott, W. M., and Fischer, J. E.: Intravenous essential L-amino acid and hypertonic dextrose in patients with acute renal failure. Effects on serum potassium, phosphate and magnesium. Am. J. Surg., *123*:632, 1972.
58. Abel, R. M. et al.: Improved survival from acute renal failure after treatment with intravenous essential L-amino acids and glucose. Results of a prospective double-blind study. N. Engl. J. Med., *288*:695, 1973.
59. Feinstein, E. I. et al.: Clinical and metabolism responses to parenteral nutrition in acute renal failure—a controlled double-blind study. Medicine, *60*:124, 1981.
60. Feinstein, E. I., Kopple, J. D., Silberman, H., and Massry, S. G.: Total parenteral nutrition with high or low nitrogen intake in patients with acute renal failure. Kidney Int., *26*: S319, 1983.
61. Mault, J. R. et al.: Starvation: a major contributor to mortality in acute renal failure. Trans. Am. Soc. Artif. Intern. Organs, *29*:390, 1983.
62. Feinstein, E. I. et al.: Nutritional hemodialysis. *In* Progress in Artificial Organs 1983. Edited by K. Atsumi, M. Makawa, and K. Ota. Cleveland, ISAO Press, 1984, p. 421.
63. Bartlett, R. H. et al.: Measurement of metabolism in multiple organ failure. Surgery, *92*:771, 1983.
64. Kresowik, T. F. et al.: Does nutritional support effect survival in critically ill patients? Surg. Forum, *35*:108, 1984.
65. Bartlett, R. H. et al.: Continuous arteriovenous hemofiltration: improved survival in surgical acute renal failure? Surgery, *2*:400, 1986.
66. Asbach, H. W. et al.: The treatment of hypercatabolic acute renal failure by adequate nutrition and haemodialysis. Acta. Anaesth. Scand., *18*:225, 1974.
67. Chang, R. W. S., Jacobs, S., and Lee, B.: Use of APACHE II severity of disease classification to identify intensive care patients who would not benefit from total parental nutrition. Lancet, *1*:1483, 1986.
68. Chima, C. S. et al.: Protein catabolic rate in patients with acute renal failure on continuous arteriovenous hemofiltration and total parental nutrition. J. Am. Soc. Nephrol., *3*: 1516, 1993.
69. Schafferhans, K., Heidbreder, E., Grimm, D., and Heidland, A.: Norepinephrine-induced acute renal failure: beneficial effects of atrial natriuretic factor. Nephron, *44*:240, 1986.
70. Shaw, S. G. et al.: Atrial natriuretic peptide protects against acute ischemic renal failure in the rat. J. Clin. Invest., *80*: 1232, 1987.
71. Conger, J. D., Falk, S. A., Yuan, B. H., and Schrier, R. W.: Atrial natriuretic peptide and dopamine in a rag model of ischemic acute renal failure. Kidney Int., *35*:1126, 1989.
72. Conger, J. D., Falk, S. A., and Hammond, W. S.: Atrial natriuretic peptide and dopamine in established acute renal failure in the rat. Kidney Int., *40*:21, 1991.
73. Humes, H. D.: Recovery phase of acute renal failure: the cellular and molecular biology of regenerative repair. Kidney, *24*:1, 1991.
74. Schulman, G. et al.: Complement activation retards resolution of acute ischemic renal failure in the rat. Kidney Int., *40*:1069, 1991.
75. Hakim, R. et al.: Use of biocompatible membrane (BCM) improves outcome and recovery from acute renal failure. Mayo Clin. Proc., *58*:729, 1983.
76. Conger, J. D.: Does hemodialysis delay recovery from acute renal failure? Semin. Dialy., *3*:146, 1990.
77. Kramer, P. et al.: Continuous arteriovenous hemofiltration: a new kidney replacement therapy. Proc. Eur. Dial. Trans. Assoc., *187*:743, 1981.
78. Magilligan, D. J.: Indications for ultrafiltration in the cardiac surgical patient. J. Thorac. Cardiovasc. Surg., *89*:183, 1985.
79. Paganini, E. P. et al.: Continuous renal replacement therapy in patients with acute renal dysfunction undergoing intraaortic balloon pump and/or left ventricular device support. Trans. Am. Soc. Artif. Int. Organs, *32*:414, 1986.
80. Mehta, R. L., McDonald, B. R., Aguilar, M. M., and Ward, D. M.: Regional citrate anticoagulation for continuous arteriovenous hemodialysis in critically ill patients. Kidney Int., *38*:976, 1990.
81. Paganini, E. P. (ed.): Acute Continuous Renal Replacement Therapy. Boston, Martinus Nijhoff, 1986.
82. Sieberth, H. G., Mann, H., and Stummvoll, H. K.: Continuous Hemofiltration. Basel, Karger, 1991.
83. Golper, T. A. et al.: Drug removal during CAVH: theory and clinical observations. Int. J. Artif. Organs, *8*:307, 1985.
84. Macris, M. P. et al.: Simplified method of hemofiltration in ventricular assist device patients. Trans. Am. Soc. Artif. Int. Organs, *34*:708, 1988.
85. Canaud, B. et al.: Pump assisted continuous venovenous hemofiltration for treating acute uremia. Kidney Int., *33(Suppl. 24)*:S154, 1988.
86. Sigler, M. H., Teehan, B. P., and Van Valkenburgh, D.: Solute transport in continuous hemodialysis: a new treatment for acute renal failure. Kidney Int., *32*:562, 1987.
87. Lauer, A. et al.: Continuous arteriovenous hemofiltration in the critically ill patient. Ann. Intern. Med., *99*:455, 1983.
88. Swann, S., and Paganini, E. P.: The practical technical aspects of slow continuous ultrafiltration (SCUF) and continuous arterio-venous hemofiltration (CAVH). *In* Acute Continuous Renal Replacement Therapy. Edited by E. P. Paganini. Boston, Martinus Nijhoff, 1986, p. 51.
89. Kramer, P. et al.: Intensive care potential of continuous arteriovenous hemofiltration. Trans. Am. Soc. Artif. Intern. Organs, *28*:28, 1982.
90. Paganini, E. P., and Nakamoto, S.: Continuous slow ultrafiltration in oliguric acute renal failure. Trans. Am. Soc. Artif. Intern. Organs, *26*:201, 1980.
91. Pallone, T. L., Hyver, S., and Petersen, J.: The simulation of continuous arteriovenous hemodialysis with a mathematical model. Kidney Int., *35*:125, 1989.
92. Silverstein, M. E., Ford, E. A., Lysaght, M. J., and Henderson, L. W.: Treatment of severe fluid overload by ultrafiltration. N. Engl. J. Med., *291*:747, 1974.
93. Neff, M. D., Sadjadi, S., and Slifkin, R.: A wearable artificial glomerulus. Trans. Am. Soc. Artif. Intern. Organs, *25*:71, 1979.
94. Shaldon, S., Beau, M. C., and Deschodt, G.: Continuous ambulatory hemofiltration. Trans. Am. Soc. Artif. Intern. Organs, *25*:71, 1979.
95. Chen, W. T. et al.: Hemodynamic studies in chronic hemodialysis patients with hemofiltration/ultrafiltration. Trans. Am. Soc. Artif. Intern. Organs, *24*:632, 1978.
96. Paganini, E. P. et al.: Hemodynamics of isolated ultrafiltration in chronic hemodialysis patients. Trans. Am. Soc. Artif. Intern. Organs, *25*:422, 1979.
97. Chaignon, M. et al.: Effect of hemodialysis on blood volume distribution and cardiac output. Hypertension, *3*:327, 1981.
98. Bosch, J. P.: Continuous arteriovenous hemofiltration. *In*

Hemofiltration. Edited by L. W. Henderson, E. A. Quellhorst, C. A. Baldamus, M. J. Lysaght. Berlin, Springer-Verlag, 1986, p. 233.
99. Paganini, E. P., O'Hara, P., and Nakamoto, S.: Slow continuous ultrafiltration in hemodialysis resistant oliguric acute renal failure patients. Trans. Am. Soc. Artif. Intern. Organs, 30:173, 1984.
100. Stott, R. B. et al.: Why the persistently high mortality in acute renal failure? Lancet, 2:75, 1972.
101. Knaus, W. A., Draper, E. A., Wagner, D. P., and Zimmerman, J. E.: APACHE II: a severity of disease classification system. Crit. Care Med., 13:818, 1985.
102. Maher, E. R. et al.: Prognosis of critically-ill patients with acute renal failure: APACHE II score and other predictive factors. Q. J. Med., 72:857, 1989.
103. Chang, R. W. S., Jacobs, S., and Lee, B.: Use of APACHE II severity of disease classification to identify intensive care patients who would not benefit from total parental nutrition. Lancet, 1:1483, 1986.
104. Velez, R. L., Woodard, T. D., and Henrich, W. L.: Acetate and bicarbonate hemodialysis in patients with and without autonomic dysfunction. Kidney Int., 26:59, 1984.
105. Sherman, R. A., Rubin, M. P., Cooly, R. P., and Eisinger, R. P.: Amelioration of hemodialysis-associated hypotension by the use of cool dialysate. Am. J. Kidney Dis., 5:124, 1985.
106. Agarwal, R. et al.: 35°C dialysis (CTD) increases peripheral resistance (PVR) and improves hemodynamic stability (HS) patients (PTS). J. Am. Soc. Nephrol., 3:35, 1992.
107. Kierdorf, H.: Continuous versus intermittent treatment: clinical results in acute renal failure. Contin. Hemofilt. Contrib. Nephrol., 93:1, 1991.
108. Baldamus, C. A., Ernst, W., Fassbinder, W., and Koch, K. M.: Differing haemodynamic stability due to differing sympathetic response: comparison of ultrafiltration, haemodialysis and hemofiltration. Proc. Eur. Dial. Trans. Assoc., 17:205, 1980.
109. Quelborst, E., Schuenemann, B., Hildebrand, U., and Falda, Z.: Response of the vascular system to different modification of haemofiltration and hemodialysis. Proc. Eur. Dial. Trans. Assoc., 17:197, 1980.
110. Kjellstrand, C. M. et al.: Complications of percutaneous femoral vein catheterizations for hemodialysis. Clin. Nephrol., 4:37, 1975.
111. Schwarzbeck, A., Brittinger, W. D., and Henning, G. E.: Cannulation of the subclavian vein for hemodialysis using Seldinger's technique. Trans. Am. Soc. Artif. Intern. Organs, 24:27, 1978.
112. Paganini, E. P., Pudelski, B., and Bednarz, D.: Dialysis delivery in the ICU—are patients receiving the prescribed dialysis dose? (Abstract.) J. Am. Soc. Nephrol., 3:384, 1992.
113. Meakins, J. L.: Etiology of multiple organ failure. J. Trauma, 30:S165, 1990.
114. Goodwin, C. W.: Multiple organ failure: clinical overview of the syndrome. J. Trauma, 30:12, 1990.
115. Sieberth, H. G., Mann, H., and Summvoll, H. K.: Pathology of multiple organ failure. Contrib. Nephrol., 93:71, 1991.
116. DeCamp, M. M., and Demling, R. H.: Post-traumatic multisystem organ failure. JAMA, 260:530, 1988.
117. Anderson, B. O., and Harken, A. H.: Multiple organ failure: inflammatory priming and activation sequences promote autologous tissue injury. J. Trauma, 30:S44, 1990.
118. Luce, J. M. et al.: Ineffectiveness of high-dose methylprednisone in preventing parenchymal lung injury and improving mortality in patients with septic shock. Am. Rev. Respir. Dis., 138:62, 1988.
119. Montgomery, A. M. et al.: Causes of mortality in patients with the adult respiratory distress syndrome. Am. Rev. Respir. Dis., 132:485, 1985.
120. Gotloib, L., Barzilay, E., Shustak, A., and Lev, A.: Sequential hemofiltration in non-oliguric high capillary permeability pulmonary edema of severe sepsis: preliminary report. Crit. Care Med., 12:997, 1984.
121. Gotloib, L. et al.: Hemofiltration in sepsis ARDS: the artificial kidney as an artificial lung. Resuscitation, 13:123, 1986.
122. Koller, W.: Continuous arteriovenous hemofiltration in ICU patients with pulmonary disorders. In International Symposium on Continuous Arteriovenous Hemofiltration. Milan, Wichtig, Editore, 1986, p. 331.
123. Romano, E., Gullo, G., and Kette, F.: Pulmonary gas exchange in critically ill patients during continuous arteriovenous hemofiltration (CAVH). In International Symposium on Continuous Arteriovenous Hemofiltration. Milan, Wichtig Editore, 1986, p. 139.
124. Cosentino, F. et al.: Continous arteriovenous hemofiltration in the adult respiratory distress syndrome: a randomized controlled trial. (Abstract.) In Second International Conference on Continuous Hemofiltration, Vienna, 1990. Berlin, Knuger, 1990.
125. Barzilay, E. et al.: Use of extracorporeal supportive techniques as additional treatment for septic-induced multiple organ failure patients. Crit. Care Med., 17:634, 1989.
126. Coraim, F. J., Coraim, H. P., Ebermann, R., and Stellwag, F. M.: Acute respiratory failure after cardiac surgery: clinical experience with the application of continuous arteriovenous hemofiltration. Crit. Care Med., 14:714, 1986.
127. McDonough, K. H., et al.: Enhanced myocardial depression in diabetic rats during E. coli sepsis. Am. J. Physiol., 253:H276, 1987.
128. Parillo, J. E. et al.: A circulating myocardial depressant substance in humans with septic shock. J. Clin. Invest., 76:1539, 1985.
129. Gomez, A. et al.: Hemofiltration reverses left ventricular dysfunction during sepsis in dogs. Anesthesiology, 73:671, 1990.
130. Hanasawa, K., Tani, T., and Kodama, M.: New approach to endotoxic and septic shock by means of polymyxin B immobilized fiber. Surg. Gynecol. Obstet., 168:323, 1989.
131. Levine, B. et al.: Elevated circulating levels of tumor necrosis factor in severe chronic heart failure. N. Engl. J. Med., 323:236, 1990.
132. Rimondini, A., et al.: Hemofiltration as short-term treatment for refractory congestive heart failure. Am. J. Med., 83:430, 1987.
133. Gollper, T. A., Jenkins, R., Wright, M., and Klein, J. B.: Tumor necrosis factor and hemofiltration membranes. Intensive Behandlung, 15:119, 1992.
134. McDonald, B. R., and Mehta, R. L.: Transmembrane flux of IL-1B and TNF-a in patients undergoing continuous arteriovenous hemodialysis. J. Am. Soc. Nephrol., 1:368, 1990.
135. Tze Kin, I. P., Aebischer, P., and Gelletti, P. M.: Cellular control of membrane permeability: implications for a bioartificial renal tubule. Trans. Am. Soc. Artif. Intern. Organs, 34:351, 1988.
136. Mortensen, J. D.: An intravenacaval blood gas exchange (IVCBGE) device: a preliminary report. Trans. Am. Soc. Artif. Intern. Organs, 33:570, 1987.
137. Bosworth, C.: SCUF/CAVH/CAVHD: critical differences. Crit. Care Nurs. Q., 14:45, 1992.
138. Paganini, E. P., and Bosworth, C. R.: Acute renal failure after open heart surgery: newer concepts and current therapy. Semin. Thorac. Cardiovasc. Surg., 3:63, 1992.

Chapter 40

SPECIAL CONSIDERATIONS IN THE PATIENT WITH CHRONIC RENAL FAILURE IN THE INTENSIVE CARE UNIT

JOSEPH ZARCONI
MELINDA S. PHINNEY

The term **chronic renal failure (CRF)** is generally defined as an irreversible reduction in renal function, a situation in which recovery of renal function is not likely. In most instances, this term is used interchangeably with "chronic renal insufficiency," by some defined as the earlier stages of chronic renal failure. **Azotemia** is simply the accumulation of nitrogenous waste products in the blood. When CRF progresses to the point beyond which the level of residual renal function is inadequate to sustain life, the patient is said to have reached **end-stage renal disease (ESRD)**. At this stage, without some form of renal replacement therapy such as dialysis or transplantation, death is imminent.

As the patient progressively loses renal function, concentrating ability is lost and nocturia often results. A reduction in erythropoietin production leads to anemia, and serum levels of 1,25 dihydroxy vitamin D_3 fall. Serum phosphorus levels rise, and calcium levels fall, resulting in secondary increases in parathyroid hormone levels in an attempt to maintain normocalcemia. Impairments in volume regulation ensue, and the kidneys progressively lose their ability to maintain the appropriate composition of the extracellular fluid. The renal clearance of acids deteriorates, resulting in acidosis. Hyperkalemia is a late manifestation, usually occurring when the glomerular filtration rate (GFR) falls below 15 to 20 ml per minute, accompanied by oliguria. Ultimately, renal failure culminates in some combination of fluid overload and **uremia,** the clinical syndrome of "symptomatic renal failure," which is fatal without renal replacement therapy. The uremic patient may complain of anorexia, nausea, vomiting, pruritus, hiccough, chest pain from pleuritis or pericarditis, dyspnea, orthopnea, or an inability to concentrate. Such a patient may manifest evidence of bleeding, friction rubs, pulmonary and peripheral edema, asterixis or obtundation, and seizures on initial presentation.

The patient with CRF presents special problems for critical care providers. Concurrent with the gradual and progressive loss of kidney function are a number of pathophysiologic derangements, which, as they accumulate, place the patient at high risk for the development of critical illness. Renal failure compromises immunity, impairs cardiovascular function, alters many endocrine functions, affects the central nervous system, and in general, places significant stress on most of the normal homeostatic mechanisms. Moreover, a large proportion of patients with CRF have diabetes mellitus as a cause, as well as hypertension, either as a cause or as a consequence of their renal disease. Diabetes and hypertension further contribute to the morbidity of these patients as a result of accelerated atherogenesis and subsequent large and small vessel vascular disease leading to the compromise of multiple organ systems.

Although it is difficult to estimate the prevalence of CRF in the population, data compiled by the United States Renal Data System[1] allow a number of important conclusions to be drawn regarding the ESRD population in the United States. It appears that continuing increases in the number of ESRD patients, as well as in their ages and acuity of illness, are likely to impact significantly on the need to be able to provide high quality critical care to this ever-growing and increasingly ill population of patients. In 1990, there were more than 195,000 ESRD patients in the Medicare system, representing some 93% of all treated ESRD patients in the United States. The age of the ESRD patient population has grown steadily since the late 1970s (Fig. 40-1), such that by 1990, nearly 44% of new ESRD patients were 65 years of age or older. The incidence of ESRD has increased most dramatically in patients whose renal disease is caused by either diabetes mellitus or hypertension (Fig. 40-2), resulting in disproportionately greater numbers of diabetics and hypertensives within this population. For example, from 1986 to 1990, while the total ESRD population grew at a rate of 8.6% per year, the population of ESRD patients with diabetic nephropathy grew at a rate of 15% per year. Finally, life expectancy among ESRD patients has been significantly prolonged by the development of dialytic therapies and transplantation.

The ESRD population and the population of patients with non-ESRD CRF—growing in size, age, life expectancy, and illness complexity—directly affect the critical care delivery system. From 1982 through 1990, the number of patients with CRF hospitalized in our ICU at Akron City Hospital grew steadily (Fig. 40-3). A summary of the diagnoses listed for these patients during their ICU admissions is shown in Table 40-1. These patients suffer from concomitant illnesses predominated by cardiovascular conditions, infectious diseases, hematologic derangements, and gastrointestinal illnesses. The diagnoses that have a direct impact on the reasons for ICU admission in these patients are summarized in Table 40-2. The prepon-

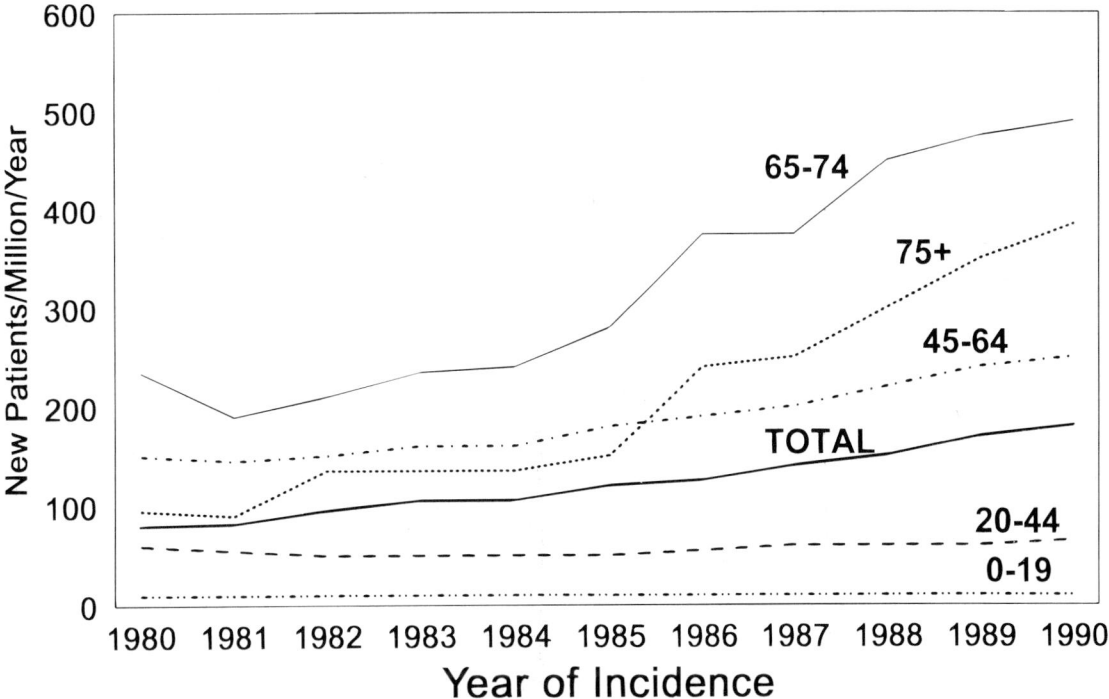

Fig. 40–1. Incidence rates per million population of reported end-stage renal disease, by age, 1977 to 1990, unadjusted. Medicare patients only. (From U. S. Renal Data System: USRDS 1993 Annual Data Report. Bethesda, MD, The National Institutes of Health, National Institute of Diabetes and Digestive and Kidney Diseases, 1993. The data reported here have been supplied by The United States Renal Data System [USRDS]. The interpretation and reporting of these data are the responsibility of the authors and in no way should be seen as an official policy or interpretation of the USRDS.)

derance of patients arrived in the critical care setting because of cardiovascular, infectious, or gastrointestinal problems. Health-care expenditures in this population of patients are immense, and mortality is sobering.

DIABETES MELLITUS

Diabetes mellitus has surfaced as the most common cause of ESRD, with the diagnosis of diabetic nephropathy accounting for approximately one third of all patients newly starting on dialysis in the United States.[1] In addition, among dialysis patients, diabetics have the highest rate of hospitalization, with diabetics averaging approximately 14 days of hospitalization per year, compared to patients whose renal disease is caused by hypertension (12 days) or glomerulonephritis (7 days), for example. Therefore, diabetics are likely to be overrepresented among hospitalized CRF patients, particularly in the critical care setting. The morbidity of diabetics with renal failure is influenced not only by their renal disease but by certain extrarenal disease processes seen in these patients as well.

Renal Disease

The nature of the diabetic renal lesion per se increases the complexity of illness in patients with diabetic nephropathy. Significant proteinuria is the hallmark of this disease, and diabetics with nephrotic syndrome present particular management problems. Further, concomitant distal tubular dysfunction, particularly with regard to the handling of potassium and the excretion of acid, is common in these patients. Hyperkalemia and metabolic acidosis frequently accompany the illnesses for which diabetics with CRF present to the ICU, and these metabolic derangements must be recognized and appropriately addressed.

Nephrotic diabetic patients characteristically demonstrate proteinuria in the range of 5 to 8 g per day, but massive proteinuria as high as 25 to 30 g per day is occasionally seen. It may be that because of the high incidence of co-morbid illnesses in these patients and the impact of these illnesses on the patients' ability to maintain adequate nutrition, diabetics tolerate nephrotic proteinuria less readily than patients who are otherwise well. As a result, hypoalbuminemia is frequent and usually more severe in this population, and nutritional supplementation is often warranted. Further, nephrotic patients suffer from a reduced effective circulatory plasma volume in the face of what can often be severe total body fluid retention. Thus, these patients may relatively underperfuse vital organs and tissues, often in the setting of an already compromised blood supply that is due to both small vessel and large vessel vasculopathy. Ischemia of the brain, heart, gastrointestinal tract, or extremities can result, and prerenal azotemia even leading to established acute renal failure can ensue if aggressive measures to optimize perfusion are either not used or are unsuccessful.

Attempts at diuresis in nephrotic patients can be complicated by reductions in both the serum albumin level and effective circulating plasma volume. Loop diuretics, given

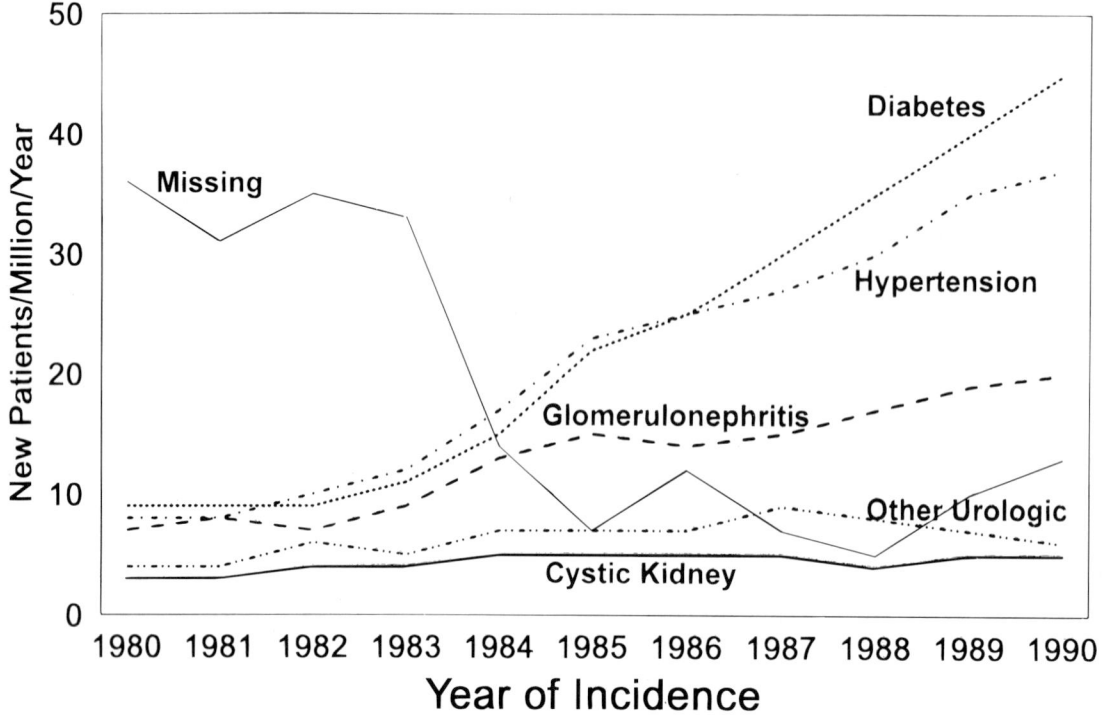

Fig. 40-2. Incidence rates per million population of reported end-stage renal disease (ESRD), by primary disease causing ESRD (diagnosis), 1977 to 1990, unadjusted. The large portion of missing information limits the usefulness of these data before 1982. Medicare patients only. (From U. S. Renal Data System: USRDS 1993 Annual Data Report. Bethesda, MD, The National Institutes of Health, National Institute of Diabetes and Digestive and Kidney Diseases, 1993. The data reported here have been supplied by The United States Renal Data System [USRDS]. The interpretation and reporting of these data are the responsibility of the authors and in no way should be seen as an official policy or interpretation of the USRDS.)

parenterally, remain the cornerstone of therapy in this setting, but these drugs require albumin binding to be effective, and in severely hypoalbuminemic patients, albumin infusion has been used to improve the efficacy of these drugs. In more resistant patients, the addition of metolazone, by virtue of its effect on the more distal nephron segment, may potentiate the diuretic effects of loop diuretics. This combination can be particularly kaliuretic, and cautious monitoring of serum potassium levels is warranted.

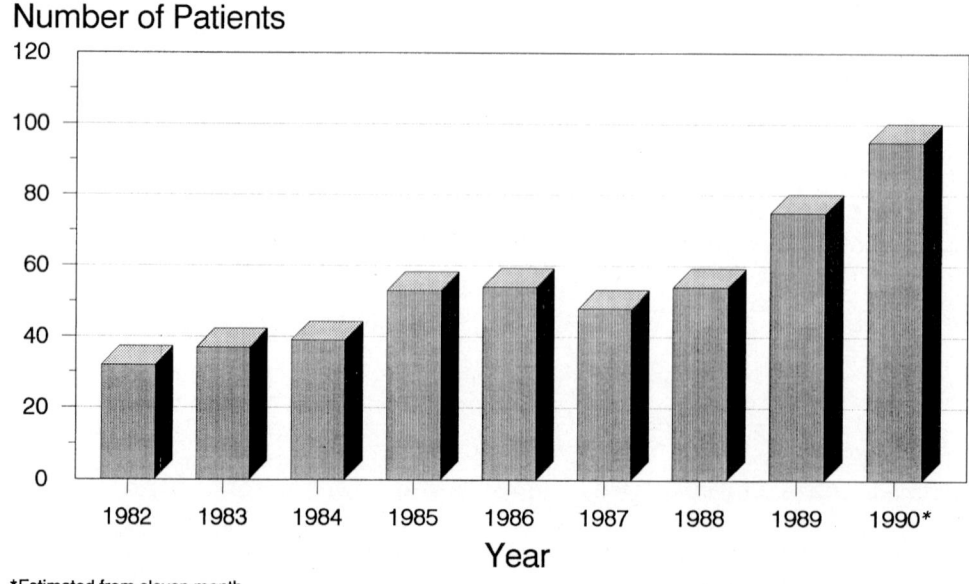

*Estimated from eleven month figure of 87 admissions

Fig. 40-3. Number of patients with chronic renal failure who were admitted to the ICU, Akron City Hospital, Akron, Ohio.

dously on critical care outcome. Clearly, CAD is more prevalent in diabetic patients and occurs at an earlier age. Most troublesome is the observation that its presence is commonly occult. An autopsy study of nine patients with type I diabetes ranging in age from 19 to 38 years demonstrated significant CAD in six.[9] In an older study, nearly half of the 21 asymptomatic patients with type I diabetes averaging 34 years of age showed angiographically documented significant CAD.[10] Krolwoski and colleagues reported that some 33% of patients with type I diabetes experience symptoms of CAD by age 59, and a third die of CAD by age 55.[11] It is therefore important to recognize that the critically ill diabetic is at high risk for the presence and complications of coronary artery disease, even if its presence is previously unrecognized or asymptomatic.

Clearly, the diabetic patient with CRF presents special challenges to the critical care provider. The nature of the renal lesion and its complications, as well as the multitude of co-morbid conditions experienced by these patients impact significantly on the outcomes of critical illness in this population. A thorough understanding of the diabetic condition as well as the early recognition and management of its consequences are pivotal to minimizing the morbidity and mortality of the patient with diabetes mellitus.

ANEMIA OF CHRONIC RENAL FAILURE

Severe normochromic, normocytic anemia is a common sequela of CRF. Many of the symptoms of uremia such as fatigue, exertional dyspnea, insomnia, generalized coldness, and depression may be in large part related to the presence of anemia.[12] This has become especially apparent since the introduction and widespread use of recombinant human erythropoietin, which has dramatically reduced the incidence and severity of the anemia in CRF patients. The significant decrement in red blood cell (RBC) mass also contributes to the morbidity of patients with CRF, especially in patients with cardiovascular disorders. The pathogenesis of the anemia associated with CRF is multifactorial and can be discussed in terms of primary and secondary mechanisms.

The primary mechanisms are those directly related to reduction in renal function. The kidneys are known to possess both excretory and endocrine functions, and anemia is a consequence of both excretory and endocrine renal failure. Failure of renal excretory function is manifested by numerous metabolic derangements. So-called "uremic toxins" accumulate and may be responsible for many of the manifestations of uremia. These toxins are also postulated to play a role in the development of anemia in these patients. The life span of circulating erythrocytes has been shown to be decreased by approximately 33% in some patients with uremia. However, RBCs from a uremic patient that are transfused into a normal, nonuremic patient have a normal life span. The opposite holds true for RBCs from healthy patients when transfused into uremic patients; that is, those cells have a shortened life span.[13] It is thus theorized that a factor or toxin is present in the plasma of patients with uremia that leads to increased destruction or diminished production of red cells. Several such toxins have been investigated, including parathyroid hormone (PTH), polyamines (spermine, spermidine), and ribonuclease, as possible inhibitors of erythropoiesis. PTH levels are known to be elevated in CRF. Extracts of parathyroid gland have been shown to inhibit early erythroid progenitor cells in vitro,[14] but purified PTH does not inhibit in vitro erythropoiesis,[15] making the role of PTH less clear as a significant factor in the development of anemia. Spermine inhibits both erythroid precursors and granulocytic and megakaryocytic precursors in vitro.[16] The absence of significant neutropenia or thrombocytopenia in uremic patients suggests that generalized hematopoietic suppression is not the primary mechanism of lowered RBC mass, and therefore spermine is unlikely to play a significant role. Studies with ribonuclease have also failed to support a causative role in erythropoietic suppression in uremic patients.[17]

Other metabolic factors have been demonstrated to be altered in the setting of uremia, which may predispose RBCs to early destruction. Transketolase activity in the hexose-monophosphate shunt is decreased with a subsequent increase in the susceptibility of erythrocytes to oxidant stressors.[18,19] Constituents of dialysate have been shown to produce such oxidant stress leading to hemolysis. Decreased activity of Na^+-K^+ adenosine triphosphatase (ATPase) has been shown in uremia as well.[20] The resultant decrease in pump activity leads to alterations in erythrocyte shape and rigidity, which in turn alters its life span. Dialysis itself can induce hemolysis secondary to chemical or mechanical means. Several substances retained in the dialyzer after cleaning may induce hemolysis, as can mechanical disruption of erythrocytes traversing dialysis needles. Significant hemolysis related to intravascular trauma has been seen most commonly in the setting of malignant hypertension.[21]

In addition to hemolysis and suppression of erythropoiesis, blood loss undoubtedly contributes to the development of anemia in hemodialysis patients. An average of approximately 20 ml of blood are lost in the dialyzer system at each dialysis treatment. In a patient who undergoes dialysis three times per week, this amounts to more than 3000 ml of blood lost over a 1-year period. Blood may also be lost through the gastrointestinal tract and into the skin as a result of a bleeding diathesis associated with uremia, which will be discussed later in this chapter.

As previously mentioned, the kidney is not only an excretory organ but has endocrine function as well. Erythropoietin is a glycoprotein produced by endothelial cells in the cortical and outer medullary peritubular capillaries in response to hypoxemia. This substance, in the presence of a diminished hematocrit leading to tissue hypoxemia, stimulates the terminal differentiation of erythroid precursors in the bone marrow, increases synthesis of hemoglobin, and promotes early release of new erythroid elements from the marrow into the peripheral blood. The kidney is the site of the production of 90% of human erythropoietin, and the remainder is synthesized in the liver. In normal individuals (normal renal function and normal hematocrit), serum erythropoietin levels are 10 to 16 U/L, and the rate of production can be increased greater than 100-fold in response to decreased RBC mass.[22] In the patient with ESRD, serum levels of erythropoietin are normal or slightly increased (19 to 30 U/L) in the face of a decreased hemoglobin, a situation in which erythropoietin levels would normally be markedly elevated. It has been shown that in patients with CRF, erythropoietin production increases only twofold to fivefold, in contrast to the 100-fold increase seen in patients with anemia and normal renal function.[23] In anephric patients, levels are markedly decreased and are clearly insufficient to maintain adequate hematocrits. Thus, before the development of recombinant human erythropoietin, many patients with CRF depended on transfusions to attain adequate circulatory RBC mass. Frequent blood product transfusion is certainly not without complications. Transmission of infections (e.g., hepatitis B and C, human immunodeficiency virus, etc.) may occur; potential transplant recipients are sensitized to many antigens, making it more difficult to find compatible donors; bone marrow is suppressed further; and if transfusions become frequent, iron overload with secondary hemochromatosis may occur. The availability of erythropoietin allows the treatment of the basic underlying mechanism of hematopoietic failure in patients with renal failure. Its administration has been shown to significantly enhance in vivo erythropoiesis, with subsequent significant rises in the hematocrits of these patients. Few complications, including iron deficiency and hypertension, may occur and are usually easily managed.[12] The use of erythropoietin has significantly lowered the incidence of severe anemia and its associated morbidity and mortality in patients with ESRD.

The bleeding diathesis seen in uremic patients may also contribute significantly to the anemia of CRF. This bleeding tendency has been investigated extensively, and although many theories have been entertained, few have been proven. Platelet counts are generally normal in these patients, as are indicators of coagulation factor activity (i.e., prothrombin time, partial thromboplastin time). Only the bleeding time has been shown to be elevated, indicating a defect in primary hemostasis. The initial hemostatic process involves local vasoconstriction, platelet aggregation, and platelet adherence at sites of membrane disruption. Bleeding times are elevated in most but not all patients with CRF and bleeding tendencies. The administration of aspirin to these patients has been shown to significantly increase bleeding time. There appear to be two mechanisms for this effect. First, as in nonuremic patients, there is irreversible inhibition of cyclo-oxygenase in platelets with a subsequent decrease in thromboxane A_2 synthesis. In uremic patients, however, aspirin administration causes a greater prolongation of bleeding time, which is transient and seems to correspond with the presence of aspirin in the blood.[24] There appears to be an imbalance between the synthesis of thromboxane A_2 and prostacycline production in vessel walls of uremic patients. The resultant decrease in thromboxane A_2 and increase in prostacycline may lead to impaired platelet thrombus formation seen in uremia and thus to a prolonged bleeding time. A decreased sensitivity of platelets to proaggregating agents such as epinephrine, adenosine diphosphate (ADP), and collagen has also been reported.[25]

Because the coagulation defect in CRF appears to be ineffective primary hemostasis, mucosal bleeding is a frequent concern in these patients. Gastrointestinal hemorrhage, epistaxis, hemorrhagic pericardial effusion with possible tamponade, and intracranial hemorrhage are potential manifestations of the bleeding diathesis of CRF. Additionally, an increased incidence of gastrointestinal telangiectasias has been seen in patients with renal disease, compounding the propensity for blood loss in these patients.[26,27]

Chronic blood loss and dietary protein restriction in patients with ESRD may aggravate iron deficiency. Given an average loss of 20 ml of blood per hemodialysis treatment, it is estimated that a patient may lose 780 mg of iron each year through the dialyzer alone.[28] Iron is also lost through the gastrointestinal tract or during menses. Iron replacement is particularly important during erythropoietin supplementation to ensure adequate iron stores for enhanced erythropoiesis. Finally, folate deficiency and aluminum toxicity may also contribute to the anemia of CRF.

Anemia in the critically ill patient with CRF impacts significantly on management and outcome. Tissue oxygen delivery—which may already be compromised dramatically as a result of peripheral vascular disease, reduced cardiac function, hypotension, or other hemodynamic derangements not uncommon in these patients—is further impaired in the presence of anemia. Thus, the risk of myocardial ischemia, as well as ischemia of the extremities and other vital vascular beds, is increased. Care should be taken to attempt to optimize the hematocrit so as to eliminate the additional morbidity associated with anemia. The exact hematocrit level to be recommended is unclear, and in any given case it must be adjusted according to the clinical circumstances. Patients at greatest risk of tissue underperfusion may require hematocrits in excess of 25 to 30% to prevent ischemic events. It is therefore important to recognize the considerable prevalence of anemia in patients with renal disease. The recognition and management of this anemia is vital in the critical care setting, because its presence may contribute significantly to the morbidity and mortality of this patient population.

CARDIOVASCULAR DISEASE IN CHRONIC RENAL FAILURE

The cardiovascular consequences of CRF deserve special consideration because cardiovascular disease is the leading cause of death in these patients.[29] The most prevalent cardiovascular complications leading to ICU admission in our hospital were hypertensive emergencies/urgencies, congestive heart failure/pulmonary edema, manifestations of CAD, and pericardial disease. Each of these conditions will be discussed with emphasis on their pathogenesis and with attention to the unique aspects of their occurrence in the patient with CRF.

Hypertension

Risk Phase

Arterial hypertension may be considered the single most important risk factor for coronary heart disease and its complications. Hypertension is a frequent finding in patients with CRF and may be either the cause or the result of the renal disease. The mechanism of hypertension in these patients is likely to be multifactorial. Patients with CRF have been consistently shown to have higher plasma volumes, higher exchangeable sodium contents, elevated plasma renin activities, and elevated catecholamine levels.[30]

Patients with CRF are also likely to have impaired feedback between the renin-angiotensin system and sodium and water balance.[31] It appears that total body sodium and volume overload is likely the dominant factor in hypertension in patients with CRF. As many as 70% of CRF patients will achieve normal blood pressure with maintenance dialysis when dialyzed to actual dry body weight and when diet, sodium, and fluid intake are controlled.[30] When dialyzing these patients, attempting to achieve dry weight is critical. Rapid, aggressive fluid removal, however, should be avoided because this practice may result in hypovolemia and reflex hypertension that is due to stimulation of the renin-angiotensin system. Approximately 30% of patients with ESRD will have refractory hypertension despite "adequate dialysis" and control of the preceding factors. It has been theorized that sympathetic nervous system hyperactivity may be involved in dialysis-refractory hypertension. Elevated catecholamine levels are found in most patients undergoing hemodialysis with refractory hypertension, and thus increased peripheral vascular resistance significantly contributes to refractory hypertension as well. The mechanism of hypercatecholaminemia is not fully understood but may involve increased intracellular calcium concentrations facilitating norepinephrine release from nerve endings, altered baroreceptor activity, altered vagal function, or reduced central dopaminergic tone.[30]

Support Phase

Patients with ESRD may present with hypertensive urgencies or emergencies much like the patient without renal failure. Manifestations of severe hypertension may range from encephalopathic or cerebrovascular events to cardiopulmonary sequelae with myocardial ischemia/infarction or pulmonary edema. As in patients without renal disease, prompt reduction of blood pressure is essential to prevent irreversible target organ damage. In patients with ESRD, volume status must be accurately determined. In a severely hypertensive patient with obvious volume overload, ultrafiltration for fluid removal may be required to control hypertension. In patients who are not anuric, loop diuretics are frequently helpful. Parenteral therapy with short-acting agents such as nitroprusside or labetalol is often the preferred therapy for hypertensive emergencies. Nitroprusside is easily titratable because of its short half-life, and thus overshooting and subsequent hypotension is less likely than with longer acting agents. However, nitroprusside is metabolized to thiocyanate, which is excreted by the kidney and thus accumulates in renal failure. The duration of its use should therefore not exceed 48 hours in such patients. Labetalol, with its combination of alpha- and beta-adrenergic receptor blockade, has several important advantages in hypertensive CRF patients. This drug, by virtue of its alpha-adrenergic receptor blockade, effects a prompt reduction in systemic vascular resistance and thus in blood pressure. In addition, the reflex tachycardia that would usually result is prevented by virtue of its beta-receptor blocking action. Additionally, this medication is hepatically metabolized so that dosage reduction is not required in renal disease. The goal of therapy in severe hypertension is to reduce blood pressure to the range of 160/100 mm Hg in a controlled fashion over the first 24 hours.[32] Intensive monitoring is essential to ensure that pressure is adequately reduced without profound, sudden hypotension. When the blood pressure has been controlled and stabilized, conversion to oral therapy is indicated. Diuretics, angiotensin-converting enzyme (ACE) inhibitors, beta blockers, and calcium-channel blockers have all been shown to be effective in treating renal parenchymal hypertension and should be selected for any given patient based on an evaluation of concomitant medical problems and the side effect profiles of the various agents. Once pressure has been adequately controlled for a 12- to 24-hour period, transfer from the critical care setting is appropriate.

Rehabilitative Phase

The goals of the rehabilitative phase of a CRF patient with hypertensive emergency are aimed at preventing recurrent hypertensive episodes and irreversible neurologic or cardiac complications. Emphasis on dietary factors (moderate salt and fluid restriction), adjustment of the dialysis prescription (accurate calculation and achievement of "dry weight"), and adjustment of antihypertensive medications are necessary to control hypertension and prevent the serious sequelae of this disease.

Pulmonary Edema/Congestive Heart Failure

Pulmonary edema and congestive heart failure account for 15 to 30% of cardiovascular deaths in patients with ESRD.[33] These patients develop complex alterations in cardiovascular physiology that are due to several interrelated factors such as salt and water retention, anemia, chronic hypertension, and the presence of arteriovenous fistulas in hemodialysis patients, all of which may contribute to the development of congestive heart failure and/or pulmonary edema.

Cardiac output is generally increased in patients with CRF.[34] Three primary mechanisms exist for this finding. First, increased blood volume (preload) causes an increase in cardiac output by Starling forces. Second, increased peripheral oxygen demand induces an increase in heart rate and stroke volume, thus increasing cardiac output. Third, as noted previously, the anemia of CRF leads to a reduction in oxygen-carrying capacity with a consequent increase in cardiac output in an attempt to maintain adequate tissue perfusion and oxygenation. The presence of an arteriovenous fistula in patients undergoing chronic hemodialysis creates a situation of apparent increase in peripheral oxygen demand because much of the blood circulating through the fistula does not contribute to tissue perfusion and oxygenation. Therefore, to meet tissue metabolic demands, an increase in cardiac output is required to compensate for the amount of blood being shunted through the fistula. The chronic increase in cardiac work seen in patients with CRF almost certainly plays a role in the potential for the development of cardiac failure.

In addition to the increased cardiac work, anatomic and physiologic changes in the myocardium are seen in these patients. Patients with CRF frequently exhibit signs and symptoms of myocardial dysfunction. Both dilated cardiomyopathy (18%) and hypertrophic cardiomyopathy (11%) are seen in this population.[35] Dilated cardiomyopathy is usually the result of chronic fluid overload that is due to some combination of chronic anemia, shunting of blood through arteriovenous fistulas, and chronic fluid retention.[36] It has been clearly shown that systemic hypertension may lead to hypertrophic myocardial changes. Because a significant proportion of patients with CRF have or have had hypertension, it is not surprising that hypertrophic cardiomyopathy is prevalent in this population of patients. Hyperparathyroidism may also predispose to left ventricular hypertrophy (LVH).[37] Patients with increased left ventricular wall thickness often have diastolic dysfunction related to decreased myocardial compliance, and in this instance, therapy directed at reducing cardiac contractility may be beneficial.

Other factors have been implicated in myocardial dysfunction. In addition to causing left ventricular hypertrophy, hyperparathyroidism—the secondary form of which is common in CRF—may result in calcification of the myocardium, which is due to elevated serum calcium levels and elevated calcium-phosphorus products. This calcification obviously causes a decrease in myocardial compliance and subsequent decline in myocardial function. Hypocalcemia and hyperkalemia, also not infrequently seen in patients with CRF, exert negative inotropic effects, thereby impairing left ventricular function. Uremic serum depresses myocardial activity, but to date, no one specific toxin has been clearly identified as the cause of this observed effect.[38,39] Ischemic heart disease with myocardial and global hypokinesis may also lead to cardiogenic decompensation and result in pulmonary edema. Finally, patients with CRF often exhibit noncompliance with medications, as well as oral salt and fluid intake restrictions, resulting in episodic and at times severe volume overload.

Risk Phase

When a patient with CRF presents with pulmonary edema, a thorough history and physical examination should be performed. The patient should be asked about previous episodes of dyspnea, congestive heart failure, or pulmonary edema, and a detailed history of the mode of onset and duration of symptoms, and any associated chest pain or ischemic symptoms should be noted. In addition, the patient undergoing dialysis should be questioned regarding treatment schedule and "dry weight," as well as any recent dietary excesses or changes in medication compliance. The physical examination should assess for hypertension and elevated jugular venous pressure, as well as the presence of an S_3 or S_4 gallop or any cardiac murmurs. In addition, evidence of hepatic congestion, hepatojugular reflux, peripheral or sacral edema, and cyanosis should be noted.

The initial diagnostic workup should include arterial blood gases, hemoglobin and hematocrit, renal profile, electrocardiogram and chest radiograph. These patients are often hypoxemic and frequently have metabolic acidosis secondary to poor tissue perfusion/oxygenation with subsequent anaerobic metabolism and development of lactic acidosis. The acidosis may be severe, especially if superimposed on the metabolic acidosis that may accompany renal failure.

Support Phase

The first step in the management of patients in pulmonary edema is to ensure adequate oxygenation. Application of oxygen by mask may be adequate in some patients, but many will require endotracheal intubation and positive pressure ventilation. It is also important to ensure that the patient has an adequate oxygen-carrying capacity by maintaining an optimal hematocrit.

The mainstay of pharmacologic therapy for pulmonary edema is diuretics, primarily those whose site of action is the loop of Henle. As would be expected, diuresis results in a decrease in extracellular fluid volume and a decrease in lung water. Surprisingly, in anuric patients with CRF, administration of furosemide also results in a decline in left ventricular filling pressures unrelated to diuresis.[40] It is hypothesized that these agents cause blood to be shifted from the central compartment to the periphery. Preload reduction with agents such as nitroglycerin and morphine, as well as afterload reduction with conventional vasodilators such as hydralazine, or ACE inhibitors may provide additional benefit.

In centers where dialysis and ultrafiltration are not readily available, other temporizing measures should be employed. Oral administration of sorbitol has been shown to produce a shift of fluid from the vascular space to the bowel with significant reduction in left ventricular filling volumes. This occurs before the onset of diarrhea and with repeated administration can result in the displacement of greater than 5 L of fluid over 12 to 15 hours.[41] The administration of furosemide seems to account for an early decrease in left ventricular filling pressures, and sorbitol helps to sustain the reduction in pulmonary capillary wedge pressures. In large centers where acute dialysis or ultrafiltration can be performed urgently, removal of extracellular water by this method will result in rapid improvement in the clinical status of the patient and may facilitate early weaning from ventilatory support, particularly if no ongoing conditions exist that would predispose to recurrent decompensation, such as myocardial ischemia. In the patient who cannot undergo ultrafiltration because of hemodynamic instability, slow continuous ultrafiltration (SCUF) is an effective alternative to decrease plasma volume, and this method is discussed in Chapter 39.

Rehabilitative Phase

Once the patient is adequately oxygenated and hemodynamically stabilized, it is important to determine the events that led to decompensation. Cardiac ischemia and infarction should be ruled out. Echocardiography should be performed to assess systolic function and left ventricular wall thickness and to estimate ejection fraction. In patients who have dilated ventricles and elevated filling pressures, therapy is directed at limiting blood volume (sodium and fluid restriction, diuretics); decreasing afterload (ACE inhibitors, certain calcium-channel blockers, vasodilators); and improving cardiac contractility. In contrast, in patients with hypertrophic cardiomyopathy, volume should be maintained, and dialyzing to an underestimated dry weight should be avoided. Medications that decrease myocardial contractility and improve compliance, such as beta blockers or calcium-channel blockers, may improve cardiac function in these patients. Anti-ischemic therapy with beta blockers, calcium-channel blockers, and nitrates is necessary in patients with significant ischemic coronary disease.

Coronary Artery Disease

Risk Phase

Atherosclerotic CAD is inordinately common in renal failure. The concept of accelerated atherogenesis in uremia has been studied extensively since the early 1970s. Early data seemed to indicate a high rate of myocardial infarction in dialysis populations.[29] It has since been shown, however, that the incidence of myocardial infarction in patients with uremia is no higher than the incidence in patients with renal failure who do not have uremia (i.e., those who undergo adequate dialysis).[42] Although cardiovascular disease is the leading cause of death in patients with ESRD, myocardial infarction accounts for only a small fraction of these deaths. These patients have a high incidence of risk factors for CAD such as hypertension, hyperlipidemia, and left LVH. Hypertension and LVH have been discussed previously in this chapter. Serum lipid abnormalities are common in CRF patients. The cause of hyperlipidemia is multifactorial and involves abnormal metabolism of lipases, abnormal apolipoprotein composition with decreased high-density lipoprotein (HDL) cholesterol and increased pre-beta-lipoprotein particles, as well as elevated triglycerides similar to type IV hyperlipoproteinemia.[43] Despite these factors that would be expected to accelerate atherogenesis, it has been shown in some experimental models that atherosclerosis is not enhanced in uremia.[44] The reason for this disparity is unclear but may involve coexisting abnormalities in platelet function and vessel wall and platelet interaction and decreased levels of vitamin D, which may serve to impede or counterbalance the atherogenic process. Recent epidemiologic and demographic data have shown no difference between the incidence of CAD in dialysis populations and in the general population.[47] Ischemic coronary disease is prevalent in dialysis populations, which is due to the increasing numbers of elderly patients and diabetics entering dialysis. As such, angina pectoris and myocardial infarction are not uncommon among these patients. It is important to identify patients with symptomatic CAD to maximize medical therapy and to adjust dialysis practices to prevent the occurrence of untoward events.

Support Phase

Many patients with ESRD have known symptomatic CAD. When such a patient develops unstable or accelerating angina or myocardial infarction, they must be evaluated and managed like any other cardiac patient. Initial therapy with platelet inhibitors (aspirin), thrombolytic, heparin, nitrates, and beta blockers or calcium channel blockers is given to reduce myocardial damage. As previously mentioned, electrocardiography (ECG) may not be sufficient to diagnose myocardial ischemia or infarction due to resting ECG abnormalities. Generally, serum creatine kinase (CK) and lactate dehydrogenase levels are determined to indicate the presence or absence of myocardial infarction. It should be kept in mind, however, that moderate CK elevations may be seen in patients with CRF in whom no cardiac disease is present. Various investigators have shown that both BB and MB fractions of CK may be elevated in the patient with CRF. The explanation for this elevation is uncertain. It has been shown, however, that the elevation of CK in the setting of acute myocardial infarction (MI) is usually significantly higher than baseline levels in these patients and therefore can still be used to diagnose acute MI if clinical data and ECG data are supportive.[45]

Once the acute event has stabilized, an assessment of the patient's coronary artery status should be performed. The evaluation of ischemic heart disease in patients with CRF is no different from that in other patients. These patients, however, frequently have poor exercise tolerance, significant anemia, and resting ECG abnormalities secondary to electrolyte abnormalities, which may limit the feasibility of exercise ECG. Thallium scanning is an alternative but may give nonspecific results in this group of patients.[46] Combining thallium imaging with dipyridamole-induced coronary vasodilatation is a useful alternative with increased sensitivity and specificity for CAD in these patients.

Coronary angiography may be required to accurately assess ischemic CAD. This procedure should be used only when the patient is at high risk for CAD, and noninvasive testing is inconclusive or abnormal, the patient has not improved with maximal medical management, and the patient is felt to be a candidate for either coronary artery angioplasty or bypass grafting.[47] Significant risks are associated with angiography in the patient with renal failure. As discussed later, the administration of radiocontrast may cause significant deterioration in renal function in the CRF patient, at times necessitating dialytic therapy. Prophylactic hydration, and loop diuretics in the hypervolemic patient to promote urine flow, have been advocated to minimize this risk. Some have recommended prophylactic dialysis following contrast administration to remove the radiocontrast agent in patients with advanced renal failure, with the hope of ameliorating the likelihood of permanent dialysis-dependent renal failure. In patients with more advanced or end-stage renal failure, large infusions of hyperosmotic contrast media may cause pulmonary edema as well. This risk can be diminished with the judicious use of smaller quantities of contrast agents or use of lower osmolality agents. In hemodialysis patients in our institution, we often attempt to arrange dialysis treatments following angiography to minimize these concerns.

Rehabilitative Phase

Once the patient has been treated for an acute cardiovascular event and the extent of CAD has been assessed, medical management is designed to control symptoms and arrest the progress of atherosclerotic disease. Modification of risk factors is essential. For patients with dyslipidemia, lipid levels should be reduced by dietary modification and pharmacologic means if necessary. Anemia should be controlled with iron supplementation, erythropoietin administration, and transfusion as appropriate. Blood pressure control should also be optimized. Agents that reduce myocardial oxygen demand such as beta blockers and calcium-channel blockers are useful in controlling hypertension was well as angina, and long-acting nitrates continue to be of proven benefit as antianginal therapy.

Hemodialysis using bicarbonate rather than acetate-based solutions may decrease the frequency of hypotensive episodes, which often lead to angina. Peritoneal dialysis offers significant advantages over hemodialysis to the ESRD patient with CAD because this therapy presents considerably less hemodynamic stress and blood pressure fluctuations. If this treatment modality is available and is feasible for a given patient, its use is certainly recommended. In patients in whom ischemic symptoms are unabated by the previously mentioned approaches, coronary artery angioplasty or bypass grafting must be considered.

Pericardial disease

Risk Phase

In addition to ischemic heart disease, pulmonary edema and hypertensive urgencies, pericarditis is another significant cardiac entity that underlies numerous critical care admissions in renal failure patients. Pericarditis has long been known to be a sequela of uremia. Before the development of dialysis, approximately 41% of patients who died with uremia were found to have pericarditis on post mortem examination.[48] It was thought for many years that pericarditis was part of the uremic syndrome and that the accumulation of nitrogenous waste was the causative process. Subsequent observations, however, demonstrated that pericarditis also occurs in patients receiving routine dialysis and whose serum urea nitrogen levels are well controlled. It has thus been hypothesized that two distinct pericarditis syndromes exist.[49] The classic syndrome of "uremic pericarditis" is seen in patients with end-stage renal failure before the institution of dialytic therapy, or in whom dialysis has been recently initiated. The cause of this form of pericarditis is uncertain, but the generalized serositis and bleeding diathesis associated with uremia may result in pericardial inflammation and hemorrhage with resultant serosanguinous effusion.[50] Although accumulated waste products such as urea, creatinine, and middle molecules have been suggested to play a role in the pathogenesis of uremic pericarditis, no data are available to substantiate this. Infection and immunologic mechanisms have also been proposed but not proven. This form of pericarditis generally responds well to the intensification of the dialysis prescription, including daily dialysis treatments using longer treatment times and higher blood flow rates. Tamponade and sudden death are said to be rare in this form of pericardial disease.

The second form of pericarditis is seen in patients who are apparently adequately dialyzed, in perhaps as many as 8 to 12% of such patients,[49] and has been called "dialysis pericarditis." The exact mechanism for the development of this form of pericarditis is also unknown. Dialysis pericarditis does not respond to intensification of the dialysis regimen,[51] and the incidence of tamponade appears to be higher, perhaps as high as 20%.[52,53]

In addition to symptomatic pericarditis, 62% of patients with ESRD in one survey had asymptomatic pericardial effusion,[54] and in these patients, volume overload may play a causative role because decreases in patient weight often correlate with a decrease in effusion size.[55]

The patient who presents with pericarditis, whether uremic or dialysis associated, generally presents with chest pain that is unrelated to exertion and often pleuritic in nature. This pain is often worse with deep inspiration and when the patient is supine and may be somewhat alleviated when the patient sits upright or leans forward. Dyspnea may be present alone or in association with chest pain. Other presenting symptoms may include cough, malaise, or a change in mental status. The physical findings vary depending on the severity of pericarditis and the presence or absence of pericardial tamponade. In 85% of patients with pericarditis, a pericardial friction rub is heard at some time during the illness.[56] Fever, although usually low grade, is also frequently seen. In the presence of tamponade, pulsus paradoxus, Kussmaul's signs, jugular venous distention, and hypotension or shock may be seen. Electrocardiographic changes are variable. The classic ECG findings of diffuse ST segment elevation (Fig. 40-4) were seen in 32% of patients in one series.[57] Supraventricular or ventricular tachydysrhythmias may also be seen. Echocardiography may serve to identify the presence of pericardial thickening, the size of the pericardial effusion if present, and signs of tamponade.

Support Phase

The management of pericarditis depends on the patient's clinical course and hemodynamic status. For patients with uremic pericarditis, intensive dialysis results in resolution of pericarditis within 2 weeks.[57] Patients with dialysis-associated pericarditis do not respond as favorably to intensive dialysis, with only 12 to 15% of patients improving. Ventura and Garella,[51] based on a retrospective review of 20 years of studies, recommend that patients with dialysis-associated pericarditis undergo intensive dialysis only if pericardial effusion is small or absent. For those patients with moderate-to-large effusions that fail to respond to initial dialysis, surgical drainage (pericardial window, pericardiostomy, or pericardiectomy), perhaps with the instillation of intrapericardial steroids, should be performed. Pericardiocentesis should be reserved for patients needing urgent drainage that is due to hemodynamically unstable tamponade, because it has been shown to have a very low success rate and high mortality. If pericardiocentesis is performed urgently, definitive surgical therapy is necessary once hemodynamic stability is achieved.

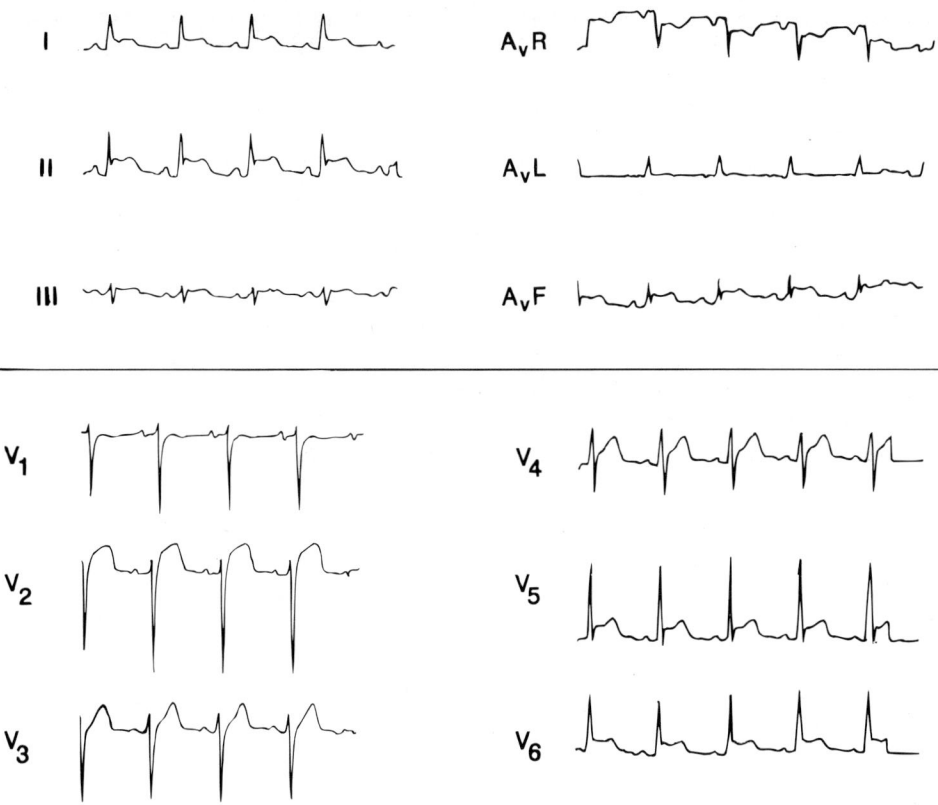

Fig. 40-4. Electrocardiogram in a hemodialysis patient with pericarditis.

For those patients with asymptomatic effusion, aggressive ultrafiltration should be instituted. If the effusion does not resolve, serial examinations and echocardiography are needed to monitor the effusion and detect early tamponade. In years past, treatment with nonsteroidal anti-inflammatory drugs (NSAIDs) and systemic steroids had been advocated. Neither of these agents appears to offer advantages over the modalities mentioned here.[51] The management of pericardial tamponade associated with these forms of pericarditis is no different from management of tamponade resulting from any other process. Hemodynamic support with volume infusion, pressor agents, and invasive monitoring may be required.

PULMONARY DISEASE IN CHRONIC RENAL FAILURE

Pulmonary complications of CRF are frequent. The two most common events, pulmonary edema and pulmonary infection, are discussed elsewhere in this chapter. Pleural disorders, specifically pleuritis and pleural effusions, are common in patients with CRF as well. Autopsy studies have demonstrated that as many as 40% of dialysis patients have evidence of pleural inflammation on post mortem examination.[58] Alterations in pleural fluid dynamics are frequently described in these patients. Volume overload, often seen in patients with renal disease that is due to poor compliance with dietary fluid restrictions or inadequate ultrafiltration during dialytic therapy, causes an increase in pleural capillary hydrostatic pressure. This, combined with the frequently seen decreased plasma oncotic pressure that results from malnutrition or urinary protein losses, results in Starling forces which favor the transudation of fluid into the pleural space with resultant accumulations of small-to-moderate pleural effusions. The pleura itself is believed to be altered in uremia, perhaps by mechanisms similar to those leading to pericardial inflammation. This so-called "uremic pleuritis," which has been described since 1836,[59] is typified by fibrinous, necrotizing pleural inflammation and may result in the leakage of cells and proteins into the pleural space. The resultant effusion may be hemorrhagic. The exact pathophysiologic mechanism that underlies uremic pleuritis is not known, but it has been postulated that "middle molecules" or low molecular weight proteins may trigger pleural inflammation. The effusions related to uremic pleuritis are generally exudative in nature, with fewer than 1500 white blood cells (WBC) per milliliter with or without a hemorrhagic competent. These effusions may become chronic and result in the development of a rigid peel, which may encase the lung, causing significant restrictive disease. In contrast, effusions that are related to volume overload are typically transudative and will often resolve with vigorous ultrafiltration and fluid restriction.

Pleural effusion may also be seen in CRF in the setting of infections as well as pulmonary embolism. Transient hydrothorax is occasionally seen in patients undergoing ambulatory peritoneal dialysis and is felt to be secondary to migration of peritoneal dialysate through diaphragmatic defects or pores. Hemothorax or pneumothorax may occur as a complication of placement of central venous dialysis catheters.

The typical presenting complaints of a patient with pleuritis or pleural effusion are pleuritic chest pain and dyspnea. Low grade fever may be present as well. A pleural friction rub may be heard over the involved hemithorax. Signs of pleural effusion including decreased breath sounds, dullness to percussion, and decreased fremitus or pectoriloquy may be noted. The evaluation of these patients differs depending on the acuity of the illness. Pleural effusions felt to be secondary to volume overload may simply be followed while vigorous ultrafiltration is performed, because these effusions often resolve with this therapy alone. If the effusion fails to improve with aggressive ultrafiltration, or if the patient is febrile or has significant pleuritic chest pain, a diagnostic thoracentesis should be performed with studies directed to determine the cause of the effusion. In the patient with exudative effusion, a thorough search for the underlying cause must be undertaken. Therapy is then directed at the primary disorder. In extreme cases of recurrent effusions or pleural thickening, decortication or pleurodesis may be required.

INFECTIOUS DISEASES IN CHRONIC RENAL FAILURE

The Immune Consequences of Chronic Renal Failure

Infection is widely accepted as a leading cause of death in patients with CRF. In hemodialysis patients, for example, the frequency of infection as a cause of death is reported to range from 10 to 40%, with little evidence that this incidence has changed appreciatively in recent years.

The immune consequences of CRF are summarized in Table 40-4. A number of factors contribute to the predisposition of patients with CRF to infection. Uremia per se is immunosuppressive. Even before the development of dialytic therapies and transplantation, infectious diseases commonly contributed to or caused death in uremic individuals. The repeated exposure of these patients to the risk of infection—either by virtue of the use of peritoneal or hemodialysis or through the immunosuppressive medications used in transplantation—places the ESRD patient at inordinate risk of infection and its consequences.

Beginning in the late 1950s, numerous investigators observed that uremic animals and humans exhibit a diminished tendency to reject skin and renal allografts.[60,61] These observations lend support to the uremic state as an immunosuppressive derangement. Since that time, various aspects of the immune system have been shown to be adversely affected in the uremic patient. It is widely accepted, for example, that patients with systemic lupus erythematosus experience a significant reduction in the serologic and systemic activity of their disease as renal failure ensues.[62] Further, patients with CRF have repeatedly been shown to have an increased incidence of malignancies, suggesting that some uremic impairment in the immune surveillance against neoplasia.[63-66]

Although measured immunoglobulin levels are normal in most patients with CRF, reductions in B-lymphocyte populations are frequently observed. In addition, investigators have noted reduced antibody response to the administration of standard influenza[67] and pneumococcal vaccines.[68,69] Finally, autoantibody production is clearly increased in patients with CRF; it was seen in as many as 70% of patients in one series.[70]

Impairment in cell-mediated immunity appears to be much more consistently observed and more clinically important in renal failure than any derangements in humoral response. Delayed hypersensitivity is decreased, as demonstrated by anergic skin test responses to a variety of antigens.[70,71] Lymphopenia, including reductions in both B-cell and T-cell populations, is consistently observed, and Hoy and co-workers showed that the institution of dialysis may partially ameliorate these deficiencies.[72] In addition, uremic lymphocytes demonstrate a decreased blastogenic response to mitogenic stimulation,[73] and uremic plasma has been shown to suppress T-cell responsiveness in vitro, suggesting a role for some accumulated uremic toxin in impairing T-cell function.[74]

With regard to monocyte-macrophage function, phagocytosis by macrophages in uremic patients has been shown to be depressed in vitro.[75,76] Recently, Ruiz and co-workers[77] demonstrated in vivo that autologous RBCs coated with immunoglobulin G (IgG) were poorly cleared from the blood of ESRD patients because of impairment in the Fc-receptor function of splenic macrophages. Moreover, in their study, the severity of this impairment correlated with the occurrence of severe infections.

Neutrophil function in the uremic environment is less clearly understood. Chemotaxis, phagocytosis, and intracellular killing by neutrophils have been shown to be reduced by some investigators, while others have failed to show consistent effects of uremia on these parameters of neutrophil function.

Finally, protein calorie malnutrition, a prevalent problem in the CRF population, may further impair immune responsiveness. Malnutrition is known to alter the function of both neutrophils and lymphocytes, and lymphocyte counts may be reduced as well.[78,79]

Modalities of treatment for ESRD compound the risk of infection in the patient already immunocompromised by uremia. The creation of angioaccess for hemodialysis as well as the frequent needle punctures of the access vessels once created provide many opportunities for the introduction of microorganisms into the circulation. Similarly, the peritoneal dialysis catheter provides a portal of entry for bacteria either into the peritoneal cavity or into the tissues surrounding the catheter exit site. Last, immunosuppressive therapies used in transplant recipients clearly magnify the risk of infection significantly.

Infections, therefore, are extremely common in the CRF patient in the critical care unit, either as the reason for admission or as a complication of the critical illness or

Table 40-4. The Immune Consequences of Chronic Renal Failure

Diminished tendency to reject allografts
Increased incidence of malignancies
Reduced B- and T-lymphocyte populations
Reduced antibody response to immunization
Increased autoantibody production
Decreased delayed hypersensitivity
Impaired lymphocyte responsiveness to mitogens
Depressed phagocytosis by macrophages
Impaired chemotaxis, phagocytosis, intracellular killing by neutrophils (?)

care. In our experience, infections were the second most common category of illness listed as diagnoses on the charts of CRF patients in the ICU during the previously mentioned 9-year period, second only to cardiovascular diseases. Among the specific infections listed, pneumonia was the most common, followed by urinary tract infection and sepsis (see Table 40-1).

Pneumonia

In addition to alterations in immunity previously discussed, CRF impairs protective mechanisms in the respiratory tract, thereby predisposing these patients to the development of pneumonia. What many years ago was referred to as "uremic lung" is now more clearly understood as several derangements in lung physiology that impair the normal mechanisms designed to protect against lung infection. Patients with renal failure have been shown to have characteristic hyaline membrane-like changes in alveoli, which appear to result from increased pulmonary capillary permeability with consequent exudation of fibrin and protein rich fluid into alveolar spaces.[80,81] The pulmonary clearance of inhaled bacteria has been shown to be markedly impaired in experimental animals with renal failure, and the degree of impairment seems to correlate with the severity of azotemia.[82] Further, Yu and co-workers demonstrated that dialysis patients exhibit an increased incidence of nasopharyngeal colonization with Staphylococcus aureus, seen in 52% of their patient population.[83] All of these findings lend support to the observation that the patient with CRF is at inordinate risk for developing pulmonary infection.

When pneumonia develops in this population, the most common causative organisms isolated differ little from the conventional organisms seen in other patient groups. Keane et al. isolated Streptococcus pneumoniae in 50% of their patients with pneumonia.[84] Gram-negative and other less common organisms are isolated with increasing frequency in patients developing pneumonia in hospitals or institutions. Finally, it should be pointed out that patients with CRF experience a 10-fold or greater incidence of tuberculosis than that seen in the normal population, thereby necessitating the consideration of this pathogen when these patients present with pneumonia.[85,86]

Risk Phase

The initial diagnostic assessment of a patient with pneumonia focuses, of course, on making the diagnosis but must also include an assessment of the patient's oxygenation and hemodynamic status. The history may reveal an antecedent or nonresolving "bad cold" with upper respiratory symptoms of nasal congestion, rhinorrhea, sore throat, myalgias, and fever. High grade fever, rigors, pleuritic chest pain, increasing dyspnea with exertion, hemoptysis, or purulent sputum production should raise concern for the presence of pneumonia, although unfortunately, many patients have more vague and generalized complaints.

The physical examination should at once include an assessment for signs of hypoxemia and hemodynamic compromise. Cyanosis, tachycardia, and tachypnea and with impending respiratory fatigue may be ominous indicators of imminent decompensation. Patients with renal failure often have baseline hypothermia, so "low grade" temperature elevation may be relatively more significant, and some of these patients will not manifest fever, even in the face of severe infection. A careful lung examination may uncover signs of consolidation, including decreased breath sounds, dullness to percussion, egophony, and increased fremitus and pectoriloquy. Evidence of pleural effusion in a patient in whom pneumonia is suspected may signal the presence of a parapneumonic effusion, which will require further investigation.

As in any critically ill patient with pneumonia, the initial diagnostic assessment should include complete blood counts (CBC), chest radiograph, sputum Gram's stain, and arterial blood gases. In interpreting these studies, one should consider several issues relating to patients with renal failure. While an elevated WBC count with a leftward shift toward less mature granulocytes is supportive of the diagnosis of significant infection, the patient with CRF may not exhibit these findings because of impairments in leukocyte response, as described previously. Further, hemodialysis patients will often exhibit a very low WBC immediately following the dialysis procedure, so that CBCs drawn at this time must be interpreted with caution. As stated previously, patients with CRF are commonly anemic, and correction of this anemia may be important in improving the patient's ability to oxygenate. The presence of pneumonia on chest radiographs may be more difficult to ascertain in the presence of congestive heart failure, fluid overload with pulmonary edema, or pleural effusion—concomitant conditions not uncommon in the renal failure patient. In cases of suspected tuberculosis, skin testing and sputum testing for acid-fast bacilli should be included in the diagnostic assessment. A negative tuberculin skin test may, however, simply be a manifestation of anergy in patients with renal failure, and further skin testing with common anergy panel antigens as well as higher strength tuberculin assays will often be warranted.

Failure or impending failure to ventilate and/or oxygenate as well as hemodynamic compromise suggesting either severe volume contraction or possible septicemia are clear indications for ICU admission. In addition, the patient who may require intensive pulmonary toilet and secretion management may be more appropriately placed in a critical care setting.

Support Phase

The successful management of the renal failure patient with pneumonia in the ICU depends on measures to optimize oxygenation, hemodynamic stability, and nutrition, as well as appropriate antimicrobial therapy.

Impairments to oxygenation in these patients include concomitant pulmonary edema as well as anemia. Transfusion therapy to correct anemia may further compound the volume status of the patient, necessitating the use of loop diuretics or dialytic fluid removal. In dialysis-dependent patients, maintenance of the ongoing dialysis regimen is important to minimize the effects of uremia and fluid overload on he patient's defense against infection. When oxygenation is compromised, care should be taken during hemodialysis to prevent further dialysis-induced reductions in Po_2 by maximizing intradialytic oxygen delivery.

In patients with renal disease, the indications for intubation and mechanical ventilation are essentially the same as for all patients. However, the hemodialysis patient who requires ventilator assistance with increasing positive end-expiratory pressures may experience hemodynamic difficulties as an extracorporeal blood volume is established during dialysis. An adequate intravascular volume must be maintained and can be supported with intradialytic colloid (e.g., 5% albumin or mannitol) or crystalloid infusion. Occasionally, intradialytic vasopressor support is necessary in these patients as well, to ensure the completion of dialysis therapy.

Efforts to assess and maximize nutrition are critically important in the renal failure patient with any serious infection. If oral intake is either not possible or not adequate to meet the patient's nutritional needs, enteral feeding (or parenteral nutrition if gastrointestinal function is impaired) is of paramount importance.

Antimicrobial therapy is made more complicated by renal failure as well. It is critically important to ascertain the level of renal function as accurately as possible in any given patient so as to permit appropriate drug dosing. It must be remembered that older patients with reduced muscle mass may have dramatic reductions in their GRFs even in the face of "normal" serum creatinine values. Before dosing with antibiotics, it is useful to estimate the GRF of the patient using the formula of Cockroft and Gault, which takes into account the patient's age, weight, and serum creatinine in the following relationship:

estimated creatinine clearance
$$= \frac{(140 - \text{age}) \times (\text{ideal body weight in kg}) \times (0.85 \text{ if female})}{72 \times (\text{serum creatinine})}$$

The ideal body weight can be estimated as:

Males

50 kg + 2.3 kg for every inch in height over 5 feet

Females

45.5 kg + 2.3 kg for every inch in height over 5 feet

The validity of any estimate of creatinine clearance (including the 24-hour urine collection) requires that the patient's renal function is at steady state such that the serum creatinine is reasonable stable.

A complete listing of the available antimicrobial agents, their pharmacokinetics, and recommendations regarding their dosage adjustment in renal failure has been published elsewhere[87,88] and is beyond the scope of this chapter.

Rehabilitative Phase

It is difficult to estimate the morbidity and mortality of pneumonia in renal failure patients, because these are affected by the severity of renal disease, treatment modality, age, concomitant medical conditions, nutritional state, and numerous other confounding variables. Keane and coworkers reported mortality rates of 12% in patients admitted with pneumonia and 57% in patients developing pneumonia while hospitalized.[84] Patients who survive to leave the hospital, particularly after prolonged hospitalizations or prolonged periods of ventilator dependency, may require intensive physical and occupational therapy during convalescence to regain maximal functional capacity.

Two vaccines are currently highly recommended to reduce the risk of developing pneumonia in patients with renal failure. Annual vaccination with influenza vaccine has impacted significantly on the incidence of influenza infections in these patients. Each year, these vaccines contain strains of viruses that are expected to surface in outbreaks during the ensuing winter. Ideally, vaccination is administered in November because peak infection rates occur in January and February. Whereas the efficacy of the vaccine is likely to be reduced in renal failure, a number of studies have shown a significant antibody response in as many as 87% of hemodialysis patients, an efficacy rate that clearly impacts positively on infection rates in this population.[89,90]

Given the significant incidence and mortality of pneumococcal disease in patients with chronic disease, the use of pneumococcal vaccine is also recommended in renal failure patients. At present, 23 pneumococcal serotypes are accounted for in the available vaccine, and these 23 (of more than 80 known) serotypes are said to be implicated in approximately 90% of serious pneumococcal infections. As is the case with influenza, the pneumococcal vaccine is less effective in patients with renal failure. Efficacy rates as high as 60 to 80% are reported in this population, but antibody titers are lower and less enduring than in otherwise well individuals. Antibody levels may fall to one third their original levels within 2 years after vaccination. In fact, the observation by Linnemann et al.[69] that revaccination of hemodialysis patients at 2-year intervals virtually eliminated the infection in these patients has led some to recommend such a revaccination schedule. Certainly, initial administration of the 23 valent vaccine should be recommended to all patients with CRF. More study is needed to clarify the usefulness of revaccination, but in high risk patients, revaccination no more often than every 2 years may be rational.

Septicemia

Little is known about the incidence of septicemia in all patients with renal failure. Most of the available data in the literature relate to patients with ESRD who are on some form of renal replacement therapy. These patients are predisposed to bacteremia by virtue not only of their underlying diseases and disease complications but by the nature of their treatment modalities per se. In most series, the majority of bacteremic episodes seems to result from infection of angioaccess sites, including temporary dialysis catheters, natural arteriovenous fistulae, or synthetic arteriovenous grafts. The majority of these infections are caused by gram-positive organisms, predominantly staphylococcal species.

When septicemia is not clearly angioaccess related,

sources of infection most commonly include the gastrointestinal, respiratory, and urinary tracts. Yet, a significant percentage will have no clearly identifiable source. The preponderance of gram-positive organisms isolated in this group, however, suggests that many of these infections may also be angioaccess related.

In addition to angioaccess sites, the urinary tract deserves special consideration as a source of infection in patients with chronic renal disease. Reductions in urine volume, urine flow rates, urinary concentrating ability, and voiding frequency combine to make the patient with renal failure particularly vulnerable to infection of the urinary tract. The high incidence of bacteruria, in some reports as high as 60%, and the pyuria that often results from bladder statis, make the diagnosis of urinary tract infection (UTI) difficult. Incidence figures in the literature vary, largely because of variations in the definition of UTI. Infection is perhaps best defined as the presence of significant (more than 10^5/ml) bacteruria and significant (more than 10 WBC per high power field) pyuria. Whether symptoms are required to diagnose infection is a matter of debate, but the fact that septicemia from the urinary tract may occur in asymptomatic individuals suggests that significant infection can occur in the absence of symptoms. Saitoh and coworkers[91] studied 182 CRF patients and reported a 27% incidence of significant bacteruria, while 19% had UTI and 7% had symptomatic UTI. Because a significant number of patients with CRF are at increased risk of infection of the upper urinary tract (including patients with polycystic disease, diabetes mellitus, neurogenic bladder dysfunction, vesicoureteral reflux, etc.), it is not surprising that the occurrence of septicemia arising from the urinary tract is not uncommon.

Risk Phase

As in any patient in whom septicemia is suspected, regardless of renal function, extremely thorough history and physical examination are vital in the search for potential sources of infection. In addition, a prompt assessment of the patient's hemodynamic status is a priority. It must be kept in mind, however, that the patient with CRF may fail to exhibit the usual manifestations of serious and even life-threatening infections. These patients often have slightly reduced baseline body temperatures, and fever in the face of infection, if present at all, may be low grade. Patients who have peripheral neuropathy with sensory impairment may not experience pain in areas of skin, soft tissue, and even osseous infections. Genital, rectal, and pelvic exams are critically important in attempting to exclude occult sites of infection in these areas.

In the assessment of hemodialysis patients, infected arteriovenous fistulae and grafts may manifest erythema, tenderness, areas of fluctuance, or purulent discharge, shunt thrombosis, pseudoaneurysm formation, and at times, direct visualization of the synthetic graft through infected tissues. Particularly problematic, however, is the observation that perhaps as many as one third of patients will lack any evidence of inflammation other than that which normally results from the regular use of the fistula.[92]

The laboratory evaluation of septic patients may provide clues to the presence of bacteremia and/or localizing infection. As mentioned previously, however, these patients may fail to demonstrate significant leukocytosis, and blood counts should not be performed immediately following hemodialysis treatments. The presence of acute respiratory alkalosis may be a valuable clue to the presence of gram-negative bacteremia and should heighten suspicion of a urinary tract or gastrointestinal source. The presence of significant bacteria and WBCs in the urine, as noted previously, particularly in the symptomatic patient, strongly suggests UTI. The presence of WBC casts and renal tubular epithelial cells in the urinary sediment indicate tubulointerstitial inflammation and suggest pyelonephritis. When arteriovenous fistula infection is suspected in the absence of local evidence of inflammation, the role of gallium and indium-labeled WBC scans remains unsettled. It is conceivable that the localized inflammation that results from normal fistula use may lead to false-positive scans, while the impairment of neutrophil function may result in false-negative examinations.

Support Phase

The management of the septic patient is described in Chapters 51 and 64 and differs little in the renal failure patient. Obviously, the hallmarks of treatment are appropriate antimicrobial therapy and hemodynamic support. It should be pointed out, however, that in the dialysis-dependent patient, the hemodynamic instability of sepsis may necessitate intradialytic vasopressor support or may even preclude conventional hemodialysis. When available and feasible, peritoneal dialysis presents less hemodynamic challenge in the septic patient and is an efficient method of fluid removal. In the most hemodynamically tenuous patient, continuous methods of ultrafiltration (SCUF) or dialysis (continuous arteriovenous hemofiltration [CAVH], continuous arteriovenous hemodialysis [CAVHD]) may be the only remaining alternatives as renal replacement therapies. These dialytic methods are discussed in Chapter 39. In addition, the choice of antimicrobial agents in patients with CRF requires special consideration, as discussed previously.

Rehabilitative Phase

The mortality of septicemia in patients with CRF has been fairly consistently reported in the 15 to 20% range,[84,92] even over the past few decades. In some series, mortality from angioaccess-related bacteremias is reported to be lower than the overall mortality rate, but these figures range from as low as 8% to as high as 18%.

Efforts to reduce the risk of recurrent infection episodes should be undertaken whenever possible. With regard to the potential for recurrent urinary tract infections, workup for anatomic or functional derangements of the urinary tract should be undertaken when indicated by previously published guidelines. Identification and treatment of neurogenic bladder dysfunction, frequent voiding routines, and at times suppressive daily antibiotic prophylaxis have been reported to be beneficial.

In patients with recurrent staphyloccocal infections, it may be useful to assess for the "carriage" of staphylococcal organisms in the nasopharynx or skin. Prophylactic measures used to decolonize these patients, including intermittent oral rifampin and topical (nasal) bacitracin, may prove useful in reducing the incidence of recurrent serious staphylococcal infections.[83]

GASTROINTESTINAL DISEASE IN CHRONIC RENAL FAILURE

Gastrointestinal Consequences of Chronic Renal Failure

The gastrointestinal consequences of CRF contribute significantly to the morbidity and mortality of patients with this diagnosis. Gastrointestinal bleeding is prevalent in this population, and in our experience it is a frequent presentation leading to ICU admission. Although the incidence of peptic ulcer disease has not been clearly shown to be increased in patients with ESRD, its associated morbidity and mortality are often increased because of concomitant malnutrition, propensity for bleeding, and impaired wound healing. Intermittent anticoagulation during hemodialysis treatment may also increase the likelihood of gastrointestinal bleeding. Derangements of gastrointestinal physiology that occur as a result of renal failure and dialytic therapy further place these patients at risk for serious bleeding from the gastrointestinal tract. Anatomic alterations in the gastrointestinal mucosa have been demonstrated in patients with CRF. Edema of the mucosa and submucosa are seen, with hyperemia, hemorrhage, and necrosis. Decreased numbers of chief cells and parietal cells seen on biopsy specimens, a decreased concentration of gastric mucus, and impaired cell renewal in the presence of uremia have all been reported.[93] In addition, an increased incidence of telangiectasias is seen in patients with CRF. These lesions may be seen throughout the gastrointestinal tract and account for as much as 20% of upper gastrointestinal bleeding and 30% of lower gastrointestinal bleeding in some studies.[26,94] Telangiectasias often present a diagnostic challenge because they are not readily visualized by radiologic contrast studies and may be located beyond the reach of the endoscope.

Physiologic alterations involving the gastrointestinal tract in uremic patients may also play a role in the development of bleeding. Renal insufficiency per se appears to have an inhibitory effect on gastric acid secretion, and treatment of uremia leads to reduction in this inhibition.[95] Some patients on maintenance hemodialysis tend to experience hypersecretion of gastric acid. Others have lower than normal rates of gastric acid stimulation, perhaps secondary to decreased numbers of parietal cells and other mucosal abnormalities. This hyposecretion may then stimulate gastrin production causing hypergastrinemia, a common finding in patients with CRF. Correction of uremia may enhance gastric mucosal integrity, with a concomitant increase in the number of parietal cells and subsequent hypersecretion of acid. Patients undergoing active and significant treatment of uremia (e.g., dialysis or transplantation) have an increased frequency of peptic ulceration and other gastrointestinal complications.

Motility abnormalities may also be seen in many renal failure patients, especially those with autonomic dysfunction secondary to diabetes mellitus. Intermittent nausea and vomiting are prevalent in this population of patients. Repeated episodes of emesis combined with the friable mucosa seen in these patients predisposes them to Mallory-Weiss tears and subsequent hemorrhage. As discussed previously, patients with CRF also have a significant bleeding diathesis and frequently have subclinical gastrointestinal hemorrhage. In one series, 1 in 10 dialysis patients was found to have hemoccult-positive stool.[96] This is higher than the incidence in azotemic patients not undergoing dialysis and may reflect the significance of intermittent heparization in increasing the risk of bleeding in these patients.

In addition, ulcerogenic drugs such as NSAIDs increase the risk of bleeding in renal failure patients by virtue of their effects on prostaglandin synthesis as well as reduction in platelet function.[97] These medications should be avoided, as should other substances known to be risk factors for the development of acid-peptic disease (e.g., alcohol, tobacco, steroids).

Risk Phase

When a patient with CRF is brought to the emergency room for evaluation of gastrointestinal blood loss, the history and physical examination are of utmost importance in determining the disposition of the patient. Important information to be elicited from the patient includes the duration and timing of symptoms. If the patient presents with hematemesis, it is important to determine whether the patient had been vomiting for several hours and then noted blood, or had suddenly vomited bloody material initially. Description of the emesis as frank blood or merely "coffee-ground" material and may help to determine the acuity of bleeding. The presence of melena, hematochezia, or abdominal pain should be noted, as well as any symptoms suggestive of intravascular volume depletion, such as dizziness, alterations in mental status, near-syncope, syncope, shortness of breath, or angina.

The goal of the physical examination is to identify the severity of bleeding as well as its source. Orthostatic reduction in blood pressure or resting tachycardia can be helpful in identifying the patient who has had hemodynamically significant blood loss. In some cases, however, orthostatic vital signs may not accurately assess hemodynamic status. In the presence of autonomic insufficiency secondary to diabetes, a patient may be "orthostatic" despite an adequate intravascular volume and RBC mass. Conversely, a patient on medications that decrease atrioventricular nodal conduction such as beta blockers may not present with resting or upright tachycardia despite significant blood loss. The presence of pallor may not be particularly useful to estimate the degree of blood loss in patients with CRF, because many of these patients have significant underlying anemia. Hemoccult testing of stool specimens and nasogastric aspirates should be performed. A patient with hematemesis and with stool that is positive for occult blood is likely to have had a more significant hemorrhage than a patient with only gastric contents or stool that has tested positively for occult blood. Signs of concomitant liver disease, such as ascites, spider angiomata, and dilated superficial venous plexes, portend a worse prognosis. The initial laboratory investigation should include complete blood counts, PT, PTT, ECG, and abdominal radiographs. Evidence of coagulopathy, myocardial ischemia, or infarction or gastrointestinal perforation require more aggressive and intensive intervention in the bleeding patient.

The decision to admit a patient with gastrointestinal bleeding to the ICU is made based on the likelihood that lifesaving intervention will be required within 24 hours of admission. This can be predicted based on several factors. First, the patient's history and physical findings are evaluated. If a patient has orthostatic vital signs suggesting intravascular volume depletion, which do not respond to initial volume repletion, ICU evaluation is warranted. The presence of involvement of a second organ system as a result of blood loss (e.g., myocardial infarction, angina, pulmonary edema, or altered levels of consciousness) mandates aggressive therapy in an intensive care setting. A patient with underlying liver dysfunction generally has higher morbidity and mortality from gastrointestinal bleeding, and therefore patients with signs of chronic liver disease and hemodynamically significant GI bleeding should be monitoring in an ICU.

Support Phase

When a patient with CRF is discovered to have hemodynamically significant gastrointestinal blood loss and is admitted to an ICU, management is similar to most patients with gastrointestinal bleeding and is discussed in depth elsewhere in this text. Parenteral access must be established, and volume replacement initiated with either crystalloid solutions or blood products if anemia is significant. Consecutive therapy with measures to reduce gastric acidity (in the case of bleeding from acid-peptic disease) and blood transfusion to maintain hemodynamic stability are the mainstay of initial management.[95] Given the bleeding diathesis and the incidence of mucosal telangiectases in patients with CRF, early endoscopy must be considered. Endoscopy may be essential in diagnosing the source of bleeding and may also provide an opportunity for therapeutic intervention. Bleeding ulcers or telangiectasias of the proximal gastrointestinal tract may be electrocoagulated or sclerosed via the endoscope. Lower gastrointestinal tract telangiectasias are not as easily treated endoscopically, but identification of their exact location may be beneficial if surgical intervention is required for persistent bleeding. For life-threatening upper or lower gastrointestinal bleeding that does not respond to conservative medical and/or endoscopic management, surgical therapy may be required.

For hemodialysis patients who are actively bleeding, care must be taken with anticoagulants during dialysis treatments. Attempts to minimize or avoid heparin usage are in order and may necessitate frequent flushing of the dialyzer system or the use of plate dialyzers in which blood is less likely to clot in the presence of reduced heparin dosages.

Rehabilitative Phase

Optimal rehabilitation following an episode of gastrointestinal bleeding allows the patient to regain his previous level of functioning once blood counts and cardiovascular status have returned to baseline. Reduction or modification of risk factors for gastrointestinal bleeding is an integral part of both rehabilitation and prophylaxis against further episodes of hemorrhage. Patients who have been demonstrated to be at high risk for gastrointestinal bleeding (previous gastrointestinal bleeding, history of peptic ulcer disease, transplant recipients) should be given prophylactic therapy with H_2 blockers, given in dosages adjusted according to level of renal function, or non-magnesium-containing antacids to minimize gastric acidity. Patient education is of utmost importance, because patients must be instructed to avoid medications or substances that may be ulcerogenic. Some investigators have shown that gastric ulceration is more common than duodenal ulceration in patients with CRF. Ulcerogenic drugs superimposed on the changes in gastrointestinal mucosa induced by uremia may be important in the pathogenesis of these gastric lesions.[97] It is thus important to counsel patients with CRF to avoid NSAIDs, aspirin, alcohol, and tobacco. They should also be instructed to watch for signs or symptoms of recurrent bleeding. Careful follow-up should include monitoring of hemoglobin or hematocrit levels, and screening for occult blood in the stool is essential to detect recurrent hemorrhage. Early detection of recurrent bleeding may significantly reduce its morbidity and mortality in patients with CRF by allowing the institution of therapy before hemodynamic instability occurs.

NEPHROLOGIC INJURY IN CHRONIC RENAL FAILURE

Acute Renal Failure

The patient with chronic renal insufficiency appears to be particularly vulnerable to insults that lead to acute deterioration in renal function. The frequency with which acute renal failure occurs in patients with underlying renal insufficiency is difficult to ascertain from the literature. Most reports detail the incidence of acute renal failure in general populations without regard to preexisting renal disease and likely underestimate the frequency of this event in CRF patients.

In a large prospective study, Hou and co-workers reported the development of acute renal failure in 4.9% of more than 2200 patients admitted to Tufts-New England Medical Center.[98] Kraman et al. studied 686 patients with respiratory failure in a respiratory ICU and observed acute renal failure in nearly 11% of these critically ill patients.[99] In a recent report of a medical-surgical ICU population of 315 patients, Menashe and co-workers noted that 15% acquired acute renal failure.[100] As will be discussed, the occurrence of acute renal failure in hospitalized patients impacts significantly on illness acuity and outcome. The patient with preexisting renal insufficiency should be seen as a patient at risk, and attention should be paid to minimizing the likelihood of the development of acute renal failure in these individuals.

Risk Phase

Table 40-5 lists the risk factors that predispose the patient to the development of acute renal failure. In the previ-

Table 40-5. Risk Factors for the Development of Acute Renal Failure

Hypovolemia
    Gastrointestinal fluid losses
    Overly aggressive diuresis
    Dehydration
    Sodium restriction
    Hemorrhage
Hypotension
Sepsis
Cardiac failure
Nephrotoxic medications
    Antimicrobial agents
    Nonsteroidal anti-inflammatory drugs
Radiocontrast agents
Trauma/major surgery

ously mentioned critical care experience reported by Menashe et al.[99] four well-known risk factors were noted, alone or in combination, to underly the occurrence of acute renal failure in all patients. These were (1) hypotension (present in 86%) and (2) sepsis and (3) administration of aminoglycoside antibiotics and (4) radiocontrast agents.

Extracellular fluid volume depletion must be considered in any patient who experiences an acute reduction in renal function. The thirsty patient with diminished skin turgor, dry mucous membranes, orthostatic hypotension and tachycardia, negative in-hospital fluid balance, and decreasing body weight is easily identified as hypovolemic. The history and physical examination findings, however, are often more subtle and less specific. In all hospitalized patients with CRF, care should be taken to monitor fluid balance and to avoid dehydration and volume losses.

Certain serum and urinary indices have been recommended as aids to diagnosing prerenal azotemia, including measurements of urine sodium concentration, osmolality, fractional sodium excretion rate, and urine/plasma ratios of creatinine and osmolality. These maneuvers have their basis in the concept that under prerenal circumstances, the normal kidney conserves sodium and concentrates the urine. These studies, however, must be interpreted with caution because numerous factors may interfere with their validity.

The presence of total body volume overload, manifested by the presence of peripheral edema, increased jugular venous pressure, rales on lung exam, and an S_3 gallop rhythm suggest cardiac failure as a potential cause of impaired renal perfusion and azotemia. Pulmonary congestion and cardiomegaly may be noted on chest radiographs, and confirmation is obtained, if necessary, by the measurement of elevated central venous and pulmonary capillary wedge pressures and reduced cardiac output during invasive hemodynamic monitoring.

With regard to nephrotoxic drugs, a thorough review of the medications to which the patient has been exposed is critically important. Aminoglycoside and beta-lactam antibiotics lead the long list of potential nephrotoxins in hospitalized patients. Careful assessment of renal function, as described previously, is essential to minimize the risk of aminoglycoside toxicity. In addition, serum aminoglycoside levels should be followed throughout the course of administration to prevent the accumulation of toxic levels that might not have been otherwise predicted by estimates of renal function and the pharmacokinetics of the drug. In addition, dosage adjustment of the beta-lactam drugs is required in renal failure. Unfortunately, serum drug levels are often less readily available for these medications. Twitching and myoclonus may be early signs of significant beta-lactam accumulation in renal failure patients, and if not addressed, seizures and coma may occur. In our experience, the occurrence of myoclonus in renal failure patients with beta-lactam toxicity has almost uniformly been associated with extremely high serum and cerebrospinal fluid (CSF) beta-lactam drug levels. Numerous reviews of nephrotoxic agents involved in acute renal failure have been published elsewhere.[101-104]

In addition to in-hospital prescribed medications, patients should be carefully questioned about the use of nephrotoxic agents before hospitalization. In particular, with the widespread availability of NSAIDs over the counter, it is important to remember that the reduction of intrarenal vasodilatory prostaglandins induced by these drugs may heighten the vulnerability of the kidneys to any number of conditions of underperfusion.

Finally, the use of radiocontrast agents deserves special consideration in the patient with CRF. A wealth of literature details the relation of radiocontrast materials to acute renal failure. The presence of chronic renal insufficiency may be the most consistently documented risk factor for the development of this problem. When acute renal failure develops in this setting, management is primarily supportive, and dialysis is occasionally indicated, at least temporarily. It is therefore vital to focus on preventive measures.

Perhaps the single most important strategy to reduce the risk of radiocontrast nephropathy in the CRF patient is to ensure adequate hydration. Adequate intravascular volumes and urine flow rates should be sought in all patients undergoing contrast procedures. A number of investigators have used mannitol to promote an osmotic diuresis, and some have demonstrated significant reductions in the incidence of acute renal failure. To date, mannitol administration has not been studied in a controlled, prospective randomized fashion, so the extent of its benefit remains unclear.[105,106] Similarly, other preventive measures have been evaluated, including the administration of loop diuretics to promote urine flow,[105] calcium channel blockers to mitigate cellular injury,[107,108] and low dose dopamine to maximize renal blood flow before or during radiocontrast administration.[109] Varying degrees of benefit have been shown in all of these reports. Until large prospective clinical trials are undertaken, however, it remains unclear which of these regimens, if any, can be uniformly recommended. Certainly, caution is warranted in hydrating patients with CRF who may also have underlying heart disease. Careful monitoring during hydration may be necessary to minimize the risk of pulmonary edema. In addition, mannitol may be dangerous in these patients if renal function and urine output are inadequate for its excretion, because under these circumstances, acute pulmonary edema can be precipitated. Finally, loop diuretics may magnify the risk of radiocontrast nephropathy if given to patients who are volume contracted.

There has been increasing interest in whether nonionic, low osmolality radiocontrast agents may be less toxic than the conventionally used ionic, high osmolality agents. Most recently, Steinberg and co-workers reported on over 200 patients receiving either low or high osmolality contrast agents during cardiac angiography and observed nephrotoxicity in 4% of each group.[110] In a simultaneously published report, Barrett and co-workers noted that of 64 patients receiving high osmolality contrast materials during cardiac catheterization, 6 (9.4%) experienced increases in serum creatinine of at least 25%, while 3 of 59 (5%) patients receiving the low osmolality agents experienced similar rises in creatinine values.[111] Because of the relatively small sample size, these differences did not reach statistical significance, and this group is engaged in a more detailed investigation of this issue for future publication. It is yet not clear that nonionic low osmolality radiocontrast agents are less likely to induce renal injury, and more study is clearly needed.

In our institution, we have recommended that patients with CRF receive carefully monitored parenteral hydration overnight before radiocontrast procedures to ensure euvolemia (if not slight hypervolemia) and adequate urine output at the time of contrast injection. Loop diuretics are used only in the hypervolemic patient, and we have not routinely recommended mannitol administration.

For cardiac angiography, a number of cardiologists in our institution have attempted to minimize radiocontrast toxicity by measuring left ventricular end-diastolic pressures at the outset of the procedure and administering volume expanding fluids before contrast injection if these pressures indicate hypovolemia. In addition, left ventriculography is performed much less commonly because noninvasive imaging techniques often provide this information fairly accurately. Biplane imaging—where images are made in two different planes with a single injection of contrast—help to minimize contrast dosage as well. At least anecdotally, these approaches seem to have substantially reduced the incidence of acute renal failure in patients at risk.

Support/Rehabilitative Phase

The management of acute renal failure is described in detail in Chapter 39 and is not appreciably altered by the preexistence of underlying chronic renal insufficiency. For any given cause of acute renal failure, the likelihood of recovery and renal function may be reduced in those with preexisting renal disease, but this has not been consistently studied. When such a difference can be shown to exist, the reduced rate of recovery of renal function may simply be a manifestation of the greater prevalence of multisystem disease in those with preexisting CRF. Clearly, the renal failure patient is uniquely predisposed to acute deterioration in renal function. It is therefore prudent to educate the patient in this regard, in an attempt to reduce the risks of exposure to nephrotoxic agents or events, and to increase the likelihood that precautions can be taken if such agents or events become unavoidable.

SUMMARY AND CONCLUSIONS

Chronic renal failure is a derangement that deleteriously affects many aspects of cellular physiology and organ function. These numerous adverse effects place the patient with CRF at particular risk for the development of serious illness. When such illness ensues, it often involves multiple organ systems and is often complex enough to necessitate care in a critical care unit. In this setting, a thorough understanding of the pathophysiology of renal disease and its impact on hematologic, cardiovascular, pulmonary, and gastrointestinal function, as well as its effects on the immune system, is vital to the care of the critically ill renal failure patient. In addition, the presence of renal failure makes a patient exquisitely vulnerable to various insults that can potentially further reduce renal function, thereby increasing the acuity of illness and the complexity of its treatment.

The anemia of CRF predisposes these patients to all of the consequences of suboptimal oxygen delivery at the tissue level. Accelerated atherogenesis, the prevalence of hypertension and dyslipidemias, and disturbances in cardiac function in the setting of uremia combine to jeopardize the cardiovascular well-being of the CRF patient. Disturbances in immune responsiveness underlie a clear increase in infection risk. Impairment in the integrity of the gastrointestinal mucosa combined with an increased tendency for blood loss result in gastrointestinal hemorrhagic events that are all too common in this patient population.

Renal failure places the patient at increased risk for developing critical illnesses, complicates the therapy necessitated by these illnesses, and increases their morbidity and mortality significantly. Efforts to preserve renal function when possible, and to use prophylactic measures to reduce the risks of developing such critical illnesses in patients with underlying renal disease are of paramount importance. When illness occurs, the appropriate management of the critically ill CRF patient depends on an awareness of the many ways in which renal failure impacts on the course of the patient's illness and its therapy.

REFERENCES

1. U.S. Renal Data System: USRDS 1993 Annual Data Report. Bethesda, MD, The National Institutes of Health, National Institute of Diabetes and Digestive and Kidney Diseases, 1993.
2. Vaamonde, C. A., and Perez, G. O.: Tubular function in diabetes mellitus. Semin. Nephrol., *10*:203, 1990.
3. Perez, G. O., Lespier, L. E., Oster, J. R., and Vaamonde, C. A.: Effect of alterations of sodium intake in patients with hyporeninemic hypoaldosteronism. Nephron, *18*:259, 1977.
4. Rastogi, S., Bayliss, J. M., Nascimento, L., and Arruda, J. A. L.: Hyperkalemic renal tubular acidosis: effect of furosemide in humans and in rats. Kidney Int., *28*:801, 1985.
5. Barbour, G. L., and Keller, A. W.: Distal renal tubular acidosis in selective hypoaldosteronism. South. Med. J., *71*:1397, 1978.
6. Robertson, W. B., and Strong, J. P.: Atherosclerosis in patients with hypertension in diabetes mellitus. Lab. Invest., *18*:538, 1968.
7. Ganda, O. P.: Pathogenesis of macrovascular disease in the human diabetic. Diabetes, *29*:931, 1980.
8. Dinerstein, C., Mason, R., and Giron, P.: Lower extremity complications of diabetes mellitus. Surg. Rounds, *7*:26, 1984.

9. Crall, F. V., and Roberts, W. C.: The extramural and intramural coronary arteries in juvenile diabetes mellitus. Analysis of nine necropsy patients aged 19 to 38 years with onset of diabetes before age 15 years. Am. J. Med., 64:221, 1978.
10. Weinrauch, L. et al.: Asymptomatic coronary artery disease: angiographic assessment of diabetics evaluated for renal transplantation. Circulation, 58:1184, 1978.
11. Krolwoski, A. S. et al.: Magnitude and determinants of coronary artery disease in juvenile-onset diabetes mellitus. Am. J. Cardiol., 59:750, 1987.
12. Eschbach, J. W.: The anemia of chronic renal failure: pathophysiology and the effects of recombinant erythropoietin. Kidney Int., 35:134, 1989.
13. Paganini, E. P.: Overview of anemia associated with chronic renal disease: primary and secondary mechanisms. Semin. Nephrol., 9(Suppl. 1):3, 1989.
14. Meytes, D. et al.: Effect of parathyroid hormone on erythropoiesis. J. Clin. Invest., 67:1263, 1981.
15. Delwiche, F. et al.: High levels of the circulating form of parathyroid hormone do not inhibit in vitro erythropoiesis. J. Lab. Clin. Med., 102:613, 1983.
16. Segal, G. M., Stueve, T., and Adamson, J. W.: Spermine and spermidine are non-specific inhibitors of in vitro hematopoiesis. Kidney Int., 31:72, 1987.
17. Freedman, M. H., Saunders, E. F., Kattran, D. C., and Rabin, E. Z.: Ribonuclease inhibition of erythropoiesis in anemia of uremia. Am. J. Kidney Dis., 11:530, 1983.
18. Yawata, Y., Howe, R., and Jacob, H. S.: Abnormal red cell metabolism causing hemolysis in uremia: a defect potentiated by tap water hemodialysis. Ann. Intern. Med., 79:362, 1973.
19. Rosenmund, A., Binswanger, U., and Straub, P. W.: Oxidative injury to erythrocytes, cell rigidity, and splenic hemolysis in hemodialyzed uremic patients. Ann. Intern. Med., 82:460, 1975.
20. Cole, C. H.: Decreased oubain-sensitive adenine triphosphatase activity in the erythrocyte membrane of patients with chronic renal disease. Clin. Sci., 45:775, 1973.
21. Capelli, J. P., Wesson, L. G., and Erslev, A. J.: Malignant hypertension and red cell fragmentation syndrome. Ann. Intern. Med., 64:128, 1966.
22. Rege, A. B., Brookins, J., and Fisher, J. W.: A radioimmunoassay for erythropoietin: serum levels in normal human subjects and in patients with hematopoietic disorders. J. Lab. Clin. Med., 100:829, 1982.
23. Besarab, A., Girone, J. F., Erslev, A., and Caro, J.: Recent developments in the anemia of chronic renal failure. Semin. Dial., 2:87, 1989.
24. Gaspari, F. et al.: Aspirin prolongs bleeding time in uremia by a mechanism distinct from platelet cyclooxygenase. J. Clin. Invest., 79:1788, 1987.
25. DiMinno, G. et al.: Platelet dysfunction in uremia: multifaceted defect partially corrected by dialysis. Am. J. Med., 79:552, 1985.
26. Eiser, A. R.: Gastrointestinal bleeding in maintenance dialysis in patients. Semin. Dial., 1:198, 1988.
27. Mitchell, C. J. et al.: Chronic function and histology in chronic renal failure. J. Clin. Pathol., 32:208, 1979.
28. Eschbach, J. W.: Hematologic problems of dialysis patients. In Replacement of Renal Function by Dialysis. Edited by W. Drukker, F. Parsons, and J. Maher. Boston, Martinus Nijhoff, 1983.
29. Lindner, A. et al.: Accelerated atherosclerosis in prolonged maintenance hemodialysis. N. Engl. J. Med., 290:697, 1974.
30. Zucchelli, P., Santoro, A., and Zuccala, A.: Genesis and control of hypertension in dialysis patients. Semin. Nephrol., 8:163, 1988.
31. Koomans, H. A. et al.: Sodium balance in renal failure. A comparison of patients with normal subjects under extremes of sodium intake. Hypertension, 7:714, 1985.
32. Perez Grovas, H., and Herrera-Acosta, J.: Mechanisms and treatment of malignant hypertension. Semin. Nephrol., 8:147, 1988.
33. Gehm, L., and Propp, D. A.: Pulmonary edema in the renal failure patient. Am. J. Emerg. Med., 7:336, 1989.
34. Ikram, H., Lynn, K. L., Bailey, R. R., and Little, P. J.: Cardiovascular changes in chronic hemodialysis patients. Kidney Int., 24:371, 1983.
35. Parfrey, P. S. et al.: Congestive heart failure in dialysis patients. Arch. Intern. Med., 148:1519, 1988.
36. London, G. M., Guerin, A. P., Marchais, S. J., and Metivier, F.: Cardiomyopathy in end-stage renal failure. Semin. Dial., 2:102, 1989.
37. Harnett, J. D. et al.: Left ventricular hypertrophy in end-stage renal disease. Nephron, 48:107, 1988.
38. Penpargkul, S., and Scheuer, J.: Effect of uremia upon the performance of the rat heart. Cardiovasc. Res., 6:702, 1972.
39. MacDonald, I. L., Uldall, R., and Buda, A. J.: The effect of hemodialysis on cardiac rhythm and performance. Clin. Nephrol., 15:321, 1981.
40. Dikshit, K. et al.: Renal and extrarenal hemodynamic effects of furosemide in congestive heart failure after acute myocardial infarction. N. Engl. J. Med., 288:1087, 1973.
41. Anderson, C. C., Shahvari, M. B. G., and Zimmeman, J. Z.: The treatment of pulmonary edema in the absence of renal function: a role for sorbitol and furosemide. JAMA, 241:1008, 1979.
42. Nicholls, A.: Atherosclerosis in chronic renal failure: A historical perspective. Scott. Med. J., 28:270, 1983.
43. Ritz, E., and Querfeld, U.: Atherogenesis—is it accelerated in uremia? Semin. Dial., 2:246, 1989.
44. Horsch, A. et al.: Atherogenesis in experimental uremia. Atherosclerosis, 40:279, 1981.
45. DeVault, G. A., Jr., and Brown, S. T., III: Creatine kinase isoenzymes in end-stage renal disease: problems in measurement and interpretation. Semin. Dial., 2:38, 1989.
46. Gelber, C. M. et al.: Thallium-201 myocardial imaging in patients on chronic hemodialysis. Nephron, 36:136, 1984.
47. Rostand, S. G., and Rutsky, Z. A.: Ischemic heart disease in chronic renal failure: Management considerations. Semin. Dial., 2:98, 1989.
48. Legendorf, R., and Pirani, L. C.: The heart in uremia: an electrocardiographic and pathologic study. Am. Heart J., 33:282, 1947.
49. Marini, P. V., and Hull, A. R.: Uremic pericarditis: a review of incidence and management. Kidney Int., 7(Suppl. 2):163, 1975.
50. Thompson, M. E., Rault, R. M., and Reddy, P. S.: Uremic pericarditis. Cardiovasc. Rev. Rep., 2:755, 1981.
51. Ventura, S. C., and Garella, S.: The management of pericardial disease and renal failure. Semin. Dial., 3:21, 1990.
52. Marini, P., and Hull, A. R.: Uremic pericarditis: a prospective echocardiographic and clinical study. Clin. Nephrol., 6:295, 1976.
53. Winney, R. J., Wright, M., Sumerling, M. D., and Lambie, A. T.: Echocardiography in uremic pericarditis with effusion. Nephron, 18:201, 1977.
54. Yoshida, K. et al.: Uremic pericardial effusion: detection and evaluation of uremic pericardial effusion by echocardiography. Clin. Nephrol., 13:260, 1980.
55. Frommer, J. P., Young, J. B., and Ayers, J. C.: Asymptomatic pericardial effusion in uremic patients: effect of long-term dialysis. Nephron, 39:296, 1985.

56. Rostand, S. G., and Rutsky, E. A.: Pericarditis in end-stage renal disease. Cardiol. Clin., 8:701, 1990.
57. Rutsky, E. A., and Rostand, S. G.: Pericarditis in end-stage renal disease: clinical characteristics and management. Semin. Dial., 2:25, 1989.
58. Fairshter, R. D., Vaziri, N. D., and Mirahmadi, M. K.: Lung pathology in chronic hemodialysis patients. Int. J. Artif. Organs, 5:97, 1982.
59. Bright, R.: Tabular view of the morbid appearance in 100 cases connected with albuminous urine, with observations. Guys Hosp. Rep., 1:380, 1983.
60. Dammin, G. J., Couch, N. P., and Murray, J. E.: Prolonged survival of skin homografts in uremic patients. Ann. NY Acad. Sci., 64:967, 1957.
61. Morrison, A. B., Maness, K., and Tawes, R.: Skin homograft survival in chronic renal insufficiency. Arch. Pathol., 75:139, 1962.
62. Coplon, N. S., Diskin, C. J., Peterson, J., and Sivenson, R. S.: The long-term clinical course of systemic lupus erythematosus in end-stage renal disease. N. Engl. J. Med., 308:186, 1983.
63. Matas, A. J. et al.: Increased incidence of malignancy during chronic renal failure. Lancet, 1:883, 1975.
64. Sutherland, G. A., Glass, J., and Gabriel, R.: Increased incidence of malignancy in chronic renal failure. Nephron, 18:182, 1977.
65. Degaauet, P., Reach, J., and Jacobs, C.: Cancer in patients on hemodialysis. N. Engl. J. Med., 300:1279, 1979.
66. Lindner, A., Farewell, Y. J., and Sherrard, D. J.: High incidence of neoplasia in uremic patients receiving long-term dialysis. Nephron, 27:292, 1981.
67. Pabico, R. C. et al.: Influence vaccination of patients with glomerular diseases. Ann. Intern. Med., 81:171, 1974.
68. Simberkoff, M. S. et al.: Pneumococcal capsular polysaccharide vaccination in adult chronic hemodialysis patients. J. Lab. Clin. Med., 96:363, 1980.
69. Linnemann, C. C., First, M. R., and Schiffman, G.: Response to pneumococcal vaccine in renal transplant and hemodialysis patients. Arch. Intern. Med., 141:1637, 1981.
70. Casciani, C. U., DeSimone, C., and Bonini, S.: Immunological aspects of chronic uremia. Kidney Int., 13(Suppl. 8):S49, 1978.
71. Selroos, O., Pasternack, A., and Virolainen, M.: Skin test sensitivity and antigen-induced lymphocyte transformation in uraemia. Clin. Exp. Immunol., 14:365, 1973.
72. Hoy, W. E., Cestero, R. V. M., and Freeman, R. B.: Deficiency of T and B lymphocytes in uremic subjects and partial improvement with maintenance hemodialysis. Nephron, 20:182, 1978.
73. Huber, H., Pastner, D., Dittrich, P. and Braunsteiner, H.: In vitro reactivity of human leukocytes in uraemia—a comparison with the impairment of delayed hypersensitivity. Clin. Exp. Immunol., 5:75, 1969.
74. Newberry, W. M., and Sanford, J. P.: Defective cellular immunity in renal failure: depression of reactivity of lymphocytes to phytohemagglutinin by renal failure serum. J. Clin. Invest., 50:1262, 1971.
75. Ringoir, S., VanLooy, L., Van de Heyning, P., and Lerous-Roels, G.: Impairment of phagocytic activity of macrophages as studied by the skin window test in patients on regular hemodialysis treatment. Clin. Nephrol., 4:234, 1975.
76. Hanicki, Z. et al.: Some aspects of cellular immunity in untreated and maintenance hemodialysis patients. Nephron, 23:273, 1979.
77. Ruiz, P., Gomez, F., and Schreiber, A. D.: Impaired function of macrophage Fc$_{gamma}$ receptors in end-stage renal disease. N. Engl. J. Med., 322:717, 1990.
78. Chandra, R. K.: Rosette-forming T lymphocytes and cell-mediated immunity in malnutrition. Br. Med. J., 3:608, 1974.
79. Schopfer, K., and Douglas, S. D.: Neutrophil function in children with kwashiorkor. J. Lab. Clin. Med., 88:450, 1976.
80. Hopps, H. C., and Wissler, R. W.: Uremic pneumonitis. Am. J. Pathol., 31:261, 1955.
81. Rackow, E. L., Fein, I. A., Sprung, C., and Grodman, R. S.: Uremic pulmonary edema. Am. J. Med., 64:1084, 1978.
82. Goldstein, E., and Green, G. M.: The effect of acute renal failure on the bacterial clearance mechanisms of the lung. J. Lab. Clin. Med., 68:531, 1966.
83. Yu, V. L. et al.: *Staphylococcus aureus* nasal carriage and infection in patients on hemodialysis. N. Engl. J. Med., 315:91, 1986.
84. Keane, W. F., Shapiro, F. L., and Raij, L.: Incidence and type of infections occurring in 445 chronic hemodialysis patients. J. Trans. Am. Soc. Artif. Intern. Organs, 23:41, 1977.
85. Andrew, O. T., Schoenfeld, P. Y., Hopewell, P. C., and Humphreys, M. H.: Tuberculosis in patients with end-stage renal disease. Am. J. Med., 68:59, 1980.
86. Belcon, M. C., Smith, E. K. M., Kahana, L. M., and Schimizu, A. G.: Tuberculosis in dialysis patients. Clin. Nephrol., 17:14, 1982.
87. Gilbert, D. N., and Bennett, W. M.: Use of antimicrobial agents in renal failure. Infect. Dis. Clin. North Am., 3(3):517, 1989.
88. Bernstein, J. M., and Erk, S. D.: Choice of antibiotics, pharmacokinetics, and dose adjustments in acute and chronic renal failure. Med. Clin. North Am., 74:1059, 1990.
89. Briggs, W. A.: Response of hemodialysis patients to bivalent influenza vaccination. Dial. Trans., 7:1011, 1978.
90. Ortbals, D. W., Marks, E. S., and Liebhaber, H.: Influenza immunization in patients with chronic renal disease. JAMA, 239:2562, 1978.
91. Saitoh, H., Nakamura, K., Hida, M., and Satoh, T.: Urinary tract infection in oliguric patients with chronic renal failure. J. Urol., 133:990, 1985.
92. Dobkin, J. F., Miller, M. H., and Steigbigel, N. H.: Septicemia in patients on chronic hemodialysis. Ann. Intern. Med., 88:28, 1978.
93. Krempien, B. et al.: Gastropathy in uremia. *In* Uremia. Stuttgart, Germany, George Thieme Verlag, 1972.
94. Clouse, R. E., Costigan, D. J., Mills, B. A., and Zuckerman, G. R.: Angiodysplasia as a cause of upper gastrointestinal bleeding. Arch. Intern. Med., 145:458, 1985.
95. Ala-Kaila, K., and Pasternack, A.: Gastrointestinal complications in chronic renal failure. Dig. Dis., 7:230, 1989.
96. Rosenblatt, S. G. et al.: Gastrointestinal blood loss in patients with chronic renal failure. Am. J. Kidney Dis., 1:232, 1982.
97. Boyle, J. M., and Johnston, B.: Acute upper gastrointestinal hemorrhage in patients with chronic renal disease. Am. J. Med., 75:409, 1983.
98. Hou, S. H. et al.: Hospital-acquired renal insufficiency: a prospective study. Am. J. Med., 74:243, 1983.
99. Kraman, S., Khan, F., Patel, S., and Seriff, N.: Renal failure in the respiratory intensive care unit. Crit. Care Med., 7:263, 1979.
100. Menashe, P. I., Ross, S. A., and Gottlieb, J. E.: Acquired renal insufficiency in critically ill patients. Crit. Care Med., 16:1106, 1988.
101. Appel, G. B., and Neu, H. C.: The nephrotoxicity of antimicrobial agents. N. Engl. J. Med., 296:663, 1977.
102. Bennett, W. M., Luft, F., and Porter, G. A.: Pathogenesis of

renal failure due to aminoglycosides and contrast media used in roentgenography. Am. J. Med., *69:*767, 1980.
103. Madias, N. E., and Harrington, J. T.: Platinum nephrotoxicity. Am. J. Med., *65:*307, 1978.
104. Clive, D. M., and Stoff, J. S.: Renal syndromes associated with nonsteroidal anti-inflammatory drugs. N. Engl. J. Med., *310:*563, 1984.
105. Brezis, M., Rosen, S., and Epstein, F. H.: Acute renal failure. In The Kidney. Edited by B. Brenner and F. C. Rector, Jr. Philadelphia, W. B. Saunders, 1986.
106. Anto, H. R., Chou, S. Y., Porush, J. G., and Shapiro, W. B.: Infusion intravenous pyelography and renal function. Effect of hypertonic mannitol in patients with chronic renal insufficiency. Arch. Intern. Med., *141:*1652, 1981.
107. Bakris, G. L., and Burnett, J. C., Jr.: Role for calcium in radiocontrast-induced reduction in renal hemodynamics. Kidney Int., *27:*465, 1985.
108. Pourrat, J. P., and Douste-Blazy, P.: Renal side effect of nifedipine. Clin. Cardiol., *7:*29, 1984.
109. Davis, R. F. et al.: Acute oliguria after cardiopulmonary bypass: renal improvement with low dose dopamine infusion. Crit. Care Med., *10:*852, 1982.
110. Steinberg, E. P. et al.: Safety and cost effectiveness of high-osmolality as compared with low osmolality contrast material in patients undergoing cardiac angiography. N. Engl. J. Med., *326(7):*425, 1992.
111. Barrett, B. J. et al.: A comparison of nonionic, low-osmolality radiocontrast agents with ionic, high-osmolality agents during cardiac catheterization. N. Engl. J. Med., *326:*431, 1992.

Chapter 41

RENAL TRANSPLANTATION, REVASCULARIZATION, AND THE HYPERTENSIVE ADRENAL PATIENT

CHARLES LEE JACKSON
ANDREW C. NOVICK

Patients who undergo renal transplantation, renal arterial reconstruction, or adrenalectomy for hypertensive adrenal tumors often require support and monitoring in a critical care unit. These patients share similar risks from the consequences of derangements in blood pressure, fluid and electrolyte balance, and renal function. Co-morbid conditions such as cardiovascular and cerebrovascular disease produce decreased physiologic reserve. Furthermore, the renal transplant patient can suffer complications as a consequence of immunosuppression, including the risk of life-threatening infection and graft rejection.

RENAL TRANSPLANTATION

Patient and graft survival following renal transplantation are now excellent. This success is due to advances in the understanding and management of post-transplant complications, improved techniques for organ harvest, and preservation and improved immunosuppressive programs. The critical care team has the opportunity to make important contributions in each of these areas. The postoperative transplant patient is frequently monitored in the ICU, and may be returned for further management in the event of surgical or immunosuppressive complications. The critical care team may also be asked to identify and manage potential organ donors or to identify patients with end-stage renal disease as possible recipient candidates for transplantation.

Pre-ICU Phase

Recipient Candidate Identification

The goal of recipient selection is to identify individuals likely to benefit from renal transplantation and who can tolerate immunosuppression with its attendant risks[1] (Table 41-1).

The primary advantage to the patient with a successful renal transplant is the ability to return to preillness activity. Therefore, the initial consideration when presented with an end-stage renal disease patient is the potential for overall recovery and rehabilitation. This situation is frequently a difficult issue to weigh and should be considered in broad, general terms with as much assistance from the family and patient as possible. The patient who is under consideration for renal transplantation should also be able to tolerate anesthesia for a major surgical procedure and should be free of malignant disease. Immunosuppressive agents impair the ability to control neoplastic processes. As a result, the patient with a malignant disease other than a simple basal cell skin cancer is advised to postpone renal transplantation for 1 year following treatment without any evidence of recurrence.[2,3]

The recipient candidate should also be free of active infections such as osteomyelitis, sinusitis, and tooth abscess. These infections should be completely resolved with appropriate antibiotics and surgical drainage to prevent recurrence. Patients with active tuberculosis should be treated for 2 years before proceeding with renal transplantation. Additionally, those patients with a remote history of tuberculosis may proceed with renal transplantation, but must be observed vigilantly for evidence of reactivation and then treated as necessary. The remainder of the evaluation of the recipient candidate is directed at the identification of medical problems that may have a negative impact on prognosis. Risk factors include:

- Patient's age
- Diabetes mellitus
- Coronary artery disease
- Diffuse atherosclerosis
- Gastrointestinal disease
- Urinary tract abnormalities

Perhaps the most important of these factors is the patient's age, because an older patient frequently has other risk factors. Nevertheless, renal transplantation in patients between 45 and 65 years of age has become commonplace over the past decade with the introduction of improved immunosuppressive protocols that reduce infectious complications.[4,5]

Other than infection, the most common cause of death in renal transplant patients is coronary artery disease. In view of this situation, patients over age 40 and diabetics are evaluated carefully for evidence of coronary artery disease.[6,7] Coronary arteriography is recommended in these patients to uncover silent occlusive disease, which is then treated with angioplasty or bypass surgery prior to renal transplantation.

The older patient is also evaluated with colonoscopy for diverticular disease. Patients with known diverticular disease should be vigilantly observed for possible post-

Table 41-1. Potential Recipient Criteria for Renal Transplantation

Surgical candidate
Age <65
Absence of malignant disease
Absence of infection
Potential for rehabilitation

transplant bowel perforation and may receive a modified immunosuppressive program to reduce the risk of bowel-related complications. Patients with active or recently treated peptic ulcer disease should also be evaluated endoscopically and considered for selective vagotomy to reduce the risk of steroid-induced gastric hemorrhage.[8] Most patients, however, can be managed conservatively with the prophylactic use of H_2 receptor blockade.

The urinary tract is evaluated to determine its suitability to receive a graft. Abnormalities such as obstruction, stone, infection, and reflux are identified by renal ultrasound, voiding cystourethrography, and urine culture. Anatomic and functional abnormalities are corrected before renal transplantation, to avoid risk to the graft.

Donor Candidate Identification

In addition to the identification and preparation of potential recipient candidates, the critical care team is often asked to identify and manage potential organ donors. The most common donor candidate is a healthy, young individual who has sustained an isolated head injury resulting in brain death. The usual criteria for potential cadaver renal donors are age of 18 months to 60 years, absence of malignant disease other than a primary brain tumor or treated skin cancer, and the absence of diabetes, renal disease, hypertension, or other systemic disease with potential renal involvement. The donor candidate should be free of viral or bacterial infection, including negative assays for hepatitis and human immunodeficiency virus (HIV). The trauma patient with multiple vascular and urinary catheters is at high risk for hospital-acquired infections and must be carefully screened with blood and urine cultures. Renal function should be normal with a creatinine less than 0.3 mg/dl unless it was known to be normal prior to injury and is resolving with hydration and diuretics[9] (Table 41-2).

Table 41-2. Donor Candidate Identification for Renal Transplantation

Brain death
Age 18 months–55 years
No malignant disease
No infection
Blood, urine, and sputum cultures
Serum HIV and hepatitis B antigen
No diabetes
No diffuse atherosclerosis
No renal disease
Creatinine <3.0 mg
Urine output >0.5 μ/kg/h
Systolic BP >90 mm Hg
Dopamine <50 μg/kg/min

Once the donor candidate is identified, the goal of donor management is preservation of organ function by maintaining adequate perfusion. The systolic blood pressure should be maintained at approximately 90 mm Hg, coupled with a urinary output of greater than 0.5 ml/kg per hour. If vasopressors are required to maintain adequate blood pressure, a dopamine infusion of less than 50 μg/kg per minute is preferred. Infusions rates of greater than 50 μg/kg per minute will produce an alpha-adrenergic renal arterial vasoconstriction with resulting renal cortical ischemia. Furosemide and mannitol are also infused to initiate and maintain a diuresis.

In most instances, the Organ Procurement Agency (OPA) coordinator participates in donor candidate management. In general, the coordinator is also best equipped to approach family members about organ donation. Federal law requires that an organ donation request be made to family members of all potential donors. Studies have indicated that the success of procurement is directly related to the skill of the person making the request. Critical care teams should have an individual or group of individuals assigned to this delicate task. They should work closely with the OPA coordinator and be prepared to help the families with this difficult decision.

ICU Phase

Circumstances requiring transplant recipient admission to the ICU include routine postoperative management and life-threatening complications from immunosuppression. Because the most common is routine postoperative management, it is important for the critical care practitioner to understand the basics of the renal transplant operation.

Intraoperative Considerations

The renal allograft is typically implanted in the iliac fossa by anastomosing the renal vein end to side to the external iliac vein. The renal artery anastomosed end to end to the recipient hypogastric artery or end to side to the external iliac artery. Before the vascular clamps are released to restore renal blood flow, the recipient is given sufficient fluids to maintain a normal central venous pressure and is given diuretics such as mannitol or furosemide (Lasix).

Adequate hydration is important to ensure good renal perfusion, and mannitol stimulates diuresis and prevents renal tubular cell edema.[10] Living related donor grafts and cadaveric grafts with short extracorporeal preservation times begin diuresis on the operating table before the urinary tract is reconstructed.

Urinary tract reconstruction is typically done with an extravesical ureteroneocystostomy.[11] In situations where this is not possible, the ureter is anastomosed to a prefashioned intestinal urinary conduit.[12]

Postoperative Monitoring

In most instances, routine critical care postoperative monitoring of the renal transplant patient is limited to 24 to 48 hours. The patient is usually extubated in the operating room at the conclusion of the procedure. All patients have a central venous line, a urethral catheter, and an arterial line. Early postoperative considerations relate to the measurement, replacement, and balance of fluids and electrolytes.

Patients with early graft function typically experience a vigorous diuresis for the first 24 to 36 postoperative hours. Urine output is measured hourly and is replaced milliliter for milliliter up to 500 ml per hour. Urine outputs in excess of 500 ml per hour are replaced with 2 to 3 ml of intravenous fluids for every milliliter of output. The central venous pressure is carefully monitored, and small boluses of colloid may be given as required to keep the central venous pressure at normal levels (5 to 8 mm Hg). It is important to avoid dehydration from the diuresis, which can impair renal perfusion and promote renal ischemic injury.

Frequent monitoring of serum electrolyte levels is also required in the presence of a brisk postoperative diuresis. Specifically, sodium, potassium, glucose, and calcium levels are measured every 4 to 6 hours and adjusted as required. Postoperative hyperglycemia may be a problem in the diabetic patient because of surgical stresses, perioperative steroids, and high volume fluid replacement with dextrose-containing fluids. If this occurs, nondextrose normal saline should be infused and an insulin drip initiated to keep glucose levels below 250 mg. Failure to control hyperglycemia adequately coupled with hyponatremic intravenous fluid replacement can produce severe hyponatremia with life-threatening consequences.

Diuresis typically begins to resolve within 24 to 36 hours postoperatively. As this occurs, replacement fluids are decreased to maintenance levels. The patient is often able to eat by this time and gradually becomes able to replace fluid losses by mouth.

Fluid and electrolyte management is more difficult for patients with delayed graft function. Ischemic renal failure may delay graft function for up to several days and is related in part to the duration of cold storage preservation before to transplantation. During this recovery phase, the patient is oliguric, and early post-transplantation dialysis may be necessary to control associated hyperkalemia. Initial management of post-transplant hyperkalemia also includes intravenous infusion of glucose, insulin, and bicarbonate. Kayexalate enemas should be avoided because of the threat of colonic necrosis precipitated by the exchange resin.[13,14] Volume status in the patient with delayed graft function is monitored closely to ensure adequate renal blood flow and to avoid additional ischemic injury to the recovering graft. Protecting the graft as it recovers from ischemic renal failure is one of the primary goals of postoperative renal transplant management.

A variety of complications that may be difficult to identify in the anuric patient can threaten the post-transplant graft. The graft and patient must therefore be constantly surveyed for indirect evidence of silent complications. Constant measurement of patient weight, blood pressure, and central venous pressure are required to estimate fluid balance in this setting. In the anuric patient with left ventricular compromise, pulmonary arterial catheterization is necessary to monitor appropriate fluid replacement accurately.

When dialysis is required in the early post-transplant period, the dialysis team should avoid aggressive fluid removal, which can cause additional ischemic injury to the graft. Antihypertensive medications should be withheld before dialysis to avoid the potential for hypotension during dialysis, and heparinization should also be minimized. Communication among the dialysis, transplant, and critical care teams will help to avoid such problems.

Table 41–3. Postoperative Complications of Renal Transplantation

Wound infection
Urinary obstruction
Urinary leak
Lymphocele
Hemorrhage
Vascular thrombosis
Graft rupture

Post-Transplantation Complications

Post-transplantation problems may be divided into those related to surgery and those related to rejection and immunosuppression. Surgical complications may be further subdivided and are briefly listed in the following discussion (Table 41–3). The many problems associated with rejection and immunosuppression are introduced along with a general discussion about goals of therapy.

Surgical Complications. Such complications include urologic disorders, lymphocele, and vascular disorders.

Urologic Complications. These complications include urinary obstruction, urinary leakage, and infection. Early urologic complications occurring within the first several hours after transplantation include anuria secondary to blood clot occluding the urinary catheter or, rarely, a kinked or twisted ureter. A catheter-induced urinary tract infection may present within the first 48 to 72 hours after renal transplantation and a urinary leak within 7 to 10 days after transplantation. Late complications are typically limited to ureteral stenosis from fibrosis and may occur months to years after transplantation. They present as:

- Increased serum creatinine level
- Fever
- Anuria

The initial approach to the anuric or oliguria patient who has undergone renal transplantation is gentle irrigation of the bladder to rule out catheter obstruction. It is not uncommon for mild bleeding to occur from the fresh ureterovesical anastomosis, which may produce small clots in the ureter or bladder. These can easily be evacuated with restoration of urinary flow. Ureteral obstruction of a more serious nature may result from inadvertent kinking or twisting of the ureter, or compression by the spermatic cord. Urine output, if present, is an unreliable measure of obstruction because the native kidneys may produce urine independent of the graft.

A urinary leak may also compromise the postoperative course presenting as decreased graft function associated with fever, graft tenderness, wound drainage, and ipsilateral thigh or genital swelling. Urinary leak is most commonly caused by compromised arterial blood supply to the transplant ureter producing ureteral infarction.

Urinary tract infections are usually catheter induced and may be prevented by prophylactic suppressive antibiotics and early catheter removal. These infections are important because of the immunosuppressed status of the patient and because infections may actually induce rejection episodes. Routine surveillance cultures are done to ensure early detection and treatment.

The investigation of urologic complications should begin with an ultrasound study, which enables one to detect dilatation of the renal pelvis secondary to obstruction or a perinephric fluid collection typical of a urinary leak. The fluid may be aspirated percutaneously and sent for electrolyte and creatinine analysis to distinguish between lymph collection and urine. Whether a leak or obstruction is discovered, the initial therapeutic step is generally percutaneous nephrostomy. This procedure provides urinary diversion and drainage to allow maximal recovery of renal function and optimization of the patient's condition.[15] Definitive operative repair using the native ureter is then performed electively.

Lymphocele. The most common perinephric fluid collection is a lymphocele. Lymphocele occurs in approximately 2% of renal transplant recipients and is rarely a significant problem. It is typically produced from leaking lymphatic channels along the recipient vessels or, less commonly, from the donor renal hilum.[16] Occasionally, one may accumulate over several weeks, to achieve sufficient size to compromise graft function by obstructing the ureter. Treatment is open operative or a laparoscopic creation of a peritoneal window to allow intraperitoneal drainage of the collected lymph fluid.

Vascular Complications. Early postoperative vascular complications occur uncommonly but with great drama and serious consequences. They include:

- Anastomotic disruption with hemorrhage
- Arterial or venous thrombosis
- Graft rupture

The causes are technical error, infection, and hyperacute rejection. The presentation typically includes pain, decreased blood pressure, absent graft function, and decreased hemoglobin and hematocrit. Investigation begins with a nuclear renal scan, arteriography, and/or venography. Because these conditions are life-threatening, the goal of treatment is to preserve the patient's life at the expense of the graft, if necessary. Although the graft may occasionally be salvaged in these situations, immediate nephrectomy is usually indicated.

Late vascular complications include arterial stenosis from technical problems at the anastomosis or intimal proliferation secondary to rejection. These patients are often difficult management problems because of the combination of severe hypertension and deteriorating renal function. As a result, they may require critical care management. The lesion is identified with intra-arterial digital subtraction angiography and an attempt at transluminal angioplasty may be made at that time. Many patients, however, require renal arterial bypass with a saphenous vein graft with considerable risk of graft loss.[17]

Rejection. The immune response to the transplanted graft produces three basic patterns of rejection: hyperacute, acute, and chronic. Hyperacute rejection occurs immediately after transplantation and is the result of circulating recipient antibodies to the new graft. It rapidly destroys the graft, causes intravascular thrombosis, and threatens graft rupture. It presents with pain, hypotension, and anuria. It is untreatable and requires emergency nephrectomy. This complication is rare today because of careful pretransplant cross-matching identifying sensitized patients. Chronic rejection, on the other hand, occurs commonly over the life of the allograft and is responsible for most long-term graft loss. It is insidious, silent, and rarely produces a condition requiring critical care.

The dominant concern in post-transplant clinical care is the prevention, identification, and treatment of acute cellular rejection. Acute rejection occurs most commonly in the first 3 months after renal transplant, less commonly in the next 6 months, and uncommonly 1 year after renal transplantation. It is characterized by a decrease in renal blood flow and deterioration in renal function. It presents with:

- Fever
- Graft tenderness
- Increased serum creatinine
- Decreased urine output

The differential diagnosis for acute cellular rejection includes ischemic acute tubular necroses, prerenal azotemia, drug-induced nephrotoxicity, ureteral obstruction, urinary leak, urinary tract infection, and arterial or venous thrombosis (Table 41-4).

The identification of acute rejection and its distinction from other elements of the differential diagnosis is fundamental to the day-to-day clinical practice of renal transplantation. An organized approach to the differential diagnosis begins with an appreciation of the subtle changes in physical examination described earlier and alterations in laboratory values (Table 41-5). Cyclosporine levels are checked to ensure therapeutic, though nontoxic cyclosporine levels. A urinalysis culture and sensitivity is performed to evaluate for urinary tract infection. A simple urinary tract infection cannot only mimic rejection, but may also initiate rejection episodes and is, therefore, important to identify and treat early in its development. Renal ultrasound demonstrates hydronephrosis of the graft as well as perirenal fluid collection secondary to a urinary leak, lymphocele,

Table 41-4. Rejection Differential Diagnosis in Renal Transplantation

Cyclosporine nephrotoxicity
Antibiotic induced nephrotoxicity
Hypovolemia
Urinary tract infection
Urinary obstruction
Urine leak
Acute tubular necrosis
Cytomegalovirus infection

Table 41–5. Evaluation of Rejection in Renal Transplantation

Repeat serum creatinine
Cyclosporine trough level
Urine culture
Renal graft ultrasound
^{123}I renal scan
Fine needle aspiration biopsy
Ultrasound guided needle biopsy

hematoma, or abscess. A renal technetium scan provides evidence of renal blood flow and an estimate of renal clearance to assist in distinguishing acute tubular nephrosis from rejection.

The most accurate method of rejection diagnosis is a percutaneous renal biopsy. Typically done with ultrasound guidance, it is especially helpful in detecting the presence of acute rejection concomitant with ischemic acute tubular necrosis (ATN). The typical signs and symptoms of rejection are absent in the presence of ischemic ATN and rejection may, therefore, silently coexist with ATN. A biopsy provides critically helpful information in this setting by identifying otherwise silent graft rejection. A biopsy is also helpful in cases of persistent poor graft function following a course of antirejection therapy. Antirejection therapy is accompanied by significant potential morbidity, and its repeated application without histologic evidence of likely benefit is unwise. Therefore, patients with apparent steroid-resistant rejection should undergo biopsy before one proceeds with additional treatment, to document potential gain, to redirect treatment programs to alternative immunosuppressive agents, or to abandon the graft in favor of the patient's survival.

Immunosuppression. The goal of immunosuppressive therapy is to modify the immune response to allow the patient to tolerate the graft. This process is done with a maintenance program of immunosuppressive drugs supplemented by aggressive antirejection therapy to arrest acute rejection episodes. The increased risk of life-threatening opportunistic infections and other complications limit the amount and frequency of antirejection treatments.

Maintenance immunosuppressive and antirejection treatment protocols vary from center to center and are further modified by graft function. Most include some combination of prednisone, azathioprine, polyclonal antilymphocyte globulin (ALG) Cyclosporine, and OKT3. A common maintenance program for a living related graft or a cadaveric graft with immediate function might include prednisone and cyclosporine with or without azathioprine. Acute rejection episodes are treated with pulses of high dose methylprednisolone. Steroid-resistant rejection episodes histologically documented by a graft biopsy are treated with monoclonal antibody OKT3 or ALG.

The nonfunctioning cadaveric graft is maintained on prednisone, azathioprine, and a polyclonal ALG preparation until the initial ischemic injury begins to resolve. Cyclosporine may then be substituted for the ALG. This delayed sequential cyclosporine therapy avoids additional renal injury by allowing recovery of renal function before the application of a potentially nephrotoxic agent. Antirejection episodes are treated initially with high dose corticosteroids and followed, if necessary, by OKT3.

Each immunosuppressive agent has characteristic immunomodulating effects accompanying a broad spectrum of potential adverse side effects. The various agents are combined simultaneously and sequentially to take advantage of the different immunosuppressive effects while attempting to minimize cumulative morbidity.

Steroids. Corticosteroids have been the cornerstone of immunosuppressive therapy since the beginning of transplantation. Steroids are used for maintenance treatment to prevent rejection episodes and in high doses as specific treatment for acute cellular rejection episodes. Steroids inhibit the release of interleukin-2 (IL-2), a lymphokine produced by helper T cells and required for lymphocyte proliferation. By inhibiting IL-2 production, steroids limit the cellular immune response. However, this nonspecific inhibition of the immune system can lead to the development of opportunistic infection and other complications. The older patient and the diabetic patient are particularly vulnerable to steroid-related complications such as infection, hyperglycemia, peptic ulcer disease, avascular necrosis, and cataracts.

Azathioprine. Azathioprine is a derivative of 6-mercaptopurine and, like corticosteroid, has been a key agent in antirejection programs since 1962. This antimetabolite interferes with nucleotide synthesis and inhibits cell division and proliferation. By inhibiting lymphocyte proliferation, it is effective in preventing acute cellular rejection. It is, therefore, included in maintenance immunosuppressive protocols, but is not used to treat acute cellular rejection episodes. Primary side effects are myelosuppression and hepatic dysfunction.

Antilymphocyte Globulin (ALG). Polyclonal ALG preparations have been used both for maintenance therapy and as specific treatment for acute rejection episodes. These substances are prepared by immunizing an animal with human lymphocytes to produce a polyclonal antisera directed against T lymphocytes. Infusion of this antisera into the transplant recipient results in antibody binding to the circulating T cells and their subsequent destruction by phagocytes. These preparations, however, contain antibodies to a wide variety of other cells and proteins that can produce inflammatory side effects such as fever, chills, phlebitis, rash, and bronchospasm. Currently, ALG is used primarily to prevent rejection in the cadaveric graft with delayed graft function. During the period of recovery from ischemic renal failure, ALG will effectively prevent rejection without nephrotoxic side effects until sufficient renal function has recovered to allow substitution with cyclosporine.[19-22]

Cyclosporine. Cyclosporine, the natural product of a fungus, has revolutionized modern organ transplantation.[13-25] In contrast to the broad immunosuppressive action of the previously described agents, cyclosporine selectively inhibits the immune response. Cyclosporine significantly reduces IL-2 synthesis and thus inhibits the activation cascade required for lymphokine production. This selective immunosuppression sufficiently reduces the incidence of rejection to allow an overall reduction in corticosteroid dose. The result is improved graft survival with a reduced incidence of steroid-related complications.

The side effects of cyclosporine have had as much impact on clinical patient management as its enhanced immunosuppressive efficacy. Most important among these side effects is Cyclosporine's nephrotoxicity.[26,27] If given immediately after renal transplantation to a cadaveric graft recovering from ischemic renal failure, cyclosporine impairs, rather than improves, renal function. This has led to the aforementioned sequential use of ALG and cyclosporine.[28] Cyclosporine also eliminates many of the symptoms previously characteristic of rejection, such as fever and graft tenderness. The first sign of rejection, therefore, is an increase in the serum creatinine level. Nephrotoxic reactions to cyclosporine are also heralded by a rise in creatinine, however, and the distinction between nephrotoxic-induced renal impairment and rejection may be difficult. In view of this, cyclosporine trough levels are followed daily to reduce the risk of nephrotoxicity while ensuring an adequate immunosuppressive effect. Rejection and nephrotoxicity may both occur, however, in spite of appropriate trough levels, and ultrasound guided needle biopsy of the graft may be required to establish a histologic diagnosis and guide treatment. Other potential side effects of cyclosporine include hyperkalemia, hirsutism, gingival hypertrophy, and malignant disease. Their impact can be reduced by dose reduction and surveillance.

Monoclonal Antibodies. Unlike the polyclonal preparation ALG, which contains antibodies to many antigen cells and cell surfaces, the monoclonal antibody preparation OKT3 contains a single antibody directed against a single antigen. The OKT3 antibody is directed against the CD3 antigen located on mature peripheral T-lymphocyte surfaces. Infusion of this antibody results in a rapid depletion of circulating T cells with subsequent reversal of acute rejection episodes. It may also be used prophylactically to prevent rejection episodes.[27-33] The side effects are fever and shaking chills, which occur with the initial dose. The older patient and the diabetic patient must be observed carefully for cardiac complications because of the increased cardiac demand caused by this first-dose effect. Patients should also be within 3% of their dry weight prior to OKT3 administration to avoid pulmonary edema produced by OKT3-induced capillary leak. Subsequent doses, however, are well tolerated and may be given via a peripheral vein in an outpatient setting.

Complications of Immunosuppressive Therapy. The sequential and combined applications of these immunosuppressive agents have improved patient and graft survival by reducing rejection episodes and infectious complications. Critical care management is often required, however, for complications of rejection and immunosuppression. Multiple rejection episodes treated with repeated courses of immunosuppressive agents produce a cumulative toxic effect with increased risk for opportunistic infections and life-threatening complications. For example, patients receiving multiple high dose steroid treatments for recurrent rejection may develop bleeding peptic ulcerations requiring immediate surgical repair and postoperative critical care support. Opportunistic bacterial fungal and viral infections may compromise vital organ systems and may require transfer to the ICU for ventilator support and cardiopulmonary monitoring until the infection is resolved. These patients have pulmonary failure, profound hypotension, mottled extremities, acidosis, and renal failure. The causes of renal failure are multiple and include hypoperfusion, toxins, sepsis, and persistent rejection resistant to immunosuppressive agents. The result may be a septic patient with one or more organ systems at risk and further complicated by ongoing graft rejection and renal failure requiring dialysis.

The approach to these complex patients centers around the goal of salvaging the patient's life primarily and the transplanted renal graft secondarily. Immunosuppressive agents are either discontinued or sharply restricted to allow recovery of the host immune system. Maintenance steroids, however, must be continued in low doses to avoid adrenal insufficiency. Appropriate antibiotics, fluids, monitoring, and organ system support are provided as for any septic patient with multiple organ failure. If necessary, the graft is removed and the patient is returned to dialysis. Subsequent retransplantation is an option when full recovery has been achieved.

Post-ICU Phase

Despite the dramatic fluid and electrolyte shifts of the first 25 to 48 hours after renal transplantation, with the potential for graft rejection and immunosuppression complications, most renal transplant patients do remarkably well. Following transfer to the transplant unit of the hospital, patients begin ambulating and often resume a normal diet within 48 hours postoperatively. During the 1 to 3 weeks of recovery, they are taught about their medications and how to monitor and record their weight, urine output, blood pressure, and diet in a journal. At our center, this period of instruction and recovery is conducted in a transitional care unit once the initial hospital recovery period is completed. The transitional care unit is a floor of the hotel at the center, staffed by transplant nursing personnel. It allows early hospital discharge and family participation in the recovery period. The patient makes a daily trip to the laboratory for blood work and regular trips to the outpatient clinic for follow-up. Following release from the transitional care unit, arrangements are made at a laboratory near the patient's home for routine blood work, including a complete blood count, electrolytes, creatinine, liver function studies, and cyclosporine levels to be mailed to the transplant coordinator's office for review. In this way, the patient is returned to the community to resume preillness activity, work, and family life as rapidly as possible. The patient, nevertheless, remains under continuous surveillance for sequelae of long-term immunosuppression.

The long-term problems of transplantation include:

- Infection
- Malignant disease
- Cardiovascular disease
- Cataracts
- Avascular necrosis[34]

The most significant of these are malignant and cardiovascular disease. Malignant disease has been found in approximately 50% of long-term transplant survivors, with lymphoma and carcinoma of the skin, lips, and uterine cervix among the other most common problems. Regular gynecologic examinations and limited sun exposure are therefore recommended.

Routine screening and dietary restraint are also recommended in light of the significant risk of cardiovascular morbidity and mortality. Long-term immunosuppression promotes many of the risk factors for cardiovascular disease, including atherosclerosis, hypertension, and hyperlipidemia. These long-term sequelae emphasize the need for further improvement in immunosuppressive programs.

Overall, a patient considering renal transplantation may expect 1-year patient and graft survival rates of 95% and 80 to 90%, respectively. The recipient may subsequently anticipate a half-life of 22, 12, and 8 years for a renal graft received from a HLA identical sibling, haploidentical parent, and cadaveric donor, respectively.[35] In the event of graft loss from acute rejection, chronic rejection or recurrent disease, the patient may return to dialysis and begin preparation for retransplantation with an almost equivalent chance of success.

RENOVASCULAR DISEASE

Admission to the ICU is routinely required in the postoperative period following renal arterial reconstruction. The goals of renal revascularization are resolution of renovascular hypertension and preservation of renal function. Renal artery stenosis is most commonly caused by atherosclerosis or one of the fibrous dysplasias. The latter disorders account for approximately 40% of cases and typically occur in younger patients without concurrent disease. Fibromuscular renal artery lesions are often amenable to angioplasty. The remaining 60% of renal artery lesions are caused by atherosclerosis and are rarely amenable to angioplasty. These patients frequently have associated coronary and cerebrovascular disease and require perioperative critical care.

Pre-ICU Phase

Atherosclerotic renal arterial occlusive disease occurs most commonly in men in their fifth through seven decades of life. It is typically a manifestation of diffuse atherosclerosis obliterans accompanied by coronary, cerebral, and peripheral vascular disease. Atherosclerosis isolated to the renal arteries is found in only 15 to 20% of cases. It is a well-known cause of renin-dependent hypertension and is increasingly recognized as a cause of renal insufficiency.

The identification of atherosclerotic renal arterial occlusive disease is important because of the natural history of progressive stenosis and complete arterial occlusion. A recent study of the natural history of atherosclerotic renal artery disease disclosed progressive obstruction in 44% of patients and complete occlusion in 16% of patients.[36] Progression of disease occurred within 2 years of disease identification in those patients with high grade renal artery stenosis. These observations indicate that atherosclerotic renal artery disease commonly progresses and is often associated with a loss of functioning renal mass and deterioration of renal function. Survival of these patients on long-term dialysis is poor as demonstrated by a median survival of 8.7 months in a review of patients with end-stage renal disease secondary to atherosclerotic occlusive disease at the Cleveland Clinic.[37] This underscores the importance of early patient identification and revascularization to preserve renal function.

Renovascular Candidate Identification

Clinical signs and symptoms suggesting renal artery disease include:

- Abrupt onset of moderate to severe hypertension before age 25
- Onset of moderate to severe hypertension after age 50
- Progressively difficult blood pressure control

Progressive atherosclerotic disease may, however, silently threaten renal function without an exacerbation of hypertension.[38] It has been observed in 33 to 47% of patients with aortic aneurysm and aortoiliac occlusive disease, and in 30% of patients with coronary artery disease.[39,40] It should be suspected, therefore, in any patient with clinical evidence of diffuse atherosclerosis with or without hypertension and especially in those patients with concurrent azotemia. Patients with unilaterally small kidneys should also be suspected of having renovascular disease. Screening studies of patients with unilateral renal atrophy have identified renal artery stenosis as the source of atrophy in 71 to 78% of cases.[41,42] More important, the contralateral normal sized kidney has been shown to have unsuspected renal artery stenosis in 42% of cases.

Evaluation of these patients may begin with a captopril stimulated nuclear renal scan and peripheral plasma renin measurement. Peripheral plasma renin is elevated in renovascular hypertension. Renin is a proteolytic enzyme found in the juxtaglomerular cells of the nephron. It is released into the lymphatics, renal tubular fluid, urine, and plasma in response to decreased perfusion pressures detected by the baroreceptors in the afferent arteriole. Renin acts on angiotensinogen to produce angiotensin I which is then converted to angiotensin II by angiotensin-converting enzyme (ACE). Angiotensin II is a powerful vasoconstrictor and has a direct sodium retaining effect on the ascending loop of Henle, in addition to stimulating adrenal production of aldosterone. The net effect is an increased blood pressure and renal perfusion and a feedback inhibition of renin production.

Manipulation of the renin-angiotensin-aldosterone mechanism may be used in combination with nuclear renography to screen for renovascular hypertension. When an ACE inhibitor such as captopril is given to a patient with suspected renovascular hypertension, the consequent inhibition of angiotensin II production will diminish glomerular efferent arteriolar vasoconstriction. The result will be a decrease in glomerular perfusion pressure and decreased renal function demonstrated on a nuclear renal scan.

Captopril stimulated renal scans are for screening purposes only and are not useful in cases of bilateral renal artery disease. Therefore, renal arteriography remains the definitive study for identifying and characterizing renal artery stenosis. This may be done with a minimum of contrast in an outpatient setting with intra-arterial digital subtraction angiography. Because most atherosclerotic renal arterial lesions are proximal lesions, aortic flush films with anterior, posterior, oblique, and lateral views are required to completely evaluate the extent of disease. Pelvic views of the iliac arteries and lateral views of the celiac origin are also included to select the appropriate operative technique for revascularization.

Patients with renin dependent hypertension secondary to unilateral renal artery stenosis may be considered for revascularization to restore normal blood pressure. Those patients that are managed medically must be closely observed for evidence of deteriorating renal function. Patients with high grade renal artery stenosis present bilaterally or in a solitary kidney should be revascularized to preserve renal function.[43] Patients with total renal artery occlusion and renal failure may still be candidates for revascularization to salvage function if there is evidence of renal viability.[44-47] Renal viability is suggested by:

- Angiographic evidence of collateral renal vessels
- Renal length of greater than or equal to 9 cm
- Function on a nuclear renal scan
- Histologic evidence of glomerular viability on renal biopsy

Patients with renal viability sustained by collateral flow may have a severe renal functional impairment and still demonstrate dramatic improvement with renal revascularization.[48] Kaylor and Novick reported successful revascularization of renal function in nine dialysis patients with end stage renal disease secondary to renal artery occlusion.[49] Recovery of renal function was immediate with a mean postoperative creatinine of 2.7 mg/dl and dialysis was no longer required. This clinical situation is unfortunately rare and again emphasizes the importance of early identification and intervention to preserve renal function.

Preoperative Preparation

Consequences of coronary artery and cerebrovascular disease comprise the majority of morbidity and mortality associated with renal revascularization. In view of this, the surgical candidate should be thoroughly evaluated with a history, physical examination, ECG and thallium cardiac stress test. If evidence of coronary artery disease is suspected, further evaluation with coronary angiography and left ventriculography is suggested. Contrast-induced renal failure following these studies may occur in the patient with a creatinine of greater than 2.0 mg/dl. It is generally transient and may be minimized with adequate hydration and mannitol infusion. Patients with severe renal impairment (creatinine greater than 5 mg/dl), require temporary dialysis immediately following these contrast studies. These studies should be done, however, in spite of the low risk of contrast induced renal failure to identify and avoid perioperative myocardial and cerebrovascular morbidity. Patients with significant, correctable coronary artery disease should undergo myocardial revascularization or angioplasty prior to renal artery reconstruction.[50]

Similarly, Doppler ultrasound evaluation of the carotid arteries is recommended. Further evaluation and surgical correction of high grade lesions should be performed before renal revascularization to protect against cerebral circulatory compromise during renal arterial reconstruction.

Preparation and anticipation of cardiovascular problems may also include preoperative admission to the ICU for flow-directed catheter placement to monitor cardiac function. Some patients will have decreased cardiac function, a diuretic induced hypovolemia, and suboptimal renal perfusion. Renal function is therefore further compromised and the associated hypertension increases cardiac work and diminishes cardiac function. Monitoring of cardiac function helps to guide pharmacologic therapy to decrease cardiac work while optimizing fluid balance to maximize cardiac reserve preoperatively and optimize intraoperative renal perfusion.

Intraoperative Considerations

The patient should be brought to the operating room well hydrated and closely monitored. An adequate intravascular volume is important to limit postischemic renal injury by ensuring optimal renal perfusion before and after renal artery clamping. Mannitol is infused prior to renal arterial clamping to further protect against ischemic renal injury.[10] Mannitol increases renal plasma flow, minimizes renal tubular intracellular edema, scavenges harmful oxygen radicals, and promotes an osmotic diuresis on renal reperfusion. Regional heparinization prior to renal artery clamping is used to prevent intrarenal vascular thrombosis.

The operation itself is selected to minimize hemodynamic alterations and reduce morbidity. Extra-aortic procedures such as splenorenal and hepatorenal bypass avoid operative manipulation and clamping of the badly diseased aorta and are designed to limit renal ischemia to the time necessary for a single vascular anastomosis.

On the left side, a single end-to-end anastomosis is all that is required for a splenorenal bypass to the left renal artery. On the right side, a hepatorenal bypass is performed by the placement of a saphenous vein graft end-to-side to the common hepatic artery just distal to the gastroduodenal artery. Renal circulation is not interrupted until this proximal anastomosis is completed. An end-to-end anastomosis of the interposition graft to the right renal artery is then completed.

Both splenorenal and hepatorenal bypass require a patent celiac axis to provide adequate blood flow for revascularization. When the celiac axis is compromised, renal revascularization from the iliac artery may be performed.[51] Atherosclerosis obliterans is a segmental disease and disease-free areas in the common iliac arteries will often be available for renal revascularization. The applicability of this procedure is limited, however, by the relatively long saphenous vein graft required and the possibility of progressive atherosclerotic compromise of the iliac arteries. Revascularization from the superior mesenteric artery is also a possibility but is rarely used to the risk of intestinal ischemia.[52] It is limited to those patients with infrarenal aortic occlusion and a significantly enlarged superior mesentera artery.

ICU Phase

Postoperative Monitoring

Postoperatively, the patient is returned to the ICU for monitoring and management. In view of the patient's generalized atherosclerotic disease and the risk of cardiovascular complications, a Foley catheter and arterial and central venous catheters are needed to monitor urine output, blood pressure, and central venous pressures. Patients with severe cardiac dysfunction will require a Swan-Ganz catheter to monitor left heart function. A central venous catheter also allows rapid fluid replacement in the event of postoperative hemorrhage and prompt infusion of antihypertensive medications. These patients are commonly hypertensive in spite of a patent renal arterial anastomosis, due to hypervolemia, hypothermic vasoconstriction, pain, or renal ischemia. A continuous infusion of nitroprusside is titrated to maintain the diastolic blood pressure between 90 and 100 mm Hg. This level ensures adequate renal perfusion to avoid thrombosis of the graft and prevents elevated pressures which can cause hemorrhage from a fresh vascular anastomosis. If hypertension persists beyond 24 to 36 hours, nitroprusside is slowly discontinued and the patient is started on labetalol, calcium-channel blockers, or other maintenance antihypertensives. A patent anastomosis is confirmed on the first postoperative day with a renal technetium scan.

A postoperative diuresis may be seen from the freshly revascularized kidney as preoperatively administered diuretics are cleared and until the once ischemic renal tubules recover their capabilities of urinary concentration. Urinary output must be measured at hourly intervals and replaced with crystalloid fluids. Electrolytes, glucose, and calcium should be measured at 4- to 6-hour intervals and replaced as required. The diuresis is typically self-limited and will resolve within 24 to 48 hours.

Pulmonary status is monitored with pulse oximetry and arterial blood gases for signs of inadequate oxygenation and ventilation. Most patients will be extubated in the operating room or on arrival to the ICU. Some patients, however, have a significant decrease in pulmonary reserve because of years of tobacco abuse and should remain intubated and mechanically ventilated until the first postoperative day.

Postoperative Complications

Because renal revascularization is performed transabdominally, it has many of the same complications as other abdominal operations. These include:

- Atelectasis
- Pneumonia
- Bowel obstruction
- Pulmonary embolus
- Myocardial infarction
- Cerebrovascular accident

Early complications specific to renal revascularization include:

- Hemorrhage
- Renal artery thrombosis
- Peripheral, visceral, and renal ischemia[53]

Hemorrhage. Early hemorrhage following renal revascularization is a consequence of a poorly performed arterial anastomosis or inadequate surgical hemostasis. Postoperative bleeding is most likely to occur from the vascular anastomosis, unsecured lumbar or collateral vessels in the renal hilum, the ipsilateral adrenal gland, or an unsecured branch of the saphenous vein graft. Bleeding from these sites may be promoted by poorly controlled postoperative hypertension, incomplete heparin reversal, or coagulopathy. Mild transient bleeding without hemodynamic consequences generally does not require treatment. More severe hemorrhage, characterized by decreased urine output and profound hypotension unresponsive to fluid challenges, will require rapid central venous replacement of blood products and immediate reoperation for hemostasis.

Renal Arterial Thrombosis. Early postoperative renal arterial thrombosis occurs in less than 5% of patients who undergo renal revascularization. Predisposing factors include hypotension, hypovolemia, a hypercoagulable state, and intrarenal arteriolar nephrosclerosis. The most common cause, however, is improper construction of the vascular anastomosis. Technical compromise of the anastomosis may be caused by traumatic injury to the vascular surface with creation of an intimal flap, embolization of atheromatous debris, or kinking and angulation of the bypass graft.

Clinical clues suggesting postoperative thrombosis are hypertension and azotemia. These are common postoperative findings and, therefore, a routine radioisotope scan on the first postoperative day to document renal blood flow is of utmost importance. Additionally, clinical suspicion should be aroused and a full evaluation initiated in the event of a sudden and persistent increase in blood pressure that is unrelated to incisional pain, hypothermia, or hypervolemia. Equivocal isotope renographic findings and a heightened clinical suspicion should be pursued with immediate angiography. Emergency reexploration for bypass graft revision and thrombectomy should be undertaken with a view towards renal salvage. More often, however, the kidney is no longer viable because of irreversible ischemic injury and must be removed. Alternatively, intra-arterial streptokinase infusion has produced successful clot lysis, but with a significant risk for hemorrhage in the early postoperative period.[54,55] Systemic heparinization is ineffective as primary therapy for thrombosis.

Aortic and Visceral Complications. Atherosclerotic renal arterial occlusive disease is commonly associated with diffuse disease of the abdominal aorta. When an aortorenal bypass is used for renal revascularization, clamping and unclamping of the diseased aorta present a significant hemodynamic challenge to an often compromised cardiovascular system. Systemic heparinization is also required to minimize risk of aortic and peripheral arterial thrombosis. The lower extremities and viscera may be further

Table 41-6. Aortic and Visceral Complications of Renovascular Disease

Aortic
  Distal embolization
  Hemorrhage
  Cardiovascular compromise
Visceral
  Hemorrhage
  Splenic capsular tear
  Pancreatitis
  Pancreatic pseudo cyst
  Gangrenous cholecystitis

---

threatened by embolic atheromatous debris or aortic intimal dissection. Vigilant postoperative observation is required to detect early signs of compromised peripheral circulation which should prompt angiographic evaluation and therapeutic thrombectomy. The potentially grave consequences of these complications underscore the wisdom of avoiding the diseased aorta using extra aortic techniques for renal revascularization.

Complications specific to these techniques include splenic, hepatic, and pancreatic injury. Splenorenal bypass exposes the spleen to possible retraction injury and hemorrhage. Splenic perfusion is preserved by short gastric and gastroepiploic arterial flow in spite of complete division of the splenic artery. Nevertheless, splenic arterial mobilization may result in injury to the splenic vein or pancreas with subsequent hemorrhage, pancreatitis, or pseudocyst formation[56] (Table 41-6).

Similarly, end-to-end hepatorenal bypass does not produce permanent hepatic ischemic injury but may yield a transient elevation in hepatic enzyme levels. Portal venous circulation and collateral hepatic arterial supply rapidly accommodate hepatic dearterialization but will not support the gallbladder. In this situation, adjunctive cholecystectomy should be performed to avoid postoperative gangrenous cholecystitis.[57,58]

Post-ICU Phase

The patient who has undergone uncomplicated renal revascularization typically stabilizes within 48 hours postoperatively and may be transferred to a regular hospital ward. Invasive monitoring catheters are removed prior to transfer and the nitroprusside infusion is replaced by maintenance antihypertensives. Patients who undergo revascularization for preservation of renal function may not demonstrate marked improvement in hypertension because of contralateral renal artery disease or coexisting essential hypertension. Those patients who undergo revascularization specifically for renovascular hypertension may demonstrate persistent hypertension for several weeks postoperatively before ultimate resolution.

Serial blood pressure measurements are continued on the ward along with routine postoperative care. Special attention is given to serum creatinine and electrolyte levels as well as overall fluid status. The patient is generally ready for discharge within 7 to 10 days postoperatively.

The patient should return 1 month postoperatively for follow-up with a serum creatinine level, blood pressure check, and isotope renal scan annual follow-up includes similar studies, as well as renal sonography to follow renal size. A deterioration in any of the above parameters is pursued with repeat intra-arterial digital subtraction angiography.

Overall, the patient undergoing renal revascularization for preservation of renal function or correction of renovascular hypertension may anticipate a successful result with relatively low risk. The operative mortality for a large series of patients with atherosclerotic renal arterial disease at the Cleveland Clinic was 2.1%, and the incidence of renal artery thrombosis or stenosis was 4.3%. Renal function was improved or preserved in 88.8% and a blood pressure benefit was achieved at 91%.[59] These results are the product of proper patient selection, aggressive preoperative preparation, proper operative approach and technique, and the vigilance of the critical care team.

HYPERTENSIVE ADRENAL TUMORS

Adrenal disease secondary to benign or malignant disorders may produce a wide range of metabolic derangements. These include alterations in corticosteroid, mineralocorticoid, androgen, and catecholamine balance. The following discussion focuses on two adrenal tumors associated with hemodynamic alterations that may require postoperative critical care management, namely, hyperaldosteronism and pheochromocytoma.

Pre-ICU Phase

Hyperaldosteronism

The most common cause of primary hyperaldosteronism is an adrenal cortical adenoma. It accounts for approximately 1% of all hypertension and occasionally requires critical care management.[60] The disease is characterized by elevated levels of aldosterone produced by an independently functioning adenoma. It is accompanied by hypertension with a low plasma renin, hypokalemia, and a metabolic alkalosis. The hypokalemia is typically severe because of the aldosterone-stimulated kaliuresis with a significant depletion of total body potassium reserves. Oral potassium supplementation alone is insufficient to restore potassium balance. Therefore, preoperative preparation includes:

- Spironolactone
- Sodium restriction to help restore total body potassium reserves

This preparation diminishes the risk of perioperative cardiac arrhythmias and helps to control hypertension.[61] It also reactivates the renin-angiotensin-aldosterone system in the contralaterally suppressed adrenal gland to avoid postoperative hypoaldosteronism. Treatment with spironolactone is typically initiated 2 months preoperatively and continued until the day of surgery. Preoperative glucocorticoid supplements are not required unless the contralateral adrenal has been previously removed or suppressed by exogenous steroids.

Pheochromocytoma

Pheochromocytoma is a catecholamine-secreting tumor most commonly occurring in the abdomen and retroperitoneum. Approximately 85% of these tumors occur in the adrenal medulla, with the remaining 10% occurring along the sympathetic chain or at the aortic bifurcation in the organ of Zuckerkandl. Another 5% occur in the posterior mediastinum, cranium, urinary bladder, or vagina. The excessive catecholamines produced by these tumors cause severe, sustained, or paroxysmal hypertension with subsequent end-organ damage including cardiomyopathy and arrhythmias. Other symptoms include lethargy, weakness, headache, and diaphoresis. The profound vasoconstriction, decreased intravascular volume, arrhythmias, and hypertension secondary to the excess catecholamines require careful preoperative preparation.

The goals of preoperative preparation in the patient with a pheochromocytoma are:

- Intravascular volume expansion
- Hypertension control
- Cardiac arrhythmia prevention

This preparation typically consists of alpha-adrenergic blockade with or without additional beta blockade. Alpha-adrenergic blockade is achieved 1 to 2 weeks preoperatively with oral phenoxybenzamine.[63] Beta blockade with propranolol is indicated for patients with significant tachycardia, a history of cardiac arrhythmias, and persistent, premature ventricular contractions. Beta blockade is initiated only after adequate alpha blockade to avoid paradoxic hypertension secondary to unopposed alpha vasoconstriction.

Unless the patient is medically unstable secondary to the hemodynamic consequences of a pheochromocytoma, preoperative preparation is typically initiated as an outpatient. Rarely, an acute pheochromocytoma may present with a severe hypertensive crisis followed by hypotension and associated cardiac arrhythmias. These patients require stabilization in the ICU, invasive cardiopulmonary monitoring, and urgent operative resection following tumor localization.[64]

Intraoperative Considerations

Pheochromocytoma. Intraoperative management of the patient with pheochromocytoma presents a significant challenge to the surgeon and the anesthesiologist. Wide and rapid hemodynamic shifts occur during anesthesia induction, surgical manipulation of the tumor, and the time of vascular ligation and tumor removal.[65] The anesthesiologist must be prepared with adequate cardiopulmonary access, including an intra-arterial catheter, central venous catheter, and pulmonary arterial catheter. Central venous access allows rapid delivery of medications for blood pressure and arrhythmia control and a rapid infusion of fluids to reexpand intravascular volume following tumor removal. A pulmonary arterial catheter helps to guide the fluid replacement and monitor left heart function. Even young, healthy patients with a pheochromocytoma may have significant cardiac dysfunction which is undetectable by the central venous catheter. This cardiac dysfunction is secondary to myocardial cellular damage from excess catecholamine exposure.[66] Sodium nitroprusside is used to manage intraoperative hypertension, whereas propranolol and lidocaine are administered as required for cardiac arrhythmias.[67,68]

The operative approach is selected to provide early access and control of the adrenal venous drainage.[69] Early ligation of the main adrenal vein prior to surgical manipulation helps to minimize sudden changes in blood pressure. Therefore, an anterior transabdominal or thoracoabdominal approach is generally most appropriate for excision of a pheochromocytoma. These incisions also allow exposure for palpation of the contralateral adrenal gland and exploration of the entire abdomen and retroperitoneum for extra adrenal pheochromocytomas.

Aldosteronoma. The posterior approach is inappropriate for surgical excision of a pheochromocytoma. It is useful, however, for the small aldosterone-producing adrenal cortical adenoma of primary hyperaldosteronism.[70] These tumors may also be removed through a standard flank incision.

ICU Phase

Postoperative Monitoring

Pheochromocytoma. Hypotension is the most common hemodynamic response to the decreased catecholamine levels that follow adrenalectomy for pheochromocytoma. Falling catecholamine levels significantly increase vascular compliance with subsequent hypotension that often requires vigorous volume expansion with two to three liters of saline and albumin. Hypotension may also be caused by residual effects of preoperative alpha-adrenergic blockade, intraoperative blood loss, or perioperative myocardial infarction.[71-73]

The change in catecholamine levels also alters glucose metabolism. Preoperative elevated circulating catecholamine levels inhibit insulin release, stimulate glycogenolysis and lipolysis, and decrease peripheral tissue glucose uptake. The subsequent hyperglycemia depletes glycogen reserves. When insulin inhibition is removed by falling catecholamine levels, glycogen reserves are unavailable to respond to the relative hyperinsulinism. This results in early postoperative hypoglycemia.[74-78] Clinical clues of hypoglycemia are lethargy and slow recovery from anesthesia. Postoperative hypoglycemia must be recognized immediately and corrected with vigorous hydration and glucose replacement to avoid encephalopathy and prolonged neurologic damage.[79]

Postoperative pulmonary status must be carefully monitored following a thoracoabdominal incision because pulmonary edema may also result from dramatic fluid shifts and catecholamine-induced cardiomyopathy. Catecholamines are potent bronchial smooth muscle dilators, and their sudden decrease may promote rebound bronchospasm requiring subcutaneous epinephrine to reverse.[80,81]

Aldosteronoma. Postoperatively, aldosterone secretion is reduced and may not respond to sodium depletion or angiotensin.[82,83] Postoperative hypoaldosteronism is typically limited and may be improved by preoperative treatment with spironolactone. Nevertheless, all antihypertensives should be eliminated postoperatively and serum electrolytes followed closely. Generally, mineralocorticoid activity is sufficient to prevent significant hyperkalemia if sodium intake is adequate. If hyperkalemia does occur, fluorohydrocortisone supplements may be required until aldosterone production recovers.

Post-ICU Phase

Metabolic and hemodynamic derangements typically stabilize within 24 to 48 hours postoperatively, and the patient can be transferred to a regular nursing floor of the hospital. Recovery proceeds as with any major surgical procedure, and the patient is ready for hospital discharge at the end of 1 week to 10 days. The patient affected by hypoaldosteronism may require mineralocorticoid supplementation with expected restoration of normal aldosterone secretion occurring within 6 to 12 months.[84]

Both the aldosteronism and pheochromocytoma patients should be followed postoperatively for evidence of persistent hypertension. Persistent hypertension in either patient group may be due to renal parenchymal damage from prolonged hypertension prior to diagnosis. Severe hypertension may also represent renal artery stenosis caused by renal artery damage occurring intraoperatively during a difficult dissection near the renal hilum.[85] Appropriate evaluation for renal artery stenosis is indicated. The patient with pheochromocytoma and persistent hypertension should also be biochemically and radiographically re-evaluated for the possibility of a missed ectopic tumor.

REFERENCES

1. Steinmuller, D. R.: Evaluation and selection of candidates for renal transplantation. Urol. Clin., *10*:217, 1983.
2. Penn, I.: Cancer as a complication of clinical transplantation. Transplant. Proc., *9*:1121, 1977.
3. Penn, I.: Transplantation in patients with primary renal malignancies. Transplantation, *24*:424, 1977.
4. Pirsch J. D., et al.: Cadaveric Renal Transplantation with Cyclosporin in Patients More than Sixty Years of Age. Transplantation, *47*:259, 1989.
5. Jordan, M. L., et al.: Renal transplantation in the older recipient. J. Urol., *134*:243, 1985.
6. Braun, W. E., et al.: Coronary arteriography and coronary artery disease in ninety-nine diabetics and non-diabetic patients on chronic hemodialysis or renal transplantation programs. Transplant. Proc., *13*:128, 1981.
7. Braun, W. D., Philips, D. F., and Vidt, D. G.: Coronary artery disease in one hundred diabetics with end stage renal failure. Transplant. Proc., *16*:603, 1984.
8. Spanos, P. K., et al.: Peptic ulcer disease in the transplant recipient. Arch. Surg., *109*:193, 1974.
9. Barry, J.: Procurement and preservation of cadaver kidneys. Urol. Clin., *10*:205, 1983.
10. Collins, C. M., et al.: Protection of kidneys from warm ischemic injury: dosage and timing of mannitol administration. Transplantation, *29*:83, 1980.
11. Ohl, D. A., et al.: Extravesicle ureteroneocystostomy in renal transplantation. J. Urol., *139*:499, 1988.
12. McGregor, P., et al.: Renal transplantation in end stage renal disease patients with existing urinary diversion. J. Urol., *135*:696, 1986.
13. Lillemoe, K. D., et al.: Intestinal necrosis due to sodium polystyrene in sorbitol enemas: clinical and experimental support for the hypothesis. Surgery, *101*:267, 1987.
14. Romolo, J. L., and Williams, G. M.: Effective kayexalate in sorbitol in colon of normal and uremic rats. Surg. Forum, *30*:369, 1979.
15. Streem, S. B., Novick, A. C., Steinmuller, D., and Musselman, P. W.: Percutaneous techniques for the management of urologic renal transplant complications. J. Urol., *135*:456, 1986.
16. Zincke, A., et al.: Experience with lymphoceles after renal transplantation. Surgery, *88*:44, 1975.
17. Sagalowski, A. I., and Peters, P. C.: Renovascular hypertension following renal transplantation. Urol. Clin., *11*:491, 1984.
18. Murray, J. E., et al.: Prolonged survival of human kidney homografts by immunosuppressive drug therapy. N. Engl. J. Med., *268*:1315, 1963.
19. Novick, A. C., et al.: Detrimental effect of cyclosporin on initial function of cadaver renal allografts following extended preservation. Transplantation, *42*:154, 1986.
20. Kupin, W. L., et al.: Sequential use of minnesota antilymphoblast globulin and cyclosporin in cadaveric renal transplantation. Transplantation, *40*:601, 1985.
21. Kupin, W. L., et al.: Use of cyclosporin in minnesota antilymphoblast globulin and early post-operative treatment of primary cadaveric renal transplant recipients. Transplant. Proc., *19*:1882, 1987.
22. Matas, A. J., et al.: Individualization of immediate post-transplant immunosuppression. Transplantation, *45*:406, 1988.
23. Kahan, B. D.: Cyclosporine. N. Engl. J. Med., *321*:1725, 1989.
24. Merion, R. M., et al.: Cyclosporin: five years' experience in cadaveric renal transplantations. N. Engl. J. Med., *310*:148, 1984.
25. Steinmuller, D. R.: Cyclosporine and organ transplantation. Cleve. Clin. Q., *52*:263, 1985.
26. Steinmuller, D. R.: Cyclosporine nephrotoxicity. Cleve. Clin. Q., *56*:89, 1989.
27. Steinmuller, D. R.: Usefulness of cyclosporine levels one to six months post-transplant. Transplant. Proc., *18*:158, 1986.
28. Barry J, M., et al.: Significance of delayed graft function in cyclosporin treated recipients of cadaver kidney transplants. Transplantation, *45*:346, 1988.
29. Thistlethwaite, J. R., et al.: "OKT3 treatment of steroid resistant renal allograft rejection. Transplantation, *43*:176, 1987.
30. Furst, M. R., et al.: "Successful re-treatment of allograft rejection with OKT3. Transplantation, *47*:88, 1989.
31. Norman, D. J., et al.: Effectiveness of the second course of OKT3 monoclonal anti-T cell antibody for treatment of renal allograft rejection. Transplantation, *46*:523, 1988.
32. Norman, D. J., et al.: Early use of OKT3 monoclonal antibody in renal transplantation to prevent rejection. Am. J. Kidney Dis., *11*:107, 1988.
33. Ortho Multicenter Transplant Study Group: A randomized trial of OKT3 monoclonal antibody for acute rejection of cadaveric renal transplants. N. Engl. J. Med., *313*:337, 1985.
34. Slavis, S. A., et al.: Outcome of renal transplantation in patients with a functioning graft of 20 years or more. J. Urol., *144*:20, 1990.
35. Cook, D. J.: Long-term survival of kidney allografts. *In* Clinical Transplants. Edited by P. I. Terasaki. Los Angeles, UCLA Tissue Typing Laboratory, 1987, p. 277.
36. Schreiber, M. J., Pohl, M. A., and Novick, A. C.: The natural history of atherosclerotic and fibrous renal artery disease. Urol. Clin. North Am., *11*:383, 1984.
37. Novick, A. C., et al.: Revascularization to preserve renal function in patients with atherosclerotic renovascular disease. Urol. Clin. North Am., *11*:477, 1984.

38. Dean, R. H., et al.: Renovascular hypertension: anatomic and renal function changes during drug Therapy. Arch. Surg., *116:*1408, 1981.
39. Olin, J., Young, J. R., Graor, R. A., and Ruschaupt, W. F.: Prevalence of atherosclerotic renal artery stenosis in patients with generalized atherosclerosis: diabetics and non-diabetics. In press.
40. Landwehr, D. M., Vetrovec, G. W., and Cowley, M. J.: Association of renal artery stenosis with coronary artery disease in patients with hypertension and/or chronic renal insufficiency. Am. Soc. Nephrol., 33A, 1983.
41. Gifford, R. W., McCormack, L. J., and Poutas, S. E.: The atrophic kidney: its role in hypertension. Mayo Clin. Proc., *40:* 834, 1965.
42. Lawrie, G. M., Morris, G. C., and DeBakey, M. E.: Long-term results of the totally occluded renal artery in 40 patients with renovascular hypertension. Surgery, *88:*753, 1980.
43. Novick, A. C.: Selection of patients with atherosclerosis for renal reconstruction to preserve renal function. World J. Urol., *7:*98, 1989.
44. Novick, A. C., et al.: Revascularization for preservation of renal function in patients with atherosclerotic renovascular disease. J. Urol., *129:*1907, 1983.
45. Dean, R. H., et al.: Revascularization of the poorly functioning kidneys. Surgery, *85:*44, 1979.
46. Schefft, P., Novick, A. C., and Stewart, B. H.: Renal revascularization in patients with total occlusion of the renal artery. J. Urol., *124:*184, 1980.
47. Libertino, J. A., et al.: Renal artery revascularization, restoration of renal function. JAMA, *244:*1340, 1980.
48. Novick, A. C.: Atherosclerotic renal artery disease: a correctable cause of renal failure. American Urologic Association Update, *6:*29, 1987.
49. Kaylor, W. M., Novick, A. C., Ziegelbaum, M., and Vidt, D. G.: Reversal of end stage renal failure with surgical revascularization in patients with atherosclerotic renal artery occlusion. J. Urol., *141:*486, 1989.
50. Novick, A. C., et al.: Diminished operative morbidity and mortality in renal revascularization. JAMA, *246:*749, 1981.
51. Novick, A. C., and Banowsky, L. H.: Ileal renal saphenous vein bypass: alternative for renal revascularization in patients with surgically difficult aorta. J. Urol., *122:*243, 1979.
52. Khauli, R., Novick, A. C., and Coseriu, G.: Superior mesenterorenal bypass for renal revascularization in patients with infrarenal aortic occlusion. J. Urol., *133:*188, 1985.
53. Novick, A. C.: Complications of renal vascular surgery and percutaneous transluminal angioplasty. In Urologic Complication. Edited by F. Marshall. Philadelphia, Mosby-Year Book, 1990.
54. Cronan, J. J., and Dorfman, G. S.: Low dose thrombolysis: a non-operative approach to renal artery occlusion. J. Urol., *130:*757, 1983.
55. Dardik, H., et al.: Lyses of arterial clot by intravenous or intra-arterial administration of streptokinase. Surg. Gynecol. Obstet., *158:*137, 1984.
56. Khauli, R., Novick, A. C., and Ziegelbaum, M.: Splenorenal bypass and the treatment of renal artery stenosis: experience with 69 cases. J. Vasc. Surg., *2:*547, 1985.
57. McElroy, J., and Novick, A. C.: Renorevascularization by end-to-end anastomosis of the hepatic and renal arteries. J. Urol., *134:*1089, 1985.
58. Chibaro, E. A., Libertino, J. A., and Novick, A. C.: Use of the hepatic circulation for renal revascularization. Ann. Surg., *199:*406, 1984.
59. Novick, A. C., et al.: Trends in surgical revascularization for renal artery disease: ten years' experience. JAMA, *257:*498, 1987.
60. Bravo, E. L.: The syndrome of primary aldosteronism and pheochromocytoma. *In* Diseases of the Kidney. Edited by R. W. Schrier and C. W. Gottschalk. Boston, Little, Brown, 1988, p. 1623.
61. Bravo, E. L., Dustan, H. P., and Tanai, R. C.: Spironolactone as a non-specific treatment for primary aldosteronism. Circulation, *48:*491, 1973.
62. Wheeler, M. H., et al.: The management of patients with catecholamine excess. World J. Surg., *6:*735, 1982.
63. Modlinger, R. S., Ertel, N. H., and Hauptman, J. B.: Adrenergic blockade in pheochromocytoma. Arch. Intern. Med., *143:* 2245, 1983.
64. Freier, D. T., Eckhouser, F. E., and Harrison, T. S.: Pheochromocytoma: a persistently problematic and still potentially lethal disease. Arch. Surg., *115:*388, 1980.
65. Bingham, W., Elliott, J., and Lions, S. M.: Management of anesthesia for pheochromocytoma. Anesthesia, *27:*49, 1972.
66. Van Vliet, P. D., Burchell, H. B., and Titus, J. L.: Focal myocarditis associated with pheochromocytoma. N. Engl. J. Med., *274:*1102, 1966.
67. Daggett, P., Vernor, I., and Caruthrs, M.: Intraoperative management of pheochromocytoma with sodium nitroprusside. Br. Med. J., *2:*311, 1978.
68. El-Naggar, M., Suerte, E., and Rosenthal, E.: Sodium nitroprusside and lidocaine in the anesthetic management of pheochromocytoma. Can. Anaesth. Soc. J., *24:*353, 1977.
69. Cullen, M. L., Staren, E. D., and Strans, A. K.: Pheochromocytoma: operative strategy. Surgery, *89:*927, 1985.
70. Novick, A. C.: Surgery for primary hyperaldosteronism. Urol. Clin. North Am., *1613:*535, 1989.
71. Burgman, S. M., et al.: Post-operative management of patients with pheochromocytoma. J. Urol., *120:*109, 1978.
72. Ross, E. J., Pritchard, E. N. C., and Kaufman, L.: Preoperative and operative management of patients with pheochromocytomas. Br. Med. J., *1:*191, 1967.
73. Temple, W. D., et al.: Phenoxybenzamine blockade in surgery of pheochromocytoma. J. Surg. Res., *22:*59, 1977.
74. Sagalowski, A., and Donahue, J. P.: Possible mechanism of hypoglycemia following removal of pheochromocytoma. J. Urol., *124:*422, 1980.
75. Costello, G. T., et al.: Hypoglycemia following bilateral adrenalectomy for pheochromocytoma. Crit. Care Med., *16:*562, 1988.
76. Chambers, S., et al.: Hypoglycemia following removal of pheochromocytoma: case report review of the literature. Postgrad. Med. J., *58:*503, 1982.
77. Meeke, R. I., O'Keefe, J. D., and Gaffney, J. D.: Pheochromocytoma removal and post-operative hypoglycemia. Anesthesia, *40:*1093, 1985.
78. Reynolds, C., et al.: Hyperinsulinism after removal of a pheochromocytoma. Can. Med. Assoc. J., *129:*349, 1983.
79. Channa, A. B., et al.: Hypoglycemic encephalopathy following surgery on pheochromocytoma. Anesthesia, *42:*1298, 1987.
80. Nishikawa, T., Dohi, S., and Azai, Y.: Recurrence of bronchial asthma after adrenalectomy for pheochromocytoma. Can. Anaesth. Soc. J., *33:*109, 1986.
81. Harvey, J. N., Deen, H. G., and Lee, M. R.: Recurrence of asthma following removal of a nor adrenalin secreting pheochromocytoma. Postgrad. Med. J., *60:*364, 1984.
82. Biglieri, E. G., et al.: Post-operative studies of adrenal function in primary aldosteronism. J. Clin. Endocrinol., *26:*553, 1966.
83. Sunsfjord, J. A., et al.: Reduced aldosterone secretion during spironolactone treatment in primary aldosteronism: report of a case. J. Clin. Endocrinol. Metab., *39:*734, 1974.
84. Bravo, E. L., Duston, H. P., and Terrazi, R. C.: Selective hypo-

aldosteronism despite prolonged pre- and post-operative hyperreninemia in primary aldosteronism. J. Clin. Endocrinol. Metab., *41*:611, 1975.

85. Julian, W. A., Cole, C. A. T., and Fried, F. A.: Renovascular hypertension: a rare complication of excision of pheochromocytoma. J. Urol., *111*:722, 1974.

SELECTED READINGS

Bravo, E. L., and Gifford, R. W., Jr.: Pheochromocytoma. Endocrinol. Metab. Clin. North Am., *22*:329, 1993.

Gokal, R.: Quality of life in patient undergoing renal replacement therapy. Kidney Int. Suppl., *40*:523, 1993.

Hayes, J. M.: The immunobiology and clinical use of current immunosuppressive therapy for renal transplantation. J. Urol., *149*:437, 1993.

Kang, J. Y.: The gastrointestinal tract in uremia. Dig. Dis. Sci., *38*:257, 1993.

Koga, S., et al.: Acute hemorrhagic cystitis caused by adenovirus following renal transplantation: review of the literature. J. Urol., *149*:838, 1993.

Paya, C. V.: Fungal infections in solid-organ transplantation. Clin. Infect. Dis., *16*:677, 1993.

Schwarz, A., et al.: The effect of cyclosporine on the progression of human immunodeficiency virus type 1 infection transmitted by transplantation—data on four cases and review of the literature. Transplantation, *55*:95, 1993.

Scott, T. R., Graham, S. M., Schweitzer, E. J., and Bartlett, S. T.: Colonic necrosis following sodium polystyrene sulfonate (Kayexalate)-sorbitol enema in a renal transplant patient. Report of a case and review of the literature. Dis. Colon Rectum, *36*:607, 1993.

Snydman, D. R., Rubin, R. H., and Werner, B. G.: New developments in cytomegalovirus prevention and management. Am. J. Kidney Dis., *21*:217, 1993.

White, J. R. Jr, and Campbell, R. K.: Treatment of post-transplant diabetic patients. Clin. Ther., *15*:261, 1993.

Chapter 42

MANAGEMENT OF THE UROLOGIC PATIENT

GABRIEL P. HAAS
EDSON J. PONTES

The object of this chapter is to review aspects of critical care that may be unique to patients with disorders of the genitourinary tract and to discuss aspects of urologic care that may have to be rendered to patients in the ICU regardless of their underlying pathophysiologic disorders. Successful treatment of these problems requires close interaction and communication between the urologist and the ICU team, with each group understanding their responsibilities with respect to management of the patient. Full understanding of urologic indications, procedures, and expected outcomes are required by all participants in care of the patient in order to provide the high standards of care which are required in the critical care setting.

Most of the principles of critical care management that apply to patients undergoing operations of similar magnitude involving any other organ system also apply to those undergoing surgery on the genitourinary tract. Nevertheless, special risk factors are present in urology patients, and some considerations are unique to this group. The significant advances in perioperative care of the past decade have increased the threshold of acceptable surgical risk and more and more high risk patients are candidates for major operative procedures. This trend is accompanied by the need for greater preoperative optimization, intraoperative monitoring, and rapid response to changing physiologic parameters, and more complex postoperative management which is often provided in the ICU.

PELVIC SURGERY

Pelvic urologic surgery involves lengthy operations with a potential for:

- Hemorrhage
- Sudden fluid shifts
- Infection
- Pelvic vein thrombosis

Disruption of the continuity of the urinary tract may make accurate monitoring of the patient's fluid status problematic, and this fact coupled with operations on high risk patients present unique challenges in the pre-, intra-, and postoperative management of a number of common disease entities.

Pre-ICU Phase

Prostate Cancer

Carcinoma of the prostate is the most common malignant tumor in men, with over 200,000 newly diagnosed cases annually which results in 38,000 deaths each year.[1] The increasing rate of diagnosis is probably not due to the increasing prevalence of prostate cancer, but is the result of more patients identified due to improved diagnostic techniques, increased awareness of the disease, and a concerted effort for earlier diagnosis. Until recently, only 25 to 30% of newly diagnosed prostate cancers were still confined to the prostate gland; with the remaining patients had either locally invasive (extracapsular or seminal vesicle involvement) or metastatic disease.

Prostate cancer is a disease of elderly men, and data from autopsy studies suggest an increase of prevalence from 40% in men 50 to 60 years old to 80 to 90% in men over 80 years of age.[2] It is evident from these data that some prostate cancers may be indolent for a long period before clinical presentation, and that even after diagnosis, the rate of progression is variable. In patients diagnosed with occult or small clinically palpable lesions, approximately 30 to 35% develop distant metastases and 20% die of prostate cancer within 5 to 10 years. Once the cancer has spread beyond the anatomic capsule of the prostate gland, 50% develop metastases and 70 to 75% die of metastases within 5 years. Once the regional lymph nodes become involved, 85% of patients develop distant metastases in 5 years, and 50% of patients who present with metastases will die of their disease in 3 years.[3–5] Metastatic disease is first treated by elimination of testosterone production, either by orchiectomy or by chemical castration. Endocrine-resistant disease has an expected survival of less than a year. Therefore, the clear goal of therapy is to diagnose patients early and render them disease free before the cancer has spread beyond the confines of the prostate gland. Once the disease has spread beyond the prostate, it is no longer considered curable.

Routine staging of prostate cancer is based on the results of digital rectal examination, transrectal ultrasound examination of the prostate gland, serum markers (e.g., prostate-specific antigen, prostatic acid phosphatase), pelvic CT scan, and bone scan. Unfortunately, none of the staging studies can accurately predict the presence of microscopic extracapsular involvement or minimal seminal vesicle involvement, and in our surgical experience, almost 50% of patients were clinically understaged.

Prostate cancer clinically localized within the prostate gland may be treated by radiation therapy (external beam or interstitial) or by radical prostatectomy. The choice of therapy is decided by the patient and physician after appropriate consideration of the expected outcome and potential risks and complications of each form of treatment.

Radical prostatectomy is the en bloc removal of the prostate, ejaculatory ducts, seminal vesicles, and a bladder cuff with re-anastomosis of the urethra and bladder neck. It may be performed via a retropubic or perineal approach, depending on the surgeon's preference. In most cases, the operation is preceded at the same setting by bilateral pelvic lymphadenectomy for staging and prognosis.

Proper patient selection is crucial for the successful outcome of the operation. The ideal candidate for radical prostatectomy is the patient who is in good health, usually under the age of 70 with at least an expected survival of 10 more years, and whose disease is confined to the prostate gland. Some centers also perform the operation on selected patients with extracapsular or even lymph node involvement,[6] and the operation, although technically much more difficult, can be performed on patients who have locally failed external beam or interstitial radiation therapy.[7] Age is not an absolute contraindication, the operation may be carried out on selected candidates older than 70 years of age, and the most important issue is physical condition and life expectancy.

Because prostate cancer is a disease of the elderly, it is not surprising that a significant proportion of the patients have hypertension, diabetes, and coexistent cardiovascular and respiratory abnormalities. Although the vast improvements in perioperative and postoperative care of the last few years have made radical prostatectomies much safer operations, these advances have also expanded the criteria for patient inclusion, and today we operate on higher risk patients who require increasingly complex preoperative preparation, intraoperative management, and postoperative care.

Bladder Cancer

New diagnoses of bladder cancer will account for over 60,000 cases in the United States this year and the diseases is four times as common in males as in females.[1] Multiple risk factors have been identified for bladder cancer, including exposure to aniline dyes, history of smoking, schistosomiasis, chronic infections, analgesic abuse, chemotherapy with cyclophosphamide, and pelvic irradiation.[8-10] Most patients present with painless hematuria. The three most common histologic types are transitional cell cancer, adenocarcinoma, and squamous cell cancer. Superficial transitional cell cancer is treated by transurethral resection, and intravesical chemotherapy, and although the lesions may recur often, only 10 to 30% actually progress to muscle invasion. Most patients found with muscle-invasive disease have this stage present at initial diagnosis. The conventional treatment of muscle-invasive bladder cancer has been radical cystoprostatectomy and urinary diversion, although neoadjuvant chemotherapy, preoperative radiation therapy, or a combination of both has been advocated.

Regardless of the form of therapy, up to 50% of patients develop metastatic disease within 2 years.[11] Patients with metastatic disease are treated with chemotherapy, but the responses are usually short term. Intractable bleeding from the bladder may have to be treated by salvage cystectomy and urinary diversion, or urinary diversion alone in patients with unresectable tumors. Patients who are not suitable candidates for a major operation may be managed by a partial cystectomy, chemotherapy, and/or radiation therapy with curative intent.

Other Major Procedures

Several other major pelvic procedures, such as pelvic exenteration for ovarian or colon cancer, bladder augmentation using segments of intestine to increase the bladder capacity, and replacement of ureteral segments by portions of bowel present similar considerations of ICU management and therefore are not individually discussed.

Preoperative Preparations

Radical Prostatectomy. The preoperative preparation for radical prostatectomy starts with evaluation of the indications for surgery and assessment of the risk of the procedure, starting with a thorough history and physical examination. Particular attention must be directed to the cardiovascular, pulmonary, and hematologic status of the patient. The significance of any abnormal findings must be assessed preoperatively. If carotid bruits are heard or if the patient has neurologic evidence of cerebral ischemia, appropriate carotid and cardiac studies should be performed. We obtain cardiac stress testing on hypertensive patients and on everyone with a prior myocardial infarction. As with any other elective surgery, anticoagulants must be discontinued in advance and any coagulopathy reversed. Because blood transfusions are frequently required in the perioperative period, many of our patients elect to donate their own blood for autotransfusion, provided sufficient time is available prior to surgery. We do not recommend lengthy delay of a cancer operation, however, to enable the patient to donate several more units of blood.

The patient who will undergo prostatectomy is hospitalized the night before surgery for hydration, mechanical, and antibiotic bowel preparation. The purpose of the bowel preparation is to decrease bowel contents, which may hinder the pelvic operation, and to minimize the chance of contamination and consequent surgery in case of unexpected injury to the rectum during dissection of Denonvillier's fascia. Rectal injury occurs in fewer than 2% of radical prostatectomies, but as long as the injury is recognized intraoperatively, is limited, and the patient has had bowel preparation, it can be treated with a two-layer primary repair. Large injuries or injury to the unprepared rectum should be treated with closure and a diverting colostomy.

Deep venous thrombosis (DVT) and pulmonary embolism (PE) are the two most common and potentially fatal complications of radical prostatectomies and pelvic surgery. The incidence of both of these conditions is higher in the cancer patient, in those undergoing pelvic operations, and in inactive patients. DVTs are reported in 5 to 12% and PE in 2 to 3% of radical prostatectomy patients, respectively.[12] Prevention starts in the preoperative period and continues during and following the operation. We use sequential compression stockings fitted in preoperative holding during the operation and continue them for the first 24 to 36 hours after surgery, until the patient starts to ambulate reasonably well. In addition, we administer minidose heparin, 5000 U preoperatively and every 12 hours following surgery to high risk patients. The benefits of heparin are controversial, because this agent may be associated with an incidence of increased postoperative lymphatic drainage and lymphocoele formation.[13]

Patients with cardiovascular compromise, who are the most likely to tolerate volume loss and any uncompensated fluid shifts poorly, should have arterial lines, central lines, or pulmonary artery catheters properly placed before anesthesia is induced.

Pulmonary care, including preoperative bronchodilation, is provided to patients with obstructive airway disease. These patients should also be monitored, however, with respect to cardiac arrhythmias, which may develop as consequence of the therapy.

Spinal or epidural anesthesia is safest for radical prostatectomy and appears to be associated with less blood loss.[14] Even when general anesthesia is used, an epidural catheter placed preoperatively and kept in place for 24 to 48 hours postoperatively can provide access for excellent pain control.

Radical Cystectomy. Unlike carcinoma of the prostate, invasive bladder cancer has no accepted therapeutic alternative to radical surgery, and therefore many elderly and high risk patients have to be adequately prepared for major pelvic surgery. Evaluation and preoperative preparation of the patient is similar to what was described for radical prostatectomy, except that formal bowel preparation is required because of the isolation of a segment of intestine to serve as the urinary conduit or reservoir. The patient is hydrated, appropriate antithromboembolic measures are taken, and hemodynamic monitoring is instituted as described previously. It is essential that the surgeon and the enterostomal therapist identify the best location for the stoma of the urinary diversion before the surgical procedure.

Surgical Technique

Radical Prostatectomy. The surgical technique of retropubic radical prostatectomy is presented briefly, to acquaint the intensive care specialist with the most salient features of the operation. Following a lower midline or transverse suprapubic incision, the lateral halves of the rectus muscle are retracted and the pericystic space is entered. The peritoneum is mobilized superiorly and should not be entered but retracted cephalad. At this point, a modified bilateral pelvic lymph node dissection is carried out from the femoral canal, the circumflex iliac artery and vein marking the distal limits of the dissection, along the adventitia of the external iliac vessels toward the proximal border of the dissection, the bifurcation of the common iliac artery and vein. The lymphatic bundle is freed en bloc from the lateral pelvic wall with great care taken not to injure the obturator nerve. Once the lymphatic tissue is removed, it may be submitted for frozen section examination, and depending on the extent of disease found in the nodes (if any), the surgeon will decide whether to proceed with the operation or to terminate the procedure and recommend an alternate form of therapy.

Removal of the prostate is initiated by bilateral incision of the endopelvic fascia. The pelvic musculature beyond this fascia can be a source of slow, but troublesome bleeding during the course of the procedure, so extreme care must be exercised to avoid injury. The puboprostatic ligaments are divided, and the dorsal vein complex, traversing over the anterolateral surface of the urethra and prostate must be ligated. Failure to adequately control these veins results in rapid, major blood loss and may be responsible for sudden hypotension. On the other hand, skillful control of these two areas of potential blood loss permits the operation to proceed with little further bleeding.

The prostatourethral junction at the apex of the prostate can now be visualized and the urethra divided around the previously placed Foley catheter. Care must be taken not to leave behind prostate tissue; on the other hand, overly generous removal of urethral tissue adversely affects continence. We prefer to place two absorbable sutures through the distal urethra anteriorly at this point, in preparation for consequent anastomosis. The Foley catheter, also divided and clamped, is now used for anterior traction while Denonvilliers' fascia is divided and the prostate is carefully separated from the rectum. Tumor involvement or fibrosis from previous resection, needle biopsy, or radiation may make this dissection extremely difficult, and hence rectal injury may occur.

The neurovascular bundles, the parasympathetic innervation to the corpora cavernosa, are located dorsolateral to the prostate and are either divided and removed with the prostate, or bluntly dissected off the gland and preserved, depending on the extent of the tumor and the intention of the surgeon to preserve the patient's potency.

Attention is now directed to the bladder neck, which is incised anteriorly over the prostatovesical junction. Once the bladder is entered, the mucosa is opened in an anterior to posterior direction, with care taken to avoid injury to the ureteral orifices. The posterior bladder wall is separated from the prostate and seminal vesicles. Prostatic branches of the inferior vesical arteries are controlled. Posterior dissection of the trigone is limited to avoid injury to the intramural portion of the ureters. The vas deferens is identified and divided in the midline, the seminal vesicles are dissected free in their entirety, and any residual vascular pedicles still holding the prostate are divided. Once the prostate gland has been removed, the presence of hemostasis is ascertained, and the anterior surface of the rectum is examined for possible injury. If everything is satisfactory, the bladder neck is reconstructed and a fresh Foley catheter is advanced into the bladder through the urethra. A tension-free anastomosis is created between the bladder neck and the stump of the urethra with four absorbable sutures placed equidistant from each other. Prior to wound closure, two pelvic drains are placed in the area of the lymph node dissection.

Table 42-1 includes some potential intraoperative complications that may not be recognized during surgery but may be present in the postoperative period.

Table 42-1. Perioperative Complications of Radical Prostatectomy

Rectal injury	1-2%
Ureteral injury	0-1%
Prolonged urine leak	1-4%
Lymphocele	1-3%
Wound infection	10-12%
Deep venous thrombosis	5-12%
Pulmonary embolus	2-3%
Myocardial infarct	1-3%
Cerebrovascular accident	1-2%

Table 42-2. Forms of Urinary Diversion

Type	Bowel Segment Used	Continent	Urethral Anastomosis
Cutaneous ureterostomy	None	No	No
Ureterosigmoidostomy	Sigmoid	No	No
Ileal loop	Ileum	No	No
Jejunal loop	Jejunum	No	No
Transverse colon loop	Transverse colon	No	No
Kock pouch	Ileum	Yes	Possible
Indiana pouch	Ileum and ascending colon	Yes	Possible
Le bag	Ileum and ascending colon	Yes	Yes
Camey	Ileum	Yes	Yes

Radical Cystectomy. Radical cystectomy in men includes pelvic lymphadenectomy and removal of the bladder, prostate, and seminal vesicles. A urethrectomy is performed either at the time of cystectomy, or at a separate time if tumor involvement of the bladder neck and prostatic fossae is present. Radical cystectomy in women includes pelvic lymphadenectomy and removal of the bladder, urethra, uterus, broad ligaments, fallopian tubes, ovaries, and the anterior vaginal wall.

Lymph node dissection is performed in a similar fashion to the procedure described in the section of this chapter on radical prostatectomy; however, the proximal margin of the dissection is extended to the aortic bifurcation. During the dissection, the superior vesical artery is ligated to decrease consequent bleeding. The ureters are ligated deep in the pelvis, and the distal ends are submitted for frozen section examination to exclude the presence of cancer or significant atypia, which if present, would necessitate resection of the ureters at a higher level. The posterior peritoneum is incised, and a plane is created between the rectum and bladder while the lateral pedicles of the bladder are divided. The dissection is carried just anterior to the rectum, behind Denonvilliers' fascia, until the bladder, seminal vesicles, and prostate are fully mobilized. The endopelvic fascia is entered laterally and distal dissection of the prostate is carried out in a similar fashion to radical prostatectomy. A potency-preserving radical cystectomy may be carried out by a modification of the technique to preserve the neurovascular bundles coursing posterolateral to the prostate gland.

In females, the bladder is mobilized in a similar fashion, but an abdominal hysterectomy and excision of the anterior vaginal wall and the urethra are performed en bloc.

At the conclusion of the radical cystectomy portion of the operation, complete hemostasis is ascertained, the pelvis is packed with surgical sponges, and attention is directed toward constructing a urinary diversion. Table 42-2 lists many alternatives for urinary diversion.

Cutaneous ureterostomy is the simplest procedure technically because no bowel resection is involved. Unless the ureter is markedly dilated, however, there is a high incidence of postoperative stenosis and obstruction requiring revision of the stoma. Ureterosigmoidostomy involves an antirefluxing anastomosis of the ureters and the sigmoid colon. This technique allows for mixing of urine and stool and has been associated with the development of colon cancer near the anastomosis after 10 or more postoperative years. Ileal loop urinary diversion is the standard treatment today because it is simple to perform and is generally free of complications such as electrolyte disorders. If, however, the patient has undergone previous radiation treatments, ureteral anastomosis into irradiated bowel should be avoided, and the patient should have a jejunal or transverse colon urinary conduit.

The last decade saw increasing demand for continent urinary diversion. This generally involves construction of a reservoir from defunctionalized small and/or larger bowel, with antirefluxing ureteral anastomoses and a nipple continence mechanism, which is either brought out to the anterior abdominal wall and will require catheterization at regular intervals, or at least in the male, anastomosis of the pouch directly to the urethral stump. As the reader can imagine, these procedures are technically much more complex than the ileal loop diversion because larger segments of bowel are needed and much more surface area has to be sutured. Although the need for revision is 15 to 20% higher, patient satisfaction is much greater. The long-term results are good; most patients have an adequate-sized, low pressure reservoir and good continence rates. Most patients with urethral anastomosis are able to void spontaneously and experience only minimal stress incontinence.

At the conclusion of surgery, the patients will have an assortment of catheters and tubes, according to the type of diversion used. Most patients have a urethral Foley catheter draining the pelvis for 24 to 48 hours. This catheter should not be irrigated and is usually removed once pelvic drainage subsides. If a urethral bowel anastomosis is created, the patient will have a Foley catheter in the neobladder, and this should not be manipulated for fear of dislodging the tube. There are usually two ureteral stents, as well as left and right drains with their tips located in the proximity of the ureteral anastomosis and in the pelvis.

ICU Phase

Radical Prostatectomy

Not all patients who undergo radical prostatectomy need to be observed in the ICU postoperatively. The decision to place the patient in the ICU, in a step-down unit, or on the surgical floor depends not only on the medical condition of the patient, but also on the set-up of the hospital, where the needed facilities and care can be provided. In most cases only observation is required, the rate of intravenous hydration determined according to input and output volumes, and the need for additional blood transfusion considered based on hemoglobin/hematocrit levels and vital signs. Pulmonary artery pressures, and central and arterial lines should be monitored until the patient is stable. Although nasogastric suction is usually not required, the patient should ingest nothing by mouth for 24 to 48 hours, until gastrointestinal function returns. The Foley catheter should be well secured to the thigh and should not be manipulated at all; if problems arise, the urology team should be notified. A dislodged Foley catheter is a major problem, and replacement should never be attempted blindly in the immediate postoperative period because of possible disruption of the anastomosis and a high rate of incontinence. Instead, the patient should undergo cystoscopy and the catheter should be placed under direct vision. If this method is unsuccessful, the incision will need to be opened, to place a suprapubic catheter. Under normal circumstances, the Foley catheter is left in place for 3 weeks.

Measures taken to prevent deep venous thrombosis should be continued in the postoperative period until the patient becomes ambulatory. These measures include: (1) Venous stasis should be avoided; (2) the patient should be ambulated as often as possible; (3) the patient should perform hourly dorsiflexion leg exercises while in bed; and (4) the patient should not be sitting with the legs in a dependent position. Early diagnosis and immediate treatment of deep venous thrombosis by anticoagulation should be initiated to prevent the potentially fatal sequela of pulmonary embolism.

Lymphocoeles are complications of the pelvic lymphadenectomy portion of the procedure and are seen in 2 to 3% of radical prostatectomies. They usually resolve spontaneously, but occasionally become large enough to impede deep venous drainage and may have to be drained. External drainage also has to be instituted if the fluid collection becomes infected. The incidence of lymphocoeles is higher in patients receiving low doses of heparin perioperatively.[13]

Hematomas may develop if incomplete hemostasis is present at the time of wound closure. Unless intractable bleeding necessitates reexploration, the process is usually self-limiting, but may require drainage if infection or venous stasis results.

If persistent high output is observed from the pelvic drains, the differential diagnoses should include lymphatic drainage or a urine leak. The latter can be confirmed by measuring the fluid creatinine. Urine may leak from the urethral anastomosis, and gentle traction of the Foley catheter for 24 to 48 hours usually improves the situation. If the patient fails to improve, a cystogram should be done to delineate the extent of the leak. If the cystogram does not reveal a leak, an intravenous pyelogram should be performed to rule out an unrecognized extravesical ureteral injury. If this extremely rare circumstance is confirmed, the patient should be treated with nephrostomy tube placement and eventual reimplantation of the ureter. The pelvic drains should be continued until the drainage resolves.

Superficial wound infection occurs in 10 to 12% of cases and is managed by incision and drainage.

Radical Cystectomy

The most common reason to admit patients undergoing radical cystectomy to the ICU is hemodynamic monitoring. Patients should undergo close evaluation of their fluid status, blood counts, electrolyte profiles, and should receive pulmonary training as well as prevention of thromboembolic phenomena. The urethral drain is usually discontinued in 1 to 2 days, once drainage has decreased. The output from the diversion and ureteral stents are monitored closely. There is no standard convention regarding the order of removal of the ureteral stents or drains. We usually remove drains when the output is less than 30 to 50 ml every 24 hours, and remove the ureteral stents in about 2 weeks. Patients who underwent previous radiation therapy may need to maintain their ureteral stents slightly longer. If there is any drop in the urine output, the first step is to gently irrigate the stents. The colostomy rod (used for Turnbull-type stomas) is removed in 7 to 10 days. Gastrointestinal function usually returns in 1 week, and the patient may be started on diet.

Post-ICU Phase

Radical Prostatectomy

Following discharge from the ICU, most patients have an uneventful recovery in the hospital and are discharged in 7 to 10 days. The Foley catheter is removed in 3 weeks, and patients start to resume their normal activity level in 4 to 6 weeks. Follow-up is performed every 3 months for the first 2 years and twice a year thereafter, and includes rectal examination and prostate-specific antigen level determination. Radiographs or bone scans are done when clinically indicated. The prognosis and potential need for further therapy are determined by the final pathology report. Patients whose prostate cancer was completely confined to the gland can expect a 50 to 75% probability of 15-year disease-free survival, and patients with extracapsular disease reportedly have an approximately 30% probability of 15-year survival; however, a 65% probability of 5-year survival was noted in individuals treated with adjuvant therapy consisting of radiation therapy and/or hormonal treatment.[6,15,16] There are insufficient data on the efficacy of radical prostatectomy combined with lymphadenectomy to control disease in patients with positive lymph nodes. In older studies, only 13 to 25% of patients survived for 15 years; however, the Mayo Clinic group reported that if early endocrine therapy is offered to this group of patients, 41% disease-free and 70% overall survival rates can be achieved.[6]

Long-term complications of radical prostatectomy include a 2% complete incontinence and an 18% mild, occasional stress incontinence rate.[17] The latter can be markedly improved by more frequent voiding and pelvic muscle exercises. Bladder neck contracture has been reported in

3 to 12% of cases and occur from a few months to years following surgery. Patients complain of decreased urinary stream and dribbling. Interestingly, patients who were originally continent may start complaining of incontinence (overflow incontinence), whereas initially incontinent patients will report improvement of their symptoms prior to the onset of urinary retention.

For years, it was assumed that 100% of patients who underwent radical prostatectomy would become impotent. Walsh[18] demonstrated that preservation of one or both neurovascular bundles results in a 60 to 86% potency rate 1 year following surgery. It should be kept in mind, however, that the primary goal of surgery is to remove all the tumor, and preservation of potency is a secondary concern.

Radical Cystectomy

Patients may be discharged from the ICU once their condition has stabilized. Following discharge, the patient should continue to ambulate, their diet may be advanced, and intravenous solutions are discontinued. The particular order in which the various stents and drains are removed varies among urologists. It is essential to the success of the operation that a close relationship develops between the patient and the enterostomal therapist, who needs to instruct the patient in the proper methods to take care of the stoma, such as irrigation of mucus and application of the proper appliances. Long-term follow-up should include not only surveillance for cancer, but also evaluation of the function of the conduit or reservoir by renal function tests, renal ultrasound, IVP, loopogram/pouchogram, and reservoir pressure studies. The expected 5-year survival for patients with muscle-invasive disease confined to the bladder wall is 60 to 70%,[19] and these figures decrease to less than 50% for extravesical disease or 25 to 30% for patients with disease in the lymph nodes.[20]

TESTICULAR CANCER

Pre-ICU Care

Approximately 6800 new cases of testicular cancer occur each year.[1] Testicular cancer is the most common solid tumor of men between the ages of 20 and 34. Seminomas are the most common histologic type, and these tumors are extremely sensitive to radiation. Nonseminomatous germ cell tumors, such as embryonal carcinoma or choriocarcinoma, are generally treated by a combination of retroperitoneal lymph node dissection and platinum-based chemotherapy. Testicular cancer is usually diagnosed as either a painful or painless testicular mass whose presence is confirmed by scrotal ultrasound. The patient undergoes a workup that includes preoperative measurement of the serum markers alpha-fetoprotein and beta-human chorionic gonadotropin. The patient undergoes an inguinal orchiectomy, and the histologic diagnosis is established. Staging studies include evaluation of the lungs, abdominal and pelvic CT scans, and repeat of the serum markers. Patients with seminomas are usually treated with radiation therapy to the ipsilateral para-aortic lymphatics, whereas those with nonseminomatous germ cell tumors are either observed, undergo chemotherapy, or undergo retroperitoneal lymph node dissection, depending on the clinical stage of the disease. The extent and type of dissection depends on the preoperative staging of the disease and is more extensive when there is evidence of grossly enlarged lymph nodes. The dissection is also technically more complicated if the patient has had previous chemotherapy. The exact type of chemotherapeutic regimen is important to know for appropriate perioperative management. Patients previously treated with bleomycin may have compromised pulmonary function due to fibrosis and are at an increased risk for developing adult respiratory distress syndrome (ARDS). To prevent this frequently fatal complication, extreme care must be exercised in the intra- and postoperative periods, patients must not be overhydrated, and the inspired oxygen concentration should not exceed 30 to 40%. Pulmonary function tests should precede any operative procedures performed when such patients are under general anesthesia, and central venous pressure monitoring is advised.

Few surgical complications are associated with retroperitoneal lymph node dissections. The procedure may involve extensive mobilization of the small intestine and colon; therefore, it is not unexpected to encounter ileus for 3 to 4 days following the operation. There may be intraoperative blood loss from the lumbar or renal vessels during the aortic or vena caval dissection, and unsecured bleeders may also result in delayed bleeding during the postoperative period. The procedure involves ligation of the inferior mesenteric artery and the spinal arteries behind the aorta; however, atherosclerotic artery disease is rare in this young age group and there have been no reports of bowel or spinal ischemia reported as the consequence of the operation. Chylous ascites, a consequence of persistent lymphatic drainage, is a rare complication manifested by marked abdominal distention, prolonged ileus, and persistent drainage through the incision site. Bed rest, diuretics, and parenteral nutrition will generally resolve the condition. In extreme cases, however, reoperation with identification and ligation of the draining lymphatics may be indicated.

ICU Care

Although limited retroperitoneal dissections for low volume disease in otherwise healthy patients may not necessitate critical care, patients with pulmonary or other systemic compromise, and those with extensive dissection of bulky disease involving major blood vessels and abdominal viscera may benefit from cardiovascular monitoring and respiratory care. Sudden hypotension, tachycardia, and increased peritoneal signs may suggest the presence of delayed intra-abdominal hemorrhage and lead to reexploration. Bowel obstruction, and unrecognized injury to retroperitoneal organs may also be evident during hospitalization in the ICU. The majority of patients, however, are expected to have an uneventful hospital course, and when it is evident that they have stabilized, they may be transferred to the regular nursing floor.

Post-ICU Care

One of the major concerns following recovery from retroperitoneal lymph node dissection is the preservation of fertility. The procedure disrupts the thoracolumbar sympathetic innervation to the seminal vesicles, vas deferens, ejaculatory ducts, bladder neck and prostatic urethra which results in failure of seminal emission, bladder neck closure, and ejaculation. Antegrade ejaculation can be improved by alpha-sympathomimetic medication, and modifications of the surgical technique in selected cases can result in preservation of the innervation at least on one side. Some patients elect to donate semen for cryopreservation prior to surgery, although evidence suggests that semen quality in patients with testicular cancer is deficient. Patients may require additional therapy following recovery from surgery. The need for further chemotherapy is usually determined by the presence of viable tumor in the pathologic specimen. Occasionally, radiation therapy may also have a role in the treatment of nonseminomatous germ cell malignancies. The overall survival is favorable (76%), even for advanced disease.[21]

KIDNEY SURGERY

Pre-ICU Phase

Renal surgery may be performed for benign or malignant disease and may involve removal of part of a kidney, an entire kidney, or both kidneys. Common indications for renal surgery include:

- Stone disease
- Obstruction
- Trauma
- Bleeding
- Infection
- Malignant disease
- Renovascular hypertension
- Renal donation
- Congenital abnormalities

The goal of surgery is usually the treatment of an abnormal area with preservation of as much function as safely possible. Table 42-3 lists many of the common renal procedures and their indications. The type of operation performed, and the surgical approach to the kidney depends on the indications for the surgery, the extent of the disease, and surgeon preference. Common open surgical approaches to the kidney include flank and retroperitoneal exposure, anterior transperitoneal approach, and thoracoabdominal access. Depending on the indications, the operation may involve resection of ribs, adjacent organs such as the spleen, ipsilateral adrenal gland, liver or colon, regional lymph nodes, vena caval thrombus which may extend as high as the right atrium, ureter, and part of the bladder. Patients may be hospitalized in the ICU following renal surgery if the magnitude of the operation and their overall medical condition require hemodynamic monitoring, or for the management of complications specifically associated with kidney surgery, such as deterioration of renal function or adrenal insufficiency. Some complications may occur after any surgical procedure, including cerebrovascular accidents, myocardial infarction, congestive heart failure, pulmonary embolism, thrombophlebitis, atelectasis, pneumonia, wound infection, and urinary in-

Table 42-3. Renal Surgery

Procedure	Indications
Radical nephrectomy	Renal cell cancer
Nephroureterectomy	Transitional cell cancer of ureter or kidney
Partial nephrectomy/enucleation	Tumor in solitary kidney, poor renal function
Bench surgery	Technical limitations on partial nephrectomy
Bilateral nephrectomy	Bilateral renal tumors, polycystic kidney disease
Extracorporeal shock wave lithotripsy	Renal stone disease
Percutaneous nephrolithotomy	Renal stone disease
Pyelolithotomy	Renal stone disease
Anatrophic nephrolithotomy	Renal stone disease
Simple nephrectomy	Symptomatic nonfunctional kidney infection, bleeding, kidney stone disease, xanthogranulomatous pyelonephritis, obstruction, transplant donation
Pyeloplasty	Ureteropelvic junction obstruction
Renovascular reconstruction	Renovascular hypertension
Renal biopsy	Renal failure

fection. Other complications may be more specific and may relate to the type of renal surgery performed and the particular surgical approach.

Radical Nephrectomy

Radical nephrectomy is the procedure of choice for the treatment of renal cell cancer (RCC) and implies the en bloc removal of the kidney and adrenal gland intact within Gerota's fascia, followed by a regional lymphadenectomy. There are approximately 30,000 newly diagnosed cases of RCC annually.[1] Most of the disease is sporadic, however numerous familial cases of RCC has been reported, and the malignancy is found at a high rate among patients with von Hippel-Lindau disease.[22] RCC is twice as common in males than females, and is much more common in smokers. Two thirds of patients present with advanced or metastatic disease, and over half of those presenting with localized disease eventually develop metastases. Hematuria, flank pain, and a palpable mass are common presenting signs. The treatment of localized disease is surgery; metastatic disease has no effective treatment modality available, and regardless of treatment, the 5-year survival is less than 10% with a median survival of 8 months. Immunotherapy appears to be a promising experimental technique for the management of metastatic disease; however, the protocols are toxic and only highly selected patients have benefited to date.[23] Therefore, the goal of surgery is to remove the tumor prior to the development of metastatic disease. Surgery is offered to patients with localized disease, but rarely to patients with metastatic disease. Patients are radiologically staged to identify the presence of metastatic disease and to determine the extent of surgery required. Knowledge of the location and size of the tumor, and the presence and extent of tumor thrombus in the vena cava is essential for the proper planning of the operative procedure. Large upper pole tumors are frequently approached through a thoracoabdominal incision, which may be either extrapleural, or transpleural, and following closure, a chest tube may be left in place to drain the chest. Vena caval involvement occurs in about 4 to 10% of patients, usually associated with right-sided lesions. Tumor involvement is manifested by the presence of an intraluminal tumor thrombus, but actual invasion of the wall of the vena cava is rare. Accurate determination of the extent of the thrombus by CT scan, MRI, ultrasound, and/or vena cavogram is essential because thrombi limited to the infrahepatic cava can be managed usually by gaining control of the vena cava and its collateral vessels above and below the thrombus with tourniquets, followed by opening of the cava, removal of the thrombus, and closure of the vessel. If the caval thrombus extends more proximally, however, particularly if it reaches into the right atrium, a much more extensive operation is required, including hypothermia, circulatory arrest, and cardiopulmonary bypass. Invasion of the wall of the vena cava is treated by cavectomy, and if extensive, major vascular reconstruction may be required.

Bilateral renal tumors occur in 2% of sporadic RCC patients, but are usually the manifestation of the disease in von Hippel-Lindau patients who have multifocal malignant disease. Treatment of bilateral RCC includes bilateral nephrectomy, partial nephrectomy on one side or another, and enucleation. The tumors frequently recur and multiple operations may be necessary.

Partial Nephrectomy

Indications for partial nephrectomy are tumor in a solitary kidney, tumor in patient with a poorly functioning contralateral kidney, bilateral renal tumors, and occasionally benign renal disease such as a symptomatic, nonfunctional duplication. Renal arteriography should be performed in the preoperative period to delineate the precise vascular anatomy. Vascular control must be established and the kidney is cooled with ice saline during the period of ischemia which should be limited as much as possible. When the operation is done for a malignant tumor, a safe margin of normal parenchyma should be resected with the tumor, regardless whether a partial nephrectomy or an enucleation is done. Following excision of the diseased segment, the collecting system of the kidney must be closed with great care to avoid formation of a urinary fistulas. If an in situ partial nephrectomy is not possible to perform due to the location of the tumor, a nephrectomy, ex vivo dissection of the tumor (bench surgery), with consequent autotransplantation of the kidney may be indicated. Because this is a technically demanding procedure with a low probability of achieving the desired preservation of renal function, the procedure is rarely indicated.

Bilateral Nephrectomy

Bilateral nephrectomy is the treatment of choice for patients with bilateral renal tumors and renal failure. The procedure is also offered to patients with polycystic kidney disease who develop hematuria, infection, or less frequently, in preparation for renal transplantation. In order to avoid the need for permanent replacement of glucocorticoids and mineralocorticoids, every effort should be made to preserve at least one adrenal gland in all patients undergoing bilateral nephrectomy.

Nephroureterectomy

Transitional cell cancer (TCC) of the renal pelvis accounts for 8% of kidney tumors and for 5% of all urothelial tumors.[11] It is even more unusual to find TCC in the ureter. Both disease entities are most common in the 50- to 70-year age group, and males outnumber females 2:1. Phenacetin abuse, Balkan nephropathy, and history of smoking have been associated with TCC.[25] Gross hematuria is the most common presentation of TCC in the renal pelvis or ureter, and the lesion appears as a negative filling defect on intravenous urogram. The tumors are often multifocal, 5% to 10% are bilateral, and over 30% of patients will eventually develop associated bladder cancer. The incidence of recurrence in the bladder is particularly high if an adequate margin of bladder surrounding the ipsilateral ureteral orifice is not removed at the time of surgery. Therefore, the procedure of choice for all high grade transitional cell cancers of the renal pelvis and ureter is radical nephroureterectomy with excision of the periureteral bladder cuff.

Treatment of Kidney Stones

With the major advances in technology, the treatment of kidney stones has experienced marked changes during the last decade. Until approximately 10 years ago, most symptomatic renal lithiasis was treated by open surgery, such as pyelolithotomy or anatrophic nephrolithotomy. Stones which were associated with nonfunctional renal segments were managed by nephrectomy or partial nephrectomy. Today, most kidney stones are treated by extracorporeal shock wave lithotripsy (ESWL) or percutaneous nephrolithotomy (PCNL), and open surgery is rarely performed. The advent of the less invasive procedures decreased the incidence of complications and ICU management is rarely required following the treatment of renal calculi.

Simple Nephrectomy

When removal of the kidney is required for benign diseases such as kidney stone disease, infection, chronic pyelonephritis, xanthogranulomatous pyelonephritis, obstruction, or donor nephrectomy, the kidney is usually approached extraperitoneally, Gerota's fascia may be entered, and the adrenal gland is preserved. These operations are usually easier to perform from a technical standpoint, however, if the underlying pathology such as infection or renal abscess is associated with immunosuppression or diabetes, the patient may represent postoperative management difficulties. Most renal infections, such as pyelonephritis, are self-limiting processes with appropriate antibiotic treatment, and do not require surgical intervention, however the combination of immunosuppression of any type, obstruction to the free flow of urine, and infection, with or without kidney stone disease, requires the establishment of prompt drainage and broad spectrum antibiotic coverage in order to avoid the untoward complications of sepsis and rapid deterioration. While percutaneous placement of a nephrostomy tube may relieve the obstruction, if adequate drainage cannot be established, or if an abscess cannot be adequately drained, the kidney has to be explored, and the decision to preserve the renal unit or perform a nephrectomy must be made based on the prevailing clinical picture. Xanthogranulomatous pyelonephritis is a chronic infectious/inflammatory condition most common in diabetic patients in association with renal calculus disease. Acute manifestations of the disease include fever, flank pain, pyuria, and signs of early sepsis. More chronic varieties may mimic the appearance of RCC. Because the disease process involves all or most of the kidney, nephrectomy is the usual treatment of choice.

Other Renal Operations

Urologists perform many other types of kidney operations, however the potential risks, complications, and management challenges are similar to the surgeries previously mentioned. Important aspects of renal transplantation and renovascular reconstruction are presented elsewhere.

ICU Phase

As is the case with most surgical procedures, patients with renal surgery are admitted into the ICU monitoring or for management of particular problems and complications. Specific management problems in the ICU may include:

- Hemorrhage
- Adrenal insufficiency
- Renal failure
- Prolonged urine leak, urinary fistulas
- Pneumothorax
- Occult GI injury

Hemorrhage

Bleeding complications following ESWL are rare, and if present, the bleeding is usually confined to and limited by Gerota's fascia. Bleeding complications following renal biopsy, nephrostomy tube placement, or open renal surgery may be immediate in the postoperative period, or may be delayed, but in either case, must be recognized and treated promptly.

When a nephrostomy tube is present, blood can often be seen as it comes through the nephrostomy tube. Clamping of the tube, or replacement with a larger caliber tube may help to tamponade the bleeding. If this is unsuccessful, selective angiographic embolization of the bleeding vessel may control the hemorrhage, otherwise prompt exploration, and possible nephrectomy may be required.

In the absence of a nephrostomy tube or a drain to alert the ICU physician to the presence of bleeding, the presenting clinical signs, physical examination, and a precise knowledge of the patient's recent medical history must be considered to make the diagnosis, and rapid intervention is mandatory. Hemorrhage is manifested by rapid onset of hypotension and shock, flank pain, increase in the girth of the abdomen, positive peritoneal signs, and development of a flank mass. This type of massive bleeding usually originates from the renal vasculature, however it may also be a consequence of unrecognized injury to an adjacent structure such as the spleen, liver, tail of the pancreas, or mesentery. Bleeding may be the consequence of an unligated renal collateral blood vessel, an uncontrolled lumbar vein, or an incompletely resected adrenal gland. Secondary bleeding may be delayed, occur even weeks following the procedure, as in cases of ruptured pseudoaneurysm of the renal artery or one of its branches. Fluid resuscitation and blood replacement should be immediately implemented. If the patient can be stabilized, angiography to identify the bleeding site, and possible infarction can be considered; however, the unstable patient should be surgically explored. In most cases, it is advisable to reopen the patient, evacuate the hematoma, and control the site of bleeding.

Adrenal Insufficiency

Adrenal insufficiency may result from the surgical excision of a solitary or bilateral adrenal glands during a nephrectomy. While every attempt is made to preserve functional adrenal tissue during such renal procedures, occasionally the location of the tumor(s) or intraoperative technical difficulties preclude the preservation of sufficient adrenal tissue to provide the necessary function. A single adrenal gland may be removed without the need for consequent hormone replacement provided there is a contralateral functioning gland present. Only 20% of functional adrenal mass is required to maintain normal plasma cortisol levels.[26] In patients who have underlying adrenal insufficiency, perioperative corticosteroids are administered for all surgical interventions and may need additional replacement in the ICU under increasingly stressful situations. Our discussion here is specifically limited to those ICU patients who had either intentional or incidental removal of all adrenal tissue. Patients who have normally functioning adrenal glands preoperatively and who undergo bilateral or solitary adrenalectomy require 100 mg of hydrocortisone intravenously during surgery and every 6 hours thereafter in the postoperative period. Eventually, a daily maintenance of 20 to 30 mg of oral cortisol in divided doses is usually sufficient; however, patients and their physician should be aware of the need to increase the dosage during periods of stress.[27] Mineralocorticoid replacement is usually unnecessary in this patient population, however, if needed, daily doses of 0.1 mg oral fluorocortisol may be administered. Inadequate replacement of adrenocortical hormones may lead to adrenal crisis, which if not properly treated, can be fatal. Acute adrenal insufficiency is characterized by lethargy, mental status changes, fever, abdominal pain, nausea, vomiting, dehydration, tachycardia, and hypotension that may rapidly progress to shock. In the early postoperative period, many of these signs may be ascribed to other, more frequent causes, so a high index of suspicion must be present to make the appropriate diagnosis. Laboratory studies may suggest evidence of hyponatremia and hyperkalemia. Immediate intervention should consist of high bolus of hydrocortisone replacement followed by continuous intravenous infusion for 24 to 36 hours before attempts are made to taper the dosage. At the same time, fluid resuscitation with isotonic saline and glucose solutions should be initiated and the patient may benefit from the administration of vasopressors. Once the patient is stabilized, the cause of increased stress, such as sepsis, which may have caused otherwise adequate levels of corticosteroid replacement to become insufficient, should be sought.

Renal Failure

Some impairment of renal function is expected anytime the kidney is manipulated, incised, subjected to warm or cold ischemia, or removed. The better the original renal function, particularly that of the contralateral kidney, the less pronounced the impairment. Living related renal transplant donors, who presumably have a healthy kidney on the other side, almost always show a transient elevation in their serum creatinine, but return to baseline function a few weeks after surgery.[28,29] On the other hand, patients undergoing partial nephrectomy often have absent or decreased renal function on the opposite side and cannot compensate as well. Acute tubular necrosis (ATN) may be the consequence of manipulation of the kidney and of prolonged ischemia time. ATN is characterized by low urine output, increasing azotemia, and electrolyte abnormalities which include hyperkalemia. Severe and prolonged ATN may have to be managed by temporary hemodialysis, but most patients ultimately recover sufficient renal function not to require it permanently. Of course, dialysis is expected for patients undergoing bilateral nephrectomy, and should be provided in the ICU during the postoperative period. Some of these patients may eventually become candidates for renal transplantation.

Patients undergoing anatrophic nephrolithotomy, partial nephrectomy, bench surgery with autotransplantation, or renovascular procedures that require manipulation and clamping of the renal vessels have an increased incidence of vascular thrombosis of the renal pedicle. A technetium renal flow scan will suggest the diagnosis of arterial occlusion and can be confirmed with a renal angiogram. Once the diagnosis is established, reexploration for thrombectomy may be attempted, however, this desperate procedure is rarely successful in recovering renal function.

Postrenal obstruction must also be considered in the differential diagnosis of anuria and renal function deterioration in a solitary kidney. The presence of blood clot in the renal pelvis or a residual stone obstructing the ureter must be overcome by instrumentation. Renal ultrasonography, which can even be performed at bedside, is a useful diagnostic modality to differentiate the causes of anuria.

Although the foregoing complications must be considered in the postoperative patient with decreased urine output and renal function, other, much more common causes should not be discounted. Hypotension, dehydration, and the use of nephrotoxic agents may all cause a similar clinical picture, and should be considered in the differential diagnosis. The goal of the ICU management of these patients should be to avoid any circumstances which may deplete the already diminished renal function, and to provide the monitoring and correction of electrolyte abnormalities resulting from renal failure.

Urinary Leak and Fistulas

A common postoperative complication, seen in 10 to 15% of partial nephrectomies and less frequently following pyelolithotomies or anatrophic nephrolithotomies is persistent urinary drainage from the wound and cutaneous fistula formation. The condition usually results from inadequate closure of the collecting system. Even large areas of leakage are expected to close spontaneously in the postoperative period, except when infection or residual obstruction is present. Should there be evidence of obstruction to the normal anatomic drainage pattern of the system, this situation has to be overcome before resolution of the nephrocutaneous fistula can be expected. Infection should be treated, and the obstruction may be overcome by placement of a ureteral stent; however, occasionally operative intervention is needed for satisfactory resolution of the complication.

Pneumothorax and Chest Tube Management

Pneumothorax in the postoperative period is usually the consequence of an unrecognized surgical complication, the inadequate pleural closure of a thoracoabdominal incision, or due to the presence of an air leak despite an intraoperatively placed chest tube. It may be diagnosed incidentally on the postoperative chest radiograph, or may be suspected due to the presence of symptoms. A small pneumothorax that does not increase on serial radiographs may be observed, a larger pneumothorax may first be treated with catheter aspiration; however, a more extensive process should be treated by chest tube placement. Chest tubes placed during surgery are usually removed 24 to 48 hours following the operation, if the lung is fully expanded and there is no air leak while off suction, if there is less than 100 ml drainage during the last 24 hours, and if the patient is not on a ventilator with high inspiratory pressures that would increase the risk of a spontaneous pneumothorax.

Gastrointestinal Complications

Although the gastrointestinal tract is not formally entered during the course of renal procedures, occasionally extensive mobilization may be required. Postoperative ileus is not unusual depending on the type of surgery performed, and patients may require nasogastric suctioning in the immediate postoperative period. Unrecognized injury to the gastrointestinal tract is rare. Cases of colonic injuries have been reported following PCNL; however, most of these spontaneously resolved after removal of the nephrostomy tube. Some enterocolic fistulas present late in the postoperative course, and these require surgical resection. Colonic or duodenal injury may occur during exposure of larger renal tumors; however, careful dissection should avoid this problem altogether. Abscess formation due to occult gastrointestinal injury usually presents with fever, elevated white count, prolonged ileus, and abdominal pain. Other sources of the fever are generally ruled out, and CT scan may demonstrate the nature of the problem. Percutaneous drainage is usually not sufficient, and open surgical drainage with resection of the involved bowel segment may have to be performed.

Another untoward complication of resection of large left sided tumors may be an injury to the tail of the pancreas. The injury usually manifests itself in the postoperative period with the onset of nausea, vomiting, abdominal pain, and a clinical picture consistent with pancreatitis. Usually, the process is self-limiting, provided the patient ingests nothing by mouth, although extreme cases may result in the formation of a pancreatic fistula. Given sufficient time, the fistula will close; however, these patients should be started on hyperalimentation. Necrosis of the tail of the pancreas, abscess formation, and recurrent problems related to unresolving fistulas may necessitate reoperation.

Splenectomy is occasionally necessary if there is an injury to the splenic capsule during mobilization of the left kidney, usually in course of surgery for a larger upper pole tumor. The approximate incidence of splenectomy associated with radical nephrectomies is 2 to 4% in most series. There has been concern regarding the potential for overwhelming pneumococcal sepsis following splenectomy in all patients, but particularly in the pediatric population. In adults, it is estimated that splenectomy increases the risk of dying from sepsis 520 times over the normal population.[30] It is therefore recommended that patients who have undergone splenectomy be given pneumococcal vaccine within 2 weeks of splenectomy, and this should take place while the patient is in the ICU.

Post-ICU Phase

Most patients after uncomplicated renal surgery can be transferred out of the critical care unit after 24 to 48 hours. Those with transient azotemia following nephrectomy, or partial nephrectomy, usually recover their renal function in a few weeks after their operation, depending on the amount of parenchyma remaining, however, as little as one fourth or one third of a kidney remaining can sustain a patient off dialysis. Patients with renal calculus disease need further workup to prevent recurrence of the nephrolithiasis. The recovered stone fragments are submitted for analysis and together with information from a consequent metabolic workup, a data base will be established that can be used for future recommendations. Depending on the type of metabolic abnormalities identified, modifications in life style may be recommended which may include improved hydration, dietary changes, or medical therapy.

Patients treated for transitional cancer of the upper urinary tract require close follow-up and evaluation for tumor recurrence in the opposite kidney or ureter, or in the urinary bladder. Our usual follow-up includes cystoscopic evaluation every 3 months for the first year, and every 6 months for the next 2 years before changing to annual examinations. In addition, radiologic evaluation of the contralateral kidney and ureter is performed annually. Patients with RCC require similar close follow-up with evaluation for local recurrence, recurrence in the opposite kidney, or at a distal metastatic site. Patients with positive lymph node involvement have a better than 50% chance for developing metastatic disease within 3 years. Those treated by a partial nephrectomy should be evaluated for local recurrence, however the prognosis is good, provided the final pathology report revealed adequate margins for the specimen.

The long-term prognosis for patients undergoing unilateral nephrectomy is good, the incidence of hypertension is no greater than in the general population, and the only dietary restriction that is suggested is the decrease of protein intake. Patients who experienced an undrained perinephric hematoma in the postoperative period may have a higher incidence of hypertension in the future, however.

TRANSURETHRAL PROSTATECTOMY

Pre-ICU Phase

Transurethral prostatectomy (TURP) is the most common surgical procedure performed by urologists. Although the mortality of TURP is less than 0.2%, the procedure does have an 18% morbidity in the immediate postoperative period,[31,32] and some of these conditions are significant enough to warrant care in the ICU. TURP is one of several alternatives available to treat bladder outlet obstruction due to the enlarged prostate. Symptoms that result in initiation of the urologic workup usually include the decreased caliber and force of the urine stream, hesitancy, dribbling, frequency, urgency, urinary tract infections, and urinary retention. Objective evidence for bladder outlet obstruction includes the presence of a low urinary flow rate in the face of normal or elevated bladder pressures, and high post-void residual urine volume.

The following options are available to treat the underlying disorder:

- Continued observation
- Catheter placement (Foley catheter or suprapubic tube)
- Medical management
- Balloon dilatation of the prostatic urethra
- Transurethral incision of the prostate
- Transurethral resection of the prostate
- Suprapubic prostatectomy
- Laser prostatectomy

The choice of treatment depends on patient and physician preference, issues of general medical condition, and size of the gland. As with so many other urologic conditions, bladder outlet obstruction is a disease of the elderly, and may be found in association with multiple medical ailments. In fact, 77% of the patients have significant preexisting medical problems.[31] Candidates for the procedure should undergo a comprehensive medical examination, should have correction of abnormalities identified, should be off all anticoagulants, and should have sterile urine. Patients are covered with prophylactic antibiotics started 1 hour prior to resection and continued for 48 hours following the procedure. The operation may be done under spinal or general anesthesia, although there seems to be less bleeding seen in association with spinal anesthesia.[14]

Transurethral prostatectomy is performed with a resectoscope introduced through the urethra. Visibility is maintained by irrigation with glycine, a near isotonic, nonhemolytic irrigant. The use of sterile water is generally avoided because of the risk of intravascular hemolysis if the fluid gets absorbed. Electric current through the resectoscope is responsible for the ability to circumferentially cut away the prostate tissue, and achieve hemostasis at the same time. Initially, the curettings flow into the bladder, but ultimately they are irrigated out and submitted to pathology. A Foley catheter, usually with a three-way system of bladder irrigation to keep the catheter patent is placed at the conclusion of the case, and is to be removed once the patient's urine is cleared. The length of the procedure is influenced by the size of the gland and is directly related to the morbidity resulting from TURP. Age and preexisting medical problems are other independent variables in the determination of risk.

ICU Phase

Certain untoward events may necessitate placement of the TURP patient in the ICU. The three most common complications are:

- Perforation
- Excessive hemorrhage
- "Post-TURP syndrome"

Although in many instances these complications can be managed with relative ease without utilization of the ICU, the combination of the physiologic instability which results from these complications superimposed on underlying medical problems may necessitate admission to the ICU.

Perforations

Small perforations of the prostatic capsule frequently occur during resection and are of no significance, provided the resection is terminated in a reasonable period. Large perforations of the prostate or of the bladder are usually detected by the onset of restlessness, nausea, vomiting, and abdominal pain despite spinal anesthesia, hypertension, respiratory changes, abdominal rigidity, and poor return of the irrigation fluid. A cystogram can confirm and demonstrate the perforation; however, this is a clinical emergency that should be treated by termination of the procedure and placement of a urinary drainage catheter. Patients with extravesical perforations may be either treated with Foley catheter drainage alone or by placement of suprapubic drains, depending on the extent of the extravasation, but intraperitoneal perforations should be explored and closed. Following the operation, patients may need to be observed in the ICU to monitor and correct the hemodynamic and electrolyte disorders. The patients may be discharged from the ICU once these parameters stabilize, and with prolonged catheter drainage for 5 to 10 days, the condition is usually self-limiting.

Hemorrhage

Intractable hemorrhage usually results from incomplete resection of the prostatic adenoma and may be either arterial or venous in origin. Arterial bleeders require meticulous hemostasis for adequate control, and the bleeding often originates in the anterior prostatic fossae. Large bleeding venous sinuses are much harder to coagulate, but these usually respond to traction by the inflated Foley catheter. Care must be taken to inflate the balloon adequately so that it places pressure on the bladder neck and does not itself slip into the resected prostatic fossae, because this can prevent collapse of the sinusoids. Patients with intractable bleeding may need to be explored, the residual adenoma removed, and the bladder packed for hemostasis. Predisposing risk factors for increased bleeding may include failure to stop or reverse the effects of anticoagulants, recent prostate infection, or irritation due to an indwelling drainage catheter. The role of the ICU in management of patients with this complication includes hemodynamic monitoring and adequate blood replacement, and vigilance to keep the catheter from developing clot obstruction. The risk of this latter event can be minimized by frequent catheter irrigation, or the use of continuous through-and-through bladder irrigation.

Post-TURP Syndrome

The most serious sequela of transurethral prostatectomy is the the post-TURP syndrome, the consequence of excessive absorption of irrigation fluid into the systemic vasculature. The patient presents either during the resection, or in the immediate postoperative period with hypertension, tachycardia, and mental status changes. Cardiovascular collapse, convulsions, and coma may develop in extreme cases. Onset of these signs should immediately alert the physician to check the electrolytes, because severe hyponatremia, sodium values below 120 mEq/L may be present and require immediate treatment. Although the occurrence of this complication usually correlates with the length (greater than one hour) and magnitude (greater than 80 to 100 g resected tissue) of the resection, rapid fluid absorption may take place within a short period if large venous sinuses open up. Patients with dilutional hyponatremia require close observation and monitoring of blood pressure, cardiac status, hematologic status, renal function and serum values of potassium, serum osmolality, and plasma sodium. Treatment includes the use of diuretics, and slow gradual infusion of hypertonic saline (3% NaCl). Rapid correction of the problem is almost as dangerous as the underlying disorder itself. Once the electrolyte abnormality is corrected and the patient's symptoms have resolved, discharge from the ICU may be implemented.

Post-ICU Phase

Once the adverse complications resolve, postoperative recovery is usually uneventful. Unless the presence of known perforation indicates the need for prolonged catheterization, the Foley catheter is usually removed in 2 to 3 days once the urine becomes free of blood. The patients need to avoid any strenuous exercise for 3 to 4 weeks. The patients should be fully continent and there should be no change in sexual potency, with the exception of the onset of retrograde ejaculation. Irritative symptoms of bladder outlet obstruction (urgency/frequency) may not resolve immediately after surgery. Moreover, approximately 10 to 15% of transurethral resection specimens reveal evidence of carcinoma, and these patients will require further workup and treatment.

SCROTAL GANGRENE

Pre-ICU Phase

Gangrene of the scrotum is a potentially life-threatening, rapid-onset, fulminant necrosis that most commonly affects debilitated, immunosuppressed individuals, such as those with diabetes, cancer, long-standing alcoholism, or other chronic diseases. Although the most popularized form of this disease is idiopathic necrotizing fasciitis, Fournier's gangrene, the process may start out as an infected urethral stricture, perirectal abscess, severe epididymitis, cellulitis, or an infected hair follicle. With an extremely rapid progression, the scrotum becomes erythematous, edematous, tense, painful, and warm. Fluctuation develops with crepitance and emphysema of the tissues rapidly spreading along fascial planes to involve the penis, and anterior abdominal wall. There is clear evidence of progressive sepsis and unless rapid intervention is initiated, high fever, decreased vascular resistance, hypotension, tachycardia sets in and the patient expires from sepsis. The microbiologic features of the disease include hemolytic staphylococci, streptococci, and anaerobic gas-forming organisms.

The most important aspect of management is rapid recognition of the clinical picture and prevention of the spread of the disease. Patients must be immediately started on broad-spectrum antibiotics offering both aerobic and anaerobic coverage, and the patient must be taken to the operating room for wide debridement of all involved areas until nothing but unequivocally healthy tissue is reached. Usually, the entire scrotal skin is necrotic and requires excision, and depending on the extent of the gangrene, the penile skin may need to be excised as well. Urinary diversion should be achieved by suprapubic catheter placement.

ICU Phase

Most patients arrive to the ICU directly from the operating room following wide debridement of scrotal, penile, and possibly abdominal skin. The intensive antibiotic therapy initiated prior to surgery must be continued. The role of hyperbaric oxygen therapy is more controversial. The combination of increased pressure and respiratory intake of 100% oxygen increases arterial oxygen content and will theoretically inactivate anaerobic organisms and their toxin production, provided adequate debridement has been implemented.[33] The role of this therapy in addition to antibiotics and surgery is unproven, treatment of the critically ill patient in hyperbaric chambers is cumbersome, and the applicability of the therapy is limited by a lack of availability in the community setting, however.

Upon arrival to the ICU, patient and ICU team have to look forward to prolonged supportive care, including vigorous fluid resuscitation, respiratory support, and vigilant wound care. Patients should be frequently evaluated for appearance of the wound edges and any evidence of gangrene progression. There should be no hesitation in returning the patient to the operating room for further debridement if indicated. Otherwise, local wound care with moist dressings and chemical debridement should be administered to allow healthy granulation and to minimize secondary wound infections. Care must be taken to keep contamination of the perineum by stool incontinence to a minimum. This condition may represent a difficult nursing problem, and placement of a diverting colostomy when the active infection has resolved has been advocated by some clinicians. In our experience, diversion of the gastrointestinal contents has not been required, but it should be considered in particularly difficult cases, or when a perirectal process was responsible for the initiation of the infection. Combination of the underlying morbid status of the patient and the prolonged immobilization during the recovery phase create a high risk for thromboembolic complications, and contribute to the greater than 50% mortality of Fournier's gangrene.

Post-ICU

Once the patient is satisfactorily recovered to be discharged from critical care, treatment of the underlying pathology responsible for onset of the infection needs to be considered, and preparations should be made for providing skin coverage of the debrided areas. The completely denuded testes may initially be placed in a thigh pouch on their respective sides, however ultimately, placement of a split thickness skin graft will be required. Large groin and abdominal wounds too large to close by granulation should be treated similarly. The results are usually satisfactory, and despite complete debridement of the scrotum and penis, an aesthetic and functional result may be achieved.

If the gangrene was due to scrotal wall infection, a perirectal abscess, or if it was idiopathic, the process was probably adequately treated during the primary operative intervention. On the other hand, if urethral stricture disease was responsible for the onset of symptoms, this should be corrected last after complete wound healing.

UROLOGIC CARE OF THE ICU PATIENT

It is not uncommon in the ICU to encounter urologic problems in patients hospitalized for other reasons. The following problems are frequently seen:

- Difficulty placing urethral catheter
- Hematuria
- Anuria
- Urinary tract infections

Catheter Placement

Pre-ICU Phase

Placement of a urinary catheter is essential for accurate fluid monitoring, or if the patient is unable to void. Signs of urinary retention may be suprapubic pain, distension, and inability to empty the bladder. Because catheter placement is considered "routine," it is often the least qualified individual on the team who is assigned the task of catheter placement. The presence of urologic abnormalities, such as urethral stricture disease, prostatic enlargement, or vesical neck contracture may prevent proper placement of the catheter. Misguided persistence and repeated attempts to force the catheter past the obstruction will not only be unsuccessful, but result in iatrogenic injury to the urethra and decrease the chance of future success by more skilled individuals. A single unsuccessful attempt by the most experienced member of the team should result in prompt urologic consultation. A good voiding history and knowledge of the patient's previous urologic symptoms should suggest who may experience difficulties in having catheters placed, and also suggest how to overcome the problem. Unfortunately, such history is not always available from patients during emergency admission to the ICU. The individual who already attempted catheter placement should convey information regarding the type of difficulty encountered, including the site of the obstruction.

Stenosis of the urethral meatus is generally visible on physical examination and may be the consequence of inflammation of the glans penis or is due to prior placement of an oversized catheter or cystoscope. Gonorrheal urethritis and previous urethral procedures, including catheterization, may predispose for stricture development. The most common site of urethral stricture disease is the bulbous urethra. Infrequently, long, irregular urethral strictures are the presenting signs of urethral cancer. Prostatic hyperplasia rarely prevents catheter placement unless the patient has a high elevation of the bladder neck. Vesical neck contracture, which is the result of previous transurethral or open prostatectomy, including radical prostatectomy, may cause obstruction at the level of the prostate gland and bladder neck.

ICU Phase

Stenosis of the urethral meatus can be dilated with a meatal dilator or with incrementally increasing caliber urethral sounds. More proximal obstruction may still be present, however. First, proper lubrication of the urethra must be accomplished. Anesthetic lubricant, such as 2% lidocaine jelly, may be introduced directly into the urethra. Adequate distention of the urethra by these means may be all that is required to pass the catheter past a wide-caliber stricture or an enlarged prostate. Coudet tip catheters with an upwardly angulated tip are suitable to negotiate an obstructing, elevated bladder neck (Fig. 42-1). Urethral strictures and vesical neck contracture may be dilated at the patient's bedside with filiforms and followers (Fig. 42-2), which are soft, flexible, narrow guide stents that can be advanced past the obstruction and are attached to wider and wider dilators suitable to stretch open the obstruction. A catheter guide can provide additional rigidity to a Foley catheter and help advance it past the obstruction, but care must be taken not to injure the urethra.

If the obstruction cannot be overcome by the foregoing methods, the urinary catheter may have to be passed under direct vision. Cystoscopy may be performed at the patient's bedside with a flexible cystoscope, or if the patient's condition is stable, he may be transferred to the cystoscopy suite for rigid cystoscopy. Once the cystoscope is manipulated into the bladder, a guide wire may be advanced through the scope, and a Foley catheter can be passed over the wire. If the cystoscope cannot be advanced into the urinary bladder by any means, placement of a suprapubic catheter should be considered (see Fig. 42-1). A percutaneous approach may be used on distended bladders in patients who have not had lower abdominal surgery in the past (Fig. 42-3). Bedside ultrasound guidance may be helpful if the bladder is not easily palpable. Alternatively, in patients with previous surgery and the potential for adherent bowel in the area, a suprapubic cutdown under local anesthesia can provide for placement of the catheter under direct vision.

Post-ICU Phase

The catheters are left in place until the patient is well enough to undergo urologic evaluation and treatment. The goal of rehabilitation is to reestablish the continuity of the urinary tract. Some of the abnormalities may already be resolved by catheter dilatation alone, in other cases, formal repair may be required. Vesical neck contracture may need

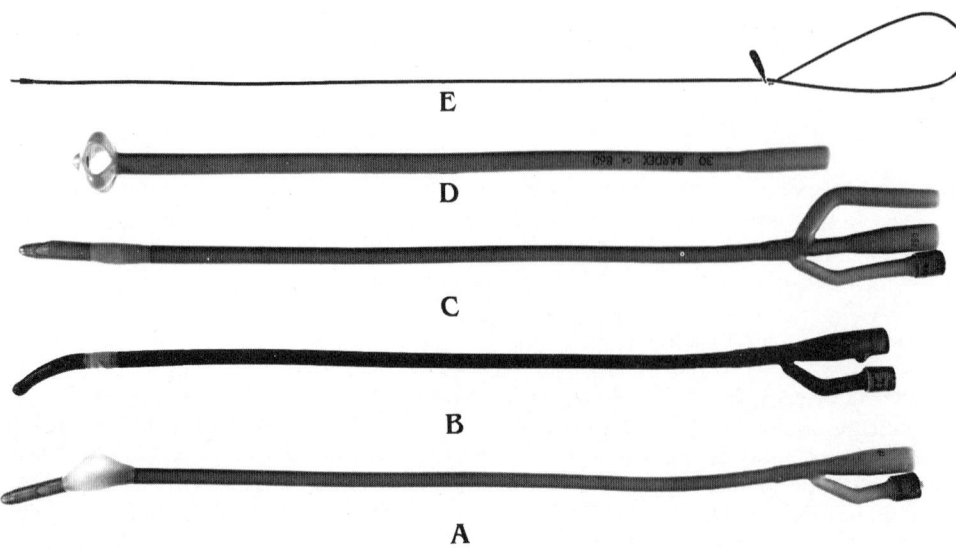

Fig. 42-1. Types of urinary catheters A Standard urethral catheter with a 5-ml balloon. B, Coude tip urethral catheter with angulation at the distal tip. C, Triple-lumen catheter used for continuous irrigation. D, Melecot suprapubic catheter E, Catheter Guide. (A through D, Courtesy of Bard Urological Division, Covington, GA.)

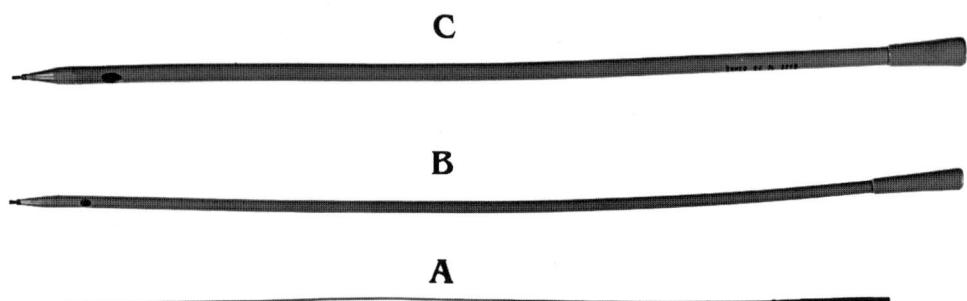

Fig. 42–2. Filiforms and followers. A, Filiforms to be advanced through urethral stricture. B and C, Various increasing caliber followers, which are attached to the filiform and dilate the stricture. (A to C, Courtesy of Bard Urological Division, Covington, GA.)

repeated dilatations; an enlarged prostate may have to be resected.

Hematuria

One of the most frustrating management problems in the ICU is gross hematuria. The hematuria may be due to a urinary tract infection, to hemorrhagic cystitis, to bleeding secondary to coagulopathy, or to previously unsuspected urinary tract abnormalities such as bladder tumors, other malignant urinary tract diseases, or stone disease. Patients with indwelling Foley catheters who have hematologic abnormalities, disseminated intravascular coagulation (DIC), or other coagulopathies may develop hematuria. Hemorrhagic cystitis remains a significant complication after systemic cyclophosphamide[34] or pelvic radiation therapy.[35] The magnitude of the bleeding may range from microscopic hematuria to massive, intractable hemorrhage associated with significant morbidity and, occasionally, death. Although microscopic hematuria or limited bleeding episodes may be observed and worked up after the patient's condition is stable enough to be discharged from the ICU, gross hematuria resulting in anemia, clot retention, or obstruction of the urinary drainage catheter require immediate intervention.

The patient's history and physical examination should suggest the cause of the hematuria. In addition, infections should be treated, existing coagulopathy should be corrected, anticoagulants should be discontinued, and bleeding diathesis should be reversed. DIC should be aggressively managed, and thrombocytopenic patients should be transfused to adequate platelet levels. Inhibition of the fibrinolytic enzyme cascade with epsilon-aminocaproic acid (Amicar) may be effective in some cases. If the patient does not have a urethral catheter in place, a wide-caliber catheter should be advanced into the bladder and any existing blood clots should be irrigated out. If the blood clots are too large to be irrigated out through the catheter, the patient may have to be transferred to cystoscopy for clot evacuation and identification of the bleeding sites. A bleeding bladder tumor may be resected; an arteriovenous fistula can be embolized.

Limited areas of hemorrhagic cystitis may be lightly fulgurated; however, diffuse hemorrhage may need to be treated by continuous irrigation. Initially, saline is the irrigant of choice, but if this does not resolve the bleeding, other, increasingly more toxic solutions may be required. Alum irrigation works by coating the bladder mucosa and binding the areas of bleeding source. Silver nitrate solution works in a similar fashion and has few side effects; however, phenol and particularly formalin are painful to the patient and require anesthesia during infusion. Formalin causes sclerosis of the bladder mucosa that may not only stop the bleeding, but may result in a permanently contracted, fibrotic, small capacity bladder. The presence of ureteral reflux should be ruled out prior to formalin use because permanent scarring and obstruction of the refluxing renal unit may occur. Extremely difficult cases may be managed by supravesical urinary diversion or ligation of the hypogastric arteries.

Anuria

Urology consultation may be obtained in the workup of sudden cessation of urine output, to differentiate urinary obstruction from other causes of acute renal failure. The

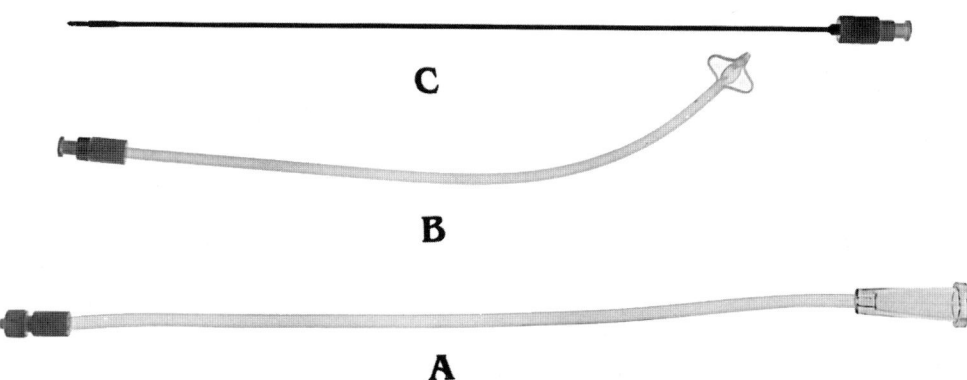

Fig. 42–3. Stamey percutaneous suprapubic catheter set. A, Drainage tube connected to closed bag drainage. B, Suprapubic drainage catheter advanced into the bladder by percutaneous trocar guidance. C, Percutaneous trocar. (A to C, Courtesy of Cook Urological, Spencer, IN.)

most common cause of the lack of urine output in the postoperative patient is severe volume depletion, and the patient is expected to respond to increased fluid administration. Obstruction of the urinary tract should be considered when appropriate fluid management does not improve the urine output, and hemodynamic monitoring suggests that fluid depletion, heart failure, sepsis, or nephrotoxic agents are not responsible for the ATN. Similarly, obstruction may have to be ruled out in a patient who is admitted to the ICU with renal failure of no apparent cause, and for whom no history is available.

Physical examination should include assessing for the presence of an indwelling Foley catheter. If the patient does not have an indwelling catheter, one should be placed. While straight catheterization and removal of the catheter after bladder drainage may be sufficient to assess the presence of urine output, it is advisable to leave the Foley catheter in place until the entire clinical picture is elucidated. If a urethral catheter is in place, but there is no drainage of any urine, the catheter should be irrigated to assess patency and appropriate placement. The presence of a distended bladder and a malfunctioning catheter indicates the need for catheter replacement. On the other hand, an empty bladder with free return of the irrigation fluid suggests that renal or prerenal azotemia, bilateral ureteral obstruction, or obstruction of a solitary renal unit is responsible for the lack of urine output. Bilateral ureteral obstruction may be caused by certain pathologic conditions that are less likely to occur simultaneously than by silent unilateral obstruction followed by the presentation of symptoms when the second side becomes completely obstructed as well. Carcinoma of the prostate may cause bilateral ureteral obstruction at the level of the distal ureter. Pelvic masses, lymphadenopathy, malignant tumors, and retroperitoneal fibrosis may obstruct the ureters at more proximal sites. Bilateral ureteral pelvic junction obstruction should also be considered in the differential diagnosis. Simultaneous obstruction by renal or ureteral calculi is much less likely; however, any of previously mentioned conditions may obstruct a solitary kidney when the other renal unit is absent or nonfunctional. Bladder cancer, ureteral tumors and strictures, and blood clots may also cause obstruction in this clinical setting.

Upper tract obstruction can usually be diagnosed by ultrasonography, which can be performed at the patient's bedside in when the patient's condition is unstable. The expected ultrosonographic finding is hydronephrosis, although we have experienced two cases of obstruction where hydronephrosis was absent. These patients had acute obstruction followed by forniceal rupture and decompression of the renal pelvis. For a more detailed study of the etiology of obstruction, CT may be helpful.

Once obstruction of the upper urinary tract is established as the cause of the anuria, steps must be taken to relieve the blockage temporarily and to reestablish renal function until a permanent solution to the problem can be achieved. Retrograde placement of a ureteral catheter to bypass the obstruction may be accomplished by cystoscopy; however, if the ureteral orifices cannot be identified or cannulated through the bladder, or if the nature of the obstruction is such that it can not be bypassed, alternate procedures are required. A typical ureteral catheter with a guide wire is illustrated in Figure 42-4. If attempts at retrograde placement of a ureteral catheter are unsuccessful, a nephrostomy tube may be introduced into the obstructed renal pelvis through the flank. If bilateral obstruction is present, it is advisable to place the nephrostomy tube in one side only, and allow the patient's condition to stabilize before making any attempts to treat the other side. The side with the better renal function, as assessed radio-

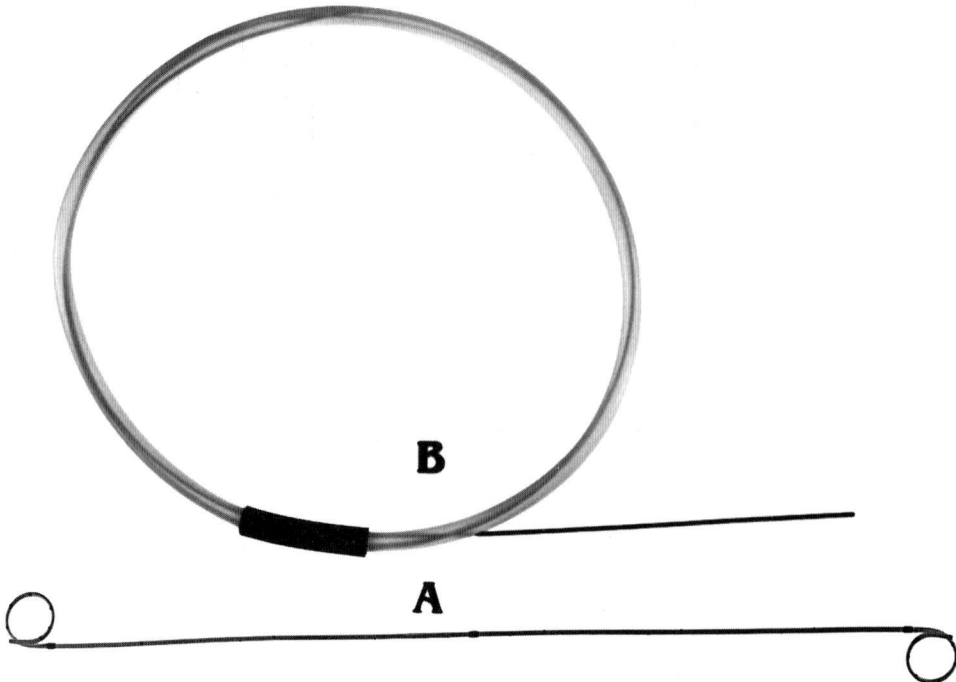

Fig. 42-4. Double pigtail ureteral stent set. *A*, Ureteral stent with proximal end to be placed in the renal pelvis and distal and curled up in the bladder. *B*, Guide wire used for placement. (*A* and *B*, Courtesy of Cook Urological, Spencer, IN.)

logically, should be selected for catheter placement. If this approach does not lead to satisfactory improvement of renal function, a nephrostomy tube should be placed in the other kidney as well. After adequate restoration of renal function and stabilization of the patient, the cause of the urinary tract obstruction can be completely evaluated, and definitive treatment can be planned.

Urinary Tract Infection (UTI)

Nosocomially acquired UTIs represent the most common hospital-acquired infections. The majority of hospital-acquired infections are related to bladder catheterization. Up to 2% of patients have bacteriuria following a single catheterization,[36] and 50% of patients develop UTI after 10 days of catheterization.[37] Because most ICU patients have a Foley catheter, it is not surprising that UTIs represent a major concern in the care of the critically ill patient. The incidence of bacteriuria is proportional to the length of catheterization and is related to catheter care. The best way to minimize the chance of infection is to minimize the period of catheterization. Clean intermittent catheterization is preferable to an indwelling Foley catheter,[38] although it may not be practical in the acute care setting. When use of an indwelling catheter cannot be avoided, as in most cases in the ICU, every attempt should be made to preserve the closed drainage system, which is the single most effective way or reducing the risk of UTI.[39] Other methods to prevent the retrograde spread of bacteria, such as antibiotic ointments applied to the urethral meatus, antibiotic bladder irrigation, or the placement of antiseptic agents into the urine collection bag, have not been effective.[40] Systemic antibiotic prophylaxis may delay the onset of infection. In the long run, however, it contributes to the development of resistant organisms that may be much harder to treat in case of symptomatic infection or sepsis. Antibiotics should ideally be reserved for treatment of symptomatic infections and should be given only for the period needed to eradicate the causative organism.

Patients in the ICU frequently require systemic antibiotics for multiple reasons. The combination of antibiotics and urinary catheters can lead not only to infection by resistant strains of bacteria, but also to fungal infections, most commonly candidiasis. If candida colonizes the urine and the patient is asymptomatic, no therapy is needed, and the problem is often resolved by discontinuating the catheter, antibiotic, or preferably both. On the other hand, if the catheter cannot be removed and the patient is diabetic or otherwise immunocompromised, candiduria may lead to serious systemic infection and treatment is required. Symptomatic candidiasis may be manifested by cystitis, ascending infection and pyelonephritis, fungus ball formation, and systemic dissemination. Candida infection in the bladder that requires treatment can be best managed by amphotericin B irrigation through a triple-lumen catheter, usually for 7 days. Irrigation of the renal pelvis can be accomplished through a nephrostomy tube, if present, and placement of such a tube is indicated if upper urinary tract obstruction develops as a consequence of the fungus infection. Patients with renal parenchymal involvement or evidence of systemic candidiasis require intravenous amphotericin B treatment.

REFERENCES

1. Boring, C. C., Squires, T. S., Tong, T., and Montgomery, S.: Cancer statistics, 1994. CA, *44*:7, 1994.
2. Sheldon, C. A., Williams, R. D., and Fraley, E. E.: Incidental carcinoma of the prostate: a review of the literature and critical reappraisal of classification. J. Urol., *124*:626, 1980.
3. Elder, J. S., and Catalona, W. J.: Management of newly diagnosed metastatic carcinoma of the prostate. Urol. Clin. North Am., *2*:283, 1984.
4. Meyers, R. P., et al.: Hormonal treatment at time of radical retropubic prostatectomy for stage D1 prostate cancer. J. Urol., *130*:99, 1983.
5. Middleton, A. W., Jr.: Pelvic lymphadenectomy with modified radical retropubic prostatectomy as a single operation: technique used and results in 50 consecutive cases. J. Urol., *125*:353, 1981.
6. Zincke, H., et al.: Bilateral pelvic lymphadenectomy and radical retropubic prostatectomy for adenocarcinoma of prostate with regional lymph node involvement. Urology, *19*:238, 1982.
7. Neerhut, G. J., Wheeler, T., Cantini, M., and Scardino, P. T.: Salvage radical prostatectomy for radiorecurrent adenocarcinoma of the prostate. J. Urol., *140*:544, 1988.
8. Wynder, E. L., Onkerdonk, J., and Mantel, N.: An epidemiological investigation of cancer of the bladder. Cancer, *16*:1388, 1963.
9. Brand, K. G.: Schistosomiasis-cancer: etiological considerations: a review. Acta Trop. (Basel), *36*:203, 1979.
10. Pearson, R. M., and Soloway, M. S.: Does cyclophosphamide induce bladder cancer? Urology, *11*:437, 1978.
11. Marshall, V. F., and McCarron, J. P., Jr.: The curability of vesical cancer: greater now or then? Cancer, *37*:2753, 1977.
12. Lieskovsky, G., and Skinner, D. G.: Technique of radical retropubic prostatectomy with limited pelvic node dissection. Urol. Clin. North Am., *10*:187, 1983.
13. Catalona, W. J., Kadmon, D., and Crane, D. B.: Effect of minidose heparin on lymphocele formation following extraperitoneal pelvic lymphadenectomy. J. Urol., *123*:890, 1980.
14. Walsh, P. C.: Radical retropubic prostatectomy. *In* Campbell's Urology. Edited by P. C. Walsh, R. F. Gittes, A. D. Perlmutter and T. A. Stamey. Philadelphia, W. B. Saunders, 1986, p. 2754.
15. De Vere White, R., et al.: Adjunctive therapy with interstitial irradiation for prostate cancer. Urology, *19*:395, 1982.
16. Flocks, R. H.: The treatment of stage C prostatic cancer with special reference to combined surgical and radiation therapy. J. Urol., *109*:461, 1973.
17. Crawford, E. D., and Kiker, J. D.: Radical retropubic prostatectomy. J. Urol., *129*:1145, 1983.
18. Walsh, P. C., and Donker, P. J.: Impotence following radical prostatectomy: insight into etiology and prevention. J. Urol., *128*:492, 1982.
19. Montie, J. R., Straffon, R. A., and Stewart, B. H.: Radical cystectomy without radiation therapy for carcinoma of the bladder. J. Urol., *131*:477, 1984.
20. Skinner, D. G., et al.: The role of adjuvant chemotherapy following cystectomy for invasive bladder cancer: a prospective comparative trial. J. Urol., *145*:459, 1991.
21. Williams, S. D., and Einhorn, L. H.: Chemotherapy of disseminated testicular cancer. *In* Testis Tumors. Edited by J. P. Donohue. Baltimore, Williams & Wilkins, 1983, p. 252.
22. Lauritsen, J. G.: Lindau's disease: a study of one family through six generations. Acta Chir. Scand., *139*:482, 1975.

23. Haas, G. P., Hillman, G. G., Redman, P. G., and Pontes, J. E.: Immunotherapy of renal cell carcinoma. CA Cancer J. Clin., 43:177, 1993.
24. Nocks, B., et al.: Transitional cell carcinoma of renal pelvis. Urology, 107:220, 1972.
25. Petkovic, S., Mutavdzic, M., Petronic, V. L., and Markovic, V.: Tumors of the renal pelvis and ureter: clinical and etiologic studies. J. Urol. Nephrol. (Paris), 77:429, 1971.
26. Hubay, C., Weckesser, E., and Levy, R.: Occult adrenal insufficiency in surgical patients. Ann. Surg., 181:325, 1975.
27. Kehlet, H., Binder, C., and Blichert-Toft, M.: Glucocorticoid maintenance therapy following adrenalectomy: assessment of dosage and preparation. Clin. Endocrinol., 5:37, 1976.
28. Wutherland, D. E. R., et al.: Information and long-term follow-up on a large number of related kidney donors at a single institution. Neth. J. Med., 28:254, 1985.
29. Steckler, R. E., Riehle, A., Jr, and Vaughan, E. D., Jr.: Hyperfiltration-induced renal injury in normal man: myth or reality. J. Urol., 144:1323, 1990.
30. O'Neal, B. J., and McDonald, J. C.: The risk of sepsis in the asplenic adult. Ann. Surg., 194:775, 1981.
31. Mebust, W. K., et al.: Transurethral prostatectomy: immediate and postoperative complications. A cooperative study of 13 participating institutions evaluating 3,885 patients. J. Urol., 141:243, 1989.
32. Holtgrewe, H. L., et al.: Transurethral prostatectomy: practice aspects of the dominant operation in American urology. J. Urol., 141:248, 1989.
33. Baker, D. J.: Hyperbaric oxygen therapy in gas gangrene: experiences and results over a 20 year period. In Seventh International Congress on Hyperbaric Medicine. Edited by S. W. Yefuni. Moscow, Academy of Science, 1982.
34. Donahue, L. A., and Frank, I. N.: Intravesical formalin for hemorrhagic cystitis: analysis of therapy. J. Urol., 141:809, 1989.
35. Liu, Y. K., et al.: Treatment of radiation or cyclophosphamide induced hemorrhagic cystitis using conjugated estrogen. J. Urol., 144:41, 1990.
36. Allo, M., and Simmons, R. L.: Surgical infectious disease and the urologist. Urol. Clin. North Am., 10:131, 1983.
37. Kunin, C. M., and McCormack, R. G.: Prevention of catheter-induced urinary tract infections by sterile closed drainage. N. Engl. J. Med., 274:1155, 1966.
38. Maynard, F. M., and Diokno, A. C.: Clean intermittent catheterization for spinal cord injury patients. J. Urol., 128:477, 1982.
39. Garibaldi, R. A., et al.: Factors predisposing to bacteriuria during indwelling urethral catheterization. N. Engl. J. Med., 291:215, 1974.
40. Burke, J. P., et al.: Prevention of catheter-associated urinary tract infections: efficacy of daily meatal care regimens. Am. J. Med., 70:655, 1981.

Section Five

THE HEMATOLOGIC SYSTEM AND ONCOLOGIC CONSIDERATIONS

Chapter 43

THROMBOTIC THROMBOCYTOPENIC PURPURA AND VARIANTS

STEVEN W. ANDRESEN
RONALD M. BUKOWSKI

Thrombotic thrombocytopenic purpura (TTP) is a rare, multisystem disorder produced by thrombotic occlusion of small vessels. It was first described by Moschcowitz in 1924 and 1925 when he described a young girl with pallor, fever, malaise, and slight paralysis of the upper extremities.[1,2] At autopsy, he found diffuse hyaline thrombi in the arterioles and capillaries and suggested that a powerful toxin that caused agglutination and hyalinization of erythrocytes produced the disease entity. In 1936, Baehr described similar patients with anemia and thrombocytopenia and postulated that the thrombi were composed of fibrin and agglutinated platelets.[3] In 1947, Singer coined the term thrombotic thrombocytopenic purpura.[4] These case reports described the complex clinical entity characterized by the triad of microangiopathic hemolytic anemia, thrombocytopenia, and fluctuating neurologic manifestations caused by small vessel occlusion resulting in tissue infarction. Fever and renal dysfunction are commonly present and complete the classic pentad.

PRE-ICU PHASE
Etiology and Pathogenesis

The etiology of TTP is unknown. It generally is an acute illness and has been associated with infection, toxins, pregnancy, and immunologic disorders. It generally occurs, however, without a discernible antecedent disease. It has been seen during the third trimester of pregnancy and may be difficult to distinguish from preeclampsia or eclampsia.[5] In this setting, fetal compromise is common and likely results from thrombotic occlusion of placental vessels.[6]

TTP has been described in association with autoimmune disorders such as systemic lupus erythematosus (SLE) and rheumatoid arthritis. These descriptions are generally in the form of anecdotal case reports, however, and a specific association between TTP and autoimmune disorders cannot be made.[7-12]

TTP has been associated with the use of drugs such as penicillin,[13] sulfonamides,[14] oral contraceptives,[15] and penicillamine.[16] It is, however, difficult to separate the effect of the medication from that of the underlying disorder for which the medication was prescribed. TTP has been associated with the use of chemotherapeutic agents such as mitomycin C, cisplatin, vinblastine, and bleomycin.[17,18]

The disorder has been reported following hypersensitivity reactions such as to insect bites,[19] and toxic exposures to hydrocarbons.[20] Twenty to 40% of patients with TTP have an antecedent illness suggesting a viral or bacterial infection. A causal relationship between infection and TTP remains elusive, however.[21,22] Table 43-1 summarizes reported clinical associations.

TTP is a rare disorder, occurring in approximately one per million population.[23] Females are affected more commonly than males; no racial preference has been observed, and the peak incidence is in the fourth decade of life.[24,25]

Hematologists agree that the small-vessel thrombi that produce the manifestations of TTP are composed of platelet aggregates and fibrin. The mechanism by which these pathologic events occur remains elusive, however. One theory proposes that endothelial cell damage initiates platelet agglutination. Antibodies cytotoxic to endothelial cells have been isolated in patients with TTP.[26] In addition, hyaline deposits containing only immunoglobulin have been observed in similar patients. Damage to vascular endothelium could produce a deficiency of prostacyclin which is an inhibitor of platelet aggregation. Prostacyclin deficiency has been described in TTP, and infusions of prostacyclin have reversed platelet aggregation.[27]

In 1977, Bukowski reported that most patients with TTP respond to plasma exchange, suggesting that a toxic substance causing platelet aggregation could be removed.[28] Lian demonstrated that therapeutic responses were seen with plasma infusion alone, however, suggesting a deficiency of a normal component that might function as an inhibitor to the platelet-aggregating activity.[29] Purification and identification of this platelet-aggregating activity is currently ongoing. An immunoglobulin inhibitor of this platelet-aggregating activity has been identified in plasma from patients with TTP.[30]

In 1982, Moake demonstrated the presence of unusually large von Willebrand (vWF) multimers in patients with TTP.[31] Moake observed that these large multimeric vWF components could cause platelet agglutination in vitro and suggested that certain initiating events could neutralize negatively charged platelet membranes and allow large multimers of vWF to be absorbed and produce agglutination. Kelton has suggested that both the platelet-aggregating activity described by Lian and the large multimers of vWF described by Moake are involved in the pathogenesis of TTP.[69]

Thus, an inciting event may induce production of platelet-aggregating activity and unusually large multimers of vWF. If insufficient immunoglobulin inhibitor is present to neutralize these substances, platelet-aggregating activity

Table 43-1. Clinical Associations with Thrombotic Thrombocytopenic Purpura

Autoimmune Disorders
  Systemic lupus erythematosus
  Rheumatoid arthritis
Drugs
  Penicillin
  Sulfonamides
  Oral contraceptives
Chemotherapeutic Agents
  Mitomycin-C
  Cisplatin
  Vinblastine
  Bleomycin
Hypersensitivity Reactions
  Infection

Table 43-3. Laboratory Values in Thrombotic Thrombocytopenic Purpura

Hematologic Features
  Anemia, microangiopathic
  Thrombocytopenia
  Reticulocytosis
  Leukocytosis (common)
  Coombs' negative
Blood Chemistry
  Blood urea nitrogen and creatinine increased
  Hyperbilirubinemia (unconjugated)
  Lactate dehydrogenase increased
Coagulation
  Prothrombin time normal
  PTT normal
  Fibrinogen normal

may neutralize the negatively charged platelet membrane, allowing the absorption of large multimers of vWF and resulting in platelet agglutination. Lian has published an in-depth review of the pathogenesis of TTP.[32]

Clinical Presentation

The triad of microangiopathic hemolytic anemia, thrombocytopenia, and neurologic symptoms is present in 74% of patients (Table 43-2). Fever and renal dysfunction complete the pentad, which is present in 40% of patients.[33] In addition to the symptoms related to specific organ-system malfunction, nonspecific constitutional symptoms are generally present. Fluctuating evanescent neurologic symptoms include altered mental status, headache, paresthesias and/or paresis, visual disturbances, seizures, and coma.[34] Renal dysfunction is common; hematuria is present in 15% of patients. In most patients abnormalities of the sediment can be found.[33] Mild azotemia is commonly present; however, oliguria and acute renal failure are unusual.[35]

Diffuse pulmonary infiltrates with or without pulmonary edema may be present, and respiratory insufficiency is not uncommon.[36] Electrocardiographic changes, heart failure, or arrhythmias may result from extensive myocardial small-vessel thrombosis. Gastrointestinal, pulmonary, and genitourinary tract bleeding are common, although blood loss is usually insignificant. Abdominal pain produced by pancreatitis or involvement of intestinal mucosa is seen in approximately 10% of patients.[37,38]

Laboratory Findings

The microangiopathic hemolytic anemia is usually moderately severe; most patients have a hemoglobin of less than 10 g/dl, and many have less than 6 g/dl. Schistocytes, or fragmented red blood cells, are present. Polychromasia and nucleated red blood cells reflect the bone marrow response to hemolysis. Unconjugated hyperbilirubinemia and elevated lactate dehydrogenase (LDH) are present. The magnitude of the increase in the LDH is an accurate indicator of the severity of the hemolysis and thus disease activity. The Coombs' test is negative. Platelets generally are less than 20,000 ml^3, and large platelets are present. A moderate leukocytosis is commonly seen. The prothrombin time, partial thromboplastin time, and fibrinogen values should be normal. Evidence of disseminated intravascular coagulation may occur, however, in the patient with TTP who develops sepsis, respiratory failure, or other severe organ dysfunction.

A bone marrow aspirate and biopsy demonstrates erythroid and megakaryocytic hyperplasia and may demonstrate the thrombotic occlusion in small vessels. Mild renal dysfunction as manifested by an elevated blood urea nitrogen and creatinine occurs commonly. Table 43-3 summarizes laboratory findings. The origin of the low grade fever commonly seen is unknown.

Variants of TTP: Differential Diagnosis

Several disease entities with many similarities to TTP occur in different settings, or affect different organ systems (Table 43-4). These include:

Table 43-2. Clinical Symptoms of Thrombotic Thrombocytopenic Purpura

Neurologic (52%)
  Confusion
  Headache
  Weakness
  Dysphasia
  Seizure
  Coma
  Visual disturbance
Bleeding (38%)
  Petechiae
  Gastrointestinal bleeding
  Pulmonary bleeding
  Genitourinary bleeding
Constitutional Symptoms (29%)
  Fatigue
  Nausea, vomiting
  Fever
Abdominal Pain (14%)

Table 43-4. Syndromes Associated with Thrombotic Thrombocytopenic Purpura

Hemolytic uremic syndrome
Preeclampsia-eclampsia
Thrombotic microangiopathy (associated with chemotherapeutic agents)

- Hemolytic uremic syndrome (HUS)
- Preeclampsia-eclampsia syndrome
- Hemolytic uremic syndrome associated with chemotherapeutic agents
- Thrombotic microangiopathy associated with organ transplantation

Adult Hemolytic Uremic Syndrome (HUS)

Many adults with thrombotic microangiopathy have lesser degrees of neurologic dysfunction and more significant renal impairment. Clinically similar to HUS of childhood, it has been termed the adult hemolytic uremic syndrome.[39,40] Although likely resulting from a similar pathogenetic mechanism as in TTP, HUS platelet fibrin thrombi occur predominantly in the kidney.

HUS may occur in the postpartum period, generally in association with a normal delivery and postpartum period. Acute renal failure and microangiopathic hemolytic anemia develops oftentimes being preceded by a flulike illness.[41] Hypertension is frequent and the renal failure generally requires dialysis.

The preeclampsia-eclampsia syndrome is a complex systemic disease with multiorgan system dysfunction. The HELLPS syndrome describes pregnant patients with severe preeclampsia who present with microangiopathic hemolysis, elevated liver enzymes, and thrombocytopenia. It may be difficult to distinguish between preeclampsia, TTP, or adult HUS. A key diagnostic feature is that preeclampsia is accompanied by laboratory evidence of disseminated intravascular coagulation (i.e., prolonged PT, PTT, thrombin time, decreased fibrogen, and elevated D-dimer), whereas TTP and HUS are not.[42] Delivery is the procedure of choice for severe preeclampsia-eclampsia syndrome.

TTP may be associated with pregnancy. The major differential diagnostic dilemma as noted earlier occurs in separating this entity from preeclampsia. The development of TTP during pregnancy produces high maternal and perinatal mortality rates. The approach to therapy of TTP during pregnancy is similar to when it occurs in other settings. This subject is discussed more extensively in the section on treatment.

HUS Associated with Chemotherapy

An HUS-like syndrome has been described in patients receiving chemotherapy. Mitomycin C is the most commonly implicated agent; however, associations with other agents such as bleomycin and cisplatin have been described.[43,44] The onset of this HUS-like illness is usually 2 to 9 weeks from the last therapy, and many of the patients are in remission from their illness. Patients present with microangiopathic hemolytic anemia, thrombocytopenia, and renal dysfunction. An illness more akin to TTP with evidence of neurologic abnormalities and fever has been described but occurs much less frequently. The anemia is frequently severe and renal failure generally progressive, and up to one third require dialysis.[43] Cardiopulmonary dysfunction is common, and exacerbations of symptoms may be related to blood transfusion. Data suggest that the drugs themselves produce renal endothelial cell injury and result in thrombotic microangiopathy.[70-72] Associated

Table 43-5. Differential Diagnosis of Thrombotic Thrombocytopenic Purpura

Hemolytic uremic syndrome
Immune cytopenias
Vasculitides
Infection/sepsis
Carcinomatosis

with a high mortality rate, some patients have survived with remissions of the hemolysis and thrombocytopenia, although some degree of renal dysfunction often persists.

Although no controlled studies are available, as with TTP or HUS, plasmapheresis or plasma exchange has been used in patients with chemotherapy-associated HUS.[45] Azathioprine, low dose cyclophosphamide, and vincristine have also been helpful in small numbers of patients.[46,47] Immunoperfusion with staphylococcal protein A filters has also resulted in hematologic improvement and stabilization of renal function in small numbers of patients.[48]

Finally, a TTP-like illness has been reported in association with renal and bone marrow transplantation.[73] As in the primary disorders, this thrombotic microangiopathy likely results from damage to endothelium produced by rejection, immunosuppressive agents in particular cyclosporine, infection, or graft versus host disease. Microangiopathic hemolysis and central nervous system dysfunction are common. When this entity occurs in recipients of marrow transplants, the prognosis is poor, whereas following renal allografting, the prognosis is somewhat better.[74-76]

Other Points of Differential Diagnosis of TTP

The differential diagnosis of TTP includes other primary hematologic disorders such as the hemolytic uremic syndrome, immune hemolysis or thrombocytopenic disorders, and disseminated intravascular coagulation. Infections such as bacterial endocarditis and meningococcemia may also be included in this differential. A thrombotic microangiopathy associated with diffuse carcinomatosis has also been described (Table 43-5). Lastly, obstetrical problems such as preeclampsia or eclampsia are often difficult to distinguish from TTP.

Clinical Course

In a review of patients thought to have TTP diagnosed between 1925 and 1964, only 13 of 271 total patients survived, demonstrating a mortality rate of 75%.[49] In patients diagnosed between the late 1960s and early 1980s, mortality rates diminished to 50 to 60%.[24,33] A review published in 1982 suggested a further diminution in mortality rate to 18%.[35] This consistent improvement in survival likely reflects improvements in therapeutic techniques. However, enhanced awareness of the disease entity, which allows for earlier detection, and improvement in general supportive measures including critical care have also contributed to this decrease in mortality. Poor prognostic indicators have included worsening anemia and progressive renal dysfunction and thrombocytopenia, despite exchange transfusion.[50] Significant renal failure and absence of response to therapy within 72 hours are also described as factors predicting poorer survival.[51]

Mild cases of TTP may be entirely stable from a cardiopulmonary standpoint and modern treatment techniques may be easily performed on a regular hospital nursing floor. Often, TTP presents as a fulminant illness with acute and rapidly progressive hemodynamic and pulmonary deterioration, however. This situation may occur as a direct result of the primary disease process involving microvascular thrombi in the heart and lungs producing dysfunction of these systems, or as a result of significant secondary problems which occur during a disease process such as sepsis. Mild to moderate degrees of hemodynamic instability may be exacerbated by modern treatment techniques which include plasmapheresis or exchange transfusion. Relatively insignificant abnormalities in gas exchange may rapidly progress to findings consistent with adult respiratory distress syndrome (ARDS). Significant bleeding is rare, yet when it occurs it may be brisk and lead to further hemodynamic instability. Although neurologic symptoms generally fluctuate, acute CNS bleeding or seizures may occur. Patients with fulminant, rapidly progressive disease and those with significant hemodynamic and/or pulmonary compromise, either secondary to the primary disease process or a complication such as infection, are best served by admission to the ICU. Here, specific therapy may be instituted, and major organ-system function monitored and abnormalities treated. The 80% survival rate seen today in patients with TTP is due in main part to improvements in supportive care measures, particularly advances in critical care medicine.

ICU PHASE

Patients with TTP may present with critical illness. Even if relatively stable at presentation, the patient's clinical situation may become progressively unstable. Because of the severity of the illness, patients often require admission to the ICU. Most frequently, this is due to hemodynamic instability, respiratory insufficiency, bleeding, or progressive neurologic dysfunction.

Treatment

At present, there is no large prospective controlled clinical trial examining therapy of TTP. Retrospective examinations are difficult because patients with TTP tend to present with fulminant life-threatening disease and are usually treated with multiple simultaneous modalities. Current data suggest that plasma exchange or plasmapheresis is the cornerstone of therapy.[52] The mechanism of therapeutic benefit of plasma exchange is unknown. It is possible that removal of a toxic substance such as platelet-agglutinating factor or large vWF multimers produces the response. Alternatively, the infusion of fresh-frozen plasma may provide immunoglobulin inhibitors to these same factors.[53,54] The concept that immunoglobulin inhibitors are replenished by the replacement with fresh-frozen plasma and plasma exchange is supported by the finding that therapeutic responses have been seen with infusions of plasma without exchange. The data available at this time suggest that when the diagnosis of TTP is made, plasma exchange with replacement with fresh-frozen plasma should be instituted as soon as possible. This therapy should be initiated even when patients are in grave clinical condition with multiple organ-system dysfunction, because this treatment has curative potential.

In exchange plasmapheresis, the patient is connected to an apheresis unit, and approximately 60 ml/kg of plasma is exchanged with fresh-frozen plasma daily. If exchange techniques are not immediately available, plasma infusion therapy should be initiated. A small amount of information suggests that the use of vincristine with plasma exchange may enhance survival rates.[55] Corticosteroids are commonly used as part of the therapeutic regimen in patients with TTP; however, data supporting their use are meager.[56] Antiplatelet agents such as aspirin, dipyridamole, and sulfinpyrazone are also commonly used, and in one retrospective study were correlated with improved survival.[57] High dose intravenous gammaglobulin infusion has also been associated with therapeutic response in patients with TTP.[58,59] Splenectomy, infusion of cryosupernatant, infusions of prostacyclin, immunosuppression with cyclophosphamide and azathioprine, and heparinization have also been associated with response in small anecdotal reports. The use of heparin, however, has generally been unsuccessful and, in fact, may be dangerous.[60] After considering all data, a reasonable initial approach to therapy would be the use of plasmapheresis and vincristine, with optional use of corticosteroids and antiplatelet agents.

The benefit of therapy is assessed by improvement in neurologic symptoms, recovering thrombocytopenia, and improvement in hemolysis as evidenced by a decreasing LDH and bilirubin. In one large series, patients who responded to plasmapheresis generally did so within 36 hours of therapy.[61] Thus, if a therapeutic benefit is not witnessed in the first 2 to 3 days of therapy, additional treatment methods such as the use of high dose intravenous gammaglobulin should be considered. Plasma exchange should be continued, however, despite the addition of other treatment modalities because delayed responses have been seen. Transfusion therapy with packed red blood cells may on occasion be required. Platelet transfusion should be avoided because it may further aggravate the pathologic process by providing more platelets for agglutination.[62]

The patient presenting with fulminant disease may improve as rapidly with response to therapy, although patients critically ill in an ICU environment may require hemodynamic monitoring for cardiovascular instability. Gas exchange may deteriorate as part of the primary disease process and may develop into ARDS requiring intensive respiratory support and monitoring. The patient's mental status will often fluctuate as part of the manifestations of the primary disease, and complications such as sepsis and drug toxicity may aggravate this situation. Fluid balance is a problem in any critically ill patient and may be aggravated by hemodynamic problems and renal insufficiency. In the event of a poor or delayed response to therapy, consideration may need to be given to nutrition support either enterally or parenterally, and dialysis or respiratory support.

TTP is a difficult disease for the patient's family. Such a

crisis is often their first exposure to the entity, and as many gaps in our knowledge of its causation and therapy become apparent, the disease remains mysterious. The fluctuating neurologic manifestations and often rapid changes in clinical status cause considerable consternation. By calm explanation and attentive listening on the part of medical and nursing personnel, however, much fear and anxiety may be allayed.

POST-ICU PHASE

A response to therapy is indicated by an improvement in neurologic symptoms, decreasing levels of LDH indicating lessening of hemolysis, and rising platelet counts. In the absence of complicating factors such as ARDS or ongoing sepsis, a response to therapy generally heralds stabilization and improvement of major organ system dysfunction. Hemodynamic parameters improve and renal and pulmonary dysfunction lessens. Most patients recover completely. Even when neurologic dysfunction is severe, most patients recover without persistent deficits.[63] Uncommonly, neurologic dysfunction may persist.[64]

Patients with severe renal and neurologic abnormalities tend to do less well with therapy and when they do respond, require longer and, perhaps, more intensive therapy to do so. As patients respond, the tempo of the disease stabilizes and cardiopulmonary function normalizes, patients may be discharged to a regular hospital nursing floor to continue specific therapy. If treatment has been protracted, or if the patient is severely ill, physical and occupational therapy may be helpful in the rehabilitative process.

As survival has increased in patients with TTP, relapse rates of 12 to 30% have been described.[65,66] Relapses may be precipitated by infections, pregnancy, and surgical procedures. Patients with relapses should receive intensive therapy similar to those who present with de novo disease. Steroids, antiplatelet agents, and vincristine may not be particularly effective in preventing relapse.[66] Although not capable of preventing relapse, splenectomy may enhance disease-free intervals.[56] Patients with relapsing TTP should be considered for prophylactic therapy with exchange or plasma infusion during episodes which have produced relapse in the past. If TTP has been associated with pregnancy, additional pregnancies may be hazardous.[67]

The unusually large vWF multimers described earlier have been detected in the plasma of patients with chronic relapsing TTP.[68] These abnormal multimers are present during times of remission and decrease during relapse, possibly being consumed in the platelet agglutination process. From a clinical standpoint, relapses of TTP tend to exhibit primary hematologic manifestations rather than neurologic or renal manifestations. Because of this risk of relapse, patients who have survived TPP should be monitored closely by platelet count and review of the peripheral smear.

Thus, TTP is a fascinating hematologic disorder, the pathogenesis of which remains elusive. Survival rates in this disorder continue to improve, largely because of the introduction of plasma exchange. The improvements in supportive care provided by modern intensive care units have allowed many patients to survive long enough to respond to primary therapy. We have come a long way since the initial description by Dr. Moschcowitz in 1925, but much is yet to be learned.

REFERENCES

1. Moschcowitz, E.: An acute febrile pleiochromic anemia with hyaline thrombosis of terminal arterioles and capillaries: an undescribed disease. Arch. Intern. Med., 36:89, 1925.
2. Moschcowitz, E.: An acute febrile pleiochromic anemia with hyaline thrombosis of terminal arterioles and capillaries: an undescribed disease. Arch. Intern. Med., 36:89, 1925.
3. Baehr, G., Klemperer, P., and Schifrin, A.: An acute febrile anemia and thrombocytopenic purpura with diffuse platelet thromboses of capillaries and arterioles. Trans. Assoc. Am. Physicians, 51:43, 1936.
4. Singer, K., Bornstein, F. P., and Wiles, A.: Thrombotic thrombocytopenic purpura. Blood, 2:542, 1947.
5. Schwartz, M. I., and Brenner, W. E.: The obfuscation of eclampsia by thrombotic thrombocytopenic purpura. Obstet. Gynecol., 131:18, 1978.
6. Wurzel, J. M.: TTP lesions in placenta but not fetus. N. Engl. J. Med., 301:503, 1979.
7. Dekken, A., O'Brien, M. E., and Cammarata, R. J.: The association of thrombotic thrombocytopenic purpura with systemic lupus erythematosus. Am. J. Med. Sci., 267:243, 1974.
8. Morey, D. A., White, J. B., and Daiy, W. M.: Thrombotic thrombocytopenic purpura diagnosed by random lymph node biopsy. Arch. Intern. Med., 98:821, 1956.
9. Myers, T. J., et al.: Thrombotic thrombocytopenic purpura: combined treatment with plasmapheresis and antiplatelet agents. Ann. Intern. Med., 92:149, 1980.
10. Berritez, L., Mathews, M., and Mallory, G. K.: Platelet thrombosis with polyarteritis nodosa: report of a case. Arch. Pathol., 77:116, 1964.
11. Steinberg, A. D., Green, W. T., and Talal, N.: Thrombotic thrombocytopenic purpura complicating Sjogren's syndrome. JAMA, 215:757, 1971.
12. Levine, S., and Shearn, M. A.: Thrombotic thrombocytopenic purpura and systemic lupus erythematosus. Arch. Intern. Med., 113:826, 1964.
13. Parker, J. C., and Barrett, D. A.: Microangiopathic hemolysis and thrombocytopenia related to penicillin drugs. Arch. Intern. Med., 127:474, 1971.
14. Case Records of the Massachusetts General Hospital. N. Engl. J. Med., 278:36, 1968.
15. Cuttner, J.: Thrombotic thrombocytopenic purpura: a 10-year experience. Blood, 56:302, 1980.
16. Speth, P. A. J., Boerbooms, A. M., and Holdrinet, R. S. G.: Thrombotic thrombocytopenic purpura associated with D-penicillamine treatment in rheumatoid arthritis. J. Rheumatol., 9:812, 1982.
17. Rabad, S. J., Khandekar, J. D., and Miller, H. J.: Mitomycin-induced hemolytic uremic syndrome: case presentation and review of the literature. Cancer Treat. Rep., 66:1244, 1982.
18. Jackson, A. M., et al.: Thrombotic microangiopathy and renal failure associated with antineoplastic chemotherapy. Ann. Intern. Med., 101:41, 1984.
19. Jones, M. B., Armitage, J. O., and Stone, D. B.: Self-limited TTP-like syndrome after bee sting. JAMA, 242:2212, 1979.
20. Pilz, P.: Moschcowitz syndrome with involvement of the central nervous system. Virchows Arch. Pathol. Histol., 366:59, 1979.
21. Brown, R. C., et al.: Thrombotic thrombocytopenic purpura after influenza vaccination. Br. Med. J., 2:203, 1973.
22. Shalev, O., et al.: Thrombotic thrombocytopenic purpura

associated with bacteriodes bacteremia. Arch. Intern. Med., *141*:692, 1981.
23. Bukowski, R. M.: Thrombotic thrombocytopenic purpura: a review. Prog. Hemost. Thromb., *6*:287, 1982.
24. Kennedy, S. S., Zacharski, L. R., and Beck, J. R.: Thrombotic thrombocytopenic purpura: analysis of 48 unselected cases. Semin. Thromb. Hemost., *6*:341, 1980.
25. Petitt, R. M.: Thrombotic thrombocytopenic purpura: a 30-year review. Semin. Thromb. Hemost., *6*:350, 1980.
26. Burns, E. R., and Zucker-Franklin, D.: Pathologic effects of plasma from patients with thrombotic thrombocytopenic purpura on platelets and cultured vascular endothelial cells. Blood, *60*:1030, 1982.
27. Fitzgerald, G. A., et al.: Intravenous prostacyclin in thrombotic thrombocytopenic purpura. Ann. Intern. Med., *95*:319, 1981.
28. Bukowski, R. M., King, J. W., and Hewlett, J. S.: Plasmapheresis in the treatment of thrombotic thrombocytopenic purpura. Blood, *50*:413, 1977.
29. Lian, E. C-Y., et al.: Presence of a platelet aggregating factor in the plasma of patients with thrombocytopenic purpura (TTP) and its inhibition by normal plasma. Blood, *53*:333, 1979.
30. Lian, E. C-Y., et al.: Inhibition of platelet-aggregating activity in thrombotic thrombocytopenic purpura plasma by normal adult immunoglobulin G. J. Clin. Invest., *73*:548, 1984.
31. Moake, J. L., et al.: Unusually large plasma factor VIII: von Willebrand factor multimers in chronic relapsins thrombotic thrombocytopenic purpura. N. Engl. J. Med., *307*:1432, 1982.
32. Lian, E. C-Y.: Pathogenesis of thrombotic thrombocytopenic purpura. Semin. Hematol., *24*:82, 1987.
33. Ridolfi, R. L., and Bell, W. R.: Thrombotic thrombocytopenic purpura: report of 25 cases and a review of the literature. Medicine, *60*:413, 1981.
34. O'Brien, J. L., and Sibley, W. A.: Neurologic manifestations of thrombotic thrombocytopenic purpura. Neurology, *8*:55, 1958.
35. Bukowski, R.: Thrombotic thrombocytopenic purpura: a review. Prog. Hemost. Throm., *6*:287, 1982.
36. Bone, R. C., et al.: Respiratory dysfunction in thrombotic thrombocytopenic purpura. Am. J. Med., *65*:262, 1978.
37. Olsen, H.: Thrombotic thrombocytopenic purpura as a cause of pancreatitis. Am. J. Dig. Dis., *18*:238, 1973.
38. Hellstrom, H. R., Nash, E. C., and Fischer, E. R.: Thrombotic thrombocytopenic purpura as a cause of massive gastrointestinal hemorrhage, report of a case. Gastroenterology, *36*:132, 1959.
39. Ponticelli, C., et al.: Hemolytic uremic syndrome in adults. Arch. Intern. Med., *140*:353, 1980.
40. Morel-Maroger, L.: Adult hemolytic-uremic syndrome. Kidney Int., *18*:125, 1980.
41. Nissenson, A. R., Krumlowsky, F. A., and del Greco, F.: Postpartum hemolytic-uremic syndrome: late recovery after prolonged maintenance dialysis. JAMA, *242*:173, 1979.
42. Byrnes, J. J., and Moake, J. L.: Thrombotic thrombocytopenic purpura and the haemolytic-uremic syndrome: evolving concepts of pathogenesis and therapy. Clin. Haematol., *15*:413, 1986.
43. Cantrell, J. E., Phillips, T. M., and Schein, P. S.: Carcinoma-associated hemolytic-uremic syndrome: a complication of mitomycin-C chemotherapy. J. Clin. Oncol., *3*:723, 1985.
44. Jackson, A. M., et al.: Thrombotic microangiopathy and renal failure associated with antineoplastic chemotherapy. Ann. Intern. Med., *101*:41, 1984.
45. Chow, S., Roscoe, J., and Cattran, D. C.: Plasmapheresis and antiplatelet agents in the treatment of hemolytic uremic syndrome secondary to mitomycin. Am. J. Kidney Dis., *7*:407, 1986.
46. Hug, V., et al.: Effect of cyclophosphamide on the mitomycin-induced syndrome of thrombotic thrombocytopenic purpura. Cancer Treat Rep., *69*:565, 1985.
47. Grem, J. L., Merrit, J. A., and Carbone, P. P.: Treatment of mitomycin-associated microangiopathic hemolytic anemia with vincristine. Arch. Intern. Med., *146*:566, 1986.
48. Korec, S., et al.: Treatment of cancer-associated hemolytic syndrome with staphylococcal protein A immunoperfusion. J. Clin. Oncol., *4*:210, 1986.
49. Amorosi, E. L., and Ultmann, J. E.: Thrombotic thrombocytopenic purpura: report of 16 cases and review of the literature. Medicine, *45*:139, 1966.
50. Pisciotta, A. V., and Gottschall, J. L.: Clinical features of thrombotic thrombocytopenic purpura. Semin. Thromb. Hemost., *6*:330, 1980.
51. Petitt, R. M.: Thrombotic thrombocytopenic purpura: a 30-year review. Semin. Thromb. Hemost., *6*:350, 1980.
52. Shapard, K. V., and Bukowski, R. M.: The treatment of thrombotic thrombocytopenic purpura with exchange transfusion, plasma infusion and plasma exchange. Semin. Hematol., *24*:178, 1987.
53. Siddiqui, F. A., and Lian, E. C-Y.: Platelet-agglutinating protein P37 from a thrombotic thrombocytopenic purpura plasma forms a complex with human immunoglobulin G. Blood, *71*:299, 1988.
54. Murphy, W. G., Moore, J. C., and Kelton, J. G.: Calcium-dependent cysteine protease activity in the sera of patients with thrombotic thrombocytopenic purpura with vincristine. JAMA, *247*:1433, 1982.
55. Gutterman, L. A., and Stevenson, T. D.: Treatment of thrombotic thrombocytopenic purpura with vincristine. JAMA, *247*:1433, 1982.
56. Bukowski, R. M., et al.: Therapy of thrombotic thrombocytopenic purpura: an overview. Semin. Thromb. Hemost., *7*:1, 1981.
57. Kennedy, S. S., Zacharski, L. R., and Beck, J. R.: Thrombotic thrombocytopenic purpura: analysis of 48 unselected cases. Semin. Thromb. Hemost., *6*:341, 1980.
58. Finn, N. G., Wang, J. C., and Hong, K. J.: High-dose intravenous immunoglobulin infusion in the treatment of thrombotic thrombocytopenic purpura. Arch. Intern. Med., *147*:2165, 1987.
59. Viero, P., et al.: Thrombotic thrombocytopenic purpura and high-dose immunoglobulin treatment. Ann. Intern. Med., *104*:282, 1986.
60. Kennedy, S. S., Zacharski, L. R., and Beck, J. R.: Thrombotic thrombocytopenic purpura: analysis of 48 unselected cases. Semin. Thromb. Hemost., *6*:341, 1980.
61. Pettit, R. M.: Thrombotic thrombocytopenic purpura: a 30-year review. Semin. Thromb. Hemost., *6*:350, 1980.
62. Gordon, L. I., Kwaan, H. C., and Rossi, E. C.: Deleterious effects of platelet transfusions and recovery thrombocytosis in patients with thrombotic microangiopathy. Semin. Hematol., *24*:194, 1987.
63. Frankel, A. E., Rubenstein, M. D., and Wall, R. T.: Thrombotic thrombocytopenic purpura: prolonged coma with recovery of neurologic function with intensive plasma exchange. Am. J. Hematol., *10*:387, 1981.
64. Ben-Yehuda, D., Rose, M., Michaeli, Y., and Eldor, A.: Permanent neurological complications in patients with thrombotic thrombocytopenic purpura. Am. J. Hematol., *29*:74, 1988.
65. Rice, L., and Vandermolen, L. A.: Recurrences of acute thrombotic thrombocytopenic purpura Blood, *66*:1070, 1985.

66. Rose, M., and Eldor, A.: High incidences of relapses in thrombotic thrombocytopenic purpura. Am. J. Med., 83:437, 1987.
67. Upshaw, J. D., Reidy, T. J., and Groshart, K.: Thrombotic thrombocytopenic purpura in pregnancy: response to plasma manipulations. South Med. J., 78:677, 1985.
68. Moake, J. L., et al.: Unusually large plasma factor VIII: von Willebrand factor multimers in chronic relapsing thrombotic thrombocytopenic purpura. N. Engl. J. Med., 307:1432, 1982.
69. Kelton, J. G., Moore, J., Santos, A., and Sheridan, D.: Detection of a platelet-agglutinating factor in thrombotic thrombocytopenic purpura. Ann. Intern. Med., 101:589, 1984.
70. Cattell, V.: Mitomycin-induced hemolytic uremic kidney: an experimental model in the rat. Am. J. Pathol., 121:88, 1985.
71. Duperray, A., et al.: The effect of mitomycin C on the biosynthesis of prostacyclin by primary cultures of human umbilical cord vein endothelial cells. In Ninth International Congress of Nephrology, Los Angeles, 1984, p. 448A.
72. Licciadello, J. T. W., et al.: Elevated plasma von Willebrand factor levels and arterial occlusive complications associated with cisplatin-based chemotherapy. Oncology, 42:296, 1985.
73. Kwann, H. C.: Miscellaneous secondary thrombotic microangiopathy. Semin. Hematol., 24:141, 1987.
74. Atkinson, K., et al.: Cyclosporin A associated nephrotoxicity in the first 100 days after allogeneic bone marrow transplantation: three distinct syndromes. Br. J. Haematol., 54:59, 1983.
75. Shulman, H., et al.: Nephrotoxicity of cyclosporin A after allogeneic marrow transplantation. N. Engl. J. Med., 305:1392, 1981.
76. Bonsib, S. M., et al.: Recurrent thrombotic microangiopathy in a renal allograft. Am. J. Med., 79:520, 1979.

Chapter 44

ONCOLOGIC TOXICITIES AND EMERGENCIES

DAVID J. ADELSTEIN
ALAN E. LICHTIN

Oncologic emergencies and the toxicities from antineoplastic interventions are frequently encountered. Many of these complications of cancer or its treatment result in morbidity rather than mortality, and most can be managed without the use of an ICU. It is important, however, that these problems be recognized early, so intervention can be successful and long-term complications avoided. A recurring problem in the management of a critically ill cancer patient is the need to balance the aggressiveness of therapeutic intervention with the natural history of the disease. Mechanical ventilation and ICU management are inappropriate in the preterminal patient. Many patients with malignancy, however, are curable, have significant survival expectations, or can look forward to long-term symptomatic palliation. Rapid, effective management of cancer-related emergencies and treatment-induced toxicities can provide such patients with major benefit.

STRUCTURAL EMERGENCIES

Superior Vena Cava Obstruction

Superior vena cava obstruction is considered one of the classic oncologic emergencies.[1-4] The clinical presentation may be dramatic and frightening and has frequently led to poor medical decision making. It has often been suggested in the past that a bedside diagnosis of superior vena cava obstruction mandates immediate radiotherapeutic intervention for symptomatic palliation of a presumed but unconfirmed malignancy.[5] More recent reviews, however, have seriously questioned this tenet, in large part because of improvements in the treatment of some of the common malignancies that produce this syndrome.[2-4]

The superior vena cava is a low pressure, thin-walled vascular structure somewhat rigidly confined in the mediastinum and surrounded by lymph nodes. It is readily compressed by any distortion of the normal architecture. Fortunately, an extensive collateral network exists, allowing for decompression and venous return. Nonetheless, in contrast to major vessels of the arterial circulation, neoplastic or traumatic occlusion or thrombosis is common.

The causes of superior vena cava syndrome have changed over the years (Table 44-1). In the past, syphilitic aneurysms and tuberculous mediastinal node involvement were common causes. More recent reviews, however, suggest that between 80 and 95% of patients presenting with superior vena cava obstruction have a thoracic malignancy and that mediastinal fibrosis occurs relatively infrequently.[1-4,6] An increasingly recognized cause of this syndrome is iatrogenic, owing to central venous catheters, pacemaker wires, and other similar interventions.[7-11] Bronchogenic carcinoma represents the most common malignancy responsible for this syndrome. In those with lung cancer and superior vena cava obstruction, up to 40% have small cell undifferentiated carcinoma.[1,4,6] Squamous cell carcinoma, adenocarcinoma, and large cell undifferentiated lung carcinoma are also represented but less commonly. Malignant lymphoma, when presenting with massive mediastinal disease, can also produce this clinical syndrome, as can other less common malignancies, such as breast cancer and germ cell neoplasms. The markedly variable prognosis of these different cancers clearly mandates the need for an accurate histologic diagnosis.

Pre-ICU Phase

Superior vena cava syndrome, although variable in severity, can usually be diagnosed at the bedside, particularly if the predisposing conditions are recognized (Table 44-2). Symptomatically patients may complain of fullness in the face and neck as well as orthopnea.[3,6,12] A cough may be present, but this may be due to the underlying disease. Swelling in the arms and upper hemibody can be quite dramatic and may be the presenting manifestation. Pain, dysphagia, syncope, lethargy, and respiratory stridor are described but are considerably less frequent.

On physical examination, distended neck veins are almost universally observed.[1,6,12] If the syndrome has developed slowly or been present for a significant period of time, a prominent venous collateral pattern on the anterior chest can be identified. Edema of the arms, face, forehead, and conjunctivae is quite characteristic.

Radiographic confirmation of the clinical diagnosis is also relatively simple. The chest radiograph may reveal mediastinal widening or a right hilar mass. Computed tomography (CT) scanning, particularly after intravenous contrast administration, clearly demonstrates a mediastinal mass with caval compression (Fig. 44-1).[13] If further delineation of the abnormality is required, contrast venography[14] or digital subtraction angiography[15] can easily be performed with little morbidity.

Although the clinical syndrome is readily identified, it is more difficult and more important to accurately determine the causes. When an indwelling venous catheter or pacemaker wire is present in a patient with caval obstruc-

Table 44-1. Causes of Superior Vena Cava Obstruction

Malignant disease	80–95%
Bronchogenic carcinoma	50–80%
Lymphoma	10–20%
Other (breast, germ cell, metastatic)	5–10%
Nonmalignant causes	5–20%
Iatrogenic	5–20%
Fibrosis	0–5%
Other (goiter, aneurysm)	0–5%

tion, the situation is clear. The diagnosis of malignancy, however, requires histologic confirmation. In the past, concern has focused on the potential for increased venous bleeding after the performance of invasive procedures in patients with superior vena cava obstruction. Despite this concern, an increased risk has not been demonstrated, and procedures such as mediastinoscopy and fiberoptic bronchoscopy have proven safe.[2-4,16]

Furthermore, death from superior vena cava obstruction alone is not well described.[3,4] Indeed, surgical ligation of the vena cava in animals is not a lethal intervention. The literature does focus on the risk of cerebral edema, laryngeal edema, and airway obstruction, which are believed to represent the sequelae of superior vena cava obstruction. In general, however, these represent other concurrent manifestations of an advanced malignancy resulting in cerebral metastases, vocal cord paralysis, or airway obstruction. In the absence of such complications, superior vena cava syndrome alone is unlikely to result in death.

As such, the concept of superior vena cava syndrome as a medical emergency must be questioned.[2-4] In the past, the rationale has been that because this syndrome represents a potentially fatal medical emergency, which carries with it an increased risk of diagnostic procedures, and because the cause is almost always neoplastic, symptomatic palliation with radiation therapy should be offered as soon as possible.[5] Although perhaps this was true at one time, the most common causes of superior vena cava syndrome at present are small cell carcinoma of the lung and malignant lymphoma, two treatable and potentially curable malignant diseases. An accurate histologic diagnosis is mandatory before treatment is started so an appropriately designed diagnostic and therapeutic plan can be followed, regardless of the presence of superior vena cava syndrome.

Table 44-2. Clinical Manifestations of Superior Vena Cava Obstruction

Symptoms
  Facial fullness
  Dyspnea
  Cough
  Upper hemibody swelling
  Dizziness/syncope
Physical Findings
  Distended neck veins
  Prominent venous collaterals
  Upper hemibody edema
  Plethora

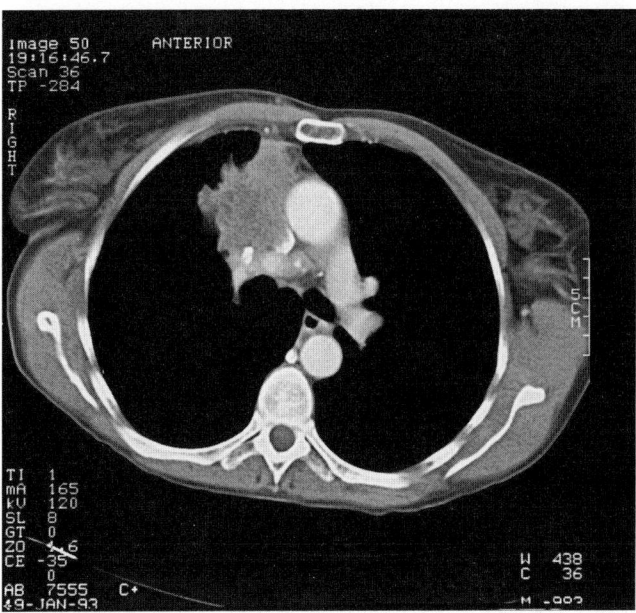

Fig. 44-1. CT chest scan demonstrating superior vena cava obstruction by a mediastinal tumor mass. Note dilated contrast-filled azygous vein.

The diagnosis should be made rapidly and a protracted evaluation discouraged. Diagnostic confusion may result from fine-needle aspirates or sputum cytology specimens. Superclavicular fullness may be mistaken for lymphadenopathy leading to fruitless attempts at node biopsy. Instead, a single, high yield procedure should be chosen to make the diagnosis rather than a series of less definitive tests.

The management of superior vena cava obstruction involves both control of the clinical symptoms and an organized approach to the underlying neoplasm. Symptoms can usually be managed with simple interventions, such as diuretics and elevation of the head of the bed. Corticosteroids have been suggested but are of unclear benefit. The roles of anticoagulation,[17,18] angioplasty,[19] surgical intervention,[6,14] and vascular stenting[20] are, as yet, incompletely defined. In the setting, however, of iatrogenic caval obstruction owing to an indwelling vascular device, strong consideration should be given to removal of the device and anticoagulation.[9,10]

ICU Phase

It is unusual for a patient with superior vena cava obstruction to require ICU management, unless other complicating features of the malignancy develop. In iatrogenic caval thrombosis, the possibility of pulmonary embolism must be recognized and might also result in a need for ICU care. Even when clinically severe manifestations prompt ICU admission, it is important that the decision making be clear. Symptomatic measures should be employed until an accurate histologic diagnosis can be made and an appropriate and organized plan for intervention undertaken.

Post-ICU Phase

The prognosis of patients with malignant superior vena cava obstruction depends on the prognosis of the underlying malignancy, not the obstruction itself. A series of patients reported from Princess Margaret Hospital in Toronto, for example, demonstrated that patients with small cell cancer of the lung have similar survivals regardless of the presence or absence of superior vena cava obstruction.[21]

The clinical manifestations of superior vena cava syndrome improve in 70 to 95% of patients.[3,4] Interestingly, venographic evidence of improvement can be demonstrated in only 55% of patients, and autopsy patency of the superior vena cava is found in less than 35%.[4] Indeed, this clinical improvement may be seen without specific therapeutic intervention. In the past, patients with benign causes for caval obstruction, such as a massive goiter or an aortic aneurysm, survived for many years without specific intervention. This suggests that symptomatic resolution occurs predominately because of the development of sufficient collateral circulation, and it again points out the importance of a focus on the underlying illness, rather than the clinical syndrome.

For patients with malignant caval obstruction, cancer surgery is generally not appropriate. Antineoplastic treatment options for non-small cell lung cancer include radiotherapy, with the expectation of clinical improvement and temporary disease control. Patients with small cell lung cancer or lymphoma, however, should be treated primarily with chemotherapy as for those patients without superior vena cava obstruction. It has been repeatedly demonstrated that primary chemotherapy for chemotherapy-sensitive diseases is a safe, appropriate intervention for patients with caval obstruction and results in rapid clinical improvement.[21-26] Any compromise in the conventional management of potentially curable malignancies to address the clinical signs and symptoms of caval obstruction should be discouraged so as not to jeopardize the possibility of disease-free, long-term survival.

Spinal Cord Compression

Spinal cord compression resulting from cancer usually occurs in patients with metastatic and incurable disease. It is responsible for serious morbidity but rarely mortality.[27-30] Indeed, treatment success is usually measured by whether a patient remains ambulatory and continent. Unfortunately, the diagnosis must be anticipated because once neurologic symptoms develop, irreversible ischemic injury has generally occurred. Furthermore, neurologic dysfunction often develops rapidly, creating a true oncologic emergency. The problem therefore is one of recognizing spinal cord compression before the development of clinical signs and symptoms.[27-30]

The pathophysiology of malignant spinal cord compression generally begins with metastatic tumor involving a vertebral body (Fig. 44-2). This metastasis extends to produce an anterior epidural cord compression. Neoplasms such as lymphoma and myeloma, may, alternatively, result in epidural cord compression by direct extension from a paravertebral mass without bone involvement.[31,32] Although epidural cord compression is the most common cause of myelopathic symptoms in a patient with malignancy, other causes, such as intradural or intramedullary tumor, carcinomatous meningitis, radiation myelopathy, and a paraneoplastic syndrome, must be considered.[34]

The thoracic spine represents the most common site of spinal cord compression, but it is important to recognize that these lesions are often multiple.[27-30] The most common neoplasms responsible are those cancers that most frequently metastasize to bone, such as lung cancer and breast cancer. Prostate cancer, myeloma, and lymphoma are also common causes. Gastrointestinal tumors, although common malignant diseases, less frequently spread to bone and are less likely to cause this complication.

Pre-ICU Phase

The symptomatic hallmark of spinal cord compression is back pain, which is present in up to 95% of patients,

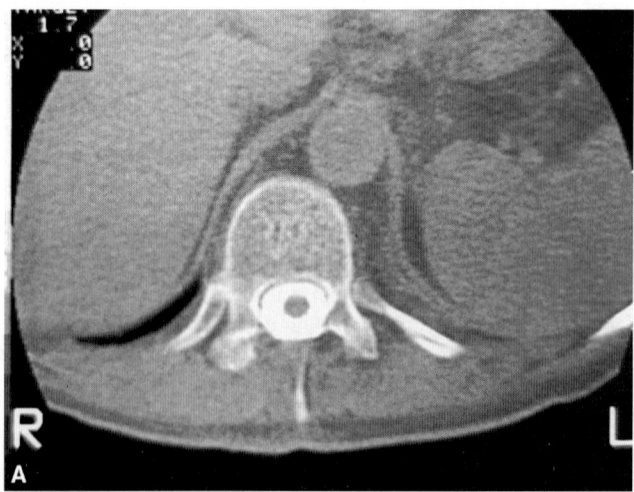
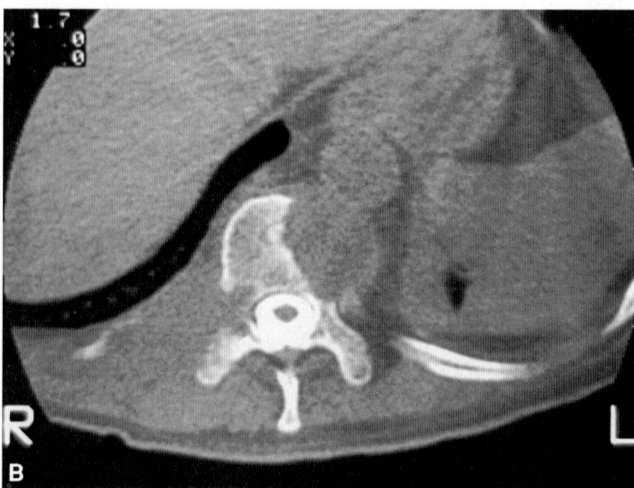

Fig. 44–2. CT scan with intrathecal metrizamide contrast material. *A*, Normal relationship of bony structures and thecal sac. *B*, Metastatic tumor involving vertebral body and pedicle but not yet compressing thecal sac.

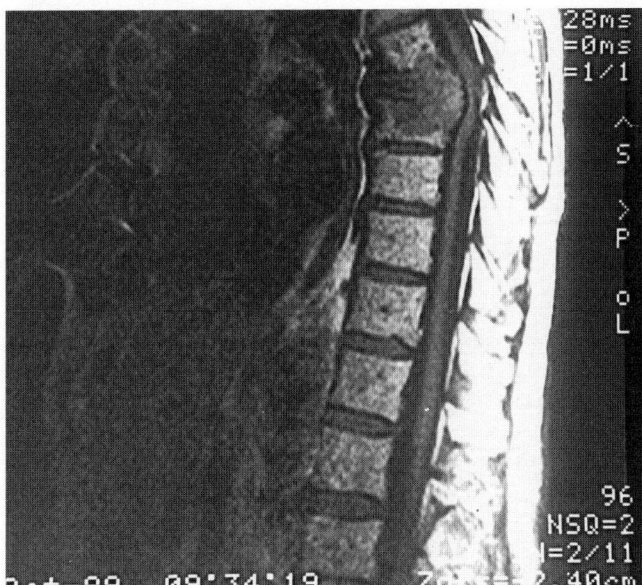

Fig. 44-3. MRI of a thoracic spinal cord compression arising from vertebral body involvement with multiple myeloma.

often for a significant period of time.[27-30] Back pain is a common symptom, but its presence in association with known spinal metastases mandates further evaluation, and its presence is the single clinical marker that allows us to intervene before irreversible neurologic damage.[27,34]

The presence of symptomatic radiculopathy or myelopathy in patients with cancer also demands a full evaluation to determine the cause because neurologic involvement is indicated. Thoracic radiculopathies are a difficult diagnostic problem in a patient with advanced malignant disease. Confusion can arise with post-thoracotomy pain, herpes zoster, malignant pleural disease, or bone metastases, and a high index of suspicion is required. The presence of a radiculopathy if often a prelude to myelopathy, and symptomatic deterioration can be rapid. Myelopathic signs and symptoms, such as incontinence, upper motor neuron dysfunction, or a sensory level, rarely improve, even with successful relief of the spinal cord compression.[27-30,35-37]

The neurologic examination is often normal in these patients. If abnormal, however, it may localize the level of cord disease. Plain spine films and a bone scan are useful in determining the presence of spinal metastases but do not define the existence of spinal cord compression. The bone scan remains the most sensitive indicator of bone metastases except in multiple myeloma, when it may be normal. The diagnosis of spinal cord compression can be made radiographically only with a magnetic resonance imaging (MRI) scan or a myelogram (Fig. 44-3). Although these procedures are either invasive or expensive, the literature is clear that up to 60% of patients with spinal metastases and back pain alone have clinically silent evidence of cord compression.[3,4] In patients with radiculopathy or myelopathy, demonstrable abnormalities are almost always found with these studies. It is also important that the myelogram be complete or that the whole spine be visualized on MRI in all circumstances because of the frequency of multiple lesions.

The immediate treatment for a patient with suspected spinal cord compression is high doses of corticosteroids.[37,38] Doses of up to 100 mg daily of dexamethasone have been recommended and demonstrated to be of value in producing pain relief and neurologic improvement. In most cases, radiation therapy is the definitive treatment of choice and has generally proved as effective as surgery, although there are few comparative data.[35,39] Surgical treatment should be reserved for an unclear diagnosis, for a radioresistant tumor, for progression or recurrence developing during or after radiation therapy, or if surgical stabilization is required.[27,30,35]

Once myelopathic signs have developed, however, the treatment of this disorder is imperfect. Data from Memorial Sloan-Kettering, gathered in a retrospective fashion, suggest that patients who are nonambulatory at presentation rarely recover the ability to walk, whereas those who retain neurologic function at diagnosis generally do not deteriorate.[35] The overall prognosis for neurologic recovery depends most on the initial neurologic status.

ICU Phase

The need for ICU management of these patients is uncommon. Close neurologic monitoring, however, is imperative in patients with high cervical spine lesions, in whom respiratory function might be threatened. If neurosurgical intervention is required, postoperative ICU care is needed. Although patients with spinal cord compression can generally be managed outside of the ICU, the urgency of their evaluation and treatment cannot be overstated. The clinical suspicion of spinal cord compression mandates immediate diagnostic evaluation and therapeutic intervention.

Post-ICU Phase

Spinal cord compression produces morbidity, not mortality, and a patient's overall prognosis depends entirely on the natural history of the malignancy. Although metastatic bronchogenic carcinoma producing spinal cord compression has a poor prognosis and a limited survival, patients with lymphoma,[31] myeloma,[32] breast cancer, or hormone-sensitive prostate cancer are more readily treatable and may survive for protracted periods of time. The preservation of neurologic function is of obvious importance in this group of patients.

Airway Obstruction

A malignant airway obstruction can result from an intrinsic mucosal lesion of the larynx, trachea, bronchus, or a smaller airway; from extrinsic airway compression; or from bilateral vocal cord paralysis (Table 44-3). The neoplasms responsible for this complication include the primary tumors of the larynx and head and neck region, which produce airway obstruction from bulky mucosal tumor or by vocal cord fixation. Bronchogenic carcinoma, with endobronchial disease involving either the trachea or major bronchi, is also frequently responsible. Extrinsic airway compression or bilateral vocal cord paralysis can

Table 44-3. Malignant Airway Obstruction

Cause	Clinical Manifestation	Treatment
Upper airway obstruction Head and neck cancer Vocal cord paralysis (mediastinal disease) Extrinsic compression	Stridor	Tracheostomy Endoscopic management Radiation therapy
Tracheal obstruction Lung cancer Extrinsic compression (mediastinal disease)	Stridor	Radiation therapy Endoscopic management Chemotherapy
Bronchial obstruction Lung cancer Extrinsic compression (mediastinal or parenchymal)	Postobstructive pneumonitis Collapse	Radiation therapy Endoscopic management Chemotherapy

result from any neoplasm that spreads to the neck or mediastinal structures, such as malignant lymphoma, thyroid cancer, metastatic bronchogenic or esophageal carcinoma, and others.[40,41]

See also Chapter 12 for further discussion of airway obstruction.

Pre-ICU Phase

The clinical symptoms depend on the location of the obstruction. In major airway obstruction, stridor is the presenting manifestation. Given the common association of these neoplasms with underlying pulmonary disease, it is important to distinguish stridor from wheezing. The inspiratory nature of the airway noise is readily apparent as well as its localization to the major airways on clinical examination. Another clue to diagnosis is its association with hoarseness. Patients with obstruction of a main stem bronchus or smaller airway may present with shortness of breath, cough, or fever related to underlying obstructive pneumonitis. Major or minor airway obstruction may be the presenting manifestation of the neoplasm or a manifestation of disease recurrence or progression.

Confirmation of airway obstruction is not difficult once the diagnosis has been considered. A chest radiograph may reveal parenchymal or mediastinal abnormality with or without associated pneumonitis or collapse. Soft tissue films of the neck can also reveal compromise in tracheal diameter. Direct visualization of the airway, however, confirms the abnormality. Laryngeal lesions can be seen in the office with indirect laryngoscopy or fiberoptic evaluation. Direct laryngoscopy and bronchoscopy almost always fully define any anatomic obstruction and allow for histologic diagnosis of an intrinsic mucosal lesion.

Treatment must be rapid and definitive. For those patients with proximal lesions in the neck, tracheostomy is often the treatment of choice. On occasion, endoscopic tumor debulking[42] or laser resection[43,44] in the larynx or proximal airway can temporize until more definitive treatment can be started. Surgical resection of laryngeal or bronchogenic carcinoma may be curative, even in the presence of airway obstruction. Radiation therapy can be used palliatively in patients with incurable lung cancer or as definitive treatment in some patients with laryngeal disease. In those patients with extrinsic airway compression, it may be the only potentially effective treatment option. Chemotherapy may prove useful for patients with extrinsic compression from chemotherapy-sensitive tumors, such as malignant lymphoma, or in patients with small cell carcinoma of the lung.[45] Given the urgent nature of this clinical problem, however, close monitoring is mandatory if a chemotherapeutic approach is chosen primarily.

ICU Phase

ICU management may be required in those patients who present with hypoxemia and respiratory failure. Ideally if the airway obstruction can be rapidly relieved, the medical emergency resolves, although intubation and mechanical ventilation may be required. Immediate improvement may not be possible, however, in those patients with extrinsic airway compression or with an obstruction that cannot be relieved by tracheostomy and that requires radiation therapy. For these patients, a protracted period of ventilatory support may be necessary. The appropriateness of such aggressive supportive efforts must be tempered against the natural history and prognosis of the underlying malignant disease.

Post-ICU Phase

The presence of malignant airway obstruction by itself does not define the overall disease prognosis. A relatively small tumor burden may be present and may be totally amenable to curative intervention if airway patency can be reestablished.[40] The prognosis instead depends entirely on the specific diagnosis and stage of the cancer. Even in those patients with incurable disease or recurrent cancer after primary treatment, the palliative importance of maintaining airway patency is obvious.

For those patients with recurrent disease after radiation therapy, other treatment approaches can be explored.[43,44,46] These include endobronchial laser therapy or brachytherapy. Although a relatively limited number of patients with airway obstruction are amenable to these interventions, significant palliation can result when applicable. Indeed, laser photoablation of airway tumors can also be an excellent initial approach for patients with airway obstruction, while awaiting completion of more definitive treatment interventions.

Postobstructive pneumonitis remains a difficult problem and is unlikely to be controlled without relief of the obstruction. Broad-spectrum antibiotics are usually given but are of only temporary benefit.

A tracheoesophageal fistula is a particularly virulent complication of esophageal cancer with airway involvement.[47,48] It is a not infrequent event in proximal esophageal cancer and can readily be explained by the proximity of the trachea to the esophagus. All treatment options are imperfect. Surgical intervention is generally limited to palliative stenting of the esophagus or a gastrostomy. Neither radiotherapy nor chemotherapy is of much benefit in this situation, and the mean survival is short.

Pericardial Tamponade

Cardiac involvement from malignant disease is often an asymptomatic autopsy finding reported in 5 to 15% of cancer patients.[49,50] It is clinically important only when it results in cardiac dysfunction, the most common manifestation being pericardial tamponade. Pericardial tamponade is rarely the first manifestation of malignancy but usually occurs as the result of progression of a known cancer.[51] As with other critical manifestations of malignancy, the overall prognosis of the patient with malignant pericardial tamponade depends more on the natural history of the underlying malignancy than on the pericardial involvement.[52]

The most common malignant diseases producing pericardial and cardiac involvement are cancers of the lung and breast, leukemia and lymphoma, melanoma, and sarcoma (Table 44-4).[50,51] Disease spread to the pericardium can reflect either direct extension from a mediastinal tumor as in lymphoma or lung cancer or widespread hematogenous disease dissemination.[50,51,53,54] Despite the dramatic presentation of patients with pericardial tamponade, several of the responsible malignancies are potentially curable, even when involving the heart. As such, an aggressive approach to diagnosis and management is imperative.

It is also important to distinguish the clinical signs and symptoms of pericardial tamponade from several antineoplastic treatment-related complications. These include the acute and chronic pericarditis that may be seen after mediastinal radiation therapy[54,55] and the cardiomyopathy that can arise after anthracycline use.[50] Careful review of radiotherapy portals as well as drug administration is important in distinguishing these entities because the clinical differences may be subtle.

Pre-ICU Phase

The symptoms of pericardial tamponade are nonspecific. Dyspnea is common, as is cough, chest pain, and orthopnea. These symptoms, however, may also reflect the underlying malignancy. Worsening dyspnea suggests a new process, such as cardiac dysfunction, and should be further evaluated.

Physical examination is notable for evidence of tachycardia, jugular venous distention, hepatomegaly, and peripheral edema. Pulsus paradoxus, the clinical hallmark of cardiac tamponade, may be found in only 30% of patients at presentation. A pericardial rub, although strongly suggestive of pericardial disease, is uncommon. Its detection in a patient with malignant disease, however, mandates further evaluation. Similarly, an enlargement in cardiac silhouette on chest radiograph may be the first sign of a pericardial effusion and impending tamponade (Fig. 44-4).[50,51,53-55]

Certain electrocardiographic abnormalities have been described in the presence of pericardial effusions and tamponade, including tachycardia, low QRS voltage, and the unusual electrical alternans pattern. The diagnostic procedure of choice, however, is the echocardiogram. This can rapidly and safely be obtained at the bedside in seriously ill individuals. Diastolic right atrial and right ventricular collapse are manifestations of tamponade in the presence of a pericardial effusion.[55] Although characteristic abnormalities are seen at right heart catheterization, this is rarely required.

ICU Phase

In contrast to most oncologic emergencies, diagnostic confirmation and further treatment of pericardial tamponade mandate ICU management. A diagnostic/therapeutic pericardiocentesis is generally indicated. This allows sampling of pericardial fluid for biochemical and cytologic analysis as well as therapeutic decompression of the pericardium. Other short-term supportive therapies include in-

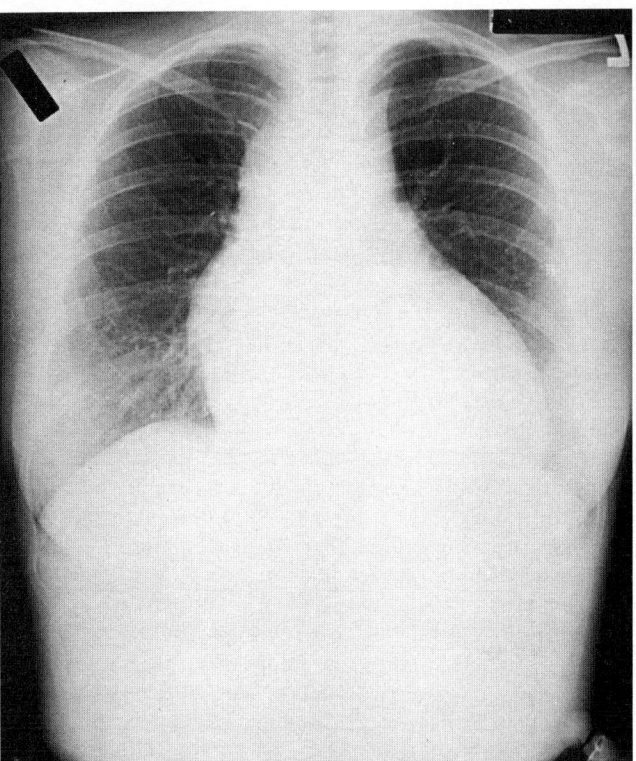

Fig. 44-4. "Water-bottle" enlargement of the cardiac silhouette in a patient with a pericardial effusion from Hodgkin's disease.

Table 44-4. Serous Effusions from Malignant Disease—Most Common Primary Tumor Sites

Pericardial Effusion	Pleural Effusion	Ascites
Lung cancer	Lung cancer	Pancreatic cancer
Breast cancer	Breast cancer	Ovarian cancer
Lymphoma/leukemia	Lymphoma	Colorectal cancer
Sarcoma	Unknown primary adenocarcinoma	Lymphoma
Melanoma		Stomach cancer

travenous fluids, oxygen, and pressors, but these are generally of only limited benefit. Pericardiocentesis can be safely performed using either echocardiographic or electrocardiographic monitoring,[55] and a drainage catheter can be left in the pericardial space after entry. Rapid return of the cardiac output to baseline usually dramatically relieves the clinical manifestations.

Cytologic evaluation of the pericardial fluid is mandatory in an effort to confirm the malignant origin and eliminate the possibility of a treatment-related pleuropericarditis. Unfortunately, in the presence of a previously irradiated mediastinum, particularly in patients with lymphoma, cytologic analysis may be negative even when the effusion is directly due to malignancy. In such a situation, a pericardial biopsy may be required.[56]

Management involves efforts to control the pericardial tamponade and prevent it from recurring as well as to treat the underlying malignancy definitively. If cytologic evidence confirms a malignant origin, catheter drainage and installation of tetracycline, talc, or any of several chemotherapeutic agents have been used with relatively good short-term success in preventing fluid reaccumulation.[50,52,54,57] For patients in whom diagnostic uncertainty exists or in whom more definitive management is required, a pleuropericardial window or subxiphoid pericardiotomy can be performed with relatively little morbidity.[50,51,53,58]

Post-ICU Phase

After clinical stabilization, it is important that definitive management of the malignant disease be considered. Patients with chemotherapy-sensitive malignant diseases, such as breast cancer, lymphoma, or small cell lung cancer, should be appropriately treated.[50] The presence of pericardial tamponade by itself does not significantly alter the underlying disease prognosis. Patients with non-small cell lung cancer or other chemotherapy-insensitive diseases are best treated with radiation therapy, in an effort to control the mediastinal manifestations of their disease. The development of pericardial involvement after definitive radiation therapy in a chemotherapy-insensitive tumor is a particularly poor prognostic sign and suggests that management efforts should be directed toward palliation.

Recurrence is uncommon after most therapeutic interventions, in part owing to the relatively poor prognosis and limited life span associated with many malignancies that produce this complication.

Pleural Effusion

Breast cancer, lung cancer, lymphoma, and adenocarcinoma of unknown primary site are the most common diagnoses in patients with malignant pleural effusions (see Table 44-4).[59] Malignant effusions may develop in one of two ways.[60] The first is the implantation of tumor metastases directly on the pleural surface with a resultant exudation of pleural fluid. The second results when tumor involves mediastinal lymph nodes and produces lymphatic obstruction and pleural fluid accumulation. This second mechanism has been more frequently described in patients with lymphoma and lung cancer. Chylous fluid may be found in this situation, particularly in patients with lymphoma, or in those with a breach in lymphatic integrity.

Pre-ICU Phase

The clinical presentation of patients with a pleural effusion includes dyspnea, cough, and chest pain,[59-61] although the effusion may be asymptomatic in up to 25%.[61] Patients may have a preexisting malignant disease, or they may have a malignant effusion as the first manifestation of disease.[59,61] The presence of bilateral pleural effusions has been noted in up to one third of patients.[61]

Accurate diagnostic confirmation and differentiation from a benign pleural effusion are of obvious prognostic and therapeutic importance.[59-62] It is particularly important to recognize that pleural effusions may develop as both an acute and a long-term complication of mediastinal or chest irradiation. A thoracentesis with pleural fluid cytology is often the easiest maneuver with the greatest diagnostic yield. Biochemical analysis of pleural fluid may be suggestive but is nonspecific. A closed pleural biopsy can be performed and may provide the diagnosis if the results of cytologic study are negative.

Unfortunately, a small percentage of patients remain undiagnosed despite several thoracenteses and pleural biopsies. Thoracoscopy or an open pleural biopsy is recommended in this situation.[59] It is important to note the diagnostic difficulty in patients with a pleural effusion from malignant mesothelioma. Pleural fluid cytology and pleural needle biopsies are often nondiagnostic or confusing in such patients, and more aggressive diagnostic measures, such as thoracoscopy, are usually required.[59]

ICU Phase

A malignant pleural effusion rarely requires ICU management, although it may complicate the management of patients in the ICU for other reasons. Although dyspnea and hypoxemia can result from massive pleural effusions, the symptom is readily relieved with thoracentesis. Pneumothorax is a relatively uncommon complication of thoracentesis but can aggravate dyspnea and temporarily mandate ICU management. This complication, however, can be rapidly relieved with chest tube insertion.

Post-ICU Phase

Patients with malignant pleural effusions are, in general, incurable, and their management strategy should be a palliative one.[59-62] Only in those patients with lymphoma does the potential for disease-free, long-term survival exist. Thoracentesis alone is of only temporary benefit, unless effective systemic treatment is available, as in breast cancer or lymphoma. Patients with non-small cell lung cancer usually require chest tube drainage and pleural sclerosis, if permanent control of the effusion is to be expected.[59-62] The intrapleural installation of agents, such as tetracycline,[59,60,63] talc,[59,62,64] quinacrine,[59] bleomycin,[59,65] and various other chemotherapeutic agents,[59,66] has been associated with a successful outcome in 70 to 85% of patients.

Those patients with continued fluid reaccumulation despite pleural sclerosis may require pleurectomy or the use of a pleuroperitoneal shunt.[59,62] Radiation therapy is, unfortunately, of only limited value except when administered to the mediastinum in patients with effusions from extensive mediastinal lymphoma.[59] As with most oncologic complications, the overall prognosis depends on the natural history of the malignancy and not on presence or absence of pleural fluid.

Malignant Ascites

The development of ascites in any patient requires a careful search for the cause. Ascites is considered malignant if it arises from the metastatic deposition of tumor on peritoneal surfaces with the resultant exudation of fluid. Ascites, however, may develop in a patient with malignancy for a variety of other reasons, including hepatic failure owing to tumor replacement or chemotherapy toxicity, myocardial or pericardial disease, vena cava or hepatic vein obstruction, lymphatic obstruction/interruption with chylous ascites, or infection.[67] The therapeutic approach taken depends on the cause of the ascites.

In patients with ovarian or gastrointestinal malignancies, malignant ascites may be the presenting manifestation of the disease or an end-stage complication. In other tumors, such as breast cancer or lymphoma, the malignant ascites usually reflects progression of an established malignancy (see Table 44-4).[67-69]

Pre-ICU Phase

The signs and symptoms of malignant ascites are well recognized. Patients present with abdominal distention, increasing abdominal girth, and complaints of "bloating."[67,68] In contradistinction to most patients with advanced malignant disease, body weight may actually increase, although loss of overall body mass may be evident in the face or extremities.

Diagnostic evaluation includes paracentesis with cultures and cytologic evaluation. CT scan of the abdomen or abdominal ultrasonography is often needed to define the presence of any hepatic abnormality. Rarely an open peritoneal biopsy is required to establish the diagnosis or to exclude the possibility of an infectious or other cause. Peritoneal mesothelioma, although an uncommon diagnosis, may be difficult to establish without such an open biopsy procedure.

The treatment options in patients with cytologically positive malignant ascites have been limited and relatively unsuccessful. In contrast to patients with malignant pleural and pericardial effusions, palliation is difficult.[67-69] Medical management, including diuresis and salt restriction, is of only marginal benefit. Repeated paracentesis is an unsatisfactory solution. It is inconvenient for patients and results in significant protein loss and a risk of infection. Intracavitary administration of radioactive colloids has been attempted in the past with mixed results.[67,70] Intracavitary sclerosing agents, such as those used for pleural effusions, make little theoretic sense and are generally not beneficial.

There has been interest in the use of intraperitoneal chemotherapy, particularly in neoplasms such as ovarian cancer.[71] Drug penetration, however, is limited, and in patients with bulky intraperitoneal tumor, this intervention has not been generally successful. In patients with breast cancer, ovarian cancer, or lymphoma, systemic chemotherapy may be effective and should be used.

ICU Phase

Malignant ascites alone is rarely a cause for ICU management. Although abdominal distention may result in respiratory embarrassment, a therapeutic paracentesis, rather than mechanical ventilation, is the appropriate intervention. Malignant ascites, however, may be a complication in a cancer patient being managed in the ICU for other reasons. The ascites may complicate fluid management and alter respiratory mechanics, but the problem is little different from patients with non-neoplastic ascites. Complications from diagnostic and therapeutic paracenteses are uncommon, although bowel perforation and peritonitis may be life-threatening.

Post-ICU Phase

A significant complication associated with malignant ascites is the development of multiple bowel obstructions from intra-abdominal carcinomatosis. This is a not infrequent complication of gastrointestinal and ovarian cancer and is difficult to palliate. It is, in general, a manifestation of extremely advanced disease, and the prognosis in such patients is limited.

For those patients with refractory ascites unresponsive to other measures, peritoneovenous shunting has had modest success. Although such patients have a limited life expectancy, they may achieve significant palliative benefit from the procedure.[67] Although shunt occlusion is frequent, the development of carcinomatosis or of a coagulopathy has not been common.[67]

HEMATOLOGIC EMERGENCIES

Hyperviscosity

Patients with cancers and benign conditions that affect blood viscosity can present in many different ways. The neoplasms and nonmalignant conditions that cause hyperviscosity are listed in Table 44-5.

The discussion of hyperviscosity is separated into those disorders that cause hyperviscosity (1) not in the presence of polycythemia and hyperviscosity (2) because of polycythemia (see under Polycythemia).

Pre-ICU Phase

Patients with hyperviscosity often present with neurologic symptoms, such as headache, fatigue, blurred vision, disorientation, and agitation. This may progress to focal findings, such as transient ischemic attack (TIA) affecting the vertebral-basilar arterial distribution with dizziness and falling to one side or TIA affecting higher cortical areas, such as aphasia, hemiparesis, or hemisensory defect.[72]

The physical examination may be completely normal or may demonstrate "sausage-shaped" retinal veins or "boxcar" alignment to the retinal vessels. Viscosity can be measured in serum or whole blood; serum viscosity is the preferred measurement because it is more reliable in

Table 44-5. Causes of Hyperviscosity

Malignant
  Paraprotein mediated
    Multiple myeloma
    Waldenström's macroglobulinemia
  Erythropoietin excess
    Renal cell carcinoma
    Hepatoma
Nonmalignant Causes
  Benign tumors causing erythrocytosis
    Large uterine myomas
    Large cerebellar hemangiomas
    Kasabach-Merritt syndrome
    Adrenal adenomas
  Iatrogenic
    Overuse of exogenous erythropoietin
    Blood "doping"
    Androgens
  Secondary erythrocytosis
    Secondary to hypoxia, high altitude
    Hemoglobinopathies with left-shifted oxyhemoglobin dissociation curves
    Secondary to diuretics
    Alveolar hypoventilation
    Cyanotic congenital heart disease
      Eisenmenger's complex (ventricular septal defect)
      Atrial septal defect secundum
      Single ventricle
      Truncus arteriosus
      Patent ductus arteriosus
      Tetralogy of Fallot
      Complete transposition of the great vessels
    Cigarette smoking
    Renal causes
      Vascular impairment
      Post-transplantation
      Polycystic kidney disease
      Hydronephrosis
Cryoglobulinemias
Cold agglutinin disease
Polycythemia vera

Disseminated Intravascular Coagulation

Disseminated intravascular coagulation (DIC) is an end result of derangement of the consumption of clotting factors and platelets in the peripheral circulation. This is associated with activation of the fibrinolytic system. A vast array of disorders causes this problem (Table 44-6). DIC may be acute and fulminant, or it may be slow in onset and indolent in clinical course.[75]

In DIC, a cascade of events leads to the foregoing derangements. First, there is activation of coagulation. Usually this is through exposure of subendothelial tissues or thromboplastic substances appearing in the circulation from whatever source. Then, events either lead to thrombosis or to bleeding. The events leading to thrombosis often lead to circulating thrombi with subsequent thrombotic occlusion of microcirculation of either an isolated organ or all organs. The events that lead to bleeding lead to the consumption of platelets and coagulation proteins. The thrombotic occlusion of the microcirculation, mentioned previously, often sets off fibrinolysis in the microcirculation, and then the circulation of fibrin degradation products is observed. The fibrin degradation products interfere with fibrinogen being converted to fibrin, so an end result of the events leading to thrombosis is a compensatory series of events leading to bleeding.

Thus, some patients with DIC have signs of microvascular thrombosis, whereas others have signs of a hemorrhagic diathesis. In general, one third of patients with DIC do not particularly bleed, one third bleed too much, and one third clot too much. This is a gross general rule of thumb and should never be relied on in any one clinical situation to guide management.

The organ systems affected by DIC can manifest different clinical syndromes and signs, depending on whether

predicting which patients actually develop neurologic problems.[73]

ICU Phase

The immediate steps one takes as the patient with hyperviscosity deteriorates may be a mechanical withdrawal from the vascular space of whatever is causing the hyperviscosity. In the case of paraproteins, plasmapheresis is an excellent, quick way to lower viscosity.[74] In patients with polycythemia, phlebotomies reduce viscosity most rapidly. This is discussed separately. The use of aspirin or pentoxifylline is of secondary importance when compared with the above-mentioned procedures.

Post-ICU Phase

In those patients with neoplasms causing hyperviscosity, the clinician must have a plan to treat the underlying neoplasm at some point. It may not be one's first treatment choice, especially in the patient in the ICU with a profound neurologic symptom. For those patients with a paraprotein causing the hyperviscosity, chemotherapy is usually necessary to control the elevated viscosity in the long term.

Table 44-6. Causes of Disseminated Intravascular Coagulation

Widespread tissue damage
Hypersensitivity reactions
Incompatible blood transfusion
Anaphylaxis
Obstetric complications
  Amniotic fluid embolism
  Premature separation of placenta
  Preeclampsia
Malignancy
  Acute promyelocytic leukemia
  Mucin-secreting tumors
Infections
  Gram-negative infections
  Meningococcemia
  Septic abortion
  Clostridial infections
Viral infections
  Purpura fulminans
Miscellaneous
  Liver failure
  Snake venoms
  Burns
  Hypothermia
  Heatstroke
  Hypoxia
  Vascular malformations

the patient with DIC has a hemorrhagic diathesis or a thrombotic diathesis.

- The **neurologic** evaluation of the patient with microvascular thrombosis might reveal multifocal findings with delirium and coma. The neurologic evaluation of a patient with hemorrhagic diathesis may demonstrate intracerebral bleeding and focal deficits.
- In a patient with microvascular thrombosis, the **skin** would demonstrate focal ischemia and superficial gangrene. In the patient with hemorrhagic diathesis, the skin would demonstrate ecchymoses and oozing at venipuncture sites.
- In patients with microvascular thrombosis associated with DIC, the **renal** system is noted for oliguria, azotemia, and cortical necrosis. In patients with hemorrhagic diathesis, the renal system is manifested by hematuria.
- **Adult respiratory distress syndrome (ARDS)** is seen in patients with the microvascular thrombotic diathesis of DIC. Tachypnea and hypoxia are observed.
- The **mucous membranes** are affected with epistaxis and gingival oozing in patients with the hemorrhagic diathesis of DIC.
- In patients with the microvascular thrombotic diathesis of DIC, the **gastrointestinal system** may be noted for acute ulceration. In patients with the hemorrhagic diathesis of DIC, there may be massive bleeding.

The laboratory evaluation of patients with DIC is notable, in general, for elevation of the prothrombin time (PT) and partial thromboplastin time (PTT), a depression of the fibrinogen level, and a depression of the platelet count. There is an elevation of the fibrin degradation products, either manifested by D-dimer elevation or direct measurement of fibrin degradation products.

Pre-ICU Phase

The treatment of DIC involves the treatment of the underlying disease. For those patients with infections, antibiotics are necessary. For those patients with obstetric complications, treatment of the underlying problem is performed, usually involving evacuating the uterus.

If the patient with DIC becomes so ill that hypotension or hypoxia arises from pulmonary thrombi or bleeding, it may be necessary to admit the patient to an ICU.

ICU Phase

All attempts at treating the underlying cause of the DIC should continue in the ICU. Further treatment with antibiotics, oxygen therapy with intubation, ventilatory support, and pressor support is necessary.

The role of heparin in DIC is controversial.[76] There are only two situations for which heparin has developed a definite role. One is the treatment of DIC associated with acute promyelocytic leukemia (APL). Even in this setting, there is controversy. Advocates of the use of heparin have demonstrated a reduction of intracerebral bleeding rates in patients with DIC associated with APL through the use of heparin infusions. Patients receive heparin at a low dose in a continuous infusion (5 to 8 U/kg/hour). Dose of heparin is titrated to raise the fibrinogen level.[76] The other setting for which heparin has a role is the treatment of thrombotic complications of those with chronic DIC in the setting of a mucin-secreting adenocarcinoma (e.g., breast, prostate, pancreas, colon). Subcutaneous heparin has been demonstrated to reduce the incidence of thrombi in such a setting. The historical name for such an entity is Trousseau's syndrome, in which there is migratory thrombi. This usually is not an issue in the ICU; however, it is more prevalent in the pre-ICU management and post-ICU management of patients with chronic DIC.

Generally infusion of platelets and cryoprecipitate to raise the platelet count and the fibrinogen count are indicated as the primary transfusion support for such patients.

Post-ICU Phase

For patients who recover from bouts of meningococcemia, for example, and who have had DIC, once out of the ICU, their management depends on whatever sequela may have resulted in the ICU. If there were no permanent neurologic damage and no permanent renal damage, the recovery is usually relatively rapid, especially in younger patients. In elderly patients, if they do survive the ICU admission, often there are sequelae because DIC can be life-threatening.

If the bone marrow is adequately nutritionally supported, it will generally respond with an erythroid hyperplasia to counterbalance the microangiopathic hemolytic anemia that occurs with DIC. Generally inhibitors of fibrinolysis, such as aminocaproic acid (Amicar), are contraindicated.

Hyperleukocytosis

Patients with acute lymphoblastic leukemia and acute myelocytic leukemia may present with white blood cell counts elevated so high that the capillaries of the brain and lungs, in particular, fill with blasts, which break down the endothelium leading to diapedesis of red cells. This can lead to bleeding. In the brain, this can lead to massive, fatal intracerebral bleeding. Generally this occurs above absolute blast counts of 100,000/mm^3. In an elderly patient, this may occur at a lower absolute blast count.

Patients with chronic phase chronic myelogenous and chronic lymphocytic leukemia do not have this problem. Even though the total white cell count of a typical patient with chronic phase chronic myelogenous leukemia might be greater than 300,000/mm^3, most of these cells are neutrophils, bands, metamyelocytes, myelocytes, and promyelocytes. These cells are pliable, not rigid. They traverse cerebral capillaries without inducing the dreaded diapedesis of red cells.

Pre-ICU Phase

Controversy surrounds the management of patients with extremely high blast counts. In the pre-ICU setting, when confronted with a newly diagnosed acute leukemia patient with an absolute blast count of greater than 100,000/mm³, one first tries to lower the count. Leukapheresis is an excellent technique to lower the blast count rapidly.[78,79] Drawbacks to this are that (1) the blast count begins rapidly rising once the procedure is finished, and (2) one must use large-bore catheters in the antecubital fossae (or even groin) to establish enough flow for the pheresis machine. If the patient has coincident DIC or poor venous access, there are hazards of bleeding with these catheters.

When the new hyperleukocytotic leukemic patient arrives, there is much diagnostic activity the aim of which is to determine which subtype of leukemia the patient has. Several days may elapse before all morphologic, immunophenotypic, and cytochemical information is collected from the laboratory. Cytogenetic analysis may take 2 to 3 weeks. Therefore the clinician must act to bring the count down before the leukemia subtype is known. There are chemotherapy drugs that lower these high counts, whether acute myelocytic leukemia or acute lymphoblastic leukemia is causing the high blast count. If the patient can take oral medicines, hydroxyurea in a dose of 1 g every 6 hours works predictably and fast. Daunorubicin or cytosine arabinose might be used as an intravenous chemotherapy drug if the patient is vomiting or has an ileus and cannot tolerate oral drugs. To reduce the risk of urate nephropathy or gout, allopurinol must be given even before the chemotherapy. An older, less beneficial technique is to radiate the brain. This disposes of the blasts that happen to be in the cerebral circulation at the time of the radiation, but these capillaries are quickly repopulated by blasts.

ICU Phase

If the patient has evidence of intracerebral bleeding and is neurologically compromised based on hyperleukocytosis with acute myelocytic leukemia or acute lymphoblastic leukemia, the prognosis is grim. Ventilatory support is usually necessary. To begin induction chemotherapy for acute leukemia in a patient who already has intracerebral bleeding and is on a ventilator, however, is almost a fruitless endeavor.

Assuming that the high blast count can be lowered rapidly with leukophoresis or chemotherapy, one may then take the necessary time to establish semipermanent intravenous access (Hickman or Broviac catheter) and proceed with more definitive chemotherapy.[80] Often by the time the high blast count has been controlled, the laboratory has confirmed which subtype of leukemia is present, and the correct definitive course of chemotherapy can be chosen.

Patients with hyperleukocytosis have a higher death rate in the first week of therapy than patients with leukemia who do not have hyperleukocytosis. If one eliminates the deaths within the first week and compares complete remission rates of hyperleukocytotic versus nonhyperleukocytotic acute leukemic patients, there are no differences. The duration of remission, however, is shorter in the former group.[80]

The previous commentary can also apply to other organ systems, usually with better outcomes than in patients with intracerebral bleeding. The pulmonary parenchyma can be affected by a high absolute blast percentage with infiltrates, hypoxia, intra-alveolar leakage of plasma and blood, and a need for ventilatory support. The pre-ICU patient usually is hypoxic with lower lobe streaky infiltrates. If hydroxyurea or leukophoresis can be effective in lowering the absolute blast count, patients may be able to avoid the ICU setting. They may progress, however, to involve all lobes, become severely dyspneic, and need to be admitted to the ICU.

A phenomenon called "pseudohypoxia" occurs when blasts sit in an arterial blood gas container for too long before being analyzed. These blasts are so hypermetabolic that they can artificially lower the P_{O_2} of the sample and misguide therapeutic decisions.[81]

Post-ICU Phase

Once the hyperleukocytosis is treated, either with leukophoresis or chemotherapy, and the patient enters the nadir of counts, the management shifts to supportive care with transfusions of platelets and red cells and the use of antibiotics to counter infections. These are the treatments used in the "induction" phase of chemotherapy in leukemia patients, designed to induce a complete remission. Specific management of the chemotherapy-induced complications of antileukemia treatment are presented later in this chapter.

Leukopenia

A patient with life-threatening leukopenia may need an ICU level of care if infection occurs. Patients with aplastic anemia, chronic neutropenia, or drug-induced or chemotherapy-induced agranulocytosis may feel perfectly well and be free of fevers or infection for months, whereas others with the same depth of neutropenia may be deathly ill with nosocomial or opportunistic infections.[82] Often a determining factor for how these patients fare is the rate of decline of neutrophils. Those individuals with a rapid decline tend to develop fevers and infections faster than those patients with a more gradual decline.

The list of drugs associated with neutropenia and agranulocytosis is long. The major groups of drugs are listed in Table 44-7. Some of these agents predictably lower all patients' neutrophil counts, whereas others cause idiosyncratic reactions.

Pre-ICU Phase

When patients present with agranulocytosis and have been receiving any medicine that could be incriminated

Table 44–7. Drug Groups Associated with Agranulocytosis

Class	Prototypic
Chemotherapy	Practically all
Anti-inflammatory	Phenylbutazone
Antithyroidal	Propylthiouracil
Anticonvulsants	Carbamazepine
Antipsychotics	Chlorpromazine
Antibiotics	Penicillins
Cardiovascular	Captopril

as its cause, it is wise to stop all medicines except those that are absolutely necessary. If patients are febrile, cultures should be done of all accessible body fluids. If there are neurologic changes, they should have a lumbar puncture to rule out meningitis. Broad-spectrum antibiotics, especially with antipseudomonal coverage, should be administered.[83-86] If patients have an absolute neutrophil count below 500/mm³ and have no fever, it is certainly prudent that cultures be done, but one need not initiate antibiotic therapy. Growth factors, especially granulocyte-colony stimulating factors (G-CSF), have been found to decrease the duration and depth of neutropenia caused by chemotherapy.[87] They are not approved by the Food and Drug Administration (FDA) for aplastic-anemia-induced or non-chemotherapy-drug-induced agranulocytosis; with their current availability, however, there are many such patients who are receiving these growth factors. It is premature to recommend their routine use in this setting without more controlled studies.

If the patient with agranulocytosis becomes febrile and septic, and broad antibacterial coverage is effective, and the neutrophil count rises, no further treatment may be necessary. If the neutrophil count remains low while the patient is receiving antibacterials and then further fevers occur, they may be due to breakthrough bacteremias with resistant bacteria, or the fevers may be due to opportunistic fungi or viruses. Amphotericin is usually added in this setting.[88,89] If a viral process becomes manifest, such as positive viral cultures of a vesicular skin or oral cavity eruption, antiviral medicines are added.

ICU Phase

If a septic neutropenic patient becomes more severely ill, such as with hypotension from bacteremia or with hypoxia from ARDS or pneumonia, the patient might require the level of care provided in an ICU. (See discussion of bone marrow transplantation for ICU management of agranulocytosis.)

Polycythemia

The discussion of polycythemia is rather similar to hyperviscosity. The reason for this is that as the red cell mass increases, viscosity rises. The causes of polycythemia, however, are usually different from the causes of hyperviscosity. As seen in Table 44-5, polycythemia may arise as a primary marrow disorder (polycythemia vera), as secondary to a malignancy, as secondary to many different medical conditions, as secondary to a hemoglobinopathy, or as a physiologic response to certain drugs.

Pre-ICU Phase

In the pre-ICU setting, polycythemia may present with vague headache, clouded sensorium, or blurred vision.[90] The physical examination depends on the cause of the polycythemia. A patient with polycythemia vera typically has plethora, suffused conjunctivae, and splenomegaly. A patient with cyanotic congenital heart disease has cyanosis and abnormalities on heart auscultation. One might be able to palpate the enlarged kidneys in patients with polycystic kidney disease.

The laboratory analysis of patients with polycythemia, again depends on the cause. Patients with polycythemia vera usually have basophilia, and often the white blood cell count and platelet count are elevated.[91,92] Patients with hypoxia-driven polycythemia have a low P_{O_2}. The patient with diuretic-induced polycythemia has a metabolic ("contraction") alkalosis.

ICU Phase

Patients are usually diagnosed with polycythemia in the outpatient setting and can be handled in such a way that they never arrive at an ICU. There may be an occasional patient, however, who arrives at the ICU or on a neurology service with TIA-like symptoms with a profound elevation of hemoglobin concentration. As stated previously, phlebotomy is the treatment of choice.[90]

Post-ICU Phase

For the patient with polycythemia vera, the post-ICU, long-term management is usually repeated phlebotomies to keep the hematocrit between 40 and 45%.[91,92] The use of ^{32}P and busulfan have fallen out of favor because of their increased risk of leukemogenesis.[93] About 15 to 20% of patients with polycythemia vera progress to acute myelogenous leukemia.[94] When they do, their prognosis is poorer than individuals who develop de novo acute myelogenous leukemia.

Anemia

Anemia is a symptom of underlying illness, not really a diagnosis. It would be rare for a patient to be admitted to the ICU only for anemia; however, anemia is a frequent finding in patients admitted to the ICU.

The marrow is the site of red cell production. The normal erythrocyte lives its first 24 to 48 hours as a reticulocyte. It then matures into a normal red cell and lives its 120-day life span traversing the vasculature serving the peripheral tissues with oxygen. The red cell senesces and dies; then the reticuloendothelial system, primarily the liver Kupffer cells, spleen, and nodes, scavenges the amino acids of the globin chains, scavenges the iron molecules of the heme moiety, and degrades the heme to bilirubin, which is then excreted in stool and urine. Any process that accelerates the destruction of red cells in the peripheral circulation signals the marrow to undergo a hyperplasia of the erythropoietic cells. Marrow production of red cells increases and a higher percentage of the peripheral red cells are reticulocytes. The reticulocyte count therefore becomes an important piece of data in determining if the anemia one is trying to diagnose is the result of a normal marrow response to a peripheral red cell injury or of a hypoproliferative marrow.

Another key part of the diagnosis of anemia is reviewing the peripheral smear. In the ICU, one often finds patients with premature peripheral destruction of red cells. The peripheral smear may demonstrate polychromasia, nucleated red blood cells, and early granulocytic precursors, such as metamyelocytes and myelocytes. This combination of findings is called a "leukoerythroblastic smear."

In the ICU, anemia from blood loss is usually treated with transfusion of red blood cells. An explanation of the practice of blood banking is beyond the scope of this chapter. Suffice it to say, the ICUs at our institution account for about 50% of all red cell transfusions. The patient who is bleeding and refuses transfusion presents a unique challenge to the intensivist.

Pre-ICU Phase

Owing to religious convictions or other reasons, some patients refuse transfusions.[95] If such a patient begins to bleed, such as with a duodenal ulcer, quick recognition and treatment are mandatory. Endoscopy with heat probes may be used. Crystalloid may dilute the hemoglobin concentration but may maintain blood pressure. If further bleeding occurs and the patient's hemoglobin drops, hypotension may ensue, prompting a transfer to the ICU. The marrow's capacity to keep up with the demand of bleeding must be supported with iron and folate. The use of vitamin B_{12} or erythropoietin does not help, unless patients are specifically deficient in them.

ICU Phase

Once such patients come to an ICU, there is the possibility of using blood substitutes. The only FDA-approved blood substitute presently available is a perfluorochemical emulsion called Fluosol. This emulsion dissolves oxygen and carbon dioxide in water.[96-98] It is approved by the FDA only for delivering oxygen to the coronary arteries during percutaneous transluminal coronary angioplasty (PTCA). It has been used systemically in severely anemic patients who refuse transfusion. Its efficacy in this latter setting is not as good as in the PTCA setting. In double-blind studies during PTCA, the use of Fluosol has preserved ventricular wall motion and global left ventricular ejection fraction better than placebo. In the ICU setting of severe anemia, it has been suggested that Fluosol has aided in the delivery of oxygen to peripheral tissues, but no survival enhancement has ever been proved with its use in this setting.

Post-ICU Phase

Once the cause of bleeding is controlled and the use of Fluosol has been discontinued, patients need to prevent a recurrence of whatever caused the bleeding. Duodenal ulcers require prolonged treatment with H_2 blockade. Colonic bleeding sites, either diverticuli or tumors, may need surgical resection to prevent recurrent bleeding. Total body iron repletion may take 6 months with oral therapy. For patients who cannot tolerate oral iron preparations, there is intravenous iron.

Thrombocytosis

Thrombocytosis either is due to a primary overproduction of platelets in the bone marrow or is caused by some other disease stimulating the bone marrow to produce too many platelets (secondary). The intensive care specialist is more likely to have trouble dealing with a patient with primary thrombocythemia (essential thrombocytosis) as opposed to the patient with a reactive process.

Essential thrombocytosis is a myeloproliferative disorder in which there is an autonomous overproduction of platelets by an increased number of megakaryocytes in the bone marrow. This disorder has many names. It is called primary thrombocythemia, essential thrombocythemia, or essential thrombocytosis. It generally occurs in older individuals. These patients have hemorrhagic manifestations or vaso-occlusive problems. Bleeding usually occurs from the mucous membranes. These patients can have devastating bleeding in the postoperative period. The patients with this disorder who have excess clotting often have erythromelalgia, with painful erythematous changes to the palms and soles with distal portions of digits demonstrating ischemic changes.[99]

The bone marrow aspirate and biopsy specimen are usually hypercellular with an increased number of megakaryocytes, and often these megakaryocytes form clusters. The distinction between polycythemia vera and essential thrombocytosis is difficult especially in their early stages. Indeed, patients may initially be considered to have one disorder and over time evolve toward a more obvious manifestation of the other. They may even take on the appearance of other myeloproliferative disorders, such as chronic myelogenous leukemia or myelofibrosis.

Reactive thrombocytosis is a condition wherein an inflammatory, neoplastic, or iron-deficient state causes a secondary thrombocytosis. Also, patients who have had a splenectomy may have a chronic thrombocytosis. Usually the underlying problem is quite obvious, and the thrombocytosis is an epiphenomenon. Platelet counts may be more than 1 million/mm^3 but usually are under this level. Defining the source of iron deficiency often involves endoscopy of the upper and lower gastrointestinal tracts. Every patient with thrombocytosis should have iron, total iron binding capacity, percent saturation, and ferritin levels drawn to discover whether a deficiency of iron is causing the thrombocytosis.

Patients with secondary thrombocytosis rarely have bleeding diathesis or excessive clotting. There are case reports in the literature of patients with high platelet counts that are secondary to some underlying disease with clotting abnormalities.[100] In general, however, these patients neither bleed nor clot. Treatment of the underlying disease usually brings the platelet count into a more normal range. Patients with secondary thrombocytosis usually have normal platelet aggregation testing. Patients with essential thrombocytosis often have abnormalities on platelet aggregation testing, such as nonresponsiveness to epinephrine.[101]

Pre-ICU Phase

Because patients with primary marrow overproduction of platelets have bleeding and clotting problems, the intensivist is more likely to be called on to deal with this population. Most patients are asymptomatic and have essential thrombocytosis discovered on routine screening with complete blood count. Hematologic evaluation discovers the cause (e.g., bone marrow examination). Some patients present to the internist or family physician with mucous membrane bleeding, soft tissue bleeding, easy bruisability, or history of excessive bleeding after dental extraction, for example, which prompts the complete blood count and hematologic evaluation.

Once these patients are followed by hematologists, attempts are usually made to bring the platelet count into a range of 400,000 to 600,000/mm^3. Patients often complain of vague neurologic symptoms, such as headache or dizziness, when their platelet count is above 600,000/mm^3.[102] Some patients with essential thrombocytosis may have absolutely no symptoms even above platelet counts of 1.5 million/mm^3. Still the literature would support the reduction of platelets to around 600,000/mm^3.

Hydroxyurea, busulfan, and anagrelide[103] (an experimental drug that lowers platelet counts) are the usual pharmacologic interventions to bring the platelet count down. If patients have an extremely high platelet count and are actively bleeding or clotting, plateletpheresis[104] is the preferred method of rapidly lowering platelet count.

The use of aspirin or other antiplatelet agents is to be avoided in patients with essential thrombocytosis because it may exacerbate the bleeding tendency. There are some clinical situations wherein the use of aspirin might be mandated. For example, a patient with excessive clotting from essential thrombocytosis who is intolerant of chemotherapy might be handled conservatively with a small dose of aspirin. Generally, however, this is not recommended.

ICU Phase

For those patients with essential thrombocytosis who have a severe bleeding tendency, there may be need for intensive treatments for gastrointestinal bleeding, bleeding into the central nervous system, or postoperative bleeding. If platelet aggregation testing has previously shown defects and the patient clearly has a bleeding tendency, there is a role for platelet transfusion during episodes of severe blood loss or bleeding into a privileged site, such as the central nervous system. It is ironic that the patient may have a platelet count over 1 million, be comatose from a central nervous system bleed, and be receiving a platelet transfusion. This may, however, need to be done.

There are some patients who, despite normalization of their platelet count with hydroxyurea, still manifest a clotting tendency. Patients who are followed on a long-term basis with essential thrombocytosis who are doing well and then suddenly develop some new problem need thorough, rapid evaluation. For example, a patient with essential thrombocytosis who is doing well on hydroxyurea but then develops abdominal pain with guaiac-positive stools must be considered a candidate for almost emergent arteriography to make sure that the patient is not having an episode of ischemic colitis from superior mesenteric artery occlusion. A patient who has sudden chest pain with electrocardiographic changes who has a platelet count even near the normal range with essential thrombocytosis must be considered as having platelet-mediated thrombi causing a myocardial infarction. If such a patient has an extremely elevated platelet count, he or she should have emergency plateletpheresis to lower the platelet count.

Post-ICU Phase

If the patient with essential thrombocytosis is first diagnosed in the ICU with a sudden change in clinical status and has weathered the storm of myocardial infarction, superior mesenteric artery occlusion, and so forth, long-term management usually requires normalization of the platelet count with hydroxyurea and other measures. Again, if demonstration of intolerance of these medicines is established, aspirin may have a limited role. Its use, as noted previously, is to be avoided if possible.

Patients with this disorder do have a risk of developing acute leukemia about 15% of the time.[105] The long-term management usually requires inspection of the bone marrow if there are some other changes in the blood counts, such as a sudden rise in white blood cell count or a worsening anemia.

Careful dental hygiene is mandatory so the need for dental extractions is lowered. Greater consideration for the risks of bleeding should lead the clinician to avoid elective surgeries, if possible. In general, these patients bleed or clot less when their platelet counts are between 400,000 and 600,000. Long-term administration of hydroxyurea to keep patients in this range would make emergency surgery safer for patients with essential thrombocytosis.

Thrombocytopenia

The patient who is bleeding and whose platelet count is extremely low is a true emergency. Determining the time course of the patient's drop in platelet count (slow or fast in onset) and the cause of the low platelet count is important. There are five broad causes of low platelet count:

- Pseudothrombocytopenia
- Poor production
- Enhanced destruction
- Sequestration
- Dilution

Pseudothrombocytopenia

Some patients' platelets clump in the presence of the ethylenediaminetetia-acetic acid (EDTA), the anticoagulant in the purple-top tube. These patients have no evidence of bleeding, such as petechiae, but the laboratory reports that their platelet count is 10,000/mm^3 or below. Simply redrawing their blood in a heparinized tube or in a citrate-containing tube should yield normal results.

Poor Production

Primary marrow disorders account for these patients. They often have some other problem with their blood besides thrombocytopenia. For example, patients with aplastic anemia have pancytopenia, patients with metastatic cancer in their marrow have a leukoerythroblastic smear and tear-drop morphology to their red blood cells, and patients with acute leukemia have circulating blasts.

In the pre-ICU setting, diagnostic tests are first done—usually a review of the peripheral smear and the bone marrow. Specific treatments are defined by the marrow disorder, e.g., daunorubicin and cytosine arabinoside for acute myelocytic leukemia, or cytoxan, adriamycin, and 5-FU for widely metastatic breast cancer. For bleeding that occurs secondary to thrombocytopenia, in the setting of ineffective marrow production of platelets, platelet transfusion is usually necessary. The level of platelets at which one transfuses depend on the clinical setting. Leukemic patients in the midst of treatment generally receive prophylactic platelet transfusions while they are at their nadir counts. Based on older studies,[106] a platelet count of 20,000/mm^3 or below was thought to be a level requiring transfusion to prevent hemorrhage. Newer studies recommend even lower counts, such as 10,000 or 15,000/mm^3. These newer studies stress that the patients should have no evidence of DIC, fever, or active infection if one is to use these lower threshold levels. It is also important not to overtransfuse platelets into these patients. Alloimmunization against platelets can occur rapidly in some patients.[107] Filters to remove leukocytes from platelets are available but are expensive. Ultraviolet irradiation of platelet products may have a role in reducing alloimmunization. In patients who are chronically thrombocytopenic (e.g., an older patient with aplastic anemia for whom bone marrow transplantation has no role) and who have no evidence of DIC, there may be a role for antifibrinolytic agents, such as epsilon-aminocaproic acid.

Enhanced Destruction

The patient's own deranged immune system, infections, and drugs are the most likely causes of increased destruction of platelets. Immune thrombocytopenic purpura (ITP) is a common reason for low platelet counts. Some individuals are never symptomatic and have platelet counts that never drop into a dangerous range, whereas others are precariously low at all times.

Pre-ICU Phase. The usual pre-ICU treatment of these patients is steroids. Most respond initially with a rise in platelet count. Most fail when the steroids are tapered. The usual recommendation at that point is splenectomy. This cures 80% of adults with ITP. For the 20% who are still thrombocytopenic, one generally uses further steroids, danazol, intravenous IgG, azathioprine, or chemotherapy to cause the platelets to rise. Practically every drug has been recorded as a cause for thrombocytopenia. Drug-induced platelet destruction may be by many mechanisms (Table 44-8).[108] Withdrawal of the offending agent usually leads to a normalization of the platelet count. This may take 1 to 2 weeks. One usually treats these patients with steroids and, in severe cases, steroids plus intravenous IgG. Again unless these patients have life-threatening intracerebral or internal bleeding, they rarely need ICU level of care.

ICU Phase. A patient with ITP or drug-induced thrombocytopenia rarely needs ICU care—the most likely reason is intracranial hemorrhage. These patients may have a rapid downhill course or may recover fairly well. Platelet transfusions are generally ineffective in ITP and should be reserved only for the most life-threatening settings.

Sequestration

Patients with certain hemoglobinopathies, particularly sickle cell syndromes, can develop splenomegaly and sequester much of their platelets in an enlarged spleen. This is more usually seen in the pediatric age group.

Other patients with liver disorders and portal hypertension have developed splenomegaly and have sequestration of their blood elements, particularly platelets, leading to problems that an intensivist might confront. Cirrhosis from whatever cause can lead to shifts of pressures in the portal circulation resulting in enlargement of the spleen. These patients usually have a mild pancytopenia and do well; however, over time, the spleen's ability to hold onto the circulating platelet pool becomes more pronounced. Patients with esophageal varices and hypersplenism can have disastrous bleeding complications.

There is no specific medical therapy to interrupt the hypersplenism and resultant thrombocytopenia. There are reports of success with splenectomy in patients with this constellation of findings. A new technique called transjugular intrahepatic portosystemic stent-shunt has been used successfully to cause a 50% reduction of the portal pressure with complete loss of variceal protrusion into the esophageal lumen. There are no reports, however, of reducing the level of thrombocytopenia using this technique. This is an area of further investigation.

Dilution

Patients who bleed extensively and require red cell replacement may have reduced platelet counts if they also do not receive platelet transfusions. The marrow recovery time to produce enough platelets to keep the platelet count normal is not quick enough in someone with extensive surgical bleeding. In some patients, even with just 2 units of red blood cells transfused during a surgical procedure, the platelet count can drop from the normal range to below 100,000. As greater than 6 units of red cells are transfused, in the vast majority of patients, platelet count drops from the normal range to below 100,000.

The best approach to such patients is to keep the platelet count as close to normal as possible using platelet transfusions. Some surgical procedures require vast amounts of red cells. Often for every 6 units of red cells, a recommendation can be made to give a pack of pooled platelets (as well as 2 to 3 units of fresh frozen plasma to replace diluted clotting factors).

Bone Marrow Transplantation

Bone marrow transplantation is a potentially curative treatment for diseases that used to be incurable.[109] The

Table 44-8. Mechanisms of Drug-Induced Thrombocytopenia

Mechanism	Prototypic Drug
Suppression of platelet production	Chemotherapy
Increased platelet consumption	
Nonimmune	Ristocetin
Drug-induced immune	Quinidine
Drug-induced nonimmune	Methyldopa

Table 44-9. Diseases for Which Bone Marrow Transplantation Has Been Defined as Standard of Care

Aplastic anemia
Myelodysplasia
Chronic myelogenous leukemia in chronic phase
Acute myelogenous leukemia
Acute lymphocytic leukemia
Relapsed (sensitive) Hodgkin's and non-Hodgkin lymphoma

---

diseases for which bone marrow transplantation has a definite role, that is those illnesses for which it is now the standard of care, are listed in Table 44-9.

Bone marrow transplantation has been applied in several diseases, and the results are quite beneficial in certain numbers of patients. It is yet not clear, however, whether the standard of care includes transplantation. These illnesses include metastatic breast cancer, multiple myeloma, ovarian cancer, testicular cancer, and certain metabolic diseases.

Transplants are divided into three types. **Allogeneic** bone marrow transplants involve taking bone marrow from a related HLA-compatible sibling or an unrelated HLA-compatible person obtained through a registry and transplanting that marrow into an ill recipient. **Autologous** bone marrow transplants involve the patient serving as his or her own donor. **Syngeneic** transplants involve taking marrow from one identical twin and giving to another.

The illnesses for which allogeneic bone marrow transplantation is applied include:

- Chronic myelogenous leukemia in chronic phase
- The acute leukemias
- Aplastic anemia
- Myelodysplasia

Illnesses for which an autologous transplant is the routine include:

- Non-Hodgkin lymphoma
- Hodgkin's disease
- Breast cancer
- Ovarian and testicular cancer

Patients who receive bone marrow transplants become extremely sick, and have prolonged nadirs of their blood counts. Complications of neutropenia and thrombocytopenia can cause infections and bleeding. These complications are similar in general to those mentioned in the sections of this chapter dealing with neutropenia and thrombocytopenia. Unique end-organ damage from high dose chemotherapy has also been discussed elsewhere in this chapter, such as veno-occlusive disease of the liver. Other unique bone marrow transplantation dose chemotherapy-related, end-organ toxicities, however, are discussed next. In the setting of allogeneic bone marrow transplantation, certain unusual infections are more prevalent, especially cytomegalovirus infection. Also in the setting of allogeneic bone marrow transplantation, there are unique problems associated with the immunosuppressed state, such as cyclosporine-induced (1) nephrotoxicity, (2) hepatotoxicity, and (3) neurologic side effects. Unique to the setting of allogeneic bone marrow transplantation is the complication of graft-versus-host disease (GVHD), which is also described subsequently.

Pre-ICU Phase

Each illness described here is treated with a unique preparative regimen of chemotherapy. Table 44-10 lists the commonly used preparative regimens for the various illnesses treated with bone marrow transplantation. Many institutions have their own unique variations on these combinations.

In general, these patients get severe mucositis, and some require hyperalimentation to maintain body weight. The use of total parenteral hyperalimentation has never been proved to be of absolute benefit to patients in the setting of bone marrow transplantation. It is often used to maintain nutrition. Its use sometimes increases the risk of infection because of the high glucose content administered. Also, metabolic derangements can occur, such as hyperglycemia requiring insulin or fatty metamorphosis of the liver with a cholestatic picture.

These patients develop agranulocytosis, which can last for 2 to 4 weeks, and they invariably need broad-spectrum antibiotics and antifungal therapy. A typical approach is to give nonabsorbable antibiotics to decontaminate the gut and either prophylactic use of an antifungal drug or early institution of amphotericin. Patients are followed through the first few days of their nadir, and at the point they develop a fever, broad cultures are done, and then the patients are started on broad-spectrum antibiotics, especially to cover enteric gram-negative organisms, pseudomonas, and staphylococcus, and streptococcus. A typical regimen would be piperacillin, tobramycin, and vancomycin. Several institutions have their own combinations, and as long as the foregoing organisms are covered, the regimens are suitable. Once patients become afebrile, then these antibiotics are maintained until the absolute neutrophil count

Table 44-10. Bone Marrow Transplantation Preparative Regimens

Aplastic anemia
  Antithymocyte globulin, 90 mg/kg, and cyclophosphamide, 200 mg/kg
Acute myelogenous leukemia
  Busulfan, 16 mg/kg, and cyclophosphamide, 200 mg/kg
  Cyclophosphamide, 200 mg/kg, and total body irradiation, 1200 rad
  VP-16, 60 mg/kg, and total body irradiation
Breast cancer
  BCNU, 600 mg/m^2, cisplatin, 165 mg/m^2, and cyclophosphamide, 5650 mg/m^2
  Cyclophosphamide, 6 g/m^2, thiotepha, 500 mg/m^2, and carboplatin, 800 mg/m^2 (STAMP V)
Multiple myeloma
  IV melphalan, 200 mg/m^2
Hodgkin's disease and non-Hodgkin lymphoma
  BCNU, 600 mg/m^2, cyclophosphamide, 1800 mg/m^2, and VP-16, 2400 mg/m^2
  BCNU, 600 mg/m^2, VP-16, 1600 mg/m^2, cytosine arabinoside, 24 g/m^2, and cyclophosphamide, 90 mg/kg

rises above 500/mm³. If the patient initially becomes febrile, then is placed on broad-spectrum antibiotics and becomes afebrile, and then becomes febrile again, the supposition is that a fungal opportunistic infection may be causing this, and amphotericin is started at a dose of approximately 0.5 mg/kg/day. Amphotericin causes renal insufficiency and potassium wastage requiring replacement.

Patients who develop thrombocytopenia from these preparative regimens often require multiple platelet transfusions. Platelet refractoriness is a major problem, and some centers rely on blood banks to give them HLA-compatible platelets, cross-match compatible platelets, or single-donor platelets.

As long as there is no evidence of DIC, antifibrinolytic agents, such as epsilon-aminocaproic acid, may also be used. These issues have also been discussed in general under Thrombocytopenia in this section.

Allogeneic bone marrow transplantation can cause a unique immunologic disorder, GVHD. Acute GVHD usually occurs during days 20 to 100 after a bone marrow transplantation. Initial onset of a diffuse macular erythematous skin rash of the torso and palms and soles heralds the onset of cutaneous GVHD. Diarrhea is a manifestation of acute gut GVHD. Liver function abnormality, especially hyperbilirubinemia, is the manifestation noted in acute liver GVHD. Histologic analysis of the liver demonstrates periductular lymphocytic infiltration.[110]

Patients receive prophylactic anti-GVHD therapy with cyclosporine and methylprednisolone, cyclosporine and methotrexate, or cyclosporine alone depending on in which institution the transplant is being performed. Once acute GVHD is noted, usually histologically by skin biopsy, high doses of steroids are administered to treat the occurrent GVHD. If no GVHD is found, there is a tapering gradually as an outpatient of the cyclosporine and other agents over a 4- to 6-month period.

If the GVHD is unresponsive to the high dose steroids, other agents and techniques may be used, such as antithymocyte globulin, infusion of OKT-3, immunoglobulin, azathioprine (Imuran), experimental agents such as thalidomide, or photopheresis.

Patients who develop resistant acute GVHD are victim to breakdown of the usual barriers, especially in the gut. Enteric organism bacteremias often result from the breakdown of the mucosal barrier in the colon. These patients are often neutropenic, and the combination of coliform sepsis and neutropenia leads to hypotension and a need for intensive care. Some authors believe that reducing gut flora may even prevent severity of acute GVHD.[111]

The causes of infection in the setting of bone marrow transplantation vary with what day after the transplant the patient is at chronologically. Usually staphylococcus, streptococcus, enteric coliforms, anaerobes, and other bacteria are noted in the first 30 days. Once the granulocyte count recovers, the risk of these infections falls. Cytomegalovirus (CMV) occurs between days 30 and 100 and is usually a result of reactivation of latent infection or emergence of CMV from the donor into a CMV seronegative recipient.[112] All donors and recipients are tested for CMV serologic status. Twenty-five percent of the general population is CMV seropositive. The blood bank screens all donors of blood products for CMV seropositivity, and all transplant patients should receive CMV negative blood products. The blood bank also irradiates all blood products delivered to bone marrow transplantation recipients to decrease the risk of infusion of immunocompetent T lymphocytes, which can react against recipient tissues. These are the cells that cause GVHD. The dose of radiation ranges among institutions from 1500 to 2500 rad.

Cytomegalovirus infection manifests itself as thrombocytopenia, pulmonary infiltrates, diarrhea, and liver function abnormalities. Culture techniques are crude, and by the time a buffy coat of blood becomes positive or urine culture becomes positive, the infection may be quite flagrant. Newer techniques using polymerase chain reaction are being increasingly used by microbiology laboratories to search for cytomegalovirus DNA, and infection may be documented earlier and antiviral therapy with gancyclovir may be administered sooner.[113] Some institutions are even using prophylactic gancyclovir in patients who are CMV seropositive or in those patients who are receiving CMV seropositive donor marrow.

The use of intravenous immunoglobulin has decreased significantly the rates of cytomegalovirus infection in bone marrow transplant patients. Generally once a week 400 mg/kg of intravenous immunoglobulin is given for the first 2 to 3 months.[112] Some centers have used CMV hyperimmune globulin, but this is expensive and difficult to find.

ICU Phase

The intensive care physician is often called on to care for a patient once sepsis has caused hypotension which cannot be handled on a bone marrow transplant unit. Dopamine or other blood pressure maintaining medicines are often required through the septic episode, giving time for antibiotics to control the infection. Patients who develop pulmonary infiltrates while in the midst of a bone marrow transplantation may be suffering from chemotherapy-induced pulmonary damage, infection, or opportunistic infection, such as cytomegalovirus, as discussed previously. Hypoxia can be handled in the bone marrow transplant unit to an extent with oxygen therapy; however, when the patient becomes so hypoxic that 100% nonrebreathing delivery systems are inadequate to maintain blood oxygen levels, or if the patient tires, he or she must be intubated. The prognosis of bone marrow transplantation recipients requiring intubation who have respiratory failure is grim. Some reports demonstrate 95% mortality.[114]

Bronchoscopy examinations either before or during the ICU phase of treatment document certain infections that cannot be established through standard sputum specimens. Particularly, Pneumocystis carinii pneumonia may be identified by bronchoscopy but not other techniques. The occurrence of this infection in the setting of bone marrow transplantation is unusual. The lymphoid malignancies are the most common settings in which one might observe this pneumocystis.

The intensivist may also care for patients who have chronic gastrointestinal bleeding either from severe acute GVHD of the gut or other cause, such as duodenal ulcer or peptic ulcer. Patients who are thrombocytopenic and bleeding often require many transfusions of red cells and platelets but still become hypotensive and need intensive care. These patients usually need endoscopy and may benefit from heat probe therapy.

Post-ICU Phase

The bone marrow transplant patient who survives an ICU stay is usually handled in the same way as patients who never needed to go to an ICU. Further antibiotics and further transfusions are necessary to support the patient. Further growth factor therapy is used to accelerate myeloid engraftment.

Chronic GVHD is another immunologic entity, which occurs beyond day 100 after the allogeneic bone marrow transplantation. These patients may develop immunologic reaction of donor T lymphocytes against any recipient tissue. Cutaneous chronic GVHD is a sclerodermalike condition with contractures and thickening and tightening of the dermis. Ulceration may occur with superinfection. The intensivist is rarely called on to aid in this setting. Bronchiolitis obliterans is a lymphocytic infiltrate of the small bronchi leading to dryness of the airways and hypoxia in bone marrow transplant recipients. These patients develop tachypnea and requirements for oxygen and unfortunately often die of infection in the lung or progressive hypoxia.

Late after the bone marrow transplantation, immunologic reconstitution slowly occurs.[115] Some bone marrow transplantation patients may develop fulminant pneumococci sepsis, pseudomonas sepsis, or other bacteremias months to years after the transplant. They may become quite ill rapidly. The bone marrow transplant physician usually is aware of this. If a patient calls not feeling well several months after a transplant, the patient needs to be evaluated rapidly, and if it appears that there is an overwhelming infection, emergent admission to an ICU may save the life of such a patient.

Cyclosporine is used prophylactically to prevent allogeneic bone marrow transplant recipients from developing GVHD. It is usually given in a relatively high dose in the hospital and then tapered over the next 6 months while the patient is followed in the clinic. It has some unique side effects, including nephrotoxicity, hypertension, seizures, neuropathy, and hepatotoxicity. The intensivist may be called on to help manage such complications. The hypertension associated with cyclosporine may be resistant to calcium channel blockers and centrally acting antihypertensive drugs. While patients are thrombocytopenic, the hypertension increases the risk for intracerebral bleeding, and for such a complication, the intensivist is usually called on.

METABOLIC AND ENDOCRINOLOGIC EMERGENCIES

Hypercalcemia

Malignant disease represents the most common cause of hypercalcemia in hospitalized patients.[116,117] The neoplasms most likely to be responsible are breast cancer and lung cancer. Multiple myeloma, although an uncommon disease, may be associated with an elevated serum calcium in as many as two thirds of patients. Lymphoma, other squamous cell cancers, prostate cancer, and kidney cancer are also associated with hypercalcemia.[116-118]

Several different mechanisms for malignant hypercalcemia have been described and are further detailed in Chapter 59.[116,117,119] The most common cause is bone destruction from metastatic bone disease. A significant percentage of patients have no evidence of bone metastases, however. In these patients, hypercalcemia is thought to be "humoral" and mediated by either a parathyroid-hormone-like substance,[120] a prostaglandin,[121] or a vitamin D metabolite.[122-124] In multiple myeloma and lymphoma, direct osteoclast activation has been demonstrated to result from one or several cytokines termed osteoclast activating factor (OAF).[125-128] Indeed, this factor may be responsible for the frequent presentation of myeloma patients with diffuse osteopenia, rather than frank lytic bone disease. In patients with bone dominant metastatic breast cancer, a transient hypercalcemia may develop after the initiation of tamoxifen or other hormonal therapy. On occasion, a hypoadrenal patient, from either iatrogenic causes or metastatic disease, may present with mild hypercalcemia.[117]

Pre-ICU Phase

In patients with malignant disease, the clinical manifestations of hypercalcemia are often dominated by neurologic symptoms (Table 44-11).[116,117,129] Indeed, hypercalcemia is one of the most common causes of a change in mental status in a patient with cancer. Malaise and fatigue may also occur. Gastrointestinal symptoms, such as nausea, vomiting, and abdominal pain, are frequent. Occasionally, patients may present with unrelenting constipation as the only manifestation of hypercalcemia. Given the frequent use of narcotic analgesics in this patient population, the relationship of the constipation to hypercalcemia may prove difficult to discern. Renal manifestations, such as hyposthenuria, polyuria, and the resulting dehydration and azotemia, are most serious and may result in death. When coupled with the nausea and vomiting that frequently results from both hypercalcemia and progressive azotemia, rapid renal deterioration often occurs. Nephrocalcinosis may result from long-standing hypercalcemia but, along with renal stones, is more common when hypercalcemia has a benign origin. Benign causes of hypercalcemia are

Table 44-11. Clinical Manifestations of Malignant Hypercalcemia

Neurologic
    Mental status changes
    Confusion
    Malaise
    Fatigue
Gastrointestinal
    Nausea, vomiting
    Constipation
    Abdominal pain
Renal
    Polyuria/hyposthenuria
    Polydipsia
    Dehydration/azotemia
    Nephrocalcinosis

Table 44-12. Management of Malignant Hypercalcemia

Acute
  Rehydration
  Saline diuresis
  Calcitonin
  Hemodialysis
Subacute
  Corticosteroids (selected patients)
  Plicamycin (mithramycin)
  Bisphosphonates
  Gallium nitrate
Chronic
  Oral phosphates
  Mobilization
  Antineoplastic therapy

---

also often associated with hypertension, pancreatitis, and peptic ulcer disease, but these are relatively infrequent when the origin is neoplastic. The key to a rapid diagnosis is a high index of suspicion when any of these nonspecific signs and symptoms are found in a cancer patient.

ICU Phase

Most patients with malignant hypercalcemia can be managed without ICU monitoring.[116,117,130] All patients with hypercalcemia, however, must be considered significantly dehydrated at presentation, and their acute management requires large volumes of isotonic fluid replacement (Table 44-12). Once rehydration has been accomplished, a saline diuresis can be started in an effort to increase calcium excretion. Efforts to promote such a diuresis before volume replacement are unwise and counterproductive, however. The vigor with which one pursues rehydration and diuresis must be tempered by the degree of calcium elevation and the patient's cardiovascular and renal function. Elderly patients with underlying heart disease and uncertain renal function may be best managed in an ICU setting with invasive monitoring. Close attention to potassium and magnesium replacement is also important. One must recognize that most hypercalcemic patients have an impaired urinary concentrating ability. As such, urine output alone is not a good indication of total body fluid status.

In the acute management of malignant hypercalcemia, parenteral calcitonin (4 IU/kg subcutaneously or intramuscularly, every 12 hours) has also proved useful. Although calcitonin is a rapidly effective intervention, patients quickly become refractory to its effects, and it is not helpful in the long-term management of hypercalcemia. In otherwise uncontrollable situations not acutely responsive to rehydration and calcitonin, hemodialysis has been effectively used. Although intravenous phosphates can also produce rapid improvement, their use is not recommended owing to the likelihood of ectopic calcification.[116,117]

Post-ICU Phase

Once the patient's hemodynamic status has been stabilized and the calcium level acutely lowered, attention can be directed to the subacute and chronic control of the problem (see Table 44-12). This involves both control of the elevated calcium level and definitive treatment of the underlying malignancy.[116,117,130] Use of high doses of glucocorticoids has been successful in patients with multiple myeloma and lymphoma and of modest value in patients with metastatic breast cancer. Because their utility is presumably related to their cytotoxic effects, they have proved relatively ineffective in most of the solid tumors, however.[117] Corticosteroids should be started immediately in patients with the appropriate diagnoses but should not be used at all for most solid tumors. A response may be expected in 48 to 72 hours.

Plicamycin (mithramycin), an antitumor antibiotic, when given intravenously in low doses (25 μg/kg), causes a significant fall in the serum calcium in most patients, regardless of cause within 24 to 48 hours. Unfortunately, repeated doses are often necessary if specific antineoplastic therapy is unavailable. Its ease of administration, however, allows for frequent outpatient use. Care must be exercised in those patients with renal dysfunction, and multiple doses of the medication can result in myelosuppression.

The newest agents found useful for the management of hypercalcemia are the bisphosphonates, a group of pyrophosphate analogs that block osteoclast bone resorption. Etidronate disodium (7.5 mg/kg per day for 3 to 5 successive days, over at least 2 hours) and pamidronate (60 to 90 mg over 24 hours) have been released in the United States and are effective with intravenous use.[131-133] Etidronate is also available in an oral formulation, which has limited, if any, value for hypercalcemia. The onset and duration of action for these agents are similar to that of plicamycin. Gallium nitrate (100 to 200 mg/m^2 per day as an intravenous continuous infusion over 5 days) has also been marketed for hypercalcemia and appears effective, although inconvenient to administer.[134,135]

The long-term management of malignant hypercalcemia is difficult. Outpatient diuretic use, although promoting a saline diuresis, aggravates intravascular dehydration and is specifically contraindicated. Repeated outpatient doses of plicamycin or bisphosphonate are inconvenient but represent a short-term solution. Oral phosphate administration may be of some value, but the cathartic activity of these agents limits their usefulness. Many of these patients, however, require narcotic analgesics for bone pain, and cathartics may be needed to counteract the resultant constipation. Patient mobilization is important but often problematic. Antineoplastic therapy with drugs such as cisplatin or with interleukin-2 has been associated with a temporary fall in serum calcium, independent of any improvement in tumor. A presumed effect on the kidney has been suggested.[136]

The overall prognosis of a patient with malignant hypercalcemia is poor. Except for those patients with chemotherapy-responsive diseases, such as lymphoma, myeloma, or breast cancer, the development of hypercalcemia generally represents an end-stage manifestation of the disease, and treatment is considered palliative.[137] When effective antineoplastic treatment is available, whether surgery, radiation, chemotherapy, or hormonal therapy, it should be rapidly initiated, with the expectation that it will result in the most satisfactory long-term control of the problem.

Table 44-13. Causes of Hyponatremia in Cancer Patients

Volume depletion
Syndrome of inappropriate secretion of antidiuretic hormone
    Lung and other neoplasms
    Pulmonary/central nervous system disease
    Medication
        Cyclophosphamide
        Vincristine
        Opiates
Chronic organ failure
    Renal disease
    Liver disease
    Cardiac disease
    Hypothyroidism
Corticosteroid deficiency
    Adrenal metastases
    Iatrogenic
        Glucocorticoid therapy
        Antiadrenal therapy
Diuretic use
Artifactual

Hyponatremia

There are multiple reasons for the development of hyponatremia in the cancer patient, and an accurate determination of cause is most important (Table 44-13).[138,139] In evaluating hyponatremia, it is first important to determine the overall fluid status of the patient.[140] Dehydration commonly results in hyponatremia, particularly when partially corrected by hypotonic volume replacement. Vomiting and diarrhea frequently accompany malignant disease and its treatment and may produce significant sodium losses.[138,139] Other signs of intravascular volume depletion should be evident in this situation.

Preexisting chronic renal disease can also result in salt wasting and hyponatremia, a condition that may be aggravated by chemotherapy administration with drugs such as cisplatin. Other medication use, especially diuretics, should be reviewed. Artifactual hyponatremia may be noted in the presence of hyperproteinemia or hyperlipidemia, and modest hyponatremia is a not infrequent finding in patients without cancer with severe cardiac and hepatic disease.[138-140]

It is important to recognize the association of glucocorticoid deficiency and hyponatremia. Patients with cancer may become hypoadrenal as a result of metastatic disease involving the adrenals, as in lung cancer, or for iatrogenic reasons. The latter is not uncommon in the patient maintained on corticosteroids who may be inadequately covered during periods of stress or in the patient treated with antiadrenal agents for metastatic breast or adrenal cancer. Hyponatremia is rarely the sole manifestation of adrenal insufficiency, but the diagnosis can be subtle. Rapid saline replacement and steroid administration are indicated.

Another problem seen in patients with malignancy is the syndrome of inappropriate secretion of antidiuretic hormone (SIADH).[138-141] The hallmark of this clinical syndrome is euvolemia and hyponatremia with a urine osmolality greater than the serum osmolality. Urinary sodium excretion is often increased as well. It is important to remember that this diagnosis cannot be made in the presence of renal, adrenal, or thyroid dysfunction. In cancer patients, SIADH is most commonly found in association with small cell carcinoma of the lung[142] and is presumed to be due to ectopic secretion of an ADH-like substance from the malignant cells. It is, however, also seen in patients with extensive non-neoplastic pulmonary disease as well as central nervous system hemorrhage, neoplasm, or infection. Cyclophosphamide and vincristine use and several nonchemotherapeutic agents, including the opiates, thiazides, and chlorpropamide, have also been reported to produce this syndrome.[138,139,143]

Pre-ICU Phase

Patients with mild hyponatremia may be asymptomatic or may complain of fatigue, anorexia, nausea, malaise, and headache. These symptoms are nonspecific, and the diagnosis may not be suspected clinically, unless serum electrolytes are measured.

Patients with more profound hyponatremia may present with an altered mental status, confusion, lethargy, psychosis, seizures, and even cerebral edema progressing to death. As in all neurologic emergencies, a metabolic evaluation, including serum electrolytes, must be obtained and should rapidly provide the correct diagnosis.

The appropriate management of patients with hyponatremia requires the correct determination of cause.[138-140] Hypovolemic patients should be treated with isotonic saline, in an effort to restore intravascular volume. Corticosteroid-deficient patients should rapidly be given appropriate stress doses of steroid hormones. In patients with SIADH and mild symptoms the initial management of hyponatremia may consist of fluid restriction alone.[138,139] If ineffective, demeclocycline, an ADH antagonist that produces nephrogenic diabetes insipidus, is an appropriate and effective intervention.[144,145] Patients who are significantly hyponatremic with serious central nervous system manifestations should receive small volumes of hypertonic (3%) saline and furosemide (to promote a hypotonic diuresis) to elevate the serum sodium more rapidly.[146]

ICU Phase

ICU management is rarely required unless serious central nervous system manifestations develop. Patients with unexplained coma or intractable seizures may well require initial ICU monitoring, until the diagnosis can be clarified and the patient stabilized. Profound dehydration and shock, which can be associated with hyponatremia, may also require short-term ICU care.

Post-ICU Phase

In most hyponatremic cancer patients, the serum sodium can be effectively controlled and the symptoms relieved. Dehydration, corticosteroid deficiency, and medication toxicity respond readily to appropriate intervention. SIADH from malignancy requires specific antineoplastic management. In patients with small cell carcinoma of the lung, combination chemotherapy is effective and often rapidly results in tumor shrinkage and normalization of serum sodium.[147] Patients with other solid tumors associated with SIADH may be more difficult to manage.

Patients with small cell carcinoma of the lung who respond to chemotherapy with resolution of SIADH should be followed closely. Recurrence of hyponatremia usually heralds tumor regrowth and may prove difficult to manage effectively.

Hypoglycemia

Tumor-induced hypoglycemia can occur in two clinical situations. The first is in patients with neuroendocrine tumors producing insulin (insulinomas). Although uncommon, the endocrinologic manifestations of this neoplasm often allow diagnosis at an early stage. The excess secretion of insulin or proinsulin produces the hypoglycemia.[148-151]

The second clinical circumstance is in patients with large, slowly growing mesenchymal tumors, particularly those involving retroperitoneum, chest, or liver, who may also develop hypoglycemia. Such neoplasms include both pleural and peritoneal mesothelioma, any of the sarcomas, adrenal cortical carcinoma, and hepatoma.[148-151,153] The mechanisms of hypoglycemia in patients with these malignancies are incompletely understood and probably multiple. Speculation centers around the production of an insulinlike substance by the neoplasm as well as the possibility of increased glucose metabolism in the tumor itself. Some evidence suggests that patients with large, particularly hepatic, neoplasms have impaired compensatory mechanisms in response to hypoglycemia. Gluconeogenesis and glycogen breakdown may be deficient, and hepatic glycogen stores are reduced.[152]

Pre-ICU Phase

Neurologic symptoms usually predominate in patients with neoplastic hypoglycemia. They may be dramatic and life-threatening or insidious and nonspecific.[148-150] Patients may present with fatigue, dizziness, and confusion, which may be relieved after a meal. Frank mental status changes, seizures, and coma may precipitously develop. The diagnosis can rapidly be made at the bedside if clinically suspected, and a rapid response to intravenous dextrose is the rule.

The cause can be determined by eliminating the other more common causes of hypoglycemia, in particular, exogenous insulin or oral hypoglycemic use, alcohol abuse, malnutrition, and adrenal or pituitary insufficiency.[148-151] If an insulinoma is suspected, insulin and proinsulin levels should be obtained because the neoplasm may be difficult to detect radiographically.

ICU Phase

ICU management may be required in those patients with a life-threatening neurologic presentation, such as seizure or coma. Effective early intervention should reverse the neurologic abnormalities, although irreversible changes can be seen. Supportive management, including large amounts of intravenous dextrose, is indicated.

Post-ICU Phase

After identifying and controlling the hypoglycemia, treatment must be directed at the primary tumor. Insulinomas can often be managed surgically[151] or, if unresectable, the hormonal manifestations treated with parenteral somatostatin.[153] Chemotherapy has also been used but remains a palliative tool.[153] Noninsulin-producing neoplasms are less successfully treated because they are often large and technically unresectable. Surgical debulking, however, may have a role, as does radiation therapy and, on occasion, chemotherapy in selected patients.[148-150,153] In general, however, a bulky tumor precludes long-term treatment success.

In such situations, nonspecific measures, such as 1increasing oral intake, the use of corticosteroids, and even parenteral glucagon, have had modest success in temporarily controlling the hypoglycemic symptoms. In patients with insulinomas, diazoxide may also have some value.[148-150,153]

TREATMENT-INDUCED EMERGENCIES
Renal and Electrolyte Complications of Treatment

A discussion of all the renal and electrolyte abnormalities induced by chemotherapeutic agents is beyond the scope of this chapter. Complications of critical concern include the acute and chronic renal failure that can result from the use of certain chemotherapeutic agents, most notably cisplatin.[154-156] A reduction in renal blood flow and glomerular filtration rate occurs commonly in patients treated with this agent and can be prevented to some extent by aggressive hydration and diuresis at the time of drug administration.[156,157] Infusion of hypertonic saline has been protective in patients treated with higher doses.[158] Renal tubular dysfunction can also develop, in particular hypomagnesemia[159,160] and sodium wasting,[161] as a result of the use of this agent. Other drugs that may cause renal failure are the nitrosoureas (including streptozotocin),[162-164] ifosfamide,[165] and high dose methotrexate, particularly if fluid management at the time of a methotrexate administration is suboptimal.[166]

Ifosfamide and to a lesser extent cyclophosphamide are agents that can produce serious cystitis, presumably owing to a drug metabolite in the urine.[154,165] This can be avoided by vigorous hydration and the use of a uroprotective agent, such as mesna. Ifosfamide has also been described as producing a profound, renal tubular acidosis and renal failure, which resolves when the drug is discontinued. As previously noted in this chapter, vincristine and to a lesser extent cyclophosphamide have been associated with hyponatremia, which may be due to SIADH.

None of these renal toxicities should result in the need for ICU management, although renal failure may require dialysis (see Chapter 39). There are two potential complications of chemotherapy administration that may result in a critically ill patient, however. The first is the tumor lysis syndrome, and the second is the chemotherapy-related hemolytic uremic syndrome.

Tumor Lysis Syndrome

One of the problems resulting from successful chemotherapy for the treatment of highly responsive neoplasms has been the need for excretion of the byproducts of tumor cell breakdown. A tumor lysis syndrome has been described that encompasses all the metabolic abnormalities seen after successful chemotherapy.[167-169] The prototype disease for this syndrome has been Burkitt's lymphoma,[168] although it has also been described after the treatment of other aggressive non-Hodgkin's lymphomas,[169] acute lymphocytic and nonlymphocytic leukemia,[170,171] and even small cell carcinoma of the lung[172] and other solid tumors.[173]

Pre-ICU Phase. The clinical setting for this syndrome is a patient with a bulky, chemotherapy-responsive neoplasm undergoing an initial course of treatment. Rapid tumor breakdown results in the release of intracellular contents into the circulation, producing hyperuricemia, hyperphosphatemia, hyperkalemia, and lactic acidosis.[167-169] Azotemia develops from both urate nephropathy and from the precipitation of calcium phosphate salts within the renal parenchyma. This aggravates the elevations in urate, phosphate, and potassium, as well as the acidosis. Hypocalcemia results from the calcium phosphate precipitation and, in the presence of hyperkalemia and acidosis, has resulted in sudden death.[174] These metabolic abnormalities are even more pronounced in patients presenting with preexisting azotemia. Not all manifestations of the tumor lysis syndrome need occur together. Patients undergoing successful chemotherapy may experience lactic acidosis without renal failure or an isolated urate nephropathy. The origin of the abnormalities and their management, however, remain the same.

The most effective treatment for this syndrome has been its anticipation and prevention.[167,168] Preexisting renal dysfunction should be corrected if possible. Particular attention should be directed to the possibility of any obstructive uropathy. Patients with chemotherapy-sensitive tumors, likely to experience tumor lysis, should be identified and chemotherapy delayed until appropriate preventive measures can be instituted. An alkaline diuresis should be started in an effort to maximize uric acid excretion, and allopurinol should be given. Patients at risk may require hospitalization and close monitoring throughout the initial days after chemotherapy, in an effort to detect the early manifestations of this syndrome.

ICU Phase. The tumor lysis syndrome is a potentially fatal complication of treatment success. It is most likely to develop in those patients with the most sensitive, potentially curable neoplasms, and ICU management would be entirely appropriate if needed. The manifestations of tumor lysis should be aggressively monitored after chemotherapy administration and appropriate treatment given. The progressive development of hyperkalemia, hyperuricemia, azotemia, or hyperphosphatemia may mandate cardiac monitoring and management in an ICU. Early hemodialysis is recommended for those patients in whom electrolyte abnormalities significantly worsen after chemotherapy. Indeed, dialysis has been suggested for patients with a serum phosphate greater than 10 mg/dl, uric acid greater than 10 mg/dl, or any hyperkalemia unresponsive to conventional management.[167,168]

Post-ICU Phase. Patients who develop the tumor lysis syndrome have highly responsive, potentially curable malignancies when managed with chemotherapy. The rapid tumor destruction rarely occurs in subsequent chemotherapy courses owing to the lack of residual bulky tumor after the initial course. It must be remembered, however, that if recurrent disease develops in such a patient, the propensity for tumor lysis again exists, as does the need for its anticipation and management.

Cancer-Associated Hemolytic Uremic Syndrome

The clinical syndrome of microangiopathic hemolytic anemia, thrombocytopenia, and renal dysfunction has been recognized in patients with malignant disease previously treated with antineoplastic agents.[175,176] The syndrome has most commonly been described in patients with adenocarcinoma, particularly gastric cancer, treated with chemotherapy regimens containing mitomycin-C.[175,177-179] Indeed, previous exposure to mitomycin-C has been noted in most patients who develop this syndrome. In general, a total dose of at least 60 mg of this medication has been required.[175] Thus the syndrome has tended to occur either in those patients given significant doses of mitomycin-C in an adjuvant setting or in those patients responding to this medication in the setting of metastatic disease. This clinical syndrome, however, has also been described in occasional patients receiving other agents, such as cisplatin or bleomycin, without mitomycin-C.[180,181]

It is extremely important to differentiate this clinical entity from other cancer-associated hematologic syndromes. Microangiopathic hemolytic anemia can be found in DIC, a condition that may occur in the setting of advanced malignant disease, most commonly adenocarcinoma. Myelosuppression from chemotherapy must also be distinguished from cancer-associated hemolytic uremic syndromes, and a bone marrow examination is usually required in these patients. Childhood hemolytic uremic syndrome and idiopathic thrombotic thrombocytopenic purpura are clinically similar but should not be considered acceptable diagnoses in a patient with malignant disease who are undergoing chemotherapy (particularly mitomycin-C-containing chemotherapy).

Pre-ICU Phase. The onset of the clinical syndrome ranges from 1 week to 15 months after chemotherapy exposure, although it usually develops within 4 months of the most recent mitomycin-C dose. Patients universally present with anemia, thrombocytopenia, and an elevation in serum creatinine. The peripheral blood smear must reveal changes of a microangiopathic hemolytic anemia for this diagnosis to be considered. Coagulation studies are usually normal, but the serum LDH is often markedly elevated. The clinical syndrome closely resembles thrombotic thrombocytopenic purpura (see Chap. 43), although fever and neurologic abnormalities are much less common. A significant percentage of patients have been recently transfused, an event that is, for unclear reasons, associated with either worsening of the hemolysis or the development of pulmonary edema.[175,176]

ICU-Phase. At presentation, patients may be asymptomatic, may note symptoms referable to their anemia, or may be clinically extremely ill. ICU monitoring may be required if renal failure results in profound metabolic aberrations or if neurologic dysfunction develops. Conventional supportive care is indicated, including hemodialysis.

Specific treatment for this syndrome is disappointing. Corticosteroids, hemodialysis, diuretics, and antiplatelet agents have been used with only limited success. Plasma exchange has been attempted, as for patients with thrombotic thrombocytopenic purpura, with perhaps 30% of patients treated in this fashion showing clinical improvement.[175,176] A small number of patients successfully treated with immunoperfusion over staphylococcal protein A columns have also been reported.[181,182]

Post-ICU Phase. Fatality in patients with the cancer-associated hemolytic uremic syndrome may be as high as 75%. Two thirds of these deaths are a direct result of the syndrome, whereas one third are from progressive malignancy.[175] A minority of patients recover. In that event, their ultimate prognosis is determined by the prognosis of their underlying malignancy.

Respiratory Complications of Treatment

Both radiation therapy and chemotherapy are well recognized to produce acute and chronic pulmonary toxicities.[183-187] When combination chemotherapy is used or when chemotherapy is combined with either sequential or concurrent radiation, the propensity to develop pulmonary complications increases. Furthermore, if such patients undergo surgery, the incidence of postoperative respiratory failure is also increased.

Radiation injury to the lung can present as either an acute radiation pneumonitis developing 1 to 6 months after completion of the radiation therapy or as a more chronic radiation fibrosis developing between 6 and 24 months after treatment.[183,184,187] The incidence of this complication is directly related to the total radiation dose administered and is uncommon with doses below 20 Gy and almost invariable when an excess of 60 Gy is given. In addition, the volume of lung treated and the dose rate appear to be important factors in the development of radiation injury. Concurrent use of chemotherapeutic agents as well as an abrupt steroid hormone withdrawal (as in patients treated for Hodgkin's disease) appears to exacerbate the potential for this problem.[188]

Multiple chemotherapeutic agents have also been implicated in the production of radiation injury (Table 44-14). Uncommonly, this is a hypersensitivity reaction, which has been described after exposure to procarbazine, methotrexate, and occasionally bleomycin.[185,186] This syndrome responds rapidly to withdrawal of the offending agent and the use of corticosteroids. It is most important to recognize the disorder and its association with chemotherapy administration because death has been described from respiratory failure.

More commonly, a progressive chemotherapy-induced fibrosis may develop after exposure to one of a number of alkylating agents,[183-186] including busulfan, cyclophosphamide, ifosfamide, chlorambucil,[189] and melphalan;[190] antibiotics, such as bleomycin,[191] and mitomycin-C;[192] and nitrosoureas, in particular carmustine.[193,194] Cytosine arabinoside has been associated with respiratory failure, although a noncardiogenic pulmonary-edema-like mechanism has been proposed and remains incompletely elucidated.[195,196]

Table 44-14. Common Chemotherapy Agents Producing Pulmonary Toxicity

Alkylating agents
 Busulfan
 Cyclophosphamide
 Chlorambucil
 Ifosfamide
 Melphalan
Antimetabolites
 Cytosine arabinoside
 Methotrexate*
Antibiotics
 Bleomycin
 Mitomycin C
Nitrosoureas
 Carmustine
 Lomustine
Miscellaneous
 Procarbazine*

* Hypersensitivity pneumonitis.

The most common offending agents, bleomycin, mitomycin-C, and carmustine, appear to be dose related in their incidence.[185] Bleomycin tends to occur at total doses above 400 units, although sporadic cases after lower doses have been reported. Mitomycin-C toxicity is rare at total doses below 50 mg, and carmustine injury appears to have an increasing incidence with doses above 800 mg/m^2.

Pre-ICU Phase

The clinical picture is relatively nonspecific. Patients usually present with dyspnea, a nonproductive cough, fatigue, and malaise. Fever may be noted, particularly after those medications associated with hypersensitivity reactions or in patients with acute radiation pneumonitis. Hemoptysis is uncommon. Physical examination may be entirely normal or may reveal rales, friction rubs, or even a pleural effusion.

The chest radiograph is also nonspecific, even in those patients with acute radiation pneumonitis in whom the infiltrate, although generally confined to the radiation therapy portal, may, on occasion, involve all lung fields (Fig. 44-5).[183,184,187] Those patients with chronic radiation fibrosis tend to have infiltrates and scarring restricted to the previous radiation therapy portal. Drug-induced injury is characteristically diffuse. The picture is usually one of a patchy nodular or interstitial infiltrate. Frank consolidation may develop as well. Early functional compromise may be present in patients with a relatively normal chest radiograph.

Pulmonary function studies often reflect underlying lung disease. The diffusion capacity (measured by the D$_{LCO}$, however, may be somewhat predictive for the development of bleomycin and perhaps mitomycin-C injury.[184-186] Baseline measurements of D$_{LCO}$ are often recommended during treatment with these agents. Any significant fall in D$_{LCO}$ should be considered a reason for discontinuation of the potentially offending drug.

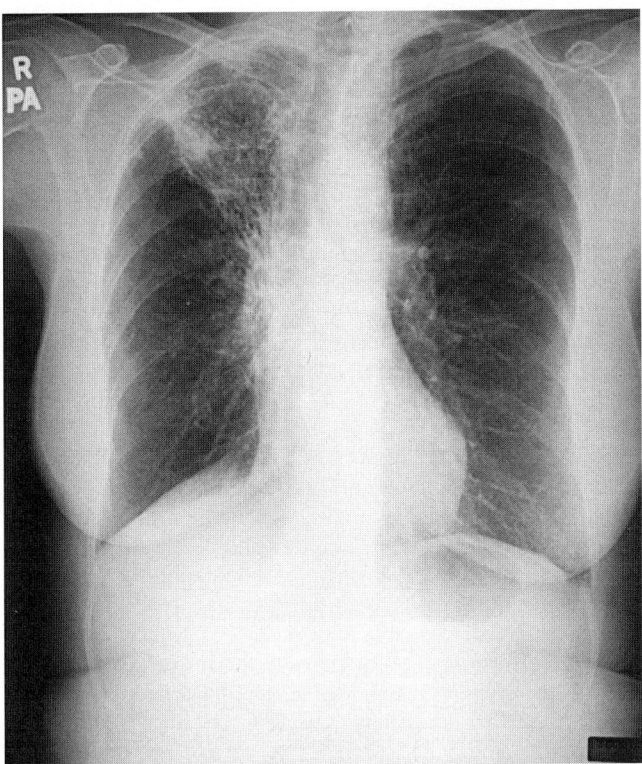

Fig. 44–5. Radiation pneumonitis. The distribution of this infiltrate correlates exactly with the radiation therapy portal.

The best management of this disorder requires its anticipation and prevention. Chemotherapeutic agents likely to produce pulmonary toxicity should be recognized and patients at risk identified. Treatment courses should be tailored to keep drug doses below those likely to produce irreversible pulmonary damage. Careful monitoring of patients with testicular cancer receiving potentially curative chemotherapy with bleomycin is important. Repeated D_{LCO} measurement should be obtained and bleomycin discontinued if abnormalities develop. In patients receiving radiation therapy, careful attention should be given to the size of the radiation therapy portal as well as the dose and dose rate and the use of concurrent chemotherapy. The risk of subsequent surgery in such patients should be recognized and appropriate plans made before surgery is contemplated.

There is an increasingly recognized risk of pulmonary dysfunction in the bone marrow transplant patient.[183,184,197,198] Clearly those patients undergoing bone marrow transplantation have multiple risk factors for respiratory failure, predominantly infectious. It is also reported, however, that the high doses of chemotherapeutic agents or the total body radiation therapy used in many transplant preparative regimens may produce early pulmonary toxicity. The exact agent or combination of agents responsible is unclear, but the D_{LCO} has proved to be a useful monitor for early pulmonary toxicity. High doses of corticosteroids have been used effectively in reversing these abnormalities.

ICU Phase

Patients requiring ICU management have a poor prognosis, and mortality is in excess of 50% once assisted ventilation is required.[183] It is most important in the management of these patients that the diagnosis of a drug-induced or radiation pneumonitis be confirmed histologically. The patient with malignancy receiving radiation therapy or chemotherapy is immunosuppressed and often myelosuppressed and as such is at risk of pneumonia from multiple infectious agents. The possibility of diffuse lymphangitic carcinomatosis mimicking a treatment-induced injury must always be considered.[183,184,199] The diagnosis of treatment-induced respiratory failure must therefore be considered a diagnosis of exclusion, particularly because the management is not specific. Bronchoscopy may yield an alternative diagnosis in a minority of cases, but often open lung biopsy is required. Unfortunately, in most, this does not result in the diagnosis of a treatable infection and only complicates the management of an otherwise critically ill patient.

High doses of corticosteroids are invariably used in these patients. Although these drugs appear to be of value in radiation pneumonitis, drug-induced hypersensitivity pneumonitis, mitomycin C injury, and the post-bone marrow transplant setting, their role in bleomycin-induced or BCNU-induced injury is limited.[183,184,187] Careful attention must be given to fluid balance and to the possibility of a secondary infection, particularly in patients who are myelosuppressed.

Post-ICU Phase

Those patients recovering from acute treatment-induced pulmonary injury often have significant residual respiratory compromise. Standard management for this disability is appropriate. It is also important to avoid further exposure to the offending agent. The ultimate prognosis, however, depends on the prognosis of the underlying malignant disease. Patients with testicular cancer after bleomycin injury or patients undergoing successful bone marrow transplantation have a significant possibility for a prolonged cancer-free survival.

Patients with chronic radiation fibrosis often have asymptomatic pulmonary infiltrates and scarring on chest radiographs. This may cause only diagnostic confusion in future years. Their functional status depends both on any underlying lung disease and on the extent of the radiation-induced injury.

Neurologic Complications of Treatment

The neurologic complications of antineoplastic therapy may be dramatic and severe but rarely result in the need for ICU management. They are briefly reviewed in this section.

Chemotherapeutic agents can produce a wide spectrum of neurologic abnormalities (Table 44–15).[200,201] Mental status changes have most notably been described after the use of ifosfamide.[202,203] This appears to be a dose-related phenomenon with confusion and lethargy, at times progressing to seizures and coma after higher doses. Cranial

Table 44–15. Neurologic Toxicities of Common Chemotherapy Drugs

Cerebral Dysfunction
    Carmustine
    Cisplatin
    Corticosteroids
    Cytosine arabinoside
    Etopside
    Hexamethylmelamine
    Ifosfamide
    L-Asparaginase
    Procarbazine

Cerebellar Dysfunction
    Cytosine arabinoside
    5-Fluorouracil
    Ifosfamide

Peripheral Neuropathy
    Cisplatin
    Etoposide
    Hexamethylmelamine
    Vinca alkaloids

nerve and cerebellar dysfunction have also been described, and the syndrome has been noted in children[203] as well as adults. The abnormalities are fully reversible when the drug is discontinued.[203] Ifosfamide-induced neurotoxicity appears to occur more frequently in those who also develop drug-induced renal dysfunction and renal tubular acidosis.[202]

Cytosine arabinoside, when given in high doses, produces both cerebellar and cerebral dysfunction.[204] The development of this toxicity is both age and dose related and is associated with specific pathologic changes in the brain.[204,205] Recovery is variable and often incomplete. 5-Fluorouracil has also been described as producing an acute cerebellar syndrome, but this has proved reversible when the drug is discontinued.[200,201]

A global encephalopathy has uncommonly been reported after the use of high doses of methotrexate, etoposide, carmustine, L-asparaginase, and procarbazine.[200,201,206,207] Hexamethylmelamine may produce depression or insomnia in occasional patients. Glucocorticoids are well recognized to cause a delirium, or "steroid psychosis," in small numbers of patients treated with higher doses. It is the recognition that a chemotherapeutic agent may be responsible that allows for an accurate diagnosis and discontinuation of the drug.

Certain chemotherapeutic agents produce peripheral neuropathies.[200,201] Although rarely life threatening, these neuropathies may prove profoundly disabling and need be recognized at the onset of symptoms. The vinca alkaloids, vincristine, vinblastine, and vindesine, are the best described drugs that produce peripheral neuropathy. Etoposide, VM-26, and hexamethylmelamine may also be culprits. Cumulative doses of cisplatin produce a particularly pernicious peripheral neuropathy, which may prove irreversible once fully established.[208,209] Similarly, ototoxicity and autonomic dysfunction[210] have been recognized after cisplatin. There is some suggestion that preexisting neurologic dysfunction may be exacerbated by these agents, but this has been difficult to verify.[200,201]

The neurologic sequelae of radiation therapy to the brain include the subacute development of fatigue, lethargy, and nausea[211] and the more chronic development of cognitive dysfunction and even frank dementia.[212] Cranial radiation therapy is often given for intracranial metastases and, in that setting, is palliative. Life expectancy is limited, and the development of delayed toxicity is not a major concern. The increasing use, however, of prophylactic cranial radiation therapy for patients with leukemia[211] and solid tumors, such as small cell carcinoma of the lung,[212] has resulted in the delayed development of irreversible neurologic damage in patients otherwise cured of their malignancy. The increasing use of intrathecal chemotherapy, particularly in patients with leukemia and lymphoma, with or without neuraxis radiotherapy, has also resulted in the development of late neurologic sequelae.[200,201]

The differential diagnosis in patients who develop neurologic abnormalities while undergoing treatment for malignant disease certainly includes treatment-induced toxicities. One must also consider the possibility of metastatic cancer (intracranial metastases, spinal cord compression, leptomeningeal metastases), a metabolic abnormality such as hyponatremia or hypercalcemia, or infection. In addition, the use of narcotics, hypnotics, or antiemetics must be addressed as well as the possibility of an acute vascular event. Concern has been expressed about a potential increase in vascular events, such as stroke and myocardial infarction, seen in otherwise healthy young men treated with cisplatin-based combination chemotherapy regimens for testicular cancer.[213] The possibility of embolic or thrombotic stroke is even higher in the older patient with underlying cerebrovascular disease.

Gastrointestinal Complications of Treatment

The cancer patient has many potential reasons to develop a gastroenterologic problem. Generally the more aggressively the patient is treated, the more hazardous the gastrointestinal complication. Because so many gastrointestinal side effects have abdominal pain as part of the constellation of clinical findings, the intensivist must work closely with consulting surgeons and endoscopists. This discussion follows the gastrointestinal tract from mouth to anus and highlights specific toxicities that may confront the critical care practitioner. No special attempt is made to focus on pre-ICU versus in-ICU versus post-ICU care.

Upper Digestive Tract

Most chemotherapy drugs cause some degree of nausea and vomiting. These drugs stimulate the chemoreceptor trigger zone and other medullary and higher centers of the brain, which causes vagal discharges, relaxation of the lower esophageal sphincter, contraction of the gastric muscles, and subsequent vomiting. Prochlorperazine, lorazepam, dexamethasone, and newer antiserotonin drugs, such as ondansetron, help. Still, patients vomit. Even the most severe vomiting and its subsequent dehydration and hypokalemia can be handled as an outpatient or with regular nursing floor admission. The one setting in which the patient may need intensive support might be a patient who ruptures the esophagus (Boerhaave's syndrome) because of prolonged or forceful emesis. These patients become hypotensive, develop left-sided pleural effusions, and usually require surgery to fix the rent in the esophagus.

The mucositis that occurs after high dose chemotherapy or radiation to the head and neck region can usually be handled with nasogastric tube feedings and pain medicines. Rinses and soft brushes can remove debris and keep the mouth "relatively" clean. Superinfection with candida and herpes usually requires some antifungal or antiviral antibiotics. The oral flora can enter the circulation and cause sepsis and hypotension, potentially requiring pressor support in the ICU. Periapical dental abscesses should be considered as sources for bacteremia in a patient with chemotherapy-induced granulocytopenia without any other overt site for infection.

Midgut and Liver

The stomach is a frequent source of bleeding in patients who are markedly thrombocytopenic for prolonged periods of time. Steroids can lead to ulcers. Patients with raised intracranial pressure, either secondary to bleeding or tumors, can develop Cushing's ulcers. Endoscopy can often elucidate the extent of the bleeding. H_2-blockade, antacids, platelet and red cell transfusions, correction of existing coagulopathy, and pressor support are necessary in severe cases. In the leukemia patient who is refractory to platelet transfusion, single-donor platelet transfusions or HLA-compatible or cross-match-compatible platelet transfusions may be necessary. As long as there is no evidence for DIC, antifibrinolytic drugs, such as epsilon-aminocaproic acid, might be of benefit.

Some patients receiving chemotherapy with autonomic neuropathy as a side effect can develop gastroparesis and ileus. The vinca alkaloids are the most commonly used chemotherapy drugs to cause this. Patients usually complain of painful constipation. Once this side effect wears off, the patients usually are able to eat satisfactorily and have bowel movements. Cathartics may be of some help. This problem is not usually so severe that it comes to the ICU physician's attention.

The liver is commonly an organ manifesting side effects of chemotherapy. The worst manifestation of this is in the setting of high dose chemotherapy with bone marrow transplantation. Depending upon the institution and preparative regimens used, veno-occlusive disease (VOD)[214] may occur in up to 20% of patients treated with transplantation. Once it occurs, it is often fatal. VOD causes jaundice, right upper quadrant pain, hepatomegaly, and ascites. The hyperbilirubinemia is usually more prominent than the transaminase elevations. In the setting of allogeneic bone marrow transplantation, the onset of full-blown VOD usually precedes liver GVHD. It can sometimes be difficult to discriminate between these two diagnoses in some patients, short of a liver biopsy. For example, the patient with acute GVHD with hyperbilirubinemia usually also has a macular skin eruption and diarrhea. Histologic evaluation of the liver in VOD demonstrates subendothelial intimal thickening, disruption of the small hepatic venules with hemorrhage, edema, and partial occlusion of the venules. Pericentral hepatocytes can have necrosis. With time, centrilobular fibrosis occurs. Patients with acute GVHD have degeneration of bile duct epithelium with cholestasis. Lymphocytes accumulate in the periductular areas.

No specific treatment exists for VOD. A report describing the use of thrombolytic therapy is of interest but not considered standard of care.[215] Pentoxifylline is thought to decrease many of the toxic manifestations of high dose therapy and may ameliorate VOD,[216] but this is not yet firmly established.

Many chemotherapy drugs cause specific types of damage to the liver. Methotrexate, often given over long periods for even nonmalignant conditions such as psoriasis, may cause fibrosis and cirrhosis. Indeed, liver biopsies are recommended periodically while patients are receiving long-term methotrexate to ensure that this complication is not occurring. High dose methotrexate, such as used in sarcoma patients, can lead to reversible elevation of transaminases. Cytosine arabinoside, used to treat acute myelogenous leukemia, leads to reversible direct hyperbilirubinemia and elevated transaminases. Certain methods of delivery of chemotherapy can cause unique liver injury. For example, intrahepatic arterial infusion of floxuridine, used to treat liver metastases from colon cancer, can cause sclerosis of bile ducts with resultant cholestasis.

The pre-ICU management of all of the aforementioned problems usually involves diagnosis of the liver injury and cessation of the drug. If VOD is diagnosed, supportive care is mandated as in any patient with liver failure. Fresh frozen plasma or cryoprecipitate may be necessary to correct the coagulopathy. Nutrition with special enteral feedings or hyperalimentation may be necessary. Cathartics to relieve hepatic encephalopathy may be used. Patients with fulminant acute GVHD require immunosuppressive treatment with steroids and cyclosporine.

Duodenitis and enterocolitis occur after x-ray therapy to the abdomen or at the nadir from chemotherapy. These patients may have crampy abdominal pain, bloody diarrhea, and histologic evidence of ulcers. Antibiotics may cause pseudomembranous colitis and enterocolitis.

Large Bowel

There are two unique problems to which the large bowel may fall victim. Typhlitis is a breakdown of the cecal wall seen in individuals with prolonged chemotherapy-induced neutropenia. Patients develop crampy abdominal pain, which may localize over time to the right lower quadrant. Bacteria from the gut lumen may invade through the mucosa of the cecal wall leading to fevers, sepsis, hypotension, and cardiovascular collapse. In the pre-ICU setting, there may be a paucity of definitive findings in these patients. They usually have no air under the diaphragms as do those patients with perforation. They may have a great deal of air in the cecum on a flat plate of the abdomen. If they become sick enough to come to the ICU, they usually need pressor support and fluid resuscitation. Surgical consultation is obtained, and eventual cecal resection may be necessary, but this is very much a procedure of last resort because the postoperative course is stormy with persistent granulocytopenia and hypotension.

Diverticular disease is a disease that many elderly patients with cancer have as a coexisting morbid condition complicating chemotherapy. As the patient with diverticulitis becomes neutropenic from chemotherapy, organisms can easily escape the diverticulum into the circulation, causing sepsis and hypotension. Bleeding, abdominal pain, and peritonitis can occur. In the pre-ICU setting, gut decontamination and a diet high in fiber may help, but these are often ineffective once the white blood cell count is low. Meglumine diatrizoate (Gastrografin) or barium enema helps establish the diagnosis. Surgery to remove the diverticular segment may be life-saving and help to avoid a repeat attack during a patient's next cycle of chemotherapy.

The large bowel has a similar tendency to be affected by drugs, such as the vinca alkaloids causing autonomic neuropathy with constipation and bleeding, as in enterocolitis, mentioned previously.

Proctitis often occurs after x-ray therapy to the pelvis. These patients may complain of rectal bleeding, bowel urgency, or tenesmus. The severity of this problem is compounded by advanced age and neutropenia.

The anus is a common location for patients with granulocytopenia to have irritation and pain, especially with bowel movements. Sitz baths with or without povidone-iodine (Betadine) and good local care with Tuck's pads and thymol iodide powder may help. A return of the granulocytes to normal helps the most. The growth factors G-CSF and GM-CSF help accelerate recovery from this and practically all of the foregoing gastrointestinal effects of chemotherapy.

Cardiac Complications of Treatment

Pre-ICU Phase

Many antineoplastic agents can affect the heart by various toxic mechanisms. Previous radiation to the heart, advanced age, or previous heart disease (e.g., coronary artery diseases, hypertension, diabetes, cardiomyopathy) accentuates any of the drug-induced toxicities on the heart discussed here.

The most widely used class of antineoplastic drugs that predictably cause heart damage is the anthracyclines.[217] Daunorubicin is used in acute leukemias, and doxorubicin is used in breast cancer, lymphomas, and sarcomas. There are anthracyclinelike drugs that are marketed as being equally effective as the two previously mentioned compounds, but with less risk of cardiotoxicity, e.g., idarubicin and mitoxantrone.

The standard method for determining damage to the heart is called the left ventricular ejection fraction using the nuclear medicine technique of multigated angiogram (MUGA) scanning. Mitochondrial disruption, myofibrillar loss, and dilatation of the sarcoplasm can be seen as the cumulative dose rises. Three percent of individuals receiving 550 mg/m^2 of doxorubicin develop congestive heart failure associated with a drop of the left ventricular ejection fraction. Patients may be completely asymptomatic, or they may complain of shortness of breath, paroxysmal nocturnal dyspnea, and peripheral edema. Patients may develop an S$_3$ or lateral displacement of the point of maximal impulse (PMI).

In the pre-ICU setting, these patients may require digitalization and diuretics and discontinuation of the anthracycline.

ICU Phase

As the congestive failure worsens, these patients may require the type of inotropic agents that may be able to be delivered only in the ICU setting. For further details on the ICU management of patients with congestive heart failure, see Chapters 26 and 31.

Higher doses of cyclophosphamide are being given (1) in the setting of bone marrow transplantation and (2) in the mobilization of stem cells (CD34$^+$) into the peripheral blood. Cyclophosphamide has a dose-dependent cardiotoxicity manifested as a hemorrhagic myopericarditis. This occurs within 1 to 2 days of receiving the drug. These patients develop peripheral and pulmonary edema, tachycardia, and tachypnea. They have electrocardiographic changes, most notably loss of amplitude of the QRS complex. Histologically, the hearts of patients who develop failure from high dose cyclophosphamide have vascular damage with small vessel plugging by microthrombi, myocardial fibrin deposition and edema in the interstitium. Hemorrhage into the myocardium with thickening of the wall occurs in the most severe cases.

Patients may rapidly die. It is important to correct any coagulopathy, i.e., to keep the platelet count close to normal, correct DIC, and raise fibrinogen using cryoprecipitate. If patients go to the ICU, treatment is again supportive but more aggressive than can be done on a regular nursing floor. Generally, if patients are adequately supported, full recovery may be seen with resolution of the histologic changes.

Post-ICU Phase

There are increasing reports[218] of some reversibility of the congestive heart failure associated with anthracyclines. In patients whose underlying cancer is cured or controlled, all attempts at supportive therapy are usually recommended, but in those individuals with congestive heart failure associated with anthracyclines whose cancers are progressive, palliation usually is the goal.

Research is being performed now to find new cardioprotective agents. These would be given with anthracyclines to counter the toxicity to the heart. One such agent, ICRF-187, holds promise.[219]

Other chemotherapy drugs known to damage the heart include Ansacrine, a not yet commercially available antileukemic agent. Ansacrine can cause ST-T wave changes and premature atrial and ventricular contractions. 5-Fluorouracil, a drug commonly used in the treatment of breast and colon cancer, causes angina pectoris in up to 5% of patients.[220]

Allergic Reactions to Chemotherapy Drugs

Pre-ICU Phase

During most anticancer treatments, patients are barraged with multiple new drugs to which they have never been exposed. Antiemetics, sedatives, and drugs to prevent gout as well as the chemotherapy drugs themselves may all produce idiosyncratic, allergic reactions. If an allergic reaction occurs, the clinician must review all medications received by the patient to prevent future exposures.

The chemotherapy drug most often associated with allergic reactions is L-asparaginase. It is used primarily in the treatment of acute lymphocytic leukemia. It is a form of enzyme therapy; i.e., its mechanism of action involves hydrolysis of L-asparagine. The antitumor effect of L-asparaginase is via depletion of circulating L-asparagine; thus tumor cells lose one of the basic building blocks they need for growth.[221] Unfortunately, allergic reactions are common with this drug. Fatal anaphylaxis has been noted with its use. Patients receiving higher doses or more frequent dosing tend to develop allergic reactions. The preferred route of administration is intramuscular. Those patients who receive it intravenously are also more prone to anaphylaxis. Commercially available L-asparaginase is derived from Escherichia coli. Patients who have allergic reactions to this form but still need the drug should be switched to L-asparaginase derived from Erwinia carotavora.[222] This may be obtained from the National Cancer Institute.

All of the alkylating agents act by binding to biologic molecules. They act as haptens and can produce allergic responses. Skin rashes, urticaria, angioneurotic edema, and anaphylaxis have been reported after the use of cyclophosphamide, mechlorethamine, and ifosfamide.[223] Patients with mycosis fungoides who receive nitrogen mustard skin cream can become sensitized such that future applications cause allergic skin eruptions.

Another drug frequently associated with allergic reactions is allopurinol. Patients at risk for tumor lysis syndrome, especially those patients with acute leukemia or bulky high grade lymphomas, almost always receive allopurinol as part of their treatment. Allopurinol is an inhibitor of xanthine oxidase; thus it prevents the formation of uric acid. As chemotherapy causes rapid tumor cell death, nucleotides are released. Without allopurinol, these patients develop hyperuricemia, gout, urate nephropathy, and renal failure. Alone allopurinol can cause a skin rash in 2% of patients who take it. If patients also are on certain antibiotics, especially ampicillin, the percentage of patients developing a skin rash can climb to 75%. A severe hypersensitivity reaction involving fever, eosinophilia, toxic epidermal necrolysis, renal failure, and hepatic failure has been reported with allopurinol.[224] This usually occurs 2 to 4 weeks after allopurinol has been started. This is about the time lymphoma or leukemic patients are at their nadir of blood counts from chemotherapy and could be developing these problems for many other reasons. Thus, once the high tumor bulk patient has received chemotherapy plus allopurinol and the risk of tumor lysis syndrome has passed, the allopurinol is stopped.

ICU Phase

Most of these patients can be treated effectively with antihistamines, epinephrine, steroids, and intravenous fluids. They never need an ICU setting. If anaphylaxis occurs, with shock, laryngospasm, or severe bronchospasm, however, these patients may need the type of support only an ICU may provide, such as dopamine or norepinephrine bitartrate (Levophed) for blood pressure support, emergent tracheostomy, or ventilatory support.

Post-ICU Phase

Once the offending drug has been stopped and the allergic reaction has subsided, patients do well. Rechallenge with the suspected allergy-causing drug should be avoided, unless its use is absolutely vital to the chemotherapeutic regimen.

REFERENCES

1. Perez, C. A., Presant, C. A., and Van Amburg, A. L., III: Management of superior vena cava syndrome. Semin. Oncol., 5:123, 1978.
2. Sculier, J. P., and Feld, R.: Superior vena cava obstruction syndrome: recommendations for management. Cancer Treat. Rev., 12:209, 1985.
3. Schraufnagel, D. E., Hill, R., Leech, J. A., and Pare, J. A. P.: Superior vena caval obstruction. Is it a medical emergency? Am. J. Med., 70:1169, 1981.
4. Ahmann, F. R.: A reassessment of the clinical implications of the superior vena caval syndrome. J. Clin. Oncol., 2:961, 1984.
5. Carabell, S. C., and Goodman, R. L.: Oncologic emergencies. In Cancer, Principles and Practice of Oncology. 2nd Ed. Edited by V. T. DeVita, S. Hellman, and S. A. Rosenberg. Philadelphia, J.B. Lippincott, 1985, p. 1855.
6. Nieto, A. F., and Doty, D. B.: Superior vena cava obstruction: clinical syndrome, etiology, and treatment. Curr. Probl. Cancer, 10:444, 1986.
7. Ryan, J. A., Jr., et al.: Catheter complications in total parenteral nutrition: a prospective study of 200 consecutive patients. N. Engl. J. Med., 290:757, 1974.
8. Chastre, J., et al.: Thrombosis as a complication of pulmonary-artery catheterization via the internal jugular vein: prospective evaluation by phlebography. N. Engl. J. Med., 306:278, 1982.
9. Gore, J. M., et al.: Superior vena cava syndrome: its association with indwelling balloon-tipped pulmonary artery catheters. Arch. Intern. Med., 144:506, 1984.
10. Bertrand, M., Presant, C. A., Klein, L., and Scott, E.: Iatrogenic superior vena cava syndrome: a new entity. Cancer, 54:376, 1984.
11. Haire, W. D., et al.: Hickman catheter-induced thoracic vein thrombosis: frequency and long-term sequelae in patients receiving high-dose chemotherapy and marrow transplantation. Cancer, 66:900, 1990.
12. Parish, J. M., Marschke, R. F., Jr., Dines, D. E., and Lee, R. E.: Etiologic considerations in superior vena cava syndrome. Mayo Clin. Proc., 56:407, 1981.
13. Schwartz, E. E., Goodman, L. R., and Haskin, M. E.: Role of CT scanning in the superior vena cava syndrome. Am. J. Clin. Oncol., 9:71, 1986.
14. Stanford, W., and Doty, D. B.: The role of venography and surgery in the management of patients with superior vena cava obstruction. Ann. Thorac. Surg., 41:158, 1986.
15. Benenati, J. F., Becker, G. J., Mail, J. T., and Holden, R. W.: Digital subtraction venography in central venous obstruction. AJR Am. J. Roentgenol. 147:685, 1986.
16. Shimm, D. S., Logue, G. L., and Rigsby, L. C.: Evaluating the superior vena cava syndrome. JAMA, 245:951, 1981.
17. Ghosh, B. C., and Clifton, E. E.: Malignant tumors with superior vena cava obstruction. N.Y. State J. Med., 73:283, 1973.

18. Adelstein, D. J., Hines, J. D., Carter, S. G., and Sacco, D.: Thromboembolic events in patients with malignant superior vena cava syndrome and the role of anticoagulation. Cancer, 62:2258, 1988.
19. Sherry, C. S., Diamond, N. G., Meyers, T. P., and Martin, R. L.: Successful treatment of superior vena cava syndrome by venous angioplasty. AJR Am. J. Roentgenol. 147:834, 1986.
20. Oudkerk, M., Heystraten, F. M. J., and Stoter, G.: Stenting in malignant vena caval obstruction. Cancer, 71:142, 1993.
21. Sculier, J. P., et al.: Superior vena caval obstruction syndrome in small cell lung cancer. Cancer, 57:847, 1986.
22. Perez-Soler, R., et al.: Clinical features and results of management of superior vena cava syndrome secondary to lymphoma. J. Clin. Oncol. 2:260, 1984.
23. Kane, R. C., Cohen, M. H., Broder, L. E., and Bull, M. I.: Superior vena caval obstruction due to small-cell anaplastic lung carcinoma: response to chemotherapy. JAMA, 235: 1717, 1976.
24. Dombernowsky, P., and Hansen, H. H.: Combination chemotherapy in the management of superior vena caval obstruction in small-cell anaplastic carcinoma of the lung. Acta Med. Scand., 204:513, 1978.
25. Maddox, A. M., et al.: Superior vena cava obstruction in small cell bronchogenic carcinoma: clinical parameters and survival. Cancer, 52:2165, 1983.
26. Pelley, R. J., Adelstein, D. J., and Hines, J. D.: Chemotherapy as initial treatment for superior vena cava obstruction in small cell carcinoma of the lung (Abstract.). Proc. ASCO 3: 215, 1984.
27. Byrne, T. N.: Spinal cord compression from epidural metastases. N. Engl. J. Med., 327:614, 1992.
28. Rodriguez, M., and Dinapoli, R. P.: Spinal cord compression: with special reference to metastatic epidural tumors. Mayo Clin. Proc., 55:442, 1980.
29. Bruckman, J. E., and Bloomer, W. D.: Management of spinal cord compression. Semin. Oncol., 5:135, 1978.
30. Willson, J. K. V., and Masaryk, T. J.: Neurologic emergencies in the cancer patient. Semin. Oncol. 16:490, 1989.
31. Haddad, P., et al.: Lymphoma of the spinal extradural space. Cancer, 38:1862, 1976.
32. Spiess, J. L., Adelstein, D. J., and Hines, J. D.: Multiple myeloma presenting with spinal cord compression. Oncology, 45:88, 1988.
33. Winkelman, M. D., Adelstein, D. J., and Karlins, N. L.: Intramedullary spinal cord metastasis. Arch. Neurol., 44:526, 1987.
34. Rodichok, L. D., et al.: Early diagnosis of spinal epidural metastases. Am. J. Med., 70:1181, 1981.
35. Gilbert, R. W., Kim, J. H., and Posner, J. B.: Epidural spinal cord compression from metastatic tumor: diagnosis and treatment. Ann. Neurol., 3:40, 1978.
36. Maranzano, E., et al.: Radiation therapy in metastatic spinal cord compression. Cancer, 67:1311, 1991.
37. Greenberg, H. S., Kim, J. H., and Posner, J. B.: Epidural spinal cord compression from metastatic tumor: results with a new treatment protocol. Ann. Neurol., 8:361, 1980.
38. Weissman, D. E.: Glucocorticoid treatment for brain metastases and epidural spinal cord compression: a review. J. Clin. Oncol., 6:543, 1988.
39. Young, R. F., Post, E. M., and King, G. A.: Treatment of spinal epidural metastases: randomized prospective comparison of laminectomy and radiotherapy. J. Neurosurg., 53:741, 1980.
40. Spain, R. C., and Whittlesey, D.: Respiratory emergencies in patients with cancer. Semin. Oncol. 16:471, 1989.
41. Kross, R.: Perioperative considerations. In Critical Care of the Cancer Patient. Edited by J. S. Groeger. St. Louis, Mosby-Year Book, 1991, p. 324.
42. Mehta, A. C., and Livingston, D. L.: Biopsy excision through a fiberoptic bronchoscope in the palliative management of airway obstruction. Chest, 91:774, 1987.
43. Mehta, A. C., et al.: Palliative treatment of malignant airway obstruction by Nd-Yag laser. Cleve. Clin. Q., 52:513, 1985.
44. Desai, S. J., et al.: Survival experience following Nd:Yag laser photoresection for primary bronchogenic carcinoma. Chest, 94:939, 1988.
45. Krupp, K. R., Adelstein, D. J., and Hines, J. D.: Efficiency of radiation therapy and/or chemotherapy for endobronchial obstruction due to small cell carcinoma of the lung (abstr.). Proc. ASCO, 4:178, 1985.
46. Mark, J. B. D., and Baldwin, J. C.: Endobronchial therapy for unresectable lung cancer. In Lung Cancer: A Comprehensive Treatise. Edited by J. Bitran, et al.: Philadelphia, Grune & Stratton, 1988, p. 401.
47. Adelstein D. J., Forman, W. B., Beavers, B.: Esophageal carcinoma: A six-year review of the Cleveland Veterans Administration Hospital experience. Cancer 54:918, 1984.
48. Lolley, D. M., et al.: Management of malignant esophagorespiratory fistula. Ann. Thorac. Surg. 25:516, 1978.
49. Okamoto, H., Shinkai, T., Yamakido, M., and Saijo, N.: Cardiac tamponade caused by primary lung cancer and the management of pericardial effusion. Cancer, 71:93, 1993.
50. Press, O. W., and Livingston, R.: Management of malignant pericardial effusion and tamponade. JAMA, 257:1088, 1987.
51. Helms, S. R., and Carlson, M. D.: Cardiovascular emergencies. Semin. Oncol., 16:463, 1989.
52. Davis, S., Rambotti, P., and Grignani, F.: Intrapericardial tetracycline sclerosis in the treatment of malignant pericardial effusion: an analysis of thirty-three cases. J. Clin. Oncol., 2:631, 1984.
53. Glover, D. J., and Glick, J. H.: Managing oncologic emergencies involving structural dysfunction. CA, 35:238, 1985.
54. Theologides, A.: Neoplastic cardiac tamponade. Semin. Oncol., 5:181, 1978.
55. Groeger, J. S., and Keefe, D.: Cardiac tamponade. In Critical Care of the Cancer Patient. Edited by J. S. Groeger. St. Louis, Mosby-Year Book, 1991, p. 250.
56. Posner, M. R., Cohen, G. I., and Skarin, A. T.: Pericardial disease in patients with cancer: the differentiation of malignant from idiopathic and radiation-induced pericarditis. Am. J. Med., 71:407, 1981.
57. David, S., Sharma, S. M., Blumberg, E. D., and Kim, C. S.: Intrapericardial tetracycline for the management of cardiac tamponade secondary to malignant pericardial effusion. N. Engl. J. Med., 299:1113, 1978.
58. Alcan, K. E., et al.: Management of acute cardiac tamponade by subxiphoid pericardiotomy. JAMA, 247:1143, 1982.
59. Hausheer, F. H., and Yarbro, J. W.: Diagnosis and treatment of malignant pleural effusion. Semin. Oncol., 12:54, 1985.
60. Sahn, S. A.: Malignant pleural effusions. Clin. Chest Med., 6:113, 1985.
61. Chernow, B., and Sahn, S. A.: Carcinomatous involvement of the pleura. Am. J. Med., 63:695, 1977.
62. Leff, A., Hopewell, P. C., and Costello, J.: Pleural effusion from malignancy. Ann. Intern. Med., 88:532, 1978.
63. Ruckdeschel, J. C., et al.: Intrapleural therapy for malignant pleural effusions: a randomized comparison of bleomycin and tetracycline. Chest, 100:1528, 1991.
64. Aelony, Y., King, R., and Boutin, C.: Thoracoscopic talc poudrage pleurodesis for chronic recurrent pleural effusions. Ann. Intern. Med., 115:778, 1991.
65. Ostrowski, M. J.: An assessment of the long-term results of

controlling the reaccumulation of malignant effusions using intracavity bleomycin. Cancer, 57:721, 1986.
66. Rusch, V. W., Figlin, R., Godwin, D., and Piantadosi, S.: Intrapleural cisplatin and cytarabine in the management of malignant pleural effusions: A Lung Cancer Study Group trial. J. Clin. Oncol., 9:313, 1991.
67. Lacy, J. H., Wieman, T. J., and Shively, E. H.: Management of malignant ascites. Surg. Gynecol. Obstet., 159:397, 1984.
68. Ringenberg, Q. S., Doll, D. C., Loy, T. S., and Yarbro, J. W.: Malignant ascites of unknown origin. Cancer, 64:753, 1989.
69. Garrison, R. N., Kaelin, L. D., Galloway, R. H., and Heuser, L. S.: Malignant ascites: clinical and experimental observations. Ann. Surg., 203:644, 1986.
70. Jackson, G. L., and Blosser, N. M.: Intracavitary chromic phosphate (^{32}P) colloidal suspension therapy. Cancer, 48:2596, 1981.
71. Markman, M.: Intraperitoneal chemotherapy. Semin. Oncol., 18:248, 1991.
72. Humphrey, P. R. D., Michael, J., and Pearson, T. C.: Management of relative polycythemia: studies of cerebral blood flow and viscosity. Br. J. Haematol., 46:427, 1980.
73. Fahey, J. L., et al.: Serum hyperviscosity syndrome. JAMA, 16:703, 1965.
74. Avnstorp, C., et al.: Plasmapheresis in hyperviscosity syndrome. Acta Med. Scand., 217:133, 1985.
75. Garcia, G. I., and Lawrence, W. D.: Disseminated intravascular coagulation in infection. Infect. Med., 7:17, 1991.
76. Feinstein, D. I.: Diagnosis and management of disseminated intravascular coagulation, the role of heparin therapy. Blood, 60:284, 1992.
77. Tallman, M. S., and Qwaan, H. C.: Reassessing the hemostatic disorder associated with acute promyelocytic leukemia. Blood, 79:543, 1992.
78. Cuttner, J., et al.: Therapeutic leukapheresis for hyperleukocytosis in acute myelocytic leukemia. Med. Pediatr. Oncol., 11:76, 1983.
79. Lichtman, M. A., and Rowe, J. M.: Hyperleukocytic leukemias: rheological, clinical, and therapeutic considerations. Blood, 60:279, 1982.
80. Dutcher, J. P., et al.: Hyperleukocytosis in adult acute non-lymphocytic leukemia: impact on remission rate and duration, and survival. J. Clin. Oncol. 5:1364, 1987.
81. Hess, C. E., et al.: Pseudohypoxemia secondary to leukemia and thrombocytosis. N. Engl. J. Med., 301:361, 1979.
82. Kyle, R. A.: Natural history of chronic idiopathic neutropenia. N. Engl. J. Med., 302:908, 1980.
83. Pizzo, P. A., et al.: A randomized study comparing Ceftazidime alone with combination antibiotic therapy in cancer patients with fever and neutropenia. N. Engl. J. Med., 315:552, 1986.
84. Rolston, K. V. I., Bodey, G. I., and Elting, L.: Aztreonam in the prevention and treatment of infection in neutropenic cancer patients. Am. J. Med., 88(Suppl. 3C):24, 1990.
85. Hughes, W. T., et al.: Guidelines for the use of antimicrobial agents in neutropenic patients with unexplained fever. J. Infect. Dis., 161:381, 1990.
86. Gucalp, R.: Management of the febrile neutropenic patient with cancer. Oncology, 5:137, 1991.
87. Lieschke, G. J., and Burgess, A. W.: Granulocyte colony—stimulating factor and granulocyte macrophage colony stimulating factor. N. Engl. J. Med., 327:28, 1992.
88. Terrell, C. L., and Hermans, P. E.: Antifungal agents used for deep-seated mycotic infections. Mayo Clin. Proc. 62:1116, 1987.
89. Talbot, G. H., Provencher, M., and Cassileth, P. A.: Persistent fever after recovery from granulocytopenia in acute leukemia. Arch. Intern. Med. 148:129, 1988.
90. Newton, L. K.: Neurologic complications of polycythemia and their impact on therapy. Oncology, 4:59, 1990.
91. Conley, C. L.: Polycythemia vera; diagnosis and treatment. Hosp. Pract., 22:181, 1987.
92. Conley, C. L.: Polycythemia vera. JAMA, 263:2481, 1990.
93. Brodsky, I.: Busulphan treatment of polycythemia vera. Br. J. Haematol., 52:1, 1982.
94. Wasserman, L. R., and Gilbert, H. S.: Complications of polycythemia vera. Semin. Hematol. 3:199, 1966.
95. Mann, M. C., Votto, J., Kambe, J., and McNamee, M. J.: Management of the severely anemic patient who refuses transfusion: Lessons learned during the care of a Jehovah's Witness. Ann. Intern. Med., 117:1042, 1992.
96. Gould, S. A., et al.: Fluosol-DA as a red cell substitute in acute anemia. N. Engl. J. Med., 314:1653, 1986.
97. Ohyanagi, H., Nakaya, S., Okumura, S., and Saitoh, Y.: Surgical use of fluosol-DA in Jehovah's Witness patients. Artif. Organs, 8:10, 1984.
98. Spence, R. K., et al.: Fluosol DA-20 in the treatment of severe anemia: a randomized, controlled study of 46 patients. Crit. Care Med., 18:1227, 1990.
99. Michiels, J. J., et al.: Erythromelalgia caused by platelet-mediated arteriolar inflammation and thrombosis in thrombocythemia. Ann. Intern. Med., 102:466, 1985.
100. Ginsburg, A. D.: Platelet function in patients with high platelet counts. Ann. Intern. Med., 82:506, 1975.
101. Kaywin, P., McDonough, M., Insel, P., and Shattil, S. J.: Platelet function in essential thrombocythemia. N. Engl. J. Med., 299:505, 1978.
102. Jabaily, J., et al.: Neurologic manifestations of essential thrombocythemia. Ann. Intern. Med., 99:513, 1983.
103. Silverstein, M. N., et al.: Angrelide: a new drug for treating thrombocytosis. N. Engl. J. Med. 318:1292, 1988.
104. Goldfinger, D., et al.: Long-term plateletpheresis in the management of primary thrombocytosis. Transfusion, 19:336, 1979.
105. Chen, Y., et al.: Blastic transformation in a case of essential thrombocythemia. South. Med. J., 80:1040, 1987.
106. Gaydos, L. A., et al.: The quantitative relation between platelet count and hemorrhage in patients with acute leukemia. N. Engl. J. Med., 226:905, 1962.
107. Schiffer, C. A.: Prevention of alloimmunization against platelets. Blood, 77:1, 1991.
108. Hackett, T., et al.: Drug induced platelet destruction. Semin. Thromb. Hemostas., 8:116, 1982.
109. Champlin, R.: Bone Marrow Transplantation. Norwell, MA, Kluwer Academic Publishers, 1990.
110. Ferrara, J. L. M., and Deeg, H. J.: Graft versus host disease. N. Engl. J. Med., 324:667, 1991.
111. Beelen, D. W., et al.: Evidence that sustained growth suppression of intestinal anaerobic bacteria reduces the risk of acute graft versus host disease after sibling marrow transplantation. Blood, 80:2668, 1992.
112. Meyers, J. D.: Management of cytomegalovirus infection. Am. J. Med., 85(Suppl. 2A):102, 1988.
113. Jiwa, N. M., et al.: Rapid detection of human cytomegalovirus DNA in peripheral blood leukocytes of viremic transplant recipients by the polymerase chain reaction. Transplantation, 48:72, 1989.
114. Afessa, B., et al.: Outcome of recipients of bone marrow transplants who require intensive care unit support. Mayo Clin., Proc., 67:117, 1992.
115. Atkinson, K.: Reconstruction of the hemotopoietic and immune systems after marrow transplantation. Bone Marrow Transpl., 5:209, 1990.
116. Silverman, P., and Distelhorst, C. W.: Metabolic emergencies in clinical oncology. Semin. Oncol., 16:504, 1989.

117. Bajorunas, D. R.: Disorders of endocrine function. *In* Critical Care of the Cancer Patient. Edited by J. S. Groeger. St. Louis, Mosby-Year Book, 1991, p. 192.
118. Muggia, F. M.: Overview of cancer-related hypercalcemia: epidemiology and etiology. Semin. Oncol. *17:*3, 1990.
119. Mundy, G. R.: Pathophysiology of cancer-associated hypercalcemia. Semin. Oncol., *17:*10, 1990.
120. Buday, A. A., et al.: Increased serum levels of a parathyroid hormone-like protein in malignancy-associated hypercalcemia. Ann. Intern. Med., *111:*807, 1989.
121. Seyberth, H. W., et al.: Prostaglandins as mediators of hypercalcemia associated with certain types of cancer. N. Engl. J. Med. *293:*1278, 1975.
122. Breslau, N. A., et al.: Hypercalcemia associated with increased serum calcitriol levels in three patients with lymphoma. Ann. Intern. Med., *100:*1, 1984.
123. Zaloga, G. P., Eil, C., and Medbery, C. A.: Humoral hypercalcemia in Hodgkin's disease. Arch. Intern. Med., *145:*155, 1985.
124. Rieke, J. W., Donaldson, S. S., and Horning, S. J.: Hypercalcemia and vitamin D metabolism in Hodgkin's disease: is there an underlying immunoregulatory relationship? Cancer, *63:*1700, 1989.
125. Mundy, G. R., et al.: Bone-resorbing activity in supernatants from lymphoid cell lines. N. Engl. J. Med. *290:*867, 1974.
126. Mundy, G. R., et al.: Evidence for the secretion of an osteoclast stimulating factor in myeloma. N. Engl. J. Med. *291:*1041, 1974.
127. Dewhirst, F. E., et al.: Purification and partial sequence of human osteoclast-activating factor: identity with interleukin-1 beta. J. Immunol. *135:*2562, 1985.
128. Garrett, I. R., et al.: Production of the bone resorbing cytokine lymphotoxin by cultural human myeloma cells. N. Engl. J. Med. *317:*526, 1987.
129. Bajorunas, D. R.: Clinical manifestations of cancer-related hypercalcemia. Semin. Oncol., *17:*16, 1990.
130. Ritch, P. S.: Treatment of cancer-related hypercalcemia. Semin. Oncol., *17:*26, 1990.
131. Singer, F. R.: Role of the biphosphonate etidronate in the therapy of cancer-related hypercalcemia. Semin. Oncol., *17:*34, 1990.
132. Jacobs, T. P., et al.: Neoplastic hypercalcemia: physiologic response to intravenous etidronate disodium. Am. J. Med., *82(Suppl. 2A):*42, 1987.
133. Gucalp, R., et al.: Comparative study of pamidronate disodium and etidronate disodium in the treatment of cancer-related hypercalcemia. J. Clin. Oncol., *10:*134, 1992.
134. Warrell, R. P., Issacs, M., Alcock, N. W., and Bockman, R. S.: Gallium nitrate for treatment of refractory hypercalcemia from parathyroid carcinoma. Ann. Intern. Med., *107:*683, 1987.
135. Warrell, R. J., Jr., et al.: A randomized double-blind study of gallium nitrate compared with etidronate for acute control of cancer-related hypercalcemia. J. Clin. Oncol., *9:*1467, 1991.
136. Lad, T. E., et al.: Treatment of cancer-associated hypercalcemia with cisplatin. Arch. Intern. Med., *147:*329, 1987.
137. Ralston, S. H., et al.: Cancer-associated hypercalcemia: morbidity and mortality. Clinical experience in 126 treated patients. Ann. Intern. Med., *112:*499, 1990.
138. Glover, D. J., and Glick, J. H.: Metabolic oncologic emergencies. CA, *37:*302, 1987.
139. Silverman, P., and Distelhorst, C. W.: Metabolic emergencies in clinical oncology. Semin. Oncol., *16:*504, 1989.
140. Berl, T., Anderson, R. J., McDonald, K. M., and Schrier, R. W.: Clinical disorders of water metabolism. Kidney Int., *10:*117, 1976.
141. Cooke, C. R., Turin, M. D., and Walker, W. G.: The syndrome of inappropriate antidiuretic hormone secretion (SIADH): pathophysiologic mechanisms in solute and volume regulation. Medicine, *58:*240, 1979.
142. Comis, R. L., Miller, M., and Ginsberg, S. J.: Abnormalities in water homeostasis in small cell anaplastic lung cancer. Cancer, *45:*2414, 1980.
143. Escuro, R. S., Adelstein, D. J., and Carter, S. G.: Syndrome of inappropriate secretion of antidiuretic hormone after infusional vincristine. Cleve. Clin. J. Med., *59:*643, 1992.
144. Forrest, J. N., et al.: Superiority of demeclocycline over lithium in the treatment of chronic syndrome of inappropriate secretion of antidiuretic hormone. N. Engl. J. Med., *298:*173, 1978.
145. Trump, D. L.: Serious hyponatremia in patients with cancer: management with demeclocycline. Cancer, *47:*2908, 1981.
146. Ayus, C. J., Olivero, J. J., and Frommer, J. P.: Rapid correction of severe hyponatremia with intravenous hypertonic saline solution. Am. J. Med., *72:*43, 1982.
147. Hainsworth, J. D., Workman, R., and Greco, F. A.: Management of the syndrome of inappropriate antidiuretic hormone secretion in small cell lung cancer. Cancer, *50:*161, 1983.
148. Bajorunas, D. R.: Disorders of endocrine function. *In* Critical Care of the Cancer Patient. Edited by J. S. Groeger. St. Louis, Mosby-Year Book, 1991, p. 192.
149. Glover, D. J., and Glick, J. H.: Metabolic oncologic emergencies. CA, *37:*302, 1987.
150. Silverman, P., and Distelhorst, C. W.: Metabolic emergencies in clinical oncology. Semin. Oncol., *16:*504, 1989.
151. Boden, G.: Insulinoma and glucoagonoma. Semin. Oncol., *14:*253, 1987.
152. Kahn, C. R.: The riddle of tumor hypoglycemia revisited. Clin. Endocrinol. Metab., *9:*335, 1980.
153. Moertel, C. G.: An odyssey in the land of small tumors. J. Clin. Oncol., *5:*1503, 1987.
154. Patterson, W. P., and Reams, G. P.: Renal toxicities of chemotherapy. Semin. Oncol. *19:*521, 1992.
155. Madias, N. E., and Harrington, J. T.: Platinum nephrotoxicity. Am. J. Med., *65:*307, 1978.
156. Blachley, J. D., and Hill, J. B.: Renal and electrolyte disturbances associated with cisplatin. Ann. Intern. Med., *95:*628, 1981.
157. Vogelzang, N. J.: Nephrotoxicity from chemotherapy: prevention and management. Oncology, *5:*97, 1991.
158. Ozols, R. F., et al.: High-dose cisplatin in hypertonic saline. Ann. Intern. Med., *100:*19, 1984.
159. Schilsky, R. L., and Anderson, T.: Hypomagnesemia and renal magnesium wasting in patients receiving cisplatin. Ann. Intern. Med., *90:*929, 1979.
160. Lam, M., and Adelstein, D. J.: Hypomagnesemia and renal magnesium wasting in patients treated with cisplatin. Am. J. Kidney Dis., *8:*164, 1986.
161. Hutchison, F. N., et al.: Renal salt wasting in patients treated with cisplatin. Ann. Intern. Med., *108:*21, 1988.
162. Schacht, R. G., et al.: Nephrotoxicity of nitrosoureas. Cancer, *48:*1328, 1981.
163. Weiss, R. B., Posada, J. G. Jr., Kramer, R. A., and Boyd, M. R.: Nephrotoxicity of semustine. Cancer Treat. Rep., *67:*1105, 1983.
164. Schein, P. S., et al.: Clinical antitumor activity and toxicity of streptozotocin. Cancer, *34:*993, 1974.
165. Antman, K. H., Elias, A., and Ryan, L.: Ifosfamide and mesna: response and toxicity at standard- and high-dose schedules. Semin. Oncol., *17:*68, 1990.
166. Frei, E.: High dose methotrexate with leucovorin rescue:

167. Silverman, P., and Distelhorst, C. W.: Metabolic emergencies in clinical oncology. Semin. Oncol., 16:504, 1989.
168. Cohen, L. F., et al.: Acute tumor lysis syndrome. A review of 37 patients with Burkitt's lymphoma. Am. J. Med., 68:486, 1980.
169. Tsokos, G. C., Balow, J. E., Spiegel, R. J., and Magrath, I. T.: Renal and metabolic complications of undifferentiated and lymphoblastic lymphomas. Medicine, 60:218, 1981.
170. Zusman, J., Brown, D. M., and Nesbit, M. E.: Hyperphosphatemia, hyperphosphaturia and hypocalcemia in acute lymphoblastic leukemia. N. Engl. J. Med., 289:1335, 1973.
171. Thomas, M. R., et al.: Tumor lysis syndrome following VP-16-213 in chronic myeloid leukemia in blast crisis. Am. J. Hematol., 16:185, 1984.
172. Vogelzang, N. J., Nelimark, R. A., and Nath, K. A.: Tumor lysis syndrome after induction chemotherapy of small-cell bronchogenic carcinoma. JAMA, 249:513, 1983.
173. Barton, J. C.: Tumor lysis syndrome in nonhematopoietic neoplasms. Cancer, 64:738, 1989.
174. Arseneau, J. C., Bagley, C. M., Anderson, T., and Canellos, G. P.: Hyperkalemia, a sequel to chemotherapy of Burkitt's lymphoma. Lancet, 1:10, 1973.
175. Lesesne, J. B., et al.: Cancer-associated hemolytic-uremic syndrome: analysis of 85 cases from a national registry. J. Clin. Oncol., 7:781, 1989.
176. Doll, D. C., and Yarbro, J. W.: Vascular toxicity associated with antineoplastic agents. Semin. Oncol. 19:580, 1992.
177. Pavy, M. D., Wiley, E. L., and Abeloff, M. D.: Hemolytic-uremic syndrome associated with mitomycin therapy. Cancer Treat. Rep., 66:457, 1982.
178. Hanna, W. T., Krauss, S., Regester, R. F., and Murphy, W. M.: Renal disease after mitomycin C therapy. Cancer, 48:2583, 1981.
179. Gulati, S. C., et al.: Microangiopathic hemolytic anemia observed after treatment of epidermoid carcinoma with mitomycin C and 5-fluorouracil. Cancer, 45:2252, 1980.
180. Jackson, A. M., et al.: Thrombotic microangiopathy and renal failure associated with antineoplastic chemotherapy. Ann. Intern. Med., 101:41, 1984.
181. Watson, P. R., Guthrie, T. H., Jr., and Caruana, R. J.: Cisplatin-associated hemolytic-uremic syndrome. Successful treatment with a staphylococcal protein A column. Cancer, 64:1400, 1989.
182. Korec, S., et al.: Treatment of cancer-associated hemolytic-uremic syndrome with staphylococcal protein A immunoperfusion. J. Clin. Oncol., 4:210, 1986.
183. White, D. A., and Levine, S. J.: Respiratory failure. In Critical Care of the Cancer Patient. Edited by J. S. Groeger. St. Louis, Mosby-Year Book. 1991, p. 13.
184. Spain, R. C., and Whittlesey, D.: Respiratory emergencies in patients with cancer. Semin. Oncol., 16:471, 1989.
185. Ginsberg, S. J., and Comis, R. L.: The pulmonary toxicity of antineoplastic agents. Semin. Oncol., 9:34, 1982.
186. Kreisman, H., and Wolkove, N.: Pulmonary toxicity of antineoplastic therapy. Semin. Oncol., 19:508, 1992.
187. Gross, N. J.: Pulmonary effects of radiation therapy. Ann. Intern. Med., 86:81, 1977.
188. Thar, T. L., and Million, R. R.: Complications of radiation treatment of Hodgkin's disease. Semin. Oncol., 7:174, 1980.
189. Lane, S. D., Besa, E. C., Justh, G., and Joseph, R. R.: Fatal interstitial pneumonitis following high-dose intermittent chlorambucil therapy for chronic lymphocytic leukemia. Cancer, 47:32, 1981.
190. Westerfield, B. T., Michalski, J. P., McCombs, C., and Light, R. W.: Reversible melphalan-induced lung damage. Am. J. Med., 68:767, 1980.
191. Bennett, J. M., and Reich, S. D.: Bleomycin. Ann. Intern. Med., 90:945, 1979.
192. Orwoll, E. S., Kiessling, P. J., and Patterson, J. R.: Interstitial pneumonia from mitomycin. Ann. Intern. Med., 89:352, 1978.
193. Weiss, R. B., Poster, D. S., and Penta, J. S.: The nitrosoureas and pulmonary toxicity. Cancer Treat. Rev., 8:111, 1981.
194. Aronin, P. A., et al.: Prediction of BCNU pulmonary toxicity in patients with malignant gliomas. An assessment of risk factors. N. Engl. J. Med., 303:183, 1980.
195. Haupt, H. M., Hutchins, G. M., and Moore, G. W.: Ara-C lung: noncardiogenic pulmonary edema complicating cytosine arabinoside therapy of leukemia. Am. J. Med., 70:256, 1981.
196. Andersson, B. S., et al.: Fatal pulmonary failure complicating high-dose cytosine arabinoside therapy in acute leukemia. Cancer, 65:1079, 1990.
197. Ettinger, N. A., and Trulock, E. P.: Pulmonary considerations of organ transplantation. Part 2. Bone marrow transplantation. Am. Rev. Respir. Dis., 144:213, 1991.
198. Seiden, M. V., et al.: Pulmonary toxicity associated with high dose chemotherapy in the treatment of solid tumors with autologous marrow transplant: an analysis of four chemotherapy regimens. Bone Marrow Transpl. 10:57, 1992.
199. Green, N., et al.: Lymphangitic carcinomatosis of the lung: pathologic, diagnostic and therapeutic considerations. Int. J. Radiat. Oncol. Biol. Phys., 2:149, 1977.
200. Weiss, H. D., Walker, M. D., and Wiernik, P. H.: Neurotoxicity of commonly used antineoplastic agents. N. Engl. J. Med., 291:75, 1974.
201. Kaplan, R. S., and Wiernik, P. H.: Neurotoxicity of antineoplastic drugs. Semin. Oncol., 9:103, 1982.
202. Antman, K. H., Elias, A., and Ryan, L.: Ifosfamide and mesna: response and toxicity at standard- and high-dose schedules. Semin. Oncol. 17:68, 1990.
203. Pratt, C. B., et al.: Central nervous system toxicity following the treatment of pediatric patients with ifosfamide/mesna. J. Clin. Oncol., 4:1253, 1986.
204. Herzig, R. H., et al.: Cerebellar toxicity with high-dose cytosine arabinoside. J. Clin. Oncol., 5:927, 1987.
205. Winkelman, M. D., and Hines, J. D.: Cerebellar degeneration caused by high-dose cytosine arabinoside: a clinicopathological study. Ann. Neurol., 14:520, 1983.
206. Willson, J. K. V., and Masaryk, T. J.: Neurologic emergencies in the cancer patient. Semin. Oncol., 16:490, 1989.
207. Burger, P. C., et al.: Encephalomyelopathy following high-dose BCNU therapy. Cancer, 48:1318, 1981.
208. Thompson, S. W., et al.: Cisplatin neuropathy. Clinical, electrophysiologic, morphologic, and toxicologic studies. Cancer, 54:1269, 1984.
209. Gregg, R. W., et al.: Cisplatin neurotoxicity: the relationship between dosage, time, and platinum concentration in neurologic tissues, and morphologic evidence of toxicity. J. Clin. Oncol., 10:795, 1992.
210. Rosenfeld, C. S., and Broder, L. E.: Cisplatin-induced autonomic neuropathy. Cancer Treat. Rep., 68:659, 1984.
211. Freeman, J. E., Johnston, P. G. B., and Voke, J. M.: Somnolence after prophylactic cranial irradiation in children with acute lymphoblastic leukemia. Br. Med. J., 4:523, 1973.
212. Fleck, J. F., et al.: Is prophylactic cranial irradiation indicated in small-cell lung cancer? J. Clin. Oncol., 8:209, 1990.
213. Doll, D. C., et al.: Acute vascular ischemic events after cisplatin-based combination chemotherapy for germ-cell tumors of the testis. Ann. Intern. Med., 105:48, 1986.

214. Woods, W. G., et al.: Fatal veno-occlusive disease of the liver following high dose chemotherapy, irradiation, and bone marrow transplantation. Am. J. Med., *68*:285, 1980.
215. Bearman, S. I., et al.: Recombinant human tissue plasminogen activator for flu treatment of severe venocclusive disease of the liver after bone marrow transplantation. Blood, *80*:2458, 1992.
216. Bianco, J., et al.: Pentoxifylline and GM-CSF decrease tumor necrosis factor—alpha levels in patients undergoing allogeneic bone marrow transplantation. Blood, *76(Suppl. 1)*: 133a, 1990.
217. Schwartz, R. G., et al.: Congestive heart failure and left ventricular dysfunction complicating doxorubicin therapy. Am. J. Med., *82*:1109, 1987.
218. Saini, J., Rich, M. W., and Lyss, A. P.: Reversibility of severe left ventricular dysfunction due to doxorubicin cardiotoxicity: report of three cases. Ann. Intern. Med., *106*:814, 1987.
219. Speyer, J. L., et al.: Protective effect of the bispiperazinedione ICRF-187 against doxorubin induced cardiac toxicity in women with advanced breast cancer. N. Engl. J. Med., *319*:745, 1988.
220. Rezkalla, S., et al.: Continuous ambulatory ECG monitoring during fluororacil therapy: a prospective study. J. Clin. Oncol., *7*:509, 1989.
221. Capizzi, R. L., et al.: L-asparginase: clinical, biochemical, pharmacological and immunological studies. Ann. Intern. Med., *74*:893, 1971.
222. Ohnuma, T., et al.: *Erwinia carotovora* asparaginase in patients with prior anaphylaxis to asparaginase from *E. Coli.* Cancer, *30*:376, 1972.
223. Weiss, R. B., and Bruno, S.: Hypersensitivity reactions to cancer chemotherapeutic agents. Ann. Intern. Med., *94*:66, 1981.
224. Singer, J., and Wallace, S. L.: The allopurinol hypersensitivity syndrome: unnecessary morbidity and mortality. Arthritis Rheum., *29*:82, 1986.

# Chapter 45

HEMATOLOGIC DISORDERS IN THE INTENSIVE CARE UNIT

ANDREA P. BALDYGA

The hematologic system can often be overlooked in the care of the critically ill ICU patient, overshadowed by disorders of solid organ systems. Hematologic dysfunction may be in itself the cause of systemic dysfunction, an aid in the diagnosis of other diseases, as well as an important contributor to the ultimate outcome of the patient. This chapter presents an overview of normal hematologic function, reviews conditions that the patient brings to the ICU that impact on management, and examines disorders that are a consequence of various ICU interventions.

NORMAL HEMATOLOGIC FUNCTION

Red Cells

The primary function of the red cell in the body is to act as the vehicle for oxygen transport, but it also has roles as the major oncotic constituent of the intravascular space and as the primary buffer for acute acidosis. The normal erythrocyte has a life span of 120 days, but this can be considerably decreased secondary to multiple factors in critically ill patients, including infection or medications. The average bone marrow production is 20 ml of red blood cells (RBCs) a day. The level of hemoglobin in any patient depends on the relationship of production to destruction or loss of RBCs. Normal hemoglobin in males is 14 to 16 g/dl, 12 to 14 g/dl in women, corresponding approximately to mean hematocrits of 47 and 42, respectively. Hemoglobin levels much lower can be well tolerated, however, by younger, healthier patients and in other situations, as proved by the practice of isovolemic hemodilution used routinely for many surgical procedures including open heart and orthopedic surgery.[1] The maintenance of an absolute hemoglobin level, therefore, is not the focus of greatest importance in most ICU patients, but rather the provision of adequate oxygen transport for cellular maintenance and recovery. This must be individualized to each patient, considering the current active disease processes present, the physiologic reserve of the patient, and coexisting systemic diseases that affect oxygen delivery and consumption, the magnitude of acute or chronic blood loss, as well as the capacity of the marrow production to respond to losses with an adequate reticulocyte response. Erythropoietin, the major stimulus for RBC production may also be deficient in ICU patients as well as in patients with other coexisting diseases such as renal failure.[2,3]

White Cells

Five different groups of white cells are present in the body with different morphology and function and include granulocytes, lymphocytes, and monocytes. The granulocyte series consists of neutrophils, basophils, and eosinophils. **Neutrophils** are phagocytic cells that ingest bacteria and fungi. This function is accomplished in several components including chemotaxis, phagocytosis, degranulation, and the intracellular production of oxygen free radicals and myeloperoxidase for organism destruction. The life span of a neutrophil is approximately 10 to 14 days. The first 6 to 9 days is spent in the marrow as the reserve pool that can be mobilized under conditions of stress such as infection. The neutrophils then pass into the circulating pool in the peripheral circulation. A considerable number of the cells are marginated on the endothelium of small vessels and can be demarginated during stress conditions but are not available to be counted in the cell count. The cells are only in the blood stream for 6 or 7 hours and then migrate through the capillary walls into the surrounding tissues, where they survive for another 2 to 4 days before destruction. **Eosinophils** are phagocytic cells involved in the digestion of antigen-antibody complexes and foreign proteins. **Basophils** are poorly phagocytic but release histamine on activation and degranulation and are thus responsible for anaphylaxis.

Lymphocytes are the next most common white cell after granulocytes. Seventy-five percent of lymphocytes are T cells, which are primarily responsible for cellular immunity and include subsets of killer, helper, suppressor, and other types that have specific functions. The rest of the lymphocyte population are B lymphocytes and are most involved in humoral immunity. To function in antibody production, B cells must first transform to plasma cells after activation. A few "null" lymphocytes have no specific characteristics as either T or B cells.

Monocytes are derived from the same cell line that produces neutrophils and are therefore phagocytic for both organisms and debris, as well as being very important in the processing of antigens for recognition by T lymphocytes. They migrate into the tissues and develop into various types of macrophages, which retain their phagocytic activity.

Normal white cell counts are very variable in the population even in the state of good health. Total white cell count ranges from 4300 to 10,000 cells per milliliter. Neutrophils compose 50 to 60% of the total; black men have a slightly lower mean count of 3700 versus 4400 for age-matched white men.[4] Therefore, there is no standardized definition of neutropenia, and each patient must be considered individually in clinical context. An absolute neutrophil count of less than 1500 to 2000 cells per milliliter is considered to be significant, with counts of less than 1000/ml having an increased chance of infection, and counts of less than 500/ml being at high risk for infection. Lymphocytes make up 30 to 40% of white cells, monocytes 5%, eosinophils 2 to 3%, and basophils 0.5%.

Platelets

Platelets have an extremely important function in the maintenance of normal coagulation function. They are produced by megakaryocytes in the marrow and have a life span of 10 days. Normal platelet count averages 250,000/mm^3, with a range of 150,000 to 400,000/mm^3. Usually, there is no significant bleeding until the platelet count reaches 50,000, and spontaneous bleeding seldom occurs before the count falls to less than 20,000.

Platelet function encompasses three major aspects:

- Adhesion
- Degranulation
- Aggregation

When there is vascular injury, subendothelial collagen and basement membrane is exposed. Platelets adhere to this surface by the von Willebrand's portion of factor VIII, which acts as a bridge between the collagen and the glycoprotein Ib (GpIb) binding site on the platelet membrane. Binding at the GpIb site causes a conformational change in the platelet membrane exposing the GpIIb/IIIa binding site, which is the site for the attachment of fibrinogen allowing for the aggregation of further platelets leading to a larger platelet plug. Exposure of the GpIIb/IIIa site also causes degranulation with release of vasoactive substances as well as thromboxane A$_2$, a product of arachidonic acid metabolism, and adenosine diphosphate (ADP), both potent stimulators of platelet aggregation. The platelet membrane serves as a surface for activation of the clotting cascade and provides some of the phospholipid co-factors necessary for clotting factor activation. The tendency for aggregation is opposed by prostacyclin, another arachidonic acid product, a potent inhibitor of platelet aggregation generated in the endothelial cells that increases the level of cyclic adenosine monophosphate (cAMP) in the platelet, thus changing calcium flux and decreasing the tendency for aggregation.

Coagulation Factors

The classic coagulation cascade is described as consisting of 12 clotting factors, some of which are procoagulants, others co-factors, which combine to make up two pathways, intrinsic and extrinsic, ending in a final common pathway. The intrinsic pathway classically operates with components contained in the blood, while the extrinsic pathway requires a tissue factor derived from tissue trauma or inflammation for activation. The cascade is well characterized and is represented in Figure 45-1. Characteristics of the clotting factors themselves are listed in Table 45-1. Factors II, VII, IX, and X are vitamin K dependent. They require vitamin K for appropriate function of the carboxylase enzyme that attaches a carboxyl group to the gamma carbon of glutamic acid in the inactive factors. The gamma carboxylation enables the factors to bind calcium and phospholipid membranes. Without this activation, the factors are present in normal quantity as measured by factor assays but are inactive.

A number of inhibitors and the fibrinolytic system are important to prevent widespread activation of the coagulation system. Antithrombin III, alpha$_2$ macroglobulin, alpha$_2$ antitrypsin, heparin cofactor II, proteins C and S, and even the activated co-factors themselves serve to modulate the coagulation cascade. The fibrinolytic system functions via plasminogen, which is bound to fibrinogen and thus made part of the organizing thrombus. The plasminogen is then activated by tissue-type plasminogen activator (t-PA) produced by the endothelial cells causing the production of plasmin that remodels the clot. Excess plasmin

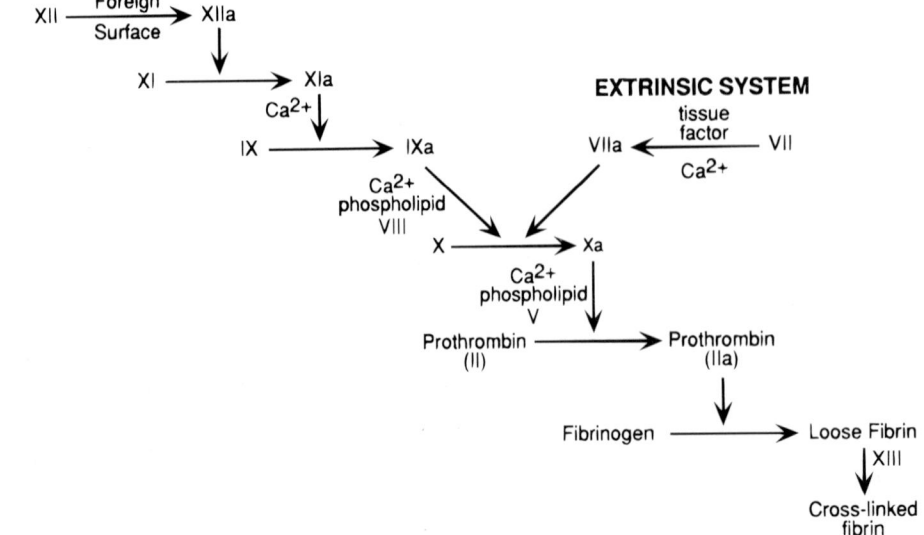

Fig. 45-1. Classic coagulation cascade.

Table 45–1. Coagulation Factor Characteristics

	Vitamin K Dependent	Half-Life (h)	Laboratory Abnormality in Deficiency	Replacement Source
I (Fibrinogen)	No	90	Fibrinogen, PT, PTT	Cryoprecipitate
II (Prothrombin)	Yes	65	PT, PTT	FFP
V (Proaccelerin)	No	15	PT, PTT	FFP
VII (Proconvertin)	Yes	5	PT, nlPTT	FFP
VII (AHF-A)	No	12	nlPT, PTT	VIII concentrate, cryoprecipitate
IX (AHF-B)	Yes	24	nlPT, PTT	IX conc., FFP
X (Stuart factor, Christmas factor)	Yes	40	PT, PTT	FFP
XI (Plasma thromboplastin antecedent)	No	45	nlPT, PTT	FFP
XII (Hageman factor)	No	120	nlPT, nlPTT Abnormal clot	FFP

Con, concentrate; FFP, fresh-frozen plasma; nl, normal; PT, prothrombin time; PTT, partial thromboplastin time.

is quickly cleared from the system by alpha$_2$ antiplasmin, preventing systemic fibrinolysis. Activators of the fibrinolytic system are in turn regulated by a series of newly identified inhibitors including plasminogen activator inhibitor 1 (PAI-1).

Function of the intrinsic pathway is measured by the partial thromboplastin time (PTT), the extrinsic pathway by the prothrombin time (PT). Activation of the fibrinolytic system is assayed by FDP (fibrin degradation products) or D-dimer.

RED CELL DISORDERS (Fig. 45–2)

Inadequate Production

Iron Deficiency Anemia

Iron deficiency is the most common cause of anemia in most parts of the world; many patients will present to the ICU with chronic anemia. This is further accentuated by the "routine" blood loss that is caused by blood drawing and other invasive procedures. Iron is normally derived exclusively from the gastrointestinal tract by absorption in the proximal small intestine. Adequate enteral nutrition is often difficult to achieve in critically ill patients; thus, iron loss may be greater than can be balanced by intake. Hypochromic, microcytic indices suggest this diagnosis, which is confirmed by measurements of serum ferritin and iron-binding capacity. Treatment involves all the measures to decrease red cell loss and institution of supplemental iron therapy.

Megaloblastic Anemias

Folate and vitamin B$_{12}$ are both necessary for DNA synthesis, and deficiencies can lead to abnormalities in cell proliferation, most marked in rapidly proliferating cell populations such as the hemopoietic tissue. Because of the reduction in DNA synthesis, there are fewer divisions of the red cell precursors at a slower rate. While under normal circumstances, red cells do not have the opportunity to regrow to their previous size between divisions, red cells in megaloblastic disorders can reach a larger size, while still possessing a normal hemoglobin concentration. More advanced varieties of the disorder result in ineffective erythropoiesis, with destruction of immature red cells in the marrow, and also affect the production of leukocytes and platelets.

Folate deficiency can be due to insufficient dietary intake relative to needs; malabsorption and diseases such as sprue; and drugs, including anticonvulsants, which cause folate deficiency by an unknown mechanism, dihydrofolate reductase inhibitors such as methotrexate, and occasionally trimethoprim. The causes of B$_{12}$ deficiency are more numerous because of the specific need for intrinsic factor secreted by the stomach for transport of B$_{12}$ to the terminal ileum for absorption. Thus, the causes include not only dietary inadequacy but also deficiency of intrinsic factor secondary to gastrectomy or pernicious anemia, disease of the terminal ileum that has eliminated the absorptive site, or bacterial overgrowth in small intestine "blind loops" with binding of B$_{12}$ by the bacteria. Diagnosis of these two disorders is made by noting megaloblastic indices. Folate and B$_{12}$ levels can be obtained to determine the factor responsible. If B$_{12}$ is determined to be the cause, a Schilling test should be done to localize the site of the problem. Folate should not be given without first determining whether a B$_{12}$ deficiency exists because of the potential for causing serious neurologic dysfunction consisting of degenerative changes of the dorsal and lateral columns of the spinal cord.

Anemias That Are Due to Low Erythropoietin Levels

Erythropoietin (EPO) has been identified as the major regulator of red cell production.[5] The majority of this glycoprotein hormone is produced in the kidney stimulated by hypoxia, although a small fraction, (less than 10%), is made by the liver, so that even anephric patients will have a very low level. Erythropoietin acts in the marrow by stimulating an increase in the number of erythroid precursors and the differentiation of these cells to mature forms. Renal disease has been found to profoundly decrease erythropoietin production even when the stimulus of significant hypoxia is present. This is due to damage by the renal disease to the cells necessary for the hormone's production. Recombinant human EPO (r-HuEPO) has been found to be exceptionally valuable in the treatment of the anemia associated with renal failure and can restore the hematocrit to normal, thus avoiding the complications of anemia, as well as significantly improving the quality of life and sense of well-being of dialysis patients.[6,7] The major side effect of this therapy is development of increased hypertension, but this can usually be controlled with careful antihypertensive management. Care must also be taken to ensure that the patient does not become relatively polycythemic and thus at risk of developing thrombotic complications, particularly in patients with atherosclerotic vascular disease. The potential for relative EPO

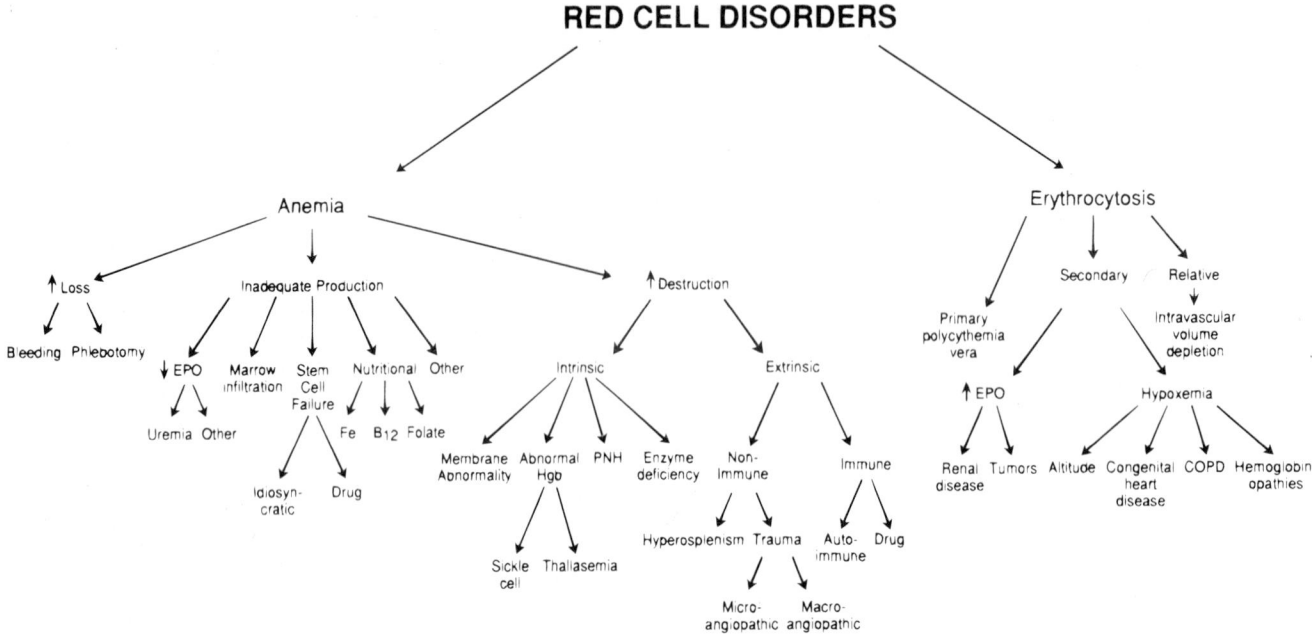

Fig. 45-2. Red cell disorders.

deficiency as a contributing factor to anemia in patients with other systemic diseases is being studied and may become of importance in critically ill patients.[3]

Other Causes of Inadequate Production

A large number of other causes of anemia are due to the inadequate production of red cells. These include the sideroblastic anemias that are due to disorders of iron metabolism; the toxic effects of chronic diseases on the marrow, such as chronic inflammatory disease; hepatic and renal insufficiency; bone marrow infiltration by neoplasm or fibrosis; and endocrine abnormalities such as hypothyroidism, hypoadrenal states; and hypopituitary diseases, all of which alter the bone marrow milieu for appropriate function. Stem cell failure, as occurs in aplastic anemia, affects all cell lines and can be idiopathic or drug induced. The leukopenia and thrombocytopenia may well be the most clinically significant aspects of the disease. Aplastic anemia can be induced by idiosyncratic reactions to some drugs such as chloramphenicol, phenylbutazone, indomethacin, tolbutamide, and chlorpropamide; the effects of chemotherapeutic agents; radiation; and viral infections, particularly hepatitis. In the case of a drug reaction, the offending drug is discontinued and supportive care given. Treatment for the idiopathic disease is mainly supportive, with component transfusion as necessary, and with androgenic steroids and corticosteroids, which may help to increase the red cell production but are generally poorly tolerated in the long term. Bone marrow transplant is offered in young, otherwise healthy patients who do not respond to conservative measures.

Increased Destruction
Hemolytic Anemias

Anemia secondary to hemolysis is classified as either intravascular or extravascular. Intravascular hemolysis is most often an acute process resulting in the release of large amounts of hemoglobin into the circulation. The hemoglobin is bound to haptoglobin, leading to markedly low levels of haptoglobin and therefore making this protein useful as a marker of hemolysis. The bound hemoglobin cannot be excreted in the urine because of its large size. If the hemoglobin load exceeds the capacity of the haptoglobin system, hemosiderin, which contains the iron processed by the kidney proximal tubular cells and complexed to storage proteins, is excreted in the urine. When the concentration of free hemoglobin exceeds this mechanism as well, hemoglobinuria occurs. Free hemoglobin can be measured in the plasma, and the indirect (unconjugated) fraction of bilirubin is elevated. Extravascular hemolysis occurs in the phagocytic cells of the spleen, liver, and bone marrow. This process is more insidious and does not result in free hemoglobin in the plasma; there is no hemoglobinuria, haptoglobin levels are minimally decreased, and the indirect fraction of bilirubin is not elevated. In either type of hemolysis, the blood smear shows polychromasia that is due to an increased number of immature red cells as well as reticulocytes. Serum lactic dehydrogenase (LDH) is elevated, which is due to the hemolysis and the increased marrow activity. In patients with a normal bone marrow and without other confounding diseases, the reticulocyte count is the most useful test in following the course of a hemolytic anemia. Table 45-2 lists some of the more important types of hemolytic anemias in ICU patients, several of which will be discussed in more detail.

Intrinsic Abnormalities
Primary Membrane Disorders

Metabolic defects affecting the red cell membrane causing it to have an abnormal shape shorten cell survival be-

Table 45–2. Classification of Hemolytic Anemia

Intrinsic abnormalities of red cells
  Membrane abnormalities
    Spherocytosis
    Elliptocytosis
  Hemoglobin abnormalities
    Sickle cell disease
    Thalassemia
  Enzyme deficiencies
    Glucose-6-phosphate dehydrogenase deficiency
    Porphyria
    Pyruvate kinase and other enzyme deficiencies
  Paroxysmal nocturnal hemoglobinuria
Extrinsic abnormalities
  Mechanical
    Traumatic cardiac hemolytic anemia
    Microangiopathic hemolytic anemia
  Chemical or drugs
  Antibody mediated
    Warm antibodies
    Cryoantibodies
    Drug related
  Hypersplenism

cause of the lack of deformability of the abnormal membrane to survive the repeated trauma of passage through capillaries. Final destruction is usually in the spleen and is therefore an extravascular disorder. The prototypic membrane disorder is hereditary spherocytosis. It is transmitted as an autosomal dominant trait. Diagnostic tests show spherocytes on the blood smear, reticulocytosis, increased osmotic fragility, and a negative Coomb's test. Splenectomy results in a clinical cure of this disease. Hereditary elliptocytosis is another membrane disorder with similar findings, but splenectomy is rarely indicated.

Hemoglobin Abnormalities

Normal adult hemoglobin is made up of a protein, globin, which contains the four iron-heme groups that carry oxygen. The globin molecule consists of four components, two alpha and two beta chains for hemoglobin A, comprising 95% of adult hemoglobin, two alpha and two gamma chains for fetal hemoglobin, hemoglobin F, making up less than 2% of adult hemoglobin, and two alpha and two delta chains for hemoglobin A_2, for up to 3% of adult hemoglobin.

Sickle Cell Disease. Abnormal hemoglobins, including hemoglobin S, and hemoglobin C, occur because of abnormal amino acid substitution in one of the hemoglobin chains.[8] In sickle cell disease, this amino acid substitution leads to polymerization of the hemoglobin when in the deoxygenated state distorting the membrane and producing the characteristic sickled cells. Inheritance is autosomal. Patients with the disease are homozygous for the gene; heterozygotes are carriers and are said to have sickle cell trait. The clinical course of sickle cell disease is severe, with a chronic, significant hemolytic anemia that begins after the level of fetal hemoglobin declines. On this chronic anemia are superimposed aplastic crises and vaso-occlusive episodes. Aplastic crises are usually precipitated by an infectious cause. The cause of vaso-occlusion are unknown but may be the end effect of chronic small vessel occlusion by the sickled cells. Tissue hypoxia occurs, leading to severe pain and ultimately tissue infarction. Although this may occur in any tissue, crises in bone, chest, abdomen, are of major clinical significance and can lead to acute mesenteric occlusion, "autosplenectomy," renal medullary infarction, osteomyelitis, pulmonary infarction, and cardiac disease. Carriers almost always have a hemoglobin S level of less than 50%, and are therefore usually totally asymptomatic. The diagnosis is made by clinical suspicion in a patient in the appropriate ethnic group and is usually evident from the family history. Laboratory confirmation is made by the visualization of sickle cells on smear, but these will not be seen in patients with sickle cell trait. Hemoglobin electrophoresis should be done to confirm the exact type of hemoglobin involved and to differentiate it from other hemoglobinopathies.

Treatment is mainly supportive, with attempts made to avoid hypoxia, acidosis, dehydration, and infection. Management of the pain of tissue infarction may be extremely difficult. Infections, particularly salmonella osteomyelitis, are common, and should be treated aggressively. Red cell transfusions are given as necessary, especially during aplastic crises but remembering that the patients chronically have a hemoglobin of only approximately 8 g/dl. Any surgery or anesthetic must be undertaken in these patient with due caution.

Hemoglobin C is another form of abnormal hemoglobin that leads to cells that are more rigid than normal, leading to decreased survival. Even homozygotes for the defect, however, have only a mild chronic hemolytic anemia. Hemoglobin SC disease occurs not infrequently and can be clinically much worse than sickle cell trait, with the same complications as sickle cell disease itself and the same potential for aplastic crises and tissue infarction.

Thalassemia. The thalassemias are a group of disorders widely distributed in populations originally from the Mediterranean, Middle East, India, and Pakistan, and throughout Southeast Asia. The pathophysiology is caused by the total absence or inadequate synthesis of one of the hemoglobin chains. Alpha thalassemia results from the lack of the alpha chain, and beta thalassemia by deficit of the beta chain. The other chain of the molecule is synthesized in normal amounts, and the resulting imbalance leads to the formation of intracellular inclusions, which lead to hemolysis by the spleen and lymphoid tissue. Inheritance is by an autosomal dominant gene, with the severe homozygous state designated thalassemia major, and the usually minimally symptomatic heterozygous condition called thalassemia minor. Beta thalassemia is characterized by an increased production of fetal hemoglobin far past the neonatal period as a compensatory mechanism for the abnormalities of hemoglobin A that are due to the decreased beta synthesis. Fetal hemoglobin has a very high oxygen affinity, however, so that patients with a high proportion of this hemoglobin suffer from chronic tissue hypoxia. The clinical course of beta thalassemia major is one of a severe transfusion-dependent hemolytic anemia usually with onset early in life. Later iron overload develops and requires attempts at chelation therapy, but death occurs in late childhood or early adolescence from the cardiac failure secondary to iron overload. Because alpha chains are part of both hemoglobin A and F, this form of the disease is much more severe, and patients with no production of alpha chains are frequently stillborn or die in infancy. Persons who are heterozygous for any of the forms of the disease do not manifest any clinical disability except during periods of stress such as pregnancy or severe infections.

Enzyme Deficiencies

The most common red cell enzyme defect is glucose-6-phosphate dehydrogenase (G-6-PD) deficiency. It is found in many patients of Mediterranean ancestry, in approximately 20% of patients of African descent, and also in Chinese and southeast Asians. Inheritance is X-linked, with males being affected, and females asymptomatic carriers except when homozygous for the gene. Patients are asymptomatic until exposed to an oxidizing drug. In absence of the enzyme, hemoglobin sulfhydryl groups are oxidized. The hemoglobin is precipitated in the cell, forming the characteristic Heinz inclusion bodies, which make the cells susceptible to destruction in the spleen and lymphoid tissue. Drugs most commonly responsible are antimalarials and sulfonamides but vitamin K, quinidine, and chloramphenicol can also be causative. Metabolic acidosis can cause oxidation and subsequent hemoglobin precipitation without drug exposure. Two varieties of the disorder exist. The Mediterranean form is more clinically significant and can result in a chronic hemolytic anemia even without drug exposure because of a near total lack of the enzyme. Hemolysis following exposure to oxidant agents or fava beans can be severe. In contrast, the variety found in black patients is less severe, which is due to enzyme deficiency only in older cells. Treatment is immediate cessation of the offending drug. Splenectomy may be useful in the treatment of the chronic hemolysis of the Mediterranean variety.

Paroxysmal Nocturnal Hemoglobinuria

Paroxysmal nocturnal hemoglobinuria (PNH) is an acquired disease of not only red cells but also platelets and granulocytes.[9] The cause is unknown, but the defect is an abnormality of the cell membrane that causes cells to be abnormally sensitive to complement. A chronic hemolysis is present, with occasional episodes of hemoglobinuria characteristically occurring after sleep, but it may also be initiated by infections, stress, or even exercise. Because of platelet involvement, hemorrhage may be a significant problem. Interestingly, venous thrombosis, particularly the Budd-Chiari syndrome of hepatic venous thrombosis, may be a frequent manifestation of the disease.[10] The diagnosis of PNH should be considered in any patient with pancytopenia of unknown cause with reticulocytosis. The urine is then examined for hemosiderin, and various in vitro tests to provoke hemolysis can be done. Therapy is supportive. Iron replacement is always necessary, and other measures—including transfusion, antibiotics, and anticoagulants—are used as necessary. Steroids are useful in raising the hemoglobin in some patients.

Extrinsic Abnormalities

Traumatic Cardiac Hemolytic Anemia (Macroangiopathic Hemolytic Anemia)

Any abnormal native cardiac valve, prosthetic valve, or other pre- or post-repair cardiac defect such as atrial or ventricular septal defect can cause a hemolytic anemia associated with reticulocytosis, the presence of schistocytes, increased plasma-free hemoglobin, hemosiderinuria, and variable hemoglobinuria.[11] The hemolysis is generally worse on the high shear arterial side and particularly with paravalvular leaks around valve prostheses. The anemia, although requiring iron, and occasionally transfusion, is usually not as important as the cardiac dysfunction that it heralds, often prompting primary or repeat cardiac surgery to repair the defect.

Microangiopathic Hemolytic Anemia

A hemolytic anemia may develop in response to trauma to the red cells occurring in the small vascular bed. Common causes are vasculitidies such as scleroderma, and allergic vasculitis, disseminated intravascular coagulation (DIC), and sepsis. More uncommon causes are thrombotic thrombocytopenic purpura (TTP) and hemolytic uremic syndrome, malignancies, and congenital vascular malformations such as cavernous giant capillary hemangiomata (Kasabach-Merritt syndrome). The laboratory findings are the same as in macroangiopathic hemolytic anemia, and as in that syndrome, the cause of the anemia rather than hemolysis itself needs to be addressed and will determine the patient's outcome.

Antibody-Mediated Hemolytic Anemia

In autoimmune hemolytic anemias, autoantibodies develop primarily, or secondary to another disease, against red cell antigens that lead to the destruction of the cells with all of the usual laboratory tests associated with hemolytic anemia, as well as evidence of the antibody cause with a positive Coomb's test. The direct Coomb's test demonstrates the presence of antibody on the red cell membrane itself, while the indirect Coomb's test determines if there are antibodies in the plasma that can be reactive against other red cells. The anemias are categorized on the basis of the thermal characteristics of the antibody. **Warm-reactive antibodies** are usually of the immunoglobulin G (IgG) class and function best at normal body temperature of 37°C. Hemolysis is most often extravascular. The disease can be idiopathic or secondary to lymphoproliferative disorders, or other autoimmune disease such as systemic lupus erythematosus (SLE). Clinical findings are widely variable, generally being slow and insidious in most patients, but with occasional episodes of severe hemolysis. In a secondary process, the symptoms of the anemia are often overshadowed by those of the primary disease. Steroids result in significant improvement in up to 80% of patients with idiopathic disease. Transfusion is often not necessary because of the chronic nature of the disease, but if required, it is associated with risk of transfusion reaction and the rapid destruction of the transfused cells. Most often, it is necessary to settle for the "least incompatible" blood unit available and monitor carefully for signs of reaction. Splenectomy has a place in the treatment of patients who require inordinate doses of steroids to control their disease, but attempts to predict which patients will benefit most from the procedure are not very accurate, and many patients will go on to relapse at variable times after splenectomy.

Cold-reactive antibodies react best at low temperatures, usually below 30°C and are most often IgM antibodies. The hemolysis is intravascular. The disorder is much less common than warm antibody disease. It occurs in a primary idiopathic form, and secondary to chronic lymphoproliferative disorders in older patients, and also as an acute, self-limited process complicating Mycoplasma pneumoniae infections or mononucleosis. The cold agglutinins may be present in high levels or for prolonged periods of time in the idiopathic disease but not be significant until the patient suffers an episode of chilling. The prognosis of the disease is usually benign, and treatment is directed at keeping the extremities warm. Steroids and splenectomy are of little value, although high dose steroids may be helpful in seriously ill patients. Transfusion should be avoided if possible, as in warm antibody disease.

Many commonly used drugs can cause **drug-related autoimmune hemolytic anemia** that is mediated by several different mechanisms.[12] Penicillin is the prototype drug that acts by a hapten mechanism. This occurs when the drug binds strongly to proteins, including those on the red cell surface. If the patient develops an antibody to the penicillin, the red cell can then be destroyed in the spleen. The anemia does not appear until the patient has been on the drug for several days and resolves slowly after the medication is discontinued. This disorder occurs quite rarely and is not related to the usual penicillin reactions but is mediated by a different class of antibody, IgG rather than the IgM responsible for most penicillin allergies. This mechanism has also been implicated with cephalosporins because of their cross-reactivity with penicillin and also with tetracyclines. Another mechanism of drug-induced hemolytic anemia is by the formation of drug-antibody complexes in the plasma, which then bind briefly to the surface of the red cell and induce hemolysis intravascularly by the binding and activation of complement. This has been termed the "innocent bystander" mechanism, because the antibodies have no affinity for the red cells themselves, and the immune complexes are not permanently fixed to the cell membrane. Common drugs that cause this type of reaction include quinine derivatives, chlorpropamide, and rifampin. The process is stopped as soon as the offending drug is eliminated. Alpha-methyldopa, L-dopa, and mefenamic acid cause the induction of autoantibodies to normal red cells. The antibodies do not develop until 3 to 6 months after the introduction of the drug. Up to 36% of patients receiving alpha-methyldopa can develop a positive antibody test, but the hemolytic anemia develops in less than 1% of these. The antibodies can cause hemolysis in the total absence of the drug and take a long time to resolve after their development. Except for the immune complex mechanism, which can produce sudden severe hemolysis, all the other mechanisms produce only a mild hemolytic anemia that simply requires discontinuation of the drug. This is absolutely necessary in the case of severe immune complex hemolytic anemia. Transfusion is rarely necessary in the majority of drug-related anemias, and cross matching is not problematic except in autoantibody-associated anemia such as occurs with alpha-methyldopa.

Disorders of Increased Production

The majority of cases of erythrocytosis are secondary to another underlying pathophysiology causing a relative tissue hypoxia that stimulates a compensatory increase in red cell mass. These include high altitude, chronic pulmonary disease, cardiac disease associated with a right-to-left shunt, or the presence of abnormal hemoglobins that have abnormal oxygen dissociation. Secondary polycythemia can also occur in an inappropriate, noncompensatory form secondary to renal disease, or with tumors or endocrine disorders such as pheochromocytomas. These are presumed to occur as the result of increased erythropoietin production. Relative polycythemia is seen as the result of intravascular volume depletion. Polycythemia vera is a stem cell disorder that causes cellular proliferation of all cell lines, not just erythrocytes. The treatment of all these disorders is phlebotomy along with iron replacement as often as necessary to keep the hematocrit below 50 to prevent the rheologic complications of polycythemia. The primary cause of secondary disorders should be treated if possible. Myelosuppressive agents can be used in polycythemia vera to control the increased marrow activity.

WHITE CELL DISORDERS

Neutrophil dysfunction, the most clinically significant of the white cell disorders, can be characterized by the same schema as the red cell abnormalities including conditions of decreased or increased production, decreased function, increased destruction, and whether drug induced or not (Fig. 45–3). It is beyond the scope of this text to consider the leukemias other than to note them as significant co-factors or primary causes of morbidity in critically ill patients. The reader is referred to any of the excellent hematology texts that are available for specific information on the leukemias.

Neutropenia

Decreased Production

A variety of congenital or acquired conditions involve neutropenia such as cyclic neutropenia, and familial neutropenia. Severe bacterial sepsis can suppress the granulocyte precursors in the marrow. Many viral illnesses can produce significant neutropenia or leukopenia. Infectious hepatitis, mononucleosis, influenza, measles, rubella, and chickenpox can demonstrate neutropenia that corresponds to the period of acute viremia. Other less common bacterial or protozoal infections can also cause neutropenia.

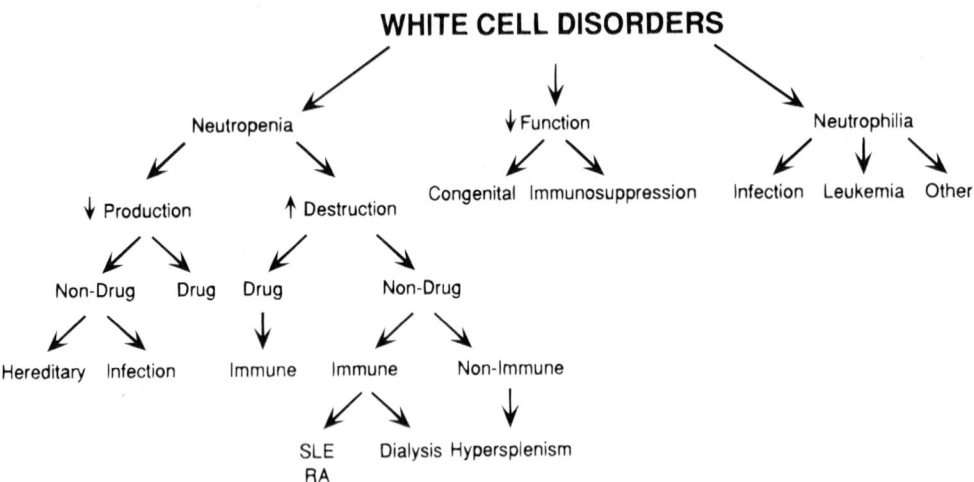

Fig. 45–3. White cell disorders.

Increased Destruction

Hypersplenism or liver disease may produce pooling of the white cells in the spleen. Some more common causes of hypersplenism include liver disease with portal hypertension, neoplasms, and inflammatory disease. Such conditions have nonimmune causes.

Collagen vascular disease, the most prominent being SLE and Felty's syndrome in rheumatoid arthritis, can be associated with a neutropenia that is mediated by antineutrophil antibodies. The majority of these patients are asymptomatic but in certain circumstances may benefit briefly from splenectomy. Hemodialysis has recently been identified as a cause of neutropenia that occurs because of the activation of complement while on dialysis, which causes the white cells to be activated and aggregate, most often in the lungs.[13] Such conditions are immune mediated.

Drug-Induced Neutropenia

Drugs are a frequent and important cause of neutropenia.[14] Chemotherapeutic agents are the most common cause of drug-induced neutropenia, which is due to their effects on stem cells. Chloramphenicol causes stem cell inhibition as well as an idiosyncratic drug effect, whereas alcohol, phenylbutazone, cimetidine,[15] and phenothiazenes act in a more dose-related fashion. Other drugs often cited in the cause of agranulocytosis are the semisynthetic penicillins such as oxacillin and methicillin, salicylazosulfapyridine (Azulfidine), quinidine, captopril, sulfonamides, propylthiouracil, and metronidazole. The majority of drug-induced neutropenias will slowly reverse after cessation of the drug, but mortality still approaches 5%.

Increased Destruction

The majority of drug-induced neutropenia is produced on an immune basis. The prototypic drug is the analgesic aminopyrene, which is no longer sold in the United States because of this effect. An antidrug antibody is induced which, when combined with the drug in an immune complex, lyses the white cell as an "innocent bystander." Quinidine may also act by the same mechanism. Penicillin may lead to neutropenia by the same hapten-mediated mechanism as in penicillin-induced hemolytic anemia. Procainamide can cause sudden peripheral destruction of neutrophils by a similar mechanism.

Evaluation and Treatment of Neutropenia

Careful attention must first be paid to the drug history and other potential neutrophil toxic factors such as infection. White cell counts with manual differential and examination of the smear are obligatory in the evaluation of a patient with neutropenia. Bone marrow examination is most often necessary in a patient not known to have a chronic neutropenia. Many sophisticated tests are available to evaluate this problem and are best coordinated with the hematologist. The first step in treatment of neutropenia is to stop all possible offending drugs. Patients with an elevated temperature and granulocyte count of less than 500 cells/mm^3 should be completely cultured and started on empiric broad-spectrum antibiotics pending the results of culture.[16] Lack of response to antibiotic therapy usually requires the addition of an antifungal agent such as amphotericin B. Reverse isolation has not been shown to be helpful in the management of neutropenic patients; only careful hand washing is necessary.[17] Granulocyte transfusion may be considered in the acutely ill, septic patient with a white cell count less than 500/mm^3 who has not responded to appropriate antibiotic therapy.[18] This must be done in consultation with hematology and infectious disease specialists. A known site of infection increases the efficacy of this treatment. The complications associated with granulocyte transfusions are significant, including severe leukoagglutinin reactions, pulmonary dysfunction, and potential for graft-versus-host disease. These will be discussed in more detail in the section on transfusion therapy later in this chapter. Immune-mediated neutropenia may benefit from infusions of intravenous gamma globulin. Recombinant human granulocyte colony-stimulating factor (G-CSF), and granulocyte-macrophage colony-stimulating factor (GM-CSF) are the most recent additions to the armamenterium of agents useful in the treatment of granulocytopenia.[19] These drugs have been used in patients with myelodysplastic syndromes, to hasten the

HEMATOLOGIC DISORDERS IN THE INTENSIVE CARE UNIT

Table 45-3. Causes of Neutrophilia

Hereditary disorders
Stress
  Exercise
  Changes in temperature
  Surgery and anesthesia[22]
  Emotional stress
Inflammation
  Tissue necrosis
  Trauma, burns
  Autoimmune diseases
  Gout
Carcinoma[23]
  Bronchogenic
  Gastric
  Renal
  Hepatic
  Pancreatic
Bleeding or hemolysis
Pregnancy[24]
Drugs
  Epinephrine
  Corticosteroids[25]
  Hydroxyethyl starch[26]
  Lithium[27]

recovery of chemotherapy-induced neutropenia, and in neutropenic patients with human immunodeficiency virus (HIV) and appears to be supplanting granulocyte transfusion as the preferred mode of treatment in most neutropenic patients.[20,21]

Neutrophilia

Although the most common cause of neutrophilia in the ICU is acute infection, there are many other causes of acute and chronic leukocytosis,[22-27] some of which are listed in Table 45-3. These diagnoses, either obtained by history or by exclusion after a careful search, have been made for the presence of an acute or chronic infection, and the complete hematologic profile has been assessed to rule out leukemia. Bone marrow examination may be required to complete the diagnostic workup.

PLATELET DISORDERS

Platelet dysfunction (Fig. 45-4) can be secondary to decrease in the absolute number of platelets that is due to either

- Decreased production
- Decreased survival
- Qualitative defects of platelet function

Because of failure of the platelet plug, bleeding secondary to platelet disorders is characteristically mucocutaneous, with petechiae and purpura, gastrointestinal bleeding, and menorrhagia often the presenting symptoms. The characteristic laboratory findings are a decreased platelet count or an increased bleeding time. It must be remembered that a platelet count of less than 100,000 can increase the bleeding time even without functional abnormalities; therefore, the test must be considered in context with the other laboratory tests.

Thrombocytopenia

Decreased Production

Decreased platelet production can be due to a decrease in the number of megakaryocytes, or a normal number of megakaryocytes, but ineffective thrombopoiesis. A number of congenital syndromes involve thrombocytopenia including Wiskott-Aldrich syndrome, maternal rubella, and cytomegalovirus infections. Megakaryocyte number can be diminished in any aplastic anemia whether idiopathic, resulting from bone marrow infiltration by malignancy, or secondary to drugs or chemicals, such as those previously mentioned in the discussion of erythrocyte disorders. The most prominent associated drugs are antimetabolites but also include chloramphenicol, phenylbutazone, tolbuta-

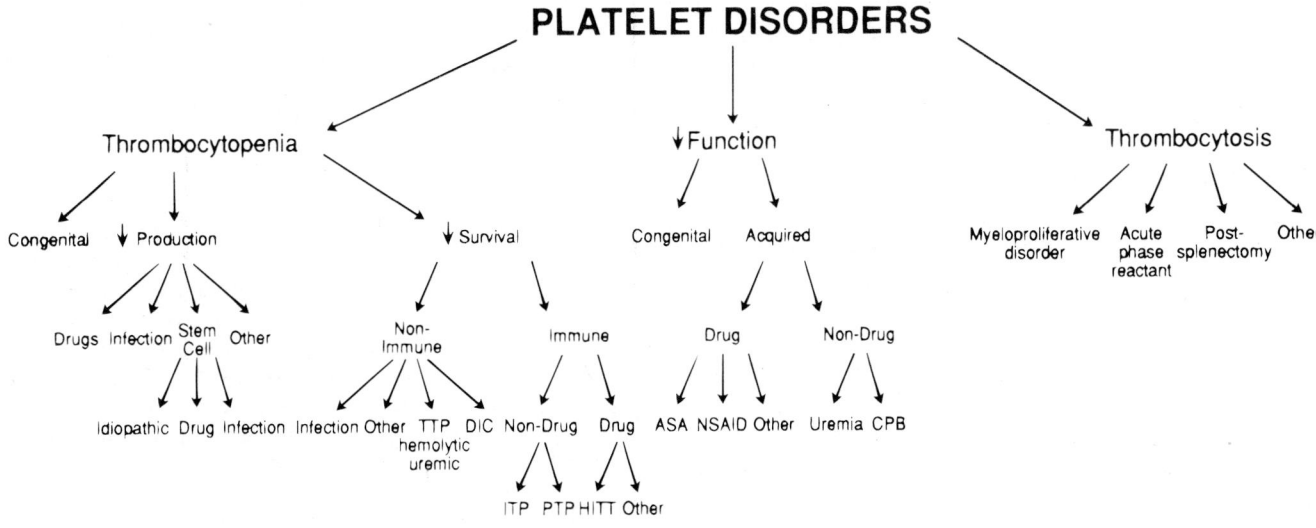

Fig. 45-4. Platelet disorders.

Table 45-4. Infectious Agents Causing Thrombocytopenia

Meningococcemia
Rocky Mountain spotted fever
Typhus
Typhoid fever
Diphtheria
Toxic shock syndrome
Disseminated tuberculosis, histoplasmosis, brucellosis
Malaria
Mumps
Varicella
Cytomegalovirus
Infectious mononucleosis

---

mide, and chlorpropamide. Alcohol, even in the absence of nutritional deficiencies,[28] thiazide diuretics, and estrogens act relatively specifically on megakaryocytes. Infectious agents such as HIV, influenza, and hepatitis can cause aplastic anemia, whereas measles, infectious mononucleosis, Mycobacterium tuberculosis, congenital rubella, and dengue fever appear to have specific effects on platelet production. A normal marrow may be present, but thrombopoiesis is ineffective, which is due to severe megaloblastic anemia or the adverse effect of alcohol on platelet production.

Decreased Survival

The characteristic finding of disorders of decreased platelet survival is a normal to increased number of megakaryocytes on bone marrow examination. Destruction of the platelets occurs in the periphery and can be secondary to direct destruction or immune-mediated effect.

Although many infections can cause thrombocytopenia by effects on the marrow, many infectious agents, as listed in Table 45-4, can cause the destruction of platelets. Thrombocytopenia should raise the possibility of sepsis in a febrile patient, even without other manifestations of DIC. Major burns frequently have a moderate thrombocytopenia several days after the injury that may be secondary to sequestration in damaged tissue. Fat embolism is also associated with thrombocytopenia. The petechiae seen with fat embolism, however, are probably due to microemboli rather than thrombocytopenia. DIC is an important cause of thrombocytopenia in the ICU and will be discussed in more detail in the section on fibrinolysis.

Thrombotic Thrombocytopenic Purpura

TTP is a disease of unknown cause that results in the destruction of platelets resulting most likely from the deposition of fibrin in small blood vessels.[29] The classic clinical findings follow:

- Thrombocytopenia
- Microangiopathic hemolytic anemia
- Fever
- Renal dysfunction
- Central nervous system (CNS) impairment

The disorder is seen most frequently in women and can occur as either a chronic or acute problem. The acute form can pursue a fulminating course and has in the past had a mortality as high as 80%. It has been associated with numerous other diseases such as connective tissue disorders and severe infections but not consistently. Theories about the cause include abnormalities in the vascular endothelium or plasma that cause defective prostacyclin synthesis or release of another factor that increases platelet aggregation. The diagnosis is most often made on clinical grounds but can be confirmed by a gingival biopsy, which is positive in 30 to 50% of patients, showing hyaline material in small vessels without inflammatory changes. The same pattern can be seen in DIC, but in TTP there are no other associated disorders of coagulation, other than thrombocytopenia. Levels of immunoglobulin and complement are normal as well. Early and aggressive plasma exchange with adjunctive high dose steroids is the present treatment of choice.[30,31] Immunosuppressive agents and splenectomy have been used in the past and in patients not responding to other therapy. Platelet transfusions are contraindicated except in the case of CNS bleeding because of potential for accelerated microvascular thrombosis (see Chap. 43).

Hemolytic Uremic Syndrome

Hemolytic uremic syndrome is closely related to TTP and may be another manifestation of the same disease. The major differences are less prominent neurologic symptoms and more severe impairment of renal function. The classic disease occurs in childhood, but a related disorder also occurs in adults. Treatment involves many of the same approaches as in TTP, but antiplatelet agents such as aspirin and dipyridamole have some utility, and dialysis frequently is needed.

Idiopathic Thrombocytopenic Purpura

Idiopathic thrombocytopenic purpura (ITP) is no longer idiopathic but is due to the autoimmune destruction of platelets, after exclusion of all other autoimmune disorders, such as infectious or drug induced. There are two forms of the disease, acute and chronic. The acute form occurs mainly in children after a viral illness and most often resolve completely within a few weeks with or without treatment. A similar pattern is seen in some adults but is rare. The predominant form of the disease in adults and in 10% of children is a chronic process.[32,33] Patients present with the insidious onset of petechiae, gingival bleeding, epistaxis, and menorrhagia. Women are affected three times as frequently as men, and the disease is rare in blacks. In most patients ITP is a chronic, potentially debilitating, but not lethal disease. Elevated levels of platelet-associated IgG are found in almost all patients. There are no other hematologic abnormalities, other than an anemia secondary to continuing blood loss. Corticosteroids are the primary mode of treatment, usually in doses of 1 to 2 mg/kg per day. This results in good response in the majority of patients. Patients who do not respond to steroids, who require large doses to achieve an effect, or who have complications associated with steroid treatment, and who are good surgical risks, are candidates for splenectomy. Removing the spleen is effective treatment because the spleen is not only the major site of platelet destruction but also may be an important site of antibody formation. The majority of patients who undergo splenectomy benefit greatly from the procedure, often with permanent return to normal platelet counts. It is not possible to predict who will be the treatment failures; however, most patients at least benefit by a significant reduction in their steroid requirements. Treatment for refractory disease includes the use of immunosuppression, vincristine, plasmapheresis, and intravenous gammaglobulin. Platelet transfusions should be given only in the setting of life-threatening bleeding, because platelet survival is very short and can increase the formation of alloantibodies, which may make later transfusion even more difficult.

Autoimmune thrombocytopenia may be the presenting symptom for other autoimmune disorders such as SLE; therefore, a thorough workup for autoimmune diseases should be performed.

Post-transfusion Purpura

Post-transfusion purpura (PTP) is a rare but significant cause of a fulminant thrombocytopenia.[34] It is caused by the induction of alloantibodies to endogenous platelets. The disorder occurs in patients who are negative for platelet antigen 1 (PLA-1). Antigen-negative status is very uncommon, occurring in only 3% of the population. The majority of patients are PLA-1 positive, and this antigen is not screened for before platelet transfusion. In some instances, when a PLA-1-negative patient is given a platelet transfusion containing PLA-1-positive platelets, the patient not only destroys the transfused platelets but also develops an alloantibody that then destroys native platelets as well. There is no proven mechanism for this occurrence, but theories include the induction of a second autoantibody, the involvement of immune complexes in the platelet destruction, and the reactivity to PLA-1-positive antibody adsorbed on the PLA-1-negative platelets. This reaction does not happen in all PLA-1-negative patients but is most frequent in those who have had previous transfusions or have been sensitized by pregnancy. The clinical course can be rapidly progressive and lethal. The most effective treatment is exchange transfusions or preferably plasmapheresis. Platelet transfusions are totally ineffective during the course of the illness. After recovery, the patient should receive only PLA-1-negative blood products if possible, although PLA-1-positive transfusions are not absolutely contraindicated, because the disease is so episodic.

Drug-Induced Thrombocytopenia

Drug-induced thrombocytopenia is quite common in the critically ill patient and is most often due to an immune mechanism.[35] The platelet membranes are known to express an Fc receptor capable of binding and removing the immune complex from the circulation. Antibodies are formed against a drug, and the drug-antibody complex binds to the platelet membrane, where it causes complement fixation and platelet destruction, the platelet being merely an "innocent bystander" to the process. The other mechanism that can lead to platelet destruction is by the drug binding to the platelet membrane as a hapten against which an antibody can form. The list of drugs that can

Table 45–5. Drugs Associated With Thrombocytopenia

Heparin
Quinidine and quinine derivatives
Chemotherapeutic agents
Antirheumatic drugs (aspirin, nonsteroidal anti-inflammatory drugs, gold)
Antibiotics (cephalosporins, penicillins, sulfonamides, isoniazid, rifampin)
Anticonvulsant drugs (carbamazepine, valproate)
Thiazide diuretics
Tranquilizers (chlorpromazine, diazepam)
Hypoglycemic drugs (tolbutamide, chlorpropamide)
Cimetidine

elicit this reaction is vast, and the drugs more important in the ICU are listed in Table 45–5. When a patient in the ICU develops thrombocytopenia, all drugs that are not absolutely necessary should be stopped, and those that are necessary should be surveyed for their potential thrombocytopenic tendency. Other drugs of the appropriate class should be substituted for those that have a high likelihood of causing thrombocytopenia. Platelet counts will gradually recover, usually within 7 days of discontinuation of the causative medication. Corticosteroids have not proven to be useful but may be somewhat helpful, especially with drugs that have a long half-life. The benefits of platelet transfusions are generally short-lived, and these transfusions should be given only if life-threatening bleeding occurs.

Heparin-Induced Thrombocytopenia

Heparin-induced thrombocytopenia, part of the heparin-induced thrombocytopenia and thrombosis syndrome (HITT) is an important subset of drug-induced thrombocytopenias that has been reported to occur in up to 30% of patients receiving heparin.[36] It can occur with beef or porcine heparin and in all forms of heparin therapy, including full-dose intravenous treatment, subcutaneous heparin for prophylaxis of deep venous thrombosis, and also heparin flushes used to maintain the patency of intravenous and arterial lines. Almost all patients develop a modest decrease in platelet counts within the first few days of heparinization, but seldom to less than 100,000/mm^3. This is most likely due to platelet sequestration along the intima of the vasculature of the capillary bed and is not due to an immunologic mechanism. This thrombocytopenia improves gradually with the continuation of heparin. The immunologic form takes several days to develop but may occur more quickly if the patient has been previously exposed to heparin. The platelet count can plummet drastically and can lead to bleeding. The more serious complication is intravascular thrombosis, usually consisting of "white clot" made up of platelets and fibrin that most commonly occurs in the arterial side of the circulation.[37] Significant morbidity consisting of limb loss, myocardial infarction, cerebrovascular occlusion, and mortality can result when this complication ensues. All patients receiving any form of heparin therapy should have monitoring of the platelet count at least every 2 days. A patient who develops thrombocytopenia in the ICU is often receiving

Table 45-6. Causes of Thrombocytosis

Chronic inflammation
    Autoimmune disorders
    Chronic infection
        Osteomyelitis
        Tuberculosis
    Chronic inflammatory diseases
        Ulcerative colitis[39]
        Regional enteritis[39]
Bleeding, hemolytic anemia
Postoperative
    Splenectomy
    Other surgical procedures[40]
Malignancy[42]
    Carcinomas
    Lymphomas
Drugs
    Epinephrine
    Vincristine
    Treatment for vitamin B_{12} deficiency

heparin and should have all forms of the drug immediately discontinued. Unfortunately, currently available tests for heparin-associated antiplatelet antibody are fairly insensitive; therefore, even if the test is negative, heparin should not be restarted in a patient with significant thrombocytopenia unless there is no alternative. Coumadin or dextran can be substituted for the patient who requires full anticoagulation, or a venacaval filter may be necessary for patients with deep venous thrombosis or pulmonary embolism. Therapy of arterial thrombosis is usually surgical, but thrombolytic agents have been used. Because of the anamnestic immune response, patients must be instructed to pursue lifelong avoidance of further heparin exposure.

Thrombocytosis

Thrombocytosis may be part of a primary myeloproliferative disease, such as polycythemia vera, or very rarely a primary thrombocythemia, but can also be increased along with other acute-phase reactants following surgery or stress or can be secondary to many other disorders,[38-40,42] some of which are listed in Table 45-6. In most patients who develop a moderate acute thrombocytosis in response to a specific insult, platelet counts will gradually normalize, and these patients will require no specific therapy. Patients with potential for prolonged thrombocytosis, such as occurs after splenectomy, or with significant thrombocytosis (platelet count greater than 750,000/mm^3) should be treated with aspirin or dipyridamole to prevent thrombosis.[41] In addition, despite an increased number of platelets, platelet function may be decreased, leading to disorders of hemostasis in the presence of bleeding.[38]

Disorders of Platelet Function

Congenital

As previously mentioned, specific platelet membrane receptors are responsible for different aspects of platelet adhesion and aggregation. Congenital deficits of these receptors cause functional platelet disorders. The common factor in the syndromes is a prolonged bleeding time in the presence of a normal platelet count. Bernard-Soulier syndrome is the congenital absence of the glycoprotein Ib (GpIb) receptor causing impaired adhesion. Platelets are noted to be abnormally large as well. The defect is inherited as an autosomal recessive disorder. Thrombasthenia, or Glanzmann's disorder, is the congenital deficit of the GpIIb/IIIa receptor and thus leads to abnormal platelet aggregation. The defect is demonstrated by abnormal clot retraction. Storage pool disorders are another rare form of qualitative platelet dysfunction that are caused by abnormalities in either the content or release of platelet granule stores. The effect on bleeding function is generally milder than that associated with the previously mentioned congenital platelet defects.

Acquired

Drugs are the major cause of qualitative platelet abnormalities.[43] Aspirin and nonsteroidal anti-inflammatory medications are the most common drugs implicated, but other agents may be responsible as well and are listed in Table 45-7. Platelet dysfunction has also been found to be a major factor responsible for the coagulopathy that can follow cardiopulmonary bypass procedures.[44,45]

Aspirin and Nonsteroidal Anti-inflammatory Drugs. Aspirin irreversibly acetylates platelet cyclo-oxygenase, which is one of the enzymes responsible for the conversion of arachidonic acid to prostaglandins with its most important effect in doses of less than approximately 1.0 to 1.5 g/day, on thromboxane A_2, the most potent mediator of platelet aggregation. The inhibition of prostaglandins is nonspecific and therefore potentially affects not only thromboxane formation but also that of the vascular endothelium prostaglandins such as prostacyclin, which could lead to an increased tendency for platelet aggregation. This effect, however, appears to be a problem

Table 45-7. Drugs Associated With Platelet Dysfunction

Anti-inflammatory agents
    Aspirin
    Nonsteroidal anti-inflammatory drugs
Phosphodiesterase inhibitors
    Dipyridamole
    Methylxanthines (theophylline, aminophylline)
Antibiotics and antiparasitic agents
    Carbenicillin and related antibiotics
    Chloroquine and derivatives
Tranquilizers and antipsychotic agents
    Phenothiazines
    Tricylic antidepressants
Sympathetic blocking agents
    Alpha blockers (hydralazine, nitroprusside)
    Beta blockers
Miscellaneous
    Ethanol
    Heparin
    Furosemide
    Antihistamines
    Clofibrate
    Reserpine
    Dextran

only at much higher doses of aspirin. The effect is irreversible; therefore, any platelet produced when the drug is in the system will be nonfunctional. Because of the life span of the platelets, 7 to 10 days are required to generate a new population of functional platelets in a patient who has been taking aspirin routinely. A large percentage of the population may be taking aspirin because it is ubiquitous in many over-the-counter medications, and because of the recent finding of the beneficial effects of aspirin in atherosclerotic disease. Nonsteroidal anti-inflammatory drugs (NSAIDs) act in the same fashion by inhibiting platelet cyclo-oxygenase, but the effect is reversible as soon as the drug is metabolized. The platelet defect usually does not cause significant clinical problems unless superimposed on another disorder such as von Willebrand's disease or hemophilia,[46] or during surgical procedures, especially procedures requiring cardiopulmonary bypass, which causes other platelet abnormalities.[47] The best treatment for problems caused by aspirin or NSAIDs is cessation of the drugs. In the setting of serious bleeding, platelet transfusions can be given, and some evidence indicates that the use of deamino-8-D-arginine vasopressin (DDAVP) may be useful in the treatment of bleeding diatheses caused by aspirin.[48]

Uremia

Although the mechanism is not well understood, uremia is associated with defects in platelet adhesion and aggregation. The improvement of platelet function after dialysis suggests that the defect is related to the presence of an uncleared metabolite, but this remains unproven. Cryoprecipitate,[49] and recently DDAVP[50] have been shown to be useful in the treatment of bleeding in association with uremia. This may implicate defects in the function of von Willebrand's factor (vWF) in the disorder, because cryoprecipitate contains large amounts of this coagulation factor, and DDAVP may increase the production or release of vWF. Platelet transfusion may be given for significant bleeding problems but with the knowledge that they will also be adversely affected by the same mechanism as native platelets.

COAGULATION FACTOR DISORDERS (Fig. 45–5)

Congenital Disorders

Hemophilia

Congenital deficiencies of all clotting factors exist but with the exception of the hemophilias are relatively rare and not generally associated with severe bleeding problems. Hemophilia A, factor VIII deficiency—also known as classic hemophilia—and hemophilia B, factor IX deficiency—or Christmas disease—are not uncommon and can cause major problems if not recognized and treated appropriately. Hemophilia A accounts for 80% of all hemophilias. Factor VIII is made up of two components, VIII:c, the procoagulant necessary for the activation of factor X, and VIII:vwF, or von Willebrand's factor, which serves as a carrier protein for VIII:c and also has a significant role of its own for normal platelet function. The two components are produced by different cells and are controlled by two separate genes. The factor VIII:Ag levels, which measure the total factor VIII, are usually normal, but a deficiency of the biologically active portion labeled as VIII:c causes hemophilia A. Hemophilia B is due to the quantitative deficiency of factor IX. The PTT is elevated in both disorders; specific factor assays or the admixture of patient plasma against various controls can be done to confirm the exact deficiency. Factor assays are necessary to assess and treat a preoperative surgical or bleeding patient to determine the level of clotting factor replacement necessary for adequate hemostasis. The two diseases are clinically indistinguishable, both presenting, in contrast to the mucocutaneous bleeding of platelet disorders, with deep hematomas in muscle or body cavities and hemarthroses, sometimes occurring spontaneously. Hemostasis of cuts and superficial abrasions is relatively normal, which is due to normal platelet function. Both diseases are transmitted as sex-linked recessive inheritance; males are affected, and females are asymptomatic carriers. Although the majority of cases are inherited, there is a 20 to 30% incidence of de novo cases of the disease, implying a new mutation. There is a spectrum of severity of the hemophilias, with affected patients ranging from mild symptoms that become significant only when stressed by surgery or trauma to spontaneous bleeding even in the absence of a precipitat-

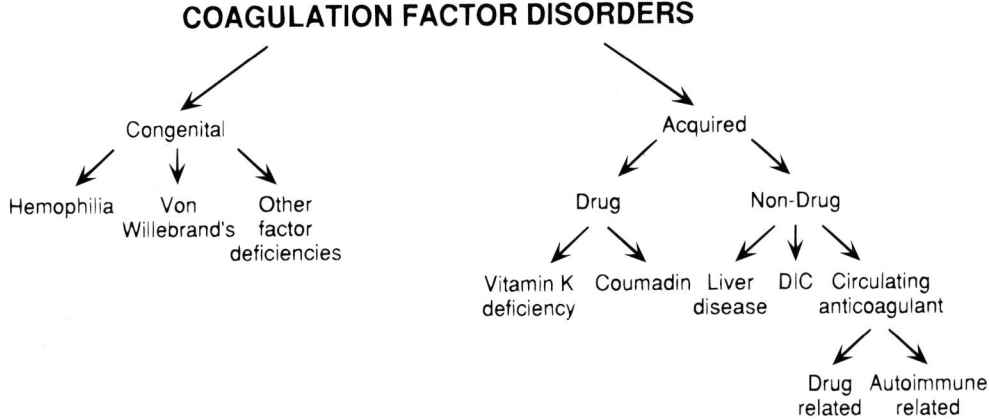

Fig. 45–5. Coagulation factor disorders.

ing event. In factor VIII deficiency, severity of disease correlates well with the levels of factor VIII:c: Disease classified as mild has levels over 5%, and patients suffer only occasional bleeding secondary to trauma; severe disease has levels less than 1%, and patients often experience spontaneous bleeding. Prophylaxis in hemophilia involves the strict avoidance of aspirin or any other agents that would have additive effects in causing bleeding.

Treatment differs for the two diseases. Non-life-threatening bleeding in patients with mild-to-moderate hemophilia A can be treated with DDAVP, which can raise the levels of VIII:c three- to sixfold. For more significant bleeding or major surgical procedures, replacement therapy is needed.[51] Cryoprecipitate was the classic form of treatment in the past, but has the major disadvantage of the unreliability of its factor VIII content, as well as the need for storage at low temperatures and a long preparation time. Commercially prepared factor VIII concentrates are now available that are accurately labeled for content of VIII and are lyophilized and stable for long periods of time in a refrigerator, allowing for home therapy. Life-threatening bleeding or major surgery require initial VIII levels of 80 to 100%, which must be maintained at levels of at least 40 to 50% for several days. After major nonorthopedic surgery, this may be necessary for 10 to 14 days, and up to several weeks following major orthopedic procedures. The biologic half-life of factor VIII is only 8 to 12 hours; the infusion therefore must be repeated at 8- to 12-hour intervals. It is useful to remember that each unit per kilogram of factor VIII infused will raise the plasma level 2%. Factor VIII:c levels must be followed and dosage adjusted for the individual patient. Approximately 10 to 20% of patients with hemophilia requiring factor replacement will develop an inhibitor, an IgG antibody to the transfused factor VIII that neutralizes the effect of the factor.[52] This develops in an unpredictable fashion but is most common in patients who have received multiple factor transfusions. Strategies for the treatment of this problem consist of massive, frequent transfusions of conventional factor VIII concentrate, plasmapheresis, or the use of large doses of activated factor IX concentrate in an attempt to bypass the need for factor VIII in the coagulation pathway. The most recent approach has been the development of a highly purified porcine factor VIII that appears to be resistant to human antibodies.[53] Treatment of hemophilia B parallels that for hemophilia A but with the use of factor IX concentrate. Major trauma or surgery requires levels of 60% for effective coagulation. Because of a larger volume of distribution, a dose of 1 U/kg will raise the plasma level by 1%. The half-life of factor IX is 24 hours; therefore, dosing is needed every 24 hours. Factor IX levels must be followed for accuracy in replacement. The side effects of replacement therapy are primarily infectious with major risk of the transmission of HIV, and hepatitis C. The infusion of large amounts of factor VIII can cause a hemolytic anemia in blood type A or B recipients, which is due to anti-A and anti-B antibodies in the concentrate. Factor IX concentrate has been associated with deep venous thrombosis and pulmonary embolism, which is due to the presence of small amounts of activated factors.[54] This problem may be diminished by the use of small doses of subcutaneous heparin simultaneous with the replacement. Disseminated intravascular coagulation has been reported in patients with cirrhosis who have received factor IX.[55]

Von Willebrand's Disease

Von Willebrand's disease (vWD) is the most common of the congenital coagulopathies and is caused by qualitative and/or quantitative deficits of von Willebrand's factor (VIII:vWF).[56] As noted previously, factor VIII consists of two components, the procoagulant VIII:c and vWF. The major contribution of vWF to the coagulation mechanism is in the initial adhesion of platelets to the damaged vascular endothelium by acting as a bridge between the endothelium and the GpIb platelet membrane receptor. Without vWF, normal adhesion cannot occur. Also, because of its role as a carrier protein for VIII:c, decreased levels of vWF cause the procoagulant to be degraded more quickly. Clinical presentation is usually bleeding early in life from mucosal and cutaneous sites, and is seldom life-threatening except in the context of major surgery or trauma. Hemarthroses and deep hematomas do occur, but only rarely, even in severe deficiencies of vWF. Laboratory findings consist of a normal platelet count, prolonged bleeding time, abnormal ristocetin cofactor assay, decreased levels of VIII:Ag, and VIII:vWF. Abnormal electrophoretic patterns of vWF are found as well, implying abnormal size and function of the molecule. The most common mode of inheritance is autosomal dominant, but a recessive form is recognized as well. Different categories of the disease are recognized and are based on the electrophoretic pattern of vWF and the relative levels of VIII:Ag, VIII:vWF, and VIII:c. Therapy for some of the less severe forms of vWD is the use of DDAVP,[50] with concomitant epsilon-amino-caproic acid for dental procedures and minor surgery. More severe deficiencies or major injury require the use of replacement treatment. Conventional VIII concentrate used in the treatment of hemophilia A is not appropriate for use in vWD, because it lacks the large vWF multimers that are the most functional. Cryoprecipitate is the treatment of choice because it is rich in vWF, but its use is hampered because there is no standardized preparation or method of measuring the concentration of vWF.[57] Therefore, response and biologic half-life are variable with each treatment. The bleeding time is the most useful test to follow in the treatment of the disorder in bleeding and planning for surgery or invasive procedures. Adequate treatment is usually 1 to 1.5 U of cryoprecipitate per 10 kg of body weight. The cryoprecipitate is then continued on an approximately daily basis for several days, depending on the magnitude of the procedure.

Acquired Disorders

Vitamin K Deficiency and Antagonists

Vitamin K has a crucial role in the production of functional factors II, VII, IX, and X. Therefore, any condition that causes a decreased availability of vitamin K will contribute to a coagulation deficit that is characterized by an abnormal PT initially, which is due to the effect on factor VII with the shortest half-life, then the development of an abnormal PTT as levels of the other factors fall. Vitamin K is obtained mainly from leafy green vegetables and is absorbed in the small intestine and stored in the liver. Inadequate dietary intake therefore can lead to deficiency. Intestinal bacteria also produce some of the vitamin; thus, broad-spectrum antibiotics that destroy the bacteria can cause the loss of this source of vitamin K. Although the liver stores of vitamin K are large, inadequate diet and the use of antibiotics in a critically ill patient can make a previously healthy patient vitamin K deficient in 1 to 2 weeks.[58] Malabsorption syndromes such as sprue, kwashiorkor, and cholestasis cause vitamin K deficiency, as well as biliary obstruction or the external drainage of bile, because as a fat-soluble vitamin, it requires the presence of bile salts for absorption. Hepatic disease causes loss of storage sites in the liver. Vitamin K antagonists, such as warfarin used as oral anticoagulants, cause a defect in the synthesis of vitamin K. Production of the biologically active form of the vitamin is decreased, and a bleeding diathesis indistinguishable from vitamin K deficiency is produced. Some of the newer broad-spectrum cephalosporins, particularly cefoperazone, moxalactam, and cefamandole, may also have an effect on the reductase enzyme and lead to decreased levels of vitamin K, especially in malnourished patients. In such patients, the use of parenteral vitamin K 10 mg once a week may avoid the potential for bleeding problems. Parenteral vitamin K is also the treatment of choice for vitamin K deficiency and to reverse overanticoagulation associated with warfarin therapy within 24 hours. If there is active and severe bleeding, the defect can be immediately corrected with fresh-frozen plasma.

Liver Disease

The liver is the source of synthesis of all coagulation factors excluding factor VIII. Therefore, any severe hepatic disease can result in a bleeding diathesis.[59] Patients with liver disease cannot store vitamin K and therefore have abnormalities of the vitamin K-associated factors II, VII, IX, and X, which are affected first, having the shortest half-lives. Factors decreased next are V, XI, and XII. The synthesis of fibrinogen is the last factor affected in liver disease, and a low level in the absence of DIC is a marker of severe hepatic failure. The liver is also the site of clearance of activated clotting factors. Therefore, the patient with severe liver disease is at higher risk of DIC secondary to an excess of activated factors. The PT and PTT are prolonged, indistinguishable from vitamin K deficiency. To distinguish between vitamin K deficiency and liver diseases, specific factor assays can be done. All levels excluding factor VIII will be depressed to a variable in liver disease, whereas only the vitamin K-dependent factors will be low in the vitamin deficiency. The other alternative is to give a single dose of vitamin K, which will at least partially correct the PT and PTT in vitamin K deficiency but not in hepatic failure. Liver disease is also associated with dysfibrinogenemia, the production of abnormal fibrinogens with abnormal biologic activity that may result in thrombotic as well as bleeding disorders. These are relatively uncommon, and the diagnosis is made by prolongation of the PT and PTT, as well as the thrombin time, then better elucidated by more sophisticated immunoassays for the component. Replacement therapy for coagulopathy associated with liver disease is frozen plasma. A large volume of plasma may be required to correct the bleeding disorder and can precipitate encephalopathy and volume overload, but it is seldom necessary to completely correct the laboratory values. Cryoprecipitate may be used in some circumstances to avoid this problem. Prothrombin complexes (factor IX concentrate) should not be used, because of the potential for causing a hypercoagulable state, which is due to the coexistent decreased synthesis of the inhibitors of coagulation including antithrombin III and proteins S and C that are also affected by severe liver disease.

Acquired Circulating Anticoagulants (Lupus Anticoagulant, Coagulation Inhibitors)

Circulating anticoagulants are inhibitors that are usually immunoglobulins that interfere with the normal coagulation mechanism. Inhibitors have been described for each of the coagulation proteins. The presence of an inhibitor is suggested by prolongation of the portion of the clotting pathway involved with the particular factor in the absence of other known anticoagulants or bleeding disorders. Factor VIII inhibitors are the most commonly occurring form. Inhibitors of factor VIII, and more rarely factor IX inhibitors, in hemophilia are a form of immune response to repeated challenges by transfusions of the deficient factor. Other factor VIII anticoagulants arise de novo in association with autoimmune diseases, as well as in patients with no other underlying disorders. Factor VIII inhibitors can occur during or following pregnancy, and as a complication of drug allergy, particularly to penicillin or betalactam antibiotics. The course of these disorders is usually self-limited, and in the case of drug-induced disorder, cessation of the drug results in improvement. These proteins can also develop in SLE, rheumatoid arthritis, ulcerative colitis, multiple myeloma, and Waldenstrom's macroglobulinemia. Another class of inhibitor, often termed lupus anticoagulant, is a nonspecific coagulation inhibitor, whose action is due to an IgG or more uncommonly IgM antibody against phopholipids.[60] This finding was first described in patients with lupus erythematosus but is found in only 5 to 10% of these patients. It also has been found to occur in patients with other autoimmune disorders, plasma cell dyscrasias, neurologic and gynecologic diseases, and in association with infections or drugs, especially procainamide, and in normal, healthy patients. The activated partial thromboplastin time (aPTT) is elevated in vitro because it involves a phospholipid emulsion as an agent in the test. Confirmation is obtained by mixing patient plasma with normal plasma. Failure to correct the aPTT with this mixture is indicative of an inhibitor. The definitive diagnosis is made by using platelets instead of the phospholipid reagent and seeing correction of the aPTT. Specific characterization of the antibody is by immunoelectrophoresis and immunoassays. Clinically, the lupus anticoagulant is not usually a problem unless there are coexistent defects of platelets or other clotting factors. Lupus anticoagulant, however, is associated with an increased incidence of thrombotic events, and the presence of lupus anticoagulant in association with episodes of thrombosis may require life-long anticoagulation.[61]

Fibrinolytic Disorders

Disseminated Intravascular Coagulation

Disseminated intravascular coagulation (DIC) is not a primary entity but is a process that occurs secondary to another disease such as trauma, neurologic or obstetric catastrophes, malignancy, or fulminant sepsis that results in the generalized activation of both the coagulation and fibrinolytic systems. It is characterized by the accelerated consumption of many of the coagulation factors and platelets, and the production of byproducts of fibrinolysis. The process can be initiated by activation of the extrinsic or intrinsic clotting pathways. The extrinsic cascade can be activated by endotoxin-mediated lysis of granulocytes in sepsis, the release of toxic products from the placenta directly into the maternal circulation, in any tissue injury, especially with the release of membrane-rich brain tissue in neurologic trauma, in major transfusion reactions, and with the necrosis of neoplastic tissue. The intrinsic pathway is involved less often in the initiation of DIC, but can be activated in patients with endothelial damage, such as acute aortic dissection or vasculitis, or with congenital vascular abnormalities such as giant hemangiomas. Once the coagulation process is begun systemically, the fibrinolytic system is activated as a secondary phenomenon. Thrombin is produced by the coagulation pathway, which is then degraded by plasminogen after it has been activated by t-PA, which is produced by thrombin stimulation or from damaged endothelial cells. The resultant fibrin degradation products then circulate in the system and act as further anticoagulants by preventing the normal polymerization of fibrin. Thrombocytopenia occurs as the result of platelet consumption in intravascular thrombi and in activation by thrombin. With the formation of intravascular fibrin strands, a microangiopathic hemolytic anemia can develop.

The laboratory findings are elevations of the PT and PTT, decreased levels of fibrinogen and platelets, and elevated fibrin degradation products (FDP or FSP) and D-dimers. The FDP assay does not differentiate between the breakdown products of fibrin and fibrinogen and is elevated in both primary and secondary fibrinolysis, whereas the D-dimer specifically quantitates fibrin fragments, thus allows the assay of fibrin converted from fibrinogen and then broken down by plasmin, as in DIC, and may therefore be a more sensitive marker of the presence of secondary fibrinolysis.[62] Specific factors, primarily II, V, VIII, and XIII are reduced. The presence of a low level of factor VIII is often useful to distinguish bleeding secondary to DIC from that of liver failure, which can also result in low levels of most of the same clotting factors. The patient with chronic DIC will generally have the same pattern of laboratory findings or will have normal-to-shortened PT and PTT, suggestive of thrombotic tendency.

DIC can be present as either an acute or chronic process. The acute syndrome can be fulminant and life-threatening and of great importance in the ICU. The clinical presentation usually consists of bleeding from the microvasculature at surgical and intravascular catheter sites, ecchymoses, and oozing from oral, gastrointestinal or urinary tract mucosa. Less often, patients present with evidence of microvascular or major vascular thrombosis with peripheral acrocyanosis and digital gangrene. The thrombotic process, however, may be present and unrecognized in the microvasculature of major organ systems that can progress to multisystem organ failure. In chronic DIC, such as that associated with malignancies, the patient may have characteristic laboratory abnormalities but be totally asymptomatic, experience bleeding problems only with trauma, or present with thrombotic events.

The most effective treatment of DIC is control of the inciting cause. Unfortunately, in critically ill patients, the secondary bleeding may be more of an acute problem, and the primary disorder may not be easily correctable. Controversy exists over the appropriate treatment for active bleeding in DIC. In the past, the use of heparin was advocated to stop the initial thrombotic process that initiates and supports the DIC cascade. This has been largely abandoned, however, except in the subset of patients with acute DIC who manifest thrombosis as their primary symptom or in some patients with chronic DIC.[63] In the past, factor replacement was not advised, because of the concern of only continuing and potentially exacerbating the fibrinolytic process by providing more substrate. This has not been proven, and appropriate blood, plasma products, and platelet replacement provide the current treatment of choice for serious bleeding. Antifibrinolytic agents, although attractive from the aspect of stopping fibrinolysis, should not be used. Although the cessation of fibrinolysis will contribute to stopping the bleeding, clearance of microthrombi from the vasculature will be decreased and, in combination with the preexisting deficit of the anticoagulant antithrombin III found in DIC, may contribute to a hypercoagulable state.

Primary Fibrinolysis

There is controversy over whether a primary fibrinolytic disorder actually exists. It may well be a form of DIC in most cases as the two disorders have many common laboratory and clinical features. The absence of significant thrombocytopenia in the presence of elevated levels of fibrin degradation products is the best differentiating factor. Primary fibrinolysis is associated with catastrophic injuries, and more recently with cardiopulmonary bypass. If the bleeding dysfunction can be conclusively attributed to primary fibrinolysis rather than DIC, the use of fibrinolytic inhibitors such as epsilon-amino-caproic acid can be considered.

TREATMENT OF THROMBOTIC DISORDERS

In addition to concerns regarding disorders that can cause an increased propensity for bleeding in ICU patients, the critical care specialist must also be concerned with the treatment of thrombotic disorders and be familiar with the use of drugs for both the prophylaxis and treatment of arterial and venous thromboembolic disorders. The major indications for the use of antithrombotic agents, primarily heparin and warfarin (Coumadin) but also aspirin and dextran, are the prevention and treatment of deep venous thrombosis and pulmonary embolism, anticoagulation for prosthetic heart valves, prophylaxis of arterial embolization secondary to atrial fibrillation, prophylaxis of cerebrovascular emboli, and maintenance of patency of diseased arteries or grafts. Patients may thus already be receiving anticoagulation agents on entering the ICU or may require the institution of such therapies during their hospital course. Recently, fibrinolytic agents are also being used more frequently for the treatment of acute, life-threatening thrombotic events.

With the recent knowledge derived from more sophisticated biochemical assays and better understanding of molecular biology, our concepts of the cause of vascular thrombosis are changing. In the past, the concept of Virchow's triad of stasis, vascular injury, and hypercoagulable state gave preeminence to the facets of stasis and vascular injury, because a hypercoagulable state could not be well defined. It has now been shown that, in addition to the circulating procoagulant factors, naturally occurring coagulation inhibitors, such as antithrombin III and the vitamin K-dependent proteins C and S, serve to modulate the coagulation response. Kindreds deficient in these factors have been shown to be at increased risk for thrombosis. Furthermore, vascular endothelial inhibitors such as thrombomodulin decrease thrombosis at the site of injury, and a complex series of activators and inhibitors of fibrinolysis including PAI-1 may be influenced, particularly during periods of physiologic stress.[64] Much of these data are still in the early stages of study, and the clinical implications are not yet entirely clear but will most likely have considerable impact on the understanding and treatment of thrombotic disorders in the future.

Heparin

Heparin is a glycosaminoglycan that acts via antithrombin III, the most important naturally occurring inhibitor of the serine proteases of the coagulation cascade. Antithrombin III in its natural state is a relatively weak anticoagulant but is necessary for normal coagulation function. Patients with congenital antithrombin III deficiencies are at risk for recurrent thrombotic episodes. Renal disease, liver disease, and oral contraceptives have been shown to lower the levels of antithrombin III as well. The presence of heparin, even in small doses, causes a conformational change in the antithrombin molecule, which markedly accelerates its activity and effectiveness as an anticoagulant. In the absence or marked deficiency of antithrombin III—as found in congenital disorders and severe liver disease or occasionally after large thrombotic events—heparin will have little effect, and there will be marked heparin resistance. The level of antithrombin III must sometimes be first repleted with fresh-frozen plasma before the reinstitution of effective heparin therapy, or the patient must be placed on warfarin therapy as an alternative anticoagulation method.[65] Patients with some forms of congenital antithrombin III deficiency may require lifelong coumadin therapy.

Full-dose heparin is used for the treatment of deep venous thrombosis and pulmonary emboli to prevent the propagation of documented clots or the formation of new thrombi in susceptible individuals. Intermittent bolus intravenous heparin is not used, because of the difficulty of maintaining adequate anticoagulation without the risk of bleeding secondary to overanticoagulation. It is important to first obtain a basic clotting screen and platelet count before the institution of therapy to rule out other bleeding disorders and to determine the baseline PTT and platelet count. A heparin bolus of 50 to 100 U/kg is given intravenously, followed by a continuous infusion of 10 to 20 U/kg per hour, with therapy monitored initially approximately every 4 hours by measurement of PTT or aPTT. The dose is then adjusted by a minimum of 100 to 200 U per hour until the PTT is 1.5 to 2 times the control or pretreatment PTT. There may be initial heparin resistance, which generally reverses over the first few days of therapy, after which the frequency of obtaining the PTT levels can be decreased. The platelet count must be monitored frequently, at least every 2 days, to note the potential occurrence of heparin-induced thrombocytopenia. Recurrent thrombosis and thromboembolism while on heparin must also raise the question of heparin-induced thrombosis in addition to the potential for failure of treatment. The intravenous heparin is usually continued for 7 to 10 days in serious thrombophlebitis or pulmonary embolism with the gradual institution of warfarin therapy to therapeutic levels to coincide with the cessation of the heparin. Full-dose heparin is also used in patients who are beginning therapy for a device such as a prosthetic heart valve until warfarin is therapeutic, or in patients who are receiving long-term warfarin therapy but require brief discontinuation to allow for normalization of clotting parameters for elective surgery. The heparin can be stopped a few hours before surgery and restarted when the risk of bleeding has subsided. The half-life of heparin is approximately 1 hour; in conventional doses, heparin therefore rapidly leaves the system. If more immediate reversal of anticoagulation is required, protamine can be given with a dose of 1 mg of protamine for each 100 U of a heparin bolus, taking into account the half-life of the drug. For neutralizing a continuous infusion, 25 to 50% of the total dose is given. Subcutaneous low dose heparin, 5000 U every 8 or 12 hours, has been shown to be effective in the prevention of pulmonary emboli and deep venous thrombosis in postoperative patients.

Oral Anticoagulants

The mechanism of action of dicoumarol and warfarin was described in detail in the discussion of vitamin K deficiency. Warfarin is the most commonly used form of oral preparation for patients requiring long-term anticoagulation. It is usually used in conjunction with heparin therapy and is begun to overlap with therapeutic heparin to allow for slow loading to achieve therapeutic PT levels. Warfarin is begun with daily doses of 10 to 15 mg per day until proper levels are obtained, a PT approximately 1.5 to 2 times the control level. Recently, a standardized international ratio (INR) has been developed to account for the variability in the sensitivity of various reagents used to determine the PT in different hospitals and countries. In the past the standard recommendation was to maintain a ratio

Table 45-8. Recommended INR Targets for Anticoagulation

Indication	Target (Range)
Prevention of DVT	2.5 (2–3)
Prevention recurrent DVT	3 (2.5–4)
Treatment of venous thrombosis	2.5 (2–3)
Prevention of arterial thrombosis (including mechanical heart valve)	3.5 (3–4.5)

DVT, Deep venous thrombosis; INR, standardized international ratio.

of 1.5 to 2 times the control. When using different reagents, this has resulted in as much as a sixfold difference using a standardized reference, with an attendant increase in the number of bleeding complications. The new system should result in more comparable results of bleeding and thrombotic complications while on anticoagulation.[66] The recommended INR values are listed in Table 45-8. Because the half-lives of the individual clotting factors vary from 6 to 48 hours, there is a time lag between the institution of therapy and a change in the PT. It generally requires a minimum of 2 to 3 days to reach therapeutic levels. Any drug or condition that affects the level of vitamin K or enhances or slows the metabolism of the warfarin will affect the level of anticoagulation in a patient on coumadin. Well-known are the effects of alcohol, cholestyramine, and barbiturates, but many other drugs interact as well, and the patient's medication list must be carefully examined when there is inappropriate response to anticoagulation.

The major complication of warfarin is hemorrhage, occurring in up to 20 to 30% of patients, but major bleeding episodes occur in less than 1%. As noted previously, vitamin K can be given, with reversal of the warfarin effect in 24 hours, and immediate correction can be obtained with fresh-frozen plasma. Another uncommon complication that occurs early in anticoagulation, usually in female patients who are heterozygous for protein C deficiency, is necrosis of the skin and subcutaneous tissue, primarily of the fatty areas of the breast, buttocks, and thighs. This is presumably secondary to induction of a hypercoagulable state. Percutaneous procedures should be avoided in patients receiving warfarin, but open procedures and some surgery can be performed if the PT is less than 1.5 times normal. If the procedure is elective and requires totally normal homeostasis, the warfarin can be stopped a few days before surgery to allow for the effect of the drug to wear off, or if anticoagulation is required in the interim, the patient can be started on intravenous heparin while the PT normalizes. The heparin can then be stopped just before surgery and reinstituted postoperatively. Anticoagulation is usually continued for 6 weeks to 3 months for uncomplicated thromboembolism, and 6 months to life for recurrent embolism.

Dextran

Dextran is a relatively uncommonly used anticoagulant for either arterial or venous disease that appears to act by decreasing platelet aggregation.[67] Its primary role is when the use of heparin is contraindicated, as in heparin-associated thrombocytopenia and thrombosis before oral anticoagulation has achieved therapeutic levels. Dextran has the problems of fluid overload and the potential for allergic reactions and is generally used only for a few days.

Aspirin

As noted earlier in the discussion of functional platelet abnormalities, aspirin is an irreversible inhibitor of cyclooxygenase, and at doses of less than 1 g per day, it tends to preferentially affect platelets, causing decreased platelet aggregation. Aspirin has been best used to prevent arterial thromboembolic events in the cerebral and cardiac circulation. Although used in the treatment of venous thromboembolic disease, aspirin is not as effective as warfarin and is generally not usually used for this indication. Usually, no significant bleeding problem is generated by use of the drug, but platelet transfusion or DDAVP may be helpful if serious bleeding occurs.

Fibrinolytic Agents

In the past several years, much work has been done to study not only preventing the formation or further propagation of thrombi with conventional antithrombotic agents heparin and coumadin but also the direct lysis of clot to achieve better short-term survival and long-term functional outcome.[68] Initially, this form of therapy was applied only to life-threatening situations such as pulmonary emboli with hemodynamic compromise, massive iliofemoral thrombosis, or acute peripheral arterial occlusion. The next field of interest was acute coronary occlusion, in which the results were so favorable that lysis in acute myocardial infarction is considered the standard of care by most centers. Currently, investigators are studying the effects of thrombolytics in non-life-threatening conditions such as smaller pulmonary emboli and deep venous thrombosis to improve long-term functional results and in cases of more chronic emboli or thrombosis and are also applying the techniques to other vascular beds such as the cerebrovascular circulation for acute nonhemorrhagic cerebrovascular events.

Streptokinase, urokinase, and recombinant t-PA are currently the most commonly used agents, although considerable effort is being made to find lytics that are more clot-specific with less chance of bleeding complications.[69] Urokinase is a naturally occurring enzyme found in the urinary tract that prevents the formation of thrombi in nephrons. It acts directly on plasminogen to form plasmin. Streptokinase, derived from beta-hemolytic streptococci, must first complex with fibrinogen; the complex then can cleave plasminogen to plasmin. Because streptokinase, unlike urokinase, is a foreign protein, allergic reactions, including anaphylaxis, are possible, and pretreatment with hydrocortisone is usually given. In addition, if a patient has had a recent streptococcal infection, a sufficient antibody titer may be present to make the streptokinase ineffective. Before starting any lytic therapy, a routine clotting screen and thrombin time should be obtained to exclude other bleeding disorders. The dosage for streptokinase is an intravenous loading dose of 250,000 U over 30 minutes followed by a continuous infusion of 100,000 U per hour for 24 to 48 hours, depending on the clinical situation. Urokinase is given with a bolus of 4400 U/kg, then an infusion of 4400 U/kg per hour for 12 to 48 hours. Intravenous therapy is generally as effective as direct intrapulmonary or intra-arterial therapy. Recombinant tissue thromboplastin is found in vascular endothelium and is one of the coagulation system's natural modulators. It has been thought to be more clot specific because of a greater affinity for fibrin polymers than for circulating fibrinogen, with less chance of generating a systemic fibrinolytic state, but this is not entirely certain. The dose of rt-PA is 100 mg given over 2 hours. After discontinuation of the lytic infusion, and after the thrombin time has decreased to less than twice normal, heparin must be started because of the potential for a hypercoagulable state as a result of depletion of the fibrinolytic system. Because of the fairly short duration and fixed dose of the therapy, monitoring of coagulation parameters is not necessary and has not been shown to correlate with clinical effectiveness. In the case of longer duration infusion, thrombin time may be obtained approximately 4 hours after the institution of therapy to ensure that a lytic state has been achieved. If this has not occurred with streptokinase, the patient should be switched to urokinase.

Bleeding is the major complication of lytic therapy. Contraindications to its use are bleeding diatheses, recent active bleeding, recent cerebrovascular accident, and trauma or major surgery, particularly in a closed space, such as cranial, spinal, or cardiac. In the setting of a potentially lethal thrombotic or embolic event, all contraindications become relative. Invasive procedures, including venipuncture, should be avoided in patients who are candidates for or are receiving thrombolytics. In the event of bleeding while undergoing lytic therapy, the agent is immediately discontinued, and because of the very short half-life of the drugs—15 minutes for streptokinase and urokinase and 5 minutes for t-PA—the effect is quickly reversed. Major hemorrhage can be treated with transfusions of cryoprecipitate and fresh-frozen plasma to replace the depleted factors (see Chap. 23).

TRANSFUSION THERAPY

Red Cells

The automatic trigger for transfusion to maintain a hemoglobin level of 10 g/dl is no longer appropriate because of the documentation of good results in patients who are allowed to have lower hemoglobin levels, the tremendous cost of transfusion therapy, and the concern for transmission of diseases, including acquired immune deficiency syndrome (AIDS) and hepatitis. Transfusion should be tailored to the individual patient, taking into account (1) the patient's general status, (2) other coexisting disease such as cardiovascular and pulmonary disease that will affect both oxygen requirements and the rate of development of the anemia, and (3) the presence of underlying hematologic disorders that may be responsible for a chronic anemia and affect the adequacy of the response to an anemic challenge. Therefore, the decision to transfuse, except in situations of obvious massive blood loss, must consider the patient's history, laboratory results, and either an evaluation of symptoms reflecting inadequate oxygen delivery or more sophisticated monitoring with calculations of oxygen delivery and consumption. Patients who are otherwise healthy and whose source of blood loss is controlled can well tolerate hemoglobin levels of 7 to 8 mg/dl.[70]

Although in the past, fresh whole blood has been advised as the best blood replacement product, especially when massive transfusion is needed, this product is seldom available except in specific instances, because of the more efficient use of a scarce resource by fractionation of a single unit of blood into multiple components. Most patients require a specific factor rather than the total contents of a unit of whole blood, and the individual factors can be banked for longer term use. In addition, the time required for the rigorous testing for infectious disease, particularly AIDS, has made the immediate delivery of blood more difficult, except in the case of known, prescreened donors, such as parents or siblings of children undergoing elective operations. Packed red cells are the most commonly used form of red cell replacement. Modern blood banking preservation techniques have extended the shelf life of RBCs to 42 days at 4°C. Cells older than 7 to 10 days will be deficient in 2,3 diphosphoglycerate levels (2,3 DPG) and thus have increased affinity for oxygen, resulting in shift of the oxygen-hemoglobin dissociation curve to the left. Except in the cases of massive transfusion, however, the levels of 2,3 DPG spontaneously replete within a few hours of transfusion. Packed RBCs are deficient in labile factors V and VIII:c, functional platelets, and functional white cells, and have elevated levels of potassium, lactate, ammonia, and microaggregate debris. Each unit of packed RBCs provides approximately 200 ml of cells with a hematocrit of 70 to 80%.

Alternatives to the use of homologous units of blood include the banking of red cells frozen in glycerol for later use. This is particularly useful for patients with rare blood types or with high levels of antibodies against antigens commonly found in the blood pool. Before elective surgery, patients may be able to bank their own blood.[71] With the addition of a short course of erythropoietin, significant increases in the number of units that can be phlebotomized over a shorter period of time are possible.[72] This has been used increasingly in orthopedic procedures, which commonly require transfusion. A newer field of use of preoperative erythropoietin is for patients who are to undergo cardiac surgery or other major surgical procedures, who may be able to either conventionally predeposit units of cells, or "prime" the marrow precursors, to be more responsive to an anemic challenge during and after surgery.[73] For procedures associated with significant blood loss, such as cardiac, major vascular, thoracic, and major orthopedic procedures, technology has been developed to allow for the collection of shed blood and the reprocessing to allow autotransfusion back to the patient during the procedure and in the early postoperative period.[74] This has become routine in large centers and helps to decrease the amount of homologous blood required by the patient.

The complications of blood transfusion, although rare, are another reason to avoid unnecessary transfusion (Table

Table 45-9. Transfusion Reactions

Reaction	Incidence	Source
Fever	1:50–1:100	Antibodies to donor leukocytes
Uticaria	1:100	Sensitization to donor plasma
Acute lung injury	1:5,000	Leukoagglutinins in donor blood
Acute hemolysis	1:6,000	ABO antibodies to donor red cells
Fatal hemolysis	1:100,000	ABO antibodies to donor red cells

(Reprinted from Marino, P.L.: The ICU Book. Philadelphia, Lea & Febiger, 1991, p. 225.)

45–9). Major hemolytic (ABO) transfusion reactions are now uncommon because of accurate means of assessing antibodies and are most often due to clerical error. They can be potentially fatal, however, with massive complement activation causing hemodynamic instability, impaired oxygenation, DIC precipitated by the lysis of red cells, and renal insufficiency. Symptoms in an awake patient include fever, headache, back pain, and chest tightness. In the operating room, the question of a hemolytic transfusion reaction should be raised by the sudden onset of abnormal bleeding and hemodynamic instability coincident with or shortly after transfusion. Treatment involves stopping the transfusion as soon as the potential of a problem is recognized and supportive measures, including respiratory support, if necessary, steroids, H_2 blockers, intravascular volume, and vasopressors. Delayed transfusion reactions are usually due to incompatibility of minor antigens. They occur 1 to 3 weeks following transfusion with the onset of symptoms of a hemolytic anemia that is self-limited and usually not of major clinical significance. They symptoms should prompt reanalysis of the patient's antibody status by repeat Coomb's tests. The majority of transfusion reactions are due to the white cell antigens present in the red cell transfusion. These are typically fever and rash but occasionally can present with noncardiogenic pulmonary edema. If a patient has a history of major nonhemolytic transfusion reactions with significant leukoagglutinating antibodies, the use of leukocyte-poor or washed cells may be considered, or frozen deglycerolized red cells, which have the lowest level of white cells of all the red cell products. All of these products are more costly and take longer to prepare than the usual packed RBCs, so their use must be planned. Common problems occurring with transfusion of large amounts of blood are volume overload, hypocalcemia, hyperkalemia, hypothermia, and pulmonary dysfunction that is due to microaggregate debris. Massive transfusion that is greater than 15 to 20 U of packed red cells can contribute to coagulopathy. Studies performed in war casualties and other trauma victims, however, have shown that this is usually due to dilutional thrombocytopenia and responds well to platelet transfusion without the need for other factor replacement despite measured abnormalities of PT and PTT.[75] Graft-versus-host disease increasingly is seen following the transfusion of red cells into immunocompromised or even normal patients, particularly the transfusion of related donor blood.[76] Brief irradiation of the red cells will destroy the lymphocytes responsible and is advisable for immunodeficient patients or related donor units. This disease can potentially cause serious morbidity and pancytopenia and can involve the skin, liver, and gastrointestinal tract.

The infectious complications of blood transfusions are well-known, sometimes causing an inordinate fear of transfusion. The risk of HIV transmission by blood transfusion is currently on the order of 1:225,000 U of blood.[77] In addition, although a donor may test negative for the HIV antibody, there is a minimum 6- to 8-week latent period after acute infection before antibody can be detected. This latent period may be much longer, up to 6 months in some patients. (HIV is discussed in greater detail in Chap. 68.) The risk of post-transfusion hepatitis (PTH) is less than 3:10,000 U of blood. Screening methods for hepatitis B are quite effective, with less than 10% of cases of PTH caused by hepatitis B. The majority of cases now are due to hepatitis C, formerly known as non-A, non-B hepatitis. New assays can detect hepatitis C antibody; thus, screening for this disease will in all likelihood decrease the incidence of PTH. PTH seldom causes a fulminant, lethal illness, but unfortunately can frequently lead to cirrhosis and chronic liver disease. Other infectious agents that can be transmitted are human T-cell lymphotrophic virus type 1 (HTLV-1), which may predispose individuals to the development of T-cell leukemia and lymphoma, cytomegalovirus, and rarely, bacterial infections that are due to contamination. Very rare transmission of yersinia, malaria, syphilis, and Lyme disease can occur.

The best prevention of any of the preceding complications is the avoidance of transfusion if at all possible, or the use of predeposited autologous blood, but this may not be possible for all patients. In addition, there are patients who have such rare blood types that they do not tolerate transfusion and patients who refuse transfusion on religious grounds, such as the Jehovah's Witnesses. For these patients, more experimental approaches may be necessary. As noted previously, many patients may tolerate very low hemoglobin levels remarkably well. Artificial colloids such as dextran or hydroxyethylstarch can be used for volume replacement in addition to crystalloid solutions.[78] Presently, no red cell substitutes are clinically available, but research is ongoing to develop a stroma-free hemoglobin product for oxygen transport. Perfluorochemicals (PFCs) are solutions that have been developed that can transport oxygen, but they are not approved by the FDA for use as a blood replacement.[79] They have been used in emergency situations but are limited by the requirement for high levels of inspired oxygen to adequately load the compound and by the limitation of the total amount of the product that can be used because of safety concerns about its metabolism. The substances appear to be taken up in the reticuloendothelial cells and stay there for prolonged periods, with their ultimate fate and long-term effects unknown.

White Cells

Granulocyte transfusions have been used to treat septic neutropenic patients.[16] It is not a simple procedure, however, and is associated with difficulties for the recipient and discomfort for the donor. Granulocytes have a short life span and must therefore be procured close to the time they are needed, making donation inconvenient. Single-donor units obtained by pheresis are used because of the large number of donors that would be required in the use of a pooled product with resulting histocompatability problems. Even with the most efficient collection methods, the number of white cells obtained is less than a normal person mobilizes in the presence of an acute infection. To increase the yield, many centers administer corticosteroids to donors before pheresis, raising questions of safety with frequent donation. Hydroxyethyl starch is used as a sedimenting agent, some of which ends up in the donor, but with few side effects.[26] White cells need only be ABO typed because of the number of red cells included with the leukocytes. More histocompatible units, however, may be needed in patients with severe reactions or those responding poorly to therapy, because some evidence indicates that more compatible units may be more effective in vivo.

The most common indication for granulocyte transfusion is severe bacterial infection in a profoundly neutropenic patient not responding to appropriate antibiotic therapy. Prognostically, patients with gram-positive infections have a better chance of recovery than those with gram-negative infections; parenchymal infections such as pneumonia are more serious than localized processes. Recovery of even minimal intrinsic neutrophil production is the most important prognostic factor. Transfusion is required at least once a day and optimally more often for maximal response. Complications of transfusions can be severe. Volume overload in a critically ill patient can be a serious problem, especially following cardiotoxic chemotherapy. Febrile reactions are common. The major clinical problem is diffuse bilateral pulmonary infiltrate, which may be due to trapping of damaged white cells in the pulmonary parenchyma or immunologically related leukoagglutinin reactions. The pulmonary dysfunction usually improves gradually and requires only supportive care. A pneumonia may be initially worsened by the migration of leukocytes to the site of inflammation. Graft-versus-host disease can develop, especially in bone marrow transplant recipients. In addition, all of the previously mentioned infectious agents can contaminate granulocyte transfusions.

The development of marrow colony-stimulating factors such as EPO, G-CSF, and GM-CSF, by recombinant DNA technology has recently revolutionized the treatment of neutropenic patients. G-CSF stimulates only neutrophil cell lines, whereas GM-CSF is more broad, affecting both neutrophils and monocytes. The question of which factor will be more useful in a particular clinical situation has yet to be defined. In addition to their effects on stem cells, the CSFs also appear to enhance the function of mature cells. Multiple clinical trials are in progress using these agents in neutropenia of diverse causes. These agents have proven useful in the neutropenia arising from AIDS and its treatment,[21] in hastening the recovery of marrow function following chemotherapy-induced myelosuppression,[20] and in the treatment of aplastic anemia. Therefore, these drugs are being used both therapeutically in established neutropenia and prophylactically to prevent the complication in those patients at high risk for the problem. The side effects of treatment are generally mild, usually low grade fever, flushing, rash, headache, myalgia, arthralgia, bone pain, fluid retention, and thrombosis around intravenous catheters. There have been reported instances of pulmonary dysfunction following the first dose of GM-CSF, which presumably are due to pulmonary sequestration of white cells. The drugs are given by intravenous or subcutaneous route. Subcutaneous administration may be the preferred method with lower dose-related toxicity and prolonged duration of action. Following the more widespread use and experience with these factors, there may be decreased incidence of patients with neutropenia that is due to prophylactic treatment and more effective and less toxic methods of dealing with the dysfunction when it occurs.

Platelets

Platelet transfusions are most appropriately indicated for thrombocytopenia secondary to decreased production such as bone marrow failure or a dilutional coagulopathy secondary to massive transfusion (more than 15 to 20 U of packed RBCs).[80] When thrombocytopenia is due to increased destruction of platelets, particularly in immune-mediated disorders, platelet transfusion will be of little benefit, because transfused platelets will be destroyed at the same rate or faster than native platelets; it therefore should be given only in the setting of life-threatening bleeding. Prophylactic transfusion may be contraindicated, as in TTP, because of the risk of accelerating microvascular thrombosis, or at least counterproductive because of the risk of inducing further alloantibodies, thus making later transfusions more problematic. Patients with DIC, a consumptive process, may require platelet transfusion, but the main focus of therapy should be treating the underlying cause of the DIC. Platelet transfusions for functional platelet disorders are seldom indicated.

As noted previously, platelet counts of 50,000/mm^3 or greater can support normal hemostasis in the absence of other coagulation defects. Except in the setting of surgery—such as intracranial procedures, where even a small amount of bleeding may be disastrous—or extensive trauma, platelet transfusions are unnecessary before this level. Platelet transfusions given to reach counts of 50,000 to 70,000/mm^3 are adequate. Prophylactic transfusion is not required unless the patient has counts of less than 20,000/mm^3 or is bleeding. Invasive procedures such as arterial or venous catheter placement, bone marrow biopsies, or other procedures during which pressure can be applied directly to a site can be performed in patients with platelet counts even less than 20,000/mm^3 if appropriate care is taken. Other procedures in which these caveats cannot be met may require transfusion before the procedure.

Platelets are prepared by centrifugation of blood from single donor units of blood and resuspended in 50 to 60 ml of plasma. Before transfusion, the appropriate number of units of platelets can be pooled to make transfusion more convenient. The alternative is to remove platelets by pheresis from a single donor, a process that can obtain between 4 and 12 U of platelets at a time. Platelets have a maximum shelf life of 5 days at room temperature in the blood bank, but once pooled, they must be used within a few hours because of the potential for bacterial contamination. Transfusion of 1 U of platelets into a normal patient can be expected to raise the platelet count by approximately 10,000/mm^3. In a patient who has thrombocytopenia that is due to increased destruction of platelets, particularly on an immune basis, or who has required multiple transfusions and may have acquired antibodies, a 1-hour and 24-hour post-transfusion platelet count should be obtained to assess the efficacy of the therapy. The problem of alloimmunization can be a difficult clinical dilemma. Antibodies are most often against many HLA antigens developed during the previous transfusions of multiple donor platelets. Siblings or single donor platelets matched as closely as possible by HLA typing are probably the best alternative. Platelet transfusions should be avoided except in the event of serious bleeding, then multiple units can be given in the hope of either removing some of the antibody, or at least giving by chance a histocompatible unit.

Transfusion reactions to platelets are usually mild, with fever and chills, sometimes hives, but usually no hemodynamic instability, except if the platelets are given rapidly by central venous access. Reactions may be due to leukocytes present along with the platelets or may occur more commonly in patients who have platelet antibodies. Some red cells are present in platelet concentrates and may sensitize patients to red cell antigens, but major transfusion reactions are rare because of the small volume of cells involved. Volume overload and all the infectious agents associated with blood products can be transmitted with platelet transfusions. Bacterial contamination, although still uncommon, happens more frequently with platelets than red cells because of the room temperature storage of the platelet concentrates. Graft-versus-host disease is a potential complication of platelet therapy. It is due to the large number of lymphocytes present in platelets and even more so in single donor units, which may contain up to 10 times as many lymphocytes as random donor units. Irradiation of platelets before use in immunocompromised patients is the obvious solution in this high-risk population, but the magnitude of the problem in other recipients is yet unknown.

Coagulation Factors

Multiple plasma products are available that contain various combinations, or single coagulation factors, each with relatively specific indications. Fresh-frozen plasma contains functional forms of all clotting and inhibitor proteins but in a dilute form, with each unit of plasma containing less than 10% of normal clotting activity.[81] Because of the low activity, large volumes of fresh-frozen plasma may be needed to treat a coagulopathy. The question of what should be the appropriate trigger level for coagulation factor replacement is not well defined. Clearly, patients who are not bleeding, and who have only moderate elevation of PT and PTT should be observed carefully, and the underlying cause of the dysfunction treated. Surgery can even be performed safely in patients who have PTs of 1.5 times normal or less. Coagulation factor replacement has been advised in patients who have PT levels greater than 1.5 times normal who are experiencing or are at high risk for bleeding. Even in that setting, however, the bleeding may not be primarily due to coagulation factor deficiency, as shown in studies of patients undergoing massive transfusion, but to another disorder such as platelet deficiency or dysfunction. Thus, the past recommendations to routinely give a combination of platelets and coagulation factors when administering large numbers of red cell units appears to be unsupported. The decision for appropriate factor replacement continues to be a difficult one that does not have a clear-cut answer. Although in the past, fresh-frozen plasma has been used for volume replacement, this is unwarranted because of the sometimes scarce supply of the product, its expense, and the potential for transmission of diseases. Other adequate colloid products are available with considerable less expense and greater safety, such as hydroxyethyl starch and other purified albumin products.[77] Fresh-frozen plasma is indicated for patients who have bleeding secondary to the deficiency of multiple clotting factors as in DIC, liver disease, and vitamin K deficiency, or overanticoagulation with warfarin when rapid correction of the coagulopathy is required. It must be remembered that vitamin K is still the treatment of choice in vitamin K-deficient states when bleeding is not life-threatening. Fresh-frozen plasma is used to treat factor deficiencies for which there is no more concentrated form of replacement. The product is also used during plasmapheresis for a variety of disorders primarily to remove pathologic plasma proteins.

Cryoprecipitate is a product that contains high concentrations of fibrinogen, factor VIII:c, and vWF. It is the treatment of choice for severe hypofibrinogenemia as occurs in DIC, or bleeding associated with fibrinolytic agents. Although it has been used for the treatment of bleeding in hemophilia A, factor VIII concentrates are a more predictable and concentrated form of replacement therapy for this disorder. Because of the high concentration of vWF, cryoprecipitate can be used in the treatment of congenital vWD,[57] or more rarely in acquired states with possible relative vWF deficiency or dysfunction such as uremia.[49] Very often, however, in the congenital disorder, and frequently in the relative dysfunction, desmopressin can be used with the avoidance of blood product use.[48]

Factor VIII and factor IX complexes are available that contain high concentrations and defined activities of the factors deficient in hemophilia A and B, respectively. They are readily available in preparations that allow for early home treatment of these bleeding disorders. Their use is described in more detail in the section on congenital coagulation disorders.

The complications associated with all of these factors are the same as for other blood products, with the risk of disease transmission, in fact, somewhat greater because of the pooled nature or requirements for large numbers of single units to achieve appropriate activity.

REFERENCES

1. Greer, A. E., Carey, J. M., and Zuhdi, N.: Hemodilution principle of hypothermic perfusion: a concept of obviating blood priming. J. Thorac. Cardiovasc. Surg., *43*:640, 1962.

2. Eschbach, J. W., and Adamson, J. W.: Anemia of end-stage renal disease. Kidney Int., 28:(1):1, 1985.
3. Levine, E. A. et al.: Erythropoietin deficiency after coronary artery bypass procedures. Ann. Thorac. Surg., 51:764, 1991.
4. Karayalcin, G., Rosner, F., and Sawitsky, A.: Pseudoneutropenia in Negroes: a normal phenomenon. N.Y. State J. Med., 72:1815, 1972.
5. Eschbach, J. W., and Adamson, J. W.: Recombinant hyman erythropoietin: implications for nephrology. Am. J. Kidney Dis., 11(3):203, 1988.
6. Eschbach, J. W. et al.: Correction of the anemia of end-stage renal disease with recombinant human erythropoietin. Results of a combined phase I and II clinical trial. N. Engl. J. Med., 316:73, 1987.
7. Lundin, A. P.: Quality of life: subjective and objective improvements with recombinant human erythropoietin therapy. Semin. Nephrol., 9(1):22, 1989.
8. Johnson, C. S.: Landmark perspective. Sickle cell anemia. JAMA, 254:1958, 1985.
9. Schrieber, A. D.: Paroxysmal nocturnal hemoglobinuria revisited. N. Engl. J. Med., 309:723, 1983.
10. Peytremann, R., Rhodes, R. S., and Hartmann, R. C.: Thrombosis in paroxysmal nocturnal hemoglobinuria (PNH) with particular reference to progressive, diffuse hepatic venous thrombosis. Semin. Haematol., 5:115, 1972.
11. Sayed, H. M., et al.: Hemolytic anemia of mechanical origin after open heart surgery. Thorax, 16:356, 1961.
12. Petz, L. D.: Drug-induced immune hemolysis. N. Engl. J. Med., 313:510, 1985.
13. Chervenick, P. A.: Dialysis, neutropenia, lung-dysfunction and complement. N. Engl. J. Med., 296:810, 1977.
14. Young, G. A., and Vincent, P. C.: Drug-induced agranulocytosis. Clin. Haematol., 9:483, 1980.
15. Posnett, D. N., Stein, R. S., Graber, S. E., and Krantz, S. B.: Cimetidine-induced neutropenia: a possible dose-related phenomenon. Arch. Intern. Med., 139:584, 1979.
16. Bodey, G. P., Bolivar, R., and Fainstein, V.: Infectious complications in leukemic patients. Semin. Hematol., 19:193, 1982.
17. Nauseef, W. M., and Maki, D. G.: A study of the value of simple protective isolation in patients with granulocytopenia. N. Engl. J. Med., 304:448, 1981.
18. Clift, R. A., and Buckner, C. D.: Symposium on infectious complications of neoplastic disease. Am. J. Med., 76:631, 1984.
19. Nienhuis, A. W.: Hematopoietic growth factors: biologic complexity and clinical promise. N. Engl. J. Med., 318:916, 1988.
20. Antman, K. S. et al.: Effect of recombinant human granulocyte-macrophage colony stimulating factor on chemotherapy-induced myelosuppression. N. Engl. J. Med., 319:593, 1988.
21. Groopman, J. E. et al.: Effect of recombinant human granulocyte-macrophage colony-stimulating factor on myelopoiesis in the acquired immunodeficiency syndrome. N. Engl. J. Med., 317:593, 1987.
22. Watkins, J., Ward, A. M., and Appleyard, T. N.: Changes in peripheral blood leucocytes following i.v. anaesthesia and surgery. (Letter.) Br. J. Anaesth. 49:953, 1977.
23. Meyer, L. M., and Rotter, S. D.: Leukemoid reaction (hyperleukocytosis) in malignancy. Am. J. Clin. Pathol., 12:218, 1942.
24. Kuvin, S. F., and Brecher, G.: Differential neutrophil counts in pregnancy. N. Engl. J. Med., 266:877, 1962.
25. Mishler, J. M., and Emerson, P. M.: Development of neutrophilia by serially increasing doses of dexamethasone. Br. J. Haematol., 36:249, 1977.
26. Mishler, J. M.: Hydroxyethyl starch as an experimental adjunct to leukocyte separation by centrifugal means: review of safety and efficacy. Transfusion. Phila., 15:449, 1975.
27. Stein, R. S., Hanson, G., Koethe, S., and Hansen, R.: Lithium-induced granulocytosis. Ann. Intern. Med., 88:809, 1978.
28. Lindenbaum, J., and Hargrove, R. L.: Thrombocytopenia in alcoholics. Ann. Intern. Med., 68:526, 1986.
29. Pettit, R. M.: Thrombotic thrombocytopenic purpura: a thirty year review. Semin. Thromb. Hemost., 6:350, 1980.
30. Lichtin, A. E. et al.: Efficacy of intensive plasmapheresis in thrombotic thrombocytopenic purpura. Arch. Intern. Med., 147:2122, 1987.
31. Breckenridge, R. L. Jr. et al.: Treatment of thrombotic thrombocytopenic purpura with plasma exchange, antiplatelet agents, corticosteroid, and plasma infusion: Mayo Clinic experience. J. Clin. Apheresis., 1:6, 1982.
32. DiFino, S. M., Lachant, N. A., Kirshner, J. J., and Gottlieb, A. J.: Adult idiopathic thrombocytopenic purpura. Clinical findings and response to therapy. Am. J. Med., 69:430, 1980.
33. Mueller-Eckhardt, C.: Idiopathic thrombocytopenic purpura (ITP): clinical and immunologic considerations. Semin. Thromb. Hemost., 3:125, 1977.
34. Abramson, N., Eisenberg, P. D., and Aster, R. H.: Post-transfusion purpura: immunologic aspects and therapy. N. Engl. J. Med., 291:1163, 1974.
35. Hackett, T., Kelton, J. G., and Powers, P.: Drug-induced platelet destruction. Semin. Thromb. Hemost., 8:116, 1982.
36. King, D. J., and Kelton, J. G.: Heparin-associated thrombocytopenia. Ann. Intern. Med., 100:535, 1984.
37. Chang, J.: White clot syndrome associated with heparin-induced thrombocytopenia: a review of 23 cases. Heart Lung, 16:403, 1987.
38. Ginsburg, A. D.: Platelet function in patients with high platelet counts. Ann. Intern. Med., 82:506, 1975.
39. Morowitz, D. A., Allen, L. W., and Kirsner, J. B.: Thrombocytosis in chronic inflammatory bowel disease. Ann. Intern. Med., 68:1013, 1968.
40. Breslow, A., Kaufman, R. M., and Lawsky, A. R.: The effect of surgery on the concentration of circulating megakaryocytes and platelets. Blood, 32:393, 1968.
41. Rodriquez-Edmann, F., Goldberg, M. E., Davey, F., and Moloney, W. C.: Treatment of symptomatic thrombocythemia. N. Engl. J. Med., 281:854, 1969.
42. Levin, J., and Conley, C. L.: Thrombocytosis associated with malignant disease. Arch. Intern. Med., 114:497, 1964.
43. Harker, L. A.: Acquired disorders of platelet function. Ann. NY Acad. Sci., 509:188, 1987.
44. Harker, L. A. et al.: Mechanism of abnormal bleeding in patients undergoing cardiopulmonary bypass: acquired transient platelet dysfunction associated with selective α-granule release. Blood, 56(5):824, 1980.
45. Mohr, R. et al.: Effect of cardiac operation on platelets. J. Thorac. Cardiovasc. Surg., 92:434, 1986.
46. Kaneshiro, M. M., Mielke, C. H. Jr., Kasper, C. K., and Rapaport, S. I.: Bleeding time after aspirin in disorders of intrinsic clotting. N. Engl. J. Med., 281:1039, 1969.
47. Bashein, G. et al.: Preoperative aspirin therapy and reoperation for bleeding after coronary artery bypass surgery. Arch. Intern. Med., 151:89, 1991.
48. Kobrinsky, N. L. et al.: Shortening of bleeding time by 1 deamino-8-D-arginine vasopressin in various bleeding disorders. Lancet, 1:1145, 1984.
49. Janson, P. A., Jubelirer, S. J., Weinstein, M. J., and Deykin, D.: Treatment of the bleeding tendency in uremia with cryoprecipitate. N. Engl. J. Med., 303:1318, 1980.
50. Mannucci, P. M.: Desmopressin (DDAVP) for treatment of disorders of hemostasis. Prog. Hemost. Thromb., 8:19, 1986.

51. Post, M., and Teffer, M. C.: Surgery in hemophilic patients. J. Bone Joint Surg. [Am.], 57:1136, 1975.
52. White, C. G. 2nd, McMillan, C. W., Blatt, P. M., and Roberts, H. R.: Factor VIII inhibitors: a clinical overview. Am. J. Hematol., 13:335, 1982.
53. Mayne, E. E., Madden, M., Crothers, I. S., and Ingles, T.: Highly purified porcine factor VIII in haemophilia A with inhibitors to factor VIII (letter). Br. Med. J. Clin. Res., 282:318, 1981.
54. Kasper, C. K.: Thromboembolic complications. Thromb. Diath. Haemorrh., 33:640, 1975.
55. Cederbaum, A. I., Blatt, P. M., and Roberts, H. R.: Intravascular coagulation with use of human prothrombin complex concentrates. Ann. Intern. Med., 84:683, 1976.
56. Bowie, E. J.: Von Willebrand's disease. Clinical picture, diagnosis, and treatment. Clin. Lab. Med., 4(2):303, 1984.
57. Weiss, H. J., and Rogers, J.: Correction of the platelet abnormality in von Willebrand's disease by cryoprecipitate. Am. J. Med., 53:734, 1972.
58. Ansell, J. E., Kumar, R., and Deykin, D.: The spectrum of vitamin K deficiency. JAMA, 238:40, 1977.
59. Kelly, D. A., and Tuddenham, E. G.: Haemostatic problems in liver disease. Gut, 27:339, 1986.
60. Love, P. E., and Santoro, S. A.: Antiphospholipid antibodies: anticardiolipin and the lupus anticoagulant in systemic lupus erythematosus (SLE) and in non-SLE disorders. Prevalence and clinical significance. Ann. Intern. Med., 112:682, 1990.
61. Mueh, J. R., Herbst, K. D., and Rapaport, S. I.: Thrombosis in patients with the lupus anticoagulant. Ann. Intern. Med., 92:156, 1980.
62. Carr, J. M., McKinney, M., and McDonagh, J.: Diagnosis of disseminated intravascular coagulation. Role of D-dimer. Am. J. Clin. Pathol., 91:280, 1989.
63. Feinstein, D. I.: Diagnosis and management of disseminated intravascular coagulation: the role of heparin therapy. Blood, 60:284, 1982.
64. Rosenfeld, B. A.: Perioperative hemostatic changes and coronary ischemic syndromes. Int. Anesth. Clin., 30:131, 1992.
65. Marciniak, E., and Gockerman, J. P.: Heparin-induced decrease in circulating anit-thrombin III. Lancet, 2:581, 1977.
66. American College of Chest Physicians and the National Heart, Lung and Blood Institute: ACC-NHLBI National Conference on Antithrombotic Therapy. Chest, 89:1S, 1986.
67. Aberg, M., Hedner, U., and Bergenta, S. E.: The antithrombotic effect of dextran. Scand. J. Haematol., 34:61, 1979.
68. Sharma, G. V., Burleson, V. A., and Sasahara, A. A.: Effect of thrombolytic therapy on pulmonary-capillary blood volume in patients with pulmonary embolism. N. Engl. J. Med., 303:842, 1980.
69. Goldhaber, S. Z.: Recent advances in the diagnosis and lytic therapy of pulmonary embolism. Chest, 99:173S, 1991.
70. Consensus conference: Perioperative red blood cell transfusion. JAMA, 260:2700, 1988.
71. AuBuchon, J. P.: Autologous transfusion and directed donations: current controversies and future directions. Transfusion Med. Rev., 3:290, 1989.
72. Goodenough, L. T. et al.: Increased preoperative collection of autologous blood and recombinant human erythropoietin therapy. N. Engl. J. Med., 321:1163, 1989.
73. D'Ambra, M. N., Lynch, K. E., Boccagno, J., and Vlahakes, G. J.: The effect of perioperative administration of recombinant human erythropoietin (r$_{HU}$EPO) in CABG patients: a double blind, placebo-controlled trial. Anesthesiology, 77(3A), 1992.
74. Hall, R. I., Schweiger, I. M., and Finlayson, D. C.: The benefit of the Hemonetics cell saver apparatus during cardiac surgery. Can. J. Anaesth., 37:618, 1990.
75. Counts, R. B., et al.: Hemostasis in massively transfused trauma patients. Ann. Surg., 190(1):91, 1979.
76. Thaler, M. et al.: The role of blood from HLA-homozygous donors in fatal transfusion associated graft-versus-host disease after open-heart surgery. N. Engl. J. Med., 321:25, 1989.
77. Dodd-Roger, Y.: The risk of transfusion-transmitted infection. N. Engl. J. Med., 327:419, 1992.
78. Diehl, J. T., Lester, J. L., III, and Cosgrove, D. M.: Clinical comparison of hetastarch and albumin in postoperative cardiac patients. Am. Thorac. Surg., 34:674, 1982.
79. Spence, R. K. et al.: Fluosol DA-20 in the treatment of severe anemia: randomized, controlled study of 46 patients. Crit. Care Med., 18:1227, 1990.
80. Consensus conference: Platelet transfusion therapy. JAMA, 257:1777, 1987.
81. Consensus conference: Fresh-frozen plasma. Indications and risks. JAMA, 253:551, 1985.

Section Six

THE INTEGUMENT

Chapter 46

SERIOUS GRAM-POSITIVE BACTERIAL INFECTIONS WITH CUTANEOUS MANIFESTATIONS

DAVID L. SNOOK

Unlike most other organ systems, the integument can be easily visualized, providing immediate information about ongoing pathologic processes. Such rapid information gathering is particularly helpful in caring for critically ill patients.

Gram-positive bacteria may cause cutaneous disease through direct invasion (erysipelas, cellulitis) or toxin production (staphylococcal scalded skin syndrome, toxic shock syndrome). In necrotizing fasciitis, subcutaneous vascular destruction may eventually cause overlying skin necrosis.

Some of the entities discussed in this chapter are not always due to gram-positive organisms alone. Cellulitis, for example, is rarely caused by gram-negative bacteria or fungi. Necrotizing fasciitis sometimes involves both gram-positive and gram-negative organisms acting in synergy.

ERYSIPELAS

Pathophysiology and Risk Factors

Erysipelas is an infection involving the dermis and upper subcutaneous tissue. The vast majority of erysipelas is caused by Streptococcus pyogenes.[1] Rare causes include group B,[2] C, and G,[3] streptococci, Streptococcus pneumoniae,[4] Staphylococcus aureus,[5] and Yersinia enterocolitica.[6] Erysipelas that is due to unusual organisms is usually seen in a setting of immunocompromise or poor lymphatic drainage.[7] Erysipelas occurs more frequently and tends to be more severe in infants, young children, and the elderly. All age groups, however, are susceptible. The portal of entry for organisms may be a microscopic or obvious traumatic wound,[8] ulcer margin, or surgical wound.

Clinical Presentation and Differential Diagnosis

Common sites of involvement include face, head, and distal limb. At the time of presentation, prominent systemic symptoms often overshadow local signs. Fever, chills, and malaise commonly precede onset of the rash. Headache and vomiting may also be present. The area of infection becomes a bright red, warm, tender, well-demarcated plaque with a peripherally spreading border. Affected skin feels slightly indurated and has a shiny, edematous appearance.[9] The plaque's sharp demarcation is usually striking and distinguishes erysipelas from the more poorly demarcated cellulitis (Fig. 46-1). With severe involvement, vesicles, bullae, petechiae, and purpura may develop within the plaque. Erysipelas devoid of erythema, but retaining the other characteristic findings, has rarely been noted in immunocompromised patients.[7]

The diagnosis of erysipelas is essentially clinical, based on the appearance of the cutaneous lesion. Most patients also have the previously mentioned systemic symptoms and a white blood cell count greater than 15,000. Because systemic symptoms may be prominent, it is important to do a complete cutaneous exam on any ill-appearing febrile patient to avoid missing erysipelas. Allergic contact dermatitis may appear identical to erysipelas but is not associated with systemic complaints or leukocytosis.

Laboratory Studies

Culturing the causative organism is quite difficult and not necessary for diagnosis. Rarely, positive and accurate culture results have been obtained from skin biopsy, vesicle fluid, or intracutaneously injected and aspirated saline.[10] Such cultures are not routinely recommended because of their low yield. Blood cultures should be done if bacteremia is suspected, but results are often negative. A rising antistreptolysin O titer is not seen in many cases, is not cost-effective, and becomes apparent only long after initial therapeutic decisions are made.[10]

Treatment and Recovery

In healthy adults, erysipelas is often a self-limited infection. Before antibiotics became available, most cases resolved spontaneously in 1 to 3 weeks. In some instances, however, erysipelas can rapidly lead to deep subcutaneous infection, sepsis, and death, particularly in the young, old, or immunocompromised.

Because almost all erysipelas is caused by streptococci, the treatment of choice is intravenous penicillin for patients who are not allergic. An appropriate dose for treating an adult with erysipelas is 1,000,000 to 2,000,000 U of aqueous penicillin G administered intravenously every 4 hours. Uncomplicated cases do not require an ICU setting. If signs and symptoms continue to progress after 24 to 48 hours of intravenous antibiotic administration, coverage should be broadened to cover rarely causative organisms and culturing should be attempted. The patient may be changed to oral antibiotics and discharged from the hospital when systemic complaints have resolved and the cutaneous lesion is substantially improved. Healing is often accompanied by superficial scaling of involved skin.

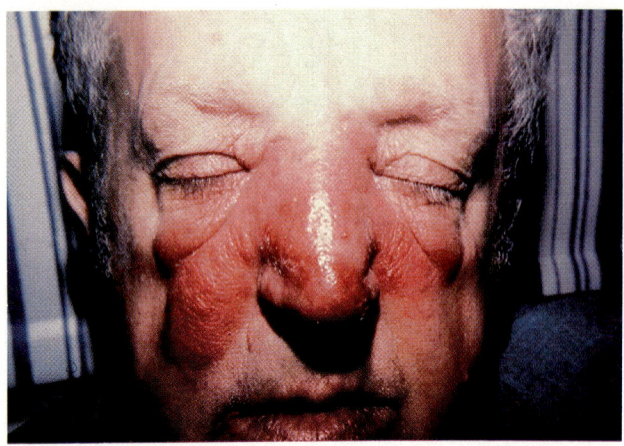

Fig. 46–1. Well-demarcated, red, warm, tender plaque of erysipelas. The face is a common site for this infection. (Courtesy of Division of Dermatology, Brown University, Providence, RI.)

Prominent dermal lymphatic involvement occurs in erysipelas and may leave permanent lymphatic damage. This may result in chronic edema of the affected area and may predispose a small minority of patients to recurrent attacks. Recurrent erysipelas then further damages lymphatics and aggravates the problem.[9] Patients with recurrent erysipelas may require long-term oral antibiotic prophylaxis.[2,11]

CELLULITIS

Pathophysiology and Risk Factors

Cellulitis is an infection involving deep subcutaneous tissue. It is similar to but distinct from erysipelas with respect to clinical appearance, responsible organisms, and treatment. Most cellulitis is caused by either group A streptococci or S. aureus.[1,12,13] Hemophilus influenza type b is a common cause of facial cellulitis in young children[14-16] but has also been described in other locations and in adults.[17]

Cellulitis that is due to group B streptococci may occur in neonates.[18] Pasturella multocida cellulitis may arise from a cat or dog bite,[19] whereas cellulitis that is due to halophilic vibrios commonly occurs in patients exposed to seawater or raw oysters.[20] Other infrequent causes of cellulitis include pneumococci[16,21,22] and Aeromonas hydrophila.[23] Immunosuppressed patients are at increased risk for cellulitis that is due to gram-negative bacteria or Cryptococcus neoformans.[24] Organisms may enter the subcutaneous tissue via a microscopic or obvious wound, ulcer, preceding pyoderma, or rarely from the blood.

Clinical Presentation and Differential Diagnosis

Cellulitis presents as a red, warm, tender, minimally elevated plaque, which, unlike the plaque of erysipelas, does not have a well-demarcated border (Fig. 46–2). The poor demarcation in cellulitis is due to the deeper location of inflammation in cellulitis than in erysipelas. The lesion spreads peripherally and usually feels infiltrated and edematous. Proximal lymphangitis or tender lymphadenopathy may be present. Occasionally, clear or hemorrhagic bullae develop within the plaque.[9] In contrast to erysipelas, fever, malaise, and leukocytosis are present in only about half of patients.[13] Infrequent complications of cellulitis include abscess formation, thrombophlebitis, sepsis, and necrotizing fasciitis.

Pediatric facial cellulitis and perianal cellulitis have some differences in presentation worth noting. A significant proportion of facial cellulitis in young children is due to Hemophilus influenza.[25] In fact, over two thirds of pediatric H. influenza cellulitis occurs on the face,[15,25] where it may be associated with otitis media, sinusitis, nasopharyngitis, or trauma.[14-16] Approximately one half of cases of pediatric H. influenza cellulitis are associated with a blue-red or violaceous color.[14,15,26] This, however, is not a specific finding, because cases of violaceous-colored pneumococcal facial cellulitis have also been described.[21]

Facial cellulitis around the eye is termed periorbital cellulitis. Patients with this disorder may develop lid cellulitis, conjunctivitis, and chemosis. Fortunately, the orbital septum usually prevents this infection from spreading posteriorly and becoming an orbital cellulitis. Orbital cellulitis, in fact, is much more likely to result from extension of a sinusitis than from a preseptal periorbital cellulitis.[16] Signs of orbital cellulitis include proptosis, ophthalmoplegia, and decreased visual acuity (Fig. 46–3).[16] Hemophilus influenza is the most commonly cultured pathogen in both periorbital and orbital pediatric cellulitis. Other significant childhood causes of periorbital or orbital cellulitis include Streptococcus pyogenes, S. aureus, and S. pneumoniae.[16,26] Potential complications of orbital cellulitis are listed in Table 46–1.

Streptococcal perianal cellulitis is usually seen in children, but may rarely occur in adults. This chronic infection may go undiagnosed for months because of a lack of systemic symptoms and confusion with other conditions. These patients present with a red, tender, perianal rash, and painful defecation. Sometimes blood-streaked stool or pruritus is present. Perianal cellulitis is frequently misdi-

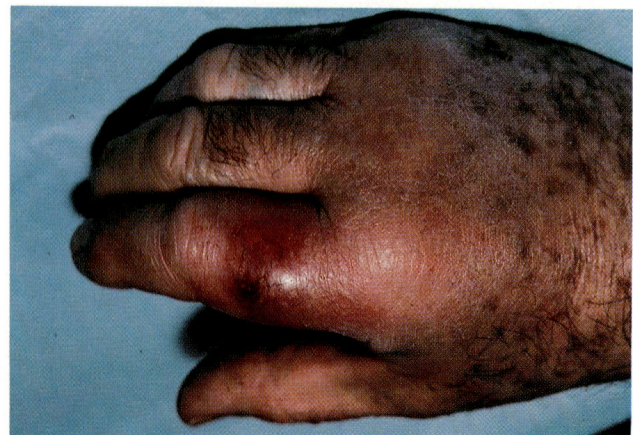

Fig. 46–2. Poorly demarcated, red, warm, tender plaque of cellulitis. (Courtesy of Division of Dermatology, Brown University, Providence, RI.)

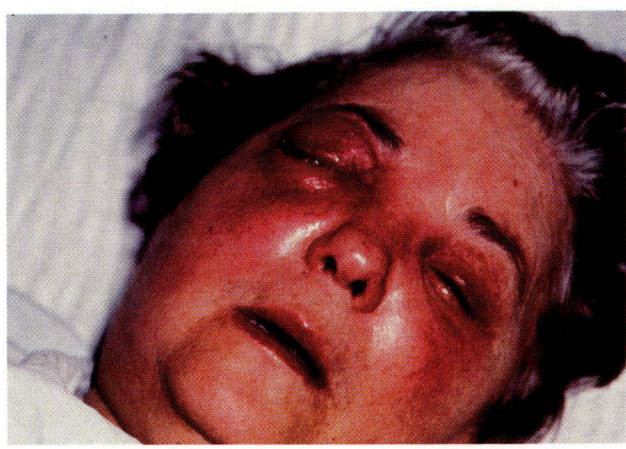

Fig. 46–3. Patient with both periorbital and orbital cellulitis. Note right eye proptosis indicating orbital cellulitis. An ethmoidal abscess was present, requiring surgical drainage. (Courtesy of Division of Dermatology, Brown University, Providence, RI.)

agnosed as diaper dermatitis, seborrheic dermatitis, moniliasis, simple anal fissure, inflammatory bowel disease, pinworm, or psychogenic stool holding.[27,28]

Laboratory Studies

In adult cellulitis, approximately 5% of patients will have positive blood cultures; 10%, positive cultures of subcutaneously injected and aspirated saline; and 20%, positive skin biopsy cultures.[12,13] Because of these low yields, patient discomfort, and the efficacy of empiric therapy, such cultures are not necessary in stable immunocompetent patients. Cultures of any contiguous wounds or pyodermas should be obtained, because these often grow the responsible organism. Even though wound cultures may also grow colonizers that are not responsible for the cellulitis, they often provide as much useful information as the more invasive skin biopsy or saline aspiration cultures.[12]

Blood cultures should always be obtained in children with facial, periorbital, or orbital cellulitis, because they often grow out the pathogen,[16,25,26] and are helpful in guiding antibiotic therapy. Cultures of injected and aspirated saline are positive in about 40% of pediatric cellulitis.[25] In perirectal cellulitis, perirectal swabbings invariably culture out S. pyogenes and should be obtained to make the diagnosis.[27]

Table 46–1. Potential Complications of Orbital Cellulitis

Orbital abscess
Subperiosteal abscess
Cavernous sinus thrombosis
Osteomyelitis
Meningitis
Epidural abscess
Subdural abscess
Brain abscess

In immunosuppressed patients, continued progression of a cellulitis despite good empiric antibiotic therapy indicates a need for fungal tests. Useful tests for fungal cellulitis include serum cryptococcal antigen titers,[24] microscopic examination of skin aspirates,[24] periodic acid Schiff-stained skin biopsy, and tissue fungal culture.

Treatment

Patients with cellulitis do not require treatment in an ICU unless the infection progresses to necrotizing fasciitis or sepsis with shock. Only a low grade cellulitis without systemic symptoms may be treated with oral antibiotics; therefore, many patients require hospital admission for intravenous therapy.

Patients with periorbital cellulitis almost always require hospitalization for intravenous antibiotics, in addition to careful ophthalmologic, otolaryngologic, and neurologic exams. Sinus films should be obtained and will disclose a sinusitis in one half of cases.[16] The presence of proptosis, ophthalmoplegia, or decreased visual acuity indicates an orbital cellulitis, which merits close attention. An orbital cellulitis accompanied by decreasing vision, worsening ophthalmoplegia, increasing proptosis, or poor response to therapy requires computed tomography scanning of the orbit and surgical intervention.[16,29] Surgery is used to drain abscesses or infected sinuses.[16]

Initial antibiotic therapy of cellulitis in adults should cover both streptococci and S. aureus. This often entails a semisynthetic penicillinase-resistant penicillin or a first-generation cephalosporin in patients who are not allergic. An alternative approach is to use penicillin, broadening coverage to treat S. aureus if the response is poor. If unusual organisms are suspected because of the clinical setting, cultures become more important, and antibiotic coverage should be broadened to cover the suspected organisms. Facial, periorbital, and orbital cellulitis in young children, but not adults, requires antibiotics that fully cover H. influenza, in addition to streptococci and S. aureus. This often consists of a semisynthetic penicillinase-resistant penicillin and chloramphenicol, or single-agent therapy with ceftriaxone or ampicillin/sulbactam.[30] In any cellulitis, if no response to intravenous antibiotics is seen within 24 to 48 hours, antibiotic coverage should be broadened, and necrotizing fasciitis considered. In a stable patient, antibiotic coverage should be narrowed if cultures identify a causative organism.

Recovery

Patients may be changed from intravenous to oral antibiotics when the cutaneous lesion has improved considerably, and the patient is without systemic symptoms. The vast majority of immunocompetent patients with cellulitis do extremely well with treatment. Even periorbital and orbital cellulitis has a good prognosis. In one series of 165 pediatric patients with periorbital or orbital cellulitis, one patient died, 9% required surgery for complications, and no patients developed permanent neurologic sequelae.[16] As with erysipelas, lymphatic damage from cellulitis may result in chronic lymphedema and recurrent attacks. If control of edema by external compressive wraps does not limit the frequency of recurrences, chronic antibiotic prophylaxis is indicated. Tinea pedis provides a site of entry for recurrent cellulitis and should therefore be treated in patients with a history of lower extremity cellulitis.

STAPHYLOCOCCAL SCALDED SKIN SYNDROME

Pathophysiology

Staphylococcal scalded skin syndrome (SSSS) is a generalized cutaneous bullous and exfoliative process caused by toxin-producing strains of S. aureus. It is most often seen in children under 5 years of age but can rarely occur in adults. Studies in mice and humans have shown the syndrome to be the direct result of a staphylococcal toxin.

The first description of SSSS was by Baron Gottfried Ritter von Rittershain (1820 to 1889), who reported nearly 300 cases of the disease affecting neonates in a Prague foundling hospital.[31] Ritter von Rittershain named the disease dermatitis exfoliativa neonatorum because of the exfoliative nature of the rash. An association with occult staphylococcal infection was soon noted. In 1956, Lyell described cases of a cutaneous syndrome resembling scalded skin, naming the condition toxic epidermal necrolysis.[32] It was subsequently shown that some of Lyell's cases were identical to Ritter's disease (SSSS), while others were a distinct disease entity, presently retaining the name toxic epidermal necrolysis. Important differences between these two syndromes will be discussed.

Not all strains of S. aureus can cause SSSS. By the early 1960s, it became apparent that most SSSS is caused by phage group 2 strains of S. aureus. In 1970 a mouse model of the disease was developed by Melish and Glasgow by injecting newborn mice with toxin-producing staphylococci.[33]

The toxin that causes SSSS has been given various names including epidermolysin, exfoliatin, and exfoliative toxin. There are two antigenic forms of the toxin, designated exfoliatins A and B. Both forms have similar molecular weights but have different stabilities in ethylenediamine tetra-acetate or when heated. Exfoliatin A is encoded for by chromosomal genes, while exfoliatin B is plasmid encoded.[34]

In the United States, exfoliative toxin is usually produced by phage group 2 S. aureus; less frequently, by organisms belonging to phage groups 1 or 3. This is in contrast to the present situation in Japan, where the majority of exfoliative toxin-producing isolates now belong to phage groups 1 or 3. In previous years, Japanese toxin-producing strains were usually phage group 2 organisms.[34-36] Implicated strains may produce exfoliatins A or B or both.[34]

The effect of exfoliative toxin is quite specific. A split in the granular layer of the skin is induced, resulting in a superficial vesicle located just beneath the stratum corneum.[33] Vesicles enlarge to form bullae, which easily rupture, giving the appearance of scalded skin.

Risk Factors

SSSS is almost invariably seen in a setting of either inadequate renal clearance of toxin or a compromised immune response. The increased susceptibility of infants and young children is due to their lower renal clearance rate compared with adults. Nephrectomized adult mice develop SSSS from toxin injection, whereas normal adult mice do not. This is in contrast to infant mice, who develop SSSS without the aid of nephrectomy.[37]

Other studies suggest that antibody production against exfoliative toxin is important in limiting the toxin's effects. Mice and humans convalescing from SSSS have a rise in anti-exfoliative toxin antibody titers.[34,38] Anti-exfoliative toxin antibody neutralizes the effect of injected exfoliative toxin in mice,[34] and adult humans with substantial levels of antiexfoliative toxin antibodies are resistant to the local effects of intracutaneously injected exfoliative toxin.[37] In one study, 14 of 16 adults without a history of SSSS showed significant anti-exfoliation A antibody titers, apparently the result of prior infections with exfoliative toxin-producing strains of staphylococci.[38] Immunocompetent adult mice do not develop SSSS after exfoliative toxin injection but do if pretreated with immunosuppressants.[39]

Clinical Presentation

In infants and young children, SSSS is usually associated with staphylococcal infection or colonization of the eyes, ears, nose, throat, or anus. The infection may be obvious but is frequently occult.[40] Cutaneous primary infections are uncommon but may occur as staphylococcal impetigo, omphalitis, or circumcision wound infection.[41,42] Fortunately, bacteremia is rare.

A child or infant with the syndrome initially presents with irritability and an erythematous, blanchable rash. Fever may or may not be present,[43-45] and leukocyte count may be normal or elevated.[43,45] The initial rash is nearly macular and may have a sandpaper texture similar to the rash of scarlet fever. This erythema begins around the mouth and in body folds and often becomes confluent over the entire skin surface within 24 hours. The rash is characteristically tender and develops superficial wrinkling followed by flaccid, ill-defined bullae. These bullae often first appear in intertriginous areas but may involve any cutaneous surface (Fig. 46-4). Friction easily causes wrinkling and displacement of the superficial epidermis, thereby initiating and extending bullae. Cultures of bullae fluid are negative for S. aureus. Because the bullae are fragile, they easily rupture, leaving red, raw, wet erosions and peeling. When first seen by a consulting physician, a patient may in fact have extensive exfoliation and many erosive lesions with few or no evident bullae (Fig. 46-5). As with toxic epidermal necrolysis (Chap. 48), Nikolsky's sign can usually be demonstrated when horizontal pressure with the examiner's finger causes or extends bullae. Patients often have a characteristic periorificial serous crusting (Fig. 46-6), but mucous membranes are never involved.[40,41,44-46]

A milder forme fruste of SSSS, frequently given the name "staphylococcal scarlet fever," has also been described. In these patients, an erythematous scarlatiniform rash develops but does not progress to bullae formation or erosions. The skin often becomes pruritic or slightly tender, and healing is accompanied by scaling and peeling. Similar-

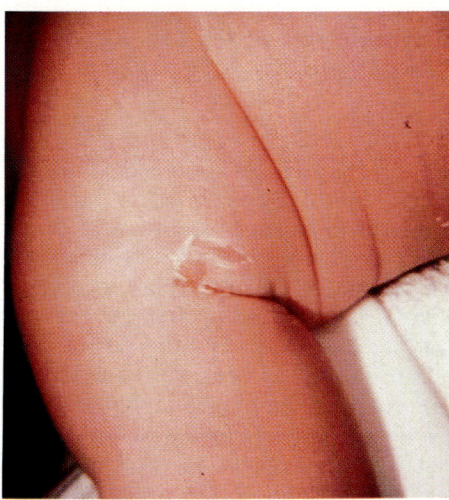

Fig. 46–4. Early staphylococcal scalded skin syndrome. A confluent macular erythema is present. In the intertriginous area near the axilla, a small bulla has formed and ruptured. (Courtesy of Division of Dermatology, Brown University, Providence, RI.)

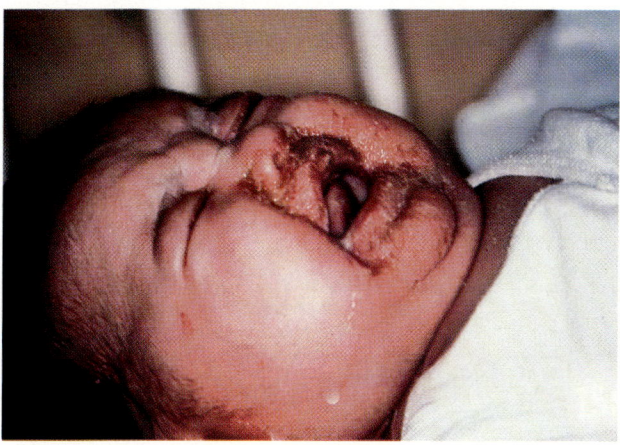

Fig. 46–6. Characteristic periorificial serous crusts of staphylococcal scalded skin syndrome. (Courtesy of Division of Dermatology, Brown University, Providence, RI.)

ities to the rash of streptococcal scarlet fever include a sandpaper texture, accentuation in skin folds, and mild-to-moderate desquamation on resolution. While staphylococcal scarlet fever is characterized by staphylococcal infection and a lack of mucous membrane involvement, the presentation of streptococcal scarlet fever includes streptococcal pharyngitis, a strawberry tongue, and submandibular lymphadenopathy.[41,44,45] The toxin responsible for staphylococcal scarlet fever is exfoliative toxin as opposed to the erythrogenic toxin of streptococcal scarlet fever. The frequency of mild forms of SSSS is not known.[41] When reviewing the literature on staphylococcal scarlet fever, it is important to realize that some cases given this name may represent different disorders that are due to staphylococcal toxins other than exfoliative toxin.

A disease akin to SSSS is bullous impetigo. In this disorder, cutaneous infection from exfoliative toxin-producing S. aureus results in local bullae formation at the site of infection. Significant amounts of toxin do not enter the blood stream, and the rash therefore remains localized to infected areas. Fever and constitutional symptoms are absent. Quite rarely, the infection will spread to much of the cutaneous surface, resulting in an appearance which is easily confused with classic SSSS.[41,45] Fluid from intact bullae, however, will be culture positive, generalized cutaneous tenderness is absent, and biopsy reveals a prominent dermal inflammatory infiltrate unlike the minimal infiltrate seen in SSSS.[37] A continuum between bullous impetigo and SSSS is also known to exist, with some cases of bullous impetigo developing erythema and bullae away from sites of infection.[41] Classic bullous impetigo is seen in patients of all ages, but more frequently in children.[47]

Adults with SSSS are invariably seen in a setting of renal insufficiency, immunosuppression, or overwhelming sepsis. Immunosuppression from leukemia, lymphoma, alcoholism, steroids, antimetabolites,[37] bone marrow transplantation,[48] and acquired immune deficiency syndrome (AIDS)-related complex[49] has been associated with adult SSSS. Immunosuppression may potentiate SSSS by inhibiting both the anti-toxin antibody response and antistaphylococcal defenses. The cutaneous signs and symptoms in adult SSSS are the same as those seen in younger patients. Unlike the setting in children, however, many reported cases of adult SSSS involve staphylococcal bacteremia and culture-positive bullae.[37] Whether such cases represent generalized bullous impetigo with local toxin production, a distant effect of toxin produced at an extracutaneous site, or both is uncertain.

Differential Diagnosis and Laboratory Studies

Whenever a patient presents with a generalized, red rash accompanied by bullae or denudation, the first step is to

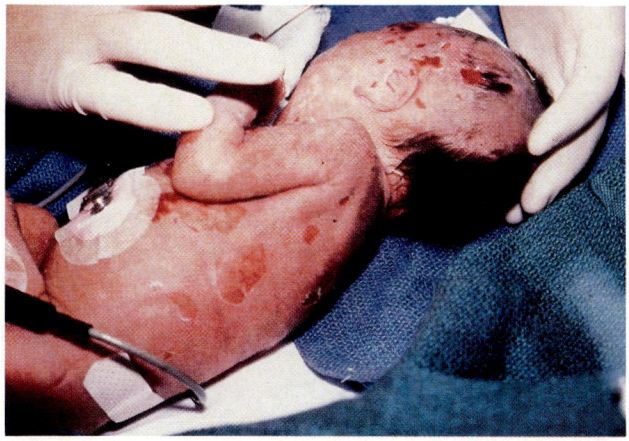

Fig. 46–5. Staphylococcal scalded skin syndrome with generalized erythroderma and numerous erosions. (From Snook, D. L., and McDonald, C. J.: The dermatologic manifestations of critical illness. J. Crit. Illness, 3:93, 1988.)

Table 46-2. Comparison of Staphylococcal Scalded Skin Syndrome (SSSS) and Toxic Epidermal Necrolysis

	SSSS	Toxic Epidermal Necrolysis
"Scalded skin" appearance	present	present
Cutaneous tenderness	present	present
Nikolsky's sign	present	present
Age	usually less than 5 years old, unless immunosuppression, renal failure, or overwhelming staphylococcal sepsis present	any age
Mucous membrane involvement	always absent	usually present
Site of split in skin	subcorneal (in stratum granulosum)	subepidermal (at dermal-epidermal junction)
Keratinocyte Necrosis	absent	present

determine if the patient has SSSS or toxic epidermal necrolysis. Both of these conditions may occur in any age group and are associated with cutaneous tenderness and a positive Nikolsky's sign. Differentiating the two is important, because toxic epidermal necrolysis has a more guarded prognosis and different treatment. Corticosteroids, which have been used to treat toxic epidermal necrolysis, increase the severity of SSSS in both mice[39] and humans.[50]

A comparison of SSSS and toxic epidermal necrolysis is presented in Table 46-2. While by no means diagnostic, age is of some statistical help because infants are more likely to have SSSS, whereas adults are more likely to have toxic epidermal necrolysis. If an adult has renal insufficiency, overwhelming staphylococcal sepsis, or immune compromise, the likelihood of SSSS increases. If characteristic mucous membrane involvement is present, a diagnosis of toxic epidermal necrolysis can be made, because SSSS does not involve mucous membranes. Definitive diagnosis, however, requires a skin biopsy.

While awaiting biopsy results, tissue frozen section or exfoliative cytology may aid in making a tentative diagnosis to guide initial therapy. Cultures of sites potentially harboring staphylococci should also be obtained, because these may later help substantiate a diagnosis or guide antibiotic selection.

Frozen section is done on Nikolsky sign-induced skin peels. In SSSS, microscopy of such tissue reveals an intact stratum corneum with adherent granular cells, whereas full thickness epidermis with necrotic keratinocytes is indicative of toxic epidermal necrolysis.[51]

Exfoliative cells for cytology are obtained by scraping a freshly denuded, Nikolsky-positive area. This material is then smeared on a glass slide, fixed, and stained, creating a Tzank preparation. Either Wright or Giemsa stains may be used. In SSSS, this preparation consists of flattened, nucleated squamous cells with a "fried egg" appearance.

In toxic epidermal necrolysis, necrotic cellular debris, polymorphonuclear leukocytes, and occasional cuboidal keratinocytes are seen.[51]

Treatment

Treatment of SSSS includes intravenous antistaphylococcal antibiotics, topical preparations, and maintenance of fluid and electrolyte balance. An intensive care setting is appropriate if extensive cutaneous denudation or sepsis are present. Neonates usually require incubator support to maintain temperature and prevent excessive fluid loss.

Although pediatric SSSS is often a self-limited process,[43,45] circumstantial evidence indicates that antibiotics may alter the course by limiting toxin production.[50] Antibiotics are of obvious use in adults, who are often immunocompromised or septic. Antibiotics probably also decrease the potential for spread of toxin-producing staphylococci to unaffected individuals.[41] Whenever a tentative diagnosis of SSSS is made, antibiotic therapy is begun immediately. Awaiting final skin biopsy results before beginning antibiotics is not advised. Good choices for intravenous antistaphylococcal antibiotics include oxacillin, nafcillin, first-generation cephalosporins, or vancomycin. Isolation precautions should be instituted, particularly in nurseries, where outbreaks have been known to occur.[45] In an epidemic, staphylococcal isolates may be tested for exfoliative toxin production by the newborn mouse bioassay[33] or a more recently developed latex agglutination technique.[52] Topical preparations are used to limit transcutaneous fluid loss and prevent superinfection. Vaseline-impregnated gauze makes a good dressing because it limits evaporation.[53] Topical antibiotics, such as silver sulfadiazine or mafenide acetate, may be used to lessen the risk of superinfection and subsequent sepsis.[41] In infants less than 2 months old, silver sulfadiazine and mafenide acetate should be avoided, because sulfonamides are known to increase the incidence of kernicterus. Infrequent side effects from transdermal absorption of sulfonamides include bone marrow suppression, metabolic acidosis from carbonic anhydrase inhibition, and hemolytic anemia in glucose-6-phosphate dehydrogenase-deficient individuals. A case of serum hyperosmolality that was due to extensive topical use of propylene glycol-containing silver sulfadiazine cream has also been reported.[54] Effective treatment without the use of topical antibiotics has been documented.[53]

Fluids and electrolytes should be monitored in all patients and replaced accordingly. Loss of fluids or electrolytes and sepsis are the most frequent factors contributing to a fatal outcome. Adult SSSS is a serious disease, with a fatal outcome in approximately one half of reported cases. The poor prognosis in adults is due to their greater incidence of immunosuppression, overwhelming sepsis, and previous debilitating illness.

Recovery

Supportive measures are usually only necessary for a few days.[41] Reepithelialization is rapid because of the superficial nature of the injury. In uncomplicated cases, complete recovery without scarring occurs in 7 to 14 days.[43,45] With recovery, erosions dry up, with a flakey exfoliation as new intact epidermis is produced from below. Topical dressings may be discontinued once an intact epidermis is reformed.

TOXIC SHOCK SYNDROME

Pathophysiology and Risk Factors

Toxic shock syndrome (TSS) is an acute serious illness characterized by fever, rash, hypotension, and functional abnormalities of several organ systems. It is most frequently seen in menstruating women but may occur at any age or in either sex. As with staphylococcal scalded skin syndrome, TSS appears to result from S. aureus toxin production.

The first description of TSS as a distinct disease entity was by Todd and colleagues in 1978.[55] They described the courses of seven children and adolescents who developed an acute syndrome consisting of fever, refractory hypotension, erythroderma, profound watery diarrhea, headache, confusion, and oliguric renal failure. It was noted that most of these patients were either colonized or infected with phage group 1 S. aureus, suggesting a causal role for the organism. Subsequently, a much larger number of similar cases was reported in menstruating women who use tampons. Again, the association with S. aureus colonization was observed, but it became apparent that strains from any phage group could be involved. Cases of nonmenstrual TSS in adults were also noted. The percentage of reported nonmenstrual TSS cases rose from 7% of TSS cases in 1980 to 29% in 1983.[56]

Over 90% of menstrual TSS-associated staphylococcal strains produce a toxin isolated independently by Schlievert et al. (pyrogenic exotoxin C),[57] and Bergdoll et al. (enterotoxin F)[58] in 1981. Both names seem to indicate the same protein, which has since been designated toxic shock syndrome toxin-1 (TST-1). A rabbit model of TSS exists in which rabbits exposed to TST-1 manifest some of the stigmata of TSS.[59] TST-1 is given the numeric designation "1" because strong evidence suggests that other TSS-producing toxins exist. For example, 40% of nonmenstrual TSS cases are associated with S. aureus strains that do not produce TST-1.[60] One of many candidates for a second TSS toxin is enterotoxin B, which is often produced by nonmenstrual TSS-associated staphylococci.[61,62] Of additional interest are reported cases of a syndrome that is similar to classic TSS but is associated with unidentified toxin(s) produced by S. pyogenes.[63-65]

The mode of action of TST-1 has not been fully elucidated. It is known, however, that TST-1 is a potent inducer of interleukin-1 production, which would explain the fever associated with the syndrome.[66] TST-1 also induced production of other mediators of fever or hypotension, including tumor necrosis factors, interleukin-2, and gamma interferon.[67] The extent to which each of these mediators is involved in the pathogenesis of TSS is presently unknown.

An adequate immune response to TST-1 seems to protect against the syndrome. Studies comparing acute, convalescent, and recovered TSS patients with healthy genital S. aureus carriers and healthy noncarriers have shown lower anti-TST-1 antibody levels in the acute, convalescent, and recovering groups versus the other two groups.[61,68] A Utah study investigating the nasal carrier rate of TST-1-producing S. aureus in healthy individuals documented an overall carrier rate of 7%, with a 22% carrier rate in persons under 20 years of age.[69]

Table 46–3. Risk Factors for TST Production

Menstruation (tampon use)
Postpartum period (childbirth, abortion)
Surgical wound infection
Nasal packing
Nonsurgical cutaneous or subcutaneous infections: abscesses, traumatic wounds, ulcers, cellulitis, insect bites, burns, abrasions

Common risk factors for TST production are presented in Table 46–3. A large variety of body sites may be colonized by TSS-producing staphylococci. The site of colonization in menstrual TSS is the vagina. Menstrual TSS begins during or immediately after menstruation and is often associated with the use of vaginal tampons, particularly superabsorbent types. It is theorized that a tampon may alter the vaginal environment in a manner that promotes growth of TST-1-producing staphylococci, or increases TST-1 production.[70] In addition, tampon-induced cervicovaginal ulceration has been postulated to provide a portal of entry for staphylococci and toxin. One histologic study of 12 fatal cases of tampon-associated TSS revealed cervicovaginal ulceration in all of 6 cases in which adequate cervicovaginal tissue specimens were received.[71]

The postpartum vaginal environment may also be conducive to toxin production. Onset of postpartum TSS may be less than 24 hours after childbirth.[72] In one reported postpartum maternal case, the patient's newborn child also become colonized with S. aureus and developed symptoms suggestive of mild TSS.[73]

Other common sites harboring TSS-associated staphylococci include cutaneous and subcutaneous lesions and surgical wounds. As elsewhere, infections in these locations may be occult, with little or no local signs of inflammation. The median interval between surgery and postoperative TSS is 2 days, but onset may occur anywhere from under 24 hours to several weeks after operation.[72] Nasal surgery has been repeatedly associated with TSS, particularly if postoperative nasal packing has been used.[74]

Situations that may infrequently result in TSS include burns, abrasions, insect bites, human bites, herpes zoster, and therapeutic abortions.[72,75] Almost any type of S. aureus infection can produce TSS, including cellulitis, lymphadenitis, bursitis, septic arthritis, nonmenstrual vaginitis, tracheitis, osteomyelitis, lung abscess, and bacteremia.[72,76]

Clinical Presentation and Laboratory Studies

The cardinal features of TSS are fever, rash, and hypotension. The rash is usually a sunburn-like, diffuse, nonpruritic, blanching, macular erythroderma. It is often scarlatiniform, with a "sandpaper" texture and accentuation in skin folds. While usually widespread, the eruption may infrequently be limited to the trunk, extremities, perineum, or vaginal area. The rash is often subtle and may be missed without a careful cutaneous exam. Petechiae are sometimes noted but not a prominent feature. Edema of the hands, face, and feet is often present. A characteristic feature in the recovering patient is a peeling desquamation of the hands and feet.[77,78] Rare cases of TSS have been described in which vesicles or bullae were present along with the more typical erythroderma.[79] Descriptions also exist of a rare papulopustular eruption that involves the lower abdomen, perineum, and thighs with sparing of skin compressed by underwear elastic. This papulopustular eruption is followed by typical hand and foot desquamation during convalescence.[77]

Mucous membranes are also often involved.[77,78] Patients may present with conjunctivitis, strawberry tongue, oral ulcerations, or pharyngitis, any of which may be accompanied by mucosal tenderness. Sometimes, these mucosal changes do not occur until several days after the exanthem has faded. Patients with menstrual TSS may develop vaginal or perineal hyperemia, which is often tender. Sometimes malodorous vaginal purulence is present.[77,78]

Common early symptoms of TSS include fever, nonrigorous chills, myalgias, nausea, vomiting, watery diarrhea, headache, and arthralgias.[77,78,80] Muscle tenderness is a nearly universal finding and is most frequently located on the trunk and proximal limbs. Abdominal muscle tenderness may mimic an acute abdomen, but peritoneal signs are absent. Some patients ache all over and complain that any motion causes pain. A minority of patients have signs of a true arthritis.[77] Cardiovascular compromise may manifest as subjective postural dizziness, orthostatic hypotension, or fulminant hypotensive shock.[77] Tachycardia and tachypnea are often present.[78]

In typical cases, toxin causes widespread organ system dysfunction. Shock is likely due to a combination of third spacing from capillary leakage, vasodilatation, cardiomyopathy, and gastrointestinal fluid loss. Adult respiratory distress syndrome or myocardial irritability may develop.[80,81] Toxic encephalopathy may manifest as confusion, agitation, or somnolence. A lumbar puncture may be needed to evaluate findings of neck stiffness and tenderness. Cerebrospinal fluid analysis reveals at most a small number of leukocytes (greater than 50% mononuclear) with normal protein and glucose concentrations.[80] Rare cases of death secondary to cerebral edema have been reported.[82] Frequently noted renal failure may be due to both acute tubular necrosis and prerenal factors.[71,81] Urine output is often in the oliguric range. Urinalysis reveals pyuria in over half of patients with TSS, but proteinuria or sizable hematuria are infrequently seen.[81] If the rash is missed, pyuria may lead the physician to make an incorrect diagnosis of pyelonephritis with septic shock.[81] Liver damage frequently occurs with elevated serum glutamic-oxaloacetic transferase and bilirubin levels. Sometimes hepatomegaly is noted on examination. Muscle damage may result in prominent elevations of serum creatinine phosphokinase.[77,81]

Complete blood cell count often shows a leukocytosis, which is usually remarkable for an increase in immature neutrophils.[77,78,81] Mild thrombocytopenia, along with increases in prothrombin time, partial thromboplastin time, and fibrin degradation products may occur, but petechiae are usually not prominent, and clinical bleeding is extremely rare.[77] Frequently occurring electrolyte and protein abnormalities include hyponatremia, hypocalcemia, hypophosphatemia (despite renal failure), hypoalbuminemia, and hypoproteinemia. Hypotensive patients often develop a lactic acidosis.[80,81] Decreases in serum albumin and protein concentrations are probably due to increased capillary permeability.[81]

Diagnosis

The Centers for Disease Control and Prevention (CDC) criteria required for a definitive diagnosis of TSS are listed in Table 46-4.[83] The cardinal features to look for on presentation are fever, typical rash, and hypotension or dizziness. It is very important to do a thorough cutaneous examination with good lighting so as to avoid missing the rash. Fortunately, the rash is usually present at time of presentation or appears within 24 hours of admission. Other previously mentioned frequent signs and symptoms are supportive evidence, as is a recent history of menstruation, tampon use, surgery, or childbirth.

Diseases that may be confused with TSS include scarlet fever, Kawasaki's disease, and staphylococcal scalded skin syndrome. All three of these conditions involve fever and rashes that share characteristics with the rash of TSS. None of these three diseases are associated with shock or hypotension.

A patient with streptococcal scarlet fever may present with a rash that is indistinguishable from the rash of TSS. Other characteristic features of scarlet fever that may occur in TSS include pharyngitis, strawberry tongue, and postrash desquamation. Nausea, vomiting, headache, mal-

Table 46-4. Centers for Disease Control Case Definition of Toxic Shock Syndrome

---

Fever: Temperature greater than or equal to 38.9°C (102°F)
Rash: Diffuse macular erythroderma
Desquamation: 1 to 2 weeks after onset of illness, particularly of palms and soles
Hypotension: Systolic blood pressure less than or equal to 90 mm Hg for adults or below fifth percentile by age of children below 16 years old, orthostatic drop in diastolic blood pressure greater than or equal to 15 mm Hg from lying to sitting, orthostatic syncope, or orthostatic dizziness
Multisystemic involvement: three or more of the following:
  gastrointestinal: Vomiting or diarrhea at onset of illness
  Muscular: Severe myalgia or creatinine phosphokinase level at least twice the upper limit of normal for laboratory
  Mucous membrane: Vaginal, oropharyngeal, or conjunctival hyperemia
  Renal: Blood urea nitrogen or creatinine at least twice the upper limit of normal for laboratory, or urinary sediment with pyuria (greater than or equal to 5 leukocytes per high-power field) in the absence of urinary tract infection
  Hepatic: Total bilirubin, SGOT, or SGPT at least twice the upper limit of normal for laboratory
  Hematologic: Platelets less than or equal to 100,000/mm³
  CNS: Disorientation or alterations in consciousness without focal neurologic signs when fever and hypotension are absent
Negative results on the following tests, if obtained:
  Blood, throat, or cerebrospinal fluid cultures (blood cultures may be positive for S. aureus)
  Rise in titer to Rocky Mountain spotted fever, leptospirosis, or rubeola

aise, and abdominal pain may also occur in both disorders. Hypotension or evidence of acute serious internal organ involvement, however, do not develop in streptococcal scarlet fever.

Characteristic features of Kawasaki's disease that may occur in TSS include fever, rash, conjunctivitis, oropharyngeal inflammation, strawberry tongue, hand and foot edema, and convalescent hand and foot desquamation. Abdominal pain, proteinuria, pyuria, and diarrhea may also be seen with both conditions. One of the many types of rashes that has been described in Kawasaki's disease is a scarlatiniform eruption similar to the rash of TSS. Unlike TSS, Kawasaki's disease presents with cervical lymphadenopathy, rarely occurs in adults, and is not accompanied by hypotension.

The diffuse erythematous rash of SSSS is similar to that of TSS but is accompanied by a positive Nikolsky's sign. Unlike the situation in TSS, hypotension, internal organ involvement, and mucous membrane inflammation do not occur in SSSS. Exfoliative toxin, which causes SSSS, is not a cause of TSS. Some cases of "staphylococcal scarlet fever" (discussed earlier in this chapter) may not be forme frustes of SSSS but instead are cases of TSS without shock. This is particularly likely in cases of staphylococcal scarlet fever, which are accompanied by mucous membrane inflammation. Such cases of probable TSS do not meet the CDC criteria for TSS (see Table 46-4).

To further complicate the situation, there are recently reported cases of an illness that is nearly identical to TSS but caused by Streptococcus pyogenes. Likely the result of streptococcal toxin, this syndrome has been called "toxic strep syndrome" or "streptococcal toxic shock."[63-65]

Treatment

When confronted with a patient who may have TSS, the first step is to check vital signs to assess if immediate support of blood pressure is needed with intravenous fluids and vasopressor agents. Then history taking and physical examination are used to gather evidence to suggest the diagnosis. If a diagnosis of TSS is likely, because of findings of fever, characteristic rash, and hypotension or orthostatic symptoms, the patient should be admitted to an ICU. Routine blood tests are obtained, including complete blood cell count, liver function tests, electrolytes, blood urea nitrogen, creatinine, calcium, phosphorus, albumin, prothrombin time, partial thromboplastin time, platelets, and creatinine phosphokinase. Continuous monitoring of cardiac electrical activity, heart rate, blood pressure, respiratory rate, and urine output is important in managing very ill, hemodynamically unstable patients.[84] Urine, when obtainable, is sent for urinalysis and culture. A chest radiograph is done, and if respiratory distress is evident, appropriate intervention is necessary (see Chap. 17). The skin is carefully inspected for wounds, abscesses, or other sites that may harbor staphylococci. Cultures and Gram's stains are obtained from such sites, in addition to nose, conjunctiva, pharynx, rectum, and vagina. Culture results are eventually used to make the definitive diagnosis, rule out streptococcal toxic shock, and guide antibiotic therapy. It is very important to remove tampons or surgical packings, drain abscesses, debride wounds, and irrigate purulent sites.[84]

The mainstay of therapy for TSS is cardiovascular support with intravenous crystalloid, supplemented by pressors as needed. Treating shock is likely to minimize damage to internal organs. In one reported series, patients required anywhere from 2.4 to 20 L of normal saline or lactate-Ringer's during the first 24 hours of hospitalization.[84] A minority of patients require pressors.[77,80,84] Use of intravenous albumin should probably be limited, because it has the theoretical potential of worsening adult respiratory distress syndrome. Patients with adult respiratory distress syndrome often require intubation, and are managed by methods described in Section II. Fortunately, many patients do not develop adult respiratory distress syndrome and may require only oxygen supplementation by nasal cannula.

Intravenous antibiotics appropriate for penicillinase-producing S. aureus should be administered, even though their efficacy in reducing morbidity or mortality has never been proven. Antibiotic treatment of an episode of TSS is, however, associated with a decreased incidence of recurrent episodes.[84] If the patient continues to deteriorate, it may be prudent to add intravenous penicillin to fully cover the rare possibility of streptococcal toxic shock.

Renal failure is minimized by treating shock. If pressors are required, dopamine may be useful in preserving renal blood flow. A minority of patients eventually require dialysis.[81,84] Electrolyte and acid/base disorders are managed using conventional methods discussed in Chapter 38. Calcium, in particular, should be aggressively replaced if the concentration of ionized calcium is low. Fortunately, hypocalcemic tetany is rare, which is perhaps due to the frequent presence of hypoalbuminemia.[81,84] In rare instances, fresh-frozen plasma or cryoprecipitate may be required to manage clinically significant disseminated intravascular coagulation.

Recovery

The first signs of patient recovery are a return of hemodynamic stability and a decrease in cutaneous erythema. The patient may be transferred out of the ICU when blood pressure no longer requires fluid or pressor support and intubation is not needed. Further hospitalization outside of the ICU is used to correct electrolyte imbalances, facilitate pulmonary recovery, manage renal failure, and make sure that toxin production has ceased. Patients with menstrual TSS should discontinue tampon use and be educated to recognize early signs of TSS, which may occur during future menses. Fortunately, most relapses are of decreased severity and do not meet the strict CDC criteria for TSS.[80]

With recovery, cutaneous erythema, extremity and facial edema, and mucosal inflammation resolve. The diffuse erythema usually fades in about 3 days. Desquamation of skin of the hands and feet is characteristically seen 5 to 12 days after the erythematous rash resolves.[77,80] Late-onset pruritic, maculopapular rashes have been described, but these may represent antibiotic drug eruptions.[83] Potential sequelae of TSS include reversible hair or nail loss, prolonged weakness, fatigue, amenorrhea, myalgias, paresthesias, chronic renal failure, and reversible vocal cord paralysis.[77,80,81,84]

Although TSS is a quite serious disease, the prognosis is good with therapy. The case fatality rate for menstrual TSS dropped from 15% before 1979 to 3.1% in 1981 and has remained the same since. This decrease in mortality likely reflects increased reporting of milder cases but may in small part be due to earlier therapeutic intervention.[83] Nonmenstrual TSS seems to have a more guarded prognosis, with a reported mortality rate of 11%.[61] Fortunately, early diagnosis and rapid institution of appropriate therapy usually results in full patient recovery.

NECROTIZING FASCIITIS

Pathophysiology and Risk Factors

Necrotizing fasciitis is an acute necrotizing infection that primarily involves superficial fascia and subcutaneous tissue, resulting in extensive undermining of overlying structures.[85] This entity was originally described by Meleney as a beta-hemolytic streptococcal infection,[86] but it eventually became apparent that necrotizing fasciitis may also be caused by other organisms, often acting in synergy. In one detailed prospective study of 16 patients, cultures from 3 patients grew group A streptococci, while the remainder grew facultative bacteria (e.g., non-group A streptococci or Enterobacteriaceae) and an anaerobe (e.g., Peptostreptococcus or Bacteroides).[87] Infrequent single-agent causes of necrotizing fasciitis include group B, C, and G streptococci;[88,89] halophilic vibrios;[90] and H. influenza.[91] The percentage of cases that is due to group A streptococci alone has varied greatly among different series.[90-94]

Predisposing factors for necrotizing fasciitis include diabetes, peripheral vascular disease, and intravenous drug abuse.[88,95] Many patients, however, have no underlying medical problems. Access of pathogenic organisms to the fascia may occur in various settings including occult or obvious trauma, surgical wounds, cutaneous ulcers, perirectal abscesses, intravenous drug use, and intestinal perforation.[93,95-97] Group A streptococcal infection tends to occur after minor trauma, whereas synergistic infections often arise from surgical wounds or perirectal abscesses.[85] This, however, is only a generalization; accurate prediction of causative agents is not possible at time of presentation. The infection easily spreads along subcutaneous fascial planes causing inflammatory edema, vascular thrombosis, and necrosis.

Clinical Presentation

During the initial stages of necrotizing fasciitis, the skin surface appears normal, but eventually a cellulitic area of poorly demarcated erythema and edema is noted. As the underlying blood supply is compromised, the cellulitic area takes on a cyanotic hue. Subsequently, bullae and cutaneous gangrene may develop (Fig. 46-7).[85] Because skin surface changes lag behind those in the fascia, the area of fascial necrosis is often much larger than that of the surface lesion. Patients often become systemically ill with fever, leukocytosis, and tachycardia.[85,90,95]

Although pain may initially be prominent,[88,95] the skin

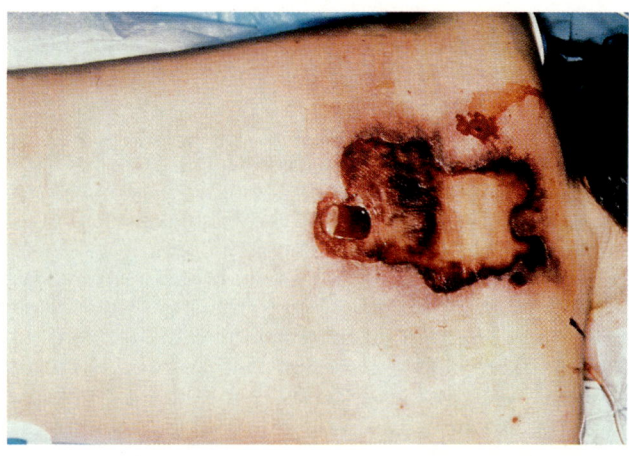

Fig. 46–7. Necrotizing fasciitis. On the upper back is a dusky, gangrenous, anesthetic plaque with an intact bulla at the inferior pole. (From Falcone, P. A., Pricolo, V. E., and Edstrom, L. E.: Necrotizing fasciitis as a complication of chickenpox. Clin. Pediatr., 27:339, 1988.)

often becomes anesthetized because its innervation is destroyed by the subcutaneous gangrene. This loss of sensation is a key feature distinguishing necrotizing fasciitis from simple cellulitis. Gangrenous crepitus is present only if there is prominent anaerobe involvement.[85] In one series of patients, 93% had evident cellulitis, 34% developed surface gangrene, 27% developed cutaneous anesthesia, 11% developed vesicles, and 5% had crepitus on examination.[92] These percentages will, of course, vary with promptness of treatment.

Necrotizing fasciitis of the male genitalia is termed Fournier's gangrene. In this location, infection advances rapidly between Buck's fascia and the dartos fascia of the genitalia, Colle's fascia of the perineum, and Scarpa's fascia of the abdominal wall. Massive genital edema and gangrene often develop (Fig. 46-8), but fortunately, the testicles are normally spared because of their separate blood supply.[96,98]

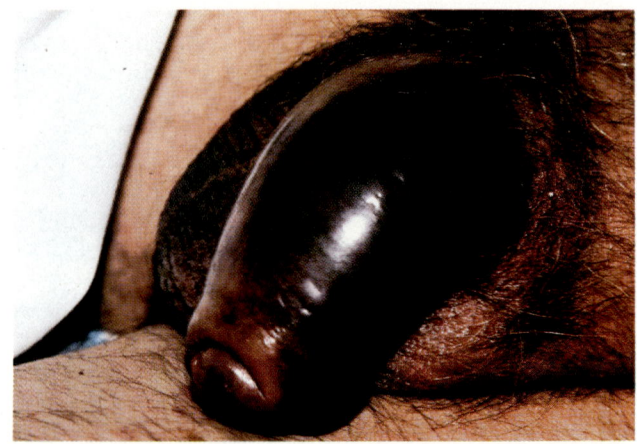

Fig. 46–8. Fournier's gangrene. Edematous penile gangrene. (Courtesy of Division of Dermatology, Brown University, Providence, RI.)

As with other necrotizing fasciitis, group A streptococcal or synergistic infection may be present, and cutaneous signs are similar.

Differential Diagnosis

Disease syndromes that may be confused with necrotizing fasciitis, because of similar cutaneous signs, include clostridial myonecrosis, progressive bacterial synergistic gangrene, and phycomycotic gangrenous cellulitis. Clostridial myonecrosis is distinguished at surgical debridement by prominent muscle necrosis and large gram-positive rods on exudate Gram's stain. Patients with clostridial myonecrosis have a fulminant course with impressive toxemia. Treatment includes debridement of necrotic muscle and intravenous penicillin. A commonly used synonym for clostridial myonecrosis is gas gangrene.[85]

Like necrotizing fasciitis, progressive bacterial synergistic gangrene was first described by Meleney. Also called Meleney's ulcer, this infection presents as a slowly but relentlessly enlarging gangrenous ulcer, usually arising around an abdominal or thoracic surgical wound. An initially cellulitic area appears one to several weeks after surgery and evolves into an undermined ulcer with gangrenous margins. Pain may be severe, but systemic symptoms are minimal. Cultures consistently grow microaerophilic streptococci from the margin of the lesion, and S. aureus or an Enterobacteriaceae sp. from the center. Meleney produced similar lesions in dogs by injecting both microaerophilic streptococci and S. aureus, confirming the synergistic nature of the lesion.[99] Treatment consists of debridement and appropriate antibiotics. In recalcitrant cases, surgical excision is required.[85]

Phycomycotic gangrenous cellulitis is an infection of subcutaneous and often fascial tissues by fungi belonging to the class Phycomycetes. Prominent vascular invasion by these organisms results in avascular tissue necrosis. Patients with this entity usually have predisposing conditions such as diabetes, burns, immunocompromise, and broad-spectrum antibiotic use. Rare cases of phycomycotic gangrenous cellulitis have a fulminant course, mimicking necrotizing fasciitis. A significant number of fulminant presentations has been due to Rhizopus sp.[100] Diagnosis may be made in several ways including fungal culture, tissue biopsy, frozen section, and potassium hydroxide preparation.[85] Tissue for these studies is best obtained from the periphery of the lesion. The fungi stain with periodic acid-Schiff (PAS) and methenamine-silver stains and appear on tissue microscopy as large, branching, mostly aseptate hyphae. Treatment includes debridement and intravenous amphotericin B.[100]

Treatment

It is important to suspect necrotizing fasciitis as early as possible, because progression may be quite rapid, and early surgical intervention results in decreased mortality.[92,95] A careful cutaneous exam is therefore extremely important. Presentation may be subtle, and spontaneous cases have been initially diagnosed as arthritis or phlebitis.[94] Any cellulitis that continues to advance despite appropriate antibiotic therapy or develops cutaneous anes-

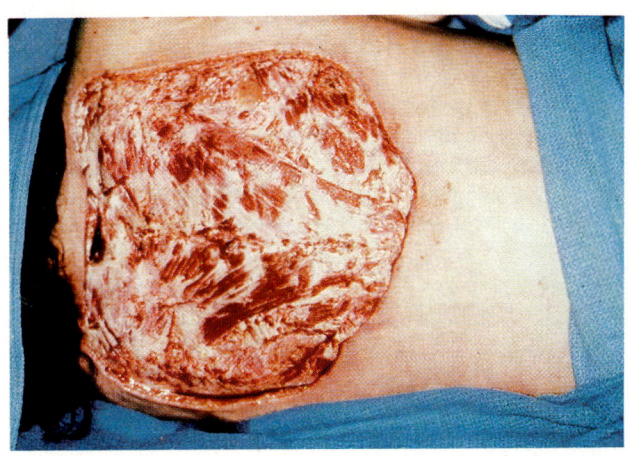

Fig. 46–9. Necrotizing fasciitis. Postdebridement wound of patient shown in Figure 46–7. Note that the area requiring debridement was larger than the overlying cutaneous changes. (From Falcone, P. A., Pricolo, V. E., and Edstrom, L. E.: Necrotizing fasciitis as a complication of chickenpox. Clin. Pediatr., 27:339, 1988.)

thesia requires immediate surgical exploration. A useful diagnostic technique for subtle cases is to obtain a bedside excisional biopsy of skin, subcutis, and fascia, and send it for frozen section. Results are rapid and may lead to earlier surgery and improved survival.[93]

All patients with necrotizing fasciitis require surgical debridement of necrotic fascia in addition to antibiotics for successful treatment. The definitive diagnosis of necrotizing fasciitis is made during surgical exploration, when necrotic fascia is visualized, and undermining is demonstrated by the ease of passing a blunt instrument along fascial planes.[85] During surgical exploration, devitalized areas are exposed and debrided. This often creates a large wound, which is left open (Fig. 46–9). Gram's stains of surgically obtained exudate are used to guide antibiotic therapy and are helpful in ruling out clostridial infection. Exudate is also sent for aerobic, anaerobic, and fungal cultures. Although the presence of necrotic muscle suggests clostridial myonecrosis, it is important to remember that other organisms can produce myonecrosis, including bacteria commonly involved in necrotizing fasciitis.[85] In most cases of necrotizing fasciitis, however, the muscle is not involved. Fungal studies should be done to rule out phycomycotic infection, even if bacteria are present on Gram's stain.[85] A foul-smelling exudate indicates the presence of facultative or obligate anaerobes.

In synergistic infections, antibiotic coverage of gram-positive, gram-negative, and anaerobic bacteria is often necessary. A pure group A streptococcal infection is treated with intravenous penicillin in patients who are not allergic. Hyperbaric oxygen therapy has been used against anaerobes but is of uncertain usefulness.[90] If a patient is receiving a nonsteroidal anti-inflammatory drug, it may be prudent to discontinue it because of recent reports of a potential association of these drugs with a fulminant course.[94]

Because severe cases may progress to muscle necrosis,

sepsis, shock, delirium, coma, and death, ICU placement is indicated for patients with necrotizing fasciitis. In the ICU, cardiovascular support, pulmonary support, perioperative care, and meticulous wound care can be provided. Repeat debridement is usually necessary and may require a repeat visit to the operating room.[95] Mortality rates ranging from 6 to 73% have been reported,[95] with most series having greater than 30% mortality.[93]

Recovery

An intensive care setting is no longer needed when the infection stops progressing and cardiopulmonary support is not required. Sterile dressings are used to prevent wound superinfection, and proper nutrition is ensured to speed healing. A large wound resulting from debridement may be covered by a skin graft after infection has resolved and granulation tissue has formed within the wound bed.[97]

REFERENCES

1. Bernard, P. et al.: Streptococcal cause of erysipelas and cellulitis in adults. Arch. Dermatol., 125:779, 1989.
2. Binnick, A. N., Klein, R. P., and Baughman, R. D.: Recurrent erysipelas caused by group B streptococcus organisms. Arch. Dermatol., 116:798, 1980.
3. Shama, S.: Atypical erysipelas caused by group G streptococci in a patient with cured Hodgkin's disease. Arch. Dermatol., 118:934, 1982.
4. Varghese, R., Melo, J. C., Chun, C., and Raff, M. J.: Erysipelas-like syndrome caused by streptococcus pneumoniae. South. Med. J., 72:757, 1979.
5. Burton, I. F., and Sosin, A.: Erysipelatous skin necrosis in a newborn infant caused by lethal toxin of staphylococcal origin. Pediatrics, 18:249, 1956.
6. Hagen, A., Lassen, J., and Berge, L. N.: Erysipelas-like disease caused by Yersinia enterocolitica. Scand. J. Infect. Dis., 6:101, 1974.
7. Cupps, T. R., Cotton, D. J., Schooley, R. T., and Fauci, A. S.: Facial erysipelas in the immunocompromised host. Arch. Dermatol., 117:47, 1981.
8. Ronnen, N., Suster, S., Schewach-Millet, M., and Modan, M.: Erysipelas: changing faces. Int. J. Dermatol., 24:169, 1985.
9. Schwartz, M. N., and Weinberg, A. N.: Infections due to gram-positive bacteria. In Dermatology in General Medicine. 3rd Ed. Edited by T. B. Fitzpatrick et al. New York, McGraw-Hill, 1987.
10. Leppard, B. J., Seal, D. V., Colman, G., and Hallas, G.: The value of bacteriology and serology in the diagnosis of cellulitis and rysipelas. Br. J. Dermatol., 112:559, 1985.
11. Bitnun, S.: Prophylactic antibiotics in recurrent erysipelas. Lancet, 1:345, 1985.
12. Hook, E. W. et al.: Microbiologic evaluation of cutaneous cellulitis in adults. Arch. Intern. Med., 146:295, 1986.
13. Newell, P. M., and Norden, C. W.: Value of needle aspiration in bacteriologic diagnosis of cellulitis in adults. Clin. Microbiol., 26:401, 1988.
14. Rasmussen, J. E.: Haemophilus influenza cellulitis: case presentation and review of the literature. Br. J. Dermatol., 88:547, 1973.
15. Nelson, J. D., and Ginsburg, C. M.: A hypothesis of the pathogenesis of hemophilus influenza buccal cellulitis. J. Pediatr., 88:709, 1976.
16. Rubinstein, J. B., and Handler, S. D.: Orbital and periorbital cellulitis in children. Head Neck Surg., 5:15, 1982.
17. McDonnell, W. M., Roth, M. S., and Sheagren, J. N.: Hemophilus influenza type b cellulitis in adults. Am. J. Med., 81:709, 1986.
18. Brady, M. T.: Cellulitis of the penis and scrotum due to group B streptococcus. J. Urol., 137:736, 1986.
19. Weber, D. J., Wolfson, J. S., Swartz, M. N., and Hooper, D. C.: Pasteurella multocida infections: report of 34 cases and review of the literature. Medicine (Baltimore), 63:133, 1984.
20. Howard, R. J., and Lieb, S.: Soft-tissue infections caused by halophilic marine vibrios. Arch. Surg., 123:245, 1988.
21. Thirumoorthi, M. C., Asmar, B. I., and Dajani, A. S.: Violaceous discoloration in pneumococcal cellulitis. Pediatrics, 62:492, 1978.
22. Mujais, S., and Uwaydah, M.: Pneumococcal cellulitis. Infection, 11:173, 1983.
23. Bateman, J. L. et al.: Aeromonas hydrophila cellulitis and wound infections caused by waterborne organisms. Heart Lung, 17:99, 1988.
24. Mayers, D. L., Martone, W. J., and Mandell, G. L.: Cutaneous cryptococcosis mimicking gram-positive cellulitis in a renal transplant patient. South. Med. J., 74:1032, 1981.
25. Fleisher, G., Ludwig, S., and Campon, J.: Cellulitis: bacterial etiology, clinical features, and laboratory findings. J. Pediatr., 97:591, 1980.
26. Powell, K. R. et al.: Periorbital cellulitis: clinical and laboratory findings in 146 episodes, including tear countercurrent immunoelectrophoresis in 89 episodes. Am. J. Dis. Child., 142:853, 1988.
27. Rehder, P. A., Eliezer, E. T., and Lane, A. T.: Perianal cellulitis: cutaneous group A streptococcal disease. Arch. Dermatol., 124:702, 1988.
28. Marks, V. J., and Maksimak, M.: Perianal streptococcal cellulitis. J. Am. Acad. Dermatol., 18:587, 1988.
29. Gold, S. C., Arrigg, P. G., and Hedges, T. R.: Computerized tomography in the management of acute orbital cellulitis. Ophthal. Surg., 18:753, 1987.
30. Kulhanjian, J. et al.: Randomized comparative study of ampicillin/sulbactam vs. ceftriaxone for treatment of soft tissue and skeletal infection in children. Pediatr. Infect. Dis. J., 8:605, 1989.
31. Ritter von Rittershain, G.: Die exfoliative dermatitis jungerer sauglinge. Zentralzeitung Kinderheilkund., 2:3, 1878.
32. Lyell, A.: Toxic epidermal necrolysis: an eruption resembling scalding of the skin. Br. J. Dermatol., 68:355, 1956.
33. Melish, M. E., and Glasgow, L. A.: The staphylococcal scalded skin syndrome: development of an experimental mouse model. N. Engl. J. Med., 282::1114, 1970.
34. Rogolsky, M.: Nonenteric toxins of Staphylococcus aureus. Microbiol. Rev., 43:320, 1980.
35. Sarai, Y. et al.: A bacteriological study on children with staphylococcal toxic epidermal necrolysis in Japan. Dermatologica, 154:161, 1977.
36. Murono, K., Fujita, K., and Yoshioka, H.: Microbiologic characteristics of exfoliative toxin-producing Staphylococcus aureus. Pediatr. Infect. Dis. J., 7:313, 1988.
37. Borchers, S. L., Gomez, E. C., and Isseroff, R. R.: Generalized staphylococcal scalded skin syndrome in an anephric boy undergoing hemodialysis. Arch. Dermatol., 120:912, 1984.
38. Baker, D. H., Wuepper, K. D., and Rasmussen, J. E.: Staphylococcal scalded skin syndrome: detection of antibody to epidermolytic toxin by a primary binding assay. Clin. Exp. Dermatol., 3:17, 1978.
39. Wiley, B. B. et al.: Staphylococcal scalded skin syndrome: potentiation by immuno-suppression in mice: toxin-mediated exfoliation in a healthy adult. Infect. Immunol., 9:636, 1974.
40. Hansen, R.: Staphylococcal scalded skin syndrome, toxic

shock syndrome, and Kawasaki disease. Pediatr. Clin. North Am., *30*:533, 1983.
41. Snyder, R. A., and Elias, P. M.: Toxic epidermal necrolysis and staphylococcal scalded skin syndrome. Dermatol. Clin. North Am., *1*:235, 1983.
42. Annunziata, D., and Goldblum, L. M.: Staphylococcal scalded skin syndrome: a complication of circumcision. Am. J. Dis. Child., *132*:1187, 1978.
43. Rasmussen, J. E.: Toxic epidermal necrolysis: a review of 75 cases in children. Arch. Dermatol., *111*:1135, 1975.
44. Melish, M. E., and Glasgow, L. A.: The staphylococcal scalded skin syndrome: the expanded clinical syndrome. J. Pediatr., *78*:958, 1971.
45. Curran, J. P., and Al-Saliki, F. L.: Neonatal staphylococcal scalded skin syndrome: massive outbreak due to an unusual phage type. Pediatrics, *66*:285, 1980.
46. Hebert, A. A., and Esterly, N. B.: Bacterial and candidal cutaneous infections in the neonate. Dermatol. Clin. North Am., *4*:3, 1986.
47. Elias, P. M., and Levy, S. W.: Bullous impetigo: occurence of localized scalded skin syndrome in an adult. Arch. Dermatol., *112*:856, 1976.
48. Goldberg, N. S. et al.: Staphylococcal scalded skin syndrome mimicking acute graft-vs-host disease in a bone marrow transplant recipient. Arch. Dermatol., *125*:85, 1989.
49. Richard, M., and Mathieu, A.: Staphylococcal scalded skin syndrome in a homosexual adult. J. Am. Acad. Dermatol., *15*:385, 1986.
50. Rudolph, R. I., Schwartz, W., and Leyden, J.: Treatment of staphylococcal toxic epidermal necrolysis. Arch. Dermatol., *110*:559, 1974.
51. Amon, R. B., and Diamond, R. L.: Toxic epidermal necrolysis: rapid differentiation between staphylococcal- and drug-induced disease. Arch. Dermatol., *111*:1433, 1975.
52. Murono, K., Fujita, K., and Yoshioka, H.: Detection of staphylococcal exfoliative toxin by slide latex agglutination. J. Clin. Microbiol., *26*:271, 1988.
53. Mirabile, R., Weiser, M., Barot, L., and Brown, A. S.: Staphylococcal scalded skin syndrome. Plast. Reconstr. Surg., *77*:752, 1986.
54. Fligner, C. L., Jack, R., Twiggs, G. A., and Raisys, V. A.: Hyperosmolality induced by propylene glycol: a complication of silver sulfadiazine therapy. JAMA, *253*:606, 1985.
55. Todd, J., Fishaut, M., Kapral, F., and Welch, T. O.: Toxic-shock syndrome associated with phage-group I staphylococci. Lancet, *2*:1116, 1978.
56. Reingold, A. L.: Toxic shock in the United States of America: epidemiology. Post. Grad. Med. J., *61*(Suppl. *1*): 23, 1985.
57. Schlievert, P. M. et al.: Identification and characterization of an exotoxin from Staphylococcus aureus associated with toxic-shock syndrome. J. Infect. Dis., *143*:509, 1981.
58. Bergdoll, M. S. et al.: An enterotoxin-like protein in Staphylococcus aureus strains from patients with toxic shock syndrome. Ann. Intern. Med., *96*:969, 1982.
59. Arko, R. J. et al.: A rabbit model of toxic shock syndrome: clinicopathologic features. J. Infect., *8*:205, 1984.
60. Garbe, P. L. et al.: Staphylococcal aureus isolates from patients with nonmenstrual toxic shock syndrome: evidence for additional toxins. JAMA, *253*:2538, 1985.
61. Crass, B. A., and Bergdoll, M. S.: Toxin involvement in toxic shock syndrome. J. Infect. Dis., *153*:918, 1986.
62. Schlievert, P. M.: Staphylococcal enterotoxin B and toxic-shock syndrome toxin-1 are significantly associated with non-menstrual TSS. Lancet, *1*:1149, 1986.
63. Cone, L. A., Woodard, D. R., Schlievert, P. M., and Tomory, G. S.: Clinical and bacteriologic observations of a toxic shock-like syndrome due to Streptococcus pyogenes. N. Engl. J. Med., *317*:146, 1987.
64. Bartter, T., Dascal, A., Carroll, K., and Curley, F. J.: "Toxic strep syndrome": a manifestation of group A streptococcal infection. Arch. Intern. Med., *148*:1421, 1988.
65. Stevens, D. L. et al.: Severe group A streptococcal infections associated with a toxic shock-like syndrome and scarlet fever toxin A. N. Engl. J. Med., *321*:1, 1989.
66. Parsonnet, J., Hickman, R. K., Eardley, D. D., and Pier, G. B.: Induction of human interleukin-1 by toxic-shock-syndrome toxin-1. J. Infect. Dis., *151*:514, 1985.
67. Parsonnet, J.: Mediators in the pathogenesis of toxic shock syndrome: overview. Rev. Infect. Dis., *11(Suppl.1)*:S263, 1989.
68. Bonventre, P. F. et al.: Antibody responses to toxic-shock-syndrome (TSS) toxin by patients with TSS and by healthy staphylococcal carriers. J. Infect. Dis., *150*:662, 1984.
69. Jacobson, J. A., Kasworm, E. M., Crass, B., and Bergdoll, M. S.: Nasal carriage of toxigenic Staphylococcus aureus and prevalence of serum antibody to toxic-shock-syndrome toxin 1 in Utah. J. Infect. Dis., *153*:356, 1986.
70. Todd, J. K. et al.: Influence of focal growth conditions on the pathogenesis of toxic shock syndrome. J. Infect. Dis., *155*:673, 1987.
71. Paris, A. L. et al.: Pathologic findings in 12 fatal cases of toxic shock syndrome. Ann. Intern. Med., *96*:852, 1982.
72. Reingold, A. L. et al.: Nonmenstrual toxic shock syndrome: a review of 130 cases. Ann. Intern. Med., *96*:871, 1982.
73. Green, S. L., and LaPeter, K. S.: Evidence for postpartum toxic-shock syndrome in a mother–infant pair. Am. J. Med., *72*:169, 1982.
74. Nahass, R. G., and Gocke, D. J.: Toxic shock syndrome associated with use of a nasal tampon. Am. J. Med., *84*:629, 1988.
75. Jacobson, J. A., Burke, J. P., Benowitz, B. A., and Clark, P. V.: Varicella zoster and staphylococcal toxic shock syndrome in a young man. JAMA, *249*:922, 1983.
76. Surh, L. S., and Read, S. E.: Staphylococcal tracheitis and toxic shock syndrome in a young child. J. Pediatr., *105*:585, 1984.
77. Tofte, R. W., and Williams, D. N.: Clinical and laboratory manifestations of toxic shock syndrome. Ann. Intern. Med., *96*:843, 1982.
78. Bach, M. C.: Dermatologic signs in toxic shock syndrome—clues to diagnosis. J. Am. Acad. Dermatol., *8*:343, 1983.
79. Elbaum, D. J., Wood, C., Abuabara, F., and Marhenn, V. B.: Bullae in a patient with toxic shock syndrome. J. Am. Acad. Dermatol., *10*:267, 1984.
80. Chesney, P. J. et al.: Clinical manifestations of toxic shock syndrome. JAMA, *246*:741, 1981.
81. Chesney, R. W., Chesney, P. J., Davis, J. P., and Segar, W. E.: Renal manifestations of the staphylococcal toxic-shock syndrome. Am. J. Med., *71*:583, 1981.
82. Smith, D. B., and Gulinson, J.: Fatal cerebral edema complicating toxic shock syndrome. Neurosurgery, *22*:598, 1988.
83. Reingold, A. L. et al.: Toxic shock syndrome surveillance in the United States, 1980 to 1981. Ann. Intern. Med., *96*:875, 1982.
84. Chesney, P. J. et al.: Toxic shock syndrome: management and long-term sequelae. Ann. Intern. Med., *96*:847, 1982.
85. Feingold, D. S.: Gangrenous and crepitant cellulitis. J. Am. Acad. Dermatol., *6*:289, 1982.
86. Meleney, F. L.: Hemolytic streptococcal gangrene. Arch. Surg., *9*:317, 1924.
87. Guiliano, A., Lewis, F., Hadley, K., and Blaisdell, F. W.: Bacteriology of necrotizing fasciitis. Am. J. Surg., *134*:52, 1977.

88. Riefler, J., Molavi, A., Swartz, D., and DiNubile, M.: Necrotizing fasciitis in adults due to group B streptococcus. Arch. Intern. Med., *148:*727, 1988.
89. Gaunt, N. et al.: Necrotizing fasciitis due to group C and G haemolytic streptococcus after chiropody. Lancet, *1:*516, 1984.
90. Pessa, M. E., and Howard, R. J.: Necrotizing fasciitis. Surg. Gynecol. Obstet., *161:*357, 1985.
91. Collette, C. J., Southerland, D., and Corrall, C. J.: Necrotizing fasciitis associated with Haemophilus influenza type b. Am. J. Dis. Child., *141:*1146, 1987.
92. Rea, W. J., and Wyrick, W. J.: Necrotizing fasciitis. Ann. Surg., *172:*957, 1970.
93. Stamenkovic, I., and Lew, P. D.: Early recognition of potentially fatal necrotizing fasciitis: the use of frozen-section biopsy. N. Engl. J. Med., *310:*1689, 1984.
94. Rimailho, A., Riou, B., Richard, C., and Auzepy, P.: Fulminant necrotizing fasciitis and nonsteroidal anti-inflammatory drugs. J. Infect. Dis., *155:*143, 1987.
95. Sudarsky, L. A., Laschinger, J. C., Coppa, G. F., and Spencer, F. C.: Improved results from a standardized approach in treating patients with necrotizing fasciitis. Ann. Surg., *206:*661, 1987.
96. Flanigan, R. C., Kursh, E. D., McDougal, W. S., and Persky, L.: Synergistic gangrene of the scrotum and penis secondary to colorectal disease. J. Urol., *119:*369, 1978.
97. Falcone, P. A., Pricolo, V. E., and Edstrom, L. E.: Necrotizing fasciitis as a complication of chickenpox. Clin. Pediatr., *27:*339, 1988.
98. Jones, R. B., Hirschmann, J. V., Brown, G. S., and Tremann, J. A.: Fournier's syndrome: necrotizing subcutaneous infection of the male genitalia. J. Urol., *122:*279, 1979.
99. Meleney, F. L.: Bacterial synergism in disease processes with a confirmation of the synergistic bacterial etiology of the abdominal wall. Ann. Surg., *94:*961, 1931.
100. Wilson, C. B., Siber, G. R., O'Brien, T. F., and Morgan, A. P.: Phycomycotic gangrenous cellulitis: a report of two cases and a review of the literature. Arch. Surg., *111:*532, 1976.

Chapter 47

SERIOUS GRAM-NEGATIVE BACTERIAL, RICKETTSIAL, AND VIRAL INFECTIONS WITH CUTANEOUS MANIFESTATIONS

GERMAINE M. CAMISHION

Gram-negative bacteria produce profound illness when they are causative agents of sepsis. Pseudomonas sepsis is usually nosocomial and may result from primary infections in various organ systems. The most common cutaneous manifestation of pseudomonal infection consists of "metastasis" involvement of the skin and is known as ecthyma gangrenosum. The meningococcus may also invade the skin, resulting in a septic vasculitis with typical lesions. Rocky Mountain spotted fever results from infection with the rickettsial organism, Rickettsia rickettsii. This results in a systemic vasculitis that is manifested in the skin by petechiae. Prognosis is related to early recognition and appropriate therapy. Herpes simplex and varicella-zoster virus infections may be benign and self-limited or life-threatening; they are particularly severe in immunosuppressed individuals.

PSEUDOMONAL INFECTIONS

Pseudomonas aeruginosa is a motile gram-negative aerobic rod that is primarily a nosocomial pathogen. It may be isolated from soil, water, plants, and animals and prefers moist environments. The organism elaborates the fluorescent pigments pyoverdin and pyocyanin, which appear blue or green at an alkaline pH and may impact these colors to exudates of cutaneous infections.

Pathophysiology

The Pseudomonas organism elaborates several extracellular substances that may directly influence pathogenicity. Proteases appear to be related to the hemorrhagic component of infections, and elastase may be responsible for dissolution of the elastic lamina of blood vessels. Protease and elastase are necrotizing in the skin, lung, cornea, and probably other organs. Hemolysins including phospholipase and heat-stable glycolipid break down lipids and lecithin. Phospholipase may be responsible for destruction of pulmonary surfactant and may thus be involved in the pathogenesis of Pseudomonas pneumonia. The outermost layer of the bacteria is known as the "slime" layer and is composed of polysaccharides, nucleic acids, hyaluronic acids, lipids, and protein. It may protect the organism from immune factors such as antibodies, complement, and phagocytic cells. Exotoxin A is an extracellular enzyme that is an inhibitor of protein synthesis and probably plays a role in necrotizing activity. Endotoxin (lipopolysaccharide) is a cell wall component related to manifestations of sepsis such as fever and hypotension. Serious, sometimes life-threatening pseudomonas infections include septicemia, pneumonia, meningitis, endocarditis, malignant otitis externa, endopthalmitis, and osteomyelitis.

Colonization by Pseudomonas spp. is uncommon in healthy persons. Only 4 to 12% of the normal population are fecal carriers, and it is seldom cultured from home environments.[1] Carriage rates increase markedly in hospitalized patients. Increased skin moisture and/or alteration of the stratum corneum may predispose to infection. The perineum, anogenital areas, axillae, and ear are frequent sites, and the organism may be cultured from urine, stool, nasal secretion, and the throat. Hospital epidemics have been traced to reservoirs such as respiratory equipment, endoscopes, and transvenous pacemakers.[2] Transmission by patient-to-patient or staff-to-patient contact may occur, but this has not been confirmed. Up to 20% of all nosocomial infections may be caused by Pseudomonas spp.[1] Colonization by the organism often precedes Pseudomonas spp. sepsis or other severe infection.[1,3] Pseudomonas is the most frequent cause of nosocomial pneumonia, the second most common isolate in burn wounds, and the third leading cause of both gram-negative bacteremia and nosocomial urinary tract infection.[4,5]

Pseudomonas septicemia is generally nosocomial or iatrogenic and often occurs at extremes of age. Predisposed persons include those immunosuppressed by malignancy (especially hematologic), those who have had chemotherapy with resultant neutropenia, those with acquired or congenital immunodeficiency states, and renal transplant patients. Patients who have received multiple antibiotics or corticosteroids or those with severe burns, chronic pulmonary disease such as cystic fibrosis, diabetes mellitus, indwelling urinary or intravenous catheters, surgical procedures, mechanical ventilation, and prematurity are also at risk. Pseudomonas sepsis may result from primary infection of the lungs, urinary tract, gastrointestinal tract or skin and soft tissue. It is clinically often indistinguishable from other gram-negative sepsis and frequently manifests with fever or hypothermia, a toxic appearance, tachycardia, tachypnea, mental status changes, and hypotension. Disseminated intravascular coagulation (DIC) is relatively uncommon in Pseudomonas septicemia.

Clinical Features and Differential Diagnosis

The skin manifestations of pseudomonas sepsis are characteristic and may consist of classic gangrene (ecthyma

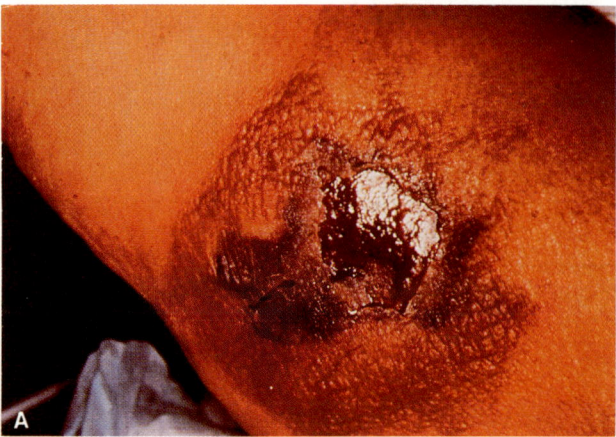 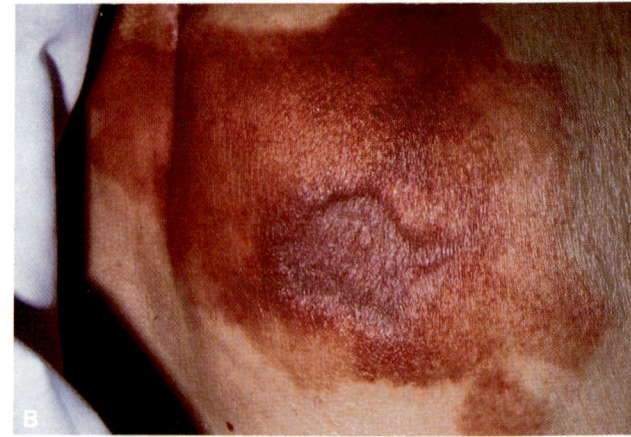

Fig. 47-1. *A,* Early lesion of ecthyma gangrenosum with characteristic bulla formation. *B,* Well-developed ecthyma gangrenosum with necrotic eschar. (Courtesy of Brown University, Providence, RI.)

gangrenosum), maculopapular or vesicular lesions, or sharply demarcated hemorrhagic cellulitis that may resemble erysipelas.[6,7] Cutaneous lesions may also be present as erythematous, indurated, poorly marginated subcutaneous nodules with or without fluctuation.[8,9] Early lesions of ecthyma gangrenosum may appear as small areas of erythema and edema or small indurated papules or nodules. Tense vesicles or bullae measuring up to 1 cm in diameter may then develop (Fig. 47-1A). These bullae become rapidly hemorrhagic and on rupture produce ulcerations that extend up to 3 cm in diameter and contain a necrotic, gray-black eschar with surrounding induration (Fig. 47-1B). They contain little, if any, purulent material. They may be ringed by a small rim of erythema or may have a concentric appearance with a central area of hemorrhage surrounded by an uninvolved area then rimmed by a narrow violaceous ring.[10,11] Lesions evolve over 12 to 24 hours and are usually present singly or in small numbers. When more than one is present, lesions of different ages are evident. The lesions have a predilection for the buttocks, perineum, axilla, and extremities. Necrotic lesions may also occur over the mucous membranes of the mouth, including the hard or soft palate, the gingiva, tongue or lips, nasal or facial areas, or the genitalia.[12,13]

Pseudomonas cellulitis may resemble typical streptococcal cellulitis except that the central area may be violaceous or hemorrhagic. The involved areas are initially macular and well demarcated. The cellulitis is often more necrotic than suppurative. Pus can be present, however, and may extend from deep-seated abscesses between facial layers down to muscle. Ecthyma gangrenosum is most frequently associated with P. aeruginosa sepsis, but identical lesions have been observed with infections due to Aeromonas hydrophilia, Pseudomonas cepacia, Pseudomonas maltophilia, Staphylococcus aureus, Serratia marcesans, aspergillus, and mucor.[1,14-17] Large, tender necrotic skin lesions with surrounding erythema that closely resemble ecthyma gangrenosum may be seen with disseminated candidiasis.[18,19] Lesions of ecthyma gangrenosum must also be distinguished from other cutaneous vasculitic lesions, such as those occurring with other bacterial septic lesions, hypersensitivity, angiitis, or polyarteritis nodosa.

Primary diffuse or localized cutaneous pseudomonal infection may occur in those predisposed by breakdown in the skin barrier such as that which occurs with trauma, burns, decubiti, or dermatitis. High moisture conditions predispose to infection. As with ecthyma gangrenosum, necrosis and hemorrhage are prominent, and microscopic vascular invasion is seen. Burn wound sepsis may occur as the rate of pseudomonal colonization increases markedly after the first 24 hours of hospitalization. Frequent manifestations of burn wound sepsis are hypotension, oliguria, hypothermia, ileus, and leukopenia. These patients are at risk for pseudomonal pneumonia, suppurative thrombophlebitis, and eye involvement when corneal damage secondary to burn is present. The burn wounds may exhibit a violaceous-to-black discoloration of the margin with hemorrhage and necrosis below the wound surface. Pseudomonal wound infections are characterized by a blue-green exudate with a fruity odor. The borders are macerated or eroded, giving a moth-eaten appearance. This infection may complicate decubiti, surgical wounds, or various dermatoses. Perirectal abscess that is due to Pseudomonas occurs most frequently in those with acute leukemia and is a frequent source of hematogenous dissemination. Pseudomonas folliculitis is a benign diffuse pruritic eruption consisting of papules and vesiculopustules localized mostly to the buttocks, hips, and axillae. It occurs in epidemics associated with contaminated swimming pools, whirlpools, and hot tubs. Associated symptoms include headache, dizziness, earache, and sore throat, breasts, eyes, and nose. Ecthyma gangrenosum developing within 24 hours after Pseudomonas folliculitis in immunocompromised patients has been described.[20,21]

Pseudomonas is the most frequent cause of a common and benign otitis externa associated with swimming. This organism also causes a sometimes life-threatening condition known as malignant otitis externa. It occurs most commonly in elderly diabetics and is characterized by purulent drainage with pain, edema, and tenderness of the soft tissue of the ear. The most important sign is presence of granulation tissue on the floor of the external auditory canal near the junction of cartilage and bone. This is an invasive necrotizing process with a mortality of up to 25% in treated patients. It may result in an osteomyelitis of the temporal bone with extension to the base of the skull, where it may cause compression and paralysis of cranial nerves with resultant dysfunction. The process may extend via the mastoid to the leptomeninges, causing meningitis or abscess.

Pseudomonal eye infections may lead to bacterial corneal ulceration. Release of pseudomonal enzymes can produce progressive destruction that may lead to eye loss. Blepharoconjunctivitis may be unilateral or bilateral and is characterized by purplish hemorrhagic appearance of the lids and periorbital areas. Endophthalmitis may follow penetrating injuries, intraocular surgery, or hematogenous spread following corneal ulcer perforation. This fulminating process requires emergency attention because visual loss may occur within hours.

Laboratory Studies

Gram's stain and culture of the ecthyma gangrenosum lesions are the most reliable methods for distinguishing it from other vasculitic lesions. Blood cultures are generally positive for the organism, though ecthyma gangrenosum has been reported in patients without bacteremia.[11] Skin biopsy is also informative and reveals vasculitis without thrombosis. Bacterial invasion of the media and adventitia of the blood vessel walls occurs, but the intima is usually spared. Histologically, it can be demonstrated that massive bacillary infiltration of the vessel walls appears to progress centripetally from involved perivascular tissue rather than progressing outward from the intimal surfaces after septic thrombosis.[22] Surrounding tissue necrosis and hemorrhage are believed to be secondary to direct bacterial injury rather than to vasculitis per se.

Treatment

Initial antibiotic therapy for pseudomonas septicemia is often empiric, with presumed diagnosis suggested by physical findings and clinical setting. Broad-spectrum synergistic combinations of intravenous antibiotics are employed, and optimal therapy often consists of aminoglycosides with semisynthetic penicillins or third-generation cephalosporins. Once the organism is isolated, sensitivities may dictate the use of alternate antibiotics. The duration of therapy is influenced by such factors as severity of infection, presence of neutropenia, and promptness of response. Patients with pseudomonal sepsis are generally profoundly ill and often require blood pressure support with fluids and pressor agents. Treatment of malignant otitis externa must be aggressive. Early recognition of the condition is important, and a high level of suspicion will lead to prompt administration of antipseudomonal drugs. Combinations of antipseudomonals, as discussed earlier, should be employed. Although monotherapy may also be curative,[23] prolonged therapy for 6 to 8 weeks or more is frequently required. Surgical debridement of granulation and necrotic tissue including bone may be necessary.

Outcome

Pseudomas septicemia carries a very poor prognosis, especially in patients with underlying immunodeficiency states. Complete resolution of skin lesions in survivors is expected.

Successful treatment of malignant otitis externa is indicated by a lack of drainage, pain, and granulation tissue. Cranial nerve deficits may be permanent where damage was significant.

MENINGOCOCCAL INFECTIONS

Neisseria meningitidis is a gram-negative endotoxin-producing diplococcus that can cause a spectrum of illnesses ranging from asymptomatic to life-threatening forms. Meningococcal disease most often presents as an acute bacterial meningitis. Acute meningococcemia, with or without meningitis, is a fulminant septicemia with a high mortality rate. Another form of the disease, chronic meningococcemia, does not usually constitute profound illness, though it may suddenly progress to overwhelming disease with shock, extensive skin necrosis, or severe endocarditis. The meningococcus can also cause localized disease including urethritis, conjunctivitis, otitis media,[24] pneumonia,[25] pericarditis,[26] arthritis,[27] and periorbital cellulitis.[28]

Pathophysiology

Acute meningococcemia is a disease of infants, children, and adolescents. Average annual age-specific attack rates per 100,000 people were 14.4 cases for infants under 1 year, 4.6 for children ages 1 to 4 years, 1.0 for children 5 to 9 years, 0.8 for those 10 to 19 years, and 0.3 for persons 20 years and older.[29] The incidence of meningococcal disease has been fairly low since the epidemics of World War II and often varies seasonally in industrialized countries, with most cases occurring in spring and autumn.[30] The case fatality rate of meningococcemia without meningeal involvement may reach as high as 19% during endemic situations in industrialized countries, though some report even higher rates, up to 70%.[30,31]

The meningococcus is transmitted from person to person by droplet spread. Nasopharyngeal colonization and a mild pharyngitis often precede sepsis. Nasopharyngeal carriage rate ranges from 2 to 11% in the general population to 30% in certain crowded situations and may approach 100% during epidemics.[30,32] The association of increased nasopharyngeal carriage rate with higher disease incidence in the population is somewhat tenuous. Persons most at risk for infection include infants and young children, especially day-care center contacts; household contacts; large populations living in close quarters such as military training camps and college dormitories; and all others who contact the oral secretions of the patient.[33] Those with secondary cases often present with signs and symptoms of an upper respiratory tract infection. Host factors that contribute to disease susceptibility include congenital or acquired deficiency of the terminal components of complement (C6-C9) and properdin deficiencies.[34-37] Compromise of host resistance that occurs with splenectomy predisposes to infection with encapsulated organisms such as the meningococcus.

942   THE HIGH RISK PATIENT: MANAGEMENT OF THE CRITICALLY ILL

Neisseria meningitidis is classified into 13 different serogroups on the basis of antigenic differences in capsular polysaccharide.[38] Outbreaks of disease are most commonly associated with groups A, B, or C, which account for at least 90% of all cases.[30] Other serogroups include D, X, Y, Z, 29E, W-135, H, I, K, and L. Most disease in the United States at this time is endemic and is caused by group B or C organisms.[32] Serogroup A organisms are usually associated with large epidemics that occur mostly in developing countries, especially in the "meningitis belt" in Africa.[39] Cyclic waves of disease caused by serogroup A organisms have been recorded approximately every decade since the early twentieth century. Organisms are further categorized according to serotypes that are based on outer membrane proteins and lipopolysaccharides. Serotypes 2 and 15 organisms are currently the predominant isolates from both military and civilian outbreaks.

Antimeningococcal antibodies of the immunoglobulin G (IgG) class may be transferred placentally and can provide protection during the first few months of life. Acquired immunity increases with increasing age, because bactericidal antibodies are produced in response to asymptomatic infection or nasal carriage of the organism. Absence of bactericidal antibody has been correlated with disease, and immunization with capsular polysaccharide can induce such antibodies.[40,41] Vaccines have been developed for the A, C, W, and Y groups. The group B capsular polysaccharide, however, is poorly immunogenic, and a vaccine against the B group has not yet been developed.[42]

Clinical Features and Differential Diagnosis

Prodromal signs are often present in acute meningococcemia. In infants, apathy, anorexia, fever, and irritability may herald a sometimes insidious onset of more specific disease manifestations.[43] Onset in children is often more abrupt, however, with fever, vomiting, and seizures. Upper respiratory tract symptoms commonly precede other disease manifestations by several days. In addition, nonspecific symptoms such as malaise, myalgias, and arthralgias may occur. Diarrhea may be the presenting symptom in some cases.[44] The rash is apparent within 36 hours of disease onset and is the most important clinical finding, occurring in 40 to 90% of patients. Petechiae, either isolated or seen within erythematous macules and papules, are the most characteristic early skin finding (Fig. 47-2). The lesions measure 1 to 2 mm and are usually present on the extremities and trunk, but they may also be seen on the head, palms, soles, mucous membranes, and palpebral conjuctivae. They are sometimes very few in number and then must be searched for carefully. They are often seen in clusters in areas of the skin where pressure is applied, for example, by elastic in underwear. The petechiae are usually palpable and are thus typical of a "palpable purpura" of inflammatory vasculitis. They often have a smudged appearance and sometimes coalesce to form purpurae with pathognomonic "gunmetal gray" centers (Fig. 47-3). Purpuric-necrotic skin lesions may result from either cutaneous vasculitis or DIC. The knees, elbows, buttocks, and face are commonly involved. Patients with this type of skin lesion tend to have more fulminant disease

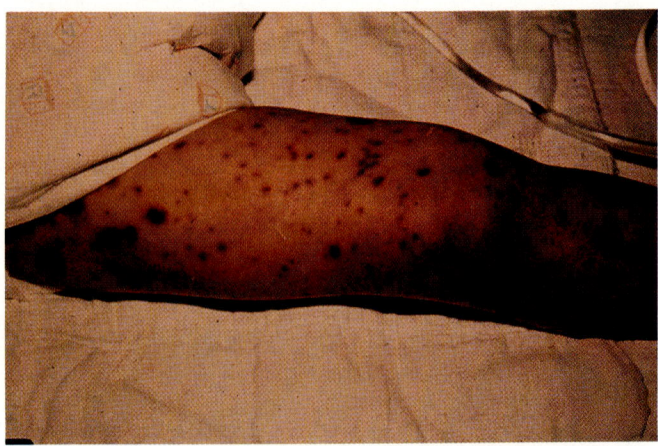

Fig. 47-2. Multiple petechiae in meningococcemia. Lesions are sometimes very few in number. (Courtesy of Brown University, Providence, RI.)

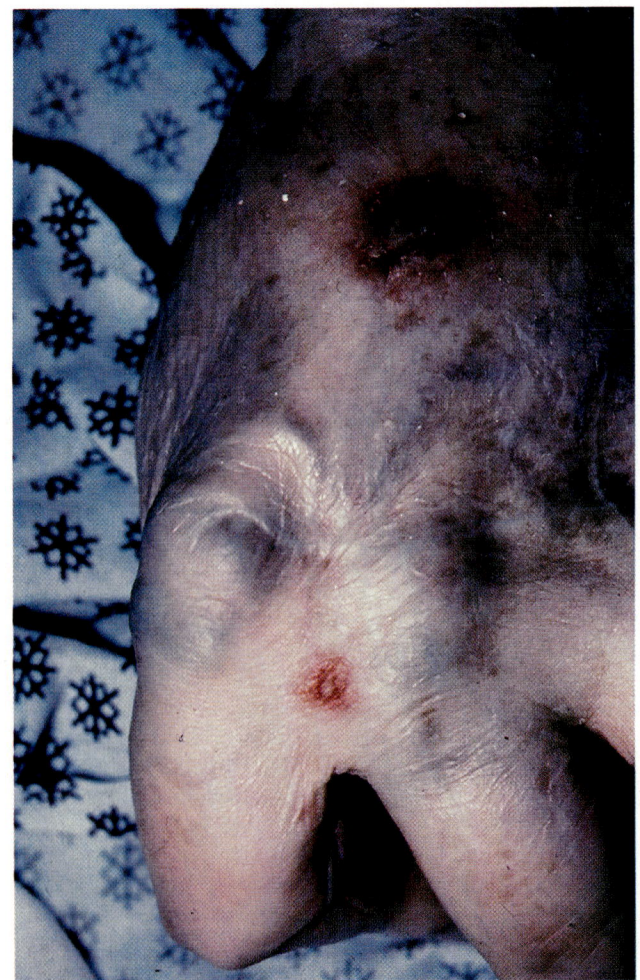

Fig. 47-3. Classic palpable purpurae of meningococcemia with "gunmetal gray" centers. (Courtesy of Brown University, Providence, RI.)

and often have little or no meningeal involvement.[45] DIC is a fairly frequent complication of meningococcemia and may cause ischemic breakdown of the skin secondary to extensive thrombosis. Necrotic lesions occasionally resolve with scarring.[30] Meningococcemia may also manifest in the skin as hemorrhagic vesicles or even as transient urticarial or morbilliform eruptions. The latter maculopapular eruption may be mistaken for a viral exanthem, especially rubella. It is asymptomatic and nonpurpuric, often resolving within 2 days.[46]

Purpuric cutaneous lesions are the result of dermal small vessel damage, which may be related to several factors. The endotoxin complex located in the outer cell wall of the organism is contributory. Endotoxin that is released from the meningococcus may produce increased permeability and dilatation of the vasculature, a Schwartzman-type reaction, and endothelial damage. Vascular inflammation occurs, tissue thromboplastin is released, and DIC with thrombotic vessel occlusion may occur. Injury of vessels is characterized by necrosis of endothelial cells as well as other elements of the vessel wall including muscle cells and pericytes.[47] Direct endothelial and perivascular invasion by the organisms results in extravasation of red blood cells and the clinical appearance of petechiae and purpurae. Such vascular damage also occurs systemically with involvement of various organs.[32]

Clinical manifestations of meningococcal disease range from transient bacteremia with upper respiratory symptoms to fulminant disease with death occurring in hours. The patient may have a septic appearance and may complain of weakness, malaise, and headache. When meningitis is present, meningeal signs with headache, fever, and altered sensorium may be observed. Patients with meningococcal meningitis may display highly aggressive behavior. Hypotension may quickly ensue, and the skin may be cool and cyanotic. Because meningococcemia is sometimes accompanied by a purulent meningitis and because a number of life-threatening complications may rapidly develop, resulting in death in approximately 12 to 16%, monitoring of the patient in an ICU is desired.[24] Among these serious complications are DIC, shock, renal failure, adult respiratory distress syndrome, and bilateral adrenal hemorrhage (Waterhouse-Friderichsen syndrome). Acute endotoxemia with shock is the major cause of death. The endotoxic shock that occurs with meningococcemia manifests as decreased cardiac output and venous return with hypotension.[48] In a study of 200 fatal cases of meningococcal infections, myocarditis often associated with congestive heart failure was the most common abnormality observed and was present in more than 75% of these cases.[49] The development of myocarditis may be indicated by the clinical picture of a low output state with a high atrial pressure.[50] Myocardial failure may be characterized by a gallop rhythm, congestive heart failure with pulmonary edema, and high central venous pressures with poor peripheral perfusion.[51] Waterhouse-Friderichsen syndrome is seen in approximately 3 to 4% of those with systemic infections and is generally not the cause of death. A small number of patients with fulminant meningococcemia also develop bilateral renal cortical necrosis resulting from thrombosis of the renal cortical glomerular capillaries that is secondary to DIC.

Petechiae are important as indicators of thrombocytopenia and DIC. The progression of petechiae should be monitored carefully early in the disease, because the number may relate to the effectiveness of therapy and the need to institute alternate or additional therapies.[45] The number of lesions in a particular area may be documented and charted on a flow sheet. DIC is sometimes indicated by increased numbers of petechiae in these areas, by gastrointestinal or gingival bleeding, or oozing at sites of venipuncture or intravenous lines. The petechiae rash usually fades within a few days. A blistering reaction (a cutaneous vasculitis) can occur, however, approximately 1 week after disease onset.[52]

Included in the differential diagnosis of fever with petechial rash are Rocky Mountain spotted fever, gonococcemia, acute hypersensitivity angiitis, subacute bacterial endocarditis, and enteroviral infections. Toxic shock syndrome should also be considered in hypotensive patients with a fever and rash. Definitive diagnosis of meningococcemia is made by culture of the organism from blood, cerebrospinal fluid (CSF), petechial lesions, or more uncommonly from the synovial, pleural, or pericardial fluids.[32] However, the 24- to 48-hour delay in obtaining results is unacceptable, because fulminant meningococcemia may progress within a matter of hours to death. Therefore, the patient must be treated based on clinical suspicion using clues such as distribution of the skin lesions and rapidity of their appearance.

Laboratory Studies

The diagnosis of meningococcemia may occasionally be quickly confirmed through direct visualization of meningococci on buffy coat smears or by Gram's stain of material obtained from petechial lesions.[53] The latter is performed by lifting off the top of the petechium, pressing a glass slide to the base, and performing a Gram's stain after drying the heat fixation. In addition, meningococci have been visualized on the peripheral blood smear, where they have been seen intracellularly and extracellularly.[54]

Culture of the organism from CSF and blood should always be attempted. Culture may be difficult, however, because the organism is fastidious in its growth, requiring specific media and optimal growth conditions. The organism may sometimes be cultured from the nose or throat. Where meningitis is present, CSF Gram's stain and culture and diagnostic in 70 to 80%, a rate that is matched by counter latex agglutination. It is notable, however, that latex agglutination often does not detect the poorly immunogenic group B meningococcus, which is the most common cause of severe disease in Western countries. A combination of culture with other diagnostic methods may improve sensitivity. When CSF microscopy and culture are accompanied by counterimmunoelectrophoresis (CIE) and latex agglutination, sensitivity may be increased by 4 to 5% and 8 to 10%, respectively. Blood cultures performed concurrently with the CSF exam may add another 3 to 10% to the diagnostic rate.[24]

Laboratory findings during the acute illness usually include a polymorphonuclear leukocytosis, although a normal white blood count with a left shift may be seen. The CSF parameters in patients with meningitis are typical of bacterial meningitis (i.e., a decreased glucose level with increased white blood cell count and protein levels). Where DIC is present, depressed levels of plasma fibrinogen, elevated fibrin degradation products, and a low erythrocyte sedimentation rate are present.

Treatment

The treatment of choice for patients with meningococcal disease is intravenous benzyl penicillin at a dosage of 14 to 18 g daily (20 to 30 megaunits) in divided doses. Such high doses may occasionally produce toxicity that is most commonly manifested as seizure during initiation of therapy with large boluses. The toxicity is facilitated in meningitis, where the brain is hyperemic and blood-brain permeability to the drug is increased. Antibiotic combinations apparently do not have increased efficacy over penicillin alone. Chloramphenicol or a second- or third-generation cephalosporin are good alternatives in those with a definite history of severe penicillin rash or anaphylaxis. Ceftriaxone, a third-generation cephalosporin, at a dosage of 80 to 100 mg/kg per day is reportedly an effective and safe treatment.[55] Most patients respond rapidly to antibiotic therapy. The use of first-generation cephalosporins is now contraindicated in treatment of meningococcal infections. Intensive supportive care for the complications of shock, DIC, cardiac failure, and/or pericarditis must be provided. When shock supervenes, monitoring of pulse and respiratory rates, blood pressure, urine output, electrocardiogram (ECG), electrolytes, acid/base studies, and right atrial pressure should be initiated. Hydrocortisone should be administered if any suspicion of acute hemorrhagic adrenal failure exist.[56]

When blistering of the skin is present, debridement with application of silver sulfadiazine may be helpful. Full-thickness skin loss should be treated by wound debridement, wet dressings, nutritional supplementation, and perhaps autografting.[57]

Outcome

Several studies have been done to identify prognostic factors in meningococcal disease. In one series, a systolic blood pressure of less than 100 mm Hg, platelet count equal to or less than 125 × 10 g/L, or extensive petechiae, and body temperature greater than 39°C, absence of meningism, a low CSF polynuclear cell count were factors that identified patients with high mortality.[58] Another study showed that such factors as coma, base excess, platelets, lack of meningism, skin and rectal temperature difference of more than 3°C, and widespread ecchymoses had discriminant power in predicting survival or death.[59] Yet another investigator's opinion is that hypotension, base deficit less than 8 mm mol/L, coma score, lack of meningism, skin and rectal temperature difference of more than 3°C, widespread ecchymoses or expanding lesions, or parental opinion that the condition had worsened were important prognostic indicators.[60]

Persons who are at risk of infection following exposure

Table 47–1. Sequelae of Meningococcal Infection

Arthritis/large joint synovitis
Cutaneous vasculitis
Episcleritis
Pericarditis
Cranial nerve dysfunction
Unilateral or bilateral deafness
Diabetes insipidis
Bone infarction and necrosis
Abnormal bone growth
Epiphyseal destruction
Premature epiphyseal-metaphyseal fusion

to those with meningococcal disease should be treated with rifampin. A throat swab may reveal growth of meningococci in such persons. The dosage is 600 mg every 12 hours for 2 days for adults and 10 mg/kg every 12 hours for 2 days in children. Approximately 50% of cases in contacts occur within 5 days of development of the index case. Polysaccharide vaccines specific for serogroups A or C should be given if there is evidence of an epidemic caused by these groups.

Following meningococcal infection, several autoimmune-like disorders and other complications can occur (Table 47–1). The most common is a symmetric large joint synovitis that appears up to 10 days after acute disease. Arthritis reportedly occurs in 4 to 10% of patients with meningococcal disease.[52,61] Cutaneous vasculitis and episcleritis are less common sequelae.[52] Pericarditis may occur early in the disease or as a late complication in its constrictive form.[62] Electrocardiograms should be examined frequently in those with pericarditis so that the development of a pericardial effusion can be recognized. Where purulent pericarditis is present, the patient must be monitored for development as tamponade both by physical examination (pulsus paradoxus) or by measurement of central venous pressure. An echocardiogram will confirm presence of fluid. Pericardiocentesis may be required if hemodynamic compromise occurs.[26] Although neurologic complications are infrequent in meningococcal meningitis, dysfunction of cranial nerves six, seven, and eight has been observed. Involvement of the sixth or seventh nerve is unilateral or bilateral, occurs late, and is usually transient. Permanent unilateral or bilateral deafness is more common, occurring in 1 to 2%.[63] Rarely, diabetes insipidus may complicate meningococcal meningitis.[64] Finally, widespread bone infarction has been reported to occur in meningococcal septicemia with DIC. Bone necrosis is to be considered in the cause of persistent fever after meningococcal septicemia.[65] Other skeletal abnormalities associated with meningococcemia and DIC as late complications include abnormal bone growth, epiphyseal destruction, and premature epiphyseal-metaphyseal fusion.[66]

The prognosis of the average case of uncomplicated meningococcal meningitis with treatment is excellent. Recovery is much less likely with meningococcemia, however, because of associated endotoxic shock and DIC.

ROCKY MOUNTAIN SPOTTED FEVER

Rocky Mountain spotted fever is the most common rickettsial disease in the United States. It is caused by Rickettsia rickettsii, a coccobacillary obligate intracellular parasite that is transmitted to humans by a tick bite.

The primary vectors are the wood tick Dermatocenter andersonii in the western United States and the dog tick Dermatocenter variabilis in the eastern United States.[67] The ticks are infected for life and act as reservoirs, transmitting the organism to their offspring transovarially. Humans usually contact the ticks outdoors or through contact with their pets.[68] A wide variety of birds and mammals have been reported as hosts to the ticks.[69] Illness is usually observed between April and September, which coincides with peak tick activity. Despite its name, Rocky Mountain spotted fever has been reported in all contiguous 48 states. The state with the highest attack rate is Oklahoma (3.0/100,000); other high incidence states are North Carolina, Kansas, Arkansas, and Missouri. In 1988, 615 cases of Rocky Mountain spotted fever were reported to the CDC, with 32.5% of the cases reported from the South Atlantic region and 24.2% from the West South Central region.[70] A history of a tick bite or exposure or travel to endemic areas is usually reported. However, in a review of 262 cases, 12% of patients recalled no tick bite or exposure. Rocky Mountain spotted fever is usually a disease of young persons with a median patient age of 15 years.[71]

Pathophysiology

Once introduced into the skin, the rickettsia enters endothelial cells. There, the organisms multiply and are released to affect other cells. The host cells are injured or killed, resulting in a necrotizing vasculitis.[72] This endothelial damage leads to abnormalities in vascular permeability and hemostasis, which are the key pathogenic mechanisms.

Clinical Features and Diagnosis

Following an incubation period of 3 to 12 days (mean, 7 days), an abrupt onset of fever, chills, headache, myalgia, and arthralgia usually occurs. The first symptom is usually fever, either alone or associated with headache or abdominal pain. In one epidemiologic study, however, fever was not among the initial symptoms in 31% of patients, thereby rendering diagnosis more difficult.[71] Other symptoms and physical findings observed on initial clinical presentation include nausea, vomiting, diarrhea, conjunctivitis, lymphadenopathy, and hepatosplenomegaly. Neurologic or neuropsychiatric manifestations including bizarre behavior, confusion such as coma, seizures, or hemiplegia are not uncommonly seen.

The rash associated with Rocky Mountain spotted fever is a cutaneous manifestation of the systemic vasculitis and is the most characteristic feature of the disease. It typically appears on the second to sixth (usually the fourth) day of fever but may be seen up to 15 days after the first symptoms. In 4 to 12% of cases, a rash may not develop.[71,73] The rash is initially comprised of blanching pink macules that are accentuated by fever. The lesions develop a deeper red color, and within 2 to 4 days, they become petechial. It is notable that all patients do not develop petechiae.[74] The regular and unique progression of the rash is a diagnostic feature. It is first seen on the wrists, ankles, and forearms, spreads after 6 to 18 hours to the palms and soles, and then moves centrally to the arms, trunk, and face. The extent and spread of the rash correlates with disease severity. Small foci of gangrene may be observed over distal areas including the fingers and toes, earlobes, nose, scrotum, or vulva.[75]

Clinical findings are the most important factors in establishing early diagnosis. A strong suspicion of disease should be present in the patient who lives in or has traveled to an endemic area during spring and summer and who presents with fever, headache, myalgias, and a rash. Delays in diagnosis may be attributable to significant variability in initial clinical presentation.[76] For example, an absent rash, gradual or late onset of fever, and no history of tick exposure may lead to incorrect conclusions. The distal extremities must be examined very carefully so an early diagnostic rash is not missed.

Included in the differential diagnosis of Rocky Mountain spotted fever are meningococcemia and enteroviral or other viral infections. Acute meningococcemia is the most important of these, and when the diagnosis is in doubt, antibiotic therapy should be instituted for both. The rash of meningococcemia occurs earlier in the disease course and does not have the orderly progression seen in Rocky Mountain spotted fever. A Gram's stain of the CSF or scraping from cutaneous lesions may be helpful in early diagnosis of meningococcemia.

Laboratory Studies

Laboratory data reflect the systemic vasculitis. Among the observed abnormalities are elevated serum glutamate oxaloacetate transaminase (SGOT), bilirubin, alkaline phosphatase and blood urea nitrogen (BUN), thrombocytopenia, anemia, hyponatremia, and hypoalbuminemia.[71] Creatine phosphokinase (CPK) may be elevated, a finding that is possibly related to myositis.[74] The chest radiograph is abnormal in approximately 25% of patients, showing cardiomegaly with pulmonary edema, interstitial or patchy alveolar infiltrates, and pleural effusion.[77] The white blood cell counts are variable and may be normal, increased, or decreased. Anemia is common. Patients with Rocky Mountain spotted fever may also exhibit hemostatic abnormalities including DIC, thrombocytopenia, complement depletion, and activation of the kallikrein-kinen system. Even in early disease, there is activation of platelets, coagulation pathways, and the fibrinolytic system.[78] Cerebrospinal fluid may show a pleocytosis with elevated protein and normal glucose levels.

The most widely used serologic test for Rocky Mountain spotted fever has been the Weil-Felix agglutination test, which uses a cross reaction between Proteus antigens OX-19, OX-2, and anti-rickettsial antibodies. This test, however, suffers from poor specificity and a failure in practice to obtain convalescent sera, which would be more sensitive than a single acute titer.[79,80] Complement fixation is another common test that is more specific but lacks sensitivity and generally requires more time to exhibit a rise in titer.[79] Other tests such as indirect fluorescent antibody, latex agglutination, indirect hemagglutination, and microagglutination have not proved suitable in acute diagnosis.

This has led to efforts to identify alternative techniques. A microliter enzyme-linked immunosorbent assay (ELISA) has been developed that has been shown to be sensitive and specific. This test utilizes R. rickettsii antigen-coated microtiter plates to test serum from patients suspected of having the disease. Its value in rapid diagnosis is unclear, however, because neither IgM nor IgG seroconversion has been demonstrated before 6 days after onset of illness.[81] Appropriate and timely antibiotic therapy reduces antibody responses, although later institution of therapy (greater than 3 days after onset of symptoms) has minimal effect on antibody production.[82] Sensitive and specific rapid diagnosis has been obtained by direct immunofluorescent staining of skin biopsy specimens, but some laboratories have found these difficult to interpret.[79,83] In any case, the decision to treat is based solely on clinical criteria, with convalescent titers serving only to confirm the diagnosis later.

Treatment

Chloramphenicol and tetracycline are both effective in treating Rocky Mountain spotted fever. The mortality associated with untreated illness may reach 70%, whereas the case fatality ratio with treatment in the last decade has hovered around 4%.[70,84] For adults and children over age 8, tetracycline is the drug of choice. An oral dosage of 20 to 40 mg/kg per 24 hours (maximum 2 g daily) given in four divided doses is recommended for those who are not seriously ill. For those with more severe illness, an intravenous dosage of 10 to 20 mg/kg per 24 hours in divided doses every 6 hours is administered. Chloramphenicol is indicated for children 8 years of age and younger. For patients with mild disease or for improving patients, the dosage is 50 mg/kg per 24 hours orally in four divided doses. The dosage is 50 to 100 mg/kg per 24 hours intravenously, in divided doses every 6 hours (maximum 3 g daily) for those more seriously ill. Therapy is continued until the patient has been afebrile for at least 48 hours, which usually occurs 5 to 7 days after initiation of therapy.[84]

Certain complications of Rocky Mountain spotted fever may require intensive supportive care. Critically ill patients may manifest confusion, delirium, diffuse petechiae, or ecchymotic lesions and tissue edema. These patients do not show a rapid response to antibiotics, as is seen in those with earlier mild disease.[84,85] The generalized rickettsial vasculitis may affect all internal organs, and resultant complications may require aggressive medical, surgical, and monitoring procedures. Continued endothelial damage results in exudation of plasma, hemorrhage, and intravascular depletion leading to shock.

Mental status should be monitored for the possibility of central nervous system (CNS) involvement and cerebral edema. Numerous CNS findings have been reported including confusion, meningismus, seizures, clonus focal motor defects, pyramidal signs, permanent deafness, and coma. Reports of retinal involvement include venous engorgement, retinal edema, papilledema, cotton-wood spots, retinal hemorrhage, anterior uveitis, and a single report of a branch retinal artery occlusion.[86]

Myocarditis, ECG abnormalities and abnormal left ventricular function with chamber enlargement may also compromise hemodynamic stability.[87,88] Observed ECG findings include sinus and nodal tachycardias, first-degree block, ST-T wave charges, low voltage, and left ventricular function. Patients are at risk for interstitial pneumonitis and for noncardiogenic pulmonary edema because of the injured pulmonary vasculature and increased pulmonary capillary permeability. Pulmonary disease may also manifest as focus infiltrates, adult respiratory distress syndrome, or secondary bacterial pneumonia.[84] Hypoalbuminemia from liver involvement and leaky vasculature frequently results in generalized edema. Impaired circulation may lead to renal insufficiency. Hyponatremia has been widely described in Rocky Mountain spotted fever. Antidiuretic hormone (ADH) levels were shown to be abnormally elevated in patients with hyponatremia and Rocky Mountain spotted fever.[89] The mechanism of the increased ADH was speculated to be attributable to hypotension and intravascular depletion. Although fluid restriction is indicated for the syndrome of inappropriate ADH secretion, patients with RMSF and hyponatremia need intravascular volume replacement with isotonic saline.[90]

Along with antibiotic therapy, supportive care is crucial in advanced cases. Hypotensive patients require fluid replacement and hemodynamic monitoring if indicated. Because patients are susceptible to noncardiogenic pulmonary edema, it is recommended that the pulmonary capillary wedge pressure be kept at the lowest possible levels that maintain cardiac output and oxygen delivery to the tissues.[91] Acute renal failure secondary to insufficient renal blood flow may require dialysis.

Outcome

The prognosis of Rocky Mountain spotted fever is excellent with appropriate antibiotic therapy initiated during the early responsive stages. The patient is usually symptomatically improved within 36 to 48 hours.

Recovery is usual with appropriate antibiotic treatment and supportive care.[84] The most important factor adversely affecting prognosis is delay in antibiotic therapy. The 3.1% case fatality ratio in 1987 was the lowest rate observed since 1970 when the CDC began monitoring the ratio. Those patients who succumbed were generally older, had no history of tick exposure, and did not receive prompt treatment.[70] Patients may be discharged from the ICU when antibiotic treatment has reversed the vasculitis and when hemodynamic stability is achieved as the endothelium heals.

Neurologic sequelae such as peripheral motor neuropathies, hemiparesis, and transverse myelitis have occurred in a small number of patients. Recrudescence of Rocky Mountain spotted fever after antibiotic therapy has been discontinued is uncommon. When it does occur, it is generally responsive to retreatment because antibiotic resistance has not been reported.[83] No vaccine is currently available.

HERPESVIRUS INFECTIONS

The herpesvirus group of viruses includes herpes simplex, varicella-zoster, cytomegalovirus, and Epstein Barr.

The herpes simplex and varicella-zoster viruses produce prominent cutaneous manifestations as well as life-threatening illness when dissemination occurs. They are the focus of this section.

The herpesviruses are enveloped, double-stranded, DNA viruses that replicate in the nucleus of affected cells. All members of this group can establish latent states, a characteristic that is important in the pathogenesis of these infections.

Herpes Simplex

The herpes simplex virus (HSV) has a worldwide distribution. Humans are the only known reservoir. Infection ranges from the recurrent, annoying but benign herpes labialis or genitalis to disseminated, life-threatening forms. Transmission of these viruses requires close, person-to-person contact that allows inoculation of virus-laden oral or genital secretions onto mucocutaneous surfaces. Transmission occurs from openly infected persons or less commonly from asymptomatic excretors. Subdivision of HSV into types I and II is based on clinical, epidemiologic, biochemical, and biologic characteristics. There is 50% homology between their genomes. HSV-I is commonly associated with herpes labialis and HSV-II with herpes genitalis, though either virus may produce infection at any cutaneous site. Antibodies to HSV-I arise during childhood, when most primary infections occur. Infection with type II generally occurs after puberty, except when the virus is transmitted to neonates via the birth canal of infected mothers.

The HSV replicates within epithelial cells, causing lysis of these cells and a local inflammatory response. Typical viral vesicles are then seen clinically. The HSV travels to the sensory nerve ganglia following infection and thus establishes the latency state. Nearly all patients who develop a primary HSV infection are thought to develop lifetime latent infections. Reactivation and secretion of the virus occurs with up to 50% developing recurrent herpes labialis lesions. Well-known triggers of such recurrent episodes include sun exposure, local trauma, menses or other hormonal changes, and stress. These triggers may operate via common cellular, humoral or neuroendocrine pathways that produce derepression of latent viral genes or interruption of the immune surveillance mechanisms that have contained activated virus.[92] It has been suggested that specific antibodies might afford some protection against the spread of HSV, but it appears that cell-mediated immunity (CMI) is more important. Patients who are immunosuppressed by hematologic and lymphoreticular malignancies, chemotherapeutic agents, or drugs administered after organ transplantation may suffer more frequent and severe infection. Dissemination to the liver, lungs, and CNS or recalcitrant progressive mucocutaneous involvement may occur in some patients.[93]

It is a common and true statement that most cutaneous HSV lesions occurring above the waist are caused by HSV-I and that those occurring below the waist involve HSV-II. Clinical manifestations of primary infection with HSV-I are usually seen in childhood. The infection often presents as a pharyngitis and gingivostomatitis and is sometimes

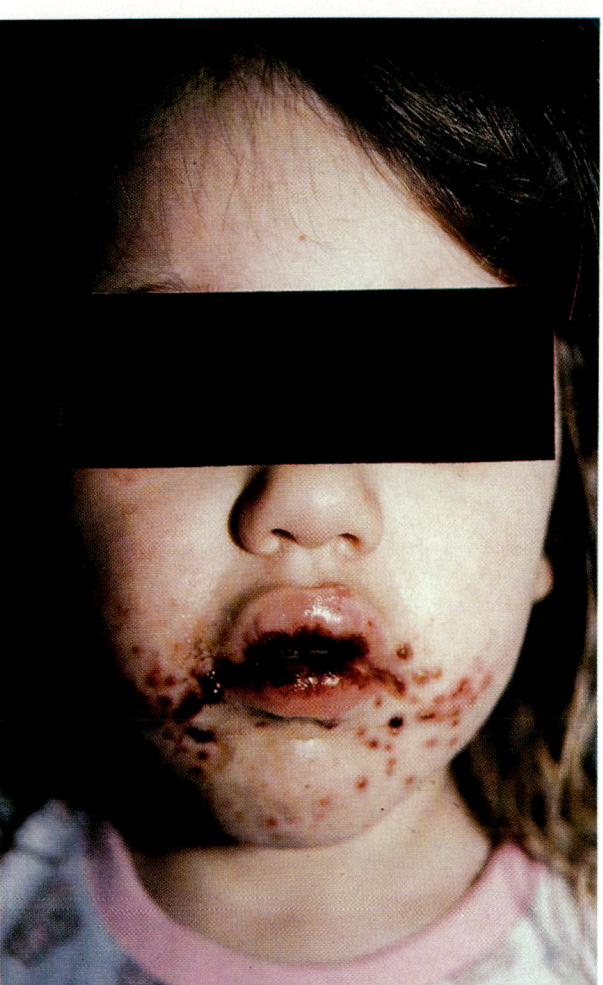

Fig. 47–4. Extensive crusting with primary herpes gingivostomatitis. (Courtesy of Brown University, Providence, RI.)

asymptomatic. The incubation period of 2 to 12 days is followed by complaints of sore throat and gums, with fever, erythema of the pharyngeal mucosa, and cervical adenopathy. Vesicles appear over the oropharyngeal mucosa, tongue and floor of the mouth, sometimes extending to the lips or cheeks. The lesions resolve with crusting (Fig. 47–4). Intraoral vesicles rupture easily and are usually seen as shallow, grayish erosions. Involvement of the eyes with HSV is usually secondary to HSV-I. Primary ocular manifestations may occur as unilateral follicular conjunctivitis and/or a blepharitis. Primary herpes genitalis infections usually develop in young adults and are caused by HSV-II in 90 to 95%. After an incubation period of 2 to 7 days, grouped vesicles on an erythematous base develop on the penile shaft or glans in men and on the vulva, perineum, buttocks, cervix, and vagina in women. Fever, malaise, anorexia, inguinal adenopathy, dysuria, and urinary retention may be present, and herpetic sacral radiculomyelitis may develop. Primary HSV infections may be rather extensive and may clinically resemble herpes zoster. The lesions of herpes zoster, however, have a distinct dermatomal distribution, and associated pain is usually greater. Recurrent herpes labialis or genitalis lesions occur in most patients after primary infection at varying intervals. Prodromal symptoms of tingling, itching, or burning may occur over the affected areas. The typical vesicles then develop in a less extensive distribution than in the primary infection and usually heal after about 10 days. Systemic complaints are generally minimal. Eye involvement may also be recurrent and may result in keratitis with dendritic ulcers or stromal involvement or as blepharitis or keratoconjunctivitis.

The remainder of this discussion will be limited to two serious and sometimes life-threatening complications of HSV infections: herpes encephalitis and eczema herpeticum (Kaposi's varicelliform eruption). The clinical manifestation, diagnosis, and treatment of each are discussed.

Herpes Simplex Encephalitis

Pathophysiology. Herpes simplex encephalitis (HSE) may occur in both immunocompromised and immunocompetent patients. It is the most common fatal endemic viral encephalitis in the United States, with frequency estimates of 250 to 500 cases per year and a mortality of greater than 50%.[92,93] HSE in adults is generally caused by HSV-I and is unaccompanied by other visceral involvement; type II is the usual pathogen in neonates, and visceral dissemination is common. There is no seasonal variation, and the age distribution is bipolar, with peaks between ages 5 and 30 years and above 50 years. Encephalitis is often preceded by primary HSV infection in children and young adults but is probably more often related to latent, recurrent HSV infection in older patients. Often, no predisposing factor is apparent. The encephalitis that develops is characterized by focal hemorrhagic necrosis. The means by which the HSV reaches the brain are not clear. It has been suggested that in primary infection the virus spreads hematogenously from infected nasopharyngeal mucosa through the cribiform plate via olfactory neurons. In latent HSV infections, the virus might spread in a retrograde fashion from affected ganglia.[94]

Clinical Manifestations and Differential Diagnosis. The presenting signs and symptoms of HSE include subacute-to-acute onset of fever, personality change, headache, irritability, mental status change, and focus neurologic deficits. The signs and symptoms may worsen progressively over several days. Temporal lobe involvement is prominent and manifests as bizarre behavior, hallucinations (including olfactory), or aphasia. Meningeal signs occur uncommonly. Focal or generalized seizures may develop. Focal signs and symptoms include hemiparesis, cranial nerve palsies, vertigo, ataxia, memory loss, and sensory deficits. The signs and symptoms of HSE are not specific, and distinction from other encephalitides may be difficult. The focal nature of the neurologic involvement is a particularly important characteristic.[95] The presence of cutaneous lesions may lead toward the suspicion of HSE, especially early in the course when other findings may be subtle. Cutaneous lesions, however, accompany the encephalitis in only 50% of affected neonates and an even smaller percentage of adults.[96] Even when cutaneous lesions are present in adults, it may be impossible to establish a relationship between the skin and neurologic findings. Typical herpetic vesicles may precede the encephalitis or may appear several days after onset. They may be present on any mucocutaneous surface. The lesions are grouped or clustered on an erythematous base, leaving oval grouped or confluent shallow ulcerations on rupture. They subsequently crust over and heal.

Differentiation of HSE from herpes zoster encephalitis (HZE) is sometimes particularly problematic. Encephalitis secondary to herpes zoster is rare; this virus is more likely to cause a self-limited meningitis. Both entities may present with similar cutaneous lesions that precede or follow onset of the neurologic symptoms by a few days. Grouped vesicles, pustules, ulcerations, and/or crusts appear in a dermatomal distribution in herpes zoster, but cutaneous dissemination may occur with several lesions outside the dermatome. Cutaneous lesions are present more commonly with HZE than HSE, but HZE may also occur without such lesions. Symptoms of HSE and HZE are similar, though temporal lobe involvement is not as prominent in HZE. The CSF findings are similar in both encephalitides. Elevation of CSF protein or lymphocytes, however, may be seen in up to 40% of uncomplicated cutaneous herpes zoster infections without encephalitis or clinical meningitis.[97] HSE must also be differentiated from other forms of viral encephalitis, tubercular and fungal meningitis, brain abscess, or tumors.

Laboratory Studies. Cutaneous lesions may be examined microscopically for a rapid confirmation of their viral nature. Tzanck smears are more sensitive than cultures for herpes zoster, but the reverse is true for herpes simplex. The Tzanck smear may be done at bedside and provides immediate results. In a recent study, false-positives were rare, whereas false-negatives were seen in approximately one fourth of culture-positive patients. Therefore, a positive smear is more informative than a negative one.[98,99] To accomplish the Tzanck smear, an intact vesicle is chosen. The roof of the vesicle is removed, and the base is scraped with a No. 15 blade using the rounded portion. The material is gently smeared on a glass slide and then air dried and stained with a Wright, Geimsa, toluidine blue, or PMS stain. A positive result is indicated by the presence of large multinucleated giant cells. The Tzanck smear produces identical findings with HSV and HZV. An equally rapid and more specific technique is direct fluorescent antibody staining. The vesicle material is prepared as described previously, and the glass slide is submitted to the laboratory. HSV may be differentiated from HZV in this way. Electron microscopy may also be used, but members of herpesvirus group cannot be differentiated, and sensitivity is variable. Culture of vesicular fluid may require up to 48 hours for a result, which is an unacceptable delay in initiation of antibiotic therapy.

Routine laboratory studies in patients with HSE are nonspecific and nondiagnostic. The CSF is abnormal in up to 97% of patients and shows a mononuclear pleocytosis with an elevated protein level and a normal glucose level.[100,101] Red blood cells appear in the CSF of 70 to 80% of patients. The organism is only rarely grown from the CSF. CSF and serum antibody levels do not rise until at least 10 days following the onset of illness and are, therefore, only useful in retrospective diagnosis.[93] Syndrome of inappropriate secretion of antidiuretic hormone (SIADH) may result from infection, and hyponatremia may be present. Computed tomographic (CT) scan may show characteristic patchy and widespread low-density areas or hemorrhage within temporal or frontal lobes, but this is not observed during the first few days of illness. Magnetic resonance imaging may show such changes earlier than CT and is a promising technique.[102] In the experience of some, the electroencephalogram (EEG) is the earliest localizing laboratory test.[103] Electroencephalogram results are often diffusely abnormal but in some cases may show temporal lobe spike activity.[104] Characteristic but not diagnostic of HSE are unilateral paroxysmal epileptiform discharges.[94] Brain biopsy is a sensitive and specific technique for diagnosis.[103,105] Antigen detection in the CSF may eventually replace brain biopsy as diagnostic technique.[106]

Treatment and Outcome. The patient with HSE generally requires admission into an ICU. Untreated patients usually deteriorate over several days, progressing to coma and death. Mortality is 60 to 80% in untreated, biopsy-proven cases, and neurologic sequelae remain in more than 90% of survivors. Antiviral therapy should be initiated empirically for any suspicion of HSE. When diagnosis remains uncertain, it is advisable to treat with broad-spectrum antibiotics as well so that purulent meningitides are covered. Vidarabine was the first drug proven effective in management of biopsy-proven herpes encephalitis.[107] It has a greater toxicity and is not as efficacious as acyclovir, which is the current drug of first choice in both HSE and HZE.[108,109] The intravenous dosage of acyclovir for HSE is 30 mg/kg per day in three divided doses for 10 to 14 days. Management of seizures, fluid, and electrolyte imbalance (with attention toward the possible development of SIADH), and increased intracranial pressure must be undertaken. Monitoring of the intracranial pressure together with attempts to lower it through the use of mannitol, steroids, and hyperventilation are of considerable importance. Frequent neurologic examination should be performed to assess progression of the disease and/or response to therapy. Hepatic and sometimes bone marrow parameters should be followed so that drug toxicity or dissemination of disease can be determined. Antipyretics may reduce the metabolic needs of the brain and may thus be useful. Respiratory support may be required in those with disseminated infection and pulmonary involvement. Cooperation among a team of physicians with expertise in critical care, neurology, neurosurgery, pulmonary care, and infectious diseases is advantageous in providing comprehensive treatment. Even with optimal care, significant morbidity and mortality occur. Variables that adversely affect outcome include increased age (those greater than 30 years have poorer prognosis), decreased level of consciousness (as rated by the Glasgow coma scale), and increased duration of disease before initiation of therapy.[97] Survivors frequently have neurologic residua that include behavioral, speech, and memory deficits.[110]

Eczema Herpeticum

Pathophysiology. Kaposi's varicelliform eruption, or eczema herpeticum (EH), is a generalized eruption caused by HSV. The most frequent causative agent is HSV-1, but HSV-2 may also be causative.[111] It occurs in those with preexisting skin diseases, including atopic dermatitis (most commonly), neurodermatitis, Darier's disease, seborrheic dermatitis, pemphigus vulgaris, congenital icthyosiform erythroderma, mycosis fungoides, and severe burns. A clinically identical entity occurs with the vaccinia virus after vaccination or by contact with a recently vaccinated person and is known as eczema vaccinatum. This entity is now fairly uncommon, because smallpox vaccination in the general population was discontinued in the 1970s. Eczema herpeticum may occur as a primary HSV infection, or it may be related to recurrent disease. The differentiation between the two is difficult and is probably of little practical significance. It has been suggested, however, that manifestations in primary disease are more severe with more widespread skin lesions and edema, fever, toxemia, and lymphadenopathy; mortality may also be higher. The predisposition of atopic patients to viral and bacterial infections of the skin is well-known. Both anergy and deficient cell-mediated immunity (CMI) have been described in these patients.[112] The predilection of EH for infants and young children probably reflects age-related susceptibility to primary HSV infection.[113] Nosocomial transmission of HSV resulting in EH may be prevented by a few simple measures. Patients with atopic or other dermatoses should not be roomed with patients who have an active viral infection. Likewise, hospital personnel with oral or other HSV lesions should not care for these patients until their lesions are crusted and dry.[114]

Clinical Manifestations and Differential Diagnosis. The diagnosis of EH may be delayed because those who are unfamiliar with its clinical presentation may assume that the findings represent an exacerbation of the underlying disease. In fact, topical steroids used in treatment of a presumed flare of dermatitis may affect local immunity and actually allow spread of the virus. The primary lesions are 1- to 3-mm vesicles found primarily over the areas of previous dermatitis but also on normal skin. A cluster of vesicles may be seen initially, which later disseminates over larger areas. The vesicles are characteristically discreet with peripheral enlargement and a tendency toward central umbilication (Fig. 47-5). Over a period of days, they progress to a pustular then crusted stage, sometimes becoming confluent. Secondary changes may include fissuring, erosions, and superficial ulcerations, purulent exudate, or a hemorrhagic appearance. Lesions often become secondarily infected with staphylococci or streptococci (most commonly S. aureus). Secondary staphylococcal infection is characterized by the development of yellowish, often varnish-like crusts. The vesicles may occur in crops over 2 to 6 weeks, but they may also appear to be in the same stage of development. Edema of the affected skin is often seen. Fever is sometimes present and may be accompanied by dehydration, electrolyte imbalance, and a toxic appearance. Localized or generalized lymphadenopathy may be present. Awareness and recognition of the clinical findings of EH in predisposed individuals is paramount in early diagnosis of the disease.

The major differential diagnosis in a patient with fever, vesicles, and atopic dermatitis is eczema vaccinatum

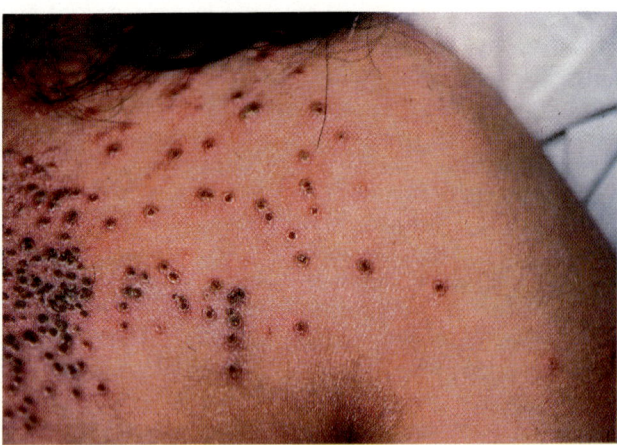

Fig. 47-5. Eczema herpeticum with discreet intact and crusted vesicles overlying an eczematous area. (Courtesy of Louis Fragola.)

which, as discussed previously, is extremely uncommon. The two may be differentiated by history, Tzanck, smear (pox virus infections show eosinophilic, intracytoplasmic inclusions), viral culture and serology, or electron microscopy. When vesicles occur in crops and are, therefore, in different stages of development, the eruption may resemble varicella. As noted previously, EH may be misdiagnosed as an exacerbation or secondary bacterial infection of the underlying skin disorder. Rarely, erythema multiforme, dermatitis herpetiformis, pemphigoid, or pemphigus may present clinical diagnostic similarities to EH. The coxsackie virus A-16 may also produce lesions not unlike those seen with EH.

Laboratory Studies. The Tzanck smear provides a rapid confirmation of the viral cause of the vesicles (see previous discussion), as does electron microscopy. Direct immunofluorescence testing of the smear is rapid and specific and differentiates HSV from the varicella zoster virus. Viral cultures and serology may also be obtained, but these clearly result in a diagnostic delay. Likewise, a skin biopsy may be diagnostic, but 24 to 48 hours are required for processing. Examination of the biopsied specimen reveals circumscribed epidermal cell "ballooning" degeneration, nuclear inclusion bodies, multinucleated giant cells, and acantholysis.

Treatment and Outcome. The course of EH varies from a mild, transient illness with recovery generally within 2 to 3 weeks (average duration 16 days) to a fulminating, life-threatening condition. Mortality rates were reported as high as 50% before the advent of antiviral therapy and adequate supportive care, but more recent reports estimate the rate at below 10%.[115,116] It appears that infants, children, and adults with deficient cellular immunity are at greatest risk for severe infection. Mortality may result from viremia with dissemination to internal organs or from secondary bacterial infection with sepsis.[117] Viremia may result in involvement of the lungs, brain, liver, and gastrointestinal tract of adrenal glands. Patients with cutaneous and/or visceral dissemination of HSV should be placed on stringent isolation precautions (wound and skin precautions at a minimum).[114] Strict isolation or even cohort nursing should be practiced when these patients are managed in the nursery, neonatal ICU, or burn unit. Antiviral therapy for EH is not well established, though there exist several reports in the literature of treatment with cytarabine, vidarabine, and acyclovir. Recently, the latter drug has been used predominantly because the others have significant toxicity.[116,117] The dosages of intravenous acyclovir in these have varied up to 30 mg/kg per day or 100 mg/m^2 per day. Treatment with acyclovir has decreased the duration of disease with no new vesicle formation. For the less ill patient who can be monitored as an outpatient, oral acyclovir at 200 mg, five times daily may be attempted.[118] Topical therapy should be initiated where numerous vesicles are present. This should consist of Burow's solution soaks to the affected areas for approximately 15 minutes, four times daily. This solution aids in faster resolution of the vesicles through its drying properties. It also has some antibacterial action and may thus prevent secondary infection. The soaks must be applied to eczematous skin with some care because the drying effects will exacerbate the eczema. The soaks should be discontinued when crusting of the vesicles is observed. Patients who have developed dissemination of the viral infection or sepsis from bacterial infection may need close monitoring in an ICU. Intravenous antiviral and antibacterial (to cover S. aureus) should be initiated, and close monitoring of blood pressure and mental status should be accomplished. If encephalitis develops, treatment guidelines as previously outlined may be followed.

Varicella-Zoster

The varicella-zoster virus (VZV) is the most contagious of the herpes viruses; like HSV, humans are the only known natural hosts. The VZV may produce both primary infection (varicella) and latent, recrudescent infection (zoster).

Clinical Manifestations, Differential Diagnosis, and Laboratory Studies: Primary Infection, Varicella. Approximately 3,000,000 cases of varicella occur each year in the United States, with more than 90% of cases occurring in those less than 14 years of age.[119] Varicella is endemic in temperate climates with peak incidence in the late winter and spring months. Adults who live in rural areas or tropical climates are less likely to have been exposed to the virus as children and are, therefore, more prone to development of primary infection. Transmission is generally airborne, though fluid from intact vesicles is infectious, and the disease might be transmitted by contact. Patients are infectious from 1 to 2 days before rash appearance to 4 to 5 days after or until all lesions are crusted. The infectious period may be longer in immunocompromised patients whose lesions tend to heal more slowly. Although less than 2% of cases occur after the second decade, up to 25% of deaths are in this group.[120] The incubation period of varicella is 14 days (median) with a range of 9 to 21 days. The primary infection consists of a vesicular eruption with fever and mild systemic signs in normal hosts. The lesions are pruritic and occur initially over the scalp, face, and trunk. Vesicles are superficial and thin-walled, measuring 2 to 3 mm in diameter. They sur-

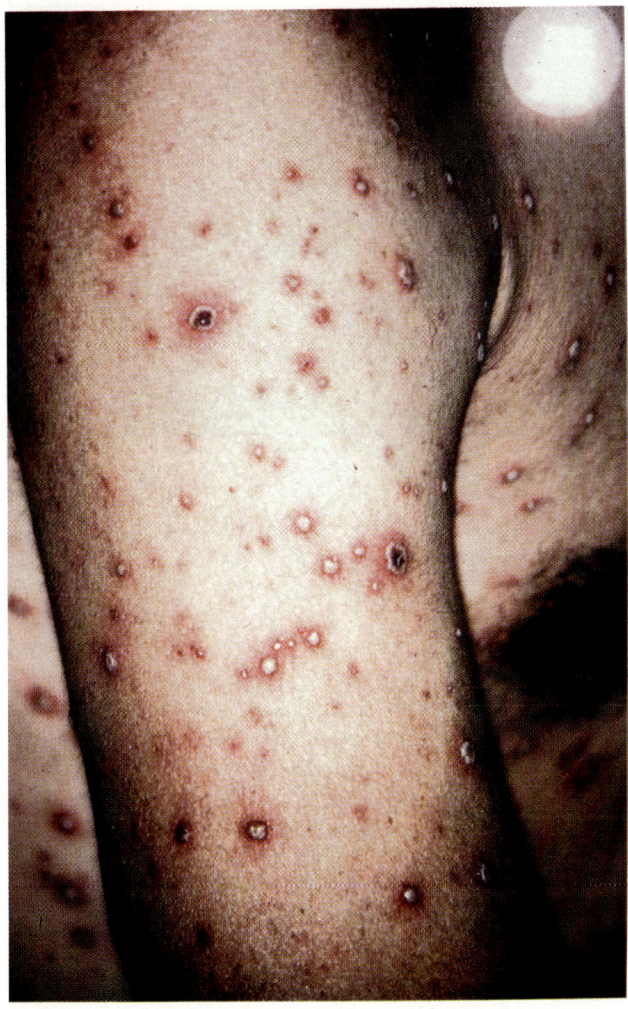

Fig. 47-6. Typical varicella with lesions of various ages. (Courtesy of Brown University, Providence, RI.)

mount an erythematous base, thus giving the "dewdrop on a rose petal" appearance (Fig. 47-6). Crops of new lesions may develop over the next 3 to 4 days, so the lesions of various ages and appearance are present at any given time. In the fully developed eruption, the lesions are most prominent over the central area of the body and in "hollow" or protected parts. Spread is from the trunk to the extremities. Numerous excoriations are usually seen. The mucous membranes including the mouth, pharynx, larynx, trachea, gastrointestinal tract, vagina, and conjunctivae are often involved. Crusting of the lesions is usually complete by day 6. Fever to 102°F, chills, malaise, arthralgias, myalgias, headache, anorexia, and sore throat may appear concurrently with the rash or may precede it by a few days.

The presentation is quite typical, and in most instances a clinical diagnosis may be made confidently. Varicella, however, may closely resemble disseminated herpes zoster or herpes simplex, eczema herpeticum, or coxsackievirus A-16 infection. Clinical setting is most important in consideration of these diagnoses. For example, a generalized vesicular eruption in an elderly person who also has a dermatomal vesicular eruption in an elderly person who also has a dermatomal vesicular eruption points to disseminated herpes zoster. A similar eruption in a person with an underlying skin disease such as atopic dermatitis may represent eczema herpeticum. A severe form of "progressive varicella" may develop in immunocompromised children. This form of the disease is estimated to occur in about 30% of leukemic children. It is characterized by a high (up to 105°F) and prolonged fever and appearance of new skin lesions into the second week of illness. The vesicles are more deep-seated than in classic varicella and often have an umbilicated appearance. They may be seen on the palms and soles late in the illness. Systemic involvement including pneumonia, meningoencephalitis, and hepatitis is frequent.[120] Viral dissemination usually occurs during the initial week of infection and coincides with peak new lesion appearance. Abdominal and back pain are often associated with visceral dissemination and are unrelated to specific organ involvement. Thus, the immunosuppressed patient with fever, abdominal or back pain, and increasing numbers of skin lesions should be considered at risk for dissemination.[121] The diagnosis of varicella may be confirmed by inoculation of vesicular fluid into cultures of human cells; virus-induced cytopathic changes may be observed after 7 to 10 days. The lesions should be cultured by aspirating one to six vesicles with a tuberculin syringe and a 25-gauge needle. The vesicle base should be gently rubbed with the needle bevel so that VZV-laden epithelial cells are withdrawn. The fluid should be inoculated into cultures of human fibroblast as soon as possible. The VZV is more difficult to culture than HSV. Serologic techniques (titers) may also provide a specific diagnosis. Skin biopsy or Tzanck smear identify the vesicle as viral, but HS and VZV cannot be distinguished. The viruses may be rapidly differentiated by smearing the vesicle contents on a glass slide and submitting this to the laboratory for direct immunofluorescence staining.

Varicella pneumonitis is the most common life-threatening complication of varicella infection in adults, neonates, and immunosuppressed children.[122,123] Pregnant women with varicella may also be at particular risk for this complication.[124] The pneumonitis may develop insidiously up to 6 days after rash onset and is characterized by cough, tachypnea, dyspnea, and fever. Pleuritic chest pain, cyanosis and hemoptysis may occur later. The chest radiograph reveals a bilateral patchy or diffuse nodular infiltrate with a prominent peribronchial distribution. Early findings may reveal 2- to 5-mm nodules, especially at the periphery. These increase in size as the disease progresses to form extensive infiltrates.[125] Diminished diffusion of gases may be present on pulmonary function studies, but ventilation is usually normal. Almost half of patients with this complication develop a superimposed bacterial infection; some also develop SIADH.[121]

Encephalitis has been said to account for 20% of hospitalizations for varicella.[121] CNS complications are rare in neonates. Encephalitis in children is often self-limited and is characterized by cerebellar findings such as ataxia and headache, nausea and vomiting, and cerebral rigidity. It usually occurs late in the first week or early in the second week after onset of rash but may occur at any time. Another form of encephalitis that is more frequent in adults has a significant mortality and is manifested by seizures, altered sensorium, and focal neurologic signs. Rapid progression to decerebrate rigidity may occur. Varicella encephalitis must be distinguished from Reye's syndrome, a noninflammatory encephalopathy with hepatic derangements that is often preceded by varicella. Clinical differentiation from HSV encephalitis may also be difficult; some differences are noted in the section on HSV. Other neurologic complications that may occur with acute varicella include aseptic meningitis, transverse myelitis, Guillain-Barré syndrome and focal neurologic damage.[126,127]

Cutaneous complications range from the common bacterial superinfection (impetiginization) of skin lesions to the rare, dramatic, and life-threatening purpura fulminans. Other cutaneous findings may include a mild febrile purpura "hemorrhagic" varicella and necrotizing faciitis. Superinfection with streptococci or staphylococci may lead to cellulitis, bullous lesions, or even gangrene.[128] Additional unusual complications of varicella include myocarditis, uveitis, hepatitis, glomerulonephritis, orchitis, arthritis, appendicitis, and pancreatitis.[97,123]

Like the HSV, the VZV maintains a latency state following primary infection. The virus resides in the sensory nerve ganglia and may reactivate as herpes zoster in up to 20% of persons during their lifetime. CMI appears most important in virus containment. Although zoster may occur at any age, there is an increased incidence with increasing age. Age-related deficits in CMI or impairment of the reticuloendothelial system may be responsible. Likewise, zoster is frequently observed in those with defective cellular immunity such as that which occurs in acquired immunodeficiency syndrome (AIDS) or following bone marrow transplantation. Patients with malignancy, especially lymphoma, are also especially prone to zoster. The incidence of zoster in patients with Hodgkin's disease may approach 40%.[129,130] The risk in these patients appears to be increased by combination radiation therapy and chemotherapy. A study of children with acute lymphocytic leukemia revealed an increased incidence of zoster with increasing number of combination chemotherapeutic agents in maintenance therapy.[121] Zoster lesions may be triggered by factors such as surgery, trauma, irradiation, or other immunosuppressive agents, arsenic or diseases such as tuberculosis, syphilis, and malaria.[97]

Clinical Manifestations, Differential Diagnosis, and Laboratory Studies: Recrudescent Infection, Zoster. Zoster is a localized vesicular eruption, often limited to dermatomes of spinal or cranial nerves. The dermatomes most frequently affected are the thoracic (50 to 55%), cranial (15 to 20%), cervical and lumbar (each 10 to 15%), and sacra (2 to 5%).[131] The cranial nerve most frequently involved is the trigeminal. Cutaneous lesions may develop abruptly or following a 1- to 4-day prodrome consisting of fever, malaise, headache, and pain or a burning, tingling sensation in the area of the affected dermatome. The earliest cutaneous finding is often a thin, erythematous plaque. At this stage, the eruption may be misdiagnosed as cellulitis. Papules and finally clusters of clear vesicles develop in a dermatomal distribution, usually

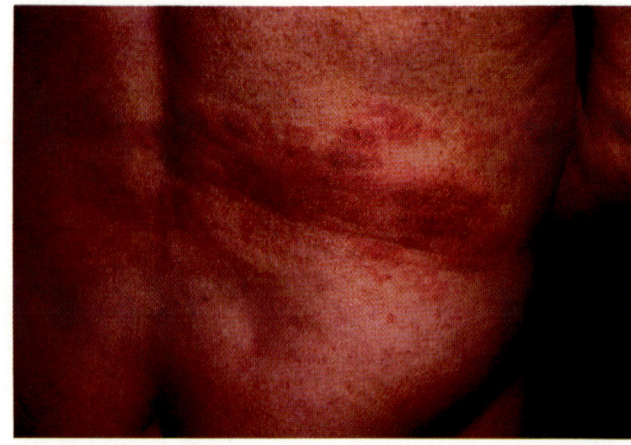

Fig. 47–7. Herpes zoster with typical dermatomal distribution. Up to three dermatomes may be involved. (Courtesy of Brown University, Providence, RI.)

unilaterally (Fig. 47–7). The clusters of vesicles may become confluent, with new vesicles developing over the next 4 days (up to 8 days). The vesicles become turbid, with a pustular appearance over the ensuing 3 to 4 days. They become dry and crusted in about 10 to 12 days. Lesions are present for longer periods and are more severe in the elderly and immunocompromised. The lesions are usually present in one dermatome but may involve up to three. Up to 10 lesions may be observed outside the dermatome if it has no evidence of cutaneous dissemination.

Dissemination is defined arbitrarily as greater than 20 lesions outside the primary and adjacent dermatomes. Dissemination is related to viremia and most often occurs in immunosuppressed patients, though it may occur in normal patients as well. Cutaneous dissemination is usually not associated with visceral involvement in immunocompetent patients. Both cutaneous and visceral dissemination may be more common with herpes zoster ophthalmicus than with herpes zoster elsewhere.[97] It occurs in up to about 25% of immunosuppressed patients, often developing 4 to 11 days following onset of the dermatomal lesions.[132] The lesions usually generalize over 3 to 5 days, but cutaneous dissemination in immunocompromised patients may persist for months. One half of patients with cutaneous dissemination have visceral, ocular, or neurologic involvement. As with varicella, the most common manifestation of visceral involvement is pneumonitis, which is also the leading cause of death. Involvement of the CNS, liver, and pancreas may also occur with viral dissemination.

HZE is an uncommon complication that usually develops between the first and second weeks after rash onset, though it may follow the skin lesions by up to 8 weeks.[132] Dermatomal and/or varicelliform skin lesions are usually present. Encephalitis is more common after trigeminal zoster than after zoster at other sites. Mortality is low in contrast with HSV encephalitis, and the majority of patients have an excellent prognosis. The initial symptoms of HZE include fever, headache, vomiting, and change in sensorium. These symptoms are usually acute, but onset may be more gradual. Examination often reveals meningeal signs. Coma and convulsions are uncommon. Other neurologic manifestations include transverse myelitis, myositis, urinary retention, polyuria, constipation or impotence when lumbosacral segments are involved, and Guillain-Barré syndrome.[133-136] The trigeminal nerve, especially the ophthalmic branch, is frequently involved in zoster infections. Involvement of any branch of the ophthalmic division of the trigeminal nerve is known as zoster ophthalmicus. The most serious consequences develop when the nasociliary branch of the ophthalmic nerve is involved. Vesicles on the nasal tip (Hutchinson's sign) indicate involvement of this nerve and is a good predictor of future ophthalmic manifestations. It occurs in about one third of patients with zoster ophthalmicus. Involvement of the second branch (maxillary) and the third branch (mandibular) of the ophthalmic nerve is indicated clinically by vesicles over the uvula and tonsillar areas and over the buccal mucosa, floor of the mouth, and anterior tongue, respectively. The viral nature of cutaneous zoster lesions may be confirmed by a Tzanck smear or skin biopsy, as described earlier in this chapter. Direct immunofluorescence may be used to identify the virus; when encephalitis is suspected, a CSF study may be undertaken. This generally reveals an increased pressure, increased white blood cell count with lymphocytes predominant, increased protein, and normal glucose levels. These findings, however, may be present in up to 40% of all patients with zoster.[127] It is difficult to recover virus from the fluid. Electroencephalogram reveals decreased voltage and increased slow wave activity.

Treatment: Varicella and Zoster. Patients who are at risk for disseminated infection with VZV must be monitored closely for appearance of visceral involvement, especially pulmonary. Assisted mechanical ventilation may be required. Serial sputum cultures should be performed so that bacterial superinfection may be detected, though antibiotic prophylaxis is not necessary. CNS involvement also necessitates admission to the ICU when seizure and coma develop. In this situation, anticonvulsant therapy and frequent neurologic monitoring should be undertaken. An additional complication of varicella that requires intensive monitoring and care is DIC (discussed in detail in Chaps. 45 and 48). Supportive treatment of VZV infection should include the administration of antipyretics (with avoidance of aspirin in varicella because of an association with Reye's syndrome), antipruritics, and analgesics. Antibiotics may be required when the skin is secondarily infected. Vesicles should be treated with four times daily compresses with Burow's solution or cool water.

Certain viral infections should be treated with acyclovir, the treatment of choice. Acyclovir shortens the duration of new lesion formation, viral shedding, and time to healing and probably decreases the rate of viral dissemination. It is indicated for varicella and zoster infections in immunosuppressed patients, for varicella in neonates, and for varicella pneumonia, disseminated zoster, and CNS and ophthalmic zoster in patients with normal immunity.[137,138] The dosage of acyclovir for treatment of severe or complicated VZV infections is 500 mg/m^2 body surface area or 10 mg/kg intravenously every 8 hours for 7 to 10 days or for 2 days after appearance of the last new lesions, whichever occurs first.[121,127,139] The acyclovir dosage should be according to creatinine clearance in patients with renal dysfunction. Vidarabine is an alternate treatment; dosage is 10 mg/kg body weight per day intravenously for 5 to 10 days.[127] Both alpha-interferon and vidarabine have significant toxicity and side effects and are not commonly used. Acyclovir must be given in a dosage approximately tenfold higher than that required for HSV treatment. High dose oral acyclovir is well tolerated, but renal toxicity may occur with intravenously administered drug. Acyclovir may crystallize in the collecting tubules and produce an obstructive nephropathy; adequate hydration will usually prevent this complication. Creatinine levels should be monitored throughout intravenous treatment; mild elevations are often seen.[140]

Varicella-zoster immune globulin (VZIG) is effective in prevention of clinical varicella infections in 60% of susceptible patients with household contacts and modifies infection in the immunosuppressed.[141] The risk of varicella pneumonia and mortality are also reduced with VZIG.[142] Those patients who are at high risk for complicated infection and who have been exposed are candidates for prophylaxis. The recommended dosage is one vial (1250) per 10 g of body weight to a maximum of five vials administered intramuscularly within 96 hours of exposure.[143]

Outcome: Varicella and Zoster. Varicella and zoster are generally benign and self-limited in immunocompetent patients. Increased morbidity and mortality often occurs in neonates, in patients with congenital or acquired immunodeficiency or malignancy, and in organ transplant patients on immunosuppressive drug regimens. Varicella sometimes may produce substantial morbidity with severe complications and even death in normal adults. Factors that lead to a high risk for complicated varicella are outlined in Table 47-2. A 7% mortality rate for children with varicella who are receiving chemotherapy has been reported.[141] Visceral dissemination occurred in about one third of these patients and were related to death in 21%. Factors that appeared to predispose patients to dissemination were chemotherapy received within 1 week of varicella onset and an absolute lymphocyte count of less than 500/mm^3 at the onset of varicella. The mortality rate for varicella in bone marrow transplant patients appears to be greater than in other immunocompromised patients; approximately one half of long-term survivors develop VZV infection as varicella or zoster. The mortality associated with zoster is low, even with disseminations, and is probably less than 5%.[132]

Table 47-2. Patients at High Risk for Complicated Varicella

Malignancy
Organ transplant recipients
Congenital or acquired immunodeficiency (defects of cell-mediated immunity)
Severe malnutrition
Severe burns
Severe dermatitis (e.g., atopic eczema)
Immunosuppressive therapy, collagen vascular disorders, rheumatic fever, psoriasis

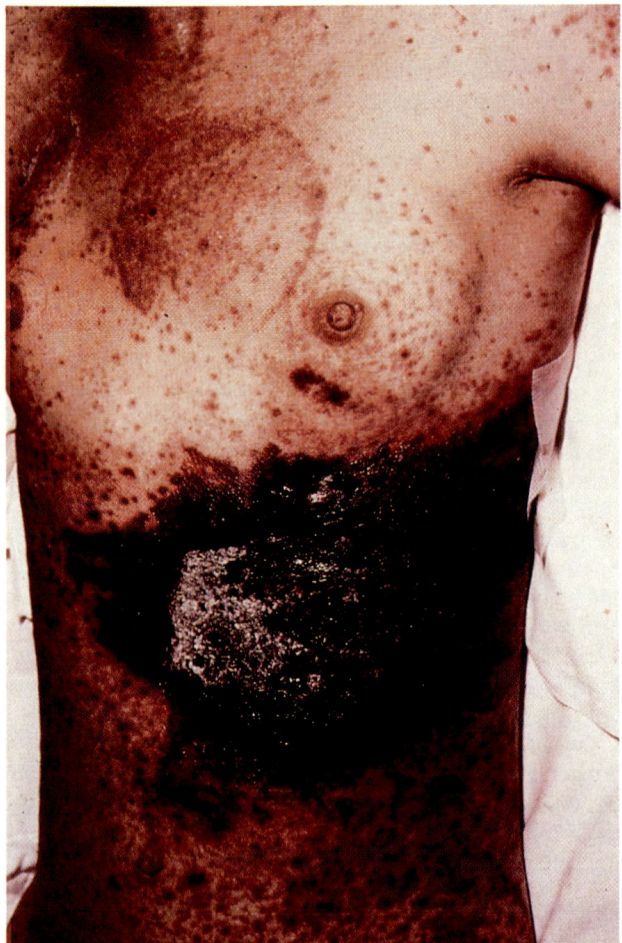

Fig. 47–8. Gangrenous zoster in a patient with lymphoma. Disseminated lesions are seen. (Courtesy of Brown University, Providence, RI.)

Zoster that occurs in association with lymphoma may be particularly severe, with hemorrhagic necrosis and scarring of the affected skin as well as cutaneous and visceral dissemination (Fig. 47–8). Following treatment of acute and severe complications of VZV infection such as pneumonia or encephalitis, attention must be directed toward residua of disease that may be incapacitating. Sequelae of VZV encephalitis may include dementia, aphasia, ataxia, and hemiplegia. Prolonged physical therapy may be required in patients who develop such conditions. Up to 72% of patients with herpes zoster ophthalmicus develop ocular complications that include keratitis and uveitis and may result in visual loss.[99,144,145] Close monitoring by an ophthalmologist is desirable in such cases. Some patients with herpes zoster ophthalmicus may develop a granulomatous arteritis up to 2 months after infection.[144] This may manifest initially with fever, headache, and confusion. A contralateral hemiplegia or aphagia, agraphia, or hemianopsia may also develop.

REFERENCES

1. Bodey, G. P., Boliver, R., Fainstein, V., and Jadeja, L.: Infections caused by Pseudomonas aeruginosa. Rev. Infect. Dis., 5:279, 1983.
2. Pollack, M.: Pseudomonas aeruginosa. In Principles and Practice of Infectious Diseases. Edited by G. L. Mandel, R. G. Douglass, Jr., and J. E. Bennett. New York, John Wiley & Sons, 1985.
3. Schimpff, S. C., Greene, W. H., Young, V. M., and Wirenik, P. H.: Pseudomonas septicemia: incidence, epidemiology, prevention and therapy in patients with advanced cancer. Eur. J. Cancer, 9:449, 1973.
4. Kreger, B. E. et al.: Gram-negative bacteremia. III. Reassessment of etiology, epidemiology and ecology in 612 patients. Am. J. Med., 68:332, 1980.
5. Centers for Disease Control: Nosocomial infection surveillance, 1980–1982. CDC Surveillance Summaries, 32:155, 1983.
6. Forkner, C. E., Frei, E. III, Edgcomb, J. H., and Utz, J. P.: Pseudomonas septicemia: observations on 23 cases. Am. J. Med., 25:877, 1958.
7. Roberts, R., Tarpay, M., Marks, M., and Nitschke, R.: Erysipelas-like lesions and hyperesthesia as manifestations of Pseudomonas aeruginosa sepsis. JAMA, 248:2156, 1982.
8. Schlossberg, D.: Multiple erythematous nodules as a manifestation of Pseudomonas aeruginosa septicemia. Arch. Dermatol., 116:446, 1980.
9. Reed, R. K., Larter, W. E., Seiber, O. F., and John, T. J.: Peripheral nodular lesions on Pseudomonas sepsis: the importance of incision and drainage. J. Pediatr., 88:977, 1976.
10. Dorff, G. J., Geimer, N. F., Rosenthal, D. R., and Rytel, M. W.: Pseudomonas septicemia. Illustrated evolution of its skin lesion. Arch. Intern. Med., 128:591, 1971.
11. Huminer, D., Siegman-Igra, Y., Morduchowicz, G., and Pitlik, S.: Ecthyma gangrenosum without bacteremia. Report of six cases and review of the literature. Arch. Intern. Med., 147:299, 1987.
12. Koopmann, C. F. Jr., and Coulthard, S. W.: Infectious facial and nasal cutaneous necrosis: evaluation and diagnosis. Laryngoscope, 92:1130, 1982.
13. Rabinowitz, R., and Lewin, E. B.: Gangrene of genitalia in children with Pseudomonas sepsis. J. Urol., 124:431, 1980.
14. Ketover, B. P., Young, L. S., and Armstrong, D.: Septicemia due to Aeromonas hydrophilia: clinical and immunologic aspects. J. Infect. Dis., 127:284, 1973.
15. Wolff, R. L., Wiseman, S. L., and Kitchens, C. S.: Aeromonas hydrophilia bacteremia in ambulatory immunocompromised hosts. Am. J. Med., 68:238, 1980.
16. Mandell, I. N., Feiner, H. D., Price, N. M., and Simbercoff, M.: Pseudomonas capacia endocarditis and ecthyma gangrenosu. Arch. Dermatol., 13:199, 1977.
17. Bottone, E. J. et al.: Pseudomonas maltophilia exoenzyme activity as correlate in pathogenesis of ecthyma gangrenosum. J. Clin. Microbiol., 24:995, 1986.
18. Fine, J. D., Miller, J. A., Harrist, T. J., and Haynes, H.: Cutaneous lesions in disseminated candidiasis mimicking ecthyma gangrenosum. Am. J. Med., 70:1133, 1981.
19. File, T. M., Marina, O. A., and Flowers, F. P.: Necrotic skin lesions associated with disseminated candidiasis. Arch. Dermatol., 115:214, 1979.
20. Gustafson, T., Band, J. D., Hutcheson, R. H., and Schaffner, W.: Pseudomonas folliculitis: an outbreak and review. Rev. Infect. Dis., 5:1, 1983.
21. El Baze, P. et al.: Pseudomonas aeruginosa 0-11 folliculitis: development into ecthyma gangrenosum in immunosuppressed patients. Arch. Dermatol., 121:873, 1985.
22. Teplitz, C.: Pathogenesis of Pseudomonas vasculitis and septic lesions. Arch. Pathol., 80:297, 1965.
23. Johnson, M. P., and Ramphal, R.: Malignant external otitis: report on therapy with ceftazidime and review of therapy and prognosis. Rev. Infect. Dis., 12:173, 1990.

24. Bannister, B.: Clinical aspects of meningococcal disease. J. Med. Microbiol., 26:161, 1988.
25. Sacks, H. S.: Meningococcal pneumonia and emphysema. Am. J. Med., 80:290, 1986.
26. Blaser, M. J., Reingold, A. L., Alsever, R. N., and Hightower, A.: Primary meningococcal pericarditis: a disease of adults associated with serogroup C Neisseria meningitidis. Rev. Infect. Dis., 6:625, 1984.
27. Schaad, U. B.: Arthritis in disease due to Neisseria meningitidis. Rev. Infect. Dis., 2:880, 1980.
28. Ferson, M. J., and Shi, E.: Periorbital cellulitis with meningococcal bacteremia. Pediatr. Infect. Dis. J., 7:600, 1988.
29. Band, J. D. et al.: Trends in meningococcal disease in the U.S. 1975–1980. J. Infect. Dis., 148:754, 1983.
30. Peltola, H.: Meningococcal disease: Still with us. Rev. Infect. Dis., 5:71, 1983.
31. Anderson, B. M. et al.: Endotoxin liberation from Neisseria meningitidis isolated from carriers and clinical cases. Scand. J. Infect. Dis., 19:409, 1987.
32. Devoe, I. W.: The meningococcus and mechanisms of pathogenicity. Microbiol. Rev., 46:162, 1982.
33. Meningococcal disease—United States 1981. MMWR, 30:113, 1981.
34. Ross, S. C., and Densen, P.: Complement deficiency states and infection; epidemiology, pathogenesis and consequences of neisserial and other infections in immune deficiency. Medicine, 63:243, 1984.
35. Ellison, R. T. et al.: Meningococcemia and acquired complement deficiency. Association in patients with hepatic failure. Arch. Intern. Med., 146:1539, 1986.
36. Ellison, R. T. et al.: Prevalance of congenital or acquired complement deficiency in patients with sporadic meningococcal disease. N. Engl. J. Med., 308:913, 1983.
37. Densen, P., Weiler, J. M., McLeod-Griffiss, J., and Hoffman, L. G.: Familial properdin deficiency and fatal meningococcemia. N. Engl. J. Med., 316:922, 1987.
38. Craven, D. E. et al.: Rapid serogroup identification of Neisseria meningitidis by using antiserum agar: prevalance of serotypes in a disease-free military population. J. Clin. Microbiol., 10:302, 1979.
39. Olyhoek, T., Crowe, B. A., and Achtman, M.: Clonal population structure of Neisseria meningitidis serogroup A isolated from epidemics and pandemics between 1915 and 1983. Rev. Infect. Dis., 9:665, 1987.
40. Goldschneider, I., Gotschlich, E. C., and Artenstein, M. S.: Human immunity to the meningococcus. I. The role of humoral antibodies. J. Exp. Med., 129:1307, 1969.
41. Gotschlich, E. C., Goldschneider, I., and Artenstein, M. S.: Human immunity to meningoccus. IV. Immunogenicity of Group A and Group C meningococcal polysaccharides in human volunteers. J. Exp. Med., 129:1367, 1969.
42. Poolman, J. T.: Meningococcal vaccines. J. Med. Microbiol., 26:170, 1988.
43. Oakley, J. R., and Stanton, A. N.: Meningoccocal infections during infancy: confidential inquiries into 10 deaths. Br. Med. J., 2:468, 1979.
44. Werne, C. S.: Gastrointestinal disease associated with meningococcemia. Ann. Emerg. Med., 13:471, 1984.
45. Toews, W. H., and Bass, J. W.: Skin manifestations of meningococcal infection. Am. J. Dis. Child., 127:173, 1974.
46. Apicella, M. A.: Neisseria meningitidis. In Principles and Practice of Infectious Disease. Edited by Mandel, G. L., Douglas, K. G., and Bennet, J. E. New York, John Wiley & Sons, 1985.
47. Sotto, M. N., Langer, B., Hoshino-Shimizu, S., and DeBrilo, T.: Pathogenesis of cutaneous lesions in acute meningococcemia in humans: light, immunofluorescent, and electron microscopic studies of skin biopsy specimens. J. Infect. Dis., 133:506, 1976.
48. May, C. D.: Circulatory failure (shock) in fulminant meningococcal infection. Pediatrics, 25:316, 1960.
49. Hardman, J. M.: Fatal meningococcal infections: the changing pathologic picture in the 60s. Milit. Med., 133:951, 1968.
50. Sheerson, J. M., and Fawcett, I. W.: The complications and management of meningococcal meningitis. Intensive Care Med., 5:5, 1979.
51. Levin, S., and Painter, M. B.: The treatment of acute meningococcal infection in adults. Ann. Intern. Med., 64:1049, 1966.
52. Whittle, H. C. et al.: Allergic complications of meningococcal disease. I. Clinical aspects. Br. Med. J., 2:733, 1973.
53. Goodall, H. B.: Evaluation of buffy coat microscopy for the early diagnosis of bacteremia-meningococcal septicemia. J. Clin. Pathol., 35:691, 1982.
54. Young, E. J., and Cardella, T. A.: Meningococcemia diagnosed by peripheral blood smear. JAMA, 260:992, 1988.
55. Tuncer, A. M. et al.: Once daily ceftriaxone for meningococcemia and meningococcal meningitis. Pediatr. Infect. Dis., 7:711, 1988.
56. Raman, G. V.: Meningococcal septicemia and meningitis: a rising tide. Br. Med. J., 296:1141, 1988.
57. Ikeda, C., and Capozzi, A.: Management of skin loss in meningococcal infection. Ann. Plast. Surg., 19:375, 1987.
58. Gardlund, B.: Prognostic evaluation in meningococcal disease. Intensive Care Med., 12:302, 1986.
59. Emparanza, J. F. et al.: Prognostic score in acute meningococcemia. Crit. Care Med., 16:168, 1988.
60. Sinclair, J. F., Skeoch, C. H., and Hallworth, D.: Prognosis of meningococcal septicemia. Lancet, 2:38, 1987.
61. Pinals, R. S., and Ropes, M. W.: Meningococcal arthritis. Arthritis Rheum., 7:241, 1964.
62. Nichols, D. A., and Peter, R. H.: Constrictive pericarditis as a late complication of meningococcal pericarditis. Am. J. Cardiol., 55:1442, 1985.
63. Weinstein, L.: Bacterial meningitis. Specific etiologic diagnosis on the basis of distinctive epidemiologic, pathogenetic and clinical features. Med. Clin. North Am., 69:219, 1985.
64. Christensen, C., and Bank, A.: Meningococcal meningitis and diabetes insipidus. Scand. J. Infect. Dis., 20:341, 1988.
65. Duncan, J. S., and Ramsay, L. E.: Widespread bone infarction complicating meningococcal septicemia and disseminated intravascular coagulation. Br. Med. J., 288:111, 1984.
66. Robinow, M., Johnson, G. F., Nanagas, M. T., and Mesghali, H.: Skeletal lesions following meningococcemia and disseminated intravascular coagulation. Am. J. Dis. Child., 137:279, 1983.
67. McDade, J. E., and Newhouse, V. F.: Natural history of Rickettsia. Ann. Rev. Microbiol., 40:287, 1986.
68. Gordon, J. C. et al.: Rocky Mountain spotted fever in dogs associated with human patients in Ohio. J. Infect. Dis., 148:1123, 1983.
69. Bozeman, M. F. et al.: Ecology of Rocky Mountain spotted fever. Natural infection of wild animals and birds in Virginia and Maryland. Am. J. Trop. Med. Hyg., 16:48, 1967.
70. Centers for Disease Control: Rocky Mountain spotted fever, United States, 1988. MMWR, 38:513, 1989.
71. Helmick, C. G., Bernard, K. W., and D'Angelo, L. J.: Rocky Mountain spotted fever: clinical, laboratory and epidemiological features of 262 cases. J. Infect. Dis., 150:480, 1984.
72. Lever, W. F., and Lever, G. S.: Histopathology of the Skin. 6th Ed. Philadelphia, J. B. Lippincott, 1983.
73. Cohen, J. I., Corson, A. P., and Corey, G. R.: Late appearance

of skin rash in Rocky Mountain spotted fever. South. Med. J., *76:*1457, 1983.
74. Kirk, J. L., Fine, D. P., Sexton, D. J., and Muchmore, H. G.: Rocky Mountain spotted fever. A clinical review based on 48 confirmed cases, 1943–1986. Medicine, *69:*35, 1990.
75. Schaffner, W.: Rickettsial and viral diseases with cutaneous involvement. In Dermatology in General Medicine. 3rd Ed. Edited by T. B. Fitzpatrick et al. New York, McGraw-Hill, 1987.
76. Tenebaum, M. J., and Markowitz, S. M.: Rocky Mountain spotted fever: diagnostic dilemma of the atypical presentation. South. Med. J., *73:*1527, 1980.
77. Lees, R. F., Harrison, R. B., Williamson, B. R. J., and Schaffer, H. A.: Radiographic findings in Rocky Mountain spotted fever. Diagn. Radiol., *129:*17, 1978.
78. Rao, A. R. et al.: A prospective study of platelets and plasma proteolytic systems during the early stages of Rocky Mountain spotted fever. N. Engl. J. Med., *318:*1021, 1988.
79. Walker, D. H., Burday, M. S., and Folds, J. D.: Laboratory diagnosis of Rocky Mountain spotted fever. South. Med. J., *73:*1443, 1980.
80. Marx, R. S., McCall, C. E., Abramson, J. S., and Harlan, J. E.: Rocky Mountain spotted fever. Serologic evidence of previous subclinical infection in children. Am. J. Dis. Child., *136:*16, 1982.
81. Clements, M. L. et al.: Serodiagnosis of Rocky Mountain spotted fever: comparison of IgM and IgG enzyme-linked immunosorbent assays and indirect fluorescent antibody test. J. Infect. Dis., *148:*876, 1983.
82. Hays, P. L.: Rocky Mountain spotted fever in children in Kansas. The diagnostic value of an IgM-specific immunofluorescence assay. J. Infect. Dis., *151:*369, 1985.
83. Linnemann, C. C.: Skin biopsy in diagnosis of Rocky Mountain spotted fever. J. Pediatr., *96:*781, 1980.
84. Woodward, T. E.: Rocky Mountain spotted fever: epidemiological and early clinical signs are keys to treatment and reduced mortality. J. Infect. Dis., *150:*465, 1984.
85. Lankford, H. V., and Glauser, F. L.: Cardiopulmonary dynamics in a severe case of Rocky Mountain spotted fever. Arch. Intern. Med., *140:*1357, 1980.
86. Duffe, R. J., and Hammer, M. E.: The ocular manifestations of Rocky Mountain spotted fever. Ann. Ophthalmol., *19:*301, 1987.
87. Marin-Garcia, J., Gooch, W. M., and Coury, D. L.: Cardiac manifestations of Rocky Mountain spotted fever. Pediatrics, *67:*358, 1981.
88. Marin-Garcia, J., and Barrett, F. F.: Myocardial function in Rocky Mountain spotted fever: echocardiographic assessment. Am. J. Cardiol., *51:*341, 1983.
89. Fishbein, D. B.: Treatment of Rocky Mountain spotted fever. JAMA, *260:*3192, 1988.
90. Kaplowitz, L. G., and Robertson, G. L.: Hyponatremia in Rocky Mountain spotted fever: role of antidiuretic hormone. Ann. Intern. Med., *98:*334, 1983.
91. Donahue, J. H.: Lower respiratory tract involvement in Rocky Mountain spotted fever. Arch. Intern. Med., *140:*223, 1980.
92. Straus, S. E.: Herpes simplex virus infections. Biology, treatment and prevention. Ann. Intern. Med., *103:*404, 1985.
93. Corey, L., and Spears, P. G.: Infections with herpes simplex viruses. N. Engl. J. Med., *314:*749, 1986.
94. Kohl, S.: Herpes simplex virus encephalitis in children. Pediatr. Clin. North Am., *35:*465, 1988.
95. Whitley, R. J.: Herpes simplex virus infections of the central nervous system. A review. Am. J. Med., *85(Suppl. 2A):*)61, 1988.
96. Brett, E. M.: Herpes simplex virus encephalitis in children. Br. Med. J., *293:*1388, 1986.
97. Leisgang, T. J.: The varicella-zoster virus. Systemic and ocular features. J. Am. Acad. Dermatol., *11:*165, 1984.
98. Solomon, A. R., Rasmussen, J. E., and Weiss, J. S.: A comparison of the Tzanck smear and viral isolation in varicella and herpes zoster. Arch. Dermatol., *122:*282, 1986.
99. Solomon, A. R., Rasmussen, J. E., Varani, J., and Pierson, C. L.: The Tzanck smear in the diagnosis of cutaneous herpes simplex. JAMA, *251:*633, 1984.
100. Koskiniemi, M., Vaheri, A., and Taskinen, E.: Cerebrospinal fluid alterations in herpes simplex virus encephalitis. Rev. Infect. Dis., *6:*608, 1984.
101. Whitley, R. J. et al.: Herpes simplex encephalitis: clinical assessment. JAMA, *247:*317, 1982.
102. Schroth, G. et al.: Early diagnosis of herpes simplex encephalitis by MRI. Neurology, *37:*179, 1987.
103. Kohl, S., and James, A. R.: Herpes simplex viral encephalitis during childhood. Importance of brain biopsy diagnosis. J. Pediatr., *107:*212, 1985.
104. Johnson, K. P., Rosethal, M. S., and Lerner, P. L.: Herpes simplex encephalitis: the course in five virologically-proven cases. Arch. Neurol., *27:*103, 1972.
105. Mahmias, A. J. et al.: Herpes simplex encephalitis: laboratory evaluations and their diagnostic significance. J. Infect. Dis., *145:*828, 1982.
106. Lakeman, F. D., Koga, J., and Whitley, R. J.: Detection of antigen to herpes simplex virus in cerebrospinal fluid from patients with herpes simplex encephalitis. J. Infect. Dis., *155:*1172, 1987.
107. Whitley, R. J. et al.: Herpes simplex encephalitis. Vidarabine therapy and diagnostic problems. N. Engl. J. Med., *304:*313, 1981.
108. Whitley, R. J., Alford, C. A., Hirsch, M. S., and Schooley, R. T.: Vidarabine vs. acyclovir therapy in herpes simplex encephalitis. N. Engl. J. Med., *314:*144, 1986.
109. Whyte, M. K. B., and Ind, P. W.: Effectiveness of intravenous acyclovir in immunocompetent patients with herpes zoster encephalitis. Br. Med. J., *293:*1536, 1986.
110. Oxbury, J. M., and McCallum, F. O.: Herpes simplex virus encephalitis. Clinical features and residual damage. Postgrad. Med. J., *49:*387, 1973.
111. Hazen, P. G., and Eppes, R. B.: Eczema herpeticum caused by herpes virus type 2. Arch. Dermatol., *113:*1085, 1977.
112. Hovmark, A.: An in vivo and in vitro study of cell-mediated immunity in atopic dermatitis. Acta Dermatol. Venereol., *55:*181, 1975.
113. Novelli, V. M., Atherton, D. J., and Marshal, W. C.: Eczema herpeticum. Clinical and laboratory features. Clin. Pediatr., *27:*231, 1988.
114. Henderson, D. K.: Nosocomial herpesvirus infections. In Principles and Practice of Infectious Diseases. Edited by G. L. Mandel, R. G. Douglass, Jr., and J. E. Bennett. New York, John Wiley & Sons, 1985.
115. Wheeler, C. E., and Abele, D. C.: Eczema herpeticum, primary and recurrent. Arch. Dermatol., *93:*162, 1966.
116. Swart, R. N. J. et al.: Treatment of eczema herpeticum with acyclovir. Arch. Dermatol, *119:*13, 1983.
117. O'Neill, J. F., and Norvell, S. S.: The role of acyclovir in the treatment of eczema herpeticum. J. Assoc. Mil. Dermatol., *15:*11, 1989.
118. Niimura, M., and Nishikawa, T.: Treatment of eczema herpeticum with oral acyclovir. Am. J. Med., *85(Suppl. 2A):*49, 1988.
119. Preblud, S. R., Orenstein, W. A., and Bart, K. J.: Varicella: clinical manifestations, epidemiology and health in children. Pediatr. Infect. Dis., *3:*505, 1984.

120. Brunell, P. A.: Varicella-zoster virus. *In* Principles and Practice of Infectious Diseases. Edited by G. L. Mandel, R. G. Douglass, Jr., and J. E. Bennett. New York, John Wiley and Sons. 1985.
121. Feldman, S.: Varicella zoster infections of the fetus, neonate and immunocompromised child. Adv. Pediatr. Infect. Dis., *1*:99, 1986.
122. Fleisher, G. et al.: Life-threatening complications of varicella. Am. J. Dis. Child., *135*:896, 1981.
123. Guess, H. A.: Population-based studies of varicella complications. Pediatrics, *78*:723, 1986.
124. Paryani, S. G., and Arvin, A. M.: Intrauterine infection with varicella-zoster virus after maternal varicella. N. Engl. J. Med., *314*:1542, 1986.
125. Triebwasser, J. H. et al.: Varicella pneumonia in adults: report of seven cases and a review of literature. Medicine, *46*:409, 1967.
126. Johnson, R., and Milbourne, P. E.: Central nervous system manifestations of chicken pox. Can. Med. Assoc. J., *102*:831, 1970.
127. Straus, S. E.: Varicella-zoster virus infections. Biology, natural history, treatment and prevention. Ann. Intern. Med., *108*:221, 1988.
128. Smith, E. W. P. et al.: Varicella gangrenosa due to group A beta hemolytic streptococcus. Pediatrics, *57*:306, 1976.
129. Wilson, J. F., Marsa, G. W., and Johnson, R. E.: Herpes zoster in Hodgkin's disease: clinical, hematologic and immunologic correlations. Cancer, *29*:461, 1972.
130. Reboul, R., Donaldson, S. S., and Kaplan, H. S.: Herpes zoster and varicella infections in children with Hodgkin's disease. Cancer, *41*:95, 1978.
131. Hope-Simpson, R. E.: The nature of herpes zoster: a long-term study and a new hypothesis. Proc. R. Soc. Med., *58*:9, 1965.
132. Dolin, R., Reichman, R. C., Mazur, M. H., and Whitley, R. J.: Herpes zoster-varicella infections in immunosuppressed patients. Ann. Intern. Med., *89*:375, 1978.
133. Hogan, E. L., and Krigman, M. R.: Herpes zoster myelitis. Arch. Neurol., *29*:309, 1973.
134. Norris, F. H. et al.: Virus-like particles in myositis accompanying herpes zoster. Arch. Neurol., *21*:25, 1976.
135. Jellenick, E. H., and Tulloch, W. S.: Herpes zoster with dysfunction of bladder and anus. Lancet, *2*:1219, 1976.
136. Singh, S., Malhotra, V., and Malhotra, R. P.: Guillain-Barre syndrome in herpes zoster. NY State J. Med., *72*:2094, 1972.
137. Prober, C. G., Kirk, L. E., and Keeney, R. E.: Acyclovir therapy of chicken pox in immunosuppressed children. A collaborative study. J. Pediatr., *101*:622, 1982.
138. Balfour, H. H. et al.: Acyclovir halts the progression of herpes zoster in immunocompromised patients. N. Engl. J. Med., *308*:1448, 1983.
139. Peterslund, N. A.: Management of varicella zoster infections in immunocompromised hosts. Am. J. Med., *85(Suppl. 2A)*:68, 1988.
140. Bean, B., and Aeppli, D.: Adverse effects of high dose intravenous cyclovir in ambulatory patients with acute herpes zoster. J. Infect. Dis., *151*:362, 1985.
141. Ross, A. H.: Modification of chicken pox in family contacts by administration of gammaglobulin. N. Engl. J. Med., *267*:369, 1962.
142. Feldman, S., Hughes, W. T., and Daniel, C. B.: Varicella in children with cancer: 77 cases. Pediatrics, *56*:388, 1975.
143. Centers for Disease Control: Varicella zoster immune globulin. MMWR, *30*:15, 1981.
144. Womack, K. W., and Leisgang, T. J.: Complications of herpes zoster ophthalmicus. Arch. Ophthalmol., *101*:42, 1983.
145. Cobo, M.: Reduction of the ocular complications of herpes zoster ophthalmicus by oral acyclovir. Am. J. Med., *85(Suppl. 2A)*:90, 1988.

Chapter 48

LIFE-THREATENING CUTANEOUS REACTIONS

DAVID L. SNOOK
GERMAINE M. CAMISHION

Patients in an intensive care setting are often receiving multiple medications, making drug eruptions a frequent complication of therapy. Stevens-Johnson syndrome and toxic epidermal necrolysis (TEN) may represent severe drug reactions or reactions to other inciting factors. Cutaneous lesions of disseminated intravascular coagulation (DIC) suggest similar changes in other organs and point to an underlying, often life-threatening illness. This chapter reviews cutaneous reaction patterns resulting from various infectious and noninfectious stimuli.

STEVENS-JOHNSON SYNDROME

Pathophysiology and Risk Factors

Stevens-Johnson syndrome is a severe form of erythema multiforme with prominent mucous membrane involvement. In contrast to the more common form of erythema multiforme, termed erythema multiforme minor, Stevens-Johnson syndrome may be life-threatening and often requires hospitalization.

Erythema multiforme is an acute, often self-limited, inflammatory skin eruption with a distinctive morphologic evolution. Although the pathogenesis of erythema multiforme is poorly understood, investigators have found evidence of immune system activity during the eruption.[1,2] Evidence for the importance of genetic factors includes association with certain HLA alleles[3] and reports of familial erythema multiforme.[4] There are a large number of implicated causes of erythema multiforme, but irrefutable proof of cause-and-effect relationships has been difficult to obtain (Table 48-1). Well-documented etiologic factors include herpes simplex infection, Mycoplasma pneumoniae infection,[5,6] and drugs.[7,8] Frequently implicated drugs include penicillins, sulfonamides, phenytoin, and phenylbutazone. Stevens-Johnson syndrome is much more likely to result from drugs or mycoplasma infection than from herpes simplex infection. Erythema multiforme has also been associated with histoplasmosis, infectious mononucleosis, vaccinia, tuberculosis, yersinia infections, malignancy, tumor radiation therapy, menstruation, pregnancy, collagen vascular disease, and occupational exposure to chemicals.[8,9]

Clinical Presentation

Erythema multiforme minor begins as erythematous round macules, which rapidly become edematous papules. Papules often enlarge to form round, erythematous, edematous plaques. The density of lesions is often greater on the distal extremities than on the trunk, with involvement of palms and soles being particularly characteristic. In contrast to urticaria, lesions of erythema multiforme persist for more than 24 hours at the same location. As papules enlarge into plaques, concentric alterations in morphology and color usually develop. The center of a plaque may become cyanotic in color, vesicular, pustular, or necrotic. Sometimes pathognomonic "target lesions," consisting of concentric rings of erythema and blanching, are noted (Fig. 48-1). The term "multiforme" refers to these many different lesion morphologies, but often only one type of morphology is present in a given patient at a particular time of evolution.[8] A minority of patients may have incomplete arcuate plaques, or lesions may coalesce to form larger polycyclic plaques. In a small percentage of cases, central vesicles enlarge into bullae, which encompass a large portion of the lesion. These bullae usually develop at the dermal-epidermal junction. This type of evolution is termed bullous erythema multiforme.

Erythema multiforme may also involve mucous membranes. Initial mucosal lesions are erythematous maculopapules, which may cause a burning sensation. If prominent mucosal involvement with bullous lesions develops, the eruption is termed erythema multiforme major or Stevens-Johnson syndrome. This is a serious form of erythema multiforme with significant morbidity and mortality.

Stevens-Johnson syndrome may occur in patients of any age.[7,10] In about one half of cases, the eruption is preceded by flu-like symptoms of fever, malaise, weakness, coryza, pharyngitis, and cough. Nausea, vomiting, myalgias, and arthralgias may also occur. About 85% of patients eventually develop fever, even in the absence of a prodrome.[7] The cutaneous rash of Stevens-Johnson syndrome is similar to that of erythema multiforme minor. The characteristic mucosal bullae may precede or follow the cutaneous eruption (Fig. 48-2). Any mucosal surface may be involved, including lips, conjunctiva, buccal mucosa, tongue, nares, pharynx, glans penis, urethra, vagina, esophagus, and anus. Mucosal bullae rapidly rupture, leaving tender erosions (Fig. 48-3). Intact vesicles are often not observed. Particularly characteristic lesions are lip erosions covered by grayish white pseudomembranes or hemorrhagic crusts (Fig. 48-4).[7,8,10,11] Conjunctival involvement is often accompanied by seromucinous, purulent, or pseudomem-

LIFE-THREATENING CUTANEOUS REACTIONS

Table 48–1. Suspected Causes of Erythema Multiforme

Infections	Cimetidine
Viral	Codeine
Herpes simplex*	Diphenylhydantoin
Infectious mononucleosis*	Ethanol
Vaccinia*	Estrogens
Adenovirus	Ethosuximide
Enterovirus	Furosemide
Hepatitis B	Glucagon
Influenza	Glucocorticoids
Milkers' nodules	Glutethimide
Mumps	Griseofulvin
Measles	Hydralazine
Orf	Meprobamate
Varicella/herpes zoster	Methotrexate
Bacterial	Minoxidil
Mycoplasma pneumoniae*	Nonsteroidal anti-inflammatory drugs
Tuberculosis*	Phenolphthalein
Yersinia*	Phenylbutazone
Bacille Calmette-Guérin vaccination	Quinine
Dental infections	Sulfonamides, including hypoglycemics
Legionnaire's disease	Sulfones
Lymphogranuloma venereum	Thiabendazole
Pneumococcus	Others
Proteus	Topical or inhaled agents
Pseudomonas	Anticholinergic eye drops
Psittacosis	Bromofluorene
Streptococcus	Fire sponge
Syphilis	Methylparathion
Tularemia	Primula
Typhoid fever	Sulfonamides
Vibrio parahaemolyticus	Trichloroethylene
Vincent's angina	Tropical woods
Fungal	*Other*
Histoplasmosis*	X-irradiation of tumors*
Coccidioidemycosis	Connective tissue disease
Dermatophyte infections	Hyposensitization therapy
Protozoan	Immunization
Trichonmonas	Inflammatory bowel disease
Drugs *	Margarine emulsifying agent
Alkylating agents	Menstruation
Antibiotics, especially penicillins and sulfonamides	Neoplasms
Arsenic	Pregnancy
Barbiturates	Sarcoidosis
Carbemazepine	

* Well-documented association.
(Adapted from Tonnesen, M. G.: Erythema multiforme: a critical review of characteristics, diagnostic criteria, and causes. J. Am. Acad. Dermatol., 6:763, 1983.)

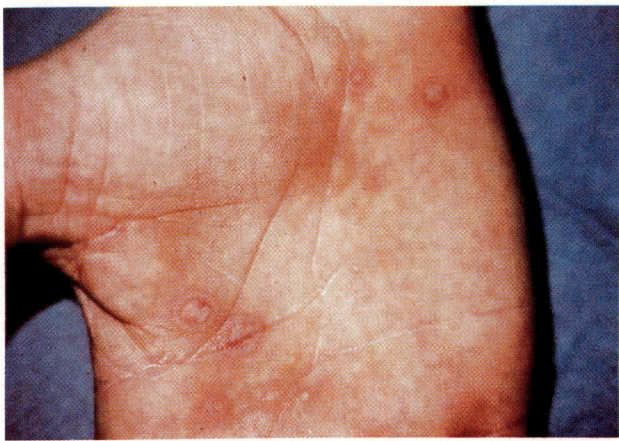

Fig. 48–1. Characteristic "target lesions" of erythema multiforme. Palmoplantar involvement by erythema multiforme is common. (Courtesy of Division of Dermatology, Brown University, Providence, RI.)

respiratory tree may occur and has been documented at autopsy.[12] In one large series, 15% of patients had roentgenographic evidence of pneumonitis, which may have been due to the syndrome itself or an infectious cause.[7] Rare reports exist of pericarditis, pericardial effusion, and atrial fibrillation associated with Stevens-Johnson syndrome.[13] Other infrequent internal manifestations include hepatitis, cystitis, and arthritis.[5,9] With severe disease, cutaneous bullae may develop and rupture, leaving extensive denuded areas similar to those seen in TEN.[8]

Diagnosis

Initial history and physical examination are used to make the diagnosis, look for possible causes, and determine extent of involvement. A diagnosis of Stevens-Johnson syndrome may be made clinically, based on the characteristic

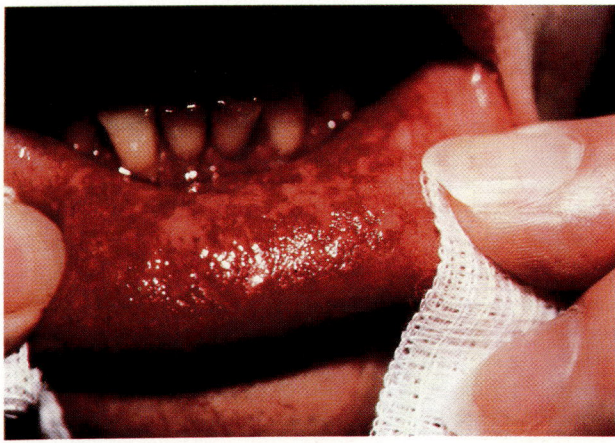

Fig. 48–2. Labial mucosal bullae in Stevens-Johnson syndrome. (From Snook, D. L., and McDonald, C. J.: The dermatologic manifestations of critical illness. J. Crit. Illness, 3(3):9, and 3(6):93, 1988.)

branous discharge; ciliary injection; and photophobia.[10] In one reported series of patients, 97% developed stomatitis, and 72% developed conjunctivitis.[7] Extramucosal cutaneous bullae may be seen in about one half of cases.[11]

Systemic derangements in Stevens-Johnson syndrome are variable (Table 48–2). Any gastrointestinal mucosa from mouth to anus may be affected, leading to signs and symptoms of dysphagia, cramps, diarrhea, or bleeding.[12] Stomach and bowel involvement has been described in the absence of more readily assessable mucosal lesions.[12] Renal involvement may result in hematuria, proteinuria, or azotemia. In one series, 50% of patients had evidence of renal disease, and 29% developed elevated serum creatinine levels.[11] Symptomatic mucosal involvement of the

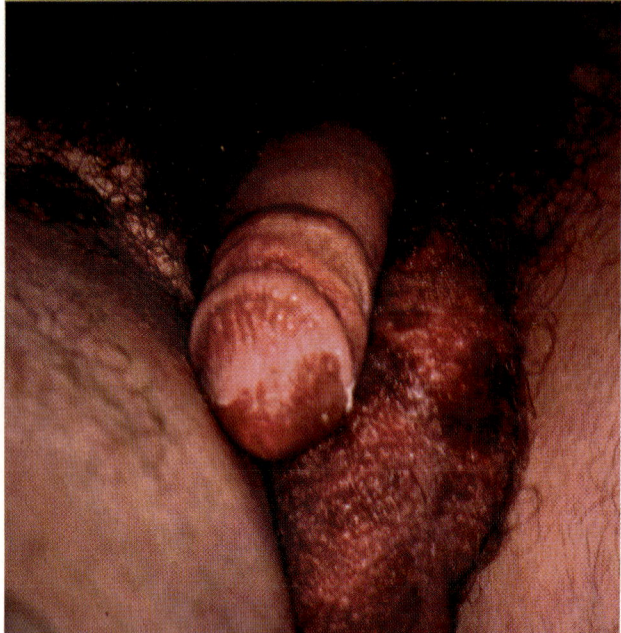

Fig. 48–3. Involvement of the glans penis in Stevens-Johnson syndrome. A periurethral bulla has ruptured, leaving an erosion. (From Snook, D. L., and McDonald, C. J.: The dermatologic manifestations of critical illness. J. Crit. Illness, 3(3):9, and 3(6):93, 1988.)

erythema multiforme rash and presence of mucosal bullae or erosions. When in doubt, a skin biopsy should be obtained to confirm the diagnosis.

In depth questioning about recent drug use is important. Any drug is suspect. Even topical ophthalmic medications have been known to cause Stevens-Johnson syndrome,[14] and over-the-counter preparations should not be overlooked. All nonessential medications should be discontinued and use of medications during hospitalization minimized.

Laboratory Studies

Initial testing includes chest film, electrolytes, liver function tests, blood urea nitrogen, creatinine, urinalysis, and complete blood cell count. These tests are supplemented by studies to evaluate any specific causes suggested by the history and physical examination. Chest film infiltrates may indicate a triggering infection, such as mycoplasma or histoplasma, or pulmonary involvement by Stevens-Johnson syndrome. If a medication is not the obvious cause, cold agglutinin titers and mycoplasma complement fixation titers should be drawn. With proper techniques, mycoplasma can sometimes be cultured from bullous cutaneous lesions of Stevens-Johnson syndrome.[6] It is important to remember that a normal chest film does not rule out the possibility of mycoplasma infection. Although herpes simplex is much more likely to cause erythema multiforme minor, it may rarely cause Stevens-Johnson syndrome;[3,10] therefore any suspicious grouped vesicles or erosions should be scraped for a Tzanck preparation.

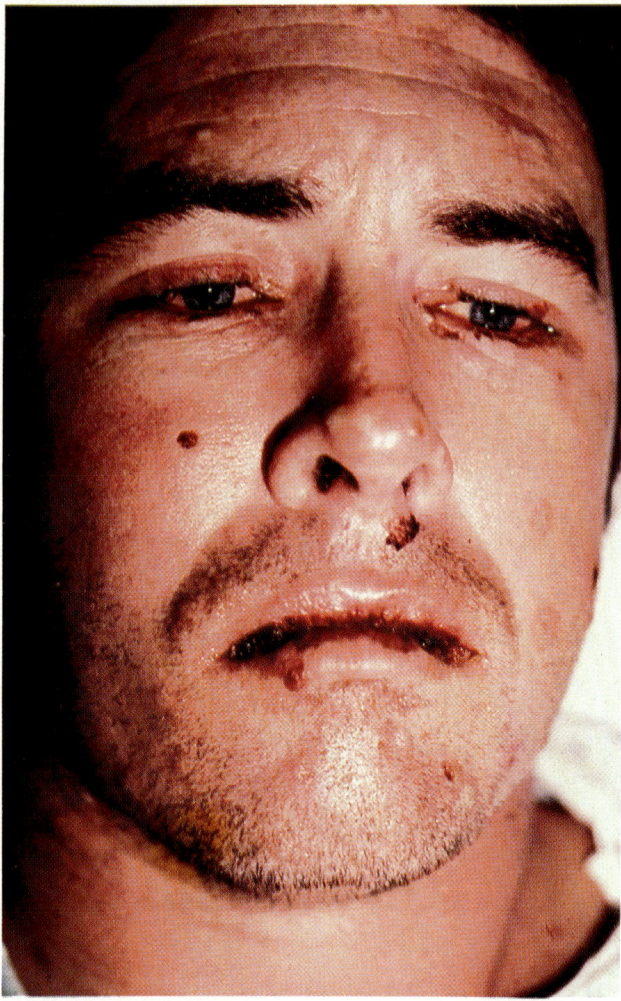

Fig. 48–4. Involvement of the conjunctiva, nares, and lips in Stevens-Johnson syndrome. Hemorrhagic lip crusts are common. (From Snook, D. L., and McDonald, C. J.: The dermatologic manifestations of critical illness. J. Crit. Illness, 3(3):9, and 3(6):93, 1988.)

Treatment

Most patients with Stevens-Johnson syndrome feel and appear quite ill and therefore should be hospitalized. Hospitalization is also advised for rapidly worsening patients, who may go on to severe involvement in less than 24

Table 48–2. Systemic Involvement in Stevens-Johnson Syndrome

Fever
Arthralgias, arthritis
Gastrointestinal: bleeding, ulceration, pain, diarrhea
Renal: hematuria, proteinuria, azotemia
Respiratory: erosions of trachea and bronchi, pneumonitis, cough, dyspnea
Hepatitis
Cystitis
Cardiac: pericarditis, pericardial effusion, atrial fibrillation

hours. Fortunately, most patients do not require admission to the ICU. If progression has definitely stopped, mucosal lesions are mild, and the patient appears nontoxic, hospitalization is not necessary. If history, physical examination, radiography, or laboratory tests uncover any causes of erythema multiforme, they should be treated or eliminated if possible. Unfortunately, in many cases, the cause is not apparent.[7]

Much of the treatment for Stevens-Johnson syndrome is supportive. Oral lesions often make eating and drinking uncomfortable or impossible. Topical viscous lidocaine may be useful in alleviating oral pain. Tap water soaks are used to soothe eroded lips and gently remove crusts. Most patients require intravenous fluids to prevent dehydration and correct electrolyte imbalances. Rarely patients require nasogastric feedings to maintain nutrition. An ophthalmology consultation should be obtained if the conjunctiva are prominently involved because conjunctival lesions may lead to synechiae, corneal ulcerations, lacrimal duct obliteration, or even blindness.[10,15] In one reported series, 15% of patients had evidence of corneal ulcerations.[11] Artificial tears, saline irrigation, topical steroids, topical antibiotics, and lysis of adhesions with glass rods have been used to treat ocular involvement, but their efficacy is unproved.[10,15] It is prudent to avoid sulfonamide-containing eye preparations because they may actually cause Stevens-Johnson syndrome.[14] Antacids are used for patients with upper gastrointestinal tract involvement or for patients who are treated with corticosteroids. Secondary bacterial infection of cutaneous lesions may require treatment to speed healing and prevent sepsis.

The use of corticosteroids to treat Stevens-Johnson syndrome is controversial because a beneficial effect has not been documented by a prospective, randomized trial. In fact, one retrospective review indicated that patients treated with corticosteroids had more complications (particularly infection and gastrointestinal bleeding) and longer hospital stays.[16] Nonrandomized, retrospective studies, however, are methodically flawed and therefore difficult to interpret. In some series, corticosteroids have been used more frequently for severe than for mild disease, thereby biasing results. Despite the concern over corticosteroid adverse effects, it has been the experience of many dermatologists that early administration of corticosteroids decreases morbidity and may avert a fulminant course. We treat patients with dosage equivalents of about 1 to 2 mg/kg of prednisone per day until clearing is achieved and then usually taper off over 1 to 2 weeks. Corticosteroids are probably not useful if the eruption has already peaked. In addition, they should probably be avoided in patients with extensive TEN-like skin lesions, or an increased risk of sepsis may result.

Treatment in an ICU is required only for extensive cutaneous denudation, supervening sepsis, pulmonary decompensation, or serious gastrointestinal bleeding. Admission criteria are according to the physiologic derangements of these clinical complications and are discussed in other chapters. Extensive cutaneous denudation is treated using methods described for TEN in this chapter. Sepsis and infectious pneumonia are the most common complications leading to death, thus necessitating monitoring for their occurrences.

Outcome

Patients who are debilitated, extremely young, or extremely old tend to do worse. Mortality rates of up to 25% have been reported for Stevens-Johnson syndrome,[5] but reports of high mortality may represent referral patterns to tertiary care centers. One comprehensive review of a large number of patients from several university hospitals documented a mortality rate of 5%.[7]

Recovery

At Brown University Affiliated Hospitals, the average hospital stay for a patient with Stevens-Johnson syndrome is about 7 days. Longer stays, however, are expected in patients who are already hospitalized for other illnesses. Some reports document hospitalizations of up to several weeks.[10,11,16] Patients without serious internal organ involvement may be discharged when mucosal inflammation has begun to subside and oral food intake is possible. Patients with drug-induced Stevens-Johnson syndrome should be instructed on which medications to avoid. Patients with mycoplasma-induced Stevens-Johnson syndrome sometimes have a recurrence owing to reinfection.[6] In one series, 13% of patients with Stevens-Johnson syndrome from various known or unknown causes had recurrence(s).[10] A minority of patients need long-term follow-up for sequelae. Conjunctival synechiae, dry eyes, corneal ulcerations, epiphora, and decreased vision require the care of an ophthalmologist. Vaginal erosions may lead to adhesions, stenosis, vaginal adenosis, vaginal endometriosis, and dyspareunia. Vaginal sequelae are treated by resecting adenosis and endometriosis, lysing adhesions, and using vaginal molds to correct stenosis.[17] Balanitis may result in adhesions between the foreskin and glans penis. Patients with esophageal strictures may require bougie dilatations.[18] Skin lesions sometimes leave temporary postinflammatory hyperpigmentation. Fortunately, cutaneous scarring does not develop in the absence of skin infection. It is thought that early intervention and good supportive care help to prevent a poor outcome.

TOXIC EPIDERMAL NECROLYSIS

Pathogenesis

TEN is an acute, severe skin eruption characterized by epidermal damage and detachment, resulting in a scalded skin appearance. The pathogenesis of TEN is thought to involve immune mechanisms but is poorly understood.[19] The association of HLA-B12 with TEN suggests that inherited factors may also play a role.[20] As with Stevens-Johnson syndrome, a large number of definite, probable, and potential causes of TEN have been reported (Table 48-3). The majority of cases of TEN are due to drugs. Frequently implicated medications include sulfonamides, other antibiotics, nonsteroidal anti-inflammatory drugs, and anticonvulsants.[19,21] Other reported causes include viral infections,[22] graft-versus-host disease,[23] airborne fumigants,[24] vaccination,[22] malignancy,[25] iodinated contrast medium,[26] pulmo-

Table 48-3. Suspected Causes of Toxic Epidermal Neurolysis

Drugs
  Allopurinol
  Antibiotics, especially sulfonamides; also penicillins, cephalosporins, tetracycline, antitubercular drugs, and others
  Barbiturates
  Carbamazepine
  Diphenylhydantoin
  Mithramycin
  Nonsteroidal anti-inflammatory drugs, e.g., aspirin, benoxaprofen, indomethacin, phenylbutazone, proxicam, sulindac
  Pentazocine
  Phenolphthalein
  Sulfones
  Others
Viral infections
  Measles
  Varicella/herpes zoster
Fungal infections
  Pulmonary aspergillosis
Other
  Fumigants
  Graft-versus-host disease
  Immunization
  Iodinated contrast medium
  Malignancy, e.g., lymphoma, leukemia
  Radiotherapy

nary aspergillosis,[27] and radiation therapy. In contrast to Stevens-Johnson syndrome, TEN has not been associated with Mycoplasma pneumoniae infections.

Clinical Presentation

TEN may be preceded by a prodrome of fever, malaise, cutaneous tenderness, arthralgias, and conjunctival burning or itching. The rash begins as a red, tender, often morbilliform eruption, which may rapidly become confluent. Flaccid, ill-defined bullae develop within areas of erythema and rupture, leaving raw, exposed dermis (Figs. 48-5 and 48-6). These bullae form at the dermal-epidermal junction, resulting in a more serious injury than that caused by the more superficial bullae of staphylococcal scalded skin syndrome. As with staphylococcal scalded skin syndrome, Nikolsky's sign can be demonstrated when horizontal pressure with the examiner's finger causes or extends bullae.[19] When first seen by a physician, only erosive lesions may be present with no evidence of intact bullae. Extension of the eruption may occur over a period ranging from 24 hours to 15 days.[28] In the most severe of cases, more than 90% of the body surface area may become devoid of epidermis.[29]

Usually prominent mucous membrane involvement occurs, with lesions identical to those seen in Stevens-Johnson syndrome. Any mucosal surface may be involved. Acute mucosal signs and symptoms include erythema, vesicles, bullae, ulcerations, burning, and pain. Commonly involved mucosae include lips, conjunctiva, buccal mucosa, nares, anogenital mucosa, pharynx, and esophagus.

Systemic manifestations of TEN are outlined in Table 48-4. Severe disease may be accompanied by tracheitis, pneumonitis, hepatitis, gastrointestinal bleeding,[19] or hypophosphatemic encephalopathy.[30] Renal changes of membranous or membranoproliferative glomerulonephritis may occur with proteinuria, hematuria, and azotemia.[31] Elevated serum amylase of pancreatic or salivary gland origin has also been reported.[32]

Differential Diagnosis

The clinical diagnosis of TEN is based on observing an acute, erythematous, tender eruption accompanied by bullous denudation, mucosal involvement, and Nikolsky's sign. Staphylococcal scalded skin syndrome may be ruled out by frozen section, exfoliative cytology, skin biopsy, or noting mucosal involvement (see Chap. 46). Adults do not develop staphylococcal scalded skin syndrome unless they are immunocompromised or have renal failure.[19] Stevens-Johnson syndrome with extensive cutaneous bullae is identical in appearance to TEN, and there has been controversy over whether or not they are separate entities. Supportive evidence for overlap between these syndromes includes identical epidermal histologic changes, similar clinical appearance, and reports of otherwise classic TEN with target lesions. Evidence supporting a distinction between the syndromes includes a lack of dermal inflammatory cells in TEN, inability to document circulating immune complexes in TEN, and absence of an association of TEN with Mycoplasma pneumoniae infection.[19] Fortunately, TEN and Stevens-Johnson syndrome with cutaneous denudation are treated similarly. Other entities that may rarely cause confusion with TEN include widespread bullous fixed drug eruption,[33] true scalding, and kerosene "burns."[34] It is always advisable to obtain a skin biopsy specimen to confirm a diagnosis of TEN.

Treatment

All patients with TEN require hospitalization for observation and therapy. Possible causes, particularly medications, should be identified and eliminated. In some cases, no cause is apparent. Admission to the ICU is indicated

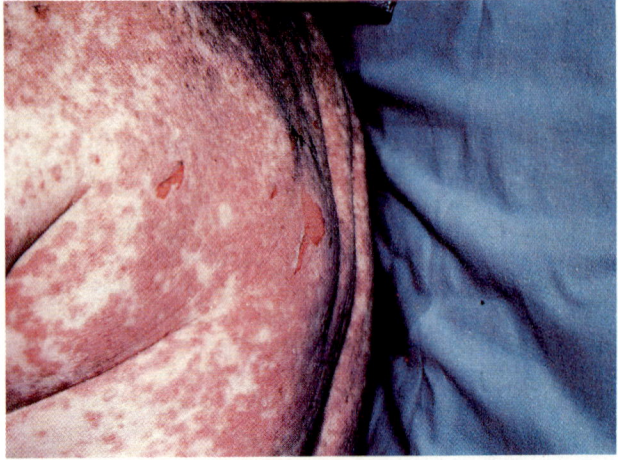

Fig. 48-5. Toxic epidermal necrolysis. Erythematous papules are coalescing into large plaques. Two erosions from ruptured bullae are present. (From Snook, D. L., and McDonald, C. J.: The dermatologic manifestations of critical illness. J. Crit Illness, 3(3): 9, and 3(6):93, 1988.)

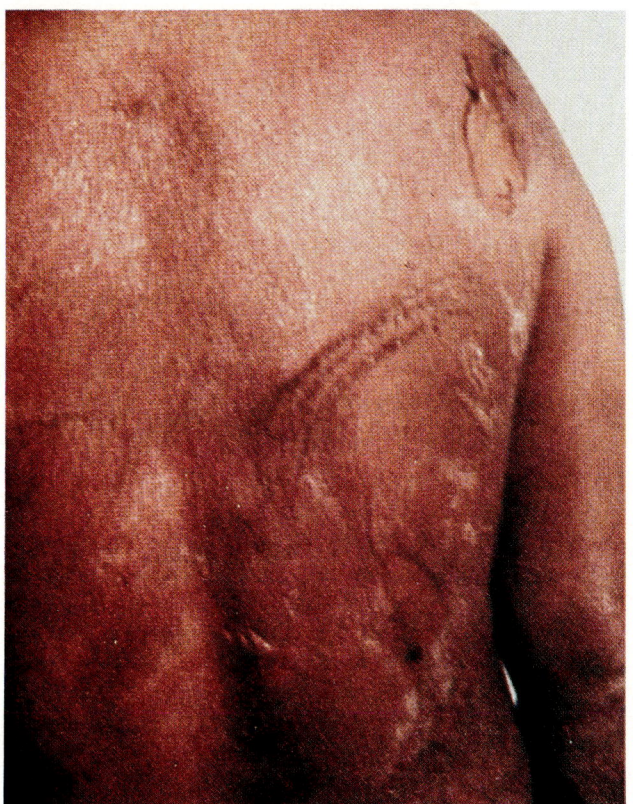 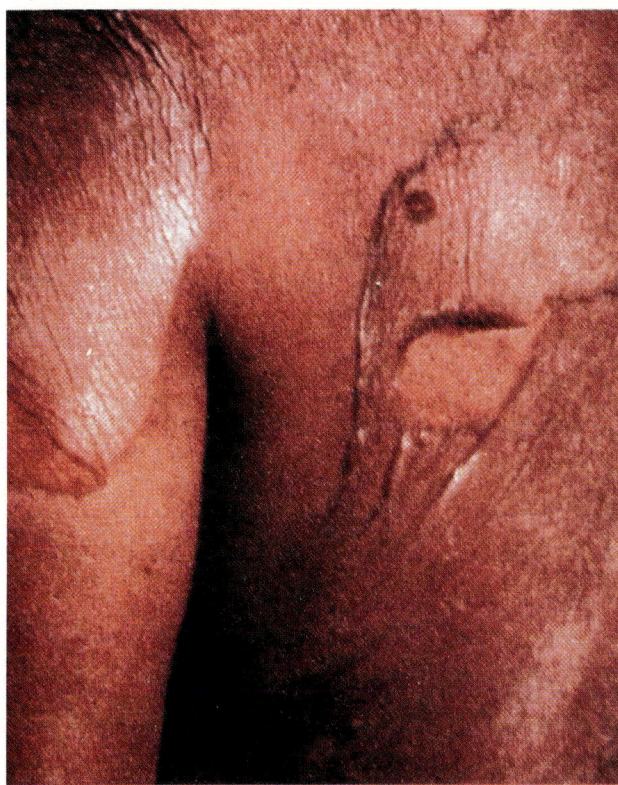

Fig. 48–6. *A* and *B,* Advanced toxic epidermal necrolysis. A generalized erytheroderma is present with several areas of denudation. Note large flaccid bulla on upper arm in *B*. (From Snook, D. L., and McDonald, C. J.: The dermatologic manifestations of critical illness. J. Crit. Illness, *3(3):*9, and *3(6):*93, 1988.)

for patients with extensive areas of cutaneous denudation, hypovolemic shock, sepsis, pulmonary decompensation, or serious gastrointestinal bleeding. Prognostic factors associated with a fatal course include old age, large area of denuded skin, and elevation of blood urea nitrogen.[28] These factors should be included in decisions to monitor patients in the ICU. Common causes of death include sepsis, gastrointestinal hemorrhage, and pulmonary embolus.[28] Extensive loss of the epidermal barrier leads to transcutaneous loss of fluid, electrolytes, and protein and provides an entry site for infection. Patients with large areas of epidermal loss are best managed using thermal burn center methods, paying particular attention to fluid replacement, infection control, nutrition, and topical

Table 48–4. Systemic Involvement in Toxic Epidermal Neurolysis

Fever
Arthralgias
Gastrointestinal: hemorrhage, nausea, vomiting
Renal: hematuria, proteinuria, azotemia
Respiratory: tracheitis, bronchitis, bronchopneumonia, pulmonary edema
Hepatitis
Elevated serum amylase (pancreatic or salivary)
Hypophosphatemic encephalopathy

dressings.[29,30,35,36] Fluids and electrolytes are replaced with crystalloid, supplemented by albumin and fresh frozen plasma as needed. Patients with extensive cutaneous involvement may present with hypotension, and often require 5 to 7 L of intravenous fluid during the first 24 hours of hospitalization.[30] Sometimes increased dermal blood flow to denuded areas results in hypothermia, which may be corrected by warming the patient's environment or by covering the patient with a survival blanket.[37] Air-fluidized beds have been used to warm patients and limit epidermal peeling owing to shear forces.[36] An air-fluidized bed may, however, increase fluid loss by as much as 6 L per day.[36]

Because sepsis is the leading cause of death from TEN,[28] prevention and treatment of infection are extremely important. Central venous lines and bladder catheters should be avoided when possible and peripheral intravenous lines discontinued as soon as they are no longer needed. When central lines are removed, the tips should be cut off and sent for culture.[28] Nystatin may be administered orally or by nasogastric tube to decrease the potential for candidal overgrowth and candidal sepsis.[29] Frequent surveillance cultures of skin, mucosa, and urine have been advocated to identify susceptibility patterns of organisms that may later cause infection.[30] Frequent chest films and blood cultures should be used during the acute illness to identify infection as early as possible. Bacterial pneumonia is a frequent complication.[36] Prophylactic antibiotics are best avoided because they serve only to select out resistant organisms. At the first sign of sepsis, patients should be placed on broad-spectrum antibiotics. Caution is in order, however, because fever is a nonspecific sign of infection, as many uninfected patients are febrile owing to the TEN itself.[28] Signs of sepsis include hypothermia or fever after the fourth day, decreased sensorial function, falling urine output, failure of gastric emptying, or any sudden change in the patient's condition.[30]

Adequate nutrition is important to replace transcutaneous nitrogen loss, speed healing, and maintain immunocompetence.[35,36] Many patients are unable to sustain adequate oral intake because of mucosal pain and therefore require nasogastric tube feedings. Fortunately, most patients have a well-functioning gastrointestinal tract and do not require intravenous hyperalimentation.[36] Treatment of ocular involvement is the same as that used for Stevens-Johnson syndrome and requires the care of an ophthalmologist.[30,36]

Topical dressings are used to prevent infection, limit transcutaneous losses, reduce pain, and speed healing. Loose, necrotic epidermis may become a nidus for infection and should be debrided before dressings are applied.[36] Whether necrotic but adherent epidermis needs to be debrided is debatable and probably not necessary.[30] Successfully used topical dressings have included Burow's soaks, silver nitrate in gauze,[29] Vaseline-impregnated gauze,[35] amnion,[38] and cadaveric or porcine grafts.[36,39] Synthetic membranes have been used for secondary coverage with varying success.[29,36] Although silver nitrate dressings have been used successfully,[29] they may cause adverse effects of wound desiccation, hyponatremia, and hypothermia.[36] Topical use of silver sulfadiazine should probably be avoided because sulfonamides are a common cause of TEN. Porcine and cadaveric skin grafts have been reported to give excellent results[36,39] and have the added benefit of not requiring frequent painful dressing changes. Although more costly than porcine xenographs, cadaveric allografts actually revascularize and "take," obviating the need for graft changes. Cadaveric allografts are simply left in place and are shed when new epidermis grows underneath them.[39]

In addition to the aforementioned therapies for TEN, standard management is used to prevent and treat complications. Subcutaneous heparin is used to prevent pulmonary embolism in bedridden patients,[30] and antacids are administered to prevent gastrointestinal ulcers.[29] Most patients require pain control. Patients with preexisting diseases, such as diabetes or congestive heart failure, require special attention to such problems.

As with Stevens-Johnson syndrome, there has been mixed enthusiasm for the use of corticosteroids in TEN. Although no randomized studies have been done, several retrospective analyses of severe cases of TEN suggest that corticosteroid use is associated with an increase in sepsis and mortality.[29,30] At one burn center, there was an impressive decrease in infection and increase in survival when corticosteroid use was eliminated from the standard care of TEN.[29] Steroids also mask signs of infection. Proponents of corticosteroids, however, believe that the incidence of sepsis is not significantly increased with corticosteroid use if dressings and topical antibacterials are properly used. Many dermatologists believe that early administration of large doses of corticosteroids may decrease morbidity and mortality. We treat patients early with an equivalent dose of about 1 to 2 mg/kg of prednisone per day. Given present knowledge, it seems reasonable to discontinue corticosteroids if a fulminant course with extensive denudation develops. Experimental modalities, such as hyperbaric oxygen[40] and plasmapheresis,[30] are presently of uncertain efficacy in the treatment of TEN.

Outcome

Although TEN may be a devastating disease, patients with loss of more than 90% total body surface area epidermis have survived with appropriate therapy.[29,38] Reported mortality rates range from 10 to 70%.[28] With present state-of-the-art therapy, using burn center techniques and avoiding steroid use in severe cases, a mortality rate of about 20% is attainable.[28,36]

Recovery

With good care, most skin wounds heal in about 14 days.[28,36] Mucosal lesions may heal more slowly.[28] Cutaneous wounds may leave transient or permanent hyperpigmentation or hypopigmentation. Rare permanent universal depigmentation has also been described.[41] Transient loss of fingernails or toenails is not uncommon.[19] Mucous membrane sequelae similar to those seen in Stevens-Johnson syndrome may also occur. As with Stevens-Johnson syndrome, ocular sequelae can be particularly devastating. TEN ocular sequelae include synechiae, entropion, ectropion, symblepharon, ankyloblepharon, distichiasis, trichiasis, loss of eyelashes, epiphora, conjunctival cysts, keratoconjunctivitis sicca, corneal neovascularization, corneal opacification, and blindness. Patients with ocular sequelae often require opthalmologic care for many years.[42]

DRUG ERUPTIONS

Cutaneous drug eruptions compose a significant proportion of adverse reactions to drugs and are encountered in about 2 to 3% of all hospitalized patients.[43] Most such eruptions pose no significant danger and resolve rapidly after discontinuation of the offending agent. Others are life-threatening, however, and as such require prompt recognition and appropriate interventions. Several types of drug eruption exist, as outlined in Table 48–5. Some are

Table 48–5. Types of Cutaneous Drug Reactions

Immune-mediated
  Urticaria/angioedema/anaphylaxis
  Serum sickness
  Purpura secondary to drug-induced thrombocytopenia
  Contact dermatitis (allergic)
Immunelike reactions (cause non–immune or uncertain)
  Erythema multiforme/Stevens-Johnson syndrome
  Morbilliform
  Toxic epidermal necrolysis
  Anaphylactoid reactions
  Contact dermatitis (irritant)

clearly immune mediated, and others simulate immune reactions but are of unclear origin. When drugs produce an immune reaction, the drug or its metabolite usually complexes with a native protein to produce a hapten. Only rarely are the native drugs immunogens, and in these cases, they are usually peptides themselves (e.g., insulin or growth hormone). Immune-mediated drug eruptions may fall into one of the four categories of the Gel and Coombs classification.

Type I (immediate hypersensitivity) reactions are mediated by reagen (IgE antibody) that is specific for a drug or drug-hapten complex. When the bound antibodies combine with mast cells, degranulation of the latter occurs, and substances such as histamine, leukotrienes, and prostaglandins are released. They mediate the ensuing clinical response, which is most often manifested in the skin by urticaria and angioedema. Anaphylaxis occurs in the most serious and dangerous cases. Urticaria occurs most commonly with penicillins; cephalosporins; polypeptide hormones, including insulin and chymopapain; and vaccines. Penicillin-sensitive patients can cross react with other beta-lactam antibiotics, including cephalosporins, cephamycins, and penems.

Type II or cytotoxic antibody reactions occur when an antigen (such as a drug) combines with normal tissue components and stimulates the formation of antibodies to these tissue components. The combination of antibody with normal cells or tissues results in destruction of the tissues. Clinical correlates may include hemolytic anemia, thrombocytopenia, and granulocytopenia. Cutaneous findings are generally secondary, such as purpura that occurs as a consequence of immune-mediated thrombocytopenia. Type II reactions have occurred with quinine, quinidine, acetaminophen, thiouracil, and sulfonamides.

Type III reactions are immune complex mediated. Here the drug or drug-hapten combines with specific IgG or IgM antibody resulting in immune complex formation. These complexes deposit in blood vessels and certain organs and result in complement fixation with subsequent damage to the organ. Clinical states associated with immune complex formation include vasculitis, some urticaria, and serum sickness. The last-mentioned is a prototype of the type III reaction and is characterized by urticaria, palpable purpura, arthralgias, fever, nephritis, and neuritis. The self-limited symptoms usually resolve after 3 to 4 days. They may develop 7 to 12 days following exposure to the antigen (here, a drug). The reaction may develop within a day, however, if the host has been previously exposed (sensitized) to the drug. Serum sickness has been described with penicillin, sulfonamides, thiouracil, phenytoin, and streptomycin, among others.

Type IV reactions (delayed-type hypersensitivity) occur most often with topical medications, such as Neosporin, topical antihistamines, parafens, and tape adhesives. Allergic contact dermatitis is to be differentiated from irritant contact dermatitis because they are clinically similar. Irritant dermatitis is dose related and occurs in a relatively large number of persons who contact the agent. It accounts for about 70% of all contact dermatitis. Allergic contact dermatitis occurs in those few who are genetically predisposed; it requires only a small amount of chemical.

It is often difficult to ascribe a particular drug to a cutaneous reaction, especially in extremely ill, often multimedicated patients. In such situations, a methodical analysis usually leads to one or two "most likely" drugs. First, a flow sheet should be constructed that lists all medications administered during the previous 6 weeks with start and stop dates. From this list, one can choose drugs that are known to produce a high incidence of cutaneous reactions. Several statistical studies can aid in this determination.[43-45] Amoxicillin, ampicillin, trimethoprim-sulfamethoxasole, and phenytoin are drugs with particularly high reaction rates. Commonly used drugs with low incidence of cutaneous reactions include acetaminophen, aluminum and magnesium hydroxide, atropine, digoxin, diphenhydramine, heparin, meperidine, potassium chloride, ferrous sulfate, and spironolactone.[46] Once the list has been narrowed, an examination of start and stop dates may further implicate a particular agent. Although most drug reactions occur within 7 days of drug initiation, several medications, including penicillin, amoxicillin, ampicillin, cephalosporins, and trimethoprim-sulfamethoxazole, may produce more delayed reactions that can be seen up to 2 weeks after initiation of therapy.[44] Age and underlying diagnosis (with a few exceptions) appear to have little effect on the propensity to develop a drug eruption. The incidence in women is reported to be 35% higher than in men when data are normalized for age, diagnosis and survival, and number of drugs administered.[45]

Urticaria is one of the two most common drug reaction patterns; the other is the morbilliform type of rash. Less common patterns include erythema multiforme and bullous drug eruptions.

Urticaria

Urticaria is most often IgE mediated and is a type I (immediate hypersensitivity) reaction. Immediate reactions often occur within minutes of drug administration. Urticaria may also be associated with type III (immune complex mediated) reactions or may be nonimmunologic. Such agents as radiocontrast dyes, certain intravenous anesthetics, opiates, and polymyxin B can cause direct nonspecific (nonimmunologic) mediator release (mast cell degranulation).

Urticaria is characterized by the presence of fairly well-demarcated pink or rosy plaques that may be large and extensive and are usually pruritic (Fig. 48-7). Urticaria alone is of little consequence, but when accompanied by angioedema and anaphylaxis, the reaction may be life-threatening. The route of administration of the drug appears to influence sensitization and risk of anaphylaxis, with the intramuscular route implicated the most followed by intravenous then oral.[47] When the patient is not already sensitized, the urticarial reactions tend to occur within 7 days of drug initiation. A dramatic response within minutes, however, can be seen in those patients who have been previously introduced to the drug. Urticarial drug reactions are defined as accelerated when they occur within hours or days following administration of the drug. When respiratory and cardiovascular compromise occur, the patient may require immediate transferral to the ICU.

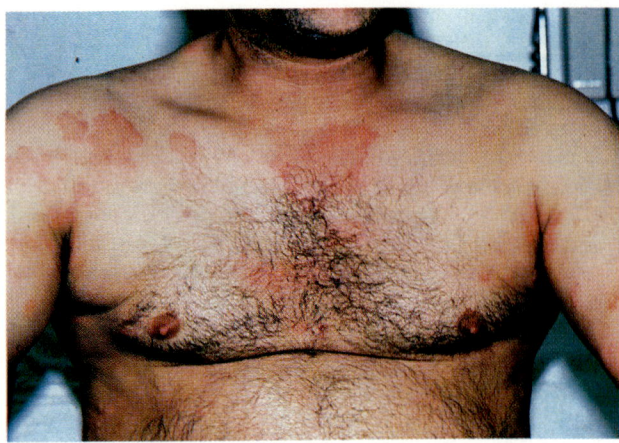

Fig. 48–7. Pink, indurated plaques or urticaria. (Courtesy of Division of Dermatology, Brown University, Providence, RI.)

Subcutaneous epinephrine, 0.3 to 0.5 ml of a 1:1000 aqueous solution, should be administered about every 15 minutes until symptoms abate. The dose for children is 0.01 ml/kg subcutaneously or intramuscularly. The epinephrine may also be administered intravenously. By this route, the drug should be administered slowly at a concentration of 1:10,000. Cardiac monitoring should be initiated because arrhythmias may occur. H_1 and H_2 antihistamines should also be used although their effect is not so immediate. Likewise, systemic corticosteroids may be useful, although their effect is not seen until 4 to 6 hours after administration. Intravenous fluids and vasopressors may be required for cardiovascular support, and aminophylline may be given if respiratory symptoms persist. Obviously the suspected drug must be discontinued. If it is absolutely necessary to continue such a drug, this may be done in the face of a minor (urticaria only) reaction under close supervision. The risk of progression to a systemic allergic reaction is reportedly lessened when the drug is maintained with frequent dosing intervals.[48] If patients are at risk for anaphylactic reactions and no alternative drug exists, desensitization may be attempted; this has been done with penicillin and insulin.[49]

Morbilliform Eruption

The morbilliform eruption is probably the most common type of drug reaction. The term "morbilliform" refers to the measleslike nature of the eruption. Although pathogenesis remains unclear, it is believed by some to be immune complex mediated. This eruption occurs with relatively high frequency with antibiotics, such as ampicillin, penicillin, sulfonamides; with anticonvulsants, such as phenytoin and barbiturates; and sometimes with blood products. Occurrence with ampicillin is even further increased when it is administered to patients with infectious mononucleosis, cytomegalovirus infections, chronic lymphocytic leukemia, and concurrent allopurinol therapy. An increased incidence of rash has also been observed in acquired immunodeficiency syndrome (AIDS) patients treated with trimethoprim-sulfamethoxasole for Pneumocystis carinii infection.[50]

Morbilliform eruptions usually occur within a week of treatment but may appear as long as 2 weeks after the medication has been discontinued. Peripheral eosinophilia is supportive of the diagnosis. The rash is often described as maculopapular and consists of numerous, often pruritic erythematous macules and papules that measure 2 to 4 mm in diameter (Fig. 48–8). These are symmetric in distribution, often starting on the trunk and dependent areas. The lesions may coalesce to a confluent erythema of the folds, especially the groin and axillae. The eruption is often more pronounced at pressure points. Involvement of the palms and soles is variable. The rash usually persists for 1 or 2 weeks after discontinuation of the drug. The lesions initially appear bright red but become brownish and dull as the eruption fades. A fine, dry desquamation often appears on resolution of the rash. The more severe morbilliform drug eruptions may progress to erythroderma or total body erythema. Erythroderma may be of significance in

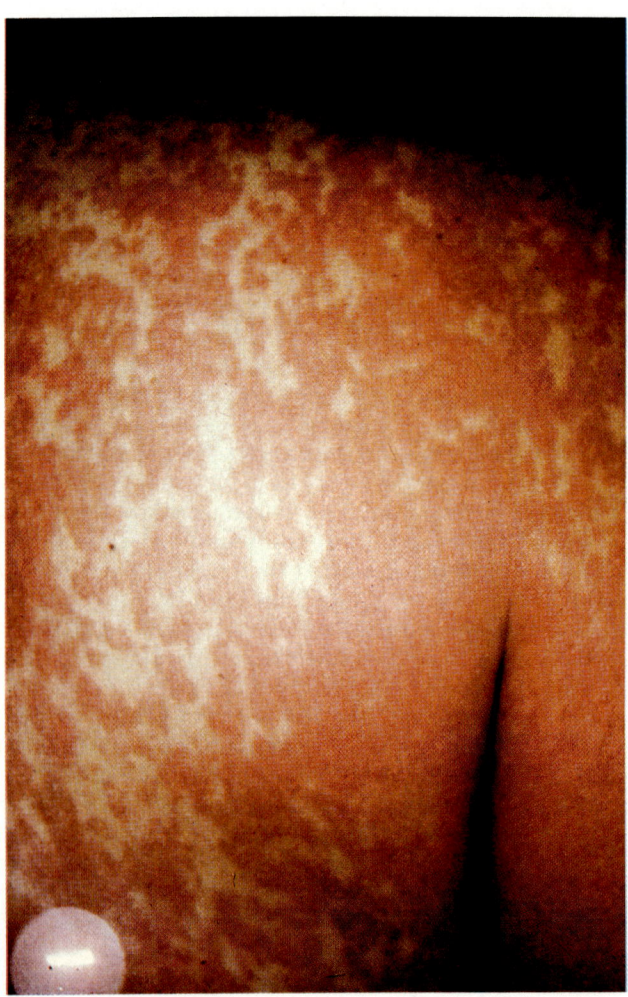

Fig. 48–8. Morbilliform drug eruption in patient with mononucleosis on ampicillin. (Courtesy of Division of Dermatology, Brown University, Providence, RI.)

patients with preexisting cardiovascular disease because high output cardiac failure may ensue because of the shunting of blood to the integument. If generalized confluent erythema occurs, there is also the possibility that the eruption might progress to TEN. In all cases of presumed morbilliform drug eruption, the differential diagnosis must include viral exanthem, miliaria rubra, and urticaria. History and careful physical examination usually point to the diagnosis. Most morbilliform eruptions are easily managed with antihistamines and topical antipruritic lotions containing menthol and phenol or pramoxine for pruritus, bland emollients, and discontinuation of the offending drug. Occasionally the eruption fades despite continuation of the drug. It is sometimes prudent to initiate prednisone therapy if the eruption is severe and no contraindication to therapy exists. Prednisone is initiated at 60 to 80 mg/day and is tapered over about 3 weeks. If erythroderma is present, fluid intake and output must be monitored because insensible loss is greatly increased. Open wet dressings with lukewarm water may induce vasoconstriction and thus aid in therapy. Hypoalbuminemia and anemia may ensue with exfoliative states, and the patient should be monitored for this development.

Erythema Multiforme

Erythema multiforme is a reaction pattern that develops after exposure to certain drugs, although it may also occur with infections, such as herpes simplex or mycoplasma. Although immune factors have been implicated, the mechanisms remain uncertain. Drugs often associated with erythema multiforme include penicillin, sulfonamides, barbiturates, anticonvulsants, salicylates, and phenothiazines. Occasionally no associated factor is recognized. This eruption is characterized by numerous well-demarcated macules that may show a dusky center with a surrounding pale halo and a peripheral ring of erythema. These are the classic "target lesions" that are often seen on the palms, soles, and distal extremities. The appearance of vesicles or bullae in the center of the lesions may indicate a propensity of the eruption to progress to Stevens-Johnson syndrome. At times, a target appearance is not present, and the lesions consist of erythematous macules and urticaria-alike plaques that measure from about 0.5 to 1 cm and may become confluent. Erythema multiforme resolves after discontinuation of the offending agent. If no contraindication is present, a course of prednisone may be initiated starting at 60 to 80 mg per day and tapering over 3 weeks. Occasionally this reaction is fulminant with involvement of the mucous membranes, conjunctivae, and internal mucosal surfaces and generalized sloughing of the skin. Mucous membrane involvement signals the development of Stevens-Johnson syndrome or erythema multiforme major. Mucous membrane involvement often limits enteral intake, and widespread skin sloughing predisposes to sepsis and fluid and electrolyte imbalance. Admission to the ICU is usually required. Some consider Stevens-Johnson syndrome a subset of TEN, which may also be drug-related. Both Stevens-Johnson syndrome and TEN are discussed in detail in previous sections of this chapter.

Bullous Drug Eruptions

Bullous drug eruptions are relatively uncommon. They have been described with several unrelated medications. Naldixic acid may produce a generalized bullous reaction that may be related to ultraviolet exposure. Furosemide may produce bullous lesions of the extremities, especially in dialysis patients. Barbiturate intoxication and coma secondary to any cause may result in bullae at pressure points that may be related to sweat gland necrosis. Erythema of the affected areas is observed initially; this progresses to bullae within about 24 hours. D-Penicillamine produces a drug-induced pemphigus with antibodies to intercellular material. Skin biopsy specimens of bullous lesions are often diagnostic. Treatment is supportive and consists of compresses with aluminum acetate or other astringent compresses as well as drug discontinuation.

Several distinct syndromes exist that are related to particular drugs. Notable among these are phenytoin hypersensitivity, coumarin necrosis, and drug-induced lupus.

PHENYTOIN HYPERSENSITIVITY SYNDROME

Adverse cutaneous reactions to phenytoin are extremely common. Morbilliform patterns are observed most often, but more serious eruptions, including erythema multiforme major (Stevens-Johnson syndrome) and TEN, occasionally occur. The incidence of mild morbilliform rashes may be as high as 10%. Most resolve after discontinuation of the drug. The rash, however, may be associated with a rare phenytoin hypersensitivity reaction. Pathogenesis of this syndrome is unknown, but an immunologic basis is suspected. This is supported by recurrence of the eruption on rechallenge and by demonstration of cell-mediated immunity and specific antibody response to phenytoin.[54,60] Others have shown depressed IgA levels in affected patients.[61,62]

Major components of the phenytoin hypersensitivity syndrome include a skin eruption, fever, lymphadenopathy, and anicteric or icteric hepatitis. Peripheral eosinophilia is not uncommon, and a leukocytosis with atypical lymphocytes may be present. Other less common manifestations include blood dyscrasias such as leukopenia, thrombocytopenia, anemia,[51] serum sickness,[52] renal failure,[53-56] interstitial pulmonary infiltrates,[57] myositis,[53] DIC,[58] lupuslike syndromes,[51] and rhabdomyolysis.[59]

The phenytoin hypersensitivity reaction may occur more commonly in blacks and can be seen at any age.[63] Fever and rash usually appear as initial symptoms 2 to 4 weeks after the drug is initiated. The reaction may appear up to 2 weeks after the drug is stopped and can progress for days after drug discontinuation.[63,64] The rash is often pruritic and generalized. It is usually morbilliform and is sometimes accompanied by striking facial and periorbital edema. The mucous membranes, including the pharynx and buccal mucosa, are sometimes erythematous. Fever may reach 40.6°C. Diffuse lymphadenopathy is usually present, and nonspecific symptoms, such as myalgias and anorexia, are experienced. The lymphadenopathy associated with the syndrome is probably distinct from that observed with phenytoin-induced pseudolymphoma, which runs a more chronic course and is not always accompanied by fever, rash, and hepatitis. The hepatitis associated with the syndrome is more concerning of all features because it is associated with significant morbidity and mortality. Massive hepatic necrosis may occur and is frequently fatal.[65] One report cites a nearly 40% incidence of fatal hepatic necrosis in cases of phenytoin hypersensitivity with hepatic involvement.[66] Phenytoin-induced hepatitis is characterized by increased transaminases and alkaline phosphatase; the levels return gradually to normal if the syndrome is recognized and the medication discontinued. If phenytoin is continued, extensive hepatic necrosis may ensue. Pathologic examination of liver tissue may show a ground-glass appearance or liver cells with hepatocellular degeneration or necrosis; granulomatous reactions with or without associated hepatocellular injury may be more frequent and severe when the drug is given intermittently.[68] Interstitial bilateral pulmonary infiltrates have been observed in association with phenytoin hypersensitivity,[57] a development that is characterized clinically by dyspnea and hypoxemia. The interstitial pneumonitis appears to be reversible on discontinuation of the drug and administration of systemic steroids.[69,70] Nephritis associated with the syndrome may be manifested by proteinuria, hematuria, polyuria, and azotemia.[71]

The cornerstone of treatment is removal of the drug. Liver function studies and creatinine should be regularly monitored. Treatment of the skin eruption is not usually necessary except when Stevens-Johnson syndrome or TEN ensues. Phenytoin is often a crucial medication in seizure control, and therefore substitution is important. It should be noted, however, that phenobarbital is a structurally related compound, and patients hypersensitive to phenytoin may show a similar rash to this drug.[72] Sodium valproate for generalized seizures or carbamazepine for partial seizures may be reasonable alternatives, although liver involvement may limit their use. The use of systemic steroids in the phenytoin-hypersensitivity syndrome has not been proved effective, but their use may be indicated in fulminant cases.

ANTICOAGULANT-INDUCED NECROSIS

The most common adverse cutaneous reaction to coumarin therapy is hemorrhage. Other more unusual complications include alopecia, urticarial or maculopapular eruptions,[73] "purple toes,"[74] and coumarin-induced necrosis.

Coumarin necrosis of the skin and subcutaneous tissue is a rare event that is sometimes, although not usually, life-threatening. More than 90% of cases occur between days 3 and 10 (usually within the first 72 hours) of drug initiation, but the reaction may occur for up to 10 days. There is no age restriction, and it is not related to underlying disease states. More than 90% of affected patients are females, often obese. Coumarin necrosis has been associated with loading dose regimens, and appearance during long-term therapy is rare.[75] The pathogenesis of coumarin necrosis remains unclear. Evidence is against an allergic or hypersensitivity reaction, and thrombosis rather than hemorrhage is the primary event. Deficiency of protein C, a vitamin-K-dependent serine protease zymogen with anticoagulant and profibrinolytic activity, has been implicated.

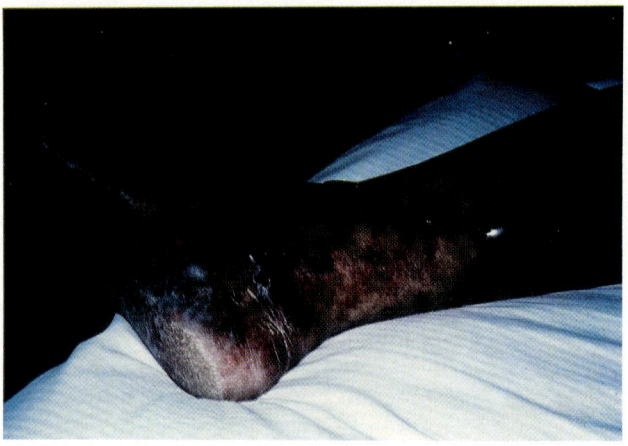

Fig. 48-9. Coumarin necrosis. The appearance of bullae indicates that necrosis has occurred. (Courtesy of Division of Dermatology, Brown University, Providence, RI.)

Patients with inherited or acquired protein C deficiency appear to have an increased risk for the development of coumarin necrosis during initial phases of treatment.[76-78] The synthesis of vitamin-K-dependent coagulation factors is suppressed by oral anticoagulant therapy, with the most rapid decline in factor VII and protein C followed by factors IX, X, and II and protein S. Pathogenesis of coumarin necrosis may involve transient imbalance between procoagulant factors (factors II, VII, IX, and X) and anticoagulant factors (protein C and protein S) that result following high initial doses of coumarin.[75]

The skin lesion is usually single but may be multiple. It appears suddenly often on the lower half of the body, especially where abundant subcutaneous fat is present, such as the thighs, buttocks, abdomen, and breasts. Involvement of the genitalia is rare, although cases of penile necrosis have been reported.[76] The face, neck, forearms, and hands are generally spared.[79] The lesion begins as a painful, erythematous, edematous, often poorly demarcated plaque. Within several hours, petechiae form within the lesion, and these become coalescent to form ecchymoses with geographic borders. Lesions continue to progress to hemorrhagic bullae, which indicate necrosis (Fig. 48-9). The necrosis may extend deeply to subcutaneous fat. The necrotic tissue sloughs, and healing occurs with scarring when involvement is deep. The extent and severity of lesions are variable; they resolve rapidly and completely when necrosis has not occurred but may require skin grafting or even amputation if deep necrosis is present. Fatalities have been reported that are related to septicemia and renal failure.[80] Progression of lesions may abort at any time despite continuation of the drug.

The onset of skin necrosis may be accompanied by an increased sedimentation rate and a decreased hemoglobin.[81] The prothrombin time is usually within the therapeutic range. Histopathologic examination reveals involvement of capillaries and venules with thrombotic occlusion and sometimes leukocytic infiltration. Hemorrhagic infarcts, dermal necrosis, and resultant subepidermal bullae are observed.[81,82]

Continuation of coumarin therapy does not appear to influence the course of the necrosis or lesion healing. Temporary discontinuation of the drug, however, is considered prudent. The process may be avoided if loading dose regimens are not used.[81] Heparin, steroids, sympathetic blockade, and local hypothermia have proved ineffective.[80] The use of vitamin K is somewhat controversial, although reports recommend parenteral vitamin K to reverse hypocoagulability.[75] The prothrombin time should be monitored daily from the time of institution of the drug. This may aid in differentiating coumarin necrosis from the much more common primary coumarin-induced hemorrhage.

Heparin necrosis is a rare event that also tends to occur in obese middle-aged women. Diabetes may predispose to this complication. It develops most often at the injection site and is heralded by the development of burning pain 1 to 2 weeks after drug initiation. Erythema is followed by bulla formation then necrosis. Thrombocytopenia may indicate a more serious course. Heparin should be discontinued and supportive therapy initiated. If anticoagulation is required, coumarin should be used.

DRUG-INDUCED LUPUS

A lupus-erythematosus-like reaction has been associated with several drugs, as outlined in Table 48-6). Approximately 50 drugs have been implicated since the 1970s, with procainamide most common and hydralazine second. Persons who are slow acetylators are more prone to suffer drug-induced lupus. Important factors in diagnosis are a lack of history of lupus before drug intake and a decline in symptoms and serologic parameters (ANA and dDNA antibodies) when the drug is discontinued.

The reaction develops at variable time intervals after initiation of the drug. It usually occurs after about 10 months of therapy with procainamide and between 6 and 24 months for hydralazine.[83] Symptoms of drug-induced lupus include fever, arthralgias or arthritis, weight loss, fatigue, and myalgias. Arthralgias are the most common finding with both procainamide-induced and hydralazine-induced lupus. Pericarditis, pleurisy, and splenomegaly are sometimes present. Renal involvement is unusual in drug-induced lupus, in contrast to the idiopathic form of the disease. The cutaneous findings are similar in drug-induced and idiopathic systemic lupus erythematosus, although purely cutaneous forms of lupus associated with drugs are uncommon. Skin manifestations are more common with hydralazine than procainamide and may appear as the typical malar (butterfly) rash consisting of multiple erythematous papules and plaques with minimal scale. Vasculitic lesions of the extremities may also be seen.[84]

The most constant laboratory feature of drug-induced lupus is a positive ANA (antihistamine antibodies) observed in greater than 95% of procainamide-induced and hydralazine-induced lupus. Lupus erythematosus cells and anti-dsDNA antibodies are present in 50 to 90% of patients treated with these drugs. Leukopenia, anemia, and thrombocytopenia may be present. Patients with idiopathic systemic lupus erythematosus show a wider variety of ANAs, including antibodies to native DNA, Smith antigen, and nuclear ribonucleoprotein.

Drug-induced lupus is reversible, with clinical symptoms and serologic abnormalities showing gradual resolution within a few months after drug discontinuation.

DISSEMINATED INTRAVASCULAR COAGULATION

DIC is a syndrome in which massive local or generalized intravascular thrombus formation leads to the irreversible aggregation and loss of platelets, consumption of specific plasma proteins, formation of fibrin, and activation of the fibrinolytic system with release of anticoagulant fibrin split product (FSP). The process is due to the presence of thrombin in the systemic circulation, which is a final common product of several initiating mechanisms. These include activation of Hageman's factor and the intrinsic clotting system secondary to endothelial cell injury, activation of the extrinsic system by tissue injury, or red cell platelet injury with release of coagulant phospholipids.[85]

Pathogenesis

Activation of Hageman's factor may result from disruption of the endothelium that may occur in gram-negative endotoxemia, including meningococcemia,[86] gram-positive endotoxemia,[87] viremia,[88] heatstroke,[89] and acute allograft rejection.[90] Activation of the extrinsic system by thromboplastic substances released after tissue injury or by certain tumors may occur in certain surgical or obstetric situations or with several carcinomas and leukemias (most commonly acute promyelocytic leukemia). A procoagulant activity in promyelocytic leukemia cells has been shown to be secondary to a substance known as tissue factor.[91-93] Damage of red blood cells or platelets with release of procoagulant phospholipids may occur with malaria or microangiopathic hemolytic anemia.[94,95] These phospholipids are necessary for proper functioning of the extrinsic and intrinsic clotting systems. In addition to the aforementioned processes, consumptive coagulopathy can occur secondary to a large, localized clotting process, such as that occurring with giant hemangiomas (Kasabach-Merritt syndrome) or dissecting arterial aneurysms.

Certain reticuloendothelial system defects predispose to or potentiate DIC. This system is responsible for removal

Table 48-6. Drugs Associated with a Lupuslike Reaction*

Procainamide
Hydralazine
Practolol
D-Penicillamine
Isoniazid
Quinidine
Prophylthiouracil
Hydantoins
Ethoxysuximide
Trimethadione
Chlorpromazine

* Arranged in decreasing order of risk.
(Adapted from Rubin, R. L.: Drug-induced lupus. Clin. Asp. Autoimmun., 2: 16, 1988.)

of fibrin, activated clotting factors, procoagulants, and endotoxins from the vascular system.[96] Thus patients with liver disease or splenectomy are more prone to the development of DIC. Two forms of DIC exist:[97] (1) The acute severe form is seen in seriously ill patients and is more frequently associated with infectious diseases, and (2) chronic DIC is a mild, protracted entity that is sometimes subclinical. A significant number of the latter patients may present with deep vein thrombosis that is sometimes migratory (Trousseau's syndrome). The chronic type of DIC has been associated with giant hemangiomata, mucin-producing carcinomas, and intracardiac thrombus.[98] DIC is always triggered by an underlying disease process. Recognition of those conditions that may predispose to DIC is of paramount importance in diagnosis and therapy (Table 48–7).[99,100]

Infection is probably the most common underlying condition associated with DIC, especially gram-negative septicemia. Obstetric complications associated with DIC include abruptio placentae, amniotic fluid embolus, retention of dead fetus, preeclampsia, eclampsia, and others.[101] Abruptio placentae occurs in about 2% of pregnancies and is the most common cause of DIC in obstetric patients.[102] Encountered less often is amniotic fluid embolism, which produces a dramatic form of DIC with a mortality of up to 80%.[103] It has been shown that nearly one third of head-injured children have laboratory parameters consistent with DIC and that a marked increase in mortality is associated with this group.[104]

Acute promyelocytic leukemia is the malignancy most often associated with DIC.[105] Low grade DIC sometimes occurs with visceral malignancy, such as gastric or pancreatic carcinoma. Warfarin (Coumadin)-induced necrosis is a special subset of DIC; it is discussed in detail in the previous section.

Clinical Presentation

The initial event in DIC is thrombosis of the microcirculation with microthrombi of fibrin or platelets. As this progresses, consumption of platelets and clotting factors lead to a hemorrhagic diathesis, which is often evident on examination of the skin. Skin findings may be secondary to either hemorrhage or thrombotic occlusion. Manifestations of the former are most common in acute DIC and include petechiae of the skin and mucous membranes, ecchymoses and occasional hemorrhagic bullae contained within the ecchymotic areas. Oozing may be present at venipuncture or cut-down sites. More uncommonly, evidence of ischemia owing to thrombosis may be seen with acrocyanosis of the extremities that can lead to gangrene.[106,107] Gangrenous purpura is usually symmetric and often involves the distal extremities, earlobes, nose, or genitalia. The characteristic purpurae, which improve only to reoccur on the digits, are clinical manifestations of intravascular coagulation and vessel occlusion. Improved perfusion with clot lysis results in reperfusion, and reoccurrence results from more clot formation. Hemorrhagic necrotic areas of the skin may reflect the cutaneous distribution of terminal arterioles. A rare but extreme form of DIC known as purpura fulminans exhibits rapidly progressive massive

Table 48–7. Acute Disseminated Intravascular Coagulation: Underlying Disease Processes

Infection
  Gram-negative septicemia
    Neisseria meningitidis*
    Neisseria gonorrheae
    Klebsiella
    Serratia
    Proteus mirabilis
    Pseudomonas aeruginosa
    Escherichia coli
    Salmonella
  Gram-positive septicemia
    Pneumococcus pneumoniae
    Staphylococcus aureus
    Staphylococcus albus
    Streptococcus
  Other infection
    Bacterial (legionnaire's disease, bacteroides, haemophilus meningitis, typhoid fever, shigella, Clostridium welchii)
    Rickettsial (Rocky Mountain spotted fever)
    Protozoal (malaria)
    Viral (congenital rubella, varicella, rubeola, dengue fever, herpes simplex, influenza)
    Mycoplasmal (tuberculosis)
    Fungal (aspergillosis, candidiasis, histoplasmosis), chlamydial (psittacosis)
Malignancy
  Carcinomas
  Leukemias (especially acute promyelocytic)*
  Other (pheochromocytoma, neuroblastoma, sarcoma, malignancy)
Obstetric complications
  Abruptio placentae*
  Placenta previa
  Amniotic fluid embolism
  Retention of dead fetus
  Septic and saline-induced abortion
  Hydatiform mole
  Preeclampsia/ecampsia
  Fatty liver of pregnancy
Shock
  Hypovolemic
  Hypoperfusion
Tissue injury
  Prolonged surgery (extracorporeal circulation, transurethral prostatectomy)
  Trauma (especially massive head injury)*
  Burns
  Heatstroke
Vascular disorders
  Giant hemangioma (Kasabach-Merritt syndrome)
  Aortic aneurysm
  Valvular heart disease
Liver disease
Other
  Transfusion reaction
  Respiratory distress syndrome in newborns
  Allograft rejection
  Necrotizing enterocolitis
  Warfarin (Coumadin)-induced necrosis

* More common associations.
(Adapted from Fruchtman, S., and Aledort, L. M.: Disseminated intravascular coagulation. J. Am. Coll. Cardiol., 8:159B, 1986; and Carr, M. E.: Disseminated intravascular coagulation: pathogenesis, diagnosis, and therapy. J. Emerg. Med., 5:311, 1987.)

ecchymoses with irregular geographic borders. Hemorrhagic blebs and areas of gangrene develop, presumably secondary to microvascular thrombosis. In addition to the skin, common sites of bleeding include the gastrointestinal and genitourinary systems and wounds.

Diagnosis

A suspicion of DIC engendered by the presence of a hemorrhagic-thrombotic diathesis in a patient with a characteristic underlying disease may be supported rapidly with results of screening laboratory tests, including platelet count, prothrombin time, and fibrinogen. A platelet count of less than 150,000 together with hypofibrinogenemia of less than 150 mg/dl and a prolonged prothrombin time (greater than 3 seconds) is strongly suggestive of DIC. Fibrinogen is an acute phase reactant and as such may be elevated in infection; levels also rise during pregnancy. Therefore a normal or even slightly elevated fibrinogen level does not exclude the diagnosis of DIC.[108] In low grade or chronic DIC, production of platelets or fibrinogen may keep up with consumption resulting in normal or increased levels. The presence of FSP is thought to be diagnostic by some. The FSP may be measured by latex particle agglutination assays,[109] by staphylococcal clumping test,[110] or by a more recently described quantitative assay.[111] It is notable that FSP may circulate in patients with liver disease; a "false-positive" may be obtained in such patients. A more specific test is the D-dimer test, which is currently used in some institutions. A prolonged thrombin clotting time reflects hypofibrinogenemia, and the presence of DIC can be confirmed by examination of a peripheral blood smear that reveals fragments of red cells, schistocytes, and helmet cells. Derangements of platelet count and coagulation factors or elevated FSP can be seen with the many disorders that accompany DIC. No single laboratory test can confirm or exclude the diagnosis, which is made by using a constellation of clinical and laboratory findings. (For additional discussion, see Chap. 45.) Other disease processes that produce abnormal coagulation screening tests are vitamin K deficiency, dilutional changes secondary to massive volume replacement, and liver disease. Severe hepatocellular liver disease is sometimes extremely difficult to differentiate from DIC; both may show prolonged prothrombin time, hypofibrinogenemia, and thrombocytopenia.[112] The presence of FSP is more common in DIC but can be present in both entities. The presence of soluble fibrin complexes or a reduction in factor VIII could confirm the diagnosis of DIC in such difficult cases.[113]

In DIC, thrombotic occlusive phenomena occur in a disseminated fashion throughout the microcirculation; all organs are therefore susceptible to injury.[97] Renal involvement may result in hematuria with acute oliguria or anuria secondary to ischemic cortical necrosis, resulting in azotemia. Hypotension may occur, further compromising renal function through acute tubular necrosis. Hemorrhagic necrosis of the adrenals (Waterhouse-Friderichsen syndrome) is a potentially life-threatening situation.

Pulmonary interstitial hemorrhage has been reported to occur in approximately 14% of patients with DIC, producing dyspnea and hemoptysis with rales on physical examination and a diffuse infiltrate on chest film.[85] The clinical picture may resemble adult respiratory distress syndrome (ARDS). DIC that accompanies heatstroke may identify a subset of patients at risk for developing ARDS.[114] DIC associated with pulmonary emboli has been reported.[115] Involvement of the gastrointestinal system may produce ulceration from submucosal necrosis, which may result in spontaneous massive bleeding. CNS dysfunction secondary to DIC may produce nonspecific changes, such as convulsions, coma, and altered mental status. Monitoring of the patient in an ICU may be required when one or more organ system demonstrates injury that is imminently or potentially life-threatening.

In the patient with DIC and sepsis with hypotension, specific, aggressive treatment with intravenous antibiotics along with fluids and sometimes pressor agents for blood passive support is indicated. Most patients with pulmonary involvement show some degree of hypoxemia, which may in some instances be sufficiently profound to require ventilatory support. When adrenal failure is suspected, hydrocortisone should be administered. Massive gastrointestinal or genitourinary bleeding requires close monitoring of the hematocrit and transfusion as indicated.

The mainstay of therapy in DIC is treatment of the underlying disease process. In many instances, this is sufficient to reverse the coagulopathy spontaneously. This includes appropriate antibiotic therapy for septic patients, cytotoxic agents for those with malignancies, and evacuation of the uterus in obstetric patients with DIC. The major cause of death in patients with the Kasabach-Merritt syndrome is bleeding owing to consumptive coagulopathy. Surgical removal of the hemangioma and cytolytic therapy are definitive forms of therapy. It is sometimes difficult, however, to excise these tumors because of their size or anatomic location. Exchange transfusion has also been used.[116] Glucocorticoids produce a variable effect on hemangioma regression and the coagulopathy. Because they may control the thrombocytopenia in some patients, their use is sometimes recommended.[117] When the underlying disease is resistant to therapy, active bleeding occurs, or surgical intervention is to take place, therapy directed at the coagulopathy may be initiated. Replacement therapy with cryoprecipitate, fresh frozen plasma, and platelet concentrates is accepted as appropriate first-line therapy in acute DIC. Maintenance of sufficient levels of these factors may be difficult, especially if the accompanying disease process remains active. Cryoprecipitate and fresh-frozen plasma contain proteins C and S and antithrombin III. These anticoagulants are depleted during DIC, and their restoration to normal levels may account for the efficacy of plasma product infusion. Because cryoprecipitate contains large amounts of fibrinogen in a small volume, it may be useful in the patient with controlled DIC who is hypofibrinogenemic. Platelet transfusions are generally not done if platelet counts exceed 50,000. The use of heparin remains somewhat controversial. A fairly well-accepted use, however, is in combination with hemostatic factors in certain settings. Here a continuous, low dose infusion at 500 U/hour serves to interfere with the action of thrombin and to prolong the half-life of circulating factors.[99] Heparin has been reported effective and even life-saving in selected situations, including amniotic fluid embolism;[118] excessive bleeding with giant hemangiomas;[112] malignancy, especially promyelocytic leukemia;[119] purpura fulminans;[108,120] and patients with evidence of thromboembolism as in Trousseau's syndrome.[121] Heparin may also be of benefit when DIC accompanies septic abortion, septicemia, and heatstroke.[100,122] Heparin increases activity of antithrombin III (AT-111). Infusion of AT-III concentrates in treatment of DIC has produced variable results.[123,124] Complete recovery without sequelae was observed in five patients with purpura fulminans after AT-III infusions.[125] It has been recommended that in DIC in which the activity of AT-III is lower than 70%, primary substitution therapy should be initiated.[126] The use of epsilon-aminocaproic acid to block the fibrinolytic component of DIC is controversial and dangerous. Its use may precipitate severe thrombosis, and it is therefore to be avoided in most situations. Glabexate mesilate is a serine protease inhibitor that exerts an inhibitory effect on the clotting activity of thrombin. In addition, it competitively inhibits the hydrolytic reactions of thrombin, factor Xa, plasmin, and kallikrein on synthetic substrates. It has an inhibitory effect on the coagulation cascade in the absence of AT-III, a situation often encountered in DIC. Initial studies with this agent are promising.[127,128] Plasma exchange should be considered in cases of severe DIC, such as that occurring with meningococcemia.

Outcome

The response to treatment of DIC should be monitored closely. In the improved patient, all bleeding should have ceased and any acrocyanosis resolved. The fibrinogen level is the single most useful parameter for following the response to therapy in patients with DIC. Fibrinogen levels should rise significantly within 1 to 3 days after treatment. The platelet count often remains low for several days after successful treatment of DIC. The FSP level declines slowly and is not helpful in monitoring. Prothrombin time and partial thromboplastin time show an early fall and are generally followed despite fluctuation. The patient requires less intensive care once the underlying disease process and coagulation factors stabilize.

Amputation of the distal extremities may be necessary in patients with severe microvascular compromise. CNS hemorrhage is fairly uncommon with DIC. Survivors of this complication may exhibit neurologic deficits. Bone infarction, abnormal bone growth, epiphyseal destruction, and premature epiphyseal-metaphyseal fusion have been reported as late complications of DIC with meningococcemia. Persistent fever after meningococcal sepsis with DIC may indicate bone necrosis.[129]

REFERENCES

1. Imamura, S., et al.: Erythema multiforme: demonstration of immune complexes in the sera and skin lesions. Br. J. Dermatol., 102:161, 1980.
2. Kazmierowski, J. A., Perzner, D. S., and Wuepper, K. D.: Herpes simplex antigen in immune complexes of patients with erythema multiforme. JAMA, 247:2547, 1982.
3. Kampgen, E., et al.: Association of herpes simplex virus-induced erythema multiforme with the human leukocyte antigen DQw3. Arch. Dermatol., 124:1372, 1988.
4. Fischer, P. R., and Shigeoka, A.: Familial occurrence of Stevens-Johnson syndrome. Am. J. Dis. Child., 137:914, 1983.
5. Sontheimer, R. D., Garibaldi, R. A., and Kruger, G. G.: Stevens-Johnson syndrome associated with Mycoplasma pneumoniae infections. Arch. Dermatol., 114:241, 1978.
6. Stutman, H. R.: Stevens-Johnson syndrome and Mycoplasma pneumoniae: evidence for cutaneous infection. J. Pediatr., 111:845, 1987.
7. Bianchine, J. R., et al.: Drugs as etiologic factors in the Stevens-Johnson syndrome. Am. J. Med., 44:390, 1968.
8. Tonnesen, M. G.: Erythema multiforme: a critical review of characteristics, diagnostic criteria, and causes. J. Am. Acad. Dermatol., 6:763, 1983.
9. Phoon, W. H., et al.: Stevens-Johnson syndrome associated with occupational exposure to trichloroethylene. Contact Dermatitis, 10:270, 1984.
10. Nathan, M. D.: Stevens-Johnson syndrome: twenty-three cases and their otolaryngologic significance. Laryngoscope, 85:1713, 1975.
11. Ting, H. C., and Adam, B. A.: Stevens-Johnson syndrome: a review of 34 cases. Int. J. Dermatol., 24:587, 1985.
12. Zweiban, B., Cohen, H., and Chandrasoma, P.: Gastrointestinal involvement complicating Stevens-Johnson syndrome. Gastroenterology, 91:469, 1986.
13. Schartum, S.: Stevens-Johnson syndrome with cardiac involvement: report of two cases. Acta Med. Scand., 179:729, 1966.
14. Gottschalk, H. R., and Orville, J. S.: Stevens-Johnson syndrome from ophthalmic sulfonamide. Arch. Dermatol., 112:513, 1976.
15. Arstikaitis, M. J.: Ocular aftermath of Stevens-Johnson syndrome: review of 33 cases. Arch. Ophthalmol., 90:376, 1973.
16. Rasmussen, J. E.: Erythema multiforme in children: response to treatment with systemic corticosteroids. Br. J. Dermatol., 95:181, 1976.
17. Wilson, E. E., and Malinak, L. R.: Vulvovaginal sequelae of Stevens-Johnson syndrome and their management. Obstet. Gynecol., 71:478, 1988.
18. Howell, C. G., Mansberger, J. A., and Parrish, R. A.: Esophageal stricture secondary to Stevens-Johnson syndrome. J. Pediatr. Surg., 22:994, 1987.
19. Snyder, R. A., and Elias, P. M.: Toxic epidermal necrolysis and staphylococcal scalded skin syndrome. Dermatol. Clin. North Am., 1:235, 1983.
20. Roujeau, J., et al.: Genetic susceptibility to toxic epidermal necrolysis. Arch. Dermatol., 123:1171, 1987.
21. Stern, R. S., and Chan, H.: Usefulness of case report literature in determining drugs responsible for toxic epidermal necrolysis. J. Am. Acad. Dermatol., 21:317, 1989.
22. Shoss, R. G., and Rayhanzadeh, S.: Toxic epidermal necrolysis following measles vaccination. Arch. Dermatol., 110:766, 1974.
23. Peck, G. L., Herzig, G. P., and Elias, P. M.: Toxic epidermal necrolysis in a patient with graft-vs-host reaction. Arch. Dermatol., 105:561, 1972.
24. Radimer, G. F., Davis, J. H., and Ackerman, B.: Fumigant-induced toxic epidermal necrolysis. Arch. Dermatol., 110:103, 1974.
25. Caldwell, I. W., Montgomery, P. R., and Peachey, R. D. G.: Toxic epidermal necrolysis and malignant lymphoma. Br. J. Dermatol., 79:287, 1967.
26. Kaffori, J., Abraham, Z., and Gilhar, A.: Toxic epidermal necrolysis after excretory pyelography: immunologic-me-

diated contrast medium reaction? Int. J. Dermatol., 27:346, 1988.
27. Rowell, N., and Thompson, H.: Toxic epidermal necrolysis in a patient with pulmonary aspergillosis. Br. J. Dermatol., 73:278, 1961.
28. Revuz, J., et al.: Toxic epidermal necrolysis: clinical findings and prognosis factors in 87 patients. Arch. Dermatol., 123:1160, 1987.
29. Halebian, P. H., et al.: Improved burn center survival of patients with toxic epidermal necrolysis managed without corticosteroids. Ann. Surg., 204:503, 1986.
30. Revuz, J., et al.: Treatment of toxic epidermal necrolysis: Cretil's experience. Arch. Dermatol., 123:1156, 1987.
31. Krumlovsky, F. A., del Greco, F., Herdson, P. B., and Lazar, P.: Renal disease associated with toxic epidermal necrolysis. Am. J. Med., 57:817, 1974.
32. Tagami, H., and Iwatsuki, K.: Elevated serum amylase in toxic epidermal necrolysis. Br. J. Dermatol., 115:250, 1986.
33. Baird, B. J., and De Villez, R. L.: Widespread bullous fixed drug eruption mimicking toxic epidermal necrolysis. Int. J. Dermatol., 27:170, 1988.
34. Barnes, R. L., and Wilkinson, D. S.: Epidermal necrolysis from clothing impregnated with paraffin. Br. Med. J., 4:466, 1973.
35. Roujeau, J., Chosidow, O., Saiag, P., and Guillaume, J.: Toxic epidermal necrolysis (Lyell syndrome). J. Am. Acad. Dermatol., 23:1039, 1990.
36. Heimbach, D. M., et al.: Toxic epidermal necrolysis: a step forward in treatment. JAMA, 257:2171, 1987.
37. Finlay, A. Y., Richards, J., and Holt, P. J. A.: Intensive therapy unit management of toxic epidermal necrolysis: practical aspects. Clin. Exp. Dermatol., 7:55, 1982.
38. Prasad, J. K., Feller, I., and Thomson, P. D.: Use of amnion for the treatment of Stevens-Johnson syndrome. J. Trauma, 26:945, 1986.
39. Birchall, N., Langdon, R., Cuono, C., and Mcguire, J.: Toxic epidermal necrolysis: an approach to management using cryopreserved allograft skin. J. Am. Acad. Dermatol., 16:368, 1978.
40. Ruocco, V., Bimonte, D., Luongo, C., and Florio, M.: Hyperbaric oxygen treatment of toxic epidermal necrolysis. Cutis, 38:267, 1986.
41. Smith, D. A., and Burgdorf, W. H. C.: Universal cutaneous depigmentation following phenytoin-induced toxic epidermal necrolysis. J. Am. Acad. Dermatol., 10:106, 1984.
42. De Felice, G. P., Caroli, R., and Autelitano, A.: Long-term complications of toxic epidermal necrolysis (Lyell's disease). Ophthalmologica, 195:1, 1987.
43. Jick, H., et al.: Comprehensive drug surveillance. JAMA, 213:1455, 1970.
44. Arndt, K. A., and Jick, H.: Rates of cutaneous reaction to drugs: a report from the Boston Collaborative Drug Surveillance Program. JAMA, 235:918, 1976.
45. Bigby, M., Jick, S., Jick, H., and Arndt, K.: Drug-induced cutaneous reactions: a report from the Boston Collaborative Drug Surveillance Program 15,438 consecutive inpatients, 1975 to 1982. JAMA, 256:3358, 1986.
46. Dunagin, W. G., and Millikan, L. E.: Drug eruptions. Med. Clin. North Am., 64:983, 1980.
47. Anderson, J. A., and Adkinson, N. F.: Allergic reactions to drugs and biologic agents. JAMA, 258:2891, 1987.
48. Wedner, H. J.: Allergic reactions to drugs. Primary Care, 14:523, 1987.
49. Blais, M. S., and deShazo, R. D.: Drug allergy. Pediatr. Clin. North Am., 35:1131, 1988.
50. Gordin, F. M., Simon, G., Wofsy, C. B., and Mills, J.: Adverse reactions to trimethoprim sulfamethoxazole in patients with acquired immunodeficiency syndrome. Ann. Intern. Med., 100:495, 1984.
51. Haruda, F.: Phenytoin hypersensitivity: 38 cases. Neurology, 29:1480, 1979.
52. Braverman, I. M., and Levin, J.: Dilantin-induced serum sickness. Am. J. Med., 35:418, 1963.
53. Michael, J. R., and Mitch, W. E.: Reversible renal failure and myositis caused by phenytoin hypersensitivity. JAMA, 236:2773, 1976.
54. Hyman, L. R., Ballow, M., and Knieser, M. R.: Diphenylhydantoin interstitial nephritis: roles of cellular and humoral immunologic injury. J. Pediatr., 92:915, 1978.
55. Sheth, J. K., Casper, J. T., and Good, T. A.: Interstitial nephritis due to phenytoin hypersensitivity. J. Pediatr., 91:438, 1977.
56. Agarwal, B. N., Cabebe, F. G., and Hoffman, B. T.: Diphenylhydantoin-induced acute renal failure. Nephron, 18:249, 1977.
57. Bayer, A. S., Targan, S. R., Pitchon, H. E., and Guze, L. B.: Dilantin toxicity: miliary pulmonary infiltrates and hypoxemia. Ann. Intern. Med., 85:475, 1976.
58. Targan, S. R., Chassin, M. R., and Guze, L. B.: Dilantin-induced disseminated intravascular coagulation with purpura fulminans: a case report. Ann. Intern. Med., 83:227, 1975.
59. Engel, J. N., Mellul, V. G., and Goodman, D. B. P.: Phenytoin hypersensitivity: a case of severe acute rhabdomyolysis. Am. J. Med., 81:928, 1986.
60. Kleckner, H. B., Yakulis, V., and Heller, P.: Severe hypersensitivity to diphenylhydantoin with circulating antibodies to the drug. Ann. Intern. Med., 83:522, 1975.
61. Aarli, J. A.: Drug-induced IgA deficiency in epileptic patients. Arch. Neurol., 33:296, 1976.
62. Seager, J., et al.: IgA deficiency, epilepsy and phenytoin treatment. Lancet, 2:632, 1975.
63. Stanley, J., and Fallon-Pellicci, V.: Phenytoin hypersensitivity reaction. Arch. Dermatol., 114:1350, 1978.
64. Chaiken, B. H., Goldberg, B. I., and Segal, J. P.: Dilantin hypersensitivity: a report of a case of hepatitis with jaundice, pyrexia and exfoliative dermatitis. N. Engl. J. Med., 242:897, 1950.
65. Lee, T. J., et al.: Diphenylhydantoin-induced hepatic necrosis. Gastroenterology, 70:422, 1976.
66. Aaron, J. S., Bank, S., and Acker, G.: Diphenylhydantoin-induced hepatotoxicity. Am. J. Gastroenterol., 80:200, 1985.
67. Mullick, F. G., and Ishak, K. G.: Hepatic injury associated with diphenylhydantoin therapy. Am. Soc. Clin. Pathol., 74:442, 1980.
68. Pezzimenti, F. J., and Hahn, A. L.: Anicteric hepatitis induced by diphenylhydantoin. Arch. Intern. Med., 125:118, 1970.
69. Michael, J. R., and Rudin, M. L.: Acute pulmonary disease caused by phenytoin. Ann. Intern. Med., 95:452, 1981.
70. Fruchter, L., and Laptook, A.: Diphenylhydantoin hypersensitivity reaction associated with interstitial pulmonary infiltrates and hypereosinophilia. Ann. Allergy, 47:453, 1981.
71. Tomsick, R. S.: The phenytoin syndrome. Cutis, 32:535, 1983.
72. Knutsen, A. P., Anderson, J., Satayaviboon, S., and Slavin, R. G.: Immunologic aspects of phenobarbital hypersensitivity. J. Pediatr., 105:558, 1984.
73. Schiff, B. L., and Kern, A. B.: Cutaneous reactions to anticoagulants. Arch. Dermatol., 98:136, 1968.
74. Feder, W., and Auerback, R.: "Purple toes": an uncommon sequela of oral coumarin drug therapy. Ann. Intern. Med., 55:911, 1961.
75. Teepe, R. G. C., et al.: Recurrent coumarin-induced skin

necrosis in a patient with acquired functional protein C deficiency. Arch. Dermatol., *122*:1408, 1986.
76. McGehee, W. G., et al.: Coumarin necrosis associated with hereditary protein C deficiency. Ann. Intern. Med., *100*:59, 1984.
77. Broekmans, A. W., et al.: Protein C and the development of skin necrosis during anticoagulant therapy. Thromb. Haemost., *49*:251, 1983.
78. Gladson, C. L., et al.: Coumarin necrosis, neonatal purpura fulminans and Protein C deficiency. Arch. Dermatol., *123*:1701a, 1987.
79. Chua, F. S., et al.: Dermal gangrene: an unpredictable complication of coumarin therapy. J. Thorac. Cardiovasc. Surg., *65*:238, 1973.
80. Lacy, J. P., and Goodin, R. R.: Warfarin-induced necrosis of skin. Ann. Intern. Med., *82*:381, 1975.
81. Jones, R. R., and Cunningham, J.: Warfarin skin necrosis: the role of factor VII. Br. J. Dermatol., *100*:561, 1979.
82. Lever, W. F., and Schaumberg-Lever, G.: Histopathology of the Skin. 3rd ed. Philadelphia, J. B. Lippincott, 1983.
83. Rubin, R. L.: Drug-induced lupus. Clin. Asp. Autoimmun., *2*:16, 1988.
84. Moschella, S., and Hurley, H.: Dermatology. 2nd ed. Philadelphia, W. B. Saunders, 1985.
85. Colman, R. W., Robboy, S. J., and Minna, J. D.: Disseminated intravascular coagulation (DIC): an approach. Am. J. Med., *52*:679, 1972.
86. Mason, J. W., Kleeburg, U., Dolan, P., and Colman, R. W.: Human plasma kallikrein and Hageman factor in endotoxic shock. Ann. Intern. Med., *3*:545, 1970.
87. Thomas, L., Denney, F. W., and Floyd, J.: Studies on the generalized Schwartzman reaction. III. Lesions of the myocardium and coronary artery accompanying the reactions in rabbits prepared by infection with group A staphylococci. J. Exp. Med., *92*:751, 1953.
88. McKay, D. G., and Margaretten, W.: Disseminated intravascular coagulation in virus diseases. Arch. Intern. Med., *120*:129, 1967.
89. Bachman, F.: Evidence for hypercoagulability in heat stroke. J. Clin. Invest., *46*:1033, 1967.
90. Colman, R. W., et al.: Coagulation studies in hyperacute and other forms of renal allograft rejection. N. Engl. J. Med., *281*:685, 1969.
91. Maekawa, T., and Gonmori, H.: Tissue thromboplastin in leukocytes from various leukemias and its localization by imminoperoxidase staining method [abstract]. Thromb. Diath. Haemorrh., *38*:151, 1977.
92. Gouault-Heilman, M., Chardon, E., Sultar, C., and Josso, F.: The procoagulant factor of leukemic promyelocytes: demonstration of immunologic cross-reactivity with human brain tissue factor. Br. J. Haematol., *30*:151, 1975.
93. Andoh, K., et al.: Tissue factor activity in leukemia cells. Special reference to disseminated intravascular coagulation. Cancer, *59*:748, 1987.
94. Dennis, L. H., Eichelberger, J. W., Inman, M. M., and Conrad, M. E.: Depletion of coagulation factors in drug resistant Plasmodium falciparum malaria. Blood, *29*:713, 1967.
95. Brain, M. C.: Microangiopathic hemolytic anemia. Ann. Rev. Med., *21*:133, 1970.
96. Walsh, R. T., and Barnhart, M. I.: Clearance of coagulation and fibrinolysis products by the reticuloendothelial system. Thromb. Diath. Haemorrh., *22*(Suppl. 36):83, 1969.
97. Colman, R. W., Hirsch, J., Marder, V. J., and Salzman, E. W., (Eds.): Hemostasis and Thrombosis. Basic Principles and Clinical Practice. Philadelphia, J. B. Lippincott, 1987.
98. McIlraith, D. M., Mant, M. J., and Brien, W. F.: Chronic consumptive coagulopathy due to intracardiac thrombus. Am. J. Med., *82*:135, 1987.
99. Fruchtman, S., and Aledort, L. M.: Disseminated intravascular coagulation. J. Am. Coll. Cardiol., *8*:159B, 1986.
100. Carr, M. E.: Disseminated intravascular coagulation: pathogenesis, diagnosis and therapy. J. Emerg. Med., *5*:311, 1987.
101. Crowley, J. P.: Coagulopathy and bleeding in the parturient patient. R. I. Med. J., *72*:135, 1989.
102. Sutton, D. M.: Intravascular coagulation in abruptio placentae. Am. J. Obstet. Gynecol., *109*:604, 1971.
103. Beller, F. K., and Uszunski, M.: Disseminated intravascular coagulation in pregnancy. Am. J. Obstet. Gynecol., *17*:250, 1974.
104. Miner, M. E., et al.: Disseminated intravascular coagulation fibrinolytic syndrome following head injury in children. Frequency and prognostic implications. J. Pediatr., *100*:687, 1982.
105. Gralnick, H. R., and Sultan, C.: Acute promyelocytic leukemia: hemorrhagic manifestations and morphologic criteria. Br. J. Haematol., *29*:373, 1975.
106. Molos, M. A., and Hall, J. C.: Symmetrical peripheral gangrene and disseminated intravascular coagulation. Arch. Dermatol., *121*:1057, 1985.
107. Stossel, T. P., and Levy, R.: Intravascular coagulation associated with pneumococcal bacteremia and symmetrical peripheral gangrene. Arch. Intern. Med., *125*:876, 1970.
108. Feinstein, D. I.: Diagnosis and management of disseminated intravascular coagulation. The role of heparin therapy. Blood, *60*:284, 1982.
109. Marder, V. J., Cruz, G. O., and Schumer, B. R.: Evaluation of a new antifibrinogen-coated latex particle agglutination test in the measurement of serum fibrin degradation products. Thromb. Haemost., *37*:183, 1988.
110. Hawiger, J., et al.: Measurement of fibrinogen and fibrin degradation products in serum by staphylococcal clumptin test. J. Lab. Clin. Med., *75*:93, 1970.
111. Sigal, S. H., et al.: Prototype quantitative assay for fibrinogen/fibrin degradation products. Arch. Intern. Med., *147*:1790, 1987.
112. Corrigan, J. J.: Disseminated intravascular coagulopathy. Pediatr. Rev., *1*:37, 1979.
113. Bick, R. L.: Disseminated intravascular coagulation: a clinical laboratory study of 48 patients. N. Y. Acad. Sci., *370*:843, 1981.
114. El-Kassimi, F. A., Al-Mashhadani, S., Abdullah, A. K., and Akhtar, J.: Adult respiratory distress syndrome and disseminated intravascular coagulation complicating heat stroke. Chest, *90*:571, 1986.
115. Pesola, G. R., and Carlon, G. C.: Pulmonary embolus-induced disseminated intravascular coagulation. Crit. Care Med., *15*:983, 1987.
116. Tanaka, K., Shimao, S., Okada, T., and Tanaka, A.: Kasabach-Merritt syndrome with disseminated intravascular coagulation treated by exchange transfusion and surgical excision. Dermatologia, *173*:90, 1986.
117. Larsen, E. C., Zinkham, W. H., Eggleston, J. C., and Zitelli, B. J.: Kasabach-Merritt syndrome: Therapeutic considerations. Pediatrics, *79*:971, 1987.
118. Sharp, A. A.: Diagnosis and management of disseminated intravascular coagulation. Br. Med. Bull., *33*:625, 1977.
119. Drapkin, R. L., et al.: Prophylactic heparin therapy in acute promyelocytic leukemia. Cancer, *41*:2484, 1978.
120. Spicer, T. E., and Tan, J. M.: Purpura fulminans. Am. J. Med., *61*:566, 1976.
121. Bell, W. R., Starksen, N. F., Tong, S., and Porterfield, J. K.:

Trousseau's syndrome. Devastating coagulopathy in the absence of heparin. Am. J. Med., *79:*423, 1985.
122. Corrigan, J. J., and Jordan, C. M.: Heparin therapy in septicemia with disseminated intravascular coagulation. N. Engl. J. Med., *283:*778, 1970.
123. Hellgren, M., Javelin, L., Hagnevik, K., and Blombach, M.: Antithrombin III concentrate as an adjuvant in DIC treatment—a pilot study in nine severely ill patients. Thromb. Res., *35:*459, 1984.
124. Blauhut, B., Kramar, H., Vinazzer, H., and Bergmann, H.: Substitution of antithrombin III in shock and DIC: a randomized study. Thromb. Res., *39:*81, 1985.
125. Fourrier, F., et al.: Meningococcemia and purpura fulminans in adults: acute deficiencies of Protein C and S and early treatment with antithrombin III concentrates. Intensive Care Med., *16:*121, 1990.
126. Vinazzer, H.: Therapeutic use of antithrombin III in shock and disseminated intravascular coagulation. Semin. Thromb. Hemostas., *15:*347, 1989.
127. Takemoto, Y., et al.: Studies on the effects of primary therapy for DIC following circulatory arrest. Am. J. Hemotol., *21:*377, 1986.
128. Umeki, S., et al.: Gabexate as a therapy for disseminated intravascular coagulation. Arch. Intern. Med., *148:*1409, 1988.
129. Duncan, J. S., and Ramsay, L. E.: Widespread bone infarction complicating meningococcal septicemia and disseminated intravascular coagulation. Br. Med. J., *288:*111, 1984.

Chapter 49

SKIN PROBLEMS OF THE CRITICALLY ILL PATIENT

EARL Z. BROWNE, JR.

Because the critically ill patient must be confined to bed and repeatedly have invasive procedures performed, the skin is placed in significant jeopardy. It is often necessary to keep patients in the same position for a prolonged period of time, have multiple areas of vascular access, and cover these areas with tape and bandages of all sorts. This makes it difficult to observe changes in the patient's skin, in addition to making the skin more vulnerable. Dealing with the problems that make patients critically ill takes much greater precedence than concern about skin integrity. The same factors that make the patient's overall condition vulnerable, however, contribute to increased vulnerability of the skin. Hypothermia, hypotension, and hypovolemia all cause decreased perfusion. Many of these patients are elderly or have poor nutritional status. All of these factors make the skin more susceptible to trauma, especially pressure, as well as diminish the ability of the skin to withstand trauma and to heal itself when that occurs. Significant injury, such as pressure sore, can occur unless care is taken to observe skin carefully and deal appropriately with any cutaneous problems that do occur. Once a pressure sore develops, the patient suffers a great deal, and a great deal of time is required for healing. In addition, open wounds become sources of added metabolic need as well as portals of entry for infection.

The most important principle to keep in mind in dealing with the skin of the critically ill patient is to prevent complications from occurring. By far, the most common significant skin problem occurring in the critically ill patient is the development of pressure sores. It has been estimated that 3 to 10% of all hospitalized patients, regardless of age or diagnosis, develop a pressure sore while in the hospital.[1] This represents a staggering economic problem as well as a medical one, causing a drain on available resources. We have found a similar incidence in our institution to those of other reports and have found that the two populations most prone to develop these sores are acutely ill patients who must be immobilized for a significant period of time flat on their back and chronically ill patients who are unable to turn and respond to ordinary painful stimuli.

The same factors that predispose to skin breakdown cause the skin to lose its ability to act as a barrier, making it susceptible to infection. In addition to the usual type of bacterial infections commonly present in the skin, the immunocompromised state that often accompanies the critically ill patient makes him or her susceptible to unusual organisms as well. The presence of edema as well as hypoperfusion causing reduced oxygenization of the skin lowers metabolism and impairs wound healing. These factors also make the skin more susceptible to trauma, and even seemingly minor problems, such as tape burns, bruises, and infiltrations, can be much more severe. In addition, the use of drugs that are toxic when infiltrated can cause severe skin problems in these acutely ill patients.

PRESSURE SORE

Pre-ICU Phase

Risk

It would seem that almost every sick patient would be at significant risk for developing a pressure sore. Certainly advanced age and debilitated status are significant risk factors, as is the deteriorated mental status that goes along with both of those conditions. Surprisingly, the incidence of pressure sore does not seem to be significantly related to these factors per se. What does seem to matter in these patients is the status of nutrition and immobility (Table 49-1). As long as the debilitated patient is kept moving and does not spend a great deal of time in one position, pressure sores need not necessarily develop. The reason that a pressure sore develops is a simple mechanical one. The amount of pressure that can be measured at any given point on a patient's surface is directly related to an underlying bony prominence. In addition to this, it depends a great deal on whether or not that prominence is rounded or tends to come to a point. The more conical the bony prominence is, the more the pressure is concentrated directly over that point. Patients who sit for a long time, such as paralyzed patients in wheelchairs, exert a great deal of pressure on the soft tissue over the ischial tuberosity. Most critically ill patients are not in that position, however, and seldom develop pressure sores except in areas that are in contact in bed in a supine position. Depending on the configuration of the sacrum and sometimes the coccyx, most patients are prone to break down this area. Other prominent areas are over the spinous processes of the vertebrae, the spine of the scapula, the occiput, and, when the patients are on their sides, the greater trochanters of the femurs. No matter what position they are in, the feet are prone to ulceration either on the heels or on the malleolae.

Despite these generalizations, it is interesting that some patients break down quickly and others can go for prolonged periods of time having to be kept immobilized flat

Table 49–1. Risk Factors of Pressure Sore Development

Absolute
    Poor nutrition
    Immobility
Relative
    Age
    Neurologic status
    Decreased skin perfusion
    Mechanical factors
    Prolonged surgical procedures

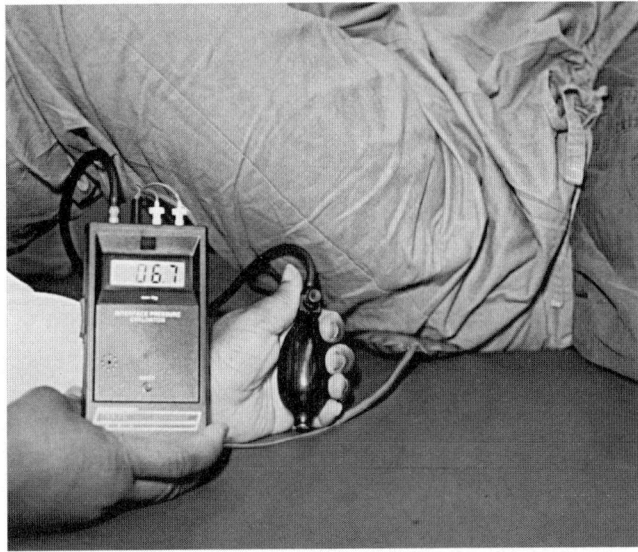

Fig. 49–2. Interstitial tissue pressure being measured under a bony prominence.

on their back and not break down. It is possible to measure the skin pressure interface by use of a pressure-sensing device connected to a monitor. The simplest of these is much like a balloon connected to a monitor, placed under the patient, and the pressure is measured much as with a blood pressure cuff (Fig. 49-1). We have found marked differences in recording pressure in different patients in areas that would appear to be significant as well as apparent insignificant pressure points. It is assumed that as long as the pressure is less than approximately 35 mm Hg that capillary pressure is not exceeded, and the skin and soft tissue will perfuse.[2] This is not an entirely valid assumption because it is known that the skin is more resistant to pressure than muscle, and it may be that deep breakdown can occur in the presence of marginal but intact skin. Seldom does breakdown occur, however, as long as the skin capillary perfusion is maintained. By using the monitoring device on patients who are lying absolutely flat on surfaces such as an operating table, we have found variations over pressure points such as the sacrum and trochanter that can vary from 30 mm Hg to as much as 90 to 100 mm Hg (Fig. 49-2). Obviously the patients who have low pressure have flat or rounded bony prominences underneath the measuring points, and those with extremely high pressures have prominent, sharply projecting bony prominences. It is difficult to determine by physical examination alone just who these patients are, but anyone who is extremely thin and appears to have obvious bony prominence must be considered to be at much greater risk than otherwise.

We have developed a pressure sore model in the pig.[3] This was done by rendering the pig anesthetic by spinal root section and placing an indenting device over the greater trochanter. To our surprise, we were not able to produce a pressure sore even after hours of the highest pressure that we could produce when the indenting device was held in place with straps. It was necessary to use an internal fixation device to apply constant pressure of hundreds of millimeters of mercury for several hours to be able to produce this lesion. Although pigs and humans are not the same, this is a reflection of skeletal shape and soft tissue mobility.

Many risk assessment tools have been developed. These are multifactorial and have generally been developed by analyzing retrospectively those factors that were present in patients who developed pressure sores.[4-6] To this point, a completely valid tool based on a prospective analysis has not been identified and brought into general use. In a series of patients who developed hospital-acquired pressure sores, we analyzed prospectively whether or not we could prevent these ulcers from worsening by use of air mattresses.[7] In analyzing the risk factors associated with this group of patients, it appeared that immobility was the only significant factor causing increased risk, although poor nutrition was a less significantly related factor. It is generally thought that if a patient's albumin is below normal levels, this is a valuable marker for the possibility of developing pressure sores. Another laboratory analysis that we have found to be of value is the transferrin level.

No matter what the risk factors are, 3 to 5% of all patients

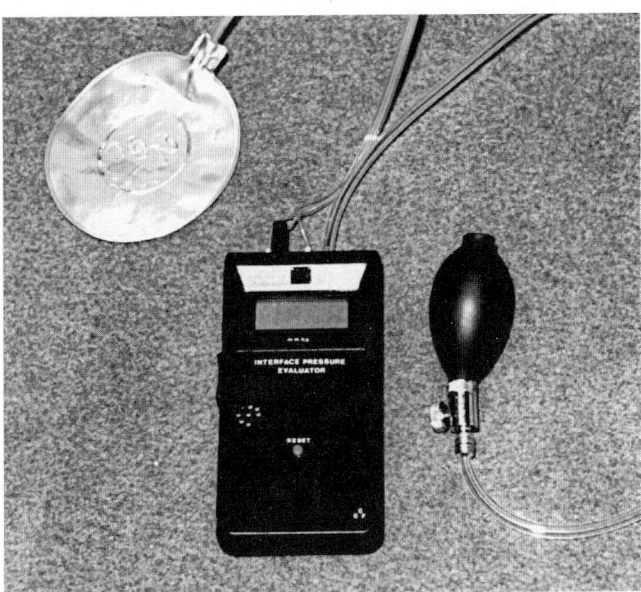

Fig. 49–1. Interface monitoring pressure device with inflatable sensor to be placed under patient.

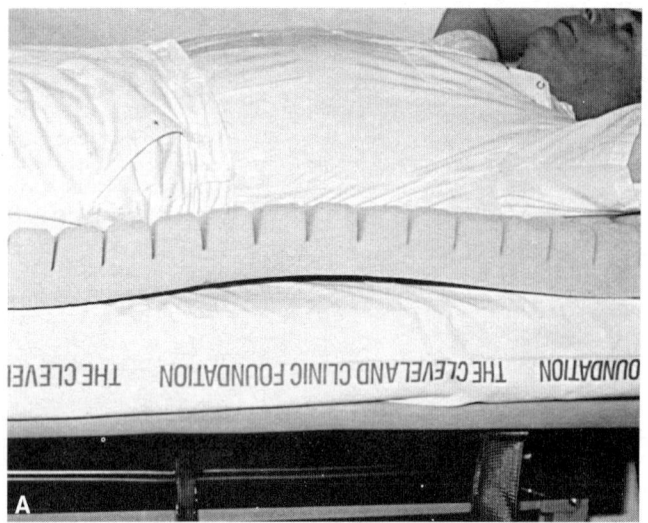 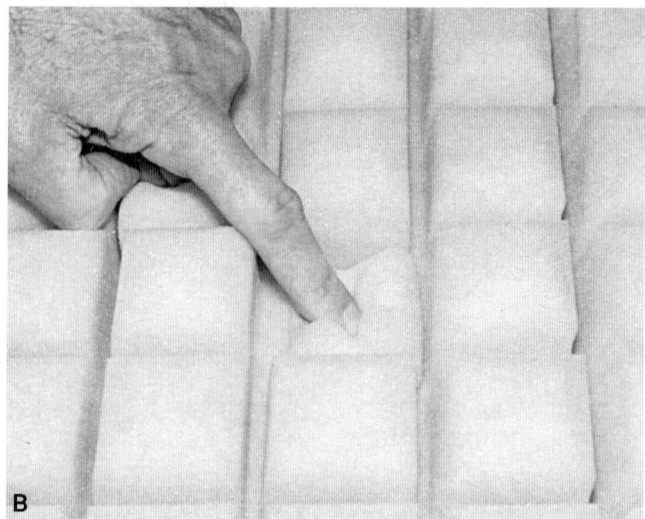

Fig. 49–3. A and B, High density foam reduces pressure under prominences. "Egg crate" is not effective.

who are admitted to hospitals develop pressure sores while they are being cared for. Clearly those patients in critical care units are the most vulnerable patients of all. In practical terms, it makes more sense not to attempt to identify which patients are at greater risk but to treat all patients in this category as if they are at significant risk of developing these sores. If real care is taken to prevent pressure sores, the incidence can be greatly diminished even in those patients who are extremely vulnerable. By far, the most important principle in prevention is simply to keep the patients turning from side to side frequently. As long as patients are awake and able to cooperate with their care, they tend to do this by themselves if not restrained. When the pressure exceeds capillary pressure and perfusion in the skin and soft tissue overlying the bony prominence is reduced, the area becomes locally ischemic. This sets up a pain response, which causes patients to roll over automatically. This is the same thing that all of us do every night while asleep. If the mental status or level of sedation gets to the point that patients can no longer move protectively, they must be moved frequently by those caring for them. Ideally the patient's position should be shifted every half hour to be absolutely sure that perfusion is intact, but certainly a maximum of 2 hours lying in any one position should not be exceeded.

In those patients who have especially prominent bony areas and in patients in whom frequent turning is not easily done, support surfaces that reduce the pressure can be valuable. An enormous number of these products are now on the market, but they fall into two basic categories: surfaces that reduce pressure sufficiently to assist in prevention of pressure sores and those that generally can reduce the pressure to a point less than the capillary pressure. Various foam mattresses are available as well as air and water surfaces, and in general these are reduction surfaces but cannot be counted on to reduce the pressure sufficiently to allow a patient to maintain the same position (Fig. 49-3). If that is necessary, the patient should be placed on a low-air-loss bed (Fig. 49-4). Although many physicians favor the use of silicone particles kept suspended in air columns, the beds that are composed of inflated chambers, which allow a slow loss of air, are effective in preventing pressure sores from developing or worsening.

Staging

A pressure sore is a wound, and it is convenient to think of it much in the same way as a thermal injury and stage the ulcer that develops in the same fashion.[8] It is convenient to use a four-stage grading method for this purpose. The first insult that is obvious in the skin is erythema. This is due to an inflammatory phase present in the skin surrounding the ischemic area. The skin becomes reddened and edematous just as does a first-degree burn and is considered to be stage 1 (Fig. 49-5). As long as the ulcer does not worsen past this stage, complete healing takes place fairly rapidly. When necrosis develops, the wound must heal first by removing all the necrotic material, then by forming a matrix of healthy tissue and epithelium from the edge of the wound and existing hair follicles. Partial-thickness skin wounds are considered stage 2 (Fig. 49-6). If the necrosis is so deep that it involves the full thickness of the skin, this is considered stage 3 (Fig. 49-7). Stage 4 ulcers are deep ones in which there is death of the underlying soft tissue. Stage 3 ulcers can extend into the fat below the skin, but if underlying muscle, fascia, or bone is involved, this is considered to be a stage 4 ulcer (Fig. 49-8). There is little functional or prognostic value associated with this classification, but it is convenient to use it when describing wounds and when communicating problems with other medical personnel. The most important principle of care is not the treatment for any of these wounds but the prevention.

Treatment

Once an ulcer does develop, there is a breakdown of the skin, and a source of infection is present. Stage 1 pressure sores have not progressed to this point and can be

SKIN PROBLEMS OF THE CRITICALLY ILL PATIENT

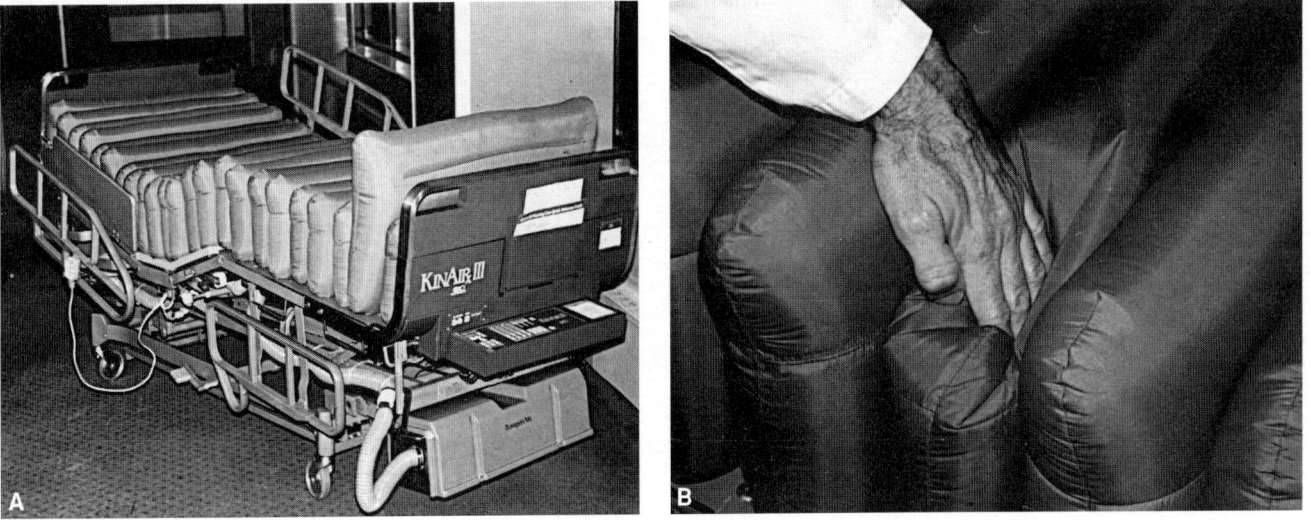

Fig. 49-4. *A* and *B,* Low-air-pressure bed provides pressure relief to safe tissue pressure levels.

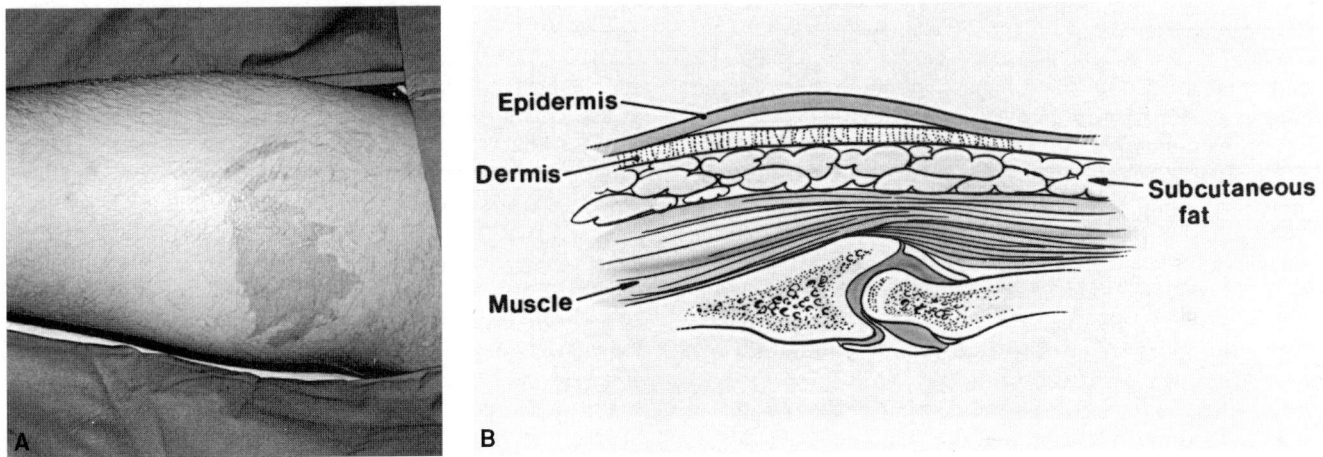

Fig. 49-5. *A* and *B,* Stage 1 pressure sore—erythema of skin—no necrosis.

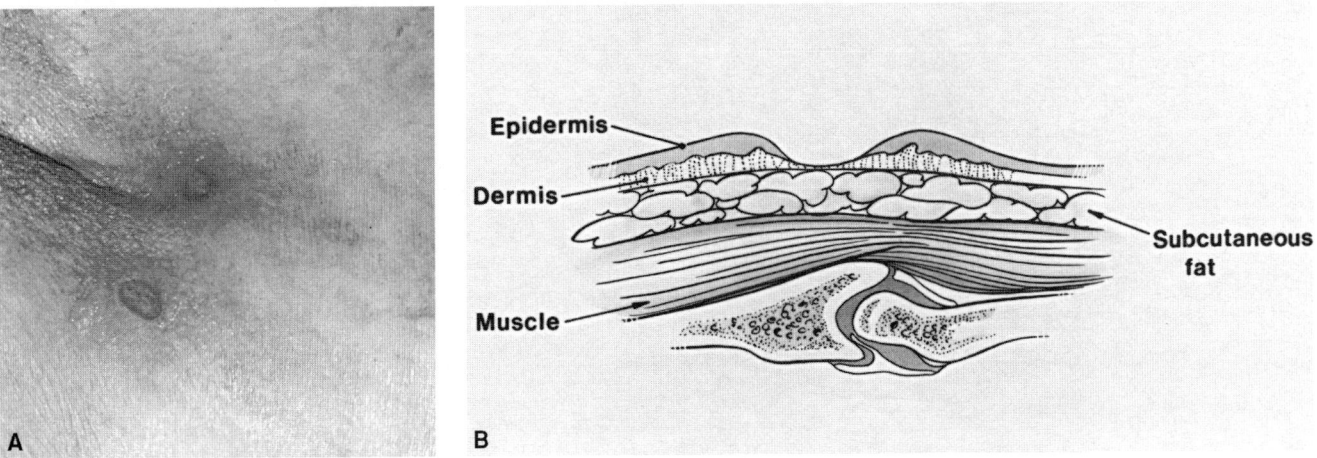

Fig. 49-6. *A* and *B,* Stage 2 pressure sore—partial-thickness necrosis of skin.

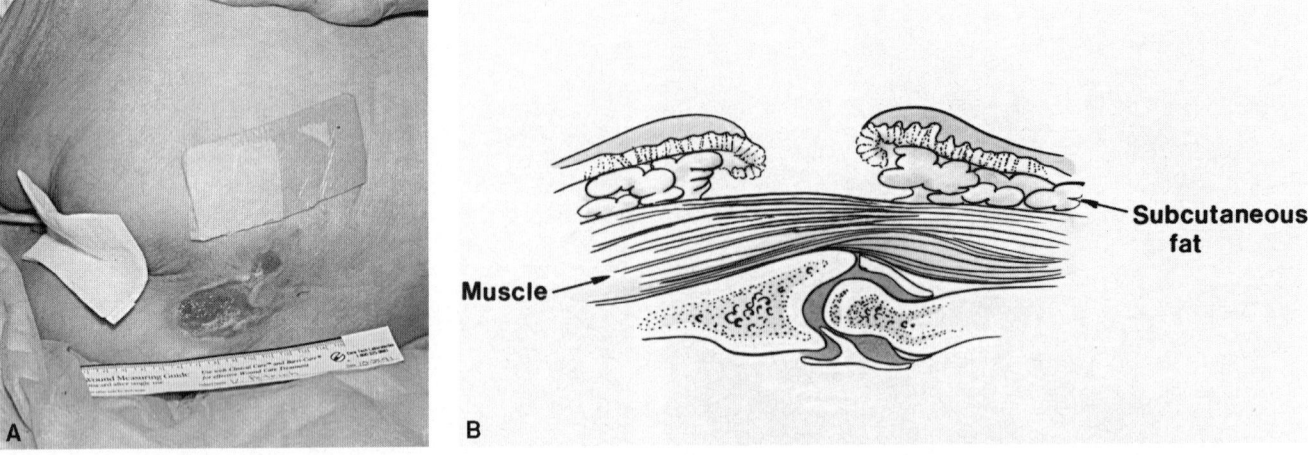

Fig. 49-7. *A* and *B*, Stage 3 pressure sore—full-thickness skin necrosis extending into subcutaneous tissue.

cared for by keeping the skin cleansed while using preventive measures. It is important to recognize, however, that erythema of the skin is present in the initial phases of any pressure sore, and these wounds evolve over a period of time. Sometimes a patient can be seen to develop a large erythematous area, and casual evaluation would make one think that this is not a significant wound. If the wound is followed over the next 24 hours or so, the full evolution of the problem becomes apparent, and the wound becomes indurated and goes on to develop necrosis with time. Even though a wound may be full thickness, it does not demonstrate necrosis for several days. Therefore all that can be said by looking at the wound is that it is at least a partial-thickness injury, and if the skin does not appear to blanch, it is most likely a full-thickness one. If the wound becomes markedly indurated, one must suspect that there is necrosis of the soft tissue deep to the skin, and these patients are candidates for surgical debridement of the wound.

As long as there is hope that the skin might heal and it is believed that there is no necrosis deep to the wound, the sore can be treated by any number of standard wound care regimens. There are a multitude of commercial products available that report to improve healing by providing a warm, moist environment. Equally efficacious is the use of frequent dressing changes with a gel or occlusive gauze. Once necrosis develops, however, the dead tissue should be debrided. This can be done surgically, or it can be done mechanically with dressings, either using wet to dry saline gauze dressings or one of the newer gel products. The method that is used is not important as long as care and diligence are used in the application. It is not acceptable to cover a necrotic, bacterially colonized wound for a few days with an occlusive dressing, hoping for something "magic" to happen, allowing the wound to become infected. If a wound has progressed to the point that there is necrotic eschar present, it is best to remove this surgically if the patient's condition permits. It is mandatory that this be done if necrosis extends into the soft tissue underlying the skin because this necrotic area can become secondarily infected and produce a source of sepsis for the patient. Because the acutely ill patient is already vulnerable to this, any additional offending source should be removed.

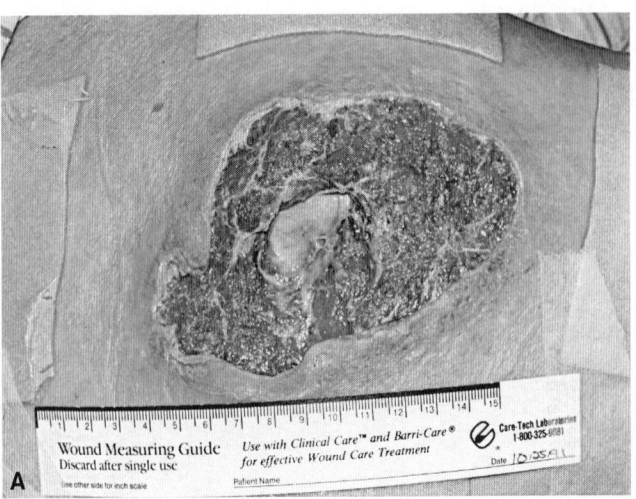
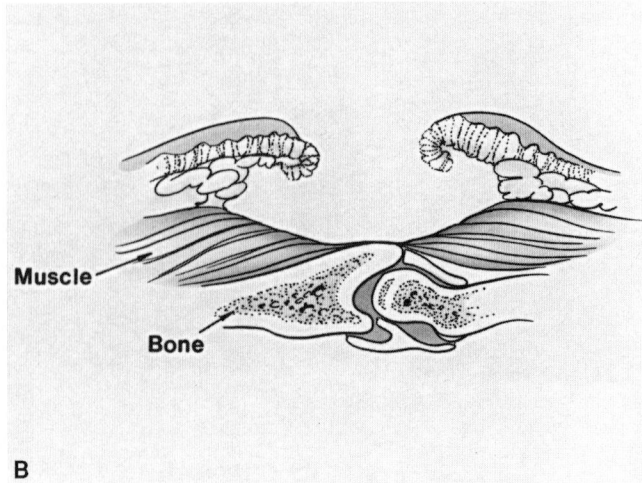

Fig. 49-8. *A* and *B*, Stage 4 pressure sore—deep extending into underlying muscle or bone.

ICU Phase

Once the patient becomes sick enough to be placed in the ICU, an even greater index of suspicion should be maintained. If the patient is hypovolemic or septic or if the cardiac mechanism is insufficient, there is physiologic shunting, and skin perfusion becomes even more diminished. As long as it is possible to move the patient frequently and observe all pressure points, that is all the treatment that is necessary. Should it not be possible to move the patient enough to assess frequently or if evidence of a pressure sore develops, the patient should be placed on a pressure reduction surface. Clearly the patient's chance of worsening justifies this, but the routine use of low-air-loss beds can become a staggering expense. At one point in our institution, we estimated that this could run up to at least a million dollars per year if all patients who were considered to be in jeopardy were treated in this fashion. A reasonable protocol for following patients is to turn them frequently and observe them carefully, and as long as no problems develop, the regular support surfaces are appropriate. Should there appear to be difficulty in doing this, a high density foam or static air overlay is indicated. Careful observation of patients continues. If, however, it appears that a pressure sore is developing despite good surveillance, the patient should be placed on a low-air-loss bed. Surgical consultation should be obtained if there is any concern that necrosis is present. In our institution, there is a Skin Care Team, whose function is to monitor carefully the progress of patients who are either at very high risk or who develop the early signs of pressure sore. All patients who develop stage 3 or 4 ulcers are seen routinely by Plastic Surgery. In general, however, while the patient is in the ICU, surgical treatment of the ulcer is given a low priority except for debridement of necrotic tissue. Once necrotic material is removed, the wound is treated with wet to dry gauze packing to maintain a clean wound until the patient's condition improves to the point that definitive closure of the wound happens. Small full-thickness wounds, of course, heal by wound contracture and epithelialization without the need for definitive surgical closure.

Post-ICU Phase

With increased ability for the patient to move around and participate in the care of the pressure sore, improvement can be expected to occur. In addition, the support surface can be modified. It is difficult for patients to get up out of bed when they are being treated with the low-air-loss therapy, and it is advantageous to down-grade the support surface to a foam or a static air overlay to assist with rehabilitation of recovering patients. Once the patient's condition is stable enough, a decision should be made whether definitive surgical closure should be done. This is based not only on the extent of the wound, but also the morbidity involved both with performing a surgical procedure and with leaving it alone. If it is thought that the wound can heal reasonably well with good quality of coverage over the bony prominence within a matter of a month or so, surgery would not be indicated. Obviously if the wound would take many months to heal and would be a chronic, open, draining, painful sore, the morbidity would be so great that a definitive closure would be indicated. It must be determined whether or not the patient's condition is strong enough to allow this closure to be done.

In general, it is not possible to treat these wounds with skin grafting because the quality of coverage that would be obtained would be poor and would be prone to break down easily. Flap procedures, which bring adjacent healthy tissue into the wound, are preferable. During this post-ICU phase, the wound care is done sufficiently to make sure that the wound stays clean and does not become a source of infection. In the past, large skin flap procedures were done, but the success of those is not as great as the use of adjacent muscle flaps (Fig. 49–9). In these procedures, a well-vascularized, healthy adjacent muscle or por-

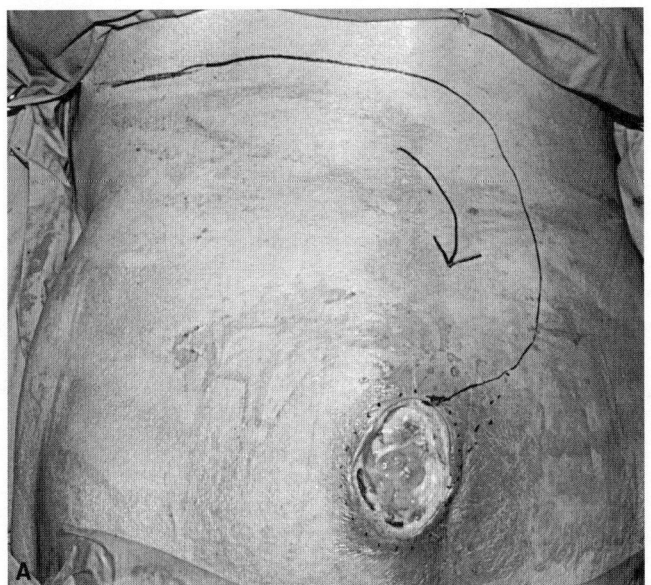 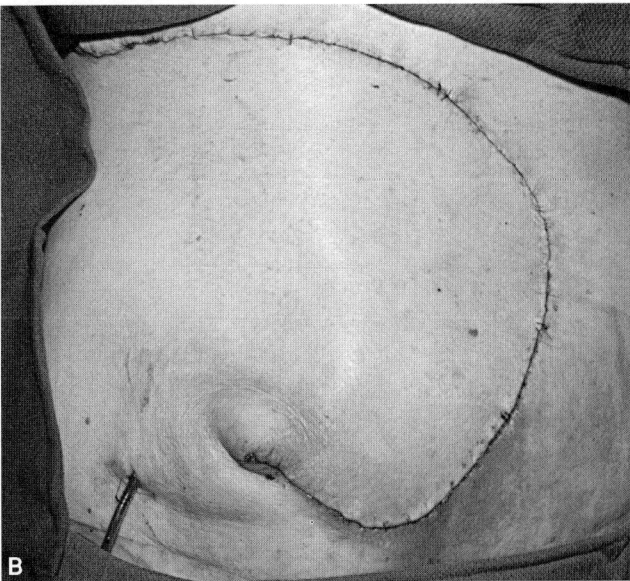

Fig. 49–9. *A* and *B*, Large rotation skin flap used for coverage of sacral ulcer.

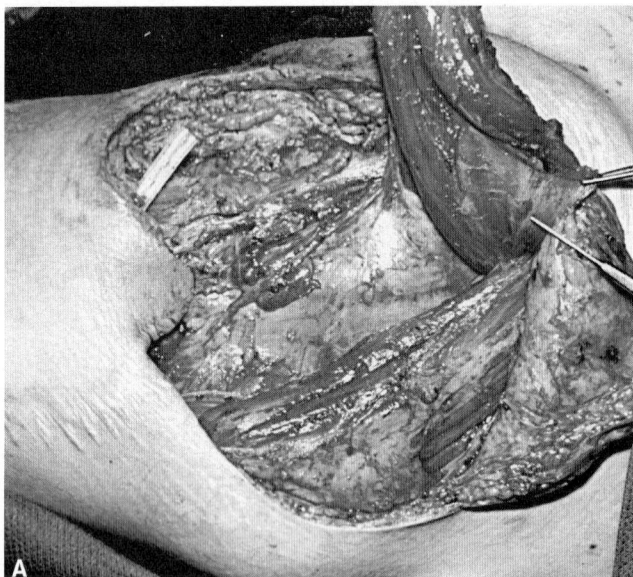
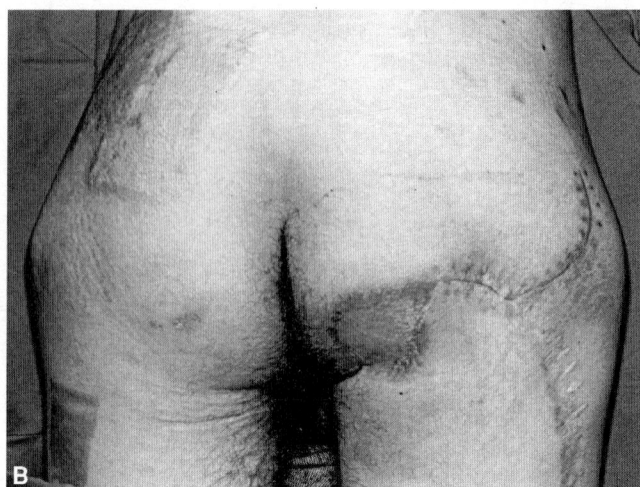

Fig. 49–10. *A* and *B,* Gluteus muscle flap covered by skin graft for coverage of ischial ulcer.

tion of a muscle is moved over to fill the defect. An example of this is the use of a portion of the gluteal muscle to fill a defect over the ischium or the sacrum (Fig. 49-10). There are many variations of this, including sometimes using skin paddles overlying the muscle or sometimes just filling the defect with muscle and then skin grafting on top of the muscle. In all of these procedures, the goal is to fill the ischemic open area with a well-nourished piece of tissue, which can improve the homeostasis of the wound and cause healing to occur rapidly. By doing this, the overall rehabilitation of the sick patient is speeded up a great deal. We believe if the patient is a reasonable surgical candidate that surgical closure is indicated in all but the small ulcers, which heal spontaneously within a month or two.

Whether the wound is open or closed, these patients all have special needs at home, and discharge planning is important. In addition to visiting nursing care and education of family members to care for the wounds, most of these patients are still in jeopardy of developing worsening pressure sores or developing recurrence of new injury. Family members must be instructed on moving the patient's position frequently as well as caring for wounds, and if the condition does not allow adequate mobility, a pressure reduction surface must be provided at home. One of the most convenient ways of doing this is to make sure that the patient is stepped-down from a low-air-loss bed to a static overlay, such as a high density foam, and then mobilized while in the hospital. This mattress overlay can then be taken home for continued use.

TRAUMA AND INFECTIONS

Pre-ICU Phase

Just as worsening of the general condition predisposes patients to pressure sore, the same problems of hypovolemia, hypotension, and so forth destroy the integrity of the skin, making it more susceptible to injury and infection. Increased permeability associated with edema is especially significant in infection because in addition to decreasing the effectiveness of the skin as a barrier, edema blocks the body's ability to deliver leukocytes and antibiotics to the site of infection once it develops. Immunocompromised patients become especially vulnerable. In addition, as invasive procedures start to be done, the wounds that are produced further compromise the skin and serve as portals for infective agents as well as for noxious substances that are toxic to the skin and subcutaneous tissue. These problems can occur during any stage of the critically ill patient but become manifest to a greater extent at the height of the illness in the ICU.

ICU Phase

Infections

Most infections occur either at the site of a wound, such as an incision, or at a puncture area from a vascular line. In addition, however, septic emboli can occur, and areas of sequestered fluid can become secondarily infected in the septic patient. Anytime there is increased capillary fragility, blood and serum extravasate in areas that are dependent for long periods of time or repeatedly traumatized. When blood is present in these areas, superoxides are produced on breakdown, further locally impairing the body's ability to heal and combat infection.[9] It is often the case that large hematomas become secondarily infected and turn into abscesses. Although most skin infections, especially those that start as a cellulitis, are caused by staphylococcus or streptococcus, almost any kind of organism can be found in infectious processes in the critically ill patient. Once these become established, they tend to respond poorly to antibiotic therapy and often progress to the point that surgical drainage is necessary. Necrotizing infections can develop, which can spread along fascial planes (Fig.

SKIN PROBLEMS OF THE CRITICALLY ILL PATIENT

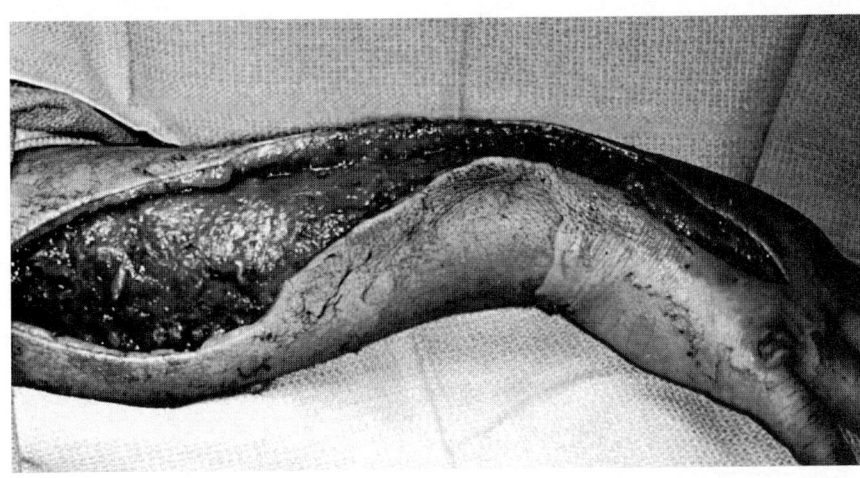

Fig. 49-11. Necrotizing fasciitis extending deep to forearm fascia from needle site in dorsum of hand.

49-11). These are deep and are not readily diagnosed because the ordinary symptoms of pain, fever, and acute illness are masked by the other acute processes that exist. Just as with pressure sore, it is important to keep a surveillance by carefully observing the skin, especially in the area of any intravenous or arterial lines, and to watch carefully for redness and induration of the soft tissue. Any drainage that occurs should be cultured, and surgical consultation should be obtained for aspiration or drainage of any area that appears to be developing into an abscess.

Some specific infections can be problematic, especially in patients who become so ill that they are immunocompromised. Necrotizing fasciitis owing to aggressive staphylococcus and streptococcus infections can spread in deep planes all the way up the extremity and can even skip deep across the groin or axilla to involve the abdominal wall. These are life-threatening infections and require wide excision and debridement. Pseudomonas can be especially problematic because the condition of ichthyma gangrenosum can develop, in which the organisms invade the capillary bed, causing thrombosis of the microcirculation (Fig. 49-12). This, in turn, causes necrosis, and it is a progressive process. Because the vessels are all thrombosed, there is no delivery of antibiotic to the involved area so the organisms are not eradicated. There is a progressive, spreading, necrotic infection surrounded by a purplish ring of vasculitis. Surgical debridement of the entire area is necessary for control of the infection.

Opportunistic infections also can develop, and any number of fungal diseases can occur in the skin and subcutaneous tissue as well as in other organs. Although these require treatment with specific drug therapy, it is usually necessary to debride the involved area completely to eradicate the process (Fig. 49-13).

Trauma

Although pressure sores are the most common traumatic problem, lacerations and avulsions of skin can occur with invasive procedures. One of the most frequently seen of these are avulsions of skin in chronically ill patients by removal of tape or occlusive dressings. This is especially bad in the patient who has thin skin owing to long-term steroid use. Large areas of skin can be easily avulsed, sometimes when just holding the patient by the leg to transfer him or her from the stretcher to the bed. This thin skin rolls up, like a piece of wet tissue paper, leaving a full-thickness loss. Although these sometimes appear to be quite large, they can be treated successfully by replacing this skin, much as is done in skin grafting. The piece of skin is usually stuck to the tape that is removed and does not look like much, but if care is taken to spread it out carefully as much as possible and replace it where it came from, the skin can be held in place with some pieces of Steri-strip and kept covered with protective bandages. It is amazing how often this skin takes completely. If this is not done, these wounds turn into chronic, open ulcerations, which may require skin grafting.

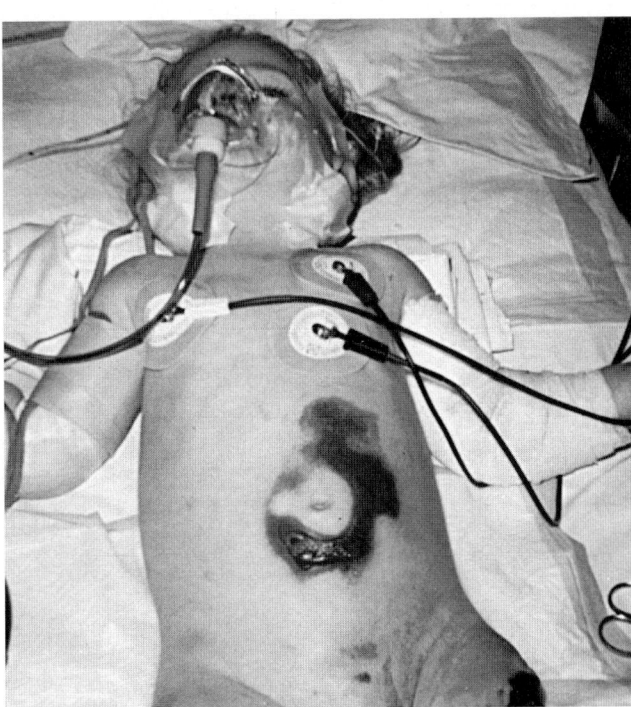

Fig. 49-12. Ichthyma gangrenosum zone of purplish discoloration (pseudomonas vasculitis) surrounding black eschar.

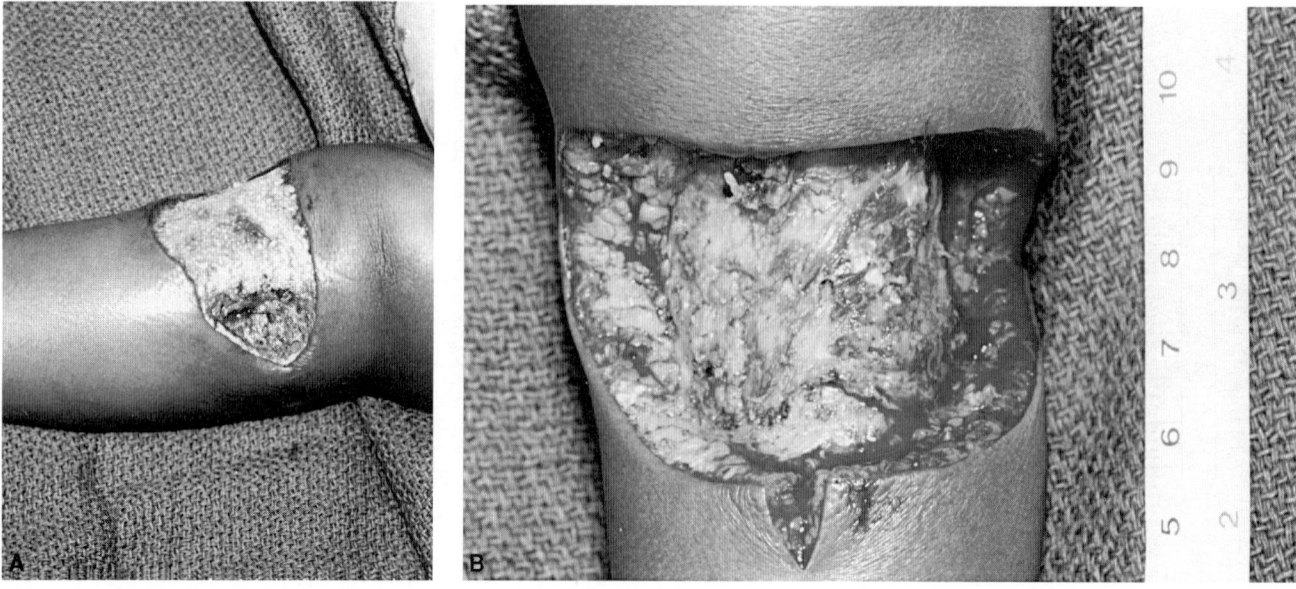

Fig. 49-13. *A* and *B,* Mucormycosis infection in the leg of an immunocompromised child.

Infiltrations

It is important to remember to administer any drug that would be toxic to the skin and subcutaneous tissue through a central line. There are some drugs that are specifically toxic just in themselves, such as cancer chemotherapy agents, but many are toxic because of high osmolarity. In addition, other drugs, such as dopamine, can cause severe necrosis owing to the effect on the blood supply of the skin.[10] If infiltration of a toxic drug can be recognized immediately, sometimes the patient can be treated with specific measures, as recommended in the individual package inserts provided by the manufacturers of these drugs. Often extravasations are not appreciated until it is too late to do this effectively, however. Under these circumstances, the patient must be watched carefully for impending necrosis of the skin. Even a large extravasation of a blood transfusion can cause necrosis, much in the same way as any hematoma, by causing rapid expansion and compromise of the circulation to the overlying skin.

If it is recognized that a significant infiltration has occurred and it appears that there is compromise, it is often appropriate to operate on this condition to remove the offending agent before a severe problem occurs. These noxious agents travel along the line of least resistance, which is generally between the superficial fascia and the subcutaneous tissue (Fig. 49-14). These infiltration areas are always larger than they appear to be and can end up with an extremely large area of necrosis compared with what appeared to be the initial area of infiltration. If the agent is allowed to stay in place and cause necrosis, the effect is that of loss of the involved area, which ultimately will have to be excised and treated. If it is possible to determine that a significant infiltration has occurred that will almost certainly result in necrosis, it is frequently possible to excise the offending agent from the subcutaneous

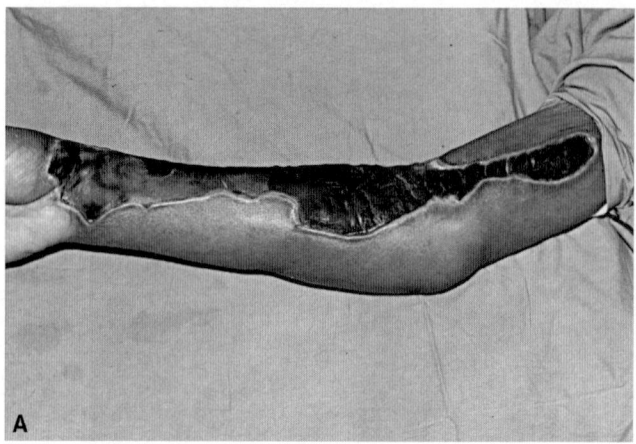
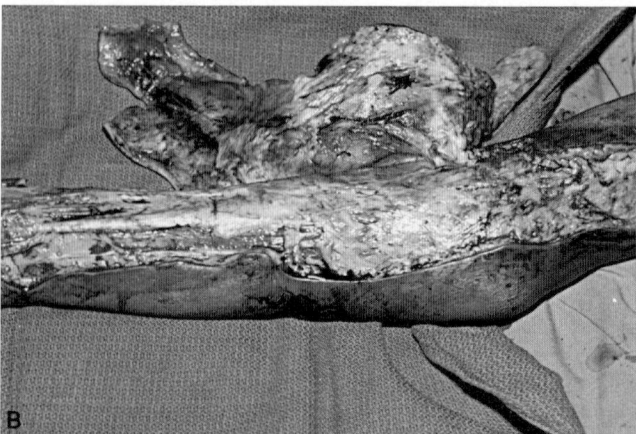

Fig. 49-14. *A* and *B,* Dopamine infiltration from cephalic vein showing necrosis of fascia and muscle.

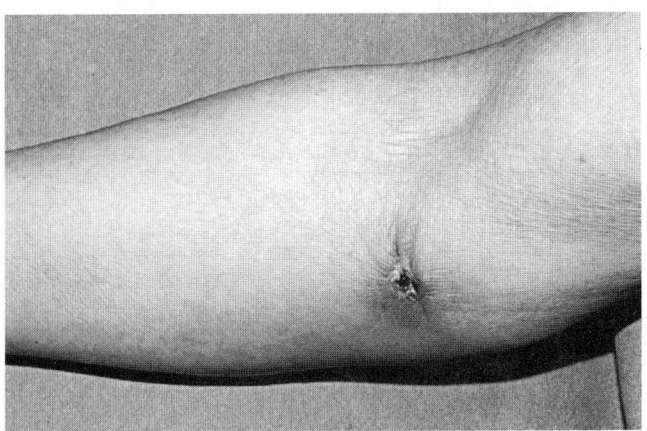

Fig. 49-15. Late contracture and chronic ulceration secondary to chemotherapy infiltration.

tissue, thus limiting the extent of spread that will take place. Signs to look for are anesthesia of the skin, loss of blanching, blistering, and especially small areas of apparent necrosis. If these signs develop over an infiltration, the area should be opened up and the offending agent removed. If this is done, often it is possible to save the skin overlying the infiltration, which would almost certainly become necrotic owing to extension of the agent or subsequent secondary bacterial infection. (Fig. 49-15). Although all cancer chemotherapy drugs can do this, doxorubicin (Adriamycin) is notorious for this kind of problem.[11] Infiltrations of this agent should be watched carefully, and if signs of progressing spread are taking place within the first day or so, the patient should be operated on to try to prevent progressive spread (Fig. 49-16).

Special consideration should be given to swelling around arterial line placement sites. Blood that leaks into the surrounding tissues under pressure may cause sufficient pressure within the muscle and neurovascular bundles to cause necrosis of their contained structures. This rare but devastating complication is often misdiagnosed by the inexperienced caregiver because the assumption is made that the presence of a pulse in the affected area implies lack of danger. In reality, these compartment syndromes are first manifested by parasthesias and other neurologic disorders. Muscle necrosis ensues later, with gangrene being the ultimate complication. These problems may be masked in the sedated patient. Under the circumstances, if there is any doubt about swelling or pain around the site of an arterial line, consultation with an experienced surgeon is warranted.

Post-ICU Phase

Sometimes surgical defects are present, which require definitive closure. Just as with pressure sore, it is generally preferable to delay any definitive treatment for these patients until their condition is stabilized and it is determined whether or not closure with skin grafts or flaps is desirable. Rehabilitation of the wounds is important because many of these types of problems occur on the extremity, and physical and occupational therapy is important to maintain motion as well as strength and function. Discharge planning should include continuing therapy for rehabilitation.

REFERENCES

1. Maklebust, J.: Pressure ulcers: etiology and prevention. Nurs. Clin. North Am., 22:359, 1987.
2. Lindan, O., Greenway, R. M., and Piazza, J. M.: Pressure distribution on the surface of the human body. Arch. Phys. Med. Rehabil., 46:378, 1965.
3. Negami, S., et al.: An experimental pressure sore model for functional electrical stimulation. In Advances in External

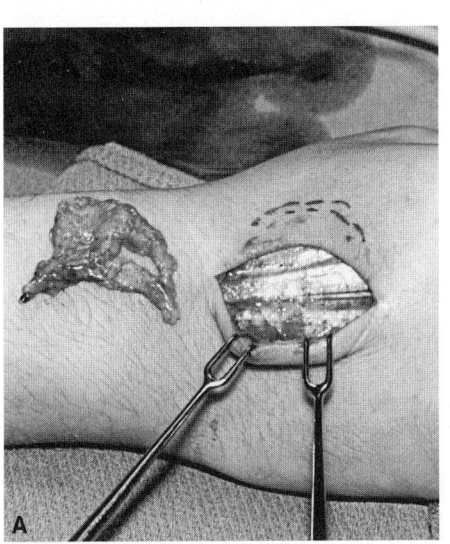
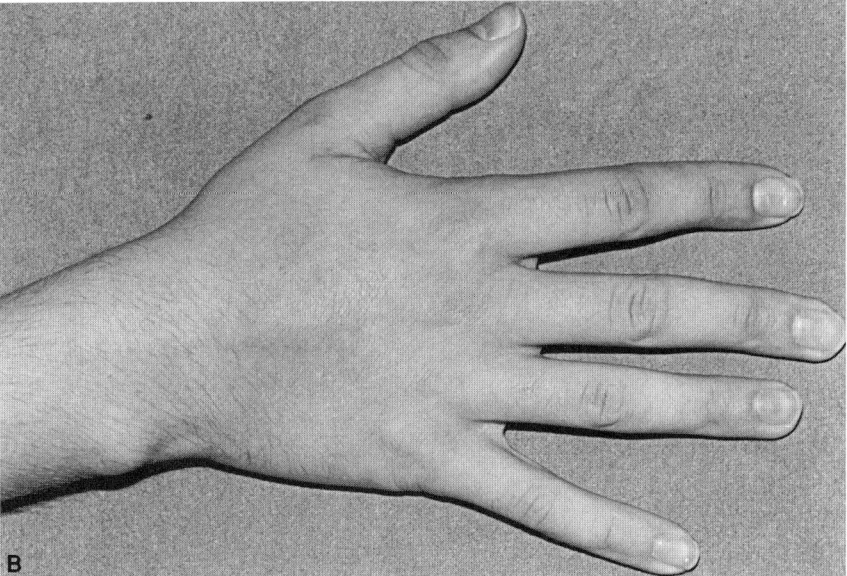

Fig. 49-16. *A* and *B*, Result of early excision of infiltration of doxorubicin (Adriamycin) into thrombosed vein and surrounding induration.

Control of Human Extremities. Vol. 10. Edited by D. Popovic. Belgrade, Yugoslavia, Nauka, 1990, p. 535.
4. Braden, B., and Bergstrom, N.: A conceptual scheme for the study of the etiology of pressure sores. Rehabil. Nurs., *12:*8, 1987.
5. Gosnell, D. J.: Assessment and evaluation of pressure sores. Nurs. Clin. North Am., *22:*399, 1989.
6. Norton, D.: Calculating the risk: reflections on the Norton scale. Decubitus, *2:*24, 1989.
7. Reyes, S. I., Browne, E. Z., and Krivanek, G.: Hospital pressure ulcer management. Submitted for publication.
8. Edberg, E. L., Cerny, K., and Stauffer, E. S.: Prevention and treatment of pressure sores. Phys. Ther., *53:*246, 1973.
9. Angel, M. F., et al.: The etiologic role of free radicals in hematoma induced flap necrosis. Plast. Reconstr. Surg., *77:*795, 1986.
10. Linder, R. M., Upton, J., and Osteen, R.: Management of extensive doxorubicin hydrochloride extravasation injuries. J. Hand Surg., *8:*32, 1983.
11. Siwy, B. K., and Sadove, A. M.: Acute management of dopamine infiltration injury with Regitine. Plast. Reconstr. Surg., *80:*610, 1987.

Section Seven

THE GASTROINTESTINAL SYSTEM

… Chapter 50

GASTROINTESTINAL BLEEDING

RAPHAEL S. CHUNG

NATURAL HISTORY OF GASTROINTESTINAL BLEEDING

The natural history of gastrointestinal bleeding is well known because it has been the subject of repeated studies. Despite dramatic progress in diagnostic and therapeutic technology and in the care of the critically ill, there is virtually no reduction in the overall mortality over several decades.[1,2] In general, 10% of all patients hospitalized with this diagnosis may succumb, a statement as true today as it was 50 years ago. The proportion of aged patients, however, was higher in more recent series. Between 70 and 80% of all patients stop bleeding spontaneously, making it hazardous to claim efficacy for any therapeutic modality without adequate control. Another common finding in these studies is that emergency surgery, when required for continued bleeding, carries a mortality of at least 15%.[3-5] In the groups with poor outcome, many studies showed that mortality is increased with the following adverse factors:

- Old age
- Massive bleeding
- Conditions prone to recurrent bleeding, including esophageal or gastric varices, giant or multiple ulcers, visible vessels on endoscopy, arteriovenous malformations
- Shock
- Coexisting diseases; including central nervous system (CNS), hepatic, renal, pulmonary, and neoplasms
- Coexisting findings; including ascites, congestive heart failure, respiratory failure, jaundice
- Medications, including steroids

These constitute adverse prognostic factors and indicate aggressive management and consideration as indicators for ICU admission. The potential interrelationships among these factors are additive because each factor taken alone may not be an expression of the true risk. From multivariate analysis of large pools of data, such as the survey of the American Society for Gastrointestinal Endoscopy of more than 2000 patients,[5] certain risk factors have been identified as being useful in predicting outcome (Tables 50-1 and 50-2).

Risk Stratification

If the clinical illness of gastrointestinal bleeding is viewed as gastrointestinal bleeding complicating a preexisting disease, two components of the illness are important in determining outcome: (1) the general condition and reserves of the patient, including cardiopulmonary, nutritional, and other system reserves, and (2) the nature of the specific bleeding process. The permutation of these two components stratifies the patients into the following clinical groups, listed in order of increasing risks, of practical importance in management:

- Known discrete bleeding lesion without systemic illness, e.g., bleeding peptic ulcer in a young man
- Obscure bleeding source in a healthy patient, e.g., colonic bleeding
- Obvious bleeding source in patients with significant system disease, e.g., variceal bleeding with poor liver function, ulcer bleeding in congestive failure
- Obscure bleeding source in patients with poor reserves, e.g., stress erosions/ulcers in sepsis with multisystem failure

Known discrete bleeding lesion without systemic illness is the least severe problem of the group. The best example is bleeding peptic ulcer in an otherwise healthy patient. A management decision is often simple. Once the lesion is identified on endoscopy and bleeding activity determined, there is little need for continued treatment in the ICU.

Bleeding from a source not readily identifiable, diffuse bleeding, bleeding from multiple locations, and bleeding in a patient without significant systemic decompensation is second in severity. An example is bleeding from arteriovenous malformation in the right colon. These patients require close monitoring because the course of the bleeding episode is less predictable and because deterioration may occur suddenly. Depending on the severity of the bleeding, ICU management may be necessary.

Gastrointestinal bleeding coming from a known source in patients with compromised cardiorespiratory or other system reserve is third. This is the most frequent presentation in a tertiary care setting. A common example is duodenal ulcer bleeding in a patient suffering from sepsis complicating a major abdominal or thoracic operation. Such patients must be monitored closely, and the bleeding episode as well as the primary illness must be managed aggressively in the ICU.

Table 50-1. Prognostic Factors in Gastrointestinal Bleeding: Relationship of Age and Transfusion Requirement to Mortality and Operation Rate

Age (years)	Mortality (%)	Operation Rate (%)
31–40	4.7	11.3
41–50	10.1	11.7
51–60	12.0	18.7
61–70	12.8	17.2
71–80	14.4	18.5

Transfusion Requirement (Units)	Mortality (%)	Operation Rate (%)
0	2.5	2.6
1–3	6.7	4.9
4–6	11.7	16.0
7–9	15.4	30.9
>10	34.2	58.7

(Modified from Silverstein, F. E., et al.: The national ASGE survey on upper gastrointestinal bleeding. II. Clinical prognostic factors. Gastrointest. Endosc., 27:80, 1981.)

Table 50-2. Prognostic Factors in Gastrointestinal Bleeding: Relationship of Mortality and Associated Conditions Expressed as % Mortality

	Positive History (%)	Negative History (%)
Coexisting Diseases		
Central nervous system	23.5	8.7
Hepatic	24.6	6.9
Neoplasm	24.3	9.6
Pulmonary	22.6	8.2
Renal	29.4	9.2
Stress	16.6	9.2
Medications		
Steroids	22.2	9.9
Aspirin	4.9	13.6
Other NSAID	6.2	11.0
Physical Findings		
Ascites	40.6	7.9
Congestive heart failure	28.4	10.1
Jaundice	42.4	7.6
Respiratory failure	58.3	10.0
Shock	29.7	9.0
Blood in nasogastric tube	17.9	6.0
Blood in stool	20.1	9.9
Final Diagnosis		
Duodenal ulcer	6.7	12.2
Erosive duodenitis	2.3	11.4
Mallory-Weiss tear	4.4	11.3
Varices	30.1	8.6

NSAID, Nonsteroidal anti-inflammatory drug.
(Modified from Silverstein, F. E., et al.: The national ASGE survey on upper gastrointestinal bleeding. II. Clinical prognostic factors. Gastrointest. Endosc., 27:80, 1981.)

Gastrointestinal bleeding from an obscure source, or from multiple sources, in patients with compromised cardiorespiratory or other system reserve is most severe. This is the group that carries the highest mortality, and the management of this group of patients calls for consummate skill and team work.

PRE-ICU ASSESSMENT

Upper or Lower Gastrointestinal Bleeding

The history and physical signs usually afford some clues as to whether the bleeding is coming from the upper or lower gastrointestinal tract, even before firmly establishing the exact location by studies. In general, upper gastrointestinal bleeding is characterized by vomiting of blood or bloody drainage from nasogastric tube, hyperactive bowel sounds, melena of foul odor, and elevation of blood urea nitrogen (BUN) ("alimentary azotemia") owing to absorption of protein components in blood. The clinical signs are, however, not infallible. In some duodenal ulcer bleeding, there may be no vomiting, and the nasogastric tube may not reveal any bloody drainage. With rapid and massive bleeding, such as bleeding from esophagal varices, the patient may have red blood per rectum. Bleeding in the small intestine, although beyond the reach of the upper endoscopic examination and usually considered as lower gastrointestinal bleeding, manifests with melena without hematemesis. In bleeding from the colon, the majority of the patients with lower gastrointestinal bleeding, there is no hematemesis, the nasal gastric aspirate is negative for blood, and the stools are red and nonodorous. Bleeding in the right colon characteristically gives rise to maroon stool, whereas rectal bleeding is bright red. These signs, however, are again far from absolute. Of more value is the observation that when solid stool is recognizable in the bloody bowel movement rather than evenly mixed with it as in melena, the bleeding location is in the distal colon, where the contents are no longer liquid.

Assessment of Bleeding Activity

The first priority in the management of gastrointestinal bleeding is assessment of bleeding activity and approximation of blood lost. When the patient is actively bleeding, the output of blood is manifest as hematemesis or bloody bowel movements or both. At a slower rate of bleeding in the upper gut, the patient may have nausea and epigastric fullness before vomiting of blood. Hyperactive bowel sounds indicate blood is being transported rapidly in the gut, a sign highly suggestive of active bleeding. The duration of bleeding and the patient's own description of the quantity give a rough but unreliable estimate of the amount of blood loss. A single reading of the hematocrit does not necessarily reflect the magnitude of blood loss because it takes several hours for equilibration to occur. Serial hematocrit measurement is more useful for quantification. Of more quantitative value is the symptom of postural hypotension. Signs of postural hypotension indicate a loss in excess of 25% of blood volume over a short time. Overt hypotension on presentation is an important prognostic sign. Not only must fluid resuscitation be carried out immediately, but also operative intervention may be required (see Chap. 60).

Table 50-3. American Society of Gastroenterology Bleeding Survey: Endoscopic Diagnoses in Upper Gastrointestinal Bleeding (2097 Patients)

Diagnosis	No. Patients	Incidence (%)
Gastric erosions	620	29.6
Duodenal ulcer	477	22.8
Gastric ulcer	457	21.9
Varices	323	15.2
Esophagitis	269	12.8
Duodenitis	191	9.1
Mallory-Weiss tear	168	8.0
Neoplasm	78	3.7
Esophageal ulcer	46	2.2
Stomal ulcer	39	1.9
Telangiectasia	10	0.5
Others	152	7.3

(Modified from Gilbert, D. A., et al.: The national ASGE survey on upper gastrointestinal bleeding. III. Endoscopy in upper gastrointestinal bleeding. Gastrointest. Endosc., 27:94, 1981.)

Search for the Source of Bleeding

Table 50-3 lists the various lesions that may bleed in the upper gastrointestinal tract, and Table 50-4 lists those that commonly cause lower gastrointestinal bleeding. History affords important clues: Familial history of bleeding or coagulation disorder, ingestion of aspirin or other nonsteroidal anti-inflammatory agents, alcoholism, ulcer disease, portal hypertension, and previous abdominal aneurysm resection are a few examples. Physical examination may reveal cutaneous or neurologic signs of liver disease, such as ascites, spider hemangiomata, palmar erythema, gynecomastia, muscle wasting, asterixis, and fetor hepaticus. Cutaneous or mucous membrane vascular lesions are found in patients with Rendu-Weber-Osler and von Willebrand's disease, whereas bruises may indicate coagulation disorder. Gastrointestinal bleeding occurring for the first time in a critically ill patient is likely to be a stress-related condition, such as erosive gastritis and duodenitis, reflux esophagitis aggravated by prolonged nasogastric tube drainage, or true peptic ulcerations. Conditions that may

Table 50-4. Lower Gastrointestinal Bleeding: Pathologic Diagnoses in 40 Patients with Emergency Colonoscopy for Massive Hematochezia

Diagnosis	Incidence (%)
Angioma	35.0
Polyps/cancer	15.0
Active diverticular bleeding	10.0
Focal colitis	5.0
Possible small bowel source	5.0
Polyp stalk	2.5
Endometriosis	2.5
Upper gastrointestinal bleeding	12.5
No sites found	12.5

(Modified from Jensen, D. M., Machicado, G. A., and Tapia, J. I.: Emergent colonoscopy in patients with severe hematochezia. Gastrointest. Endosc., 29:177, 1983.)

Table 50-5. Indications for ICU Admission for Management of Gastrointestinal Bleeding

Adverse prognostic factors
  Massive bleeding (>2 L/24 hours) with hemodynamic instability
  Old age (>60); shock on presentation
  Large (>2 cm) or multiple ulcers
  Vessel endoscopic sign
  Visible
Concomitant systemic illness: heart, renal, liver, respiratory failure
Portal hypertension
Source(s) of bleeding unknown

bleed in the lower gastrointestinal tract are less numerous, but telangiectasia, polyps, cancer, and active diverticular bleeding account for 70% of cases.[8] Others include colitis (inflammatory bowel disease, radiation proctitis, ischemic colitis), endometriosis, and miscellaneous lesions. In one study, more than 10% of patients undergoing emergency colonoscopy for massive hematochezia actually had upper gastrointestinal bleeding (see Table 50-4). Lesions in the small bowel, considered after exclusion of a source in the upper or lower tract, include Meckel's diverticulum, leiomyoma, carcinoid, and other less common tumors, with few clues from symptoms and signs.

Indications for ICU Admission and Management

The indications for ICU admission are based on consideration of a patient's general condition and the activity of bleeding (Table 50-5). If a patient is suffering from a primary illness with significant impairment of system reserves, response to hemorrhage is also impaired. For example, in severe aortic stenosis, resuscitation cannot be optimally done without monitoring. If the bleeding is massive or active or if the source is obscure and activity unpredictable, close monitoring and aggressive resuscitation in the ICU are essential. The presence of adverse prognostic factors mentioned previously, such as old age (>60), massive bleeding, shock on presentation, anemia, large ulcers (>2 cm), and ingestion of steroids, also influence the decision for management in the ICU. The uncommon gastrointestinal bleeder who does not require management in the ICU is the patient for whom simple clinical monitoring is adequate: for example, a young patient with a moderate blood loss from a source that has been adequately treated endoscopically.

MANAGEMENT IN THE ICU

Monitoring Parameters

Continuous electrocardiogram display and blood pressure taken at frequent intervals are the minimal basic parameters to be followed. In an elderly patient with unknown cardiac reserve, a Swan-Ganz catheter should be inserted for pulmonary capillary wedge pressure to guide volume replacement. This need is particularly evident when postural hypotension, tachycardia, and decreased urine output failed to improve with initial infusion of fluids. Continuous recording of urinary output by Foley catheter insertion is important. The peripheral cutaneous circulation gives important information as to adequacy of fluid replacement. A flow chart must be kept of the vital signs, blood loss in the form of bloody stool, hematemesis or bloody nasogastric tube drainage, infusion of blood products and other fluids, and laboratory results. Arterial line for continuous blood pressure determination and for facilitated blood gas sampling and other laboratory tests is indicated in the high risk patient. The trends of heart rate and pulse pressure often provide reliable guides to the status of circulating volume.

Volume Replacement

Volume replacement is the first treatment to be considered (see Chap. 60). Large-bore intravenous catheters, two or more, may be required depending on the need for rapid infusion. Crystalloids are generally used before blood is available from the blood bank. A general indication for blood transfusion is hemodynamic instability persisting after infusion of more than 50 ml/kg of crystalloids. Albumin may be considered, but the marginal theoretical advantage probably does not justify the expense because albumin may be lost into the extravascular space from the damaged and leaky endothelium owing to shock. Hetastarch as volume expander has the advantage of lower cost. Fresh frozen plasma is used only when there is significant coagulopathy. Pressure infusion may be required to administer packed cells and should be resorted to if blood loss continues to outpace replacement. The adequacy of replacement is clinically determined by widened pulse pressure, decreased heart rate, improved peripheral perfusion, and increased urine output.

Correction of Coagulopathy

Coagulopathy should be corrected as soon as possible to limit the ongoing blood loss. Fresh frozen plasma corrects most of the defects and is expeditious when the patient is being prepared for an emergency operation. Specific treatment may be possible if a cause has been found. If aspirin-induced gastric bleeding is suspected, bleeding time should be determined. Aspirin-induced gastric bleeding often has a characteristic endoscopic appearance, such as multiple bleeding gastric erosions with fragments of aspirin adherent to the eroded mucosa. Administration of platelets to correct the thrombocytopathy is an essential part of the treatment.

Emergency Endoscopy

The next priority, after stabilization of vital signs, is preparation for emergency endoscopic examination. Although many prospective studies showed that emergency endoscopy conferred no advantage in outcome even though accuracy in diagnosis has been enhanced, those studies were done without regard to the treatment used.[1] Another cogent argument for emergency endoscopy is the advent of therapeutic endoscopy. The National Institute of Health (NIH) Consensus Development Conference[2] summarized available data and strongly supported the use of hemostatic probes in bleeding peptic ulcers manifesting with stigmata of bleeding.

Emergency endoscopic approaches differ somewhat depending on whether upper or lower gastrointestinal endoscopy is performed.

Upper Gastrointestinal Bleeding (Other than Variceal)

Bleeding from the nasopharynx, esophagus, stomach, and small intestine proximal to the ligament of Treitz is conventionally regarded as upper gastrointestinal bleeding. If the patient has just vomited blood, the stomach is effectively cleared of the clots and lavage may not be necessary. If the patient has much nausea, the stomach is likely to be full of blood and clots, and oral insertion of a large-bore gastric tube for lavage of the contents is necessary. A method for rapid, effective lavage is to instill 300 to 400 ml of saline and allow the contents to be drained out by siphonage and then repeated until nearly clear. Even large clots can be evacuated this way. Some endoscopists, however, do not lavage at all but rely on changing the patient's position to shift the clots for total inspection of the gastric mucosa during endoscopy.

Before insertion of the endoscope, oral suction must be standing by to prevent aspiration. Frequently in massive bleeding from esophageal varices, it may be necessary to perform endotracheal intubation for airway protection before endoscopy. The use of sedation requires considerable judgement. In the cooperative patient, sedation may not be necessary, but for most patients, some short-acting sedation with, for instance, midazolam is useful, particularly if the patient is vomiting bright red blood. Meperidine should be avoided if hypotension is a problem, even when the effect can be rapidly reversed with opiate antagonists. Topical pharyngeal anesthesia may also be used, but it may enhance the risk of aspiration. Monitoring of oxygenation by pulse oximetry is now universally adopted as a safety standard.

Endoscopic Technique

The patient lies on the left side, and the endoscope is expeditiously inserted, preferably under direct vision into the cricopharyngeal sphincter. The aim is to reach the second or third portion of the duodenum and then inspect carefully as the instrument is withdrawn. The stomach always contains blood or irrigant, but the exposed area can be adequately inspected because liquid blood only stains but does not adhere to the normal mucosa. After inspection of the exposed mucosa, the patient is turned on to the right side, and the previously submerged areas are now exposed. Complete examination is thus possible without complete cleansing.

Interpretation of Findings

Experience is required in interpretation of findings, particularly in avoiding confusion by artifacts. Dark blood stains between the folds are of no localizing value. They indicate that blood had been acted on by gastric acid. Either the bleeding has been relatively slow, or the blood has been in the stomach for a while. Small clots are easily washed away, to be clearly differentiated from the adherent clot, which resists even vigorous jets of water and which indicates an underlying bleeding lesion. Although ulcerations are relatively simple to recognize, erosions have to be distinguished from blood staining, often calling for much irrigation. In contrast to blood staining, erosions cannot be washed away. The epithelium is eroded, with a surrounding rim of erythema. Fresh red blood in the stomach is a sign of active bleeding, indicating that a careful search is likely to yield the positive source. Other stigmata of bleeding are not only of therapeutic importance, but also prognostic importance. The visible vessel sign has been much debated; the term is applied to a raised nodule in the bottom of an ulcer, mostly red or black, indicating an exposed blood vessel, a small but densely adherent blood clot on top of the vessel, or a pseudoaneurysm of a vessel recently bled.[9] Oozing may be seen around this raised lesion indicating active bleeding. The prognostic significance of the visible vessel sign is that recurrent hemorrhage from the ulcer is high, ranging from 30 to 100%, depending on the series reviewed.[10,11] An ulcer with a clean base or with one or two flat spots of red or brown indicates low likelihood of rebleeding. A Mallory-Weiss tear of the lower esophageal mucosa is often without stigmata of bleeding. Recurrent bleeding from the tear is unlikely, unless the patient has been anticoagulated.

Many sources of error may confound the endoscopist: Artifacts from trauma of suction, blood clots in various forms and colors, multiple sources of bleeding, and incomplete examination are the main sources of difficulty. The endoscopist must carefully analyze the data and resolve all inconsistencies before coming up with the best diagnosis. In the event of no certain diagnosis, it is vitally important for subsequent management to state the pertinent negatives. For example, knowing that the patient is not bleeding from esophageal varices alone is worth the examination. Similarly, in the absence of erosive gastritis or varices, the surgeon tends to search for duodenal sources (e.g., aortoduodenal fistula) even though no definite duodenal ulcer is seen at endoscopy.

Therapeutic Endoscopic Techniques

Local therapeutic measures directed at the bleeding lesions are now generally part of the emergency endoscopy, but they are successful only when the sources of bleeding have been accurately identified. Thus, if bleeding comes from discrete lesions at a rate commensurate with good visualization, effective treatment can usually be delivered. Therapeutic endoscopy has been shown to reduce recurrent bleeding by 70%, emergency surgery rate by 60%, and in-hospital mortality by 30%.[12] Many portable modalities are available, the selection of which depends on user familiarity and to a lesser extent the nature of the lesions.

Heater Probe. The heater probe is a flexible probe with a Teflon-coated tip (a miniature branding iron) that can be heated in 5 seconds to a temperature of 150° Celsius and maintained at the level to deliver a calibrated amount of heat energy (Joules). For convenience, a water pump is attached to the device to give more vigorous clot-dislodging irrigation, quite helpful in exposing the bleeding artery preparatory to delivering the heat. To apply the probe, it is essential that pressure be used to coapt the walls of the vessel to create a heat seal. Tangential applications usually are not effective, and bleeders in areas allowing only a tangential approach are not suitable for this or any other modality using probes (such as the BICAP; see next).

BICAP Probe. This is similar to the heater probe except that a bipolar electrocoagulation of the tissue takes place on activation. It also has an irrigating pump for the probe to be used as an irrigating catheter to expose the vessel before application of bipolar electrocoagulation. In bipolar electrocoagulation, electric current flows through the tissue between the probe and delivers heat until the tissue is dessicated. At this state, the tissue is no longer conductive, and the flow of current stops. This serves as a built-in, current-limiting safety factor. Just as in the use of the heater probe, pressure application is also essential for efficacy and so may not be optimally used for tangential application. Both BICAP and heater probes are useful for similar situations: discrete bleeding from erosions and ulcerations in the stomach or duodenum allowing a direct (en face) approach.

Injection. Injection of dehydrated ethanol has been shown to be effective for hemostasis in bleeding ulcers. Intramucosal injection of minute amounts (0.2 to 0.4 ml), not exceeding a total of 1 to 1.5 ml, successfully treats bleeding in more than 90% of cases.[13] Provided that the dose is kept small, the risks of perforation from full-thickness necrosis can be kept low. Because an en-face approach is not essential, this technique works well for lesions regardless of location, but the injections must be given with accuracy. For larger areas of bleeding, 1:10,000 epinephrine injected submucosally in larger volumes (1 to 5 ml, up to 10 to 15 ml) rapidly tamponades bleeding areas resulting in temporary hemostasis. A second injection of epinephrine 24 hours later is sometimes necessary to prevent rebleeding.[14]

Other Endoscopic Methods. Monopolar electrocoagulation was the first well-studied modality in endoscopic hemostasis. The equipment is simple to operate, but the safety margin is small because depth of injury is difficult to predict. Adhesion of the coagulator to the eschar is another problem. Laser photocoagulation (argon, Nd:YAG) is also effective, but the equipment is bulky, has special electrical and plumbing requirements, and cannot be moved to the ICU, where most of the therapeutic work for bleeding is done.

Ancillary Measures. Antacids and H_2-blockers are effective in prevention of stress erosive gastritis and are effective treatment for ulcer disease. All endoscopic modalities (heater probe, BICAP probe, injections) tend to aggravate or create ulcers, and the postprocedure treatment must include an intensive regimen of antacids and H_2-blockers.

Variceal Bleeding in Portal Hypertension

Variceal bleeding is considered a special case because the bleeding is liable to be persistent and recurrent owing to high venous pressure and because the patient often suffers from hepatic decompensation, malnutrition, coagulopathy, massive ascites, renal failure, and other complicated metabolic problems.

After endoscopic diagnosis of bleeding esophageal varices, two major options are open. If bleeding is not massive and if required expertise is available, emergency endoscopic sclerosis of the varices is the option of choice.[15,16] This has the advantage of assured hemostasis (albeit temporary) so attention can be devoted to management of hepatic insufficiency and other metabolic ills. If emergency sclerosis is not possible, temporizing measures may be used to stabilize the patient and sclerosis done semielectively. One such regimen is to start intravenous infusion of vasopressin, up to 0.4 unit per minute (20 units in 50 ml of D5W, at 1 ml per minute) via a central venous catheter, but many patients may not be suitable for this treatment because of atherosclerotic heart disease. Simultaneous administration of nitroglycerin has been shown to enhance the reduction of portal pressure. A promising new analog of vasopressin, triglycyl lysine vasopressin (terlipressin) is relatively free of the side effects on the coronary arteries[17] and may be useful in these patients. Clinical effects of vasopressin include a prominent antidiuretic action, enhanced peristaltic activity of the gut, hypertension, bradycardia, and skin pallor. Many of the signs may interfere with monitoring of the patient's blood volume, and due allowance should be made. (*Editor's note:* Caution is advised when simultaneous administration of vasopressin and blood transfusion is underway. Flash pulmonary edema may occur with rapid precipitation of respiratory failure.)

Sengstaken-Blakemore Balloon Tamponade

Besides being an uncomfortable procedure for the patient, the use of this tube carries considerable risks of massive aspiration pneumonitis from salivary or blood aspiration and gastric or esophageal rupture from the balloons. Most clinicians prefer a four lumen tube (Minnesota tube), one for gastric balloon, one for esophageal balloon, and one each for gastric and esophageal lumen aspiration—the last-mentioned serving to reduce the risks of aspiration pneumonitis. The balloons are first tested for integrity, then totally collapsed by aspiration. The tube is passed either nasally or orally. Topical anesthetic should be applied to the oral and nasal pharynx. After passage, the position of the tube can be determined clinically by auscultation over the stomach when air is instilled into the gastric lumen. The gastric balloon is then inflated with 400 ml of air. If excessive resistance is encountered during inflation, the clinician should be mindful that the tube could be located in the esophagus. Traction against the cardia is applied (Fig. 50-1) and held at 1 to 1.5 lb force, usually accomplished by taping the tube to a football helmet or similar apparatus worn by the patient. If bleeding stops as monitored by gastric aspiration, the esophageal balloon need not be used. The correct position of the gastric balloon must then be verified by a plain film of the abdomen. If bleeding continues, the esophageal balloon should be inflated to 35 mm Hg, using a sphygmomanometer. Even though the patient is instructed not to swallow, continuous suction should be applied to the esophageal lumen to recover the saliva trickled into the esophagus. The esophageal balloon must be deflated after 18 to 24 hours to prevent ischemic necrosis. The tube (with the balloons down) may be removed if bleeding remains controlled after 12 hours; in any case, continuous use of the tube over 36 hours incurs a high risk of ischemic pressure necrosis of the stomach and esophagus.

Sclerotherapy

Sclerotherapy has become the emergency treatment of choice for bleeding esophageal varices.[15,16] In most instances, repeated injections after a long-term regimen lead to eradication of the varices after months of therapy. Direct injection of sclerosants (e.g., 1.5% tetradecyl sulfate, 5% sodium morrhuate, 5% ethanolamine oleate) into the varices induces venous thrombosis of the varices. Injections are first performed at the gastroesophageal junction and then at a higher level as well if the varices are large and the columns are long. Postprocedure care includes nothing by mouth for 24 hours, continued monitoring for bleeding (serial hematocrit, rectal output, nausea), and avoidance of a nasogastric tube to reduce mechanical trauma to the varices. Rebleeding should be immediately investigated by endoscopy and be treated with further sclerotherapy if it proves to be variceal.

Endoscopic Variceal Ligation. Varices may be ligated endoscopically with a variceal ligator, which is a device attached to the tip of the conventional end-viewing endoscope.[18,19] The principle is identical to that of rubber banding of the hemorrhoids: Tiny rubber bands are released onto the neck of the varix, which has been sucked into the ligating chamber. The advantage of this method is that there is no chemical inflammation, and, therefore, it is free of many of the undesirable side effects of sclerotherapy, such as necrosis, ulceration, stenosis, and needle puncture bleeding.

Emergency Surgery for Bleeding Esophageal Varices. This option is taken as a last resort owing to a prohibitively high mortality. In a few patients who do not respond to the less invasive measures, however, the clinician is left with little choice. Devascularization procedures, such as stapler transection of the lower esophagus for interruption of the variceal channels, may prove lifesaving if done expeditiously.[20] When used alone, however, the incidence of late recurrent bleeding is high and should be followed by elective sclerotherapy. Emergency portasystemic shunting is used much less often than formerly but may occasionally be a procedure of choice for the better risk patients, usually those classified as Child's A or B in terms of hepatic reserve (see Chap. 54).

Ancillary Management. Massive and tense ascites must be treated, using paracentesis if necessary, because the intra-abdominal pressure may contribute to the portal pressure. Hepatic failure must be treated aggressively. Nu-

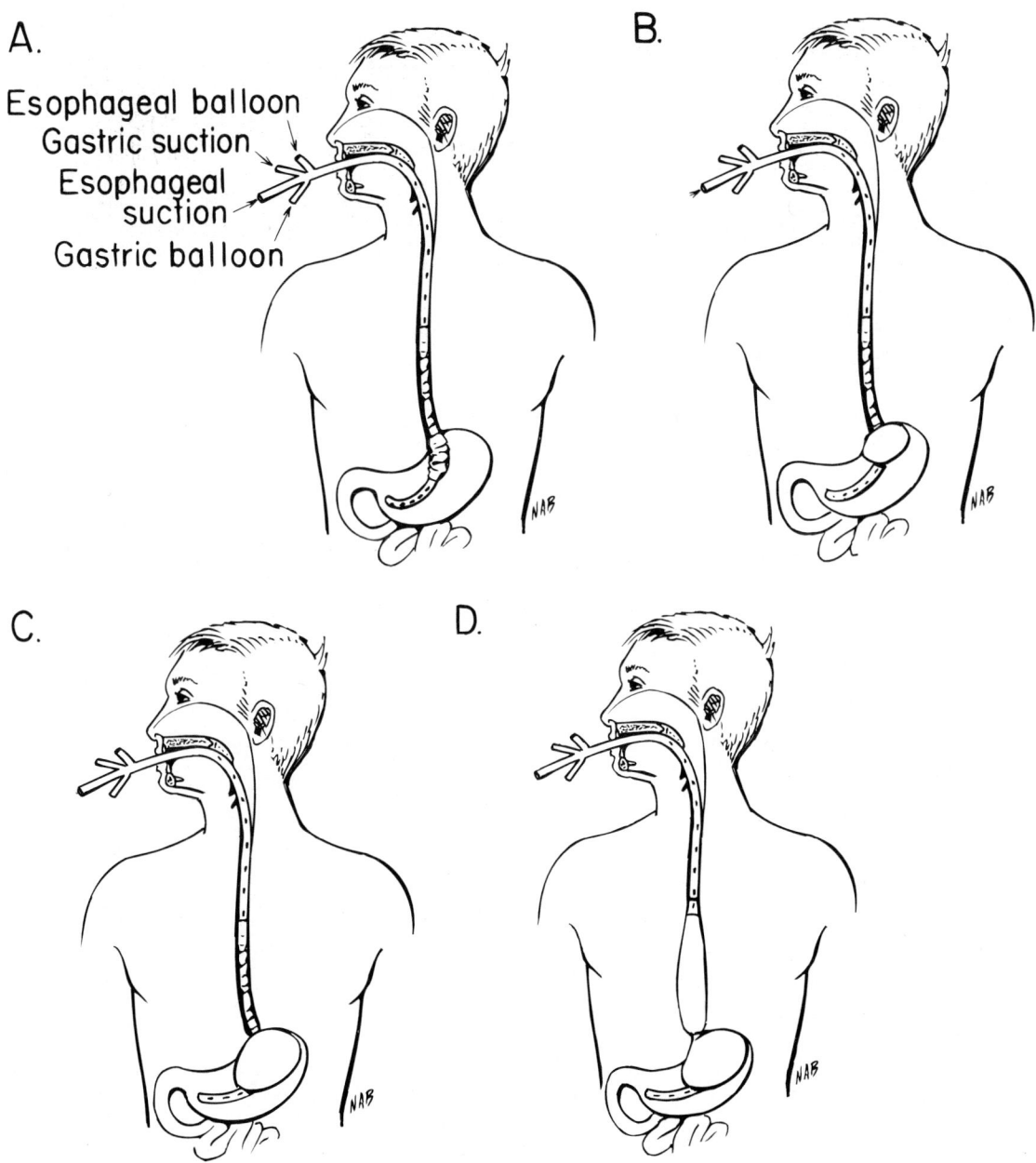

Fig. 50–1. The Minnesota Four Lumen Esophagogastric Tamponade Tube for the control of bleeding from esophageal varices. *A*, The approximate position of the tube after passage through the nasopharynx or oral pharynx. Either route may be used, but the nasopharyngeal route is the preferred route. *B*, After positioning of the tube, the gastric balloon is inflated to about 150 ml of volume, and an x-ray film of the lower chest and upper abdomen is obtained to check the position of the stomach balloon. *C*, After confirmation of tube and balloon position in the stomach, the stomach balloon is inflated to a volume of 400 to 500 ml, and then gentle traction is placed on the tube to "snug" the stomach balloon up against the cardia of the stomach. Traction of the inflated balloon may be sufficient for hemostasis. *D*, If inflation and traction of the gastric balloon are insufficient for hemostasis, inflation of the esophageal balloon should be undertaken. The esophageal balloon should never be inflated without proper inflation of the gastric balloon. If done, there is risk of dislocation of the tube into the posterior pharynx and the potential for total obstruction of the upper airway in the nonintubated patient. The esophageal balloon should be inflated to a pressure of no more than 45 mm Hg. Less pressure is desirable if hemostasis occurs at a lesser pressure. Sustained pressure above 25 to 30 mm Hg is associated with ulceration of esophageal mucosa. Therefore the esophageal balloon should be periodically deflated for 5 minutes every 6 hours.

tritional care is critical, and treatment of hepatorenal syndrome requires the input of multispecialties.

Lower Gastrointestinal Bleeding

Lower gastrointestinal bleeding includes all bleeding sites distal to the ligament of Treitz, but the preponderance of the lesions occur in the colon, rectum, and lower ileum. Although passage of bright red blood per rectum is a sign indicating bleeding in the lower gastrointestinal tract, massive bleeding from the upper tract can manifest in this manner and must first be excluded. A quick upper gastrointestinal endoscopy accomplishes this in minutes.

The difficulties with diagnosis in lower gastrointestinal bleeding is the fact that bleeding tends more to be intermittent and that a large territory (the small bowel) is not readily accessible to the usual diagnostic tests. Fortunately bleeding in the small bowel is infrequent. A coordinated sequential use of endoscopy and radiography is most important to cover the territory adequately.

Endoscopic Technique

An initial sigmoidoscopy with either the flexible or the rigid instrument should be performed. The rigid instrument has the advantage of much better suction and washing capability but does not give as good a view. If active bleeding is identified in the rectum and sigmoid, it can be treated endoscopically (such as heater probe or BICAP or resnaring of a bleeding stalk after polypectomy) and further investigation postponed pending further bleeding activity. A rather frequent cause of massive bleeding is that following polypectomy. Typically it presents either within 24 hours after the procedure (inadequate coagulation) or 6 to 8 days later (septic necrosis). If blood is seen to come continuously from above the limit of sigmoidoscopy, colonoscopy should be undertaken after bowel preparation depending on the bleeding activity. For continuous active bleeding, a small enema may be given to clear the sigmoid lumen to facilitate insertion of the colonoscope. Visualization of the entire colon may then be possible in most instances because fresh blood does not become adherent to the mucosa and is easily irrigated, in contrast to melena, in which water absorption renders the stool tenacious to washing. The instrument is passed to above the highest section of blood staining, followed by withdrawal and inspection for stigmata of bleeding, irrigating and removing the clots as necessary. Most often this means passing into the terminal ileum because the entire colon is blood stained owing to the segmentation movement of the colon, and blood may be found as high as the cecum even if location of bleeding is in the sigmoid. With careful inspection and irrigation, however, the active bleeding segment may be discernible, and bleeding lesions, such as arteriovenous malformations, diverticula, and Crohn's disease, can be identified by means of this technique.

If the patient has recently bled but is not actively bleeding, a full colon preparation is necessary. This is most expediently accomplished by whole-gut lavage, using Colyte solution at 2 L/hour either by mouth or by nasogastric tube.

Therapeutic Endoscopy for Colonic Bleeding

The modalities available are those developed for upper gastrointestinal bleeding but caution must be exercised to avoid full-thickness burn because the bowel may be thinned out from air or blood distention. Insufflation with carbon dioxide to prevent explosion before electrocoagulation is advisable if the colon is full of stool. There are not enough data to establish the efficacy of these modalities, but many series of small experience indicate a beneficial effect.[21]

If endoscopy fails to uncover significant leads, a labeled red cell scan should be performed. Sequential imaging over the next 24 hours may demonstrate extravasation if the scanning interval is appropriately short. Inference from the scan as to the location of extravasation is always tentative and takes into account the peristaltic activity of the gut. When the labeled red cells appear in the small bowel, distal transport can be seen outlining more small bowel with sequential scanning, but in the colon, segmentation and mixing tend to outline the entire colon. A positive scan should be followed by angiography (see later) or repeat colonoscopy if bleeding has been localized in the colon.

Nonendoscopic Workup of Lower Gastrointestinal Bleeding

Instead of sigmoidoscopy followed by colonoscopy as the initial investigation, an alternative is to proceed directly to technetium 99m sulfer colloid scan for rapid confirmation of active bleeding and tentative localization of bleeding sites. The scan can be completed in 15 minutes to be followed immediately by angiography if the scan is positive. The combined procedures give a good yield, but the colloid scan is also subject to the same caveats in interpretation as the red cell scan. A major disadvantage is that the patient has to be sent out of the ICU frequently, necessitating additional manpower and placing the patient in an area not primarily equipped for monitoring or resuscitation.

Other Therapeutic Methods

Angiography

Endoscopy has replaced radiologic contrast studies in the diagnosis of gastrointestinal bleeding, not only because of better accuracy, but also because of its ready availability, portability to the bedside, and therapeutic potential. Angiography is still of great value, however, when bleeding is not identifiable by endoscopy. In the "no man's land," the jejunum and ileum, for example, angiography is the diagnostic tool of choice. A bleeding rate of 0.5 to 2 ml/min is required for angiographic demonstration of bleeding. A major advantage of diagnostic angiography is that it can be therapeutic at the same time. The visible bleeding vessel identified angiographically may be treated by occlusive or constrictive techniques—an indication for angiography over endoscopy when bleeding is too rapid to be controlled by endoscopic means. Another major indication is failure to demonstrate the bleeding site by endoscopy and suspicion of bleeding outside of the territory covered by endoscopy.

Two broad categories of techniques may be used. The choice depends on anatomy of the circulation as well as other factors.

Occlusive Technique. Selective angiography and selective embolization of the feeding vessel is generally feasible in the upper gastrointestinal tract, where the richness of the collaterals make ischemic necrosis less likely. By contrast, many bleeding vessels in the colon are end vessels, and embolization may result in necrosis. By the same token, because of the rich collaterals, many vessels, such as the gastroduodenal, require embolization at both directions (the inflow proximal and distal to the feeding vessel) to be effective. Even so, occluding one side of the collateral is helpful in many instances even when hemostasis is temporary. Many innovative techniques of embolization have been introduced; the more commonly used material includes miniature steel coils, Gelfoam, cyanoacrylate, and detachable balloons.

Constrictive Technique. The systemic infusion of vasoconstrictors originally developed for bleeding esophageal varices has been modified for selective intra-arterial infusion after catheterization of the bleeding artery. Although superior mesenteric arterial infusion of vasopressin does not confer any advantage over systemic venous infusion in treating bleeding esophageal varices, selective infusion into a catheterized visceral artery causes selective vasoconstriction of the territory supplied and is effective in treatment of bleeding conditions, such as peptic ulcer bleeding, stress erosions, and so forth. The vasoconstrictor is delivered to the site of action, and the total dose used is less than systemic administration. Constrictive intervention via selective angiography is preferred over occlusive technique in lower gastrointestinal bleeding because there is less risk of ischemic necrosis. It is also useful in the upper gut, where devascularization may have occurred with previous surgery or atherosclerosis.

SURGICAL TREATMENT

Indication for Surgery

In the era of therapeutic endoscopy, one pitfall is to persist too long with an ineffective modality to the detriment of the patient. In the presence of continued bleeding despite support, when the lesion is judged unsuitable for endoscopic therapy, or when the patient rebleeds after an adequate trial of endoscopic therapy, surgery must be considered and the patient must be prepared for it without delay. Indications for surgery are:

- Failure of endoscopic therapy (failure to achieve hemostasis or recurrent bleeding after an adequate trial)
- Presence of adverse prognostic factors (see earlier)
- Patient not deemed to be a prohibitive surgical risk

Many clinicians use an arbitrary volume of blood transfusion as an incontrovertible indication of failure of nonsurgical treatment, but it is important to note that it is not the volume of blood required but the resolution not to procrastinate that is the underlying merit of this practice. Because there is no scientific method to define surgical risks (it varies to a substantial degree with the skill of the surgeon), conjoint assessment by the entire team (intensivist, endoscopist, surgeon) is essential. (See under integrated care.)

Localization of the exact bleeding site is crucial to the success of surgical treatment. Operative endoscopy is a last resort, which, although useful, may not substitute for a good preoperative endoscopic examination. Before incision is made after the patient is under anesthesia, an expeditious endoscopic examination may be undertaken to confirm the findings for the benefit of the surgeon. It is crucial to avoid air distention of the bowel because it interferes with the operation.

The principle of operation consists of direct exposure of the bleeding artery for its ligation. Operative management can be expeditiously rendered if a preoperative diagnosis has been firmly established. For bleeding gastric ulcers, a gastrectomy if possible should be undertaken. Vagotomy and pyloroplasty with transfixion of the bleeding vessel generally suffices for duodenal ulcer. In the past 10 years or so, however, proximal gastric vagotomy (without accompanying gastric operations) has been performed for bleeding duodenal ulcer because the ulcer, after accurate localization by preoperative endoscopy, can be plicated by a separate small incision in the duodenum.[22] Diffuse gastric erosions, such as in severe stress-related mucosal disease, may require near total gastrectomy for successful hemostasis.

In patients with an undiagnosed source of bleeding, some preliminary operative maneuver may be necessary to locate the source. The stomach is opened in the body and the clots evacuated. After the pylorus and the cardia are packed with sponges, detailed inspection of the mucosa becomes possible. The packs are removed one side at a time. If bleeding comes from the pyloric side, further inspection by duodenotomy is warranted. If bleeding comes from the cardia, attention is directed toward the lower esophagus and upper cardia. Definitive surgical operation then follows once the diagnosis is made.

Surgical operations for colonic bleeding differ from that for upper tract bleeding in that direct ligation of the exposed bleeding vessel is not practical because a colotomy in the unprepared bowel may lead to septic complications owing to contamination. Instead, the involved segment is resected followed by either a temporary colostomy or reanastomosis. In a patient bleeding massively with known arteriovenous malformations in the right colon and diverticulosis in the left, without certain indication which is bleeding, a subtotal colectomy with ileorectal anastomosis may be life-saving.[23,24]

Postoperative complications to watch for after gastric surgery for bleeding include wound infection and dehiscence, leakage with intra-abdominal infections and recurrent bleeding from the suture line, inadequately ligated artery, or stress erosions.

NUTRITIONAL SUPPORT

Anticipation is the key to prevent malnutrition and the adverse effect on recovery. When the duration of illness is expected to last more than 10 days and the patient is already without food intake for 5 to 7 days, nutritional intervention must be considered. Whenever possible, the gastrointestinal tract should be used. Placing a feeding tube does not necessarily interfere with monitoring of the gastric output. In postoperative ileus, parenteral nutrition should be considered, switching back to the enteral route as soon as the gut function returns.

POST-ICU CARE

Discharge from ICU

The decision to discharge is based on a consideration of the bleeding status, how likely or imminent is recurrence, and what the patient's requirements are for monitoring and stabilization. For the patient whose bleeding appeared to have stopped spontaneously, 24 hours of continued vigilance is necessary before such a judgement can be made. The following conditions are high risks for recurrent hemorrhage:

- Giant or multiple ulcers
- Visible bleeding vessels at endoscopy
- Esophageal or gastric variceal bleeding
- Bleeding from arteriovenous malformations, particularly in patients with coagulopathy

For patients whose bleeding has been arrested with effective endoscopic therapy, including sclerotherapy, a similar period of close observation is beneficial, although it may be shortened if the level of confidence of the procedure is high. After a major surgical operation for arrest of bleeding, the patient should be cared for in the ICU in the early recovery phase, usually 3 to 4 days, but the postoperative course can be variable owing to complications.

After discharge from the ICU, routine surveillance should include daily physical examination for bleeding activities, hematocrit determination at appropriate intervals, stool charting, and repeat endoscopy, if necessary. For sclerotherapy or ligation of varices, a second injection or ligation is usually scheduled within 7 days of the initial session.[15,25] For bleeding ulcers, maximal medical therapy is continued until healing.

INTEGRATED CARE

Gastrointestinal bleeding can be a difficult condition to treat not only because the patient is often critically ill, the diagnosis is obscure, and the treatment is uncertain, but also because optimal care involves coordination of multispecialties, which often hold divergent views. For example, many surgeons believe that if high risk patients can be optimized quickly and operated on early, mortality can be reduced.[26,27] Nonsurgeons, however, point to the fact that mortality is often due to complications, such as leakage from anastomosis and infection, so early surgery is not the sole answer. The reluctance of nonsurgeons to recommend surgery may well be based on an unrealistic assessment of hazards of the operation, which are best assessed by surgeons. Persistence at in ineffective modality, often the plight of the superspecialist working in isolation, is to be avoided at all cost. It is therefore vital that the decision for surgery be made conjointly, and the surgeon should be involved early rather than called in as the last resort. In many centers with outstanding success in management of gastrointestinal bleeding, surgical consultation is obtained as soon as the patient is admitted into the hospital, a policy that pays handsome dividends.[27-29] To attain the best survival in the ICU setting, the intensivist, the gastroenterologist/endoscopist, and the surgeon should work as an integral team with constant communication.[27-29]

REFERENCES

1. Bronfield, N. W., et al.: Outcome of endoscopy and barium radiography for acute upper gastrointestinal bleeding: controlled trial in 1037 patients. Br. Med. J., *284:*545, 1982.
2. Consensus Conference: Therapeutic endoscopy and bleeding ulcers. JAMA, *262:*1369, 1989.
3. Avery-Jones, F.: Hematemesis and melena with special reference to causation and to factors influencing the mortality from bleeding ulcers. Gastroenterology, *30:*166, 1956.
4. Read, R. C., Hubel, H. C., and Thal, A. P.: Randomized study of massive bleeding from peptic ulceration. Ann. Surg., *162:*561, 1965.
5. Silverstein, F. E., et al.: The national ASGE survey on upper gastrointestinal bleeding. II. Clinical prognostic factors. Gastrointest. Endosc., *27:*80, 1981.
6. Clason, A. E., MacLeod, D. A. D., and Elton, R. A.: Clinical factors in the prediction of further hemorrhage or mortality in acute upper gastrointestinal hemorrhage. Br. J. Surg., *73:*985, 1986.
7. Bornman, P. C., et al.: Importance of hypovolemic shock and endoscopic signs in predicting recurrent hemorrhage from peptic ulceration: a prospective evaluation. Br. Med. J., *291:*245, 1985.
8. Boley, S. J., et al.: Lower intestinal bleeding in the elderly. Am. J. Surg., *13:*57, 1979.
9. Swain, C. P., et al.: Nature of the bleeding vessel in recurrently bleeding gastric ulcers. Gastroenterology, *90:*595, 1986.
10. Wara, P.: Endoscopic prediction of major rebleeding—a prospective study of stigmata of hemorrhage in bleeding ulcer. Gastroenterology, *88:*1209, 1985.
11. Storey, D. W., et al.: Endoscopic prediction of recurrent bleeding in peptic ulcers. N. Engl. J. Med., *305:*915, 1981.
12. Sacks, H. S., Chalmer, T. C., and Blum, A. L.: Endoscopic hemostasis: an effective therapy for bleeding peptic ulcers. JAMA, *264:*494, 1990.
13. Lane, L.: Multipolar electrocoagulation versus injection therapy in the treatment of bleeding peptic ulcers. Gastroenterology, *99:*1303, 1990.
14. Chung, S. C., et al.: Endoscopic injection of adrenaline for actively bleeding ulcers: a randomized trial. Br. Med. J., *296:*1631, 1988.
15. Chung, R. S.: The role of sclerotherapy in management of esophageal variceal bleeding. *In* Therapeutic Endoscopy in Gastrointestinal Surgery. Edited by R. S. Chung. New York, Churchill Livingstone, 1987, p. 61.
16. Westaby, D., et al.: Controlled clinical trial of injection sclerotherapy for active variceal bleeding. Hepatology, *9:*274, 1989.
17. Freeman, J. G., et al.: Controlled trial of terlipressin (glypressin) versus vasopressin in the early treatment of esophageal varices. Lancet, *2:*66, 1982.
18. Stiegmann, G. V., Cambre, A., and Sun, J. H.: A new endoscopic elastic band ligating device. Gastrointest. Endosc., *32:*230, 1986.

19. Steigmann, G. V., et al.: Endoscopic elastic band ligation for active variceal hemorrhage. Am. Surg., *55:*124, 1989.
20. Burroughs, A. K., et al.: A comparison of sclerotherapy with staple transection of the esophagus for the emergency control of bleeding from esophageal varices. N. Engl. J. Med., *321:*857, 1989.
21. Waitman, A. M., Grant, D. Z., and Chateau, F.: Endoscopic management of vascular lesions. *In* Therapeutic Gastrointestinal Endoscopy. Edited by S. E. Silvis. New York, Igaku-Shoin, 1984, p. 126.
22. Herrington, J. L., and Davidson, J.: Bleeding gastroduodenal ulcers: choice of operations. World J. Surg., *11:*304, 1987.
23. Alexander-Williams, J.: Surgical management of acute intestinal bleeding. *In* Gastrointestinal Hemorrhage. Edited by P. W. Dykes and M. R. B. Keighley. Bristol, Wrights, PSG, 1981, p. 357.
24. Drapanas, T., et al.: Emergency subtotal colectomy: preferred management of massive diverticula disease. Ann. Surg., *177:*519, 1973.
25. Chung, R. S., Lewis, J. W., and Camera, D.: A technique of sclerotherapy. Surg. Gastroenterol., *2:*303, 1983.
26. Himal, H. S., Perralt, C., and Mzabi, R.: Upper gastrointestinal hemorrhage: aggressive management decreases mortality. Surgery, *84:*448, 1978.
27. Morris, D. L., et al.: Optimal timing of operation for bleeding peptic ulcer: prospective randomized trial. Br. Med. J., *288:*1277, 1984.
28. Hunt, P. S., et al.: Bleeding duodenal ulcer: reduction of mortality with a planned approach. Br. J. Surg., *66:*633, 1979.
29. Hunt, P. S.: Bleeding gastroduodenal ulcers: selection of patients for surgery. World J. Surg., *11:*289, 1987.

Chapter 51

SEVERE INTRA-ABDOMINAL INFECTION

GAIL S. LEBOVIC
LORI J. MORGAN
KATHERINE HODGE
ADAM SEIVER

Sepsis is defined as the "systemic inflammatory response to infection."[1] In the United States, there are an estimated 70,000 to 500,000 cases of sepsis each year.[2,3] Considering all sources, the most reasonable estimate is approximately 300,000 cases per year. Mortality rates for the septic patient vary from 25 to 70% depending on the patient population and their risk factors (e.g., age, underlying disease, source and type of infection).[4]

Severe intra-abdominal infection is a common cause of sepsis syndrome (multiple organ failure) necessitating intensive medical therapy in an appropriate tertiary facility. Most studies indicate that mortality from intra-abdominal sepsis is greater than 60%. In fact, within the setting of the surgical ICU, intra-abdominal infection followed by sepsis is the most common cause of death.[5] Management of these patients requires early diagnosis and treatment of the underlying problem, appropriate administration of antibiotics, and provision of adequate nutrients to support the hypermetabolic state associated with sepsis. Unfortunately, despite adequate medical intervention, a persistent inflammatory response frequently develops, which may lead to multiple organ dysfunction, organ failure, and ultimately death.

Despite advances in critical care technology, organized intensive care treatment protocols, and a new armamentarium of powerful antibiotics, the death rate from sepsis has not significantly improved over the past decade. A more thorough understanding of the pathophysiology of sepsis and the humoral response to the inflammatory reaction will, it is hoped, result in innovative therapies that can be used to improve survival in the face of this challenging problem.

The following discussion begins with a number of case histories presented to introduce the pre-ICU phase and criteria for determining ICU admission. The pathophysiology of the systemic inflammatory response syndrome resulting from severe intra-abdominal infection is then described in detail, and useful guidelines for the clinical management of these patients are outlined. Definitive surgical intervention, optimal support of oxygen transport, and investigational therapies now on the horizon are also briefly discussed. Finally, the post-ICU rehabilitation of these patients is discussed.

PRE-ICU PHASE

A wide variety of diseases and injuries may lead to severe intra-abdominal infection. This is reflected in the multiplicity of ways in which patients with severe intra-abdominal infections present to the clinician. In most cases, patients with an intra-abdominal infection present with symptoms consistent with an "acute abdomen." The "acute abdomen" implies a need for surgical intervention and clinically is characterized by signs of peritoneal irritation (tenderness, guarding, rebound, and referred pain). In addition, gastrointestinal dysfunction (distention, nausea, vomiting, diarrhea, lack of flatus), fever, or leukocytosis may accompany the aforementioned physical findings. Establishing an accurate diagnosis depends on prompt patient evaluation, a detailed history, and a thorough physical examination (Table 51-1). These either lead to the diagnosis or direct further diagnostic workup of the problem. The following scenarios characterize possible presentations of critically ill patients presenting with an "acute abdomen" and intra-abdominal sepsis.

Case I

A. S., a senior citizen with a history of Alzheimer's disease, was "found down" by his visiting family on the bathroom floor. When discovered, he was minimally arousable and was surrounded by emesis and urine. His past medical history was significant for two previous myocardial infarctions, peptic ulcer disease, and diverticular disease. A record of current medications was unavailable. He had no history of any previous operations.

He was transported to the emergency room by ambulance, where initial evaluation revealed an elderly man who was arousable but unresponsive to commands. His skin was cool and clammy with poor turgor. Pertinent physical findings included a systolic blood pressure of 90 mm Hg, a heart rate of 120 beats/minute, and a respiratory rate of 30 breaths/minute. Examination revealed normal heart sounds, bilateral breath sounds, a tense and silent abdomen, and trace heme-positive stool on rectal examination.

Initial resuscitation included the placement of two large-bore intravenous lines and administration of 2 L of lactated Ringer's solution. An endotracheal tube was placed and

Table 51–1. History and Examination for the Acute Abdomen

Medical/Surgical History
  Any major medical problems?/previous hospitalizations?
  Any previous surgeries?/postoperative problems?
  Medications?
  History of bowel disease?
  Blood dyscrasia?
  Sexual history?
  Gynecologic/birth control history (women)?
  When did you last feel normal?
Pain
  When and how did it start?.
  Does it radiate?/Is it constant?
  Location at start and now?
  Is it better or worse now?
  Quality of the pain?
  Have you ever had this pain before?
Gastrointestinal/Renal Function
  When/what did you last eat?
  Did anyone else eat the same thing? Are they sick too?
  Any nausea/vomiting/diarrhea/constipation?
  What are your usual bowel habits?
  Are you still passing flatus/stool?
  When did you last have a bowel movement?
  Are you hungry now?
  Can you tolerate solids/liquids?
  Any dysuria/hematuria/pneumaturia?
  When is the last time you urinated?
  Any history of kidney stones, urinary tract infections, urologic problems?
Abdominal Examination
  Is your abdomen distended/Is this what it always looks like?
  Are there bowel sounds/What type?
  Where is the pain?
  Where is it tender to palpation?
  Is there referred pain?
  Is there percussion tenderness/guarding/rebound?
  Are there any masses?
Rectal Examination
  Is there tenderness?
  Any masses?
  Is there stool in the rectum/What is the stool guaiac?
Gynecologic Examination (women)
  Is there any vaginal discharge?/cervical motion tenderness?
  Are there any masses?
  Can you palpate the pelvic organs?/are they tender?

mechanical ventilation instituted. In addition to ongoing fluid resuscitation, monitoring devices, including a urinary bladder catheter and oxygen saturation monitor, were placed.

Significant laboratory values included a white blood cell count of 18,000, a hematocrit of 48, serum amylase of 35, and a total bilirubin of 1.4. Arterial blood gas indicated hypercarbia, a combined severe metabolic and respiratory acidosis, and moderate hypoxemia. Electrocardiogram showed evidence of old myocardial infarcts, but no acute changes were seen. A portable chest radiograph was significant only for a mildly enlarged cardiac silhouette. Radiographs of the abdomen revealed a small amount of bowel gas in the right lower quadrant and a lack of air and stool in the left colon and rectum. Several air-fluid levels were present throughout the small bowel, and a rim of free air was noted along the abdominal wall on the cross-table lateral film.

Consultation with the general surgeons yielded a clinical impression consistent with septic shock secondary to a perforated viscus, and exploratory celiotomy was recommended. The patient, however, remained hypotensive and acidotic after his initial resuscitation. Therefore he was transferred to the ICU for stabilization before operation.

At exploration, an obstructing tumor mass was found in the transverse colon at the hepatic flexure. Dilatation of the bowel proximal to the obstruction had caused the cecum to perforate with a moderate amount of peritoneal soiling. A right hemicolectomy with end ileostomy was performed, and the patient was admitted to the ICU for postoperative management.

Case II

Mrs. I. H. had recently completed a course of chemotherapy for lymphoma and had been neutropenic, requiring protective isolation. Her medical team became concerned when her appetite did not return several days after her chemotherapy. She began having persistent low grade fevers and complained of mild abdominal pain with melanotic stools. Clinical examination revealed a soft, mildly distended, diffusely tender abdomen with hypoactive bowel sounds. Examination did not reveal rebound tenderness. Blood cultures were pending.

Radiographs of the abdomen revealed several dilated loops of small bowel with air-fluid levels and a minimal amount of air in the colon and rectum. A computed tomography (CT) scan did not yield other findings. Surgical consultants recommended an abdominal exploration. At laparotomy, the distal ileum was noted to be necrotic, but without gross perforation. A small bowel resection was performed, and the patient was transferred to the ICU.

Case III

Mr. A. T. was admitted to the emergency department following a motor vehicle accident. The rate of speed of the car on impact was unknown. It was unclear from the patient if there had been a loss of consciousness. The patient was found with a lap belt but no shoulder harness on. The patient was transported to the emergency department by ambulance, and on initial evaluation he was noted to be intoxicated and combative. Vital signs were stable.

A complete survey was performed. The patient complained of chest wall tenderness and right leg pain but denied neck, abdominal, or other extremity pain. Significant injuries included facial lacerations, several rib fractures, unilateral pneumothorax, and an open femur fracture. There was a small abrasion noted on the lower abdomen attributed to the patient's seat belt, but the patient denied abdominal tenderness and had no other significant abdominal findings. Genital, rectal, and prostatic examinations were all normal. CT scans of the abdomen and pelvis with oral and intravenous contrast material were normal. After placement of a chest tube, the patient was taken to the operating room for debridement, open reduction, and internal fixation of the femur fracture.

Postoperatively the patient was maintained on antibiotics, chest tube suction, and pulmonary toilet and was kept at bed rest. He noted vague abdominal pain and was kept at bowel rest for several days. Serial abdominal examinations were performed. On the fourth postoperative day, he developed a low grade fever. Workup included blood cultures, urinalysis, chest x-ray film, wound checks, changing of all intravenous lines, and inspection of the chest tube and surgical sites. There was a slightly increased white blood cell count, but other studies were noncontributory. The following day, the patient developed a fever to 102°F and complained of increased abdominal pain. Surgical consultation was obtained, and the patient was found to have guarding and rebound tenderness. Abdominal radiographs showed a mild ileus but no free air. The patient was taken to the operating room for abdominal exploration.

At laparotomy, diffuse peritonitis with a significant amount of bowel contents was noted. Careful examination revealed a small bowel perforation, which was repaired, and the abdominal cavity was irrigated. The fascia was closed, but the subcutaneous tissue and skin were left open so as to heal by secondary intention. Wet-to-dry dressing changes were used to promote granulation tissue and debride the wound.

The patient's postoperative course was marked by persistent fever, ileus, and abdominal pain. He was maintained throughout this period on parenteral nutrition and antibiotics. One week after surgery, the patient remained unable to tolerate even small amounts of a liquid diet. One morning, the patient sat up in bed and on straining, his abdominal incision dehisced, and a loop of small bowel was extruded. In addition, drainage of a significant amount of seropurulent, foul-smelling fluid was noted.

Immediate reexploration in the operating room revealed an abscess in the right subdiaphragmatic space. Anaerobic and aerobic cultures were taken, the abscess was drained, and copious abdominal lavage was performed. Once again, the midline fascia was closed, leaving the subcutaneous tissue layers packed open.

In anticipation of respiratory deterioration secondary to the systemic inflammatory response, he was transferred to the ICU intubated and maintained on full ventilatory support.

Indications for ICU Admission

The previous case presentations illustrate clinical scenarios that should prompt ICU admission. Candidates for ICU care are not always easy to identify, and often clinical "intuition" anticipating impending organ dysfunction motivates the physician to admit the patient to the ICU. This section details guidelines that can be helpful to the clinician debating the need for a patient's admission to the ICU.

Patients with severe intra-abdominal infection typically have a problem that requires definitive surgical management at some point during their hospitalization. Frequently these patients need at least brief postoperative ventilatory support. In some cases, the patient(s) requires intensive care management before operation. This situation applies to the patient who presents in the emergency department with a surgical abdomen that has progressed to shock with associated hemodynamic instability. These patients require rapid resuscitation before an expeditious operation. If this is not accomplished, the patient may suffer severe hypotension on induction of anesthesia. In many cases, the resuscitation can be accomplished in the emergency department or in the operating room. Some patients, however, particularly the elderly with underlying respiratory or cardiac disease, require invasive hemodynamic monitoring and life-support equipment, which in most institutions is best instituted in the ICU.

If significant peritoneal soiling is found at operation or if signs of sepsis were apparent preoperatively, admission to the ICU postoperatively should be strongly considered. Such patients require life-support measures guided by invasive monitoring to optimize oxygen transport. In cases in which the patient is managed with an "open abdomen" technique (see Fig. 51–5), the patient requires ICU management to allow anesthesia and mechanical ventilation and to provide the extensive nursing care required for management of these complicated abdominal wounds.

Many other special clinical situations arise that should prompt ICU admission. It is essential to evaluate patients critically on presentation and determine the underlying risk for increased morbidity. Certainly patients with evidence of single or multiple organ dysfunction/failure are considered as "high risk" and should be monitored in the ICU. This includes patients with respiratory, cardiac, gastrointestinal, renal, or metabolic compromise.

Immunocompromised patients present an entire "class" of patients that deserve ICU admission for close observation because these patients lack the ability to mount an adequate response to acute inflammatory processes, and the early clinical signs of sepsis and shock may be virtually absent. Similarly, alcoholic and chronically ill patients are somewhat immunocompromised and may present with signs of infection from an unknown source that can prove to be devastating (i.e., spontaneous bacterial peritonitis).

Mentally obtunded, debilitated, and elderly patients represent another subgroup of patients deserving of ICU admission in the face of severe illness. The clinician must be hypervigilant in these cases and admit even those patients who may appear hemodynamically stable to the ICU if clinical suspicion of underlying sepsis is high. These patients may not manifest a febrile response to a septic insult but rather may present with hypothermia, tachypnea, tachycardia, hypotension, or an unexplained confusional state.

Patients with known or presumed peritonitis with early or ongoing sepsis syndrome should be managed in an ICU setting with hemodynamic monitoring, maximization of oxygen delivery, and, when possible, monitoring of clinical parameters with the metabolic cart. This can help guide the clinician through prolonged seemingly static periods in the patient's recovery and can help maximize the patient's nutritional status as well.

Patients with peritonitis provide a model for studying the pathophysiology and management of sepsis. These patients have widely varying presentations, and many develop a systemic inflammatory response syndrome (SIRS).[1] Of this group, a subset of patients goes on to develop multiple system organ failure, and this group of patients historically has had little chance of survival.

Multiple system organ failure, almost universally fatal, is

to be avoided if at all possible. As clinicians, we must have a thorough understanding of the pathophysiology and cellular mechanisms that create such an overwhelming and catastrophic event. Many questions remain unanswered; however, aggressive resuscitation and treatment of patients with early sepsis in an ICU setting may help salvage patients before the irreversible damage created by the inflammatory response.

The following sections of this chapter are intended to enrich the clinician's understanding of the pathophysiology of sepsis syndrome and multiple organ system failure using severe intra-abdominal infection (peritonitis) as an example of an inciting inflammatory process.

Pathophysiology of Sepsis

The pathophysiology of infection and sepsis can serve as a guide for the management of severe intra-abdominal infection. Correction of the physiologic derangements in these patients should lead to eventual recovery; thus it is essential that the cascade of events following infection is understood, recognized, and treated appropriately.

Invasion of the normally sterile peritoneal cavity by microbial organisms results in severe intra-abdominal infection. These microbes can gain access to the peritoneal cavity without a clearly defined antecedent pathologic process involving an intra-abdominal organ. The resulting inflammation of the peritoneal lining is termed primary peritonitis. Examples of primary peritonitis include spontaneous bacterial peritonitis, hematogenous spread of bacteria, translocation of intraluminal bacteria, and contamination via foreign bodies. More commonly, peritonitis is secondary to underlying intra-abdominal pathology. The primary process may be inflammatory, mechanical, vascular, traumatic, or iatrogenic/operative (Table 51-2).

Table 51-2. Pathology of Primary and Secondary Peritonitis

Primary peritonitis
    Spontaneous bacterial peritonitis
        Translocation of bacteria from the intestine
    Hematogenous spread of bacteria
        Peritoneal tuberculosis
    Foreign bodies
        Peritoneal dialysis catheter
Secondary Peritonitis
    Inflammatory
        Diverticulitis
        Appendicitis
        Necrotizing enterocolitis
        Inflammatory bowel disease
    Mechanical
        Obstruction
        Obstruction with perforation
        Volvulus
        Intussusception
    Vascular
        Arterial occlusion
        Venous stasis
    Traumatic
        Blunt (hollow viscous injury)
        Penetrating
    Operative
        Failed bowel anastomosis
        Unrecognized enterotomy
        Intraoperative spillage

Table 51-3. Criteria for Systemic Inflammatory Response Syndrome[1]

Two or more of the following:
    Temperature > 38°C or 36°C
    Heart rate > 90 beats/min
    Respiratory rate > 20 breaths/min
    or
    $Paco_2$ < 32 torr
    WBC > 12,000 cells/mm^3
    or
    WBC > 10% bands

The systemic inflammatory reaction initiated by an intra-abdominal infection presents a difficult clinical challenge. This systemic response is typically manifest by two or more of the following signs: fever, tachycardia, tachypnea, or leukocytosis (Table 51-3). This has been termed the **systemic inflammatory response syndrome (SIRS)** and is diagramatically illustrated in Figure 51-1.[1] When this syndrome is associated with infection, the condition is termed **sepsis**. Sepsis generally involves the presence of organisms in the bloodstream—**bacteremia**; however, this is not a prerequisite for the diagnosis.

SIRS begins with an initial "insult" or event leading to intra-abdominal infection, which sets the inflammatory process in motion. If the infection remains localized to a small area within the abdominal cavity, few inflammatory mediators are released into the systemic circulation, thereby limiting the systemic response. In this fashion, prompt drainage of abscesses and correction of the underlying intra-abdominal problem can help to avert the systemic inflammatory response.

In contrast, if the process cannot be contained or is not treated in a timely fashion, inflammatory mediators are dispersed and begin to circulate systemically, thereby activating numerous humoral factors. These mediators ac-

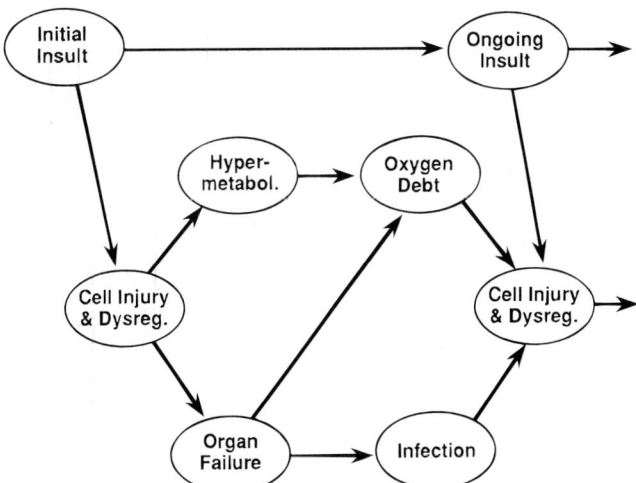

Fig. 51-1. Pathophysiology of the systemic inflammatory response syndrome. In the systemic inflammatory response syndrome, there is loss of homeostasis with the development of self-perpetuating cellular injury and dysregulation.

tivate various "cascades," which ultimately can lead to organ dysfunction. Many of these cascades have been described, and they are known to affect and interact with one another.

It is important to note that SIRS may be seen following a significant degree of tissue injury (i.e., in trauma, pancreatitis, and large burns), and therefore the severe clinical course associated with this entity is not exclusively linked to underlying infection.

The onset of sepsis, with its associated morbidity and mortality, certainly complicates the management of patients with severe intra-abdominal infection. As described previously, sepsis can progress and lead to single or multiple organ dysfunction. The mechanism underlying this frequently lethal progression is complex, with many important interconnecting "feedback loops," some of which are self-perpetuating. If it were possible to control or modify these events, organ dysfunction or failure might be averted, and the high mortality rates associated with sepsis might decrease.

The cellular pathophysiology occurring during sepsis is quite complex but offers some insight into the end product—organ failure. Endotoxin, a well-studied protein derived from gram-negative bacteria, is known to activate the humoral factors responsible for the "septic response." Endotoxin, when present in the bloodstream, even in small amounts, directly activates the complement and coagulation mechanisms within the body. This, in turn, activates neutrophils, which release oxygen radicals and proteases. Platelet activation leads to platelet aggregation. Macrophage-derived cytokines trigger arachidonic acid metabolism, producing prostaglandins and leukotrienes. T cells are activated, leading to the production of tumor necrosis factor, interleukins, gamma interferon, and granulocyte and macrophage colony stimulating factors. The collection of circulating activated factors, including oxygen radicals, proteases, aggregated platelets, prostaglandins, leukotrienes, and cytokines, causes endothelial damage and microvascular thrombosis. Ultimately this damage and thrombosis leads to tissue injury and destruction, which manifests as organ dysfunction or organ system failure (Fig. 51-2).

Each vital organ system of the body has its own finite ability to sustain function in the face of, or recuperate from, significant microvascular injury. The delicate pulmonary tissues are the most sensitive to these critical changes, and intrapulmonary damage is the first to manifest with the onset of sepsis.[6,7]

Early lung injury is characterized by tachypnea and hypoxemia followed by x-ray changes, which tend to "lag" behind the clinical impact of intrapulmonary endothelial cell injury. Destruction of alveolar type I pneumocytes, the onset of an acute inflammatory response, and microcirculatory coagulopathy directly damage the pulmonary endothelium. This causes an increased permeability of the lung tissue, resulting in exudation of fluid into the pulmonary interstitium. The lymphatic drainage of the interstitium is rapidly overwhelmed, causing fluid to shift into the alveoli. In addition to being filled with fluid, the interstitium becomes infiltrated with inflammatory cells. The combined effect leads to a decrease in pulmonary compliance, ventilation-perfusion abnormalities, and impaired gas exchange. Clinically this is noted as hypoxemia and, when severe, manifests as hypercarbia as well. Radiographically this is seen as an increase in the interstitial pulmonary markings progressing to diffuse patchy infiltrates. When these symptoms are "mild," the injury is referred to as **acute lung injury.** When severe, this constellation of findings is termed **adult respiratory distress syndrome (ARDS).**

As mentioned previously, each of the body's vital organ systems may become dysfunctional during the septic state. Monitoring patients in the ICU setting allows for close observation and immediate management of these problems, which are most often life-threatening. The clinical signs associated with each organ system are listed in Table 51-4.

In addition to organ dysfunction and failure, SIRS is associated with a marked increase in metabolic demand. The body's response to overwhelming infection can be considered as a "hypermetabolic" state. This hypermetabolism may be prolonged and can persist for weeks in the critically ill patient. During this time, there is a marked increase in energy expenditure, oxygen consumption and carbon dioxide production.[8-10]

The energy source, in the form of adenosine triphosphatase (ATP), is not derived from glucose alone but instead from carbohydrate, fat, and amino acid. To provide adequate resuscitation of cellular function, energy expenditure may be more than doubled. The hypermetabolic state involves both anabolic and catabolic processes; however, the catabolic rate predominates, with resultant overall diminution of lean body mass. This process has been termed "autocatabolism."

Anabolic and catabolic processes of gluconeogenesis, glycogenolysis, and glycolysis are responsible for carbohydrate energy sources—glucose, glycerol, and lactate—which are used mainly by cardiac muscle. Most of these processes occur in the liver; however, skeletal muscle has large stores of protein, which can provide an additional source of substrates, such as alanine, glutamine, glycine, and serine. There are many metabolic mediators during the septic response, including glucagon and insulin. Although insulin increases the peripheral uptake of glucose, it does not seem to have an effect on its oxidative use in sepsis.

During the hypermetabolic phase of sepsis, fat oxidation provides another source of energy using short, medium, and long chain fatty acids as substrates. For example, linoleic and arachidonic acid are commonly metabolized and produce oleic and arachidonic acid metabolites as well as hepatic ketones as byproducts. Lipolysis occurs at a low level initially, but with increasing beta-adrenergic stimulation, the rate of lipolysis greatly increases, and the liver becomes the major site for fat oxidation.

Amino acids contribute the largest fraction of substrate for energy extraction during the hypermetabolic phase of sepsis. Protein metabolism is significantly altered under these extreme circumstances, and autocatabolism accounts for the greatest source of amino acid production. Hepatic protein synthesis is insignificant compared with the rate of autocatabolism. Major sites of catabolic activity include skeletal muscle, connective tissue, and unstimu-

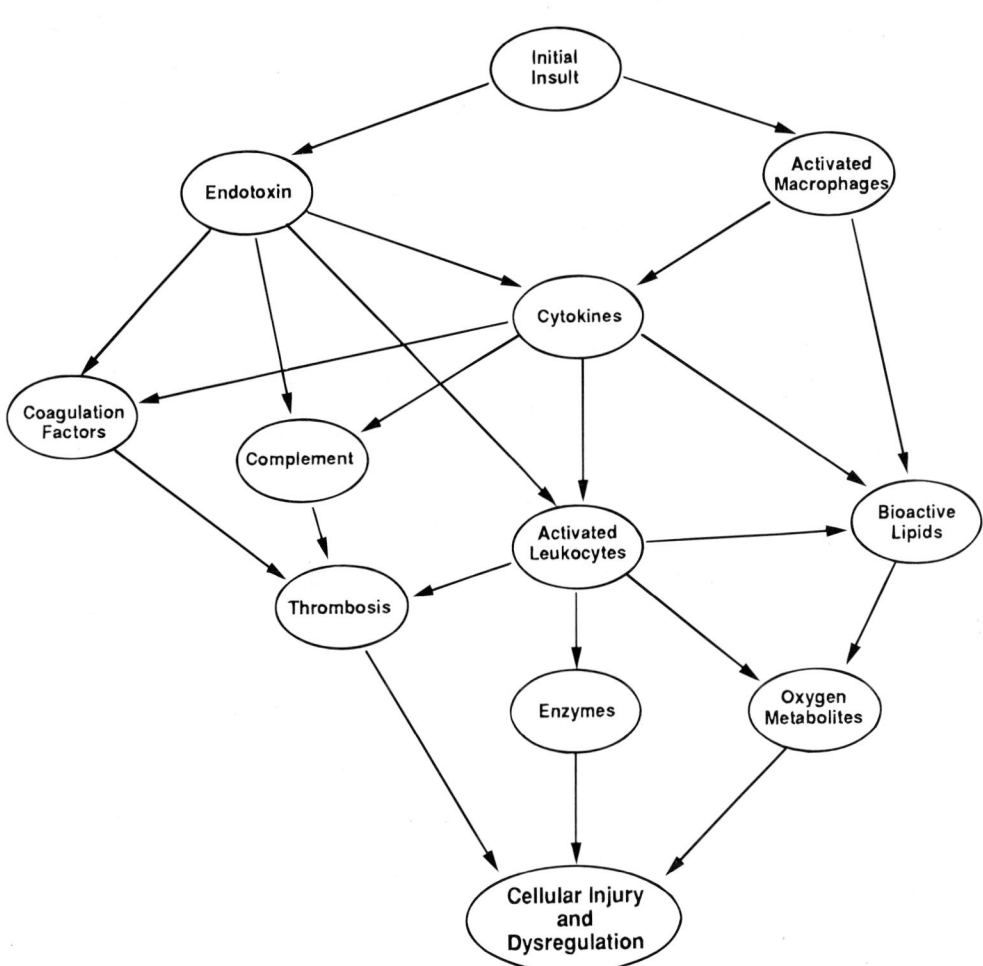

Fig. 51–2. Mediators of the systemic inflammatory response syndrome. Activation of inflammatory mediators leads to cellular injury and dysregulation. This diagram highlights only a few of the key pathways and components of an extremely complex mechanism. For example, the activated leukocytes include platelets, neutrophils, and endothelial cells. Missing are the many feedback loops that result in amplification and self-perpetuation.

lated intestinal protein stores. Branched-chain amino acids, such as leucine, isoleucine, and valine, serve as the primary substrates.

The altered protein metabolism, characteristic of the hypermetabolic phase of sepsis, appears to be controlled by circulating factors secreted by activated macrophages. These include: interleukin, prostaglandin E$_2$, tumor necrosis factor, peptides, cortisol, and endotoxin. Decreased amino acid uptake and catabolism of protein stores are apparent in skeletal muscle. Meanwhile, (within the liver) production of proteins, such as albumin and transferrin, is decreased, and production of acute phase reactant proteins and antiproteases is increased. Presumably this is done in an attempt to regulate the inflammatory response.

The increased turnover of various amino acids leads to increased ureagenesis. The nitrogen produced is used to form alanine and glutamine. These products, in turn, are transferred from muscle, viscera, and other peripheral tissues to vital tissues, such as the heart, liver, and inflammatory cells. Autocatabolism refers to the net body catabolism occurring during the hypermetabolic phase of sepsis and corresponds to a markedly depleted lean body mass after 7 to 10 days, with a high urinary nitrogen excretion (up to 20 g/day).[11,12]

The demands of hypermetabolism combined with organ failure lead to an inability to supply the body's vital tissues with adequate nutrients. On a cellular level, oxygen is the most critical nutrient. Tissue oxygen consumption is limited by oxygen transport. Oxygen debt develops when the increased oxygen demand is not met by an increased oxygen consumption.[13,14] Oxygen consumption is a function of the amount of oxygen delivered and extracted. Endothelial injury, microvascular thrombosis, and other microvascular changes seen with the inflammatory response are associated with impaired vasoregulation and an inability to match perfusion to metabolic needs. This results in supply-dependent oxygen consumption unless the critical higher level of oxygen delivery can be attained (Fig. 51–3). The patient's oxygen extraction curve thus demonstrates a diminished slope in the face of an increased plateau of need.

To compensate for the impaired extraction, markedly increased oxygen delivery is necessary. Delivery is a function of arterial oxygen content and cardiac output. The arterial oxygen content may be diminished by anemia and by the hypoxemia of respiratory dysfunction. Cardiac output may be diminished by hypovolemia or by cardiac dysfunction. Thus multiple organ dysfunction contributes to the inability to provide the necessary increase in oxygen delivery.

In the face of an increasing oxygen debt, a recurring

Table 51–4. Clinical Signs of Organ System Dysfunction

Systemic
  Hyperthermia or hypothermia
  Mental status changes
  Leukocytosis or severe leukopenia
  Thrombocytopenia
  Lactic acidosis
  Coagulopathy
Cardiac
  Hypotension
  Biventricular failure
  Bradycardia in the face of hypotension
  Ventricular arrhythmias
Pulmonary
  Hypoxia
  Hypercarbia
  Ventilation-perfusion mismatch
  Elevated wedge pressure
Gastrointestinal
  Gastric, small or large bowel "ileus"
  Hyperbilirubinemia
  Elevated transaminase levels
Renal
  Oliguria
  Azotemia
  Decreased creatinine clearance
Endocrine
  Hyperglycemia
  Insulin resistance

temic effects. For these reasons, management of the septic patient must be directed in a multileveled fashion if the patient is to survive.

Unfortunately, the original locus is not always the only ongoing source of infection. Organ failure can lead to secondary sites of infection distant and distinct from the initiating source. For example, gastrointestinal failure secondary to hypoperfusion and inadequate nutrition is associated with an ileus that enables bacterial overgrowth in the normally sterile stomach and small bowel.[15] These bacteria—particularly the virulent organisms selected by antibiotics—may migrate up the intestinal lumen or through the intestinal wall (bacterial translocation). Migration into the upper gastrointestinal tract can colonize the pharynx and then the trachea leading to nosocomial pneumonias. Translocation may lead to seeding of the peritoneal cavity and the portal circulation. The hepatic macrophages (Kupffer's cells) may not be able to clear the portal circulation, and systemic bacteremia may occur. Under these conditions, the risk of translocation is high given the large reservoir of infected material within the intestinal lumen. Wet fecal material is half bacteria by weight, and each gram of bacteria contains a milligram of endotoxin. The LD50 known to cause sepsis and activation of the humoral cascades in clinical models is 3 to 10 mg/kg of endotoxin.[16-18]

The inflammatory response is then sustained or even heightened by secondary infection, creating an even greater oxygen debt. If the initial intra-abdominal infection is not completely controlled, there may be an additional ongoing insult providing stimulus for the perpetuation of the inflammatory response. Thus, the inflammatory re-

cycle of ischemic damage, increased oxygen demand, failure to fulfill the demand, and continuing damage occurs. Although this entire cascade may begin in response to an infected locus, it can swiftly develop into far-reaching sys-

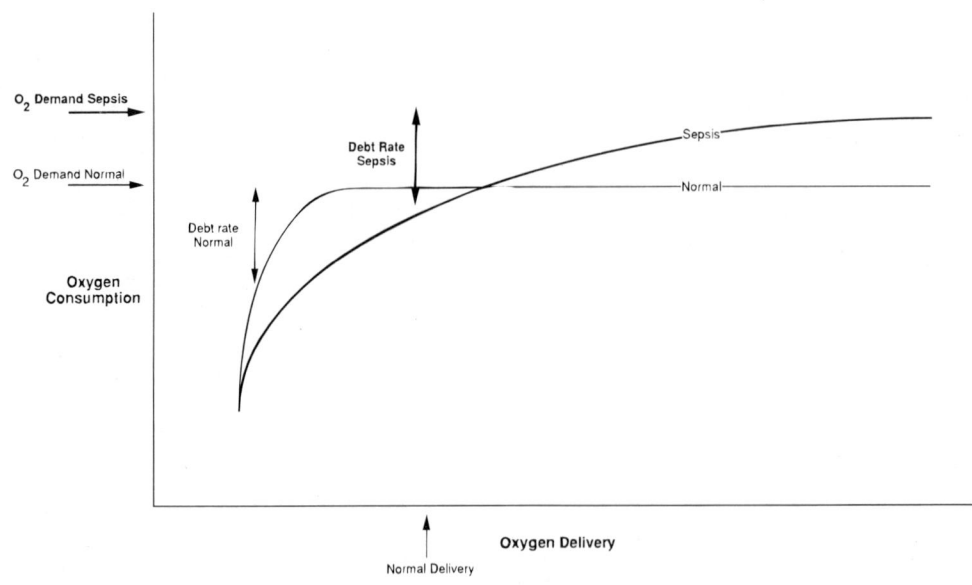

Fig. 51–3. Graphs of the relationship between oxygen delivery and oxygen demand in septic and normal patients. Septic patients have a capability to extract oxygen that is lower than that of normal patients. The oxygen demand, however, is higher for septic patients. The rate at which oxygen debt develops is the difference between the oxygen consumption and the oxygen demand. Note that septic patients may accumulate oxygen debt even at a normal delivery because the rate of extraction is lower and the demand is higher. The normal patient would exhibit an equivalent debt rate only at a much lower than normal oxygen delivery. This provides a rationale for supranormal values for oxygen delivery as a therapeutic goal in sepsis.

sponse can become increasingly severe with magnified deleterious effects. The phrase "inflammatory anarchy" has been used to describe these events.

Severe intra-abdominal infections incite an uncontrolled, destructive, self-perpetuating inflammatory response that manifests in the high morbidity and mortality rates associated with this process. Initial humoral activation leads to endothelial injury, hypermetabolism, and tissue nutrient deprivation, each of which contributes to organ dysfunction, secondary infection, and a continued humoral activation with a recurring cycle of insult and injury. Ultimately, this cycle of ongoing tissue injury, organ dysfunction, and organ failure leads to the patient's demise.

The following sections outline various avenues for clinical intervention in the management of sepsis and severe intra-abdominal infection. Special attention is given to clinical parameters, and dosages for specific pharmaceutical agents are noted when applicable.

ICU MANAGEMENT OF SEVERE INTRA-ABDOMINAL INFECTION

The goal of managing patients with severe intra-abdominal infection during the ICU phase is complex and focuses on several key areas: (1) prevention and early operative intervention, (2) interruption of the cycle of destructive inflammation (as described in the previous section on pathophysiology), and (3) supportive care in the face of multiple organ dysfunction. Figure 51-4 presents an overview of therapeutic options and integrates them into the inflammatory cycle initially presented in Figure 51-1. Patients who are at risk for or who have developed SIRS must be treated with multiple modalities, each designed to break a link in the cycle.

Crucial elements in the management of these patients include hemodynamic monitoring and support, nutritional support, maximization of oxygen transport and delivery, and careful control of additional or ongoing infection.

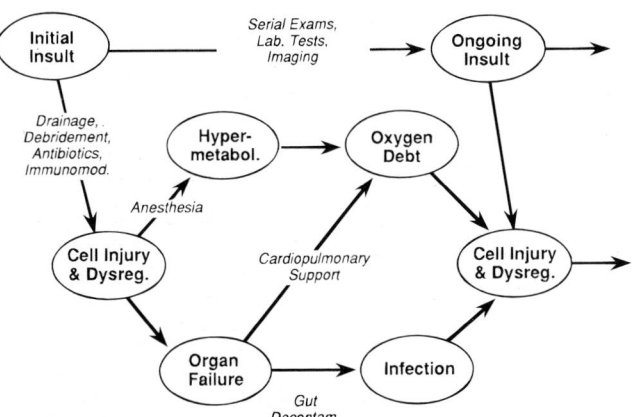

Fig. 51-4. The management of the systemic inflammatory response syndrome comprises multiple therapies directed at breaking the cycle of self-perpetuating cellular injury and dysregulation.

Prevention

The preferred management of intra-abdominal infection is prevention. An all too common initial insult is an inflamed viscus that has progressed to necrosis or perforation. A failed anastomosis may also be the source of intra-abdominal contamination that progresses to severe infection. Thus, sound clinical (surgical) judgment and technique are important in avoiding many cases of intra-abdominal infections. A patient presenting with acute abdominal pain and tenderness should be considered to have a surgical problem until proved otherwise. Such a patient should receive an expeditious workup ending in exploratory surgery if a surgical condition cannot be excluded.

With respect to surgical technique, a good blood supply should be ensured for healing of an anastomosis. If viability is questionable at the time of operation, the anastomosis shoud be revised or a proximal diversion performed. Careful closure of the fascia and sterile technique are essential for prevention of wound infections and dehiscence. Postoperatively increasing abdominal pain, tachycardia, tachypnea, oliguria, or leukocytosis should prompt evaluation for possible intra-abdominal infection.

Source Control

CT scanning can be extremely useful in the diagnosis and treatment of intra-abdominal infection.[19,20] Abdominal imaging can detect and localize septic foci and provide an avenue for intervention as well. CT guidance allows for expeditious percutaneous drainage of abscesses, promoting rapid intervention in critically ill patients who may experience significant hemodynamic instability with operative drainage. Timely abscess drainage can significantly improve survival. Immediate drainage is associated with mortality rates of only 5 to 15%, whereas delayed drainage is associated with mortality rates between 55 and 60%.[21,22] A comparison of surgical and percutaneous drainage techniques showed the two interventions as being equal in regards to success rate, length of hospital stay, and mortality.[22] Successful surgical drainage was accomplished in 78% of patients, with average hospital stay being 33 days and a mortality rate of 22% Successful percutaneous drainage was achieved in 72% of patients, with average hospital stay being 36 days and a mortality rate of 21%.[23-25] Not all studies have been as successful with percutaneous catheter drainage, but it is clear that it is a valuable technique for the management of some intra-abdominal abscesses.[26] Unsuccessful drainage requiring further intervention is determined by poor initial patient response and radiographic evidence (abdominal CT scan) of persistent intra-abdominal abscess. Regardless of drainage technique, all patients must have careful follow-up studies to assess for a continuing source of infection.

Optimal management of intra-abdominal abscesses requires careful consideration of several factors. Percutaneous drainage can be performed when a safe, direct drainage route is available. Single, multiple, or complex abscesses can be drained using this method. In contrast, surgical drainage is preferred for abscesses with complex drainage routes that may require traversing uninvolved intra-abdominal structures or large loculated abscesses with necrotic debris that will not drain through catheters. On occasion, the infection is so severe and necrotic that only by leaving the abdomen open with one of several "open abdomen" techniques can adequate drainage be obtained (see Appendix). This is notably the case with severe pancreatic abscesses.

Cardiopulmonary Support and Oxygen Transport

Frequently the physician needs to manage a patient after organ dysfunction or failure has become established. This can occur quite early in the course of shock, and patients may present initially with a significant amount of organ dysfunction. The physician should quickly establish effective means to assume pulmonary, cardiac, renal, and nutritional support. Patients in shock with signs of systemic inflammation should be intubated and ventilated early in the course of their treatment even if pulmonary dysfunction is moderate. Often times this may be the subtle predictor of impending pulmonary failure. Positive pressure ventilation with mechanical assistance decreases the "work" associated with breathing, thereby decreasing the overall metabolic demands and oxygen requirements. Hemodynamic parameters of these patients must be closely monitored using arterial lines, central venous pressure lines, and intracardiac pressure monitors (Swan-Ganz catheters).

The overall goal of cardiopulmonary support is to meet the oxygen demands of the hypermetabolic patient. This is achieved by increasing oxygen delivery until oxygen consumption plateaus. The increase in delivery is complemented by an effort to decrease demand as much as possible. Oxygen demands can be decreased with adequate pain control, sedation, and chemical paralysis of the patient. Multiple combinations of drugs are effective for this purpose. We have seen up to a 20% decrease in oxygen demand with epidural anesthesia combined with narcotics and intravenous propofol.[27] Once therapy to reduce oxygen demand in the septic patient has been initiated, a concentrated effort is made to meet the oxygen requirement. Again, in these patients, the overall metabolic demands are far higher than in the normal state or even in the nonseptic postoperative state. *Therefore, until the patient's metabolic demands are met, the patient must be considered to be inadequately resuscitated.*

The following criteria, based on Shoemaker's work,[13,28-31] can be used as a guide to determine adequacy of resuscitative efforts: cardiac index greater than 4.0 L/min/m^2, oxygen delivery greater than 600 ml per minute, and oxygen consumption greater than 160 ml per minute. The initial goals are refined by an ongoing assessment of whether there is more than a 20 ml per minute change in oxygen consumption with changes in oxygen delivery that result from volume resuscitation or changes in inotropic medications.

Efforts to improve oxygen exchange across the pulmonary capillaries are important. One key therapy for improving pulmonary gas exchange is positive end-expiratory pressure (PEEP). PEEP prevents alveolar collapse with subsequent intrapulmonary shunting and decreases ventilation-perfusion mismatch secondary to atelectasis. At high levels, however, PEEP can reduce cardiac output by decreasing venous return to the heart and increases the risk of barotrauma to the alveoli. Thus, subsequent risk of pneumothorax is increased. Moderate levels of PEEP (5 to 10 cm H$_2$O) are appropriate for most patients, although in extreme cases, such as in patients with severe ARDS, higher levels may be required for adequate oxygenation.

In addition to PEEP, pressure support ventilation can be helpful in increasing oxygenation by decreasing the work of breathing—particularly when weaning patients from mechanical ventilation. To be advantageous, patients must be able to initiate spontaneous breathing effort. Not all ventilators are capable of this relatively new mode of ventilation.

In addition to ventilatory support, aggressive cardiac support is essential. This is guided by continuous monitoring of oxygen transport variables. Here again, the goal of cardiac support is to maintain oxygen delivery to meet the patient's oxygen demand. If this demand is not met, the availability of oxygen to the end organs is diminished, and oxygen debt results.

Oxygen debt has a negative impact on organ function. Oxygen debt is ascertained by following organ dysfunction. Therefore, by monitoring urine output, serial lactates, extremity perfusion, and intramucosal gastric pH, the clinician can follow accumulating oxygen debt. The appearance of organ dysfunction, as evidenced by acidosis, oliguria, and cyanosis, suggests an overall oxygen debt. Of these parameters, only the intramucosal gastric pH can be directly measured to follow end organ function.

Intramucosal gastric pH is measured with a special nasogastric tube that has a gas-permeable balloon at its tip. The balloon is filled with saline, which rests against the gastric mucosa. As it rests, gas exchange takes place, and CO$_2$ diffuses across the membrane. After a period of calibration (30 to 60 minutes), the saline is removed and a Pco$_2$ is measured. This value is used along with the arterial HCO$_3$ to calculate a pH for the gastric mucosa. Early clinical studies have shown that an acid mucosal pH can be used as a predictor of inadequate resuscitation and oxygen debt.[32] The mucosal pH is used together with other less direct measurements of oxygen debt and cellular dysfunction to assess the patient's overall metabolic status.

In our ICU, if the patient has accumulated a significant oxygen debt or if oxygen delivery seems to be inadequate, the patient is placed on a metabolic monitor to measure oxygen consumption and the respiratory quotient continuously. The metabolic monitor is hooked in line to the patient's ventilator and provides minute-by-minute measurements of oxygen consumption, carbon dioxide production, respiratory quotient, and caloric requirements. This provides a precise method of monitoring the patient's metabolic status and allows us to evaluate the effectiveness of interventions quickly.

In addition to the metabolic monitor, a pulmonary artery catheter with mixed venous monitoring is placed. These monitors are used to guide and evaluate therapy. If there appears to be oxygen debt, the patient is initially given a volume challenge. Typically crystalloid is used, but colloid or other blood products are used as indicated by abnormal hematologic laboratory tests. The response to a fluid challenge is evaluated by studying how the pulmonary artery diastolic pressure, wedge pressure, arterial blood pressure, and urine output change. Of particular importance is whether or not oxygen consumption increases. If it does increase, this indicates that "flow-dependent oxygen consumption" is present, and the patient's oxygen consumption was not meeting his oxygen demand. In other words, oxygen debt was accumulating secondary to inadequate resuscitation. The patient is considered adequately resuscitated only when flow-dependent oxygen consumption is abolished; at that time, increased delivery is not accompanied by increased consumption. This state is shown graphically in Figure 51-3 as the plateau of the oxygen consumption curve.

If flow-dependent oxygen consumption cannot be abolished with fluid alone without jeopardizing the patient's pulmonary status, inotropes are used. Dobutamine is started at 5 to 10 μg/kg/min to improve cardiac output. This can increase myocardial oxygen demand—an important issue in patients with possible ischemic heart disease. In general, the overall benefits from increased cardiac output (e.g., better perfusion, decreased acidosis) balance the risk to the myocardium itself. Continuous ST segment monitoring can be used to titrate the dose of inotropic agents and achieve a balance between delivering adequate oxygen to the tissues while avoiding iatrogenic myocardial ischemic injury. If hypotension is severe, other ionotropic and alpha agents may be considered. It is important to recognize, however, that the peripheral vasoconstriction and acidosis caused by alpha agents may exacerbate the systemic inflammatory response.

The use of vasodilators has been considered in light of their potential to increase cardiac output and improve regional blood flow at the precapillary level. In general, this has not proved beneficial in the face of sepsis or shock because the peripheral vascular resistance is already low, and these agents exacerbate the hypotension associated with shock. In addition, the most commonly used agent, nitroprusside, tends to increase intrapulmonary shunting by affecting hypoxic vasoconstriction. Experimental data with other agents, such as prostacyclines, show improved oxygen transport and uptake in addition to decreasing pulmonary hypertension in the face of congestive heart failure.[33,34] Unfortunately, however, these data are limited, and the use of such agents in the septic patient should be considered on an individual basis.

Nutritional Support

In addition to oxygen delivery, other critical nutrients must be delivered to maintain the patient. Severe malnutrition can become a prominent problem within a few days of the onset of shock owing to the hypermetabolic state. Although nutritional support does not appear to have an impact on overall mortality, it does avert starvation. Starvation is a comorbid condition that depletes lean body mass and results in nutrient deficiencies, visceral malnutrition, and disabled immune function. Nutritional support should be structured to provide adequate amounts of substrate so body stores are not exhausted during the hypermetabolic phase of shock.

If possible, nutrients should be given via the enteral route. It is important that feedings be made into the small bowel (preferably past the ligament of Treitz) and not the stomach to avoid the hazard of aspiration. These feedings can be given in the presence of an ileus because these are principally gastric and colonic with the small bowel retaining peristalsis. Feedings can be given through a fluoroscopically placed nasoenteric tube, a percutaneous gastrostomy with a Moss tube, or an operatively placed jejunostomy feeding tube. Enteral feeds (particularly fat emulsions) not only provide a source of calories, but also assist in the maintenance of the gastrointestinal mucosal barrier and enteral immunologic function and may offer protection against gastrointestinal hemorrhage.[35,36]

In the critically ill patient, it may be necessary to provide nutritional support via the parenteral route. The last two decades have seen an explosion of advances in this area of medicine.[37,38] Optimal parenteral formulations should include decreased caloric and glucose loads with the bulk of caloric energy being provided from protein. Guidelines for parenteral nutrition should include 30 to 35 cal/kg per day of nonprotein calories and 2 g/kg per day of amino acids.[39] Fat emulsions are an excellent source of nonprotein calories and should account for 30 to 40% of the nonprotein calories per day.[39]

This regimen is designed to reduce glucose administration, prevent essential fatty acid deficiency, and avert hepatic steatosis from excess fat emulsion use. The use of branched-chain amino acids may supply those amino acids that are in increased demand. Patients with renal insufficiency require special attention because excess nitrogen may worsen already existing azotemia. Tissue catabolism can be avoided by providing adequate nutrition, and, if necessary, hemodialysis can be used to assist with nitrogen accumulation secondary to amino acid metabolism. Further adjustments in hyperalimentation composition can be accomplished by determining respiratory quotient values and basal energy expenditure rates. The metabolic monitor detailed previously is particularly useful in determining nutritional requirements.

As with any intervention, there are complications that can arise when nutrition is supplied parenterally to the patient. One of the major complications associated with parenteral hyperalimentation is catheter-related sepsis, seen in 5 to 20% of patients.[40,41] Fever and leukocytosis of unexplained origin may be the first signs of catheter sepsis, and central lines proved to be infected or highly suspected of infection should be immediately removed, cultured, and replaced at an alternate site. Peripheral blood cultures should also be obtained if line sepsis is suspected. The incidence of line infections can be decreased by using the minimum number of necessary ports on a catheter[42] and by using an attached cuff impregnated with silver nitrate.[43,44] The other major complication associated with parenteral nutrition is the development of a pneumothorax when central access is obtained. This can be minimized by using precise technique and having experienced personnel oversee or perform line placement. All of these complications must be avoided in these patients because their metabolic balance is tenuous at best, and any new setback can further fuel the inflammatory state and lead to further organ dysfunction or failure. In addition to these complications, "overfeeding" can occur and should be avoided because it may result in increased carbon dioxide production, thereby complicating respiratory weaning.[45]

To maintain metabolic balance, management of the gastrointestinal tract is critical. The various portions of the upper and lower intestine must be protected from direct and indirect injury, such as ulcer formation with hemorrhage or gastrointestinal ischemia with translocation of bacteria, necrosis, or perforation. Regimens to protect the gastric mucosa from ulcer formation use antacids or histamine (H_2) blockers to keep the gastric pH at a level of 4.0 or greater.[46,47] Omeprazole therapy can be considered for those patients with high gastric pH despite H_2 blockers. Antacids can be as effective and less expensive than H_2 blockers.

When the pH of the stomach is alkalinized, the environment facilitates the overgrowth of gastric bacteria. Aspiration of stomach contents or migration of bacteria into the pharynx can cause an aspiration pneumonia. Some physicians choose to treat high risk patients prophylactically with sucralfate, a barrier method that protects the gastric mucosa but has no effect on gastric pH and does not alter normal gastric flora. Patients treated with antacids and H_2 blockers have a greater incidence of nosocomial pneumonia than those treated with sucralfate.[48,49]

Renal Dysfunction

If renal failure becomes evident, hemodialysis may be required but is often poorly tolerated by the hypotensive patient. Alternatively, continuous arterial venous hemofiltration (CAVH)[50] or continuous venovenous hemofiltration (CVVH) can be used.[51] This allows for gradual removal of waste products and fluid with the slow adjustment of acid-base abnormalities having minimal hemodynamic impact. Mild metabolic acidosis can be corrected by ventilatory adjustments rather than dialysis. In the extreme cases, bicarbonate may be necessary; however, this can lead to other cardiac and respiratory complications.

Antibiotic Therapy

Antibiotics are used as an adjunct to the definitive surgical management of the initiating problem. Studies have shown that, on average, 3.9 microbial species can be isolated in cases of intra-abdominal abscess.[52] Of the anaerobic organisms, bacteroides species were the most common, with the B. fragilis species isolated in 36% of patients. Clostridium was found in 19% and gram-positive anaerobic cocci in 16%. E. coli infections were found in 53% of the isolates of the aerobic gram-negative category. Also, klebsiella species composed 10% of isolate growth, with 7% proteus, and 15% Pseudomonas aeruginosa. Gram-positive aerobic organisms were cultured from the isolates in 27% of cases, including Staphylococcus aureus, Staphylococcus epidermidis, Streptococcus viridans, and enterococci.

Because most cases involve multiple organisms with varying antibiotic sensitivity, it is important to provide both aerobic and anaerobic antibiotic coverage. In the ideal situation, antibiotic agents can be selected according to the results of bacterial cultures from the suspected site of infection. Without such information, various empiric antibiotic combinations are recommended depending on the suspected focus of infection.[53] For patients with intra-abdominal sepsis, an aminoglycoside is nearly always included in the drug combination, along with anaerobic coverage. Recommended drugs for anaerobic coverage are clindamycin, metronidazole, and chloramphenicol. In patients with renal insufficiency or aminoglycoside sensitivity, other antibiotics that provide aerobic coverage include aztreonam, cefoperazone, cefotaxime, cefotetan, cefoxitin, ceftizoxime, and the quinolones. For granulocytopenic patients, an antipseudomonal penicillin is added, such as ticarcillin, mezlocillin, or piperacillin.[54] If methicillin-resistant S. aureus is suspected or there is a penicillin allergy, vancomycin can be added to the previously determined two-drug regimen.

Once culture results have been obtained, antibiotic therapy should be tailored appropriately. If possible, a single drug should be used; however, in most cases, this does not provide adequate coverage. Regardless, the least toxic drug combinations should be given. Consideration should be given to cost. For example, if equally effective and toxic, the least expensive drug(s) should be used. In most patients, the presence of several gram-negative organisms requires a minimum of two-drug antibiotic coverage.

The current pharmaceutical trend is to develop "superpotent" single agents. Studies have shown these agents to be effective in the treatment of many infections.[52,55] In the septic patient with probable resistant organisms, however, multiple-drug therapy remains the standard. The immunocompromised host presents a particular challenge, and special antibiotic combinations may be required to treat unusual or resistant bacteria. Consultation with an infectious disease specialist can be particularly helpful in these difficult cases.

The choice of antibiotics depends upon whether a primary or secondary infection is being treated. Patients with severe intra-abdominal infection who develop organ failure frequently have prolonged critical care stays. The systemic inflammation and hypermetabolism often last for weeks. During this period, the patient may develop secondary infection(s)—perhaps with resistant organisms selected for by the antibiotics treating the primary intra-abdominal infection. Making the diagnosis of secondary infection is extremely difficult. It may be heralded by fever and leukocytosis. Unfortunately, these may simply be reflections of the systemic inflammatory response triggered by the primary infection, and distinguishing these two possibilities can be difficult. Cultures of wounds, urine, blood, and intravascular devices may identify a secondary source and organism. Sputum cultures from routine endotracheal tube suctioning are often not helpful because of difficulties differentiating between colonizing and invading organisms. Specimens obtained bronchoscopically using a protected brush directed at new infiltrates seen radiographically provide more reliable cultures.[56]

Selective decontamination of the gut has been suggested for the prevention of nosocomial infections, with some studies showing a significant decrease in the incidence of pulmonary infections.[57] The benefit and efficacy of this therapy, however, have not been fully proved.[57] The primary goal of decontamination is to minimize colonization of the upper respiratory tract as well as the oropharynx and stomach by decontaminating the gut. The presence of the normal gut flora as a protective resistance factor is thought to prevent or minimize the likelihood of the colonization by pathogens. The existence and proliferation of normal flora can be encouraged by using enteral feedings.[58] A second method involves the administration of protective anaerobic flora during and after the use of systemic antibiotics. Treatment of patients with lactobacillus to eradicate pathogenic bacteria has also been a successful therapy.[59]

In addition to developing secondary bacterial infections, the critically ill patient undergoing treatment with broad-spectrum antibiotics is susceptible to developing fungemia, particularly with Candida albicans. In general, the presence of fungemia, or the colonization of three sites by fungal isolates, is sufficient to warrant antifungal therapy. Multiple sites of colonization predispose the patient to fungemia. Studies indicate that those patients treated before overt fungemia have a better survival rate.[60] As would be expected, survival also depended on whether therapy was instituted before the onset of organ failure. In another study, patients with preexisting organ failure and fungemia had a survival rate of 18%, whereas those without apparent organ failure had a survival rate of 78%.[61]

Before colonization, antifungal prophylaxis can include the use of local control measures, such as ketoconizole, miconazole, or nystatin liquids and suppositories in the oral cavity, vaginal orifice, and stomach via nasogastric tube. Antifungal powders can be used in the intertriginous sites and groin. These local control treatments are best applied several times a day. Antifungal prophylaxis is important in all critically ill patients, particularly immunocompromised patients on broad-spectrum antibiotics. For the patient with widespread fungemia, amphotericin B remains the antifungal drug of choice, although other agents, such as fluconazole, are being studied. There is some evidence that prophylactic treatment of the immune-suppressed patient with fluconazole therapy can decrease the incidence of fungal infection, but randomized trials with a large number of patients have yet to be completed.[62]

Another method of treating the septic patient that will soon be available is immunomodulation. Monoclonal antibodies are being tested against each of the elements in the humoral cascade that is activated by infection.[63-65] These include monoclonal antibodies against endotoxin (HA-1A and E5), tumor necrosis factor, and interleukins. The use of these agents is controversial because they have not yet been shown to improve survival, although clinical trials are underway. Additionally, the drugs are expected to be extremely expensive. Randomized trials now being conducted should provide valuable information about the role of these agents in systemic inflammation.

Ongoing Infection

A rising bilirubin level, rising creatinine level, worsening pulmonary gas exchange, or other deterioration in organ system function should prompt a search for continued source of infection. CT can be most useful and has markedly decreased the need for exploratory laparotomy, previously used to search for such abscesses. Historically abdominal exploration has been recommended for patients who are deteriorating clinically without an obvious source of infection. The widespread use of CT has nearly eliminated the need for such explorations. Theory suggests that organ failure may be progressive secondary to the systemic inflammatory response even after the initiating infection has been controlled.

The patient surviving severe intra-abdominal infection and sepsis is often significantly weakened owing to the prolonged period of mechanical ventilation. A program of reconditioning the respiratory musculature is therefore necessary for weaning the patient from the ventilator. Before initiating the weaning process, several conditions should be met: (1) The initiating surgical problem and any complicating factors should be controlled and resolving, (2) the patient's period of hypermetabolism should be nearing an end, and (3) the patient should have evidence of anabolic metabolism and be in positive nitrogen balance with a rising albumin and wounds that are healing. In addition, pulmonary and cardiac organ dysfunction should be minimal, and the patient should be close to his or her dry weight or be actively mobilizing all third-spaced fluids. If there is irreversible renal failure, the patient should be tolerating hemodialysis without hemodynamic instability.

In this setting, the use of pressure support ventilation can be most helpful. Once the aforementioned conditions are met, the patient is switched from the intermittent mandatory ventilation (IMV) mode of ventilation to continuous positive airway pressure (CPAP) with a high level of pressure support over a 1-hour period. If necessary, up to 30 cm H_2O of pressure support is provided to offset the patient's work of breathing and make CPAP sustainable indefinitely. This level of support should consistently achieve tidal volumes of greater than 600 ml per breath and an adequate minute ventilation. Weaning is then accomplished simply by progressive, monotonic reduction in the level of pressure support. Progression is slow, usually weaning 1 to 4 cm H_2O per day. Frail elderly patients tolerate weaning only 1 or 2 cm H_2O per day, whereas younger patients with greater cardiopulmonary reserve can be weaned more rapidly. The patient's breathing mechanics, respiratory rate, arterial blood gases, and metabolic measurements are followed closely; if the patient is tiring or ventilation or oxygenation is inadequate, the wean is either slowed or an IMV can be added for rest.

Occasionally a patient may require a more prolonged wean from ventilation. This most often occurs in patients with significant premorbid pulmonary or neuromuscular disease. For such patients, transfer to a stepdown unit with a precisely defined weaning schedule is most appropriate. These patients benefit from consultation with pulmonologists to design an effective weaning schedule. In this case, the patient's respiratory rehabilitation takes place along with their general rehabilitation.

POST-ICU PHASE

Patients who survive a prolonged ICU course require a period of rehabilitation. The length of this period depends on the patients age, premorbid health, and the existence of any permanent deficits resulting from the prolonged illness (e.g., renal failure, amputation). Each rehabilitation program must be tailored to the individual's needs.

All these patients, however, suffer from their prolonged period of bed rest and immobilization. Immobilization can cause a wide variety of system deficits, from muscle weakness and atrophy to cardiovascular deconditioning or even renal calculi. The most profoundly affected is the musculoskeletal system.

Prolonged inactivity and immobilization lead to muscle weakness, atrophy, contractures, and osteoporosis. When patients are at complete bed rest, they can lose 50% of their muscle strength in just 3 to 5 weeks.[66] This affects a patient's ability to sit, walk, and attend to activities of daily living. A gradual program of intensive physical therapy is necessary to regain muscle mass and increase strength. Disuse weakness can be reversed at a rate of 6% per week when a program of submaximal (65 to 75%) exercise is used.[66]

Contractures can generally be prevented with prophylactic flexibility exercises several times a week. Once they are present, mild contractures are treated with passive range of motion for 20 to 30 minutes two times per day. Severe contractures require prolonged stretching for 20 to 30 minutes each day.[67] Prolonged stretching is usually accompanied by the application of heat with either ultrasound or a waterbath. In addition to muscular dysfunction, the musculoskeletal system can be severely damaged by osteoporosis secondary to increased bone resorption during immobilization. In a 30- to 36-week period, approximately 4% of total body calcium is lost.[68]

Unfortunately, bone resorption of calcium not only causes osteoporosis, but also can cause renal calculi. The calcium that is resorbed is excreted in the urine causing stones,[69,70] increasing susceptibility to urinary tract infections and urosepsis. This is compounded by the fact that bed rest decreases the ability to drain the urinary system completely, leading to urine stagnation and greater propensity to stone formation.[71]

The cardiovascular system is also severely affected by prolonged immobilization. The normal compensatory mechanisms of vasoconstriction, increased heart rate, and increased blood pressure that should occur on standing are not active. This causes severe postural hypotension, which can be a difficult problem in the early phase of rehabilitation.[72] Cardiac reconditioning should begin with a program that induces 65% or less of maximal heart rate with gradual increases in heart rate as conditioning improves. A program with this approach should show approximately a 30% increase in endurance and work capacity each week.[67]

As the patient's conditioning and strength improve, attention must be given to specialized training needs of individual patients. If possible, patients with permanent tracheostomies should learn to suction themselves and to dress and care for the tracheostomy site. These patients also need training and assistance with speech communication and swallowing skills.[73]

Patients with enteral stomas need to learn stomal care. This is greatly facilitated by the consultation of a stomal therapist or nurse specialist, who can provide training and

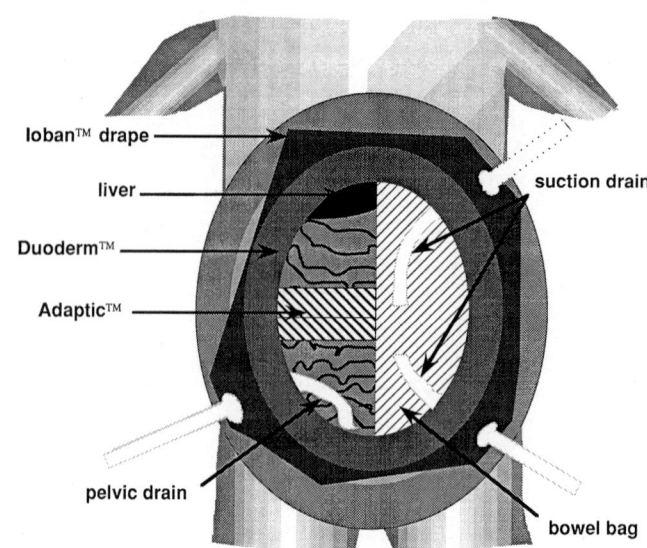

Fig. 51–5. Open abdomen technique. The infected abdomen can be left open for drainage and frequent, repeated debridement by dressing with impregnated gauze (Adaptic), bowel bags, drains, and "sticky drapes" (Ioban). Pliable skin protection, such as that used for stoma appliances (Duoderm), prevents shear injury from the drape.

advice on the most appropriate appliance for an individual stoma. As the specialized training is pursued, arrangements should be made for continued rehabilitation and perhaps occupational therapy in the nonacute setting. Many patients are able to be discharged to home. Elderly patients may require care in a short-term care facility before they are able to live independently.

In summary, severe intra-abdominal infection is a major cause of sepsis and death. The infection initiates a self-perpetuating systemic inflammatory process that can lead to severe metabolic derangement and progressive multisystem organ dysfunction. Management of these patients emphasizes source control aimed at the identification and eradication of the cause of SIRS and its sequelae. This requires rapid diagnosis and assessment for surgical or interventional procedures necessary to drain abscesses and control intra-abdominal soilage. During the resuscitation of patients with SIRS, the support of oxygen transport and the reduction of oxygen demand are essential to minimize oxygen debt. Metabolic support, providing adequate nutrition and gastrointestinal maintenance, supplies essential nutrients, prevents overwhelming catabolism, and maintains normal gut homeostasis. These supportive measures have proved to be successful when implemented early in the course of SIRS or sepsis. Once a patient has survived a prolonged ICU stay, extensive rehabilitation and training are required to return to a healthy, active life.

APPENDIX: MANAGEMENT OF THE OPEN ABDOMEN

Managing the open abdomen requires a significant committment from all members of the critical care team. In the operating room, no fascial closure of any type is attempted initially, and the abdomen is closed by other means. Some techniques use Marlex mesh or zippers to enclose the abdominal contents. We cover the viscera with a layer of petrolatum (Vaseline)-impregnated gauze and bowel bags for protection and then place large drains on top of the bags. Next the abdomen is sealed with several adhesive Ioban drapes. The skin at the wound edges is protected from the shear force generated by the Ioban drapes by using a continuous lining of Duoderm or other stoma-type skin protector (Fig. 51-5). The patient is kept paralyzed, sedated, and narcotized for several days to minimize intra-abdominal pressure and to allow the intestines to heal and granulate, avoiding evisceration. The abdominal dressing is changed every day for approximately 1 week then every other day until the infection is controlled. Dressing changes are usually conducted in the operating room. If patient transport presents some difficulty, the dressing changes can be performed in the ICU, given the availability of adequate light and suction at the bedside. The drains are used to remove collections of fluid from underneath the drapes and in cases of particularly severe infection can be used for continuous irrigation of the abdomen.

REFERENCES

1. Consensus Conference Committee, American College of Chest Physicians/Society of Critical Care Medicine Consensus Conference: Definitions for sepsis and organ failure and guidelines for the use of innovative therapies in sepsis. Crit. Care Med., 20:864, 1992.
2. Bone, R. C., et al.: Sepsis syndrome: a valid clinical entity. Crit. Care Med., 17:389, 1989.
3. Bone, R. C.: Let's agree on terminology: definitions of sepsis. Crit. Care Med., 19:973, 1991.
4. Smith, C. R., Straube, R. C., and Zeigler, E. J.: HA-1A: a human monoclonal antibody for the treatment of gram negative sepsis. Infect. Dis. Clin. North Am., 6:253, 1992.
5. Hackford, A. W.: Intra-abdominal sepsis: a medical-surgical dilemma. Clin. Ther., 12:43, 1990.
6. Simmons, D. H., Nicoloff, J., and Guze, L. B.: Hyperventilation and respiratory alkalosis as signs of gram-negative bacteremia. JAMA, 174:2196, 1960.
7. Vito, L., et al.: Sepsis presenting as acute respiratory insufficiency. Surg. Gynecol. Obstet., 138:896, 1974.
8. Siegel, J. H., et al.: Physiological and metabolic correlations in human sepsis. Surgery, 86:409, 1979.
9. Cerra, F. B.: Hypermetabolism, organ failure, and metabolic support. Surgery, 101:1, 1987.
10. Cerra, F. B.: Hypermetabolism-organ failure syndrome: a metabolic response to injury. Crit. Care Clin., 5:289, 1989.
11. Cuthbertson, D., and Tilstone, W.: Metabolism during the post-injury period. Adv. Clin. Chem., 12:1, 1977.
12. Cerra, F. B., et al.: Autocannibalism, a failure of exogenous nutritional support. Ann. Surg., 192:570, 1980.
13. Shoemaker, W. C., Appel, P., and Kran, H. B.: Role of oxygen debt in the development of organ failure, sepsis, and death in the high risk surgical patient. Chest, 102:208, 1992.
14. Weg, J. G.: Oxygen transport in adult respiratory distress syndrome and other acute circulatory problems: relationship of oxygen delivery to oxygen consumption. Crit. Care Med., 19:650, 1992.
15. Deitch, E. A.: Bacterial translocation. In Multiple System Organ Failure. Edited by D. E. Fry. St. Louis, Mosby-Yearbook, 1992, p. 57.
16. Outzen, H. C., Corrowd, D., and Schultz, L. D.: Attenuation of exogenous murine mammary tumor virus virulence in the C3H/HeJ substrain bearing the LPS mutation. J. Natl. Cancer Inst., 75:917, 1985.
17. Hamill, R., and Maki, D.: Endotoxin shock in man caused by gram-negative bacilli. Etiology, clinical features, diagnosis, natural history and prevention. In Handbook of Endotoxin. Edited by R. A. Proctor. Amsterdam, Elsevier, 1986, p. 55.
18. Cavaillon, J., et al.: Cytokine response by monocytes and macrophages to free and lipoprotein-bound lipopolysaccharide. Infect. Immunol., 58:2375, 1990.
19. Hamilton, S. H.: Monitoring and investigation of intra-abdominal sepsis. Can. J. Surg., 31:327, 1988.
20. Adam, E. J., and Page, J.: Intra-abdominal sepsis: the role of radiology. Baillieres Clin. Gastroenterol., 5(3 Pt 1):587, 1991.
21. Pitcher, W. D., and Musher, D.: Critical importance of early diagnosis and treatment of intra-abdominal infection. Arch. Surg., 117:328, 1982.
22. Deveney, C., Lurie, K., and Deveney, K.: Improved treatment of intra-abdominal abscess. A result of improved localization, drainage and patient care, not technique. Arch. Surg., 123:1126, 1988.
23. Aeder, M., Wellman, F., Haaga, F., and Hau, T.: Role of surgical and percutaneous drainage in the treatment of abdominal abscesses. Arch. Surg., 146:112, 1983.
24. Glass, C., and Cohn, I.: Drainage of intra-abdominal abscess. A comparison of surgical and computerized tomography catheter drainage. Am. J. Surg., 147:315, 1984.
25. Lurie, D., Plazk, L., and Deveney, C.: Management of intra-abdominal abscesses. Infect. Surg., 7:477, 1988.
26. Lent, W. M., Goldman, M., and Bizer, L. S.: An objective appraisal of the role of computed tomographic (CT) guided drainage of intra-abdominal abscesses. Am. Surg., 56:688, 1990.
27. Barr, J., Seiver, A., and Morgan, L.: Unpublished data. 1992.
28. Shoemaker, W. C., Appel, P., and Kram, H. B.: Prospective trial of supranormal values of survivors and therapeutic goals in high risk surgical patients. Chest, 94:1176, 1988.
29. Shoemaker, W. C., Appel, P., and Kram, H. B.: Incidence, physiologic description, compensatory mechanisms, and therapeutic implications of monitored events. Crit. Care Med., 17:1277, 1989.
30. Shoemaker, W., Appel, P., and Kram, H. B.: Therapy of shock based on pathophysiology, monitoring and outcome prediction. Crit. Care Med., 18(1 of 2):S19, 1990.
31. Shoemaker, W. C., Appel, P., and Kram, H. B.: Oxygen transport measurements to evaluate tissue perfusion and titrate therapy: dobutamine and dopamine effects. Crit. Care Med., 19:672, 1991.
32. Guillermo, R. D., et al.: Gastric mucosal pH as a prognostic index of mortality in critically ill patients. Crit. Care Med., 19:1037, 1991.
33. Scott, J. P., Higgenbottom, T., Smyth, R. L., and Wallwork, J.: Acute pulmonary hypertensive crisis in a patient with primary pulmonary hypertension treated by both epoprostenol (prostacyclin) and nitroprusside. Chest, 99:1284, 1991.
34. Rubin, L. J.: Primary pulmonary hypertension. Practical therapeutic recommendations. Drugs, 43:37, 1992.
35. Berg, R. D., Wommack, E., and Deitch, E. A.: Immunosuppression and intestinal bacterial overgrowth synergistically promote bacterial translocation. Arch. Surg., 123:1359, 1988.
36. Pingleton, S. K.: Role of enteral feeding in stress ulcer protection. In The Gastrointestinal Response to Injury, Starvation, and Enteral Nutrition. Edited by A. F. Roche. Columbus, Ross Laboratories, 1988, p. 59.
37. Campos, A. C., Paluzzi, M., and Meguid, M. M.: Total nutritional admixtures. Nutrition, 6:347, 1990.

38. Koea, J. B., and Shaw, J.: Total parenteral nutrition in surgical illness: How much? How good? Nutrition, *8*:275, 1992.
39. Cerra, F. B.: Nutritional Support. Multiple Organ Failure Symposium. Costa Mesa, CA, Merck, Sharp & Dohme, 1988, p. 16.
40. Putterman, C.: Central venous catheter-related sepsis: a clinical review. Resuscitation, *20*:1, 1990.
41. Manglano, R., and Martin, M.: Safety of triple lumen catheters in the critically ill. Am. Surg., *57*:370, 1991.
42. Rose, S. G., Pitsch, R. J., Karrer, F. W., and Moor, B. J.: Subclavian catheter infections. J. Parenteral Enteral Nutr., *12*:511, 1988.
43. Maki, D. G., et al.: An attachable silver-impregnated cuff for prevention of infection with central venous catheters: a prospective randomized multicenter trial. Am. J. Med., *85*:307, 1988.
44. Norwood, S., Hajjar, G., and Jenkins, L.: The influence of an attachable subcutaneous cuff for preventing triple lumen catheter infections in critically ill surgical and trauma patients. Surg. Gynecol. Obstet., *175*:33, 1992.
45. Talpers, S. S., Romberger, D., Bunce, S. B., and Pingleton, K. S.: Nutritionally associated increased carbon dioxide production. Excess total calories vs. high proportion carbohydrate calories. Chest, *102*:551, 1992.
46. Hastings, P. R., et al.: Antacid titration in the prevention of acute gastrointestinal bleeding: a controlled, randomized trial in 100 critically ill patients. N. Engl. J. Med., *298*:1041, 1978.
47. Vorder Bruegge, W. F., and Peura, D. A.: Stress-related mucosal damage: review of drug therapy. J. Clin. Gastroenterol., *12(Suppl. 2)*:S35, 1990.
48. Driks, M. R., et al.: Nosocomial pneumonia in intubated patients given sucralfate as compared with antacids or histamine type 2 blockers: role of gastric colonization. N. Engl. J. Med., *317*:1376, 1987.
49. Cook, D. J., Laine, L., Guyatt, G. H., and Raffin, T. A.: Nosocomial pneumonia and the role of gastric pH. A meta-analysis. Chest, *100*:7, 1991.
50. Hoton, M. V., and Godley, P.: Continuous arteriovenous hemofiltration: an alternative to hemodialysis. Am. J. Hosp. Pharm., *45*:361, 1988.
51. Macias, W., Mueller, H. A., and Scarim, S. K.: Continuous venovenous hemofiltration: an alternative to continous arteriovenous hemofiltration and hemodiafiltration in acute renal failure. Am. J. Kidney Dis., *8*:451, 1991.
52. Hackford, A., et al.: Prospective study comparing imipenum-cilastin with clindamycin and gentamicin for the treatment of serious surgical infections. Arch. Surg., *123*:322, 1988.
53. Reed, R. L.: Antibiotic choices in surgical intensive care patients. Surg. Clin. North Am., *71*:765, 1991.
54. Klastersky, J., et al.: Empiric antimicrobial therapy for febrile granulocytopenic cancer patients: lesson from four EORTC trials. Eur. J. Cancer Clin. Oncol., *24(Suppl. 1)*:S35, 1988.
55. Pokorny, W. J., Kaplan, S., and Mason, E. O.: A preliminary report of ticarcillin and clavulanate versus triple antibiotic therapy in children with ruptured appendicitis. Surg. Gynecol. Obstet., *172(Suppl.)*:54, 1991.
56. Broughton, W. A., et al.: Bronchoscopic protected specimen brush and bronchoalveolar lavage in the diagnosis of bacterial pneumonia. Infect. Dis. Clin. North Am., *5*:437, 1991.
57. Hammond, J. M., Potgeiter, P. D., Saunders, G. L., and Forder, A. A.: Double-blind study of selective decontamination of the digestive tract in intensive care. Lancet, *340*:5, 1992.
58. Offenbartl, K., and Bengmark, S.: Intra-abdominal infections and gut origin sepsis. World J. Surg., *14*:191, 1990.
59. Gorbach, S. L., Chang, T., and Goldin, B.: Successful treatment of relapsing clostridium difficile colitis with lactobacillus GG. Lancet, *2*:1519, 1987.
60. Solomkin, J. S., et al.: The role of *Candida* in intraperitoneal infections. Surgery, *88*:524, 1980.
61. Solomkin, J. S., Flohr, A., and Simmons, R. L.: *Candida* infections in surgical patients. Dose requirements and toxicity of amphotericin B. Ann. Surg., *202*:166, 1982.
62. Denning, D. W., et al.: Antifungal prophylaxis during neutropenia or allogenic bone marrow transplantation: what is the state of the art? Chemotherapy, *38(Suppl. 1)*:43, 1992.
63. Distasio, J. A., and Cheung, N. K.: Current therapies using monoclonal antibodies: I. organ transplantation, bacterial sepsis, and bone marrow transplantation. Compr. Ther., *18*:33, 1992.
64. Fisher, C. J., and Bellingan, G.: Immunotherapy of sepsis syndrome: a comparison of the available treatments. Klinische Wochenschrift *69(Suppl. 26)*:162, 1992.
65. Christman, J. W.: Potential treatment of sepsis with cytokine-specific agents. Chest, *102*:613, 1992.
66. Muller, E. A.: Influence of training and inactivity on muscle strength. Arch. Phys. Rehabil. Med., *51*:449, 1970.
67. Halar, E. M., and Bell, K. R.: Rehabilitation's relationship to inactivity. *In* Krusen's Handbook of Physical Medicine and Rehabilitation. 4th Ed. Edited by F. J. Kottke and J. F. Lehmenn. Philadelphia, W. B. Saunders, 1990, p. 1113.
68. Schneider, V. S., and McDonald, J.: Skeletal calcium homeostasis and counter measures to prevent disuse osteoporosis. Calcif. Tissue Int., *36*:S151, 1984.
69. Ledbetter, W. F., and Engster, H.: Problems of renal lithiasis in convalescent patients. J. Urol., *53*:269, 1945.
70. Issekutsz, B., et al.: Effect of prolonged bedrest on urinary calcium output. J. Appl. Physiol., *21*:1013, 1966.
71. Stewart, A. F., et al.: Calcium homeostasis in immobilization: an example of resorptive hypercalciuria. N. Engl. J. Med., *306*:1136, 1982.
72. Taylor, H. L., Henschel, A., Porozek, J., and Keys, A.: Effects of bedrest on cardiovascular function and work performance. J. Appl. Physiol., *2*:223, 1949.
73. Godwin, J., and Heffner, J.: Special critical care considerations in tracheostomy management. Clin. Chest Med., *12*:573, 1991.

Chapter 52

ACUTE PANCREATITIS

CHARLES F. FREY
TATSUO ARAIDA

Acute pancreatitis morphologically ranges in severity from edema to necrosis. Its initiation and progression are only partially understood. The development of pancreatic necrosis and infection are the main determinants of mortality following acute pancreatitis. Morbidity and mortality are largely related to the extent of peripancreatic and pancreatic parenchymal necrosis, to the presence or absence of bacterial contamination of the necrotic tissue,[1] the adequacy of the initial fluid resuscitation, and the development or nondevelopment of multiple organ failure. The management of patients with pancreatitis is directed at confirming the diagnosis of pancreatitis, determining its etiology and severity, providing resuscitation and supportive care, and intervening operatively in patients developing septic complications.

ETIOLOGY OF PANCREATITIS

Alcoholism and biliary tract disease account for 75 to 80% of all episodes of clinically acute pancreatitis. The relative frequency of these two associations depend on the prevalence of alcoholism in the population studied. Among patients treated in large city hospitals in the United States there is a high incidence of alcohol abuse and alcoholic pancreatitis. In community hospitals, gallstone pancreatitis is most common.[2,3]

Postoperative pancreatitis is more common than often appreciated. Imrie[4] reviewed 15 reports from 1962 to the present, each of which included between 13 and 30 patients. The incidence of postoperative pancreatitis was 7.5% (291/3874 patients). Probably, only the most severe cases are recognized.[5] Therefore, the mortality rate is high (32.6%). Delay in recognition of postoperative pancreatitis is common. The pain associated with pancreatitis is often mistaken for postoperative pain.

Endoscopic retrograde cholangiopancreatography (ERCP) pancreatitis is now a common cause of pancreatitis occurring in 2 to 5% of all patients undergoing ERCP. In one report on ERCP, pancreatitis, one third of all deaths from pancreatitis were from ERCP pancreatitis.[6] Other causes of acute pancreatitis are listed in Table 52-1 and include hyperlipidemia, injury, drugs, hyperparathyroidism, hypercalcemia, transplantation, cardiac bypass surgery, pancreas divisum, pregnancy, congenital abnormalities of the pancreatic ductal system, or cancer.

Drugs linked to pancreatitis include diuretics,[7,8] steroids,[9,10,11] sulindac,[12] sulfonamide,[13,14] azathioprine,[7,15] isotretinon (Accutane),[16] tetracycline,[17,18] estrogen, or estrogen-containing contraceptives,[19] organophosphate insecticides[20] and anticholinesterases.[21]

Acute pancreatitis is the initial presentation in roughly 2% of patients with pancreatic cancer. When pancreatitis develops in a person older than 50 years in the absence of the history of alcoholism or gallbladder disease, the possibility of pancreatic cancer should be considered.[22]

PATHOGENESIS OF ACUTE PANCREATITIS

Despite extensive research with experimental models of acute pancreatitis, both the cause and the factors that determine the severity of the disease still remain unclear in humans. Acute inflammation develops when natural safeguards fail and proteolytic enzymes are activated. As such, a number of initiators and mediators are involved in the progression of edema to necrosis.

Initiators and Mediators of Injury

A variety of mechanisms either involving the pancreatic vasculature or acinar intracellular events have been proposed as initiators of acute interstitial and necrotizing pancreatitis.

Vascular

In patients with ischemic pancreatitis (cardiac bypass), primary hypertriglyceridemia, or secondary hypertriglyceridemia due to alcohol abuse or isotretinon (Accutane), the initial injury is believed to be vascular, not acinar and is localized to capillaries where platelet and fibrin thrombi and swollen endothelium are noted. In animal models simulating ischemic pancreatitis and hypertriglyceridemia, adenosine triphosphate (ATP) levels were 30% of normal, and the acini were normal. The vascular changes were believed mediated by oxygen-derived free radicals and ameliorated by free radical scavengers, superoxide dismutase, and catalase.[23]

Work from the Hopkins group[24] confirmed by others[25,26] has shown the importance of oxygen-derived free radicals in both the initiation of some forms of pancreatitis by capillary injury and its role as a mediator in other forms of pancreatitis in which the primary event is acinar cell injury.[27] In the ethionine mouse model, Rutledge and Steer noted that free radical scavengers reduced edema forma-

Table 52–1. Etiologic Factors in Acute Pancreatitis

Most common causes
    Biliary tract disease
    Ethyl alcohol abuse
Common causes
    Tumors of the pancreas
    Endoscopic retrograde cholangiopancreatography
    Hyperlipoproteinemias (type I, IV, V)
    Hypercalcemia (especially in hyperparathyroidism and multiple myeloma)
    Peptic ulcer disease
    Surgery
    Trauma
Uncommon causes
    Drug use (such as azathioprine, estrogens, corticosteroids and thiazides, isotretinoin, sundilac)
    Hereditary pancreatitis
    Infectious agents
    L-asparaginase administration
    Methyl alcohol poisoning
    Pancreas divisum
    Pregnancy (third trimester)
    Scorpion bites
    Transplantation
    Vascular factors
    Cardiopulmonary bypass surgery, hypotensive shock
Rare or only recently reported causes
    Infection with campylobacter, legionella, or mycoplasma organisms
    Kawasaki disease (mucocutaneous lymph node syndrome)

tion, but not the mortality, morphologic severity, or biochemical changes.[28]

Oxygen free radicals have also been incriminated in the pulmonary injury associated with acute pancreatitis.[29,30] The oxygen-derived free radicals associated with pancreatitis appear to be tissue-derived and xanthine oxidase-dependent, as well as phagocyte driven and NADPH oxidase-dependent. Free radicals are byproducts of the oxidation that accompanies an inflammatory reaction. They have been implicated as mediators of cell injury and edema in bacterial infection. They have also been shown to play an important role in promoting cell injury during ischemia, post ischemia perfusion, and oxygen toxicity.[20,31-33]

A free radical is a molecule containing a single unpaired electron occurring in its outer shell. Oxygen-derived free radicals, including the superoxidase free radical (O^{2-}), hydrogen peroxidase (H_2O_2) hydroxy radical (H^+) and single oxygen (O_2) can cause tissue injury by degrading hyaluronic acid and collagen in the extracellular matrix.[34] They may directly damage cell membranes through the peroxidation of structurally important lipids within the phospholipid structure of the membrane itself,[35] and cause disruption of lysosomes and mitochondria by injuring the membrane surrounding these intracellular organelles. They also attack nucleic acids within the nucleus and cytoplasm. Some events, such as the destruction of lysosome membranes, result in the release of enzymes. These events in turn potentiate the free radical induced injury by propagating further formation of free radicals.[36] Biologic mechanisms for the detoxification of these oxygen-derived free radicals include the use of superoxide dismutase and catalase, glutathione peroxidase, vitamin E, cysteine, and cysteamine.[34,36,37] Superoxide radical to hydrogen peroxide and oxygen, and catalyze promotes the further reduction of hydrogen peroxide to water and oxygen. Under a variety of pathologic conditions, oxygen-derived free radical production may exceed this scavenging capability, and tissue injury is produced.[26]

Intracellular

Koike[39] and Watanabe[40] have reported that the duct obstruction models of pancreatitis, the CDE mice diet, and the hypersecretory model utilizing cerulein excess inhibit intracellular transport and discharge of secretory proteins stimulate autophagocytose and crinophagy of membrane-bound secretory compartments.

Normally, the synthesis of enzymes proceeds by the physiologic pathway in the cisternae of rough-surface endoplasmic reticulum (RER) and transport to the Golgi complex and condensing vacuoles. Subsequently, there is secretion by lysosomal hydrolyses into lysosomes with maturation of condensing vacuoles into zymogen granules that contain digestive enzymes and discharge of the digestive enzymes into the acinar lumen by fusion of the zymogen limiting membrane and the luminal plasmalemma. During enzyme cotransplantation within the cisternal space of RER, degradation of secretory proteins by lysosomal enzymes does not occur because lysosomal enzymes only operate in the acidic environment of lysosomes (pH 3.5 to 4.5).[41] Leach has postulated that manipulation of subcellar pH by chloroquine may inhibit the action of lysosomes by increasing subcellar pH.[42]

Pathologic conditions that inhibit the intracellular transport and discharge of secretory proteins autophagocytose and crinophagy of membrane-bound secretary compartments. These abnormal pathways were demonstrated by Koike[39] and Watanabe[40] in the three models of pancreatitis described (i.e., CDE diet in mice, duct obstruction, and cerulein hypersecretion). On electron microscopy, they observed pathologic pathways of secretion in the CDE diet and cerulean hyperstimulation model. Intracytoplasmic digestion of the contents of secretory vacuoles after the vacuoles fused with lysosome was noted in diet-induced pancreatitis, a process called crinophagy.

In hyperstimulation-cerulein induced pancreatitis, the condensing vacuoles failed to mature normally and instead large vacuoles containing both lysosomal hydrolyses and digestive enzymes developed. These developments result in leakage and disruption of lysosomal structures and deposition of activated enzymes into the cystolic space. These studies indicated that during the development of these forms of pancreatitis cytoplasmic vacuoles, often of large size, form which contain both digestive enzymes and lysosomal hydrolyses. This colocalization of digestive enzyme zymogens and lysosomal hydrolyses could lead to the intracellular activation of digestive enzymes.[41] At least one lysosomal hydrolase (cathepsin B) is capable of activating trypsinogen. These studies indicate that intracellular changes in the transport, storage, and secretion of enzymes have moved the possible activation of these enzymes back from the duct and duodenum to inside the cell. Colocalization of digestive enzyme zymogen and lysosomal hydrolyses, intravacuolar activation, and increased fragility and rupture of the vacuoles initiating pancreatitis has also been reported using the pancreatic duct obstruction model of pancreatitis in rabbits.[43] These effects can be prevented by esterase inhibitors according to Ohshio,[44] and by chloroquine in ethonine pancreatitis which raises the pH of the acidic subcellular model inhibiting lysosomal enzyme activity.[42]

Janes and colleagues[45] found in a duct obstruction model and the cerulein hyperstimulation model on electron microscopy and high energy phosphate metabolism studies that acinar cell changes consisting of depletion of zymogen granulates condensing vacuole formation and dilatation of the RER occurred prior to any blood vessel changes. In these models of pancreatitis, the ATP and inorganic phosphate levels were unchanged. These findings were the reverse of the findings in the ischemic and oleic acid perfusion model in which ATP and inorganic phosphate levels fell and vascular capillary changes preceded any acinar cell changes.

In the case of alcoholic pancreatitis, it has been proposed that a combination of acetaldehyde and ischemia play a role in initiating pancreatitis. Acetaldehyde, a product of oxidative ethanol metabolism may act as a substrate for xanthine oxidase which when oxidized releases oxygen-derived free radicals.[46]

Progression of Edema to Necrosis

It is generally assumed that edema and inflammation are due to digestive enzyme activation and autodigestion of the acinar cell.[47] Investigators have suggested that the lesion may progress from interstitial pancreatitis, a relatively mild form of pancreatitis, to a more severe form characterized by widespread necrosis and hemorrhage. Little is known about the factors that influence the evolution from edematous to hemorrhagic pancreatitis. Intralobular pancreatic ducts are accompanied by a rich plexus of veins and arteries. Leakage of enzymes from damaged cells or a permeable ductal system may result in vasculitis involving these vessels with secondary rupture or thrombosis. Individuals in whom the blood supply to the pancreas is compromised are predisposed to develop pancreatic necrosis, infection, and severe systemic complications of pancreatitis.

Harvey[48] and Wedgwood[49] studied the process by which acute edematous pancreatitis might be converted to acute hemorrhagic pancreatitis in their low pressure perfusion model of pancreatitis in the cat. Their early studies in this model suggested that hemorrhagic changes developed when pancreatic parenchymal microvascular permeability was increased by agents such as prostaglandin and histamine, substances known to be present in the serum or ascites fluid of patients with necrotizing pancreatitis. Prostaglandins are released into the ascitic fluid[50] and portal venous blood, and some probably enter the systemic circulation. Histamine is thought to be released from the mucosal mast cell and is known to be present in ascites fluid.[51-53] These substances increase microvascular permeability by causing endothelial cell contraction and the formation of gaps in the vascular wall.[54,55] Recently, Karanjia and colleagues[56] theorized that conversion of an interstitial form of pancreatitis to necrotizing pancreatitis depended not only on increased microvascular permeability but the presence of activated enzymes within the main pancreatic duct and interstitium of the pancreas. He has also reported that terbutalline and dopamine reduce the severity of pancreatitis without affecting blood flow to the pancreas.

PATHOPHYSIOLOGY OF NECROTIZING PANCREATITIS AND MULTIPLE ORGAN FAILURE

The extent of necrosis of pancreatic and peripancreatic tissue in general is correlated with multiple organ failure. Whether multiple organ failure actually results may depend in large part on how vigorously the patient has been fluid resuscitated. Multiple organ failure is seen most often in patients with necrotizing pancreatitis who have been inadequately resuscitated. Acute pancreatitis is frequently associated with hypotension and organ hypoperfusion. Transudation as well as exudation of intravascular fluid into the peripancreatic retroperitoneum is common and may be of great magnitude. In our experience, on the day of hospital admission, the positive fluid balance in seven patients who died averaged 9 L.[6] Frequently, there is evidence of a diffuse microvascular leak in which fluid is lost into interstitium in areas remote from the pancreas (e.g., subcutaneous tissue, pulmonary interstitium, peritoneal cavity, etc.). The mechanism by which this leak occurs is unclear. It may reflect a hypoalbuminemia-related decrease in intravascular colloid osmotic pressure but is more likely caused by disruptions of the microvascular endothelium with extravasation of protein rich plasma into the interstitium. In addition, it has been suggested that vasoactive agents released into the circulation from the inflamed pancreas may play an important role in this process[27,29,51] (Fig. 52-1).

The entire process can result in the following disruption or alteration in the functions or organ systems:

- Hemodynamic instability
- Renal failure
- Respiratory insufficiency and ARDS
- Liver function and morphology
- Diabetes mellitus
- Hypocalcemia
- Alteration in coagulation
- Alteration in macrophage function

Hemodynamic Changes

Most hemodynamic studies in humans have shown that there is a hyperdynamic cardiovascular state in severe pancreatitis similar to that noted in cirrhosis and septicemia (Table 52-2). When it occurs, hypotension is usually related to an inadequate cardiac response to diminished peripheral resistance and decreased intravascular volume.[57-59] Vasoactive agents, including activated enzymes released from the pancreas, have been implicated in this hypotension and various myocardial depressant factors have been sought.[60-62] During the course of this disease, trypsin and other pancreatic proteases are released from the pancreas to the surrounding tissues and into the sys-

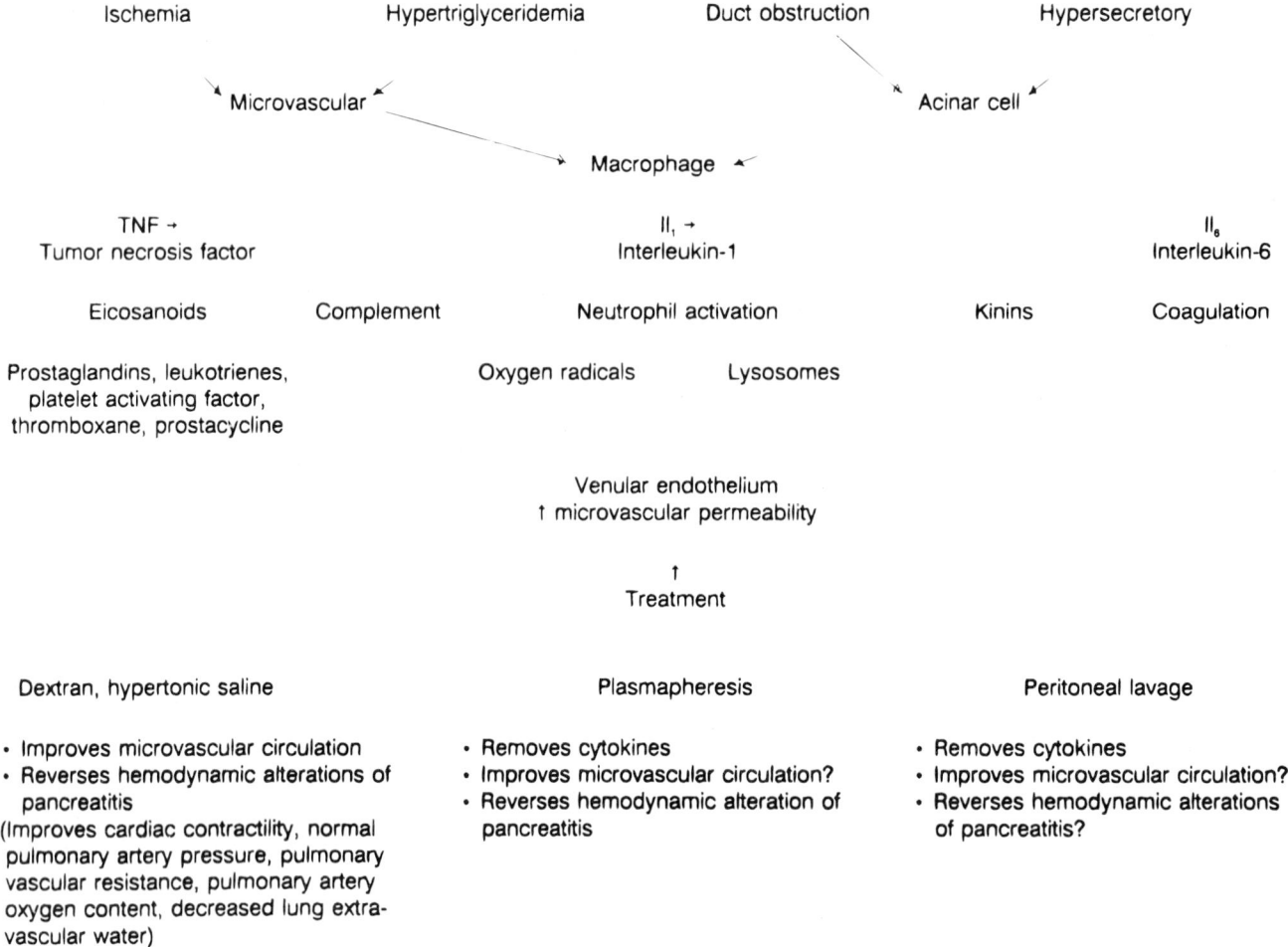

Fig. 52–1. Pancreatitis: initiating factors.

temic circulation.[63] These proteases may act as triggers of the complement cascade by proteolytic cleavage at the third and fifth complement components, C3a and C5.[64,65] When complement is activated, the anaphylatoxin C3a and C5a are formed.[66] C3a and C5a increase vascular permeability, induce smooth muscle contractions, and release histamine from most cells and basophils (inflammatory reaction). C5a is a chemotactic agent for polymorphonuclear leukocytes and causes leukocyte activation, aggregation, and sequestration. The leukocyte activation will result in production and release of substances toxic to vascular endothelium such as oxygen-derived free radicals and leukocyte proteases. A complete activation of the complete cascade will also result in formation of the terminal complexes.[67] These exit in two forms. The membrane-associated C5b9 is the so-called membrane attack complex which is responsible for the complement cystolytic activity. The other one presents as inactivated, monolytic analogue (Fig. 52–2). Roxvall[68] reported that complement activation and anaphylatoxin generation (C3a, C5a) play a role in developing multiple organ failure in severe acute pancreatitis in humans. In experimental animals, hypotension can be induced by intravenous infusion of hemorrhagic ascitic fluid obtained from patients or experimental animals with pancreatitis.[52,53] The role of resuscitation in preventing the systemic manifestations of necrotizing pancreatitis is under scrutiny in our laboratory. What has been considered an adequate volume of fluid replacement in necrotizing pancreatitis is being reevaluated. Using dogs as a study group, Knol[69] was unable over a 4-hour period to completely reverse the hemodynamic changes associated with necrotizing pancreatitis to prepancreatic levels by either his high volume, 6.5 ml/kg per hour, or low volume, 1.75 ml/kg per hour, resuscitation. Mean arterial pressure was unchanged in all groups. Central venous pressure decreased in both groups and pancreatic blood flow was

Table 52–2. Hemodynamic Changes in Human Necrotizing Pancreatitis

	CI	SVRI	PVRI	AVDO₂	Shunt Fraction
Bradley[29]	↑↑	↓↓	↑↑	—	—
Berger[31]	↑↑	↓↓	—	↑↑	↑↑
Cobo[30]	↑↑	↓↓	↑↑	—	↑↑

CI, cardiac index; SVRI, systemic vascular resistance index; PVRI, pulmonary vascular resistance index; AVDO, alveolar versus oxygen difference.

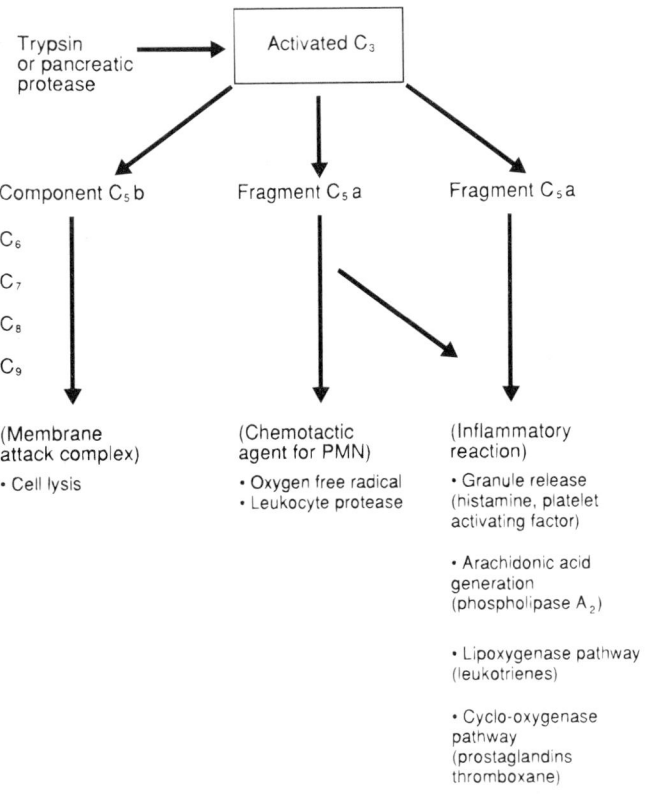

Fig. 52–2. The pathway of activation of the complement system in pancreatitis.

23% in the high volume group and 73% in the low volume group. Oxygen consumption was reduced in both groups.

In our experience with pigs with necrotizing pancreatitis given a low volume of 6 ml/kg per hour or normal saline and a high volume of 25 ml/kg per hour or normal saline for 48 hours, there was no difference in SVRI in either group compared to prepancreatitis values. Cardiac index was approximately twice prepancreatitis levels. Heart rate increased by one third in both groups. Central venous pressure (CVP) and pulmonary artery wedge pressure (PAWP) were not significantly different from preoperative levels in both the low and high fluid volume groups. Pulmonary artery pressure was slightly higher in the high fluid groups and comparable to prepancreatitis levels in the low volume group. Peripheral vascular resistance index (PVRI) values were double prepancreatitis levels in the high volume group, whereas those of the low volume group were unchanged.

Donaldson,[70] using dextran 40 in dogs showed pancreatic blood flow was better maintained than with saline or plasma despite the fact cardiac output was better maintained with plasma. The beneficial effects were attributed to dextran's role in plasma expansion and antithrombotic properties.

Klar[71] using dextran 60 in rabbits showed a marked improvement in microcirculatory perfusion over a 6 hour period compared to undiluted controls—60% versus 10%. These changes in microcirculatory perfusion resulting from increased vascular permeability were apparent 30 minutes after the onset of necrotizing pancreatitis and attributed by us to hemodilution.

Using a pig model of necrotizing pancreatitis Lehtola[72] compared Dextran 70 5.7 ml/kg per hour and saline 7.5 ml/kg per hour to a saline group 26 ml/kg per hour followed over a 5-hour period. During the 5 hours cardiac output fell 6% in the dextran-saline group and 58% in the saline group. There was no significant change in the blood pressure and pulse rate in the dextran-saline group. Pancreatic blood flow in the dextran saline group decreased 10% from prepancreatic levels while the fraction of cardiac output (CO) going to the pancreas was unchanged. In the saline group, pancreatic blood flow decreased more than 70% while the CO decreased slightly.

Horton[73] using a 6% dextran 70 solution and 2400 mOsm of sodium solution infused at 17 ml/kg per hour in dogs with necrotizing pancreatitis followed for 4 hours was compared with an infusion of lactated Ringer's solution at 65 ml/kg per hour. These rates of infusion were those necessary to maintain CO and mean arterial pressure at prepancreatitis levels. The volume of fluid required to achieve this goal was 1879 ml in the dextran-saline group and 6857 ml in the lactated Ringer's group. The dextran hypertonic saline infusion also improved cardiac contractibility, maintained normal pulmonary artery pressure, pulmonary vascular resistance and pulmonary artery oxygen content, and decreased lung extravascular lung water. At the cellular level, the dextran hypertonic saline mixture is known to reduce cellular swelling associated with shock.[74]

Renal Failure

Severe attacks of acute pancreatitis may be associated with renal failure. The etiology of renal insufficiency in patients with acute pancreatitis is still obscure. The kidneys receive approximately 20 to 25% of the CO, or 1300 ml blood flow per minute. Because both kidneys weigh only 250 g, the ratio of blood flow to weight is high. With a normal hematocrit, the expected effective renal plasma flow averages 650 ml per minute of which 20% to 125 ml per minute is filtered through the glomerular tufts. Assuming that hypovolemia and hemoconcentration occurs early during the course of pancreatitis, Lucas[75] postulated that mild degrees of hypovolemia probably cause postglomerular vasoconstriction, which reduced renal plasma flow without altering glomerular filtration. Greater degrees of plasma volume deficit cause both pre- and postglomerular vasoconstriction leading to reduction of renal plasma flow and glomerular filtration. Concomitant renin release augments renal vasoconstriction through its action on angiotensin I and as a stimulus for aldosterone release.

Werner[76] also studied the renal response to edematous acute pancreatitis shortly after admission in 11 patients with an alcohol-related attack. During the acute illness, the kidneys demonstrated both pre- and postglomerular vasoconstriction as reflected by modest falls in glomerular filtration rate and renal plasma flow. On the basis of increased mean arterial pressure, total peripheral resistance, renal vascular resistance, normal extracellular fluid space, low CO, low normal blood volume and the results of other investigations, these authors suggested the presence of a suppressor mechanism with both systemic and renal effects. Gupta[77] postulated that localized intravascular coagulation was important in the pathogenesis of renal insufficiency and failure. The histologic finding of localized intravascular coagulation in the capillaries of the renal glomeruli in patients who died of acute pancreatitis and associated renal failure has been noted at autopsy. Oxygen-derived free radicals may have a role in acute renal failure in pancreatitis as they have been implicated in other causes of renal failure associated with ischemia.[78]

A related but separate issue to renal failure is renal handling of low molecular weight protein in mild to moderately severe pancreatitis. Warshaw[79] has reported the ratio of clearance of amylase to creatinine clearance (CAM/CCR) to be useful in distinguishing patients with acute pancreatitis from abdominal pain of other causes. Mock and colleagues[80] have shown, however, that the elevated CAM/CCR ratios associated with mild to severe acute pancreatitis are seen primarily in patients with alcoholism or alcoholic pancreatitis and much less frequently in nonalcoholic pancreatitis. The elevated CAM/CCR ratios were attributed to impaired tubular reabsorption of amylase and other low molecular weight proteins. Increased urinary excretion of amylase, lysosomal enzymes and beta$_2$ microglobulin were noted in patients with alcoholism or alcoholic pancreatitis indicating the phagolysosomal system of the renal tubules was not functioning normally and there was a defect in reabsorption perhaps mediated in part by glucagon known to be elevated in acute pancreatitis.

Respiratory Complications and ARDS

The most frequent complications found in severe acute pancreatitis are respiratory, 15 to 55%[81,82] (Table 52–3).

Table 52–3. Pre- and Postoperative Complications Associated With Necrotizing Pancreatitis in Survivors

Complications	No (%) of Patients Who Survived (n = 359)
Prolonged ileus (including gastric or duodenal obstruction)	82 (22.8)
Adult respiratory distress syndrome (and other pulmonary complications)	110 (30.6)
Renal failure	44 (12.3)
Enteric fistulas (including large and small bowel)	44 (12.3)
Pancreatic fistula	56 (15.6)
Bleeding (including retroperitoneal and gastrointestinal bleeding)	35 (9.7)
Sepsis	19 (4.5)
Shock (including cardiogenic failure)	14 (3.9)
Incisional hernia (including wound infection and dehiscence)	38 (10.6)
Splenic vein thrombosis	7 (1.9)
Diabetes (postoperative insulin dependent)	7 (1.9)
Secondary and recurrent abscess	54 (15.4)
Urinary tract infection	12 (3.3)
Others	

(Data from references 5, 83–91.)

Table 52–4. Complications of Necrotizing Pancreatitis in Patients Who Died

Complications	No (%) of Patients Who Survived (n = 87)
Prolonged ileus (including gastric or duodenal obstruction)	4 (4.6)
Adult respiratory distress syndrome (and other pulmonary complications)	32 (36.8)
Renal failure	27 (31.0)
Enteric fistulas (including large and small bowel)	5 (5.7)
Pancreatic fistula	5 (5.7)
Bleeding (including retroperitoneal and gastrointestinal bleeding)	32 (36.8)
Sepsis	26 (29.9)
Shock (including cardiogenic failure)	10 (11.5)
Incisional hernia (including wound infection and dehiscence)	2 (2.3)
Secondary and recurrent abscess	11 (12.6)
Urinary tract infection	11 (12.6)
Others	

(Data from references 5, 83–91.)

and often a cause of death (Table 52–4). Impaired ventilation results from large pleural effusions, elevation of the diaphragm and limited excursion of the diaphragm from abdominal distension, inflammation and ileus, as well as pain.

Other pulmonary events observed in acute pancreatitis include pulmonary hypertension, evidence of thromboembolic damage, endothelial damage from circulating free fatty acids, the catabolic products of complement and ARDS.

The biochemical sequence of events that leads to adult respiratory distress syndrome (ARDS) is complex and not fully understood. Certainly, complement-induced neutrophil aggregation in the lung releases oxygen-derived free radicals that cause capillary injury; one also sees involvement of various eicosanoids, which appear to cause airway dysfunction and pulmonary vasoconstriction.[27,29,92,93] Fibrin is deposited as the plasminogen system is overwhelmed and the lymphatics become blocked. The pathophysiologic lung changes in ARDS include interstitial pulmonary edema (the result of increased microvascular permeability), alveolar flooding and hemorrhage, atelectasis, vascular microthrombi, hyaline membranes, and progression to interstitial fibrosis.[94] The whole process may continue inexorably.[82] These ARDS changes occurring early after the onset of severe pancreatitis are to be distinguished from the ARDS associated with sepsis.[95] Sepsis-related ARDS occurs later in the course of necrotizing pancreatitis if the necrosis becomes infected.

The extent to which the ARDS observed early after the onset of severe pancreatitis is a reflection of inadequately treated hypovolemic shock or features unique to severe pancreatitis is not known. Features thought to be unique to pancreatitis include alveolar surfactant destruction induced by phospholipase A$_2$ which has been demonstrated in experimental and human pancreatitis[96-98] and results in fluid exudation and atelectasis. Levels of C-reactive proteins are known to be markedly elevated in patients with necrotizing pancreatitis but less so in interstitial pancreatitis.[99] C-reactive protein (CRP) has been shown to bind to liposomes containing surfactant (dipalmitoyl phosphatidycholine and phosphorycholine) and inhibits the surface activity of the complex in a dose-dependent manner.[100] The lung edema of pancreatitis is an exudation fluid with a high protein content supporting the belief that it results from increased pulmonary microvascular permeability and is not a pressure-related transudate unbound.[101] As a result of lipolysis in patients with hypertriglyceridemia secondary to alcoholism or primary hyperlipoproteinemia, free fatty acids are liberated which are believed to be capable of injuring the capillary endothelium.[102] Even in the cerulein-induced rat pancreatitis model producing a mild form of pancreatitis, Guice[29] was able to demonstrate both physiologic and morphologic evidence of capillary injury and increased capillary permeability. The alveolar capillary endothelial cell injury induced by cerulein hyperstimulation model in rats induced microvascular permeability, leading to interstitial edema, intra-alveolar hemorrhage, and fibrin deposition. Both neutrophil and complement depletion or inhibition or catalase or superoxide dismutance prevented the endothelial injury. They proposed that in acute pancreatitis complement activation causes neutrophil recruitment, sequestration and adherence to alveolar capillary endothelium and results in endothelial cell injury from oxygen-free radicals released from neutrophils.[103] Importantly, Horton[73] has shown that the hemodynamic derangements of the pulmonary capillary associated with ARDS, increased pulmonary vascular resistance, decreased bronchial blood flow, pulmonary endothelial permeability and minimal extracellular fluid can be avoided in dogs with necrotizing pancreatitis by vigorous resuscitation with 6% dextran 70 solution and 2400 mOsm of sodium solutions. In patients with necrotizing pancreatitis who have become septic, elevated levels of TXB_2 (average 410 pg/ml) have been associated with the development of ARDS whereas those without ARDS average TXB_2 levels of 120 pg/ml.[93]

Liver Function and Morphologic Alterations

Acute pancreatitis is known to affect liver function and morphology.[104] Andrzejewska and Pawlicka have shown that liver mitochrondria responsible for cell respiration and energy formation through ATP are adversely effected by necrotizing pancreatitis[105,106,107] with reduced mitochondrial ATP synthesis probably due to decreased cytochrome A and B. As reported by Kitamura, these effects may be mediated by ischemia or phospholipase A_2 or lysolecithin.[108] Prostacylin (PGI_2) has been shown to have a protective effect.[105]

Diabetes Mellitus

The incidence of hyperglycemia (serum glucose 130 to 200 mg) in patients with acute pancreatitis is between 50 and 75%.[109] Glycosuria is not as common and occurs in only 30% of these patients. Ketoacidosis in patients without a previous history of diabetes is rare. Although mild hyperglycemia is common, blood glucose concentrations occasionally are higher than 200 mg/dl. Ranson[110] has used an elevation of 200 mg/dl of blood as one of his signs of severity in patients with acute pancreatitis. The mortality in acute pancreatitis rarely is the result of hyperglycemia or diabetic complications alone, however.

In patients with acute pancreatitis, the physiology of insulin and glucagon secretion appears to be different than that in patients with other pathologic forms of stress such as trauma or sepsis. Drew[111] demonstrated markedly increased glucagon levels in the initial 24 hours after hospitalization with acute pancreatitis which were significantly elevated in comparison to a suitable control group of patients with other illness of similar severity. He also postulated that high levels of insulin but low relative to the elevation of blood cortisol and glucagon levels, were responsible for a significant rise in nonesterified fatty acid levels. Both serum growth hormone and cortisol concentrations were higher in patients with pancreatitis than in patients with other forms of stress. The serum glucagon concentration was 10 times higher in pancreatitis patients than in other stressed patients. Serum insulin and blood glucose concentrations were elevated in both groups, but twice as high in the stressed group as compared to the pancreatitis patients. Thus, patients with pancreatitis had elevated serum glucagon concentrations with inappropriate levels of insulin and glucose.[111] A more prolonged study of glucose response in acute pancreatitis was carried by Solomon[112] who examined the effect of arginine infusion at three stages after the onset of pancreatitis. The infusion was initially performed at 48 to 72 hours, then between 7 and 10 days, and finally between 18 and 21 days. Arginine stimulation early in the disease demonstrated high glucose and glucagon responses which became normal by three weeks. Both phases of the typical biphasic insulin response to arginine were decreased during the initial assessment. By 3 weeks, the first phase was completely normal whereas the second phase of insulin secretion remained depressed.[46] The first phase is characterized by a rapid release and the second phase by a more prolonged release. Primary diabetes most commonly affects the early-release phase. These authors came to the same conclusion that glucose intolerance occurred as a result of high levels of glucagon and relatively low levels of insulin. Thus, not only the exocrine but also the endocrine pancreas is significantly altered during pancreatitis. Because glucagonemia may resolve precipitously, administration of insulin should be administered with care to avoid dangerous levels of hypoglycemia.[113]

Hypocalcemia

Hypocalcemia, sometimes severe enough to cause tetany, may occur with pancreatitis. For the most part, the decrease in serum calcium is merely a reflection of the hypoalbuminemia that occurs and in this case ionized (i.e., nonprotein-bound) calcium levels remain at normal or near normal levels.[114,115] Although the exact incidence is unknown, occasionally in severe pancreatitis a reduction in the level of ionized calcium may occur. Several explanations have been proposed: (1) loss of calcium by precipitation of calcium salts into areas of fat necrosis;[116] (2) a decrease in parathyroid hormone (PTH) release from parathyroid glands;[117] (3) diminution of the activity of the parathyroid hormone as a result of serum proteases and alpha$_2$-macroglobulin complexes; (4) failure of bony tissues to respond to released parahormone;[118] and (5) enhanced release of thyrocalcitonin.[119] The issue remains unsettled.[120]

Coagulation Response

Clinically significant coagulopathy is uncommon in patients with acute pancreatitis but is reported.[121] In patients with severe acute pancreatitis, it is common, however, to find evidence of fibrinogen degradation production in the blood for a few days.[121-123] A drop in platelet count during the initial phase of acute pancreatitis which, together with a shortening of the clotting time compared to controls has been taken to indicate a degree of intravascular coagulation.[121,122] The behavior of plasminogen as an indicator of activation of the fibrinolytic system has been documented by Lasson and associates[122] with the levels being below 75% of normal in the first 6 days of severe attacks.

Immune Response

The macrophage produces alpha$_2$-macroglobulin which is responsible for binding circulatory trypsin. The alpha$_2$-macroglobulin complex retains some proteolytic activity but is rapidly removed from the circulation by the reticuloendothelial system. Marked depletion of alpha$_2$-macroglobulin occurs in necrotizing pancreatitis and has been used as a screening test to identify patients with necrotizing pancreatitis.[99] The macrophage is also responsible for clearance from the peripheral circulation of the alpha$_2$-macroglobulin trypsin complex, which has a half-life of 8 to 10 minutes. Stimulation of the macrophages with glycan which increases its secretory phagocytic activity has been reported to increase survival in ethionine pancreatitis when administered as late as 12 hours after initiation of the ethionine diet.[124]

PRE-ICU PHASE—"RISK PHASE"

The three diagnostic objectives in the management of pancreatitis include:

- Confirmation of the diagnosis of pancreatitis
- Establishment of the etiology of pancreatitis
- Definition of the severity of pancreatitis

Confirmation of the Diagnosis (Differential Diagnosis)

In the patient who presents with abdominal pain, nausea, and vomiting and is suspected of having pancreatitis, the differential diagnosis must include perforated peptic ulcer and acute cholecystitis. Less frequently hepatic abscess, cholangitis, right lower lobe lung abscess or pneumonia, ureteral calculus, myocardial infarction expanding abdominal, aortic, or visceral aneurysm may simulate acute pancreatitis.

History

The epigastric pain of acute pancreatitis is likely to radiate straight through to the back whereas in patients with acute cholecystitis the pain often radiates around to the back. With perforated ulcer, the onset of pain is usually abrupt and immediately disabling. A history of alcoholism or biliary disease is seen both in patients with acute pancreatitis, perforated ulcer, or acute cholecystitis.

Physical Examination

Eighty percent of patients with acute pancreatitis have a rather mild course and on abdominal palpation are found to have only deep abdominal tenderness.[125] In contrast, patients with perforated ulcer usually have a diffusely tender abdomen with guarding spasm and rebound. Patients with acute cholecystitis usually have either a mass in the right upper quadrant or guarding and tenderness limited to that region. The 20% of patients with severe pancreatitis will usually have abdominal distension, guarding, and tenderness. Tympany over the liver, of course, establishes the presence of a perforated viscus.

Ancillary Studies

Although pancreatitis may be suspected based on the history and physical examination, objective studies are needed to confirm the diagnosis of acute pancreatitis and rule out other conditions. Formally, this was a process of elimination in which other surgically correctable causes of abdominal pain such as perforated viscus and acute cholecystitis were ruled out before the diagnosis of pancreatitis could be entertained. Now with the use of the CT scan, the diagnosis of pancreatitis can be established directly. The workup of the patient with abdominal pain suspected to be pancreatitis should include a flat plate and upright film of the abdomen, WBC, serum amylase and urine analysis. The flat plate and upright of the abdomen or upright chest radiograph will show free air in 80% of patients with a perforated ulcer. Should no free air be apparent on the flat plate and upright of the abdomen and the diagnosis of perforated ulcer still be suspected, then a water soluble contrast swallow should be performed to settle the issue. The chest film may also provide other information about some of the complications of pancreatitis including pleural effusions or fistulas, mediastinal extension of a pseudocyst, atelectasis, and noncardiac pulmonary edema. On the abdominal film, gas bubbles are associated with an abscess; an isolated air-filled loop of small bowel (Sentinel loop) and cut off of air in the transverse colon may indicate a localized ileus secondary to pancreatitis; an absent left psoas shadow may indicate retroperitoneal peripancreatic inflammation and intraductal calcification indicates the pancreatitis is an acute exacerbation of chronic pancreatitis.[126]

Serum Amylase

The serum amylase test often helps in establishing the pancreas as the source of the patient's pain. The serum amylase test is nonspecific for pancreatitis, however, and may be both falsely negative and falsely positive. The level of serum amylase is not an indication of severity of pancreatitis but reflects the summation of three independent factors. The serum level of amylase is dependent on amylase production by a viable acinar cell, the degree of ductal obstruction, and renal clearance of amylase. Ductal obstruction impedes secretion into the ductal lumen and results in amylase being diverted into the interstitium of the gland where it is picked up by the venous capillaries or extravasated through the capsule of the pancreas into the abdominal cavity where it is picked up by the abdominal lymphatics and returned to the thoracic duct. False-positive amylase elevations can occur from nonpancreatic amylase (e.g., parotitis secondary to mumps) or from macroamylasemia in which amylase is bound to a larger molecule not cleared by the glomerulus or in instances of perforated peptic ulcer when pancreatic juice exists in the duodenum of the abdominal cavity and is returned to the venous blood through the abdominal lymphatics and thoracic duct. Intestinal obstruction, ruptured ectopic pregnancy, and mesenteric ischemia may also cause elevated levels of amylase.[127]

False-negative amylase determinations may result from necrosis of a large portion of the pancreas so that even in the presence of ductal obstruction, serum levels of amylase do not become elevated. Hypertriglyceridemia interferes in the colorometric determination of serum amylase and may cause a falsely negative test. Either diluting the serum if it shows evidence of lipemia or obtaining a urinary amylase or serum lipase may unmask the problem. Acute exacerbations of chronic pancreatitis may not be associated with elevated levels of serum amylase because there may be few remaining viable acinar. The sensitivity of the serum amylase test is generally reported to be around 90%, although in one series of alcoholic pancreatitis, for reasons already mentioned (hyperlipidemia, destruction of acinar tissue), it was as low as 68%.[128] Typically, serum amylase increases very early in the course of the disease, reaching a peak that is at least five times the upper limit of normal. The serum amylase often declines rapidly, however, returning to normal within 24 to 72 hours. An amylase elevation may be missed if the assessment is made after the first day or two of the illness. In such an event, an increased urinary amylase which persists longer than serum amylase, can be helpful in the diagnosis.[129] Pancreatic isoamylase is seldom readily available and has no great advantage over total amylase. The amylase creatine ratio is unreliable. Serum elevations of lipase are thought by some to persist longer than amylase elevations. Like amylase, lipase can be elevated in cholelithiasis and choledocholithiasis. There seems to be no major advantage to utilizing lipase rather than or in addition to serum amylase.

Although the CT scan has shown its greatest usefulness in the identification of patients with necrotizing pancreatitis through the vascular enhancement, it has also proven useful in establishing the diagnosis of pancreatitis. Pancreatic enlargement, peripancreatic inflammation, ascites, and pleural fistulas are findings which not only substantiate the diagnosis of pancreatitis but provide information about the severity of the disease.

Assessing the Etiology of Pancreatitis

The second diagnostic objective in assessing patients with pancreatitis is to identify the etiology of pancreatitis. The distinction regarding etiology is important to make in order to institute specific and appropriate therapy (e.g., insecticide-induced pancreatitis, gallstone pancreatitis, hyperlipidemic pancreatitis). Of the two most frequent causes of pancreatitis alcoholism is treated nonoperatively and gallstone disease operatively. The patient's history is important in recognizing the role of alcohol, but some patients may have both a history of alcoholism and gallstone disease. Biochemical studies of liver function show some statistically significant differences when groups of patients with alcoholic and gallstone pancreatitis are compared.[130-132] Elevations of bilirubin over 4 mg/dl and elevated alkaline phosphatase values in the presence of normal serum albumin are more compatible with gallstone pancreatitis.

The presence of lipemic serum from markedly elevated levels of triglycerides identifies a high risk group for severe pancreatitis. Hypertriglycerdemia is seen in some alcoholics after a drinking binge and as a primary inherited hyperlipoproteinemia in others. Occasional cases are associated with the use of isoretonin (Accutane), which is used in the treatment of acne and which may cause a marked and usually reversible hypertriglyceridemia in some patients.

In individual patients when the decision to operate is being weighed, precise information is required regarding the etiology of pancreatitis. Although ultrasound is not useful in assessing the pancreas in patients with acute pancreatitis,[133] it is useful in identifying patients with gallstone disease and providing information about the size of the stones. The smaller (2 to 4 mm) stones are most likely to precipitate gallstone pancreatitis.[134] Larger stones seldom reach the ampulla whereas smaller ones pass without causing symptoms. In the absence of ultrasound evidence of gallstones and a history of alcoholism, operations on the biliary tract are not indicated in acute pancreatitis.

The distinction between gallstone pancreatitis and acute cholecystitis may be difficult to make clinically and biochemically, or by ultrasound. Both show evidence of gallstones on ultrasound and the thickness of the gallbladder wall is not always a reliable indicator of acute cholecystitis. The HIDA scan if it shows function of the gallbladder rules out cystic duct obstruction, the sine qua non of acute cholecystitis. Some patients with unobstructed cystic ducts with acute pancreatitis have gallbladders that are not visible on an HIDA scan for several weeks after the pancreatitis attack has subsided.[135,136] These patients may or may not have gallstones. The patients that do not have gallstones will be identified on ultrasonography and an unnecessary operation will be avoided. Regarding the patients with gallstones, the distinction as to whether they have gallstone pancreatitis or acute cholecystitis is not as important as that the biliary disease should be corrected operatively in either case before they leave the hospital. Patients having both a history of alcoholism and biliary tract disease should have their biliary tract disease eliminated. In such patients it is impossible to know with certainty, in the absence of changes compatible with chronic pancreatitis, whether the patient's symptoms were due to alcoholism or gallstones. Patients leaving the hospital without their biliary being corrected have a 30% chance of having another attack of pancreatitis from another stone passing from the gallbladder and the ampulla within 3 months of hospital discharge.[135-137]

There has been much written about the timing of operative or endoscopic intervention in gallstone pancreatitis. While there is uniform agreement that patients should not go home without correction of their biliary pathology,[136] there is disagreement as to whether urgent (24 to 48 hours after onset of symptoms) choledocholithotomy or endoscopic sphincterotomy reduces the mortality and morbidity of gallstone pancreatitis.[130]

Evidence indicates that the earlier operative or endoscopic sphincterotomy is initiated after the onset of gallstone pancreatitis, the higher will be the evidence of common duct stones (0 to 75%) at 24 to 48 hours.[136,138,139] Within 5 to 7 days, however, 85 to 90% of stones will pass spontaneously through the ampulla into the duodenum.[134] Acosta[138] postulated that operative intervention within 24 to 48 hours after the onset of symptoms would reduce the incidence of necrotizing pancreatitis and lower the mortality of gallstone pancreatitis by eliminating any stones impacted at the ampulla. When compared to his historical controls, he reduced the mortality of gallstone pancreatitis from 16 to 2.9%. This is admirable; however, the incidence of necrotizing pancreatitis in his early operation series was not reduced. When his historical controls (86 patients) were compared with the early operative group (46 patients) the incidence of necrosis found at operation was 10.5% versus 18%, respectively. Clearly, the reduction in mortality that Acosta reported in his early operative group compared to his historical controls group was not achieved by reducing the incidence of necrotizing pancreatitis by early operative intervention but probably attributable to improved surgical ICU management of the severely ill patient according to Frey.[135] The only purpose served by early or late operation is the prevention of a second attack of pancreatitis not the prevention of necrotizing pancreatitis, which Acosta's own data show is already present at 24 to 48 hours following the onset of symptoms. Kelly,[140] in a randomized study of gallstone pancreatitis, comparing only less than 48 hours versus more than 48 hours operative intervention also confirmed that the incidence of edematous and necrotizing pancreatitis occurred with the same frequency in the early and late group.

Stone[99,139] has also reported a low mortality rate (2.7%) with early operative intervention in patients with gallstone pancreatitis. Sphincterotomy was performed in all his patients in addition to cholecystectomy. Endoscopic sphincterotomy has been recommended by Safrany and Cotton[141] as a less invasive method than operative sphincterotomy and Neoptolemos reported favorably on a prospective experience with endoscopic sphincterotomy. Safrany's and Cotton's study,[141] the Neoptolemos study,[142,143] and Stone's study[139] while randomized took little account of the severity of illness of the patients with gallstone pancreatitis. Of even greater concern is the lack of evidence presented by any of these authors to justify sphincterotomy. Sphincterotomy for removal of stones of the common bile duct performed less than 48 hours does not prevent necrotizing pancreatitis. It is already present according to the literature. The patients with necrotizing pancreatitis infrequently have an impacted stone at the ampulla. How then does sphincterotomy help these patients? In all probability it does not,[144] but it does subject them to the risk of other complications. Kelly[140] found that only 2 of 13 patients who died after early surgery had an impacted stone whereas 8 of the 13 had necrotizing pancreatitis. Ranson[145] has opposed early operative intervention on the biliary tract in patients who are severely ill citing an increased mortality in patients operated on "early" for gallstones pancreatitis versus an initially nonoperative group. Among 74 patients his operative and nonoperative group of 14 patients had a Ranson score of 3.5, however. Therefore, his conclusion that early operation is associated with a higher mortality than nonoperation or delayed operation has lost some of its force because the 2 groups were not comparable in severity.

As we have come to know more about the natural history of gallstone pancreatitis and the onset of the necrotizing process, however, the so-called early operation 24 to 48 hours is probably already too late to prevent the development of the necrotizing process nor in the preponderance of patients who die of pancreatitis do we find an impacted stone. In patients with gallstone pancreatitis in whom necrosis is evident on CT scan with vascular enhancement performed on admission, priority should be given to managing the necrotizing process by vigorous fluid resuscitation.[136] Operative or endoscopic elimination of the biliary tract disease should be put on hold until the patient has recovered from the local and systemic complications associated with necrotizing pancreatitis. An exception to this recommendation would be the patient with documented common bile duct obstruction and cholangitis. The reason operation or endoscopic elimination of the biliary tract pathology takes a low priority in the patient with necrotizing pancreatitis is that the only purpose served by eliminating the biliary tract pathology is prevention of a recurrent attack of gallstone pancreatitis. Elimination of the biliary tract pathology will not reverse or ameliorate the pancreatic necrosis already present. The folly of early operative intervention in patients with severe pancreatitis was documented by Kelly[140] in 165 patients graded for severity. Among 83 patients operated on (< 48 hours), there was a 15% mortality whereas those operated on 3 to 7 days had a mortality of 2.4%. When only the severe cases were analyzed, Ranson's score greater than 3, the mortality was 38.8% and for delayed surgery, 11%. Kelly confirmed that the incidence of necrotizing pancreatitis was the same in the early and late operative group. Mortality was attributed not to the impacted stone but to necrotizing pancreatitis.

In summary, patients with alcoholic pancreatitis biliary tracts who are operated on are receiving unnecessary and meddlesome surgery. The 80 to 90% or more of patients with gallstone pancreatitis without severe pancreatitis should have their biliary tract pathology eliminated before leaving the hospital. Operations on the biliary tract during the initial management of patients with gallstone pancreatitis and evidence of necrosis on CT scan with vascular enhancement serve no useful purpose and should be delayed until the patient has recovered from the episode of necrotizing pancreatitis.

Table 52-5. Systemic Signs of Severe Acute Pancreatitis

Unusual systemic signs
　Coma
　Body wall ecchymosis (Cullen sign, Grey Turner sign)
　Severe hypocalcemia
　Subcutaneous fat necrosis
　Disseminated intravascular coagulation
Common systemic signs
　Abdominal pain radiating to back
　Vomiting
　Jaundice
　Paralytic ileus and abdominal distention
　Capillary leak (Hypovolemia, hemoconcentration, hypotension)
　Tachypnea
　Pleural effusion
　Multiple organ failure (respiratory insufficiency, renal insufficiency, cardiac insufficiency)
　Liver failure

Table 52-6. Eleven Ranson's Signs Used to Classify the Severity of Pancreatitis (Death or Complications)

At admission or diagnosis
　Age over 55 years
　White blood cell count over 16,000/mm³
　Blood glucose over 200 mg/100 ml
　Serum lactic dehydrogenase over 350 IU/L
　Serum glutamic oxaloacetic transaminase over 250 Sigma-Frankel U %
During the initial 48 hours
　Hematocrit fall greater than 10 percentage points
　Blood urea nitrogen rise more than 5 mg/100 ml
　Arterial PO_2 below 60 mm Hg
　Base deficit greater than 4 mEq/L
　Estimated fluid sequestration more than 6000 ml
　Serum calcium level < 8 mg/ml

Assessing the Severity of Pancreatitis

The third diagnostic objective in the assessment of patients is determining the severity of the pancreatitis. Roughly 80% of patients with acute pancreatitis will have edematous or interstitial pancreatitis. Ten percent of patients with acute pancreatitis will develop pseudocysts and 10% pancreatic and peripancreatic necrosis.[87] Signs of clinical severity are listed in Table 52-5. Our objective is to identify the 10 to 20% of patients with pancreatitis and peripancreatic necrosis. This is best achieved in pancreatitis by anatomic and physiologic indices of severity which in part reflect the local complications of pancreatitis including pancreatic and peripancreatic necrosis, infected pancreatic and peripancreatic necrosis, fluid collections, pseudocysts, and fat sequestra. The definitions and descriptions are detailed by Frey, Beger, and Bradley.[146]

Severity of illness indices serve several functions. They are important in predicating various outcomes such as death, infection of necrotic pancreas, complications, comparing results of various therapies or results of treatment between institutions or as a quality assurance tool.

Severity of illness predictors is essential in the management of patients with pancreatitis as the clinical assessment at the time of hospital admission regarding survival[147] and development of infection[91] are inaccurate. McMahon[147] found the initial clinical assessment of pancreatitis identified only 39% of those with severe attacks. Fink[91] reported that 72% of patients who subsequently developed pancreatic infections had at the time of hospital admission a rather benign clinical appearance and course initially and less than three Ranson signs and were not thought to be at risk of serious complications such as infection. Ranson's signs were not predictive of death in this series (fewer than three Ranson signs, 65% of deaths and 74% of survivors). Ranson has identified seven signs of severity which he feels are more likely to be predictive of sepsis than his 11 signs.[148]

Physiologic Indices

Ranson's signs[110] are an important contribution to our ability to assess the severity of pancreatitis and are widely used by clinicians in the United States, Europe, and Japan (Tables 52-6 and 52-7). Five observations are made on admission, (i.e., the age of the patient, white blood cell count, blood glucose and liver functions); six observations are made 48 hours later (i.e., the fall of the hematocrit following hydration and the amount of fluid required to produce this fall, the degree of metabolic acidosis reflecting the degree of shock, inadequate tissue perfusion and an assessment of renal and pulmonary function).

In a group of 450 patients with acute pancreatitis, Ranson observed a mortality rate of 9% when there were fewer than 3 positive signs, 16% for patients with 3 or 4 prognostic signs, 40% when 5 or 6 signs were present and 100% in patients with 7 or more signs. The frequency with which patients survived but required more than a week of intensive care was 3% for 2 or fewer signs, 24% for 3 or 4 signs, and 53% for 5 or 6 signs.[110] Most of these patients (70%) were alcoholics. Ranson later modified the criteria for the predictors of severe pancreatitis in gallstones,[149] (see Table 52-7) and in predicting sepsis.

Other investigators including Blamey[150] and Banks[151] have developed physiologic criteria with similar characteristics and ability to predict mortality as the Ranson signs.

The Acute Physiology and Chronic Health Evaluation (APACHE) II score developed by Knaus (Fig. 52-3), is a widely used predictor of the severity of illness.[152] The power of the score to predict mortality is greatest when applied to patients with the same disease process. Various investigations have applied the APACHE II score on hospital admission, daily on surgical ICU admission or immediately prior to operation. Misapplication of the score gives

Table 52-7. Ranson's Prognostic Signs in Patients Known to Have Pancreatitis Due to Biliary Stones

At admission or diagnosis
　Age over 70 years
　White blood cell count over 18,000/mm³
　Serum lactic dehydrogenase over 400 IU/L
　Glutamic oxaloacetic transaminase over 250 Sigma-Frankel U %
During the initial 48 hours
　Hematocrit fall greater than 10 percentage points
　Blood urea nitrogen rise more than 2 mg/100 ml
　Base deficit greater than 5 mEq/L
　Fluid sequestration more than 4000 ml

PHYSIOLOGIC VARIABLE	HIGH ABNORMAL RANGE					LOW ABNORMAL RANGE			
	+4	+3	+2	+1	0	+1	+2	+3	+4
TEMPERATURE rectal (°C)	≥41°	39°–40.9°		38.5°–38.9°	36°–38.4°	34°–35.9°	32°–33.9°	30°–31.9°	≤29.9°
MEAN ARTERIAL PRESSURE — mm Hg	≥160	130–159	110–129		70–109		50–69		≤49
HEART RATE (ventricular response)	≥180	140–179	110–139		70–109		55–69	40–54	≤39
RESPIRATORY RATE (non ventilated or ventilated)	≥50	35–49		25–34	12–24	10–11	6–9		≤5
OXYGENATION A-aDO$_2$ or PaO$_2$ (mm Hg) a. FIO$_2$ ≥ 0.5 record A-aDO$_2$	≥500	350–499	200–349		<200				
b. FIO$_2$ < 0.5 record only PaO$_2$					PO$_2$ >70	PO$_2$ 61–70		PO$_2$ 55–60	PO$_2$ <55
ARTERIAL pH	≥7.7	7.6–7.69		7.5–7.59	7.33–7.49		7.25–7.32	7.15–7.24	<7.15
SERUM SODIUM (mMol/L)	≥180	160–179	155–159	150–154	130–149		120–129	111–119	≤110
SERUM POTASSIUM (mMol/L)	≥7	6–6.9		5.5–5.9	3.5–5.4	3–3.4	2.5–2.9		<2.5
SERUM CREATININE (mg/100 ml) (Double point score for acute renal failure)	≥3.5	2–3.4	1.5–1.9		0.6–1.4		<0.6		
HEMATOCRIT (%)	≥60		50–59.9	46–49.9	30–45.9		20–29.9		<20
WHITE BLOOD COUNT (total/mm3) (in 1,000s)	≥40		20–39.9	15–19.9	3–14.9		1–2.9		<1
GLASGOW COMA SCORE (GCS) Score = 15 minus actual GCS									
A Total ACUTE PHYSIOLOGY SCORE (APS) Sum of the 12 individual variable points									
Serum HCO$_3$ (venous mMol/L) (Not preferred, use if no ABGs)	≥52	41–51.9		32–40.9	22–31.9		18–21.9	15–17.9	<15

B AGE POINTS:
Assign points to age as follows:

AGE (yrs)	Points
≤ 44	0
45-54	2
55-64	3
65-74	5
≥ 75	6

C CHRONIC HEALTH POINTS
If the patient has a history of severe organ system insufficiency or is immuno-compromised assign points as follows:
a. for nonoperative or emergency postoperative patients — 5 points
or
b. for elective postoperative patients — 2 points

DEFINITIONS
Organ insufficiency or immuno-compromised state must have been evident prior to this hospital admission and conform to the following criteria:

LIVER: Biopsy proven cirrhosis and documented portal hypertension; episodes of past upper GI bleeding attributed to portal hypertension; or prior episodes of hepatic failure/encephalopathy/coma.

CARDIOVASCULAR: New York Heart Association Class IV.

RESPIRATORY: Chronic restrictive, obstructive, or vascular disease resulting in severe exercise restriction, i.e., unable to climb stairs or perform household duties; or documented chronic hypoxia, hypercapnia, secondary polycythemia, severe pulmonary hypertension (>40mmHg), or respirator dependency.

RENAL: Receiving chronic dialysis.

IMMUNO-COMPROMISED: The patient has received therapy that suppresses resistance to infection, e.g., immuno-suppression, chemotherapy, radiation, long term or recent high dose steroids, or has a disease that is sufficiently advanced to suppress resistance to infection, e.g., leukemia, lymphoma, AIDS.

APACHE II SCORE
Sum of A + B + C
A APS points
B Age points
C Chronic Health points
Total APACHE II

Fig. 52–3. The APACHE II severity of disease classification system. (From Knaus, W. A., et al.: APACHE II: a severity of disease classification system. Crit. Care Med., *13*:818, 1985.)

erroneous information. Civetta[153] has pointed out some of the limitations of the APACHE II, particularly with regard to the timing of its application and to its use for "cost containment and quality assurance" when applied to surgical patients. He found the APACHE II when applied to patients in the surgical ICU immediately postoperatively did not account sufficiently for the effect of the recent therapeutic intervention by surgeon and anesthesiologist. He concluded the APACHE II was not designed to predict problems after surgical ICU admissions of high risk postoperative surgical patients, and was not predictive of outcome for patients with long-term stays among surgical ICU patients.

The score has been validated, however, in more than 6000 ICU patients from multiple institutions and when applied appropriately provides an accurate reproducible prognostic index which permits identification of patients needing aggressive monitoring and therapy is predictive of mortality and permits interinstitutional comparison of treatment results and can be used for internal quality assurance.

The APACHE II score when applied as we have done on the day of admission has several advantages over the Ranson score. The Ranson score has only been validated for use in the first 48 hours after the onset of symptoms. Therefore, it is of no value in determining the severity of illness in patients who are transferred from other hospitals 48 or more hours after the onset of illness. The greatest advantage of the APACHE II score is that the information to calculate the score is available on the day of admission whereas only 5 of the 11 Ranson signs are available at that time. Even at 48 hours, Larvin and McMahon[154] in 290 patients with acute pancreatitis found that the APACHE II score is a more accurate predicator of the outcome than the Ranson's signs. APACHE II correctly predicted the outcome in 88% of attacks, the Ranson score 69% and the Imrie score 84%. Larvin and McMahon[154] reported that they had no survivors with an APACHE II score over 20. Other investigators have applied the APACHE II to their patients with acute pancreatitis and have found it highly predictive of outcome with regard to survival. Using the APACHE II score, Demmy[155] reported a 33% mortality rate for patients with a score of 16 to 20. No survivors had a score higher than 20.

Among a group of 50 consecutive patients with necrotizing pancreatitis admitted to our surgical ICU, data on the APACHE II score was available on 45 at the time of admission.[156] All seven deaths were predicted on the day of hospital admission by the APACHE II score. The range of scores for survivors was 4 to 27 and 25 to 43 for nonsurvivors. Of the 8 patients with a score greater than or equal to 25, 7 died. All patients with a score less than 25 survived. Using a score of 25 or greater to predict mortality, all 7 deaths would have been accurately predicted and a single survivor would have been predicted to die. All patients with a score of less than 25 would have been accurately predicted to survive. The APACHE II system can be used for quality assurance purposes as a screen assisting in the identification of patients predicted to survive that did not. Last, by applying this system as a uniform index of severity, meaningful evaluation of alternative therapies and comparison of interinstitutional results can be undertaken.

Anatomic Predictors of Severity

The physiologic severity of illness predictors are notoriously inaccurate when identifying patients with necrosis, the group at risk of developing infection. Using Ranson's criteria, Fink[70] found only 28% of patients developing a pancreatic abscess were identified on admission as having severe pancreatitis by Ranson's criteria. Applying the APACHE II score at 48 hours, Larvin and McMahon[154] found that the APACHE II predicted 73% of pancreatic collections. Ranson's signs predicted 65%[4,110] and Imrie's signs 58%.[78,156]

Peritoneal lavage has been evaluated as a technique for predicting the severity of acute pancreatitis by McMahon[241] who compared the accuracy of lavage with clinical assessment. Aspiration of 20 ml of free fluid, aspiration of dark free fluid, or return of infused fluid that was straw-colored or darker was considered an indication of severe pancreatitis by McMahon. Lavage and clinical assessment were carried out at the time of hospital admission. Clinical assessment correctly predicted only 39% of severe attacks compared with a 72% success rate for diagnostic lavage. The mild attacks were correctly predicted by clinical assessment while lavage was wrong in 3 of 61 patients (95% success rate).

Diagnostic peritoneal lavage is an accurate early guide to the severity of pancreatitis but because it is an invasive procedure it has little chance of acceptance by many physicians. It would have to be employed on all hospitalized patients with pancreatitis, many of whom do not appear to be seriously ill by clinical criteria. Peritoneal lavage would be useless if used selectively by physicians whose ability to clinically identify severely ill patients on hospital admission is only 28%.

The CT scan with vascular enhancement, a technique developed by Kivisaari, Somer[157] and widely used in Europe[83,158] and the United States[136,160,161] makes it possible to identify all patients with pancreatic necrosis and peripancreatic inflammation fluid and fat necrosis on the day of hospital admission. This group of patients constitutes approximately 15 to 20% of all patients presenting with acute pancreatitis. Of those patients with necrotizing pancreatitis identified by CT scan with vascular enhancement, between 40 to 80% will become infected.[6,83,159] In general, the greater the extent of necrosis the greater the risk of infection. This technique, however, while highly accurate in identifying patients with pancreatic necrosis[160] and peripancreatic alterations is unable to reliably distinguish the nature of the peripancreatic collections which may consist of necrotic or liquified fat, fluid, pancreatic juice, or inflammation.

We have further graded the peripancreatic fluid collections from 1 to 5, depending on their extent but neither the presence of necrosis or the extent of the peripancreatic fluid collection had a direct bearing on survival, but did successfully predict those patients at risk of infections.

Table 52-8. Balthazar's CT Grades of Severity

Grade A: normal
Grade B: focal or diffuse pancreatic edema with no peripancreatic disease
Grade C: pancreatic abnormality with inflammation restricted to peripancreatic fat
Grade D: a phlegmon present or fluid collection within or adjacent to the pancreas
Grade E: two or more fluid collections

The relationship between the extent of the peripancreatic inflammatory process and infection was recognized by Balthazar[161] (Table 52-8) even before the CT scan with vascular enhancement began to be used widely. In a grading system from A to E based on the extent of the peripancreatic process, he found infectious complications most common in his patients with extensive peripancreatic fluid and inflammation accumulations which he designated grades D and E.

CT scan with vascular enhancement is also predicative of diabetes. When there is failure of enhancement of the entire pancreas then diabetes will develop in patients who have been nondiabetic (Fig. 52-4). Two of our 50 patients were accurately predicted to become diabetic[6] on the basis of the CT scan with vascular enhancement showing virtually total necrosis. Similarly, this technique is also predictive of those patients who will develop pancreatic fistulas or pseudocysts. When a segment of the body of the pancreas is necrosis and the tail viable, then we can safely predict that a pancreatic fistula or pseudocyst will develop if the patient does not become infected (Fig. 52-5).

Authors such as Gebhardt[162] have recommended the use of endoscopic retrograde cholangiopancreatography (ERCP) early in the course of necrotizing pancreatitis to identify patients with pancreatic fistulas, a predictor of necrosis. In their institution, patients with extravasation of contrast from the main duct are considered to be operative candidates for resection of the pancreas distal to the fistula. We do not subscribe to this belief. A large percentage of patients with main duct extravasation do not become infected. Managing a pseudocyst or pancreatic fistula at a later time is associated with less morbidity and mortality than resecting a portion of the pancreas in an acutely ill or septic patient.

Applying CT scan with vascular enhancement to all patients in order to identify the 20% with pancreatic necrosis is expensive. The immediate availability and accuracy of screening measures for pancreatic necrosis leave something to be desired, however. C-reactive protein and levels of alpha$_2$-macroglobulin are two tests that in European reports have shown significant differences among patients with interstitial or edematous pancreatitis as compared to those with necrotizing pancreatitis[163,164] (Figs. 52-6 and 52-7). Ferguson[165] was unable to duplicate their results, however, based on CT scan evidence of pancreatic necrosis. Il-6 and PMN elastase have also been found to be elevated in the serum of patients with pancreatic necrosis.[166,167] PMN elastase peaks hours after the onset of necrotizing pancreatitis, Il-6 within 24 hours, and CRP within 72 hours. Correlation of these serum tests with the

1028   THE HIGH RISK PATIENT: MANAGEMENT OF THE CRITICALLY ILL

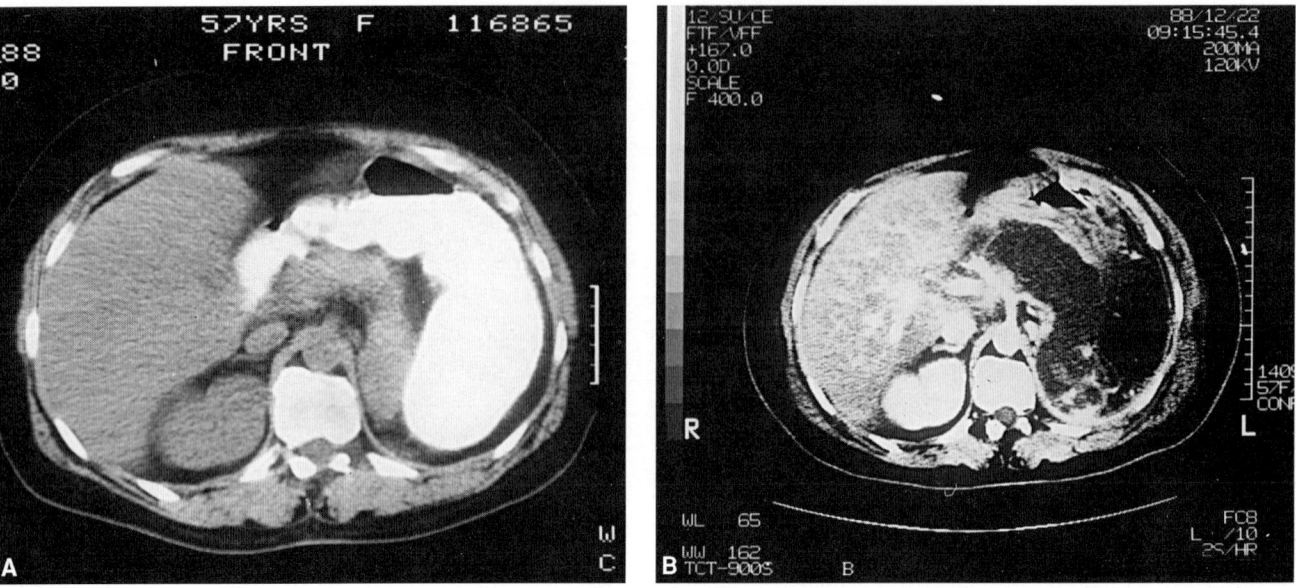

Fig. 52–4. A, Oral contrast only. B, Contrast enhancement shows virtually complete nonopacification of the pancreas.

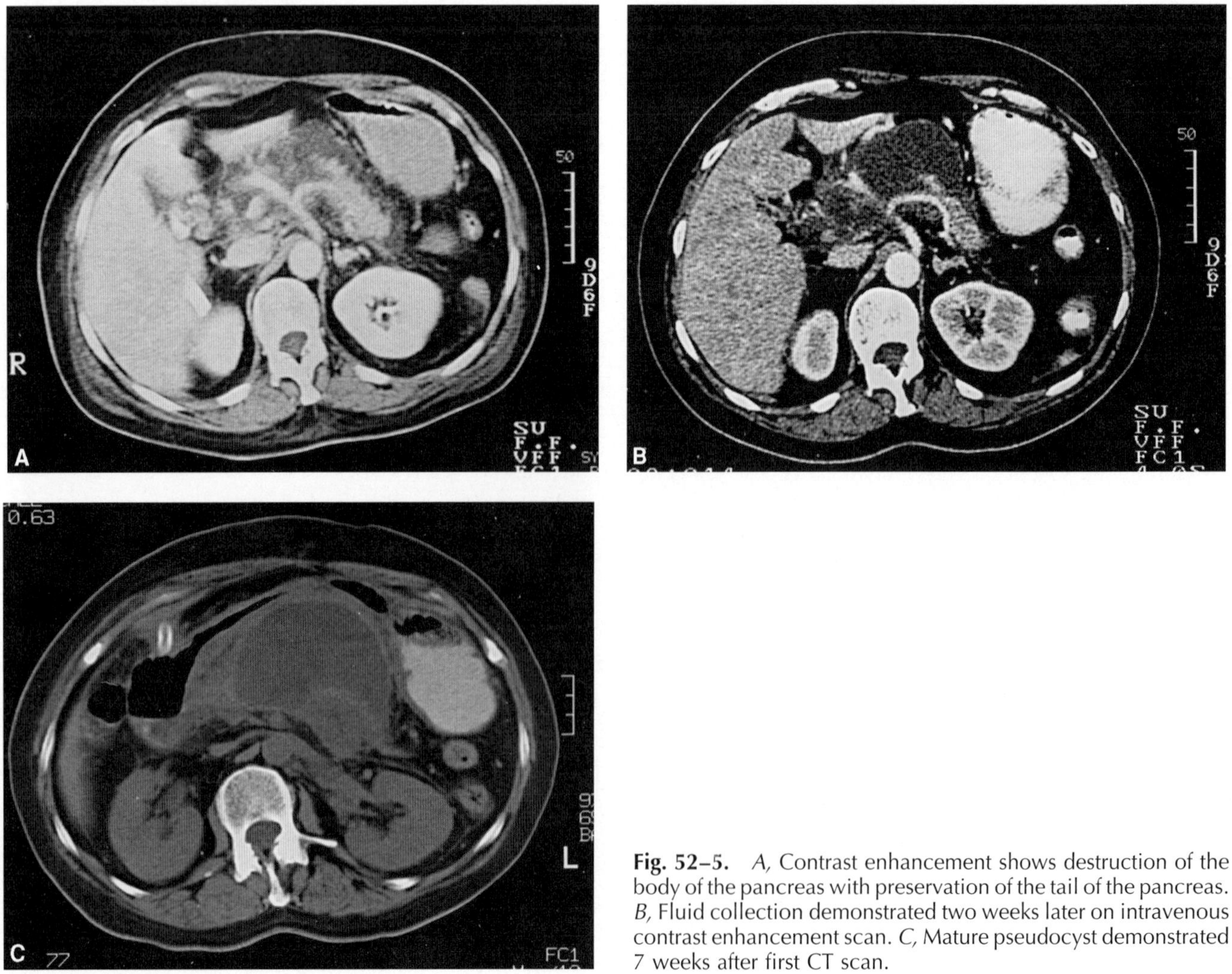

Fig. 52–5. A, Contrast enhancement shows destruction of the body of the pancreas with preservation of the tail of the pancreas. B, Fluid collection demonstrated two weeks later on intravenous contrast enhancement scan. C, Mature pseudocyst demonstrated 7 weeks after first CT scan.

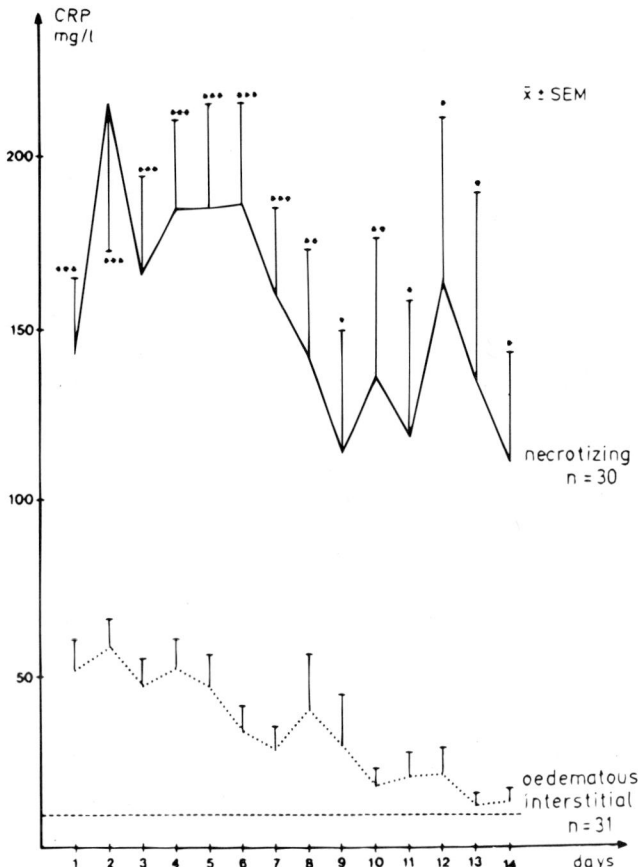

Fig. 52–6. Serum values for C-reactive protein (CRP) in 61 patients with acute pancreatitis.

extent of pancreatic and peripancreatic necrosis as evidenced by CT scan findings needs to be studied.

There is not an immediate solution to the problem of identifying patients with necrotizing pancreatitis the day they come to the hospital. Peritoneal lavage is an invasive study that would have to be performed on all patients with pancreatitis because clinical identification of patients with necrosis is highly inaccurate. The procedure, while accurate in identifying patients with necrosis, does not provide information about the extent and location of pancreatic and peripancreatic necrosis. Serum methemalbumin by the calorimetric technique has not proven to be highly accurate because of overlapping spectra with other breakdown products of hemoglobin. The stoichiometric method overcomes these technical problems, but has not been sufficiently validated in a group of patients having both mild and severe acute pancreatitis.[168] While accurate in predicting survival, the physiologic indices of severity may not be as helpful in identifying patients with necrotizing pancreatitis, some of whom have a relatively benign clinical presentation. At present, the only option other than performing CT scan with vascular enhancement on all patients with acute pancreatitis, a practice which can be criticized on the basis of cost and the fact that only 20% of patients tested will have necrosis is to compromise and use some less than perfect method of assessing the presence or absence of necrosis. As a start, perhaps, all patients with APACHE II scores of seven or above should have CT scan with vascular enhancement. If this had been done it would have identified 44 of our 46 patients with necrotizing pancreatitis in whom we had APACHE scores. We have no data on how many patients would be subjected to CT scan with vascular enhancement without evidence of necrosis.

Assessment of Infection in Pancreatic Necrosis

The manifestations of pancreatic necrosis and those of sepsis may be difficult to differentiate as both can be associated with a capillary leak, large fluid losses, a hyperdynamic circulation, increased insulin requirements, and multiple organ failure.

Temporally, systemic manifestations of necrosis occur at the outset of pancreatitis and tend to diminish with time, so by 7 to 14 days they are usually on the wane. Manifestations of sepsis seldom become clinically apparent until 7 days after the onset of symptoms of pancreatitis. The highest incidence of infection and sepsis occur 2 to 3 weeks after the onset of symptoms. Infection of necrotic pancreatic and peripancreatic tissue can occur, however, as late as 6 to 8 weeks after the onset of symptoms (Table 52–9; Beger[169]).

Concern about the presence of infection of necrotic pancreatic or peripancreatic tissue should be raised in any patient in whom fever develops or persists a week or more after the onset of pancreatitis, or if there is an increase in leukocytosis, increased insulin requirement, evidence of a capillary leak, positive fluid balance, deterioration of pulmonary or renal function, coagulation abnormalities, persistent ileus, and increased or persistent tachycardia. The source of the bacterial infection in the necrotic pancreatic and peripancreatic tissue is believed to be the patient's own gastrointestinal tract.[170-174]

Because of the difficult in clinically distinguishing symptoms associated with pancreatic necrosis from those due to sepsis, as well as the need to identify patients with infections so that appropriate therapy can be instituted before they develop septic shock, the technique of CT scan guided aspiration of areas of necrosis has been a welcome addition to our diagnostic armamentarium. This technique of guided aspiration of areas of necrotic pancreatic and peripancreatic tissue for gram stain and culture was developed by Gerzof and Banks.[175]

CT scan with percutaneous aspiration is the earliest and best method of determining the presence of infection in necrotizing pancreatitis. Gerzhof and his colleague reported on 41 episodes with pancreatic sepsis and documented all episodes by the initial aspiration. There were neither false-positive nor false-negative results of needle aspiration. Gram stains revealed organisms in 41 of 42 infected aspirates, and cultures were positive from all 42 infected aspirates. Furthermore, percutaneous aspiration was performed safely in all instances. There were no complications, exacerbations of symptoms, or introduction of infection by this procedure.[175]

Roughly half the patients with more than 10 to 15%

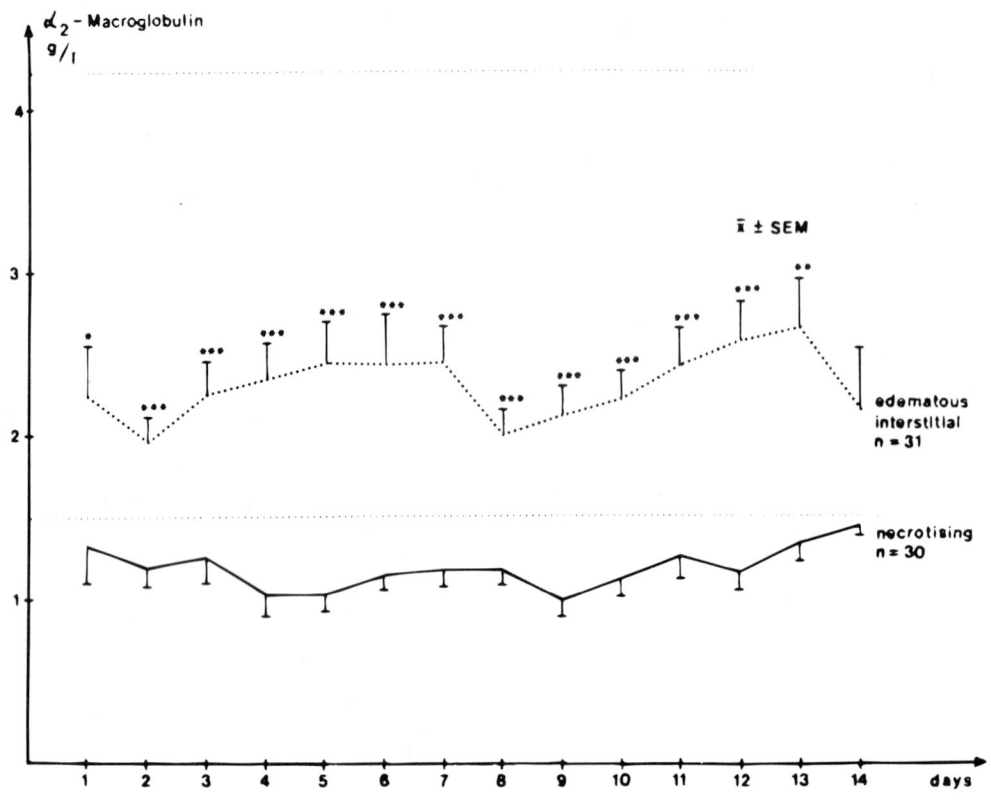

Fig. 52–7. Serum values for alpha₂-macroglobulin in 61 patients with acute pancreatitis.

necrosis as judged by CT scan with vascular enhancement become infected range 40 to 80%.[6,83,159]

ICU PHASE

Admissions Criteria to Surgical ICU

- Clinical assessment of severity
- Evidence of necrosis on CT scan with vascular enhancement
- APACHE II score seven or more

- Infected necrosis
- Pancreatic abscess

Patients with pancreatitis may enter the ICU under a variety of circumstances including: deterioration of their condition following hospitalization; directly from the emergency department; following hospital transfer; from the operating room following drainage or debridement of pancreatic abscess or necrosis.

Criteria for entering the surgical ICU on hospital admission include:

Table 52–9. Clinical Morphologic Parameters in Relation to Bacteriology and the Duration of the Disease at the Time of Operation

Parameters	Duration of Disease at Time of Operation (days)*			
	1–7	8–14	15–21	>21
Bacteriologically positive patients				
Total number of patients	5	8	10	22
Early objective signs (median)	7.0	4.0	3.5	3.0
No. (%) of patients with subtotal or total pancreatic necrosis	3 (60)	3 (38)	3 (30)	6 (27)
No. (%) of patients with extrapancreatic necrosis	4 (80)	7 (88)	8 (80)	8 (36)
No. (%) of deaths	5 (100)	4 (50)	5 (50)	3 (14)
Bacteriologically negative patients				
Total number of patients	16	14	4	35
Early objective signs (median)	4.0	3.0	3.0	2.0
No. (%) of patients with subtotal or total pancreatic necrosis	5 (31)	3 (21)	1 (25)	5 (14)
No. (%) of patients with extrapancreatic necrosis	11 (69)	8 (57)	1 (25)	8 (23)
No. (%) of deaths	2 (13)	—	—	4 (11)

* Since onset of symptoms.
(From Beger, H.G., et al.: Bacterial contamination of pancreatic necrosis: a prospective clinical study. Gastroenterology, 9:433, 1986.)

- All patients with pancreatitis who are septic or requiring mechanical ventilation
- An APACHE II score of 7 or over
- Two or more Ranson's signs
- Infected necrosis
- Pancreatic abscess

Of 50 patients with necrotizing pancreatitis at our institution, 44 of 46 patients who had an APACHE score configured had an APACHE II score of 7 or above. A Ranson score of 2 or above included 40 of 46 patients with necrotizing pancreatitis. A Ranson score of 3 or above would have only identified 34 of 46 patients with necrotizing pancreatitis.[6] Patients who have been operated on for abscesses or infected pancreatic necrosis will usually require intensive care. Additionally, hospital transfers are a high risk category. We have found these patients often more seriously ill than appreciated on the basis of a phone conversation with the referring physician. This may result from the deterioration of the patient en route in a rapidly evolving illness or the gravity of the situation may not have been sufficiently conveyed or understood by the referring physician.

Initial management of the patient includes assessment of the severity of illness by CT scan with vascular enhancement and calculation of the physiologic severity of injury by the APACHE II and Ranson scores if they have not already been performed prior to coming to the ICU. The CT scan with vascular enhancement identifies the patients who are at risk of infection, development of pseudocysts, or diabetes. The physiologic indices identify the patients at risk of death.

Management objectives vary depending on the status of the patient on arrival in the ICU (i.e., whether the patient is septic, nonseptic, post drainage or admitted early after the onset of pancreatitis). For patients with necrotizing pancreatitis whether the etiology be biliary, alcoholic, or hyperlipidemia, the management is virtually identical.

The management objective for the patient with recent onset of symptoms or who is not septic is to maximize supportive care in the hope of avoiding multiple organ failure or infection of the necrotic pancreatic or peripancreatic tissue. In general, the longer operative intervention can be avoided following the onset of symptoms, the lower the mortality. The more time that elapses after the onset of symptoms and the initial insult to the pancreatic tissue, the more complete the delineation between what is viable and nonviable will be apparent if operation is required. While we have seen evolution of the peripancreatic lesions and fluid collections over time we have not seen extension of pancreatic necrosis following the initial CT scan in patients with uninfected necrosis. When early operative observations of the pancreas have been made at 24 to 48 hours, pancreatic necrosis is already present.[138,140] While there is not conclusive proof yet available, we theorize that pancreatic necrosis when it occurs develops concomitant with or within hours of the onset of symptoms. Whether pancreatic or peripancreatic necrosis in the human extends over succeeding days as a result of inadequate fluid resuscitation is unknown. On the other hand, we believe there is extension of pancreatic necrosis in patients with infected pancreatic and peripancreatic necrosis due to the combined action of enzymes and bacteria.

The patient's condition permitting, it is important to convey to the patient and family the likelihood of a long surgical ICU and hospital stay, on the average 45 to 60 days, often requiring mechanical ventilation and one or more operations.[6] If the patient and family are not appraised of the need for patience at the outset of hospitalization, they may develop unrealistic expectations that could result in low patient morale and disaffection of the family.

The elements of supportive care we commonly employ in patients with necrotizing pancreatitis include vigorous fluid resuscitation, the use of antibiotics prophylactically and mechanical ventilation, Swan-Ganz, TPN, nasogastric suction, low dose dopamine, digitalization and H_2-blocker therapy. No evidence indicates that atrophine, antifibrinolytics, apoprotinin (Traysylol) glucagon, calcitonin, somatostatin, and vasopressin are of benefit in the management of patients with pancreatitis.[176]

Fluid Management

Early vigorous fluid management is, we believe, the single most important therapeutic intervention in preventing multiple organ failure and infection in necrotizing pancreas. Our objective is to maximize cardiac output in spite of the large capillary leak known to be present in most patients with necrotizing pancreatitis and that requires Swan-Ganz monitoring. We keep pulmonary wedge pressure high at 16 to 20 cm H_2O. We have in some patients given as much as 18 to 25 L of electrolyte solution the first several days of the onset of pancreatitis. Cardiac support is provided by digitalizing the older patients and in cases of severe capillary leak and hypotension by the use of dopamine in low doses of 3 to 4 mg/kg per minute.

Most of the patients we have seen with multiple organ failure have been referred. Review of their hospital records often shows initial inadequate fluid resuscitation. Those in charge of their management have focused on monitoring the adequacy of urine output rather than cardiac output. Use of furosemide (Lasix) and administration of intravenous fluid volumes of 3 to 5 L in patients with a significant capillary leak creates organ hypoperfusion and leads to multiple organ failure.

Due to the appreciation that there is significant plasma volume sequestration in acute pancreatitis, few patients die in classic hypovolemic shock (3.7%) (see Table 52-4) during the first 4 to 5 days of necrotizing pancreatitis. Many patients still die of the sequelae of inadequate fluid resuscitation, however, the inadequacy of which we believe is only now becoming appreciated. It is our belief that many patients with necrotizing pancreatitis develop multiple organ failure and secondary infection of necrotic pancreas as a result of insufficiently vigorous and appropriate fluid resuscitation which must maximize cardiac output, return pulmonary hemodynamics to normal, and avoid hypoorgan perfusion.

Historically, some lesions thought to be unique to the inciting event on further study prove tractable to improved, more vigorous fluid replacement (e.g., crush injuries of the extremities with renal failure from myoglobinuria, fat emboli, and pulmonary failure from long bone fractures). We believe necrotizing pancreatitis may be another example. We believe through improved fluid resuscitation, the incidence of renal failure, ARDS, intravascular coagulation, and infection may either be reduced or ameliorated. Based on work in experimental animals of Horton[73] and ourselves, hypertonic saline-dextran fluid combination appears to be a significant improvement in resuscitating dogs and pigs with necrotizing pancreatitis. We are now using the hypertonic saline-dextran resuscitation fluids in humans. In patients with a marked capillary leak from pancreatitis (early after onset of symptoms) or sepsis (late after onset of symptoms) associated with metabolic acidosis and decreased systemic vascular resistance, low dose dopamine may be of some benefit.

Peritoneal Lavage

No evidence indicates that pancreatitis causes a unique renal lesion or can cause acute renal failure in patients with necrotizing pancreatitis who have undergone vigorous fluid resuscitation. Acute renal failure is frequent, however, in patients with necrotizing pancreatitis who have not been adequately fluid resuscitated. Later in the course of necrotizing pancreatitis, acute renal failure may also occur in the patient with infected pancreatic necrosis who becomes septic. Those patients who develop renal failure are best treated by peritoneal lavage rather than hemodialysis which is hazardous in the hemodynamically unstable patient with pancreatitis. Lankisch[177] recommends institution of peritoneal lavage when the hourly urine falls below 50 ml per hour and serum creatinine exceeds 25 mg/100 ml.[80]

Peritoneal lavage may have a role in the management of patients with necrotizing pancreatitis aside from the management of renal failure or as a diagnostic technique to assess the severity of pancreatitis. Peritoneal lavage has been proposed as a therapy to ameliorate the course of necrotizing pancreatitis in the absence of renal complications by Gebhardt in 1965[224] and other presumably by the removal of large amounts of ascites fluid which is known to contain bradykinin, myocardial depressant factor, prostaglandins, histamine and large quantities of pancreatic enzymes.[50,52,83,178-180] The sterile hemorrhagic ascitic fluid has shock-like, often fatal, effect.[52,53,178] If the hemorrhagic ascitic fluid is infected, the lethality of the fluid is markedly increased. The addition of a protease inhibitor to the ascites decreases the mortality of the fluid when it is given to other dogs or mice without pancreatitis.[180,181]

In 1985, Mayer and colleagues[182] reported the results of a multicenter controlled trial of peritoneal lavage in 91 patients with severe acute pancreatitis who were randomized to receive standard supportive care or 3 days of peritoneal lavage. There was no statistical difference in either the mortality rate or the incidence of major complications between the 2 groups.[182] Ranson[183] described 29 patients who received nonoperative treatment for severe acute pancreatitis. In those patients with 3 or more + Ranson signs, a 7-day course of peritoneal lavage using large volumes of fluid 18 to 24 L per 24 hours reduced the frequency of pancreatic sepsis from 40 to 22% and the mortality rate secondary to sepsis from 20 to 0% compared to a group of patients receiving 2 days of peritoneal lavage. Despite the conflicting results of these studies, the rapid and dramatic clinical improvement accompanied by pain which follows peritoneal lavage in some patients with severe acute pancreatitis is impressive to many clinicians.

What has yet to be determined is whether the beneficial affects of lavage reflect removal of toxic substances or simply improved fluid management. The experimental work of Niederau[180] and associates shows that either vigorous fluid replacement or lavage improve survival but do not modify the severity of the pancreatic lesion.

Mechanical Ventilation

Many factors contribute to respiratory failure and ARDS in necrotizing pancreas. The presence of pleural effusions, a subdiaphragmatic inflammatory process, ileus and abdominal distention all limit pulmonary ventilation anatomically or as a result of pain. Loss of surfactant[29] and damage to the pulmonary endothelium also contribute to impaired respiratory function.[184] Therefore, it is not surprising that 50 to 70% of patients with necrotizing pancreatitis have major lung complications.[82,95] The early changes in the lung as noted by Burnweit[184] include a rise in pulmonary vascular resistance, a fall in nutritive blood flow to the lung, and increase in pulmonary vascular resistance. These were attributed to capillary alveolar membrane injuries leading to an increase in extravascular lung water. These changes precede blood gas abnormalities. Burnweit[184] concluded that the lungs were responding to humoral or reflex effects emanating from the injured pancreas rather than from impaired circulation to the lung. Two years later, however, some of the same authors found that a more vigorous resuscitation regimen consisting of hypertonic saline-dextran reversed the accumulation of extracellular lung water and avoided the increased pulmonary vascular resistance, rise in pulmonary artery pressure, changes in pulmonary artery oxygen content, and decreased nutritive blood flow to the lung seen in the earlier experiments in a canine bile-induced pancreatitis. These results reported by Horton[216] tend to reinforce the belief that ARDS associated with acute pancreatitis can be reversed or ameliorated by improving the circulation to the lung and other organs through vigorous fluid resuscitation.

The mechanical obstacles to ventilation are of some consequence but difficult to treat. Diaphragmatic splinting from pain or abdominal distention is not easily avoided, although epidural anesthesia may improve ventilatory function. Large pleural effusions may have to be tapped. Humidified oxygen should be delivered by nasal prongs and mask at a flow rate of 2 to 5.2 L per minute.[82] Imrie[156] reported that this step reduced mortality from 26.7 to 12.2% in a prospective study.[78] If the P_{O_2} falls below 60 mm Hg despite oxygen therapy, intubation and mechanical ventilation with positive end expiratory pressure (PEEP) is essential.[185]

It may be trite to say all patients with pancreatitis requiring intensive care should have blood gases obtained at least every 3 to 6 hours and their respiratory rate closely observed for the initial 3 to 5 days after the onset of symptoms. Ignorance of the incidence and severity of pulmonary failure in necrotizing pancreatitis or complacency kills, however. We recommend intubation for any patient with pancreatitis having a P_{O_2} of 60 mm Hg or below, or a respiratory rate of 30 or more.

Pain Control

Meperidine H_2 (Demerol) IM or IV and hydroxyzine (Vistaril) IM or morphine or patient-controlled analgesic (PCA) may be of help in controlling pain. All narcotics cause spasm of the sphincter of Oddi, but in patients in whom the pancreas is already necrotic, this should not be considered a contraindication or limitation on their use. Epidural anesthesia may be necessary and desirable in some patients.

Antibiotics

Major pancreatic necrosis (over 10%) of the pancreas occurs in 8 to 10% of patients with acute pancreatitis. Approximately half these patients become infected.[6,159,169,234] Eighty percent of the deaths in acute pancreatitis are associated with infectious sequelae.[186-196] Beger[169] found that the highest mortality occurs in the patients with infected pancreatic necrosis early after the onset of symptoms—100% the first week, 50% the second and third weeks, and 14% after 21 days. Beger[169] operated on 114 patients with pancreatic necrosis and found positive tissue cultures in 40%. The frequency of positive cultures correlated with the extent of necrosis and peripancreatic necrosis. Among patients with necrosis, approximately 25% of those coming to operation the first week following onset of symptoms were infected, 33% the second week, 72% the third week, and 39% thereafter.

An improvement in overall mortality of necrotizing pancreatitis would follow if necrosis could be prevented, the host reaction to the necrosis ameliorated or pancreatic or peripancreatic infection prevented. With regard to the latter goal, antibiotic prophylaxis has been evaluated in several studies. Four controlled prospective studies were unable to document a statistically significant benefit of prophylactic antibiotic therapy in acute pancreatitis.[197-200] These studies were flawed, however. They randomized patients with all degrees of severity into their studies which, therefore, included only a few patients with necrotizing pancreatitis who are the only patients at risk of infection. None of these series had more than 100 patients. Knowing that the usual incidence of necrotizing pancreatitis to be 10%, there could not be more than 5 patients each at risk of infection in the treated and control group. Also knowing that only half of the patients with necrosis become infected in the absence of antibiotics leaves us comparing 2 to 3 patients in the control and antibiotic group. Not surprisingly no differences were noted. Equally as disconcerting was the failure to use in these 4 studies antibiotics with a spectrum likely to be active against the organisms most commonly found in pancreatic infections.

The favorable effect of antibiotics on reducing mortality of experimental pancreatitis was first shown by Hermann.[201] We have performed experimental studies using a retrograde pancreatic duct injection technique with bile salts and trypsin in dogs and pigs. Antibiotics reduced morality in this model.

Unfortunately, no current clinical studies address the value of antibiotic prophylaxis in patients at risk (i.e., those with necrotizing pancreatitis). Some investigators believe, however, and support the use of antibiotics on the presumptive theory that, in patients with necrotizing pancreatitis,[225] antibiotics may reach therapeutic levels in pancreatic tissue and pancreatic juice may have value in preventing or delaying the onset of infection in the necrotic tissue.[203] A number of issues remain unresolved. Infectious complications of necrotizing pancreatitis are not limited to pancreatic tissue but include peripancreatic tissue, principally retroperitoneal fat. Do antibiotics in high concentration in pancreatic tissue and juice also have a high concentration in peripancreatic tissue? We could find no references addressing this issue. Are all patients with necrotizing pancreatitis at the same risk of infection (e.g., do patients with gallstones have a higher risk of infection than those with a history of alcoholism?). What is the proper timing of antibiotic prophylaxis in necrotizing pancreatitis? The danger of infection among patients with necrotizing pancreatitis persists for many weeks.[169] Should antibiotic prophylaxis be started early after the onset of necrotizing pancreatitis in hopes of avoiding secondary infectious complications known to occur in 25% of those operated on the first week of pancreatitis? If so, how long should antibiotic prophylaxis be continued knowing that the risk of infection persists for 5 to 7 more weeks? Prolonged use of prophylactic antibiotics increases the risk that infections with resistant organisms, particularly candida infections, may emerge. Candida organisms are seen quite frequently in patients, 6 of 50 patients at our institution have been treated with broad spectrum antibiotics for pancreatic infections for prolonged periods.[6] Calandra reported candida was significantly more likely to cause infection in patients who had surgery for acute pancreatitis than in those with gastrointestinal perforations (90 versus 32%, $p = 0.005$), or with other disorders (90 versus 17%, $p = 0.003$).[202]

Candida was seen as the primary organism in 6 (13%) of our 45 patients with infected necrosis, some of whom had received antibiotics prior to referral. Finally, we know that not all patients with pancreatic and peripancreatic necrosis will become infected (33 to 71%). In the absence of a controlled trial performed in patients at risk (i.e., those with necrotizing pancreatitis), there is no way of knowing for certain whether prophylactic antibiotics are of benefit. The multicenter Italian trial using imipenem showed a statistically significant decrease in the incidence of infection in patients with necrotizing pancreatitis, but the mortality was not statistically reduced by the therapy.[225]

Based on these considerations, and in the absence of data to resolve all issues, it seems prudent to initiate antibiotic presumptive theory to reduce the risk of secondary infections in the group of patients with necrotizing pancreatitis at greatest risk of death (i.e., those patients with necrotizing pancreatitis at greatest risk of death, which are those patients who become infected within the first one to three weeks following onset of symptoms. If we can avoid infection and thus avoid operation at this early stage when the distinction between what is viable and nonviable tissue is more difficult to determine, when bleeding complications are greater, and when the patient is likely to be hemodynamically unstable, then we should be able to decrease the 100% mortality found in patients operated on by Beger within the first 2 weeks after onset of necrotizing pancreatitis.[203] Therefore, we recommend a 14 to 28-day course of antibiotic prophylaxis in patients with necrotizing pancreatitis demonstrated by CT scan with vascular enhancement starting the day of hospital admission. We are less concerned about infections that become evident 4 or more weeks after the onset of symptoms because the mortality is less than those of patients whose infections present earlier. In our experience, the organisms most commonly found in pancreatic infections are aerobic, gram-negative rods, enterococci, and candida. Fifty percent of the infections were polymicrobial.[6] These bacteria are similar to those reported by Lumsden and Bradley[204] in their review of pancreatic infections.

It has been assumed that the bacteria grown from the infected pancreas are secondary invaders coming from the colon based on their resemblance to colonic flora. It has been postulated that bacteria from the colon reach the necrotic pancreas by either an increase in their normal translocation to lymph nodes accelerated by shock and endotoxins and perhaps even the macrophage or by direct passage into the circulation from the intestine.[170-174]

The role of sterilizing the colon with antibiotics or diverting the fecal stream to avoid secondary infections in patients with necrotizing pancreatitis has been considered by some investigators.[171,173]

Those antibiotics which are found in therapeutic concentrations (Mic-90 value) in pancreatic tissue and juice for colonic bacteria flow based on ERCP and fistula collections have been reviewed by Bradley[204] and include cefotaxime, ceftazidime, clindamycin, ciprofloxacin, metronidazole, trimethoprim sulfate, methoxazole, and rifampin and netilmicin. Bradley recommends a regimen of ceftazidine and clindamycin, but does not make a recommendation regarding coverage of enterococcus. The penetration, activity, and protein binding of these antibiotics in inflammatory and necrotic pancreatic and peripancreatic tissue may be altered and affect their efficacy. In general, lipid-soluble drugs may have greater penetration (e.g., metronidazole, chloramphenicol and trimethoprim) than water-soluble drugs such as the aminoglycosides and beta-lactams. Much work is still needed to define those antibiotics most efficacious in avoiding secondary infections of necrotic pancreas.

The number of patients and the number of antibiotics on which these conclusions by Bradley were based is small, 22 antibiotics and 83 patients. Most had only the pancreatic juice measured not actual pancreatic tissue levels. The most well-designed and comprehensive study on human pancreatic tissue levels of antibiotics was presented by Buchler.[205] His study included 97 patients in whom antibiotic levels were measured in tissue, juice and cyst fluid at the time of operation in patients receiving a variety of intravenous antibiotics 30 minutes before celiotomy. An efficacy factor was calculated taking into account the percentage and type of bacteria found in pancreatic infections, the median pancreatic tissue concentrations found after 120 minutes, and the minimal antibiotic concentrations of the respective drug. His results are shown in the table reproduced from his abstract at the Pancreas Club meeting (Table 52-10). They concluded, "Imipenum, ofloxacin, ciprofoxacin, or cefotaxime are the antibiotics of choice. Aminoglycosides do not reach sufficient concentrations in the human pancreas, although they are widely used in these patients." In the few patients with necrotizing pancreatitis where we have had an opportunity to treat early in the course of pancreatitis, we have used standard combination therapy of ampicillin, gentamicin, and metronidazole. This regimen is not ideal, based on the review by Bradley and the work of Buchler, but in changing it we are also concerned we know so little about tissue concentrations of these antibiotics in retroperitoneal and peripancreatic fat. In addition to pancreatic tissue, the necrotic peripancreatic tissue is at risk of infection. Antibiotics known to have penetrance and activity in pancreatic tissue may not be active in peripancreatic tissues.

Nasogastric suction

Despite theoretic considerations to the contrary, studies have shown that nasogastric suction has no value in modifying the course of mild or moderate pancreatitis.[206] In patients with severe or necrotizing pancreatitis who are vomiting, however, nasogastric suction is a necessity. H_2-blocker therapy is indicated in patients with necrotizing pancreatitis and infected necrosis to prevent gastric and duodenal ulceration and bleeding. Ph levels should be maintained at five or above. Should pH levels fall, the dose of H_2 blockers should be doubled. Intravenous infusion of the H_2 blockers is the most effective route of administration. Daily maximum doses of cimetidine, 2400 mg, ranitidine, 1000 mg, or famotidine, 200 mg, are usually well tolerated.

Table 52-10. Human Pancreatic Tissue Levels of Antibiotics

	NET	TOB	MEZ	PIP	CFI	CTX	CIP	OFX	IMI
Tissue conc. (mg/kg)	0.4	0.4	17.7	20.3	7.8	9.1	0.9	1.7	3.7
(%)*	21.4	21.8	67.2	68.9	76.2	81.9	86.5	87.5	98.1

* 100% would be an optimal drug to treat pancreatic infection; 30 minutes prior to laparatomy, one of the following drugs was given intravenously. PIP, Piperacillin 4 gm; MEZ, mezlocillin 4 gm; CTX, cefotaxime 2 gm; CFI, ceftrixozime 2 gm; NET, netilmicin 150 mg; TOB, tobramycin 80 gm; IMI, imipenem/cilastatin 500 mg; OFX, ofloxacin 200 mg; CIP, ciprofloxacin 20 mg.
(From paper presented by Buchler, M., Friess, H., Isemann, R., and Beger, H. G.: In 24th Annual Meeting of the Pancreas Club, Inc., San Antonio, May 14, 1990.)

TPN

The metabolism of the patients with necrotizing pancreatitis is similar to that of patients with sepsis[207] (i.e., protein catabolism, impaired glucose oxidation). Goodgame[208] demonstrated that total parenteral nutrition has only a supportive role in patients with necrotizing pancreatitis and in the absence of appropriate operative intervention is of no benefit in reducing mortality or complications.

Enteral feedings instituted by means of tube jejunostomy performed in those patients requiring celiotomy for management of complications of necrotizing pancreatitis has been advocated. This technique can usually but not always be performed in patients with infected pancreatic necrosis and does not stimulate pancreatic secretion.[209] Jejunal contents can leak around the jejunal tube, however, or the tube may become misplaced and require reoperation. Those patients most at risk of leaking jejunal contents about the tube are those patients with necrotizing pancreatitis having marked edema of the small bowel and its mesentery. Such conditions preclude the safe placement of a jejunostomy tube.[231a]

Comprehensive Surgical ICU Management of the Patient with Necrotizing Pancreatitis

On admission to the surgical ICU, needs of the patient with necrotizing pancreatitis should be rapidly established regarding the necessity for mechanical ventilatory support, Swan-Ganz monitoring, vigorous fluid resuscitation, exogenous insulin, antibiotic prophylaxis, total parenteral nutrition, and correction of electrolytes and calcium abnormalities. Concomitantly, if not already performed, the anatomic and physiologic assessment of the severity of pancreatitis through the use of the CT scan with vascular enhancement and the APACHE II score and Ranson's signs should be obtained.

Our philosophy regarding the management of patients with pancreatic and peripancreatic necrosis is that necrosis alone in the absence of infection or clinical deterioration is not an indication for operative intervention.[6,86,145,210,211] On the other hand, we believe that all patients with infected pancreatic and peripancreatic necrosis should have the necrosis removed operatively.

Uninfected Pancreatic and Peripancreatic Necrosis

Some patients with pancreatic and peripancreatic necrosis will not become infected. This figure is said to be somewhere between 30 to 60% of all patients with necrotizing pancreatitis identified by CT scan with vascular enhancement or at operation.[6,83,159] While the greater the extent of the pancreatic and peripancreatic necrosis the more likely infection, it is by no means inevitable that all patients with more than 50% necrosis will become infected.[159]

Most patients with infected pancreatic and peripancreatic necrosis are hemodynamically stable and can be treated nonoperatively with supportive care until they recover or develop some noninfected complication of pancreatitis such as a pseudocyst or pancreatic fistula, which may require later operative intervention.

A small subset of patients in the uninfected group of patients may benefit from operative intervention.[231b] These are patients who after 3 to 10 days of maximum supportive care fail to improve and show progressive deterioration in cardiopulmonary function, persistent signs of an acute abdomen, and the development of multiple organ failure. At operation, all necrotic pancreatic and peripancreatic tissue and fluid collections were removed. This approach was successful in the three patients in whom we tried it. We had two patients, however, with uninfected peripancreatic necrosis who came to operative lavage both of whom died. These patients had experienced a rapid fulminant pancreatitis. Both had been inadequately fluid resuscitated at the referring hospital and were in multiple organ failure on arrival at our hospital. One patient was in coma and suffered a myocardial failure, the other had severe ARDS required 1.00 F_{IO_2} and 20 cm PEEP to maintain an arterial oxygen saturation of 80%. In each, at operation a triple-lumen Davol catheter was placed in the lesser sac and was followed by vigorous lavage (1 L per hour), but neither patient improved. We are uncertain as to what, if anything, should have been done other than continue supportive care in these patients who appeared terminally ill on arrival.

Infected Pancreatic and Peripancreatic Necrosis

There is general agreement that patients with infected pancreatic and peripancreatic necrosis require prompt operative removal of all infected necrotic tissue. These patients may be identified on the basis of clinical signs of sepsis and signs of an acute abdomen. Signs of sepsis include evidence of a capillary leak, shock, tachycardia, positive fluid balance, deterioration of pulmonary function, increased insulin requirement, metabolic acidosis, leukocytosis, thrombocytopenia and persistent fever, or on the basis of CT scan guided aspiration for Gram stain culture and biopsy, looking for aerobic, anaerobic, and fungal organisms. The latter technique developed by Gerzhof and Banks[213] has proven helpful in identifying some patients with infected pancreatic and peripancreatic necrosis before sepsis had become clinically evident. We performed this procedure on 31 of our 50 patients. We have had two patients who had negative Gram stain and cultures but the clinical course dictated operative intervention. At operation, cultures were positive. CT scan guided aspiration should be performed on all patients with pancreatic and peripancreatic necrosis in whom there are signs of sepsis, persistent fever, or failure to improve. In some patients the procedure may need to be repeated several times every 2 to 3 days depending on the clinical course. Unlike Banks and Gerzhol,[213] we found that in patients with more than one collection, not all collections of necrosis and fluid were inevitably infected if one was infected.

Those patients with pancreatic necrosis who become infected early after the onset of symptoms have the highest mortality (e.g., the mortality, in spite of operative intervention, was 100% among Beger's patients who became infected the first week).[169] These patients will all have evidence of major systemic abnormalities reflected in high APACHE II scores or Ranson's signs. We believe it may be possible to diminish the likelihood of infection or delay its onset in this high risk group of patients by maximizing supportive care at the outset of their illness. Whether "long" (7 days) peritoneal lavage advocated by Ranson[183] has any advantage over vigorous fluid resuscitation with hypertonic saline-6% dextran solution needs to be determined.

Operative Management

A spectrum of pancreatic infection ranges from infected pancreatic necrosis seen early after onset of symptoms and associated with high APACHE II scores and a high number of Ranson's signs to well walled off collections (abscesses) with low APACHE II scores and few positive Ranson's signs consisting primarily of fluid from liquification of necrotic pancreatic or peripancreatic tissue or both, or a pancreatic pseudocyst which has become secondarily infected. These infected collections are usually not clinically apparent before the fifth week after the onset of symptoms and after the subsidence of the acute hemodynamic phase of pancreatitis.[214] Fink[91] found that such patients constituted 72% of his 100 patients with infectious complications of pancreatitis. These 72 patients had fewer than 3 or more Ranson's signs on hospital admission whereas some had no fever, leucocytosis, or abdominal tenderness. If the diagnosis is not missed and drainage instituted promptly, the mortality should be low in this patient group. If the infected collection consists of liquid pus in the absence of infected tissue, percutaneous drainage rather than operative drainage can be considered.[215,216]

Between these two extremes are many patients with a combination of liquid pus and necrotic tissue and others in which both infected necrotic tissue and infected fluid are present but one predominates over the other. Any patients with more than 10 to 15 g of necrosis will require operative debridement rather than percutaneous drainage suitable only for pure liquid collections. We have found as little as 10 to 15 g of necrotic infected tissue will inhibit a patient's recovery.

We favor open packing and continuous catheter irrigation with chloropactin in high risk patients with extensive infected pancreatic and peripancreatic necrosis and in those patients who become infected soon after the onset of symptoms in whom it is difficult at operation to distinguish between viable and nonviable tissue and in whom debridement is inevitable. We performed open packing and irrigation in 12 of our 50 patients with necrotizing pancreatitis. These patients averaged 7.1 trips to the operating room for surgical procedures and 9 out of the 12 survived. The open technique popularized by Bradley[84,217] and used by others[75,218,219] evolved from the marsupialization technique that Booloki[220] described in the 1960s.

Following removal of all necrotic pancreatic and peripancreatic tissue performed through a subcostal incision, two to four triple-lumen Davol drains are inserted for irrigation purposes. Formerly, we suctioned and irrigated through the same drains, but found that constant suctioning may result in hemorrhage from vessels pulled against the suction ports. We rely now on dependent drainage for fluid return from large soft siliconized chest tubes and use the Davol drains for irrigation only.[221] We use chloropactin for our irrigant as recommended by Bradley and maintain a flow rate of 1 L per hour. Others have used antibiotic solutions[200,222,223] or antiprotease[180] solutions for their peritoneal lavage. Xeroform gauze is laid over the drains and the bowel and Kerlex rolls are used to pack the wound open from the anterior surface of what is left of the pancreas to the anterior abdominal wall. The irrigant chloropactin is antibacterial and antifungal, keeps the dressings wet and from adhering to the bowel, and removes necrotic particulate matter, pancreatic enzymes, and bacteria. Beger[83] has demonstrated high levels of active pancreatic enzymes in lavage fluid up to 3 weeks after drainage. In addition to removing enzymes, the lavage also carries out necrotic debris. Many surgeons advocate its use.[6,83,84,224,225] Another advantage of lavage is in managing patients with renal failure. We have not had to employ hemodialysis in any patient with renal failure, a procedure which carries major risk in patients who are hemodynamically unstable. The lavage functions much as peritoneal dialysis. The open packing technique permits access to the retroperitoneum and lesser sac above the transverse mesocolon. The abdominal cavity otherwise remains virgin territory in most patients. For those patients with extension of the infected necrosis behind the ascending and descending colons, small (6 to 8 cm) separate incisions are made in the flank and these areas debrided and drained retroperitoneally without entering the abdominal cavity.

We have found that our results with open packing improved when we returned to the operating room to change the packing and debride further the necrotic pancreatic and peripancreatic tissue on an every 2- to 3-day schedule rather than waiting for a change in the patient's condition. CT scans with vascular enhancement are periodically repeated to ensure that all necrotic pancreatic and peripancreatic tissue have been removed. Among our 50 patients, the average patient underwent 3.3 CT scans during their hospitalization. We quantitated the total infected necrotic tissue removed on 24 of our patients. The total grams of infected necrotic tissue removed averaged 227 g, with a range of 430 to 2000 g.

Not all patients with infected pancreatic or peripancreatic necrosis require open packing. When 3 to 4 weeks have elapsed after the onset of symptoms, even though the necrosis may be extensive, the body has defined better what is viable from nonviable tissue and a single debridement and closed drainage and irrigation is often sufficient. However, 42% of our patients with closed drainage required reoperation for complications or persistent sepsis. Persistent sepsis is an absolute indication for reoperation.[89,191,226] An attempt should be made to identify the sites of residual necrotic tissue on CT scan with vascular enhancement prior to reoperation.

Pre- and Postoperative Complications

Pre- and postoperative complications are common in patients with necrotizing pancreatitis (Table 52-11). Persistent ileus and the requirement for parenteral or enteral nutrition is the most common. Over 80% of patients in our experience required TPN and the average number of days of therapy was 50. Pulmonary, renal, and cardiac failure

ACUTE PANCREATITIS

Table 52–11. Preoperative and Postoperative Complications of Necrotizing Pancreatitis

Complications	No. of Patients
Prolonged ileus	41
Adult respiratory distress syndrome	26
Renal failure	15
Cardiac failure or arrhythmia	11
Enteric fistula	10
Pancreatic fistula	10
Hepatic failure	1

were the next most common complications. The patients in which infected pancreatic and peripancreatic necrosis predominated over the liquid component had the highest incidence of these complications. These findings were similar to the observations by Bittner.[214] Elimination of any septic source should be the overriding priority in the correction of ARDS, renal failure, and cardiac failure.

Enteric fistulas are not an uncommon complication of necrotizing pancreatitis. Some are iatrogenic; others are a result of the necrotizing process itself. Particularly vulnerable to spontaneous necrosis is the left transverse colon, although we have seen spontaneous massive duodenal and right transverse colon necrosis as well. A proximal colostomy or ileostomy is the operation of choice for colonic necrosis. Others[227-229] have reported mortality rates as high as 22 to 58% associated with the development of enteric fistulas. We had one death following spontaneous necrosis of the colon and duodenum but none after iatrogenic injury.[230]

Pancreatic fistulas are common. Some surgeons recommend ERCP early in the course of necrotizing pancreatitis to identify patients with necrosis interrupting the major pancreatic duct, and have used ductal rupture as an operative indication for resection of the distal pancreas.[230]

Twenty percent of our patients with necrotizing pancreatitis were identified as having a pancreatic fistula. This complication can be expected when the area of necrosis involves the head or midportion of the gland while a viable, juice secreting tail remains. Instead of operative resection of the distal gland as advocated by Gebhardt,[230] we rely initially on adequate drainage of these fistulas. Their long-term management is addressed in the section of this chapter on post-ICU care.

In summary, achieving mortality rates in patients with necrotizing pancreatitis is possible by employing a comprehensive management plan to address the problem. The central components of the strategy include:

- Rapid evaluation and assessment of the degree of physiologic and anatomic derangement; the latter by prompt use of the vascular enhanced CT scan
- Vigorous fluid resuscitation; the adequacy of which should be determined by Swan-Ganz monitoring
- Attempts to identify and document infected foci by means of CT scan guided percutaneous aspiration
- Aggressive and frequent (when indicated) surgical debridement

Close adherence to these policies allowed us to achieve a mortality of 14% in this seriously ill group of patients with Ranson signs and an average APACHE II score of 17.5. Most deaths (6 of 7) occurred in patients transferred to our service late in the course of their disease with an average APACHE II score of 33.6. Although our mortality rates compare favorably with those reported by others, mortality rates have greater significance when the severity of illness is taken into account (Table 52-12).

Table 52–12. Mortality Rate for Severe Acute Pancreatitis

	No. of Patients	Severity Ranson Score* (APACHE II)	No. of Deaths	Mortality (%)
Shaak[231] (1963–1980)	127	—	30	24
Stone[83] (1964–1981)	22	—	2	9
Howard[86] (1962–1989)	36	6.1	1	3
Katsohis[127] (1962–1982)	8	—	3	37.5
(1982–1989)	10	—	0	0
Gebhardt[235] (1981–1984)	62	—	14	22
Warshaw[88] (1974–1978)	26	—	10	38
(1979–1983)	19	—	1	5
(1984–1989)†	—	—	—	14
Pemberton[218] (1979–1984)	14	—	3	21
Fink[91] (1973–1985)	100	1.6	20	20
Roher[212] (1979–1985)	32	—	12	37
Malangoni[89] (1975–1980)	10	—	6	60
(1980–1985)	17	—	3	17.5
Nicholson[90] (1974–1985)	11	4.7	3	27.3
Bradley[84] (1976–1986)	28	5.3	3	11
(1976–1990)†	59	—	—	14
Beger[83] (1982–1988)	74	4.5	6	8.5
Wilson[232] (1980–1986)	21	—	8	38
Garcia-Sabrido[220] (1982–1988)	49	5.9 (25)	13	27
Ivatury[233] (1982–1987)	5	— (8.4)	2	40
Larvin[154] (1985–1987)	59	— (17)	22	37
Al-Hadeedi[234] (1986–1989)	91	— (11.1)	20	21
Stanten[6] (1982–1989)	50	6.6 (33.5)	7	14
	871	115	152	21.9

* Average of the score.
† Personal communication.

Table 52-13. Evaluation of Major Duct Pathology Following Necrotizing Pancreatitis as Visualized on Endoscopic Retrograde Cholangiopancreatography (ERCP)

Author	First Check (% Ductal Abnormality)	Postpancreatitis	Second Check (% Ductal Abnormality)	Postpancreatitis
Martin[242]	15/28 (53.6%)	1–2 yr	15/28 (53.6%)	1–5 yr
Buchler[243]				
Alcohol	19/20 (95.0%)	<12 mo	17/19 (89.5%)	>12 mo
Biliary	13/16 (81.3%)	<12 mo	7/12 (58.8%)	>12 mo
Angelini[245]	5/12 (41.7%)	1–2 yr	5/12 (41.7%)	1–3 yr
Total:	52/76 (68.4%)		44/71 (62.0%)	

Discharge from the ICU can be considered in patients with uninfected pancreatic and peripancreatic necrosis when the capillary leak phase of the illness has resolved as indicated by a negative fluid balance, and when the patient has demonstrated adequate pulmonary function off the mechanical ventilator.

New treatment modalities whose efficacy have not yet been verified include various types of hemofiltration or plasmapheresis. It has been hypothesized by Bodeker[236] and his co-workers that removal of low molecular weight proteins (up to mol. wt. 30,000) including activated components of complement C3a AND C5a, by hemofiltration is helpful in patients with severe pancreatitis having multiple organ failure. Zirngible and co-workers[237] have used plasmapheresis techniques in patients with acute pancreatitis and removed protein molecules much larger than the 30,000-mol. wt. proteins removed by hemofiltration (see Figure 52-2). The hemodynamic changes of acute pancreatitis are reversed by plasmapheresis just as they are by vigorous fluid resuscitation with the hypertonic saline Dextran solutions.[73]

Unresolved Issues

- Although presumptive antibiotics are useful in preventing infection in pancreatic and peripancreatic necrosis, it has not yet been demonstrated that mortality can be reduced.
- Does pancreatic necrosis which seems to occur in the first hours after onset of symptoms progress over a period of days in the absence of vigorous fluid replacement?
- Is the principal benefit of vigorous fluid replacement prevention of further extension of pancreatic necrosis or improved hemodynamics which reduces the incidence and severity of multiple organ failure and infection allowing the patient to better cope with his pancreatic necrosis?
- Does the apparent benefit of peritoneal lavage and plasmapheresis result from removal of activated complement and other noxious substances from peritoneal fluid and plasma, or simply because of improved hemodynamics associated with improved fluid management?

Discharge Criteria for the Surgical ICU

- Hemodynamic stability
- Resolution of sepsis
- Lack of need for mechanical ventilation

POST-ICU "REHABILITATION PHASE"

The post-ICU problems which require assessment and treatment include:

- Failure to thrive
- Delayed gastric emptying
- Pancreatic exocrine and endocrine insufficiency
- Pancreaticocutaneous fistula
- Pseudocysts
- Colostomy closure
- Operations on the biliary tract

Failure to Thrive

Recovery from necrotizing pancreatitis is usually rapid after leaving the ICU. TPN can usually be tapered and the patient started on oral intake. A persistent failure to thrive indicates the need to search for a residual infected necrotic foci. We have found a persistent failure to thrive may be the only sign of a residual foci of infections and that as little as 10 g of infected necrosis may impede recovery.

Table 52-14. Exocrine Function Assessed by Cholecystoleinin and Secretin Challenge: Long-Term Follow-Up After Necrotizing Pancreatitis

Author	First Check (% dysfunction)	Postpancreatitis	Second Check (% dysfunction)	Postpancreatitis
Martin[242]	10/24 (41.7%)	1–3 yr	5/24 (20.8%)	3–5+ yr
Buchler[243]				
Alcohol	20/21 (95.2%)	<12 mo	13/19 (68.4%)	>12 mo
Biliary	13/18 (72.2%)	<12 mo	3/10 (30.0%)	>12 mo
Angelini[245]	6/14 (42.9%)	1–2 yr	1/14 (7.1%)	1–3 yr
Total:	49/77 (63.6%)		22/67 (32.8%)	

Delayed Gastric Emptying

On the other hand, delayed gastric emptying may occur in patients without residual infected necrosis but in whom the periduodenal inflammatory response from the pancreatitis may alter gastric motility. Jejunal feedings or home TPN may be required if the problem does not resolve within two to three weeks.

Assessment of Exocrine and Endocrine Functions

Resumption of oral intake requires evaluation of the adequacy of exocrine and endocrine function. Many of these patients have lost significant amounts of pancreatic mass. The pancreas has great reserve and as little as 10% of the normal gland may be sufficient to avoid exocrine or endocrine insufficiency.[238] The remaining pancreas may not be normal, however, or the patient may have a family history of diabetes. Therefore, blood sugars should be followed closely in all patients with necrotizing pancreatitis on resumption of oral intake. A 72-hour stool fat collection should also be obtained to access exocrine function. On a 100-g fat diet per day, fecal fat loss should not exceed 7%. Clinically evident steatorrhea is often not apparent, however, unless stool fat loss exceeds 20 g. A rough guide for enzyme replacement is to supply 1000 U of lipase for each gram of fat ingested. The average American diet has 25 g of fat with each meal. Therefore, 25,000 U of lipase need to be administered. In the absence of enteric-coated enzymes such as pancreas and creon, H_2-blockers should be administered to maintain a pH in the stomach sufficiently high to permit the enzymes safe transit through the stomach to the duodenum.

Another reason for providing pancreatic enzymes in the form of trypsin and chymotrypsin is to reduce the cholecystokinin stimulation of pancreatic enzyme secretion especially with patients known to have a major duct disruption or obstruction. These proteases must be active in the duodenum to cleave the CCK release factor in order to be effective.[239]

Pancreatic Fistulas and Pseudocysts

Many patients, 20% in our experience, with necrotizing pancreatitis develop pancreatic fistulas or pseudocysts. This complication can be expected when the area of necrosis involves the head or midportion of the gland while a viable juice secreting distal portion of pancreas persists. The juice either exits through a drain site in the form of a pancreatic fistula in the case of infected necrosis or if the patient's necrosis was uninfected and did not require operation, the extravasated pancreatic juice may be contained as a pseudocyst. Ten percent of patients with acute pseudocysts may develop pseudoaneurysms associated with visceral vessels. The vessels most frequently involved are the splenic and gastroduodenal artery. Massive hemoductal hemorrhage may occur.[240,241] Initial control of hemorrhage may be achieved by angiographic embolization.[242]

Pancreaticocutaneous fistulas may close spontaneously. In our experience with 10 such fistulas, this happened in 3 patients. Closure occurred spontaneously as late as 11 months after the attack of necrotizing pancreatitis. The fistula persists in 3 patients after an average of 8 months. Surgical drainage was required in 4 patients. Three of these patients stopped draining from their pancreaticocutaneous fistulas, but the fluid continued to accumulate internally and evolved into a pseudocyst.

Colostomy Closure and Operations on the Biliary Tract

It is best to allow 6 to 12 months to pass before reentering the abdomen after operative management of major pancreatic infections. This interval of time allows edema and inflammation to subside to the point the procedure can be performed safely.

Splenic Vein Thrombosis

Splenic vein thrombosis, a complication of acute pancreatitis or pseudocysts formation, may have long-term sequelae (i.e., left-sided portal hypertension and bleeding from gastric varices).[242]

Long-Term Morphologic Changes After Necrotizing Pancreatitis

Long-term morphologic changes after necrotizing pancreatitis based on ERCP assessment of the major pancreatic duct showed little reversal of structural abnormalities over a 1- to 2-year period in patients with either alcoholic or biliary pancreatitis (Table 52-13).

Long-Term Changes in Exocrine Function After Necrotizing Pancreatitis

Long-term changes in exocrine function based on stimulation of the pancreas by CCK and secretin showed statistically significant improvement over a 1- to 2-year period in patients with biliary pancreatitis as well as those with alcoholic pancreatitis though the improvement was more moderate in the latter group (Table 52-14).

Table 52-15. Necrotizing Pancreatitis: Endocrine Follow-Up of Pathologic Results by Glucose Tolerance Test

Author	First Check (% intolerance)	Postpancreatitis	Second Check (% intolerance)	Postpancreatitis
Martin[242]	18/31 (58.1%)		12/24 (50.8%)	
Buchler[243]				
Alcohol	12/20 (60.0%)	<12 mo	7/16 (43.8%)	>12 mo
Biliary	7/16 (43.8%)	<12 mo	2/9 (22.2%)	>12 mo
Angelini[245]	14/19 (73.7%)	1–2 yr	9/19 (47.4%)	1–3 yr
Total:	51/86 (59.3%)		30/68 (44.1%)	

Long-Term Changes in Endocrine Function After Necrotizing Pancreatitis

Long-term changes in endocrine function were observed based on the glucose tolerance test after 1 to 2 years follow-up. Whereas endocrine function improved in patients with biliary and alcoholic pancreatitis, the changes were not statistically significant (Table 52–15).

REFERENCES

1. Beger, H. G., et al.: Results of surgical treatment of necrotizing pancreatitis. World J. Surg., 9:972, 1985.
2. Howard, J. M.: Pancreatitis in the United States of America. In Surgical Diseases of the Pancreas. Edited by J. M. Howard, G. L. Jordan, Jr., and H. A. Reber. Philadelphia, Lea & Febiger, 1987.
3. Ranson, J. H. C.: Acute pancreatitis. In Surgery of the Pancreas. Edited by J. R. Brooks. Philadelphia, W. B. Saunders, 1983.
4. Imrie, C. W., and Dickson, A. P.: Postoperative pancreatitis. In Surgical Disease of the Pancreas. Edited by J. M. Howard, G. L. Jordan, Jr., and H. A. Reber. Philadelphia, Lea & Febiger, 1987.
5. Frey, C. F., and Beal, J. M.: Pancreatitis as a complication of operation. Arch. Surg., 87:1053, 1963.
6. Stanten, R., and Frey, C. F.: Comprehensive management of acute necrotizing pancreatitis and pancreatic abscess. Arch. Surg., 125:1269, 1990.
7. Scarpelli, D. G.: Toxicology of the pancreas. Toxicol. Appl. Pharmacol., 101:534, 1989.
8. Eckhauser, M. L., Dokler, M., and Imbembo, A. L.: Diuretic-associated pancreatitis: a collective review and illustrative case. Am. J. Gastroenterol., 82:865, 1987.
9. Vane, D. W., Grosfeld, J. L., West, K. W., and Rescorla, F. J.: Pancreatic disorders in infancy and childhood: experience with 92 cases. J. Pediatr. Surg., 24:771, 1989.
10. Sitges-Serra, A., et al.: Pancreatitis and hyperparathyroidism. Br. J. Surg., 75:158, 1988.
11. Levine, R. A., and McGuire, R. F.: Corticosteroid-induced pancreatitis: a case report demonstrating recurrence with rechallenge. Am. J. Gastroenterol., 83:1161, 1988.
12. Zygmunt, D. J., Williams, J. H., and Bienzi, S. R.: Acute pancreatitis associated with long-term sulindac therapy. West. J. Med., 144:461, 1986.
13. Brazer, S. R., and Medoff, J. R.: Sulfonamide-induced pancreatitis. Pancreas, 3:583, 1988.
14. Albert-Flor, J. J., et al.: Fulminant liver failure and pancreatitis associated with the use of sulfamethoxazole-trimethoprim. Am. J. Gastroenterol., 84:1577, 1989.
15. Mallory, A., and Kern, F.: Drug-induced pancreatitis. Baillieres Clin. Gastroenterol., 2:293, 1988.
16. Flynn, W. J., Freeman, P. G., and Wickboldt, L. G.: Pancreatitis associated with isotretinoin-induced hypertriglyceridemia. Ann. Intern. Med., 107:63, 1987.
17. al-Awadhi, N. Z., Ashkenani, F., and Khalaf, E. S.: Acute pancreatitis associated with brucellosis. Am. J. Gastroenterol., 84:1570, 1989.
18. Torosis, J., and Vendor, R.: Tetracycline-induced pancreatitis. J. Clin. Gastroenterol., 9:580, 1987.
19. Tiscornia, O. M., et al.: Estrogen effects on exocrine pancreatic secretion in menopausal women: a hypothesis for menopause-induced chronic pancreatitis. Mt. Sinai J. Med., 53:356, 1986.
20. Marsh, W. H., Vukov, G. A., and Conrad, E. C.: Acute pancreatitis after cutaneous exposure to an organophosphate insecticide. Am. J. Gastroenterol., 83:1158, 1988.
21. Frick, T. W., et al.: Effect of insecticide, diazinon, on pancreas of dog, cat and guinea pig. J. Environ. Pathol. Toxicol. Oncol., 7:1, 1987.
22. Frey, C. G., Gerzof, S. G., Greenberger, N. J., and Vennes, J. A.: Progress in acute pancreatitis. Patient Care, 15:38, 1989.
23. Nordback, I., et al.: Effect of free radical scavengers on energy metabolism and cellular structure in acute experimental pancreatitis. Presented at the 24th Annual Meeting of the Pancreas Club, Inc., San Antonio, May 14, 1990.
24. Sanfey, H., Bulkley, G. B., and Cameron, J. L.: The role of oxygen-derived free radicals in the pathogenesis of acute pancreatitis. Ann. Surg., 200:405, 1984.
25. Del Maestro, R. F.: An approach to free radicals in medicine and biology. Acta Physiol. Scand. Suppl., 192:153, 1980.
26. Del Maestro, R. F., Bjork, J., and Arfors, K. E.: Increase in microvascular permeability induced by enzymatically generated free radicals (II): role of superoxide anion radical, hydrogen peroxide and hydroxyl radical. Microvasc. Res., 22:255, 1981.
27. Guice, K. S., et al.: Superoxide dismutase and catalase: a possible role in established pancreatitis. Am. J. Surg., 151:163, 1986.
28. Rutledge, P. L., et al.: Role of oxygen-derived free radicals in diet-induced hemorrhagic pancreatitis in mice. Gastroenterology, 93:41, 1987.
29. Guice, K. S., et al.: Neutrophil-dependent, oxygen-radical mediated lung injury associated with acute pancreatitis. Ann. Surg., 210:740, 1989.
30. Crapo, J. D., et al.: The failure of aerosolized superoxide dismutase to modify pulmonary oxygen toxicity. Am. Rev. Respir. Dis., 115:1027, 1977.
31. Baker, G. L., Corry, R. J., and Autor, A. P.: Oxygen free radical induced damage in kidneys subjected to warm ischemia and reperfusion: protective effect of superoxide dismutase. Ann. Surg., 202:628, 1985.
32. Parks, D. A., Bulkley, G. B., and Granger, D. N.: Role of oxygen derived free radicals in digestive tract disease. Surgery, 94:415, 1983.
33. Parks, D. A., and Granger, D. N.: Ischemia-induced vascular changes role of xanthine oxidase and hydroxyl radicals. Am. J. Physiol., 245:G285, 1983.
34. Brawn, K., and Fridovich, I.: Superoxide radical and superoxide dismutases: threat and defense. Acta Physiol. Scand., 492:9, 1980.
35. Fridovich, I.: The biology of oxygen radicals. Science, 201:875, 1978.
36. McCord, J. M.: The superoxide free radical: its biochemistry and pathophysiology. Surgery, 94:412, 1983.
37. Frank, L., and Massaro, D.: Oxygen toxicity. Am. J. Med., 69:117, 1980.
38. Bulkley, G. B.: The role of oxygen free radicals in human disease processes. Surgery, 94:407, 1983.
39. Koike, H., Steer, M. L., and Meldolesi, J.: Pancreatic effects of ethionine: blockade of exocytosis and appearance of crinophagy and autophagy precede cellular necrosis. Am. J. Physiol., 242:G297, 1982.
40. Watanabe, O., Baccino, F. M., Steer, M. L., and Meldolesi, J.: Supramaximal caerulein stimulation and ultrastructure of rat pancreatic acinar cell: early morphological changes during development of experimental pancreatitis. Am. J. Physiol., 246:G457, 1984.
41. Niederau, C., and Grendell, J. H.: Intracellular vacuoles in experimental acute pancreatitis in rats and mice are an acidified compartment. J. Clin. Invest., 81:229, 1988.
42. Leach, S. D., et al.: Manipulation of subcellar pH during experimental acute pancreatitis. Surgery. (In press.)

43. Saluja, A., et al.: Pancreatic duct obstruction in rabbits causes digestive zymogen and lysosomal enzyme colonization. J. Clin. Invest., *84*:1260, 1989.
44. Ohshio, G., et al.: Esterase inhibitors prevent lysosomal enzyme redistribution in two noninvasive models of experimental pancreatitis. Gastroenterology, *96*:853, 1989.
45. Janes, N., Clemens, J. A., Glickson, J. D., and Cameron, J. L.: Phosphorus-31 nuclear magnetic resonance spectroscopic study of the canine pancreas: applications to acute alcoholic pancreatitis. Adv. Alcohol Subst. Abuse, *7*:213, 1988.
46. Nordback, I., MacGowan, S., and Cameron, J. L.: Does Acetaldehyde play a role in the pathogenesis of acute pancreatitis? Presented at the 24th Annual Meeting of the Pancreas Club, Inc., San Antonio, May 14, 1990.
47. Kloppel, G., et al.: Human acute pancreatitis: its pathogenesis in the light of immunocytochemical and ultrastructural findings in acinar cells. Virchows Arch. A, *409*:791, 1986.
48. Harvey, M. H., Wedgwood, K. R., and Reber, H. A.: Vasoactive drugs, microvascular permeability and hemorrhagic pancreatitis in cats. Gastroenterology, *93*:1296, 1987.
49. Wedgwood, K. R., Farmer, R. C., and Reber, H. A.: A model of hemorrhagic pancreatitis in cats: the role of 16, 16-dimethyl prostaglandin E2. Gastroenterology, *90*:32, 1986.
50. Farias, L. R., Frey, C. F., Holcroft, J. W., and Gunther, R.: Effect of prostaglandin blockers on ascitic fluid in pancreatitis. Surgery, *98*:571, 1985.
51. Guice, K. S., Bognasco, J. M., and Oldham, K. T.: Histamine and pancreatic edema. Presented at the 24th Annual Meeting of the Pancreas Club, Inc., San Antonio, May 14, 1990.
52. Traverso, L. W., Pullos, T. G., and Frey, C. F.: Hemodynamic characterization of porcine hemorrhagic pancreatitis ascites fluid. J. Surg., Res., *34*:254, 1983.
53. Frey, C. F., Wong, H. N., Hickman, D., and Pullos, T.: Toxicity of hemorrhagic ascitic fluid associated with hemorrhagic pancreatitis. Arch. Surg., *117*:401, 1982.
54. Grega, G., Svensjo, E., and Haddy, F. J.: Macromolecular permeability of the microvascular membrane: physiological and pharmacological regulation. Microcirculation, *1*:325, 1981/1982.
55. Majno, G., Shea, S. M., and Leventhal, M.: Endothelial contraction induced by histamine type mediators: an electron microscopic study. J. Cell. Biol., *42*:647, 1969.
56. Karanjia, N. D., et al.: A study of the time course of conversion of edematous to hemorrhagic pancreatitis. Int. J. Pancreatol., *8*:133, 1991.
57. Bradley, E. L. III, et al.: Hemodynamic consequences of severe pancreatitis. Ann. Surg., *198*:130, 1983.
58. Cobo, J. C., Abraham, E., Bland, R. D., and Shoemaker, W. C.: Sequential hemodynamic and oxygen transport abnormalities in patients with acute pancreatitis. Surgery, *95*:324, 1984.
59. Beger, H. G., et al.: Hemodynamic data pattern in patients with acute pancreatitis. Gastroenterology, *90*:74, 1986.
60. Lefer, A. M., and Glenn, T. M.: Role of the pancreas in the pathogenesis of circulatory shock. *In* The Fundamental Mechanisms of Shock. Edited by L. B. Hinshaw and B. G. Cox. New York, Plenum Press, 1972, p. 311.
61. Lefer, A. M., et al: Inotropic influence of endogenous peptides in experimental hemorrhagic pancreatitis. Surgery, *69*:220, 1971.
62. Lefer, A. M., and Martin, J.: Origin of the myocardial depressant factor in shock. Am. J. Physiol., *218*:1423, 1970.
63. Ohlsson, K., and Tegener, H.: Experimental pancreatitis in the dog. Demonstration of trypsin in ascitic fluid, lymph and plasma. Scand. J. Gastroenterol., *8*:129, 1973.
64. Bokisch, V. A., Muller-Eberhard, H. J., and Cochrane, C. G.: Isolation of fragment (C3a) of the third component of human complement containing anaphylatoxin and chemotactic activity and description of an anaphylatoxin inactivator of human serum. J. Exp. Med., *129*:1109, 1969.
65. Wetsel, R. A., and Kolb, W. P.: Complement-independent activation of the fifth component (C5) of human complement: limited trypsin digestion resulting in the expression of biological activity. J. Immunol., *128*:209, 1982.
66. Cochrane, C. G., and Muller-Eberhard, H. J.: The derivation of two distinct anaphylatoxin activities from the third and fifth components of human complement. J. Exp. Med., *127*:371, 1968.
67. Muller-Eberhard, H. J.: The membrane attack complex. Springer Semin. Immunopathol., *7*:93, 1984.
68. Roxvall, L., Bengston, A., and Heideman, M.: Anaphylatoxin generation and multisystem organ failure in acute pancreatitis. Prog. Clin. Biol. Res., *308*:265, 1989.
69. Knol, J. A., Inman, M. G., Strodel, W. E., and Eckhauser, K. E.: Pancreatic response to crystalloid resuscitation in experimental pancreatitis. J. Surg. Res., *43*:387, 1987.
70. Donaldson, L. A., Williams, R. W., and Schenk, W. G.: Experimental pancreatitis: effect of plasma and dextran on pancreatic blood flow. Surgery, *84*:313, 1978.
71. Klar, E., Herforth, C., and Messmer, K.: Therapeutic effect of isovolemic hemodilution with dextran 60 on the impairment of pancreatic microcirculation in acute biliary pancreatitis. Ann. Surg., *211*:346, 1990.
72. Lehtola, A.: Effects of dextran 70 vs. crystalloids in the microcirculation of porcine hemorrhagic pancreatitis. Surg. Gynecol. Obstet., *162*:556, 1986.
73. Horton, J. W., Dunn, C. W., Burnweit, C. A., and Walker, P. B.: Hypertonic saline-dextran resuscitation of acute canine bile-induced pancreatitis. Am. J. Surg., *158*:48, 1989.
74. Halverson, L., Blaisdell, F. W., and Holcroft, J. W.: Recent advances in prehospital fluid resuscitation. *In* Advances in Trauma. Edited by H. Cleveland. Chicago, Year Book, 1990.
75. Lucas, C. E., and Ledgerwood, A. M.: Shock and renal failure. *In* Complications of Pancreatitis: Medical and Surgical Management. Edited by E. L. Bradley. Philadelphia, W. B. Saunders, 1982.
76. Werner, M. H., Hayes, D. F., Lucas, C. E., and Rosenberg, I. K.: Renal vasoconstriction in association with acute pancreatitis. Am. J. Surg., *127*:185, 1974.
77. Gupta, R. K.: Immunohistochemical study of glomerular lesions in acute pancreatitis. Arch. Pathol. *92*:267, 1971.
78. Canavese, C., Stratta, P., and Vercellone, A.: The case for oxygen free radicals in the pathogenesis of ischemic acute renal failure. Nephron, *49*:9, 1988.
79. Warshaw, A. L. and Fuller, A. F., Jr.: Specificity of increased renal clearance of amylase in diagnosis of acute pancreatitis. N. Engl. J. Med., *292*:325, 1975.
80. Mock, D. M., Grendell, J. H., Cello, J., and Morris, R. C.: Pancreatitis and alcoholism disorder the renal tubule and impair reclamation of some low molecular weight proteins. Gastroenterology, *92*:161, 1987.
81. McKenna, J. M., et al.: The pleuropulmonary complications of pancreatitis. Clinical Conference in pulmonary disease from Northwestern University, McGaw Medical Center and Veterans Administration Lakeside Hospital, Chicago. Chest, *71*:197, 1977.
82. Imrie, C. W., Ferguson, J. C., Murphy, D., and Blumgart, L. H.: Arterial hypoxia in acute pancreatitis. Br. J. Surg., *64*:185, 1977.
83. Beger, H. G., et al.: Necrosectomy and postoperative local lavage in patients with necrotizing pancreatitis: results of a prospective clinical trial. *In* Acute Pancreatitis. Edited by H. G. Beger and M. Buchler. Berlin, Springer-Verlag, 1987.

84. Bradley, E. L., III: Management of infected pancreatic necrosis by open drainage. Ann. Surg., *206*:542, 1987.
85. Stone, H. H., Strom, P. R., and Mullins, R. J.: Pancreatic abscess management by subtotal resection and packing. World J. Surg., *8*:340, 1984.
86. Howard, J. M.: Delayed debridement and external drainage of massive pancreatic or peripancreatic necrosis. Surg. Gynecol. Obstet., *168*:25, 1989.
87. Katsohis, C. D., et al.: Pancreatic abscess following acute pancreatitis. Am. Surg., *55*:427, 1989.
88. Warshaw, A. L., and Jin, G. L.: Improved survival in 45 patients with pancreatic abscess. Ann. Surg., *202*:408, 1985.
89. Malangoni, M. A., et al.: Factors contributing to fatal outcome after treatment of pancreatic abscess. Ann. Surg., *203*:605, 1986.
90. Nicholson, M. L., Mortensen, N. J., and Espiner, H. J.: Pancreatic abscess: results of prolonged irrigation of the pancreatic bed after surgery. Br. J. Surg., *75*:89, 1988.
91. Fink, A. S., et al.: Indolent presentation of pancreatic abscess. Arch. Surg., *123*:1067, 1988.
92. Brigham, K. L.: Mechanisms of lung injury. Clin. Chest Med., *3*:9, 1982.
93. Deby-Dupont, G., et al.: Thromboxane and prostacyclin release in adult respiratory distress syndrome. Intensive Care Med., *13*:167, 1987.
94. Ranson, J. H., Roses, D. F., and Fink, S. D.: Early respiratory insufficiency in acute pancreatitis. Ann. Surg., *178*:75, 1973.
95. Ranson, J. H., et al.: Respiratory complications in acute pancreatitis. Ann. Surg., *179*:557, 1974.
96. Aho, H. J., Ahda, R. A., Tolvanen, A. M., and Nevalainen, T. J.: Experimental pancreatitis in the rat: changes in pulmonary phospholipid during sodium taurocholate-induced acute pancreatitis. Res. Exp. Med. (Berl.), *182*:79, 1983.
97. Buchler, M., et al.: Phospholipase: an activity determines the severity of human acute pancreatitis. Digestion, *35*:11, 1986.
98. Zieve, L., and Vogal, W. C.: Measurement of lecithinase A in serum and other body fluids. J. Lab. Clin. Med., *57*:586, 1961.
99. Buchler, M., et al.: Sensitivity of antiproteases, complement factors and C-reactive protein in detecting pancreatic necrosis: results of a prospective clinical study. Int. J. Pancreatol., *1*:227, 1986.
100. Li, J. J., et al.: Impact of C-reactive protein (CRP) on surfactant function. J. Trauma, *29*:1690, 1989.
101. Warshaw, A. L., Lesser, P. B., Rie, M., and Cullen, D. J.: Pathogenesis of pulmonary edema in acute pancreatitis. Ann. Surg., *182*:505, 1975.
102. Kimura, T., et al.: Respiratory failure in acute pancreatitis: a possible role for triglycerides. Ann. Surg., *189*:509, 1979.
103. Guice, K. S., et al.: Pancreatitis-induced acute lung injury. Ann. Surg., *208*:71, 1988.
104. Anderson, M. C.: Hepatic morphology and function: alterations associated with acute pancreatitis. Arch. Surg., *92*:664, 1966.
105. Pawlicka, J. E., Dlugosz, J., Andrzejewska, A., and Gabryelewicz, A.: The functional and ultrastructural changes of hepatic mitochondria in acute experimental pancreatitis in dogs treated with prostacyclin. Exp. Pathol., *22*:157, 1982.
106. Andrzejewska, A., Dugosz, J., and Kurasz, S.: The ultrastructure of the liver in acute experimental pancreatitis in dogs. Exp. Pathol., *28*:167, 1985.
107. Dlugosz, J., Pawlicka, E., and Gabryelewicz, A.: Lysosomal-mitochondrial interrelationships in damage to the liver in acute experimental pancreatitis in dogs: treatment with prostacyclin (PGI2). Int. J. Pancreatol., *3*:343, 1988.
108. Kitamura, O., Oazawa, K., and Honjo, I.: Alterations in liver metabolism associated with experimental acute pancreatitis. Am. J. Surg., *126*:379, 1973.
109. Wellman, K. F., and Volk, B. W.: Pancreatitis, pancreatic lithiasis and diabetes mellitus. *In* The diabetic pancreas. Edited by K. F. Wellman, and B. W. Volk. New York, Plenum Press, 1977.
110. Ranson, J. H., et al.: Prognostic signs and the role of operative management in acute pancreatitis. Surg. Gynecol. Obstet., *139*:69, 1974.
111. Drew, S. E., et al.: The first 24 hours of acute pancreatitis. Changes in biochemical and endocrine homeostasis in patients with pancreatitis compared with those in control subjects undergoing stress for reasons other than pancreatitis. Am. J. Med., *64*:795, 1978.
112. Solomon, S. S., et al.: The glucose intolerance of acute pancreatitis: hormonal response to arginine. Diabetes, *29*:22, 1980.
113. Wedgwood, K., and Reber, H. A.: Pathogenesis of acute pancreatitis. *In* Surgical Diseases of the Pancreas. Edited by J. M. Howard, G. L. Jordan, Jr., and H. A. Reber. Philadelphia, Lea & Febiger, 1987.
114. Allam, B. F., and Imrie, C. W.: Serum ionized calcium in acute pancreatitis. Br. J. Surg., *64*:665, 1977.
115. Imrie, C. W., Allam, B. F., and Ferguson, J. C.: Hypocalcaemia of acute pancreatitis: the effect of hypoalbuminaemia. Curr. Med. Res. Opin., *4*:101, 1976.
116. Edmondson, H. A., and Fields, I. A.: Relation of calcium and lipids to acute pancreatic necrosis. Arch. Intern. Med., *69*:177, 1942.
117. Condon, J. R., Ives, D., Knight, M. J., and Day, J.: The aetiology of hypocalcaemia in acute pancreatitis. Br. J. Surg., *62*:115, 1975.
118. Weir, G. C., et al.: The hypocalcemia of acute pancreatitis. Ann. Intern. Med., *83*:185, 1975.
119. Bardenheier, J. A., Kaminski, D. L., and Willman, V. L.: Pancreatitis after biliary tract surgery. Am. J. Surg., *116*:773, 1968.
120. Steer, M. L.: Etiology and pathophysiology of acute pancreatitis. *In* Exocrine Pancreas: Biology, Pathobiology and Disease. Edited by V. L. W. Go, et al. New York, Raven Press, 1986.
121. Murphy, D., Imrie, C. W., and Davidson, J. F.: Haematological abnormalities in acute pancreatitis: a prospective study. Postgrad. Med. J., *53*:310, 1977.
122. Lasson, A., and Ohlsson, K.: Consumptive coagulopathy fibrinolysis and protease-antiprotease anteractions during acute human pancreatitis. Thromb. Res., *41*:167, 1986.
123. Lasson, A.: Acute pancreatitis in man: a clinical and biochemical study of pathophysiology and treatment. Scand. J. Gastroenterol., *19(Suppl. 99)*:1, 1984.
124. Browder, I. W., et al.: Protective effect of glucan-enhanced macrophage function in experimental pancreatitis. Am. J. Surg., *153*:25, 1987.
125. Frey, C. F.: Hemorrhagic pancreatitis. Am. J. Surg., *137*:616, 1979.
126. Blake, R. L., Jr.: Acute pancreatitis. Prim. Care, *15*:187, 1988.
127. Salt, W. B., II and Schenker, S.: Amylase-its clinical significance: a review of the literature. Medicine, *55*:269, 1976.
128. Spechler, S. J., et al.: Prevalence of normal serum amylase levels in patients with acute alcoholic pancreatitis. Dig. Dis. Sci., *28*:865, 1983.
129. Moossa, A. R.: Current Concepts. Diagnostic tests and pro-

cedures in acute pancreatitis. N. Engl. J. Med., *311*:639, 1984.
130. Neoptolemos, J. P., et al.: The urgent diagnosis of gallstones in acute pancreatitis: a prospective study of three methods. Br. J. Surg., *71*:230, 1984.
131. Neoptolemos, J. P., et al.: The role of clinical and biochemical criteria and endoscopic retrograde cholangiopancreatography in the urgent diagnosis of common bile duct stones in acute pancreatitis. Surgery, *100*:732, 1986.
132. Davidson, B. R., et al.: Biochemical prediction of gallstones in acute pancreatitis: a prospective study of three systems. Br. J. Surg., *75*:213, 1988.
133. Freeny, P. C.: Radiology of acute pancreatitis: diagnosis, detection of complications and interventional therapy. *In* Acute Pancreatitis. Edited by G. Glazer, and J. H. C. Ranson. London, Bailliere Tindall, 1988.
134. Acosta, J. M., and Ledesma, C. L.: Gallstone migration as a cause of acute pancreatitis. N. Engl. J. Med., *290*:484, 1974.
135. Frey, C. F.: Gallstone pancreatitis. Surg. Clin. North Am., *61*:923, 1981.
136. Frey, C. F.: A strategy for the surgical management of gallstone pancreatitis. *In* Acute Pancreatitis. Edited by H. G. Beger and M. Buchler. Berlin, Springer-Verlag, 1987.
137. Glenn, F., and Frey, C. F.: Re-evaluation of the treatment of pancreatitis associated with biliary tract disease. Ann. Surg., *160*:723, 1964.
138. Acosta, J. M., et al.: Early surgery for acute gallstone pancreatitis: evaluation of a systemic approach. Surgery, *83*:367, 1978.
139. Stone, H. H., Fabian, T. C., and Dunlap, W. E.: Gallstone pancreatitis: biliary tract pathology in relation to time of operation. Ann. Surg., *194*:305, 1981.
140. Kelly, T. R., and Wagner, D. S.: Gallstone pancreatitis: a prospective randomized trial of the timing of surgery. Surgery, *104*:600, 1988.
141. Safrany, L., and Cotton, P. B.: A preliminary report: urgent duodenoscopic sphincterotomy for acute gallstone pancreatitis. Surgery, *89*:424, 1981.
142. Neoptolemos, J. P., et al.: Controlled trial of urgent endoscopic retrograde cholangiopancreatography and endoscopic sphincterotomy versus conservative treatment for acute pancreatitis due to gallstones. Lancet, *2*:979, 1988.
143. Neoptolemos, J. P., and Carr-Locke, D. L.: ERCP in acute cholangitis and pancreatitis. *In* ERCP Diagnostic and Therapeutic Applications. Edited by I. M. Jacobson. New York, Elsevier Science Publishing, 1989.
144. Farias, L. R., Frey, C. F., French, S., and Gunther, R.: The role of ductal obstruction on the course of hemorrhagic pancreatitis in the pig. Int. J. Pancreatol., *1*:51, 1986.
145. Ranson, J. H.: The role of surgery in the management of acute pancreatitis. Ann. Surg., *211*:382, 1990.
146. Frey, C. F., Bradley, E. L., III, and Beger, H. G.: Progress in acute pancreatitis. Surg. Gynecol. Obstet., *167*:282, 1988.
147. McMahon, M. J., Playforth, M. J., and Pickford, I. R.: A comparative study of methods for the prediction of severity of attacks of acute pancreatitis. Br. J. Surg., *67*:22, 1980.
148. Ranson, J. H. C.: Management of pancreatic abscess. *In* Progress in Hepatic, Biliary and Pancreatic Surgery. Edited by J. S. Najarian, and J. P. Delaney. Chicago, Year Book Medical Publishers, 1990.
149. Ranson, J. H.: The timing of biliary surgery in acute pancreatitis. Ann. Surg., *189*:654, 1979.
150. Blamey, S. I., et al.: Prognostic factors in acute pancreatitis. Gut, *25*:1340, 1984.
151. Banks, S., Wise, L., and Gersten, M.: Risk factor in acute pancreatitis. Am. J. Gastroenterol., *78*:637, 1983.
152. Knaus, W. A., Draper, E. A., Wagner, D. P., and Zimmerman, J. E.: APACHE II: a severity disease classification system. Crit. Care Med., *13*:818, 1985.
153. Civetta, J. M., Hudson-Civetta, J. A., and Nelson, L. D.: Evaluation of APACHE II for cost containment and quality assurance. Ann. Surg. *212*:266, 1990.
154. Larvin, M., and McMahon, M. J.: APACHE II score for assessment and monitoring of acute pancreatitis. Lancet, *2*:201, 1989.
155. Demmy, T. L., et al.: Comparison of multiple parameter prognostic systems in acute pancreatitis. Am. J. Surg., *156*:492, 1988.
156. Imrie, C. W., and Blumgart, L. H.: Acute pancreatitis: a prospective study on some factors in mortality. Bull. Soc. Int. Chir., *34*:601, 1975.
157. Kivisaari, L., et al.: Early detection of acute fulminant pancreatitis by contrast-enhanced computed tomography. Scand. J. Gastroenterol., *18*:39, 1983.
158. Clavien, P. A., et al.: Value of contrast-enhanced computerized tomography in the early diagnosis and prognosis of acute pancreatitis: a prospective study of 202 patients. Am. J. Surg., *155*:457, 1988.
159. Bradley, E. L., III, and Allen, K.: A prospective longitudinal study of observation versus surgical intervention in the management of necrotizing pancreatitis. Am. J. Surg., *161*:19, 1991.
160. Bradley, E. L. III, Murphy, F., and Ferguson, C.: Prediction of pancreatic necrosis by dynamic pancreatography. Ann. Surg., *210*:495, 1989.
161. Balthazar, E. J., et al.: Acute pancreatitis: prognostic value of CT. Radiology, *156*:767, 1985.
162. Gebhardt, C., Kraus, D., Schonekas, H., and Muschweck, H.: Early endoscopic retrograde cholangiopancreatography in acute pancreatitis. Leber Magen Darm, *19*:125, 1989.
163. Buchler, M., Uhl, W., and Malfertheiner, P.: Biochemical staging of acute pancreatitis. *In* Acute Pancreatitis. Edited by H. G. Beger and M. Buchler. Berlin, Springer-Verlag, 1987.
164. Wilson, C., et al.: C-reactive protein, antiproteases and complement factors as objective markers of severity in acute pancreatitis. Br. J. Surg., *76*:177, 1989.
165. Ferguson, C. M., and Bradley, E.: Can serum markers for pancreatic necrosis be used as indicators for surgery? Am. J. Surg., *160*:459, 1990.
166. Murata, A., et al.: Serum Interleukin 6, C-reactive protecin and pancreatic secretory trypsin inhibitor (PSTI) as acute phase reactants after major thoraco-abdominal surgery. Immunol. Invest., *19*:271, 1990.
167. Dominguez-Munoz, E., et al.: PMN elastase: an effective marker in early prognostic evaluation on acute pancreatitis: results of Spanish multicenter study. Presented at the Fourth Meeting of the International Association of Pancreatology, Nagasaki, August 20, 1990.
168. Andres, S. F., et al.: Clinical determination of methemalbumin. Clin. Chem., *21*:1506, 1975.
169. Beger, H. G., et al.: Bacterial contamination pancreatic necrosis: a prospective clinical study. Gastroenterology, *91*:433, 1986.
170. Hancke, E., and Marklein, G.: Bacterial contamination of the pancreas with intestinal germs: a cause of acute suppurative pancreatitis. *In* Acute Pancreatitis. Edited by H. G. Beger and M. Buchler. Heidelberg, Springer-Verlag, 1987.
171. Deitch, E. A., Berg, R., and Specian, R.: Endotoxin promotes the translocation of bacteria from the gut. Arch. Surg., *122*:185, 1987.
172. Baker, J. W., et al.: Hemorrhagic shock induces bacterial translocation from the gut. J. Trauma, *28*:896, 1988.
173. Wells, C. L., Maddaus, M. A., and Simmons, R. L.: Role of

the macrophage in the translocation of intestinal bacteria. Arch. Surg., *122:*48, 1987.
174. Sori, A. J., et al.: The gut as source of sepsis after hemorrhagic shock. Arch. Surg., *155:*187, 1988.
175. Gerzof, S. G., et al.: Early diagnosis of pancreatic infection by computed tomography-guided aspiration. Gastroenterology, *93:*1315, 1987.
176. Creutzfeld, W., and Lankisch, P. G.: Intensive medical treatment of severe acute pancreatitis. World J. Surg., *5:*341, 1981.
177. Lankisch, P. G.: Peritoneal lavage in the treatment of acute pancreatitis. *In* Acute Pancreatitis: Advances in Pathogenesis, Diagnosis and Treatment. Edited by P. A. Banks, and P. G. Bianchi. Milan, Masson, 1984, p. 115.
178. Pullos, T., Frey, C. F., and Zaiss, C.: Toxicity of ascitic fluid from pigs with hemorrhagic pancreatitis. J. Surg. Res., *33:* 136, 1982.
179. Mayer, A. D., Airey, M., Hodgson, J., and McMahon, M. J.: Enzyme transfer from pancreas to plasma during acute pancreatitis: the contribution of ascitic fluid and lymphatic drainage of the pancreas. Gut, *26:*876, 1985.
180. Niederau, C., et al.: Therapeutic regimens in acute experimental hemorrhagic pancreatitis. Gastroenterology, *95:* 1648, 1988.
181. Satake, K., Koh, I., Nishiwaki, H., and Umeyama, K.: Toxic products in hemorrhagic ascites fluid generated during experimental acute hemorrhagic pancreatitis in dogs and treatment which reduces their effect. Digestion, *32:*99, 1985.
182. Mayer, A. D., et al.: Controlled clinical trial of peritoneal lavage for the treatment of severe acute pancreatitis. N. Engl. J. Med. *312:*399, 1985.
183. Ranson, J. H., and Berman, R. S.: Long peritoneal lavage decreases pancreatic sepsis in acute pancreatitis. Ann. Surg., *211:*708, 1990.
184. Burnweit, C. A., and Horton, J. W.: Extravascular lung water as an indicator of pulmonary dysfunction in acute hemorrhagic pancreatitis. Ann. Surg., *207:*33, 1988.
185. Hayes, M. F., Jr., Rosenbaum, R. W., Zibelman, M., and Matsumoto, T.: Adult respiratory distress syndrome in association with acute pancreatitis. Am. J. Surg., *127:*314, 1979.
186. Holden, J. L., Berne, T. V., and Rosoff, L., Sr.: Pancreatic abscess following acute pancreatitis. Arch. Surg., *111:*858, 1976.
187. Camer, S. J., Tan, E. G., Warren, K. W., and Braasch, J. W.: Pancreatic abscess. A critical analysis of 113 cases. Am. J. Surg., *129:*426, 1975.
188. Frey, C. F., Lindenauer, S. M., and Miller, T. A.: Pancreatic abscess. Surg. Gynecol. Obstet., *149:*722, 1979.
189. Becker, J. M., et al.: Prognostic factors in pancreatic abscess. Surgery, *96:*455, 1984.
190. Beger, H. G., Block, S., and Bittner, R.: The significance of bacterial infection in acute pancreatitis. *In* Acute Pancreatitis. Edited by H. G. Beger and M. Buchler. Berlin, Springer-Verlag, 1987.
191. Aranha, G. V., Prinz, R. A., and Greenlee, H. B.: Pancreatic abscess: an unresolved surgical problem. Am. J. Surg., *144:* 534, 1982.
192. Altemeier, W. A., and Alexander, J. W.: Pancreatic abscess. Arch. Surg., *87:*80, 1963.
193. Evans, F. C.: Pancreatic abscess. Am. J. Surg., *117:*537, 1969.
194. Farringer, J. L. Jr., Robbins, L. B. II, and Pickens, D. R. Jr.: Abscesses of the pancreas. Surgery, *60:*964, 1966.
195. Jones, C. E., Polk, H. C., and Fulton, R. L.: Pancreatic abscess. Am. J. Surg., *129:*44, 1975.
196. Warshaw, A. L.: Pancreatic abscesses. N. Engl. J. Med., *287:* 1234, 1972.
197. Craig, R. M., Dordal, E., and Myles, L.: Letter: the use of ampicillin in acute pancreatitis. Ann. Intern. Med., *83:*831, 1975.
198. Howes, R., Zuidema, G. D., and Cameron, J. L.: Evaluation of prophylactic antibiotics in acute pancreatitis. J. Surg. Res., *18:*197, 1975.
199. Finch, W. T., Sawyer, J. L., and Schenker, S.: A prospective study to determine the efficiency of antibiotics in acute pancreatitis. Ann. Surg., *183:*667, 1976.
200. Stone, H. H., and Fabian, T. C.: Peritoneal dialysis in the treatment of acute pancreatitis. Surg. Gynecol. Obstet., *150:*878, 1980.
201. Hermann, R. E., and Knowles, R. C.: Lethal factors and response to therapy in experiment bile-reflex pancreatitis. Ann. Surg., *161:*456, 1965.
202. Calandra, T., et al.: Clinical significance of candida isolated from peritoneum in surgical patients. Lancet, *2:*1437, 1989.
203. Beger, H. G., Bittner, R., Block, S., and Buchler, M.: Bacterial contamination of pancreatic necrosis. Gastroenterology, *91:*433, 1986.
204. Lumsden, A., and Bradley, E. L., III: Secondary pancreatic infections. Surg. Gynecol. Obstet., *170:*459, 1990.
205. Buchler, M., et al.: Human pancreatic tissue concentration of bactericidal antibiotics. Gastroenterology, *103:*1902, 1992.
206. Sarr, M. G., Sanfrey, H., and Cameron, J. L.: Prospective randomized trial of nasogastric suction in patients with acute pancreatitis. Surgery, *100:*500, 1986.
207. Shaw, J. H., and Wolfe, R. R.: Glucose, fatty acid and urea kinetics in patients with severe pancreatitis. The response to substrate infusion and total parenteral nutrition. Ann. Surg., *204:*665, 1986.
208. Goodgame, J. T., and Fischer, J. E.: Parenteral nutrition in the treatment of acute pancreatitis: effect on complications and mortality. Ann. Surg., *186:*651, 1977.
209. Ryan, J. A., and Page, C. P.: Intrajejunal feeding: development and current status. JPEN J. Parenter. Enteral Nutr., *8:* 187, 1984.
210. Howard, J. M.: Treatment of acute pancreatitis. Principles of Management: conservative attitude. *In* Surgical Diseases of the Pancreas. Edited by J. M. Howard, G. L. Jordan, Jr., and H. A. Reber. Philadelphia, Lea & Febiger, 1987.
211. Reber, A. H., and Smale, B. F.: Planned operation for acute pancreatitis: the American experience. *In* Surgical Diseases of the Pancreas. Edited by J. M. Howard, G. L. Jordan, Jr., and H. A. Reber. Philadelphia, Lea & Febiger, 1987.
212. Roher, H. D., and Maroske, D.: Timing and indications for surgical treatment in necrotizing pancreatitis in acute pancreatitis. Edited by H. G. Beger and M. Buchler. Berlin, Springer-Verlag, 1987.
213. Gerzof, S. G., et al.: Percutaneous catheter drainage of abdominal abscesses: a five-year experience. N. Engl. J. Med., *305:*653, 1981.
214. Bittner, R., et al.: Pancreatic abscess and infected pancreatic necrosis: different local septic complications in acute pancreatitis. Dig. Dis. Sci., *32:*1082, 1987.
215. Freeny, P. C., Lewis, G. P., Traverso, L. W., and Ryan, J. A.: Infected pancreatic fluid collections: percutaneous catheter drainage. Radiology, *167:*435, 1988.
216. Pickleman, J., and Moncada, R.: The role of percutaneous drainage of pancreatic abscesses. Am. Surg., *53:*451, 1987.
217. Davidson, E. D., and Bradley, E. L., III: Marsupialization: in the treatment of pancreatic abscess. Surgery, *89:*252, 1981.
218. Bolooki, H., Jaffe, B., and Gliedman, M. L.: Pancreatic abscesses and lesser sac collections. Surg. Gynecol. Obstet., *126:*1201, 1968.

219. Pemberton, J. H., et al.: Controlled open lesser sac drainage for pancreatic abscess. Ann. Surg., *203*:600, 1986.
220. Garcia-Sabrido, J. L., et al.: Treatment of severe intra-abdominal sepsis and/or necrotic foci by an open-abdomen approach: zipper and zipper-mesh techniques. Arch. Surg., *123*:152, 1988.
221. Buchler, M., et al.: Necrotizing pancreatitis: peritoneal lavage (PL) or local lavage (LL) of the lesser sac. Dig. Dis. Sci., *29*:944, 1984.
222. Ranson, J. H., and Spencer, F. C.: The role of peritoneal lavage in severe acute pancreatitis. Ann. Surg., *187*:565, 1978.
223. Balldin, G., and Ohlsson, K.: Demonstration of pancreatic protease-antiprotease complexes in the peritoneal fluid with acute pancreatitis. Surgery, *85*:451, 1979.
224. Gebhardt, C., and Gall, F. P.: Importance of peritoneal irrigation after surgical treatment of hemorrhagic necrotizing pancreatitis. World J. Surg., *5*:379, 1981.
225. Pederzoli, P., et al.: Retroperitoneal and peritoneal drainage and lavage in the treatment of severe necrotizing pancreatitis. Surg. Gynecol. Obstet., *170*:197, 1990.
226. Frey, C. F., Lindenauer, S. M., and Miller, T. A.: Pancreatic abscess. Surg. Gynecol. Obstet., *149*:722, 1979.
227. Fielding, G. A., et al.: Acute pancreatitis and pancreatic fistula formation. Br. J. Surg., *76*:1126, 1989.
228. Doberneck, R. C.: Intestinal fistula complicating necrotizing pancreatitis. Am. J. Surg. *158*:581, 1989.
229. Aldridge, M. C., et al.: Colonic complications of severe acute pancreatitis. Br. J. Surg. *76*:362, 1989.
230. Meister, R.: Treatment of biliary pancreatitis: approach, technique and results. *In* Acute Pancreatitis. Edited by H. G. Beger and M. Buchler. Berlin, Springer-Verlag, 1987.
231. Shaak, T. V., Zinevich, V. P., and Ivanova, R. M.: Treatment experiences with acute pancreatitis. Vestn. Khir. (Eng. Abstr.), *125*:63, 1980.
231a. McCarthy, M. C., and Dickerman, R. M.: Surgical management of severe acute pancreatitis. Arch. Surg., *117*:476, 1982.
231b. Ruttner, D. W., et al.: Early surgical debridement of pancreatic necrosis is beneficial irrespective of infection. Am. J. Surg., *163*:105, 1992.
232. Wilson, C., et al.: Surgical treatment of acute necrotizing pancreatitis. Br. J. Surg., *75*:1119, 1988.
233. Ivatury, R. R., et al.: Open management of the septic abdomen: therapeutic and prognostic considerations based on APACHE II. Crit. Care Med., *17*:511, 1989.
234. Al-Hadeedi, S., Fan, S. T., and Leaper, D.: APACHE II score for assessment and monitoring of acute pancreatitis. (Letter.) Lancet, *2*:738, 1989.
235. Gebhardt, C.: Indications for surgical intervention in necrotizing pancreatitis with extrapancreatic necrosis. *In* Acute Pancreatitis. Edited by H. G. Beger and M. Buchler. Berlin, Springer-Verlag, 1987, p. 310.
236. Bodeker, H., et al.: Conservative treatment of severe necrotizing pancreatitis using continuous hemofiltration. Presented at the 24th Annual Meeting of the Pancreas Club, Inc., San Antonio, May 14, 1990.
237. Zirngible, H., Mannis, S., and Braun, G.: Plasma separation in acute pancreatitis: animal experiments and first clinical results. Presented at the 24th Annual Meeting of the Pancreas Club, Inc., San Antonio, May 14, 1990.
238. Wittinger, J., and Frey, C. F.: Islet concentration in the head, body and tail and uncinate process of the pancreas. Ann. Surg., *179*:412, 1974.
239. Owyang, C., Louie, D. S., and Tatum, D.: Feedback regulation of pancreatic enzyme secretion: suppression of cholecystokinin release by trypsin. J. Clin. Invest., *77*:2042, 1986.
240. Stanley, J. L., et al.: Major arterial hemorrhage: a complication of pancreatic pseudocysts and chronic pancreatitis. Arch. Surg., *111*:435, 1976.
241. Frey, C. F., Eckhauser, F., and Stanley, J. C.: Hemorrhage. *In* Complications of Pancreatitis. Edited by E. L. Bradley, III. Philadelphia, W. B. Saunders, 1982.
242. Vujic, I., Anderson, M. C., Meredith, H. C., and Cullom, J. W.: Successful embolization of the dorsal pancreatic artery to control massive upper gastrointestinal hemorrhage. Am. Surg., *46*:184, 1980.
243. Martin, F., Pederzoli, P., and Marzoli, G. P.: Short- and long-term results after necrotizing pancreatitis. *In* Acute Pancreatitis. Edited by H. G. Beger and M. Buchler. Heidelberg, Springer-Verlag, 1987, p. 375.
244. Buchler, M. B., Hauke, A., and Malfertheiner, P.: Follow-up after acute pancreatitis: morphology and function. *In* Acute Pancreatitis. Edited by H. G. Beger and M. Buchler, Heidelberg, Springer-Verlag, 1987, p. 367.
245. Angelini, G., et al.: Long-term outcome of acute necrohemorrhagic pancreatitis: a four-year follow-up. Digestion, *30*:131, 1984.

Chapter 53

BILIARY SEPSIS

THOMAS A. BROUGHAN

In Western culture, 15 to 20% of adults harbor gallstones, and 500,000 to 600,000 cholecystectomies per year are performed. The current populations of aged and critically ill patients have presented new challenges to the physician interested in hepatobiliary diseases. Older, more infirm patients may not show the characteristic symptoms and signs of right upper quadrant inflammation. Further, sepsis in these groups of patients with comorbid disease is less well tolerated. Other organ system derangements make treatment increasingly hazardous. Patients may not even be conscious enough to talk to their doctors. Cholecystitis without gallstones has appeared as a result of our ability to sustain critical patients who would have succumbed in earlier years. Sophisticated antibiotics, improved imaging technology, endoscopy, and percutaneous access to the biliary tract are more recent advances to refine management. With such advances in technology, all patients do not require surgery, at least not immediately. Despite more than a century of technological development, however, since John Bobbs performed the first cholecystostomy (1867), Carl Langenbuch the first cholecystectomy (1882), and Ludwig Courvoisier the first common bile duct exploration (1890), clinical suspicion and seasoned judgment are the most valuable aids in making a timely diagnosis. The abdomen remains a "black box" without precise testing or imaging to alert the physician to all that brews within it.

PRE-ICU PHASE

Asymptomatic Gallstones

With gallstones so prevalent, it is important to realize that all gallstones do not require treatment.[1] Biliary colic, which is abdominal pain that can be related to gallstones, is the only incontrovertible evidence of symptomatic gallstones. Nonspecific symptoms like indigestion, "gas," belching, food intolerance, nausea and vomiting, and heartburn likely relate to other nonspecific gastrointestinal disorders. Two studies have estimated the risk of asymptomatic gallstone patients becoming symptomatic to be 10 to 18% at 20 years.[2,3] Prophylactic cholecystectomy has largely become a thing of the past (this will be discussed later in this chapter).

Concomitant Cholecystectomy

Should a patient with gallstones undergoing abdominal operation for other reasons have concomitant cholecystectomy? The addition of a cholecystectomy to another operative procedure is not felt to increase operative risk.[4] The main argument on this point concerns patients undergoing intra-abdominal vascular operations requiring the implantation of synthetic graft material. In this instance, opinion is fairly evenly divided between removing the gallbladder or leaving it in-situ at the time of vascular repair.[5,6] Two points should be made about these vascular patients. When the gallbladder is to be removed at the time of aneurysmectomy, the vascular operation should be completed, the retroperitoneum closed, and then the gallbladder should be excised. Second, vascular and other surgical patients who have undergone large operations with known gallstones in their gallbladder should be watched closely postoperatively for cholecystitis if their gallbladders have not been removed. One study suggested that the incidence of immediate postoperative cholecystitis in vascular patients was 18%.[7] Ottinger reported a 47% mortality rate for postoperative cholecystitis in a group of patients with gallstones after various operations.[8]

Concomitant cholecystectomy in nonvascular operations seems more clearly worthwhile. Two papers report a 54 to 70% incidence of cholecystitis in patients with gallstones remaining after nonvascular operations, and 22% of the instances of cholecystitis occurred within 30 days of operation.[9,10] Thus, cholecystectomy at the time of other abdominal surgery appears to be prudent, particularly if planned preoperatively.

Morbidity and Mortality

Before one can understand the adverse effects of various factors impacting on the outcome of biliary surgery, a knowledge of the usual morbidity and mortality is necessary (Table 53-1).[11] The mortality rate for cholecystectomy for chronic cholecystitis is 0.5% in the general population, including all age groups. Cholecystostomy for chronic cholecystitis carries an 8% mortality rate. The anticipated mortality rate of cholecystectomy and common bile duct exploration is 3.2%. Common duct exploration alone has a mortality rate of 2.1%. If one excludes common duct exploration for cholangitis and pancreatitis, the mortality rate is 1.2%. Most deaths result from operations for acute cholecystitis, and most of the deaths are cardiovascular in origin with cirrhosis, infection, pancreatitis, gastrointestinal bleeding, and renal dysfunction also contributing. The mortality rates for acute cholecystitis are 1.3% for cholecystectomy and 10.6% for cholecystostomy. These mortality rates have significantly decreased over time. In a

Table 53–1. The Mortality Rates Attendant on the Operative Procedures for Chronic Disease of the Biliary Tract

	No. of Cases	No. of Deaths	Mortality Rate (%)
Cholecystectomy	7,413	35	0.5
Cholecystostomy	92	7	7.6
Choledochotomy plus cholecystectomy or cholecystostomy	1,378	48	3.5
Choledochotomy alone	341	7	2.1
Procedures for strictures and miscellaneous conditions	237	20	8.4
Total operations	9,461	117	1.2

(From McSherry, C.K., and Glenn, F.: The incidence and causes of death following surgery for nonmalignant biliary tract disease. Ann. Surg., *191:* 271, 1980.)

more recent report on cholecystectomy by Traverso, the overall morbidity rate was 4.5%, and procedure-related morbidity rate was 2.2% with no mortality (Table 53-2).[12] Therefore, it is important that new therapies like lithotripsy, oral dissolution, and laparoscopic cholecystectomy be judged in comparison with the excellent results obtained with open surgery. These three new therapies remain unproven.

Special Risk Groups

The growing size of the aged population and many more patients with associated medical problems make preoperative risk assessment important. Four groups of patients have been mentioned prominently in the literature:

- Elderly patients
- Patients with diabetes mellitus
- Patients with jaundice
- Cirrhotic patients

Elderly Patients

The incidence of gallstones in the gallbladder and common bile duct increases with age. Studies estimate that 35

Table 53–2. Morbidity from Cholecystectomy

Complication	Overall	Procedure Related
Wound problems	9	9
Urinary retention	5	
Urinary infection	3	
Biliary injury	3	3
Atelectasis	2	
Atrial fibrillation	2	
Subhepatic fluid collection	2	2
Cerebrovascular accident	1	
Clostridium difficile colitis	1	
Superficial leg vein phlebitis	1	
Total	29 (4.5)*	14 (2.2)*

* Numbers in parentheses are percentages
(From Gilliland, T.M., and Traverso, L.W.: Modern standards for comparison of cholecystectomy with alternative treatments from symptomatic cholelithiasis with emphasis on long term relief of symptoms. Surg. Gynecol. Obstet., *170:*39, 1990.)

to 50% of 75-year-old patients have gallstones, and almost 50% have common bile duct stones at cholecystectomy.[13,14] Further, older patients too often fail to display classic signs and symptoms of gallbladder inflammation and biliary sepsis.[15] A delayed diagnosis of cholecystitis in the over 60-year-old group was reported in 33% of patients by Morrow.[15] In patients over age 65, the mortality rate for elective cholecystectomy ranges from 0.8 to 4.4%, but increases to 10 to 19% in cases requiring emergent cholecystectomy.[14] The morbidity rates are 20% for elective cholecystectomies and 32 to 44% for emergency operations.[15,16]

Unfortunately, the incidence of an acute rather than chronic presentation of cholecystitis rises from 20% in the general population to 35 to 48% in the 65-year-old and older group.[14,15] Bile cultures are positive in 27% of the elderly patients undergoing elective cholecystectomy and in 65% having emergency surgery.[17] Morrow reported a series of 39 patients over age 60 with acute cholecystitis of whom 44% had simple acute cholecystitis, 21% purulent cholecystitis, 18% gangrenous or perforated cholecystitis, and 15% subphrenic or liver abscess.[15] In Morrow's group of patients, 38% had heart disease, 26% had severe pulmonary disease, 15% had hypertension, and 13% had diabetes.[15]

The aerobic bacteria involved in biliary sepsis are, in descending order of frequency:

- Escherichia coli
- Klebsiella species
- Enterococcus
- Enterobacter species[16]

Anaerobes are more common in patients with advanced age, a history of prior biliary surgery, or biliary obstruction, and the two groups organisms to remember are Bacteroides fragilis and clostridium species.[16] Older patients with chronic cholecystitis should be offered operation unless their medical condition is prohibitive. Intravenous hydration and preoperative broad spectrum antibiotics should be employed. Elderly patients with acute cholecystitis should undergo operation within 24 hours, if possible.

Operation for cholelithiasis is not undertaken in the current era unless a history of biliary colic, cholangitis, or gallstone pancreatitis is evident. This philosophy has also been extended to diabetics with asymptomatic gallstones. Older studies by Rabinowitz (1932),[18] Eisele (1943),[19] Turrill (1961),[20] Mundth (1962),[21] Schein (1969),[22] and Turner (1969)[23] described the greater morbidity and mortality among diabetics with cholecystitis. Routine gallbladder studies and prophylactic cholecystectomy were suggested for diabetic patients. Walsh and co-workers identified the special concerns in diabetics with cholecystitis: acute onset, insulin dependence, renal disease, and atherosclerosis obliterans.[24] Noninsulin-dependent diabetics with acute cholecystitis had a 5.9% mortality and 58.5% morbidity; insulin-dependent diabetics had a 16.7% mortality and 66.7% morbidity.[24]

Patients with Diabetes Mellitus

If one proposes routine cholecystectomy for all diabetics with gallstones in order to avoid the increased mor-

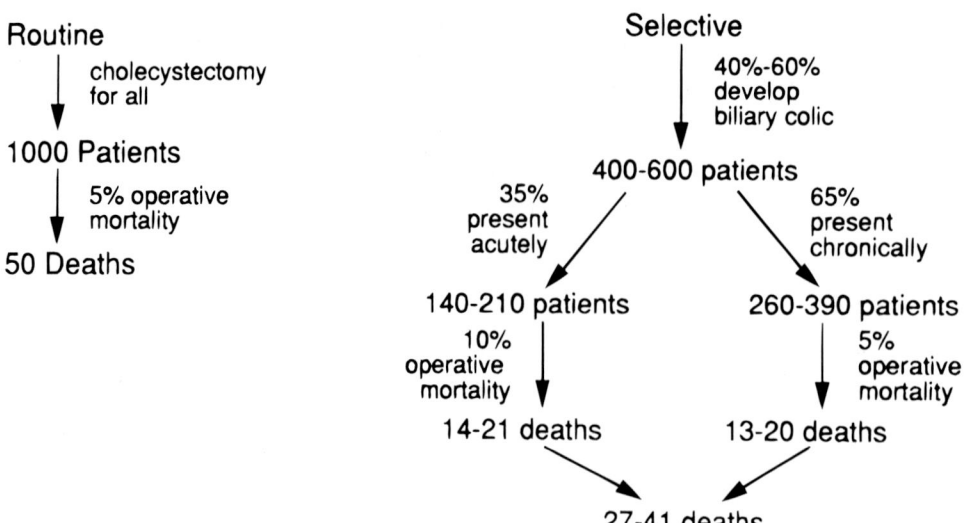

Fig. 53-1. Hypothetic model demonstrating an advantage in operative mortality from selective cholecystectomy for biliary colic vs routine prophylactic cholecystectomy in 1000 diabetic patients with gallstones. (Adapted from Hermann, R. E.: Biliary disease in the aging patient. In The aging gut. Edited by E. C. Texter Jr. New York, Masson, 1983, p. 27; and Reiss, R., Dutsch, A. A., and Nudelmann, J.: Biliary Surgery in diabetic patients: statistical analysis of 189 patients. Dig. Surg., 4:37, 1987.)

bidity and mortality of operation for acute cholecystitis, the resultant mortality rate can be hypothesized to be greater (Fig. 53-1). Hickman and associates present several points to remember in comparing cholecystectomy for acute cholecystitis in diabetic and nondiabetic patients as summarized in Table 53-3.[26] Finally, currently available data are not conclusive regarding the role of prophylactic cholecystectomy in diabetes.

Patients with Jaundice

Experimentally in animals, hyperbilirubinemia has been demonstrated to hamper renal, immunologic, and cardiovascular functions.[27-33] An increased incidence of renal failure, coagulation disorders, gastrointestinal hemorrhage, and delayed wound healing have been recorded in cholemic patients.[34] Although early reports suggested increased morbidity and mortality for jaundiced patients undergoing surgery,[35-37] more recent reports have not consistently demonstrated an advantage for jaundiced patients undergoing preoperative biliary decompression.[34,38-40] The presence of comorbid disease in jaundiced patients and the complications associated with preoperative percutaneous biliary drainage have thus far outweighed any benefits from preoperative biliary drainage.[41] Obstructive jaundice leads to the absence of bile in the gut and a decrease in hepatocyte and Kupffer cell function.[42] It is suggested that with no bile salts in the intestine to interfere, more endotoxin is absorbed into the portal venous blood.[34] The mechanical obstruction of the bile duct has also been demonstrated to decrease reticuloendothelial cell function.[42] Therapeutically, lactulose and bile salts have been given preoperatively and have raised the possibility that they may reduce the postoperative incidence of renal failure.[43,44]

Cirrhotic Patients

Cirrhosis of the liver is the final risk factor to be considered. In cirrhotic patients, Garrison and co-workers reported mortality rates of 21% for biliary operations, 35% for peptic ulcer operations, and 55% for colectomies.[45] Prolonged prothrombin time, large operative blood loss, common duct exploration, and emergency surgery lead to increased morbidity and mortality rates.[45-48] Elective cholecystectomy should be undertaken, however, for genuinely symptomatic patients. Jaundice in cirrhotic patients is usually due to hepatocellular dysfunction, and should be investigated carefully prior to proceeding to operation because of this finding alone.[49] Careful preoperative preparation with correction of coagulation defects, antibiotics, hemodynamic monitoring, control of ascites and encephalopathy, and minimization of intraoperative blood loss have been reported to decrease operative morbidity and mortality for major abdominal procedures to 28 and 8%, respectively.[48] Vasopressin infusions have been administered perioperatively to decrease blood loss.[48] Cirrhotic patients with jaundice secondary to common duct stones are better managed with endoscopic retrograde cholangiopancreatography (ERCP) and sphincterotomy rather than open common duct exploration.[47]

Microbiology

Bile in the gallbladder is considered sterile.[50] There are rare reports that demonstrate cultured bacteria from the

Table 53-3. Characteristics of Acute Cholecystitis in Diabetic Versus Nondiabetic Patients

	Diabetics	Non-Diabetics
Co-morbid disease	34.7%	15.3%
Positive bile cultures	75.5%	43.9%
Postoperative complications	38.9%	20.8%
Infection-related complications	19.4%	6.9%

(From Hickman, M.S., Schwesinger, W.H., and Page, C.P.: Acute cholecystitis in the diabetic. Arch. Surg., 100:15, 1986.)

bile and liver of normal patients.[51] Infections of the biliary tract are considered in two basic categories: cholecystitis and cholangitis. Cholecystitis is thought to be a disease of high morbidity but low mortality.[52] It is felt to begin as inflammation of the gallbladder that becomes infected, secondarily.[50] Cholangitis is a disease of high mortality that begins as an infection of the bile in an obstructed bile duct.[52] The portal of entry for bacteria to enter the obstructed biliary tract is somewhat puzzling. Classically, enteric organisms are thought to emanate from the duodenum, therefore the term "ascending cholangitis." The mechanism of infecting gallbladder bile in lieu of a normal bile duct is not known, however.[50] In a collected series encompassing 22 studies of chronic cholecystitis, gallbladder bile cultures were positive in 16 to 32%.[50] Escherichia coli, Enterobacteriaceae, and enterococcus comprised 75% of cultured organisms. Anaerobic bacteria were cultured in 0 to 9%.[50] Patients with bactibilia have a 40-fold increased incidence of postoperative sepsis.[51] Patients with bactibilia characteristically develop infections composed of organisms found in the bile. Patients having a low risk for bactibilia characteristically develop wound infections formed by gram-positive skin organisms like the staphylococcus species.[50]

Acute cholecystitis carries a higher rate of bactibilia than chronic cholecystitis. Patients who have surgery within 48 hours of the onset of acute cholecystitis have an 81% incidence of bactibilia which decreases to 50% when surgery is delayed beyond 6 days.[50] The bacterial spectrum present in acute cholecystitis is the same as that for nonacute situations. Multiple risk factors for bactibilia have been identified:

- Age 60 or older
- Emergency surgery
- Obstructive jaundice
- Recent rigors
- Biliary operation within the prior 4 weeks
- Choledocholithiasis
- Type of bile duct disease
- Immunosuppressed conditions
- Morbid obesity
- Diabetes mellitus[50,52]

Most of the complications ascribed to bactibilia are wound infections, but the rates of endotoxic shock, acute renal failure, and intraabdominal abscess formation are also increased.

The bacteria involved in cholangitis are once again dominated by the Enterobacteriaceae. Anaerobes are more frequent (33%) in cholangitis than cholecystitis whereas Bacteroides species dominate in contrast to clostridia and other anaerobes in cholecystitis.[50] Bactibilia is present in 80 to 100% of cases of benign bile duct obstruction compared to 10 to 15% of malignant cases.[50] Benign obstructions are more apt to be partial rather than total, probably contributing to the higher rate of bactibilia. Bile can be colonized with bacteria, and signs of sepsis need not be present.[50] In cases of cholangitis, the increased pressure generated in the bile ducts plays a significant role in the pathogenesis leading to bacteria entering the bloodstream.[50]

McDonald and Howard presented a collected series of 885 patients with pyogenic liver abscesses due to the following causes:

- Biliary source in 33%
- Intra-abdominal in 22%
- Cryptogenic in 21%
- Hematogenous in 13%
- Others 11%[54]

The bacteria involved in hepatic abscesses are listed in order of frequency: E. coli, other Enterobacteriaceae, streptococci, anaerobes, and staphylococci.[50] Sterile cultures are obtained in 20 to 27% of cases.[50] Hepatic abscesses are often polymicrobial, and mortality rates are increased when more than one organism is involved.[50]

The use and selection of antibiotics for infections of the biliary tract and liver can be complicated. Prophylactic antibiotics are chosen and given with the knowledge of the pathologic situation at hand and the potential for subsequent infection. It is difficult to obtain cultures of the biliary tract and liver short of an invasive procedure or operation. Therefore, antibiotics are given according to expectations and not actual culture results. Three conclusions can be gathered about the use of prophylactic antibiotics in biliary surgery.[52] First, the concentration of an antibiotic in blood and tissue are of prime importance rather than the concentration of the antibiotic in the bile. Studies indicate that antibiotics heavily concentrated in the bile enjoy no advantage. Proper use of an antibiotic is more important than an antibiotic covering every cultured organism as long as most of the usual biliary organisms are covered by the antibiotic chosen. Second, antibiotics must be given pre-operatively, and have no advantage when continued postoperatively unless a complicated situation exists.[55] Finally, cephalosporins are commonly used for prophylaxis because of their broad spectrum of activity, low toxicity, favorable kinetics, and established efficacy in multiple trials. In a collected series, prophylactic antibiotics reduced the incidence of wound infection in biliary surgery in high risk patients from 27 to 42% to 0 to 4%.[52] Although the literature is sparse, antibiotics in the intraabdominal irrigation solution used at operation may be as effective in the prophylactic sense as parenteral drug.[56] Prophylactic antibiotics are also important before ERCP and percutaneous transhepatic cholangiography. Pseudomonas infections can originate from the instruments used in ERCP and should be considered as a potentially offending organism.[57] Antibiotics covering enterococcus, gram negative aerobes, and anaerobes are indicated in cases of cholangitis, gallbladder empyema, gallbladder perforation, and emphysematous cholecystitis.

ICU PHASE

Patients with biliary problems may be transferred to the ICU because of their comorbid diseases or have the biliary situation develop while they are confined in the ICU for other reasons. In the first instance, the biliary condition is

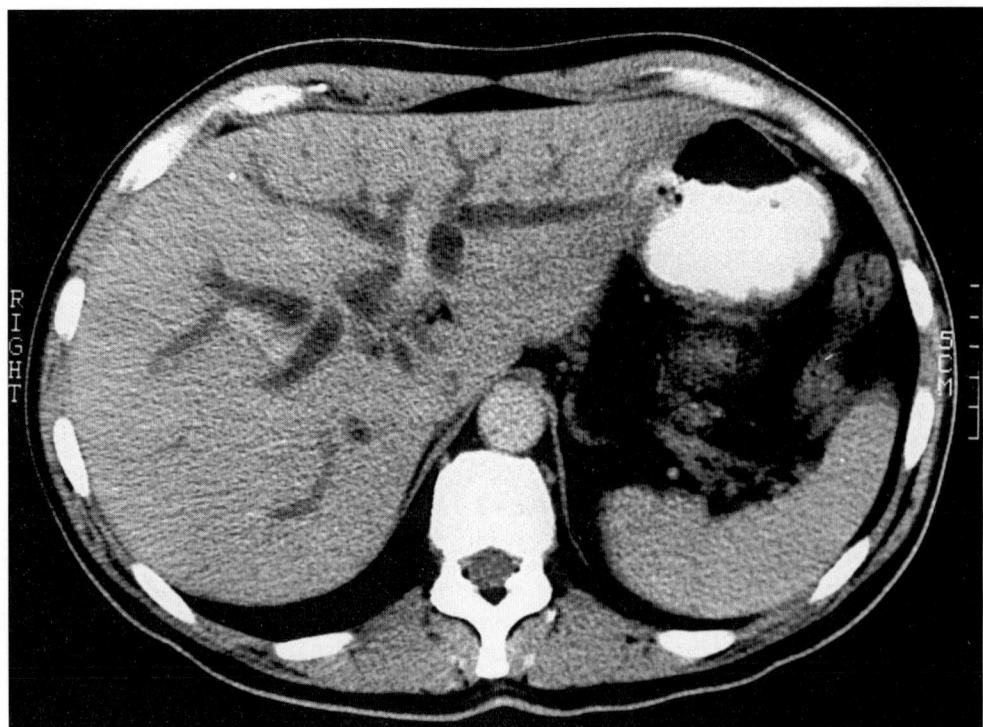

Fig. 53-2. CT scan demonstrating dilated intrahepatic ducts.

known, and it is the other parts of the patient's medical condition that remain to be defined. In the latter circumstance, patients who are already very ill must be watched carefully for the development of biliary sepsis.

Jaundice

Jaundice and sepsis may coexist in the ICU patient, but they are not necessarily related etiologically. The usual circumstance is that a patient on a ventilator with several organ systems failing develops an elevated bilirubin. A bedside ultrasound is performed, gallstones are identified, and the surgeon is consulted. History, physical examination, and blood work will identify the cause of hyperbilirubinemia in 90% of cases.[58] Ultrasound and computerized tomography are useful in excluding dilated ducts, and therefore, extrahepatic biliary obstruction (Fig. 53-2). It has been well documented, however, that bile duct diameter will remain normal in 11 to 17% of patients with biliary obstruction.[59,60] This means that ERCP or percutaneous transhepatic cholangiography may need to be undertaken to exclude mechanical obstruction of the biliary tract in clinically suspected patients despite what appears to be normal-sized bile ducts.

Hyperbilirubinemia can also be a byproduct of prolonged intensive care. te Boekhorst and colleagues reported on the development of **medical** jaundice in 96 severely ill postoperative patients on mechanical ventilation.[61] The exact etiologic factors involved in the production of hyperbilirubinemia (plasma total bilirubin greater than 3 mg/dl) were not identified, but higher bilirubin levels, greater number of organ failures, and increased mortality rates all correlated. Sicker patients have higher bilirubin levels, and they have mortality rates approaching 100%.[61] Morgenstern reported on 1000 patients with postoperative jaundice.[62] The jaundice was rarely obstructive in origin. More commonly, sepsis, renal failure, multiple transfusions, and retained hematomas accounted for such elevations in serum bilirubin.

Acalculous Cholecystitis

Acalculous cholecystitis has been the focus of a large amount of literature in recent years. Increasingly sophisticated intensive care management of critically ill patients has been responsible for the evolution of this disease which now accounts for 2 to 10% of all cases of acute cholecystitis.[63] These are patients who have significant comorbid diseases or have had recent trauma or surgery. Acute calculous cholecystitis presents with persistent, severe, upper right quadrant pain and tenderness, fever, and leukocytosis. In contrast, many patients who develop acute acalculous cholecystitis are unconscious, and 25% may initially manifest themselves only by the new onset of a fever.[64] In a report from the Shock Trauma Center of the Maryland Institute for Emergency Medical Services Systems by Flancbaum, all patients had a fever, 11% had less than 10,000 white blood cells/mm³, 39% did not have right upper quadrant pain, and 38.5% had unexplained sepsis.[65] Calculous cholecystitis is felt to be caused by a stone occluding the cystic duct. Acalculous cholecystitis seems to arise when the gallbladder and its bile are stagnant. Fasting or an adjacent inflammatory condition (e.g., pancreatitis or peptic ulcer disease) can render the gallbladder static and produce a functional obstruction of the cystic duct. The events that transpire between stasis and the appearance of a necrotizing inflammation of the gallbladder wall are unknown. It is clear, however, that the process moves quickly. Johnson reported a collected series that showed 40 to 100% of patients with acute acalculous cholecystitis will have gangrene, empyema, or perforation of the gallbladder at operation.[64] In Flancbaum's personal series, only 8% of patients with acalculous cholecystitis who underwent operation within 48 hours of onset of symptoms had a gallbladder perforation; whereas, 40% had a perforation of their gallbladder when operation was delayed beyond 48 hours.[65]

Although arguments are raised regarding the superiority of cholescintigraphy (e.g., HIDA, PIPIDA, DISIDA scans), CT, or ultrasound in diagnosing acute acalculous or calculous cholecystitis, the first and commanding weapon in the diagnostic armamentarium must be clinical suspicion. Sick patients with fever or sepsis regardless of clinical and laboratory findings must always be considered candidates to contract this disease. Mirvis and associates compared sonography, cholescintigraphy, and CT in 56 patients with acute acalculous cholecystitis.[66] The sensitivity for sonography and CT were 92% and 100%. The specificity for sonography and CT were 96% and 100%. Cholescintigraphy had a false positive rate of 54%. These statistics seem to favor ultrasonography and CT, but one must remember that cholescintigraphy cannot be expected to work if the gallbladder has not recently had reason to function (i.e., the patient has not been eating for several days). A false-positive scan, therefore, can be expected. Others report accurate gallbladder scans in over 90% of patients.[67] False-negative results are uncommon, and many false-positive results can be eliminated by using cholescintigraphy in the appropriate clinical context. In a clinically suspicious patient, ultrasound might be followed by cholescintigraphy if the patient has eaten recently (Figs. 53-3 and 53-4). A CT scan would exclude most other sources of intra-abdominal sepsis.

A small group of patients will arise in whom the diagnosis is still uncertain, and these are the patients one would least like to take to surgery for a negative exploratory laparotomy. Percutaneous needle aspiration of the gallbladder and insertion of a cholecystostomy tube are appropriate in these situations.[68,69] A few patients with acute acalculous cholecystitis have no leukocytes or organisms in their bile upon aspiration and Gram stain, but routine placement of a percutaneous catheter into the gallbladder after aspiration covers all patients. The procedure has few risks, and relieves biliary sepsis in almost all patients in which it is used.[68,69] Open cholecystostomy and cholecystectomy are further options in managing acute cholecystitis of any type.

Fig. 53-4. Radioisotope uptake by the liver and excretion into the duodenum are seen, but the gallbladder fails to visualize.

Cholecystectomy or open/percutaneous cholecystostomy for acute cholecystitis should be undertaken expeditiously.[70] The advantages of early versus delayed cholecystectomy are technical ease of operation, decreased total duration of illness and disability, decreased costs, and a decrease in the complications of acute cholecystitis.[70] Patients with a worsening clinical condition, diabetes, advanced age, significant co-morbid disease, immunosuppression of any sort, and suspected acalculous cholecystitis should undergo a procedure as soon as they can reasonably be prepared. Patients who are watched and develop empyema,[71] gangrene,[72] or perforation[73] of the gallbladder suffer mortality rates up to 20% or greater.

Acute Cholangitis

Charcot described acute cholangitis in 1877 and noted three clinical findings: jaundice, chills and fever, and right upper quadrant abdominal pain. A pentad of clinical findings was formed when Reynolds and Dargan described shock and mental stupor as being indicative of advanced cholangitis and added these findings to Charcot's triad.[74] It is important to realize that Charcot's triad is completely present in only 54 to 70% of patients with cholangitis.[59,75]

Cholangitis is part of the differential diagnosis whenever the signs and symptoms of infection and bile duct obstruction are present. The diagnosis of infection is usually not

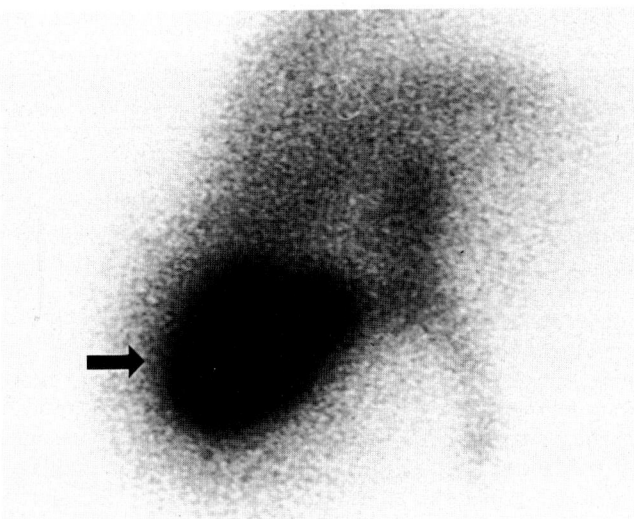

Fig. 53-3. The healthy gallbladder (arrow) fills with radioisotope on cholescintigraphy.

difficult, but the demonstration of bile duct obstruction may be more so. Bile ducts may be normal in diameter despite obstruction.[59,60] When ultrasound and CT do not show ductal dilation, percutaneous transhepatic cholangiography or ERCP may need to be undertaken to directly visualize the ductal system. Cholangitis has been separated into nonsuppurative and suppurative forms. This separation is artificial and probably meaningless. It has not been shown that suppurative cholangitis (i.e., pus in the bile duct) presents in a different manner clinically, requires different treatment, or has a different outcome.[75] Depending on the series, stones and strictures account for the majority of bile duct obstructions. Bactibilia is present in 80 to 100% of cases of benign bile duct obstruction compared to 10 to 15% of malignant cases.[50]

Cancer composes a minority, albeit troublesome minority of cases with cholangitis. The problem with malignant obstructions of the intrahepatic biliary tract is the occurrence of multiple segmental and subsegmental bile duct obstructions can occur with resultant cholangitis that no technique, open or closed, can completely drain (Fig. 53-5). Patients with acute cholangitis need resuscitation with fluids and broad-spectrum antibiotics. Conservative therapy will result in improvement in 70 to 85% of patients.[61] If clinical improvement is not prompt and continuous, placement of a percutaneous biliary stent, endoscopic papillotomy with stone extraction or positioning of an internal or nasobiliary stent, or open surgery should be performed.

Surgery has been relegated to the least desirable option acutely due to reported mortality rates of 17 to 50%, but it remains an important element in the definitive treatment of the bile duct obstruction.[61] Percutaneous transhepatic biliary drainage had a high morbidity and mortality in the past. Studies like that reported by Pessa and colleagues, however, which recorded a 7% morbidity in 42 patients using a 22-gauge "skinny" needle and an "accordion" catheter have changed the outlook on this procedure.[59] In this series, only 2 patients (5%) died of septic shock within 8 hours of admission despite resuscitation and percutaneous biliary drainage. Percutaneous transhepatic stenting provides drainage of proximal biliary obstructions, access to take high quality cholangiograms in order to plan definitive bile duct surgery, and access to perform percutaneous dilation of bile duct strictures which may be final therapy in itself. Endoscopic papillotomy with stone extraction or placement of a nasobiliary stent are the final options in the management of cholangitis. Endoscopic techniques can be expected to be successful if the bile duct obstruction is distal in location or caused by small- to medium-sized common duct stones.

Classen summarized his results in the endoscopic management of 115 patients with acute, obstructive cholangitis; 45% had choledocholithiasis, 45% malignant obstruction, and 10% benign stricture.[76] Endoscopic sphincterotomy successfully treated 90% of patients with stones and 73% with a malignant obstruction. The mortality rates were 8% for stones and 27% for malignant obstructions. When ERCP is performed and the stone or other bile duct obstruction cannot be relieved, a nasobiliary stent should be placed to decompress the bile duct until another therapeutic maneuver can be planned and performed. When poor risk patients present with cholangitis and choledocholithiasis, but have their gallbladders intact, a growing number of reports is accumulating regarding the success of endoscopic sphincterotomy, clearance of stones from the bile duct, and maintenance of the gallbladder in-situ. Siegel and co-workers report on 1272 patients having duodenoscopic sphincterotomy with the gallbladder in place.[77] Prior to endoscopy, 25% of patients had cholangitis, and 10.5% had gallstone pancreatitis. Postprocedure, cholecystitis developed in 8.6%. The 30-day mortality was 0.15%. Long-term follow-up of 337 patients revealed only 2 deaths secondary to recurrent cholecystitis. Thus, treatment of cholangitis presents multiple options, and each has its own clinical utility.

Hepatic Abscess

A pyogenic hepatic abscess may complicate the clinical situation of a patient with biliary or other intra-abdominal site of sepsis. A few hepatic abscesses also arise from hematogenous seeding or cryptogenic sources. Fever and chills, upper abdominal pain, vomiting, malaise, and weight loss are common clinical findings.[78] Leukocytosis, anemia, and elevated alkaline phosphatase are each present in more than half of cases.[78] An ultrasound or CT scan of the liver is the usual mode of diagnosis (Fig. 53-6). The essence of treatment for a pyogenic hepatic abscess is drainage. Although controlled studies comparing CT- or ultrasound-guided percutaneous and open, operative drainage of hepatic abscesses do not exist, each method has its practical applications. Severely ill or recent postoperative patients

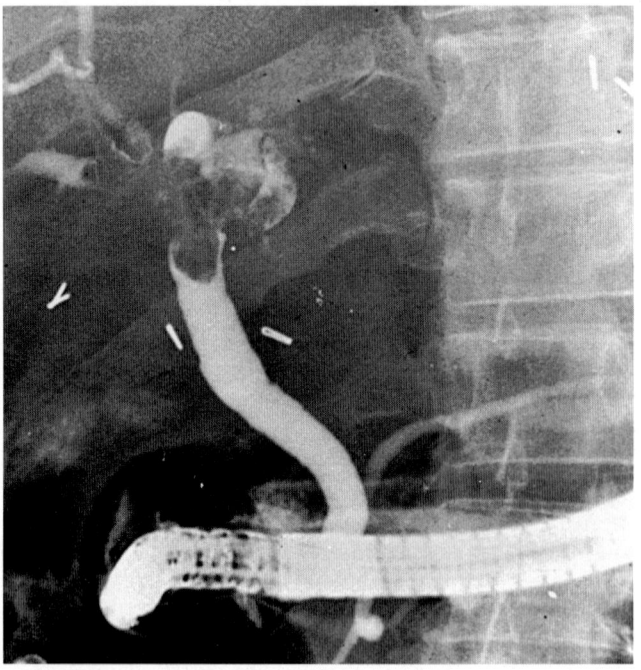

Fig. 53-5. A proximal cholangiocarcinoma is shown by ERCP to be obstructing several right hepatic segmental ducts and the entire left hepatic biliary tract.

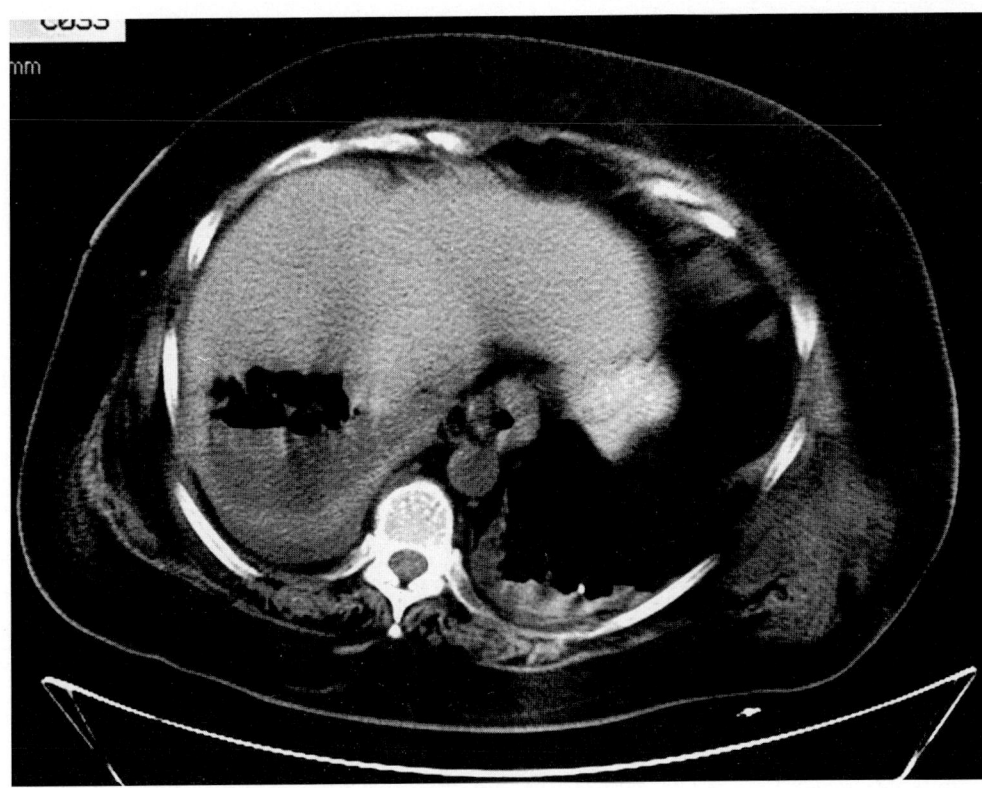

Fig. 53-6. CT scan of a large right hepatic lobe abscess with an air-fluid level.

with an isolated hepatic abscess might be better drained percutaneously. Incomplete percutaneous drainage or concomitant intra-abdominal disease make laparotomy necessary. Percutaneous drainage fails in approximately 10 to 30% of cases.[78] The mortality rates for percutaneous drainage average 3 to 4%; surgical mortality ranges from 4 to 13%.[78] Because most hepatic abscesses are secondary to another infectious focus, an earnest attempt should be made to find the source once the patient's condition permits.

Once a liver abscess has been identified and prior to draining it by any means, broad-spectrum antibiotics should be started. Preferably, a percutaneous stent(s) can be placed in the abscess cavity. A search is undertaken for the origin of the abscess. A CT scan will exclude most intra-abdominal sources. ERCP is undertaken if biliary disease is suspected. Drainage is maintained for several weeks until the abscess cavity collapses around the catheter, and it can safely be removed.

Total Parenteral Nutrition (TPN)

Many critically ill patients are placed on parenteral nutrition. Roslyn and associates reviewed 109 patients receiving TPN for at least 3 months.[79] Twenty-three percent developed gallstones. Resection or disease of the ileum led to an increased incidence of gallstones: 7% in the group without ileal resection or disorder, and 29% in those with ileal resection or disorder. Sludge may be observed in 6% of patients during the first 3 weeks of TPN, which increases to 100% of patients receiving TPN for 6 to 13 weeks.[80] This sludge will disappear after 4 weeks of oral feeding.[80] All of these considerations lead to an increased incidence (up to 45% of adults) of acute calculous and acalculous cholecystitis in patients receiving long-term TPN.[81] The morbidity and mortality of cholecystitis in patients receiving TPN is 54% and 11%, respectively, because 40% of these patients require emergency surgery.[82] This has prompted some to recommend that patients receiving long-term TPN be regularly screened for gallstones and have cholecystectomy when stones first appear or anytime laparotomy is undertaken for other reasons.[82] A proposal has also been made to use cholecystokinin-octapeptide (CCK-OP) prophylactically after 3 weeks of TPN to prevent the development of gallbladder sludge.[83] Prophylactic use of CCK-OP in a small, prospective, randomized study of 15 patients showed that CCK-OP was effective in preventing gallbladder sludge.[83]

TPN may also produce deranged liver function tests to further confuse the picture in deciphering some of these complicated patients. After a median of two weeks of TPN, Lindor reported that 21% of bilirubin, 54% of alkaline phosphatase, and 68% of SGOT values were more than 50% greater than pre-TPN values.[84] As many as 15% of home TPN patients display chronic liver dysfunction.[85] Laboratory confirmation of acute biliary tract disease is, therefore, difficult when overlaid with these chronic enzyme changes.

Sclerosing Cholangitis

Sclerosing cholangitis can present two challenges to the clinician, sepsis and liver failure (Fig. 53-7). Most patients have multiple intrahepatic strictures, which make surgical access impossible. Emperic courses of broad-spectrum antibiotics for sepsis can be a recurring theme in some pa-

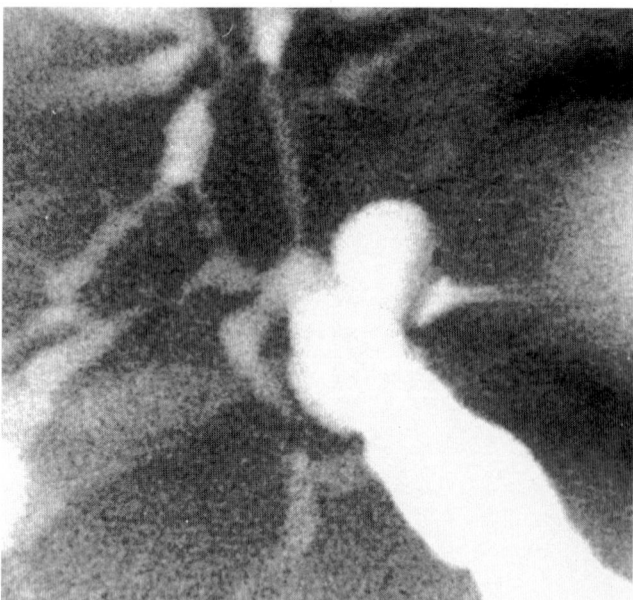

Fig. 53–7. Cholangiogram of a patient with extensive intrahepatic sclerosing cholangitis.

tients and may promote the consideration of liver transplantation in much the same way that the development of liver failure does. Percutaneous ductal dilatation has provided limited short-term bile duct patency in some patients. When sepsis is recurrent, patients may benefit from chronic antibiotic suppression with ampicillin, trimethoprim/sulfamethoxazole, or ciprofloxacin. AIDS patients have now been recognized to develop what appears to be sclerosing cholangitis biochemically and radiologically, and it is found in association with papillary stenosis.[86] The likely etiology is some sort of opportunistic infection, (e.g., CMV or cryptosporidia).[87] Endoscopic papillotomy may be of some help.

POST-ICU PHASE

Once biliary sepsis has been controlled, the patient's care focuses on treatment of the co-morbid diseases. If the biliary sepsis has been successfully managed, the co-morbid diseases should then determine survival. Adequate antibiotic therapy and decompression of the gallbladder and/or biliary tract comprise the basis of biliary therapy. Gallstones, strictures, and neoplasms may remain, but are not important acutely. In the post-ICU phase, however, the fate of the gallstones, strictures, or neoplasms must now be decided. Dogma has it that a gallbladder should always be removed at some point if a cholecystostomy tube has been placed for cholecystitis. Despite various studies showing the incidence of recurrent gallstones after cholecystostomy to be between 37 and 83%, it is unknown what percentage of patients with recurrent gallstones will become symptomatic again.[88] This has suggested to some that patients whose gallstones have been removed can be followed after cholecystostomy without the routine need for cholecystectomy.[88] In patients who recover from acalculous cholecystitis after open/closed cholecystostomy, the requirement for cholecystectomy is not widely reported, and should be no greater and perhaps less than that for patients with calculi as the cause for their cholecystitis.[69]

Recovery from open cholecystectomy with or without common bile duct exploration is relatively straightforward. The acute pain of the operation and the postoperative ileus lasts for 3 to 4 days if performed open. Food is offered once the ileus begins to resolve. Patients are discharged 2 to 7 days after surgery. Laparoscopic cholecystectomy attempts to minimize both pain and ileus allowing discharge in a day or so. If a common bile duct exploration has been performed, a T-tube is usually positioned in the bile duct, and the stem of the T-tube exits the skin. A T-tube cholangiogram is taken 5 to 7 days after surgery to confirm ductal integrity and exclude retained stones. The patient can be discharged with the T-tube in place and tied off. It can then be removed in the office in several weeks providing no retained stones are present. If retained stones are present, they can be removed via the T-tube tract in 6 weeks, or endoscopically.

A percutaneous transhepatic biliary stent can remain in place as long as it is needed. When a temporary blockage, like a stone, is subsequently removed, the percutaneous catheter can safely be removed. If ductal pathology remains, however, the catheter should probably be maintained until the definitive procedure or operation is performed. In patients who are too infirm for surgery or have widespread cancer, these percutaneous catheters can be kept in place indefinitely. Regular catheter changes every 6 to 8 weeks minimize the occurrence of cholangitis.

When these patients develop upper gastrointestinal bleeding, hemobilia should be considered. An angiogram

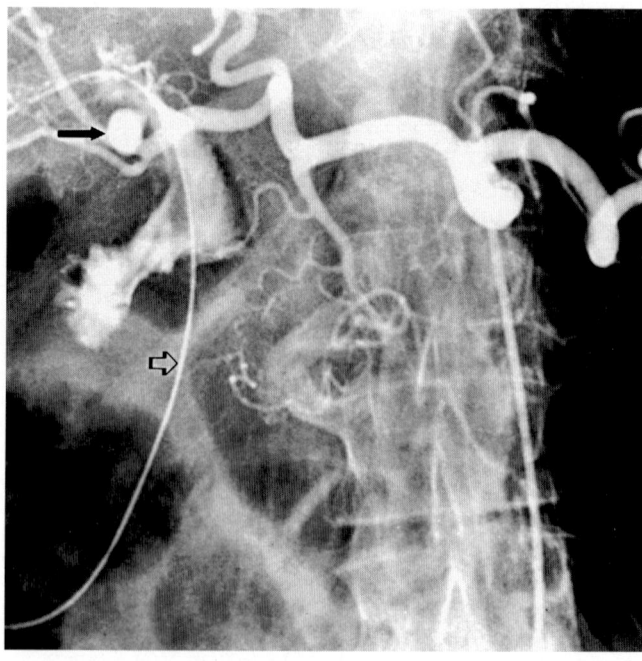

Fig. 53–8. A celiac axis angiogram reveals a right hepatic artery pseudoaneurysm (closed arrow) bleeding into the biliary tract after placement of a percutaneous biliary stent (open arrow).

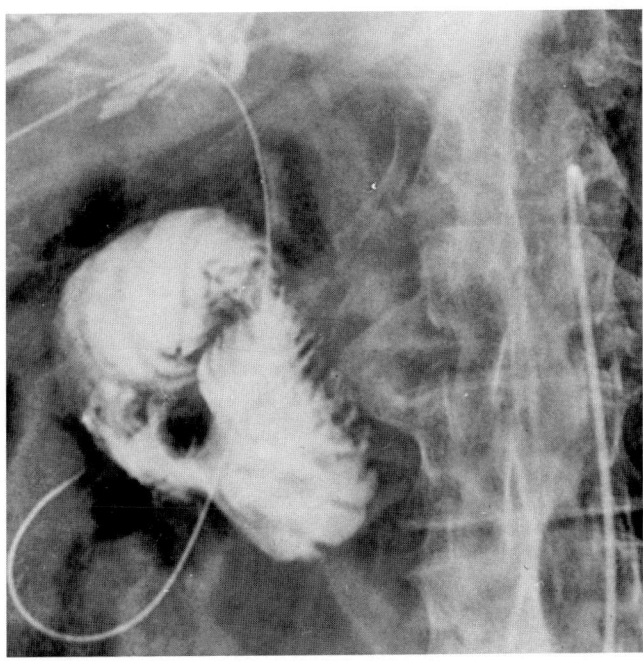

Fig. 53–9. A later phase of the arteriogram shown in Figure 53–7 showing contrast in the biliary tract and bowel.

should be performed unless another obvious source of bleeding can be demonstrated (Figs. 53–8 and 53–9).

Surgically placed biliary stents can also be maintained for a prolonged period and can be replaced under fluoroscopy as needed. In successful biliary operations, stents can be safely removed after 1 to 3 months.[89] Reports touting the benefits of prolonged (6 to 12 months) biliary stenting have not been widely accepted.[90] The current trend is to stent only precarious biliary-enteric anastomoses briefly.

Armed with appropriate suspicion, a host of diagnostic techniques, and versatile temporary and permanent treatment options, the physician has much to offer the patient with biliary sepsis. Biliary sepsis can be the primary cause for admission to the ICU, or it can become manifest in the already ICU-bound patient. The propagation of an aged and ill population and the greater appreciation of diseases like sclerosing cholangitis and AIDS-related cholangitis promise to provide fresh challenges to physicians interested in hepatobiliary disease.

REFERENCES

1. Ransohoff, D. F., Gracie, W. A., Wolfenson, L. B., and Neuhauser, D.: Prophylactic cholecystectomy or expectant management for silent gallstones. Ann. Intern. Med., 99:199, 1983.
2. McSherry, C. K., et al.: The natural history of diagnosed gallstone disease in symptomatic and asymptomatic patients. Ann. Surg., 202:59, 1985.
3. Gracie, W. A., and Ransohoff, D. F.: The natural history of silent gallstones. N. Engl. J. Med., 307:798, 1982.
4. McSherry, C. K., and Glenn, F.: Biliary tract surgery concomitant with other intra-abdominal operations. Ann. Surg. 193:169, 1981.
5. String, S. T.: Cholelithiasis and aortic reconstruction. J. Vasc. Surg., 5:664, 1984.
6. Fry, R. E., and Fry, W. J.: Cholelithiasis and aortic reconstruction: the problem of simultaneous surgical therapy. J. Vasc. Surg., 4:345, 1986.
7. Ouriel, K., Ricotta, J. J., Adams, J. T., and DeWeese, J. A.: Management of cholelithiasis in patients with abdominal aortic aneurysm. Ann. Surg., 198:717, 1983.
8. Ottinger, L. W.: Acute cholecystitis as a postoperative complication. Ann. Surg., 184:162, 1976.
9. Thompson, J. S., Philben, V. J., and Hodgsons, P. E.: Operative management of incidental cholelithiasis. Am. J. Surg., 148:821, 1984.
10. Bragg, L. E., and Thompson, J. S.: Concomitant cholecystectomy for asymptomatic cholelithiasis. Arch. Surg., 124:460, 1989.
11. McSherry, C. K., and Glenn, F.: The incidence and causes of death following surgery for nonmalignant biliary tract disease. Ann. Surg., 191:271, 1980.
12. Gilliland, T. M., and Traverso, L. W.: Modern standards for comparison of cholecystectomy with alternative treatments from symptomatic cholelithiasis with emphasis on long term relief of symptoms. Surg. Gynecol. Obstet., 170:39, 1990.
13. Hermann, R. E.: Biliary disease in the aging patient. In The aging gut. Edited by E. C. Texter Jr. New York, Masson, 1983, p. 27.
14. Margiotta, S. J., Willis, I. H., and Wallack, M. K.: Cholecystectomy in the elderly. Am. Surg., 54:34, 1988.
15. Morrow, D. J., Thompson, J., and Wilson, S. E.: Acute cholecystitis in the elderly. Arch. Surg., 113:1149, 1978.
16. Norman, D. C., and Yoshikawa, T. T.: Intraabdominal infection: diagnosis and treatment in the elderly patient. Gerontology, 30:327, 1984.
17. Huber, D. F., Martin, E. W., Jr., and Cooperman, M.: Cholecystectomy in elderly patients. Am. J. Surg., 146:719, 1983.
18. Rabinowitch, I. M.: On the mortality resulting from surgical treatment of chronic gallbladder disease in diabetes mellitus. Ann. Surg., 96:70, 1932.
19. Eisele, H. E.: Results of gallbladder surgery in diabetes mellitus. Ann. Surg., 118:107, 1943.
20. Turrill, F. L., McCarron, M. M., and Mikkelsen, W. P.: Gallstones and diabetes: an ominous association. Am. J. Surg., 102:184, 1961.
21. Mundth, E. D.: Cholecystitis and diabetes mellitus. N. Engl. J. Med., 267:642, 1962.
22. Schein, C. J.: Acute cholecystitis in the diabetic. Am. J. Gastroenterol., 51:511, 1969.
23. Turner, R. J. III, Becker, W. F., Coleman, W. O., and Powell, J. L.: Acute cholecystitis in the diabetic. South Med. J., 62:228, 1969.
24. Walsh, D. B., Eckhauser, F. E., Ramsburgh, S. R., and Burney, R. B.: Risk associated with diabetes mellitus in patients undergoing gallbladder surgery. Surgery, 91:254, 1982.
25. Reiss, R., Dutsch, A. A., and Nudelmann, J.: Biliary surgery in diabetic patients: statistical analysis of 189 patients. Digestive Surg., 4:37, 1987.
26. Hickman, M. S., Schwesinger, W. H., and Page, C. P.: Acute cholecystitis in the diabetic. Arch. Surg., 123:409, 1988.
27. Green, J., et al.: The "jaundiced heart": a possible explanation for postoperative shock in obstructive jaundice. Surgery, 100:15, 1986.
28. Bomzon, A., et al.: Systemic hypotension and decreased pressor response in dogs with chronic bile duct ligation. Hepatology, 6:595, 1986.
29. Cioffi, W. G., DeMeules, J. E., Kahng, K. U., and Wait, R. B.: Renal vascular reactivity in jaundice. Surgery, 100:356, 1986.
30. Green, J., et al.: Jaundice, the circulation and the kidney. Nephron, 37:145, 1984.

31. Warren, R. S., et al.: Impaired metabolic response to endotoxin in obstructive jaundice. Surgery, 100:349, 1986.
32. Roughneen, P. T., et al.: Impaired specific cell-mediated immunity in experimental biliary obstruction and its reversibility by internal biliary drainage. J. Surg. Res., 41:113, 1986.
33. Katz, S., et al.: Impaired hepatic bacterial clearance is reversed by surgical relief of obstructive jaundice. J. Pediatr. Surg., 26:401, 1991.
34. Pain, J. A., Cahill, C. J., and Bailey, M. E.: Perioperative complications in obstructive jaundice: therapeutic considerations. Br. J. Surg., 72:942, 1985.
35. Blamey, S. L., et al.: Prediction of risk in biliary surgery. Br. J. Surg., 70:535, 1983.
36. Dixon, J. M., Armstrong, C. P., Duffy, S. W., and Davies, G. C.: Factors affecting morbidity and mortality after surgery for obstructive jaundice: a review of 373 patients. Gut, 24:845, 1983.
37. Hatfield, A. R. W., et al.: Preoperative external biliary drainage in obstructive jaundice. Lancet, 2:896, 1982.
38. McPherson, G. A. D., et al.: Pre-operative percutaneous transhepatic biliary drainage: the results of a controlled trial. Br. J. Surg., 71:371, 1984.
39. Pitt, H. A., et al.: Does preoperative percutaneous biliary drainage reduce operative risk of increase hospital cost? Ann. Surg., 201:545, 1985.
40. Smith, R. C., Pooley, M., George, C. R. P., and Faithful, G. R.: Preoperative percutaneous transhepatic internal drainage in obstructive jaundice: a randomized, controlled trial examining renal function. Surgery, 97:641, 1985.
41. Pellegrini, C. A., Allegra, P., Bongard, F. S., and Way, L. W.: Risk of biliary surgery in patients with hyperbilirubinemia. Am. J. Surg., 154:111, 1987.
42. Diamond, T., Dolan, S., Thompson, R. L. E., and Rowlands, B. J.: Development and reversal of endotoxemia and endotoxin-related death in obstructive jaundice. Surgery, 108:370, 1990.
43. Pain, J., and Bailey, M. E.: Experimental and clinical study of lactulose in obstructive jaundice. Br. J. Surg., 73:775, 1986.
44. Cahill, C.: Prevention of postoperative renal failure in patients with obstructive jaundice: the role of bile salts. Br. J. Surg., 70:590, 1983.
45. Garrison, R. N., Cryer, H. M., Howard, D. A., and Polk, H. C. Jr.: Clarification of risk factors for abdominal operations in patients with hepatic cirrhosis. Ann. Surg., 199:648, 1984.
46. Schwartz, S.: Biliary tract surgery and cirrhosis: a critical combination. Surgery, 90:577, 1981.
47. Aranha, G.: Therapeutic options for biliary tract disease in advanced cirrhosis. Am. J. Surg., 155:374, 1988.
48. Sirinek, K. R., Burk, R. R., Brown, M., and Levine, B. A.: Improving survival in patients with cirrhosis undergoing major abdominal operations. Arch. Surg., 122:271, 1987.
49. Dunnington, G., et al.: Natural history of cholelithiasis in patients with alcoholic cirrhosis. Ann. Surg., 205:226, 1987.
50. Claesson, B. E. B.: Microflora of the biliary tree and liver clinical correlates. Dig. Dis., 4:93, 1986.
51. Dye, M., MacDonald, A., and Smith, G.: The bacterial flora of the biliary tract and liver in man. Br. J. Surg., 65:285, 1974.
52. Kanter, M. A., and Geelhoed, G. W.: Biliary antibiotics: clinical utility in biliary surgery. South. Med. J., 80:1007, 1987.
53. Chetlin, S. H., and Elliott, D. W.: Biliary bacteremia. Arch. Surg., 102:303, 1971.
54. McDonald, V. P., and Howard, R. J.: Pyogenic liver abscess. World J. Surg., 4:369, 1980.
55. Stone, H. H., et al.: Prophylactic and preventive antibiotic therapy. Ann. Surg., 189:691, 1979.
56. Freischlag, J., McGrattan, M., and Busuttil, R. W.: Topical versus systemic cephalosporin administration in elective biliary operations. Surgery, 96:686, 1984.
57. Allen, J. I., et al.: Pseudomonas infection of the biliary system resulting from use of a contaminated endoscope. Gastroenterology, 92:759, 1987.
58. Scharschmidt, B., Goldberg, H. I., and Schmid, R.: Current concepts in diagnosis: approach to the patient with cholestatic jaundice. N. Engl. J. Med., 308:1515, 1983.
59. Pessa, M. E., Hawkins, I. F., and Vogel, S. B.: The treatment of acute cholangitis. Ann. Surg., 205:389, 1987.
60. Frank, B. B., and Members of the Patient Care Committee of the American Gastroenterological Association. Clinical evaluation of jaundice. JAMA, 262:3031, 1989.
61. te Boekhorst, T., et al.: Etiologic factors of jaundice in severely ill patients. J. Hepatol., 7:111, 1988.
62. Morgenstern, L.: Postoperative jaundice. Am. J. Surg., 128:255, 1974.
63. Sievert, W., and Vakil, N. B.: Emergencies of the biliary tract. Gastroenterol. Clin. North Am., 17:245, 1988.
64. Johnson, L. B.: The importance of early diagnosis of acute acalculus cholecystitis. Surg. Gynecol. Obstet., 164:197, 1987.
65. Flancbaum, L., Majerus, T. C., and Cox, E. F.: Acute posttraumatic acalculous cholecystitis. Am. J. Surg., 150:252, 1985.
66. Mirvis, S. E., et al.: The diagnosis of acute acalculous cholecystitis: a comparison of sonography, scintigraphy, and CT. AJR, 147:1171, 1986.
67. Swayne, L. C.: Acute acalculous cholecystitis: sensitivity in detection using technetium-99m iminodiacetic acid cholescintigraphy. Radiology, 1:33, 1986.
68. Klimberg, S., Hawkins, I., and Vogel, S.: Percutaneous cholecystostomy for acute cholecystitis in high-risk patients. Am. J. Surg., 153:125, 1987.
69. Werber, G. B., et al.: Percutaneous cholecystectomy in the diagnosis of treatment of acute cholecystitis in the high-risk patient. Arch. Surg., 124:782, 1989.
70. Sharp, K. W.: Acute cholecystitis. Surg. Clin. North Am., 68:269, 1988.
71. Fry, D. E., Cox, R. A., and Harbrecht, P. J.: Empyema of the gallbladder: a complication in the natural history of acute cholecystitis. Am. J. Surg., 141:366, 1981.
72. Ahman, M. M., Macon, W. L. IV: Gangrene of the gallbladder. Am. Surg., 49:155, 1983.
73. Felice, P. R., Trowbridge, P. E., and Ferrara, J. J.: Evolving changes in the pathogenesis and treatment of the perforated gallbladder. Am. J. Surg., 149:466, 1985.
74. Reynolds, B. M., and Dargan, E. L.: Acute obstructive cholangitis. Ann. Surg., 150:299, 1959.
75. Boey, J. H., and Way, L. W.: Acute cholangitis. Ann. Surg., 191:264, 1980.
76. Classen, M.: Endoscopic papillotomy—new indications, short- and long-term results. Clin. Gastroenterol., 15:456, 1986.
77. Siegel, J. H., et al.: Duodenoscopic sphincterotomy in patients with gallbladders in situ: report of a series of 1272 patients. Am. J. Gastroenterol., 83:1255, 1988.
78. Frey, C. F., Zhu, Y., Suzuki, M., and Isaji, S.: Liver abscesses. Surg. Clin. North Am., 69:259, 1989.
79. Roslyn, J. J., et al.: Gallbladder disease in patients on long-term parenteral nutrition. Gastroenterology, 84:148, 1983.
80. Messing, B., Bories, C., Kunstlinger, F., and Bernier, J. J.: Does total parenteral nutrition induce gallbladder sludge foundation and lithiasis? Gastroenterology, 84:1012, 1983.
81. Pitt, H. A., et al.: Increased risk of cholelithiasis with prolonged total parenteral nutrition. Am. J. Surg., 145:106, 1983.
82. Roslyn, J. J., et al.: Parenteral nutrition-induced gallbladder

disease: a reason for early cholecystectomy. Am. J. Surg., *148*:58, 1984.
83. Sitzmann, J. V., et al.: Cholecystokinin prevents parenteral nutrition induced biliary sludge in humans. Surg. Gynecol. Obstet., *170*:25, 1990.
84. Lindor, K. D., Fleming, C. R., Abrams, A., and Hirschkorn, M. A.: Liver function values in adults receiving total parenteral nutrition. JAMA, *241*:2398, 1979.
85. Bowyer, B. A., et al.: Does long-term home parenteral nutrition in adult patients cause chronic liver disease? Abstracts of Papers *86*:1033, 1984.
86. Dolmatch, B. L., et al.: AIDS-related cholangitis: radiographic findings in nine patients. Radiology, *163*:313, 1987.
87. Schneiderman, D. J.: Hepatobiliary abnormalities of AIDS. Gastroenterol. Clin. North Am., *17*:615, 1988.
88. Skillings, J. C., Kumai, C., and Hinshaw, J. R.: Cholecystostomy: a place in modern biliary surgery? Am. J. Surg., *139*:865, 1980.
89. Genest, J. F., et al.: Benign biliary strictures: an analytic review. Surgery, *4*:409, 1986.
90. Pitt, H. A., et al.: Factors influencing outcome in patients with postoperative biliary strictures. Am. J. Surg., *144*:14, 1982.

SUPPLEMENTAL READINGS

Aucott, J. N., Copper, G. S., Bloom, A. D., and Aron, D. C.: Management of gallstones in diabetic patients. Arch. Intern. Med., *153*:1053, 1993.
Babb, R. R.: Acute acalculous cholecystitis: a review. J. Clin. Gastroenterol., *15*:238, 1992.
Baek, S. Y., et al.: Therapeutic percutaneous aspiration of hepatic abscesses: effectiveness in 25 patients. Am. J. Roentgenol., *160*:799, 1993.
Bender, J. S., and Talamini, M. A.: Diagnostic laparoscopy in critically ill intensive-care-unit patients. Surg. Endosc., *6*:302, 1992.
Bonacini, M.: Hepatobiliary complications in patients with human immunodeficiency virus infection. Am. J. Med., *92*:404, 1992.
Friedman, G. D.: Natural history of asymptomatic and symptomatic gallstones. Am. J. Surg., *165*:399, 1993.
Hansen, N., and Vargish, T.: Pyogenic hepatic abscess: a case for open drainage. Am. Surg., *59*:219, 1993.
Ishizaki, U., et al.: Management of gallstones in cirrhotic patients. Surg. Today, *23*:36, 1993.
Jacobson, A. F., et al.: Frequent occurrence of new hepatobiliary abnormalities after bone marrow transplantation: results of a prospective study using scintigraphy and sonography. Am. J. Gastroenterol., *88*:1044, 1993.
Khardori, M., et al.: Infections associated with biliary drainage procedures in patients with cancer. Rev. Infect. Dis., *13*:587, 1991.
Lai, E. C., et al.: Severe acute cholangitis: the role of emergency nasobiliary drainage. Surgery, *107*:268, 1990.
Landau, O., et al.: Multifactorial analysis of septic bile and septic complications in biliary surgery. World J. Surg., *16*:962, 1992.
Ponsky, J. L.: Alternative methods in the management of bile duct stones. Surg. Clin. North Am., *72*:1099, 1992.
Reiss, R., and Deutsch, A. A.: State of the art in the diagnosis and management of acute cholecystitis. Dig. Dis., *11*:55, 1993.
Sauter, G., et al.: Antibiotic prophylaxis of infectious complications with endoscopic retrograde cholangiopancreatography: a randomized controlled study. Endoscopy, *22*:164, 1990.
Strasberg, S. M., and Clavien, P. A.: Overview of therapeutic modalities for the treatment of gallstone diseases. Am. J. Surg., *165*:420, 1993.
Sugiyama, M., Atomi, Y., Kuroda, A., and Muto, T.: Treatment of choledocholithiasis in patients with liver cirrhosis. Ann. Surg., *218*:68, 1993.
Vauthey, J. N., et al.: Indications and limitations of percutaneous cholecystostomy for acute cholecystitis. Surg. Gynecol. Obstet., *176*:49, 1993.

Chapter 54

DISORDERS OF HEPATIC FUNCTION

EUGENE I. WINKELMAN

Hepatitis is classically defined as an inflammatory process of the liver indicated by clinical, biochemical, and histologic evidence of hepatocellular injury and necrosis; the term has become virtually synonymous with a viral origin, although other causes may be indistinguishable. Although the presentation may be similar, the spectrum of symptoms, physical findings, and biochemical abnormalities varies from patients who are asymptomatic or have vague transient findings to those who develop hepatic failure and death. The underlying disease may be classified as either acute or chronic based on the history or histologic changes, which can be as dissimilar as massive hepatic necrosis or cirrhosis (Table 54-1).

EVALUATION

The ability to diagnose liver disease accurately and estimate its severity depends on the interpretation of specific biochemical and other laboratory studies that evaluate hepatocellular damage and its effect on hepatic function. These are of value only when used in conjunction with a detailed history, careful and complete physical examination, and, when indicated, special imaging techniques or liver biopsy.

History

Jaundice is an objective finding and the observation most apt to call attention to underlying liver disease. Its accompanying symptoms, the circumstances under which the symptoms occurred, and their duration supply important information in formulating a diagnosis. A jaundiced drug user with a short prodromal history of malaise and anorexia is a prime suspect for acute viral hepatitis, whereas a jaundiced alcoholic with similar symptoms and signs is diagnosed as having alcoholic hepatitis; however, the possibility (10%) of infectious mononucleosis should not be ignored in the adolescent with the same complaints.[1] A history of intermittent jaundice in an otherwise well young person may be the result of a congenital hyperbilirubinemia (Table 54-2),[2] whereas recurrent episodes of intrahepatic cholestasis may be manifestations of the unusual syndrome of benign recurrent cholestasis.[3] Jaundice and fever in a middle-aged woman with recurrent or acute biliary colic is recognized as calculous biliary tract disease; a similar individual with painless jaundice, weight loss, and alcoholic stools probably has a pancreatic carcinoma. If the jaundice does not clear after surgery, there must be bile duct injury, an obstructive lesion above the cystic duct, or hepatocellular disease. If it returns within a few weeks, the possibilities are a retained stone, bile duct injury, pancreatitis, hepatotoxicity from the anesthetic agent, medication, or sepsis. If 4 to 6 weeks or later jaundice recurs, a search for biliary tract pathology as well as hepatocellular disease is indicated. The sudden onset of jaundice in the immediate postoperative period prompts questions of shock with subsequent hepatic ischemia, transfusion reaction, or previously undetected hepatocellular disease.

Information regarding the use of drugs, now and in the past, both prescription and over-the-counter, cannot be omitted nor can use of other substances:[4] i.e., pyrrolizidine alkaloids in "bush teas" available in health food stores and an excess use of vitamin A, either of which can produce veno-occlusive disease.[5,6] Women, who tend not to consider oral contraceptives as medicine, must be queried specifically about their use. A history of blood transfusion, parenteral or other street drugs, tattoos, and travel, both abroad and within the United States, should be documented. Also, an occupational history might provide a cause: carbon tetrachloride used by mechanics,[4] polyvinyl chloride exposure in chemical workers,[7] leptospirosis as a risk in sanitation workers,[8] and the increased incidence of hepatitis A in workers at day care centers[9] or hepatitis B in health care workers.[10]

A medical history includes diseases past and present, hospitalizations and surgery, and their diagnoses. Further surgical history should necessarily include the diagnosis and procedure. The family history, often unobtainable because of adoption, divorce, family separation, or lack of diagnosis, can never be ignored. A review of all systems may provide clues to the liver disease:

Table 54-1. Diseases that May Present as Acute Viral Hepatitis

Viral hepatitis (hepatitis A, B, C, D, E)
Other viral infections
   Yellow fever
   Herpetic viruses; i.e., Epstein-Barr, cytomegalovirus, herpes simplex
Alcoholic hepatitis
Autoimmune hepatitis
Drug-induced hepatitis
Wilson's disease
Ischemia
Sepsis
Systemic disease
Veno-occlusive disease

Table 54-2. Abnormalities of Bilirubin Metabolism

Unconjugated Hyperbilirubinemia
  Increased production
    Hemolysis (intravascular, hematoma)
    Ineffective erythropoiesis
  Decreased hepatic clearance of bilirubin
    Neonatal (physiologic)
    Breast-milk jaundice
    Drug
  Defects in bilirubin conjugation
    Crigler-Najjar type I syndrome (chronic nonhemolytic jaundice with absent glucuronyl transferase activity)
    Crigler-Najjar type II syndrome (chronic nonhemolytic jaundice with decreased glucuronyl transferase activity)
    Gilbert's syndrome (chronic low grade unconjugated hyperbilirubinemia)
Conjugated hyperbilirubinemia
  Dubin-Johnson syndrome
  Rotor's syndrome

(Modified from Crawford, J. M., and Gollan, J.: Bilirubin metabolism and the pathophysiology of jaundice. In Diseases of the Liver. 7th Ed. Edited by L. Shiff and E. R. Shiff. Philadelphia, J. B. Lippincott, 1993.)

- Chronic ulcerative colitis and primary sclerosing cholangitis or cholangiolar carcinoma[11]
- Extrahepatic malignancy and metastasis
- Paraneoplastic phenomena[12,13]
- Associated autoimmune diseases (rheumatoid arthritis, Raynaud's phenomenon, CREST syndrome) and autoimmune hepatitis
- Hypothyroidism and primary biliary cirrhosis[14]
- Polycythemia and Budd-Chiari syndrome[15]

Obviously the potential for sexually transmitted disease and sexual practice, although seemingly unimportant in critical care settings, is of importance.

Physical Examination

History taking allows evaluation of the general and mental status. An unusual affect, poor memory, confusion, or obtundation of varying degrees can be a clue to the presence of hepatic encephalopathy. Asterixis may be spontaneous but is most often elicited. Simultaneously the patient's physical appearance can be assessed: neat versus disheveled, well nourished versus malnourished. Jaundice is not always detectable, either in acute or chronic disease, but actual excoriation, skin pigmentation, and possibly xanthelasma or xanthomas are highly suggestive of chronic cholestatic disease (Fig. 54-1). Hemochromatosis may present with a slate gray skin, more so than the classic "bronze diabetes".

Spider angiomas, found predominantly on the face, upper trunk, shoulders, and upper arms, may also be visible in normal and pregnant women and in nonhepatic disorders (Fig. 54-2). Multiple needle scars or injection sites identify parenteral drug abuse. Clubbing of the fingers and toes, the "white nails of Terry" (leukonychia), liver palms (palmar erythema), and Dupuytren's contracture suggest chronic liver disease but are nonspecific (Fig. 54-3). Common findings in the hepatic diseases, especially those associated with alcohol, are a decrease in muscle mass, particularly the shoulder girdle; gynecomastia; testicular atrophy; and loss of body hair.[16]

A Kaiser-Fleischer ring, although possibly absent, should be confirmed by slit-lamp examination because younger people with Wilson's disease may masquerade as chronic liver disease or fulminant hepatic failure.[17] Cervical adenopathy may be present with acute viral hepatitis, but infectious mononucleosis and lymphoma are suggested by systemic adenopathy. Distended pulsatile neck veins in an icteric patient call attention to the presence of right-sided heart failure or constrictive pericarditis.

Examination of the abdomen should include a search for prominent abdominal veins. These may be present in a thin abdominal wall stretched by abdominal distention, but in the collateral circulation associated with portal hypertension, the blood flow in dilated veins should radiate outward from the umbilicus (Fig. 54-4). Pathognomonic of inferior vena cava obstruction, the blood flows cephalad in the dilated veins visualized on the flank and/or the back (Fig. 54-5).[18] A normal liver may be felt 2 to 4 cm below the right costal margin on deep inspiration. The upper border is normally percussed at the fifth intercostal space to the right of the midclavicular line. The edge is smooth,

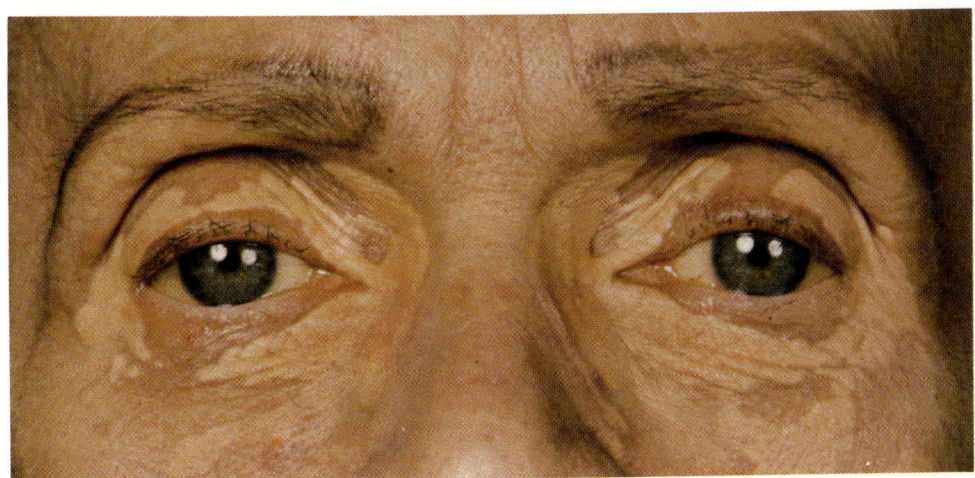

Fig. 54-1. Xanthelasma associated with primary biliary cirrhosis.

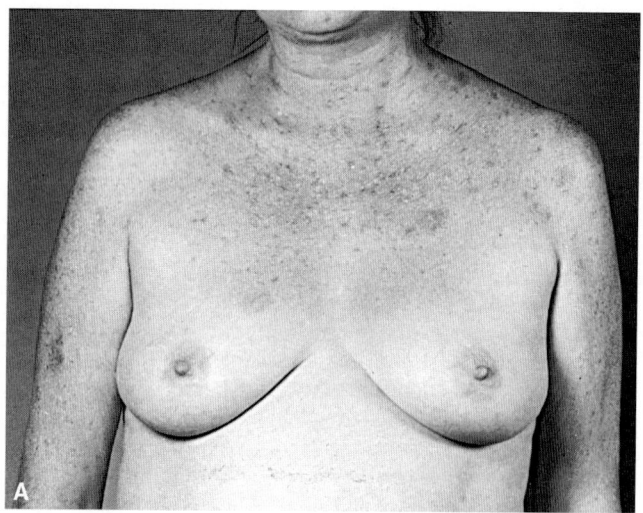
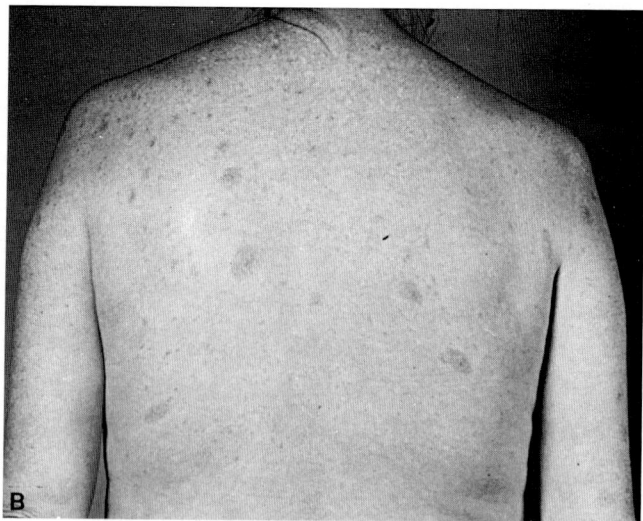

Fig. 54–2. *A,* Spider angiomas on chest, neck, shoulders, and arms in a patient with alcoholic cirrhosis. *B,* Spider angiomas on back, shoulder, and arms. (From Achkar, E. A., Farmer, R., and Fleshler, B. (eds.): Clinical Gastroenterology. Philadelphia, Lea & Febiger, 1992, p. 98.)

sharp, and nontender. A false impression of hepatomegaly is the result of downward displacement by pulmonary emphysema, prolongation of the right lobe (Riedel's lobe), or severe scoliosis. The right lobe of the cirrhotic liver may be moderately enlarged with a rounded or irregular nontender edge but is often too atrophic to be felt. Palpation of the left lobe should not be ignored because it may be difficult to distinguish a hypertrophied cirrhotic left lobe from an abdominal mass. It is unusual to feel nodularity in micronodular cirrhosis, whereas in macronodular cirrhosis, the liver may be hard, irregular, and confused with a neoplasm. Congenital polycystic liver disease may be mistaken for cirrhosis and/or neoplasm (Fig. 54–6). Livers that are palpable 10 cm or more below the right costal margin are most commonly associated with alcoholic hepatitis, fatty infiltration, other infiltrative disorders, amyloidosis, tumor, or congestive heart failure. Hepatic pulsation is a specific clue to constrictive pericarditis, chronic cardiac failure, or a valvular disease. Tender minimal-to-moderate hepatomegaly is seen with viral hepatitis, drug toxicity, or extrahepatic biliary disease. Hepatic tenderness or a lack of pain is not diagnostic, although in patients with acute

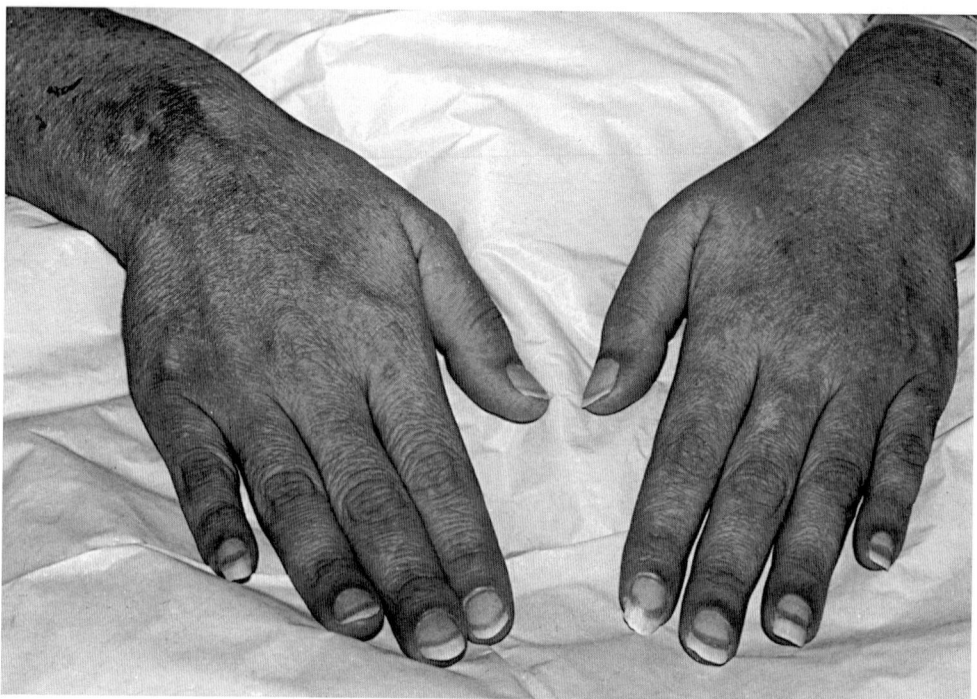

Fig. 54–3. "White nails of Terry" (leukonychia), absent lunula, opaque nail bed, erythematous zone at tip of nail in a patient with alcoholic cirrhosis. (From Achkar, E. A., Farmer, R., and Fleshler, B. (eds.): Clinical Gastroenterology. Philadelphia, Lea & Febiger, 1992, p. 97.)

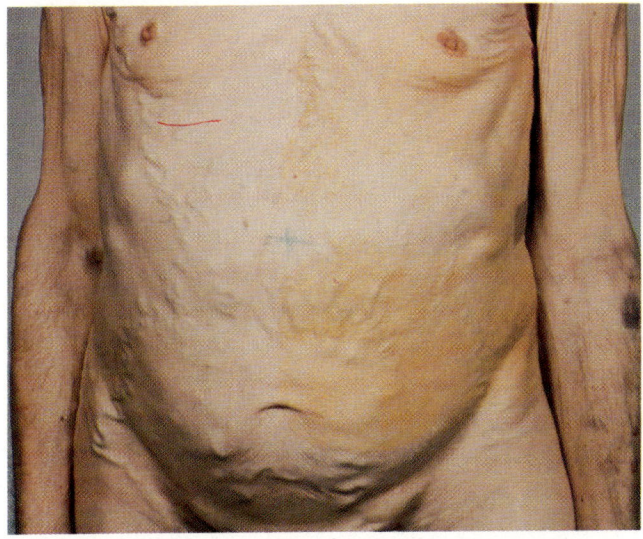

Fig. 54-4. Dilated abdominal veins of collateral circulation in portal hypertension secondary to alcoholic cirrhosis. Note radial outward flow from umbilicus. (From Achkar, E. A., Farmer, R., and Fleshler, B. (eds.): Clinical Gastroenterology. Philadelphia, Lea & Febiger, 1992, p. 99.)

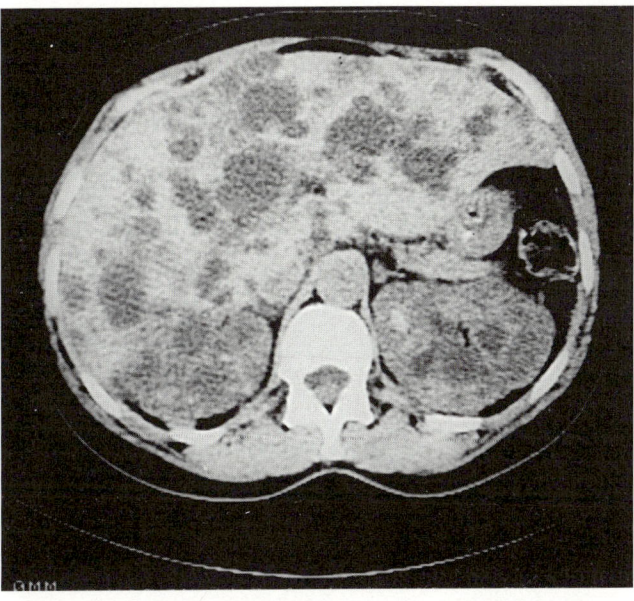

Fig. 54-6. CT scan of the liver in an adult with polycystic liver and kidney disease. Hepatomegaly (nodular) involved the entire upper abdomen with normal liver function. Note renal cysts.

congestive failure, viral hepatitis, or alcoholic hepatitis, the liver is usually exquisitely painful. Auscultation rarely reveals the friction rub associated with a carcinoma or the harsh murmur of vascular tumors of the liver. Occasionally a bruit may be heard over the xiphosternal junction and/or periumbilically. This is secondary to the collateral circulation through a recanalized umbilical vein (Cruveilhier-Baumgarten syndrome).

An enlarged gallbladder may actually be seen on examination, particularly when the abdomen is visualized obliquely. It cannot be seen or palpated unless distended, but in these circumstances, it is hard, circumscribed, tender, and easily mistaken for a hepatic, renal, or colonic tumor. Lacking a history of cholecystectomy, the presence of hydrops should be considered (Fig. 54-7). According to Courvoisier's law, jaundice in association with a palpable gallbladder is diagnostic of a malignant obstruction in the pancreatic head or ampulla of Vater 90 to 95% of the time.[19] A wall thickened by the inflammation associated with biliary calculi is unable to distend as opposed to the distensibility of the normal thin gallbladder wall; hence the differentiation between an extrinsic malignant obstruc-

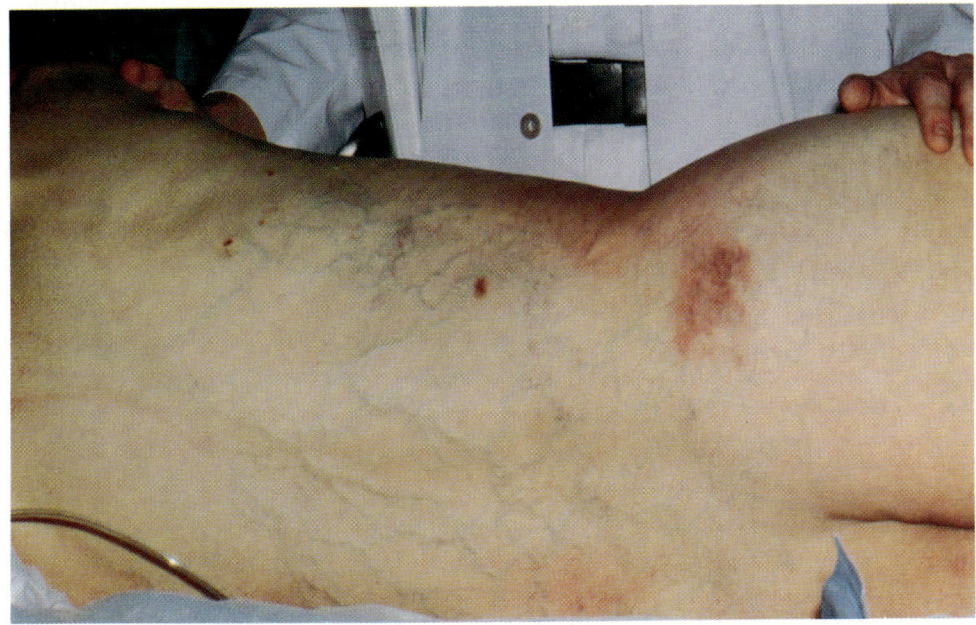

Fig. 54-5. Dilated back and flank veins pathognomonic of inferior vena cava obstruction in a patient with hepatocellular carcinoma with tumor thrombosis of inferior vena cava.

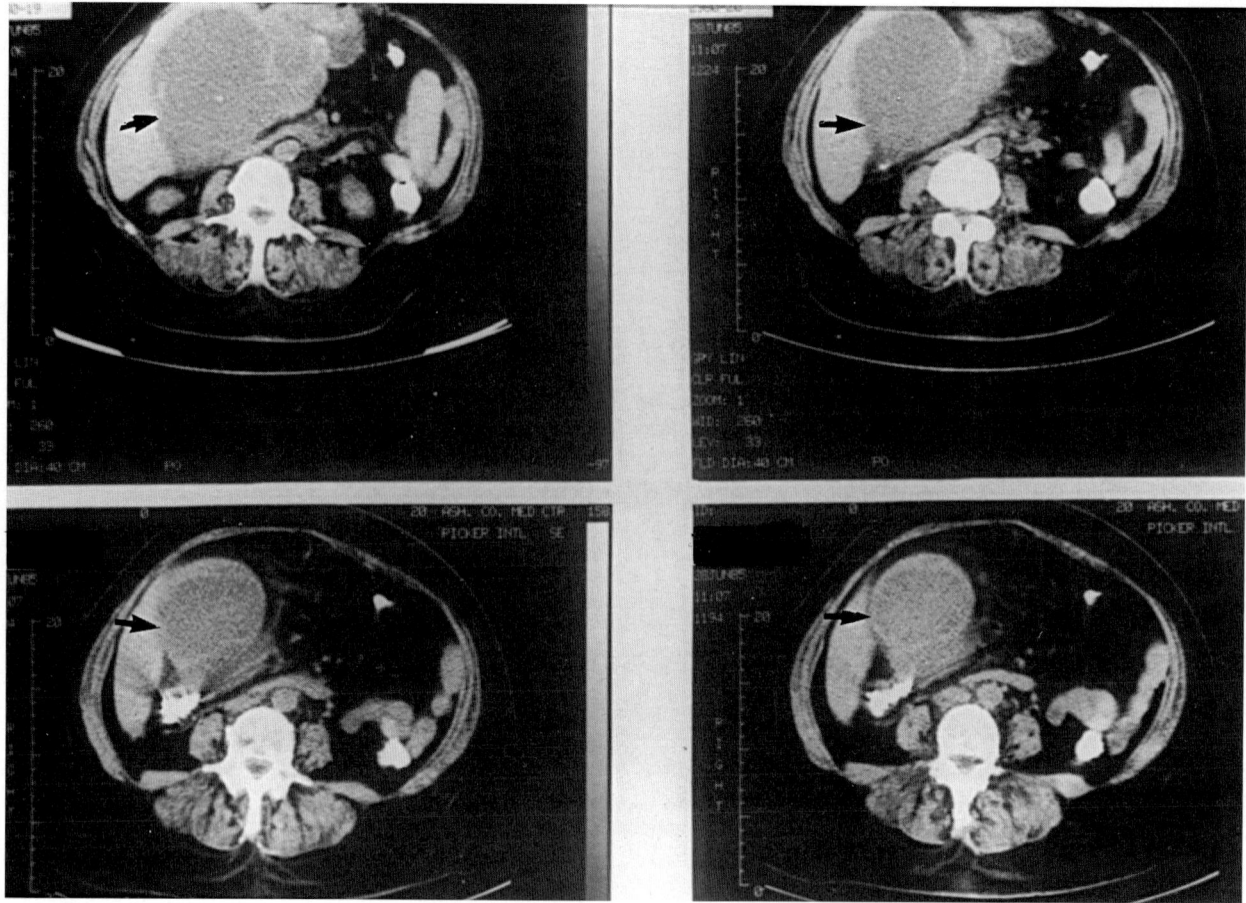

Fig. 54–7. Abdominal CT scan demonstrates hydrops of gallbladder *(arrows)*. Note oral contrast in small intestine.

tion as opposed to calculous disease.[19] A distended gallbladder may also be the result of a stone impacted in the common duct distal to the cystic duct.[20]

Marked tenderness on deep inspiration when the examining fingers palpate the area below the liver edge (Murphy's sign) characterizes acute cholecystitis. On rare occasion, hyperesthesia may be elicited posteriorly between the ninth and eleventh ribs on the right (Boas's sign).[21] The absence of splenomegaly does not exclude portal hypertension, but an enlarged spleen may not only be indicative of cirrhosis, but also may be the result of a splenic vein thrombosis or an associated hemolytic disorder. Ascites, with or without peripheral edema, is most often associated with cirrhosis but must be differentiated from other causes: intra-abdominal fluid, infection, peritoneal implants, hepatoma, the nephrotic syndrome, hepatic vein obstruction, or even uroascites, the last-mentioned seen following urologic procedures. A pleural effusion is found in 10% of patients with ascites and liver disease.[22]

Laboratory Evaluation

Enzyme abnormalities indicate ongoing hepatocellular damage, but the routine biochemical means of characterizing hepatic function are limited to measurements of the bilirubin and albumin levels and prothrombin time. True tests of quantitative function, i.e., galactose tolerance elimination capacity (GEC),[23] and aminopyrine breath test, have not achieved widespread use.[24] Dye tests are no longer used clinically other than bromosulphalein (BSP) for differentiating between Dubin-Johnson and Rotor's syndromes.[25] Indocyanine green (ICG) is used primarily in the determination of hepatic blood flow.[26]

The Child-Turcotte classification and its Pugh modification were conceived to forecast the outcome of portal systemic shunting in patients with esophageal varices.[27,28] Composed of components that are readily available, discriminating, noninvasive, and inexpensive, this combination of biochemical and clinical observation evaluates hepatic function at a specific time (Tables 54–3 and 54–4). These classifications are now used as prognostic indices for survival in patients with liver disease requiring surgery for reasons other than varices, and its status as the gold standard by which risk and outcome are predicted has been demonstrated to be as effective as any other combination of studies.[29-32]

Bilirubin

Jaundice becomes clinically apparent when the plasma concentration of bilirubin surpasses 3.0 mg/dl. The classification of jaundice (Table 54–5) is based on abnormalities encountered secondary to abnormality of bilirubin metabolism, hepatocellular damage, or cholestasis.[2] Hepatocellu-

Table 54–3. Child-Turcotte Classification of Hepatic Functional Reserve*

Chemical and Biochemical Measurements	A	B	C
Bilirubin (mg/dl)	<2	2–3	>3
Albumin (g/dl)	>3.5	3.0–3.5	<3.0
Ascites	None	Easily controlled	Difficult to control
Encephalopathy	None	Minimal	Advanced
Nutrition	Excellent	Good	Poor, wasting
Risk	Good	Moderate	Poor

* Patients are classified by assigning a unit number to each of the five factors (points in column A = 1, B = 2, C = 3) with Class A = 5–8 points, Class B = 9–11 points, and Class C = 12–15 points.
(From Child, C. G., III, and Turcotte, J.: Surgery and portal hypertension. In The Liver and Portal Hypertension. Edited by C. G. Child, III. Philadelphia, W. B. Saunders, 1964.)
(Operative mortality: A–7.7%, B–25.9%, C–51.8%. Five-year survival [life table]: A–51.8%, B–28.4%, C–17.3%. Data from Turcotte, J. G., and Lambert, M. J.: Variceal hemorrhage, hepatic cirrhosis and portacaval shunts. Surgery, 73:810, 1973.)

lar pathology may be a secondary result of systemic disease as well as primary hepatic disease, whereas cholestasis, although commonly assumed as synonymous with obstruction of the extrahepatic biliary tree, is defined as "the result of an impaired formation and low flow of bile"[33] caused by a variety of intrahepatic and extrahepatic disorders, many of which remain unexplained. It is obligatory to distinguish between the causes of extrahepatic cholestasis that are potentially surgically correctable ("surgical jaundice") and intrahepatic cholestasis ("medical jaundice").[33,34] The latter may be secondary to injury of the canalicular membranes and/or organelles (hepatocyte, interlobular), associated with bile secretion without demonstrable evidence of biliary obstruction, or intralobular, in which a mechanical cause is discernible but not surgically accessible. With progression and greater involvement of

Table 54–4. Pugh Modification of Child-Turcotte Classification

Chemical and Biochemical Measurements	Points for Increasing Abnormality		
	1	2	3
Encephalopathy	None	1 and 2	3 and 4
Ascites	Absent	Slight	Moderate
Bilirubin (mg/dl)	1–2	2–3	>3.0
Albumin (g/dl)	>3.5	2.8–3.5	<2.8
Prothrombin time (seconds prolonged)	1–4	4–6	>6
For primary biliary cirrhosis (bilirubin—mg/dl)	1–4	4–10	>10
Died in hospital	2/7 (28.6%)	5/13 (38.5%)	14/18 (77.8%)
Died within 6 months	0/7	4/13 (30.7%)	4/18 (12.5%)
Survived 24 months	3/7 (43%)	4/13 (30.7%)	0/18

(Modified from Pugh, R. N. H., et al.: Transection of the esophagus for bleeding esophageal varices. Br. J. Surg., 60:646, 1973.)

Table 54–5. Classification of Jaundice

Intrahepatic jaundice ("medical jaundice")[33,34]
  Hepatocellular dysfunction
    Hepatic disease with systemic manifestations (e.g., viral hepatitis)
    Hepatic disease with manifestations secondary to systemic disease (e.g., sarcoidosis)
Cholestasis without demonstrable biliary obstruction
  Primary abnormality of hepatocyte injury[34]
    Drugs, hormones[35,36]
    Sepsis[76]
    Total parenteral nutrition[38]
    Cholestasis of pregnancy[39]
    Benign postoperative intrahepatic cholestasis[40]
    Infiltrative disease[41]
    Benign recurrent cholestasis
  Primary abnormality of intralobar bile duct injury
    Primary biliary cirrhosis[42]
    Graft-versus-host disease[43]
    Posthepatic transplant rejection[44]
    Vanishing bile duct syndrome[45,46]
  Intrahepatic ductal (interlobular) bile duct injury[34]*
    Primary sclerosing cirrhosis (intrahepatic)[11]
    Intrahepatic ductal calculi (Caroli's disease and biliary calculi)[47]
    Malignancy (cholangiolar, hepatocellular, metastatic)
    Cirrhosis
Cholestasis (extrahepatic) ("surgical jaundice")
  Choledocholithiasis
  Malignant tumor
    Ampulla of Vater
    Duodenal
    Cholangiolar
    Gallbladder
    Pancreas
  Benign tumors
    Adenoma
    Papilloma
  Inflammatory
    Stricture, secondary to choledocholithiasis
    Pancreatitis
    Sclerosing cholangiolitis (extrahepatic) (suppurative, primary)
  Miscellaneous
    Choledochal cyst[48]
    Duodenal diverticulum[49]
    Parasites (Ascaris lumbricoides, Fasciola hepatica, Clonorchis sinensis, Echinococcus granulosus, Schistosoma mansoni)[50]
    Hemobilia

* Cholestasis with demonstrable intrahepatic biliary obstruction.
(From Winkelman, E. I.: Cirrhosis. In Clinical Gastroenterology. 2nd Ed. Edited by E. A. Achkar, R. Farmer, and B. Fleshler. Philadelphia, Lea & Febiger, 1992.)

the liver, the differential diagnosis of pure cholestasis becomes more difficult, if not impossible.

Although high performance lipid chromatography affords the most sensitive, accurate measurements of conjugated (direct) and unconjugated (indirect) bilirubin, it is not routinely available for clinical use. Routine laboratory measurements are based on the method of van den Bergh, in which total bilirubin is determined colorimetrically 30 minutes after the addition of a diazo reagent and then alcohol to the plasma. The rapid color change occurring 1 minute after the diazo reagent alone is added becomes the end point for the determination of conjugated bilirubin, and the concentration of the unconjugated bilirubin is determined by subtracting the conjugated from the total.[51]

Normal values of the total bilirubin vary from 0.03 to 1.5 mg/dl, but increased levels furnish neither a sensitive index of liver function nor a discriminating assessment of hepatic damage. The ability to detect mild biliary disease is low, and the "overlap" between the icterus of "medical" and "surgical" jaundice prevents separation of the two. The total measurement is considered an adverse prognostic factor when persistently elevated in primary biliary cirrhosis, alcoholic hepatitis, or fulminant hepatic failure, but when applied as an individual variable in cirrhosis, a bilirubin level of 1 mg/dl or less is a favorable prognostic sign.[52]

The concentration of conjugated bilirubin in normal individuals is 0.1 to 0.3 mg/dl. The fractionation is helpful only when the total bilirubin level is normal or mildly elevated. In these situations, a conjugated bilirubin greater than 0.5 mg/dl is a sensitive marker of hepatic dysfunction except as an isolated abnormality in congenital conjugated hyperbilirubinemia, i.e., Dubin-Johnson syndrome.[53]

Unconjugated bilirubin comprises almost all the circulating bilirubin in normal individuals. A total bilirubin greater than 1.2 mg/dl with a conjugated level less than 20% of that indicates an unconjugated hyperbilirubinemia.[54] Causes of this may be defects in the bilirubin metabolism secondary to a congenital or acquired defect of impaired hepatic uptake, impaired bilirubin conjugation, or the overproduction of bilirubin, primarily by intravascular hemolysis.[2] The normal liver's ability to excrete bilirubin beyond ordinary requirements is explained by the excessive hepatic excretory capacity, which far exceeds the maximum production of conjugated bilirubin; therefore the plasma bilirubin in the healthy person remains normal even with a 50% acute reduction of the red blood cell survival and is unlikely to surpass a level of 4 to 5 mg/dl even if the hemolysis increases by a factor of six. This also explains why intrahepatic focal ductal obstruction in a normal person does not present with jaundice as long as there is adequate intrahepatic drainage.[55] In normal individuals with hemolysis, unconjugated bilirubin is the major component of the circulating bilirubin. However, greater than 15% of its total may be conjugated when hemolysis is superimposed on acute or chronic disease.[54] In this instance, mild abnormalities of liver function may produce marked hyperbilirubinemia because the liver, although able to conjugate the increased unconjugated bilirubin, cannot normally excrete the excess amount of conjugated bilirubin, which then refluxes back into the plasma. Clinically the greatest increase in bilirubin is registered when excessive hemolysis occurs in the presence of both hepatic and renal dysfunction, the latter because the kidney is the main means of excretion in cases of biliary obstruction or hepatocellular disease.[56]

A less frequently recognized portion of circulating bilirubin, also reacting biochemically as conjugated bilirubin, is identified by high performance lipid chromatography and referred to as the "delta fraction." Undetectable in normal patients or those with unconjugated bilirubinemia, this bilirubin is tightly bound to albumin and may constitute 8 to 90% of the total bilirubin elevation associated with hepatobiliary disease. Its relative proportion increases with the duration of the disease. Because the albumin bond prevents glomerular filtration, it is not excreted by the kidney, and the rate of clearance is dictated by the 20-day half-life of its covalent bond, explaining the prolonged icterus present without associated bilirubinuria in patients whose underlying hepatobiliary pathology has resolved.[2,57]

Albumin

Although considered a major biochemical determinant of liver synthetic function, albumin is actually an insensitive indicator of hepatic dysfunction. The liver's enormous reserve capacity allows the albumin level to become abnormal only in advanced liver disease and so does not reflect the lesser, although significant, hepatic damage present in many cirrhotic patients. Produced solely by the liver, albumin has a half-life of 20 to 21 days, accounting for the normal levels usually seen in acute hepatitis or early in fulminant disease as opposed to the decrease in levels found in severe chronic hepatocellular disease and decompensated cirrhosis.[58] The normal albumin concentration may be affected by extrahepatic causes: capillary leakage, dilution secondary to fluid retention, poor nutrition, or an increased rate of degradation. Gamma globulin, synthesized by the hepatic reticuloendothelial cells, is a nonspecific indicator of inflammation, although an increase in the gamma globulin to twice normal or more is a hallmark of chronic active autoimmune hepatitis.

Prothrombin Time

Critical components of the coagulation cascade are elaborated only by hepatocytes. Measurement of the prothrombin time alone provides a practical means of assessing hepatic synthetic capacities; thus there is no need to measure individual clotting factors routinely. Most individual coagulation components have a circulating half-life of less than 12 hours, and a decrease in their synthesis can quickly prolong the prothrombin time to antedate other evidence of liver decompensation. Vitamin K is essential for the synthesis of factors II, VII, IX, and X, and failure to absorb this fat-soluble vitamin because of cholestasis or other causes of steatorrhea increases the prothrombin time.[59] In this instance, parenterally administered vitamin K rapidly corrects the prothrombin time, whereas in hepatic cell failure, the abnormality remains unchanged; however, in the presence of significant cholestasis secondary to severe hepatocellular damage, vitamin K administered parenterally may minimally decrease an abnormal prothrombin time but does not correct it. The activated partial thromboplastin time does not supersede the prothrombin time as a satisfactory index to the clotting process.

Aminotransferases

Serum alanine aminotransferase (ALT) and the serum aspartate aminotransferase (AST), formerly labeled SGPT and SGOT respectively, are sensitive indicators of liver cell injury. Increased plasma levels represent leakage via increased permeability of a damaged cell membrane. Elevation of both enzymes may be present in all types of hepatic disorders: infection, congestion, steatosis, infiltrative and granulomatous diseases, drug and chemical injury, neoplasm, and acute and chronic biliary tract disease. An elevated AST can be present in both cardiac and skeletal muscle injury, but the increase in ALT seen after a myocardial infarction is usually the result of hepatic ischemia, secondary to congestive failure or shock.[60] Levels may rise to greater than 1000 IU in acute hepatic necrosis induced by viruses, toxins, drugs, chemicals, shock, and acute rhabdomyolysis.[60] These are not always interpreted as ominous prognostic signs because they define hepatocellular injury, not necessarily necrosis. Conversely, in patients with uremia, values may be lower than normal or even absent, presumably as a result of a serum inhibiting factor.[61] Enzyme levels greater than eight times normal are almost always associated with hepatocellular disease, but any type of acute disorder may exhibit an elevation of that degree. A minimal increase of three times or less may seem to be trivial but can have significant implications in deciding whether further diagnostic studies are necessary or therapy is indicated.

The elevation of the ALT is a more specific and sensitive indicator of hepatocellular injury, preceding jaundice by 1 to 2 weeks in patients with acute hepatitis and usually exceeding the level of the AST. Both diminish in parallel during recovery, but their decrease in the face of increasing bilirubinemia suggests massive hepatic necrosis.

The natural history of hepatitis C is characterized by AST and ALT, which fluctuate from normal to several times that level over a period of months to years. Acute biliary obstruction can also cause elevation of both aminotransferases to greater than eight times normal, but within the next 24 to 72 hours, sequential testing reveals a decrease of 58 to 76%.[62] In these instances, a ratio of AST to ALT is less than 1, but according to Williams and Hoofnagle,[63] a ratio greater than 1 occurring in nonalcoholic liver disease should suggest the presence of cirrhosis. An AST-to-ALT ratio of 2:1 or greater is usually seen in alcoholic hepatitis, especially when the values do not exceed 200 to 300 IU.[64] Serum lactic dehydrogenase (LDH) is neither sensitive nor specific in the diagnosis of liver disease and offers no advantages over the aminotransferases.

Alkaline Phosphatase

An elevated serum alkaline phosphatase is the most constant abnormality associated with cholestasis and the end result of an increased synthesis of the enzyme, which is then regurgitated into the bloodstream.[58] Contrary to belief, it does not differentiate extrahepatic from intrahepatic cholestasis because the highest values seen with complete biliary obstruction are rivaled by those recorded in some cases of primary biliary cirrhosis or drug-induced cholestasis.[65] An increase greater than three times normal should also raise a question of hepatocellular carcinoma, primary sclerosing cholangitis, obstruction of a major duct, partial or complete obstructing choledocholithiasis common bile duct stone, infiltrative disease, sarcoidosis, tuberculosis, or metastatic carcinoma. Values less than three times the normal limit are nonspecific and seen not only with cholestatic lesions, but also with hepatitis or other noncholestatic disorders. A cholestatic picture simulating extrahepatic biliary tract obstruction may be present in the occasional person with hepatitis A[66] or as a paraneoplastic manifestation in those without liver disease as reported with hypernephroma (Stauffer's syndrome) or Hodgkin's lymphoma.[12,13]

Osteoblasts and placenta also produce alkaline phosphatase and explain the abnormal elevation found in children, adolescents, or women in late pregnancy. Heat fractionation or electrophoresis can identify the appropriate fraction in those situations when it is necessary to differentiate the source. Gamma-glutamyl transpeptidase (GGTP) levels remain normal in disorders of the bone and can indirectly provide the same information as the isoenzymes. Because it is an inducible enzyme, an isolated increase in GGTP may result from the use of certain drugs, most commonly alcohol, phenobarbital, or hydantoin.[67]

Routine Laboratory Studies

Abnormalities in routine studies can raise suspicion of liver disease in an otherwise asymptomatic individual. Microcytic and macrocytic anemia are commonly seen with cirrhosis. Because alcohol affects folate metabolism, macrocytic anemia in conjunction with an elevated GGTP and no other abnormalities suggests continued or excess use of alcohol. Microcytic anemia necessitates a search for blood loss usually secondary to esophageal varices, portal hypertensive gastropathy, or peptic ulcer disease, all entities that are best diagnosed endoscopically. Leukopenia and thrombocytopenia secondary to hypersplenism may be the sole indication of compensated liver disease.

Urinary urobilinogen is colorless and must be detected chemically, but its presence is evidence that bile has entered the intestinal tract.[2,51] Bilirubinuria, detectable by observation or chemically, is present only when conjugated bilirubin is elevated.[2,51] The presence of both hyperbilirubinuria and increased urobilinogen is compatible with hepatocellular dysfunction. A normal-appearing urine in a patient with jaundice indicates hemolysis, unconjugated hyperbilirubinemia, or the presence of a "delta fraction" whereas bilirubinuria in the absence of urobilinogen is strong evidence for complete exclusion of the bile from the gut; however, absence of the intestinal flora secondary to antibiotic treatment, rapid intestinal transit, and renal insufficiency can also eliminate urinary urobilinogen. Clinically, the determination of urinary urobilinogen is of little value.[51]

Renal tubular acidification defects are common in cirrhosis and may be responsible for hypokalemia and hepatic encephalopathy.[68]

Miscellaneous Markers

Abnormalities of ferritin, ceruloplasmin or alpha$_1$-antitrypsin are respectively suggestive of hemochromatosis, Wilson's disease, or alpha$_1$-antitrypsin deficiency. Alpha-fetoprotein levels are elevated late in pregnancy, but their increase in severe hepatitis is thought to be a favorable prognostic sign because it is considered to represent hepatocellular regeneration; however, its greatest value is for screening or detection of hepatocellular carcinoma.[69] Antimitochondrial antibodies, not seen in extrahepatic or intrahepatic cholestasis, are found in almost all patients with primary biliary cirrhosis but are not specific because they are present in 30% of patients with chronic active autoimmune hepatitis.[70] Elevation of the antinuclear and smooth muscle antibodies is suggestive of autoimmune liver disease.

Serologic testing has now identified five separate types of hepatitis viruses. These include hepatitis A (HA), hepatitis B (HB), hepatitis C (HC) (formerly non-A, non-B hepatitis), hepatitis D (HD) (only diagnosed in the presence of the hepatitis B surface antigen), and hepatitis E (HE).[71-73] The last-mentioned, a water-borne-epidemic with negative serologic tests for HA and HB and differing clinically from non-A, non-B hepatitis (HC), is seen exclusively in the underdeveloped countries of the world. It may have affected those who have visited these areas within proximity to the onset of their hepatitis. The incidence is higher throughout pregnancy but has a conspicuously high mortality of approximately 20% in the last trimester.[73] Observations on the syndrome hepatitis-associated aplastic anemia implicates a new non-A, non-B, non-C agent in both this and fulminant hepatitis, suggesting a yet to be defined hepatitis F.[74]

Imaging

Abdominal Radiography

Plain abdominal films are commonly ordered in jaundiced patients looking for biliary calculi. The yield is low because only 10 to 20% of gallstones are visualized[75] (Fig. 54-8). Other calcific densities, i.e., granulomas, calcified metastatic neoplasms or primary hepatomas, hemangiomas, hydatid cysts, and the "porcelain gallbladder," are more unusual causes of right upper quadrant calcification and may be misleading, raising the questions of intrahepatic duct calculi as in Caroli's disease (Fig. 54-9).

The plain film may reveal other abnormalities. The presence of a distended gallbladder in a nonicteric patient with acute right upper abdominal pain and no prior history of gallbladder disease strongly suggests an acute obstruction of the cystic duct (Fig. 54-10). Pancreatic calcium is diag-

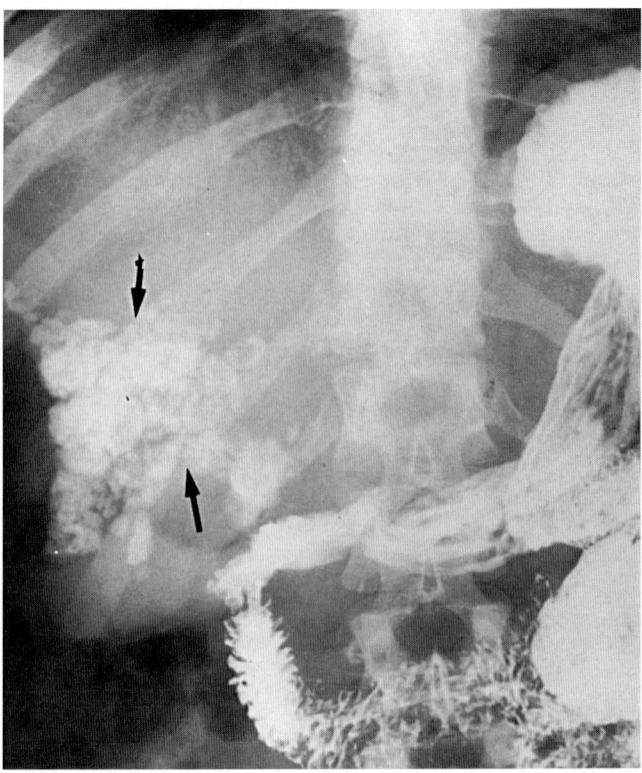

Fig. 54-9. Right upper quadrant calcification in cholangiocarcinoma (arrows). Incidental finding.

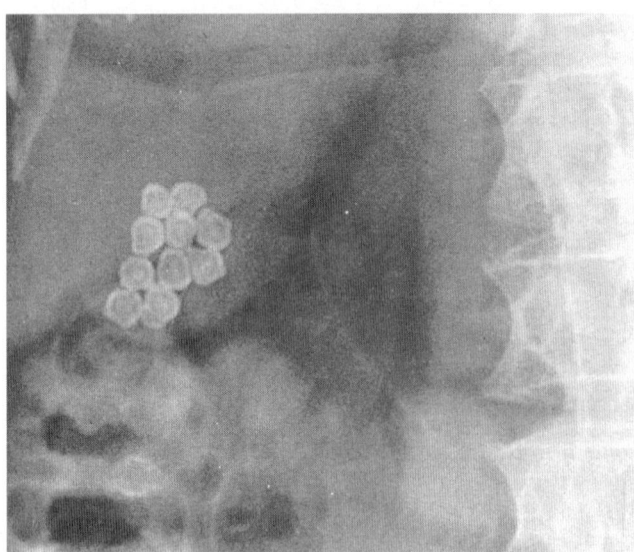

Fig. 54-8. Plain abdominal film with calcified gallstones.

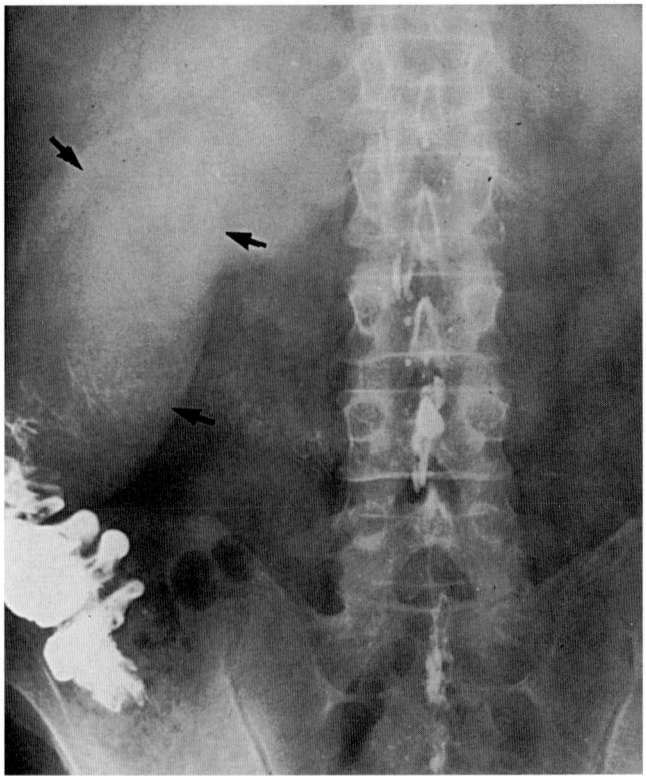

Fig. 54-10. Plain film. Hydrops of gallbladder (arrows).

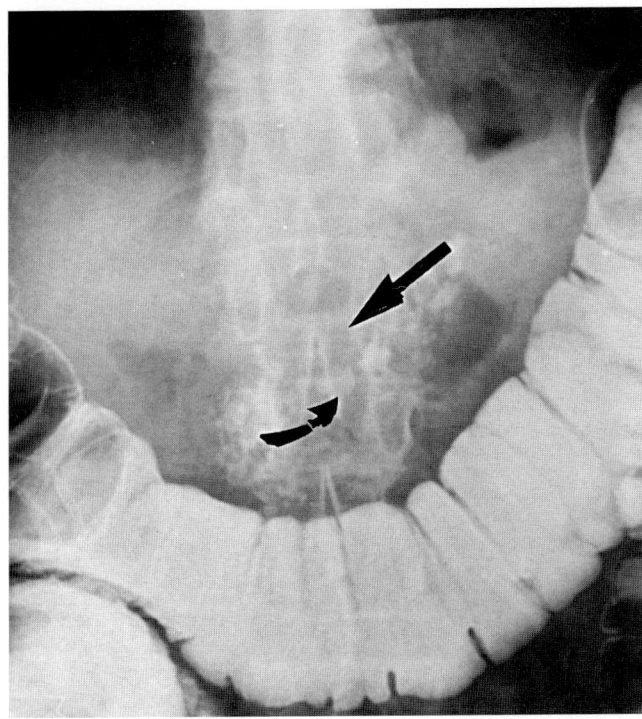

Fig. 54-11. Pancreatic calcification (area of arrows) was an incidental finding on this film.

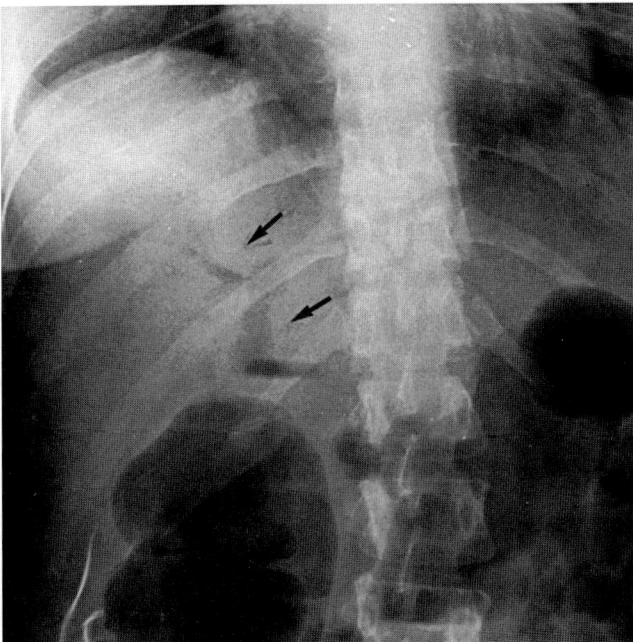

Fig. 54-12. Plain abdominal film. Air in biliary tree (arrows). Note choledochostomy to the patient's right side.

nostic of chronic pancreatitis, and large calcium stones in infants and adolescents represent hereditary pancreatitis (Fig. 54-11). Air in the biliary tree is easily identified as it follows the branching pattern of the major ducts, dispersing as the ramifications become finer. The usual causes of pneumobilia are enterobiliary anastomosis, sphincterotomy, or a spontaneous fistula resulting from the perforation of gallstones into the gastrointestinal tract or the perforation of an ulcer into the biliary tree, but the possibility of pyogenic cholangitis and emphysematous cholecystitis cannot be ignored (Fig. 54-12). Branching radiolucencies extending peripherally to the capsule indicate air in the portal venous system and are easily overlooked (Fig. 54-13). Most frequently, this is secondary to sepsis accompanying acute cholecystitis, biliary tract surgery, or necrotic bowel and carries an ominous prognosis.[76] Intrahepatic abscesses are seen as pockets of gas within the substance of the liver, although they can present as either round or irregular lucencies with or without an air-fluid level.

Scintigraphy

The liver spleen scan uses a gamma-emitting [99m]techetium-labeled sulfur colloid (^{99m}Tc-sulfur colloid), which is taken up by the reticuloendothelial system in the liver, spleen, and bone marrow of the sternum, ribs, and vertebral bodies. Highly effective in detecting hepatic and splenic enlargement and diffuse liver disease, it lacks the ability to characterize focal defects, i.e., hemangiomas, cysts, abscesses, and metastatic or primary hepatic neoplasms, or to define the cause of diffuse hepatocellular dysfunction. The most distinctive patterns are seen in alcoholic cirrhosis (Fig. 54-14) and in one third to two thirds of patients with Budd-Chiari syndrome (Fig. 54-15). Despite a 80 to 85% sensitivity that serves well as a screening examination, it has fallen from favor owing to the inability to identify the nature of its abnormal findings.[77]

Single-photon emission computed tomography (SPECT)

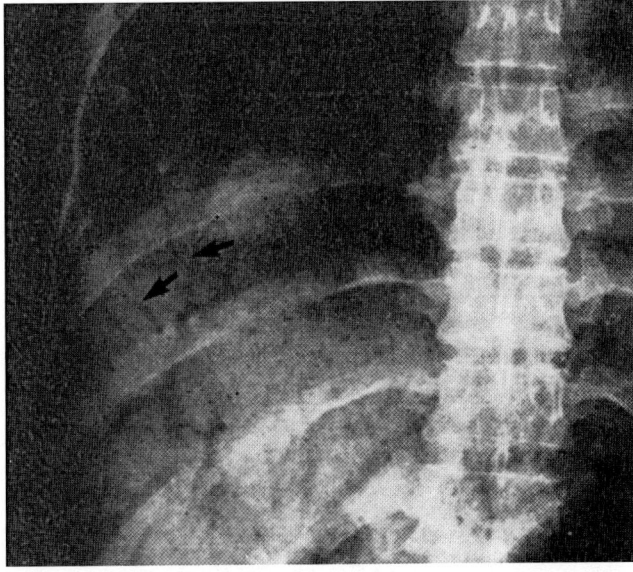

Fig. 54-13. Plain abdominal film. Gas within the portal vein and intrahepatic branches. Radiolucencies extended to periphery of capsule (arrows). (From Fred, H. L., Mayhall, C. G., and Harle, T. S.: Hepatic portal venous gas: a review and report on six new cases. Am. J. Med., 44:557, 1968.)

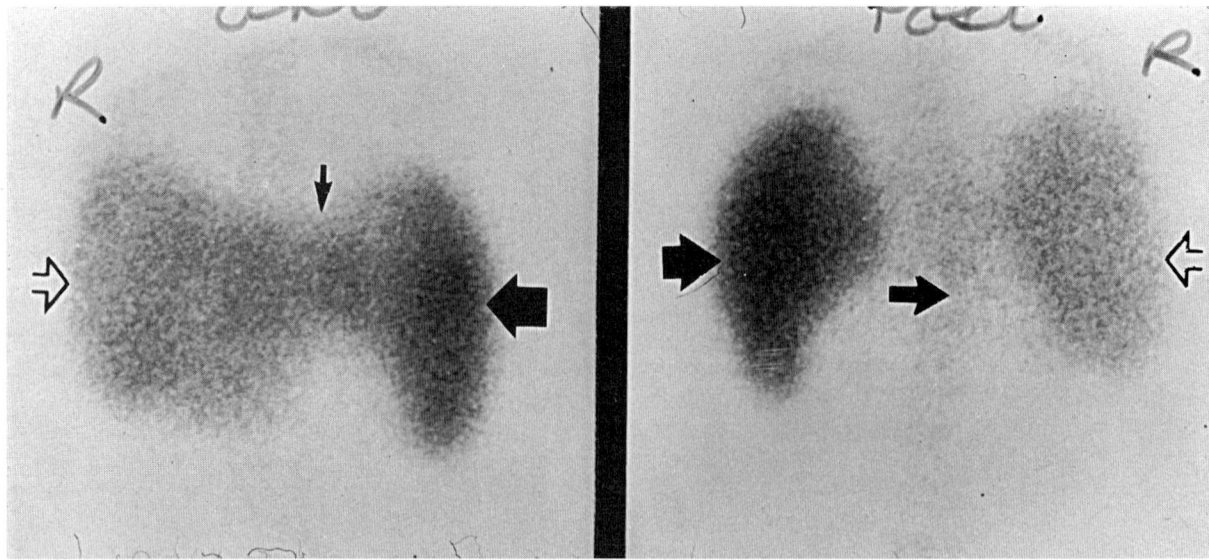

Fig. 54–14. Liver-spleen scan (^{99m}Tc-sulfur colloid, anterior view on the left) in a patient with alcoholic cirrhosis. Small right lobe with decreased heterogeneous uptake *(white arrow)* and left lobe *(small arrow)* and spleen *(large arrow)* with increased uptake. Posterior view on right. Increased uptake over spleen *(large arrow)* and vertebral body *(small arrow)*. Liver is small with decreased uptake *(white arrow)*.

combines conventional radiopharmaceutical and nuclear imaging equipment to obtain transaxial tomographic imaging. This produces a three-dimensional image and improves the accuracy of lesion detection. Standard ^{99m}Tc sulfur colloid allows a more accurate evaluation of abnormalities of size and shape of focal defects. ^{99m}Tc-radiolabeled red blood cells which visualize the intravascular blood pool in the liver has become the method of choice to differentiate hemangioma from other hepatic lesions. Localization of hepatocellular carcinoma and inflammatory lesions has been improved by the use of ^{67}gallium citrate, and ^{111}indium-labeled white blood cells. As both gallium and indium accumulate normally in liver tissue and the bowel, the three-dimensional ability of SPECT permits the separation of the abnormal from normal tissue, allowing a more precise detection of intra-abdominal pathology.[78]

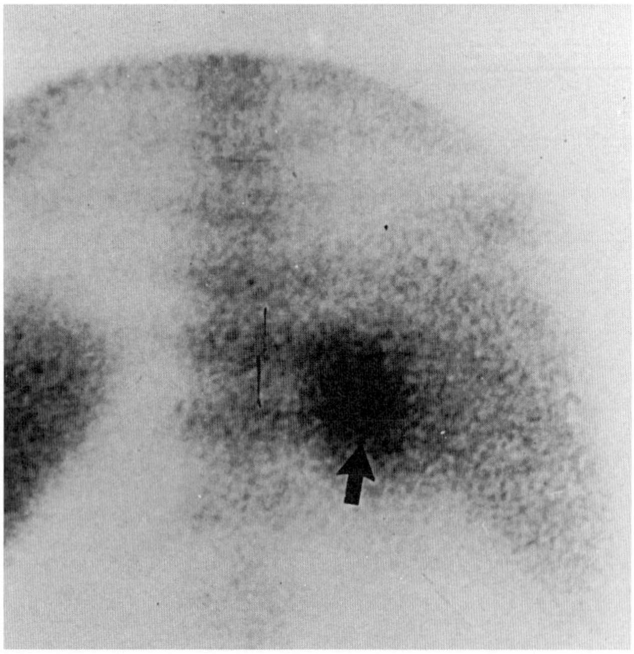

Cholescintigraphy

Cholescintigraphy makes use of derivatives of technetium 99-labeled iminodiacetic acid (HIDA, PIPDA, DISIDA). By virtue of maintaining its rate of hepatic extraction even when the bilirubin is >5 mg/dl, DISDA has become the agent of choice.[79] Once excreted into the bile, it images the liver, extrahepatic ducts, and gallbladder and normally is seen in the small intestine within 1 hour (Fig. 54–16). Failure to visualize the gallbladder in the presence of this agent is diagnostic in 98% of cases of cystic duct obstruction, the primary cause of acute cholecystitis, whereas visualization of the gallbladder excludes the diagnosis of acute cholecystitis in 99% (Fig. 54–17). False-positive scans can be seen in patients with prolonged fasting both with and without total parenteral nutrition, acute pancreatitis, heavy alcoholic intake, chronic cholecystitis, and acalculous cholecystitis.[80] It is the sole noninvasive technique that can confirm the patency of biliary enteric anastomoses or a bile leak.[77,81] It also provides a means to detect obstruction before duct dilatation or to demonstrate a patent bile duct in the presence of obstruction.[82]

Fig. 54–15. Liver-spleen scan (^{99m}Tc-sulfur colloid). Posterior scan. Budd-Chiari syndrome. Increased uptake in spleen, vertebral bodies, and caudate lobe of liver *(arrow)*. Minimal heterogeneous uptake in remaining liver.

Ultrasonography

By virtue of its ability to visualize and assess the gallbladder and bile ducts rapidly, plus its low cost, real-time ultrasonography is the method of choice initially to evaluate patients with jaundice and/or right upper quadrant pain. Noninvasive and quickly performed at the bedside, it is completed without the use of contrast material or exposure to radiation. Additionally, it can evaluate the hepatic parenchyma and pancreas detect a hepatic laceration, hematoma or unsuspected ascites, and other intra-abdominal pathology. Focal lesions within the liver can be identified, and, when necessary, it provides a means for obtaining directed biopsy or aspiration.

Hyperechoic foci that move with a change in position and cast an acoustic shadow predict gallstones with a 98 to 100% accuracy. Nonvisualization of the gallbladder is diagnostic of biliary calculi 88 to 96% of the time.[83-85] "Sludge" lacks both movement and an acoustic shadow, but gallstones must move with a change in position.

Acute cholecystitis is associated with gallstones in 98%

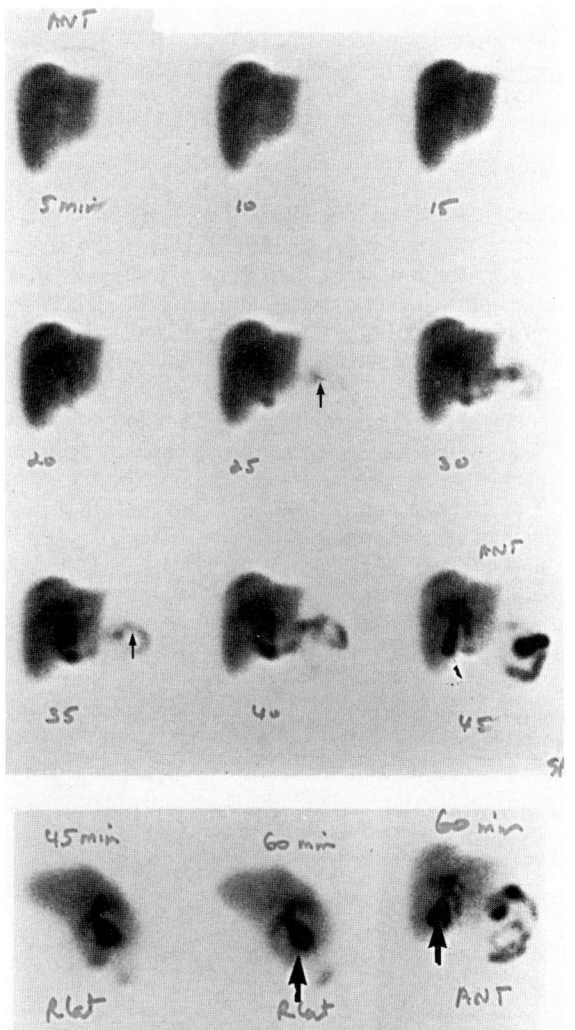

Fig. 54–16. Normal DISDA cholescintigram. Prompt visualization of the liver with migration of the isotope into the duodenum (small arrows) at 25 and 35 minutes. Definite visualization of the gallbladder (large arrow) at 45 minutes. Right lateral views at 60 minutes demonstrate relationship of liver and biliary tree. (Courtesy of S. A. Cook, M.D.)

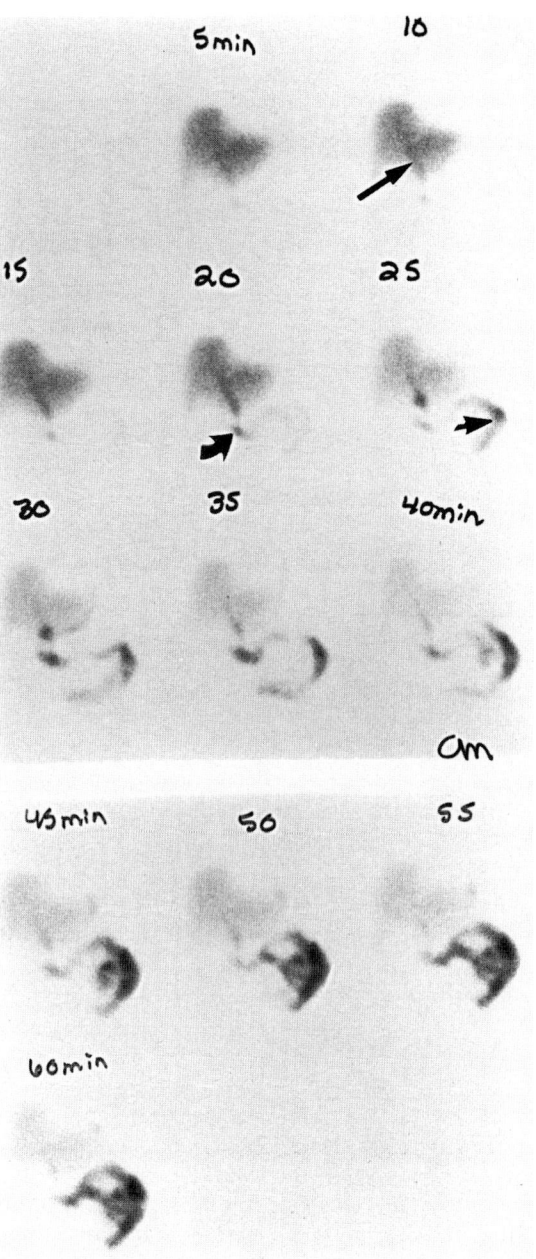

Fig. 54–17. DISDA cholescintigram. Prompt visualization of liver with nonvisualization of gallbladder at 60 minutes (the longer the nonvisualization, the more sensitive the scan). Arrows indicate extrahepatic biliary tree, duodenum, and intestine. (Courtesy of S. A. Cook, M.D.)

of all cases, and acute calculous cholecystitis is diagnosed with almost 100% accuracy when stones are present, the gallbladder is greater than 5 cm in any dimension and its wall is thicker than 5 mm, pericholecystic fluid is seen, and there is tenderness directly over the gallbladder ("sonographic Murphy's sign").[85] The criteria for the diagnosis of acalculous cholecystitis (2 to 10% of all cases of acute cholecystitis) are variable, but the primary components are the sonographic Murphy's sign, an enlarged gallbladder without stones, a thickened wall, and (in the absence of

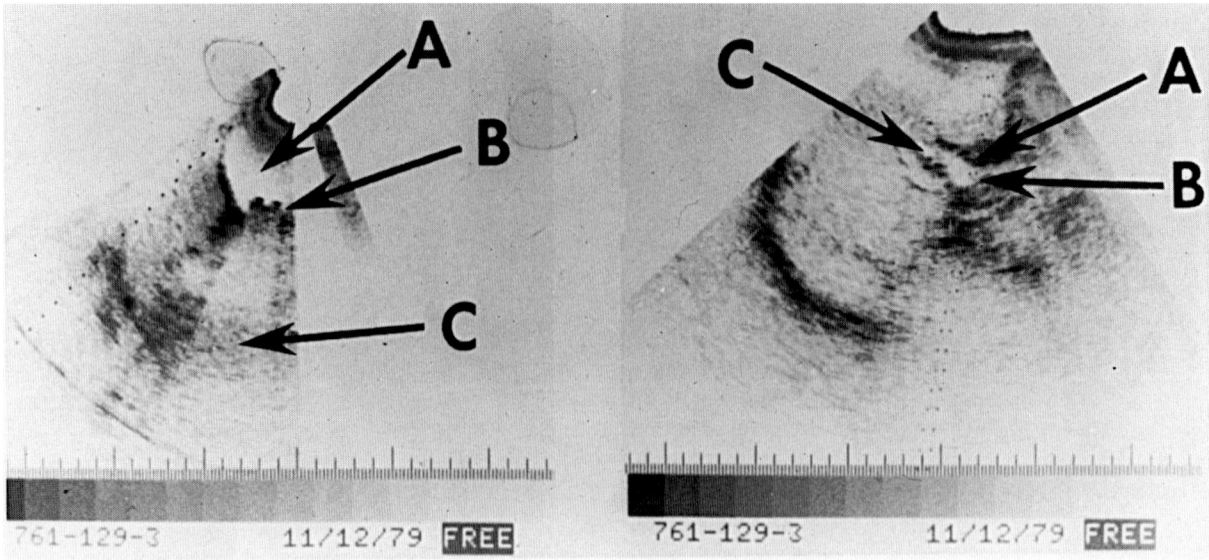

Fig. 54-18. Ultrasound examination of a jaundiced man with biliary colic. The figure on the right reveals a dilated bile duct (A) and implies gallstones (B) but lacks an acoustic shadow. Portal vein (C) is posterior to the common bile duct. The oblique sector scan on the left confirms the diagnosis by visualization of the distended gallbladder (A), gallstones (B), and a sharp acoustic shadow (C). (From Winkelman, E. I.: The differential diagnosis of jaundice. Prim. Care, *8*:215, 1981.)

ascites) pericholecystic fluid. The sensitivity is less than that of calculous cholecystitis.[85]

Biliary tract obstruction is demonstrated by the appearance of dilated extrahepatic and/or intrahepatic ducts, which may reflect the levels at which obstruction occurs:

- Within the pancreatic head
- Superior to the pancreas
- At the porta hepaticus
- Intrahepatic ducts

It cannot always determine the cause but differentiates between extrahepatic biliary obstruction and intrahepatic cholestasis 65 to 99% of the time (Fig. 54-18); however, the ability to detect early partial biliary tract obstruction is lacking, and detection of choledocholithiasis is poor as demonstrated by the significant number of patients who have choledocholithiasis and a normal-sized common bile duct.[86-88] Although providing the most accurate measurement of the diameter of the common bile duct, ultrasonography cannot discriminate between the dilatation secondary to previous resolved obstruction, prior biliary tract surgery, or an active process.

Color Doppler sonography is now available to evaluate both the patency and pattern of blood flow in the hepatic artery and hepatic and portal venous circulation.

Computed Tomography

Computed tomography (CT) scanning of the liver and biliary tree is routinely performed after administration of both intravenous and oral contrast material allowing visualization of both blood vessels and hollow viscera. The ability to visualize extrahepatic and extraperitoneal structures may lead to an explanation of hepatobiliary abnormalities.

Neither obesity nor gaseous distention interferes with definition, but patients must be able to cooperate and hold their breath for at least 1 to 2 seconds. An inability to give contrast material either orally or intravenously decreases detection and definition.

Although used extensively for the initial staging and follow-up of patients with metastatic hepatic disease, the principal use of CT scanning is to detect and characterize focal and diffuse parenchymal abnormalities, to differentiate the origin of jaundice, or to evaluate biliary obstruction (Figs. 54-19 and 54-20).[89] It has little role in the diagnosis of cholelithiasis, although it is highly sensitive to the presence of calcium. An accurate diagnosis of choledocholithiasis is achieved in 70% but depends on identification of a calcified or a rounded density surrounded by water density bile within the distal duct. The level of obstruction, highly suggestive of its origin, is reported with accuracy; however, 25% of patients with obstruction secondary to common duct stones will not have dilated ducts. The ability to examine multiple abdominal organs rapidly and reliably makes it invaluable in the initial evaluation of patients with acute abdominal trauma (Fig. 54-21).[90]

Magnetic Resonance Imaging

Magnetic resonance imaging (MRI) plays a minor role in hepatic imaging except in the diagnosis of hemangiomas, in which it is superior to other imaging methods.[91] It is a reliable, noninvasive means of establishing the diagnosis of portal vein thrombosis and Budd-Chiari syndrome and is reported to be as sensitive as CT and sonography in determining hepatocellular carcinoma and hepatic metastases;[91,92] however, other modalities are less expensive and more readily available.

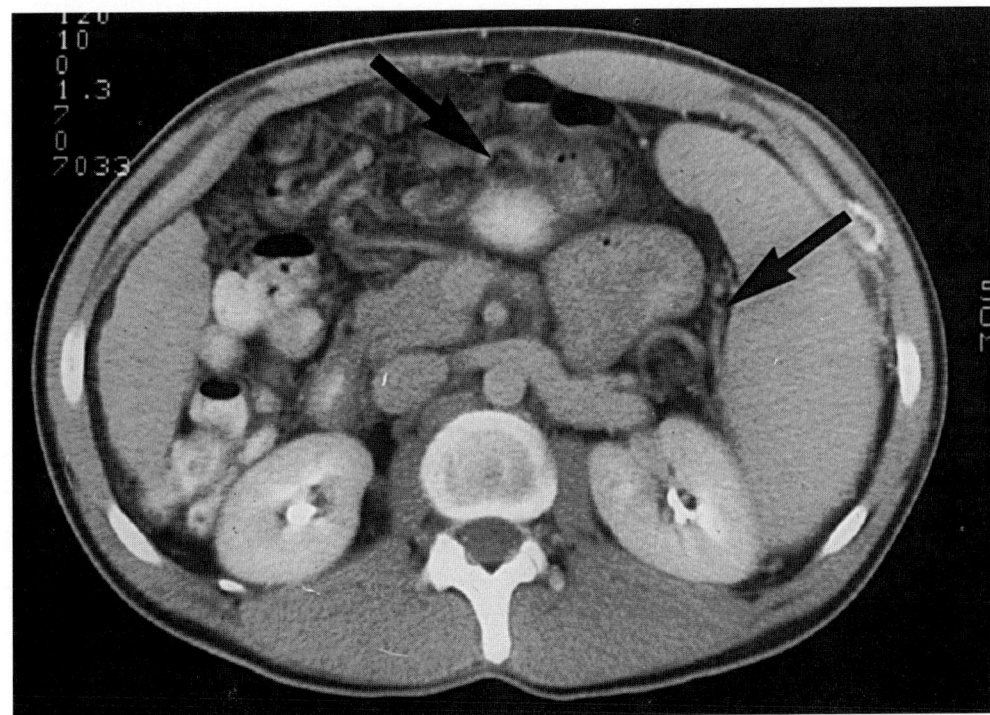

Fig. 54-19. Abdominal CT scan in a patient with alcoholic cirrhosis. Arrows indicate intra-abdominal varices compatible with portal hypertension. Note small irregular right lobe of liver and splenomegaly (oral and intravenous contrast material).

Cholangiography

Visualization of the biliary tree is obtained by the direct injection of contrast material either transcutaneously or endoscopically. Endoscopic retrograde cholangiopancreatography (ERCP) and percutaneous transhepatic cholangiography (PTHC) have comparable rates of morbidity (3 to 6%) and mortality (less than 1%). Complications of ERCP are cholangitis, pancreatitis, hemorrhage, and perforation, all usually related to the extent and nature of the manipulation of the duct and the ampulla. ERCP also allows the endoscopist to evaluate the upper gastrointestinal tract for

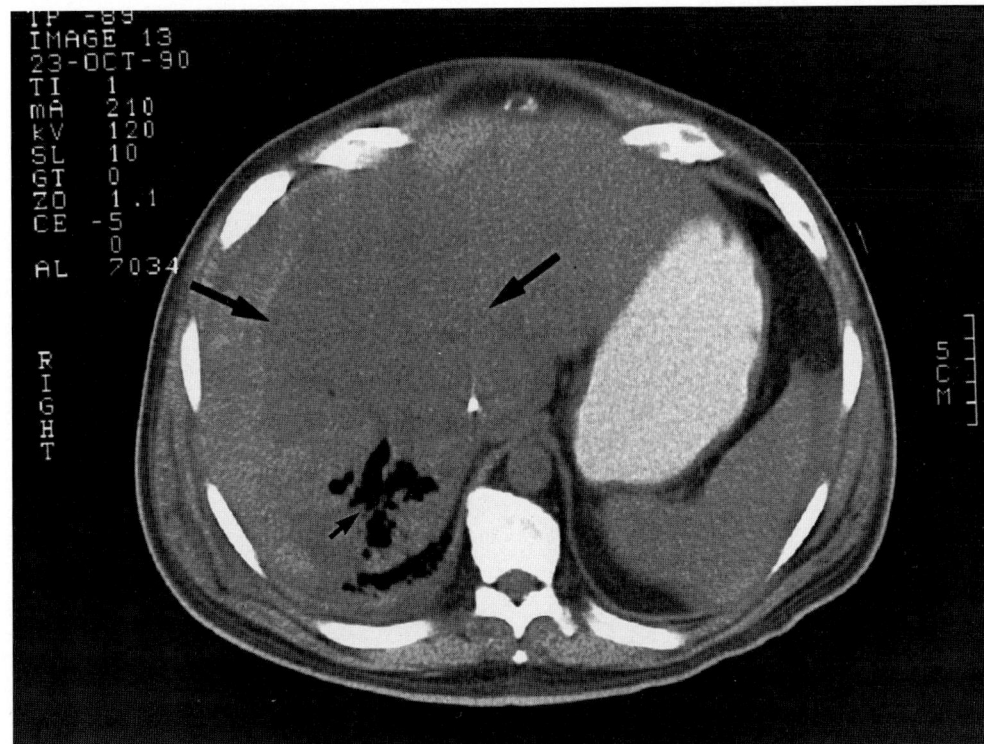

Fig. 54-20. Abdominal CT scan. Patient was an acutely ill jaundiced febrile man with acute necrosis in the right lobe of the liver *(large arrows)* and air containing abscesses in posterior aspect of right lobe *(small arrow)*. Infection secondary to Clostridium welchii and acute calculous cholecystitis (oral contrast only).

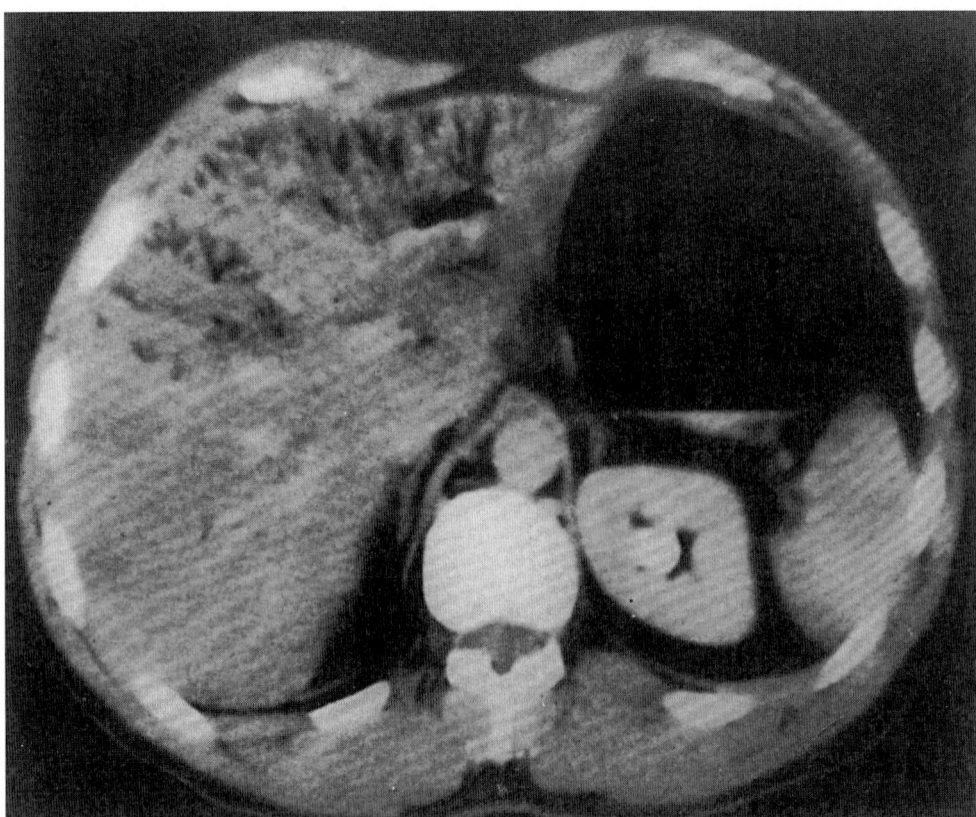

Fig. 54-21. Abdominal CT scan demonstrating hepatic vein gas secondary to necrotic bowel 24 hours following trauma to the abdomen. Note air at the hepatic periphery. (From Friedman, D., Flancbaum, L., Ritter, E., and Trooskin, S. Z.: Hepatic portal venous gas identified by computed tomography in a patient with blunt abdominal trauma: a case report. J. Trauma, 31:290, 1991.)

coexisting disease (varices, tumors, peptic ulcer disease) and especially to view the duodenum and ampulla of Vater (ulcer, tumor, diverticula, hemobilia, or stricture). Any anatomic lesion that impedes visualization of the ampulla is reason to use PTHC. These include obstruction of the pylorus, duodenum, duodenal diverticula, and other obstructive lesions as well as the varied gastroenterostomies performed following gastric resection, in which it is difficult or impossible to view and cannulate the ampulla (Fig. 54-22). Contraindications to PTHC are coagulopathies, ascites, and peritonitis. Percutaneous instrumentation of the biliary tree is transhepatic, traversing both the vascular and the biliary systems allowing bile, a potential source of sepsis, direct access to the bloodstream. Similar reasoning dictates that this is not a routine procedure in those with known sensitivity to contrast material. The uncommon complications of PTHC are hemorrhage, bile leakage, and pneumothorax. Obviously, in the face of an obstructed biliary system, either procedure is preceded and followed with antibiotic coverage, usually ampicillin and gentamicin.[91]

Diagnostically, direct cholangiography by either method is the gold standard when cause of cholestasis, duct dilatation, and partial or incomplete obstruction is not discernible by other modalities. Although visualization is accomplished by PTHC in all patients with dilated ducts, only 70 to 80% of those patients with normal ducts can be cannulated;[92] hence, ERCP is the procedure of choice in those with cholestasis without dilatation (Figs. 54-23 and 54-24).

An additional advantage of both techniques is the ability to decompress a distal obstruction of the common bile duct. External drainage is much more successful with proximal lesions and when the distal obstruction cannot

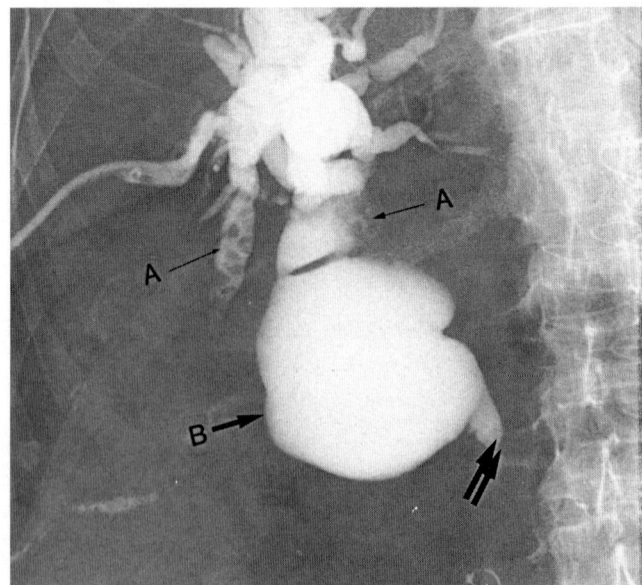

Fig. 54-22. Choledochal cyst with intrahepatic calculi (A), proximal dilatation of duct (B), and cyst and local stenosis of distal bile duct (double arrow) postcholedochostomy.

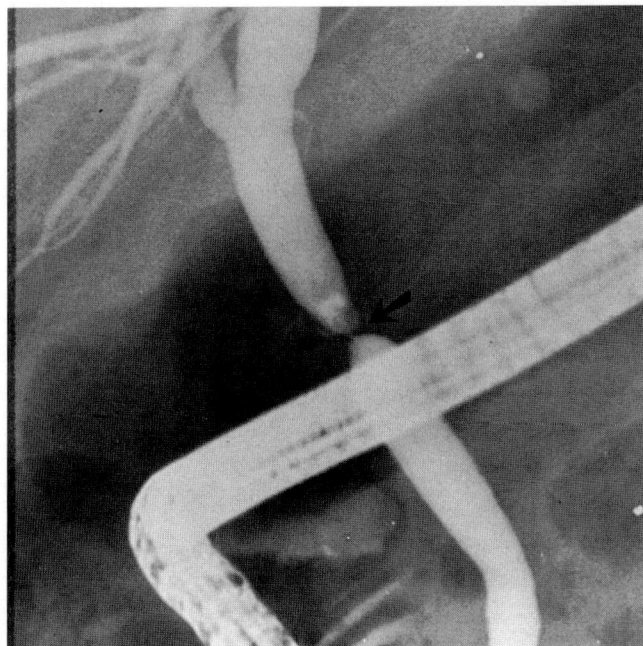

Fig. 54–23. Endoscopic retrograde cholangiography. Prior cholecystectomy for gallstones. Recurrent bouts of "Charcot's triad." Stricture without ductal dilatation with bits of calculous material proximal to it. (From Starling, J. R., and Matallana, R. H.: Benign mechanical obstruction of the common hepatic duct (Mirizzi syndrome). Surgery, *88*:737, 1980.)

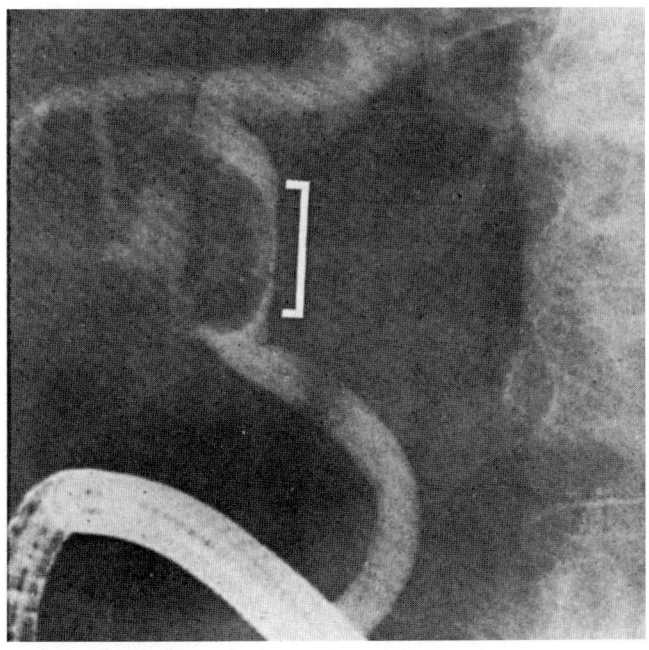

Fig. 54–24. Endoscopic retrograde cholangiopancreatogram illustrating severe mechanical obstruction of common hepatic duct by impacted gallstone in fundus of gallbladder. The bracket shows the 3-cm-long benign obstruction (Mirizzi syndrome). (From Winkelman, E. I.: The differential diagnosis of jaundice. Prim. Care, *8*:215, 1981.)

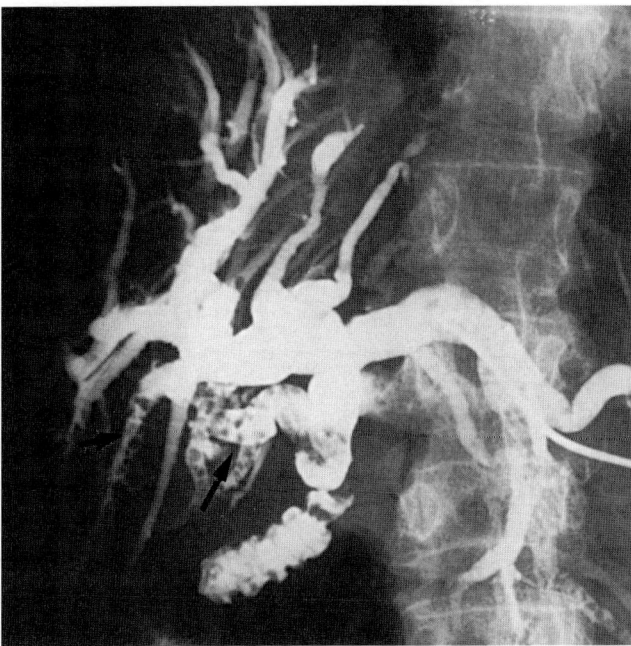

Fig. 54–25. Percutaneous transhepatic cholangiography. The patient had a history of cholecystectomy for gallstones and recent jaundice. A common duct stricture is present. Ductal dilatation is obvious. Arrows indicate areas of recurrent intrahepatic calculi.

be relieved from below (Fig. 54-25). If the obstruction is secondary to choledocholithiasis, ERCP, sphincterotomy and extraction of the stones by various methods are successful; however, a small papillotomy followed by the passage of a nasal biliary catheter to a point above the obstruction can also deal immediately with the problem when the obstruction cannot be circumvented. Stones may also be removed by PTHC, but this requires additional time to establish a tract that will admit the basket used to extract the stone. Brushings for cytology are obtained with both. Strictures can be dilated or stents placed from above or below, but repeated procedures are more easily accomplished via an external catheter.

Angiography

Angiography is rarely necessary for the diagnosis of liver lesions. It is accurate in the differential diagnosis of cavernous hemangioma but remains an invasive procedure, as opposed to MRI, which is superior to it. Other mass lesions lend themselves to diagnosis by other noninvasive techniques. The venous phase of selective splenic artery catheterization allows visualization of the portal vein, collateral circulation, and the patency of portal systemic shunts (Fig. 54-26). Because the blood supply of hepatocellular carcinoma is arterial, these lesions are best seen with hepatic arteriography, which also becomes necessary in liver transplantation when the patency of the hepatic artery is questioned. Pressure studies of the portal tract require hepatic venography, and the diagnosis of Budd-Chiari syndrome relies on venography of the hepatic veins and inferior vena cava (Fig. 54-27). A major use of angiography is to diagram the vascular anatomy of those for whom resection of he-

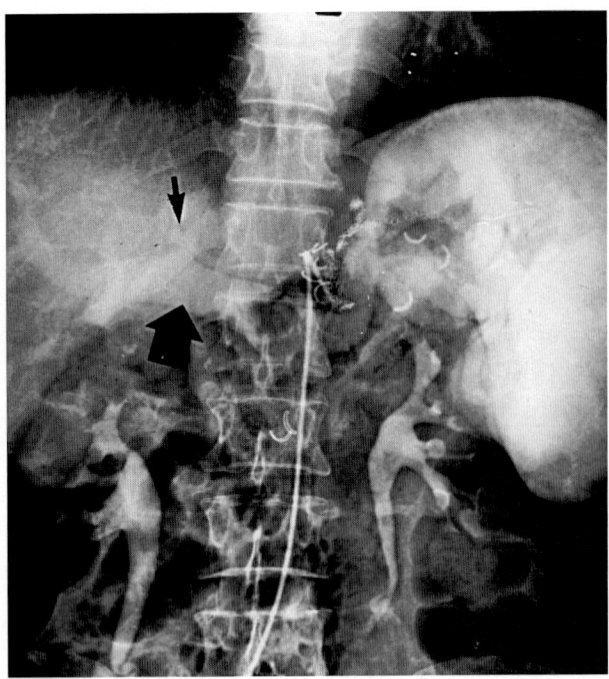

Fig. 54-26. Venous phase of a selective celiac angiogram. Intrahepatic block (cirrhosis) with enlarged spleen, patent splenic and portal vein *(large arrow)*, and varices *(small arrow)*. (From Achkar, E. A., Farmer, R., and Fleshler, B. (eds.): Clinical Gastroenterology. Philadelphia, Lea & Febiger, 1992, p. 587.)

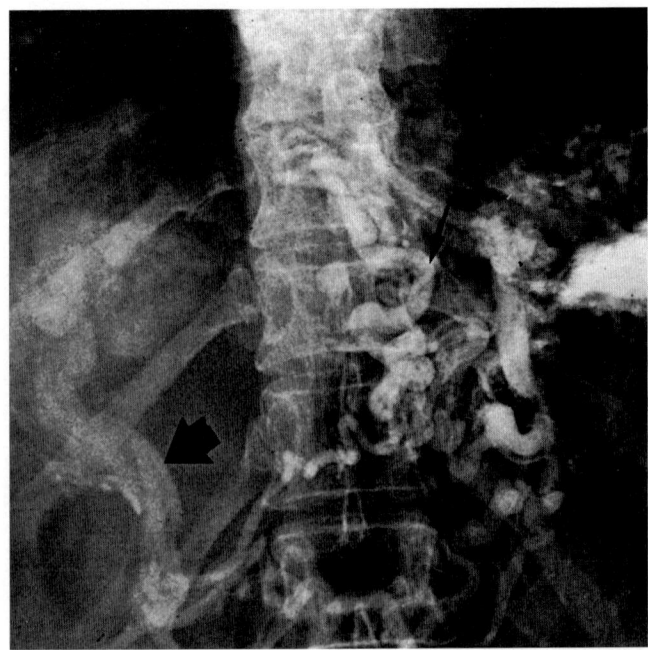

Fig. 54-28. Splenoportography. Cavernomatous transformation with massive gastroesophageal varices *(small arrow)*. Bridging collateral circulation via the gastroduodenal vein *(large arrow)*.

patic lesions is contemplated or to provide access for the interarterial infusion of chemotherapy or embolization of bleeding vessels and aneurysms. CT has superseded angiography in the evaluation of patients with abdominal trauma. Splenoportography is rarely used except in unusual instances when the portal system or shunts cannot be visualized angiographically (Fig. 54-28).

Liver Biopsy

Percutaneous liver biopsy has become a routine procedure in the diagnosis of hepatic disease. It is indicated when extrahepatic biliary obstruction has been ruled out and doubt remains as to the nature of the disease. Seldom is there need to perform a biopsy in the presence of biliary tract obstruction, but if necessary the risk is acceptable.[91] Other indications include unexplained hepatomegaly (Fig. 54-29), chronically abnormal liver studies (Fig. 54-30), and imaging abnormalities; biopsy of the last-mentioned, if discrete, is better performed under direct vision using either ultrasonography or CT. When used appropriately, it allows the physician to follow the progression of disease and its response to therapy as well as diagnose storage and multisystem diseases and investigate fevers of unknown origin (Fig. 54-31). In many of these instances, the results of culture or special strains of the biopsy are helpful. It is unnecessary to perform a biopsy in cases of acute viral hepatitis, no matter how severe the jaundice or abnormal the enzymes.[91] A successful biopsy yield depends on procurement of an adequate specimen, avoidance of a sampling error, and the availability of pathologists who can properly interpret the specimens and avoid drawing erro-

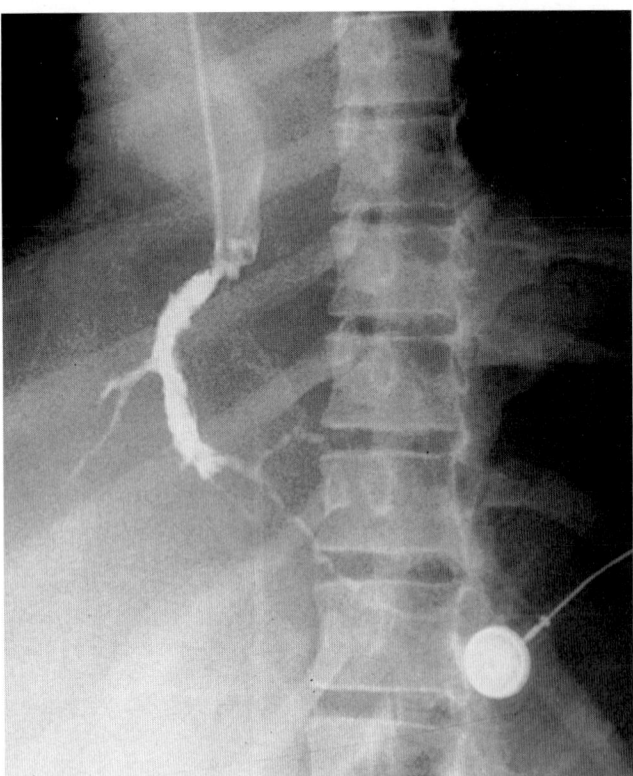

Fig. 54-27. Hepatic venogram. Budd-Chiari syndrome with luminal thrombosis.

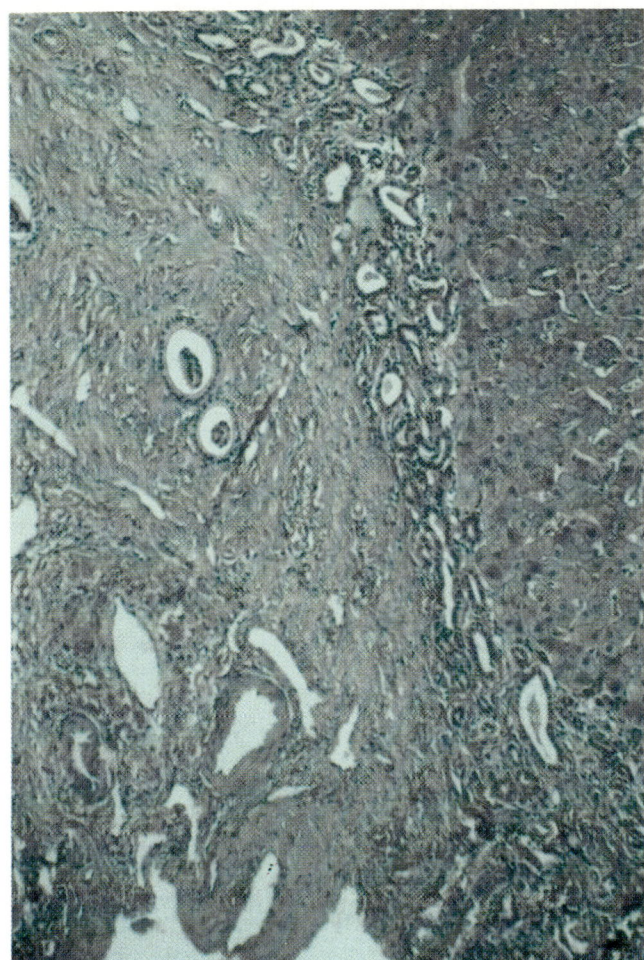

Fig. 54-29. Congenital hepatic fibrosis. Variceal hemorrhage in an asymptomatic 18-year-old patient with hepatosplenomegaly and normal liver studies. Increased fibrous tissue in a portal tract area is associated with increased numbers of variably dilated marginal cholangioles. Portal vein triads are present and appear to be small in caliber. Hematoxylin and eosin × 31.2. (Courtesy of Ralph J. Tuthill, M.D.)

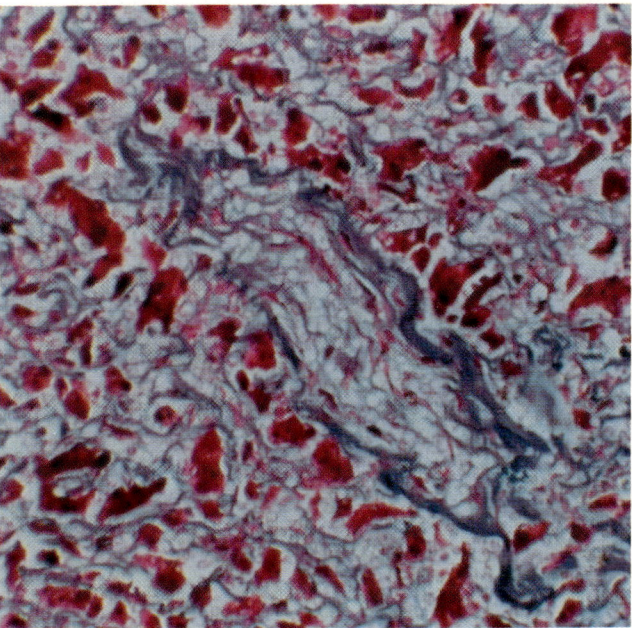

Fig. 54-30. Veno-occlusive disease. Six weeks after radiation therapy for carcinoma of hepatic flexure. Perivenular fibrosis of an obstructed terminal hepatic vein with centrilobular congestion and hepatic cell atrophy. Masson stain × 100. (Courtesy of Ralph J. Tuthill, M.D.)

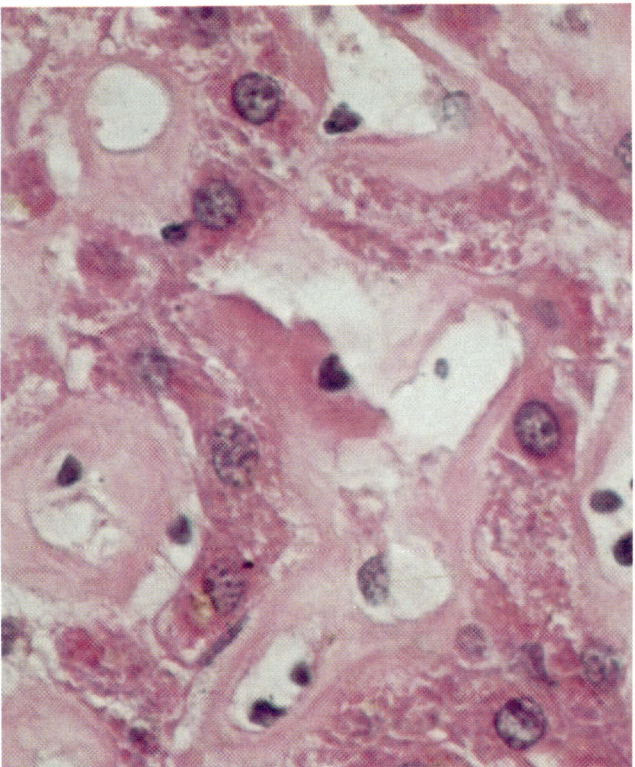

Fig. 54-31. Amyloidosis in a 67-year-old cachectic man with hepatomegaly and minimally abnormal liver tests. There is prominent deposition of eosinophilic hyaline amyloid material along the sinusoids separating hepatocytes from the sinusoidal lumen. There is variable atrophy and loss of hepatocytes. Hematoxylin and eosin × 128. (Courtesy of Ralph J. Tuthill, M.D.)

neous conclusions from inadequate tissue or misinterpreting artifacts or reactive or nonspecific changes.

Contraindications are a prothrombin time more than 3 to 4 seconds greater than normal and/or platelets less than 75,000, but these are correctable with fresh frozen plasma and platelet transfusions. Hemophiliacs should not undergo biopsy unless factor VIII is adequate. The procedure must be explained to the patient who is able to cooperate and be aware of the potential complications. Tense ascites makes it difficult to obtain an adequate biopsy specimen. Biopsy should not be done without consideration of these factors as well as the presence of localized infection in the right upper quadrant or right lower chest and, in the case of directed biopsy, the question of hemangioma, or a hydatid cyst. A series of studies, each of which included 10,000 or more biopsies, revealed a mortality of 0.009 to 0.17% (Table 54-6). Significant hemorrhage, the most frequent cause of serious biopsy complications, is

Table 54–6. Fatalities from Needle Liver Biopsy

Author	Source	Date	Biopsies	Mortality (%)
Zamcheck*	United States	1953	20,016	0.17
Thaler†	Europe combined	1964	23,382	0.01
Lindner‡	Germany	1967	80,000	0.015
Piccinino§	Italy	1986	68,276	0.009
McGill‖	United States	1990	9212	0.11

* Zamcheck, N., and Sidman, R. L.: N. Engl. J. Med., *249*:1020, 1953; Zamcheck, N., and Klausenstock, O.: N. Engl. J. Med., *249*:1062, 1953.
† Thaler, H.: Wein. Klin. Wochenschr., *29*:533, 1964.
‡ Lindner, H.: Dtsch. Med. Wosenchr., *92*:1751, 1967.
§ Piccinino, F., et al.: J. Hepatol., *2*:165, 1986.
‖ McGill, D. B., et al.: Gastroenterology, *99*:1396, 1990.
(From Sherlock, S., and Daoley, J.: Diseases of the Liver and Biliary Tree. 9th Ed. London, Blackwell Scientific Publications, 1993, p. 37.)

Table 54–8. Causes of Acute Hepatic Failure

Acute viral hepatitis
Drug hepatotoxicity
Chemicals, poisons
Hypoxia, ischemia
Metastatic liver disease
Metabolic liver disease
Miscellaneous

rare with an incidence of 0.001 to 1.0%.[93] Most recently, the results of 9212 procedures, performed according to a definite protocol, revealed 10 (0.11%) fatal and 22 (0.24%) nonfatal hemorrhagic episodes. The risk of fatal bleeding was estimated to be 0.4% in those with nonmalignant disease, but in nonfatal bleeding episodes, the risk was 0.16%, whereas the risk was 0.57% in those with carcinoma.[94]

In those few situations in which percutaneous liver biopsy is contraindicated or has failed, the transjugular approach is available. The major indications for its use are coagulopathy; massive ascites; and, to a lesser degree, marked obesity and, it is hoped, evaluation of prognosis in fulminant hepatic failure.[95,96] Biopsy specimens are also obtained when procedures are done to measure hepatic venous pressure or during transjugular cholangiography. Adequate tissue was obtained in 77 to 97% of cases but was fragmented in 20 to 64% of those patients with fibrosis or cirrhosis.[95,96] In the earlier series, the tissue was considered only marginal in 23%,[95] but multiple specimens can be obtained by this technique.

Complications vary between 0 and 20%, but only perforation of the liver capsule with intraperitoneal hemorrhage and induction of arrhythmias were considered major, occurring in 2.7, and 6% of procedures.[95,96] Among seven centers, the mortality ranged from 0 to 0.5%. Transjugular liver biopsy was time-consuming and expensive, requiring a greater number of hospital days and, despite an experienced interventional radiologist, was plagued by smaller and fragmented specimens, particularly in cirrhosis (Table 54–7).

FULMINANT HEPATIC FAILURE

Fulminant hepatic failure (FHF) is the result of massive hepatocellular injury and/or necrosis in patients without a history of prior liver disease but may also present as the initial manifestation of a previously undiagnosed chronic liver disease: i.e., Wilson's disease or chronic active hepatitis. Bernuau and colleagues[97] define acute liver disease as severe acute liver disease with a 50% or greater decrease in factor V and prothrombin time but do not consider it to be fulminant until the development of hepatic encephalopathy, which does not always follow. It is presently almost universally accepted that hepatic encephalopathy occurring within 8 weeks after the onset of abnormal liver function defines FHF, although others consider time intervals of 2 to 6 weeks before classifying it as such.[97-100] A more protracted course of an 8- to 24-week period of time before the appearance of hepatic encephalopathy is now referred to as "late-onset hepatic failure," or subfulminant hepatic failure.[97,101]

Causes

Universally, acute viral hepatitis (AVH) accounts for 40 to 94% of all cases of FHF. Drug hepatotoxicity is the second most common cause, occurring in 20 to 25% except in London, where acetaminophen accounts for approximately 60%. Poisons, chemicals, hypoxia and ischemia, metastatic disease, metabolic disorders, and miscellaneous factors are responsible for all but a few of the remainder (Table 54–8).[97,99,102-104]

Table 54–7. Major Reported Series of Transjugular Liver Biopsy

Author, year (ref)*	Location	No. Patients	Adequate Tissue (%)	Complications (%)	Death
McAfee, 1991	Portland, OR	146	92†	16.4‡	0
Goldman, 1978 (12)	Atlanta, GA	76 (?)	83	6.3	0
Lebrec, 1982 (15)	Clichy, France	1033	97§	9.8	0.1
Bull, 1983 (16)	London, UK	193	97	20.2	0.5%
Velt, 1984 (17)	Bridgeport, CT	160	81	1.3	0
Gamble, 1985 (18)	Toronto, Canada	461	92	18.4‖	0.2%
Steadman, 1988 (19)	Brisbane, Australia	67	93	6.0	0

* References refer to McAfee article (see credit line below).
† Tissue was adequate for diagnosis in 69% of patients and marginal in 23% of patients.
‡ Minor complications in 13.7% and major complications in 2.7%.
§ Tissue was adequate for diagnosis in 64% of patients with fibrosis or cirrhosis and in 99% of patients with liver disease and no fibrosis.
‖ Minor complications in 17.1% and major complications in 1.3%.
(From McAfee, J. H., et al.: Transjugular liver biopsy. Hepatology, *15*:726, 1992.)

Table 54-9. Relative Frequencies of Viral Etiologies in Series of Patients with Fulminant Hepatic Failure

	Hepatitis A Virus (%)	Hepatitis B Virus (%)	Non-A, Non-B Hepatitis Virus (%)
United Kingdom	20	44	36
France	6	60	34
Denmark	20	32	48
Greece	2	74	24
United States	2	60	38
Japan	2	74	24

(Modified from O'Grady, J., and Williams, R.: Acute liver failure. Bailliere's Clin. Gastroenterol., 3:75, 1989.)

Acute Viral Hepatitis

The incidence of FHF secondary to AVH varies both among the geographic areas of the world and the inciting agents (Table 54-9).[105]

Hepatitis A (HA) is diagnosed serologically by the presence of the IgM antibody to hepatitis A virus (HAV). The titer of this acute-phase antibody increases rapidly over the 4 to 6 weeks following the onset of clinical signs and symptoms, declining to undetectable levels within the next 3 to 6 months, although it may persist for longer than 200 days in approximately 13 to 14% of patients.[71] The IgG antibody may be detected simultaneously or within 1 to 2 weeks of the acute illness and remain for years without evidence of chronicity or long-term sequelae. It confers immunity.[71,92]

The disease is mild, particularly in children, although on occasion it is prolonged and severe in adults. Hospitalization is necessary only for prolonged anorexia, nausea, and vomiting that require such support. Steroids, antibiotics, and immune serum globulin are of no help at this time. The risk of FHF is rare, ranging from 0.01 to 0.35%, and a survival rate of 43 to 62% predicts a better prognosis than the other causes of FHF (Fig. 54-32).[97,100,104-106]

Because a vaccine is not yet universally available, sound hygienic measures must be routine. Postexposure prophylaxis is recommended only for those health care workers unknowingly exposed and all household members and sexual contacts. Immune serum globulin is given according to the published guidelines, but causal contacts need not be treated.[71]

Hepatitis B (HB) is the most common cause of FHF. The hepatitis B surface antigen (HBsAg) indicates an actual infection but may be absent in 12 to 25% of cases because the blood is sampled too early in the convalescent stage when the HBsAg is undectable, producing a "window" period, or there is an excessive immune response with prior clearance of the antigen. In these, as in all cases of acute HB, the diagnosis depends on the identification of IgM antibody to HB core antigen (anti-HBc) because anti-HBc initially increases both IgM and IgG anti-HBc. The IgM anti-HBc develops simultaneously with the increased enzyme abnormalities but generally decreases in 6 to 8 months, regardless of the evolution of the disease.[107] The IgG anti-HBc gradually increases, stabilizes, and remains indefinitely, conferring immunity.[107] A 1.4% risk of FHF secondary to acute hepatitis B virus (HBV) is reported with a survival rate of 14 to 33%.[100,103,105,108]

Active immunization is available, efficacious, safe, and strongly advised for all health care givers, particularly those in contact with patients and exposed to blood and other body fluids. Household members and other intimate contacts of patients who are persistently HBsAg positive should also be vaccinated if they are not immune.[107]

Hepatitis B immunoglobulin (HBIG) should be given immediately when a person without known immunity is exposed to a potential or known source of HBsAg (i.e., needlestick, eczema, inadvertent ingestion of blood in the laboratory). Blood should be collected from the exposed individual before the administration of HBIG and if the person is immune, (positive serology for anti-HBs, anti-HBc) or HBsAg is present, nothing further is required. As soon as possible after HBIG, the nonimmune person should begin active immunization and does not require further HBIG. If the donor source (which also must be tested, if possible) is not found to be positive, additional HBIG is unnecessary, unless the life style of either donor or recipient indicates a high risk situation.[107] Sexual partners of patients with acute HBV should also receive HBIG if they lack evidence of immunity.[109]

Hepatitis D (HD) is an incomplete RNA virus that cannot replicate in the absence of HBsAg. It is acquired either simultaneously with HB (coinfection) or at a later date from a chronic HB carrier (superinfection).[110] Principally transmitted by blood or blood products, it should be considered in the differential diagnosis of patients who are HBsAg positive or superinfected with HA or HC, have a flare of chronic HB or coinfection of HA, HB, or HC.

Coinfection is associated with two bouts of hepatitis, IVS, HB, then HD, which may occur concurrently or as two separate closely related episodes. Although acute, they are usually self limited. Superinfection is most often associated with FHF and accounts for approximately 10 times greater incidence of FHF than the other forms of viral hepatitis, with a mortality of close to 80%. It is also responsible for the presence of chronic HD in 70% of the cases.[110]

The antibody to HD develops late in the convalescent stage of HBV and then is only transiently positive in low titer, but the more reliable marker is the anti-IgM HD.[111] Evidence of anti-HD Ag may be absent within months to years. Superinfection is characterized by the presence of IgM and IgG anti-HD in the acute phase which persists with chronicity. There is no known treatment other than prevention of HBV.

Hepatitis C (HC) a diagnosis of exclusion before the advent of serologic testing for the antibody to hepatitis C virus (HCV), was previously called non-A, non-B hepatitis. The antibody has now been found in 70 to 100% of patients with post-transfusion hepatitis as well as 50 to 70% of those with community-acquired (episodic) hepatitis, but to date no commercial means are available to differentiate acute from chronic or the active from the resolved HCV.[112,113] Only a few cases of FHF after transfusion or parenteral drug abuse were considered to be the result of HCV after testing serologically or by polymerase chain reaction (PCR), but non-A, non-B hepatitis is deemed the major cause of late-onset hepatic failure, with a mortality of 81

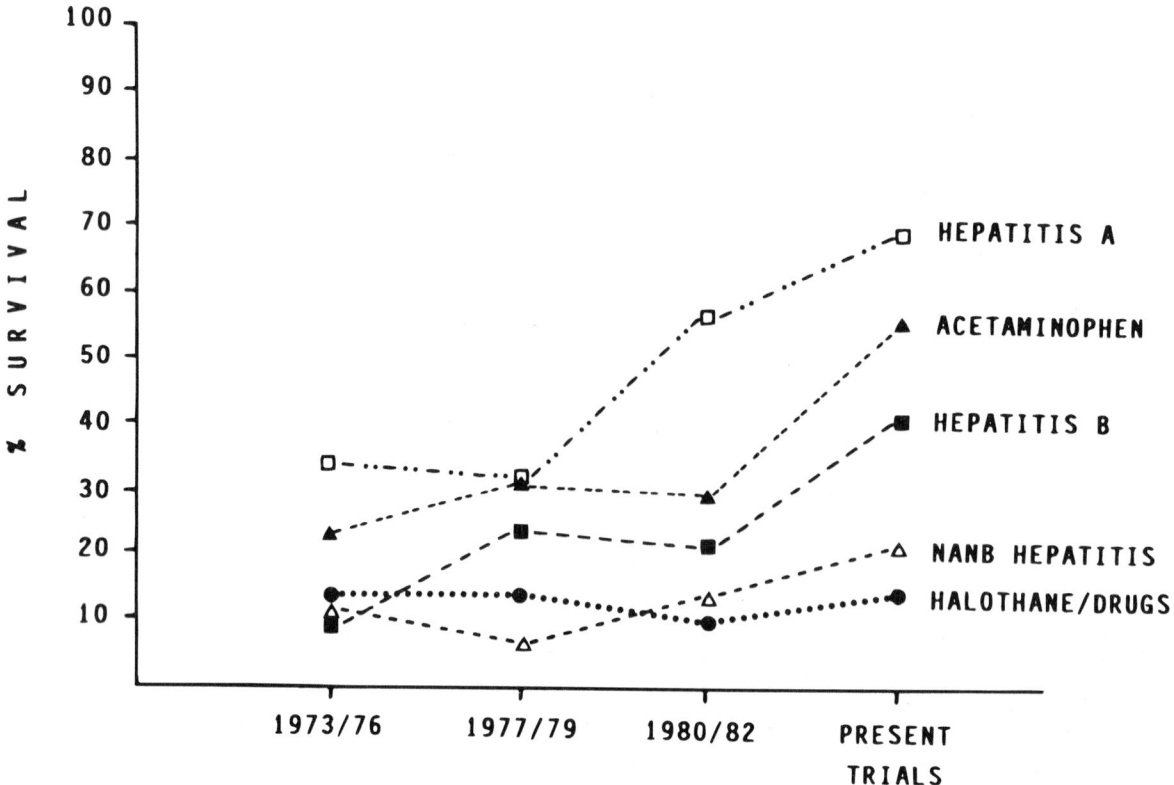

Fig. 54-32. Serial survival rates in the main etiologic subgroup of fulminant hepatic failure treated from 1973 through 1985. There is steady increase in survival in those with acetaminophen overdose, hepatitis A virus, and hepatitis B virus, but no significant increase in non-A, non-B (NANB) hepatitis, halothane, or drug reaction. (From O'Grady, J. C., et al.: Controlled trials of charcoal hemoperfusion and prognostic factors in fulminant hepatic failures. Gastroenterology, 94:1186, 1988.)

to 91%.[101,108,114] Serious speculation given to the cause of FHF in non-A, non-B hepatitis has raised the question of the role of various noninfectious causes as well as other viruses.[115]

HCV is predominantly spread via a parenteral route, both apparent and nonapparent. Numerous studies have shown the incidence of chronic hepatitis with and without cirrhosis in post-transfusion hepatitis to vary between 44 and 97%, thus its importance is the propensity to progress to different degrees of chronicity, including cirrhosis and possibly hepatocellular carcinoma (Table 54-10).[113,116]

Hepatitis E, an enteric transmitted non-A, non-B hepatitis, has now been identified and characterized. It is endemic in Third World countries and found elsewhere only in those individuals who have been in endemic areas. Pregnant women in the third trimester are particularly suscepti-

Table 54-10. Prevalence of Anti-HCV Among Patients with HCC in Selected Countries

Senior Author (ref.)*	Area Studied	Year	Percentage of Overall anti-HCV Positivity rate in HCC Patients	anti-HCV According to HBsAg Status HBsAb-positive	HBsAg-negative	Anti-HCV in Blood Donors (ref.)*
Colombo (10)	Milano	1989	65 (86/132)	54 (22/41)	70 (64/91)	
Simonetti (11)	Palermo	1989	76 (152/200)	58 (18/31)	79 (134/169)	
Caporaso (30)	Naples	1991	72 (63/88)			0.87 (17)
Levrero (20)	Roma/Padua	1991	58 (97/167)	28 (15/53)	72 (82/114)	
Nalpas (14)	Paris	1991	58 (32/55)	75 (9/12)	57 (20/35)	0.68 (18)
Bruix (12)	Barcelona	1989	75 (72/96)	56 (5/9)	77 (67/87)	0.5
Kiyosawa (13)	Matsumoto, Japan	1990	73 (61/83)	35 (10/29)	94 (51/54)	1.3 (16)
Chen (21)	Taipei	1990	33 (22/66)	17 (7/42)	63 (15/24)	0.95
Hasan (15)	Miami	1990	53 (31/59)	61 (11/18)	49 (20/41)†	0.5 (15)–1.4 (19)
Kew (23)	Johannesburg	1990	29 (110/380)	26 (47/184)	32 (63/196)	0.7

† Anti-HBc st
* References are from the article in *Hepatology* (see credit line below).
(From Okuda, K.: Hepatocellular carcinoma: recent progress. Hepatology, 15:949, 1992.)

ble, with a mortality rate of 20%.[73] Other viral causes of FHF are herpes simplex I, II, and VI; varicella zoster; cytomegalovirus, and Epstein-Barr virus.[117]

Drug-Induced Hepatic Failure

Drugs produce a broad range of clinical syndromes that are easily overlooked or confused with other causes of FHF. These patterns are categorized as:

- Hepatocellular necrosis
- Cholestasis
- Mixed

Drug-induced acute hepatocellular necrosis may be indistinguishable from that seen with AVH and is characterized by an increase in aminotransferases ranging as high as several hundred beyond normal. The degree of hyperbilirubinemia and coagulopathy correlate with the severity of hepatocyte damage. Liver biopsy cannot define a specific etiologic agent and may not differentiate between drug and viral injuries; however, in a clinical pathologic classification, two types of injury are described. Type I is characterized by a variable degree of necrosis and liver cell loss, whereas the findings in type II are microvesicular steatosis with minimal evidence of necrosis attributed to failure of the intracellular organelles.[75] Viral hepatitis, halothane, acetaminophen and phenytoin hepatotoxicity, exhibit changes typical of type I, whereas tetracycline, acute fatty liver of pregnancy, and hepatotoxic changes of tetracycline and valproate are associated with type II. Cholestasis may mimic biliary tract obstruction, necessitating the use of ultrasonography and cholangiography to exclude extrahepatic disorders. Histologically, the changes of intracellular cholestasis (portal triaditis with mild parenchymal changes) or actual duct destruction can be present. Mixed forms present predominant features of hepatocellular disease with cholestatic aspects or vice versa.[118]

The estimated frequency of overt jaundice in hepatitis from drugs is less than 1%, but in general the presence of clinical icterus in association with drug hepatotoxicity has a mortality of 10%.[118] Acetaminophen hepatotoxicity from suicidal intent is the most common cause of FHF in the United Kingdom, but the normal prescribed dose may produce hepatotoxicity in those with chronic alcoholic liver disease and even chronic illness[118-120] (see Chap. 70). Hepatotoxicity and fatalities are seen commonly with a number of other analgesic and anti-inflammatory drugs. Halothane and other halogenated anesthetic agents, isoniazid, alpha-methyldopa, various antidepressants, and various anticonvulsants are common offenders.[6,91,118] Less frequent occurrences are seen with tetracycline,[121] antithyroid drugs,[122] ketoconazole,[123] niacin,[124] cocaine,[125] and flutamide.[126]

Chemicals and Poisons

Exposure to chlorinated hydrocarbons, i.e., carbon tetrachloride and trichloroethane, can result in hepatic necrosis. Alcohol greatly increases susceptibility to the hepatotoxic effects of carbon tetrachloride, which also produces renal changes and renal failure.[6,91,118,127] With carbon tetrachloride, the severity of the hepatic injury correlates with the degree of jaundice. Hepatic deaths are seen within the first week, and those from renal failure occur in the following weeks. Patients who recover from these hepatic diseases largely have no residual changes, although fibrosis is seen on occasion. Deaths occur from trichloroethane following both exposure to the organic solvent and "glue sniffing."[6,91,118,128] Occupational exposure is now unusual but has been reported with 2-nitropane.[128]

Ingestion of yellow phosphorus, a component of rat and roach poison, has a mortality rate of 75%. Histologically the salient finding is extreme periportal fatty infiltration.[6,91,118,127]

Although a common problem in Europe, mushroom poisoning has become better recognized in the United States. Amanita phalloides is the major cause of fatal mushroom poisoning. Its ingestion becomes a medical emergency requiring immediate recognition and aggressive treatment. The first symptoms, which appear within 6 to 24 hours, are usually seen 10 to 12 hours after ingestion. These mimic severe gastroenteritis with marked abdominal pain, nausea and vomiting, and choleralike, diarrhea. This is followed by a 24 hour latent period, which is succeeded by increasing jaundice and renal failure, which from this point may progress to coma and death. Patients may be categorized as having mild, moderate, or severe disease, with death occurring primarily in those who have marked hyperbilirubinemia, prolongation of the prothrombin time, and extreme elevation of the aminotransferase levels. Extreme prolongation of the prothrombin time and a precipitous drop of the aminotransferase level are associated with a poor prognosis. Death occurs in approximately 80% of patients within 6 to 18 days after the ingestion of mushrooms. Therapy is primarily supportive in KUs, with aggressive replacement of underlying fluid and electrolyte disturbances. To eliminate the enterohepatic circulation of the toxin, gastric lavage is immediately performed followed by continuous gastroduodenal drainage. Cathartics are administered regularly along with activated charcoal and forced diuresis (urinary output >300 ml/hour), whereas centers have used plasmapheresis or dialysis.[129,130] This vigorous attack program has reduced mortality to 11.3%.[129] Liver transplantation has been used successfully, but the disease must be identified quickly to hasten procurement of an organ.[130]

Ischemia and Hypoxia

FHF secondary to hypoxia is associated with either hypoperfusion or venous stasis and invariably is the result of disease involving other organs or systems. Acute left ventricular failure or right-sided congestive failure, hypotension, or shock dramatically increases aminotransferase levels to startling heights, but despite a 3- to 5-day rapid drop toward normal, both jaundice and hypoprothrombinemia may follow.[131] Often confused with acute viral hepatitis it is histologically identified by centrolobular congestion and necrosis. Its mortality correlates with the underlying cause of disease.[132]

Centrilobular congestion and cell necrosis are also caused by hepatic outflow obstruction. The Budd-Chiari syndrome describes hepatic vein obstruction principally caused by thrombosis but also reflects nonthrombotic obstruction from a number of local lesions.[133] A literature review cites 42% of well-documented cases of hepatic vein thrombosis caused by myeloproliferative disorders, with the remainder labeled as idiopathic or from miscellaneous cause.[15] Less frequent causes are hypercoagulable states; hepatocellular, renal cell, and adrenal malignancy; pregnancy; oral contraceptive use; and other even less frequent events.[133] The acute presentation of abdominal pain, hepatomegaly, and ascites can lead to other diagnoses and miss the opportunity for surgical correction: i.e., portocaval shunt, mesoatrial shunt, or transplantation.[134]

Veno-occlusive disease is a nonthrombotic occlusion of the central and sublobular hepatic veins with centrolobular necrosis, which is now most commonly seen as a complication of bone marrow transplantation.[135-137] Twenty percent to 54% develop a pathognomonic clinical syndrome within the first 20 days. The typical initial symptoms are weight gain, hepatomegaly, and acute abdominal pain usually within the first 10 days followed 2 days later by hyperbilirubinemia greater than 2 mg/dl, edema, and ascites.[136,137] Encephalopathy occurred between the first and third week in 21 to 54%.[136,137] Jones and associates[136] reviewed 235 patients who underwent bone marrow transplantation. Twenty-two percent developed veno-occlusive disease, and 47% of these died, with deaths attributed to liver failure. In others dying with persistent veno-occlusive disease, their death was not liver induced but was labeled multifactorial.[136] MacDonald and associates[137] noted that 69% of the deaths in patients with veno-occlusive disease were attributable to liver dysfunction, which did not play a role in the deaths of the remaining 31%. In both the series of Jones and MacDonald, multiple organ failure was common.

"Bush teas," which are commonly used as folk remedies in rural and undeveloped areas, contain pyrrolizidine alkaloids, and similar substances are also present in remedies available in urban health food stores.[4] Antimetabolites, alkylating agents, arsphenamine, urethane, and radiation are other causes of veno-occlusive disease (see Fig. 54–30).[91]

Metastatic Liver Disease

Eras and Sherlock[138] reported that 21 of 427 (7.2%) of autopsied patients with hepatic metastases had died in hepatic coma. The primary lesions were attributed to gastric, colonic, and breast neoplasms, but reports of metastatic small lung tumors and massive lymphoblastic infiltration have also been published.[138-141] Massive tumor cell infiltration of the sinusoids and hepatic venules resulting in ischemic hepatocellular necrosis were suggested as the cause of the fulminant course.[139,140]

Metabolic Causes

FHF is an unusual presentation of Wilson's disease but must be considered particularly in adolescents and those with concomitant acute hemolytic anemia.[142] A high index of suspicion is necessary because low normal ceruloplasmin levels can be found in 15% of patients with Wilson's disease. Kaiser-Fleischer rings are not always present. Elevation of hepatic and serum copper levels has been reported as the most usual parameters of copper metabolism in this disease.[143] Microscopy reveals massive hepatic necrosis, nodular regeneration, Mallory bodies, and microvesicular fat. The response to medical treatment is poor, and death is the usual outcome without hepatic transplantation.

The acute fatty liver of pregnancy is seen in patients in their third trimester who also have clinical evidence consistent with preeclampsia. It may progress to FHF but if promptly recognized improves in response to delivery. Recovery is at times prolonged and complicated but complete. Liver histology shows cholestasis, a fatty liver with predominantly centrolobular microvesicular fat, portal inflammation, lobular disorientation, and hepatocyte dropout. If the disease needs clarification, a liver biopsy stained with the appropriate fat stain is indicated. Liver transplantation has been described as successful.[144]

Miscellaneous Causes

Sepsis has been described as the cause of FHF in four patients: meningitis, gangrenous appendicitis with Escherichia coli septicemia, diverticulitis, and intrahepatic abscess. The latter two patients recovered after surgical drainage and antibiotic therapy.[145] Heatstroke results in massive hepatic necrosis and rhabdomyolysis and has been treated successfully with transplantation.[146]

Complications

Hepatic Coma

Hepatic coma (portal systemic encephalopathy [PSE]) is the result of the diversion of portal venous blood from the liver directly into the systemic circulation. It is seen principally in the cirrhotic patient who has developed portal hypertension and a collateral circulation or in whom a portal systemic shunt has been surgically created. Intrahepatic shunting plays a role in both chronic and acute hepatic failure when hepatocellular damage is so great as to compromise the ability of the hepatocyte to function.[91] Encephalopathy is uncommon in the presence of normal liver function but has been reported in idiopathic noncirrhotic portal hypertension,[147] extrahepatic hypertension,[148] and congenital or spontaneous shunts without liver disease.[149]

Clinical Picture. The diagnosis is readily made in the patient with known liver disease who develops neuropsychiatric changes. It is at times unsuspected when seen in patients not suspected of having hepatic pathology: i.e., well-compensated cirrhotics or unsuspected shunts. The differential diagnosis must include intracranial hemorrhage, space-occupying lesions, psychiatric disorders, and drugs or other metabolic encephalopathies.

A grading of clinical observation classifies four stages: prodrome, impending coma, stupor, and coma (Table 54–11).[150] Subclinical PSE has been recognized and defined as "a condition in which patients with cirrhosis, regardless of the etiology, demonstrate a number of quantifiable neuropsychiatric defects yet have a normal mental and neurological status to clinical examination."[151] These

Table 54–11. Stages of Hepatic Encephalopathy

Stage	Clinical Status	Neurologic Signs
Subclinical	Recognized only by impaired psychometric testing	Normal
Stage I (Prodrome)	Personality change Euphoria, depression Intermittent mild confusion Irritability, untidiness Lack of attention to detail Intellectual deterioration Sleep inversion (night into day)	Deterioration of writing Constructional apraxia
Stage II (Impending Coma)	Increasing intellectual and personality deterioration Increasing confusion Inappropriate behavior Lethargy	Asterixis Worsening of prior problem
Stage III (Stupor)	Sleeping, but arousable Confused, incoherent Possibly combative	Asterixis Fluctuating reflexes and muscle tone
Stage IV (Coma)	Asleep, response to noxious stimuli Asleep, does not respond	Areflexia, absent reflexes Dilated pupils

(Modified from Davidson, C. S.: Hepatic coma. *In* Gastroenterology. Vol. III. 3rd Ed. Edited by H. L. Bockus. Philadelphia, W. B. Saunders, 1976.)

are demonstrated by simple psychometric testing that can be done with relative ease and quickness revealing the presence of subclinical PSE in 60 to 70% of patients with cirrhosis.[151] Cortical atrophy and edema, demonstrated by CT scan, have been correlated with the abnormalities found by psychometric testing.[152] Forty patients with chronic liver disease and portal hypertension without PSE were extensively evaluated with psychometric testing, and only 15% were deemed fit to drive.[153] As yet this is not readily accepted, and its impact remains undocumented.[154] Treatment of hepatic encephalopathy and liver transplantation improve subclinical PSE but do not completely abolish the abnormalities.[155,156]

The **prodromal stage (stage I)** may be so subtle as to be viewed only in retrospect. Personality changes manifest themselves intermittently with irritability, exaggeration of usual behavior, garrulousness, and untidiness. Inversion of the sleep pattern with insomnia and daytime napping bring the patient to a physician for a "sleeping pill," often worsening the situation. Intellectual deterioration, forgetfulness, an inability to do simple mathematics, decreased attention to detail, and change in handwriting are gradual and may go unnoticed. Asterixis, the "liver flap," is not a part of this stage.[157]

Stage II further emphasizes the previous changes but is characterized by marked lethargy, inappropriate behavior, and confusion as well as continuing deterioration of intellectual function. Asterixis can be elicited. This is usually bilateral, but the typical tremor may involve only one side and may be present not only in the wrist and hand, but also on the tongue, jaw, eyelids, and feet. It is not specific for hepatic encephalopathy but is seen in other encephalopathies, most notably uremia.[157]

Stage III (stupor) consists of long periods of restful sleep. When aroused, there is confusion, slurred speech, and sufficient agitation to necessitate restraint occasionally, even raising the question of alcoholic withdrawal. Neurologic changes fluctuate rapidly from flaccidity to rigidity and hyperreflexia to absent deep tendon reflexes. Convulsions are unusual but do occur.[158]

In **stage IV (coma),** the semistupor has progressed to coma, in which noxious stimuli may or may not provoke a response. Pupils dilate; decorticate and decerebrate posturing appear and may disappear within hours.[159] The deeper and more profound the coma, the worse the prognosis; however, on recovery, patients return to their previous normal functional state. Exceptions to this are few and seen in those who develop cerebral edema and intracranial hypertension.[160]

The diagnosis is made by clinical observations. A thorough neuropsychiatric evaluation is required and observation and reevaluation done at frequent intervals. Fluctuating neurologic findings may be confusing, but these are typical and may aid by suggesting the diagnosis as well as confirming it. Measurements of ammonia done on arterial blood are more reliable than venous samples, which are contaminated by the products of muscular metabolism. Regardless, ammonia levels, which can be of assistance in cases in which the nature of the encephalopathy is doubtful, do not correlate well with the clinical status and are of little, if any, use in following the patient's course.[161] The findings of a normal electroencephalogram (EEG) are valuable because they usually exclude the diagnosis, but as the neuropsychiatric status fluctuates, so does the EEG. The earliest changes are seen symmetrically over the temporal lobes with progression to involve both hemispheres, at which time large slow waves become more random. These changes are nonspecific and are reported as changes compatible with metabolic encephalopathy. Imaging of the brain eliminates overt intracranial pathology, and even though the CT scan may show changes of cerebral edema or cortical atrophy, they correlate with the increased intracranial pressure measurements only 27 to 33% of the time.[162,163] Cerebrospinal fluid analysis aids in identifying or eliminating vascular accidents and infection. Although it has not achieved regular use, possibly owing to the need for a lumbar puncture, an elevated spinal fluid glutamine level provides the best correlation with clinical severity.[161,164]

Patients with liver disease develop a wide spectrum of neuropsychiatric disorders. The rapid deterioration of hepatocellular function in FHF may bypass the earlier stages of encephalopathy to exhibit agitation, confusion, or stupor as the initial manifestations of the fulminant disease. Cerebral edema, intercranial hypertension, and herniation of the brain are a common cause of death. The presence of cerebral edema and the aforementioned sequence of events in end-stage chronic liver disease is rare but has been reported.[165]

Hepatic encephalopathy seldom occurs without a precipitating cause, which may arise from either an endogenous or exogenous source. Ammonia is the principal endogenous cause, entering the renal vein as a result of renal tubular acidosis or hypokalemia.[68] The elevated concentrations of urea in azotemia readily diffuse into the gut, where bacterial production of ammonia increases.[166] Constipation also plays a major role, as does hypoxia, metabolic alkalosis, hypokalemia, and electrolyte depletion, in predisposing to the development of encephalopathy in the cirrhotic patient. The most prominent exogenous source of ammonia is an increased nitrogen load provoked by gastrointestinal bleeding or a protein-rich diet, supplying the substrate in ammonia formation. Narcotics (opiate derivatives), sedation (barbiturates and paraldehyde), and tranquilizing agents (benzodiazepines, chlordiazepoxide, phenothiazines) further depress the central nervous system and have a prolonged effect resulting from decreased hepatic clearance. Although they are reasonably well tolerated in those without decompensated cirrhosis,[161] diuretics of any type are considered by many to be the major precipitant by inducing hypovolemia and electrolyte depletion, particularly hypokalemia. Sepsis, surgery, trauma, and vomiting and diarrhea are other causes not to be ignored. Once identified and the offending cause or causes eliminated or treated, the response is rapid and accompanied by return to the patient's usual preencephalopathic state. Hepatocyte insufficiency, whether due to massive necrosis or end-stage liver disease, must be included in the differential diagnosis and seldom responds to treatment (Table 54-12).

Chronic Hepatic Encephalopathy. A chronic type of hepatic encephalopathy occurs in conjunction with an extensive collateral circulation and is usually seen within months of a portal systemic shunt. Changes in personality, mood swings, and intellectual deterioration are intermittent and fluctuate in severity. Psychotic and neurotic reactions occur and often require psychiatric care. Motor abnormalities can also occur. There may be no discernible precipitating event. Proper treatment may reverse these changes, which are also reflected by the return of EEG changes toward normalcy. Recurrent episodes over years may precede a state of mild dementia and symptoms compatible with cerebellar disease, pyramidal tract disorders, and parkinsonism. This acquired, nonwilsonian, hepatocerebral degeneration develops slowly. Pathologic changes are found in the cortex, basal ganglion, and cerebellum.[167,168] Treatment may allow the patient to function normally but does not ensure total remission of the chronic changes. These individuals may survive for up to 7 years after the onset of neurologic symptoms.[167,168]

Spastic paraparesis occurs within months to years after portacaval shunt but has been reported with a huge spontaneous portal systemic shunt. Demyelinating changes are limited to the corticospinal tracts. The rate of progression is variable and is virtually unaltered by treatment.[167,169,170]

Pathogenesis. Despite the general consensus that the clinical syndrome is a result of a failure of neurotransmission, the mechanism remains debatable. Four major hypotheses have been postulated:

- Ammonia neurotoxicity
- Gamma-aminobutyric acid (GABA) and endogenous benzodiazepines
- Synergism of interacting toxins augmented by nonspecific metabolites
- False neurotransmitters

Historically, clinically, and experimentally the argument made for ammonia neurotoxicity remains the strongest. Ammonia, which is generated primarily in the colon by the action of colonic bacterial urease on protein, urea, and amino acids, is then transported via portal circulation to the liver, where it is converted to urea. Failure of this, whether caused by bypassing the hepatic parenchyma or hepatocyte insufficiency, or both, increases the plasma level of ammonia. Evidence exists that the cerebral metabolic rate of ammonia is increased in patients with portal systemic encephalopathy, and its association with the increased permeability of the blood-brain barrier in PSE allows easier access to the brain.[171,172] These findings help explain the heightened sensitivity of the cirrhotic to those conditions conducive to increased production of ammonia as well as the discordance between ammonia levels in the clinical stages of hepatic encephalopathy: i.e., low levels of blood ammonia with severe hepatic encephalopathy.[171,172] Lacking a urea cycle, cerebral ammonia removal depends on the production of glutamine, catalyzed by glutamine-synthetase from tissue glutamate. Cerebrospinal fluid glutamine provides the best correlation with the severity of encephalopathy and EEG changes. It also relates well to the increased concentration of glutamine found in the brains of autopsied cirrhotic patients who died with hepatic encephalopathy or FHF as well as to the known effects of ammonia on inhibitory and excitatory neurotransmission.[172] Finally, the keystone of treatment continues to be directed at decreasing the production of ammonia by eliminating the intestinal substrate and inhibiting the growth of colonic urease-producing organisms.

Experimentally, mercaptopurine, fatty acids, phenols, and ammonia in combination with hypoglycemia and hypoxia produce hepatic coma in smaller doses than when each is given alone.[161] "False neurotransmitters" (octopamine, phenol, ethanolamine), also produced in the gut,

Table 54–12. Precipitants of Hepatic Encephalopathy

Exogenous
Drugs
 Diuretic
 Sedatives, analgesics, tranquilizers
Increased nitrogen load
 Gastrointestinal bleeding (blood in gut)
 Excess dietary protein
Volume contraction
Infection
Surgery
Trauma

Endogenous
Hepatic failure (acute and/or chronic)
Azotemia
Constipation
Renal tubular acidosis
Metabolic alkalosis
Volume contraction (vomiting, diarrhea)

were theorized to replace neurotransmitters,[173] but these postulates have been replaced by enthusiasm for the GABA mechanism.

The GABA theory proposes GABA, the major inhibitory neurotransmitter, to be the principal factor in the pathogenesis of hepatic encephalopathy.[174] Earlier studies in experimentally induced FHF in rabbits proposed that enteric derived GABA, following the same route as ammonia, produced an interaction between GABA and its receptors that inhibited neurotransmission.[174] Later, increased serum levels of GABA-like activity in patients with cirrhosis or FHF were found in patients with and without hepatic encephalopathy and did not correlate with either the stage of encephalopathy or plasma ammonia concentration.[175] In the absence of strong supporting evidence, the emphasis has shifted to the role of endogenous benzodiazepines, which stimulate the benzodiazepine receptors. These are coupled to the postsynaptic GABA receptors, and therefore mediate their action.[176,177] This concept is promulgated on clinical observations that cirrhotics are unusually susceptible to the action of benzodiazepines and the response of hepatic encephalopathy to benzodiazepine receptor agonists and antagonists.[177,178,179] Experimentally, benzodiazepine agonists, given to rabbits with FHF, provoke the behavioral changes and visual evoked responses of hepatic encephalopathy, whereas their antagonists normalized electrophysiologic changes and induced transient but improved behavioral response.[176,180] Benzodiazepinclike substances have been demonstrated in the cerebrospinal fluid.[181] Brain tissue obtained at autopsy in patients with FHF secondary to acetaminophen overdose but without a history of benzodiazepine treatment contained diazepam and its metabolite in a sufficiently greater concentration than that found in control patients who had died from nonhepatic causes, but these levels were compatible only with those in other patients who had used small tranquilizing doses of diazepam that were far less than a sedating dose. It is also possible that benzodiazepines have a synergistic reaction with other neurotoxins or metabolites, with their enhanced effect actually increasing the GABA-ergic tone;[182] however, in the absence of an exogenous benzodiazepine, the source of an endogenous benzodiazepine substance remains unknown. Because hepatic encephalopathy was characterized before the advent of these pharmaceutical preparations, demonstration of the endogenous substances remains critical for this thesis.

The use of flumazenil, a benzodiazepine antagonist, has been reported in a number of uncontrolled studies all describing patients who remained unchanged or were only partially improved.[183,184] The changes occurred quickly but were transient, with evidence of exogenous benzodiazepines in some. Conversely, in those patients with benzodiazepine-induced hepatic encephalopathy, the results obtained with flumazenil were excellent.[185] Continuing investigation raises further questions, but until the advent of a definite answer, treatment remains directed at the gut flora, restoration of normal portal flow, or replacement of the defective organ.

Cerebral Edema. Cerebral edema leading to increased intracranial pressure (ICP) is reported to have been present in up to 80% of patients with FHF and stage IV hepatic encephalopathy.[163] Autopsies on patients dying from FHF revealed the presence of cerebral edema, and of these, 25 to 81% had evidence of brain stem herniation or temporal lobe coning.[186-188] Although the mortality of late-onset hepatic failure (81%) is similar to that of FHF (90.5%), the incidence of cerebral edema in late-onset hepatic failure was only 9%.[101]

The basic pathology in cerebral edema consists of an increase in tissue water secondary to altered intracellular osmoregulation (cytotoxic brain edema) and vasogenic brain edema, the result of damage to the cerebral capillary endothelial cells allowing protein-rich fluid to pass the blood-brain barrier and enter the extracellular space of the brain.[182,187,189] Different pathogenic mechanisms have been proposed, but the precise cause remains undetermined.

Increased ICP refers to the elevated pressure produced within an unyielding brain case by the edematous brain. Cerebral perfusion pressure (CPP), the difference between the mean arterial pressure and ICP, must be maintained above 40 to 60 mm Hg to avoid brain ischemia.[163,190] Hypotension, the result of the peripheral vasodilatation seen in FHF, can decrease the threshold at which ICP retards cerebral perfusion, and although the occurrence of hypertension implies an elevated ICP, the use of hypotensive drugs could only further increase the CCP.[187,190]

Neurologic changes may not be manifested until an ICP of 30 mm Hg and as high as 60 mm Hg.[187,191] Papilledema is rarely observed, but dilated or irregular pupils or those that react abnormally to light, increased muscle tone and mild clonus, hypertension, spontaneous hyperventilation, decerebrate positioning, and seizures are ominous prognostic findings.[105,187] Initially these may be paroxysmal when precipitated by various somatic stimuli before becoming more sustained. Although neither an EEG or CT scan of the brain can reliably evaluate the presence of ICP,[163,190] the loss of the occulovestibular reflex is the most reliable clinical index of herniation.[187,188,191] An unsuspected respiratory arrest may also be the result of brain stem compression.[191]

Abnormal neurologic findings are neither sensitive nor specific indications of ICP because they are often absent or abolished by mechanical ventilation and paralysis. ICP transducers are capable of monitoring ICP and are placed when the patient develops stage III to IV encephalopathy.[163,187,190] They provide the opportunity to manage treatment objectively and to decide if or when liver transplantation is indicated.[163,190] If transplantation is undertaken, their input is continued during surgery and postoperatively.[163,190] Epidural, subdural, and intraparenchymal transducers have been used, but the frequent complications seen with the latter two have favored the use of the epidural site, particularly when they are placed in the security of the operating room.[163,190,191] Hypoprothrombinemia should be corrected and maintained within 3 to 5 seconds of the control, platelets transfused when less than 75,000, and cryoprecipitate infused when the fibrinogen concentration is less than 100 mg/dl.[163] Although the transducer is left in place for a relatively short period of time and infection is uncommon, antibiotic coverage is ordered; however, hemorrhage remains a major complication.[191]

With the transducer in place, the head of the bed is raised to 45 degrees and the ICP and CPP continually monitored to ensure an optimum ICP less than 20 to 25 mm Hg and CPP greater than 40 to 60 mm Hg.[163,187,190] Movements of the head and stimulation produced by nursing care, medical examination, chest physiotherapy, and other machination may produce transient rises, but it is the sustained increase that is an indication to begin a specific protocol. In the absence of an intracranial monitoring device, an ongoing neurologic evaluation by an experienced member of the staff, with particular attention to the pupillary reflexes and continuous measurement of the arterial blood pressure, substitutes clinical acumen for objective data. In these situations, a sustained arterial pressure of greater than 150 mm Hg that peaks to 200 or more or neurologic changes are the most reliable signals of an increased ICP.[105]

Initially a bolus of 20% mannitol (0.5 to 1.0 g/kg) is given with expectations of a reduction of 20 to 30 mm Hg in the ICP.[188,192] This is more effective when it has been started before a marked rise in the ICP.[187] The dose may be repeated hourly, but the serum osmolality must remain between 310 and 320 mOsm/L. An adequate diuresis needs to be maintained, and, if not, ultrafiltration should be started. In those cases with accompanying renal failure, hemodialysis with ultrafiltration is necessary because fluid overload and hyperosmolality worsen the ICP. Hemodialysis may precipitate hypo-osmolar edema, and in patients at risk for developing cerebral edema, hemodialysis should also be preceded by evaluation and, if necessary, correction of the serum osmolality.[187] Neither furosemide nor corticosteroids are of use.[187,192] Short-term hyperventilation to produce hypocapnia to 30 to 32 mm Hg is helpful but of limited value over a prolonged period.[187,191]

The presence of stage IV hepatic encephalopathy with evidence of increased ICP refractory to treatment with mannitol implies death within 30 hours.[163,188] Despite conflicting studies concerning the use of barbiturates in the treatment of head injuries, Forbes and associates[193] studied the effects of pentobarbital in 13 patients with stage IV encephalopathy, renal failure, and intractable increased ICP. While monitored by an intracranial transducer and treatment with mannitol, ultrafiltration, and hyperventilation was continued, pentobarbital was slowly infused, and following 3 to 5 mg/kg given over 15 minutes, the ICP and CPP decreased by 10 to 29 mm Hg and were maintained by a continuous infusion of 1 to 3 mg/kg as necessary to maintain optimum ICP. The infusion was discontinued if controlled for more than 4 hours or if hypotension occurred. ICP returned to normal in eight patients, five (38%) of whom recovered completely. The other three died of unrelated causes (two with sepsis). Two others also died of sepsis despite maintaining a normal ICP, and the deaths of the remaining three resulted from increased ICP after transient control; hence an overall survival of 38% was achieved in a group whose predicted survival was less than 5%.[104]

Lidofsky and associates,[163] using intracranial monitoring, reported the outcome of 23 patients with stage IV PSE awaiting liver transplantation. If the ICP rose above 25 mm Hg, mannitol was given, and if this failed to control the ICP or oliguria ensued, pentobarbital was added. Thirteen patients whose ICP remained less than 25 mm Hg required no further intervention. One recovered spontaneously, 10 others survived and received transplants, but 2 with other medical complications died before a donor organ could be found. Ten patients required further treatment to control ICP. Four responded, three to mannitol alone, and the fourth required the addition of pentobarbital. Of these, one recovered without transplantation, two were successfully transplanted, and the remaining patient died of sepsis, again before an organ could be procured. Six received no benefit from either mannitol or pentobarbital despite the lack of a significant difference between the ICP and that of the four responders. Therefore deemed refractory to treatment and judged unlikely to recover neurologically, they were removed from the waiting list, and all died with brain stem herniation within 2 to 30 hours. Neurologic function was normal in the 12 patients who were monitored and underwent transplantation procedures. All monitored patients who underwent transplantation procedures survived the initial hospitalization with the return of full neurologic function.[163]

Treatment. Treatment begins with recognition of hepatic encephalopathy and the identification and therapy of the precipitating event. Unless extenuating circumstances are present, stage I is treated on an outpatient basis by restricting dietary protein to 40 g per day, an amount to be increased or decreased as dictated by the clinical response. Lactulose, the keystone of therapy, is also prescribed. A nonabsorbable disaccharide, it passes unchanged into the colon to be metabolized by colonic bacteria into organic acids and carbon dioxide, thereby decreasing the intracolonic pH. In the induced acidic environment, the absorbable ammonia is reduced to the ammonium ion, which is unable to escape the intestinal lumen. The newly created gradient between tissue and intestinal contents facilitates passage of extraluminal ammonia into the colon.[91] Lactulose also stimulates the incorporation of urea, ammonia, and other nitrogenous compounds into the fecal bacteria as demonstrated by increased fecal and soluble nitrogen excretion.[194] As an osmotic cathartic, it decreases colonic transit time, with a subsequent increase in fecal nitrogen elimination, but can also be the cause of diarrhea, severe enough to induce hypovolemia and electrolyte depletion. The dose varies from 10 to 30 ml three to four times a day, with the end point of three to four stools daily and a rapid (24 to 72 hours) remission of the encephalopathy. The frequent stools, flatulence, abdominal distress, and innate sweetness of the sugar can result in noncompliance. Recurrent encephalopathy, failure to maintain or attain remission, and normal or constipated stools imply an inadequate dose or disregard for lactulose or protein restriction.

Lactitol, a more palatable and less expensive nonabsorbable disaccharide, is as effective as lactulose. It is derived from lactulose, but its gastrointestinal effects (flatulence and diarrhea) are less, and resolution of the acute encephalopathy is quicker than with lactulose alone, although a meta-analysis of chronic encephalopathy revealed no significant difference between the therapeutic effect of either.[195,196] Although available elsewhere, at this time it cannot be obtained in the United States. A similar effect is obtained with the use of lactose in lactase-deficient individuals.[197] Lactose and lactulose enemas have also been satisfactorily used.[198,199]

Before the introduction of lactulose, neomycin was used to suppress urease-splitting bacteria. This fell into disuse when lactulose was demonstrated to be effective without the side effects of ototoxicity, nephrotoxicity, and malabsorption, but in many patients resistant to lactulose, the addition of neomycin has been effective.[200,201] The success of this apparent contradictory combination was explained by demonstrating that neomycin inhibits aerobic organisms, which are less effective urea splitters than the bacteroides and other anaerobes that metabolize lactulose. Metronidazole and vancomycin are effective in lactulose-resistant patients because they also attack anaerobic urea-splitting bacteria.[202,203] The long-term use of metronidazole can produce peripheral neuropathy, and vancomycin is almost prohibitively expensive.

Controlled studies of corticosteroids have shown no benefit but rather serious side effects. Their use is not advocated.[204-206]

The inability of the failing liver to metabolize aromatic amino acids (AAAs), as contrasted to the continued catabolism of branched-chain amino acids (BCAAs) in skeletal muscles, alters the BCAA-to-AAA ratio from 3:1 to 1:1. In FHF, the total of all amino acids is elevated to 700 to 800% of normal, mainly as the result of an increase in the AAAs and maintenance of a steady level of BCAAs.[207] The false neurotransmitter theory is based on the marked increase in AAAs, which enter the brain overwhelming the true neurotransmitters; therefore supplemental BCAAs, in themselves a useful energy source that decreases muscle breakdown and increases protein synthesis and ammonia metabolism, should normalize this ratio.[173] Other studies have weakened support for this hypothesis, and despite multiple trials, there remains much disagreement regarding the efficacy of BCAAs in improving recovery and survival in both FHF and chronic liver disease.[208,209] Some evidence exists for its effectiveness when given orally, but this should be used only in the absence of improvement with standard therapy in those tolerant of enteral feedings and intolerant of protein. The role of BCAAs in parenteral nutrition remains uncertain, and BCAAs are not recommended for general use, particularly in regard to their cost. In patients unresponsive to other measures, BCAAs may be of help.

Protein provided in a vegetable diet in hepatic encephalopathy has been demonstrated to be beneficial in the animal model. Fecal nitrogen excretion is increased primarily via the bacterial portion of the stool, which has been incorporated into the additional fiber component of the diet. The amount of vegetable protein necessary to be efficacious, however, is the cause of poor acceptance by patients, not only because of the ensuing flatulence and diarrhea, but also because of its bulk and unpalatable nature.[194]

Other treatments have been used only infrequently but lack the legitimacy accompanying controlled trials and experience. Zinc deficiency, predicated on a decreased dietary intake, poor intestinal absorption, and an increased urinary excretion, is a common finding in cirrhotics. It appears to correlate with the severity of the disease and to be more common in patients with encephalopathy than those without it.[211] The first of two controlled short-term studies using an oral zinc supplement in patients with portal systemic encephalopathy, unresponsive to diet and lactulose, showed improvement on the number correction test, whereas the second study noted no change.[212,213] A single well-documented case report wherein zinc acetate was used to correct zinc deficiency in a patient with encephalopathy presents supporting evidence, but the use of zinc requires further investigation.[214]

Sodium benzoate has been described as a safe, effective treatment for chronic encephalopathy. It is a nontoxic, easily available, and inexpensive substance that is taken orally. In a single large series, when tested against lactulose in patients with acute encephalopathy, it was as effective in improving the mental status as in two previously reported experiences.[215-217]

The action and utility of the benzodiazepine receptor antagonist flumanezil was discussed previously.[178,179,181-183] Bromocriptine, a long-acting dopamine receptor antagonist, was used on the premise that hepatic encephalopathy was secondary to a defect in dopaminergic neurotransmission. Responses have occurred in patients resistant to the usual treatment regimen.[92]

Based on early experience and uncontrolled studies, charcoal hemoperfusion was initially thought to be beneficial to patients with FHF.[106] Two controlled trials involving 137 patients revealed that the correlation between survival and cause was unrelated to either the use or duration of hemoperfusion. Patients with HA, HB, and acetaminophen hepatotoxicity had similar rates of survival, which were significantly higher than those of non-A, non-B hepatitis, halothane, and other drug reactions. Charcoal perfusion was confirmed to be of no importance to the outcome in the latter group, whereas the better outcome in the former was more influenced by the absence of cerebral edema, oliguria, renal failure, and uncompensated metabolic acidosis (Fig. 54-33).[102]

At present, liver transplantation is accepted as treatment for hepatic encephalopathy in patients with FHF. Earlier workers in the late 1950s to the early 1970s espoused radical and exotic techniques ranging from dialysis, exchange transfusion and plasmapheresis, cross circulation with volunteers, cadaveric livers, pigs or baboons, and the "total body washout" (asanguineous hypothermic total body perfusion), all of which have been abandoned.[219-224] The previous double-blind studies of corticosteroids had also revealed the lack of efficacy in treating FHF.[204-206]

Established medical means control most cases of encephalopathy, which are usually associated with portal systemic encephalopathy; however, a small number of patients are intractable to the routine measures, unable to tolerate them, or develop side effects. These cases manifest as frequent bouts of encephalopathy requiring lengthy complicated hospitalizations or permanent, progressively severe mental or neurologic deterioration.

Occlusion of the portasystemic shunt by either spontaneous thrombosis or surgical or radiologic intervention is effective in eliminating systemic encephalopathy, thus al-

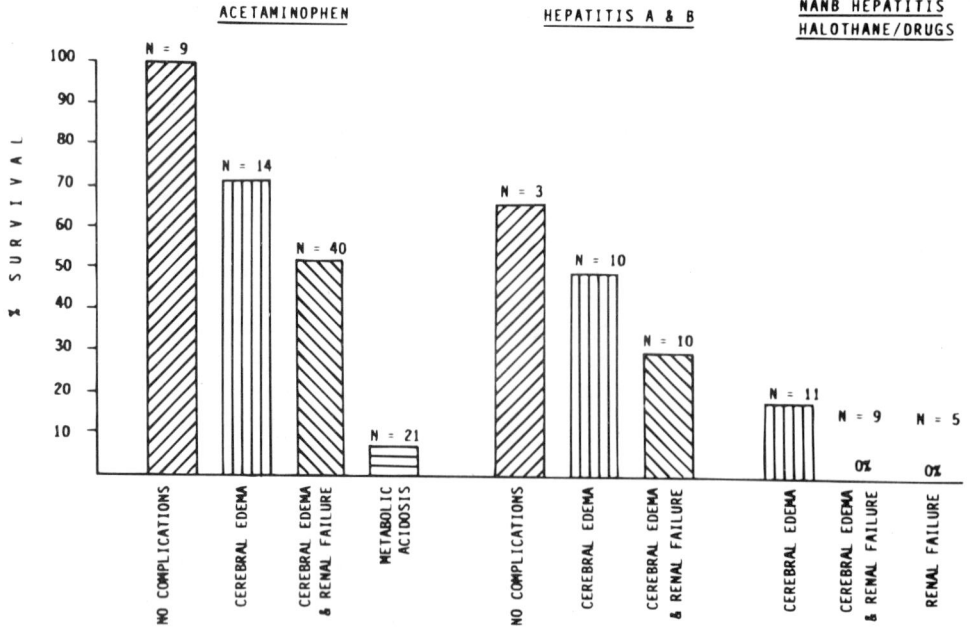

Fig. 54-33. Survival rates in acetaminophen and hepatitis A and B patients correlate with the pattern of complications present. In hepatitis and halothane or drug reaction non-A, non-B (NANB) patients, the survival rates are too low to detect a significant influence of clinical complications of outcome. (From O'Grady, J. C., et al.: Controlled trials of charcoal hemoperfusion and prognostic factors in fulminant hepatic failure. Gastroenterology, 94: 1186, 1988.)

lowing the patient to return to a normal life without protein restriction with or without lactulose.[225-227] The potential for recurrent variceal bleeding must be considered, and although extensive prophylactic procedures can be used, other measures of less magnitude are available for prophylaxis and treatment of varices that recur and bleed.[226]

Elimination of the site of the bacterial enzymatic activity, the major source of ammonia, provided the rationale for colonic exclusion, which consists of an ileosigmoid or ileorectal anastomosis with ligation of the distal ileal stump and creation of a sigmoid mucous fistula to vent the colon. A variation exploits a distal ileostomy to allow lavage of the colon. The reported cases were few in number but the results remarkable, particularly the reversal of mental and neurologic changes previously unresponsive to medical therapy.[227-230] A controlled trial published in 1965 reported a mortality of 26% in a randomized series of 38 patients who had advanced liver disease, i.e.,[230] Child-Pugh classification C, emphasizing previous observations that the procedure should be limited only to patients with relatively good hepatic function (Child-Pugh A and B) but with incapacitating hepatic encephalopathy.[229] Despite the absence of significant differences in the patients, the surgically treated survivors appeared to have benefited more than those treated medically.[230] Excellent results were reported in four of five patients with the Child B classification treated by colonic exclusion. The lone fatality was secondary to hepatic failure in a Child C candidate.[227] Colonic exclusion and shunt occlusion provide an option for those excluded from liver transplantation.

Hemodynamic Complications

A systolic blood pressure less than 80 mm Hg is common, occurring in 87% of 94 patients with FHF and grade IV encephalopathy. Hemorrhage and respiratory arrest were responsible for death in 25%, another 11% died during the preterminal period, and 4% of deaths occurred in patients undergoing extracorporeal hemoperfusion. Hypotension in the other 60% was unexplained by hypovolemia, bacteremia, or many of the aforementioned causes. Liver damage was more severe in those with unexplained hypotension than in those who remained normotensive or who had a definable cause. The survival rate of patients without a defining cause was less than 10%. Fifty percent of those patients without an explanation for their hypotension who were autopsied had evidence of temporal cloning or cerebellar herniation as opposed to those who remained normotensive.[231]

The circulation is hyperdynamic and simulates that seen in septic shock or systemic arteriovenous shunting. It is characterized by an increased cardiac output, a low blood pressure with decreased diastolic levels, and bounding pulses.[91] Decreased peripheral vascular resistance and vasomotor tone produce a relative hypovolemia as documented by a low pulmonary capillary pressure that is corrected by either whole blood or albumin.[232] Bradycardia that occurs with hypotension is highly suggestive of cerebral edema and increased ICP.[231]

Weston and colleagues[233] noted that cardiac arrhythmias occurred in 92% of 106 patients who had FHF with stage IV hepatic encephalopathy. Sinus tachycardia was present in 79% but was the sole abnormality in only 24%. Atrial fibrillation, supraventricular tachycardia, ventricular tachycardia, and atrial or nodal arrhythmias were common. These lasted only a short time, at the most only a few hours, and reverted either spontaneously or responded to standard specific treatment.[233] They were explained by electrolyte abnormalities, acidosis, hypoxemia, increased ICP, or even irritation of the myocardium by an aberrant Swan-Ganz catheter.[105] Cardiac arrest occurred in 27%. Autopsies on 76 of the 84 patients found cardiac abnormalities in 42 (67%). Eleven (26%) had a pale, flabby, fatty myocardium, and another 26% had small pericardial effusions. Dilatation of the ventricles without other organic causes was present in 17%, and scattered petechial hemorrhages were seen in a little over one third.[232]

The outlook is poor with the appearance of hypotension, particularly when the blood pressure cannot be maintained even with the correction of hypovolemia. Caution must be exercised during volume expansion in regards to the potential for pulmonary edema and is a greater problem in the face of renal failure. Inotropes are of little use, although vasoconstricting agents (norepinephrine, vasopressin, or epinephrine) are effective for a short time, i.e., for maintaining CPP in severely hypotensive patients with increased ICP. Long-term use does not alleviate the accompanying tissue hypoxemia.[105] It is hypothesized that the hypotension reflects only the underlying liver disease and is not responsible for the mortality rate, which is due to inappropriate vasodilatation rather than primary cardiac failure.[231]

Pulmonary Complications

Hypoxemia frequently complicates FHF as a result of infection, aspiration, fluid overload, noncardiac pulmonary edema, adult respiratory distress syndrome, intrapulmonary hemorrhage, ventilation-perfusion mismatch, or intrapulmonary shunting. Intrapulmonary shunting is well documented in chronic liver disease but is not always due to a true anatomic shunt but rather a "diffusion perfusion" impairment.[234] Deoxygenated blood, which resembles that of a functioning arteriovenous shunt, is the result of inadequate diffusion of oxygen into the center of the blood column flowing within abnormally dilated pulmonary vessels at the capillary level (Fig. 54-34).[234] The nature and source of the vasodilating agent or agents remain unknown, but the perfusion defect can be corrected temporarily with 100% oxygen and eventually with liver transplantation.[235] Intrapulmonic shunts of up to 39% of the cardiac output have been described in association with the peripheral dilatation of FHF, and diffuse dilatation of intra-acinar vessels has been demonstrated in autopsy specimens obtained from patients with FHF, encephalopathy, and significant shunting.[236,237]

The obvious pulmonary abnormalities are treated appropriately. Oxygen is given, but endotracheal intubation is indicated with deterioration of the P_{O_2} and/or stage III to IV encephalopathy. This provides ventilatory control, prevents aspiration of gastric content, and simplifies access for pulmonary toilet. Positive end-expiratory pressure (PEEP) may be necessary if the P_{O_2} cannot be corrected to greater than 60 mm Hg.

Renal Failure

As reported in different studies, a discrepancy exists regarding the frequency of renal failure in FHF. This range of 55 to 73% may be explained by the lack of uniformity in defining renal failure: i.e., serum creatinine of 1.5 to 3.4 mg/dl, the stage of encephalopathy at which time renal failure occurred, and the inclusion or exclusion of the immediate preterminal state.[238-241] Direct renal toxicity is ascribed to acetaminophen, and these patients commonly develop renal failure before entering stage III or IV coma; however, there is no statistical difference between the incidence of renal abnormalities associated with acetaminophen toxicity and other causes of FHF.[105,232,242]

The pathogenesis of renal failure in FHF includes:

- Prerenal azotemia
- Functional renal failure (the hepatorenal syndrome)
- Acute tubular necrosis[243]

Prerenal azotemia is the result of dehydration from nausea and vomiting, diarrhea, the aggressive use of diuretics, or absorption of a large nitrogen influx following gastrointes-

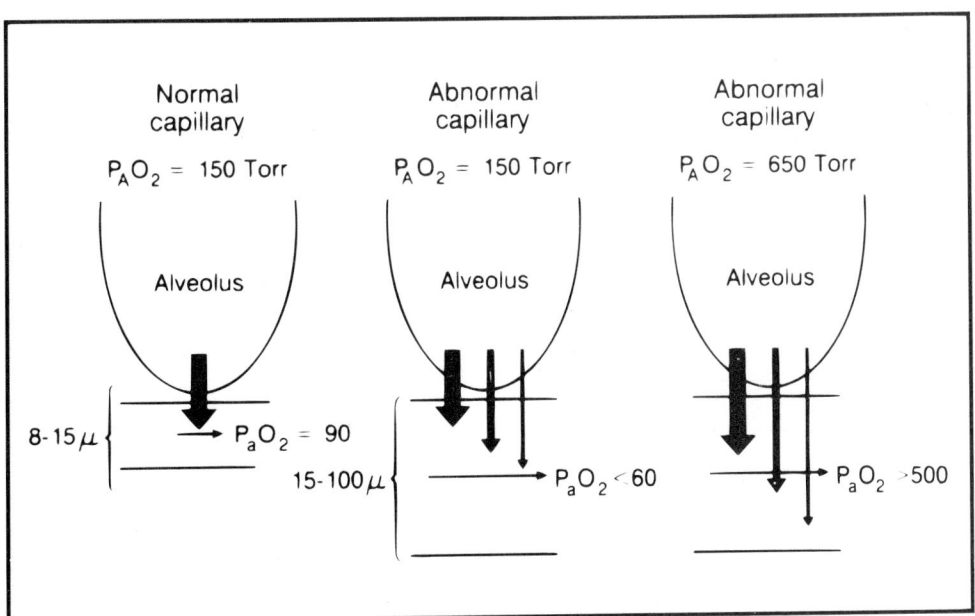

Fig. 54-34. Diagram of capillary level pulmonary vessel abnormality in chronic liver disease. Driving pressure of Pa_{O_2} is depicted by arrows. This concept was originally proposed by Benovesi and associates. (From Krowka, M. J., and Cortese, D. A.: Severe hypoxemia associated with liver disease and the experimental use of almitrine bisnesylate. Mayo Clin. Proc., 62:164, 1987.)

tinal bleeding. The causative factors of functional renal failure, defined as "kidney failure in patients with severely compromised liver function in the absence of clinical laboratory or anatomical evidence of other known causes of renal failure"[243] remain unknown. Only minor anatomic changes are noted at necropsy, glomerular filtration rate (GFR) and renal blood flow are decreased, and angiographic studies show marked vasoconstriction of the renal circulation, which is not seen on postmortem angiography (Figs. 54-35 and 54-36).[244] The presence of this intense vasoconstriction amidst a hyperdynamic circulation is a paradox in the presence of an increased cardiac output and adequate plasma volume. Prostaglandins and endotoxins are major candidates as a causative agent or agents but appear to be only part of a complex involving the sympathetic nervous system, vasoactive polypeptides, and the renin-angiotensin-aldosterone and kallikrein systems.[245,246] Acute tubular necrosis is associated with hypotensive episodes, most of them following gastrointestinal bleeding. It is a commonplace occurrence in the 24 hours before death and has been considered to be the end result of a prolonged period of ischemia secondary to renal constriction. There is wide variation in reports of the frequency of functional renal failure (32.7 to 73%) and acute tubular necrosis (20 to 42%), once again reflecting the different criteria for diagnosis and preterminal appearance of acute tubular necrosis.[231,239,240]

Treatment is mainly supportive. Because of hypotension and vasodilatation, measurement of the pulmonary capillary wedge pressure is necessary to assess adequately and

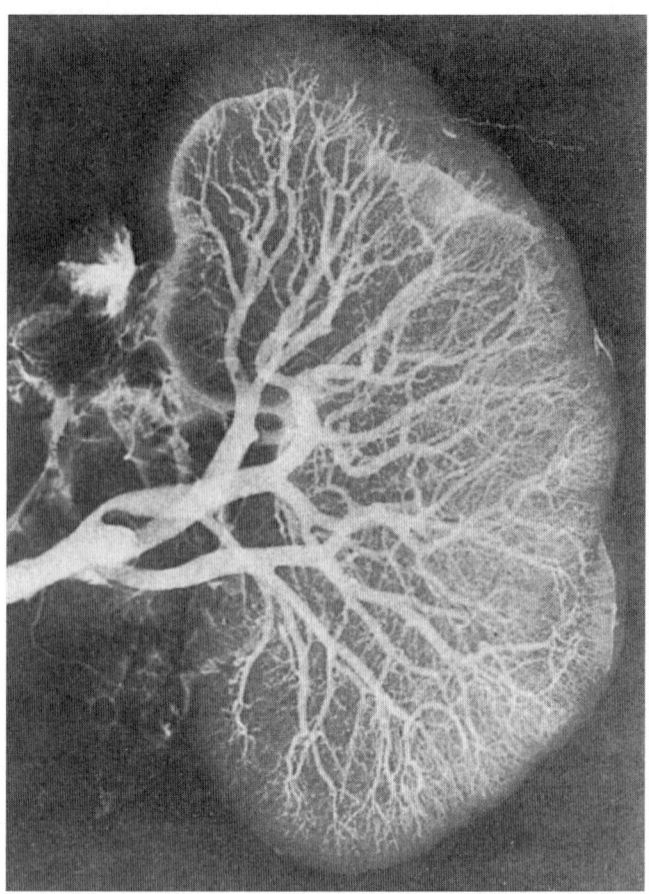

Fig. 54-36. Postmortem angiogram of kidney in Figure 54-35. Note filling of the entire renal vasculature, which is normal and extends to the periphery of the renal cortex. (From Epstein, M., et al.: Renal failure in the patient with cirrhosis: the role of active vasoconstriction. Am. J. Med., *49*:175, 1970.)

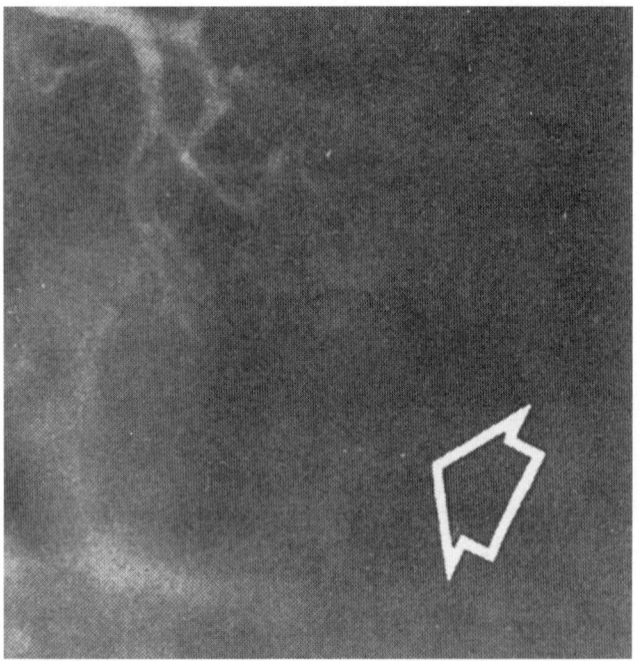

Fig. 54-35. Selective renal angiogram in a patient with oliguric renal failure and liver disease. Note the abnormality of the infrarenal arteries and the lack of the arcuate and cortical arteries. The arrow is at the periphery of the kidney. (From Epstein, M., et al.: Renal failure in the patient with cirrhosis: the role of active vasoconstriction. Am. J. Med., *49*:175, 1970.)

correct any volume deficits. Blood plasma, albumin, and crystalloid solution are used as necessary to achieve a pulmonary capillary wedge pressure within the normal range. Nephrotoxic drugs, which include neomycin, contrast media, and mannitol, are to be given only after great and careful consideration, and nonsteroidal anti-inflammatory drugs are to be avoided. Rapid, large changes in volume loss should be avoided; hence tense ascites should be treated with slow 500 to 750 ml paracentesis every 8 to 12 hours as indicated, and high dose furosemide is not advocated. A continuous infusion of low dose dopamine may produce a transient increase in renal blood flow and GFR but not a prolonged change or diuresis.[105] In the presence of irreversible liver failure, dialysis is of no help, although it is used to gain time when the cause of renal failure is not known. Hemodialysis has been done without significant complication in patients with acidosis, hyperkalemia, or a fluid overload and when combined with ultrafiltration, has allowed the use of mannitol in cerebral edema in the presence of oliguria.[105] Hypernatremia has been reported as a result of dehydration secondary to the osmotic diuresis provoked by infusions of hypertonic dextrose or fructose or the excess amount of sodium contained in multiple transfusions of fresh frozen plasma given in the presence of oliguria.[246] The mortality figures are high, ranging from 70 to 100%, although when induced by acetaminophen, it is only 50%.[106,240] Liver transplantation can reverse these changes.[106,238]

Electrolyte and Acid/Base Balance Abnormalities

Electrolyte disturbances are common. Hyponatremia is dilutional secondary to the inability of the kidney to excrete water despite an increase in total body sodium. Hypokalemia contributes to the dilution by inducing the migration of intracellular water into the extracellular fluid, and diuretics decrease the actual serum sodium concentration.[247] Hypertonic sodium is contraindicated in the treatment of dilutional hyponatremia, unless there is strong suspicion that profound hyponatremia has produced neurologic and EEG changes that are indistinguishable from those of hepatic encephalopathy.[248] Treatment begins with discontinuation of diuretics and fluid restriction. Correction of the hypokalemia may be necessary to correct resistant hyponatremia and requires up to 200 mEq of potassium chloride per day. If it does not respond to this, the addition of up to 400 mEq per day of magnesium may be necessary.[248] Persistent hyponatremia is a poor prognostic sign but may be secondary to the use of dextrose and water, particularly in the preterminal stage.[247]

Hypokalemia is a common occurrence resulting from the increased urinary excretion of potassium secondary to hyperaldosteronism or usage of a diuretic and a decreased intake induced by anorexia, nausea, and vomiting, particularly in patients with ascites. Both subclinical renal tubular acidosis and respiratory mediated alkalosis can contribute to potassium loss and precipitate encephalopathy by the increased renal production of ammonia. In the presence of normal renal function, up to 120 mEq per day is the usual minimal requirement.[68,248]

Hypocalcemia, hypomagnesemia, and hypophosphatemia can also occur in FHF. Hypocalcemia may be related to hypoalbuminemia or concomitant pancreatitis. The mechanisms of hypomagnesemia and hypophosphatemia are unclear, but both should be corrected cautiously in the presence of renal failure, in which increased levels of both phosphorus and potassium are seen.[248]

FHF can be an exercise in the diagnosis and treatment of acid/base disturbances. All perturbations are possible. Respiratory alkalosis, the usual abnormality, occurs as the result of the hyperventilation associated with cerebral edema, whereas hypokalemia and increased bicarbonate are responsible for a metabolic alkalosis. Tissue damage, increased lactic acid concentration, hypoxemia, and hypotension predispose to metabolic acidosis, whereas carbon dioxide retention from either pulmonary disease or depression of the respiratory center secondary to increased ICP is associated with a respiratory acidosis. Combinations of the above-mentioned are frequent, and the interaction between the multiple system involvement provides a constant challenge.

Infection

An increased incidence of bacterial infection is seen in patients with FHF. Published reports cite a frequency of infection ranging from 12 to 80% in all patients with grade III and IV encephalopathy.[249-254] Different investigators have enumerated a number of defects in the host's defenses: faulty function of the Kupffer cells and neutrophils, a decrease in opsonization, and a deficiency of fibronectin and components of the complement cascade.[254-259]

In the series of 50 patients described by Rolando and colleagues,[254] most infections involved the respiratory and urinary tracts and were usually associated with the need for endotracheal tubes and indwelling catheters. Staphylococcus aureus and Staphylococcus epidermidis (considered a pathogen in compromised hosts, particularly when present on repeated culture[260]) and gram-negative bacilli were the most common isolates in pneumonia and urinary tract infections. Bacteremia was frequent, with and without a known source, but this was less seldom than expected in patients with indwelling vascular catheters.[253]

Infections in blood, respiratory tract, and urine occurred within 3 to 5 days of admission to an ICU. The diagnosis was difficult because fever and leukocytosis were absent in a fourth of these patients, who later had culture-proven infections (Fig. 54-37). This emphasized the need to obtain daily cultures of the blood, sputum, urine, and catheters as well as to institute an aggressive treatment program using an antibiotic combination directed against staphylococcus and gram-negative bacilli based on a heightened clinical suspicion rather than a culture.[254] Bacterial infection is a major complication and the cause of death in apparently 20% of all cases of FHF. Thirty percent to 50% of patients with renal failure are infected, and 75 to 80% of these patients die.[254] Conversely, six of seven patients with septicemia who underwent emergency liver transplantation survived.[253]

Fungal infections were diagnosed in 16 of 50 patients (32%) within 1 to 14 days after antibiotics had been started to treat bacterial infection.[261] Candida albicans was cultured from the blood, respiratory tract, urine, gastric aspirate, nose, and skin. Eleven patients infected with fungus died, 7 from an overwhelming fungal infection. Infection during the second week of hospitalization, established renal failure, a fever unresponsive to antibiotics, leukocytosis, and, despite initial improvement, regression in coma status and prolongation of the prothrombin time strongly suggested a fungal infection. Amphotericin B was the drug of choice, and those not treated died, whereas the mortality was much less in those receiving the drug.[261]

The Liver Failure Unit at Kings College Hospital reported a prospective, controlled trial of selective parenteral and enteral antimicrobial treatment in FHF demonstrating that prophylaxis with systemic antimicrobials with or without enteral decontamination was effective in reducing infection rates, even though it did not affect mortality; however, they believed that reduction in infection was an important consideration in situations in which active sepsis was considered a contraindication to liver transplantation.[262]

Coagulopathy

Because factors I (fibrinogen), II (prothrombin), V, VII, IX, X, fibrinolytic factor, and antithrombin III are synthesized in the liver, it is inevitable that coagulopathy is en-

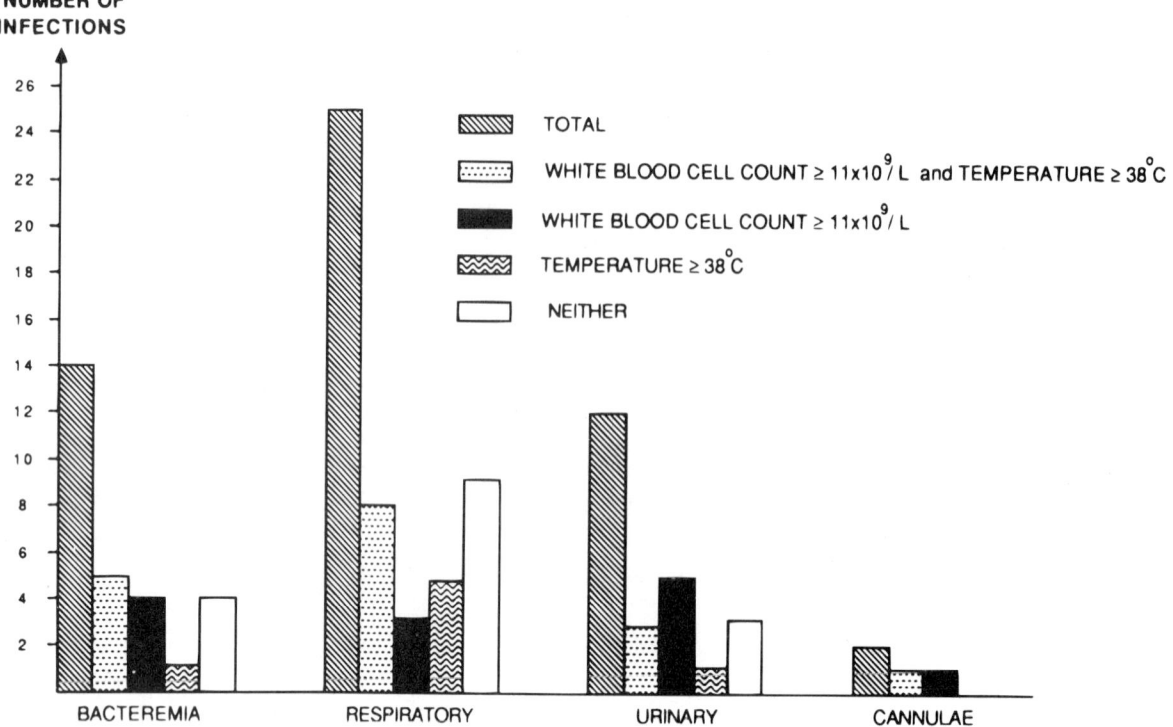

Fig. 54–37. Clinical signs of bacterial infection related to significant microbiologic cultures in acute liver failure patients. (From Rolando, N., et al.: Prospective study of bacterial infection in acute liver failure: an analysis of fifty patients. Hepatology, 11:49, 1990.)

countered as a complication of FHF. The decrease in their plasma levels is the result of reduced synthetic function (unresponsive to vitamin K and treated with fresh frozen plasma) and to a lesser degree intravascular consumption. These abnormalities are responsible for prolonged prothrombin time and activated partial thromboplastin time (APTT), both of which measure the common pathway of the coagulation cascade. The prothrombin time also measures the function of the extrinsic pathway whereas APTT abnormalities are usually on the basis of a mild deficiency of one of the clotting factors of the intrinsic pathway. Both are invariably abnormal in FHF. Their abnormal values become the initial and most significant indications of hepatic deterioration, which may predict hepatic encephalopathy. Because factors V and VII have the shortest half-life, they are considered the most sensitive manifestation of the degree of liver failure.[263–265] Bernuau and associates[269] have used a factor V level of less than 50% as a major criterion to determine which patients with FHF are candidates for liver transplantation. Clinically significant disseminated intravascular coagulation (DIC) is rare, but a low grade process exists in almost all.[105] Overt DIC may be precipitated by sepsis, the infusion of clotting factor concentrate, peritoneovenous shunts or the decreased level of antithrombin III.[105,266]

Platelets are not only reduced, but also are structurally and functionally abnormal. Thrombocytopenia is attributed to bone marrow depression, hypersplenism, DIC, and the use of extracorporeal perfusion devices. Electron microscopic studies revealed ultrastructural abnormalities, and the smaller size of platelets is postulated to be the result of their impaired release from the bone marrow or lack of clearance by the abnormal liver, or both.[266] An increase in platelet adhesiveness has been associated with elevated levels of factor VIII, the only clotting factor that has been noted to be increased in FHF.[105,266]

Marked coagulation defects do not necessarily imply overt hemorrhage, nor is hemorrhage always related to them, but injury to blood vessels, i.e., gastric erosions, is the most common course of clinically significant bleeding in FHF. Platelets and fresh blood are transfused in these instances, and fresh-frozen plasma may be used if hemostasis cannot be obtained. Fresh-frozen plasma and platelets have also been infused before any planned invasive procedures, but neither the fresh-frozen plasma nor clotting concentrate should be used prophylactically because they have not been beneficial and may have dire side effects.[105] A H_2 receptor blocking agent is routinely given and is effective in decreasing the incidence of gastrointestinal bleeding.[267] The value of routinely administered intravenous heparin to treat low grade DIC has not been demonstrated even though the half-life of heparin has been shortened by the reduced levels of antithrombin III.[264,266]

Metabolism

Severe hypoglycemia is attributed to the inability to mobilize liver glycogen, impaired gluconeogenesis, and an increased level of circulating insulin.[105] Massive hepatocellular necrosis has both depleted glucagon stores and compromised the ability to bind insulin to its hepatocyte receptors, the principal sites of insulin degradation.[268] Forty percent of adults with hepatic coma have been reported to have had at least one episode of hypoglycemia.[269]

Encephalopathy may obscure hypoglycemia or be intensified by it. It may occur precipitously, even in stage II, presenting as an abrupt worsening of the patient's neuropsychiatric status.[105] If undetected and untreated, irreversible brain damage and brain death are possible. Despite an infusion of 5 or 10% dextrose and water, the blood glucose level should be monitored at least every 12 hours and in some protocols as often as every hour. When hypoglycemia occurs, 50% glucose is given and once detected monitored closely, potentially requiring up to 2 kg of glucose per day.[270]

Portal Hypertension

The hepatic venous pressure gradient, used as an index of portal pressure, is elevated in 50 to 60% of patients with FHF.[241,271] Because none of the accepted causes of portal hypertension are present, the most plausible explanation for the increased portal pressure is the amplified intrahepatic resistance resulting from the massive hepatocellular necrosis and collapse of the reticulum framework.[241] Portal hypertension is absent in typical cases of viral hepatitis, which show limited necrosis, and the subsequent disappearance in those who survive FHF lends further credence to the documented studies.[241,271]

Ascites was a common occurrence in 60 to 70% of those studied and was related to the severity of the portal hypertension.[241,271] Renal failure was impaired in 64% of those with an abnormally high hepatic venous gradient but absent in those with a gradient less than 12 mm Hg. The mortality in these patients, most of whom had viral hepatitis, was 60 to 65%.[241,271]

Pancreatitis

Because of difficulty interpreting clinical findings and the serum amylase, the association between FHF and pancreatitis has most often been described postmortem. Death is seldom a result of pancreatitis, but moderate-to-severe pancreatitis was identified in 7 to 36% of postmortem examinations.[250,272-275] Ham and Fitzpatrick[272] reported pancreatitis in 33% of 42 patients, although the number of necropsies was not specified. Hepatitis serology was not available in 1968, when four cases of acute pancreatitis were reported and associated with "infectious hepatitis." Two patients developed FHF, and severe pancreatitis was found at autopsy. The serum amylase was normal in the only three in whom pancreatitis was considered. Upper gastrointestinal series were done in two patients, one with FHF, and those both suggested pancreatitis.[275]

In a prospective study of 60 patients with FHF, 14 had raised levels of serum amylase, and of the 11 patients autopsied, 10 had acute pancreatitis.[273] The use of the (P_3) isoenzyme in conjunction with marked elevation of serum lipase revealed biochemical pancreatitis in 12 of 35 patients; however, the mortality of that group was no greater than those who lacked this abnormality.[274] In none of the studies was the use of corticosteroid therapy or the etiologic agent a factor. The cause remains unknown, although there is a possibility this could have been viral or part of a multiple organ dysfunction system.[275]

Prognosis

Between 1969 and 1986, the overall mortality of FHF ranged from 70 to 97%. In 1969, Ritt and associates[250] described 31 deaths in 32 patients (97%), and 1 year later, Trey and colleagues[102] published a mortality rate of 78% among the 318 patients reported to the FHF Surveillance Study, an outcome influenced by age, the depth of coma, cause, and complications. The greatest mortality was in those older than 45 and the least in the patients with viral hepatitis.[102] Serologic tests for HA and HB eventually allowed the identification of non-A, non-B hepatitis, and in 1983, Gimson and associates[108] noted that the illness associated with HA was less severe and its survival with FHF was significantly greater. Bernuau and his coworkers investigated 15 patients with HB which they defined by the presence of IgM antibody to HBcAg. Factor V, age, the absence of HBsAg and the concentration of alpha fetoprotein were significantly different in survivors when compared to those who died. A univariate analysis showed age and the factor V level to be the most significant determinant between the survivors and those who died. A decreased factor V level was a more sensitive measurement of liver failure than the degree of coma present on the day of admission. Comparison between those with and without circulating HBsAG showed a significant higher rate of survival in patients who lacked the surface antigen. This appeared to indicate an exaggerated immune response with recovery from the acute infection resulting in a more limited necrosis and more efficient hepatocyte regeneration.[263]

O'Grady and associates evaluated the results of medical therapy in 588 patients with FHF (1973-85) in order to elicit factors that projected a poor prognosis.[104] They then retrospectively tested the value of their results in another 175 patients amassed between 1986 and 1987 and constructed criteria which indicated a prognosis so poor that medical therapy no longer was feasible and transplantation was necessary. Patients with acetaminophen induced FHF were considered separately and within this cohort, the presence of metabolic acidosis (pH < 7.3) indicated a 95% mortality, no matter the degree of encephalopathy. A prothrombin time greater than 100 seconds combined with a serum creatinine greater than 3.4 mg/dl and a Grade III-IV hepatic encephalopathy also predicted a fatal outcome and 77% of the deaths but a mortality of only 11.4% in the other acetaminophen-induced cases. Among those with nonacetaminophen-related FHF, a prothrombin time greater than 100 seconds alone was the most ominous. Any three of the following—prothrombin time greater than 50 seconds, FHF induced by non-A, non-B hepatitis, halothane or idiosyncratic drug reactions, age less than 10 or greater than 40, more than 7 days of jaundice before the onset of encephalopathy, or a bilirubin level greater than 17.5 mg/dl— predicted 95.5% of fatalities, with survival of 81.8% in the remaining cases (Table 54-13).[104]

Overall survival in those patients treated medically has

Table 54–13. Criteria Adopted in Kings College Hospital for Liver Transplantation in Fulminant Hepatic Failure

---
Acetaminophen
　pH <7.30 (regardless of grade of encephalopathy)
　or
　Prothrombin time >100 sec and serum creatinine >300 μmol/L in patients with grade III or IV encephalopathy.
Nonacetaminophen patients
　Prothrombin time >100 sec (regardless of grade of encephalopathy)
　or
　Any 3 of the following variables (regardless of grade of encephalopathy):
　　Age <10 or >40 years
　　Etiology—non A, non B hepatitis, halothane hepatitis, idiosyncratic drug reactions
　　Duration of jaundice before onset of encephalopathy >7 days
　　Prothrombin time >50 sec
　　Serum bilirubin >300 μmol/L

(From O'Grady, J. G., et al.: Early indicators of prognosis in fulminant hepatic failure. Gastroenterology, 97:439, 1989.)

varied from 3 to 30%; however, Brems and associates[276] compiled the results of transplantation done for FHF before 1987. Forty-one (including 6 operated on by us) patients had been transplanted with a 61% survival. Eight series, including that of Brems, reported transplantation for FHF from 1987 through 1992 (Table 54-14). A total of 197 patients were accepted as candidates. The greatest number were adults affected with viral hepatitis and considered for transplantation primarily because of cerebral edema. Twenty-one recovered spontaneously (11%), and 33 (17%) died either of complications making them unsuitable candidates or while awaiting a donor organ. Posttransplantation survival in individual series varied from 67 to 100%, a total of 71% (102/143); of those originally listed for transplantation 62.5% (123/197) survived. Most postoperative deaths resulted from complications of sepsis. Neurologic causes and graft loss were present to a lesser extent.

Because transplantation has become a definite option for treatment, every patient with acute hepatic failure should be transferred to a center where liver transplantation is done. Criteria for transplantation vary, but there is agreement that evidence of cerebral edema and increased ICP is an indication to begin to search for a donor organ. The Kings College criteria provide a means for early identification of transplant candidates before they develop advanced encephalopathy (see Table 54-13).[104] Bernuau and colleagues[265] reported the result of transplantation using coma and a factor V less than 20% to select those who require transplantation as opposed to those who will survive without it. Other transplant centers use the presence of coma, a rising bilirubin greater than 17.6 mg/dl, and uncorrectable coagulopathy as indications for proceeding. Survival of patients with halothane or idiosyncratic drug reaction (12.5%), non-A, non-B hepatitis (20%), and HB (39.5%) is definitely improved by liver transplantation.[106] FHF owing to Wilson's disease is almost invariably fatal within days to weeks, and early transplantation is indicated for these patients.

Ritt and associates[250] noted that despite the severity of liver disease, all deaths were not necessarily the result of "a critical decrease in functional hepatic mass alone" and "major complications or accompanying diseases were documented with surprising frequency and may have been the factors that prevented recovery in some instances." Assessment of hepatocyte loss by determination of the hepatocyte volume fraction (HVF) was made in 83% of 96 patients on whom autopsy was performed.[251] Death was ascribed to complications in 75% and solely to hepatic necrosis in the remaining 25%. The lowest HVF was calculated in the latter group, as opposed to levels in a range that could be considered compatible with recovery in the almost two thirds dying from cerebral edema, sepsis, or bleeding. FHF may in some be so severe as to obscure any hope of regeneration recovery, but in others recovery could occur if complications have not occurred.[251] A marked decrease in survival in those with complications has been shown graphically by O'Grady and coworkers (see Fig. 54-33).[106] The hyperdynamic circulation, increased cardiac output, and decreased systemic vascular resistance of FHF have a striking similarity to that of the "sepsis syndrome" or the multiple organ dysfunction syndrome.[281] Although started by any process that activates the systemic inflammatory response syndrome, i.e., bacteria, fungi, virus, endotoxin, or tissue injury, it may also be incited without evidence of infection in those who die from this. The inflammatory response ultimately damages the vascular endothelium, contributing to cerebral edema, adult respiratory distress syndrome, renal failure, and hepatic and gastrointestinal failure.[281] Bacterial translocation occurs when intestinal bacteria escape the lumen and in-

Table 54–14. Liver Transplantation in Fulminant Hepatic Failure

Author	Year	Number of Patients for Transplantation	Recovered without Transplantation, N (%)	Died Before Transplantation, N (%)	Survived Operation, N (%)
Brems[276]	1987	6			4/6 (66.7)
Bismuth[253]	1987	17			12/17 (71)
O'Grady[238]	1988	33			23/33 (70)
Emond[277]	1989	37	10 (27)	8 (21.6)	14/19 (74)
Iwatsuki[278]	1989	42			25/42 (61)
Van de Stadt[279]	1990	12	3 (25)	3 (25)	4/6 (66.7)
Sheil[280]	1991	27	6 (22)	13 (48)	8/8 (100)
Lidofsky[163]	1992	23	2 (8.7)	9 (39)	12/12 (100)
Total		197	21 (10.6)	33 (16.8)	102/143 (71)

vade the lymph nodes and portal system. It is absent in the presence of a healthy immune system, a normal intestinal tract, or a normal microflora but is described in those who are immunoincompetent with an altered intestinal epithelial barrier and a microflora modified by a variety of therapeutic agents. Endotoxin may also be absorbed from an injured gut into the portal blood.[282] Although a dysfunctional reticuloendothelial system has been demonstrated in FHF, patients with the same severe hepatocyte dysfunction but without hepatic encephalopathy had normal Kupffer cell function, raising the possibility that a normal reticuloendothelial system either removed or blocked the entry of unknown cerebral toxins into the systemic circulation.[283] The same authors also noted severe impairment of the reticuloendothelial system in patients who developed renal failure complicating FHF.[283] Deitch[284] postulated that gut endotoxin may be the link between gut failure in multiple organ dysfunction syndrome in those without obvious infection. Immunoincompetence in FHF, disruption of the epithelial barrier by manipulation or the inability to provide enteral nutrition, and inhibition of anaerobes by antibiotics provide the opportunity for overgrowth by fungi and gram-negative enteric bacteria; thus emphasizing another role of the gut in FHF apart from that of a source of significant blood loss or elaborator of cerebral toxins.

CIRRHOSIS

Cirrhosis is the end result of a variety of causes that produce chronic inflammatory change in liver cell injury with eventual distortion of the normal architecture. Anatomically it is "widespread hepatic fibrosis with nodule formation" resulting in parenchymal cell injury with a loss of hepatic function and fibrotic distortion producing portal hypertension.[91]

Cirrhosis is classified based on morphology and cause (Table 54-15). Anatomically the cirrhotic pattern is based on the size of the nodule:

Table 54-15. Classification of Cirrhosis

Morphology
  Micronodular
  Macronodular
  Mixed
Cause
  Established
    Alcohol
    Viral hepatitis
    Bile duct obstruction (intra, extra)
    Autoimmune
    Metabolic
    Drugs and toxin
    Venous outflow obstruction
    Jejunoileal bypass
  Debatable
    Nonalcoholic steatonecrosis
    Malnutrition
  Unknown
    Cryptogenic
Functional[4]

(Modified from Winkelman, E. I.: Cirrhosis. *In* Clinical Gastroenterology. 2nd Ed. Edited by E. A. Achkar, R. Farmer, and B. Fleshler. Philadelphia, Lea & Febiger, 1992.)

- Micronodular (diffuse uniform nodules 3 mm in diameter or less)
- Macronodular (nodules 3 mm to 5 cm in diameter)
- Mixed (an approximately equal number of micronodules and macronodules).[285]

The categories of cause are broad and characterized as to whether they are known, debatable, or unknown. Sherlock[91] attempts a functional assessment, which includes aspects of liver failure and portal hypertension and the status regarding whether the disease is progressive, regressive, or stable. The Child-Pugh classification is an attempt to characterize liver failure[27,28] (see Tables 54-3 and 54-4).

Cirrhosis becomes clinically apparent in the presence of hepatic insufficiency and portal hypertension. Portal hypertension without clinical evidence of liver disease is not diagnostic of cirrhosis but may be the presenting feature by virtue of splenomegaly and bleeding varices. Abnormalities of liver biochemistry associated with splenomegaly imply cirrhosis, and chronic changes in liver function require further investigation. Many cases are diagnosed by serendipity or found incidentally in 11 to 50% of patients at autopsy.[286] The definitive diagnosis is made by histologic evidence of diffuse fibrosis and nodule formation. Peritoneoscopy is indicated when portal hypertension is prominent with little or no evidence of liver disease, as seen in patients with compensated cirrhosis or noncirrhotic causes. European authors, however, have shown that biopsies done in conjunction with laparoscopy significantly decrease the number of false-negative results.[287,288] Using microscopic changes, special stains, cultures, and quantitative measurements of heavy metal, the biopsy findings can lead to etiologic diagnoses, evaluate activity, and provide the differential between two similar clinical presentations: i.e., fibrosis and cirrhosis, cirrhosis and alcoholic hepatitis, chronic active hepatitis and Wilson's disease. There is no therapy to reverse established cirrhosis other than to withdraw the toxin (alcohol, drug), remove the offending agent (copper, iron), or treat hepatitis B or C to halt progression. Treatment is supportive in the asymptomatic patient, but complications require directed care. These complications are primarily:

- Hepatic encephalopathy
- Portal hypertension and bleeding esophageal varices
- Ascites
- Spontaneous bacterial peritonitis
- Hepatorenal syndrome

Clinical Presentation

The signs and symptoms of cirrhosis are caused by hepatocellular dysfunction, portal hypertension, or both. Nonspecific complaints of fatigue, malaise, weakness, dyspepsia, and nausea and vomiting are the most common. Unexplained right upper quadrant pain is a problem in one third of patients. Fluid retention may disguise weight loss. Ascites occurs in 30 to 70% and is associated with a right pleural effusion in 10%. Edema precedes ascites in 20% but may be minimal or absent. Jaundice is seen in 65% of patients at one time or another, but persistent clinical icterus is indicative of a decompensating cirrhotic. The liver is palpable in 28 to 78%, and the spleen can be felt in 20 to 70% of patients; however, a nonpalpable spleen does not exclude the possibility of portal hypertension.[286] A friction rub over the liver suggests neoplasm, whereas a pulsatile liver and distended neck veins indicate right-sided cardiac failure or constrictive pericarditis.[286] Clubbing and cyanosis are nonspecific, but the presence of dyspnea in the upright position relieved by recumbency (platypnea) suggests a hepatopulmonary syndrome, which is accompanied by a Po_2 less than 70 mm Hg.[234] Thirty percent to 60% of patients manifest a hyperdynamic circulation, the cause of which remains unknown. Fever, seldom greater than 38°C, present for weeks without explanation and unresponsive to antibiotics, is seen in one third of patients with decompensated cirrhosis.[286] Epistaxis occurs in up to 40% but is secondary to capillary fragility and not coagulopathy.[16]

More than 80% of patients have carbohydrate intolerance, defined as a 2-hour postprandial glucose level of greater than 120 mg/dl, which does not require treatment nor develop significant clinical problems. True diabetes in cirrhotics is defined as a 2-hour postprandial blood glucose level of greater than 200 mg/dl.[268]

The incidence of peptic ulcer disease is no different than that seen in the noncirrhotic patient, but the number of patients with cirrhosis and cholelithiasis is twice that of others.[286]

Cirrhosis cannot be diagnosed by biochemical means, which only determine the degree of synthetic function, possibly confirm a cause, or characterize the clinical state at that specific point in time. Despite histologically proven cirrhosis, laboratory determinations may all be normal. The occurrence or persistence of hyperbilirubinemia strongly suggests worsening of the liver disease or superimposition of another disorder: i.e., alcoholic hepatitis, viral hepatitis, or hemolysis. Aminotransferase levels greater than 200 units raise similar questions, particularly in the presence of jaundice. Albumin concentration and prothrombin time are markers of synthetic function. Anemia may be secondary to blood loss, hemolysis, or interference in folic acid metabolism. Galactose elimination capacity and ^{14}C-aminopyrine breath test may be used to measure functioning liver cell mass quantitatively.[289]

Complications

Portal Hypertension and Esophageal Varices

Portal hypertension is the result of increased resistance to an increased portal blood flow, the latter secondary to a hyperdynamic splanchnic circulation, which in turn is the result of a hyperdynamic systemic circulation. As noted previously, a collateral circulation diverts the portal blood from the liver directly into the superior and inferior cava systems. The gastroesophageal junction, where the coronary vein and short gastric veins communicate with the azygous system to form esophageal varices, is clinically the most significant of these anastomoses. Superior, middle, and inferior hemorrhoidal veins come together to form rectal and sigmoid varices, whereas remnants of the fetal circulation pass through the falciform ligament to mesh with abdominal wall veins and produce a caput medusae, distended veins, and rarely an epigastric venous hum (Cruveilhier-Baumgarten syndrome). Varices are also found in the retroperitoneum, parietal peritoneum, omentum, adhesions, scars, colon, and about ostomies. Decompression via a spontaneous shunt into the left renal vein from splenic and adrenal veins may occur.[18]

Approximately 50% of all cirrhotics develop varices, but only 20 to 40% hemorrhage, 25 to 70% doing so within 2 years of the discovery.[290] Varices that develop in the gastric fundus, duodenum, anorectum, and colon may also bleed. Hoskins and coworkers[291] believe that anorectal varices and hemorrhoids coexist but are separate entities, suggesting that the development of anorectal varices reflects severe portal hypertension that can bleed significantly; however, the prevalence of hemorrhoids is greater than that of rectal varices by a wide margin, even though portal hypertension can be present in most patients with hemorrhoids but who lack rectal varices. Significant bleeding has been reported in a few cases of varices elsewhere in the colon and intestine.[291] Ruptured abdominal varices producing hemoperitoneum have been reported in only six patients but should be suspected whenever sudden abdominal pain and distention occur.[292]

Diagnosis of Esophageal Varices. Esophageal varices are best diagnosed by fiberoptic endoscopy. Gastric varices can be visualized but are often mistaken for large gastric folds and neither recognized nor visualized. Barium studies of the esophagus are seldom, if ever, ordered but when done with expertise and care can demonstrate serpiginous filling defects, mainly in the lower third but that may also fill the entire esophagus (Fig. 54-38). Rarely, a routine chest film may show a retrocardiac paravertebral density, which represents paraesophageal collateral vessels. Endoscopic ultrasound studies can define the disease as well as differentiate gastric varices from other gastric abnormalities (Fig. 54-39). Splenoportography has been replaced by selective celiac and superior mesenteric angiography, whose venous phase demonstrates the splenic and portal veins as well as the collateral circulation (see Fig. 54-26). Excellent visualization of the portal system and collaterals is available with percutaneous transhepatic portography, but this is seldom necessary. Doppler ultrasound provides a means of evaluating the presence or absence and direction of blood flow as well as identifying thrombosis and intraluminal masses. The enhanced CT scan and MRI are also available but seldom necessary because they add little but additional cost.

Diagnosis of Portal Hypertension. Portal venous pressure is measured indirectly by catheterization of the hepatic vein. The catheter is wedged into an intrahepatic vein and the recorded hepatic vein wedge pressure equals that of the sinusoidal venous pressure. A zero reference point of intra-abdominal pressure is determined by withdrawing the catheter into the hepatic vein or vena cava, and this value subtracted from the hepatic vein wedge pressure determines the hepatic vein portal gradient, which is a more accurate measure of the portal pressure.[293] If necessary, umbilical vein catheterization or transhepatic portal catheterization can directly measure the portal vein pressure.[294] The normal pressure is 3 to 6

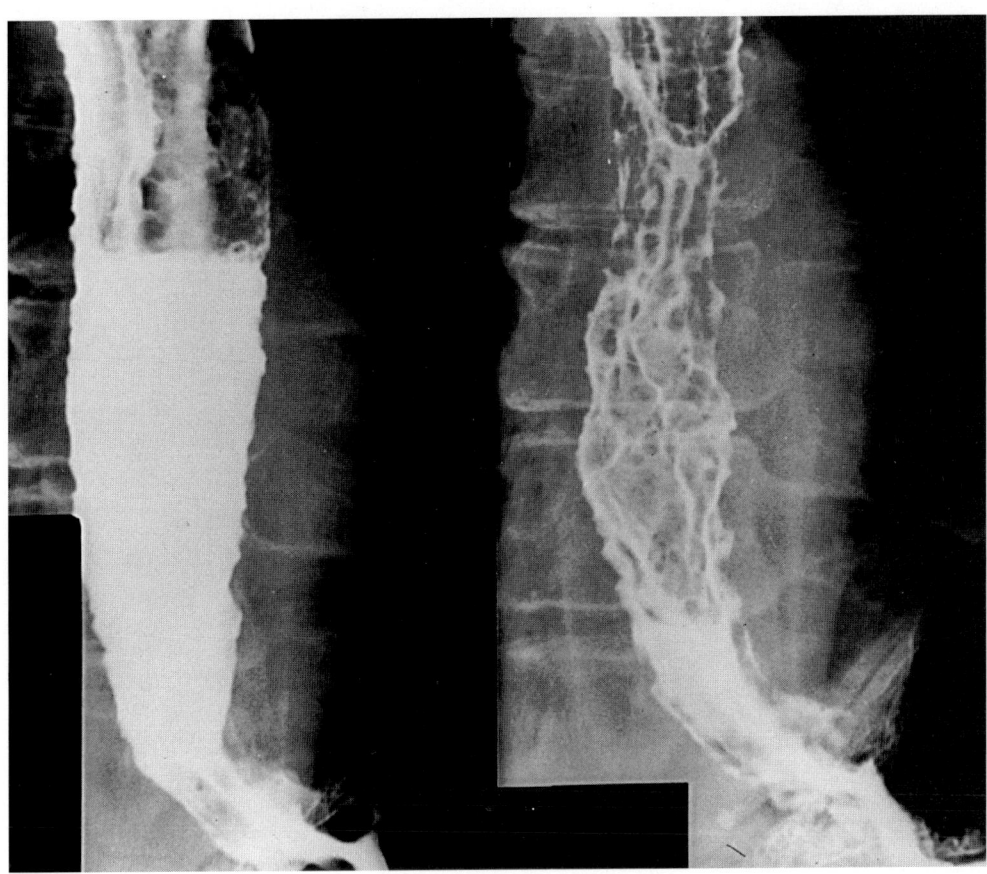

Fig. 54-38. Barium swallow of the esophagus. Filled study shows irregularity of walls with varices superior to the barium. In the air-contrast study, the multiple serpiginous filling defects represent another view of esophageal varices.

mm Hg; higher values are those of portal hypertension;[91] however, variceal bleeding occurs only when the hepatic vein portal gradient is 12 mm Hg or greater, although hemorrhage does not necessarily occur at higher levels.[295,296]

Portal hypertension is clinically classified by the anatomic site of increased resistance (Table 54-16). Prehepatic (extrahepatic) portal hypertension is the result of a partial or complete obstruction of the portal system at any point proximal to entry into the liver: i.e., splenic or portal vein thrombosis, or an increased splanchnic blood flow from arteriovenous fistula. Posthepatic (suprahepatic) portal hypertension is caused by interference in the venous outflow beyond the central vein: i.e., veno-occlusive disease, Budd-Chiari syndrome. The liver remains the major point of obstruction (intrahepatic, hepatic). Once attributed to distortion and compression of the postsinusoidal drainage by regenerating nodules, there is now evidence that the increased resistance lies within the sinusoid, secondary to collagenization of the space of Disse, pressure of enlarged hepatocytes, and contractile myofibroblasts that surround sinusoids and venules.[297,298] Sherlock[91] characterizes portal hypertension by the value of the hepatic vein portal gradient, defining a presinusoidal type in which the level is normal or less than normal as seen in splenic vein thrombosis. Any measurement greater than 6 mm Hg is indicative of a hepatic cause: i.e., intrahepatic or postsinusoidal.[91] A more complicated hemodynamic classification relates portal venous pressure and hepatic vein wedge pressure in different areas of the liver and portal system, but this is not generally used because of its complexity and overlap.[293]

Variceal Rupture. The actual cause of variceal rupture and bleeding remains undecided. Esophagitis secondary to gastric reflux, once a prominent theory, has never been confirmed. Although varices are understood not to bleed when the hepatic vein portal gradient is 12 mm Hg or less, not every patient with this level hemorrhages.[295,296,299] Lebrec and associates[300] reported a series of 100 patients with alcoholic cirrhosis in whom the pressure and size of varices were not related to the degree of portal hypertension, but rather the risk of bleeding was significantly related to the size of the varices. Reynolds[301] noted that his group has never been able to relate portal pressure to bleeding in those patients with established portal hypertension and has used the hepatic vein portal gradient only to eliminate candidates for shunt surgery when this number was such as to indicate that the patient had not bled from varices. Conversely, Conn[302] cites volcanic eruption as an illustration in that "although both volcanoes and varices bulge before they erupt, it is the pressure within that is the ultimate determinant" to display his disbelief. Polio and Groszman[299] suggest that the inability to identify a single factor implies an interaction between local factors, portal pressure, and variceal size as demonstrated by LaPlace's law: $(T = TPr/w)$, where T = tension, TP = transmural pressure, r = radius, and w = thickening of the wall. The tension within the vessel wall remains in equilibrium with the expanding force, and if exceeded the

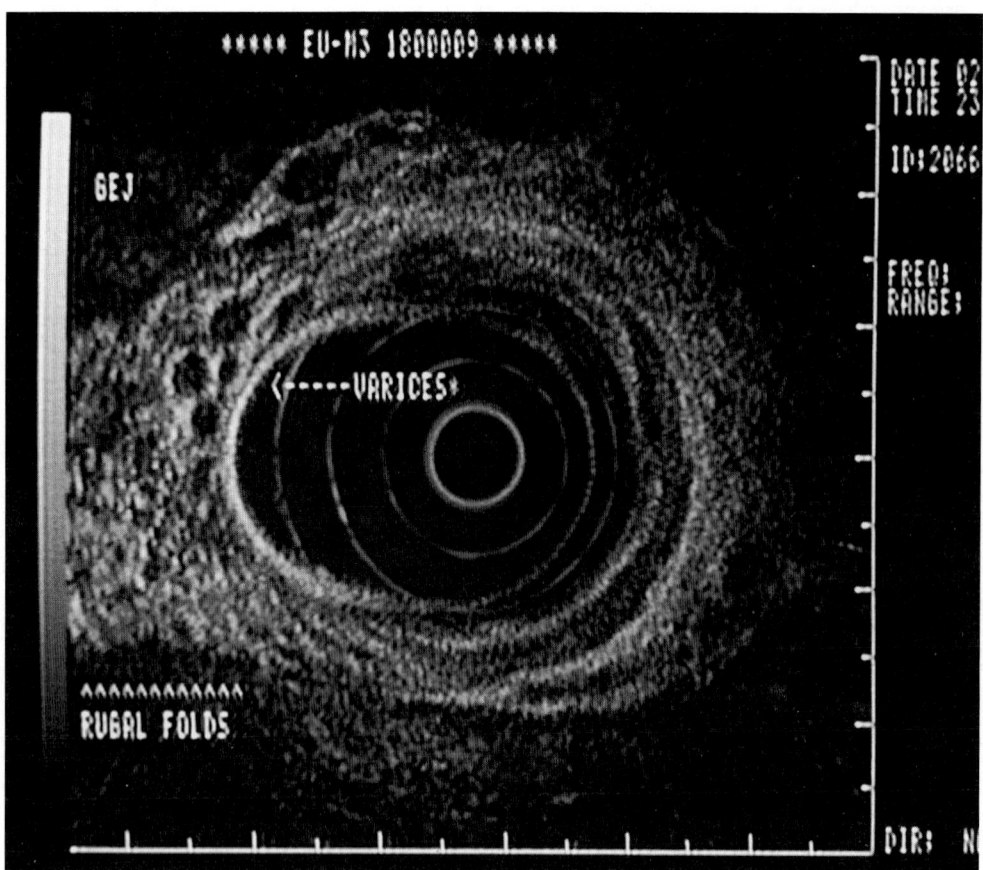

Fig. 54-39. Endoscopic ultrasonography of cardioesophageal junction demonstrating varices. (From Achkar, E. A., Farmer, R., and Fleshler, B. (eds.): Clinical Gastroenterology. Philadelphia, Lea & Febiger, 1992, p. 588.)

wall bursts. In this theory, the presence of support to the vessel wall is also important, because its absence places the varix at greater risk for rupture.[299]

Treatment of Bleeding in Portal Hypertension. Hematemesis is the initial symptom in 5 to 30% of cirrhotic patients and, although present in 20 to 40% of all cases, is not always the result of variceal hemorrhage.[290,303,304] Identification of the bleeding site is the first priority after resuscitation because 20 to 60% bleed from lesions other than esophageal varices.[305] Most are attributed to portal hypertensive gastropathy.[306,307] Peptic ulcer disease, mostly gastric ulcer, plays a minor role, constituting 6 to 10%, whereas esophagitis and Mallory-Weiss tears account for 3 to 4.5% of bleeding lesions. Gastric and duodenal erosions are seen but may be difficult to distinguish from bleeding secondary to portal hypertensive gastropathy.[308-310] Gastric varices, found in association with esophageal varices in 16% of all cases, occurred alone 12% of the time.[311] Gastric varices, which remain undiscovered despite endoscopy, may be the source of repeated bouts of gastrointestinal bleeding until diagnosed by the venous phase of selective splenic arterial angiography.[311] Portal hypertensive gastropathy may also go unrecognized until evaluated by a more experienced endoscopist.

Bleeding varices are an emergency not only because of the blood loss, but also their presence in decompensated cirrhosis has the potential to create liver failure. Contrary to general understanding, varices do not always bleed catastrophically and can ooze or bleed slowly. Thirty percent to 48% of variceal bleeding will stop spontaneously.[305,312] These individuals nevertheless require skilled, meticulous care, both medical and nursing, and initially should be afforded this in an ICU with appropriate treatment facilities. Blood volume should be restored using whole blood, and the coagulopathy, worsened by multiple transfusions, may require fresh-frozen plasma, platelets, and calcium. If the prothrombin time is unduly prolonged, a trial of vitamin K (10 mg) is administered for 3 days. Initially a large-bore Ewald tube is placed to evacuate blood clots and is then replaced by a nasogastric tube to provide continuous suction. Magnesium sulfate and enemas cleanse the gut, but in

Table 54-16. Classification of Portal Hypertension

Prehepatic (extrahepatic)
   Obstruction of portal system to porta hepatis
   Increased splanchnic blood flow (rare)
Hepatic (intrahepatic)
   Clinical—major point of obstruction
   Physiologic—anatomic zone of obstruction measured hemodynamically by relationship between portal venous pressure and wedged hepatic venous pressure
      Presinusoidal (could include prehepatic)[91]
      Sinusoidal
      Postsinusoidal
Posthepatic (suprahepatic)
   Obstruction of inferior vena cava and/or hepatic veins
   Right-sided cardiac failure

the absence of encephalopathy, lactulose is not necessarily ordered. Although there is no evidence that H₂ antagonist receptors prevent recurrent variceal bleeding, these are given in the hope of preventing hemorrhage from acute ulceration, erosive gastroduodenitis, or portal hypertensive gastropathy.[313] Sedation should be avoided, but when indicated chlordiazepoxide may be used, particularly in alcoholics. When liver studies are not grossly abnormal, sedation may be used more liberally.

Acute Variceal Rupture. This complication may be controlled by:

- Pharmacologic agents
- Balloon tamponade
- Injection sclerotherapy
- Endoscopic variceal ligation
- Portosystemic shunt created surgically or transhepatically (TIPS)
- Esophageal Transection

Pharmacologic Agents. Because of its availability and ease of administration, vasopressin is widely used as the first-line treatment. Its vasoconstricting action decreases the splanchic circulation, reducing the flow into the portal system with subsequent lessening of the portal pressure. Alternatively, it may affect the contractile myofibroblasts in the sinusoids.[314] Originally given selectively into the superior mesenteric artery to avoid its systemic effects, it controlled hemorrhage in 27 of 28 patients.[315] When compared with peripheral intravenous infusion in randomly controlled trials, both routes were found to be equally effective with similar complications but no increase in survival.[316] A continuous infusion of 0.4 U per minute was effective in controlling hemorrhage in only 53%. Complications of its vasoconstricting action are hypertension, ventricular arrhythmias, myocardial ischemia and infarction, cerebrovascular accidents, mesenteric angina, lower extremity pain, and skin necrosis. Abdominal colic and profuse diarrhea are so common that their absence suggests a lack of therapeutic effect. The addition of the vasodilator nitroglycerin, 300 µg per minute, to an infusion of vasopressin controlled hemorrhage in 68% as opposed to 40% receiving vasopressin (Pitressin) alone. There was only a single complication as opposed to seven in the vasopressin group.[317] Sublingual nitroglycerin plus intravenous vasopressin studied against vasopressin alone also favored the combination with a statistically significant less number of complications; however, mortality remained the same.[318] Transdermal administration of nitroglycerin alone in the absence of bleeding was studied hemodynamically, and the results strongly suggested that it decreased the hepatic vein portal gradient by reducing vascular resistance without a change in the hepatic blood flow; however, it did decrease the mean arterial pressure by 13%.[319] Although still used as an initial procedure, there are questions as to the efficacy, and it should still be considered only as an emergency treatment.

Somatostatin has been as successful as vasopressin in the control of bleeding but without the complications;[320,321] however, not all studies have agreed to its efficacy, and its cost is almost prohibitive.[322]

Balloon Tamponade. Esophageal tamponade with the two-balloon (gastric and esophageal), multilumen Sengstaken-Blakemore tube (SB), modified by an aspirating lumen above the esophageal balloon or the Linton-Nachlas (single gastric balloon) tube (LN), has been effective in stopping variceal hemorrhage in greater than 90% of the patients,[323-326] although in two other studies, success was limited to 40 and 73%.[327,328] Both tubes were effective in controlling variceal hemorrhage, but the SB was more successful with esophageal varices, whereas the LN was better suited to bleeding gastric varices.[324] Unfortunately, one fourth to two thirds rebled after removal of the tube. If bleeding continues or recurs after successful placement and the tube has remained properly placed, repeat endoscopy is indicated to ensure the absence of another bleeding site.[305,323,325-328] Chojkier and Conn[327] noted that tamponade was more successful in those proved to be bleeding from varices endoscopically than in those diagnosed clinically.[327]

The presence of skilled, experienced ICU personnel is extremely important because balloon tamponade is traumatic and painful to the majority of patients. Sedation while passing the tube and during its use is invariably necessary. A new tube is used for each patient, and before insertion it is inspected to ensure the patency of the channels and integrity and capacity of the balloons (Fig. 54-40). The stomach is emptied to avoid aspiration, and if the patient exhibits stage III or IV hepatic encephalopathy, endotracheal intubation is indicated to protect the airway further. The head of the bed is raised and the well-lubricated tube passed through the nose (or mouth) into the stomach. The gastric balloon is filled with 100 to 130 ml of air and then withdrawn until resistance is felt at the gastroesophageal junction. After auscultatory and radiologic evidence that the balloon is seated properly in the fundus, the gastric balloon is filled to its predetermined capacity and fixed firmly to the nose (or corner of the mouth) without using external fixation. A pad is placed between the tube and nares and upper lip to prevent pressure necrosis. The esophageal balloon is then inflated to a pressure of 20 to 30 mm Hg (a value greater than the expected portal vein pressure). This is not a universal practice because the esophageal balloon is not always inflated if there is evidence that bleeding has stopped. Someone should always be at the bedside to observe closely and, if respiratory distress occurs, immediately cut and remove the tube. Balloon pressure and traction are checked frequently, and after 24 to 48 hours, the esophageal balloon is deflated and traction decreased, leaving the gastric balloon inflated for another 24 hours. If bleeding recurs, the process is repeated for another 24 to 48 hours, and if not successful, either sclerotherapy or surgery should be undertaken. Although balloon tamponade is considered by most to be only temporary and a prelude to prompt sclerotherapy or portal systemic shunt, Panes and colleagues[325] and Paquet and Foussher[328] report sustained hemostasis in 47 and 59%. Factors that affect the eventual outcome are control of the bleeding, liver function, and the degree of hypovolemia when the tamponade was begun. Death occurs more frequently from liver failure rather than from hemorrhage itself.

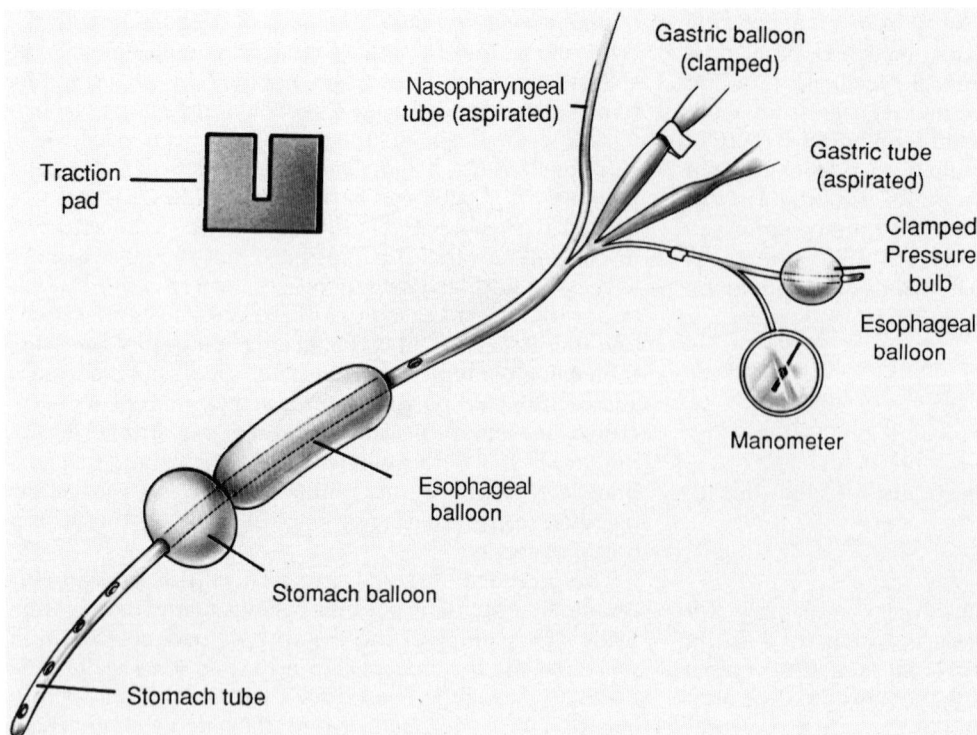

Fig. 54-40. Senstaken-Blakemore tube with nasogastric aspirating tube. (From Achkar, E. A., Farmer, R., and Fleshler, B. (eds.): Clinical Gastroenterology. Philadelphia, Lea & Febiger, 1992, p. 590.)

The hazards are considerable, with asphyxia by pharyngeal or tracheal obstruction secondary to upward migration of the balloon and esophageal rupture of perforation the most dreaded.[324,326,327] Aspiration is common but can be eliminated by the use of intubation and the esophageal port, which is placed on suction to drain secretions that pool above the proximal balloon.[325]

Sclerotherapy. Sclerotherapy is successful in controlling acute variceal hemorrhage 75 to 95% of the time.[329] These results plus the availability of skilled endoscopists have made it the emergency treatment used in most hospitals. After initial control, which may be obtained at the time of the diagnostic endoscopy, two to three further sessions of sclerotherapy are done 2 to 3 days apart during the first hospitalization. Sclerotherapy has been shown to be more effective than conservative medical therapy, the latter defined as vasopressin or balloon tamponade.[328,330,331]

If significant bleeding does recur within hours to days of the initial sclerotherapy, balloon tamponade is reinstituted, and this is followed by another trial of sclerotherapy. If uncontrolled, a shunting procedure should be considered.[305] Cello and co-workers[332] have agreed that sclerotherapy is the first line of treatment, followed thereafter by surgical shunting if sclerotherapy fails.

Complications may be classified as side effects or local systemic complications. Chest pain in 25 to 50% and low grade fever without an obvious cause are the most common side effects, whereas esophageal ulceration, a potential source of bleeding in 40 to 60%, usually occurs 1 to 5 days after a procedure. Esophageal perforation may happen 5 to 7 days later in 1 to 2%, and esophageal stricture is a later phenomenon that occurs in 3%. Pulmonary function is undisturbed despite nonspecific changes in chest radiographs and exudative pleural effusions that are seen in otherwise well patients. These resolve without difficulty in approximately 50%. Various isolated systemic complications have been reported.[333]

Percutaneous transhepatic venography provides access to the coronary vein through which varices can be embolized with Gelfoam or thrombin. Hemorrhage is controlled in 80%, but this is a procedure of last resort in poor risk patients. It requires a high degree of technical expertise and is associated with a high incidence of rebleeding and complications.[334]

Endoscopic variceal ligation is the newest method for the control of variceal bleeding. A technique similar to rubber band ligation of hemorrhoids allows the endoscopist to place a small rubber band around the bleeding site to control the hemorrhage. In a randomized trial, endoscopic sclerotherapy and endoscopic ligation were compared in 129 patients, demonstrating control of active bleeding to be equally effective in 75 and 86%. Of these, 48 and 36% had recurrent bleeding, but neither this nor the number of procedures, transfusions, or length of hospitalization was significantly different. Patients rated as Child A and B treated with ligation had an overall better rate of survival, but no difference was noted in those classified as Child C. Significantly fewer complications were noted.[335]

Shunt Procedures. All types of shunts have been used in emergency situations, but the end-to-end shunt has been the most used; however, because the surgical shunts as emergency treatment are associated with as much as 50% mortality, it has been avoided, particularly in the poor risk patient.[336-338] Nevertheless, Orloff and colleagues[339] have continued to operate on all patients with alcoholic cirrhosis and bleeding varices notwithstanding their risk status. Within 8 hours of admission, they undergo an end-to-side portacaval shunt. The operative mortality of 180 patients was 42%, 60% of whom died of hepatic failure.[339] Cello et al.,[332] in a controlled study comparing esophageal sclerotherapy with portacaval shunt in 64 patients classified as Child C, reported a 50% mortality for esophageal sclerotherapy and 56% mortality for portacaval shunt, noting that one half of the survivors of sclerotherapy eventually required a portacaval shunt ("surgical rescue") because of recurrent bleeding. Villeneuve and associates[337] operated on 36 patients characterized as having mild-to-moderate disease, with seven deaths (19%), whereas in the three patients with severe disease, the mortality was 100%.

Because the mesocaval (H graft) shunt can be done with greater technical ease, more quickly with less blood loss, and more effective control of bleeding and can be used in patients with massive ascites, it was considered by some as the preferred procedure in the acute situation. Although still used by many in modified forms, the increased incidence of hepatic encephalopathy, propensity for spontaneous thrombosis, and recurrent bleeding have limited its indications to catastrophic variceal bleeding or to those whose anatomy does not allow the use of other more standard shunts.[340]

Transjugular Intrahepatic Portal Systemic Shunt Anatomically the transjugular intrahepatic portal systemic shunt (TIPS) represents the nonoperative creation of a portal systemic shunt, whereas dynamically it is an intrahepatic small-caliber interpositional shunt with partial portal decompression.[341] To date, published series of 25 and 60 patients and two as yet unpublished series (cited with the author's permission by Conn) have documented the following:[341-343]

- Safe, reliable creation of an intrahepatic shunt
- Effective control of portal pressure and variceal hemorrhage
- Low incidence of complications

Thus far, candidates for the TIPS procedure have been those with cirrhosis, the majority alcoholic Child class B and C with active or chronic variceal hemorrhage resistant to sclerotherapy. Many were awaiting transplantation. Coagulopathy was not a contraindication. The catheter is placed via either the right jugular or the femoral vein. Using a transjugular needle, it is advanced beyond the hepatic vein into the hepatic parenchyma and directed toward the right portal vein under the guidance of ultrasonography. The portal vein is opacified and an angiographic wire passed into the main portal vein and the stent advanced to cover the entire parenchymal tract from the hepatic vein into the portal vein, diverting portal blood from the collateral circulation (Fig. 54-41). Two types of shunt are available: the Palmaz, a relatively rigid metal stent expandable by a balloon to a diameter of 12 to 16 mm (Fig. 54-42), and the Walstent, a more flexible wire mesh stent self-expanding to a maximum diameter of 10 mm

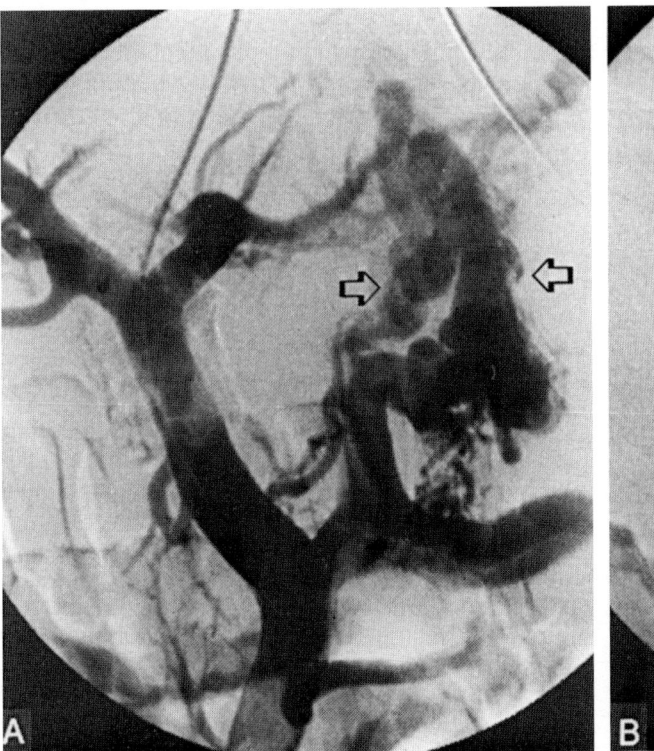
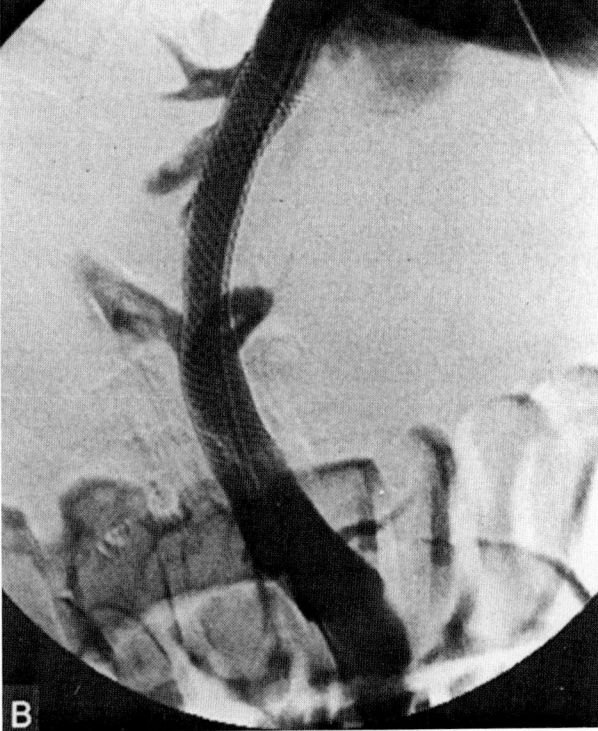

Fig. 54-41. *A,* Portal venogram before transjugular intrahepatic shunt (TIPS) (arrow indicates esophageal varices). *B,* Portal venogram following TIPS reveals total diversion through shunt and no flow into varices. (From LaBerge, J. M., et al.: Transjugular intrahepatic shunt: preliminary results in 25 patients. J. Vasc. Surg., *16:*258, 1992.)

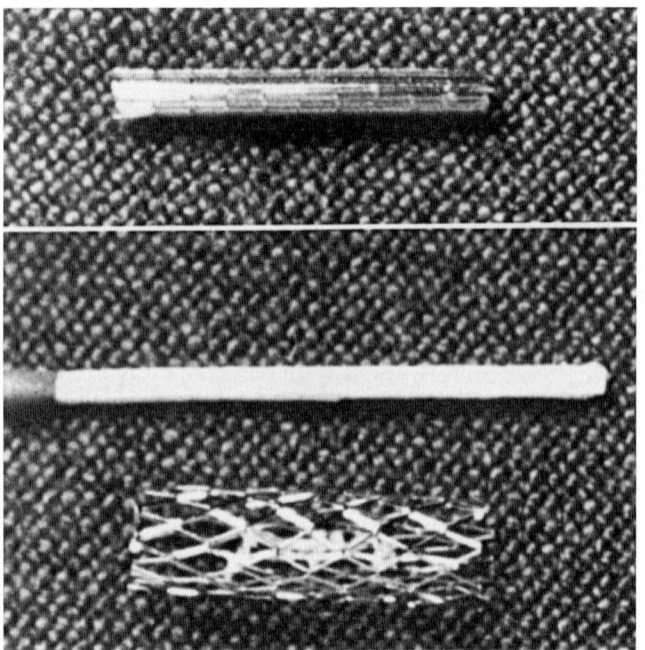

Fig. 54-42. The Polmaz stent. *Top,* Undistended. *Bottom,* Distended in comparison with a matchstick. (From Conn, H. O.: Transjugular intrahepatic portasystemic shunt: the state of mind. Hepatology, *17*:148, 1993.)

(Fig. 54-43). Both have pros and cons, but the Wallstent is placed with less technical difficulty, and its use has decreased the time required for the procedure.[343,344] The coronary vein is not embolized routinely because this carries an inherent risk. Follow-up is by duplex Doppler ultrasound or angiography. This radiologic intervention requires a highly skilled angiographer who, when using state-of-the-art equipment, can complete the procedure in 1 to 3 hours.

The shunt is localized successfully in 92 to 100% with a 30-day mortality of 2 to 28%. Only 3% of these deaths were related to hepatic failure or hemorrhage. The overall mortality ranged from 6 to 26% but encompassed months to a few years.[341-343] Variceal bleeding was controlled in 88 to 100% and was associated with decreased portal pressure in all, although not always to less than 12 mm Hg. Ascites, when present, was controlled in 70 to 100% of cases, and refractory ascites in a single case secondary to the Budd-Chiari syndrome cleared following TIPS.[341-345]

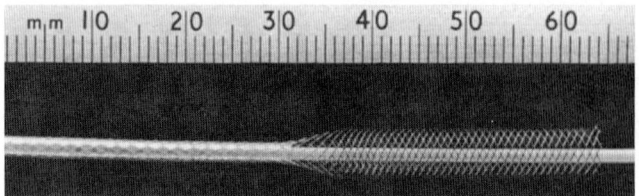

Fig. 54-43. The Wallstent stent undistended on the left and partially distended on the right. (From Conn, H. O.: Transjugular intrahepatic portasystemic shunt: the state of mind. Hepatology, *17*:148, 1993.)

Additional advantages are the extra time gained to increase the well-being of the transplant candidate and the use of an intrahepatic site, which spares the transplant surgeon the extra effort of dealing with an intra-abdominal surgical shunt.[343]

Hepatic encephalopathy, the most commonly reported complication, occurred in 3 to 20% of cases, mostly in patients with a prior history of encephalopathy.[341,343] Most were easily controlled medically. Stenosis or occlusion of the shunt occurred in 5 to 15% of cases but was corrected by re-expansion of the stent or insertion of a larger one.[343] Other infrequent complications have been reported: perforation of either gallbladder or liver capsule, hemobilia, septic shock, fever, intravascular hemolysis, and pulmonary emboli and partial portal vein obstruction occlusion.[343]

A randomized, prospective study of sclerotherapy versus TIPS in 39 patients concluded that both were equally effective in treatment of variceal hemorrhage but lacked the numbers in follow-up to finalize any conclusions.[346]

Esophageal transection using an auto suture stapling device has been employed in both emergency and elective settings. The mortality in elective procedures ranges from 10.5 to 20% and in emergencies 28 to 73%. Ninety percent of the 73% deaths were patients with severe decompensation, again stressing the importance of hepatic function. Recurrent bleeding was noted in 2% of patients so treated.[347-349]

Recurrent Variceal Bleeding. Because 70% of patients surviving a variceal hemorrhage will most likely rebleed within 2 years with a high mortality rate, prevention of recurrent bleeding is a continuing and important part of therapy.[305]

Sclerotherapy. The goal of sclerotherapy is to eradicate variceal channels by producing fibrosis. This requires an individualized program of repeated endoscopic sessions extending over several months, which my or may not completely eliminate all varices. Once accomplished, surveillance is required every 3 to 6 months, but this has not been standard practice. Japanese workers reported a 9-year prospective study on 1000 patients consecutively treated with sclerotherapy. *Esophageal varices were completely eradicated* in 77.8%. Sclerotherapy was done weekly until varices were eradicated with follow up endoscopy every 3 months. The cumulative nonbleeding rate at 5 years was 94.5%. Other independent factors influencing survival rate were the Child status, eradication, and whether the indication for sclerosis was acute, elective, or prophylactic.[350] Survival at 5 years was 54.1% in those without hepatoma.[350] Multiple trials of sclerotherapy have compared it with supportive medical treatment and beta-adrenergic blocking agents. These studies have shown sclerotherapy to decrease the risk of bleeding but overall not to affect definitely survival;[351-355] however, although a large Danish study showed no significant difference between conservative treatment and sclerotherapy, as indicated by the duration of bleeding, number of transfusions, and immediate mortality, when patients receiving sclerotherapy were stratified to account for the degree of encephalopathy and ascites, improved survival became statistically significant albeit a weak trend.[356] When compared with surgical shunting, recurrent bleeding was significantly greater, again without a long-term difference in survival.[332,357,358] To compare the relative efficacy of sclerotherapy and the dissplenorenal shunt (DSRS) in the prevention of recurrent variceal bleeding, Henderson and colleagues randomized 72 patients to receive one or the other. Patients treated with sclerotherapy had a significantly better survival than those receiving the shunt (p = 0.02); however, only 3% of the shunt group rebled, whereas sclerotherapy failed to control bleeding and 35% required "surgical rescue" by DSRS. Almost 60% of these had bleeding from either gastric varices or portal hypertensive gastropathy.[359] By consensus, endoscopic sclerotherapy is an acceptable therapy for control of variceal hemorrhage, both emergency and elective, and although there is rarely a significant difference in survival with any of the methods, sclerotherapy with surgical rescue is the optimal approach.[332,357-359]

Surgical Treatment. Before undertaking surgical therapy to control recurrent variceal bleeding, it is necessary to be sure that variceal decompression is necessary, the anatomy suitable for a shunting procedure, and the reserve hepatic function sufficient. Once decided, this is achieved in a number of ways:

- End-to-side portacaval shunt
- Side-to-side portacaval shunt
- Distal splenorenal shunt (DSRS)
- Interposition mesocaval shunt
- Partial portal decompression

The **end-to-side portacaval shunt** (Fig. 54-44) is a direct anastomosis between the portal vein and inferior vena cava that diverts all portal blood flow from the liver, whereas the **side-to-side shunt** is designed to allow a portion of the portal flow to perfuse the hepatic circulation (Fig. 54-45); unfortunately, this is seldom achieved because the sinusoidal blood flows retrograde into the vena cava, producing a totally diverting shunt in 65 to 80% of these patients.[18] This provides the physiologic rationale for the use of the portal vein as an outflow tract to decompress the liver in patients with refractory ascites or the Budd-Chiari syndrome. Four randomized, controlled studies were reported between 1971 and 1981 comparing conventional medical therapy with the portacaval shunt.[360-363] Variceal bleeding was significantly decreased in all those treated with portacaval shunts, and although survival was longer in the postsurgical patients, neither it nor the incidence of encephalopathy (20 to 49%) was statistically significant. Although there remain staunch supporters of the portacaval shunt, it has largely been displaced by the distal splenorenal shunt when applicable.

The **DSRS (Warren shunt)** was devised to decompress gastroesophageal varices via the short gastric veins, spleen, and splenic vein by anastomosis of the distal splenic vein to the left renal vein.[364] Hepatic perfusion is maintained by the hypertensive splanchnic blood flow maintained through the superior mesenteric vein and portal vein. Gastric devascularization and coronary azygous disconnection are an essential part of the entire procedure (Fig. 54-46).[364] Although the survival curves of Child class A and B patients when comparing the DSRS and nonselective shunt did not differ statistically, survival was better in the nonalcoholic than the alcoholic patient.[366] After several years, angiography revealed the evolution of transpancreatic, colonic, and transgastric collateral vessels, which siphoned blood from the high pressure portal circulation into the lower pressure splenorenal anastomosis. The original procedure was then modified by dissecting the complete splenic vein from the pancreas, interrupting the splenocolic ligament and ligating the left gastric venous system resulting in an increased survival of the alcoholic patient. Bleeding is controlled in 88 to 97% of cases, and although rebleeding secondary to thrombosis of the shunt

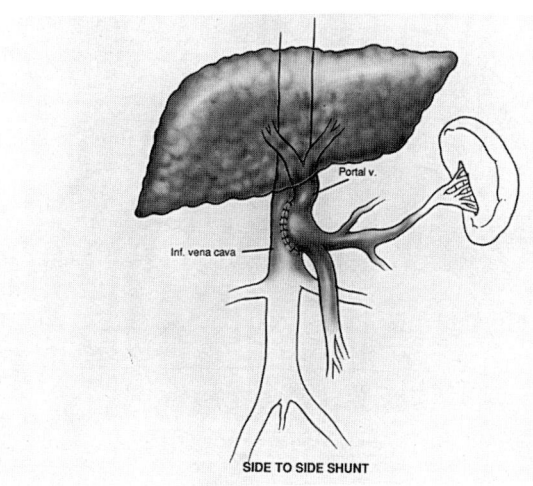

Fig. 54-45. Partial diversion of portal blood into the inferior vena cava while continuing to perfuse the liver. (From Achkar, E. A., Farmer, R., and Fleshler, B. (eds.): Clinical Gastroenterology. Philadelphia, Lea & Febiger, 1992, p. 592.)

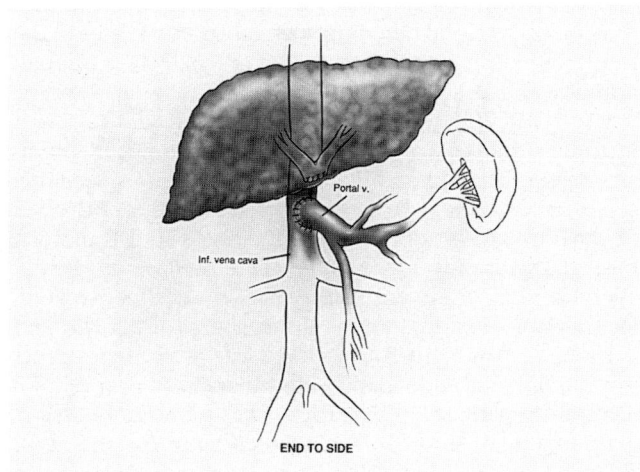

Fig. 54-44. Complete division of portal blood directly into inferior vena cava. (From Achkar, E. A., Farmer, R., and Fleshler, B. (eds.): Clinical Gastroenterology. Philadelphia, Lea & Febiger, 1992, p. 591.)

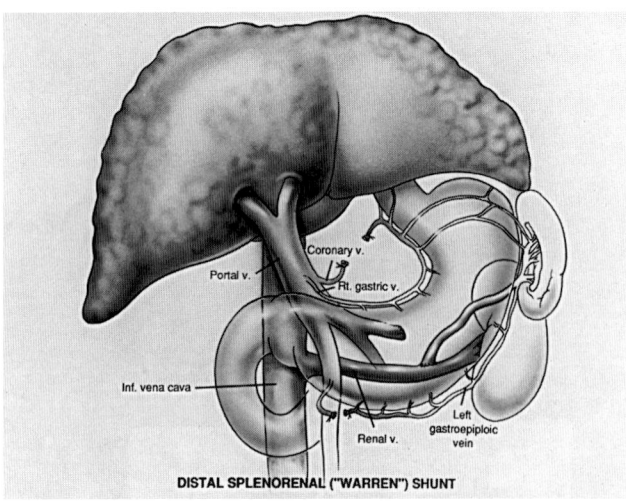

Fig. 54–46. Diversion of a portion of the portal blood into the vena cava, but the remainder continues to perfuse the liver. (From Achkar, E. A., Farmer, R., and Fleshler, B. (eds.): Clinical Gastroenterology. Philadelphia, Lea & Febiger, 1992, p. 592.)

occurs in 3 to 14%, the thrombosis can be surgically corrected if noted within 2 weeks. Thrombosis over the long-term follow-up is present less than 2% of the time. Shunt stenosis in the late follow-up period is suspected with the recurrence of bleeding and diagnosed and treated with catheterization and balloon dilatation.[364] Milliken and coworkers[365] followed Child class A and B patients with DSRS for 10 years and reported encephalopathy in 3% at 2 years, 12% at 3 to 6 years, and 27% at 10 years, significantly less than in those with nonselective shunts. Surgical skill plays a major role in the success of this procedure, which is related to the technical difficulty of the splenic vein dissection. The DSRS has been accepted by most as the treatment of choice.

The **interposition mesocaval shunt (H-graft)** uses a large-diameter prosthesis to shunt blood from the superior mesenteric vein to the inferior vena cava (Fig. 54–47).

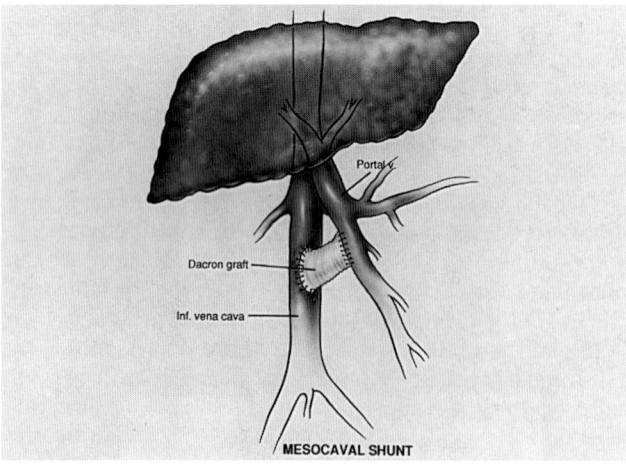

Fig. 54–47. Mesocaval Shunt. See text. (From Achkar, E. A., Farmer, R., and Fleshler, B. (eds.): Clinical Gastroenterology. Philadelphia, Lea & Febiger, 1992, p. 593.)

Originally conceived as a selective shunt, it was later shown to divert portal blood totally giving it no advantage over the portacaval shunt, resulting in a comparable incidence of portal systemic encephalopathy and mortality.[340] Over the long term, a 24 to 58% rate of thrombosis has been reported.[340,366] A variation of the H-graft, now called the mesocaval C shunt, is even less demanding technically and has made thrombosis less likely. Those who champion it use it as a procedure of choice in emergency and semi-emergency situations and in lieu of other shunts when they are not possible.[366]

Rypins and Sarfeh[367] used a small-diameter portacaval H-graft and demonstrated that the portal flow pattern was an independent predictor of surgical mortality and correlated with long-term survival better than did the Child classification. When combined, both factors predicted survival in emergency and nonemergency operations as well as for long-term survival ($P < 0.001$).[367] They also noted a significantly lower incidence of encephalopathy than seen in those with total shunts, illustrating the importance of hepatic perfusion as well as hepatic reserve.

Johansen[368] constructed a side-to-side shunt with a 10- to 12-mm diameter **(partial portal decompression)**. One of the four who bled again bled from varices. All patients had patent shunts, but despite this, encephalopathy was seen in only 6%. Six patients (12%) died during the follow-up averaging 26 months.[368]

Medical Treatment. Propranolol, a nonselective beta-adrenergic blocking agent, given orally at a dose titrated to decrease the resting pulse rate by 25%, decreases and sustains portal pressure in cirrhotics.[369] It also reduces the blood flow in the azygous system, the main drainage of the esophageal veins.[370] The most important action is splanchnic vasoconstriction and with it a resulting decrease in portal blood flow; hence, a reduction in intrahepatic resistance now also in part attributed to relaxation of the myofibroblasts in the sinusoids and dilatation of the portal collateral circulation.[296,314]

Lebrec and colleagues[37] reported the results of a 2-year propranolol versus placebo controlled trial in 74 patients who were mainly good risk alcoholic cirrhotics. Control of recurrent variceal bleeding was statistically better in the propranolol group at 1 and 2 years ($P < 0.001$). Although mortality did not differ after the first year, at 2 years, survival with the active drug was greater ($P > 0.02$).[371] Burroughs and coworkers[372] found no significant difference between propranolol and a control group. Their subjects were recruited from patients with differing causes for cirrhosis, of whom 40% were either Child B or C. A third trial with only 11% Child A patients showed slightly less rebleeding at the end of the first year in those treated, but this was even less and still not significant at the end of 2 years.[373] When propranolol alone was tried against propranolol plus endoscopic sclerotherapy or propranolol plus transhepatic sclerotherapy, it was found to be inadequate treatment for esophageal bleeding in patients with advanced liver disease.[374] Reichen[375] compared seven randomized, controlled trials of nonselective beta-adrenergic blockers against placebo and found, at best, the effects of the drug to be small; however, some patients did respond. Westaby and associates[354] noted that a pretreatment pulse of 90 or more could signify a predilection to bleeding, and the ability to reduce the resting pulse rate by 25% may indicate success. This observation is based on the pulse rate and its response to a blocking agent as a marker of adrenergic activity. In this particular trial a well-compensated group of patients proved propranolol to be the only long-term therapy needed.[354] Fleig and co-workers[352] found no difference between the use of sclerotherapy and propranolol regarding rebleeding or survival and concluded that both were of comparable value.

Portal Hypertensive Gastropathy

Acute gastric lesions are reported to be the source of bleeding in 10 to 50% of patients with known esophageal varices.[306,376] Endoscopy describes a spectrum of macroscopic changes in the gastric mucosa of cirrhotic patients ranging from a scarlatinalike appearance or a white reticular network surrounding erythematous areas (mosaic pattern) (Fig. 54–48) to the presence of cherry red spots that may or may not bleed spontaneously.[306] These same gross changes, although seen at times in patients without portal hypertension, are microscopically different. The most diagnostic findings are focally dilated ectatic capillaries, vascular congestion, and edema.[306,377-379] Few inflammatory cells are seen, thus negating previous theories of an inflammatory lesion. Injection studies revealed submucosal arteriovenous anastomoses as well as dilatation of precapillaries, capillaries, and veins.[380] Ultrastructural studies showed endothelial abnormalities and thickening of submucosal arteries and veins, all suggesting a mucosal vascular abnormality.[381] Earlier experimentation in animals with portal hypertension and cirrhosis had demonstrated a marked increase in submucosal vascular communications with a decrease in effective mucosal flow, correlating with the finding of both decreased mucosal oxygen saturation and gastric acid concentration.[381] Although in contrast with expectations of an increased gastric circulation secondary to the hyperdynamic general circulation, this could reflect shunting elsewhere in the stomach, but the cause remains unknown.

Sarfeh and associates,[382] reported that hemorrhage from the gastritis associated with varices could not be controlled without variceal decompression and referred to the studies of other authors who also indicated that bleeding from erosive gastritis was rare following portacaval shunt for bleeding varices. Other authors have corroborated this observation and have also noted the failure of H_2 receptor blocking agents or antacids to treat significant gastric mucosal bleeding successfully.[359,377,378]

In Lebrec's study[371] of propranolol, the risk of recurrent bleeding was reduced not only in those with varices, but also acute gastric erosions. Propranolol, used by Hoskins et al.[376] in an open study, stopped gastric mucosal bleeding in 13 of 15 patients with portal hypertension and nonbleeding varices. Follow-up endoscopy showed a return to normal in five and a decrease in the number of cherry red spots in four. These uncontrolled observations all suggest that portal decompression and propranolol are effective in the treatment of gastric mucosal bleeding from portal hypertensive gastropathy, whereas the traditional methods are lacking.

Liver Transplantation

Portal hypertension and esophageal varices occur in patients whose pathology does not impair liver function to the degree necessitating liver transplantation: i.e., splenic vein thrombosis, idiopathic portal hypertension, or congenital hepatic fibrosis. Varices are also present in patients with compensated cirrhosis (Child-Pugh A and B); therefore, before considering transplantation, a treatment specifically designated to replace the diseased failing liver, it is mandatory to determine the exact cause of the varices and the precise source of bleeding. Determination of the liver's functional capacity is aided by quantitative testing (galactose elimination capacity). Certain centers routinely incorporate hemodynamic studies in their evaluation, and the Child-Pugh classification plays a major role in the decision to transplant.

Sclerotherapy is successful in the control of bleeding from esophageal varices in 75 to 95% and is the consensus choice in the management of both emergency and recurrent variceal bleeding. In situations in which bleeding is not controlled, the options become selective or nonselective portal systemic shunts, esophageal transection, TIPS, or transplantation. A Child class A individual or one with known contraindications to transplantation should not be considered for transplantation and the bleeding controlled by the procedure done most often and best, locally or at a referral center. If otherwise indicated, a transplant evaluation is possible at a later date; however, Iwatsuki and colleagues[383] state that "patients in whom long-term sclerotherapy has failed should be considered for liver transplantation" and that "shunt or nonshunt operations are not the treatment for bleeding varices unless there are

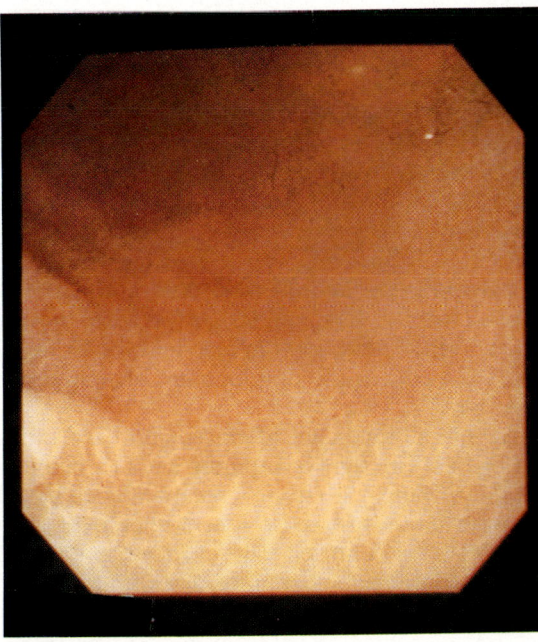

Fig. 54–48. Gastroscopic photograph of the mosaic pattern of portal hypertensive gastropathy.

clear contraindications to it" (i.e., liver transplantation). Survival in Child-Pugh A and B patients who receive sclerotherapy is 95 and 80% at the end of 1 and 5 years and 70 and 90% and 50 to 65% with either selective or nonselective shunts over the same period. Wood and associates[384] compared these figures with the University of Nebraska transplant actuarial rate of 89% at 1 and 4 years. They also noted that in their series most transplantation mortality occurred within the first year regardless of the Child-Pugh classification, but that fatalities related to transplantation were unlikely to occur in succeeding years, whereas in comparable previously shunted groups, survival continually decreased as time contributed to continuing erosion of their liver function.[384] In these situations, the decision should be individualized.

Liver transplantation is the logical choice in patients with end-stage liver disease and uncontrolled bleeding varices. In those for whom a donor organ is not available or who have not yet been evaluated for transplantation, TIPS, with an almost negligible mortality, has shown the ability to bridge the time gap until transplantation can be accomplished and in some patients has postponed the need for transplantation.[343] At this time, because of limited experience, TIPS should not be done routinely and then only by a well-qualified team.

Complications of liver transplantation in patients who have had shunts have led to a reluctance to consider such patients as transplant candidates. Data from the University of Pittsburgh reveal no statistical difference in the actuarial 9-year survival between those transplanted with or without a prior shunt; however, previous shunts that required no hilar dissection were done more safely. The mesocaval shunt and DSRS were preferable, but the presence of a previous shunt or portal vein abnormalities did not preclude successful transplantation, albeit more difficult and time-consuming.[383,385] At the University of Nebraska 9 of 11 (81%) adult patients who underwent liver transplantation who had had earlier shunts survived to leave the hospital, whereas survival in a similar group at University of California, Los Angeles, was 13 of 15 patients (87%).[384,386] Forty percent of the latter group had a previous portocaval shunt, and both deaths occurred in patients with portocaval shunts. On the average, hospital stay of those with a portocaval shunt was prolonged to 62 days versus 35 days in those with a mesocaval or DSRS.[386]

Alcoholic Hepatitis

A precise diagnosis may be difficult because the spectrum of alcoholic liver disease runs the gamut from the asymptomatic patient with hepatomegaly or abnormal enzyme levels found on routine examination to end-stage liver disease. In between these extremes are the patients with a fatty liver, cholestatic hepatitis, and mild-to-severe alcoholic hepatitis. The differentiation between florid alcoholic hepatitis and end-stage cirrhosis is often blurred clinically and biochemically, making it difficult to separate a potentially reversible disorder from an active cirrhosis.

Complaints are nonspecific: fatigue, weakness, anorexia, nausea and vomiting, weight loss, chills and fever, and almost invariably right upper quadrant pain. A long history of excessive alcohol use is elicited but may be denied, and at times it becomes necessary to query family and friends. Hepatomegaly is a constant finding, and in its absence the diagnosis must be questioned. Jaundice, spider angiomas, and ascites, common in the acute form, mimic decompensated cirrhosis, and the spontaneous appearance of hepatic encephalopathy strongly suggests that the disease is life-threatening. A cholestatic picture with icterus, pruritus, light stools, leukocytosis, and a tender palpable liver is easily confused with cholecystitis or extrahepatic biliary obstruction, the latter possibly the result of chronic pancreatitis.

Aminotransferase levels of up to 300 units, invariably present with a 2:1 ratio of AST to ALT, are typical of alcoholic hepatitis but may also be present in nonalcoholic steatonecrosis.[62] Williams and Hoofnagle[63] have demonstrated that a ratio greater than 1 in nonalcoholic hepatitis should raise the question of underlying cirrhosis and when associated with markedly elevated aminotransferase levels should imply a superimposed viral infection, acetaminophen hepatotoxicity, or other insults. Alkaline phosphatase levels are usually elevated, mostly less than twice normal, but may be greatly increased in the cholestatic form. The GGTP is high. Jaundice is present in up to 90% of cases and suggests severe involvement. Hypoalbuminemia also indicates serious disease. The prothrombin time, generally prolonged 1 to 3 seconds beyond normal, becomes a signpost of advanced disease when it is 4 seconds or greater than normal.

Normochromic normocytic anemia is common, but macrocytosis is a clue to continued alcoholic use, particularly when reinforced by an increased GGTP. Leukocytosis ranges from 10 to 40,000, often with an accompanying left shift, and platelets may be decreased, secondary to either alcohol or hypersplenism. Antibodies to HBV were found in approximately 30% of all patients with alcoholic liver disease, and HBsAG was present in 3%, both of which are much greater than the percentages in normal blood donors, implicating the high exposure rate of alcoholics to HBV.[387] There was no relationship between the presence of HBV antibodies and the severity of long-term results of liver disease in alcoholics.[387,388] The presence of antibodies to HCV in alcoholic liver disease of varying degrees (24.3%) was greater than that in alcoholics without liver disease (2.2%) or their controls (1.2%), and the presence of anti-HCV antibodies correlated with both the severity of liver disease and microscopic features similar to those of chronic viral infections. At present, the prevalence of anti-HCV antibodies in alcoholics with liver disease implies a role in the development of significant hepatic disease.[389,390]

Because of its broad clinical presentation and the poor correlation between signs, symptoms, and biochemical parameters, liver biopsy is strongly recommended to define and stage the illness. Just as severe acute alcoholic hepatitis (steatonecrosis) is confused with cirrhosis, profound microscopic changes can exist in the asymptomatic or relatively asymptomatic patient. This is a necrotizing inflammatory disease characterized by ballooning hepatocytes, hepatocellular necrosis and infiltration of polymorphonuclear leukocytes, steatosis of varying degree, Mallory bodies, and perivenular and perisinusoidal fibrosis. Neither steatosis nor Mallory bodies are essential for the diagnosis of steatonecrosis, also referred to as steatohepatitis. There is no morphologic difference between the nonalcoholic steatonecrosis, found predominantly in middle-aged obese women; amiodarone hepatotoxicity, the liver disease of postoperative jejunal ileal bypass; or Indian childhood cirrhosis. Involvement of the terminal hepatic venules with a histologic picture of veno-occlusive disease was observed in 14.6% of cases of precirrhotic alcoholic hepatitis. The clinical relevance of this finding is its relationship to portal hypertension in noncirrhotic alcoholic patients.[391] Cholestatic changes in biopsies were found in 22% of 306 male alcoholics, whose survival was significantly less and correlated well with other predictors of decreased survival.[392] The mortality of acute alcoholic hepatitis varies from 10 to 60%.[393] No one specific abnormality has been shown to predict outcome, although most deaths occur in patients with prothrombin times so prolonged as to preclude biopsy. Encephalopathy and a bilirubin level of 10 mg/dl or more are both ominous prognostic signs. Maddrey and associates[394] developed a "discriminant factor" (DF = 4.6 × prothrombin time + bilirubin) in which a product greater than 93 identified those most severely ill and likely to die. Orrego and colleagues[395] devised the combined clinical laboratory index (CCLI). They thought that by using the seven clinical and five laboratory findings most often associated with the high risk of death (Table 54-17), the outlook would be less liable to be improperly influenced by a nonspecific effect of treatment.[395] The bar graph with Table 54-17 shows the scale of 1 to 25, divided into five equal ranges. There were no deaths at scores of zero. Unfortunately, it is more cumbersome, and the clinical observations are subject to individual interpretation. Despite emphasis on the need for biopsy, none of the prognostic indices (DF, CCLI and Child-Pugh classification) includes histologic findings, suggesting the lack of their prognostic significance.

Treatment is based on withdrawal and abstinence from alcohol (Fig. 54-49). The diet is restricted only when clinically indicated by hepatic encephalopathy, fluid retention, and electrolyte deficiencies. Gastrointestinal bleeding and infections are treated specifically as are the replacement of nutritional, vitamin, and mineral deficiencies. Be wary

Table 54-17. Combined Clinical and Laboratory Index (Range 0-25)

Clinical Abnormalities	Grade	Score*	Laboratory Abnormalities	Grade	Score*
Encephalopathy	1–3	2	Prothrombin (seconds over control)	4–5	1
				>5	2
Collateral circulation	1–2	1	Hematocrit (% of normal)	75–89.9	1
	3	3		<75	3
Edema	1	1	Albumin (g/dl)	2.5–2.9	2
	2–3	2		<2.5	3
Ascites	1–3	2	Bilirubin (mg/dl)	2.1–8	2
				>8	3
Spider nevi	>10	1			
Weakness	—	1	Alkaline phosphatase (IU/dl)	>330	2
Anorexia	—	1			

* Σ scores = combined clinical and laboratory index.

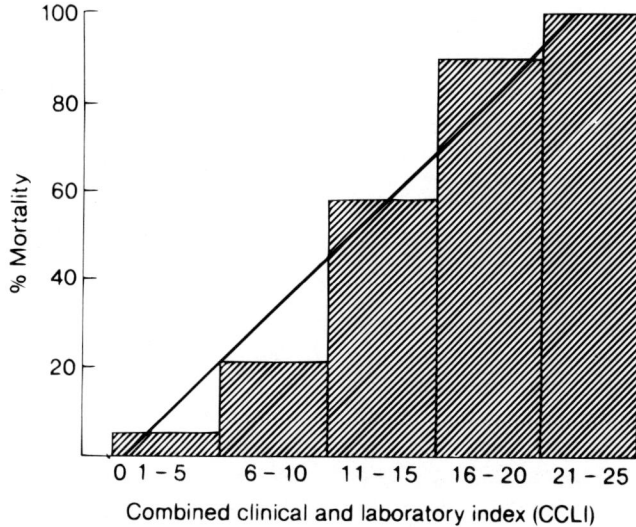

(Orrego, H., et al.: Assessment of prognostic factors in alcoholic liver disease: toward a global quantitative expression of severity. Hepatology, 3; 896, 1983.

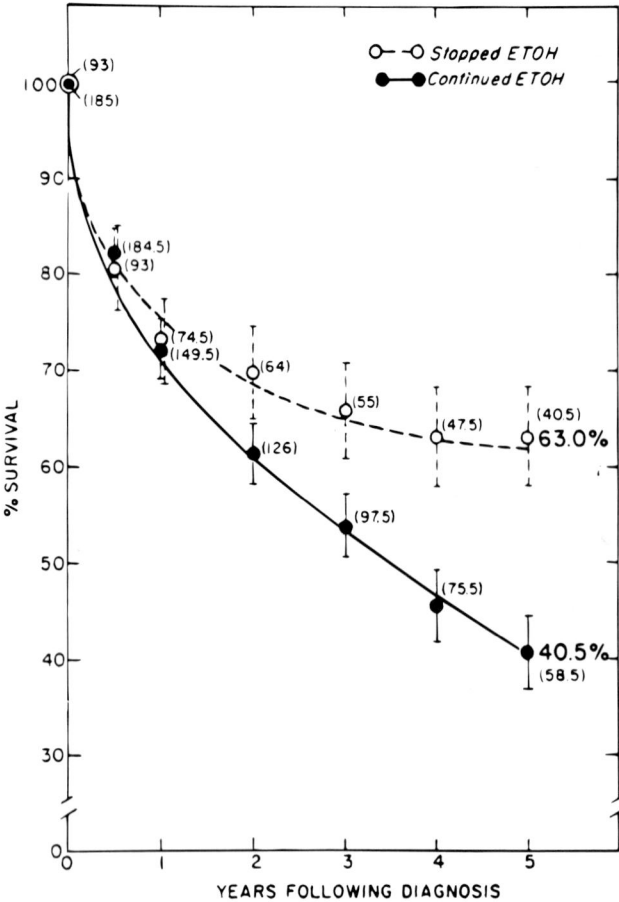

Fig. 54-49. Duration of survival in patients with alcoholic cirrhosis. Influence of alcohol withdrawal and possible effects of changes in management. (From Powell, W. J., Jr., and Klatskin, G.: Duration of survival in patients with Laennec's cirrhosis: influence of alcohol withdrawal, and possible effects of recent changes in general management of the disease. Am. J. Med., 44: 406, 1968.)

of withdrawal symptoms, which can be misconstrued as encephalopathy or vice versa, and if the patient has been actively drinking until admission, the use of chlordiazepoxide prophylactically is suggested. Recovery may be prolonged and require weeks to months.

No treatment is universally considered effective in severe alcoholic hepatitis. Corticosteroids have been widely and extensively studied with conflicting results. The rationale for their use is diverse: to decrease inflammation and collagen formation, to suppress any existing immunologic mediation, and to increase serum albumin and appetite. A meta-analysis of 11 studies concluded that corticosteroids are not effective in mild-to-moderate disease but do decrease short-term mortality in the subcategory of patients with spontaneous hepatic encephalopathy.[396] Carithers and associates,[393] using methylprednisolone in patients manifesting either spontaneous encephalopathy or a markedly increased determinant factor but without gastrointestinal hemorrhage requiring transfusion, active infection, or persistent renal disease, demonstrated a decreased short-term mortality (6%) as opposed to that in a placebo group (35%). In those with spontaneous hepatic encephalopathy, the cumulative mortality in the placebo group was 47% compared with 7% in those receiving the active drug. The question of long-term survival or the development of cirrhosis remains unanswered.[393] A similar study in France used the same criteria as Carithers, including only those patients with biopsy-proven disease but excluding those patients with gastrointestinal bleeding or infection.[397] The results of these two studies were remarkably similar. The latter study suggests that treatment be started immediately in the severely ill and to be discontinued only if the diagnosis is not confirmed by biopsy. The only variables correlating with survival were treatment, ascites, and bilirubin. At 6 months, the survival rate was significantly greater ($P < 0.002$) in those treated.[397]

In 1979, Orrego and associates[398] reported the use of prophylthiouracil (PTU) in the treatment of severe alcoholic hepatitis. The clinical trial was based on animal experiments using animals fed alcohol on a long-term basis; these experiments had previously demonstrated evidence of a hepatic hypermetabolic state characterized by increased oxygen consumption that was abolished by PTU. Similar animal models developed centrilobular necrosis and changes compatible with hypoxia when exposed to low oxygen states, and these changes were reduced or prevented when PTU was administered. The initial short-term trial demonstrated no difference in survival between those receiving the active drug and placebo; however, when using the CCLI to discern the severity of the disease, the PTU was shown to have a significant effect in the sicker individual.[398] A similar controlled study from Los Angeles showed no difference between treated patients and the controls.[399]

Eight years later, a larger long-term study by the Toronto group, using a revised CCLI, reported a 2-year 48% decrease in the cumulative mortality rate ($P < 0.05$) with the greatest effect seen in the most seriously ill.[400] Alcohol use was determined by monitoring urinary alcohol levels, revealing that those with moderate levels receiving PTU were almost completely protected (mortality 2.8%) versus placebo (mortality 25%). The drug did not help patients with higher urine alcohol levels, who had a mortality of 22%, similar to the mortality of the placebo group. Side effects were not of statistical significance, but leukopenia and thrombocytopenia are not uncommon.[400] PTU has not been widely accepted or used in the treatment of alcoholic hepatitis.

Agents that promote hepatic regeneration have been tried to recoup the regenerative power inhibited by the excess alcoholic intake. Insulin and glucagon used together have been studied, but the results conflict and at this time play little if any role in the treatment of acute alcoholic hepatitis. Hypoglycemia has been a fatal side effect.[401-404]

Protein calorie malnutrition is common and, when quantified with the Blackburn criteria,[405] was present in all 273 patients studied in a VA cooperative study.[406] Ninety-six percent of these patients are categorized as either moderately or severely malnourished. Nutritional support was given in an attempt to correct and prevent further injury and to promote hepatic regeneration. Precipitation of encephalopathy was a major concern, but standard amino acids as part of a nutrient solution have no significant effect on encephalopathy but do improve protein retention.[407] These patients were evaluated during and after a 90-day protocol in which oxandralone and an enteral high calorie, high protein nutritional supplement were compared with a placebo and a low calorie, low protein supplement in a control group. Forty percent drank again following hospital discharge, but that did not significantly affect the 6-month mortality rate; however, further analysis concluded that protein calorie malnutrition is a critical complication, and patients with the most severe protein calorie malnutrition and greater DF have the worst prognosis. An adequate caloric intake is a significant factor associated with improved survival in patients with moderate and severe protein calorie malnutrition, making a strong argument for aggressive nutritional support, particularly because oxandralone was not effective when caloric intake was inadequate.[406] Although intravenous administration is best for those with encephalopathy, transition to enteral feeding should be made as soon as possible to maintain small intestinal mucosal integrity and avoid bacterial translocation with its subsequent morbidity.[408]

Multiple studies using solutions of dextrose and amino acids have shown no effect on short-term survival, although these patients do show an increase in nitrogen balance with improved levels of bilirubin and albumin and a better nutritional status. Bonkovsky and coworkers[409,410] evaluated the short-term effects of the anabolic steroid oxandralone, intravenous nutritional supplements of dextrose plus amino acids, or a combination of these against standard treatment in 39 patients with moderate-to-severe alcoholic hepatitis. The combination of oxandralone and supplemental nutrition significantly improved galactose and aminopyrine metabolism as well as albumin and transferrin levels and prothrombin time. Nutritional supplements with or without the steroid significantly increased the prealbumin level, total protein, lymphocyte count, and nitrogen balance. Anthropomorphic measurements were not significantly affected.[409,410]

End-stage alcoholic liver disease has been the fastest-growing indication for transplantation since 1991. The actual survival of these patients is no different than that of nonalcoholics, but the biggest problem remains how to select the patient who will stay free of addictive behavior and be compliant with the demands of care for the new organ.[411-413] The Pittsburgh experience reports the rate of recidivism to be 43% in patients with 6 or less months of abstinence pretransplantation and 6.7% with a period greater than 6 months of sobriety, although this is not universally accepted. Patient selection requires a definite diagnosis of alcohol dependence, the assessment of the acceptance of the disease by the patient and the family, and an assessment of social stability and the other factors dealing with the changes in lifestyle that influence the outlook for a long-term remission. Proper selection results in low rates of long-term relapse.[414,415] Experience with the patient with acute severe alcoholic hepatitis is limited, but these patients are so ill with severe protein calorie malnutrition and other factors commensurate with an increased mortality (DF, CCLLI, and the Child-Pugh classification) as to mitigate a successful result. Additionally, unless they have previously confronted their alcoholism and have begun a treatment program, there is usually not time for the proper evaluation of their psychologic and social stability. In view of the growing numbers of patients approved for liver transplantation and the increasing number of those patients who die awaiting a donor liver organ, acceptance of patients with acute severe alcoholic hepatitis for transplantation should await a greater experience.

Ascites

The appearance of ascites in the cirrhotic is evidence of decompensated cirrhosis. Cirrhosis is the most common cause of ascites, occurring in 30 to 78% of all cirrhotics.[286] According to Runyon and Reynolds,[416] patients with cirrhosis and alcoholic hepatitis constituted 81.4% of 576 patients who underwent paracentesis between 1982 and 1988. Malignancies were a distant second with 10% and heart failure 3%, the latter a sign of the times, as in 1912 it made up greater than 50% of all cases of ascites (Table 54-18).[416]

Ascitic fluid is in dynamic equilibrium with other fluid compartments, as shown by the rapid diffusion of an intravenous marker into the ascitic fluid and the rapid appearance in the bloodstream of a marker placed in the ascites. The amount of ascites mobilized in a 24-hour period is limited to approximately 900 ml.[417]

Pathogenesis. The exact pathogenesis of ascites is debated among two long-standing theories and a newcomer:

- Classic (underfilled)
- Overflow (primary renal sodium retention)
- Peripheral arterial vasodilatation

The classic (underfilled) theory is based on the presence of increased portal hydrostatic pressure with or without hypoalbuminemia promoting transudation of fluid into the peritoneal cavity, resulting in a decreased intervascular volume. The ensuing hypovolemia activates vasopressin, nor-

Table 54-18. Causes of Ascites (576 Cases)*

Cause	Number	% of Total
Cirrhosis, alcoholic hepatitis	469	81.4
Malignancy	57	10.0
Heart failure	17	3.0
Tuberculosis	10	1.7
Nephrogenic ("dialysis ascites")	6	1.0
Pancreatic	5	0.9
Fulminant hepatic failure	4	0.7
Biliary	2	0.5
Lymphatic tear	2	0.3
Chlamydia	2	0.3
Nephrotic syndrome	1	0.2

* 1196 paracenteses in 576 patients—general medical and gastroenterology wards of three academic institutions. 10 (1.7%) were chylous (2 surgical "tears"), 3 lymphoma, 5 "cirrhotic chylous ascites," 25 (4.3%) mixed ascites (2 cases of ascites)—e.g., cirrhosis and malignancy.
(Modified from Runyon, B. D., and Reynolds, T. B.: Approach to the patient with ascites. *In* Textbook of Gastroenterology. Edited by T. Yamada, et al. Philadelphia, W. B. Saunders, 1991.)

epinephrine, renin, angiotensin, and aldosterone, leading to renal sodium and water retention, which returns plasma, volume, and osmotic pressure toward normal levels; however, continual ascites formation does not allow plasma volume to return to normal, and the baroceptors continue to maintain hormonal production and perpetuate the vicious circle. The increase in sodium excretion when the central blood volume is increased by "head-out" water emersion or the expanded blood volume as a result of peritoneal venous shunting is further evidence favoring this theory.[418]

The overflow theory is based on the finding that there is no difference between the mean levels of plasma volume in patients with liver disease, with or without ascites. Even the lowest plasma volume found is consistently greater when compared with normal controls. An unknown stimulus in patients with liver disease is theorized to incite renal sodium retention, resulting in a primary increase in plasma volume, which, in association with an increased portal pressure, "spills over" to create ascites.[419]

The latest postulate is that of peripheral arterial vasodilatation, proposing that the primary event in the initiation of sodium and water retention is an enlarged vascular compartment resulting not only from the arterial dilatation in the skin, lungs, and muscle, but also principally from marked vasodilatation in the splanchnic circulation. This essentially decreases the effective plasma volume and activates the hormonal mechanisms responsible for renal vasoconstriction and sodium and water retention. The active agent(s), although seemingly related to the liver disease and its resulting in portal-systemic shunting, remains unknown, and none of the known bioactive substances have qualified for that role. As hepatic decompensation increases, there is a continued increase in peripheral and splanchnic vasodilatation, and the relative decrease in blood volume is accompanied by arterial hypotension, tachycardia, increased cardiac output, increased concentration of products of hormonal stimulation with renal vasoconstriction, and increased body sodium and water. This progresses to the hepatorenal syndrome, refractory ascites, and eventually renal failure.[420]

Conflicting data concerning all three abound, and without a proven specific causative agent or physiologic event, these cannot be considered mutually exclusive and may even operate together.

Clinical Evaluation. Clinically, ascites is diagnosed by the appearance of a symmetrically distended abdomen with bulging flanks, shifting dullness, and the presence of a fluid wave. The absence of flank dullness predicts either little or no ascites with a 90% accuracy.[421] With tense ascites, the umbilicus may be effaced or protuberant. When clinically in doubt, particularly in the presence of minimal ascites or an obese abdomen, ultrasound provides a simple and definitive answer and can even direct the paracentesis needle. This is a safe, rapid, and relatively inexpensive means of making or confirming a diagnosis.[422] Only the most profound coagulopathy, i.e., fibrinolysis or DIC, should impede this, and fresh-frozen plasma and platelets are not necessary in otherwise worrisome situations. The safest site, after having had the patient void, is midline, midway between umbilicus and suprapubic area. Surgical scars and their immediate areas are to be avoided because loops of bowel may adhere to the abdominal wall, which in patients with portal hypertension may contain large venous channels. Leakage of the ascitic fluid and abdominal wall hematoma are the most common complications but occur in less than 1%.[422]

Causes. Approximately 5% of patients may have another cause other than cirrhosis for ascites; hence the presence of liver disease in patients with ascites should not be assumed to exclude other pathology (see Table 54–18).[416] In malignant disease, peritoneal metastases with or without hepatic metastases are responsible for 63% of the ascites. Chylous ascites, massive hepatic metastases, and hepatocellular carcinoma with portal hypertension constitute the rest.[416] Heart failure should be considered in the context of the clinical findings. Bile ascites is secondary to a ruptured gallbladder or iatrogenic or traumatic injury of the liver or biliary tree. Ascites, secondary to persistent leakage from trauma to the pancreatic duct or a persistent pseudocyst in chronic alcoholic pancreatitis is not inflammatory, but that accompanying acute pancreatitis has dire implications. Patients with FHF develop ascites secondary to the presence of portal hypertension, whereas those with acute and chronic Budd-Chiari syndrome have both portal hypertension and venous outflow obstruction. Myxedema as a cause of ascites is easily overlooked but, once a diagnosis is established, resolves with treatment of the hypothyroid state. Ascites in essentially well, sexually active women should raise the question of chlamydial peritonitis. Chylous ascites is found primarily in patients with lymphoma or solid tumor carcinoma, inflammatory and traumatic ruptures of the thoracic duct, and, on rare occasions, cirrhosis. Fluid occurring in patients who recently underwent urologic procedures should be suspected of being urine. Clinical correlation should allow the diagnosis in patients with nephrotic syndrome, which may be chylous in 50%, but ascites occurring in patients on hemodialysis is more difficult to explain after elimination of liver disease.[416]

Ascitic Fluid Analysis. Diagnostic paracentesis is part of the initial evaluation of all patients with a recent onset of ascites. The gross appearance must be recorded. Usually straw-colored and clear, the presence of a cloudy fluid is due to an increased number of polymorphonuclear leukocytes. Opalescent or milky fluid represents the presence of lipid-laden lymph, which on standing, while refrigerated, separates into layers. Biochemically the triglyceride level is greater than that of plasma, and this differentiates it from "pseudochylous fluid," the opalescence of which is due to degenerating inflammatory, neoplastic, or mesothelial cells.[423] Bloody ascitic fluid that clots mostly represents a traumatic tap, whereas in nontraumatic instances, the blood cells have already hemolyzed. The former is most common in neoplasm, abdominal trauma, or following invasive procedures. Bloody chylous ascites may resemble chocolate milk. It is important to realize that the extravasation of sterile bile may cause distention but seldom inflammatory change. The result of trauma or invasive procedures of the liver, it can be treated conservatively. Acute bile peritonitis is the result of a ruptured gangrenous gallbladder. The diagnosis of bile in the peritoneal cavity is easily made when the ascitic fluid bilirubin is greater than that of the serum level. A yellow gelatinous fluid is seen in 3 to 4% of cases of myxedema ascites.[424]

In the past, ascites has been characterized as an exudate, when the total protein was greater than 3.0 g/dl or the specific gravity greater than 1.016, and, if these values were less, a transduate. These terms and definitions are being replaced by the use of the serum-ascites-albumin-gradient (SAAG), in which the albumin concentration of ascites is subtracted from the serum albumin concentration; however, both biochemical determinations must be done within minutes to a few hours of each other. This indirect measurement of portal pressure is based on the concept of oncotic-hydrostatic balance. A high SAAG (greater than or equal to 1.1 g/dl) represents portal hypertension with a 90% reliability; a gradient of less than 1.1 g/dl is also 90% reliable in predicting the absence of portal hypertension (Table 54-19).[425,426] Some difficulties in interpretation result from a high protein ascites, which is present in one fifth of cirrhotics, an increase in ascitic protein occurring in two thirds during diuresis, unreliability in a nonsteady-state condition, and a falsely low gradient when the serum albumin is less than 1.1 g/dl. Chylous ascites interferes with the albumin assay.[425]

Determination of the absolute number of polymorphonuclear leukocytes (PMN) is the best single, most important means to detect infection.[426,427] The upper limit of cells found normally in ascitic fluid is less than or equal to 250 PMNs/mm³, and any number greater is presumptive evidence of infection. This, used in conjunction with the results of bacterial culture, can characterize ascitic fluid infection. The previously low percentage of positive cultures in patients with spontaneous bacterial peritonitis (SBP) has cast doubt on the conventional method of ascitic fluid culture, which uses a small volume inoculate taken to the microbiology laboratory where agar plates are then inoculated. When compared with a bedside inoculation of 10 ml of fluid into blood culture bottles, the conventional method was positive in only 42 to 57% of instances of neutrocytic ascites as opposed to positive results of 77 to 92% using the beside technique.[427,428] Both were statistically significant. The frequent false-negative cultures obtained "conventionally" were related to the minimal number of bacteria present in 1 to 2 ml of fluid.[427]

Amylase is elevated in both pancreatic ascites and free perforation of the gastrointestinal tract. Cytology is almost 100% positive in cases of peritoneal metastases but far less in those without peritoneal involvement.[416]

Complications. Cirrhotics, particularly with decompensated cirrhosis, are considered immunoincompetent as a result of decreased complement activity and the neutrophilic and reticuloendothelial system (RES) dysfunction. Rimola studied RES phagocytic activity and found bacterial infection to be a major problem when the phagocytic activity was decreased. Bacteremia and urinary tract infection were the major sites of infection, but bacteremia was found only in those patients with decreased RES phagocytic activity.[429] Survival correlated with normal RES activity (Fig. 54-50).

Spontaneous Bacterial Peritonitis (SBP). This disorder is the model on which classification of infected ascitic fluid infection is based (Table 54-20). A serious complication of cirrhotics with ascites, its importance was not recognized until Conn's report in 1964.[430] It is now defined by a positive ascitic fluid culture and absolute PMN cell count of greater than 250 cells/mm³ in the absence of an intra-abdominal cause requiring surgery.[431] SBP or a variant has been reported in 10 to 27% of all cirrhotics with ascites at the time of hospitalization.[427,432-434] Recognition of this has made paracentesis a routine procedure for all such patients when hospitalized.

Clinical Picture. Although primarily a complication of alcoholic cirrhosis, SBP has been reported in 22% of patients with nonalcoholic cirrhosis and 32% of those with severe acute hepatitis with ascites.[416,434,435] As many as

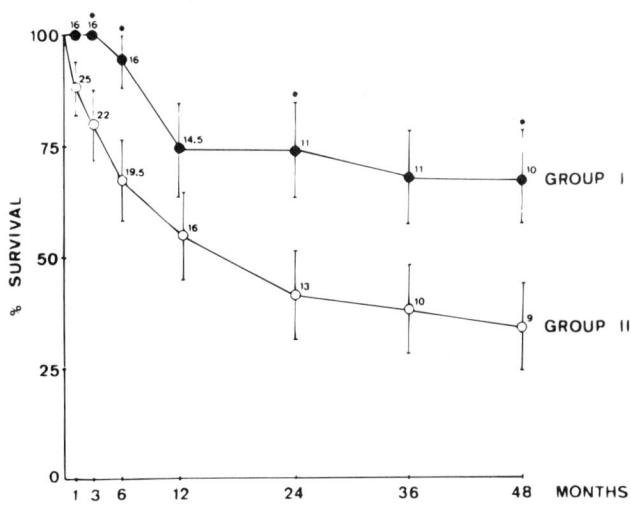

Fig. 54-50. Survival curves of patients with normal (group I, solid circles) and depressed reticuloendothelial system phagocytic activity (group II, open circles). The *vertical line* at each time interval represents ± 1 standard error. The figures over the curves are the numbers of patients on which the survival rates are based. *, $P < 0.05$. (From Rimola, A., et al.: Reticuloendothelial system phagocytic activity in cirrhosis and its relation to bacterial infection and prognosis. Hepatology, *4*:53, 1984.)

Table 54-19. Wide and Narrow Albumin Gradient Ascites*

Wide (>1.1 g/dl)	Narrow (<1.1 g/dl)
Chronic liver disease	Peritoneal carcinoma
Massive hepatic metastasis	Peritoneal inflammation
Veno-occlusive disease	Hollow organ leak
Budd-Chiari syndrome	Pancreatic, bilous, chylous, ureteric
Cardiac	Oncotic
Hemodialysis with fluid overload	Nephrotic syndrome, protein-losing enteropathy, chronic disease
Myxedematous (?)	Idiopathic

* A wide gradient ascites is present in patients with portal hypertension in conjunction with disorders that typically produce narrow gradient ascites (portal hypertension plus another cause of ascites).
(Modified from Hoefs, J. C.: Diagnostic paracentesis; a potent clinical tool. Gastroenterology, *98*:230, 1990.)

Table 54–20. Classification of Infected Ascites

Category	Ascitic Fluid Analysis
Spontaneous bacterial peritonitis	PMN ≥250/mm³, single organism
Culture-negative neutrocytic ascites	PMN ≥500/mm³, negative culture
Secondary bacterial peritonitis	PMN ≥250/mm³, usually multiple organisms
Monomicrobial bacterascites	PMN <250/mm³, single organism
Polymicrobial bacterascites	PMN <250/mm³, multiple organisms

PMN, Polymorphonuclear neutrophils.
(From Runyan, B. A.: Paracentesis and ascitic fluid analysis. In Textbook of Gastroenterology. Edited by T. Yamada, et al. Philadelphia, W. B. Saunders, 1991.)

88% have been classified as either Child-Pugh class C or described as severely ill. Fever, abdominal pain, tenderness and rebound, mental confusion, with or without hepatic encephalopathy were the most common findings at the time of diagnosis. Ascitic fluid may not be easily detected, but as its presence is necessary for the diagnosis, and any suspicion or any abrupt change in clinical status should prompt ultrasound examination with directed paracentesis.

Pathogenesis. Acute bacterial infections are common in decompensated cirrhotics who have been shown to be immunologically incompetent and have intrahepatic and extrahepatic shunting of portal blood. Hoefs[433] cites reports of SBP in 5 to 30% of all infections in cirrhotics, 19% of all documented bacteremic episodes, and 60 to 70% of all serious infections. Spontaneous bacteremia was found in 42% of only those patients with a documented decrease in RES phagocytic activity, and SBP was present in 27% of these. Rimola and associates[429] noted that only single organisms were cultured from the ascitic fluid, and these were overwhelmingly representative of the normal aerobic enteric gram-negative bacilli, i.e., E. coli, Klebsiella pneumoniae, a finding shared by others.

Cirrhotic ascites has a significantly lower concentration of total protein, complement, and opsonic (endogenous antimicrobial activity) than noncirrhotic ascites.[436] There is close correlation between the ascitic opsonic activity and ascitic concentration of total protein; thus, ascitic fluid with less than 1 g/dl of protein lacking bactericidal and opsonic activity allows an existing bacteremia to seed the immunoincompetent ascites.[436] The combination of liver spleen scanning to detect intrahepatic shunting and the total protein concentration of ascites may be a means of identifying those patients most likely to develop SBP.[437]

That the poor opsonic activity could be secondary to dilution of the ascitic antimicrobial protein suggests that control of the ascites could be prophylactic.[438] Unfortunately, therapeutic paracentesis decreases not only fluid, but also protein;[433] however, diuresis has been shown to increase opsonic activity in proportion to the increase in protein concentration.[438] This is also difficult to achieve because control of ascites by diuretics is frustrated by the refractory nature of the ascites in these severely ill patients, but even when accomplished, the incidence of SBP is not decreased.[433] Intravenously administered albumin also increases ascitic fluid protein but is not economically feasible.[433]

Treatment. Cultures of ascitic fluid and blood should be obtained simultaneously, even in the asymptomatic patient. The presence of greater than 250 cells/mm³ is the indication to begin empiric antibiotic therapy immediately without awaiting the culture report. Because of the difficulty in dosing patients with ascites and the nephrotoxic effects of the aminoglycoside, the previously recommended antibiotic combination of ampicillin and gentamicin has been replaced. Cefatoxime was demonstrated to be more effective than an ampicillin-tobramycin combination in 73 patients, 96% of whom had either bacteremia or SBP. Seven of 11 patients unresponsive to this combination were cured by cefatoxime, and two thirds of those unresponsive to cefatoxime responded to the ampicillin-tobramycin combination.[439] Toledo et al.[440] treated 213 consecutive episodes in 185 patients, 74% of whom were Child-Pugh class C. Two grams of cefatoxime adjusted for the renal status were given intravenously every 6 hours. Seventy-seven percent responded; however, in 11 episodes, there was no response to the cefatoxime or other antibiotics. Death occurred in another 37 (18%) episodes within the first 4 days of treatment, even though three of these patients had clinical resolution of infection.[440] Death was due to liver failure, gastrointestinal bleeding, or septic shock. Of interest were the findings that the in vitro susceptibility of the isolated bacteria did not predict resolution of the SBP, and cefatoxime cured infections in 82% of those resistant in vitro to that particular antibiotic.[440]

Fong and associates,[441] using mostly ampicillin and cefatoxime, demonstrated both the sterility of a previously culture-positive ascitic fluid and an exponential fall in the PMN count 48 hours after treatment had begun; thus, the number of PMNs is less than that noted in pretreatment specimens when appropriate treatment is used. Although the usual length of treatment had been 10 to 14 days, there was no difference in mortality between the patients treated only until the PMN count was less than 250 (4.5 days) and those treated empirically (9.6 days).[441]

In an attempt to establish the most effective duration of antibiotic treatment, a randomized, controlled study of 90 patients with SBP or culture-negative neutrocytic ascites received either 5 or 10 days of intravenous cefatoxime. Fever and pain responded quickly, mostly within 24 hours. No significant difference was found between the groups regarding infection-related mortality, hospitalization-related mortality, bacteriologic cures, or recurrence of SBP. The authors concluded that short-term therapy was adequate and less costly. An infection-related mortality of only 2.2%, despite the 87.8% who were classified as Child-Pugh class C, was attributed to the awareness and immediate treatment espoused by the University of Southern California Liver Unit; however, 37.8% of all patients died secondary to liver failure or gastrointestinal bleeding.[442]

Mortality. Hospital mortality as opposed to infection-related mortality varies from 37.8 to 91%.[432,440,443] In 1982, Hoefs[431] differentiated two groups of patients with SBP who were clinically and prognostically different. A lack of previous hospitalization for chronic liver disease, hepatomegaly, bilirubin greater than 8 mg/dl or creatinine greater than 2.1 mg/dl, and white blood cell count greater than 25,000 characterized a group with a 75% mortality within 7 days of the onset of SBP, suggesting superimposition of an acute event. The second group who survived their initial bout of SBP had a small liver, minimal elevation of bilirubin, and little or no evidence of renal impairment, which implied advanced but relatively inactive liver disease. The 1-year survival for the more seriously ill was 5% as opposed to 18% in the second category.[431] Felisart and associates[439] noted the hospital mortality to be the same in those receiving cefatoxime (despite its greater cure rate) as those treated with the ampicillin-tobramycin combination, further evidence that survival from SBP does not lessen the impact of the underlying liver disease. Fong and co-workers[441] also reported that those who died were significantly more ill with a higher Child-Pugh score. Toledo et al.[440] used a multivariant analysis and found an elevated blood urea nitrogen (BUN) to be the most powerful independent indicator of infection resolution and survival, further substantiating others who had previously noted kidney function to be a poor prognostic sign.[430,439,444]

Hospital-acquired infections were also associated with a poor response and a high mortality rate, reinforcing the concept of the need for selective intestinal decontamination in these patients.[429,440,443-445] Carey and co-workers related an increased incidence in SBP to hospitalization and its more common occurrence in those requiring and undergoing invasive procedures.[444] A randomized, controlled trial evaluating the effectiveness of nonabsorbable oral antibiotics in preventing bacterial infections in cirrhotics who were hospitalized for gastrointestinal bleeding revealed a significantly lower rate of infection in the prophylactically treated patients than in controls. These infections included bacteremia, SBP, and urinary tract infection, but those caused by nonenteric bacteria were similar in both groups. Infections played a major role in mortality only among the controls, but again no significant difference existed in the overall hospital mortality of both groups.[445]

Recurrence. Tito and colleagues[443] reported that of 75 patients who recovered from SBP, 38 suffered one or more recurrences, with the probability of recurrence estimated to be 43% at 6 months, 69% at 1 year, and 74% at 2 years. Seventy-nine percent of those who recovered from their initial bout died during follow-up: 44% from hepatic failure; 31% from SBP; and the remainder from gastrointestinal hemorrhage, hepatocellular carcinoma, or other infections. Enteric-type bacteria were the most frequent organisms found in both the first and recurrent episodes. Ascitic fluid protein less than 1 g/dl and a prothrombin time equal to or greater than 45% correlated with recurrences.[443]

To evaluate the effect of norfloxacin in preventing recurrence, Gines and co-workers,[446] in a double-blind, placebo-controlled trial, studied 80 patients who had recovered from SBP. In the 40 patients receiving norfloxacin, the recurrence rate was 12% as opposed to 35% in controls ($P = 0.014$). Organisms associated with recurrence in controls were primarily aerobic gram-negative enteric bacilli, whereas four of the five recurrences in the prophylactically treated patients were gram-positive cocci. Ten percent developed other infections (bacteremia, pneumonia, urinary tract infection, soft tissue, and orchitis) but without a significant difference between groups. The probability of recurrence after 1 year was 68% for controls and 20% for those treated prophylactically. Among the 19 with recurrences, the infection resolved with proper antibiotics, but 4% died of hepatic failure. The sole side effect was an easily resolved case of oral and esophageal candidiasis.[446] Selective decontamination of the gut with norfloxacin did prevent recurrence, but the number of hospitalizations and survival was similar to that accomplished by "perspective detection in treatment of SBP;" hence the cost-benefit issue is debatable.[433,447]

Because of the frequency of recurrence and decreased survival, recovery from an episode of SBP should prompt early referral for consideration of transplantation, and once accepted prophylaxis should be available to those on the waiting list. It should not go unnoticed that gram-positive cocci were the organisms that precipitated recurrence in those on norfloxacin, and treatment of a recurrence should be the antibiotic of choice for those particular organisms.[446]

It has been suggested that patients with an ascitic protein concentration of less than or equal to 1 g/dl should be considered for transplantation before developing SBP. In such instances, prophylaxis would be in order.

Culture-Negative Neutrocytic Ascites (CNNA). This diagnosis is made in the presence of a PMN count greater than 250 cells/mm^3, the absence of a positive culture lacking a history of prior antibiotics, and the lack of another explanation for the neutrocytic ascites. The severity of the liver disease, clinical presentation, and course is similar to SBP. One third have simultaneous bacteremia and evidence of ascitic fluid infection. As noted earlier, an inadequate technique can explain the negative culture, but regardless empiric treatment is started in the presence of the increased number of PMNs. A repeat paracentesis in 48 hours that shows a decrease in PMNs is considered as a response to treatment, whereas no change strongly suggests another nonbacterial cause, and a search for this should be initiated.[448]

Monomicrobial Neutrocytic Bacterascites (MNB). As described by Runyon,[449] the diagnosis of this common variant of SBP is characterized by the growth of a single organism, and a PMN count less than 250 cells, both in the absence of an intra-abdominal source of infection. Of 138 episodes of ascitic fluid infection, 32% were classified as monomicrobial neutrocytic bacteriascites (MNB) and the remainder SBP. Fever was present in similar percentages, but abdominal pain was significantly less than that seen in SBP. Those with MNB had a significantly better LDH level and prothrombin time but were otherwise similar demographically, clinically, and with regard to the infecting organism. Bacteremia and peritonitis occurred simultaneously in 40% of SBP and MNB, multiple recurrences were present in both, and 16% of the total number of patients had previously had both SBP and MNB. A second paracentesis in those with MNB before the institution of antibiotic therapy revealed negative cultures without significant neutrophils in 62%, whereas in the remaining 38%, the original organism was recultured. The PMN count had increased to greater than 250, and these patients were considered to have progressed to SBP; however, despite the hospital mortality of 46 and 32% for SBP and MNB, the difference was not statistically significant.[449]

Secondary Bacterial Peritonitis. Clinical signs and symptoms are absent in approximately 30% of patients with infected ascites, and clinical evaluation by itself cannot differentiate SBP from secondary bacterial peritonitis; therefore this must be a consideration in any instance of patients with both ascites and peritonitis.[450] An ascitic fluid with a positive culture usually of multiple organisms, a PMN count greater than 250, and at least two of the following criteria—protein greater than 1 g/dl, glucose less than 50 mg/dl, and LDH greater than the upper limit of normal for serum—is characteristic of a perforation of the gut.[425,450] Gram stains may reveal multiple organisms, and all findings indicate the need for emergency radiologic and surgical consultation. Nonperforating lesions, i.e., abscesses or inflammatory gut lesions, can present in a similar manner and are suggested when a paracentesis done 48 hours later to assess the results of the antibiotic therapy reveals the same or greater cell count and continued positive cultures. This negates the possibility of SBP and requires further evaluation to seek the source of the infection. The importance of a proper diagnosis cannot be underestimated because secondary bacterial peritonitis treated solely by antibiotics has a mortality nearing 100%, and the mortality of laparotomy in SBP was 80%.[427,451]

Polymicrobial Bacterascites. The diagnosis of polymicrobial bacterascites is made when the ascitic fluid contains less than 250 cells, but a culture grows multiple organisms. This diagnosis, which assumes an inadvertent perforation of the gut by a paracentesis needle, is rare, occurring in only 10 of 1578 paracenteses (0.6%).[452] Six of these were considered traumatic taps containing blood or feces, and positive Gram stains showed multiple bacteria. Clostridial organisms and enterococcus were the most frequent growths among the 34 types identified by culture, but only one patient (0.06%) developed clinical peritonitis. Individuals with higher ascitic protein concentration in their ascitic fluid did not develop a neutrocytic response or peritonitis and possibly were protected by this. Eight of ten patients were treated conservatively without antibiotics, one underwent laparotomy without localization of a perforation and survived, and the last received antibiotics but died with hepatorenal syndrome. Laparotomy does not appear necessary, and most require only follow-up paracentesis.[452]

Hernia. Both umbilical and inguinal hernias are common in patients with cirrhosis and ascites. The 1931 study of Chapman, cited by other authors, reported that 42% of 47 abdominal wall hernias in 112 cirrhotic patients with ascites were umbilical.[453,454] Umbilical hernias in ascitic cirrhosis were present in 17% of 162 patients admitted to a French hospital over a 3-year period.[455] Of the 92 patients in a VA hospital who underwent umbilical herniorrhaphy repair,[39] (42%) were cirrhotics who had or had had ascites.[453] Most repairs in the cirrhotic patients were elective, but 20% were for incarceration, ulceration, strangulation, or rupture. A second VA study of 85 umbilical hernia repairs documented no significant difference between those with and without ascites who required emergency repair because of incarceration.[456] Kirkpatrick and Schubert[454] reviewed 56 reported cases of ruptured umbilical hernias, noting that all but one had alcoholic liver disease, and most had severely decompensated cirrhosis. Complications of the rupture were mainly peritonitis (23%) and renal failure (11%). Staphylococcus aureus was the most frequently isolated organism (46%).[454] Massive fluid loss caused minimal hypodynamic instability. Spontaneous rupture had an overall mortality of 16 to 31%, a mortality of 60 to 88% in those not surgically repaired, and a surgical mortality varying from 0 to 38%.[454] The 38% (6 of 16 patients) appears to be an aberration because the closest mortality to that was 11%, and among the many other individual reports, there were no deaths.[457] Recurrence depended on the presence of ascites (16.6 to 73%) as opposed to those without (0.12%). Prevention of rupture is achieved by controlling ascites by diuretics, paracentesis, or LeVeen shunt and recognizing that ulceration is a prelude to rupture. Once an overt rupture or an ascitic leak occurs, antibiotics, sterile dressings, and restoration of fluid and electrolyte equilibrium are instituted until herniorrhaphy can be done. The timing of surgical repair varied from within 48 hours up to 28 days after admission.[454] Abdominal binders and pressure dressings are used postoperatively because ascites does recur. Eighty-six percent survived hospitalization, and although long-term survival data are incomplete, this follow-up may be as long as 45 months, although Kirkpatrick in his review reports a mean survival of 6 months.[454] Most surgical repairs were done using local anesthetic when possible. Repairs varied from closing the fascial plane to simple closure of the skin and control of ascites. In elective situations, ascites should be eliminated, and in those with refractory ascites, a LaVeen shunt has been helpful.

Hepatic Hydrothorax. Pleural effusions are not unusual in patients with cirrhosis and ascites. Predominantly occurring on the right, they vary from small to moderate and are presumed to be secondary to reaction produced by the underlying ascites. In a cirrhotic with ascites, a large effusion that obscures most, if not all, the right lung and is not associated with primary pulmonary or cardiac disease is considered a hepatic hydrothorax. It has been reported in up to 10% of all patients with cirrhosis and ascites and is the result of a diaphragmatic defect.[4] The pressure exerted intra-abdominally by the ascites and the negative intrathoracic pressure combine to exploit a congenital weakness in the tendinous part of the diaphragm or mesothelial lined blebs on the dome that rupture. This can be demonstrated using methylene blue injected into the ascites and observing it later in the pleural fluid. Intraperitoneally injected ^{99m}Tc sulfur colloid also passes into the pleural cavity, as does air from an induced pneumoperitoneum.[458,459] Rarely patients present with hepatic hydrothorax and no clinical ascites, indicating a unidirectional flow into the chest.[459] The major clinical findings are shortness of breath and an obviously large pleural effusion. Many do not respond to medical management of the ascites or else develop the complications of diuretic-induced fluid and electrolyte abnormalities when therapy is intensified. The mobilization of pleural fluid depends on control of ascites, and a peritoneovenous shunt may be of help. Unfortunately, these may clot spontaneously, particularly when the hemodynamics are not right, and shunt failure as well as the high rate of other complications makes this an unreliable treatment. Chest tubes and repeat large-volume thoracentesis are seldom successful, resulting in the loss of large volumes of fluid, protein depletion, and long hospital stays. Tetracycline pleurodesis with chest tube drainage has been attempted both with and without success. Thoracotomy with localization and repair of the defect has been used but is undertaken with trepidation in these severely ill people.[459] Despite satisfactory treatment of the hydrothorax, ascites may continue or in cases without ascites appear. Liver transplantation was successful in one of our patients refractory to all attempts, conservative and surgical.

Treatment of Ascites. The main indications for treatment are cosmetic and relief of discomfort, dyspnea, or tense ascites. Identification and treatment of the underlying disease should precede the institution of specific therapeutic steps to relieve the ascites: i.e., discontinuation of a hepatotoxic drug, cessation of alcoholic intake, treatment of active liver disease and congestive cardiac failure, and diagnosis and appropriate treatment of the Budd-Chiari syndrome.

Cirrhotic patients with ascites retain sodium and have both an excess of total body sodium and water. Restriction of sodium intake is the key to successful management and may, in 20%, be sufficient alone to produce a diuresis.[460,461] In the days before effective diuretics, limitation of physical activity and hospitalization with bed rest did produce spontaneous diuresis in 40%, which is explained in part by the demonstration that the upright position activates both the sympathetic nervous and renin-angiotensin-aldosterone systems to decrease GFR and increase sodium reabsorption.[461,462] Other than in the most resistant ascites, a no-added-salt diet (1 to 2 g sodium) is practical and effective for outpatient use, but this requires a dietitian who can interact with the patient and whoever prepares the food to alert them to the pitfalls of both hidden and obvious salt in ordinary foods. Various home remedies and prescription drugs can also present a similar hazard. Restriction of liquids is not necessary unless there is significant hyponatremia. Daily weights at the same time of day on the same scale are adequate to monitor outpatients, but hospitalized patients require these plus a reliable measurement of 24-hour urine output. There is no need to measure urinary sodium routinely other than in those situations in which diuretics have not been effective. When weight increases and urine output decreases, a search for the source of an increased sodium intake should be undertaken. Cirrhotic patients exhibiting ascites for the first time who are recovering from a reversible hepatic disease or an acute complication (bleeding) and who have a normal serum creatinine and a 24-hour urine sodium greater than 10 mEq demonstrate the best response to a conservative regimen.[91]

Diuretics. Diuretics are started when indications have become acute or there has been no response after a week of conservative treatment. These drugs are only as effective as their ability to block renal reabsorption of sodium and are classified according to their site of action:

- Ascending loop of Henle (loop diuretic)
- Distal nephron

The most powerful are the loop diuretics (furosemide, bumetanide, ethacrynic acid), which block the reabsorption of sodium chloride and potassium. Spironolactone acts in the distal nephron by primarily opposing the action of aldosterone and its inhibition of sodium reabsorption but still exhibits a natriuretic effect, although considerably less than that of the loop diuretic; however, it conserves potassium. Triamterene and ameloride act directly on the renal tubules and are weak natriuretic agents that are used principally for their ability to conserve potassium.[460]

Spironolactone was shown to more effective (95%) than furosemide (52%) in the diuresis of nonazotemic cirrhotics with ascites.[463] Those patients unresponsive to furosemide developed a diuresis within 48 hours after administration of spironolactone, whereas furosemide had no effect on the lone patient not responding to spironolactone. The patients unresponsive to furosemide had significantly higher levels of aldosterone than the responders; hence in these, a similar pharmacologic effect was overridden by higher levels of aldosterone, which allowed the markedly increased sodium concentration reaching the distal nephron to be reabsorbed. Patients who responded to low-dose spironolactone (150 mg per day) had a normal or moderate increase in baseline renin and aldosterone concentration as opposed to those whose baseline levels were greatly increased and required 300 mg per day.[463] Spironolactone, with a half-life of 24 hours, can be given in a single dose and is started at 100 to 150 mg daily, with increases to 300 to 400 mg if not effective;[460] however, the usual schedule is a combination of furosemide, 40 mg daily, plus 100 mg of spironolactone, with an increase in dose to as much as 160 mg of furosemide and 400 mg of spironolactone when necessary. In those patients who use salt substitutes containing potassium, hyperkalemia may complicate the use of spironolactone, and patients must be forewarned. Prostaglandin inhibitors, such as nonsteroidal anti-inflammatory drugs, should be prohibited because of their adverse effect on diuresis.[460]

Complications of diuretic therapy are considerable. These are primarily:

- Hypovolemia with prerenal azotemia
- Hyponatremia
- Hypokalemia
- Precipitation of hepatic encephalopathy
- Miscellaneous

Hypovolemia, a cause of prerenal azotemia, occurs in approximately 25% of those receiving diuretics but is easily treated by stopping the precipitating drug.[460] Shear and co-workers reported the maximum absorption of ascites to be near 900 ml a day, equal to about a 2-pound weight loss.[417] Any decrease greater than 2 pounds is the result of a fluid contribution from the intravascular compartment and is responsible for a decreased blood volume and resulting decreased GFR.[417] The presence of edema, which is more easily mobilized, allows a quicker, safer diuresis, but following correction of the interstitial edema, the diuretic program should be readjusted to maintain a daily weight loss of 2 pounds or less.

Hyponatremia results from an inability to excrete free water. Hypovolemia, engendered by the diuretic agents, increases water and solute reabsorption in the proximal tubule, decreasing the amount of sodium, chloride, and water in the loop of Henle, thus decreasing free water formation. Antidiuretic hormone (ADH) secretion is also induced by the hypovolemia.[460] This is not sodium deficiency but dilutional hyponatremia and is treated by restricting fluid intake and discontinuing or readjusting the diuretic dosage.

Hypokalemia can be severe. Sodium reabsorption in the distal and collecting tubules fosters potassium secretion, and this, plus the potassium excretion, induced by loop diuretics, increases urinary excretion of potassium and decreases serum potassium concentration.

The failure to respond to a maximum dose of diuretics is generally the indication to move on to more aggressive procedures; however, thiazide diuretics and metolazone, which act similarly to inhibit sodium reabsorption, may be used in combination with both a loop diuretic and potassium-sparing diuretic. This must be done carefully, preferably in a hospital situation with frequent determination of electrolytes, BUN, and creatinine as well as close clinical observation. These produce marked potassium excretion, and hypokalemia is a frequent complication. Ethacrynic acid is an extremely potent diuretic, which requires constant and frequent monitoring with adjustments as indicated by its effect on renal function, electrolytes, weight, and clinical state. Deafness is a reversible side effect.

A study reported the successful use of captopril, an inhibitor of angiotensin-converting enzyme, to supplement furosemide and spironolactone in eliciting diuresis in unresponsive ascites. Four of eight patients responded with complete remission of ascites and edema without side effects or complications. Weight loss began 1 to 6 days after starting the captopril, and the dosage of both furosemide and spironolactone was later decreased by approximately one third.[464]

Conversely, those potassium-sparing diuretics that directly inhibit sodium reabsorption are responsible for decreasing both potassium secretion and its urinary excretion. Used together with loop diuretics, they promote an increase in sodium excretion with minimal change in serum potassium concentration.

Spontaneous or diuretic-induced azotemia was the principle cause of hepatic encephalopathy among 100 patients.[465] Included among other causes were a significant number of cases of alkalosis and hypokalemia. A distressing side effect of spironolactone in men is the development of gynecomastia. Decrease in sexual desire and performance in men and menstrual irregularities in women have been attributed to spironolactone, but these symptoms are commonplace in patients with decompensated cirrhosis. Neither amelioride nor triamterene is associated with these problems.

Paracentesis for Ascites. Before the mid-1950s, large-volume paracentesis was the conventional mode of therapy for symptomatic or refractory ascites. The availability of potent diuretics and increasing fear of consequences of paracentesis, mainly hypovolemia, renal impairment, and hepatic encephalopathy, led to its discard except in cases of tense ascites with severe discomfort, dyspnea, or ascitic leakage. Because of the need for longer hospitalization, complications, and the failure of approximately 20% of patients to respond to diuretics, paracentesis was resurrected to provide an alternate treatment. In 1985, both Kao et al.[466] and Quintero et al.[467] demonstrated large-volume paracentesis to be safe and effective in relieving ascites. Quintero et al.[467] and later Gines et al.[468] compared 4- to 6-L paracentesis followed by intravenous albumin with combination treatment with furosemide and spironolactone and demonstrated paracentesis to be more effective ($P > 0.05$) with a lower incidence of complication and shorter hospital stay than those treated with diuretics. Over an approximately 45-week follow-up, 68% of all people were readmitted. The number of readmissions, reasons for admissions, and probability of survival were almost identical in both groups. The following year, Gines and associates[469] published the results of a randomized study of paracentesis with and without intravenous albumin. In 105 patients, there was almost complete elimination of ascites and a marked reduction or disappearance of peripheral edema in both groups; however, hyponatremia and renal impairment were present in a significant number of those not receiving the albumin, even though the number of serious complications between the two was not statistically significant.[469] The occurrence of hyponatremia, renal impairment or both following initial paracentesis or the manifestation of hepatic encephalopathy, gastrointestinal bleeding, or severe infection during the first hospitalization were the only predictors of a lessened survival. Almost one third of the total number died during follow-up, and approximately 20% required readmission regardless of whether or not albumin was given. Despite the inability to improve survival, large-volume paracentesis with a subsequent infusion of albumin is proved to be an effective treatment for ascites without impairing systemic hemodynamic or renal function.[469]

Peritoneovenous Shunts. The peritoneovenous shunt (PVS), as reported by LeVeen[470] in 1974, drains ascitic fluid from the peritoneal cavity into the superior vena cava. An external peritoneal pressure-sensitive one-way valve connects a perforated intraperitoneal catheter to a silicon, tube which is tunneled beneath the skin of the chest into the neck, where it is placed at the junction of the superior vena cava and right atrium, allowing ascitic fluid to pass into the systemic circulation and maintain the circulating plasma volume. Its function depends on the pressure gradient between the peritoneal cavity and superior vena cava, created simultaneously by the increased intra-abdominal and decreased intrathoracic pressure during inspiration. When the gradient is inadequate, the valve closes, and blood is unable to reflux into the peritoneal cavity. The LeVeen shunt is prone to become occluded, and this high incidence of obstruction led to the development of the Denver shunt, a valve that is activated at a lower pressure gradient with a pump chamber that can be compressed manually, the latter theoretically to prevent regurgitation and thrombosis. Twenty-one patients were randomly assigned to receive either the LeVeen or Denver shunt, and comparison between the two revealed a superior function (patency) of the LeVeen shunt.[471] Within a few hours after proper shunt placement and aided by intravenous furosemide, a profuse diuresis begins; however, some patients require several days to respond, and some do not diurese at all. Some centers also use an abdominal constricting band to increase intra-abdominal pressure. Diuretics and sodium restriction are continued and adjusted as dictated by weight loss and decreasing ascitic volume. Long-term survivors may require continued sodium restriction with or without a diuretic or no longer require treatment. Greenlee and colleagues[472] noted the general improved physical state and the ability of the patient to be self-sufficient. The mean survival time of the 44% survivors in that study was 46 months. Smadya and Franco[473] reported a 1-year survival of 61.4% in the 140 patients operated on, but when survival was classified according to risk, the 1-year survival was 77% in those with good liver function, 61.3% in those with moderate failure, and 24.7% in those with severe failure (Fig. 54-51).

Operative mortality ranged from 10 to 26%.[91,472,473] Pulmonary edema, attributed to the rapid expansion of intravascular volume, has occurred within hours of shunt insertion, and bleeding from varices has been reported early in the postoperative course. DIC of varying degrees was seen in almost all patients and has been responsible for some deaths. Replacement of ascites with saline before shunting was considered useful in preventing DIC, as was preshunt paracentesis to reduce the volume of ascites.[470,473,474] Maintenance of a marked diuresis (5 to 10 lb in 24 hours) immediately postoperative was also used to avert overloading the circulation.[472] Infection, mainly peritonitis and septicemia, was a major complication and cause of death, usually occurring within the first year.[473,475] Intestinal obstruction secondary to a thickened fibrotic peritoneum has been reported.[472] Migration of the venous catheter into the right ventricle produced runs of ventricular tachycardia.[476] Shunt occlusion in 30% or more is secondary to thrombosis of the superior vena cava or fibrin deposition around the catheter or in the valve.[477] This is the most common postoperative problem and usually the cause of recurrent ascites. Injection of water-soluble contrast dye into the venous limb can localize the obstruction, but on occasion venography is necessary to evaluate the superior vena cava for thrombosis.

The VA Cooperative Study of alcoholic cirrhosis with massive ascites initially evaluated 2565 patients with grade three to four ascites, classified according to their clinical status. Of the total, 299 individuals with intractable or recurrent severe ascites were eventually randomized to receive either a more intense medical regimen or PVS. The ascites was relieved more quickly, the length of stay decreased, and recurrence delayed within each group. Survival and complication rate, however, were not affected. This study reiterated that the severity of the disease at randomization reliably predicted survival. Although the early mortality (30-day) was significantly lower in those treated medically in the "healthiest" group, in the others, it was no different. Almost one quarter of those randomized died during hospitalization. If the ascites cannot be controlled by adequate medical treatment or large-volume paracentesis and the patient is an acceptable operative risk, PVS should be considered; however, of particular interest is that standard medical therapy for ascites succeeded in 90% of all the patients with cirrhotic ascites (Fig. 54-52).[474]

Franco and co-workers,[478] unhappy with the results of PVS, treated 57 cirrhotics with resistant ascites using in almost all cases a side-to-side portasystemic shunt. Of these, 98% became ascites free, but there were three operative deaths, and severe and disabling side effects occurred in 12 of 27 patients who developed hepatic encephalopa-

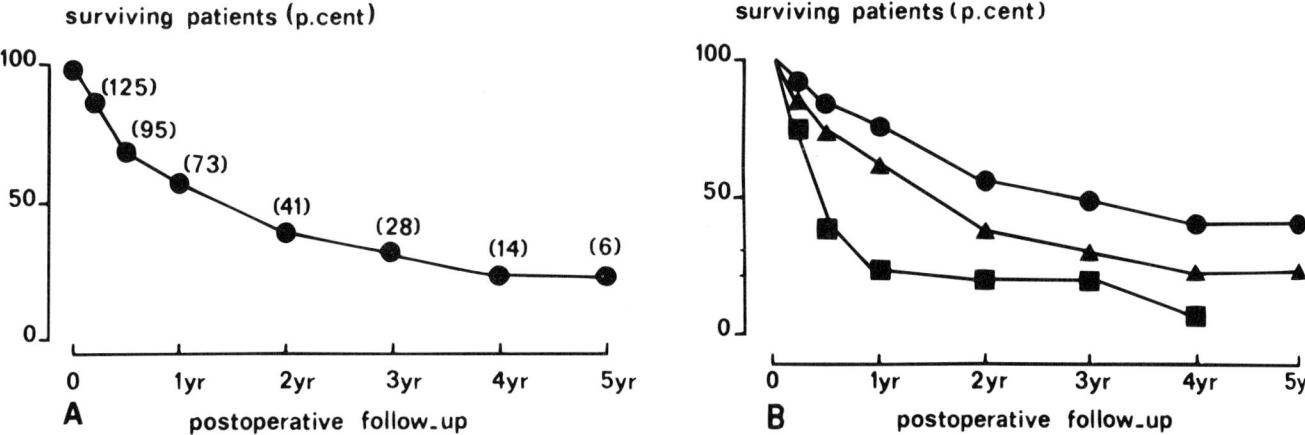

Fig. 54-51. *A,* Postoperative actuarial survival curve of 140 cirrhotic patients with intractable ascites treated by peritoneovenous shunt (PVS). *B,* Postoperative actuarial survival curve of cirrhotic patients with good liver function *(circle),* moderate liver failure *(triangle),* and severe liver failure *(box),* following PVS for the treatment of intractable ascites. (From Smadja, C., and Franco, D.: The LeVeen shunt in the elective treatment of intractable ascites in cirrhosis: a prospective study on 140 patients. Ann. Surg., *201:*488, 1985.)

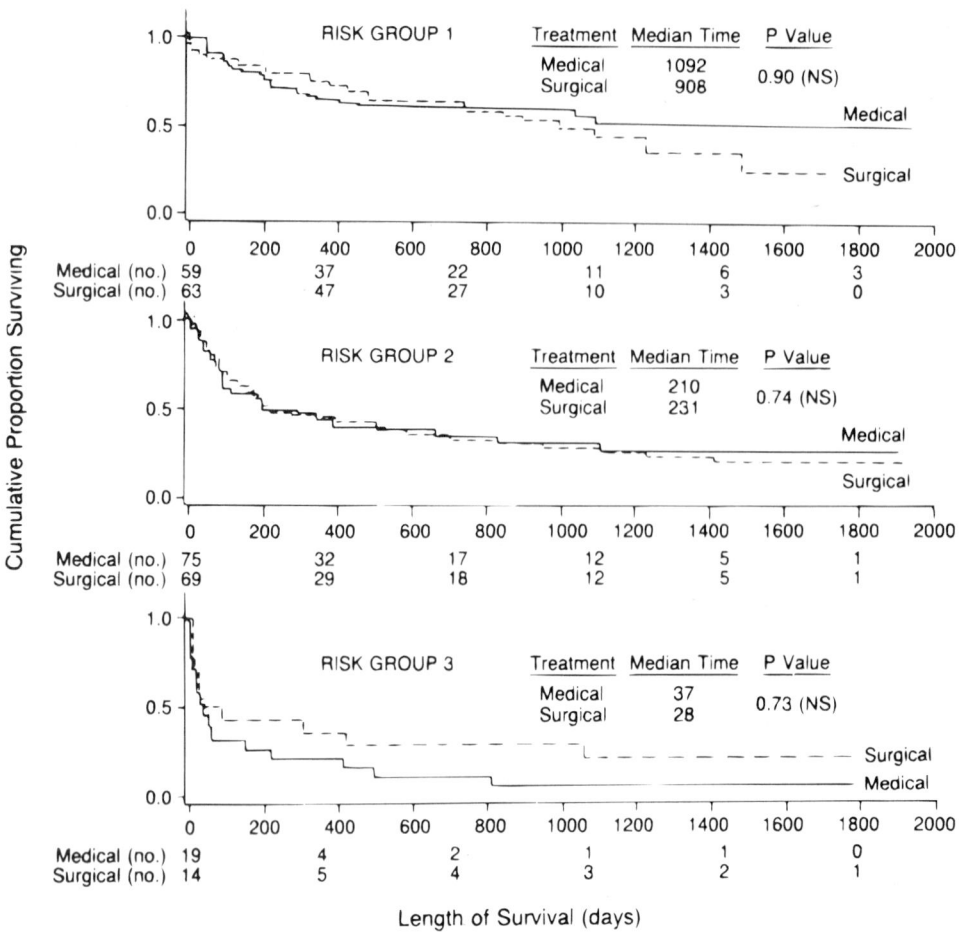

Fig. 54–52. Survival curves for patients treated medically or surgically in the three risk group. Survival was not changed by treatment. The median length of survival, however, differed significantly between risk groups ($P = 0.01$). NS, Not significant. (From Stanley, M. M., et al.: Peritoneovenous shunting as compared with medical treatment in patients with alcoholic cirrhosis and massive ascites. N. Engl. J. Med., 321:1632, 1989.)

thy. It was concluded that this should be done as a last resort to treat resistant ascites.[478]

Miscellaneous. A randomized trial of extracorporeal filtration of ascitic fluid with intravenous infusion of the ascitic protein concentrate versus large-volume paracentesis and intravenous albumin revealed both procedures to be safe and effective in 35 patients treated because of tense ascites.[479] Ascitic fluid was drained by a catheter passed through a polyamide fiber hemofilter, with gravity providing the transmembrane pressure necessary for separation of proteins from the water and solute. After the filtrate was discarded, the protein-containing fluid was reinfused into the peritoneal cavity used as a mixing chamber. On completion of several cycles 2 to 10 hours later, the concentrated protein was infused intravenously. The volume of ascitic fluid removed was similar to that of both ultrafiltration and large-volume paracentesis. Minimal changes in fibrinogen and platelets resolved by the eighth day and were the only significant side effects. The cost was one half that of large-volume paracentesis with albumin infusion.

Conclusions that can be drawn are:

- 90% of cirrhotics respond to an adequate program of sodium restriction and appropriate diuretics.
- All treatment programs have complications.
- Successful treatment survival is related to the severity of the underlying liver disease.
- Patients with intractable (resistant) ascites with or without spontaneous bacterascites should be considered for liver transplantation.

Hepatorenal Syndrome

The term hepatorenal syndrome, originally used in 1932 to describe renal failure occurring in jaundiced patients after surgery for biliary obstruction, is still entrenched in medical usage; however, today it is realistically labeled functional renal failure because the kidney is anatomically normal, but its physiology is awry.[243] Further evidence of functional failure is the return of renal function when these organs are transplanted into patients with end-stage renal disease, just as normal kidney function returns after successful liver transplantation.[480,481]

With the exception of those with FHF, all these patients had decompensated cirrhosis and ascites. The onset can occur gradually over weeks to months, but many happen within days. Progressive oliguria, of 500 ml/day or less, and azotemia are the earliest manifestations. Urinary sodium is less than 10 mEq/L, osmolality is two to three times that of plasma, and a routine urinalysis is normal. The accompanying hyponatremia is dilutional. A sudden increase in bilirubin increases the suspicion of renal failure resulting from the decreased GFR, which decreases bilirubin excretion.

Ascites becomes more refractory, and encephalopathy may appear. Patients die with azotemia, but their deaths are due to liver failure and its consequences.[243]

The cause remains unknown, and for that reason all possible reversible causes are sought out and eliminated. The onset, most often occurring after hospitalization, infers an iatrogenic effect. An acute change in plasma volume brought on by overly aggressive diuresis or large-volume paracentesis has been implicated. Other causes of volume depletion are gastrointestinal bleeding or lactulose-induced diarrhea. Because the urinary findings and circumstances are so similar, the differential diagnosis between hepatorenal syndrome and prerenal azotemia is usually made by a fluid challenge. Monitoring by central venous pressure or Swan-Ganz catheter attempts to maintain an 8 to 10 mm Hg or 10 mm Hg pressure without precipitating pulmonary edema or causing a massive increase in ascites. Packed red blood cells, salt-free albumin, and normal saline are the solutions of choice to be infused as necessary. Those with prerenal impairment show improvement by demonstrating an increased urine output and decreased azotemia. Acute tubular necrosis is a common accompaniment of cirrhosis because of hypotension from sepsis or gastrointestinal bleeding. It may also be the result of nephrotoxicity from aminoglycocides, cyclosporin, and rarely demeclocycline.[482] A nonsteroidal anti-inflammatory drug may inhibit the synthesis of renal prostaglandin E_2, a vasodilator, thus increasing the unopposed effect of thromboxane, a potent renovasoconstrictor and mediator of decreased GFR.[483] Attempts to improve renal function by intrarenal infusion of prostaglandin E_2 or thromboxane inhibitors have not been successful.[484] Other causes to be considered are obstructive uropathy, urinary tract infections, and pyelonephritis.

The pathogenesis remains obscure, but despite decreased systemic vascular resistance, peripheral vasodilatation, arterial hypotension, and increased cardiac output, there is intense renal vasoconstriction resulting in decreased glomerular filtration and renal blood flow. Tubular function remains normal, allowing the normal concentration of urine, but acute tubular necrosis may eventually occur, although more often the patient dies before this. Angiography demonstrates severe renal cortical vasoconstriction of the renal artery and its main branches as well as renal cortical ischemia (see Figs. 54-35 and 54-36). This decrease in effective renal blood flow occurs in the presence of marked vasodilatation of the splanchnic circulation despite the powerful vasoconstricting effect of an activated renin-angiotensin-aldosterone system, increased alpha-adrenergic tone, and other neurohumoral events. Endotoxemia has been implicated as well, but the precise bioactive agent or agents remain as yet undetermined.[246] The majority theory at present suggests that profound splanchnic vasodilatation plays a major role and that endogenous vasodilators are the catalytic agent for this complex phenomenon.[485]

The outlook is poor, and almost all die unless liver function returns after recovery from an acute superimposed event, liver transplantation is successfully accomplished, or a reversible cause is recognized and adequately treated. Further aggressive diuresis is of little help, and hemodialysis should be considered only in an attempt to tide the patient over the acute episode or until a donor organ can be obtained. Acute changes in plasma volume should be avoided, and if tense ascites necessitates paracentesis, it should be followed by an albumin infusion. Paracenteses should never be greater than 500 ml, be done slowly, and no more than a few times daily. Peritoneal dialysis to control fluid and electrolyte balance, while managing renal failure and decreasing ascites in patients with potential reversible liver disease, i.e., acute alcoholic hepatitis being supplemented with nutritional support, has been reported.[246] Drug therapy affords only a temporary effect. Portacaval shunting, which decreases the splanchnic volume and corrects the diminished circulating systemic volume, has been successful on occasion but not in all patients. Obviously the associated mortality and morbidity constitute a great risk. Peritoneal venous shunting may dramatically mobilize refractory ascites, but in hepatorenal syndrome, the experience is limited and attended by a 20% mortality and complications in two thirds of patients.[486] Neither surgical procedure is recommended.

Prognosis

Survival in compensated and uncompensated cirrhosis has been addressed in the literature. In an Italian survey, 37% (435 patients) were asymptomatic, whereas the remaining 63% (720 patients) had complications. The overall 5-year survival of these 1155 consecutive patients was 40%. Only 21% of those with complications survive for 6 or more years, whereas the 6-year survival rate for the compensated group was 54%, albeit 10% of these decompensated annually.[487] A total of 293 compensated cirrhotics were studied in Spain. The overall survival time was 8.9 years, but once complications arose, this dropped to 1.6 years. The probability of a 10-year survival was 47%.[52] In England, 35% of 454 cirrhotic patients had a 5-year survival rate of 50%. Cirrhosis was an unsuspected finding in 58 patients on whom autopsy was performed.[488] Over a 26-year period, 582 Japanese patients with compensated cirrhosis had the following survival rates: 62% in 5 years, 42% in 10 years, 30% in 15 years, and 19% in 20 years.[489]

The variation in the survival as well as other statistics reflect the differences among the different populations studied. In particular, this included the clinical status of the individual, the cause of the liver disease, the histologic appearance of the liver, both the length and completeness of the follow-up, the capability of treatment of disease, and the epidemiology of the area studied as well as the role of alcohol. Although cirrhotics die from causes other than liver disease, the hepatic function is the ultimate determinant of survival.

SURGERY IN CIRRHOSIS

Intra-abdominal surgery in cirrhotic patients is a high risk procedure. Although the mortality rate of biliary tract surgery in the more than 10,000 patients reported by McSherry and Glenn,[490] was 1.7% (0.5% of cholecystectomies, 3.5% of cholecystectomy plus common bile duct explorations and 8.4% of common bile duct repairs), retrospective analysis of the mortality in cirrhotics undergoing all types of biliary surgery ranged from 8.3 to 35%.[491-495] Those classified as Child A, however, range from 0 to 9%.[451,491-495] In a VA hospital series, the mortality associated with a prothrombin time less than 2.5 seconds above the normal limit was 9.3% but was 83% when greater than 2.5 seconds.[491] Doberneck and colleagues[492] stratified patients with cirrhosis and operative procedures according to the level of bilirubin; i.e., those with a bilirubin less than 3.5 mg/dl had a 13.7% mortality, but at levels beyond that, the mortality was 41.2%.[492] Using the Child classification, Bloch and associates[493] demonstrated no deaths in those classified A, 9% in B, and 23.5% in C. Schwartz[494] reported that of 21 cirrhotic patients undergoing cholecystectomy, 2 of 3 had a significant coagulation abnormality, and 2 died of sepsis from infected subhepatic hematomas; however, when cholecystectomy was done at the same time as portal decompressive surgery, 2 of 7 (28.6%) died, and death occurred in all 5 patients who had common bile duct exploration and repair, 4 from hemorrhage and 1 with sepsis. Costaing and associates[495] did cholecystectomies on 14 patients with symptomatic gallbladder disease and cirrhosis with only one death that was unrelated to liver disease. The three deaths that occurred in 33 patients with simultaneous portal systemic shunts and incidental cholecystectomy (8) or cholecystolithotomy (23) were percentage wise no different than the deaths in 170 patients who underwent portal tract shunting without cholecystectomy. Unfortunately, the hepatic function reserve was not defined.

The major causes of mortality were hemorrhage and sepsis. These occurred with and without hepatic or renal failure and led to multiple organ dysfunction.[281] A number of indicators of prognosis exist, but those that indicate hepatic decompensation dominate a list headed by the Child-Pugh classification, which includes the presence of ascites, prolongation of prothrombin time, hypoalbuminemia, and hyperbilirubinemia. As noted earlier, the Child-Pugh classification, although initially proposed to predict operative risk in portal systemic shunting, is also applicable to all major surgical procedures.[493] The presence of concomitant infection is also to be highly feared.

Of particular interest are those patients whose surgery was in search of a cause for jaundice but who at operation were most commonly found to have hepatocellular disease and not an underlying ductal lesion.[491,493] Powell-Jackson and colleagues[496] discussed 36 patients referred for further diagnosis or treatment of unsuspected liver disease found at laparotomy. Sixteen of these had a preoperative diagnosis of common bile duct obstruction, and the remainder were referred for postoperative complications of liver disease or treatment of an underlying lesion. Jaundice, rapidly developing ascites, and right upper quadrant pain were the major symptoms leading to operation, in which the Budd-Chiari syndrome, primary biliary cirrhosis, chronic active hepatitis, and alcoholic hepatitis were eventually the major diagnoses. Sixty-one percent developed complications, predominantly hepatic failure and sepsis, and 30.5% died within 1 to 31 days, each from the precipitation of hepatic failure. Seven of these had acute viral or alcoholic hepatitis.[496] Garrison and associates[451] noted that exploratory laparotomy was responsible for four deaths when it was done searching for a correctable source of infection, but open liver biopsy was without mortality in five others. Aranha and Greenlee[497] reported that two of six patients who died following elective exploration for jaundice, but five of six cirrhotics (83%) did not survive a celiotomy done for treatment of an acute abdomen. The impact of a mortality rate of 58% (7 of 12) in patients with alcoholic hepatitis undergoing open liver biopsy is somewhat modified by the knowledge that 5 of these patients had a simultaneous procedure done with biopsy.[498] These included two patients who underwent a portal systemic shunt and one with splenectomy. A statistically significant difference differentiated open biopsy from the 10% death rate of 4 of 39 patients who had a percutaneous biopsy and in whom death was due to hepatic failure.[498]

Other intra-abdominal procedures carry the same, if not greater, risk than that involving the liver and biliary tree. Lehnert and Herfarth[499] reported a 54% mortality in 69 patients operated on for complications of gastroduodenal disease, of whom 81% were done as an emergency, mostly for bleeding. Infection and postoperative bleeding constituted the major complications seen in 78%. Gastric surgery had a 35 to 70% mortality as cited by Garrison and Aranha.[451,497] Eighty-three percent to 100% died when surgery was done in emergency situations, almost always the result of nonvariceal hemorrhage.[451,507] In 1974, Wirthlin and associates reported a surgical mortality of 57% among 63 patients who underwent emergency gastric surgery to control hemorrhage from peptic ulceration or gastritis. Four components of the Child-Pugh classification were included in an empiric 5-point system that predicted individual mortality with near linearity.[500] Surgical treatment of gastroduodenal ulcer perforation in 22 cirrhotic patients was associated with an overall mortality of 50%. Ten of the 16 patients with ascites (62.5%) died, as opposed to only 16.6% (1 of 6) without ascites ($p < 0.05$).[501] Esophagogastrectomy in noncirrhotic patients was quoted to have a 1.5 to 10% mortality rate by Belghiti and co-workers,[502] who reported deaths in 7 of 32 patients (21%) with cirrhosis and esophageal cancer treated by esophagogastrectomy. Sixty-eight percent developed ascites, which was associated with the death of six of seven patients. Sepsis was present in 11, including all those who died.[502]

The Mayo Clinic reported a mortality of 41% in 54 patients with cirrhosis undergoing colectomy primarily for resection of carcinoma or ulcerative colitis. This mortality and the accompanying 48% morbidity were related to intraoperative complications or the underlying hepatic disease.[503] Three other series consisting of a variety of colonic procedures combined to yield a 60% mortality.[451,497,504] Of the 23 patients with primary sclerosing cholangitis who underwent colectomy at the Cleveland Clinic for complications of inflammatory bowel disease, 7 were cirrhotics. Three of these died within 60 days of surgery (43%), whereas all the noncirrhotic patients survived ($p = 0.02$).[505]

The cirrhotic patient is unable to tolerate emergency surgery, and the victim of trauma, regardless of the cause, is no different. Among 40 patients, the mortality in 22 with ascites, hyperbilirubinemia, and increased prothrombin time was 50% versus the 6% in patients lacking any of these. Twelve fatalities (30%), with nine the direct result of hepatic failure, constituted a significantly greater mortality rate than that predicted in relationship to the severity of the injury in a group that was less severely injured than the norm found in the multiple trauma outcome study.[506] This finding correlates well with the statistical demonstration that cirrhosis was the preexisting chronic condition that most increased the risk of adult trauma patients dying as inpatients. The greater mortality that resulted from the presence of a preexisting chronic condition was generally greater among patients who had less severe injuries.[507]

Ascites after abdominal surgery in cirrhotic patients without a previous portacaval shunt or ascites was initially reported in 1982 in 14 of 33 patients.[508] Intractable ascites occurred in four of these, 8% of those who had biliary surgery and 40% following partial gastrectomy. The presence of a high ascitic fluid protein (mean 4.5 g) suggested a lymphatic injury, as also noted by Belghiti.[502] Those whose ascites responded to conservative treatment were less ill than those with intractable ascites, who required either peritoneal venous shunting or side-to-side portacaval anastomosis for control.[508]

The report of Doberneck,[492] besides recording a 46% mortality in patients with alimentary and intraperitoneal surgery, reported mortality rates of 8.3% in genitourinary and gynecologic procedures, 8.7% for herniorrhaphies and operations on extremities, and 11.1% for neurosurgical and thoracic operative procedures. Despite the report of Bell and co-workers[509] that negates the risk of portacaval shunt in patients with acute alcoholic hepatitis and variceal bleeding, consensus still regards any operative procedure in patients with acute alcoholic hepatitis as a high risk procedure.[502,510]

In view of the excessive mortality and morbidity of surgery in cirrhotics, particularly intra-abdominal surgery, a complete, thorough evaluation using the modalities available today should precede surgical intervention on any jaundiced or cirrhotic patient to rule out a nonsurgical diagnosis and especially in an emergency to correct as many of the underlying complications of cirrhosis as time allows. The use of prophylactic antibiotics, not only because of the risk of operative infection, but also for selective decontamination of the intestine, should be considered and the most limited possible surgical procedure performed. The patient and family should be made completely aware of the risk. Criteria for elective cholecystectomy and common bile duct surgery should be more restrictive and adhered to even more strictly than in those without hepatocellular disease and should be reserved for patients with the most serious complications, i.e., empyema, gangrene of the gallbladder or common bile duct obstruction. The impact of laparoscopic cholecystectomy has yet to be evaluated, but patients classified as a Child-Pugh class C or with ascites or abnormal coagulation remain the highest risk until proved otherwise. ERCP to rule out common duct disease or endoscopic or interventional radiology to diagnose and treat obstructed biliary tract disease allows a nonsurgical approach to most such problems. The most conservative approach possible should be the treatment of choice in all decompensated cirrhotics as well as those without evidence of active liver disease.

POSTOPERATIVE JAUNDICE

Postoperative jaundice is the end result of hepatocellular dysfunction, cholestasis, or abnormalities of bilirubin metabolism. A diagnosis is considered within the framework of these pathophysiologic mechanisms, even though, at times, the multiple variables present in postoperative patients make a definitive diagnosis impossible. The primary need to identify a cause is particularly important to be able to differentiate between intrahepatic and extrahepatic cholestasis to determine whether an invasive procedure or conservative approach is appropriate.

Abnormal Bilirubin Metabolism

Hemolysis is an unusual cause of postoperative jaundice but may occur secondary to sickle cell disease or a hemolytic transfusion reaction. Multiple unit transfusions of stored blood, each with a decreased half-life of red blood cells, can increase the pigment load beyond the liver's ability to process it, particularly when hepatic function has been compromised by hypoxia, hypovolemia, sepsis, or anesthesia. Reabsorption of blood sequestered in body cavities, retroperitoneum, or in muscle following multiple fractures or severe crush injuries when absorbed can also overwhelm the functional capacity of the liver and produce jaundice under similar circumstances. In these instances, unconjugated bilirubin constitutes the major portion of the bilirubin, but greater than 15% may be conjugated in patients with acute or chronic liver disease.[54,511]

Sulfonamides, aspirin, nitrofurantoin, and chloramphenicol may cause hemolysis in patients with G-6-PD deficiency, a congenital deficiency of glucose-6-phosphate dehydrogenase. Clostridium welchii septicemia is another source of hemolysis, and Coombs-positive autoimmune hemolytic anemia has been reported in some instances of cardiac valve replacement. Congenital unconjugated hyperbilirubinemia (Gilbert's syndrome) may become overt with the stress of surgery as well as with fasting.[511]

Hepatocellular Dysfunction

The hepatitislike picture prominent in postoperative jaundice may be related to drugs, the most prominent being the anesthetic agent, halothane. Halothane hepatitis has been evaluated extensively, and use of halothane has been dramatically decreased, even though it has been vindicated by the National Halothane Study; however, this study has been criticized based on inadequate case collection, the percentage and inadequacy of autopsies, and the difference of opinion among several pathologists in this small number of cases.[512] It has also been argued that there is other evidence that is more incriminating than that used to make the conclusions of the national study.

Halothane-induced hepatitis mimics viral hepatitis both clinically and biochemically and is histologically indistinguishable from it. It is rare after an initial exposure, and in that circumstance a fever of unknown cause is usually the first manifestation, occurring 6 to 14 days postoperatively. After more than a single exposure, evidence of hepatotoxicity may be present as early as the first day but more often within the week. Jaundice may not occur for several days, and some patients remain anicteric. Eosinophilia and a variety of autoantibodies may be present. Death occurs in 16 to 42%, possibly within a few weeks, not unlike other forms of FHF. Those most at risk are greater than age 60, are obese, have a history of jaundice after the previous use of halothane, or have had multiple exposures to halothane over a short period of time. There is no specific treatment. Other fluorinated anesthetic agents (methoxyflurane, isoflurane, and enflurane) have also been mentioned as causes of hepatitis.[513]

Ischemic hepatitis (shock liver) is the result of prolonged hypoxia following decreased hepatic profusion secondary to hypovolemia and hypoxemia. It is not unknown for it to happen in the absence of documented hypovolemia as portal venous flow decreases to a greater extent than hepatic arterial flow and is not necessarily related to systemic blood pressure.[514,515] The diagnosis is made in the appropriate clinical setting, particularly as a complication of cardiac surgery or severe congestive heart failure.[131,132] Jaundice is mild but bilirubin can rise to 10 to 20 times greater than normal. There is a marked, almost overnight, increase in the serum transaminase levels to 8 to 260 times greater than normal followed by a rapid fall to normal over the next 3 to 11 days.[131,132] Ischemic hepatic injury is difficult to differentiate clinically and biochemically from viral hepatitis, and differentiation may be made only after a liver biopsy. The histologic changes in ischemia occur in the region of the central vein and manifest themselves as venous congestion and centrolobular cellular necrosis.[514,515] The associated mortality reflects the underlying disease and not liver failure.[132]

Viral hepatitis is not seen in the immediate postoperative period because the incubation of post-transfusion hepatitis, previously called non-A, non-B hepatitis and now HC, may be as little as 2 weeks after exposure but most often is 5 to 12 weeks later. The incubation period of other hepatitis viruses is also longer. Harville and Summerskill[516] reported a 9.5% mortality in 42 patients with acute viral hepatitis who had had surgery. Emergency surgery in cirrhotic patients, particularly those with decompensated cirrhosis, carries a high morbidity and mortality, in patients with underlying liver disease, operated on for suspected biliary tract disease or to obtain a diagnosis in those with unexplained ascites or sepsis.[451,491,493,496]

Cholestasis

Systemic infections may produce biochemical and histologic changes even though the liver is not the primary site of infection.[37,517,518] The biochemical changes (increased conjugated bilirubin, alkaline phosphatase less than three times normal, and normal or minimally elevated D-amino transferase) may suggest extrahepatic obstruction, but the medical staff must not be misled to overuse various imaging techniques to rule out this possibility. Many organisms have been associated with septic jaundice: E. coli, salmonella species, K. pneumoniae, P. aeruginosa, H. influenzae, bacteroides, and proteus species. Staphylococcus aureus, in toxic shock syndrome, and Streptococcus pneumoniae are well known as causes of jaundice. Mild cholestasis with little or no parenchymal abnormality is the most commonly seen histologic abnormality. The acute onset of fever with jaundice, and normal to unusually increased aminotransferase and alkaline phosphatase levels, should lead one to consider septic jaundice, but it remains necessary to exclude extrahepatic biliary obstruction or hepatic abscess. There appears to be no correlation between the degree of enzyme and bilirubin levels and prognosis.[37,517,518] Drugs may also produce a cholestatic picture, with erythromycin estolate, phenothiazines, and contraceptive steroids as particular examples.[4]

The most anxiety-producing jaundice is that which develops within the first 4 postoperative days in a patient who typically has undergone a difficult abdominal procedure under general anesthesia. Most have required multiple transfusions with evidence of hypotension and hypoxemia. Bilirubin may reach levels of 40 mg/dl and with light stools and dark urine mimic extrahepatic obstruction. Despite only mild-to-moderate increases in alkaline phosphatase and minimal changes in the transaminases, albumin, and prothrombin time, it provokes a variety of imaging studies and often exploratory laparotomy with findings of a normal gallbladder of biliary sludge and, despite this, cholecystectomy or exploration of a normal biliary tree. The maximum bilirubin level is usually reached by the 10th day and then decreases to normal usually within the following 2 to 3 weeks. Liver biopsy specimens, when available, lack the changes associated with hepatocyte inflammation or necrosis but show bile plugs and enlarged canaliculi with bile staining of the centrolobular hepatocytes. Although associated with certain aspects usually seen with ischemic hepatitis, this is not an accepted cause, and most evidence now indicates it to be an acquired disorder of the hepatic bilirubin transport system.[40,511,519] Dutch workers have retrospectively studied ICU patients with severe trauma or intra-abdominal complications postoperatively and concluded that developing cholestatic jaundice reflects multiple organ dysfunction syndrome and a poor prognosis.[520] Prognosis for the liver disease is good; however, the mortality is high, with deaths related to the associated illnesses but not hepatic failure because liver synthetic function remains intact, and hepatic encephalopathy does not occur.[520]

Extrahepatic Biliary Obstruction

Postoperative jaundice as a result of extrahepatic biliary obstruction is uncommon but when present is usually caused by retained common duct stones, operative biliary tract injury, or acute pancreatitis. When present after an open cholecystectomy or common duct exploration for biliary calculi, residual stones are the major consideration. Bile duct abnormalities are usually erroneously identified, and surgical injury to the duct has an incidence of 0.1 to 0.2% at major medical centers.[521] A bile duct leak is suspected in the presence of bilious drainage or in a patient with bile ascites, presenting as abdominal distention, a possible fluid wave, and minimal clinical and chemical jaundice. Bile peritonitis, the result of bacterial contamination, presents with fever, abdominal and occasionally shoulder pain, peritoneal irritation, and even septic shock as well as clinical jaundice. Both are best identified by ultrasound or CT scan of the abdomen and can be drained percutaneously and treated with the appropriate supportive care. A persistent cutaneous fistula heals in due time unless there is distal obstruction, but one that continues with a high output can be treated successfully with ductal dilatation or stinting by either ERCP or PTHC. Biliary obstruction is typified by alcoholic stool and biochemical changes highlighted by significant elevation of bilirubin and alkaline phosphatase. The presence of a T-tube allows cholangiography, but in its absence, PTHC or ERCP can delineate the injury, and possible treatment by dilating or stinting the obstruction; otherwise, surgical intervention is indicated.

Laparoscopic cholecystectomy has been widely accepted by patients and physicians, and although the true incidence of bile duct injury is not yet available, published reports indicate a rate of injury two to three times higher than that of the conventional method.[521] The National Institutes of Health (NIH)[521] consensus conference of 1992 reports this to be 0.2 to 0.6%, a figure that has decreased with necessary surgical experience. These injuries are also characterized, localized, and treated by the same judicious use of noninvasive and invasive studies and even repeat laparoscopy. Surgery may also again be required, and the potential or recurrence of obstructive symptoms and signs secondary to stricture or obstruction in months to years after the original insult must not be ignored.

Pancreatitis with obstruction of the common duct as it passes through its intrapancreatic portion can occur not only after surgery on the pancreas, biliary tree, duodenum, or stomach, but also from more distant organs. Chronic alcoholism and recurrent bouts of hyperlipidemia cause chronic pancreatitis that can result in biliary duct obstruction demonstrated by ERCP. Transient edema, the result of various infections and drugs, can produce transient pancreatic edema and cholestasis.[522]

Previously unrecognized obstructive hepatic disease can be seen postoperatively. The most common of these is the neoplasm occurring at the bifurcation of the common bile duct (Klatskin tumor), producing abnormal liver studies but overlooked at the time of cholecystectomy when operative cholangiography is not routine or is inadequate. Suspicion should be high when no stones are found or the common bile duct and gallbladder are normal. Residual stones in both the common bile duct and intrahepatic ducts can be overlooked, particularly if no other cause for jaundice can be elicited. As noted earlier, the liver should always be evaluated at the time of the exploration to rule out the possibility of hepatic disease. Obstructing tumor emboli from hepatoma, cholangiocarcinoma, colonic carcinoma, and malignant melanoma have been rarely reported.[523]

Acute Acalculus Cholecystitis

Acute acalculus cholecystitis is seen in trauma, after surgery unrelated to the biliary tree, trauma, or in other critically ill patients. Right upper quadrant pain, unexplained fever, leukocytosis, and jaundice may be typical of acute cholecystitis, but the diagnosis is often delayed because of confusing findings related to the other problems.[524] Both ultrasound and CT scans have a greater than 90% specificity when, in the absence of gallstones, the following findings are present:

- Thickened gallbladder wall
- Enlarged tender gallbladder
- Pericholecystic collection in the absence of ascites[525]

Recognition is important because 40 to 100% of patients with acute acalculus cholecystitis have advanced disease with gangrene, empyema, or perforation and require surgical intervention.[524]

In cases of postoperative gastrointestinal bleeding, it is imperative to rule out bleeding varices, portal hypertensive gastropathy, or peptic ulceration; however, hemobilia, although unusual, must be considered, particularly following liver biopsy, invasive endoscopic or radiologic intervention, and surgical procedures on the liver or biliary tree. This diagnosis is best made by endoscopic evaluation of the esophagus, stomach, and duodenum with particular attention to the ampulla of Vater.

Help in making a diagnosis is available from a careful evaluation of the clinical features: a relationship of the onset of jaundice to the surgical procedure, the surgery itself, anesthetic agent, need for transfusion, operative course, postoperative course, drugs, and a review of the previous medical history and preoperative studies. A thorough examination, basic laboratory and biochemical studies, and abdominal ultrasound study resolve most problems.

In summary, the usual consultation for evaluation of a hepatic problem, particularly in an ICU, is requested for an opinion regarding jaundice or abnormal liver studies that have appeared suddenly or have remained unexplained. Other frequent questions, which should be succinctly presented, deal with the treatment of upper gastrointestinal bleeding, abdominal pain or masses, the risk of procedures (particularly surgical), short-term and long-term prognosis, suggestions for further medical and nutritional treatment, and even consideration of limitations of therapeutic intervention.

Obviously a diagnosis is necessary, but the answer becomes available only after a tedious review of an often illegible, incomplete, and disorganized medical and treatment record, previous operative and anesthetic records, laboratory reports, and nursing notes. At times, additional information is lacking and requires further communication with former treating physicians and even their hospitals to review past records. Other members of the family may have additional information and need to be contacted. Further consultation with the pathologists and review of pathologic specimens and even a literature search may be necessary. It may be difficult, it can be exasperating and unfortunately at times fruitless.

Because not everyone sees the same things or thinks along similar lines, cooperation between the attending staff and the consultant is imperative. The problem must be precisely stated as well as answered, questions and criticism accepted as constructive, and mutual respect exhibited. An orderly approach to the problem, as stated initially, will determine, as best as possible, the contribution of the consultant.

REFERENCES

1. Fuhrman, S. A., et al.: Marked hyperbilirubinemia in infectious mononucleosis. Arch. Intern. Med., *38:*850, 1987.
2. Crawford, J. M., and Gollan, J.: Bilirubin metabolism and the pathophysiology of jaundice. *In* Diseases of the Liver. 7th Ed. Edited by L. Schiff and E. R. Schiff. Philadelphia, J. B. Lippincott, 1993.
3. Summerskill, W. H. J.: The syndrome of benign recurrent cholestasis. Am. J. Med., *38:*298, 1965.
4. Zimmerman, H. J.: Hepatoxicity: The Adverse Effects of Drugs and Other Chemicals in the Liver. New York, Appleton-Century-Crofts, 1978.
5. Stuart, K. L., and Bras, C.: Veno-occlusive disease of the liver. Q. J. Med. NS, *26:*291, 1957.
6. Russell, R. M., et al.: Hepatic injury from chronic hypervitaminosis A resulting in portal hypertension and ascites. N. Engl. J. Med., *291:*435, 1971.
7. Popper, H., et al.: Development of hepatic angiosarcoma in man inducted by vinyl chloride, thorotrast, and arsenic. Am. J. Pathol., *92:*349, 1978.
8. Heath, C. W., Jr., and Alexander, A. D.: Leptospirosis in the United States: analysis of 483 cases in man, 1949–61. N. Engl. J. Med., *273:*377, 1965.
9. Hadler, S. C., et al.: Hepatitis A in day-care centers: a community-wide assessment. N. Engl. J. Med., *302:*1222, 1980.
10. Lewis, T. L., et al.: A comparison of the frequency of hepatitis B antigen and antibody in hospital and non-hospital personnel. N. Engl. J. Med., *289:*647, 1973.
11. La Russo, N. F., et al.: Primary sclerosing cholangitis. N. Engl. J. Med., *310:*899, 1984.
12. Perera, D. R., Greene, M. L., and Fenster, L. F.: Cholestasis associated with extrabiliary Hodgkins disease. Gastroenterology, *67:*680, 1975.
13. Stauffer, M. H.: Nephrogenic hepatosplenomegaly. Gastroenterology, *40:*694, 1961.
14. Beswick, D. R., Klatskin, G., and Boyer, J. E.: Asymptomatic primary biliary cirrhosis. Gastroenterology, *89:*267, 1985.
15. Valla, D., et al.: Primary myeloproliferative disorder and hepatic vein thrombosis. Ann. Intern. Med., *103:*329, 1985.
16. Martini, G. A.: Extrahepatic manifestations of cirrhosis. Clin. Gastroenterol., *4:*438, 1975.
17. Scott, J., et al.: Wilson's disease presenting as chronic active hepatitis. Gastroenterology, *74:*645, 1978.
18. Reynolds, T. B.: Portal hypertension. *In* Diseases of the Liver. 4th Ed. Edited by L. Schiff and E. R. Schiff. Philadelphia, J. B. Lippincott, 1975.
19. Elman, R.: The gallbladder and pancreas. *In* Pathologic Physiology. Edited by W. A. Sodeman. Philadelphia, W. B. Saunders, 1956.
20. Flood, C. A., et al.: The differential diagnosis of jaundice. A study of 235 cases of non-hemolytic jaundice due to carcinoma, calculus in the common duct and liver degeneration. Am. J. Med. Sci., *185:*358, 1953.
21. Karran, S., and Lane, R. H. S.: Calculus disease and cholecystitis. *In* Liver and Biliary Disease. Edited by R. Wright, K. G. Alberti, S. Karran, and G. H. Millward-Sadler. London, W. B. Saunders, 1979.
22. Johnson, R. F., and Loo, R. B.: Hepatic hydrothorax: studies to determine the source of fluid and report of thirteen cases. Ann. Intern. Med., *61:*385, 1964.
23. Tystrup, N.: The galactose elimination capacity in control subjects and patients with cirrhosis of the liver. Acta Med. Scand., *175:*281, 1964.
24. Hepner, G. W., and Vessel, E. S.: Quantitative assessment of hepatic function by breath analysis after oral administration of ^{14}C-aminopyrine. Ann. Intern. Med., *83:*632, 1975.
25. Shani, M., et al.: Sulfobromophthalein tolerance test in patients with Dubin-Johnson syndrome and their relatives. Gastroenterology, *59:*842, 1970.
26. Grosszmann, R. J.: The measurement of liver blood flow using clearance techniques. Hepatology, *3:*1031, 1982.
27. Child, C. G., III, and Turcotte, J.: Surgery and portal hypertension. *In* The Liver and Portal Hypertension. Edited by C. G. Child, III. Philadelphia, W. B. Saunders, 1964.
28. Pugh, R. N. H., et al.: Transection of the esophagus for bleeding esophageal varices. Br. J. Surg., *60:*646, 1973.
29. Villeneuve, J. P., et al.: Prognostic value of the aminopyrine test in cirrhotic patients. Hepatology, *6:*928, 1986.
30. Infante-Rivard, C., Esanaola, S., and Villeneuve, J. P.: Clinical and statistical validity of conventional prognostic factors in predicting short term survival among cirrhotics. Hepatology, *7:*660, 1987.
31. Christensen, E., et al.: Prognostic value of Child-Turcotte classification in medically treated cirrhosis. Hepatology, *4:* 430, 1984.
32. Albers, I., et al.: Superiority of the Child-Pugh classification to quantitative liver function tests for assessing prognosis of liver cirrhosis. Scand. J. Gastroenterol., *24:*269, 1989.
33. Schaffner, F., and Popper, H.: Classification and mechanisms of cholestasis. *In* Liver and Biliary Disease. Edited by R. Wright, K. G. Alberti, S. Karran, and G. H. Millward-Sandler. London, W. B. Saunders, 1979.
34. Zimmerman, H.: Intrahepatic cholestasis. Arch. Intern. Med., *139:*1038, 1979.
35. Ishak, K. G., and Irey, N. S.: Hepatic injury associated with phenothiazines. A clinical and pathological follow-up of 36 cases. Arch. Pathol. Lab. Med., *93:*283, 1972.
36. Zimmerman, H. J., and Ishak, K. G.: Drug-induced and toxic liver injury. *In* Pathology of the Liver. Edited by R. M. N. MacSween, A. P. Anthony, and P. Scheuer. Edinburgh, Churchill Livingstone, 1979.
37. Miller, D. J., et al.: Jaundice in severe bacterial infection. Gastroenterology, *71:*94, 1976.
38. Klein, S., and Nealon, H.: Hepatobiliary abnormalities associated with total parenteral nutrition. Semin. Liver Dis., *8:* 237, 1988.
39. Holzbach, R. T., Sivak, D. A., and Braun, W. E.: Familial recurrent intrahepatic cholestasis of pregnancy: a genetic study. Gastroenterology, *85:*175, 1983.
40. Schmid, M., et al.: Benign postoperative intrahepatic cholestasis. N. Engl. J. Med., *272:*545, 1965.
41. Cohen, J. A. E.: Amyloidosis. N. Engl. J. Med., *277:*522, 1967.
42. Kaplan, M. D.: Primary biliary cirrhosis. N. Engl. J. Med., *316:*521, 1987.
43. McDonald, G. B., et al.: Intestinal and hepatic complications of human bone marrow transplantation. Gastroenterology, *90:*450, 1986.
44. Vierling, J., and Fennell, R.: Histopathology of early and late human allograft rejection, evidence of progressive destruction of interlobular bile ducts. Hepatology, *5:*1076, 1985.
45. Brugera, M., Llach, J., and Rodes, J.: Nonsyndromic paucity of intrahepatic bile ducts in infancy and idiopathic ductopenia in adulthood: the same syndrome? Hepatology, *15:* 830, 1992.
46. Hubscher, S. G., Lumley, M., and Elias, E.: Vanishing bile duct syndrome: a possible mechanism for intrahepatic cholestasis in Hodgkin's lymphoma. Hepatology, *17:*70, 1992.
47. Benhamou, J. P.: Congenital hepatic fibrosis and Caroli's

syndrome. *In* Diseases of the Liver. 7th Ed. Edited by L. Schiff and E. R. Schiff. Philadelphia, J. B. Lippincott, 1993.
48. Deziel, D. J., et al.: Management of bile duct cysts in adults. Arch. Surg., *121*:410, 1986.
49. Pinotti, H. W., et al.: Juxta-ampullar duodenal diverticula as a cause of biliopancreatic disease. Digestion, *4*:353, 1971.
50. Ong, G. B.: Helminthic diseases of the liver and biliary tract. *In* Liver and Biliary Disease. Edited by R. Wright, K. G. Alberti, S. Karran, and G. H. Millward-Sadler. London, W. B. Saunders, 1979.
51. Billing, B. H.: Bilirubin metabolism. *In* Diseases of the Liver. 6th Ed. Edited by L. Schiff and E. R. Schiff. Philadelphia, J. B. Lippincott, 1987.
52. Gines, P., et al.: Compensated cirrhosis: natural history and prognostic factors. Hepatology, *7*:122, 1987.
53. Muraca, M., Fevery, J., and Blanckaert, N.: Analytic aspects and clinical interpretation of serum bilirubin. Semin. Liver Dis., *8*:137, 1988.
54. Tisdale, W. A., Klatskin, G., and Kinsella, E.: The significance of the direct-reacting fraction of serum bilirubin in hemolytic jaundice. Am. J. Med., *26*:214, 1959.
55. Powell, L. H., Billing, B. H., and Williams, H. S.: The assessment of red blood cell survival in idiopathic unconjugated hyperbilirubinemia (Gilbert's syndrome) by the use of radioactive diisopropylfluorophosphate and chromium. Australas. Ann. Med., *16*:221, 1967.
56. Fulop, M., Katz, S., and Lawrence, C.: Extreme hyperbilirubinemia. Arch. Intern. Med., *127*:254, 1971.
57. Weiss, J. S., et al.: The clinical importance of a protein-bound fraction of serum bilirubin in patients with hyperbilirubinemia. N. Engl. J. Med., *309*:147, 1983.
58. Kaplowitz, N., Eberle, D., and Yamada, T.: Biochemical tests in liver disease. *In* Hepatology: A Textbook of Liver Disease. Edited by D. Zakim, and T. A. Boyer. Philadelphia, W. B. Saunders, 1982.
59. Friedman, R. A.: Vitamin K dependent proteins. N. Engl. J. Med., *310*:1458, 1984.
60. Reichling, J. J., and Kaplan, M. M.: Clinical use of serum enzymes in liver disease. Dig. Dis. Sci., *33*:1601, 1988.
61. Cohen, G. A., et al.: Observations on decreased serum glutamine oxaloacetic transaminase (SGOT) activity in azotemic patients. Ann. Intern. Med., *84*:275, 1976.
62. Patwardhan, R. V., Smith, O. J., and Farmelant, M. H.: Serum transaminase levels and cholescintigraphic abnormalities in acute biliary tract obstruction. Arch. Intern. Med., *147*:1249, 1987.
63. Williams, A. L. B., and Hoofnagle, J. H.: Ratio of serum aspartate to alanine aminotransferase in chronic hepatitis. Relationship to cirrhosis. Gastroenterology, *95*:734, 1988.
64. Cohen, J. A., and Kaplan, M. M.: The SGOT/SGPT ratio; an indicator of alcoholic liver disease. Dig. Dis. Sci., *24*:835, 1979.
65. Elibol, T., Winkelman, E. I., and King, J. W.: Lack of diagnostic significance of serum alkaline phosphatase in differentiating hepatocellular and obstructive jaundice. Cleve. Clin. J. Med., *35*:159, 1968.
66. Gordon, S. C., et al.: Prolonged intrahepatic cholestasis secondary to acute hepatitis A. Ann. Intern. Med., *101*:635, 1984.
67. Lumeng, L.: New diagnostic markers of alcohol abuse. Hepatology, *4*:742, 1986.
68. Shear, L., Bonkowsky, H. L., and Gabuzda, G. J.: Renal tubular acidosis in cirrhosis. A determinant of susceptibility to recurrent hepatic precoma. N. Engl. J. Med., *280*:1, 1969.
69. Karvountzis, G. G., and Redeker, A. G.: Relation of alpha-fetoprotein in acute hepatitis to severity and prognosis. Ann. Intern. Med., *80*:156, 1974.
70. Walker, J. G., et al.: Serological tests in diagnosis of primary biliary cirrhosis. Lancet, *1*:827, 1965.
71. Hollinger, B. F., and Ticehurst, J.: Hepatitis A virus. *In* Viral Hepatitis. 2nd Ed. Edited by B. F. Hollinger, et al. New York, Raven Press, 1991.
72. Alter, H. J.: The hepatitis C virus and its relationship to the clinical spectrum of non-A, non-B hepatitis. J. Gastroenterol. Hepatol., *5*:(Suppl. 1):78, 1990.
73. Khuroo, M. S.: Study of an epidemic of non-A, non-B hepatitis. Possibility of another human hepatitis virus distinct from past transfusion non-A, non-B hepatitis. Am. J. Med., *68*:818, 1980.
74. Hibbs, J. R., et al.: Aplastic anemia and viral hepatitis, non-A, non-B, non-C? JAMA, *267*:2051, 1992.
75. Karran, S., et al.: Investigation of the jaundiced patient. *In* Liver and Biliary Disease. Edited by R. Wright, K. G. M. M. Alberti, S. Karran, and G. H. Millward-Sadler. London, W. B. Saunders, 1979.
76. Liebman, P. R., et al.: Hepatic-portal venous gas in adults. Ann. Surg., *187*:281, 1978.
77. Drane, W. E.: Nuclear medicine techniques for the liver and biliary system. Update for the 1990s. Radiol. Clin. North Am., *29*:1129, 1991.
78. Alazroki, N. P., Fajman, W. A., and Christian, P. E.: Gastrointestinal imaging procedures. *In* Textbook of Gastroenterology. Edited by T. Yamada, et al. Philadelphia, W. B. Saunders, 1991.
79. Frietas, J. E.: Cholescintigraphy in acute and chronic cholecystitis. Sem. Nucl. Med., *12*:18, 1982.
80. Weissman, H. S., et al.: Spectrum of 99m-Tc-IDA cholescintigraphic patterns in acute cholecystitis. Radiology, *138*:167, 1981.
81. Weissman, H. S., et al.: Evaluation of the postoperative patient with 99m-Tc-IDA cholescintigraphy. Sem. Nucl. Med., *12*:27, 1982.
82. Zeman, R. K., et al.: Hepatobiliary scintigraphy and sonography in early biliary obstruction. Radiology, *153*:793, 1984.
83. Crade, M., et al.: Surgical and pathologic correlation of cholecystosonography and cholecystography. Am. J. Gastroenterol., *13*:227, 1978.
84. McIntosh, D. M. F., and Penney, H. F.: Gray-scale ultrasonography as a screening procedure in the detection of gallbladder disease. Radiology, *136*:725, 1980.
85. Marton, K. I., and Doubilet, P.: How to image the gallbladder in suspected cholecystitis. Ann. Intern. Med., *109*:722, 1988.
86. Grossman, S. J., and Joyce, J. M.: Hepatobiliary imaging. Emerg. Med. Clin. North Am., *9*:853, 1991.
87. Einstein, D. M., et al.: The unsensitivity of sonography in the detection of choledocholithiasis. Am. J. Roentgenol., *142*:725, 1984.
88. Cohen, S. M., and Kurtz, A. B.: Biliary sonography. Radiol. Clin. North Am., *29*:1171, 1991.
89. Foley, W. D., and Jochem, R. J.: Computed tomography. Focal and diffuse liver disease. Radiol. Clin. North Am., *29*:1213, 1991.
90. Baron, R. L.: Computed tomography of the biliary tree. Radiol. Clin. North Am., *29*:1235, 1991.
91. Borkowski, G. P.: Hepatobiliary and pancreatic imaging. *In* Clinical Gastroenterology. 2nd Ed. Edited by E. Achkar, R. G. Farmer, B. Fleshler. Philadelphia, Lea & Febiger, 1992.
92. Sherlock, S.: Disease of the Liver and Biliary System. 8th Ed., London, Blackwell Scientific Publications, 1989.
93. Edmondson, H. A., and Schiff, L.: Needle biopsy of the liver. *In* Diseases of the Liver. 4th Ed. Edited by L. Schiff. Philadelphia, J. B. Lippincott, 1975.
94. McGill, D. B., et al.: A 21 yr. experience with major hemor-

rhage after percutaneous liver biopsy. Gastroenterology, 99:1396, 1990.
95. McAfee, J. H., et al.: Transjugular liver biopsy. Hepatology, 15:726, 1992.
96. Corr, P., Beningfield, S. J., and Davey, N.: Transjugular liver biopsy: a review of 200 biopsies. Clin. Radiol., 45:238, 1992.
97. Bernuau, J., Rueff, B., and Benhamou, J. P.: Fulminant and subfulminant liver failure: definition and cause. Semin. Liver Dis., 6:97, 1986.
98. Mathiesen, L. R., et al.: Hepatitis A, B, and non-A, non-B in fulminant hepatitis. Gut, 21:72, 1979.
99. European Association for the Study of Liver Disease: Randomized trial of steroid therapy in acute liver failure. Gut, 20:620, 1979.
100. McNeil, M., et al.: Etiology of fatal viral hepatitis in Melbourne. Med. J. Aust., 141:637, 1984.
101. Gimson, A. E. S., et al.: Late onset hepatic failure: clinical serological and histological features. Hepatology, 6:288, 1986.
102. Trey, E., Lipworth, L., and Davidson, C. S.: Parameters influencing survival in the first 318 patients reported to the Fulminant Hepatic Surveillance Study. Gastroenterology, 58:306, 1970.
103. Rakela, J., and Acute Hepatic Failure Study Group: Etiology and prognosis in fulminant hepatitis. Gastroenterology, 77: A3, 1979.
104. O'Grady, J. G., et al.: Early indicators of prognosis in fulminant hepatic failure. Gastroenterology, 97:439, 1989.
105. O'Grady, J., and Williams, R.: Acute liver failure. Bailliere's Clin. Gastroenterol., 3:75, 1989.
106. O'Grady, J. C., et al.: Controlled trials of charcoal hemoperfusion and prognostic factors in fulminant hepatic failure. Gastroenterology, 94:1186, 1988.
107. Hollinger, B. F.: Hepatitis B virus. In Viral Hepatitis. 2nd Ed. Edited by F. B. Hollinger, et al. New York, Raven Press, 1991.
108. Gimson, A. E. S., et al.: Clinical and prognostic difference in fulminant hepatitis A, B and non-A, non-B. Gut, 24:1194, 1983.
109. Redecker, A. G., et al.: Hepatitis B immune globulin as a prophylactic measure for spouses exposed to acute type B hepatitis. N. Engl. J. Med., 293:1055, 1975.
110. Purcell, R. H., and Gerin, J. L.: Hepatitis delta virus. In Viral Hepatitis. 2nd Ed. Edited by B. F. Hollinger, et al.: New York, Raven Press, 1991.
111. Farci, P., et al.: Diagnostic and prognostic significance of the IGM antibody to the hepatitis delta virus. JAMA, 255: 1443, 1986.
112. Alter, M. J.: Non-A, non-B hepatitis: sorting through a diagnosis of exclusion. Ann. Intern. Med., 110: 583, 1989.
113. Hollinger, F. B.: Non-A, non-B hepatitis virus. In Viral Hepatitis. 2nd Ed. Edited by F. B. Hollinger, et al. New York, Raven Press, 1991.
114. Wright, T. L., et al.: Hepatitis C virus not found in fulminant non-A, non-B hepatitis. Ann. Intern. Med., 115:111, 1993.
115. Wright, T. L.: Etiology of fulminant hepatic failure: is another virus involved? Gastroenterology, 104:640, 1993.
116. Kiyosawa, K., et al.: Interrelationship of blood transfusion. Non-A, non-B hepatitis and hepatocellular carcinoma: analysis by detection of antibody to hepatitis C virus. Hepatology, 12:671, 1990.
117. Fagan, E. A., and Williams, R.: Fulminant viral hepatitis. Br. Med. Bull., 46:462, 1990.
118. Lewis, J. H., and Zimmerman, H.: Drug induced liver disease. Med. Clin. North Am., 73:775, 1989.
119. Seef, L., et al.: Acetaminophen hepatoxicity in alcoholics. Ann. Intern. Med., 87:299, 1977.
120. Eriksson, L. S., et al.: Hepatotoxicity due to repeated intake of low doses of paracetamol. J. Intern. Med., 123:567, 1992.
121. Schultz, J. C., et al.: Fetal liver disease after intravenous administration of tetracycline in high dosage. N. Engl. J. Med., 269:999, 1963.
122. Jonas, M. M., and Eidson, M. S.: Propylthiouracil hepatotoxicity: two pediatric cases and review of the literature. J. Pediatr. Gastroenterol. Nutr., 7:776, 1988.
123. Brusko, C. S., and Marten, J. T.: Ketoconazole hepatoxicity treated for environmental illness and systemic candidiasis. DICP Ann. Pharmacother., 25:1321, 1991.
124. Hodis, H. N.: Acute hepatic failure with the use of low-dose sustained-release niacin. JAMA, 264:181, 1990.
125. Wanless, I. R., et al.: Histopathology of cocaine hepatotoxicity. Gastroenterology, 98:497, 1990.
126. Wysowski, D. K., et al.: Fatal and nonfatal hepatotoxicity associated with flutamide. Ann. Intern. Med., 118:860, 1993.
127. Klatskin, G.: Toxic and drug-induced hepatitis. In Diseases of the Liver. 4th Ed. Edited by L. Schiff. Philadelphia, J. B. Lippincott, 1975.
128. Harrison, R., et al.: Fulminant hepatic failure after occupational exposure to 2-nitropropane. Ann. Intern. Med., 107: 466, 1987.
129. Vesconi, S., et al.: Therapy of cytoxic mushroom intoxication. Crit. Care Med., 13:402, 1985.
130. Pinson, C. W., et al.: Liver transplantation in severe Amanita phylloides mushroom poisoning. Am. J. Surg., 159:493, 1990.
131. Nouel, O., et al.: Fulminant hepatic failure due to transient circulatory failure in patients with chronic heart disease. Dig. Dis. Sci., 25:49, 1980.
132. Gibson, P. D., and Dudley, F. J.: Ischemic hepatitis: clinical features, diagnosis and prognosis. Aust. N.Z. J. Med., 14: 822, 1984.
133. Tavill, A. S.: The Budd-Chiari syndrome: correlation between hepatic scintiography and the clinical, radiological and pathological findings in nineteen cases of hepatic venous outflow obstruction. Gastroenterology, 68:509, 1975.
134. Powell-Jackson, P. R., Ede, R. J., and Williams, R.: Budd-Chiari syndrome presenting as fulminant hepatic failure. Gut, 27:1101, 1986.
135. Rollins, B. J.: Hepatic veno-occlusive disease. Am. J. Med., 81:297, 1986.
136. Jones, R. J., et al.: Veno-occlusive disease of the liver following bone marrow transplantation. Transplantation, 44:778, 1987.
137. McDonald, G. B., et al.: Veno-occlusive disease of the liver and multiorgan failure after bone marrow transplantation: a cohort study of 355 patients. Ann. Intern. Med., 118:255, 1993.
138. Eras, P., and Sherlock, P.: Hepatic coma secondary to metastatic disease. Ann. Intern. Med., 74:591, 1971.
139. Zafrani, E. S., et al.: Massive metastatic infiltration of the liver: a cause of fulminant hepatic failure. Hepatology, 3: 428, 1983.
140. Schneider, R., and Cohen, A.: Fulminant hepatic failure complicating metastatic breast carcinoma. South. Med. J., 77:84, 1984.
141. Colby, T., and LaBrecque, D. R.: Lymphoreticular malignancy presenting as fulminant hepatic disease. Gastroenterology, 82:339, 1982.
142. Roche-Sicot, J., and Benhamou, J. P.: Acute intravascular hemolysis and acute liver failure associated as a first manifestation of Wilson's disease. Ann. Intern. Med., 86:301, 1977.

143. McCullough, A. J., et al.: Diagnosis of Wilson's disease presenting as fulminant hepatic failure. Gastroenterology, 84: 161, 1983.
144. Riely, C. A., et al.: Acute fatty liver of pregnancy. Ann. Intern. Med., 106:703, 1987.
145. Prix, L. Y., et al.: Primary sepsis presenting as fulminant hepatic failure. Q. J. Med. N. S., 73:1037, 1989.
146. Hassanein, T., et al.: Liver failure occurring as a component of exertional heat stroke. Gastroenterology, 100:1442, 1991.
147. Kingham, J. G. C., et al.: Non-cirrhotic intrahepatic portal hypertension: a long term follow-up study. Q. J. Med. N. S., 50:259, 1981.
148. Mikkelsen, W. P.: Extrahepatic portal hypertension in children. Am. J. Surg., 111:333, 1966.
149. Raskin, N. H., Pierce, J. B., and Fishman, R. A.: Portal-systemic encephalopathy due to congenital intrahepatic shunts. N. Engl. J. Med., 270:225, 1964.
150. Davidson, C. S.: Hepatic coma. In Gastroenterology. Vol. III. 3rd Ed. Edited by H. L. Bockus. Philadelphia, W. B. Saunders, 1976.
151. Gitlin, N.: Subclinical portal-systemic encephalopathy. Am. J. Gastroenterol., 83:8, 1988.
152. Bernthal, P., et al.: Cerebral CT scan abnormalities in cholestatic and hepatocellular disease and their relationship to neuropsychologic test performance. Hepatology, 7:107, 1987.
153. Shomerus, H., et al.: Latent portasystemic encephalopathy: nature of cerebral functional defects and their effect on fitness to drive. Dig. Dis. Sci., 26:622, 1981.
154. Srivastana, A., et al.: Fitness to drive in compensated cirrhosis. Hepatology, 14:89A, 1991.
155. Mullen, K. D.: New approaches to the management of chronic hepatic encephalopathy. American Association for the Study of Liver Disease Post graduate course. Chicago, 1992.
156. Tarter, R. E., et al.: Subclinical hepatic encephalopathy—comparison before and after orthotopic liver transplantation. Transplantation, 50:632, 1990.
157. Conn, H. O.: Asterixis in non-hepatic disorders. Am. J. Med., 29:647, 1960.
158. Adams, R. C., and Foley, J. M.: The neurological disorder associated with liver disease. Res. Publ. Assoc. Res. Nerv. Ment. Dis., 32:198, 1953.
159. Conomy, J. P., and Swash, M.: Reversible decerebrate and decorticate posture in hepatic coma. N. Engl. J. Med., 278: 876, 1968.
160. O'Brien, C. J., et al.: Neurological sequelae in patients recovered from fulminant hepatic failure. Gut, 28:93, 1987.
161. Zieve, L.: Hepatic coma. In Diseases of the Liver. 6th Ed. Edited by L. Schiff and E. R. Schiff. Philadelphia, J. B. Lippincott, 1987.
162. Munoz, S. J., et al.: Elevated intracranial pressure and computed tomography of the brain in fulminant hepatocellular failure. Hepatology, 13:209, 1991.
163. Lidofsky, S. D., et al.: Intracranial pressure monitoring and liver transplantation for fulminant hepatic failure. Hepatology, 16:1, 1992.
164. Hourani, B. T., Hamlin, E. M., and Reynolds. T. B.: Cerebrospinal fluid glutamine as a measure of hepatic encephalopathy. Arch. Intern. Med., 127:1033, 1971.
165. Donovan, J. P., et al.: Cerebral edema as a complication of chronic liver disease. Hepatology, 12:860(A), 1990.
166. Brown, C. L., Hill, M. J., and Richards, P.: Bacterial ureases in uremic men. Lancet, 2:406, 1971.
167. Read, A. E., et al.: The neuro-psychiatric syndromes associated with chronic liver disease and an extensive portal-systemic collateral circulation. Q. J. Med., 141:135, 1962.
168. Victor, M., Adams, R., and Cole, M.: The acquired (non-Wilsonian) type of chronic hepatocerebral degeneration. Medicine, 44:345, 1965.
169. Powell, E. E., et al.: Improvement in chronic hepatocerebral degeneration following liver transplantation. Gastroenterology, 98:107, 1990.
170. Lebovics, E., et al.: Portal systemic myelopathy after portacaval shunt surgery. Arch. Intern. Med., 145:1921, 1985.
171. Lockwood, A. H., Yap, E. W. H., and Wong, W. H.: Cerebral ammonia metabolism in patients with severe liver disease and minimal encephalopathy. J. Cerebr. Blood Flow Metab., 11:331, 1991.
172. Butterworth, R. F.: Pathogenesis and treatment of portal systemic encephalopathy: an update. Dig. Dis. Sci., 37:321, 1992.
173. Fischer, J. E.: Hepatic coma in cirrhosis, portal hypertension and following portacaval shunt. Arch. Surg., 108:325, 1974.
174. Schafer, D. E., and Jones, E. A.: Hepatic encephalopathy and gamma aminobutyric acid. Lancet, 1:18, 1980.
175. Ferenci, P., et al.: Serum levels of gamma-aminobutyric acid-like activity in acute and chronic hepatocellular disease. Lancet, 2:811, 1983.
176. Jones, E. A., Skolnick, P., and Gammal, S.: The gamma-aminobutyric acid (GABA) receptor complex. Ann. Intern. Med., 110:532, 1989.
177. Mullen, K. D., et al.: Could an endogenous benzodiazepine contribute to hepatic encephalopathy? Lancet, 1:457, 1988.
178. Scollo-Lavizzari, G., and Steinmann, E.: Reversal of hepatic coma by benzodiazepine antagonist (RO15-1788). Lancet, 1:1324, 1985.
179. Bansky, G., et al.: Reversal of hepatic coma by benzodiazepine antagonist (RO15-1788). Lancet, 1:1324, 1985.
180. Bassett, M. L., et al.: Amelioration of hepatic encephalopathy by pharmacologic antagonism of GABA-benzodiazepine receptor complex in a rabbit model of fulminant hepatic failure. Gastroenterology, 93:1069, 1987.
181. Mullen, K. D., Szauter, K. M., and Kaminsky-Russ, K.: Endogenous benzodiazepine activity in body fluids of patients with hepatic encephalopathy. Lancet, 336:81, 1990.
182. Basile, A. S., et al.: Elevated brain concentration of 1-4 benzodiazepine in fulminant hepatic failure. N. Engl. J. Med., 325:473, 1991.
183. Bansky, G., et al.: Effect of the benzodiazepine receptor antagonist flumazenil in hepatic encephalopathy in humans. Gastroenterology, 99:744, 1989.
184. Grimm, G., et al.: Improvement of hepatic encephalopathy treated with flumazenil. Lancet, 2:1392, 1988.
185. Mejer, R., Gyr, K., and Scholer, A.: Persisting benzodiazepine metabolites responsible for the reaction to the benzodiazepine antagonist flumazenil in patients with hepatic encephalopathy. Gastroenterology, 101:274, 1991.
186. Ware, A. J., D'Agostino, A. N., and Combes, B.: Cerebral edema: a major complication of massive hepatic necrosis. Gastroenterology, 61:877, 1971.
187. Ede, R., and Williams, R.: Hepatic encephalopathy and cerebral edema. Semin. Liver Dis., 6:107, 1986.
188. Hanid, M. A., et al.: Clinical monitoring of intracranial pressure in fulminant hepatic failure. Gut, 21:866, 1980.
189. Blei, A. T.: Cerebral edema and intracranial hypertension in acute liver failure: distinct aspects of the same problem. Hepatology, 13:376, 1991.
190. Schafer, D. F., and Shaw, B. W., Jr.: Fulminant hepatic failure and orthotopic liver transplantation. Semin. Liver Dis., 9: 187, 1989.
191. Blei, A. T.: Brain edema in fulminant hepatic failure (FHF).

The importance of intracranial pressure monitoring. Postgraduate course, American Association for the Study of Liver Disease. Chicago, 1992.
192. Canalese, J., et al.: Controlled trial of dexamethasone and mannitol for the cerebral edema of fulminant hepatic failure. Gut, 23:625, 1982.
193. Forbes, A., et al.: Thiopental infusion in the treatment of intracranial hypertension complicating fulminant hepatic failure. Hepatology, 10:306, 1989.
194. Weber, F. L., Jr., et al.: Nitrogen in fecal bacteria, fiber, and soluble fractions of patients with cirrhosis. Effect of lactulose and lactulose and neomycin. J. Lab. Clin. Med., 110:259, 1987.
195. Morgan, M. V., and Hawley, K.: Lactitol vs. lactulose in the treatment of acute hepatic encephalopathy in cirrhotic patients: a double-blind randomized trial. Hepatology, 6:1278, 1987.
196. Blanc, P., et al.: Lactilol or lactulose in the treatment of chronic hepatitic encephalopathy: results of a meta-analysis. Hepatology, 15:222, 1992.
197. Uribe, M.: Treatment of chronic portal-systemic encephalopathy with lactose in lactase difficient patients. Dig. Dis. Sci., 25:924, 1980.
198. Kersh, E. S., and Rifkin, H.: Lactulose enemas. Ann. Intern. Med., 78:81, 1973.
199. Uribe, M., et al.: Lactose enemas plus placebo tablets vs. neomycin tablets plus starch enemas in acute portal systemic encephalopathy. Gastroenterology, 81:101, 1981.
200. Conn, H. O., et al.: Comparison of lactulose and neomycin in the treatment of chronic portal-systemic encephalopathy. Gastroenterology, 72:573, 1972.
201. Pirotte, J., Guffens, J. M., and Devos, J.: Comparative study of basal arterial ammonemia and of orally-induced hyperammonemia in chronic portal systemic encephalopathy treated with neomycin, lactulose, and an association of neomycin and lactulose. Digestion, 10:435, 1974.
202. Morgan, M. H., Read, A. E., and Speller, D. C. E.: Treatment of hepatic encephalopathy with metronidazole. Gut, 23:1, 1982.
203. Tarao, K., et al.: Successful use of vancomycin hydrochloride in the treatment of lactulose resistant chronic hepatic encephalopathy. Gut, 31:702, 1990.
204. Ware, A. J., et al.: A controlled trial of steroid therapy in massive hepatic necrosis. Am. J. Gastroenterol., 62:130, 1974.
205. Redeker, A. G., Schweitzer, I. L., and Yamahiro, H. S.: Randomization of corticosteroid therapy in fulminant hepatic failure. N. Engl. J. Med., 294:728, 1976.
206. Rakela, J., et al.: A double-blinded randomized trial of hydrocortisone in acute hepatic failure. Dig. Dis. Sci., 36:1223, 1991.
207. Rosen, H. M., et al.: Plasma aminoacid pattern in hepatic encephalopathy of differing etiology. Gastroenterology, 72:483, 1977.
208. Naylor, C. D., et al.: Parenteral nutrition with branched-chain aminoacids in hepatic encephalopathy. A meta-analysis. Gastroenterology, 97:1033, 1989.
209. Munoz, S. J.: Nutritional therapies in liver disease. Semin. Liver Dis., 11:278, 1991.
210. Mullen, K. D., and Weber, F. L., Jr.: Role of nutrition in hepatic encephalopathy. Semin. Liv. Dis., 11:292, 1991.
211. Prasad, A. S., and Rabbani, P.: Nucleoside phosphorylase in zinc deficiency. Trans. Am. Assoc. Phys., 94:314, 1981.
212. Redding, P., Duchateau, J., and Bataille, C.: Oral zinc supplementation improves hepatic encephalopathy. Lancet, 2:493, 1984.
213. Riggio, O., et al.: Short-term oral zinc supplementation does not improve chronic hepatic encephalopathy: results of a double-blind cross-over trial. Dig. Dis. Sci., 36:1204, 1991.
214. van der Rijt, C. P. A., et al.: Overt hepatic encephalopathy precipitated by zinc deficiency. Gastroenterology, 100:1114, 1991.
215. Mendenhall, C. L., et al.: A new therapy for portal systemic encephalopathy. Am. J. Gastroenterol., 81:450, 1986
216. Uribe, M., et al.: Sodium benzoate versus dissacharides: a controlled multicenter clinical trial [abstr.]. Biennial Scientific Meeting of International Association for the Study of Liver Disease, Gold Coast, Australia, 1990.
217. Sushma, S., et al.: Sodium benzoate in the treatment of acute hepatic encephalopathy: a double-blind randomized trial. Hepatology, 16:138, 1992.
218. O'Grady, J. C., et al.: Controlled trials of charcoal hemoperfusion and prognostic factors in fulminant hepatic failure. Gastroenterology, 94:1186, 1988.
219. Burnell, J. M., et al.: Acute hepatic coma treated by cross-circulation or exchange transfusion. N. Engl. J. Med., 276:935, 1967.
220. Saunders, S. J., et al.: Acute hepatic coma treated by cross-circulation with a baboon and by repeated exchange transfusions. Lancet, 2:585, 1968.
221. Lepore, M. J., and Martel, D. J.: Plasmapheresis with plasma exchange in hepatic coma. Ann. Intern. Med., 72:165, 1970.
222. Sen, P. K., et al.: Use of isolated cadaver liver in the management of hepatic failure. Surgery, 59:774, 1966.
223. Eiseman, B., Liem, D. S., and Rafucci, I. F.: Heterologous liver perfusion in treatment of liver failure. Ann. Surg., 162:329, 1965.
224. Klebanoff, G., et al.: Resuscitation of a patient in stage IV hepatic coma using total body washout. J. Surg. Res., 13:159, 1972.
225. Hanna, S. S., et al.: Reversal of hepatic encephalopathy after occlusion of total portasystemic shunt. Am. J. Surg., 142:285, 1981.
226. Bismuth, H., Houssin, D., and Grange, D.: Suppression of the shunt and esophageal transection: a new technique for the treatment of disabling post shunt encephalopathy. Am. J. Surg., 146:392, 1983.
227. Dagenais, M. H., et al.: Surgical treatment of severe post shunt hepatic encephalopathy. World J. Surg., 15:109, 1991.
228. McDermott, W. V., Jr., Victor, M., and Point, W. W.: Exclusion of the colon in the treatment of hepatic encephalopathy. N. Engl. J. Med., 267:850, 1962.
229. Walker, J. G., et al.: Treatment of chronic portal-systemic encephalopathy by surgical exclusion of the colon. Lancet, 2:861, 1965.
230. Resnick, R. H., et al.: Controlled trial of colon bypass in chronic hepatic encephalopathy. Gastroenterology, 51:1057, 1968.
231. Trewby, P. N., and Williams, R.: Pathophysiology of hypotension in patients with fulminant hepatic failure. Gut, 18:1021, 1977.
232. Bihari, D. J., Gimson, A. E. S., and Williams, R.: Cardiovascular, pulmonary and renal complications of fulminant hepatic failure. Semin. Liver Dis., 6:119, 1986.
233. Weston, M. J., et al.: Frequency of arrhythmias and other cardiac abnormalities in fulminant hepatic failure. Br. Heart J., 38:1179, 1976.
234. Krowka, M. J., and Cortese, D. A.: Severe hypoxemia associated with liver disease and the experimental use of almitrine bismesylate. Mayo Clin. Proc., 62:164, 1987.
235. Stoller, J. K., et al.: Reduction of intrapulmonary shunt and resolution of digital clubbing associated with primary biliary cirrhosis after liver transplant. Hepatology, 11:54, 1990.

236. Trewby, P. N., et al.: Intrapulmonary vascular shunts in fulminant hepatic failure. Digestion, *14*:466, 1970.
237. Williams, A., et al.: Structural alterations to the pulmonary circulation in fulminant hepatic failure. Thorax, *34*:447, 1979.
238. O'Grady, J. G., et al.: Outcome of orthotopic liver transplantation and etiological and clinical variables of acute liver failure. Q. J. Med., *69*:817, 1988.
239. Wilkinson, S. P., et al.: Pathogenesis of renal failure in cirrhosis and fulminant hepatic failure. Postgrad. Med. J., *51*: 503, 1975.
240. Ring-Larsen, H., and Palazzo, U.: Renal failure in fulminant hepatic failure and terminal cirrhosis: a comparison between incidence, types and prognosis. Gut, *22*:585, 1981.
241. Navasa, M., et al.: Portal hypertension in acute liver failure. Gut, *33*:965, 1992.
242. Wilkinson, S. P., et al.: Frequency of renal impairment in paracetamol overdose compared with other causes of acute liver damage. J. Clin. Pathol., *30*:141, 1977.
243. Papper, S.: The hepatorenal syndrome. *In* The Kidney and Liver Disease. 2nd Ed. Edited by M. Epstein. New York, Elsevier Biomedical, 1983.
244. Epstein, M., et al.: Renal failure in the patient with cirrhosis. The role of active vasoconstriction. Am. J. Med., *49*:175, 1970.
245. Guarner, R., et al.: Renal function in fulminant hepatic failure: hemodynamics and renal prostaglandins. Gut, *28*:1643, 1987
246. Better, O., and Schrier, R. W.: The hepatorenal syndrome. In Diseases of the Kidney. 5th Ed. Edited by R. W. Schrier and C. W. Gottshalk. Boston, Little, Brown & Co., 1993.
247. Wilkinson, S. P., Blendis, L. M., and Williams, R.: Frequency and type of renal and electrolyte disorders in fulminant hepatic failure. Br. Med. J., *1*:186, 1974.
248. Wilkinson, S. P., and Williams, R.: Ascites, electrolytes and renal failure. *In* Liver and Biliary Disease. Edited by R. Wright, K. G. M. N. Alberti, S. Karran, and G. H. Millward-Sadler. London, W. B. Saunders, 1979.
249. Pampligionie, G.: The effect of metabolic disorders on brain activity. J. R. Coll. Phys. (Lond.), *7*:347, 1973.
250. Ritt, D. J., et al.: Acute hepatic necrosis with stupor or coma. Medicine, *48*:151, 1969.
251. Gazzard, B. G., et al.: Causes of death in fulminant hepatic failure and relationship to quantitative histological assessment of parenchymal change. Q. J. Med. N. S., *54*:615, 1975.
252. Rakel, J., et al.: Fulminant hepatitis: Mayo Clinic experience with thirty-four cases. Mayo Clin. Proc., *60*:289, 1985.
253. Bismuth, H., et al.: Emergency liver transplantation for fulminant hepatitis. Ann. Intern. Med., *107*:337, 1987.
254. Rolando, N., et al.: Prospective study of bacterial infection in acute liver failure: an analysis of fifty patients. Hepatology, *11*:49, 1990.
255. Canalese, J., et al.: Reticuloenohelial system and hepatocyte function in fulminant hepatic failure. Gut, *23*:265, 1982.
256. Imawari, M., et al.: Fibronectin and Kupffer cell function in fulminant hepatic failure. Dig. Dis. Sci., *30*:1028, 1985.
257. Larcher, V. F., et al.: Bacterial and fungal infection in children with fulminant hepatic failure: possible role of opsonization and complement deficiency. Gut, *23*:1037, 1982.
258. Wyke, R. J., et al.: Defective opsonization and complement deficiency in serum from patients with fulminant hepatic failure. Gut, *21*:643, 1980.
259. Altin, M., et al.: Neutrophil adherence in chronic liver disease and fulminant hepatic failure. Gut, *24*:746, 1983.
260. DeLeon, S. P., and Wenzel, R. P.: Hospital-acquired bloodstream infections with staphylococcus epidermidis. Am. J. Med., *77*:639, 1984.
261. Rolando, N., et al.: Fungal infection: a common unrecognized complication of acute liver failure. J. Hepatol., *12*:1, 1991.
262. Rolando, N., et al.: Prospective controlled trial of selective parenteral and enteral antimicrobial regimen in fulminant hepatic failure. Hepatology, *17*:196, 1993.
263. Bernuau, J., et al.: Multivariate analysis of prognostic factors in fulminant hepatitis B. Hepatology, *6*:648, 1986.
264. Williams, R., and Gimson, A. E. S.: Intensive liver care and management of acute hepatic failure. Dig. Dis. Sci., *36*:820, 1991.
265. Bernuau, J., et al.: Criteria for emergency liver transplantation in patients with acute viral hepatitis and factor V (FV) below 50% of normal: a prospective study. Hepatology, *14*: 49A, 1991.
266. Hughes, R. D., Wendon, J., and Gimson, A. E. S.: Acute liver failure. Gut, *5(Suppl.)*:86, 1991.
267. MacDougall, B. R. D., and Williams, R.: H₂ receptor antagonist in the prevention of acute upper gastrointestinal hemorrhage in fulminant hepatic failure. Gastroenterology, *74*: 164, 1978.
268. Stone, B. G., and Van Thiel, D. H.: Diabetes mellitus and the liver. Semin. Liver Dis., *5*:8, 1985.
269. Saunders, S. J., et al.: Acute liver failure. *In* Liver and Biliary Disease. Edited by R. Wright, K. G. M. N. Alberti, S. Karrau, and G. H. Millward-Sadler. London, W. B. Saunders, 1979.
270. Samson, R. I., et al.: Fulminant hepatitis with recurrent hypoglycemia and hemorrhage. Gastroenterology, *53*:291, 1967.
271. Valla, D., et al.: Portal hypertension and ascites in acute hepatitis: clinical hemodynamic and histologic correlations. Hepatology, *10*:482, 1989.
272. Ham, J. M., and Fitzpatrick, P.: Acute pancreatitis in patients with acute hepatic failure. Am. J. Dig. Dis., *18*:1079, 1973.
273. Parbhoo, S. P., Welch, J., and Sherlock, S.: Acute pancreatitis in patients with fulminant hepatic failure. Gut, *14*: 428(A), 1973.
274. Ede, R. J., et al.: Frequency of pancreatitis in fulminant hepatic failure using isomzyne markers. Gut, *29*:778, 1988.
275. Achord, J. L.: Acute pancreatitis with infectious hepatitis. JAMA, *205*:837, 1968.
276. Brems, J. J., et al.: Fulminant hepatic failure: the role of liver transplantation as primary therapy. Am. J. Surg., *154*:137, 1987.
277. Emond, J. C., et al.: Liver transplantation in the management of fulminant hepatic failure. Gastroenterology, *96*:1582, 1989.
278. Iwatsuki, S., et al.: Liver transplantation for fulminant hepatic failure. Transplant. Proc., *21*:2431, 1989.
279. Van de Stadt, J., et al.: Liver transplantation for fulminant and subacute viral hepatitis failure in adults. Transplant. Proc., *22*:1505, 1990.
280. Sheil, A. G., et al.: Acute and subacute fulminant hepatic failure: the role of liver transplantation. Med. J. Aust., *154*: 724, 1991.
281. Bone, R. C., and the ACCP/SCCM Concensus Conference Committee: Definitions for sepsis and organ failure and guidelines for the use of innovative therapies in sepsis. Chest, *101*:1644, 1992.
282. DeCamp, M. M., and Demling, R. H.: Post-traumatic multisystem organ failure. JAMA, *260*:530, 1988.
283. Canalese, J., et al.: Reticuloenthial system and hepatocyte function in fulminant hepatic failure. Gut, *23*:265, 1982.
284. Deitch, E. A.: The role of the intestinal barrier failure and bacterial translocaiton in the development of systemic in-

fection and multiple organ failure. Arch. Surg., *125*:403, 1990.
285. Anthony, P. O., et al.: The morphology of cirrhosis. J. Clin. Pathol., *31*:395, 1978.
286. Winkelman, E. I.: Cirrhosis. In Clinical Gastroenterology. 2nd Ed. Edited by E. A. Achkar, R. Farmer, and B. Fleshler. Philadelphia, Lea & Febiger, 1992.
287. Lindner, H. Y.: Laparoscopy? Gastrointest. Endosc., *19*:176, 1973.
288. Orlando, R., Lirussi, F., and Okolicsanyi, L.: Laparoscopy and liver biopsy: further evidence that the two procedures improve the diagnosis of liver cirrhosis. J. Clin. Gastroenterol., *12*:47, 1990.
289. Merkel, C., et al.: Prognostic value of galactose elimination capacity, aminopyrine breath test and indocyanine green clearance in patients with cirrhosis: comparison with the Pugh score. Dig. Dis. Sci., *36*:1197, 1991.
290. Burroughs, A. K., D'Hygere, F. D., and McIntyre, N.: Pitfalls in studies of prophylactic therapy for variceal bleeding in cirrhotics. Hepatology, *6*:1407, 1986.
291. Hoskins, S. W., et al.: Anorectal varices, hemorrhoids and portal hypertension. Lancet, *1*:349, 1989.
292. Shapero, T. F., Bourne, R. H., and Goodall, R. G.: Intra-abdominal bleeding from variceal bleeding in cirrhosis. Gastroenterology, *74*:129, 1978.
293. Groszmann, R. J., and Atterbury, C. E.: The pathophysiology of portal hypertension: a basis for classification. Semin. Liver Dis., *2*:177, 1982.
294. Boyer, T. D., et al.: Direct transhepatic measurement of portal vein pressure using a thin needle. Gastroenterology, *72*:584, 1977.
295. Viallet, A., et al.: Hemodynamic evaluation of patients with intrahepatic portal hypertension. Gastroenterology, *69*:1297, 1975.
296. Garcia-Tsao, et al.: Portal presure, presence of gastroesophageal varices and variceal bleeding. Hepatology, *5*:419, 1985.
297. Schaffner, F., and Popper. H.: Capillarization of hepatic sinusoids in man. Gastroenterology, *44*:239, 1963.
298. Blendis, L., et al.: The role of hepatocyte enlargement in hepatic pressure in cirrhotic and non-cirrhotic alcoholic liver disease. Hepatology, *2*:539, 1982.
299. Polio, J., and Groszmann, R. J.: Hemodynamic factors involved in the development and rupture of esophageal varices: a pathophysiologic approach to treatment. Semin. Liver Dis., *6*:318, 1986.
300. Lebrec, D., et al.: Portal hypertension, size of esophageal varices and risk of gastrointestinal bleeding in alcoholic cirrhosis. Gastroenterology, *79*:1139, 1980.
301. Reynolds, T. B.: Interrelationships of portal pressure, variceal size and upper gastrointestinal bleeding. Gastroenterology, *79*:1332, 1980.
302. Conn, H. O.: The varix volcano connection. Gastroenterology, *79*:133, 1980.
303. MacDonald, R. A., and Mallory, C. K.: The natural history of post necrotic cirrhosis: a study of 221 autopsy cases. Am. J. Med., *24*:334, 1955.
304. Stone, W. D., Isham, N. R. K., and Paton, A.: The natural history of cirrhosis. Q. J. Med., *37*:119, 1968.
305. Terblanche, J., Burroughs, A. K., and Hobbs, K. E. F.: Controversies in the management of bleeding esophageal varices. N. Engl. J. Med., *320*:1393 and 1469, 1989.
306. McCormack, T. T., et al.: Gastric lesions in portal hypertension: inflammatory gastritis or congestive gastropathy? Gut, *26*:1226, 1985.
307. Rabinowitz, M., et al.: Combined upper and lower gastrointestinal endoscopy: a prospective study in alcoholic and non-alcoholic cirrhosis. Alcoholism: Clin. Exp. Res., *13*:790, 1989.
308. Kirk, A. D., Dooley, J. S., and Hunt, R. N.: Peptic ulceration in patients with chronic liver disease. Dig. Dis. Sci., *25*:756, 1980.
309. Sutton, F. M.: Upper gastrointestinal bleeding in patients with esophageal varices. What is the most common? Am. J. Med., *83*:273, 1987.
310. Pinto, H. C., et al.: Long-term prognosis of patients with cirrhosis of the liver and upper gastrointestinal bleeding. Am. J. Gastroenterol., *84*:1239, 1989.
311. Sarin, S. K., et al.: Endoscopic sclerotherapy in the treatment of gastric varices. Br. J. Surg., *75*:747, 1988.
312. Fleischer, D.: Etiology and prevalence of severe persistent upper gastrointestinal bleeding. Gastroenterology, *84*:538, 1983.
313. MacDougall, B. R. D., and Williams, R.: A controlled trial of cimetidine in the recurrence of variceal hemorrhage: implication about the pathogenesis of hemorrhage. Hepatology, *3*:69, 1983.
314. Bhathal, P. S., and Groszmann, R. J.: Reduction of the increased portal vascular resistance of isolated perfused cirrhotic rat liver by vasodilation. J. Hepatol., *1*:325, 1985.
315. Baum, S., and Nusbaum, M.: The control of gastrointestinal hemorrhage by selective mesenteric arterial infusion of vasopressin. Radiology, *98*:497, 1971.
316. Chojkier, M., et al.: A controlled comparison of continuous intra-arterial and intravenous infusions of vasopressin in hemorrhage from esophageal varices. Gastroenterology, *77*:540, 1979.
317. Gimson, A. E. S., et al.: A randomized trial of vasopressin and vasopressin and nitroglycerin in the control of acute variceal hemorrhage. Hepatology, *6*:410, 1986.
318. Tsai, Y., et al.: Controlled trial of vasopressin and nitroglycerin vs. vasopressin alone in the treatment of bleeding esophageal varices. Hepatology, *6*:406, 1986.
319. Iwao, T., et al.: Hemodynamic study during transdermal application of nitroglycerin tape in patients with cirrhosis. Hepatology, *13*:124, 1991.
320. Kravetz, D., et al.: Comparison of intravenous somatostatin and vasopressin infusions in treatment of acute variceal hemorrhage. Hepatology, *4*:442, 1984.
321. Burroughs, A. K., et al.: Randomized double-blind placebo controlled trial of somatostatin for variceal bleeding. Gastroenterology, *99*:1388, 1990.
322. Valenzuela, J. E., et al.: A multicenter randomized double-blind trial of somatostatin in the management of acute hemorrhage from esophageal varices. Hepatology, *10*:958, 1989.
323. Hunt, P. S., et al.: An 8 year prospective experience with balloon tamponade in emergency control of bleeding esophageal varices. Dig. Dis. Sci., *27*:413, 1982.
324. Teres, J., et al.: Esophageal tamponade for bleeding varices: controlled trial between Sengstaken-Blakemore tube and Linton-Nachlas tube. Gastroenterology, *75*:566, 1978.
325. Panes, J., et al.: Efficacy of balloon tamponade in treatment of bleeding gastric and esophageal varices. Dig. Dis. Sci., *33*:454, 1988.
326. Feneyrou, B., et al.: Initial control of bleeding from esophageal varices with the Sengstaken-Blakemore tube. Am. J. Surg., *155*:509, 1988.
327. Chojkier, M., and Conn, H. O.: Esophageal tamponade in the treatment of bleeding varices: a prospective controlled randomized trial. Dig. Dis. Sci., *25*:267, 1980.
328. Paquet, K. J., and Feussner, H.: Endoscopic sclerosis and esophageal balloon tamponade in acute hemorrhage from

328. esophageal varices: a prospective controlled randomized trial. Hepatology, 5:580, 1985.
329. Allison, J. G.: The role of injection sclerotherapy in the emergency and definitive management of bleeding esophageal varices. JAMA 249:1484, 1983.
330. Larson, A. W., et al.: Acute esophageal variceal sclerotherapy: result of a prospective randomized controlled trial. JAMA 255:497, 1986.
331. Westaby, D., et al.: Injection sclerotherapy for active variceal bleeding: a controlled trial. Gut, 7:A1246, 1986.
332. Cello, J. P., et al.: Endoscopic sclerotherapy vs. portal-caval shunt in patients with severe cirrhosis and acute variceal hemorrhage. Long-term follow-up. N. Engl. J. Med., 316: 11, 1987.
333. Sivak, M. V., Jr.: Esophageal varices. In Endoscopy. Edited by M. V. Sivak, Jr. Philadelphia, W. B. Saunders, 1987.
334. Smith-Laing, G., et al.: Role of percutaneous transhepatic obliteration of varices in the management of hemorrhage from gastroesophageal varices. Gastroenterology, 80:1031, 1981.
335. Stiegman, G. V., et al.: Endoscopic sclerotherapy as compared with endoscopic ligation for bleeding esophageal varices. N. Engl. J. Med., 326:1527, 1992.
336. Prandi, D., et al.: Life threatening hemorrhage of the digestive tract in cirrhotic patients: an assessment of the postoperative mortality after emergency portacaval shunt. Am. J. Surg., 131:204, 1976.
337. Villeneuve, J. P., et al.: Emergency portacaval shunt for variceal hemorrhage. A prospective study. Ann. Surg., 206:48, 1987.
338. Malt, R. A., et al.: Randomized trial of emergency mesocaval and portacaval shunts for bleeding esophageal varices. Am. J. Surg., 135:584, 1978.
339. Orloff, M., et al.: Long-term results of emergency portacaval shunt for bleeding esophageal varices in unselected patients with alcoholic cirrhosis. Ann. Surg., 201:325, 1980.
340. Smith, R. B., et al.: Dacron interposition shunts for portal hypertension. Ann. Surg., 192:9, 1980.
341. Richter, G. M., et al.: Transjugular intrahepatic portasystemic shunts. Bailliére's Clin. Gastroenterol., 6:403, 1992.
342. LaBerge, J. M., et al.: Transjugular intrahepatic shunt: preliminary results in 25 patients. J. Vasc. Surg., 16:258, 1992.
343. Conn, H. O.: Transjugular intrahepatic portasystemic shunt: the state of mind. Hepatology, 17:148, 1993.
344. Vinel, J. P., et al.: Transjugular intrahepatic portacaval shunt (TIPS) using the Wall stent endoprothesis: prospective study in 66 patients. Hepatology, 16:85A, 1992.
345. Rossle, M., et al.: Feasibility of transjugular intrahepatic portasystemic stent shunt (TIPS) in the treatment of fulminant Budd-Chiari syndrome. Hepatology, 14:75A, 1992.
346. Sanyal, A. J., et al.: Transjugular intrahepatic portasystemic shunt (TIPS) vs. sclerotherapy for variceal hemorrhage: results of a randomized prospective study. Hepatology, 16: 88A, 1992.
347. Wanamaker, S. R., Cooperman, M., and Carey, L. C.: Use of the E.E.A. stapling instrument for control of bleeding esophageal varices. Surgery, 94:620, 1983.
348. Huizinga, W. K. J., Angorn, I. B., and Baker, L. W.: Esophageal transection vs. injection sclerotherapy in the management of bleeding esophageal varices in patients at high risk. Surg. Gynecol. Obstet., 160:539, 1985.
349. Spence, A. J., and Johnston, C. W.: Results in 100 consecutive patients with stapled esophageal transection for varices. Surg. Gynecol. Obstet., 160:323, 1985.
350. Hashizume, M., et al.: Endoscopic injection sclerotherapy for 1000 patients with esophageal varices: a 9 year prospective study. Hepatology, 15:69, 1992.
351. Westaby, D., MacDougall, B. R. D., and Williams, R.: Improved survival following injection sclerotherapy for esophageal varices: final analysis of a controlled trial. Hepatology, 5:827, 1985.
352. Fleig, W. E., et al.: Prevention of recurrent bleeding in cirrhotics with recent variceal hemorrhage: prospective, randomized comparison with sclerotherapy. Hepatology, 7: 355, 1987.
353. Dosarothy, S., et al.: A prospective randomized trial comparing repeated esophageal sclerotherapy and propranolol in decompensated (child B and C) cirrhotic patients. Hepatology, 16:89, 1992.
354. Westaby, D., et al.: A controlled trial of oral propranolol compared with injection sclerotherapy for the long-term management of variceal bleeding. Hepatology, 11:353, 1990.
355. Korula, J., et al.: A prospective randomized clinical trial of chronic esophageal variceal sclerotherapy. Hepatology, 5: 584, 1985.
356. Copenhagen Esophageal Varices Sclerotherapy Project: Sclerotherapy after the first variceal hemorrhage in cirrhosis: a randomized multicenter trial. N. Engl. J. Med., 311: 1594, 1984.
357. Rikkers, L. F., et al.: Shunt surgery vs. esophageal sclerotherapy for long-term treatment of variceal bleeding. Ann. Surg., 206:261, 1987.
358. Teres, J., et al.: Sclerotherapy vs. distal splenorenal shunt treatment in the elective treatment of variceal hemorrhage: a randomized controlled trial. Hepatology, 7:430, 1987.
359. Henderson, M., et al.: Endoscopic variceal sclerosis compared with distal splenorenal shunt to prevent recurrent variceal bleeding in cirrhosis. Ann. Intern. Med., 112:262, 1990.
360. Jackson, F. C., et al.: A clinical investigation of the portacaval shunt. V. Survival analysis of the therapeutic operation. Ann. Surg., 174:672, 1971.
361. Resnick, R. H., et al.: A controlled study of the therapeutic portacaval shunt. Gastroenterology, 67:843, 1974.
362. Reuff, B., et al.: A controlled study of therapeutic portacaval shunt in alcoholic patients. Lancet, 1:655, 1976.
363. Reynolds, T. B., et al.: Results of a 12 year randomized trial of portacaval shunt in patients with alcoholic liver disease and bleeding varices. Gastroenterology, 80:1005, 1986.
364. Henderson, J. M., Milliken, W. J., Jr., and Galloway, J. R.: The Emory perspective of the distal splenorenal shunt in 1990. Am. J. Surg., 160:54, 1990.
365. Milliken, W. J., Jr., et al.: The Emory prospective randomized trial: selective versus non-selective shunts to control variceal bleeding. Ann. Surg., 201:712, 1984.
366. Lillimoe, K. D., and Cameron, J. L.: The interposition-mesocaval shunt. Surg. Clin. North Am., 70:379, 1990.
367. Rypins, E. B., and Sarfeh, I. J.: Small diameter portacaval H-graft for variceal hemorrhage. Surg. Clin. North Am., 70: 395, 1990.
368. Johansen, K.: Partial portal decompression. Am. J. Surg., 157:479, 1989.
369. Lebrec, D., et al.: The effect of propranolol on portal hypertension in patients with cirrhosis. Hepatology, 2:523, 1982.
370. Bosch, J., et al.: Effects of propranolol on azygous venous blood flow and hepatic systemic hemodynamics in cirrhosis. Hepatology, 4:1200, 1984.
371. Lebrec, D., et al.: A randomized controlled study of propranolol for prevention of recurrent gastrointestinal bleeding in patients with cirrhosis. Hepatology, 4:355, 1984.
372. Burroughs, A. K., et al.: Controlled trial of propranolol for the prevention of recurrent variceal hemorrhage in patients with cirrhosis. N. Engl. J. Med., 309:1539, 1983.

373. Villeneuve, J. P., et al.: Propranalol for the prevention of recurrent variceal hemorrhage: a controlled study. Hepatology, 6:1239, 1986.
374. O'Connor, K. W., et al.: Comparison of three non-surgical treatments in bleeding esophageal varices. Gastroenterology, 96:899, 1989.
375. Reichen, J.: Pharmacology of portal hypertension. American Association for the study of Liver Disease Post Graduate Course. Chicago, 1989.
376. Hoskins, S. W., et al.: The role of propranolol in congestive gastropathy of portal hypertension. Hepatology, 7:437, 1987.
377. Quintero, E., et al.: Gastric mucosal vascular ectasias causing bleeding in cirrhosis. Gastroenterology, 93:1054, 1987.
378. D'Amico, G., et al.: Natural history of congestive gastropathy in cirrhosis. Gastroenterology, 99:1558, 1990.
379. Vargo, J. J., et al.: Portal hypertensive gastropathy: an endoscopic and histomorphic study (A). Am. J. Gastroenterol., 85:1242, 1990.
380. Hashizume, M., Tanaka, K., and Inokuchi, K.: Morphology of gastric microcirculation in cirrhosis. Hepatology, 3:1008, 1983.
381. Sarfeh, I. J., and Tarnawski, A.: Gastric mucosal vasculopathy in portal hypertension. Gastroenterology, 93:1129, 1987.
382. Sarfeh, I. J., et al.: Results of surgical management of hemorrhagic gastritis in patients with gastroesophageal varices. Surg. Gynecol. Obstet., 155:167, 1982.
383. Iwatsuki, S., et al.: Liver transplantation in the treatment of bleeding esophageal varices. Surgery, 104:697, 1988.
384. Wood, H. P., Shaw, B. W., Jr., and Rikkers, L. T.: Liver transplantation for variceal hemorrhage. Surg. Clin. North Am., 70:449, 1990.
385. Mazzaferro, V., et al.: Liver transplantation in patients with previous portasystemic shunt. Am. J. Surg., 160:111, 1990.
386. Brems, J. J., et al.: Effect of a prior portasystemic shunt on subsequent liver transplantation. Ann. Surg., 209:51, 1988.
387. Gludd, C., et al.: Hepatitis B and A virus antibodies in alcoholic steatosis and cirrhosis. J. Clin. Pathol., 35:693, 1982.
388. Mendenhall, C. L., et al.: Antibodies to hepatitis B virus and hepatitis C virus in alcoholic hepatitis and cirrhosis: their prevalence and clinical relevance. Hepatology, 14:581, 1991.
389. Pares, A., et al.: Hepatitis C virus antibodies in chronic alcoholic patients: association with severity of liver injury. Hepatology, 12:1295, 1990.
390. Caldwell, S. H., et al.: Antibody to hepatitis C is common among patients with alcoholic liver disease with and without risk factors. Am. J. Gastroenterol., 86:1219, 1991.
391. Goodman, Z. D., and Ishak, K. G.: Occlusive venous lesions in alcoholic liver disease. Gastroenterology, 83:786, 1982.
392. Nissenbaum, M., et al.: Prognostic significance of cholestatic hepatitis. Dig. Dis. Sci., 35:891, 1990.
393. Carithers, R. L., et al.: Methylprednisolone therapy in patients with severe alcoholic hepatitis: a randomized multicenter trial. Ann. Intern. Med., 110:685, 1989.
394. Maddrey, W. C., et al.: Corticosteroid therapy of alcoholic hepatitis. Gastroenterology, 75:193, 1978.
395. Orrego, H., et al.: Assessment of prognostic factors in alcoholic liver disease: toward a global quantitative expression of severity. Hepatology, 3:896, 1983.
396. Imperiale, T. F., and McCullough, A. J.: Do corticosteroids reduce mortality from alcoholic hepatitis? A meta-analysis of the randomized trials. Ann. Intern. Med., 113:299, 1990.
397. Ramond, M.-J., et al.: A randomized trial of prednisone in patients with severe alcoholic hepatitis. N. Engl. J. Med., 326:507, 1992.
398. Orrego, H., et al.: Effect of short-term therapy with propylthiouracil in patients with alcoholic liver disease. Gastroenterology, 76:106, 1979.
399. Halle, P., et al.: Double-blind controlled trial of propylthiouracil in severe acute alcoholic hepatitis. Gastroenterology, 82:925, 1982.
400. Orrego, H., et al.: Long-term treatment of alcoholic liver disease with propylthiouracil. N. Engl. J. Med., 317:1421, 1987.
401. Baker, A. L., et al.: A randomized controlled trial of insulin and glucagon infusion for treatment of alcoholic hepatitis. Gastroenterology, 80:1410, 1981.
402. Fehrer, J., et al.: A prospective multi-center study of insulin and glucagon in acute alcoholic hepatitis. J. Hepatol., 5:2243, 1987.
403. Bird, G., et al.: Insulin and glucagon infusion in acute hepatitis: a perspective randomized controlled trial. Hepatology, 14:1097, 1991.
404. Trinchet, J. C., et al.: Treatment of severe alcoholic hepatitis by infusion of insulin and glucagon: a multi-center sequential trial. Hepatology, 15:76, 1992.
405. Blackburn, G. L., et al.: Nutritional and metabolic assessment of the hospitalized patient. J. Parenter. Enteral. Nutr., 1:11, 1977.
406. Mendenhall, C. L.: A study of oral nutritional support with oxadrolone in malnourished patients with alcoholic hepatitis: results of a department of Veterans Affairs Cooperative Study. Hepatology, 17:564, 1993.
407. O'Keefe, S. J. D., et al.: Short term effects of an intravenous infusion of a nutrient solution containing amino-acids, glucose and insulin on leucine turnover and aminoacid metabolism in patients with liver failure. J. Hepatol., 6:101, 1988.
408. Steffen, E., Berg, R. D., and Deitch, C. A.: Comparison of translocation rate of various indigenous bacteria from the gastrointestinal tract to the mesenteric nodes. J. Infect. Dis., 157:1032, 1987.
409. Bonkovsky, H. L., et al.: A randomized controlled trial of treatment of alcoholic hepatitis with parenteral nutrition and oxandrolone. I. Short-term effects on liver function. Am. J. Gastroenterol., 86:1200, 1991.
410. Bonkovsky, H. L., et al.: A randomized controlled trial of treatment of alcoholic hepatitis with parenteral nutrition and oxandrolone. II. Short-term effects on nitrogen metabolism, metabolic imbalance and nutrition. Am. J. Gastroenterol., 86:1209, 1991.
411. Kumar, S., et al.: Orthotopic liver transplantation for alcoholic liver disease. Hepatology, 11:159, 1990.
412. Bird, G., et al.: Liver transplantation in patients with alcoholic cirrhosis: selection criteria and rate of survival and relapse. Br. Med. J., 301:15, 1990.
413. Schenker, S., Perkins, H. S., and Sorrell, M. F.: Should patients with end-stage alcoholic disease have a new liver? (edit.) Hepatology, 11:314, 1990.
414. Lucey, M. R., et al.: Selection for outcome of liver transplantation in alcoholic liver disease. Gastroenterology, 102:1763, 1992.
415. Beresford, T. P.: Psychiatric evaluation of alcoholics for liver transplantation. American Association for the Study of Liver Disease; Postgraduate Course. Chicago, 1992.
416. Runyon, B. A., and Reynolds, T. B.: Approach to the patient with ascites. In Textbook of Gastroenterology. Edited by T. Yamada, et al. Philadelphia, W. B. Saunders, 1991.
417. Shear, L., Ching, S., and Gabuzda, G. J.: Compartmentalization of ascites and edema in patients with hepatic cirrhosis. N. Engl. J. Med., 282:1391, 1970.
418. Epstein, M.: Deranged sodium homeostasis in cirrhosis. Gastroenterology, 76:622, 1979.

419. Lieberman, F. L., et al.: The relationship of plasma volume, portal hypertension, ascites and renal sodium retention in cirrhosis: the overflow theory of ascites formation. Ann. N. Y. Acad. Sci., *170:*202, 1970.
420. Schrier, R. W., et al.: Peripheral arterial vasodilatation hypothesis: a proposal for the initiation of renal sodium and water retention in cirrhosis. Hepatology, *8:*1151, 1988.
421. Cattau, E. L., et al.: The accuracy of the physical exam in the diagnosis of suspected ascites. JAMA, *247:*1164, 1982.
422. Runyan, B. A., et al.: Paracentesis of ascitic fluid: a safe procedure. Arch. Intern. Med., *146:*259, 1986.
423. Bender, M. D., and Ockner, R. K.: Ascites. *In* Gastrointestinal Disease: Pathophysiology, Diagnosis, Management. 3rd Ed., Edited by M. H. Sleisenger and J. S. Fordtran. Philadelphia, W. B. Saunders, 1983.
424. Runyan, B. A.: Paracentesis and ascitic fluid analysis. *In* Textbook of Gastroenterology. Edited by T. Yamada, et al. Philadelphia, W. B. Saunders, 1991.
425. Hoefs, J. C.: Diagnostic paracentesis; a potent clinical tool. Gastroenterology, *98:*230, 1990.
426. Abillos, A., et al.: Ascitic fluid polymorphonuclear cell count and serum to ascites albumin gradient in the diagnosis of bacterial peritonitis. Gastroenterology, *98:*134, 1990.
427. Runyon, B. A.: Spontaneous bacterial peritonitis: an explosion of information. Hepatology, *8:*171, 1988.
428. Castellote, J., et al.: Comparison of two ascitic fluid culture methods in cirrhotic patients with subacute bacterial peritonitis. Am. J. Gastroenterol., *85:*1605, 1990.
429. Rimola, A., et al.: Reticuloendothelial system phagocytic activity in cirrhosis and its relation to bacterial infection and prognosis. Hepatology, *4:*53, 1984.
430. Conn, H. O.: Spontaneous bacterial peritonitis and bacteremia in Laennec's cirrhosis caused by enteric organisms. A relatively common but rarely recognized syndrome. Ann. Intern. Med., *60:*568, 1964.
431. Hoefs, J. C.: Spontaneous bacterial peritonitis. Hepatology, *2:*399, 1982.
432. Llach, J., et al.: Incidence and predictive factors of first episode of spontaneous bacterial peritonitis in cirrhosis with ascites: relevance of ascitic fluid protein concentration. Hepatology, *16:*724, 1992.
433. Hoefs, J. C.: Spontaneous bacterial peritonitis: prevention and therapy. Hepatology, *12:*776, 1990.
434. Pinzello, G., et al.: Spontaneous bacterial peritonitis: a prospective investigation in predominantly non-alcoholics. Hepatology, *3:*545, 1983.
435. Chu, C-M., Chu, K-W., and Liaw, Y-F.: The prevalence and prognostic significance of spontaneous bacterial peritonitis in severe acute hepatitis with ascites. Hepatology, *15:*799, 1992.
436. Runyon, B. A., et al.: Opsonic activity of human ascitic fluid: a potentially important protective mechanism against spontaneous bacterial peritonitis. Hepatology, *5:*634, 1985.
437. Jonas, G., et al.: Liver-spleen scan reticuloendothelial shift of sulfur colloid predicts the development of spontaneous bacterial peritonitis (abstr.). Hepatology, *8:*1351A, 1988.
438. Runyan, B. A., Antillon, M. R., and Montano, A. A.: Effect of diuresis versus therapeutic paracentesis on ascitic fluid opsonic activity and serum complement. Gastroenterology, *97:*158, 1989.
439. Felisart, J., et al.: Cefotaxime is more effective than is ampicillin-tobramycin in cirrhotics with severe infections. Hepatology, *5:*457, 1985.
440. Toledo, C., et al.: Spontaneous bacterial peritonitis in cirrhosis: predictive factors of infection resolution and survival in patients treated with cefotaxime. Hepatology, *17:*251, 1993.
441. Fong, T-L., et al.: Polymorphonuclear cell count response and duration of antibiotic therapy in spontaneous bacterial peritonitis. Hepatology, *9:*423, 1989.
442. Runyon, B. A., et al.: Short-course versus long-course antibiotic treatment of spontaneous bacterial peritonitis. Gastroenterology, *100:*1737, 1991.
443. Tito, L., et al.: Recurrence of spontaneous bacterial peritonitis in cirrhosis: frequency and predictive factors. Hepatology, *8:*27, 1988.
444. Carey, W. D., Boayke, A., and Leatherman, J.: Spontaneous bacterial peritonitis: clinical and laboratory features with reference to hospital-acquired cases. Am. J. Gastroenterol., *81:*1156, 1986.
445. Rimola, A., et al.: Oral, nonabsorbable antibiotics prevent infection in cirrhotics with gastrointestinal hemorrhage. Hepatology, *5:*463, 1985.
446. Gines, P., et al.: Norfloxacin prevents spontaneous bacterial peritonitis recurrence in cirrhosis: results of a double-blind placebo-controlled trial. Hepatology, *12:*716, 1990.
447. Schubert, M. L., Sanyal, A. J., and Wong, E. S.: Antibiotic prophylaxis for prevention of spontaneous bacterial peritonitis. Gastroenterology, *101:*550, 1991.
448. Runyon, B. A., and Hoefs, J. C.: Culture negative neurocytic ascites: a variant of spontaneous bacterial peritonitis. Hepatology, *4:*1209, 1984.
449. Runyon, B. A.: Monomicrobial non-neutrocytic bacterascites: a variant of spontaneous bacterial peritonitis. Hepatology, *12:*710, 1990.
450. Akriviadis, E. A., and Runyon, B. A.: The utility of an algorithm in differentiating spontaneous from secondary bacterial peritonitis. Gastroenterology, *98:*127, 1990.
451. Garrison, R. N., et al.: Clarification of risk factors for abdominal surgery in patients with hepatic cirrhosis. Ann. Surg., *199:*648, 1984.
452. Runyon, B. A., Hoefs, J. C., and Canawati, H. N.: Polymicrobial bacterascites: a unique entity in the spectrum of infected ascitic fluid. Arch. Intern. Med., *146:*2173, 1986.
453. Leonetti, J. P., et al.: Umbilical herniorrhaphy in cirrhotic patients. Arch. Surg., *119:*442, 1984.
454. Kirkpatrick, S., and Schubert, T.: Umbilical hernia rupture in cirrhotics with ascites. Dig. Dis. Sci., *33:*762, 1988.
455. Belghiti, J., Rueff, B., and Fekete, F.: Umbilical hernia in cirrhotic patients with ascites: prevalence, cause and management. (abstr.) Gastroenterology, *84:*1363A, 1983.
456. Runyon, B. A., and John Juler, G. L.: Natural history of repaired umbilical hernia in patients with and without ascites. Am. J. Gastroenterol., *80:*38, 1985.
457. Baron, H. C.: Umbilical hernia secondary to cirrhosis of the liver. N. Engl. J. Med., *263:*824, 1960.
458. Lieberman, F. L., et al.: Pathogenesis and treatment of hydrothorax complicating cirrhosis with ascites. Ann. Intern. Med., *64:*341, 1966.
459. Rubinstein, D., McInnes, I. E., and Dudley, F. J.: Hepatic hydrothorax in the absence of clinical ascites: diagnosis and management. Gastroenterology, *88:*188, 1985.
460. Arroyo, V., et al.: Management of patients with cirrhosis and ascites. Semin. Liver Dis., *6:*353, 1986.
461. Arroyo, V., and Rodes, J.: A rational approach to the treatment of ascites. Postgrad. Med. J., *51:*558, 1975.
462. Bernardi, M., et al.: Renal function impairment induced by change in posture in patients with cirrhosis and ascites. Gut, *26:*629, 1985.
463. Perez-Ayuso, R. M., et al.: Randomized comparative study of efficacy of furosemide versus spironolactone in nonazotemic cirrhosis with ascites. Gastroenterology, *84:*961, 1983.
464. van Vliet, A. A., et al.: Efficacy of low dose captopril in

addition to furosemide and spironolactone in patients with decompensated liver disease during blunted diuresis. J. Hepatol., *15:*40, 1992.
465. Fessel, J. M., and Conn, H. O.: An analysis of cause and prevention of heptic coma (A). Gastroenterology, *61:*191, 1972.
466. Kao, H. W., et al.: The effect of large volume paracentesis on plasma volume: a cause of hypovolemia? Hepatology, *5:* 403, 1985.
467. Quintero, E., et al.: Paracentesis versus diuretics in the treatment of cirrhotics with tense ascites. Lancet, *1:*611, 1985.
468. Gines, P., et al.: Comparison of paracentesis and diuretics in the treatment of cirrhotics with tense ascites. Gastroenterology, *93:*234, 1987.
469. Gines, P., et al.: Randomized comparative study of therapeutic paracentesis with and without intravenous albumin in cirrhosis. Gastroenterology, *94:*1493, 1988.
470. LeVeen, H. H., et al.: Peritoneovenous shunting for ascites. Ann. Surg., *180:*580, 1974.
471. Fulenwider, J. T., et al.: LeVeen vs. Denver peritoneovenous shunts for intractable ascites of cirrhosis. Arch. Surg., *121:* 351, 1986.
472. Greenlee, H. B., Stanley, M. M., and Reinhardt, G. F.: Intractable ascites treated with peritoneovenous shunt (LeVeen). Arch. Surg., *116:*518, 1981.
473. Smadya, C., and Franco, D.: The LeVeen shunt in the elective treatment of intractable ascites in cirrhosis. Ann. Surg., *201:*448, 1985.
474. Stanley, M. M., et al.: Peritoneovenous shunting as compared with medical treatment in patients with alcoholic cirrhosis and massive ascites. N. Engl. J. Med., *321:*1632, 1989.
475. Greig, P. A., et al.: Complications after peritoneovenous shunting for ascites. Am. J. Surg., *139:*125, 1980.
476. Bournigal, D. R., et al.: Recurrent ventricular tachycardia in a patient with a peritoneovenous catheter. (left.) Ann. Intern. Med., *106:*474, 1987.
477. Fry, P. D., Hallgren, R., and Robertson, M. E.: Current status of the peritoneovenous shunt for the management of intractable ascites. Can. J. Surg., *22:*557, 1979.
478. Franco, D., et al.: Should portosystemic shunt be reconsidered in the treatment of intractable ascites? Arch. Surg., *123:*987, 1988.
479. Bruno, S., et al.: Comparison of spontaneous ascitic filtration and reinfusion with total paracenteses with intravenous albumin infusion in cirrhotic patients with ascites. Br. Med. J., *304:*1655, 1992.
480. Koppel, M. H., et al.: Transplantation of cadaveric kidneys from patients with hepatorenal syndrome: evidence for the functional nature of renal failure in advanced liver disease. N. Engl. J. Med., *280:*1367, 1969.
481. Iwatsuki, S., et al.: Recovery from "hepatorenal syndrome" after orthotopic liver transplantation. N. Engl. J. Med., *289:* 1155, 1973.
482. Miller, P. D., Linas, S. L., and Schrier, R. W.: Plasma demeclocycline levels and nephrotoxicity: correlation in hyponatremic cirrhotic individuals. JAMA, *243:*2513, 1980.
483. Zipser, R. D., et al.: Urinary thromboxane B2 and prostaglandin E2 in the hepatorenal syndrome: evidence for increased vasoconstrictor and decreased vasodilator factors. Gastroenterology, *84:*697, 1983.
484. Zipser, R. D., et al.: Therapeutic trial of thromboxane synthesis inhibition in the hepatorenal syndrome. Gastroenterology, *87:*1228, 1984.
485. Fernandez-Seara, J., et al.: Systemic and regional hemodynamics in patients with liver cirrhosis and ascites with and without functional renal failure. Gastroenterology, *97:* 1304, 1989.
486. Linas, S. L., et al.: Peritovenous shunt in the management of the hepatorenal syndrome. Kidney Int., *30:*736, 1986.
487. D'Amico, G., et al.: Survival and prognostic indications in compensated and uncompensated cirrhotics. Dig. Dis. Sci., *31:*468, 1986.
488. Saunders, J. B., et al.: A twenty year prospective study of cirrhosis. Br. Med. J., *282:*263, 1981.
489. Tanaka, R., Itoshima, T., and Nagashima, H.: Follow-up study of 582 liver cirrhotic patients for 26 years in Japan. Liver, *7:*316, 1987.
490. McSherry, C. K., and Glenn, F.: The incidence and causes of death following surgery for non-malignant biliary tract disease. Ann. Surg., *191:*271, 1980.
491. Aranha, G. V., Sontog, S. J., and Greenlee, H. B.: Cholecystectomy in morbidity and mortality after cirrhotic patients: a formidable operation. Am. J. Surg., *143:*55, 1982.
492. Doberneck, R. C., Sterling, W. A., and Allison, D. C.: Morbidity and mortality after operation in non-bleeding cirrhotic patients. Am. J. Surg., *146:*306, 1983.
493. Bloch, R. S., Allaben, R. D., and Walt, A. J.: Cholesystectomy in patients with cirrhosis. Arch. Surg., *120:*669, 1985.
494. Schwartz, S. I.: Biliary tract surgery and cirrhosis: a critical condition. Surgery, *90:*577, 1981.
495. Castaing, D., et al.: Surgical management of gallstones in cirrhotic patients. Am. J. Surg., *146:*310, 1983.
496. Powell-Jackson, P., Greenway, B., and Williams, R.: Adverse effects of exploratory laparotomy in patients with unsuspected liver disease. Br. J. Surg., *69:*449, 1982.
497. Aranha, G. V., and Greenlee, H. B.: Intra-abdominal surgery in patients with advanced cirrhosis. Arch. Surg., *121:*275, 1986.
498. Greenwood, S. M., Leffler, C. T., and Minkowitz, S.: The increased mortality rate of open liver biopsy in alcoholic hepatitis. Surg. Gynecol. Obstet., *134:*600, 1972.
499. Lehnert, T., and Herfarth, C.: Peptic ulcer surgery in patients with liver cirrhosis. Ann. Surg., *217:*338, 1993.
500. Wirthlin, L. S., et al.: Predictors of surgical mortality in patients with cirrhosis and nonvariceal gastro-duodenal bleeding. Surg. Gynecol. Obstet., *139:*65, 1974.
501. Mosnier, H., et al.: Gastroduodenal ulcer perforation in the patient with cirrhosis. Surg. Gynecol. Obstet., *174:*297, 1992.
502. Belghiti, J., et al.: Esophagogastrectomy for carcinoma in cirrhotic patients. Hepatogastroenterology, *37:*388, 1990.
503. Metcalf, A. M., et al.: The surgical risk of colectomy in patients with cirrhosis. Dis. Colon Rectum, *30:*529, 1987.
504. Griffin, W. O., Jr.: Discussion of clarification of risk factors for abdominal operations in patients with hepatic cirrhosis. Ann. Surg., *199:*654, 1984.
505. Post, A. B., et al.: Surgical risk of colectomy in patients with primary sclerosing cholangitis. (abstr.) Am. J. Gastroenterol., *86:*1335A, 1991.
506. Tinkoff, G., et al.: Cirrhosis in the trauma victim. Ann. Surg., *211:*172, 1990.
507. Morris, J. A., MacKenzie, E. J., and Edelstein, S. L.: The effect of preexisting conditions on mortality in trauma patients. JAMA, *263:*1942, 1990.
508. Brown, M. W., and Burk, R. F.: Development of intractable ascites following upper abdominal surgery in patients with cirrhosis. Am. J. Med., *80:*879, 1986.
509. Bell, R. H., Miyai, K., and Orloff, M. J.: Outcome in cirrhotic patients with acute alcoholic hepatitis after emergency portacaval shunt for bleeding esophageal varices. Am. J. Surg., *147:*78, 1984.
510. Mikkelsen, W. R., Turril, F. L., and Kern, W. H.: Acute hya-

line necrosis of the liver: a surgical trap. Am. J. Surg., *116:* 266, 1968.
511. LaMont, J. T., and Isselbacher, K.: Postoperative jaundice. *In* Liver and Biliary Disease. 2nd Ed. Edited by R. Wright, C. H. Millward-Sadler, K. G. M. N. Alberti, and S. Karran. London, Balliere Tindall, 1985, p. 1087.
512. Bunker, J. P.: Final report of the national halothane study. Anesthesiology, *29:*231, 1968.
513. Moult, P. J. A., and Sherlock, S.: Halothane related hepatitis: a clinical study of 26 cases. Q. J. Med. N.S., *44:*99, 1975.
514. Nunes, G., Blaisdell, W., and Margaretten, W.: Mechanism of hepatic dysfunction following shock and trauma. Arch. Surg., *100:*546, 1970.
515. Bynum, T. E., Boitnott, J. K., and Maddrey, W. C.: Ischemic hepatitis. Dig. Dis. Sci., *24:*129, 1979.
516. Harville, D., and Summerskill, W. H. J.: Surgery in acute hepatitis. JAMA *184:*258, 1963.
517. Abernathy, C. O., et al.: Jaundice of systemic infection. *In* Current Perspectives in Hepatology. Edited by L. B. Seefi, and J. H. Lewis. New York, Plenum Medical Book, 1989, p. 337.
518. Sikuler, E., et al.: Abnormalities in bilirubin and liver enzyme levels in adult patients with bacteria. Arch. Intern. Med., *149:*2246, 1989.
519. Kantrowitz, P. A., et al.: Severe postoperative hyperbilirubinemia simulating obstructive jaundice. N. Engl. J. Med., *276:*591, 1967.
520. Boekhorst, Th., et al.: Etiologic factors of jaundice in severely ill patients. J. Hepatol., *7:*111, 1988.
521. National Institutes of Health consensus development conference statement on gallstone and laparoscopic cholecystectomy. Am. J. Surg., *165:*390, 1993.
522. Mallory, A., and Kern, F.: Drug-induced pancreatitis: a critical review. Gastroenterology, *78:*813, 1980.
523. Kartsonis, A., et al.: Postoperative jaundice as a clue to unrecognized biliary tract obstruction. J. Clin. Gastroenterol., *9:*666, 1987.
524. Johnson, B. B.: The importance of early diagnosis of acute acalculous cholecystitis. Surg. Gynecol. Obstet., *164:*197, 1987.
525. Mirvis, S. E., et al.: The diagnosis of acute acalculous cholecystitis: a comparison of sonography, scintigraphy and CT. Am. J. Roentgenol., *147:*1171, 1986.

Chapter 55

INTENSIVE CARE ASPECTS OF LIVER TRANSPLANTS

DAVID P. VOGT
WILLIAM D. CAREY

For the first two decades after Starzl described orthotopic liver transplantation (OLT), it remained an operation infrequently performed with disappointing results. In the early 1980s improved survival rates were achieved due to improvements in surgical techniques, management of complications, and most important, immunosuppression regimens. One-year survival rates of 70% are now commonplace, and many centers claim 80 to 90% one year survival in selected good risk patients. At least 70 centers in the United States perform this operation. Despite formidable problems of organ procurement, cost, demands on hospital personnel and facilities, most acknowledge that liver transplantation is the "standard of care" for end-stage liver disease and certain other conditions. The degree to which the shortage of donor organs impedes application of this lifesaving operation is reflected in the fact that over 1300 patients were on the national United Organ Sharing (UNOS) waiting list in February, 1991.[1] In this chapter, we explore the problems likely to be faced in the ICU by the patient with advanced liver disease, a detailed discussion of the operative phase, and problems encountered in the postoperative period.

Current selection criteria for OLT candidacy are broad. Contraindications are few and are diminishing each year. In general, patients are selected for OLT candidacy if one or more of the following apply:

- End-stage liver disease with a life expectancy of less than one year
- Quality of life judged sufficiently poor that the risks appear justified
- A liver-based metabolic disease with lethal implications

Age, per se, is usually not considered a contraindication to OLT, although the chance of a disqualifying coexistent disease (e.g., heart damage from coronary artery disease, advanced pulmonary disease, cancer, etc.) is greater with advancing age. Those with acute liver failure are suitable for OLT. Unfortunately, it is often logistically difficult to obtain a suitable donor organ in the short "window of opportunity" available in such patients. Table 55-1 defines current indications and contraindications for liver transplantation. Prior surgery in the right upper quadrant poses an additional technical burden to the transplant surgeon. Extensive adhesions, which are likely to contain collateral venous channels in the cirrhotic patient, require meticulous dissection and increase operative time.

PRETRANSPLANT PERIOD

Patients awaiting liver transplantation may be either well enough to wait for a donor organ at home, or ill enough to spend the entire wait in a hospital. Patients selected for liver transplantation usually have common problems related to end-stage cirrhosis (or to fulminant liver failure) regardless of the etiology of the disease. Even those waiting at home may have episodes which require hospitalization. Many of these are of an emergency nature. The most frequent reasons for ICU admission for advanced cirrhotic patients are acute gastrointestinal (GI) bleeding and portosystemic encephalopathy (PSE). Infection, especially spontaneous bacterial peritonitis, may add more burden to these already sick patients.

Gastrointestinal Bleeding

Clinically, significant bleeding in the cirrhotic patient is a consequence of portal hypertension. Most frequently, major GI bleeding is caused by varices in either the distal esophagus, or proximal stomach (or both), or from portal hypertensive gastropathy. Of course, ulcers, Mallory-Weiss tears, and other lesions may cause upper GI bleeding in the cirrhotic patient. Occasionally, major bleeding will occur from varices at other sites in the digestive tract, such as rectal varices (frequently mistaken for large hemorrhoids), or from stomal varices in a patient with an ileostomy. Coagulation abnormalities are frequent because the synthetic function of the liver (the site of production of coagulation proteins except factor VIII) is impaired. Thrombocytopenia from hypersplenism may be present. Coagulation defects alone do not account for brisk bleeding in the cirrhotic patient, although they may account for easy bruisability, nosebleeds, and occult GI bleeding, and may compound bleeding problems caused by mucosal defects. Superior management of bleeding rests on early diagnosis and aggressive volume replacement as in bleeding patients without cirrhosis (see Chap. 54).

Vasoactive Therapy

Bleeding varices are managed initially by intravenous vasopressin. This agent appears to work by constricting the splanchnic arterioles through vasopressinergic recep-

Table 55–1. Current Indications and Contraindications for Liver Transplantation

INDICATIONS
Advanced cirrhosis: primary biliary cirrhosis, chronic active hepatitis and cirrhosis, cryptogenic, secondary biliary, sclerosing cholangitis, hepatitis B or C
Metabolic disorders: Wilson's Disease, protoporphyrin, hemochromatosis with cirrhosis, alpha-1 antitrypsin deficiency, Type IV hyperlipidemia, hemophilia A and B, primary hyperoxaluria
Vascular disease: thrombosis of hepatic veins (Budd-Chiari syndrome)
Neoplastic disease: hepatoma (especially fibrolamellar variant), life-threatening adenomas, large symptomatic APUDomas
Fulminant or submassive hepatic necrosis (drugs, toxins, infections)
Pediatric disorders: biliary atresia, congenital biliary cirrhosis, congenital hepatic fibrosis, tyrosinemia, galactosemia, Crigler-Najjar, urea enzyme deficiency, C-protein deficiency, glycogen storage disease I and IV, Byler's disease, Sea Blue histiocyte disease, Alagille's syndrome, cystic fibrosis, Niemann-Pick

CONTRAINDICATIONS
HIV positive status
Active infection outside the biliary tree
Malignant disease outside liver/biliary tree (except APUDomas)
Advanced extrahepatic organ damage (particularly heart or lung disease)
Active alcoholism or other chemical dependence
Insufficient personal strength and/or social resources to adapt to the demands of life with a liver transplant

tor (V1-receptor) stimulation. Many years ago, studies suggested that vasopressin is effective in controlling variceal hemorrhage. In a comparison of vasopressin to ice water lavage, bleeding was controlled with vasopressin 87% of the time, compared to 47%.[2] Other studies indicate control of variceal bleeding in 28 to 70% of cases.[3-6] The design of many of these early studies would be unacceptable by today's standards. In some studies, there was no endoscopic verification of a variceal source for bleeding. Not all studies have shown a benefit of vasopressin. In one study there was no significant advantage of vasopressin over a placebo in controlling upper GI hemorrhage, although these patients were often bleeding from nonvariceal sources.[7]

Vasopressin causes severe vasoconstriction in many arterial beds. Prolonged systemic vasoconstrictor effects are commonly seen in the cirrhotic patient and may produce ischemic effects in the coronary and general circulation. The cirrhotic patient appears to be unable to neutralize vasopressin normally, which may account for this prolonged effect.[8] Abdominal pain, lower extremity ischemia, thoracic discomfort, and bradycardia are common side effects. Attempts have been made to reduce side effects and, therefore, allow a more generous dose of vasopressin to be used safely. Several series have demonstrated control of bleeding in 55 to 83% of cases.[9-12] Table 55-2 shows details of several trials of vasopressin, plus nitroglycerin in the management of variceal hemorrhage.

The search for improved pharmacologic agents to reduce intravariceal pressure and affect cessation of bleeding from varices continues. Somatostatin and somatostatin analogues have been reported to decrease blood flow and pressure in the portal system.[13,14] Unfortunately, a recent randomized clinical trial of somatostatin for emergency control of variceal bleeding suggested that somatostatin is ineffective.[15] Other studies are in progress and some suggest a role for somatostatin.[16]

Tamponade

Esophageal tamponade has been available for the control of bleeding esophageal and gastric varices for many decades. Tamponade remains unsurpassed for the emergency control of variceal bleeding and may be superior to vasopressin. It appears to be just as effective as sclerotherapy in the urgent case. Several different balloon-tube configurations are available. Some configurations (such as the Sengstaken-Blakemore and Minnesota tubes) have two balloons, one at the distal end, which is designed to be inflated in the stomach to obliterate gastric varices, and the other which is a sausage-shaped balloon along the shaft of the tube that is used to compress esophageal varices. Other devices (e.g., Linton tube) have a single gastric balloon. Inflation of this device will compress gastric varices only. In some cases, this may be sufficient to decrease blood flow to esophageal varices and so is occasionally helpful for bleeding esophageal varices as well.

The technique of tube insertion and management has been well described.[17] Absolute contraindications include patients in whom bleeding has stopped, and patients with recent surgery involving the esophagogastric junction. The exact instructions for each type of tube vary and details usually accompany a new tube. It is important to test-inflate the balloons for leakage prior to insertion. After deflating the balloon completely, and preparing the patient, the tube is lubricated and inserted through the mouth. When the gastric balloon has reached the stomach, a test inflation with a relatively small volume of air is attempted. A pressure rise of more than 15 mm Hg after 100 ml of air (in a 500 ml capacity Minnesota tube) suggests that the balloon is still within the esophagus. In this event, the tube must be deflated and repositioned. When the physician is confident that the tube is within the stomach, inflation with 450 to 500 ml of air is accomplished, and over the bed traction with a one pound weight is applied. If bleeding does not cease with inflation of the gastric balloon, then the esophageal balloon is inflated.

Table 55–2. Regimens Using Vasopressin Plus Vasodilator Therapy to Control Variceal Hemorrhage

Author	Year	Vasopressin Dose (U/min)	Nitroglycerin Type/Dose	Initial Control of Bleeding
Gimson[10]	1986	20 units in 15 min initial; then 0.4 µg/min	IV 40 µg/min initial; 400 µg/min max	68%
Tsai[12]	1986	0.6 µg/min initial; then 0.33 µg/min	Sublingual 0.6 mg q 30 min	55%
Bosch[9]	1989	0.4 µg/min initial; 0.8 µg/min max	Transdermal 2 patches 25 mg each	83%
Teres*	1990	0.4 initial; 0.6–0.8	IV 40 µg/min initial; 400 µg/min max	—

* Teres, et al.: Vasopressin/nitroglycerin infusion vs esophageal tamponade in the treatment of acute variceal bleeding. Hepatology, *11*:964, 1990.

Table 55-3. Trials of Tamponade to Control Variceal Bleeding

Author	Year	Number of Patients	Initial Control of Bleeding
Teres[22]	1990	52	87%
Hernomo[19]	1983	30	87%
Panes[20]	1988	151	91%
Teres[23]	1978	52	92%

The position of the tube should be verified by portable radiograph. The esophageal balloon should be deflated for 10 to 15 minutes every 3 to 4 hours. Care must be taken to ensure that proximal migration of the tube does not occur because asphyxiation could occur. Provision must be made to remove blood and secretions that may accumulate proximal to the inflated balloon. Otherwise, aspiration may occur. If sudden respiratory difficulty occurs the balloon must be deflated and removed at once. Ordinarily, the balloon is left inflated for 24 hours. If no bleeding occurs, then the esophageal balloon is deflated and the patient observed for 6 to 12 more hours, after which the gastric balloon is deflated. The deflated apparatus can be left in place for an additional 12 hours. If rebleeding occurs another 24 hours of therapy can be administered. The success of balloon tamponade is over 80% in most modern series[18-20] (Table 55-3). Although tamponade is of unquestioned value in controlling hemorrhage for the first several hours, immediate plans need to be made to begin treatment of varices to prevent recurrent hemorrhage. When esophageal varices are the source of bleeding, obliteration sclerotherapy is usually the therapy of choice.

Variceal Obliteration

There are several techniques and agents for injecting varices. Many endoscopists in this country choose to inject the sclerosing solution directly into the varix. Others perform paravariceal injection. Quinine, sodium morrhuate, ethanolamine polidocanol, and sodium tetradecyl plus 50% dextrose are some of the sclerosing agents. We usually employ direct variceal injection of sodium tetradecyl plus 50% dextrose, using 1 to 2 ml per injection. Up to 6 ml may be injected at one site if needed, although with more volume injected, the risk of complications such as esophageal ulceration occurs. This is the preferred method for both initial control of bleeding and prevention of subsequent bleeding.[21] Careful analysis reveals that endoscopic sclerotherapy has never been shown to be more effective than tamponade for initial control of hemorrhage.[22]

Endoscopic ligation of esophageal varices has recently been described. In this approach the varix and surrounding mucosa are aspirated into the suction channel of the endoscope and an elastic O ring is slipped over the tissue which strangulates the tissue and obliterates the bleeding varix. Repeated sessions allowed for complete obliteration of varices in 68% of patients who survived to their index hospitalization. Control of bleeding was comparable to that with injection sclerotherapy. Although no direct comparisons of these two techniques are available, it appears that endoscopic ligation is a promising new tool in the control of bleeding esophageal varices. Whether or not there are fewer complications with this technique remains to be seen.[24]

When neither pharmacologic infusions, mechanical compression, or endoscopic obliteration controls bleeding, emergency surgery needs to be considered, especially if the patient is still a candidate for liver transplantation. Such situations are far from ideal and the mortality rate is very high. The choice of operation ranges from esophageal transection and reanastomosis to a shunt constructed between the portal venous system and the systemic circulation. The subject is beyond the scope of this chapter.

Ascites

The cirrhotic patient in the ICU is at risk for the development or worsening of sodium and water retention which produce an increase in extracellular space fluid and hyponatremia. The pathogenesis of fluid retention is incompletely understood. There is a direct correlation between renal sodium retention and liver function as measured by clearance of antipyrine, caffeine, and cholate, but no apparent relationship between sodium retention and degree of portosystemic shunting.[25] The kidney of the cirrhotic patient behaves as if it were receiving a decreased blood flow, even though when measured, renal blood and plasma flow are normal in stable cirrhotic patients with ascites. The signal to which the kidney is responding has been elusive, but is non-neurogenic and therefore, is probably a humoral factor. Recently, deficiency of atrial natriuretic factor deficiency has been hypothesized, yet levels of this hormone are increased in cirrhotics with ascites.[26] Whatever the signal, the kidney avidly retains sodium and water, through the renin-aldosterone angiotensin mechanisms, producing ascites and edema.

The critically ill patient in the ICU frequently requires substantial amounts of colloid, crystalloid, and water either during resuscitation (e.g., from bleeding) or as a vehicle for the administration of medicines (e.g., antibiotics). Because the kidney's ability to excrete sodium and water is already compromised, and additional renal impairment may occur due to hypotension or nephrotoxic drugs, ascites may become a major problem. Diuretic administration may worsen renal function and may thereby limit this therapeutic option. Increasing ascites may impair pulmonary dynamics, and even right ventricular function.

Ascites and edema can be minimized by careful attention to the volume of fluid and sodium delivered to such patients. If renal function is satisfactory, diuretics such as spironolactone and furosemide may be administered with caution. If renal dysfunction limits this approach, fluid can be removed by repeated large volume paracentesis. Removal of 4 to 6 (or more) L at a time has been shown to be safe and effective therapy for ascites and may be safer than diuretic therapy.[27] Removal of substantial amounts of protein may ensue with repeated paracentesis. Infusion of albumin protein (20 to 60 g per paracentesis) will replace this loss, allowing for repeated large volume removal. Because of the expense and occasional difficulty in obtaining albumin for infusion, synthetic plasma volume expanders

Table 55–4. Pathogenesis of Spontaneous Bacterial Peritonitis[31-34]

Spontaneous Bacteremia in Association With Immunologic Deficiencies:
Decreased ascitic fluid proteins
Decreased complement (ascitic fluid and serum)
Decreased ascitic fluid opsonic activity
Impaired neutrophil function
Impaired reticuloendothelial system function

(Data from references 31–34.)

such as 3.5% hemaccel (150 ml/L of ascites evacuated) appears to be an effective substitute.[28] Previous concerns of cardiovascular collapse or renal failure as a consequence of large volume ascitic fluid removal have not been borne out by experience.[29,30] In some situations, continuous ultrafiltration or other dialytic techniques may be necessary.

Infections

The patient with advanced cirrhosis is immune compromised and is susceptible to a number of infections. Urosepsis frequently sets the stage for additional infected sites. Pneumonia may occur with increased frequency. In patients with biliary tract problems, especially sclerosing cholangitis which has been stented or otherwise manipulated, biliary sepsis is common. A frequent infection in hospitalized cirrhotic patients is spontaneous bacterial peritonitis. It usually occurs in the cirrhotic patient with marked ascites. Table 55–4 indicates some of the pathophysiologic features of this disorder.[31-35]

The diagnosis of SBP may be obvious in the stable cirrhotic patient who suddenly develops fever and prominent abdominal pain. More commonly, however, the presentation is subtle. The most frequent manifestation is a *change* in clinical state in the cirrhotic patient. A high index of suspicion for the cirrhotic patient who "isn't doing well" will improve diagnostic accuracy. The diagnosis of SBP rests on the findings in peritoneal fluid (Table 55–5). Both the cell count and the culture are important. A suggestive cell count and a negative culture still warrant treatment. The cell count almost always reveals >250 polymorphonuclear cells (PMNs)/mm³. Usually the count is higher (e.g., over 1000); however, an occasional patient may have a much lower ascitic fluid PMN count.[36] The results of ascitic fluid culture are variable depending on the care with

Table 55–5. Ascitic Fluid Analysis in Spontaneous Bacterial Peritonitis

CORE TESTS
White blood cell count and differential > 250 neutrophils/mm³ = presumption of infection
Culture
 Traditional plating technique results in 42–65% diagnostic yield
 Inoculation of blood culture bottle results in 90% diagnostic yield
ANCILLARY TESTS (high specificity, variable sensitivity)
pH
Lactate
Arterial tests: ascitic pH, glucose, lactate gradients

Table 55–6. Typical Organisms Causing Spontaneous Bacterial Peritonitis

Gram-Negative	Percentage (%)	Gram-Positive	Percentage (%)
Escherichia coli	37	Pneumococcus	12
Klebsiella pneumoniae	17	Streptococcus viridans	9
Enterobacter	6	Gamma hemolytic streptococcus	4
Other	5	Enterococcus	3
		Other group D streptococcus	1
		Other	5

(From Barnes, P. F., et al.: A prospective evaluation of bacteremic patients with chronic liver disease. Hepatology, 8:1099, 1988.)

which the aspirated fluid is handled. When ascitic fluid is sent to the bacteriology laboratory to be plated the positive yield in cases of established or strongly presumed SBP is approximately 50%. This yield can be increased to 90% by pouring 10 ml or more into a blood culture bottle at the bedside[37,38] (Table 55–6). Blood cultures obtained at the same time may also be positive.

Treatment of SBP requires intravenous antibiotics. Because aerobic gram-negative organisms and Streptococcus pneumoniae are the predominate organisms, empiric selection of an antibiotic before cultures are available is possible. Usually, a third-generation cephalosporin such as cefotaxime is used. The combination of ampicillin and an aminoglycoside (tobramycin or gentamicin) is also effective, although recent studies indicate that the kidneys of cirrhotic patients are particularly susceptible to toxicity from aminoglycosides.[39] We do not consider aminoglycosides as first-choice therapy for SBP. Recently, amoxicillin-clavulanic acid therapy was found to eradicate SBP in 85% of cases.[40]

Duration of treatment may vary depending on the clinical course of the patient. Because this is a serious, sometimes life-threatening, infection, 10 to 14 days of treatment formerly was standard. Recent studies indicate that 5 days of antibiotics is sufficient and as effective as 10 days both for initial cure and for freedom from recrudescence of infection.[41]

Prevention of some cases of SBP appears possible. We and others have found that a significant number of cases of SBP occur after cirrhotic patients with sterile ascites are admitted to the hospital.[42] As Table 55–6 indicates, most organisms that cause SBP are part of the normal aerobic gut environment. One possibility is that the bacteremia which frequently occur with invasive procedures (e.g., sclerotherapy, endoscopy, etc.) may seed the peritoneal fluid. Low protein ascites are also low in antibacterial properties, such as opsonic activity, and may be fertile grounds for infection. Selective gut decontamination by norfloxacin has been shown to be effective in reducing the likelihood of a second bout of SBP from 35 to 12% over a mean follow-up period of approximately 6 months.[43] Although the major mechanism of action of norfloxacin is likely to be reduction of gut flora, which serves as a reservoir for ascitic contamination, it has recently been shown that the antibacterial activity of ascitic fluid (ascitic fluid total protein, and C3 component of complement) increases after norfloxacin therapy.[44] Although these results need to be confirmed, it seems prudent to attempt infection control in all cirrhotic patients with ascites admitted to the ICU by selective gut decontamination. Norfloxacin, 400 mg per day, is reasonably inexpensive and well tolerated and is currently our drug of choice. Whether this regimen should be continued in a patient receiving multiple antibiotics for established infection is unclear. This subject has been recently reviewed.[45]

Hepatic Encephalopathy

Cirrhotic patients are vulnerable to deranged central nervous function. This is called hepatic encephalopathy, or portosystemic encephalopathy (PSE). The pathogenesis is incompletely understood. The degree of hepatic reserve plays a role, but it is not nearly as important as the fact that blood draining the gut is highly toxic to the central nervous system (CNS). In normal individuals, the liver extracts the toxins which produce encephalopathy so that in the first pass through the liver portal blood is virtually stripped of neurotoxic substances. Cirrhotic patients with portal hypertension develop shunts, and this allows some portal blood to gain access to the general circulation prior to passing through the liver. Hence, the shunted blood perfuses the brain and the neurotoxins exert their deleterious effects. The degree to which portosystemic shunts exist will determine, in part, the patient's susceptibility to cephalopathy. The search for the neurotoxin(s) has been long and controversial. Ammonia, aromatic amino acids, and short chain fatty acids may all work together to produce the CNS dysfunction. There is accumulating evidence that unidentified substances accumulate in the brain that bind to gamma aminobutyric acid (GABA)-benzodiazepine receptors. Whether these observations are central or epiphenomena is not yet clear.[46]

Dietary protein is a strong inducer of encephalopathy in the predisposed patient. Proteins rich in aromatic amino acids are more toxic than those which are high in branched-chain amino acids (BCAA). On a gram-for-gram basis, blood protein is the most toxic, hence the frequent worsening of encephalopathy in the cirrhotic patient with intestinal bleeding. Red meat protein is more toxic than white meat protein, which generally correlates with levels of aromatic amino acids in the different protein sources. Substitution of amino acids with their alpha ketoanalogues reduces PSE.

The diagnosis of encephalopathy is usually simple. A cirrhotic patient with disordered brain function may have other problems, such as a subdural hematoma, CNS infection, or generalized sepsis causing confusion. The diagnosis of PSE, therefore, needs to be made with caution and with a full awareness that alternative diagnoses needs to be entertained. The stages of hepatic encephalopathy are described in the Table 55-7. In all but the earliest and latest stages of encephalopathy, asterexis can be elicited by having the patient hold the arm outstretched and pull back the separated fingers. Failure of ability to sustain tone in the antigravity muscles results in a quick drop of the fingers followed by recovery. Although the appearance is characteristic of asterexis, it needs to be distinguished from a tremor which has much faster oscillations. Asterexis is not pathognomonic of hepatic encephalopathy; it may be seen in liver disease, renal failure, and carbon dioxide narcosis. While not pathognomonic, in the right clinical setting (e.g., the cirrhotic patient in the ICU with bleeding varices who develops obtundation), asterexis is highly suggestive of hepatic encephalopathy.

Treatment of PSE is usually not too difficult in the short run. Review of medications is essential and hypnotics, sedatives, and tranquilizers should be discontinued. A search for infection (e.g., SBP) is undertaken. Cleansing the bowel of protein (especially blood protein) is critical. It is critical to educate the nursing staff that gut cleansing of this complication will be most helpful to treatment. Additional control of gut protein comes from dietary protein restriction, and by control of GI bleeding. Bowel cathartics typically consist of 300 ml of 50% lactulose added to 700 ml of tap water, used as an enema. Alternatively, neomycin, 500 mg to 1.0 g, can be put in 200 ml of saline and given as a retention enema. In the conscious patient, oral lactulose 30 to 45 ml per hour is given initially until diarrhea develops and then the dose is tapered until there are two soft stools per day. Oral neomycin, 500 mg to 1.0 g, can also be given orally every 4 to 6 hours. The rigor of the treatment can be tailored to the severity of the problem, of course.

The value of therapy with branched chain amino acid-enriched solutions in patients with PSE has been repeatedly documented. A recent meta-analysis of several randomized controlled trials confirmed a highly significant improvement in the degree of encephalopathy. Some, but not all, studies have also demonstrated improved survival for those treated with intravenous BCAA.[47-50] Some advocate use of BCAA in PSE;[51] others heed caution in the use of BCAA therapy because of the conflicting data regarding survival.[52] We do not usually use BCAA therapy in patients with PSE.

Acute Liver Failure

Intensive care physicians are likely to see all patients who undergo liver transplantation for acute liver failure

Table 55-7. Stages of Hepatic Encephalopathy

	Clinical	Neurologic	EEG
Stage 0	Subtle personality changes (apparent only to family or sophisticated neuropsychiatric testing)	Alert, no asterexis	Normal
Stage 1	Definite personality changes; alteration of sleep pattern	Asterexis present	Delta waves
Stage 2	Sleepy; abnormal behavior	Asterexis present	Delta waves
Stage 3	Somnolent but arousable	Asterexis present	Delta waves
Stage 4	Comatose (may respond to painful stimuli)	Asterexis present	Delta waves

both before and after the operation. There are important differences in the problems encountered prior to liver transplantation in the patient with fulminant acute liver failure compared to the cirrhotic patient. Many of these differences have direct therapeutic implications.

Acute liver failure occurs because of either massive or submassive hepatic necrosis. The common causes for acute liver failure are severe viral hepatitis (A, B [sometimes complicated by delta virus] or C), drug intoxication (especially acetaminophen taken in a suicide attempt), and, occasionally, mushroom poisoning (usually amanitia species). An excellent overview has been published.[53] The main difference between massive hepatic necrosis and submassive necrosis is the speed with which liver failure and death develop. In the former, the entire disease may express itself in a matter of days; in the latter the duration is a month or two. In either case the urgency to control complications and find a suitable donor liver is great. Problems posed by acute liver failure include:

- Sepsis
- Coagulopathy
- Renal failure
- Encephalopathy
- Acute cerebral edema
- Metabolic disorders

Each time a patient is admitted to the ICU with acute liver failure an inventory of these (remember SCREAM) should be made and systematically addressed.

Sepsis is likely, in part because the acute liver failure patient is immunocompromised. Bacterial infections occur in more than four out of five patients; Staphylococcus aureus, streptococci, and enteric coliform bacteria predominate.[54] In patients who survive for more than a few days, invasive fungal infections (typically candida or aspergillus) may occur, but may be hard to diagnose with certainty ante mortem. A patient who appears to get better and then relapses may well have developed invasive fungal infection. Those with renal insufficiency are at particularly high risk. An unexplained temperature elevation (or one that persists after all identified bacterial infections are being treated appropriately) particularly if the white blood cell count is elevated, should raise the index of suspicion for a fungal coinfection.[55] Our approach in all patients with acute liver failure is to administer norfloxacin and mycostation to achieve selective gut decontamination (discussed later in this chapter) even in the absence of established infection. Daily chest radiographs and pan culture for bacteria and fungi are done. The threshold to begin broad-spectrum antibiotics is quite low. In a patient not responding to antibiotics, further search for fungal infection is considered on a case-by-case basis.

Coagulation disorders occur because all coagulation proteins except factor VIII are produced in the liver, and its failure to do so results in abnormal coagulation. Superimposed infection may lead to disseminated intravascular coagulation. Prophylactic administration of fresh-frozen plasma is not necessary or desirable, although it is usually given at least to cover the neurosurgical placement of a CNS pressure measuring device (see the following discussion). Gastrointestinal bleeding may be due either to coagulation abnormalities or to erosive gastritis. The incidence of upper GI bleeding in acute hepatic failure has been reduced by administration of H_2-receptor antagonists.[56] Where intravenous omeprazole is available, this will likely be the agent of choice.

Renal failure in acute hepatic failure is usually functional, i.e., reversible. It frequently is oliguric, and the urine sediment is bland unless there is deep jaundice, in which case "dirty brown casts" may be seen. Avid sodium retention (urine sodium < 10 mEq/L) is the rule. It can just as easily develop in those normal or even high intravascular volumes, and does not respond to either further volume challenge or to diuretics. Renal failure in the ICU may also develop due to the administration of nephrotoxic drugs, or from acute volume loss from GI bleeding. Rigorous studies demonstrating the value of "renal dose" dopamine (2 to 4 µg/kg per hour) are lacking. Nevertheless, this agent is frequently employed in our ICU. Ultrafiltration or hemodialysis may be required in severe cases.

The patient with acute liver failure has some degree of hepatic **encephalopathy,** depletion of coagulation proteins, frequently intestinal bleeding, and sometimes renal insufficiency. The encephalopathy has at least in part a different basis from that described in the cirrhotic patient. In acute liver failure there frequently is not an association with aromatic amino acids; gut cleansing is generally ineffective. Recent studies indicate an association, however, between the level of ammonia levels in experimental acute liver failure and decreases in brain function, suggesting that ammonia is of key importance in the encephalopathy that develops after both acute and chronic liver injury.[57] In addition, there is a substantial risk of **acute cerebral edema,** which frequently produces tonsillar herniation and death of the patient from brain stem compression. The frequency of cerebral edema occurring in fulminant hepatic failure may be as high as 85%. The pathophysiology of cerebral edema in acute liver failure has been reviewed.[58] This complication needs to be prevented when possible.

Recognition of significant cerebral edema is difficult clinically. Headache, projectile vomiting, bradycardia, and papilledema are usually absent.[59] Other noninvasive measures such as CT scanning are relatively insensitive in identifying this rapidly progressing complication. In one center in which routine placement of an epidural pressure transducer was placed in 15 patients with fulminant hepatic failure, elevated intracranial pressure (>15 mm Hg) was identified in 11 (73%). Routine CT scans showed evidence of effacement or flattening of cortical sulci, reduction in size, or narrowing or obliteration of the cerebral ventricles or cisterns, or presence of generalized decreased attenuation of the hemispheres in only 27% of cases where increased intracranial pressure had been identified by pressure measurement.[60]

Several different systems are being used to record intracranial pressure. Epidurally placed transducers may be safer to place in the patient with severe coagulopathy. Technical problems are more frequent in getting reliable information over time. "Bolts" or extremely thin brain parenchymal transducers provide better fidelity but are riskier.[61] We rely on direct measurement of intracranial pressure in the setting of acute liver failure. This involves the placement of an intracranial transducer, which can be done with safety despite markedly disordered coagulation studies. Treatment of cerebral edema caused by acute liver failure involves attempts to dehydrate the brain. Mannitol intravenously is given unless renal function is inadequate. Intubation and deliberate hyperventilation sufficient to maintain an P_{CO_2} of less than 30 mm Hg may also be used. Corticosteroids such as dexamethasone are uniformly unhelpful.

A variety of **metabolic disorders** may be seen. A centrally mediated respiratory alkalosis is common and should not be corrected. Metabolic acidosis, particularly in the patient with acetaminophen liver failure, is an ominous finding with a 90% mortality rate if the arterial pH is less than 7.30. Hypoglycemia due to impaired gluconeogenesis and depleted glycogen stores may have disastrous consequences when severe. Blood sugars must be monitored frequently and hypoglycemia treated aggressively.

Search for a Liver

Considerable frustration on the part of patient, family, and physician occurs as the wait for a liver donor lengthens from days to weeks or months. Not all centers performing liver transplantation can readily obtain a suitable liver in a short period for even their sickest patients. Approximately 23% of patients die before receiving a liver transplant. In February, 1991, 1334 patients were waiting for a liver.[1]

There is a national policy of organ donation. Through the UNOS, federal law administers a national organ procurement and transplantation network. The policy is ever-changing. The current rules are as follows:

1. All potential recipients of livers must be listed with UNOS.
2. Listing of a single patient on more than one local waiting list is permissible. Because prioritization for liver transplantation depends on medical factors, the number of times a patient is listed is a minor factor in obtaining a liver.
3. Each transplant center must record with UNOS their minimum criteria for an acceptable liver. This ensures that livers will not be offered to a center which are clearly unacceptable to that center.

UNOS liver allocation criteria are complicated and necessarily imperfect because no manageable scheme can encompass all possible situations. Nevertheless, there is a logic to assigning different priorities to patients with different severities of liver failure. Most patients in the ICU will be listed as a status 4 or 3 (see Table 55–8).

Allocation of donor livers is also determined by the geographic region from which the organ is recovered, and in part by the medical urgency of the patient. Status 4 patients, for example, take precedence over all other according to the following plan:

- Local, status 4
- Local, all other

Table 55–8. Priority Levels for Allocation of Donor Livers

Status	Points	Definitions
0	0	Temporarily inactive; continues accruing waiting time. UNOS staff confirms status at 30 days. Patients who are considered to be temporarily unsuitable transplant candidates can be temporarily inactive in Status 0. The patient continues to accrue waiting time as his/her disease is deteriorating further.
1	6	At home, functioning normally. Patients in Status 1 are considered to be elective patients, for whom an excellent donor will be accepted.
2	12	Continuous medical care. These patients are all other patients who need liver transplants soon. The patient can be followed at home or near the transplant center. Short hospitalizations for intercurrent problems are not an indication for a change in status.
3	18	Continuously hospitalized. These patients are in such a medical condition that they cannot leave the hospital. Therefore, continuous hospitalization is necessary.
4	24	ICU patient. Acute and chronic liver failure. A maximum of 7 days with a one time, 7 day extension on request is the total allowable time at Status 4. Only waiting time on Status 4 counts for donor allocation. The patient is considered in critical condition in the ICU due to acute or chronic liver disease. Patients requiring urgent retransplant for nonfunctioning grafts will usually be in this category.

- Regional status 4
- Regional, all other
- National, status 4
- National, all other

The development of effective local procurement agencies will have great bearing on the number of transplants done within each region.

General factors predicting outcome following liver transplantation include the specific type and stage of disease and the status of the recipient. Several investigators have reported analyses of certain risk factors that may predict outcome and therefore aid in patient selection. The predictors analyzed include serum creatinine, bilirubin, ascites, encephalopathy, prior upper abdominal surgery, albumin, malnutrition, variceal hemorrhage, spontaneous bacterial peritonitis, age, and coagulopathy (Table 55–9).[62-68]

The factors associated with a higher postoperative morbidity and mortality are an elevated serum creatinine, severe coagulopathy, coma, ascites, and having a prior portacaval shunt.[62,64-68] The serum creatinine is the most reliable predictor of outcome. Prior nonshunt upper abdominal surgery does increase red cell usage and may increase the incidence of intra-abdominal infections, but it does not adversely impact survival.[65] In contrast, a prior portacaval shunt results in more intraoperative blood loss (13 blood volumes versus 3 blood volumes), a longer hospital stay (62 days versus 35 days), more septic complications, and a higher operative mortality (34% versus 0%).[64]

Table 55-9. Risk Factors Predicting Outcome in Liver Transplantation

Creatinine*
Ascites*
Bilirubin
Encephalopathy*
Prior Upper Abdominal Surgery**
Serum Albumin
Malnutrition
Variceal Hemorrhage
Spontaneous Bacterial Peritonitis
Age
Coagulopathy*

* Denotes factors that increase postoperative morbidity and mortality.
** Such surgery does not, per se, increase mortality. A prior portacaval shunt, however, does increase operative mortality.
(Data from references 62 to 68.)

Table 55-10. Criteria for Organ Donation[71,72]

General Criteria	Liver-Specific Criteria
Age (varies with organ)	Relative normal liver function
No history of preexisting disease in the organ	bilirubin < 2 md/dl
No malignant tumors except primary brain	transaminases < 200 U
Absence of sepsis	normal prothrombin time
Absence of transmissible diseases (e.g., AIDS, hepatitis)	No history of liver injury or disease
No history of alcohol or IV drug abuse	No history of alcohol abuse
No prolonged hypotension or cardiac arrest	P_{O_2} > 70 torr
No evidence of DIC	No acidosis
	CVP < 15 cm H_2O
Prolonged vasopressors (limits vary with organ)	Dopamine < 10 µg/kg/min

ICU PHASE AND CONSIDERATIONS RELATING TO THE POTENTIAL ORGAN DONOR

The number of donor organs available remains one of the most limiting factors in liver transplantation. There are approximately 4000 to 10,000 potential candidates for liver transplantation in the United States each year.[69] Currently, the maximum donor organ availability meets about one third of that need.[69] Several states have passed "required request" legislation in an effort to increase the number of donors. The law "requires" that hospitals provide documentation that the families of all patients who are potential donors were "requested" to donate their loved one's organs. Unfortunately, according to a 1989 report from the Ohio Department of Health, only 10% of families informed of their opportunity to donate consented to anatomic donation.[70] Therefore, the impact of "required request" legislation has fallen far short of the expectations. Educational campaigns which dispel the myths about organ donation and emphasize the success of transplantation directed at both the medical community and the lay public may help realize more donors.

All potential cadaveric organ donors are ICU patients. They are usually young, healthy people who have suffered a tragic, unexpected death from either trauma or spontaneous intracranial hemorrhage. The general criteria for organ donation and specific criteria for liver donation are given in Table 55-10.[71,72] The "ideal" potential liver patient is a brain-dead patient who:

- Is less than 50 years of age
- Has been in the hospital for a short period (1 to 2 days)
- Is hemodynamically stable on no or minimal pressor agents
- Has normal liver function tests

In an effort to expand the donor pool, some centers accept potential liver donors up to 60 years of age; their results are comparable to those obtained with younger donors.[73]

Current criteria for donor evaluation and selection does not accurately predict early graft function in a significant percentage of cases. Makowka and colleagues retrospectively analyzed their donor selection criteria relative to predicting graft function.[74] These criteria included bilirubin, transaminase, prothrombin time, arterial blood gases, blood pressure, and dose of dopamine. Good donors were defined as those in whom these criteria were normal or almost normal. Poor donors had abnormal liver functions, were hypotensive (systolic blood pressure < 60 mm Hg), hypoxic (P_{O_2} < 60 torr), and required greater than 15 µg/kg per minute of dopamine for pressor support. Fourteen percent of the good donors had poor initial function; 6% did not function at all. Conversely, 51% of the poor donors demonstrated good initial function; 10% did not function. Makowka concluded that the current criteria used to select donors were not good indicators of graft function, especially in the poor donor group.[74] He advised a more liberal selection criteria to increase the donor pool.

More recently, a new assay which measures a "single pass" metabolite of lidocaine has demonstrated some promise in predicting early graft function. The potential donor is injected with 1 mg/kg of lidocaine; 15 minutes later a blood sample is drawn and the amount of monoethyl glycine xylidide (MEGX) is determined. Values above a certain range are associated with excellent initial graft function and a very low incidence of primary nonfunction irrespective of the other donor criteria.[75,76] In addition to its value in predicting graft function, this assay is available in kits and can be performed at most hospitals in less than 30 minutes.

Excellent donor management both in the ICU and the operating room is essential for successful organ recovery. The local organ procurement agency becomes responsible for management once the donor has been declared brain dead, and consent for organ donation has been obtained from the next of kin. The majority of donors require hydration and correction of electrolyte abnormalities (especially hypernatremia) incurred as a result of keeping the patient dry in an effort to minimize cerebral edema. Most are receiving dopamine for pressure support and many need vasopressin to control diabetes insipidus. Ventilatory support should be optimized as well.

Careful management must be continued in the operating room until the organs are removed by the various transplant teams. A single donor may provide a heart, lungs, liver, pancreas, and kidneys. Most of the time several surgical teams are involved in the retrieval endeavor, which may last 3 to 4 hours. Therefore, timing, cooperation, and good anesthesia support are necessary for a successful outcome.

Preoperative Preparation

The degree of preoperative preparation required depends on the severity of the illness of the recipient. Patients called in from home need a brief history and examination, chest radiograph, ECG, routine blood studies, type and cross for 20 U each of packed red blood cells, freshly frozen plasma and platelets and overnight hydration. Half the quantity of each blood product is reserved for children. Prophylactic antibiotics are given on call in the operating room. A loading dose of cyclosporine is no longer given preoperatively because of its associated renal toxicity. Non-ICU hospital-bound patients may benefit from being transferred to the ICU the evening prior to transplantation. A pulmonary artery catheter and arterial line are inserted to allow optimal resuscitation which often requires the administration of blood products. Renal dose dopamine is also begun if the patient's renal function has deteriorated as a consequence of their liver disease.

Timing of the Recipient Procedure

With some exceptions, the recipient operation may be started at 8:00 A.M. Recipients who are well enough to wait at home are called to the hospital as soon as a potential donor has been identified. Before the introduction of the University of Wisconsin (UW) preservative solution, the maximum allowable cold ischemia time was 10 to 12 hours.[77,78] This time constraint mandated precise timing of the donor and recipient procedures, so the diseased liver was ready for removal when the new organ arrived. Therefore, both portions of the transplant effort were often performed at night. The extended ischemia time of 20 to 24 hours afforded by the UW solution allows the recipient team to be fresh for the long operation.[77,78] A patient with acute liver failure or a patient who requires urgent retransplantation are the exceptions that cannot wait until the following morning to begin the recipient operations.

Intraoperative Predictors of Survival

Hemorrhage and technical problems are the intraoperative factors which affect morbidity and mortality.[69] Portal hypertension, coagulopathy, and prior upper abdominal surgery (especially a portacaval shunt) all contribute to intraoperative blood loss. During the anhepatic and reperfusion stages of the procedure, fibrinolysis may develop and have a major impact on transfusion requirements.[79] Analysis of coagulation factors during liver transplantation has revealed that both a consumption coagulopathy and fibrinolysis occur to varying degrees in the latter two states of the procedure.[79] Replacement of blood components including plasma, platelets, and cryoprecipitate helps correct the bleeding. Occasionally, specific antifibrinolytic (Amicar) therapy is necessary.[79] A graft that functions promptly virtually prevents the development of fibrinolysis.

Intraoperative Monitoring

As with any major operative procedure, a liver transplant requires extensive intraoperative monitoring. When the recipient arrives in the operating room, further intravenous lines and an arterial line are started. After the induction of anesthesia, two large-bore (8 French) intravenous introducers are inserted, as well as a pulmonary artery catheter, if not previously placed. The introducers are connected to a "rapid infusion device" which consists primarily of a roller pump which is capable of delivering between 2 to 3 L of fluid per minute should the need arise. Hemodynamic parameters monitored throughout the procedure include mean arterial pressure (MAP), central venous pressure (CVP), cardiac output (CO), systemic vascular resistance (SVR), and wedge pressure (PCWP). Renal dose dopamine is begun shortly after the induction of anesthesia; urine output is measured hourly for the duration of the operations.[80]

Laboratory studies that are checked frequently throughout the procedure include arterial blood gasses, ionized calcium, hematocrit, and coagulation profiles. In addition to the prothrombin time, partial thromboplastin time, platelet count and fibrinogen, coagulation is monitored with the thromboelastogram (TEG). This device measures the mechanical properties of a clot and is particularly helpful for determining which coagulation components should be replaced or if fibrinolysis is present.[81]

Body temperature requires constant monitoring to minimize hypothermia. The length of the procedure and the size of the incision promote significant loss of body heat. Hypothermia adversely affects both cardiac function and coagulation. Measures to maintain body temperature include a heating blanket, wrapping the arms, legs, and head in plastic bags, periodically instilling warm saline into the peritoneal cavity, and raising the ambient temperature in the operating room.

Operative Procedure

Orthotopic liver transplantation (OLT) has become a relatively standardized, although demanding operative procedure.[82] The operation may be thought of in three stages:

- Dissection
- Anhepatic stage
- Reperfusion

The dissection is the most demanding portion of the procedure because of the presence of coagulopathy and portal hypertension, especially in the patients who have had prior right upper quadrant surgery. After the portal structures are skeletonized, the liver including the retrohepatic vena cava is mobilized from the diaphragm to just above the renal veins. The importance of maintaining hemostasis throughout this first stage of the transplant cannot be overemphasized. The donor organ is prepared for implantation on the back table as the recipient dissection is completed.

Most centers routinely use venovenous bypass during the anhepatic stage of the operation.[82] Heparin-bonded tubing is inserted into the saphenous and portal veins; the blood is returned to the axillary vein by a centrifugal pump (Bio-medicus) (Fig. 55-1). Clamps are placed on the hepatic artery and the vena cava both above and below the liver. The liver is then excised, often leaving the vena cava in situ. The cited advantage of bypass includes hemodynamic stability, less blood loss, tailoring of excision of the diseased liver, and less postoperative renal dysfunction.[83] Some centers, however, including our own, use bypass only in those patients who do not maintain hemodynamic stability despite additional volume loading. Bypass is necessary in approximately 10% of patients undergoing liver transplantation.[84] Cardiac output decreases approximately 40% and systemic vascular resistance increases approximately 80% if bypass is not used (unpublished data from our center). Review of our own data and reports from other centers reveal that these hemodynamic changes are temporary and do not adversely impact on transfusion requirements, renal function, or survival.[80]

The preservation solution is flushed from the graft with normal saline (approximately 500 ml in an adult) through the portal vein cannula while the lower cava anastomosis is performed so sudden hyperkalemia and possible cardiac arrest do not occur when the clamps are removed. After completion of the venous anastomoses, the clamps are removed, restoring systemic and portal return. The arterial and biliary reconstruction are carried out next (Fig. 55-2). When hemostasis is adequate, a cholecystectomy and cholangiogram are performed. Drains are placed in both subphrenic spaces and in the subhepatic space. The abdomen is closed and the patient is transported directly to the ICU.

Immediate Postoperative Monitoring and Care

After the transplant procedure is completed, the patient is transported directly to the ICU. Hemodynamic monitoring includes MAP, CVP, CO, SVR, PCWP, and heart rate. Over the first 12 to 24 hours the patient may require a large volume of crystalloid and blood products to maintain filling pressures and urine output. Cardiac output is characteristically high, which is a manifestation of the previous cirrhotic state.

The volume of urine, bile, drain output, and nasogastric drainage is closely monitored. Urine output may be low as a result of preoperative renal dysfunction, sustained intraoperative hypotension, fluid shifts, and inadequate volume replacement. Renal dose dopamine is maintained for at least the first 24 to 36 hours postoperatively to maximize renal perfusion.[80] Because of its nephrotoxic effects, cyclosporine is withheld for the initial 12 hours; it is usually started the next morning if the urine output remains adequate and the BUN/creatinine remain stable.

Patients with intractable ascites prior to liver transplantation can be expected to continue to generate large volumes of drainage for several days postoperatively. Efforts to replace the ascitic losses on a volume for volume basis are unnecessary and will result in fluid overload. Bloody drainage is anticipated in the first 12 to 24 hours. The combination of large amounts of grossly bloody drainage, hemodynamic instability, and relatively normal coagulation studies points to surgical bleeding that requires immediate exploration, however. Drainage of 100 to 200 ml per

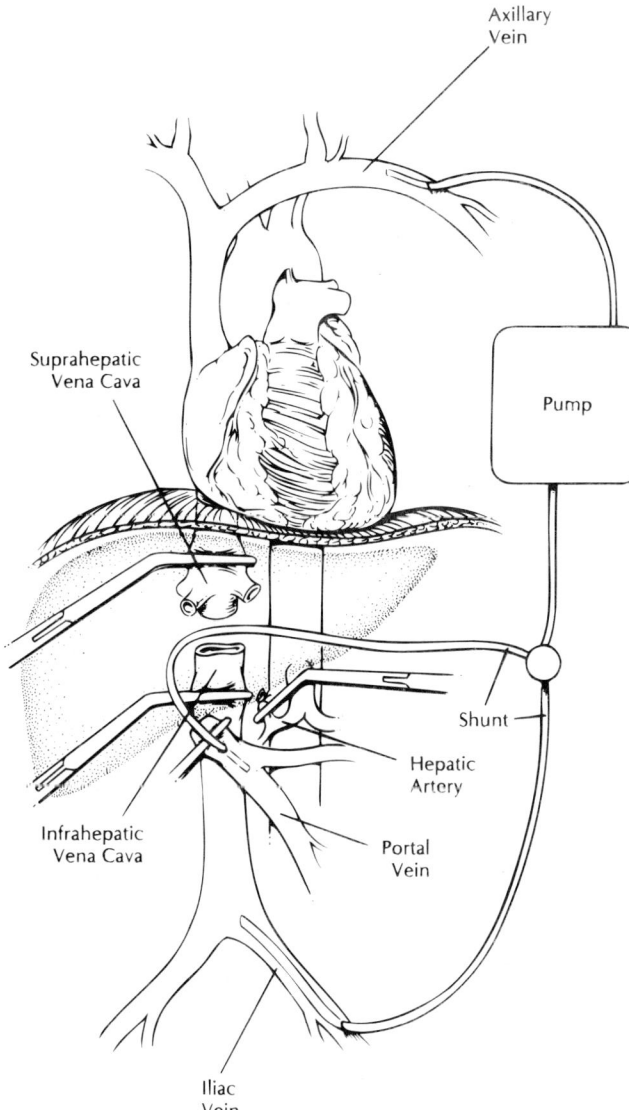

Fig. 55-1. Venovenous bypass can buy time and cardiovascular stability for transplant recipient after the diseased liver has been removed. The centrifugal pump circulates blood from the iliac and portal veins, bypassing the clamped-off area, and shunting blood into the axillary vein for return to the heart. Before the bypass procedure was developed, clamping of the portal vein and vena cava would cause rapid pooling of blood in leg and abdominal veins, compromising venous return. Note also the long segments of vena cava that have been dissected free and left in place after excision of the diseased liver. These can be fashioned to meet reconstruction requirements at reimplantation. (Adapted from Starzl, T. E., et al.: Refinements in the surgical technique of liver transplantation. Seminars in Liver Disease, 5: 349, 1985.)

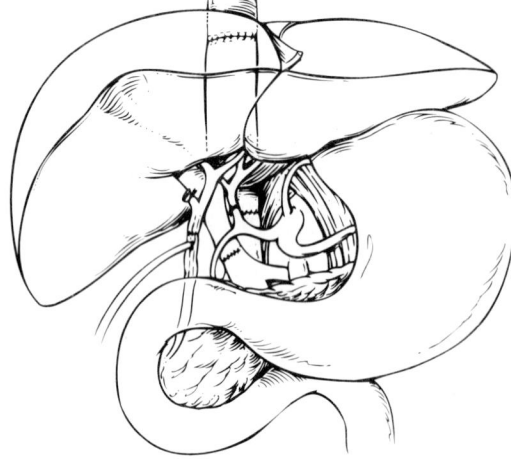

Choledochocholedochostomy

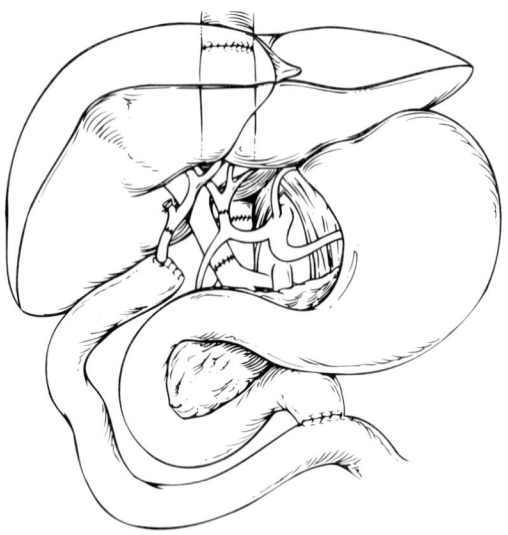

Choledochojejunostomy

Fig. 55-2. Techniques of biliary tract reconstruction were improved in the mid-1970s to ensure adequate biliary drainage. Preferred anastomosis is duct-to-duct (choledochocholedochostomy). In situations where the recipient duct is diseased, absent, or too small, Roux-en-Y choledochojejunostomy provides an equally safe alternative (Adapted from Starzl, T. E., et al.: Refinements in the surgical technique of liver transplantation. Seminars in Liver Disease, 5:349, 1985).

day of dark bile is reassuring because bile production is one of the most accurate indicators of early graft function.[85]

Frequent laboratory studies are necessary for optimal management of the postoperative liver transplant patient. Upon arrival in the ICU, a full battery of tests are obtained including liver and renal function, complete blood count (CBC), platelet count, and coagulation profile. The CBC, prothrombin time, and platelet count are measured every 6 hours for the first 24 hours; renal function is checked every 12 hours; liver tests are obtained daily. Once cyclosporine is started, trough levels are obtained every day.

Efforts are not made to correct a prothrombin time of 18 seconds or less, especially in small children who have a higher incidence of hepatic artery thrombosis.[85] Fresh-frozen plasma is given liberally when the prothrombin time is more than 18 seconds. Production of bile, normalizing coagulation parameters, and appropriate mental status are the best early indicators of adequate graft function.[85]

Thrombocytopenia is common for the first several days following liver transplantation, especially in patients with preoperative hypersplenism.[85] Platelet counts of 20,000 to 25,000 are not unusual. Despite these low counts, clinical bleeding is rarely a problem. Efforts to maintain the platelet count above 25,000 may require pooled platelet transfusions for the first few days, however. The platelet count usually begins to rise to normal levels by the end of the first postoperative week. The mechanism for the profound thrombocytopenia seen in the immediate post-transplant period is not well understood.

The liver functions which are measured daily include the AST (SGOT), ALT (SGPT), bilirubin, alkaline phosphatase (AP) and gamma glutamyl transpeptidase (GGTP). The transaminase reflect ischemic hepatocyte injury and are elevated from 200 to 1000 U or greater in the first 24 to 48 hours post-transplant. The AST and ALT usually normalize by the seventh postoperative day. Initially, the bilirubin may drop dramatically, depending on the severity of the jaundice preoperatively. This initial decrease is primarily a "washout" phenomenon associated with the large volumes of fluid and blood products administered during the operative procedure. The bilirubin slowly rises but should level off by the end of the first week. The canalicular enzymes (AP, GGPT) reflect damage to the cells of the biliary tree; they are normal immediately postoperatively and rise slowly over the next several days as rejection becomes more likely.

Postoperative ICU Course

The two major determinants of the initial postoperative course are the preoperative condition of the recipient and the conduct of the operation.[69] As with any major operative procedure, an intraoperative effort free of technical problems, major blood loss, and hypotension results in a relatively uncomplicated postoperative course. Recipients well enough to wait at home for their transplant are usually awake within a few hours of completion of the operation, extubated within 12 hours of the procedure, and discharged from the ICU on the second or third day. A prolonged ICU stay should be anticipated in patients who were hospital-bound before they underwent liver transplantation, especially patients in the ICU either because of sudden deterioration of chronic disease or because of acute liver failure. These debilitated patients may require prolonged ventilatory assistance, aggressive nutritional support, and dialysis.

Surgical bleeding and primary graft nonfunction (PNF) are two immediate, severe postoperative complications of liver transplantation.[69] Voluminous bloody drainage, hemodynamic instability in spite of continuous volume replacement, and relative normal coagulation parameters indicate surgical bleeding. Prompt exploration is mandatory to correct the problem.

Primary graft nonfunction is a disastrous complication that usually results in death unless immediate retransplantation is possible.[86,87] Approximately 10% of patients develop PNF; the etiology is not clear but may be related to preservation injury of the sinusoidal endothelium of the graft.[86,87] The clinical manifestations of PNF include:

- Scant bile production
- Encephalopathy
- Extremely high transaminases
- Rapidly rising bilirubin
- Severe coagulopathy
- Acute renal failure
- Respiratory insufficiency
- Hypoglycemia
- Death[86]

Mortality without retransplantation is 80% at 6 months.[86] Greig and colleagues reported the efficacy of prostaglandin E₁ (PGE₁) in reversing PNF in 8 of 10 patients; 2 required retransplantation.[86] Ninety percent of the patients treated with PGE₁ survived in contrast to a 33% survival in patients not treated with PGE₁.[86,87] Although our experience has been limited, we have seen dramatic improvements in transaminase levels and prothrombin time in a few patients given PGE₁ who had evidence of severe graft dysfunction.

POST-ICU PHASE

Postoperative Course

The average length of hospitalization following a relatively uncomplicated liver transplantation is 3 to 4 weeks. Status 1 or 2 recipients (see Table 55-8) are usually stable enough to transfer to a regular nursing floor on the second or third postoperative day. Vital signs and urine output are monitored closely for the first few days; then on a routine basis. Approximately 60 to 70% of the patients require treatment for hypertension, which is primarily a manifestation of cyclosporine.[88] Ambulation is permitted and encouraged as the patient becomes stronger and more comfortable.

Oral intake is resumed by the third day and advanced as tolerated. Laboratory studies including liver and renal function and cyclosporine trough levels are obtained on a daily basis until the patient is discharged from the hospital. Methylprednisolone (Solu-medrol) is replaced by oral prednisone after the initial steroid taper is completed. Oral cyclosporine is added once the patient is eating. The bowel decontamination regimen, begun when the patient was first identified as needing a liver transplant, is continued for 1 month postoperatively or until the patient is discharged from the hospital. Gamma globulin prophylaxis for cytomegalovirus is administered every 2 weeks until 3 months after liver transplantation.

A protocol liver biopsy and cholangiogram are obtained on the seventh post-transplant day. Repeat biopsies are performed as necessary thereafter; especially after the completion of therapy for an episode of acute rejection.[89] If the cholangiogram is normal, the T tube or biliary stent (if a Roux-en-Y choledochojejunostomy was constructed) is shortened and tied off, and the abdominal drains are removed. Intravenous cyclosporine is weaned once adequate blood levels with oral cyclosporine are obtained. The remainder of the hospitalization is spent primarily adjusting cyclosporine dosage, convalescing, and in patient education. Once discharged from the hospital, the patient receives weekly blood studies for the first 1 to 2 months, and they return to the outpatient department in 2 weeks. Eventually, the blood studies are performed monthly and the patient returns yearly.

Postoperative Complications

Only 10 to 15% of patients do not develop a significant complication following OLT.[88] Complications may generally be categorized as either graft related or extrahepatic. Graft-related problems include:

- Primary nonfunction
- Retrieval injury
- Rejection
- Vascular thrombosis
- Infection
- Biliary tract difficulties
- Hemolysis
- Drug injury[90]

Every extrahepatic organ can manifest a complication as well; pulmonary, cardiovascular, GI, renal, neurologic, and infection (Table 55-11).[88] Some of the extrahepatic problems particularly germane to liver transplantation are renal dysfunction, neurologic toxicity, and opportunistic infection.[88]

Graft Dysfunction

Graft dysfunction occurs in 66% of organs transplanted.[90] The causes of graft dysfunction are listed in Table 55-11. Several studies are necessary to evaluate graft dysfunction including a liver biopsy, cholangiogram, duplex scanning of the hepatic artery, and cyclosporine levels (Table 55-12). Further investigation that may be required includes computed tomography of the abdomen and celiac arteriography. As discussed earlier, primary nonfunction is evident immediately postoperatively and results in a mortality of at least 80% without urgent retrans-

Table 55-11. Complications After Liver Transplantation

Graft-Related	Non-Graft Related (Extrahepatic)
Primary nonfunction	Pulmonary: infection, pleural effusion, respiratory failure
Harvest-induced injury	Gastrointestinal: bleeding, perforation, pancreatitis
Vascular thrombosis	Renal dysfunction: ATN, drug induced, hypoperfusion
Infection	Neurologic: tremors, seizures, ataxia
Bile duct complications	Infection: bacterial, fungal, viral
Hemolysis	Cardiovascular: hypertension, arrhythmias, myocardial infarction
Drug-induced injury	Malignant: de novo skin, lymphoma, or recurrence

Table 55-12. Studies to Evaluate Liver Graft Dysfunction

Liver biopsy
Cholangiogram
Hepatic artery patency
    Duplex ultrasonography
    Arteriography
Cyclosporine levels

---

plantation.[86,87] The etiology of primary nonfunction is now known and the role of PGE_1 in its treatment remains to be determined.[86,87]

Rejection is the most frequent cause of graft dysfunction in the first 3 months after transplantation.[90] The reported incidence ranges from 40 to 100%;[29] approximately 80 to 85% of our patients develop graft rejection. Acute rejection usually presents by day 7 to 10 after liver transplantation; the patient may experience malaise and mild graft tenderness. Most often, however, rejection is asymptomatic, but is always evident by deranged liver function and a typical histologic appearance on biopsy.[89] The initial therapy is to repeat the 5-day course of a steroid taper. "Steroid resistant" rejection is treated with a 10 to 14 day course of monoclonal antibodies (OKT3).[91] A small percentage of patients (2 to 5%) require liver retransplantation in the perioperative period because of uncontrolled graft rejection.[91] Although acute rejection occurs in the majority of patients, it is responsible for only 8 to 10% of deaths.[87,92]

Vascular complications associated with liver transplantation result from thrombosis of the hepatic artery, portal vein, or hepatic veins.[94-97] Of these, hepatic artery thrombosis (HAT) is the most frequent with an overall incidence of 10%: 5% in adults, and 5% in children.[94] Technical errors such as using a recipient vessel with inadequate inflow, development of an intimal flap, and a substandard anastomosis may result in HAT.[98] Nontechnical factors contribute as well, however.[98] Rejection has been shown to dramatically diminish arterial blood flow through the graft.[39] A hematocrit above 45% is another predisposing factor.[98] Children have a higher incidence of HAT in part because of the small diameter of the vessels.[94] Doppler ultrasound and arteriography are the screening and definitive diagnostic studies, respectively.

HAT presents with equal frequency in one of three ways:

- Fulminant hepatic necrosis
- Relapsing bacteremia[94]
- Delayed bile leak

Fulminant liver necrosis occurs an average of 16 days after liver transplantation; fever, markedly elevated transaminase, and multiorgan failure are the clinical manifestations. Urgent retransplantation is the only recourse; approximately 25% of patients survive. A delayed bile leak, which usually manifests 1 month postoperatively, results from necrosis of the donor bile duct. Bile peritonitis, subhepatic abscess, and bacteremia are the associated manifestations. Initial therapy consists of controlling the bile leak by draining it externally; this may be accomplished by either percutaneous or operative means. Retransplantation is inevitable once the sepsis has resolved, and only 50% of patients survive.[94]

Relapsing bacteremia is the most insidious presentation of HAT.[94] It does not become symptomatic until 4 to 6 weeks after liver transplantation. The liver function remains normal and antibiotics are temporarily effective in controlling the recurrent sepsis. Arteriography may be necessary to confirm the diagnosis. Most of the 50% of patients who survive require retransplantation.[94]

Meticulous operative technique, aggressive treatment of rejection, and prophylactic anticoagulation in small recipients may help prevent HAT. Immediate exploration, thrombectomy, and arterial reconstruction may salvage the graft if HAT is diagnosed shortly after it occurs.[99] Most of these patients still develop a biliary stricture, however, or leak several days to weeks later which may require further surgery including retransplantation.[99] Overall, HAT carries a 50% mortality.[94]

The biliary anastomosis is no longer the "Achilles' heel" of liver transplantation. The decreased incidence of biliary tract complications results from standardization of techniques of reconstruction; primary duct-to-duct (choledochocholedochostomy) and Roux-en-Y choledochojejunostomy (Fig. 55-2). A bile leak or stricture still occurs in 20 to 24% of patients with equal frequency between the two types of reconstruction.[100,101] Bile leaks tend to occur within a week or two following liver transplantation and usually result from a technically poor anastomosis or a thrombosed hepatic artery.[90] Immediate exploration is required to control or repair the leak. Strictures occur late in the postoperative course and are more frequent with a choledochojejunostomy. An attempt at percutaneous dilatation is worthwhile; surgical revision, however, may be necessary.[100]

Infection, hemolysis, and drug-induced injury may cause graft dysfunction.[90] Bacterial and fungal sepsis can cause hyperbilirubinemia in nontransplant, as well as liver transplant, patients.[90] Herpes simplex, herpes zoster, and cytomegalovirus may directly infect the graft and result in severe dysfunction.[90] Treatment consists of lowering the immunosuppression and adding either acyclovir (herpes) or ganciclovir (CMV).[102] Hemolysis may occur if a mismatch is present between the donor and recipient blood types; an O blood group liver is placed into a patient who is either an A or B blood type. The passenger lymphocytes in the donor liver are capable of producing isohemagglutinins that hemolyze the recipient's red blood cells which results in anemia and hyperbilirubinemia.[86] This problem is self-limiting and resolves in several weeks. Transfusion replacement should be of the donor's blood type. Both cyclosporine and amphotericin B may cause cholestasis, which resolves if the dose of the drug is reduced.[90]

Surgical Complications

OLT has a reoperation rate of 43 to 55%.[103,104] The complications requiring surgical intervention include:

- Bleeding
- Sepsis

- Biliary tree problems
- Gastrointestinal bleeding or perforation
- Vascular thrombosis
- Retransplantation

Starzl reported that the 6-month mortality in patients with a surgical complication was 32%, in contrast to a 11% mortality in those patients who did not require reoperation.[104] Shaw, however, found no difference in survival between patients who did (76%) and did not (80%) need post-transplant operative intervention.[103] Although survival was not significantly less in the reoperated group, the length of hospitalization was considerably longer.[103] Prior biliary operations, the status of the recipient pretransplant, operating time of 12 hours or greater, and severe rejection did not predict the probability for reoperation.[103] Survival was lower (63 versus 77%), and surgical complications were higher (63 versus 43%) in patients who underwent liver retransplantation.[103]

Infection

Infection is the major cause of death following liver transplantation. Seventy to 80% of patients develop an average of 2.5 infections in the post-transplant period.[105] Of the 85% of deaths associated with sepsis, 50% occur in the first postoperative month and 90% have occurred by 2 months.[69] The condition of the donor liver, technical problems, preexisting infection, and immunosuppression are factors that determine the frequency and type of septic complications that may develop after liver transplantation.[69]

Post-transplant infections may be classified as to their etiologic agent or the timeframe in which they occur (Table 55–13).[106] Bacterial and fungal infections are seen in the early postoperative course and often result from technical problems such as HAT, bile leaks, intraabdominal abscesses, GI complications, and wound sepsis. Gram-negative organisms, including pseudomonas, are largely responsible for bacterial infections, which are associated with a mortality significantly higher than in those patients who do not develop early bacterial sepsis (71% versus 18%).[69]

Candida and aspergillosis account for 42% of postoperative fungal infections.[107,108] A culture from either blood, the peritoneal cavity, or both, that is positive for candida is presumptive evidence that a GI perforation has occurred and exploration is indicated. Overall, fungal infections carry a 50% mortality.[107-109]

Recent reports and our own experience have shown that selective bowel decontamination significantly reduces the incidence of postoperative bacterial and fungal infections.[110,111] Our regimen for bowel decontamination consists of norfloxacin and mycostatin, which are begun when the patient is placed on the donor list. Both of these agents are continued for four weeks or until discharge from the hospital.

Viral infections are endemic in transplant patients. Cytomegalovirus, herpes simplex and zoster, and Epstein-Barr viruses are encountered on a regular basis. Viral infections are frequent from one to six months post-transplant. Although up to 70% of liver transplant patients develop positive cultures for CMV in the buffy coat, urine, or throat swab, only 10 to 15% develop CMV disease manifested by fever, pneumonia, hepatitis, or multiorgan failure. A patient with no prior exposure to CMV who received an organ from a CMV serologically positive donor has an 80% risk of developing CMV infection.[112,113] All our patients receive gamma globulin, 500 mg per kg every 2 weeks for the first 3 months in an effort to reduce the severity of CMV. Review of our data suggests that the gamma globulin may be somewhat effective.[111] Once CMV disease occurs, however, treatment consists of reducing the immune suppression and introduction of ganciclovir. Herpes simplex or zoster infections are treated with acyclovir.

Other infections which occur weeks to months after transplantation are Pneumocystis and Legionella.[69] The former is particularly lethal and is associated with marked hypoxemia, which precedes radiographic changes by several hours. Bronchoscopy and bronchoalveolar lavage provides material for special stains and culture; the former are important in providing rapid diagnostic information which allows prompt institution of therapy. Pneumocystis is treated primarily with trimethoprim-sulfamethoxazole, and legionella with erythromycin. Because the latter agent slows the metabolism of cyclosporine, dosage adjustments based on frequent blood levels must be made. We have a high index of suspicion for Pneumocystis carinii pneumonia in any transplant patient with respiratory symptoms, particularly breathlessness, dyspnea, fever, and headache. Early determination of arterial oxygen desaturation, followed by bronchoalveolar lavage for definitive diagnosis, has allowed us to identify and treat all of our patients who have P. carinii before they have become ill enough to require admission to the ICU. Nevertheless, some patients will develop respiratory failure.

Table 55–13. Classification of Post-Transplantation Infections

Phase 1 First Transplant Month	Phase 2 Month 2–6	Phase 3 After 6 Months
Bacterial		
Typical postoperative infections; reactivation of tuberculosis	Continuation of earlier infections, pneumocystis, Listeria, Nocardia	Community acquired, (e.g., pneumococcal pneumonia, Legionella, pneumocystis)
Viral		
Hepatitis B, C, or HIV (from donor organ or blood)	Cytomegalovirus, Epstein-Barr virus, hepatotrophic viruses	Chronic viral hepatitis, CMV
Fungal		
Candida, aspergillus, others	—	Cryptococci
Parasitic		
Parasitic: activation of preoperative infestation (e.g., stercolaris), others.	Rare	Rare

Treatment with parenteral trimethoprim-sulfamethoxazole has been our initial treatment, although pentamidine may occasionally be needed. For more severe cases (PaO$_2$ < 70 mm Hg or an A-a gradient > 35 mm Hg) adjunctive corticosteroids should be used (e.g., oral or parenteral prednisone 40 mg twice a day for 5 days, then 40 mg daily for 5 days, followed by 20 mg daily for the duration of anti-infective therapy).[114] Whether these data apply to liver transplant patients is unknown.

Extrahepatic Complications

Renal Dysfunction

Renal dysfunction occurs in as many as 30% of patients after OLT.[88] Manifestations include oliguria, serum creatinine of 2.2 mg/dl for 48 hours, or both. Early renal dysfunction is seen in the first postoperative week and probably results largely from cyclosporine toxicity.[1] Other independent predictors of early postoperative renal impairment include preoperative renal dysfunction as a result of severe hepatocellular disease, ascites, hypoalbuminemia, and intraoperative hypotension.[62] Cyclosporine-sparing immunosuppressive regimens which use either antilymphocyte globulin (ALG) or OKT3 for the first 7 to 10 days post-transplant allow for resolution of hepatic-induced renal dysfunction.[115] Renal dysfunction that occurs after the first postoperative week has a less favorable prognosis and is associated with shock, graft failure, sepsis, and nephrotoxic drugs such as cyclosporine, aminoglycosides, and amphotericin.[71] The mortality in patients requiring dialysis ranges from 41 to 73%.[68,88]

Neurologic Toxicity

Neurologic complications occur in 20 to 30% of patients after OLT.[116,117] These complications include seizures, tremor, coma, paresthesias, confusion, visual hallucinations and ataxic and cerebellar syndromes.[116,117] Meningitis may result from infection, or as an aseptic variety associated with administration of OKT3.[118] Brachial plexus and peroneal nerve injuries may result from improper positioning during the lengthy procedure.[84] Neurologic problems were seen in OLT patients before the introduction of cyclosporine; however, this drug is felt to play at least some role in the development of some of the problems listed above.[117,119] Other etiologic factors cited include hypomagnesemia, high dose steroids, fluid overload, hypocholesterolemia, and demyelination.[120]

Evaluation of neurologic problems requires a thorough neurologic examination, lumbar puncture, CT scan, MRI scan, and EEG. In many patients, this exhaustive battery of studies does not provide either a definitive diagnosis or point to a specific etiologic agent. Seizures are treated with either phenytoin (Dilantin) or phenobarbital; both drugs accelerate cyclosporine metabolism so that more may be required to maintain an adequate blood level. Since cyclosporine is incriminated in many of the more severe neurologic syndromes, the dosage is often reduced or the drug eliminated.[116,117] Four of our patients suffered severe neurologic complications manifested by seizures impaired in spite of cessation of cyclosporine.

Malignancy

Transplant patients have an increased risk of developing de novo malignancies.[121] Among the cancers encountered are carcinoma of the skin, cervix, and, most importantly lymphoproliferative disorders (LPD) including lymphomas.[122] Since the introduction of cyclosporine, the incidence of lymphomas and LPD has increased to 18%, in contrast to a 4% incidence in the general public.[117] Patients on triple drug therapy are at the highest risk of developing LPD.[121,123,124] Several centers have reported a strong association between the Epstein-Barr infection and the development of lymphomas in the post-transplant period.[123,124] Multiple courses of OKT3 also appear to increase the risk of EBV-related LPD.[123,124] Fortunately, EBV-related lymphomas often respond favorably to reducing the dosage of cyclosporine and giving acyclovir.[123,124] We have had two patients develop malignant disease: an adult with a basal cell carcinoma of the skin, and a teenager who died of lymphoblastic lymphoma after a prolonged course of OKT3 failed to reverse a severe rejection episode that resulted from noncompliance.

Miscellaneous Issues for the Intensivist

Certain health care issues encountered in the liver transplant recipient do not, by themselves, require ICU admission. The intensive care physician needs to be aware of these because those admitted to such units with other problems will need these details attended to. Hypertension and relative renal insufficiency are common in patients receiving cyclosporine. Antihypertensive agents will need to be adjusted in the unit, and sometimes converted to intravenous agents. Relative renal insufficiency due to cyclosporine is common, and appropriate adjustment of drug dosages needs to be made with this in mind. Animal studies suggest a protective effect of calcium-channel blockers (nifedipine) against the acute renal toxicity of cyclosporine.[125] Clear documentation that this effect is seen in humans after liver transplantation is lacking.

Cyclosporine may make the patient particularly susceptible to renal insults of diverse natures. In addition, cyclosporine must frequently be given intravenously. Adjustment of dosage from oral to IV requires about one third the oral dosage. The drug is given every 12 hours as a continuous infusion. Frequent trough blood levels are obtained to allow for appropriate fine-tuning of dosage. Cyclosporine is metabolized by the hepatic cytochrome P-450 family enzymes. Many other commonly used agents share this degradation pathway. Co-administration of such agents may result in slower metabolism of each agent and much higher blood levels which can result in toxicity. Caution should therefore be employed when considering such drugs. Table 55–14 indicates some of these.

An important drug-drug interaction not related to the cytochrome P-450 system is that between azathioprine and allopurinol. Many transplant patients will have an elevated uric acid level. Administration of allopurinol interferes with the principal pathway for detoxification of allopurinol. If these drugs need to be given together, reduce the dosage of azathioprine to one third to one fourth the usual.

Table 55-14. Drug Alteration of Cyclosporine Metabolism

Impeded Cyclosporine Metabolism	Enhanced Cyclosporine Metabolism
Ketaconazole	Phenobarbital
Amphotericin B	Phenytoins
Erythromycin	Rifampin
Aminoglycosides	
Anti-inflammatory drugs	
Trimethoprim/Sulfamethoxazole	

Survival

The survival after OLT has improved dramatically in the last decade. Starzl reported a one year survival rate of 33% in 11 transplants performed from 1963 to 1976.[126] In a comprehensive report which included all centers in the United States, UNOS reported an average 1-year survival rate of 76% for first time transplants performed in 1988.[127] The range of 12-month survival varies from 54 to 84%.[69] Factors cited for improved results of OLT include cyclosporine, standardized arterial and biliary reconstruction, better organ preservation, venovenous bypass, appropriate patient selection, and training of surgeons to perform the procedure.[69] Pittsburgh reported a 5-year survival of 60 to 65% for over 800 patients transplanted since the introduction of cyclosporine.[128] Our overall survival in 83 patients, in whom 93 transplants were performed, is 69%; the mean follow-up is 20 months, with a range of 3 to 67 months.

Several factors are responsible for outcome in liver transplantation. These include the specific disease for which the transplant was performed, the stage of disease, the immune response mounted by the patient, and the general state of health of the patient at the time of OLT.[69] Clearly, sicker patients in a more advanced stage of disease have a higher operative morbidity and mortality. The patients with the lowest survival are those with terminal disease who precipitously decompensate and require life support measures such as mechanical ventilation and dialysis. The emergency of rejection that necessitates heavy immunosuppression or retransplantation is associated with a high incidence of septic-related complications and mortality.[69]

Survival in liver transplantation correlates with the primary disease for which transplantation is performed (Table 55-15).[69] The best results are obtained in patients who undergo liver transplantation for cholestatic liver disease, which includes primary biliary cirrhosis (PBC) and scleros-ing cholangitis (PSC). The 1- and 5-year survival rates range from 80 to 70%, respectively.[68] Transplantation for cirrhosis from chronic active hepatitis (CAH), either autoimmune or from non-A and non-B hepatitis, carries a survival rate just slightly less than for cholestatic liver disease.[129] The outcome in patients with cirrhosis as a result of chronic B virus infection is significantly less, with a 1- and 5-year survival rate of 57 and 38%, respectively.[98] The major reason for the decreased survival is the virtual 100% incidence of reinfection of the new liver with the B virus.[102,130]

Patients who undergo liver transplantation for primary hepatic cancer, either hepatocellular carcinoma or bile duct in origin, have the poorest long-term outlook.[69] These patients initially do well because their transplant procedures are relatively easy to perform, because they do not have chronic liver disease and its associated portal hypertension and coagulopathy. The likelihood of tumor recurrence is extremely high, however. The 42% 1-year and 30% 3-year survival rates primarily reflect deaths from recurrent tumor and metastatic disease.[131,132] Early results suggest that neoadjuvant chemotherapy with a regimen of doxorubicin (Adriamycin) may improve the results of liver transplantation for hepatocellular carcinoma.[133] Currently, all patients undergoing liver transplantation for malignant disease should be given neoadjuvant chemotherapy as part of a protocol in which chemotherapy is given before the transplant in an effort to reduce the high recurrence rate of malignant disease.

Retransplantation

The frequency of retransplantation ranges from 8 to 30% with a mean of 10%.[134] The three most common reasons for retransplantation are rejection, technical problems, and primary graft nonfunction (Table 55-16).[134] Rejection refractory to immunosuppression is the most frequent indication (41%) and it carries the highest survival (64%).[134] Technical problems such as HAT and biliary complications account for one third, with a 1-year survival of 40%.[135] Retransplantation for primary graft nonfunction has a 30% 1-year survival.[134] Overall, retransplantation salvages at least half the patients in whom it is performed.[135] Ten of our 83 patients (12%) have undergone liver retransplantation, primarily for chronic rejection and hepatic artery thrombosis; 55% are still alive.

Late Graft Dysfunction

Late graft dysfunction may result from rejection, viral infection, biliary stricture, and recurrence of the primary liver disease.[102] Acute rejection is encountered infre-

Table 55-15. Survival in Adults After Liver Transplantation

Cause of Disease	1-Year Survival	5-Year Survival
Cholestatic diseases		
Primary biliary cirrhosis	77	70
Sclerosing cholangitis	80	85
Postnecrotic cirrhosis (HBsAG −)	60–80	70
Postnecrotic cirrhosis (HBsAG +)	58	38
Malignancy	25–90	0–30

Table 55-16. Retransplantation Indications and Survival

Indication (%)		1-Year Survival (%)
Rejection	(41)	64
Technical	(33)	40
Primary Nonfunction	(24)	30

quently greater than three months after transplantation and usually responds to standard immunosuppressive strategies.[102] Chronic rejection, however, results in relentless, progressive graft dysfunction that requires retransplantation and carries a 25% mortality.[102] Viral infections responsible for late graft dysfunction include cytomegalovirus, and de novo B or non-A/non-B hepatitis.[102] Anastomotic biliary strictures typically occur several months after liver transplantation. Strictures that do not respond to either percutaneous or endoscopic dilatation do well after surgical revision.[50]

Many of the disorders leading to end-stage liver disease remedied by transplantation have been shown to recur in allografts; primary biliary cirrhosis, primary sclerosing cholangitis, hepatitis B, malignant tumors, Budd-Chiari syndrome, and autoimmune hepatitis.[69,102] A few mild cases of PBC have been reported 3 to 5 years after liver transplantation.[136] One of our patients has developed PSC 3 years after liver transplantation for the same disease.

Recurrent infection of the allograft with hepatitis B varies from 50 to 100%.[102] Low recurrence rates may be anticipated when the transplant is done for fulminant hepatitis B, but when chronic B hepatitis with cirrhosis is the indication for transplantation, virtually all have reinfections in their grafts. The administration of hyperimmune gamma globulin and interferon have not reduced the incidence of reinfection.[102] The 5-year survival is only 38% in this group of patients.[102] The frequency of recurrent non-A/non-B hepatitis is much lower than with B virus patients and the survival rates almost match those of cholestatic diseases.[102] As mentioned earlier, malignant disease is associated with the highest rate of recurrence. In one report, 80% of hepatocellular carcinomas recurred by 18 months, and virtually all cholangiocarcinomas recurred by 1 year.[132]

Quality of Life

The quality of life after liver transplantation is of considerable interest, but data are limited and inconsistent. Some studies have shown the restored physical and emotional well-being that is possible in infants and children.[102,137] Over 90% of adults who require a single liver transplant have no or minimal health problems 2 years later.[102] Eighty-five percent return to work or full-time activities in the home.[102] In contrast, only 43% of those who require more than one liver transplant are able to return to work, for a variety of disabilities.[102] In our own series, 80% of adults have returned to work or a full life style, and all children and teenagers have returned to school.

REFERENCES

1. UNOS Update; 7:18, 1991.
2. Hernomo, K., et al.: Sengstaken tube for bleeding varices: a prospective randomized controlled trial. Hepatology, (abstract) 3:1058, 1983.
3. Merigan, T., Plotkin, G., and Davidson, C.: The effect of intravenous pituitrin on hemorrhage from bleeding varices. N. Engl. J. Med., 266:134, 1962.
4. Conn, H. Q., et al.: Intraarterial vasopressin in the treatment of upper gastrointestinal hemorrhage: a prospective controlled trial. Gastroenterology, 68:211, 1975.
5. Johnson, W., et al.: Control of bleeding varices by vasopressin: a prospective randomized study. Ann. Surg., 186:369, 1977.
6. Chojkier, M, et al.: A controlled comparison of continuous intraarterial and intravenous infusion of vasopressin in hemorrhage from esophageal varices. Gastroenterology, 77:540, 1979.
7. Fogel, M., et al.: Continuous intravenous vasopressin in active upper gastrointestinal bleeding: a placebo-controlled trial. Ann. Intern. Med., 96:556, 1982.
8. Moreau, R., et al.: Abnormal pressor response to vasopressin in patients with cirrhosis: evidence for impaired buffering mechanisms. Hepatology, 12:7, 1990.
9. Bosch, J., et al.: Association of transdermal nitroglycerin to vasopressin infusion in the treatment of variceal hemorrhage: a placebo controlled trial. Hepatology, 10:962, 1989.
10. Gimson, A. E. S., et al.: Randomized trial of vasopressin and vasopressin plus nitroglycerin in the control of acute variceal hemorrhage. Hepatology, 6:410, 1986.
11. Teres, J., et al.: Vasopressin/nitroglycerin infusion versus esophageal tamponade in the treatment of acute variceal bleeding: a randomized controlled trial. Hepatology, 11:964, 1990.
12. Tsai, Y-T., et al.: Controlled trial of vasopressin plus nitroglycerin versus vasopressin alone in the treatment of bleeding esophageal varices. Hepatology, 6:406, 1986.
13. Yates, J., et al.: Effects of somatostatin, sandostatin, and vasopressin on portal pressure and collateral blood flow in portal hypertensive rates. Gut, (abstract) 30:A1498, 1989.
14. Bosch, J., et al.: Azygous blood flow in cirrhosis; effects of balloon tamponade, vasopressin, somatostatin and propranolol. Hepatology, (abstract) 3:855, 1983.
15. Valenzuela, J. E., et al.: A multicenter randomized double-blind trial somatoastatin in the management of acute hemorrhage from esophageal varices. Hepatology, 10:958, 1989.
16. Burroughs, A. K., et al.: Randomized double-blind placebo controlled trial of somatostatin for variceal bleeding. Gastroenterology (in press).
17. Levinson, S. L.: Insertion of the Minnesota tube. In Manual of Gastroenterologic Procedures. Edited by D. Drossman. New York, Raven Press, 1987.
18. This reference has been deleted.
19. Hernomo, K., et al.: Sengstaken tube for bleeding varices: a prospective randomized controlled clinical trial. Hepatology, 3:1058, 1983.
20. Panes, J., et al.: Efficacy of balloon tamponade in treatment of bleeding gastric and esophageal varices: results of 151 consecutive episodes. Dig. Dis. Sci., 33:454, 1988.
21. Moreta, M., et al.: A randomized trial of tamponade or sclerotherapy as immediate treatment for bleeding esophageal varices. Surg. Gynecol. Obstet., 167:331, 1988.
22. Teres, J.: Balloon tamponade vs endoscopic sclerotherapy in the management of active variceal hemorrhage. (Correspondence) Hepatology, 11:898, 1990.
23. Teres, J., et al.: Esophageal tamponade for bleeding varices: controlled trial between Sengstaken-Blakemore tube and Linton-Nachlas tube. Gastroenterology, 75:566, 1978.
24. Steigmann, G. V., et al.: Endoscopic ligation of esophageal varices. Am. J. Surg., 159:21, 1990.
25. Rector, W. G., et al.: Renal sodium retention complicating alcoholic liver disease: relation to portosystemic shunting and liver function. Hepatology, 12:455, 1990.
26. La Villa, G., et al.: Natriuretic hormone activity in the urine of cirrhotic patients. Hepatology, 12:467, 1990.
27. Gines, P., et al.: Comparison of paracentesis and diuresis in the treatment of tense ascites: results of a randomized study. Gastroenterology, 93:234, 1987.
28. Salerno, F., et al.: Randomized comparative studies of hem-

accel versus albumin infusion after total paracentesis in cirrhotic patients with cirrhotic ascites. Hepatology, 13:707, 1991.
29. Carey, W. D., et al.: Ascitic fluid removal: does it cause renal or hemodynamic compromise? Cleve. Clin. Qt., 50:397, 1983.
30. Tito, L., et al.: Total paracentesis associated with intravenous albumin management of patients with cirrhosis and ascites. Gastroenterology, 98:146, 1990.
31. Clark, J. H., Fitzgerald, J. F., and Kleiman, M. B.: Spontaneous bacterial peritonitis. J. Pediatr., 104:495, 1984.
32. Wilcox, C. M., and Dismukes, W. E.: Spontaneous bacterial peritonitis, a review of pathogenesis, diagnosis and treatment. Medicine, 66:447, 1987.
33. Barnes, P. F., et al.: A prospective evaluation of bacteremic patients with chronic liver disease. Hepatology, 8:1099, 1988.
34. Crossley, I. R., and Williams, R.: Spontaneous bacterial peritonitis. Gut, 26:325, 1985.
35. Runyon, B. A.: Patients with deficient ascitic fluid opsonic activity are predisposed to spontaneous bacterial peritonitis. Hepatology, 8:632, 1988.
36. Runyon, B.: Monomicrobial nonneutrocytic bacterascites: a variant of spontaneous bacterial peritonitis. Hepatology, 12:710, 1990.
37. Runyon, B. A., Umland, E. T., and Merlin, T.: Inoculation of blood culture bottles with ascitic fluid. Arch. Intern. Med., 147:73, 1987.
38. Runyon, B. A., Canawati, H. N., and Akriviadis, E. A.: Optimization of ascitic fluid culture technique. Gastroenterology, 95:1351, 1988.
39. Felisart, J., et al.: Cefotaxime is more effective than is ampicillin-tobramycin in cirrhotics with severe infections. Hepatology, 5:457, 1985.
40. Grange, J. D., et al.: Amoxicillin-clauvulanic acid therapy of spontaneous bacterial peritonitis: a prospective trial of 27 cases in cirrhotic patients. IIcpatology, 11:360, 1990.
41. Runyon, B. A., et al.: Short course versus long course therapy of spontaneous bacterial peritonitis: a randomized trial of 100 patients. Gastroenterology, 100:1737, 1991.
42. Carey, W. D., Boayke, A., and Leatherman, J.: Spontaneous bacterial peritonitis: clinical and laboratory features with reference to hospital-acquired cases. Am. J. Gastroenterol., 81:1156, 1986.
43. Gines, P., et al.: Norfloxacin prevents spontaneous bacterial peritonitis recurrence in cirrhosis: results of a double-blind placebo-controlled study. Hepatology, 12:716, 1990.
44. Such, J., et al.: Selective intestinal decontamination increase serum ascitic fluid C3 levels in cirrhosis. Hepatology, 12:1175, 1990.
45. Hoefs, J. C.: Spontaneous bacterial peritonitis: prevention and therapy. Hepatology, 12:776, 1990.
46. Butterworth, R. F., and Layrargues, G. P.: Benzodiazepine receptors and hepatic encephalopathy. Hepatology, 11:499, 1990.
47. Rossi-Fanelli, F., Riggio, O., and Cangiano, C.: Branched chain amino acids versus lactulose in the treatment of hepatic coma: a controlled study. Dig. Dis. Sci., 27:929, 1982.
48. Wahren, J., et al.: Is intravenous administration of branched chain amino acids effective in the treatment of hepatic encephalopathy? A multicenter study. Hepatology, 3:475, 1983.
49. Michel, H., et al.: Treatment of hepatic encephalopathy by infusion of a modified amino acid solution: results of a controlled study in 47 cirrhotic patients. In Hepatic encephalopathy in chronic liver failure. Edited by L. Capocaccia, J. E. Fischer, and F. Rossi-Fanelli. New York, Plenum, 1984, p. 323.
50. Cerra, F. B., et al.: Disease-specific amino acid infusion (FO80) in hepatic encephalopathy: a prospective randomized double blind controlled trial. J. Parenter. Enteral. Nutr., 9:288, 1985.
51. Naylor, C. D., et al.: Parenteral nutrition with branched-chain amino acids in hepatic encephalopathy: a meta analysis. Gastroenterology, 97:1033, 1989.
52. Erickson, L. S., and Conn, H. O.: Branched chain amino acids in the management of hepatic encephalopathy: an analysis of variants. Hepatology, 10:228, 1989.
53. Williams, R., and Gimson, A. E. S.: Intensive liver care and management of acute hepatic failure. Dig. Dis. Sci., 36:820, 1991.
54. Rolando, N., et al.: Prospective study of bacterial infection in acute liver failure: an analysis of 50 patients. Hepatology, 12:49, 1990.
55. Rolando, N., et al.: Fungal infection: a common unrecognized complication of acute liver failure. J. Hepatol., 12:1, 1991.
56. Macdougall, B. R. D., and William, R.: H-2 receptor antagonist in the prevention of acute upper gastrointestinal hemorrhage in fulminant hepatic failure. Gastroenterology, 74:164, 1978.
57. Bosman, D. K., et al.: Changes in brain metabolism during hyperammoniemia and acute liver failure: results of a comparative 1H-NMR spectroscopy and biochemical investigation. Hepatology, 12:281, 1990.
58. Blei, A. T.: Cerebral edema and intracranial hypertension is acute liver failure; distinct aspects of the same problem. Hepatology, 13:376, 1991.
59. Norma, L. M., and Bleck, T. P.: Increased intracranial pressure complicating hepatic failure. J. Crit. Illness, 4:87, 1989.
60. Munoz, S., et al.: Elevated intracranial pressure and computed tomography of the brain in fulminant hepatocellular failure. Hepatology, 13:209, 1991.
61. Allen, R.: Intracranial pressure: a review of clinical problems, measurement, techniques, and monitoring methods. J. Med. Eng. Tech., 10:299, 1986.
62. Maddrey, W., et al.: Liver transplantation: an overview. Hepatology, 89:948, 1988.
63. Bontempo, F., et al.: The relation of preoperative coagulation findings to diagnosis, blood usage, and survival in adult liver transplantation. Transplantation, 39:532, 1985.
64. Brems, J., et al.: Effect of a prior portasystemic shunt on subsequent liver transplantation. Ann. Surg., 209:51, 1989.
65. Cuervas-Mons, V., et al.: Does previous abdominal surgery alter the outcome of pediatric patients subjected to orthotopic liver transplantation? Gastroenterology, 90:853, 1986.
66. Shaw, B., et al.: Influence of selected patient variables and operative blood loss on six month survival following liver transplantation. Semin. Liver Dis., 5:385, 1985.
67. Shaw, B., et al.: Stratifying the causes of death in liver transplant recipients. Arch. Surg., 125:895, 1989.
68. Brems, J., et al.: Variables influencing the outcome following orthotopic liver transplantation. Arch. Surg., 122:1109, 1987.
69. Goldstone, D., and Clinton, J.: Assessment of liver transplantation. AHCPR Health Technology Assessment Reports, 1990.
70. Fletcher, R.: "Required Request": its impact on organ/tissue donation and transplantation in Ohio, 1989. Columbus, State of Ohio, 1989.
71. Wood, R. P., and Shaw, B. W., Jr.: Multiple organ procure-

ment. *In* Organ Transplantation and Replacement. Edited by G. J. Cerelli. Philadelphia, J. B. Lippincott, 1988.
72. Klintmalm, G., et al.: The liver donor; special considerations. Transplant. Proc., *20:*9, 1988.
73. Wall, W., Mimeault, D., Grant, D., and Bloch, M.: The use of older donor livers for hepatic transplantation. Transplantation, *49:*377, 1990.
74. Makowka, L., et al.: Analysis of donor criteria for the prediction of outcome in clinical liver transplantation. Transplantation Proceedings, *19:*2378, 1987.
75. Schroeder, T., et al.: Lidocaine metabolism as an index of liver function in hepatic transplant donors and recipients. Transplant Proceedings, *21:*2299, 1989.
76. Burdelski, M.: Donor rating in human liver transplantation; correlation of oxygen consumption after revascularization with MEGX formation in donors. Transplant Proceedings, *21:*2392, 1989.
77. Cofer, J., et al.: A comparison of UW with Eurocollins preservation solution in liver transplantation. Transplantation, *49:*1088, 1990.
78. Olthoff, K., et al.: Comparison of UW solution and Eurocollins solutions for cold preservation of human liver grafts. Transplantation, *49:*284, 1990.
79. Harper, P., et al.: Coagulation changes following hepatic revascularization during liver transplantation. Transplantation, *48:*603, 1989.
80. Polson, R. J., et al.: The prevention of renal impairment in patients undergoing orthotopic liver grafting by infusion of low dose dopamine. Anesthesia, *42:*15, 1987.
81. Kang, Y., et al.: Intraoperative changes in blood coagulation and thromboelastogram monitoring in liver transplantation. Anesth. Analg., *64:*888, 1985.
82. Starzl, T. E., et al.: Refinements in the surgical technique of liver transplantation. Semin. Liver Dis., *5:*349, 1985.
83. Shaw, B. W., et al.: Advantages of venous bypass during orthotopic transplantation of the liver. Semin. Liver Dis., *5:*344, 1985.
84. Wall, W. J., et al.: Liver transplantation without venous bypass. Transplantation, *43:*56, 1987.
85. Starzl, T. E., Demetris, A. J., and Van Theil, D.: Liver transplantation. N. Engl. J. Med., *321:*1014, 1989.
86. Greig, P. D., et al.: Treatment of primary liver graft nonfunction with prostaglandin E1. Transplantation, *48:*477, 1989.
87. Greig, P. D., et al.: Prostaglandin E1 and primary nonfunction following liver transplantation. Transplantation Proceedings, *21:*3360, 1989.
88. Wood, R. P., Shaw, B. W., and Starzl, T. E.: Extrahepatic complications of liver transplantation. Semin. Liver Dis., *5:*369, 1985.
89. Ray, R. A., et al.: The role of liver biopsy in evaluating acute allograft dysfunction following liver transplantation: a clinical histologic correlation of 34 liver transplantations. Human Pathol., *19:*835, 1988.
90. Esquivel, C. O., et al.: Liver rejection and its differentiation from other causes of graft dysfunction. Semin. Liver Dis., *5:*369, 1985.
91. Klintmalm, G. B., et al.: Rejection in liver transplantation. Hepatology, *10:*978, 1989.
92. Bismuth, H., et al.: Hepatic transplantation in Europe: first report of the European Liver Transplant Registry. Lancet, *2:*674, 1987.
93. Scharschmidt, B. F.: Human liver transplantation: analysis of data on 540 patients from four centers. Hepatology, *4:*95, 1984.
94. Tzakis, A. G., et al.: Clinical presentation of hepatic artery thrombosis after liver transplantation in the cyclosporine era. Transplantation, *40:*667, 1985.
95. Wozney, P., et al.: Vascular complications after liver transplantation. Am. J. Radiol., *147:*137, 1986.
96. Blumhardt, G., et al.: Vascular problems in liver transplantation. Transplantation Proceedings, *19:*2412, 1987.
97. Lerut, J., et al.: Complications of venous reconstruction in human orthotopic liver transplantation. Ann. Surg., *205:*259, 1987.
98. Yanaga, K., Makowka, L., and Starzl, T. E.: Is hepatic artery thrombosis after liver transplantation really a surgical complication? Transplantation Proceedings, *21:*3511, 1989.
99. Langnas, A. N., et al.: Hepatic allograft rescue following arterial thrombosis. Role of urgent revascularization. Transplantation, *51:*86, 1991.
100. Stratta, R. J., et al.: Diagnosis and treatment of biliary tract complications after orthotopic liver transplantation. Surgery, *106:*674, 1989.
101. Busuttil, R. V., et al.: The first 100 liver transplants at UCLA. Ann. Surg., *206:*397, 1987.
102. Starzl, T. E., Demetris, A. J., and Van Theil, D.: Liver transplantation. N. Engl. J. Med., *321:*1092, 1989.
103. Wood, R. P., et al.: Complications requiring operative intervention after orthotopic liver transplantation. Am. J. Surg., *156:*513, 1988.
104. Leneau, G., et al.: Analysis of surgical complications after 397 hepatic transplantations. Surg. Gynecol. Obstet., *179:*317, 1990.
105. Colonna, J. O., et al.: Infectious complications after 397 hepatic transplantations. Surg. Gynecol. Obstet., *170:*317, 1990.
106. Rubin, R. H.: Infectious disease problems. *In* Transplantation of the Liver. Edited by W. C. Maddrey. New York, Elsevier Press, 1988, p. 11.
107. Colonna, J. O., et al.: Infectious complications in liver transplantation. Arch. Surg., *123:*360, 1988.
108. Dummer, J. S., et al.: Early infections in kidney, heart and liver transplant recipients on cyclosporine. Transplantation, *36:*259, 1983.
109. Wajszczuk, C. P., et al.: Fungal infections in liver transplant recipients. Transplantation, *40:*347, 1985.
110. Wiesner, R. H., et al.: Selective bowel decontamination to decrease gram-negative aerobic bacterial and candida colonization and prevent infection after orthotopic liver transplantation. Transplantation, *45:*570, 1988.
111. Gorensek, M. J., et al.: Selective bowel decontamination (SBD) with quinoline antimicrobials and mycostatin reduces gram negative and fungal infections in orthotopic liver transplantation recipients. (Submitted.)
112. Gorensek, M. J., et al.: A multivariant analysis of risk factors for CMV infection following liver transplantation. Gastroenterology, *98:*1326, 1990.
113. Rakela, J., et al.: Incidence of cytomegalovirus infection and its relationship to donor-recipient serologic status in liver transplantation. Transplantation Proceedings, *19:*2399, 1987.
114. Bozzette, S. A., et al.: A controlled trial of early adjunctive treatment with corticosteroids for pneumocystis carinii pneumonia in the acquired immunodeficiency syndrome. N. Engl. J. Med., *322:*1451, 1990.
115. Millis, J. M., et al.: Preservation of renal function using OKT3 in liver transplant patients. Transplantation Proceedings, *21:*3551, 1989.
116. Adams, D. H., et al.: Neurologic complications following liver transplantation. Lancet, *1:*949, 1987.
117. De Groen, P. C., et al.: Central nervous system toxicity after liver transplantation. The role of cyclosporine and cholesterol. N. Engl. J. Med., *371:*861, 1987.

118. Martin, M. A., et al.: Nosocomial aseptic meningitis associated with administration of OKT3. JAMA, 259:2002, 1988.
119. Starzl, T. E., et al.: Acute neurologic complications after liver transplantation with particular reference to intraoperative air embolus. Ann. Surg., 87:236, 1978.
120. Vogt, D. P., et al.: Neurologic complications of liver transplantation. Transplantation, 45:1057, 1988.
121. Wilkinson, A. H., et al.: Increased frequency of post transplant lymphomas in patients treated with cyclosporine azathioprine and prednisone. Transplantation, 47:293, 1989.
122. Penn, I.: Lymphomas complicating organ transplantation. Transplantation Proceedings, 15:2790, 1983.
123. Hanto, D. W., et al.: Epstein Barr virus induced B cell lymphoma after renal transplantation. N. Engl. J. Med., 306:913, 1982.
124. Ho, M., et al.: The frequency of Epstein-Barr virus infection and associated lymphoproliferative syndrome after transplantation and its manifestation in children. Transplantation, 45:719, 1988.
125. McNally, P. G., et al.: Effect of nifedipine on renal hemodynamics in an animal model of cyclosporine. A nephrotoxicity. Clin. Sci., 79:259, 1990.
126. Starzl, T. E., et al.: Immunosuppression and other nonsurgical factors in the improved results of liver transplantation. Semin. Liver Dis., 5:334, 1985.
127. Benenson, E.: National survival rates for organ transplantation. UNOS Update, 7:2, 1991.
128. Gordon, R. D., and Starzl, T. E.: Long term survival after liver transplantation. Transplantation and Immunology Ltr., 4:2, 1988.
129. Transplantation of the Liver Health Technology Assessment Report. National Center for Health Services Research and Health Care Technology Assessment. 1983; 16.
130. Iwatsuki, S., et al.: Experience in 100 liver transplants under cyclosporine-steroid therapy; a survival report. Transplantation Proceedings, 20:498, 1988.
131. Iwatsuki, S., et al.: Role of liver transplantation in cancer therapy. Ann. Surg., 202:401, 1985.
132. Ringe, B., et al.: The role of liver transplantation in hepatobiliary malignancy. A retrospective analysis of 95 patients with particular regard to tumor stage and recurrence. Ann. Surg., 209:88, 1989.
133. Klintmalm, G., et al.: Neoadjuvant chemotherapy and orthotopic liver transplantation for hepatocellular carcinoma. Transplantation, 48:344, 1989.
134. Shaw, B. W., et al.: Hepatic retransplantation. Transplantation Proceedings, 17:264, 1985.
135. Gordon, R. D.: Clinical efficacy of human orthotopic liver transplantation: experience with 1000 cases treated with cyclosporine and prednisone with special emphasis on results of patients over 18 years of age (unpublished report).
136. Neuberger, J., et al.: Recurrence of primary biliary cirrhosis after liver transplantation. N. Engl. J. Med., 306:1, 1982.
137. Starzl, T. E., et al.: The quality of life after liver transplantation. Transplantation Proceedings, 11:252, 1979.

Section Eight

THE ENDOCRINE SYSTEM

Chapter 56

THE DIABETIC PATIENT

BYRON J. HOOGWERF

Several problems are encountered in the management of diabetes mellitus which may predispose admission to an ICU. These include:

- Diabetic ketoacidosis
- Hyperosmolar, nonketotic states
- Management of the diabetic patient who needs surgery
- Treatment of profound hypoglycemia

Diabetes mellitus is characterized by hyperglycemia. There are a number of different types of diabetes, however.[1] Type I or insulin-dependent diabetes mellitus (IDDM; formerly called juvenile-onset diabetes) is characterized by insulinopenia, and insulin is necessary for survival. The overall prevalence in the United States and most Northern European countries is about 0.2 to 0.4%. Type II diabetes mellitus is characterized by insulin resistance as the pathophysiologic mechanism for hyperglycemia. This type which is noninsulin-dependent diabetes mellitus (NIDDM; formerly called adult-onset diabetes) has an overall incidence of about 6.6% between the ages of 20 and 74.[2] About one half of all such patients do not know that they have the disease. Many such patients require insulin administration for adequate glycemia control, but they do not need insulin under most circumstances for survival. These are the two types of diabetes addressed particularly in this chapter. The other major types of diabetes include gestational diabetes and secondary forms of diabetes which occur as a result of pancreatitis, pancreatectomy, or administration of certain agents toxic to the beta cell. Some of the problems considered in this chapter may be applicable to these latter two groups of diabetic patients.

Diabetic ketoacidosis (DKA) occurs almost exclusively in type I diabetic subjects (because absolute or relative insulinopenia is a requisite condition for ketosis), whereas the hyperglycemic, hyperosmolar nonketotic states occur almost exclusively in type II diabetes.[3-6] Although these two conditions have certain similar predisposing risk factors and similarities in their management, they occur in fundamentally different patient populations. Furthermore, the fluid management may be quite different at the outset and the mortality is much higher in hyperglycemic, hyperosmolar nonketotic coma (HHNKC), probably because of the underlying problems in the patient population at risk. Therefore, DKA and HHNKC should be considered separate entities.

Most diabetic patients undergoing surgery are not hospitalized in an ICU situation. Both type I and type II diabetic subjects may have, however, an underlying urgent surgical problem necessitating ICU management and, therefore, require aggressive preoperative management. Similarly, most diabetic patients with hypoglycemia are treated on an outpatient basis. There are two high risk groups which may be admitted to an ICU, however. First, diabetic patients who have hypoglycemia as a result of administration of long-acting sulfonylureas may need a few days of ICU management. (In fact, occasional cases of drug substitution of sulfonylurea agents for other drugs in nondiabetic subjects may result in ICU admissions.) Second, occasionally patients with hypoglycemia from very high doses of insulin administration may require ICU-based treatment. These are most frequently type I diabetic subjects (or in some cases nondiabetic subjects) who have deliberately administered potentially lethal doses of insulin. Each of these entities will be discussed separately.

DIABETIC KETOACIDOSIS

Diabetic ketoacidosis (DKA) may be defined in several ways, but a reasonable working definition includes the following elements:

- Blood glucose > 250 mg/dl
- Serum pH < 7.3
- Serum bicarbonate < 15 mg/dl
- Ketonemia and serum ketones present at 1:2 dilution

DKA is characterized by three major interrelated metabolic abnormalities:[7-11] hyperglycemia, accumulation of ketones (organic acids), and dehydration. The initial step in the evolution of ketoacidosis is hyperglycemia. This is always the result of relative or absolute underinsulinization and consequently the failure to deliver glucose to the cells. Second, this relative insulinopenia also results in ketone formation; such ketone formation is regulated by the relative concentrations of glucagon and insulin and their effect on malonyl Co-A.[12-14] The accumulation of ketones in the form of acetoacetate and betahydroxybutyrate results in a reduction in pH or acidosis and an associated anion gap.[15,16] Finally, hyperglycemia usually results in glycosuria with attendant obligate free water loss, and the net result is usually dehydration. This combination of events is usually accompanied by a net loss of potassium and phosphate. Hyperkalemia as the result of intercellular to extracellular cationic shifts frequently characterizes DKA, however.[17]

Not all patients with DKA require admission to an ICU. Very mild cases may be treated on an outpatient basis. Most patients are admitted to the hospital with the severity of the DKA and the type and number of associated problems determining the need for ICU management. Prior risk factor assessment and initial therapy may help reduce the need for transfer to the ICU in some cases.

Pre-ICU Management (See Table 56–1)

Risk Factors

Risk factors associated with the development of diabetic ketoacidosis and severity of presentation most commonly include combinations of the following:

- Underinsulinization
- Associated illness including infections, cardiac events, or surgical intervention
- Administration of medications that may elevate blood glucose
- Dehydration

There is always a relative underinsulinization. Frequently, this is a result of a reduction in insulin administration. As the result of viral illness or feeling symptomatic with nausea from early diabetic ketoacidosis, many patients withhold insulin. They make the false assumption they did not need insulin because they were unable to eat or have reduced food intake. This underinsulinization may, in fact, accelerate the progression to DKA. Other events that constitute "stress" may play a role in increasing glucose production as a result of counterregulatory hormones including glucagon, epinephrine, growth hormone, and cortisol. These "stress events" include such things as infection, myocardial infarction, bowel infarction, or surgery. Administration of medications which may increase blood glucose levels such as glucocorticoids may also be an inciting factor in the development of DKA. Both endogenous glucocorticoid production and exogenous administration of glucocorticoids increase glucagon production and effectively change the internal milieu into a ketotic mode. In general, hyperglycemia would not supervene in the face of adequate hydration. As soon as plasma glucose concentrations exceed the renal threshold, the body can eliminate it providing there is sufficient free water. The overall "illness" generally reduces free water intake, however, and marked hyperglycemia occurs.

The four key factors in the pre-ICU management of diabetic ketoacidosis are:

- Assessment of underlying causes and factors associated with increased mortality and morbidity
- Assessment of the level of hydration
- Assessment of the overall degree of dysmetabolism (hyperglycemia, level of acidosis, degree of hyperkalemia)
- Assessment of associated risk factors that may affect the management or outcome (e.g., impaired renal function or impaired cardiac function, both of which may affect fluid and electrolyte administration)

Assessment of Causes

Assessment of etiologies which predispose to diabetic ketoacidosis begins with a good history. In known diabetic patients, evaluation for "missed" insulin doses or reduction in insulin intake is most common. Assessment of clues to underlying infections including viral infections, urinary tract infections, pneumonia, or other more subtle forms such as periodontal abscesses, perinephric abscesses or occult osteomyelitis need to be specifically elicited. Johnson and colleagues, in a community-based study, found infections were the most common predisposing cause for DKA.[18] Furthermore, infections may present without fever, or even with hypothermia, presumably because of decreased substrate availability for thermogenesis.[19] A history of "missed" menses suggesting pregnancy, abdominal pain suggesting a possible appendicitis or bowel infarct, or exercise-induced chest discomfort suggesting coronary heart disease should also be sought. The last is particularly important with long-standing diabetes and the fact that silent myocardial ischemia may be more common in diabetes should not be forgotten. In fact, myocardial infarctions are the most common cause of death within 48 hours of a diagnosis of DKA.[18] The use of medications that may have an adverse effect on glucose control include such things as decongestants, glucocorticoids and, less commonly, antiarthritic agents. Each of these variables (with the exception of reduced insulin dose) may be associated with the development of DKA in patients not previously known to have diabetes. Johnson and colleagues reported that 23% of their patients had DKA as the initial presentation of diabetes mellitus.[18] Older patients may also be more likely to have DKA as a presenting condition.[20] There are other features that may predict overall mortality in patients with DKA. These include increasing age, degree of blood glucose elevation, osmolality, and blood urea nitrogen.[21-23] The change from high dose insulin administration to the current widespread use of "low dose" insulin therapy did not affect mortality.[24]

Table 56–1. Pre-ICU Management of Diabetic Ketoacidosis

Risk factor assessment
   History of underinsulinization
   Infection
   Myocardial infarction
   Pregnancy
Baseline clinical and laboratory determinations
   Vital signs, cardiac status
   Glucose, electrolytes, pH, renal function, ketones
   Level of dehydration (10% of total volume is typical)
Initial treatment
   Fluids—0.9% saline; or D5W/0.45% saline if plasma glucose <250 mg/dl (replace 25% of total fluid needs in first 2 to 3 hours)
   Insulin administration—0.1U/kg/hr
   Possible correction of other metabolic abnormalities
      bicarbonate
      potassium
      phosphorus

Assessment of Hydration

Assessment of level of hydration again begins with historical evidence of increased thirst and urine output. Comparison of body weight with previously known body weight may be helpful. Both resting tachycardia and orthostatic blood pressure drops may be confirmatory. In patients with long-standing diabetes mellitus, these both may occur, however, as a result of autonomic neuropathy. Therefore, in such patients they may be less useful clinical parameters than in someone without autonomic neuropathy. The level of hyperglycemia is an indirect measure of dehydration as previously noted. Blood urea nitrogen gives some measure of prerenal azotemia. Patients with long-standing diabetes may have elevations of BUN and creatinine as a result of diabetic nephropathy with early renal failure. Furthermore, creatinine determinations done by the alkaline picrate (Jaffe) method may be falsely elevated because of cross-reactivity with acetoacetate.[25,26] Thus, there are no absolute guidelines that will clearly define the exact volume loss in the acute setting.

Assessment of Metabolic Status

Assessment of the associated dysmetabolism besides hyperglycemia and level of hydration needs to take into account the degree of acidosis. There is not a consistent relationship between the amount of hyperglycemia and the degree of acidosis.[27] Usually, arterial blood gas pH determinations can be obtained most rapidly. Serum bicarbonate determinations are also a good reflection of the degree of diabetic acidosis especially for values between 5 and 25 mEq/L which correlate with pH levels between 7.1 and 7.4. The degree of acidosis is only crudely determined by urine ketones as these are directly related to total urine output. Serum ketone determinations done by dilution give a reflection of the total amount of organic acids. Low levels of ketones can be best determined by direction determinations of betahydroxybutyrate, which is formed first. Acetoacetate is measured by nitroprusside reactions.[15,28] In most cases these differences do not have a significant impact on the overall management. Finally, measurements of serum potassium are necessary at baseline. "Normal" serum potassium levels in the face of marked acidosis actually represent a relative hypokalemia since potassium is driven out of cells as hydrogen is taken into the cells and insulin therapy also results in lower intracellular potassium levels. Timely determinations of potassium are important because of associated risk for cardiac arrhythmias or respiratory arrest with abnormal values.[29-31]

Assessment of Other Risk Factors

Assessment of other risk factors can frequently be done by history. As noted previously, these may include infectious causes for which treatment may need to be initiated, consideration of possible diseases requiring surgical intervention, e.g., appendectomy, bowel infarct or complications of diabetes which may affect fluid and electrolyte management. The two most common such complications include impaired renal function in which there may be difficulty handling volume and/or potassium or evidence of impaired cardiac function in which there is increased risk for volume overload or arrhythmias as a result of metabolic abnormalities including acidosis and hyper- and hypokalemia. A baseline electrocardiogram and continuous cardiac monitoring as dictated by the clinical circumstances should be undertaken. As noted above, myocardial infarction and impaired renal function are both predictors of mortality.

Initial Treatment

Initial treatment of DKA should focus on three key features: (1) rehydration; (2) insulin administration; and (3) correction of other metabolic abnormalities. These are listed in the relative order of importance for initiating treatment in most patients. Whereas underlying contributing problems, such as infections, may need to be treated as well, usually this can be initiated after rehydration and insulinization have been started.

In general, the assumption can be made that most patients who come in with DKA have about a 10% volume deficit. The exact extent of volume depletion may be difficult to assess, but several guidelines including tachycardia, orthostatic blood pressure drops, elevated BUN, and level of hyperglycemia are all crude but readily available as guides. The fact that many patients with long-standing diabetes mellitus may have autonomic neuropathy (resulting in resting tachycardia and orthostatic blood pressure changes) and renal dysfunction makes the evaluation of dehydration somewhat more difficult.

Initial fluid replacement is usually undertaken with 0.9% saline with the intent of replacing half the volume deficit in the first 8 hours and approximately 25% of the total estimated replacement in the first 2 to 3 hours. Adequate hydration may have a benefit to reduce hyperglycemia by facilitating clearance of glucose via the kidney. Rehydration is the most effective way to lower the glucose initially. For patients with only modest elevations of glucose, the initial solution may be D5W/0.45% saline (see discussion later in this chapter). With less dehydration, slower rates of infusion of 0.9% saline may be associated with more rapid correction of the acidosis.[32] Less commonly, colloid is recommended as a replacement fluid.[33] Improvement in vital signs and the rate of fall of glucose and BUN may be used to monitor hydration status. Finally, slower rates of fluid administration may be advisable in younger patients to reduce the risks of cerebral edema (see discussion later in this chapter).

Insulin therapy is necessary to reverse gluconeogenesis and lipolysis which are the sources of the organic acids. It is also necessary to correct the peripheral tissue caloric deficit. Therefore, adequate insulin administration will reverse the hyperglycemia by decreasing hepatic glucose production[34] and lipolytic (ketosis producing) state. Initial insulin doses can be targeted as a constant rate infusion of approximately 0.1 U/kg per hour given in saline.[34-40] Ease of administration is achieved if the concentration is 1 U/ml of 0.9% saline. Small amounts of the solution may be run through the tubing to ensure that any tubing related binding of insulin is "saturated." Intravenous boluses of insulin have been recommended in the past, however, there appears to be little advantage to such administration and, in fact, it may entail some risk especially in patients in whom there is acute reduction in serum potassium levels. In patients in whom IV access is difficult or not readily available, insulin administration may be initiated in comparable doses given intramuscularly every hour (i.e., 0.1 U/kg). Adjustment of insulin dosages is made on the basis of subsequent blood glucose response (see discussion later in this chapter).

Additional metabolic abnormalities need to be considered in the pre-ICU state. These include whether to administer bicarbonate, evaluation of the need for potassium replacement, and the possible role of hypophosphatemia. The first consideration is whether to administer intravenous bicarbonate. Several studies have now demonstrated no particular advantage of acute bicarbonate administration as long as the serum pH is greater or equal to 7.1.[40,41] Few studies have dared to limit bicarbonate administration at lower pH levels because of the increased risk for cardiac dysfunction and arrhythmias. Intravenous bolus bicarbonate administration as well as adding bicarbonate to the initial infused solutions is recommended for individuals with low pH values (i.e., pH < 7.1).

The next major consideration is administration of potassium. Because the combination of glucose and insulin results in a potassium influx into cells, especially as acidosis is corrected, consideration for immediate administration of potassium should be given when the serum potassium concentration is midrange of normal or below (e.g., <4.0 mEq/L). Only rarely is there profound hypokalemia, but risk of respiratory arrest highlights the need for immediate replacement under this circumstance.[31] In hyperkalemic patients, potassium does not need to be administered until there is a drop of serum values to normal. Potassium should be administered cautiously until there is evidence of urine output and until preliminary assessment of renal function (BUN/creatine) has been obtained. Administration of phosphate is still controversial. In spite of clear evidence of hypophosphatemia in most patients with DKA, administration of phosphate does not seem to have any significant effect on the rate at which the dysmetabolic state improves whether measured by normalization of glucose, clearing of ketones, or improvement in acidotic state.[40,42] With marked hypophosphatemia either sodium phosphate or potassium phosphate may be added to the intravenous solutions. If sodium phosphate is used, then one or two 45-mEq vials may be added to 0.45% saline to make a solution approximately equivalent to 0.71% (1 vial) or 0.97% (2 vials) saline. Potassium phosphate may be given when there is a need for potassium replacement.

In all patients with DKA, a flow sheet which monitors the key variables should be initiated prior to admission to the ICU. This flow sheet (see Fig. 56-1) should include vital signs, type and quantity of fluid administered, urine output, and serial determinations of blood sugar, potassium, and measurement of ketones as well as some sequential determination of acid/base status (pH or serum bicarbonate). Flow sheets should also include some assessment of level of consciousness and neurologic status.

Plasma glucose levels should fall by about 1 to 2 mg/dl per minute or 60 to 120 mg/dl per hour. Plasma ketone bodies should fall by about 1 mm/hr initially with rehydration, but it may take 12 to 24 hours for them to clear completely. Most patients will require glucose-containing solutions within the first 4 to 8 hours and should be out of ketoacidosis in about 12 to 18 hours.

ICU Management (Table 56-2)

Patients with mild ketoacidosis may be treated on an outpatient basis (if adequate facilities and skilled personnel are available), or on the regular nursing floor. Patients with more severe DKA as defined by profound dehydration, altered level of consciousness, significant underlying disease (e.g., cardiac or renal infection, neuropathy) or significant metabolic abnormalities (e.g., hyperkalemia or marked acidosis) usually require ICU management. The ICU management of the patient with ketoacidosis includes the following key features:

- Clinical monitoring of the patient
- Monitoring of the fluid status (intake and output)
- Serial laboratory determinations of blood (plasma/serum) glucose, potassium, bicarbonate and ketones

Clinical status measures must first take into account the level of consciousness. This fact is especially true for patients who are comatose. Levels of consciousness should improve with correction of volume and acid/base status. Hypotension and tachycardia should also improve. As comatose patients become more alert, careful clinical evaluation looking for historical causes of the DKA as well as repeated physical examination looking for sources of infection should be undertaken. For example, abdominal pain indicating underlying infections such as appendicitis may become evident, or clinical evidence of pneumonia that was not obvious in the face of dehydration may become evident. Cerebral edema, a complication of DKA that may characterize the later stages of treatment, is seen more commonly in children with DKA. The first clinical sign of such cerebral edema is usually deterioration in the level of consciousness anytime during the course of treatment. Although computed tomography (CT) scan studies suggest cerebral edema may be present before treatment of DKA and occur to a limited extent in most patients with DKA, the mechanism for development is unknown.[43,44] Rate of fluid administration[45] and ionic/osmotic exchange may be important.[46] Decreased rates of fluid administration may ameliorate this problem in the early stages and preclude a comatose condition from cerebral edema.

Slower rates of fluid infusion may slow the rate at which glucose is excreted through the kidney and the rate at which ketones are cleared, but should not have a significant impact on overall outcome. There are no good comparative studies, however, on rates of fluid administration and their impact on the correction of DKA. Serial determinations of blood glucose, potassium, and bicarbonate, as well as serum or urine ketones, will help to determine the success of the therapy and the need for changes in the regimen. Blood glucose values should be checked hourly, and the other biochemical determinations (potassium, bi-

THE DIABETIC PATIENT

FLOW SHEET

DIABETES FLOW SHEET		NAME		HOSPITAL NO.	
DATE					
TIME					
Weight					
Pulse					
BP					
Temp					
LOC					
Intake					
Type IV fluid					
I.V. intake					
P.O. intake					
Running total					
Output					
Blood glucose					
Lab					
Fingerstick					
Na					
K					
Cl					
Bicarb					
BUN					
Creatinine					
Urine ketones					
pH					
Insulin dose					
Other measures					

Fig. 56–1. Example of a flow sheet for diabetic ketoacidosis. BP, Blood pressure; LOC, level of consciousness; U/O, urinary output; FSBS, fingerstick blood sugar, PG/PS, plasma glucose/serum glucose.

Table 56–2. ICU Management of Diabetic Ketoacidosis

Clinical monitoring
  Vital signs
  Intake and output
  Cardiac status
  Level of consciousness
Laboratory monitoring
  Serial glucose, potassium, bicarbonate (or pH), ketones
Treatment
  Fluids
    0.9% saline (replace 50% of total fluid needs in first 8 hours and 100% of total fluid needs in 24 hours)
    D5W/0.45% saline (when plasma glucose <250 mg/dl)
    Potassium, bicarbonate, phosphorus as needed
  Insulin
    Intravenous—adjust doses based on blood glucose
    Change to subcutaneous when
      Blood glucose stabilized
      Ketones have cleared
      Patient tolerating oral intake of nutrients
  Treatment of underlying causes (e.g., infection)

carbonate and ketones) every 2 to 4 hours as determined by the clinical circumstances. This degree of monitoring is usually necessary for at least the first 6 to 12 hours of treatment (and sometimes longer in more difficult cases). If blood glucose values do not continue to drop by 1 to 2 mg/dl per minute or 60 to 120 mg/dl per hour during the course of therapy, then adequacy of hydration needs to be evaluated and insulin infusion rates need to be increased. It is usually safe to double the insulin infusion rate if no significant change in blood glucose occurs over a 1- to 2-hour period. If glucose levels fall as the rates noted previously, the infusion rates for insulin may be decreased to maintenance rates of 1 to 2 U per hour until the ketosis is cleared. When blood sugar levels approach 250 to 300 mg/dl, then the intravenous infusion fluid should be changed to include 5% dextrose and 0.45% saline. Intravenous insulin should be maintained until ketosis has cleared at which time subcutaneous insulin can be initiated (see discussion later in this chapter). Use of 10% dextrose has been compared to 5% and was associated with a need for increased insulin and a correspondingly more rapid clearance of ketones, but no differences in rate of change of pH.[47] Therefore, more concentrated glucose solutions do not yet offer any clear advantage. Potassium infusion should be determined by levels of serum potassium. Both the reduction in blood glucose and increasing pH cause a reduction in serum potassium levels. Failure of the bicarbonate levels to increase usually indicates a need to look for some other cause of acidosis (e.g., from lactic acid or aspirin ingestion).

In uncomplicated cases of ketoacidosis, the switch to subcutaneous insulin can be made when the urine ketones have cleared. This usually occurs 12 to 24 hours after the start of therapy. Usually acid/base abnormalities will have corrected by this time and patients will be able to take oral fluids. The initial injection of subcutaneous insulin should be given at least 1 to 2 hours before discontinuing the insulin drip. In patients whose prior insulin doses are known, and whose oral intake has been reinitiated, the starting dose(s) of insulin may be based on these prehospitalization insulin requirements. For newly diagnosed diabetics or in patients in whom there is not prior information on insulin doses, the projected daily dose of subcutaneous insulin will likely be in the range of 0.5 U/kg per 24 hours. A starting dose of regular insulin targeted to control blood glucose in the next 4 hours would be about one sixth this dose. For example, a person weighing 60 kg will likely require about 30 U of insulin per day and a starting dose of 5 U would be appropriate. A simple rule of thumb is to start the first dose of subcutaneous regular insulin at about 0.1 U/kg. This will prevent the patient from becoming insulinopenic during the transition period from IV to subcutaneous insulin. Overlap of the IV and subcutaneous insulin is based on the fact that intravenous insulin has a half-life of about 10 minutes and the absorption of subcutaneous insulin will not be effective for at least an hour or two after injection depending on the type of insulin being administered. It is frequently easiest to make this transition in the morning and begin insulin administration with doses which approximate the preadmission insulin requirements. This assumes that the patient will be able to eat the usual number of calories. Dosages may be adjusted for anticipated lower caloric intake. Some intermediate or long-acting insulins should be incorporated into this regimen as well as regular insulin.

When the patient has no previous history of insulin use or it is evident that the previous insulin administration schedule represented underinsulinization sufficient to result in DKA, then some general guidelines for administration can be used to get patients on subcutaneous insulin regimens. Synthetic or semisynthetic human insulins are recommended for patients who have not previously received insulin. Most regimens include a combination of short-acting insulin (regular), and intermediate-acting insulins (NPH, lente) or longer-acting insulin (ultralente). All human insulins are relatively shorter acting than their animal counterparts and this is most evident with ultralente for which the human form has a duration of action which is closer to "intermediate"-acting than to the long-acting beef ultralente. Usually about one half to two thirds of the insulin will be given as intermediate-acting insulin and the remaining one third to one half as regular insulin. Furthermore, in many patients approximately two thirds is given in the morning and the remaining one third in the evening. The most common insulin administration schedules include combinations of NPH and regular in these approximate ratios. (The selection of NPH over lente is largely based on the observations that mixtures of regular human insulin with lente or ultralente human insulin result in marked changes in the insulin kinetics.) Therefore, a person weighing 60 kg will be expected to require about 30 U insulin per day. This patient could be started on a regimen of about 14 U NPH and 6 U regular insulin in the morning (two-thirds of 30 U = 20 U), and 6 U NPH and 4 U regular before the evening meal. (Many physicians and patients prefer to use even numbers since this is the usual division on insulin syringes.) Regular insulin may need to be added to "cover" markedly elevated glucoses (e.g., >200 mg/dl) in the early stages. When such insulin coverage is required, the dose should be incorporated into the

Table 56–3. Post-ICU Management of Diabetic Ketoacidosis

Review and treatment of precipitating causes of DKA
Adjustment of subcutaneous insulin administration
Diabetes education
    Insulin administration
    Self-glucose monitoring
    "Sick day" management of blood sugars

next day's insulin schedule. Conversely, if insulin reactions occur in the face of normal caloric intake, insulin dosages should be correspondingly reduced. Both physician and patient should recognize that refining this insulin schedule will take place after discharge.

In cases of ketoacidosis which are complicated by a need for surgical intervention, it is best to continue intravenous insulin and carbohydrate containing fluids throughout the proposed surgery. The stress of surgery may be associated with increased insulin requirements largely as the result of counterregulatory hormone responses to anesthesia and surgery. The transition to subcutaneous insulin is generally made in conjunction with the capability to take nutrients orally.

Post-ICU Management (Table 56–3)

Transfer from the ICU can be made when the patient's clinical status is stable. If ICU beds are at a premium and there is adequate nursing/physician observation available on regular nursing floors this should be done about the time that blood glucoses are under 250 mg/dl, ketone levels are diminishing and bicarbonate levels are over 20 mg/dl. Transition to subcutaneous insulin is made as outlined in the foregoing discussion.

Management in the intermediate post-ICU period should focus on a review of the precipitating causes for DKA and future management of diabetes. In known diabetic patients, special emphasis on the need to take insulin even with limited oral intake needs to be made to patients whose DKA came as the result of stopping insulin therapy in the face of nausea or vomiting. Review of "sick day" management of diabetes also should be provided for the patient. The transition to maintenance doses of insulin, review of diet, and activity can be initiated in the hospital. Attempts at rigorous blood sugar control are usually better carried out in the outpatient setting with the usual daily activities and dietary schedule in conjunction with home glucose monitoring. Obviously, in newly diagnosed diabetic patients, a full program of diabetes education is necessary.

HYPERGLYCEMIC HYPEROSMOLAR NONKETOTIC STATES/COMA (HHNKC)

Hyperglycemic, hyperosmolar nonketotic coma, like DKA does not have a rigid definition. The definition proposed by Kitabchi[40] and others is generally accepted to include the following:

- Plasma glucose > 500 mg/dl
- Serum osmolarity > 330 mOsm
- Absence of serum ketones by Acetest
- Arterial pH > 7.3
- Serum bicarbonate > 20 mEq/L
- Moderate to severe mental obtundation
- Negative urine ketones by Acetest

Whereas DKA usually occurs in type I diabetes mellitus, HHNKC occurs in type II diabetes mellitus. Many of the patients have not been previously diagnosed as diabetic patients, however. The overall morbidity is high because of associated illnesses and mortality rates in the range of 40% have been reported.

Pre-ICU Management (Table 56–4)

Risk Factors

The major metabolic abnormalities which predispose to hyperglycemic nonketotic states are similar to those which predispose to ketoacidosis including associated illness, relative underinsulinization and dehydration. Hyperglycemia occurs in diabetic patients as the result of too little medication or a stress event which increases the intrinsic insulin need. Similarly, nondiabetic patients (or more likely, patients with unrecognized diabetes mellitus or glucose intolerance) may become hyperglycemic in conjunction with a number of known predisposing factors. These factors include infection (especially with gram-negative organisms), dehydration, administration of diabetogenic drugs, and surgical procedures. Other reported risk factors include female sex, impaired renal function, and use of hyperalimentation.[48-54] Most cases of hyperosmolar coma occur in the elderly and most of the patients have underlying diabetes mellitus, frequently being treated with diet alone or diet and oral hypoglycemic agents. In many cases (36%), the diabetes had not been recognized before the hyperosmolar state occurred.[53]

As with DKA, dehydration is a characteristic feature of these hyperosmolar states. With adequate hydration, the hyperglycemia could be ameliorated by renal excretion of

Table 56–4. Pre-ICU Management of Hyperglycemic, Hyperosmolar Nonketotic Coma (HHNKC)

Risk factors
    Dehydration
    Inadequate administration of glucose regulating drugs (insulin, oral agents)
    Infection
    Use of diabetogenic drugs (e.g., glucocorticoids, thiazides)
    Surgery
    Use of parenteral nutrition
    Impaired renal function
    Female sex
Baseline clinical and laboratory determinations
    Vital signs
    Glucose, electrolytes, BUN, creatinine, osmolality, urinalysis
    Electrocardiogram
    Chest radiograph
Management
    Fluids
        0.45% saline, or
        0.9% saline (if patient is hypotensive or hyponatremic)
    Insulin—0.1 U/kg/hr IV

glucose. Ketosis does not occur presumably because low levels of insulin are sufficient to prevent significant lipolysis and, in turn, the formation of acetoacetate and beta hydroxybutyrate. Although HHNKC is much less common than DKA, it is associated with a very high mortality with reported rates in the range of 20 to 40%. Risk of mortality is increased with gram-negative infections, impaired renal function, and delayed initiation of treatment. Surgical procedures, especially cardiac, are associated with increased risk to develop HHNKC. This is associated with a high mortality (42%) especially with previously undiagnosed diabetes.[51]

A large number of people are actually at risk of developing HHNKC because more than 5% of the population between the ages of 20 and 74 years has diabetes mellitus.[2] Furthermore, the predisposing associated risk factors are also common in this group of people because the incidence of diabetes is more common with increasing age and such patients are more likely to develop infections, need surgery, take diabetogenic drugs such as glucocorticoids and thiazides, or have impaired renal function. In most cases, the hyperosmolar state develops insidiously over days to weeks outside of the hospital setting. Consequently, there is often little to be done by way of direct risk factor reduction prior to the development of the coma short of broad-based regular self-glucose monitoring.

Pre-ICU Evaluation and Treatment

Pre-ICU evaluation and treatment are frequently initiated in the emergency room. Key features of the pre-ICU assessment include clinical evaluation to look at evidence for dehydration and for underlying precipitating causes such as infections, drugs, coronary heart disease, and evidence for central nervous system insults (such as strokes), which may impair the thirst mechanism. Documentation of the degree of coma should be made at this time. Because elderly diabetic patients are at increased risk for coronary heart disease careful cardiac examination is warranted. Supporting laboratory determinations must include measures of the degree of dysmetabolism including plasma glucose, electrolytes, serum osmolality, and measures of renal function. This will also permit some measure of the degree of dehydration. In addition, urinalyses and chest radiographs are usually justified looking for specific sources of infection. A surface electrocardiogram should be obtained to help determine whether there is evidence for preexisting coronary heart disease or an acute myocardial infarction.

Initial therapy should focus on correcting the major metabolic problem, that of dehydration. Initial fluid therapy may be selected on the basis of the degree of dehydration. Initial fluid therapy may be selected on the basis of the degree of dehydration (especially if patient is hypotensive), serum sodium levels, and the serum osmolality. In most cases with hypernatremia and hyperosmolar states, a hypotonic (0.45%) saline solution should be started at rates up to 2 to 3 L over the first 2 to 3 hours. If there is severe dehydration with risk of marked hypotension, risk of acute renal failure[50] or poor cardiac perfusion, isotonic (0.9%) saline may be preferable as an initial solution. Volume replacement may be more critical than correcting the hyperosmolar state. In very severe cases, administration of colloid solutions has also been recommended. Dextrose infusions should be avoided early in the treatment period. In patients in whom the serum osmolality is less than 330 mOsm and in whom serum sodium levels may be low, initial fluid therapy may be started with 0.9% saline. Fluid administration rates may need to be lower in patients with evidence of impaired cardiac function. Because serum potassium levels are usually normal, and because most patients are total body potassium depleted, addition of potassium to the intravenous fluids is usually initiated early in the course of therapy. This must be initiated very cautiously if there is any evidence of impaired renal function. Insulin administration should be done at starting doses similar to those used for DKA beginning at a rate of about 0.1 U/kg body weight per hour. Overall insulin requirements are usually less than in patients with DKA.

ICU Management (Table 56–5)

Admission to the ICU is to minimize existing risks by continuous monitoring of therapeutic interventions. Key parameters to monitor in the early ICU phase include status of hydration, plasma glucose levels, and serum potassium. Hydration can be followed clinically with measurements of intake and output, pulse and blood pressure responses, as well as periodic cardiopulmonary examinations to help prevent volume overload. Because hydration itself will help to lower blood glucose levels, the expected rate of decline of glucose initially should be in the range of 1 to 2 mg/dl per minute of therapy or in the range of 100 mg/dl per hour. Failure to achieve this rate of glucose decline in the face of adequate rehydration necessitates reevaluating volume status and increasing the insulin infusion. Insulin infusion can be doubled hourly until there is evidence of correction of the hyperglycemia as evidenced by appropriate decline in serum/plasma glucose levels. It is rare that such high doses of insulin are necessary to achieve continued improvement in the plasma glucose levels. Hyperglycemia and type II diabetes mellitus are both characterized, however, by insulin resistance.

In addition to key parameters (i.e., glucose, electrolytes, and osmolality), the ICU staff need to serially monitor men-

Table 56–5. ICU Management of Hyperglycemic, Hyperosmolar, Nonketotic Coma

Clinical monitoring
   Vital signs
   Intake and output
   Mental status
   Cardiac status
Laboratory monitoring
   Serial glucose, electrolytes, osmolality
Treatment
   Fluids
      0.9% or 0.45% saline (see above)
      0.45% saline/D5W (when plasma glucose <250 mg/dl)
   Insulin
      Intravenous—adjust doses based on plasma glucose
      Change to subcutaneous when plasma glucose is stabilized
   Treatment of underlying causes (e.g., antibiotics for infections)

tal status, cardiac status, and be attentive to anything that suggests underlying infection. Any adverse change needs to be treated aggressively to reduce the mortality and morbidity associated with the hyperosmolar state.

As the hyperglycemia improves, dextrose should be added to the intravenous infusion along with the insulin. Nondiabetic patients, as well as some diabetic patients may maintain near normoglycemia without insulin infusion after correction of the acute hyperosmolar state and correcting any underlying predisposing conditions.

The late ICU phase involves transition from intravenous fluid administration to oral intake. This is obviously affected by factors such as whether underlying problems necessitated mechanical ventilation, NPO status in anticipation of surgery, or full recovery of swallowing capability in the face of permanent CNS deficits. In diabetic patients or some patients on drugs such as glucocorticoids, there may be a need to make this transition by converting them over to subcutaneous insulin administration. Initially, this may be done only by using "coverage" schedules of regular insulin given subcutaneously until some measure of insulin requirements are determined. There is much variation in insulin requirements for such a coverage schedule, but most are based on insulin requirements in the range of 0.5 to 1 U/kg per 24 hours. For patients who are not eating (and there is constant IV nutrient administration), "coverage" schedules are usually based on blood sugars obtained every 4 hours. A typical schedule would have the following doses of regular insulin based on blood sugar determinations made every 4 hours:

Blood Sugar (mg/dl)	Insulin Dose (units)
<80	0
81–150	4
151–200	6
201–250	8
251–300	10
301–350	12
>350	notify physician

Such coverage schedules always administer insulin "too late" because a high glucose indicates underinsulinization in the preceding period. Therefore, a practice of administering some intermediate-acting insulin along with this schedule helps to prevent profound hyperglycemia and facilitates the transition to dosages compatible with a home insulin regimen. Insulin requirements, including the "coverage" schedules will vary widely because of varying degrees of insulin resistance that characterize type II diabetes mellitus and the predisposing factors to HHNKC. In fact, some diabetic patients may be able to be adequately controlled on oral glucose lowering agents or diet alone after initial insulin treatment.

When coma and the underlying metabolic and precipitating medical problems have stabilized, the patient may be transferred from the ICU to a regular nursing floor. Unless serious underlying problems that necessitate surgical therapy have been identified, the patient may go directly to the operating room from the ICU and postopera-

Table 56–6. Post-ICU Management of Hyperglycemic, Hyperosmolar, Nonketotic Coma

Diabetic education
    Full instruction for newly diagnosed diabetes mellitus
    Glucose monitoring instructions
    Review of precipitating causes
    Initiation of glucose-lowering agents as appropriate
Treatment of precipitating causes (e.g., infection, myocardial infarction, medication regimen)

tive management may require a return to the ICU. (See the discussion later in this chapter.)

Post-ICU Management (Table 56–6)

The post-ICU period must include the final stages of stabilization of the metabolic problems which precipitated the admission, as well as a review of the precipitating risk factors with an eye to preventing recurrence. Some risk factors for recurrence such as impaired renal function may not always be amenable to change. During this phase, decisions regarding the need for long-term management of the diabetes need to be made. These include decisions about the need for insulin or oral agent therapy, and corresponding appropriate instruction prior to discharge. Many times the change from insulin to oral agent therapy will be made after discharge from the hospital. Underlying risk factors such as infections will be followed and treated as appropriate. Any patient who has the capability to learn self-glucose monitoring (using capillary blood obtained by fingerstick) should be taught to do so. Regular blood glucose determinations should be obtained after discharge. Insulin requiring patients may require frequent determinations (e.g., up to four times a day), whereas patients on diet only may require only one or two tests per week. Such monitoring, when performed accurately, will pick up the insidious hyperglycemia that precedes the hyperosmolar state. Patients may then be in a position to contact their physician while problems are not life-threatening and can be managed on an outpatient basis.

SURGICAL HYPERGLYCEMIC PATIENT

Pre-ICU Management (Table 56-7)

In the surgical patient, the pre-ICU phase constitutes the preoperative, intraoperative and immediate postoperative

Table 56–7. Pre-ICU Management of the Surgical Patient with Diabetes Mellitus (preoperative, intraoperative, and immediate postoperative period)

Insulin administration
    Subcutaneous insulin: half or two-thirds or usual insulin doses of intermediate acting insulin preoperatively
    Intravenous insulin
        Chronic poor glycemic control
        Blood glucose >300 mg/dl
Anticipation of increased insulin needs
    Administration of glucocorticoids, adrenergic agents
    Cardiac surgery with bypass and hypothermia (see text)
    Total parenteral nutrition

(postanesthesia recovery area) period. Presurgical management of diabetes includes attempts to control blood glucose as rigorously as the preoperative period permits. Furthermore, anticipating the effects of surgery on blood glucose levels will help to determine insulin needs. Various approaches to insulin administration in the preoperative state are used. For insulin-requiring diabetic patients, administration of insulin is individualized to the proposed procedure and patient insulin needs.[54-57] Typically, in patients with stable glycemic control, one half to two thirds of usual insulin doses may be given preoperatively as intermediate-acting (NPH, lente) or longer-acting (ultralente) insulin for many procedures. In some cases, glucose levels may be regulated by constant insulin infusions with adjustments based on intraoperative glucose determinations. Intravenous insulin may be more advisable whenever there is significant risk of marked hyperglycemia such as in patients with chronically poor outpatient glycemic control or in whom glucoses obtained preoperatively are markedly elevated (e.g., >300 mg/dl). The clinician should be mindful that intravenous insulin is associated not only with lower levels of glucose, but also with an increased risk for hypoglycemia. Synthetic or semisynthetic human insulins are preferred in any patient who will be newly started on insulin in conjunction with the surgery or in whom insulin use is intermittent (e.g., used with previous surgery). Intraoperative intravenous solutions should contain dextrose and usually a 5% solution is satisfactory, regardless of which method of insulin administration is selected.

Some patients who need urgent surgery are in DKA. DKA should be largely corrected before taking such patients to the operating room using approaches described earlier. The acidemia usually takes longer to correct than hyperglycemia.[58] If patients are taken to the operating room before all metabolic parameters have corrected or stabilized, the use of fluids and IV insulin is essentially the same as that for ICU management of DKA. The possibility of lactic acidosis must also be considered and confirmed in many such patients especially those with major soft tissue injury, hypoxia, surgical problems in the abdomen, or associated sepsis.

The severity of preoperative diabetes mellitus is somewhat determinant of risk factors for postoperative hyperglycemia. **First,** type I diabetic patients and insulin-requiring type II diabetic patients are more likely to have marked hyperglycemia postoperatively. **Second,** anesthesia and surgery are associated with release of counterregulatory hormones including epinephrine growth hormone and glucocorticoids which increase glucose levels.[59-63] In addition, some surgical procedures such as coronary artery bypass procedures are associated with marked hyperglycemia even in nondiabetic persons, perhaps because pump oxygenator membranes may bind insulin, including endogenously secreted insulin.[64] **Third,** some patients undergoing surgery need high dose glucocorticoid administration which increases the risk for hyperglycemia. This group includes patients on chronic glucocorticoid therapy preoperatively for adrenal disease, asthma, or collagen vascular disease as well as those for whom glucocorticoids are therapy for a problem associated with the need for surgery, e.g. dexamethasone administration for brain tumors or methylprednisolone (Solu-medrol) administration in organ transplant recipients.

The immediate pre-ICU period is that of the postanesthesia recovery area. Because the management here is similar to that in the ICU, these phases are discussed together.

ICU Management (Table 56–8)

When the patient arrives in the ICU, management of blood glucose must take into account several variables that may affect therapy (Table 56-9):

- The amount and type of insulin administered preoperatively;
- The amount and type of insulin administered intraoperatively;
- The quantity and type of intravenous solutions containing calories;
- Administration of any drugs that may have an effect on blood glucose, including glucocorticoids and adrenergic agents;
- The degree of blood pressure instability or hypothermia;
- Nature and type of projected nutrient intake while in the ICU, especially whether total parenteral nutrition will be incorporated into the patient's schedule;[65]
- The blood/plasma glucose at the time of arrival
- Presence of infection (peritonitis, soft tissue infections, etc.)

When these variables have been assessed, decisions about the nature of insulin administration can be made. Intravenous insulin administration is usually necessary

Table 56–8. ICU Management of the Surgical Patient with Diabetes Mellitus (postoperative period)

Insulin administration
  Intravenous insulin
    Marked hyperglycemia (e.g., >300 mg/dl)
    Unstable blood pressure; use of pressor agents
    Hypothermia
    Total parenteral nutrition
  Subcutaneous insulin
    Stable patients on oral intake, enteral feeding, or parenteral feeding
    Insulin regimen tailored to nutrient intake (see text)

Table 56–9. Variables to Consider in the Postsurgical, ICU Management of Diabetic Patients

Amount and type of insulin administered preoperatively
Amount and type of insulin administered intraoperatively
Quantity and type of intravenous solutions containing calories
Administration of any drugs that may affect blood glucose (e.g., glucocorticoids, adrenergic agents)
Evidence of blood pressure instability or hypothermia (hypotension and hypothermia may affect the absorption of insulin administered subcutaneously)
Nature and type of projected nutrient intake
Blood/plasma glucose level on arrival in the ICU
Presence of infection

under circumstances in which the initial blood glucose is greater than 300 mg/dl:

- When large amounts of counterregulatory drugs have been administered (glucocorticoids, pressor agents)
- When there is hypotension or hypothermia which may result in erratic absorption of subcutaneously administered insulin
- When the patient needs total parenteral nutrition to meet caloric needs

Management of the moderate hyperglycemic state (e.g., blood glucose concentrations of 150 to 300 mg/dl), in the ICU following surgery is essentially the same as the intermediate management of glucose levels in patients with DKA or hyperosmolar states (see earlier discussion). The type of intravenous fluids and the transition to subcutaneous insulin require a similar approach.

Management of total parenteral nutrition (TPN) or total enteral nutrition (TEN) in the ICU requires special consideration (Table 56–10). TPN solutions usually contain quantities of dextrose, frequently final concentrations are in the range of 10 to 35%, amino acids, and soluble lipids.[59] The large number of calories from carbohydrate and protein require adequate insulin to facilitate insulin-mediated glucose disposal. Two major considerations are frequently ignored. First, the total number of calories infused and the body's capability to dispose of the total nutrient load must be considered when looking at blood glucose levels. Second, approximately 30 to 50% of the total administered calories are used by the body via noninsulin mediated mechanisms. The central nervous system, formed blood components (red blood cells, white cells, platelets), and liver use glucose through such noninsulin mediated mechanisms. Therefore, there is a nonlinear relationship between total calories administered and total insulin requirements.

When patients become markedly hyperglycemic in the ICU while on TPN (especially if they are getting insulin doses which should be adequate), the first consideration is whether the total caloric intake provided by the TPN exceeds the body's capability to dispose of the nutrients. In general, caloric intakes above 50 kcal/kg body weight per 24 hours are approaching the limits of nutrient disposal. If the caloric infusion rates (including the calories from all sources including lipids and other IV solutions) approach or exceed this rate, the treatment of choice is to reduce caloric intake to a more modest level. Usually 35 to 40 kcal/kg per 24 hours will improve blood glucose levels. When patients are normoglycemic (e.g., blood glucoses of 80 to 120 mg/dl) or near normoglycemic (e.g., blood glucose up to 150 mg/dl) on TPN with a specific quantity of insulin in the TPN solution, any change in the rate of TPN administration must be accompanied by appropriate adjustments of the insulin in the solution must also be reduced. This occurs because the proportion of calories used by the central nervous system, bone marrow, and liver remains reasonably constant and this utilization is via a noninsulin mediated mechanism. For example, if a patient receiving 3000 kcal per day via TPN has a corresponding insulin dose of 40 units of IV insulin and we assume that about 2000 kcal of nutrients are handled via insulin-mediated mechanisms, then the remaining 1000 kcal require no insulin for nutrient disposal. If we assume for simplicity that there is no effect of endogenously secreted insulin then about 10 units of insulin are necessary for each 500 kcal of nutrient disposal mediated by insulin. If the caloric load is cut to 2500 kcal, the total number of calories requiring insulin for tissue disposal will be 1500 kcal and the dose of insulin in that solution should be cut to 30 U. Such formulas are too simplistic, but the concept generally helps to estimate insulin needs. Finally, when patients on TPN become hypoglycemic, there is frequently a tendency to discontinue the TPN fluid (which contains insulin) and administer 10% dextrose. It is much easier simply to increase the TPN infusion rate. Small increases will frequently raise blood glucoses into the normoglycemic range.

Although some patients can be maintained on subcutaneous insulin while on TPN, this is usually only possible in stable patients who need long-term TPN therapy. In most patients, the transition to subcutaneous insulin is made as they are changed from TPN to oral nutrient intake.

Insulin administration during enteral feeding needs to take three main factors into account. The **first** consideration is the total number of calories being administered. The **second** consideration is whether the calories are administered continuously or as bolus feedings. A **third** consideration is whether there are likely to be unexpected interruptions in the administration of nutrients because of

Table 56–10. Blood Glucose Management During the Use of Total Parenteral Nutrition (TPN) and Total Enteral Nutrition (TEN) in Diabetic Patients

Total parenteral nutrition
  Nutrients
    Dextrose, amino acids, lipids
    Total calories; 30–40 kcal/kg/24 hr
    Nutrient disposal
      50–70% via insulin-mediated mechanisms
      30–50% via noninsulin-mediated mechanisms
  Insulin
    Continuous IV in TPN or as separate drip
    Target blood glucose: 80–150 mg/dl
  Treatment of hyperglycemia
    Decrease TPN rate (if total calories exceed glucose disposal rate of 50 kcal/kg/24 h)
    Increase insulin
  Treatment of hypoglycemia
    Increase TPN rate
    Decrease insulin
Total enteral nutrition
  Major nutrient intake considerations
    Continuous feeding
    Bolus feeding
    Interruption of feedings (for surgery, studies, delayed gastric emptying)
  Insulin administration
    Continuous feeding
      IV drip, or
      Multiple doses of intermediate and regular insulin subcutaneously (typical ratio is 70:30)
    Bolus feeding
      Basal: intermediate or long-acting insulin subcutaneously
      Bolus: "premeal" regular insulin subcutaneously

Table 56–11. Post-ICU Management of the Surgical Patient with Diabetes Mellitus

Diabetes education
    Nutrition instruction
    Self-glucose monitoring
    Insulin administration (patient newly started on insulin)
Adjustment of oral glucose lowering agents or insulin

---

radiographic studies, additional surgery, or impaired gastric emptying. With stable continuous enteral feeding, insulin should be administered in such a way as to provide essentially constant plasma insulin levels. This may be done by constant insulin infusion. Alternatively, frequent administration of intermediate acting and regular insulin will achieve a nearly constant insulin effect. For example, giving NPH and regular insulin in fixed doses (typically a 70:30 ratio is appropriate) every 6 to 8 hours works well in many patients. When enteral feedings are given in bolus fashion, the insulin administration may follow any of the patterns typically followed on an outpatient basis with maintenance of basal insulin via intermediate or long-acting insulin and "premeal" boluses of regular insulin. Where frequent interruptions are expected, intravenous insulin (or in some cases, regular insulin administered subcutaneously), makes regulation of blood glucose easier.

Post-ICU Management (Table 56–11)

The post-ICU phase of the surgically treated diabetic patient usually involves decisions about progressive return to oral intake and whether there will be a need for pharmacotherapy of the hyperglycemia. Many times patients are discharged with instructions to keep taking insulin even when they are expected to return to oral glucose lowering agents in the future. This is especially true when patients are receiving tapering doses of glucocorticoids. Most patients who are likely to have changes in their blood glucose levels as a result of changing diet, activity, and drugs should either be taught to do self-glucose monitoring at home, or else arrangements should be made for a visiting health-care professional to help the patient with blood glucose monitoring. If they have not been taking insulin prior to hospitalization, proper instruction in insulin administration must also be initiated well before discharge to ensure competence in this procedure.

For patients who require long-term TPN or TEN therapy, insulin administration methods and doses generally need to be stabilized prior to discharge or transfer. Self-monitoring of blood glucose is necessary for satisfactory outpatient management of blood sugars. Such discussion might be included in ICU discharge planning.

HYPOGLYCEMIA

Pre-ICU Management (Table 56–12)

Although hypoglycemia has multiple causes, this discussion will focus on hypoglycemia associated with diabetes mellitus and hypoglycemia associated with administration of glucose lowering agents in nondiabetic individuals. Other causes such as hypoglycemia associated with liver disease, malignant disease, insulinomas, or nondiabetes-associated renal disease will not be discussed.

Table 56–12. Pre-ICU Management of the Hypoglycemic Patient

Risk factors
  Diabetic patient
    Diminished oral intake
    Increased exercise
    Excess insulin or oral sulfonylurea administration
    Associated risk factors
      Autonomic neuropathy with decreased awareness of hypoglycemia
      Worsening renal function
      Adrenal or pituitary insufficiency
  Nondiabetic patient
    Deliberate insulin or oral agent administration
    Inadvertent drug substitution of sulfonylurea for another drug
    Endocrine causes including insulinoma, adrenal insufficiency, hypopituritarism
    Nonendocrine causes including liver disease, renal disease, tumors, inanition
Treatment
  Oral nutrients (for alert patients)
  D50W bolus; D5W or D10W infusions
  Glucagon

The diabetic patient who takes insulin has certain common risk factors for hypoglycemia. Most episodes occur as a result of alterations in life style in which a missed meal or increased exercise occur in the face of normal insulin administration. Most such episodes are managed on an outpatient basis. Severe hypoglycemia may occur, however, in persons with long-standing type I diabetes who may have hypoglycemic unawareness. This is the result of a reduction or loss of counterregulatory hormone secretion including glucagon and epinephrine.[63] The loss of an adrenergic response limits the capability of such diabetic patients to detect insulin reactions (because of the loss of typical adrenergic symptoms) in addition to the intrinsic loss of the body's capability to respond to hypoglycemia. The diabetic patient who receives a beta-blocking agent for blood pressure control or angina pectoris may also be at risk for unrecognized hypoglycemia with an impaired counterregulatory response. Such patients may have profound hypoglycemia resulting in loss of consciousness as well as temporary or permanent neurologic deficits sufficient to necessitate hospitalization and ICU-based management. Other predisposing risk factors for hypoglycemia in the insulin-requiring diabetic patient include inadvertent administration of the wrong dose of insulin because of visual impairment. Diabetic nephropathy with impaired renal function results in a reduction in insulin requirements. (Insulin is cleared by the kidneys and any alteration in renal function is associated with an increased half-life of administered insulin.) Under this circumstance, patients may be at increased risk for significant hypoglycemia. Finally, occasionally patients have associated adrenal insufficiency or hypopituitarism in conjunction with diabetes mellitus.

Diabetic patients on oral agents are always at increased risk for hypoglycemia.[66,67] The most significant hypoglycemia is associated with chlorpropamide which has the longest duration of action. The frequency of hypoglycemia is increased with glyburide as well as chlorpropamide when compared to other sulfonylureas. The duration of hypoglycemia is usually not so prolonged with glyburide as with chlorpropamide, however. Elderly patients are at greatest risk for serious hypoglycemia. Some of the sulfonylurea compounds have active metabolites that are cleared by renal mechanisms, and renal insufficiency becomes another risk factor for hypoglycemia in patients taking such agents.

In nondiabetic persons who become hypoglycemic as a result of the administration of pharmacologic agents, there are two common causes. First is inadvertent drug substitution, in which a sulfonylurea is inadvertently given to a patient in the place of another agent. Usually, this may be ascribed to factors including illegible handwriting and similar sounding names (e.g., chlorpromazine/chlorpropamide, tolazamide/tolbutamide/tolectin). The increasing use of generic drugs reduces the capability of patients to detect such drug substitutions. Second, either sulfonylureas or insulin may be administered by the patient or someone else as a suicide gesture/homicide attempt. The former are perhaps more common, or at least somewhat easier to identify. The cause of hypoglycemia is usually more difficult to identify in nondiabetic patients who present to emergency rooms with low blood sugars because the appropriate history may be lacking. Furthermore, serum/plasma levels of insulin or C-peptide which may be helpful to determine whether insulin or sulfonylureas have been administered are not usually available from the laboratory for a matter of days. Sulfonylurea determinations may take a matter of weeks. Therefore, initial treatment requires empiric guidelines. Less common causes of hypoglycemia from pharmacologic agents include other sulfa-containing compounds such as sulfonamides (including topical preparations), aspirin, or beta blockers.

Initial treatment of the noncomatose patient is oral nutrients, usually in the form of carbohydrates. In comatose patients, the initial forms of therapy may be glucagon (kits exist for home use) or concentrated dextrose IV solutions such as 50% dextrose. In many cases patients do not need to be admitted to an ICU. General indications for in-hospital observation and treatment include:

- Inability to maintain adequate caloric intake in diabetic patients (i.e. when they will be unable to deal with ongoing hypoglycemia at home)
- Hypoglycemia associated with long-acting sulfonylurea administration, either in known diabetic patients or where drug substitution is suspected, but the drug is unknown
- Suspected high dose insulin administration, either deliberate or inadvertent

ICU Management (Table 56–13)

ICU management of hypoglycemia must focus on maintaining blood glucose levels in the near normoglycemic range. Usually, this can be done by constant infusion of 5 or 10% dextrose containing solutions frequently by peripheral venous access. In patients with renal failure the total volume of administered fluid may be a consideration and higher concentrations of dextrose may be necessary. These solutions usually need to be given via a central venous access. Oral nutrients may supplement intravenous nutrient administration. Intravenous dextrose may need to be maintained for at least 48 to 72 hours in some cases of long-acting sulfonylurea administration, routine doses of insulin in the face of renal failure or with high dose insulin administration associated with suicide attempts.

Table 56–13. ICU Management of the Severely Hypoglycemic Patient

Serial glucose monitoring
Parenteral glucose administration
Removal of offending agent
   Gastric lavage for sulfonylureas
   Surgical removal of high dose insulin site (if known)
Administration of counterregulatory hormones
   Glucagon
   Glucocorticoids

Additional therapeutic maneuvers may include such things as gastric lavage to remove high dose oral agents taken in suicide attempts. When high doses of insulin have been administered, and the site of injection is known, surgical removal of the injection site may also be considered. Finally, although rarely necessary, administration of high dose glucocorticoids may help to control profound, long-lasting hypoglycemia.

In each case, as the hypoglycemia improves, noncomatose patients can be transferred from the ICU for reevaluation of their treatment regimen. Most comatose diabetic patients whose comatose state persists because of neurologic damage need parenteral nutrients and insulin (IV or subcutaneous) until the coma resolves or stable conditions prevail.

Post-ICU Management (Table 56–14)

Insulin-requiring diabetic patients who have had significant hypoglycemic episodes usually need reevaluation of their homegoing regimens with reeducation about the relationship of insulin, diet, and exercise. Additional education may be necessary to deal with the need to adjust for factors such as reduced hypoglycemic awareness and renal failure. Patients with reduced awareness for hypoglycemia can be educated to be attentive to neuroglycopenic symptoms. Spouses, co-workers, and friends must also be taught to recognize early subtle mental status changes that accompany hypoglycemia. Instructions should be given on home use of parenteral glucagon.

Diabetic patients on oral agents who have become hypoglycemic, need to have appropriate adjustments made in

Table 56–14. Post-ICU Management of the Hypoglycemic Patient

Review of precipitating causes
Treatment of underlying causes (e.g., adrenal insufficiency, tumor)
Adjustment of oral glucose lowering agents/insulin

their medication regimen. This may involve a change to another agent, reduction in dose of the current agent, or a change to insulin (especially in the face of renal compromise or liver disease).

Nondiabetic patients who have inadvertently received sulfonylureas must be trained to pay careful attention to the drugs they receive. Patients who have received excess insulin or sulfonylureas by virtue of self-administration should have appropriate psychiatric evaluation during the hospitalization. Sometimes this can be initiated in the ICU.

GENERAL CONSIDERATIONS OF GLUCOSE MANAGEMENT IN THE ICU

In several stages in the management of the ICU patients described earlier, accurate and timely blood glucose determinations are essential to the proper management of the patient. Features of obtaining such blood glucose levels that deserve consideration include:

- Use of small-machine capillary glucose determinations employing reflectance meters or other similar devices
- Problems that may occur with glucose determinations using glucose oxidase methods in the laboratory in selected ICU situations

The popularity of the small-machine glucose determinations is directly related to the fact that glucose levels can be rapidly obtained, and the quantity of blood necessary for the determination is small.[68,69] A drop of blood can be obtained by fingerstick, from an arterial line, or from a tip of a needle for venous sampling. Usually within 30 seconds to 2 minutes (depending on the device used), a glucose determination is available. Coefficients of variation for such devices are usually in the range of 10%. Most of this variation is a function of the operator accuracy. This degree of accuracy is sufficient for most clinical situations. In most hospital settings, nursing personnel are responsible for such determinations. Proper training on the device is necessary to maintain accuracy of results.[70,71] Routine quality control checks of the bedside meters are necessary to ensure accuracy of results.[72]

Alternatives to bedside monitoring with reflectance meters include capillary tube glucoses or samples obtained from arterial lines, venous lines, or venipuncture. Most such samples are run on autoanalyzers with coefficients of variation of less than 2%. Analyzers in or near the laboratory usually provide for timely responses that are directly dependent on transport and reporting mechanisms used by the particular hospital. Even with these devices, some specific considerations may affect the accuracy of "blood" glucose determinations. Plasma glucose determinations obtained from samples drawn into tubes containing sodium fluoride generally maintain their stability from the time of sample acquisition to the time that it is run in the laboratory. Serum glucose determinations may be artifactually low, especially in the face of very high white blood cell counts. This situation results from glucose consumption by the cellular components of blood. Rapid transfer and separation of the cells, as well as cooling the tubes, helps to reduce this risk.

In any patient whose capillary or blood glucose determinations are suspected to be inaccurate, repeat determinations must be obtained before major changes in therapy are initiated. This is especially true with capillary-based determinations with small machines in which laboratory confirmation should be obtained periodically during the patient's stay in the ICU and anytime there is concern about the accuracy of values.

REFERENCES

1. National Diabetes Data Group. Classification and diagnosis of diabetes mellitus and other categories of glucose intolerance. Diabetes, 28:1039, 1979.
2. Harris, M. I., Hadden, W. E., Knowler, W. C., and Bennett, P. H.: Prevalence of diabetes and impaired glucose levels in U.S. population ages 20–74 years. Diabetes, 36:523, 1987.
3. Fleckman, A. M.: Diabetic ketoacidosis. Endocrinol. Metabol. Clin. North Am., 22:181, 1993.
4. Kecskes, S. A.: Diabetic ketoacidosis. Pediatr. Clin. North Am., 40:355, 1993.
5. Siperstein, M. D.: Diabetic ketoacidosis and hyperosmolar coma. Endocrinol. Metabol. Clin. North Am., 21:415, 1992.
6. Cefalu, W. T.: Diabetic ketoacidosis. Crit. Care. Clin., 7:89, 1991.
7. Kreisberg, R. A.: Diabetic ketoacidosis: new concepts, trends and pathogenesis of treatment. Ann. Intern. Med., 88:681, 1978.
8. Halperin, M. L., Bear, R. A., Hannaford, M. C., and Goldstein, M. B.: Selected aspects of the pathophysiology of metabolic acidosis in diabetes mellitus (review). Diabetes, 30:781, 1981.
9. Schade, D. S., and Eaton, P. R.: Diabetic ketoacidosis—pathogenesis, prevention and therapy. Clin. Endocrinol. Metabol., 12:321, 1983.
10. Foster, D. W., and McGarry, J. D.: The metabolic derangements and treatment of diabetic ketoacidosis. N. Engl. J. Med., 309:159, 1983.
11. Keller, U.: Diabetic ketoacidosis: current view of pathogenesis and treatment. Diabetologia, 29:87, 1986.
12. McGarry, J. D., Wright, P. H., and Foster, D. W.: Hormonal control of ketogenesis: rapid activation of hepatic ketogenic capacity in fed rats by anti-insulin serum and glucagon. J.C.I., 55:1202, 1975.
13. McGarry, J. D., and Foster, D. W.: Hormonal control of ketogenesis. Arch. Intern. Med., 137:495, 1977.
14. McGarry, J. D.: New perspectives in the regulation of ketogenesis. (Lilly Lecture 1978). Diabetes, 28:517, 1979.
15. Stephens, J. M., Sulway, M. J., and Watkins, P. J.: Relationship of blood acetoacetate and beta-hydroxybutyrate in diabetes. Diabetes, 20:485, 1971.
16. Emmett, N., and Narina, R.: Clinical use of the anion gap. Medicine, 56:38, 1977.
17. Van Gaal, L. F., DeLeeuw, I. H., and Bekaert, J. L.: Diabetic ketoacidosis-induced hyperkalemia: prevalence and possible origin. Intensive Care Med., 12:416, 1986.
18. Johnson, D. D., Palumbo, P. J., and Chu, C-P.: Diabetic ketoacidosis in a community-based population. Mayo Clin. Proc., 55:83, 1980.
19. Guerin, J. M., Meyer, P., and Segrestaa, J. M.: Hypothermia in diabetic ketoacidosis. Diabetes Care, 10:801, 1988.
20. Malone, M. L., Gennis, V., and Goodwin, J. S.: Characteristics of diabetic ketoacidosis in older versus younger adults. J. Am. Geriatr. Soc., 40:1100, 1992.

21. Sanson, T. H., and Levine, S. N.: Management of diabetic ketoacidosis. Drugs, *38:*289, 1989.
22. Keller, U., Berger, W., Ritz, R., and Truog, P.: Course and prognosis of 86 episodes of diabetic coma: a five-year experience with a uniform schedule of treatment. Diabetologia, *11:*93, 1975.
23. Basu, A., et al.: Persisting mortality in diabetic ketoacidosis. Diabet. Med., *10:*282, 1993.
24. Sheppard, M. C., and Wright, A. D.: The effect on mortality of low-dose insulin therapy for diabetic ketoacidosis. Diabetes Care, *5:*111, 1982.
25. Molitch, M. E., Rodman, E., Hirsch, C. A., and Dubinsky, E.: Spurious serum creatinine elevations in ketoacidosis. Ann. Intern. Med., *93:*280, 1980.
26. Mascioli, S. R., Bantle, J. P., Freier, E. G., and Hoogwerf, B. J.: Artifactual elevation of serum creatinine level due to fasting. Arch. Intern. Med., *144:*1575, 1984.
27. Brandt, K. R., and Miles, J. M.: Relationship between severity of hyperglycemia and metabolic acidosis in diabetic ketoacidosis. Mayo Clin. Proc., *63:*1071, 1988.
28. Felts, P. W.: Ketoacidosis. Med. Clin. North Am., *67:*831, 1983.
29. Soler, N. G., Bennett, M. A., Fitzgerald, M. G., and Malins, J. M.: Electrocardiogram as a guide to potassium replacement in diabetic ketoacidosis. Diabetes, *23:*610, 1974.
30. Leventhal, R. I., and Goldman, J. M.: Immediate plasma potassium levels in treating diabetic ketoacidosis. Arch. Intern. Med., *147:*1501, 1987.
31. Donn, R. I., and Crapo, L. M.: Hypokalemic respiratory arrest in diabetic ketoacidosis. JAMA, *257:*1515, 1987.
32. Adrogue, J. J., Barrero, J., and Eknoyan, G.: Salutary effects of modest fluid replacement in the treatment of adults with diabetic ketoacidosis: use in patient without extreme volume deficit. JAMA, *262:*2108, 1989.
33. Hillman, K.: Fluid resuscitation in diabetic emergencies—a reappraisal. Intensive Care Med., *13:*4, 1987.
34. Luzil, L., et al.: Metabolic effects of low-dose insulin therapy on glucose metabolism in diabetic ketoacidosis. Diabetes, *37:*1470, 1988.
35. Kitabchi, A. E.: Low-dose insulin therapy in diabetic ketoacidosis: fact or fiction? Diabetes Metab. Rev., *5:*337, 1989.
36. Padilla, A. J., and Loeb, J. N.: "Low-dose" versus "high-dose" insulin regimens in the management of uncontrolled diabetes. Am. J. Med., *63:*843, 1977.
37. Sherwin, R.: Low-dose insulin therapy in diabetic ketoacidosis. Arch. Intern. Med., *137:*1361, 1977.
38. Heber, D., Molitch, M., and Sperling, M.: Low dose continuous insulin therapy for diabetic ketoacidosis. Arch. Intern. Med., *137:*1377, 1977.
39. Kitabchi, A. E., Matteri, R., and Murphy, M. B.: Optimal insulin delivery in diabetic ketoacidosis (DKA) and hyperglycemic, hyperosmolar nonketotic coma (HHNC). Diabetes Care, *5(Suppl 1):*78, 1982.
40. Kitabchi, A. E., and Murphy, M. B.: Diabetic ketoacidosis and hyperosmolar hyperglycemic nonketotic coma. Med. Clin. North Am., *72:*1545, 1988.
41. Lever, E., and Jaspan, J. B.: Sodium bicarbonate therapy in severe diabetic ketoacidosis. Am. J. Med., *75:*263, 1983.
42. Kebler, F., McDonald, F. D., and Cadnapaphornchai, P.: Dynamic changes in serum phosphorus in diabetic ketoacidosis. Am. J. Med., *79:*571, 1985.
43. Krane, E. J., Rockoff, M. A., Wallman, J. K., and Wolfsdorf, J. L.: Subclinical brain swelling in children during treatment of diabetic ketoacidosis. N. Engl. J. Med., *312:*1147, 1985.
44. Hoffman, W. H.: Cranial CT in children and adolescents with diabetic ketoacidosis. AJNR, *9:*733, 1988.
45. Duck, S. C., and Wyatt, D. T.: Factors associated with brain herniation in the treatment of diabetic ketoacidosis. J. Pediatr., *113:*10, 1988.
46. Van der Muelen, J. A., Klip, M., and Grinstein, S.: Possible mechanism for cerebral oedema in diabetic ketoacidosis. Lancet, *2:*306, 1987.
47. Krentz, A. J., Hale, P. J., Singh, B. M, and Natrass, M.: The effect of glucose and insulin infusion on the fall of ketone bodies during treatment of diabetic ketoacidosis. Diabetic Med., *6:*31, 1989.
48. Gerich, J. E., Martin, M. M., and Recant, L.: Clinical and metabolic characteristics of hyperosmolar nonketotic coma. Diabetes, *20:*228, 1971.
49. Arieff, A. E., and Carroll, H. J.: Nonketotic hyperosmolar coma with hyperglycemia: clinical features, pathophysiology, renal function, acid-base balance, plasma-cerebrospinal fluid equilibria and the effects of therapy in 37 cases. Medicine, *51:*73, 1972.
50. Wachtel, T. J., Silliman, R. A., and Lamberton, P.: Predisposing factors for the diabetic hyperosmolar state. Arch. Intern. Med., *147:*499, 1987.
51. Jordan, R. M.: Endocrine emergencies. Med. Clin. North Am., *67:*1193, 1983.
52. Brenner, W. I., Lensky, Z., Engelman, R. M., and Stahl, W. M.: Hyperosmolar coma in surgical patients: an iatrogenic disease of increasing incidence. Ann. Surg., *178:*651, 1973.
53. Seki, S.: Clinical features of hyperosmolar hyperglycemic nonketotic diabetic coma associated with cardiac operations. J. Thorac. Cardiovasc. Surg., *91:*867, 1986.
54. Grenfall, A.: Acute renal failure in diabetics. Intensive Care Med., *12:*6, 1986.
55. Taitelman, U., Reece, E. A., and Bessman, A. N.: Insulin in the management of the diabetic surgical patient: continuous intravenous infusion vs. subcutaneous administration. JAMA, *237:*658, 1977.
56. Goldberg, N. J., et al.: Insulin therapy in the diabetic surgical patient: metabolic and hormone response to low dose insulin infusion. Diabetes Care, *4:*279, 1981.
57. Rosenstock, J., and Raskin, P.: Surgery: practical guidelines for diabetes management. Clin. Diabetes, *5:*181, 1988.
58. Johnston, D. G., and Alberti, K. G. M. M.: Diabetic emergencies: practical aspects of the management of diabetic ketoacidosis and diabetes during surgery. Clin. Endocrinol. Metabol., *9:*437, 1980.
59. Daykin, A. P.: Anesthetic and surgical stress in the diabetic patient: carbohydrate homeostasis. Int. Anesthesiol. Clin., *26:*206, 1988.
60. Kuntschen, F. R.: Alterations of insulin and glucose metabolism during cardiopulmonary bypass under normothermia. J. Thorac. Cardiovasc. Surg., *89:*97, 1985.
61. Hoogwerf, B. J., Sheeler, L. R., and Licata, A. A.: Endocrine management of the open heart surgical patient. Semin. Thorac. Cardiovasc. Surg., *3:*1, 1991.
62. Vanderwoude, M. F., Van Gaal, L. F., and DeLeeuw, I. H.: Perioperative parenteral nutrition in the stressed diabetic patient. World J. Surg., *10:*72, 1986.
63. Gerich, J. E.: Glucose counterregulation and its impact on diabetes mellitus. Diabetes, *37:*1608, 1988.
64. Mandelbaum, I., and Morgan, D. R.: Effect of extracorporeal circulation upon insulin. J. Thorac. Cardiovasc. Surg., *55:*526, 1968.
65. Mauritis, F. J., Vandewoude, M. D., Van Gaal, L. F., and De Leeuw, I. H.: Perioperative parenteral nutrition in the stressed diabetic patient. World J. Surg., *10:*72, 1986.
66. Gerich, J. E.: Drug therapy—oral hypoglycemic agents. N. Engl. J. Med., *321:*1231, 1989.

67. Selzer, H. S.: Drug-induced hypoglycemia: a review based on 473 cases. Diabetes, *21:*955, 1972.
68. American Diabetes Association: Consensus statement: self-monitoring of blood glucose. Diabetes Care, *10:*95, 1987.
69. American Diabetes Association: Policy statement: self-monitoring of blood glucose. Diabetes Care, *8:*515, 1985.
70. Lawrence, P. A.: Accuracy of nurses in performing capillary blood glucose monitoring. Diabetes Care, *12:*298, 1989.
71. Kucler, M., Goormastic, M., and Hoogwerf, B. J.: Influence of frequency, time interval from initial instruction and method of instruction on performance competency for blood glucose monitoring. Diabetes Care, *13:*488, 1990.
72. Joint Commission perspectives: standards on decentralized lab testing and approval. Chicago, IL, Joint Commission on Accreditation of Hospitals, 7, March/April, 1989.

Chapter 57

THE PITUITARY-ENDOCRINE AXIS

LESLIE R. SHEELER

PRE-ICU PHASE

Normal Function of the Hypothalamic Pituitary-Endocrine Axis

A brief review of normal endocrine function will facilitate understanding both the endocrine changes with stress and the pituitary, adrenal, and thyroid diseases that may cause serious illness for patients.

The hypothalamic pituitary (HP) unit regulates the function of three principal target glands via meticulous feedback control: the thyroid, the adrenal, and the gonad. The general physiology in health is similar: hypothalamic-releasing hormones or factors cause the secretion of their trophic polypeptide from the pituitary. The pairs which have all been isolated, purified, synthesized and used for testing or therapy are corticotropin-releasing factor (CRF) and adrenocorticotropic hormone (ACTH), thyrotropin-releasing hormone (TRH), thyroid-stimulating hormone (TSH), luteinizing hormone-releasing hormone (LHRH or GNRH), luteinizing hormone (LH), and follicle-stimulating hormone (FSH). Table 57-1 summarizes these hormones and some of their current uses in diagnostic testing and in therapy.

The trophic hormone then has multiple effects on the target gland, including the secretion of the principal steroid hormone (thyroxine, cortisol, estradiol, or testosterone) which, in turn, modulates the hypothalamic pituitary's further secretion of trophic hormone. The details of the modulation of the steroid on the HP unit vary slightly. High levels of T_4 or the other active thyroid hormone triiodothyronine (T_3) thoroughly suppress TSH secretion. Table 57-2 details the normal ranges of endocrine tests. High cortisol levels only relatively suppress ACTH output. LHRH, LH and FSH, and testosterone or estradiol interactions are far more complex. At times, negative feedback occurs as in the other two systems. At other times enhancing or positive feedback results, for example, the LH surge at ovulation.

Growth hormone secretion is primarily regulated by growth hormone releasing hormone (GHRH) secreted by the hypothalamus. Growth hormone probably effects nearly all its biologic activity through the production of somatomedin C by the liver and other tissues. Somatomedin C mediates most of growth hormone's metabolic effects on tissues including bone, cartilage, fat, liver, and muscle.

Prolactin is unique among these major anterior pituitary hormones because its control is primarily through chronic inhibition by prolactin-inhibiting factor (dopamine) rather than by a releasing factor. Lesions that interrupt the flow of dopamine from the hypothalamus down the stalk to the anterior pituitary cause elevations in serum prolactin levels. In normal physiology, prolactin primarily facilitates lactation. Other putative effects in humans, for example, in water balance or as another growth factor, seem questionable or at least of minor significance.

Response of the Hypothalamic-Pituitary-Peripheral Gland Unit to the Stress of Illness

There are many adverse effects on the body during critical illness. An understanding of the response to stress serves as a model for understanding problems encountered in the ICU. The acuity and severity of illness and the nutritional status of the patient modulate the responses of the hypothalamic pituitary-target gland axis to stress. These reactions to stress are complex and vary in patients without primary or secondary endocrine disease. Growth hormone, prolactin, ACTH, and cortisol[6,7] levels tend to rise with most stressful stimuli including critical illness. The other two systems, the HP thyroid axis[8,9] and the HP gonadal axis,[10,11] tend to be suppressed by the same sort of stresses that stimulate the other systems. The most studied and most complex of all the systems is the HP thyroid axis, which shows several different patterns in response to illness depending on acuity, severity, nutritional status, and other factors.

Cortisol Output and Stress

In normal patients, the output of cortisol from the adrenal gland often increases in a dramatic fashion in response to stress. Multiple illnesses and stresses have been shown to alter the hypothalamic pituitary adrenal axis in this manner.[12] A few of the many common clinical conditions that often lead to increased cortisol secretion include psychiatric illness, anesthesia and surgery, serious infections, blood loss, hypotension, myocardial infarction, and heart failure. The rise in cortisol output can be quite dramatic. In patients with severe heart failure, plasma cortisol levels may rise to approximately 100 µg/dl (normal 5 to 25). The urine free cortisol levels with the stress of anesthesia and open heart surgery for coronary artery disease are about 10 times the upper limit of normal.[13]

Most of the drugs known to block cortisol production (i.e., ortho-para DDD, aminoglutethimide, and metyrapone) are usually only used long term as medical therapy

Table 57-1. Hypothalamic and Pituitary Hormones

Hypothalamic Releasing Hormone	Pituitary Hormone	Uses of Releasing Factor
Luteinizing hormone-releasing hormone (LHRH) or gonadotropin Releasing hormone (GNRH)	Luteinizing hormone (LH)	Test for LH deficiency Induce puberty in patients with GNRH deficiency Induce ovulation Cause hypogonadism to treat uterine fibroids, precocious puberty, or prostatic cancer.
Thyrotropin-releasing hormone (TRH)	Thyroid-stimulating hormone (TSH)	Test for TSH or prolactin deficiency Test to confirm hyperthyroidism in an equivocal case
Corticotropin-releasing factor (CRF)	Adrenocorticotropic hormone (ACTH)	Test for ACTH deficiency To sort out different causes of Cushing's syndrome
Growth hormone-releasing hormone (GHRH)	Growth hormone (GH)	Test for GH deficiency Treat children with GH deficiency due to GHRH deficiency

(Data from references 1 to 4.)

for cortisol excess. An exception is the antifungal agent ketoconazole which blocks the production of cortisol well enough to be useful as medical therapy for Cushing's syndrome.[14] Otherwise few drugs besides high dose glucocorticoid treatment[15] are known to block the stress induced rises in cortisol output.

This makes screening tests for cortisol deficiency on critically ill patients relatively easy. If none of the above drugs are being given, the more ill the patient, the more one would tend to find high serum cortisol levels on sampling. Because ACTH and cortisol are secreted in bursts, a tentative diagnosis of presumed adrenal failure in a critically ill patient should be based on two or three cortisol levels drawn 20 to 40 minutes apart. Normal values in ill patients would be 20 to 100 mg/dl.

"Euthyroid Sick Syndromes"

The HP thyroid axis in illness is the best studied and, in many ways, the most complex of the pituitary endocrine systems. The interpretation of thyroid function tests in patients with critical illness may at times be confusing to the clinician. The changes in thyroid function tests that occur with illness while the patient presumably remains normal

Table 57-2. Normal Values for Endocrine Studies

Laboratory Study	Normal Value
ACTH	5–50 pg/ml
Cortisol, serum	AM: 15.9 ± 5.0 µg/dl (range 8.2–29.0) PM: 8.6 ± 2.6 µg/dl (range 3.3–15.0)
Prolactin HPRL	1.0–17.4 ng/ml
TSH	0.4–5.5. uU/ml
FTI	6.4–10.7 µg/dl
T_4	5.0–10.5 µg/dl
T_4U	0.7–1.2
T_3, RIA	94–170 ng/dl
Free T_4 by RIA	0.76–2.0 ng/dl
Total testosterone in men, RIA	220–1000 ng/dl
FSH	2–18 µg/ml Postmenopausal = 20–100
LH	1–12 µg/ml Menopausal = >mIU/ml
Urine free cortisol	7–70 µg/24 hr

in thyroid function are frequently termed "euthyroid sick." Alteration in thyroid function tests with illness occurs in several different patterns summarized in Table 57-3.

In health, much of the circulating triiodothyronine (T_3) is formed via conversion of T_4 to T_3 in the periphery. There is a lesser contribution to total circulating T_3 levels via direct secretion of T_3 by the thyroid gland. This peripheral deodination reaction which converts T_4 to T_3 is often thoroughly blocked as patients become more ill. T_3 levels in severely ill patients are often reported as less than 25 mg/dl (normal 90 to 170 mg/dl). The T_4 and TSH levels often remain normal. Acute psychiatric illness[21] and HIV infection[22] tend to be the only exception to this low T_3 euthyroid sick syndrome.

Especially in the first stages of severe illness or an acute event such as fever or acute psychiatric events, total serum T_4 levels may rise to above the upper limit of normal. Since more than 99% of the total T_4 and T_3 levels represent bound hormone, changes in thyroid binding proteins can cause large changes in the total T_4 and T_3 levels. The major thyroid hormone binding proteins are thyroid-binding globulin (TBG), albumin, and prealbumin. Hospital laboratories estimate and correct for binding protein changes by measuring T_3 resin uptake which corrects for TBG changes, or T_4 resin uptakes which corrects for TBG as well as albumin and prealbumin changes. The total T_4 level then is adjusted for binding protein levels by multiplying or dividing the T_4 by the T_3 or T_4 resin value. This adjusted total T_4 termed free thyroxine index (FTI, T_7, or corrected T_4) better reflects the actual circulating T_4 level than the total T_4 level. The total T_3 levels should be approached in the same way correcting for binding protein changes. Most laboratories do not provide corrected T_3 levels, but the clinician can easily calculate the value by using the T_3 or T_4 resin uptake level. For example, if the total T_3 is 185 mg/dl and a T_4 resin is 0.8, the corrected T_3 would be 185/.80, which equals 231 mg/dl.

The new ultrasensitive TSH assays now available make further evaluation of this high T_4 euthyroid sick state relatively easy. Almost all hyperthyroid patients, except for the rare ones with TSH-driven hyperthyroidism, would have TSH levels of less than 0.05 mg/ml. Thus, an ill patient

Table 57-3. Patterns of Alterations in Thyroid Function Tests with Nonthyroidal Illness

Laboratory Finding	Probable Explanation	Clinical Conditions
Low total serum T_3 level with a normal total T_4; usually, TSH is normal	Decreased peripheral conversion of T_4 to T_3	Most ill hospitalized patients including febrile illness, renal failure, malnutrition
Low total T_4 and low total T_3 levels; usually, TSH is normal	Multiple factors—decreased TRH, TSH, thyroid output of T_4, increased clearance of T_4	Nearly any severe illness
High T_4; TSH is normal	Increased TBG levels, decreased clearance of T_4, and decreased T_4 to T_3 conversion	Liver disease, psychiatric illness; acute nonthyroidal illness

(Data from references 16 to 20.)

with a high corrected T_4, but with a measurable TSH, almost always would be euthyroid.[23,24]

Despite all these changes in total T_4 and T_3 levels these patients are probably euthyroid.[9] Although different assay systems may give varying estimates of free T_4 levels in critically ill patients,[25] the actual free levels for T_4 and T_3 measurements often are normal[9,26] in patients with "euthyroid sick" alterations in thyroid function tests.

Pituitary-Gonadal Axis

When patients are in negative caloric balance or seriously ill, the hypothalamic pituitary-gonadal axis tends to decline. This happens in critical illnesses as well as in a variety of caloric deprivation stages such as anorexia nervosa, starvation, and in female athletes with low body fat percentage. This hypogonadotropic hypogonadism reverses as refeeding or recovery from serious illness occurs. The astute reader will now be aware that this pattern complicates the evaluation of the hypothalamic pituitary endorgan axis in critical illness. If a menopausal woman has a critical illness with a low T_4 euthyroid sick-state, gonadotropin measurements may be misleadingly low.[10,11]

Pituitary, Thyroid, or Adrenal Disorders That May Cause Critical Illness

Adrenal Failure

Primary adrenal failure (Addison's disease), is a rare endocrine disorder that may cause critical life-threatening illness.[27] A patient with known adrenal failure who receives inadequate replacement therapy when stressed,[28] resulting in adrenal crisis is less of a diagnostic problem than the patient with previously unrecognized adrenal failure, presenting in adrenal crisis.

Primary adrenal failure may be caused by numerous pathologic conditions that injure adrenal cortical tissue,[29] and lead to failure of the adrenals to make enough cortisol and aldosterone to sustain normal health. "Idiopathic" or autoimmune adrenal failure is now the most common cause of adrenal failure in the United States. The association of this condition with injury to other endocrine and nonendocrine tissues in the polyendocrine deficiency syndromes is frequent and may provide the clinician with some important clues to the diagnosis of Addison's disease. Thus, patients with type I diabetes, immune thyroid disease, vitiligo, alopecia, vitamin B_{12} deficiency, sprue, or primary gonadal failure should be especially suspect for Addison's disease if signs and symptoms begin. The other causes of adrenal failure include chronic infections such as cryptococcosis, histoplasmosis, and especially tuberculosis,[30] replacement of the adrenal by metastatic cancer,[31] and hemorrhagic destruction of the adrenals.[32] Patients in the late stages of illness from HIV have recently been reported to develop adrenal failure, presumably because of chronic infections.

Patients who slowly develop primary adrenal failure due to one of the foregoing pathologic processes often have several of the classic signs and symptoms: increased pigmentation, weakness anorexia, nausea and vomiting, weight loss, and postural hypotension (Table 57-4). The preceding features are present 70 to 90% of the time. About half the time, patients will admit to salt craving or unusually frequent or severe hiccups. Approximately 80% of the patients with primary adrenal failure will have either hyponatremia or hyperkalemia or both at the time of diagnosis.[29] Hyponatremia is the more common electrolyte disturbance at the time of diagnosis.

Table 57-4 outlines two simple ways to document the diagnosis of adrenal failure. If one has access to a good ACTH assay, this measurement can be helpful. A high level (6 to 10 times the upper limit of normal), with a low plasma

Table 57-4. Major Symptoms and Signs of Primary Adrenal Failure*

Symptoms
  Often present
    Anorexia
    Nausea
    Vomiting
    Extreme weakness
    Hyperpigmentation
    Hypotension or postural hypotension
    Myalgias, arthralgias
  Present about 50%
    Hiccups
    Salt craving
Laboratory clue
  Hyponatremia
  Hyperkalemia
Diagnostic Testing (Diagnostic procedures to confirm diagnosis)
  Obtain an ACTH level
  Obtain a plasma cortisol level
  Give 0.25 mg; synthetic ACTH IM or IV; measure plasma cortisol before and 1 hour later

* Consider diagnosis of primary adrenal failure if several of the foregoing symptoms are present with any combination of electrolyte disturbance.

cortisol level, especially with a compatible history is virtually diagnostic. Alternatively, a short ACTH stimulation test showing no response or a markedly blunted response (e.g., baseline plasma cortisol less than 3 µg/dl and post-stimulation value only 8 µg/dl is diagnostic. For cases where these initial studies are equivocal, a longer ACTH infusion, lasting up to 48 hours can be done. (See reference 31 for details of this longer test.)

Once the diagnosis of Addison's disease is suspected and the aforementioned tests are done, treatment should be begun. If the results turn out normal, glucocorticoid therapy can then be stopped. Initial therapy would be with IV normal saline, 2 to 3 L over the first few hours of treatment, parenteral hydrocortisone (e.g., semisuccinate) 100 mg, IM or IV push every 8 hours for the first day, and if needed for hypotension or hyperkalemia, flurocortisone, 0.1 mg orally once or more in the first 24 hours. This treatment will resuscitate patients ill from adrenal failure alone. Patients ill with Addison's disease plus another serious illness will need support and therapy for the other illness or illnesses. Maintenance therapy for newly diagnosed adrenal failure patients will be reviewed in the post-ICU phase of this chapter.

If the diagnosis of adrenal failure has not been made by the time a patient is seriously ill, recognition and therapy by the ICU physician may be lifesaving. By the time adrenal failure has reached the critical illness stage, the patient will usually have impending circulatory collapse, with a declining blood pressure that is difficult to maintain. Some patients have been reported to have high output circulatory failure that can mimic sepsis.[33]

Thyroid Disorders

Hyperthyroidism. Hyperthyroidism usually presents with the following characteristic signs and symptoms:

- Nervousness
- Insomnia
- Tachycardia
- Weight loss
- Heat intolerance
- Weakness
- Thirst
- Tremor
- Excessive sweating
- Irritability
- Diminished ability to concentrate

Atypical presentations of hyperthyroidism, with weight gain, which occurs about 20% of the time, or with only one dominant symptom such as weakness or heart failure, are fairly common. Elderly patients are especially prone to nonclassic presentations when they develop hyperthyroidism. The term "apathetic hyperthyroidism" has been applied to this clinical syndrome in older patients.[34] When patients with organic heart disease due to valvular disease, coronary artery disease, or cardiomyopathy, develop hyperthyroidism, marked exacerbation of cardiac symptoms will almost invariably occur.

The laboratory diagnosis of hyperthyroidism is usually straightforward. Corrected total T_4 or T_3 levels are usually high, whereas the TSH levels are low (≤ 0.05 uU/ml). If a patient with untreated or unrecognized hyperthyroidism develops a second major illness such as pneumonia, perforated ulcer, sepsis, or myocardial infarction or has anesthesia[35] and surgery,[36] the severe life-threatening endocrine emergency of hyperthyroid crisis or thyroid storm may eventuate.

The most common form of hyperthyroidism is Graves' disease, which is an autoimmune disease accompanied by obvious thyroid ocular disease in roughly one half of the affected patients. Sometimes the eye changes of proptosis, periorbital swelling, lid retraction, or extraocular muscle dysfunction are so striking that a clinician can instantly consider Graves' disease as the diagnosis. About one half of the patients with Graves' disease do not have obvious thyroid ocular disease, although most Graves' disease patients without obvious eye changes do have eye muscle swelling which would be detectable with orbital ultrasound or CT or MRI imaging.

Numerous other forms of hyperthyroidism have been characterized and defined. These include: multinodular goiter, solitary hyperfunctioning adenoma, lymphocytic thyroiditis with spontaneously resolving hyperthyroidism, subacute thyroiditis, ingestion of excessive amounts of thyroid hormone, TSH producing pituitary tumors or pituitary resistance to thyroid hormone and amiodarone or iodine-induced hyperthyroidism. Thyroid storm is rarely due to any disorder other than Graves' disease.

Hypothyroidism. Primary hypothyroidism is most often due to auto-immune injury to the thyroid gland from lymphocytic thyroiditis. Other causes include:

- Radioiodine therapy for hyperthyroidism
- Thyroidectomy
- Various medications including iodine, amiodarone, and lithium
- Antithyroid drugs such as methimazole or propylthiouracil (PTU)

If unrecognized and untreated, severe hypothyroidism, usually along with other stress or illness such as hypothermia, infection, or the use of medications that suppress the central nervous system, the life-threatening condition of myxedema coma may develop. Numerous signs and symptoms may occur in hypothyroidism. These include:

- Dry skin
- Hair loss
- Cold intolerance
- Constipation
- Muscle aches and muscle cramps
- Carpal tunnel syndrome
- Fatigue
- Sluggishness
- Facial puffiness
- Deepening of the voice
- Delayed relaxation of the deep tendon reflexes

Corrected T_4 levels in primary hypothyroidism are low or low normal, whereas TSH levels are high.

Severe hypopituitarism when undiagnosed and untreated may lead to critical illness due to cortisol deficiency and to a lesser extent thyroid hormone deficiency. The most common cause of hypopituitarism is a primary pituitary tumor, usually a large (i.e., macro) adenoma. When hypopituitarism develops secondary to a slowly expanding mass, growth hormone and LH and FSH deficiency usually occur first, followed later by ACTH and TSH deficiency. With an acute injury, however, such as postpartum pituitary infarction (Sheehan's syndrome) or with pituitary apoplexy or with physical injury to the gland such as head trauma or pituitary surgery, selective deficiency of ACTH or TSH will occur more commonly. Thus, a patient with Sheehan's syndrome might have normal menses, but may be ill from ACTH or TSH deficiency. A patient ill from hypopituitarism from a pituitary adenoma would almost always have hypogonadotropic hypogonadism in addition to ACTH or TSH deficiency. Besides the aforementioned causes, numerous other parasellar lesions including late effects from pituitary or cranial radiation therapy, sarcoidosis, aneurysms meningioma or craniopharyngioma, metastatic carcinoma, and infections such as tuberculosis or viral meningitis may cause hypopituitarism. Autoimmune pituitary failure appears to be rare, as does lymphocytic hypophysitis. A confirmed diagnosis of hypopituitarism thus frequently will lead to the discovery of other health threatening or vision threatening intracranial conditions that may require diagnosis and therapy.

As patients become ill with panhypopituitarism, the major symptoms will be similar to Addison's disease: nausea, vomiting, anorexia, myalgia, and weakness. However, instead of hyperpigmentation, skin pallor is usually noted. Hypogonadism is usually present and may be a helpful clue on the physical examination. Similar to primary adrenal failure, hyponatremia may be a helpful laboratory finding.[37]

ICU PHASE

Thyroid Disease

Euthyroid Sick Syndrome

As previously discussed, thyroid function tests may be altered in nonthyroidal illness (see Table 57-3). As patients develop more serious illness and a catabolic state develops as nutrition worsens, the final euthyroid sick pattern develops, a low T_4 state.[38] The T_4 level may fall to unmeasurable (less than 1.0 µg/dl) levels with severe or prolonged illness. Current TSH assays can help one to sort this out. With primary hypothyroidism and low T_4 levels, the TSH would be many times the upper limits of normal (5.0 to 5.5 uU/ml in most assays). In euthyroid sick syndrome with low T_4 levels, the TSH value is usually normal, but occasionally slightly high.[9] The TSH level is virtually never as high as it would be with primary hypothyroidism and such a low T_4. The remaining possibility that clinicians always should be mindful of is the consideration of secondary hypothyroidism when an ill patient has a low T_4 and a low TSH. Secondary hypothyroidism is relatively rare (less than 5% of ICU patients with low T_4 and normal TSH have true secondary hypothyroidism), the remainder have "euthyroid sick syndrome" (unpublished data E. Sivak, L. Sheeler). It would be rarer still to have isolated TSH deficiency.[39] Thus, if pituitary function is normal otherwise, the chance of true hypothyroidism with a low T_4 and normal TSH would be exceedingly low.

The low T_4 euthyroid sick state correlates well with the severity of illness. The nadir of the T_4 level and the failure to rise as an illness continues[40-42] are both negative prognostic factors for survival. This leads to an as yet unanswered clinical question. Should these patients with low T_4 euthyroid sick be treated with thyroid hormone? If one decides to treat these patients, conservative doses such as 0.05 to 0.1 mg of L-thyroxine daily given orally or parentally seem reasonable.

Thyroid Storm

Thyroid storm[43] is a rare medical emergency characterized by severe hyperthyroidism, most often in the setting of a second severe illness, or post-thyroid surgery, or nonthyroid surgery, accompanied by fever. There is some uncertainty about one of the alleged causes of thyrotoxic crisis, namely, the role of ^{131}I therapy for thyrotoxicosis.[44] Acute decompensation of numerous organ symptoms including cardiovascular, central nervous system, hepatic, renal, and gastrointestinal may occur. The clinical features of thyroid storm include those of uncomplicated hyperthyroidism mentioned earlier, as well as confusion and lethargy progressing to stupor and coma. Many thyrotoxic patients who progress to thyroid storm have lost a good deal of weight and are poorly nourished. Important clues on the physical examination include signs of thyroid ocular disease, a goiter, tremor, warm, smooth moist skin, and tachycardia. Early detection and prompt intervention are imperative. Historically, thyroid storm causes a high mortality, approximately 30% to as high as 100%.[45]

Treatment of thyroid storm is designed to:

- Alleviate the underlying intercurrent illness
- Decrease the synthesis and release of more thyroid hormone from the thyrotoxic gland
- Antagonize the effect of existing thyroid hormone
- Provide supportive care until the hyperthyroidism is improved or corrected

Like many rare conditions, we lack exact natural history data for thyroid storm, save the presumption that most untreated patients would die. No controlled studies show whether certain aspects of currently available therapy are more important than others.

Therapy directed at the thyroid gland begins with an antithyroid drug such as methimazole or PTU to decrease thyroid hormone synthesis. PTU has the added benefit of decreasing the conversion of T_4 to T_3 in the periphery. The doses for thyroid storm are 1200 to 1500 mg per day for PTU and 80 to 120 mg per day for methimazole. Because no IV form of these drugs is available, either oral (via nasogastric tube) or rectal suppository administration is necessary. After several doses of antithyroid drug have been administered stable iodine (as SSKI 10 gtt orally twice daily, or sodium iodide 1 g IV every 24 hours, or the contrast material iodate 3 g per 24 hours) should be given to block the release of stored thyroid hormones. If iodine is given too soon, thyroid hormone synthesis may actually increase.

The detection and therapy (if possible) of underlying precipitating causes should be a major concern of the clinician treating a patient with thyroid storm. Controlling fever, replacing fluids as needed, and monitoring hemodynamic parameters are important supportive measures. Improving nutritional status is another aspect of treating thyroid crisis which most likely is important. Glucocorticoids are used by many clinicians as ancillary treatment. The equivalent of 300 mg of hydrocortisone semisuccinate per 24 hours should be sufficient. Beta-blocking drugs, which have been reported to control many of the manifestations of hyperthyroidism, are also used for thyroid crises. These drugs do not interfere with thyroid hormone synthesis or release, although they do seem to inhibit peripheral T_4 to T_3 conversion. The dosage of beta blockers should be titrated to control manifestations such as tachycardia. An oral dose might vary from the equivalent of 160 to several hundred milligrams of propranolol per 24 hours. IV therapy would be equivalent to 1 to 2 mg of propranolol every 3 to 6 hours. If we can deliver a therapeutic dose of radioiodine before we give stable iodine, we sometimes will do so. Some authorities would disagree strongly with giving ^{131}I therapy to a patient already seriously ill with hyperthyroidism.

Illustrative Case. A 54-year-old woman was admitted to our hospital after her family noted confusion and brought her in for an evaluation. Because of social problems, she had not had previous medical attention, despite more than a 1-year illness. Her symptoms included a 12-kg weight loss, weakness, heat intolerance, sweating, palpitations, and nervousness. She had been treating herself with multivitamins and kelp. On physical examination, her weight was 48 kg, her pulse rate was 150, blood pressure 214/100, and temperature 37°C. Bilateral lid retraction, proptosis, and periorbital edema were present. Mild scleral icterus, warm skin, and a fine rapid tremor were also noted. She was confused on admission. Within 16 hours, her mental status markedly deteriorated to stupor with responsiveness only to noxious stimuli. Admitting laboratory values showed numerous abnormalities including a hemoglobin of 11 g/dl, hematocrit of 32%, platelet count of 62,000, prothrombin time (PT) of 23.3 sec, control (11 to 13), a partial thromboplastin time (PTT) was 41 (23–33.5), and abnormal liver function tests including a bilirubin of 4.4 mg/dl (normal ≤ 1.5) and SGOT of 84 IU/L (7 to 40), an LDH of 368 IU/L (50 to 210) and an alkaline phosphatase of 246 IU/L (20 to 120). Thyroid function tests showed a total T_4 of 36.6 µg/dl with an FTI of 38.5 µg/dl (6.4 to 10.7) a total T_3 of 533 with a corrected T_3 calculated as follows:

$$\frac{\text{Total } T_3}{T_4 \text{ Uptake}} \frac{533}{.95} = 561$$

The TSH level was <0.05 uU/ml (0.4 to 5.5). When stupor developed, asterixis was noted. At that time a blood ammonia level was obtained 184 µmol/L (normal is 11 to 35).

Treatment was begun on admission with methimazole, propranolol, hydrocortisone, and IV fluids. Lactulose was added when the high blood ammonia levels were found 24 hours after admission. Thiamine and vitamin K also were given. Numerous diagnoses were considered, but excluded, including thrombotic thrombocytopenic purpura, idiopathic thrombocytopenic purpura, and vitamin A or vitamin E intoxication.

The patient improved considerably over a 10-day stay in the hospital. At the time of discharge, laboratory studies showed a PT of 16 sec, PTT of 31.9, alkaline phosphatase 229 IU/L, SGOT 64 IU/L, bilirubin 2.8 mg/dl and platelet count of 97,000. A radioactive iodine uptake done during the hospitalization was low (7%), undoubtedly because of the iodine content of kelp. Discharge medications included methimazole, 60 mg per day, atenolol, 100 mg per day, and lactulose, 200 mg per day. One month later, the radioiodine uptake was high enough to allow administration of a therapeutic dose of ^{131}I. The hyperthyroidism eventually was controlled by this treatment. Five months after her admission, a liver biopsy showed "mild nonspecific chronic portal inflammation" and "mild stellate portal and parenchymal fibrosis."

Untreated hyperthyroidism led to this severe illness in this woman, with both the hepatic[46] and hematologic[47] manifestations likely related to the hyperthyroidism. One year after the severe illness, the patient's CBC was normal and liver function tests were near normal.

Although most cases of hyperthyroid crisis or thyroid storm would occur with Graves' disease, other causes of hyperthyroidism might rarely do this.[36] Once a patient with hyperthyroidism is critically ill, the euthyroid sick alterations in thyroid tests may be seen and might be confusing to the clinician. Hyperthyroidism with normal T_3 by RIA due to euthyroid sick syndrome has been well documented.[48] Even more impressive is the report of patients with known hyperthyroidism who became seriously ill, accompanied by falls in the T_4 and T_3 levels to values of nearly zero.[49]

Myxedema Coma

Of all the endocrine emergencies, myxedema coma seems to be the least common. The last case seen at our thousand-bed institution was in 1971. At least two conditions need to be present to allow the development of myxedema coma: severe untreated hypothyroidism and an underlying precipitating event. The precipitating cause of coma may be hypothermia due to cold exposure (probably the main factor in the world's literature),[50] or any severe medical or surgical illness.

A comatose patient with clinical features of myxedema including typical facies, dry skin, prolonged relaxation of deep tendon reflexes, and hypothermia would obviously suggest the diagnosis. Mortality is estimated to be 60%.[45] As in thyroid storm, multiple systems may fail. There may be cardiovascular and respiratory failure. Many patients would have hyponatremia, hypercapnia, and hypoxia on testing. Most would have pericardial effusion.[50] Underlying coronary artery disease or other organic heart disease would be fairly common. A detailed case report by Mazonson and colleagues[51] describes a fatal episode of myxedema coma due to amiodarone. This case matches the general profile described earlier.

Far more common than myxedema coma would be the situation described earlier of the hypothyroxinemic variant of euthyroid sick in a seriously ill patient in an ICU. As mentioned, the TSH assay helps to sort this out. I have found that when consulted for a low T_4 in an ICU patient, before the TSH result is available, the most I can do for the consulting physician is decide whether the patient indeed does or does not have severe hypothyroidism clinically. It seems unlikely that a patient could have myxedema coma, even as impure an entity as it seems to be, without having myxedema.

Probably the most important aspect in managing a patient with myxedema coma is general supportive care. Measures include:

- Warming the hypothermic patient
- Treating infections
- Managing heart failure
- Correcting electrolyte disturbances
- Correcting ventilatory disturbances

The majority of articles or textbook chapters advocate roughly the same approach to thyroid hormone replacement, an exceedingly large loading dose of L-thyroxine 300 to 500 μg IV.[45,48,49] In every other clinical setting besides coma, this would most likely be therapeutically neutral[52] in the absence of coronary artery disease. If heart disease is present this would be deleterious, however. One might wonder if this large dose of thyroid hormone is really proper. A fascinating article in this respect by Impallomeni[53] describes five patients treated with supportive care initially and given 0.05 mg of T_4 orally when they recovered from coma. Three patients fully recovered to leave the hospital, whereas two died of their underlying illnesses (rectal carcinoma and pneumonia). In essence, all five patients survived "myxedema coma" without the high dose T_4 therapy advocated in many articles.

Adrenal Disease

Adrenal Crisis

Patients with previously undiagnosed adrenal failure often present the ICU physician the final opportunity to make the correct, lifesaving diagnosis. Patients with Addison's disease will have either the insidious onset of the illness characterized earlier in the section on pre-ICU phase (see Table 57–4), or acute adrenal failure usually due to acute hemorrhagic destruction of the gland. In either case, by the time a patient is in the ICU for an episode of adrenal crisis, the findings would likely include:

- Circulatory collapse
- Hyperpigmentation (the acute onset variety usually would not have time to develop this)
- Thready pulse
- Obtundation
- Hyponatremia and/or hyperkalemia

Well-documented adrenal failure can occur without either classic electrolyte disturbance. In the first 30 patients I cared for with primary adrenal failure, the sodium and potassium levels were normal in half of the patients at the time the diagnosis was made.

If one has reasonable grounds to suspect the diagnosis in an ICU patient, one should order the simple studies such as a baseline plasma cortisol and aldosterone level and an ACTH level (if the laboratory is prepared to properly handle the sample), followed by treatment. If one wishes to do the 1-hour ACTH stimulation test, dexamethasone, which does not interfere with cortisol measurements, can be given in a dose of 2 to 4 mg as soon as the baseline values have been obtained.

Acute therapy can then be administered as outlined earlier with the parenteral administration of 100 mg of hydrocortisone semisuccinate every 8 hours and as much normal saline as the patient's status warrants (usually 1 to 2 L quickly and 3 to 5 L over the first 24 hours). With these doses of this steroid preparation mineralocorticoid therapy with fluorocortisone acetate is rarely necessary.[54] By the time the laboratory studies are available, one usually has a strong suspicion about the results. If adrenal failure, without much else wrong, has been diagnosed, the patient will have gone from in extremis to well in 24 hours.

Illustrative Case. A 27-year-old woman was admitted to our hospital for evaluation of possible recurrent pulmonary emboli. This admission was prompted by complaints of dyspnea, tachypnea, and chest pain in the preceding 24 hours. She had had a well-proven diagnosis of pulmonary embolus 1 month prior to this admission. She was on coumarin therapy with a prothrombin time of 18 seconds (control 12). Approximately 2 months before she developed the acute onset of chest pain dyspnea and hemoptysis which led to the discovery of the pulmonary embolus, she began to feel ill. Her symptoms included nausea, vomiting, anorexia, a 15-kg weight loss in 3 months, unusually frequent hiccups, and noting that her skin looked darker. In addition she complained of marked weakness, frequent myalgia and frequent dizziness. Her examination on admission showed a pulse of 130, BP of 96/60 mm Hg reclining and 70/50 mm Hg standing, respirations of 30, and temperature of 38.4°C. Hyperpigmentation of the skin was noted. Laboratory studies included a serum sodium of 124 mEq/L and potassium of 5.0 mEq/L. Addison's disease was suspected when the aforementioned findings were noted. Both a 1-hour ACTH stimulation test and a 48-hour test were done. The short test showed plasma cortisol levels of 8.1 μg/dl and 8.7 μg/dl 1 hour after the injection of ACTH.

The highest plasma cortisol level during the 48-hour ACTH infusion was 26 mg/dl (normal ≥ 60), while a urine free cortisol was 68 μg/24 hours (normal ≥ 1000). With cortisone therapy, all related symptoms resolved.

Because of anticoagulant usage and the possibility of adrenal hemorrhage, a CT of the adrenal glands was obtained. The adrenal glands were normal in size, making a recent hemorrhage seem unlikely. Thyroid function tests revealed a positive microsomal antibody test, an FTI of 7.0 (normal 6.4 to 10.7 μg/dl) and a TSH of 22 μg/ml (normal 0.4 to 5.5).

Thus, the patient probably had idiopathic adrenal failure as her initial diagnosis. Perhaps the pulmonary embolus was related partly to dehydration and other abnormalities associated with the adrenal failure.

Hypopituitarism

Patients occasionally become so ill from previously unrecognized, untreated hypopituitarism that they are admitted to an ICU. Predominantly the illness would be driven by ACTH and cortisol deficiency with perhaps a minor contribution from secondary hypothyroidism. Thus, the illness will be much like primary adrenal failure. Important clues would include pallor, loss of sexual hair, small testes, hyponatremia, circulatory collapse, obtundation, and especially in men, anemia, related to androgen deficiency. An acute onset of hypopituitarism from pituitary apoplexy, or Sheehan's syndrome, or metastatic cancer to the hypothalamic pituitary area obviously would not allow time for some of the these manifestations to develop. A clinically important distinction needs to be recalled when examining patients: the physical findings of hypogonadism would be normal in a postmenopausal woman. Hypogonadism in a man always should be regarded as abnormal no matter how old the patient might be. This sometimes can lead to rapidly and correctly considering hypopituitarism as the diagnosis (see the following illustrative case).

A special consideration is the iatrogenic development of isolated ACTH deficiency from large dose glucocorticoid therapy.[28,53] Knowlton has an excellent discussion of this condition (see reference 54 and accompanying editorial).[55] The ICU physician should always at least consider this possibility in patients who have received large doses of glucocorticoids in the past. Again in the setting of serious illness, simple measurements of plasma cortisol followed by the glucocorticoid therapy described earlier should be strongly considered if the patient's illness all has components that at all resemble adrenal failure. Unless the plasma cortisol measurements reflect previously administered steroids (e.g., prednisone or hydrocortisone) the values will be appropriately low if iatrogenic ACTH deficiency is the correct diagnosis.

Illustrative Case. A 68-year-old black man was admitted to our hospital on April 1, 1984 for evaluation of recurrent syncope of 2 years' duration. Over the past 6 to 18 months, he had experienced numerous symptoms including fatigue, nausea, anorexia, occasional vomiting, and an 11-kg weight loss over the last 6 months. Admitting examination showed a reclining BP of 130/70 with a fall to 110/66 while standing. He also had pallor and decreased pubic, axillary, and body hair with small testes. Admitting routine laboratory studies showed a sodium of 110 mEq/L, potassium of 5.2 mEq/L, and chloride of 82. Hemoglobin was 12.3, hematocrit 37.5. Within 24 hours of admission he was transferred to our medical ICU because he experienced syncope with a blood pressure of 50/0 mm Hg.

The admitting ICU resident, noting the earlier findings, immediately suspected hypopituitarism and obtained the following: plasma cortisol levels 5 µg/dl and 8 µg/dl cortrosyn test; plasma cortisol 8.0 µg/dl before, 18 µg/dl 1 hour after the injection, T_4 level 4.2 µg/dl, TSH 2.0 µg/ml, testosterone 10 ng/dl, LH 5 µg/ml, baseline plasma aldosterone level 9.8 ng/dl. Therapy with hydrocortisone semisuccinate as detailed earlier was begun as soon as the synthetic ACTH stimulation test was completed. Within hours the patient felt incredibly better. His blood pressure was consistently 130/80 mm Hg with no postural change. Twelve hours after glucocorticoid therapy was begun, the serum sodium was 131 mEq/L. Subsequent studies showed mild elevations of prolactin, 23 to 32 (normal < 17.0 ng/ml). A CT scan of the parasellar area showed a moderate-sized macroadenoma with a slight suprasellar extension. The patient had normal visual fields and no other detectible mass effects from the tumor. After discussion he preferred therapy for the tumor to be radiation therapy which subsequently was given. He has remained well on treatment with testosterone injections, thyroxine, and cortisone acetate. The tumor has regressed following the radiation therapy.

This man had sought help elsewhere for his illness for 2 years. An observant resident, taking advantage of the clues of signs and symptoms of adrenal failure, hypogonadism, and hyponatremia, correctly assessed and treated him in a few moments, undoubtedly both saving his life and restoring him to good health. The mildly high prolactin level likely was from an effect on the stalk, rather than a prolactin-secreting tumor. Only cytochemical staining of the tumor for prolactin would answer this question

POST-ICU PHASE

Thyroid Disease

Euthyroid Sick Syndrome

As patients recover from nonthyroidal illness, abnormal thyroid function tests related to the illness return to normal. Patients who have had the hypothyroxinemic variant of euthyroid sick may exhibit slight elevation of TSH levels as T_4 levels return to normal.[42] Patients who have both intrinsic thyroid disease and euthyroid sick will again have thyroid tests which better fit their true status.[49]

Hyperthyroidism

Once the patient has recovered from thyroid storm, the hyperthyroidism will require further therapy. We usually recommend ^{131}I therapy rather than surgery or home antithyroid drug therapy. In the United States, drug therapy and ^{131}I are about equally favored by "experts" with surgery as the preferred therapy a very distant third choice (about 1%). Depending on the therapy chosen by the treating physician, follow-up will be necessary until the hyperthyroidism resolves.

Hypothyroidism

Once primary hypothyroidism has been diagnosed, therapy is relatively simple. The patient needs to be taught that thyroid hormone therapy likely will be necessary for their lifetime. An initial therapeutic probable replacement dose would be roughly 0.18 µg. L-thyroxine 1 kg of body weight. The dose can be specifically titrated to an individual patient depending on thyroid function test results. Periodic assessment of therapy using TSH and T_4 measurements will be necessary.

Addison's Disease

The long-term therapy of this endocrine disease is relatively simple. A major feature of therapy also is patient education. The need for compliance almost cannot be overemphasized to the patient. We advise the patient to obtain a medic alert bracelet or tag noting the need for chronic glucocorticoid use. We teach them to give or make sure they are given an injection of glucocorticoid if they have nausea and vomiting and thus might not really absorb an oral dose of glucocorticoid. We stress that they double their usual therapeutic dose if they are ill or feel they might have symptoms of adrenal insufficiency.

An obvious further problem with adrenal failure is the cause of the illness. If the underlying problem is metastatic cancer to the adrenal,[31] the ultimate prognosis likely is grave. If autoimmune factors have caused the problem, other related illnesses (e.g., vitamin B_{12} deficiency, Hashimoto's thyroiditis, Graves' disease, type I diabetes, etc.) might develop. If the problem has been an infection such as tuberculosis or cryptococcosis, specific therapy for the infection might well be necessary.

Hypopituitarism

Most often hypopituitarism will be due to a potentially significant problem that essentially is a totally separate issue from the patient's endocrine illness. There are many potential questions the discovery of hypopituitarism might provoke. Is there a primary pituitary tumor? If so, is there a threat to vision or health that would require some therapy? How should a given tumor best be treated? Radiation? Surgery? Medication (bromocriptine, somatostatin analogue, etc.)? It is likely that these and similar important clinical questions have to be approached on a "one-on-one" basis. I doubt that only one standard approach to all patients with pituitary disease could be correct.

REFERENCES

1. Hofman, A. R., and Crowley, W. F.: Induction of puberty in men by long-term pusatile administration of low-dose gonadotropin-releasing hormone. N. Engl. J. Med., *307:*1237, 1982.
2. Hurley, D. M., et al.: Induction of ovulation and fertility in amenorrheic women by pulsatile low-dose gonadotropin-releasing hormone. N. Engl. J. Med., *310:*1069, 1984.
3. Comite, F., et al.: Short-term treatment of idiopathic precocious puberty with a long-acting analogue of luteinizing hormone-releasing hormone. N. Engl. J. Med., *305:*1546, 1981.
4. Hammond, C. B., and Ory, S. J.: Diagnostic and therapeutic uses of gonadotropin-releasing hormone. Arch. Intern. Med., *145:*1690, 1985.
5. Newmark, S. R.: Can the pituitary release adrenocorticotropic hormone during stress? Arch. Intern. Med., *143:*2248, 1983.
6. Chernow, B., et al.: Hormonal responses to graded surgical stress. Arch. Intern. Med., *147:*1273, 1987.
7. Jurney, T. H., et al.: Spectrum of serum cortisol response to ACTH in ICU patients. Chest, *92:*292, 1987.
8. Chopra, I. J., Hershman, J. M., Pardridge, W. M., and Nicoloff, J. T.: Thyroid function in nonthyroidal illnesses. Ann. Intern. Med., *98:*946, 1983.
9. Kaplan, M. M., et al.: Prevalence of abnormal thyroid function test results in patients with acute medical illnesses. Am. J. Med., *72:*9, 1982.
10. Woolf, P. D., et al.: Transient hypogonadotropic hypogonadism caused by critical illness. J. Clin. Endocrinol. Metabol., *60:*444, 1985.
11. Quint, A. R., and Kaiser, F. E.: Gonadotropin and determinations and thyrotropin-releasing hormone and luteinizing hormone-releasing hormone testing in critically ill postmenopausal women with hypothyroxinemia. J. Clin. Endocrinol. Metabol., *60:*464, 1985.
12. Finlay, W. E., and McKee, J. I.: Serum cortisol levels in severely stressed patients. Lancet, *1:*1414, 1982.
13. Hoogwerf, B. J., Sheeler, L. R., and Licata, A. L.: Endocrine management of the open heart surgical patient. Sem. Thorac. Cardiovasc. Surg., *3:*75, 1991.
14. Sheperd, F. A., Hoffert, B., and Evans, W. K.: Ketoconazole. Use in the treatment of ectopic adrenocorticotropic hormone production and Cushing's syndrome in small-cell lung cancer. Arch. Intern. Med., *145:*863, 1985.
15. Cunningham, S. K., Moore, A., and McKenna, T. J.: Normal cortisol response to corticotropin in patients with secondary adrenal failure. Arch. Intern. Med., *143:*2276, 1983.
16. Bermudez, F., Surks, M. I., and Oppenheimer, J. H.: High incidence of decreased serum triiodothyronine concentration in patients with nonthyroidal disease. J. Clin. Endocrinol. Metabol., *41:*27, 1975.
17. Wehmann, R. E., et al.: Suppression of thyrotropin in the low-thyroxine state of severe nonthyroidal illness. N. Engl. J. Med., *312:*546, 1985.
18. Kaptein, E. M., et al.: Thyroxine metabolism in the low thyroxine state of critical nonthyroidal illnesses. J. Clin. Endocrinol. Metabol., *53:*764, 1981.
19. Gardner, D. F., Carithers, R. L., and Utiger, R. D.: Thyroid function tests in patients with acute and resolved hepatitis B virus infection. Ann. Intern. Med., *96:*450, 1982.
20. Jackson, J. A., Verdonk, C. A., and Spiekerman, A. M.: Euthyroid hyperthyroxinemia and inappropriate secretion of thyrotropin. Arch. Intern. Med., *147:*1311, 1987.
21. Spratt, D. I., Pont, A., and Miller, M. B.: Hyperthyroxinemia in patients with acute psychiatric disorders. Am. J. Med., *73:*41, 1982.
22. LoPresti, J. S., Fried, J. C., and Spencer, C. A.: Unique alterations of thyroid hormone indices in the acquired immunodeficiency syndrome (AIDS). Ann. Intern. Med., *10:*970, 1989.
23. Bayer, M. F., Macoviak, J. A., and McDougall, I. R.: Diagnostic performance of sensitive measurements of serum thyrotropin during severe nonthyroidal illness: their role in the diagnosis of hyperthyroidism. Clin. Chem., *3:*2178, 1987.
24. Schutte, D. P., Vermaak, J. H., Zakolski, W. J., and Kalk, W. J.: High sensitivity thyrotrophin assays in patients with severe non-thyroidal illnesses: a first-line screening test. Med. Lib. Sci., *44:*312, 1987.
25. Slag, M. F., et al.: Free thyroxine levels in critically ill patients. JAMA, *246:*2702, 1981.
26. Faber, J., Kirkegaard, F. C., et al.: Pituitary-thyroid axis in critical illness. J. Clin. Endocrinol. Metab., *65:*315, 1987.
27. Vasely, D. L.: Recognizing and managing acute adrenal insufficiency. J. Crit. Illness, *3:*101, 1988.
28. Jacobs, T. P., Whitlock, R. T., Edsall, J., and Holub, D. A.: Addisonian crisis while taking high-dose glucocorticoids. JAMA, *260:*2082, 1988.
29. Nerup, J.: Addison's disease—clinical studies. A report of 108 cases. Acta. Endocrinol., *76:*127, 1974.

30. Vita, J. A., et al.: Clinical clues to the cause of Addison's disease. Am. J. Med., 78:461, 1985.
31. Sheeler, L. R., Myers, J. H., Eversman, J. J., and Taylor, H. C.: Adrenal insufficiency secondary to carcinoma metastatic to the adrenal gland. Cancer, 52:1312, 1983.
32. Liu, L., Haskin, M. E., Rose, L. I., and Bemis, C. E.: Diagnosis of bilateral adrenocortical hemorrhage by computed tomography. Ann. Intern. Med., 97:720, 1982.
33. Dorin, R. I., and Kearns, P. J.: High output circulatory failure in acute adrenal insufficiency. Crit. Care Med., 16:296, 1988.
34. Thomas, F.B., Mazzaferri, E. L., and Skillman, T. G.: Apathetic thyrotoxicosis: a distinctive clinical and laboratory entity. Ann. Intern. Med., 72:679, 1970.
35. Bennett, M. H., and Wainwright, A. P.: Acute thyroid crisis on induction of anaesthesia. Anaesthesia, 44:28, 1989.
36. Blum, M., Kranjac, T., and Park, C. M.: Thyroid storm after cardiac angiography with iodinated contrast medium. Occurrence in a patient with a previously euthyroid autonomous nodule of the thyroid. JAMA, 235:2324, 1976.
37. Oelkers, W.: Hyponatremia and inappropriate secretion of vasopressin (antidiuretic hormone) in patients with hypopituitarism. N. Engl. J. Med., 321:492, 1989.
38. Silberman, H., et al.: The relation of thyroid indices in the critically ill patient to prognosis and nutritional factors. Surg. Gynecol. Obstet., 166:223, 1988.
39. Gharib, H., and Abboud, C. F.: Primary idiopathic hypothalamic hypothyroidism. Am. J. Med., 83:171, 1987.
40. Arem, R., and Deppe, S.: Fatal nonthyroidal illness may impair nocturnal thyrotropin levels. Am. J. Med., 88:258, 1990.
41. Slag, M. F., et al.: Hypothyroxinemia in critically ill patients as a predictor of high mortality. JAMA, 245:43, 1981.
42. Hamblin, P. S., et al.: Relationship between thyrotropin and thyroxine changes during recovery from severe hypothyroxinemia of critical illness. J. Clin. Endocrinol. Metabol., 62:717, 1986.
43. Mackin, J. F., Canary, J. J., and Pittman, C. S.: Thyroid storm and its management. N. Engl. J. Med., 291:1396, 1974.
44. Sheller, L. R., Skillern, P. G., Schumacher, O. P., and Eversman, J. J.: Radioiodine-induced thyroid storm: a point of controversy. Am. J. Med., 76:A98, 1984.
45. Ehrmann, D. A., and Sarne, D. H.: Early identification of thyroid storm and myxedema coma. J. Crit. Illness, 3:111, 1988.
46. Yao, J. D., Gross, J. B., Ludwig, J., and Purnell, D. C.: Cholestatis jaundice in hyperthyroidism. Am. J. Med., 86:619, 1989.
47. Adrouny, A., Sandler, R. M., and Carmel, R.: Variable presentation of thrombocytopenia in Graves' disease. Arch. Intern. Med., 142:1460, 1982.
48. Caplan, R. H., Pagliara, A. S., and Wickus, G.: Thyroxine toxicosis. A common variant of hyperthyroidism. JAMA, 244:1934, 1980.
49. Lum, S., Kaptein, E. M., and Nicoloff, J. T.: Influence of nonthyroidal illnesses on serum thyroid hormone indices in hyperthyroidism. West. J. Med., 138:670, 1983.
50. Senior, R. M., Birge, S. J., Wessler, S., and Avioli, L. V.: The recognition and management of myxedema coma. JAMA, 217:61, 1971.
51. Mazonson, P. D., et al.: Myxedema coma during long-term amidarone therapy. Am. J. Med., 77:751, 1984.
52. Kaptein, E. M., et al.: Acute hemodynamic effects of levothyroxine loading in critically ill hypothyroid patients. Arch. Intern. Med., 146:662, 1986.
53. Impallomeni, M. G.: Unusual presentation of myxoedema coma in the elderly. Age Ageing, 6:71, 1977.
54. Knowlton, A. I.: Adrenal insufficiency in the intensive care setting. J. Intensive Care Med., 4:35, 1989.
55. Melby, J. C.: Adrenal insufficiency: a resurgence. J. Intensive Care Med., 4:2, 1989.

SUPPLEMENTAL READINGS

Arem, R., and Deppe, S.: Fatal nonthyroidal illness may impair nocturnal thyrotropin levels. Am. J. Med., 88:258, 1990.
Baeza, A., Aguayo, J., Barria, M., and Pineda, G.: Rapid perioperative preparation in hyperthyroidism. Clin. Endocrinol. Metabol., 35:439, 1991.
Behr, R., Hildebrandt, G., Koca, M., and Bruck, K.: Modifications of thermoregulation in patients with suprasellar pituitary adenomas. Brain, 114:697, 1992.
Butcher, G. P., Zambon, M., Moss, S., and Walters, J. R. F.: Addisonian crisis presenting with a normal short tetracosactrin stimulation test. Postgrad. Med. J., 68:465, 1992.
Hardy, K., Mead, B., and Gill, G.: Adrenal apoplexy after coronary artery bypass surgery leading to Addisonian crisis. J. R. Soc. Med., 85:577, 1992.
Kidess, A. I., et al.: Transient corticotropin deficiency in critical illness. Mayo Clin. Proc., 68:435, 1993.
Midgely, J. E. M., et al.: Concentration of free thyroxin and albumin in serum in severe nonthyroidal illness: assay artifacts and physiological influences. Clin. Chem., 36:765, 1990.
Naito, Y., et al.: Biphasic changes in hypothalamo-pituitary-adrenal function during the early recovery period after major abdominal surgery. J. Clin. Endocrinol. Metabol., 73:111, 1991.
Romijn, J. A., and Wiersinga, W. M.: Decreased nocturnal surge of thyrotropin in nonthyroidal illness. J. Clin. Endocrinol. Metabol., 70:35, 1990.
Span, L. F. R., et al.: Adrenocortical function: An indicator of severity of disease and survival in chronic critically ill patients. Intensive Care Med., 18:93, 1992.
Toshiaki, S., Kovacs, K., Scheithauer, B., and Young, W.: Aging and the human pituitary gland. Mayo Clin. Proc., 68:971, 1993.

Chapter 58

CALCIUM AND MAGNESIUM IN SERIOUS ILLNESS: A PRACTICAL APPROACH

PAUL L. MARINO

Consider what sodium is to a nephrologist, and potassium to a cardiologist, and that is what calcium and magnesium represent to critical care physicians. These electrolytes have been adopted by ICUs because they are abnormal in the majority of patients in these areas,[1] but these electrolyte abnormalities are shared by many patient populations. In fact, calcium and magnesium are now regarded as the leading two sources of abnormal electrolyte balance in hospitalized patients. The material in this chapter is taken mostly from the encyclopedia of observations on calcium and magnesium generated over the past decade, and it represents the practical aspects that can be useful at the bedside. As you will learn in the chapter, we have created as many problems as the illnesses (i.e., we have overlooked magnesium, creating a nuisance called magnesium deficiency, and have overused calcium, adding a risk for ischemia to a group of patients who already are at risk for ischemia). The goal of this chapter is to help correct these tendencies.

MAGNESIUM

Magnesium plays an important part in the aerobic energy cycle, participating in both the production of oxygen by plant photosynthesis, and the use of oxygen by aerobic life forms. In mammalian cells, magnesium is a catalyst for alkyl enzyme reactions that involve high energy phosphate compounds with at least 3009 different enzyme reactions using magnesium as a cofactor.[1] One of the magnesium-dependent enzyme systems is the ion pump in cells membranes that creates the electrical gradient across cell membranes and is responsible for generating all electrical impulses in excitable tissues.[2,3] Magnesium also regulates the movement of calcium into smooth muscle cells by acting as an antagonist to calcium inflow,[2,3] which gives magnesium a pivotal role in the control of vascular dynamics.

Magnesium Balance

The average adult contains about 24 g (1 mol) of magnesium, 1% of which is located in the interior of cells. The nonuniform distribution of magnesium in the adult human body shown in Table 58-1.[1] The bulk of these magnesium is in bone and soft tissue, whereas less than 1% is located in plasma.[1] The small fraction of total body magnesium found in the plasma indicates the limited value that monitoring serum magnesium levels will have for assessing total body magnesium content. This limits out knowledge of magnesium balance in pathologic states, since many of the clinical reports on magnesium have reported only the plasma values. The plasma magnesium is particularly limited as a marker of magnesium deficiency, and numerous reports exist of patients with normal serum magnesium levels who have evidence of magnesium deficiency by tissue levels.[1,4] In an effort to improve the assessment of magnesium stores, intracellular magnesium assays have been developed for erythrocytes and leukocytes, but these assays offer little advantage over the plasma for predicting total body magnesium status.[4]

Plasma Magnesium

The magnesium in plasma is present in three forms:

- An ionized form, which represents the functionally active form of the electrolyte
- A fraction that is bound to serum proteins, most of which is bound to albumin
- A fraction that forms chelates divalent anions in the plasma (e.g., phosphates and sulfates)

The relative contribution of each fraction to the total plasma magnesium pool is shown in Figure 58-1. The height of the column on the left indicates the total plasma magnesium, which is given a representative value of 1.7 mEq/L,[5] and the subdivisions are used to indicate the relative contribution of each fraction to the total plasma magnesium. The largest fraction is the ionized magnesium which accounts for 60% of the total plasma pool. The protein-bound fraction is the next largest at 25%, followed by the 15% that represents the chelate fraction of plasma magnesium.

The standard assay for magnesium in blood is based on light transmission (spectrophotometry), which measures all three fractions of magnesium in the blood. Therefore, when the magnesium level is reduced, it will be impossible to determine if the problem is a decrease in the ionized magnesium (the active form) or a decrease in the bound fractions (e.g., hypoproteinemia). Fortunately, there is little of the total body magnesium in the plasma, and this should limit the potential for error in hypoproteinemic states.[6] There are methods being developed to measure the ionized magnesium levels with ion-specific electrodes[7] and with ultrafiltration techniques,[8] but neither is available for clinical use at the present time. Since such a small fraction of magnesium is in the plasma, it seems that efforts to measure ionized magnesium will have little impact,

Table 58–1. Magnesium Distribution in the Adult

Tissue	Wet Weight (kg)	Mg Content (mmol)	Total Body Mg (%)
Bone	12.3	530	52.9
Muscle	30	270	27
Soft tissue	22.7	193	19.3
RBC	2.0	5.0	0.5
Plasma	3.0	2.6	0.3
TOTAL	70	1000.6	100

(From Elin, R.J.: Magnesium metabolism in health and disease. Dis. Mon., 34:161, 1988.)

Table 58–2. Reference Values for Magnesium and Calcium

Test	Normal Range
Serum magnesium*	0.7–1.0 mmol/L
	1.4–2.0 mEq/L
Urine magnesium	5–15 mEq/24h
Magnesium retention test	$\dfrac{\text{Urinary Mg}}{\text{Intravenous Mg}} > 0.8$
1. Add 15 mEq mg to 500 ml saline	
2. Infuse at 0.8 ml/min for 12 h	
3. Collect urine for 24 h	
Plasma calcium†	2.1–2.5 mmol/L
	8.5–10.2 mg/dl
Ionized calcium	1.1–1.3 mmol/L
	4.8–7.2 mg/dl

* Conversion factors 1mEq = 0.5 mmol = 12 mg
† Conversion factors: 1mEq = 0.5 mmol = 20 mg

however, in improving the reliability of the plasma magnesium as a measure of total body magnesium status.

Regulatory Mechanisms

The average intake of magnesium is 300 to 350 mg per day in healthy adults, but only 30 to 40% of the oral intake will be absorbed from the gastrointestinal tract.[9] When intake is altered, fractional absorption of magnesium changes in the opposite direction (i.e., fractional absorption can increase to 75% when intake is low, or can decrease to 25% when intake is excessive).[9] This helps control total body magnesium levels when intake is altered, but the amounts involved are small, and the bowel is not considered to play a major role in magnesium hemostasis.

The kidneys play a major role in magnesium regulations, and do so by adjusting urinary magnesium excretion to match the amount absorbed from the bowel each day.

When the magnesium balance is normal, urinary excretion will be 0.4 × (300 to 350 mg) or 120 to 140 mg per day. The normal range for urinary magnesium excretion is shown in Table 58-2 (note the conversion factors at the bottom of the table). Only small amounts of magnesium are excreted under normal circumstances, with most reabsorbed along the renal tubules. When magnesium intake is deficient, the kidneys conserve magnesium, and urinary excretion falls to negligible levels. This is shown in Figure 58-2, which is taken from a study where healthy adults were placed on a magnesium diet for 1 week.[10] Note that urinary magnesium excretion falls over the first days until it reaches negligible levels and remains there for the remainder of the study. Note also that the serum magnesium level remains normal in each subject throughout the study. This study illustrates the relative merits of the urine versus the blood for early detection of magnesium deficiency. The renal response to magnesium excess is also prompt, and will be described in more detail later in this chapter.

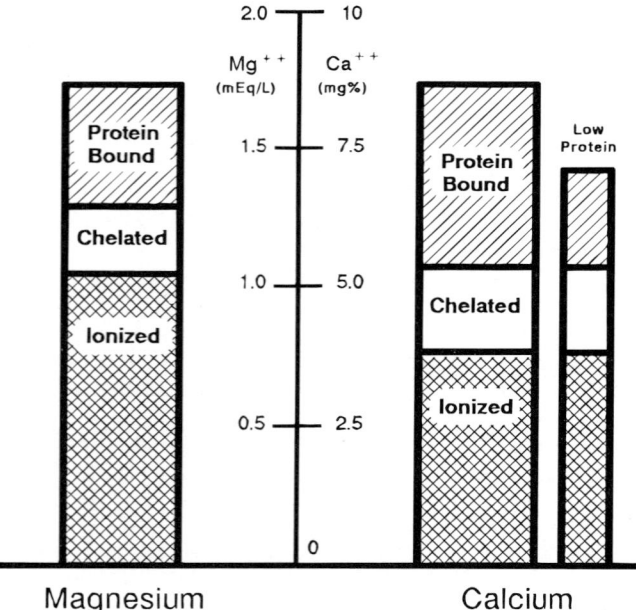

Fig. 58–1. Bar diagrams illustrating the fractions of plasma magnesium (left) and plasma calcium (right). The narrow column on the right illustrates the effect of hypoproteinemia. See text for explanation.

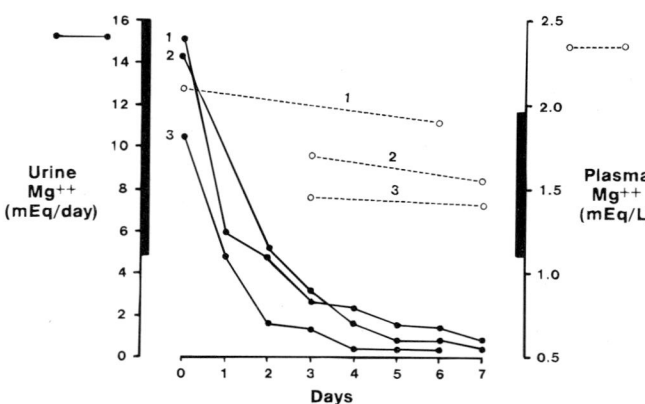

Fig. 58–2. Plasma and urine magnesium measured in three healthy adults during seven days of magnesium-free diet. Numbers identify individual subjects. Solid bars indicate the normal range for the urine and plasma magnesium. (From Shils, M. E.: Experimental human magnesium depletion. Medicine, 48:61, 1969.)

Laboratory Tests

The laboratory tests for assessing total body magnesium are limited, but the available tests are shown in Table 58-2 along with the normal values for each (note the conversion factors at the bottom of the table; they can be a source of confusion).

Serum Magnesium Concentration

Serum is favored over plasma for the magnesium assay because the anticoagulant used for plasma collections can be contaminated with citrate or other anions that bind magnesium. The normal range for the serum magnesium concentration in adults is 1.4 to 2.0 mEq/L or 0.7 to 1.0 mmol/L, as listed in Table 58-2.[5] The daily intake of magnesium differs in various parts of the world, and this can influence the range of normal values used as the standard reference range. Thus, the normal range in Table 58-2 is taken from a survey of healthy adults in the United States.[5] The serum magnesium also shows a circadian rhythm, with peak levels at 1200 hours, but the changes are small and should not push the serum levels outside the normal range.[11]

The magnesium concentration in erythrocytes is about three times greater than the serum concentration,[1] so that hemolysis can cause an increase in the serum magnesium. This can occur either in vivo from a pathologic process, or in vitro from trauma and cell disruption imposed by the blood collection. The pathologic variety of hemolysis can raise the serum magnesium by 0.05 mmol/L for each unit of red blood cells lysed,[1] so that massive hemolysis would be necessary to push the serum magnesium out of the normal range.

Urine Magnesium

In healthy adults with normal magnesium balance, the daily excretion of magnesium in the urine will be about the same as the dietary magnesium that is absorbed from the bowel. Assuming a magnesium intake of 300 mg daily and 40% absorption from the bowel, the range should be 120 mg or 10 mEq of magnesium excreted daily in the urine. The normal range for urinary magnesium is shown in Table 58-2. When magnesium intake is reduced, this urinary excretion will become even smaller (see Fig. 58-2), and in the proper patient population, urinary magnesium excretion can be a sensitive marker of magnesium intake. The test requires normal renal function, however, and the absence of other factors that could promote urinary magnesium losses, which is unlikely to occur in the patient population served by this text. The urinary levels can be used, however, to monitor daily magnesium losses to help design replacement protocols, or the urinary levels can be measured in response to an intravenous magnesium load, as described next.

The urinary magnesium excretion in response to intravenous infusion of magnesium can be a valuable test for uncovering magnesium deficiency.[12,13] As indicated in Table 58-2, the **magnesium retention test** involves the infusion of a known quantity of magnesium intravenously for 12 hours, and the percentage recovered in the urine is used to identify a magnesium deficient or "magnesium avid" state. As explained earlier, because the normal rate of magnesium reabsorption is close to the maximum tubular reabsorption rate (Tmax), most of the infused magnesium will be excreted in the urine in normal subjects. In magnesium deficiency, however, the baseline reabsorptive rate is much lower than Tmax, so more of the infused magnesium will be reabsorbed and less excreted in the urine. The cutoff in the test is 80%, so recovery of less than 80% of the infused dose in the urine would indicate a magnesium deficient state. This test has proven valuable for identifying patients who are magnesium deficient,[12,13] but the clinical experience with this test is limited at the present time.

Magnesium Deficiency

Magnesium is one of the more common electrolyte abnormalities encountered in hospitalized patients, and has also been described as "the most underdiagnosed electrolyte abnormality in current medical practice."[14] The problem has several causes, but like most deficiency states, it represents a "physician deficiency" that allowed the condition to develop.

Pre-ICU Phase

Surveillance studies have uncovered hypomagnesemia in as many as 50% of hospitalized patients,[15] and up to 65% of admissions to ICUs.[16,17] Assuming the magnesium depletion is not always accompanied by hypomagnesemia (as explained earlier), this means that magnesium depletion may be universal in hospitalized patients, particularly those in ICUs. This emphasizes the importance of recognizing magnesium deficiency and promptly replacing any deficits that are uncovered.

Predisposing Conditions. Most cases of magnesium deficiency are caused by an increase in magnesium excretion that is allowed to continue without replacement therapy. The following clinical conditions or situations will signal high risk patients that need to be monitored carefully and (unless contraindicated) started on magnesium replacement. These disorders are listed at the top of Figure 58-3.

Diuretic Therapy. Diuretics are considered by many to be the leading cause of magnesium deficiency in clinical practice. The agents that block sodium reabsorption also interfere with magnesium reabsorption, and the resultant loss of magnesium in the urine can parallel urinary sodium losses. The most potent of the diuretics in this regard are the "loop diuretics" (e.g., furosemide). At least 50% of patients receiving long-term therapy with furosemide for heart failure will develop magnesium deficiency if magnesium losses are not replaced.[18] As a result magnesium replacement is recommended for all patients receiving loop diuretics (unless they have renal insufficiency) to prevent significant deficits in total body magnesium. This is the same strategy that is currently used to prevent potassium depletion during diuretic therapy. The thiazide diuretics are not as prone to produce magnesium deficiency except in elderly patients,[19] and the "potassium-sparing" agents (e.g., triamterene) are not considered to pose a risk for magnesium depletion.[20]

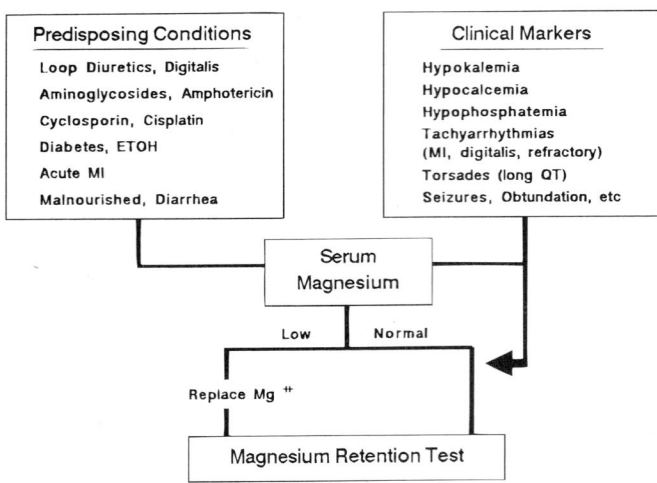

Fig. 58-3. Chart showing the risk factors used to justify serum magnesium testing, and the use of the urine retention test in select patients. See text for explanation.

Antibiotic Therapy. The antibiotics that pose a risk are the aminoglycosides,[21] amphotericin,[22] or pentamidine.[23] Aminoglycosides can block magnesium reabsorption in the ascending loop of Henle, and hypomagnesemia has been reported in 38% of patients during aminoglycoside therapy.[18] The other risk from antibiotics is their propensity for producing diarrhea, which can lead to significant magnesium losses in the stool (see discussion later in this chapter).

Other Drugs. A variety of drugs have been associated with magnesium depletion including digitalis,[24] adrenergic agents,[25] and chemotherapy with cisplatin[26] and cyclosporine.[27] The first two agents shift magnesium into cells, whereas the later two increase renal magnesium excretion.

Alcohol-Related Illness. Alcohol is a common cause of magnesium deficiency, and this is often apparent on admission or early in the hospital stay. Hypomagnesemia is reported in 30% of hospital admissions or early in the hospital stay. Hypomagnesemia is reported in 30% of hospital admissions associated with alcohol abuse, and in 85% of admissions for delirium tremens.[28,29] The magnesium depletion in these conditions is due to a number of factors, including a generalized malnutrition and a tendency to chronic diarrhea. In addition, there is an association between magnesium deficiency and thiamine deficiency.[30] Magnesium is required for the transformation of thiamine into thiamine pyrophosphate, so magnesium deficiency can promote a thiamine deficient state, even in the face of adequate thiamine intake. In fact, magnesium depletion can cause a thiamine deficiency which is refractory to thiamine replacement therapy until the magnesium deficit is replenished. For this reason, any patient with thiamine deficiency should have a thorough search for magnesium deficiency and should receive immediate magnesium replacement when indicated.

Secretory Diarrhea. Diarrhea can lead to significant losses as a result of the high concentration of magnesium (10 to 14 mEq/L) in secretions from the lower intestinal tract.[31] Upper tract secretions are not rich in magnesium (1 to 2 mEq/L), so that vomiting does not pose the same risk for magnesium depletion as diarrhea. Osmotic diarrhea should not be associated with exaggerated magnesium loss, but diarrhea from tube feedings might aggravate a magnesium deficient state by limiting magnesium absorption from the intestinal tract.

Diabetes Mellitus. Insulin-dependent diabetes mellitus is almost always associated with magnesium depletion, with the magnitude of magnesium depletion being inversely proportional to the degree of glucose control.[32] Hypomagnesemia is reported in only 7% of admissions for diabetic ketoacidosis, but can increase to 50% over the first 12 hours after admission,[33] probably as a result of insulin-induced movement of magnesium into cells or solute-induced magnesium excretion in urine.

Clinical Markers. In addition to the predisposing conditions just described, certain clinical signs can be markers of an underlying magnesium deficiency. Many of the clinical signs that follow will either represent a magnesium deficient state or will benefit from magnesium infusion. Therefore, the presence of these signs should prompt a search for magnesium deficiency, or a trial of magnesium therapy, or both. Many of the signs described are listed in Figure 58-3.

Hypokalemia. Hypokalemia has been reported in 40% of patients with hypomagnesemia,[34] and is considered to be the result rather than the cause of the magnesium deficit. Intracellular magnesium blocks the outward movement of potassium from cells,[2-4] and deficient intracellular magnesium will lead to potassium egress from cells. In renal tubular cells, this leads to potassium movement into the tubular fluid and loss in the urine. The final result will be a reduction in total body potassium. The hallmark of hypokalemia from magnesium depletion is its refractory behavior when attempting repletion (because potassium will not stay in cells) despite even the most aggressive regimens for potassium repletion.[35] Magnesium deficits must be replenished first to hold the potassium in the cells which will permit repletion of the potassium deficit.

Hypocalcemia. Hypocalcemia is reported in 20 to 30% of patients with hypomagnesemia[34] and is due to impaired parahormone release[36] combined with impaired endo-organ response to parahormone.[37] In addition, magnesium deficiency may act directly on bone to reduce calcium release, independent of parathyroid hormone.[38] The hypocalcemia from magnesium depletion behaves like the hypokalemia in that it is difficult to correct unless magnesium deficits are repleted. Thus, whenever hypocalcemia is identified, a serum magnesium should be obtained. If the hypocalcemia is associated with hypomagnesemia, the magnesium deficit should be replaced first and often the hypocalcemia will correct spontaneously without calcium supplementation.

Hypophosphatemia. Hypophosphatemia is reported in 30% of patients with hypomagnesemia.[36] The primary disorder in this setting is the phosphate depletion, which enhances renal magnesium excretion.[39] Therefore, when hypophosphatemia and hypomagnesemia coexist, replenish phosphate stores before attempting to correct the magnesium deficit.

Neurologic Syndromes. The neurologic manifestations of magnesium deficiency include:

- Altered mentation (from delirium to coma)
- Generalized seizures
- Tremors
- Chvostek and Trousseau signs

All are uncommon, nonspecific, and of relatively little value in heightening suspicion for magnesium deficiency.

A neurologic syndrome has been described recently that can abate with magnesium therapy, and this deserves mention. The clinical presentation is characterized by ataxia, slurred speech, metabolic acidosis, excessive salivation, diffuse muscle spasms, generalized seizures, and progressive obtundation.[40,41] The clinical features are often brought out by loud noises or bodily contact, and thus the term "reactive central nervous system magnesium deficiency."[40] A similar syndrome called "grass tetany" has been described in grazing cattle after ingesting large quantities of calcium-rich grass. The mechanism is complex, and is believed result from prolonged magnesium depletion aggravated by a sudden increase in serum calcium, which leads to deposition of plasma magnesium in bone. This further reduces the plasma magnesium and leads to compensatory movement of magnesium out of the cerebrospinal fluid. This leads to a decline in magnesium in cerebrospinal fluid, and is considered to be the trigger for the neurologic syndrome. This explanation is supported by reports of low cerebrospinal fluid magnesium levels in this syndrome, and by the clinical benefit seen after infusion of magnesium.[40] The prevalence of this neurologic syndrome is unknown at the present time, as is the validity of the proposed mechanism.

ICU Phase

The last group of clinical markers are conditions that appear in an ICU setting, and so the discussion of them is included in the ICU phase section. All involve cardiac events.

Cardiac Manifestations. These manifestations include myocardial infarction, digitalis toxicity, and refractory cardiac arrhythmias.

Acute Myocardial Infarction. Myocardial infarction has an interesting association with hypomagnesemia that may have therapeutic implications. As many as 80% of patients with acute myocardial infarction will have hypomagnesemia in the first 48 hours after the event.[42] The mechanism is not clear, but may be due to an intracellular shift of magnesium produced by catecholamines released in the peri-infarction period.[43] Intravenous magnesium given in the early period after infarction has been successful in reducing the incidence of serious arrhythmias,[42-45] and has been associated with a decrease in mortality.[44] The arrhythmia suppression seen with magnesium has been independent of the serum magnesium level,[43-45] suggesting that magnesium may be working as a nonspecific membrane stabilizer, in keeping with its actions as a cofactor for the ion pump that maintains the polarity across cell membranes and prevents spontaneous depolarization.

The experience with magnesium in acute MI is exciting in light of the improved survival associated with magnesium infusions in the early peri-infarction period. One possible mechanism for the benefit is the vasodilator action of magnesium, particularly if they involve the coronary arteries. As mentioned early in this chapter, magnesium blocks calcium influx into vascular smooth muscle,[2,3] which can produce significant vasodilatation. This makes magnesium a potential coronary vasodilator. Magnesium deficiency has been associated with coronary artery spasm[46] and a recent study has uncovered magnesium deficiency in patients with variant angina,[13] so it is possible that magnesium has benefits via coronary vasodilator actions. Another benefit might come from systemic vasodilatation since magnesium has been shown to dilate arteries but not veins,[47] which would reduce left ventricular afterload and reduce myocardial stroke work.

Digitalis Cardiotoxicity. This disorder is much more prominent in the setting of magnesium deficiency because both digitalis and magnesium deficiency inhibit the ATPase pump in cardiac cell membranes. This means that magnesium deficiency will always magnify the digitalis effect and promote toxicity. Hypomagnesemia has been reported in 20% of patients on digitalis therapy,[24] which is twice the frequency of hypokalemia in combination with digitalis therapy.[24] Intravenous magnesium is well known for being effective in suppressing digitalis-toxic arrhythmias, even when serum magnesium levels are normal.[48,49] Although it is impossible to determine if this is a specific or nonspecific effect, magnesium is effective in this setting, and should be considered in patients with suspected digitalis-associated arrhythmias, even when serum magnesium levels are normal.

Refractory Arrhythmias. Arrhythmias that are unresponsive to traditional therapeutic agents have been abolished by intravenous magnesium,[50] and this effect is also independent of the serum magnesium level. A serious arrhythmia for which magnesium has proven to be of value is "polymorphous ventricular tachycardia" (torsades de pointes), which is easily abolished by intravenous magnesium if it is associated with a prolonged QT interval.[51] In fact, magnesium has been suggested as the therapy of choice for torsades,[45] because it is much safer and less involved than the traditional approach to this arrhythmia that uses heart rate acceleration with either isoproterenol or cardiac pacing.

Diagnosis. The serum magnesium is not used as a screening test for all patients coming into the ICU, but is reserved for patients with a risk of magnesium deficiency, and particularly for patients who have clinical manifestations of magnesium deficiency (see Fig. 58-3). The serum magnesium test is not used as a screening test because it lacks the features required of a successful screening test. That is, a screening test should detect all patients with an illness, and to do this it must have a very high "sensitivity" (i.e., always abnormal in the presence of disease). A test with a low sensitivity, like the serum magnesium test, can be normal in the presence of disease, so that it can miss patients with the illness and will not function as an effective screening test. On the other hand, the serum magnesium test has a high "specificity" (only abnormal in the presence of disease), and this type of test is well suited for groups of patients with a high probability of disease. Thus, the correct use of the serum magnesium test is to reserve it for patients who are at risk for magnesium deficiency. When a patient has a normal serum magnesium level but has other signs of magnesium deficiency, the magnesium retention test should be considered (see Fig. 58-3).

Magnesium Replacement Therapy. The magnesium preparations available for oral and parenteral use are listed in Table 58-3.[52,53] Oral replacement can be associated with erratic absorption, and intravenous replacement is always favored when prompt replacement is desirable. The intravenous preparation favored in most situations is the magnesium sulfate ($MgSO_4$), available as a 50% solution (500 mg/ml) that must be diluted to a strength of 10% (100 mg/ml) or 20% (200 mg/ml) to minimize local irritation from extravasation. Magnesium chloride is recommended when hypocalcemia is also present, because the sulfate in $MgSO_4$ can bind calcium and aggravate the hypocalcemia.[51] Magnesium solutions should not be diluted with Ringer's solution because the calcium in Ringer's solution will counteract the actions of the magnesium, thereby erasing the benefit.

Replacement Protocols. Specific suggestions for magnesium replacement are shown in Table 58-4.[53] These are designed only for patients with normal renal functions. When renal insufficiency is present, it is wise not to infuse magnesium aggressively unless there are life-threatening reactions. The doses suggested can be reduced by 50% in renal insufficiency,[53] but acute replacement is not wise unless absolutely necessary.

Patients with mild hypomagnesemia (i.e., serum Mg > 1 mEq/L) and no clinical manifestations of a deficiency state can be treated with an oral regimen using a dose of 0.5 mEq/kg ideal body weight. Patients with a more severe deficiency state (i.e., serum Mg < 1 mEq/L) should receive parenteral replacement therapy. In the absence of clinical signs of severe deficiency, a standard regimen starting with 1 mEq/kg on the first day (see Table 58-4) should suffice.

Table 58-3. Oral and Parenteral Magnesium Preparations

	Elemental Magnesium	
	mg	mEq
Oral Tablets		
Magnesium chloride enteric-coated tablets	64	5.3
Magnesium oxide (400 mg)	241	19.8
Magnesium oxide (140 mg)	85	6.9
Magnesium gluconate (500 mg)	27	2.3
	mg/ml	mEq/L
Parenteral Solutions		
Magnesium sulfate* (20%)	0.2	16.6
Magnesium chloride (20%)	1.9	23.6

* Stocked as 50% solution, and must be diluted to 20% before intravenous administration.

Table 58-4. Magnesium Therapy

Condition	Regimen
	Oral
Asymptomatic and serum Mg* = 1–2 mEq/L	0.4 mEq/kg/d or 2 mEq/g Nitrogen/d
	Parenteral
Asymptomatic and serum Mg* <1 mEq/L	1 mEq/kg IV over first 24 h, then 0.5 mEq/kg IV every 24 h × 5 d
Hypomagnesemia plus hypocalcemia or serum K = 3–3.5 mEq/L	6 g IV over 3 h, then 5 g IV over next 6 h, then 5 g IV every 12 h × 5 d
Seizures or ventricular arrhythmias* or hypomagnesemia plus serum K <3 mEq/L	2 g IV over 2 min, then 5 g IV over next 6 h, then 5 g IV every 12 h × 5 days

* Refractory, polymorphous (prolonged QT), associated with acute MI or digitalis IV regimens (From Oster, J. R., and Epstein, M.: Management of magnesium depletion. Am. J. Nephrol., *8*:349, 1988.

Ongoing losses should also be determined with a urine magnesium on the first day. The serum level may correct in 1 to 2 days, but it will take about 5 days to completely replenish ion stores.[53]

Then hypomagnesemia is complicated by life-threatening conditions, rapid intravenous administration (e.g., 2 g $MgSO_4$ over 2 to 3 minutes) is effective and has proven safe.[53] The bolus dose lasts only 15 minutes, and must be followed with a continuous infusion. There is a risk for hypotension with rapid infusion of magnesium,[54] but it is uncommon. In fact, there is little agreement at the present time on what infusion rate is acceptable, and recommended rates have varied widely from 10 to 40 g per hour.[54,55] The recommendations in Table 58-4 have been used in my ICUs for the past 3 or 4 years without a single instance of a deleterious effect.

Monitoring Replacement Therapy. The serum magnesium should be monitored periodically, but valves can be misleading because serum levels will often correct in the first day or two of replacement, yet total body stores will require 5 days or longer to replenish.[53] The "magnesium retention test" can become a valuable aid in this setting, and is recommended at the end of the 5-day regimen to determine if the replacement is complete (as in Fig. 58-3). Once completed, maintenance therapy should be started to avert another bout of magnesium depletion.

Post-ICU Phase

Maintenance Therapy. Daily provision of magnesium is a requirement for all patients with adequate renal functions, and the Food and Nutrition Board sets the recommended dietary requirement (RDA) at 5 mg/kg ideal body weight (or 0.4 mEq/kg) for adults.[55] The RDA has been adjusted upward to 10 mg/kg/per day for optimal results,[56] but this has been tested only in healthy outpatients, and does not seem advised for ill hospitalized patients who are prone to cardiovascular and renal compromise.

Nutritional Support Methods. Enteral tube feedings that have a standard caloric density of 1 kcal/ml will contain about 200 mg (16 mEq) magnesium in each liter, and this should provide the daily requirement if the daily volume of feeding solution is 1.5 L or higher. The problem with enteral replacement is the risk for inadequate absorption, particularly in ICU patients, who are prone to atrophy of the bowel mucosa from prolonged bowel rest or prior hemodynamic compromise.

Parenteral nutrition solutions have commercial electrolyte mixtures added in fixed amounts, and they provide magnesium at 5 mEq/L, which for most nutritional regimens corresponds to 8 to 10 mEq per day if standard calories were delivered. This is adequate for daily requirements in normal adults, but may be inadequate for replacing deficits or ongoing losses. Supplements can be added to the feeding solutions as needed.

Oral Supplements. When possible, oral supplements should be used for hospitalized patients on full oral feedings to correct the erratic intake that is so often seen in hospitalized patients. Some oral magnesium preparations that are currently available are listed in Table 58-3. The comparative absorption of different magnesium salts is not studied, and there is no preferred oral preparation at the present time.

Hypermagnesemia

Magnesium excess is much less common than magnesium deficiency, with one study reporting 5.7% of hospitalized patients with hypermagnesemia versus 47% of the same population with hypomagnesemia.[15] Hypermagnesemia also has fewer sources, fewer clinical manifestations, and has a serum magnesium test that is a reliable marker of magnesium status.

Pre-ICU Phase

Renal Insufficiency. The dominant risk factor for hypermagnesemia is renal insufficiency, and the problem begins to appear when the creatinine clearance dips below 30 ml per minute.[57] The renal insufficiency is usually combined with excessive intake of magnesium, classically in the form of magnesium-containing antacids or cathartics. The therapy of preeclampsia often produces hypermagnesemia, at least transiently, because of the large doses of magnesium that are used (4 to 6 g MgSO$_4$ as an IV bolus, followed by an infusion 1 to 4 g per hour). Other predisposing conditions include:[57]

- Diabetic ketoacidosis
- Pheochromocytoma
- Adrenal insufficiency
- Hyperparathyroidism
- Lithium

ICU Phase

Hypermagnesemia often goes unsuspected on clinical grounds, and the diagnosis is first suspected when a laboratory test result is abnormal. The serum magnesium is reliable as a marker of magnesium excess, which is very different from the poor performance of blood levels in magnesium deficiency.

Clinical Markers. Hypermagnesemia is defined as a serum magnesium of 2.0 mEq/L (1.0 mmol/L) or higher. Clinical events can occur in relationship to the serum level as follows:[57]

- Hyporeflexia at levels of 2.0 mEq/L (1.0 mmol/L) and higher
- Hypotension at levels of 5.0 mEq/L (2.5 mmol/L; only transiently at this level)
- Prolonged QT interval and atrioventricular block at 10 mEq/L (5 mmol/L)
- Complete heart block at 12.5 mEq/L (6.25 mmol/L)
- Respiratory depression at 13 mEq/L (6.5 mmol/L)

Management. Hemodialysis is recommended by many as the first line of therapy, but intravenous calcium gluconate (1 g IV over 2 to 3 minutes) can reverse the cardiovascular and respiratory toxicity temporarily. An infusion of calcium gluconate (15 mg/kg elemental calcium infused over 4 hours) will help temporarily, until dialysis is available.[54,57] If fluids are permissible, aggressive volume infusion combined with furosemide may be effective in reducing the serum magnesium levels acutely. Dialysis should be anticipated in any case of severe complications, regardless of improvement during short-term therapy, because the toxicity tends to be prolonged, and there is a risk for recurrence that can be prevented by eliminating magnesium with dialysis.

CALCIUM

Calcium is similar to magnesium in that it is often deficient, but is also often without any clinical consequence. When one infuses calcium, however, the margin of safety may not be the same as calcium infusion, which can promote vasoconstriction and ischemia (see discussion later in this chapter). Calcium has a central role in muscle contraction where it links contractile elements together and permits muscle fibers to shorten during active contraction.[58,59] Smooth muscle contraction requires calcium movement into cells from extracellular fluid. Although there have been occasional reports of calcium levels correlating with cardiac contraction[60] or vascular smooth muscle contraction,[57] these reports are uncommon. The lack of influence of hypocalcemia and hypercalcemia on muscle contraction remains an enigma.

Calcium also participates in neuromuscular transmission as a cofactor in the coagulation cascade, blood coagulation, and is partly responsible for the structural integrity of bone. There is no documented ability for these actions to become expressed as clinically significant other than the role of these actions on bone rigidity.[58] The influence that calcium exerts on muscle contraction, however, overshadows any other effect in the seriously ill patient.

Plasma Calcium

Calcium differs from magnesium in favoring the extracellular fluid, with a ratio of 10,000:1 defining extracellular to intracellular concentration.[59] The plasma calcium is present in three forms (the same ones described earlier for magnesium):

- Free or ionized fraction
- Protein-bound fraction

- Fraction representing calcium chelates with sulfates and phosphates

The relative size of each plasma fraction is illustrated in Figure 58-1, using 9.0 mg/dl as a representative plasma calcium. The largest fraction (45%) is the biologically active ionized fraction, with the protein-bound fraction close behind (40%). As with magnesium, the laboratory assay for plasma calcium measures all three fractions, and it can be misleading when protein binding is altered. The influence of protein binding on the plasma calcium is shown in Figure 58-1. The column indicating hypoproteinemia shows an equivalent decrease in the protein-bound calcium and the "total" plasma calcium, with no change in the ionized fraction. Because only the ionized fraction is biologically active, the drop in total calcium in this case does not represent true hypocalcemia, and could be misinterpreted without a specific measure of ionized calcium. Raising the total calcium 0.8 mg/dl for each 1 mg/dl decrease in serum albumin below 4.0 mg/dl has been recommended as a correction factor,[58,59] but this has not proven reliable.[60]

Ionized calcium, an ion-specific electrode for calcium, is available in many clinical laboratories, with this method being the gold standard for identifying hypo- and hypercalcemia. The normal range for total and ionized calcium is shown in Table 58-2. Ionized calcium is usually expressed in mmol/L, whereas total calcium is mg/dl. The following conditions can cause spurious reading of ionized calcium:

- Acid pH (alkaline pH has the opposite effect)
- Anticoagulants that bind calcium
- Plasma sodium concentrations
- Temperature of blood sample

Acid pH will decrease calcium binding to serum proteins thereby increasing the ionized fraction, whereas alkaline pH will have the opposite effect.[58,59] Therefore, a blood sample that is allowed to sit and accumulate carbon dioxide from blood cell metabolism will generate a spurious increase in ionized calcium. To minimize the influence of carbon dioxide, the blood sample should be collected in anaerobic containers and transported directly to the laboratory, where cells are separated by centrifugation.

Anticoagulants like citrate can bind calcium and cause a spurious decrease in ionized calcium.

Plasma sodium concentration (i.e., hyponatremia increases calcium binding to proteins and will decrease the ionized calcium, whereas hypernatremia has the opposite effect).[59]

Temperature of the blood sample can increase the ionized calcium if it approaches room temperature. The ionized calcium measurement must not sit for any length of time prior to the assay.

Calcium Homeostasis

The ionized calcium is maintained within a narrow range in the blood, through the interplay of three processes:

- Calcium absorption from the gut
- Calcium exchange with bone
- Calcium excretion

These processes are controlled by parathyroid hormone and vitamin D, and are influenced by a host of other factors, some of which are described in the following paragraphs. Bowel absorption plays a minor role in calcium homeostasis, as only 10 to 15% of the calcium ingested orally is absorbed from the bowel.[58] Altered bone exchange and renal calcium excretion are responsible for most cases of hypo- and hypercalcemia.

Hypocalcemia

Pre-ICU Phase

As many as two thirds of patients admitted to ICUs have a subnormal total serum calcium concentration.[61-63] Ionized hypocalcemia may be much less common, with one study reporting ionized hypocalcemia in only 12% of ICU admissions.[62] As with magnesium, the first stage in the evaluation of hypocalcemia is to identify high risk patients with the following condition being most common:

- Magnesium depletion
- Alkalosis
- Sepsis
- Renal failure

Note that parathyroid disease is not included as a common cause of hypocalcemia in hospitalized patients.

Magnesium Depletion. Magnesium deficiency produces hypocalcemia by reducing both the secretion and the end-organ efficacy of parahormone (see earlier discussion). Because magnesium depletion enhances renal calcium excretion, calcium given as replacement therapy will be excreted in the urine. As a result, the hypocalcemia from magnesium depletion is refractory to calcium replacement therapy, thus this observation can provide the diagnosis. Repletion of the magnesium often corrects the serum calcium spontaneously.

Alkalosis. A rapid rise in plasma pH increases the anionic equivalency of albumin thereby promotes calcium binding to the albumin. This can reduce ionized calcium by as much as 0.2 mg/dl for each 0.1 unit rise in pH.[58] Alkalosis is common in the ICU with the common culprits for metabolic alkalosis being diuretics and nasogastric suction, while respiratory alkalosis arises from mechanical ventilation and sepsis.

Sepsis. Sepsis can produce hypocalcemia through several mechanisms, including alkalosis, calcium loss from the microcirculation, and depressed parahormone secretion.[64] The hypocalcemia is usually mild (0.8 to 1.0 mm/L) and should not be replaced unless there is hypotension requiring pharmacologic support. Replacement is probably unwise unless necessary because calcium can accumulate in cells during sepsis, and calcium replacement might aggravate the problem and lead to calcium-mediated cell destruction. The prognosis in sepsis is worse when hypocalcemia is also present.[64]

Renal Failure. The hypocalcemia of renal failure is primarily the result of phosphorous retention, with a minor component from reduced absorption of calcium from the gut. The acidosis that accompanies renal failure will decrease calcium binding to serum proteins which tends to maintain the ionized calcium fraction and protect against symptomatic hypocalcemia. Since calcium infusion is not advised in the face of hyperphosphatemia because of the risk of precipitation of calcium phosphate, hypocalcemia associated with renal failure is never corrected if there are no life-threatening signs of hypocalcemia.

Miscellaneous. The other causes of hypocalcemia that deserve mention are:[59]

- Pancreatitis
- Burns
- Fat embolism syndrome
- Massive blood transfusion
- Cardiopulmonary bypass
- Burns
- Drugs

Pancreatitis and burns are associated with depressed parahormone secretion, and the mechanism in fat embolism syndrome is calcium binding by free fatty acids that are abundant in the blood. Calcium binding by the citrate preservative in banked blood is the presumed culprit in massive transfusion. The medications that can be involved[65] act either by suppressing parahormone secretion (e.g., nitroprusside, propranolol, and cimetidine), or by interfering with bone resorption (e.g., steroids, theophylline, indomethacin, protamine).

ICU Phase

Clinical Signs. The harmful effects of hypocalcemia are confined to the cardiovascular and neuromuscular systems. Fortunately, most patients with mild or moderate hypocalcemia tolerate the condition without apparent ill effect.

Cardiovascular Signs. A few clinical studies have shown the expected relationship between blood pressure, myocardial contractility, and plasma-ionized calcium in hospitalized patients.[66,67] Plasma calcium levels have little influence, however, on cardiac output or vascular tone in most patients, and there is no consistent response to calcium infusion which can be demonstrated.[68] Hypocalcemia also prolongs the QT interval which can pose a risk for ventricular dysrhythmia, but documentation is lacking in this area.

Neuromuscular Signs. Calcium participates in transmission of electrical impulses across the neuromuscular junction, but muscle weakness is not a prominent feature in hypocalcemia, at least weakness that is demonstrable in the ICU setting. Hypocalcemia can also depolarize cell membranes and could produce neuromuscular excitability. Exaggerated deep tendon reflexes and the Chvostek and Trousseau signs are invariably mentioned as manifestations of hypocalcemia, but these are overemphasized. The Chvostek sign can be absent in 30% of patients with hypocalcemia, whereas it is present in 25% of patients without hypocalcemia.[60] Trousseau sign is equally insensitive and nonspecific. The presence of these signs should prompt a search for hypocalcemia and prompt therapy if needed, however.

Calcium Replacement The intravenous infusion of calcium can promote unwanted ischemia and organ damage in seriously ill patients, particularly those with hemodynamic compromise and ongoing ischemia. In the seriously ill patient population, calcium replacement should be reserved for patients with a documented need for replacement. The potential for harm from calcium is presented here briefly.

Postresuscitation Syndrome. Successful resuscitation of cardiac arrest or hemorrhagic shock, usually defined as restoration of blood pressure, does not always indicate return to premorbid organ function. Organ injury that is sustained during the ischemic period can persist or progress in the postresuscitation period, culminating in the syndrome of "multi-organ system failure" which is often fatal. Two explanations have been proposed for this postresuscitation injury response, and calcium is implicated in both.

The No-Reflow Phenomenon. The earliest explanation for postresuscitation organ injury is called the no-reflow phenomenon,[70] which is a persistent vasoconstriction in the systemic circulation that persists after the blood pressure is resuscitated in patients with hypotension or cardiopulmonary arrest. The mechanism is believed to be due to intense vasoconstriction produced by calcium influx into vascular smooth muscle cells across cell membranes that have been damaged by ischemia.[71] The final result is prolonged ischemia to all organs and multiorgan failure. This theory is supported by reports of intracellular calcium accumulation during periods of shock,[72] by the observed association between intracellular calcium accumulation and multiorgan failure,[73] and by reports showing that calcium-channel blocker therapy can reduce the severity of postresuscitation organ damage.[74] The existence of postresuscitation vasoconstriction is far from proven, however, and the benefit from calcium blockers is not consistent.[75]

Reperfusion Injury. The other mechanism for postresuscitation injury involves toxins like the metabolites of oxygen, which are believed to accumulate in areas of ischemia and, when flow is resumed, are carried to distant sites and produce widespread damage. This mechanism is called reperfusion injury,[76] which differs from the no-reflow phenomenon in that blood flow is restored after the resuscitation period. Calcium influx across damaged smooth muscle membranes may also play a role in this process because calcium can promote the formation of oxygen metabolites.[77] Reperfusion injury is largely unproven at the present time, but it is an area of intense interest and will certainly be clarified in the next few years.

Intravenous Replacement. The risks associated with calcium infusion in patients with ongoing or recent ischemia should limit the use of calcium in these patients. In addition, patients with hypocalcemia and hyperphosphatemia should not receive intravenous calcium because of the risk for precipitation of calcium phosphate crystals. Table 58–5 shows the parenteral calcium solutions available and the infusion rates that should correct the serum calcium in 12 hours. Calcium solutions should be administered through large central veins to limit local irritation which is characteristic of these solutions. If given through a peripheral vein, the line should be free flowing. Neither calcium chloride nor calcium gluconate should be given intramuscularly. When the hypocalcemia is corrected,

Table 58–5. Parenteral Calcium Therapy

Solution	Unit Size (ml vials)	Calcium Content (mg)	(mEq)	Max Infusion Rate (ml/min)
Calcium chloride	10	272	13.6	1.0
Calcium gluconate	10	90	4.5	0.5
Calcium gluceptate	5	90	4.5	0.5

Preparation:
  Dilute one vial in 100 ml D5W, and warm to body temperature to minimize precipitation
Dosage:
  Initial dose: 250 mg infused over 10 minutes (30 min during digitalis Rx)
  Maintenance dose: 1–2 mg/kg/h

daily maintenance doses of calcium should be started in all patients except those with hyperphosphatemia. The intravenous route is advised when patients are seriously ill because calcium absorption from the bowel is erratic and incomplete. The daily intravenous dose is 4 to 7 mg/kg, which corresponds to an oral dose of 15 to 20 mg/kg.[65]

Hypercalcemia

Pre-ICU Phase

Hypercalcemia (>2.55 mmol/L) has a reported incidence of 0.6 to 4% in the hospital setting.[75] The most likely sources of an individual case of hypercalcemia are determined by the patient population. In outpatients, parathyroid disease is the leading cause, whereas in hospitalized patients malignancy is identified most often.[79-81] A variety of malignancies can produce a hypercalcemia state, and the ones most often implicated are squamous cell carcinoma of the lung, breast carcinoma, leukemia, lymphoma, and multiple myeloma. The mechanism is not clear, and several factors may contribute in individual patients. Bone metastases are not present in at least 30% of patients with hypercalcemia.[82]

The **clinical appearance** in hypercalcemia is extremely variable and nonspecific. Symptoms and signs include:

- Altered mental status (agitation, confusion, obtundation, coma)
- Ileus
- Hypotension
- Short QT interval
- Ventricular arrhythmias
- Renal failure

Severe hypercalcemia (17 to 20 mg/dl) can produce a constellation of signs called "hypercalcemic crisis" that includes obturation and coma, ileus, ventricular arrhythmias, heart failure, and renal failure.

ICU-Phase

Management Strategies. The acute management of severe hypercalcemia has a well-defined sequence of

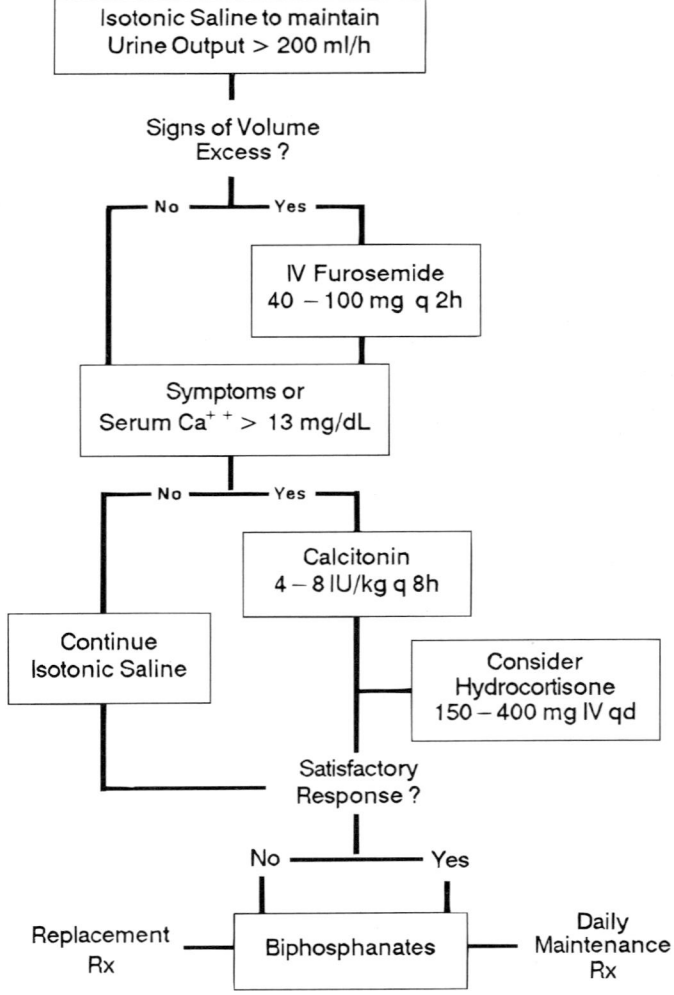

Fig. 58–4. Flow diagram for the parenteral therapy of hypercalcemia. See text for explanation.

events which is shown in the flow diagram in Figure 58–4. The specific drugs and dosing recommendations are then listed in Table 58–6.

Saline Infusion. Volume depletion is common in patients with severe hypercalcemia, and is the result of an osmotic diuresis produced by the hypercalciuria the culprit with resultant hypercalciuria. This condition will promote a volume depletion thereby aggravating the hypercalcemia. Infusion of isotonic saline will help maintain the intravascular volume and, since sodium and calcium share the same reabsorption site in the proximal renal tubule, the natriuresis from saline infusion will promote urinary calcium excretion. A 48-hour course of saline infusion can be expected to reduce the serum calcium by 1 to 2 mg/dl.[83] This is a rather small effect, and hydration alone rarely is enough to return the serum to normal levels.

Furosemide. Furosemide blocks calcium reabsorption in the thick ascending loop of Henle and promotes calcium loss in the urine.[78] Intravenous furosemide in doses of 20 to 100 mg every 2 hours has been successful in alleviating

Table 58-6. Parenteral Therapy for Hypercalcemia

Agent	Dose	Response
0.9% NaCL	1 L in the first h, then 200 ml/h or match urine output, whichever is higher	Expect a drop in serum calcium of as much as 2.5 mg/dl after 48 h
Furosemide	20–100 mg IV q 2h to maintain urine output at 200 ml/hr	The higher doses can drop serum calcium 4 mg/dl in 24 h
Calcitonin	4–8 IU/kg q 12h (×2) given IV or subcutaneously	Rapid response (2–4 h) and rapid tolerance (72–96 h); can prolong effect to 7 days by adding steroids in a dose equivalent to 30–50 mg/day of prednisone
Mithramycin	25 μg/kg as IV bolus	Takes 1–2 days for full effect; toxic side effects include hepatitis, renal failure, coagulopathy
Biphosphanates	Etidronate: 7.5 mg/kg IV over 20 min, given daily for 3 days. Pamidronate: 45–60 mg IV over 4 h	Both agents require days for full effect. Pamidronate may be preferred because only a single dose is required

hypercalcemia. The higher doses can reduce the serum calcium by as much as 4 mg/dl in just 24 hours.[82] The risk for volume depletion has tempered the enthusiasm for aggressive diuretic administration, however, and, as indicated in Figure 58-4 furosemide is usually reserved for cases where saline infusion leads to worrisome volume expansion.

Calcitonin. Thyrocalcitonin is a potent inhibitor of bone resorption, and synthetic calcitonin can return the serum calcium to normal in just 2 to 3 hours.[81] The usual dose is 4 to 8 IU/kg every 12 hours for two doses, and the drug can be given via the intravenous or subcutaneous route (intravenous administration may be preferred in patients who are volume depleted from osmotic diuresis of hypercalcemia), subcutaneously every 12 hours for two doses. If this is ineffective, the dose can be doubled after 2 days have elapsed. Calcitonin is well tolerated, but can cause nausea and vomiting.

Mithramycin. Mithramycin is an antineoplastic agent that inhibits bone resorption. It is more effective than calcitonin, but the response takes 24 to 36 hours to appear.[9] The usual dose is 25 μg/kg given intravenously, either as bolus or a 6-hour infusion. The dose of mithramycin for hypercalcemia is lower than the antineoplastic dose, and bone marrow depression should not develop. The drug is well tolerated if 2 to 3 days is allowed between doses.

Phosphonates. The phosphonates are structurally similar to inorganic phosphate and they inhibit bone resorption. One agent in this class, etidronate sodium, is approved for intravenous therapy of hypercalcemia from malignancy, and another, pamidronate, was recommended to the FDA for approval in October, 1990. Pamidronate is given as a single dose (30 mg in saline infused over 4 hours), whereas etidronate is given in three daily doses (7.5 mg/kg each day), and the response to each agent is 60 and 63%, respectively.[85,86] Repeat therapy can be given at 7 days as necessary. The newer agent, pamidronate, may be preferred because of ease in dosing.

Dialysis. Hemodialysis is very effective for removing calcium from the blood, but is not practical for routine therapy. Dialysis is indicated only when the other measures are ineffective. Hemodialysis is much more effective than peritoneal dialysis,[9] and is preferred whenever possible.

Maintenance Therapy. Oral etidronate has been effective for maintaining normocalcemia after the acute phase of therapy. One report claims 35% of the subject patients were able to maintain normocalcemia for 30 days when given etidronate at a dose of 20 mg/kg each day.[87]

REFERENCES

1. Elin, R. J.: Magnesium metabolism in health and disease. Dis. Mon., *34*:161, 1988.
2. Reinhart, R. A.: Clinical correlates of the molecular and cellular actions of magnesium on the cardiovascular system. Am. Heart J., *121*:1513, 1991.
3. Shattock, M. J., Hearse, D. J., and Fry, C. H.: The ionic basis of the anti-ischemic and anti-arrhythmic properties of magnesium in the heart. J. Am. Coll. Nutr., *6*:27, 1987.
4. Reinhart, R. A.: Magnesium metabolism: a review with special reference to the relationship between intracellular content and serum levels. Arch. Intern. Med., *148*:2415, 1988.
5. Lowenstein, F. W., and Stanton, M. F.: Serum magnesium levels in the United States 1971-1974. J. Am. Coll. Nutr., *5*:399, 1985.
6. Kroll, M. H., and Elin, R. J.: Relationship between magnesium and protein concentration in serum. Clin. Chem., *31*:244, 1985.
7. Alvarez-Lefmans, F. J., Giraldez, F., and Gamino, S. M.: Intracellular free magnesium in excitable cells: its measurement and its biologic significance. Can. J. Physiol. Pharmacol., *65*:915, 1987.
8. Munoz, R., et al.: Ionized hypomagnesemia: a frequent problem in critically ill neonates. Crit. Care Med., *19*:S48, 1991.
9. Graham, L. A., Caesar, J. J., and Burgen, A. S. V.: Gastrointestinal absorption and excretion of magnesium in man. Metabolism, *9*:646, 1960.
10. Shils, M. E.: Experimental human magnesium depletion. Medicine, *48*:61, 1969.
11. Touitou, Y., et al.: Serum magnesium, circadian rhythm in human adults with respect to age, sex and mental status. Clin. Chim. Acta., *87*:35, 1978.
12. Rasmussen, H. S., et al.: Magnesium deficiency in patients with ischemic heart disease with and without acute myocardial infarction uncovered by an intravenous loading test. Arch. Intern. Med., *148*:329, 1988.
13. Goto, K., et al.: Magnesium deficiency detected by intravenous loading test in variant angina pectoris. Am. J. Cardiol., *65*:709, 1990.
14. Whang, R.: Magnesium deficiency: pathogenesis, prevalence, and clinical implications. Am. J. Med., *82*:22, 1987.
15. Whang, R., and Ryder, K. W.: Frequency of hypomagnesemia and hypermagnesemia: requested vs routine. JAMA, *263*:3063, 1990.
16. Ryzen, E., Wagers, P. W., Singer, F. R., and Rude, R. K. Magnesium deficiency in a medical ICU population. Crit. Care Med., *13*:19, 1985.

17. Chernow, B., et al.: Hypomagnesemia in patients in postoperative intensive care. Chest, 95:391, 1989.
18. Dykner, T., and Wester, P. O.: Potassium/magnesium depletion in patients with cardiovascular disease. Am. J. Med., 82(Suppl. 3A):11, 1987.
19. Hollifield, J. W.: Thiazide treatment of systemic hypertension: effects on serum magnesium and ventricular ectopic activity. Am. J. Med., 63:22G, 1989.
20. Ryan, M. P.: Diuretics and potassium/magnesium depletion. Am. J. Med., 82:38, 1987.
21. Zaolga, G., et al.: Hypomagnesemia is a common complication of aminoglycoside therapy. Surg. Gynecol. Obstet., 158:561, 1984.
22. Barton, C. H., Pahl, M., Vaziri, N. D., and Cesario, T.: Renal magnesium wasting associated with amphotericin therapy. Am. J. Med., 77:471, 1984.
23. Shah, G. M., Alvarado, P., and Kirshchenbaum, M. A.: Symptomatic hypocalcemia and hypomagnesemia with renal magnesium wasting associated with pentamidine therapy in a patient with AIDS. Am. J. Med., 898:380, 1990.
24. Whang, R., Oci, T. O., and Watawabe, A.: Frequency of hypomagnesemia in hospitalized patients receiving digitalis. Arch. Intern. Med., 145:655, 1985.
25. Whyte, K., Addis, G. J., Whitesmith, R., and Reid, J. L.: Adrenergic control of plasma magnesium in man. Clin. Sci., 72:135, 1987.
26. Ashraf, M., et al.: Cis-platinum-induced hypomagnesemia and peripheral neuropathy. Gynecol. Oncol., 16:309, 1983.
27. Thompson, C. B., June, C. H., Sullied, K. M., and Themes, E. D.: Associated between cyclosporin neurotoxicity and hypomagnesemia. Lancet, ii:1116, 1984.
28. Balesteri, F. J.: Magnesium metabolism in the critically ill. Clin. Crit. Care Med., 5:217, 1985.
29. Martin, H. E.: Clinical magnesium deficiency. Ann. N.Y. Acad. Sci., 162:891, 1969.
30. Dyckner, T., Ek, B., Nyhlin, H., and Wester, P. O.: Aggravation of thiamine deficiency by magnesium depletion. Acta Med. Scand., 218:129, 1985.
31. Kassirer, J. P., Hrick, D. E., and Cohen, J. J.: Repairing body fluids: principles and practice. Philadelphia, W. B. Saunders, 1989.
32. Sjogren, A., Floren, C. H., and Nilsson, A.: Magnesium deficiency in IDDM related to level of glycosylated hemoglobin. Diabetes, 35:459, 1986.
33. Lau, K.: Magnesium metabolism: normal and abnormal. In Fluids, Electrolytes, and Acid-Base Disorders. Edited by A. L. Arieff and R. A. Defronzo. New York, Churchill Livingstone, 1985, p. 575.
34. Whang, R., et al.: Predictors of clinical hypomagnesemia. Arch. Intern. Med., 144:1794, 1984.
35. Whang, R., et al.: Magnesium depletion as a cause of refractory potassium repletion. Arch. Intern. Med., 145:1686, 1985.
36. Anast, C. S., Winnacker, J. L., and Forte, L. R.: Impaired release of parathyroid hormone in magnesium deficiency. J. Clin. Endocrinol. Metab., 42:707, 1976.
37. Rude, R. K., Oldham, S. B., and Singer, F. R.: Functional hypoparathyroidism and parathyroid hormone end-organ resistance in human magnesium deficiency. Clin. Endocrinol., 5:209, 1976.
38. Graber, M. L., and Schulman, G.: Hypomagnesemic hypocalcemia independent of parathyroid hormone. Ann. Intern. Med., 104:804, 1986.
39. Dominiquez, J. H., Gray, R. W., and Lemann, J. Jr. Dietary phosphate deprivation in women and men: Effects on mineral and acid balances, parathyroid hormone and metabolism of 25-OH-vitamin D. J. Clin. Endocrinol. Metab., 43:1056, 1976.
40. Langley, W. F., and Mann, D.: Central nervous system magnesium deficiency. Arch. Intern. Med., 151:593, 1991.
41. Langley, W. F., and Mann, D. J.: Skeletal buffer function and symptomatic magnesium deficiency. Med. Hypotheses, 34:62, 1991.
42. Abraham, A. S., et al.: Magnesium in the prevention of lethal arrhythmias in acute myocardial infarction. Arch. Intern. Med., 147:753, 1987.
43. Rasmussen, H. S., et al.: Magnesium infusion reduces the incidence of arrhythmias in acute myocardial infarction: a double-blind placebo-controlled study. Clin. Cardiol., 10:351, 1987.
44. Schecter, M., et al.: Beneficial effect of magnesium sulfate in acute myocardial infarction. Am. J. Cardiol., 66:271, 1990.
45. Tsivoni, D. T., and Keren, A.: Suppression of ventricular arrhythmias by magnesium. Am. J. Cardiol., 65:1397, 1990.
46. Iseri, L. T.: Magnesium in coronary artery disease. Drugs, 28(Suppl 1): 151, 1984.
47. Rasmussen, H. S., Larsen, O. G., Meier, K., and Larsen, J.: Hemodynamic effects of intravenously administered magnesium on patients with ischemic heart disease. Clin. Cardiol., 11:824, 1988.
48. Cohen, L., and Kitzes, R.: Magnesium sulfate and digitalis-toxic arrhythmias. JAMA. 239:2808, 1983.
49. French, J. H., et al.: Magnesium therapy in massive digoxin intoxication. Ann. Emerg. Med., 13:562, 1984.
50. Borris, M. N., and Pap, L. Magnesium: a discussion of its role in the treatment of ventricular dysrhythmia. Crit. Care Med., 16:292, 1988.
51. Tsivoni, D., et al.: Treatment of torsades de pointes with magnesium sulfate. Circulation, 77:392, 1988.
52. Dipalma, J. R.: Magnesium replacement therapy. Am. Fam. Physician, 42:173, 1990.
53. Oster, J. R., and Epstein, M.: Management of magnesium depletion. Am. J. Nephrol., 8:349, 1988.
54. Fassler, C. A., et al.: Magnesium toxicity as a cause of hypotension and hypoventilation. Arch. Intern. Med., 145:1604, 1985.
55. Recommended Dietary Allowances. 9th Ed. Washington, D.C., National Academy of Sciences, 1980, p. 134.
56. Seelig, M. S.: Magnesium requirements in human nutrition. Magnesium. Bull., 3(Suppl 1A):26, 1981.
57. Van Hook, J. W.: Hypermagnesemia. Crit. Care Clin., 7:215, 1991.
58. Feldman, H. I., and Wolfson, A. B.: Disorders of calcium and magnesium metabolism. In Endocrine and Metabolic Emergencies. Edited by A. B. Wolfson. New York, Churchill Livingstone, 1990, p. 45.
59. Zaloga, G. P., and Chernow, B.: Calcium and calcium channels: implications in intensive care. Crit. Care, 10:79, 1989.
60. Ladenson, J. H., Levius, J. W., and Boyd, J. C.: Failure of total calcium corrected for protein, albumin and pH to correctly assess free calcium status. J. Clin. Endocrinol. Metab., 46:986, 1978.
61. Desai, T. K., Carlson, R. W., and Geheb, M. A.: Hypocalcemia and hypophosphatemia in acutely ill patients. Crit. Care Clin., 5:927, 1987.
62. Chernow, B., et al.: Hypocalcemia in critically ill patients. Crit. Care Med., 10:848, 1982.
63. Desai, T. K., Carlson, R. W., and Geheb, M. A.: Prevalence and clinical implications of hypocalcemia in acutely ill patients in a medical intensive care unit. Am. J. Med., 84:209, 1988.
64. Zaloga, G. P., and Chernow, B.: The multifactorial basis for hypocalcemia during sepsis: studies of the parathyroid hormone-vitamin D axis. Ann. Intern. Med., 107:36, 1987.

65. Baldwin, T. E., and Chernow, B.: Hypocalcemia in the ICU: coping with the causes and consequences. J. Crit. Illness, 2: 9, 1987.
66. Lang, R. M., et al.: Left ventricular contractility varies directly with blood ionized calcium. Ann. Intern. Med., 108:524, 1988.
67. Desai, T. K., Carelson, R. W., Thill-Baharozian, M., and Geheb, M.: A direct relationship between ionized calcium and arterial pressure among patients in an intensive care unit. Crit. Care Med., 16:578, 1988.
68. Steinhorn, D. M., Sweeney, M. F., and Layman, L. K.: Pharmacodynamic response to ionized calcium during acute sepsis. Crit. Care Med., 18:851, 1990.
69. Zaloga, G. P., and Chernow, B.: Calcium metabolism. In Endocrine Aspects of Acute Illness. Clinics in Critical Care Medicine. Vol. 5. Edited by G. W. Geelhoed and B. Chernow. New York, Churchill Livingstone, 1985, p. 169.
70. Ames, A., et al.: Cerebral ischemia, II: the no-reflow phenomenon. Am. J. Pathol., 52:437, 1968.
71. Seisjo, B. K.: Historical overview: calcium, ischemia, and death of brain cells. Ann. N.Y. Acad. Sci., 522:638, 1988.
72. Trunkey, D., Holcrofte, J., and Carpenter, M. A.: Calcium flux during hemorrhagic shock in baboons. J. Trauma., 16: 633, 1976.
73. Zaloga, G. P., and Washburn, D.: Multiorgan failure is associated with elevated free intracellular calcium in human sepsis. Chest, 94(Suppl):6S, 1988.
74. Vaagenes, P., et al.: Amelioration of brain damage by lidoflazine after prolonged ventricular fibrillation cardiac arrest in dogs. Crit. Care Med., 12:846, 1984.
75. Dean, J. M., et al.: Effect of lidoflazine on cerebral blood flow following 12 minutes of total cerebral ischemia. Stroke, 15: 531, 1984.
76. Hallenbeck, J. M., and Dutka, A. J.: Background review and current concepts of reperfusion injury. Arch. Neurol., 47: 1245, 1990.
77. Halliwell, B., and Gutteridge, J. M. C.: Free Radicals in Biology and Medicine. Oxford, Clarendon Press, 1989, p. 299.
78. Neville, W. E.: Intensive Care of the Surgical Cardiopulmonary Patients. 2nd Ed. Chicago, Yearbook Medical Publishers, 1983, p. 77.
79. Shek, C. C., et al.: Incidence, causes and mechanism of hypercalcemia in a hospital population in Hong Kong. Q. J. Med., 284:1277, 1990.
80. Keating, F. R. J., Jones, J. D., and Elevback, L. R.: Distribution of serum calcium and phosphorous values in unselected ambulatory patients. J. Lab. Clin. Med., 74:507, 1969.
81. Roswell, R. H.: Severe hypercalcemia: causes and specific therapy. J. Crit. Illness, 2:14, 1987.
82. Green, L., and Ringenberg, Q. S.: Current concepts in the management of hypercalcemia and malignancy. Hosp. Formul., 23:268, 1988.
83. Hosking, D. J., Cowley, A., and Bucknall, C. A.: Rehydration in the treatment of severe hypercalcemia. Q. J. Med., 200: 473, 1981.
84. List, A.: Malignant hypercalcemia: choice of therapy. Arch. Intern. Med., 151:437, 1991.
85. Singer, F. R., et al.: Treatment of hypercalcemia of malignancy with intravenous etidronate: a controlled multicenter trial. Arch. Intern. Med., 151:471, 1991.
86. Kirkwood, C. F.: Pamidronate: a new bi-phosphanate. Pharmacol. Ther., 16:472, 1991.
87. Ringenberg, Q. S., and Ritch, P. S.: Efficacy of oral administration of etidronate disodium in maintaining normal serum calcium levels in previously hypercalcemic cancer patients. Clin. Ther., 9:318, 1987.

Section Nine

GENERAL SUPPORT CONSIDERATIONS

Chapter 59

SURGICAL RISKS, PREOPERATIVE ASSESSMENT, AND PREVENTIVE STRATEGIES FOR THE CRITICALLY ILL PATIENT

EDWARD M. CORDASCO, JR.
JOSEPH A. GOLISH

Critically ill patients pose many management challenges to those responsible for their care. The stress of surgery and invasive procedures may inadvertently compromise organ function in fragile patients. Recognition of those critically ill patients with well-defined "risk factors" for the development of postoperative complications, as well as possible "risk modification" should be the objective of the medical team, including the critical care practitioner. It is mandatory that the critical care specialist be aware of patient risk factors predicting poor postoperative outcome and modify these same risk factors, thus minimizing postoperative complications. Therefore, preoperative assessment should have the following goals:

- Identification of high risk surgical patients
- Definition of strategies to modify those factors in a favorable fashion
- Emphasis on prevention of postoperative pulmonary, cardiovascular, and cerebrovascular complications through this risk factor modification

PULMONARY COMPLICATIONS

Factors predisposing to the development of major pulmonary complications (Table 59-1) following both upper abdominal and thoracic surgery are well defined. Upper abdominal surgery as opposed to lower abdominal surgery has been shown to independently place patients at increased risk of pulmonary complications by altering respiratory mechanics.[1-6] Within 10 to 12 hours of upper abdominal surgery, the vital capacity drops by 50%,[3,7] and the tidal volume is reduced by 25%.[8,9] To maintain minute ventilation to preoperative levels and balance off the fall in tidal volume, a 20% increase in the respiratory rate above resting values also occurs.[8,9] Late postoperative changes (16 to 24 hours beyond upper abdominal surgery) include a 30% reduction of both functional residual capacity and residual volume. These measurements return to within 90% of their preoperative value by the fifth postoperative day.[7,10] Similar reductions of vital capacity, tidal volume, and functional residual capacity have been noted following thoracic surgery. These changes tend to persist, however, for longer periods and may not return to preoperative values for 3 to 4 months.[7,10-12]

Diaphragm dysfunction following surgery, as suggested by reduced transdiaphragmatic pressure, contributes to the postoperative reduction of functional residual capacity and vital capacity.[9] Pain and voluntary splinting which contribute to reduction of thoracic volume are not major contributors to this dysfunction. Simmoneau and co-workers[13] studying patients who underwent upper abdominal surgery noted that epidural anesthesia sufficient to relieve postoperative pain was not accompanied by increases in the transdiaphragmatic pressure during either quiet and maximal voluntary breathing. Dureuil and colleagues[14] noted no difference in pre- or postsurgical diaphragmatic contractility as assessed by transdiaphragmatic pressure measurements on maximal external phrenic nerve stimulation. They concluded that postoperative diaphragm dysfunction was not due to impaired muscle contractility per se, but related to submaximal central nervous system phrenic nerve stimulation.

In contrast to patients undergoing abdominal surgery, patients with lateral thoracotomies display better preservation of diaphragmatic function but incur dysfunction of other muscles of respiration. Maeda and associates[15] studied diaphragm function in 20 patients following resectional thoracic surgeries for lung neoplasma with transdiaphragmatic and mouth occlusion pressures and phrenic nerve stimulation. These authors were unable to demonstrate altered diaphragm function postoperatively but found evidence for dysfunction of other respiratory muscles. As a result of these studies, it would appear that postoperative "diaphragm dysfunction" responsible for changes in vital capacity and functional residual capacity may be on the basis of altered central nervous system output, rather than altered diaphragm contractility. Postoperative pain, although not directly linked to altered diaphragm function, nonetheless produces voluntary splinting which may aggravate the reduction of vital capacity and functional residual capacity.

Surgically induced reduction of functional residual capacity has certain physiologic consequences. Normally, the end-tidal point of the functional residual capacity exceeds or lies above the closing volume (Fig. 59-1). The closing volume defines that volume of lung above the residual volume at which small peripheral airways collapse. When the functional residual capacity is reduced, the end-tidal point may drift below the closing volume, thus allowing small airways to collapse and produce atelectasis. Sighing (a breath three times the tidal breath), which normally

Table 59-1. Major Pulmonary Complications Following Surgery

Respiratory failure requiring intervention
  Increasing oxygen requirement
    Aggressive bronchopulmonary hygiene
      Postural drainage/clapping
      Frequent airway suctioning
      Control of airway with oral nasotracheal tube
  Mechanical ventilation
Pneumonia
Lobar Collapse
Atelectasis
Pneumothorax
Bronchopleural fistula
Pleural space infection

prevents airway closure, is also reduced postoperatively and thus contributes further to this problem.[16] In addition to these two factors, the typical postoperative breathing pattern (characterized by tachypnea and low tidal volumes), promotes alveolar and airway collapse. Generous fluid administration in the perioperative period and impaired lymphatic flow following disruption of mediastinal structures during thoracic surgery increase the extravascular water content of the lung.[19] Extravascular water, by altering thoracic compliance, also reduces functional residual capacity, promotes alveolar and airway collapse, and increases the work of breathing.[18,19] As a consequence of these changes, ventilation and perfusion relationships are altered, and thus, shunting and hypoxemia develop.

The magnitude of postoperative hypoxemia has been characterized by Parfrey and colleagues[20] who noted:

- 30% reduction in the arterial oxygen for the first 48 hours after upper abdominal surgery
- 10 to 18% reduction in arterial oxygen within the first 48 hours after lower abdominal surgery
- 5 to 10% reduction following nonabdominal surgery

These changes in the oxygen level occurred despite aggressive measures to prevent atelectasis, which suggested the possibility of "nonatelectatic" causes for ventilation-perfusion mismatch and resultant hypoxemia. Evaluation of extravascular lung water or measurements of alteration in thoracic compliance were not performed in this study.

Anesthetic agents produce alteration of the pulmonary system that may predispose patients to the development of postoperative complications. General anesthetics and analgesic agents, particularly narcotics, reduce mucociliary transport and clearance.[21] It appears that all the general anesthetic agents including enflurane, halothane, and isoflurane are equally potent in this regard.[22] Mucociliary inhibition by anesthetic agents may be additive to other factors that impair mucous clearance, namely, endotracheal intubation, postoperative immobilization, and ineffective coughing. As a result, airway secretions accumulate impairing airflow, and go on to produce mucous plugs, obstruct airways, promote atelectasis, and alter ventilation-perfusion relationships. Other effects of general anesthetic agents on pulmonary mechanical and gas exchange function include reduction of the functional residual capacity, alteration of regional functional residual capacity to total lung capacity ratios, and an increase in the dead space to tidal volume ratio.[23] These changes, coupled with dampened airway clearance, impair gas exchange producing hypoxemia and impaired carbon dioxide elimination.

Retained secretions, impaired mucociliary clearance, and airway collapse following surgery provide an opportunity for the growth and proliferation of "colonizing" gram-negative bacterial agents in the lower airways, producing nosocomial pneumonia and sepsis.[24] Impairment of gas exchange through the physiologic alterations induced by surgery and general anesthesia alter carbon dioxide elimination and oxygen transport and thus may compromise multiple organ systems. In critically ill patients with limited physiologic reserves and who frequently have preexisting multisystem organ dysfunction, these additional adverse

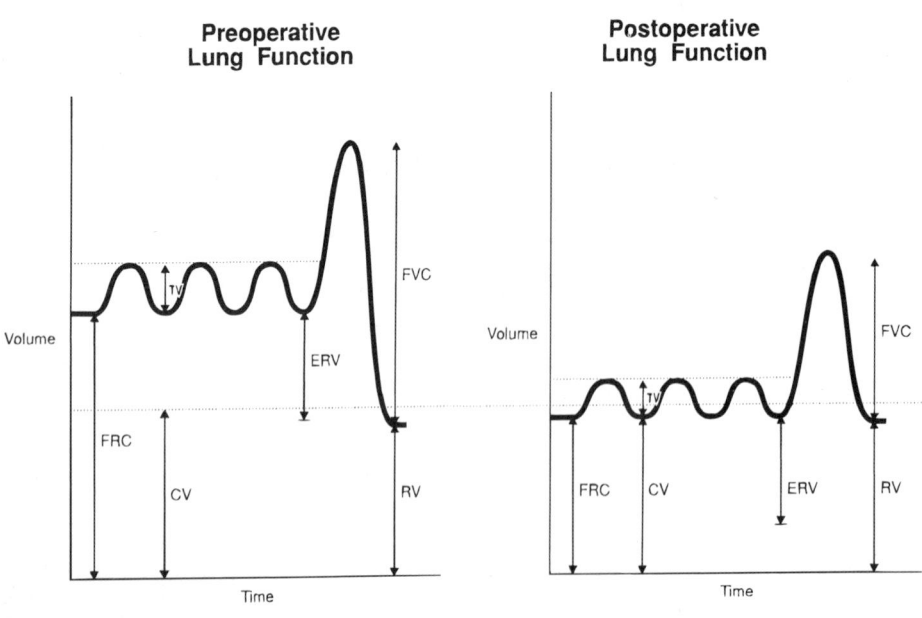

Fig. 59-1. Postoperative changes in lung function graphically compared to preoperative situation. Note a fall of the FRC allowing tidal breathing to occur in the closing volume range, thus promoting atelectasis. Reduction in tidal volume accompanied by concomitant increase in respiratory rate and reduction of forced vital capacity are also depicted. TV, Tidal volume; CV, closing volume; FRC, functional residual capacity; ERV, expiratory reserve volume; FVC, forced vital capacity; RV, residual volume. (Courtesy of ACT/PC.)

physiopathologic factors may favor development of multisystem organ failure syndrome.

Pre-ICU Phase: Identification and Evaluation of Pulmonary Risk

To prevent postoperative respiratory complications, the clinician must proactively identify the factors that predispose patients to these complications. These risk factors can be divided into those peripheral to pulmonary disease (nonpulmonary risk factors) and those directly related to pulmonary disease (pulmonary risk factors). The principal reason for identification is to implement strategies to reduce risks. The key to these is objective quantification of these risks by invasive and noninvasive pulmonary function studies.

Nonpulmonary Surgical Risk Factors

Specific nonpulmonary risk factors identifying patients at increased risk of postoperative pulmonary complications have been enumerated in the literature (Table 59-2).

Obesity. Obese patients have a highly variable rate of postoperative pulmonary complications estimated to be as low as 3.9% and as high as 95%.[25] These complication rates are extracted from retrospective studies in which factors besides the degree of obesity may have influenced outcome. Dureuil and associates[26] attributed the marked reduction in vital capacity in the obese compared to the nonobese patient to impaired diaphragm function following upper abdominal surgery. Hypoxemia after jejunal bypass surgery is more severe in markedly obese patients compared to nonobese "control" patients undergoing the same surgery.[27] Latimer and colleagues noted a 53% rate of atelectasis in obese patients after upper abdominal surgery versus a 9% atelectatic rate in nonobese subjects.[3] Meyers and co-workers[10] similarly noted an increased rate of atelectasis with concomitant reduction in vital capacity of obese patients following upper abdominal surgery.

Sleep Apnea/Hypoventilation. Both hypoventilation and sleep apnea syndrome, which may accompany obesity, have been considered to add additional risk because of accompanying derangements of cardiovascular and pulmonary function, although in one study these risks may have been offset by prior tracheostomy in 19 of 30 patients.[28] All efforts to reduce weight should be undertaken preoperatively. Measures to reduce atelectasis and hypoxemia should be instituted given the high frequency of these postoperatively in this patient population. Discovery of the obese patient with either obstructive sleep apnea syndrome or hypoventilation producing impaired cardiopulmonary function appears warranted. The ultimate preoperative treatment of these latter patients (i.e., nasal, constant positive airway pressure versus tracheostomy or other surgeries), however, it has not been directly assessed in a rigorous fashion and needs to be better defined.

Cigarette Smoking. This factor has also been associated with an increased rate of postoperative pulmonary complications. A history of 20 pack years[29] or consumption of more than 20 cigarettes on a daily basis[30] are threshold levels of smoking thought to increase the rate of postoperative complications. Cigarette smoke causes small airways dysfunction,[31,32] hypersecretion of mucus,[33] and reduced closing volume[34] thus predisposing to atelectasis and impaired tracheobronchial mucociliary clearance.[30] It has been stated that 8 weeks' cessation from smoking[31,32] prior to the anticipated surgery is required to effectively eliminate the adverse effects of cigarette smoke on airways function. Hence, this has been the usual recommendation given to patients undergoing abdominal or thoracic surgery. A recent study by Warner and associates[21] in 192 prospectively studied patients who had undergone open heart surgery noted that smoking cessation within 8 weeks of surgery actually increased the risk of postoperative complications (bronchospasm, lobar collapse, pneumothorax, and pneumonia). This finding may be accounted for by the increased sputum production noted to occur in long-term cigarette smokers who suddenly stop smoking. During this smoke-free interval, mucous gland hypersecretion is responsible for an increase in the baseline phlegm and sputum production. Impaired ciliary activity secondary to prior cigarette smoking, anesthesia, and endotracheal intubation hinder effective elimination of respiratory secretions. As a result of impaired airway clearance and hypersecretion, mucus plugging, and atelectasis may lead to gas exchange abnormalities and the development of pneumonia.

It would appear that the time-accepted adage of cessation from smoking for at least 8 weeks prior to surgery may still hold. For those patients who stop smoking for lesser periods of time, pulmonary risk may be increased, given the data from Warner and colleagues.[21] Although the results of this well-controlled, prospective trial are intriguing, they need to be verified by other similarly designed trials for patients undergoing thoracic and nonthoracic surgeries before further conclusions can be drawn.

Anesthesia. The type and duration of anesthesia administered during surgery may also influence the development of postoperative pulmonary complications. General anesthesia may affect pulmonary function by reducing mucociliary clearance and altering regional ventilation-perfusion matching. Similar postoperative complication rates have been noted for both spinal and general anesthesia,[35-37] but regional blocks appear to be associated with lower risk[8] than either of the two aforementioned anesthetic methods. Prolonged surgery and anesthesia times longer than 3.5 hours have also been associated with an increased rate of postoperative pulmonary complications. Although regional anesthetic techniques cannot always be used as the sole anesthetic perioperatively, local anesthetic agents can be used to advantage. Thoracic nerve blocks

Table 59-2. Nonpulmonary Surgical Risk Factors

Obesity[10,25-27]
Hypoventilation/sleep apnea
Cigarette smoking[29-32]
Type of anesthesia[8,35-38]
Type of incision[40-42]
Cardioplegic agents[44,45]
Nasogastric tubes[24,47]
Age[48,49]

reduce the amount of discomfort and splinting and thus improve deep breathing, cough, and airway clearance. Less reduction of post-thoracotomy FEV₁ (forced expiratory volume in 1 second) has been noted with use of intercostal blocks compared to parenteral narcotics.[38] The improvement in bronchopulmonary toilet an preservation of airway mechanics may reduce the potential for atelectasis and other respiratory complications. Epidural patient-controlled narcotic administration may also provide improved postoperative comfort while minimizing respiratory depression and impairment of airway clearance.[39]

Incision. The specific type of surgical incision influences postoperative pulmonary complication rate. Lower magnitude of postoperative fever, less severe reduction in vital capacity, and lesser degrees of hypoxemia have been noted with the subcostal as opposed to the midline incision for cholecystectomy.[40] Ventral laparotomy produces more atelectasis and hypoxemia than the horizontal approach for upper abdominal surgery.[41,42] In patients undergoing esophageal resection, separate incision for laparotomy and thoracotomy produce less impairment of pulmonary function than single incision thoracolaparotomy.[43] Anterolateral as opposed to posterolateral thoracotomy produces less postoperative pain and, therefore, may reduce the incidence of splinting and atelectasis associated with lateral thoracotomy.[38]

Cardioplegia. Phrenic nerve injury can contribute to respiratory failure by producing either unilateral or bilateral diaphragm dysfunction postoperatively.[44] Ice slush for cardioplegia can produce phrenic nerve damage during open heart surgery and manifest in some patients as diaphragmatic dysfunction or paralysis with impaired ventilatory function.[45] Postoperative respiratory failure requiring a prolonged course of mechanical ventilatory support with its associated complications may result, and full resolution may require up to 70 weeks.[46]

Nasogastric Tubes. The use of nasogastric tubes in the postoperative period is an underappreciated risk factor for the development of postoperative pulmonary complications, especially for nosocomial pneumonia.[24,47] Nasogastric tubes, like endotracheal tubes, may impair mucociliary clearance of the upper airway and also serve as a conduit for the transport of bacteria from the gastrointestinal tract to the lower airways promoting colonization and thus increasing the risk of nosocomial pneumonia.[24] Judicious use of these devices and removal as early as possible following surgery are the easiest means of reducing the potential respiratory risk.

Age. Increasing age as an isolated risk factor for postoperative pulmonary complications has not been well defined because older patients also tend to have multiple coexisting medical problems. Boushy and colleagues[48] noted that patients older than 60 years had an increased rate of post-thoracotomy pulmonary complications. However, these patients also had moderate airflow obstruction with FEV₁ values of less than 2 L. Didolkar and co-workers[49] also noted a high complication rate and mortality after thoracotomy for older patients in their study population, but these patients also had concomitant cardiovascular abnormalities reflected by ECG changes (left or right ventricular hypertrophy, premature ventricular contrac-

Table 59–3. Pulmonary Surgical Risk Factors

Chronic Obstructive Pulmonary Disease[3,4,50,51]
Hypercapnia (PCO_2 > 45 mmHg)[53,54]
Asthma[57,58]

tions, nonspecific ST and T wave changes) and airflow obstruction as evidenced by maximal voluntary ventilation (MVV) values less than 60% of predicted. Both Tarhan and associates[37] and Mitchell and colleagues[47] noted no increased mortality in older patients undergoing general surgery despite the presence of concomitant moderate airflow obstruction.

Pulmonary Surgical Risk Factors

Postoperative respiratory complications directly related to specific pulmonary "risk factors" are due to preexisting disorders of pulmonary function (Table 59-3). In general, both the patterns and severity of deranged pulmonary function can be categorized into either restrictive or obstructive types depending upon the magnitude of reduction of FVC, FEV₁ or FEV₁/FVC ratio (Fig. 59-2). Of note, patients with significant airflow obstruction producing air trapping may have reductions of FVC and normal FEV₁/FVC ratios, thus mimicking restriction. However, determination of total lung capacity (TLC) and residual volume (RV) which are both increased in the case of air trapping (and either reduced or normal in restriction) can help clarify the situation.

Chronic Obstructive Pulmonary Disease. The presence of chronic airflow obstruction has been noted as an underlying factor in the development of postoperative pulmonary complications for all types of surgeries compared to patients with purely restrictive impairment in whom flow rates and cough are well preserved. Stein and co-workers[50] noted pulmonary complications in 21 of 30 patients with abnormal preoperative pulmonary function but in only 1 of 33 patients with normal function.[50] In another study by Stein and Cassara,[51] a 60% postoperative compli-

	Obstructive	Restrictive
FVC	reduced or normal	reduced
FEV₁	reduced	reduced
FEV₁/FVC	reduced	normal
Magnitude of Obstructive or Restrictive Impairment		
FEV₁/FVC	>75%	normal
	75–65%	mild
	65–50%	moderate
	<50%	severe
FVC or FEV₁	>80%	normal
	80–60%	mild
	60–50%	moderate
	<50%	severe

Fig. 59–2. Characteristic spirometric obstructive and restrictive patterns. FVC, Forced vital capacity; FEV₁, forced expiratory volume in 1 second.

cation rate was noted in a population of patients with chronic airflow obstruction, as determined by three well-defined "risk factors":

- FEV_1/FVC ratio < 0.7
- End tidal $CO_2 > 45$ mm Hg
- Maximal expiratory flow rate (MEFR) < 200 L per minute

These patients did not receive preoperative bronchodilators, chest physical therapy, or postural drainage. Those patients not receiving preoperative pulmonary interventions and in whom only one of these risk factors was present had a 25% postoperative complication rate compared to a "normal population" complication rate of 10%. Latimer and colleagues[3] noted a 100% complication rate in a study of postoperative patients with chronic obstructive pulmonary disease if the FEV_1/FVC ratio was less than 0.65 and the forced vital capacity was less than 70% of predicted. An increased postoperative complication rate for patients with preexisting airflow obstruction who failed to improve the maximum voluntary ventilation, forced expiratory flow 25 to 75, and forced vital capacity 48 to 72 hours after surgery to preoperative values was noted by Gracey and co-workers.[4] Additionally, those patients with a maximum voluntary ventilation or forced expiratory flow 25 to 75 of less than 50% of predicted or a forced vital capacity less than 75% of predicted maximum were at "high risk" of postoperative respiratory failure and prolonged mechanical ventilation. Therefore, it would appear as a result of these studies that the degree of airflow obstruction correlates with and is predictive of the development of postoperative pulmonary complications.

Although surgical risk and postoperative complication rates are increased in patients with chronic airways disease, there has not been a single study defining the lower limit of FEV_1 or FVC below which a patient should not be subjected to surgery or anesthesia. Patients undergoing surgery with values of lung function considered by Miller and co-workers[52] to be "prohibitive" for surgery were noted by Cain and associates,[53] Milledge and Nunn,[54] and Williams and Brenowitz[55] to tolerate both upper abdominal and thoracic surgery. Cain and co-workers[53] studied patients undergoing abdominal or thoracic cardiovascular surgery and found no direct correlation between complication rates and values of FEV_1 as low as 450 ml but did note that all patients with an arterial carbon dioxide level of greater than 45 mm Hg either died or developed pulmonary complications. Similarly, Milledge and Nunn[54] found carbon dioxide levels of greater than 45 to 50 mm Hg more specific predictors of postoperative complications than FEV_1. Williams and Brenowitz[55] studied 16 patients with severe "prohibitive" chronic airflow obstruction who underwent thoracotomies and upper abdominal surgeries. A 19% incidence of postoperative complications (pulmonary and cardiovascular), and a 6% mortality rate were noted from this study population. Hypercapnia more accurately predicted the development of postoperative pulmonary complications than FEV_1 values ranging from approximately 1.3 to 0.39/L. Unlike hypercapnia, hypoxemia has been an inconsistent marker of increased postoperative risk for both the development of cardiovascular and pulmonary complications.[4,11,53,54,56]

Therefore, although patients with chronic airflow obstruction have an increased risk of complications following thoracic and upper abdominal surgeries, there is no degree of spirometric impairment which should solely be considered prohibitive of anesthesia and surgery. Hypercapnia, rather than the degree of airflow obstruction quantitated by pulmonary function testing, is a more specific marker for the high risk patient.

Asthma. Patients with bronchial asthma and reactive airways have been shown to have an increased risk of postoperative complications compared to the nonasthmatic.[57] Airway irritation accompanying intubation is probably the most common factor precipitating bronchospasm during the administration of a general anesthetic.[58] Postoperative complications in one study of asthmatic patients most closely correlated to the duration of anesthesia and site of surgery rather than the magnitude of airflow obstruction.[57] Because the general anesthetic agents enflurane, isoflurane, and halothane are equally effective in preventing[59] and reversing[60] bronchospasm in asthmatics, no one agent appears superior. Halothane should not be given to patients using theophylline perioperatively given the arrhythmic potential of this drug combination.[61] In experimental animal models, both enflurane[61] and isoflurane[62] appear not to enhance theophylline arrhythmogenic potential. Some authors[37] recommend avoiding the neuromuscular relaxant D-tubocurarine because of its potential histamine releasing effect, although the clinical significance of this effect is unknown. Other agents such as morphine sulfate and neostigmine have been shown to increase the incidence of bronchospasm and should be used with caution or avoided altogether.[57] High spinal and epidural anesthesia (above T6) may allow unopposed vagal tone and lead to bronchospasm by blocking sympathetic efferent to the pulmonary plexus.[37]

Measurements of Pulmonary Function and Objective Quantitation of Postoperative Risks

In an attempt to quantify pulmonary risk in postoperative thoracic surgical patients, some investigators have performed noninvasive and invasive preoperative assessment of lung function.

Noninvasive Pulmonary Studies. Specific pulmonary mechanics identifying the patient at increased risk of respiratory complications following resectional lung surgery have been defined in the literature. As summarized in Table 59-4, a variety of mechanical pulmonary factors and various degrees of respiratory derangement as depicted by these factors have been associated with increased postoperative morbidity and mortality. Early investigations by Gaensler and associates[63] and Mittman,[64] primarily used reduction of maximal breathing capacity as an indicator of increased post-thoracic surgical risk. Later studies, most notably by Boushy and co-workers,[48] Lockwood,[65] and Boysen and colleagues[66] emphasized the importance of reduced vital capacity and expiratory flow as accurate predictors of postoperative complications.

As an extension of the observations in Table 59-4, calcu-

Table 59–4. Measurements of Pulmonary Function Indicating Increased Operative Risk

MBC (MVV)	<50%[4,63,64]
	<28 L/min[65]
FVC	<75%[4]
	<70%[3,63]
	<1.7 L[65]
FEV$_1$	<2 L[48]
	<1.2 L[65]
FEV$_1$/FVC	<50%[48]
	<0.65%[3]
	<0.7[51]
MEFR	<200 L/min[51]
FEF$_{25-75}$	<50%[4]
D$_{LCO}$	<60%[74]
	<40%[75]

MBC, maximal breathing capacity; MVV, maximal voluntary ventilation; FVC, forced vital capacity; FEV$_1$, forced expiratory volume in one second; MEFR, maximal expiratory flow rate; FEF$_{25-75}$, forced expiratory flow at 25–75; D$_{LCO}$, diffusion capacity.

lation of postresectional lung function has been undertaken to determine the patient's capacity to tolerate the anticipated degree of resection based on prediction of postoperative pulmonary function. The objective of this type of determination is to define the tolerable level of postresectional lung capacity which will allow normal functionality and minimal postoperative complications. In the 1940s and 1950s, bronchospirometry (in which separate lung intubation is performed to measure the contribution of each lung to total ventilation and oxygen uptake), was the most accurate method of predicting postpneumonectomy FEV$_1$ and MVV. Later, lateral position testing, which is less cumbersome, became a more popular technique. Changes in tidal respiration and FRC are measured in both supine and right/left decubitus positions using an oxygen-filled spirometer. This technique allows measurement of individual lung function and, thus, can be used to estimate postresectional pulmonary mechanics. Walkup and associates[67] found good correlation between the predicted postoperative FEV$_1$, bilateral decubitus position testing, and the actual measured postoperative value in patients with preoperative FEV$_1$ values of greater than 2 L. Jay and associates[68] and Schoonover and co-workers,[69] however, both noted a high degree of day-to-day variability among normal subjects and intersubject variability with this method when the FEV$_1$ was less than 2 L. Given the variability of lung function estimation by the lateral position technique and limitation to accurately assess patients with FEV$_1$ of approximately 2 L, the present usefulness of this testing technique is limited.

Quantitative ventilation-perfusion scanning is a newer method allowing accurate prediction of postoperative lung function. Calculation of postoperative FEV$_1$ and FVC is based on the fractional radionuclide uptake by the nonresected lung. Determination of postoperative FEV$_1$ and FVC is obtained by multiplying the preoperative FEV$_1$ and FVC by the percentage of radionuclide activity in the non-operated lung or lobes. For example, in a patient anticipated to undergo left pneumonectomy with a preoperative FEV$_1$ for 1.5 L and a differential perfusion scan demonstrating 55% uptake by the right lung and 45% by the left, the predicted postoperative FEV$_1$ would be 0.825 L.

Studies have been performed to verify the accuracy of predicted postoperative lung mechanics estimated by radionuclide scanning. Kristersson and associates[70] using ^{133}xenon ventilation scans, demonstrated differential quantitative correlations of 0.73 and 0.63 between the actual and predicted postoperative FEV and FVC. Olsen and colleagues,[71] using ^{99m}technetium macroaggregate perfusion scanning, noted respective correlation coefficients of 0.75 and 0.72 for postoperative FVC and FEV predicted from preoperative values. Additionally, these authors noted a tendency for perfusion scanning to underestimate the true postoperative FEV volume and FVC values.

Ali and co-workers[72] found a correlation of 0.83 for prediction of postoperative pulmonary function involving four or more lung segments using ^{133}xenon scanning. Patients undergoing lobectomy had a greater than predicted loss of lung function compared to the estimated value from this scanning technique, which eventually resolved with time. Thus, those individuals undergoing limited resectional surgery (lobectomy) because of marginal lung function may unexpectedly lose more lung function than anticipated.

Wernly and co-workers,[73] reaffirming the accuracy of quantitative ventilation-perfusion scanning for the prediction of postoperative FEV and FVC, derived "prediction formulas" frequently used today for postlobectomy pulmonary function estimation:

expected loss of function = the preoperative forced expiratory volume × the number of functional segments in lobe to be resected ÷ total number of segments in both lungs

These noninvasive, scintigraphic techniques are most frequently performed in the preoperative assessment of ambulatory outpatients. Their usefulness in patients who are acutely, critically ill would seem to be limited since few of these patients would be candidates for elective resectional lung surgery. Should resectional surgery be required, however, for critically ill patients in select situations (i.e., for control of massive hemoptysis), operative candidacy and tolerability of the anticipated procedure could be estimated in particular by ventilation-perfusion radionuclide scanning.

Finally, the utility of diffusion capacity, another noninvasive indicator of lung function, to predict postoperative morbidity and mortality has also been studied in the literature. Ferguson and associates[74] retrospectively reviewed lung resection results in 237 patients to identify factors predicting postoperative complications and mortality. The preoperative single breath diffusion capacity was the best predictor of outcome compared to clinical markers for atherosclerotic cardiovascular disease or other determinants of lung function. Preoperative values of diffusion capacity below 60% of predicted maximum were especially predictive of adverse outcome. Markos and colleagues[75] compared lung function, exercise capacity, and preoperative pulmonary scintigraphic estimation of postoperative lung function in 55 patients undergoing lung resection for suspected malignancy. Of these, 18 patients underwent pneumonectomy and 29 patients lobectomy; 6 patients were unresectable at the time of thoracotomy. Complications occurred in 16 patients including 3 deaths within 30 days of surgery. A high correlation between the estimated and measured postoperative FEV$_1$ predicted from ventilation-perfusion scanning and diffusion capacity (R = 0.86 and R = 0.80, respectively) was noted from the study. The overall mortality rate was 5.7%; 16.7% for the group undergoing pneumonectomy. A postoperative estimated FEV$_1$ of less than 40% predicted identified all cases of mortality in pneumonectomy patients but not for those who underwent lobectomy. A postoperative predicted diffusion capacity (based upon preoperative perfusion data) of less than 40% overall was the single best predictor of mortality and morbidity for the entire group. Other lung function variables and exercise variables including maximal oxygen consumption were not useful discriminators for predicting outcome.

Invasive Pulmonary Vascular Studies and Exercise Testing. Invasive pulmonary vascular studies and exercise testing may be used to assess patient operability for thoracic surgical procedures (Table 59-5). Of these two methods, invasive measurements of hemodynamic parameters appear to have greater potential usefulness for preoperative assessment of the critically ill patient. Harrison and co-workers[76] correlated elevations of resting and exercise pulmonary arterial pressure with increasing degrees of patient disability following pneumonectomy. Exercise-induced reduction of cardiac output accompanied by pulmonary hypertension in postpneumonectomy patients was also noted by DeGaff and colleagues.[77] Most likely, these hemodynamic changes occurred on the basis of a reduction in the cross-sectional area of the pulmonary capillary bed following lung resection. Reduction of exercise capacity in these patients appeared to be limited by these hemodynamic alterations and did not correlate well with postresectional diffusion capacity or ventilatory mechanics.

The development of pulmonary hypertension and hypoxemia during temporary unilateral pulmonary artery occlusion has been used by some authors to identify the "physiologically unresectable" patient. During the technique, the pulmonary artery of the lung to be resected is temporarily balloon occluded, and measurements of pulmonary arterial pressure and pulmonary arterial oxygen levels are performed at rest and during exercise. Pulmonary arterial pressures of greater than 35 mm Hg systolic or room air pulmonary arterial oxygen levels of less than 45 mm Hg during occlusion have been used to define unresectability.[78-80] Using these criteria as permissive of surgery, Olsen and associates[81] noted an "acceptable" postoperative complication rate of 7.7% for lobectomy and 17.6% following pneumonectomy. Although this technique may allow the identification of surgical candidates who would be denied resection on the basis of other less invasive methods and has potential usefulness in evaluation of "resection candidates," it has major problems. Technical failure rates of up to 26%, lack of catheter availability, and a high degree of technical expertise limit its availability to a few tertiary centers and, thus, have inhibited the widespread use of this technique in the preoperative assessment of patients.

Reichel[82] retrospectively reviewed 31 patients who had undergone treadmill exercise testing before pneumonectomy. Of the patients who had completed all 6 stages of the exercise, 100% experienced no complications, whereas 57% of patients unable to complete the exercise test experienced postoperative complications (i.e., respiratory failure requiring mechanical ventilation, chest infections, arrhythmias, congestive heart failure, and cardiac arrest). Pulmonary function tests inaccurately predicted the development of these complications. The results of this study are tainted by a selection bias, however. An unknown number of patients were automatically excluded from surgery and, hence, exercise testing on the basis of poor lung function values alone. Therefore, only patients with "acceptable" preoperative lung function underwent treadmill testing. As a result of this study, one can only conclude that individuals demonstrating excellent "global" function of the cardiorespiratory system as determined by treadmill testing will successfully tolerate pneumonectomy.

Preoperative measurements of arterial blood gases, pulmonary mechanics, and pulmonary arterial vascular resistance measurements during treadmill exercise testing were performed in 45 patients by Fee and co-workers.[83] Of these patients, 30 subsequently underwent resectional surgery. Factors deemed predictive of "low risk" candidates included an arterial oxygen level of greater than 50 mm Hg on room air, a FEV$_1$ and FVC of greater than 50% of maximum predicted, and exercise pulmonary vascular resistance of less than 190 dyne·sec·cm^{-5}. Eighteen operated patients identified by these characteristics survived surgery. Five patients who underwent varying degrees of pulmonary resectional surgery died postoperatively of respiratory failure and cor pulmonale. All of the patients who died were noted to have exercise pulmonary vascular resistances of greater than 190 dyne·sec·cm^{-5}. The positive predictive value of this cutoff value of pulmonary vascular resistance is 43%; however, the negative predictive value is 100%. Therefore, pulmonary vascular resistance determination of less than 190 dyne·sec·cm^{-5} accurately identified patients at lower risk for lung resection. Elevation of the

Table 59-5. Invasive Pulmonary Vascular Studies and Exercise Testing

Unilateral pulmonary arterial occlusion pressure
  PAP systolic >35 mmHg[78-80] (high risk)
  Pulmonary arterial O$_2$ <45 mmHg[78-80] (high risk)
Treadmill testing
  PVR >190 dyne·sec·cm^{-5} [83] (high risk)
  V̇O$_2$ <1 L/min[85] (high risk)
      <15 ml/kg/min[86] (high risk)
      <10 ml/kg/min[87] (high risk)
      >10 ml/kg/min[89] (low risk)
  CI   >4.0 L/kg/m^2 [89] (low risk)

PAP, Pulmonary arterial pressure; PVR, pulmonary vascular resistance; V̇O$_2$, oxygen consumption; CI, cardiac index.

pulmonary vascular resistance above 190 dyne·sec·cm^{-5} may indicate loss of a critical amount of pulmonary vascular bed beyond which respiratory failure and cor pulmonale may possibly develop. This cutoff value unpredictably identifies high risk patients, however. Pulmonary artery measurements in critically ill patients may be potentially useful to identify high risk, unresectable patients by virtue of elevated vascular resistance. This issue has not been formally studied, however, in a clinical trial.

Measurement of peak oxygen consumption during exercise testing has been used to identify patients at increased risk of complications of lung resection. Peak exercise oxygen consumption from cycle ergometry testing did not predict the development of post-lung resection complications in a study of 47 patients by Colman and colleagues.[84] However, a significant relationship between the degree of mechanical pulmonary impairment as determined by FEV$_1$, FVC, and postoperative complications was noted. These complications included wound infections, excessive blood loss, gastrointestinal hemorrhage, prolonged air leaks, and empyema. Although the authors concluded that exercise testing was not predictive of postoperative complications for lung resection candidates, this conclusion may be unfounded. Surgical complications per se as opposed to postoperative cardiorespiratory complications may not, in the strictest sense, be "predicted" by a test designed to determine "fitness" of the cardiovascular and respiratory systems. The listed complications do not appear to be directly attributable to either cardiovascular or respiratory dysfunction detected by exercise testing. Hence, the authors conclusion that there is no utility to the measurement of oxygen consumption during exercise testing in preoperative evaluation of patients for lung resection surgery is invalid.

Eugene and colleagues[85] measured prelung resection pulmonary function and maximum oxygen consumption during cycle ergometry and noted a direct correlation between values of maximal oxygen consumption and postoperative mortality. Patients with maximal oxygen consumption of less than 1 L per minute had a 75% mortality rate postoperatively, whereas all patients with a value greater than 1 L per minute survived surgery.

To determine which test could best predict the development of postlung resection complications, Smith and co-workers[86] performed pulmonary function tests, quantitative ventilation-perfusion radionuclide lung scanning, and cycle ergometry preoperatively on 22 patients undergoing lung resection. Specific cardiorespiratory events (e.g., respiratory failure requiring mechanical ventilatory support, pneumonia, atelectasis, myocardial infarction, arrhythmia, pulmonary embolism, and death) within the first 30 days of surgery comprised the "complications" in the study. Measured preoperative values of FEV$_1$, FVC, diffusion capacity, MVV, and residual volume to total lung capacity ratio, as well as predicted postoperative lung mechanics by quantitative ventilation-perfusion scanning failed to discriminate between those who did or did not develop postoperative complications. Nine of 10 patients with a maximal oxygen consumption during cycle ergometry of >20 ml/kg per minute experienced no complications, however. Six of six patients with maximal oxygen consumption of <15 ml/kg per minute developed postoperative complications, and 66% of patients (4 of 6) with a maximal oxygen consumption of 15 to 20 ml/kg per minute also developed complications. Therefore, maximal oxygen consumption during exercise testing in comparison to other preoperative tests appeared to be the most accurate or best global estimator of patient candidacy for lung resection by virtue of its ability to predict postoperative tolerance.

Bechard and Wetstein[87] also noted the power of preoperative maximal oxygen consumption to accurately predict those patients undergoing lung resection who would develop complications and fatalities. These authors found that mortality and complications occurred only if the patient's preoperative maximal oxygen consumption was less than 10 ml/kg per minute. Both pulmonary function testing and determination of static respiratory muscle strength failed to predict poor outcome.

Miyoshi and associates[88] performed cycle ergometry and pulmonary function tests on 33 patients undergoing lung resection. Complications (atelectasis, pneumonia, respiratory failure, and pulmonary edema) occurred in 45% of patients, and those developing complications had a lower percent predicted FEV$_1$, diffusion capacity to alveolar volume ratio, vital capacity to body surface area ratio, and MVV to body surface area ratio compared to the noncomplication group. Only the ratio of maximal oxygen consumption to body surface area, however, could discriminate between survivors (471 ± 53 ml/min/m^2) and nonsurvivors (296 ± 72 ml/min/m^2); the resting pulmonary function tests failed to do so.

Olsen and associates[89] studied the preoperative utility of pulmonary function testing, quantitative ventilation-perfusion scanning, and invasively monitored hemodynamics during submaximal exercise cycle ergometry in a group of patients undergoing lung resection. All patients were considered by conventional criteria at "increased risk" by virtue of FEV$_1$ values of less than 2 L and MVV of less than 50% of maximum predicted. Patients were to undergo various degrees of lung resection according to the anticipated or predicted postoperative lung function. Pneumonectomy was to be performed if the postoperative FEV$_1$ was predicted to be greater than 800 ml or if the pulmonary vascular resistance at the highest workload was less than 190 dyne·sec·cm^{-5}. Lobectomy would be performed for those patients with predicted postoperative values of FEV$_1$ of less than 800 ml or if pulmonary vascular resistance was greater than 190 dyne·sec·cm^{-5} at maximal work level. Postoperatively, 22 patients survived surgery (13 developed complications), and 7 patients either died or developed ventilatory dependency. Pulmonary function testing using quantitative ventilation-perfusion scanning to predict postoperative function failed to predict survivors as well as those who either developed complications or ventilator dependency. Similarly, the measured pulmonary vascular resistance value of 190 dyne·sec·cm^{-5}, unlike the data from Fee and associates[83] failed to identify those who did or did not tolerate resection. However, a cardiac index obtained during exercise of greater than 4 L/min/m^2 and a maximal oxygen consumption of greater than 10 ml/kg per minute identified all the survivors. Therefore, the best

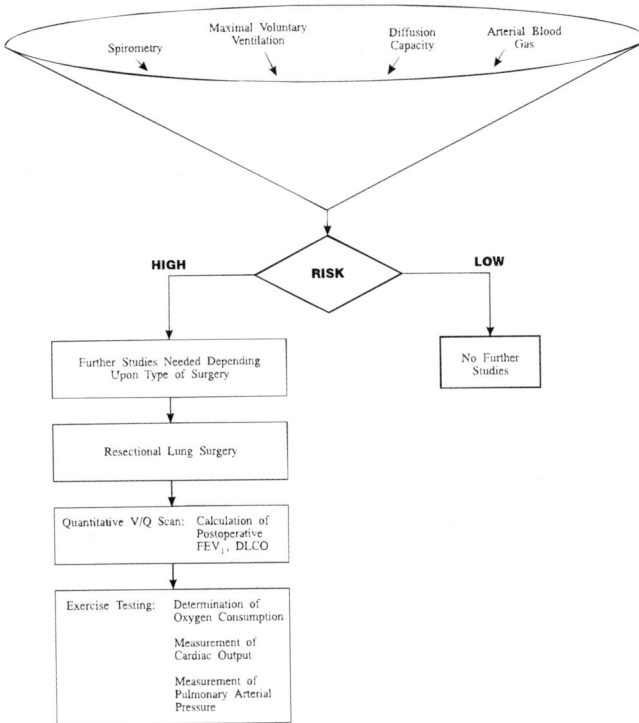

Fig. 59-3. Algorithm for preoperative assessment of pulmonary risk. (Courtesy of George Morrison, CD, Inc.)

predictor of survivability after varying degrees of resectional lung surgery appeared to be maximal oxygen consumption and cardiac index.

In summary, spirometry and pulmonary function testing have conventionally served to identify those patients at increased risk of postoperative pulmonary complications. An algorithm for preoperative assessment of pulmonary risk is presented in Figure 59-3. The ability of these tests to accurately identify those who will develop complications has been inconsistent, however. Individuals with baseline hypercapnia, regardless of the anticipated surgery, are extremely poor candidates with a "prohibitive" complication and mortality rate. Nonhypercapnic patients with borderline or marginal pulmonary function undergoing resectional lung surgery need further studies. There is no universal agreement on the estimated lower limit level of postoperative FEV_1 that is permissive of resection. Values greater than 800 ml or 30 to 40% of maximal predicted appear to approximate a tolerable level of lung function that allows normal patient function postoperatively. Quantitative ventilation perfusion lung scanning is a noninvasive method that allows accurate estimation of postoperative lung function. This technique may overestimate, however, the actual postoperative lung function in patients with "marginal" preoperative respiratory mechanics. As a result, an unanticipated degree of adverse respiratory or cardiovascular events may occur postoperatively in these high risk patients and thus increase morbidity and mortality disproportionately to the gains anticipated by the surgical intervention.

Invasive testing of patients with pulmonary artery catheters at rest and during exercise to obtain pulmonary vascular resistance measurements and cardiac output may identify those patients at high risk of mortality for lung resection. Oxygen consumption measured during exercise testing, although not yet studied, in a validated fashion, may also serve as a sensitive indicator of tolerability for lung resection. Determination of pulmonary vascular resistance, cardiac output, and oxygen consumption in critically ill patients may similarly identify "high risk" patients; however, this hypothesis has not been studied nor validated. Perhaps more attractive, determination of diffusion capacity in those critically ill patients able to tolerate such testing may also serve as a useful means of identifying those at increased risk for surgery. Thus, by identifying the high risk patient prior to surgery, candidacy for the anticipated procedure can be more accurately determined. Lung resection, even for chest malignancy, should not be performed under the premise that any degree of mortality or morbidity is acceptable in an attempt to cure a uniformly fatal illness. Patients must be adequately evaluated so that risk of a procedure can be weighed against the morbidity and mortality of the illness.

ICU Phase: Strategies to Modify Pulmonary Risks

Once those patients at high risk of developing postoperative complications have been identified and adequately evaluated for the anticipated surgery, the clinician should direct attention to the preparation of the patient for surgery. To optimize patient outcome, preoperative preparation must include modification of pulmonary risk factors (Table 59-6). Patients undergoing upper abdominal and thoracic surgery should be instructed in the use of **incentive spirometry** preoperatively. **Sitting** and **early ambulation** after surgery can increase the FRC by 10 to 20%[10,90] and thus may reduce atelectasis and the potential for pneumonia. In one study,[91] healthly patients who had undergone cholecystectomy and who had ambulated early had a lower incidence of atelectasis than those failing to do so, even though the patients who ambulated failed to use incentive spirometry as frequently as the nonambulators.

Other methods have been used to promote "lung expansion" postoperatively besides incentive spirometry. Celli and associates[36] in a prospective study of 172 healthy patients following upper abdominal surgery divided patients into four separate categories to observe the effect of lung expansion methods. Patients received **intermittent positive pressure breathing** treatments or incentive spirometry or were coached in the use of deep breathing exercises.

Table 59-6. Strategies to Modify Pulmonary Risk Factors

Early ambulation, IS[10,36,90,91]
IPPB, deep breathing exercises[36]
CPAP[92,93]
Chest physiotherapy, postural drainage[94]
Pharmacologic optimization of pulmonary function
Cessation of cigarette smoking

IS, Incentive spirometry; IPPB, intermittent positive pressure breathing; CPAP, continuous positive airway pressure.

These maneuvers were performed for 15 minutes 4 times daily for each of these 3 groups. Patients who received no lung expansion interventions served as controls. These authors noted no difference between the control group and any of the treatment groups with regard to the development of radiographic appearance of atelectasis. In all three treatment groups, however, a lower incidence of fever and a shorter hospital stay compared to the control group was noted. There appeared to be no one treatment among the 3 that was superior in its ability to prevent fever and atelectasis and, thus, shorten duration of hospitalization.

Stock and colleagues[92] compared the administration of CPAP of 7.5 cm H_2O to both incentive spirometry and deep breathing exercises in 65 patients following upper abdominal surgery. Maneuvers were performed every 2 hours for 15-minute intervals. At 72 hours postoperatively, there was a 23% incidence of radiographic atelectasis in the CPAP treated group versus a 41% and 42% incidence for the deep breathing and incentive spirometry groups, respectively. These values did not achieve statistical significance, however.

Rickstern and co-workers[93], in 50 patients after upper abdominal surgery, compared 10 cm H_2O pressure of CPAP, 15 cm H_2O of positive expiratory pressure, and incentive spirometry for atelectasis prevention. These authors noted a decreased incidence of atelectasis and higher measured FRC and oxygenation in either the CPAP or positive expiratory pressure treated groups compared to the group using incentive spirometry.

Chest physical therapy has generally not proven as useful a "prophylactic" expander of thoracic volume as the other techniques previously discussed. There appears, however, to be a role for chest physical therapy accompanied by postural drainage in the treatment of lobar atelectasis or in other conditions characterized by copious phlegm production of greater than 30 mL per day.[94]

Patients with chronic obstructive pulmonary disease, as in other patients undergoing abdominal and thoracic surgical procedures, should undergo **instruction preoperatively** on proper technique of incentive spirometry. In addition, preoperative spirometry may detect clinically-silent bronchospasm (increase of either FVC or FEV_1 by 15% after bronchodilator administration) amenable to pharmacologic intervention. In those patients with a significant increase in either the FEV_1 or FVC after **bronchodilator administration,** inhaled beta-agonists and ipratropium bromide metered dose inhaler should be considered. In more severe airflow obstruction and reactive airway disease, oral steroids may be used preoperatively and intravenously during the perioperative period. In those cases where patients by conventional determination have "marginal candidacy" for thoracic surgical resection, concomitant oral theophylline, inhaled beta agonists, ipratropium bromide, and steroids can be used in an attempt to improve pulmonary function to a level that may more safely allow surgery. Antibiotics are not given routinely to patients unless signs and symptoms are suggestive of active infection. If such is the case, surgery is postponed until the infection is cleared.

Asthmatic patients who had received steroids within 1 year, even if these patients are stable and without symptoms, routinely receive steroids pre- and perioperatively in addition to their other maintenance medications. Asthmatics with active bronchospasm do not undergo surgery until medical management is optimized and bronchospasm is relieved. Aminophylline in both asthmatic patients and in individuals with chronic airflow obstruction is not routinely administered perioperatively given its arrhythmogenic potential and rather weak bronchodilator effects. **Cigarette smoking** is discouraged preoperatively, preferably for 8 weeks. Patients should be encouraged to rid themselves of this habit completely, especially because many cases of thoracic surgical intervention are for the treatment of malignant chest disease.

CARDIOVASCULAR COMPLICATIONS

Pre-ICU Phase: Identification and Evaluation of Cardiovascular Risk

The estimated perioperative incidence of myocardial infarction from pooled data of individuals without evidence of underlying cardiovascular disease undergoing major noncardiac operations approximates 0.15%.[95-97] Mortality rates from these same series vary from 32 to 69% for those patients developing perioperative myocardial infarctions.[95-97] Patients with a history of prior myocardial infarction have an incidence of reinfarction during major noncardiac surgery of 2.8 to 17.7%.[95-97] This risk for reinfarction[97] is unrelated to prior Q-wave or non-Q-wave infarction but does appear to correlate best with the time interval between the prior infarction and the noncardiac surgery. Reinfarction incidence is highest when surgery is performed within three months of the cardiac event, approximately 27 to 32%.[95,98] An incidence of 11 to 16% has been noted when the interval between surgery and infarction is 3 to 6 months.[95,98] Beyond 6 months of an infarction, reinfarction incidence associated with major noncardiac surgery falls to approximately 5%.[95,98] Given the high mortality rate from perioperative infarctions, the need clearly exists to identify those patients at risk for the development of this complication. Once identified, the goal of the clinician assessing preoperative risk is to reduce the likelihood of poor outcome, if possible, through risk modification. This is particularly pertinent to critically ill high risk patients requiring emergent or urgent surgical interventions.

Studies Defining Cardiovascular Risk Factors

In an attempt to identify the patient at risk of adverse perioperative cardiovascular complications, Goldman and colleagues[99] performed multivariate analysis of 39 variables in 1001 patients undergoing noncardiac surgery. These authors found that 9 variables (Table 59-7) were independent predictors for the development of perioperative cardiac events. The multivariate discriminant function coefficient from each variable (Table 59-8) was used to derive a weighted "point value score" for each variable. A multifactorial "cardiac risk index" (Table 59-9) could then be estimated from the sum of the variables' weighted value: the higher the summated point value score, the

Table 59-7. Variables Suggesting Increased Risk of Life-Threatening/Fatal Postoperative Complications

Factors (in Order of Decreasing Significance)	Stepwise Significance Level when Added to Previous Factors in Column
1. S₃ gallop or jugular vein distention on preoperative examination	$P < 0.001$
2. Myocardial infarction in preceding 6 months	$P < 0.001$
3. Rhythm other than sinus, or premature atrial contractions on preoperative electrocardiogram	$P < 0.001$
4. >5 premature ventricular contractions/min documented at any time before operation	$P < 0.001$
5. Intraperitoneal, intrathoracic or aortic operation	$P < 0.001$
6. Age >70 years	$P = 0.001$
7. Important valvular aortic stenosis	$P = 0.007$
8. Emergency operation	$P = 0.007$
9. Poor general medical condition*	$P = 0.027$

* Partial pressure of oxygen < 60 mm Hg, partial pressure of carbon dioxide > 50 mm Hg, potassium > 3.0 or bicarbonate < 20 mEq/L, blood urea nitrogen > 50 or creatinine > 3.0 mg/dl, elevated transaminase, signs of chronic liver disease or patient bedridden from noncardiac causes.
(From Goldman, L., et al.: Multifactorial index of cardiac risk in noncardiac surgical procedures. N. Engl. J. Med., *297*:845, 1977.)

Table 59-9. Cardiac Risk Index

Class	Point Total	No or Only Minor Complication (N = 943)	Life-Threatening Complication* (N = 39)	Cardiac Deaths (N = 19)
I (N = 537)	0–5	532 (99)†	4 (0.7)	1 (0.2)
II (N = 316)	6–12	295 (93)	16 (5)	5 (2)
III (N = 130)	13–25	112 (86)	15 (11)	3 (2)
IV (N = 18)	≥26	4 (22)	4 (22)	10 (56)

* Documented intraoperative or postoperative myocardial infarction, pulmonary edema or ventricular tachycardia without progression to cardiac death.
† Figures in parentheses denote percentages.
(From Goldman, L., et al.: Multifactorial index of cardiac risk in noncardiac surgical procedures. N. Engl. J. Med., *297*:845, 1977.)

greater the risk of an adverse event. Four classes of risk using the point system were defined: class I (0 to 5 points), class II (6 to 12 points), class III (13 to 25 points), and class IV (>26 points). From their study population, 19 postoperative cardiac deaths and 39 life-threatening cardiac complications (pulmonary edema, myocardial infarction, and ventricular tachycardia) occurred. The incidence of morbid and fatal cardiac events for each risk class is summarized in Table 59-9.

Zeldin[100] validated the "hypothesis generating" findings of Goldman and associates[99] in a prospective study of 1140 patients undergoing various noncardiac surgeries. These authors noted an 8-fold increased risk of life-threatening cardiac events in patients deemed "high risk" by Goldman's[99] risk classification scheme. Perioperative cardiovascular death occurred in 9.3% of class III and class IV patients compared to 0.5% of class I or class II patients. Notably, 43% of all cardiac deaths occurred in class IV patients.

On the other hand, Jeffery and co-workers[101] in their study of 99 patients undergoing elective abdominal aortoiliac procedures for either aneurysmal or occlusive disease were unable to validate the predictive power of the cardiac risk index, noting poor correlation between the index and patient outcome. Those patients considered low risk by Goldman's[99] criteria had a 9% incidence of adverse cardio-

Table 59-8. Multivariate Discriminant Function Coefficient and Point Assignment for each Variable

Criteria*	Multivariate Discriminant-Function Coefficient	"Points"
1. History		
(a) Age > 70 years	0.191	5
(b) MI in previous 6 months	0.384	10
2. Physical examination		
(a) S₃ gallop or JVD	0.451	11
(b) Important VAS	0.119	3
3. Electrocardiogram		
(a) Rhythm other than sinus or PACs on last preoperative ECG	0.283	7
(b) >5 PVC/min documented at any time before operation	0.278	7
4. General Status		
Po₂ < 60 or Pco₂ > 50 mm Hg, K < 3.0 or HCO₃ < 20 mEq/L, BUN > 50 or Cr > 3.0 mg/dl, abnormal SGOT, signs of chronic liver disease or patient bedridden from noncardiac causes	0.132	3
5. Operation		
(a) Intraperitoneal, intrathoracic or aortic operation	0.123	3
(b) Emergency operation	0.167	4
Total possible points		53

* MI, Myocardial infarction; JVD, jugular vein distention; VAS, valvular aortic stenosis; PACs, premature atrial contractions; ECG, electrocardiogram; PVCs, premature ventricular contractions; Po₂, partial pressure of oxygen; Pco₂, partial pressure of carbon dioxide; K, potassium; HCO₃, bicarbonate; BUN, blood urea nitrogen; Cr, creatinine; and SGOT, serum glutamic oxalacetic transaminase.
(From Goldman, L., et al.: multifactorial index of cardiac risk in non-cardiac surgical procedures. N. Engl. J. Med., *297*:845, 1977.)

vascular events, higher than the 3% rate predicted by the risk index. These authors surmised that the risk index was unreliable in separating low risk from high risk patients undergoing abdominal aortic procedures. The inability of the cardiac risk index to predict adverse cardiovascular events in patients with peripheral vascular disease most likely reflects the difference of coronary artery disease prevalence between the general population from which the index was derived and the patient population with diffuse vascular disease.

Routine preoperative coronary angiography performed by Taylor and colleagues[102] in patients undergoing vascular surgical procedures demonstrated severe multivessel coronary disease in 59% of patients. Respective coronary artery disease rates of 95%, 71%, and 84% were noted by these authors in patients undergoing surgical procedures for aortic aneurysms, carotid, and aortoiliac disease. Hertzer and associates[103] studied 1000 patients undergoing various types of vascular surgical procedures and also noted a high incidence of coronary artery disease. Of 554 patients who had evidence of coronary artery disease by history and clinical parameters, 34% were proven to have angiographically severe operable coronary disease. Of the 446 patients without clinical evidence of coronary disease, 22% were found to have "advanced but compensated" coronary disease and 14% had severe, operable disease.

Given the prevalence of severe coronary disease in the population of patients with peripheral vascular disease, it is not surprising that coronary events have been found to strongly influence survival in these patients. Brown and associates[104] and Hollier and co-workers[105] noted that 70 and 38% of adverse events in their respective abdominal aortic surgical populations were directly related to coronary ischemia and infarctions. Aortic surgical procedures in particular are associated with a higher risk of prolonged intraoperative hypotension which has been implicated as a cause of perioperative aortic cardiac complications.[96,99,106] In addition, large fluid shifts and subsequent hemodynamic alterations may produce hypoxemia that could aggravate severe occult coronary disease, thus potentiating the development of myocardial ischemia. Therefore, the presence of risk factors as elucidated by Goldman[99] may serve to identify patients at increased risk for cardiovascular perioperative events. In addition, patients undergoing vascular surgical procedures should especially be considered at increased risk of cardiac complications given the high prevalence of both symptomatic and asymptomatic coronary artery disease in this population.

To improve the predictive capability of preoperative risk factor assessment beyond that demonstrated by the Goldman[99] index, Detsky and associates[107,108] derived a modified risk index ("modified multifactorial index") which incorporated the presence and severity of angina as well as the type of surgical procedure into a "post-test probability" estimate of potential cardiac complications. Four hundred and fifty-five patients with known coronary, valvular, or myocardial disease undergoing noncardiac operations were separated preoperatively into risk classes according to the presence and number of weighted cardiac risk factors (Table 59-10). Three risk classes (Table 59-11) based on the sum of these weighted variables were derived: class I (0 to 15 points), class II (16 to 30 points), class III (>30 points). Forty-three perioperative severe or serious cardiac events occurred including 15 episodes of left ventricular failure, 13 myocardial infarctions, 6 episodes of unstable angina, and 9 cardiovascular related deaths. Likelihood ratios of adverse cardiovascular events (Table 59-11) were calculated for each of the risk classes depending on the type of surgery (major surgery; class I = 0.42, class II = 3.58, class III = 14.93) and plotted on a nomogram (Fig. 59-4) along with the "pretest probability" (actual cardiac complication rate) to estimate post-test probability ("risk" of perioperative cardiac complications). These same values plotted in a graphic form (Fig. 59-5) clearly indicate increasing risk of postoperative complication for higher risk classification and for surgical

Table 59-10. Variables Suggesting Increased Risk of Postoperative Complications from Modified Multifactorial Index

Variables	Points
Coronary artery disease	
Myocardial infarction within 6 months	10
Myocardial infarction more than 6 months	5
Canadian Cardiovascular Society angina	
Class III	10
Class IV	20
Unstable angina within 6 months	10
Alveolar pulmonary edema	
Within 1 week	10
Ever	5
Valvular disease	
Suspected critical aortic stenosis	20
Arrhythmias	
Rhythm other than sinus or sinus plus atrial premature beats on last preoperative electrocardiogram	5
More than five premature ventricular contractions at any time prior to surgery	5
Poor general medical status	5
Age over 70	5
Emergency operation	10

* As defined in original multifactorial index in Goldman, L., et al.: Multifactorial index of cardiac risk in non-cardiac surgical procedures. N. Engl. J. Med., 297:845, 1977.
(From Detsky, A. S., et al.: Predicting cardiac complications in patients undergoing non-cardiac surgery. J. Gen. Intern. Med., 1:211, 1986.)

Table 59-11. Risk Classes and Corresponding Likelihood Ratios for Adverse Cardiovascular Events

Risk Classes (Points)	Major Surgery	Minor Surgery	All Surgery
I (0-15)	0.42	0.39	0.43
II (15-30)	3.58	2.75	3.38
III (>30)	14.93	12.20	10.60

(Adapted from Detsky, A. S., et al.: Predicting cardiac complications in patients undergoing non-cardiac surgery. J. Gen. Intern. Med., 1:211, 1986.)

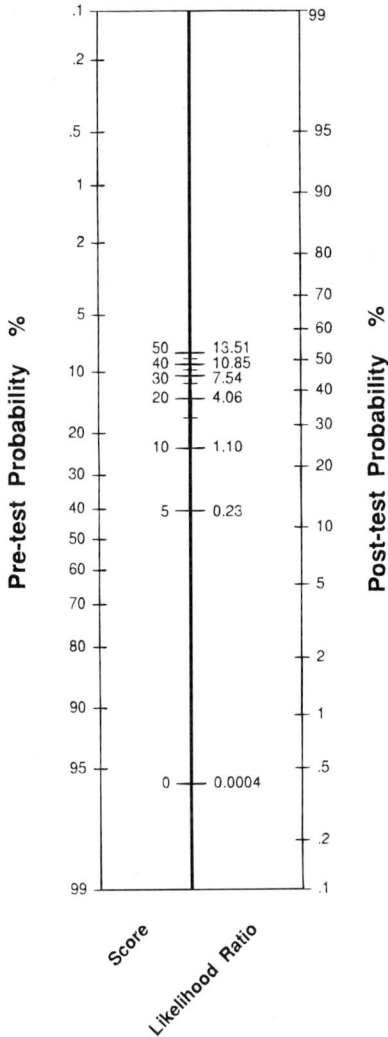

Fig. 59-4. Nomogram for predicting likelihood of perioperative cardiac complication. Likelihood ratio nomogram. Anchor a straight edge at the value on the pretest side of the nomogram determined by the surgical procedure. Direct the straight edge through the point in the center column reflecting the patient's index score and associated likelihood ratio. The point where the straight edge meets the right-hand column denotes the post-test probability for the patient (i.e., his risk of perioperative cardiac complication). (Redrawn by ACT/PC from Detsky, A. S., et al.: Predicting cardiac complications in patients undergoing noncardiac surgery. J. Gen. Intern. Med., 1:211, 1986.)

procedures associated with greater complication rates. This modified risk index has yet to be prospectively validated before its predictive capability is established.

Although preoperative risk stratification indices are useful "yardsticks" to approximate the degree of risk, low scores merely indicate the probability of "low risk" and do not guarantee an event-free postoperative course. Other factors beside the "patient profile" including the magnitude and type of surgery, expertise of the anesthesiologist,[109] and the patient population undergoing the surgery may also influence risk stratification and, thus, outcome in a less predictable, quantifiable fashion.

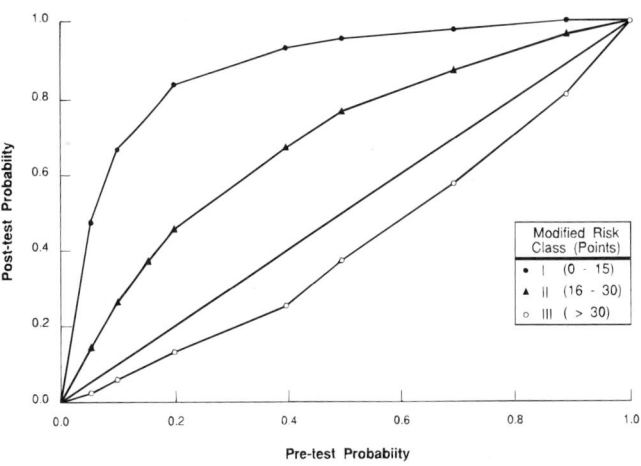

Fig. 59-5. Graphic Representation of Pre- and Post-Test Probability for Each Modified Risk Class. (Data from Detsky, A. S., et al.: Predicting cardiac complications in patients undergoing noncardiac surgery. J. Gen. Intern. Med., 1:211, 1986.; redrawn by ACT/PC from Freeman, W. K., Gibbons, R. J., and Shub, C.: Preoperative assessment of cardiac patients undergoing surgical procedures. Mayo Clin. Proc., 64:1105, 1989.)

Objective Quantification of Cardiovascular Risk Factors

The presence of left ventricular dysfunction and ischemic heart disease are important "markers" of preoperative cardiovascular risk. Studies have been performed to evaluate the significance of these risk factors.

Left Ventricular Function. Ventricular performance is an important preoperative risk variable influencing patient outcome as summarized by studies in Table 59-12. The level of function has been shown to be the single most important prognostic indicator of survival in patients with coronary artery disease. Evidence of left ventricular dysfunction preoperatively predicts the occurrence of cardiac events during noncardiac surgery.[99,107,108] Correlation of risk to the magnitude of ventricular dysfunction has not been determined since most studies have used indirect, nonquantitative clinical markers (S3 gallop, rales, and jugular venous distention) of ventricular impairment.

Table 59-12. Left Ventricular Function and Cardiovascular Risk

---

Nonquantitative clinical evidence of left ventricular dysfunction predicts adverse perioperative cardiac events[99,107,108]
Angiographic evidence of left ventricular dysfunction correlates with occurrence of perioperative cardiac events[110]
Nuclear ejection fraction values suggesting increased risk
 <55% (high risk)[111]
 <35% (high risk)[112]
 <40% (high risk)[113]
Pressure/volume measurements of left ventricle suggesting increased risk
 LVEDV > 120 ml/m² [113]
 LVESV > 60 ml/m² [113]
 LVEDP > 15 mm Hg[113]

LVEDV, Left ventricular end diastolic volume; LVESF, left ventricular end systolic volume; LVEDP, left ventricular end diastolic pressure.

In an attempt to better define risk directly attributable to impaired ventricular function, Foster and colleagues[110] studied the influence of angiographically defined coronary disease and left ventricular function in 1600 patients undergoing noncardiac surgery. Thirteen cardiac deaths, 4 episodes of congestive heart failure, and 10 perioperative myocardial infarctions occurred. Operative outcome and mortality by univariate analysis were noted to be related to age, male sex, presence of diabetes, exertional dyspnea, left ventricular hypertrophy, preoperative use of nitrates, and angiographic wall motion abnormalities. Multivariate analysis showed, however, that only exertional dyspnea and left ventricular wall motion abnormality independently predicted cardiac related morbidity and mortality.

History of prior myocardial infarction within 6 months of surgery was not an independent predictor of postoperative cardiac complications or mortality. Prior coronary revascularization reduced mortality to 0.9% which was similar to the mortality rate for patients without angiographic evidence of severe coronary disease. Those patients with significant angiographically proven coronary disease who had not undergone prior revascularization had a mortality rate of 2.4%. No statistically significant difference between those individuals with and without prior coronary revascularization was noted, however, for the development of perioperative myocardial infarction, stroke, heart failure, or major rhythm disturbance. The authors concluded that their results supported the direct link between preoperative ventricular performance and surgical outcome. In addition, reduction of operative mortality can be realized for those individuals with significant coronary disease who undergo "preoperative" coronary revascularization.[110]

In a retrospective study of 100 patients undergoing lower extremity revascularization procedures, Pasternack and associates[111] noted a strong correlation between left ventricular function as determined by resting nuclear studies and perioperative myocardial infarction and death. None of the patients with ejection fractions greater than 56% developed perioperative myocardial infarction. Of patients with ejection fractions between 55 and 36%, 19% developed perioperative infarctions including one cardiac death. Six of eight patients with ejection fractions of less than 35% developed perioperative infarctions. One patient also died from this latter group of patients as a direct result of a cardiac event.

Kazmers and co-workers[112] similarly noted the influence of left ventricular function on adverse outcome in patients undergoing vascular surgery. Nuclear ejection fractions were obtained preoperatively in a series of patients undergoing carotid endarterectomies. Overall, 12.2% of the surgeries were accompanied by perioperative cardiac complications (myocardial infarction, congestive heart failure, ventricular arrhythmia). Perioperative complications were more frequent in patients with ejection fractions of less than 35% (43% incidence of complications), as opposed to patients with ejection fractions of greater than 35% (9% complication rate). The same "cutoff" value of ejection fraction was unable to discriminate between those who did and did not develop fatal perioperative events. However, cumulative mortality differed significantly for these two groups of patients separated by an ejection fraction of 35 to 57% mortality for those with ejection fractions less than 35 versus 11% for the group with ejection fractions greater than 35%.

Goenen and co-workers[113] studied 183 patients undergoing coronary bypass surgery to determine the influence of preoperative left ventricular dysfunction on patient outcome and operative risk. One hundred and twenty-seven patients with impaired ventricular function were divided into 4 risk groups based on the cumulative presence of 4 indicators of deranged left ventricular function (ejection fraction <40%, left ventricular end diastolic volume >120 ml/m^2, left ventricular end systolic volume > 60 ml/m^2, and left ventricular end-diastolic pressure > 15 mm Hg). The remaining 56 patients without evidence of ventricular dysfunction served as the control population. Only one perioperative death in a patient stratified to group IV risk class was noted. More perioperative arrhythmia and circulatory assist interventions were required for patients with greater degrees of ventricular dysfunction as determined by risk stratification compared to those with lesser degrees of ventricular impairment. Neither circulatory assist nor arrhythmia control was required for those with normal left ventricular function. The authors also noted a difference in 2-year mortality according to group risk classification (5.6% for control versus 8% for group IV patients). Therefore, regardless of the type of surgery, impaired left ventricular performance is a potent marker identifying those patients at increased risk for adverse perioperative cardiovascular events.

Exercise Testing. Exercise testing has also been used as an objective supplemental means to assess preoperative cardiovascular status (Table 59–13). Cutler and co-workers[114] investigated 130 patients undergoing arm ergometry or treadmill testing before vascular surgical procedures and noted a correlation between the electrocardiographic evidence of exercise-induced ischemia and subsequent adverse postoperative cardiac events. Nonfatal postoperative myocardial infarction occurred in 43% of patients with exercise-induced ischemia. A subgroup of patients who demonstrated ischemic electrocardiographic changes at only 75% of predicted maximal heart rate had a 25.9% incidence of perioperative myocardial infarctions with a 71% mortality rate. Postoperative cardiac death, myocardial infarction, ischemia, and injury occurred in 27% of patients with abnormal preoperative exercise tests, compared to 14% of patients with normal preoperative exercise tests in a prospective study of 200 noncardiac surgery patients by Carliner and associates.[115] These authors also noted a higher complication rate (21%) in patients able to achieve only 5 METS workload as opposed to a 12% complication rate for

Table 59–13. Exercise Testing to Assess Cardiovascular Risk

Increased incidence of perioperative cardiovascular events and mortality in patients with exercise-induced ischemia[114,115]
Exercise workload values suggesting increased risk
    4.5 METS[117]
    5.0 METS[115]
    inability to exercise > 2 min with maximal heart rate > 99 bpm[116]

patients achieving higher workloads. Multivariate analysis of multiple preoperative risk factors indicated that an abnormal preoperative electrocardiogram as defined by evidence of left ventricular hypertrophy, left bundle branch block, nonspecific ST-segment and T-wave changes, or Q-wave myocardial infarction was the single best predictor of adverse cardiovascular events.

Gerson and co-workers[116] evaluated 100 patients undergoing elective abdominal aortic or thoracic surgery with exercise radionuclide angiography preoperatively. Independent risk factors predictive of cardiac events were the inability to exercise for 2 minutes to a heart rate of greater than 99 beats per minute and regional left ventricular wall motion abnormalities. An ejection fraction of less than 50% in the presence of a "Goldman risk index"[99] variable was also a significant univariate predictor. In the absence of a "Goldman variable,"[99] the inability to exercise for 2 minutes and achieve a maximal heart rate of greater than 99 beats per minute was associated with a 19.4% incidence of perioperative cardiac events versus a 1.5% complication rate for those able to exceed this level of exercise. Kopeckey and associates[117] studied 148 patients undergoing symptom-limited exercise radionuclide angiography before peripheral vascular surgery. Eleven perioperative cardiac events including 5 deaths, 5 myocardial infarctions, and 1 cardiac arrest occurred in patients who were unable to exceed more than a very low level of energy expenditure (4.5 METS) during exercise testing. Neither resting nor exercise induced changes in left ventricular ejection fraction correlated with the development of adverse cardiovascular events.

Dipyridamole Thallium Testing. Many patients with peripheral vascular disease, orthopedic, or neurologic disease or severe debilitation from combinations of illnesses are unable to undergo stress testing. Limited ambulatory abilities frequently do not allow these patients to achieve maximal or near-maximal heart rates, thus reducing the prognostic value of cardiovascular stress testing. In these patients who are unable to exercise adequately, dipyridamole thallium imaging may serve as an alternative to conventional stress testing. Intravenous dipyridamole produces vasodilatation of nonstenotic coronary vessels increasing blood flow to the myocardium supplied by these vessels. Blood flow to areas supplied by stenotic vessels is not similarly affected. The resultant heterogeneity of blood flow produces thallium perfusion defects on immediate images that later resolve on delayed images. These reversible redistribution defects suggest the presence of ischemic myocardium, whereas nonreversible thallium defects are compatible with myocardial scarring.[118,119]

Dipyridamole-induced coronary vasodilatation, coupled with thallium imaging, has been shown to have a sensitivity and specificity for the detection of coronary disease approaching that of conventional thallium stress testing. Several studies have been performed to determine the utility of this technique for the prediction of adverse perioperative cardiovascular events (Table 59-14). Boucher and associates[120] prospectively studied the ability of dipyridamole thallium testing to predict adverse cardiac events in patients undergoing peripheral vascular surgeries. Forty-eight patients were studied of which 16 had redistribution defects on preoperative dipyridamole thallium testing. Of these patients, 50% had a subsequent perioperative cardiac even (death, infarction or ischemia). All patients with either normal scans or scans showing persistent thallium defects representing old scars had no cardiac events. The authors concluded that patients without thallium redistribution defects are at low risk for postoperative ischemic events when undergoing vascular surgery. Those with redistribution defects have an increased incidence of postoperative ischemic events and should be considered for preoperative angiography and coronary revascularization surgery.

Leppo and co-workers[121] noted a 33% incidence of cardiac events, either myocardial infarction or death, in 42 patients with preoperative thallium dipyridamole redistribution defects undergoing either aortic or peripheral vascular surgeries. Only 2% of the total study population without thallium redistribution defects suffered cardiac events perioperatively. The negative predictive value of the thallium scan without redistribution defects was extremely high at 96%. Similarly, a 96% positive predictive value for scans demonstrating redistribution defects was noted. A positive redistribution thallium scan yielded only a 62% negative predictive value, however. The presence of diabetes or ST segment depression induced by dipyridamole was shown by regression analysis to increase the risk of cardiac events to over 30 times the risk observed in patients without a thallium redistribution defect.

Similar to the study of Leppo and associates,[121] Eagle and co-workers,[122] utilizing dipyridamole thallium imaging in patients undergoing vascular surgery, noted comparable

Table 59-14. Dipyridamole Thallium Testing to Assess Cardiovascular Risk

		Prediction of Adverse Perioperative Cardiovascular Events via Presence of Redistribution Defects		Predictive Value of Positive Redistribution Defects	
Author	# Patients with Redistribution Defects	Adverse Cardiovascular Events	Incidence of Adverse Events in Patients with Redistribution Defects	Positive	Negative
Boucher et al.[120]	16	cardiac death, myocardial infarction, unstable angina	8/16 (50%)	100%	80%
Leppo et al.[121]	42	cardiac death, myocardial infarction	14/42 (33%)	96%	62%
Eagle et al.[122]	18	cardiac death, myocardial infarction, pulmonary edema, unstable angina	8/18 (44%)	100%	81%

positive and negative predictive values for "positive" and "negative" scans. The presence of positive redistribution thallium defects, coupled with one or more clinical cardiac risk factors (angina, prior myocardial infarction, congestive heart failure, electrocardiographic evidence of Q waves, or diabetes) was associated, however, with a perioperative complication rate of 44% compared to a 0% complication rate in patients with "positive scans" without risk factors. As a result of this finding, the authors recommended that dipyridamole thallium tests in patients undergoing peripheral vascular surgery be performed only if cardiac risk factors are present.

ICU Phase: Strategies to Modify Cardiovascular Risk

Strategies to modify cardiovascular risk factors and reduce adverse perioperative and postoperative events are summarized in Table 59-15. The principal logic in these strategies is identification of the high risk patient and optimization of hemodynamic status by guaranteeing satisfactory cardiac rhythm, valvular integrity, and ventricular performance.

Identification of the High Risk Patient

To reduce and modify operative risk for patients undergoing surgery, it is necessary to identify the high risk cardiovascular patient. From the history, the presence of well-defined risk factors for atherosclerosis as well as symptoms suggestive of atherosclerosis (claudication, transient ischemic attacks, angina or prior myocardial infarction) serve as screening markers identifying high risk patients. Signs and symptoms suggestive of left ventricular dysfunction given the high complication rate of these patients are also key historical features identifying those patients at increased risk. Functional limitation of patients with ischemic heart disease as determined by stress testing has a significant impact on prediction of cardiac risk in noncardiac surgical patients. Patients with functional class II angina pectoris by the New York Heart Association classification will most likely tolerate the stress of noncardiac surgery.[123] In these patients, therefore, there is probably no need to "routinely" perform preoperative stress testing unless the patient will undergo upper abdominal, vascular, or thoracic surgery. If, however, patients with functional class II angina have other factors placing them at increased risk (left ventricular dysfunction, diabetes, or prior myocardial infarction), stress testing may uncover significant, unsuspected ischemic coronary disease requiring further evaluation. Patients with class III or class IV New York Heart Association angina or unstable angina should undergo coronary angiography and revascularization surgery if necessary prior to the noncardiac surgery.

In those patients whose anginal functional class or status is unknown, especially if they will undergo either thoracic, upper abdominal, or vascular surgery, then performance of exercise testing seems prudent. A level of exercise approximately 5 to 6 METS without electrocardiographic evidence of ischemia signifies a rather low cardiac risk for noncardiac surgeries. Those patients demonstrating ischemic changes or unable to exercise beyond a low level without the development of ischemic changes should undergo coronary angiography and revascularization prior to surgery. Critically ill patients, usually unable to exercise, who have significant cardiovascular risk factors and who require surgery can be screened by dipyridamole thallium "stress" testing. No clinical trials demonstrate the utility or usefulness of this technique in these patients at present, however.

Those patients who have a history of prior myocardial infarction, congestive heart failure, angina, or diabetes and who are unable to perform exercise stress testing should undergo dipyridamole thallium stress testing prior to major abdominal, peripheral vascular, or intrathoracic surgery. Those patients demonstrating no redistribution defects given the high negative predictive value of the test should be considered at low risk for the development of perioperative cardiac complications. Those patients with reversible thallium defects given the 30% incidence of adverse perioperative myocardial events[120-122] in this group of patients should undergo coronary angiography. The high incidence of coronary artery disease in patients with peripheral and cerebrovascular disease has led some authorities[124] to recommend routine preoperative coronary angiography with the intent to perform coronary bypass surgery prior to peripheral revascularization.[124-127] At the least, these patients must be considered high risk for perioperative cardiac events and perhaps should undergo dipyridamole thallium testing if no other risk factors are present.

Along these same lines, "prophylactic" coronary revascularization in patients with significant coronary disease undergoing elective noncardiac surgery can reduce the perioperative mortality to approximately 1.1% compared to 2.4% for similar medically treated patients.[110] Therefore, these patients should be evaluated for such a treatment strategy. To minimize the risks and maximize the benefit of noncardiac surgery, the risk-to-benefit ratio of bypass surgery for those patients requiring such surgery preoperatively must be acceptably low. The overall operative mortality rate for coronary bypass surgery varies from 1 to 8% depending on the institution and surgical population. In one CASS report, bypass surgical mortality rate was 2.3%.[128] The presence of left ventricular impairment with an ejection fraction below 50% increased this mortality to 2.9%, as did age of greater than 70 years.[128] The role of preoperative angioplasty in the same group of high risk patients has not been well defined by clinical studies. In general, the overall mortality for coronary angioplasty approximates 1% and increases to approximately 2.8% in

Table 59–15. Strategies to Modify Cardiovascular Risk Factors

---

Identification of the high risk patient
  presence of risk factors for atherosclerotic cardiovascular disease
  severity of atherosclerotic cardiovascular disease as assessed by:
    New York Heart Association functional class
    exercise/dipyridamole/thallium testing
    magnitude of left ventricular dysfunction
Optimizing hemodynamic status of high risk patient
Control of arrhythmia and utility of pacemaker
Management of valvular heart disease
Management of hypertrophic cardiomyopathy

those with triple vessel disease.[125] The reported 4.3% incidence of nonfatal myocardial infarction and a need for emergent bypass graft surgery in 3.4% of those undergoing angioplasty tend to reduce the potential usefulness of this modality as a preoperative risk modifier.[129]

Optimizing Hemodynamic Status

Preoperatively, individuals with impaired ventricular function should receive medical treatment aimed at optimizing cardiac function. Overdiuresis may produce volume depletion and possibly lead to hypotension during induction of anesthesia or in the intraoperative period. Invasive hemodynamic monitoring allows for the determination of optimal ventricular filling and performance in patients with known ventricular impairment and is especially important in those individuals undergoing major vascular, thoracic, or upper abdominal surgeries. Hemodynamic measurements with pulmonary artery catheters facilitate the administration of fluids, vasoactive, and inotropic agents intra- and postoperatively. This is especially important in the postoperative period when large fluid shifts may adversely affect cardiac performance, producing maldistribution of flow and thus impair organ perfusion and predispose to multisystem failure.

Alteration of perioperative cardiac performance as assessed by changes in the pulmonary occlusion pressure may be a more sensitive reflection of myocardial ischemia than the electrocardiogram. In addition, close monitoring of hemodynamic status postoperatively is important in the early detection of ischemic events since approximately 50% of patients will not have typical symptoms or electrocardiographic evidence of myocardial ischemia.[97,99,100] Meticulous postoperative care aided in part by hemodynamic monitoring and ventricular optimization has been shown to reduce the incidence of perioperative reinfarction (from 7.7 to 1.9%) and mortality (from 57 to 36%) in one series of patients.[106] Therefore, intraoperative hemodynamic monitoring to optimize ventricular function should be considered in the following patients:

- Severe, nonoperable coronary disease
- Left ventricular dysfunction
- History of, and electrocardiographic evidence suggestive of, prior myocardial infarction
- Severe mitral or aortic stenosis
- Patients undergoing aortic aneurysmal repair
- Emergent or urgent surgeries performed under conditions in which the cardiac status is either unknown or considered suboptimal

Currently, there are no randomized, controlled trials substantiating a reduction in either cardiac mortality or morbidity by use of intraoperative hemodynamic monitoring in these "high risk" patients. Our experience and that of others[106,130] would tend to support this management scheme, however.

Arrhythmia Control

Patients using medications for control of arrhythmias should, in general, be maintained on the medications up until the time of surgery and resumed on the same regimen postoperatively. Beta blockers have not posed a major problem by producing either bradyarrhythmias or hypotension during general anesthesia. They should be continued in the preoperative period, especially in patients with coronary atherosclerosis to prevent "rebound ischemia" from sudden beta-blocker withdrawal.[131]

Both supraventricular and ventricular arrhythmias developing in the perioperative period have been independently associated with increased risk of adverse cardiac events reflecting the presence of either valvular or underlying myocardial disease.[97,99] Prophylactic lidocaine infusions preoperatively may have a role for patients who historically have symptomatic ventricular ectopy or in patients with a prior history of cardiac arrest.[123] Preoperative pacing specifically for patients with preexisting bundle branch block, bifascicular or trifascicular heart block is unnecessary (pacing should only be performed in those situations for which it is usually indicated).[132] Patients with underlying left bundle branch block who require preoperative insertion of a pulmonary artery catheter are not at increased risk of developing complete heart block.[133,134] Therefore, temporary pacemaker insertion is unnecessary in these patients.

Hypertension Control

Patients with a history of hypertension have a 25% incidence of significant perioperative hypertension unrelated to the degree of preoperative blood pressure control.[135] This appears to be especially true in patients undergoing either abdominal aortic aneurysmal repair or other peripheral vascular surgeries including carotid endarterectomy.[135] Ultrashort-acting agents by continuous intravenous infusion (osmolal) may be especially useful in these patients. The medical regimen successful in control of preoperative hypertension should be reinstituted as soon as possible in the postoperative period.

Valvular Heart Disease

Patients with severe, symptomatic aortic, or mitral valvular disease should undergo correction of those conditions prior to the noncardiac surgery.[130] Those individuals with severe, asymptomatic aortic stenosis can be safely managed with the guidance of intraoperative hemodynamic monitoring. Optimization of fluid status and ventricular performance may reduce the risk of perioperative cardiac events to that of the age-matched population without aortic stenosis undergoing noncardiac operations.[136]

Those patients with mechanical valves receiving anticoagulation have been managed pre- and perioperatively in a number of ways. Oral anticoagulants may be discontinued one to three days preoperatively and safely resumed approximately 48 to 72 hours postoperatively without an excessive risk of bleeding or thromboembolic events.[137] Others[138] have recommended full dose intravenous heparin infusion until 6 hours prior to surgery in addition to cessation of oral anticoagulants for a 48-hour preoperative period. Heparin infusion is usually resumed 24 hours after surgery, and oral anticoagulants are subsequently used. Low thromboembolic and bleeding rates similar to that for the other management scheme have been noted using this protocol.

Antibiotic prophylaxis for patients with valvular heart disease has been recently outlined in the American Heart Association's 1990 statement.[139] Patients with previous bacterial endocarditis, congenital cardiac malformations, rheumatic or acquired valvular dysfunction, surgically constructed systemic pulmonary shunts, mitral valve prolapse with insufficiency, and those with hypertrophic obstructive cardiomyopathy undergoing upper respiratory/dental procedures or genitourinary and gastrointestinal procedures are candidates for prophylaxis. Standard antibiotic regimens are outlined in Chapters 67 and 75.

Hypertrophic Cardiomyopathy

Patients with hypertrophic cardiomyopathy generally tolerate major noncardiac surgery well without increased cardiac related mortality or arrhythmia events.[140] Vasodilators, hypovolemia, and tachycardia all of which aggravate the dynamic left ventricular outflow obstruction noted in this illness should be avoided when possible.

In summary, identification of the high risk cardiovascular patient hinges on key historical information and physical findings suggestive of diffuse atherosclerosis, valvular disease, or ventricular decompensation. Other well-defined risk factors as suggested by several "risk indices" may also serve to define the risk for the patient of the anticipated surgery. Patients with evidence of ventricular failure and those with peripheral vascular atherosclerosis require special preoperative attention for optimization of ventricular function and detection of severe, operable coronary artery disease. Exercise testing and dipyridamole thallium testing are useful techniques to define the presence of significant coronary atherosclerosis that may otherwise not be suspected preoperatively. To reduce surgical risk, patients with severe coronary artery disease should undergo preoperative bypass surgery. Careful perioperative monitoring of patients with severe valvular disease and left ventricular dysfunction may serve to reduce adverse effects of perioperative medications and fluid shifts, thus improving operative outcome.

NEUROLOGIC COMPLICATIONS

Major postoperative neurologic complications include:

- Cerebrosvascular deficits (transient and fixed)
- Peripheral neuropathies/plexopathies
- Spinal cord infarction

The postoperative incidence for each of these complications has been defined in the literature. Neuropathy and plexopathy incidence following cardiac, noncardiac, and orthopedic surgery varies from 0.02 to 5%.[141-145] Paraplegia as a result of ischemic spinal cord injury occurs in 1 to 22% of patients after thoracoabdominal aortic aneurysm repair.[146] The largest pool of information is available for neurovascular events following open heart surgery and carotid endarterectomy. The rate of postoperative vascular deficits after coronary artery bypass grafting approximates 1 to 2%,[147-150] whereas a 4% rate[151,152] has been noted for patients undergoing valvular heart surgery. Following carotid endarterectomy, the incidence of transient and fixed neurologic vascular events has been quite variable. Older series have noted rates varying from 5 to 21%,[153,154] whereas more recent authors report rates of approximately 2 to 3%.[155] Stroke rate accompanying more "remote" peripheral vascular and thoracoabdominal aortic surgery as well as other noncardiac surgeries have not been well summarized by the literature.

The mortality rate in those patients who develop postoperative strokes is high, noted by one set of investigators to approximate 23%[156] and by another set 45%.[153] A major cause of death in these patients is directly related to myocardial coronary events rather than neurologic devastation.[157] Therefore, patients who develop postoperative strokes or reversible neurologic deficits are at higher risk for subsequent lethal myocardial events.

Identification and Evaluation of Cerebrovascular Risks

Certain clinical characteristics as summarized in Table 59-16 serve to identify the patient population at increased risk of postoperative cerebrovascular events.

Pre-ICU Phase

Coronary Artery Disease. Because cardiac events are a major source of mortality, studies have been performed to determine the incidence of coronary disease in patients with neurovascular disease. Rokey and associates[158] studied 50 patients with symptoms suggestive of cerebral insufficiency in order to determine the presence of concomitant coronary disease. Patients were divided into two groups based on clinical suspicion for the presence or absence of coronary disease. Resting and exercise ventriculography estimated by gated wall motion studies and thallium perfusion scintigraphy were performed in each of these patients. Of 16 patients suspected to have coronary disease by history and electrocardiography, 15 had abnormal thallium or ventriculography scans. In addition, 14 of 34 patients without suspicion for coronary disease had abnormal scans. Of these 14 patients, 8 were subsequently noted by coronary angiography to have "significant" coronary disease.

Hertzer and co-workers[159] noted a 35% overall incidence of coronary artery disease in 506 patients with cerebrovascular disease undergoing corrective cerebrovascular surgery. Of this group, 306 patients had clinical evidence of coronary disease either by history of electrocardiography, and 200 patients were without evidence of coronary atherosclerosis. Coronary angiography performed in all 506

Table 59–16. Neurovascular Surgical Risk Factors

Coronary artery disease[158,159]
Age[160-162]
Preexisting cerebral vascular disease[164,165]
Inoperative hypotension[166]
Prolonged cardiopulmonary bypass time[167]
Aortic sclerosis
Left ventricular thrombi[168]

patients demonstrated severe correctable disease in 37% of those suspected to have coronary insufficiency and in 16% of patients not suspected to have coronary disease. Inoperable, diffuse coronary atherosclerosis was noted in 9 and 2% of these patient groups, respectively. Therefore, the presence of cerebrovascular disease should serve as a marker to identify patients with coronary artery disease. These patients may have significant asymptomatic and unsuspected coronary atherosclerosis which requires further evaluation to determine the need for surgical intervention.

Age. The rate of stroke for patients undergoing coronary bypass grafting has been defined by the literature at approximately 2%.[147-150] Cosgrove and associates[160] noted an overall 1.7% rate of stroke from 1970 through 1973 and a 1.5% stroke rate from 1980 through 1983 on a retrospective review of coronary revascularization performed on 25,000 patients. These authors also noted a trend toward increasing stroke incidence and increasing patient age (4.5% stroke rate in patients 70 years or older). Increasing stroke incidence commensurate with increasing age has also been noted by other authors in coronary bypass surgery populations. For patients over 70 years of age, Hall and colleagues[161] noted a 5.8% stroke rate compared to a 2.8% incidence overall, whereas Faro and coworkers[162] found a 10.5% stroke incidence for patients 70 years or older. Older patients undergoing valvular replacement are also at increased risk for the development of adverse cerebrovascular events. Craver and co-workers[151] noted a neurologic event rate of 8.4% for those patients over 70 years of age compared to 3% for younger patients. By multivariate analysis, increasing age was the only variable predicting development of neurologic vascular events from this study.

Gardner and colleagues[156] retrospectively studied the stroke rate over a 10-year period for 3279 patients undergoing coronary revascularization. Of this group, 56 patients developed strokes, yielding an overall incidence of 1.7%. Yearly variability in the stroke rate was noted with a low of 0.57% for 1979 and a high value of 2.4% for 1983. The overall mortality rate for the 10-year period was 3.7% with a trend to lower rate (6% in 1975 versus 2.6% in 1983) in spite of the rising yearly stroke rate. Factors identifying those patients at risk of developing stroke by univariate analysis included increasing age, evidence by history and examination for preexisting cerebrovascular disease, severe atherosclerosis of the ascending aorta noted at the time of surgery, protracted cardiopulmonary bypass time, and severe perioperative hypotension (systolic blood pressure of 40 mm Hg or less for at least 5 minutes while normothermic). History of diabetes mellitus, hypertension, and prior myocardial infarction were not significant variables identifying patients at increased stroke risk.

Underlying Cerebral Vascular Disease. The presence of cerebrovascular atherosclerosis has intrigued clinicians as a potential preoperative stroke risk factor in particular for patients undergoing open heart surgery. A history of cerebrovascular events and the presence of carotid bruits have been the usual factors identifying these "high risk" patients. The degree of carotid stenosis has been most often delineated initially by noninvasive screening studies and is frequently followed by angiography in patients considered as operable candidates. Breslau and associates[163] used noninvasive duplex scanning to ascertain the incidence of significant (>50% stenosis) cerebrovascular disease in 102 patients undergoing coronary revascularization. Twenty-four patients had either asymptomatic carotid bruits or remote symptoms suggestive of cerebrovascular disease, where 78 patients were without evidence of cerebrovascular disease by history or physical examination. Stenosis was noted in 54 and 6% of patients in these groups, respectively. One postoperative stroke and TIA occurred in 2 patients from the group without historical or physical evidence of cerebrovascular atherosclerosis, whereas no cerebrovascular complications were noted in the group with evidence of stenosis. As a result, the authors concluded that detection of asymptomatic carotid disease in a population undergoing coronary surgery did not identify a "high risk" population for adverse cerebrovascular events and, therefore, was unnecessary.

In contrast to these findings, Jones and colleagues[164] noted an increased incidence of stroke (3.3% compared to 0.9% overall) in patients with asymptomatic carotid bruits undergoing coronary bypass surgery. Furthermore, patients with a prior history of stroke or a transient ischemic attack had an 8.6% stroke rate, whereas those with prior carotid endarterectomy had a 5.1% stroke rate. Although these patients with historical evidence of cerebrovascular disease demonstrated a trend toward higher cerebrovascular complication rates, given the small patient numbers, the results were not statistically significant. Of those patients who developed strokes postoperatively, only advanced age, presence of carotid bruits, and extensive aortic atherosclerosis at the time of surgery were variables predictive of postoperative stroke.

In a retrospective series of 4047 patients who underwent cardiac surgery and were screened for the presence of asymptomatic carotid disease with noninvasive studies, Brener and co-workers[165] noted a 3.8% incidence of significant (>50% stenosis) carotid disease. Similar to the findings of Jones and associates[164] patients without any evidence of carotid disease had a lower incidence (1.9%) of fixed and reversible cerebrovascular events following surgery, whereas a 9.2% incidence was noted in those patients with significant stenosis. Patients with complete inoperable unilateral or bilateral carotid occlusion had a 15.6% incidence of postoperative neurologic events. A subset of patients with operable carotid disease underwent combined carotid and coronary revascularization surgery, whereas another group of patients with a similar magnitude of carotid atherosclerosis were only subjected to open heart surgery. The incidence of postoperative neurologic events, both permanent and reversible, in these two groups were 8.8 and 6.3%, respectively. Permanent deficits were noted in 1.8 and 1.6% of patients in each of these groups. A group of 12 patients with complete occlusion of a single carotid artery and concomitant significant obstruction of the opposite internal carotid artery were noted to have the highest incidence (33%) of postoperative neurologic events, with the majority of these events occurring in those undergoing combined carotid and cardiac surgery. As a result of these findings, the authors suggested that patients with asymptomatic carotid disease, although at increased risk of postoperative stroke, need not undergo either simultaneous or precardiac surgery carotid endarterectomy.

Intraoperative Hypotension. Intraoperative brain hypoperfusion may also place patients at increased risk for the development of perioperative cerebrosvascular insufficiency. Stockard and co-workers[166] studied 75 patients undergoing cardiovascular surgery and noted the development of cerebral dysfunction in 8 of 15 patients who were subjected to significant intraoperative hypotensive stress (drop of the mean cerebral perfusion pressure to <40 mm Hg). Of these 8 patients, 2 developed irreversible cerebral dysfunction, and 6 patients developed transient reversible ischemic events. None of the other 7 patients who were exposed to a similar level of brain hypoperfusion suffered neurologic dysfunction. Both advanced age and a history of cerebrovascular insufficiency were the key factors separating those patients developing neurologic dysfunction from those who did not. Kolkka and associates[167] studied the incidence of neurologic and neuropsychologic dysfunction following low flow, low pressure, cardiopulmonary bypass in 204 patients who underwent various types of heart surgery. Of this group, 6 patients developed new discrete motor deficits postoperatively, and an additional 35 patients exhibited global neurologic or neuropsychologic dysfunction. Patients developing these complications were older, had a higher mortality rate, a lower incidence of coronary artery bypass grafting as the sole surgical procedure, and a more prolonged time on cardiopulmonary bypass compared to patients not developing postoperative neurologic dysfunction. Mean arterial pressure during cardiopulmonary bypass was similar between the two groups (51 ± 7 mm Hg versus 49 ± 7 mm Hg), and an index of time at low pressure (torr × minutes below 50 torr) was also comparable between these two groups. As a result of these findings, the authors concluded that cardiopulmonary bypass pressure appeared not to influence neurologic outcome per se, but that prolonged cardiopulmonary bypass time, advanced age, and the type of cardiac procedure strongly influence neurologic outcome.

Aortic Sclerosis. Severe aortic sclerosis noted at the time of revascularization may be a "risk factor" related to stroke as a result of atheromatous debris embolization at the time of aortic cannulation, aortic cross-clamping or construction of the proximal vein graft anastomosis. This surgical observation has not been verified, however, in any clinical trials to date and has not been universally identified in all studies of cerebrovascular risk.

Left Ventricular Thrombi. Large left ventricular thrombi may be another source of emboli that potentially produces strokes perioperatively in open heart surgeries. In a study of 155 patients with known left ventricular clot at the time of open heart surgery, Breuer and colleagues[168] noted a 10% stroke rate in those patients versus a 2% rate in patients without evidence of ventricular clot. Manipulation of the heart during surgery may serve to dislodge micro- or macroscopic portions of clot, thus producing the cerebral insult.

In contrast to all previously outlined studies, Breuer and co-workers[169] evaluated 451 variables in a prospective analysis of 421 patients undergoing coronary revascularization to assess the frequency of central nervous system complications. Of this group, 22 patients developed central nervous system infarction, 8 of which resulted in major functional disability including 1 death; 49 additional patients were encephalopathic at the fourth postoperative day but did not have focal neurologic deficits. These authors were unable to identify by univariate analysis any specific preoperative or intraoperative risk factors predicting the development of neurovascular complications. Specifically, advanced age, history of cerebrovascular events, presence of cervical bruits, prolonged cardiopulmonary bypass time, intraoperative hypotension, and the magnitude of aortic atherosclerosis noted at the time of surgery were not variables predictive of adverse neurologic outcome, contrary to the results of previous studies.

ICU Phase: Strategies to Modify Cerebrovascular Risk

To reduce the incidence of adverse, postoperative cerebrovascular events, management strategies must include identification of factors responsible for postoperative morbidity and mortality and modification of these factors (Table 59-17). The development of perioperative stroke and transient neurologic events serve to identify patients with coronary artery disease. Given these patients' high cardiovascular mortality, it would seem prudent to evaluate these patients for the presence of surgical correctable coronary lesions prior to any anticipated surgery. Purported mechanisms responsible for these neurologic events include atheromatous debris embolization and reduced perfusion across critically stenosed cerebral vessels. Variables that may identify the open heart surgery patient with an increased risk of developing postoperative neurologic complications include:

- Advanced age
- Prolonged cardiopulmonary bypass time
- Presence of severe aortic atherosclerosis
- Left ventricular clot

Previous history of cerebrovascular events and the presence of asymptomatic cerebrovascular disease are controversial risk factors but may also serve to help identify high risk patients. Improved operative technique and avoidance of the severely sclerotic portion of the aorta during cannulation for bypass surgery may help to reduce perioperative atherosclerotic embolization. Minimizing cardiopulmonary bypass time during surgery would seem to be a prudent measure. Presence of asymptomatic cerebrovascular disease does not appear to warrant more invasive testing; however, patients should be informed of an increased risk for postoperative stroke. Patients with symptomatic neuro-

Table 59–17. Strategies to Modify Cerebrovascular Risk Factors

---
Define presence/severity of concomitant coronary atherosclerosis
Minimized cardiopulmonary bypass time/hypotension
Avoid manipulating severely sclerotic portion of aorta
Staged cerebral/coronary bypass grafting
---

vascular disease or patients in whom a history of stroke exists should undergo angiographic evaluation of the cerebral circulation to determine the presence of disease requiring surgery. In the absence of significant coronary disease, most authorities would perform surgical correction in a staged fashion completing carotid revascularization prior to any other surgery.[157,164] In patients with unstable angina, triple vessel or left main coronary disease and transient ischemic attacks, simultaneous carotid/coronary surgery can be safely performed.[157,164,170]

Identification and Evaluation of Peripheral Nerve Surgical Risk

Well-defined factors increasing the risk of peripheral nerve damage in postoperative patients have been enumerated in Table 59–18.

Pre-ICU Phase

Positioning. Brachial plexus injury during general anesthesia was noted to occur in three separate cases among 15000 cases by Cooper and colleagues[141] yielding an incidence of 0.02%. Others[142] have reported incidence of brachial plexus injury of approximately 0.06% for various types of surgery. Damage most likely results from nerve stretching due to positioning of the arms. Upper plexus lesions tend to occur during abduction, whereas lower plexus lesions tend to occur when the arm lies close to the side.[171] Wrist suspension in the Trendelenburg position stretches the lower trunk of the plexus. Abduction of the arms while in the Trendelenburg position as may happen with lateral placement of arm pads drives the humeral head downward towards the wrists and stretches the plexus around it.[171]

Perioperative ulnar nerve damage may also occur, attributable to injury produced by pronation and adduction of the arm. Miller and Camp[172] studied 8 patients who developed ulnar injuries after abdominal and thoracic surgery. The electrophysiologic data supported injury at the level of the cubital tunnel. The authors hypothesized that injury was due to pressure from either the side rail of the bed used to attach appliances or pressure from a sharp edge of the operating room table.

Surgical/Invasive Procedures. The frequency of brachial plexus injuries following median sternotomy during open heart surgery has been quite variable. Graham and co-workers[173] noted that 5 patients among 940 developed injury to the lower root of the brachial plexus, whereas Lederman and associates[144] and Hanson and colleagues[145] found that 26 patients from 531 undergoing open heart surgery sustained plexus injury. Pain was not a prominent feature in most of these patients, and recovery within six to eight weeks occurred frequently. Cannulation of the jugular vein producing "needle trauma" may play a role in the injury, since the authors were able to correlate the site of jugular line placement with brachial injury. In addition, left internal mammary artery dissection which requires a greater degree of chest wall retraction and, thus, nerve stretching may also be another co-factor in the development of brachial injury.

Rib resection for thoracic outlet syndrome has also been noted to produce brachial injury. Wilbourn[174] described 8 patients who underwent surgery for thoracic outlet syndrome who subsequently developed severe causalgia and neurologic deficit. Electromyelographic findings performed 6 to 7 years after surgery were compatible with severe axonal injury, especially in the median nerve territory. Kline and Judice,[175] in a series of 171 patients with diverse types of brachial injury described 4 patients with brachioplexopathy following first rib resection. Cherington and associates[176] described 5 patients with brachial plexus injury after thoracic outlet surgery, 3 of whom developed postoperative causalgia. Stretching injury to the plexus is the most likely clinical explanation for injury; however, the nature of the clinical finding did not support this mechanism. Kline and Judice[175] suggested that surgical trauma (nerve avulsion) may be the culprit, whereas Wilbourn[174] argued that reduction of sensory and motor action potentials on electromyelography was not compatible with avulsion injury

Ischemic injury to nerve due to invasive catheter placement, angiography, and other similar procedures may also produce nerve damage. Hematoma formation at the site of cannulation may compromise blood supply to the nerve. Carroll and Wilkins[177] described two cases of brachial plexopathy following axillary artery puncture as a result of hematoma compression. Honet and colleagues[178] noted that 6 patients following femoral vein cannulation developed neurologic deficits to the legs and suggested hematoma formation may be responsible. That several patients demonstrated bilateral injury argues, however, against a purely compressive phenomenon and suggests embolic vascular lesions. In a study of patients receiving renal transplantation, 8 patients were noted to develop ulnar neuropathies.[179] The presence of the arteriovenous fistula in the same arm may have played a role in the development of the neuropathy. Follow-up electromyelographic studies by Wilbourn and associates[180] were performed on 14 patients who had ischemic neuropathy of diverse types. Distal burning pain and sparing of muscular power were the main clinical features. Axonal loss without muscle damage was demonstrated on the electrophysiologic studies of these patients.

Rose and colleagues[181] noted a 0.88% incidence of peroneal palsy following arthroplasties. Etiologies possibly accounting for the injury included soft tissue surgical dissection and postoperative positioning in the continuous passive motion machine applied to the knee.[182] Surgical trauma, bleeding, or stretching of nerves have been the

Table 59–18. Peripheral Nerve Surgical Risk Factors

Positoning during surgery[171,172]
Surgical/invasive procedures
    following median sternotomy[144,145,178]
    following thoracic outlet syndrome surgery[174-176]
    following vascular catheter placement[177-178]
    following arteriovenous fistula[179]
    following arthroplasty[181-183]
    following abdominal surgery[184,185]

most frequently cited etiologies for sciatic, femoral or obturator nerve damage following hip arthroplasty.[183]

Abdominal surgery, hernia repair, and gynecologic surgery may damage local nerves traversing the abdominal wall. The ilioinguinal nerve is probably the most frequently damaged of the cutaneous nerves supplying the area. Nerve damage produces pain, sensory loss of the inguinal canal as well as the scrotum or labia and the base of the penis. Similarly, damage to the ilioinguinal nerve and genitofemoral nerve may, respectively, produce sensory loss and causalgia over the area of the greater trochanter, the lower abdominal wall above the pubis, the medial thigh, and the majority of the scrotum or labia.[184,185]

Post ICU Phase: Recovery from Peripheral Nerve Injury

The prognosis and recovery from nerve injury depends on the nature of the mechanism producing the deficit. Therefore, it becomes important to identify whether the etiology is due to compression, traction, or ischemia. Electrophysiologic studies performed early after the insult usually are able to accurately localize the damage and differentiate between axonal loss or conduction block.[186] Electromyelography may show evidence of denervation only one to three weeks following nerve injury, whereas conduction studies revealing axonal loss may demonstrate abnormalities within the first week of injury.[186] Studies performed weeks beyond the insult may demonstrate more clearly axonal loss or suggest regeneration and reinnervation.[186] In the absence of this latter finding, some recommend surgical exploration to determine whether the nerve trunk is in continuity and in need of reconstructive repair.[175]

In summary, perioperative peripheral neuropathy may result from a number of insults. Nerve stretching, avulsion, compression, and ischemia may occur from various procedures during surgery or in the postoperative period. Certain operations (i.e., sternotomy or first rib resection) appear to place patients at increased risk for nerve damage; however, other risk factors have not been clearly defined by the literature.

Spinal Cord Surgical Risk Factors and Modification of Risk

The development of spinal cord infarction producing paraplegia following thoracicoabdominal aortic aneurysm surgery is unpredictable.[155] The occurrence of this complication is probably most closely related to the extent and nature of the aneurysm itself, rather than the operative technique.[187] The incidence is directly related to the extensiveness of the aneurysm as summarized in Table 59-19.

In order to reduce the rate of this complication, several authors[188] recommend careful monitoring of cerebrospinal fluid pressure during surgery to detect elevated pressure. Drainage of the spinal fluid may facilitate lowering of pressure and may promote improved anterior spinal artery blood flow and, thus, prevent vascular injury to the cord.[188,189] Another approach uses regional spinal cord hypothermia to protect the cord during surgery from ischemic and metabolic insult.[190] Both techniques have not

Table 59–19. Incidence of Spinal Cord Ischemic Injury in Relation to Type of Aorta Aneurysm

Type I	8%
Type II	21%
Type III	2%
Type IV	1%

(Data from Crawford, E. S., et al.: Thoracoabdominal aortic aneurysms: preoperative and intraoperative factors determining immediate and long term results of operation in 605 patients. J. Vasc. Surg., *3*:389, 1986.)

been studied in a prospective fashion and await further studies before acceptance into routine clinical practice.

Post- and perioperative control of blood pressure with sodium nitroprusside may promote spinal fluid hypertension and increase the potential for ischemic cord injury. Therefore, other agents, particularly the calcium-channel blockers, may eventually replace sodium nitroprusside for the control of blood pressure perioperatively if trials verify improved outcome in reduction of paraplegia.

REFERENCES

1. Stein, M., Koota, G. M., Simon, M., and Frank, H. A.: Pulmonary evaluation of surgical patients. JAMA, *181:*765, 1962.
2. Meneely, G. R., Ferguson, J. L.: Pulmonary evaluation and risk in patient preparation for anesthesia and surgery. JAMA, *175:*1074, 1961.
3. Latimer, R. G., et al.: Ventilatory patterns and pulmonary complications after upper abdominal surgery determined by preoperative and postoperative computerized spirometry and blood gas analysis. Am. J. Surg., *122:*622, 1971.
4. Gracey, D. R., Divertie, M. B., and Didier, E. P.: Preoperative pulmonary preparation of patients with chronic obstructive pulmonary disease. Chest, *76:*123, 1979.
5. Claque, M. B., Collin, J., and Fleming, L. B.: Prediction of postoperative respiratory complications by simple spirometry. Ann. R. Coll. Surg. Eng., *61:*59, 1979.
6. Tahir, A. H., et al.: Effects of abdominal surgery upon diaphragm function and regional ventilation. Int. Surg., *48:*337, 1973.
7. Ali, J., et al.: Consequences of postoperative alterations in respiratory mechanics. Am. J. Surg., *128:*376, 1974.
8. Tisi, G. M.: Preoperative evaluation of pulmonary function. Am. Rev. Respir. Dis., *119:*293, 1979.
9. Ford, G. T., et al.: Diaphragm function after upper abdominal surgery in humans. Am. Rev. Respir. Dis., *127:*431, 1983.
10. Meyers, J. R., Lembeck, L., O'Kane, H., and Baue, A. E.: Changes in functional residual capacity of the lung after operation. Arch. Surg., *110:*576, 1975.
11. Gass, G. D., and Olsen, G. N.: Preoperative pulmonary function testing to predict postoperative morbidity and mortality. Chest, *89:*127, 1986.
12. Woltering, E. A., Flye, M. W., and Huntley, S.: Evaluation of bupivacaine nerve blocks in the modification of pain and pulmonary function after thoracotomy. Ann. Thorac. Surg., *30:*122, 1980.
13. Simmoneau, G., et al.: Diaphragm dysfunction induced by upper abdominal surgery. Am. Rev. Respir. Dis., *128:*899, 1983.

14. Dureuil, B., et al.: Diaphragmatic contractility after upper abdominal surgery. J. Appl. Physiol., 61:1775, 1986.
15. Maeda, H., et al.: Diaphragm function after pulmonary resection. Am. Rev. Respir. Dis., 137:678, 1988.
16. Bartlett, R. H., Gazzaniga, A. B., and Geraghty, T. R.: Respiratory maneuvers to prevent postoperative pulmonary complications. JAMA, 224:1017, 1973.
17. Pett, S. B., and Wernly, J. A.: Respiratory function in surgical patients: Perioperative evaluation and management. Surg. Annu., 20:311, 1988.
18. Hales, C. A., and Kazemi, H.: Small airways function in myocardial infarction. N. Engl. J. Med., 290:761, 1974.
19. Harken, A. H., and O'Connor, N. E.: The influence of clinically undetectable edema on small airway closure in the dog. Ann. Surg., 184:183, 1976.
20. Parfrey, P. S., Harte, P. J., Quinlan, J. P., and Brady, M. P.: Pulmonary function in the early postoperative period. Br. J. Surg., 64:384, 1977.
21. Warner, M. A., et al.: Role of preoperative cessation of smoking and other factors in postoperative pulmonary complications: a blinded prospective study of coronary artery bypass patients. Mayo Clin Proc., 64:609, 1989.
22. Stevens, W. C., and Kingston, H. G. G.: Inhalation anesthesia. In Clinical Anesthesia. Edited by P. G. Barash, B. F. Cullen, and R. K. Stoelting. Philadelphia, J. B. Lippincott, 1989, p. 293.
23. Rehader, K., Sessler, A., and Marsh, H. M.: General anesthesia and the lung. Am. Rev. Respir. Dis., 112:541, 1975.
24. Niederman, M. S., Craven, D. E., Fein, A. M., and Schultz, D. E.: Pneumonia in the critically ill hospitalized patient. Chest, 97:170, 1990.
25. Pasulka, P. S., Bistrian, B. R., Benotti, P. N., and Blackburn, G. L.: The risks of surgery in obese patients. Ann. Intern. Med., 104:540, 1986.
26. Dureuil, B., Cantineau, J. P., and Vogel, J.: Vital capacity and diaphragm function after abdominal surgery (abstract). Anesthesiology, 61:A478, 1984.
27. Vaughan, R. W., Engelhart, R. C., and Wise, L.: Postoperative hypoxemia in obese patients. Ann. Surg., 180:877, 1974.
28. Sugerman, H. J., Fairman, R. P., Baron, P. L., and Kwentus, J. A.: Gastric surgery for respiratory insufficiency of obesity. Chest, 90:81, 1986.
29. Warner, M. A., Divertie, M. B., and Tinker, J. H.: Preoperative cessation of cigarette smoking and pulmonary complications in coronary artery bypass patients. Anesthesiology, 60:380, 1984.
30. Camner, P., and Philipson, K.: Some studies of tracheobronchial clearance in man. Chest, 63:23S, 1973.
31. Martin, R. R., et al.: The early detection of airway obstruction. Am. Rev. Respir. Dis., 111:119, 1975.
32. Buist, A. S., Sexton, G. J., Nagy, J. M., and Koss, B. B.: The effect of smoking cessation and modification on lung function. Am. Rev. Respir. Dis., 114:115, 1976.
33. Mitchell, C., Garrahy, P., and Peake, P.: Postoperative respiratory morbidity: identification and risk factors. Aust. N. Z. J. Surg., 52:203, 1982.
34. Bode, F. R., Dosman, J., Martin, R. R., and Macklem, P. T.: Reversibility of pulmonary function abnormalities in smokers: a prospective study of early diagnostic tests of small airways disease. Am. J. Med., 59:43, 1975.
35. Ravin, M. B.: Comparison of spinal and general anesthesia for lower abdominal surgery in patients with chronic obstructive pulmonary disease. Anesthesiology, 35:319, 1971.
36. Celli, R. B., Rodriguez, K. S., and Snider, G. L.: A controlled trial of intermittent positive pressure breathing, incentive spirometry and deep breathing exercises in preventing pulmonary complications after abdominal surgery. Am. Rev. Respir. Dis., 130:12, 1984.
37. Tarhan, S., et al.: Risk of anesthesia and surgery in patients with chronic bronchitis and chronic obstructive pulmonary disease. Surgery, 74:720, 1973.
38. de la Rocha, A. G., and Chambers, K.: Pain amelioration after thoracotomy: a prospective, randomized study. Ann. Thorac. Surg., 37:239, 1984.
39. Gustafsson, L. L., Schildt, B., and Jacobsen, K. J.: Adverse effects of extradural and intrathecal opiates: report of a nationwide survey in Sweden. Br. J. Anaesth., 54:479, 1982.
40. Ali, J., and Khan, T. A.: the comparative effects of muscle transection and median upper abdominal incisions on postoperative pulmonary function. Surg. Gynecol. Obstet., 148:863, 1979.
41. Vaughan, R. W., and Wise, L.: Choice of abdominal operative incision in the obese patient. Ann. Surg., 181:829, 1975.
42. Halasz, N. A.: Vertical vs. horizontal laparotomies. Arch. Surg., 88:911, 1964.
43. Black, J., Kalloor, G. J., and Collis, J. L.: The effect of the surgical approach on respiratory function after oesophageal resection. Br. J Surg., 64:624, 1977.
44. Tita, J., et al.: Clinical correlations of diaphragmatic paralysis associated with heart surgery. Chest, 88(Suppl):2S, 1985.
45. Esposito, R., and Spencer, F. C.: The effect of pericardial insulation on hypothermic phrenic nerve injury during open heart surgery. Ann. Thorac. Surg., 43:303, 1987.
46. Abd, A. G., et al.: Diaphragmatic dysfunction after open heart surgery: treatment with a rocking bed. Ann. Intern. Med., 111:881, 1989.
47. Mitchell, C., Garrahy, P., and Peake, P.: Postoperative respiratory morbidity: identification and risk factors. Aust. N. Z. J. Surg., 52:203, 1982.
48. Boushy, S. F., Billig, D. M., North, L. B., and Helgason, A. H.: Clinical course related to preoperative and postoperative pulmonary function in patients with bronchogenic carcinoma. Chest, 59:383, 1971.
49. Didolkar, M. S., Moore, R. H., and Takita, H.: Evaluation of risk in pulmonary resection for bronchogenic carcinoma. Am. J. Surg., 127:700, 1974.
50. Stein, M., Koota, G. M., Simon, M., and Frank, H. A.: Pulmonary evaluation of surgical patients. JAMA, 181:765, 1962.
51. Stein, M., and Cassara, E. L.: Preoperative pulmonary evaluation and therapy for surgery patients. JAMA, 211:787, 1970.
52. Miller, W. F., Wu, N., and Johnson, R. L.: Convenient method of evaluating pulmonary ventilatory function with a single breath. Anesthesiology, 17:480, 1956.
53. Cain, H. D., Stevens, P. M., and Adoniya, R.: Preoperative pulmonary function and complications after cardiovascular surgery. Chest, 76:130, 1979.
54. Milledge, J. S., and Nunn, J. F.: Criteria of fitness for anesthesia in patients with chronic obstructive lung disease. Br. Med. J., 3:670, 1975.
55. Williams, C. D., and Brenowitz, J. B.: Prohibitive lung function and major surgical procedures. Am. J. Surg., 132:763, 1976.
56. Hodgkin, J. E., Dines, D. E., and Didier, C. P.: Preoperative evaluation of the patient with pulmonary disease. Mayo Clin. Proc., 48:588, 1973.
57. Gold, M. I., and Helrich, M.: A study of the complications related to anesthesia in asthmatic patients. Anesth. Analg., 42:283, 1963.
58. Oh, S. H., and Patterson, R.: Surgery in corticosteroid-dependent asthmatics. J. Allergy Clin. Immunol., 53:345, 1974.

59. Hirshman, C. A., and Bergman, N. A.: Halothane and enflurane protect against bronchospasm in an asthma dog model. Anesth. Analg., 57:629, 1978.
60. Hirshman, C. A., et al.: Mechanism of action of inhalational anesthesia on airways. Anesthesiology, 56:107, 1982.
61. Stirt, J. A., et al.: Safety of enflurane following administration of aminophylline in experimental animals. Anesth. Analg., 60:871, 1981.
62. Stirt, J. A., Berger, J. M., and Sullivan, S. F.: Lack of arrhythmogenicity of isoflurane following administration of aminophylline in dogs. Anesth. Analg., 62:568, 1983.
63. Gaensler, E. A., et al.: The role of pulmonary insufficiency in mortality and invalidism following surgery for pulmonary tuberculosis. J. Thorac. Cardiovasc. Surg., 29:163, 1955.
64. Mittman, C.: Assessment of operative risk in thoracic surgery. Ann. Rev. Respir. Dis., 84:197, 1961.
65. Lockwood, P.: Lung function test results and the risk of post-thoracotomy complications. Respiration, 30:539, 1973.
66. Boysen, P. G., Block, A. J., and Moulder, P. V.: Relationship between preoperative pulmonary function tests and complications after thoracotomy. Surg. Gynecol. Obstet., 52:813, 1981.
67. Walkup, R. H., Vossel, L. F., Griffin, J. P., and Proctor, R. J.: Prediction of postoperative pulmonary function with the lateral position test: a prospective study. Chest, 77:24, 1980.
68. Jay, S. J., Stonehill, R. B., Kiblani, S. O., and Norton, J.: Variability of the lateral position test in normal subjects. Am. Rev. Respir. Dis., 121:165, 1980.
69. Schoonover, G. A., et al.: Lateral position test and quantitative lung scan in the preoperative evaluation for lung resection. Chest, 86:854, 1984.
70. Kristersson, S., Lindell, S., and Sranberg, L.: Prediction of pulmonary function loss due to pneumonectomy using 133Xe radiospirometry. Chest, 62:694, 1972.
71. Olsen, G. N., Block, A. J., and Tobias, J. A.: Prediction of postpneumonectomy pulmonary function using quantitative macroaggregate lung scanning. Chest, 66:13, 1974.
72. Ali, M. L., et al.: Predicting loss of pulmonary function after pulmonary resection for bronchogenic carcinoma. Chest, 77:337, 1980.
73. Wernly, J. A., et al.: Clinical value of quantitative ventilation-perfusion lung scans in the surgical management of bronchogenic carcinoma. J. Thorac. Cardiovasc. Surg., 80:535, 1980.
74. Ferguson, M. K., et al.: Diffusing capacity predicts morbidity and mortality after pulmonary resection. J. Thorac. Cardiovasc. Surg., 96:894, 1988.
75. Markos, J., et al.: Preoperative assessment as a predictor of mortality and morbidity after lung resection. Am. Rev. Respir. Dis., 139:902, 1989.
76. Harrison, R. W., et al.: The clinical significance of cor pulmonale in the prediction of cardiopulmonary reserve following extensive pulmonary resection. J. Thorac. Surg., 36:352, 1958.
77. DeGaff, A. C., et al.: Exercise limitation following extensive pulmonary resection. J. Clin. Invest., 44:1514, 1965.
78. Laros, C. D., and Swierenga, J.: Temporary unilateral pulmonary artery occlusion in the preoperative evaluation of patients with bronchial carcinoma. Med. Thorac., 24:269, 1967.
79. Rams, J. J., et al.: Operative pulmonary artery pressure measurements as a guide to postoperative management and prognosis following pneumonectomy. Dis. Chest, 41:85, 1962.
80. Uggla, L. G.: Indications for and results of thoracic surgery with regard to respiratory and circulatory function tests. Acta Chir. Scand., 111:197, 1956.
81. Olsen, G. N., et al.: Pulmonary function evaluation of the lung resection candidate: a prospective study. Am. Rev. Respir. Dis., 111:379, 1975.
82. Reichel, J.: Assessment of operative risk of pneumonectomy. Chest, 62:570, 1972.
83. Fee, J. H., et al.: Role of pulmonary vascular resistance measurements in preoperative evaluation of candidates for pulmonary resection. J. Thorac. Cardiovasc. Surg., 75:519, 1975.
84. Colman, N. C. Schraufrasel, D. E., Rivington, R. N., and Purdy, R. J.: Exercise testing in evaluation of patients for lung resection. Am. Rev. Respir. Dis., 125:604, 1982.
85. Eugene, J., et al.: Maximum oxygen consumption: a physiology guide to pulmonary resection. Surg. Forum, 33:260, 1982.
86. Smith, T. P., et al.: Exercise capacity as a predictor of post-thoracotomy morbidity. Am. Rev. Respir. Dis., 129:730, 1984.
87. Bechard, D., and Wetstein, L.: Assessment of exercise oxygen consumption as preoperative criterion for lung resection. Ann. Thorac. Surg., 44:344, 1987.
88. Miyoshi, S., et al.: Exercise tolerance test in lung cancer patients: the relationship between exercise capacity and post-thoracotomy hospital mortality. Ann. Thorac. Surg., 44:487, 1987.
89. Olsen, G. N., et al.: Submaximal invasive exercise testing an quantitative lung scanning in the evaluation for tolerance of lung resection. Chest, 95:267, 1989.
90. Anscombe, A. R., and Buxton, R. S.: Effect of abdominal operations on total lung capacity and its subdivisions. Br. Med. J., 2:84, 1958.
91. Schwieger, I., et al.: Absence of benefit of incentive spirometry in low risk patients undergoing elective cholecystectomy. Chest, 89:652, 1986.
92. Stock, M. C., et al.: Prevention of postoperative pulmonary complications with CPAP, incentive spirometry and conservative therapy. Chest, 87:151, 1985.
93. Ricksten, S., et al.: Effects of periodic positive airway pressure by mask on postoperative pulmonary function. Chest, 89:774, 1986.
94. Kiriloff, L. H., Owens, G. R., Rogers, R. M., and Mazzocco, M. C.: Does chest physical therapy work? Chest, 88:436, 1985.
95. Tarhan, S., Moffitt, E. A., Taylor, W. F., and Giuliani, E. R.: Myocardial infarction after general anesthesia. JAMA., 220:1451, 1972.
96. Van Knorring, J.: Postoperative myocardial infarction: a prospective study in a risk group of surgical patients. Surgery, 90:55, 1981.
97. Goldman, L., et al.: Cardiac risk factors and complications in non-cardiac surgery. Medicine, 57:357, 1978.
98. Steen, P. A., Tinker, J. H., and Tarhan, S.: Myocardial reinfarction after anesthesia and surgery. JAMA, 239:2566, 1978.
99. Goldman, L., et al.: Multifactorial index of cardiac risk in non-cardiac surgical procedures. N. Engl. J. Med., 297:845, 1977.
100. Zeldin, R. A.: Assessing cardiac risk in patients who undergo noncardiac surgical procedures. Can. J. Surg., 27:402, 1984.
101. Jeffery, C. C., Kunsman, J., Cullen, D. J., and Brewster, D. C.: A prospective evaluation of cardiac risk index. Anesthesiology, 58:462, 1983.
102. Taylor, P. C.: Evaluation and surgical management of patients with severe combined coronary artery disease and

peripheral vascular atherosclerosis. Cleve. Clin. Q., 48:172, 1981.
103. Hertzer, N. R., et al.: Coronary artery disease in peripheral vascular patients: a classification of 1,000 coronary angiograms and results of surgical management. Ann. Surg., 199: 223, 1984.
104. Brown, O. W., et al.: Abdominal aortic aneurysm and coronary artery disease: a reassessment. Arch. Surg., 116:1484, 1981.
105. Hollier, L. H., et al.: Late survival after abdominal aortic aneurysm repair: influence of coronary artery disease. J. Vasc. Surg., 1:290, 1984.
106. Rao, T. L. K., Jacobs, K. H., and El-Etr, A. A.: Reinfarction following anesthesia in patients with myocardial infarction. Anesthesiology, 59:499, 1983.
107. Detsky, A. S., et al.: Predicting cardiac complications in patients undergoing non-cardiac surgery. J. Gen. Intern. Med., 1:211, 1986.
108. Detsky, A. S., et al.: Cardiac assessment for patients undergoing noncardiac surgery: a multifactorial clinical risk index. Arch. Intern. Med., 146:2131, 1986.
109. Slogoff, S., and Keats, A. S.: Does perioperative myocardial ischemia lead to postoperative myocardial infarction? Anesthesiology 62:107, 1985.
110. Foster, E. D., et al.: Risk of noncardiac operation in patients with defined coronary disease: the Coronary Artery Surgery Study (CASS) Registry experience. Ann. Thorac. Surg., 41: 42, 1986.
111. Pasternack, P. F., et al.: The value of the radionuclide angiogram in the prediction of perioperative myocardial infarction in patients undergoing lower extremity revascularization procedures. Circulation, 72(Suppl. II):II13, 1985.
112. Kazmers, A., Cerqueira, M. D., and Zierler, R. E.: The role of preoperative radionuclide left ventricular ejection fraction for risk assessment in carotid surgery. Arch. Surg., 123: 416, 1988.
113. Goenen, A., et al.: Preoperative left ventricular dysfunction and operative risk of coronary artery bypass surgery. Chest, 92:804, 1987.
114. Cutler, B. S., Wheeler, H. B., Paraskos, J. A., and Cardullo, P. A.: Applicability and interpretation of electrocardiographic stress testing in patients with peripheral vascular disease. Am. J. Surg., 141:501, 1981.
115. Carliner, N. H., et al.: Routine preoperative exercise testing in patients undergoing major noncardiac surgery. Am. J. Cardiol., 56:51, 1985.
116. Gerson, M. C., et al.: Cardiac prognosis in noncardiac geriatric surgery. Ann. Intern. Med., 103:832, 1985.
117. Kopecky, S. L., Gibbons, R. J., and Hollier, L. H.: Preoperative supine exercise radionuclide angiogram predicts perioperative cardiovascular events in vascular surgery (abstract). J. Am. Coll. Cardiol., 7(Suppl A):226A, 1986.
118. Leppo, J. A., et al.: Serial thallium-201 myocardial imaging following dipyridamole infusion: diagnostic utility in detecting coronary stenosis and relationship to regional wall motion. Circulation, 66:649, 1982.
119. Josephson, M. A., et al.: Noninvasive detection and localization of coronary stenoses in patients: comparison of resting dipyridamole and exercise thallium-201 myocardial perfusion imaging. Am. Heart J., 103:1008, 1982.
120. Boucher, C. A., et al.: Determination of cardiac risk by dipyridamole-thallium imaging before peripheral vascular surgery. N. Engl. J. Med., 312:389, 1985.
121. Leppo, J., et al.: Noninvasive evaluation of cardiac risk before elective vascular surgery. J. Am. Coll. Cardiol., 9:269, 1987.
122. Eagle, K. A., et al.: Dipyridamole-thallium scanning in patients undergoing vascular surgery: optimizing preoperative evaluation of cardiac risk. JAMA, 257:2185, 1987.
123. Goldman, L.: Assessment and management of the cardiac patient before, during and after noncardiac surgery. In Cardiology. Vol. 2. Edited by W. W. Parmley, K. Chatterjee. Philadelphia, J. B. Lippincott, 1988, p. 1.
124. Hertzer, N. R., et al.: Routine coronary angiography prior to elective aortic reconstruction: results of selective myocardial revascularization in patients with peripheral vascular disease. Arch. Surg., 114:1336, 1979.
125. DeBakey, M. E., and Lawrie, G. M.: Combined coronary artery and peripheral vascular disease: recognition and treatment (editorial). J. Vasc. Surg., 1:605, 1984.
126. Hertzer, N. R.: Fatal myocardial infarction following lower extremity revascularization: two hundred seventy three patients followed six to eleven postoperative years. Ann. Surg., 193:492, 1981.
127. Ennix, C. L., Jr., et al.: Improved results of carotid endarterectomy in patients with symptomatic coronary disease: an analysis of 1,546 consecutive carotid operations. Stroke, 10:122, 1979.
128. Kennedy, J. W., et al.: Clinical and angiographic predictors of operative mortality from the Collaborative Study in Coronary Artery Surgery (CASS). Circulation 63:793, 1981.
129. Detre, K., et al.: Percutaneous transluminal coronary angioplasty in 1985-1986 and 1977-1981: The National Heart, Lung and Blood Institute Registry. N. Engl. J. Med., 318: 265, 1988.
130. Freeman, W. K., Gibbons, R. J., and Shub, C.: Preoperative assessment of cardiac patients undergoing noncardiac surgical procedures. Mayo Clin. Proc., 64:1105, 1989.
131. Goldman, L.: Cardiac risk and complications of noncardiac surgery. Ann. Intern. Med., 98:504, 1983.
132. Frye, R. L., et al.: Guidelines for permanent cardiac pacemaker implantation. May 1984: a report of the Joint American College of Cardiology/American Heart Association Task Force on Assessment of Cardiovascular Procedures (Subcommittee on Pacemaker Implantation). Circulation, 70: 331A, 1984.
133. Sprung, C. L., et al.: Risk of right bundle branch block and complete heart block developing pulmonary artery catheterization. Crit. Care Med., 17:1, 1989.
134. Morris, D., Mulvihill, D., and Lew, W. Y. W.: Risk of developing complete heart block during bedside pulmonary artery catheterization in patients with left bundle branch block. Arch. Int. Med., 147:2005, 1987.
135. Goldman, L., and Caldera, D. L.: Risks of general anesthesia and elective operation in the hypertensive patient. Anesthesiology, 50:285, 1979.
136. O'Keefe, J. H., Shub, C., and Rettke, S. R.: Can patients with severe aortic stenosis safely undergo noncardiac surgery? (abstract). Circulation, 78(Suppl. II):II-132, 1988.
137. Tinker, J. H., and Tarhan, S.: Discontinuing anticoagulant therapy in surgical patients with cardiac valve prostheses: observations in 180 operations. JAMA, 239:738, 1978.
138. Katholi, R. E., Nolan, S. P., and McGuire, L. B.: The management of anticoagulation during noncardiac operations in patients with prosthetic heart valves: a prospective study. Am. Heart J., 96:163, 1978.
139. Dajani, A. S., et al.: Prevention of bacterial endocarditis: recommendations by the American Heart Association. JAMA, 264:2919, 1990.
140. Thompson, R. C., Liberthson, R. R., and Lowenstein, E.: Perioperative anesthetic risk of noncardiac surgery in hypertrophic obstructive cardiomyopathy. JAMA, 254:2419, 1985.
141. Cooper, D. E., Jenkins, R. S., Bready, L., and Rockwood, C.

A.: The prevention of injuries of the brachial plexus secondary to malposition of the patient during surgery. Clin. Orthop., *228*:33, 1988.
142. Parks, B. J.: Postoperative peripheral neuropathies. Surgery, *74*:348, 1973.
143. Po, B. T., and Hansen, H. R.: Iatrogenic brachial plexus injury: a survey of the literature and pertinent cases. Anesth. Analg., *48*:915, 1969.
144. Lederman, R. J., et al.: Peripheral nervous system complications of coronary artery bypass graft surgery. Ann. Neurol., *12*:297, 1982.
145. Hanson, M. R., et al.: Mechanism and frequency of branchial plexus injury in open heart surgery: a prospective analysis. Ann. Thorac. Surg., *36*:675, 1983.
146. Crawford, E. S., et al.: Thoracoabdominal aortic aneurysms: preoperative and intraoperative factors determining immediate and long term results of operation in 605 patients. J. Vasc. Surg., *3*:389, 1986.
147. Ashor, G. W., et al.: Coronary artery disease surgery in 100 patients 65 years of age or older. Arch. Surg., *107*:30, 1973.
148. Breuer, A. C., et al.: Neurologic complications of open heart surgery: computer assisted analysis of 531 patients. Cleve. Clin. Q., *48*:205, 1981.
149. Loop, F. D., et al.: An 11 year evolution of coronary artery surgery (1967–1978). Ann. Surg., *190*:444, 1979.
150. Reul, F. J., et al.: Current concepts in coronary artery surgery: a critical analysis of 1,287 patients. Ann. Thorac. Surg., *14*:243, 1972.
151. Craver, J. M., et al.: Predictors of mortality, complications, and length of stay in aortic valve replacement for aortic stenosis. Circulation, *78*:185, 1988.
152. Gallo, I., Artiano, E., and Nistal, F.: Four to seven year follow-up of patients undergoing Carpentier-Edwards porcine heart valve replacement. Thorac. Cardiovasc. Surg., *33*:347, 1985.
153. Easton, J. D., and Sherman, D. G.: Stroke and mortality rate in carotid endarterectomy: 228 consecutive operations. Stroke, *8*:565, 1977.
154. Bouchier-Hayes, D., DeCosta, A., and Macgowan, A. L.: The morbidity of carotid endarterectomy. Br. J. Surg., *66*:433, 1979.
155. Callow, A. D.: Cerebrovascular insufficiency. *In* Haimovici's Vascular Surgery Principles and Practices, 3rd Ed. Edited by H. Haimovici, et al. East Norwalk, CT, Appleton & Lange, 1989, p. 734.
156. Gardner, T. J., et al.: Stroke following coronary artery bypass grafting: a ten year experience. Ann. Thorac. Surg., *40*:574, 1985.
157. Graor, R. A., and Hertzer, N. R.: Management of coexisting carotid artery and coronary artery disease. Stroke, *19*:1441, 1988.
158. Rokey, R., et al.: Coronary artery disease in patients with cerebrovascular disease: a prospective study. Ann. Neurol., *16*:50, 1984.
159. Hertzer, N. R., et al.: Coronary angiography in 506 patients with extracranial cerebrovascular disease. Arch. Intern. Med., *145*:848, 1985.
160. Cosgrove, D. M., et al.: Primary myocardial revascularization trends in surgical mortality. J. Thorac. Cardiovasc. Surg., *88*:673, 1984.
161. Hall, R. J., et al.: Coronary artery bypass: long term followup of 22,284 consecutive patients. Circulation, *68*:II-20, 1983.
162. Faro, R. S., et al.: Coronary revascularization in septuagenarians. J. Thorac. Cardiovasc. Surg., *86*:616, 1983.
163. Breslau, P. J., et al.: Carotid arterial disease in patients undergoing coronary artery bypass operations. J. Thorac. Cardiovasc. Surg., *82*:765, 1981.
164. Jones, E. L., et al.: Combined carotid and coronary operations: When are they necessary? J. Thorac. Cardiovasc. Surg., *87*:7, 1984.
165. Brener, B. J., et al.: The risk of stroke in patients with asymptomatic carotid stenosis undergoing cardiac surgery: a follow-up study. J. Vasc. Surg., *5*:269, 1987.
166. Stockard, J. J., et al.: Hypertension induced changes in cerebral function during cardiac surgery. Stroke, *5*:730, 1974.
167. Kolkka, R., and Hiberman, M.: Neurologic dysfunction following cardiac operation with low-flow, low-pressure cardiopulmonary bypass. J. Thorac. Cardiovasc. Surg., *79*:432, 1980.
168. Breuer, A. C., Franco, I., Marzewski, D., and Soto-Velasco, J.: Left ventricular thrombi seen by ventriculography are a significant risk factor for stroke in open heart surgery. (Abstract.) Ann. Neurol., *10*:103, 1981.
169. Breuer, A. C., et al.: Central nervous system complications of coronary artery bypass graft surgery: prospective analysis of 421 patients. Stroke, *14*:682, 1983.
170. Hertzer, N. R., Loop, F. D., Taylor, P. C., and Beven, E. G.: Combined myocardial revascularization and carotid endarterectomy. J. Thorac. Cardiovasc. Surg., *85*:577, 1983.
171. Britt, B. A., Joy, N., and Mackay, M. B.: Positioning trauma. *In* Complications in Anesthesiology. Edited by F. K. Orkin, L. H. Cooperman. Philadelphia, J. B. Lippincott, 1983, p. 646.
172. Miller, R. G., and Camp, P. E.: Postoperative ulnar neuropathy. JAMA, *242*:1636, 1979.
173. Graham, J. G., Pye, I. F., and McQueen, I. N. F.: Brachial plexus injury after median sternotomy. J. Neurol. Neurosurg. Psychiatry, *44*:621, 1981.
174. Wilbourn, A. J.: Thoracic outlet syndrome surgery causing severe brachial plexopathy. Muscle Nerve, *11*:66, 1988.
175. Kline, D. G., and Judice, D. J.: Operative management of selected brachial plexus lesions. J. Neurosurg., *53*:631, 1983.
176. Cherington, M., Happer, I., Mechanic, B., and Parry, L.: Surgery for thoracic outlet syndrome may be hazardous to your health. Muscle Nerve, *9*:632, 1986.
177. Carroll, S. E., and Wilkins, W. W.: Two cases of brachial plexus injury following percutaneous arteriograms. Can. Med. Assoc. J., *102*:861, 1970.
178. Honet, J. C., et al.: Neurological abnormalities in the leg(s) after use of intra-aortic balloon pump. Arch. Phys. Med. Rehabil., *56*:346, 1975.
179. Zylicz, Z., Nuyten, F. J. J., Notermans, S. L. H., and Koene, R. A. P.: Postoperative ulnar neuropathy after kidney transplantation. Anesthesia, *39*:1117, 1984.
180. Wilbourn, A. J., Furlan, A. J., Hulley, W., and Ruschhaupt, W.: Ischemic monomelic neuropathy. Neurology, *33*:447, 1983.
181. Rose, H. A., et al.: Peroneal nerve palsy following total knee arthroplasty. A review of The Hospital for Special Surgery experience. J. Bone Joint Surg. (Am), *64*:347, 1982.
182. James, S. E., and Wade, P. J. F.: Lateral popliteal nerve palsy as a complication of the use of a continuous passive motion knee machine. Injury, *18*:72, 1987.
183. Weber, E. R., Daube, J. R., and Conventry, M. B.: Peripheral neuropathies associated with total hip arthroplasty. J. Bone Joint Surg. (Am), *58*:66, 1976.
184. Starling, J. R., Harms, B. A., Schroeder, M. E., and Eichman, P. L.: Diagnosis and treatment of genitofemoral and ilioinguinal entrapment neuralgia. Surgery, *102*:581, 1987.
185. Sippo, W. C., and Gomez, A. C.: Nerve entrapment syn-

dromes from lower abdominal surgery. J. Fam. Pract., 25: 585, 1987.
186. Dawson, D. M., and Krarup, C.: Perioperative nerve lesions. Arch. Neurol., 46:1355, 1989.
187. Livesay, J. J., et al.: Surgical experience in descending thoracic aneurysmectomy with and without adjuncts to avoid ischemia. Ann. Thorac. Surg., 39:37, 1985.
188. Berendes, J. N., Bredee, J. J., Schipperheyn, J. J., and Mashhour, Y. A.: Mechanisms of spinal cord injury after cross-clamping of the descending thoracic aorta. Circulation, 66: I-112, 1982.
189. Oka, Y., and Miyamoto, T.: Prevention of spinal cord injury after cross-clamping of the thoracic aorta. J. Cardiovasc. Surg., 28:398, 1987.
190. Colon, R., Frazier, O. H., Cooley, D. A., and McAllister, H. A.: Hypothermic regional perfusion for protection of the spinal cord during periods of ischemia. Ann. Thorac. Surg., 43:639, 1987.

Chapter 60

FLUID RESUSCITATION OF THE CRITICALLY ILL PATIENT

JOHN T. OWINGS
JAMES W. HOLCROFT

The concept of replacing body fluid losses parenterally originated in England during a cholera pandemic in 1831. Latta wrote an eloquent description in the *Lancet* of both hypovolemic shock and the response of the shock patient to parenteral fluid administration. Once his patient had "... reached the last moment of her earthly existence...," he administered a mixture consisting roughly of 58 mEq/L sodium, 49 mEq/L chloride, and 9 mEq/L bicarbonate into her basilic vein. He saw a dramatic change in her condition as "... she began to breath less laboriously, soon the sharpened features and sunken eye, and fallen jaw, pale and cool, bearing manifest impress of death's signet, began to glow with returning animation; the pulse, which had long ceased, returned to the wrist...." This patient eventually succumbed to her underlying pathology as the "... vomiting and purging recurring soon reduced her to her former state of disability."[1] Many of the day thought that the rehydration had caused the return of diarrhea and vomiting, so intravenous fluid administration was abandoned until late in the nineteenth century.

In 1891, Lane wrote in a eulogy about the canine experiments of Wooldridge: "He thereby showed after an animal has sustained a loss of blood sufficient to terminate its life, there was left in the blood enough haemoglobin to sustain life, if only enough fluid be added to keep it in circulation." Lane in the same report published his experience with the administration of saline to a 13-year-old girl who had suffered a significant hemorrhage during a cleft palate repair. His description closely paralleled that of Latta except that his patient survived. This led him to quote his deceased mentor: "No person should die of hemorrhage."[2] Crile later found that the administration of intravenous saline into the shock animal increased the central venous pressure, leading to restoration of cardiac output, blood pressure, and organ perfusion.[3]

During the last part of the nineteenth and the early portion of the twentieth century, Starling shed an important light on capillary dynamics. He stated that there is an equilibrium of forces that determine the net flux of fluid into or out of the capillary bed. These forces are determined by the content and hydrostatic pressure of the plasma, the content and hydrostatic pressure of the interstitial space, and the permeability of the capillary membrane. He found that, in general, there is a slight net flux of free water out of the capillary and into the interstitium. This fluid is then drained by the lymphatic channels out of the interstitium and back into the great veins.[4]

Over the next 40 years, a debate raged as to the cause of the shock state, and the leading theories supposed a toxic factor to be primarily responsible. This issue was decisively addressed by Blalock in 1943 and quoted by Moss:[5] "Since the major single cause of shock seems to be a decrease in the volume of circulating blood, treatment should be based on checking such loss and replacing body fluids by the best means at hand." In response to this, whole blood transfusion was used widely as a means of resuscitation in hemorrhagic shock. Wiggers gave support to this theory and advanced the concept of reversible and irreversible shock with his experimental work in dogs. He found that the shock state could be reproduced by simple hemorrhage and that after enough blood was shed, the animal could not be resuscitated by reinfusing the anticoagulated blood that had been let.[6] By late in the Korean War, it was realized that patients previously thought to have suffered irreversible shock, with resulting renal failure, could be salvaged with the administration of increased volumes of saline. Shires et al.[7] furthered the work of Wiggers by bleeding dogs to the point of irreversible shock and then infusing one group of dogs with only the shed blood and a second group of dogs with both the shed blood and a supplemental electrolyte solution. He found, as Wiggers had, that the dogs that received only their own blood died. In addition, he found that those that had received their blood plus additional cystalloid volume survived.[7] Shires et al.[8] later showed that in shock fluid shifted from the extracellular to the intracellular space and created a debt in the interstitium that had to be repaid by further depleting the intravascular space. This laid the groundwork for the current approach to resuscitation of the volume-depleted patient.

The resuscitation of patients potentially bound for the ICU must be directed toward correcting fluid and electrolyte abnormalities. This resuscitation must be modified by the underlying medical history and should be aimed at the prevention of future derangements. Here we examine conditions that lead to fluid volume derangements and electrolyte changes. We look at the methods of their diagnosis, consider individual patient circumstances that alter diagnosis and treatment, and outline an approach to therapy.

INITIAL MANAGEMENT ISSUES BEFORE ICU ADMISSION

The first step in treating any patient is defining the pathologic condition to be treated. Here one considers the pathologic states of patients with fluid derangements and decides which are significant enough to warrant ICU admission. Unless the patient is in extremis, a detailed history should be taken. Subsequently, a physical examination and selection of laboratory and diagnostic studies are in order. Almost simultaneously, monitoring is initiated with the intent of selecting fluids and initiation of resuscitation with them.

History

The patient's medical history should be taken to identify the primary fluid abnormalities, to determine their cause, and to consider the underlying medical conditions that may affect their treatment. The key point of history usually begins with the physician evaluating a patient for an altered hemodynamic status. Because there are many different causes of altered hemodynamic and fluid status, it may be helpful to group them into three major groups. First, true hypovolemia, when there is an actual decrease in the intravascular fluid volume, as would be seen in hemorrhagic shock. Second, relative hypovolemia, which occurs when there has been a change in the capacitance of the vascular tree, as in neurogenic or late septic shock. Third, nonvolume-related causes, such as those that occur with primary cardiac pump failure or cardiac dysfunction caused by compression (Table 60-1). Questions should be directed toward systemic signs and symptoms of hypovolemia and toward individual organ systems that may be at the root of the problem. To identify the systemic signs and symptoms of hypovolemia, one should include questions about a history of decreased urine output, orthostatic or frank hypotension, drying of mucous membranes, unexplained confusion, agitation, lethargy, decreased oral intake, increased thirst, fever, infection, medications, trauma, ongoing disease processes, or recent surgery. Special attention should be given to the possibility of blood loss. Questions about specific organ systems should be directed at identifying the signs or symptoms of any of the aforementioned causes, such as gastrointestinal bleeding, diarrhea, or presence of fistulas. One should consider intracavitary causes of blood loss from vessel rupture, splenic rupture, and intramuscular hematoma that may be somewhat obscure to the clinician. These causes should be considered when causes of an altered hemodynamic status are not apparent. In most cases, the history directs the physician to the cause of the volume derangement. Several of the nonvolume-related causes may mimic true fluid disorders; physical examination is helpful in distinguishing these.

Physical Examination

Although a full physical examination should usually be performed, in cases of patient instability, an abbreviated examination may be necessary until the patient can be stabilized. It is important to examine the neck veins early in the patient's evaluation. Distended neck veins should alert the physician to the possibility of a cardiac (nonvolume-related) cause of hypotension. There are many physical signs of hypovolemia, which may include postural changes in the blood pressure; hypotension; dry mucous membranes; poor skin turgor; and cool, clammy, pale skin. One can get a general idea of the degree of hypovolemia from the signs present (Table 60-2). In an attempt to compensate for volume loss, blood is initially shunted away from organ systems that tolerate ischemia well, to provide perfusion for those that do not. During the loss of the first 20% of a patient's blood volume, blood is shunted away from the skeletal muscle, skin, fat, and bone. This results in pale, cool, clammy skin and postural pressure changes. Tachycardia may be manifest; however, it may also be absent—even in severe shock—and therefore is not a reliable sign.[9] When 20 to 40% of the blood volume is lost, the body's ability to compensate is impaired, and blood must be shunted away from organ systems that do not tolerate ischemia well. These include the visceral organs (such as the kidneys, pancreas, spleen, and liver). The patient is thirsty, urine output falls unacceptably low, and hypotension may be seen, even when the patient is in the supine position. Children, however, may maintain a relatively normal blood pressure until they have lost more than 40% of blood volume, and so caution must be used when interpreting blood pressure values in children. Once greater than 40% of the blood volume is lost, decompensation re-

Table 60-1. Conditions Requiring Resuscitation

Hypovolemia	Relative Hypovolemia	Cardiac or Nonvolemic Related
Hemorrhage	Spinal cord injury	Cardiac failure
Abnormal gastrointestinal losses	Neurogenic shock	Tension pneumothorax
	Regional anesthesia	Cardiac tamponade
Abnormal urinary losses	Early septic shock	Mechanical ventilation
	Adrenal dysfunction	Large pulmonary emboli
Abnormal sensible losses		
Redistribution of fluids		

Table 60-2. Manifestations of Hypovolemia

Mild hypovolemia: < 20% blood volume loss
  Compensation—blood shunted from organs that tolerate ischemia well (bone, skin, skeletal muscle)
  Patient is thirsty and feels cool, early orthostatic changes, neck veins are flat, urine is concentrated, and patient is pale
Moderate hypovolemia: 20–40% volume loss
  Early decompensation—blood shunted from organs that tolerate ischemia poorly (visceral organs, gut, liver, spleen)
  Patient feels weak, may have hypotension in supine position, urine output low
Severe hypovolemia: > 40% volume loss
  Decompensation—blood flow to heart and brain reduced
  Patient becomes disoriented or obtunded, frank hypotension, arrhythmias, ashen color

(From Holcroft, J. W.: Surgical intensive care: shock and adult respiratory distress syndrome. In Current Surgical Diagnosis and Treatment. Vol. 1. Edited by L. W. Way. Norwalk, CT, Appleton & Lange, 1988.)

sults. Perfusion is not high enough to supply the most vital organs—the heart and brain. These patients have an altered sensorium, with hypotension in the supine position.[10] The detailed physical examination should attempt to identify any of the possible causes of hypoperfusion we have identified here (for the physical diagnosis of the specific disorders, refer to the appropriate chapters). In a few cases, the cause of the hypotension may be elusive even after a history and physical examination. Laboratory studies must then be considered, especially when intracavitary (chest, abdomen, intramuscular areas) or intraluminal (gastrointestinal tract) pathology is the cause of volume loss.

Laboratory and Diagnostic Studies

A complete battery of laboratory tests should be obtained when the question of hypovolemia is being entertained. In most cases, a blood sample can be obtained when intravenous access is secured, and urine can be retrieved when a Foley catheter is placed. Depending on the circumstances, blood should be sent for complete blood count, electrolytes, chemistries, amylase, coagulation studies, alcohol level, toxicology screen, and cultures (if infection is in the differential diagnosis). Urine should be sent for analysis, toxicology screen, and culture.[11] Some caution must be used when reviewing these studies. In the acute situation of hemorrhage, for example, the hemoglobin concentrations may be normal because plasma refill typically shows little effect until an hour has passed. Insensitivity of some laboratory measurements under certain circumstances should not discourage the use of these tests, however, because most of these studies are of value in following trends. In the previous example, one might well find a normal hemoglobin initially, but reexamination in 2 hours might reveal a significant change. Conversely, one might find a low hemoglobin initially, as in a menstruating female, that shows no change over time. One should review laboratory studies in the light of the organization of Table 60-1 to determine whether abnormal studies elucidate a type of hypovolemia, which might heighten suspicion of a particular diagnosis.

It is important to examine a chest roentgenogram and, in some cases, a pelvic film. The chest roentgenogram, if normal, rules out the chest as a site of internal hemorrhage and eliminates tension pneumothorax as a cause of cardiac decompensation.[11] Patients with extensive trauma, especially the elderly, should undergo a pelvic roentgenogram. When pelvic fracture is present, the possibility of exsanguinating retroperitoneal hemorrhage must be considered. Other radiologic studies may be of great value in identifying a specific source of fluid loss (e.g., angiogram for gastrointestinal hemorrhage) but are of limited value in the initial workup of the hypotensive patient. Because of the ability to visualize chest, abdomen and pelvis in a third dimension, computed tomography (CT) scans provide additional information (see Chap. 71).

Initial Monitoring

Although multiple laboratory studies may provide a source of monitoring, they are usually too slow to return with data that will help in the minute-to-minute management of the patient. Here we look at those monitoring devices placed before the patient's arrival in the ICU. One of the simplest—a Foley catheter—should be placed in all patients suspected of being hypovolemic. In general, we accept 0.5 ml·kg^{-1}·hr^{-1} urine output in the adult patient as adequate but only in the absence of glycosuria. The urine must be regularly checked for glucose because when the serum glucose exceeds the renal tubular maximum, glucose is spilled into the urine and results in an osmotic diuresis. Under these circumstances, the hypovolemic patient can actually manifest a brisk diuresis.[12] In the absence of glycosuria, urine output can be an excellent way to follow hourly changes in the patient's hemodynamic status. The arterial line is another simple device that allows for rapid assessment of hemodynamic changes. It is minimally invasive and should be placed in most patients who are initially hypotensive. Placement, however, may be initially difficult in the severely volume-contracted patient, especially if vasopressors are being used (see Chap. 65). Central venous lines can be useful in assessing the volume status of the patient, and similar to arterial lines, show changes minute by minute. For these reasons, some advocate their use as the primary access for resuscitation. Volume depletion contracts the venous system, however, making blind cannulation of the subclavian or the internal jugular vein more difficult than normal. Because of this, the incidence of serious complications is increased in hypovolemic patients over nonhypovolemic patients (see Chap. 65). Some clinicians use the femoral vein as a site of venous access. This, similar to the great veins, is a blind cannulation, and in the shock patient, it may be difficult to distinguish an accidental arterial puncture from a venous puncture for two reasons. First, because of hypotension, the femoral artery may have poor return as opposed to the usual brisk pulsatile flow, and second, frequently these patients are hypoxic, and the arterial blood may be quite dark resembling venous blood. In most cases, an unintentional femoral arterial cannulation used for resuscitation results in no significant morbidity, and hence use of femoral venous catheters is generally acceptable. In the rare case a late pseudoaneurysm or arteriovenous fistula may occur. In addition, vasoactive medications (as used in neurogenic shock) must never be given arterially. We prefer a saphenous vein cut-down technique. The skin over the medial ankle is cleansed, and the saphenous vein is exposed with a scalpel. A nick is then made in the vein, and a piece of intravenous extension tubing cut at an angle is threaded up the vein. This technique has several advantages. The risk of serious complications, such as those associated with central venous lines, is nil. The procedure requires minimal training. Because the added resistance of an angiocatheter is not added, this infusion system can deliver fluids at rates exceeded only by cardiopulmonary bypass. Finally, there is no question as to the venous location of the line because direct visualization is used.

Fluids for Resuscitation

Many solutions have been used for resuscitation over the years. Currently two crystalloid solutions predominate,

Table 60-3. Composition of Parenteral Electrolyte Solutions

Solution	Osm (mOsm)	Na⁺ (mEq/L)	Cl⁻ (mEq/L)	K⁺ (mEq/L)	Ca²⁺ (mEq/L)	Lactate (mEq/L)	Dextrose (g/L)
Normal saline	308	154	154	0	0	0	0
Lactated Ringer's	273	130	109	4	3	28	0
Dextrose 5% in water	252	0	0	0	0	0	50
D5½ normal saline	406	77	77	0	0	0	50
D5 lactated Ringer's	525	130	109	4	3	28	50
7.5% hypertonic saline	2567	1283	1283	0	0	0	0

with some interest given to several colloid solutions (discussed later). The first crystalloid solution is normal saline, which is a mixture of sodium chloride in water. One liter of normal saline contains 154 mEq of sodium and 154 mEq of chloride. It exerts an osmotic load of 308 Osm and has a pH of approximately 4. Lactated Ringer's solution has an electrolytic composition more closely resembling that of normal plasma. One liter of lactated Ringer's contains 130 mEq of sodium, 109 mEq of chloride, 4 mEq of potassium, and 3 mEq of calcium and is buffered with 28 g of lactate. The pH of lactated Ringer's solution is roughly 6.8 (Table 60-3).

Several standard colloid solutions are also available as a resuscitation fluid. These include albumin 5% and 25%, low and high molecular dextran, and hetastarch (Table 60-4). Table 60-4 lists several of the distinguishing features between the various colloids. All of these solutions differ from standard isotonic solutions in four ways. First, they supply a colloid osmotic pressure to the intravascular space that, because of Starling forces, promotes the shift of fluid from the interstitium to the intravascular space in the periphery. Second, significantly less fluid is required to resuscitate to a desired blood pressure when using colloid than crystalloid. Third, occasionally anaphylactic reactions occur with the colloid solutions that do not occur with the crystalloids. Fourth, resuscitation using a colloid is between 10 and 50 times the cost of that using a crystalloid solution. It has been theoretically argued that the decrease in the colloid osmotic pressure, which results from large volume isotonic resuscitation, causes pulmonary edema and leads to "shock lung." If this were the case, by maintaining the colloid osmotic pressure, one should be able to reduce the incidence of, or prevent, these complications, and colloid solutions should be the resuscitation fluid of choice.

Substantial debate, however, has existed as to whether colloid solutions should be used in resuscitation to maintain the colloid osmotic pressure. The concept that it is important to maintain the colloid osmotic pressure to prevent pulmonary edema is based on the Starling forces and the observation that when the plasma colloid osmotic pressure falls during crystalloid resuscitation, peripheral edema results. This supposes that the capillary dynamics of the peripheral and pulmonary capillary beds are the same. This, however, does not seem to be the case. The peripheral tissue oncotic pressure is 15 to 20% of the peripheral capillary, whereas pulmonary interstitial oncotic pressure is 70 to 80% of that in the pulmonary capillary.[13] Also, the rate of pulmonary lymph flow, during resuscitation, may be as high as 5 to 10 times that of normal peripheral lymph flow, thus protecting the lung from edema formation. Some investigators have suggested that during the shock state, a change occurs in the permeability of the pulmonary capillary bed. The pulmonary microvasculature may become more permeable and allow the egress of albumin (or other colloid) into the pulmonary interstitium, thus paradoxically causing the condition that the solutions are supposed to protect against. In the baboon shock model, Holcroft and Trunk[14] found that colloid-resuscitated animals were more likely to suffer pulmonary edema than those resuscitated with an isotonic solution. In a randomized human trial, Virgilio et al.[15] placed abdominal aortic surgery patients into two different resuscitation groups. The first group received isotonic fluid for resuscitation, and the second received albumin in an isotonic fluid. They found that despite increased volume requirements and a decreased plasma colloid osmotic pressure, those patients receiving the isotonic solution alone had no increase in incidence of pulmonary edema.[15] Of the two cases of "shock lung" that occurred, both occurred in the albumin group and seemed to be related more to the onset of sepsis than to the colloid osmotic pressure. Although a decrease

Table 60-4. Characteristics of Colloid Solutions

	Albumin		Dextran		Hetastarch	Normal Saline
Concentration	5%	25%	Low	High	6%	0.9 Normal
Molecular weight	69,000		40,000	70,000	450,000 avg	58.4
Source	Human donor		Bacteria		Synthetic	Naturally occurring crystal
Duration of expansion	16–24 hours		1.5 hours	4 hours	24–36 hours	0.5–1 hour
Excretion	Hepatic		Renal		Hepatic and renal	Renal
Anaphylaxis[36]	0.011%		0.05%		0.08%	0%
Cost to hospital*	$75/500 ml	$34.94/100 ml	$15/500 ml	$7/500 ml	$36/500 ml	$1.20/L

* Based on 1990 estimates.

in the colloid osmotic pressure does seem to correlate with peripheral edema formation, it does not seem to be the critical factor in the development of either pulmonary edema or "shock lung." The expense of albumin, nearly 50 times that of saline, and the increased risk of adverse reactions do not seem warranted.[15,16]

We recommend the use of normal saline as the initial resuscitation fluid for several reasons:

- It is isotonic.
- It maintains a slight acidemia.
- It contains no dextrose.
- It is compatible with the administration of blood transfusions through the same intravenous line.

We also have found that for patients in shock (systolic blood pressure less than 90 mm Hg), 250 ml of 7.5% (hypertonic) saline with dextran administered as a prehospital (ambulance) resuscitation fluid can improve patient survival over traditional isotonic solutions.[17] Prolonged administration of hypertonic solutions, however, may lead to serious electrolyte abnormalities and also fail to yield the improved survival seen with the prehospital administration.[18] Hypotonic solutions given to the hypovolemic patient promote the shift of free water from the extracellular to the intracellular space because of osmotic forces.[19] Studies have demonstrated that transiently maintaining a slightly acidic environment during the resuscitative effort may protect against cellular injury.[20] In general, dextrose-containing solutions are not appropriate for resuscitation because large volumes produce both hyperglycemia and an osmotic diuresis. Lactated Ringer's solution contains calcium. Many blood banks recommend against using intravenous extension tubing run simultaneously with lactated Ringer's solution for blood transfusion because the calcium in the lactated Ringer's can cause deactivation of the citrate anticoagulant leading to clotting of the administered blood.

Fluid Resuscitation

When beginning fluids for resuscitation, the clinician should consider the differential diagnosis and the type of the hemodynamic alteration that is being treated (hypovolemia, relative hypovolemia, or cardiac or nonvolume related; see Table 60-1). Further expansion of this differential suggests that volume resuscitation is curative only in true states of hypovolemia. In states of relative hypovolemia, fluid resuscitation plus pharmacologic intervention is usually in order. Finally, in cardiac or nonvolume-related hypotension, further intervention with volume, pharmacologic agents (pressors, inotropes), and possible mechanical intervention (pericardiocentesis or lytic therapy) may be mandatory (Table 60-5).

We have designed an algorithm for the initial fluid resuscitation of the hypotensive patient (Fig. 60-1). The first question to be answered concerns the cause of the hypotension: Is the hypotension caused by a true hypovolemia, a relative hypovolemia, or a cardiac cause? A review of a 12-lead electrocardiogram and a brief look at the electrocardiac monitor should reveal the presence of infarc-

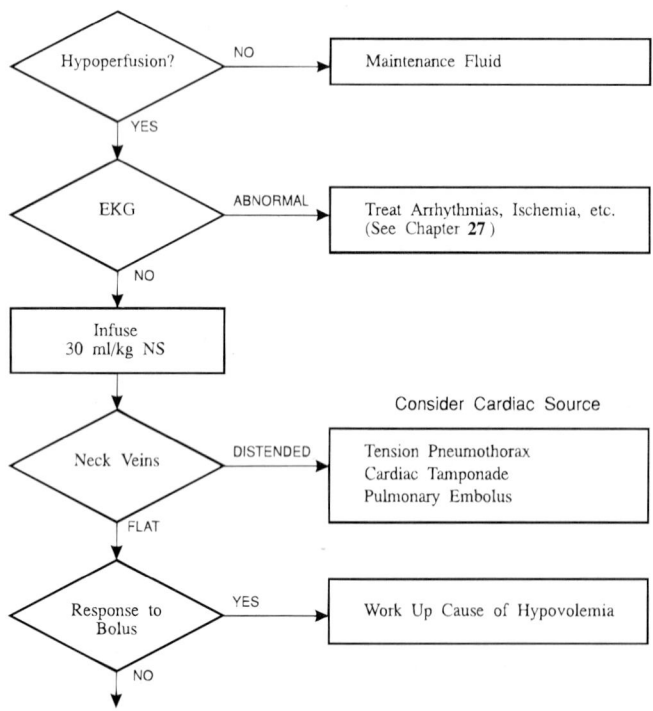

Fig. 60-1. Resuscitation. (Drawing, Courtesy, George Morrison, CD, Inc.)

Table 60–5. Therapeutic Tools of Resuscitation

Hypovolemia	Relative Hypovolemia	Cardiac
Crystalloids	Crystalloids	Mechanical
Blood	Vasopressors	Thoracostomy
Colloids	Colloids	Pericardiocentesis
		Crystalloids
		Thrombolytics
		Inotropic drugs

tion or ischemia and most major arrhythmias that might be responsible for hypotensive crisis (see Chaps. 27 and 29). Any arrhythmias should be treated appropriately (see Chaps. 27 and 29). The clinician must be mindful, however, that supraventricular tachycardia or atrial fibrillation with rapid ventricular response may be due to hypovolemia. If the cardiac rhythm is not responsible for the hypotension, 30 ml/kg of normal saline should be infused. While this fluid is being infused, the cause of the hypotension must be found. Examination of the neck veins is helpful in identifying a cause. If the neck veins are distended, one of the causes of cardiac compression should be sought (e.g., myocardial muscle dysfunction from ischemia, pneumothorax, cardiac tamponade, or pulmonary embolus). These conditions should be treated immediately. The patient's response to the fluid bolus should then be evaluated. If there has been a good response, a systematic workup and therapeutic plan can be carried out. If the patient remains hypotensive despite the bolus, a second bolus should be started. At this time, the algorithm should be reentered at the top. In the trauma patient, surgical consultation and operative exploration for ongoing hemorrhage is appropriate.[10] In the patient who has not suffered trauma, the possibility of occult blood loss (e.g., ruptured thoracic or abdominal aneurysm, pathologic splenic rupture, or gastrointestinal hemorrhage) should be considered because continued resuscitation without correction of the underlying source of blood loss is futile. Patients with possible primary cardiac dysfunction, or other causes, should have a pulmonary artery catheter inserted for determination of the filling pressures and cardiac indices. These patients require admission to the ICU simply to perform the monitoring functions.

Some of the patients who are resuscitated without the need of a pulmonary artery catheter may not need to be admitted to the ICU. The threshold, however, for admission to the ICU for a patient who presents with hypotension should be low. Disease processes, such as myocardial infarction, gastrointestinal hemorrhage, or septic shock, necessitate ICU admission regardless of fluid status of the patient. We believe that unless the patient has a self-limited, easily correctable cause for hypotension, such as simple dehydration or food poisoning, ICU admission is warranted.

ICU MANAGEMENT OF FLUIDS FOR RESUSCITATION

In the majority of cases in which a significant fluid replacement is required, the diagnosis is known before the patient's admission to the ICU. Under such circumstances, monitoring the hemodynamic status takes on the function of assessing therapeutic intervention.

Monitoring of Therapeutic Intervention

Several basic monitoring devices were mentioned in the last section, including the Foley catheter, arterial line, electrocardiogram, and central venous line. The first three of these should, with few exceptions, be placed in all ICU patients with any question of fluid volume abnormality. As stated earlier, the Foley catheter may be the most helpful monitor of perfusion hour by hour, and the arterial line gives more immediate information but requires more careful interpretation. The central venous catheter, although not appropriate for placement in a hypovolemic emergency room patient, is of great value once the patient is resuscitated and in the ICU. This catheter provides access for the administration of medications and nutrition not compatible with peripheral lines. It may also be used for the monitoring of volume status in a patient with normal left ventricular function. The strength of these data is improved when correlated with other information, such as urine output. For example, if a patient has low urine output and the central venous pressure is low, it is likely that hypovolemia is present and fluid challenge is warranted. If, however, the central venous pressure is high in a patient with oliguria, cardiac compression or congestive heart failure must be considered. There are key questions that must be answered from the monitored parameters. If the hypovolemia is manifested by tachycardia, hypotension, and narrowed pulse pressure, initial response to resuscitation should include widened pulse pressure and slowing heart rate. (This correlates with increasing efficiency of the heart—an increased stroke volume and maintenance of cardiac output at a lower heart rate.) Subsequent to this response, increased urine output may be seen. If a patient requires volume plus vasoactive agents, one is likely to see a reduction in the requirements for such agents before the above-mentioned events take place. Finally, if such events do not take place, clearly further analysis of cardiac function with a pulmonary artery catheter is in order.

We believe that pulmonary artery catheterization is indicated in a patient with questionable cardiac function or when large fluid shifts are expected. The catheter allows for the measurement of central venous pressure, pulmonary artery pressures, pulmonary artery wedge pressure, cardiac output, and the mixed venous oxygen saturation. In addition, many other helpful pieces of information can be calculated from these parameters. The calculated data include stroke volume, oxygen consumption, systemic vascular resistance, left atrial pressure (by inference from the wedge pressure), and the cardiac index (cardiac output divided by the total body surface area). With all of these measurements and calculations comes an increase in diagnostic power but also an increase in the chance for error. Hypovolemia may be manifest in many of the parameters provided by the catheter. Decreases are typically seen in the central venous pressure, left atrial pressure, wedge pressure, and cardiac index, whereas there is an increase in the systemic vascular resistance and decreased stroke

Table 60–6. Clinical and Physiologic Changes Associated with Disorders Requiring Fluid Resuscitation

Disorder	Neck Veins	ECG	Urine Output	Blood Pressure	CVP	PCWP	Cardiac Index	SVR
Mild hypovolemia	Flat	Normal	Low	Normal	Low	Low	Low	Increased
Severe hypovolemia (shock)	Flat	ST wave changes	Oliguria	Low	Low	Low	Low	High
Early high output sepsis	Flat	Normal	Low	Normal	Low	Low	High	Low
Low output septic shock	Flat	Normal	Oliguria Low	Low	Low	Low	Low	High
Neurogenic shock	Flat	Normal	Low	Low	Low	Low	Low	Low
Cardiac compression	Distended	Variable	Low	Low	High	High	Low	High
Cardiac failure	Distended	Specific changes	Low	Low	High	High	Low	High

CVP, Central venous pressure; SVR, systemic vascular resistance; PCWP, pulmonary capillary wedge pressure.

volume (Table 60–6). When a deviation from this pattern is seen, the clinician should suspect something other than pure hypovolemia and should review other diagnostic possibilities.

The Swan-Ganz catheter can provide information not only on the presence or degree of hypovolemia, but also on the adequacy of resuscitation. The central venous pressure and pulmonary artery wedge pressure indicate the volume status but should not be used as the sole guide for volume replacement. The goal of fluid resuscitation is to maximize perfusion (i.e., to reverse shock). The Frank-Starling law of the heart states that as the diastolic filling volume of the heart increases and as cardiac fibers stretch, the force of contraction increases. The central venous pressure is an indirect measure of the right heart filling volumes, whereas the pulmonary artery wedge pressure (PAWP) is indirectly related to the left ventricular end diastolic volume (LVEDV). The relationship of PAWP to the LVEDV is not one-to-one or linear but is a curvilinear line (Fig. 60–2).[21] Because of this, a Starling curve constructed by plotting the stroke volume against the PCWP should only be used with caution when resuscitating a patient.

The reason that PAWP is not directly proportioned to LVEDV is that PAWP also depends on the ventricular compliance. That is, a given volume may have many different wedge pressure values associated with it depending on the ventricular compliance at the time of the measurement. An example of how this fact might be misleading is found in the patient with an extremely compliant heart secondary to cardiomyopathy. Even though the ventricular volumes might be extremely high, the wedge pressure would be normal or low; hence seemingly appropriate continued fluid administration might result in less efficient cardiac function (decomposition), decreased cardiac index, and urine output.

By looking at Figure 60–2, one can see that at low filling volumes, a fluid bolus results in a small increase in the PAWP. At high filling volumes, the same fluid bolus results in a large increase in the PAWP. This large rise in the PAWP signals the point at which the filling volumes of the heart are excessive and further increases will decrease rather than increase the efficiency of the heart. Knowing this allows the clinician to use the PAWP correctly. For a patient in a low flow state, the PAWP is measured, then a small isotonic fluid bolus is given. If this results in a small increase in the PAWP with a corresponding increase in the cardiac index, fluid therapy is appropriate. If, however, in response to the small fluid challenge there is a large

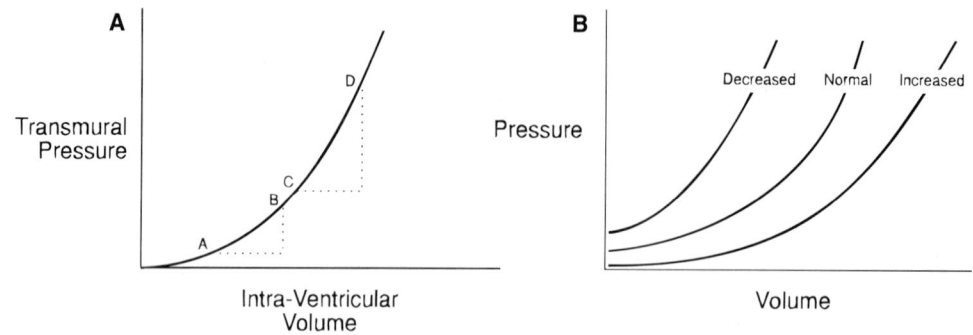

Fig. 60–2. *A*, The small rise in pressure, point A to point B, for a given change in end-diastolic volume, is in contradistinction to the large increase in pressure, point C to point D, for similar or smaller changes in end-diastolic volume. Therefore the ventricle described by A to B is more distensible (i.e., more compliant) than the ventricle described by C to D. *B*, The "family" of ventricular compliance curves. Not only may compliance fall along an ascending curve, but also disease and drugs may effect a change in the compliance curve, up and to the left (reduced compliance) or shifting it down and to the right (increased compliance). Conditions such as pericardial effusion, myocardial ischemia, and hyperkalemia cause decreased compliance and shift to the left. Congestive cardiomyopathy causes increased ventricular compliance. (Redrawn, George Morrison, CD, from Sibbald, W. J., and Driedger, A. A.: Right and left ventricular pre-load and diastolic ventricular compliance: implications for therapy in critically ill patients. *In* Textbook of Critical Care. Edited by W. C. Shoemaker, W. J. Thompson, and P. R. Holbrook. Philadelphia, W. B. Saunders, 1984.)

rise in the PAWP, without a significant increase in cardiac index, the clinician knows that the patient is reaching the limits of preload, and diuretic therapy may be appropriate. In either case, the end point of therapy is to maximize tissue perfusion, and the clinician rarely goes wrong adjusting the fluid therapy to maximize cardiac and urine output.

Fluid Replacement and Maintenance in the ICU (General Considerations)

The approach to fluid replacement should be as simple as possible. The fluid that is lost must be replaced both in volume and in content. Earlier in this chapter, we described the algorithm for the initial resuscitation. Fluid volumes administered subsequently should be given based on the monitoring information available. If the patient becomes significantly hypovolemic after resuscitation has restored normal hemodynamic parameters, volumes of 7 to 14 $ml \cdot kg^{-1} \cdot hour^{-1}$ of isotonic (normal saline or lactated Ringer's) solution should be administered. Throughout this process, the monitoring data should be scrutinized and volume replacement titrated to provide adequate urine output (0.5 $ml \cdot kg^{-1} \cdot hour^{-1}$) with acceptable hemodynamic parameters. Once the patient becomes euvolemic, a maintenance rate based on body mass is acceptable.

A well-accepted maintenance formula is as follows:

- 100 $ml \cdot kg^{-1} \cdot day^{-1}$ for each of the patient's first 10 kg of body mass
- 50 $ml \cdot kg^{-1} \cdot day^{-1}$ for the next 10 kg
- 20 $ml \cdot kg^{-1} \cdot day^{-1}$ for each kilogram after

For a 70-kg man, this would give 1000 ml per day for the first 10 kg, 500 ml per day for the second 10 kg, and 1000 ml per day for the remaining 50 kg. Thus, the patient would be given 2500 ml per day or roughly 105 ml per hour. This rate may be adjusted up or down depending on the patient's individual circumstances. The next issue concerns which type of fluid to administer.

If the patient requires significant volume replacement, it is best to run two different solutions through different lines. The first is the maintenance solution, which should be run at the rate calculated previously. This solution should contain at least 5% dextrose, even in diabetics. The administration of glucose in the otherwise starved patient decreases the catabolism of proteins for use in gluconeogenesis. In diabetics, who are not able to take enteral nutrition, it is critical to give them glucose and have their blood glucose levels checked at regular intervals. No patient should be allowed to go more than 24 hours without a glucose-containing solution. If this does occur, the patient is at risk for increased protein catabolism and ketosis. In addition to the maintenance fluid, a second fluid should be hung for future resuscitation or volume-for-volume replacement of lost bodily fluids. Tables 60–3 and 60–7 illustrate our approach to choosing the appropriate parenteral replacement fluid. Table 60–3 lists the composition of many of the parenteral electrolyte solutions available

Table 60–7. Composition of Various Bodily Fluids

	Na+ (mEq/L)	K+ (mEq/L)	Cl− (mEq/L)	HCO3 (mEq/L)	Volumes/24 Hours (ml/day)
Gastric secretion					
High acid	20	10	120	0	1000–9000
Low acid	80	15	90	5–25	1000–2500
Pancreatic secretion	140	5	75	80	500–1000
Bile	148	5	100	35	300–1000
Small bowel secretion	110	5	105	30	300–1000
Distal ileum drainage	80	8	45	30	1000–3000
Diarrhea	120	25	90	45	500–1700
Sweat	30	5	20	7	0–2000/hour
Normal urine	125	60	130	15	0–2000/hour

today. Table 60–7 lists the fluid composition of various bodily fluids that may be lost. By estimating the composition of the fluid lost, one can choose a parenteral replacement solution to give. When long-term fluid replacement is required, the patient should be monitored with regular laboratory studies, including measurement of serum and bodily fluid electrolytes. The composition of the replacement solution should be adjusted to meet the specific and changing needs of the patient.

When formulating an approach to fluid resuscitation, individual clinical entities should be kept in mind. Generally, these entities can be typed as:

- Hemorrhage
- Gastrointestinal fluid loss
- Urinary fluid loss
- Sensible or insensible volume loss
- Distributional fluid loss

Hypovolemia

True hypovolemia may occur in any state in which there has been a loss of fluid from the intravascular space. This is not an entity of its own but rather a condition that is the result of some underlying pathologic process. Here we review the therapy of hypovolemia caused by hemorrhage, gastrointestinal losses (including gastric, small bowel, and colonic), urinary losses, increased insensible losses, and redistributional losses (Table 60–8). The therapy of any of these disorders must be directed both at correcting the factors responsible for the process and replacing the fluid lost (see Tables 60–3, 60–7, and 60–8).

Hemorrhage

The loss of fluid secondary to hemorrhage may be due to a number of causes. The primary concerns should be to stop the blood loss and provide the initial resuscitation. In some cases, such as gastrointestinal bleeding, a significant period of time may pass between admission and correction of the lesion responsible for the blood loss. There-

Table 60-8. Approach to Hypovolemia Based on Source of Volume Lost

Hemorrhage
    External (visible)
        Traumatic
        GI upper: varices, PUD, gastritis, arteriovenous malformation, Mallory-Weiss tear
        GI lower: arteriovenous malformation, diverticulitis, cancer
    Internal (nonvisible)
        Vascular: aneurysm, tumor
        Traumatic
Gastrointestinal Fluid Loss
    Stomach: intractable vomiting, nasogastric suction
    Biliary: fistulas
    Small bowel: fistulas
    Colon: diarrhea
Urinary Loss
    Primary renal: high output failure, postobstructive diuresis, diabetes insipidus (due to renal insensitivity)
    Secondary renal: diabetes mellitus, diabetes insipidus (decreased ADH)
Sensible and Insensible Fluid Loss
    Heat exhaustion
    Fever
Redistribution of Fluid
    Sepsis
    Pancreatitis
    Trauma

PUD, Peptic ulcer disease; ADH, antidiuretic hormone.

fore, there may be a requirement for prolonged fluid resuscitation with ongoing hemorrhage. Acute hemorrhage is actually the simplest of the hypovolemic states to conceptualize because all blood elements (cells, proteins, and electrolytes) are lost in their normal concentrations. Replacement should be directed first at resuscitation (correction of the shock state and return of acceptable hemodynamic parameters) and then at replacement of fluid, electrolytes, cells, and clotting factors as needed. Because normal saline is the intravenous fluid that is compatible with transfusions, at least one large-bore intravenous line should be kept open with this solution as long as ongoing hemorrhage is present or recurrent hemorrhage is possible. For patients in whom ongoing massive hemorrhage is expected and in whom multiple simultaneous transfusions may be required, all lines should be maintained with normal saline. Patients lose all electrolytes in this disorder, so once the initial resuscitation has been accomplished, all but the potential transfusion line may be switched to lactated Ringer's solution.[6] Lactated Ringer's solution contains a more normal concentration of various electrolytes and has been shown in numerous studies not to cause or contribute to lactic acidemia.[24] Once past the initial 24-hour period, dextrose should be added to one line. This decreases the breakdown of muscle protein for gluconeogenesis. If no enteral nutrition is expected for 5 or more days, total parenteral nutrition should be considered. Patients, such as those with gastrointestinal hemorrhage, who are resuscitated with large volumes of crystalloids and packed red cells may rapidly develop a coagulopathy because of the depletion of clotting factors. These may be replaced as depletion occurs with fresh-frozen plasma platelets (see Chap. 61).

Gastrointestinal Fluid Loss

Many disorders lead to the loss of fluid from the gastrointestinal tract. Under such circumstances, it is convenient to divide these into gastric, small intestinal, and colonic fluid loss. Fluid is commonly lost from the stomach by vomiting or nasogastric suction. Shown in Table 60-7 is the typical concentration of gastric fluid. Note that there is slight difference in the electrolyte composition of the high and low acidity fluids, as might be seen in someone on H_2-blocking agents versus someone who is not.[22] The electrolytes likely to be depleted in this situation are chloride and potassium. Once the volume status of the patient has been restored with isotonic solutions, the replacement solution may be chosen. Because the sodium loss is roughly 50 mEq/L and the chloride loss is 90 to 120 mEq/L, half normal saline supplies the sodium lost and slightly more than half of the chloride lost. Chloride and potassium are disproportionately lost, so potassium chloride should be added at 30 mEq/L.[23] Dextrose may be added at a concentration of 5%; however, if more than 3.5 ml·kg^{-1}·hr^{-1} of fluid is required, the dextrose should be removed from the amount in excess of that to prevent creating an osmotic diuresis.[23] Regular measurement of a patient's electrolyte deficits should be made and correction based on these values.

Fluid may be lost from the small bowel, pancreas, or biliary tree through fistulas, from an ileostomy, or from an improperly placed nasogastric tube. The compositions of the various fluids are shown in Table 60-7. The one area of note is the pancreas, because it has a relatively high concentration of bicarbonate. Otherwise all of these fluids have similar electrolyte concentrations and may be replaced with lactated Ringer's solution with the addition of a single ampule of sodium bicarbonate (44.6 mEq NaHCO$_3$) per liter of infused lactated Ringer's. In the case in which pancreatic drainage is high, it may be necessary to administer an additional ampule of sodium bicarbonate for each liter of replacement fluid because of the high concentration of bicarbonate in these secretions. Again, dextrose should be added to one of the lines and then run at a constant rate as the maintenance fluid.[23] Volume replaced should be based on volume lost on a nursing shift-per-shift basis.

Fluid lost from the colon in the form of diarrhea is rich in potassium and bicarbonate and varies widely in its sodium chloride concentration. This fluid may also be replaced with lactated Ringer's solution with the addition of 20 mEq/L of potassium chloride and administration of 1 ampule of sodium bicarbonate for each liter of infused replacement solution. In this situation, the patient must be monitored for hypernatremia or hyperchloremia. If these are a problem, use dextrose 5% in water, either with or without the addition of 30 mEq/L of potassium chloride and with or without the administration of bicarbonate. Again, volume replaced should equal volume lost on a nursing shift-per-shift basis. If volumes are excessive and electrolyte balance is distributed, it is not unreasonable to measure the concentrations of electrolye in the fluids lost to define the composition of replacement fluids accurately.

Table 60-9. Causes of Inappropriate Renal Fluid Loss

Intrinsic (Renal)	Extrinsic (Nonrenal)
Diabetes insipidus (ADH insensitive)	Diabetes insipidus (decreased ADH production)
Diuretic overuse	Diabetes mellitus
Postobstructive diuresis	Diabetic ketoacidosis
	Hyperosmolar coma

ADH, Antidiuretic hormone.

Urinary Fluid Losses

The kidneys are the primary organs responsible for the regulation of fluid and electrolytes. We briefly highlight a few conditions associated with abnormal fluid loss from the urinary system. It may be helpful to group these disorders into two types. In the first type—caused by either direct renal pathology or by hormonal or drug influences—the kidneys produce an inappropriate diuresis in the face of initially normal plasma chemistry. The second type occurs when the change in the composition of the plasma and diuresis is caused by an increase in a normal plasma component, such as glucose, or due to the presence of an agent that acts as a diuretic, such as mannitol (Table 60-9). The composition of the urine must be examined in any state in which there is an inappropriate diuresis. Initial volume repletion with an isotonic solution (normal saline) to correct hypovolemia while the urine is analyzed for electrolytic content is appropriate. The further medical and fluid management must be based on correcting the underlying disorder and replenishing the electrolytes lost in the urine.

Diabetes insipidus is caused either by an abnormally low level of antidiuretic hormone (ADH) or by renal insensitivity to the hormone. Either abnormality causes a voluminous diuresis of hypotonic urine with a specific gravity less than 1.006, resulting in a serum osmolality frequently greater than 320 mOsm/kg. Diabetes insipidus may be brought on by trauma, surgery, drugs, tumors, or genetic causes. The underlying cause should be identified and corrected, if possible. Initial volume deficits should be corrected with an isotonic solution. Subsequent fluids should be 5% dextrose in water because the serum sodium during this disease is frequently elevated. Pharmacologic treatment is provided by administration of 5 to 10 U of aqueous vasopressin (Pitressin) intramuscularly or intravenously every 3 to 4 hours. Care must be taken during fluid resuscitation to avoid cerebral edema, caused by correcting the serum sodium concentration or osmolality too quickly. The serum sodium should be brought down no faster than 1 mEq/L/hour and the osmolality no faster than 2 mOsm/kg/hour.[25] The urine should be monitored for the presence of glucose to avoid the creation of an osmotic diuresis.

When overadministration of diuretics is the cause of the polyuria, the drug should be temporarily withheld. Although by looking at the type of diuretic used (loop, thiazide, or potassium sparing), one can get an idea of the serum deficits to be expected, it is best to base therapeutic interventions on laboratory analysis of the serum and urine.

Occasionally, after the relief of a urinary tract obstruction, the kidneys appropriately diurese the abnormal concentrations of serum electrolytes and fluid volumes but then continue with an abnormal diuresis. As in the previous cases, volume losses should be corrected with normal saline. A hypotonic solution with electrolytes added based on measurements of urine electrolytes should then be administered. The rule of "volume replaced should equal at least volume lost" applies here also.

Both diabetic ketoacidosis and nonketotic hyperosmolar coma present with fluid losses that are largely caused by osmotic diuresis. The fluid deficit in hyperosmolar coma tends to be greater (an average of about 10 L) than that of ketoacidosis, averaging 3 to 5 L.[25] Restoration of normal hemodynamic parameters should be accomplished with the bolus administration of 30 ml/kg normal saline (see Fig. 60-1). Because these patients generally have an elevated serum sodium, once the hemodynamics have returned to normal, the replacement fluid should be changed to ½ normal saline. The hyperglycemia should be brought under control with the administration of intravenous insulin. Attenuation in the rate of fall in the serum glucose should be provided, once the serum glucose falls to about 300 mg/dl, by changing the replacement fluid to a dextrose-containing solution, such as 5% dextrose in ¼ normal saline. If severe hypernatremia exists with a serum concentration that exceeds 155 mM/L, 5% dextrose in water may be used as the means of replenishing the free water deficit. Both of these conditions have the potential for specific electrolyte abnormalities. Each may present with hyperkalemia, even though total body stores are depleted as a consequence of acidosis (mild in hyperosmolar coma) and extracellular volume contraction. In both conditions, as the hyperglycemia is corrected with insulin, potassium is shifted to the intracellular space. This shift is more pronounced in hyperosmolar coma because in ketoacidosis the more severe acidosis helps to counteract the shift of potassium to the intracellular space. This shift may result in serious hypokalemia, and 20 to 40 mEq/L of potassium should be added to the maintenance solution once the serum potassium falls to normal. In ketoacidosis, the phosphate is usually depleted; therefore potassium should initially be given as the phosphate salt. The phosphate, however, mandates a slower rate of administration than if potassium chloride were used. Ketoacidosis may also result in a severe acidosis (pH <7.0). When this occurs, sodium bicarbonate should be administered to bring the pH up to 7.2 and then discontinued. Overuse of bicarbonate decreases the oxygen delivery to the tissues and compounds the intracellular acidosis (see Chap. 38).

Sensible and Insensible Fluid Losses

Sensible fluid loss is the fluid lost in sweat, whereas insensible fluid loss is that lost to nonsweat evaporation, both from the skin and the respiratory tract. Sweat volumes can vary widely, from zero in resting nonstressed situations to 2 L per hour in the stressed individual. The most potent stimulator of sweat production is an increase in the core

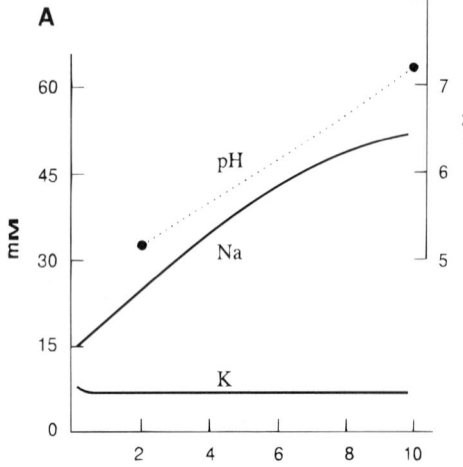
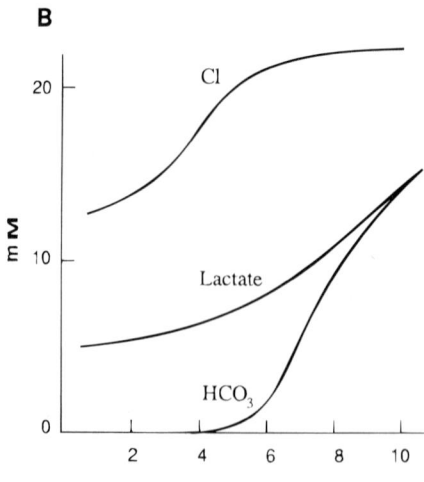

Fig. 60-3. Concentration versus single gland sweat rate of Na and K (A) and Cl, HCO$_3$, and lactate (B). Dashed line for pH drawn for convenience, not to represent function. (Redrawn by George Morrison, CD, from Quinton, P. M.: Physiology of sweat secretion. Kidney Int., 32:5102, 1987.)

body temperature. Increased core temperature stimulates the hypothalamus to cause a cutaneous vasodilatation, which shifts blood flow through capillaries surrounding the sweat follicles. This results in increased sweat production causing heat loss and body cooling. The electrolyte composition of the sweat varies with the volume and with the cardiovascular conditioning of the individual. When the volumes of sweat are small, the sweat is relatively acidic and hypotonic. As the volume of sweat increases, its pH increases, and its concentration of sodium, chloride, and bicarbonate rises (Fig. 60-3).[26] Interestingly, the potassium concentration remains constant at approximately 5 mEq/L through all these changes. It has been estimated that a normal adult at 23.5°C loses about 400 ml per day in the form of sweat.[26] If fever is present, the patient may have periods of sweating in an attempt to return core temperature to normal. During these periods, patients can increase their sweat production to six to eight times normal. These periods of increased sweating occur for 4 to 7 hours per day and can increase fluid losses by approximately 600 ml per day.[27] In the patient with sustained fever, it is reasonable to use the maintenance formula provided earlier with the addition of up to 600 ml per day to compensate for sweat losses. These losses should be replaced with half normal saline with some attention paid to the serum potassium concentration. The extreme case of sensible fluid loss occurs in heat exhaustion, in which prolonged massive losses have occurred. These patients should be resuscitated, according to the protocol in the previous section, with normal saline. Any remaining electrolyte abnormalities should be corrected based on laboratory studies.

Insensible fluid loss is caused by the evaporation of moisture from the skin—roughly 60%—and from the respiratory tract—roughly 40%. A calculation of 170 ml/m^2 BSA per day is arrived at when the effects of sweating are eliminated. Because the body surface area-to-body weight ratio does not change significantly in adulthood, this estimate may be given as 10 ml/kg per day, which would result in 700 ml per day in the average 70-kg man. This figure has been calculated into the maintenance formula. Although sensible losses increase with fever, insensible losses are constant. Endotracheal intubation with mechanical ventilation using 100% humidified air (with varying concentrations of oxygen) eliminates the respiratory tract as a course of evaporative loss. In these cases, the 40% ascribed to this source is subtracted. Thus the intubated 70-kg patient loses 420 ml per day.[28]

Distributional Fluid Losses

Although hemorrhage may be the simplest of the hypovolemic states to recognize and conceptualize, fluid loss caused by redistribution may be the most difficult. Distributional losses occur when fluid is shifted from the intravascular space to the intracellular, interstitial, or the so-called third space. This form of intravascular fluid loss is unfortunately common in the ICU and may be seen in pancreatitis, sepsis, trauma, peritonitis, or in patients following a major abdominal operation, such as an aneurysmectomy. The subtlety of these disorders arises because there is no increase or else a decrease in excreted or shed fluids. Such patients may be treated as having renal failure with diuretics rather than with the aggressive fluid support they require. Under such circumstances, one can expect large fluid shifts, and therefore attention must be paid to intravascular volume. Resuscitation should be started with normal saline and, as the diagnosis is elucidated and ongoing hemorrhage is ruled out, changed to lactated Ringer's solution. Foley catheters and arterial lines should be standard, and we advocate the use of pulmonary artery catheterization early in the disease process to facilitate maintenance and management of hemodynamic status. Clearly, from the studies done, it is of paramount importance to ensure adequate intravascular fluid volume and hemodynamic status. In some cases, this may require up to 20 L of isotonic fluid in a 24-hour period.

Pancreatitis, whether edematous or hemorrhagic, is caused by the activation of inactive pancreatic enzymes, trypsinogen, chymotrypsinogen, and carboxypolypeptidase. The active enzymes autodigest the pancreas and retroperitoneum with sequestration of large fluid volumes there and in the peritoneal cavity. As autodigestion occurs, the motility of the overlying bowel comes to a halt. With this ileus, more fluid is lost into the lumen of the bowel because of the cessation of normal motility and reabsorptive processes. The fluid lost is typically rich in protein, which may lead to the loss of more intravascular volume as the Starling forces equilibrate in the periphery. In uncomplicated pancreatitis, the treatment is supportive, and at least two large intravenous lines should be in place. One line should be used for fluid replacement with lactated Ringer's solution. The fluids given through this line can be adjusted to maintain adequate urine output and cardiac index. The second line should be used to deliver a dextrose-containing solution, such as lactated Ringer's with 5% dextrose, at a constant rate of 100 to 125 ml per hour. This second line supplies the small amount of sugar needed to decrease the breakdown of protein for gluconeogenesis. Because these patients may not be able to take enteral feedings for an extended period of time, total parenteral nutrition should be instituted early. Patients with pancreatitis must be watched for hypocalcemia. Lactated Ringer's solution does contain calcium, but supplementation with 1 to 2 ampules of calcium gluconate per liter may be necessary and should be based on serum laboratory studies. Alcohol abuse is a common cause of this disease and is associated with several electrolyte abnormalities and vitamin deficiencies so it is important to check and monitor the serum magnesium level and consider folate and vitamin B$_{12}$ replacement.[29]

Sepsis is another condition that results in the redistribution of significant amounts of the intravascular fluid volume. In contrast to pancreatitis, however, supportive treatment alone usually results in the patient's demise. The initial insult in sepsis is infection. While the diagnosis and treatment of the infection are ongoing, initial resuscitation with 30 ml/kg of normal saline should be started. Sepsis has two distinct phases: early or high output sepsis and late or low output septic shock. In early sepsis, the body attempts to fight off the hypothalamic setpoint; reflexes originating from the preoptic hypothalamic nucleus result in shunting of blood flow to the cutaneous vessels to promote cooling through sweating. This causes a drop in the central intravascular volume and a decrease in the blood flow to the kidneys, where, in response, the urine output is decreased. The heart compensates for the volume loss by dramatically increasing the cardiac output. This patient appears pink. As long as the heart is able to compensate for the degree in central intravascular volume, the blood pressure is maintained. The infection must be identified and treated at this point—either surgically, if possible, or pharmacologically—to avoid the progression to septic shock. If the infection progresses, bacterial toxins lead to the intravascular release of inflammatory mediators, which cause increased capillary permeability with leakage of fluid into the interstitium. This signals the decompensation and onset of late or low output septic shock. As the intravascular volume continues to decrease, the heart can no longer compensate, adrenergic tone is increased, and peripheral vasoconstriction occurs, in an attempt to shunt blood flow to the brain and heart. When the peripheral perfusion drops to the shock level, cellular membrane function is impaired. As the cell allows the inward flux of free water, sodium, and chloride, the normal resting transmembrane potential of -90 mV deteriorates to approximately -60 mV. Extrapolating from experimental data, this shift to the intracellular space accounts for an extracellular fluid loss of up to 4 L.[31] Even with peripheral vasoconstriction, coronary blood flow is inadequate, and cardiac decompensation occurs. The patient appears pale and has a low blood pressure and low cardiac output. The inflammatory mediators may activate the clotting cascade and cause disseminated intravascular coagulation. These patients can require fluid quantities similar to those with pancreatitis, up to 20 L per day. Once the question of hemorrhage has been eliminated, the fluid for resuscitation and ongoing capillary leak should be lactated Ringer's solution. Lactated Ringer's is recommended because the fluid lost across the leaky capillary membrane is isotonic with the same electrolytic composition as plasma.

As with pancreatitis, and in contrast to many of the other disorders we have examined, there are no direct ways to measure the fluid lost. Indirect measures include monitoring the urine output, blood pressure, central venous pressure, pulmonary artery wedge pressure, and cardiac indices, and should all be used. With these massive fluid shifts to the extravascular space, the patient becomes edematous, and the temptation occurs to correct their oliguria and anasarca with diuretic therapy. This must be avoided, unless the cardiac filling pressures have exceeded those required for the maximum cardiac output. In most cases, these patients do not have the increased central venous pressures of right-sided cardiac failure but low pressures indicating that continued or increased fluid support is required. The underlying infection must be found. All body fluids should be cultured. Lines should be changed and cultured regularly. Radiologic exploration of the abdomen (CT scan) is warranted when a source of infection is not identifiable.[30]

In trauma, a condition similar to sepsis and septic shock occurs except that the initial intravascular volume loss is caused by hemorrhage and not cutaneous vasodilatation. For this reason, we recommend the extended use of normal saline rather than Ringer's lactate to allow for emergent transfusions with maximum efficiency. Tissue factors act much in the same way that the bacterial toxin acted in septic shock, to cause the release of inflammatory mediators. These mediators lead to the same increased microvascular permeability and leak with the possibility of disseminated intravascular coagulation. In trauma, a vigilant search must be carried out for continuing sources of blood loss, and if found, they must be corrected. All fractures should be stabilized early to prevent continued release of tissue fragments. As with the septic patient, vigorous monitoring and fluid support are required to maintain maximal cardiac output and tissue perfusion.

POST-ICU PHASE

The discharge from intensive monitoring of any patient may be a difficult decision to make. In many cases, the fluid status of the patient heralds the first signs of recovery; yet in most cases, the decision to discharge from the ICU is based on the underlying pathology of the condition that led to ICU admission. In this section, we examine the signs of return to normal fluid status.

Recovery

One of the first signs of improvement in any disease process that has required the administration of large amounts of fluid is a spontaneous diuresis. If the patient is receiving vasopressor agents, a reduction in the dosage while maintaining blood pressure may precede the diuresis. The urine must be checked for glucose, and, if present, the urine production should be disregarded as a sign of improvement. If there is no glucose in the urine and if diuretics have not been given, the progressive increase in urine output or decreasing fluid requirements to maintain adequate urine output is an excellent sign that on a cellular level healing is occurring. Preceding these responses may be a decreased requirement for vasopressors.

In the shock state, one sees disruption in the normal cellular membrane function with a transmembrane potential change from its resting level of about -90 mV to a more positive level of -60 mV. This change represents an influx of sodium, chloride, and free water and an afflux in potassium. As the shock state is reversed and adequate tissue perfusion is regained, the cellular membrane function normalizes. The transmembrane potential is returned to its resting level as the increased intracellular water, sodium, and chloride are shifted to the extracellular space. This is one aspect of the mobilization of fluid responsible for the recovery phase diuresis.[6,31,32]

On another scale, the repair of the leaky microvasculature has a similar effect. In the section on volume redistribution, we described the release of inflammatory mediators that lead to endothelial damage and a leaky microvasculature.[30,33] This resulted in a shift of intravascular fluid to the interstitium, causing peripheral edema. As the supply of inflammatory mediators decreases and the oxygen tension (among other things) increases, the capillary endothelial cells regain their integrity. Intravascular hydrostatic and oncotic pressures are restored, and the kidney is again able to function properly. This same process may be observed as the weight and the percentage of inspired oxygen required decrease while the cardiac index increases. In rare cases, even after this healing process occurs, there is a prolonged requirement for parenteral fluid or nutritional support.

Home Venous Access

In 1973, Broviac introduced a Silastic right atrial catheter designed to allow patients requiring extended courses of vein sclerosing chemotherapy to leave the hospital. Since that time, the Broviac or Hickman (slightly larger) catheters have provided outpatient central venous access for many types of therapy not compatible with peripheral administration.[34,35] Total parenteral nutrition is given for those with intractable malabsorption or short bowel syndrome. Chemotherapy is available for outpatients with numerous malignant processes. The semipermanent central venous catheter is also appropriate for use when long-term intravenous access is needed. Normal hydration of some short bowel patients is not possible enterally, even though small bowel hyperplasia has allowed for adequate enteral nutrition. Rarely total colectomy results in a similar condition. These catheters are appropriate for weeks of parenteral antibiotics. These devices now allow for a more rapid, smooth transition of selected patients from ICU to ward and on to the outpatient setting.

These catheters are associated with a complication rate of between 15 and 50%. The most common complications are related to infection—up to 20%. This underscores the importance of adequate training in the sterile technique for ICU personnel who care for these lines. Each entry or break into the system must be performed with great care and the strictest sterile technique. These entries must be made only as truly necessary. These catheters should not be treated simply as another intravenous access. Venous thrombosis also occurs in up to 10% of cases. This seems to be related to size of the catheter, its rigidity, and internal catheter tip location. Owing to this potentially serious complication, most authors recommend the use of heparin in low doses (2000 to 5000 U/L) to be mixed with total parenteral nutrition or ongoing infusion. Also, it seems that positioning the internal catheter tip at or more central to the superior atriocaval junction reduces the risk of thrombosis.[37] With appropriate care, these lines provide much needed access in a patient population with poor access and greatly improves their quality and duration of life. Proper precautions should be instituted in the event that patients with these catheters require ICU admission. Although not just regarded as another intravenous access, when no other appropriate sites are available, they can be used for fluid replacement, antibiotic therapy, and so forth.

REFERENCES

1. Cosnett, J. E.: The origins of intravenous fluid therapy. Lancet, 1:768, 1989.
2. Lane, W. A.: A surgical tribute to Dr. Wooldridge. Lancet, 2: 620, 1891.
3. Crile, G. W.: Experimental Research into Surgical Shock. Philadelphia, J. B. Lippincott, 1899.
4. Guyton, A. C.: Textbook of Medical Physiology. 6th Ed. Philadelphia, W. B. Saunders, 1981.
5. Moss, G. S.: An argument in favor of electrolyte solution for early resuscitation. Surg. Clin. North Am., 52:3, 1972.
6. Holcroft, J. W., and Blaisdell, F. W.: Shock: causes and management of circulatory collapse, pp 19–33. In Textbook of Surgery. Edited by D. C. Sabiston. Philadelphia, W. B. Saunders, 1991.
7. Shires, G. T., et al.: Fluid therapy in hemorrhagic shock. Arch. Surg., 88:688, 1964.
8. Shires, G. T., et al.: Alterations in cellular membrane function during hemorrhagic shock in primates. Ann. Surg., 176:288, 1972.
9. Little, R. A.: 1988 Fitts Lecture: heart rate changes after hemorrhage and injury—a reappraisal. J. Trauma, 29:903, 1989.
10. Holcroft, J. W. and Wisner, D. H.: Surgical intensive care: shock and adult respiratory distress syndrome. In Current Surgical Diagnosis and Treatment. 10th Ed. Edited by L. W. Way. Norwalk, CT, Appleton & Lange, 186, 1994.
11. Wisner, D. H.: General assessment, resuscitation and exploration of penetrating and blunt abdominal trauma. In Trauma Management. Vol. 14. Edited by F. W. Blaisdell and D. D. Trunkey. New York, Thieme-Stratton, 1993.
12. Sullivan, L. P., and Grantham, J. J.: Physiology of the Kidney. Philadelphia, Lea & Febiger, 1982.
13. Gammage, G.: Crystalloid vs. colloid: is colloid worth the cost? Int. Anesth. Clin., 25:37, 1987.
14. Holcroft, J. W., and Trunk, D. D.: Extravascular lung water

following hemorrhagic shock in the baboon: comparison between resuscitation with Ringer's lactate and plasmanate. Ann. Surg., *180:*408, 1974.
15. Virgilio, R. W., et al.: Crystalloid versus colloid resuscitation: is one better? Surgery, *85:*129, 1979.
16. Lowe, R. J., Moss, G. S., Jilek, J., and Levine, H. D.: Crystalloid versus colloid in the etiology of pulmonary failure after trauma: a randomized trial in man. Surgery, *81:*676, 1977.
17. Holcroft, J. W., et al.: 3% NaCl and 7.5% NaCl/Dextran 70 in the resuscitation of severely injured patients. Ann. Surg., *206:*29, 1987.
18. Gunn, M. L., et al.: Prospective, randomized trial of hypertonic sodium lactate versus lactated Ringer's solution for burn shock resuscitation. J. Trauma, *29:*1261, 1989.
19. Carrico, C. J., Canizaro, P. C., and Shires, G. T.: Fluid resuscitation following injury: rationale for the use of balanced salt solutions. Crit. Care Med., *4:*46, 1976.
20. Kitakaze, M., Weisfeldt, M. L., and Marban, E.: Acidosis during early reperfusion prevents myocardial stunning in perfused fetter hearts. J. Clin. Invest., *82:*920, 1988.
21. Sibbald, W. J., and Driedger, A. A.: Right and left ventricular pre-load and diastolic ventricular compliance: implications for therapy in critically ill patients. *In* Textbook of Critical Care. Edited by W. C. Shoemaker, W. J. Thompson, and P. R. Holbrook. Philadelphia, W. B. Saunders, 1984.
22. Humphreys, M. C.: Fluid and electrolyte management. *In* Current Surgical Diagnosis and Treatment. 10th ed. Edited by L. W. Way. Norwalk, CT, Appleton & Lange, 129–142, 1994.
23. Kohan, D. E.: Fluid and electrolyte management. *In* Manual of Medical Therapeutics. Edited by W. C. Dunagan and M. L. Ridner. Boston, Little, Brown, 1989.
24. Canizaro, P. C., Prager, M. D., and Shires, G. T.: The infusion of Ringer's lactate solution during shock. Am. J. Surg., *122:*494, 1971.
25. Foster, D. W.: Diabetes mellitus. *In* Harrison's Principles of Internal Medicine. Edited by E. Braunwald, et al. New York, McGraw-Hill Book Company, 1987.
26. Quinton, P. M.: Physiology of sweat secretion. Kidney Int., *32:*S102, 1987.
27. Lamke, L., Nilsson, G., and Reithner, L.: The influence of elevated body temperature on skin perspiration. Acta Chir. Scand., *146:*81, 1980.
28. Cox, P.: Insensible water loss and its assessment in adult patients: a review. Anesth. Scand., *31:*771, 1980.
29. Reber, H. A., and Way, L. W.: Pancreas. *In* Current Surgical Diagnosis and Treatment. Edited by L. W. Way. Norwalk, CT, Appleton & Lange, 567–594, 1994.
30. Holcroft, J. W.: Shock. *In* American College of Surgeons: Care of the Surgical Patient. Vol. 1, Critical Care. Edited by D. W. Wilmore, et al. A publication of the Committee on Pre- and Postoperative Care. New York, Scientific American, 1994.
31. Campion, P. S., et al.: Effect of hemorrhagic shock on transmembrane potential. Surgery, *66:*1051, 1969.
32. Cunningham, J. N., Carter, N. W., Rector, F. C., and Seldin, D. W.: Resting transmembrane potential difference of skeletal muscle in normal subjects and severely ill patients. J. Clin. Invest., *50:*49, 1989.
33. Blaisdell, F. W.: Traumatic shock: the search for toxic factor. Bull. Am. Coll. Surg., *68:*1, 1983.
34. Broviac, J. W., Cole, B. S., and Schribner, M. D.: A silicone rubber right atrial catheter for prolonged parenteral alimentation. Surg. Gynecol. Obstet., *136:*602, 1973.
35. Hickman, R. O., et al.: A modified right atrial catheter for access to the venous system on marrow transplant patients. Surg. Gynecol. Obstet., *148:*871, 1979.
36. Ring, J., Messmer, K.: Incidence and severity of anaphylactoid reactions to colloid volume substitutes. Lancet, *1:*466, 1977.
37. Owings, J. T., and Wolfe, B. M: Prevention of complications associated with semipermanent silastic central venous catheters. JPEN J. Parenter. Enteral. Nutr., *18:*345, 1994.

Chapter 61

PRINCIPLES OF BLOOD REPLACEMENT

JOHN C. ALVERDY
EDWARD LEVINE
STEVEN A. GOULD

The real and perceived risks of blood product administration have forced a reassessment of transfusion practice (Table 61-1). This new appreciation of the morbidity associated with homologous transfusion has led to an unprecedented decline in blood use. These risks tend to be higher in the critical care setting, where urgent and multiple transfusion of blood products is often necessary. Although the screening of blood for infectious agents should make homologous transfusion safer, it seems clear that the risk of infectious disease related to transfusion and the resulting fears will never be nonexistent.[1] For this reason, each unit of transfused blood should be administered based on physiologic need rather than by mere tradition or unstudied guidelines.

In patients undergoing surgical procedures, homologous red blood cell transfusions may be particularly hazardous. Allergic and hemolytic transfusion reactions as well as alloimmunization remain important sequelae of homologous blood exposure. Blood transfusions have been shown to be immunosuppressive in a variety of laboratory and clinical settings. The immunosuppressive effects of transfusion are associated with an increase in the incidence of perioperative septic complications, burn sepsis,[2] and multisystem organ failure.[3] Furthermore, increased recurrence and decreased survival rates following resections of sarcomas[4] and carcinomas[5] have been reported. Although the mechanism of transfusion-related immunosuppression has not been completely elucidated, it appears that homologous blood exposure is of particular risk to the surgical patient. Therefore, it is important to consider blood conservation practices and physiologic need when attempting to minimize the morbidity of blood transfusion in the critically ill. Quite often simple blood conservation measures and a working understanding of the physiology of oxygen-carrying capacity can significantly reduce the requirements for homologous transfusion.

PRE-ICU CONSIDERATIONS FOR BLOOD USE

Blood Conservation Techniques

It is important to consider the striking reports of iatrogenic anemia that occur in the ICU from phlebotomy alone. In support of this, Smoller and Kruskall[6] reviewed the records of 100 patients admitted to a tertiary care institution and reported that patients in the ICU had a mean blood volume of 944 ml withdrawn and were phlebotomized a mean of four times a day during their ICU stay. Therefore an important pre-ICU consideration for patients is that strategies for blood conservation be developed. These include:

- Routine use of microchemical techniques for the determination of blood gases, electrolytes, and hematocrit so the amount of blood required for the serial multianalyte determination does not exceed 1 ml
- The use of sterile reservoirs attached to indwelling arterial catheters to avoid the need to discard blood as a consequence of "clearing the line" before blood sampling
- The use of "cell saver" techniques in traumatically injured patients, selected operative cases, and postoperative critically ill patients
- The use of erythropoietin in appropriately selected patient populations, particularly those with chronic renal failure
- Routine consideration of preoperative autologous donation or hemodilution in those undergoing elective operative procedures

Preoperative Programs for Autologous Blood Donation

This technique was repopularized in the 1960s as a means of obtaining autologous blood for patients with rare antibodies that were difficult to crossmatch. The risks of blood-borne infection transmission from homologous transfusions has led to an exponential rise in the use of autologous blood donation (ABD) programs before elective operations. In a national survey of transfusion practices in the United States during the 1980s, autologous blood donations increased from 30,000 U in 1982 to 397,000 U in 1987.[7] This figure continues to rise into the 1990s. Nevertheless, the application of this procedure to the treatment of patients in the ICU is limited to those situations in which acute blood loss is anticipated, such as planned high risk surgical procedures, and therefore limits its use before ICU admission.

The criteria used for donor acceptability for ABD programs are variable from institution to institution. The American Association of Blood Banks recommends a minimum hematocrit value of 34% and a hemoglobin of 11 g/dl for autologous donation. Donations are most commonly scheduled 7 days apart. A review has shown that, following

Table 61-1. Estimated Risks of Blood Transfusion

Factor	Risk
Human immunodeficiency virus	1:40,000–1,000,000
Hepatitis B	≤1:200–300
Non-A, non-B hepatitis	≤1:100
Fever, chills, urticaria	1:100
Hemolytic transfusion reactions	1:6000
Fatal hemolytic transfusion reactions	1:100,000

(From NIH Consensus Development panel: Perioperative red blood cell transfusion. JAMA, *260*:2700, 1988.)

the aforementioned criteria, 96% of patients could donate at least 3 units of blood before operative intervention. The most common reasons cited for the limitation of this procedure in the elective surgical setting are physician underuse, insufficient time intervals for collection before surgery, and limited erythropoietic reserve of patients subjected to repeated phlebotomy.[8]

Hemodilution

This technique is based on the cardiovascular changes that occur during the induction of normovolemic anemia. Blood is withdrawn to reduce the hematocrit reading acutely to 30% or less, while blood volume is maintained with Ringer's lactate, dextran, or other volume expanders. A healthy individual maintains oxygen delivery during this period of normovolemic anemia. Messmer[9] has suggested that tissue oxygenation remains normal during hemodilution, and advocates of purposeful hemodilution have suggested that a hematocrit reading of 30% is optimal for ideal microcirculatory rheology. Furthermore, by reducing the hematocrit, the number of red cells lost during surgical procedures is decreased because the hematocrit of the shed blood is lower.

This method can provide several units of whole blood from intraoperative use. Although the technique has been used widely in Europe, in the United States it has been primarily limited to patients undergoing open heart operations. Because heart operations are responsible for a large proportion of our homologous blood demand, wider use of this method could have a substantial influence on the availability of blood.[10]

Intraoperative Autotransfusion

Autotransfusion represents an efficient means of reducing homologous blood requirements through the recycling of red cells lost during intraoperative hemorrhage.[11] This technique has been known for many years but has experienced renewed interest. The technique has been extended to the ICU setting with newer devices, including chest tube recovery systems and other means of recovery for ongoing blood loss. The problem of contamination limits its use in a variety of settings in which it might be most helpful, such as major trauma and gastrointestinal bleeding. Contamination with tumor cells limits the use of this technique for cases involving major cancer resections. Another concern is the required logistic support necessary to implement this expensive technique on a 24-hour basis.

Lastly, air embolism during reinfusion of shed blood is a rare but important complication to avoid.

Acceleration of Erythropoiesis

Approximately two thirds of all red cell transfusions are administered in the perioperative period. Effective preoperative autologous donation and rapid postoperative recovery from anemia both depend on intense erythropoietic responses. Consequently, the pharmacologic stimulation of erythropoiesis represents an attractive potential means of increasing red cell recovery after acute blood loss. The advent of recombinant DNA technology has led to the isolation and cloning of numerous hematopoietic growth factors, which promote bone marrow cellular proliferation. Erythropoietin, a glycoprotein normally released by the kidney in response to tissue hypoxia, is known to be the primary regulator of red cell proliferation. Preclinical and clinical studies with exogenously administered recombinant-human erythropoietin (rHuEPO) have demonstrated its efficacy both in increasing the number of autologous units collected before elective operations and in enhancing erythropoietic recovery when given before acute blood loss.[12,13] When rHuEPO is administered following acute blood loss, however, clinically significant effects are not evident until approximately 1 week after therapy is initiated.[14] Accordingly, in the setting of nonanticipated blood loss, rHuEPO's therapeutic potential is limited. One exception is the patient who, for religious reasons, refuses blood. The use of rHuEPO in this setting can be life-saving if blood loss has ceased and oxygen delivery can be maintained. The use of rHuEPO in this setting can permit earlier recovery of red blood cell mass and may improve survival.

In the pre-ICU setting, all efforts should be made to minimize blood loss, correct coagulopathies, and encourage preoperative donation. Each unit of red cells, fresh frozen plasma, and platelets must be viewed as drugs with significant side effects.

ICU—DEFINING THE INDICATION FOR BLOOD BASED ON PHYSIOLOGIC NEED

Red Blood Cells

To guide transfusion of red blood cells based on physiologic need, it is important to have a working understanding of normal oxygen delivery and consumption relationships. It is equally important to understand the limitations of the present technologies for measuring oxygen need, especially in light of the growing complexities of critically ill patients. Although whole-body oxygen transport dynamics may be useful in guiding red blood cell repletion, it is important to recognize that a variety of clinical disease states may interact to perturb oxygen transport at the cellular level. Present technologies are limited in assessing these abnormalities in individual organs.

The introduction of the Swan-Ganz catheter allowed measurement of the mixed venous oxygen content, permitting a better understanding of the alterations in oxygen dynamics during shock. Advances in our understanding of the imbalance of oxygen supply versus demand during critical illness have focused therapy in this regard. Yet a healthy skepticism persists in "maximizing" oxygen delivery with inotropes, vasodilators, and red blood cell transfusion because normalization of whole-body oxygen dynamics may not necessarily reflect amelioration of the microcirculatory disturbance of oxygen transport.

Oxygen Delivery/Oxygen Consumption

Oxygen delivery (D_{O_2}) is defined as the amount of gaseous oxygen that is pumped from the left ventricle each minute and is therefore the product of the cardiac output (CO) and the arterial oxygen content (Ca_{O_2}). Thus:

$$D_{O_2} = (CO)(Ca_{O_2}) \qquad (1)$$

is the equation for oxygen delivery (Equation 1). A normal cardiac output for a 70-kg man is 5 L per min. Ca_{O_2} is defined by equation 2:

$$\text{(Hemoglobin g/dl)(\% saturation of } O_2 \qquad (2)$$
$$\text{of arterial blood) (1.34)} + Pa_{O_2} (0.003)$$

and is approximately 20 ml/dl in patients with a hemoglobin of 15 g/dl and whose hemoglobin is 100% saturated with oxygen. Therefore, the oxygen delivery in a patient with a hemoglobin of 15 g/dl, an Sa_{O_2} of 100%, and a CO of 5 L per minute would be 1000 ml per minute.

The other component determining the balance of oxygen is the oxygen consumption ($\dot{V}_{O_2}$). Oxygen consumption is the amount of gaseous oxygen that is actually used by the body each minute and is calculated using the Fick equation. The Fick equation states that the amount of oxygen consumed is equal to the CO times the arterial venous oxygen content difference. Oxygen consumption is defined by equation 3:

$$\dot{V}_{O_2} = CO \, (Ca_{O_2} - Cv_{O_2}) \qquad (3)$$

where Cv_{O_2} = Hemoglobin (% saturation of the mixed venous blood) (1.34) + Pv_{O_2} (0.003). The normal oxygen consumption for a 70-kg man is approximately 250 ml per minute.

Oxygen utilization defines the fraction of oxygen delivered that is actually used and is also known as the oxygen extraction ratio (O_2ER). O_2ER is expressed by equation 4:

$$O_2ER = \dot{V}_{O_2}/D_{O_2} \qquad (4)$$

The normal resting oxygen extraction ratio is between 0.2 and 0.3. Therefore only 20 to 30% of the oxygen normally delivered is actually consumed by the body, indicating the enormous reserve that exists in case of sudden demand. Values of O_2ER that exceed 0.35 are thought to be in a range that compromises the reserve capacity to meet demand in a short period of time and therefore imposes significant stress on the normal balance of oxygen. O_2ER values of greater than 50% result in anaerobic metabolism, hemodynamic instability, and death.

Oxygen demand is the volume of oxygen that is needed by the tissue to function aerobically. Presently there is no technology to measure oxygen demand, and therefore we must rely on indicators that measure need versus consumption. When the demand for oxygen exceeds consumption ($O_2ER > 50\%$), anaerobic metabolism must take over to supply the tissues with adequate energy.

Monitoring Oxygen Transport

The balance of oxygen supply and demand depends on the relative relationship between those factors that determine supply (cardiac output, hemoglobin concentration, arterial oxygen saturations) and oxygen consumption. Monitoring of this balance currently involves invasive monitoring so the pulmonary artery blood oxygen content (mixed venous oxygen) can be determined. Although traditionally the Pv_{O_2} has been used, the $Satv_{O_2}$ is the key variable (see later), and therefore reliance on fiberoptic oximetry catheters permits precise and continual measurement of this important oxygen parameter. In addition, changes in the position of the O_2 dissociation curve can make the Pv_{O_2} an unreliable indicator of tissue oxygenation (Fig. 61-1). The importance of monitoring $Satv_{O_2}$ can be best understood when the Fick equation is solved for $Satv_{O_2}$.

The real determinants of oxygen utilization can be observed by mathematically rearranging the oxygen extraction ratio equation (Equation 4).

$$O_2ER = \frac{\dot{V}_{O_2}}{D_{O_2}} \qquad (5)$$

substituting equation 1 for D_{O_2}, the following is obtained:

$$O_2ER = \frac{\dot{V}_{O_2}}{(CO)Ca_{O_2}} \qquad (6)$$

Substituting equation 3 for $\dot{V}_{O_2}$, the following is obtained:

$$O_2ER = \frac{CO(Ca_{O_2} - Cv_{O_2})}{(CO)Ca_{O_2}} \qquad (7)$$

Canceling CO and eliminating the Pa_{O_2} and Pv_{O_2} from equations 2 and 3 because they represent a trivial amount of oxygen, the following is obtained (Equation 8):

$$O_2ER = \frac{Hb(Sata_{O_2})1.34 + Hb(Satv_{O_2})1.34}{Hb(Sata_{O_2})1.34} \qquad (8)$$

Canceling out the numerator and denominators' common variables, the following is obtained (Equation 9):

$$O_2ER = \frac{Sata_{O_2} + Satv_{O_2}}{Sata_{O_2}} \qquad (9)$$

One can now see that the oxygen extraction ratio is determined primarily by the change in the mixed venous oxygen saturation (not Pv_{O_2}) because clinically the arterial oxygen saturation is usually maintained constant with supplemental oxygen. The determinates of Satv can be easily seen by combining equations 6 and 9 and solving for $Satv_{O_2}$:

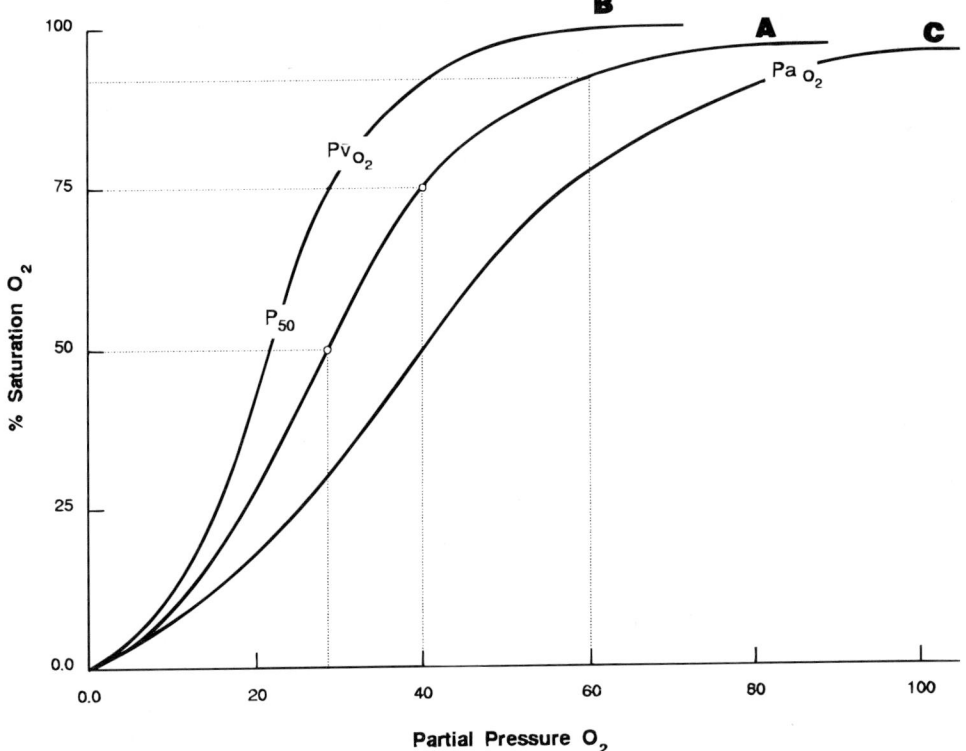

Fig. 61–1. The hemoglobin dissociation curve illustrates the nonlinear relationship between oxygen saturation of hemoglobin and the partial pressure of oxygen in plasma. The P50 is the point at which 50% of the hemoglobin is saturated under the laboratory conditions of 37°C, P_{CO_2} 40 mm Hg, and pH 7.40 *(Curve A)*. If the P50 decreases, affinity of hemoglobin for oxygen increases, and the partial pressure of oxygen in plasma decreases, making less oxygen available to the tissues. In other words, the hemoglobin is 50% saturated at a lower P_{O_2}. Increased affinity or decreased P50 is shown by *Curve B* (shift to the left) and represents clinical conditions of alkalemia, hypothermia, hypocarbia, and decreased 2,3-diphosphoglycerate (2,3-DPG). The opposite or an increased P50 (shift to the right) represents a decreased affinity of hemoglobin for oxygen *(Curve C)*. Clinical conditions of acidemia, hyperthermia, hypercarbia, and increased 2,3-DPG decrease hemoglobin affinity for oxygen. Oxygen content is reduced at any given P_{O_2}, and thus oxygen transport to the tissues is reduced.[23] (Drawn by: George Morrison, C.D., Madison, WI.)

$$\frac{\dot{V}_{O_2}}{C_{aO_2}} = \frac{Sa_{tO_2} + Sa_{tvO_2}}{Sa_{tO_2}} \quad (10)$$

Substituting equation 4 for C_{aO_2} and solving for Sa_{tvO_2}, one obtains the following (Equation 11):

$$Sa_{tvO_2} = Sa_{tO_2} - \frac{\dot{V}_{O_2}}{CO(Hb)1.34} \quad (11)$$

Substituting normal values for $\dot{V}_{O_2}$, CO, Hb, and Sa_{tO_2} and maintaining the units constant (10 dl = 1 L), the following is obtained (Equation 12):

$$Sa_{tvO_2} = 1 - \frac{250 \text{ ml/min}}{5 \text{ L/min } (15 \text{ g/dl}) \ 1.34(10_{\text{conversion factor}})} \quad (12)$$

Satv = 0.75, which is the normal mixed venous oxygen saturation.

When the venous oxygen saturation (Sa_{tvO_2}) decreases, significant stress is placed on the balance between oxygen supply and consumption. As the resting Sa_{tvO_2} approaches 0.50, or the extraction ratio nears 50%, critically ill patients develop anaerobic metabolism, and mortality rates are high if venous desaturation persists and is unable to be corrected. Following are four case histories that illustrate the importance of monitoring the mixed venous saturation and extraction ratio as guides to transfusion therapy. This can be performed either with continuous mixed venous fiberoptic oximetry or by intermittent blood gas sampling from the pulmonary artery port of the Swan-Ganz catheter.

Case 1. A 53-year-old Jehovah's witness with a previous history of myocardial infarction is admitted to the hospital with an upper gastrointestinal hemorrhage. The patient is alert and mentally competent and refuses any blood products. The patient is taken to the operating room and undergoes an ulcer operation. On postoperative day 3, the patient develops an aspiration pneumonia and is intubated and mechanically ventilated. His problems include anemia (hemoglobin 5.5 g/dl), sepsis (temperature 39.5°C, white blood cell count = 24,000/mm³), and respiratory failure (on 80% oxygen, the patient's Pa_{O_2} = 75, O_2 saturation = 93%). The patient's cardiac output is 4.2 L/mm, and his

Satvo$_2$ = 53%. Substituting this patient's pulmonary artery catheter values into equation 8, one can solve for oxygen consumption:

$$0.53 = 1 - \frac{\dot{V}o_2}{6.2(5.5)1.34} = 217 \text{ ml/min}$$

This patient has an abnormally low Satvo$_2$. Furthermore, substituting the Satao$_2$ and Satvo$_2$ into equation 9, the extraction ratio for this patient is 47%, placing this patient at risk for inadequate oxygen delivery should a sudden increase in oxygen consumption occur. This most likely has occurred because this patient was unable to compensate adequately for the present level of anemia owing to his previous history of coronary artery disease. Because this patient cannot receive blood owing to religious objections, strategies for this patient would be to (1) increase the cardiac output with volume, vasodilators, or inotropes. Because the variables in the denominator of equation 4 are all multiplicative, increasing the cardiac output by 30% (CO = 8), the Satvo$_2$ would be 65%, a much safer range for the patient. (2) Sedate and induce muscular paralysis to decrease oxygen consumption. Referring to equation 11, if oxygen consumption were reduced by 30% ($\dot{V}o_2$ = 152 ml/min) with pharmacologic sedation, then the Satvo$_2$ would be 67%, again a much safer range for the critically ill patient. To what extent the patient should have either component (consumption or delivery) manipulated must be individualized. Maximizing preload with volume, however, or simply sedating the patient can be easily performed, is metabolically an inexpensive maneuver, and can be rapidly accomplished. Once these have been performed, the oxygen variables can be reevaluated, and further therapy, such as muscular paralysis or inotropic pressor support, can be considered. A final strategy to consider if the Satvo$_2$ remains below 50% and the extraction ratio greater than 50% is the use of red blood cell substitutes. These are addressed in a later section of this chapter.

Case 2. An 84-year-old, extremely thin woman is admitted to the hospital after a fall and is diagnosed with a hip fracture. The patient is known to have severe aortic stenosis. Surgery is planned to replace her hip for early mobilization. Preoperatively a Swan-Ganz catheter is placed, and the patient's CO is 2.3 L per minute. The hemoglobin is 10.0 g/dl, and the Satvo$_2$ is 60% with an extraction ratio of 40% and a $\dot{V}o_2$ of 120 ml per minute. This patient's borderline extraction ratio and Satvo$_2$ are of immediate concern because her CO is fixed by aortic stenosis. Using equation 8, one can see that any small increase in oxygen consumption results in immediate venous desaturation. Furthermore, surgery results in some blood loss. Again using equation 11, if she is transfused to a hemoglobin of 15 g/dl, she should be able to tolerate up to a 35% increase in oxygen consumption (120 to 166 ml/min) without a further fall in her mixed venous saturation. Thus, in this particular setting, red blood cell transfusion may be valuable, despite a quite acceptable hemoglobin of 10 g/dl.

Case 3. A 28-year-old man is admitted to the ICU with a history of a gunshot wound to the right groin area and shock (blood pressure = 70 systolic). The patient is given 3 L of Ringer's lactate solution, and the blood pressure immediately is reestablished to the normal range (120/80 mm Hg). The groin wound is explored, and an injury to the femoral artery is primarily repaired. The patient is brought to the ICU, and the following data are obtained from the Swan-Ganz pulmonary artery catheter: CO = 9.0 L per minute, heart rate = 88, pulmonary capillary wedge pressure (PCWP) = 10 mm Hg, Satvo$_2$ = 70%, Satao$_2$ = 100%, $\dot{V}o_2$ = 230 ml per minute, hemoglobin = 6.4 g/dl. Substituting the arterial and venous saturation values in equation 9, the extraction ratio is in the normal range at 30%. Therefore despite a low hemoglobin, this patient does not require red blood cell transfusion because the anemia is compensated completely by the elevated cardiac output. Furthermore, this patient's elevated CO is not due to rate alone but rather reflects a high stroke volume and efficiently operating myocardium (CO = HR × SV). This point is of particular note in patients with coronary artery or valvular disease. If compensation to anemia demands an elevated heart rate because stroke volume is fixed owing to underlying or ongoing myocardial dysfunction, red blood cell transfusion may be necessary to decrease myocardial oxygen demand. Because there is no technology currently available to measure myocardial oxygen demand clinically, heart rate is often used. It should be noted, however, that the cause of tachycardia in the critically ill is usually multifactorial (e.g., pain, anxiety, drugs), and therefore one should make every attempt to treat these disorders before administration of red blood cells. It is our experience that tachycardia in the euvolemic, mildly anemic critically ill patient (8 to 10 g/dl) is rarely responsive to red blood cell transfusion. The reason for this response is not well understood. This may be due to the microcirculatory disturbances that occur during critical illness. Nonetheless, in the critically ill patient with myocardial ischemia, it is common practice to maintain the hemoglobin concentration near 10 g/dl. Although this practice seems to "make sense," it should be recognized that there are no studies that demonstrate efficacy in preventing myocardial ischemia with red blood cell transfusion for anemia in the patient with a normal mixed venous oxygen concentration without tachycardia.

Case 4. A 39-year-old woman is admitted with pancreatitis. The patient is administered intravenous fluids and is given nothing by mouth. Ultrasound study reveals gallstones and several small stones in a dilated common bile duct. The patient is taken to the operating room and undergoes a cholecystectomy and common bile duct exploration with extraction of several stones and manipulation of the distal common bile duct. Over the next several days, the patient develops severe adult respiratory distress syndrome and hypotension and is mechanically ventilated and placed on an arterial pressor to maintain mean arterial pressure at approximately 85 mm Hg. A Swan-Ganz catheter is placed, and the following data are generated: CO = 9.8 L per minute, heart rate = 108, Satvo$_2$ = 80%, PCWP = 12 mm Hg, Satao$_2$ = 95%, and hemoglobin = 7.9 g/dl. The patient extraction ratio using equation 6 is 18%, and the $\dot{V}o_2$ using equation 8 is 177 ml per minute. The patient's serum arterial lactate level is 3.8 mEq/L. Several important questions must be addressed relative to this patient's need for oxygen.

First, why is the lactate level elevated in this patient when the extraction ratio is actually lower than normal and clearly below the anaerobic threshold? The apparent reason for the abnormally low extraction ratio in this patient is perturbed oxygen uptake at the cellular level. Both infection and inflammation have been reported to result in significant impairment in cellular oxygen uptake. The main clinical evidence for this has been demonstration of pathologic supply-dependent oxygen consumption.[15] That is, in the patient with a normal oxygen extraction ratio and a normal Satvo$_2$, supplying greater amounts of oxygen (i.e., increasing oxygen delivery) actually results in increased oxygen consumption, suggesting the presence of continued oxygen need despite apparent normal delivery. When lactate levels are elevated, as is present in this particular case, increasing oxygen delivery, and thereby increasing oxygen consumption, may decrease the blood lactate level, perhaps reflecting an improvement in cellular oxygenation (Fig. 61-2).

Second, how should oxygen delivery be increased? Oxygen delivery, the product of the CO and arterial oxygen content (Cao$_2$), can be increased by either improving the CO with volume expansion and inotropes, or alternatively the Cao$_2$ can be increased by red blood cell transfusion. Note: Cao$_2$ = hemoglobin (% saturation) 1.34 + Pao$_2$ (0.003); because the patient is 95% saturated, the only meaningful increase in Cao$_2$ will occur by increasing the hemoglobin concentration. Therefore the question arises as to whether one approach is more efficacious than the other. Several randomized, prospective studies have asked this question and have failed to show an increase in oxygen consumption when oxygen delivery is increased with red blood cell transfusion during states of pathologic supply-dependent oxygen consumption.[16] In fact, these studies by Dietrich et al. demonstrated that volume-resuscitated anemic shock patients did not benefit in terms of oxygen consumption after red blood cell transfusion. Other investigators have demonstrated an increase in oxygen consumption following packed red blood cell transfusion in surgical sepsis, yet neither oxygen consumption increased nor blood lactate levels correlated favorably with outcome.[17] These findings are in contradistinction to studies that clearly suggest that oxygen consumption can be increased by increasing the CO component of oxygen delivery during clinical states, in which pathologic supply-dependent oxygen consumption can be demonstrated. These studies in addition demonstrated a distinct survival advantage with inotropes and volume support to achieve "supranormal" oxygen deliveries in the patient with demonstrable pathologic supply-dependent oxygen consumption. It should be noted, however, that there is not universal acceptance of the maximum oxygen delivery concept. The hypothesis that cellular hypoxia and bioenergetic failure are common findings during sepsis has been questioned. Using extremely sensitive markers for cellular hypoxia, including in vivo[31] phosphorus nuclear magnetic resonance spectroscopy, studies by Hotchkiss and Karl[17] demonstrated elevated lactate levels in sepsis without cellular hypoxia. Studies such as these may force a complete reevaluation of the role of maximizing oxygen delivery in sepsis. This "cloud of doubt" on supernormalization of all parameters of oxygen transport during sepsis must attenuate the clinician's zeal for excessive use of blood and inotropes. Consideration of the real risks of transfusion of packed red blood cells must be weighed against the theoretic benefit of transfusion to achieve superphysiologic oxygen delivery levels. Therefore, based on the real risks of homologous blood exposure and the potential for increasing myocardial oxygen demand when supply is limited (coronary artery disease) with inotropes, we recommend the following transfusion guidelines:[19]

- If the hemoglobin is greater than 10 g/dl, transfusion is rarely indicated.
- If the hemoglobin is less than 7 g/dl, transfusion is usually indicated.
- If the hemoglobin is greater than 7 g/dl, but less than 10 g/dl, the clinical status, Satvo$_2$, and the O$_2$ extraction ratio will be helpful in assessing transfusion need.

Platelet Transfusion and Fresh-Frozen Plasma

The diagnosis and treatment of abnormalities of the coagulation cascade are covered elsewhere. The post-ICU effects, however, of massive transfusion on the coagulation profile of the critically ill deserves mention. Studies of patients receiving massive transfusion following traumatic injury have shown that dilutional thrombocytopenia is the most frequent cause for deranged hemostasis.[19] It is unlikely that a patient with a platelet count of 50,000/mm^3

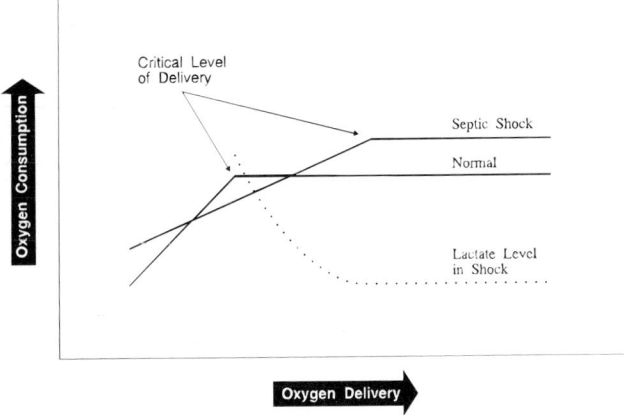

Fig. 61-2. The relationship between oxygen delivery and oxygen consumption. Normally an increase in oxygen consumption (for example, with an increase in workload) is associated with an increase in oxygen delivery (increased cardiac output). There is a point at which any further increase in oxygen delivery is not associated with increased oxygen consumption (critical level of delivery). In septic shock, as illustrated, this point is shifted, owing to impaired cellular uptake of oxygen. Under these circumstances, an increased oxygen delivery (via an increase in cardiac output) is associated with increased oxygen uptake. As oxygen delivery increases, oxygen uptake increases, and anaerobic metabolism (depicted by lactate levels) decreases. (Redrawn by George Morrison, C.D., Madison, WI, from Dietrich, K. A., et al.: Cardiovascular and metabolic response to red blood cell transfusion in critically ill volume-resuscitated non-surgical patients. Crit. Care Med., 18:940, 1990.)

or higher will benefit from platelet transfusion if thrombocytopenia is the sole abnormality. Therefore no definite trigger platelet count can be identified for transfusion. The coagulopathy that may accompany massive transfusion is often multifactorial. Hypothermia, thrombocytopenia, and deficiencies of circulating procoagulants secondary to dilution may interfere with all three phases of normal coagulation. Furthermore, significant disseminated intravascular coagulation may complicate the care of any patients following significant injury or shock.

Treatment of hemostatic defects complicating resuscitations may require the administration of homologous blood products. Platelets and fresh-frozen plasma (FFP) may transmit viral infectious disease. Exposure to these blood products carries risks to similar homologous red cell exposure. The risk is likely to be the same as for whole blood. These components should therefore be used with the same precautions used for any other blood components.

Successful treatment of coagulopathy associated with massive transfusion is most commonly accomplished with rewarming and platelets alone, suggesting that elevated prothrombin time (PT) and activated partial thromboplastin time (PTT) in the presence of a coagulopathy are not evidence that administration of FFP will correct the hemostatic defect. It is well known that normal clotting can still occur when the various clotting protein concentrations are substantially reduced. Furthermore, the infusion of FFP in patients who develop microvascular hemorrhages or so-called oozing after massive transfusion and who have abnormal PT and PTT values frequently fails to stop bleeding despite attempts at normalizing the PT and PTT times.

Prophylactic use of FFP and platelets has failed to reduce the incidence of coagulopathy after massive transfusion. Therefore the practice of prophylactic blood product transfusion to avoid possible coagulopathy should be abandoned. Current practice parameters for use of platelets are listed in Table 61-2, and practice parameters for cryoprecipitate are shown in Table 61-4.

A National Institutes of Health (NIH) consensus conference on the use of FFP concluded that the majority of FFP transfusions may be unnecessary.[20-22] Although FFP is frequently used clinically, its recommended indications are few, as shown in Table 61-3.

Red Blood Cell Substitutes

Efforts to develop a safe and effective red cell substitute have continued for many decades. The goal has been to obtain a product that would transport oxygen and carbon dioxide adequately enough to replace the primary function of the red cell in the setting of temporary unavailability of blood. The focus on the risks associated with homologous transfusion has accelerated the efforts to develop a sterile red cell substitute as an alternative to homologous blood. Perfluorochemical emulsions and hemoglobin solutions are the two potential products that have been most extensively studied.

Perfluorochemical Emulsions

Considerable progress has been made in research with perfluorochemicals since they were first described by Clark and Gollan in 1966. Perfluorochemicals are organic

Table 61-2. Practice Parameter for the Use of Platelets

Clinical Indications	Example	Recommendation
Decreased platelet production with or without increased platelet destruction	Aplastic anemia; acute leukemia; following chemotherapy or radiation to the bone marrow	• Counts of 5000/mm^3 or below—administer platelets regardless of apparent bleeding • Counts between 5000 and 30000/mm^3—platelets may be given prophylactically on the basis of risk of bleeding (e.g., gastrointestinal or central nervous system hemorrhage)
Enhanced platelet destruction: transfusions are of limited usefulness where platelet destruction, either by antibodies or by consumption, is the cause of thrombocytopenia	Patients undergoing major surgery who start with intact hemostatic systems (there must be evidence of microvascular bleeding—usually visualized in surgical field) Prolonged bleeding after heart surgery; similarly with neurologic or ophthalmologic surgery	• Counts below 50000/mm^3 with evidence of microvascular bleeding • Counts below 100000/mm^3 following heart surgery when major unexplained bleeding occurs with normal coagulation values • Contraindicated in thrombotic thrombocytopenic purpura; with idiopathic thrombocytopenic purpura—limited major surgery with excessive bleeding • Other destructive states—counts 20000 to 50000/mm^3 with unexpected excessive bleeding
Platelet dysfunction	Platelet transfusions are useful in some instances	

(Adapted from: Fresh-frozen Plasma, Cryoprecipitate and Platelets Administration Practice Guidelines Development Task Force of the College of American Pathologists: Practice parameter for the use of fresh-frozen plasma, cryoprecipitate, and platelets. JAMA, 271:777, 1994.)

Table 61-3. Practice Parameter for the Use of Fresh-Frozen Plasma

Clinical Indications	Documentation
History or clinical course suggestive of a coagulopathy due to a congenital or acquired deficiency of coagulation factors, with: active bleeding; prior to an operative or other invasive procedure	• Prothrombin time (PT) greater than 1.5 times the midpoint of normal range • Activated partial thromboplastin time (aPTT) greater than 1.5 times the top of the normal range (usually > 55 to 60 sec) (Fibrinogen must be normal; specimen must be free of heparin) • Coagulation factor assay of less than 25% of activity
Massive blood transfusion	• Replacement of more than 1 blood volume (e.g., 5000 ml in a 70-kg adult) within several hours with evidence of a coagulation deficiency
Reversal of warfarin effect	• Immediate hemostasis required to stop active bleeding or prior to emergency surgery or invasive procedure (PT > 18 seconds; international normalized ratio > 1.6 seconds)
Documented congenital or acquired coagulation factor deficiency when used for bleeding or prophylactically for surgery of an invasive procedure	• Congenital deficiency of factor II, V, VII, X, XI, or XIII • von Willebrand's disease (if desmopressin acetatevDDAVP [1-desamino-8-D-arginine vasopressin] is not effective and cryoprecepitate or vWF-containing factor VIII concentrate is not available) • Congenital or acquired deficiency of factor VIII or factor IX • Acquired deficiency of multiple factors such as seen in severe liver disease, disseminated intravascular coagulation, or vitamin K depletion
Deficiency of antithrombin III, heparin cofactor II, protein C or protein S	• For antithrombin III deficiency when concentrate is not available
Hypoglobulinemic states in rare instances	• Generally, intravenous immune globulin is preferable
Plasma exchange for thrombotic thrombocytopenic purpura or hemolytic uremic syndrome	
The use of fresh-frozen plasma as a plasma expander is contraindicated	

(Adapted from: Fresh-frozen Plasma, Cryoprecipitate and Platelets Administration Practice Guidelines Development Task Force of the College of American Pathologists: Practice parameter for the use of fresh-frozen plasma, cryoprecipitate, and platelets. JAMA, 271:777, 1994.)

liquids that have the unique property of carrying large amounts of oxygen in physically dissolved form. The solubility for oxygen in the pure perfluorochemicals is actually 10-fold to 20-fold greater than in water. It was Clark and Gollan's liquid breathing experiment with mice that so vividly demonstrated this remarkable property and led to the potential application of perfluorochemicals as clinically useful oxygen carriers. The next important event was the report by Geyer et al. They demonstrated that rats could survive a total exchange with perfluorochemicals to a zero hematocrit reading. The important stipulation was that the rats were required to breathe a high concentration of oxygen. This requirement continues to be a limiting factor with all perfluorochemicals. Considerable efforts were then devoted to developing a product that would be suitable for clinical testing. The commercially prepared product Fluosol-DA, 20% (Green Cross Corporation, Japan) was the first product to be introduced into clinical testing. Several preclinical studies eventually led to clinical studies with Fluosol-DA in the United States.

Table 61-4. Practice Parameter for the Use of Cryoprecipitate

- Hypofibrinobenemia
- von Willebrand's disease
- Hemophilia A
- Fibrin surgical adhesive (derived from cryoprecipitate) has not been standardized

(Adapted from: Fresh-frozen Plasma, Cryoprecipitate and Platelets Administration Practice Guidelines Development Task Force of the College of American Pathologists: Practice parameter for the use of fresh-frozen plasma, cryoprecipitate, and platelets. JAMA, 271:777, 1994.)

In the trial at Michael Reese Hospital and Medical Center, the safety and efficacy of Fluosol-DA as a red cell substitute in acute anemia were assessed. Twenty-three surgical patients with blood loss and religious objections to receiving blood transfusions were evaluated. Fifteen moderately anemic patients with a mean hemoglobin level of 7.2 ± 0.5 g/dl had no evidence of a physiologic need for increased arterial oxygen content and did not receive Fluosol-DA. Eight severely anemic patients with a mean hemoglobin of 3.0 ± 0.4 g/dl met criteria of need and received the drug until the physiologic need disappeared or a maximal dose of 40 ml/kg of body weight was reached. All patients breathed supplemental oxygen. No adverse reactions to Fluosol-DA were observed. The average peak increment in arterial oxygen content with the drug was only 0.7 ± 0.1 ml/dl. This was equivalent to an increase in hemoglobin concentration of only 0.5 g/dl. There were no appreciable beneficial effects of Fluosol-DA, perhaps because of the small increase in arterial oxygen content, the brief half-life of the drug, and the limited total dose. Six of the 8 patients receiving Fluosol-DA died. One of the survivors received red cell transfusions against his wishes, under a court order, after his total Fluosol-DA dose. Fourteen of the 15 moderately anemic patients lived.

These data suggest that after blood loss, Fluosol-DA is unnecessary in moderate anemia and ineffective in severe anemia. Efforts are continuing to develop other modifications that would have higher concentrations of perfluorochemicals and a longer intravascular biologic half-life. In the near future, however, there does not appear to be any perfluorochemical that will likely be an effective red cell substitute.

Hemoglobin Solutions

Hemoglobin solutions are prepared from outdated blood. Various techniques have been used to separate the hemoglobin from the red cell membrane to prepare this stroma-free hemoglobin (SFH) solution. The first generation of this unmodified tetrameric form or "stripped" hemoglobin had a hemoglobin concentration of only 7 g/dl, and a P_{50} of 12 to 14 mm Hg (normal = 26 mm Hg). Although SFH can be prepared with a concentration of 14 g/dl, it has a colloid oncotic pressure of greater than 60 mm Hg. Despite these limitations, SFH supports life in primates at a zero hematocrit reading documenting effective oxygen transport in the absence of red cells. The problem of the hemoglobin concentration was to use a polymerized product that would permit a normal hemoglobin concentration and a normal colloid oncotic pressure. Polymerized stroma free hemoglobin (SFH-P) is initially prepared with a hemoglobin concentration and a normal colloid oncotic pressure. Polymerization of this product reduces the total number of molecules while increasing the average molecular size. No hemoglobin mass, however, is lost in this process. Polymerized pyridoxylated hemoglobin solution, Poly SFH-P, therefore achieves the goal of both a hemoglobin concentration of 15 g/dl and a normal colloid oncotic pressure of 20 mm Hg. The P_{50} is 20 to 22 mm Hg. Thus a product that has virtually the same properties as a bag of red cells is available. In addition to these physiologic improvements, the product has a half-life of 24 to 48 hours.

The efficacy of Poly SFH-P has been evaluated in both nonhuman primates and in a phase I trial in humans.[23] The results document that Poly SFH-P supports life in a primate at a zero hematocrit reading. In addition, the first clinical evaluation of Poly SFH in healthy human volunteers has been completed. In this study, no significant differences between preinfusion and postinfusion measures of renal function occurred. There were no clinically significant abnormalities in routine chemical and hematologic variables throughout a 6-week follow-up. Although these results are encouraging, the efficacy of this therapy depends on future studies in anemic patients. Until completion of those studies, red cell substitutes remain a promising but experimental therapy.

POST-ICU CONSIDERATIONS

Once patients are well enough to be discharged from the ICU, the main issue regarding transfusion practices is the indication for red blood cell transfusion in the anemic (hemoglobin 5 to 8 g/dl) but completely stable patient. The indications for red blood cell transfusion in the stable, nonbleeding patient still conform to the physiologic principles outlined previously. When patients begin to ambulate and increase their oxygen consumption, transfusion of red blood cells to patients in anticipation of this "increased demand" must be weighed against the potential infectious risks. The experience of the authors has been that this is rarely necessary. Transfusion of red blood cells to the traditional end point of a hemoglobin of 10 g/dl is not warranted in the absence of physiologic need. If a safe, efficacious blood substitute that is virus free becomes available, reconsideration of the transfusion trigger may be appropriate.

REFERENCES

1. Zuck, T. F.: Transfusion-transmitted AIDS reassessed. N. Engl. J. Med., *381*:511, 1988.
2. Graves, T. A., et al.: Relationship of transfusion and infection in a burn population. J. Trauma, *29*:948, 1989.
3. Maetani, S., Nishikawa, T., Hirakawa, A., and Tobe, T.: Role of blood transfusion in organ system failure following major abdominal surgery. Ann. Surg., *203*:275, 1986.
4. Rosenberg, S. A., Seipp, C. A., White, D. E., and Wesley, R.: Perioperative blood transfusions are associated with increased rates of recurrence and decreased survival in patients with high grade soft tissue sarcomas of the extremities. J. Clin. Oncol., *3*:693, 1985.
5. Blumberg, N., et al.: Further evidence supporting a cause and effect relationship between blood transfusion and earlier cancer recurrence. Ann. Surg., *207*:410, 1988.
6. Smoller, B. R., and Kruskall, M. J.: Phlebotomy for diagnostic lab tests in adults. N. Engl. J. Med., *314*:1233, 1986.
7. Toy, P. T. C. Y., et al.: Predeposited autologous blood for elective surgery. N. Engl. J. Med., *316*:517, 1987.
8. Chambers, L. A., and Kruskall, M. S.: Preoperative autologous blood donation. Trans. Med. Rev., *4*:35, 1990.
9. Messmer, K.: Hemodilution. Surg. Clin. North Am., *55*:659, 1975.
10. Stehling, L., and Zauder, H. L.: Acute normovolemic hemodilution. Transfusion, *31*:857, 1991.
11. Popovsky, M. A., Devine, P. A., and Taswell, H. F.: Intraoperative autologous transfusion. Mayo Clin. Proc., *60*:125, 1985.
12. Levine, E. A., et al.: Perioperative recombinant human erythropoietin. Surgery, *106*:932, 1989.
13. Goodnough, L. T., et al.: Increased preoperative collection of autologous blood with recombinant human erythropoietin therapy. N. Engl. J. Med., *321*:163, 1989.
14. Levine, E. A., et al.: Treatment of acute postoperative anemia with recombinant human erythropoietin. J. Trauma, *29*:1134, 1989.
15. Steffes, C. P., Bender, J. S., and Levinson, M. A.: Surgical sepsis. Crit. Care Med., *19*:512, 1991.
16. Dietrich, K. A., et al.: Cardiovascular and metabolic response to red blood cell transfusion in critically ill volume-resuscitated non-surgical patients. Crit. Care Med., *18*:940, 1990.
17. Hotchkiss, R. S., and Karl, I. E.: Re-evaluation of the role of cellular hypoxia and bioenergetic failure in sepsis. JAMA *267*:1503, 1992.
18. NIH Consensus Development panel: Perioperative red blood cell transfusion. JAMA, *260*:2700, 1988.
19. Counts, R. B., et al.: Hemostasis in massively transfused trauma patients. Ann. Surg., *190*:91, 1979.
20. NIH Consensus Development panel: Platelet transfusion therapy. JAMA, *257*:1777, 1987.
21. NIH Consensus Development panel: Fresh frozen plasma indications and risks. JAMA, *253*:551, 1985.
22. Gould, S. A., Sehgal, L. R., Rosen, A. L., and Sehgal, H. L.: Efficacy of polymerized pyridoxylated hemoglobin solution as an O_2 carrier. Ann. Surg., *211*:394, 1990.
23. Finch, C., and Lenfant, C.: Oxygen transport in man. N. Engl. J. Med., *286*:407, 1972.

Chapter 62

NUTRITION SUPPORT IN THE MANAGEMENT OF THE CRITICALLY ILL

LAURA E. MATARESE
EZRA STEIGER
BRYAN E. JEWETT

The evaluation and management of critically ill patients can be organized into three phases: (1) the pre-ICU phase (risk phase), (2) the ICU phase (support phase), and (3) the post-ICU phase (rehabilitation phase). The nutrition assessment and support of these patients can also be considered in three phases:

- The routine assessment and maintenance support required for hospitalized patients
- The modified nutrition (metabolic) support required for acutely stressed patients in the ICU (catabolic phase)
- The standard, long-term nutrition support needed to replenish body mass and function (anabolic phase)

PRE-ICU PHASE (RISK PHASE)

Diagnosis of Malnutrition

The prevalence of malnutrition as a clinical diagnosis in the hospital setting has become more apparent in recent years. Bistrian et al.[1,2] found a significant prevalence of protein calorie malnutrition in both general medical and surgical patients in the urban hospital setting in the range of 40 to 50%. The diagnosis of malnutrition was based on information regarding weight loss, anthropometrics, and visceral protein measurements and measurement of lymphocyte count and hematocrit. Weinsier and co-workers[3] noted a 48% incidence of malnutrition in general medical patients using eight nutrition-related parameters that correlated with an increase in hospital stay and increased mortality. It was also noted that the incidence of malnutrition in this group of patients increased during hospitalization (69%) even in patients with normal parameters on admission. Hill and associates[4] noted that malnutrition in surgical patients was common (50%) and often went clinically unrecognized and untreated.

From a quality assurance standpoint, malnutrition has been correlated with increases in morbidity and mortality in various clinical settings. Reviews have underscored the fact that nutrition is directly related to the patient's ability to survive a major illness[5] and that the debilitated patient usually dies from sepsis and organ failure associated with abnormal protein metabolism and a failed immune system.[6]

Thus, given the prevalence of the problem and its significant role in patient outcome, prevention and appropriately timed intervention are required. The initial problem becomes one of defining specific criteria for the diagnosis of malnutrition. To make such a definition requires the understanding of certain terminology used to quantitate nutritional status of a patient. These terms include anthropometry, visceral and somatic protein stores, total lymphocyte count, and delayed hypersensitivity skin tests (Table 62-1).

Nutrition Assessment

The primary objectives of nutrition assessment include:

- Identifying high risk patients
- Establishing the severity and type of malnourished state and its possible causes
- Identifying specific aspects of nutritional deficit that result in increased morbidity or mortality
- Reassessing to establish a response to nutritional therapy[7]

The initial assessment should be completed as part of the general medical workup on all patients admitted to the hospital. There is no single clinical or laboratory parameter that can be used to define malnutrition specifically.[7-9] Thus a variety of tests and procedures are used. Controversy exists over the approach to assessment (whole body versus individual organs), the validity of multivariable indices (e.g., prognostic nutrition index) to assess nutrition status accurately, and whether objective criteria from clinical and laboratory analyses are more predictive than the global nutritional assessment. Reviews suggest that the global clinical assessment when done by a trained observer is at least as good as the individual objective traditional measurements of nutritional status in predicting outcome in some patients. These traditional measures include a history and physical examination, anthropometric measurements, and laboratory studies.[10-13]

History and Physical Examination

In the clinical assessment, a thorough medical, social, and dietary history should include a history of unexplained weight loss, abnormal or inadequate nutrient intake, abnormal losses (diarrhea, malabsorption), recent major sur-

Table 62–1. Components of a Nutrition Assessment

History and physical examination
Anthropometry
    Triceps skinfold (adipose tissue)
    Midupper arm muscle circumference (lean muscle)
    Weight history
Visceral proteins
    Albumin
    Transferrin
    Thyroxine-binding prealbumin
    Retinol-binding protein
    Fibronectin
    Somatomedin C
Urine studies
    Nitrogen balance
    Creatinine/height index
    3-Methylhistidine
    Urea kinetics
Immunocompetence
    Total lymphocyte count
    Delayed hypersensitivity skin tests

gery or illness, chronic illnesses, and hypermetabolic states (Table 62–2). Physical findings include end-organ responses that constitute deficiencies in macronutrients or micronutrients (Table 62–3) and cutaneous manifestations of malnutrition.

Weight loss is often used as a gross indicator of lean body mass and has also been used as a prognostic parameter in nutrition studies. Ideal body weight is calculated based on height allowing 100 lb for the first 5 ft in height for women and 5 lb for every inch thereafter and 106 lb for men for the first 5 ft in height and 6 lb for every inch thereafter. The weight is then adjusted by adding or subtracting 10% based on frame size.[14]

Table 62–2. Clinical Assessment of Nutrient Status

MEDICAL HISTORY
    Medications
    Diagnostic procedures
    Chronic illness
    Surgical procedures
    Therapies
    Weight history
NUTRITION HISTORY
    Factors affecting intake
        Nausea/vomiting
        Anorexia
        Early satiety
        Dysgeusia
        Psychosocial
    Factors relating to eating habits
        Previous dietary modifications and compliance
        Living conditions
        Ability to purchase and prepare food
        Food preference
        Allergies
        Use of vitamin/mineral supplements
        Elimination habits
        Activity level
        Cultural and religious limitations

Table 62–3. Organ Function Alterations Secondary to Nutrient Deficiencies

Organ System	Alteration
Cardiovascular	Decreased red blood cell production, decreased blood volume, decreased cardiac output, stroke volume and contractility, decreased blood pressure, decreased heart muscle mass, diminished venous return, bradycardia, postural hypotension, hemodilution, anemia
Cutaneous	Cheilosis, glossitis, ecchymosis, dermatosis, follicular hyperkeratosis, petechiae
Gastrointestinal	Decreased brush border enzymes, maldigestion and malabsorption, decreased transit time, decreased mucosal cell integrity, decreased bile production, intestinal villi atrophy
Hepatic	Decreased liver weight, decreased visceral protein synthesis, hepatic insufficiency, fatty infiltration
Pulmonary	Respiratory infections, decreased functional, vital, and maximum breathing capacities, decreased response to hypoxia
Renal	Decreased plasma flow, reduced glomerular filtration rate, decreased tubular function, polyuria, metabolic acidosis

(Data from Keys, A.: Biology of human starvation; and Torum, B., and Viteri, F. E.: Protein-calorie malnutrition. *In* Modern Nutrition in Health and Disease. Edited by M. Shils and V. Young. Philadelphia; Lea & Febiger, 1988, pp. 746–773; and Baker, J. P., et al.: Nutritional assessment: a comparison of clinical judgement and objective measurements. N. Engl. J. Med., *306*:969, 1982.

Actual weight is compared with the patient's usual (pre-illness) body weight (Table 62–4). In general, an unintentional weight loss of more than 10% in a 6-month period is considered significant.[9]

Body mass index (BMI) indicates the presence of obesity and is highly correlated with body fat:[15,16]

$$BMI = \frac{Weight\ (kg)}{Height\ (m^2)}$$

Table 62–4. Calculations of Body Weight

Percentage of ideal body weight (IBW):

$$\%\ IBW = \frac{Actual\ Weight}{Ideal\ Body\ Weight} \times 100$$

Percentage of usual body weight (UBW):

$$\%\ IBW = \frac{Actual\ Weight}{Usual\ Weight} \times 100$$

Percentage of weight change:

$$\%\ Weight\ Change = \frac{Usual\ Weight - Actual\ Weight}{Usual\ Weight} \times 100$$

BMI is interpreted as follows:

Women BMI <18.5 (lean)
       BMI = 18.5-23.5 (normal)
       BMI >23.5-29.5 (excess weight)
       BMI >29.5 (obese)

Men   BMI <19.5 (lean)
       BMI = 19.5-24.5 (normal)
       BMI >24.5-29.5 (excess weight)
       BMI >29.5 (obese)

Anthropometric Measurements

Compartmental nutrition analysis involving individual assessment of portions of the body cell mass is known as anthropometry. It is a useful technique for assessing fat stores (energy reserves) with a triceps skinfold (TSF) measurement and assessing somatic protein stores with the midupper arm muscle circumference (MUAMC). These measurements are simple, inexpensive, noninvasive, and easy to obtain. They are only gross estimates, however, and may lack specificity and sensitivity when applied to individual patients. These measurements can also be inaccurate when applied to acute situations and especially when there are changes in extracellular fluid volume. They can be helpful in the initial assessment of patients and in the long-term (weeks) follow-up.

Approximately 50% of total body fat is located in the subcutaneous tissue.[17] The TSF measurement is a tool for assessing subcutaneous fat. Because the degree of subcutaneous fat is related to the amount of total body fat, TSF indirectly reflects adipose tissue and energy reserves. There is little agreement as to which side of the body to measure. Some clinicians measure the right side because many of the standards are based on right arm measurements. Others select the nondominant arm because it is thought that these measurements may be larger. The difference, however, between the dominant and nondominant arm has been shown to be about 0.2 to 0.3 standard deviation units.[18-21] Consequently, it matters little whether the left or right side is chosen. For the critically ill patient, care must be taken to select the nonedematous arm. To obtain TSF, the distance between the lateral tip of the acromion and the olecranon process is measured, and the midpoint is marked. A double fold of skin and fat tissue is grasped, lifting it away from the underlying muscle tissue; the calipers are applied at the midpoint; and a reading is obtained after 3 seconds. Three consecutive measurements are taken, and the mean from these measurements is used for the TSF value.[22]

The MUAMC is a number derived from the measurement of the TSF and the midarm circumference (MAC):[22]

$$\text{MUAMC (cm)} = \text{MAC (cm)} - 0.314 \times \text{TSF (cm)}$$

The MUAMC provides a gross estimation of the muscle mass of the upper arm and is used to evaluate somatic protein stores.

Laboratory Studies

The biochemical assessment of nutritional status includes measurement of **visceral protein parameters** (i.e., serum proteins), urine nitrogen studies, and parameters of immune function. The utility of plasma protein levels as nutrition and prognostic parameters has been demonstrated in several studies.[23-25] The tacit assumption is that serum levels reflect steady-state synthesis in the liver that is directly dependent on provision of adequate substrate; thus decreased levels would be indicative of malnutrition. Reduced levels of plasma proteins, however, may be affected by other factors, which include:

- Changes in the extracellular fluid compartment secondary to illness
- Stress
- Trauma
- Burns
- Altered liver function secondary to disease or altered hepatic perfusion, redistribution of liver synthetic activity (e.g., increased production of acute phase proteins with injury or stress), changes in peripheral catabolism of plasma proteins, abnormal loss (e.g., renal failure)
- Protein-losing enteropathy
- Administration of blood products

For example, Dahn and Jacobs[26] reviewed the possible causes of decreased albumin levels in injury and sepsis, noting the variability in albumin synthesis as one of several factors involved. Individual plasma proteins are also affected by changes related to their primary function (e.g., increased transferrin levels with iron deficiency anemia). Plasma proteins with shorter half-lives (more rapid turnover) are generally more sensitive than albumin in detecting acute changes in synthetic rates and substrate requirements (Table 62-5). There are other plasma proteins that may be more predictive of nutritional status and patient outcome.[27-31] These include fibronectin, somatomedin-C, and various cytokines. They are currently under investigation and are not used routinely as clinical tools at present.

Nitrogen balance has been used as both a nutrition therapeutic monitor and a prognostic parameter. Nitrogen output is based on 24-hour measurement of urinary urea nitrogen, which represents approximately 80% of the nitrogenous breakdown products of protein metabolism. A constant of 4 g N_2 per 24 hours is added to this output to account for fecal and nonurinary urea nitrogen loss. This constant factor may not be accurate in all situations (i.e., abnormal renal function, ileus, gastrointestinal bleed, open wounds and fistulas).

Nitrogen balance is calculated in most patients by the following formula:

Nitrogen balance = Nitrogen intake − nitrogen output

Nitrogen intake = Enteral or parenteral grams of amino acids ÷ 6.25

Nitrogen output = Urine urea nitrogen in mg ÷ 100 × liters of urine

Nitrogen balance = (Enteral or parenteral grams of amino acid or protein ÷ 6.25) (urine urea nitrogen ÷ 100 × urine volume) + 4

Table 62–5. Plasma Proteins

Protein	Characteristics	Elevated Levels	Decreased Levels
Albumin	21-day half-life; hepatic synthesis	Exogenous albumin, dehydration, corticosteroids, insulin, blood transfusion	Trauma, sepsis, nephrotic syndrome, fluid overload, multiple myeloma, inflammation, renal insufficiency, rheumatoid arthritis, hepatic failure, protein-losing enteropathy, diarrhea, draining fistulas and wounds, infections, burns, congestive heart failure, malabsorption, zinc deficiency, post-operatively, fluid overload, malnutrition
Transferrin	7- to 8-day half-life; hepatic synthesis	Iron deficiency anemia, pregnancy, dehydration, hypoxia, blood transfusions	Trauma, inflammation, liver disease, protein-losing enteropathy, iron overload, post-operatively, fluid overload, malnutrition
Thyroxin-binding prealbumin	2- to 3-day half-life; hepatic synthesis	Renal failure, dehydration	Trauma, acute catabolic states, post-operatively, hepatic insufficiency, infection, dialysis, fluid overload, hyperthyroidism, malnutrition
Retinol-binding protein	12- to 24-hour half-life; hepatic synthesis	Renal failure, dehydration, vitamin A supplementation	Trauma, vitamin A deficiency, postoperatively, hepatic failure, fluid overload, cystic fibrosis
Fibronectin	12- to 24-hour half-life		Malnutrition, suppressed host defense
Somatomedin-C	2- to 8-hour half-life		Malnutrition

Negative nitrogen balance occurs when protein intake is less than excretion and when not enough carbohydrate and fat have been provided to meet energy needs and spare protein. Each gram of nitrogen lost translates into 6.25 g of protein or 31.5 g of lean body mass when you consider lean body mass to be 20% protein and 80% water. Herein lies the clinical significance of negative nitrogen balance. Although it may be difficult to replete lean body mass in an acute hospital setting, knowledge of the nitrogen balance may make estimates of protein requirements more precise, and appropriate nutrition support may prevent further loss of lean body mass.

Although a positive nitrogen balance has been held as the gold standard by which to measure efficacy of nutrition support in hospitalized patients, research has suggested that other functional parameters may be a more sensitive measure.[32–37]

The **excretion rate of urinary creatinine** as reflected in the creatinine/height index has also been used as a measure of muscle protein stores.[38,39] It requires an accurate 24-hour urine specimen for analysis. The actual creatinine excretion is then divided by the expected 24-hour creatinine excretion of a normal adult of the same height. There are many limitations of creatinine excretion evaluation. Controversy exists as to its value in predicting complications, its correlation with measured changes in body composition, and its usefulness in critically ill patients in whom muscle creatinine flux increases out of proportion to true muscle mass in situations of increased muscle catabolism.

Urinary 3-methylhistidine (3-MEH) excretion has been used as an index of the rate of muscle catabolism but is currently used primarily as a research tool.[40,41] During muscle catabolism, 3-MEH is released from muscle protein and is proportional to muscle mass. It does not represent, however, all muscle breakdown. In addition, factors such as age, sex, trauma, starvation, protein intake, infection, and the accuracy of the 24-hour urine collection affect the validity of the test.

Body composition determinations use various techniques (i.e., multiple isotope dilution methods, proton-gamma-analysis, and neutron activation) to obtain objective measurements of different body compartments.[42–50] Total body potassium and nitrogen measurements have been found to parallel the clinical appearance of the patient and reflect changes in lean body mass.[51–54] The ratio of total body sodium and potassium has been identified as a parameter for diagnosing clinically relevant malnutrition.[43] Controversy exists as to the correlation of anthropometric and biochemical evaluations with body composition data. At present, these methods are available in some centers for measurement of short-term (acute) changes.

Functional tests have been investigated as possibly better parameters for assessing acute changes in nutritional status. Clinical studies have noted improved outcome (less morbidity and mortality) after a short period of nutrition support before significant changes in body composition or total body nitrogen were documented (i.e., no change in traditional nutrition parameters).[32–37] Studies have suggested that tests of the functional component, such as muscle strength and fatigue, and clinical parameters noting return to normal activity may have value in predicting clinical outcome.[55] The electrical stimulation of the ulnar nerve at the wrist and measurement of contraction-relaxation characteristics of the abductor pollicis muscle in the hand have been found by Jeejeebhoy's group to be a useful clinical test correlation between anergy and increased sepsis and mortality and with improvement in these areas with nutritional support. Unfortunately, many conditions can contribute to anergy (Table 62–6). Without the ability to separate the effects of malnutrition from those of disease, it becomes difficult to justify the utilization of these tests as independent indicators of nutritional deficiency.[62]

The identification of patients at a high risk for the development of complications related to malnutrition depends on an accurate and complete nutrition assessment. Although there is presently no single independent parameter that has proved to be ideal, a combination of nutrition assessment parameters has been used to assess a patient's nutritional status. Our present approach combines the input from several sources of data (e.g., laboratory, immune) with the clinical picture and natural history of various disease processes into a global assessment.

Table 62-6. Non-Nutritional Influences on Skin Test Response

Technical	Immune alterations
Antigen source and batch	Congenital
Preparation and storage	DiGeorge syndrome
Method of administration	Thymic aplasia
Site or test	Acquired
Booster effect	Systemic lupus erythematosus
Criteria of positivity	Rheumatoid arthritis
Reader variability	Trauma, burns, hemorrhage
Patient factors	Diseases—malignant
Age	Most solid tumors, especially advancing stages
Race	Lymphomas
Geographic location	Leukemias
Prior exposure to antigen	Prior malignancy, especially squamous cancer, lymphoma
Circadian rhythm	Iatrogenic—Drugs
Psychologic state	Immunosuppressants
Diseases—benign	Most antineoplastics
Infections	Anti-inflammatory
Viral	Anticoagulants
Bacterial	H_2 blockers (cimetidine)
Fungal	Aspirin (?)
Metabolic	X-ray therapy
Uremia	General anesthesia
Liver diseases	Surgery
Inflammatory	
Crohn's disease	
Ulcerative colitis	
Sarcoid	

(From Twomey, P., Ziegler, D., and Rombeau, J.: Utility of skin testing in nutritional assessment: a critical review. JPEN, 6:50–58, 1982.

Prognostic Use of Nutrition Assessment Parameters

The principle purpose of early nutrition assessment is to minimize the morbidity and mortality associated with malnutrition. There have been several attempts to correlate improvement in nutritional status with improved patient outcome. The main problems have been defining sensitive and specific criteria for (1) the method of diagnosis of malnutrition and (2) the clinical effects of malnutrition in various disease processes. Most studies have used the likelihood of developing complications and the risk of death from disease as end points.

Studley[63] noted that preoperative weight loss is correlated with an increase in postoperative mortality in patients undergoing elective operation for peptic ulcer disease. Other studies have noted a correlation between the extent of weight loss over a specified period of time (i.e., 10% weight loss over a 6-month period[9]) and the incidence of malnutrition. More recent studies have also found preoperative weight loss to be a useful predictor of surgical mortality[64] as well as a risk factor for postoperative complications and length of hospital stay, especially when associated with clinically obvious physiologic impairment.[65]

Serum albumin and other plasma proteins have been proposed as nutrition prognostic parameters. Decreased albumin levels in hospitalized veterans have been correlated with an increased mortality.[66] Several studies have found that the serum albumin level on admission was an independent predictor of morbidity and mortality, with a decreased level being associated with an increased incidence of anergy, sepsis, longer hospitalization, and death.[27,55,67,68] One study has noted a decreased incidence of sepsis with exogenous supplementation of albumin, although there was no significant change in mortality or length of hospital stay.[69] Still other reviews[30,44] have discussed the ability of several plasma proteins that have a shorter half-life than albumin to be used as predictors of morbidity and mortality. Unfortunately, there is still much controversy as to the specificity of these proteins as true indicators of malnutrition. More recently, various acute phase proteins, including somatomedin-C and fibronectin, have been correlated with the clinical response to nutritional therapy in injured and critically ill patients.[29-31,70]

The occurrence of anergy as determined by the lack of cutaneous response to injected antigens has also been used as a predictor of malnutrition and patient outcome, with an improved response correlating with an improved prognosis.[27,67] As noted previously, there is still controversy regarding the utility of this parameter as a guide in the acute illness and as a specific indicator of malnutrition (see Table 62-6).

Thyroid indices have also been correlated with survival and an increased mortality associated with a decreased triiodothyronine (T_3) and thyroxine (T_4) or an increased T_3UR or rT_3.[28] Whether these changes are related to the severity of the disease process or to nutritional deprivation remains to be determined.

In an attempt to predict more accurately patient outcome as a function of nutritional factors, different investigators developed multiple regression equations from a combination of nutritional indices (Table 62-7). Harvey and colleagues[67] developed the hospital prognostic index (HPI), which was based on the serum albumin, skin test response, presence of sepsis, and the diagnosis of cancer. This parameter had a predictive accuracy of 72% for subsequent mortality. Mullen et al.[71] developed the prognostic nutritional index (PNI) based on serum albumin, TSF, serum transferrin, and delayed cutaneous hypersensitivity response. He demonstrated this parameter to be predictive of a reduction in postoperative morbidity and mortality with the supplementation of preoperative nutrition support. The main problem with this type of mathematical analysis is that it is only as good as the parameters from which it is derived and is subject to the same inadequacies and criticisms.

Although current research has documented several possible associations between various proposed nutritional indices and their predictive value in patient outcome, definitive prospective, randomized studies providing proof that nutrition support independently reduces morbidity and mortality in hospitalized medical and surgical patients remain to be completed. In a multi-institutional clinical trial conducted by the Department of Veterans Affairs to assess the efficacy of perioperative total parenteral nutrition (TPN), there was no benefit of TPN in borderline malnourished patients. The study also provided strong evidence against clinically relevant efficacy in mildly or moderately malnourished patients but did suggest that there may be some benefit in the severely malnourished patient.[72] Buzby and Muller[73] have reviewed general criticisms of prior research:

Table 62-7. Prognostic Indices

Prognostic Nutrition Index (PNI)

PNI% = 158 − 16.6(ALB) − 0.78(TSF) − 0.20(TFN) − 5.8(DH)

ALB = Serum albumin (g/dl)
TSF = Triceps skinfold (mm)
TFN = Serum transferrin (mg/dl)
DH = Delayed cutaneous hypersensitivity skin test (% positive reaction)

Interpretation:

PNI <40%   Low risk for postoperative complications
PNI 40–49% Intermediate risk for postoperative complications
PNI >50%   High risk for postoperative complications

Hospital Prognostic Index (HPI)

HPI% = 0.92(ALB) − 1.00(DH) − 1.44(SEP) + 0.98(DX) − 1.09

ALB = Serum albumin (g/dl)
DH = Delayed cutaneous hypersensitivity skin test
   Positive response to one or more = 1
   Positive response to all = 2
SEP = Sepsis
   Present = 1
   Not present = 2
DX = Diagnosis
   Cancer = 1
   No cancer = 2

Interpretation:

HPI −2: 10% probability of survival
HPI 0: 50% probability of survival
HPI +1: 75% probability of survival

Nutrition Risk Index (NRI)

NRI = 1.519 × ALB + 0.417 × (Current Weight/Usual Weight) × 100

ALB = Serum Albumin in Grams Per Liter

Interpretation: Score ≤100 = Malnutrition

- Defects in statistical design
- Inappropriate patient selection
- Inappropriate treatment regimens
- Inadequate definition of end point criteria

He and colleagues have also outlined the direction of future research to prove the above-mentioned hypothesis. In general, however, early recognition of altered nutritional status is mandatory for reducing the associated morbidity and mortality.

Determining Nutrient Needs

Following nutrition assessment, energy requirements should be estimated before nutrition support is initiated. The basal energy expenditure (BEE) provides an estimation of the amount of energy required to maintain minimal body processes. It does not account for the increase in energy expenditure caused by illness and injury. The BEE must be multiplied by additional factors to derive an estimate of the patient's total energy expenditure (TEE). BEE can be calculated using the Harris-Benedict[74] equation:

Males BEE = (66.47 + 13.75W + 5H − 6.76A)
Females BEE = (655.1 + 9.56W + 1.85H − 4.68A)

W = Weight in Kilograms
H = Height in Centimeters
A = Age in Years

Actual body weight is used in the formula so that energy requirements are not overestimated in the ectomorph or underestimated for the overweight patient. For those patients who are obese, that is greater than 120% of ideal body weight (IBW), BEE may be calculated using an adjusted body weight (ABW):[75]

ABW = [(Actual Weight − IBW) × 0.25] + IBW

There are many equations that have been used to estimate energy expenditure.[76] Depending on the severity of the illness, BEE is multiplied by various factors to obtain the TEE. Factors may range from 1.1 to 2.0 × BEE. It is important to distinguish between total and nonprotein kilocalories. The difference is generally 15 to 20%.

Predictive equations provide a reasonable estimate of caloric need. There are occasions, however, in which it would be advantageous to measure energy expenditure. This can be done directly, by placing an individual in a calorimeter and measuring the amount of heat given off by the body mass. This equipment is expensive and has limited clinical applicability.

Energy expenditure may also be measured indirectly with an indirect calorimeter (metabolic cart). Indirect calorimetry is a technique that measures oxygen consumption ($\dot{V}O_2$) and carbon dioxide production ($\dot{V}CO_2$) to calculate resting energy expenditure (REE). One liter of oxygen consumed generates 3.9 kcal, whereas 1 L of carbon dioxide produced generates 1.1 kcal. The Weir equation is then used to calculate energy expenditure (EE):[77]

EE = [(3.941 ($\dot{V}O_2$) + 1.106 ($\dot{V}CO_2$)] 1.44 − 2.17 (UN)

Where: $\dot{V}O_2$ = Oxygen Consumption (ml/min)
$\dot{V}CO_2$ = Carbon Dioxide Production (ml/min)
UN = Urinary Nitrogen (g/day)

The number derived, EE, is the REE. REE is often used interchangeably with BEE. By definition, BEE is the energy required to perform essential body functions, such as respiration, cardiac function, and maintenance of body temperature. It is measured 12 to 15 hours after absorption, at rest and in a thermoneutral environment.[78] REE is usually not measured under basal conditions. The difference between REE and BEE, however, is that REE is only 10 to 15% greater than BEE.[79] TEE is the amount of heat eliminated from the body plus external work performed. It includes REE, accounting for approximately 70% of TEE, and physical activity and thermogenesis of food, each accounting for approximately 15% of TEE. TEE is also influenced by illness and injury. In the ICU setting where the patient

Table 62-8. Stoichiometry for Substrate Oxidation*

1 Ethanol + 6 O$_2$ → 4 CO$_2$ + H$_2$O
1 Palmatate + 230 O$_2$ → 160 CO$_2$ + 16 H$_2$O
1 Amio acid + 5.1 O$_2$ → 4.1 CO$_2$ + 2.8 H$_2$O + 0.7 Urea
1 Glucose + 6 O$_2$ → 6 CO$_2$ + 6 H$_2$O
13.5 Glucose + 3 O$_2$ → C$_{55}$H$_{104}$O$_6$ + 26 CO$_2$ + 29 H$_2$O

*Utilization of oxygen and release of carbon dioxide during the oxidation of ethanol, fat, protein, and carbohydrate.

Table 62-10. Respiratory Quotient Interpretation

Possible Causes of RQ < 0.070
  Oxidation of ethanol
  Oxidation of ketones
  Lipolysis
  Underfeeding
  Diabetes mellitus
  Technical error
Possible Causes of RQ > 1.0
  Overfeeding
  Lipogenesis
  Hyperventilation
  Excess CO$_2$ production
  Hydrogen buffering by bicarbonate
  Non-steady-state ventilation
  Technical error

is sedated, the REE obtained from indirect calorimetry closely approximates the TEE. To account for minimal physical activity and diurnal variation, however, REE may be multiplied by 1.1 to 1.3 to derive the TEE.[80]

The respiratory quotient (RQ) can also be determined from indirect calorimetry to ascertain substrate utilization:

$$\text{Total RQ} = \frac{\dot{V}_{CO_2}}{\dot{V}_{O_2}}$$

The energy equivalents and respiratory quotients are based on the stoichiometry for oxidation of various substrates (Table 62-8).[81] The respiratory quotient can be useful in altering the patient's nutrition prescription (Table 62-9). The RQ should be in physiologic range and consistent with the patient's history and feeding. In general, if the RQ is greater than 1.0, lipogenesis is occurring, and the total caloric load should be decreased. If the RQ is equal to 1.0, decrease carbohydrate or increase lipid calories (or both) for ventilator weaning. If RQ is less than 0.82, increase total calories.[82-87]

Care must be taken when interpreting the RQ. There are many circumstances in which RQ does not reflect substrate oxidation (Table 62-10). The RQ does not reflect substrate utilization during hyperventilation, during metabolic alkalosis, 6 to 8 hours after general anesthesia, and with changing gas stores (i.e., changes in F$_{IO_2}$). There are also some normal or expected variations in RQ. Immediately after a meal, the RQ is generally 1.0 to reflect carbohydrate oxidation. Eight to 10 hours postprandially, the RQ is 0.71 as oxidation of fuels converts to fat. In diabetes mellitus, the RQ is approximately 0.71 because little carbohydrate is used by the body.[88]

Indirect calorimetry may be used for ventilated or spontaneous breathing patients. In general, the test is not valid for patients receiving F$_{IO_2}$ greater than 0.60. Expired gas is collected via a mask, canopy, mouthpiece, or tracheostomy tube and ventilator into a Douglas bag or spirometer. The inspired and expired gas concentrations of oxygen and carbon dioxide are then analyzed using a chemical gas analyzer, mass spectrometry, or Haldane techniques. When the volume of gas collected and the composition are known, the REE can be calculated. Spontaneously breathing patients may be measured with a hood or canopy, face mask, or mouthpiece and nose clip. Each has its own set of limitations. When using a mouthpiece and nose clip or mask, the breathing patterns may be altered. It requires a complete seal and should be done for a short period of time. The canopy cannot be used for patients with tracheostomies or supplemental oxygen. The canopy offers some theoretical advantages in that it should not alter the subject's breathing pattern. Some individuals, however, feel claustrophobic.

The measurement conditions greatly influence the validity of the test. Patients should be at rest for at least 30 minutes. The test should be done 2 hours after absorption and in a quiet, thermoneutral environment. There should be no patient movement during the study and no system leaks. There must be steady-state data analysis and a stable F$_{IO_2}$.[89]

Protein Requirements

Although it is conventional to speak of protein requirements, the actual requirement is not for protein but rather for specific amino acids and for nonessential amino acid nitrogen. Most unstressed individuals require 0.8 to 1.0 g protein/kg body weight per day.[90] In moderate stress, the requirements increase to 1.0 to 1.5 g; for more severe stress, 1.5 to 2 g/kg body weight (Table 62-11).[91] In some

Table 62-9. Substrate Utilization

Substrate Oxidation	Respiratory Quotient
Ethanol	0.67
Fat	0.71
Protein	0.82
Mixed fuels	0.85
Carbohydrate	1.0
Carbohydrate (lipogenesis)	1.01–1.20

Table 62-11. Protein Requirements During Stress

Stress Level	Protein (g/kg)
Unstressed	0.8–1.0
Mild	1.0–1.5
Moderate	1.5–2.0
Severe	2.0–2.5

Table 62-12. Daily Electrolyte and Mineral Requirements for Adults

Electrolyte	RDA[a]	Grant[b]	Shils[c]	Silberman[d]
Sodium (mEq)	45–145	80–100	≤60	100–300 (typical intake)
Potassium (mEq)	45–145	80–100	≥60	50–150 (typical intake)
				5–6/g Nitrogen[e]
				120–160[f]
Chloride (mEq)	45–150	80–100	—	100–300 (typical intake)
Calcium (mEq)	40	0.2–0.3 kg/day body weight	10–25	0.25 kg[g]
Magnesium (mEq)	Males: 29	0.25–0.35 kg/day body weight	12–20	2/g nitrogen[e]
	Females: 25			
Phosphorus (mM)	25.5	7–9/1000 kcal	450 mg	15/1000 nonprotein kcal[h,i]

[a] The National Research Council: Recommended Dietary Allowances. 10th Ed. Washington, D.C., National Academy of Science, 1989.
[b] Grant, J.: Handbook of Total Parenteral Nutrition. Philadelphia, W.B. Saunders, 1992, p. 180.
[c] Shils, M. E.: Parenteral nutrition. In Modern Nutrition in Health and Disease. 7th Ed. Edited by M. E. Shils and V. R. Young. Philadelphia, Lea & Febiger, 1988, p. 1052.
[d] Silberman, H., and Morris, J. A., Jr.: Parenteral and Enteral Nutrition for the Hospitalized Patient. Norwalk, CT, Appleton-Century-Crofts, 1989, p. 104.
[e] Lee, H. A., and Hartley, T. F.: Postgrad. Med. J., 51:441–445, 1975.
[f] Sheldon, G. F., Kudsk, K. A., and Morris, J. A. Jr.: Electrolyte requirements in total parenteral nutrition. In Nutrition in Clinical Surgery. Edited by M. Deitel. Baltimore, Williams & Wilkins, 1985, p. 161.
[g] Wittine, M. F., and Freeman, J. B.: JPEN, 1:152–155, 1977.
[h] Conner, C. S.: Drug Intell. Clin. Pharm., 18:594, 1984.
[i] Thompson, J. S., and Hodges, R. E.: JPEN J. Parenter. Enteral Nutr., 8:137, 1984.

instances, such as severe thermal burns or major traumas, the protein requirements may be even greater. Nitrogen balance studies may be used to determine the exact requirement.

Fluid and electrolyte requirements must be individualized. To determine fluid requirements, extrarenal losses, such as vomiting; diarrhea; fistula and drainage output; and insensible losses secondary to fever, ventilation and wounds, and nasogastric suction, must be considered. An approximation of the patient's fluid requirements is derived from Keiswetter[92] formula, which applies to any patient weighing more than 5 kg:

$$\text{1st 10 kg of weight} = 100 \text{ ml/kg}$$
$$\text{2nd 10 kg of weight} = 50 \text{ ml/kg}$$
$$\text{Weights above 20 kg} = 20 \text{ ml/kg}$$

Electrolyte requirements must also be individualized. Patients receiving nutrition support often require higher amounts of electrolytes owing to the infusion of glucose and amino acids. As the patient becomes anabolic, requirements for potassium, magnesium, and phosphorus increase (Table 62-12).

Adequate quantities of **vitamins and trace minerals** are necessary for the utilization of nutrients. Many patients requiring nutrition support have borderline nutritional status when therapy is initiated. Deficiencies can develop rapidly if these nutrients are not supplemented. Guidelines for parenteral vitamin supplementation have been developed (Table 62-13).[93]

Trace minerals are required by the body in "trace" amounts. They generally function as metalloenzymes and cofactors. Deficiencies may result from decreased intake, increased excretion, increased requirements, and decreased plasma binding. Multiple trace element products are available commercially for intravenous use (Table 62-14).[94]

Table 62-13. Parenteral Vitamin Supplementation

Vitamin	AMA/NAG* Guidelines	RDA†‡
Vitamin A	3300 IU	1000 IU
Vitamin D	200 IU	400 IU
Vitamin E	10 IU	10 IU
Ascorbic acid	100 mg	60 mg
Folic acid	400 μg	200 μg
Niacin	40 mg	20 mg
Riboflavin	3.6 mg	1.8 mg
Thiamine	3.0 mg	1.5 mg
Pyridoxine	4.0 mg	2.0 mg
Cyanocobalamin	5.0 μg	2.0 μg
Pantothenic acid	15 mg	4–7 mg§
Biotin	60 μg	30–100 μg§

* American Medical Association Nutrition Department of Foods and Nutrition: Multivitamin preparations for parenteral use. A statement by the Nutrition Advisory Group. JPEN, 3:258, 1979.
† The National Research Council: Recommended Dietary Allowances. 10th ed. Washington, D.C., National Academy of Sciences, 1989.
‡ Highest recommended dosage for age range 11–51 years.
§ No RDA established. Values provided are estimated safe and adequate.

Table 62-14. Parenteral Trace Minerals

Mineral	AMA/NAG* Guidelines	RDA†‡
Zinc	2.5–4.0 mg/day	15 mg/day
Copper	0.5–1.5 mg/day	1.5–3.0 mg/day
Chromium	10–15 μg/day	50–200 μg/day
Manganese	0.15–0.8 mg/day	2.0–5.0 mg/day
Selenium	—	70 μg/day
Iodine	150 μg	150 μg

* American Medical Association Department of Foods and Nutrition: Guidelines for essential trace element preparations for parenteral use. A statement by an expert panel. JAMA, 241:2051, 1979.
† The National Research Council Recommended Dietary Allowances. 10th Ed. Washington, D.C., National Academy of Sciences, 1989.
‡ Highest recommended dosage for age range 11 to 51 years.

The goal of nutrition support is to maintain lean body mass and optimize nutrition status to accelerate healing and resist infection. Thus, the efficacy of therapy should be documented. All patients receiving nutritional support should have a comprehensive nutrition assessment at the initiation of therapy to document baseline nutrition status (Fig. 62-1). This assessment should be repeated at regular intervals to document the efficacy of therapy and reassess nutrient requirements (Fig. 62-2).[95]

Cleveland Clinic Foundation
Department of General Surgery
Nutrition Support Team

9-999-999-4
JANE DOE
10-Jul-1991
9806

Nutritional Assessment Consultation Report

Referring Physician: STEIGER
Diagnosis: ENTEROCUTANEOUS FISTULA
Operation: RESECTION, ENTEROCUTANEOUS FISTULA 12/25
Age (years): 71
Sex: F
Height (cm): 158.0
Frame type: M
Usual weight (Kg): 63.6
Ideal weight (Kg): 50
BEE (Kcal): 1179
ECR (Kcal): 2064 to 2358
Protein Req (gms): 89 to 118

Date	Act Wt (Kg)	% Wt Change	BMI	TSB (mm)	MUAMC (cm)	Alb	Tfn	Pre Alb	TLB	BUN	Creat	Gluc	Skin Test	PNI
11/28/81	53.0	−17%	21.2	7	20.8	2.6	156	3.1	600	17	1.3	95	0/4	78%
12/12/83	56.0	−12%	22.4	10	21.9	3.0	190	4.0	900	42	1.3	85	0/0	
01/03/84	59.0	−7%	23.6	12	23.2	3.5	247	10.1	1000	33	1/3	112	1/4	30%

Body Mass Index (BMI):　　　　　　　　　　　Excess Weight

Upper Arm Anthropometry
　Adipose Stores (SFT);　　　　　　　　　　 6%ile Severe Deficit
　Somatic Protein (MUAMC):　　　　　　　　60%ile Adequate

Visceral Protein:
　Albumin (Alb):　　　　　　　　　　　　　　Adequate
　Transferrin (Tfn):　　　　　　　　　　　　 Adequate
　Pre-Albumin (Pre/Alb):　　　　　　　　　 Mild Deficit

Immune Function:
　Total Lymph. Count (TLC):　　　　　　　　Moderate Deficit
　Skin Tests:　　　　　　　　　　　　　　　 Relatively Anergic

Prognostic Nutr. Index (PNI):　　　　　　　　30% Low Risk for Postoperative Complications

SUGGESTED GOAL:
CENTRAL USE ONLY　　　　　TOTAL KCAL/L　　GM PRO/L　　NON-PRO KCAL:N2　　%KCAL

D50	500 ml	1020	42.5	119:1	83% CHO
Standard AA 8.5	500 ml				17% PRO

84 to 96 ml/hr

Improved nutritional status.

Fig. 62-1. Example of nutritional assessment. (Courtesy of the Cleveland Clinic Foundation, Cleveland, OH.)

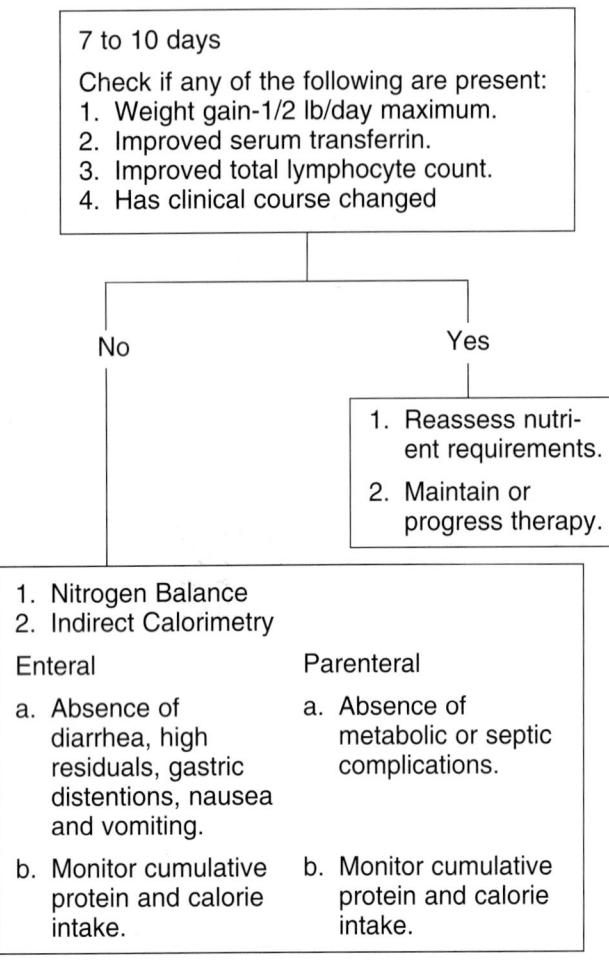

Fig. 62-2. Algorithm for reassessment.

Methods of Nutrition Support

There are several methods of providing nutrition support. The choice is made based on the patient's nutritional status, ability to eat, and functional capability of the gastrointestinal tract (Fig. 62-3).

All patients should be screened within 24 hours of admission. Not all patients require a full nutrition assessment but should be checked for weight loss, abnormal laboratory data, and chronic illness. There are some patients who present so malnourished that one's clinical impression is that they will require TPN. The changes in nutritional status, however, are often subtle and difficult to recognize. If there are no nutritional risk factors, such as low visceral proteins or chronic illness, and there is adequate oral intake and gastrointestinal absorption, the patient should receive usual dietary treatment. If there are risk factors present, however, the patient should be fed enterally. As long as adequate appetite is present, the patient should be al-

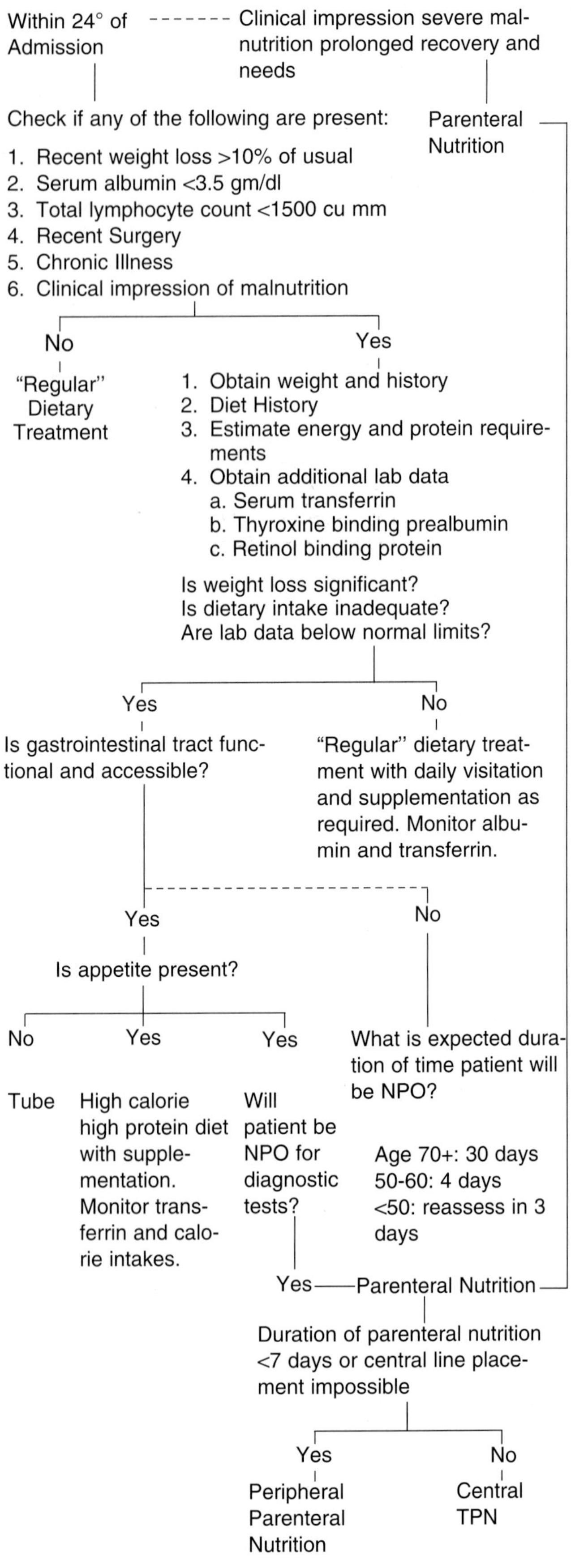

Fig. 62-3. Algorithm for nutrition support. (From Mugglia-Sullam, M., and Fischer, J. E.: Current concepts of indications for preoperative parenteral nutrition. Clin. Anaesthesiol., 1:583, 1983.)

lowed to eat but monitored carefully. If the patient is anorectic or cannot ingest nutrients adequately, enteral feeding by tube should be initiated. If the gastrointestinal tract is not functional, the patient is malnourished, or is going to be nulla per os (NPO) status for an extended period of time, the patient may require parenteral nutrition. The duration of NPO status should be evaluated with reference to age and nutritional status. Elderly patients generally have limited reserves and may require nutrition support sooner. If parenteral nutrition is not possible, peripheral parenteral nutrition may be used.

Commercial products have been formulated to provide essential nutrient components. They can be combined in varying amounts to form nutritionally complete solutions for enteral as well as parenteral feedings (Table 62-15).

Total Parenteral Nutrition Prescription

The TPN prescription should be tailored to meet the individual needs of the patient. The solution should be designed only after assessing the patient's requirements for energy, protein, fluid, and electrolytes. Orders should be written on a daily basis to reflect the patient's changing needs.

Amino Acids

Crystalline amino acids are available in concentrations ranging from 3.5 to 15% (Table 62-16). They generally contain 40 to 50% essential amino acids and 50 to 60% nonessential amino acids. Solutions containing modified amino acids for specific disease states are also available and are discussed later.

Dextrose

Dextrose is generally the primary energy source in TPN regimens. Dextrose solutions are available in concentrations ranging from 5 to 70% (Table 62-17). A final dextrose concentration of 25 to 35% is infused through a central line. A maximum concentration of 10% can be comfortably administered through a peripheral vein. One gram of anhydrous dextrose used in intravenous solutions provides 3.4 kcal. To avoid hyperglycemia, the initial dextrose concentration should be 20% and gradually increased using 50 or 70% dextrose.

Lipids

Commercially available lipid emulsions can be used to provide calories and essentially fatty acids. Fat emulsions are available in 10 and 20% concentrations supplying 1.1 and 2.0 kcal/ml. These emulsions are isotonic and may be administered either peripherally or centrally. They may be used to prevent essential fatty acid deficiency (usually by giving 500 ml of a 10% emulsion two to three times per week) and can be used as a major calorie source for patients with glucose intolerance or carbon dioxide retention. Intravenous lipids may be combined with dextrose and amino acids to form a total nutrient admixture (TNA) or 3-in-1 solutions (see Table 62-15).

Enteral Formulas

As a result of the proliferation of commercially available enteral formulas, selection of appropriate formulas has become more complicated and is based on several factors (Fig. 62-4).[96] Digestive capability and absorptive capacity must be evaluated. Those patients with an impaired ability to digest or absorb nutrients may require a predigested formula. Nutrient requirements should be assessed. Patients in hypermetabolic states may require high caloric density and high protein formulas. The feeding route should be considered. Feedings delivered directly into the small intestine may necessitate the use of isotonic formulas on initiation. Those patients who are fluid restricted require a high-nutrient-density formula. Medical conditions such as renal or hepatic failure may necessitate the use of specialized formulas.

Tube feedings should be initiated at isotonic concentration. In general, they are started at 50 ml per hour and advanced according to administration site and patient tolerance. If the feedings are delivered intragastrically, the concentration is advanced first and then the volume. For intestinal feedings, the volume should be increased by 25 ml per hour every 8 to 12 hours as tolerated, and then concentration can be increased because the small bowel is less capable of handling the osmotic loads. Rate and concentration should not be altered simultaneously.[96]

Clearly there are many methods of nutrition support available to the clinician to prevent and correct malnutrition in critically ill patients. The high risk patient must be identified and supported aggressively.

Complications of Nutrition Support

Life-saving techniques are not without potential complications (Table 62-18). Prevention and early recognition, however, reduce the morbidity associated with nutritional support. One way to ensure safe, accurate delivery of enteral and parenteral feedings is to use standing order sheets (Figs. 62-5 and 62-6).

Sepsis is a serious potential complication of parenteral nutrition.[97-102] Many patients who require parenteral nutrition are already predisposed to infectious complications owing to malnutrition, presence of other infections, and use of antibiotics. The presence of fever may indicate catheter sepsis. More often, it is associated with other concomitant infections, such as pneumonia, wound and intra-abdominal abscesses, urinary tract infections, and peripheral venous thrombophlebitis. If the patient does not have an obvious source of infection, the catheter should be suspected. Central and peripheral blood cultures should be obtained. The parenteral nutrition solution should be changed. If the patient's fever does not decrease after changing the solution, blood cultures should be obtained through the catheter and the catheter changed over a guidewire or removed.

Pneumothorax can occur during placement of the subclavian venous catheter.[97,103-106] The barrel of the syringe should be kept parallel to the patient's chest wall during insertion. A chest x-ray film should be obtained to ensure that there is no pneumothorax and that the catheter tip is in the superior vena cava and pointing downward toward

Table 62-15. Stable Total Parenteral Nutrition Formulas

	Central Use Only		Total kcal/L	Protein (g/L)	Nonprotein kcal:N₂	% kcal
1.	D50*	500 ml	1020	42.5	119:1	83% CHO
	Standard AA 8.5%	500 ml				17% Protein
2.	D50*	500 ml	1050	50	103:1	81% CHO
	Standard AA 10%	500 ml				19% Protein
3.	D70	500 ml	1360	42.5	166:1	87% CHO
	Standard AA 8.5%	500 ml				13% Protein
4.	D70	500 ml	1390	65	144:1	86% CHO
	Standard AA 10%	500 ml				14% Protein
5.	D70	350 ml	1093	65	78:1	76% CHO
	Standard AA 10%	650 ml				24% Protein
6.	D70	400 ml	1192	60	96:1	80% CHO
	Standard AA 10%	600 ml				20% Protein
7.	D70	450 ml	1291	55	118:1	83% CHO
	Standard AA 10%	550 ml				17% Protein
8.	D50*	500 ml	975	31.3	164:1	87% CHO
	Standard AA 8.5%	250 ml				13% Protein
	RF† AA 5.4%	250 ml				
9.	D70	500 ml	1315	31.3	230:1	90% CHO
	Standard AA 8.5%	250 ml				10% Protein
	RF† AA 5.4%					
10.	D50*	500 ml	1187	13.3	531:1	96% CHO
	RF AA 5.4%	250 ml				4% Protein
11.	D70	500 ml	1640	13.3	744:1	97% CHO
	RF AA 5.4%	250 ml				3% Protein
12.	D50	500 ml	1002	38	142:1	85% CHO
	LF† AA 8%	500 ml				15% Protein
13.	D50*	250 ml	1095	42.5	129:1	39% CHO
	Standard AA 8.5%	500 ml				15% Protein
	Fat emulsion 20%	250 ml				46% Fat
14.	D50*	250 ml	1125	50	112:1	38% CHO
	Standard AA 10%	500 ml				18% Protein
	Fat emulsion 20%	250 ml				44% Fat
15.	D70	250 ml	1265	42.5	153:1	47% CHO
	Standard AA 8.5%	500 ml				13% Protein
	Fat emulsion 20%	250 ml				40% Fat
16.	D70	250 ml	1295	50	133:1	46% CHO
	Standard AA 10%	500 ml				15% Protein
	Fat emulsion 20%	250 ml				39% Fat
17.	D50	200 ml	980	60	75:1	35% CHO
	Standard AA 10%	600 ml				24% Protein
	Fat emulsion 20%	200 ml				41% Fat
18.	D70	200 ml	1116	60	88:1	43% CHO
	Standard AA 10%	600 ml				21% Protein
	Fat emulsion 20%	200 ml				36% Fat
19.	D50	250 ml	1050	31.3	179:1	40% CHO
	Standard AA 8.5%	250 ml				12% Protein
	RF AA 5.4%	250 ml				48% Fat
	Fat emulsion 20%	250 ml				
20.	D70	250 ml	1220	31.3	212:1	49% CHO
	Standard AA 8.5%	250 ml				10% Protein
	RF AA 5.4%	250 ml				41% Fat
	Fat emulsion 20%	250 ml				
CENTRAL OR PERIPHERAL USE						
21.	D20	250 ml	840	42.5	94:1	20% CHO
	Standard AA 8.5%	500 ml				20% Protein
	Fat emulsion 20%	250 ml				60% Fat
22.	D20	250 ml	870	50	81:1	20% CHO
	Standard AA 10%	500 ml				23% Protein
	Fat emulsion 20%	250 ml				57% Fat

* D50W with electrolytes may be used.
† These formulas have been tested and are stable for 48 hours at room temperature. LF AA, Liver failure amino acids; RF AA, Renal failure amino acids.
D50, dextrose 50%; D70, dextrose 70%; CHO, carbohydrate.

Table 62-16. Approximate Composition of Amino Acid Solutions

Concentration (%)	3	3.5	5.0	7.0	8.5	10	11.4	15
Amino Acids (g)/L	30	35	50	70	85	100	114	150
Nitrogen (g)/L	4.8	5.6	8	11.2	13.6	16	18.2	24

Table 62-17. Dextrose Solutions

Concentration (%)	5	10	20	50	70
Anhydrous dextrose (g)	5	10	20	50	70
kcal/L	170	340	680	1700	2380

the heart. Catheter tips positioned outward against the side wall of the vena cava can perforate it and should be repositioned.

Air embolism is a potential complication of central venous catheter insertion and care.[107-110] Patients should be in Trendelenburg position during catheter insertion. If air embolism is suspected, the patient should be placed in reverse Trendelenburg position with the left side down.

Subclavian artery laceration may occur during placement.[111,112] The needle should be removed and pressure applied. A hemothorax may occur as a result of subclavian artery laceration. This may also be a delayed complication associated with catheterization, especially when the tip of the catheter is probing against the side wall of the superior vena cava.

Subclavian vein thrombosis may occur in patients with central catheters.[113-118] There is ipsilateral arm swelling and fullness in the thorax and supraclavicular area of the affected side. Distended prominent chest wall veins may be noted on the affected side, and there may be sore throat and axillary tenderness. The diagnosis must be confirmed with a venogram and treated immediately with thrombolytic agents if possible or heparin.

There are a variety of **metabolic complications** that can occur in patients receiving parenteral nutri-

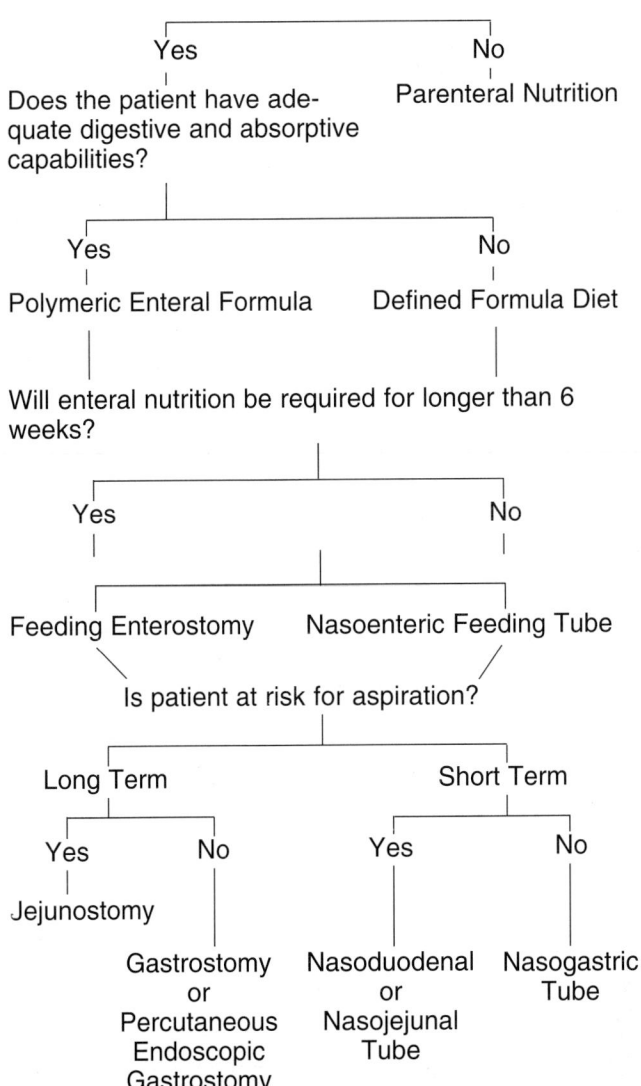

Fig. 62-4. Algorithm for enteral nutrition by tube.

Table 62-18. Complications of Nutrition Support

Parenteral Nutrition
  Mechanical
    Pneumothorax
    Air embolism
    Subclavian artery laceration
    Subclavian vein thrombosis
  Metabolic
    Sepsis
    Hypokalemia
    Hyperkalemia
    Hypophosphatemia
    Hyperphosphatemia
    Hypomagnesemia
    Hypermagnesemia
Enteral Nutrition
  Mechanical
    Tube misplacement
    Perforation
    Pulmonary aspiration
  Gastrointestinal
    Diarrhea
    Abdominal cramps
    Nausea
    Vomiting
    Distention
  Metabolic
    Fluid and electrolyte imbalance
    Fever

THE CLEVELAND CLINIC HOSPITAL
CLEVELAND, OHIO
PHYSICIAN'S ORDERS

ALLERGIES AND SENSITIVITIES: ______

IMPRINT

DATE	TIME	USE BALLPOINT PEN ONLY	C	K	R
		TPN ANCILLARY ORDERS (REVISED 8/3/87)			
PHYSICIAN:		**Please complete the following section:**			
		1. CHECK APPROPRIATE INDICATION(S) FOR TPN: ☐GI Obstruction ☐GI Fistula ☐Ileus			
		☐I.B.D. ☐Intractable Diarrhea ☐Intractable Vomiting ☐Malignancy ☐Other: ______			
		2. CHECK ONE: ___ Pre-op TPN Post-op TPN ___ Neither			
		3. HAS ENTERAL NUTRITION BEEN CONSIDERED AND RULED OUT? ___ Yes No			
PHARMACY:		1. If patient has no egg allergy, infuse 500 ml. IV Fat Emulsion 10% (Intralipid) I.V. over 4-6 hrs. every			
		Monday, Wednesday and Friday starting with the initiation of T.P.N.			
NURSING:		1. Vital signs and temperature every 4 hours - notify M.D. if a sudden change in temperature or			
		shaking chills occur.			
		2. Strict intake and output (Record TPN fluid in separate column.)			
		3. Daily weights.			
		4. Urine reductions every 6 hours – notify M.D. if greater than 2+.			
		5. Encourage ambulation.			
		6. Change I.V. tubing every Sunday, Monday, Wednesday and Friday.			
		7. Notify T.P.N. Nurses (page #122-1827, 122-1111, 122-1277, or 122-2688) to schedule regular			
		catheter care.			
		8. Notify Nutritional Support Team (x46667) to perform initial nutritional assessment, & 2nd assessment			
		in 7-10 days.			
		9. Infuse D10W at same rate as TPN solution if next TPN admixture is not available. Notify physician			
		if D10W is expected to infuse for more than 1 hour			
LABORATORY:		1. SMA-17 every Sunday.			
		2. Blood Glucose and KP-6 every Tuesday and Thursday.			
		3. CBC, Pro-Time, Serum Mg++, and Serum Transferrin every Tuesday			
		DATE: ______ ORDERED BY: ______			

PWO 875 6/87 ALL ORDERS MUST BE SIGNED BY PHYSICIAN

Fig. 62–5. Example of standing order sheet for total parenteral nutrition. (Courtesy of the Cleveland Clinic Foundation, Cleveland, OH.)

THE CLEVELAND CLINIC HOSPITAL
CLEVELAND, OHIO
PHYSICIAN'S ORDERS

ALLERGIES AND SENSITIVITIES: ______

IMPRINT

DATE	TIME	USE BALLPOINT PEN ONLY	C	K	R
		INITIATING ADULT TUBE FEEDING			
		PHYSICIAN: Please complete. Check appropriate indication(s) for enteral feeding:			
		☐ Neurological Disorder ☐ Functional Disability ☐ Psychological Factors ☐ Hypermetabolic State Other ______			
		Tube Placement (circle): Nasogastric Naso-duodenal Naso-jejunal Gastrostomy Jejunostomy Needle catheter jejunostomy			
		Has tube tip been confirmed ______ yes ______ no			
		Initial tube feeding order:			
		1. Initiate ______ (product) at ______ strength at ______ ml/hr for 24 hours (if less than 1/2 strength, advance on Daily Physician Order Sheet).			
		2. If tolerated, increase to full strength at above rate.			
		3. If above tolerated increase volume by 25 cc's every 24° until maximum feeding of ______ ml/hr is reached.			
		NURSING:			
		1. Check rate of tube feeding every hour. Keep flow rate within 20% (+ or −) of that ordered. (See nursing procedure manual #4.06.)			
		2. Urine reductions every 6 hours.			
		3. Notify physician for urine sugar 3+ or greater.			
		4. Vital signs every 8 hours.			
		5. Daily I and O: Record amount of undiluted formula and fluids for flush and/or dilution in separate column.			
		6. Daily weights.			
		LABORATORY:			
		1. Initially and every Monday: SMA-17, prothrombin time, CBC with Diff, transferrin			
		2. Every Thursday: KP_6			
		NUTRITION SERVICE:			
		1. Notify Floor Dietitian that tube feeding has been started.			
		Date ______ Ordered by ______			

F361 6/85 ALL ORDERS MUST BE SIGNED BY PHYSICIAN

Fig. 62–6. Example of standing order sheet for initiating adult tube feeding. (Courtesy of the Cleveland Clinic Foundation, Cleveland, OH.)

tion.[111,112,119-121] Depending on the patient's age, insulin secretion, peripheral insulin resistance, and the presence of sepsis, most nondiabetic adults can use between 0.8 and 1.0 g of glucose per minute. If administration of hypertonic dextrose results in hyperglycemia, adjustments have to be made in the rate of administration or the amount of insulin added. In some instances, the patient may have to be switched to a TNA containing lipids. If insulin has been added to the parenteral nutrition solution and the requirements change, hypoglycemia may ensue.

Potassium is the principal intracellular cation. **Hypokalemia** can develop rapidly, especially as the patient becomes anabolic and potassium moves intracellularly.[122-124] Patients may require 3 to 6 mEq potassium per gram of nitrogen infused during anabolism. An intracellular ratio of potassium to nitrogen of 3.5:1 should be maintained for optimal protein synthesis. Additional potassium may be required during glucose and insulin administration. Certain conditions of excessive losses (i.e., diarrhea, intestinal fistulas, diuretic therapy, amphotericin B) may necessitate additional potassium supplementation. The amount of potassium excreted is a function of acid-base balance, sodium intake, fluid volume reaching the renal tubules, and medications. **Hyperkalemia** can result if potassium levels are not monitored and adjusted.[122-124] Potassium may have to be limited in renal failure and during the administration of certain medications (i.e., cyclosporin, diuretics, antineoplastics). Hyperkalemia may occur rapidly in the catabolic patient whose TPN solution is abruptly stopped, especially if renal insufficiency or failure is an accompanying problem.

Ninety-nine percent of the body's calcium stores are found in bone and 1% in the extraskeletal pool. Total serum calcium levels depend on total plasma protein concentration because half of the total calcium is bound to albumin. The other fraction exists as the ionized or metabolically active form. The clinically relevant ionized calcium concentration may be calculated as:

$$(\text{Albumin deficit} \times 0.8) + \text{serum calcium}$$

$$[(4.0\ \text{g/dl} - \text{patient's albumin level}) \times 0.8] + \text{serum calcium}$$

Phosphorus is the principal ion in bone. Approximately 85% of the total body stores are located in the skeleton and 15% in soft tissue. Phosphorus acts as an extracellular buffer, a component of phospholipids and nucleic acids, and mediator of energy transport and is required for action of B-complex vitamins. Phosphate levels are regulated by parathyroid hormone, growth hormone, and vitamin D.

Symptomatic hypophosphatemia may develop in

patients receiving phosphate-free TPN or as a result of anabolism. This is referred to as the refeeding syndrome. Refeeding syndrome occurs once refeeding begins after a period of starvation.[125,126] There may be profound deficits of electrolytes. Hypophosphatemia can develop quickly, within 48 hours if not supplemented or within the first 10 days if inadequately supplemented. Hypophosphatemia is associated with decreased levels of 2, 3-DPG and left-shifted oxyhemoglobin dissociation curve with an increase in hemoglobin oxygen affinity, which decreases tissue oxygen transfer. To avoid the consequences of refeeding syndrome in the malnourished patient, nutritional requirements should be gradually increased over several days. **Hyperphosphatemia** may occur in patients with impaired renal function or neoplastic disease.[122-124] Intravenous lipid emulsions contain 47 mg of phosphorus per 100 ml of lipid and should be considered for those patients with hyperphosphatemia.

Magnesium, an intracellular cation, plays a key role in cellular metabolism. **Magnesium deficiency** can develop rapidly in malnutrition, alcoholic cirrhosis, pancreatitis, increased renal losses, chronic diuretic therapy, and during anabolism.[119,123,124] Hypomagnesemia may result in muscle cramps, tremors, and seizures. About 0.5 mEq of magnesium is required for 1 g of nitrogen used for protein synthesis. Magnesium deficiency is prevented by supplying at least 0.35 to 0.45 mEq/kg per day. During anabolic periods, patients may require at least 2 mEq of magnesium per gram of nitrogen. Magnesium requirements are also increased with increased glucose infusions and alcohol consumption. **Hypermagnesemia** may occur in patients with impaired renal function.[119,123,124]

Many of the complications associated with parenteral nutrition can be avoided with enteral nutrition. Enteral nutrition, however, is not totally innocuous and carries its own set of complications.[96,126-129]

Tube misplacement and perforation can be a serious and life-threatening complication. Care should be exercised during intubation. Tube tip location should be confirmed by x-ray film. Polyvinylchloride stiffens when exposed to gastric acid. There have been numerous reports of perforation.[130-135] The use of soft, pliable, small-bore feeding tubes decreases the potential for this complication.

Pulmonary aspiration is the most serious risk of enteral nutrition. It is most likely to occur in weak, debilitated patients, especially if the cardia is intubated and free reflux into the esophagus occurs. Olivares et al.[136] examined 720 autopsy cases of the neurologic patients. Lethal aspiration occurred in 9.5% of the cases, and gastric tubes increased the risk sixfold.[136] Transpylorically directed feeding tubes may decrease the potential for aspiration because two sphincters, the pylorus and lower esophageal, can theoretically prevent or lessen the potential for aspiration. Patients should not be left flat in bed during feedings. Gastric residuals should be checked frequently. The position of the tube should be checked radiographically. Food coloring may be added to the tube feeding for those patients at risk of aspiration to facilitate determination of aspiration. Tracheal aspirates may be checked for glucose.[137]

Diarrhea is the most common complication of tube feeding. It can result when one or a combination of factors is present:

- Hypertonic solutions
- Hypoalbuminemia
- Rapid delivery rate
- Bacterial contamination
- Lactose intolerance
- Concurrent drug therapy[138]

Thus, it is important to determine the cause and initiate treatment.

Administration of hypertonic tube feedings has been associated with distention, hypermotility, dumping syndrome and osmotic diarrhea.[139,140] Initial dilution of hyperosmolar solutions to isotonic concentration with a gradual increase in concentration as tolerated may reduce the incidence of this problem. Administration of formulas by continuous infusion rather than by bolus delivery also allows the gut to adapt to the osmolar load.

Hypoalbuminemia has also been associated with tube feeding intolerance.[141,142] Albumin maintains colloidal osmotic pressure, which increases the absorptive capacity of the villous capillaries. Many patients requiring enteral feedings have a lowered serum albumin as a result of malnutrition or the disease process. The serum albumin level should be raised either by parenteral administration of albumin or nutrition support if the serum albumin is less than 2.7 g/dl. When albumin is administered parenterally, nutrition support should be given concurrently so albumin is not used as a nutrient substrate.

Many individuals lack the ability to absorb various disaccharides, the most prevalent being lactose.[143-147] In addition, protein calorie malnutrition often results in loss of brush border enzymes, particularly lactase. Undigested lactose creates a hyperosmolar load in the gut that precipitates dumping syndrome and osmotic diarrhea. Because clinically there is a high incidence of lactose intolerance, enteral formulas containing lactose should be avoided.

Diarrhea associated with bacterial contamination of tube feedings is preventable.[148-150] Commercially prepared formulas are sterile before opening. These solutions are excellent media for bacterial growth. Consequently, clean technique should be used during the preparation, storage, and administration of these solutions. Changing the feeding container every 12 to 24 hours reduces the risk of bacterial growth. There is little agreement as to the appropriate amount of time an enteral feeding should be allowed to hang at room temperature. Most institutions, however, allow hang times only of 8 hours or less.

Concomitant drug therapy may induce diarrhea.[151] Medications may have to be altered or discontinued. If treatment cannot be discontinued, the use of antidiarrheal agents may be necessary. When diarrhea is a result of antibiotic therapy, the normal flora of the gastrointestinal tract may have to be restored before tolerance of the tube feeding can be demonstrated.

Fluid and electrolyte imbalances may also occur with the administration of enteral formulas, particularly in those patients who are unable to express thirst.[152-158] Patients receiving enteral nutrition by tube should have the same metabolic monitoring that parenterally fed patients receive.

Patients receiving enteral nutrition by tube may also complain of gastrointestinal disturbances, such as abdominal cramps, distention, nausea, and vomiting.[159-161] These problems are generally avoided when feedings are administered by continuous drip as opposed to bolus delivery.

Additional problems may occur with medications or supplemental potassium when administered by a feeding tube. If theophylline preparations are given, abdominal cramping or diarrhea may occur. Potassium should not be administered in bolus form, especially if the feeding tube is placed in the small intestine. If intestinal mobility is decreased, concentrated solutions or tablet particles may cause ulcerations and inflammation with possible obstruction.

ICU PHASE (SUPPORT PHASE)

Normal Nutritional Biochemistry and Physiology

The 70-kg man, unstressed, requires approximately 2400 kcal per day. The average 58-kg woman requires approximately 1800 kcal per day. Protein requirements are approximated at 0.8 g/kg per day.[90] These requirements increase with illness and injury.[162] Fever increases energy expenditure by 7% per degree Fahrenheit. There is little increase in energy expenditure for a minor operation. For more severe forms of trauma and major operative procedures, however, there is a substantial increase in energy requirements. These requirements are increased further when the patient is septic or has other complicating factors.[163,164]

Glycogen stores are depleted within 24 hours during acute starvation. Substrate requirements must then be met from muscle or adipose stores. Glucose is formed from amino acids released by muscle and converted by the liver by gluconeogenic processes into glucose. Glucose is required by the central nervous system. The heart, kidney, liver, and other viscera can use ketone bodies or fatty acids as fuels.

Hypermetabolic State

During prolonged starvation, the body enters into an adaptive phase in which there is a marked decrease in gluconeogenesis, an increase in lipolysis, and a decrease in metabolic rate. Urinary nitrogen excretion decreases after 2 weeks of starvation. In illness or injury, however, this adaptive process does not occur. Lipolysis is inhibited, muscle breakdown and gluconeogenesis are accelerated, and urea nitrogen excretion is increased. The gluconeogenic substrates are not only derived from peripheral skeletal muscle, but also visceral proteins, such as cardiac muscle, diaphragm, and other critical organs. Thus muscle function, particularly ventilation, may be affected. This hypermetabolic state may be self-limiting and resolve, or it may progress to multisystem organ failure (MSOF). Intensive nutrition support lessens the net protein loss.

Determining Nutrient Needs of the Hypermetabolic Patient

The nutrient needs of the hypermetabolic patient can be defined using various tests and procedures. A 24-hour urine sample may be collected to determine the degree of catabolism by measuring urinary urea nitrogen loss. A factor of 4 g is generally added to account for nonurinary urea nitrogen losses. To perform nitrogen balance studies in patients with compromised renal function, urea kinetic modeling may be used as outlined by Murray[165] (Table 62-19).

Energy expenditure may be measured using indirect calorimetry. If a 24-hour urea nitrogen value is available, the nonprotein respiratory quotient may be derived from substrate partitioning (see Table 62-9).

Problems with Meeting the Nutrient Needs of the Hypermetabolic Patient

Certain factors may complicate the provision of nutrition to the hypermetabolic patient. In some instances, the patient may be fluid restricted, necessitating the use of concentrated dextrose and amino acid solutions. Patients receiving parenteral nutrition may exhibit metabolic complications, such as elevated blood glucose levels and rising liver function test results. In those instances when blood glucose levels are difficult to control, additional insulin may be necessary or the use of total nutrient admixtures containing dextrose, amino acids, and lipid (or both). When liver function test results rise, the caloric load of the parenteral nutrition may have to be decreased if it is excessive (i.e., RQ > 1.0, total kilocalories given exceeded

Table 62-19. Urea Kinetic Modeling

Stable; No Dialysis

$$KrUn = \frac{UUN}{BUN} \times \frac{Uv}{t}$$

$$GUN = BUN \times KrUN$$

$$PCR = (GUN + 1.2) \times 9.35$$

Catabolic; No Dialysis

$$KrUn = \frac{UUN}{BUN} \times \frac{Uv}{t}$$

$$GUN = \frac{(BUN_2 - BUN_1)(Vu)}{0} + (KrUN \times BUN)$$

$$PCR = (GUN + 1.2) \times 9.35$$

No Urine Urea; Dialysis

$$GUN = \frac{(Vu_2 \times BUN_2) - (Vu_1 \times BUN_1)}{0}$$

$$PCR = (GUN + 1.2) \times 9.35$$

Urine Urea; Dialysis

$$KrUn = \frac{UUN}{BUN} \times \frac{Uv}{t}$$

$$GUN = \frac{(Vu_2 \times BUN_2) - (Vu_1 \times BUN_1)}{0} + (KrUN \times BUN)$$

$$PCR = (GUN + 1.2) \times 9.35$$

Abbreviation Key: KrUN, Residual urea clearance by kidney (ml/min); UUN, urine urea nitrogen (g/ml); BUN, serum urea nitrogen (mg/ml); GUN, urea nitrogen generation (mg/min); Uv, volume of urine (ml); t, time interval of urine collection (min); Vu, estimated urea volume of body water (ml); 0, time interval between blood samples (min); BUN_1, postdialysis BUN (mg/L); BUN_2, predialysis BUN (mg/L); Vu_1, urea volume of dry body weight (ml); Vu_2, Vu_1 = interdialytic weight gain (ml); BUN, Mean BUN = $\frac{BUN_1 + BUN_2}{2}$ (mg/ml).

(From Murray, R. L.: Protein and energy requirements. *In* Dynamics of Nutrition Support. Edited by S. H. Krey and R. L. Murray. Norwalk, CT, Appleton-Century-Crofts, 1986, pp. 185-217.

calculated needs). There is a transient increase in the function tests that generally return to normal within 1 week of cessation of hypertonic glucose infusion.

Fat emulsions can be used to supply up to 60% of the total caloric requirements. They are isotonic and are available in a 10 and 20% concentration. When fat emulsions are used as a TNA, the components must be mixed in certain concentrations and in a certain sequence to ensure stability of the emulsion. These solutions can be useful in controlling blood glucose and decreasing the carbon dioxide generated from the oxidation of glucose. There is some concern, however, that lipids may suppress the immune response.[166-171] There are several disadvantages to the TNA system. Lipid emulsions support the growth of a variety of microorganisms better than dextrose and cannot be filtered through a 0.22-μm bacterial filter. These solutions must be compounded carefully in a particular mixing order and within certain guidelines to avoid cracking the emulsion and other unstable conditions (see Table 62-15, formulas 13 to 22). They are also difficult to inspect for particulate matter.

There are problems associated with the use of enteral feedings as well. Critically ill patients often do not have functioning gastrointestinal tracts and may present with ileus or marginally functioning gastrointestinal tracts. Glutamine may play a vital role in maintaining gastrointestinal tract mucosal integrity and preventing bacterial translocation from the gut to the mesenteric tissue and then to the vascular system.[172-176] Glutamine is a major energy source for the gut and processes nitrogen and carbon into precursors for hepatic ureagenesis and gluconeogenesis. In critical illness, protein catabolism is associated with markedly diminished muscle glutamine pools, reduced plasma levels of glutamine, and increased intestinal glutamine utilization. Thus glutamine may be conditionally essential in stress and trauma.

Bacteria from the gastrointestinal tract have been implicated as a source of sepsis.[177-179] Animal studies have demonstrated an increase in translocation when the gastrointestinal tract is subjected to stress, such as hemorrhagic shock, intestinal handling, and administration of endotoxin.[180-182] Glutamine may be conditionally essential to strengthen the mucosal barrier and prevent translocation in humans. Hypoalbuminemia has been implicated as a reason for intolerance to enteral feedings.[183-186] Enteral feedings should be initiated slowly and at isotonic concentration.

Enteral nutrition may be the superior mode of nutrition therapy in the critically ill patient if it can be done safely. There are many physiologic advantages to using enteral nutrition, including better substrate utilization and maintenance of gastrointestinal mucosa integrity.[187-191] Enteral nutrition in the critically ill, however, is often complicated by diarrhea or ileus rendering the gastrointestinal tract nonfunctional and a minimally functioning gastrointestinal tract. Also, if pulmonary aspiration were to occur, it may hasten the demise in an already compromised patient. The risks and benefits of this therapy must be weighed carefully and administered and monitored appropriately.

Importance of Reassessment of Nutritional Status

The importance of assessing nutritional status and nutrient requirements cannot be overemphasized. Nutrients must be delivered safely, accurately, and in amounts adequate to meet the patient's requirements. As the clinical course progresses, therapy can be altered and progressed, and an end point of therapy can be established (see Fig. 62-2).

Writing the Total Parenteral Nutrition Prescription

Case 1

A 58-year-old woman, 5'6" tall and weight 70 kg, is transferred to the ICU with fever, abdominal pain and decreased urine output. A serum amylase elevation and a computed tomography scan of the pancreas confirm the diagnosis of pancreatitis. A chest radiograph reveals elevated hemidiaphragm and atelectasis. She is obtunded and requires intubation to correct hypoxemia. Within the first 24 hours, urine output improves with fluid resuscitation, but because of fever and agitation, the patient requires continued mechanical ventilation and sedation. Her serum chemistries are as follows: sodium 130 mEq/L, potassium 3.7 mEq/L, chloride 95 mEq/L, carbon dioxide 19 mEq/L, blood urea nitrogen (BUN), 12 mg/dl, creatinine 1.0 mg/dl. The patient's energy requirements are estimated by calculating the BEE using the Harris-Benedict equation:

$$BEE = 655.1 + 9.56W + 1.85H - 4.68A$$

Where W = weight in kilograms, H = height in centimeters, and A = the patient's age in years. Thus, for this patient:

$$BEE = 655.1 + (9.56 \times 70) + 1.85 \times 66 \times 2.54)$$
$$- (4.68 \times 58)$$
$$= 1363 \text{ kcal/day}$$

The BEE must be adjusted to represent total estimated caloric requirement (ECR):

$$ECR = 1363 \times 1.76 \text{ to } 2.0$$
$$= 2399 \text{ to } 2726 \text{ kcal/day}$$

The patient's protein requirements are estimated at 1.5 to 2.0 g/kg per day:

$$70 \text{ kg} \times 1.5 - 2.0 = 105 \text{ to } 140 \text{ g Protein/day}$$

Thus, the TPN prescription would read:

D50	500 ml =	850 kcal
Amino Acids, 10%	500 ml =	200 kcal and 50 g Protein
	1000 ml	1050 kcal and 50 g Protein

If the solution is infused at a rate of 100 ml per hour for 24 hours, the patient will receive 2520 kcal and 120 g protein. This is within the range of her estimated requirements. This solution provides:

1050 kcal/L
50 g protein/L
103:1 nonprotein kcal:nitrogen ratio
81% carbohydrate
19% protein

The electrolytes that should be added initially to each liter of TPN should include 9 mEq of calcium gluconate, 50 mEq of sodium chloride, 25 mEq of sodium acetate, 20 mEq of potassium chloride, 10 mEq of potassium phosphate, and 4 mEq of magnesium sulfate. Multiple vitamins (MVI), 10 ml, and trace elements, 1 ml, are added to 1 L per day.

The TPN order is written as follows:

Bottle #1
Amino acids 10% 500 ml
Dextrose 50% 150 ml
Sterile water 250 ml
Electrolytes as above
Rate = 100 ml/hour

Bottle #2
Amino acids 10% 500 ml
Dextrose 50% 375 ml
Sterile water 125 ml
Electrolytes as above
Rate = 100 ml/hour

Bottle #3
Amino acids 10% 500 ml
Dextrose 50% 500 ml
Electrolytes as above
Rate = 100 ml/hour

Case 2

A 67-year-old man, 5'10" tall, weight 82 kg, undergoes resection of the descending colon for removal of a carcinoma. Forty-eight hours after the procedure, he is obtunded and febrile. He develops a distended abdomen and is returned to surgery, at which time an anastomotic leak is found. A diverting colostomy is required, and the patient is returned to the ICU in stable condition. His serum chemistries are as follows: sodium 138 mEq/L, potassium 40 mEq/L, chloride 100 mEq/L, carbon dioxide 22 mEq/L, BUN 20 mg/dl, creatine 0.9 mg/dl. The patient's energy requirements are estimated:

$$BEE = 66.47 + 13.75W$$
$$+ 5H - 6.76A$$
$$BEE = 66.47 + (13.75 \times 82)$$
$$+ (5 \times 70 \times 2.54)$$
$$- (6.76 \times 67)$$
$$= 1630$$
$$ECR = 1630 \times 1.76 \text{ to } 2.0$$
$$= 2869 \text{ to } 3260$$
$$\text{Protein Requirements} = 82 \times 1.5 \text{ to } 2.0$$
$$= 123 \text{ to } 164 \text{ g/day}$$

Thus, the TPN prescription would read:

D50 500 ml = 850 kcal
Amino Acids, 500 ml = 200 kcal and 50 g Protein
10% 1000 ml 1050 kcal and 50 g Protein

If the solution is infused at a rate of 125 ml per hour for 24 hours, the patient will receive 3150 kcal and 150 g protein. This is within the range of his estimated requirements. This solution provides:

1050 kcal/L
50 g protein/L
103:1 nonprotein kcal:nitrogen ratio
81% Carbohydrate
19% Protein

The electrolytes that should be added initially to each liter of TPN should include 6.0 mEq of calcium gluconate, 25 mEq of sodium chloride, 25 mEq of sodium acetate, 20 mEq of potassium chloride, 10 mEq of potassium phosphate, and 4 mEq of magnesium sulfate. MVI, 10 ml, and trace elements, 1 ml, are added to 1 L per day. TPN is advanced as previously described.

Case 3

A 62-year-old man, 5'11" tall, weight 70 kg, develops respiratory failure at another hospital and is transferred to a tertiary care ICU after 5 days of mechanical ventilation. He is persistently febrile. Bronchoscopy studies reveal that legionella species are the cause of the pneumonia. He requires sedation and mechanical ventilation for at least 7 to 10 more days.

His serum chemistries are within normal limits. The patient's energy requirements are estimated by calculating the BEE:

$$BEE = 66.47 + 13.75$$
$$+ 5H - 6.76A$$
$$BEE = 66.47 + (13.75 \times 70)$$
$$+ (5 \times 71 \times 2.54) - (6.76 \times 62)$$
$$= 1511 \text{ kcal}$$
$$ECR = 1511 \times 1.76 \text{ to } 2.0$$
$$= 2659 \text{ to } 3022 \text{ kcal/day}$$
$$\text{Protein Requirements} = 70 \times 1.5 \text{ to } 2.0 = 105 \text{ to } 140 \text{ g/day}$$

Thus, the TPN prescription would read:

D50 250 ml = 425 kcal
Amino acids, 8.5% 500 ml = 170 kcal and 42.5 g protein

Fat emulsion, 20% $\dfrac{250 \text{ ml}}{1000 \text{ ml}} = \dfrac{500 \text{ kcal}}{1090 \text{ kcal and}}$
42.5 g Protein

If the solution is infused at a rate of 110 ml per hour for 24 hours, the patient will receive 2891 kcal and 112 g protein. This is within the range of his estimated requirements. This solution provides:

1095 kcal/L
42.5 g protein/L
129:1 nonprotein kcal:nitrogen ratio
39% Carbohydrate
15% Protein
46% Fat

The patient should receive standard electrolytes, vitamins, and trace minerals. The TPN order is written as follows:

Bottle #1
Dextrose   50% 250 ml
Amino acids 8.5% 500 ml
Fat emulsion 20% 250 ml
Rate = 50 ml/hour

Bottle #2
Dextrose   50% 250 ml
Amino acids 8.5% 500 ml
Fat emulsion 20% 250 ml
Rate = 75 ml/hour

Bottle #3
Dextrose   50% 250 ml
Amino acids 8.5% 500 ml
Fat emulsion 20% 250 ml
Rate = 110 ml/hour

Specialized Nutrition Support

The development of disease-specific solutions has been a major advancement in the care of critically ill patients.

Renal Failure

There is little disagreement that renal failure patients tend to be malnourished.[192-195] These patients are often unable to eat secondary to anorexia, early satiety, nausea, or vomiting. There may be increased losses from fistulas or dialysis therapy. In addition, there are increased requirements imposed by illness and injury. The mortality associated with renal failure is high.

The concept of providing solutions composed of essential amino acids (EAA) to patients with oliguria or anuria was based on the work of Rose.[196] In 1963, Giordano[197] reported that uremic patients fed 2 g of EAA nitrogen as the sole source of nitrogen with adequate calories, vitamins, and minerals showed lowered BUN levels. Patients were maintained in positive nitrogen balance, and there was a net decrease in endogenous protein catabolism. Similar results were reported by Giovannetti and Maggiore.[198]

Intravenous EAAs were first used for treating renal failure in a single patient by Wilmore and Dudrick.[199] They reported weight gain; improved wound healing; positive nitrogen balance; and decreased levels of urea nitrogen, potassium, and phosphorus. EAAs were used in acute renal failure by other researchers.[200-202]

In 1973, Abet[203] demonstrated decreased mortality in a prospective, double-blind study administering EAA and 70% dextrose compared with the administration of dextrose alone. The duration of the acute renal failure was decreased, and there was a reduction in serum potassium, phosphorus, and magnesium.[203]

In contrast to the above-mentioned studies, other studies have not confirmed these advantages. In a double-blind, randomized, prospective study, Feinstein et al.[204] compared three parenteral nutrition regimens in patients with acute renal failure. Patients received glucose alone, glucose plus EAAs, or glucose plus essential and nonessential amino acids. There was no difference in recovery of renal function or survival rate between any of the groups.[204] Similar findings were reported by Mirtallo et al.[205]

Recommendations for protein needs in renal failure vary among clinicians. Many restrict according to glomerular filtration rate (GFR):[206]

GFR ml/min	Protein g/kg/day
25–70	0.6–0.7 (continuing at least 0.35 g/kg high biologic value)
<25	0.28 (supplemented with essential amino acids)
<5	1.0–1.2 w/dialysis (50% high biologic value)

The protein may have to be adjusted according to the patient's clinical condition, associated therapies, and tolerance. Thus, a patient with acute renal failure, multiple trauma, or sepsis may have high protein needs, which would necessitate the use of dialysis. Patients with chronic renal failure receiving hemodialysis generally require 1.0 g protein/kg per day.[207] Recommendations during peritoneal dialysis are higher, generally 1.2 to 1.5 g/kg per day.[208]

Nutrition management of the patient with acute renal failure is affected by the superimposed illness. Adequate energy and nitrogen should be supplied to support the patient. This is often complicated by fluid and electrolyte restrictions. For those patients in whom dialysis may be difficult, specialized solutions containing EAAs may be indicated for limited periods of time. Once dialysis is initiated, standard enteral or parenteral solutions may be used to provide a full complement of amino acids. Long-term use of EAAs only should be discouraged because they do not adequately meet nutrition needs.

Patients undergoing peritoneal dialysis may be absorbing glucose through the dialysis solution. It has been reported that peritoneal dialysis results in a 500 kcal load, as much as 600 to 800 kcal for continuous ambulatory peritoneal dialysis.[209-213] This should be considered for maintaining normal blood glucose levels as well.

Example: Patient on cycle for four 2 L exchanges all 2.5% solutions
Ultrafiltrate: 914 ml
Glucose: 1404 mg/dl
Total drain volume: 8 L from exchanges
+914 ml ultrafiltrate
8914 ml
Initial glucose: 8 L 2.5% glucose = 200 g
Glucose remaining: $\frac{1.404 \text{ g/dl} \times 8914 \text{ ml}}{100} = 125 \text{ g}$

Absorbed: 75 g

Hepatic Failure

The liver plays a central role in nutrient synthesis, secretion, metabolism, and detoxification. Hepatic failure is common in intensive care settings and can have catastrophic effects on the patient's nutritional status and overall morbidity and mortality. These patients are a nutritional paradox—protein requirements for regeneration are high, but tolerance to the substrate is reduced owing to the damaged organ.

Hepatic failure may be acute as in fulminant hepatic failure owing to viral or toxic hepatitis. Fortunately, these patients are generally well nourished before the insult. Conversely, patients with chronic liver insufficiency, such as that caused by alcohol abuse, are usually malnourished. Nutrition support is probably most beneficial in the patient with chronic liver insufficiency who sustains an acute insult.

Owing to the metabolic derangements associated with liver insufficiency, alterations in nutrition support are necessary. Carbohydrate metabolism is affected by decreased glycogen storage and synthesis, accelerated gluconeogenesis, and subsequent glucose intolerance. Lipid metabolism is altered as well. The damaged liver is unable to absorb adequately and metabolize long-chain triglycerides. Circulating levels of nonesterified fatty acids are elevated owing to the liver's inability to metabolize them. Enteral lipids may not be tolerated owing to reduced bile salt and lipoprotein synthesis. Parenteral lipids, however, are usually cleared if there is adequate lipoprotein lipase.

Fluids often are restricted. Lymphatic blockage and hypoalbuminemia contribute to the patient's inability to handle fluid. Ascites and anasarca result. The problem is further compounded by the increased secretion of aldosterone, which results in sodium retention.

By far, the most deleterious derangements occur in protein metabolism. Nutrition support for liver failure patients has been based on normalization of plasma amino acids. In hepatic failure, there is an elevation of the aromatic amino acids, tryptophan, tyrosine and phenylalanine, as well as methionine, glutamate, aspartase, and ornithine. The branched-chain amino acids, valine, leucine, and isoleucine, are decreased as a result of increased muscle metabolism.[214,215] Normally the plasma molar ratio of the branched-chain amino acid to aromatic amino acid is 3:1 to 3.5:1. In hepatic encephalopathy, this ratio is reduced to 1:1 to 1.5:1 allowing increased influx of aromatic amino acids across the blood-brain barrier, which results in a derangement of neurotransmitter function with resultant encephalopathy.[216-218]

The amount and type of protein selected depend on the degree and type of liver failure. Unless encephalopathy is present, standard amino acids may be used at 1.0 to 1.5 g/kg dry body weight. If the patient is protein intolerant or becomes encephalopathic, specialized liver failure solutions may be necessary. Hepatamine (McGaw Laboratories) contains 36% branched-chain amino acids and is low in aromatic amino acids. There is no tyrosine and a reduced amount of methionine. Arginine has been increased because it is the amino acid responsible for the processing of ammonia in the urea cycle. Hepatamine, administered at 1.0 g/kg to encephalopathic patients, has resulted in improved nitrogen balance and improvement in encephalopathy.[219,220]

Case Example. A 50-year-old man, 6′ tall, weight 91 kg, 81 kg dry weight, is admitted with end-stage liver disease from alcoholic cirrhosis. He is cachectic with extreme muscle wasting and ascites. He is encephalopathic and has no bowel sounds. His serum chemistries are as follows: sodium 129 mEq/L, potassium 4.5 mEq/L, BUN less than 45 mg/dl, creatinine 0.9 mg/dl. The patient's energy requirements are estimated by calculating the BEE:

$$BEE = 66.47 + 13.75W + 5H - 6.76A$$

$$BEE = 66.47 + (13.75 \times 81) + (5 \times 72 \times 2.54) - (6.76 \times 50)$$

$$= 1756 \text{ kcal/day}$$

$$ECR = 1756V \times 1.76 \text{ to } 2.0$$

$$= 3090 \text{ to } 3512 \text{ kcal/day}$$

Protein Requirements $= 81 \text{ kg} \times 1.0 \text{ to } 1.5 = 81 \text{ to } 121 \text{ g/day}$

Thus, the TPN prescription would read:

D50	500 ml =	850 kcal
Liver failure amino acids, 8%	500 ml =	152 kcal and 38 g Protein
	1000 ml =	1002 kcal and 38 g Protein

If the solution is infused at a rate of 125 ml per hour for 24 hours, the patient will receive 3006 kcal and 114 g protein. This is within the range of his estimated requirements.

Pulmonary Failure

The effects of malnutrition on pulmonary function have been well documented.[221-224] There is a reduction of total lean muscle mass, including the diaphragm, abdominal muscles, and intercostal muscles. Muscle atrophy, whether induced by malnutrition or prolonged mechanical ventilation, can result in compromised respiratory function and complications such as pneumonia and atelectasis.

Although respiratory failure, especially with malnutrition, is an indication for nutrition support, excessive carbohydrate infusion can be detrimental to these patients.[225,226] In the unstressed starved patient, excessive carbohydrate loads result in increased lipogenesis and increased carbon dioxide production with a shift in the RQ from 0.7 to 1.0.[227] In stressed patients, excessive carbohydrate infusions stimulate catecholamine release without a significant net increase in lipogenesis. There is an increase in both carbon dioxide and oxygen production, and the RQ shifts from 0.7 to 0.9.[228] This increases the demand on an already compromised respiratory function. Askanazi has proposed the substitution of 50% of carbohydrate calories with lipid to decrease the carbon dioxide production. Intravenous infusion of parenteral lipids is not without potential risk. Decreased pulmonary diffusion capacity in adults and fat accumulation in infants has been reported.[228-231] Thus, both pulmonary function and lipid tolerance need to be monitored carefully.

Case Example. A 70-year-old man is admitted to the ICU with respiratory failure and adult respiratory distress syndrome. He requires mechanical ventilation for at least 2 weeks. He has bowel sounds, and a decision is made to initiate tube feeding. The patient is 5'7" tall and weighs 68 kg. The patient's energy requirements are estimated:

$$BEE = 66.47 + 13.75W + 5H - 6.76A$$

$$BEE = 66.47 + (13.75 \times 68) + (5 \times 67 \times 2.54) - (6.76 \times 70)$$

$$= 1379 \, kcal/day$$

$$ECR = 1379 \times 1.76 \, to \, 2.0$$

$$= 2427 \, to \, 2758 \, kcal/day$$

$$\text{Protein requirements} = 68 \, kg \times 1.5 \, to \, 2.0 + 102$$

$$- 136 \, g/day$$

The enteral feeding prescription should read:

Standard Isotonic Formula	1000 ml = 1000 kcal + 34 g Protein
Protein Module	3 TBSP + 45 kcal + 9 g Protein
	1045 kcal + 43 g Protein

If the formula is infused at a rate of 100 ml per hour, the patient would receive 2508 kcal and 103 g protein. This is within the range of his estimated requirements. This solution provides:

1045 kcal/L
43 g protein/L
126:1 non-protein kcal:nitrogen ratio
50% carbohydrate
16% protein
39% fat

Because the formula is isotonic, it is initiated at full strength 50 ml per hour and advanced by 25 ml per hour as tolerated.

Neurologic Disease

Nutrition support of the neurologic patient can be complex owing to the metabolic demands and clinical restrictions. Many of these patients, particularly those with head trauma and closed head injuries, are extremely catabolic with excessive urinary nitrogen excretions.[232,233] Thus, they have extremely high protein requirements. Supplying the neurologic patient with adequate nutrition is often complicated by intolerance to glucose and fluid. This often necessitates the use of concentrated solutions or TNA.

The use of enteral feedings in this patient population is possible because the gastrointestinal tract is generally functional and accessible. The risk of pulmonary aspiration, however, should be carefully evaluated. Those patients who are unable to protect their airway are probably best nourished parenterally.

Postoperative Complications

Nutrition support may be necessary postoperatively to support patients who will be unable to eat for an extended period of time.[234-237] Critically ill patients often have prolonged ileus. This, coupled with increased requirements, leads to deteriorating nutrition status and its functional consequences. If a patient is in negative nitrogen balance by 1 g, the loss of lean body mass is approximately 31 g. If this net nitrogen loss is allowed to continue for a week, the loss of lean body mass exceeds 200 g. Although it may be difficult to replete patients who are hypermetabolic or septic, provision of adequate nutrition may prevent further loss. Patients with large wounds, decubitus ulcers, fistulas, or abscesses have large nitrogen losses. The provision of adequate nutrition support is imperative to promote healing and reduce infectious complications.

Sepsis

Nutritional requirements during sepsis can be significant.[238-241] Yet there is sometimes a reluctance to initiate parenteral nutrition owing to concern over seeding a central line. The septic patient experiences accelerated gluconeogenesis and inhibition of lipolysis. These patients are generally glucose intolerant owing to increased peripheral insulin resistance. Owing to the peripheral insulin resistance, energy requirements are met through protein catabolism. Because the skeletal muscle uses branched-chain amino acids for energy, parenteral nutrition solutions containing increased amounts of branched-chain amino acids have been shown to improve nitrogen balance in severe stress.[240,241] No difference in clinical outcome, however, has been demonstrated.

POST-ICU PHASE (REHABILITATION PHASE)

Transitional Feedings

After prolonged illness or injury, return of gastrointestinal function may be impaired. Parenteral nutrition should not be discontinued until the patient can be adequately

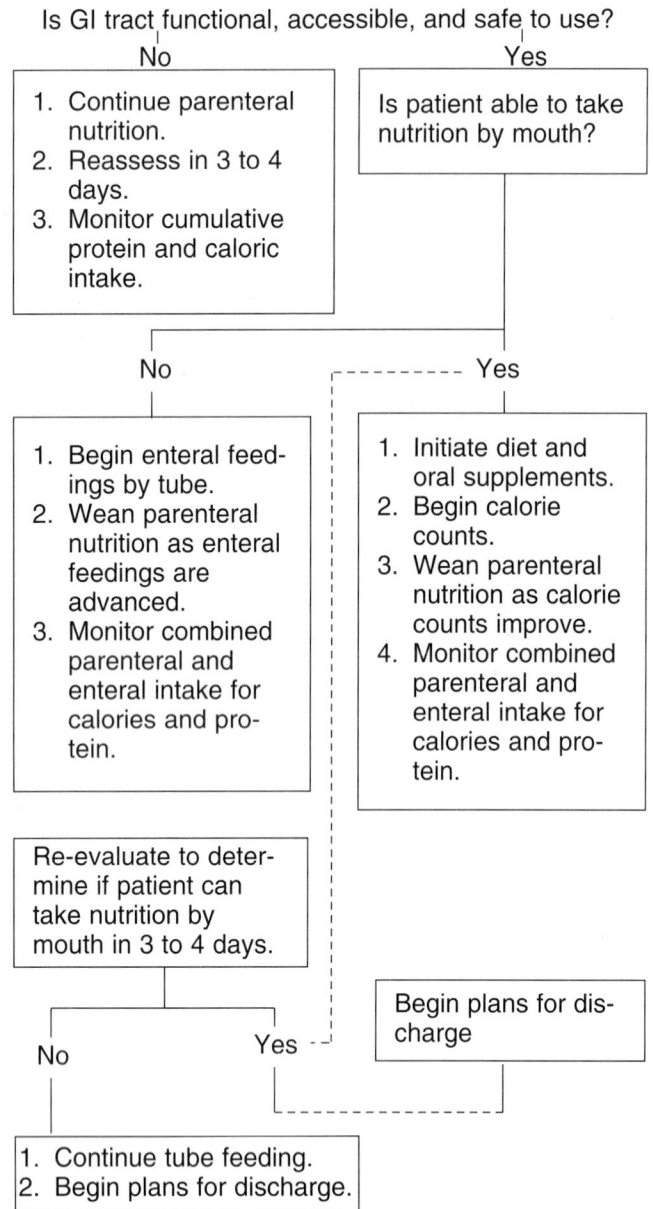

Fig. 62-7. Algorithm for advancing nutrition support.

nourished by tube feedings, diet, oral supplements, or a combination of these techniques (Fig. 62-7).

For the patient who is being nourished parenterally, a determination of adequate gastrointestinal function has to be made. The best signs of adequate gastrointestinal function are normal upper gastrointestinal and small bowel x-ray contrast studies and normal flatus or bowel movements. The presence of bowel sounds and hunger may also indicate the return of gastrointestinal function.

Once gastrointestinal tract function has been assessed, the patient's ability to consume diet or oral supplements should be evaluated. If appetite is not present or the patient is incapable of self-feeding, tube feedings should be initiated. Patients receiving enteral feedings by tube should receive close monitoring to document the safety and efficacy of therapy. Tube feedings should not be discontinued until the patient can consume adequate nutrition by mouth. During the weaning process from parenteral feeding, it may be necessary to provide supplemental tube feedings at night while allowing the patient to eat during the day.

Throughout the weaning process, it is necessary to document calorie and protein intake and monitor nutritional status. It should be noted that many patients will not return to "normal" or even premorbid nutritional status until well after discharge.[94] Consequently, there is no one laboratory value or nutrition parameter that can determine the end point of therapy. It is important to look for general trends in the patient's progress.

Effect of Prolonged Parenteral Nutrition on Gut Function

During prolonged periods of parenteral nutrition, atrophy of the gut mucosa may occur.[242,243] This may complicate the initiation of tube feedings or oral diet. The introduction of nutrients into the gastrointestinal tract may have to be slowed to avoid or minimize diarrhea, abdominal cramping, and distention. In some cases, predigested nutrient formulas may be necessary.

Consideration for Prolonged Enteral and Parenteral Support

In some instances, it may be necessary to continue enteral or parenteral nutrition in the home setting. The patient with a functioning gastrointestinal tract who cannot take adequate nutrition by mouth may be a candidate for home tube feeding. Home enteral nutrition has been used to manage a variety of disorders, including glycogen storage disease; gastrointestinal disorders; cancer; neurologic disorders; psychologic disorders; and chronic systemic disorders such as renal, cardiac, pulmonary, and liver disease.[244] Patients without adequate gastrointestinal function may require home parenteral nutrition (HPN). HPN has been used to nourish patients with Crohn's disease, radiation enteritis, superior mesenteric artery or vein thrombosis resulting in short bowel syndrome, enterocutaneous fistulas, volvulus of the small bowel, and pseudoobstruction.[245] Plans for discharge should be made early in the patient's hospital stay.

The decision to initiate home parenteral or enteral nutrition depends on the functional capacity of the gastrointestinal tract and the patient's ability to eat. Some patients may require specialized nutrition support to supplement oral intake. Commercial supplements should be palatable and easily obtained in the home setting.

For those patients who are unable to consume nutrition by mouth but have a functioning gastrointestinal tract, enteral feedings by tube are indicated. The choice of feeding route depends on the anticipated length of duration of feeding and the risk of aspiration. If the enteral feedings are required only for 6 weeks or less, a nasoenteric tube can be used. If aspiration is a concern, however, a nasoduodenal or nasojejunal tube should be used. For long-term enteral feedings, a permanent enterostomy has to be considered.

Those patients who are not at risk for aspiration can use

a gastrostomy for nutritional support. This allows the most flexibility for administration techniques. Those patients who are at risk for aspiration, however, should have a jejunostomy. A percutaneous gastrostomy or jejunostomy may be used in those patients who are unable to undergo general anesthesia.

Home Total Parenteral Nutrition

The decision to place a patient on HPN support should be made after all other possibilities are explored. Most candidates for HPN have short bowel syndrome, radiation enteritis, or some malabsorption syndrome refractory to medical management.[246] This therapy requires careful planning and teaching and is best accomplished through a multidisciplinary approach involving the dietitian, nurse, pharmacist, physician, psychiatrist, social worker, and home health-care provider.[247]

Many factors must be considered before a patient is deemed to be a good candidate for HPN. These can be divided into several categories: nutritional, medical, psychosocial, and financial. Nutritionally the patient may be unable to meet fluid and nutrient requirements through the gastrointestinal tract. The parenteral nutrition formulas are designed to meet the requirements of each individual patient.

A permanent catheter (i.e., Hickman or Broviac) must be placed for central venous access. The extravascular portion of the catheter is tunneled under the skin and exits at a point in the chest wall where the patient can easily see and care for it. In some instances, an implanted vascular access device (i.e., Port-A-Cath) is used. In either case, the catheter or device can be used if the patient is rehospitalized.

There are many medical issues that need to be addressed, including the underlying illness and its effect on the patient and the HPN therapy. There may be other medications and therapies that alter the type and method of HPN delivery. In addition, it is important to know the patient's prognosis because this may influence the nutritional, medical, social, and financial aspects of the HPN treatment.

Although HPN is a lifesaving therapy, many psychosocial issues need to be addressed, particularly if the patient is unable to take anything by mouth. Other issues, such as body image and lifestyle changes, need to be addressed. These issues are generally handled by the psychiatrist and social worker.[248]

Often the patient's biggest concern is financial. Does the patient have adequate insurance to cover the HPN therapy as well as nursing visits if needed? Is the patient the primary or sole provider, and will he or she be able to continue in this capacity?

In conclusion, the nutrition management of the critically ill patient is complex and multifaceted. The patient's nutritional requirements change as he or she progresses. The therapeutic approach should be comprehensive with consideration given to all phases of care: risk, support, and rehabilitation.

The patient should be assessed for risk level. Nutrition support should be initiated as soon as the patient is hemodynamically stable. Reassessment of nutritional status should occur every 7 to 10 days to document the efficacy of therapy. The patient should be monitored for potential complications. As soon as the gastrointestinal tract is functional and accessible, it should be used.

REFERENCES

1. Bistrian, B. R., Blackburn, G. L., Hallowell, E., and Heddle, R.: Protein status of general surgical patients. JAMA, *230*: 858, 1974.
2. Bistrian, B. R., et al.: Prevalence of malnutrition in general medical patients. JAMA, *235*:1567, 1976.
3. Weinsier, R. L., Hunker, E. M., Krumdieck, C. L., and Butterworth, C. E.: Hospital malnutrition: a prospective evaluation of general medical patients during the course of hospitalization. Am. J. Clin. Nutr., *32*:418, 1979.
4. Hill, G. L., et al.: Malnutrition in surgical patients: an unrecognized problem. Lancet, *1*:689, 1977.
5. Apelgren, K. N., and Wilmore, D. W.: Nutritional care of the critically ill patient. Surg. Clin. North Am., *63*:497, 1983.
6. Jeejeebhoy, K. N.: Nutrition in critical illness. *In* Critical Care. State of the Art. Edited by W. C. Shoemaker. Philadelphia, Society of Critical Care Medicine, 1989.
7. Bistrian, B. R.: Nutritional assessment of the hospitalized patient: a practical approach. *In* Nutritional Assessment. Edited by R. A. Wright and S. Heymsfield. Boston, Blackwell Scientific Publications, 1984.
8. Shaw, J. H. F.: Recent advances in the nutritional and metabolic management of critically ill surgical patients. N. Z. Med. J., *99*:665, 1986.
9. Blackburn, G. L., et al.: Nutritional and metabolic assessment of the hospitalized patient. JPEN J. Parenter. Enteral Nutr., *1*:11, 1977.
10. Baker, J. P., et al.: Nutritional assessment: a comparison of clinical judgement and objective measurements. N. Engl. J. Med., *306*:969, 1982.
11. Detsky, A. S., et al.: Evaluating the accuracy of nutritional assessment techniques applied to hospitalized patients: methodology and comparisons. JPEN J. Parenter. Enteral Nutr., *8*:153, 1984.
12. Detsky, A. S., et al.: Predicting nutrition associated complications for patients undergoing gastrointestinal surgery. JPEN J. Parenter. Enteral Nutr., *11*:440, 1987.
13. Detsky, A. S., et al.: What is subjective global assessment of nutritional status? JPEN J. Parenter. Enteral Nutr., *11*:8, 1987.
14. Hamwi, G. J.: Therapy: changing dietary concepts. *In* Diabetes Mellitus: Diagnosis and Treatment. Edited by T. S. Danowski. New York, American Diabetes Association, 1964: 73-78.
15. Roche, A. F., Siervogel, R. M., Chumlea, W. C., and Webb, P.: Grading body fatness from limited anthropometric data. Am. J. Clin. Nutr., *34*:2831, 1981.
16. Bray, G. A., Jordan, H. A., and Sims, E. A.: Evaluation of the obese patient. I. An algorithm. JAMA, *235*:1487, 1976.
17. Divkovics, A.: The nutrition interview. *In* Case Study Methods Nutritional Assessment. Philadelphia, George F. Stickley, 1987.
18. Damon, A.: Notes on anthropometric techniques: II. skinfolds—right and left sides, held by one or two hands. Am. J. Phys. Anthropol., *23*:305, 1965.
19. Laubach, L. L., and McConville, J. T.: Notes on anthropometric technique: anthropometric measurements, right and left sides. Am. J. Phys. Anthropol., *26*:367, 1967.
20. Schell, L. M., Johnson, F. E., Smith, D. R., and Paolone, A. M.:

Directional asymmetry of body dimensions among white adolescents. Am. J. Phys. Anthropol., 67:317, 1985.
21. Reynaldo, M., Mendoza, F., Mueller, W., and Pawson, I. G.: Which side to measure, right or left? In Anthropometric Standardization Reference Manual. Edited by T. G. Lohman, A. F. Roche, and R. Martorell. Champaign, IL; Human Kinetics Books, 1988.
22. Grant, A., and DeHoog, S.: Anthropometric assessment. In Nutritional Assessment and Support. 4th Ed. Seattle, Grant & DeHoog, 1991.
23. Church, J. M., and Hill, G. L.: Assessing the efficacy of intravenous nutrition in general surgical patients: dynamic nutritional assessment with plasma proteins. JPEN J. Parenter. Enteral Nutr., 11:135, 1987.
24. Miller, S. F., Morath, M. A., and Finley, R. K.: Comparison of derived and actual transferrin: a potential source of error in clinical nutritional assessment. J. Trauma, 21:548, 1981.
25. Forse, R. A., and Shizgal, H. M.: Serum albumin and nutritional status. JPEN J. Parenter. Enteral Nutr., 4:450, 1980.
26. Dahn, M. S., and Jacobs, L. A.: The significance of hypoalbuminemia following injury and infection. Am. Surg., 51:340, 1985.
27. Christou, N. V., and Tellado-Rodriguez, J.: Estimating mortality risk in preoperative patients using immunologic, nutritional, and acute-phase response variables. Ann. Surg., 210:69, 1989.
28. Silberman, H., and Eisenberg, D.: The relation of thyroid indices in the critically ill patient to prognosis and nutritional factors. Surg. Gynecol. Obstet., 166:223, 1988.
29. Hawker, F. H., and Stewart, P. M.: Relationship of somatomedin-C/insulin-like growth factor I levels to conventional nutritional indices in critically ill patients. Crit. Care Med., 15:732, 1987.
30. Powand, M. C., and Moyer, E. D.: Plasma proteins and wound healing. Surg. Gynecol. Obstet., 153:749, 1981.
31. Linden, C. J. U., and Buur, W. A.: Fibronectin levels in stressed and septic patients fed with total parenteral nutrition. JPEN J. Parenter. Enteral Nutr., 10:360, 1986.
32. Russell, D. Mc. R., et al.: Skeletal muscle function during hypocaloric diets and fasting: a comparison with standard nutritional assessment parameters. Am. J. Clin. Nutr., 37:133, 1983.
33. Russell, D. Mc. R., et al.: A comparison between muscle function and body composition in anorexia nervosa: the effect of refeeding. Am. J. Clin. Nutr., 38:229, 1983.
34. Russell, D. Mc. R., et al.: The effect of fasting and hypocaloric diets on the function and metabolic characteristics of rat gastrocnemius muscle. Clin. Sci., 67:185, 1984.
35. Russell, D. Mc. R., et al.: Metabolic and structural changes in skeletal muscle during hypocaloric dieting. Am. J. Clin. Nutr., 39:503, 1984.
36. Brough, W., et al.: Effect of nutrient intake, surgery, sepsis and long term administration of steroids on muscle function. Br. Med. J., 293:983, 1986.
37. Lenmarken, C., Sandstedt, S., Schenck, H. V., and Larsson, J.: The effect of starvation on skeletal muscle function in man. Clin. Nutr., 5:99, 1986.
38. Bistrian, B. R., Blackburn, G. L., Sherman, M., and Scrimshaw, N. W.: Therapeutic index of nutritional depletion in hospitalized patients. Surg. Gynecol. Obstet., 141:512, 1975.
39. Smith, L. C., and Mullen, J. L.: Nutritional assessment and indications for nutrition support. Surg. Clin. North Am., 71:11, 1991.
40. Long, C. L., et al.: Urinary excretion of 3-methylhistidine: an assessment of muscle protein catabolism in adult normal subjects and during malnutrition sepsis and skeletal trauma. Metabolism, 30:756, 1981.
41. Kim, C., and Okada, A.: Urinary 3-methylhistidine as an index of protein nutrition in total parenteral nutrition. JPEN J. Parenter. Enteral Nutr., 12:198, 1988.
42. Hill, G. L., King, R. F. G., and Smith, R. C.: Multi-element analysis of the living body by neutron activation analysis—application to critically ill patients receiving intravenous nutrition. Br. J. Surg., 66:868, 1979.
43. Tellado, J. M., and Garcia-Sabrido, J. L.: Predicting mortality based on body composition analysis. Ann. Surg., 209:81, 1989.
44. Mequid, M. M., Campos, A. C., and Hammond, W. G.: Nutritional support in surgical practice: part I. Ann. J. Surg., 159:345, 1990.
45. Heymsfield, S. B., et al.: Dual photon absorptiometry: accuracy of bone mineral and soft tissue mass measurement in vivo. Am. J. Clin. Nutr., 49:1283, 1989.
46. Cohn, S. H.: Non-invasive techniques for measuring body elemental composition. Biol. Trace Elem. Res., 13:179, 1987.
47. Vartsky, D., Ellis, K. J., and Cohn, S. H.: In vivo quantification of body nitrogen by neutron capture prompt gamma-ray analysis. J. Nucl. Med., 20:1158, 1963.
48. Mazess, R. B., Peppler, W. W., and Gibbons, M.: Total body composition by dual-photon (153Gd) absorptiometry. Am. J. Clin. Nutr., 40:834, 1984.
49. Harrison, G. G., and Van Itallie, T. B.: Estimation of body composition: a new approach based on electromagnetic principles. Am. J. Clin. Nutr., 32:524, 1982.
50. McNeill, K. G., et al.: In vivo measurements of body protein based on the determination of nitrogen by prompt gamma analysis. Am. J. Clin. Nutr., 32:1955, 1979.
51. Forbes, G. B., Gallop, J., and Hursh, J. B.: Estimation of total body fat from potassium-40 content. Science, 133:101, 1961.
52. Pierson, R. N., Lin, D. H. Y., and Phillips, R. A.: Total body potassium in health: effects of age, sex, height and fat. Am. J. Physiol., 226:206, 1974.
53. Shizgal, H. M., Spainer, A. H., Humes, J., Wood, C. D.: Indirect measurement of total exchangeable potassium. Am. J. Physiol., 233:253, 1977.
54. Anderson, E. C.: Three-component body composition analysis based on potassium and water determination. Ann. N. Y. Acad. Sci., 110:189, 1963.
55. Apelgran, K. N., and Rombeau, J. L.: Comparison of nutritional indices and outcome in critically ill patients. Crit. Care Med., 10:305, 1982.
56. Abraham, E.: Immune mechanisms underlying sepsis in critically ill surgical patients. Surg. Clin. North Am., 65:991, 1985.
57. McIrvine, A. J., and Mannick, J. A.: Lymphocyte function in the critically ill surgical patient. Surg. Clin. North Am., 63:245, 1983.
58. MacLean, L. D.: Delayed type hypersensitivity testing in surgical patients. Surg. Gynecol. Obstet., 166:285, 1988.
59. Meakins, J. L., Pietsch, J. B., and Bubenick, O.: Delayed hypersensitivity: indicator of acquired failure of host defenses in sepsis and trauma. Ann. Surg., 186:241, 1977.
60. Meakins, J. L., and Shizgal, H. M.: Therapeutic approaches to anergy in surgical patients. Ann. Surg., 190:286, 1979.
61. O'Mahony, J. B., McIrvine, A. J., and Paler, S. B.: The effect of short term postoperative intravenous feeding upon cell-mediated immunity and serum suppressive activity in well nourished patients. Surg. Gynecol. Obstet., 159:27, 1984.
62. Twomey, P., Ziegler, D., Rombeau, J.: Utility of skin testing

in nutritional assessment: a critical review. JPEN J. Parenter. Enteral Nutr., 6:50, 1982.
63. Studley, H. O.: Percentage of weight loss. A basic indicator of surgical risk in patients with chronic peptic ulcer. JAMA, 106:458, 1936.
64. Seltzer, M. H., and Slocum, B. A.: Instant assessment: absolute weight loss and surgical mortality. JPEN J. Parenter. Enteral Nutr., 6:218, 1982.
65. Windsor, J. A., and Hill, G. L.: Weight loss with physiologic impairment: a basic indicator of surgical risk. Ann. Surg., 207:290, 1988.
66. Reinhardt, G. F., Myscofski, J. W., and Wilkins, B.: Incidence of mortality of hypoalbuminemic patients in hospitalized veterans. JPEN J. Parenter. Enteral Nutr., 4:357, 1980.
67. Harvey, K. B., Moldawer, L. L., and Bistrian, B. R.: Biological measures for the formation of a hospital prognostic index. Am. J. Clin. Nutr., 34:2013, 1981.
68. Anderson, C. F., and Moxness, K.: The sensitivity and specificity of nutrition-related variables in relationship to the duration of hospital stay and the rate of complications. Mayo Clin. Proc., 59:477, 1984.
69. Brown, R. O., and Bradley, J. E.: Effect of albumin supplementation during parenteral nutrition on hospital morbidity. Crit. Care Med., 16:1177, 1988.
70. Young, G. A., Chem, C., and Zeiderman, M. R.: Influence of preoperative intravenous nutrition upon hepatic protein synthesis, plasma proteins and amino acids. JPEN J. Parenter. Enteral Nutr., 13:596, 1989.
71. Mullen, J. L., et al.: Reduction of operative morbidity and mortality by combined preoperative and postoperative nutritional support. Ann. Surg., 192:604, 1980.
72. Buzby, G. P., et al.: Perioperative total parenteral nutrition in surgical patients. N. Engl. J. Med., 325:525, 1991.
73. Buzby, G. P., and Mullen, J. L.: Analysis of nutritional assessment indices—prognostic equations and cluster analysis. In Nutritional Assessment. Edited by R. A. Wright and S. Heymsfied. Boston, Blackwell Scientific Publications, 1984.
74. Harris, H. A., and Benedict, F. G.: Biometric Studies of Basal Metabolism in Man. Washington, D.C., Carnegie Institute, Publication No. 279, 1919.
75. Wilkens, K. (Ed.): Suggested Guidelines for Nutrition Care of Renal Patients. Chicago, American Dietetic Association, 1990.
76. Foster, G. D., Knox, L. S., Dempsey, D. T., and Mullen, J. C.: Caloric requirements in total parenteral nutrition. J. Am. Coll. Nutr., 6:231, 1987.
77. Weir, J. B. de V.: New methods for calculating metabolic rate with special reference to protein metabolism. J. Physiol., 109:1, 1949.
78. Boothby, W. M., and Sandiford, I.: Laboratory Manual of the Technique of Basal Metabolic Rate Determinations. Philadelphia, W. B. Saunders, 1920.
79. Elwyn, D. H., Kinney, J. M., and Askanazi, J.: Energy expenditure in surgical patients. Surg. Clin. North Am., 61:545, 1981.
80. Goran, M. I., Peters, E. J., Herndon, D. N., and Wolfe, R. R.: Total energy expenditure in burned children using the doubly-labeled water techniques. Am. J. Physiol., 259:E576, 1990.
81. Lusk, G. L.: The Elements of the Science of Nutrition. 4th Ed. Philadelphia, W. B. Saunders, 1928.
82. Kleiber, M.: The Fire of Life: An Introduction to Animal Energetics. Melbourne, Fla, Robert E. Krieger Publishing, 1975.
83. Schutz, Y., and Ravussin, E.: Respiratory quotients lower than 0.70 in ketogenic diets [letters to the editor]. Am. J. Clin. Nutr., 33:1317, 1980.
84. Ireton-Jones, C. S., and Turner, W. W.: The use of respiratory quotient to determine the efficacy of nutritional support regimens. J. Am. Diet. Assoc., 87:180, 1987.
85. Askanazi, J., et al.: Influence of total parenteral nutrition on fuel utilization in injury and sepsis. Ann. Surg., 191:40, 1980.
86. Askanazi, J., et al.: Respiratory changes induced by the large glucose loads of total parenteral nutrition. JAMA, 243:1444, 1980.
87. Giovannin, I., et al.: Respiratory quotient and patterns of substrate utilization in human sepsis and trauma. JPEN J. Parenter. Enteral Nutr., 7:226, 1983.
88. Guyton, A. C.: Dietary balances, regulation of feeding; obesity and starvation. In Textbook of Medical Physiology. 8th Ed. Philadelphia, W. B. Saunders, 1991.
89. Feurer, I., and Mullen, J. L.: Bedside measurement of resting energy expenditure and respiratory quotient via indirect calorimetry. Nutr. Clin. Pract., 1:43, 1986.
90. The National Research Council: Recommended Dietary Allowances. 10th Ed. Washington, D.C., National Academy of Sciences, 1989.
91. Cerra, F. B.: Pocket Manual of Surgical Nutrition. St. Louis: C. V. Mosby, 1984.
92. Randall, H. T. (Ed.): Manual of Preoperative and Postoperative Care. Philadelphia, W. B. Saunders, 1967.
93. American Medical Association Nutrition Department of Foods and Nutrition: Multivitamin preparations for parenteral use. A statement by the Nutrition Advisory Group. JPEN J. Parenter. Enteral Nutr., 3:258, 1979.
94. American Medical Association Department of Foods and Nutrition: Guidelines for essential trace element preparations for parenteral use. A statement by an expert panel. JAMA, 241:2051, 1979.
95. Matarese, L. E.: Reassessment and determining an endpoint of therapy. In Dynamics of Nutrition Support. Edited by S. H. Krey, and R. L. Murray. Norwalk, CT, Appleton-Century-Crofts, 1986.
96. Matarese, L. E.: Enteral alimentation. In Surgical Nutrition. Edited by J. E. Fischer. Boston, Little, Brown, 1983.
97. Sitzmann, J. V., Townsend, T. R., Siler, M. C., and Bartlett, J. G.: Septic and technical complications of central venous catheterization: a prospective study of 200 consecutive patients. Ann. Surg., 202:766, 1985.
98. Bjornson, H. S., et al.: Association between micro-organism growth at the catheter insertion site and colonization of the catheter in patients receiving total parenteral nutrition. Surgery, 92:720, 1982.
99. Bozzetti, F., et al. Blood cultures as a guide for the diagnosis of central venous catheter sepsis. JPEN J. Parenter. Enteral Nutr., 8:396, 1985.
100. Williams, W. W.: Infection control during parenteral nutrition therapy. JPEN J. Parenter. Enteral Nutr., 9:735, 1985.
101. Bozzetti, F., et al.: A new approach to the diagnosis of central venous catheter sepsis. JPEN J. Parenter. Enteral Nutr., 15:412, 1991.
102. Curtas, S., and Tramposch, K.: Culture methods to evaluate central venous catheter sepsis. Nutr. Clin. Pract., 6:43, 1991.
103. Wolfe, B. M., et al.: Complications of parenteral nutrition. Am. J. Surg., 152:93, 1986.
104. Ryan, J. A.: Complications of total parenteral nutrition. In Total Parenteral Nutrition. Edited by J. E. Fischer. Boston, Little, Brown, 1976.
105. Bernard, R. W., and Stahl, W. M.: Subclavian vein catheterizations: a prospective study. I: non-infectious complications. Ann. Surg., 173:184, 1971.
106. Blackett, R. L.: A prospective study of subclavian vein cathe-

ters used exclusively for the purpose of intravenous feeding. Br. J. Surg., 65:393, 1978.
107. Armstrong, R. F., Peters, J. L., and Cohen, S. L.: Air embolism caused by fractured central venous catheter. Lancet, 1:954, 1977.
108. Feliciano, D. V., et al.: Major complications of percutaneous subclavian vein catheters. Am. J. Surg., 138:869, 1979.
109. Peters, J. L., and Armstrong, R.: Air embolism occurring as a complication of central venous catheterization. Ann. Surg., 187:375, 1978.
110. Haavik, P. E., and Steen, P. A.: Air embolism caused by rupture of a silicone central venous catheter. JPEN J. Parenter. Enteral Nutr., 8:579, 1984.
111. Grant, J. P.: Handbook of Total Parenteral Nutrition. 2nd Ed. Philadelphia, W. B. Saunders, 1992.
112. Fischer, J. E., and Freund, H. R.: Central hyperalimentation. In Surgical Nutrition. Edited by J. E. Fischer. Boston, Little, Brown, 1983.
113. Bozzetti, F., et al.: Subclavian venous thrombosis due to indwelling catheters: a prospective study on 152 patients. JPEN J. Parenter. Enteral Nutr., 7:560, 1983.
114. Curnow, A., et al.: Urokinase therapy for silastic catheter-induced intravascular thrombi in infants and children. Arch. Surg., 120:1237, 1985.
115. Fabri, P. T., et al.: Incidence and prevention of thrombosis of the subclavian vein during total parenteral nutrition. Surg. Gynecol. Obstet., 155:238, 1982.
116. Fleming, C. R., et al.: Analytical assessment of broviac catheter occlusion. JPEN J. Parenter. Enteral Nutr., 9:314, 1985.
117. Gale, G. B., et al.: Restoring patency of thrombosed catheters with cryopreserved urokinase. JPEN J. Parenter. Enteral Nutr., 8:298, 1984.
118. Macoviak, J. A., et al.: The effect of low-dose heparin on the prevention of venous thrombosis in patients receiving short-term parenteral nutrition. Curr. Surg., 41:98, 1984.
119. Silberman, H.: Parenteral nutrition: non-nutritional effects and metabolic complications. In Parenteral and Enteral Nutrition. 2nd Ed. Edited by H. Silberman. Norwalk, CT, Appleton & Lange, 1989.
120. Ashworth, C. J., Sach, K., Williams, L. F. Jr.: Hyperosmolar hyperglycemic non-ketotic coma: its importance in surgical problems. Ann. Surg., 167:556, 1968.
121. Dormal, N. M., and Canter, J. W.: Hyperosmolar hyperglycemic non-ketonic coma complicating intravenous hyperalimentation. Surg. Gynecol. Obstet., 136:729, 1973.
122. Moore, F. D.: Two dozen syndromes: pattern recognition in diagnosis and treatment of fluid and electrolyte disorders. In Surgical Nutrition. Edited by J. E. Fischer. Boston, Little, Brown, 1983.
123. Ang, S. D., and Daly, J. M.: Potential complications and monitoring of patients receiving total parenteral nutrition. In Parenteral Nutrition. Edited by J. Rombeau and M. Caldwell. Philadelphia, W. B. Saunders, 1986.
124. Aalyson, M.: Metabolic complications of parenteral nutrition. In Dynamics of Nutrition Support. Edited by S. H. Krey and R. L. Murry. Norwalk, CT, Appleton-Century-Crofts, 1986.
125. Weinsier, R. L., and Krumdieck, C. L.: Death from overzealous total parenteral nutrition: the refeeding syndrome revisited. Am. J. Clin. Nutr., 34:393, 1980.
126. Solomon, S. M., and Kirby, D. F.: The refeeding syndrome: a review. JPEN J. Parenter. Enteral Nutr., 14:90, 1990.
127. Lysen, L. K.: Metabolic complications during enteral nutrition support. In Dynamics of Nutrition Support. Edited by S. H. Krey and R. L. Murry. Norwalk, CT, Appleton-Century-Crofts, 1986.
128. Bernard, M., and Forlaw, L.: Complications and their prevention. In Enteral and Tube Feeding. Edited by J. Rombeau and M. Caldwell. Philadelphia, W. B. Saunders, 1986.
129. Silberman, H.: Enteral nutrition. In Parenteral and Enteral Nutrition. 2nd Ed. Edited by H. Silverman. Norwalk, CT, Appleton & Lange, 1989.
130. Hayhurst, E. G., and Wyman, M.: Morbidity associated with prolonged use of polyvinyl feeding tubes. Am. J. Dis. Child., 129:72, 1975.
131. Siegle, R. L., Rabinowitz, J. G., and Surasuhn, C.: Intestinal perforation secondary to nasojejunal feeding tubes. Am. J. Roentgenol. 126:1229, 1976.
132. Sun, S. C., Samuels, S., Lea, J., and Marquis, J. R.: Duodenal perforation. A rare complication of neonatal nasojejunal feeding. Pediatrics, 55:371, 1975.
133. Boros, S. F., and Reynolds, J. W.: Duodenal perforation. A complication of neonatal nasojejunal feeding. J. Pediatr., 85:107, 1974.
134. Chen, J. W., and Wong, P. W. K.: Intestinal complication of nasojejunal feeding in low-birth weight infants. J. Pediatr., 85:109, 1974.
135. Fogel, R. S., Smith, W. L., and Gresham, E. L.: Perforation of feeding tube into right renal pelvis. J. Pediatr., 93:122, 1978.
136. Olivares, L., Segovia, A., and Revuetta, R.: Tube feeding and lethal aspiration in neurological patients: a review of 720 autopsy cases. Stroke, 5:654, 1974.
137. Jacobs, S., Chang, R. W. S., Lee, B., and Bartlett, F. W.: Continuous enteral feeding: a major cause of pneumonia among ventilated intensive care unit patients. JPEN J. Parenter. Enteral Nutr., 14:353, 1990.
138. Heimburger, D. C.: Diarrhea with enteral feeding: will the real cause please stand up? Am. J. Med., 88:89, 1990.
139. Edes, T. E., Walk, B. E., and Austin, J. L.: Diarrhea in tube-fed patients: feeding formula not necessarily the cause. Am. J. Med., 88:91, 1990.
140. Keohane, P. P., et al.: Relation between osmolarity of diet and gastrointestinal side effects in enteral nutrition. Br. Med. J., 288:678, 1984.
141. Patterson, M. L., et al.: Enteral feeding in the hypoalbuminemic patient. JPEN J. Parenter. Enteral Nutr., 14:362, 1990.
142. Schwartz, D. B., and Darrow, A. K.: Hypoalbuminemia-induced diarrhea in the enterally alimented patient. Nutr. Clin. Pract., 3:235, 1988.
143. Simoons, F. J.: Primary adult lactose intolerance and the milking habit. A problem in biological and cultural interrelations. Dig. Dis., 14:819, 1969.
144. Gudmand-Hoyer, E., Dahlquist, A., and Jarnun, S.: The clinical significance of lactose malabsorption. Am. J. Gastroenterol., 53:460, 1970.
145. Dahlquist, A., et al.: Intestinal lactase deficiency and lactose intolerance in adults: preliminary report. Gastroenterology, 45:488, 1963.
146. Beline, M. S., and Bayless, T. L.: Intolerance of small amounts of lactose by individuals with low lactose levels. Gastroenterology, 65:735, 1973.
147. Necomer, A. D.: Disaccharide deficiencies. Mayo Clin. Proc., 48:648, 1973.
148. Anderson, K. R., et al.: Bacterial contamination of tube-feeding formulas. JPEN J. Parenter. Enteral Nutr., 8:673, 1984.
149. Baldwin, B. A., Zagoren, A. J., and Rose, N.: Bacterial contamination of continuously infused enteral alimentation with needle catheter jejunostomy—clinical implications. JPEN J. Parenter. Enteral Nutr., 8:30, 1984.
150. Mickschl, D. B., et al.: Contamination of enteral feedings and diarrhea in patients in intensive care units. Heart Lung, 19:362, 1990.
151. White, K. C., and Harbavy, K. L.: Hypertonic formula result-

ing from added oral medications. Am. J. Dis. Child., *136:* 931, 1982.
152. Vanlandingham, S., Simpson, S., Daniel, P., Newmark, S. R.: Metabolic abnormalities in patients supported with enteral tube feeding. JPEN J. Parenter. Enteral Nutr., *5:*322, 1981.
153. Primrose, J. N., Carr, K. W., Sim, A. J. W., and Shenkin, A.: Hyperkalemia in patients on enteral feeding. JPEN J. Parenter. Enteral Nutr., *5:*130, 1981.
154. Engle, F. L., and Jaeger, C.: Dehydration with hypernatremia, hyperchloremia and azotemia complicating nasogastric tube feeding. Am. J. Med., *17:*196, 1954.
155. Cramer, L. M., Haverback, C. Z., and Smith, R. R.: Hypertonic dehydrating complicating high protein nasogastric tube feeding. Med. Ann. DC, *27:*331, 1958.
156. Gault, M. H., Dixon, M. E., Doyle, M., and Cohen, W. M.: Hypernatremia, azotemia and dehydration due to high-protein tube feeding. Ann. Intern. Med., *68:*778, 1968.
157. Walike, J. W.: Tube feeding syndrome in head and neck surgery. Arch. Otolaryngol., *89:*117, 1969.
158. Wilson, W. S., and Meinert, J. K.: Extracellular hyperosmolarity secondary to high-protein nasogastric tube feeding. Ann. Intern. Med., *47:*585, 1957.
159. Heymsfield, S. B., et al.: Enteral hyperalimentation: an alternative to central venous hyperalimentation. Ann. Intern. Med., *90:*63, 1979.
160. Bury, K. D., and Jambunathan, G.: Effects of elemental diets on gastric emptying and gastric secretion in man. Am. J. Surg., *127:*59, 1974.
161. Heitkemper, M. E., et al.: Rate and volume of intermittent enteral feeding. JPEN J. Parenter. Enteral Nutr., *5:*125, 1981.
162. Long, C. L.: The energy and protein requirements of the critically ill patient. *In* Nutritional Assessment. Edited by R. A. Wright and S. Hesymsfield. Boston, Blackwell Scientific Publications, 1984.
163. Clowes, G. H. A., et al.: Energy metabolism and proteolysis in traumatized and septic man. Surg. Clin. North Am., *56:* 1169, 1976.
164. Cuthbertson, D. P.: The metabolic response to injury and its nutritional implications: retrospect and prospect. JPEN J. Parenter. Enteral Nutr., *3:*108, 1979.
165. Murray, R. L.: Protein and energy requirements. *In* Dynamics of Nutrition Support. Edited by S. H. Krey and R. L. Murray. Norwalk, CT, Appleton-Century-Crofts, 1986.
166. Saba, T. M., and Luzio, N. R.: Reticuloendothelial blockage and recovery as a function of opsonic activity. Am. J. Physiol., *216:*197, 1979.
167. Sobrado, J., et al.: Lipid emulsions and reticuloendothelial system function in healthy and burned guinea pigs. Am. J. Clin. Nutr., *42:*855, 1985.
168. Hamaway, K. J., et al.: The effect of lipid emulsions on reticuloendothelial system function in the injured animal. JPEN J. Parenter. Enteral Nutr., *9:*559, 1985.
169. Lanser, M. E., and Saba, T. M.: Neutrophil-mediated lung localization of bacteria: a mechanism for pulmonary injury. Surgery, *90:*473, 1981.
170. Fischer, G. W., Hunter, K. W., Wilson, S. R., and Mease, A. D.: Diminished bacterial defenses with intralipid. Lancet, *2:*819, 1980.
171. Locniskar, M., Nauss, K. M., and Newberne, P. M.: The effect of quality and quantity of dietary fat on the immune system. J. Nutr., *113:*951, 1983.
172. Souba, W. W., Smith, R. J., and Wilmore, D. W.: Glutamine metabolism by the intestinal tract. JPEN J. Parenter. Enteral Nutr., *9:*608, 1985.
173. Wilmore, D. W., et al.: The gut: a central organ after surgical stress. Surgery, *104:*917, 1988.
174. Proceedings of an International Glutamine Symposium—Glutamine Metabolism in Health and Disease: Basic science and clinical aspects. JPEN J. Parenter. Enteral Nutr., *14(Suppl.):*39, 1990.
175. Bulus, N., Cersosimo, E., Ghishan, F., and Abumrad, N. N.: Physiologic importance of glutamine. Metabolism, *38(Suppl.):*1, 1989.
176. Lacy, J. M., and Wilmore, D. W.: Is glutamine a conditionally essential amino acid? Nutr. Rev., *48:*297, 1990.
177. Cerra, F. B.: Hypermetabolism, organ failure and metabolic support. Surgery, *101:*1, 1987.
178. Deitch, E. A., Winterton, J., and Li, M.: The gut as a portal of entry for bacteremia. Role of protein malnutrition. Am. Surg., *205:*681, 1987.
179. Border, J. R., Hassett, J., and LaDuca, J.: The gut origin septic states in blunt multiple trauma (ISS + 40) in the ICU. Ann. Surg., *206:*427, 1987.
180. Kudsk, K. A., et al.: Enteral and parenteral feeding influences mortality after hemoglobin–E coli peritonitis in normal rats. J. Trauma, *23:*605, 1983.
181. Suito, H., et al.: The effect of route of nutrient administration on the nutritional state, catabolic hormone secretion, and gut mucosal integrity after burn injury. JPEN J. Parenter. Enteral Nutr., *11:*1, 1987.
182. Deitch, E. A., et al.: Hemorrhagic shock-induced bacterial translocation is reduced by xanthine oxidase inhibition or inactivation. Surgery, *104:*191, 1988.
183. Ford, E. G., Jennings, L. M., and Andrassy, R. J.: Serum albumin (oncotic pressure) correlates with enteral feeding tolerance in the pediatric surgical patients. J. Pediatr. Surg., *22:* 597, 1987.
184. Brinson, R. R., and Kolts, B. E.: Hypoalbuminemia as an indicator of diarrheal incidence in critically ill patients. Crit. Care Med., *15:*506, 1987.
185. Brinson, R. R., and Kolts, B. E.: Diarrhea associated with severe hypoalbuminemia: a comparison of a peptide-based chemically defined diet and standard enteral alimentation. Crit. Care Med., *16:*130, 1988.
186. Brinson, R. R., Anderson, W. M., and Singh, M.: Hypoalbuminemia-associated diarrhea in critically ill patients. J. Crit. Ill., *2:*72, 1987.
187. Allardyce, D. B., and Groves, A. C.: A comparison of nutritional gains resulting from intravenous and enteral feedings. Surg. Gynecol. Obstet., *139:*180, 1974.
188. Hindmarsh, J. T., and Clark, R. G.: The effects of intravenous and intra-duodenal feeding on nitrogen balance after surgery. Br. J. Surg., *60:*589, 1973.
189. Lickley, H. L. A., Track, N. S., Vranic, M., and Bury, K. D.: Metabolic responses to enteral and parenteral nutrition. Am. J. Surg., *135:*172, 1978.
190. Bark, S.: Amino acid concentration in plasma after gastrointestinal intraportal and intravenous administration of crystalline amino acids. Acta Chir. Scand., *466(Suppl.):*38, 1976.
191. Higgs, S. D.: A comparison of oral feeding and total parenteral nutrition in infants of very low birth weight. S. Afr. Med. J., *48:*2169, 1974.
192. Coles, G. A.: Body composition in chronic renal failure. Q. J. Med., *41:*25, 1972.
193. Kopple, J. D., and Swendseid, M. E.: Protein and amino acid metabolism in uremic patients undergoing maintenance hemodialysis. Kidney Int., *2(Suppl.):*S64, 1975.
194. Blumenkrantz, M. J., and Kopple, J. D.: Incidence of nutritional abnormalities in uremic patients entering dialysis therapy. Kidney Int., *10:*514, 1976.
195. Kopple, J. D., et al.: Nutritional status of patients with different levels of chronic renal insufficiency. Kidney Int., *36(Suppl. 127):*5185, 1989.

196. Rose, W. C.: Amino acid requirements of man. Fed. Proc., 8:546, 1949.
197. Giordano, C.: Use of exogenous and endogenous urea for protein synthesis in normal and uremic subject. J. Lab. Clin. Med., 62:213, 1963.
198. Giovannetti, S., and Maggiore, Q.: A low nitrogen diet with protein of high biological valve for severe chronic uremia. Lancet, 1:1000, 1964.
199. Wilmore, D., and Dudrick, S.: Treatment of acute renal failure with intravenous essential L-amino acids. Arch. Surg., 99:669, 1969.
200. Dudrick, S. J., Steiger, E., and Long, J. M.: Renal failure in surgical patients: treatment with intravenous essential amino acids and hypertonic glucose. Surgery, 68:180, 1970.
201. Abel, R. M., Abbott, W. M., and Fischer, J. E.: Acute renal failure: treatment without dialysis by total parenteral nutrition. Arch. Surg., 103:513, 1971.
202. Abbott, W. M., Abel, R. M., and Fischer, J. E.: Treatment of acute renal insufficiency after aortoiliac surgery. Arch. Surg., 103:590, 1971.
203. Abel, R. M.: Improved survival from acute renal failure after treatment with intravenous essential L-amino acids and glucose. N. Engl. J. Med., 288:695, 1973.
204. Feinstein, E. I., et al.: Clinical and metabolic responses to parenteral nutrition in acute renal failure. Medicine, 60:124, 1981.
205. Mirtallo, J. M., et al.: A comparison of essential and general amino acid infusions in the nutritional support of patients with compromised renal function. JPEN J. Parenter. Enteral Nutr., 6:109, 1982.
206. Life Sciences Research Office, Federation of American Societies for Experimental Biology: Guidelines for the scientific review of enteral food products for special medical purposes. Edited by J. M. Talbot. JPEN J. Parenter. Enteral Nutr., 15:995, 1991.
207. Burton, B. T., and Hirschman, G. H.: Current concepts of nutritional therapy in chronic renal failure: an update. J. Am. Diet. Assoc., 82:359, 1983.
208. Bodnar, D. M.: Rationale for nutritional requirements for patients on continuous ambulatory peritoneal dialysis. J. Am. Diet. Assoc., 80:247, 1982.
209. Miller, D.: Use of total parenteral nutrition in patients with renal failure. Nutr. Suppl. Serv., 1:14, 1981.
210. Nolph, K. D., et al.: Peritoneal glucose transport and hyperglycemia during peritoneal dialysis. Am. J. Med. Sci., 259:272, 1970.
211. Grodstein, G. P., et al.: Glucose absorption during continuous ambulatory peritoneal dialysis. Kidney Int., 16:888, 1979.
212. Wathen, R. L.: The metabolic effects of hemodialysis with and without glucose in the dialysate. Am. J. Clin. Nutr., 31:1870, 1978.
213. Manji, N., et al.: Peritoneal dialysis for acute renal failure: overfeeding resulting from dextrose absorbed during dialysis. Crit. Care Med., 18:29, 1990.
214. Fischer, J. E., et al.: The effect of normalization of plasma amino acids on hepatic encephalopathy in man. Surgery, 80:77, 1976.
215. James, J. H., et al.: Hyperammonemia, plasma amino acid imbalance, and blood-brain amino acid transport: a unified theory of portal-systemic encephalopathy. Lancet, 2:772, 1979.
216. Fischer, J. E., et al.: The role of plasma amino acids in hepatic encephalopathy. Surgery, 78:276, 1975.
217. Fischer, J. E., and Baldessarini, R.: False neurotransmitters and hepatic failure. Lancet, 2:75, 1971.
218. Fischer, J. E., and James, J. H.: Treatment of hepatic coma and hepatorenal syndrome: mechanism of actin of L-dopa and aramine. Am. J. Surg., 123:222, 1972.
219. Freund, H., et al.: Infusion of branched-chain enriched amino acid solution in patients with hepatic encephalopathy. Ann. Surg., 196:209, 1982.
220. Cerra, F. B., et al.: Disease-specific amino acid infusion (F080) in hepatic encephalopathy: a prospective randomized, double-blind, controlled trial. JPEN J. Parenter. Enteral Nutr., 9:288, 1985.
221. Doekel, R. C., et al.: Clinical semi-starvation: depression of hypoxic ventilatory response. N. Engl. J. Med., 295:358, 1976.
222. Arora, N. S., and Rochester, D. F.: Respiratory muscle strength and maximal voluntary ventilation in undernourished patients. Am. Rev. Respir. Dis., 126:5, 1982.
223. Hunter, A. M. B., Carey, M. A., and Larsh, H. W.: The nutritional status of patients with chronic obstructive pulmonary disease. Am. Rev. Respir. Dis., 124:376, 1981.
224. Rochester, D. F.: Malnutrition and respiratory muscles. Clin. Chest Med., 7:91, 1986.
225. Askanazi, J., et al.: Respiratory changes induced by the large glucose loads of total parenteral nutrition. JAMA, 243:1444, 1980.
226. Covelli, H. D., et al.: Respiratory failure precipitated by high carbohydrate loads. Ann. Intern. Med., 95:579, 1981.
227. MacFie, J., et al.: Effect of the energy source on changes in energy expenditure and respiratory quotient during total parenteral nutrition. JPEN J. Parenter. Enteral Nutr., 7:1, 1983.
228. O'Shea, R.: Altering parenteral nutrition for specific disease states. In Dynamics of Nutrition Support. Edited by S. H. Krey and R. L. Murray. Norwalk, CT, Appleton-Century-Crofts, 1986.
229. Sundstrom, G., Zauner, C. W., and Mans, A.: Decrease in pulmonary diffusing capacity during lipid infusion in healthy men. J. Appl. Physiol., 34:816, 1973.
230. Dahms, B. B., and Halpin, T. C.: Pulmonary arterial lipid deposit in newborn infants receiving intravenous lipid infusion. J. Pediatr., 97:800, 1980.
231. Shulman, R. J., Langston, C., and Schanler, R. J.: Pulmonary vascular lipid deposition after administration of intravenous fat to infants. Pediatrics, 79:99, 1987.
232. Twyman, D., et al.: High protein enteral feedings: a means of achieving positive nitrogen balance in head injured patients. JPEN J. Parenter. Enteral Nutr., 9:679, 1985.
233. Clifton, G. L., et al.: The metabolic response to severe head injury. J. Neurosurg., 60:687, 1984.
234. Detsky, A. S., Baker, J. P., O'Rourke, K., and Goel, V.: Perioperative parenteral nutrition: a meta-analysis. Ann. Intern. Med., 107:195, 1987.
235. Buzby, G. P., et al.: A randomized clinical trial of total parenteral nutrition in malnourished surgical patients: the rationale and impact of previous clinical trials and pilot study on protocol design. Am. J. Clin. Nutr., 47:357, 1988.
236. Buzby, G. P., et al.: Study protocol: a randomized clinical trial of total parenteral nutrition in malnourished surgical patients. Am. J. Clin. Nutr., 47(Suppl. 2):366, 1988.
237. Shaw, J. H. F.: Influence of stress, depletion and/or malignant disease on the responsiveness of surgical patients to total parenteral nutrition. Am. J. Clin. Nutr., 48:144, 1988.
238. Goldstein, S. A., and Elwyn, D. H.: The effects of injury and sepsis on fuel utilization. Annu. Rev. Nutr., 9:445, 1989.
239. Nelson, K. M., and Long, C. L.: Physiological basis for nutrition in sepsis. Nutr. Clin. Pract., 4:6, 1989.
240. Bower, R. H., et al.: Branched chain amino acid-enriched solutions in the septic patient: a randomized, prospective trial. Ann. Surg., 203:13, 1986.

241. Cerra, F. B., et al.: Branched chain metabolic support: a prospective, randomized, double-blind trial in surgical stress. Ann. Surg., *199:*286, 1984.
242. Cameron, I. L., Paulat, W. A., and Urban, E.: Adaptive responses to total intravenous feeding. J. Surg. Res., *17:*45, 1974.
243. Koga, Y., et al.: The digestive tract in total parenteral nutrition. Arch. Surg., *110:*742, 1975.
244. Bastian, C., and Driscoll, R. H.: Enteral tube feeding at home. *In* Enteral and Tube Feeding. Edited by J. L. Rombeau and M. D. Caldwell. Philadelphia, W. B. Saunders, 1984.
245. Steiger, E., et al.: Home parenteral nutrition. *In* Parenteral Nutrition. Edited by J. L. Rombeau and M. D. Caldwell. Philadelphia, W. B. Saunders, 1986.
246. Howard, L., et al.: Four years of North American registry home parenteral nutrition outcome data and their implications for patient management. JPEN J. Parenter. Enteral Nutr., *15:*384, 1991.
247. Marein, C., et al.: Home parenteral nutrition. Nutr. Clin. Pract., *1:*179, 1986.
248. Gulledge, A. D., et al.: Psychosocial issues of home parenteral and enteral nutrition. Nutr. Clin. Pract., *2:*183, 1987.

SUPPLEMENTAL READINGS

Borlase, B. C., et al.: Tolerance to enteral tube feeding diets in hypoalbuminemic critically ill, geriatric patients. Surg. Gynecol. Obstet., *174:*181–188, 1992.

Brasztein, S., et al.: Measured and predicted energy expenditure in critically ill patients. Crit. Care Med., *21:*363–367, 1993.

Claxton, B.: The prognostic inflammatory and nutrition index in traumatized patients receiving enteral nutrition. JPEN J. Parenter. Enteral Nutr., *16:*85–86, 1992.

de Chalain, T. M., et al.: The effect of fuel source on amino acid metabolism in critically ill patients. J. Surg. Res., *52:*1767–1776, 1992.

Gentilello, L. M., et al.: Enteral nutrition with simultaneous gastric decompression in critically ill patients. Crit. Care Med., *21:*392, 1993.

Haglund, U.: Systemic mediators released from the gut in critical illness. Crit. Care Med., *21(Suppl. 2):*515–518, 1993.

Jeevanandan, M., et al.: Substrate efficiency in early nutrition support of critically ill multiple trauma victims. JPEN J. Parenter. Enteral Nutr., *16:*511, 1992.

Kelly, K. G., et al.: Advances in perioperative nutritional support. Med. Clin. North Am., *77:*465–475, 1993.

Kemper, M., et al.: Caloric requirements and supply in critically ill surgical patients. Crit. Care Med., *20:*344–348, 1992.

Kudsk, K. A., et al.: Enteral versus parenteral feeding: effects on septic morbidity after blunt and penetrating abdominal trauma. Ann. Surg., *215:*503–511, 1992.

Levinson, M., et al.: Enteral feeding, gastric colonization and diarrhea in the critically ill patient: is there a relationship? Anaesth. Intens. Care, *21:*85–88, 1993.

Mariam, M., et al.: The failure of conventional methods to prevent spontaneous transpyloric feeding tube passage and the safety of intragastric feeding in critically ill ventilated patients. Surg. Gynecol. Obstet., *176:*475–479, 1993.

McClave, S. A., et al.: Immunonutrition and enteral hyperalimentation of critically ill patients. Dig. Dis. Sci., *37:*1153–1561, 1992.

The Veteran Affairs Total Parenteral Nutrition Cooperative Study Group: Perioperative total parenteral nutrition in surgical patients. N. Engl. J. Med., *325:*525–532, 1991.

Weissman, C., et al.: Assessing hypermetabolism and hypometabolism in the postoperative critically ill patient. Chest, *102:*1566–1571, 1992.

Chapter 63

SEDATION, PAIN RELIEF, AND NEUROMUSCULAR BLOCKADE IN THE CRITICALLY ILL

THOMAS L. HIGGINS
JOSEPH P. COYLE

The management of pain, sedation, and paralysis in the critically ill patient is a significant challenge. These patients are exposed to a variety of noxious stimuli (intubation, mechanical ventilation, line placement, cardioversion, endoscopy), which can trigger a stress response, with autonomic and hormonal sequelae that complicate management and contribute to morbidity. Patients with invasive monitors on mechanical ventilation pose a significant risk to themselves if they thrash and dislodge vital support equipment. Hemodynamically unstable patients are most susceptible to the cardiovascular side effects of opioids, sedatives, and muscle relaxants used to attenuate stress response, keep patients calm, or produce immobility. Dysfunction in other organ systems affects both the pharmacokinetic and pharmacodynamic response to these drugs. Effective control of pain improves patient comfort, facilitates respiratory care, and decreases the stress response to traumatic interventions. With the use of intravenous agents, pharmacologic management in the critically ill patient must be balanced, using specific drugs to achieve specific components of the anesthetic state (Fig. 63-1). By using specific agents for sedation, pain control, paralysis, and control of autonomic reflexes, less total drug is given, which reduces the severity of side effects and allows for quicker emergence when the drugs are discontinued. Before initiating any of these drugs, a careful assessment of the patient should be done to ensure that the patient's agitation or hypertension is not the result of inadequate ventilation, low cardiac output, sepsis, or a specific irritant that might be addressed, such as a distended bladder.

Clinical goals in a critically ill patient include:

- Maintenance of a comfortable, relaxed state and decreasing stress response
- Pain relief during procedures or after surgery
- Preservation of the day-night sleep cycle allowing daytime usefulness for neurologic assessment and cooperation with therapy
- Reduction of barotrauma and facilitation of mechanical ventilation
- Conservation of energy
- Preventing shivering
- Control of agitation, delirium, or withdrawal
- Preventing dislodgment of critical life support devices

Therapeutic goals should be defined for each of the drugs used so therapy can be titrated to achieve the desired effect (Tables 63-1 and 63-2). Although hypertension is a marker of pain in the intubated, neuromuscularly blocked patient, opioid administration should not necessarily become a reflex response to treatment of elevated blood pressure. Care should be taken to distinguish between hypertension caused by pain from that due to a hyperdynamic circulation. Although nonspecific application of an antihypertensive lowers the pressure, optimal care would provide specific pain relief in the first situation and perhaps adrenergic blockade in the second.

The line between sedation and general anesthesia is easily crossed. Thus sedation and pain relief, and particularly use of neuromuscular blocking agents, should be supervised by individuals experienced in airway control and hemodynamic resuscitation and in a location where adequate monitoring of oxygenation and ventilation and the ability to control the airway are immediately available.

RISK PHASE

Population Differences Affecting Pain Response

A number of factors influence the sedation and pain relief needs of patients in the ICU, including age, concurrent drug therapy, smoking and alcohol history, prior experiences, personality traits, and education level and, in operative patients, preoperative teaching, site of operation, and amount of tissue damage that has occurred (Table 63-3). Advancing age is associated with numerous physiologic changes in the central nervous system (CNS),[1] circulatory system,[2] and hepatic and renal systems.[3] Decreases in cardiac output, total body water, lean body mass, and serum albumin affect the distribution of therapeutic agents.[4] Metabolism and excretion of agents in the elderly is delayed by decreased hepatic mass and hepatic blood flow, decreased renal blood flow, glomerular filtration rate, and tubular secretion. In general, the elderly require smaller initial doses of therapeutic agents, more careful titration to effect with subsequent doses, and a close watch for delayed effects as the result of accumulation of active metabolites.

Interactions between multiple therapeutic agents complicate sedative therapy in the critically ill. Investigators suggest that the analgesic effects of opioids such as fen-

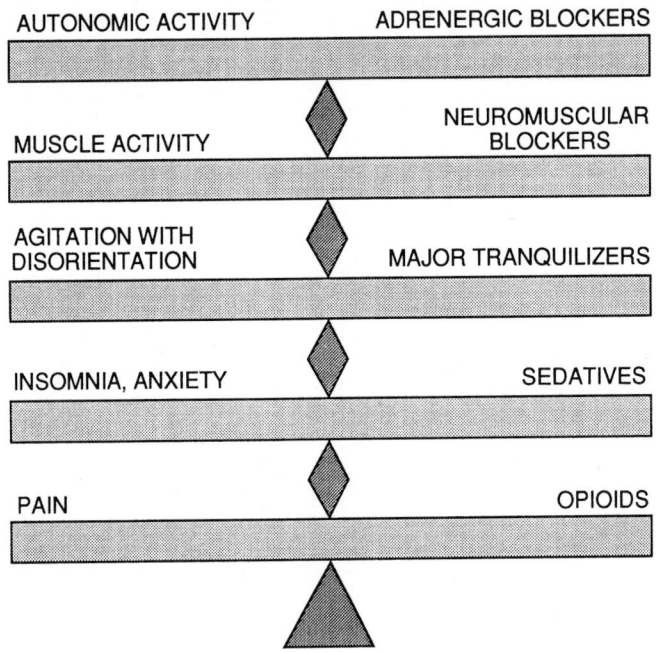

Fig. 63-1. Balanced approach to ICU sedation.

Table 63-2. Indications for Neuromuscular Blockade

Shivering not responsive to other measures
Uncontolled seizure activity
Prevention of barotrauma with high peak ventilation pressures
Facilitation of ventilation
Deliberate hypothermia
Decerebrate rigidity/posturing
Multisystem organ failure

tanyl can be enhanced by alpha-adrenergic agonists such as clonidine and calcium-channel blockers such as verapamil.[5]

Changes in protein binding or body fat that occur during illness may also have an effect on drug requirements. Adaptation to chronic stimulation or blockade occurs with adrenergic agents and opioids. The increasing dosage requirements during therapy with opioids is well recognized; increasing requirements for neuromuscular blocking agents such as vercuronium have also been reported.[6]

Indications for Intervention

Sedation and pain relief are indicated in patients with postoperative pain, severe respiratory failure, systemic sepsis, and shivering on rewarming from anesthesia and in individuals intolerant of the endotracheal tube. Certain procedures in the ICU, such as elective cardioversion, require sedation to the point of general anesthesia. Most postsurgical patients experience some degree of pain, depending in large measure on the operative site, amount of tissue trauma, and effects of residual anesthetic. Although many patients are awakened and extubated in the operating room or shortly after arrival in the recovery room, there is a growing trend to extending anesthetic care and ventilation well into the postoperative period in complex patients, particularly those at risk of ischemia. Some evidence indicates that controlling the stress response in these patients may improve outcome, specifically by reducing the incidence of myocardial infarction.[7] In these patients, a smooth transition is accomplished by extending the effects of anesthetic drugs until the patient has fully rewarmed, is hemodynamically stable, has minimal chest tube drainage (in thoracic cases) and is ready for weaning from mechanical ventilation.

Pain in the critically ill patient has implications beyond the discomfort and psychologic trauma inflicted on the patient because it can play a role in early morbidity. Pain is associated with activation of the sympathetic nervous system, which can lead to hypertension, tachycardia, dysrhythmias, and a greater need for vasodilators. Splinting and ineffective cough as a result of pain can lead to loss of lung volume and subsequent respiratory complications. The stress response to pain includes elevated catecholamines and serum cortisol, which can aggravate metabolic problems and complicate recovery, and pain can interfere with return of gastrointestinal function. In high risk patients undergoing a variety of procedures, effective pain control has been shown to reduce the postoperative complication rate significantly, decrease the incidence of cardiac failure, reduce the infection rate, and shorten hospital stay.[8]

The critically ill patient is faced with an unfamiliar, stressful, often chaotic environment. The typical critically ill, mechanically ventilated patient lacks control over his or her environment, down to such basic bodily functions as eating, elimination, and the ability to take a deep breath. Normal circadian rhythm is disturbed by noise, the effects of medication, and lack of environmental cues, such as

Table 63-1. Indications for Pain Relief in the ICU

Surgical pain
Cancer pain
Diagnosed abdominal pain (i.e., pancreatitis)
Invasive devices (i.e., chest tubes)
Painful procedures
    Debridement, packing, irrigation
    Cardioversion
    Insertion of chest tubes

Table 63-3. Factors Affecting Patient's Response to the ICU Environment

Age
Prior experience
Education level
Personality traits
Neurologic status
Type of illness
Drug and alcohol consumption
Length of time in ICU

Table 63-4. Ramsay Sedation Scale

1. Anxious, agitated, or restless
2. Cooperative, oriented, and tranquil
3. Drowsy but responsive to commands
4. Asleep, brisk response to stimulus
5. Asleep, no response

(Adapted from Ramsay, M. A. E., Savege, T. M., Simpson, B. R. J., and Goodwin, R.: Controlled sedation with alphaxalone-alphadolone. Br. Med. J., 22:656, 1974.)

daylight and regular meals. Sleep loss tires the patient, inhibits cooperation with therapy, and may result in a situational psychosis. With the uncertainties of outcome from a serious medical illness, it is easy to understand why patients in the ICU become anxious, agitated, or even psychotic. Sequelae of anxiety and agitation include tachycardia, hypertension, and difficulty with medical and nursing management. Critically ill patients who are still aware of their surroundings generally benefit from moderate sedation, and sedation becomes mandatory when the patient endangers his or her own care with nonpurposeful movement or agitation to the point of pulling out monitoring lines, chest tubes, or indwelling catheters. Provision of a good night's sleep each evening facilitates restoration of a normal sleep-wake cycle, leaving the patient awake and better able to cooperate with physical and respiratory care during the day. Level of sedation can be quantitated using the scale developed by Ramsay and colleagues (Table 63-4).[9]

Specific Agents

Benzodiazepines and Benzodiazepine Antagonists

The most commonly used sedative/hypnotic medications in the ICU are the benzodiazepines (diazepam, midazolam, and lorazepam) (Table 63-5). These drugs allay anxiety and in higher doses produce sedation and hypnosis by engaging receptors in the brain, which enhance the activity of the neurotransmitter gamma-aminobutyric acid (GABA) in a dose-dependent fashion.[10] Benzodiazepines can be titrated to achieve a level of consciousness from mild anxiolysis to unresponsiveness, although side effects increase with increasing dose. They are most useful in making the patient sedate and comfortable from the time the patient first becomes responsive in the ICU until he or she can be safely extubated. Continued administration after extubation is occasionally required in the extremely anxious patient or the patient with a history of heavy use of alcohol, benzodiazepines, or other sedatives. The benzodiazepines have useful secondary effects in preventing and treating seizures and in relieving muscle spasm.

The most significant problems with benzodiazepine use in the critically ill patient relate to the potential for respiratory depression and to their hemodynamic effects. Both diazepam and midazolam have been shown to decrease blood pressure up to 15% primarily by decreasing systemic vascular resistance with little effect on heart rate or contractility.[11,12] Left ventricular filling pressures decrease, and circulating catecholamine levels are reduced.[13] These effects are transient and not usually deleterious; however, patients who are hypovolemic or those dependent on endogenous catechols to support the circulation may have an exaggerated hemodynamic effect from these drugs. In addition, the combination of benzodiazepines with narcotics has been shown occasionally to lead to significant hypotension as a result of systemic vasodilation, thought to be related to decreased catecholamines.[14]

Respiratory depression with benzodiazepine administration is dose dependent, and although it is not usually a problem in healthy patients, it can be a significant problem

Table 63-5. Sedative/Hypnotics

Drug	Dosing	Comments
Diazepam (Valium)	2.0–5.0 mg q 1–4 h intravenously prn; may be slowly titrated up to 20 mg intravenously	Accumulation with repeated doses; active metabolites Irritating to veins Do not mix or dilute with other drugs
Midazolam (Versed)	0.5–2.0 mg intravenously initial 1.0–4.0 mg/hr infusion	Shorter half-life than diazepam Water-soluble/nonirritating
Lorazepam (Ativan)	1.0–4.0 mg intravenously, 0.5–2 mg orally 2 to 3 times a day	Must be diluted before intravenous use Longer acting (6 to 8 h) Good amnestic Renal excretion—not recommended with renal or hepatic failure
Chlordiazepoxide (Librium)	25–100 mg intravenously/intramuscularly; repeat in 2–4 h p.m. up to 300 mg/24 h	Classically used for alcohol withdrawal Blood dyscrasias reported with protracted use Active metabolites
Propofol	10–100 μg/kg/min by infusion	Short-acting—must be infused Cardiac depressant at high doses Supplied in lipid emulsion, which supports bacterial growth if contaminated
Haloperidol (Haldol)	1.0–2.0 mg intravenously q 4–6 h Much higher in acute delirium	Very long half-life Intravenous usage not FDA approved but supported by literature and clinical experience Useful in delirium Extrapyramidal reactions possible
Droperidol (Inapsine)	0.6–10 mg intravenously Action lasts 2–4 h	Antiemetic at low doses Mild alpha-adrenergic blockade Alteration of alertness for 12–24 h

in the critically ill. Respiratory depression may be accentuated in the elderly, patients with chronic obstructive pulmonary disease,[15] and those who have received narcotics; means to support ventilation should be available when benzodiazepines are administered to these patients. Ventilatory depression can be minimized by slow administration of the drug or titration in small incremental doses until the desired effect is achieved.

Choice of benzodiazepine is usually determined by duration of action, method of clearance of the drug, or route of administration. **Diazepam** has a relatively long clinical duration of action based on its long elimination half-life (2 to 8 days) and the production of several metabolic products that also have hypnotic effects, such as *n*-desmethyl diazepam.[16] Diazepam is administered intravenously in doses of 2.0 to 4.0 mg at intervals of 1 to 4 hours depending on the patient's response. Patients with a history of heavy alcohol or sedative use before their illness may require considerably more drug to achieve the desired response. An important drug interaction to consider in the ICU setting is the antagonism of the sedative effect of benzodiazepines by aminophylline.[17] The initial effects of diazepam are terminated by redistribution of the drug in tissues; with continued administration, the tissues become saturated, and clearance of the drug from the blood becomes dependent on hepatic metabolism with a subsequent prolongation of clinical effect. Diazepam is not water soluble and is available for parenteral administration suspended in propylene glycol; this preparation is irritating to veins and can cause pain on administration via peripheral intravenous lines or when given intramuscularly.

Midazolam is a relatively new water-soluble benzodiazepine with two to three times the potency of diazepam. The clinical duration of action of midazolam is short, based both on redistribution and a higher rate of hepatic and renal clearance than diazepam, with an elimination half-life of approximately 2 hours.[18] Hydroxymidazolam, the primary metabolite of midazolam, does not appear to have clinically significant hypnotic effects. These pharmacologic properties make midazolam an excellent drug for sedation in the ventilator-dependent patient, particularly when used by continuous infusion.[19,20] Midazolom is also an excellent choice as a short-term anesthetic for painful procedures, such as cardioversion.[21] Continuous delivery allows for a more constant blood level, minimizing hemodynamic side effects and allowing for easy titration of the drug based on the patient's level of consciousness. Midazolam is given in incremental doses of 0.5 to 1.0 mg intravenously until the desired effect is achieved, and then an infusion is started at 1.0 to 4.0 mg/hour with subsequent adjustment of the rate based on the patient's responsiveness. In general, patients awaken promptly after discontinuation of the infusion,[22] although prolonged effects of midazolam have been reported in patients with impaired hepatic function and in patients with chronic renal failure.

Other benzodiazepines may be useful in certain select clinical circumstances in the intensive care patient. **Lorazepam** is a potent long-acting benzodiazepine that does not cause pain on injection and does not have active metabolites. Although clearance is not dependent on hepatic microsomal enzymes, lorazepam must be used cautiously with combined hepatic and renal failure. When administered in doses of 2 to 4 mg orally or intramuscularly, patients experience 6 to 8 hours of sedation, making it useful for nighttime sedation in the chronically ventilated patient. **Oxazepam** is an orally available benzodiazepine (and is also a major metabolic product of diazepam) that has sedative properties. The clearance of oxazepam depends entirely on renal elimination, making this a useful drug for sedation in the patient with impaired hepatic function. **Chlordiazepoxide** has been administered intramuscularly in doses of 50 to 200 mg to control the excitatory symptoms associated with alcohol withdrawal, although its use in this setting has been largely replaced by diazepam and midazolam.

Reversal of benzodiazepine sedation can be accomplished in several ways. Nonspecific and less predictable reversal has been reported with the use of physostigmine in doses of 1.0 to 2.0 mg intravenously or with aminophylline in doses of 50 to 100 mg. **Flumazenil** is a specific benzodiazepine receptor antagonist recently released in the United States that when given intravenously consistently reverses sedation within 2 minutes of intravenous administration.[23] The duration of action of flumazenil is somewhat shorter than many of the benzodiazepines, making resedation a possibility particularly when used in benzodiazepine overdose. Physostigmine acts nonspecifically to reverse effects of benzodiazepines and may be used diagnostically in the workup of the somnolent patient.[24] Withdrawal of benzodiazepines should be gradual, to avoid excitatory symptoms similar to those of alcohol withdrawal.[25]

Propofol is a short-acting intravenous anesthetic that is prepared in a lipid emulsion and is rapidly cleared from the circulation and does not result in accumulation. In higher doses (up to 200 μg/kg/min), propofol has been shown to result in significant decreases in systemic arterial blood pressure as a result of myocardial depression in patients with coronary artery disease.[26] When used in low doses (13 μg/kg/min), propofol has been shown to be comparable to midazolam in providing sedation for patients in the ICU after cardiac surgery.[27] In the low dose range, there was no demonstrable effect on hemodynamic performance, and patients receiving propofol had better overall sedation, required less narcotic, needed somewhat less nitroprusside, and awakened promptly on discontinuation of the drug.[28] Concern has been raised about the potential for contamination of the lipid emulsion, and this concern should be addressed to treating propofol with the same degree of caution as total parenteral nutrition solutions, minimizing use of stopclocks in the line, and changing the infusion at regular intervals.

Control of Acute Confusional States

Delirium, or acute confusional state, is a common problem in the ICU, particularly for elderly patients.[29] Risk factors for delirium in hospitalized elderly patients (age >65 years) include prior cognitive impairment, age over 80 years, fracture on admission, symptomatic infection, and male gender.[30] Neuroleptic and narcotic use, but not anticholinergic use, was also independently associated with

Table 63–6. Selected Causes of Agitation

Sepsis
Hypoxia
Cerebral/ischemia
Hypercapnia
Alcohol and sedative withdrawal
Delirium tremens
Hepatic encephalopathy
Uremic encephalopathy
Hypoglycemia
Hyponatremia
Viral encephalitis
Subarachnoid hemorrhage

---

delirium. Delirium may be overlooked in the intubated, ventilated patient until it presents as uncontrolled thrashing, self-extubation, or accidental disconnection of monitoring lines and devices. Common findings in the delirious patient include an acute onset and fluctuating course, inattention, disorganized thinking, altered level of consciousness, disorientation, memory impairment, perceptual disturbances, abnormal psychomotor activity, and altered sleep-wake cycle. Criteria have been established by Inouye and colleagues[31] to provide a simple checklist that enables nonpsychiatric clinicians to detect delirium quickly in high risk settings. The presence of acute onset with a fluctuating course plus inattention, plus either disorganized thinking or an altered level of consciousness, has high sensitivity (>95%), specificity (>90%), and positive predictive accuracy (>91%) when compared with formal validation by psychiatrists.

New onset of agitation requires a quick examination to rule out common, remediable causes (Table 63–6). Occasionally, delirium can be managed with simple reassurance and reorientation of the patient, a process helped by the presence of familiar faces of family or friends. When pharmacologic intervention is required, the choices are antipsychotic and neuroleptic drugs, which include the phenothiazines or butyrophenones.

Phenothiazines

The phenothiazines act by antagonizing dopamine-mediated neurotransmission at CNS synapses. Reduction of psychotic symptoms is accompanied by anxiolysis, reduced initiative, and blunted emotions, with preservation of higher intellectual function and spinal reflexes. Reduced neurotransmission at the basal ganglia produces extrapyramidal effects, and partial alpha-adrenergic blocking activity and muscarinic blockade can interfere with inotropic and vasoactive drugs commonly used in the ICU setting. Orthostatic hypotension and reflex tachycardia are common after intravenous administration of phenothiazines. The electrocardiogram may be altered with prolonged QT and RR intervals and nonspecific ST-T wave changes.

The phenothiazines can be thought of as psychic filters, which both sedate and reduce sensory overload, leaving the patient better able to focus on reality without conflicting, nonsensical messages. The therapeutic index of these agents is unfortunately narrow. **Chlorpromazine** (Thorazine), the prototypical phenothiazine, may be administered intravenously, beginning with 2-mg doses at 2-minute intervals, titrating to desired effect. Intramuscular administration requires a much larger dose (25 to 50 mg initially with up to 400 mg daily) and a longer time to effect. Other available major tranquilizers, including **thiethylperazine** (Torecan) and **prochlorperazine** (Compazine) are typically used more for antiemetic effects than antipsychotic effects.

Butyrophenones

The butyrophenones, haloperidol and droperidol, are neuroleptic agents rather than true antipsychotics. The butyrophenones have minimal CNS, cardiac, and respiratory depressive effects and blunt spontaneous movement without producing marked incoordination or ataxia. In contrast to the phenothiazines, which can precipitate seizures, the butyrophenones do not appear to increase seizure activity, making them useful in head trauma patients and in the setting of acute alcohol withdrawal.[32] Both drugs are metabolized in the liver, with mostly inactive metabolites excreted in the urine.

Haloperidol (Haldol) has effective calming and sleep-inducing effects useful in the agitated critically ill patient. Its precise method of action is unknown but likely involved alterations of neurotransmitter reuptake and blunting of catecholamine receptor response in the midbrain. The package insert for the drug describes oral and intramuscular uses, but intravenous use is accepted practice[33] in the ICU, where intramuscular absorption may be unreliable. Using the intravenous route, haloperidol can be administered in increasing doses starting with 2 mg, doubling the dose with repeated administration every 15 to 20 minutes until the symptoms of delirium are controlled. One half of the total dose used to achieve initial control can then be given either at bedtime or with return of agitation. If a third dose is needed, one quarter of the initial total dose can be administered. Subsequent doses of 2 to 4 mg at bedtime then facilitate sleep. Although this dosage schedule has not been approved by the Food and Drug Administration (FDA), it seems to provide superior early response, while avoiding the late oversedation seen when small amounts are given at 6-hour intervals. Haloperidol has a long duration of action, with an elimination half-life of up to 35 hours, making a daily bedtime dose practical once control of symptoms has been achieved.

The most common side effect of haloperidol is extrapyramidal reactions, which usually occur early in treatment and may be manifest as Parkinson-like symptoms, drowsiness, or lethargy. These symptoms are generally mild and rapidly reversible with withdrawal of the drug. Other complications—oculogyric crisis, torticollis, trismus—are dose related and easily treated with diphenhydramine (Benadryl) and uncommonly seen in the ICU setting. Tardive dyskinesia, which has no effective treatment if it occurs, fortunately appears to be unusual in the ICU setting. Neuroleptic malignant syndrome, a rare, potentially fatal idiosyncratic reaction to antipsychotic medications, is characterized by fever, muscle rigidity, autonomic dysfunction, and altered consciousness. It may be misdiagnosed as sepsis syndrome and can be complicated by rhabdomyolysis.

If the syndrome is promptly recognized, it responds to discontinuing the offending agent, hydration, supportive care, and administration of dantrolene sodium.

Droperidol (Inapsine), an anxiolytic closely related to haloperidol, is often used in combination with fentanyl for neuroleptic anesthesia. Its antiemetic and sedative effects are greater than those of haloperidol, but the chances of extrapyramidal effects are similar.[34] Droperidol in doses of 0.6 to 6.0 mg intravenously causes a state of indifference to environmental stimuli, dysphoria, and a sensation of restlessness, which may be manifest as akathisia (inability to hold still). It is an unpleasant drug to receive when given alone but in combination with a narcotic or benzodiazepine provides useful anxiolysis within 10 minutes, with sedative effects for 2 to 4 hours and altered consciousness for 12 hours or longer. The respiratory effects of droperidol are minimal, but its alpha-adrenergic blocking activity affects the cardiovascular system.

Barbiturates

The barbiturates cause dose-related CNS depression, respiratory depression, and cardiac depression, with no analgesic or even hyperalgesic effect. Respiratory depression is produced by loss of CNS, hypercapnic, and eventually hypoxic respiratory drives.[35] Cardiovascular effects at low doses are minimal, but hypotension may be seen in hypertensive patients. Higher doses of barbiturates diminish cardiac output and provoke hemodynamic instability. Duration of action varies from very short to very long. Short-acting agents such as thiopental sodium (Pentothal; 3 to 5 mg/kg intravenously) or methohexital (Brevital; 1 mg/kg intravenously) are primarily used as anesthetic induction agents for dressing changes or cardioversion. Medium-acting agents such as pentobarbital (Nembutal) or phenobarbital may be used in an initial adult dose of 30 mg for sedation or 100 mg for sleep. Longer-acting agents, such as phenobarbital, 150 to 300 mg, are preferred as anticonvulsants or for inducing barbiturate coma. Hypotension is a common sequela of intravenous barbiturate administration, and these agents have by and large been supplanted by the benzodiazepines for ICU use except for induction of anesthesia and the specific indication of barbiturate coma.

Barbiturate coma has been extensively used to reduce elevated intracranial pressure secondary to head trauma or hemorrhagic stroke despite controversy about its effect on outcome. The underlying concept is to give enough barbiturate to reduce cerebral metabolism (and thus cerebral oxygen consumption) during a period of compromised perfusion. Because the doses of barbiturate necessary to accomplish electroencephalogram evidence of diminished activity are also likely to cause reductions in cardiac output and blood pressure, this therapy is a double-edged sword and should be used with full hemodynamic and intracranial pressure monitoring. In the critically ill, barbiturates are best avoided except for the specific indication listed because the hyperalgesic effect seen with low doses may cause excitement, restlessness, or delirium, and the hemodynamic instability makes high dose therapy more difficult to control.

PAIN CONTROL

Patterns of pain vary greatly in different intensive care units depending on the patient population. Narcotic needs are typically less in the elderly medical patient than in the young trauma patient. The pattern of pain after median sternotomy and cardiac surgery can be surprisingly benign by virtue of forces contributing to pain, the effects of intraoperative high dose narcotic anesthesia, and factors related to the patient profile. Pain after median sternotomy itself may be somewhat less than pain after major abdominal or thoracic surgery owing to fixation of the sternotomy with wires resulting in less movement of the incision. More troublesome pain may be secondary to chest or mediastinal tubes,[36] musculoskeletal trauma from sternal spread, the site of internal mammary dissection, or the leg wounds when saphenous veins are harvested. Most often, the sum total of these sources contributes to overall patient discomfort.[37]

A variety of **routes of administration** are available for analgesic drugs, including intravenous, intramuscular, oral, transcutaneous, intrathecal, and epidural. The route chosen depends on the drug to be given, the degree of pain, and the portals available. This discussion is limited to the parenteral and peridural use of commonly used narcotics targeted for opiate receptors in the brain and spinal cord and the parenteral nonsteroidal drug ketorolac. **Opiate** receptors have been identified in many places throughout the neuraxis, particularly the substantia gelatinosa of the spinal cord and the periaqueductal gray area of the midbrain; they are also found in other tissues, such as the adrenal medulla and the gastrointestinal tract.[38] A number of different types of opiate receptors have been identified (mu$_1$, mu$_2$, kappa, sigma, delta, and epsilon), which have varying affinity for different endogenous and exogenous ligands and modulate many of the effects associated with opiate administration, such as analgesia, euphoria, dysphoria, respiratory depression, dependence, and vasomotor stimulation.

Parenteral Narcotics

The opioids most commonly used as parenteral narcotics in the critically ill patient are listed in Table 63-7. **Morphine** produces reliable analgesia in a dose-dependent manner as well as providing some sedation and euphoria. It is considered a relatively long-acting narcotic with an analgesic effect lasting 3 to 5 hours after a 10-mg dose intramuscularly. When given intramuscularly, peak blood

Table 63–7. Narcotics

Drug	Dosing	Comments
Morphine	5.0–10.0 mg IM q3–4 h	Vasodilation
	2.0–4.0 mg/h IV	Effective by patient-controlled analgesia
Meperidine	50–75 mg IM	Effective for shivering
	25–50 mg IV	Less biliary spasm
Fentanyl	50–100 μg IV bolus	Hemodynamic stability
	50–200 μg/h by drip	Rigidity possible
Sufentanil	1.0 μg/kg/h by drip	Shorter half-life than fentanyl

levels are attained in 15 to 20 minutes; in the blood, morphine is rapidly redistributed to tissues and converted by the liver to the glucuronide, which is renally excreted with an elimination half-life of 2 to 3 hours.[39] Blood levels of morphine do not appear to correlate with analgesic effect, with passage into and out of the blood-brain barrier being the major determinant of clinical effect.[40] Like all opiates, morphine is a potent respiratory depressant with a relatively narrow therapeutic window. Morphine has little effect on myocardial performance and produces vasodilation in systemic venous, arterial, and pulmonary vascular beds by both a direct effect on smooth muscle and an indirect effect via histamine release.[41] The clinical effect is a net reduction in afterload and preload with no effect on contractility, making morphine a useful adjunct in the management of congestive heart failure. Secondary effects of morphine that can limit usefulness include decreased gastrointestinal motility, biliary spasm, nausea and vomiting, urinary retention, and pruritus.

Intermittent intramuscular or intravenous dosing of morphine can lead to peaks and valleys in both the desired analgesic effect and the hemodynamic, respiratory depressant, and other side effects of the drug. Continuous infusion or **patient-controlled analgesia** (PCA), with smaller, more frequent doses administered by the patient, has been shown to lead to better analgesia with fewer side effects and less total drug.[42] PCA with morphine or meperidine has been shown to be effective in both the trauma setting and in postoperative patients. Effective use of PCA requires a cooperative patient with the ability to understand the use of the pump and carry out the maneuvers to self-administer the narcotic. In hemodynamically unstable patients who are unable to use PCA, such as the patient on an intra-aortic balloon, the use of continuous infusion of morphine can allow for excellent control of analgesia without the alternating periods of hypertension and hypotension that often accompany intermittent dosing.

Meperidine is a synthetic opioid with approximately one tenth the potency of morphine and a slightly shorter clinical duration of action. Meperidine is metabolized by the liver into several active and inactive metabolites that are renally excreted. In the presence of renal disease, meperidine metabolites may accumulate. Normeperidine, the major breakdown product of meperidine, is a proconvulsant that can cause tremors, myoclonus, or grand mal seizures.[43] The hemodynamic effects of meperidine include a slight increase in heart rate as a result of its anticholinergic effect with little direct effect on contractility or vascular tone in the usual clinical doses. At higher doses, meperidine can exhibit significant myocardial depression. Meperidine has less effect on biliary tone than morphine and may produce less depression of gastrointestinal function. Meperidine has been shown to have a specific effect on decreasing the severity of shivering associated with the administration of amphotericin,[44] and in doses of 25 to 50 mg intravenously, it appears to be useful in decreasing the intensity of shivering in postoperative surgical patients who are actively rewarming.

Fentanyl and sufentanil are extremely potent synthetic opioids that have gained widespread use in cardiac anesthesia by virtue of their ability to produce profound analgesia and modest sedation with minimal effects on hemodynamic performance, producing only modest increases in vagal tone.[41] Fentanyl in doses of 2 to 5 µg/kg intravenously can provide analgesia for 60 to 90 minutes in intubated surgical patients, and continuous infusion of fentanyl at 2 to 5 µg/kg per hour are useful in maintaining analgesia in patients who are hemodynamically unstable and intolerant of the transient hypotension occasionally seen with other narcotics. Fentanyl is a lipid-soluble drug whose short clinical duration of action depends on redistribution of the drug to tissues. When patients have received large doses of fentanyl in the operating room, the tissues become saturated, and clearance becomes dependent on hepatic elimination with a markedly prolonged duration of analgesia, respiratory depression, and sedation. Delayed respiratory depression after large doses of fentanyl has been reported, possibly owing to tissue release and possibly owing to sequestration in the acid medium of the stomach with subsequent reabsorption from the small intestine.[45] Clearance of fentanyl may also be prolonged in the elderly[46] and in patients receiving beta blockers.[47] An additional problem with fentanyl relates to its ability to induce musculoskeletal rigidity in some patients, which can interfere with effective ventilation, and tolerance to the analgesic effect has been seen in the ICU population.[48] Sufentanil is more potent than fentanyl, with a slightly shorter duration of action with a similar profile of hemodynamic effects and side effects. Sufentanil has been shown to have slightly less respiratory depression than fentanyl and somewhat longer duration of analgesia. Fentanyl and sufentanil have analgesic and anxiolytic effects, useful in bolus administration just before painful procedures. For long-term use, the sedative action is less than the analgesic action, and combination with benzodiazepine is often used. The sum effect of opioids with benzodiazepine is greater than either drug alone, particularly with reference to hemodynamic changes.[49] Other factors influencing opioid pharmacokinetics are listed in Table 63-8.

Agonist/antagonist narcotic agents may be useful in the critically ill; however, their use has been limited by their potential for producing dysphoria and deleterious hemodynamic effects, such as elevated pulmonary vascular resistance and systemic hypertension.[50,51] Specific indications include patients who are particularly susceptible to the respiratory depressant effects of pure opioid agonist narcotics; in that setting, butorphanol in a dose of 2 mg intravenously or intramuscularly produces analgesic comparable to morphine with only modest depression of venti-

Table 63-8. Factors Influencing Narcotic Pharmacokinetics

Age (increased sensitivity in elderly)
Acid-base status (increased arterial pH increases brain penetration)
Cardiopulmonary bypass (prolongs elimination half-life)
Liver disease
Renal disease (active metabolites may accumulate)
Other CNS depressants
Acute and chronic tolerance

lation. Nalbuphine in doses of 1 to 10 mg partially reverses respiratory depression associated with fentanyl, while maintaining a stable level of analgesia. In the setting of life-threatening respiratory depression or when neurologic status must be acutely assessed, naloxone may be used specifically to reverse CNS depression associated with narcotics; however, extreme care must be taken with its use. Acute reversal of narcotics with naloxone can be accompanied by extreme agitation, severe hypertension, dysrhythmias, hypertension, cardiac failure, and cardiac arrest.[52-54] Reversal is best accomplished with small incremental doses of naloxone (20 to 40 μg at a time) in a monitored setting until the desired effect is achieved.

Peridural Narcotics

Experience in surgical patients has demonstrated that placing opioids in the vicinity of opiate receptors in the substantia gelatinosa of the spinal cord by intrathecal or epidural administration allows for superior pain control without sedation, respiratory depression, and hemodynamic sequelae seen with parenteral administration. A growing body of information supports the use of the peridural route of administration in high risk patients to provide superior analgesia, with less sedation, less decrement in pulmonary function,[55] less requirement for vasodilators,[56] and a decreased stress response.[57] Morphine has been used intrathecally in doses of 0.5 to 4.0 mg with effective analgesia for up to 36 hours after a single dose; doses above 1.0 mg do not appear to increase the quality of analgesia but do increase the incidence and degree of respiratory depression.[58] Morphine, fentanyl, and meperidine[59] have all been used in the epidural space with similar results. Epidural narcotics may be used alone or combined with local anesthetics (Table 63-9). Catheters may be placed in either the thoracic or lumbar epidural space with equal effectiveness as long as sufficiently large volumes are administered via the lumbar route.

Table 63-9. Drugs Used in the Epidural Space

Drug	Concentration	Comments
Local Anesthetic		
Bupivacaine	0.0625 to 0.125%	Numbness and weakness at higher concentrations Sympathectomy with high thoracic level
Lidocaine	1.5% usually used as test loading dose	
Narcotic		
Fentanyl	2–10 μg/ml	Analgesia without neural blockade Pruritus Nausea Urinary retention Side effects reversible with systemic naloxone
Morphine (Duramorph)	0.04 mg/ml by infusion 2–10 mg by bolus q 8–12 h	Same as above Only preservative-free preparations should be used

Placement of the epidural catheter should be accomplished by an anesthesiologist experienced in the technique. Pain relief may be more effective if the first dose of epidural analgesic is given in the operating room, before systemic anesthesia and analgesia has dissipated. Complications of the catheter include migration into an epidural vein or the subarachnoid space. Therefore, before each dose of epidural narcotics, the placement of the catheter should be checked by aspiration. Before the first dose, and whenever there is a question about catheter location, a **test dose** of 3 ml of 2% lidocaine mixed with epinephrine 1:100,000 should be given. If the catheter is subarachnoid, a moderate spinal level results, and if the catheter is intravascular, tachycardia is noted from the epinephrine. If both tests are negative, analgesic or anesthetic agents are given in a total volume of 5 to 15 ml (depending on operative site and level of epidural placement). Careful attention must be paid to keeping the injection part of the catheter sterile. If there is any doubt about proper placement of the catheter, the test dose is repeated or the catheter removed and replaced. Preservative-free morphine, being less lipophilic, can cause respiratory depression as late as 6 hours after the epidural dose, so monitoring must extend well past the final dose. There is less concern of late effects when using fentanyl as the epidural narcotic agent. Epidural narcotics may also be given by continuous infusion. A common protocol for continuous infusion is to dilute bupivacaine with fentanyl and saline to achieve a final concentration of 0.0625% bupivacaine and 5 μg/ml of fentanyl. This mixture can be infused at 4 to 12 ml per hour depending on patient size and site of desired pain relief. Side effects of this mode of administration include infrequent respiratory depression, which is reversible with intravenous naloxone, without reversing analgesia and without the untoward side effects seen with naloxone in other settings. Occasional but less troublesome side effects include pruritus, urinary retention, and nausea and vomiting, which can also be mitigated with naloxone. More research needs to be done in this area to define which patients will most benefit from these interventions and how best to apply them in the critically ill.

Intercostal Nerve Blocks

Post-thoracotomy pain is effectively relieved and respiratory function improved by placing local anesthetic along the neurovascular bundle at the low rib margin of the incision level and two intraspaces above and below that level.[60] The patient is positioned prone with a pillow under the midabdomen, laterally, or leaning over the bedside table, to increase the size of the intercostal spaces and to widen the distance between the scapula and the midline. To include the lateral cutaneous division of the intercostal nerve, the block must be performed at or posterior to the midaxillary line (about four fingerbreadths from the spine). Under sterile conditions, 30 ml of local anesthetic is drawn up in three 10-ml syringes. The patient's back is prepared with a sterile iodine-containing solution, and a 1.5-inch, 23-gauge needle is gently walked off the lower rib border. After aspirating for blood, 3 to 5 ml of local anesthetic is used to the point of entry for the chest tubes. Either lidocaine (1 to 2%) or bupivacaine (0.25 to 0.5%) may be used, with epinephrine added to prolong duration if the patient is free of significant heart disease.

This technique is best suited to patients with lateral chest wall incisions and chest tubes after lobectomy because effective pain relief results in better expansion of the remaining lung segments. Intercostal nerve blocks may also be used after pneumonectomy, but the benefit of pain relief must be balanced against the potential of introducing infection into a devascularized closed space. Cutaneous infection at the site of entry is a contraindication to intercostal nerve block. Duration of pain relief varies with choice of anesthetic, but most patients require retreatment at 8 to 12 hours even with long-acting bupivacaine. Potential adverse effects include:

- Local anesthetic toxicity
- Inadvertent intravascular injection
- Injection directly into the nerve
- Pneumothorax

The most common problem encountered in inexperienced hands is incomplete block owing to misplacement of the anesthetic.

Other Methods of Pain Relief

Interpleural catheters have been used as a conduit for local anesthetic solutions to relieve both post-thoracotomy pain and visceral abdominal pain.[61] Potential complications of this technique include loss of anesthetic via chest tubes and local anesthetic toxicity. Clinicians should also be aware that preoperative instruction and postoperative encouragement from the medical and nursing staff go a long way toward reducing the need for postoperative analgesia.[62]

Ketorolac tromethamine is a recently released potent parenteral nonsteroidal analgesic without opioid-related side effects, such as respiratory depression.[63] Intramuscular doses of 30 to 90 mg appear to be equivalent to 12 mg of morphine or 100 mg of meperidine for up to 3 hours after administration.[64] Ketorolac has an elimination half-life of 5 to 6 hours, with clinical dosing every 8 hours effective in most circumstances. Advantages of ketorolac include potent analgesia without respiratory or hemodynamic side effects and minimal sedation and nausea. Gastrointestinal function may recover more rapidly than with opioids. Disadvantages appear to be a ceiling effect similar to that seen with agonist/antagonist drugs and the potential for impaired platelet function and gastrointestinal mucosal breakdown seen with other nonsteroidal analgesics. It is probably best to avoid ketorolac in patients with a history of allergy to aspirin products. Other non-narcotic options for pain relief include rectal indomethacin[65] and enteral ibuprofen.[66]

NEUROMUSCULAR BLOCKING AGENTS

The use of muscle relaxants is generally relegated to situations in which sedative/hypnotics or narcotics have not been sufficient to keep the patient immobile in the presence of invasive devices, especially when the patient becomes a threat to himself or herself from agitation and movement. This scenario most often occurs in the hemodynamically unstable patient who may tolerate only low doses of sedatives or narcotics and requires mechanical ventilation and invasive monitoring. The use of relaxants may also be indicated to allow for adequate ventilation of patients in whom activity of the chest wall muscles is interfering with ventilation or when high peak airway pressures (greater than 50 to 60 cm H_2O) make barotrauma a risk. Muscle relaxation may also be indicated to control severe shivering during rewarming or to facilitate invasive procedures, such as intubation or bronchoscopy. Clinically available muscle relaxants induce paralysis by blocking acetylcholine receptors at the neuromuscular junction in skeletal muscle, and they have no intrinsic sedative or narcotic properties and therefore must be used in concert with other medications. Relaxants should be titrated to minimal patient movement, or their use should be monitored with a peripheral nerve stimulator to prevent overdosage.

The paralyzed patient requires full mechanical ventilation and ventilator disconnects can be disastrous (Table 63-10). Careful monitoring of ventilation should be used, and means to support the airway, such as a bag and mask, should be at the bedside. The use of paralysis removes the patient's ability to communicate, protect himself or herself from noxious stimuli, and perform simple but important maneuvers such as coughing, swallowing, and blinking. Care must be taken to reassure patients, provide sedation, protect the eyes, turn frequently, and suction secretions from the oropharynx and trachea (Table 63-11). The risk of pressure necrosis can be minimized by placing paralyzed patients on an air mattress or specialized ICU bed. The paralyzed patient is unable to communicate physical discomfort, such as dyspnea, chest pain, or abdominal pain, which may have important clinical implications, and physical examination can become unreliable because neu-

Table 63-10. Hazards of Neuromuscular Blockade in the ICU

Ventilator disconnect
Hemodynamic changes
Pressure necrosis
Corneal drying
Inability to communicate
Ability to hear bedside conversations

Table 63-11. Checklist Before Instituting Neuromuscular Blockade

Determine minute ventilation adequate to prevent hypercarbia and acidosis
Increase ventilator support to compensate for loss of patient's spontaneous ventilation
Have appropriate monitors available:
   Train-of-four nerve stimulator, ventilator disconnect alarm pulse oximeter and end-tidal CO_2
Reassure and instruct patient
Provide adequate sedation

Table 63-12. Clinical Signs of Inadequate Sedation in a Neuromuscularly Blocked Patient

Dilated pupils
Copious tears
Diaphoresis
Tachycardia
Systemic hypertension
Elevated pulmonary artery pressure
Ineffective/thrashing movement

rologic examination is impossible, and peritoneal signs cannot be elicited. The ability to mount a temperature elevation in the presence of sepsis may be impaired by prevention of shivering caused by paralysis. Most importantly, the patient may not be able to signal distress and must rely on the clinician to detect inadequate sedation (Table 63-12).

Depolarizing Relaxants

Choice of muscle relaxants is usually based on duration of action, hemodynamic side effects, and mode of excretion of the drug (Table 63-13).[67] **Succinylcholine** is the only clinically available depolarizing muscle relaxant, engaging the acetylcholine receptor and activating it with a subsequent blocking effect. This is clinically manifest as muscular contraction in the form of fasciculations with subsequent paralysis. Succinylcholine has the advantage of having the most rapid onset (45 to 60 seconds) and shortest duration of action (5 to 15 minutes) of the relaxants, making it ideal for emergency endotracheal intubation. The disadvantages of succinylcholine stem from muscular contraction occurring with onset of the drug, which can cause release of potassium from cells thus increasing serum potassium. This is usually of little consequence in most patients with potassium increases of 0.5 mEq/L; however, patients with burns, head injuries, or other neurologic problems may have exaggerated increases in potassium with resultant cardiac arrest. Fasciculations can also result in increased intra-abdominal pressure and regurgitation, increased intracranial and intraocular pressure, and muscle pain. The secondary effects of fasciculation can all be minimized by pretreatment with a small dose of a nondepolarizing muscle relaxant (commonly 3 mg of D-tubocurarine), which reduces the severity of fasciculations. Succinylcholine is also capable of activating muscarinic acetylcholine receptors with resultant bradycardia, particularly in children and on repeat dosing in adults; this can be prevented by pretreatment with atropine. Succinylcholine is rapidly cleared from the blood by plasma cholinesterase; in certain patients with hereditary or drug-induced abnormalities of plasma cholinesterase, the duration of action of succinylcholine may be markedly prolonged.

Nondepolarizing Relaxants

Nondepolarizing muscle relaxants are most commonly used in the intensive care setting. These drugs are competitive antagonists of acetylcholine at the neuromuscular junction and have no agonist activity; therefore they do not produce fasciculations. The most commonly used drugs in this class are the medium-duration relaxants vecuronium and atracurium and the long-acting agents pancuronium, metocurine (Metubine), D-tubocurarine, and recently released long-acting drugs pipecuronium and doxacurium.

Vecuronium has been popular as a relaxant in this setting because of its relatively short duration of action, and it has no hemodynamic side effects in clinical doses.[67] It is usually given with a loading dose of 0.1 mg/kg with subsequent doses of 2 to 4 mg every 30 to 45 minutes or a continuous infusion of 3 to 6 mg per hour.[68] Vecuronium is metabolized by the liver and renally excreted and does appear to accumulate over time, and prolonged infusion has been shown to lead to prolonged paralysis in a few patients with hepatic or renal compromise.[69] **Atracurium** has a duration of action that is similar to that of vecuronium and a method of clearance from the blood that is unique; it undergoes hydrolysis by esterases in the blood as well as spontaneous breakdown by a process called Hoffman elimination. Atracurium therefore has the advantage of

Table 63-13. Muscle Relaxants

Drug	Intubating Dose	Infusion	Comments
Succinylcholine	1.0–1.5 mg/kg	Not recommended owing to phase II block with infusion	Hyperkalemia, bradycardia with repeat dose. Prolonged effect with atypical plasma cholinesterase activity
Mivacurium	0.15–0.2 mg/kg bolus	0.25–0.6 mg/kg/hr	
Vercuronium	0.07–0.1 mg/kg	0.06–0.14 mg/kg/hr	Minimal hemodynamic effects, accumulation with infusion
Atracurium	0.3–0.6 mg/kg	0.4–0.6 mg/kg/hr	Cleared by Hoffman elimination, slight risk of histamine release
Pancuronium	0.06–0.1 mg/kg	Repeat intubating dose q1–2h based on clinical response	Medium duration of action, tachycardia (vagolytic effect)
Doxacurium	0.03–0.05 mg/kg	Repeat intubating dose q1–3h based on clinical response	Medium-to-long action, minimal hemodynamic effects
Pipercuronium	0.06–0.1 mg/kg	Repeat intubating dose q1–3h based on clinical response	Medium-to-long action, minimal hemodynamic effects
Metocurine	0.3 mg/kg	Not recommended	Renal excretion, histamine release
D-Tubocurarine	0.5–0.6 mg/kg	0.1–0.15 mg/kg/hr	Likely to accumulate, hypotension, histamine release

being independent of renal and hepatic function and is useful in patients with impaired function in these systems.[70] It is given in a loading dose of 0.3 to 0.4 mg/kg followed by a continuous infusion of 0.4 to 0.7 mg/kg per hour.[71] The drawbacks to the use of atracurium are its expense, and it can infrequently cause hypotension owing to histamine release with bolus administration. Laudaunosine, a breakdown product of atracurium, can cause CNS activation and seizures in the laboratory setting, although this has never been shown to be a problem in clinical use in intensive care.

Pancuronium has a long history of use as a muscle relaxant in critically ill patients. It has a relatively long duration of action (60 to 90 minutes from an intubating dose), and it can be cleared both by hepatic elimination and renal clearance with modest prolongation of effect in patients with impairment in one or the other organ system.[72] Pancuronium is given as a loading dose of 0.1 mg/kg, which can be followed by intermittent dosing of 2 to 4 mg per hour or continuous infusion of 2 to 4 mg per hour. The major limiting factor to the use of pancuronium is tachycardia, particularly with bolus administration; this results from a vagolytic effect of the drug as well as a release of endogenous catecholamines.[73] D-Tubocurarine is another long-acting relaxant with a long history of use in critical care, although its use has been largely supplanted by other relaxants with less hemodynamic side effects. D-Tubocurarine can cause significant hypotension owing to histamine release and ganglionic blockade; this can usually be avoided by slow administration of the drug.[73] **Metocurine** is chemically related to D-tubocurarine, is twice as potent, has a similar duration of action, and causes less hypotension. Metocurine can also cause hypotension from histamine release with bolus administration and is entirely dependent on renal excretion with a markedly prolonged effect in patients with compromised renal function.

The two recently released long-acting nondepolarizing muscle relaxants pipecuronium and doxacurium may become useful in the critical care setting. These drugs have a duration of action of up to 100 minutes and little or no effect on hemodynamics. **Pipecuronium** is an agent with structural similarity to pancuronium and vecuronium; doses of 70 to 100 μg/kg result in effective paralysis in 3 minutes lasting up to 70 minutes with no effect on heart rate or blood pressure.[74] **Doxacurium** in doses of 50 to 80 μg/kg provides relaxation for up to 100 minutes with no effect on hemodynamics.[75]

In most clinical circumstances, neuromuscular function is restored by simply discontinuing the drug and waiting until the relaxant effect has dissipated; however, reversal of neuromuscular blockade can be accomplished acutely by administering anticholinesterase drugs, which increase the amount of acetylcholine available at the end plate and overcome competitive blockade. The reversal agents have potent muscarinic side effects (bradycardia, bronchoconstriction, bronchorrhea, and increased bowel motility) and must be administered concurrently with a vagolytic drug. Neostigmine, an anticholinesterase, can be used in this fashion in a dose of 0.03 to 0.07 mg/kg given with atropine 0.8 mg per milligram of neostigmine administered. The adequacy of reversal can be assessed by use of a peripheral

Table 63-14. Factors Potentiating the Action of Neuromuscular Blocking Agents

Respiratory acidosis
Metabolic alkylosis
Hypokalemia
Hyponatremia
Hypocalcemia
Hypermagnesemia
Preexisting neurologic disease, particularly myasthenia gravis
Antiarrhythmics
Antibiotics, particularly aminoglycosides

nerve stimulator demonstrating sustained tetanus and minimal fade on train-of-four stimulation. Clinical adequacy of reversal can be assessed by bedside spirometry and the ability to sustain a head lift for longer than 5 seconds. Common clinical conditions, such as the use of aminoglycosides, may potentiate the effect of neuromuscular blocking agents (Table 63-14). Extreme prolongation of neuromuscular blockade, possibly owing to neurogenic atrophy, can occur.[76] For this reason, it is our clinical practice to stop neuromuscular blocking agents periodically to allow return of neuromuscular function.

Induced Hypothermia

Patients with severe respiratory failure may reach a point at which, despite toxic levels of oxygen, high levels of positive end-expiratory pressure, and various adjustments in ventilatory pattern, adequate tissue oxygenation cannot be sustained. Evidence of this state would include A-aDo$_2$ (alveolar-arterial oxygen difference) of 500 mm Hg or more or shunt greater than 40% on 100% oxygen. Initial efforts should include reduction of fever, avoidance of overfeeding, and appropriate sedation. Further decreases in metabolism can be achieved by deliberate cooling to temperatures of about 32°C. This mode of therapy is controversial and is justified primarily as a means of buying time by reducing oxygen consumption and carbon dioxide production while any reversible processes are treated or spontaneous improvement in lung function occurs. Cooling may also be used in the treatment of massive bronchopleural fistulas to reduce the inspired oxygen concentration to less than 60% to delay oxygen toxicity. Induced hypothermia is of unproven efficacy with regard to outcome and introduces many potential complications, including a rise in systemic vascular resistance, hyperglycemia, increased blood viscosity, left-sided shift of the oxygen-hemoglobin dissociation curve, acid-based abnormalities, masking of febrile response to infection, decreased gastric motility, and inability to assess mental status.

Hypothermia is accomplished in a patient on full ventilatory support by first inducing sleep with opioids, propofol, barbiturates, or benzodiazepines and then inducing neuromuscular blockade to prevent shivering. With the patient placed on a cooling blanket, the temperature is gradually lowered to approximately 32°C. At this temperature, oxygen consumption and carbon dioxide production decrease by 40 to 50%, with minimal hemodynamic instability.

Lower temperatures offer little additional benefit but increase the risk of ventricular irritability and hemodynamic instability because there appears to be a "switch-off" of the adrenergic system at around 29°C.[77] Monitoring of temperature is essential, using core temperature measured from the thermistor tip of the pulmonary artery catheter when available or posterior nasopharyngeal, esophageal, rectal, or thermocouple-containing Foley catheter temperature probes.

While in a hypothermic state, the patient needs appropriate protection against pressure sores, nerve injury, stress ulceration, and eye trauma. All signs of intracranial, intra-abdominal, or intrathoracic catastrophe may be masked, so special vigilance is needed, particularly in looking for pneumothorax. Surveillance cultures must be drawn daily because the patient is unable to mount a hyperthermic response to infection. Rewarming is attempted as soon as clinical conditions permit and is best achieved by passive rewarming while maintaining sedation.

FUTURE DIRECTIONS

Many new drugs and novel routes of administration have greatly increased our ability to improve patient comfort and safety in the face of tremendous stresses imposed by critical illness and modern technology. The stress response of the patient in this setting has significant physiologic consequences that have an impact on respiratory, cardiopulmonary, gastrointestinal, immunologic, and metabolic recovery. Research must be directed at ameliorating the stress response to facilitate return to normal function in all body systems. Some exciting areas of investigation include the use of peridural narcotics to deal with postoperative pain, the use of central alpha$_2$-agonists such as clonidine to blunt the sympathetic nervous system response and provide analgesia, and the use of new delivery systems such as PCA and transdermal patches that better match the administration of drug to the need.

REFERENCES

1. Melamed, E., et al.: Reduction in regional cerebral blood flow during normal aging in man. Stroke, *11*:31, 1980.
2. Van Brummelen, P., Buhler, F. R., Kiowski, W., and Amann, F. W.: Age-related decrease in cardiac and peripheral vascular responsiveness to isoprenaline: studies in normal subjects. Clin. Sci., *60*:571, 1981.
3. Epstein, M.: Effects of aging on the kidney. Fed. Proc., *38*:168, 1979.
4. Montamat, S. C., Cusack, B. J., and Vestal, R. E.: Management of drug therapy in the elderly. Med. Intell., *321*:303, 1986.
5. Horvath, G., Benedek, G., and Szikszay, M.: Enhancement of fentanyl analgesia by clonidine plus verapamil in rats. Anesth. Analg., *70*:284, 1990.
6. Coursin, D. B., Klasek, G., and Goelzer, S. L.: Increased requirements for continuously infused vercuronium in critically ill patients. Anesth. Analg., *69*:518, 1989.
7. Mangano, D. T.: Perioperative cardiac morbidity. Anesthesiology, *72*:153, 1990.
8. Yeager, M. P., et al.: Epidural anesthesia and analgesia in high-risk surgical patients. Anesthesia, *66*:729, 1987.
9. Ramsay, M. A. E., Savege, T. M., Simpson, B. R. J., and Goodwin, R.: Controlled sedation with alphaxalone-alphadolone. Br. Med. J., *22*:656, 1974.
10. Costa, E., and Guidotti, A.: Molecular mechanisms in the receptor action of benzodiazepines. Ann. Rev. Pharmacol. Toxicol., *19*:531, 1979.
11. Samuelson, P. N., et al.: Hemodynamic responses to anesthetic induction with midazolam or diazepam in patients with ischemic heart disease. Anesth. Analg., *60*:802, 1981.
12. Marty, J., et al.: Effects of midazolam on the coronary circulation in patients with coronary artery disease. Anesthesiology, *64*:206, 1986.
13. Marty, J., et al.: Effects of diazepam and midazolam on baroreflex control of heart rate and on sympathetic activity in humans. Anesth. Analg., *65*:113, 1986.
14. Tomicheck, R. C., et al.: Diazepam-fentanyl interaction—hemodynamic and hormonal effects in coronary artery surgery. Anesth. Analg., *62*:881, 1983.
15. Gross, J. B., et al.: Time course of ventilatory depression after thiopental and midazolam in normal subjects and in patients with chronic obstructive pulmonary disease. Anesthesiology, *58*:540, 1983.
16. Greenblatt, D. J., et al.: Benzodiazepines: a summary of pharmacokinetic properties. Br. J. Clin. Pharmacol., *11*:11S, 1981.
17. Stirt, J. A.: Aminophylline is a diazepam antagonist. Anesth. Analg., *60*:767, 1981.
18. Allonen, H., Zeigler, G., and Klotz, U.: Midazolam kinetics. Clin. Pharmacol. Ther., *30*:653, 1981.
19. Westphal, L. M., et al.: Use of midazolam infusion for sedation following cardiac surgery. Anesthesiology, *67*:257, 1987.
20. Shapiro, J. M., et al.: Midazolam infusion for sedation in the intensive care unit: effect on adrenal function. Anesthesiology, *64*:394, 1986.
21. Khan, A. H., and Malhotra, R.: Midazolam as intravenous sedative for electrocardioversion. Chest, *95*:1068, 1989.
22. Lowery, K. G., et al.: Pharmacokinetics of diazepam and midazolam when used for sedation following cardiopulmonary bypass. Br. J. Anaesth., *57*:883, 1985.
23. Forster, A., et al.: Effect of a specific benzodiazepine antagonist (RO 15-1788) on cerebral blood flow. Anesth. Analg., *66*:309, 1987.
24. Bidwai, A. V., Stanley, T. H., Rogers, C., and Riet, E. K.: Reversal of diazepam-induced postanesthetic somnolence with physotigmine. Anesthesiology, *51*:256, 1979.
25. Busto, U., et al.: Withdrawal reaction after long-term therapeutic use of benzodiazepines. N. Engl. J. Med., *315*:854, 1986.
26. Stephan, H., et al.: Effects of propofol on cardiovascular dynamics, myocardial blood flow and myocardial metabolism in patients with coronary artery disease. Br. J. Anaesth., *58*:969, 1986.
27. Grounds, R. M., et al.: Propofol for sedation in the intensive care unit: preliminary report. Br. Med. J., *294*:397, 1987.
28. Higgins, T. L., et al.: ICU sedation following CABG: propofol vs midazolam. Crit. Care Med. In press.
29. Levkoff, S. E., Besdine, R. W., and Wetle, T.: Acute confusional states (delirium) in the hospitalized elderly. Ann. Rev. Gerontol. Geriatr., *6*:1, 1986.
30. Schor, J. D., et al.: Risk factors for delirium in hospitalized elderly. JAMA., *267*:827, 1992.
31. Inouye, S. K., et al.: Clarifying confusion: The confusion assessment method. Ann. Intern. Med., *113*:941, 1990.
32. Clintol, J. E., et al.: Haloperidol for sedation of disruptive emergency patients. Ann. Emerg. Med., *16*:319, 1987.
33. Tesar, G. E., and Stern, T. A.: Rapid tranquilization of the agitated intensive care unit patient. J. Intens. Care Med., *3*:195, 1988.
34. Smith, T. C., and Wollman, H.: Preanesthetic medication. *In* The Pharmacological Basis of Therapeutics. 5th Ed. Edited

by L. S. Goodman and A. Gilman. New York, Macmillan, 1975, p. 66.
35. Harvey, S. C.: Hypnotics and sedatives. The Pharmacological Basis of Therapeutics p. 102.
36. Higgins, T. L., et al.: Influence of pleural and mediastinal tubes on respiration following coronary artery bypass grafting. Chest, *96:*237S, 1989.
37. Coyle, J. P., et al.: Patient controlled analgesia after cardiac surgery. Anesth. Analg., *70:*S1, 1990.
38. Akil, H., et al.: Endogenous opioids: biology and function. Ann. Rev. Neurosci., *7:*223, 1984.
39. Stanski, D. R., Greenblatt, D. J., and Lowenstein, E.: Kinetics of intravenous and intramuscular morphine. Clin. Pharmacol. Ther., *24:*52, 1978.
40. Hug, C. C., et al.: Pharmacokinetics of morphine injected intravenously into the anesthetized dog. Anesthesiology, *54:*38, 1981.
41. Bovill, J. G., Sebel, P. S., and Stanley, T. H.: Opioid analgesics in anesthesia: with special reference to their use in cardiovascular anesthesia. Anesthesiology, *61:*731, 1984.
42. White, P. F.: Use of patient-controlled analgesia for management of acute pain. JAMA, *259:*243, 1988.
43. Chauvin, M., et al.: Morphine pharmacokinetics in renal failure. Anesthesiology, *66:*327, 1987.
44. Burks, L. C., et al.: Meperidine in the treatment of shaking chills and fever. Arch. Intern. Med., *140:*483, 1980.
45. Caspi, J., et al.: Delayed respiratory depression following fentanyl anesthesia for cardiac surgery. Crit. Care Med., *16:*238, 1988.
46. Bentley, J. B., et al.: Age and fentanyl pharmacokinetics. Anesth. Analg., *61:*968, 1982.
47. Roerig, D. L., et al.: Effect of propranolol on the first pass uptake of fentanyl in the human and rat lung. Anesthesiology, *71:*62, 1989.
48. Shafer, A., White, P. F., Schuttler, J., and Rosenthal, M. H.: Use of fentanyl infusion in the intensive care unit: tolerance to its anesthetic effect? Anesthesiology, *59:*215, 1983.
49. Bailey, P. L., et al.: Differences in magnitude and duration of opioid-induced respiratory depression and analgesia with fentanyl and sufentanil. Anesth. Analg., *70:*8, 1990.
50. Baily, P. L., et al.: Antagonism of postoperative opioid-induced respiratory depression: nalbuphine versus naloxone. Anesth. Analg., *66:*1109, 1987.
51. Blaise, G. A., Nugent, M., McMichan, J. C., and Durant, P. A. C.: Side effects of nalbuphine while reversing opioid-induced respiratory depression: report of four cases. Can. J. Anaesth., *37:*794, 1990.
52. Flacke, J. W., Flacke, W. E., and Williams, G. D.: Acute pulmonary edema following naloxone reversal of high-dose morphine anesthesia. Anesthesiology, *47:*376, 1987.
53. Michaelis, L. L., et al.: Ventricular irritability associated with the use of naloxone hydrochloride. Ann. Thorac. Surg., *18:*608, 1974.
54. Andree, R. A.: Sudden death following naloxone administration. Anesth. Analg., *59:*782, 1980.
55. Fitzpatrick, G. J., and Moriarty, D. C.: Intrathecal morphine in the management of pain following cardiac surgery: a comparison with morphine i.v., Br. J. Anaesth., *60:*639, 1988.
56. Vanstrum, G. S., Bjornson, K. M., and Ilko, R.: Postoperative effects of intrathecal morphine in coronary artery bypass surgery. Anesth. Analg., *67:*261, 1988.
57. El-Baz, N., and Goldin, M.: Continuous epidural infusion of morphine for pain relief after cardiac operations. J. Thorac. Cardiovasc. Surg., *93:*878, 1987.
58. Melendez, J. A., Cirella, V. N., and Delphin, E. S.: Lumbar epidural fentanyl analgesia after thoracic surgery. J. Cardiovasc. Anesth., *3:*150, 1989.
59. Robinson, R. J. S., et al.: Epidural meperidine analgesia after cardiac surgery. Can. Anaesth. Soc. J., *33:*550, 1986.
60. Coleman, D. L.: Control of postoperative pain—nonnarcotic and narcotic alternatives and their effect on pulmonary function. Chest, *92:*520, 1987.
61. Durrani, Z., Winnie, A. P., and Ikuta, P.: Interpleural catheter analgesia for pancreatic pain. Anesth. Analg., *67:*479, 1988.
62. Egebert, L. D., Battit, G. E., Welch, C. E., and Barlett, M. K.: Reduction of postoperative pain by encouragement and instruction of patients—a study of doctor-patient rapport. N. Engl. J. Med., *270:*825, 1964.
63. Litvak, K. M., and McEvoy, G. K.: Ketorolac, an injectable nonnarcotic analgesic. Clin. Pharm., *9:*921, 1990.
64. O'Hara, D. A., Fragen, R. J., Kinzer, M., and Pemberton, D.: Ketorolac tromethamine as compared with morphine for treatment of postoperative pain. Clin. Pharmacol. Ther., *41:*556, 1987.
65. Kennan, D. J. M., Cave, K., Langdon, L., and Lea, R. E.: Comparative trial of rectal indomethacin and cryoanalgesia for control of early postthoracotomy pain. Br. Med. J., *287:*1335, 1983.
66. Iles, J. D. H.: Relief of postoperative pain by ibuprofen: a report of two studies. Can. J. Surg., *23:*288, 1980.
67. Coyle, J. P., and Cullen, D. J.: Anesthesia pharmacology in critical care. In The Pharmacologic Approach to the Critically Ill Patient. Edited by B. Chernow and C. R. Lake. Baltimore, Williams & Wilkins, 1989.
68. Coursin, D. B., Klasek, G., and Goelzer, S. L.: Increased requirements for continuously infused vecuronium in critically ill patients. Anesth. Analg., *69:*518, 1989.
69. Segredo, V., et al.: Prolonged neuromuscular blockade after long-term administration of vecuronium in two critically ill patients. Anesthesiology, *72:*566, 1990.
70. Griffiths, R. B., Hunter, J. M., and Jones, R. S.: Atracurium infusions in patients with renal failure on an ITU. Anaesthesia, *41:*375, 1986.
71. Wadon, A. J., Dogra, S., and Anand, S.: Atracurium infusion in the intensive care unit. Br. J. Anaesth., *58:*64S, 1986.
72. Stoelting, R. K.: The hemodynamic effects of pancuronium and d-tubocurarine in anesthetized patients. Anesthesiology, *36:*612, 1972.
73. Savarese, J. J., and Philbin, D. M.: Cardiovascular effects of neuromuscular blocking agents. Int. Anesthesiol. Clin., *17:*13, 1979.
74. Larijani, G. E., et al.: Clinical pharmacology of pipecuronium bromide. Anesth. Analg., *68:*734, 1989.
75. Stoops, C. M., et al.: Hemodynamic effects of doxacurium chloride in patients receiving oxygen sufentanil anesthesia for coronary artery bypass grafting or valve replacement. Anesthesiology, *69:*365, 1988.
76. Gooch, J. L., et al.: Prolonged paralysis after treatment with neuromuscular junction blocking agents. Crit. Care Med., *19:*1125, 1991.
77. Chernow, B., et al.: Sympathetic nervous system "switch off" with severe hypothermia. Crit. Care Med., *11:*677, 1983.

Chapter 64

MULTIPLE ORGAN SYSTEM FAILURE: A SPECTRUM OF RISK AND OF DISEASE

FRANK S. RUTLEDGE
WILLIAM J. SIBBALD

Multiple organ system failure (MOF) is a term used to describe a syndrome characterized by the sequential dysfunction and eventual failure of vital organs in critically ill patients.[1-3] It is a nonspecific expression and frequently the final complication of critical illness.[4] In part, it is a product of our ability to prolong the process of dying such that the complete natural history of many disease processes can be observed, unobscured by earlier death.[5] Although MOF is a major cause of late mortality in surgical patients[6] and in patients with adult respiratory distress syndrome (ARDS),[7-9] sepsis is its most frequent clinical association.[10,11]

The development of MOF is dynamic and usually follows a definite identifiable event such as bacterial infection, trauma, hypotension, or a persistent inflammatory focus[1,3] (Fig. 64-1). The development of MOF usually follows one of two patterns:[6]

- Developing quickly and directly following a particular insult
- Developing insidiously and more remote in time from the initial insult

Although the causes of the syndrome appear to be multifactorial and potentially synergistic, it is possible to identify patients at risk for the development of MOF. These risk factors are frequently operative before admission to an ICU and remain important concerns throughout the ICU and rehabilitative phases of a patient's care. Other risk factors arise de novo and may interact with preexisting risk factors to perpetuate and propagate the progression from organ dysfunction to organ failure. An understanding of these risk factors and how they interrelate with the currently known pathophysiology of MOF allows the clinician to anticipate the need for appropriate monitoring and close observation of these patients. Further, this should facilitate the judicious use of appropriate preventative or adjunctive therapies early in the course of organ dysfunction when they may be more efficacious.[11-15]

In this chapter we examine the interaction and contribution of preexisting, concurrent, and propagating risk factors to the development of multiple organ system dysfunction (MOD) and MOF. We focus on recognizing conditions that may hasten the development of MOF and on situations for which the conditions may be favorably modified. In this context, we also examine more closely the effects on individual organ systems and the expression of this dysfunction. First, however, the epidemiology and pathogenesis of MOF are discussed.

EPIDEMIOLOGY OF MULTIPLE ORGAN SYSTEM FAILURE

MOF is an acute and dynamic process that includes a spectrum of disease with a spectrum of morbidity and mortality. Less figuratively, any particular definition of failure will, by design, miss mild cases of organ dysfunction that may be important contributors to the patient's ultimate prognosis. Knaus et al.[16] and others[5,17] have proposed and published definitions of organ failure that represent an extreme end of the dysfunction-failure spectrum (Table 64-1). In contrast, Marshall and Meakins[12] have categorized organ dysfunction as mild, moderate, or severe, which may represent an earlier and therefore more sensitive method of recognizing the potential for progression from dysfunction to failure (Table 64-2). Using these categories, MOF scores have been created and related to mortality.[11]

Because uniform criteria for the definition of "dysfunction" or "failure" of individual organ systems have not been clearly established, the incidence of natural history of MOF is variously reported. In association with ARDS, however, Dorinsky and Gadek[18] have reported the following incidence of individual organ failure, representing a summary incidence from individual reports:

- Renal, 40 to 55%
- Hepatic, 12 to 95%
- Central nervous system (CNS) 7 to 30%
- Gastrointestinal, 7 to 30%
- Hematologic, 0 to 26%
- Cardiac, 10 to 23%

Despite the lack of agreement or consensus on definitions of MOF, a growing literature allows the following observations:

- The more organ systems that are affected and the longer they are dysfunctional, the greater the mortality (Table 64-3).[16]
- It is axiomatic that preexisting organ dysfunction places the patient at greater risk, given a new insult.[16]
- Some organ systems are more frequently injured than others.[11,16,17]

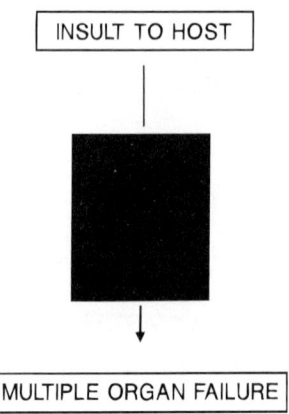

Fig. 64–1. The process leading to multiple organ system failure (MOF). Following an insult to the host, a complicated series of events may occur, which may ultimately lead to MOD and/or MOF.

- The progression of MOF appears to follow a temporal course that is frequently characteristic (Table 64–4).[6,11,19,20]
- The dysfunction of one organ system may contribute to the dysfunction of another organ system in a process of poorly understood organ-to-organ interactions.[3,7]

Given the poor prognosis associated with MOF, the best management strategies that may be employed require efforts directed to prevent its development. These include efforts to prevent the triggering insult and/or to modify the contributions that particular risk factors bring to the process. Before examining particular risk factors, we first discuss the pathogenesis of MOF.

PATHOGENESIS

The progression from a state of relative health and homeostasis to one of organ dysfunction and ultimately organ failure begins with an insult to the host in general and to individual organs in particular. This insult may result in a direct injury to a specific organ or may result in an indirect injury secondary to the host's response to the original insult. This frequently occurs in a setting where physiologic reserve is limited by prior organ dysfunction. Infection, pancreatitis, necrotic tissue, and shock can all produce an identical hyperdynamic, hypermetabolic systemic host response.[3,4,6,19,20] This response may be considered appropriate if it contains the process; it may also be considered inappropriate if it becomes generalized such that other organs suffer as relatively "innocent bystanders." Pinsky[4] has employed the term "malignant inflammation" to describe this latter situation: Inflammatory cells and their mediators are activated and recruited; the mediators are not contained and are therefore free to exert their inflammatory effects on a more widespread and unrestricted basis.

MOF can be produced by any process that activates the inflammatory cascade, which may become manifest clinically as the sepsis syndrome (Table 64–5).[21] This syndrome is defined using clinical criteria and although frequently initiated or perpetuated by a documented infection or inflammatory focus, it does not require confirmation with positive cultures.

In the next section, concepts are introduced that will be required in subsequent sections of discussions of factors that predispose the patient to the risks of developing MOF. Emphasis is placed on the role of infection and the metabolic regulation of tissue oxygen delivery (Do_2) in the overall pathogenesis of MOF.

Role of Infection and the Host's Septic Response

Tilney et al.[22] first characterized the clinical findings of MOF, and Baue[1] popularized the term MOF. Baue[1] described patients who sustained a metabolic insult secondary to trauma or surgery and then developed sequential organ failure. In particular, he noted that the septic response and particularly peritonitis were a concomitant oc-

Table 64–1. Definitions of Individual Organ Failure

Organ System	Clinical Signs, Symptoms, or Conditions

Cardiovascular	Presence of one or more
	  Heart rate ≤ 54 bpm
	  Mean arterial pressure ≤ 49 mm Hg
	  Congestive heart failure with chest radiograph and clinical evidence of pulmonary edema
	  Evidence of hypoperfusion with serum pH < 7.30 with normal $Paco_2$ or cardiac index < 2.2 l/min/m^2
	  Occurrence of ventricular tachycardia or ventricular fibrillation

Respiratory failure	Presence of one or more
	  Respiratory rate ≤ 5 or ≥ 40
	  $Paco_2$ ≥ 50 with pH < 7.35
	  A-aDo_2 ≥ 350
	  Dependent on mechanical ventilation or CPAP > 3 days

Renal failure	Presence of one or more
	  Serum creatinine > 300 μmol/L
	  Twice pre-admission creatinine in cases of chronic renal failure

Hepatic failure	Inclusive
	  Elevated prothrombin time (not associated with vitamin K deficiency, DIC, or hemorrhage) with at least twice-normal elevation of total bilirubin and elevated AST
	  Associated with metabolic encephalopathy

Hematologic failure	White blood cell levels ≤ 1000 mm^3 Platelets ≤ 20,000 Hematocrit ≤ 20% without active bleeding
Neurologic failure	Glasgow coma scale ≤ 6 in the absence of sedation or paralytic drugs Polyneuropathy of critical illness Encephalopathy

Gastrointestinal failure	Presence of one or more
	  Stress ulceration
	  Acalculous cholecystitis
	  Pancreatitis

* If the patient has one or more of the preceding during a 24-hour period, then organ system failure has occurred on that day. A-a, Alveolar-arterial oxygen gradient; AST, aspartate aminotransferase; CPAP, Continuous positive airway pressure; Do_2, oxygen delivery.
(Modified from Knaus W. A. et al.: Prognosis in acute organ system failure. Ann. Surg., 202:685, 1985.)

Table 64–2. Recognition and Assessment of Organ System Dysfunction

Organ System	Indicators of Dysfunction	Mild	Moderate	Severe
Respiratory	Pa_{O_2}, F_{IO_2}, Pa_{O_2}/F_{IO_2}, PEEP, number of days on ventilator, peak airway pressure, use of high-frequency ventilation or ECMO	$Pa_{O_2}/F_{IO_2} > 250$	Pa_{O_2}/F_{IO_2} 150–250	$Pa_{O_2}/F_{IO_2} < 150$
Renal	Creatinine level, creatinine clearance, BUN, need for dialysis to regulate serum potassium and bicarbonate	Creatinine < 150 µmol/L	Creatinine 150–300 µmol/L	Creatinine > 300 µmol/L; need for dialysis
Hepatic	Bilirubin, albumin, cholesterol, ALT, AST, glutamyltransferase, alkaline phosphatase, ammonia	Bilirubin < 30 µmol/L	Bilirubin 30–80 µmol/L: Elevation of transaminases or alkaline phosphatase to > 2 times normal values	Bilirubin > µmol/L: Evaluation of serum ammonia
Gastrointestinal	Stress-related mucosal ulceration and bleeding, mucosal acidosis, failure of pH regulation, volume of nasogastric drainage, ileus, diarrhea intolerance of enteral feeding, acalculous cholecystitis, pancreatitis	Nasogastric drainage < 300 ml/24 hr; diarrhea in response to enteral feeding	Nasogastric drainage 300–1,000 ml/24 hr; visible blood in drainage fluid	Nasogastric drainage > 1,000 ml/24 hr; upper GI bleeding necessitating transfusion, acalculous cholecystitis, pancreatitis
Cardiac	Supraventricular arrhythmias, elevated PAWP and mean pulmonary arterial pressure, reduced ventricular stroke work index, requirement for inotropes or vasopressors to maintain adequate mean arterial pressure	Development of supraventricular tachycardias with heart rate < 140 beats/min and no fall in mean arterial pressure	PAWP 16–20 mm Hg: Requirement for dopamine or dobutamine at dosage of < 10 µg/kg/min to maintain satisfactory cardiac output and PAWP	Requirement for vasopressors (e.g., dopamine, epinephrine, norepinephrine, phenylephrine) to maintain mean arterial pressure > 80 mm Hg
Central nervous system	Glasgow coma scale score, especially on components reflecting level of consciousness	Glasgow coma scale score 13–14	Glasgow coma scale score 10–12	Glasgow coma scale score ≤ 9
Hematologic	Thrombocytopenia, elevated PT and PTT, elevated fibrin degradation products	Platelet count > 60,000/mm^3	Platelet count 20,000–60,000/mm^3; mild elevation of PT or PTT in absence of anticoagulation	Platelet count < 20,000–mm^3; DIC
Metabolic/endocrine	Insulin requirements, levels of T_4 and reverse T_3	Insulin requirements ≤ 1 U/hr	Insulin requirements ≥ 2–4 U/hr	Insulin requirements ≥ 5 U/hr
Immunologic	Impaired DTH responsiveness, reduced in vitro lymphocyte proliferation, infection with ICU pathogens (e.g. S. epidermidis, Candida, Pseudomonas, enterococci)	Reduced DTH reactivity	Cutaneous anergy	Cutaneous anergy, recurrent infection with ICU pathogens
Wound healing	Wound infection, impaired formation of granulation tissue, wound dehiscence	Wound infection	Impaired formation of granulation tissue	Decubitus ulcers, wound dehiscence

ECMO, extracorporeal membrane oxygenation; ALT, alanine aminotransferase; AST, aspartate aminotransferase; BUN, blood urea nitrogen; PAWP, pulmonary arterial wedge pressure; PT, prothrombin time; PTT, partial thromboplastin time.
(Reprinted from Marshall, J. C.: Multiorgan failure: care of the surgical patient. Sci. Am., 13:1, 1991. © 1991 Scientific American, Inc. All rights reserved.)

currence. Fry et al.[23] emphasized the importance of infection in the development of MOF and further demonstrated that failure of four or more organ systems was associated with 100% mortality. Numerous other reports have demonstrated that infection is the most frequently associated factor that underlies the development of MOF.[11,20,24] Late deaths in patients with ARDS have been attributed to MOF. Of interest is the observation that in this series the infection was in the lungs.[25]

It is important to discriminate between infection and a host's response to it. Infection is a microbial phenomenon that involves the invasion of sterile tissues with micro-organisms. Under normal circumstances, infection elicits a host (septic) response by generating the release of mediator substances (see following discussion). Not all clinical sepsis, however, is due to established foci of infection, and the host's septic response is not always uniform in its expression or static in its progression.

Much confusion exists with respect to the use of terms such as sepsis, sepsis syndrome, and septic shock, and

Table 64-3. Prognosis in Multiorgan Failure

Number of Failing Systems	Mortality (%)
0	3
1	30
2	50–60
3	85–100
4	72–100
5	100

(From Marshall, J. C., and Meakins, J. L.: Multiorgan failure. In Scientific American Medicine. American College of Surgeons Care of the Surgical Patient, Vol. 1. Edited by N. Ehrlich. New York, Scientific American, 1989, p. 1.

attempts to agree on definitions are the focus of recent editorials.[26,27] For the purpose of this discussion, **sepsis** is defined as the host response to both infectious and noninfectious stimuli, and as such it is by definition a syndrome. **Septic shock** is defined as sepsis associated with inadequate tissue perfusion and as such reflects a more severe manifestation of sepsis.[26]

This distinction between infection and the septic response is critical. Therapy for infection is directed at the eradication of the infecting organism, whereas therapy for the septic response is directed toward support of the host. Measures used to treat infection include surgical debridement and drainage and the use of antimicrobial therapy. Measures used to treat the septic response include the use of fluids, inotropes, and vasopressors to maintain organ function through the insurance of adequate systemic oxygen transport (see following discussion). If the septic response is due to infection, then eradication of the infection will attenuate the host response; if it is not, then anti-infective therapy will be unproductive.[26]

As discussed, sepsis may be clinically evident without a clinically proven infection. This has been described by Meakins and Marshall[28] as nonbacteremic sepsis. They described a series of patients with multiple organ impairment as manifest by the following:

- Hypoxemia
- Hyperbilirubinemia
- Gastric bleeding
- Renal failure
- Thrombocytopenia

Table 64-4. Temporal Course of Multiorgan Failure

System	Median Interval of Onset of Failure, 6, 10 Days
Respiratory	2–3
Hematologic	3–5
Renal	4–5
Hepatic	6–7
Central Nervous	7–9

(From Marshall, J. C., and Meakins, J. L.: Multiorgan failure. In Scientific American Medicine. American College of Surgeons. Care of the Surgical Patient, Vol. 1. Edited by N. Ehrlich. New York, Scientific American, 1989, p. 1.)

Table 64-5. Definition of Septic Syndrome

Clinical evidence of infection
Fever or hypothermia
Tachypnea
Tachycardia
Impaired organ system function or perfusion
  Altered orientation
  Hypoxemia
  Elevated plasma lactate
  Oliguria

(Reprinted from Balk, R. A., and Bone, R. C.: The septic syndrome. Crit. Care Clin., 5:1, 1989.)

- Altered mentation
- Transient hypotension

In this series of patients, only 22 of 42 patients had positive cultures.[28] This concept has been confirmed by other studies,[29-31] including a large multicentered trial of high dose methylprednisolone in which only 45% of patients with presumed sepsis or septic shock had positive cultures.[32] These results must be interpreted with the knowledge that proportion of these patients without positive cultures will have clinically silent septic foci. Even in the original paper by Tilney et al.,[22] a significant percentage of patients had undetected intraperitoneal disease, and Bell et al.[29] found that 40% of nonsurvivors had autopsy-proven foci of infection, most commonly in the lungs or peritoneum.

Controlled Versus Malignant Inflammation

The usual response to infection includes the host's attempt to contain, restrict, suppress, and eliminate infecting organisms and their products.[2] Thus, monocytes, lymphocytes, tissue macrophages, and complement are activated.[11,33-36] Each of these defensive systems releases secretory products in an attempt to contain the process and facilitate tissue repair. Within this environment, fibroblasts, proteases, reactive oxygen species (ROS), neutrophils, and complement act to eliminate the microbial insult.[33-38] As many of the systemic mediators are blood borne, the effects of these mediators may continue to be noted on remote organ systems and may continue to be noted until the initiating insult is eliminated or the abscess is drained. Unfortunately, if this process is not controlled or contained, widespread inflammation and diffuse microcirculatory injury may occur, ultimately leading to cell injury and organ dysfunction or failure (Fig. 64-2).

Antiproteases, albumin, ROS, scavengers, and phagocytes serve as host defenses.[2,11,38] The resolution of the initial insult depends on the ability of these host defenses to balance and contain the potential systemic response to the blood-borne systemic inflammatory mediator effects.

In gram-negative sepsis, the lipopolysaccharide component of the cell wall (endotoxin) induces production and release of a proinflammatory mediator, tumor necrosis factor (TNF) from resident tissue macrophages or circulating polymorphonuclear leukocytes (PMNL).[35,39,40] This substance in turn may promote neutrophil adherence to endothelial cells and participates in the further activation of

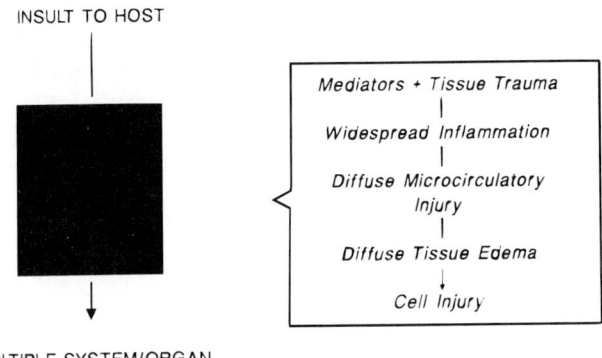

Fig. 64-2. Some of the events that occur following an insult to the host. Mediators released as a result of, or in conjunction with, tissue trauma may result in widespread or malignant inflammation. Local and diffuse tissue injury occur and result in tissue edema and cellular injury.

tissue macrophages, PMNL, and T-lymphocytes.[39-42] TNF also stimulates endothelial cells to synthesize and release interleukin 1 (IL1),[43-45] Interferon-gamma,[46] platelet-activating factor (PAF),[47] endothelium-derived relaxant factor (EDRF),[48] and cyclo-oxygenase and lipo-oxygenase metabolites of arachidonic acid (the eicosanoids).[49]

These inflammatory mediators have many potential direct and indirect effects, which include direct cell toxicity, complement activation, kinin synthesis, coagulation, and fibrinolytic system activation. Together the effects may contribute to microthrombus formation.[2,11] Teleologically, this may be to help limit the arena of activity for these many mediators, but the microthrombus formation might also contribute to tissue injury. Platelets are activated and consumed, and leukocytes are attracted and begin to aggregate. Damage to endothelial cells follows and is consequent on release of ROS, both initially and on reperfusion.[37,50]

A systemic endothelial injury appears to be the critical and typical lesion underlying the tissue injury in MOF[41-48] (Fig. 64-3). This injury contributes to the observed increased permeability and altered vascular reactivity. As the process becomes generalized (malignant inflammation), widespread interstitial edema and altered oxygen delivery (through altered microcirculatory perfusion) occur. With altered microcirculatory flow and oxygen delivery, ischemic tissue injury and subsequent organ dysfunction follow. The now dysfunctional organs interact with other dysfunctional organs or therapies required to support individual organ systems. The process is thus amplified and perpetuates itself.

The process described previously can also be initiated by trauma, burns, pancreatitis, and so on. The acute inflammatory response to these insults is identical in many respects to that caused by infectious insults. Necessary supportive therapies are required for these patients, and these therapies place the patient at a variable risk for a nosocomial acquired infection, which may sustain and perpetuate the process begun by a noninfectious insult (see following discussion).

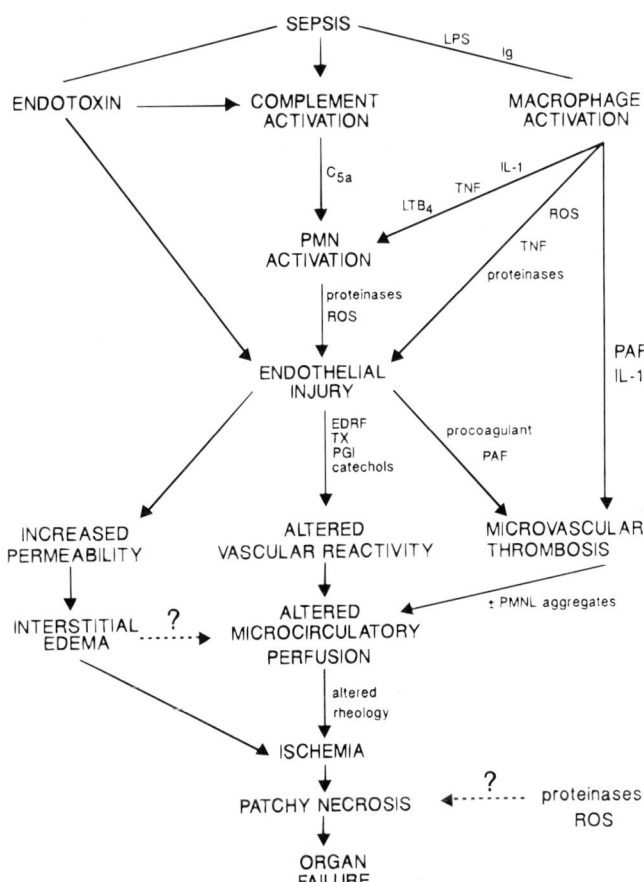

Fig. 64-3. The possible interaction of sepsis, endotoxemia, and numerous mediators to effect the microvasculature. Endothelial injury, altered permeability, and altered vascular reactivity or perfusion may ultimately result in patchy ischemic changes in multiple end organs. These ischemic changes are believed to play a role in altered organ function, which may progress to organ failure. LPS, lipopolysaccharide; IL-1, interleukin 1; TNF, tumor necrosis factor; LTB_4, leukotriene B_4; C_{5a}, activated complement; ROS, reactive oxygen species; PAF, platelet-activating factor; EDRF, endothelial-derived relaxing factor; TX, thromboxanes; PGI, prostacycline; PMNL, polymorphonuclear leukocytes.

Why do some patients handle this acute inflammatory response well, while in others the process becomes a generalized pansystemic injury that progresses to MOF (Fig. 64-4).? It has been suggested[2,11] that for the process to progress, ongoing inflammation or superimposed and recurrent nosocomial infections are required. This progression to a pansystemic injury appears to be more likely in those with impaired host defenses (e.g., the immunosuppressed, those with hepatic impairment, or those with chronic underlying disease.[2,11,51-53]

Role of Tissue Hypoxia

It has been repeatedly suggested that decreased tissue oxygen availability is the ultimate cause of the tissue injury that (manifest as tissue ischemia) results in the progression of organ dysfunction to organ failure. With sepsis, tissue oxygen needs are increased and reflect the systemic hyper-

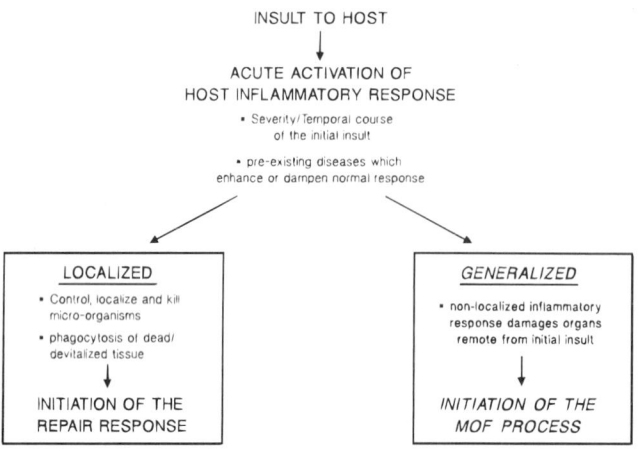

Fig. 64-4. Following the initial insult and the acute activation of the host inflammatory response, a localized and possibly generalized process is initiated. The localized inflammatory process is designed to initiate tissue repair and is considered a normal response. A more generalized (malignant) inflammatory process may occur whereby organ systems remote from the initial insult become involved and possibly damaged. Preexisting, concurrent, and propagating risk factors interact to determine in part whether the normal and appropriate repair response becomes more generalized and potentially more destructive.

metabolic response and increased oxygen consumption that follow a systemic insult or injury.[2,6,11,19,54] This increased oxygen use is required to support attempts at tissue repair in the face of altered metabolic regulation. If these needs are not met by increased oxygen delivery, tissue hypoxia results.[54] Potential causes for this demand–supply imbalance include direct cytotoxicity, systemic hypoxia, anemia, or circulatory dysfunction resulting in decreased oxygen delivery.[54-56]

The metabolic theory of local circulatory control proposes that the primary function of the circulation is to couple blood flow and hence oxygen delivery to tissue and cellular needs.[54,55] This autoregulation of blood flow is accomplished, in health, by alterations in the following:

- Global cardiac output
- Arteriolar tone and consequently, regional blood flow, provided that arterial perfusion pressures are not depressed
- Precapillary sphincter tone and, consequently, changes in the numbers of perfused capillaries at the microcirculatory level

In sepsis, the host's response to inflammation may demonstrate altered regulation of tissue Do_2 at all levels of the circulation. A depression in vascular responsiveness and ventricular performance may contribute, at a central level, to a reduction in arterial perfusion pressure and in systemic Do_2. In animal models of sepsis, abnormalities of the control of tissue Do_2 have been demonstrated at both the regional[54] and microregional levels of the circulation.[54-59] Patchy tissue ischemia is, however, characteristic of these models. It therefore follows that widespread metabolic dysregulation is an important feature of this syndrome.[60]

Evidence to support this position comes from several sources. Supranormal Do_2 levels have been correlated with survival.[56,61-64] High arterial lactate levels, however, indicating anaerobic metabolism and perhaps inadequate Do_2, have been correlated with death.[56,65] Oxygen consumption ($\dot{V}o_2$) depends on Do_2 at lower levels of Do_2 (pathologic supply dependency),[66-70] and covert oxygen debts have been unmasked by the use of vasodilators.[71,72] Ultrastructural[60] and functional studies[73] suggest that a systemic vascular lesion and widespread cell injury precede and accompany both pulmonary and nonpulmonary organ dysfunction and MOF. These studies show an increase in mitochondrial destruction of various cell types including the vascular endothelium. Endothelial cell swelling, decreased capillary luminal diameter, and an increased interstitial space and volume, which has an increased protein content, have been noted.[60] These ultrastructural changes were not due to a falling cardiac output, regional blood flow, or regional Do_2; therefore, these observed changes apparently were due to changes occurring at the microregional level.[54,74]

Figure 64-3 depicts events that occur in sepsis and illustrates how these events might interact to affect the microcirculation and ultimately lead to the patchy ischemia shown in the preceding studies. Endotoxin, complement, and macrophage activation and a host of mediators interact to damage the capillary endothelium. Increased microvascular permeability, altered vascular reactivity, vasodilatation, redistribution of blood volume with intravascular pooling, and microvascular thrombosis all contribute to altered rheology within many vascular beds.

Given the probable relationship of a relative inadequate tissue Do_2 to the onset and/or progression of MOD/MOF, a number of risk factors (see following discussion) impact on the ability of the host to augment tissue Do_2.

PRE-ICU PHASE: RISK FACTORS AND MULTIPLE ORGAN SYSTEM DYSFUNCTION/FAILURE

By definition, a risk factor is a condition that increases the likelihood that a patient will encounter a physiologic injury given the occurrence of any event that is an insult to the patient. In the context of MOF, risk factors can be defined as conditions that exist before an initial physiologic insult, those that develop concurrent with patient's illness, and those that arise during the management of a patient's illness that are in many ways unique to this phase of a patient's care.

Preexisting Risk Factors

As discussed, the cascade of changes that culminate in MOF begins with an inciting event. The host's ability to meet this challenge depends to a large extent on the state of general health at the time of the insult and also on the type of insult that any particular patient might face. The elderly, the immunocompromised, the malnourished, and those with chronic disease have reduced functional reserve and are thus less able to tolerate single (initial) or

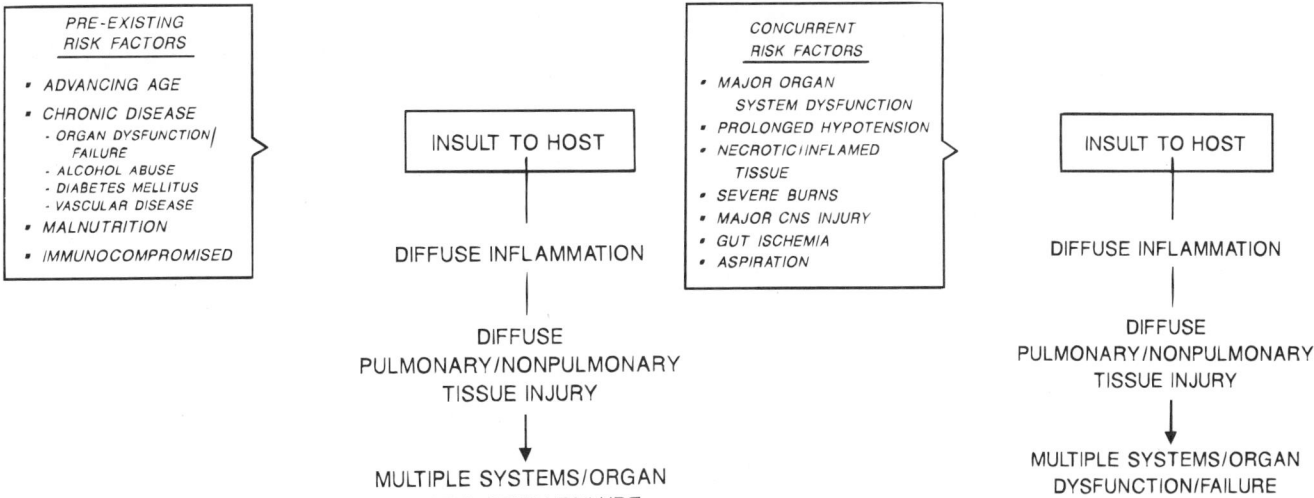

Fig. 64–5. Preexisting risk factors are present before the initial insult and are essentially unalterable. These risk factors continue to be present and operative throughout the patient's entire illness.

Fig. 64–6. Concurrent risk factors become operative at the time of the initial insult and may in fact be the initial insult itself. They potentially interact with each other and with preexisting risk factors to influence the inflammatory response and its potential progression to a more diffuse tissue injury. CNS, central nervous system.

multiple insults (Fig. 64–5). They are disadvantaged from the start, and this disadvantage persists throughout their illness.

All the risk factors detailed in Figure 64–5 potentially reduce the patient's ability to increase metabolic response to any given insult. Patients with these conditions are less able to resist infection or to increase tissue Do_2 under times of stress. Further, those patients with preexisting disease appear to be more susceptible to the risks associated with the necessary therapies required to support these patients. For example, the patient with chronic lung disease, in addition to tolerating a pulmonary insult (e.g., pneumonia) more poorly, may recover from respiratory failure more slowly and require more support (more positive end expiratory pressure (PEEP), higher fraction of impaired oxygen (Fio_2) for a longer period of time. Consequently, they may experience more complications from the therapy. Similarly, Matuschak and Martin[51] have detailed in a retrospective review how global hepatic function is a major determinant of the patient's host defense and how hepatic reticuloendothelial function is critical in determining the potential for recovery from ARDS.[51-53]

Concurrent Risk Factors

The conditions listed in Figure 64–6 could also be entitled "initial insults." They may occur concurrent with the patient's illness and may have additive detrimental effects in patients with preexisting disease. Each condition can trigger the diffuse inflammatory process discussed previously. Whether or not this process is contained or becomes generalized depends on both the relative severity of the initial insult and the ability of the host to meet the challenge. Knaus et al. have identified that the single strongest predictor of subsequent MOF is the severity of disease for which the patient is admitted to the ICU.[16] Following this, the diagnosis of sepsis and the presence of a respiratory infection appear to be critical factors.[16] All too frequently, several of these insults occur simultaneously in a patient with several preexisting risk factors. For example, an elderly patient with ischemic heart disease and chronic renal failure may incur multiple injuries in a motor vehicle accident. Prolonged hypotension, the need for massive blood transfusions, and/or required and repeated surgical procedures would all contribute to an increased likelihood of MOF and possible death. In this example, little can be done to alter the sequence of events before presentation; however, because these risks can be additive and contribute to morbidity and mortality, our efforts should be directed to aggressive resuscitation, early control of hemorrhage, and timely operative intervention to minimize the impact of these multiple insults.[75]

In other situations, a similar high risk patient may require a complex or major surgical procedure. For example, an elderly patient with a recent anterior wall myocardial infarction might require urgent surgery for a rapidly expanding abdominal aortic aneurysm. We know that this patient's prognosis will be better if the aneurysm is not allowed to rupture and that the chance of rupture increases with time.[76] On the other hand, we know that the risk of a serious myocardial event is increased with major surgery occurring recently after a myocardial infarction and that this risk is reduced with time.[15,77]

In this type of less emergent situation, strategies can be employed to minimize or prevent additional factors from affecting the patient's outcome. Rao et al.[15] suggested that invasive intravascular monitoring with a pulmonary artery catheter (PAC) and aggressive treatment of circulatory aberrations might significantly reduce the risk of reinfarction and/or death. Others have suggested that data obtained from the PAC is useful in detecting myocardial ischemia during intra-abdominal or aortic surgery[78,79] and in reducing the incidence of acute renal failure after surgery.[80]

Thus, aggressive monitoring can be used to guide therapy to minimize or prevent the effects of additional insults consequent on significant hemodynamic alterations.[15]

The dysfunction of a major organ system is arguably the most important preexisting and/or concurrent risk factor for the development of MOF. Preexisting dysfunction reduces functional reserve and the ability to tolerate additional insults. Dysfunction that occurs concurrent with an insult to the host similarly restricts the patient's ability to defend itself against that insult. Dysfunctional organ systems interact with other dysfunctional organs to propagate the process.[7,52] Figure 64-7 depicts a schema for the organ interactions that are thought to occur between the lung and the kidney, gut, and liver. Similarly, impaired organ systems require support that may be easily tolerated by healthy organ systems but that may be poorly tolerated if the organ system is already dysfunctional. For example, gut blood supply and function, which may already be limited, may be further compromised by the use of dopamine or noradrenalin when these agents are used to support blood pressure and other organ perfusion.

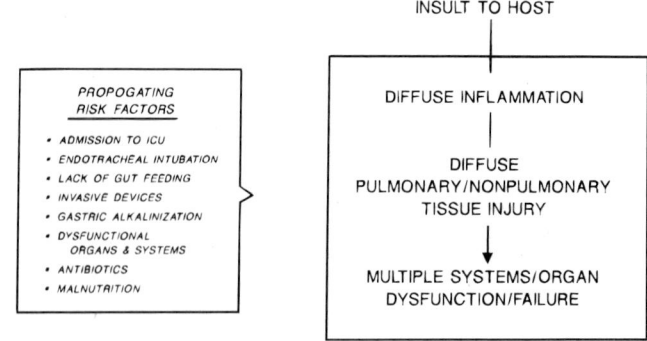

Fig. 64-8. Propagating risk factors occur as a result of the patient's need for intensive care. These factors are frequently required supportive therapies that may have both beneficial and detrimental effects on different organ systems. They may also interact with preexisting and concurrent risk factors and may influence organ system interactions. Efforts to minimize the detrimental aspects of these therapies coupled with careful support of all organ systems constitute a central strategy in our efforts to prevent the progression to multiple organ system failure.

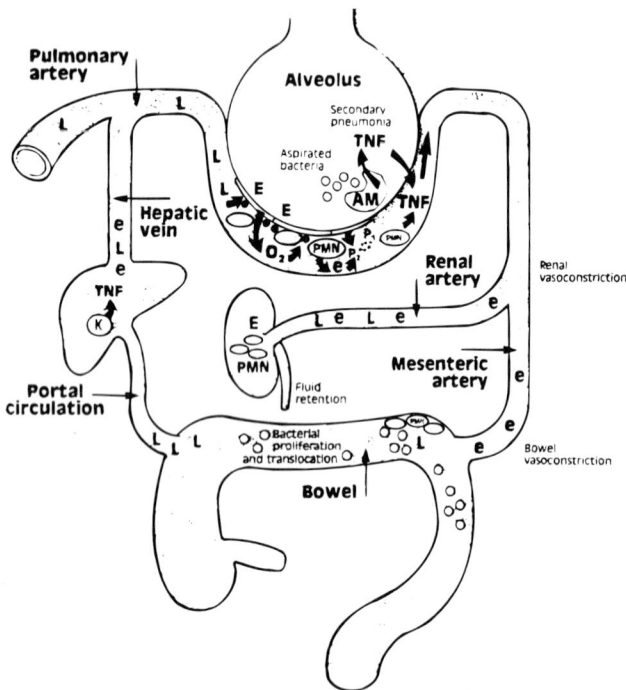

Fig. 64-7. A unifying hypothesis explaining the relationship between adult respiratory distress syndrome (ARDS) and extrapulmonary organ system failure. Infection and mediator activation occurring in the lungs may affect organ systems downstream (e.g., kidney or gut). Similarly, insults resulting in bowel or liver dysfunction can ultimately affect organs downstream (e.g., lung). Risk factor and organ system interactions occur and may accelerate the progression to multiple organ system failure. TNF, tumor necrosis factor; K, Kupffer cells; E, endothelial cells; e, eicosanoids; L, LPS (endotoxin); open circle, bacteria; PMN, polymorphonuclear leukocytic activation; AM, alveolar macrophage; P_1, platelets; P_2, procoagulants; solid circle, new surface glycoprotein (for PMN attachment). (Reprinted from Rinaldo, J., and Heyman, S. J.: ARDS—a multisystem disease with pulmonary manifestations. Crit. Care Rep., *1*:174, 1990.)

Propagating Risk Factors

Propagating risk factors (Fig. 64-8) occur during the management of a patient's illness. They reflect the requirement for specific monitoring techniques or specific therapies that have the potential to increase the chance that the patient may encounter further injury. Admission to an ICU and the need for supportive therapy thus become risk factors for the critically ill patient.

Endotracheal intubation may be necessary but increases the likelihood of nosocomial pneumonia. Central venous access may be required, but its establishment may result in a pneumothorax or facilitate the development of a bacteremia. Superinfection may follow appropriate antibiotic use, and gastric alkalization may protect the stomach from stress ulceration at the expense of increasing the incidence of significant bacterial aspiration.[81]

Because dysfunctional organs may interact to cause further dysfunction in organ systems remote from those involved in the initial process, so too might different therapies interact with dysfunctional organ systems to aggravate the situation. For example, PEEP therapy may affect lung function through barotrauma and may alter hepatic and renal blood flow through direct and/or indirect effects on cardiac output.[74] Therapies required to support individual organ systems may thus damage that system and impair the function of more remote systems.

ICU PHASE ORGAN-BASED APPROACH TO RISK FACTOR ANALYSIS

To appreciate how these risk factors interrelate with the host's response after an insult, we must look at individual organ systems and review the effects on these systems, expression of dysfunction (or failure) of these systems (Fig. 64-9), and attempts to support the organ's function without contributing to further dysfunction.

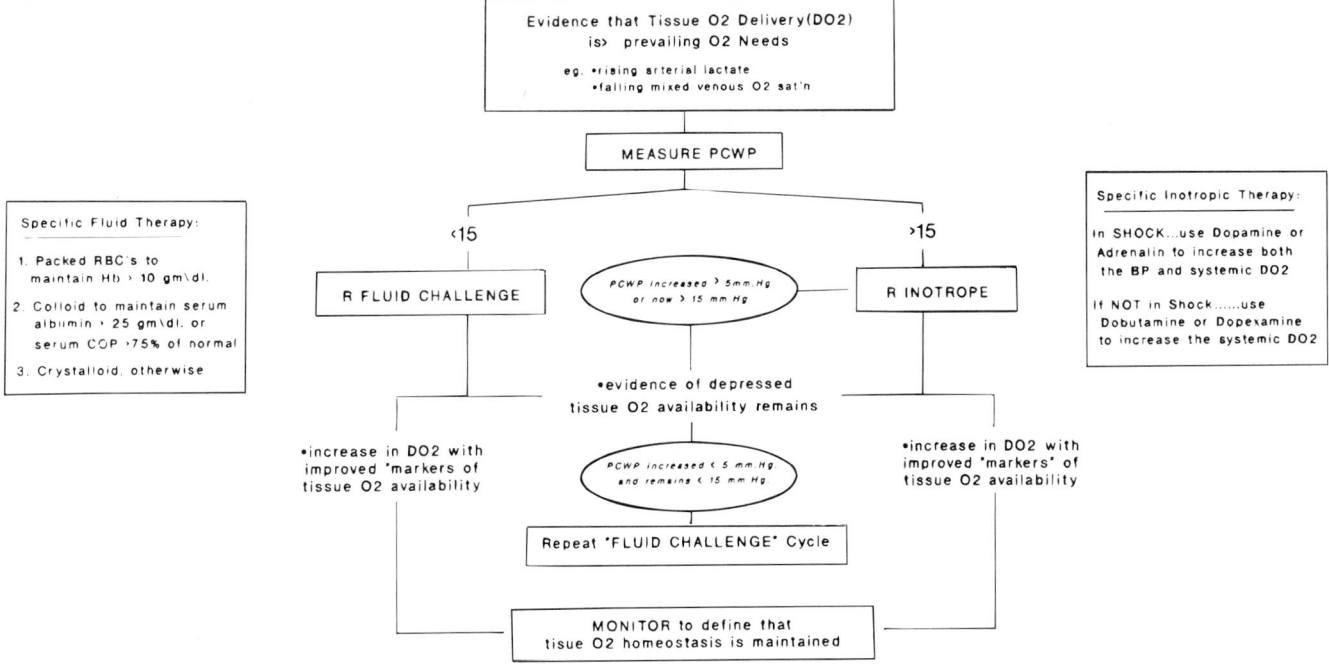

Fig. 64-9. Sequential therapeutic decisions that may be made when providing hemodynamic support. The adequacy of tissue oxygen delivery is assessed by review of mixed venous oxygen saturation and arterial lactate. If the pulmonary capillary wedge pressure (PCWP) is less than 15 mm, then appropriate fluid therapy is selected. If the PCWP is greater than 15 mm Hg, then appropriate inotropic or inodilator therapy is considered. Repeated assessment of the chosen therapy and the markers of tissue oxygen availability are required to guide further therapy. Do_2, delivery of oxygen; RBC, red blood cell transfusion; Hb, hemoglobin; COP, colloid oncotic pressure.

Circulatory Dysfunction

With an insult to the host, such as a bacterial infection, the acute inflammatory response and a subsequent malignant inflammation that frequently follow result in a hyperdynamic, hypermetabolic response.[6,19,54] This response increases tissue oxygen needs and, if homeostasis is to be maintained, dictates appropriate changes in Do_2. The hyperdynamic response that occurs in this setting is characterized by the following:

- Increase in cardiac index
- Normal systolic pressure
- Normal pulmonary capillary wedge pressure
- Decrease in systemic vascular resistance

With these hemodynamic changes, Do_2 and $\dot{V}o_2$ increase. These changes occur at a global level, at a regional level, and at a microregional level.[54]

At a central level, global cardiac performance may be compromised in sepsis.[54,82-85] Cardiac failure may be defined as in Table 64-1 and Table 64-2 or more simplistically by the need for vasopressor or inotropic therapy. Indeed, it may be argued that cardiac dysfunction is present even in the presence of an increased cardiac output if it can be shown that the increase cardiac output is insufficient to meet the need for Do_2. Impaired global cardiac performance may be translated into impaired global Do_2. It may also require alteration of regional blood flow to some organs (e.g., gut) in an attempt to perfuse other more vital organs (e.g., heart, brain, etc).

Conclusions concerning the adequacy or inadequacy of Do_2 are drawn from the following:

- Clinical assessment of peripheral perfusion
- An interpretation of arterial lactate levels
- Interpretation of mixed venous oxygen tensions (Pvo_2)

A cool, shut-down periphery implies that the patient may not be as hyperdynamic as could be expected or as may be required. Rashkin et al.[65] found a correlation between death and elevated arterial lactate and depressed Do_2. Elevated lactate levels reflect an inadequate oxygen supply and may predict an increase in the systemic $\dot{V}o_2$ in response to an increase in Do_2.[86,87]

Pvo_2 is a single index that reflects the many components of the oxygen supply-demand relationship. It is also a measurement that is least subject to technical variation. It represents the flow-weighted mixture of end capillary Po_2 and as such reflects changes in arterial content of oxygen (Cao_2) local blood flow, local $\dot{V}o_2$, and the affinity of hemoglobin for oxygen.[68,88] The Pvo_2 does not accurately reflect single tissue oxygenation. Tissue beds that are not perfused are not represented in the Pvo_2 value. Perfusion of some vascular beds on the other hand may be artificially high. The Pvo_2 is, therefore, a reflection of the total body oxygen supply-demand status but gives no valid information regarding individual tissues or organs. An abnormal Pv_{O_2} (e.g., Pv_{O_2} less than 30 mm Hg) indicates that there is a problem but does not indicate where the problem is or what therapy might be required. Thus, an abnormal Pv_{O_2} should prompt a determination of the other parameters of the oxygen supply–demand equation.

Risk factors that might limit the patient's ability to make appropriate changes in D_{O_2} include the following:

- Preexisting ischemic heart disease
- Peripheral vascular disease

In these patients, physiologic reserve may be limited, and their ability to increase global cardiac output may be impaired. The ability to alter regional blood flow might also be limited. Diabetic patients will have microvascular disease, which may affect both myocardial performance and regional organ perfusion.

It has been previously shown that survivors of high risk surgical operations have significantly higher D_{O_2} levels than nonsurvivors.[56,62] Further, it has been shown that protocolized therapies designed to reach these higher, supranormal D_{O_2} levels significantly reduce mortality in high risk surgical patients.[61] These supranormal D_{O_2} levels can be accomplished through a number of combined strategies. The maintenance of oxygen saturation, in excess of 95%, can usually be accomplished by the judicious use of nontoxic levels of F_{IO_2} (less than 0.5 to 0.6) and PEEP. Transfusions of packed red cells to a target hemoglobin of 11 to 12 g/dl will assist in increasing the Ca_{O_2} while avoiding the potential reduction in blood flow that follows the increase in blood viscosity associated with higher hemoglobin or hematocrit levels. With these components of D_{O_2} optimized, attention can be directed to improving cardiac index toward the supranormal levels described by Shoemaker et al.[61] This may require using the Frank-Starling relationship, whereby an increase in cardiac output (CO) can be accomplished by an increase in right and left ventricular end-diastolic volumes. Increased filling pressures, however, may aggravate pulmonary or peripheral edema and may therefore require that the desired increase in cardiac output be accomplished by the use of inotropic agents (e.g., dobutamine or amrinone). This type of therapy may have side effects that may limit its use (e.g., tachycardia) and therefore may force a consideration of therapy designed to reduce vascular resistance further to increase CO. Practically speaking, the goal of increasing D_{O_2} is accomplished by careful administration of combinations of all of these therapies. The extent to which these therapies are successful in increasing D_{O_2}, however, is limited in those with preexisting cardiac disease.

Concurrent and propagating risk factors also affect the circulatory dysfunction that is seen in association with MOF. Serum from septic patients can depress myocardial contraction in vitro, and this effect appears to be related to the depression of left ventricular ejection fraction (LVEF) that is seen in vivo.[82-85,89] It has been postulated that this effect is due to the production of a myocardial depressant substance in sepsis.[90] Therapeutically, recent work has suggested that this substance may be filtered by membranes as simple as those employed in continuous arterial venous hemofiltration systems (CAVH).[91] Ventricular dilatation, diminished right and left ventricular ejection fractions, altered Frank-Starling relationships, and altered diastolic pressure volume relationships have been observed in sepsis and MOF.[82,83,92] Although survivors and nonsurvivors of septic shock may have similar hemodynamic variables, survivors present with a left ventricular dilatation and a lower left ventricular ejection fraction that returned to normal with resolution of the septic shock. Reversible left ventricular dysfunction thus appears to be common in these patients. The important effects of sepsis on cardiovascular performance is underscored with the observation that ventricular volumes are larger and ejection fractions are lower in septic patients than in traumatized patients.[93] Pulmonary hypertension (increased right ventricular afterload) and right ventricular dilatation can interact to limit right ventricular coronary perfusion and reduce left ventricular preload, distensibility, and function, through the phenomenon of ventricular interdependence.[94]

Sepsis is also associated with a decrease in vascular responsiveness.[54,55] Microvascular abnormalities and decreased redistribution have been demonstrated in models of sepsis.[54,60,75] An increase in interstitial edema and the all too frequent inadequate volume resuscitation may also affect myocardial performance subsequent to an insult to the host. All of these changes may culminate in a reduced ability to mount an appropriate change in oxygen delivery to meet the increased oxygen needs. As previously discussed, this may be translated into a patchy ischemia within organs and contribute to the multiorgan dysfunction that is frequently observed.

Splanchnic Organ Dysfunction

It is becoming increasingly apparent that the gastrointestinal tract, the liver, and the pancreas play central roles in the perpetuation (if not the initiation) of the processes leading to the development of MOF. The gastrointestinal tract is felt to be important as a potential reservoir for infection.[37,95-97] As an organ that is susceptible to ischemia, it is thus an important potential portal for the translocation of bacteria and/or endotoxin.[37,95-97] Some authors therefore have suggested that the gut may be the "motor of MOF."[98]

As the motor of MOF, the gut augments the effects of the initial insult and may become of primary importance in the perpetuation of this process. It appears that with gut failure the intestinal integrity is lost such that bacterial and endotoxin translocation may occur. This is particularly true if the gut becomes ischemic. Further, the gastrointestinal microflora are frequently disturbed, and bacterial overgrowth with aerobes (especially gram-negative aerobes) and facultative anaerobes occurs and facilitates this translocation.

Gut-related factors that potentially contribute to impaired host defense in this population include the following:[99]

- Loss of the protective swallowing mechanism
- Decrease in secretory immunoglobulin A (IgA) from salivary glands or gallbladder

- Suppression of gastric acidity (through illness or pharmacologic means)
- Reduced intestinal motility
- Overgrowth of potentially resistant bacteria subsequent to the use of broad-spectrum antibiotics
- Overall impaired infection defense

Gut failure may be defined as the presence of an ileus, the intolerance to enteral feeding, stress ulceration and/or gastrointestinal bleeding, or acalculous cholecystitis (see Tables 64–1 and 64–2).

The liver, on the other hand, is felt to play a pivotal role in its dual capability to both produce and remove from the circulation a variety of mediators involved in the development of MOF.[51] Cytokines, especially TNF, have been implicated as significant mediators of infectious injury, with TNF being frequently detected in the circulation of patients with sepsis.[40] The hemodynamic and endocrine disturbances commonly observed in patients with sepsis have been produced with high dose infusions of TNF.[39,100-103] Hepatic macrophages have been demonstrated to be capable of production many inflammatory mediators including TNF.[52] The release of TNF has been demonstrated in the splanchnic circulation in response to endotoxin infusion. The TNF efflux accounted for approximately one half of the estimated total body TNF response in this study.[104] Further, pretreatment with anti-TNF antiserum completely inhibited the subsequent development of a pulmonary injury.[105]

The liver also synthesizes vitamin K-dependent procoagulant proteins, and abnormalities in prothrombin time (PT) and partial thromboplastin time (PTT) are frequent, early indicators of impaired synthetic function. The liver synthesizes fibronectin, which is a nonspecific opsonin that assists in removal of particulate aggregates from the bloodstream. Fibronectin depletion has been demonstrated in patients with sepsis and in those with liver disease.[106]

The liver also has an extremely important reticuloendothelial function. Endotoxin, fibrin aggregates, the eicosanoids, and TNF are all cleared by the liver. It has been demonstrated that endotoxin-induced mortality is increased if liver injury has been induced with a specific hepatotoxin. The liver contains a large reservoir of Kupffer cells, which comprise the majority of the body's reticuloendothelial system. In critical illness, this system is charged with the clearance of a large amount of translocated enteric organisms and proinflammatory monokines such as IL-1 and TNF. Thus, with endotoxemia, hepatocyte dysfunction may result in prolonged circulation of these mediators, which amplifies the inflammatory response that may occur downstream from this process. Thus, the lung, as the next organ downstream, is at greatest risk for manifestation of these remote effects (see Fig. 64–7). As previously mentioned, Matuschak et al.[52,53] suggested that the efficiency of the hepatic reticuloendothelial system appears to be a critical factor in modulating the severity and potential for recovery from ARDS.[53]

The pancreas also appears to play a role in the development of multiorgan failure.[95] Pancreatitis has been described as a frequent and unexpected finding in patients with MOF and we have observed that pancreatic blood flow is reduced in an animal model of hyperdynamic sepsis.[74] Nicod et al.[107] have demonstrated pancreatic enzymes are increased in ARDS, and pancreatitis is felt to be a not infrequent cause of this syndrome.

Preexisting risk factors that may amplify the contribution of splanchnic organs to the development of multiorgan failure, therefore, include the following:

- Intestinal ischemia
- Chronic liver disease, such as cirrhosis
- Chronic pancreatitis

Vascular disease places the gut at increased risk for ischemia. The various circulations of the gut are normally subservient to the requirements of the coronary and cerebral circulations during states of global reduced oxygen availability.[95] Animal studies have shown that mesenteric flow is reduced.[60] Pathologic evidence of pancreatic injury during sepsis, perhaps on an ischemic basis, has been previously demonstrated in both clinical[107] and animal studies.[60] Hepatic blood supply, on the other hand, appears to be maintained, with systemic flow compensating for alterations in portal venous flow.[74]

Patients with cirrhosis or preexisting liver dysfunction or those who develop hepatic dysfunction during their illness will have reduced synthetic, excretory, and reticuloendothelial reserve. They are thus at greater risk for coagulation disorders, infection, and central or peripheral edema secondary to hypoalbuminemia.

Concurrent and propagating risk factors can also modify or influence the contribution of the splanchnic organs to the process leading to the development of MOF. Thus, prolonged hypotension or bowel ischemia that develops during the patient's illness can contribute to the dysfunction of the splanchnic organs. Conversely, therapy that is designed to support global cardiac function and, by inference splanchnic Do_2, may reduce the risk of an ischemic contribution to the overall process. Therapy designed to protect against ongoing malnutrition can also aggravate the situation if the injudicious use of fat-containing solutions results in fatty infiltration and liver dysfunction. Here, once again, the beneficial effects of some therapies may carry a cost to other organ systems that may be failing or impaired or that interact directly with the function of the splanchnic organs.

Given the importance of the splanchnic organs and the potential role of either pre-existing or concurrent/propagating risk factors, strategies have been developed to reduce the contribution of the splanchnic organs to the development of MOF. These include the following:

- Maintenance of Do_2
- Selected decontamination of the digestive tract (SDD)
- Gut-directed nutritional support

It has been demonstrated that with decreased superior mesenteric arterial (SMA) blood flow that tissue edema is increased and is associated with mucosal disruption.[108] In similar models increased systemic and portal endotoxin levels have been observed.[109] Efforts directed at increasing the gut DO_2 have demonstrated decreased bacterial translocation.[109]

In an attempt to enhance the colonization defense of these patients, efforts are directed at preventing oral pharyngeal and gastrointestinal carriage of potentially pathogenic micro-organisms. It is speculated that this will reduce the endotoxin load and reduce the incidence of nosocomial pneumonia. This is achieved by using bactericidal, nonabsorbable, enteral antibiotics. This process has been termed SDD and includes the use of oral polymyxin E, oral tobramycin, oral amphotericin, and intravenous cefotaxime.[99,110-118] This group of antibiotics has been chosen specifically so that the spectrum of activity includes all aerobic, gram-negative, potentially pathogenic microorganisms such as the Enterobacteria and in particular, species of Pseudomonas and Acinetobacter. It also covers Staphylococcus aureus. The spectrum of activity is also designed to exclude indigenous anaerobic flora. The antibiotics are all bactericidal because the absence of intestinal luminal leukocytes dictates that bacteriostatic antibiotics would be of little use. Polymyxin E is used because it fulfills the preceding criteria and because it has the capacity to bind and neutralize endotoxin. Tobramycin is employed because of its spectrum of activity in synergy with polymyxin E. Amphotericin is used for its antimycotic effect. Systemic antibiotics such as intravenous cefotaxime are used for two reasons: (1) to treat overt or subclinical infections contracted before admission or after failure of SDD and (2) to offer a supplementary prophylaxis during the establishment of SDD, for ICU-acquired infections.[99] It has been shown that SDD significantly reduces nosocomial infection[99,111,118] without the emergence of multiresistant bacteria. Although no published study has shown an overall reduction in mortality, several have made claims that infection-related mortality has been reduced.[112,116,118] Almost all studies agree that colonization and infections due to Enterobacter or Pseudomonas spp. are dramatically reduced and would agree that if SDD is employed a heightened microbiologic surveillance should be employed.[99,111-118] Furthermore, some subgroups of patients such as trauma patients, those with moderate APACHE II scores (10 to 20), liver transplant patients, and perhaps long-stay patients may benefit from SDD.[111,114,118] The exact role of this therapy in the routine care of critically ill patients awaits further elucidation. Large, stratified, concurrent, controlled studies are underway and should help in this regard.[110]

Bacterial or endotoxin translocation, stress ulceration, and hemorrhage contribute significantly to the outcome of critically ill patients. Nutritional support has been documented to reduce the incidence of these complications and to modify the stress response to injury.[119] The method of administration of nutritional support is also relevant. Enteral nutrition attenuates the endocrine and hypermetabolic response to stress more than with total parenteral nutrition (TPN) and has a significantly lower incidence of major infections as compared with TPN.[120] This difference has been attributed to villous atrophy and to increase bacterial translocation. Enteral nutrition, on the other hand, is beneficial in maintaining mucosal integrity. Further, enteral nutrition stimulates the secretion of bile salts, which bind endotoxin. It helps to eliminate cholestasis and gallbladder sludge and, therefore, reduces the risk of acalculus cholecystitis. It also promotes the replication of enterocytes. These beneficial affects are seen only if enteral feeding is commenced early; it has been suggested that feeding should begin immediately through an enterostomy if abdominal surgery is required.[120,121]

Accumulating evidence suggests that the maintenance of gut mucosal integrity is beneficial. In this regard, intestinal glutamine metabolism has assumed a central role. Glutamine has a trophic affect on mucosal cellularity, and it promotes the proliferation of crypt enterocytes.[122-127] With sepsis, a marked reduction in glutamine metabolism occurs with a consequent reduction in mucosal integrity. Bacterial and endotoxin translocation are thus facilitated. The addition of glutamine to enteral nutrition has been shown to reduce bacterial translocation. On the other hand, current TPN solutions are glutamine free. This may be part of the reason why villous atrophy occurs in those patients receiving TPN.[122-127]

Stress ulcer prophylaxis is frequently required in the treatment of critically ill patients. Antacids, histamine$_2$ antagonists, and sucralfate have all been shown to be effective, although the incidence of pulmonary infections secondary to increased gastric colonization with bacteria is higher with antacids and histamine$_2$ antagonists.[81,128,129] We therefore currently use sucralfate for prophylaxis to reduce gastric and subsequent tracheal colonization with potential pathogens.[81,128,129]

Hematologic Dysfunction

Definitions of hematologic failure are given in Tables 64-1 and 64-2 and are discussed, in part, in Chapter 45. All components of the hematologic system become important in the host's response to critical illness; dysfunction of any one part of the hematologic system can thus contribute to the development MOF. Red blood cells and the hemoglobin contained within are thus important to carry oxygen. White blood cells and granulocytes are important in the defense against infection. Platelets and coagulation factors are required defenses against bleeding, and all of these components may be affected during critical illness.

Thus, patients with anemia, white cell dysfunction, or thrombocytopenia are at increased risk even before the initial insult to the host. Anemia that develops during the critical illness will reduce the ability to maintain adequate DO_2. Critical illness may also affect red blood cell function through an altered red blood cell deformability.[130] Microvascular DO_2 may therefore be compromised. Profound leukocytosis or leukocytopenia and an absolute lymphopenia may also occur, and the ability to defend against exogenous or endogenous bacterial or endotoxin loads is reduced in these situations. Thrombocytopenia is a frequent companion of sepsis and in this setting reflects a consumption of platelets. If associated with an elevation in PT or PTT, the syndrome of disseminated intravascular coagulation should be considered (see Chap. 45).

Leukocyte or platelet function may be affected by other organ system dysfunction such as renal failure. Platelet dysfunction may complicate the management of these patients. Thus, gastrointestinal bleeding may become a larger problem, and the need for invasive monitoring or therapeutic vascular devices may place the patient at additional risk.

Given that preexisting or concurrent dysfunction of any component of the hematologic system places the patient at risk, therapy must be directed at minimizing the role of any singular component dysfunction in the process culminating in MOF. Adequate oxygen carrying capacity can be maintained with the judicious use of packed red blood cell infusions. The risk of bleeding can be minimized by appropriate efforts to minimize the use of intravascular monitoring devices, by appropriate stress ulcer prophylaxis, and by judicious use of platelet transfusions. Aggressive treatment of infection and appropriate use of antibiotics can help to protect the patient who may be at increased risk for infection given the white blood cell abnormalities that may precede illness or subsequently develop.

Respiratory Dysfunction

Respiratory failure and the respiratory distress syndrome are discussed in Chapters 10 and 17, respectively. Definition of respiratory failure include alterations in respiratory frequency, an increase in the alveolar-arterial oxygen difference, abnormalities in carbon dioxide elimination and acid/base balance, and the requirement for prolonged mechanical ventilatory support (see Tables 64-1 and 64-2). In its most severe form, profound respiratory failure is associated with profound hypoxemia, respiratory acidosis, decreased pulmonary compliance, and radiologic abnormalities. Hemodynamic correlates of the ARDS include the absence of an elevated pulmonary arterial wedge pressure. Pathologic correlates include injury to alveolar epithelial cells and capillary endothelial cells. Accumulation of a protein exudate and the deposition of hyaline material have also been noted.[131]

As with all other organ systems, patients with pre-existing pulmonary disease are less able to tolerate any pulmonary insult and require more intensive therapy to support this system. The degree of support required is dictated by the degree of respiratory failure and the amount of underlying pulmonary function or pulmonary reserve that the patient has at the time of presentation. The FIO_2 and the requirement for different levels of PEEP are dictated by levels of the partial pressure of oxygen in arterial blood (PaO_2). Tidal volume and respiratory rate are dictated by the need to provide adequate carbon dioxide elimination in a setting where carbon dioxide production is frequently increased. Each of these therapies carry a cost to both lung and to remote organ systems. High FIO_2 levels can be toxic, and high levels of PEEP therapy invite the complication of barotrauma. PEEP may decrease venous return and may thus affect cardiac output and DO_2. Regional flows may be altered by PEEP, and this relationship is, in itself, altered in the presence of sepsis.[74] Prolonged intubations increase the likelihood of a pulmonary nosocomial pneumonia, and this is aggravated by the concomitant need to provide stomach alkalization therapy or by the need for the patient to remain supine.

When confronted with a patient with pulmonary dysfunction, every effort should be made to optimize this system before surgery (the pre-ICU phase). As such, cessation of smoking, bronchodilator administration, and physiotherapy should be administered. Once the patient is in established respiratory failure, attention should be directed to minimizing further insults and to aggressively treating complications as they occur. PaO_2 requirements should be met with the use of nontoxic FIO_2 and a minimal level of PEEP. Respiratory muscle tone should be maintained by the employment of a ventilatory strategy that requires the patient to do some ventilatory work. Respiratory muscle fatigue, on the other hand, should be avoided by ensuring proper nutrition and adequate rest. Nosocomial pneumonia is an ever-present threat and should be aggressively sought and treated with appropriate antibiotics. SDD and cytoprotection of gastric mucosa with sucralfate should be considered, because both have been shown to reduce the incidence of nosocomial pneumonia, as previously discussed.

Renal Dysfunction

Definitions of renal dysfunction are given in Tables 64-1 and 64-2. This topic is also discussed in Chapters 39 and 40. Essentially, renal dysfunction is defined as an impairment in renal concentrating ability or excretory function. Intravascular volume depletion, as may occur in sepsis, and acute tubular necrosis, as may follow an acute hypotensive event or an insult that is due to myoglobinuria following trauma, are frequent causes of this syndrome in the population that develops MOF. Histologically, disruption of basement membranes, patchy necrosis of tubules, and interstitial edema with tubular casts have been noted. These changes do not correlate well, however, with functional impairment.

Patients with renal failure are at great risk for the development of MOF for a number of reasons. In the face of complete anuria, fluid management is complicated. Pulmonary edema is more likely, and the ability to freely use TPN solutions is restricted. Host defense is depressed, and bleeding is more likely, which is due to the platelet dysfunction that occurs with uremia.

Fluid and TPN therapies are facilitated by the use of dialysis or CAVH, but these technologies are not without complications. Invasive intravascular access is required, and as such, line-related complications including line-related sepsis may occur. The dialysis membrane may activate PMNL, and complement and pulmonary hypertension and hypoxemia may result.

Patients with widespread atherosclerosis are at greater risk for the development of the acute renal failure, because they are less able to adjust renal blood flow with changes in perfusion pressure (e.g., hypotension). In sepsis, the kidney may not participate proportionately in the increased CO that is observed.[74] With preexisting renal failure, thromboxane (a potent vasoconstrictor) production and release is increased, and consequently, increments in renal blood flow may be difficult to achieve. Dopamine is sometimes used prophylactically to optimize renal blood flow in these patients through the selective dopaminergic effect, which occurs in low doses, on the mesenteric and renal vascular beds.[132] Intravascular volume depletion with or without shock and the use of potentially nephrotoxic drugs may all aggravate this process.

Given these concerns, it becomes critical to attempt to avoid hypotension and intravascular volume depletion. For example, prophylactic monitoring of abdominal aortic aneurysm patients with the use of a PAC has been shown to reduce the incidence of postoperative renal failure.[80] To the extent that this experience can be generalized to other situations, it follows that the PAC might facilitate aggressive yet tightly controlled volume administration or removal with dialysis or CAVH.

Preexisting or developing renal failure is identified by a rising blood urea nitrogen (BUN) and serum creatinine. Creatinine clearance is, however, a more sensitive indicator of the adequacy of renal function, and it correlates better with the outcome for the patient. Aggressive clearance of urea and creatinine can be obtained with the use of dialysis. Volume management may be obtained with concomitant ultrafiltration. Recently, CAVH, with or without the use of a dialysate fluid (CAVHD), has greatly facilitated the management of renal failure, especially in hemodynamically unstable critically ill patients. This form of therapy may be continuous, and although large volumes of fluid may be removed per unit time, it is frequently better tolerated in patients with marginal perfusion pressures. With CAVH or CAVHD, however, the clearance of solutes, BUN, and creatinine is slower; the effect of this therapy on the clearance of many drugs is more unpredictable.[133] Nevertheless, it has greatly facilitated the care of these patients and is occasionally the only option for some patients who would not tolerate dialysis.

Neurologic Dysfunction

Nervous system dysfunction is a common feature of MOF. It is manifest primarily as a peripheral polyneuropathy and/or as an encephalopathy and is objectively scored with the Glasgow coma scale (see Tables 64-1 and 64-2). These two entities are most frequently seen in patients who have been in the ICU for longer periods (mean onset of 28 days), and they are thus most frequently seen in association with sepsis and other organ dysfunction.

Peripheral Neuropathy

The polyneuropathy of critical illness was first described in 1983.[134] It is a syndrome of peripheral nerve dysfunction that is frequently seen in critically ill, septic ICU patients, and often in patients with MOF. Indeed, it is in itself an organ system failure (see Table 64-1). The incidence of this neuropathy, as defined electrophysiologically, is approximately 70% in a population with MOF.[135]

This neuropathy is characteristically painless. Clinically, it is manifest as distal weakness of limb muscles, reduced deep tendon reflexes, and difficulty weaning from mechanical ventilation.[134-137] Electrophysiologic studies show essentially normal conduction velocities and distal latencies but reduced compound muscle and sensory nerve action potential amplitudes. Needle electromyography (EMG) studies show abnormal spontaneous activity in muscle.[135] This constellation of observations suggests axonal degeneration, and it is thus clearly different from the Guillian-Barré syndrome, which affects primarily the myelin sheath with relative sparing of the nerve axons.[135] The neuropathy has been observed in peripheral nerves and in more central nerves such as the phrenic nerve. It has been correlated with EMG abnormalities in the intercostal muscles and in the diaphragm and has been confirmed with autopsy studies showing axonal degeneration of the phrenic nerve and denervation atrophy of the diaphragm and intercostal muscles. The neuropathy does not appear to be associated with significant or sustained elevations in creatinine phosphokinase levels or with the use of neuromuscular blocking drugs or particular antibiotics such as aminoglycosides or metronidazole.[134-137]

This syndrome can be identified by having a high index of suspicion and by performing EMG and electrophysiologic studies in a population with MOF, sepsis, or prolonged ICU admissions. In our experience, it is also frequently discovered in the attempt to explain why some patients fail to wean from mechanical ventilation. A typical scenario includes a patient in whom every physiologic variable has been corrected or optimized and the conclusion that the patient is not currently disadvantaged by any particular disease process. Such a patient would be hemodynamically stable without administration of inotropes or vasopressors and would have normal or adequate gas exchange as defined by a Pa_{O_2} of greater than 60 mm Hg or an F_{IO_2} of less than 40%. Further, the patient would have many of the predictive criteria for successful weaning[138,139] (see Chap. 24). The patient would be adequately nourished and have no evidence of metabolic alkalosis, CNS depression, or significant electrolyte abnormalities.

By all of these criteria, many of these patients should be successfully weaned from mechanical ventilation. Frequently, however, a failure to wean is observed. In these circumstances, the spontaneous respiratory rate climbs to levels more than 30 breaths per minute. The pH frequently falls, and patients develop a respiratory acidosis with a pH of less than 7.3 and a blood pressure level higher than 50 mm Hg. With the tachypnea, a fall in the spontaneous tidal volume is observed (a typical extraparenchymal restrictive pattern). The clinical signs of respiratory muscle fatigue, respiratory alternans, abdominal paradox, or asynchronous breathing may also be observed. Why then do these patients fail to wean? It is possible that occult cardiac failure is a factor, but this should be ruled out by use of a chest radiograph and Swan-Ganz catheterization. The other possibilities include an unsuspected increased work of breathing, respiratory muscle fatigue, respiratory muscle weakness, an inadequate ventilatory drive or excessive carbon dioxide production. Estimates for the work of breathing or of excessive carbon dioxide production can be obtained through the use of a metabolic measurement monitor (indirect calorimetry). A change in the EMG frequencies might also suggest respiratory muscle fatigue that frequently accompanies the clinical pattern of respiration mentioned previously. Respiratory muscle weakness can be postulated if the respiratory muscles have not been used adequately before the weaning attempt or if the muscle glycogen stores are hypothesized to be depleted as a result of inadequate nutrition.

In the day-to-day activity of the ICU, not all of these potential reasons for failure to wean can be investigated. However, if it is assumed that the circuitry of the ventilator has been optimized; if the resistances provided by the endotracheal tube or ventilator tubing have been minimized, and if there is no significant change in the work of breathing, then the following questions must be asked:

- Is a neuropathy present?
- Is a myopathy present?
- Is evidence of fatigue present?
- Is (by exclusion) a central problem with ventilatory drive present?

EMG and electrophysiologic studies can provide hard evidence in an attempt to answer these four questions.

The clinical relevance of these potential diagnoses lies in the natural history of this neuropathy of critical illness. Should the patient survive, then recovery from this polyneuropathy may be complete when the neuropathy is felt to be mild or even moderately severe. Those with severe polyneuropathy, however, may have prolonged recoveries and, in those patients who have been studied, may have a higher mortality rate.[135] The diagnosis of a polyneuropathy dictates, however, that we continue to support the patient, knowing that the prognosis for significant improvement is good. Establishing this diagnosis thus allows us to be patient and directs our attention to continuing to treat the complications of critical illness and to provide adequate nutrition and rest for these patients. As the patients begin to recover, strategies at respiratory muscle training may be introduced. Repeated EMG and electrophysiologic studies can further document the improvement in the neuropathy.

Encephalopathy

Almost all patients with a critical illness polyneuropathy suffer from a degree of encephalopathy.[140,141] The dysfunction of the brain is diffuse and is without either focal signs, cranial nerve dysfunction, decerebrate posturing, or paralysis. The major clinical abnormality is an alteration in the level of consciousness that may range from simple confusion to deep coma.[140,141] This abnormality characteristically fluctuates. When it is suspected, conditions such as meningitis, encephalitis, bacterial endocarditis, nonconvulsive seizures, and fluid or electrolyte disorders must be ruled out as a cause for this encephalopathy.

The disturbance in cerebral function yields typical electroencephalogram (EEG) changes. The degree of EEG changes reflects the clinical severity of the encephalopathy. Characteristically, slowing, triphasic waves, or intermittent rhythmic delta activity are observed. Some patients will show a burst suppression pattern.[141] The EEG cannot, however, be used to predict irreversibility. Indeed, no evidence suggests that the encephalopathy is irreversible. Observations of patients with MOF and the sepsis-associated encephalopathy have shown that the brain fails in parallel with other organs.[140,141] The brain thus appears to be a sensitive indicator of severe or generalized septic illnesses, and the presence of encephalopathy thus should be taken as a serious sign.

Computed tomographic head scans are frequently unremarkable, and the cerebral spinal fluid analysis is essentially normal with the exception of a mild increase in protein. Autopsy series have demonstrated disseminated microabscesses in the brain, most commonly in the cerebral cortex and subcortical white matter. There is also evidence of surrounding reaction within the brain, indicating that these microabscesses are not an agonal phenomenon. Some patients, however, have had only microglial nodules, and this suggests a purely metabolic cause rather than a primary infective cause.[140,141]

It has been hypothesized that the encephalopathy associated with sepsis is at least in part due to alterations in the function of the cerebral vasculature. It has been shown that cerebral blood flow is reduced in both human sepsis[142] and septic animal models.[143] This is apparently not due to a reduction in cerebral metabolic rate or consumption of oxygen, because this has been shown to be maintained or even increased in sepsis.[144] It has been shown that in animal models of sepsis the cerebral vascular resistance to blood flow is increased and that there is evidence of ischemia or insufficient blood flow for metabolic needs. This is supported by the observed increase in cerebral arterial venous oxygen difference of total carbon dioxide bicarbonate or oxygen saturation.[143]

Reduction in cerebral perfusion may be due to cerebral edema, which in turn may be due to increased capillary permeability. This could compromise both the microvasculature as well as impaired diffusion of oxygen to the brain cells. It has been shown that following intravenous injection of Escherichia coli endotoxin in dogs there is a rapid rise in cerebral spinal fluid (CSF) pressure.[145] With this increase in pressure, there is also an increase in CSF protein concentration, which may reflect an increase in blood-brain barrier permeability. Because this increase in CSF or intra-cranial pressure was not due to an increase in cerebral blood flow (this being decreased) and because it is unlikely that CSF production is increased, it may be hypothesized that reduction in cerebral perfusion is due to vasogenic edema.

The encephalopathy of sepsis may be due to either altered metabolism or altered clearance of toxic substances, as may occur in hepatic or renal failure. In hepatic failure, the encephalopathy has been attributed to ammonia, gamma amino butyric acid (GABA), short chain fatty acids, mercaptens (sulfur-containing compounds derived from the effect of colonic bacteria on methionine), or to a combination of all of these substances.[146,147]

An increase in aromatic amino acids (AAA) and a decrease in branched chain amino acids (BCAA) have also been implicated as a cause of hepatic encephalopathy.[146] In hepatic failure and in sepsis, increased glucagon initiates muscle catabolism and the release of amino acids. Hyperinsulinemia that is due to decreased hepatic clearance of insulin facilitates the uptake of BCAA by peripheral tissues while decreased hepatic metabolism of AAA occurs. This results in a net increase in AAAs and a relative decrease in BCAAs. These amino acids are transported across the blood-brain barrier by a common carrier, and as such, the altered AAA/BCAA ratio favors the accumulation of AAAs in the CNS. The increase in CNS AAA results in an increase in false neurotransmitters such as octopopamine or phenylethanolamine, a decrease in normal neurotransmitters such as dopamine or noradrenalin, and an increase in neuroinhibitors such as serotonin.[146].

Attempts to modify the encephalopathy associated with liver failure with BCAA infusions have met with various degrees of success. As a therapy for the encephalopathy, it is perhaps equal to the use of lactulose or neomycin in effectiveness.[146] It does, however, have the advantage over these two agents in allowing these patients to receive more nutrition than would otherwise be possible.

The consideration of septic encephalopathy is important. First, it requires exclusion of other conditions such as primary CNS infections, drug intoxications, or primary hepatic or renal failure. Following these exclusions, the presence of a septic encephalopathy suggests the possibility of occult sepsis, which must then be investigated and treated. As with the polyneuropathy of critical illness, a diagnosis of a septic encephalopathy suggests that patience and continued support are required because the condition is reversible, given time.

CLINICAL MANAGEMENT ISSUES
Metabolic Support

Metabolic support is an important adjunct to the hemodynamic support discussed previously (see Chap. 62). Here, the goals of therapy are to provide adequate substrate to correct malnutrition, reverse catabolism, and permit tissue repair. This is accomplished by providing a balanced caloric support of protein, carbohydrate, and fat and by attempts to reverse catabolism, which includes drainage of abscesses, fixation of fractures, and removal of necrotic tissue.[11]

The details of nutritional support are discussed elsewhere (see Chap. 62). Several elements of nutritional therapy, however, warrant emphasis:

- A minimum amount of carbohydrate is required by the brain, blood elements, and wound tissue (approximately 150 g of glucose), and this cannot be replaced by the administration of fat.
- Adequate amounts of amino acids are required to achieve position nitrogen balance (1.5 to 3 g of nitrogen per day).
- The enteral route is the preferred route if gut function permits.

Attempts to optimize host defenses and/or to prevent infection also require attempts to reverse catabolism (see preceding discussion) and attention to nutrition and tissue oxygenation. Additionally, attention needs to be directed to support mucosal and epithelial integrity. Thus, efforts should be directed to use invasive monitoring or support devices conservatively. Enteral nutrition supports gut mucosal integrity, and coupled with the sparing use of antibiotics or alkalinization agents, it minimizes the risk of bacterial overgrowth and consequently nosocomial pneumonia.

General Support

In addition to the physiologic support discussed previously, other principals of critical care support should be consistently and repeatedly applied. We must continue to look for and treat correctable problems such as occult infections and unrecognized operative complications or injury. We must continue to monitor organ system function so that the beneficial or detrimental effects of various therapies can be identified and/or modified. This requires that we remain cognizant of the numerous potential iatrogenic effects that may compromise a patient's or an organ's ability to recover. As such, we must guard against the inappropriate use of FIO_2, nephrotoxic, hepatotoxic, antibiotic, or sedative drugs and attempt to limit any exacerbation of preexisting chronic disease.

Endotoxin is a lipopolysaccharide component of the cell walls of gram-negative bacteria. In patients with sepsis and gram-negative bacteremia, endotoxin is believed to be the trigger that initiates many of the adverse system reactions that occurs in sepsis and septic shock (see previous discussion). Immunotherapy with human polyclonal antiserum, which is directed against endotoxin, has been shown to reduce mortality in patients with gram-negative bacteremia and to protect high risk surgical patients from septic shock.[148,149]

Recently, human monoclonal IgM antibody against endotoxin (HA-1A) has been developed. In a multicenter trial, HA-1A has been shown to reduce mortality by 39% in patients with gram-negative bacteremia. In patients with gram-negative bacteremia and septic shock, mortality was reduced by 42%. In a subgroup, patients with gram-negative bacteremia, septic shock, and MOF showed a reduction in mortality of 51% when given the human monoclonal antibody. No benefit was observed for patients who were septic who did not have gram-negative bacteremia.[150] In this study, the antibody was safe, well tolerated and nonimmunogenic. In addition to the reduced mortality discussed previously, a greater rate of resolution of major complications of sepsis (shock, desseminated intravascular coagulation, acute renal failure, acute hepatic failure, or ARDS) occurred in the group of patients receiving HA-1A.[150]

Murine IgM monoclonal antibody appears to protect patients with the sepsis syndrome, whether they are bacteremic or not. For those in shock, however, this particular monoclonal antibody does not appear to be protective.[151] The human IgM monoclonal antibody, on the other hand, appear to be protective.[151] The human IgM monoclonal antibody, on the other hand, appears to protect similar patients whether or not they are in shock, but only if they are bacteremic (with gram-negative organisms) at the time the antibody is given.[150] Exact clinical application of this new technology awaits more precise definition and many questions, such as the following, remain to be answered:

- Are there subgroups of patients that could be expected to benefit more than others and are there predictors that allow identification of these subgroups?
- Is it safe to use the agent more than once and, if so, is there an added benefit?
- Is there an optimal dose?
- Could it be used in conjunction with other antibodies?

Many developments are occurring in this area and include the use of antibodies against cytokines such as TNF. As discussed previously, TNF has been incriminated as a central mediator, and antibodies against TNF have been demonstrated to reduce mortality in different animal models of sepsis.[152-155] The effect of TNF and antibodies to TNF appear, however, to differ in different models of sepsis.[152-155] Indeed, low-dose recombinant TNF has also been demonstrated to protect animals against the lethality of sepsis.[152] The exact role of antibodies to TNF in the treatment of septic patients awaits the completion of multicenter trials that are presently ongoing.

Similarly, there are now antagonists to IL1 receptors (IL-1ra), which have been demonstrated to decrease mortality in a dose-dependent manner in endoxemic conditions.[156] Phase II trials are currently underway and are expected to further define the role of these new agents in the treatment of septic patients.

Further developments in addition to these blocking antibodies are expected to include technologies to stimulate biologic control systems, such as growth factors, colony stimulating factors, and so on, or technologies to replace deficits such as occurs in ARDS (surfactant). At present, current management strategies are not yet using these new technologies. Our therapies therefore remain directed at both diagnosing and aggressively treating infection, removing devitalized or necrotic tissue, and stabilizing fractures, while continuing to guard against the potential negative effects of what might be required therapies to support specific organ dysfunction.

Hemodynamic Support

Normally, local blood flow, tissue oxygen demand, and tissue Do_2 are closely coupled.[54] As previously discussed, data support the thesis that elevated tissue oxygen needs, which are characteristic of the host's septic response, are not adequately matched by increases in tissue oxygen availability.[56,62] Increased mortality in critical illness has been correlated with a relative depression in systemic Do_2 and rising arterial lactates,[65] and vasodilators have uncovered a covert oxygen debt in some septic patients.[71,72] It has also been demonstrated that outcome from critical illness is improved by the maintenance of supranormal oxygen delivery.[61]

Clinically, there are few available predictors that significant ischemia exists at the level of individual organs at least until the process is severe enough to cause systemic manifestation. In the presence of hypotension, we must assume that oxygen needs exceed Do_2. In normotensive patients, the identification of the presence of tissue oxygen needs in excess of delivery is imprecise and requires a synthesis of clinical and laboratory data in an appropriate situation. For example, tissue oxygen needs will be elevated in patients suffering major trauma or surgery. If there is also evidence that Pvo_2 is falling and/or arterial lactate is rising, then it is reasonable to assume that tissue oxygen needs are not being met, regardless of the level of systemic Do_2. In these patients, supranormal levels of Do_2 may be required, and a therapeutic challenge designed to augment Do_2 is warranted to reduce or reverse subtle indicators of tissue ischemia.

When systemic Do_2 is felt to be inadequate, therapeutic efforts should be altered, as discussed previously and as outlined in Figure 64-9. Thus, Cao_2 and CO should be augmented. This can be accomplished by several strategies, and each strategy raises several controversies. It is not the purpose of this chapter to review these controversies, but they are listed here as background for those strategies presented in Figure 64-9:

- Is there an optimal hemoglobin or hematocrit, and if so, are these levels the same for all organs?
- Is there a hydrostatic pressure that should not be exceeded during fluid resuscitation?
- Are there advantages or disadvantages to the use of sympathomimetic agents for different regional circulations (e.g., dopaminergic effects on mesenteric or renal blood flow)?

In summary, given the relatively high incidence and poor prognosis of MOF, it is important to attempt to prevent its development. Once MOF has developed, therapies designed to support individual organ systems become extensions of those strategies that were used to attempt to prevent its occurrence in the first place.

The most important step in the prevention of MOF is the identification of those patients at risk. With this identification, preventive efforts may be commenced in an effort to prevent organ system dysfunction or to provide support for already dysfunctional organ systems. In many cases, this may require admission to an ICU, which is the only place where some of these therapies may be given or where adequate monitoring of these therapies and organ system function may be done. It must be emphasized that the need for admission to an ICU is in itself a risk factor. The need for endotracheal intubation, forced immobility, broad-spectrum antibiotics, invasive intravascular devices, and so on, all place the patient at risk for the development of complicating factors.

Management of MOF thus involves stopping and controlling the injury or insult, improving blood flow, maintaining a high or supranormal oxygen consumption, supporting metabolism, and preventing or aggressively treating infection should it occur. These strategies should be introduced early, and a need for these strategies should be anticipated in those patients who are felt to be at high risk for the development of MOF.

REFERENCES

1. Baue, A. D.: Multiple, progressive, or sequential systems failure: a syndrome of the 1970s. Arch. Surg., *110*:779, 1975.
2. Pinsky, M. R., and Matuschak, G. M.: A unifying hypothesis of multiple systems organ failure: failure of host defense homeostasis. J. Crit. Care, *5(2)*:108, 1990.
3. Pinsky, M. R., and Matuschak, G. M.: Multiple systems organ failure: failure of host defense homeostatis. Crit. Care Clin., *5(2)*:199, 1989.
4. Pinsky, M. R.: Multiple system organ failure: malignant intravascular inflammation. Crit. Care Clin., *5(2)*:195, 1989.

5. Marsh, H. M.: Metabolic integrity of specific organ systems. Clin. Chem., 36:1547, 1990.
6. Cerra, F. B.: Hypermetabolism-organ failure syndrome: a metabolic response to injury. Crit. Care Clin., 5:289, 1989.
7. Rinaldo, J. E., and Heyman, S. J.: ARDS—a multisystem disease with pulmonary manifestations. Crit. Care Rep., 1:174, 1990.
8. Rinaldo, J. E., and Rogers, R. M.: Adult respiratory-distress syndrome. N. Engl. J. Med., 315:578, 1986.
9. DeCamp, M. M., and Demling, R. H.: Post-traumatic multisystem organ failure. JAMA, 260:530, 1988.
10. Marshall, J. C., and Sweeney, D.: Microbial infection and the septic response in critical surgical illness. Sepsis, not infection, determines outcome. Arch. Surg., 125:17, 1990.
11. Marshall, J. C.: Multiorgan failure. Care of the surgical patient. Sci. Am. 13:1, 1991.
12. Marchall, J. C., and Meakins, J. L.: Multiorgan failure. In Scientific American Medicine. American College of Surgeons. Care of the Surgical Patient, Vol. 1. Edited by N. Ehrlich.New York, Scientific American, Inc., 1989, p. 1.
13. Goldman, L.. Cardiac risks and complications of non-cardiac surgery. Ann. Intern. Med., 98:504, 1983.
14. Goldman, L., et al.: Multifactorial index of cardiac risk in non-cardiac surgical procedures. N. Engl. J. Med., 297:845, 1977.
15. Rao, T. L. K., Jacobs, K. H., and El-Etr, A. A.: Reinfarction following anesthesia in patients with myocardial infarction. Anesthesiology, 59:499, 1983.
16. Knaus, W. A., et al.: Prognosis in acute organ-system failure. Ann. Surg., 202:685, 1985.
17. Goris, R. J. A., Hans, K. S., and Nuytinck, Redl, H.: Scoring systems and predictors of ARDS and MOF. First Vienna shock forum, part B: monitoring and treatment of shock. Edited by G. Schlag and H. Redl. New York, Alan R. Liss, 1987, p. 3.
18. Dorinsky, P. M., and Gadek, J. E.: Mechanisms of multiple nonpulmonary organ failure in ARDS. Chest, 96: 885, 1989.
19. Cerra, F. B.: Multiple organ failure syndrome. Perspect. Crit Care, 1:1, 1988.
20. Baue, A. E.: Clinical manifestations and sequences of organ failure. In Shock, Sepsis and Organ Failure. Edited by G. Sclag, et al. New York, Springer-Verlag, 1990.
21. Balk, R. A., and Bone, R. C.: The septic syndrome. Crit. Care Clin., 5:1, 1989.
22. Tilney, N. L., et al.: Sequential system failure after rupture of abdominal aortic aneurysms: an unresolved problem in postoperative care. Ann. Surg., 178:117, 1973.
23. Fry, D. E., Pearstein, L., Fulton, R. L., and Polk, H. C.: Multiple system organ failure: the role of uncontrolled infection. Arch. Surg., 115:136, 1980.
24. Polk, J. C. Jr., and Shields, C. L.: Remote organ failure: a valid sign of occult intra-abdominal infection. Surgery, 81: 310, 1977.
25. Montgomery, A. B., Stager, M. A., Carrico, J. C., and Hudson, L. D.: Causes of mortality in patients with the adult respiratory distress syndrome. Am. Rev. Respir. Dis., 132:485, 1985.
26. Canadian Multiple Organ Failure Study Group: Sepsis—clarity of existing terminology . . . or more confusion? Crit. Care Med., 19:996, 1991.
27. Bone, R. C.: Sepsis, the sepsis syndrome, multiorgan failure: a plea for comparable definitions. Ann. Intern. Med., 114: 332, 1991.
28. Meakins, J. L., and Marshall, J. C.: The gastrointestinal tract: the "motor" of MOF (part of SIS panel discussion). Arch. Surg., 121:197, 1986.
29. Bell, R. C., Coalson, J. J., Smith, J. D., and Johanson, W. G.: Multiple organ system failure and infection in adult respiratory distress syndrome. Ann. Intern. Med., 99:293, 1983.
30. Sprung, C. L., et al.: The effects of high dose corticosteroids in patients with septic shock: a prospective controlled study. N. Engl. J. Med., 311:1137, 1984.
31. Goris, R. J. A., et al.: Multiple-organ failure and sepsis without bacteria. Arch. Surg., 121:897, 1986.
32. Bone, R. C., et al.: Controlled clinical trial of high dose methylprednisolone in treatment of severe sepsis and septic shock. N. Engl. J. Med., 317:653, 1987.
33. Craddock, P. R., et al.: Complement and leukocyte-mediated pulmonary dysfunction in hemodialysis. N. Engl. J. Med., 296:769, 1977.
34. Jacob, H. S., Craddock, P. R., Hammerschmidt, D. E., and Moldow, C. F.: Complement-induced granulocyte aggregation. N. Engl. J. Med., 302:789, 1980.
35. Michie, H. R., et al.: Detection of circulating tumor necrosis factor after endotoxin administration. N. Engl. J. Med., 318: 1482, 1988.
36. Wewers, M. D., Herzyk, D. J., and Gadek, J. E.: Alveolar fluid neutrophils elastase activity in the adult respiratory distress syndrome is complexed to alpha-2-macroglobulin. J. Clin. Invest., 82:1260, 1988.
37. Deitch, E. A., et al.: Hemorrhagic shock-induced bacterial translocation: the role of neutrophils and hydroxyl radicals. J. Trauma, 30:942, 1990.
38. McCord, J. M.: Oxygen-derived radicals: a link between reperfusion injury and inflammation. Fed. Proc., 46:2404, 1987.
39. Beutler, B., and Cerami, A.: The history, properties, and biological effects of cachectin. Biochemistry, 27:7575, 1988.
40. Colletti, L. M., et al.: Role of tumor necrosis factor-α in the pathophysiologic alterations after hepatic ischemia/reperfusion injury in the rat. J. Clin. Invest., 86:1936, 1990.
41. Nawroth, P. P., and Stern, D. M.: Modulation of endothelial cell hemostatic properties by tumor necrosis factor. J. Exp. Med., 163:740, 1986.
42. Mathison, J. C., Wolfson, D., and Ulevith, R. J.: Participation of tumor necrosis factor in the mediation of gram negative bacterial lipopolysaccharide-induced injury in rabbits. J. Clin Invest., 81:1925, 1988.
43. Cybulsky, M. I., Colditz, I. G., and Movat, H. Z.: The role of interleukin-1 in neutrophil leukocyte migration induced by endotoxin. Am. J. Pathol., 124:367, 1986.
44. Neta, R.: Why should internists be interested in interleukin-1? Ann. Intern. Med., 109:1, 1988.
45. Okusawq, S., and Gelfand, J. A.: Interleukin 1 induces a shock-like state in rabbits. J. Clin. Invest., 81:1162, 1988.
46. Beutler, B., et al.: Effect of gamma interferon on cachectin expression by mononuclear phagocytes. J. Exp. Med., 164: 1791, 1986.
47. Sun, X. M., and Hsueh, W.: Bowel necrosis induced by tumor necrosis factor in rats is mediated by platelet activating factor. J. Clin. Invest., 81:1328, 1988.
48. Palmer, R. M. J., Ferrige, A. G., and Moncada, S.: Nitric oxide release accounts for the biological activity of endothelium-derived relaxation factor. Nature, 327:524, 1987.
49. Stotman, G. J., et al.: Interaction of prostaglandins, activated complement, and granulocytes in clinical sepsis and hypotension. Surgery, 99:744, 1986.
50. Hinder, R. A., and Stein, H. J.: Oxygen-derived free radicals. Arch. Surg., 126:104, 1991.
51. Matuschak, G. M., and Martin, D. J.: Influence of end-stage liver failure on survival during multiple systems organ failure. Transplant. Proc., 9:40, 1987.
52. Matuschak, G. M., and Rinaldo, J. E.: Organ interactions in

the adult respiratory distress syndrome during sepsis: role of the liver in host defense. Chest, 94:400, 1988.
53. Matuschak, G. M., et al.: Effect of end-stage liver failure on the incidence and resolution of the adult respiratory distress syndrome. J. Crit. Care, 2:162, 1987.
54. Bersten, A., Ffaracs, B. S., and Sibbald, W. J.: Circulatory disturbances in multiple systems organ failure. Crit. Care Clin., 5:233, 1989.
55. Shepherd, A. P., et al.: Local control of tissue oxygen delivery and its contribution to the regulation of cardiac output. Am. J. Physiol., 225:747, 1973.
56. Shoemaker, W. C., Appel, P. L., and Kram, H. B.: Tissue oxygen debt as a determinant of lethal and nonlethal postoperative organ failure. Crit. Care Med., 16:1117, 1988.
57. Chernow, B., and Roth, B.: Pharmacologic manipulation of the peripheral vasculature in shock: clinical and experimental approaches. Circ. Shock, 18:141, 1986.
58. Cryer, H. G., Richardson, J. D., Longmine-Cook, S., and Brown, C. M.: Oxygen delivery in patients with adult respiratory distress syndrome who undergo surgery. Arch. Surg., 124:1378, 1989.
59. Cryer, H. M., et al.: Skeletal microcirculatory responses to hyperdynamic Escherichia coli sepsis in unanesthetized rats. Arch. Surg., 122:86, 1987.
60. Hersch, M., et al.: Histologic and ultrastructural changes in non-pulmonary organs during early hyperdynamic sepsis in sheep. Surgery, 107:397, 1990.
61. Shoemaker, W. C., et al.: Prospective trial of supranormal values of survivors as therapeutic goals in high-risk surgical patients. Chest, 6:1176, 1988.
62. Shoemaker, W. C., Montgomery, E. S., Kaplan, E., and Elwyn, D. H.: Physiologic patterns in surviving and nonsurviving shock patients. Arch. Surg., 106:630, 1973.
63. Shoemaker, W. C.: Relation of oxygen transport patterns to the pathophysiology and therapy of shock states. Intensive Care Med., 13:230, 1987.
64. Bland, R. D., Shoemaker, W. C., Abraham, E., and Cobo, J. C.: Hemodynamic and oxygen transport patterns in surviving and nonsurviving patients. Crit. Care Med., 13:85, 1985.
65. Rashkin, M. C., Bosken, C., and Baughman, R. P.: Oxygen delivery in critically ill patients relationship to blood lactate and survival. Chest, 87:580, 1985.
66. Cain, S. M.: Supply dependency of oxygen uptake in ARDS: myth or reality? Am. J. Med. Sci., 288:119, 1984.
67. Cain, S. M.: Peripheral oxygen uptake and delivery in health and disease. Clin. Chest Med., 4:139, 1983.
68. Cain, S. M.: Assessment of tissue oxygenation. Crit. Care Clin., 2:537, 1986.
69. Danek, S. J., et al.: The dependence of oxygen uptake on oxygen delivery in the adult respiratory distress syndrome. Am. Rev. Respir. Dis., 122:287, 1980.
70. Dantzker, D. R.: Role of oxygen supply dependence in ARDS. Crit. Care Rep., 1:260, 1990.
71. Bihari, D., Smithies, M., Gimson, A., and Tinker, J.: The effects of vasodilation with prostacyclin on oxygen delivery and uptake in critically ill patients. N. Engl. J. Med., 317:397, 1987.
72. Bihari, D. J., and Tinker, J.: The therapeutic value of vasodilator prostaglandins in multiple organ failure associated with sepsis. Intens. Care Med., 15:2, 1988.
73. Hersch, M., et al.: PEEP increases non-pulmonary microvascular fluid flux in healthy and septic sheep. Chest, 96:1142, 1989.
74. Bersten, A. D., Gnidec, A. A., Rutledge, F. S., and Sibbald, W. J.: Hyperdynamic sepsis modifies a PEEP-mediated redistribution in organ blood flows. Am. Rev. Respir. Dis., 141:1198, 1990.

75. Baue, A. E.: Multiple organ failure: a reappraisal. Intens. Care World., 7:23, 1990.
76. Diehl, J. T., Cali, R. F., Hertzer, N. R., and Beven, E. G.: Complications of abdominal aortic reconstruction. Ann. Surg., 197:49, 1983.
77. Tarhan, S., Moffitt, E. A., Taylor, W. F., and Giuliam, E. R.: Myocardial infarction after general anesthesia. JAMA, 220:1451, 1972.
78. Attia, R. R., et al.: Myocardial ischemia due to infrarenal aortic cross clamping during aortic surgery in patients with severe coronary artery disease. Circulation, 53:961, 1976.
79. Silverstein, R. R., et al.: Avoiding the hemodynamic consequences of aortic cross clamping and unclamping. Anesthesiology, 50:462, 1979.
80. Hesdorffer, C. S., et al.: The value of Swan-Ganz catheterization and volume loading in preventing renal failure in patients undergoing abdominal aneurysmectomy. Clin. Nephrol., 28:272, 1987.
81. Tryba, M.: Sucralfate versus antacids or H_2-antagonists for stress ulcer prophylaxis: a meta-analysis on efficacy and pneumonia rate. Crit. Care Med., 19:942, 1991.
82. Parker, M. M., et al.: Profound but reversible myocardial depression in patients with septic shock. Ann. Intern. Med., 100:483, 1984.
83. Parker, M. M., et al.: Response of left ventricular function in survivors and nonsurvivors of septic shock. J. Crit. Care, 4:19, 1989.
84. Parrillo, J. E.: Cardiovascular dysfunction in human septic shock and endotoxemia. In Perspectives in Shock Research: Metabolism Immunology, Mediators, and Models. Proceedings of the Eleventh Annual Conference on Shock, Fontana, W. I., June, 1988. Edited by J. C. Passmore. New York, Alan R. Liss, 1989, p. 107.
85. Parrillo, J. E., et al.: A circulating myocardial depressant substance in humans with septic shock. J. Clin. Invest., 76:1539, 1985.
86. Vincent, J. L.: The relationship between oxygen demand, oxygen uptake, and oxygen supply. Intensive Care Med., 16(Suppl. 2):S145, 1990.
87. Haupt, M. T., Gilbert, E. M., and Carlson, R. W.: Fluid loading increases oxygen consumption in septic patients with lactic acidosis. Am. Rev. Respir. Dis., 131:912, 1985.
88. Snyder, J. V.: Assessment of systemic oxygen transport. In Oxygen Transport in the Critically Ill. Edited by J. V. Snyder and M. R. Pinsky. Chicago, Year Book Medical Publishers, 1979, p. 179.
89. Reilly, J. M., et al.: A circulating myocardial depressant substance is associated with cardiac dysfunction and peripheral hypoperfusion (lactic acidemia) in patients with septic shock. Chest, 95:1072, 1989.
90. Haglund, U.: Myocardial depressant substances in septic shock. In Septic Shock—European View. Edited by J. L. Vincent and L. G. Thijs. New York, Springer, 1987, p. 129.
91. Gomez, A., et al.: Hemofiltration reverses left ventricular dysfunction during sepsis in dogs. Anesthesiology, 73:671, 1990.
92. Thijs, L. G., Schneider, A. J., and Groenveld, A. B. J.: The haemodynamics of septic shock. Intensive Care Med., 16(Suppl. 3):S182, 1990.
93. Raper, R., Sibbald, W. J., Driedger, A. A., and Gerow, K.: Relative myocardial depression in normotensive sepsis. J. Crit. Care, 4:9, 1989.
94. Weber, K. T., et al.: Contractive mechanics and interaction of the right and left ventricals. Am. J. Cardiol., 47:686, 1981.
95. Dahn, M. S., et al.: Splanchnic and total body oxygen consumption differences in septic and injured patients. Surgery, 101:69, 1987.

96. Deitch, E. A., Berg, R., and Specian, R.: Endotoxin promotes the translocation of bacteria from the gut. Arch. Surg., *122:*185, 1987.
97. Deitch, E. A., and Bridges, R. M.: Effect of stress and trauma on bacterial translocation from the gut. J. Surg. Res., *42:*536, 1987.
98. Carrico, C. J., et al.: Multiple-organ failure syndrome. Arch. Surg., *121:*196, 1986.
99. Van Saene, H. F. K., Stoutenbeek, C. P., and Zandstra, D. F.: Concept of selective decontamination of the digestive tract in the critically ill. *In* Update in Intensive Care and Emergency Medicine: Infection Control by Selective Decontamination. Vol. 7. Edited by H. F. K. Van Saene, C. P. Stoutenbeek, P. Lawin, and I. Ledingham. New York, Springer-Verlag, Heidelberg, 1989, p. 88.
100. Tracey, K. J., et al.: Shock and tissue injury induced by recombinant human cachectin. Science, *234:*470, 1986.
101. Beutler, B., Milsark, I. W., and Cerami, A.: Passive immunization against cachectin/tumor necrosis factor protects mice from lethal effect of endotoxin. Science, *229:*869, 1985.
102. Tracey, K. J., Lowry, S. F., and Cerami, A.: Cachectin/TNF-α in septic shock and septic adult respiratory distress syndrome. Am. Rev. Respir. Dis., *138:*1377, 1988.
103. Ziegler, E. J.: Tumor necrosis factor in humans. N. Engl. J. Med., *318:*1533, 1988.
104. Fong, Y., et al.: The acute splanchnic and peripheral tissue metabolic response to endotoxin in humans. J. Clin. Invest., *85:*1896, 1990.
105. Tracey, K. J., et al.: Anti-cachectin/TNF monoclonal antibodies prevent septic shock during lethal bacteremia. Nature, *330:*662, 1986.
106. Proctor, R. A.: Fibronectin: a brief overview of its structure, function, and physiology. Rev. Infect. Dis., *9:*S317, 1987.
107. Nicod, L., et al.: Evidence for pancreas injury in adult respiratory distress syndrome. Am. Rev. Respir. Dis., *131:*696, 1985.
108. Deitch, E. A., Morrison, J., Berg, R., and Specian, R. D.: Effect of hemorrhagic shock on bacterial translocation, infestinal morphology and intestinal permeability in conventional and antibiotic-decontaminated rats. Crit. Care Med., *18:*529, 1990.
109. Cevas, P., and Fine, J.: Route of absorption of endotoxin from the intestine in nonseptic shock. J. Reticulo. Endothelial. Soc., *11:*535, 1972.
110. de-Champs, C. L., et al.: Selective digestive decontamination by erythromycin-base in a polyvalent intensive care unit. Intensive Care Med., *19:*191, 1993.
111. Blair, P., et al.: Selective decontamination of the digestive tract: a stratified, randomized propsective study in a mixed intensive care unit. Surgery, *110:*303, 1991.
112. Kerver, A. J. H., et al.: Prevention of colonization and infection in critically ill patients: a prospective randomized study. Crit. Care Med., *16:*1087, 1988.
113. Ledingham, I. Mc. A., et al.: Triple regimen of selective decontamination of the digestive tract, systemic cefotaxime, and microbiological surveillance for prevention of acquired infection in intensive care. Lancet, *1:*785, 1988.
114. Ramsay, G., Newman, P. M., McCartney, A. C., and Ledingham, I. Mc. A.: Endotoxemia in multiple organ failure due to sepsis. *In* Bacterial Endotoxins: Pathophysiological Control. New York, Alan R. Liss, 1988, p. 237.
115. Tetteroo, G. W. M., Wagenvoort, J. H. T., Ince, C., and Bruining, H. A.: Effects of selective decontamination on gram-negative colonisation, infections and development of bacterial resistance in esophageal resection. Intensive Care Med., *16(Suppl. 3):*S224, 1990.
116. Ulrich, C., et al.: Selective decontamination of the digestive tract with norfloxacin in the prevention of ICU-acquired infections: a prospective randomized study. Intensive Care Med., *15:*424, 1989.
117. van der Waaij, D., Manson, W. L., Arends, J. P., and de Vries-Hospers, H. G.: Clinical use of selective decontamination: the concept. Intensive Care Med., *16(Suppl. 3):*S212, 1990.
118. van Saene, H. K. F., Stoutenbeek, C. P., and Gilberton, A. A.: Review of available trials of selective decontamination of the digestive tract (SDD). Infection, *18(Suppl. 1):*S5, 1990.
119. Cerra, F., et al.: The effect of stress level, amino acid formula, and nitrogen dose on nitrogen retention in traumatic and septic stress. Ann. Surg., *205:*282, 1987.
120. Moore, F. A., et al.: TEN versus TPN following major abdominal trauma—reduced septic morbidity. J. Trauma, *29:*916, 1989.
121. Moore, E. E., and Jones, T. N.: Benefits of immediate jejunostomy feeding after major abdominal trauma—a prospective randomized study. J. Trauma, *26:*874, 1986.
122. Jacobs, D. O., et al.: Combined effects of glutamine and epidermal growth factor on the rat intestine. Surgery, *104:*358, 1988.
123. Salloum, R. M., Copeland, E. M., and Soube, W. W.: Brush border transport of glutamine and other substrates during sepsis and endotoxemia. Ann. Surg., *213:*401, 1991.
124. Souba, W. W., et al.: The effects of sepsis and endotoxemia on gut glutamine metabolism. Ann. Surg., *211:*543, 1990.
125. Souba, W. W., et al.: The role of glutamine in maintaining a healthy gut and supporting the metabolic response to injury and infection. J. Surg. Res., *48:*383, 1990.
126. Hardy, P. E., Fedorak, R. N., Thomson, A. B. R., and Thurston, O. G.: Glutamine and its effects on the intestine. Can. J. Gastroenterol., *5:*94, 1991.
127. Detsky, A. S.: Parenteral nutrition—is it helpful? N. Engl. J. Med., *325:*573, 1991.
128. Cook, D. J., Laine, L. A., Guyatt, G. H., and Raffin, T. A.: Nosocomial pneumonia and the role of gastric pH: a meta-analysis. Chest, *100:*7, 1991.
129. Driks, M. R., et al.: Nosocomial pneumonia in intubated patients randomized to sucralfate versus antacids and/or histamine type 2 blockers: the role of gastric colonization. N. Engl. J. Med., *317:*1376, 1987.
130. Hurd, T. C., et al.: Red cell deformability in human and experimental sepsis. Arch. Surg., *123:*217, 1988.
131. Ashbaugh, D. G., et al.: Adult respiratory distress in adults. Lancet, *2:*319, 1967.
132. Szerlip, H. M.: Renal-dose dopamine: fact and fiction. Ann. Intern. Med., *115:*153, 1991.
133. Merrill, R. H.: the technique of slow continuous ultrafiltration. J. Crit. Ill., *6:*289, 1991.
134. Bolton, C. F., Brown, J. D., and Sibbald, W. J.: The electrophysiologic investigations of respiratory paralysis in critically ill patients. Neurology, *33:*186, 1983.
135. Witt, N. J., et al.: Peripheral nerve function in sepsis and multiple organ failure. Chest, *99:*176, 1991.
136. Zochodne, D. W., et al.: Critical illness polyneuropathy. Brain, *110:*819, 1987.
137. Roelofs, R. I.: Critical illness polyneuropathy. Chest, *99:*5, 1991.
138. Marini, J. J.: Weaning from mechanical ventilation. N. Engl. J. Med., *324:*1496, 1991.
139. Yang, K. L., and Tobin, M. J.: A prospective study of indexes predicting the outcome of trials of weaning from mechanical ventilation. N. Engl. J. Med., *324:*1445, 1991.

140. Young, G. B.: The encephalopathy associated with sepsis. Ann RCPSC, *19*:279, 1986.
141. Young, G. B., et al.: The encephalopathy associated with septic illness. Clin. Invest. Med., *13*:297, 1990.
142. Bowton, D. L., Bertels, N. H., Prough, D. S., and Stump, D. A.: Cerebral blood flow is reduced in patients with sepsis syndrome. Crit. Care Med., *17*:399, 1989.
143. Parker, J. L., and Emerson, T. E. Jr.: Cerebral hemodynamics, vascular reactivity, and metabolism during canine endotoxin shock. Circ. Shock, *4*:41, 1977.
144. Ekstrom-Jodal, B., Haggendahl, E., and Larsson, L. E.: Cerebral blood flow and oxygen uptake in endotoxin shock. An experimental study in dogs. Acta Anaesthesiol. Scand., *26*: 163, 1982.
145. Ekstrom-Jodal, B., Haggendahl, J., Larsson, L. E., and Westerlind, A.: Cerebral hemodynamics, oxygen uptake and cerebral arteriovenous differences in catecholamines following E. coli endotoxin in dogs. Acta Anaesthesiol. Scand., *26*:446, 1982.
146. Alexander, W. F., Spindel, E., Harty, R. F., and Cerda, J. J.: The usefulness of branched chain amino acids in patients with acute or chronic hepatic encephalopathy. Am. J. Gastroenterol., *84*:91, 1989.
147. Freund, H. R., Maggia-Sullam, M., Peiser, J., and Melamed, E.: Brain neurotransmitter profile is deranged during sepsis and septic encephalopathy in the rat. The effect of amino acid infusions. Arch. Surg., *121*:209, 1986.
148. Ziegler, E. J., et al.: Treatment of gram-negative bacteremia and shock with human antiserum to a mutant Escherichia coli. N. Engl. J. Med., *307*:1225, 1982.
149. Baumgartner, J. D., et al.: Prevention of gram-negative shock and death in surgical patients by antibody to endotoxin core glycolipid. Lancet, *2*:59, 1985.
150. Ziegler, E. J., et al.: Treatment of gram-negative bacteremia and septic shock with Ha-1A human monoclonal antibody against endotoxin. N. Engl. J. Med., *324*:429, 1991.
151. Greenman, R. L., et al.: A controlled clinical trial of E5 murine monoclonal IGM antibody to endotoxin in the treatment of Gram-Negative sepsis. JAMA, *266*:1097, 1991.
152. Sheppard, B. C., Fraker, D. L., and Norton, J. A.: Prevention and treatment of endotoxin and sepsis lethality with recombinant human tumor necrosis factor. Surgery, *106*:156, 1989.
153. Bagby, G. J., Plessala, K. J., Wilson, L. A., and Thompson, J. J.: Divergent efficacy of antibody to tumor necrosis factor-α in intravascular and peritonitis models of sepsis. J. Infect., *163*:83, 1991.
154. Evans, G. F., Snyder, Y.M., Butler, L.D., and Zuckerman, S. H.: Differential expression of interleukin-1 tumor necrosis factor in marine shock models. Circ. Shock, *29*:279, 1989.
155. Bone, R. C.: A critical evaluation of new agents for the treatment of sepsis. JAMA, *266*:1686, 1991.
156. Ohlsson, K., et al.: An interleukin-1 receptor antagonist reduces mortality from endotoxin shock. Nature, *348*:550, 1990.

SUPPLEMENTAL READINGS

Appelmelk, B. J., Degraaff, J., Thijs, L. G., and Maclaren, D. M.: Reappraisal of endotoxin in gram-negative sepsis. Lancet, *41*:1662, 1993.
Arnow, P. M., Quimosing, E. M., and Beach, M.: Consequences of intravascular catheter sepsis. Clin. Infect. Dis., *16*:778, 1993.
Astiz, M. E., et al.: Oxygen delivery and consumption in patients with hyperdynamic septic shock. Crit. Care Med., *15*:26, 1987.
Ayala, A., et al.: Differential alterations in plasma IL-6 and TNF levels after trauma and hemorrhage. Am. J. Physiol., *260*:R167, 1991.
Bone, R. C.: Monoclonal antibodies to endotoxin: new allies against sepsis. JAMA, *266*:1125, 1991.
Bone, R. C.: A critical evaluation of new agents for the treatment of sepsis. JAMA, *266*:1686, 1991.
Bone, R. C., Sprung, C. L., and Sibbald, W. J.: Definitions for sepsis and organ failure. (Editorial). Crit. Care Med., *20*:724, 1992.
Bone, R. C.: A new therapy for the adult respiratory distress syndrome. N. Engl. J. Med., *328*:431, 1993.
Bone, R. C.: Why new definitions of sepsis and organ failure are needed. Am. J. Med., *95*:348, 1993.
Carrico, C. J.: The elusive pathophysiology of the multiple organ failure syndrome. Ann Surg., *218*:109, 1993.
Caset, L. C., Balk, R. A., and Bone, R. C.: Plasma cytokine and endotoxin levels correlate with survival in patients with the sepsis syndrome. Ann. Intern. Med., *119*:771, 1993.
Celli, B.: Respiratory muscle strength after upper abdominal surgery. Thorax, *48*:683, 1993.
Cipolle, M. D., Pasquale, M. D., and Cerra, F. B.: Secondary organ dysfunction: from clinical perspectives to molecular mediators. Crit. Care Clin., *9*:261, 1993.
Coalson, J. J.: Pathology of sepsis, septic shock and multiple organ failure. In Perspectives on Sepsis and Septic Shock. Edited by W. J. Sibbald and C. L. Sprung. Fullerton, CA, Society of Critical Care Medicine, 1986, p. 27.
Cohen, J.: Clinicial studies of anti-tumor necrosis factor in sepsis. In Tumor Necrosis Factor: Molecular and Cellular Biology and Clinical Relevance. Basel, S. Karger, 1993, p. 172.
Deitch, E. A., Maejima, K., and Berg, R.: Effect of oral antibiotics and bacterial overgrowth on the translocation of the GI tract microflora in burned rats. J. Trauma, *25*:385, 1985.
Deitch, E. A., and Berg, R. D.: Endotoxin but not malnutrition promotes bacterial translocation of the gut flora in burned mice. J. Trauma, *27*:161, 1987.
Demling, R., Lalonde, C., Saldinger, P., and Knox, J.: Multiple-organ dysfunction in the surgical patient: pathophysiology, prevention and treatment. Curr. Probl. Surg., *30*:345, 1993.
Gianotti, L., Alexander, J. W., Pyles, T., and Fukushima, R.: Arginine-supplemented diets improve survival in gut-deprived sepsis and peritonitis by modulating bacterial clearance: the role of nitric oxide. Ann. Surg., *217*:644, 1993.
Hebert, P. C., et al.: A simple multiple system organ failure scoring system predicts mortality of patients who have sepsis syndrome. Chest, *104*:230, 1993.
Hersch, M., et al.: Histopathological evidence of tissue ischemia in a hyperdynamic and non-hypotensive septic animal mode. Surgery, *107*:397, 1990.
Johnson, B. D., and Sieck, G. C.: Differential susceptibility of diaphragm muscle fibers to neuromuscular transmission failure. J. Appl. Physiol., *75*:341, 1993.
Lang, C. H., Bagby, G. J., Ferguson, J. L., and Spitzer, J. J.: Cardiac output and redistribution of organ blood flow in hypermetabolic sepsis. Am. J. Physiol., *246*:R331, 1984.
Livingston, D. H.: Management of the surgical patient with multiple system organ failure. Am. J. Surg., *165(2A Suppl.)*:8S, 1993.
Michie, H. R., et al.: Detection of circulating tumor necrosis factor after endotoxin administration. N. Engl. J. Med., *318*:1418, 1988.
Pullicino, E. A., et al.: The relationship between the circulating concentrations of interleukin 6, TNF and the acute phase

response to elective surgery and accidental injury. Lymphokine Res., 9:231, 1990.

Siafakas, N. M., et al.: Effect of aminopohylline on respiratory muscle strength after upper abdominal surgery: a double-blind study. Thorax, 48:693, 1993.

Suffredini, A. F., et al.: the cardiovascular response of normal humans to the administration of endotoxin. N. Engl. J. Med., 321:280, 1989.

Tracey, K. J., et al.: Shock and tissue injury induced by recombinant human cachectin. Science, 234:470, 1986.

Walmrath, D.: Aerosolised prostacyclin in adult respiratory distress syndrome. Lancet, 342:961, 1993.

Weissman, C.: The metabolic response to stress: an overview and update. Anesthesiology, 73:308, 1990.

West, M. A., Manthei, R., and Bubrick, M. P.: Autoregulation of hepatic macrophage activation in sepsis. J. Trauma, 34:473, 479, 1993.

Wilmore, D. W., et al.: The gut: a central organ after surgical stress. Surgery, 104:917, 1988.

Chapter 65

RECEPTOR PHYSIOLOGY AND PHARMACOLOGY IN CIRCULATORY SHOCK

THOMAS L. HIGGINS
BART CHERNOW

Shock is a syndrome of circulatory dysfunction characterized by inadequacy of tissue perfusion and oxygen delivery (Do_2). Management of circulatory shock is an important function of the critical care practitioner, because untreated shock progresses rapidly to death. Investigations over the past decade suggest that maximal benefits are attained with prompt initiation of treatment, which highlights the importance of early recognition and intervention. The final common pathway of shock results in hypotension and organ hypoperfusion, but because the initial events differ, an understanding of both homeostatic compensation and pharmacologic manipulation is essential. Such understanding includes knowledge of receptor physiology and the pharmacology of the vasoactive drugs.

In this chapter we discuss the physiology of the shock state, review the circumstances in which shock states are likely, and review the causes and diagnostic characteristics of four types of shock: distributive, cardiogenic, hypovolemic, and obstructive. The factors that increase a patient's risk for shock are discussed, as are the factors that modulate the expected homeostatic compensation and therapeutic responses to catecholamines and other vasoactive agents.

DEFINITION AND CLINICAL PRESENTATION OF SHOCK

Circulatory shock exists when perfusion to tissues is inadequate to maintain normal cellular function. Diminished perfusion is typically accompanied by severe hypotension, abnormalities of circulation, and lactic acidosis. Shock may be present, however, even with normal blood pressure, at any level of cardiac output, and with any value of peripheral vascular resistance. If abnormalities exist in the distribution of cardiac output, some organ systems may remain in a low perfusion state, while total cardiac output and oxygen transport appear normal. Thus, it is important to clinically assess individual organ systems for evidence of hypoperfusion (Table 65-1). Clinical findings associated with shock include the following:

- Mean arterial blood pressure less than 60 mm Hg
- Cardiac index of less than 2.1 L/min/m^2
- Urinary output of less than 0.5 ml/kg per hour
- Diminished cerebral perfusion resulting in confusion
- Decreased toe temperature[1]

Laboratory findings include an increase in the gradient between arterial and venous oxygen content, venous hypercarbia,[2] a metabolic acidosis, and increases in venous and arterial blood lactate concentrations.[3] Analysis of oxygen transport typically shows low oxygen consumption (Vo_2) and Do_2 with cardiogenic shock.[4] With distributive shock, however, Vo_2 may be increased, inappropriately normal, or diminished in the face of increased demand because of inadequate Do_2. In the early, compensated stages of shock, actions of endogenous catecholamine release are prominent. The patient may be anxious, pale, diaphoretic, and have a thready pulse as arterial vasoconstriction shifts blood from the peripheral to the central compartment. In the next, or progressive stage of shock, vasoconstriction cannot be maintained, and the vascular space enlarges secondarily from peripheral vasodilatation. Pulmonary, hepatic, and renal congestion occurs, and increased lung water in this phase can precipitate respiratory failure and the need for endotracheal intubation and mechanical ventilation. Arterial and central venous pressures decrease as does peripheral blood flow. Acidosis, ileus, and a hypercoagulable state are often present. Hematologic abnormalities include consumptive coagulopathy, microembolization, and fibrinolysis; these abnormalities can present clinically as "oozing" from needle puncture sites or gastrointestinal bleeding. The final stage of shock is characterized by irreversible multiple organ system failure from prolonged inadequate tissue perfusion. At this stage, mortality from shock is likely in most if not all patients.

CATEGORIES OF SHOCK

Shock states can be categorized as follows:

- Hypovolemic
- Distributive
- Cardiogenic
- Obstructive

Hypovolemic shock occurs with acute or subacute bleeding caused by trauma, surgery, or occult blood loss into body cavities. Severe dehydration as a result of glucosuria, diaphoresis, inadequate fluid intake, and intestinal losses from diarrhea and vomiting can also precipitate hypovolemic shock. Experimental animals tolerate 30% loss of blood volume; but, when the blood loss exceeds 40%, timely intervention is necessary to prevent irreversible pro-

Table 65–1. Clinical Presentation of Shock

Organ System	Effect
Brain	Obtundation, infarction
Heart	Ischemia, arrythmias, low output
Lungs	Hypoxemia, hypercardia
Gastrointestinal tract	Intraluminal pH decrease; gastrointestinal bleeding; failure of antacids to neutralize pH
Liver	Enzyme elevation, decreased synthesis
Kidney	Oliguria, anuria, decreased clearance
Skin	Mottling, temperature change

gression to death.[5] Hemorrhagic shock activates the sympathetic nervous system, as evidenced by markedly increased plasma concentrations of epinephrine and norepinephrine.[6] The hypothalamic-pituitary-adrenocortical axis is also stimulated. Demedullation of the adrenal glands eliminates the epinephrine response and blunts the norepinephrine response to hemorrhagic shock, suggesting that the adrenals are a major source of this catecholamine release.[7]

Distributive shock occurs as a result of sepsis syndrome (particularly in the setting of gram-negative bacteremia with release of endotoxin), spinal cord injury, anaphylactic and anaphylactoid reactions, and other conditions in which the blood volume, no longer contained by reflex vasoconstriction distributes over a much larger space. Distributive shock is called "warm shock," because in the early phases capillary beds are wide open, resulting in increased skin blood flow. The early clinical presentation of distributive shock includes tachypnea, warm dry skin, low central venous pressures, and arterial hypotension. Patients with distributive shock with good myocardial function may have a cardiac index in excess of 5 L/per minute per m^2 and a systemic vascular resistance, which is correspondingly low (less than 600 dynes per second per cm^5). This phase of shock is transient if untreated and progresses to the more typical presentation of "cold, clammy shock" as capillary leakage occurs, resulting in further hypovolemia and decreased venous return to the heart, or as the heart fails from ischemia or the effects of direct myocardial depressant factors.

Cardiogenic shock results from loss of functioning myocardium, for example, after massive myocardial infarction or following cardiopulmonary bypass for open heart surgery. Clinically important, impairment of ventricular function occurs with loss of more than 40% of left ventricular myocardium but can also be precipitated by lesser amounts of myocardial compromise when prior dysfunction, valvular disease, or concomitant rhythm disturbances are present. Hallmarks of cardiogenic shock include a reduction in the arterial blood pressure, accompanying arrhythmias, pulmonary edema, reduced shock volume, and increased vascular filing pressures. The initial compensatory response to decreased stroke volume is tachycardia, which can further exacerbate ischemia. Peripheral vasoconstriction, another compensatory response, also impairs myocardial performance through increased afterload. Because cardiogenic shock is a form of pump failure that results in a mismatch between the body's oxygen supply and demand, a reduction in cardiac afterload through pharmacologic vasodilatation is often part of the therapeutic strategy. This approach is in contrast to other forms of shock where the systemic vascular resistance is already low and afterload reduction would be ineffective or contraindicated.

Obstructive shock is caused by pericardial tamponade dissecting aortic aneurysms, vena caval obstruction, valvular heart disease, and embolization of air, fat, or thrombus to major vessels such as pulmonary arteries. Cardiovascular collapse occurs secondary to either diminished preload or abrupt increases in afterload as a result of mechanical obstruction. Volume expansion temporarily augments cardiac filling in obstructive shock, allowing time for definitive surgical or thrombolytic therapy of the responsible lesion. Initial compensation for obstructive shock is similar to that of cardiogenic shock, but initial therapy differs markedly, as volume expansion (increased preload) is indicated with obstructive shock.

PRE-ICU PHASE: RISK FACTORS FOR CLINICAL SHOCK

Bacteremia and Nosocomial Infections

Any seriously ill patient is at risk for developing shock, but certain conditions increase the risk. Patients in ICUs are at risk for developing secondary infections, with nearly one quarter of patients in one prospective study developing nosocomial infections during their ICU stay.[8] It has been suggested that bacteremia in hospitalized patients may be predicted by the following factors:[9]

- Rapidly or ultimately fatal disease
- Shaking chills
- Intravenous drug abuse
- Acute abdominal process
- Major co-morbidity

Abnormalities of membrane receptors in neutrophils and monocytes have been noted in ICU patients who develop nosocomial infections.[10] The presence of indwelling central venous catheters breaches the defense of intact skin,[11] and contamination of intravenous infusion delivery systems occurs. This risk can be minimized by use of a 0.22-μm bacterial retention filter on intravenous catheters.[12] Factors that may influence the rate of catheter-related sepsis include the following:

- Limiting period of catheterization to 6 days[13]
- Use of dry gauze rather than transparent plastic dressings[14]
- Use of a silver-impregnated cuff at the catheter entry site[15]
- Hand-washing practices of hospital personnel[16]

Contaminated condensate in mechanical ventilatory circuits increases the risk of nosocomial pneumonia, and special care must be taken to minimize "rain out" and prevent any potentially contaminated condensate from entering the patient's tracheobronchial tree.[17] The incidence of nosocomial pneumonia can be decreased by the use of sucralfate (as compared to antacids or histamine$_2$ blockers) for gastric cytoprotection in ventilated patients, possibly by preserving the bacteriostatic activity of an acid stomach pH.[18] Use of a polymyxin-tobramycin paste on the buccal mucosa may prevent lower airway colonization and infection in mechanically ventilated patients.[19] Daily monitoring of respiratory mucous pH may be of benefit in early detection of the change from colonization to pneumonia in intubated patients.[20] The presence of an indwelling bladder catheter is an important risk factor for the subsequent development of cystitis and ascending urinary tract infections. Measurement of urinary leukocyte esterase activity can screen for the presence of clinically important bacteriuria.[21] Although the patient's underlying disease state is possibly the most important risk factor for bacteremia, it is the ICU physician's responsibility to be aware of these other risk factors and take appropriate managerial steps to minimize the occurrence rate of nosocomial bacteremias and pneumonias.

Anaphylactic and Anaphylactoid Reactions

Hypersensitivity reactions are common in the ICU and may range from mild urticaria to fatal anaphylactic shock. Anaphylactic reactions result from reactions between a specific allergen and cell-fixed antibodies. Anaphylactic reactions are immunoglobulin E (IgE) mediated. Anaphylactoid reactions manifest in a similar way but are caused by non-IgE-mediated release of mediators. Although not presently routine, measurement of the plasma or serum tryptase concentration may be predictive of mass cell-related events in a susceptible population.[22] Anaphylactoid reactions are associated with the administration of a number of drugs, including narcotics, sedatives, and muscle relaxants commonly used in the ICU (Table 65-2). Intravenous contrast material may also precipitate an anaphylactoid reaction, and pretreatment with corticosteroids may minimize these reactions.[23] Protamine, used to reverse heparin anticoagulation, is associated with life-threatening reactions, and the risk is increased in patients with measurable protamine IgG antibodies.[24]

Loss of Functioning Myocardium

Cardiogenic shock is common after acute myocardial infarction, and early identification of patients at high risk for postinfarct complications can be accomplished using clinical variables such as systolic blood pressure, heart rate, age, presence of intraventricular conduction disturbances, site of myocardial infarction, and degree of obesity.[25] Primary ventricular fibrillation, when present, increases the risk of early mortality in patients with acute myocardial infarction.[26] Serial tomographic imagery with radionucleotides may prove useful in identifying patients with ST-segment changes whose myocardium is at risk and can be salvaged by reperfusion therapy.[27] Ventricular septal rupture is an important cause of postinfarction shock and may dictate surgical intervention.[28] Even infarction without ventricular septal rupture markedly increases the risk of perioperative mortality in both cardiac[29] and noncardiac operations.[30]

Limitations to Blood Flow

Prolonged bed rest or immobilization increases the risk for pulmonary embolism, an important cause of obstructive shock. Congestive heart failure, extensive trauma, surgery to the pelvis or lower extremities, thrombophlebitis, obesity, malignant neoplasms, or debilitating illnesses, hemiplegia or hemiparesis, coagulation abnormalities, or history of previous pulmonary embolism are other important risk factors for obstructive shock secondary to pulmonary embolism.[31] Risk factors for sudden hemodynamic compromise also include idiopathic hypertrophic subaortic stenosis (IHSS), intracardiac tumors, and aneurysms with potential for dissection.

Mediators in Shock States

Regardless of the initial cause of circulatory failure, release of vasoactive mediators eventually results in a final common pathway of vasodilatation, myocardial depression, and organ system failure as homeostatic mechanisms are overwhelmed (Fig. 65-1). About 30 mediators with important clinical effects have been described in shock states (Table 65-3).

The transition from homeostatic response to injury to multisystem organ failure occurs with persistent perfusion deficits, and in the presence of dead or injured tissue, uncontrolled infection, respiratory distress syndrome, persistent hypermetabolism, and preexisting fibrotic liver disease.[32] Failure of the liver is an important marker for this transition, and monokines are felt to have a role in altering hepatic metabolism in sepsis.[32] Other mediators associated with circulatory collapse and progression to multiple organ failure include plasma endotoxin levels,[33] and circulating phospholipase A_2 levels[34] and tumor necrosis factor (TNF).[35]

Increased plasma endotoxin and vasoactive intestinal polypeptide concentrations correlate with poor outcome in septic shock.[36] D-erythroneopterin plasma levels[37] and serum phospholipase A_2 levels[34,38] are among the markers proposed for early assessment of severity in septic shock, although the clinical relevance is uncertain until rapid assays are widely available. Early reports on the use of antiendotoxin monoclonal IgM antibodies were favorable.[39,41] However, questions have been raised about the reproducibility of these studies and whether antiendotoxin mono-

Table 65-2. ICU Pharmacologic Agents Commonly Associated With Anaphylactic or Anaphylactoid Reactions

Anaphylactic Reactions
  Antibiotics (Beta-lactam drugs, vancomycin, sulfonamides, nitrofurantoin)
  Blood products
  Contrast media
  Egg protein (foods, antisera)
  Hormones: insulin, adrenocorticotropic hormone, thyroid-stimulating hormone
  Local anesthetics
Anaphylactoid Reactions
  Antibiotics: vancomycin
  Barbiturates: thiopental, thioanylal
  Contrast media
  Muscle relaxants: D-tubocurarine, atracurium
  Opioids: morphine, meperidine

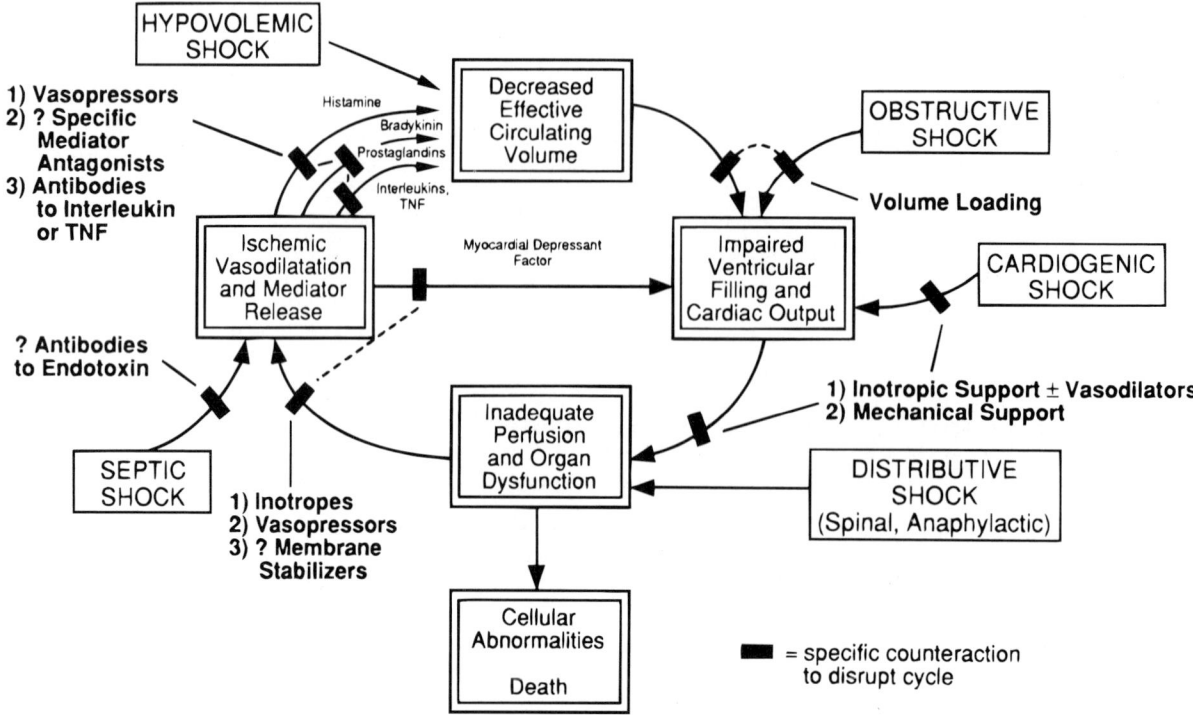

Fig. 65–1. Regulatory systems in shock. Regardless of the entry point, untreated shock eventually results in cellular dysfunction and death. Homeostatic mechanisms to break this downward spiral include endogenous catecholamines and other mediators. Physicians can disrupt the spiral at a number of points with volume loading, inotropic and mechanical support, vasopressors, membrane-stabilizing agents, and specific antagonists of endogenous mediators such as histamine, prostaglandins, beta endorphin, endotoxin, and tumor necrosis factor. (From Higgins, T. L.: Current concepts in inotropic support. Hosp. Form. 25:966, 1990.)

clonal therapy will be cost effective.[41a,41b] At this writing, these therapies remain experimental.

Eicosanoids

Monokines—regulatory proteins that mediate endocrine mechanisms—are released as part of the nonspecific host defense to inflammation. The macrophage system is thought to be responsible for the secretion of monokines, which if unchecked, contribute to the metabolic derangements of septic shock.[42] Platelets, granulocytes, mast cells, and monomacrophages are responsible for the generation of eicosanoids, a class of endogenous mediators derived from arachidonic (eicosatetraenoic) acid.[43] After arachidonic acid is released, some is transformed by cyclo-oxygenase into a variety of vasoactive substances, including prostaglandins, thromboxanes, endoperoxides, and hydroperoxides[44] (Fig. 65–2). Arachidonic acid is also transformed by lipoxygenase to form leukotrienes, and the balance between cyclo-oxygenase and lipoxygenase products determines the overall vasoactive effects. Eicosanoids include prostaglandin E_2 (PGE_2), a vasodilator and bronchodilator; $PGF_{2\alpha}$, a broncho and vasoconstrictor; thromboxane A_2 (TxA_2), a vasoconstrictor and platelet aggregator; and PGI_2, which has effects opposite those of TxA_2.

Tumor necrosis factor, produced in large quantities by endotoxin-activated monocytes,[45] is released following exogenous endotoxin administration[46] and also in septic shock. TNF, also called cachectin, is thought to be responsible for the severe wasting seen with chronic infectious and neoplastic diseases.[35] Increased circulating TNF levels are found in patients with septic shock, and increased TNF levels correlate with mortality rate.[47] When administered to laboratory animals, in quantities similar to those concentrations produced in response to endotoxin, TNF causes hypotension, metabolic acidosis, hemoconcentration, and death as a result of respiratory arrest within minutes to hours.[47] A single injection of TNF in healthy volunteers activates the common pathway of coagulation, probably by the extrinsic route,[48] suggesting that this mediator plays a role in the early activation of the hemostatic mechanism in septicemia as well. TNF may also be important in mobilization of host energy stores and depletion of intravascular volume. Because TNF is thought to be responsible for the severe wasting seen in chronic infections and neoplastic diseases,[35] speculation can be raised that these patients may be at higher risk for shock by virtue of existing low grade TNF activation. The administration of monoclonal antibodies to TNF prevents septic shock following induced bacteremia in animals,[49] but clinical studies have been less conclusive, because the entry points are less clear and matching for severity of illness more difficult.

Other Mediators

Other mediators present in shock states include myocardial depressant factor (MDF), leukotriene D4 (LTD_4), and platelet-activating factor (PAF). They mediate potent

Table 65-3. Mediators in Shock States

Mediator	Effect
Arachidonic acid metabolites	Vasoconstriction or dilatation
Bradykinin	Vasodilatation
	Inflammatory response
Beta endorphin	Hypotension, sedation
Catecholamines	Alterations in regional blood flow
Complement	Neutrophil aggregation
Corticosteroids	Inhibition of mediator release
Endotoxin	Monokin release; "triggering" agent?
Hageman factor	Activation of clotting and fibrinolysis
Interleukin 1	Altered temperature
	Breakdown of muscle
	Pituitary and hypothalamic stimulation (see Table 65-4)
Interleukin 6 (Interleukin β-2)	Fever, synthesis of acute phase proteins, activation of B and T lymphocytes, stimulation of hematopoietic progenitor and stem cells
Interleukin 2	Ventricular dysfunction
Leukotrienes	Vasoconstriction
	Bronchoconstriction
	Capillary permeability
Monokines	Cellular activation
Myocardial depressant factor	Negative inotropy
Platelet-activating factor	Platelet activation (adherence)
	Ventricular dysfunction
	Capillary permeability
	Bronchoconstriction
Prekallikrein and histamine	Hypotension
	Capillary permeability
Prostaglandins	Multiple effects (see text)
Serotonin	Capillary leakage
Thromboxane A_2	Vasoconstriction
	Platelet aggregation
Tumor necrosis factor (TNF/Cachexin)	Coagulability
	Endothelial changes
	Necrosis
	Hypotension
	Metabolic acidosis
	Hemoconcentration

Table 65-4. Effects of Interleukin 1[55,56]

Target Organ/Tissue	Effect
Pituitary	Release of adrenocorticotropic hormone
Hypothalamus	Fever
Bone marrow	Leukocytosis, activation of T and B cells, proliferation of antigen-stimulated lymphocytes
Liver	Acute-phase reactants synthesis of fibrinogen and iron-binding proteins
	Downregulates hepatocyte glucocorticoid receptors and gluconeogenesis
Muscle	Autocannibalism
Fibroblasts	Proliferation
Endothelium	Change in cell shape
Pancreas	Inhibits insulin release

changes in the vascular system, including vasoconstriction, platelet aggregation, changes in membrane permeability, bronchial constriction, depression of cardiac output, and enhanced fluid leakage from the intravascular compartment.[50] Profound, but reversible, myocardial depression is noted in patients with septic shock[51] and circulating cardiodepressant substances have been implicated.[52] Serum of patients with septic shock contains a myocardial depressant substance (called MDF) associated with reversible decreases in left ventricular ejection fraction.[53,54]

Fever is a common finding, particularly in bacteremia and septic shock, and results from the release of endogenous pyrogen from phagocytic cells. This pyrogen seems identical with interleukin 1, which exerts a variety of other biologic activities including release of multiple hormones by direct action on pituitary cells,[55] and secretion of corticotropin-releasing factor (CRF) from the hypothalamus[56] (Table 65-4). Other interleukins have direct myocardial effects[57] and appear to increase acute phase protein synthesis in the liver. The growing knowledge of mediators in shock states suggests that specific inhibitors and modulators of monokines and other humoral agents might well be used in the treatment of shock. Ongoing investigation of antiendotoxin antibodies, platelet aggregating factor antagonists, interleukin receptor antagonists, and antioxidants such as N-acetylcysteine and tocopherol may eventually demonstrate how to counteract mediator release in shock states. Nevertheless, it may be difficult to find a single "silver bullet" because of multiple causal factors. Mediators also may interact in a way that administration of a single inhibitor (e.g., a prostaglandin antagonist) directly or indirectly influences other factors. Readers are referred to a recent review of new strategies in nonantibiotic treatment of gram-negative sepsis,[57a] as well as editorials cautioning tempered enthusiasm for these agents.[41a,41b]

Adrenergic Receptors and Their Function

The concept of a single "adrenoreceptor," first identified through the action of adrenal gland concentrate, has given way to knowledge of multiple adrenergic receptors, now that pharmacologic agents are available to identify types and even subtypes of receptors. The adrenergic receptor system can be broadly divided into alpha, beta, and dopaminergic receptors. The alpha-adrenergic receptors are responsible for control of blood pressure by action on the peripheral vasculature, primarily arterioles. Alpha-adrenergic receptors also exist in the heart and are implicated in the genesis of cardiac arrhythmias, because alpha-adrenergic receptor blockade increases the threshold for epinephrine-induced arrhythmias.[58] Other effects of alpha receptors in various tissues are summarized in Table 65-5. Beta-adrenergic receptors abound in the heart, especially within the sinoatrial node and the atrioventricular node, and are responsible for control of heart rate, rhythm, and contractility. Beta receptors are also found in bronchioles and arterioles, where they mediate bronchodilatation and vasodilatation, respectively. The target tissues and responses of beta-adrenergic receptors are summarized in Table 65-6. Dopaminergic receptors are widely distributed, not only in the renal and mesenteric vessels, but also in the brain and in peripheral tissues. Measurable concentrations of dopamine occur in the plasma, with only some

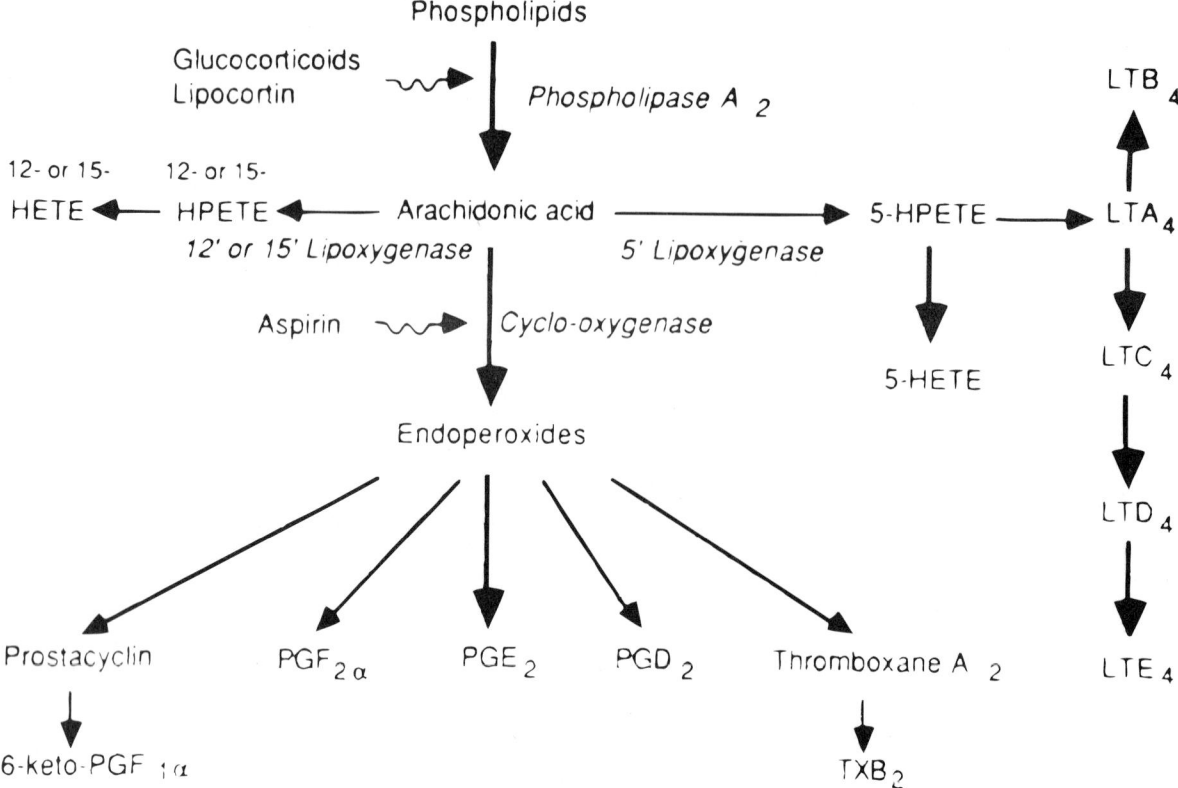

Fig. 65–2. The Arachidonic acid cascade: metabolism of arachidonic acid (AA). Prostacyclin and other prostaglandins are formed from arachidonic acid by cyclo-oxygenase via cyclic endoperoxide intermediates. Prostacyclin breaks down chemically to the stable 6-keto-prostaglandin F_1 alpha (6-keto-$PGF_{1\alpha}$). Glucocorticosteroids, through induction of the synthesis of the protein lipocortin, inhibit phospholipase A_2, thus preventing the liberation of AA from phospholipids. Aspirin-like drugs block cyclo-oxygenase and thereby prevent prostacyclin generation. Hydroperoxyeicosatetrenoic acids (HPETE) and hydroxyeicosatetrenoic acids (HETE) are generated from AA by a number of lipogenase enzymes. One of these, 5-HPETE, is the precursor of the potent chemotactic and bronchoconstrictor leukotrienes (LTA_4, LTB_4, LTC_4 and LTD_4). (From Vane, J. R., and Botting, R. M.: Prostaglandins, prostacyclin, thromboxane and leukotrienes: the arachidonic acid cascade. In Critical Care—State of the Art. Edited by B. P. Fuhrman and W. C. Shoemaker. Fullerton, CA, Society of Critical Care Medicine, 1989, p. 4.)

originating from the adrenal glands, suggesting there is a widely distributed peripheral dopaminergic system.[59] The best known action of the dopamine[1] receptor occurs in the renal and mesenteric arteries and produces vasodilatation, natriuresis, and inhibition of aldosterone secretion. Dopamine[2] receptors, however, also exist on the presynaptic membrane, where they may inhibit norepinephrine release. Dopamine is also a precursor of norepinephrine and can have indirect effects on the alpha-adrenergic system if insufficient dopamine is available for genesis of norepinephrine (substrate depletion).

Receptor Subtypes

The varied target tissues and responses of subtypes of adrenergic receptors are presented in Tables 65–5 and 65–6. Recognition sites distinct from the currently defined alpha, beta, and dopaminergic receptors have also been postulated. A response to isoproterenol, unrelated to alpha- and beta-adrenoreceptor activity has been observed.[60] A variant of the beta-adrenoreceptor that does not fit into the current beta[1]/beta[2] classification also exists in experimental animals.[61] It has been theorized that these atypical beta adrenoreceptors, which selectively stimulate lipolysis in brown fat cells, have an important role in the regulation of energy balance and may potentially serve as a target for antiobesity drugs.[62] Agonists to this third subtype of beta adrenoreceptor have been synthesized and are potent stimulators of metabolic rate, adipose tissue thermogenesis, ileum relaxation, and muscle glycogen synthesis.[63]

Activation of the Adrenergic System

Decreases in systemic arterial blood pressure from acute blood loss, pump failure, or reduction in peripheral vascular resistance from sepsis, anaphylaxis, and loss of spinal sympathetic tone, trigger the baroreceptor reflex and sympathetic nervous system-mediated outflow of catecholamines. Norepinephrine and epinephrine then bind to specific cell membrane-associated glycoproteins, (i.e., alpha- and beta-adrenergic receptors). The function of the adrenergic system is to translate a sympathetic nervous system impulse into an end-organ result. The sequence of events for the alpha-adrenergic system is demonstrated in Figure 65–3. Depolarization of the sympathetic nerve produces fusion of the norepinephrine vesicle to the membrane of

Table 65-5. Target Tissues and Responses of Alpha-Adrenergic Receptors

Receptor Subtype	Tissue	Response
Alpha$_1$ adrenergic	Smooth muscle: vascular, uterus, trigone, pilomotor, ureter, sphincters (gastrointestinal and bladder), eye (iris), radial, vas deferens	Contraction
	Smooth muscle (gastrointestinal)	Relaxation
	Liver*	Glycogenolysis, gluconeogenesis, ureogenesis
	Myocardium	Increased force of contraction
	Central nervous system	Increased locomotor activity, neurotransmission
	Salivary glands	Secretion (K$^+$, H$_2$O)
	Kidney (proximal tubule)	Glucogenesis
	Adipose tissue	Glycogenolysis
Alpha$_2$ adrenergic	Sympathetic nerve terminal	Inhibition of norepinephrine release
	Vascular smooth muscle	Contraction
	Platelets	Aggregation, granule release
	Central nervous system	Sedation, inhibition of sympathetic outflow, neurotransmission
	Adipose tissue	Inhibition of lipolysis
	Eye	Decreased intraocular pressure
	Endothelium	Release of vasodilator substance
	Jejunum	Inhibition of secretion
	Kidney	Inhibition of renin release
	Pancreatic islet cells	Inhibition of insulin release
	Cholinergic neutrons and cell bodies of noradrenergic neurons	Inhibition of firing
	Melanocytes	Inhibition of MSH-induced granule dispersion

* Applies mainly to the rat; in humans, beta$_2$ adrenergic responses predominate.
(From Graham, R. M.: Adrenergic receptors: structure and function. Cleve. Clin. J. Med., 57:481, 1990.)

binding of guanine residues), phospholipase-C, diacylglycerol (DAG), and inositol triphosphate (IP3).[65] Binding at the alpha$_1$ receptor promotes intracellular calcium flux and an increase in cytosolic calcium, which activate calmodulin kinase. In addition, the calcium plus the diacylglycerol activates protein kinase C, which catalyzes the phophoralation of myosin light chain.[64]

Signal transduction by the alpha$_2$- and beta-adrenergic receptors uses yet another system involving G proteins guanosine triphosphate (GTP), guanosine diphosphate (GDP), adenosine triphosphate (ATP), cyclic adenosine monophosphate (cAMP), and protein kinase A (Fig. 65-5).[66] Activation of the receptors by an agonist causes an alteration in the confirmation of the receptor and its G protein resulting, in dissociation of GDP and association of GTP by the alpha subunits of the receptor. With beta-

Table 65-6. Target Tissues and Responses of Beta-Adrenergic Receptors

Receptor Subtype	Tissue	Response
Beta$_1$ adrenergic	Myocardium	
	Sinoatrial node	Increase in heart rate
	Atria	Increase in contractility and conduction velocity
	Atrioventricular node	Increase in automaticity and conduction velocity
	His-Purkinje system	Increase in automaticity and conduction velocity
	Ventricles	Increase in contractility, conduction, velocity, automaticity, and rate of idioventricular pacemakers
	Kidney	Renin secretion
	Adipose tissue	Lipolysis
	Posterior pituitary	Antidiuretic hormone secretion
	Sympathetic nerve terminal	Increased neurotransmitter release
Beta$_2$ adrenergic	Smooth muscle: vascular uterus, gastrointestinal (stomach, intestine, gall bladder and bile ducts), bladder (detrusor), lung (tracheal and bronchial)	Relaxation
	Skeletal muscle	Increased contractility, glycogenolysis, K$^+$ uptake
	Liver	Glycogenolysis and gluconeogenesis
	Pancreas	Insulin secretion
	Splenic capsule	Relaxation
	Salivary glands	Amylase secretion
	Lung: bronchial glands	Increased secretion
Beta$_3$ adrenergic	Ileum (guinea pig)	Relaxation
	Fat cells (rat)	Lipolysis

(From Graham, R. M.: Adrenergic receptors: structure and function. Cleve. Clin. J. Med., 57:481, 1990.)

the sympathetic nerve varicosity, releasing norepinephrine into the synaptic cleft. Some of the norepinephrine binds to a postsynaptic alpha$_1$ receptor, while some norepinephrine acts on the presynaptic alpha$_2$ receptor to inhibit the further norepinephrine release.[64] The chain of events occurring at the cellular level when an alpha$_1$-adrenergic agonist binds to an effector cell is shown in Figure 65-4. Signal transduction is accomplished through a number of proteins, including the G-protein (named for its

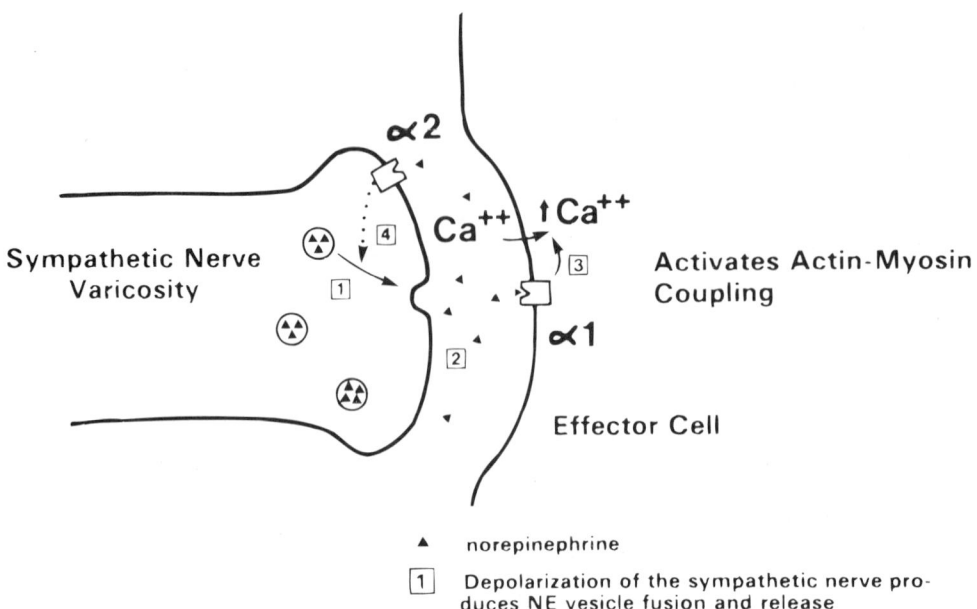

Fig. 65–3. Effect of norepinephrine (NE) in the sympathetic nervous system. Peripheral circulatory control is achieved via alpha-adrenergic receptors. The sequence of events includes sympathetic nerve stimulation, release of NE across the synaptic cleft, binding at the postsynaptic effector cell, calcium influx, and feedback inhibition of further NE release via alpha$_2$ receptors on the presynaptic membrane. (From Zaritsky, A., and Chernow, B.: Catecholamines, sympathomimetics. *In* The Pharmacologic Approach to the Critically Ill Patient. Edited by B. Chernow and C. R. Lake. Baltimore, Williams & Wilkins, 1983, p. 484.)

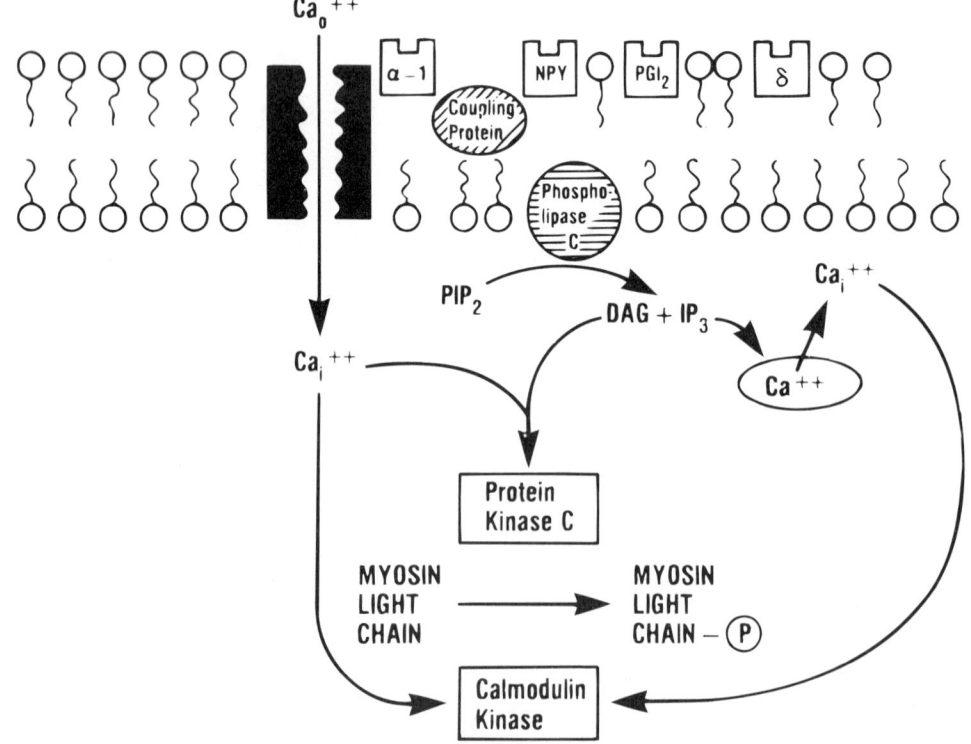

Fig. 65–4. The phosphatidylinositol/protein kinase C cascade. The external cell membrane accommodates receptors for alpha-adrenergic agents and also neuropeptide Y (NPY), prostaglandin I$_2$ (PGI$_2$), and the delta-opioid peptide. Extracellular calcium (Ca^{++}) moves into the cell via the calcium channel. Effects that are mediated through coupling proteins include hydrolysis of phosphatidylinositol 4,5 biphosphate (PIP$_2$) and generation of diacylglycerol (DAG) and inositol 1,4,5-triphosphate (IP$_3$). The increase in intracellular calcium (CA$_i^{++}$) allows vasoconstriction to occur. (From Chernow B., and Roth, B. L.: Pharmacologic support of the cardiovasculature in septic shock. *In* New Horizons Perspectives on Sepsis and Septic Shock. Edited by W. J. Sibbald and C. L. Sprung. Fullerton, CA, Society of Critical Care Medicine, 1986, p. 173.)

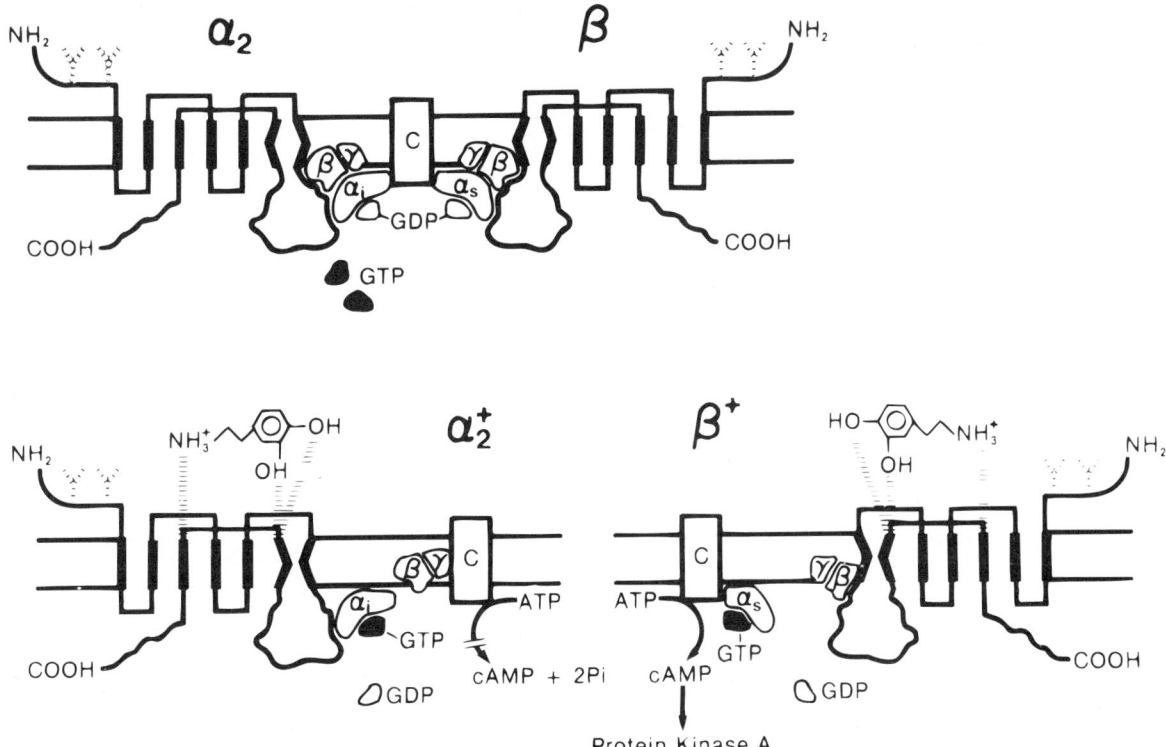

Fig. 65-5. Signal transduction by alpha- and beta-adrenergic receptors. The receptors are represented as single polypeptides that span the plasma membrane (horizontal lines) seven times, with the amino terminus (NH$_2$) located extracellularly and the carboxyl terminus (COOH) located intracellularly. The third intracellular loop connecting the fifth and sixth transmembrane spanning regions is depicted as interacting with the receptor coupled G-proteins, each of which consists of three subunits (α, β, and γ). The transmembrane spanning regions are most likely alpha-helical in structure, and some of these regions may be kinked, as shown, because they contain prolyl residues. In the basal state (upper panel), guanosine diphosphate (GDP) is bound to the alpha subunits of the G-proteins. Activation of the receptors (α^+, β^+) by an agonist (lower panel) such as norepinephrine causes an alteration in the conformation of the receptor and its G-protein leading to dissociation of the GDP and association of guanosine triphosphate (GTP) by the alpha subunits. As a result, the alpha subunits dissociate from the beta-gamma subunits. With the beta-adrenergic receptor, the resulting GTP-activated α_s subunit then activates the membrane-bound enzyme adenylyl cyclase (C) leading to cyclic adenosine monophosphate (cAMP) formation. The cAMP thus formed activates protein kinase A. With the alpha$_2$-adrenergic receptor, the beta-gamma subunits released with receptor activation prevents α_{zGTP} stimulation of C and thus inhibits cAMP formation. (From Graham, R. M.: Adrenergic receptors: structure and function. Cleve. Clin. J. Med., 57:481, 1990.)

adrenergic activation, membrane-bound adenyl cyclase promotes the formation of cAMP from ATP. At the alpha$_2$-adrenergic receptor, stimulation of adenyl cyclase is prevented, thus inhibiting cAMP formation.[64] Cyclic AMP is broken down to 5′ AMP by the enzyme phosphodiesterase. Phosphodiesterase inhibitors such as amrinone effectively increase the amount of cAMP within the cell, thus explaining their synergism with beta-adrenergic agents. cAMP is thought to be involved in diastolic relaxation of the heart, and preliminary data now suggest that drugs that augment cAMP, such as beta-adrenergic agents and phosphodiesterase inhibitors, may improve lusitrophic function (diastolic relaxation) by reducing the diastolic intracellular calcium.[67]

Factors Affecting Adrenergic Responses

The expected response of adrenergic receptors to endogenous and exogenous catecholamines is influenced by a variety of factors (Table 65-7). Acidosis increases catecholamine synthesis and secretion but is possibly accompanied by end-organ resistance to exogenous catecholamines. Severe acidosis may be associated with decreased cardiac contractility, cardiac output, and a systemic vasoconstrictive response. Acidosis also inhibits presynaptic

Table 65-7. Selected Influences on Catecholamine Response

Acid/base status	Downregulation (chronic stimulation)
Age	Electrolytes
Alpha-adrenergic blockers	Ethnicity/race/individual variation
Anesthetics/opioids	Hemodilution
Beta-adrenergic blockers	Hypothermia
Calcium channel blockers	Sepsis
Congestive heart failure	Substrate depletion
Denervation	Surgical stress
Diabetes mellitus	Upregulation (chronic blockade)
Drug therapy	

norepinephrine uptake and may produce difficulty with defibrillation.[68] Alkalosis may decrease catecholamine secretion, inhibits sympathetic nervous system activity, and results in decreased vasoconstrictive ability, accentuated vasodilatation, and a propensity to ventricular dysrhythmias.[68] In untreated shock states, acidosis is more common, but alkalosis can result from overaggressive bicarbonate therapy. Many clinicians choose to treat metabolic acidosis when arterial pH values are less than 7.25 but allow mild degrees of acidosis to be corrected with definitive therapy rather than risk overcorrection and alkalosis. Acidosis represents an adaptive response to stress, and mild degrees of acidosis may result in improved catecholamine response.

Catecholamine depletion may contribute to a diminished endogenous catecholamine response to stress. Oral levodopa, administered to patients with severe congestive heart failure, produces a sustained improvement in cardiac function attributed to activation of beta-adrenergic and dopamine receptors. Because levodopa is the precursor of dopamine and thus norepinephrine (in the endogenous biosynthetic pathway of catecholamines), it represents restoration of depleted substrate.[69]

Individual Differences in Adrenergic Response

Young subjects have a much smaller blood pressure response and corresponding release of norepinephrine than subjects over the age of 40 years, as judged by cold pressor testing.[70] Studies of the kinetics of plasma norepinephrine indicate that the appearance rate of norepinephrine is higher and clearance rate lower in elderly individuals.[71] Increased concentrations of circulating catecholamines may be present in the elderly, because of declining end-organ responsiveness, presumably at the level of the receptor. Evidence for this concept includes markedly increased catecholamine levels, but significantly less chronotropic response to the stress of intubation, in elderly patients.[72] Reduced receptor affinity for agonist may play a role in altered beta-adrenergic sensitivity in the elderly.[73,74] Parallel reductions in cardiac, peripheral vascular, and renal responses to catecholamines are noted with increasing age.[75,76]

Significant interindividual differences in the density of adrenergic receptors may also contribute to the variability in response to adrenergic medication. The density of beta-adrenergic receptors is one of the principal factors controlling beta-receptor response in humans,[76] and a relationship has been demonstrated between myocardial and lymphocyte beta-adrenoreceptor density,[77] raising the possibility that drug- or disease-induced receptor changes may be easily monitored in the future. Racial or ethnic differences may also exist. Men of Chinese descent have greater sensitivity than white men to the effects of propranolol on heart rate and blood pressure, an effect that is partly, but incompletely, explained by changes in protein binding.[78]

Patients receiving beta-adrenoreceptor-blocking drugs demonstrate an altered hemodynamic response to dobutamine.[79] Dobutamine is supplied as a racemic mixture of (+) and (−) isomers, which are beta- and alpha-adrenergic receptor agonists, respectively. In congestive heart failure, as loss of functional beta-adrenoreceptors occurs, the effects of alpha stimulation become more prominent.[80] Calcium-entry blockers may also interfere with the pressor response to alpha-adrenergic stimulation,[81] although verapamil does not affect the ability of dopamine to augment cardiac output in clinical relevant doses.[82] The response to a phenylephrine bolus in patients undergoing open heart surgery, however, decreases with increasing serum nifedipine levels, even though baseline hemodynamics are unchanged.[83] Beta-adrenergic receptor blockade potentiates the degree of coronary artery vasoconstriction seen with cocaine administration,[84] presumably by blocking the beta$_2$-vasodilating response to cocaine-induced vasoconstriction.

Alterations With Cardiac Disease

A number of alterations in sympathetic nervous system activity are noted during coronary artery bypass surgery and are thought to be related to hypothermia and/or hemodilution. Pressor responses are markedly reduced in hindlimb experimental animal preparations subjected to hemodilution. Retransfusion of packed red cells, or increased blood flow to the hindlimb preparation, restores this pressor responsiveness to normal.[85] Pressor hyperresponsiveness has also been demonstrated in saline-infused rabbits, implicating atrial natriuretic hormone involvement in the pressor response.[86] Alterations in sympathetic nervous system activity are noted during intraoperative hypothermia for coronary artery bypass surgery.[87] Other studies indicate that the sympathetic nervous system can compensate for a fall in core temperature from 37 to 31°C, but that below levels of about 29°C, a "switch-off" of the endogenous sympathetic nervous system occurs.[88] Beta-adrenergic receptor function abruptly changes in surgical patients,[89] possibly because of substrate depletion during surgical stress.

Cardiac and peripheral vascular responses are altered following denervation, whether from cardiac transplantation[90] or as a result of long-standing diabetic autonomic neuropathy.[91] Insulin-dependent diabetic subjects are less sensitive to beta-adrenergic stimulation, and the magnitude of this decrease corresponds with the duration of diabetes mellitus.[92] Autoantibodies to the beta$_2$-adrenergic receptor have been identified both in normal individuals and in patients with a history of atopic disease.[93]

Markedly altered myocardial and peripheral vascular responses to catecholamines are observed in patients with congestive heart failure.[94] The initial compensatory response to diminished cardiac output is increased release of endogenous circulating catecholamines to sustain cardiac output. Long-term exposure to these high levels of catecholamines eventually results in decreased catecholamine sensitivity and decreased beta-adrenergic receptor density.[94] Although some authors maintain that plasma norepinephrine levels correlate with hemodynamic evidence of cardiac dysfunction,[95] others have concluded that catecholamine levels do not reflect the severity of heart failure.[96] Experimental studies have demonstrated that beta-adrenergic receptors are not functionally coupled to the

G proteins in dogs with congestive heart failure.[97] Congestive heart failure patients with cachexia demonstrate increased circulating levels of TNF, which is associated with activation of the renin-angiotensin system.[98] Reduced affinity and increased beta-adrenergic receptor number are also seen in experimentally induced left ventricular hypertrophy.[99] Net myocardial norepinephrine release is approximately 20-fold greater in congestive heart failure than in patients with angina pectoris but without heart failure.[100] Increased circulating catecholamine concentrations are thought to play a role in the reduced alpha-adrenergic receptor responsiveness seen in patients with poor ventricular function.[101] Clinically, patients with moderately severe left ventricular dysfunction require greater alpha-adrenergic support during "weaning" from cardiopulmonary bypass.[102]

Sepsis and the Adrenergic Response

The hypoglycemia seen in conjunction with sepsis suggests the presence of specific effect on hepatic alpha receptors in the septic state. In an experimental study examining Sprague-Dawley rats 24 hours after cecal ligation and puncture, a 40% reduction in $alpha_1$-adrenergic responsiveness could be demonstrated without corresponding change in antagonist affinity for receptors.[103] This finding suggests either an alteration in the number of alpha-adrenergic receptors or in receptor-effector coupling in the septic state.

Tachyphylaxis, or a reduction in the expected response to an agonist with repeated use, is a familiar consequence of overuse of phenylephrine nasal spray. The phenomenon of tachyphylaxis was experimentally noticed by Bendixen and colleagues studying the effect of respiratory acidosis on the circulation.[104] These effects appear to be mediated either by uncoupling of receptors from G proteins, or possibly repetitive internalization of hormone-receptor complexes within the cell, with inadequate generation of replacement receptors,[64] a process called "downregulation." Upregulation, an increase in the number of receptors per cell, occurs following chronic receptor blockade. For example, when propranolol therapy has been withdrawn, a markedly increased response to isoproterenol can be seen during the next 12 to 48 hours. Other agents known to affect adrenergic function include thyroid hormones, estrogen and progesterone, ischemia, alcohol withdrawal, and psychotropic agents.[105] Absolute catecholamine levels vary from species to species,[106] mandating careful attention to species studied in comparing influences.

Electrolyte Disorders and Adrenergic Response

Because adrenergic receptor action is known to be a calcium-dependent process, it is not surprising that the level of serum electrolytes is important in modulating the activity of the endogenous sympathetic system and exogenous pharmacologic agents. Calcium is essential for normal cardiac and neuromuscular functioning, and calcium regulates a number of intracellular mechanisms necessary for cellular homeostasis. Both total serum hypocalcemia and ionized hypocalcemia are common in critically ill medical and surgical patients.[107] Hypocalcemic patients spend a longer time in the ICU and have an increased frequency of complications, including renal failure and sepsis, and a higher mortality rate than normocalcemic patients.[107] The Hastings-McClean normgram,[108] which relates ionized calcium levels to total serum calcium levels, probably underestimates protein-dependent changes in calcium concentrations in critically ill patients.[109] In the ICU population, increases in free fatty acids alter binding of calcium by increasing the number of binding sites on albumin.[110] Normally, circulating calcium concentrations are maintained within a narrow range by parathyroid hormones in a vitamin D-dependent process. Patients with gram-negative infection, however, may develop parathyroid gland dysfunction and/or vitamin D insufficiency with consequent systemic arterial hypotension.[111] Direct relationships have been demonstrated between the ionized calcium level and left ventricular contractility[112] and arterial pressure.[113] Concerns have been raised, however, about Ca^{++} administration in sepsis, because increased mortality has been noted in Ca^{++}-treated animals with endotoxic shock.[114]

Hypophosphatemia is also common in critically ill patients and contributes to pulmonary insufficiency, erythrocyte and leukocyte dysfunction, metabolic acidosis, and central nervous system dysfunction.[115] Maintenance of normal levels of 2,3-diphosphoglycerate requires normal phosphate metabolism. Experimentally, phosphate depletion is associated with lower mean arterial pressure and cardiac index, with increased norepinephrine and renin secretion. Correction of hypophosphatemia improves myocardial function possibly via improving intracellular availability of ATP.[116] Severe hypophosphatemia may be seen with diabetic ketoacidosis, hyperosmolar nonketotic coma, chronic alcoholism, and the use of phosphate-binding antacids.

Hypomagnesemia is another common finding in the critically ill. Magnesium has a permissive action on parathyroid hormone (PTH) release, and thus, hypomagnesemia may contribute to hypocalcemia.[117] Hypomagnesemia results from gastrointestinal loss, renal loss, inadequate replacement via total parenteral nutrition, and following hypothermia, cardiopulmonary bypass, and burns. Plasma levels of magnesium appear to be influenced by the adrenergic system.[118] The magnitude of hypomagnesemia following cardiopulmonary bypass is influenced by the type of cardioplegia used for myocardial preservation.[119] Other risk factors for magnesium deficiency include congestive heart failure, diabetic ketoacidosis, acute and chronic alcoholism, delirium tremens, and diuretic phase of acute tubular necrosis, primary aldosteronism, and pancreatitis.[120] Hypomagnesemia may also complicate aminoglycoside therapy because the neuromuscular weakness induced by hypomagnesemia is potentiated by aminoglycosides.[121] Deficiency of magnesium, like deficiency of potassium, predisposes to tachyarrhythmias, digitalis toxicity, sudden death, and congestive heart failure.[117] Because diuretic therapy causes the renal loss of both magnesium and potassium, frequent determination of the levels of these electrolytes and adequate replacement therapy are essential in the critically ill. Intracellular shifts of magnesium may also occur as a result of inotropic therapy.[118] Magnesium administration is helpful with occasional arrhythmias refractory to conventional therapy.[120]

Other Environmental Influences

Hyperlipidemia and clinical jaundice are both associated with increased vascular sensitivity to norepinephrine.[122] Drug therapy with prostaglandin inhibitors, specifically indomethacin, can influence the blood pressure response in endotoxic and hemorrhagic shock.[123,124] Anesthetic and sedative drugs including opioids, barbiturates,[125] and benzodiazepines[126] can inhibit sympathetic nervous system activity and block sympathetic recruitment in response to stress. Only the anesthetic induction agent ketamine increases plasma and urine catecholamine levels.[127]

THE ICU PHASE OF SHOCK STATES

ICU admission is justified for patients in shock and for patients at high risk for developing hemodynamic instability. In many institutions, ICU admission is a necessary prerequisite to placement of invasive monitoring devices for the diagnosis and treatment of shock states.

Diagnosis

The classic hemodynamic picture of the circulatory shock state includes low mean arterial pressure and evidence of diminished perfusion, including peripheral vasoconstriction, diminished urine output, changes in mentation, and other organ system dysfunction. Although shock is easy to recognize in the late stages, many barriers obstruct the *early* recognition of shock. Peripheral vasoconstriction may prevent accurate blood pressure readings, particularly when a blood pressure "cuff" is employed. Arterial catheters in peripheral blood vessels such as the radial artery may cause underestimation of mean aortic pressure with vasodilatation of the forearm. The circumstance has been documented following cardiopulmonary bypass;[128] its relevance in septic shock is speculative.

Inadequate organ perfusion may exist even with a cardiac index greater than 2.1 L per minute per m^2 when peripheral autoregulation is impaired by trauma, sepsis, or pheochromocytoma. The maldistribution of blood flow in these situations is difficult to measure, and presently, no clinically available monitoring devices allow assessment of individual organ oxygen consumption. At present, the best measures of the adequacy of perfusion are determinations of oxygen transport[4,129] and examination of individual organ function, particularly urine output (see Chap. 64).

Measurement of the blood lactate concentration is valuable in the diagnosis of hypoperfusion,[3] even though lactate levels may be transiently high during the washout phase of recovery from shock following circulatory arrest.[130] Increased lactate levels are occasionally seen early in the ICU course of patients recovering from cardiothoracic surgery as vasodilatation begins. Although increased lactate levels are a reliable indication of shock, they are not necessarily predictive of mortality.[131]

Seventy percent of patients with gram-negative sepsis show a decrease in blood phosphate levels to less than 0.6 mmol (1.6 mg%).[132] Great toe temperature correlates moderately ($r = 0.71$) with cardiac output and correctly predicts outcome in about 66% of patients.[1] While toe temperature is useful in following cardiac output trends in pediatric patients, it is less reliable in adult patients with peripheral vascular disease. Other early indications of shock include failure of antacids or cimetidine to control the gastric pH.[133] Conjunctival and mixed venous oximeters may provide early warning of cardiopulmonary compromise.[134]

Resuscitation

The "ABCs" of resuscitation (airway, breathing, and circulation) always apply in the treatment of the patient in shock. Death in shock states often occurs from respiratory failure, and thus, intubation and controlled mechanical ventilation should be an early consideration in the hemodynamically unstable patient. Adequate volume expansion must be accomplished before institution of inotropic therapy. There is little justification for the use of exogenous catechols in situations (e.g., hemorrhagic shock) in which endogenous circulating catecholamine levels are already increased.[6] Resuscitation from hemorrhagic shock is best accomplished with fluid therapy, including blood and blood product replacement, as indicated.

In the presence of right ventricular failure that is due to increased right ventricular afterload, inotropic support may occasionally be preferred to fluid loading. One experimental study demonstrated that in the presence of normal peripheral vascular resistance, the addition of 6% dextran increased both stroke volume and mean arterial pressure.[135] If the pulmonary vasculature resistance was experimentally increased by glass bead embolization, volume expansion then resulted in a decrease in stroke volume and mean arterial pressure despite a decrease in pulmonary artery pressure. In this situation norepinephrine both increased the stroke volume and decreased end diastolic pressure. The authors of the study[135] concluded that in the presence of pulmonary hypertension as in respiratory failure, small increases in blood volume may result in right ventricular dysfunction and inotropic pressure agents might be preferred to volume expansion.

Right ventricular dysfunction is common in septic shock.[136] This finding may be of therapeutic importance because treatment of right ventricular failure may rely on both catecholamine support and volume resuscitation. Evidence suggests that catecholamines with beta-adrenergic (dilating) properties are preferred in right ventricular failure, and a shift from dopamine to dobutamine in this setting may improve right ventricular function.[137] Caution must be exercised with concurrent tricuspid regurgitation and right ventricular dysfunction because increasing right ventricular contractility can also increase the regurgitant fraction.[138]

Catecholamines

The choice of a catecholamine should take into consideration the expected functioning of the adrenergic receptors (Table 65-8) as well as specific patient factors that might influence catecholamine response (Table 65-7).

Table 65-8. Selectivity of Catecholamines for Adrenergic Receptors

	Alpha$_1$	Alpha$_2$	Beta$_1$	Beta$_2$	Dopamine$_1$	Dopamine$_2$
Phenylephrine	+ +	0	0	0	0	0
Norepinephrine	+ + +	+ +	+ + +	+	0	0
Epinephrine	+ + +	+ + +	+ + +	+ +	0	0
Dopamine	0 to + + +	0 to +	0 to + + +	0 to + +	+ + +	+ +
Dobutamine	0 to +	0	+ + +	+ +	0	0
Fenaldopam	0	0	0	0	+ +	+ +
Dopexamine	0	0	+	+ +	+ +	+ +

+ to + + + = Relative amounts of stimulation; these are not necessarily to scale between drugs. Some agents, particularly dopamine, have dose-dependent effects with alpha activity increasing at higher doses.
0 = no effect
(From Higgins, T. L., and Chernow, B.: Pharmacotherapy of shock. Dis. Month, 23:311, 1987.)

Typical dosages of inotropic agents are listed in Table 65-9. After deciding which agent to employ, the next consideration is basically whether an increase or a decrease in afterload will best serve the patient's needs. In general, if the patient has both a low cardiac output and low mean arterial pressure, then volume loading and/or stimulation of both the alpha- and beta-adrenergic systems would be appropriate. Drugs that act on both alpha and beta receptors include epinephrine, norepinephrine, and high dose dopamine. On the other hand, if low cardiac output is associated with a high systemic vascular resistance, then afterload reduction is indicated. This reduction can be accomplished pharmacologically with agents that have primarily beta-adrenergic activity (isoproterenol, dobutamine, low dose dopamine) or with a combination of inotropic support plus peripheral vasodilatation with a direct-acting vasodilator such as sodium nitroprusside or hydralazine.

Dopamine

Dopaminergic receptors mediate vasodilatation in the renal, mesenteric, coronary, and cerebral arterial beds. "Classic" infusion rates of the drug dopamine described in experimental animals do not reliably reflect the activation range in critically ill patients. As a general guide, dopamine infused intravenously at rates between 0.5 and 3 µg/kg per minute activates first the dopamine$_2$ receptor and then the dopamine$_1$ receptor. Beta$_1$-adrenergic receptor activation occurs usually at rates of approximately 5 to 10 µg/kg per minute. Alpha activation may occur at infusion rates as low as 5 µg/kg per minute, but in shock states response may require 50 µg/kg per minute or more. Part of this observed variability may be due to the earlier described alterations in receptor physiology in septic states.[103] Dopamine is presently the only catecholamine with specific renal vasodilating effects. The renal vasodilating effect of dopamine is mediated through calcium-dependent mechanisms and prostaglandin release[139] and may persist even when other, vasoconstricting agents are added to the regimen. Schaer and colleagues[140] demonstrated that renal blood flow during combination therapy with norepinephrine and low dose dopamine was markedly increased over that observed with norepinephrine alone and that renal vascular resistance decreased with the combination therapy (Fig. 65-6). Even when renal blood flow is indexed

Table 65-9. Dosages of Inotropic Agents

Agent	Usual Preparation	Usual Adult Dosages
Epinephrine	Ampules of 1:1000 mix 1–4 1-mg ampules in 250 mg of D5W or NS (4–16 µg/ml)	5 µg/kg SQ (0.3 ml of 1:1,000) 100 µg IV bolus followed by 1–16 µg/min infusion; in extremis: 1 mg IV or intratracheally
Norepinephrine	1 or 2 4-mg ampules in 250 ml of D5W or NS (16–32 µg/ml)	0.05 µg/kg/min to >0.30 µg/kg/min
Dopamine	1–4 200-mg ampules in 250 ml of D5W (800 µg/ml) (800–3200 µg/ml)	0.5–3 µg/kg/min (dopaminergic range) 5–10 µg/kg/min (beta range) >20 µg/kg/min (alpha range)
Dobutamine	1–2 250-mg vials in 250 ml of D5W or NS to make 1000–2000 µg/ml	
Isoproterenol	1–4 1-mg ampules in 250 ml of D5W or NS (4–16 µg/min)	0.05–0.50 µg/kg/min
Phenylephrine	10-mg ampule in 250 ml of D5W or NS	0.15–5 µg/kg/min
Amrinone	5 mg/ml ampule (20 ml) 200 mg in 250 NS (*not* D5W)	0.75–1.5 mg/kg bolus; repeat at 30 min 5–10 µg/kg/min
Milrinone	40 mg in 250 ml D5W or NS	50–75 µg/kg bolus 0.3 to 0.75 µg/kg/min infusion
Naloxone*	0.4 mg/ml ampule 4–10 mg in 250 D5W	0.01–0.80 mg/kg IV bolus 0.2–8 µg/kg/min infusion
Glucagon*	1-mg vial 5–10 mg in 250 D5W	0.01–0.05 mg/kg IV 1–3 mg/hr infusion

* Naloxone and glucagon have not received FDA approval for use in shock; the dosage recommendations are based on case reports referenced in the test. Dosages of all drugs must be titrated to effect. In most cases, more concentrated mixes can be prepared if volume loading is of concern.
D5W, Dextrose 5% in water; NS, normal saline; SQ, subcutaneously.
(Adapted from Higgins, T. L., and Chernow, B.: Pharmacotherapy of circulatory shock. Dis. Mon., 33:351, 1987.)

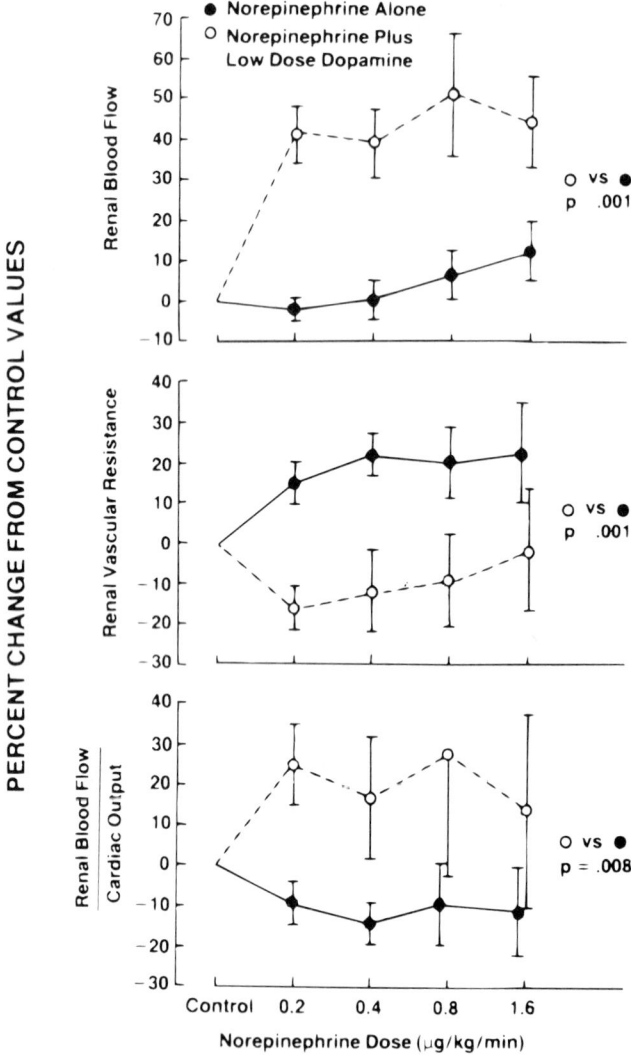

Fig. 65–6. Renal vascular effects of norepinephrine alone or in combination with low dose dopamine. Renal blood flow improves by 40% when dopamine is added (top), which is due to dopamine's effect on renal vascular resistance (middle). This effect is independent of improved cardiac output (bottom). (From Schaer, G. L., Fink, M. P., and Parrillo, J. E.: Norepinephrine versus norepinephrine plus low dose dopamine: enhanced renal blood flow with combination pressor therapy. Crit. Care Med., 13:494, 1985.)

by cardiac output, up to a 30% increase in renal blood flow occurred with the combination versus norepinephrine alone. Many clinicians employ "renal dose" dopamine in the presence of oliguria despite limited evidence of efficacy in improving outcome.[141] Dopamine, because of its beta-adrenergic activity, may precipitate tachycardia, and as the dose of dopamine increases, more and more alpha-adrenergic activity and hence increased afterload is seen. This vasoconstriction could be beneficial in the setting of decreased peripheral vascular resistance in shock states and following cardiopulmonary bypass but may be deleterious in a patient in whom afterload is already increased, as in acute myocardial infarction. Expected cardiovascular actions of dopamine when infused at rates of 2 to 8 μg/kg per minute may include an increase in cardiac output and stroke volume; an increase in heart rate, particularly at rates above 6 μg/kg per minute; increased pulmonary capillary "wedge" pressure at rates greater than 4 μg/kg per minute; and markedly increased systemic vascular resistance at high infusion rates.[142]

Dobutamine

Dobutamine increases cardiac output with less tachycardia and less effect on arterial and pulmonary pressures than dopamine. It may be better tolerated than dopamine in the setting of heart failure, perhaps because of its potential pulmonary vasodilating effects. Dobutamine augments myocardial blood flow more than dopamine after open heart surgery[143] and has a more favorable effect than dopamine on right ventricular function,[137] probably because of afterload reduction. The expected hemodynamic responses of dobutamine are altered by preoperative beta-adrenergic blockade.[79] The explanation for this phenomenon lies in the chemical composition of the drug. Dobutamine is supplied as a 50:50 racemic mixture. The (−) isomer is selected for the alpha$_1$ receptor, while the (+) isomer is selected for the beta$_1$ and beta$_2$ receptors. In vivo, a physiologic antagonism occurs between the alpha$_1$ and beta$_2$ receptors, so that only the beta$_1$ action (inotropy) is clinically predominant.[144] The response to dobutamine, however, may be modified by previous alpha- or beta-adrenergic receptor blockade as this balance is upset. In addition, the major metabolite of dobutamine (3-O-methyldobutamine) is an alpha$_1$ antagonist, which may further contribute to vasodilatation with prolonged use.[145] The expected hemodynamic actions of dobutamine at infusion rates of 2 to 10 μg/kg per minute include an increase in cardiac output and stroke volume, little or no change in heart rate, and a decrease in pulmonary capillary wedge pressure and systemic vascular resistance.[142] Dobutamine may thus produce substantial vasodilatation in the clinical setting, an effect that can be used to advantage in patients with pulmonary hypertension or right ventricular failure. Dobutamine is also preferred in the setting of hypoxemic respiratory failure and with normotensive left ventricular failure, especially after myocardial infarction, because additional vasoconstriction is not necessary in these situations and may actually worsen right ventricular function. Dobutamine is preferred to dopamine when tachycardia is a particular concern, such as postmyocardial infarction. Dobutamine at an infusion rate of 5 μg/kg per minute increases both oxygen supply and consumption in septic shock.[146] Some investigators have recently reported use of massive doses of dobutamine (greater than 40 μg/kg per minute) in the treatment of cardiogenic shock.[4] From the earlier discussion, we know that tachyphylaxis to catecholamines may develop, and thus, the initial dosage guidelines need not be adhered to in the face of minimal or no response and adequate hemodynamic monitoring. It is worth noting, however, that none of the patients treated with doses of dobutamine greater than 40 μg/kg per minute survived their episode of septic shock.[4]

Fenaldopam

Fenaldopam is a new presently experimental selective dopamine$_1$ agonist that increases renal blood flow, lowers blood pressure, and causes slight increases in heart rate.[147] It is effective as an antihypertensive at intravenous infusion rates of 0.025 to 0.50 µg/kg per minute. Fenaldopam does not activate the alpha or beta receptors, and a limiting effect to its use may be hypotension rather than tachycardia or cardiac stimulation.

Dopexamine

Dopexamine is a new synthetic catecholamine typically infused at rates of 1 to 6 µg/kg per minute. Dopexamine acts on the dopamine$_1$, dopamine$_2$, and beta$_2$-adrenergic receptors with little effect on the beta$_1$ receptor and no effect on alpha receptors.[148] Dopexamine decreases mean arterial pressure and systemic vascular resistance; increases heart rate by reflex action; improves organ blood flow to cardiac, hepatic, splanchnic, and renal beds; and increases inotropy via beta$_2$ cardiac stimulation.[149] Favorable hemodynamic responses to dopexamine have been reported in cardiorespiratory failure and following open heart surgery.[148,149]

Epinephrine

Epinephrine is the prototypical adrenergic agent, a potent vasopressor, and the drug of choice for treatment of cardiac arrest, hypersensitivity drug reactions, and cardiogenic shock. At lower dosages, epinephrine acts primarily on the beta-adrenergic receptor to increase blood pressure by positive inotropic and chronotropic cardiac effects. At higher dosages, alpha-agonist activity occurs, resulting in vasoconstriction of the peripheral vasculature. Epinephrine is rapidly metabolized by catechol-O-methyltransferase (COMT) and monoamine oxidase (MAO). Epinephrine is indicated in cardiopulmonary resuscitation both for inotropic support and to convert fine ventricular fibrillation refractory to cardioversion to coarse fibrillation.[150] The potent beta-adrenergic actions of epinephrine make it useful in the treatment of shock beginning with dosages of 0.01 µg/kg per minute. Doses exceeding 0.02 µg/kg per minute result in both alpha- and beta-adrenergic stimulation. Many clinicians shy away from epinephrine therapy because of the belief that it is potentially more dangerous than other inotropic agents in causing ventricular arrhythmias or cerebral hemorrhage. With the widespread availability of infusion pumps, however, epinephrine can be safely administered, as always, titrating to effect. In fact, recommended doses of epinephrine may in certain instances be too low. Case reports have documented the utility of high dose epinephrine in the resuscitation of a patient with cardiac arrest who fails to respond to standard therapy.[151] Experimental evidence indicates that epinephrine in larger doses than currently recommended may improve regional cerebral blood flow compared to equipotent doses of mexthoxamine during cardiopulmonary resuscitation.[152] Complications of epinephrine therapy include hyperglycemia, hypophosphatemia, and reduced granulocyte adherence. Because epinephrine is well absorbed after intratracheal administration, it can be used to initiate therapy in a patient who is intubated but not yet equipped with intravascular lines.[153]

Norepinephrine

Norepinephrine is another extremely useful catecholamine that until recently has seen relatively limited use because of concern for detrimental effects on renal function and other adverse peripheral effects. Recent reappraisals of norepinephrine therapy have concluded that it is often useful in the therapy of intractable shock[154] and may improve arterial blood pressure and urine flow when volume replacement and dopamine therapy alone have failed to reverse the hypotension of septic shock.[155] Experimental[135] and clinical evidence[156] suggest that norepinephrine may be the treatment of choice for volume-resuscitated septic shock associated with pulmonary hypertension and impaired right ventricular performance. While one recent study indicates that norepinephrine may be used in the treatment of human septic shock without deleterious renal effects,[157] it has also been shown that norepinephrine increases urine flow only when serum lactate levels are in the normal range, suggesting that when norepinephrine is used in shock with oliguria, both lactate and renal function should be carefully monitored.[158] Many clinicians add "low dose" dopamine for its renal vasodilating effect when using norepinephrine therapy, based on evidence that renal blood flow is enhanced in shock patients receiving combination pressor therapy.[140] On the other hand, experimental animal studies during endotoxic shock indicate that renal, splanchnic, and skeletal blood flow are unchanged during vasopressive therapy with either norepinephrine, dopamine, or phenylephrine.[159] While norepinephrine is considered by many as a "pure" alpha-adrenergic agent, in low doses, norepinephrine stimulates the beta-adrenergic receptor.[7] Pure alpha-adrenergic effect may be achieved through the use of the sympathominetic phenylephrine, which occasionally offers an advantage over norepinephrine therapy when beta stimulation results in undesirable tachycardia. Experimental data suggest that following coronary bypass, phenylephrine may produce a decrease in blood flow to both internal mammary and saphenous vein grafts while norepinephrine produces an increase in both types of grafts.[160]

Isoproterenol

Isoproterenol is a potent agonist that acts almost exclusively on the beta-adrenergic system. Because it increases cutaneous and muscular vasodilatation, it may redistribute blood to nonessential areas, resulting in lowered blood pressure. Isoproterenol is indicated for therapy of cardiac failure because of its effects on inotropic activity and its potential for increasing cardiac output by augmenting preload and reducing afterload. Animal evidence indicates that isoproterenol function is augmented in cardiomyopathic hearts to a degree not seen in normal control hearts.[161]

Phosphodiesterase Inhibitors

The phosphodiesterase inhibitors prevent the breakdown of cAMP, thus increasing effective intracellular cAMP levels. Aminophylline is a nonselective phosphodiesterase inhibitor but is not clinically used for its inotropic action, because other side effects supervene. More selective phosphodiesterase inhibitors include amrinone, milrinone, enoximone and a number of experimental agents. Amrinone acts by an inhibition of phosphodiesterase F3 and augments the action of beta-adrenergic agents by raising intracellular cAMP levels (see Fig. 65–4). Because it acts intracellularly and bypasses both the adrenergic receptor and the calcium channel, it may be beneficial in reversing cardiodepressant effects of drugs such as verapamil and propranolol.[162] Administration of amrinone results in significant improvements in cardiac index, pulmonary capillary wedge pressure, right atrial pressure, systemic vascular resistance, and pulmonary vascular resistance in low output states after open heart surgery.[163] Combination therapy with dopamine and amrinone has been described in the setting of refractory low output syndrome after open heart surgery.[164] Amrinone may also have advantages over the alpha-adrenergic agents in restoring intracellular calcium levels toward normal.[67] The bolus dose of 750 µg/kg recommended by the manufacturer may be at the lower end of the effective range, but higher doses may precipitate substantial vasodilatation. Administering the bolus dose over several minutes allows an effective response while minimizing hypotension. The maintenance infusion of amrinone should be started at 5 µg/kg per minute and titrated as clinically appropriate. An additional bolus injection may be necessary 30 minutes after initiation of therapy or when increasing the infusion rate. The manufacturer recommends that the total daily dose, including boluses, should not exceed 10 µg/kg per day, although a limited number of patients have tolerated amounts up to 18 µg/kg per day for shortened durations of therapy.[165] Amrinone may cause clinically important hypotension in the setting of septic shock because of its vasodilatating effects. Norepinephrine can counteract the vasodilatation, and clinical experience suggests the two agents in combination are useful with right ventricular failure, although formal studies of this approach are lacking.

Dobutamine and amrinone at equipotent doses in patients with heart failure produce similar effects on cardiac index, pulmonary capillary wedge pressure, mean right atrial pressure, heart rate, systemic vascular resistance, and mean arterial pressure[166] (Fig. 65–7). The addition of amrinone to 15 µg/kg per minute of dobutamine has an additional synergistic effect, resulting in continued increases in ejection fraction,[167] suggesting this combination with refractory congestive failure.

Milrinone (2-methyl, 5-carebonitrile amrinone) is 20 times as potent as amrinone. It is given as a 50- to 75- µg/kg intravenous bolus, followed by a 0.3- to 0.75- µg/kg per minute infusion. Hypotension, tachycardia, atrial fibrillation, and atrial bigeminy occur, as with amrinone, but milrinone is associated with a lower incidence of fever and thrombocytopenia. In a study of the systemic and coronary effects of intravenous milrinone and dobutamine in patients with congestive heart failure, either drug produced

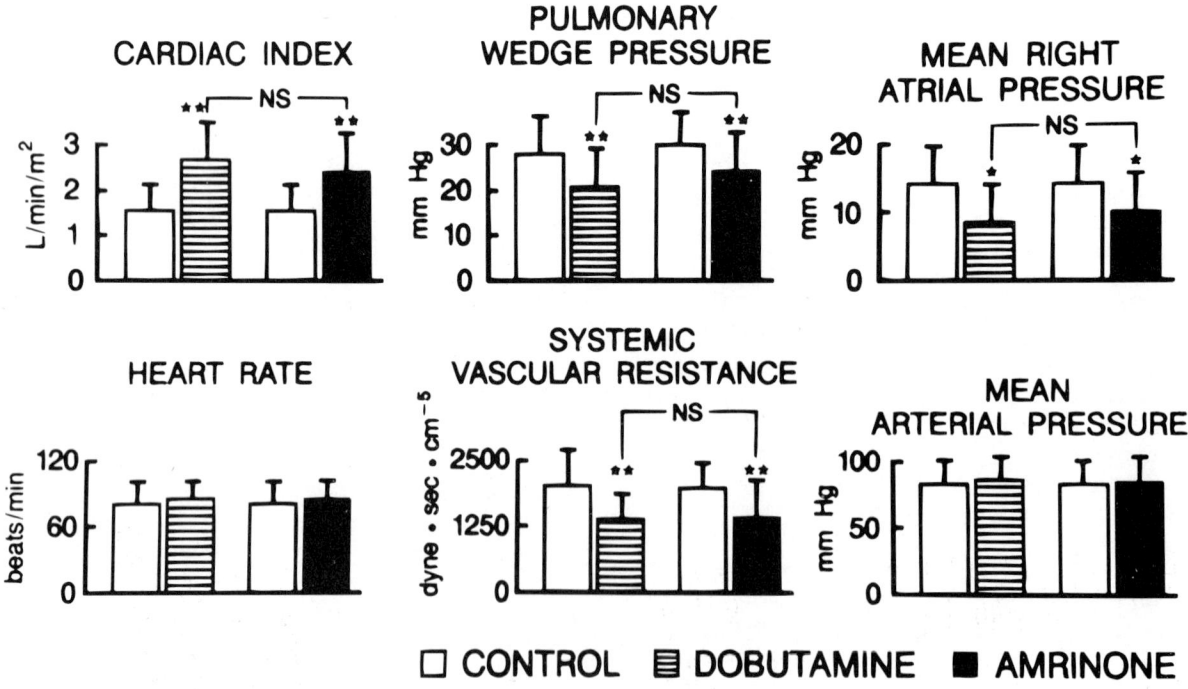

Fig. 65–7. Comparative effects of dobutamine and amrinone on hemodynamic parameters. The initial response is compared with control values in 15 patients with heart failure admitted to a coronary care unit. Patients received infusion of 2.5 µg/kg per minute of dobutamine initially, increased by 2.5 µg/kg per minute each hour until 15 µg/kg per minute was reached, after which therapy was terminated. After a washout period, amrinone was administered with a loading dose of 1.5 mg/kg followed by constant infusion of 10 to 30 µg/kg per minute. Comparisons are maximal response relative to control; *, $p \leq 0.01$; **, $p \leq 0.001$; NS, not significant. (From Benotti, J. R., McCue, J. E., and Alpert, J. S.: Comparative vasoactive therapy for heart failure. Am. J. Cardiol., 56:19B, 1985.)

similar improvements in cardiac index, but dobutamine increased myocardial oxygen consumption, whereas milrinone did not.[167a] Milrinone is increasingly used in the treatment of low cardiac output following cardiac surgery, for which it has been shown to be well tolerated and effective.[167b,167c]

Enoximone is another selective phosphodiesterase type III inhibitor. It increases cardiac output, decreases pulmonary capillary and pulmonary arterial pressures, and assists in "weaning" patients with impaired myocardial function from cardiopulmonary bypass.[168]

Calcium

Calcium is essential for normal cardiac and neuromuscular function and can act as both a vasopressor and inotrope. Left ventricular contractility varies directly with blood-ionized calcium levels.[112] Normal circulating calcium concentrations are needed for myocardial performance and maintenance of vascular tone.[169] As previously noted, critically ill patients are commonly hypocalcemic, possibly because of abnormalities in the PTH-vitamin D access. Opinions vary, however, on whether the hypocalcemia of sepsis is pathologic or adaptive and whether it should be treated.[170] Pending more definitive studies on this subject, the clinician should be aware of the ionized serum calcium level and may choose to administer calcium chloride or calcium gluconate in the setting of circulatory dysfunction. Calcium administration has been associated with an increased risk of pancreatitis when used for inotropic support after cardiopulmonary bypass.[171]

UNCONVENTIONAL APPROACHES TO THE THERAPY OF SHOCK

Naloxone

Pro-opiomelanocortin is a 31,000 molecular weight substance released in response to stress.[172] One fragment of the pro-opiocortin becomes adrenocorticotropin (ACTH), and another fragment becomes beta endorphin, which presumably acts at endogenous opiate receptors and contributes to the hypotension seen in patients with shock. Animal research has suggested that blockade of beta endorphin by naloxone might be a benefit in reversing the hypotension of shock states.[173-175] Some early clinical reports demonstrated remarkable increases in blood pressure in patients given naloxone even in small doses.[176-178] More controlled studies have reported that naloxone does not reliably change physiologic variables[179] and have demonstrated that the dose, the timing of the dose, and the patient's renal function all affect the response.[180,181] Naloxone in the postoperative patient reverses any narcotic anesthesia that has been given and often provokes extreme agitation and/or hypertension. While the latest studies suggest naloxone is efficacious in improving the hemodynamic profile of patients with early hyperdynamic septic shock, improvement in survival has not been demonstrated.[181] Thyrotropin-releasing hormone, a physiologic opiate antagonist, may provide the same blood pressure effects as naloxone without reversal of opiate-induced pain relief.[182] More research needs to be done with both of these agents before they can be recommended for routine clinical use in shock.

Glucagon

Glucagon is another endogenous hormone released following shock or trauma. The effects of glucagon are altered by verapamil, suggesting that its effects are mediated via calcium channels.[183] Glucagon in intravenous doses of 1 to 4 mg has been reported to be useful in beta-blocked patients for reversal of intractable hypotension or bradycardia.[184] In an experimental model of postcountershock asystole and electromechanical dissociation, glucagon had little effect on blood pressure, cerebral perfusion pressure, or coronary sinus flow. In 14 of the 19 animals, however, glucagon restored effective circulation by increasing the intrinsic discharge rate of the animals' hearts. The authors speculate that the probable mechanism is a nonadrenergic effect on cAMP.[185] Clinical reports describe responses to intravenous glucagon infusion in patients with heart failure unresponsive to conventional therapy.[186,187] Glucagon also is an effective antagonist of calcium channel blockers in the clinical setting.[188]

Digoxin

Clinicians have avoided the use of digoxin in the setting of acute hemodynamic instability because of fear of toxicity with acute electrolyte shifts. Recent information, however, suggests that digoxin is useful in a subset of patients with left ventricular dysfunction and severe heart failure.[189] In one study of 20 patients with severe sepsis and left ventricle dysfunction manifested by systemic hypoperfusion, digoxin as a bolus of 10 µg/kg over 3 minutes led to increases in mean arterial pressure, stroke volume index, and left ventricular stroke work index (LVSWI).[190] This study must be interpreted with caution, because 55% of the patients died before ICU discharge. The increase in LVSWI was 74 ± 16% in the digoxin-treated patients versus 13 ± 10% in dopamine-treated (5 to 12 µg/kg per minute) patients.[190] The authors speculate that beta-adrenergic receptor downregulation, which occurs in sepsis, may have caused the lack of response to dopamine in this population. Digoxin also augments pressor responsiveness to both norepinephrine and angiotensin in normal volunteers.[191] The positive inotropic effect of cardiac glycosides may result from the sodium-current-induced release of calcium from cardiac sarcoplasmic reticulum.[192]

Prostaglandin Inhibitors

As noted earlier, inhibition of the cyclo-oxygenase pathway alters the relationship between vasoconstricting arachidonic acid metabolites. In an experimental endotoxic shock model in dogs, intravenous doses of ibuprofen (1, 5, 10, or 20 mg/kg) resulted in significant increases in systolic and diastolic blood pressure, mean arterial pressure, and systemic vascular resistance.[193] Pulmonary artery pressure and pulmonary vascular resistance were also increased. There was a lack of a dose–response relationship, suggesting that low dose ibuprofen may be beneficial. Because high dose ibuprofen is known to have adverse renal effects, caution must be exercised in applying this information to humans; some actions of the nonsteroidal anti-inflammatory drugs are species specific. Other animal studies have documented improved hemodynamics with ibuprofen-treated sheep given live Escherichia coli[194] and indomethacin-treated cats given endotoxin.[195]

Prostaglandin E₁

Animal studies demonstrate membrane-stabilizing effects and reduced myocardial depressant factor production in experimental traumatic shock.[196] Prostaglandin E₁ (at doses of 30 to 150 ng/kg per minute) is effective in reducing pulmonary hypertension and thus relieving refractory right heart failure following mitral valve replacement. Prostaglandin E is a profound system vasodilator, and norepinephrine, given via a left atrial line, may be necessary to reverse the severe hypotension caused by prostaglandin E.[197]

The Role of Corticosteroids in Shock

Because mediator release with resulting vasodilatation is part of the common final pathway of shock states, considerable interest centered on preventing mediator release by stabilizing cell membranes with corticosteroids. A number of anecdotal reports prompted the conduct of numerous studies. One of the earlier studies, a prospective randomized, double blind study of 172 patients, showed that the mortality rate in saline-treated patients was 33 of 86 (38.4%), while mortality rate was only 9 of 86 (10.4%) in the steroid-treated group.[198] Further retrospective analysis of 328 patients by the same author demonstrated a mortality rate of 42.5% in those patients not treated with corticosteroids but 14% in those patients treated with steroids. The complication rate of superinfection was reported at 6% in the steroid-tested groups. This landmark study[198] prompted many clinicians to adopt "steroids" as a routine therapy in shock states during the late 1970s and early 1980s. Further examination of this controversy, however, has changed the prevailing opinion. A study by Sprung and colleagues[199] demonstrated that steroid-treated patients had a lower mortality rate early in the hospital course but that over the entire hospital stay there was no difference in mortality. Patients in this study treated with methylprednisolone had a mortality rate of 76%, those patients treated with dexamethasone a mortality of 77%, and those in the control group 69% mortality rate. The authors concluded that corticosteroids were of no benefit in late septic shock but may be helpful early in the course of shock and in certain subgroups. The methylprednisolone sepsis study group led by Bone and colleagues[200] was a multicenter study involving 382 patients who were entered into the study at the onset of sepsis (not shock). Mortality in the methylprednisolone group was 31/79 (39%); the mortality rate in the placebo group was only 28%. A subgroup of patients with increased serum creatinine concentrations showed increased mortality rate (59%) when compared to the placebo group (29%). The Veterans Administration sepsis study group[201] was another multicenter study with 223 patients entered at the onset of sepsis with a normal sensorium. In this study, the glucocorticoid mortality and placebo mortality were nearly identical, but resolution of secondary infection was better in the placebo group. Because numerous animal studies indicate that pretreatment with corticosteroids clearly reduces the mortality rate in experimental shock, it is still possible that corticosteroids could have a role in the treatment of human septic shock if the appropriate population could be determined earlier. The issue remains the focus of intense investigation by numerous researchers. Although the current standard of care is to avoid administration of steroids in septic shock, perhaps subgroups of patients that benefit will be identified in the future. One study suggests that vasopressin maintains cardiovascular function in early endotoxic shock and that corticosteroids may be beneficial when vasopressin is absent.[202]

Other Agents in Shock

Space permits only a passing mention of fructose 1-6 diphosphate,[203] lidocaine,[204] and charcoal hemoperfusion[205] as experimental countermeasures in shock therapy. The methylxanthine derivative pentoxifylline, currently in clinical use in the treatment of peripheral vascular disease, may improve flow through constricted microcirculation by (1) its effects on red blood cell deformability, (2) release of prostacyclin, (3) decrease of adhesiveness of activated polymorphonuclear leukocytes, and (4) inhibition of production of TNF.[206] Pretreatment with pentoxifylline in experimental septic syndrome attenuated differences in systemic vascular resistance (SVR) and pulmonary vascular resistance (PVR) without other hemodynamic effects and markedly decreased neutrophil adhesiveness.[207] Active clinical investigation of pentoxifylline is currently underway. Glucose-insulin-potassium infusion is also readily available in the clinical setting and has been demonstrated to enhance left ventricular function in the setting of acute myocardial infarction in patients with impaired ejection fractions[208] in septic shock[209] and following separation from bypass in open heart surgery.[210] A typical dosage regimen consists of D50, regular insulin 80 IU/L, and potassium 100 mEq/L at a rate of 1 mL/kg per hour for up to 48 hours.[210] Further experimental support is needed before this drug combination can be recommended as routine therapy. The roles of antibodies to endotoxin[39,40] and TNF[49] similarly need to be refined.[211] Early reports suggest that human recombinant interleukin-1 receptor antagonist[212] and leukotriene B-4 receptor antagonists[213] will have a role in therapy of sepsis syndrome.

THE POSTRESUSCITATION PHASE

Weaning Pharmacologic Support

The rapidity with which pharmacologic support can be weaned from the patient in shock relates to the length of time of hemodynamic support and the expected level of receptor downregulation and substrate depletion. Most clinicians would choose to begin titrating pressors in 10 to 25% increments on a half-hour or hourly basis, relying on clinical monitoring (hemodynamics and oxygen transport) to determine the end point of weaning. Because the end point is to increase Do_2 to optimize Vo_2, vasopressors needing early temporary blood pressure for support during rehydration may become undesirable in later stages of support if they depress D_{O_2} and V_{O_2}. Response to therapy is best evaluated by end-organ functional exam and oxygen transport variables.[4]

ICU Discharge Criteria Following Shock

The extremely high mortality rate with circulatory shock results in very few patients in whom discharge criteria must be considered. Generally, these patients have multiorgan system dysfunction. Before these patients can be discharged from the unit, they must demonstrate adequate neurologic, cardiac, respiratory, renal, metabolic, and hepatic function and be free of ongoing infectious processes. Many clinicians discontinue hemodynamic monitoring in stages, removing the pulmonary artery catheter when the cardiac index has been stable and the information gained from the catheter no longer outweighs the risk of leaving it in place. Under stable conditions, patients can be weaned from inotropic support without a pulmonary artery catheter in place, although continued central venous monitoring and arterial monitoring are essential. Removal of central venous lines often hinges on vascular access requirements for medications and total parenteral nutrition rather than the need for hemodynamic monitoring per se. Arterial decannulation requires the patient to be stable from a respiratory standpoint (i.e., not requiring multiple daily blood gases) and can be accomplished more easily if accurate noninvasive monitoring is available in the ICU. Because the apparent risks of arterial catheterization are small, this level of monitoring is often left in until unit discharge.

The patient is ready for ICU discharge when all systems are stable and when the likelihood of emergent return to the ICU from the "floor" is small. This approach depends on the hospital's facilities, including availability of monitoring on the floor or in a stepdown unit.

In summary, circulatory shock is a major therapeutic problem that may be difficult to recognize by clinical findings alone. Hypotension, inadequate tissue perfusion, lactic acidosis, oliguria, increased arterial venous oxygen content difference, and decreased toe temperature may all be valuable early warning signs. The cause of the shock state must be identified as one of four major categories (hypovolemic, distributive, cardiogenic, obstructive) to determine the therapeutic approach. As always, the ABCs of resuscitation must be considered (airway, breathing, circulation), and only after adequate fluid repletion has been accomplished should pharmacologic support be initiated. Hypovolemic shock is best treated with hemostatic control and repletion of intravascular volume. Distributive shock may require volume loading and concurrent institution of inotropic support as well as attention to the precipitating cause (sepsis, anaphylaxis, spinal injury). Volume loading and restoration of blood flow, often by surgical means, are required for obstructive shock. Cardiogenic shock may be the most difficult to evaluate without hemodynamic monitoring to optimize preload and afterload. Pharmacologic support is not effective when intravascular volume is repleted and the patient's acid/base status is normal. Catecholamines are chosen on the basis of inotropic and peripheral vasoconstrictive effects and may often require combination therapy or use of an inodilating drug such as amrinone milrinone or dobutamine. Catecholamine response may be altered by the patient's premorbid condition, acidosis, prolonged drug therapy (downregulation), and hypothermia. While the catecholamines and phosphodiesterase inhibitors are presently the major therapeutic options, increased attention is being paid to use of digoxin, and specific inhibitors of the endorphin, prostaglandin, and other systems. Promising therapeutic advances include monoclonal antibodies to endotoxin, leukotriene and interleukin receptor antagonists, glucose-insulin-potassium infusions, PGE, and pentoxyphylline. Although these unconventional therapies are still at the stage of research findings as of this writing, some of these modalities may become clinically relevant in the near future. The postresuscitation phase involves gradual withdrawal of support while maintaining adequate monitoring to ensure continued stability.

REFERENCES

1. Joly, H. R., and Weil, M. H.: Temperature of the great toe as an indication of the severity of shock. Circulation, 39:131, 1969.
2. Mecher, C. E., Rackow, E. C., Astiz, M. E., and Weil, M. H.: Venous hypercarbia associated with severe sepsis and systemic hypoperfusion. Crit. Care Med., 18:585, 1990.
3. Weil, M. H., Michaels, S., and Rackow, E. C.: Comparison of blood lactate and concentrations in central venous, pulmonary artery, and arterial blood. Crit. Care Med., 15:489, 1987.
4. Creamer, J. E., Edwards, J. D., and Nightingale, P.: Hemodynamic and oxygen transport variables in cardiogenic shock secondary to acute myocardial infarction, and response to treatment. Am. J. Cardiol., 65:1297, 1990.
5. Hess, M. L., Warner, M., and Okabe, E.: Hemorrhagic shock. In Handbook of Shock and Trauma. Vol. 1. Basic Science. Edited by B. M. Altura, A. M. Lefer, and W. Schumer. New York, Raven Press, 1983.
6. Chernow, B. et al.: Sympathetic nervous system sensitivity to hemorrhagic hypotension in the subhuman primate. J. Trauma, 24:229, 1984.
7. Chernow, B., Rainey, T. G., and Lake, C. R.: Endogenous and exogenous catecholamines in critical care medicine. Crit. Care Med., 10:409, 1982.
8. Potgieter, P. D., Linton, D. M., Oliver, S., and Forder, A. A.: Nosocomial infections in a respiratory intensive care unit. Crit. Care Med., 15:495, 1987.
9. Bates, D. W., Cook, E. F., Goldman, L., and Lee, T. H.: Predicting bacteremia in hospitalized patients. A prospectively validated model. Ann. Intern. Med. 113:495, 1990.
10. Martin, C. et al.: Abnormalities of some phagocyte membrane receptors during nosocomial infections. Crit. Care Med., 15:467, 1987.
11. Bozzetti, F.: Central venous catheter sepsis. Surg. Gynecol. Obstet., 161:293, 1985.
12. Quercia, R. A. et al.: Bacteriologic contamination of intravenous infusion delivery systems in an intensive care unit. Am. J. Med., 80:364, 1986.
13. Gil, R. T., Kruse, J. A., Thill-Baharozian, M. C., and Carlson, R. W.: Triple- vs single-lumen central venous catheters. A prospective study in a critically ill population. Arch. Intern. Med., 149:1139, 1989.

14. Craven, D. E. et al.: A randomized study comparing a transparent polyurethane dressing to a dry gauze dressing for peripheral intravenous catheter sites. Infect. Control, 6: 361, 1985.
15. Maki, D. G. et al.: An attachable silver-impregnated cuff for prevention of infection with central venous catheters: a prospective randomized multicenter trial. Am. J. Med., 85: 307, 1988.
16. Albert, R. K., and Condie, F.: Hand-washing patterns in medical intensive-care units. N. Engl. J. Med., 304:1465, 1981.
17. Craven, D. E., Goularte, T. A., and Make, B. J.: Contaminated condensate in mechanical ventilator circuits. A risk factor for nosocomial pneumonia? Am. Rev. Respir. Dis., 129:625, 1984.
18. Driks, M. R. et al.: Nosocomial pneumonia in intubated patients given sucralfate as compared with antacids or histamine type 2 blockers. The role of gastric colonization. N. Engl. J. Med., 317:1376, 1987.
19. Van Uffelen, R., Rommes, J. H., and Van Saene, H. K. F.: Preventing lower airway colonization and infection in mechanically ventilated patients. Crit. Care Med., 15:99, 1987.
20. Karnad, D. R., Mhaisekar, D. G., and Moralwar, K. V.: Respiratory mucus pH in tracheostomized intensive care unit patients: effects of colonization and pneumonia. Crit. Care Med., 18:699, 1990.
21. Chernow, B. et al.: Measurement of urinary leukocyte esterase activity: a screening test for urinary tract infections. Ann. Emerg. Med., 13:150, 1984.
22. Schwartz, L. B. et al.: Tryptase levels as an indicator of mast-cell activation in systemic anaphylaxis and mastocytosis. N. Engl. J. Med., 316:1622, 1987.
23. Lasser, E. C. et al.: Pretreatment with corticosteroids to alleviate reactions to intravenous contrast material. N. Engl. J. Med., 317:845, 1987.
24. Weiss, M. E. et al.: Association of protamine IgE and IgG antibodies with life-threatening reactions to intravenous protamine. N. Engl. J. Med., 320:886, 1989.
25. Willems, J. L., Pardaens, J., and DeGeest, H.: Early risk stratification using clinical findings in patients with acute myocardial infarction. Euro. Heart J., 5:130, 1984.
26. Volpi, A. et al.: In-hospital prognosis of patients with acute myocardial infarction complicated by primary ventricular fibrillation. N. Engl. J. Med., 317:257, 1987.
27. Pellikka, P. A., Behrenbeck, T., Huber, K. C., and Gibbons, R. J.: Measurement of myocardium at risk and salvage in myocardial infarction with ST-segment depression. Mayo Clin. Proc., 65:1222, 1990.
28. Radford, M. J. et al.: Ventricular septal rupture: a review of clinical and physiologic features and an analysis of survival. Circulation, 64:545, 1981.
29. Slogoff, S., and Keats, A. S.: Does perioperative myocardial ischemia lead to postoperative myocardial infarction? Anesthesiology, 62:107, 1985.
30. Becker, R. C., and Underwood, D. A.: Myocardial infarction in patients undergoing noncardiac surgery. Cleve. Clin. J. Med., 54:25, 1987.
31. Moser, K. M.: Pulmonary embolism. Am. Rev. Respir. Dis., 115:829, 1977.
32. Cerra, C. B. et al.: Role of monokines in altering hepatic metabolism in sepsis. In Molecular and Cellular Mechanisms of Septic Shock. Edited by B. L. Roth, T. B. Nielsen, and A. E. McKee. New York, Alan R. Liss, 1988, p. 265.
33. Brandtzaeg, P. et al.: Plasma endotoxin as a predictor of multiple organ failure and death in systemic meningococcal disease. J. Infect. Dis., 159:195, 1989.
34. Vadas, P. et al.: Pathogenesis of hypotension in septic shock: correlation of circulating phospholipase A_2 levels with circulatory collapse. Crit. Care Med., 16:1, 1988.
35. Beutler, B., and Cerami, A.: Cachectin: more than a tumor necrosis factor. N. Engl. J. Med., 316:379, 1987.
36. Brandtzaeg, P., Oktedalen O., Kierulf, P., and Opstad, P. K.: Elevated VIP and endotoxin plasma levels in human gram-negative septic shock. Reg. Pep., 24:37, 1989.
37. Strohmaier, W., Redl, H., Schlag, G., and Inthorn, D.: D-erythro-neopterin plasma levels in intensive care patients with and without septic complications. Crit. Care Med., 15: 757, 1987.
38. Heath, M. F., Tighe, D., Moss, R., and Bennett, E. D.: Relevance of serum phospholipase A_2 assays to the assessment of septic shock. Crit. Care Med., 18:766, 1990.
39. Ziegler, E. J. et al: Treatment of gram-negative bacteremia and septic shock with HA-1A human monoclonal antibody against endotoxin. A randomized, double-blind, placebo-controlled trial. N. Engl. J. Med., 324:429, 1991.
40. Fisher, C. J. et al.: Initial evaluation of human monoclonal anti-lipid A antibody (HA-1A) in patients with sepsis syndrome. Crit. Care. Med., 18:1311, 1990.
41. Greenman, R. L. et al.: A controlled clinical trial of E5 murine monoclonal IgM antibody to endotoxin in the treatment of gram-negative sepsis. JAMA, 266:1097, 1991.
41a. Wenzel, R. P.: Anti-endotoxin monoclonal antibodies: a second look. N. Engl. J. Med., 326:1151, 1992.
41b. Warren, H. S., Danner, R. L., and Munford, R. S.: Sounding board: anti-endotoxin monoclonal antibodies. N. Engl. J. Med., 326:1153, 1992.
42. Filkins, J. P.: Monokines and the metabolic pathophysiology of septic shock. Fed. Proc., 44:300, 1985.
43. McGiff, J. C.: Thromboxane and prostacyclin: implications for function and disease of the vasculature. Adv. Intern. Med., 25:199, 1980.
44. Lefer, A. M.: Eicosanoids as mediators of ischemia and shock. Fed. Proc., 44:275, 1985.
45. Tracey, K. J. et al.: Shock and tissue injury induced by recombinant human cachectin. Science 234:470, 1986.
46. Michie, H. R. et al.: Detection of circulating tumor necrosis factor after endotoxin administration. N. Engl. J. Med., 318: 1481, 1988.
47. Damas, P. et al.: Tumor necrosis factor and interleukin-1 serum levels during severe sepsis in humans. Crit. Care Med., 17:975, 1989.
48. van der Poll, T. et al.: Activation of coagulation after administration of tumor necrosis factor to normal subjects. N. Eng. J. Med., 322:1622, 1990.
49. Hinshaw, L. B. et al.: Survival of primates in LD_{100} septic shock following therapy with antibody to Tumor Necrosis Factor (TNFα). Circ. Shock, 30:279, 1990.
50. Lefer, A. M.: Interaction between myocardial depressant factor and vasoactive mediators with ischemia and shock. Am. J. Physiol., 252:R193, 1987.
51. Parker, M. M. et al.: Profound but reversible myocardial depression in patients with septic shock. Ann. Intern. Med., 100:483, 1984.
52. Goldfarb, R. D.: Cardiac dynamics following shock: role of circulating cardiodepressant substances. Circ. Shock, 9: 317, 1982.
53. Reilly, J. M. et al.: A circulating myocardial depressant substance is associated with cardiac dysfunction and peripheral hypoperfusion (lactic acidemia) in patients with septic shock. Chest, 95:1072, 1989.
54. Parrillo, J. E.: A circulating myocardial depressant substance in humans with septic shock. Septic shock patients with a reduced ejection fraction have a circulating factor that

depresses in vitro myocardial cell performance. J. Clin. Invest., 76:1539, 1985.
55. Bernton, E. W. et al.: Release of multiple hormones by a direct action of interleukin-1 on pituitary cells. Science, 238:519, 1987.
56. Sapolsky, R. et al.: Interleukin-1 stimulates the secretion of hypothalamic corticotropin-releasing factor. Science, 238:522, 1987.
57. Ognibene, F. P. et al.: Interleukin-2 administration causes reversible hemodynamic changes and left ventricular dysfunction similar to those seen in septic shock. Chest, 94:750, 1988.
57a. Cohn, J., and Bone, R. C.: New strategies in nonantibiotic treatment of gram-negative sepsis. Cleve. Clin. J. Med., 59:608, 1992.
58. Maze, M., Haywood, E., and Gaba, D. M.: Alpha-1 adrenergic blockade raises epinephrine arrhythmic threshold in halothane anesthetized dogs in a dose dependent fashion. Anesthesiology, 63:611, 1985.
59. Lackovic, A., and Relja, M.: Evidence for a widely distributed peripheral dopaminergic system. Fed. Proc., 42:3000, 1983.
60. Bond, R. A., and Clarke, D. E.: A response to isoprenaline unrelated to alpha- and beta-adrenoceptor agonism. J. Pharmacol., 91:683–686 1987.
61. Wilson, C. et al.: The rat lipolytic beta-adrenoceptor: studies using novel beta-adrenoceptor agonists. Euro. J. Pharmacol., 100:309, 1984.
62. Arch, J. R. S.: Atypical beta-adrenoceptor on brown adipocytes as target for anti-obesity drugs. Nature, 309:163, 1984.
63. Emorine, L. J.: Molecular characterization of the human beta3-adrenergic receptor. Science, 245:1118, 1989.
64. Lefkowitz, R. J., and Caron, M. G.: Adrenergic receptors: molecular mechanisms of clinically relevant regulation. Clin. Res., 33:395, 1985.
65. Berridge, M. J., and Irvine, R. F.: Inositol triphosphate, a novel second messenger in cellular signal transduction. Nature, 312:315, 1984.
66. Graham, R. M.: Adrenergic receptors: structure and function. Cleve. Clin. J. Med., 57:481, 1990.
67. Aufferman, W. et al.: Influence of positive inotropic agents on intracellular calcium transients. Part I. Normal rat heart. Am. Heart J., 118:1219, 1991.
68. Barton, M., Lake, C. R., Rainey, T. G., and Chernow B.: Is catecholamine release pH mediated? Crit. Care Med., 10:751, 1982.
69. Rajfer, S. I., Anton, A. H., Rossen J. D., and Goldberg, L. I.: Beneficial hemodynamic effects of oral levodopa in heart failure. Relation to the generation of dopamine. N. Engl. J. Med., 310:1357, 1984.
70. Palmer, G. J., Ziegler, M. G., and Lake, C. R.: Response of norepinephrine and blood pressure to stress increases with age. J. Gerontol., 33:482, 1978.
71. Veith, R. C., Fetherstone, J. A., Linares, O. A., and Halter, J. B.: Age differences in plasma norepinephrine kinetics in humans. J. Geronotol., 41:319, 1986.
72. Bullington, J. et al.: The effect of advancing age on the sympathetic response to laryngoscopy and tracheal intubation. Anesth. Analg., 68:603, 1989.
73. Feldman, R. D. et al.: Alterations in leukocyte beta-receptor affinity with aging: a potential explanation for altered beta-adrenergic sensitivity in the elderly. N. Engl. J. Med., 310:815, 1984.
74. Pan, H. Y.-M., Hoffman, B. B., Pershe, R. A., and Blaschke, T. F.: Decline in beta adrenergic receptor-mediated vascular relaxation with aging in man. Am. Soc. Pharmacol. Exp. Ther., 239:802, 1986.
75. Van Brummelen, P., Buhler, F. R., Kiowski, W., and Amann, F. W.: Age-related decrease in cardiac and peripheral vascular responsiveness to isoprenaline: studies in normal subjects. Clin. Sci., 60:571, 1981.
76. Zhou, H. H., Silberstein, D. J., Koshakji, R. P., and Wood, A. J. J.: Interindividual differences in B-receptor density contribute to variability in response to B-adrenoceptor antagonists. Clin. Pharmacol. Ther., 45:587, 1989.
77. Brodde, O. E. et al.: Human beta-adrenoceptors: relation of myocardial and lymphocyte beta-adrenoceptor density. Science, 231:1584, 1986.
78. Zhou, H.-H. et al.: Racial differences in drug response. Altered sensitivity to and clearance of propranolol in men of chinese descent as compared with american whites. N. Engl. J. Med., 320:565, 1989.
79. Tarnow, J., M. D., and Komar, K.: Altered hemodynamic response to dobutamine in relation to the degree of preoperative β-adrenoceptor blockade. Anesthesiology, 68:912, 1988.
80. Hayes, J. S., Bowling, N., and Pollock, G. D.: Effects of beta adrenoceptor down-regulation on the cardiovascular responses to the stereoisomers of dobutamine. J. Pharmacol. Exp. Ther., 235:58, 1985.
81. Pedrinelli, R., and Tarazi, R. C.: Interference of calcium entry blockade in vivo with pressor responses to β-adrenergic stimulation: effects of two unrelated blockers on responses to both exogenous and endogenously released norepinephrine. Circulation, 69:1171, 1984.
82. Sturm, J. T.: The influence of verapamil on dopamine's ability to augment cardiac output. Ann. Emerg. Med., 14:945, 1985.
83. Massagee, J. T. et al.: Effects of peroperative calcium entry blocker therapy on a-adrenergic responsiveness in patients undergoing coronary revascularization. Anesthesiology, 67:485, 1987.
84. Lange, R. A. et al.: Potentiation of cocaine-induced coronary vasoconstriction by beta-adrenergic blockade. Ann. Intern. Med., 112:897, 1990.
85. Estafanous, F. G. et al.: Hemodilution affects the pressor response to norepinephrine. J. Cardiothorac. Anesth., 1:36, 1987.
86. Sakamaki, T. et al.: Pressor hyperresponsiveness in saline-infused rabbits. Hypertension, 6:503, 1984.
87. Reed, H. L. et al.: Alterations in sympathetic nervous system activity with intraoperative hypothermia during coronary artery bypass surgery. Chest, 95:616, 1989.
88. Chernow, B. et al.: Sympathetic nervous system "switch off" with severe hypothermia. Crit. Care Med., 11:677, 1983.
89. Marty, J. et al.: β-Adrenergic receptor function is acutely altered in surgical patients. Anesth. Anagl., 71:1, 1990.
90. Borow, K. M., Neumann, A., Arensman, F. W., and Yacoub, M. H.: Cardiac and peripheral vascular responses to adrenoceptor stimulation and blockade after cardiac transplantation. J. Am. Cardiol., 14:1229, 1989.
91. Hilsted, J. et al.: Metabolic and cardiovascular responses to epinephrine in diabetic autonomic neuropathy, epinephrine and diabetic autonomic neuropathy. N. Engl. J. Med., 317:421, 1987.
92. Berlin, I., Grimaldi, A., Bosquet, F., and Puech, A. J.: Decreased β-adrenergic sensitivity in insulin-dependent diabetic subjects. J. Clin. Endocrinol. Metab., 63:262, 1986.
93. Fraser, C. M., Venter, J. C., and Kaliner, M.: Autonomic abnormalities and autoantibodies to beta-adrenergic receptors. N. Engl. J. Med., 305:1165, 1981.
94. Bristow, M. R. et al.: Decreased catecholamine sensitivity

and β-adrenergic-receptor density in failing human hearts. N. Engl. J. Med., *307*:205, 1982.
95. Levine, T. B. et al.: Activity of the sympathetic nervous system and renin-angiotensin system assessed by plasma hormone levels and their relation to hemodynamic abnormalities in congestive heart failure. Am. J. Cardiol., *49*:1659, 1972.
96. Viquerat, C. E. et al.: Endogenous catecholamine levels in chronic heart failure. Am. J. Med., *78*:455, 1985.
97. Vatner, D. E., Vatner, S. F., Fujii, A. M., and Homcy, C. J.: Loss of high affinity cardiac beta adrenergic receptors in dogs with heart failure. J. Clin. Invest., *76*:2259, 1986.
98. Levine, B. et al.: Elevated circulating levels of tumor necrosis factor in severe chronic heart failure. N. Engl. J. Med., *323*:236, 1990.
99. Vatner, D. E. et al.: Effects of pressure overload, left ventricular hypertrophy on β-adrenergic receptors, and responsiveness to catecholamines. J. Clin. Invest., *73*:1473, 1984.
100. Swedberg, K. et al.: Comparison of myocardial catecholamine balance in chronic congestive heart failure and in angina pectoris without failure. Am. J. Cardiol., *54*:783, 1984.
101. Schwinn, D. A. et al.: α-Adrenergic responsiveness during coronary artery bypass surgery: effect of preoperative ejection fraction. Anesthesiology, *69*:206, 1988.
102. Smith, C. E. et al.: α-Adrenergic agonist drugs, left ventricular function, and emergence from cardiopulmonary bypass. J. Cardiothorac. Anesth., *4*:681, 1990.
103. McMillan, M., Chernow, B., and Roth, B. L.: Hepatic alpha1-adrenergic receptor alteration in a rat model of chronic sepsis. Circ. Shock, *19*:185, 1986.
104. Bendixen, H. H., Laver, M. B., and Flacke, W. E.: Influence of respiratory acidosis on circulatory effect of epinephrine in dogs. Circ. Res., *13*:64, 1963.
105. Lefkowitz, R. J., Caron, M. G., and Stiles, G. L.: Mechanisms of membrane-receptor regulation. N. Engl. J. Med., *310*:1570, 1984.
106. Hart, B. B. et al.: Catecholamines: study of interspecies variation. Crit. Care Med., *17*:1203, 1989.
107. Chernow, B., et al.: Hypocalcemia in critically ill patients. Crit. Care Med., *10*:848, 1982.
108. McLean, F. C., and Hastings, A. B.: The state of calcium in the fluids of the body: the conditions affecting the ionization of calcium. J. Biol. Chem., *108*:285, 1935.
109. Zaloga, G. P. et al.: Assessment of calcium homeostasis in the critically ill surgical patient. Ann. Surg., *202*:587, 1981.
110. Zaloga, G. P., and Chernow, B.: Stress-induced changes in calcium metabolism. Semin. Respir. Med., *7*:52, 1985.
111. Zaloga, G. P., and Chernow, B.: The multifactorial basis for hypocalcemia during sepsis. Ann. Intern. Med., *107*:36, 1987.
112. Lang, R. M. et al.: Left ventricular contractility varies directly with blood ionized calcium. Ann. Med., *108*:524, 1988.
113. Desai, T. K., Carlson, R. W., Baharozian, M., and Geheb, M. A.: A direct relationship between ionized calcium and arterial pressure among patients in an intensive care unit. Crit. Care Med., *16*:578, 1988.
114. Malcolm, D. S., Zaloga, G. P., and Holaday, J. W.: Calcium administration increases the mortality of endotoxic shock in rats. Crit. Care Med., *17*:900, 1989.
115. Janson, C., Birnbaum, G., and Baker, F. J.: Hypophosphatemia. Ann. Emerg. Med., *12*:107, 1983.
116. O'Connor, L. R., Wheeler, W. S., and Bethune, J. E.: Effect of hypophosphatemia on myocardial performance in man. N. Engl. J. Med., *297*:901, 1977.
117. Chernow, B., Smith, J., Rainey, T. G., and Finton, C.: Hypomagnesemia: implications for the critical care specialist. Crit. Care Med., *10*:193, 1982.
118. Whyte, K., Addis, G. J., Whitesmith, R., and Reid, J. L.: Adrenergic control of plasma magnesium in man. Clin. Sci., *72*:135, 1987.
119. Coyle, J. P., Kamath, G., Licina, M. G., and Higgins, T. L.: Factors affecting magnesium levels after cardiac surgery. Anesthesiology, *71*:A192, 1989.
120. Iseri, L. T., Freed, J., and Bures, A. R.: Magnesium deficiency and cardiac disorders. Am. J. Med., *58*:837, 1975.
121. Zaloga, G. P. et al.: Hypomagnesemia is a common complication of aminoglycoside therapy. Surg. Gynecol. Obstet., *158*:561, 1984.
122. McCalden, T. A., Bloom, D., and Rosendorff, C.: The effects of jaundiced plasma and hypercholesterolaemic plasma on vascular sensitivity to injected noradrenaline. Experientia, *31*:1173, 1975.
123. Feuerstein, G. et al.: Effect of indomethacin on the blood pressure and plasma catecholamine responses to acute endotoxaemia. J. Pharm. Pharmacol., *33*:576, 1981.
124. Montgomery, S. B., Jose, P. A., and Eisner, G. M.: The role of anesthesia and catecholamines in the renal response to mild hemorrhage. Circ. Shock, *9*:433, 1982.
125. Baum, D. et al.: Pentobarbital effects on plasma catecholamines: temperature, heart rate, and blood pressure. Am. J. Physiol., *248*:E95, 1985.
126. Goldstein, D. S. et al.: Circulatory, plasma catecholamine, cortisol, lipid and psychological responses to real-life stress (third molar extractions): effects of diazepam sedation and of inclusion of epinephrine with the local anesthetic. Psychosom. Med., *44*:259, 1982.
127. Chernow, B. et al.: Plasma, urine, and CSF catecholamine concentrations during and after ketamine anesthesia. Crit. Care Med., *10*:600, 1982.
128. Bazaral, M. G., Welch, M., Golding, L. A. R., and Badhwar, K.: Comparison of brachial and radial arterial pressure monitoring in patients undergoing coronary artery bypass surgery. Anesthesiology, *73*:38, 1990.
129. Astiz, M. et al.: Oxygen delivery and consumption in patients with hyperdynamic septic shock. Crit. Care Med., *15*:26, 1987.
130. Leavy, J. A., Weil, M. H., and Rackow, E. C.: Lactate washout following circulatory arrest. JAMA, *260*:662, 1988.
131. Weil, M. H., and Afifi, A. A.: Experimental and clinical studies on lactate and pyruvate as indicators of the severity of acute circulatory failure (shock). Circulation, *41*:989, 1970.
132. Craddock, P. R., Yawata, Y., and Van Santen, L.: Acquired phagocytic dysfunction: a complication of hypophosphatemia. N. Engl. J. Med., *290*:1403, 1974.
133. Martin, L. F., Max, M. H., and Polk, H. C.: Failure of gastric pH control by antacids or cimetidine in the critically ill: a valid sign of sepsis. Surgery, *88*:59, 1980.
134. Kram, H. B., Appel, P. L., Fleming, A. W., and Shoemaker, W. C.: Conjunctival and mixed-venous oximeters as early warning devices of cardiopulmonary compromise. Circ. Shock, *19*:211, 1986.
135. Ghignone, M., Girling, L., and Prewitt, R. M.: Volume expansion versus norepinephrine in treatment of a low cardiac output complicating an acute increase in right ventricular afterload in dogs. Anesthesiology, *60*:132, 1984.
136. Kimchi, A.: Right ventricular performance in septic shock: a combined radionuclide and hemodynamic study. J. Am. Coll. Cardiol., *4*:945, 1984.
137. Vincent, J.-L., Reuse, C., and Kahn, R. J.: Effects on right ventricular function of a change from dopamine to dobutamine in critically ill patients. Crit. Care Med., *16*:659, 1988.

138. Dhainaut, J.-F. et al.: Role of tricuspid regurgitation and left ventricular damage in the treatment of right ventricular infarction-induced low cardiac output syndrome. Am. J. Cardiol., 66:289, 1990.
139. Manoogian, C., Nadler, J., Ehrlich, L., and Horton, R.: The renal vasodilating effect of dopamine is mediated by calcium flux and prostacyclin release in man. J. Clin. Endocrinol. Metab., 66:678, 1988.
140. Schaer, G. L., Fink, M. P., and Parrillo, J. E.: Norepinephrine alone versus norepinephrine plus low-dose dopamine: enhanced renal blood flow with combination pressor therapy. Crit. Care Med., 13:492, 1985.
141. Davis, R. F. et al.: Acute oliguria after cardiopulmonary bypass: renal functional improvement with low-dose dopamine infusion. Crit. Care Med., 10:852, 1982.
142. Leier, C. V. et al.: Comparative systemic and regional hemodynamic effects of dopamine and dobutamine in patients with cardiomyopathic heart failure. Circulation, 58:466, 1978.
143. Fowler, M. B. et al.: Dobutamine and dopamine after cardiac surgery: greater augmentation of myocardial blood flow with dobutamine. Circulation, 70(Suppl. 1):1, 1984.
144. Ruffolo, R. R., Jr., and Yaden, E. L.: Vascular effects of the stereoisomers of dobutamine. J. Pharmacol. Exp. Ther., 224:46, 1983.
145. Ruffolo, R. R., Jr., Messick, K., and Horng, J. S.: Interactions of the enantiomers of 3-O-methyldobutamine with α- and β-adrenoceptors in vitro. Naunyn-Schmiedeberg's Arch. Pharmacol., 329:244, 1985.
146. Vincent, J.-L., Roman, A., and Kahn, R. J.: Dobutamine administration in septic shock: addition to a standard protocol. Crit. Care Med., 18:689, 1990.
147. Goldberg, L. I.: Dopamine and new dopamine analogs: receptors and clinical applications. J. Clin. Anesth., 1:66, 1988.
148. Vincent, J.-L., Reuse, C., and Kahn, R. J.: Administration of dopexamine, a new adrenergic agent, in cardiorespiratory failure. Chest, 96:1233, 1989.
149. Poelaert, J. I. T., Mungroop, H. E., Koolen, J. J., and Van den Berg, P. C. M.: Hemodynamic effects of dopexamine in patients following coronary artery bypass surgery. J. Cardiothorac. Anesth., 3:441, 1989.
150. Pearson, J. W., and Redding, J. S.: The role of epinephrine in cardiac resuscitation. Anesth. Analg., 42:599, 1963.
151. Koscove, E. M., and Paradis, N. A.: Successful resuscitation from cardiac arrest using high-dose epinephrine therapy. Report of two cases. JAMA, 259:3031, 1988.
152. Brown, C. G., Davis, E. A., Werman, H. A., and Hamlin, R. L.: Methoxamine versus epinephrine on regional cerebral blood flow during cardiopulmonary resuscitation. Crit. Care Med., 15:682, 1987.
153. Chernow, B. et al.: Epinephrine absorption after intratracheal administration. Anesth. Analg., 63:829, 1984.
154. Meadows, D., Edwards, J. D., Wilkins, R. G., and Nightingale, P.: Reversal of intractable septic shock with norepinephrine therapy. Crit. Care Med., 16:663, 1988.
155. Desjars, P. et al.: A reappraisal of norephinephrine therapy in human septic shock. Crit. Care Med., 15:134, 1987.
156. Schreuder, W. O., Schneider, A. J., Groeneveld, A. B. J., and Thijs, L. G.: Effect of dopamine vs. norepinephrine on hemodynamics in septic shock. Emphasis on right ventricular performance. Chest, 95:1282, 1989.
157. Desjars, P., Pinaud, M., Bugnon, D., and Tasseau, F.: Norepinephrine therapy has no deleterious renal effects in human septic shock. Crit. Care Med., 17:426, 1989.
158. Fukuoka, T. et al.: Effects of norepinephrine on renal function in septic patients with normal and elevated serum lactate levels. Crit. Care Med., 17:1104, 1989.
159. Breslow, M. J. et al.: Effect of vasopressors on organ blood flow during endotoxin shock in pigs. Am. J. Physiol., 252:H291, 1987.
160. Jett, G. K. et al.: Vasoactive drug effects on blood flow in internal mammary artery and saphenous vein grafts. J. Thorac. Cardiovasc. Surg., 94:2, 1987.
161. Camacho, S. A. et al.: Improvement in myocardial performance without a decrease in high-energy phosphate metabolites after isoproterenol in Syrian cardiomyopathic hamsters. Circulation, 77:712, 1988.
162. Makela, V. H. M., and Kapur, P. A.: Amrinone and verapamil-propranolol induced cardiac depression during isoflurane anesthesia in dogs. Anesthesiology, 66:792, 1987.
163. Goenen, M., Pedemonte, O., Baele, P., and Col, J.: Amrinone in the management of low cardiac output after open heart surgery. Am. J. Cardiol., 56:33B, 1985.
164. Olsen, K. H., Kluger, J., and Fieldman, A.: Combination high dose amrinone and dopamine in the management of moribund cardiogenic shock after open heart surgery. Chest, 94:503, 1988.
165. Physicians Desk Reference. 44th Ed. Oradell, NJ, Medical Economics, 1990, p. 2315.
166. Benotti, J. R., McCue, J. E., and Alpert, J. S.: Comparative vasoactive therapy for heart failure. Am. J. Cardiol., 56:19B, 1985.
167. Sundram, P. et al.: Myocardial energetics and efficiency in patients with idiopathic cardiomyopathy: response to dobutamine and amrinone. Am. Heart J., 119:891, 1990.
167a. Grose, R., Strain, J., Greenberg, M., and LeJemtel, T. H.: Systemic and coronary effects of intravenous milrinone and dobutamine in congestive heart failure. J. Am. Coll. Cardiol., 7:1107, 1986.
167b. Copp, M. V., Hill, A. J., and Feneck, R. O.: Overview of the effects of intravenous milrinone in acute heart failure following surgery. Eur. J. Anaesth., 5(Suppl.):35, 1992.
167c. Feneck, R. O., and the European Milrinone Multicentre Trial Group: Intravenous milrinone following cardiac surgery: effects of bolus infusion followed by variable dose maintenance infusion. J. Cardiothorac. Vasc. Anesth., 6:554, 1992.
168. Boldt, J., Kling, D., Moosdorf, R., and Hempelmann, G.: Enoximone treatment of impaired myocardial function during cardiac surgery: combined effects with epinephrine. J. Cardiothorac. Anesth., 4:462, 1990.
169. Drop, L. J.: Ionized calcium, the heart, and hemodynamic function. Anesth. Analg., 64:432, 1985.
170. Chernow, B. (ed.): Calcium: Does it have a therapeutic role in sepsis? Crit. Care. Med., 18:895, 1990.
171. Fernandez-Del Castillo, C. et al.: Risk factors for pancreatic cellular injury after cardiopulmonary bypass. N. Engl. J. Med., 325:382, 1991.
172. Adler, M. W.: Minireview. Opioid peptides. Life Sci., 26:497, 1980.
173. Holaday, J. W., and Faden, A. I.: Naloxone reversal of endotoxin hypotension suggests role of endorphins in shock. Nature, 275:450, 1978.
174. Gahhos, F. N.: Endorphins in septic shock. Ann. Surg., 117:1053, 1982.
175. Vargish, T. et al.: Naloxone reversal of hypovolemic shock in dogs. Circ. Shock, 7:31, 1980.
176. Higgins, T. L., and Sivak, E. D.: Reversal of hypotension with naloxone. Cleve. Clin. Q., 48:283, 1981.
177. Peters, W. P., Johnson, M. W., Friedman, P. A., and Mitch, W. E.: Pressor effect of naloxone in septic shock. Lancet, 1:529, 1981.

178. Higgins, T. L., and Sivak, E. D.: Reversal of hypotension by continuous naloxone infusion in ventilator-dependent patients. Ann. Intern. Med., 98:47, 1983.
179. Rock, P. et al.: Efficacy and safety of naloxone in septic shock. Crit. Care Med., 13:28, 1985.
180. DeMaria, A. et al.: Naloxone versus placebo in treatment of septic shock. Lancet, 1:1363, 1985.
181. Safani, M. et al.: Prospective, controlled, randomized trial of naloxone infusion in early hyperdynamic septic shock. Crit. Care Med., 17:1004, 1989.
182. Zaloga, G. P. et al.: Diagnostic dosages of protirelin (TRH) elevate BP by noncatecholamine mechanisms. Arch. Intern. Med., 144:1149, 1984.
183. Chernow, B. et al.: Glucagon: endocrine effects and calcium involvement in cardiovascular actions in dogs. Circ. Shock, 19:393, 1986.
184. Zaloga, G. P., Delacey, W., Holmboe, E., and Chernow, B.: Glucagon reversal of hypotension in a case of anaphylactoid shock. Ann. Intern. Med., 105:65, 1986.
185. Niemann, J. T. et al.: Postcountershock pulseless rhythms: hemodynamic effects of glucagon in a canine model. Crit. Care Med., 15:554, 1987.
186. Wilcken, D. E. L., and Lvoff, R.: Glucagon in resistant heart-failure and cardiogenic shock. Lancet, 1:1315, 1970.
187. Lvoff, R., and Wilcken, D. E. L.: Glucagon in heart failure and in cardiogenic shock. Experience in 50 patients. Circulation, 45:534, 1972.
188. Zaritsky, A. L., Horowitz, M., and Chernow, B.: Glucagon antagonism of calcium channel blocker-induced myocardial dysfunction. Crit. Care Med., 16:246, 1988.
189. Lewis, R. P.: Digitalis: a drug that refuses to die. Crit. Care Med., 18:S5, 1990.
190. Nasraway, S. A. et al.: Inotropic response to digoxin and dopamine in patients with severe sepsis, cardiac failure, and systemic hypoperfusion. Chest, 95:612, 1989.
191. Guthrie, G. P. Jr.: Effects of digoxin on responsiveness to the pressor actions of angiotensin and norepinephrine in man. J. Clin. Endocrinol. Metab., 58:76, 1984.
192. Leblanc, N., and Hume, J. R.: Sodium current-induced release of calcium from cardiac sarcoplasmic reticulum. Science, 248:372, 1990.
193. Balk, R. A. et al.: Low dose ibuprofen reverses the hemodynamic alterations of canine endotoxin shock. Crit. Care Med., 16:1128, 1988.
194. Bone, R. C., Jacobs, E. R., and Wilson F. J. Jr.: Increased hemodynamic and survival with endotoxin and septic shock with ibuprofen treatment. In First Vienna Shock Forum. Part A: Pathophysiological Role of Mediators and Mediator Inhibitors in Shock. New York, Alan R. Liss, 1987, p. 327.
195. Feuerstein, G., Dimicco, J. A., Ramu, A., and Kopin, I. J.: Effect of indomethacin on the blood pressure and plasma catecholamine responses to acute endotoxaemia. J. Pharm. Pharmacol., 33:576, 1981.
196. Levitt, M. A., and Lefer, A. M.: Beneficial effects of prostaglandin E₁ infusion in experimental traumatic shock. Crit. Care Med., 15:769, 1987.
197. D'Ambra, M. N. et al.: Prostaglandin E₁. A new therapy for refractory right heart failure and pulmonary hypertension after mitral valve replacement. J. Thorac. Cardiovasc. Surg., 89:567, 1985.
198. Schumer, W.: Steroids in the treatment of clinical septic shock. Ann. Surg., 184:333, 1976.
199. Sprung, C. L. et al.: The effects of high-dose corticosteroids in patients with septic shock. A prospective, controlled study. N. Engl. J. Med., 311:1137, 1984.
200. Bone, R. C. et al.: A controlled clinical trial of high-dose methylprednisolone in the treatment of severe sepsis and septic shock. N. Engl. J. Med., 317:653, 1987.
201. Hinshaw, L. et al.: Effect of high-dose glucocorticoid therapy on mortality in patients with clinical signs of systemic sepsis. N. Engl. J. Med., 317:659, 1987.
202. Brackett, D. J., Schaefer, C. F., and Wilson, M. F.: The role of vasopressin in the maintenance of cardiovascular function during early endotoxin shock. Adv. Shock Res., 9:147, 1983.
203. Markov, A. K.: Hemodynamics and metabolic effects of fructose 1-6 diphosphate in ischemia and shock—experimental and clinical observations. Ann. Emerg. Med., 15:1470, 1986.
204. Fletcher, J. R., and Ramwell, P. W.: Lidocaine treatment following baboon endotoxin shock improves survival. Adv. Shock Res., 2:219, 1979.
205. Bende, S., and Bertok, L.: Elimination of endotoxin from the blood by extracorporeal activated charcoal hemoperfusion in experimental canine endotoxin shock. Circ. Shock, 19:239, 1986.
206. Waxman, K.: Pentoxifylline in septic shock. Crit. Care Med., 18:243, 1990.
207. Tighe, D. et al.: Pretreatment with pentoxifylline improves the hemodynamic and histologic changes and decreases neutrophil adhesiveness in a pig fecal peritonitis model. Crit. Care Med., 18:184, 1990.
208. Whitlow, P. L. et al.: Enhancement of left ventricular function by glucose-insulin-potassium infusion in acute myocardial infarction. Am. J. Cardiol., 49:811, 1982.
209. Bronsveld, W., Van Den Bos, G. C., and Thijs, L. G.: Use of glucose-insulin-potassium (GIK) in human septic shock. Crit. Care Med., 13:566, 1985.
210. Gradinac, S. et al.: Improved cardiac function with glucose-insulin-potassium after aortocoronary bypass grafting. Ann. Thorac. Surg., 48:484, 1989.
211. Fisher, C. J. et al.: Influence of an anti-tumor necrosis factor monoclonal antibody on cytokine levels in patients with sepsis. Crit. Care Med., 21:318, 1993.
212. Fisher, C. J. et al.: Initial evaluation of human recombinant interleukin-1 receptor antagonist in the treatment of sepsis syndrome: a randomized, open-label, placebo-controlled multicenter trial. Crit. Care Med., 22:12, 1994.
213. Fink, M. P. et al.: A novel leukotriene B₄-receptor antagonist in endotoxin shock: a prospective, controlled trial in a porcine model. Crit. Care Med., 21:1825, 1993.

SUPPLEMENTAL READINGS

Brown, C. G., et al.: A comparison of standard-dose and high-dose epinephrine in cardiac arrest outside the hospital. N. Engl. J. Med., 327:1051, 1992.

Burstein, S., et al.: Positive inotropic and lusitropic effects of intravenous flosequinan in patients with heart failure. J. Am. Coll. Cardiol., 20:822, 1992.

Butterworth, J. F. et al.: Calcium inhibits the cardiac stimulating properties of dobutamine but not of amrinone. Chest, 101:174, 1992.

Callaham, M., et al.: A randomized clinical trial of high-dose epinephrine and norepinephrine vs. standard-dose epinephrine in prehospital cardiac arrest. JAMA, 268:2667, 1992.

Devins, S. S., et al.: Effects of dopamine on T-lymphocyte proliferative responses and serum prolactin concentrations in critically ill patients. Crit. Care Med., 20:1644, 1992.

Giroir, B. P.: Mediators of septic shock: new approaches for interrupting the endogenous inflammatory cascade. Crit. Care Med., 21:780, 1993.

Levy, J. H., and Bailey, J. M.: Amrinone: its effects on vascular resistance and capacitance in human subjects. Chest, *105*: 62, 1994.

Lucas, C. E.: A new look at dopamine and norepinephrine for hyperdynamic septic shock. Chest, *105*:7, 1994.

Royster, R. L., et al.: Combined inotropic effects of amrinone and epinephrine after cardiopulmonary bypass in humans. Anesth. Analg., *77*:662, 1993.

Safar, P.: Cerebral resuscitation after cardiac arrest: research initiatives and future directions. Ann. Emerg. Med., *22*:324, 1993.

Silverman, H. J., Penaranda, R., Orens, J. B., and Lee, N. H.: Impaired β-adrenergic receptor stimulation of cyclic adenosine monophosphate in human septic shock: association with myocardial hypo responsiveness to catecholamines. Crit. Care Med., *21*:31, 1993.

Smiley, R. M., Pantuck, C. B., Chadburn, A., and Knowles, D. M.: Down-regulation and desensitization of the β-adrenergic receptor system of human lymphocytes after cardiac surgery. Anesth. Analg., *77*:653, 1993.

Stiell, I. G., et al.: High-dose epinephrine in adult cardiac arrest. N. Engl. J. Med., *327*:1045, 1992.

Wortsman, J. O., et al.: Functional responses to extremely high plasma epinephrine concentrations in cardiac arrest. Crit. Care Med., *21*:692, 1993.

Wright, E. M., and Sherry, K. M.: Clinical and haemodynamic effects of milrinone in the treatment of low cardiac output after cardiac surgery. Br. J. Anaesth., *67*:585, 1991.

Chapter 66

ANTIBIOTIC PHARMACOKINETICS

MARCUS T. HAUG, III
PETER H. SLUGG

PHARMACOKINETIC MODELS

Antibiotic dosage requirements and dosage alterations, in the treatment of the critically ill, require a basic understanding of the pharmacokinetic principles that describe drug disposition. Antibiotic disposition can usually be described by one- and two-compartment linear, open models. In the one-compartment model, the antibiotic is introduced into the central volume of distribution (Vd) (Fig. 66-1), and the concentration is considered to be the same throughout the body. An analogy can be made by representing this as "the bathtub concept," where a drug added to a bathtub partially full of water is then instantaneously mixed and gives a certain concentration (Fig. 66-2). Disease states and other patient factors may alter the Vd. For example, the "normal" Vd of aminoglycosides (AGSs) is approximately 0.20 to 0.25 L/kg (AGSs distribute primarily to extracellular fluid). A severely dehydrated patient may have an AGS Vd of less than 0.1 L/kg. On the other hand, a severely septic surgical patient who has received fluid resuscitation may readily have a Vd of 0.3 to 0.6 L/kg based on actual body weight. The Vd is a mathematic relationship between dosage and concentration achieved:

$$Vd = \frac{\text{amount of drug in the body}}{\text{concentration of drug in body}} = \frac{\text{dose}}{\text{Cp0}} \quad (1)$$

Volume of distribution does not usually correspond to a certain portion of the anatomy (the drug does not, e.g., specifically reside in an arm, a leg, or the body trunk). Antibiotics with large volumes of distribution on a liter or L/kg basis (greater than 1.4 L/kg) are said to have "deep" tissue peripheral concentrations of drug. Usually, one does not know the patient's individual tissue antibiotic concentrations, and one uses the mathematic relationship between plasma concentration and dose. On the other hand, an antibiotic with a small Vd indicates certain characteristics of the drug. In a 70-kg individual, an antibiotic Vd of 0.04 L/kg, 0.07 L/kg, 0.14 to 0.28 L/kg, 0.36 to 0.43 L/kg, 0.57 L/kg may mean the drug is confined to plasma volume only (possibly very highly protein bound); blood volume only (possibly highly protein bound or distributes highly into white or red blood cells); extracellular fluid; intracellular fluid; and total body water, respectively.[1-4] These are still only generalizations about antibiotic Vd. Again, the same antibiotic under widely different patient conditions may have a remarkably different Vd.

Elimination of the antibiotic from the body may occur with a monoexponential decline of concentration in the characteristic first-order elimination pattern, as shown in Figure 66-3. Analogously, one should think about drug elimination from "the bathtub"—a little different from draining a real bathtub. The water (the Vd) is never really emptied out of the tub. Instead, the drain (the organ for antibiotic elimination) acts as a sieve such that only the antibiotic molecules are filtered out, and these go "down the drain" (elimination). This concept also helps define the pharmacokinetic term clearance. **Clearance** is the hypothetic volume of plasma that is cleared of antibiotic per unit time (clearance measurements take on the units of volume per time such as milliliters per minute, liters per hour, etc.). It is somewhat similar to having the water of "the bathtub" rotate by the drain (organ of elimination) where antibiotic molecules are extracted for elimination. Again, the water is not necessarily eliminated, only the antibiotic molecules. The elimination rate of a linear first-order system is measured in inverse time (hour − 1, minute − 1, etc.). Elimination in a first-order linear elimination system is not measured as an amount per unit time loss (e.g., milligrams per minute or per hour that can occur for drugs undergoing zero-order elimination, e.g., with ethanol) but rather as a percentage of the total drug eliminated per time. If we look at Figure 66-3, the elimination rate (kel) can be described by Equation 2, and the mathematic relationship of clearance (Cl) is given in Equation 3.

$$kel = \text{slope of the time concentration line} = \frac{\ln Cp2 - \ln Cp1}{t2 - t1} \quad (2)$$

$$Cl = (kel) \times (Vd) \quad (3)$$

Elimination of antibiotics can also be described by half-life (t1/2). In a linear first-order one-compartment system, the half-life is the time necessary for the concentration to drop in half and the amount of drug in the body to be reduced 50%. Half-life is measured in units of time such as minutes, hours, and days and is represented mathematically in Equation 4.

$$t1/2 = \frac{0.693}{kel} \quad (4)$$

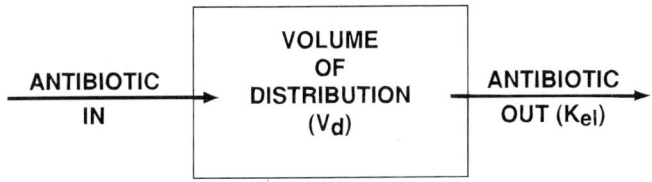

Fig. 66-1. The open, one-compartment pharmacokinetic model.

For many antibiotics, use of a one-compartment model has had to suffice for pharmacokinetic dosing considerations. Aminoglycosides and vancomycin have commonly been dosed with the one-compartment model in the past. Replacement of simplified pharmacokinetic models by more complex models that better describe an antibiotic's disposition is readily achievable with various computer programs that have been developed.[5,6] In addition, portable computers make it possible to bring the use of these pharmacokinetic control programs to the patient's bedside.

The two-compartment, open linear model (Fig. 66-4) may better explain the mathematic disposition of antibiotics. The simplistic one-compartment model may initially suffice for guiding therapy but may lose its ability to identify appropriate pharmacokinetic parameters needed to predict antibiotic concentrations. Additionally, the antibiotic's inherent pharmacokinetic characteristics and/or blood level collection strategy may require pharmacokinetic analysis and dose calculation with a two-compartment model.[7]

The characteristics of a natural log concentration versus a time plot of an open, two-compartment antibiotic are represented in Figure 66-5. A distinct antibiotic distribution phase and elimination phase occur. The elimination phase is analogous to the elimination phase of the one-compartment model. Sampling during the distribution phase may result in greater than expected concentrations and place error in the one-compartment model pharmacokinetic calculations resulting in inappropriate dose regi-

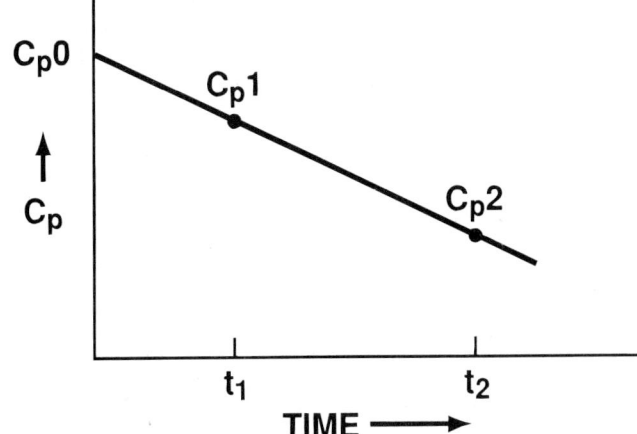

Fig. 66-3. Characteristic first-order concentration versus time plot of a linear, open, one-compartment antibiotic model. Cp, is the natural log of the antibiotic concentration (ln Cp); t, unit of time.

mens. Alternatively, use of a two-compartment model may alleviate the need to wait until the distribution phase is finished before sampling of the peak level. Some error may be interjected with the drawing of a peak level during the elimination phase, but if the population pharmacokinetic model adequately represents your patient, calculating a dosage for the patient should be no problem. The utility of the two-compartment model is its ability to use blood levels drawn at various times after a dose without having to rigidly control sample timing in the clinical setting. Our goal is to control the antibiotic therapy, not the people who deliver patient care. This is not to say that appropriate antibiotic drawing times should not be optimized to obtain the most accurate pharmacokinetic information. Other patient care needs must be met, and the antibiotic drawing time may be delayed or moved to a time immediately after the infusion. As long as the times of antibiotic administration and antibiotic level sampling are noted, analysis using a Bayesian two-compartment fitting model will help in de-

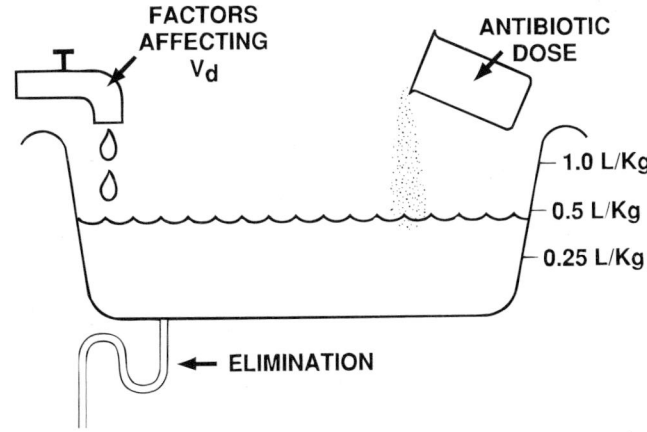

Fig. 66-2. Volume of distribution (Vd), "the bathtub concept."

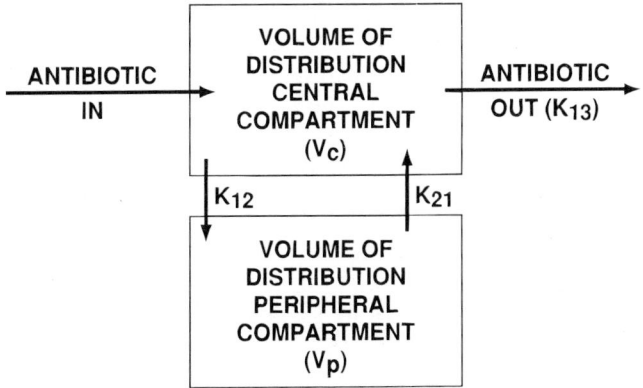

Fig. 66-4. The open, two-compartment model of antibiotic disposition.

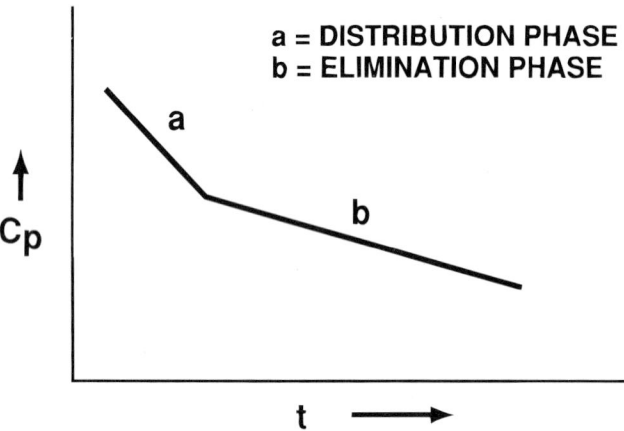

Fig. 66-5. Characteristic first-order concentration versus time plot of a linear, open two-compartment antibiotic model. Cp, is the natural log of the antibiotic concentration (ln Cp); t is the unit of time.

Table 66-1. Modes of Bacterial Antibiotic Action and Representative Antibiotics

Inhibition of Cell Wall Formation	
Bacitracin	D-cycloserine
Carbepenems	Cephalosporins
Vancomycin	Novobiocin
Penicillins	
Inhibition of Protein Biosynthesis	
Bacitracin	Oleandomycin
Gentamicin	Tobramycin
Neomycin	Tetracylines
Streptomycin	Erythromycin
Amikacin	Clindamycin
Flucytosine	Paromomycin
Chloramphenicol	Netilmicin
Kanamycin	Viomycin
Disruption of Deoxyribonucleic Acid Metabolism	
Norfloxacin	Griseofulvin
Actinomycin D	Enoxacin
Ciprofloxacin	Novobiocin
Disruption of Ribonucleic Acid Metabolism	
Griseofulvin	Rifampin
Streptomycin	Neomycin
Netilmicin	Gentamicin
Kanamycin	Amikacin
Tobramycin	
Alteration in Cellular Membrane Function	
Amphotericin B	Ketoconazole
Nystatin	Novobiocin
Miconazole	Vancomycin
Bacitracin	Fluconazole
Polymyxin	

termining dosage needs. Clinicians who deal with pharmacokinetic adjustment of antibiotic doses realize that they are dealing with all types of possible errors in the clinical setting in calculation of antibiotic pharmacokinetics and dosage. The science of population Bayesian pharmacokinetics hclps deal with these errors. Clinicians need not be paralyzed or frightened into making no decision on dosage because of clinical setting errors. Additional patient expense can be avoided by being able to use almost any antibiotic blood level(s) in pharmacokinetic calculations by use of the Bayesian pharmacokinetic techniques.

Mode of Action of Antibiotics

Antimicrobial therapy of severe infections generally revolves around the use of antibiotics that demonstrate the five general modes of action listed in Table 66-1.[8] Furthermore, various structure activity relationships are involved in ensuring that an antibiotic is more active against certain organisms (e.g., Pseudomonas aeruginosa, Staphylococcus aureus, and others).

Penicillins and cephalosporins attach to binding proteins that inhibit cell wall mucopeptide synthesis and cause cell wall rupture. These binding proteins are called cephalosporin-binding proteins and penicillin-binding proteins. There are eight cephalosporin-binding proteins (penicillin-binding proteins [PBPs]). Usually, binding proteins 1 and 3 are most involved in cell wall destruction. All cephalosporins (first-, second-, and third-generation cephalosporins), penicillins, extended spectrum penicillins, and antistaphylococcal penicillins are bactericidal through binding protein inhibition of mucopeptide synthesis. The monobactam aztreonam (a beta-lactam antibiotic) also binds with PBPs 1 and 3, much like the cephalosporins and penicillins. Vancomycin is bactericidal by blockage of cell wall glycopeptide polymerization. This causes inhibition of cell wall synthesis and cytoplasmic membrane damage. Carbapenems, of which only imipenem is available, binds to PBP 1 and 2, causing cell wall destruction and rupture through inhibition of mucopeptide synthesis.

The macrolide antibiotics erythromycin and troleandomycin along with the nonrelated antibiotics clindamycin and lincomycin both bind to the 50s ribosome and inhibit peptide bond formation, thus preventing protein synthesis. Metronidazole is bactericidal, amebicidal, and trichomonacidal from its reduction by low-redox-potential electron transport proteins to unidentified polar products. These products appear to be responsible for the cytotoxic and antimicrobial effects. The beta-lactamase inhibitors clavulanic acid, sulbactam and tazobactam inhibit beta-lactamase destruction of the antibiotics ticarcillin, amoxicillin, ampicillin, and piperacillin. Aminoglycosides are active against aerobic gram-negative organisms, S. aureus and Staphylococcal epidermidis and enterococcus. These drugs bind irreversibly to the 30s ribosome, causing faulty protein synthesis resulting in cell death. Quinolones (ciprofloxacin, enoxacin, ofloxacin, norfloxacin, etc.) are bactericidal and bind to DNA-gyrase with disruption of DNA metabolism. The antifungal amphotericin B binds to sterols in cell walls, causing the membrane not to function as a selective barrier, causing loss of potassium and other cellular components. Ketoconazole, fluconazole, and miconazole alter membrane permeability, resulting in increased leakage of cell contents. They inhibit cytochrome P-450 14-alpha-desmethylase in fungi and usually are fungistatic in action.

CLINICAL INTERDEPENDENCY OF PHARMACOKINETICS AND DISEASE STATES

Pre-ICU Considerations

Factors operative in the pre-ICU phase of hospitalization may determine the dose needs of patients in a number of different ways. If the patient has been chronically ill or has a severely catabolic infection, dehydration may exist. **Dehydration** affects both kidney function and Vd of some antibiotics. Therefore, dose intervals may need to be lengthened and dose size reduced initially for renally excreted antibiotics (especially for those antibiotics with a narrow margin of safety). This is a dynamic process and after rehydration kidney function may improve dramatically even if the patient is receiving "nephrotoxic" antibiotics. Increases in dosage and shortening of the dose interval now may be required. Of course, this is most important for the antibiotics that are renally excreted and require antibiotic level measurement, such as the AGSs and vancomycin. Penicillins and cephalosporins may require dosage alterations with increases or decreases in kidney function. Most other non-AGS or non-vancomycin antibiotics have a wide range of safety; dose alterations, however, may be required, because excess antibiotic has no greater antibacterial efficacy and accumulation may cause unwanted side effects.

Many times infections affect the elderly who already have a reduced renal or cardiac function that compromises renal blood flow. Any improvement of their medical problems could help facilitate kidney and liver elimination of the antibiotics prescribed. Additionally, severe catabolism may leave the patient with a low albumin level. Theoretically, those highly protein-bound antibiotics should then have increased free antibiotic levels. This will either increase Vd and/or increase antibiotic elimination, but clinical consequences of these changes are hard to quantify.

An infection may occur in a patient who has been in the hospital for some time. Most likely, the patient's fluid balance has already been stabilized and maximized by the clinician. These are the patients who should have their antibiotic doses maximized when treated for an infection to effect cure and prevent an ICU admission that is due to inadequate treatment of an infection. Appropriate antibiotic therapy is associated with reduced mortality in nosocomial-acquired bacteremias as well as a twofold reduction in shock, as suggested by Kreger and associates.[9]

Kidney function and Vd changes have the greatest effect on antibiotic dosage size and dose intervals for pre-ICU, ICU, and post-ICU antibiotic care. Patients who are elderly, pregnant (or postpartum), have renal and/or liver disease, have burns or cystic fibrosis, or are receiving drugs that reduce kidney and/or liver function will experience alterations in clearance of antibiotics (Table 66-2).

ICU Considerations

The risk factors for alterations in antibiotic pharmacokinetics are greatest in patients in the ICU. With all the manipulations and acute patient changes, a plethora of direct or indirect pharmacokinetic alterations occurs. Again, antibiotic elimination and volume of distribution changes are the factors most involved, but protein binding changes may occur also, and this may directly or indirectly affect the first two factors (see Table 66-2).

Once an infectious diagnosis is entertained, appropriate treatment should be given. The optimal dose of an antibiotic(s) is one of the few things that can be manipulated to ensure that the optimal effect is obtained (assuming the right antibiotic or right combination of antibiotics has been prescribed). For the patient with gram-negative infection and good renal function (as reflected by increased cardiac output, normal serum creatinine, increased urine output, and/or increased measured creatinine clearance), antibiotic doses should be pushed to the maximum. This could be accomplished with AGSs by using initial starting guidelines for therapy for the type of patient being treated. Initial doses may vary between surgical (SICU), neurologic (NICU), medical (MICU), and cardiothoracic (CTICU) intensive care units. Levels of these drugs can be measured, and doses can be adjusted to prevent toxicity yet give the patient the optimum treatment. Dosage of other antibiotics can be adjusted, based on package insert or other reference guidelines. Again, we should not rely on a "standard" dosage for this type of patient but need to push doses to the upper end of the dosage spectrum that these guidelines suggest. This involves using guidelines for severely ill patients (not moderately ill). These guidelines are also somewhat specific for handling reduced renal function dosing. Table 66-2 lists the various physiologic or pathophysiologic states that may result in altered elimination and/or Vd. These processes generally require the need for antibiotic dose and dose-interval alterations.[10-22]

The ICU patient may be receiving concomitant drug therapy that is directly nephrotoxic (AGSs, vancomycin, amphotericin B, contrast, etc.) or drugs that themselves affect kidney function (levophed, dopamine, angiotensin-converting enzyme inhibitors, diuretics, metoclopramide, etc.). The pharmacologic effects of these and various disease states can alter antibiotic pharmacokinetics and must be taken into account when making dose adjustments. Drug-induced interstitial nephritis (e.g., caused by penicillins, cephalosporins, etc.) must be watched for also, because this renal dysfunction can alter dose needs but more

Table 66-2. Pathophysiologic States Associated With Altered Disposition of Antibiotics

Increased Elimination	Increased Volume of Distribution
Warm sepsis	Sepsis/infection
Cystic fibrosis	Fever
Pregnancy/postpartum	Pregnancy/postpartum
Burns	Burns
Neurotrauma	Hematologic disorders
Young adult	Stress
Spinal cord injury	Spinal cord injury
Dialysis	Septic shock
Multiple organ dysfunction	Ascites
Decreased Elimination	**Decreased Volume of Distribution**
Severe preeclampsia	Dehydration
High dose pressors	Major amputations
Renal failure	Improvement in infection
Elderly patient	Diuretic use
Multiple organ dysfunction	Mannitol use
Severe shock	Uncontrolled diabetes insipidus
Septic	Diuresis from glycosuria
Cardiogenic	
Concomitant nephrotoxins	
Liver disease	
Dialysis stopped	
Ascites	

Table 66-3. Drugs That May Cause Nephrotoxicity and Decrease Elimination of Renally Eliminated Antibiotics

Direct Nephrotoxins
  Aminoglycosides
  Amphotericin B
  Mannitol
  Vancomycin
  Radiocontrast agents
  Certain cephalosporins
  Dextran
  Foscarnet
  Cisplatin
  Cyclosporine A
  Methoxyflurane
  Pentamidine

Immunologic Nephrotoxins
  Penicillins
  Fluoroquinolones
  Penicillamine
  Cephalosporins
  Analgesics
  Allopurinol
  NSAIDs
  Gold salts

Indirect Nephrotoxins
  NSAIDs
  Diuretics
  Metoclopramide
  ACE inhibitors
  Pressors

Obstructive Nephrotoxins
  Methotrexate
  Sulfonamides

Pseudonephrotoxicity (Creatinine Secretion/test Interference)
  Flucytosine
  Androgens
  Levodopa
  Trimethoprim
  Cimetidine
  Ascorbic acid
  Methyldopa
  Co-trimoxazole
  Cefoxitin
  Cephalothin
  Penicillin

NSAIDs, Nonsteroidal anti-inflammatory agents; ACE inhibitors, angiotensin-converting enzyme inhibitors.

importantly may be interpreted inappropriately as AGSs or vancomycin toxicity. See Table 66-3 for a list of drugs that may cause decreased kidney function.[23-43]

Infection itself can cause renal dysfunction in patients and has been reported with all types of infection including viral, fungal, gram-negative, and gram-positive infections. This is very important to note because uncontrolled infection is usually accompanied by an increase in serum creatinine requiring dosage alterations. Dose alterations for the AGSs and vancomycin is especially important because these medications can accumulate and cause toxicity themselves. At the same time, we must not blame these agents for the initial rise in serum creatinine if uncontrolled infection is present.[44-53]

Post-ICU Considerations

Post-ICU care of the infected patient can be just as important as pre-ICU or ICU care. Renal function may improve, requiring assessment of dosage when the patient leaves the ICU. This is the critical phase because the patient may be well enough for admission to a regular nursing floor but still require antibiotic therapy. To prevent a relapse, certain factors must be taken into account to ensure a complete course of adequate drug therapy. Again, renal function improvement may require dose increases and/or dose-interval decreases. The patient who is discharged from the ICU may not have as much attention placed on fluid status and could become dehydrated, thus requiring dose reductions. Worse yet, this dehydration can cause renal dysfunction through a prerenal mechanism causing decreased elimination of renally eliminated drugs.

An additional area of post-ICU care of the infected patient involves the use of AGSs. When the patient is well enough to leave the ICU, he may still require combination therapy that was initiated in the ICU. We have seen a number of SICU cases where the patient infection relapsed on the regular nursing floor when the AGS was discontinued (this is referred to as the "tapering" of antibiotic therapy). These patients were participating in their own care and rehabilitation when they left the ICU, and later they succumbed to recurrent infection. Our initial experience in the SICU indicated that, the longer the course of high dose AGSs (in combination with other appropriate antibiotics), the greater the percentage of patients who survived both SICU and were discharged from the hospital.[54]

One additional area of post-ICU care involves the antibiotic treatment of "recyclers"—for example, ventilator-dependent and/or pulmonary disease patients who are considered "colonized" and are treated for 7 to 10 days only to relapse again and again. Their clinical condition improves while on antibiotics only to have a relapse 7 to 14 days later after antibiotics are discontinued. These patients are just starting to make strides in weaning, physical therapy, nutrition, and assisting in daily decisions about their care. When antibiotics are discontinued, they revert to a hospital care-dependent state and all strides are lost. Some of these patients are "colonized" with P. aeruginosa and have received AGSs. In the clinician's zeal to remove nephrotoxic antibiotics, we find antibiotic therapy has been shortened once the patient "looks" cured. Aminoglycoside and/or vancomycin pharmacokinetic monitoring, along with recognition of all the factors that affect renal function, should be able to guide a patient through an extended course of therapy without AGS or vancomycin toxicity. In this manner, a 3- to 6-week course of antibiotic therapy may allow the patient to rehabilitate himself enough to be discharged home or to an extended care facility thus limiting excessive resource use.

AMINOGLYCOSIDE PHARMACOKINETICS

Aminoglycoside antibiotics still play a major role in the treatment of serious and life-threatening infections in the hospital. Although one might expect that newer antibiotics would replace the AGSs, this has not occurred for a number of reasons,[55-57] including:

- Aminoglycosides have remained active against a wide variety of gram-negative organisms in spite of heavy use over the last 10 years.
- Aminoglycosides have proved effective for serious gram-negative infections.
- Aminoglycosides are consistently bactericidal, even in the presence of a large inocula of bacteria.
- Aminoglycosides are synergistic when combined with a beta-lactam.
- Aminoglycosides have a long postantibiotic effect (PAE).
- Aminoglycosides acquisition cost is much less than the newest penicillins or cephalosporins.
- The higher the AGS peak concentration to the minimum (MIC), the higher the rate of bacterial killing (which does not occur with other beta lactams).

Disadvantages of AGSs include their "perceived" extreme nephro- and ototoxicity. "Perceived" toxicity is used because clinicians have been so conditioned that these agents cause toxicity, that they shy away from these effective antibiotics for less effective regimens in the seriously infected patient. Additionally, any negative change in renal function is termed AGS toxicity but in fact may be related to the infection itself, or other clinical factors, and not the use of the AGS. Additionally, the measurement of AGS levels is looked on as an unpleasant task. This, plus the interpretation of the results has been enough to discourage clinicians from using these vitally needed antibiotics. Measurement of AGS blood levels is mostly undertaken to determine if potentially toxic levels are present. Many do not worry about achieving adequate peak concentrations that are needed for optimizing clinical cure of the infection. If doses and levels are pharmacokinetically adjusted, little nephrotoxicity directly attributed to AGSs is obtainable.[58-60]

The mechanism of action of the AGSs makes them very powerful antibiotics when compared to the beta lactams (Table 66-4). AGSs irreversibly bind to the RNA 30S ribosome, creating genetic flaws that are universally and irrevocably fatal for that organism. There is no way for that organism to survive once the AGS binds to the 30S ribosome. Beta lactams on the other hand, bind reversibly to PBPs. PBPs cause alterations of the bacterial wall glycoprotein matrix, resulting in cell wall opening and destruction. Unfortunately, these cell wall alterations can be reversed when antibiotic concentrations fall below the minimum inhibitory concentration (MIC) of the organism. Bacterial cell wall repair can occur, and the log growth phase can begin again. Therefore, the AGSs have a long postantibiotic effect and a high log kill rate because of their irrevocable killing effect, whereas most beta lactams have a short postantibiotic effect and low log kill profile. Additionally, AGSs can inhibit exotoxin A production (the necrotizing substance released during severe P. aeruginosa infections) and can inhibit endotoxin release at below MIC concentrations.[61-64]

Table 66-4. Comparison of Aminoglycoside to Penicillin/Cephalosporin Mechanism of Action

Aminoglycosides	Penicillins or Cephalosporins
Binds to 30S ribosome	Binds to penicillin binding proteins (PBPs)
Irreversible binding to 30S ribosome causes fatal flaws in RNA/DNA machinery; if drug reaches 30S ribosome, there is no chance of survival	Cell wall destruction by opening cell wall through alteration in glycoprotein matrix
Inhibits endotoxin release at below MIC concentrations	Unfortunately, the binding to PBPs is reversible, and cell wall repair can occur
Inhibits exotoxin A production (Pseudomonas aeruginosa)	When antibiotic concentrations approach the MIC log, growth phase can begin again
Long postantibiotic effect, high log kill	Short, postantibiotic effect, low log kill

MIC, Minimum inhibitory concentration; PBPs, penicillin binding proteins.

In 1971, reports and studies began to appear in the literature concerning the efficacy (as measured by mortality, infectious cure, "favorable clinical response," negative cultures, and others) of AGSs being related to various pharmacokinetic indices and appropriate AGS levels. The common thread that runs through these reports is that attainment of adequate peak AGS levels was associated with enhanced survival of the infectious episode. Additional measures included higher doses than the control group, high peak AGS level/MIC ratios of minimally 4:1 to 8:1 (preferably, 16:1 in neutropenic patients); more intensive therapy programs based on achieving levels above the MIC during a greater percentage of the dosage interval; and a higher total dose of AGS.[65-80]

Appropriate AGS therapy dictates that peak levels must overcome certain "barriers" that must be bypassed to get the "drug" to the "bug." Such barriers include the following:

- Various tissues of the body may receive limited AGS penetration depending on the tissue (e.g., bronchial secretions, bile, spinal fluid, bone, etc.).[81-86]
- Low pH of infected sites: AGSs are less active in areas of low pH.[87]
- Purulent material present at the site of infection binds to AGSs, inactivating the drug.[88]
- The ICU patient may have a large volume of distribution for AGSs, which requires increased dosage to obtain therapeutic peak levels.[89-98]

Thus, higher peak levels are necessary for clinical response. The peak AGS level is the driving force to ensure that adequate levels are achieved at the site of infection.

Zaske et al. reported on the pharmacokinetic variability of gentamicin in 1640 patients.[58,60,99] The half-life of gentamicin varied from 0.4 to 32.7 hours in 1369 patients who had normal serum creatinine and from 0.4 to 7.6 hours in 331 patients who had normal creatinine clearance. The volume of distribution varied from 0.04 to 0.74 L/kg, and doses ranged from 0.5 to 25.8 mg/kg per day. Only 13 patients (0.9%) had a significant change in baseline serum creatinine that "possibly" could be related to gentamicin "toxicity." These patients were pharmacokinetically dosed, and nephrotoxicity was markedly low. Cochlear or vestibular toxicity did not occur. Zaske and co-workers noted this same pharmacokinetic variability of gentamicin in 417 elderly patients who were pharmacokinetically dosed. Gentamicin dose requirements varied from 0.3 to 22.0 mg/kg per day. The half-life of gentamicin varied from 0.3 to 32.7 hours, and Vd ranged from 0.07 to 0.53 L/kg. No ototoxicity was noted, and 2% of patients may have had nephrotoxicity. The elderly do not necessarily have long gentamicin half-lives; although increased age is considered a risk factor for nephrotoxicity, appropriate dosing did not result in appreciable toxicity in this population.[58,60,99]

Volume of Distribution Considerations

Volume of distribution determines the dose size needed to obtain therapeutic AGS blood levels. The Vd for critically ill patients is generally larger than the normal 0.2 to 0.25 L/kg. Various reports have indicated an average Vd of 0.29 L/kg to 0.41 L/kg for these patients. Possible reasons for this larger volume of distribution in the ICU patient include the following:

- Fever
- Altered vascular integrity
- Increased use of colloids and crystaloids for volume resuscitation
- Enhanced fluid retention

AGSs distribute to extracellular fluid (ECF), so that factors increasing ECF can be expected to increase Vd.[89-92,95,96] Some patients may have a "collapse" of their AGS Vd when they are recovering from their infection. A small percentage have a marked reduction in volume of distribution as they respond to antibiotic therapy. Major, life-threatening infection, appears to be one factor associated with increased Vd. When Vd is compared in the same patient for a less severe infection, Vd and doses are generally smaller in comparison. A recent study suggested that AGS volume of distribution decreased as patients were weaned off ventilators, and doses had to be decreased.[100]

Renal Function Considerations

Aminoglycosides are eliminated renally, and decreases in renal function will mainly increase the drug's half-life. Aminoglycoside half-life, in total renal shutdown, can vary from 40 to greater than 100 hours. The use of extended spectrum penicillins, such as carbenicillin, ticarcillin, mezlocillin, azlocillin, and piperacillin, will reduce AGS half-life in renal failure. Interaction of extended spectrum penicillins with gentamicin, tobramycin, amikacin, and sisomicin have all been reported. The interaction is initiated by the nucleophilic opening of the beta-lactam ring by the amino group of the aminoglycoside forming an inactive complex. This inactive complex has no toxicity or therapeutic effect.[101-105] This interaction may be important both from an in vitro and an in vivo standpoint. The in vitro study of this interaction between penicillins and AGSs reveals that it is time, temperature, and concentration dependent and that amikacin is least likely to undergo this interaction.[106-117] Aminoglycoside levels that are drawn while a patient receives extended spectrum penicillins require prompt attention by the laboratory so that in vitro inactivation does not give a falsely low AGS concentration. These specimens should be transported promptly to the laboratory, and beta-lactamase should be added to neutralize the penicillin and frozen if immediate analysis does not take place.

The in vivo inactivation of tobramycin by piperacillin in patients with normal renal function was studied by Lau et al.[118] There was no difference in half-life, volume of distribution, or area under the curve between those receiving tobramycin alone versus those receiving tobramycin and piperacillin. Elimination of the AGS is dependent on the fastest process of removal. Tobramycin half-life was 2.8 to 2.9 hours in these patients with normal renal function, rather than the 6 to 20 hours reported in patients with renal failure. Renal elimination of AGSs is the predominant factor for drug elimination in patients with fairly normal kidney function. When renal function is markedly impaired, then the complexation interaction is the fastest mode of elimination. This interaction is abrupt in onset, with an immediate reduction in AGS half-life within the first 24 hours of therapy. Likewise, discontinuation of the extended spectrum penicillin results in marked prolongation of half-life within the first 24 hours after the penicillin is stopped. The use of extended spectrum penicillins has been stated to attenuate AGS renal toxicity.[119-121]

Various dialysis methods have been employed in renal failure to control fluid and waste solutes. Continuous arterial venous hemofiltration (CAVHF), continuous arterial venous hemodialysis (CAVHD), and hemodialysis all remove AGSs. Aminoglycosides are not protein bound, with 95% of the drug free. Sieving coefficients are high at 73 to 88%, and this indicates that AGSs are dialyzable.[122-126] Our SICU patients who received high dose AGSs for severe infections required 20% shorter dose intervals when receiving CAVH/CAVHD compared to hemodialysis (these patients were not receiving extended spectrum penicillins). A continuous removal of AGS occurs during continuous therapy compared to hemodialysis, which may have accounted for these results. This was hard to explain considering that AGS half-life and volume of distribution were similar between the two groups. An additional study by Ernest and Cutler indicated minor and variable contribution of gentamicin total body clearance by CAVHD (about 25%) and that measurement of gentamicin levels was mandatory for guiding dosage.[127] Analysis of our patients' pharmacokinetic profiles who received hemodialysis, CAVHF, or CAVHD revealed that dose intervals and half-lives were reduced 29 to 37% and 32 to 48%, respectively, when patients received extended spectrum penicillins during these dialyses (compared to the same dialysis methods without concomitant extended spectrum penicillins). Volume of distribution did not differ among these patients.

Practical Points: Dosage of Aminoglycosides in Hemodialysis

First, the decision to use an AGS is made with the belief that the patient may benefit from use of these antimicrobials. Therefore, therapy in the first 24 hours of therapy is very important in producing a therapeutic effect; therapy thereafter is important for toxicologic reasons and therapeutic effect. The toxicity of these drugs appears to be related more to repeat dosing at intervals that do not allow the levels to drop into an acceptable range, and toxicity is not related to their use in renal dysfunction. Therefore, the old rule that these drugs should be avoided in renal failure is an oversimplification of a disease-drug interaction that has little basis if appropriate monitoring is done.

The first dose of an AGS in renal dysfunction is the most important dose the physician can give the patient for therapeutic effect, especially if the patient is anuric. Because these compounds have a high log kill related to peak concentration, sufficient drug must be given to reach acceptable peak AGS concentrations on that first dose, because the physician may not get a chance to give another dose for a few days, especially in the anuric patient. On the other hand, we have seen anuric surgical ICU patients dosed with the standard 80 mg of gentamicin or tobramycin dose (one-time dose) and have achieved peak concentrations of 2.5 µg/ml after the first dose. After assessment of these situations, we were still able to give the next dose 12 hours later, because the levels at that time were 1.9 µg/ml as a result of tissue distribution and some elimination in anuria. We then targeted therapeutic doses to reach high peak levels, but it would have been optimal to give the appropriate dose initially. The initial gentamicin and tobramycin doses in ICU patients have been referenced as 3 mg/kg.[91] By work at our institution, to achieve average peak gentamicin levels of 10 µg/ml (the peak immediately after infusion of the drug), an extremely ill surgical ICU patient should receive a gentamicin dose of 3.8 mg/kg of actual body weight (ABW), whereas the tobramycin loading dose should be 3.4 mg/kg ABW. Neurologic and medical ICU loading doses for gentamicin and tobramycin should be 3.4 mg/kg and 3.0 mg/kg of ABW to achieve immediate peaks of 10 µg/ml.

Hemodialysis removes AGSs, but the role of supplemental doses of AGSs after hemodialysis needs to be clarified. Most textbooks state that an additional dose of AGS should be given after hemodialysis. This is probably only true when the dose has been the standard 80 mg of gentamicin or tobramycin, the peak level was 2.5 µg/ml, and dialysis was done. The dose can be given again, because the level will be below 2 µg/ml; this would have occurred, however, even without dialysis. When we use high dose AGS therapy in the anuric hemodialysis patient, we find it is the exception and not the rule that a dose needs to be given after hemodialysis. Three, four, or five dialysis sessions may be required before the gentamicin or tobramycin levels fall to acceptable levels for redosing (redose at levels of 1 to 2 µg/ml or 2 to 2.5 µg/ml if the patient has extremely serious infection). An analysis of the gentamicin or tobramycin concentrations after hemodialysis when the predialysis AGS concentration was 10 µg/ml would show quite a dramatic drop in concentration of about 2 to 4 µg/ml. When dialysis is accomplished at a concentration of 5 µg/ml, concentrations may drop only 1 to 2 µg/ml; if dialysis is done at concentrations of 3 µg/ml, the concentrations may be lucky to drop 0.5 to 1 µg/ml. At times AGS levels rebound after dialysis, probably as a result of redistribution from tissue stores, and this keeps AGS levels higher than expected. Additionally, use of the extended spectrum penicillins result in inactivation of the AGSs in anuria, resulting in shorter dosage intervals. Addition or subtraction of these drugs from the antibiotic regimen should be considered when evaluating dosage intervals and measurement of AGS levels in hemodialysis patients. Generally speaking, the dose interval from the first high dose of an AGS to the second high dose of an AGS regimen in a hemodialysis patient is fairly short at 24 to 48 hours. The dose intervals prolong, however, after the second dose. One strategy to handle this situation is to give the 3- to 3.8-mg/kg loading dose and then take a peak level after this first dose and a level the next day. Pharmacokinetic analysis should then help predict when the second dose will be due and the appropriate dose size needed for therapeutic peak levels.

Infection-Induced Renal Dysfunction

Gram-negative, gram-positive, fungus and viral, and tuberculous infections can cause renal dysfunction for which AGS should not automatically be implicated.[44-53,128-136] Additionally, numerous literature reports have indicated that treatment with appropriate antibiotics (which may include AGS, vancomycin, and/or amphotericin—supposedly nephrotoxic drugs) results in improvement of kidney function.[137-142] A number of articles deal with the issue of AGS use in patients with reduced renal function or renal failure. A common observation made by the authors concerned the effect of infection on renal function. Infection, superinfection, and inadequately treated infections resulted in renal dysfunction, and adequate infection treatment resulted in improved kidney function.[143-149] A report by Keller et al.[150] reported that peak and trough netilmicin levels were significantly greater in the patients who lived (8.2 ± 2.5 and 3.8 ± 1.2 µg/ml, respectively, in 28 patients), compared to the 22 patients who died (5.9 ± 1.7 µg/ml and 3.0 ± 0.9 µg/ml, respectively). From this information, it appears that the use of AGSs in renal dysfunction needs to be totally reevaluated. Much of the reported nephrotoxicity could very well be related to infection.

Mechanism of Gram-Negative-Related Renal Dysfunction

A possible mechanism for gram-negative infection related renal dysfunction has been proposed. Gram-negative bacteria produce endotoxin, which in turn elicits tumor necrosis factor (TNF) production. If endotoxin or TNF is injected in animals, reduction in kidney function occurs. TNF may reduce kidney blood flow up to 50%. Additionally, TNF destroys endothelial tissues, producing a substance called endothelin. Endothelin has five to ten times the effect on reducing kidney function and may produce 100% renal blood flow shutdown. The role of AGS is to reduce the inherent number of organisms, thus lowering the amount of endotoxin, TNF, and endothelin produced. Aminoglycosides also inhibit endotoxin release, and this may be an additional mechanism of renal function improvement with the AGSs. Although this mechanism is conjecture at this time, it could very well explain why 61% of our SICU patients had improved or no change in renal function while dialysis for acute renal failure (ARF) declined 44% the year that high dose AGS dosing was started in SICU.[151-161]

Major Aminoglycoside Toxicities

Nephrotoxicity of the AGS antibiotics has been reported in 0.9 to 30% of the patients receiving these drugs and is more common when trough AGS levels are allowed to rise (troughs greater than 2.0 µg/ml for gentamicin and tobramycin and greater than 5 to 10 µg/ml for amikacin).[7,58,60,162-168] Nephrotoxicity usually requires a minimum of 3 to 5 days of therapy to develop and produces a clinical picture of acute tubular necrosis with casts in the urine, increased urinary *N*-acetyl-beta-D-glucosaminidase (NAG), beta$_2$ microglobulin, and increased serum creatinine. Proximal tubular damage occurs with AGS nephrotoxicity and is due to lysosomal destruction. This nephrotoxic reaction is reversible on discontinuation of the AGS. Some patients have required dialysis until return of renal function. Previous studies of pharmacokinetic dosing of AGSs indicate a reduced incidence of nephrotoxicity, compared to other literature reports, when this method of dosing AGSs is used.[169-180] Zaske and co-workers[58,60] reported gentamicin nephrotoxicity of 0.9% of 1640 patients and 2% in 417 elderly patients. A number of these patients required high dose AGS therapy (doses up to 22.0 to 25.8 mg/kg per day) to obtain therapeutic peak concentrations.

The great majority of the literature describes nephrotoxicity of AGSs by increases in serum creatinine of greater than or equal to 0.5 mg/dl from baseline values when baseline is less than 3.0 mg/dl. When baseline creatinine is greater than 3.0 mg/dl, an increase of 1.0 mg/dl is required for definition of nephrotoxicity. Although AGSs can cause nephrotoxicity if not monitored appropriately, increases in serum creatinine are invariably blamed on the AGS, or the AGS is the heavily favored clinical contender when other factors are at work. If the AGS is appropriately monitored and serum creatinine still increases, this may be a sign that the infectious process has changed and that other factors should receive rigorous attention. Has the patient developed a new site of an infection? Must a prior abscess be redrained? Has the organism become resistant to the present beta-lactam, and must a new agent be selected for combination therapy?

The past literature describing AGS nephrotoxicity has numerous problems including the lack of control of AGS levels in these studies and the presence of known factors that can cause renal dysfunction such as septicemia, hypotension, shock, continued infection, and elevated trough AGS levels. The last disturbing factor is that most, if not all, of the reports say nothing about the patients who have improvements of renal function during administration of AGS.

Aminoglycoside ototoxicity causes great concern and anxiety for the clinician. It is a toxicity that pushes the clinician into choosing alternative therapies that are less effective. In the not too distant past, AGS ototoxicity was thought to occur at a 10 to 20% incidence and to be irreversible. Infectious disease experts feel that this high incidence is overstated, because they rarely see this in their patients.[181] Cochlear toxicity was found to be reversible in 55% of patients who received AGS antibiotics by Fee.[182] A study by Powell et al.[183] of 52 cystic fibrosis patients receiving tobramycin with maximal concentrations of 40-60 μg/ml found no ototoxicity when audiologic and speech reception thresholds were tested. Much attention has been paid to this area lately because earlier literature was poorly controlled with respect to documentation of ototoxicity.[184,185] Recent studies have been made of hospitalized patients receiving no ototoxic drugs; these studies have indicated both increases and decreases in audiometry thresholds (an increase in audiometry threshold of 15 dB at any frequency is considered clinically significant) when tested over time.[186] Studies have compared placebo to regimens of cefotaxime monotherapy compared to tobramycin-combination therapy.[187] Placebo-treated patients were reported to have moderate hearing loss. Cefotaxime monotherapy resulted in 13% ototoxicity, whereas the tobramycin-combination therapy group had 7.4% ototoxicity, as documented by audiometry changes. An additional study by Smith[188] found no ototoxicity when placebo, netilmicin, or gentamicin were given to normal volunteers. Brummett and Morrison[189] looked at changes in auditory thresholds of 20 volunteers three times at 1-week intervals. This was done to simulate baseline results before and after 1 week of AGS therapy (but no drug was given) and results 1 week after AGS therapy ended. They found 27 differences between tests indicating worsened thresholds and 26 differences between retests indicating hearing improvement (improvement defined as improvement of at least 15 dB in hearing at any frequency, and worsening defined as worsening of at least 15 dB in hearing at any frequency).

To summarize, audiometry tests have had high false-positive results for ototoxicity. Additionally, patients will experience changes in auditory tests that are interpreted as ototoxicity when patients are not receiving drugs known to be ototoxic or are not receiving drugs. In other words, the incidence of ototoxicity has been greatly overestimated, and past work does not reflect the influence of AGSs on hearing.

Clinical Experience With High Dose Aminoglycoside Therapy

We initially released a preliminary report on the use of high dose AGS therapy in SICU patients treated for a variety of infections.[54] In 51 patients both gram-positive and gram-negative organisms were isolated, in 13 only gram-negatives, in 10 only gram-positives, and 10 patients had negative cultures or were positive for yeast alone. A total of 51 patients survived the SICU for a survival rate of 62.2%. The average APACHE II score for all patients was 20.65 ± 5.99 (7 to 35), and the average mortality risk was .3539 ± .2056 (0.0505 to 0.8744). The patients with renal dysfunction were dosed with the same peak and trough level goals as those without renal dysfunction. The average dose size was 192 mg, and the average dose interval was 18.9 ± 18.19 hours (6 to 260 hours). The average daily dose was 294.9 mg (50 to 1200 mg). The average initial serum creatinine (2.11) was not considered clinically or significantly ($p > 0.05$) different from the last treatment day creatinine (2.52 ± 1.81). Twenty patients had decreases in serum creatinine; in 33 patients creatinine remained the same; and 31 patients had increases in serum creatinine, and this was more prevalent in patients who expired. The 31 patients with a decrease in renal function had a survival rate of only 16.13% from the SICU and 3.2% from the hospital compared to survival rates of 89.5 to 90.63% from the SICU and a 78.57 to 88.9% from the hospital for patients with improved or stable renal function. Increased serum creatinine was related to multiple organ dysfunction and/or dying with continued infection and not to AGS therapy. The average total bilirubin in the increased serum creatinine group with high mortality was 6.48 mg/dl. Further analysis of the three renal function groups by patients who survived and patients who died indicated that those who expired had an average total bilirubin that was two to three times higher than those who survived. We have used both serum creatinine and bilirubin as indicators of infectious response in the SICU patient (the use of bilirubin as an indicator in other ICUs does not seem to follow this pattern). If after prolonged therapy we cannot decrease total bilirubin, then the chance of patient mortality is high. On the other hand, when an infected patient's total bilirubin is high and begins a downward trend, this is an extremely good sign that the infection is responding to efforts to maximize antibiotic therapy.

Clinical ototoxicity may have occurred in two patients, but they both died, and both had received vancomycin and loop diuretics. The greatest dose was 660 mg of tobramycin, and the highest daily dose was 1200 mg of gentamicin without nephrotoxicity or ototoxicity. The two patients who received these maximum doses both had improvements in creatinine clearance, eradication of their infection, and survived.

Antibiotics used in the SICU setting require a prolonged course of intensive therapy to be of benefit to these patients. Survival from the SICU increased from 53.3 to 57.1% to 61.1 to 72.7% as total days of AGS therapy increased from 4 to 10, 11 to 14, 15 to 21, and greater than 21 days of therapy, respectively. This may indicate that a prolonged course of high dose AGS therapy (in combination with the appropriate other antibiotics) is needed for effective infection control in these severely ill SICU patients.

Large-Dose Once-a-Day Aminoglycoside Dosing

Once-a-day AGS dosing is the recent fad that is being praised as an alternative to small daily divided doses. Ter-Braak and co-workers[190] reported that once-a-day doses of netilmicin resulted in peak levels of 12 to 16 μg/ml and troughs of 1 to 2 μg/ml (whereas divided doses result in peaks of 4 to 8 μg/ml). Two other papers reported use of once-a-day gentamicin, tobramycin, or netilmicin. The work by Nordstrom et al.[191] used peak levels of up to 18.6 μg/ml, and Powel et al.[183] used peaks of 40 to 60 μg/ml. Experimentation with this method is being promoted because of the evidence linking peak levels with improved response of infection, as discussed earlier, and the possibility of decreased toxicity. The results of these few limited clinical studies indicate no difference in clinical response to the infection or incidence of nephrotoxicity or ototoxicity between divided daily or daily doses.

When reported, the trough levels were 1 to 2 μg/ml when daily doses were used, but the populations were composed of the elderly, who have an age-related reduction in renal function. These trough levels would be normally targeted for any AGS dosage regimen, whether 4-hour, 72-hour, or other. The young patient with excellent renal function may have nonmeasurable AGS levels by 6 to 8 hours after dosing. Waiting an additional 16 to 20 hours to obtain a daily AGS dose may not be expected to benefit these patients and may be possibly detrimental, because they are without antibiotic for a prolonged portion of the day. This may be the very reason why some authors caution about use of this method and state that more clinical studies are needed to determine the validity of this approach. Until this method is proved in both the young and elderly, with good and poor renal function, once-daily dosing should be reserved only for those patients who would normally require daily doses. Our recommendation is to use individualized doses and dose intervals determined pharmacokinetically (dose intervals of 6, 8, 12, 18, 24, 36, 48, 72 hours etc., rather than once a day) for peak levels of 10 to 16 μg/ml and trough levels of 1 to 2 μg/ml. The auditory study by these authors is excellent in that they have provided the proof that high peak AGS peak levels do not result in any different ototoxic potential than those obtained by small divided doses. This gives us the chance to push for the more effective higher peak concentrations.[183,190,191]

VANCOMYCIN PHARMACOKINETICS

Vancomycin has become a widely used antibiotic in ICUs as methicillin-resistant staphylococcus organisms have become more frequent pathogens, especially with the advent of invasive technology. Numerous controversies surround the use of this drug, including the relationships of vancomycin concentration to efficacy or toxicity, as well as time of plasma level sampling and which pharmacokinetic model should be used in formulating vancomycin dosage regimens.[191,192]

Vancomycin renal clearance correlates well with indices of renal function such as inulin, iothalamate, and creatinine clearance. Normal vancomycin half-life is 4 to 8 hours and may be prolonged to greater than 100 hours with anuria. Protein binding of vancomycin may vary from 0 to 60%, and the volume of distribution varies depending on pharmacokinetic model chosen and subject type. One-compartment volume of distribution varies from 0.04 L/kg to 1.9 L/kg, with most running 0.47 to 0.84 L/kg.[192-194] Two-compartment volume of distribution varies from 0.04 to 0.70 L/kg.

Confusion exists as to sampling times most appropriate for the peak level. Because the distribution phase of elimination requires approximately 3 hours, it would be wrong to use the one-compartment model for dose predictions when peak levels are drawn less than 3 hours after infusion. Using the one-compartment model in this manner would underestimate the terminal vancomycin half-life. This may lead to shorter dose intervals, which could result in achieving toxic vancomycin concentrations. The more appropriate pharmacokinetic dosing model would be the open two-compartment model when levels are drawn less than 3 hours after infusion. Our pharmacokinetic service uses the two-compartment model (USC PACK), which results in excellent dosage control and does not require us to retrain the phlebotomy and nursing staff for a new peak drawing time. We feel it is more important to control the patient's drug therapy than to put controls on the people who deliver the patient's care.

The normal therapeutic ranges for vancomycin before (trough) and after (peak) plasma levels are commonly listed as 5 to 10 μg/ml and 30 to 40 μg/ml (peak drawn 1 hour after the vancomycin infusion is finished). The relationships between efficacy and toxicity and plasma vancomycin levels are less established than the AGSs.[195-197] We generally have found that vancomycin trough levels of 10 to 15 μg/ml have been more useful in producing a clinical response to infection. Of all the patients we have dosed, our average trough vancomycin level registers 13.02 μg/ml. This contrasts with the stated normal trough level of 5 to 10 μg/ml. So in contrast to the AGSs, for which clinical response is related to peak concentrations, we have noted from clinical experience that response to vancomycin therapy may be related to obtaining a trough of 10 to 15 μg/ml (or 15 to 20 μg/ml with central nervous system infections). One report states that minimal vancomycin levels should remain in the 10- to 15-μg/ml trough range for maximum response.[198] Trough levels of greater than 20 to 30 μg/ml seem to be associated with more nephrotoxicity in our experience and other's.[199]

Vancomycin Dosing Considerations in the Elderly

Vancomycin elimination in the elderly is decreased, partially due to the normal reduction in renal function that occurs with aging. Additionally, volume of distribution is generally increased, which also promotes prolongation of drug half-life. The disposition changes in the elderly may also depend on altered vancomycin tissue distribution volume and/or tissue binding.[200] In an elderly patient with normal serum creatinine, we often administer a dose of 1 g every 12 hours. Predose and postdose levels in the first 3 to 5 days of the first week of therapy are almost always in the accepted therapeutic ranges. By the first to second half of the second week, however, it is the trough levels commonly have accumulated to greater than 15 μg/ml with a proportional increase in peak levels. Serum creatinine in these patients remains unchanged. Marked prolongations in vancomycin dose interval are needed to bring trough levels down to the therapeutic range to avoid toxicity. The reasons for these changes are not known at present but may be related to the altered tissue binding/distribution and possible accumulation in multiple body organs. Use of a two-compartment model has been instrumental in determining the changes in kinetics and predicting the possible accumulation that can occur in these elderly patients.

Practical Points: Dosing Vancomycin in Dialysis Patients

Vancomycin is not considered to be removed by hemodialysis,[201-203] but this should be qualified with the statement that the type of dialysis membrane influences removal. Cuprophane and cellulose acetate membranes do not result in an appreciable removal of vancomycin because of their limited permeability of the large vancomycin molecule. Vancomycin is cleared relatively easily when the polyamide filters are used, which is due to their permeability to larger drug molecules. The removal is so efficient with the polyamide filters that there may be a rebound increase in vancomycin levels after dialysis, which is due to tissue redistribution.[204-206]

CAVHF and CAVHD are becoming popular methods to control solute and fluid status. These methods contrast with hemodialysis in that hemodialysis is accomplished intermittently with 3- to 5-hour dialysis sessions. CAVHF and CAVHD are continuous processes that may be less hemodynamically compromising to the patient. These processes are important from the drug removal viewpoint in that CAVHF/CAVHD filters are constantly being presented for drug removal, whereas increased hemodialysis removal of drug can occur only during the intermittent dialysis process. Thus, CAVHF/CAVHD may potentially have greater effects on vancomycin removal in general. The filters are usually of the polyamide or polyacrylonitrile type, which as mentioned, have a greater permeability to larger drug molecules than do the commonly used cuprophane or cellulose acetate HEMO filters. Which of these two factors contributes most to vancomycin elimination is not known. A few papers have appeared documenting vancomycin pharmacokinetics during CAVHF or CAVHD. The increased clearance of vancomycin, in renal failure, by CAVHF accounts for about 66% of total vancomycin clearance. Additional work indicates that CAVHD removes vancomycin twice as effectively as CAVHF. We have not noticed this difference clinically based on the dose-interval and dose-size needs of our patients. An additional paper by Dupuis et al. confirms a short dose interval of approximately every three days when on CAVHF.[207-210] This does not differ significantly from our results for both CAVHF or CAVHD, as explained later.

Work from our institution indicates that there are markedly different kinetics and dose interval needs when pharmacokinetic differences between patients receiving hemodialysis versus patients receiving CAVHF or CAVHD are compared. Average beta-elimination half-life for hemodialysis was 158.94 ± 131.68 hours versus 70.69 ± 24.49 hours for CAVHF/CAVHD ($p < 0.001$). Central volume of distribution averaged 0.297 ± 0.127 L/kg ABW) for hemodialysis versus 0.253 L/kg ± 0.117 L/kg ABW) for CAVHF/CAVHD ($p > 0.05$). The average dose size and dose interval for hemodialysis was 961.29 ± 255.491 mg and 123.14 ± 72.65 hours versus 1121.4 mg ± 204.2 mg ($p < 0.05$) and 63.09 ± 28.30 hours ($p < 0.001$) for CAVHF/CAVHD. The peak/trough levels for HEMO patients averaged 32.40 ± 6.36 μg/ml and 14.15 ± 6.005 μg/ml, whereas peak/trough levels for CAVHF/CAVHD averaged 28.83 ± 3.62 μg/ml and 11.08 μg/ml ± 2.748 μg/ml). Both peak and trough vancomycin levels tested significantly different between hemodialysis and CAVHF/CAVHD ($p < 0.005$ for both) and may be the reason for significantly different doses between hemodialysis and CAVHF/CAVHD.[211]

We have discussed the influence of renal function and dialytic methods on vancomycin elimination. Numerous attempts have been made to characterize the patterns of elimination and present dosage guidelines for initial vancomycin dosages.[212,213] The preponderance of literature indicates once-a-week dosing of vancomycin is necessary in total anuria or end-stage renal disease. As mentioned earlier, we redose our patients when trough levels of 10 to 15 μg/ml are reached. We feel we have better clinical success with this regimen with little or no renal toxicity and/or ototoxicity. The initial fast distribution phase of vancomycin will generally bring the levels of vancomycin down to 10 to 15 μg/ml in the first 12 to 24 hours even in total anuria (after a 1-g dose). Although it may take a week to reach levels of 5 µg/ml after a 1-g dose, we wish to give the most aggressive antimicrobial regimen as early as possible. This requires that the ICU patient receive an additional 1-g dose within the first 24 hours of therapy. After these two doses are administered, the second compartment apparently has been repleted with enough drug to allow prolonged dosage intervals. This is applicable to the ICU patient but has not been as thoroughly tested clinically in the regular-floor patient.

Of the literature describing the relationships of combined AGS/vancomycin to renal dysfunction, most put causal relationship to combined use of the two drugs. A recent article by Pauly et al.[214] described associations between renal toxicity and age, AGS and vancomycin trough/peak levels, liver disease, duration of AGS/vancomycin therapy, concomitant amphotericin B therapy and a few others. A significant finding was the association of peritonitis with decreases in renal function. This again brings up the role of infection causing kidney dysfunction.

ANTIBIOTIC DOSING IN RENAL AND/OR LIVER DYSFUNCTION

The clinician needs to be aware of organ dysfunction and its relationship to antibiotic dosage alterations. Table 66-5 lists the antibiotics and their major route of elimination. The reader can readily use this list to see if a patient's present regimen contains an antibiotic that matches the patient's organ dysfunction.[215-223] Specific dosage recommendations are listed for degree of renal impairment and liver disease where available. For a few antibiotics, elimination is by both renal and liver elimination; if one organ of elimination is impaired, the remainder of drug elimination is picked up by the other route of elimination. Cefoperazone is one such drug.

The information from all the previously mentioned sources may present different doses for the same antibiotic. This brings us to the fact that we probably do not know as much as we need to know concerning antibiotic dosage in many of our ICU patients. Most hospitals do not have readily available assays to measure all types of antibiotic blood levels, and this may impede progress in determining more exact dosage needs. Much work is left to be done in this area, although most physicians feel comfortable with the "normal" dose recommendations currently available. If the AGSs and vancomycin have a wide range of pharmacokinetic parameters in the ICU patient, there is no reason that the other antibiotics will not have the same variability. This, combined with the fact that different bacteria are considered sensitive to the same antibiotic at different MICs, brings up the point that our dose regimens in renal dysfunction may be fine for one organism and not for another, even though the same trough antibiotic concentrations were achieved. Remember that, when a beta-lactam antibiotic level falls below the MIC, ready repair of bacterial cell wall damage and re-entry into log growth phase can occur. Allowing the antibiotic blood level to fall below the MIC for too long is not in the best interest of the patient care.[224]

Antibiotic dosage modifications for various dialysis methods are presented in much the same sources as quoted previously. Additionally, further information on the CAVHF/CAVHD removal of antibiotics is presented by Bickley.[225] Again, this area of therapeutics is very imprecise, and dosage recommendations based on sieving coefficients and ultrafiltrate rates cannot always be extrapolated to dosage needed. Much more is involved, such as blood/dialysate flow rate, filter material and type, filter surface area, and size of the drug molecule. As an example, we have mentioned that vancomycin is removed by CAVHF/CAVHD. By use of equations, sieving coefficients, and so on, it has been determined that approximately 100 mg of vancomycin is removed daily by CAVHF. The replacement of this amount daily is not the way vancomycin dosing is generally handled; it may be the way a beta-lactam antibiotic dosage is handled, because antibiotic blood levels are not readily available. As mentioned, knowledge of vancomycin pharmacokinetics has been useful in identifying dosages needed for this type of therapy. The equations using sieving coefficients and so on are not useful in targeting therapy for specific vancomycin or AGS concentration goals but are useful in the general investigation that determines if the drug is removed by various dialysis methods. Hemodialysis guidelines are mentioned in previously cited references.[215,218,220-223,225,226] Table 66-6 is a list of antibiotics and indicates whether hemodialysis and/or CAVHF/CAVHD affect drug disposition.[225,226]

Reduction of doses of antibiotics may be needed to prevent adverse reactions that may be associated with accumulation related to changes in antibiotic pharmacokinetics that are due to renal dysfunction (Table 66-7). The change incurred is usually the prolongation of drug half-life and drug accumulation. Table 66-7 presents those antibiotics that need to be thought of when renal dysfunction arises; the adverse reactions may be avoided by appropriate dosage reduction or switching to an alternative agent.[227-230]

Antibiotic Pharmacokinetics in Multiple Organ System Dysfunction

Antibiotic pharmacokinetic studies on patients with multiple organ system dysfunction (MOD) are virtually nonexistent, and the studies available involve single organ failure (renal or liver failure). Altered patterns of absorption, distribution, metabolism, and excretion (ADME processes) are sure to exist in the patient with MOD, but these have not been quantified with any single antibiotic. Absorption of antibiotics by the oral or intramuscular route should be considered unpredictable in MOD, and therefore the intravenous route should be employed. Distribution processes in MOD can be altered, and lipid-soluble antibiotics' distribution to tissue sites from the plasma may be inhibited by conditions that promote low blood flow or perfusion such as hypotension and/or shock. Poor capillary integrity for antibiotics that tend to distribute into total body water (TBW) can lead to larger than normal volumes of distribution (e.g., with AGSs).

A complex relationship exists between antibiotics that are highly protein or tissue bound and volume of distribution. Generally, only the free drug is available for clearance. Decreases in albumin concentration (e.g., with severe infections, other ICU catabolic conditions, or malnutrition)

Table 66–5. Dosage Adjustments for Intravenous Antibiotics Whose Disposition Is Altered by Renal or Liver Dysfunction

				Dosage Based on Creatinine Clearance or Hepatic Disease				
Antibiotic	ROE/% RE	P.B.% Vd(L/kg)	T1/2NRF T1/2RF	<10 ml/min	10–50 ml/min	50–100 ml/min	Hepatic Disease	Daily Dosage
Acyclovir	R/70	25/0.70	2.9/19	2.5 mg/kg q24h	5 mg/kg q12–24h	5 mg/kg q8h	—	—
Amantidine	R/90	60/4–5	12/500	0.2 g q168h	0.2 g × 1, 0.1 g q48–72h	0.1 g q8–12h	—	—
Amdinocillin	R/70	15/0.23	0.9/3.3	0.5 g q8–12h	0.5–1 g q6–8h	0.5–1 g q4h	—	—
Aminoglycosides	R/95	<5/0.1–0.6	2/40–150	Follow levels	Follow levels	Follow levels	—	Normal dose
Amphotericin	?/5	90/4	24/24	0.25–0.5 mg/kg q24–48h max 50 mg to 1 mg/kg daily	0.25–0.5 mg/kg q24–48h max 50 mg to 1 mg/kg daily	0.25–0.5 mg/kg q24h max 50 mg–1 mg/kg daily	—	—
Ampicillin	R/90	20/0.30	1.5/15	1–2 g q12–24h	1–2 g q6–12h	1–2 g q4–6h	Cirrhosis	Normal dose
Azlocillin	R/65	25–45/0.22	0.9/6.5	1–3 g q12h	2–3 g q8–12h	2–3 g q4–6h	—	—
Aztreonam	R/75	56/0.18	1.5–2/8.4	0.25 g q8–12h	0.25–0.5 g q8–12h	0.5 g–1 g q6–12h	Primary biliary cirrhosis / Cirrhosis / Various	Normal dose / Normal dose / Normal dose
Carbenicillin	R/95	50/0.15	1.5/15	2 g q8–12h	2–4 g q6h	4–6 g q4h		
Cefamandole	R/70	75/0.22	1.0/11	0.5 g q8–12h	1–2 g q6–8h	1–2 g q4–6h	—	—
Cefazolin	R/90	80/0.14	2.0/25	0.5–1 g q24–48h	0.5–1 g q12h	0.5–1 g q6–8h	—	—
Cefmetazole	R/85	85/0.18	1.4/20.8	0.5–1 g q24–48h	1 g q12–24h	1 g q8h	—	—
Cefonicid	R/90	90/0.12	4–10/60	0.25–1 g q72h	0.25–1 g	1–2 g q24h	—	—
Cefoperazone	H/25	90/0.18	2.0/2.0	0.5–1 g q12h	1–2 g q12h	1–2 g q12h	Biliary obstruction / Cirrhosis	Dec. 25–50% / Dec. 25–50%
Cefuranide	R/80	81/0.14	4.0/15	1 g q24–48h	1 g q24h	1 g q12h	—	—
Cefotaxime	H/20	35/0.25	1.5/2.5	1–2 g q12–24h	1–2 g q6–12h	1–2 g q4–8h	Cirrhosis	Dec. 25–50%
Cefotetan	R/72	90/0.14	3.7/11.5–16.5	1 g q24–48h	1 g q8–12h	1 g q8h	—	—
Cefoxitin	R/80	55/0.16	0.7/20	0.5–1 g q12–48h	1–2 g q8–12h	1–2 g q4–6h	—	—
Ceftazidime	R/89	20/0.20	1.8/>8	0.5–2 g q36h	0.5–2 g q12–24h	0.5–2 g q8h	Intrahepatic cholestasis / Chronic liver disease	Normal dose / Normal dose
Ceftizoxime	R/80	35/0.36	1.8/19	0.5 g q24–48h	0.5–1 g q12h	0.5–2 g q8h	—	—
Ceftriaxone	H/45	95/0.18	8/12–15	1–2 g q24h	1–2 g q12–24h	1–2 g q12–24h	Cirrhosis	Normal dose
Cefuroxime	R/90	33/0.22	1.5/18	0.75 g q24–48h	0.75 g q12–24h	0.75–1.5 g q8h	Cirrhosis	Normal dose
Cephalothin	R-H/52	60/0.26	0.7/3–18	1 g q8–12h	1 g q6h	1–2 g q4–6h	—	—
Cephapirin	H-R/49	45/0.20	0.6/2.4	1 g q6–12h	1 g q6h	1–2 g q4–6h	—	—
Cephradine	R/86	10/0.33	1.3/13	1 g q8h	1 g q6h	1 g q4–6h	—	—
Chloramphenicol	H/10	60/1.4	2–4/2–4	0.5–1 g q6h Follow levels	0.5–1 g q6h Follow levels	0.5–1 g q6h Follow levels	Cirrhosis / Acute hepatitis / Budd-Chiari / Portal hypertension / Extrahepatic obstruction	Dec. 50–75% / Dec. 50–75% ?avoid use / Dec. 25–75% / Dec. 25–50% / Dec. 25–50%
Cilastatin*	R-H/65	44/.23	0.9/11.6	0.25 g q12h	0.25–0.5 g q12h	0.25–0.5 g q6h	—	—
Ciprofloxacin	R-H/51	20–40/2.59–2.73	4.6/7.9–8.3	0.2–0.4 g q12–24h	0.2–0.4 g q12–24h	0.2–0.4 g q12h	—	—
Clavulonic* acid	H/40	9–30/0.32	1.3/2.9	67 mg q12h	67 mg q12h	100 mg q12h	—	—
Clindamycin	H/10	94/0.66	2.7/4.3	0.3–0.6 g q6–8h	0.6–0.9 g q6–8h	0.6–0.9 g q6–8h	Cirrhosis / Acute hepatitis / Chronic hepatitis	Normal dose / Normal dose / Normal dose

(continued)

Table 66–5. Dosage Adjustments for Intravenous Antibiotics Whose Disposition Is Altered by Renal or Liver Dysfunction—*(Continued)*

Antibiotic	ROE/% RE	P.B.% Vd(L/kg)	T1/2NRF T1/2RF	<10 ml/min	10–50 ml/min	50–100 ml/min	Hepatic Disease	Daily Dosage
Co-trimoxazole	\multicolumn{3}{Dose based on trimethoprim 2–5 mg/kg/day}		4–10 mg/kg/day q8–12h	8–20 mg/kg/day q6–8h	See trimethoprim and sulfamethoxazole	
Erythromycin	H/15	72/0.72	2.5/5	0.25–0.5 g q6–8h	0.25–1 g q6h	0.25–1 g q6h	Cirrhosis	Normal to Dec. 50%
Doxycycline	R-?/50	73/.58–.67	17.3/24.2	0.1 g q12h	0.1 g q12h	0.1 g q12h	—	—
Fluconazole	R/60–80	11/0.7–1	20/50	Load then 25% of load q24h	Load then ½ of load q24h	100–400 mg load ×1, then ½ load q24h	—	—
Flucytosine	R/80	5/0.6	4/70	10–35 mg/kg/day q24–48h Follow levels	25–75 mg/kg/day q12–24h Follow levels	50–150 mg/kg/day q6h Follow levels	—	—
Foscarnet	R/80–90	14–17/0.3–0.6	3/?	See package insert: dose based on creatinine clearance in ml/min/kg			—	—
Gancyclovir†	R/91	2/17–59 l/1.73 m (2)	3.6/30	1.25 mg/kg q24h	1.25–2.5 mg/kg q24h	‡2.5 mg/kg q8h ‡5 mg/kg q12h §2.5 mg/kg q12h	—	—
Imipenem	R/80	15–25/0.20	0.7–1/3.5	0.25–.5 g q12h	0.25–0.5 g q6–8h	0.5–1 g q6–8h	—	—
Isoniazid	H/3–11	4–30/.71	2.3/4.3	0.3 g q24h	0.3 g q24h	0.3 g q24h	—	—
Methicillin	R-H/90	50/0.30	0.5/4	1–2 g q12h	1–2 g q6h	1–2 g q4h	—	—
Metronidazole	H/20	20/0.90	6–8/12	0.5 g q8–24h	0.5 g q8–12h	0.5 g q6h	Cirrhosis (severe) Cirrhosis (mild)	Dec. 50% Normal Dose
Mezlocillin	H-R/50	35/0.26	0.85/2.2	1–3 g q8h	2–4 g q8h	2–4 g q4–6h	Cirrhosis	Dec. 25–50%
Miconazole‖	H/20	90/2.1	22/22	0.2–3 g/day	0.2–3 g/day	0.2–3 g/day	—	—
Minocycline	H-R/12	76/0.99	15.5/20.1	0.1 g q12h	0.1 g q12h	0.1 g q12h	—	—
Moxalactam	R/60	45/0.32	2.5/20	1 g q24h	1–2 g q8–12h	1–4 g q8h	—	—
Nafcillin	H/50	90/0.9	0.5/1.2	1–2 g q4–6h	1–2 g q4h	1–2 g q4h	Cirrhosis Biliary obstruction	Dec. 25–50% Dec. 25–50%
Oxacillin	H-R/50	92/0.8	0.4/1.0	1–2 g q4–6h	1–2 g q4h	1–2 g q4h	—	—
Penicillin G	R-H/60	40/0.36	0.5/13	1–2 mU q6h	2–4 mU q4h	4 mU q4h	?	—
Pentamidine	?/4–29	69/55–165	29/73–118	4 mg/kg q48h	4 mg/kg q24–36h	4 mg/kg q24h	—	—
Piperacillin	R/75	16/0.26	1.0/4.2	3 g q12h	3 g q8h	3–4 g q4–6h	—	—
Sulbactam***	R/84	38/.26–.59	1.1/4.1–15.2	1 g q24h	1 g q8–12h	1 g q6h	Cirrhosis	Normal Dose
Sulfamethoxazole	R/30	65/0.40	8.6/24	0.25–0.8 g q24h	0.5–.8 g q12h	0.8–1 g q12h		
	See Co-trimoxazole							
Teicoplanin	R/100	93/1.08–1.14	85.8/206.8	Follow levels	Follow levels	Follow levels	—	—
Tetracycline	R/48	65/1.3	7/48	Try not to use	0.25 g q24h	0.25–0.5 g q6h	—	—
Ticarcillin	R/90	45/0.17	2.4/16	3 g q24h	3–4 g q6–8h	3–4 g q4–6h	—	—
Trimethoprim	R/70	70/1.8	11/24	40 mg q12h	80 mg q12h	160 mg q12h	Cirrhosis	Normal Dose
	See Co-trimoxazole							
Vancomycin	R/90	10–50/0.47–0.84	6–8/100–350	Follow plasma levels	Follow levels	Follow levels	Undefined liver disease	Dec. 60%
Vidarabine	R-H/50	20–30/0.7	3.5/—	5–10 mg/kg q24h	10 mg/kg q24h	15 mg/kg q24h	—	—
Zidovudine	H/15	35/1.5	1.0/1.4	1–2 mg/kg q4h	1–2 mg/kg q4h	1–2 mg/kg q4h	—	—

* These agents are not antibiotics themselves but are combined with some antibiotics as enzyme inhibitors to enhance antibiotic action.
† Gancyclovir dosages are listed for induction doses. Maintenance doses use either a prolonged dose interval or approximate 50% dose reduction. This depends on site of disease and other factors. Refer to most recent dose recommendations.
‡ Doses are for creatinine clearances >70 ml/min.
§ Doses are for creatinine clearances of 50–79 ml/min.
‖ Dosage depends on the fungal infection treated. See manufacturer's recommendations.
ROE, route of elimination being renal (R) or hepatic (H), major route of elimination appears first; %RE, percentage renally eliminated; PB%, percentage protein bound; Vd (l/kg), volume of distribution in l/kg; T1/2NRF, half-life with normal renal function; T1/2RF, half-life with creatinine clearance less than 10 ml/min; Dec, decrease.

Table 66–6. Antibiotic Pharmacokinetics and Dosing During CAVHF/CAVHD and Hemodialysis

Antibiotic	ROE/% RE	PB%/Vd (l/kg)	T1/2 CrCl <10 ml/min	T1/2 During Hemodialysis	Dose After Dialysis?	Seiving Coefficient	Removed by CAVH/CAVHD?	Comments
Acyclovir	R/70	25/0.70	19 hr	5.4 hr	Y	?	?	
Amantidine	R/90	60/4–5	500 hr	199.2 hr	N	?	?	≤ 5% Removed by hemodialysis
Amdinocillin	R/70	15/0.23	3.3 hr	2.3 hr	?	?	?	Parameters indicate probably dialyzed out
Aminoglycosides	R/95	<5/0.1–0.6	40–150 hr	2.9–9.1 hr	Sometimes	0.73–0.89	Y	Follow plasma levels: give dose if level low
Amphotericin	?/5	90/4	24–360 hr	24–360 hr	N	0.4	N	
Ampicillin	R/90	20/0.30	15 hr	2.7 hr	Y	0.60 ± 0.21	Y	
Azlocillin	R/65	25–45/0.22	6.5 hr	2.2 hr	Y	?	?	Probably removed by dialysis
Aztreonam	R/75	56/0.18	8.4 hr	2.6 hr	Y	?	?	
Carbenicillin	R/95	50/0.15	18.2 hr	5.5 hr	Y	?	?	
Cefamandole	R/70	75/0.22	11 hr	5.0 hr	Y	?	?	
Cefazolin	R/90	80/0.14	25 hr	5–28 hr	Y	?	?	Parameters do not indicate dialyzable but reported as hemodialyzed
Cefmetazole	R/85	85/0.18	20.8 hr	2.1 hr	Y	?	?	
Cefonicid	R/90	90/0.12	60 hr	?	Y	?	?	Parameters do not indicate dialyzable but reported as hemodialyzed
Cefoperazone	H/25	90/0.18	3.7 hr	2.4 hr	N	0.27	N	
Ceforanide	R/80	81/0.14	20.7 hr	4.1 hr	Y	?	?	
Cefotaxime	H/20	35/0.25	2.5 hr	2.1 hr	Y	0.51	?	
Cefotetan	R/72	90/0.14	16.5 hr	6.5 hr	?	?	?	
Cefoxitin	R/80	55/0.16	20 hr	3.9 hr	Y	?	?	
Ceftazidime	R/89	20/0.20	23 hr	3.2 hr	Y	1.0	Y	
Ceftizoxime	R/80	35/0.36	19 hr	2.1 hr	Y	?	?	
Ceftriaxone	H/45	95/0.18	15 hr	5–16 hr	?	0.10	N	Parameters indicate probably not removed by dialysis
Cefuroxime	R/90	33/0.22	18 hr	3.6 hr	Y	?	?	
Cephalothin	R-H/52	60/0.26	3–18 hr	3.4 hr	?	?	?	
Cephapirin	H-R/49	45/0.20	2.4 hr	2.4 hr	N	0.7	Y	
Cephradine	R/86	10/0.33	13 hr	?	?	?	?	
Chloramphenicol	H/10	60/1.4	5.6 hr	3.2 hr	?	?	?	Follow plasma levels
Cilastatin*	R-H/65	44/.23	11.6 hr	3.5 hr	Y	?	?	
Ciprofloxacin	R-H/51	20–40	7.9 hr	5.3 hr	N	?	?	
Clavulanic* acid	H/40	9–30/0.32	2.9 hr	?	Y	?	?	
Clindamycin	H/10	94/0.66	4.3 hr	2.5 hr	N	0.98	?	Conflicting parameters for dialysis
Co-Trimoxazole	See trimethoprim and sulfamethoxazole							
Erythromycin	H/15	72/0.72	5 hr	?	N	0.37	N	
Doxycycline	R-?/50	73/.58	24.2 hr	18.5 hr	N	0.4–1.0	?	Conflicting parameters for dialysis
Fluconazole	R/60–80	11/0.7–1	50 hr	3 hr	Y	?	?	Give daily dose after dialysis to prevent having to give additional dose
Flucytosine	R/80	5/0.6	70–200 hr	?	Y	?	?	Give that day's dose after hemodialysis or supplement with 20–50 mg/kg after dialysis: follow levels
Foscarnet	R/90	14–17/0.3–0.6	?	?	?	?	?	

(continued)

Table 66–6. Antibiotic Pharmacokinetics and Dosing During CAVHF/CAVHD and Hemodialysis—*(Continued)*

Antibiotic	ROE/% RE	PB%/Vd (l/kg)	T1/2 CrCl <10 ml/min	T1/2 During Hemodialysis	Dose After Dialysis?	Seiving Coefficient	Removed by CAVH/CAVHD?	Comments
Gancyclovir*	R/91	2/17–59 l/1.73 m(2)	30 hr	4 hr	Y	0.69	Y	Suggest following levels: give that day's dose after dialysis; do not exceed 1.25 mg/kg/24 hrs
Imipenem	R/80	15–25	3.4 hr	1.6 hr	Y	?	?	
Isoniazid	H/3–11	4–30/.71	4.3 hr	?	Y	?	?	
Methicillin	R-H/90	50/0.30	4 hr	?	N	?	?	
Metronidazole	H/20	20/0.90	12 hr	2.7 hr	Y	0.86	Y	Parameters suggest dialysis can occur
Mezlocillin	H-R/50	35/0.26	2.2 hr	1.8 hr	N	0.68	Y	Parameters indicate possible removal by dialysis
Miconazole	H/20	90/2.1	22 hr	22 hr	N	?	?	
Minocycline	H-R/12	76/0.99	20.1 hr	?	N	?	?	
Moxalactam	R/60	45/0.32	20 hr	4.1 hr	?	?	?	
Nafcillin	H/50	90/0.9	2.1 hr	1.7 hr	N	0.19–0.54	?	
Oxacillin	H-R/50	92/0.8	1.0 hr	?	N	0.02	N	
Penicillin G	R-H/60	40/0.36	13 hr	2.3 hr	Y	?	?	
Pentamidine	?/4–29	69/55–165	73–118 hr	10.6 hr	N	?	?	Conflicting parameters do not predict dialysis
Piperacillin	R/75	16/0.26	4.2 hr	1.3 hr	Y	0.78–0.84	Y	Parameters suggest dialysis can occur
Sulbactam*	R/84	38/0.26–.59	15.2 hr	2.3 hr	Y	?	?	Parameters suggest dialysis can occur
Sulfamethoxazole	R/30	65/0.40	24 hr	3.1 hr	Y	0.90	?	Parameters suggest dialysis can occur
Teicoplanin	R/100	93/1.14	206.8 hr	?	N	?	?	Follow levels
Tetracycline	R/48	65/1.3	48 hr	?	N	?	?	Try not to use in renal failure
Ticarcillin	R/90	45/0.17	16 hr	2.7 hr	Y	?	?	
Trimethoprim	R/70	70/1.8	24 hr	6.0 hr	Y	0.30–0.70	?	
Vancomycin	R/90	10–50	100–350 hr	24 hr	Sometimes	0.66–0.79	Y	Follow plasma level for dosing
Vidarabine	R-H/50	20–30/0.7	3.5/— hr	?	?	?	?	
Zidovudine	H/15	35/1.5	1.4 hr	1.0 hr	N	?	?	Reduce dose for anemia and/or granulocytopenia. GAZT metabolite may accumulate in renal failure but not known to be toxic

* These agents are not antibiotics themselves but are combined with some antibiotics as enzyme inhibitors to enhance antibiotic action.
CAVH, Continuous arterial venous hemofiltration; CAVHD, continuous arterial venous hemodialysis; GAZT, 3'-azido-3'-deoxy-5'O-β-D-glucopyranuronosyl/thynidine. ROE, route of elimination being renal (R) or hepatic (H), major route of elimination appears first; %RE, percentage renally eliminated; PB%, percentage protein bound; Vd (l/kg), volume of distribution in l/kg.

may very well result in increased free fractions of highly bound drugs initially and a fall in total drug concentration with increased clearance if volume of distribution does not change. If the decreased binding results in more free drug, allowing greater tissue distribution, clearance may be reduced and drug volume of distribution may be increased. Supplementation of albumin solutions in the ICU situation may reverse the previously mentioned changes. High blood urea nitrogen (BUN) levels in renal failure may alter protein binding molecular structure. Accumulated substances may interfere with or compete for antibiotic protein binding. Liver failure may result in decreased protein production and low protein binding. High bilirubin may displace acidic drugs from protein binding, leading to the complex problems mentioned at the beginning of this paragraph.

Other factors that can alter physiology and antibiotic disposition include capillary leak that is due to elevated BUN, decreased plasma volume that is due to cirrhosis with tissue retention of drug, cardiac failure-induced kidney dysfunction, and hepatic congestion with hypoperfusion and/or hypoxemia. Mechanical ventilation with positive end-expiratory pressure (PEEP) may cause increased venous pressures and cause attendant decreased hepatic blood flow. PEEP-induced secretion of antidiuretic hormone (ADH) may increase, thus increasing antibiotic vol-

Table 66-7. Adverse Antibiotic Reactions That May Have Some Relationship to Pharmacokinetic Alterations and Accumulation in Renal Dysfunction

Neurotoxicity: Causes Neuropsychiatric Symptoms	
Acyclovir	Foscarnet
Amantidine	Gancyclovir
Neurotoxicity: Seizures	
Penicillin G	Cefazolin
Ciprofloxacin	Metronidazole
Other penicillins	Ceftazidime
Imipenem	
Ototoxicity	
Aminoglycosides	Erythromycin
Vancomycin	
Bleeding	
Piperacillin	Mezlocillin
Ticarcillin	Azlocillin
Carbenicillin	
Bone Marrow suppression	
Gancyclovir	

ume of distribution. All the previously mentioned possibilities may affect the pharmacokinetic disposition of antibiotics; these are not quantified, however, for the MOD patient.[231-241]

BETA-LACTAM PHARMACOKINETICS

Pharmacokinetics of Penicillins, Carbapenems, and Monobactams

The penicillins (amdinocillin, ampicillin, azlocillin, carbenicillin, penicillin G, piperacillin, ticarcillin) are all predominantly renally excreted. Antibiotic half-lives increase from 0.5 to 2 hours in normal renal function to 3 to 15 times the normal renal function half-life with creatinine clearances less than 10 ml per minute. Dose intervals need to be prolonged when renal dysfunction is encountered (see Table 66-5). Most of these agents are hemodialyzed and may require dose supplementation after hemodialysis. Extra dose supplementation can be avoided by scheduling doses after dialysis on days of hemodialysis. Doses should not be administered just before or during dialysis, because this will excessively remove antibiotic. Mezlocillin has only 50% renal elimination and 50% liver elimination, and therefore, little is considered dialyzed, but in reality, the liver elimination compensates for the renal dysfunction. Renal excretion therefore is not the rate-limiting step to elimination of this antibiotic. The same reasoning for not administering the other penicillin doses just before or during hemodialysis is true for mezlocillin also. Less is known about CAVH removal of these agents, but ampicillin, mezlocillin, and piperacillin are removed. More information needs to be gathered on the others. The protein binding of less than 50% and volumes of distribution less than 0.36 L/kg indicate they may well be removed by CAVH.

The carbapenem, imipenem, and monobactam aztreonam, although not penicillins, have very similar pharmacokinetic parameters to the penicillins, are renally excreted, and are hemodialyzed. Little is known, however, about CAVH removal of these agents.

Pharmacokinetics of Antistaphylococcal Penicillins

The antistaphylococcal penicillins as a class generally differ from the penicillins. Two of the three agents (oxacillin and nafcillin) are predominantly dependent on hepatic elimination whereas methicillin is 90% renally eliminated. Protein binding is greater than the other penicillins, at 50 to 92%. Even with this greater protein binding of the antistaphylococcal penicillins, the volume of distribution is greater, at 0.3 to 0.9 L/kg, rather than 0.15 to 0.36 L/kg for the other penicillins. Renal dysfunction has little effect on antibiotic half-life except for methicillin, which requires the greatest prolongation of dose intervals in renal dysfunction. The agents are not considered to be removed by hemodialysis, which is possibly related to the higher protein binding and/or the fact that two of the three agents are removed by the liver and renal elimination or dialysis is not the rate-limiting step. No doses are needed after hemodialysis, but it is still not advisable to administer these antibiotics just before or during dialysis. Based on the pharmacokinetic parameters of oxacillin and nafcillin, one would not expect CAVH removal of these drugs. Although the effect of CAVH on methicillin is not known, the kinetic parameters indicate that this drug may be more susceptible to removal by CAVH.

Pharmacokinetics of Cephalosporin Antibiotics

The cephalosporins have a number of similarities and differences when compared to the penicillins. Of the 17 cephalosporins listed earlier, in Table 66-5, 10 (cefazolin, cephalothin, cefamandole, cefonicid, ceforanide, cefotetan, cefoxitin, cefmetazole, cefoperazone, and ceftriaxone) have protein binding in excess of 50% while penicillin protein binding is less than 50%. This probably accounts partially for the lower volume of distribution of these 10 cephalosporins at 0.12 to 0.26 L/kg. The other seven cephalosporins (cephapirin, cephradine, cefuroxime, cefotaxime, ceftazidime, moxalactam, and ceftizoxime) have protein binding values less than 50% with a generally larger volume of distribution range of 0.2 to 0.36 L/kg, which is much the same as the penicillins. Most cephalosporins are considered removed by hemodialysis even with high protein binding and after hemodialysis doses are usually recommended except for the four agents that undergo hepatic elimination (cephapirin, cefoperazone, cefotaxime, and ceftriaxone). Cephalosporin half-lives in normal renal function range from 0.6 to 10 hours and increase to 3 to 60 hours when creatinine clearance is less than 10 ml per minute. The hepatically eliminated cephalosporins have minimal renal dysfunction changes in half-life, requiring less dose-interval adjustments than those that are eliminated renally. Second- and third-generation cephalosporins generally have longer drug half-lives (and many longer dose intervals) than the penicillins or first-generation cephalosporins in normal renal function. The hepatically eliminated cephalosporins either are not hemodialyzed or pharmacokinetic parameters indicate that little dialysis should occur. Cephapirin and ceftazidime are removed by CAVH, and little or no information is available on the other 15 cephalosporins.

PHARMACOKINETICS OF ANTIFUNGALS

Two of the four commercially available intravenous antifungals (amphotericin, miconazole) have minimal renal excretion; both are not considered to be removed by hemodialysis and most likely also are not removed by CAVH. The high volume of distribution of these agents (2.1 to 4.0 L/kg) indicates distribution and binding to deep tissue compartments. These agents do not require dose adjustments for renal failure because of alteration in pharmacokinetic parameters. Amphotericin dose intervals are prolonged (see Table 66-5) in an attempt to stem nephrotoxicity from the drug. In clinical practice, every-other-day amphotericin has been used to prevent further renal dysfunction. Again, it is hard to determine which patient factors are involved with this renal dysfunction; and increasing amphotericin doses in serious fungal infections may improve renal function. The antifungals fluconazole and flucytosine are highly renally eliminated with great prolongations of drug half-life in renal failure, and they require dose-interval adjustments. Protein binding of these agents is minimal at 5 to 11%, and volume of distribution is 0.6 to 1 L/kg, indicating these drugs are not distributed as deeply in tissue as amphotericin or miconazole. The influence of this on clinical outcome is not known.

PHARMACOKINETICS OF ANTIVIRALS

The antiviral agents acyclovir, amantadine, foscarnet, and ganciclovir are highly renally eliminated, with marked prolongations of drug half-life in renal dysfunction. Although amantadine is not available in the intravenous preparation, it is included here because the drug is administered through nasogastric tubes and has a high incidence of central nervous system toxicity if the dose is not reduced appropriately. This drug has the greatest volume of distribution of these three agents at 4 to 5 L/kg, indicating deep tissue distribution. Although half-life of amantadine is reduced markedly during hemodialysis, no additional doses are needed after dialysis, probably because of the deep tissue stores of the drug.

Both acyclovir and ganciclovir require doses after hemodialysis, but again, this may be avoided by administering that day's dosage after hemodialysis and by not giving the dose just before or during hemodialysis.

Foscarnet is 90% renal excreted with a normal half-life of 3 hours. The drug itself can cause renal dysfunction. The drug is 14 to 17% protein bound, and volume of distribution is only 0.3 to 0.6 L/kg. Induction and maintenance dosages are based on creatinine clearance per kilogram body weight. The creatinine clearance formula is a modified Cockcroft and Gault formula, and package insert recommendations should be followed closely.

Vidarabine undergoes approximately 50% kidney and 50% liver elimination. It is not known if doses are needed after hemodialysis. Because vidarabine is administered every 24 hours, this dose should be scheduled after that day's dialysis and not before or during hemodialysis.

Zidovudine is an antiviral that is 85% liver metabolized with the GAZT metabolite predominating. Little prolongation of zidovudine half life occurs with renal dysfunction; GAZT, however, which is renally excreted, has a marked prolongation of half-life. It is not believed that zidovudine requires an extra dose after hemodialysis, and removal by CAVH is not known. Paoli and colleagues[221] recently measured zidovudine and GAZT levels in three patients with end-stage renal disease undergoing hemodialysis three times weekly and one patient with a creatinine clearance of 20 ml per minute. These patients received zidovudine 100 mg three times daily (rather than six times daily) and maintained adequate trough zidovudine levels. Confirmation of their work may be needed. Dose reductions in liver disease are not known.

THE USE OF COMPUTER PROGRAMS FOR AMINOGLYCOSIDE/VANCOMYCIN DOSING

Computer programs for AGS and vancomycin dosing are readily available for programmable hand calculators, MS-DOS computers, and a few for Apple computers. These programs take the drudgery out of calculating volume of distribution, elimination rates, and drug half-lives. They also save time involved in the calculations and standardize the procedure in determination of the various pharmacokinetics parameters used in calculating dose and dosage interval. A personal computer is needed for the more complex two-compartment modeling that some programs can perform because of the complexity of the math and the extra time required in computation. An extremely inexpensive and reliable set of clinical pharmacokinetic programs[5,242] is available as the USC PACK clinical and research pharmacokinetic adaptive control programs from Dr. Roger Jelliffe at the Laboratory of Applied Clinical Pharmacokinetics, University of Southern California School of Medicine, CSC 135D, 2250 Alcazar Street, Los Angeles, CA 90033 (213-342-1300). A one-time fee is required for the technical booklets and phone support (there is no charge for the computer program itself). This is an MS-DOS program that requires a math co-processor, and the math chips run anywhere in price from $75.00 to $500 depending on the type of computer used.[243]

Pharmacokinetic Computer Guidance Systems

Aminoglycoside and Vancomycin Case Study in Good Renal Function

Patient 1 was a 32-year-old 66.4-kg white man admitted to Cleveland Clinic Foundation Hospital after a brick was thrown through his car window, causing a depressed skull fracture and epidural hematoma. The patient was taken to surgery for a craniotomy and drainage of the hematoma and admitted to the NICU. On the seventh postoperative day, he developed fever, severe sinusitis, aspiration pneumonia, and staphylococcal and gram-negative bacteremia. He was started on gentamicin 80 mg every 8 hours and vancomycin 1000 mg every 12 hours. Serum creatinine was 0.7 mg/dL, calculated creatinine clearance was 141 ml per minute per 1.73 m² urine output averaged 101 ml per hour, and white blood cell counts were 11,900/ml. The ICU population model indicated that 80 mg of gentamicin every 8 hours would be inadequate, and a dosage of 250 mg every 8 hours was instituted. Predose and postdose gentamicin levels were returned at 0.5 μg/ml and 5.6 μg/ml, respectively, with actual immediate predose trough and immediate postdose peak gentamicin levels of 0.49 μg/ml and 6.90 μg/ml, respectively. The gentamicin pharmacokinetic parameters obtained included a half-life of 1.926 hours, Vd of 0.48 L/kg ABW. Actual peak gentamicin levels of 10 to 12 μg/ml were targeted, and the gentamicin dose was increased to 400 mg every 8 hours.

Predose and postdose vancomycin levels were 5.10 μg/ml and 21.2 μg/ml while receiving a vancomycin dosage of 1000 mg every 8 hours on the second day of therapy (drawn on the sixth dose). Vancomycin two-compartment pharmacokinetic parameters indicated that the half-life beta was 4.99 hours, volume of the central compartment (Vc) = 0.18 L/kg, KCP was 0.4681 hours−1, KPC was 0.2676 hours−1 where KCP is the rate constant central to the peripheral compartment and KPC is the rate constant peripheral to the central compartment. Vancomycin dosage was increased to 1200 mg every 6 hours to obtain predose vancomycin levels of 10 to 15 μg/ml. Antibiotics were discontinued on day 4 of antibiotic therapy after the third dose of gentamicin, 400 mg every 8 hours, and after the third dose of vancomycin, 1200 mg every 6 hours, and urine output had been maintained and serum creatinine had decreased to 0.6 mg/dl. Maximum daily temperature had declined from 38.7°C to 37.6°C.

Therapy was stopped because hearing loss was noted, and an audiogram test was ordered. The official report, 3 days later, showed a bilateral conductive hearing loss confirmed by audiogram, which indicated that the hearing loss was not due to AGSs or vancomycin. During this lapse in antibiotic coverage, the patient's fever had climbed to 39.6°C, serum creatinine increased to 0.8 mg/dl, and white blood cell counts were 26,560/ml, which indicated an uncontrolled infection. Antibiotics were reinstituted with ceftazidime, 2 g every 8 hours; tobramycin, 400 mg every 8 hours; and vancomycin, 1200 mg every 6 hours. Two days later metronidazole, 500 mg every 4 hours, was added, and the ceftazidime dosage was increased to 2 g every 6 hours (these high doses were instituted knowing the patient was excreting the AGS and vancomycin very quickly, so he was assumed to also be excreting these antibiotics quickly). Serum creatinine was 0.7 mg/dl, urine output was greater than 100 ml per hour, and temperature maximum was 38.8°C. Tobramycin predose and postdose levels of 400 mg every 8 hours were 0.2 μg/ml and 6.8 μg/ml (Fig. 66-6). Actual immediate postinfusion peak tobramycin levels were 10.53 μg/ml. Tobramycin kinetics indicated a shorter half-life of 1.2 hours and a large Vd of 0.48 L/kg. Because of the severity of the infection, a new immediate postinfusion target peak of 15 μg/ml was set, and a tobramycin dose of 500 mg every 6 hours was instituted, with maximum temperature decreasing to below 38°C 4 days later and serum creatinine declining to 0.4 mg/dl.

Vancomycin predose and postdose levels on day 3 of therapy with 1200 mg every 6 hours were 10.8 μg/ml and 28.0 μg/ml (Fig. 66-7). Vancomycin pharmacokinetic parameters at this time indicated that the half-life beta was 3.52 hours, and Vc was 0.41 L/kg. A dosage of 1200 mg every 6 hours was continued until day 10 of therapy, when dosage was reduced to 1 g every 8 hours. Repeat predose and postdose tobramycin levels on the regimen of 500 mg

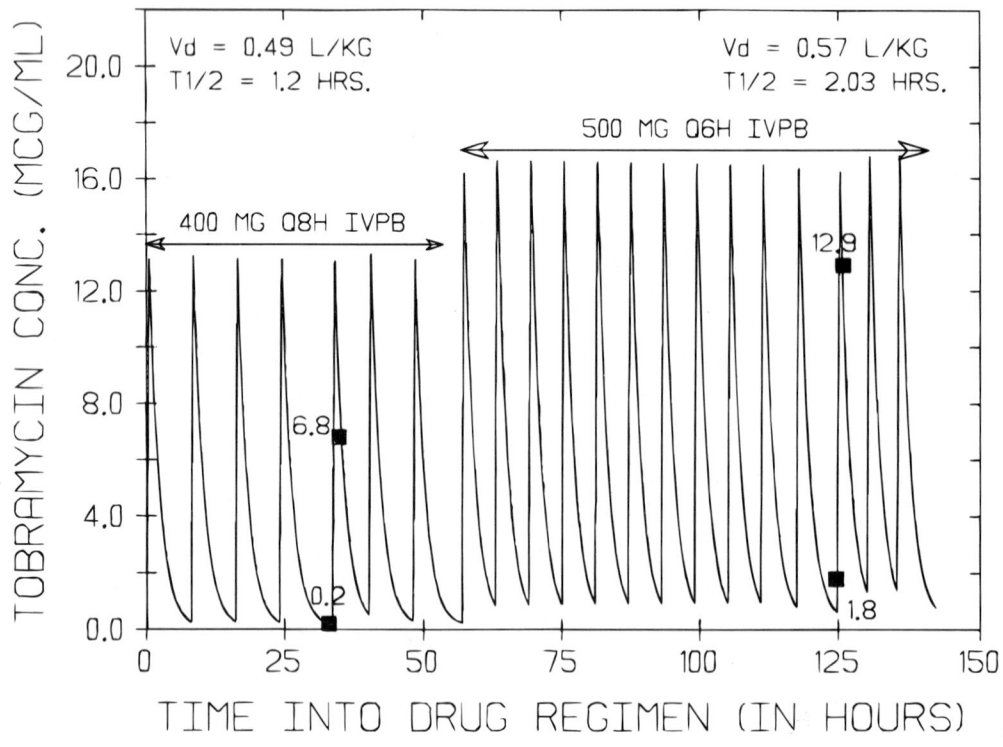

Fig. 66-6. Tobramycin concentration versus time in patient B. B. with good renal function. Closed squares represent measured tobramycin concentrations, and solid lines show the patient B. B.'s pharmacokinetic model-generated tobramycin concentration. Because of the large volume of distribution (Vd) of 0.49 to 0.57 L/kg and short half-life (T½) of 1.2 to 2.0 hours, large tobramycin doses at short-dose intervals were needed to achieve therapeutic levels. Serum creatinine never exceeded 0.7 mg% during or after tobramycin therapy. IVPB, Intravenous "piggyback."

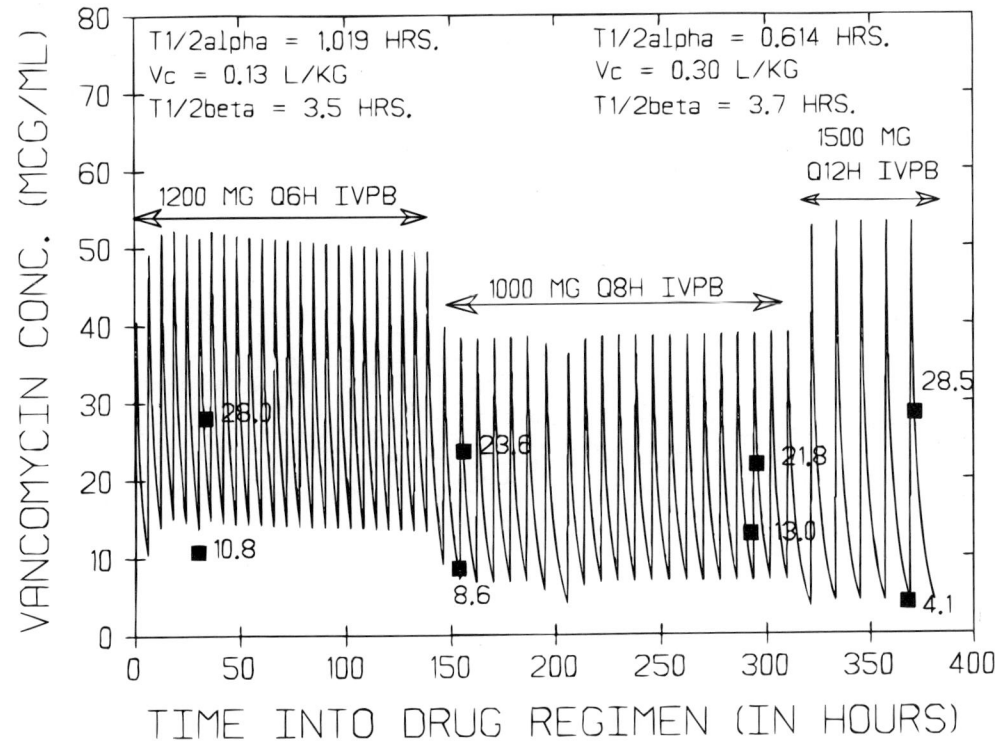

Fig. 66-7. Vancomycin concentration versus time in patient B. B. with good renal function. Closed squares represent measured vancomycin concentrations, and solid lines show the patient B. B.'s pharmacokinetic model-generated vancomycin concentration. Pharmacokinetic analysis indicated a short vancomycin half-life (T½) beta of 3.5 to 3.7 hours. Based on an earlier course of vancomycin therapy, and the short half-life beta, an initial dosage of 1200 mg q6h was chosen to obtain predose vancomycin levels of 10 to 15 μg/ml. The dose interval was prolonged as the patient's clinical condition improved. Serum creatinine never exceeded 0.7 mg/dl. IVPB, Intravenous "piggy back;" Vc, volume of central compartment.

every 6 hours (day 6) indicated levels of 1.8 μg/ml and 12.9 μg/ml, respectively. Actual immediate predose trough levels were 1.76 μg/ml, and actual immediate postdose peak levels were 15.05 μg/ml. The dosage was reduced to 500 mg every 8 hours, and a total of 7 days of tobramycin was given. Vancomycin predose and postdose levels on day 14 of the second course of therapy were 13 μg/ml and 21.8 μg/ml, respectively. Vancomycin was continued at a dose of 1000 mg every 8 hours and, finally, 1500 mg every 12 hours, when the patient improved (total of 23 days of vancomycin). Serum creatinine never exceeded 0.7 mg% during the balance of the antibiotic treatment course. The patient was discharged to an extended care facility for rehabilitation after 48 days in the hospital.

Aminoglycoside and Vancomycin Case Study in Anuric Renal Failure and Hemodialysis

Patient 2 was a 37-year-old 74.5-kg white man admitted for right shoulder pain and fever that began 2 days before admission. He was anuric (from prior bilateral nephrectomy) and being hemodialyzed three times a week. He was admitted to the surgical ICU with a fever of 39.4°C and a diagnosis of S. aureus sepsis, septic arthritis, possible pneumonia, respiratory failure, and slight left ventricular dysfunction. Staphylococcal aureus was isolated from blood, sputum, the right shoulder abscess, and right shoulder fluid. The patient was started on one dose each of tobramycin 140 mg and vancomycin 1000 mg. The patient received hemodialysis on the second day of antibiotic therapy for 3 hours. An additional dose of tobramycin 140 mg was given after dialysis with predose and postdose tobramycin levels of 1.70 and 4.00 μg/ml (Fig. 66-8). The peak immediately after infusion was 5.24 μg/ml, and the immediate predose level was 1.47 μg/ml. Tobramycin pharmacokinetic parameters indicated a half-life of 30.66 hours and Vd of .42 L/kg ABW. The next dose of vancomycin 1 g was given 36 hours after the first dose, but the vancomycin level measured 27 hours after the first dose was 10.7 μg/ml even in total anuria. The postdose vancomycin level was measured at 29.4 μg/ml, but the immediate postinfusion level was 64.45 μg/ml (Fig. 66-9). Vancomycin kinetics on day 3 of treatment indicated a half-life alpha of 1.014 hours, half-life beta of 160.2 hours, Vc of 0.151 L/kg, KPC of .4560 hour-1, and KPC of .1107 hour-1. The patient was discharged from the ICU on day 6 of antibiotic therapy and received intermittent hemodialysis sessions on days 3, 6, 8, 10, 11, 13, 16, 18, 19, 20 of antibiotic therapy. The third dose of tobramycin 250 mg was given 40.5 hours after the second dose of tobramycin (day 4 of antibiotics) with predose/postdose measured levels of 2.50 μg/ml and 8.2 μg/ml, respectively. The actual peak level was 8.46 μg/ml immediately after infusion, the tobramycin half-life had prolonged to 52.7 hours, and Vd was 0.52 L/kg. The dose interval to the next dose was not expected for over a week, and the half-life showed another prolongation to 112 hours. Figure 66-8 indicates the removal of tobramycin by hemodialysis also. Vancomycin was continued, and now the dose intervals between the second and third dose were 124 hours, and between dose 3 and 4, 132 hours. Vancomycin half-life beta then began to prolong to greater than 550 hours. The last dose of vancomycin was on day 13 of antibiotics, and the vancomycin level was still 16.4 μg/ml on day 45 of antibiotic therapy. This clearly

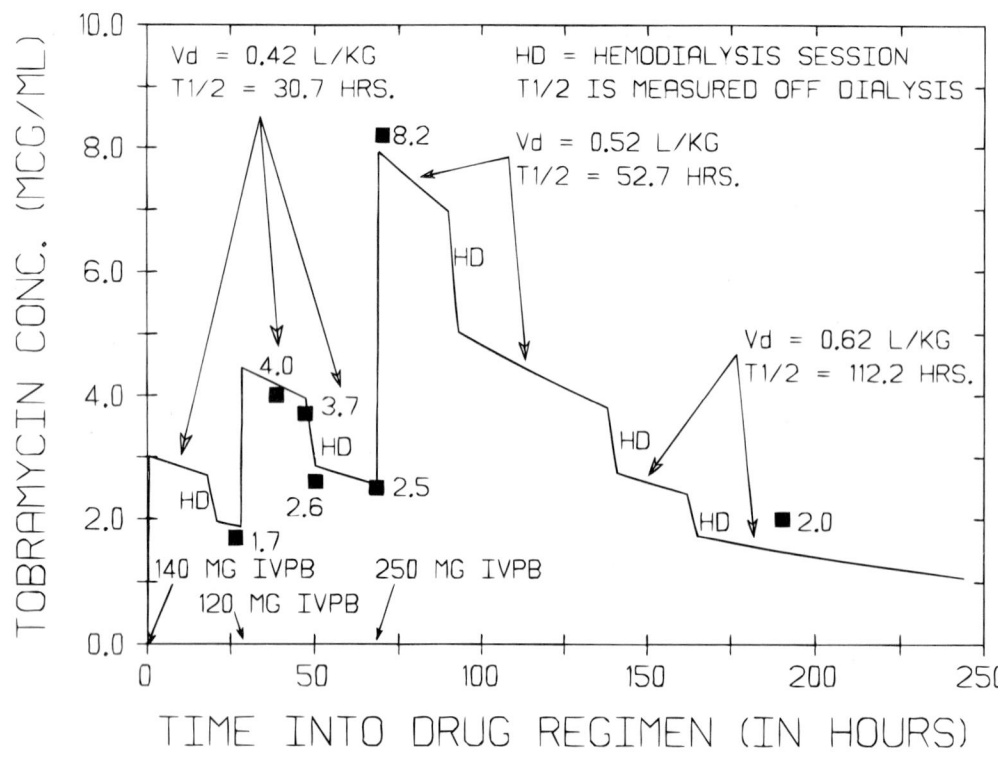

Fig. 66–8. Tobramycin concentration versus time in patient G. T. with anuria and hemodialysis. Closed squares represent measured tobramycin concentrations, and solid lines show the patient G. T.'s pharmacokinetic model-generated tobramycin concentration. The tobramycin half-life increased from 30.7 to 52.7 to 112.2 hours as dosing continued. This is a characteristic prolongation of half-life (T½) that occurs in anuric patients that results in prolongation of dose intervals with continued therapy. Hemodialysis readily reduces tobramycin concentrations, but additional doses were not needed after each hemodialysis session, as most literature would have us believe. Vd, Volume of distribution.

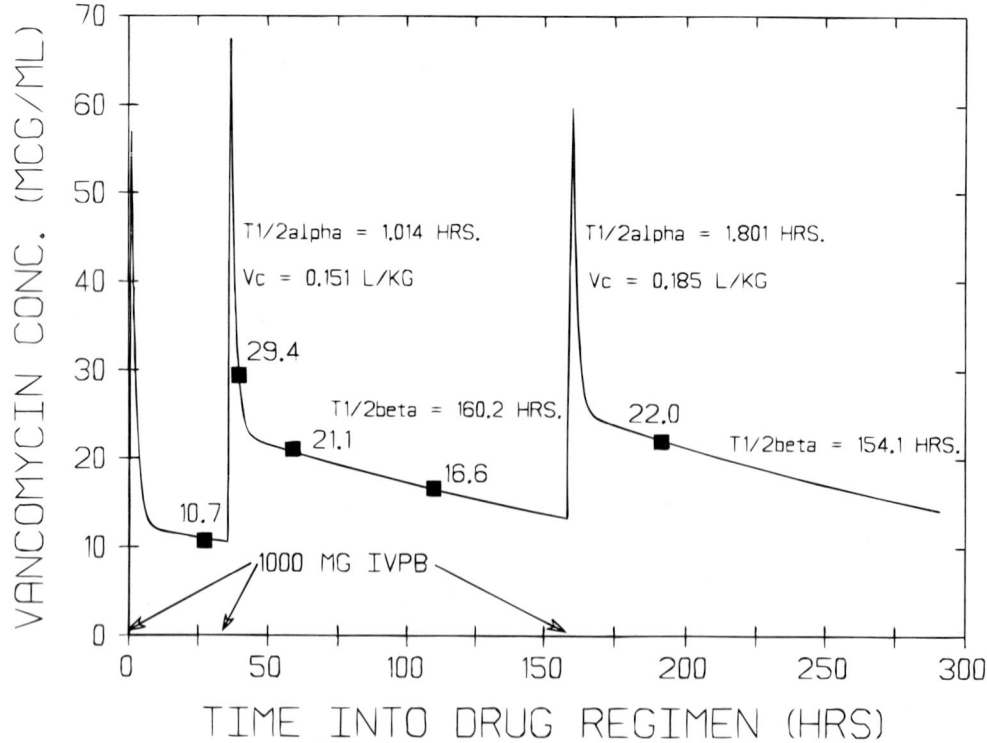

Fig. 66–9. Vancomycin concentration versus time in patient G. T. with anuria and hemodialysis. Closed squares represent measured vancomycin concentrations, and solid lines show the patient's G. T.'s pharmacokinetic model-generated vancomycin concentration. The figure points out that in the ICU patients with anuric renal failure can be readministered an additional dose of vancomycin 12 to 24 hours after the initial dose when levels are 10 to 15 μg/ml. This is in contrast to the accepted once-a-week dosing rule for hemodialysis patients. After the second dose, a prolongation of dose interval should occur as half-life (T½) beta becomes prolonged, and eventually half-life beta was greater than 550 hours. After one more dose of 1000 mg of vancomycin (not shown on graph) on day thirteen, there was no need for further doses until after day 45, when a measured level was 16.4 μg/ml. IVPB, Intravenous "piggy back;" Vc, volume of central compartment.

indicates the phenomenon of increasing dosage interval with vancomycin that can occur with aggressive dosing in anuria. This patient had no influence of dialysis removal of vancomycin because the cuprophane filter type was used, and it was not necessary to build hemodialysis into the dosing model. The patient was discharged after 20 days of hospitalization with plenty of vancomycin to last for an additional 25 days as an outpatient.

REFERENCES

1. Gibaldi, M., and Perrier, D.: Pharmacokinetics. 2nd Ed. Philadelphia, Lea & Febiger, 1982.
2. Benet, L. Z., and Massoud, N.: Pharmacokinetics. In Pharmacokinetic Basis for Drug Treatment. Edited by L. Z. Benet, N. Massoud, and J. G. Gambertoglio. New York, Raven Press, 1984.
3. Gibaldi, M.: Biopharmaceutics and Clinical Pharmacokinetics. 2nd Ed. Philadelphia, Lea & Febiger, 1977.
4. Niazi, S.: Textbook of Biopharmaceutics and Clinical Pharmacokinetics. Norwalk, CT: Appleton-Century-Crofts, 1979.
5. Jelliffe, R. W., and Schumitsky, A.: Modeling, adaptive control, and optimal drug therapy. Med. Prog. Technol., *16:*95, 1990.
6. D'Argenio, D. Z., and Schumitzky, A.: A program package for simulation and parameter estimation in pharmacokinetic systems. Comp. Prog. Biomed., *9:*115, 1979.
7. Schentag, J. J. et al.: Aminoglycoside nephrotoxicity in critically ill surgical patients. J. Surg. Res., *26:*270, 1979.
8. Brumfitt, W., and Hamilton-Miller, J. M. T.: Principles and practice of antimicrobial chemotherapy. In Avery's Drug Treatment: Principles and Practice of Clinical Pharmacology and Therapeutics. 3rd Ed. Edited by T. M. Speight. Auckland, ADIS Press, 1987.
9. Kreger, B. E., Craven, D. E., and McCabe, W. R.: Gram-negative bacteremia. IV. Re-evaluation of clinical features and treatment of 612 patients. Am. J. Med., *68:*344, 1980.
10. McNeeley, S. et al.: Delayed gentamicin elimination in patients with severe preeclampsia. Am. J. Obstet. Gynecol., *153:*793, 1985.
11. Zaske, D. E. et al.: Rapid gentamicin elimination in obstetric patients. Obstet. Gynecol., *56:*559, 1980.
12. Lazebnik, N. et al.: Gentamicin serum half-life: a comparison between pregnant and non-pregnant women. Postgrad. Med., *61:*979, 1985.
13. Philipson, A.: Pharmacokinetics of antibiotics in pregnancy and labour. Clin. Pharmacokinet., *4:*297, 1979.
14. Zaske, D. E., Sawchuk, R. J., Gerding, D. N., and Strate, R. G.: Increased dosage requirements of gentamicin in burn patients. J. Trauma, *16:*824, 1976.
15. Zaske, D. E., Bootman, J. L., Solem, L. B., and Strate, R. G.: Increased burn patient survival with individualized doses of gentamicin. Surgery, *9:*142, 1982.
16. Segal, J. L. et al.: Pharmacokinetics of gentamicin in patients with spinal cord injury. Clin. Pharm., *3:*418, 1984.
17. Meyers, B. R., and Wilkinson, P.: Clinical pharmacokinetics of antibacterial drugs in the elderly: implications for selection and dosage. Clin. Pharmacokinet., *17:*385, 1989.
18. Bonate, P. L.: Pathophysiology and pharmacokinetics following burn injury. Clin. Pharmacokinet., *18:*118, 1990.
19. Morgan, D. J., and Smallwood, R. A.: Clinical significance of pharmacokinetic models of hepatic elimination. Clin. Pharmacokinet., *18:*61, 1990.
20. Segal, J. L., and Brunnemann, S. R.: Clinical pharmacokinetics in patients with spinal cord injuries. Clin. Pharmacokinet., *17:*109, 1989.
21. Durnas, C., Loi, C. M., and Cusack, B. J.: Hepatic drug metabolism and aging. Clin. Pharmacokinet., *19:*359, 1990.
22. deGroot, R., and Smith, A. L.: Antibiotic pharmacokinetics in cystic fibrosis: differences and clinical significance. Clin. Pharmacokinet., *13:*228, 1987.
23. Manoogian, C., Naler, J., Ehrlich, L., and Horton, R.: The renal vasodilating effect of dopamine is mediated by calcium flux and prostacyclin release in man. J. Clin. Endocrinol. Metab., *66:*678, 1988.
24. Kincaid-Smith, P.: Effects of non-narcotic analgesics on the kidney. Drugs, *32(Suppl. 4):*109, 1986.
25. Halton, J., and Haagensen, D.: Renal dysfunction associated with ciprofloxacin. Pharmcotherapy, *10:*337, 1990.
26. Blackshear, J. L., Davidman, M., and Stillman, M. T.: Identification of risk for renal insufficiency from nonsteroidal anti-inflammatory drugs. Arch. Intern. Med., *143:*1130, 1983.
27. Clive, D. M., and Stoff, J. S.: Renal syndromes associated with nonsteroidal anti-inflammatory drugs. N. Engl. J. Med., *310:*563, 1984.
28. Linton, A. L. et al.: Acute interstitial nephritis due to drugs. Ann. Intern. Med., *93:*735, 1980.
29. Cohen, D. J. et al.: Cyclosporine: a new immunosuppressive agent for organ transplantation. Ann. Intern. Med., *101:*667, 1984.
30. Moyer, T. P. et al.: Cyclosporine nephrotoxicity is minimized by adjusting dosage on the basis of drug concentration in blood. Mayo Clin. Proc., *63:*241, 1988.
31. Finley, R. S., Fortner, C. L., and Grove, W. R.: Cisplatin nephrotoxicity: a summary of preventative interventions. Drug Intell. Clin. Pharm., *19:*362, 1985.
32. Berns, A. S.: Nephrotoxicity of contrast media. Kidney Int., *36:*730, 1989.
33. Solez, K., Racusen, L. C., and Olsen, S.: The pathology of drug nephrotoxicity. J. Clin. Pharmacol., *23:*484, 1983.
34. Lieberthal, W., and Leninsky, N. G.: Treatment of acute tubular necrosis. Semin. Nephrol., *10:*571, 1990.
35. Berad, K., Perera, D. R., and Jich, H.: Drug-induced parenchymal renal disease in outpatients. J. Clin. Pharmacol., *28:*431, 1988.
36. Cooper, K., and Bennet, W. M.: Nephrotoxicity of common drugs used in clinical practice. Arch. Intern. Med., *146:*1213, 1987.
37. Paller, M. S.: Drug-induced nephropathies. Med. Clin. North Am., *74:*909, 1990.
38. Abraham, P. A., and Matzke, G. R.: Drug-induced renal disease. In Dipiro, J. T. et al. (eds.). Pharmacotherapy: a pathophysiologic approach. New York, Elsevier Science, 1989.
39. Moran, M., and Kapsner, C.: Acute renal failure associated with elevated plasma oncotic pressure. N. Engl. J. Med., *317:*150, 1987.
40. Mason, N. A.: Angiotensin-converting enzyme inhibitors and renal function. DICP. Ann. Pharmacother., *24:*496, 1990.
41. Interferences seen on ASTRA systems chemistries. Astra Advisor, *16:*1, 1982.
42. Larsson, R., Bodemer, G., Kagedal, B., and Walan, A.: The effects of cimetadine (Tagamet) in patients with renal failure. Acta. Med. Scand., *208:*27, 1980.
43. Berglund, F., Killander, J., and Pompeius, R.: Effect of trimethoprim-sulfamethoxazole on the renal excretion of creatinine in man. J. Urol., *114:*802, 1975.
44. Davis, J. P. et al.: Tri-state toxic-shock syndrome study. II. Clinical and laboratory findings. J. Infect. Dis., *145:*441, 1982.
45. Slotki, I. N., MacIver, J. E., Mallick, N. P., and Palmer, H. M.: Acute intravascular hemolysis with minimal renal impairment in Clostridium perfringins infection. Clin. Nephrol., *6:*451, 1976.

46. Sinnassamy, P., Landthaler, G., and Vasmant, D.: Acute renal insufficiency of glomerular origin and staphylococcal infection. A report of two cases in pediatric patients. Ann. Pediatr., *33*:191, 1986.
47. Cone, L. A., Woodard, D. R., Schlievert, P. M., and Tomory, G. S.: Clinical and bacteriologic observations of a toxic shock-like syndrome due to Streptococcus pyogenes. N. Engl. J. Med., *317*:146, 1987.
48. Scully, R. E., Mark, E. J., McNeely, W. F., and McNeely, B. U.: Weekly clinicopathological exercises—Case 4-1988. N. Engl. J. Med., *318*:234, 1988.
49. Hagemann, V. I. et al.: Nierenfunktion, bakteriologische un histologische untersuchungen bei therapie der experimentellen E.-coli pyelonephritis mit trimethoprim-sulfamethoxazol (TMP-SMO). Z. Urol. Nephrol., *78*:681, 1985.
50. Hagemann, V. I. et al.: Bakteriologische, histologische und Funktionsuntersuchungen der Niere bei 5tagiger Therapie der experimentellen E. coli pyelonephritis mit gentamycin. Vergleich mit 9tagiger therapie. Z. Urol. Nephrol., *78*:625, 1985.
51. Cockram, C. S., and Bax, R. P.: The safety of cefuroxime and gentamicin in patients with reduced renal function. Curr. Med. Res., *6*:398, 1980.
52. Leunk, R. D., and Moon, R. J.: Physiological and metabolic alterations accompanying systemic candidiasis in mice. Infect. Immunol., *26*:1035, 1979.
53. Sobel, J. D.: Candida infections in the intensive care unit. Crit. Care Clin., *4*:325, 1988.
54. Haug, M., Slugg, P., Lockrem, J., and Brynes, J.: High dose aminoglycoside (AGS) therapy in surgical ICU patients. Clin. Pharmacol. Ther., *47*:208, 1990.
55. Barriere, S. L.: Aminoglycosides: a reassessment of their therapeutic role. Clin. Pharm., *7*:385, 1988.
56. Killilea, T.: Happy birthday gentamicin. Hosp. Pharm., *25*:55, 1990.
57. Murphy, J. E.: Aminoglycosides: another look at current and future roles in antimicrobial therapy. Pharmacotherapy, *10*:217, 1990.
58. Zaske, D. E. et al.: Gentamicin pharmacokinetics in 1,640 patients: method for control of serum concentrations. Antimicrob. Agents Chemother., *21*:407, 1982.
59. Tablan, O. C., Reyes, M. P., Rintelmann, W. F., and Lerner, A. M.: Renal and auditory toxicity of high-dose, prolonged therapy with gentamicin and tobramycin in pseudomonas endocarditis. J. Infect. Dis., *149*:257, 1984.
60. Zaske, D. E. et al.: Wide interpatient variations in gentamicin dose requirements for geriatric patients. J. Am. Med. Assoc., *248*:3122, 1982.
61. Shenep, J. L., Barton, R. P., and Mogan, K. A.: Role of antibiotic class in rate of liberation of endotoxin during therapy for experimental gram-negative bacterial sepsis. J. Infect. Dis., *151*:1012, 1985.
62. Grimwood, K., To, M., Rabin, H. R., and Woods, D. E.: Inhibition of Pseudomonas aeruginosa exoenzyme expression by subinhibitory antibiotic concentrations. Antimicrob. Agents Chemother., *33*:41, 1989.
63. Snell, K., Holder, I. R., Leppla, S. A., and Saelinger, C. B.: Role of exotoxin and protease as possible virulence factors in experimental infections with Pseudomonas aeruginosa. Infect. Immun., *19*:839, 1978.
64. Ogaard, A. R., Bjoro, K., Bukholm, G., and Berdal, B. P.: Pseudomonas aeruginosa virulence factors: modifications by sub-inhibitory concentrations of carbenicillin or gentamicin. Acta Pathol. Microbiol. Immunol. Scand., *94*:63, 1986.
65. Jackson, G. G., and Riff, L. J.: Pseudomonas bacteremia: pharmacologic and other basis for failure of treatment with gentamicin. J. Infect. Dis., *124*:S185, 1971.
66. Noone, P. et al.: Experience in monitoring gentamicin therapy during treatment of serious gram-negative sepsis. Br. Med. J., *1*:477, 1974.
67. Hall, W. H., and Gerding, D. N.: Penetration of tobramycin into infected extravascular fluids and its therapeutic effectiveness. J. Infect. Dis., *135*:957, 1977.
68. Zaske, D. E., Bootman, J. L., Solem, L. B., and Strate, R. G.: Increased burn patient survival with individualized dosages of gentamicin. Surgery, *91*:142, 1982.
69. Moore, R. D., Smith, C. R., and Lietman, P. S.: The association of aminoglycoside plasma levels with mortality in patients with gram-negative bacteremia. J. Infect. Dis., *149*:443, 1984.
70. Moore, R. D., Smith, C. R., and Lietman, P. S.: Association of aminoglycoside levels with therapeutic outcome in gram-negative pneumonia. Am. J. Med., *77*:657, 1984.
71. Williams, P. J. et al.: Factors associated with nephrotoxicity and clinical outcome in patients receiving amikacin. J. Clin. Pharmacol., *26*:79, 1986.
72. Deziel-Evans, L., Murphy, J. E., and Job, M. L.: Correlation of pharmacokinetic indices with therapeutic outcome in patients receiving aminoglycosides. Clin. Pharm., *5*:319, 1986.
73. Gill, M. A. et al.: Matched case-control study of adjusted versus nonadjusted gentamicin dosing in perforated and gangrenous appendicitis. Ther. Drug Monit., *8*:451, 1986.
74. Anderson, E. T., Young, L. S., and Hewitt, W. L.: Simultaneous antibiotic levels in "breakthrough" gram negative rod bacteremias. Am. J. Med., *61*:493, 1976.
75. Moore, R. D., Lietman, P. S., and Smith, C. R.: Clinical response to aminoglycoside therapy: importance of the ratio of peak concentration to minimal inhibitory concentration. J. Infect. Dis., *155*:93, 1987.
76. Moore, R. D., Lietman, P. S., and Smith, C. R.: Reply—clinical response and peak concentrations of aminoglycosides. J. Infect. Dis., *157*:395, 1988.
77. The EORTC International Antimicrobial Therapy Cooperative Group: Ceftazidime combined with a short or long course of amikacin for empirical therapy of gram-negative bacteremia in cancer patients with granulocytopenia. N. Engl. J. Med., *317*:1692, 1987.
78. Johnson, D. E., Thompson, B., and Calia, F. M.: Comparative activities of piperacillin, ceftazidime, and amikacin, alone and in all possible combinations, against experimental Pseudomonas aeruginosa infection in neutropenic rats. Antimicrob. Agents Chemother., *27*:736, 1985.
79. Stratton, C. W.: Combating Pseudomonas resistance with multidrug therapy. J. Crit. Illness, *5*:215, 1990.
80. Hilf, M. et al.: Antibiotic therapy for Pseudomonas aeruginosa bacteremia: outcome correlations in a prospective study of 200 patients. Am. J. Med., *87*:540, 1989.
81. Alexander, M. R. et al.: Bronchial secretion concentrations of tobramycin. Am. Rev. Respir. Dis., *125*:208, 1982.
82. Klastersky, J., Thys, J. P., and Mombelli, G.: Comparative studies of intermittent and continuous administration of aminoglycosides in the treatment of bronchopulmonary infections due to gram-negative bacteria. Rev. Infect. Dis., *3*:74, 1981.
83. Hall, W. H., Gerding, D. N., and Schierl, E. A.: Penetration of tobramycin into infected extravascular fluids and its therapeutic effectiveness. J. Infect. Dis., *135*:957, 1977.
84. Wong, G. A., Peirce, T. H., Goldstein, E., and Hoeprich, P. D.: Penetration of antimicrobial agents into bronchial secretions. Am. J. Med., *59*:219, 1975.
85. McCrae, W. M., Raeburn, J. A., and Hanson, E. J.: Tobramycin therapy of infections due to Pseudomonas aeruginosa in patients with cystic fibrosis: effect of dosage and

concentration of antibiotic in sputum. J. Infect. Dis., *128:* S191, 1976.
86. Pennington, J. E., and Reynolds, H. Y.: Concentrations of gentamicin and carbenicillin in bronchial secretions. J. Infect. Dis., *128:*63, 1973.
87. Bryant, R. E., and Hammond, D.: Interaction of purulent material with antibiotics used to treat Pseudomonas infections. Antimicrob. Agents Chemother., *6:*702, 1974.
88. Potter, J. L., Matthews, L. W., Spector, S., and Lemm, J.: Complex formation between basic antibiotics and deoxyribonucleic acid in human pulmonary secretions. Pediatrics, *36:*714, 1965.
89. Fuhs, D. W., Mann, H. J., Kubajak, C. A. M., and Cerra, F. B.: Intrapatient variation of aminoglycoside pharmacokinetics in critically ill surgery patients. Clin. Pharm., *7:*207, 1988.
90. Dasta, J. F., and Armstrong, D. K.: Variability in aminoglycoside pharmacokinetics in critically ill surgical patients. Crit. Care Med., *16:*327, 1988.
91. Chelluri, L., Warren, J., and Jstremski, M. S.: Pharmacokinetics of a 3 mg/kg body weight loading dose of gentamicin or tobramycin in critically ill patients. Chest, *95:*1295, 1989.
92. Fuhs, D. W., Mann, H. J., Kubajak, C. A. M., and Cerra, F. B.: Intrapatient variation of aminoglycoside pharmacokinetics in critically ill surgery patients. Clin. Pharm., *7:*207, 1988.
93. Pennington, J. E., Dale, D. C., Reynolds, H. Y., and MacLowry, J. D.: Gentamicin sulfate pharmacokinetics: lower levels of gentamicin in blood during fever. J. Infect. Dis., *132:*270, 1975.
94. Summer, W. R., Michael, J. R., and Lipsky, J. J.: Initial aminoglycoside levels in the critically ill. Crit. Care. Med., *12:*948, 1983.
95. Niemiec, P. W., Allow, M. D., and Miller, C. F.: Effect of altered volume of distribution on aminoglycoside levels in patients in surgical intensive care. Arch. Surg., *122:*207, 1987.
96. Triginer, C. et al.: Gentamicin volume of distribution in critically ill septic patients. Intensive Care Med., *16:*303, 1990.
97. Martin, C. et al.: Tobramycin dosing in mechanically ventilated patients: inaccuracy of a "rule of thumb." J. Antimicrob. Chemother., *22:*505, 1988.
98. Phillips, J. K., Spearing, R. L., Crome, D. J., and Davies, J. M.: Gentamicin volumes of distribution in patients with hematological disorders. N. Engl. J. Med., *319:*1290, 1988.
99. Smith, T. R.: Risk factors for aminoglycoside nephrotoxicity. *In* The Aminoglycosides: Microbiology, Clinical Use, and Toxicology. Edited by W. A. Whelton and H. C. Neu. New York, Marcel Dekker, 1982.
100. Triginer, C. et al.: Gentamicin pharmacokinetic changes related to mechanical ventilation. DICP. Ann Pharmacother., *23:*923, 1989.
101. Noone, P., and Pattison, J. R.: Therapeutic implications of interaction of gentamicin and penicillins. Lancet, *2:*575, 1971.
102. McLaughlin, J. E., and Reeves, D. S.: Clinical and laboratory evidence for the inactivation of gentamicin by carbenicillin. Lancet *1:*261, 1971.
103. Schentag, J. J. et al.: Complexation versus hemodialysis to reduce elevated aminoglycoside concentrations. Pharmacotherapy, *4:*374, 1984.
104. Benveniste, R., and Davies, J.: Structure-activity relationships among the aminoglycoside antibiotics: role of hydroxyl and amino groups. Antimicrob. Agents Chemother., *4:*402, 1973.
105. Waitz, J. A., Drube, C. G., Moss, E. L., and Oden, E. M.: Biological aspects of the interaction between gentamicin and carbenicillin. J. Antibiot. (Tokyo), *25:*219, 1972.
106. Wallace, S. M., and Chan, L.: In vitro interaction of aminoglycosides with beta-lactam penicillins. Antimicrob. Agents Chemother., *28:*274, 1985.
107. Ervin, F. R., Bullock, W. E., and Nuttall, C. E.: Inactivation of Gentamicin by penicillins in patients with renal failure. Antimicrob. Agents Chemother., *9:*1004, 1976.
108. Adam, D., and Haneder, J.: Studies on the inactivation of aminoglycoside antibiotics by acylureidopenicillins and piperacillin. Infection, *9:*182, 1981.
109. Kradjan, W. A., and Burger, R.: In-vivo inactivation of gentamicin by carbenicillin and ticarcillin. Arch. Intern. Med., *140:*1668, 1980.
110. Blair, D. C., Duggan, D. O., and Schroeder, E. T.: Inactivation of amikacin and gentamicin by carbenicillin in patients with end-stage renal failure. Antimicrob. Agents Chemother., *22:*376, 1982.
111. Kampf, D., Schurig, R., and Forster, D.: Interactions between mezlocillin and sisomicin in vitro and in patients with normal and various degrees of impaired renal function. Clin. Nephrol., *19:*37, 1983.
112. Matzke, G. R., Luckham, D. R., Collins, A. J., and Halstenson, C. E.: Effect of ticarcillin on gentamicin and tobramycin pharmacokinetics in a patient with end-stage renal disease. Pharmacotherapy, *4:*158, 1984.
113. Chow, M. S., Quintiliani, R., and Nightingale, C. H.: In-vivo inactivation of tobramycin by ticarcillin: a case report. JAMA, *247:*658, 1982.
114. Weibert, R., Keane, W., and Shapire, F.: Carbenicillin inactivation of aminoglycosides in patients with severe renal failure. Trans. Am. Soc. Artif. Intern. Organs, *22:*439, 1976.
115. Murillo, J., Standiford, H. C., Schimpff, S. C., and Tatem, B. A.: Gentamicin and ticarcillin serum levels. JAMA, *241:* 2401, 1979.
116. Kradjan, W. A., and Burger, R.: In-vivo inactivation of gentamicin by carbenicillin and ticarcillin. Arch. Intern. Med., *140:*1668, 1980.
117. Ervin, F. R., Bullock, W. E., and Nuttall, C. E.: Inactivation of gentamicin by penicillins in patients with renal failure. Antimicrob. Agents Chemother., *9:*1004, 1976.
118. Lau, A. et al.: Effect of piperacillin on tobramycin pharmacokinetics in patients with normal renal function. Antimicrob. Agents Chemother., *24:*533, 1983.
119. Hayashn, T. et al.: Protective effect of piperacillin against nephrotoxicity of cephaloridine and gentamicin in animals. Antimicrob. Agents Chemother., *32:*912, 1988.
120. English, J. et al.: Attenuation of experimental tobramycin nephrotoxicity by ticarcillin. Antimicrob. Agents Chemother., *27:*897, 1985.
121. Katahira, J. et al.: Protective effect of piperacillin on the renal toxicity of aminoglycosides. Chemotherapy (Tokyo), *36:*946, 1988.
122. Paganini, E. P., O'Hara, P., and Nakamoto, S.: Slow continuous ultrafiltration in hemodialysis resistant oliguric acute renal failure patients. Trans. Am. Soc. Artif. Intern. Organs, *30:*173, 1984.
123. Golper, T. A. et al.: Drug removal during continuous arteriovenous hemofiltration: theory and clinical observations. Int. J. Artif. Organs, *8:*307, 1985.
124. Lehman, M. E., and Kolb, K. W.: Gentamicin elimination in a patient undergoing continuous ultrafiltration. Clin. Pharm., *4:*327, 1985.
125. Akahoshi, S. K., Bollish, S. J., and Kerr, L. E.: Clearance of aminoglycosides by continuous arteriovenous hemofiltration. Paper presented to 19th Annual ASHP Midyear Clinical Meeting. Dallas, TX, 1984.

126. Bickley, S. K.: Drug dosing during continuous arteriovenous hemofiltration. Clin. Pharm., 7:198, 1988.
127. Ernest, D., and Cutler, D. J.: Gentamicin clearance during continuous arteriovenous hemodiafiltration. Crit. Care Med., 20:586, 1992.
128. Beaufils, M. et al.: Acute renal failure of glomerular origin during visceral abscesses. N. Engl. J. Med., 295:185, 1976.
129. Bismuth, H., Kuntziger, H., and Corlette, M. B.: Cholangitis with acute renal failure. Ann. Surg., 181:881, 1975.
130. Jaresko, G. S. et al.: Risk of renal dysfunction in critically ill trauma patients receiving aminoglycosides. Clin. Pharm., 8:43, 1989.
131. Lewandowski, A., Kozaczek, W., Orlowski, T., and Weuta, H.: Kidney function of pyelonephritis patients with impaired renal function treated with mezlocillin. Arzneimittelforschung, 36:1148, 1986.
132. Isaac, V., and Hemalatha, H.: Abortion and renal failure. J. Obstr. Gynaecol. India, 26:657, 1976.
133. Bodaghi, E., Kheradpir, M. H., and Maddah, M.: Vasculitis in acute streptococcal glomerulonephritis. Int. J. Pediatr. Nephrol., 8:69, 1987.
134. Charton, M. et al.: Upper urinary tract obstruction associated with primary urinary tract infection. Ann. Urol., 21:168, 1987.
135. Jadav, S. K., Sant, S. M., and Acharya, V. N.: Bacteriology of urinary tract infection in patients of renal failure undergoing dialysis. J. Postgrad. Med., 23:10, 1977.
136. Verrier-Jones, K. et al.: Glomerular filtration rate in schoolgirls with covert bacteriuria. Br. Med. J., 285:1307, 1982.
137. Solomkin, J. S., Flohr, A., and Simmons, R. L.: Candida infections in surgical patients. Dose requirements and toxicity of amphotericin B. Ann. Surg., 195:177, 1982.
138. Lasater, J., Hyde, C., Aldridge, G. A., and King, R. W.: Acute reversible renal failure secondary to renal candidiasis. J. Urol., 122:386, 1979.
139. Ramsay, A. G., Olesnicky, L., and Pirani, C. L.: Acute tubulointerstitial nephritis from candida albicans with oliguric renal failure. Clin. Nephrol., 24:310, 1985.
140. Staib, F. et al.: Amphotericin B and flucytosine therapy in aspergillus pneumonia and acute renal failure. Simultaneous infection by A. flavus and A. fumigatus. Klin. Wochenschr., 65:40, 1987.
141. Zappacosta, A. R., and Ashby, B. L.: Gram-negative sepsis with acute renal failure: occurrence from acute glomerulonephritis. JAMA, 238:1389, 1977.
142. Kljucar, S. et al.: A comparison of intravenous ciprofloxacin dosage regimens in severe nosocomial infections. Infect. Med., 9(Suppl. B):58, 1992.
143. Brogard, J. M., Conraux, C., Collard, M., and Lavillaureix, J.: Ototoxicity of tobramycin in humans—influence of renal impairment. Int. J. Clin. Pharmacol. Ther. Toxicol., 20:408, 1982.
144. Frimodt-Moller, N., Maigaard, S., and Madsen, P. O.: Netilmicin treatment of complicated urinary tract infection in patients with renal function impairment. Antimicrob. Agents Chemother., 16:406, 1979.
145. Jonsson, M., Julander, I., Tunevall, G., and Haeger, K.: Netilmicin treatment of serious infections in patients with renal insufficiency. J. Int. Med. Res., 6:226, 1978.
146. Baron, D., Drugeon, H., Nicolas, F., and Courtieu, A.: The use of tobramycin in the management of severe infections. Clinical and pharmacological data. Euro. J. Intensive Care Med., 2:89, 1976.
147. Atukorala, S. D. F., and SherFiff, M. H. R.: Aminoglycoside in advanced renal failure. Ceylon Med. J., 29:101, 1984.
148. Schwab, S. et al.: Ph-Dependent accumulation of clindamycin in a polycystic kidney. Am. J. Kidney Dis., 3:63, 1983.
149. Bennett, W. M. et al.: Gentamicin concentrations in blood, urine, and renal tissue of patients with end-stage renal disease. J. Lab. Clin. Med., 90:389, 1977.
150. Keller, F. et al.: Therapeutic aminoglycoside monitoring in renal failure patients. Ther. Drug Monit., 9:148, 1987.
151. Tarao, K. et al.: Effect of paromomycin sulfate on endotoxemia in patients with cirrhosis. J. Clin. Gastroenterol., 4:263, 1982.
152. Thompson, J. N. et al.: Endotoxemia in obstructive jaundice: observations on cause and clinical significance. Am. J. Surg., 155:314, 1988.
153. Wilkinson, S. P. et al.: Relation of renal impairment and haemorrhagic diathesis to endotoxaemia in fulminant hepatic failure. Lancet, 1:521, 1974.
154. Nitsche, D., Kriewitz, M., Rossberg, A., and Hamelmann, H.: The quantitative determination of endotoxin in plasma samples of septic patients with peritonitis using the chromogenic substrate and its correlation with the clinical course of peritonitis. In Detection of Bacterial Endotoxins with the Limulus Lysate Test. New York, Alan R. Liss, 1987, p. 417.
155. Tune, B. M., and Hsu, C. Y.: Augmentation of antibiotic nephrotoxicity by endotoxemia in the rabbit. J. Pharmacol. Exp. Ther., 234:425, 1985.
156. Tune, B. M., Hsu, C. Y., Bieber, M. M., and Teng, N. N. H.: Effects of anti-lipid A human monoclonal antibody on lipopolysaccharide-induced toxicity to the kidney. J. Urol., 141:1463, 1989.
157. Ohkawa, S. I. et al.: Hepatic arterial infusion of human recombinant tumor necrosis factor-alpha. Cancer, 63:2096, 1989.
158. Gaskill, H. V. III: Continuous infusion of tumor necrosis factor: mechanisms of toxicity in the rat. J. Surg. Res., 44:664, 1988.
159. Miller, W. L., Redfield, M. M., and Burnett, J. C.: Integrated cardiac, renal, and endocrine actions of endothelin. J. Clin. Invest., 83:317, 1989.
160. Tomita, K., Nakanishi, T., Matsuda, O., and Shichiri, M.: Plasma endothelin levels in patients with acute renal failure. N. Engl. J. Med., 321:1127, 1989.
161. Firth, J. D., Ratcliffe, P. J., Raine, A. E. G., and Ledingham, J. G. G.: Endothelin: an important factor in acute renal failure? Lancet, 2:1179, 1988.
162. Smith, C. R. et al.: Nephrotoxicity induced by gentamicin and amikacin. Johns Hopkins Med. J., 142:85, 1978.
163. Smith, C. R. et al.: Controlled comparison of amikacin and gentamicin. N. Engl. J. Med., 296:349, 1977.
164. French, M. A. et al.: Amikacin and gentamicin accumulation pharmacokinetics and nephrotoxicity in critically ill patients. Antimicrob. Agents Chemother., 19:147, 1981.
165. Moore, R. D., Smith, C. R., and Lietman, P. S.: Increased risk of a renal dysfunction due to interaction of liver disease and aminoglycosides. Am. J. Med., 80:1093, 1986.
166. Schentag, J. J., Cerra, F. B., and Plaut, M. E.: Clinical and pharmacokinetic characteristics of aminoglycoside nephrotoxicity in 201 critically ill patients. Antimicrob. Agents Chemother., 21:721, 1982.
167. Schentag, J. J.: Specificity of renal tubule damage criteria for aminoglycoside nephrotoxicity in critically ill patients. J. Clin. Pharmacol., 23:473, 1983.
168. Schentag, J. J. et al.: Aminoglycoside nephrotoxicity in critically ill patients. J. Surg. Res., 26:270, 1979.
169. Destache, C. J., Meyer, S. K., Bittner, M. J., and Hermann, K. G.: Impact of a clinical pharmacokinetic service on patients treated with aminoglycosides: a cost benefit analysis. Ther. Drug Monit., 12:419, 1990.
170. Destache, C. J., Meyer, S. K., and Rowley, K. M.: Does ac-

171. Crist, K. D., Nahata, M. C., and Ety, J.: Positive impact of a therapeutic drug-monitoring program on total aminoglycoside dose and cost of hospitalization. Ther. Drug Monit., 9: 306, 1987.
172. Bootman, J. L., Zaske, D. E., Wertheimer, A. I., and Rowland, C.: Cost of individualizing aminoglycoside dosage regimens. Am. J. Hosp. Pharm., 36:368, 1979.
173. Taylor, W. J., Robinson, J. D., and Slaughter, R. L.: Establishing a pharmacy based therapeutic drug monitoring service. Drug Intell. Clin. Pharm., 19:818, 1985.
174. Rietscha, W. J. et al.: Collaborative clinical pharmacokinetics service in a community hospital. Am. J. Hosp. Pharm., 41:473, 1984.
175. Vozeh, S.: Cost-effectiveness of therapeutic drug monitoring. Clin. Pharmacokinet., 13:131, 1987.
176. Sveska, K. J., Roffe, B. D., Solomon, D. K., and Hoffmann, R. P.: Outcome of patients treated by an aminoglycoside pharmacokinetic dosing service. Am. J. Hosp. Pharm., 42: 2472, 1985.
177. Kimelblatt, B. J. et al.: Cost-benefit analysis of an aminoglycoside monitoring service. Am. J. Hosp. Pharm., 43:1205, 1986.
178. Mathews, A., and Bailie, G. R.: Clinical pharmacokinetics, toxicity and cost effectiveness analysis of aminoglycosides and aminoglycoside dosing services. J. Clin. Pharamcol. Ther., 12:273, 1987.
179. Gill, M. A. et al.: Matched case-control study of adjusted versus nonadjusted gentamicin dosing in perforated and gangrenous appendicitis. Ther. Drug Monit., 8:451, 1986.
180. Destache, C. J., Meyer, S. K., Padomek, M. T., and Ortmeier, B. G.: Impact of a clinical pharmacokinetic service on patients treated with aminoglycosides for gram negative infections. DICP. Ann. Pharmacother., 23:33, 1989.
181. Brummett, R. E.: Drug induced hearing loss—an update. PharmIndex, 32:11, 1990.
182. Fee, W. E.: Aminoglycoside toxicity in the human. Laryngoscope, 90(Suppl. 24):1, 1980.
183. Powell, S. H. et al.: Once-daily vs. continuous aminoglycoside dosing: efficacy and toxicity in animal and clinical studies of gentamicin, netilimicin, and tobramycin. J. Infect. Dis., 147:918, 1983.
184. Davey, P. G. et al.: The use of pure-tone audiometry in the assessment of gentamicin auditory ototoxicity. Br. J. Audiol., 16:151, 1982.
185. Davey, P. G. et al.: A controlled study of the reliability of pure-tone audiometry for the detection of gentamicin auditory toxicity. J. Laryngol. Otol., 97:27, 1983.
186. Worning, A. M. et al.: Antibiotic prophylaxis in vascular restructive surgery: a double-blind placebo-controlled study. J. Antimicrob. Chemother., 17:105, 1986.
187. Smith, C. R. et al.: Cefotaxime compared with nafcillin plus tobramycin for serious bacterial infections. Ann. Intern. Med., 101:467, 1984.
188. Smith, C. R.: Review of studies evaluating the pathophysiological effects of aminoglycosides in normal human volunteers. In Current Chemotherapy and Immunotherapy: Proceedings 12th International Congress of Chemotherapy. Edited by P. Periti and G. Grassi. Washington, DC, The American Society for Microbiology, 1981, p. 2.
189. Brummett, R. E., and Morrison, R. B.: The incidence of aminoglycoside antibiotic-induced hearing loss. Arch. Otolaryngol. Head Neck Surg., 116:406, 1990.
190. TerBraak, E. W. et al.: One-daily dosing regimen for aminoglycoside plus beta-lactam combination therapy of serious bacterial infections: comparative trial with netilmicin plus ceftriaxone. Am. J. Med., 89:58, 1990.
191. Nordstrom, L. et al.: Does administration of an aminoglycoside in a single daily dose affect its efficacy and toxicity? J. Antimicrob. Chemother., 25:159, 1990.
192. Rotschafer, J. C.: Vancomycin. In A Textbook for the Clinical Application of Therapeutic Drug Monitoring. Edited by W. J. Taylor and M. H. Diers Caviness. Irving, TX, Abbott Laboratories, 1986.
193. Matzke, G. R.: Vancomycin. In Applied Pharmacokinetics: Principles of Therapeutic Drug Monitoring. Edited by W. E. Evans, J. J. Schentag, and W. J. Jusko. Spokane, WA, Applied Therapeutics, 1986.
194. Bennett, W. M. et al. (eds.): Drug Prescribing in Renal Failure: Dosing Guidelines for Adults. Philadelphia, American College of Physicians, 1987.
195. Rodvold, K. A., Zokufa, H., and Rotschafer, J. C.: Routine monitoring of serum vancomycin concentrations: can waiting be justified? Clin. Pharm., 6:655, 1987.
196. Edwards, D. J., and Pancorbo, S.: Routine monitoring of serum vancomycin concentrations: waiting for proof of its value. Clin. Pharm., 6:652, 1987.
197. Sayers, J. F., and Shimasaki, R.: Routine monitoring of serum vancomycin concentrations: the answer lies in the middle. Clin. Pharm., 7:18, 1988.
198. Schaad, U. B., Nelson, J. D., and McCracken, G. H. Jr.: Pharmacology and efficacy of vancomycin for staphylococcal infection in children. Rev. Infect. Dis., 3(Suppl.):459, 1981.
199. Farber, B. F., and Moellering, R. C.: Retrospective study of the toxicity of preparations of vancomycin from 1974 to 1981. Antimicrob. Agents Chemother., 23:138, 1983.
200. Culter, N. R. et al.: Vancomycin disposition: the importance of age. Clin. Pharmacol. Ther., 36:803, 1984.
201. Bierman, M. H., and Needham-Walker, C. A.: Vancomycin therapy for serious staphylococcal infections in chronic hemodialysis patients. J. Dial., 4:179, 1980.
202. Edell, L. S., Westby, G. R., and Gould, S. R.: An improved method of vancomycin administration to dialysis patients. Clin. Nephrol., 29:86, 1988.
203. Tan, C. C., Lee, H. S., Ti, T. Y., and Lee, E. J. C.: Pharmacokinetics of intravenous vancomycin in patients with end-stage renal failure. Ther. Drug Monitor., 12:29, 1990.
204. Lanese, D. M., Alfrey, P. S., and Molitoris, B. A.: Markedly increased clearance of vancomycin during hemodialysis using polysulfone dialyzers. Kidney Int., 35:1409, 1989.
205. Matzke, G. R., O'Connell, M. B., Collins, A. J., and Keshaviah, P. R.: Disposition of vancomycin during hemofiltration. Clin. Pharmacol. Ther., 40:425, 1986.
206. Bastani, B. et al.: In vivo comparison of three different hemodialysis membranes for vancomycin clearance: cuprophan, cellulose acetate and polyacrylonitrile. Dial. Transplant, 17:527, 1988.
207. Lau, A. H., and John, E.: Elimination of vancomycin by continuous arteriovenous hemofiltration. Child. Nephrol. Urol., 9:232, 1988–1989.
208. Lau, A. H., Kronfol, N. O., and John, E.: Increased vancomycin elimination with continuous hemofiltration. Trans. Am. Soc. Artif. Intern. Organs, 33:772, 1987.
209. Bellomo, R., Ernest, D., Parkin, G., and Boyce, N.: Clearance of vancomycin during continuous arteriovenous hemodiafiltration. Crit. Care Med., 18:181, 1990.
210. Dupuis, R. E., Matzke, G. R., Maddux, F. W., and O'Neil, M. G.: Vancomycin disposition during continuous arteriovenous hemofiltration. Clin. Pharm., 8:371, 1989.
211. Slugg, P. H., Haug, M. T., Bosworth, C., and Paganini, E. P.: Comparative vancomycin kinetics in intensive care unit patients with acute renal failure: intermittent hemodialysis

versus continuous hemofiltration hemodialysis. *In* Continuous Hemofiltration. Contributions Nephrology. Edited by H. G. Sieberth, H. Mann, and H. K. Stummvoll. Basel, Karger, 1991.

212. Matzke, G. R., McGory, R. W., Halstenson, C. E., and Keane, W. F.: Pharamcokinetics of vancomycin in patients with various degrees of renal function. Antimicrob. Agents Chemother., 25:433, 1984.

213. Brown, D. L., and Mauro, L. S.: Vancomycin dosing chart for use in patients with renal impairment. Am. J. Kidney Dis., 11:15, 1988.

214. Pauly, D. J. et al.: Risk of nephrotoxicity with combination vancomycin-aminoglycoside antibiotic therapy. Pharmacotherapy, 10:378, 1990.

215. McEvoy, G. K. et al. (eds.): American Hospital Formulary Service (AHFS) Drug Information. Bethesda, MD, American Society of Hospital Pharmacists, 1992.

216. Cipolle, R. J., and Solomkin, J. S.: Amphotericin B. *In* A textbook for the Clinical Application of Therapeutic Drug Monitoring. Edited by W. J. Taylor and M. H. Diers Caviness. Irving, TX, Abbott Laboratories, 1986.

217. Zaske, D. E., and Lesar, T.: Other anti-infective agents. *In* A textbook for the Clinical Application of Therapeutic Drug Monitoring. Edited by W. J. Taylor and M. H. Diers Caviness. Irving, TX, Abbott Laboratories, 1986.

218. Yuk-Choi, J. H., Nightingale, C. H., and Williams, T. W.: Considerations in dosage selection for third generation cephalosporins. Clin. Pharmacokinet., 22:132, 1992.

219. McLean, A. J., and Morgan, D. J.: Clinical pharmacokinetics in patients with liver disease. Clin. Pharmacokinet., 21:42, 1991.

220. St. Peter, W. L., Redic-Kill, K. A., and Halstenson, C. E.: Clinical pharmacokinetics in patients with impaired renal function. Clin. Pharmacokinet., 22:169, 1992.

221. Paoli, I., Dave, M., and Cohen, B. D.: Pharmacodynamics of zidovudine in patients with end-stage renal disease. N. Engl. J. Med., 326:839, 1992.

222. Bennett, W. M. et al. (eds.): Drug Prescribing in Renal Failure: Dosing Guidelines for Adults. Philadelphia, American College of Physicians, 1987.

223. Mammen, G. J. (ed.): Clinical Pharmacokinetics: Drug Data Handbook. Auckland, New Zealand, 1990.

224. Lorian, V., and Burns, L.: Predictive value of susceptibility tests for the outcome of antibacterial therapy. J. Antimicrob. Chemother., 25:175, 1990.

225. Bickley, S. K.: Drug dosing during continuous arteriovenous hemofiltration. Clin. Pharm., 7:198, 1988.

226. Rello, J. et al.: Effect of continuous arteriovenous hemodialysis on ganciclovir pharmacokinetics. DICP. Ann. Pharmacother., 24:544, 1990.

227. Slaker, R. A., and Danielson, B.: Neurotoxicity associated with ceftazidime therapy in geriatric patients with renal dysfunction. Pharmacotherapy, 11:351, 1991.

228. Ballard, J. O., Barnes, S. G., and Sattler, F. R.: Comparison of the effects of mezlocillin, carbenicillin, and placebo on normal hemostasis. Antimicrob. Agents Chemother., 25:153, 1984.

229. Fass, R. J. et al.: Platelet-mediated bleeding caused by broad-spectrum penicillins. J. Infect. Dis., 155:1242, 1987.

230. Swanson, D. J. et al.: Erythromycin ototoxicity: prospective assessment with serum concentrations and audiograms in a study of patients with pneumonia. Am. J. Med., 92:61, 1992.

231. Jacobs, J. R., and Watkins, W. D.: Pharamcokinetics in Multiple Organ Failure. Crit. Care, 9:163, 1988.

232. Krishaswamy, K.: Drug metabolism and pharmacokinetics in malnutrition. Clin. Pharmacokinet., 3:216, 1978.

233. Bidlack, W. R., Brown, R. C., and Mohan, C.: Nutritional parameters that alter hepatic drug metabolism, conjugation and toxicity. Fed. Proc., 45:142, 1986.

234. Richard, C. et al.: Effect of mechanical ventilation on hepatic drug pharmacokinetics. Chest, 90:837, 1986.

235. Hug, C. C.: Pharmacokinetics of drugs administered intravenously. Anesth. Analg., 57:704, 1978.

236. Paxton, J. W.: Elementary pharmacokinetics in clinical practice. 5: The effect of pathological condition on pharmacokinetics. N. Z. Med. J., 95:116, 1982.

237. Maher, J. F.: Adjustment of medications in renal failure. *In* The Pharmacologic Approach to the Critically Ill Patient. Edited by B. Chernow and C. R. Lake. Baltimore, Williams & Wilkins, 1983, p. 65.

238. Reidenberg, M. M., and Drayer, D. E.: Alteration of drug-protein binding in renal disease. Clin. Pharmacokinet., 9(Suppl. 1):18, 1984.

239. Wedlund, P. J., and Branch, R.A.: Adjustment of medications in liver failure. *In* The Pharamcologic Approach to the Critically Ill Patient. Edited by B. Chernow and C. R. Lake. Baltimore, Williams & Wilkins, 1983, p. 84.

240. Benowitz, N. L., and Meister, W.: Pharmacokinetics in patients with cardiac failure. Clin. Pharmacokinet., 1:389, 1976.

241. Dunn, G. D. et al.: The liver in congestive heart failure: a review. Am. J. Med. Sci., 265:174, 1973.

242. D'Argenio, D. Z., and Schumitzky, A.: A program package for simulation and parameter estimation in pharmacokinetic systems. Comp. Prog. Biomed., 9:115, 1979.

243. Robischon, T.: Pharmacokinetic guidance systems optimize patient care. Intern. Med. World Rep., 7:12, 1992.

SUPPLEMENTAL READINGS

Austinx, N. M., and Hoepelman, I. M.: Aminoglycoside dosage regimens: is once a day enough? Clin. Pharmacokinet., 25:427, 1993.

Chan, G. L. C.: Alternative dosing strategy for aminoglycosides: impact on efficacy, nephrotoxicity, and ototoxicity. Ann. Pharmacother., 23:788, 1989.

Fausti, S. A., et al.: High-frequency monitoring for early detection of cisplatin ototoxicity. Arch. Otolaryngol. Head Neck Surg., 119:661, 1993.

Hickling, K. G. et al.: Serum aminoglycoside clearance is predicted as poorly by renal aminoglycoside clearance as by creatinine clearance in critically ill patients. Crit. Care Med., 19:1041, 1991.

Konrad, F. et al.: Studies on drug monitoring in thrice and once daily treatment with aminoglycosides. Intensive Care Med., 19:215, 1993.

Korvick, J. A. et al.: Prospective observational study of klebsiella bacteremia in 230 patients: outcome for antibiotic combinations versus monotherapy. Antimicrob. Agents Chemother., 36:2639, 1992.

McGrath, B. J., Bailey, E. M., Lamp, K. C., and Ryback, M. J.: Pharmacodynamics of once-daily amikacin in various combinations with cefepime, aztreonam, and ceftazidime against Pseudomonas aeruginosa in an in vitro infection model. Antimicrob. Agents Chemother., 36:2741, 1992.

Prins, J. M. et al.: Once versus twice daily gentamicin in patients with serious infections. Lancet, 341:335, 1993.

Rotschafer, J. C., Zabinski, R. A., and Walker, K. J.: Pharmacodynamic factors of antibiotic efficacy. Pharmacotherapy, 12:645, 1992.

Spivey, J. M.: The postantibiotic effect. Clin. Pharm., 11:865, 1992.

Chapter 67

CRITICAL CARE ANTIMICROBIALS: CHOICE AND USE

BURTON C. WEST
GEORGE L. DRUSANO

Physicians' age-old authority in treating fever and purulence has been enhanced by antibiotics, but the use of these agents has not kept pace with the science of them. A cause is known, prevention exists, and a cure can be prescribed for more infectious diseases than any other kind of illness. Because we expect the "magic bullets" will cure, only the rare ICU patient does not get antimicrobials. Dictating the scientific selection and use of antimicrobial agents should be a rational examination of the conditions, epidemiology, indications, microbial agents, complications, and special ICU considerations. The high risk patient is "easy to treat," but hard to cure. Antimicrobials come with a biologic cost. They change the skin and mucous membrane microbial flora, thus predisposing healthy persons and much more so the nutritionally deficient, postoperative, or multiple-organ-damaged critically ill patient to infections with nonvirulent and saprophytic organisms. Allergies, cytopenias, hepatic and renal dysfunction, euphoria, and other toxicities increase with increasing numbers of antimicrobials. Not all critical care patients should receive antimicrobials. We must choose and use them with great care.

PRINCIPLES OF ANTIMICROBIAL SELECTION

Selection of the best antimicrobial agent(s) for a definite or presumed infection is based on criteria outlined in Table 67-1. Establishing a clinical diagnosis of an infection is the first task. The anatomic site of infection is the focus of the clinical evaluation (Table 67-2). So much is assumed in the phrase "thorough history and physical examination" and so much is needed. Defining the bacteria and other organisms presumably responsible is a fundamental of scientific treatment (Table 67-3). The microbiologic diagnosis is objectively rooted in the Gram's stain and other smears and stains, cultures, and serologic and immunologic testing, but usually without a defined bacterium, empiric antimicrobial therapy must be instituted. It should be guided by the likely organisms present at an infection site if they cannot be proved. Although gram-positive bacteria commonly caused hospital infections in the preantibiotic era, bacteremic episodes with gram-negative bacilli have steadily increased.[1,2] Moreover, gram-positive bacteria, e.g., methicillin-resistant Staphylococcus aureus (MRSA), are important once again. Table 67-4 lists the common sites of infection frequently proved by diagnostic evaluations and the likely pathogens at those sites at which empiric therapy should be directed.[2] The antimicrobials that are available should be known to clinicians and are outlined in Tables 67-5, 67-6 and 67-7. Specific knowledge of the expected blood level after a given dose of any antimicrobial is useful.[3] The empiric choice should also be influenced by the epidemiology or the setting in which the patient developed the infection. Susceptibility patterns—some, not all—are quite different in community-acquired infections from those acquired in the hospital. Knowledge of one's hospital's antimicrobial resistance patterns for common bacteria helps the clinician focus on the correct empiric antimicrobials, and the hospital formulary narrows the selection to antibiotics approved by the medical staff based on scientific merit and cost analysis. Selection of the classes and specific antimicrobial(s) is broadly determined at this point in the process (Table 67-8). What remains, however, is highly important. It is individualization of therapy.

Patients respond differently to treatment because of clinical variables (Table 67-9). Renal failure, hepatic dysfunction, shock, and two simultaneous infections complicate antimicrobial selection and make more difficult optimal therapy and the prevention of adverse effects. The most effective, least toxic therapy is always the goal. A cookbook approach to complexity, however, may substitute ineffective, toxic choices for what is desired. By frequent follow-up and revisions of management, individualization of therapy should prevent iatrogenic omissions, commissions, and failure.

Critical care is defined by the patients by their acuity and complexity, by the ICU setting itself, by various justifications for its use, and, through circular logic, by what is done by intensivists. Patients progress through three phases, the pre-ICU phase, the ICU phase, and the post-ICU phase. The pre-ICU phase is a defined period during which the disease process developed that resulted in critical illness. The following examples illustrate the phases.

Example 1 is a 30-year-old woman with excessive weight gain during her first pregnancy who develops diabetic ketoacidosis as a complication of gestational diabetes and in whom acute pyelonephritis prompted the admission. Her weight gain triggered diabetes. Because she thought polydipsia, polyphagia, and polyuria were normal in pregnancy, ketoacidosis was advanced before she sought care. By then she had flank pain and fever. The pre-ICU phase was her pregnancy and particularly the recent

1365

Table 67-1. Principles of Antimicrobial Selection

Establishing a diagnosis
Identifying responsible microorganisms
Antimicrobial selection
Individualization of therapy

---

period of clinical hyperglycemia. The symptomatic duration of her infection began in the pre-ICU phase and extended through the course of antimicrobial therapy until her renal function and bladder epithelium returned to normal. Although her ICU phase lasted only 2 days, the post-ICU phase was clearly the duration of her pregnancy, not limited to her recovery from pyelonephritis, but extending into the postpartum period until her diabetes resolved.

Example 2 is a 40-year-old man who was admitted for pneumonia because of severe hypoxemia. His PO_2 of 52 on room air was low in proportion to minimal interstitial infiltrate by chest radiograph and his nonproductive cough. Although he denied risk factors for acquired immunodeficiency syndrome (AIDS), following residents' report empiric therapy for Pneumocystis carinii pneumonia was administered. Human immunodeficiency virus (HIV) testing proved positive. The pre-ICU phase began when he acquired HIV an unknown number of years earlier, possibly from a prostitute. The ICU phase lasted 3 days, for he responded nicely to trimethoprim/sulfamethoxazole therapy and oxygen. The post-ICU phase will be the rest of his life, the duration of his infection with HIV.

Example 3, a 72-year-old man admitted to the ICU following coronary artery bypass surgery, has a pre-ICU phase that is hard to quantify. As in other men with chronic obstructive pulmonary disease whose admission to the ICU follows coronary artery bypass grafting, and whose course is complicated by nosocomial gram-negative bacillary pneumonia, this man's diseases began in his teens with his first cigarette and arterial intimal plaque. The ICU phase was 3 weeks long. The post-ICU phase will last the remainder of his life because of arterial disease and lung disease that preceded his complicated hospital course.

Admission to intensive care is a clinical judgment. The major criteria for admission are summarized in Table 67-10. The general medical/surgical ICU may have patients with:

- Acute infectious diseases
- Acute or severe or complicated medical illnesses

Table 67-2. Principles of Establishing a Diagnosis

History
Clinical epidemiology
Risk assessment
Physical examination
Other anatomic assessments
    All imaging techniques
    All endoscopic methods
Laboratory, nonmicrobiologic

Table 67-3. Identifying Responsible Microorganisms

Gram's stain
  Of suspected source fluid or tissue
  Of common or easy to get fluid, e.g., urine
Other stains and smears, e.g., direct wet preparation, Kinyoun acid-fast stain
  Of suspected source fluid or tissue
  Of common or easy to get fluid, e.g., urine, malarial smears of blood
Cultures
  Blood, the final common pathway
    Aerobic and anaerobic
    Neutralize or bind antibiotics if present in blood (several methods available)
    Mycobacterial and fungal in selected cases
  Suspected fluid or tissues, e.g., CSF, abscess contents, urine, sputum, pleural fluid, pleura, or endometrium
  Of common or easy to get fluid, e.g., urine
Serologic tests
  For common diseases, e.g., syphilis (the rapid plasma reagin test)
  For suspected diseases, e.g., HIV with HIV antibody testing *or* deep fungal infection with complement fixing antibody tests for histoplasmosis and coccidioidomycosis and the antigen test of serum and CSF for cryptococcosis
  For rare diseases, e.g., Rocky Mountain spotted fever (Weil-Felix agglutinins) or brucellosis (agglutinins)

CSF, cerebrospinal fluid; HIV, Human immunodeficiency virus.

- Acute psychiatric emergencies
- Acute neurologic emergencies
- Acute surgical conditions pending a decision to operate
- Acute surgical patients, postoperatively
- Acute patients with multiple organ crisis, serious injuries, e.g., blunt trauma, radiation, chemical injury, and burns
- Acute patients in need of intense observation, not treatment

Each category presents specific risks for infection. These risks can precipitate decisions derived either from a commitment to an assumed or specific diagnosis, e.g., for the treatment of infection loosely diagnosed as a fever (of undetermined origin) or a commitment to a specific antimicrobial regimen for the treatment of a definite or presumed infection.

The risks for infection can be logically associated forward from a diagnosis or backward from a complication. For example, abdominal surgery predisposes to decreased excursion of the diaphragm and thereby atelectasis and pneumonia. A yeast superinfection in the urine of a catheterized patient may suggest previously undetected diabetes mellitus or steroid-induced diabetes mellitus.

Most febrile critical care patients should be treated with antimicrobial therapy, although only some require it, and a few should not. Specific viral, bacterial, mycobacterial, fungal, and parasitic infections should be treated with specific antimicrobial agents. Our focus is on empiric and special considerations for use of antimicrobial agents in the ICU.

HOW TO MAKE ANTIMICROBIALS WORK

Definitive, supportive, and supplemental care are essential to effective antimicrobial therapy. The whole patient

Table 67–4. Site and Predicted Common Organisms

Site	Gram-positive	Gram-negative	Other
Blood	Streptococcus pneumoniae Staphylococcus aureus Enterococcus spp. Streptococci, Group A, B, D, or other Viridans streptococci Staphylococcus epidermidis Coagulase staphylococci Listeria monocytogenes Anaerobic bacteria	Haemophilus influenzae Neisseria meningitidis Neisseria gonorrhoeae Escherichia coli Klebsiella pneumoniae Enterobacter spp. Proteus mirabilis Proteus vulgaris Providentia stuartii Providentia rettgeri Morganella morganii Citrobacter freundii Serratia spp. Pseudomonas aeruginosa Bacteroides fragilis Bacteroides spp Other anaerobes Salmonella spp. Shigella spp. Yersinia spp.	Mycobacterium avium–intracellulare Deep fungi
Cerebrospinal fluid	S. pneumoniae	N. meningitis H. influenzae Enterobacteriaceae	Mycobacterium tuberculosis Cryptococcus neoformans
Joint fluid	S. aureus S. pneumoniae	N. gonorrhoeae N. meningitidis	M. tuberculosis
Pleural fluid	S. pneumoniae Group A beta-hemolytic streptococci Anaerobic streptococci S. aureus	Bacteroides melaninogenicus Bacteroides fragilis Bacteroides spp. Fusobacterium spp. Other anaerobes	M. tuberculosis
Skin	Group A, beta-hemolytic streptococci S. aureus S. epidermidis Coagulase staphylococci Corynebacterium diphtheriae		
Sputum	S. pneumoniae S. aureus	H. influenzae Moraxella catarrhalis K. pneumoniae Legionella spp. N. meningitidis B. melaninogenicus Other anaerobes Enterobacteriaceae	Mycoplasma pneumoniae M. tuberculosis Cryptococcus neoformans
Stool		Shigella spp. Salmonella enteritidis Other salmonella Yersinia enterocolitica Campylobacter spp. Vibrio spp. Helicobacter pylori	Cryptosporidium Entamoeba histolytica Giardia lamblia M. avium–intracellulare
Throat	Group A beta-hemolytic streptococci C. diphtheriae	N. meningitidis N. gonorrhoeae	
Urethra		N. gonorrhoeae	Chlamydia spp.
Urine	Enterococcus spp. Staphylococcus saprophyticus	E. coli K. pneumoniae Enterobacter spp. P. mirabilis P. vulgaris P. stuartii P. rettgeri M. morganii C. freundii Serratia spp. P. aeruginosa	Candida spp. M. tuberculosis
Urine-, blood-borne	S. aureus	Enterobacteriaceae, in neonatal sepsis	Candida spp. M. tuberculosis Disseminated deep fungal infections
Uterine cervix		N. gonorrhaeae Gardnerella vaginalis Mobiluncus spp.	Chlamydia spp. Trichomonas vaginalis

Table 67-5. Therapeutic Choices Against Bacteria

Class	Name
Penicillin G and Related Beta-Lactam Antibiotics	
Penicillins	Penicillin G and V, ampicillin, amoxicillin
	Semisynthetic penicillins: methicillin, oxacillin, nafcillin, cloxacillin, dicloxacillin
	Carboxypenicillins: carbenicillin, ticarcillin
	Ureidopenicillins: mezlocillin, azlocillin, piperacillin
	Penicillins combined with beta-lactamase inhibitors: ampicillin/sulbactam, amoxicillin/clavulanic acid, ticarcillin/clavulanic acid, piperacillin/tazobactam
Cephalosporins	First-generation: cefazolin, cephalothin, cephapirin, cephalexin
	Second-generation: cefuroxime, cefoxitin, cefotetan
	Third-generation: cefotaxime, ceftriaxone, ceftazidime
	Special drugs
Special cases	Monobactams: aztreonam
	Imipenem/cilastatin
	Amdinocillin (mecillinam)
Non-Beta-Lactam Antibiotics	
Macrolide antimicrobials	Erythromycin
	Clarithromycin
	Azithromycin
Clindamycin and lincomycin	
Vancomycin and teicoplanin	
Aminoglycosides	Gentamicin
	Tobramycin
	Netilmicin
	Amikacin
	Streptomycin
	Spectinomycin
	Neomycin
	Paromomycin
Quinolones	Ciprofloxacin
	Norfloxacin
	Ofloxacin
	Enoxacin
	Nalidixic acid
Metronidazole	
Chloramphenicol	
Tetracyclines	Doxycycline
	Tetracycline
Sulfa drugs	Trimethoprim/sulfamethoxazole
	Sulfadiazine
	Dapsone
Antituberculous drugs	Isoniazid
	Rifampin
	Pyrazinamide
	Ethambutol
	Others
Miscellaneous agents	Rifabutin (ansamycin)
	Cycloserine
	Clofazimine
	Nitrofurantoin
	Novobiocin
	Polymyxins
	Bacitracin

Table 67-6. Therapeutic Choices Against Viruses

Agents for Human Immunodeficiency Virus
Zidovudine
Didanosine (ddI)
Zalcitabine (ddC)
Miscellaneous Antiviral Agents
Adenine arabinoside
Acyclovir
Ganciclovir
Foscarnet
Interferon
Amantadine
Ribavirin

Table 67-7. Therapeutic Choices Against Fungi and Parasites

Antifungal Antimicrobial Agents
  Nystatin
  Imidazole and triazole derivatives
    Ketoconazole
    Miconazole
    Clotrimazole
    Fluconazole
    Itraconazole
  Amphotericin B
  Flucytosine
Antiparasitic Antimicrobial Agents
  Antiprotozoans
    Antimalarials
    Anti-leishmania and anti-trypanosoma agents
    Amebicides and other agents for intestinal protozoans
    Agents for tissue protozoans
  Antihelmintics
  Miscellaneous

Table 67-8. Antimicrobial Selection

Knowledge of core antimicrobials, classes of antimicrobials, toxicities, and pharmacokinetics
Antimicrobial resistance
  Usual patterns, as published
  Hospital susceptibility patterns, e.g., MRSA: Does it account for 5% or 50% of the hospital's Staphylococcus aureus isolates? What percentage of Pseudomonas aeruginosa and Enterobacteriaceae are resistant to gentamicin and tobramycin?
Formulary considerations: What is available?
  Scientific arguments
  Controlled antimicrobials: Those limited to prescription by infectious diseases consultants
  Rare diseases and orphan drugs: How would you treat cerebral malaria?
  Cost

MRSA, Methicillin-resistant Staphylococcus aureus.

must be attended. Selecting the correct antimicrobial(s) must be complemented by the more general knowledge of medicine and the principles of management.

Definitive antimicrobial care is outlined in Table 67-11. With few exceptions, undrained pus thwarts any otherwise appropriately chosen and dosed antibiotic. Correct dosing is essential. Blood levels are readily available for the glycopeptide vancomycin and for aminoglycosides gentamicin, tobramycin, and amikacin. Others are not. Except for these directly measured levels, the clinician correctly assumes that standard doses of antimicrobials, as adjusted for renal and other functions, will yield blood and tissue

Table 67-9. Individualization of Therapy Using Predictions of Patient Response

Allergy
Immunosuppression
  Neutropenia
  Leukopenia
  Thrombocytopenia
  Humoral deficits
  Reversible versus irreversible
  Drug-induced
  Tumor-associated
  Metabolism-induced
  Infectious
  Postoperative
  Nutritional
Hepatic function
Renal function
Other organ dysfunction
Pharmacokinetics
  Administration
    Route
    Rate
    Dose
    Frequency
  Distribution
  Elimination and metabolism
  Accumulation
  Toxicities
    Organ damage
    Drug interaction
    Allergies
    Adverse effects
    Nonantimicrobial drug actions
Pregnancy and lactation
Superinfection

Table 67-10. Major Functional Criteria for Admission to a Critical Care Unit

Real or potential deterioration in mental function
Real or potential deterioration in hemodynamic function
Real or potential deterioration in respiratory function
Real or potential deterioration in metabolic function

Table 67-11. How to Make Antimicrobials Work: Definitive Care

Drainage of pus (whenever appropriate)
  Surgery
  Debridement
  Foreign body: Identification and removal, including intra-arterial and intravenous devices
  Obstruction: Identification and relief
Selection of antimicrobial agent(s)
Monitoring effectiveness of antimicrobial dosing with blood levels:
  Blood levels are standardized and related to tissue levels and effectiveness everywhere except the CNS
  Blood levels are assumed based on published data
  Blood levels are easily gotten for:
    aminoglycosides: Gentamicin, tobramycin, and amikacin
    Vancomycin
  Blood levels for other drugs and measuring levels in other body fluids may be done, but the result usually is not immediately available and therefore is not clinically useful, and levels usually are neither indicated nor done

Table 67-12. How to Make Antimicrobials Work: Supportive Care

Nonspecific therapy
  Nursing
  Nutrition
  Behavioral or attitudinal or spiritual—the will to live
  Family visits, friends, letters, and flowers
  Prevention of decubitus ulcers
Temporary mechanical assistance
  Dialysis
  Ventilators
  Aortic balloon pump
  Chest tubes
  Cranial bolts for monitoring and pressure reduction

levels comparable to those that are published. If indicated for a particular infection, the published dose schedule should be adequate to accomplish the clinical purpose.

Supportive care is the essence of critical care units (Table 67-12).

Supplemental care is what scientific physicians wish to offer: the individualization of care or the act of making each patient a clinical experiment in the finest sense of that conceptual tradition. Direct observation of the patient (the text) and ancillary data (from the laboratory) are synthesized, formulated, and then expressed as a tactical plan for the diagnosis and cure of that individual. The initial plan must be modified by daily observations, a key part of clinical science, and by new conclusions based on the new data, new conceptualization, and insight (Table 67-13).

CLINICAL PRESENTATIONS, PATIENT ASSESSMENT, AND SPECIFIC SYNDROMES

General Considerations

Risk and the Pre-ICU Phase of Infectious Diseases

The languages and ideas of anatomy, physiology, microbiology, pharmacology, molecular biology, pathology, and pathophysiology are integrated with practical bedside experience by physicians to learn and to know risk. Clinical judgment is clinical epidemiology applied to one patient, a synonym for blending complex probability, measurement, and experience into personal advice to a patient. Because the proprietary interest of a physician is his or her individual patient, a physician's knowledge of risk does not exist

Table 67-13. How to Make Antimicrobials Work: Supplemental Care

Use of the laboratory in critical care
Thinking like a *clinical investigator:*
  Data-based decision making
  Each decision must be followed over time and critically reviewed for patient value and benefit
  Time is needed to assess each consultant's opinion, recommendations, and contribution to the patient's progress
  Reassessing treatment:
    "Every *treatment is an experiment:*" Its benefit is not preordained but must be witnessed, measured, verified, and confirmed
  Changing one's mind: How to do it for the patient's benefit

apart from a patient. Risk is inherent in medical decisions. To treat or not to treat is always the question. Despite best efforts, management with a drug or a procedure is a decision always made with an inadequate database. The best decisions are fully informed, made by physicians with the largest and best knowledge base and whose concern is inseparable from the patient through full knowledge of that human being. Risk of death, risk of infection, risk of uncontrolled susceptibilities to infection and critical illness, and risk of not knowing the full clinical epidemiology of specific patients are objective exterior forces we wish to understand and control.

All patients who enter the ICU, by virtue either of the acute illness or the predisposition to the acute illness, are immunocompromised in the larger sense. HIV, diabetes mellitus, and alcoholism are obvious, established causes of immunosuppression. More recently, nutritional deficiency has been attributed to acute illnesses and the postoperative state, and, in turn, to these recently recognized nutritional deficiencies is attributed the biologic evidence of immunosuppression. Immunosuppression ranges from evidence for diminished skin test reactivity to elevated biologic mediators of inflammation, notably tumor necrosis factor or cachectin. Nutritional deficiency may be cause or effect in any given person, but the association has given rise to substantial new therapeutic efforts in clinical nutrition.

The ICU Phase

The Febrile Patient. Assessment for infection usually is prompted by fever. The ICU evaluation should proceed along the classic lines established for any patient with fever as listed in Tables 67-2 and 67-14. There is no substitute for a detailed history and physical examination, which then guide the clinician. The entire database is used analytically to construct a differential list of likely infectious sites, including disseminated infections not limited to any site, that might be causing fever. Empiric antimicrobial therapy can then be chosen from clinical knowledge of the most likely pathogens isolated from each of these sites and the known antimicrobial susceptibility profiles determined for one's hospital (Table 67-14).

It is dangerous, however, for the clinical algorithm to be too cumbersome. It is essential for the clinician not to delay the institution of appropriate antimicrobial therapy in the patient in whom one seriously entertains the diagnosis of sepsis. At one time, infectious disease specialists were considered the epitome of the deliberate, organized clinician, who "always" waited for the results of thorough collection and testing of pus and other body fluids and tissues for evidence of specific bacterial or other infectious agents before making the "right" therapeutic choice. Using this pseudosophisticated mind-set, which was never true for the best clinicians, some physicians unnecessarily delayed empiric therapy while awaiting the answer. These physicians have used the threat of criticism to delay therapy while obtaining cultures and other proof. Conversely, the popular "local medical doctor" was derided for selecting antimicrobials totally empirically from the outset. Although practical and empiric, the "local doctor" too was "wrong" because he or she had not done any scientific workup. **In the ICU, executive decision making combining science and empiricism is the correct approach.** The database should be obtained, but empiric therapy must be promptly initiated, or else the critically ill patient can die or have irreversible organ damage while the physician awaits a comprehensive database, especially cultures. Empiricism is correct in the ICU but only until the database is known and the response to the initial clinical therapeutic trial has been observed. At that point, all assumptions about the initial diagnosis and treatment are reassessed in the light of objective information and the interim clinical outcome.

In the ICU, drawbacks to establishing the traditional complete history and physical examination are numerous and may limit their use. Intubated or unconscious patients cannot give a history. In acute patients, old records and family members may not be available. Reliance on emergency squad members, police officers, or passersby increases but only for the circumstances of a medical event, injury, or assault; such people do not provide a history. The physical examination may similarly be difficult because of apparatus, dressings, splints, open or closed wounds, monitors, and, in ventilator patients, neuromuscular blockade. Noise may preclude an accurate cardiac or abdominal auscultation. Why is it that most ICU rooms are yellow? It would appear just to make the diagnosis of jaundice more difficult.

Treatment with narcotics, sedatives, and anticonvulsants may alter mood, level of consciousness, and behavior, but surprisingly so may many antimicrobial agents, including acyclovir, amantadine, amphotericin B, cephalosporins, quinolones (e.g., ciprofloxacin), ethionamide, ganciclovir, isoniazid, mefloquine, metronidazole, procaine penicillin G (the procaine), penicillins (high dose), quinacrine, and sulfa drugs, including dapsone.[4] Treatment with adrenal corticosteroids, interferon alfa, nonsteroidal anti-inflammatory agents, monoclonal antibodies to endotoxin, and antimicrobials will definitely modify the evidence of clinical

Table 67-14. Algorithm for Assessment and Initial Empiric Therapy in the ICU.

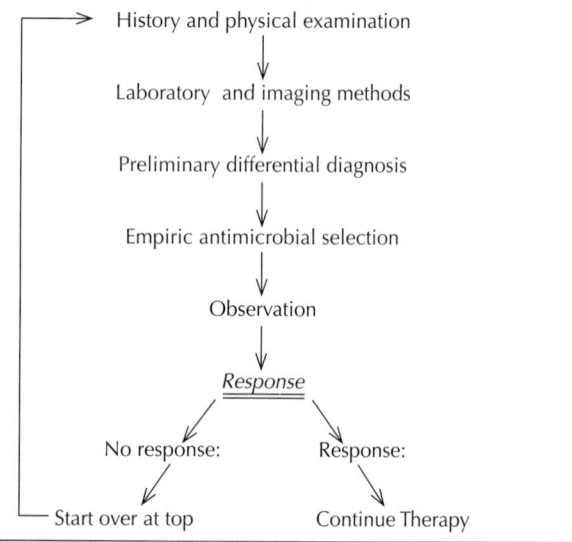

inflammation if treatment is administered. Treatment with antimicrobial agents may obscure or even hide evidence for infection that might have been present without them. Understandably, in such circumstances, greater reliance must be placed on laboratory evaluations, noninvasive and invasive diagnostic procedures, and, ironically, empiricism. Furthermore, the presence of antimicrobial agents may cause specimens containing organisms to have negative cultures; for example, isoniazid may cause urine containing sensitive Mycobacterium tuberculosis to be negative on culture despite their presence on smear. Current or recent therapy with antimicrobial agents actually increases the value and importance of direct methods of observation, such as Gram's stain, and the importance of empiricism.

Nonlocalized Infections. Antimicrobial selection initially should be based on the anatomic location of the definite or presumed infection (Table 67-15). Some patients with fever have no localizing findings and are presumed to have a bacteremia or sepsis. Although this may be true or at least a good working hypothesis, the differential diagnostic considerations should be much more extensive (Table 67-15). Systemic viral infections (as varied as systemic cytomegalovirus infection and Lassa fever), typhoid or another enteric fever, typhoidal tularemia, brucellosis, disseminated Mycobacterium avium–intracellulare, miliary tuberculosis, pre-eruptive exanthematous infections (such as the rickettsioses), disseminated histoplasmosis or another deep fungal infection, recurrent fever (Borrelia recurrentis), endocarditis, and malaria can present without focal findings. These diseases constitute a small number of critical care unit patient admissions, however, in the United States.

Drug-induced fever is an important, usually nonlocalizing diagnostic consideration in every febrile critical care patient. It is usually associated with no focus of infection and no physical findings except an occasional rash. Rarely pruritus is present. Evidence of hepatic, renal, bone marrow, and occasionally other organ dysfunction consistent with an antigen-antibody reaction is present. The findings may be nonspecific showing moderate evidence of hepatocellular damage; renal insufficiency; or allergic neutropenia, thrombocytopenia, or anemia. Acute hepatic or renal failure, however, may occur, as may severe cytopenia requiring blood component therapy. Resolution of the abnormality by withdrawing the drug is the empiric clinical method of diagnosis. Hepatic or renal dysfunction, however, may persist for some time. The anemia may be Coombs'-test positive, but no good tests proving immune neutropenia or thrombocytopenia are available. Generally, the diagnosis is established by clinical inference: The suspected offending drug is proved toxic when the impaired function or cytopenia resolves on its withdrawal. Only some drug reactions have an associated eosinophilia. Often it is so mild as to be missed—in the 3 to 4% range. Because bacterial and other serious infections tend to cause eosinopenia, 3% is significant in the puzzling febrile patient. The most allergenic and possibly least well-rationalized empiric or sustained drug therapies should be stopped in this setting of puzzling fever but mild illness, especially with eosinophilia.

Occasionally, a systemic vasculitis presents with no focal findings as a fever of undetermined origin but typically not to the ICU.

"Sepsis," as distinguished from provable bacteremic illness, is commonly diagnosed in persons with multiple organ crisis or failure syndrome (See Chaps. 51 and 64). It has ample correlates of actual bacteremic diseases, such as elevation in levels of circulating tumor necrosis factor and other biologically active substances, which are both markers and vehicles of inflammation. Therapy to reverse immediately the toxic effects of bacterial endotoxin on endothelium and organ function remains experimental but holds promise.[5,6]

In contemplating the meaning of unusual blood isolates, consider that sentinel infections for AIDS have continued to expand to organisms not previously associated with immunosuppression. Septicemia from Haemophilus influenzae or Salmonella enteritidis in adults should raise the consideration of HIV and AIDS.

Infection without fever or localization may be present, making the possibility of empiric therapy in the absence of typical clinical markers of infection a particularly difficult judgment. Bacteroides species may be present in the blood without fever being present. Other single and polymicro-

Table 67–15. Major Specific Clinical Syndromes to Be Considered in a Critical Care Unit

Nonlocalized or generalized infections
  Sepsis (see Chaps. 51 and 64)
    Bacteremia
      Enteric fevers
      Typhoidal tularemia
      Brucellosis
      Miliary tuberculosis and other mycobacterioses
      Recurrent fever
      Endocarditis
    Systemic viral infections
    Generalized fungal infections
    Malaria
    Noninfections mimicking generalized infections
      Drug fever
      Vasculitis
      Collagen vascular disease
CNS infections (see Chap. 7)
Upper respiratory infections
Chest infections
Endocarditis
Genitourinary tract infections
  Septic abortion
  Prostatitis
Gastrointestinal and diarrheal infections
Cutaneous infections
Nosocomial infections
Infections complicating aspects of critical care
  "Line sepsis"
  Open fractures; basilar skull fracture
  Gunshot wounds, other penetrating wounds
  Multiple trauma; burns
Parasitic, tropical, and exotic infections
  Travelers' diseases
Infections usually incidental to critical care
  Sexually transmitted diseases, PID, HIV
  Bone, joint, and muscle infections
  Tuberculosis

PID, Pelvic inflammatory disease; HIV, human immunodeficiency virus.

bial bacteremias may occasionally be associated with a normal temperature or hypothermia. In advanced septic shock or so-called cold shock, cold, clammy extremities with cooling even of core structures, e.g., the rectum and the centrally concentrated blood flow, may occur, thus deceiving the clinician, who counts on temperature elevation to point to the diagnosis of a serious infection. Advanced age or diabetes mellitus is occasionally associated with a muted response to pyrogens. Thus, infection without fever is a well-recognized entity. In contrast to popular medical knowledge, adrenal corticosteroid and antipyretic drug therapies do not usually keep a significant fever from being expressed, although they may delay or mute the febrile response until the underlying inflammatory or infectious disease is more advanced than it otherwise would be.

Localized Infections. These disorders include infections of the central nervous system and other organ systems.

Infections of the Central Nervous System (See also Chap. 7). Bacterial meningitis is a devastating medical emergency. Subdural empyema, brain abscess, spinal cord collections of pus (from epidural to intramedullary), retropharyngeal abscess, cervical spondylitis, Ludwig's angina, diphtheritic bull neck, botulism, and tetanus enter the differential for meningitis. Inflammation of the surface of the brain and spinal cord may also be due to mycobacteria, fungi, protozoans, viruses, and mycoplasmas as well as drugs (e.g., ibuprofen), lead, systemic lupus, and vasculitis, not to mention unusual bacteria, such as spirochetes. Recognizing bacterial meningitis early, performing the lumbar puncture within 30 minutes of the patient's arrival, and in the same time, providing intravenous antibiotic therapy directed at the most likely pathogens should be every physician's goal (Table 67-16). By thus acting decisively, and usually not delaying the judgments involved for computed tomography (CT), early therapy may be provided. The first dose of empiric therapy for bacterial meningitis should be given within 30 minutes of arrival. At the first evidence of bacterial meningitis, if the patient is not allergic to penicillin G, the order should immediately be given to prepare an intravenous dose of 3 million units of aqueous benzyl penicillin G potassium. Today such initial treatment should usually be administered in the emergency room before the patient is transferred to the ICU. If possible, the cerebrospinal fluid (CSF) should be obtained within that time frame, but if there is any delay in evaluation once a clinical diagnosis is suspected, empiric therapy should be given before or without CSF examination. If CSF is quickly obtained by lumbar puncture, antimicrobial therapy should be given immediately, and there should be no waiting for the Gram's stain, protein, or glucose results. Therapy may be changed to a more suitable agent as soon as any result (Gram's stain, culture, India ink preparation) is known.

The usual causes of acute bacterial meningitis in adults are Streptococcus pneumoniae, Neisseria meningitidis, and gram-negative aerobic bacilli. The former two classic causes of bacterial meningitis are currently best treated with high dose intravenous penicillin G (24 million units per day, administered as 3 million units every 3 hours), thus the empiric recommendation. Gram-negative aerobic bacillary meningitis is usually a complication of trauma or neurosurgery. It may complicate a congenital dural sinus. Medically the major (and rare) predisposition is hyperinvasive strongyloidiasis.[7] Therefore patients at risk for gram-negative aerobic meningitis can be identified without great difficulty. In those situations, the drug of choice is a third-generation cephalosporin, e.g., 2 g of ceftriaxone or 3 g of cefotaxime, given as an immediate intravenous dose as soon as CSF is obtained and without waiting for the result of the Gram's stain.

In children, indicated empiric therapy is one of these third-generation cephalosporins because in children under the age of 7 years, Haemophilus influenzae is common, and these agents are effective. The index of suspicion for Listeria monocytogenes should be increased in immunosuppressed persons, in alcoholics, in newborns, and occasionally in parturient women. Therapy is with ampicillin and an aminoglycoside. If suspected, ampicillin may be given empirically pending Gram's stain and culture results. Ampicillin in a dose of 8 to 12 g per day is comparable to high dose penicillin therapy and is interchangeable with penicillin G in the treatment of pneumococcal or meningococcal meningitis. Special problems, such as management of tuberculous meningitis, fungal meningitis, Lyme disease meningitis, and penicillin-resistant pneumococcal meningitis, are beyond the scope of this chapter. In the penicillin-allergic patient, the choices for empiric therapy include the third-generation cephalosporins, provided that there is no history of anaphylaxis or immediate hypersensitivity to penicillins, in which cross-reactions with the cephalosporins are more likely. Regarding the potential risk of allergic reaction, a safer, effective choice for pneumococcal or meningococcal meningitis is chloramphenicol, administered intravenously in a dose of 0.5 to 1.0 g every 6 hours. Vancomycin may be used to treat pneumococcal

---

Table 67-16. Initial Therapy of Suspected or Proven Bacterial Meningitis*

Adults
Not immunosuppressed and no neurosurgery: Presumption is Streptococcus pneumoniae or Neisseria meningitidis
  Initial *stat* treatment (within 30 min of arrival):
    If not allergic to penicillin, **3 million units of aqueous benzyl penicillin G potassium,** and then q 3 h (24 megaunits/day)
    If allergic to penicillin, **ceftriaxone** 2 g or **cefotaxime** 3 g
    If penicillin anaphylaxis or allergy to all beta-lactams, **chloramphenicol** 1 g
If head trauma, especially neurosurgery, or dural sinus or strongyloidiasis: Presumption is gram-negative aerobic bacilli and possible S. pneumoniae
  Ceftriaxone 2 g or **cefotaxime** 3 g
If immunosuppressed: Consider Listeria monocytogenes, Cryptococcus neoformans, and the common oganisms S. pneumoniae and N. meningitidis
  If not allergic to penicillin, **ampicillin** 2 g q 4 h
  If allergic to penicillin, **ceftriaxone** 2 g or **cefotaxime** 3 g
  If penicillin anaphylaxis or allergy to all beta-lactams, **chloramphenicol** 1 g

Children
In addition to above, Haemophilus influenzae is possible < age 7 years
Treatment: Ceftriaxone or cefotaxime

* All recommendations are immediate intravenous treatments.

meningitis. Treatment of gram-negative aerobic bacillary meningitis without third-generation cephalosporins is difficult and requires the input of an infectious diseases specialist.

The contagious nature of certain ICU infections is often underplayed or overdramatized. Meningococcal meningitis is spread from person to person by the respiratory route. Because some such patients are coughing from a respiratory site of infection as well as having the systemic and CNS infection, they may expose 20 to 30 hospital personnel within the first 24 hours, before antimicrobial therapy may be expected to stifle respiratory tract N. meningitidis enough to reduce or eliminate its virulence. Therefore isolation of such patients is appropriate to protect the personnel. Careful selection by a physician specialist of highly or definitely exposed persons for prophylaxis should be implemented as soon as the diagnosis is confirmed. Therapy with 600 mg of rifampin twice daily for 2 days is indicated. In especially severe exposures, such as mouth-to-mouth resuscitation efforts, rifampin prophylaxis may be followed by a course of minocycline. Minocycline has also been shown to be effective in prophylaxis by itself but is a second-line drug because of the relatively common vestibular disturbances that may accompany its use.

Contagion from CNS infections is a serious concern in encephalopathic patients. Rabies is an encephalitis of human beings that, although typically spread by the bite of a infected mammal, may be spread by human bite. The virus is present in saliva, and patients' behavior is unpredictable. Precautions must be implemented in the care of such patients. Creutzfeldt-Jakob disease is caused by a transmissible agent, that, in contrast to rabies, is not thought to pose a risk to family or medical or nursing personnel. These rare diseases are often misdiagnosed until late, with rabies being erroneously considered an intercurrent arborvirus encephalitis and Creutzfeldt-Jakob disease mistaken for Alzheimer's disease with myoclonus. Emphatically, caution to prevent needle sticks with blood and CSF from these possible diseases is strongly urged. Brain, eye, and other CNS tissues in addition to blood and CSF pose a threat of serious disease that should alert neurosurgeons, anesthesiologists, critical care specialists, and neurointensive care personnel to be especially careful.

Upper Respiratory Tract Infections. **Pharyngitis** occurring in critical care is usually not from a specific infecting organism, but rather it is a mechanical irritation from endotracheal intubation required for anesthesia, a ventilator, or resuscitation. An intercurrent infection from an incubating viral upper respiratory tract infection or an incubating gonococcal or group A beta-hemolytic streptococcal pharyngitis can emerge during the stay in the critical care unit. A concurrent infection with infectious mononucleosis or a N. meningitidis respiratory tract infection should be considered most typically in the adolescent or young adult admitted to the critical care unit for another diagnosis, e.g., an overdose, a ruptured spleen, or meningitis. Diphtheria, blastomycosis, adenovirus, and retropharyngeal abscess are rare.

Occasionally, there is nosocomial acquisition of an upper respiratory tract infection from other patients or from medical personnel or even visitors during the patient's stay in the ICU. Usually this is a viral infection, the classic being the nosocomial transmission and acquisition of influenza during an epidemic.[8]

Nosocomial acquisition through colonization of the pharynx by hospital strains of gram-negative aerobic bacilli is an ordinary occurrence in persons admitted to the hospital. These bacteria do not in themselves cause throat disease but are situated to be the bacteria aspirated into the lungs during hospitalization. Such enteric organisms from the hospital environment are often multiresistant and constitute a threat.

In the presence of HIV infection with or without AIDS, pharyngitis and stomatitis from Candida albicans are a predictable concurrent infection. Candida mouth and throat infection or thrush, however, should not be equated with HIV infection because critical care patients are predisposed to thrush. Thrush without HIV occurs in the uncontrolled diabetic, the postoperative patient, the burned patient, the corticosteroid-treated patient, the patient with multiple or prolonged courses of antimicrobials, and the otherwise immunosuppressed or malnourished patient. Such patients may be treated with traditional swirl and swallow nystatin mouthwash three times daily either with their cooperation or by nursing application of the drug to the oral and pharyngeal mucosa. Treatment of the gastrointestinal reservoir of C. albicans is recommended because this source is likely to colonize and infect the perianal skin, vagina, and urinary tract. Swallowing nystatin mouthwash or tablets or receiving treatment with nystatin mouthwash through a nasogastric tube would complement topical mouth treatment. Oral clotrimazole troches or nystatin vaginal suppositories, placed in the mouth and allowed to melt (if the patient can hold one in his mouth), are effective for treatment of oropharyngeal and esophageal candidiasis and for suppression of the intestinal reservoir of these yeasts. An oral suspension of amphotericin B has been used, although other treatments are preferred. Systemic therapy may be needed in severe cases, especially in AIDS, and in patients unable to take topical oral therapy. Current effective systemic therapy includes fluconazole or itraconazole, and if this is contraindicated or not available, intravenous amphotericin B is recommended.

Sinusitis is a well-recognized complication of prolonged nasotracheal or nasogastric intubation. It results from obstruction of drainage from the maxillary sinus or ethmoid air cells. Usually it does not happen until after several days of nasal intubation, typically with a large-bore tube. Although relatively uncommon, it has been recognized as a complication of nasal intubation at least since the 1950s. Observations about this complication have sparked reports[9,10] but there is no sentinel paper that "originally" described the entity about which authorities agree.

Confirmation of sinusitis is classically accomplished with an upright Waters' view of the skull. This lordotic anteroposterior x-ray film shows the maxillary sinuses with fluid levels and other lesions and much of the ethmoid and frontal sinuses. CT scan is preferred, but portable x-ray films may be all that can be obtained. Not needed is the lateral view because sphenoid sinusitis is not considered a complication of intubation. A lateral decubitus Waters' view (suspected side down) was reported in abstract to demonstrate a layered fluid level in maxillary sinuses better than other methods. This x-ray technique is useful for bedside examination of patients unable to be moved or to have a CT scan. If necessary, nasogastric or nasotracheal tubes may be moved to the opposite side. A nasotracheal tube could be changed to an orotracheal tube or tracheostomy. A replacement nasogastric tube, if for feeding, should be small bore and inserted on the opposite side.

How to treat a nosocomial sinusitis in a critically ill person is similar to treating any sinusitis, for at present, there is no information proving that resistant bacteria cause ICU-acquired sinusitis. This is in contrast to nosocomial lower respiratory tract infections. Agents that are active against pneumococci and ordinary mouth flora are usually effective for sinusitis. Proof is lacking that S. aureus and multiresistant gram-negative aerobic bacilli are usually present and need to be treated. Occasionally, such organisms cause sinusitis, but with no proven greater frequency than in ordinary sinusitis. Short of a sinus puncture, moreover, pus uncontaminated by the mucosal flora is not available for bacteriologic study, making unlikely an accurate bacteriologic diagnosis. When sinus pus is available, the importance of the Gram stain increases dramatically because the stain should reflect the actual infecting organism and should be accepted as the most useful test in the empiric selection of an antimicrobial agent. Because most ICU patients receive antimicrobials, the culture may be negative or show organisms resistant to current therapy. Such a culture result is altered away from clinical utility. The recovered organism usually is not the pathogen and is not pathogenetically important but grows because it is all that can grow in the presence of empiric antimicrobial(s). Thus, the Gram stain is more important than the culture. This principle applies to significant pus obtained during antimicrobial therapy from any site.

Because most ICU patients are receiving antimicrobials, at the time sinusitis is suspected or diagnosed the patient may already be receiving antimicrobial therapy that is reasonable for the treatment of sinusitis. There is not just one correct treatment.

Recommended for the treatment of sinusitis is amoxicillin/clavulanic acid (Augmentin) orally or intravenous administration of ampicillin/sulbactam (Unasyn). The rationale for treatment is that the common organisms here are airway flora: pneumococci, other streptococci, haemophilus species, mouth anaerobes, and the possibility of S. aureus methacillin-sensitive Staphylococcus aureus (MSSA). When there is no improvement, surgical drainage is indicated.

Chest or Lower Respiratory Tract Infections. Pulmonary infections are commonplace in the ICU because of the patient population and because of the use of anesthesia and ventilators.[11] An endotracheal tube, whatever the indication, is a foreign body and acts more like one the longer it is left in place. Increasingly with time, an endotracheal tube adversely changes the mucosa and tracheal epithelium with mild-to-moderate damage owing to scraping and pressure. A lower respiratory tract flora becomes established, at least to the level of the carina, consisting of pharyngeal organisms, including hospital strains of gram-negative bacilli. Tracheostomies are associated with alterations in the mucosa and a chronic tracheal and bronchial flora. Mechanisms normally at work to cleanse the airway are impaired by the foreign body, by reduced humidification, and by the combination of a bacterial flora in the presence of damaged mucosa. The mucosal inflammation generates enzyme and free radical release that may lead to a continuing adverse cycle of damage.

On hospitalization (or ICU admission), even without antimicrobial therapy, the throat bacterial flora change promptly to hospital flora. Well understood is that the hospital flora are resistant to more antimicrobials and are distinguished from normal flora. Typically, patients receive antimicrobials that accelerate the change in the upper airway flora. Even before admission, antimicrobials may be self-administered or prescribed with the intent to prevent serious disease requiring admission, e.g., the broadly active drug amoxicillin/clavulanic acid. Comparable agents may be prescribed on admission or as perioperative prophylaxis, e.g., the first-generation cephalosporin cefazolin. Therefore, without and especially with antimicrobials, when aspiration into the trachea occurs, the upper airway mucosal surface bacteria include hospital-acquired gram-negative bacilli. When these organisms or MRSA are aspirated into the lung and result in disease, therapy must take the hospital's resistance pattern into account.

Bronchitis and pneumonia are the two types of pulmonary infection to which ICU patients are predisposed. If a good chest film can be obtained with portable technique or if the patient is well enough, rare as that might be, to travel to the radiology department for good posteroanterior and lateral chest films, combined with a careful clinical examination of the chest, one can be fairly confident in distinguishing bronchitis from pneumonia, given a purulent sputum specimen aspirated through the endotracheal tube. The presence of purulent sputum grossly and microscopically combined with a normal chest examination and x-ray film indicates bronchitis. Because a single abnormal x-ray film might be pneumonia or another chronic or acute abnormality, a previous x-ray film can be invaluable. Even with such a "control" film, however, typical ICU patients already have abnormal chest radiographs, the classic example of which is the post-cardiac surgery patient with pleural effusions, making the firm radiographic establishment or confirmation of the diagnosis of pneumonia problematic.

Purulent sputum, however, in this critical care unit setting is usually an indication for antimicrobial treatment, whether the initial diagnosis is bronchitis or pneumonia. This is particularly true in the patient with fever, leukocytosis, and no other or better explanation for the newly diagnosed fever.

Multiresistant gram-negative bacilli are a common part of the hospital flora in ICUs especially. Reports with varying degrees of drama and alarm have been recounted repeatedly for over 20 years and there is no let-up.[12] MRSA and organisms with unusual resistance patterns commonly reside in the hospital.[13,14] Accurate clinical microbiologic identification is essential. Because of the emergence of resistance, e.g., to imipenem, even the identification of bacteria by common laboratory criteria might not be accurate, thus further confusing the therapeutic algorithm.[15] Resis-

Table 67-17. Treatment of Nosocomial Pneumonia*

Usual treatment
    Aminoglycoside and a third-generation cephalosporin, e.g., cefotaxime, ceftriaxone, ceftazidime
Alternates
    Aminoglycoside and piperacillin/tazobactam
    Aminoglycoside, ciprofloxacine, and clindamycin
    Aminoglycoside, aztreonam, clindamycin
    Aminoglycoside, third-generation cephalosporin, and clindamycin
    Aminoglycoside and imipenem (if imipenem not reserved)
Note:
    Vancomycin may be added or substituted for clindamycin's aerobic gram-positive therapy, if MRSA or MRSE is likely.
    Metronidazole may be added or substituted for clindamycin's anaerobic therapy
    Other possible substitutions: See text

* Choose drugs based on hospital susceptibility patterns.
MRSA, Methicillin-resistant Staphylococcus aureus; MRSE, Methicillin-resistant Staphylococcus epidermitis

tance is often worse the longer a group of patients is present, e.g., in a neurosurgical ICU, and the more immunosuppressed the patients are, especially in a transplant unit.[16]

Recommended for treatment of nosocomial pneumonia is a combination of, e.g.; amikacin and either a third-generation cephalosporin, such as cefotaxime, ceftriaxone, or ceftazidime, or a fluoroquinolone and occasionally a specific antistaphylococcal agent or a specific antianaerobic agent (Table 67-17). Exceptions to these generic recommendations must be made locally, where, for example, Enterobacter aerogenes is resistant to all of the third-generation cephalosporins. These generally suggested drugs are selected to combat, anticipate, and prevent the emergence of multiple antimicrobial resistance patterns. Resistance rates for a single agent equal the predicted single antimicrobial agent failure rate. The most widely used antimicrobials in a hospital gradually gain the worst resistance profile among the hospital's flora (Figure 67-1). This is not limited to any class of antimicrobials, although amikacin is a relative exception. Hospital isolates retain or regain susceptibility among antimicrobials not in use over time.

Amikacin is preferred in some hospitals because resistance to gentamicin of recent isolates of P. aeruginosa exceeds 20 to 30%, and resistance to tobramycin of recent isolates of P. aeruginosa exceeds 10 to 15%. The aminoglycosides are bactericidal. When susceptibility tests, however, show greater than 5% resistance for one agent, physicians must find another mainstay empiric agent for ICU use. Currently in many hospitals, amikacin has retained its low (<2 to 4%) are of resistance to sentinel organisms, such as pseudomonas. Resistance has emerged less so for amikacin apparently because its structure is susceptible to one less bacterial resistance enzyme compared with other aminoglycosides and because it is used less widely. Its use is less because (1) its pharmacokinetics are less familiar to physicians than gentamicin and tobramycin, and physicians shy away from it; (2) it is restricted in some hospitals to the prescription of an infectious diseases specialist; and (3) it is the most expensive of aminoglycosides.

A **third-generation cephalosporin** continues to complement amikacin or another aminoglycoside for treating nosocomial pneumonia, provided that isolates resistant to the one commonly used within a hospital have not emerged to a worrisome degree of prevalence, arbitrarily defined as more than 5%. When that happens, another beta-lactam, such as imipenem/cilistatin, piperacillin/tazobactam, or ticarcillin/clavulanic acid may be substituted, although many hospitals experiencing the emergence of drug resistance have taken a different approach. A common one is to use intravenous **ciprofloxacin** instead of an advanced spectrum beta-lactam to complement the aminoglycoside. Ciprofloxacin, although an excellent choice for certain gram-negative bacillary infections, is not considered optimal therapy for certain other, especially gram-positive, organisms. Another approach is to complement amikacin by using the monobactam, **aztreonam,** and add to that an agent that would kill gram-positive organisms against which aztreonam has no activity. Organisms such as pneumococci, mouth anaerobes, and staphylococci may be undetected in sputum cultures from patients already receiving other antimicrobials but be predictably present in the aspiration of mouth and throat contents into the lungs in the ICU patient. Complementing aztreonam for this purpose could be penicillin, ampicillin, ampicillin/sulbactam, nafcillin, erythromycin, clindamycin, or vancomycin. Penicillin, ampicillin, ampicillin/sulbactam, and nafcillin could conceivably interfere with the action of the monobactam and are generally not used, although clinical proof of an interaction preventing successful therapy has not to our knowledge been reported. **Erythromycin** is not a good choice as a narrower spectrum antistaphylococcal agent because about 10% of S. aureus are frankly resistant and better agents exist. Erythromycin remains the alternate or second-choice therapy for pneumococcal pneumonia behind penicillin G. Erythromycin is the drug of choice for **legionellosis** at 4 g intravenously per day. When legionella is a consideration, it is the only drug to prescribe, and the combination of erythromycin, amikacin, and aztreonam is logical. In most instances in which

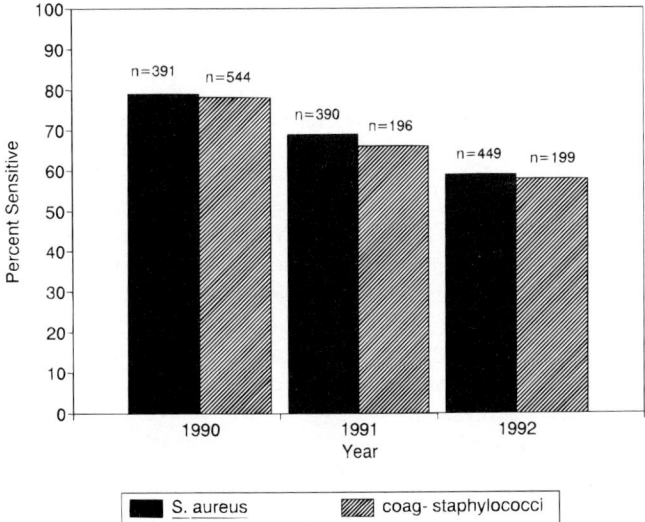

Fig. 67-1. The decline in susceptibility to ciprofloxacin of Staphylococcus aureus and coagulase-negative staphylococcal isolates in Meridia Hillcrest Hospital, Cleveland, Ohio.

aztreonam and amikacin are selected for nosocomial pneumonia, vancomycin would be the logical accompanying drug for gram-positive organisms. If anaerobic infections are considered, however, clindamycin usually is preferred to metronidazole for the anaerobes (despite occasional resistant organisms), and because clindamycin is a good antistaphylococcal drug, it is preferred to vancomycin for the gram-positive organisms, including S. aureus, unless S. aureus is the major suspected organism. Thus the addition of clindamycin to amikacin and aztreonam is more sensible than the addition of both metronidazole and vancomycin to amikacin and aztreonam treatment.

Addition of a potent antistaphyloccal drug to the basic regimen for nosocomial pneumonia is sometimes indicated. For example, vancomycin, nafcillin, or clindamycin should be considered if the sputum Gram's stain shows gram-positive cocci in clusters in addition to gram-negative rods. If the Gram's stain demonstrates a single organism consistent with **staphylococcal pneumonia,** the patient should be isolated and placed on the appropriate antistaphylococcal agent. The two types of staphylococcal pneumonia are bronchopneumonia, typically following influenza, and hematogenous, the latter having little sputum and the diagnosis made from blood cultures. Even with sputum, the Gram's stain might be misleading because of the absence of neutrophils; staphylococcal leukocidin may destroy the neutrophils. Therapy is vancomycin if the organism is MRSA and nafcillin, cefazolin, or vancomycin if the organism is MSSA. MRSA is somewhat less virulent than MSSA but may be community acquired and cannot be distinguished reliably by clinical observation. Therefore initial therapy of staphylococcal pneumonia should be vancomycin. Semisynthetic penicillins, cephalosporins, erythromycin, and clindamycin are not recommended for MRSA. These agents may be used for MSSA, but erythromycin is inferior, and clindamycin may be considered inferior to semisynthetic penicillins and vancomycin for MSSA. The emergence of vancomycin-resistant staphylococci and enterococci is discussed later. Management of these cases requires special expertise. Teicoplanin, which is similar to vancomycin, does not appear to offer much. Agents now receiving special attention are the rediscovered novobiocin combined with rifampin[17] and combination therapy including an aminoglycoside, a fluoroquinolone, rifampin, and trimethoprim/sulfamethoxazole.

Similarly, a more potent antianaerobic drug should be considered for addition to the treatment of nosocomial pneumonia if significant anaerobic pulmonary infection is strongly considered. This could occur in the hospitalized patient with grossly infected teeth and gums, who aspirates mouth contents at surgery or early in the ICU sojourn. Clindamycin is usually recommended because of its other activities, but metronidazole or another agent is an appropriate consideration in certain circumstances.

Multiresistant M. tuberculosis is a constant threat to the public and to those who suffer from susceptibility to tuberculosis, especially HIV-infected individuals, and to those exposed to tuberculosis, especially ICU personnel and other patients. No longer is resistance to isoniazid likely to occur alone. Typically, it is the undiagnosed patient or the truly secretive or uncooperative patient who constitutes a threat to others. Patients with severe tuberculosis can be admitted and even experience cardiopulmonary arrest with extensive pulmonary infiltrates or tuberculous pneumonia before the diagnosis is known. Sometimes, patients are aware of the diagnosis but are too sick to provide the information to physicians. Thus, periodically, urban ICUs place employees on notice that they have been exposed to an undiagnosed case of tuberculosis and that appropriate skin testing and chest films must be done. In HIV-positive patients and in persons suspected of having become infected with multiresistant tuberculosis, four drugs are recommended: isoniazid (INH), rifampin, pyrazinamide, and either ethambutol or streptomycin.[18] Therapy in the ICU setting should be started immediately when the diagnosis is made by history, by smear, by radiologic criteria, or by any method having clinical validity. Clinical validity often does not mean bacteriologic proof. It cannot. Smears are frequently negative, and cultures take 3 to 10 weeks. Immediate means just that, not daily therapy that happens to start the next day at 10 A.M. because that is when the daily treatments such as antituberculous drugs are usually provided by the pharmacy and administered by nurses. It means immediate. Most experienced clinicians have seen measurable clinical improvement in moribund patients with tuberculosis in as little as 24 hours, so it is important to the outcome and not just to the beginning of prevention of spread to others that tuberculosis must be treated immediately on the diagnosis.

Other chest infections, such as mediastinitis and empyema require drainage. The diagnosis and management of serious specific pneumonias, such as anthrax, tularemia, and nocardia, are beyond the scope of this chapter.

Endocarditis and Infections of the Heart and Great Vessels (See also Ch. 75) Empiric therapy for possible endocarditis would include consideration of the presence or absence of a prosthetic valve. Surprisingly, there is no evidence that coronary artery bypass grafting causes endocarditis, microbial coronary endarteritis, or graft infections at all. Therapy in the presence of a prosthetic valve and without other risk factors, such as intravenous drug abuse, must include vancomycin for the treatment of the likely organism: coagulase-negative staphylococci, resistant to methicillin. Staphylococci virtually do not cause endocarditis with negative blood cultures. Without a prosthetic valve and without a positive blood culture, the presumption is that the other worst organism would be present: enterococcus species. In this case, gentamicin and high dose penicillin or ampicillin would be recommended, unless the patient has an allergy to penicillin, in which case vancomycin would be substituted for the penicillin.

Occasionally the presentation of chest pain with fever is diagnosed as atypical unstable angina or acute myocardial infarction with fever instead of acute purulent pericarditis. Because bacterial pericarditis is rare by comparison and because patients mask fever with self-prescribed nonsteroidal anti-inflammatory drugs and antimicrobials, the clinician should remain alert to the symptoms of pericarditis.

Whenever S. aureus is isolated from the blood, a presumed diagnosis of acute endocarditis should be made.[19] Therapy pending susceptibility should be immediate with vancomycin; generally 2 g per day in two to four divided doses should be administered intravenously to persons without allergy and with normal renal function. Radical reduction in dose is needed in renal insufficiency. Vancomycin is more ototoxic than nephrotoxic, but it accumulates rapidly in renal insufficiency. Each infusion should be for 90 minutes to avoid the alarming red neck syndrome. If the organisms are MSSA instead of MRSA and the patient is not allergic to penicillin, the switch to nafcillin therapy, 12 g daily, is recommended. With or without identifying a source for the bacteremia (a site of staphylococcal infection), acute staphylococcal endocarditis must be considered and, if made, is a major diagnosis. Intravenous treatment must extend 6 weeks. Right-sided staphylococcal endocarditis, associated with intravenous drug abuse and multiple septic pulmonary emboli, may require surgical excision of the tricuspid valve without replacement, in addition to 6 weeks of intravenous therapy. Endocarditis from other organisms, e.g., viridans streptococci, is less frequently encountered in the ICU.

The classics of infected vessels are (1) salmonella species infecting an aneurysm of the abdominal aorta or another major vessel and (2) syphilitic aortitis. The question of a mycotic or a syphilitic aneurysm occasionally occurs in critical care units of hospitals that perform a high volume of vascular surgery.

More commonly seen in the ICU is the development of septic thrombophlebitis. In addition to well-chosen antimicrobial(s), surgical excision is recommended.

Intra-abdominal Infections. The distinction between medical and surgical intra-abdominal infections is blurred in the ICU. Some diseases for which surgery would normally be indicated and performed are treated medically or are not precisely diagnosed with an exploratory laparotomy because the patients are "too sick." Many intra-abdominal infections are surgical in nature because cure includes therapy with surgery. Such patients are admitted to the ICU only when they are seriously ill, in unstable condition, undiagnosed, or being groomed for surgery. More obvious are the persons with blunt or penetrating trauma to the abdomen. The latter category is sadly all too common in urban critical care units, where preoperative or postoperative management crises of knife and gunshot wounds are routine. Most complex are patients with multiple trauma that includes the abdomen with the potential for nondiagnosis, delayed diagnosis, or misdiagnosis. The autopsy remains the fine arbiter of our best but failed efforts.

The common nontraumatic causes of intra-abdominal infections are cholecystitis and ascending cholangitis; perforation of a viscus, such as a Mallory-Weiss esophageal tear leading to mediastinitis, a peptic ulcer leading to a subhepatic abscess, and diverticulitis leading to an adjacent intra-abdominal abscess and portal bacteremia with liver abscess formation; an eroding malignant tumor; and abscesses. Abscesses in the liver (bacterial versus amebic); in the subphrenic or subhepatic space following a perforated viscus; in the pelvis from colonic diverticulitis, perirectal abscess dissection, or pelvic inflammatory disease; and in the retroperitoneal areas from a renal cortical or perinephric abscess or a posteriorly lying ruptured appendix, have many common features. They may be indolent or acutely symptomatic. Liver and perinephric abscesses are hematogenous, whereas a diverticular abscess is contiguous.

Confusing, even paradoxic, associated diagnoses include pancreatitis, possibly due to alcohol, a penetrating peptic ulcer, or a toxic drug effect (e.g., didanosine), with its associated pain, fever, leukocytosis, and clinical findings. Others, fortunately rare but worthy of frequent consideration, are familial Mediterranean fever and porphyria. Both are associated with periodic attacks of abdominal pain and fever. Typically, patients with one of these diseases have multiple abdominal scars evidencing previous efforts at surgical treatment. Also confusing are the presentations of lead colic and of abdominal rigidity from a black widow spider bite. A thoughtful internist working with a good general surgeon together can usually establish the diagnosis. Many diagnoses are obvious to the experienced clinician.

Therapy depends upon knowing the likely bacteria. The gut and therefore intra-abdominal abscesses and biliary infections typically include anaerobic bacteria, gram-negative aerobic bacilli, and streptococci (occasionally S. bovis) and enterococcus species. Abscesses typically contain predominantly anaerobic bacteria that do not kill through virulence and septicemia but debilitate the patient. In the colon, approximately 99.9 to 99.99% of bacteria are anaerobic; thus, 1 bacterium in 1000 to 10,000 is an aerobe. Rapid death may result from acute bacterial infection following acute perforation of the gastrointestinal tract. Because the relatively rare aerobic bacteria are the virulent potential pathogens, blood is invaded, and septicemia results. With direct and widespread endotoxin-induced damage to endothelium and the resulting total body organ damage and malfunction, we as clinicians see hypotension, pooling, encephalopathy, diarrhea, renal failure, myocardial dysfunction, adult respiratory distress syndrome, and essentially microbiologic multiple organ damage before death. Anaerobic bacteria may cause sepsis, but as a rule they are isolated from blood as part of a polymicrobial bacteremia when gross fecal spillage into the blood occurs. Aerobes cause sepsis and death, and as a rule anaerobes cause abscess formation.

Historically, several regimens have been effective when combined with appropriate surgical drainage. From the beginning, single-drug therapies have been observed to have higher failure rates than combinations of antimicrobials. High dose penicillin combined with streptomycin or with chloramphenicol were early successful combinations. First-generation cephalosporins were shown to save lives from an impending appendiceal rupture and to reduce abscess formation; however, their relative ineffectiveness against anaerobes and enterococci did not permit their being accepted as single-drug regimens.

Antimicrobial treatment of intra-abdominal infections continues to require multiple agents for optimal therapy. There is no single prescription. Both aerobic gram-negative bacilli and anaerobic bacteria must be treated (Table 67-18). Therapeutic recommendations must be individualized for allergy and renal function. Hepatic function, gastrointestinal tract functioning, and drug interactions should be considered.

Table 67–18. Empiric Treatment of Intra-Abdominal Infections, Excluding Diarrhea

Therapy directed against sepsis causing aerobic gram-negative bacilli
  Aminoglycoside: gentamicin or tobramycin or amikacin
  Alternates to aminoglycosides (*note:* none is comparable against enterococci):
    Ampicillin/sulbactam, piperacillin/tazobactam
    Fluoroquinolones, e.g., ciprofloxacin
    Aztreonam
    Third-generation cephalosporin, e.g., cefotaxime, ceftriaxone, ceftazidime
    Imipenem/cilistatin
Therapy directed against anerobic bacteria
  Metronidazole or
  Clindamycin (choose if aztreonam is selected) or
  Rarely today, chloramphenicol
Therapy directed against enterococci
  Treatment of presumed enterococci is recommended but not required at the onset
  Combination of aminoglycoside and
  A selected beta-lactam from among the following choices:
    Ampicillin (or penicillin G) (includes ampicillin/sulbactam),
    Piperacillin (includes piperacillin/tazobactam)
    Imipenem
Therapy directed against *Staphylococcus aureus,* which may cause peritonitis and, through sepsis, intra-abdominal foci of infection
  Not always necessary to treat
  For MSSA: Nafcillin 12 g daily (or first-generation cephalosporin). If penicillin allergic, vancomycin, not over 2 g daily
  For MRSA: Vancomycin, not over 2 g daily
  In initial therapy, if clindamycin, ampicillin/sulbactam, piperacillin/tazobactam, or imipenem/cilistatin is chosen, there is no need to add nafcillin
  If penicillin allergic, choose clindamycin or metronidazole plus vancomycin

MSSA, methacillin-sensitive Staphylococcus aureus
MRSA, methicillin-resistant Staphylococcus aureus.

To treat threatened or impending sepsis from the broadest group of aerobic gram-negative bacilli, an **aminoglycoside** is the preferred bactericidal "master." The rationale for using an aminoglycoside includes its important action against enterococci when combined with a cell-wall-active agent, such as high dose penicillin G, ampicillin, amoxicillin, piperacillin, or imipenem. Although enterococci do not frequently kill people quickly from sepsis originating in an intra-abdominal abscess, they are a potential longer term cause of endocarditis, other distant site infections, and failure to cure the abscess. Gentamicin is the preferred selection against non-nosocomial aerobic gram-negative bacilli. It is slightly more effective than tobramycin against Enterobacteriaceae but not against P. aeruginosa. P. aeruginosa is rarely a cause of sepsis from an intra-abdominal source except in immunosuppressed, transplant, or oncologic patients, whose real predisposition is neutropenia, and in part the recent use of multiple antimicrobials, thus causing an unusual organism such as P. aeruginosa to become a dominant member of the diminished flora of gram-negative aerobic bacilli in the gut. Pseudomonas is usually not important. Gentamicin is active against most P. aeruginosa, but if this is a serious consideration because of the predispositions, tobramycin or amikacin should be selected. Amikacin is selected in some hospitals because it often has retained its activity against a higher percentage (usually >96%) of all of the gram-negative aerobic bacilli than the other aminoglycosides. The drugs have generally comparable toxicity, despite the mountain of data about renal toxicity from aminoglycosides. They are all dangerous if not used with frequent attention to the serum creatinine and blood levels for the entire duration of the course of therapy. Gentamicin and tobramycin may be dosed in adults at 5 mg/kg per 24 hours in 8-hour dosing intervals, or 1.7 mg/kg per 8 hours. With normal renal function, the loading dose and the interval dose are the same and trough and peak serum concentrations should be checked around the third or fourth dose. The trough is drawn literally just before the next dose, preferably exactly 8 hours after the previous dose infusion was begun. The infusion should run for 30 minutes, and precisely 30 minutes after the infusion ends, the serum should be drawn for peak level determination. The latter interval is important to measure and record. For amikacin, the principle is the same, but the dose and interval are different. Recommended in normal renal function is amikacin 15 mg/kg per 24 hours in 12-hour dosing intervals, administered as 7.5 mg/kg per 12 hours. Infusion should be over 30 minutes and levels obtained as above. Asymptotic approach to steady-state is approximated after four doses but does not occur until later. Given the instability of ICU patients, even those with ostensibly normal renal function should have serum aminoglycoside levels at a minimum of every other day over the course of their therapy.

Renal insufficiency must be judged by every direct and indirect method. Tiny, frail persons with a serum creatinine value greater than 0.9 mg/dl have renal insufficiency. Robust, muscular men may have normal renal function with a creatinine of 2.0 mg/dl. Estimates and measurements of creatinine clearance must be conducted to dose aminoglycoside antibiotics after the first dose. Sepsis, surgery, volume depletion including blood loss (e.g., fracture), and cardiogenic shock may reduce renal function with nonoliguric or oliguric renal failure and may reduce or vastly increase the volume of distribution of all drugs. Clinical judgment must be integrated into aminoglycoside dosing decisions, making it inappropriate for the nonphysician to control or dictate this critical aspect of patient care (see Chap. 66).

The penicillin-sensitive anaerobic bacteria and as noted the cell-wall-active component of action against enterococci are adequately treated by high dose penicillin G, ampicillin, piperacillin, or imipenem. The penicillin-resistant anaerobes, such as most Bacteroides fragilis, some Bacteroides melaninogenicus, and some Bacteroides species, must also be treated. Most but not all of the resistance of these organisms is mediated by a beta-lactamase. Therefore inhibition of beta-lactamases by treating with a combination of clavulanic acid, sulbactam, or tazobactam, with ticarcillin (Timentin), ampicillin (Unasyn), or piperacillin (Zosyn) may be accomplished. Because the ticarcillin component of Timentin is not particularly active against enterococci, it may be considered less frequently now. It is active, however, as a second agent (in addition to an aminoglycoside) against P. aeruginosa, if that is a serious consideration (see earlier). Because the ampicillin component of Unasyn is excellent against most enterococci, it may be the favored agent in this group, provided that P. aeruginosa is not seriously considered likely. Ampicillin has no activity against P. aeruginosa. Although new and relatively untested, the combination of **piperacillin/tazobactam** does address both of these points: It is active as a component in the therapy of sensitive enterococcal infections, and it generally is active against P. aeruginosa. Clinical experience with it, however, is limited, especially in treating large numbers of proven beta-lactamase-positive B. fragilis infections. The advantage of all three of these agents—ticarcillin/clavulanic acid, ampicillin/sulbactam, and piperacillin/tazobactam—is their activity against penicillin-resistant S. aureus, a sometimes deceitful pathogen, and some but not all other beta-lactamases. S. aureus rarely causes intra-abdominal infection, but causes sepsis with abdominal signs and symptoms and possibly incidental abscess formation, such as in the liver, with or without jaundice.

When combined with an aminoglycoside, piperacillin/tazobactam is the least used but shows the greatest promise; ampicillin/sulbactam is outstanding against anaerobes and against most enterococcal cell walls in combination but is not active against P. aeruginosa; and ticarcillin/clavulanic acid is not effective against enterococcal cell walls, is active against 90% of B. fragilis, a lesser percentage than the other two combinations, and hence appears to be the least desirable of these three choices. Note that MRSA and methicillin-resistant Staphylococcus epidermitis (MRSE) are not susceptible to these beta-lactamase inhibitor-containing combinations.

Imipenem may be used, but it should not be used alone. Many experts continue to try to withhold this outstanding drug from daily routine use. The reasons for caution are (1) its routine use is unnecessary in most hospitals, and (2) new multidrug resistance patterns emerge constantly in ICUs, occasionally making obvious the wisdom of withholding the drug and thereby having a backup agent available for the organisms that are susceptible only to it.

Alternative drugs against **anaerobic bacteria**, especially B. fragilis, are metronidazole, clindamycin, and chloramphenicol. The great advantage of each of these is that each drug is active against the penicillin-sensitive and the penicillin-resistant anaerobic bacteria. Metronidazole is the most effective followed closely by chloramphenicol and clindamycin. The quinolones are not active and are not recommended against B. fragilis and other anaerobes.

Metronidazole is not effective against aerobes. Because aminoglycosides are inactive against pneumococci and not indicated in treatment of aerobic gram-positive cocci, the combination of an aminoglycoside and metronidazole must be supplemented by an agent active against gram-positive aerobes. Also note that this combination relies totally on the aminoglycoside for treatment of all aerobic gram-negative bacilli, a plausible, but not always correct, assumption. Therefore the combination of an aminoglycoside and metronidazole may be excellent in the worst anaerobic infections and in the penicillin-allergic patient, but it should be supplemented by an agent for aerobic gram-positive cocci. Penicillin G or ampicillin would suffice in most instances, or in the case of penicillin allergy, vancomycin could be administered. An alternative for the penicillin-allergic patient or in whom multiple agents for gram-negative aerobic bacilli appear indicated is to use a quinolone, such as ciprofloxacin. This agent is not ideal for streptococci and staphylococci but in this circumstance should be adequate, and it adds hefty activity against gram-negative rods. Therefore an aminoglycoside and metronidazole should not be used without the addition of penicillin G, ampicillin, vancomycin, or ciprofloxacin.

Clindamycin is an excellent anaerobic agent except for resistance in a few strains of clostridia and certain anaerobic streptococci. It has the advantage not shared by metronidazole of being a first-rate agent against MSSA, streptococci, and pneumococci. The combination of an aminoglycoside and clindamycin is acceptable treatment of intra-abdominal abscess if concern about the possible deficiencies in treatment of the aerobic gram-negative bacilli and its ineffectiveness in treatment of enterococci and a few clindamycin-resistant anaerobes is not great. This combination may be considered in the penicillin-allergic patient.

Chloramphenicol is not generally used for this indication today because of the concern that approximately 1 in 20,000 persons treated with it are at risk for developing aplastic anemia. That statistic is from oral courses of the drug, not generally used in intensive care. Ten cases of aplastic anemia associated with parenteral chloramphenicol, however, were reviewed by one of us, confirming the existence of this risk.[20]

Cefoxitin or cefotetan are active against about 80 to 90% of B. fragilis, but these and cephalosporins in all classes are not recommended for the cell wall growth inhibition component of treating enterococci. Because cephalosporins are excreted by the liver in part, choosing one in the treatment of cholecystitis and cholangitis is appropriate; because of anaerobic bactibilia, cefoxitin remains the favored agent, sometimes as a single agent in uncomplicated cases, or in combinations with an aminoglycoside. The other combinations for intra-abdominal infection outlined previously, however, are also effective.

Doxycycline (or another tetracycline) is not used for intra-abdominal infections except to treat chlamydia, an important cause of pelvic inflammatory disease and an occasional cause of peritonitis and perihepatitis (Fitz-Hugh-Curtis syndrome). The antibiotic management of gonococcal infections, including pelvic inflammatory disease, peritonitis, and perihepatitis, should include ceftriaxone. Although some of the other combinations noted previously would also be active against Neisseria gonorrhoea, ceftriaxone should be administered if that is the clinical diagnosis.

Acutely, excessive concern about every possible organism is unwarranted. Many of the combinations, including some of the simpler ones presented, are highly effective. Treatment directed against enterococci presumed to be present may be postponed and addressed later, but it should not be ignored. A characteristic of good management is to refine and readdress therapy as necessary. There is no reason that appropriate additions, substitutions, and deletions of antimicrobials cannot be accomplished whenever medically indicated. Caution, of course, should be exercised in changes, for if there is no consistent therapeutic course for a few days, clinical assessment of a favorable or a clearly unfavorable response becomes impossible. Effective therapy, as judged clinically, should not automatically be changed if contrary information is received from the microbiology laboratory. Generally, however, ignoring culture and susceptibility results from properly obtained and labeled specimens performed in a competent laboratory is a risky judgment. Once there is established an anatomic and a microbiologic diagnosis, a full course of antimicrobial therapy coupled with skilled surgical intervention in some cases cures a remarkable number of desperately ill patients. The following examples illustrate aforementioned points about intra-abdominal infections.

In **Example 1** a 60-year-old woman enters the hospital with an enlarged gallbladder in which a huge stone was seen with outpatient imaging techniques. She is afebrile but develops fever and is transferred to the ICU for stabilization before surgery because of multiple unstable medical problems of hypertension, diabetes mellitus (glucose 474 mg/dl), and a supraventricular tachyarrhythmia. Therapy with cefoxitin alone was given before surgery, but at surgery, purulent exudate was found on the surface of the inflamed gallbladder. What therapy should then be given? Gram-stained smears revealed gram-positive cocci in chains and pairs and gram-negative nonencapsulated rods having two different morphologies. Cefoxitin was discontinued. Gentamicin and ampicillin/sulbactam (Unasyn) were selected to treat the presumed aerobic gram-negative bacilli, anaerobic bacteria, including possible B. fragilis, and enterococci. No bacteria were recovered, and she recovered uneventfully.

Example 2 is a febrile patient who has adult respiratory distress syndrome following a stormy coronary artery bypass graft operation requiring the aortic balloon pump to "get off the table" and will probably not have abdominal surgery for a newly diagnosed "surgical abdomen." Medical treatment based on the aforementioned principles would be amikacin and piperacillin/tazobactam with the possible addition of vancomycin, considering the percutaneous use of intravascular hardware, and possibly metronidazole depending on the clinical diagnosis.

Example 3 is a 25-year-old nurse with a known history of peptic ulcer disease who presented to the hospital having vomited blood in the hospital parking lot. The endoscopy showed blood, but fresh blood was not apparent. After transfusion, she stabilized and was discharged on medical therapy. Two weeks later she began feeling as if she would not recover and did not return to work. She said she still had a little discomfort, not like she had before, in the left upper quadrant. She tried to ignore it. She had no fever recorded. A CT scan showed a small fluid collection in the left subdiaphragmatic region. A decision to explore the area was abandoned when at surgery a large volume of green pus flowed from the incision. Antibiotic therapy because of her penicillin allergy was with gentamicin and clindamycin. Mixed aerobic (E. coli) and anaerobic bacteria (B. fragilis) were recovered, and she recovered rapidly and completely.

Thus, multiple drugs are nearly always indicated for intra-abdominal infections, and specific considerations must be carefully thought through at the time of initial therapy and periodically thereafter.

Gastrointestinal Infection and Diarrheal Illnesses. Gastrointestinal infection is not usually acquired in the critical care unit, although rarely an enteric pathogen is distributed to patients through a hospital's food service. Patients may be incubating an infectious diarrhea or gastroenteritis at the time of admission and have it become symptomatic after admission. More commonly, enteral feeding induces osmotic diarrhea in ICU patients. Customarily it is managed by varying the volume or prescription for liquid enteral food.

Occasionally, diarrhea is accompanied by toxicity and septicemia and is so severe that ICU admission is needed for management and treatment. Examples include diseases of travelers or endemically acquired infections, such as toxigenic or nontoxigenic strains of Vibrio cholerae or severe bacillary dysentery from Shigella species. If coupled with signs of toxicity and septicemia, such patients certainly have an indication for critical care. In the United States, V. cholerae have endemic foci on the Gulf coast, and shigellosis occurs in every city, more commonly in association with young children or those who care for young children, such as parents, grandparents, and day care workers. Anyone living in or coming from an area where food or water might be fecally contaminated is a candidate for a long list of specific agents that cause traveler diarrhea. Water-borne and food-borne illnesses regularly occur in developed countries.

The evaluation of diarrhea is through a single "good" stool specimen for culture and a fecal leukocyte smear with Wright's stain. Because stool is cultured with many media containing various inhibitors and nutrients, it is an expensive test, and properly done, it needs to be done only once.

Consideration of intestinal parasites should be less frequent. Unless there is chronic diarrhea that might be Giardia lamblia or travelers' diarrhea that might be amebiasis, stool examination for ova, cysts, and parasites is usually not indicated in the ICU. Typically, in the United States, one's patient must have an exposure (certain travel) or be high risk (e.g., AIDS), have diarrhea for 7 to 10 days or more, or have unexplained eosinophilia to justify a workup for intestinal parasites. When ordered, however, the best approach is to start with a minimum of three specimens of stool to be trichrome-stained for ova, cysts, and parasites as well as the direct and flotation methods in common use. Fresh warm stool is essential for seeing motile trophozoites, e.g., in amebiasis. If your patient is or might be infected with HIV, also order that stool be examined with an acid-fast stain to look for cryptosporidia and M. avium–intracellulare.

Toxin-induced diarrhea, e.g., from S. aureus enterotoxin or Clostridium perfringens, does not usually destabilize basic hemodynamic functioning to result in admission to the ICU. Typically, individual cases that form a cluster and are traced to a common point source rarely require critical care. Antibiotic-induced diarrhea is considered common in the ICU. With regularity, the toxin produced by C. difficile is considered and many times causes diarrhea in the ICU. False-positive and false-negative test results occur, meaning that therapy must be given empirically and sometimes continued based on the positive clinical response when the assay result is negative. Antibiotic-induced diarrhea is not all caused by C. difficile toxin. For example, small numbers of salmonella are far more likely to cause disease in persons receiving antimicrobials than a much larger number of salmonella organisms consumed by an untreated control. Because there are numerous other causes of diarrhea in humans, a quixotic search for C. difficile toxin is not warranted. Therapy with oral vancomycin, usually 250 mg orally every 6 hours for 14 days, is recommended. Oral metronidazole is recommended by some.

Botulism is not a diarrheal illness but most certainly results from ingestion (except for rare wound botulism) of preformed neurotropic toxin. As such, a patient with botulism might be admitted to the ICU misdiagnosed as an unusual stroke or acute neurologic disease. The usual method of recognition is that the patient's thinking remains intact, while sensitive muscle functions are lost. The alert old man with the sudden onset of ophthalmoplegia would be one classic example. When this is diagnosed, management includes a cathartic to remove preformed but unabsorbed toxin from the gut (see Chap. 8).

Genitourinary Tract Infections. Nosocomial infection of the urinary tract during the nearly invariable use of an indwelling Foley catheter is common. Closed systems if maintained properly help to prevent infection, but through one or more mechanisms, the urine in critical care patients eventually gets infected. Prevention or at least postponement of infection is accomplished by keeping the system closed. To obtain a specimen of urine, the port on the catheter must be treated as if it were a vein. The port must be thoroughly and repeatedly cleansed, including waiting the time required for antisepsis to work, before aspirating urine with a sterile syringe and needle. Preventing infection is best accomplished by minimizing use of urinary catheters and removing them as soon as possible. All ICU patients do not require a catheter.

Discussions as to the significance of organisms recovered from the urine of catheterized patients have split. The strict constructionists have asserted that any organisms recovered under conditions of indwelling catheterization constitute a urinary tract infection and must receive serious consideration for treatment. Practical clinicians have noted that a small number of organisms from the urine of an afebrile, critical care patient may be gracefully ignored and treated only if these organisms become "symptomatic."

Caring for the catheter remains an art of bedside nursing rather than a science. Meatal care, meticulously prescribed and carried out, has been shown not to prevent organisms from gaining access to the urine. Hygiene and cleanliness to the urinary meatus make good sense, but a precise prescription of nonspecific antimicrobials, e.g., povidone-iodine gel, is not of proven benefit. In prostatitis and following laser resection of the prostate, there may be sloughing and buildup of tissue in the space around the catheter. Concretions may collect on the external surface of the catheter, making its removal painfully traumatic. Periodic changing of the catheter is indicated. Instead of using a fixed schedule, the catheter should be changed more frequently in the acute situation than in the chronic and when inspection shows slime exuding from around the catheter or deposits building up on the external part of the catheter and when its functioning deteriorates.

Treatment of urinary tract infection should be undertaken if a symptomatic infection is documented in the uncatheterized or catheterized patient. Documentation usually is with the recovery of any microorganism from urine culture, including cultures of as few as 1000 colonies/ml of urine from a catheter, in contrast to the "standard" midstream criterion that places 100,000 colonies/ml of urine as significant. Typically, multiple organisms from the midstream collection suggest a faulty collection but must be taken more seriously from a catheterized specimen. Rarely, multiple organisms suggest an enteric or vaginal fistula to the urinary tract. Therapy with ampicillin or a first-generation cephalosporin early in the ICU course is appropriate for patients who have not lived long in the hospital. Others, however, should be empirically treated for potential multiresistant hospital-acquired bacteria in the urine or with infection at another site given equal consideration in the choice of antimicrobial. The presence of a urinary tract infection should not delay the removal of the urinary catheter if that can be accomplished. Provided no mechanical or anatomic abnormality is present, resolution is faster without the catheter. The Foley catheter represents an irritating foreign body in the bladder, leading to damage to the urothelium having contact with it. The urinary tract does not return to normal until the catheter is out and the urothelium healed.

One of the puzzles of the ICU is how to manage the patient with candida urinary tract infection. A rational recommendation has been put forward to use a 2- to 3-day trial of amphotericin B, periodically infused into the bladder through a triple-lumen catheter, with clamping periodically to hold the solution in place. The concentration of amphotericin B recommended is 20 mg/L of sterile water (not saline and not glucose), which is lower than the previous recommendation of 50 mg/L. Similarly, the recommended duration of the irrigation treatment is shorter than the conventional 7 to 10 days of treatment, and the rationale is good.[21] Women having candida infections should receive a course of intravaginal nystatin, clotrimazole, or miconazole to suppress this source of reinfection.

Genitourinary tract infections are not limited to the lumen containing urine. Older men who are lying in bed, as in the ICU, are prone to urinary retention and to require drainage. Prostatic enlargement and urinary retention with or without prostatitis are a common combination. Prostatitis, if not present as a part of the urinary retention, may develop conversely, making prostatitis a complication of catheterization. Blastomyces dermatitidis may reside in the prostate and become symptomatic and even disseminate during prostate manipulation that can occur with catheterization, rectal examination, or sigmoidoscopy.

Chlamydia infections in women may result in critical illness. Chlamydia may infect any part of the male genital tract, but rarely cause life-threatening disease. In contrast, serious illness may be caused by chlamydia infecting the female genital tract, contributing to pelvic inflammatory disease or coexisting with N. gonorrhoeae peritonitis. Occasionally, pelvic inflammatory disease or sexually transmitted diseases are associated with septicemia and require intensive care. Most cases of disseminated gonorrhea, syphilitic meningitis, and other serious or complicated sexually transmitted diseases, however, may be effectively treated without intensive care.

Septic abortion is a major obstetric, critical care, and infectious diseases catastrophe. Recognition of the major pathogens to be treated must include anaerobic bacteria, including C. perfringens; the beta-hemolytic streptococci of abortion, which in the female genital tract are usually group B; aerobic gram-negative bacilli; and other organisms. Endometritis associated with pregnancy may be treated with intensive care with fetal monitoring, to optimize the potential for saving the fetal life as well as hastening the parturient mother's improvement.

Cutaneous Infections (See Chaps. 46 to 48). Skin infections can be considered in two basic groups: those that are part of systemic infections and those that are local. Although many systemic infections are manifested in the skin, many, such as leprosy, do not deserve discussion under critical care. There are three exanthematous diseases in adult medicine that well deserve consideration because knowing them can firmly establish the early diagnosis and correct treatment of the patient. The three are meningococcemia, Rocky Mountain spotted fever (RMSF) and a small percentage of cases of gram-positive coccal septicemia.

N. meningitidis infections have a range of manifestations that are beyond the scope of this discussion, but a principal finding is macular erythematous lesions of various sizes that are first found in the axilla and later spread centrally and distally to involve most areas of the body. Although palm and sole lesions are rare, they have been described. These lesions may become confluent or grow to significant size, although they may be 1 to 3 mm in diameter and not change. They may be purplish from internal hemorrhage or become so later; usually this is associated with thrombocytopenia as a manifestation of disseminated intravascular coagulation. Organisms have been isolated from these skin lesions, although blood culture and cerebrospinal fluid culture are better ways to make the bacteriologic diagnosis. Early treatment, essential to making a difference, depends on early diagnosis. The clinical diagnosis is sufficient.

Therapy of meningococcemia with or without meningitis is intravenous high dose aqueous benzyl penicillin G potassium (24 million units daily, administered as 3 million units every 3 hours. Alternate therapies include intravenous ampicillin (8 to 12 g daily) or one of several third-generation cephalosporins that is approved for this indication. Not one of these therapies is effective against rickettsia. Chloramphenicol, although effective, is no longer recommended.

RMSF is the main endemic rickettsiosis of the United States and is the prototype of rickettsial infection for North American physicians. Rickettsioses are all similar, with murine or endemic typhus being generally milder, and epidemic typhus, perhaps partly because of the persons in whom it occurs, being a worse and more likely fatal disease. Presenting with a rash sometimes after 2 to several days of significant fever, RMSF is not usually fulminantly fatal as a significant minority of meningococcal infections are. It kills more slowly when unrecognized and untreated.

The palm is commonly the first place an exanthem is seen. Initially the lesions blanch on pressure or with heat the same way that meningococcal lesions do. They become fixed, nonblanching maculas, however, after less than 1 day of existence. The lesions appear to spread proximally and may involve the extremities and entire trunk. Because headache and nonspecific inflammation of the cerebral vessels are a part of every severe rickettsial infection, not uncommonly the patients have a lumbar puncture for evaluation for bacterial meningitis early in the course, with the special fear and differential diagnosis being meningococcal meningitis.

Currently recommended for rickettsial infection is intravenous doxycycline as the preferred tetracycline preparation, although chloramphenicol is also effective. Doxycycline would be effective for meningococcal infections only if they remained outside of the central nervous system. Although the lipid-soluble doxycycline might penetrate the blood-brain barrier, there is too little experience in using tetracyclines for meningococcal meningitis, and they are not recommended.

If both diseases must be treated initially, a combination of drugs is indicated. One must bear in mind that administering tetracycline with penicillin in the treatment of pneumococcal meningitis resulted in a much higher death rate and implied in vivo antagonism between these drugs. Therefore, that combination is usually avoided. Therapy with ceftriaxone and doxycycline is reasonable pending a diagnosis. Some authorities would use or continue to recommend chloramphenicol alone. Deleting the unneeded drug should be done as soon as a microbiologic diagnosis is established.

Disseminated pustules, indicating bacteremia, occur in some patients with significant abscesses or other pus collections containing S. aureus or group A beta-hemolytic streptococci. Rare patients with viridans streptococcal endocarditis may have them. Why most people with bacteremia do not develop numerous small cutaneous pustules as does this minority is unknown. The reason may be an undescribed cutaneous virulence factor or an unrecognized acquired or genetic host factor. These lesions are usually on an erythematous base and are firm initially, not frankly draining pus. They may be yellow or white in color and may crust. The crops of pustules are literally the sign of disseminated bacterial infection with cutaneous seeding and the beginnings of innumerable cutaneous abscesses. A vigorous search for the source is strongly indicated. A presumed diagnosis of acute endocarditis should be made whenever S. aureus is the causative bacterium, with or without identifying another source site. Although consideration to immunosuppression should be given, evaluation for underlying diseases may be completed after management of the acute infectious disease. An example is a teenage boy with pain in the hip. He sought help and got many x-ray films of the hip from the emergency department, but nothing showed up. Close examination showed a slight bulge in the buttock, but the evaluation did not progress before he developed more obvious fever and disseminated pustules. Blood and pustule cultures grew S. aureus. Definitive therapy was immediate incision of the deep buttock abscess, supplemented by intravenous nafcillin treatment, 8 g daily.

Disseminated gonococcemia commonly has somewhat larger distal pustules. Several other disseminated infections are associated with metastatic pustules in late stages, such as candida.

Patients with severe pemphigus or toxic epidermal necrolysis or desquamating drug reactions covering much of the skin of the body or burns should be treated in critical care units or in specialized burn units. Because the origin of toxic epidermal necrolysis is staphylococcal, therapy with nafcillin or in the penicillin-allergic patient with vancomycin should be administered.

The toxic shock syndrome, also a manifestation of a staphylococcal toxin, is managed as if it were a bacteremic sepsis from S. aureus, although it is not. Therapy with nafcillin or in the penicillin-allergic patient vancomycin in addition to the management of sepsis is indicated. Occasionally the clinical picture is similar in rare patients with cutaneous manifestations of a streptococcal infection, but initial therapy is the same. If a scarlet fever variant is confirmed by isolation of group A beta-hemolytic streptococci from an infected site, antimicrobial therapy may be changed to penicillin G and benzathine penicillin G after the toxicity has cleared.

The most common **localized** skin lesion in critical care units is skin trauma. Skin trauma of various kinds results in breakdown lesions of the skin. Some are from rubbing skin on sheets. Some are from tape removal ripping skin away. Others are from pressure on sensitive tissues, such as the nares under pressure from a nasotracheal tube or the heels from prolonged nonmovement. Each lesion must be individually assessed and treated (see Chap. 49).

Surgical wounds are a common site of infection in an ICU. Following Petersdorf's rule, "Look where the surgeons have been," has been good advice for a generation of infectious diseases consultants in the assessment of fever.

Skin structure infections are not strictly skin infections but usually have changes in the overlying skin, and some break through and drain. Several dramatic, related, and potentially fatal diseases include overlapping syndromes partly characterized by the bacteriology, e.g., clostridia and other gas-forming organisms, such as E. coli; streptococci; and mixed anaerobic as well as synergistic, which refers to a "witch's brew" of mixed aerobic and anaerobic bacteria. Clinical characterizations include gas-forming cellulitis, synergistic necrotizing gangrene, necrotizing fasciitis, infected vascular gangrene, streptococcal gangrene, and clostridial or gas gangrene. Streptococcal gangrene is separated from streptococcal myonecrosis, in that the latter may spare the skin. Therapy is principally surgical, but medical management includes Gram's stain and anaerobic and aerobic culture of available fluids (blood, vesicular fluid, wound drainage) and tissue. Not infrequently, gram-positive rods consistent with clostridia are seen only on Gram's stain because of the difficulty in obtaining either true anaerobic conditions without exposing the specimens to air or because the patient has received antibiotics. Antimicrobial therapy must include the best agent for anaerobes, i.e., **metronidazole,** 0.5 g every 6 hours. Clindamycin is a potential alternate. Chloramphenicol, although active against anaerobes, is not recommended. Therapy must also include the best agent for streptococci and penicillin-sensitive anaerobes, i.e., **penicillin G,** in high dose, meaning 24 million units per day, given as 3 million every 3 hours. Therapy for the other likely organisms, which could be nafcillin or vancomycin for staphylococci, and gentamicin and a fluoroquinolone should also generally be given. The latter two drugs for gram-negative bacilli suspected or proved to be present should definitely be administered to patients with gas-forming cellulitis, infected vascular gangrene, necrotizing fasciitis, synergistic necrotizing gangrene, and septic patients. Hyperbaric oxygen may be beneficial. All of the support of the ICU services is needed to bring these patients to, through, and past surgery to healing.

Most ICU patients with skin lesions are at risk for tetanus. Their management should include tetanus prophylaxis if indicated (Td [tetanus-diphtheria] toxoid ± tetanus immune globulin).

Nosocomial Infections. Nosocomial infections are infectious diseases that are not present or incubating at the time of admission to the hospital. Nosocomial infections are a major consideration in the ICU but are hardly unique to it. As noted, typically the intubated patient who becomes febrile should first be thought of as having developed a pneumonia or bronchitis that by definition is nosocomial. "Line sepsis," discussed next, is an important ICU problem. Most urinary tract infections in the ICU are nosocomial. Many of the skin breakdown lesions are hospital associated if not iatrogenic. Common major viral respiratory infections, including influenza, measles, chickenpox, and others, may be spread from patient to patient by the airborne route. The majority of viral infections, however, are spread nosocomially from and by personnel who do not wash their hands between patients. The latter group includes the causes of the common cold and enteroviruses.

Occasionally, insects including flies or mosquitoes gain access to critical care units, spreading a variety of infections, an astonishing example for a long-term ICU patient being the development of maggots in a wound. Mosquitoes can bring arbovirus infections and malaria into the hospital. Historically an important nosocomial infection was typhus, occasioned by fleas leaving an infected corpse to bite a live human being, although some have emphasized the rats (and the fleas they carry) that can be found near the outside garbage storage areas of some hospitals even today. Physicians must continue to take an interest in insect and rodent control.

Infections Complicating Special Aspects of Critical Care. Two infections in this category require special attention. One is common. That is "**line sepsis.**" This name is apt for the bacterial and fungal infections that occur around and inside intravenous and occasionally intra-arterial catheters. Despite an enormous effort by investigators from 1970 to the present, the goal of prevention is not achieved. Present wisdom is:

- To use aseptic technique when placing any line, with special efforts when a line is placed in a deep or hard-

to-stick vein that might be used either for more than 72 hours or for parenteral nutrition,
- To use clorhexidine for prevention of infection at the site[22]
- To use catheters impregnated with an effective antimicrobial substance[23]
- To avoid the femoral vein because of the proximity to the perineum
- To attend the external appearance of the skin puncture site

If local purulence develops, remove the catheter, culture the site and the contents of the catheter, and attempt the semiquantitative method for culturing the catheter. If local infection is obvious or if systemic fever is present and infection is suspected, perform blood cultures through the catheter before removing it and obtain them from peripheral sites, preferably two separate sites. If there is no local infection, the catheter must still be removed, unless there is another obvious source for fever. Noting whether or not manipulation of the intravascular catheter was made before or during the peripheral blood cultures makes sense because physical manipulation might shower the blood with organisms, but the significance of the manipulation has been nearly impossible to quantitate. The presence of organisms only from the catheter suspected of infection or from both that site and the peripheral sites supposedly adds credence to the localized versus systemic infection hypothesis and might help in treatment. A blood isolate of S. aureus, however, should invoke the rule of thumb that infective endocarditis is present. S. aureus from the catheter site should raise the suspicion of infective endocarditis, but that cannot result in a conclusion without ancillary information, especially peripheral blood cultures. There may be no other method other than the isolation of S. aureus of confirming S. aureus endocarditis because clinical examination, teichoic acid antibodies, and transesophageal echocardiogram are not definitive when negative. When in doubt, the conservative approach is to treat with effective intravenous antistaphylococcal therapy for the full standard 6 weeks.

Coagulase-negative staphylococci when isolated from blood do not provide such an easy basis for generalization. They are less virulent and are more likely to be interpreted as contaminants, instead of intravascular pathogens, in the absence of a prosthetic valve or intravenous drug abuse. This approach is practical. Such blood isolates should be managed in the same manner as S. aureus, but a high threshold for deciding to treat empirically for infective endocarditis for 6 weeks is indicated.

C. albicans is another common isolate from intravenous catheters and their sites. Sick patients should be treated. A rule of thumb regarding such candida species isolates is that it might be cured by the removal of the catheter, if there is no evidence of diabetes mellitus, corticosteroid therapy, AIDS, systemic candidiasis, or candidiasis localized as endophthalmitis, nephritis, endocarditis, or hepatosplenic disease. If the patient is sick, however, or he or she has one of the above-mentioned conditions, the recommendation is to treat the fungemia in addition to removing the intravascular device. Some experts now would choose fluconazole or itraconazole, although the standard is amphotericin B. The pathogenesis of catheter-associated infections has focused on the existence of organisms in the biofilm before physiologic studies.[24,25]

Therapy with intravenous amphotericin B must be individualized for the dose and the duration of treatment. The general principles of treatment with amphotericin B are:

- Daily intravenous infusion dosing
- Dilute in D5W (approximately 1 mg per 20 ml)
- Infuse slowly (preferably not >10 mg per hour or over 4 hours)
- Most organisms cannot be treated with less than 15 mg
- Give test dose of 1 mg in 50 to 100 ml D5W over 1 hour
- Give first therapeutic dose of 5 to 20 mg, increasing daily dose up to desired amount
- Treat deep fungal infections with a total duration or total dose, using 25 to 35 mg daily
- Treat candida fungemia for 10 to 14 days of 15 to 25 mg daily
- Treat disseminated candida infections longer
- Treat infusion-related fever with antipyretic
- Treat infusion-related nausea and vomiting with antiemetic

Tetanus is a special disease consideration. Such rare patients require well-experienced specialists for their successful management. The site of the wound, laceration, abrasion, cutaneous ulcer, burn, or iatrogenic obstetric or surgical incision that is the inferred source of tetanus must be treated surgically. Penicillin G is indicated. A primary series of three injections of tetanus toxoid, given to adults as Td toxoid (0.5 ml intramuscularly immediately, then in 1 month, then in 6 to 12 months) is indicated. Wound management of tetanus or the tetanus-prone wound in the unimmunized, the incompletely immunized, or those whose status is unknown or uncertain should include human tetanus immune globulin. Typically a benzodiazepine drip is needed to settle the periodic spasms. It is all too frequent an experience for such patients to have an apparent successful recovery from tetanus only to die of a pulmonary embolism shortly after ambulation. Prevention of tetanus is preferred.

Other infections relatively specific to the ICU include several complications of surgery and of trauma, such as open fractures (e.g., S. aureus, S. epidermidis), basilar skull fracture (S. pneumoniae), gunshots and other penetrating wounds (Clostridium tetani), multiple trauma, and burns (P. aeruginosa).

Parasitic, Tropical, Exotic, and Travelers' Infections. Parasitic, tropical, exotic, and so-called travelers' infections can occasion an admission to a critical care unit in a developed country. Some are infections in AIDS patients that may necessitate intensive care because of immunosuppression and multiorgan disease. Others are travelers or visitors from endemic areas.

Malaria is one of the most common infections in the world. It is typically associated with fever, splenomegaly, and leukopenia. The internist and critical care specialist should know more than that. Delirium, pulmonary edema, and a multiple organ crisis or "sepsis" in the patient at risk should prompt consideration of **falciparum** malaria. This medical emergency is diagnosed by a personal, not an electronic, examination of the peripheral blood smear. Because multiple organs are being damaged by vascular compromise in small arterioles from the intravascular infection, multiple organ crisis may be the presentation. Chloroquine resistance in Plasmodium falciparum is widespread. When severe falciparum malaria is diagnosed, immediate intravenous quinidine therapy, 10 mg/kg of quinidine gluconate, over 1 to 2 hours, followed by a constant infusion of 0.02 mg/kg per minute is recommended. This therapy is available in hospitals, and it may be given without delay. If the history favors malaria acquisition in an area of the world free of chloroquine resistance, chloroquine therapy can follow intravenous quinidine.[26] If chloroquine resistance is likely, alternative therapies are recommended. Lacking other advice, an oral tetracycline is recommended because it is safe (except in pregnancy) and available, although by itself it acts slowly in the treatment of malaria. Therapy with corticosteroids may worsen or prolong coma in cerebral malaria. The blood glucose must be monitored closely because intravenous quinidine and intravenous quinine stimulate the pancreas to release insulin and may cause hypoglycemia. Therapy should be administered, information collected, and decisions made about which additional antimalarial agents and about whether the parenteral route for that therapy of falciparum malaria is required. Choice of agent depends on where malaria was acquired, the most recent susceptibility of organisms from that area, and sometimes late-breaking developments in therapy. For this information, physicians are strongly advised to contact the Centers for Disease Control, Atlanta, Georgia, malaria information service: 404-332-4555 or 404-488-4196. Moreover, a few patients have more than one kind of malaria and are difficult to diagnose. If malaria is unsuspected, the exoerythrocytic phase of Plasmodium vivax or Plasmodium ovale may relapse later.

Infections Usually Incidental to Critical Care. For infections not generally managed in the critical care unit and recalling that the scope of this chapter is not intended to substitute for a textbook of infectious diseases, the reader is referred to other major sources for consideration of infections not usually requiring critical care. These include sexually transmitted diseases; pelvic inflammatory disease; HIV infection; bone, joint, and muscle infections; tuberculosis, and many others.[27-29]

INFECTIOUS DISEASES BASIS OF ANTIMICROBIAL CHOICE

Mechanisms of Antibiotic Resistance Among Bacteria

When looking at large collections of organisms, nosocomially acquired pathogens, whether gram-positive or gram-negative, are frequently resistant to multiple classes of antimicrobial agents. Resistance mechanisms are seen among both gram-positive and gram-negative organisms.[30]

The ICU **setting** is extremely conducive to the selection of resistant organisms. Patients often develop the most severe infections, with large organism loads. This means that there is a high probability that some of the organisms in this dense population will, by chance, have acquired a mutation that will allow them to be more resistant to some of the antibiotics frequently used clinically. Further, because the ICU is also a place in which there is heavy use of many different antibiotics, there will be strong selective pressure for the more resistant organisms to grow freely and thus take over the population. This becomes clinically manifest either as colonization of the patient with resistant organisms or, less frequently, as failure of therapy owing to the emergence of these resistant pathogens.[31,32]

Beta-Lactam Antibiotics

Beta-lactam antibiotics normally act by interruption of cell wall synthesis and cell division by binding to penicillin-binding proteins (PBPs), which are naturally occurring enzymes required to build normal bacterial cell walls. Beta-lactam antibiotics, in other words, are enzyme inhibitors. The major mechanism of resistance is that bacterial beta-lactamases destroy beta-lactam antibiotics. In addition, bacteria may produce altered PBPs, which resist beta-lactam antibiotics' inhibition of PBPs naturally occurring enzymatic function. Third, bacteria may decrease their accumulation of or become impermeable to beta-lactam antibiotics.

Among **gram-positive organisms,** elaboration of beta-lactamase active against the early penicillins (see Table 67-5) is the most common resistance mechanism with which most clinicians are familiar. This can be seen in S. aureus and more recently has been demonstrated in enterococcus species resistant to penicillin and ampicillin.[33] Enterococcus faecium is resistant to virtually all beta-lactam antibiotics because of target site resistance. That is, beta-lactam agents have a difficult time binding to the PBPs of E. faecium except at high, nonphysiologic concentrations. For S. aureus, methicillin resistance has been increasingly described throughout the United States.[34] Although most of these cases are nosocomially acquired, community acquisition of MRSA infection among intravenous drug abusers has been described from Detroit.[35,36] The mechanism for this resistance is usually production of an unusual PBP (PBP 2A or sometimes referred to as PBP2'), which binds the penicillin only at extremely high concentrations. Most recently, E. faecalis and E. faecium have been isolated that are resistant to vancomycin.[37-39] These strains all contain a relatively large plasmid whose transcription results in the elaboration of a 38 to 39 Kd cell wall protein.

Among **gram-negative bacilli,** the outer membrane of these organisms adds another layer of complexity to the problem of antimicrobial resistance. In contrast to gram-positive organisms, in which resistance mechanisms for beta-lactam drugs are usually limited to alteration of target site (PBPs) and beta-lactamase-mediated hydrolysis, the gram-negative organisms also have an outer membrane, which restricts the passage of hydrophilic molecules such as the beta-lactam class of drugs, thus setting up a diffusion barrier. The anatomy of the gram-negative organisms as displayed in Figure 67-2 allows resistance to beta-lactam drugs at three levels: (1) penetration across the outer mem-

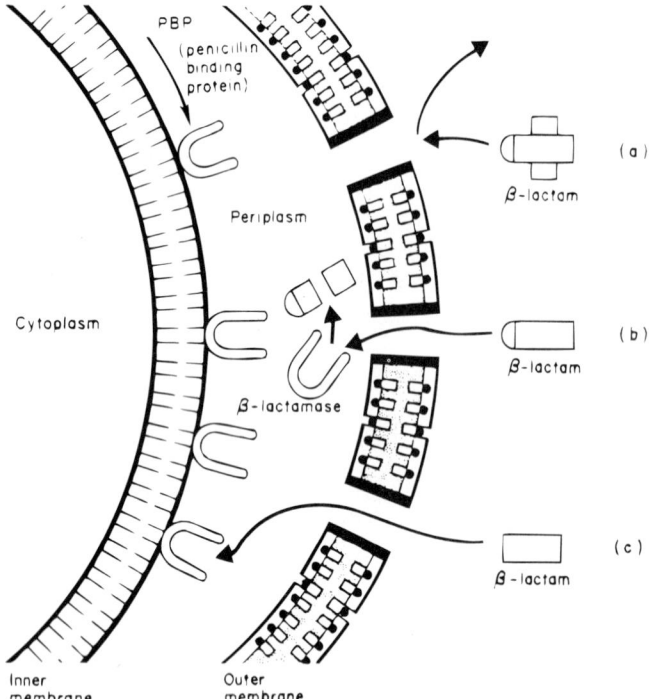

Fig. 67–2. The three mechanisms of resistance to beta-lactamases: (a) Penetration across the outer membrane, (b) beta-lactamase-mediated hydrolysis in the periplasm; and (c) failure to acylate the target site, the penicillin binding proteins.

brane; (2) beta-lactamase-mediated hydrolysis in the periplasm; and (3) failure to acylate the target site, the PBPs.

Much new information is available regarding beta-lactam resistance among gram-negative organisms. Patients with nosocomially acquired infection are more likely to have organisms bearing a Sykes class 1 chromosomal beta-lactamase as the causative pathogen. This beta-lactamase is under the control of a repressor and is produced in small amounts under normal conditions. In the presence of a strongly inducing beta-lactam antibiotic, however, the production of beta-lactamase can rise manyfold. More troublesome with regard to beta-lactam resistance, moreover, are the mutants that arise from these organisms. With a mutational frequency of the order of $1/10^7$ to $1/10^8$, these organisms (e.g., P. aeruginosa, enterobacter species, serratia species, citrobacter species, and indole-positive proteus species) acquire a mutation in which their repressor ceases to work, and the organisms produce large amounts of beta-lactamase all the time regardless of the presence of beta-lactam drugs in the environment. These organisms are referred to as constitutive or stably derepressed mutants. They are selected from dense populations of organisms with relatively high efficiency by weak induction beta-lactam agents (e.g., most third-generation cephalosporins, monobactams, and acylampicillin derivatives). Once selected, these organisms can take over the population and cause not only failure of therapy, but also resistance to a wide variety of beta-lactam agents.[40] Indeed, only agents such as the carbapenems, such as imipenem or meropenem, and cephalosporins, such as cefipime and cefpirome (both experimental agents) that are stable to the Sykes class I chromosomal beta-lactamases are suitable as therapy for these organisms among the beta-lactams. Selection of stably depressed mutants is a particular problem for the intensive patient care setting. Nosocomial pneumonia is a common problem in the ICU. Organism densities frequently run from $1/10^{10}$ to $1/10^{11}$. Consequently, considering the mutational frequency, there are already 10^3 to 10^4 stably derepressed organisms in the population before the institution of antimicrobial therapy. It is, therefore, a relatively easy task for a weak induction agent to select for these organisms, which are at a survival advantage relative to normal organisms. Strong induction beta-lactam drugs usually do not have this problem of selection because all of the organisms in the population have their beta-lactamase production turned up nearly to maximum. Therefore the drug is either stable to the beta-lactamase, in which case the drug wins and the organisms lose or it is labile to the chromosomal beta-lactamase, in which case the organisms win and the drug loses, but no selection of resistant mutants has taken place. The clinically important point is that patients who acquire their infection nosocomially are at much higher risk for these types of organisms, many of which may be resistant to a wide variety of beta-lactam antibiotics.

Other mechanisms of beta-lactamase-mediated resistance have also come to light in the recent past. Some organisms, such as E. coli and K. pneumoniae, normally sensitive to beta-lactam combinations with beta-lactamase inhibitors (e.g., ticarcillin/clavulanate and ampicillin/sulbactam) have acquired high copy number plasmids.[41] These high copy number plasmids produce such a large amount of traditional beta-lactamases such as TEM-1 and TEM-2 that they are able to overwhelm the beta-lactam inhibitors and hydrolyze the companion drug, leading to resistance. Finally, a troublesome new mechanism of resistance has been described for beta-lactamases referred to as the "extended TEM type of beta-lactamase."[42] These beta-lactamases are derived from classic TEM-1 and TEM-2 type beta-lactamases with two to four point mutations, which allow many of the newer beta-lactam agents (e.g., ceftazidime, ceftriaxone, cefoperazone, cefotaxime, or ceftizoxime) to fix into the hot spot of the enzyme and be hydrolyzed into microbiologic inactivity. These enzymes may be substrate specific and thus may express resistance only to a subset of these drugs, thus making empiric selection of therapy difficult. Currently, these beta-lactams are relatively uncommon but are on easily transmissible plasmids, and the implication of their spread for empiric therapy in the ICU setting is considerable. Epidemiology of these resistance plasmids bears careful monitoring over the next several years.

Aminoglycosides

Aminoglycosides normally work by binding to ribosomes and thus interrupting translation. Without translation of instructions to produce, the bacterial cell dies. Bacteria resist aminoglycoside antibiotics by producing enzymes that destroy the aminoglycoside's structure. A single bacterium might produce one or more than one enzyme. The enzymes perform phosphorylation, acetylation, or nucleotidylation to the aminoglycoside destroying its effectiveness. Cleverly, bacteria may resist action by altering the target ribosomal proteins, so the aminoglycoside cannot bind to its usual site, thus blocking the antimicrobial action. Third, bacteria may decrease their accumulation of or become impermeable to aminoglycoside antibiotics.

For aminoglycosides, little is new in the way of resistance mechanisms, with decreased penetration and aminoglycoside inactivating enzymes accounting for the vast majority of the resistance among gram-negative bacilli.[43] What has been appreciated, however, is the relative frequency of high levels of aminoglycoside resistance (greater than 500 µg/ml) among enterococci.[44] This is beginning to be an important clinical problem. Occasionally, such strains harbor not only aminoglycoside resistance, but also the beta-lactamase necessary to mediate penicillin and ampicillin resistance or, in a few cases, a plasmid-mediating vancomycin resistance. In the near future, patients with serious enterococcal infections may literally not have an active drug with which to be treated. Furthermore, aminoglycoside resistance alone is a serious issue because patients with enterococcal endocarditis cannot receive bactericidal therapy in the absence of an active aminoglycoside.

Fluoroquinolones

Fluoroquinolones kill bacteria by preventing replication of DNA through the mechanism of enzyme inhibition. The enzyme targeted by fluoroquinolones is DNA gyrase. Without replication, DNA is not copied, and the bacteria cannot divide into progeny cells. The principal mechanism of antimicrobial resistance is in bacterial alteration of the target enzyme structure, preventing a good fit between the fluoroquinolone and DNA gyrase. Bacteria, moreover, may become impermeable to or decrease their accumulation of fluoroquinolone antibiotics.

Fluoroquinolones have more recently been introduced into the physician's therapeutic armamentarium. We are starting to note, however, the rise of resistance to the clinically available fluoroquinolone agents, particularly among P. aeruginosa and S. aureus (see Fig. 67–1).[45,46] Resistance mechanisms among organisms to fluoroquinolones are most commonly two in number. Organisms may produce an altered target site, the DNA gyrase enzyme.[47] The A subunit of this enzyme no longer binds fluoroquinolone as avidly, leading to an increase in minimal inhibitory concentration (MIC), usually of the range of eightfold. In addition, organisms may delete outer membrane protein porins, which decreases the penetration of the fluoroquinolones across the outer membrane of the organisms and causes an increase in MIC, usually of approximately fourfold for these agents.[48] The first mechanism is restricted to fluoroquinolones, but the second mechanism of resistance causes an increase in MIC not only to quinolones, but also to many beta-lactam drugs.[48]

P. aeruginosa and S. aureus are the organisms for which this is seen most frequently as a clinical problem with resistance. The reason for this is straightforward. MICs for staphylococci and pseudomonas are generally higher than for other common microorganisms. MIC_{90}s (minimal inhibitory concentration for 90% of the isolates) for ciprofloxacin for P. aeruginosa and S. aureus are 0.5 µg/ml and 1.0 µg/ml. These numbers are near the limits of clinically achievable plasma concentrations. Acquisition of a mutation that mediates an altered DNA gyrase enzyme increases MICs by eightfold. This pushes the MICs for these two organisms above clinically achievable plasma concentrations. For E. coli, in which the MIC_{90}s are much lower (e.g., 0.06 µg/ml), a single point mutation still increases the MIC eightfold, but this new MIC is still within the range of clinically achievable plasma levels.

Plasmids containing genetic information that can be acquired by bacteria are the vehicles transmitting the molecular/genetic information that transfers resistance from one bacterium to another. Plasmids may not be genus or species specific, thus giving rise to bacteria having multiple types of resistance, acquired in plasmids originating in numerous other bacteria and selected in a classic darwinian sense by wide use of antimicrobials in the ICU. Plasmids may be partly thwarted through use of more than one antimicrobial at once, provided that the agent acts at different sites or through different mechanisms. This principle has been used in tuberculosis therapy for two generations, but in the ICU, the principle of two-drug therapy is not so fully rationalized. The resulting organisms have become more highly selected for multiple resistance factors. This principle has been contrasted with the trend toward using a single effective agent for the purposes of elegance, cost cutting, and avoidance of toxicity. It appears that for the present, the best therapy is rationalized in its benefit to the individual and not to the pool of organisms lying in the hospital environment.

Clearly then, there is considerable resistance among many of the microorganisms frequently seen in the setting of nosocomial infection. The ICU patient thus should have antimicrobial agents empirically chosen with care, taking the increased resistance of nosocomial pathogens to multiple classes of antimicrobials into account.

Application of Bacterial Resistance Patterns to the ICU Phase of Patient Management

Obviously once in the ICU and once the patient has been approached as described in the preceding sections of this chapter, specific management is determined based on the location of the infection and many other criteria. The appropriate management strategy for all possible infectious sites cannot be detailed. The data that follow explain the optimal mode of administration of different classes of drugs: (1) beta-lactams, (2) aminoglycosides, and (3) fluoroquinolones.

Beta-Lactam Antibiotics

In the test tube, beta-lactam drugs are not concentration dependent in the rate of kill for aerobic or facultative gram-negative bacilli.[49] This means that kill rates are not appreciably different at different multiples of the MIC. Consequently, high peak concentrations as are obtained near the

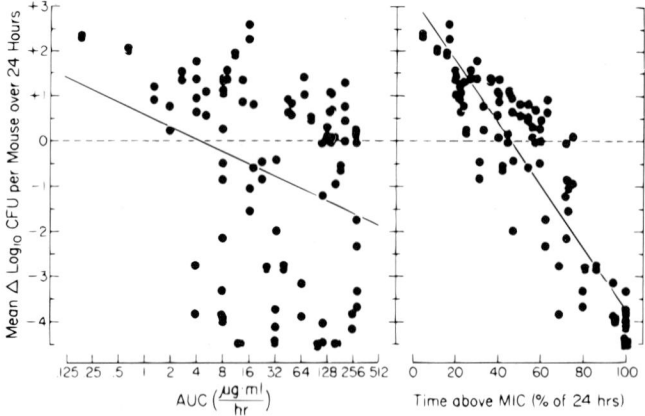

Fig. 67–3. Relationship between pharmacokinetic parameters and therapeutic efficacy of penicillin against Streptococcus pneumoniae (clinical isolate VA 180). The results of univariate regression analysis were as follows (AUC, area under the curve): For the $\log_{10}$ AUC, $y = 0.60 - 0.923 \times$, and $R^2 = 10\%$, and for time above the minimal inhibitory concentration (MIC), $y = 3.16 - 0.0693 \times$ and $R^2 = 84\%$. (From Vogelman, B., et al.: correlation of antimicrobial pharmacokinetic parameters with therapeutic efficacy in an animal model. J. Infect. Dis., *158*:831, 1988.

end of infusion do not kill appreciably faster than concentrations down lower on the curve near the MIC. This has important implications for the appropriate dose and schedule of this class of drugs. Gerber, Vogelman, and colleagues[50,51] have examined the behavior of beta-lactam drugs in the cure of infection in a neutropenic mouse thigh infection model. As can be seen in Figures 67–3 and 67–4,

where killing of the pneumococcus is examined with differing doses and schedules of penicillin G, and where killing of E. coli and S. aureus was examined with differing doses and schedules of cefazolin, it is clear that there is a highly significant linear correlation between an increased time that concentrations remain above the MIC of the infecting pathogen and the number of organisms killed at the primary infection site. Prior studies from Gerber and Craig have examined differing doses and schedules of ticarcillin for P. aeruginosa infection. These data are presented in Figure 67–5. The number of organisms at the primary infection site after therapy with a large dose of ticarcillin given every 3 hours was compared with that of one third the dose given hourly. The animals, therefore, were receiving the same total daily dose. If peak concentration had been important, the larger dose less frequently would have proved more efficacious. If total exposure were the variable most closely linked to organism kill at the primary infection site, both regimens would have been equally effi-

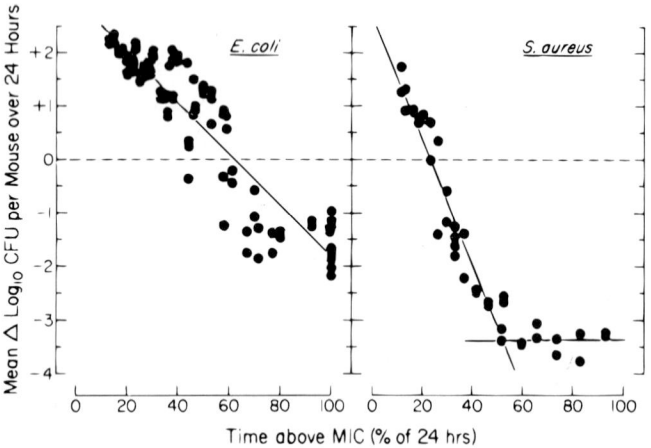

Fig. 67–4. Relationship between the duration of time that serum levels exceeded the minimal inhibitory concentration (MIC) and the efficacy of cefazolin against Escherichia coli ATCC 25922 and against Staphylococcus aureus ATCC 25923. *Left,* The results of regression analysis for cefazolin against E. coli were as follows: $y = 2.98 - 0.0477 \times$ and $R^2 = 84\%$. *Right,* The results of regression analysis for cefazolin against S. aureus were as follows: For those regimens with a time above the MIC of $0\% - 55\%$, $y = 2.75 - 0.117 \times$ and $R^2 = 92\%$; for those regimens with a time above the MIC of $55\% - 100\%$, $y = -3.42 + 0.0006 \times$ and $R^2 = 0.1\%$.[51]

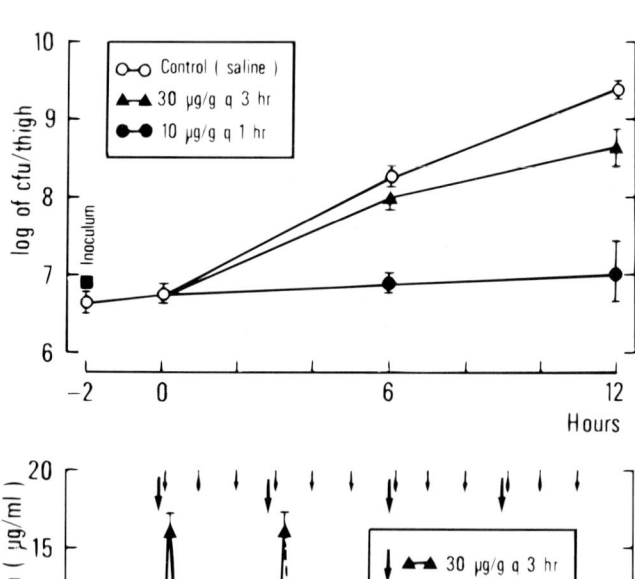

Fig. 67–5. Kinetics of sub-minimal inhibitory concentrations of ticarcillin and the corresponding effect on Pseudomonas aeruginosa ATCC 27853 in the same granulocytopenic mice. *Top,* Growth kinetics of P. aeruginosa in vivo. Each point represents the geometric mean ± standard deviation of the number of colony forming units (CFU) per thigh in three mice. The differences among the three growth curves are significant ($P < 0.01$). *Bottom,* Plasma kinetics after repeated 3 hour and 1 hour subcutaneous injections of ticarcillin (30 and 10 μg/g, respectively). Each point stands for the mean ± standard deviation of the plasma level in three mice. Limit of detectability (dotted line), 1 μg/ml.[50]

cacious. If time above the MIC were the important variable determining outcome, the smaller dose more frequently would produce the best results. As can be seen from Figure 67-5, the small dose more frequently, which produces the longest times above the MIC, had a significantly better control of organism growth at the primary infection site. This is consistent with other animal model data.[52]

These in vitro and animal model observations have clinical analogies, supported by three lines of evidence developed in patients. (First, a definition: Serum bactericidal activity or titer refers to the concentration of serially diluted serum containing antimicrobial(s) [that got there through clinical administration] required to kill the clinically recovered or experimental index organism.) The first line of evidence comes from studies of serum bactericidal titers in which a magic number has been identified using a peak titer (i.e., drawn 1 hour after the end of a half-hour infusion) of 1 to 8 or 1 to 16.[53-55] Although the timing of the serum titers is associated with the peak, it is actually powerful evidence that, for beta-lactam drugs, it is the time above the MIC, which is more closely linked to outcome. This conclusion is supported by the data of Platt and colleagues.[55] That investigator used the drug moxalactam as a single agent in the therapy of seriously ill patients with nosocomial infections. The dosing interval for this study was 8 hours. This drug has a terminal half-life observed in patients on the order of 2 to 3.5 hours.[56] One twofold dilution of serum halves the drug concentration. The same change in concentration takes place physiologically over one terminal elimination half-life. We assume the vast majority of distribution has taken place by 1 hour into the dosing interval, and therefore the drug is in "pseudodistribution equilibrium," which is to say that we are observing the terminal half-life at this time. Therefore a titer of 1 to 8 only means that we can go through three sequential halvings of drug concentration and still kill 99.9% of an initial inoculum of 10^5 to 10^6 microorganisms. Physiologically, this translates into the ability to maintain plasma concentrations greater than the MIC over three terminal half-lives or, in the case of moxalactam, for 6 to 10.5 hours. As the serum is drawn 1 to 1½ hours into the dosing interval, this means coverage for 7 to greater than 8 hours, essentially the entire dosing interval. Consequently, we are merely restating the lessons of animal model systems that it is time above the MIC or minimal bactericidal concentration (MBC), which is important for the outcome with beta-lactam drugs.

The second line of evidence was developed at the University of Maryland.[57] Investigators studied the use of cefoperazone (1.5 g intravenously every 6 hours) as empiric therapy for patients thought to be septic in a randomized trial. Cefamandole and tobramycin served as the comparator regimen. A total of 120 patients were randomized. Ten of the 60 cefoperazone-treated patients had a single-organism gram-negative rod bacteremia documented. A pharmacokinetic evaluation of this drug[58] enabled the investigators to perform a simulation that predicted a free drug concentration at trough of approximately 2 μg/ml. Consequently, we predicted that if the patients had an organism in their blood that had a cefoperazone MIC less than or equal to 2 μg/ml, we would predict success. If the MIC

Table 67-19. Patients Treated Empirically with Cefoperazone: Response Prediction in Patients with Single-Organism Gram-Negative Rod Bacteremia*

Prediction	6 successes	4 failures
Matched observation	5 successes	5 failures

* $P = 0.014$ by the Kappa statistic.
Patients were treated with 1.5 g of cefoperazone q 6 hours.
Predictions of "success' were based on the minimal inhibitory concentration (MIC) of the bacteremic organism being less than or equal to the predicted trough free drug concentration of cefoperazone (2 μg/ml). (Data from Standiford, H. C., et al.: Comparative pharmacokinetics of moxalactam, cefoperazone and cefotaxime in normal volunteers. Rev. Infect. Dis., 4(Suppl.):S585, 1982.)

were greater than 2 μg/ml, we would predict failure. Of the 10 patients, we predicted 6 successes and four failures (Table 67-19). Clinical results showed 5 successes and 5 failures. The one mispredicted patient was 85 years old, in septic shock at entry with renal failure and acidosis, and succumbed less than 24 hours after hospital admission. This appeared to be a physiologic and not a pharmacologic failure. Of further interest, if there had not been a correction for protein binding (total drug troughs of 20 μg/ml), we would have predicted nine successes and one failure. These results must be viewed with some caution because the number of patients was small, and actual concentrations of cefoperazone were not measured. Nonetheless, these data are compatible with the lessons learned from the animal model systems: It is time above the MIC or MBC that is important for the outcome with beta-lactam drugs.

There are other data from the clinical arena (third line of evidence) addressing the concept that for beta-lactam drugs, the time plasma concentration remains above the MIC is of prime importance so as to optimize clinical outcome. These data were developed by Schentag and colleagues.[59] This trial had both a learning portion and a validation portion. In the learning part of the trial, patients diagnosed as having gram-negative bacillary pneumonia received a fixed dose of the cephalosporin, cefmenoxime. Patient-specific pharmacokinetic parameters were estimated from serum concentrations determined during the early portion of each patient's clinical course. The causative organisms had cefmenoxime susceptibilities determined. The lower respiratory tract was sampled every 24 to 48 hours, through an endotracheal tube, when possible, and the day of bacterial eradication determined (two successive cultures without the original pathogen). Day to bacterial eradication served as the dependent variable. Univariate linear regressions were performed with **AUC/MIC**, where AUC means area under the curve of time/concentration plots, **and time greater than MIC**, "time greater than MIC," serving as the independent variables. The "time greater than MIC" provided an excellent correlation to the day of bacterial eradication (Fig. 67-6). The prospective validation portion used the AUC/MIC pharmacodynamic parameter as the guide to dose alteration (Fig. 67-7). An exposure was chosen that would cause eradication at day 4. These prospectively studied patients, when their data are analyzed with time above the MIC as the independent variable, fit the original regression line quite

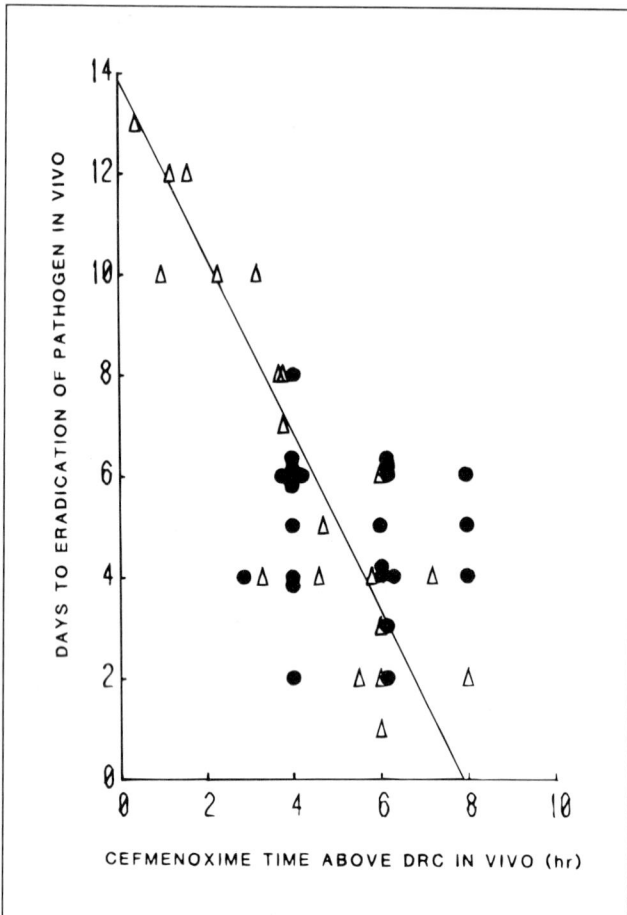

Fig. 67-6. Relationship between the time cefmenoxime serum concentrations exceeded the dynamic response concentration (DRC) for retrospectively (open triangle) and prospectively (solid circle) treated patients and the days to bacterial eradication in vivo. Each data point represents one pathogen. The regression line describing the retrospective data took the form of the equation: Days to eradication = 13.86 − 1.78 (time over dynamic response concentration), r = 0.89, $P < 0.001$. The dual individualized dosage method clustered the eradication day tightly around days 4 and 6. (From Schentag, J. J., et al.: Role for dual individualization with cefmenoxime. Am. J. Med., 77(Symp. 6A): 43, 1984.)

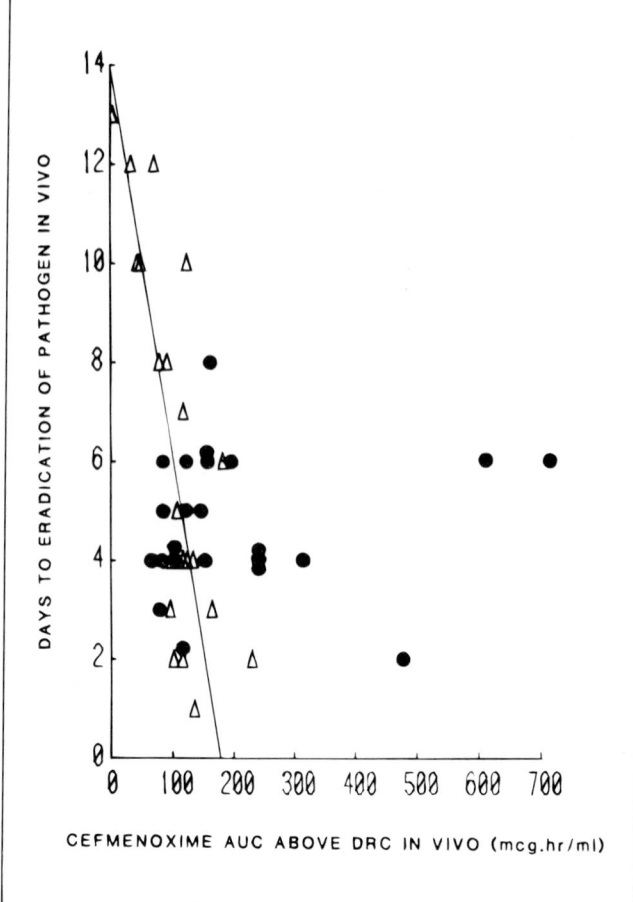

Fig. 67-7. Relationship between cefmenoxime area under the curve (AUC) over the dynamic response concentration (DRC) and days to bacterial eradication in vivo for retrospective (open triangle) and prospective (solid circle) patients. Each data point represents one pathogen. The regression line shows the relationship used to apply dual individualization prospectively. (From Schentag, J. J., et al.: Role for dual individualization with cefmenoxime. Am. J. Med., 77(Symp. 6A): 43, 1984.)

nicely (see Fig. 67-6) and better than the original AUC/MIC regression (see Fig. 67-7), wherein a number of the prospective patients became outliers.

There are reasonable data derived form human investigation that provide direct support to the hypothesis that the time plasma concentrations exceed the threshold of bacterial inhibition will have a direct relationship to the ultimate patient outcome from serious bacterial infections. A corollary to this statement is that, for beta-lactam drugs, the "time above the MIC" can be maximized by using shorter rather than longer dosing intervals. Consequently, for any daily dose of drug, using smaller doses more frequently will tend to maximize the time plasma concentrations exceed the MIC of the infecting pathogen.

This principle also provides a mechanism to allow comparison of differing beta-lactam drugs to allow a rational choice of doses and schedule in the empiric therapy setting. One need only examine the time that the nonprotein-bound drug remains above the MICs of relevant clinical pathogens at the specific institution where the choice of agent is being made. A group at the University of Maryland including one of us produced a series of publications examining the time greater than MIC for a series of beta-lactam antibiotics for aerobic or facultative gram-negative bacilli (Table 67-20).[60-63] The success of this approach may be judged by its ability to predict the clinical utility of these compounds. Clearly, all are highly active against E. coli and K. pneumoniae. The time periods in hours that free drug concentration equalled or exceeded the MIC for 90% of the isolates for P. aeruginosa shows a greater range among the compounds evaluated. Clearly the early third-generation cephalosporins have not become drugs of choice as single agents for patients with serious pseudomonas infections because clinical outcome has been subopti-

Table 67-20. Duration That Free Drug Concentrations of New Beta-Lactams Exceed the Minimum Inhibitory Concentration (μg/ml) for 90% of Strains of Important Gram-Negative Pathogens in Volunteers

		Hours of Free Drug Concentration >MIC for:				
Antibiotic	Dose (g)	Escherichia coli	Klebsiella pneumoniae	Enterobacter cloacae	Serratia marcescens	Pseudomonas aeruginosa
Moxalactam	2	>12.0	>12.0	>12.0	>12.0	0.4
Cefotaxime	2	8.9	8.9	6.5	6.5	0.2
Cefoperazone	2	5.3	5.3	3.6	0.6	0.6
Ticarcillin	5	0.0	0.0	0.0	0.0	0.1
Piperacillin	5	1.4	4.4	0.6	0.0	3.3
Mezlocillin	5	2.0	3.8	2.0	0.0	1.1
Ceftazidime	2	>12.0	>12.0	>12.0	>12.0	5.8
Imipenem	1	>6.0	>6.0	>6.0	5.6	4.5

(Data from Drusano, G. L.: Role of pharmacokinetics in the outcome of infections. Antimicrob. Agents Chemother., *32*:289, 1988.)

mal. This is reflected in short time periods in hours of free drug concentration above the MIC for 90% of the isolates for these compounds. This is so even for a drug such as cefoperazone, which has a reasonably low MIC for 90% of the isolates of pseudomonas but is extensively protein-bound at approximately 90%, resulting in low free drug concentrations and a short "time above the MIC." Drugs that have shown better clinical utility against pseudomonas include piperacillin, ceftazidime, and imipenem. Once again, this is reflected in the "time above the MIC$_{90}$," relative to their respective dosing intervals (every 4 to 6 hours for piperacillin, every 8 hours for ceftazidime, and every 6 hours for imipenem; see Table 67-20). Interestingly, imipenem has 4 hours above the MIC$_{90}$ but also possesses a postantibiotic effect of 1 to 3 hours for this pathogen, which may contribute to its performance against this organism. The simple exercise of determining the time in hours that plasma concentrations of free drug exceed the MIC of clinically important pathogens allows the clinician to select the most rational beta-lactam agent in the empiric therapy setting, keeping in mind the likely pathogens based on the infection site and the antimicrobial susceptibility profile of the hospital (or, more appropriately, the specific unit in which the patient developed the infection because this can differ within an institution).

Aminoglycosides

In contrast to the beta-lactam class of drugs, where the in vitro animal model and clinical data are in close accord, there are differences in these data as to which pharmacodynamic variable is most closely linked to outcome for the aminoglycosides (peak concentration versus AUC).[51,64-66] Vogelman and associates[51] examined the ability of aminoglycosides to inhibit or kill E. coli or P. aeruginosa in their mouse thigh infection model. Their evaluation demonstrated that kill of these gram-negative rods at the primary infection site was associated with the AUC of drug exposure in the plasma (Figs. 67-8 and 67-9).

In clinical trials, however, peak concentrations of aminoglycoside or peak-to-MIC ratios have been linked to favorable outcome when serious gram-negative rod infections have been treated with single-agent aminoglycoside therapy. There are a number of reasons for this. The most likely is that there is a great deal of covariance between peak and AUC. For any specific half-life of drug, higher peaks must then translate into higher AUC. Consequently, in a clinical sense, it is difficult to differentiate peak from AUC in linking either one of these variables to organism kill or ultimate patient outcome. Further, because of the limitations of obtaining appropriate plasma concentrations in the clinical setting, study designs have made robust determination of the area under the plasma concentration versus time curve difficult, whereas determination of an isolated peak and trough concentration is clinically achievable.

Moore and colleagues[65,66] have addressed the relationship between aminoglycoside plasma concentrations and the outcome of infections. The data reported were compi-

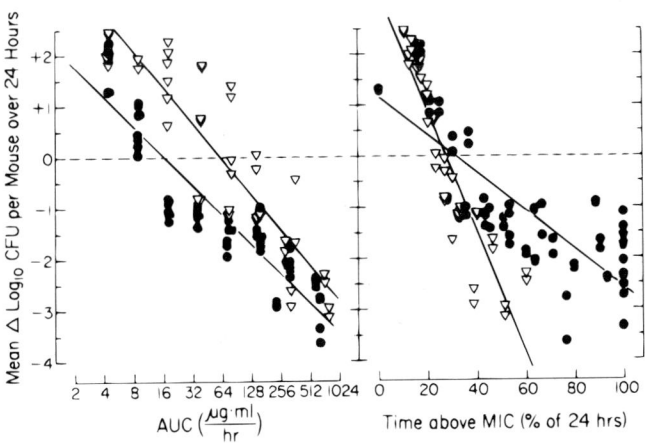

Fig. 67-8. Relationship between pharmacokinetic parameters and efficacy for gentamicin against Escherichia coli ATCC 25922. The results of univariate regression analysis for the 1 to 4 hour regimens (solid circle) were as follows: for the log$_{10}$ area under the curve (AUC), $y = 2.29 - 1.89 \times$ and $R^2 = 83\%$, and for the time above the minimum inhibitory concentration (MIC), $y = 1.18 - 0.0377 \times$ and $R^2 = 62\%$. The results of univariate regression analysis for the 6 to 12 hour regimens (open upside-down triangle) were as follows: for the log$_{10}$ AUC, $y = 4.18 - 2.33 \times$ and $R^2 = 80\%$, and for the time above the MIC, $y = 3.30 - 0.120 \times$ and $R^2 = 85\%$.[51]

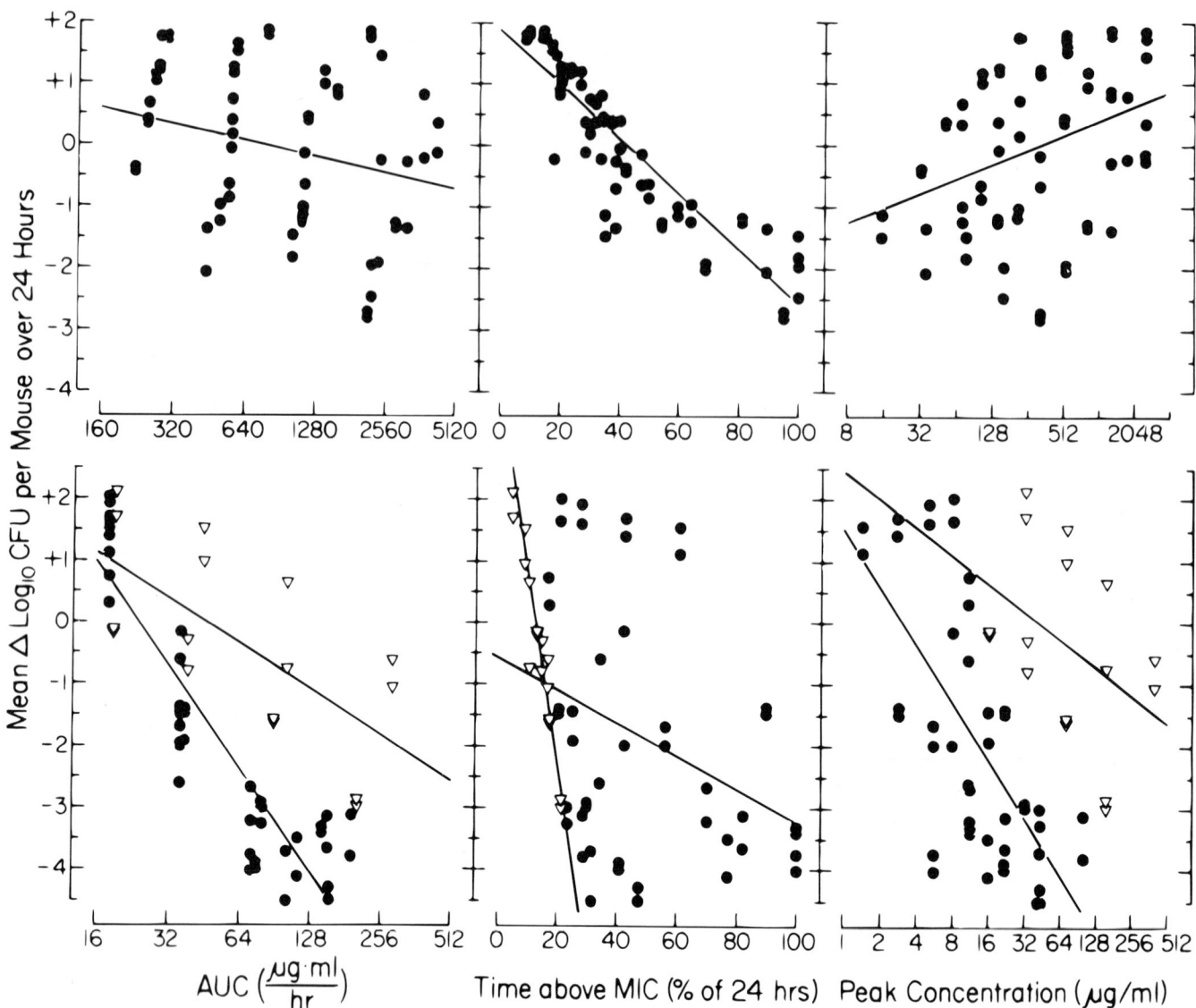

Fig. 67-9. Relationship between pharmacokinetic parameters and therapeutic efficacy for ticarcillin and tobramycin against Pseudomonas aeruginosa ATCC 27853. Each data point represents the difference between the mean number of cfu in the two thighs from a mouse at the end of 24 hours of therapy and in the thighs from control mice at the onset of therapy. *Upper panels,* The results of univariate regression analysis for ticarcillin were as follows: for the $\log_{10}$ area under the curve (AUC), $y = 2.52 - 0.878 \times$ and $R^2 = 7\%$; for the time above the minimal inhibitory concentration (MIC), $y = 1.85 - 0.0446 \times$ and $R^2 = 81\%$; and for the $\log_{10}$ peak level, $y = -2.03 + 0.811 \times$ and $R^2 = 13\%$. *Lower panels,* The results of univariate regression analysis for 1 to 8 hour regimens (solid circle) of tobramycin were as follows: for the $\log_{10}$ AUC, $y = 7.69 - 5.57 \times$ and $R^2 = 83\%$; for time above the MIC, $y = -0.06 - 0.0272 \times$ and $R^2 = 12\%$; and for $\log_{10}$ peak level, $y = 1.53 - 3.12 \times$ and $R^2 = 44\%$. The results of univariate regression analysis for the 12 to 24 hour regimens (upside-down open triangle) were as follows: for the $\log_{10}$ AUC, $y = 4.08 - 2.45 \times$ and $R^2 = 48\%$; for time above the MIC, $y = 4.00 - 0.314 \times$ and $R^2 = 91\%$; and for the $\log_{10}$ peak level, $y = 2.42 - 1.49 \times$ and $R^2 = 18\%$.[51]

lations of patients from three prospective, randomized trials of the empiric therapy of patients suspected of suffering from serious gram-negative infections. Aminoglycosides studied were gentamicin, tobramycin, and amikacin.

In the first paper, 37 patients with gram-negative pneumonia who received an aminoglycoside for therapy of their infection were analyzed. Those patients who achieved peak aminoglycoside concentrations **(one half hour after the end of a half-hour infusion)** of 7 μg/ml for gentamicin or tobramycin or 28 μg/ml for amikacin had a significantly improved outcome (Table 67-21). In the second paper, 236 patients with a variety of well-documented gram-negative infections (including the above-mentioned pneumonias) were analyzed. Clearly, both pharmacologic and microbiologic data are important in an analysis of outcome in patients with differing infections. These investigators included both types of information in their analysis. They found that there was a significant rela-

Table 67–21. Peak Plasma Concentrations of Aminoglycosides and the Relationship to Outcome of Gram-Negative Pneumonia

	≥7 μg/ml* ≥28 μg/ml†	<7 μg/ml* <28 μg/ml†
Success	14 (70%)	6 (32%)
Failure	6 (30%)	13 (68%)

* For gentamicin and tobramycin.
† For amikacin.
P <0.006, by Fisher's exact test.
(Data from Moore, R. D., Smith, C. R., and Lietman, P. S.: Association of aminoglycoside plasma levels with therapeutic outcome in gram-negative pneumonia. Am. J. Med., 77:657, 1984.)

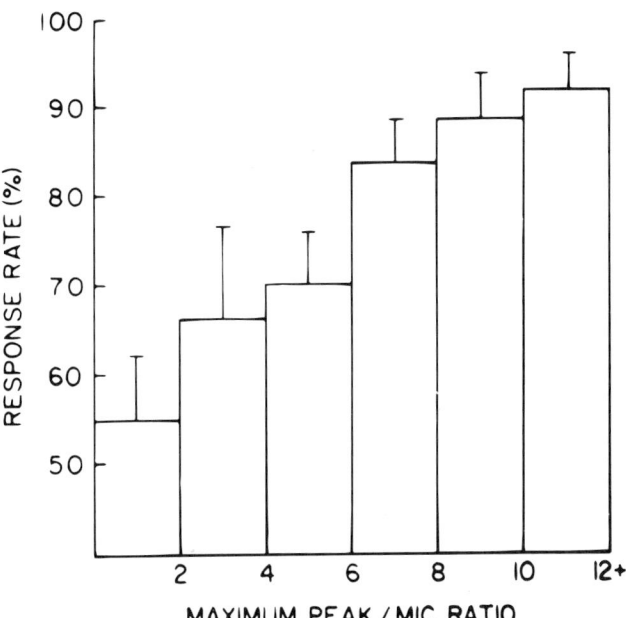

Fig. 67–10. Relationship between the maximal peak level-to-minimal inhibitory concentration (MIC) ratio and the rate of clinical response. Vertical bars represent SE values. (Data from Moore, R. D., Lietman, P. S., and Smith, C. R.: Clinical response to aminoglycoside therapy: importance of the ratio of peak concentration to minimal inhibitory concentration. J. Infect. Dis., 155:93, 1987.)

tionship between the ratio of peak concentration to MIC and outcome. This relationship held up even when other important patient variables were considered in a multiple logistic regression analysis. With an increasing peak-to-MIC ratio, there was an increasing likelihood of a positive outcome. The actual odds ratios and their 95% confidence intervals are presented in Table 67–22. The response rates as a function of this ratio are presented in Figure 67–10.

For aminoglycosides, the time plasma concentrations remain above the MIC is far less important to patient outcome. Rather, larger doses of drug less frequently, obtaining higher peak-to-MIC ratios, may optimize outcome of patients with serious gram-negative rod infections. All the clinical data developed to support this hypothesis have been with a fixed dosing interval. Whether giving larger doses less frequently to obtain a greater peak-to-MIC ratio (e.g., once or twice daily aminoglycoside dosing) will result in improved clinical outcomes is an area of active, ongoing investigation. At the least, we can say that **a low peak-to-MIC ratio** on a more traditional dosing schedule should be a signal to the clinician to increase the drug dose, if that is possible to do safely. Failing that, a low ratio should cause the clinician to consider a change or addition of antimicrobial(s) to a more active class of drugs.

Fluoroquinolones

Fluoroquinolone antimicrobials are additions to the physician's quiver. Their microbiologic properties are similar to aminoglycosides in that they are highly concentration dependent in their rate of kill. Consequently, it is not surprising that, similar to the aminoglycosides, both "AUC" and "peak-to-MIC ratio" have been identified as being the factors most closely linked to infection outcome.[51,64,67,68]

Blaser and colleagues[64] examined the relationship between plasma concentration time profile and the ability to kill a strain of K. pneumoniae in an in vitro model system that simulates plasma concentration time profiles seen in patients (Figs. 67–11 and 67–12). They compared a large dose of enoxacin, a fluoroquinolone, given once daily to half the dose given every 12 hours. In one of their experiments, they noted breakthrough growth with the half-dose-every-12-hour regimen (see Fig. 67–11). When they examined all of their data (see Fig. 67–12), they noted that virtual sterilization of their in vitro system occurred only when the "peak-to-MIC ratio" for the fluoroquinolone exceeded 10:1. Dudley and colleagues[67] used this same system to examine the mechanism by which this occurred. In this experiment, the investigators examined the use of ciprofloxacin against a strain of P. aeruginosa. They simulated a dose of 200 mg intravenously every 12 hours. They examined the number of resistant organisms present in their in vitro system at the start of therapy and at 12 hours and at 24 hours after initiation of the experiment. As can be seen by examining Figure 67–13, the use of relatively low doses of this fluoroquinolone caused selection of resistant mutants from the population of pseudomonads. Of interest, as stated earlier, gyr A mutants have approximately an eightfold increase in their MICs relative to the

Table 67–22. Association Between Maximal Peak-to-Minimal Inhibitory Concentration Ratio and Relative Odds to Clinical Response to Aminoglycoside Therapy

Maximal Peak/Minimal Inhibitory Concentration	Relative Odds	95% Confidence Interval
<2	1.00	—
2 to <4	1.63	0.84–3.16
4 to <6	1.83	1.09–3.03
6 to <8	4.35	2.53–7.46
8 to <10	6.49	3.56–11.82
≥10	8.41	4.62–15.33

(Data from Moore, R. D., Lietman, P. S., and Smith, C. R.: Clinical response to aminoglycoside therapy: importance of the ratio of peak concentration to minimal inhibitory concentration. J. Infect. Dis., 1:55:93, 1987.)

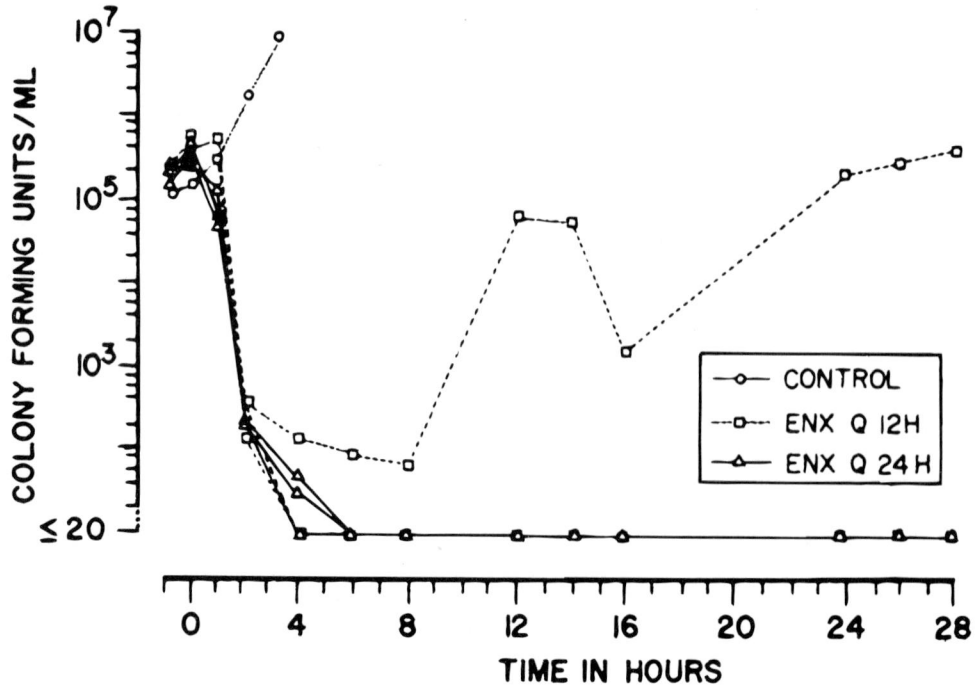

Fig. 67-11. Bactericidal activity of two enoxacin regimens against Klebsiella pneumoniae in the pharmacokinetic model. Cultures were eradicated in three of three experiments when the total daily dose was given as one dose every 24 hours but in only two of three experiments when the same total daily dose was given as equal doses every 12 hours.[64]

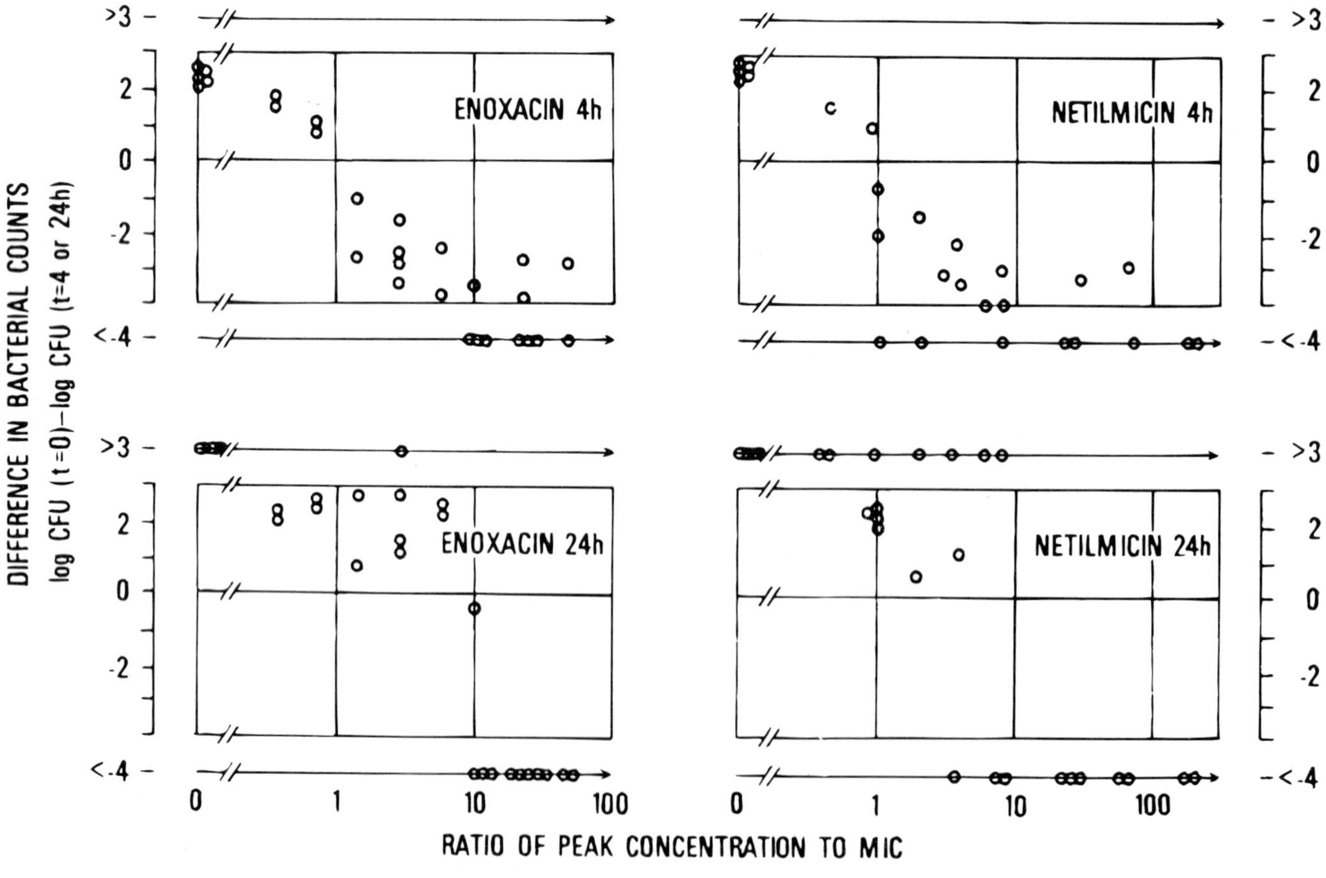

Fig. 67-12. Antibacterial effect of multiple-dose regimens of enoxacin and netilmicin against five organisms. Changes in bacterial numbers during treatment periods of 4 and 24 hours are plotted against the ratios of peak concentration to minimal inhibitory concentration (MIC).[64] t, Time.

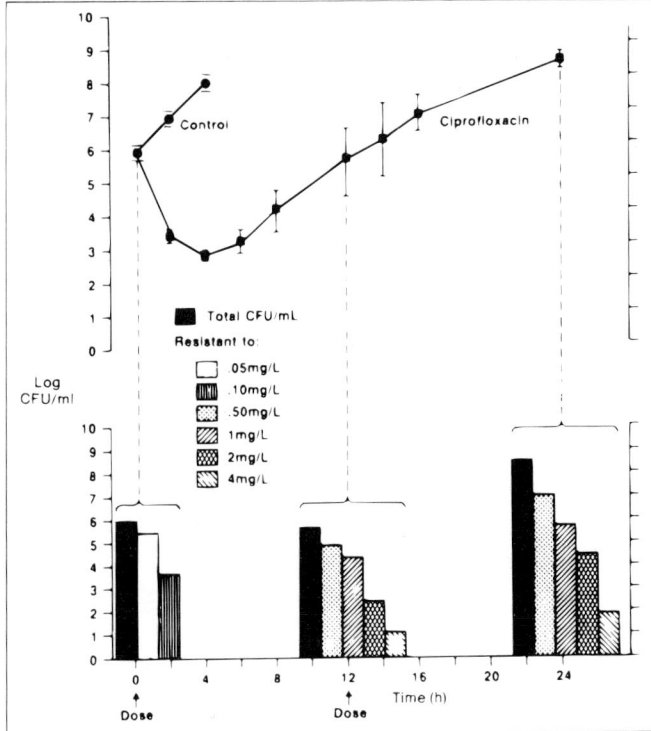

Fig. 67–13. Bactericidal activity of ciprofloxacin and subpopulation analysis for Pseudomonas aeruginosa 810 in an in vitro model following two simulated 200-mg doses. Values are mean ± SD.[67]

parent strain. Consequently the findings seen by Blaser and associates as well as Dudley and colleagues may be explained by having high peak-to-MIC ratios (>10:1) being able to suppress not only the parent strain, but also the gyr A mutants in the population.

This was examined by one of us in a neutropenic rat model of pseudomonas sepsis.[69] Indeed, the investigators were able to verify that peak to MIC ratios greater than 10:1 were associated with far better outcomes in this animal model system and further that there was a relationship between peak-to-MIC ratio and survivorship in this set of experiments. Also found was that when peak-to-MIC ratios did not exceed 10:1, it appears as if area under the plasma concentration time curve is most closely linked to outcome, explaining some of the findings reported by Craig and colleagues.

Pelloquin and colleagues[70] have performed a study with ciprofloxacin in their ICU among patients with gram-negative rod pneumonia similar to the study performed and mentioned previously for beta-lactam drugs. In that study, however, a large number of organisms were noted to emerge resistant to the fluoroquinolone during therapy. This occurred statistically significantly more frequently when peak-to-MIC ratios were below 10:1. The original conclusion from this study was that response among patients treated with fluoroquinolones was related to the time plasma concentrations exceeded the MIC, but emergence of resistance may be related to peak-to-MIC ratio. Further analysis performed on the same data set, but with more elegant and appropriate statistical methodology, indicates that AUC was most directly linked to outcome.[71]

Consequently, there are in vitro, animal model, and human data with fluoroquinolones that seem to indicate that peak-to-MIC ratio or AUC plays an important role in the determination of outcome for seriously infected patients. Once again, a corollary of this finding is that to optimize the administration of fluoroquinolone antibiotics for seriously infected patients in the ICU, larger doses less frequently (i.e., on an every 12 or even 24 hour schedule) should be administered.

Differing classes of drugs have differing pharmacodynamic parameters linked to outcome. For beta-lactam drugs, which are nonconcentration dependent in their rate of kill, time above the MIC is of utmost importance, which would indicate smaller doses of drug given on a more frequent schedule. For both aminoglycosides and fluoroquinolone antimicrobials, which are both concentration dependent in their rates of kill for gram-negative organisms, peak-to-MIC ratio and the total area under the concentration time curve are most closely linked to outcome. For these agents then, larger doses of drug less frequently, obtaining higher peak-to-MIC ratios are most likely to obtain the best patient outcome.

Application of Principles to Antimicrobial Therapy in the Post-ICU Phase

Little is known with molecular clarity about exactly when to stop antimicrobial treatment. The optimal duration of therapy for serious infections has been determined largely by empiric observation. Relapse rates can be measured and used to establish courses that are long enough to prevent relapse. Some patients (and physicians) stop therapy as soon as there is improvement, sometimes with a poor result and sometimes without penalty. The most that can be said is that major signs and symptoms of infection should be seen to have returned to baseline. Further, fever should have also returned to baseline. Cultures, if indicated during therapy, of the infected fluid or tissue, should be negative. A plan to obtain cultures of the infected fluid or tissue following clinical cure and the end of antimicrobial therapy should be developed with the patient's involvement and the explicit invitation to the patient to contact you immediately if symptoms, including fever, recur. That culture should be taken following an antimicrobial-free interval of at least 1 to 2 weeks, i.e., until the body is free of antimicrobials, antimicrobial metabolites, and antimicrobials stored in tissues. The return of surrogate markers of infection to baseline, such as elevated white blood cell count and elevated erythrocyte sedimentation rate, may also be useful in determining the length of therapy. When one considers bacterial persistence, seeding to distant sites, late recurrence, and other complications of incomplete therapy, most physicians think that a "full" or established course of therapy makes sense and is good insurance at a low cost compared with the complications of inadequate foreshortened treatment. The cost of antimicrobials is low compared with the cost of any of the diseases for which they are indicated.

Several investigators are exploring the possibility of

switching seriously ill patients to oral therapies once the patient's condition has stabilized. Obviously such a decision is predicated on the presence of an intact, normally functioning gastrointestinal system. With a stable patient and the return of appropriate data from the clinical microbiology laboratory, investigators such as Quintiliani and coworkers[72] have discontinued costly intravenous antibiotic therapy and have placed the patient on fluoroquinolone antimicrobials, such as ciprofloxacin or ofloxacin. They have termed this practice streamlining of antimicrobial therapy. Although such a practice is attractive because of the possibilities of major cost savings, its true place in clinical practice still needs to be defined, and the patients that are selected for such practice should be chosen extremely conservatively.

Infection in the ICU patient is a tremendous challenge to the clinician. The severity of patient illness, previous therapies, and frequent acquisition of infection in the hospital all make treatment of such patients difficult. Knowledge of the probable site of infection along with probable organisms at such an infection site and knowledge of the microbiologic susceptibility data for that hospital's ICU should allow the rational choice of antimicrobial agents for the therapy of the infection. Knowledge of the underlying relationships between drug exposure and infection outcome should allow the clinician to choose doses and schedules of differing classes of antimicrobials, which will provide optimal outcomes for this seriously ill and impaired patient population.

REFERENCES

1. Centers for Disease Control and Prevention: Increase in national hospital discharge survey rates for septicemia—United States, 1979–1987. M.M.W.R., *39:*31, 1990.
2. Martin, M. A.: Epidemiology and clinical impact of gram-negative sepsis. Infect. Dis. Clin. North Am., *5:*739, 1991.
3. Moellering, R. C., Jr., Yao, J. D. C., and Thornsberry, C.: Approximate concentrations of antimicrobial agents achieved in blood. *In* Manual of Clinical Microbiology. 5th Ed. Edited by A. Balows, et al. Washington, D.C., American Society for Microbiology, 1991, p. 1201.
4. Drugs that cause psychiatric symptoms. Med. Lett., *35:*65, 1993.
5. Danner, R. L., et al.: Therapeutic trial of lipid X in a canine model of septic shock. J. Infect. Dis., *167:*378, 1993.
6. Quezado, Z. M., et al.: A controlled trial of HA-1A in a canine model of Gram-negative septic shock. JAMA, *269:*2221, 1993.
7. West, B. C., and Wilson, J. P.: Subconjunctival corticosteroid therapy complicated by hyperinfective strongyloidiasis. Am. J. Ophthalmol., *89:*854, 1980.
8. Blumenfeld, H. L., Kilbourne, E. D., Louria, D. B., and Rogers, D. E.: Studies on influenza in the pandemic of 1957–1958. I. An epidemiologic, clinical and serologic investigation of an intrahospital epidemic, with a note on vaccination efficacy. J. Clin. Invest., *38:*199, 1959.
9. Caplan, E. S., and Hoyt, N.J.: Nosocomial sinusitis. JAMA, *247:*639, 1982.
10. Lum-Cheong, R. S., and Cornwell, E. E., III: Suppurative sinusitis in critically ill patients: a case report and review of the literature. J. Natl. Med. Assoc., *84:*1057, 1992.
11. Rello, J., et al.: Pneumonia due to Haemophilus influenzae among mechanically ventilated patients. Incidence, outcome, and risk factors. Chest, *102:*1562, 1992.
12. Meyer, K. S., et al.: Nosocomial outbreak of Klebsiella infection resistant to late-generation cephalosporins. Ann. Intern. Med., *119:*353, 1993.
13. Fang, F. C., et al.: Value of molecular epidemiologic analysis in a nosocomial methicillin-resistant Staphylococcus aureus outbreak. JAMA, *270:*1323, 1993.
14. Back, N. A., et al.: Recurrent epidemics caused by a single strain of erythromycin-resistant Staphylococcus aureus. The importance of molecular epidemiology. JAMA, *270:*1329, 1993.
15. Ehrhardt, A. F., et al.: Emergence of resistance to imipenem in Enterobacter isolates masquerading as Klebsiella pneumoniae during therapy with imipenem/cilastatin. Clin. Infect. Dis., *17:*120, 1993.
16. Kramer, M. R., et al.: Infectious complications in heart-lung transplantation. Analysis of 200 episodes. Arch. Intern. Med., *153:*2010, 1993.
17. Walsh, T. J., et al.: Randomized double-blinded trial of rifampin with either novobiocin or trimethoprim-sulfamethoxazole against methicillin-resistant Staphylococcus aureus colonization: prevention of antimicrobial resistance and effect of host factors on outcome. Antimicrob. Agents Chemother., *37:*1334, 1993.
18. Iseman, M. D.: Treatment of multidrug-resistant tuberculosis. N. Engl. J. Med., *329:*784, 1993.
19. Wilson, R., and Hamburger, M.: Fifteen years' experience with staphylococcus septicemia in large city hospital: analysis of fifty-five cases in Cincinnati General Hospital 1940–1954. Am. J. Med., *22:*437, 1957.
20. West, B. C., DeVault, G. A., Jr., Clement, J. C., and Williams, D. M.: Aplastic anemia associated with parenteral chloramphenicol: review of 10 cases, including the second case of possible increased risk with cimetidine. Rev. Infect. Dis., *10:*1048, 1988.
21. Sanford, J. P.: The enigma of candiduria: evolution of bladder irrigation with amphotericin B for management—from anecdote to dogma and a lesson from Machiavelli. Clin. Infect. Dis., *16:*145, 1993.
22. Maki, D. G., Ringer, M., and Alvarado, C. J.: Prospective randomized trial of povidone-iodine, alcohol, and chlorhexidine for prevention of infection associated with central venous and arterial catheters. Lancet, *338:*339, 1991.
23. Mermel, L. A., Stolz, S. M., and Maki, D. G.: Surface antimicrobial activity of heparin-bonded and antiseptic-impregnated vascular catheters. J. Infect. Dis., *167:*920, 1993.
24. Klotz, S. A.: Fungal adherence to the vascular compartment: a critical step in the pathogenesis of disseminated candidiasis. Clin. Infect. Dis., *14:*340, 1992.
25. Klotz, S. A., et al.: Adherence of *Candida albicans* to immobilized extracellular matrix proteins is mediated by calcium-dependent surface glycoproteins. Microb. Pathogen., *14:*133, 1993.
26. Strickland, G. T.: Malaria. *In* Hunter's Tropical Medicine. 7th Ed. Edited by G. T. Strickland. Philadelphia, W. B. Saunders, 1991. p. 586.
27. Drugs for AIDS and associated infections. Med. Lett., *35:*79, 1993.
28. Warren, K. S., and Mahmoud, A. A. F. (Eds.): Tropical and Geographic Medicine. 2nd Ed. New York, McGraw-Hill, 1990.
29. Mandell, G. L., Douglas, R. G., and Bennett, J. E. (Eds.): Principles and Practice of Infectious Diseases. 3rd Ed. New York, Churchill Livingston, 1990.
30. Cooksey, R. C.: Mechanisms of resistance to antimicrobial agents. *In* Manual of Clinical Microbiology. 5th Ed. Edited

by A. Balows, et al. Washington, D.C., American Society for Microbiology, 1991, p. 1099.
31. Stillwell, M., and Caplan, E. S.: The septic multiple-trauma patient. Infect. Dis. Clin. North Am., *3*:155, 1989.
32. Sanders, W. E., Jr., and Sanders, C. C.: Inducible beta-lactamases: clinical and epidemiologic implications for use of newer cephalosporins. Rev. Infect. Dis., *10*:830, 1988.
33. Murray, B. E.: The life and times of the Enterococcus. Clin. Microbiol. Rev., *3*:46, 1990.
34. Mylotte, J. M., McDermott, C., and Spooner, J. A.: Prospective study of 114 consecutive episodes of Staphylococcus aureus bacteremia. Rev. Infect. Dis., *9*:891, 1987.
35. Crane, L. R., Levine, D. P., Zervos, M. J., and Cummings, G.: Bacteremia in narcotic addicts at the Detroit Medical Center. I. Microbiology, epidemiology, risk factors, and empiric therapy. Rev. Infect. Dis., *8*:364, 1986.
36. McGowan, J. E., Jr.: Gram-positive bacteria: spread and antimicrobial resistance in university and community hospitals in the USA. J. Antimicrob. Chemother., *21(Suppl. C)*:49, 1988.
37. Johnson, A. P., Uttley, A. H., Woodford, N., and George, R. C.: Resistance to vancomycin and teicoplanin: an emerging clinical problem. Clin. Microbiol. Rev., *3*:280, 1990.
38. al-Obeid, S., Collatz, E., and Gutmann, L.: Mechanism of resistance to vancomycin in Enterococcus faecium D366 and Enterococcus faecalis A256. Antimicrob. Agents Chemother., *34*:252, 1990.
39. Watanakunakorn, C.: Mode of action and in-vitro activity of vancomycin. J. Antimicrob. Chemother., *14(Suppl. D)*:7, 1984.
40. Drusano, G. L.: Bacterial pathogens for the 1990's: a case for new drug development. *In* Emerging Targets in Antibacterial and Antifungal Chemotherapy. Edited by J. A. Sutcliffe and N. H. Georgopapadakou. New York, Chapman & Hall, 1991, p. 24.
41. Sanders, C. C., Iaconis, J. P., Bodey, G. P., and Samonis, G.: Resistance to ticarcillin-potassium clavulanate among clinical isolates of the family Enterobacteriaceae: role of PSE-1 beta-lactamase and high levels of TEM-1 and SHV-1 and problems with false susceptibility in disk diffusion tests. Antimicrob. Agents Chemother., *32*:1365, 1988.
42. Mabilat, D., et al.: Direct sequencing of the amplified structural gene and promoter for the extended-broad-spectrum beta-lactamase TEM-9 (RHH-1) of Klebsiella pneumoniae. Plasmid, *23*:27, 1990.
43. Mitsuhashi, S., and Kawabe, H.: Aminoglycoside antibiotic resistance in bacteria. *In* The Aminoglycosides: Microbiology, Clinical Use and Toxicology. Edited by A. Whelton and H. C. Neu. New York, Marcel Dekker, 1982, p. 97.
44. Patterson, J. E., and Zervos, M. J.: High-level gentamicin resistance in Enterococcus: microbiology, genetic basis, and epidemiology. Rev. Infect. Dis., *12*:644, 1990.
45. Peterson, L. R., et al.: Emergence of ciprofloxacin resistance in nosocomial methicillin-resistant Staphylococcus aureus isolates. Resistance during ciprofloxacin plus rifampin therapy for methicillin-resistant S. aureus colonization. Arch. Intern. Med., *150*:2151, 1990.
46. Sreedharan, S., et al.: DNA gyrase gyrA mutations in ciprofloxacin-resistant strains of Staphylococcus aureus: close similarity with quinolone resistance mutations in Escherichia coli. J. Bacteriol., *172*:7260, 1990.
47. Wolfson, J. S., Hooper, D. C., and Schwartz, M. N.: Mechanisms of action of and resistance to quinolone antimicrobial agents. *In* Quinolone Antimicrobial Agents. Edited by J. S. Wolfson and D. C. Hooper. Washington, D.C., American Society for Microbiology, 1989, p. 5.
48. Sanders, C. C., and Watanakunakorn, C.: Emergence of resistance to beta lactams, aminoglycosides, and quinolones during combination therapy for infection due to Serratia marcescens. J. Infect. Dis., *153*:617, 1986.
49. Craig, W. A., and Ebert, S. C.: Killing and regrowth of bacteria in vitro: a review. Scand. J. Infect. Dis., *74*:63, 1990.
50. Gerber, A. U., et al.: Impact of dosing intervals on activity of gentamicin and ticarcillin against Pseudomonas aeruginosa in granulocytopenic mice. J. Infect. Dis., *147*:910, 1983.
51. Vogelman, B., et al: Correlation of antimicrobial pharmacokinetic parameters with therapeutic efficacy in an animal model. J. Infect. Dis., *158*:831, 1988.
52. Roosendaal, R., Bakker-Woudenberg, I. A., van den Berghe-van Raffe, M., and Michel, M. F.: Continuous versus intermittent administration of ceftazidime in experimental Klebsiella pneumoniae pneumonia in normal and leukopenic rats. Antimicrob. Agents Chemother., *30*:403, 1986.
53. Klastersky, J., Daneau, D., Swings, G., and Weerts, D.: Antibacterial activity in serum and urine as a therapeutic guide in bacterial infections. J. Infect. Dis., *129*:187, 1974.
54. Sculier, J. P., and Klastersky, J.: Significance of serum bactericidal activity in gram-negative bacillary bacteremia in patients with and without granulocytopenia. Am. J. Med., *76*:429, 1984.
55. Platt, R., et al.: Moxalactam therapy of infections caused by cephalothin-resistant bacteria: influence of serum inhibitory activity on clinical response and acquisition of antibiotic resistance during therapy. Antimicrob. Agents Chemother., *20*:351, 1981.
56. Swanson, D. J., et al.: Steady-state moxalactam pharmacokinetics in patients: noncompartmental versus two-compartmental analysis. J. Pharmacokinet. Biopharm., *11*:337, 1983.
57. Warren, J. W., et al.: A randomized, controlled trial of cefoperazone vs. cefamandole-tobramycin in the treatment of putative, severe infections with gram-negative bacilli. Rev. Infect. Dis., *5(Suppl. 1)*:S173, 1983.
58. Standiford, H. C., et al.: Comparative pharmacokinetics of moxalactam, cefoperazone and cefotaxime in normal volunteers. Rev. Infect. Dis., *4(Suppl)*:S585, 1982.
59. Schentag, J. J., et al.: Role for dual individualization with cefmenoxime. Am. J. Med., *77(Symp. 6A)*:43, 1984.
60. Drusano, G. L., et al.: Integration of selected pharmacologic and microbiologic properties of three new beta-lactam antibiotics: a hypothesis for rational comparison. Rev. Infect. Dis., *6*:357, 1984.
61. Drusano, G. L., et al.: Comparison of the pharmacokinetics of ceftazidime and moxalactam and their microbiological correlates in volunteers. Antimicrob. Agents Chemother., *26*:388, 1984.
62. Drusano, G. L., et al.: Multiple-dose pharmacokinetics of imipenem-cilastatin. Antimicrob. Agents Chemother., *26*:715, 1984.
63. Drusano, G. L.: Role of pharmacokinetics in the outcome of infections. Antimicrob. Agents Chemother., *32*:289, 1988.
64. Blaser, J., Stone, B. B., Groner, M. C., and Zinner, S. H.: Comparative study with enoxacin and netilmicin in a pharmacodynamic model to determine importance of ratio of antibiotic peak concentration to MIC for bactericidal activity and emergence of resistance. Antimicrob. Agents Chemother., *31*:1054, 1987.
65. Moore, R. D., Smith, C. R., and Lietman, P. S.: Association of aminoglycoside plasma levels with therapeutic outcome in gram-negative pneumonia. Am. J. Med., *77*:657, 1984.
66. Moore, R. D., Lietman, P. S., and Smith, C. R.: Clinical response to aminoglycoside therapy: importance of the ratio of peak concentration to minimal inhibitory concentration. J. Infect. Dis., *155*:93, 1987.
67. Dudley, M. N., et al.: Pharmacokinetics and pharmacodynam-

ics of intravenous ciprofloxacin. Studies in vivo and in an in vitro dynamic model. Am. J. Med., *82 (Symp. 4A):*363, 1987.
68. Leggett, J. E., Ebert, S., Fantin, B., and Craig, W. A.: Comparative dose-effect relations at several dosing intervals for beta-lactam, aminoglycoside, and quinolone antibiotics against gram-negative bacilli in murine thigh-infection and pneumonitis models. Scand. J. Infect. Dis., *74(Suppl.):*179, 1991.
69. Drusano, G. L., Johnson, D. E., Risen, M., and Standiford, H. C.: Use of a wild type and derived mutant strains of P. aeruginosa with differing MIC's to elucidate the effect on survivorship of changing fluoroquinolone peak/MIC ratio in a neutropenic rat sepsis model. Program and Abstracts of the 31st Interscience Conference on Antimicrobial Agents and Chemotherapy, Chicago, 1991. Washington, D.C., American Society for Microbiology, 1991, Abstract 1203.
70. Peloquin, C. A., et al.: Evaluation of intravenous ciprofloxacin in patients with nosocomia lower respiratory tract infections. Impact of plasma concentrations, organism, minimum inhibitory concentration, and clinical condition on bacterial eradication. Arch. Intern. Med., *149:*2269, 1989.
71. Forrest, A., et al.: Population pharmacodynamics of ciprofloxacin. Program and Abstracts of the 31st Interscience Conference on Antimicrobial Agents and Chemotherapy, Chicago, 1991. Washington, D.C., American Society for Microbiology, 1991, Abstract 602.
72. Quintiliani, R., Cooper, B. W., Briceland, L. L., and Nightingale, C. H.: Economic impact of streamlining antibiotic administration. Am. J. Med., *82(Symp. 4A):*391, 1987.

Chapter 68

ACQUIRED IMMUNODEFICIENCY SYNDROME

SUSAN J. REHM

As the human immunodeficiency virus (HIV) epidemic enters its second decade, significant advances have been made in diagnostic methodology and, to a lesser extent, in therapeutics. By the spring of 1985, isolation of the virus led to the capability for widespread screening for infection. Testing of azidothymidine (AZT, zidovudine) proceeded rapidly; treatment and prophylaxis of the most common infectious complication, Pneumocystis carinii pneumonia, has improved considerably in the past 10 years. Nonetheless, there are massive deficits in education of both the public and health-care professionals, and significant problems remain in recognition and appropriate primary management of people infected with HIV.

CASE STUDY

A 66-year-old farmer was evaluated by his family physician for complaints of weight loss, nonproductive cough, and low grade fevers. Thrush was noted on physical examination, and a chest radiograph revealed subtle interstitial changes. He was treated with oral erythromycin. Three weeks later he was admitted to the hospital because of progressive respiratory distress. The patient was intubated on arrival; a chest radiograph revealed a five-lobe interstitial process, and therapy was initiated with parenteral erythromycin. After he was extubed, his physician elicited a history of multiple male sexual partners. Trimethoprim-sulfamethoxazole and methylprednisolone were added to the therapeutic regimen after he again required intubation. As soon as he was extubated for the second time, he was transferred to a tertiary-care hospital.

At the time of transfer, he was extremely dyspneic at rest despite high concentrations of oxygen delivered by nonrebreather mask. Seborrheic dermatitis and perirectal ulcerations were noted. The probable diagnosis of HIV-related P. carinii pneumonia and the impending need for reintubation was discussed; the patient requested full supportive measures, at least until a diagnosis could be confirmed. He underwent endotracheal intubation, bronchoscopy, and transfer to the medical ICU. Therapy with parenteral trimethoprim-sulfamethoxazole and methylprednisolone was continued; examination of the bronchoalveolar lavage fluid revealed cysts of P. carinii. The diffuse interstitial pulmonary infiltrates progressed, and pentamidine was substituted for trimethoprim-sulfamethoxazole. Both enzyme-linked immunosorbent assay (ELISA) and Western blot testing revealed antibodies to HIV. The $CD4^+$ (T-helper) lymphocyte count was $33/mm^3$.

Within 4 days of admission, the patient was extubated and transferred out of the ICU. He requested that no further invasive diagnostic tests or extraordinary support measures be undertaken. One week after discharge from the ICU, he developed lower gastrointestinal bleeding. As his steroid therapy was tapered, fever and dyspnea recurred; the chest radiograph again worsened. The methylprednisolone dose was restored to 20 mg every 6 hours, and ganciclovir was added to the therapeutic regimen because of the finding of cytomegalovirus on culture of the bronchoalveolar lavage fluid. A few days later, ticarcillin/clavulanate and tobramycin were added because of suspected intra-abdominal sepsis. The patient continued to refuse repeat bronchoscopy, colonoscopy, and surgical evaluation. He died of progressive respiratory failure, 3 weeks after transfer. His brother refused permission for an autopsy.

The afternoon after the patient died, the microbiology laboratory reported growth of acid-fast bacilli from the bronchoalveolar lavage fluid obtained the day after admission. The isolate was later identified as Mycobacterium tuberculosis. As a result, more than 100 health-care workers underwent skin testing for tuberculosis.

The preceding case brings to light a number of issues commonly encountered in the care of individuals with advanced infection that is due to HIV. Perhaps foremost is the patient's initial refusal to disclose his risk for HIV infection to his longitudinal care physician and his lack of awareness of the potential relevance of HIV infection to his illness. This undoubtedly led to some delay in the establishment of a diagnosis and appropriate therapy for his pneumonia. Likewise, the primary physician's index of suspicion for opportunistic infection and underlying immune deficiency was low despite the presence of thrush, substantial weight loss, dermatologic abnormalities, and an atypical chest radiograph. Once the diagnosis of acquired immunodeficiency syndrome (AIDS) and P. carinii pneumonia was suspected, personnel at the local hospital were anxious to transfer him to another facility, citing concerns about spread of infection and lack of experience with treatment of HIV infection and its attendant complications.

Physicians at the tertiary-care hospital to which the patient was transferred were skeptical about reintubating the patient in the face of apparent treatment failure and advanced HIV infection but elected to institute a full treatment trial because the diagnosis had not been proven, and the previous antibiotic doses were subtherapeutic. When the patient survived the ICU stay and subsequently refused further diagnostic and therapeutic measures, his competence was questioned. His decision was allowed to stand after he was interviewed by experienced social workers and psychiatrists. The finding of pulmonary tuberculosis, revealed just after the patient died, led to consternation on three counts: first, the history of tuberculosis exposure had been sought from and was denied by the patient, leading to lack of consideration of tuberculosis as an explanation for his respiratory deterioration; second, the patient had died of a condition that usually responds well to standard therapy; and third, respiratory precautions had not been instituted, placing a number of people at risk for tuberculosis.

Emergent situations will inevitably occur when individuals are unaware of HIV infection and physicians do not recognize subtle signs of HIV infection and its complications. As physicians and patients gain insight into the natural history and therapy of HIV infection, management evolves from "crisis management" to a model of longitudinal care for a person with a chronic, gradually progressive illness. Even when HIV infection has been documented, however, unanticipated events and severe illnesses sometimes lead to consideration of admission to the ICU. In this situation, the physician, patient, friends, and family depend on their understanding of the patient's health-care priorities and the likelihood of full recovery when making decisions.

In this chapter, the epidemiology, immunopathogenesis, and natural history of HIV infection are reviewed. Testing for HIV is discussed in detail, as are the sequelae of HIV infection. Medical and psychosocial considerations, both for previously diagnosed and newly diagnosed patients, are emphasized. Through growth in understanding of HIV infection and its complications, patient care will be enhanced and practitioners will be able to use hospital resources, and particularly the resources of ICUs, more efficiently.

PRE-ICU PHASE

The Spectrum of HIV Infection

Epidemiology

In the first decade of the HIV epidemic in the United States, over 160,000 individuals were diagnosed with AIDS, and an estimated 1,000,000 Americans have been infected with the virus.[1] AIDS has emerged as the leading cause of death among young adults in the United States.[2] By the end of 1990, more than 100,000 deaths were due to HIV infection; nearly three quarters of the deaths occurred in individuals between the ages of 25 and 44. Projections indicate that an additional 165,000 to 215,000 HIV-infected people would die during 1991 to 1993.[3] An estimated $1 billion was paid by private insurers for AIDS-related life and health insurance claims in 1989.[4]

HIV is spread through sexual intercourse and through exposure to infected blood or body fluids via intravenous drug use, transfusions of blood or blood products, or perinatal interactions. The proportion of individuals in the major exposure groups remained stable for the first 5 years of the epidemic, but new trends are being recognized. Homosexual and bisexual males originally accounted for nearly three quarters of AIDS cases; by 1990 they constituted 59% of the total. Intravenous drug users, heterosexual contacts of those at risk, and neonatal patients make up an increasing share of HIV-infected people in the United States. From 1990 to 1991, a 28% increase in the number of cases of heterosexually acquired AIDS occurred, compared to an 11 to 12% increase in cases among homosexual/bisexual men and injecting drug users.[5] The prevalence of HIV infection is highly variable in various communities and regions in the United States, ranging from 0.1 to 7.8%.[6] African-Americans and Hispanics are disproportionately represented among people with AIDS; that is, the proportion of AIDS patients who are African-American or Hispanic is higher than the proportion of these groups in the population as a whole.

The HIV epidemic is particularly significant with regard to the health of women and children. More than 20,000 American women have been diagnosed with AIDS; many thousands of women may be infected with HIV and unaware of their infection. The growth in AIDS cases is more rapid in women than in any other epidemiologic group.[7] The risk for continued perinatal spread of infection is obvious: more than three quarters of women with AIDS are 13 to 39 years of age.

The number of patients with AIDS that is due to transmission of HIV infection through transfusion of blood or blood products is declining. Since the spring of 1985, all blood in the United States has been screened for HIV antibody before transfusion, making the blood supply much safer, but there is still a chance (estimated at 1 in a million) of HIV transmission via transfusion with seronegative blood; in these cases, the blood was tested during the "window" period after infection, before antibody was detectable.[8] Approximately three dozen health-care workers have been infected in workplace accidents.

Transmission of Infection

HIV has been isolated from a number of body fluids, including blood, semen, vaginal secretions, breast milk, saliva, urine, cerebrospinal fluid, and tears. In addition, tissues such as the brain, lymph nodes, and other organs with large numbers of infected lymphocytes and macrophages are considered potentially infectious. Transmission of virus potentially occurs with parenteral or mucosal contact with body fluids that contain high concentrations of virally infected cells, such as semen, blood, or cervical secretions. Clearly, sexual contact and inoculation with infected blood through IV drug use, perinatal exposure, and transfusion are the primary modes of spread of HIV.[9,10] An infected mother has a 30 to 50% chance of transmitting infection to her child perinatally, either during gestation or during the birth process.[11] A few cases in infants have been linked to ingestion of infected breast milk.

Thus, intravascular mucous membrane, or broken skin contact with infected fluid can result in transmission of HIV. The concentration and variety of virus, duration and type of exposure, and unknown host factors probably determine whether infection takes place. Several reports have been made of seroconversion after a single sexual encounter or needlestick. On the other hand, some regular sexual partners of infected individuals have inexplicably remained seronegative. The risk of seroconverting after receiving a unit of HIV-positive blood is close to 100%.

Studies have demonstrated that HIV is not spread to household contacts of an infected patient.[12] Surveys of health-care personnel with intense exposure to AIDS patients demonstrate no increased incidence of HIV infection unless there was a significant parenteral exposure (intramuscular injection or deep cut) with HIV-infected materials[13] or a nonoccupational risk for infection.[14] Overall, the risk of transmission of HIV after parenteral exposure to infected blood is estimated at 0.3%; when simple needlesticks are analyzed separately, the risk is even less. Six patients of an HIV-infected dentist became infected by unknown routes during dental care.[15,16] Testing of over 16,000 patients[17] of HIV-infected surgeons has not revealed additional cases of patient transmission.

The Virus and Immunopathogenesis

HIV was described in 1983 by Montagnier, who called it LAV (lymphadenopathy-associated virus), and Gallo, who named his isolate HTLV-III (human T-lymphotrophic virus). Subsequently, it was shown that the isolates were essentially the same. In 1986 a subcommittee of the International Committee for the Taxonomy of Viruses recommended HIV-1 as the standard name for the causative agent of AIDS. HIV-2 is a related retrovirus, primarily isolated from individuals in West Africa, which causes a syndrome similar to AIDS.[18]

HIV is one of a family of viruses that contain a unique enzyme, reverse transcriptase, which can translate viral RNA into DNA. Like other retroviruses, the HIV genome contains three major genes coding for the viral structural proteins *(gag)*, reverse transcriptase *(pol)*, and envelope glycoproteins *(env)* (Table 68-1).[19] Analysis of HIV isolates from different patients has shown that the genome differs substantially from one person to another, particularly in the portion that encodes the viral envelope. Thus, different strains of HIV have biologically important differences in their envelope antigens. Strains in individual patients appear to mutate with time; in addition, patients may be infected with several HIV strains. These factors, coupled with the apparent lack of development of effective neutralizing antibody during the course of infection, complicate attempts to develop effective vaccines.

HIV preferentially infects CD4$^+$ cells, primarily T-helper/inducer lymphocytes, but it may also infect other cells, including monocytes and macrophages.[20] Infected monocytes are felt to act as important cellular reservoirs for HIV-1, allowing viral infection to spread to the brain and other organs. HIV attaches to the CD4 receptor via its gp120 envelope protein. The viral DNA is incorporated into the host cell DNA and is reproduced, along with normal cellular components, every time the cell divides. Using host cell components, HIV produces a DNA copy of its RNA genome through its unique enzyme, reverse transcriptase. Production of HIV virions usually proceeds at a low level for long periods after establishment of infection, but there is progressive loss of CD4$^+$ lymphocytes with time because of the cytopathic effect of viral reproduction.[21] It is postulated that at some point in the infection, an event (possibly an intercurrent infection) may trigger rapid HIV production and subsequent development of severe immunodeficiency. AIDS-defining illnesses usually develop in proportion to the degree of immune compromise.

The protean clinical manifestations of HIV infection are related to its devastating effect on the immune system, which is primarily due to a selective infection of the CD4$^+$ lymphocytes. These lymphocytes are responsible for the generation of most specific human immune responses, so functional defects occur in virtually all limbs of the system (Table 68-2).[21] The severity of the defects depends on the host, the stage of infection, and unknown variables.[22]

Natural History of HIV Infection

At least 50% of patients infected with HIV will develop an infectious mononucleosis-like syndrome now recognized as acute HIV infection.[23] This is observed 3 to 6 weeks after exposure, is associated with high viral titers in blood,[24] and resolves spontaneously. Transverse myelitis, lymphocytic pneumonitis, and other syndromes have also been described in the setting of acute HIV infection. HIV seroconversion occurs approximately 10 to 12 weeks after exposure to the virus. Most, if not all, seropositive individuals will eventually develop long-term sequelae of infection, with an incubation period ranging from 18 months to more than 10 years.

Most HIV-infected individuals look and feel well. There is progressive depletion of the CD4$^+$ T-lymphocyte subset, expansion of the CD8$^+$ T lymphocytes, and polyclonal B

Table 68-1. The HIV Virion

Gene	Product	Proteins
gag	Core	p24, p17, p9, p7
pol	Enzymes	p66/51, p31
env	Viral coat	gp120, gp41

Table 68-2. Immune Dysfunction in HIV Infection

Lymphopenia—predominantly due to a selective defect in the CD4-lymphocyte subset
Decreased in vivo T-cell function
   Susceptibility to neoplasms and opportunistic infections
   Decreased delayed hypersensitivity
Altered in vitro T-cell function
   Decreased blast transformation
   Decreased alloreactivity
   Decreased specific and nonspecific cytotoxicity
   Decreased ability to provide help to B lymphocytes
Polyclonal B-cell activation
   Elevated levels of total serum immunoglobulins and circulating immune complexes
   Inability to mount a de novo serologic response to a new antigen
   Increased numbers of spontaneous immunoglobulin-secreting cells
   Refractoriness to the normal in vitro signals for B-cell activation

(From Fauci, A. S., et al.: Acquired immunodeficiency syndrome: epidemiologic, clinical, immunologic, and therapeutic considerations. Ann. Intern. Med., *100*:92, 1984.)

cell stimulation.[25] Minor infections such as shingles, thrush, mucocutaneous herpes simplex, and condyloma acuminata (human papilloma virus infection) appear with greater frequency and severity than in the general population. HIV-related disease of the central nervous system, intestinal tract, liver, kidney, or other major organs may be present without major infection. The CD4+ lymphocyte count (normal range, 500 to 1600 cells/mm^3, or 35–62%), p24 antigen level, and beta$_2$-microglobulin level may serve as "surrogate markers" for the progression of immune deficiency, but they are poorly predictive of the clinical course in individual patients.[26,27] When the CD4+ lymphocyte count is less than 200/mm^3 (less than 14%), major infectious complications occur with greater frequency. The risk of death increases considerably after the CD4+ lymphocyte count drops below 50/mm^3.[28]

Testing for HIV Infection

Well over 95% of patients develop detectable antibody to HIV within 12 weeks of infection. The ELISA currently used for screening carries a false-negative rate of less than 1%; the false-negative results are usually found in individuals who are in the "window period" (first 6 to 8 weeks) of infection.[29] ELISA results should not be reported to the patient until they have been confirmed by Western blot or other confirmatory testing. False-positive rates vary, depending on the prevalence of infection in the population studied and the type of ELISA used, but up to 70% of initially reactive tests are not confirmed by the second ELISA.[29] The most common causes of a false-positive ELISA are multiparity, multiple blood transfusions, infections, and autoimmune diseases.

A rapid latex agglutination test for antibodies to HIV-1 was designed for use in areas lacking adequate laboratory facilities. Its sensitivity and specificity are 63.6 and 96.2%, respectively, compared with the 98 to 99% sensitivity and specificity of ELISA methodology. The result is a greater probability of false-negative results, which is probably related to technical difficulties in reading low levels of latex agglutination. False-positive tests also occur. Because of these problems, the latex test is not recommended for screening low exposure populations.

The Western blot test, radioimmunoprecipitation, or immunofluorescent antibody studies are used to confirm the results of screening tests.[30,31] The Western blot assay, the most commonly used confirmatory test, is a much more specific method for detection of HIV antibodies. The assay is technically difficult and interpretation is challenging; laboratories performing Western blot assays must maintain rigid quality standards and maintain competence through experience.[32]

Various methods for HIV antigen detection, such as the p24 antigen determinations and polymerase chain reaction (PCR) studies, may be used to evaluate suspected false-positive and false-negative test results. The p24 antigen test and PCR techniques may be used to detect HIV infection before antibody has formed, and they may be useful for diagnosis in infants less than 15 months of age.[33] In this population, the presence of maternal antibody would obscure the diagnosis in the child through methods that rely on antibody detection. The p24 antigen determination is not frequently used as a diagnostic test in adults, however, because the levels of antigen fluctuate during the course of infection. The antigen level is high in the first 3 months of HIV infection, but it usually becomes undetectable shortly thereafter. As HIV infection progresses, p24 antigen may be intermittently present; in advanced disease, there are high antigen levels, especially in when opportunistic conditions are active.

Table 68–3. Classification System for HIV Infection and Expanded Surveillance Case Definition for AIDS Among Adolescents and Adults

CD4+ T-cell Categories	A. Asymptomatic, Acute HIV or PGL	B. Symptomatic, Not A or C Conditions	C. AIDS-indicator Conditions
1. ≥500/μL	A1	B1	C1
2. 200–499/μL	A2	B2	C2
3. <200/μL	A3	B3	C3

PGL, Persistent generalized lymphadenopathy.
(From Centers for Disease Control: 1993 Revised classification system for HIV infection and expanded surveillance case definition for AIDS among adolescents and adults. M.M.W.R., 41:1, 1993.)

Classification of HIV Infection and the Centers for Disease Control and Prevention Surveillance Definition of AIDS

The Centers for Disease Control and Prevention (CDC) classification system for AIDS was modified in 1993 to include the CD4+ lymphocyte count as well as various clinical conditions associated with HIV infection[34] (Table 68–3). The CD4 lymphocyte categories are to be used in conjunction with one of three clinical categories (Tables 68–4 to 68–6) to assess morbidity associated with the infection. The categories are hierarchical: once a more advanced category has been reached, the person remains in the higher category.

The CDC surveillance definition of AIDS is designed to identify individuals with the most severe manifestations of HIV infection. In January 1993, the definition was changed; now any HIV-infected individual whose CD4+ lymphocyte count is less than 200/μl is classified as having AIDS (subcategories 3A, 3B, and 3C). The presence of one of the specified "indicator diseases" (see Table 68–6) is also diagnostic of AIDS, regardless of the CD4 count (subcategories 1C, 2C, and 3C). Invasive cervical cancer, recurrent bacterial pneumonia, and pulmonary tuberculosis were recently added to the list of indicator diseases.

Table 68–4. Clinical Category A

Acute (primary) HIV infection or history of acute HIV infection
Asymptomatic HIV infection
Persistent generalized lymphadenopathy (PGL)

PGL, Persistent generalized lymphadenopathy.
(From Centers for Disease Control: 1993 Revised classification system for HIV infection and expanded surveillance case definition for AIDS among adolescents and adults. M.M.W.R., 41:1, 1993.)

Table 68–5. Clinical Category B: Non-AIDS-Defining HIV-Related Conditions

Bacillary angiomatosis
Candidiasis: oropharyngeal, vaginal (persistent, frequent)
Cervical dysplasia (moderate or severe)/carcinoma in situ
Constitutional symptoms (fever >38.5°C, diarrhea lasting >1 month)
Hairy leukoplakia, oral
Herpes zoster (shingles), involving at least two distinct episodes or >1 dermatome
Idiopathic thrombocytopenic purpura
Listeriosis
Pelvic inflammatory disease, particularly if complicated by tubo-ovarian abscess
Peripheral neuropathy

PGL, Persistent generalized lymphadenopathy.
(From Centers for Disease Control: 1993 Revised classification system for HIV infection and expanded surveillance case definition for AIDS among adolescents and adults. M.M.W.R., 41:1, 1993.)

Table 68–7. Antiretroviral Treatment of HIV Infection

Drug	Dose*	Potential Adverse Effects
AZT	100 mg, 3 to 5 times daily	Anemia, Leukopenia, thrombocytopenia Nausea Restlessness, irritability, insomnia Abnormal liver function tests Myositis Nail dyschromia
ddI	Weight ≥60 kg: 200-mg tablet or 250 mg powder, b.i.d. Weight <60 kg: 125-mg tablet or 167 mg of powder, b.i.d.	Pancreatitis Peripheral neuropathy Abnormal liver function tests Nausea, abdominal pain, diarrhea
ddC + AZT	0.750 mg t.i.d. plus 200 mg t.i.d.	Peripheral neuropathy Mucosal ulcerations Pancreatitis Rash (See adverse effects of AZT)

* Dose for patients with normal renal function.
AZT, Azidothymidine; ddC, dideoxycytidine; ddI, dideoxyinosine.

Used together, the CD4+ lymphocyte and clinical categories can help to guide clinical decision making. For example, an individual with a CD4+ lymphocyte count of 435/µl and thrush would fit in subcategory 2B; he would be a candidate for antiretroviral therapy. Individuals in subcategories 3A, 3B, and 3C (CD4+ lymphocyte count less than 200/µl, various clinical stages) would all meet the CDC surveillance definition for AIDS; prophylaxis against P. carinii pneumonia should be instituted.

Therapies and Their Impact

The availability of suppressive antiretroviral agents, increasing use of prophylactic antibiotic regimens to prevent opportunistic infections, and development of advanced antimicrobial treatments for established infections have changed the natural history of HIV infection. Although

Table 68–6. Clinical Category C: AIDS-Defining Conditions

Candidiasis, invasive
Cervical cancer, invasive
Coccidioidomycosis, extrapulmonary
Cryptococcosis, extrapulmonary
Cryptosporidiosis of >1-month duration
Cytomegalovirus disease outside lymphoreticular system
Encephalopathy, HIV-related
Herpes simplex infection of >1-month duration or visceral
Salmonella bacteremia, recurrent
Histoplasmosis, extrapulmonary
Isosporiasis of >1-month duration
Kaposi's sarcoma
Lymphoma: primary central nervous system, immunoblastic, or Burkitt's
Myobacterial disease, disseminated or extrapulmonary
Mycobacterium tuberculosis infection
Pneumocystis carinii pneumonia
Pneumonia, recurrent (>1 episode in a year)
Progressive multifocal leukoencephalopathy
Toxoplasmosis, cerebral
Wasting syndrome due to HIV

PGL, Persistent generalized lymphadenopathy.
(From Centers for Disease Control: 1993 Revised classification system for HIV infection and expanded surveillance case definition for AIDS among adolescents and adults. M.M.W.R., 41:1, 1993.)

some patients may present in extremis from opportunistic infections secondary to previously unrecognized HIV infection, access to testing and therapies reduces the frequency of this scenario. Those who are undergoing antiretroviral therapy and appropriate prophylaxis are more likely to present with subacute syndromes or neurologic problems.

When the diagnosis of HIV infection is made before complications of immunosuppression become apparent, a "chronic illness" model is appropriate. Compliant individuals who have access to care undergo regular monitoring of their clinical status and CD4+ lymphocyte count; therapeutic and prophylactic agents are administered based on the results. For example, when the CD4+ lymphocyte count is 500/mm³ or less, antiretroviral therapy may be indicated. A recently convened National Institutes of Health (NIH) panel, however, stated that for patients with counts between 200 and 500 CD4+ lymphocytes, careful monitoring without drug therapy is an acceptable option.

The regimens currently available include AZT, ddI (dideoxyinosine), and the combination of AZT and ddC (dideoxycytidine). All three antiviral drugs inhibit the reproduction of HIV through reverse transcriptase, resulting in partial preservation of immune function and a reduction in the frequency of opportunistic infections. Table 68–7 summarizes treatment regimens and potential adverse effects. Concerns about the development of resistance to antiretroviral agents[35,36] and recently released data from a European study group[37] will have an impact on the use of reverse transcriptase inhibitors.

Antiretroviral Therapies

Azidothymidine (AZT, zidovudine, Retrovir), the first antiretroviral agent released, remains the prototype for this group of drugs.[38] It is a nucleoside analog that acts as a chain terminator when it is incorporated into the developing strand of HIV DNA, where it is substituted for thymidine, the naturally occurring nucleoside. It also inhibits reverse transcriptase through mechanisms that are not well understood. Early trials showed that AZT treated HIV-infected individuals with a CD4 lymphocyte count less than 200/mm³ gained weight, maintained higher CD4 lymphocyte counts, and had fewer opportunistic infections than a comparable group who received placebo.[39] However, 25% of the AZT group required transfusions because of the marrow-suppressive effect of the treatment. Subsequent studies indicated that lower doses of AZT (300 to 500 mg per day as opposed to the 1200-mg daily dose in the initial trials)[40,41] and initiation of AZT therapy when the CD4 lymphocyte count was less than or equal to 500/mm³ resulted in similar benefits.[42,43] The use of lower doses of AZT and initiation of therapy earlier in the course of HIV infection greatly reduces the likelihood of severe anemia.[44] Virtually every patient will develop macrocytosis, unrelated to folate or vitamin B_{12} deficiency, during the course of AZT therapy.

Several other clinically relevant side effects of AZT are not dose related. Some individuals develop headaches, restlessness, irritability, or insomnia early in the course of AZT therapy; these symptoms usually abate as treatment continues. Muscle aches with laboratory findings of myositis may occur during the course of therapy. Although this problem may be related to HIV infection alone, AZT has also been causally linked, and symptoms may resolve with discontinuation of AZT. Hepatic function abnormalities have been reported in AZT-treated patients, but elevated hepatic enzymes are so prevalent in HIV-infected persons that it is often difficult to distinguish AZT effects from conditions such as viral hepatitis, disseminated Mycobacterium avium-intracellulare infection, and reactions to other drugs.

Long-term follow-up of AZT-treated patients has clouded the picture in terms of the efficacy of AZT therapy, particularly in asymptomatic HIV-infected individuals. Two studies indicate that AZT delays progression to AIDS,[45,46] but no survival benefit was associated with therapy in one of the studies.[45] A study of patients who received AZT therapy after AIDS was diagnosed demonstrated improved survival, compared with patients studied before AZT was available.[47] As in untreated patients, deaths in patients who have received AZT tend to occur in individuals with a CD4+ lymphocyte count of less than 50 cells.[48]

ddI (dideoxyinosine, didanosine, Videx)[49] and ddC (dideoxycytidine, zalcitabine, HIVID)[50,51] have mechanisms of action similar to that of AZT, but the side effects are different. ddI is used as a single agent or in combination with AZT, but ddC is presently recommended for use only in combination with AZT. Both agents/regimens are useful for patients whose condition has deteriorated during AZT therapy; the ddI regimen can be used in patients who are intolerant to AZT. The most important adverse reactions are pancreatitis and painful peripheral neuropathy; pancreatitis is more common in ddI-treated patients, and peripheral neuropathy is seen more frequently in patients treated with ddC. The neuropathy is indistinguishable from that due to HIV infection itself; it may be irreversible despite discontinuation of therapy. ddC may also produce mucosal ulcerations and rash.

Despite the use of antiretroviral therapies, immunosuppression (specifically, loss of CD4 lymphocytes) usually progresses. Regimens that alternate antiretroviral drugs in a effort to slow or abort the development of viral resistance are underway. A full description of HIV therapies in development is beyond the scope of this discussion. Immunostimulants, vaccines, novel antiretroviral drugs, and other agents are being studied in a variety of settings; the use of combination therapy is a promising strategy.[52,53]

The Impact of Prophylaxis and Treatment of Opportunistic Infections

In addition to the influence of antiretroviral therapy, prophylactic antibiotic regimens designed to prevent certain opportunistic infections have changed the spectrum and presentation of HIV-related complications.[54] Table 68-8 summarizes current recommendations for primary and secondary prophylaxis. The percentage of individuals who develop P. carinii pneumonia (PCP) as their initial manifestation of AIDS has diminished from nearly 80 to approximately 40%. This can be ascribed to greater awareness of the HIV epidemic, resultant HIV testing, and the use of prophylaxis against Pneumocystis when the CD4 lymphocyte count is less than 200/mm³. Although some authors have suggested that trimethoprim-sulfamethoxazole prophylaxis against PCP also reduces the incidence of toxoplasmosis,[55] this has not been corroborated in subsequent reports. Cryptococcal meningitis, previously associated with much morbidity and mortality, is managed

Table 68-8. Prophylaxis Against Common Opportunistic Infections in HIV-Infected Patients

Infection	Prophylactic Drug(s)	Dose*
Primary prophylaxis		
Pneumocystis carinii pneumonia	Trimethoprim-sulfamethoxazole	160/800 mg p.o. daily or q.o.d.
	Pentamidine aerosol	300 mg monthly
	Dapsone	50–100 mg p.o. daily
Mycobacterium avium complex†	Rifabutin	300 mg p.o. daily
Secondary prophylaxis		
Oral candidiasis	Nystatin	Mouthwash: 5 ml q.i.d.
	Clotrimazole	One troche 3 to 5 times daily
	Ketoconazole	200–400 mg p.o. daily
	Fluconazole	50–100 mg p.o. daily
Vaginal candidiasis	Clotrimazole	1% vaginal cream or 100-mg suppositories, daily
	Ketoconazole	200–400 mg p.o. daily
	Fluconazole	50–100 mg p.o. daily
Herpes simplex	Acyclovir	200–400 mg p.o. b.i.d. to q.i.d.
Cryptococcosis†	Fluconazole	100 mg p.o. daily
Toxoplasmosis†	Trimethoprim-sulfamethoxazole	160/800 mg p.o. daily

* For patients with normal renal function.
† Indication not well established or incompletely tested.

more easily subsequent to the availability of potent oral antifungal agents. Cytomegalovirus (CMV) disease is now more effectively controlled, with the availability of ganciclovir and foscarnet therapy.

In the second decade of the HIV epidemic, other infections have become more prominent.[56-58] Pneumonia and extrapulmonary infections with M. tuberculosis (both drug-resistant and -sensitive strains) are becoming more frequent as populations with latent tuberculosis become immunosuppressed as a result of HIV infection. HIV-infected individuals may develop pulmonary tuberculosis long before other opportunistic infections become apparent; in many cases, the appearance of tuberculosis is the first clue that HIV infection might be present. Subtle clinical manifestations and a lack of awareness of the resurgence of tuberculosis in HIV patients have led to several nosocomial outbreaks.

Disseminated infection that is due to M. avium-intracellulare and other nontuberculous mycobacteria, usually manifesting as a febrile wasting process, is a more common source of morbidity than a direct cause of mortality. Nonetheless, it is important to mention this entity in the context of a discussion of changes in the natural history of HIV infection: More patients are living long enough to allow emergence of these infections. As previously mentioned, suppressive therapy is now available, but adverse reactions are a significant problem.[59]

Central nervous system manifestations continue to plague HIV-infected individuals. Recommendations for prophylaxis against toxoplasmosis and cryptococcosis should be standardized in the near future. The incidence of primary CNS lymphoma may increase as HIV-infected persons live longer. Aside from this factor, it remains to be seen whether antiretroviral chemotherapy directly increases the likelihood of the development of lymphoma.

Infections and Other Sequelae of HIV Infection

Patients with advanced HIV infection experience a variety of concomitant infections. Some are due to opportunistic pathogens; others are related to infection with common organisms that cause severe disease in the face of underlying immune abnormalities. Infections may be diagnosed in an isolated organ system, but disseminated disease is often present. No matter the cause of infection, there is considerable overlap in symptoms. To add to the confusion, noninfectious conditions may cause the same clinical syndromes.

Respiratory Tract Disease

Cough, dyspnea, and sinus congestion are very common symptoms in persons with AIDS.[60] Despite major advances in prophylaxis and therapy, P. carinii continues to be the most frequent cause of pneumonia in this patient population.[61,62] In the past, the organism has been classified as a protozoan, but recent evidence indicates it is more closely related to the fungi. It is a ubiquitous pathogen with which most people have become infected by the age of 5 years. Reactivation of infection occurs in the presence of profound suppression of T lymphocytes; in persons with AIDS, the risk of pneumonia increases significantly when the CD4 lymphocyte count dips below 200/mm³.[63] Clinically, PCP usually presents insidiously, with progressive fever, nonproductive cough, weight loss, and dyspnea on exertion. The chest radiograph typically shows a diffuse interstitial process, but a variety of radiographic changes (or no changes) may be observed.[64] Individuals who have received aerosol pentamidine prophylaxis may present with bilateral upper lobe disease, reflecting the preferential distribution of the aerosol to the middle and upper lobes of the lung. The diagnosis is established by the demonstration of typical cysts on silver stain of induced sputum or material obtained through bronchoscopy. Chest films, diffusion capacity of carbon monoxide (DLCO) measurements, and gallium scans may be useful adjuncts to diagnosis but do not provide definitive information.[65]

Treatment with either trimethoprim-sulfamethoxazole or pentamidine for 21 days appears to be equally effective; there is no benefit to using the agents concomitantly.[66] Patients with milder cases of PCP may be treated with oral trimethoprim/sulfamethoxazole or the combination of dapsone and trimethoprim.[67] The rate of significant cutaneous or systemic reaction to trimethoprim/sulfamethoxazole is over 50% when high doses are used to treat persons with AIDS. Renal dysfunction and abnormalities of serum glucose regulation (either hyperglycemia or hypoglycemia) may accompany pentamidine therapy. In sulfa-hypersensitive patients who cannot take pentamidine and for patients unresponsive to other therapies, clindamycin-primaquine,[68] atovaquone,[69,70] and trimethrexate/leukovorin[71] are alternative regimens.

Patients with moderate-to-severe PCP may benefit from the adjunctive administration of corticosteroids.[72] Because recurrent pneumonia is common, patients who have had one episode of PCP should receive prophylaxis against recurrence with low-dose trimethoprim/sulfamethoxazole, aerosol pentamidine, or dapsone.[73] Most HIV-infected patients receive "primary prophylaxis" (prophylaxis before the first clinical episode of PCP) when the CD4 lymphocyte count drops below 200/mm³. Survival is improved in patients with advanced HIV infection who are treated with AZT while receiving prophylaxis against PCP.[74] Pneumonia confined to the upper lobes of the lung and extrapulmonary pneumocystis infection has been described in patients receiving aerosol pentamidine prophylaxis. These facts, and concerns about the costs of therapy and the potential for spread of airborne pathogens such as M. tuberculosis, have led to preferential use of oral trimethoprim-sulfamethoxazole prophylaxis by many practitioners.[75,76] Newer oral trimethoprim-sulfamethoxazole prophylaxis regimens, which use very low doses, may be tolerated in individuals who were unable to complete courses of therapeutic trimethoprim-sulfamethoxazole therapy because of mild-to-moderate adverse reactions.[77,78]

PCP is by no means the only type of pneumonia seen in HIV-infected persons. Bacterial pneumonia that is due to Hemophilus influenzae, Streptococcus pneumoniae, Staphylococcus aureus, Branhamella catarrhalis, and other common pathogens is being recognized with increasing frequency.[79] In contrast to PCP, the onset of bacterial pneumonia is usually more sudden and the cough is often productive; the chest radiograph may show a well-defined infiltrate, but radiographic abnormalities may lag behind clinical findings. Examination of the sputum Gram's stain and culture, along with blood cultures, usually establishes the diagnosis. Nocardia pneumonia, which is less common than the other bacterial pneumonias, can also be diagnosed by these methods.

The incidence of pulmonary tuberculosis is rising in the face of the AIDS epidemic. The clinical and radiographic presentation is often atypical, leading to delays in diagnosis and to potential spread to persons in contact with the patient.[80,81] Even in a profoundly immunosuppressed patient, the PPD is occasionally positive; it is always worthwhile to perform skin testing.[82] The CDC suggest that the presence of 5 mm of induration after the administration of an intermediate strength (5TU) skin test is indicative of infection.[83,84] All PPD-positive persons with HIV infection should receive at least 12 months of prophylaxis with isoniazid. Because of the high prevalence of tuberculosis exposure in injecting drug users, Selwyn and colleagues recommend administration of INH prophylaxis to HIV-infected injecting drug users who are anergic.[85] Patients with active disease usually respond well to standard two- or three-drug regimens (isoniazid, rifampin, and pyrazinamide for the first 2 months of therapy, followed by isoniazid and rifampin), but in most cases, the duration of therapy should be longer than the currently recommended 6 to 9 months. Noncompliance with treatment regimens may lead to relapses and drug resistance.[86]

Tuberculosis is a particularly vexing problem because of the ease with which the bacteria becomes drug resistant. More than 200 cases of tuberculosis that were due to drug-resistant strains were reported in 1992. Infection with multiple-drug-resistant M. tuberculosis (MDR-TB) is usually rapidly fatal in HIV-infected patients; even HIV-seronegative contacts, such as family members and health-care workers, may rapidly succumb to primary infection with MDR-TB.[87,88] Institutional spread within hospitals, jails, and shelters for the homeless has been a particular problem.[89-91] Recommendations to prevent spread of tuberculosis in the health-care setting will be discussed in the section on infection control, which follows.

The role of M. avium-intracellulare and other nontuberculous mycobacteria in producing pulmonary symptomatology remains controversial. Likewise, CMV seems to be associated with pulmonary disease less frequently than would be predicted by its prevalence. Although it is often isolated from the bronchoalveolar lavage fluid of patients with PCP, it does not appear to cause clinical pneumonitis in the majority of patients, and its presence has no effect on survival in the face of PCP. A positive bronchoalveolar lavage (BAL) culture for CMV may have the same significance as positive urine or saliva cultures in immunosuppressed patients: It often represents reactivation of viral secretion, without parenchymal invasion.

Fungal pneumonias that are due to Histoplasma capsulatum, Cryptococcus neoformans, and Coccidioides immitis have been described in persons with HIV infection and AIDS. Pulmonary aspergillosis is quite uncommon, but it has been observed in HIV-infected individuals who are neutropenic and/or receiving corticosteroid therapy. Last, several noninfectious disorders such as visceral Kaposi's sarcoma and various lymphocytic pneumonitis syndromes may be associated with respiratory tract symptoms.

Sinusitis has been recognized as another serious respiratory tract complication of HIV infection.[92] Both allergic and infectious sinusitis have been described; high levels of immunoglobulin E (IgE) are common in HIV-infected patients. Intranasal steroid therapy combined with topical and systemic decongestants is effective for most patients. When infection complicates sinusitis, it is frequently caused by common bacteria, but unusual fungal pathogens or suprainfection with resistant bacteria may complicate treatment. A sector computed tomography (CT) scan of the sinuses is a quick and relatively cost-effective way to evaluate this area. Parenteral antibiotic therapy and/or surgical drainage may be required in serious cases of sinusitis. The availability of sinus endoscopy has reduced the need for extensive surgical procedures.

Neurologic Disorders

Neurologic symptoms in HIV-infected patients may be related to HIV infection itself[93] or to conditions (primarily infections) that arise as a result of profound immunosuppression. HIV infects the central nervous system early in the course of disease.[94-96] Up to 90% of persons with AIDS have evidence of HIV encephalopathy at autopsy, and rigorous testing reveals that 70% of AIDS patients develop mental deterioration consistent with AIDS dementia complex. Severe HIV-associated dementia is observed in a minority of patients. It is an "indicator disease" and is diagnostic of AIDS in an otherwise healthy HIV-infected patient. In its early stages, HIV encephalopathy may be confused with depression. Memory loss, changes in effect and judgment, and disruption of normal sleep patterns progress at variable rates. The diagnosis is established when dementia is present in an HIV-infected person and all other causes have been ruled out via brain imaging, lumbar puncture, and appropriate serologic tests.

Peripheral neuropathy is also a common manifestation of HIV infection of the nervous system.[97,98] The prevalence increases as HIV infection progresses, but neuropathy may be observed at any stage of illness. Acute inflammatory demyelinating polyneuropathy, sensory ganglioneuritis, and acute cranial nerve palsy have been observed with primary HIV infection. Guillan-Barré syndrome has been observed in this setting and in patients with established HIV infection. Asymptomatic or minimally symptomatic HIV-infected individuals may develop acute or chronic inflammatory demyelinating polyneuropathy, polyradiculopathy, or mononeuritis multiplex. The latter condition is probably autoimmune in nature; it responds to steroid therapy and/or plasmapheresis. Polyradiculopathy may be related to CMV infection; a trial of ganciclovir therapy may be warranted. The most common neuropathy associated with AIDS is a distal symmetric polyneuropathy; it is observed in more than 70% of individuals with AIDS. Therapy with ddI or ddC is associated with peripheral neuropathy that mimics HIV-related neuropathy; whether this represents a separate syndrome or an exacerbation of subclinical HIV peripheral neuropathy is not clear.

Central nervous system conditions related to advanced immunosuppression are either infections or neoplasms. Toxoplasmosis is the most common cause of cerebral mass lesions in HIV-infected persons;[99,100] in fact, empiric treatment for toxoplasmosis (either sulfa or clindamycin in conjunction with pyramethamine) is recommended when no other diagnosis has been confirmed.[101] If the patient has not responded to therapy for toxoplasmosis in 2 to 3 weeks, brain biopsy should be performed. Biopsy should be considered earlier in the course of empiric therapy if the serum toxoplasma antibody titer is found to be negative. Short-term use of dexamethosone may be necessary if the lesion produces symptoms related to cerebral edema. Even in the presence of profound neurologic dysfunction as presentation, the prognosis for recovery and sustained restoration of function is excellent (Figs. 68-1 and 68-2). Lifelong suppressive antibiotic therapy is indicated to prevent reactivation of CNS toxoplasmosis. Cryptococcal meningitis may produce a paucity of symptoms, and a high index of suspicion is warranted (see section entitled Disseminated Infections).[102] Because treatment failures have been reported with primary fluconazole therapy, initial therapy with intravenous amphotericin B (with or without 5-FC) should be followed with long-term oral fluconazole suppression.[103]

Syphilis is now recognized as an important cause of neurologic and systemic symptoms in HIV-infected persons, and it is clear that HIV infection profoundly influences the individual's response to treatment. Many who develop symptoms during the course of their HIV infection were treated for syphilis years earlier; the infection is reactivated in the nervous system because of inadequate CNS penetration of benezathine penicillin. Serologic tests in patients with profound immunosuppression may be unreliable;[104] lumbar puncture and intravenous penicillin therapy are indicated when there is a high degree of suspicion for neurosyphilis. Tuberculous meningitis, another CNS infection that may be difficult to diagnose, has been documented in approximately 10% of HIV-infected individuals with tuberculosis.[105]

Progressive multifocal leukoencephalopathy (PML),[106] primary CNS lymphoma,[107] and lymphomatoid angiomatosis[108] are other conditions that produce cerebral mass lesions in patients with advanced HIV infection. PML is characteristically associated with nonenhancing lesions in the periventricular white matter on cerebral imaging studies. Mass effect is uncommon; the lesions usually spare the cerebral cortex. The condition is due to reactivation of infection with a polyomavirus, the JC virus (not to be confused with the causative agent of Jacob Creutzfeldt disease). There is no effective therapy. Central nervous system lymphoma and lymphomatoid granulomatosis will be discussed later, in the section describing neoplastic diseases.

If a central nervous system abnormality is suspected, the physician should determine whether an intracranial mass

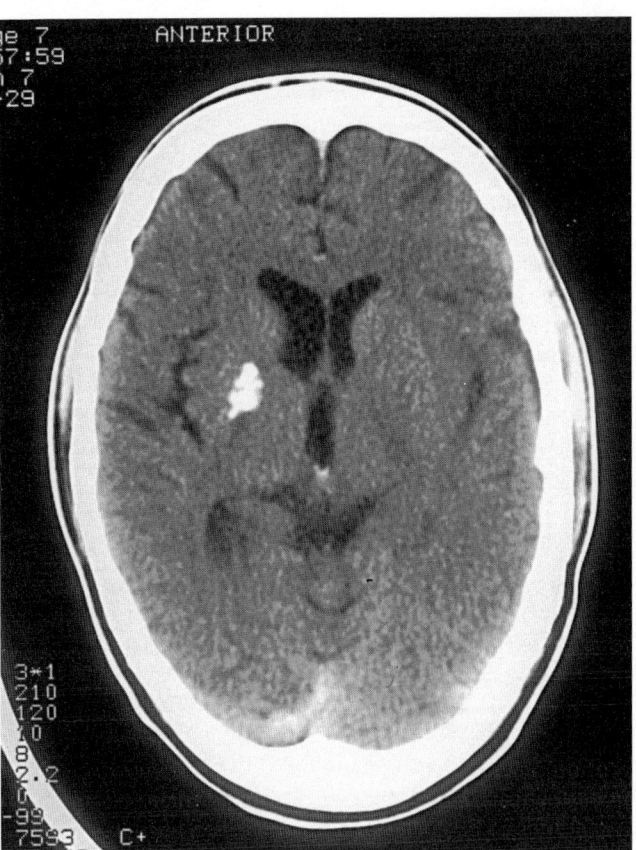

Fig. 68-2. Computed tomography scan of the same patient, 1 year later. Clindamycin and pyrimethamine therapy were maintained at a lower dose. The patient had no residual neurologic symptoms.

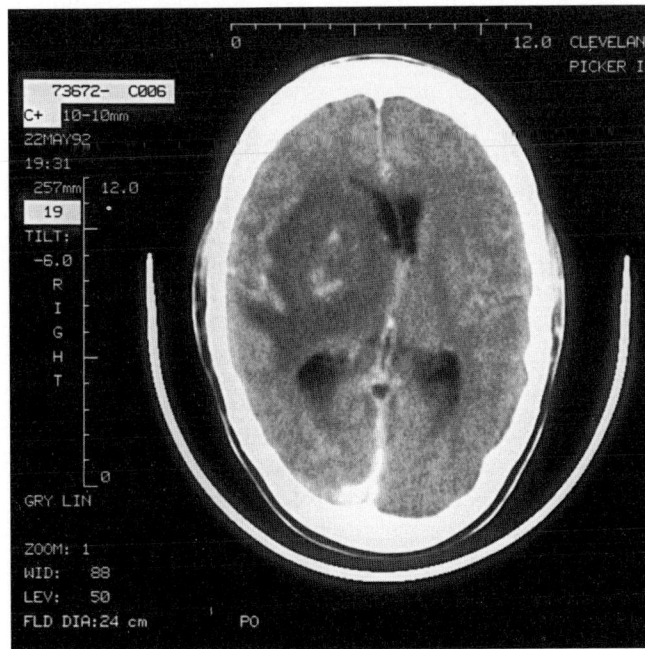

Fig. 68-1. Pretreatment computed tomography scan of the head for a patient with toxoplasmosis who presented with left hemiparesis. Because of sulfa allergy, he was treated with clindamycin and pyrimethamine; massive edema around the lesion led to concomitant dexamethasone therapy for the first 3 weeks.

lesion is present, because further diagnostic and therapeutic considerations depend on the result of the initial CT or magnetic resonance imaging (MRI) scan of the brain. In the absence of mass lesions that cause a midline shift, lumbar puncture is indicated as part of the evaluation of HIV-infected patients with significant neurologic symptoms. Cerebrospinal fluid cell counts; protein and glucose determinations; routine, fungal, and mycobacterial cultures; and cryptococcal antigen and VDRL titers should be performed. Because many central nervous system infections in HIV-infected patients are manifestations of disseminated infections, determination of peripheral blood Venereal Disease Research Laboratories test (VDRL) and fluorescent treponemal antibody (FTA), cryptococcal antigen titers, and toxoplasmosis antibodies may be helpful during the evaluation.

Gastrointestinal Disease

Oral Lesions. Oral manifestations of HIV infection are underrecognized; they may serve as a clue to the presence of immunosuppression in individuals who have not been HIV tested.[109] Thrush (oral candidiasis) is a well-recognized complication of HIV infection, but it is not diagnostic of AIDS. Therapy with clotrimazole or nystatin topical preparations (troches or mouthwash) is usually adequate; ketoconazole or fluconazole therapy should be reserved for patients with recalcitrant disease. Severe gingivitis and periodontitis, related to impaired local immunity in the gingivae, is quite common. Cases of acute necrotizing ulcerative gingivitis have been described. Some of these disorders can be avoided or ameliorated by careful attention to daily dental hygiene and regular dental prophylaxis.

Hairy leukoplakia is a characteristic heaped-up, white lesion on the lateral borders of the tongue.[110] Epstein-Barr viral particles have been identified within these lesions. This disorder is of some clinical significance in that it indicates significant immune dysfunction. No treatment is necessary, but acyclovir has been shown to reduce the bulk of the lesion. Patients with AIDS sometimes experience severe aphthous ulcers; when antiseptic mouthwashes fail, topical steroid therapy may be of benefit. "Noninfectious" diseases of the mouth are less common. Therapy with ddC may produce oral ulcerations or stomatitis. Macular or papular purple lesions in the oral cavity should raise the suspicion of Kaposi's sarcoma.

Esophageal Disorders. Dysphagia is a frequent complaint among patients with AIDS. Although candida esophagitis is its most frequent cause, CMV and herpes simplex infections may also be observed.[111] Ulcers that are due to AZT, ddC,[112] and "giant aphthous ulcers" of uncertain origin may cause the same symptoms.[113] If the patient does not respond to empiric antifungal therapy, endoscopy and biopsy are indicated.

Gastrointestinal Diseases. All parts of the gastrointestinal tract may be involved with HIV disease and immunosuppression-related infection.[114] Candidiasis and herpesvirus infections may involve the stomach separately or as an extension of esophageal disease. Other disorders, such as lymphoma and Kaposi's sarcoma, may be diagnosed on upper endoscopy in patients presenting with a variety of symptoms. Most HIV-infected individuals eventually develop hypochlorhydria, which may increase susceptibility to infection with enteric pathogens.[115] Elevated gastric pH levels may also impair absorption of medications, with ketoconazole being a noteworthy example.[116]

Whether it is due to opportunistic infection, neoplasms, or HIV infection itself, diarrhea is a ubiquitous problem in HIV-infected individuals. Intestinal infections with opportunistic pathogens such as Cryptosporidium, Isospora belli, cytomegalovirus, nontuberculous mycobacteria, and microsporidia are frequent and document the diagnosis of AIDS.[117] Other more common microorganisms such as Salmonella, Shigella, and Campylobacter spp., Yersinia enterocolitica, Clostridium difficile, Giardia lamblia, and Entamoeba histolytica may also cause diarrhea in HIV-infected patients, but their presence does not imply immunodeficiency.

Noninfectious causes of diarrhea in this patient population include gastrointestinal lymphomas and Kaposi's sarcoma. Many patients with HIV infection, however, experience gastrointestinal symptoms in the absence of infections or malignancy. This appears to be due to HIV infection of the gastrointestinal tract itself, known as HIV enteropathy.[118] A spectrum of clinical manifestations of HIV enteropathy are observed. The gastrointestinal tract involvement is asymptomatic in some patients, whereas others experience varying degrees of diarrhea, malabsorption, weight loss, or abdominal pain. Stool analysis is frequently diagnostic for infectious disorders: stool stains for acid-fast bacteria (which also reveals the presence of cryptosporidium organisms) and for ova and parasites, cultures for enteric bacterial pathogens and acid-fast bacteria, and C. difficile toxin determination should be performed. Patients with negative stool studies should undergo colonoscopy and biopsy with cultures, because CMV colitis and gastrointestinal neoplasms are most effectively diagnosed in this manner. Antibiotic treatment of common enteric pathogens is usually curative; the response to therapy for opportunists is less successful. Ganciclovir therapy has been demonstrated to reduce diarrhea and promote weight gain in treated patients.[119] There is no effective treatment for cryptosporidiosis. Octreotide administration may reduce symptoms in patients with HIV enteropathy.

Hepatic, Biliary Tract, and Pancreatic Disease. Many patients with HIV infection have abnormal liver function parameters, even in the absence of infection with hepatitis A, B, or C virus. The reasons for baseline liver dysfunction have not been elucidated fully. Patients with advanced HIV infection, fevers, and elevated alkaline phosphatase levels may be infected with M. avium complex or CMV; bacillary peliosis hepatitis has also been described (see next section, entitled "Disseminated Infections").[120] A wide variety of medications may cause abnormal hepatic function tests; Kaposi's sarcoma or lymphoma may also produce these abnormalities. Liver biopsy may provide diagnostic help in patients who have not yet developed severe immunodeficiency,[121] but those with advanced AIDS often develop hepatic involvement with an opportunistic infection that can be diagnosed via blood cultures. Biliary tract disease has been described, usually in association with CMV, mycobacterial, or microsporidial

Table 68-9. Disseminated Infections

Bacteria*	Fungi	Viruses	Protozoa
Mycobacterium spp.	Cryptococcus neoformans	Cytomegalovirus	Pneumocystis carinii
Salmonella spp.	Histoplasma capsulatum	Parvovirus B19	Strongyloides stercoralis
Rochalimaea spp.	Coccidioides immitis	Adenovirus	Leishmania donovani
Treponema pallidum	Aspergillus spp.	Vaccinia	Microsporidia
Listeria monocytogenes	Blastomyces dermatitidis		
Rhodococcus equi	Fusarium spp.		
Shigella spp.	Pseudoallescheria boydii		
Bacille Calmette-Guérin			

* Excluding bacteremias with common bacteria: see text.
(From Gradon, J. D., Timpone, J. G., and Schnittman, S. M.: Emergence of unusual opportunistic pathogens in AIDS: a review. Clin. Infect. Dis., 15:134, 1992.)

infection.[122,123] Kaposi's sarcoma may involve the hepatobiliary system and pancreas.[124] Currently, drug-induced inflammation that is due to ddI, ddC, or pentamidine is the most common cause of pancreatitis in HIV-infected individuals.

Disseminated Infections

Nearly any of the infections described for individual organ systems can disseminate; likewise, many infections, such as CMV retinitis, which are recognized in a single organ system, are actually manifestations or disseminated infection. They tend to occur in patients with advanced HIV infection and profound immunosuppression. The infection may represent reactivation of a dormant organism, or it may be related to exposure to a new microbe.[58] Table 68-9 lists some of the common and unusual infections that may disseminate in the setting of HIV infection. Fever and rash may be associated with any disseminated infection; appropriate blood cultures and skin biopsies for cultures and histopathology are vital in establishing the diagnosis in many cases. Biopsy and culture of bone marrow and/or liver may be helpful in cases where less invasive tests have not been successful.

Bacterial Infections. Disseminated infection that is due to M. avium complex (MAC) or other nontuberculous mycobacteria occurs most frequently in HIV-infected patients with advanced immunodeficiency.[125] In one study, 43% of patients who survived 2 years after the diagnosis of AIDS was established developed MAC bacteremia; 39% of patients surviving 1 year after the CD4+ lymphocyte count dropped below 10/mm^3 were found to have MAC bacteremia.[126] A wasting syndrome, associated with fevers, chills, and anorexia is observed; reemergent lymphadenopathy and hepatosplenomegaly are sometimes found on examination.[127] Bone marrow involvement is common, leading to the expected leukopenia, anemia, and thrombocytopenia. Elevation of alkaline phosphatase is commonly associated with hepatic involvement.

The diagnosis is established by culturing the blood for acid-fast bacteria; cultures of lymph nodes, bone marrow, and other targets of dissemination serve as adjuncts to the diagnostic process but are not necessary in most cases. The significance of MAC in sputum or bronchoscopy cultures is debatable: if the organism is isolated from no other site and if there are alternative explanations for the pulmonary symptoms that prompted the culture, it is likely that the tracheobronchial tree is colonized rather than infected. Likewise, the significance of MAC in stool cultures is variable, dependent on the clinical situation. MAC is very resistant to most of the drugs used to treat M. tuberculosis infections; the availability of newer antibiotics for treatment of MAC infection has improved the once-dismal prognosis (Table 68-10).[127a] Due to the profound immunosuppression of patients who develop MAC disease, antibiotic therapy may suppress symptoms without clearing the infection.

Extrapulmonary infection with M. tuberculosis occurs at least as frequently as pulmonary tuberculosis in patients with HIV infection.[128] Shafer and co-workers, studying a group of patients with extrapulmonary tuberculosis, found a 38% rate of disseminated disease among HIV-infected individuals, as compared to an 8% rate in seronegative controls.[129] The rates of bacteremia and primary drug resistance were increased in the HIV-infected patients. The diagnosis is established with the techniques listed for diagnosis of MAC; in addition, a chest radiograph demonstrating miliary, lobar, or diffuse infiltrates may suggest tuberculosis.[130] As previously discussed, PPD testing should always be performed, but a negative result does not exclude the diagnosis of tuberculosis.[82] Hematogenous dissemination of tuberculosis may be a marker for particularly fulminant disease.

Bacteremia that is due to S. pneumoniae, S. aureus, Pseudomonas spp., and other gram-negative organisms may be seen in isolation or in association with an identified source such as pneumonia, infected intravenous catheters, cellulitis, or urinary tract infections.[131] Fever may be absent in half of the patients with AIDS and bacteremia. Community-acquired bacteremias are usually responsive to the prompt institution of appropriate antimicrobial therapy; pneumococcal sepsis, however, may cause rapid death.

Treponema pallidum has reemerged as an important pathogen in HIV-infected patients. In sexually active persons, primary or secondary manifestations of infection may appear; the more difficult problem, however, is the development of neurosyphilis in previously infected and treated patients.[132,133] Reports of a variety of unusual manifestations of recurrent disease have been published in recent years.[134] HIV-infected individuals should undergo routine serum RPR testing at least yearly. Serum testing, however, may be unreliable in HIV-infected patients who are severely immunocompromised. A high index of suspicion,

Table 68–10. Treatment of MAC and CMV Infections

Infection	Antibiotic(s)	Dose*	Adverse Effects†
Mycobacterium avium complex	Ethambutol	15–25 mg/kg/day	Nausea, optic neuritis, acute gout
	+ Rifabutin	450–600 mg p.o. b.i.d.	Nausea, vomiting; uveitis; orange-colored secretions
	+ Ciprofloxacin	750 mg p.o. b.i.d.	Nausea, vomiting, rash
	+ Clarithromycin	500 mg p.o. b.i.d.	Nausea
	or Azithromycin	500 mg p.o. b.i.d.	
	± Amikacin	7.5 mg/kg IV q12h or 15 mg/kg IV/day	Auditory and vestibular toxicity, renal dysfunction
Cytomegalovirus disease	Ganciclovir	5 mg/kg IV q12h for 2–3 weeks, then 5 mg/kg IV q24 h	Leukopenia, anemia, renal dysfunction
	or Foscarnet	60 mg/kg IV q8h for 2–3 weeks, then 90 mg/kg IV q24h	Renal dysfunction, electrolyte abnormalities, fatigue, malaise, nausea

* Doses for patients with normal renal function.
† Other adverse effects have been reported for each antimicrobial agent.
CMV, Cytomegalovirus; MAC, Mycobacterium avium complex.

careful history taking, and lumbar puncture are necessary for the establishment of the diagnosis of patients with suspected syphilis.[104] Knowledge of the presence of CNS lues also influences therapeutic decisions, because a 10-day course of intravenous penicillin G rather than intramuscular benzathine penicillin would be prescribed for treatment of neurosyphilis.

Cutaneous bacillary angiomatosis and bacillary peliosis hepatitis in HIV-infected patients have received much attention despite their apparent rarity. The causative organism, Rochalimaea henselae, is a member of the order Rickettsiales.[135] The cutaneous and hepatic disorders are manifestations of disseminated disease. Bacillary angiomatosis in HIV-infected patients clinically resembles but is histologically different from classic cat scratch disease. Cutaneous disease is characterized by multiple angiomatous nodular lesions; bacillary angiomatosis mimics Kaposi's sarcoma in some cases. Patients with pelosis hepatitis present with fever, abdominal pain, and weight loss.[136] Hepatomegaly is always present; splenomegaly and/or lymphadenopathy may also be observed. Cerebral involvement has also been reported.[137] The diagnosis can be established with Warthin-Starry staining of the causative bacilli in tissue specimens. Special cultures of blood or tissue may reveal growth of the organism after 10 to 14 days of incubation.[138] Serologic tests are under development. Treatment with erythromycin, quinolone antibiotics, trimethoprim-sulfamethoxazole, aminoglycosides, or other antimicrobials to which the organism is susceptible has been effective, but prolonged or repeated courses of therapy may be necessary.

Given the profound cellular immunodeficiency of individuals with advanced HIV infection, one would expect that infection due to Listeria monocytogenes would be quite common. As of 1991, only 20 cases had been reported; the authors of a review suggested that high tumor necrosis factor (TNF) levels found in patients with AIDS might be protective against listeriosis. Bacteremia and CNS infection are the most common manifestations of infection; in many cases, gastrointestinal symptoms precede the development of systemic symptoms.[139] Treatment with ampicillin and gentamicin is optimal. Penicillin-allergic patients have received trimethoprim-sulfamethoxazole therapy, but little information is available about the results of therapy with alternative agents.

Fungi. The risk for development of fungal infection in HIV-infected patients depends on both the stage of disease and on the individual's exposure to fungi, which is often highly related to geography. Cryptococci are found throughout the United States; histoplasmosis[140,141] and blastomycosis[142] cases tend to be found around river valleys; and coccidioidomycosis[143] is found in the Southwest. In most cases, the infection is acquired through inhalation of contaminated dust; in immunocompetent hosts the infection is usually confined to the lungs. Thus, isolation of one of these fungi from an extrapulmonary focus must be considered diagnostic of fungemia and disseminated infection. The finding should arouse suspicion of the presence of immunodeficiency. Disseminated aspergillosis has been described, primary in the setting of corticosteroid therapy and/or neutropenia.[144]

Cryptococcal meningitis is probably the most common manifestation of disseminated fungal infection in patients with HIV infection in the United States.[102] The clinical manifestations are often subtle because patients who are profoundly immunocompromised may not mount a cellular response to central nervous system invasion by cryptococci. Meningeal symptoms will not be present unless there is a cellular response. Fever, headache, and/or cranial neuropathies may be present; some patients are entirely asymptomatic.[145] Because cerebral cryptococcosis may cause cerebral mass lesions and edema, a brain imaging study should be performed before lumbar puncture. Serum and cerebrospinal fluid (CSF) cryptococcal antigen determinations (CAD) quickly establish the diagnosis. More than 95% of patients with cryptococcal meningitis have a positive serum CAD. Abnormal mental status and hyponatremia have been cited as bad prognostic signs in patients with HIV infection and cryptococcosis;[102] others have noted that a CSF cryptococcal CAD level above 1:1024 and a CSF white blood cell count below 20 as risk factors for death.[146] It has a mortality rate of up to 30% despite aggressive therapy; most of the deaths occur within 2 weeks of presentation. Initial therapy with intravenous amphotericin B is still the standard because of concerns that fluconazole therapy results in slower sterilization of the CSF. Patients who are at lower risk for poor outcome may respond to high dose fluconazole therapy.[146] All HIV-infected patients with cryptococcosis should receive long-term suppressive therapy with oral fluconazole to prevent relapses.[103] During therapy, serum and CSF CADs can be followed to assess adequacy of response.

Viruses. Recognition of one of the well-known "localized" infections with CMV, namely CMV retinitis or colitis, establishes the diagnosis of disseminated CMV infection. The diagnostic utility of positive blood, urine, or BAL cultures for diagnosis of significant CMV infection is poor, because the majority of HIV-infected patients are latently infected with CMV and intermittently secrete the virus is the absence of invasive disease.[147] Treatment with either ganciclovir or foscarnet is instituted with a higher dose, "induction" course, followed by maintenance therapy at a lower dose (see Table 68-10), often for the rest of the patient's life. The lack of oral antibiotic therapy for treatment of CMV disease is a significant problem.

Protozoal Infections. In the United States, disseminated protozoal infections are uncommon. In patients receiving aerosol pentamidine prophylaxis, however, extrapulmonary P. carinii infection may develop because systemic pentamidine levels are not achieved with aerosol doses. Involvement of the retina, spleen, liver, and numerous other sites has been described.[148-151] Treatment with trimethoprim-sulfamethoxazole, parenteral pentamidine, or other systemic agents is necessary. Disseminated toxoplasmosis is occasionally found at autopsy in patients with AIDS; premortem diagnosis depends on recognition of an involved organ or system.

Ophthalmologic Manifestations

The most common retinal manifestation of AIDS is CMV retinitis.[152] Affected patients, most of whom have advanced immune dysfunction, may notice progressive "floaters," visual field deficits, or cloudiness in the field of vision. Usually, one eye is more involved than the other, but bilateral disease may be found in the absence of symptoms when the periphery is involved. Characteristic fluffy white lesions associated with hemorrhage are visualized along blood vessels of the retina. Early lesions must be distinguished from cotton wool spots. Uveitis is usually mild compared to the degree of retinitis; severe retinal disease, however, may be associated with diffuse vitreal inflammation. Progression of the lesions results in retinal necrosis. CMV retinitis usually responds to therapy with ganciclovir[153] or foscarnet,[154] but lifelong suppressive antibiotic therapy is required to prevent recurrent disease. Blindness often develops despite aggressive treatment.

Toxoplasma retinitis and P. carinii choroiditis are less common causes of visual symptoms in patients with AIDS. Pneumocystis choroiditis is a manifestation of disseminated infection, which may complicate aerosol prophylaxis for pneumonia.[155] Toxoplasma retinitis usually responds well to treatment with sulfonamides. Experience with treatment of Pneumocystis choroiditis is limited, but some patients have responded to infusions of intravenous pentamidine.

Several forms of keratitis may also complicate the course of a patient with AIDS. Bacterial keratitis has been observed in individuals who wear contact lenses when the lenses are not cleansed properly. Corneal infection with herpes simplex or varicella zoster may lead to blindness. Microsporidian (protozoal) keratitis, for which there is no known effective antimicrobial therapy, has been described.[156] Luetic or tuberculous uveitis serve as markers for disseminated disease and call for aggressive therapy.

Dermatologic Disease

Most patients with HIV infection experience several types of skin lesions in the course of their illness, and dermatologic changes are an important early clue to the presence of HIV infection.[157,158] Many conditions, such as herpes simplex infections, shingles, warts, condyloma acuminata, and molluscum contagiosum, represent reactivation of old infections that is due to immunosuppression. Many patients require continuous suppressive therapy with acyclovir for herpes simplex infection; rarely, acyclovir resistance may emerge.[159] Established herpes varicella-zoster infections often require parenteral acyclovir therapy. In association with chronic shingles, eruptions, or recurrent zoster, acyclovir resistance may emerge; foscarnet has been used successfully in such situations.[160]

Other eruptions may be associated with cutaneous manifestations of systemic disease: cryptococcosis, bacillary angiomatosis/cat scratch disease, CMV, nontuberculous mycobacteria, and other causes have been identified. In addition, a number of common skin disorders (most notably, seborrheic dermatitis, folliculitis, and psoriasis) may become severe as HIV infection progresses.[161] Most of these skin disorders can be distinguished from Kaposi's sarcoma without difficulty, but clinical manifestations may overlap, making skin biopsy and cultures useful adjuncts to the usual battery of diagnostic tests. In the context of HIV infection, Kaposi's sarcoma is primarily a disease of individuals who acquired infection sexually; as safer sex practices were used more frequently in the gay population, the incidence of Kaposi's sarcoma has fallen dramatically, leading to speculation that it is a manifestation of a sexually transmitted disease. A full discussion of Kaposi's sarcoma is found in the neoplastic diseases section, later in this chapter.

Gynecologic Manifestations and Considerations

Until recently, the unique manifestations of HIV infection in women were underrecognized.[162,163] Clearly many of the infectious complications are the same in men and women, but the frequency with which each occurs may be different. For example, Carpenter's study indicated that candida esophagitis was the most common AIDS-defining illness in HIV-infected women, but that P. carinii pneumonia was more common in men.[164] Vaginal candidiasis,[165] sexually transmitted diseases, pelvic inflammatory disease,[166,167] and gynecologic neoplasms[168] tend to occur more frequently and progress more rapidly in HIV-infected women; vigilance is necessary to diagnose and treat these conditions. Aggressive cervical carcinoma, related to human papilloma virus (HPV) infection, is of particular concern.[169] Pap smears should be performed every 6 months in HIV-infected women; some authors even recommend routine colposcopy.[170] Invasive cervical cancer has been added to the list of conditions that establish the CDC definition of AIDS in the presence of HIV infection.[34]

A complete discussion of the manifestations of HIV infection in children and the management of HIV infection in pregnant women is beyond the scope of this chapter. Preliminary reports of AZT use in pregnant women suggest that the treatment is well tolerated; anemia and growth retardation were observed in a minority of the infants.[171]

Hematologic Disorders

Major and minor abnormalities of the hematopoietic system occur at all stages of HIV infection.[172] Primary infection with HIV may be associated with leukopenia and atypical lymphocytes in the peripheral blood. Parameters then normalize until the infection progresses; most patients have a mild leukopenia and moderate-to-marked lymphopenia. Therapeutic agents such as sulfonamide antibiotics and antiviral agents will exaggerate the leukopenia, as will disseminated processes such as MAC infection when the marrow is involved. Patients with advanced HIV infection may become granulocytopenic, which is due to disseminated infection, progressive HIV disease, or therapies (particularly ganciclovir). The risk of infection associated with granulocytopenia in HIV-infected patients has not been defined, but the observed rate of overwhelming sepsis in this population in no way approximates the experience with sepsis in patients who become granulocytopenic during cancer chemotherapy. Empiric antibiotic therapy therefore is not recommended for stable HIV-infected patients. When aggressive treatment of CMV infection is limited by granulocytopenia, recombinant granulocyte colony-stimulating factor (G-CSF) or granulocyte-macrophage colony-stimulating factor (GM-CSF) therapy has been used to raise white blood cell levels.[173]

With time, anemia usually develops in HIV-infected patients; it may be exacerbated by therapies such as AZT, which is associated with a macrocytic anemia as a result of its action on erythrocyte precursors. Disseminated infections are associated with a normocytic, normochromic anemia (anemia of chronic disease). Long-term management of anemia may include use of recombinant erythropoietin therapy.[174] Hemolytic drug reactions (particularly those due to sulfonamides, dapsone, and related drugs, even in patients with normal levels of G6PD) and gastrointestinal bleeding that is due to involvement with Kaposi's sarcoma may result in rapidly progressive anemia. Vitamin B_{12} deficiency resulting from HIV gastropathy and inadequate intrinsic factor production has been reported.[175] Profound anemia related to persistent infection of the marrow with parvovirus can be treated with intravenous immunoglobulin.[176]

Thrombocytopenia is not unusual in HIV infected patients. Isolated thrombocytopenia may be observed early in infection and may respond to antiretroviral therapy and/or intravenous immunoglobulin therapy.[177] Immunologic and thrombocytopenic purpura (ITP and TTP) have been described in patients with HIV infection.[178,179] Low dose splenic irradiation or splenectomy have been used to treat ITP;[180,181] TTP has been treated with plasma exchange (plasmapheresis with fresh-frozen plasma infusions).[179]

Neoplasms

Kaposi's sarcoma is a neoplasm of the endothelial lining of blood vessels. It manifests as ecchymotic macules that evolve into purple nodules. Both skin and mucosal surfaces such as the mouth may be affected; primary lymph node involvement may develop; and visceral Kaposi's sarcoma, involving the lungs, gastrointestinal tract, and liver, has also been observed. The clinical course is highly variable. Kaposi's sarcoma may present early in the course of HIV infection and behave as an indolent condition, or it may explode and rapidly disseminate. Kaposi's sarcoma has been found primarily in individuals who acquired HIV infection through intercourse with gay or bisexual men. It is not as common in the 1990s as it was during the early part of the AIDS epidemic, when more than 20% of patients developed Kaposi's sarcoma. It is thought that the condition is related, at least in part, to infection with a transmissible agent. Therefore, as individuals began to use safer sex techniques, the incidence of Kaposi's sarcoma has declined.[182] In vitro, growth of AIDS-associated Kaposi's sarcoma can be stimulated by various cytokines, including interleukin 6 (IL^6), IL 1B, gamma interferon, and TNF.[183] Another growth factor, oncostatin M, may be a factor in the development of Kaposi's sarcoma.[184]

These observations have led to changes in strategies for the treatment of AIDs-associated Kaposi's sarcoma. Indolent or limited disease may require no therapy or local therapy such as radiation, cryotherapy, laser surgery, or intralesional injections with vinblastine or alpha interferon. Disseminated Kaposi's sarcoma, defined as visceral disease, disease in an individual whose $CD4^+$ lymphocyte count is less than 200/µl, the presence of more than 25 lesions, or formation of 10 or more new lesions in a month, is best treated with systemic agents.[185] Therapy with a variety of chemotherapeutic drugs, used alone or in combination, produces response rates in excess of 30%.[186] The combination of adriamycin, bleomycin, and vincristine is commonly used; single agents include these drugs and etoposide, doxyrubicin, vinblastine, and mitxantrone. Toxicity (granulocytopenia, fever, diarrhea, nausea, and vomiting) limits therapy in some cases. Alpha interferon has been used alone or in combination with AZT; the major side effect is a flu-like illness, which is dose-related.[187] Alpha-interferon therapy appears to be more effective in patients who immune system is relatively intact. Liposomally packaged chemotherapeutic drugs, antiangiogenesis agents, and other novel therapies may offer improved response rates for future patients with Kaposi's sarcoma.

HIV-related lymphomas are usually B-cell type or Burkitt-like lymphomas.[188] Histologic subtypes include immunoblastic and small noncleaved cell (high grade) tumors; large cell diffuse (intermediate grade) lymphomas have also been described.[189] Extranodal primary disease, particularly primary central nervous system non-Hodgkin's lymphoma (NHL), is quite common. Approximately 25% of patients with HIV-related NHL have disease confined to the central nervous system. One third of patients with generalized lymphoma have central nervous system involvement at diagnosis; one investigator reported a 63% rate of central nervous system involvement when all stages of illness are considered.[186] Investigators have speculated that more patients will develop lymphoma as antiretroviral therapies allow HIV-infected patients to live longer.[190,191]

Signs and symptoms of lymphoma in HIV-infected patients are nonspecific. Primary central nervous system lymphoma may manifest as headache, lethargy, confusion, seizures, cranial nerve palsy, or hemiparesis; similar symptoms may be observed in patients with toxoplasmosis or cerebral cryptococcosis. An MRI or a CT scan reveals single or multiple hypodense or isodense contrast-enhancing lesions, which are not easily distinguishable from those of toxoplasmosis. Empiric therapy directed at toxoplasmosis, with reassessment in 10 to 14 days, is warranted. Patients who do not respond should undergo brain biopsy for histologic diagnosis. Patients with negative toxoplasma serologies may be candidates for brain biopsy earlier in the course of therapy. Fever, isolated elevation of lactic dehydrogenase (LDH) levels, or biliary obstruction may accompany intra-abdominal NHL. In these cases, abdominal CT scanning is helpful in localizing disease in preparation for biopsy. Involvement of peripheral lymph nodes is relatively uncommon, and routine biopsy of enlarged nodes in an HIV-infected person is not indicated. If, however, a patient develops asymmetric lymphadenopathy, rapidly progressive adenopathy, bulky nodes, or in the setting of advanced HIV infection, new lymphadenopathy, biopsy may be helpful.

The prognosis of HIV-related NHL seems to be correlated with the patient's overall condition at the time the lymphoma develops. Poor performance status, bone marrow involvement, CD4+ lymphocyte count less than 200/mm³, and a diagnosis of AIDS before the development of lymphoma have been cited as poor prognostic factors. Survival rates of 2.5 to 4.5 months after diagnosis of primary central nervous system lymphoma have been reported.[186] Palliative whole-brain irradiation with a boost to the primary site of involvement produces a clinical or radiographic response in most patients,[192] but the prognosis remains poor. Chemotherapy for other forms of HIV-related central nervous system lymphoma has been limited by the development of opportunistic infections in patients with advanced AIDS at the time of diagnosis. Regimens such as CHOP, M-BACOD, and MACOP-B* have produced responses,[193] particularly in patients with a good performance status whose CD4+ lymphocyte count exceeds 100/mm³.

A wide variety of other neoplasms that occur less frequently than Kaposi's sarcoma and NHL has been described in HIV-infected patients. Lymphomatoid granulomatosis, which is probably a form of lymphoma, has been reported; radiation therapy may be effective. Cervical and anal neoplasms, related to human papilloma virus infection, are found with increased frequency in HIV-infected individuals.[169,194]

Miscellaneous

Metabolic and Endocrinologic Abnormalities. Studies suggest that resting energy expenditure is elevated in HIV-infected individuals and that energy expenditure increases with advanced disease.[195,196] This metabolic derangement has been linked to elevated levels of interferon-alfa found in response to HIV infection. Triglyceride levels are elevated even in asymptomatic patients whose weight is stable.

Rapid weight loss and wasting are found primarily in the setting of secondary infections. In this situation, the combination of illness-induced reduction in caloric intake and rising basal energy expenditures may produce a drop in weight averaging 5% of body weight in 28 days.[195] Cytokines released in response to secondary infections, such as TNF, IL1, and acute-phase proteins may act synergistically to produce the weight loss; alternatively, they may act as paracrine mediators. In patients with severe diarrhea that is due to enteric pathogens or HIV enteropathy, malabsorption may contribute to low caloric intake and accelerated weight loss. The wasting syndrome and its attendant loss of muscle mass is perpetuated by illness-imposed inactivity.

Therapeutic strategies for prevention or reversal of HIV wasting syndrome are limited. Prophylaxis against and/or prompt treatment of secondary infections is vital.[197] Medications that stimulate appetite, such as megestrol acetate and dronabinol, may promote weight gain; it is not yet clear whether this results in replenishment of muscle mass. Patients with AIDS who are hyperalimented tend to increase fat deposits, rather than rebuild muscle mass. Pentoxyfylline therapy, which may reduce TNF levels, is attractive but unproven. Likewise, the use of growth hormone has been associated with positive nitrogen balance and weight gain in limited studies, but the long-term effects of such therapy are unknown.

Disorders of fluid and electrolytes related to HIV-related illnesses and their treatment are very common. For example, chronic diarrhea results in the expected hypokalemia and dehydration; amphotericin B therapy produces hypokalemia and hypomagnesemia. In a prospective study of hospitalized individuals with AIDS, 56% were hyponatremic.[198] In many cases, pulmonary or cerebral lesions cause syndrome of inappropriate secretion of antidiuretic hormone (SIADH), but a few patients retain free water solely on the basis of non-volume-mediated, nonosmolar vasopressin release. Lactic acidosis in the absence of sepsis, malignancy, or other causes of systemic hypoxemia

---

* CHOP, Cyclophosphamide, doxorubicin, vincristine, prednisone; M-BACOD, Bleomycin, doxorubicin, vincristine, dexamethasone, methotrexate, calcium leukovorin; MACOP-B, Methotrexate, calcium leukovorin, doxorubicin, cyclophosphamide, vincristine, bleomycin, prednisone.

has been reported; the authors postulate that the disorder is related to intercurrent infection or AZT myopathy with overproduction of lactate.[199]

Endocrine abnormalities are fairly common as HIV infection advances, but the clinical significance of the disorders is variable. Up to 50% of men with AIDS are hypogonadal;[200] the development of hypogonadism may correspond with wasting. Thyroid dysfunction, manifesting as declining rT3 levels and elevated thyroxine-binding globulin, accompanies progressive HIV infection; wasting may be promoted by persistently normal T3 levels.[201] Declining T3 levels have been observed in patients who subsequently develop opportunistic infections. Hypopituitarism secondary to toxoplasmosis has been reported.[202]

Dobs found abnormal responses to adrenocorticotropic hormone (ACTH) stimulation in 8% of the 39 AIDS patients he tested.[200] Vitting et al.[198] found extensive adrenal abnormalities in all eight hypontremic patients who underwent postmortem examination. Mycobacterial or CMV infection are the most common causes of adrenal insufficiency. In McKenzie's series, CMV adrenalitis was found in 59% of HIV-infected individuals who underwent autopsy; in no case was the disorder diagnosed or presumptively treated before death.[203] Ketoconazole therapy is associated with hypogonadism and adrenal insufficiency through inhibition of steroid hormone synthesis. Thus, in a marginally insufficient adrenal gland, ketoconazole therapy may precipitate adrenal crisis.[204] Pentamidine therapy may be associated with profound and sustained hypoglycemia; it may also cause diabetes mellitus, and ketoacidosis has been reported.[205] patients who develop pentamidine-induced hyperglycemia may require life-long insulin therapy.

Renal Complications. Several types of renal involvement have been described in HIV-infected patients: HIV-associated nephropathy, acute renal failure that is due to acute tubular necrosis, and a variety of glomerular, vascular, and tubulointerstitial diseases.[206-208] HIV-associated nephropathy is characterized by focal and segmental glomerulosclerosis, tubular and interstial changes, ultrastructurally defined cytoplasmic and nuclear damage, heavy proteinuria, and rapidly progressive renal impairment. It may appear at any stage of HIV infection. HIV nephropathy occurs more frequently in black patients and in men.[209] Although the cause of the disease has not been proven, it is possibly related to HIV infection of various renal cells; concomitant secondary infections such as CMV disease may contribute to the changes. Rarely, patients recover renal function. Most patients with HIV nephropathy die within a year despite dialysis, but this depends on the stage of HIV infection at the time nephropathy develops.[206]

Acute tubular necrosis in HIV-infected patients is observed in relationship to toxic or ischemic insults, as would be seen in noninfected patients. Renal involvement in disseminated processes such as cytomegalovirus disease, cryptococcosis, histoplasmosis, or mycobacterial infection has been reported. There is a single case report of renal amyloidosis in an HIV-infected person.[210]

Cardiac Manifestations. An HIV-related cardiomyopathy may be observed in patients with advanced HIV infection; symptoms of congestive heart failure predominate.[211,212] Cases of pericarditis that are due to bacteria, mycobacteria, fungi, and CMV, some of which were associated with cardiac tamponade, have been reported. In patients with preterminal conditions, nonbacterial thrombotic endocarditis may develop. Myocardial infection with Toxoplasma gondii has been diagnosed at postmortem examination, as have focal cardiac metastases of Kaposi's sarcoma.

Musculoskeletal and Rheumatologic Disorders. Myalgia is a common symptom, and myositis may be found in HIV-infected persons; whether this is due to HIV infection itself, or to therapy such as AZT, is not clear.[213-215] Pyomyositis has been described in patients with AIDS, and careful examination is necessary to detect mass lesions within muscles. MRI, followed by aspiration and culture of the material in the mass lesion, will aid in the diagnosis of pyomyositis. Staphylococcus aureus has been the most common isolate.

The Influence of HIV Status on ICU Admission

For both the patient and the physician, perceptions about the prognosis of HIV infection and its complications determine whether an HIV-infected individual is admitted to an ICU. Wachter et al. have published a superb review of the literature related to critical care of patients with AIDS.[216] They conclude that an HIV-infected patient's ability to recover from various events depends on his overall health status. In fact, the outcome of ICU care for many HIV-related complications is equal to or better than that of non-HIV-related conditions for which such care is routinely administered.

Prognosis of Various Conditions Leading to ICU Care

Physicians who have not had the opportunity to care for HIV-infected patients may be unenthusiastic about admitting a patient with AIDS to the ICU. After all, AIDS is frequently described as a "uniformly fatal illness;" is the physician merely delaying the inevitable by committing the resources of an ICU to someone with AIDS? In reality, such resources are used very frequently by patients whose long-term prognosis is similar to if not worse than that of individuals with advanced HIV infection. This point is illustrated by a study[217] comparing the presence of "DNR" orders in the charts of patients with one of four different conditions with similar prognoses: unresectable non-small cell lung cancer, AIDS, cirrhosis with esophageal varices, and severe congestive heart failure (CHF) with a history of coronary artery disease. The length of stay was similar for each diagnosis, and the in-hospital mortality was 3% for patients with CHF, 12% for those with AIDS, 14% for patients with lung cancer, and 18% for patients with cirrhosis. Fifty-two percent of the patients with AIDS had a DNR order written during the hospitalization; none of the HIV-infected patients in the study was in an ICU at the time, and the authors were unable to identify precipitating events that prompted the discussion about resuscitation. Similarly, a DNR order was written for 47% of the lung cancer patients, usually without apparent changes in patient status. In contrast, only 16% of the patients with cirrhosis received a DNR order, and the order was usually written after clinical deterioration during the hospital stay. Four percent of the patients admitted for treatment of severe CHF received a DNR order, despite the fact that many patients were in functional categories with poor prognoses. Several studies in the last decade suggest that an AIDS diagnosis should not be the deciding factor when ICU care is under consideration.

Respiratory Failure. Much has been written about life-sustaining therapies for patients with HIV-related PCP. For patients with AIDS, approximately two thirds of ICU admissions are precipitated by respiratory failure, and the overwhelming majority of cases of respiratory failure have been due to PCP. In patients requiring mechanical ventilation for respiratory failure, fatality rates of up to 87% were cited in the early years of the epidemic.[218] By the late 1980s, the overall 1-month mortality had dropped to approximately 25%,[219] and the mortality among patients admitted to an ICU for treatment of PCP was approximately 50%.[220-225]

Outcome studies of ICU care for PCP that compare patients treated before 1986 with those hospitalized in subsequent years have provided further optimism.[216,221,226] Statistically significant differences in hospital survival were attributable to higher serum albumin level on admission and admission to the ICU during 1986 to 1988. The availability of effective antiretroviral therapy and earlier recognition of the diagnosis of PCP may have influenced both the nutritional status and the survival of patients treated in the late 1980s.[227] A trend toward better survival was observed in intubated patients who received adjunctive corticosteroid therapy. In a separate review, Friedman et al. found a statistically significant benefit for the use of steroids.[222] Preliminary data indicate that the length of ICU stay does not correlate with outcome.[216] At present, there is little information about the outcome of treatment for respiratory failure in AIDS patients with recurrent PCP; Efferen's group reported a 25% survival rate for patients intubated for a second bout of PCP.[223]

Other causes of respiratory failure are far less common than PCP. Bacterial pneumonia that is due to S. pneumoniae, S. aureus, H. influenzae or other isolates may be associated with sepsis and respiratory failure; in HIV-infected patients, bacterial pneumonia may occur before other AIDS-defining conditions are present. Similarly, pulmonary tuberculosis may occur in HIV-infected persons with a $CD4^+$ lymphocyte count more than $200/\mu l$. Under the new criteria for the diagnosis of AIDS, HIV-infected individuals with two or more bouts of bacterial pneumonia and those with pulmonary tuberculosis are categorized as having AIDS.[34] The changes in the definition for AIDS point out the wide variation in clinical conditions within the group and the need for individual assessment for ICU admission. The prognosis for recovery from bacterial pneumonia or drug-sensitive pulmonary tuberculosis in HIV-infected persons with a relatively preserved CD4 lymphocyte count is excellent, provided that the diagnosis is established and treatment instituted promptly.

Respiratory failure that is due to opportunistic pathogens other than P. carinii, such as CMV, nontuberculous Mycobacteria, T. gondii, and C. neoformans, accounted for approximately 12% of ICU admissions in Wachter and coworkers' summary.[216] The patient's outcome will depend on his level of immune function, nutritional status, and the responsiveness of the infection to antimicrobial therapy. The isolation of CMV from BAL fluid does not necessitate antiviral therapy; the short- and long-term prognosis of patients with PCP and CMV in BAL fluid who do not receive antiviral therapy does not differ from that of patients with PCP alone. In one study, early deterioration in oxygenation and use of ICUs was less common in the CMV-infected patients.[228] Last, pulmonary Kaposi's sarcoma or lymphoma may cause respiratory failure. The prognosis for HIV-infected patients with pulmonary neoplasms, which are usually manifestations of disseminated visceral neoplasms, is poor.

Other Conditions. Events such as hypotension, sepsis, intractable seizures, and procedure-related complications may precipitate admission of an HIV-infected patient to an ICU. In these situations, the immediate outcome of treatment is unlikely to be influenced by the patient's HIV status. A meta-analysis of four studies[218,220,229,230] that addressed the question of ICU admission for conditions other than respiratory failure revealed an overall in-hospital survival rate of 58%.[216]

Cardiopulmonary Resuscitation. The reported outcome of cardiopulmonary resuscitation (CPR) in patients with AIDS has been dismal. A 1988 study comparing the results of CPR in patients with and without AIDS showed initial revival rates of 23 and 42%, respectively.[231] Only 2.3% of the AIDS patients survived to hospital discharge, compared to 6.5% of non-AIDS patients. The cause of arrest was respiratory failure in 23% of the AIDS patients and in 9.5% of the control group. The authors were unable to demonstrate differences in length of resuscitation efforts or use of technology between the two groups that would explain the marked differences in outcome.

Patient Preferences

As the natural history and prognosis of AIDS were studied in the 1980s, HIV-infected persons became more proactive in their medical care planning. Perhaps the most visible activities related to lobbying for improved treatment for HIV and related conditions, but interest in directing all phases of care was widespread. Many patients and physicians became aware of the value of developing mutually agreed-on guidelines for use of various therapies, including life-sustaining treatments, well in advance of the need for such actions. In 1985, a survey of 118 homosexual men with AIDS revealed that two thirds of the respondents had thought "a lot or a moderate amount" about whom they wanted to designate to make medical decisions for them if they were unable to do so.[232] In many same-sex relationships, the patient preferred that partners or friends make surrogate decisions; this may lead to tension between relatives and the patient/partner.[233] Formalization of patient preferences via execution of advance directives statements and designation of durable power of attorney for medical care help to reduce problems of this nature during times of crisis.[234]

Patients' interest in and expectations of intensive care have varied throughout the past decade. Because of improved therapies for HIV infection and its complications, determination of expected outcomes has been a moving target. For example, participants in Steinbrook's 1986 study overestimated the survival rate of patients with P. carinii pneumonia who required ventilation; their estimates, however, are lower than the survival rate of similar patients who were treated with steroids in the early 1990s.[232] Patients and physicians need to stay informed of developments in therapies. More importantly, they need to maintain a dialogue with patients about life-style priorities, which will help to guide specific decisions in a variety of situations.[235]

ICU PHASE

Diagnostic and Support Measures

The overall care of an HIV-infected patient in the ICU does not differ significantly from that of other patients requiring special supervision and support. If the cause for clinical deterioration is not known at the time of ICU admission, every effort should be made to establish a diagnosis as rapidly as possible. For HIV-infected patients with respiratory failure, bronchoscopy with bronchoalveolar lavage is usually diagnostic for most opportunistic infections; noninfectious intrabronchial or parenchymal disease may require transbronchial biopsy for diagnosis. Open lung biopsy is rarely required.

Patients whose ICU admission is precipitated by rapid changes in mental status or intractable seizures will often require empiric therapy and support for several days or weeks before a definitive diagnosis is made. MRI or CT scans of the head should be completed, and a lumbar puncture should be performed if possible. Routine CSF studies in this setting include cell count and differential, protein, glucose, bacterial and cryptococcal antigen tests, VDRL, and cultures for bacteria and fungi. A patient with advanced HIV infection and typical cerebral or cerebellar mass lesions should be treated empirically for toxoplasmosis for 2 to 3 weeks. If the patient does not respond to therapy, brain biopsy may be necessary for diagnosis. In patients with impending herniation, corticosteroid therapy may be necessary for a short time, along with mannitol infusions and other measures designed to reduce intracranial pressure.

Fever is a common problem in patients with HIV infection. In evaluating the cause of fever in a patient without other specific symptoms, it is helpful to determine the duration (i.e., acute or chronic) and intensity of the fever. Disseminated infections due to M. avium-intracellulare, M. tuberculosis, CMV, or C. neoformans are usually characterized by the gradual onset of low grade fevers. M. avium-intracellulare and CMV infection typically occur in patients with very advanced AIDS. Rarely, individuals with long-standing HIV infection will develop subacute bacteremia that is due to S. aureus. Acute fevers in patients with HIV infection may be associated with bacteremic pneumonias that are due to S. pneumoniae, H. influenzae, or S. aureus; line-associated sepsis may be a factor in patients with Hickman catheters or other indwelling intravenous devices. It is useful to obtain two or three sets of routine blood cultures from febrile individuals. Repeated blood cultures with temperature spikes, however, are not likely to be helpful. Blood cultures for acid-fast bacteria and CMV may be useful in evaluating the patient with chronic fevers, and serum cryptococcal antigen titers should also be performed in this population. Recent studies, however, indicate that blood and urine CMV cultures are poorly predictive of visceral or invasive CMV infection.[147]

Infection Control Concerns

In the ICU setting, concerns about the possibility of transmission of infection—either HIV or an opportunistic infection—may persist despite ongoing educational efforts.[236] The use of "universal" or "blood and body substance" precautions should be routine in all health-care settings.[237-240] In this system, individualized, encounter-specific measures are used; the health-care worker is responsible for anticipating which devices (i.e., gloves, mask, goggles) will be appropriate for use during the procedure. Occupational Health and Safety Act provisions reinforce the requirement that workers use appropriate personal safety devices in the workplace. When universal precautions are properly used, transmission of infection is reduced dramatically.[241] Other components of daily infection control practice include frequent hand washing and proper disposal of needles and other sharps. All health-care workers whose duties involve exposure to body fluids should receive hepatitis B vaccination.

These infection control measures are designed to reduce the risk of mucosal or percutaneous contact with contaminated devices or body fluids. The risk of needlestick is not eliminated by use of universal precautions, and this remains a concern. The chance of transmission of HIV infection after percutaneous exposure to HIV-positive blood is a 0.3%. This compares to a 30% chance of hepatitis B infection after percutaneous exposure to HBeAg-positive blood.[12] AZT prophylaxis has been offered to exposed health-care workers, but the efficacy of AZT in preventing HIV infection after percutaneous exposure is not known.[242,243] Transmission of HIV has occurred in several cases after percutaneous exposure to relatively large volumes of infected blood despite immediate and aggressive administration of AZT.

Transmission of tuberculosis in the ICU is a particular concern. The manifestations of pulmonary tuberculosis in a critically ill patient may be minimal; symptoms are usually nonspecific, mimicking those of many other infections commonly observed in HIV-infected patients. Increasing numbers of patients infected with MDR-TB strains have added to the anxiety of health-care workers. The major preventive measure is the use of masks by individuals caring for immunocompromised patients with productive coughs; these individuals should be housed in hospital rooms with negative pressure compared with the surrounding corridors.[244] Routine bacille Calmette-Guérin vaccination is not recommended for adult health-care workers, because of the limited immunogenicity of the preparation and its effect on tuberculin skin tests. Recommendations for drug prophylaxis of health-care workers exposed to patients with MDR-TB include the possible use of combination therapy with pyrazinamide and ethambutol for 12 months.[245] An investigational trial of prophylactic pyrazinamide and a fluoroquinalone antibiotic is being organized by the Clinical Research Branch of the CDC.

Reassessment and Decision Making

The question of the appropriate duration of ICU care (in particular, the question of how long to continue mechanical ventilation) has not been addressed comprehensively. The data of Wachter et al., which specifically addressed the HIV-infected patient with PCP and respiratory failure, suggests that length of ICU admission is unrelated to eventual outcome.[216] According to this group, a trial of mechanical ventilation that is shorter than 10 days is probably inadequate to predict the outcome for the treatment of PCP and respiratory failure.

In general, decisions about the continuation of intensive care center around the perceived utility of the treatment: What are the chances of survival? If the patient survives, what quality of life can he expect? As in other critical care situations, the prospects for survival depend as much on the individual's underlying nutritional status and premorbid level of function as they on the immediate cause of ICU admission.

POST-ICU PHASE/REHABILITATION

Recovery

After discharge from the ICU, most patients will require several additional days of supervised therapy. The goals of this period are to plan a transition from hospital to home and to establish long-term treatment regimens. If antiretroviral therapy has not been given before, the post-ICU period may be a good time to start it. All patients whose CD4+ lymphocyte count is less than 200/μl should receive prophylactic antibiotic therapy to prevent PCP. Other preventive regimens should also be considered (see Table 68-8). Specific information about antiretroviral therapy and prophylaxis against infectious complications has been provided in an earlier section of this chapter.

Site of Care

Increasingly, care for HIV-infected patients is delivered outside the hospital. There are many reasons for this phenomenon: the availability of "high tech" therapies in the ambulatory clinic, home, and other alternative settings;[246] cost considerations; and most importantly, patient preferences to avoid hospitalization. Discussions about site of care may catalyze the patient's understanding of care goals. Patients with profound neurologic dysfunction may have difficulty finding either skilled or custodial care. The availability of rehabilitation and extended care beds is highly variable, reflecting the lack of familiarity that institutions may have with the care of HIV-infected patients.

Psychosocial and Ethical Considerations

Support from friends, family, social workers, pastoral care personnel, volunteers, and the hospital staff is crucial, both during the transition from ICU to regular nursing floor, and also during the transition from hospital to home. These individuals are essential in helping the patient to frame his health-care priorities for times of crisis in the future. Because, in some cases, the ICU admission will mark the revelation of risk behavior for HIV infection and the initial diagnosis of AIDS, patients and families may have special counseling needs. Above all, the consistent provision of accurate information and an ongoing educational effort will help patients and their loved ones to cope with the acute situation and make decisions about their future.

In summary, HIV infection is a chronic, complex illness that may, primarily because of opportunistic infectious complications, be associated with acute respiratory failure, seizures, coma, hypotension, and other events that precipitate ICU admission. The diagnosis of AIDS (CDC clinical categories C1, C2, C3, A3, or B3) does not preclude admission to the ICU, because underlying nutritional status and immune function will influence outcome more than the disease category. The prognosis for recovery from PCP is good, particularly when steroids are used in conjunction with antipneumocystis chemotherapy. For patients with other conditions, the outcome of their treatment does not appear to differ from that of noninfected patients with similar complications. Most HIV-infected patients will survive several opportunistic infections despite the presence of profound immunodeficiency. Quality of life issues may supervene in patients with dementia, blindness, or profound wasting. The initiation of discussions about healthcare priorities will guide patients and physicians in considerations of the appropriateness of ICU care.

REFERENCES

1. Centers for Disease Control: Update: Acquired immunodeficiency syndrome—United States, 1981-1990. M.M.W.R., 40:358, 1991.
2. Selik, R. M., Chu, S. Y., and Buehler, J. W.: HIV infection as leading cause of death among young adults in US cities and states. JAMA, 269:2991, 1993.
3. Centers for Disease Control: HIV prevalence estimates and AIDS case projections for the United States: report based on a workshop. M.M.W.R., 39(RR-16):30, 1990.
4. Carroll, W.: AIDS-Related Claims Survey: Claims Paid in 1989. Washington, DC, American Council of Life Insurance/Health Insurance Association of America, September 1989.
5. Centers for Disease Control: Projections of the number of persons diagnosed with AIDS and the number of immunosuppressed HIV-infected persons-United States, 1992-1994. M.M.W.R., 41(RR-18):1, 1992.
6. St. Louis, M. E. et al.: Seroprevalence rates of human immunodeficiency virus infection at sentinel hospitals in the United States. N. Engl. J. Med., 323:213, 1990.
7. Chin, J.: Current and future dimensions of the HIV/AIDS pandemic in women and children. Lancet, 336:221, 1990.
8. Cohen, H. D. et al.: Transmission of retroviruses by transfusion of screened blood in patients undergoing cardiac surgery. N. Engl. J. Med., 320:1172, 1989.
9. Friedland, G. H., and Klein, R. S.: Transmission of the human immunodeficiency virus. N. Engl. J. Med., 317:1125, 1987.
10. Padian, N. S., Shiboski, S. C., and Jewell, N. P.: Female-to-male transmission of human immunodeficiency virus. JAMA, 266:1664, 1991.
11. Nanda, D., and Minkoff, H. L.: HIV in pregnancy—transmission and immune effects. Clin. Obstet. Gynecol., 32:456, 1989.

12. Friedland, G. H. et al.: Lack of transmission of HTLV-III infection to household contacts of patients with AIDS or AIDS-related complex with oral candidiasis. N. Engl. J. Med., 314:344, 1986.
13. Henderson, D. et al.: Risk for occupational transmission of human immunodeficiency virus type 1 (HIV-1) associated with clinical exposures: a prospective evaluation. Ann. Intern. Med., 113:740, 1990.
14. Chamberland, M. E. et al.: Health care workers with AIDS: national surveillance update. JAMA, 266:3459, 1991.
15. Centers for Disease Control: Update: transmission of HIV infection during an invasive dental procedure—Florida. M.M.W.R., 40:21, 1991.
16. Centers for Disease Control: Update: investigations of persons treated by HIV-infected health-care workers—United States. M.M.W.R., 42:329, 1993.
17. Rogers, A. S. et al.: Investigation of potential HIV transmission to the patients of an HIV-infected surgeon. JAMA, 269:1795, 1993.
18. Markovitz, D. M.: Infection with the human immunodeficiency virus type 2. Ann. Intern. Med., 118:211, 1993.
19. Greene, W. C.: The molecular biology of human immunodeficiency virus type 1 infection. N. Engl. J. Med., 324:308, 1991.
20. Fauci, A. S. et al.: Immunopathogenic mechanisms in human immunodeficiency virus infection. Ann. Intern. Med., 114:678, 1991.
21. Fauci, A. S.: The human immunodeficiency virus: infectivity and mechanisms of pathogenesis. Science, 239:617, 1988.
22. Levy, J. A.: Human immunodeficiency viruses and the pathogenesis of AIDS. JAMA, 261:2997, 1989.
23. Tindall, B., and Cooper, D. A.: Primary HIV infection: host responses and intervention strategies. AIDS, 5:1, 1991.
24. Clark, S. J. et al.: High titers of cytopathic virus in plasma of patients with symptomatic primary HIV-1 infection. N. Engl. J. Med., 324:954, 1991.
25. Pantaleo, G., Graziosi, C., and Fauci, A. S.: The immunopathogenesis of human immunodeficiency virus infection. N. Engl. J. Med., 328:327, 1993.
26. Polis, M. A.: Predicting the progression to AIDS. Am. J. Med., 89:701, 1990.
27. Anderson, R. E. et al.: Use of β2-microglobulin level and CD4 lymphocyte count to predict development of acquired immunodeficiency syndrome in persons with human immunodeficiency virus infection. Arch. Intern. Med., 150:73, 1990.
28. Phillips, A. N. et al.: Immunodeficiency and the risk of death in HIV infection. JAMA, 268:2662, 1992.
29. Sloand, E. M., Pitt, E. Chiarello, R. J., and Nemo, G. J.: HIV testing: State of the art. JAMA, 266:2861, 1991.
30. Davey, R. T., and Lane, H. C.: Laboratory methods in the diagnosis and prognostic staging of infection with human immunodeficiency virus type 1. Rev. Infect. Dis., 12:912, 1990.
31. Centers for Disease Control: Update: serologic testing for antibody to human immunodeficiency virus. M.M.W.R., 36:833, 1988.
32. Centers for Disease Control: Interpretation and use of the Western blot assay for serodiagnosis of human immunodeficiency virus type 1 infections. M.M.W.R., 38(S-7):1, 1989.
33. Stramer, S. L. et al.: Markers of HIV infection prior to IgG antibody seropositivity. JAMA, 262:64, 1989.
34. Centers for Disease Control: 1993 Revised classification system for HIV infection and expanded surveillance case definition for AIDS among adolescents and adults. M.M.W.R., 41(RR-17):1, 1993.
35. Erice, A. et al.: Primary infection with zidovudine-resistant human immunodeficiency virus type 1. N. Engl. J. Med., 328:1163, 1993.
36. Larder, B. A., Darby, G., and Richman, D. D.: HIV with reduced sensitivity to zidovudine (AZT) isolated during prolonged therapy. Science, 243:1731, 1989.
37. Aboulker, J.-P., and Swart, A. M.: Preliminary analysis of the Concorde trial. Lancet, 341:889, 1993.
38. McLeod, G. X., and Hammer, S. M.: Zidovudine: five years later. Ann. Intern. Med., 117:487, 1992.
39. Fischl, M. A. et al.: The efficacy of azidothymidine (AZT) in the treatment of patients with AIDS and AIDS-related complex. N. Engl. J. Med., 317:185, 1987.
40. Collier, A. C. et al.: A pilot study of low-dose zidovudine in human immunodeficiency virus infection. N. Engl. J. Med., 323:1015, 1990.
41. Fischl, M. A. et al.: A randomized controlled trial of a reduced daily dose of zidovudine in patients with the acquired immunodeficiency syndrome. N. Engl. J. Med., 323:1009, 1990.
42. Volberding, P. A. et al.: Zidovudine in asymptomatic human immunodeficiency virus infection: a controlled trial in persons with fewer than 500 CD4-positive cells per cubic millimeter. N. Engl. J. Med., 322:941, 1990.
43. Fischl, M. A. et al.: The safety and efficacy of zidovudine (AZT) in the treatment of subjects with mildly symptomatic human immunodeficiency virus type 1 (HIV) infection: a double-blind, placebo-controlled trial. Ann. Intern. Med., 112:727, 1990.
44. Moore, R. D. et al.: Long-term safety and efficacy of zidovudine in patients with advanced human immunodeficiency virus disease. Arch. Intern. Med., 151:981, 1991.
45. Hamilton, J. D. et al.: A controlled trial of early versus late treatment with zidovudine in symptomatic human immunodeficiency virus infection: results of the Veterans Affairs Cooperative Study. N. Engl. J. Med., 326:437, 1992.
46. Graham, N. M. H. et al.: The effects on survival of early treatment of human immunodeficiency virus infection. N. Engl. J. Med., 326:1037, 1992.
47. Moore, R. D. Hidalgo, J., Sugland, B. W., and Chaisson, R. E.: Zidovudine and the natural history of the acquired immunodeficiency syndrome. N. Engl. J. Med., 324:1412, 1991.
48. Yarchoan, R. et al.: CD4 count and the risk for death in patients infected with HIV receiving antiretroviral therapy. Ann. Intern. Med., 115:184, 1991.
49. Kahn, J. O. et al.: A controlled trial comparing continued zidovudine with didanosine in human immunodeficiency virus infection. N. Engl. J. Med., 327:581, 1992.
50. Meng, T.-C. et al.: Combination therapy with zidovudine and dideoxycytidine in patients with advanced human immunodeficiency virus infection: a phase I/II study. Ann. Intern. Med., 116:13, 1992.
51. Skowron, G. et al.: Alternating and intermittent regimens of zidovudine and dideoxycytidine in patients with AIDS or AIDS-related complex. Ann. Intern. Med., 118:321, 1993.
52. Connolly, K. J., and Hammer, S. M.: Antiretroviral therapy: strategies beyond single-agent reverse transcriptase inhibition. Antimicrob. Agents. Chemother., 36:509, 1992.
53. Sachs, M. K.: Antiretroviral chemotherapy of human immunodeficiency virus infections other than with azidothymidine. Arch. Intern. Med., 152:485, 1992.
54. Jewett, J. F., and Hecht, F. M.: Preventive health care for adults with HIV infection. JAMA, 269:1144, 1993.
55. Carr, A. et al.: Low-dose trimethoprim-sulfamethoxazole prophylaxis for toxoplasmic encephalitis in patients with AIDS. Ann. Intern. Med., 117:106, 1992.
56. Kaplan, L. D. et al.: Treatment of patients with AIDS and associated manifestations. JAMA, 257:1367, 1987.

57. Glatt, A. E., Chirgwin, K., and Landesman, S. H.: Treatment of infections associated with human immunodeficiency virus. N. Engl. J. Med., *318*:1439, 1988.
58. Gradon, J. D., Timpone, J. G., and Schnittman, S. M.: Emergence of unusual opportunistic pathogens in AIDS: a review. Clin. Infect. Dis., *15*:134, 1992.
59. Lee, B. L., and Safrin, S.: Interactions and toxicities of drugs used in patients with AIDS. Clin. Infect. Dis., *14*:773, 1992.
60. Meduri, G. U., and Stein, D. S.: Pulmonary manifestations of acquired immunodeficiency syndrome. Clin. Infect. Dis., *14*:98, 1992.
61. Masur, H. et al.: Pneumocystis pneumonia: from bench to clinic. Ann. Intern. Med., *111*:813, 1989.
62. Glatt, A. E., and Chirgwin, K.: *Pneumocystis carinii* pneumonia in human immunodeficiency virus-infected patients. Arch. Intern. Med., *150*:271, 1990.
63. Phair, J. et al.: The risk of *Pneumocystis carinii* pneumonia among men infected with human immunodeficiency virus type 1. N. Engl. J. Med., *322*:161, 1990.
64. Kennedy, C. A., and Goetz, M. B.: Atypical roentgenographic manifestations of *Pneumocystis carinii* pneumonia. Arch. Intern. Med., *152*:1390, 1992.
65. Davey, R. T., and Masur, H.: Recent advances in the diagnosis, treatment, and prevention of *Pneumocystis carinii* pneumonia. Antimicrob. Agents Chemother., *34*:499, 1990.
66. Masur, H.: Prevention and treatment of pneumocystis pneumonia. N. Engl. J. Med., *327*:1853, 1992.
67. Medina, I. et al.: Oral therapy for *Pneumocystis carinii* pneumonia in the acquired immunodeficiency syndrome: a controlled trial of trimethoprim-sulfamethoxazole versus trimethoprim-dapsone. N. Engl. J. Med., *323*:776, 1990.
68. Noskin, G. A., Murphy, R. L., Black, J. R., and Phair, J. P.: Salvage therapy with clindamycin/primaquine for *Pneumocystis carinii* pneumonia. Clin. Infect. Dis., *14*:183, 1992.
69. Hughes, W. T. et al.: Safety and pharmacokinetics of 566C80, a hydroxynaphthoquinone with anti-*Pneumocystis carinii* activity: a phase I study in human immunodeficiency virus (HIV)-infected men. J. Infect. Dis., *163*:843, 1991.
70. Falloon, J. et al.: A preliminary evaluation of 566C80 for the treatment of pneumocystis pneumonia in patients with the acquired immunodeficiency syndrome. N. Engl. J. Med., *325*:1534, 1991.
71. Allegra, C. J. et al.: Trimetrexate for the treatment of *Pneumocystis carinii* pneumonia in patients with the acquired immunodeficiency syndrome. N. Engl. J. Med., *317*:978, 1987.
72. The National Institutes of Health–University of California Expert Panel for Corticosteroids as Adjunctive Therapy for Pneumocystis Pneumonia: Consensus statement on the use of corticosteroids as adjunctive therapy for Pneumocystis pneumonia in the acquired immunodeficiency syndrome. N. Engl. J. Med., *323*:1500, 1990.
73. Centers for Disease Control: Recommendations for prophylaxis against *Pneumocystis carinii* pneumonia for adults and adolescents infected with HIV. M.M.W.R., *41(RR-4)*:1, 1992.
74. Chaisson, R. E. et al.: Pneumocystis prophylaxis and survival in patients with advanced human immunodeficiency virus infection treated with zidovudine. Arch. Intern. Med., *152*:2009, 1992.
75. Schneider, M. M. E. et al.: A controlled trial of aerosolized pentamidine or trimethoprim-sulfamethoxazole as primary prophylaxis against *Pneumocystis carinii* pneumonia in patients with human immunodeficiency virus infection. N. Engl. J. Med., *327*:1836, 1992.
76. Hardy, W. D. et al.: A controlled trial of trimethoprim-sulfamethoxazole or aerosolized pentamidine for secondary prophylaxis of *Pneumocystis carinii* pneumonia in patients with the acquired immunodeficiency syndrome. N. Engl. J. Med., *327*:1842, 1992.
77. Ruskin, J., and LaRiviere, M.: Low-dose co-trimoxazole for prevention of *Pneumocystis carinii* pneumonia in human immunodeficiency virus disease. Lancet, *337*:468, 1991.
78. Wormser, G. P. et al.: Low-dose intermittent trimethoprim-sulfamethoxazole for prevention of *Pneumocystis carinii* pneumonia in patients with human immunodeficiency virus infection. Arch. Intern. Med., *151*:688, 1991.
79. Polsky, B. et al.: Bacterial pneumonia in patients with the acquired immunodeficiency syndrome. Ann. Intern. Med., *104*:38, 1986.
80. Barnes, P. F., Bloch, A. B., Davidson, P. T., and Snider, D. E. Jr.: Tuberculosis in patients with human immunodeficiency virus infection. N. Engl. J. Med., *324*:1644, 1991.
81. Kramer, F. et al.: Delayed diagnosis of tuberculosis in patients with human immunodeficiency virus infection. Am. J. Med., *89*:451, 1990.
82. Johnson, M. P. et al.: Tuberculin skin test reactivity among adults infected with human immunodeficiency virus. J. Infect. Dis., *166*:194, 1992.
83. Centers for Disease Control: Tuberculosis and human immunodeficiency virus infection: recommendations of the Advisory Committee for the Elimination of Tuberculosis (ACET). M.M.W.R., *38*:236, 1989.
84. Graham, N. M. H. et al.: Prevalence of tuberculin positivity and skin test anergy in HIV-1-seropositive and -seronegative intravenous drug users. JAMA, *267*:369, 1992.
85. Selwyn, P. A. et al.: High risk of active tuberculosis in HIV-infected drug users with cutaneous anergy. JAMA, *268*:504, 1992.
86. Small, P. M. et al.: Treatment of tuberculosis in patients with advanced human immunodeficiency virus infection. N. Engl. J. Med., *324*:289, 1991.
87. Frieden, T. R. et al.: The emergence of drug-resistant tuberculosis in New York City. N. Engl. J. Med., *328*:521, 1993.
88. Fischl, M. A. et al.: Clinical presentation and outcome of patients with HIV infection and tuberculosis caused by multiple-drug-resistant bacilli. Ann. Intern. Med., *117*:184, 1992.
89. Beck-Sagué, C. et al.: Hospital outbreak of multidrug-resistant *Mycobacterium tuberculosis* infections: factors in transmission to staff and HIV-infected patients. JAMA, *268*:1280, 1992.
90. Edlin, B. R. et al.: An outbreak of multidrug-resistant tuberculosis among hospitalized patients with the acquired immunodeficiency syndrome. N. Engl. J. Med., *326*:1514, 1992.
91. Dooley, S. W. et al.: Nosocomial transmission of tuberculosis in a hospital unit for HIV-infected patients. JAMA, *267*:2632, 1992.
92. Small, C. B., Kaufman, A., Armenaka, M., and Rosenstreich, D. L.: Sinusitis and atopy in human immunodeficiency virus infection. J. Infect. Dis., *167*:283, 1993.
93. Gabuzda, D. H., and Hirsch, M. S.: Neurologic manifestations of infection with human immunodeficiency virus. Ann. Intern. Med., *107*:383, 1987.
94. Ho, D. D., Brfedesen, D. E., Vinters, H. V., and Daar, E. S.: The acquired immunodeficiency syndrome (AIDS) dementia complex. Ann. Intern. Med., *111*:400, 1989.
95. Price, R. W. et al.: The brain in AIDS: central nervous system HIV-1 infection and AIDS dementia complex. Science, *239*:586, 1988.
96. Koralnik, I. J. et al.: A controlled study of early neurologic

abnormalities in men with asymptomatic human immunodeficiency virus infection. N. Engl. J. Med., *323*:864, 1990.
97. Parry, G. J.: Peripheral neuropathies associated with human immunodeficiency virus infection. Ann. Neurol., *23 (Suppl.)*:S49, 1988.
98. Dalakas, M. C., and Pezeshkpour, G. H.: Neuromuscular disease associated with human immunodeficiency virus infection. Ann. Neurol., *23(Suppl.)*:S38, 1988.
99. Cimino, C. et al.: The evaluation of patients with human immunodeficiency virus-related disorders and brain mass lesions. Arch. Intern. Med., *151*:1381, 1991.
100. Porter, S. B., and Sande, M. A.: Toxoplasmosis of the central nervous system in the acquired immunodeficiency syndrome. N. Engl. J. Med., *327*:1643, 1992.
101. Cohn, J. A. et al.: Evaluation of the policy of empiric treatment of suspected *Toxoplasma* encephalitis, in patients with the acquired immunodeficiency syndrome. Am. J. Med., *86*:521, 1989.
102. Chuck, S. L., and Sande, M. A.: Infections with *Cryptococcus neoformans* in the acquired immunodeficiency syndrome. N. Engl. J. Med., *321*:794, 1989.
103. Bozzette, S. A. et al.: A placebo-controlled trial of maintenance therapy with fluconazole after treatment of cryptococcal meningitis in the acquired immunodeficiency syndrome. N. Engl. J. Med., *324*:580, 1991.
104. Matlow, A. G., and Rachlis, A. R.: Syphilis serology in human immunodeficiency virus-infected patients with symptomatic neurosyphilis: case report and review. Rev. Infect. Dis., *12*:703, 1990.
105. Berenguer, J. et al.: Tuberculous meningitis in patients infected with the human immunodeficiency virus. N. Engl. J. Med., *326*:668, 1992.
106. Chaisson, R. E., and Griffin, D. E.: Progressive multifocal leukoencephalopathy in AIDS. JAMA, *264*:79, 1990.
107. So, Y. T., Beckstead, J. H., and Davis, R. L.: Primary central nervous system lymphoma in acquired immune deficiency syndrome: a clinical and pathological study. Ann. Neurol., *20*:566, 1986.
108. Anders, K. H. et al.: Lymphomatoid granulomatosis and malignant lymphoma of the central nervous system in the acquired immunodeficiency syndrome. Hum. Pathol., *20*:326, 1989.
109. Schulten, E. A. J. M., tenKate, R. W., and van der Waal, I.: The impact of oral examination on the Centers for Disease Control classification of subjects with human immunodeficiency virus infection. Arch. Intern. Med., *150*:1259, 1990.
110. Greenspan, D. et al.: Relation of oral hairy leukoplakia to infection with the human immunodeficiency virus and the risk of developing AIDS. J. Infect. Dis., *155*:475, 1987.
111. Bonacini, M., Yound, T., and Laine, L.: The causes of esophageal symptoms in human immunodeficiency virus infection: a prospective study of 110 patients. Arch. Intern. Med., *151*:1567, 1991.
112. Indorf, A. S., and Pegram, P. S.: Esophageal ulceration related to zalcitabine (ddC). Ann. Intern. Med., *117*:133, 1992.
113. Bach, M. C. et al.: Aphthous ulceration of the gastrointestinal tract in patients with the acquired immunodeficiency syndrome. Ann. Intern. Med., *112*:465, 1990.
114. Smith, P. D. et al.: Gastrointestinal infection in AIDS. Ann. Intern. Med., *116*:63, 1992.
115. Belitsos, P. C. et al.: Association of gastric hypoacidity with opportunistic enteric infections in patients with AIDS. J. Infect. Dis., *166*:277, 1992.
116. Lake-Bakarr, G. et al.: Gastropathy and ketoconazole malabsorption in the acquired immunodeficiency syndrome (AIDS). Ann. Intern. Med., *109*:471, 1988.
117. Smith, P. D. et al.: Intestinal infections in patients with acquired immunodeficiency syndrome (AIDS): etiology and response to therapy. Ann. Intern. Med., *108*:328, 1988.
118. Kotler, D. P. et al.: Enteropathy associated with the acquired immunodeficiency syndrome. Ann. Intern. Med., *101*:421, 1984.
119. Dieterich, D. T. et al.: Ganciclovir treatment of cytomegalovirus colitis in AIDS: a randomized, double-blind, placebo-controlled multicenter study. J. Infect. Dis., *167*:278, 1993.
120. Schneiderman, D. J. et al.: Hepatic disease in patients with the acquired immunodeficiency syndrome (AIDS). Hepatology, *7*:925, 1987.
121. Cappell, M. S., Schwartz, M. S., and Biempica, L.: Clinical utility of liver biopsy in patients with serum antibodies to the human immunodeficiency virus. Am. J. Med., *88*:123, 1990.
122. Cello, J. P.: Acquired immunodeficiency syndrome cholangiopathy: spectrum of disease. Am. J. Med., *86*:539, 1989.
123. Pol, S. et al.: Microsporidia infection in patients with the human immunodeficiency virus and unexplained cholangitis. N. Engl. J. Med., *328*:95, 1993.
124. Schwartz, M. S., and Brandt, L. J.: The spectrum of pancreatic disorders in patients with the acquired immune deficiency syndrome. Am. J. Gastroenterol., *84*:459, 1988.
125. Horsburgh, C. R.: *Mycobacterium avium* complex infection in the acquired immunodeficiency syndrome. N. Engl. J. Med., *324*:1332, 1991.
126. Nightingale, S. D. et al.: Incidence of *Mycobacterium avium-intracellulare* complex bacteremia in human immunodeficiency virus-positive patients. J. Infect. Dis., *165*:1082, 1992.
127. Jacobson, M. A. et al.: Natural history of disseminated *Mycobacterium avium* complex infection in AIDS. J. Infect. Dis., *164*:994, 1991.
127a. Masur, H., and the Public Health Service Task Force on Prophylaxis and Therapy for Mycobacterium avium Complex: Recommendations on prophylaxis and therapy for disseminated complex disease in patients infected with human immunodeficiency virus. N. Engl. J. Med., *329*:898, 1993.
128. Braun, M. N. et al.: Acquired immunodeficiency syndrome and extrapulmonary tuberculosis in the United States. Arch. Intern. Med., *150*:1913, 1990.
129. Shafer, R. W. et al.: Extrapulmonary tuberculosis in patients with human immunodeficiency virus infection. Medicine, *70*:384, 1991.
130. Clark, R. A. et al.: Hematogenous dissemination of *Mycobacterium tuberculosis* in patients with AIDS. Rev. Infect. Dis., *13*:1089, 1991.
131. Krumholz, H. M., and Sande, M. A.: Community-acquired bacteremia in patients with acquired immunodeficiency syndrome: clinical presentation, bacteriology, and outcome. Am. J. Med., *86*:776, 1989.
132. Musher, D. M., Hamill, R. J., and Baughn, R. E.: Effect of human immunodeficiency virus (HIV) infection on the course of syphilis and on the response to treatment. Ann. Intern. Med., *113*:872, 1990.
133. Berry, C. D., Hooton, T. M., Collier, A. C., and Lukehart, S. A.: Neurologic relapse after benzathine penicillin therapy for secondary syphilis in a patient with HIV infection. N. Engl. J. Med., *316*:1587, 1987.
134. Johns, D. R., Tierney, M., and Felsenstein, D.: Alteration in the natural history of neurosyphilis by concurrent infection with the human immunodeficiency virus. N. Engl. J. Med., *316*:1569, 1987.
135. Slater, L. N., Welch, D. F., and Min, K.-W.: *Rochalimaea*

135. *henselae* causes bacillary angiomatosis and peliosis hepatitis. Arch. Intern. Med., *152:*602, 1992.
136. Perkocha, L. A. et al.: Clinical and pathological features of bacillary peliosis hepatitis in association with human immunodeficiency virus infection. N. Engl. J. Med., *323:*1581, 1990.
137. Spach, D. H. et al.: Intracerebral bacillary angiomatosis in a patient infected with human immunodeficiency virus. Ann. Intern. Med., *116:*740, 1992.
138. Koehler, J. E. et al.: Isolation of rochalimaea species from cutaneous and osseous lesions of bacillary angiomatosis. N. Engl. J. Med., *327:*1625, 1992.
139. Decker, C. F., Simon, G. L., DiGiolia, R. A, and Tauzon, C. U.: *Listeria monocytogenes* infections in patients with AIDS: report of five cases and review. Rev. Infect. Dis., *13:*413, 1991.
140. Zarabi, C. M., Thomas, R., and Adesokan, A.: Diagnosis of systemic histoplasmosis in patients with AIDS. South Med. J., *85:*1172, 1992.
141. Neubauer, M. A., and Bodensteiner, D. C.: Disseminated histoplasmosis in patients with AIDS. South Med. J., *85:*1166, 1992.
142. Pappas, P. G. et al.: Blastomycosis in patients with the acquired immunodeficiency syndrome. Ann. Intern. Med., *116:*847, 1992.
143. Bronnimann, D. A. et al.: *Coccidiodomycosis* in the acquired immunodeficiency syndrome. Ann. Intern. Med., *106:*872, 1987.
144. Klapholz, A., Salomon, N., Perlman, D. C., and Talavera, W.: Aspergillosis in the acquired immunodeficiency syndrome. Chest, *100:*1614, 1991.
145. Clark, R. A. et al.: Spectrum of *Cryptococcus neoformans* infection in 68 patients infected with human immunodeficiency virus. Rev. Infect. Dis., *12:*768, 1990.
146. Saag, M. S. et al.: Comparison of amphotericin B with fluconazole in the treatment of acute AIDS-associated cryptococcal meningitis. N. Engl. J. Med., *326:*83, 1992.
147. Zurlo, J. J. et al.: Lack of clinical utility of cytomegalovirus blood and urine cultures in patients with HIV infection. Ann. Intern. Med., *118:*12, 1993.
148. Telzak, E. E. et al.: Extrapulmonary *Pneumocystis carinii* infection. Rev. Infect Dis., *12:*380, 1990.
149. Raviglione, M. C.: Extrapulmonary pneumocystosis: the first 50 cases. Rev. Infect. Dis., *12:*1127, 1990.
150. Northfelt, D. W., Clement, M. J., and Safrin, S. L.: Extrapulmonary pneumocystosis: clinical features in human immunodeficiency virus infection. Medicine, *69:*392, 1990.
151. Cohen, O. J., and Stoeckle, M. Y.: Extrapulmonary *Pneumocystis carinii* infections in the acquired immunodeficiency syndrome. Arch. Intern. Med., *151:*1205, 1991.
152. deSmet, M. D., and Nussenbatt, R. B.: Ocular manifestations of AIDS. JAMA, *266:*3019, 1991.
153. Jacobson, M. A. et al.: Retinal and gastrointestinal disease due to cytomegalovirus in patients with AIDS: prevalence and natural history, and response to ganciclovir therapy. Q. J. Med., *67:*473, 1988.
154. Palestine, A. G. et al.: A randomized, controlled trial of foscarnet in the treatment of cytomegalovirus retinitis in patients with AIDS. Ann. Intern. Med., *115:*665, 1991.
155. Sneed, S. R. et al.: *Pneumocystis carinii* choroiditis in patients receiving inhaled pentamidine. N. Engl. J. Med., *322:*936, 1990.
156. Lowder, C. Y. et al.: Microsporidia infection of the cornea in an HIV-positive man. Am. J. Ophthalmol., *109:*242, 1990.
157. Zalla, M. J., Su, W. P. D., and Fransway, A. F.: Dermatologic manifestations of human immunodeficiency virus infection. Mayo Clin. Proc., *67:*1089, 1992.
158. Kaplan, M. H. et al.: Dermatologic findings and manifestations of acquired immunodeficiency syndrome (AIDS). J. Am. Acad. Dermatol., *16:*485, 1987.
159. Erlich, K. S. et al.: Acyclovir-resistant herpes simplex virus infections in patients with the acquired immunodeficiency syndrome. N. Engl. J. Med., *320:*293, 1989.
160. Safrin, S. et al.: Foscarnet therapy in five patients with AIDS and acyclovir-resistant varicella-zoster infection. Ann. Intern. Med., *115:*19, 1991.
161. Buchness, M. H. et al.: Eosinophilic pustular folliculitis in the acquired immunodeficiency syndrome: treatment with ultraviolet B phototherapy. N. Engl. J. Med., *318:*1183, 1988.
162. Allen, M. A.: Primary care of women infected with the human immunodeficiency virus. Obstet. Gynecol. Clin. North Am., *17:*557, 1990.
163. Minkoff, H. L., and Dehovitz, J. A.: Care of women infected with the human immunodeficiency virus. JAMA, *266:*2253, 1991.
164. Carpenter, C. C. J. et al.: Human immunodeficiency virus infection in North American women: experience with 200 cases and a review of the literature. Medicine, *70:*307, 1991.
165. Rhoads, J. L. et al.: Chronic vaginal candidiasis in women with human immunodeficiency syndrome. JAMA, *257:*3105, 1987.
166. Hoegsberg, B. et al.: Sexually transmitted diseases and human immunodeficiency virus infection among women with pelvic inflammatory diseases. Am. J. Obstet. Gynecol., *163:*1135, 1990.
167. Safrin, S. et al.: Seroprevalence and epidemiologic correlates of human immunodeficiency virus infection in women with acute pelvic inflammatory disease. Obstet. Gynecol., *75:*666, 1990.
168. Centers for Disease Control: Risk for cervical disease in HIV-infected women-New York City. M.M.W.R., *39:*846, 1990.
169. Vermund, S. H. et al.: High risk of human papillomavirus infection and cervical squamous intraepithelial lesions among women with symptomatic human immunodeficiency virus infection. Am. J. Obstet. Gynecol., *165:*892, 1991.
170. Maiman, M. et al.: Colposcopic evaluation of human immunodeficiency virus-seropositive women. Obstet. Gynecol., *78:*84, 1991.
171. Sperling, R. S. et al.: A survey of zidovudine use in pregnant women with human immunodeficiency virus infection. N. Engl. J. Med., *326:*857, 1992.
172. Groopman, J. E.: Management of the hematologic complications of human immunodeficiency virus infection. Rev. Infect. Dis., *12:*931, 1990.
173. Donahue, R. E. et al.: Suppression of *in vitro* haematopoiesis following human immunodeficiency virus infection. Nature, *326:*200, 1987.
174. Spivak, J. L., Barnes, D. C. Fuchs, E., and Quinn, T. C.: Serum immunoreactive erythropoietin in HIV-infected patients. JAMA, *261:*3104, 1989.
175. Harriman, G. R. et al.: Vitamin B12 malabsorption in patients with acquired immunodeficiency syndrome. Arch. Intern. Med., *149:*2039, 1989.
176. Frickhofen, N. et al.: Persistent B19 parvovirus infection in patients infected with human immunodeficiency virus type I (HIV-1): a treatable cause of anemia in AIDS. Ann. Intern. Med., *113:*926, 1990.
177. Pollack, A. N., Janinis, J., and Green, D.: Successful intravenous immune globulin therapy for human immunodeficiency virus-associated thrombocytopenia. Arch. Intern. Med., *148:*695, 1988.
178. Karpatkin, S., Nardi, M. A., and Hymes, K. B.: Immunologic

thrombocytopenic purpura after heterosexual transmission of human immunodeficiency virus (HIV). Ann. Intern. Med., *109*:190, 1988.
179. Segal, G. H. et al.: Thrombotic thrombocytopenic purpura in a patient with AIDS. Cleve. Clin. J. Med., *57*:360, 1990.
180. Needleman, S. W., Sorace, J., and Poussin-Rosillo, H.: Low-dose splenic irradiation in the treatment of autoimmune thrombocytopenia in HIV-infected patients. Ann. Intern. Med., *116*:310, 1992.
181. Kin, H. C., Raska, K. Trooskin, S., and Saidi, P.: Immune thrombocytopenia in hemophiliacs infected with human immunodeficiency virus and their response to splenectomy. Arch. Intern. Med., *149*:1685, 1989.
182. Beral, V., Peterman, T. Z., Berkelman, R. L., and Jaffe, H. W.: Kaposi's sarcoma among persons with AIDS: a sexually transmitted infection? Lancet, *335*:123, 1990.
183. Miles, S. A. et al.: AIDS KS-derived cells produce and respond to IL-6. Proc. Natl. Acad. Sci., *87*:4068, 1990.
184. Miles, S. A.: Oncostatin M as potent mitogen for AIDS-KS-derived cells. Science, *255*:1432, 1992.
185. Chachoua, A. et al.: Prognostic factors and staging classification of patients with epidemic Kaposi's sarcoma. J. Clin. Oncol., *7*:774, 1989.
186. Levine, A. M.: Therapeutic approaches to neoplasms in AIDS. Rev. Infect. Dis., *12*:938, 1990.
187. Kovacs, J. A. et al.: Combined zidovudine and interferon-alpha therapy in patients with Kaposi's sarcoma and the acquired immunodeficiency syndrome (AIDS). Ann. Intern. Med., *111*:280, 1989.
188. Beral, V. et al.: AIDS-associated non-Hodgkins lymphoma. Lancet, *337*:805, 1991.
189. Rabkin, C. S. et al.: Incidence of lymphomas and other cancers in HIV-infected and HIV-uninfected patients with hemophilia. JAMA, *267*:1090, 1992.
190. Pluda, J. M. et al.: Development of non-Hodgkin's lymphoma in a cohort of patients with severe human immunodeficiency virus (HIV) infection on long-term antiretroviral therapy. Ann. Intern. Med., *113*:276, 1990.
191. Moore, R. D. et al.: Non-Hodgkin's lymphoma in patients with advanced HIV infection treated with zidovudine. JAMA, *265*:2208, 1991.
192. Baumgartner, J. E. et al.: Primary central nervous system lymphomas: natural history and response to radiation therapy in 55 patients with acquired immunodeficiency syndrome. J. Neurosurg., *73*:206, 1990.
193. Levine, A. M. et al.: Low-dose chemotherapy with central nervous system prophylaxis and zidovudine maintenance in AIDS-related lymphoma: a prospective multi-institutional trial. JAMA, *266*:84, 1991.
194. Palefsky, J. M. et al.: Anal intraepithelial neoplasia and anal papillomavirus infection among homosexual males with group IV HIV disease. JAMA, *263*:2911, 1990.
195. Grunfeld, C., and Feingold K. R.: Metabolic disturbances and wasting in the acquired immunodeficiency syndrome. N. Engl. J. Med., *327*:329, 1992.
196. Hommes, M. J. et al.: Increased resting energy balance in human immunodeficiency syndrome. Metabolism, *39*:1186, 1990.
197. Kotler, D. P. et al.: Body mass repletion during ganciclovir treatment of cytomegalovirus infections in patients with acquired immunodeficiency syndrome. Arch. Intern. Med., *149*:901, 1989.
198. Vitting, K. E. et al.: Frequency of hyponatremia and nonosmolar vasopressin release in the acquired immunodeficiency syndrome. JAMA, *263*:973, 1990.
199. Chattha, G., Arieff, A. I., Cumming, C., and Tierney, L. M.: Lactic acidosis complicating the acquired immunodeficiency syndrome. Ann. Intern. Med., *118*:37, 1993.
200. Dobs, A. S. et al.: Endocrine disorders in men infected with human immunodeficiency virus. Am. J. Med., *84*:611, 1988.
201. LoPresti, J., Gried, J. C., Spencer, C. A., and Nicoloff, J. T.: Unique alterations of thyroid hormone indices in the acquired immunodeficiency syndrome (AIDS). Ann. Intern. Med., *110*:970, 1989.
202. Milligan, S. A. et al.: Toxoplasmosis presenting as panhypopituitarism in a patient with the acquired immune deficiency syndrome. Am. J. Med., *77*:760, 1984.
203. McKenzie, R. et al.: The causes of death in patients with human immunodeficiency virus infection: a clinical and pathologic study with emphasis on the role of pulmonary diseases. Medicine, *70*:326, 1991.
204. Khosla, S., Wolfson, J. S., Demerjian, Z., and Godine, J. E.: Adrenal crisis in the setting of high-dose ketoconazole therapy. Arch. Intern. Med., *149*:802, 1989.
205. Lambertus, M. W. et al.: Diabetic ketoacidosis following pentamidine therapy in a patient with the acquired immunodeficiency syndrome. West. J. Med., *149*:602, 1988.
206. Glassock, R. J., Cohen, A. H., Danovitch, G., and Parsa, K. P.: Human immunodeficiency virus (HIV) infection and the kidney. Ann. Intern. Med., *112*:35, 1990.
207. Rao, T. K. S., Friedman, E. A., and Nicastri, A. D.: The types of renal disease in the acquired immunodeficiency syndrome. N. Engl. J. Med., *316*:1062, 1987.
208. Bourgoignie, J. J.: Renal complications of human immunodeficiency virus type 1. Kidney Int., *37*:1571, 1990.
209. Cantor, E. S., Kimmel, P. L., and Bosch, J. P.: Effect of race on expression of acquired immunodeficiency syndrome-associated nephropathy. Arch. Intern. Med., *151*:125, 1991.
210. Cozzi, P. J., Abu-Jawdeh, G. M., Green, R. M., and Green, D.: Amyloidosis in association with human immunodeficiency virus infection. Clin. Infect. Dis., *14*:189, 1992.
211. Acierno, L. J.: Cardiac complications in the acquired immunodeficiency syndrome (AIDS): a review. J. Am. Coll. Cardiol., *13*:1144, 1989.
212. Cohen, I. S. et al.: Congestive cardiomyopathy in association with the acquired immunodeficiency syndrome. N. Engl. J. Med., *315*:628, 1986.
213. Buskila, D., and Gladman, D.: Musculoskeletal manifestations of infection with human immunodeficiency virus. Rev. Infect. Dis., *12*:223, 1990.
214. Berman, A. et al.: Rheumatic manifestations of human immunodeficiency virus infection. Am. J. Med., *85*:59, 1988.
215. Kaye, B. R.: Rheumatologic manifestations of infection with human immunodeficiency virus (HIV). Ann. Intern. Med., *111*:158, 1989.
216. Wachter, R. M., Luce, J. M., and Hopewell, P. C.: Critical care of patients with AIDS. JAMA, *267*:541, 1992.
217. Wachter, R. M., Luce, J. M., Hearst, N., and Lo, B.: Decisions about resuscitation: inequities among patients with different diseases but similar prognoses. Ann. Intern. Med., *111*:525, 1989.
218. Wachter, R. M. et al.: Intensive care of patients with the acquired immunodeficiency syndrome: outcome and changing patterns of utilization. Am. Rev. Respir. Dis., *134*:891, 1986.
219. Kovacs, J. A., and Masur, H.: *Pneumocystis carinii* pneumonia: therapy and prophylaxis. J. Infect. Dis., *158*:254, 1988.
220. Rogers, P. L., et al.: Admission of AIDS patients to a medical intensive care unit: causes and outcome. Crit. Care Med., *17*:113, 1989.
221. Wachter, R. A. et al.: *Pneumocystis carinii* pneumonia and respiratory failure in AIDS: improved outcomes and in-

creased use of intensive care units. Am. Rev. Respir. Dis., *143*:251, 1991.
222. Friedman, Y., Franklin, C., Freels, S., and Weil, M. H.: Long-term survival of patients with AIDS, *Pneumocystis carinii* pneumonia, and respiratory failure. JAMA, *266*:89, 1991.
223. Efferen, L. S., Nadarajah, D., and Palat, D. S.: Survival following mechanical ventilation for *Pneumocystis carinii* pneumonia in patients with the acquired immunodeficiency syndrome: a different perspective. Am. J. Med., *87*:401, 1989.
224. El-Sadr, W., and Simberkoff, M. S.: Survival and prognostic factors in severe *Pneumocystis carinii* pneumonia requiring mechanical ventilation. Am. Rev. Respir. Dis., *137*:1264, 1988.
225. Friedman, Y., Franklin, C., Rackou, E. C., and Weil, M. H.: Improved survival in patients with AIDS, *Pneumocystis carinii* pneumonia, and severe respiratory failure. Chest, *96*:862, 1989.
226. Harris J. E.: Improved short-term survival of AIDS patients initially diagnosed with *Pneumocystis carinii* pneumonia, 1984 through 1987. JAMA, *263*:397, 1990.
227. Lemp, G. F. et al.: Survival trends for patients with AIDS. JAMA, *263*:402, 1990.
228. Bozzette, S. A. et al.: Impact of *Pneumocystis carinii* and cytomegalovirus on the course and outcome of atypical pneumonia in advanced human immunodeficiency virus disease. J. Infect. Dis., *165*:93, 1992.
229. Rosen, M. J., Cucco, R. A., and Tierstein, A. S.: Outcome of intensive care in patients with the acquired immunodeficiency syndrome. J. Intensive Care Med., *1*:55, 1986.
230. Schein, R. M., Fischl, M. A., Pitchenick, A. E., and Sprung, C. L.: ICU survival of patients with the acquired immunodeficiency syndrome. Crit. Care Med., *14*:1026, 1986.
231. Raviglione, M. C., Battan, R., and Taranta, A.: Cardiopulmonary resuscitation in patients with the acquired immunodeficiency syndrome: a prospective study. Arch. Intern. Med., *148*:2602, 1988.
232. Steinbrook, R. et al.: Preferences of homosexual men with AIDS for life-sustaining treatment. N. Engl. J. Med., *314*:457, 1986.
233. Steinbrook, R. et al.: Ethical dilemmas in caring for patients with the acquired immunodeficiency syndrome. Ann Intern. Med., *103*:787, 1985.
234. Mangione, C. M., and Lo, B.: Beyond fear. Resolving ethical dilemmas regarding HIV infection. Chest, *95*:1100, 1989.
235. Haas, J. et al.: Discussion of preferences for life-sustaining care by persons with AIDS: predictors of failure in patient-physician communication. Arch. Intern. Med., *153*:1241, 1993.
236. Berbert, B. et al.: Why fear persists: health care professionals and AIDS. JAMA, *260*:3481, 1988.
237. Gerberding, J. L., and Henderson, D. K.: Design of rational infection control policies for human immunodeficiency virus infection. J. Infect. Dis., *156*:861, 1987.
238. Lynch, P., Jackson, M. M., Cummings, M. J., and Stamm, W. E.: Rethinking the role of isolation practices in the prevention of nosocomial infections. Ann. Intern. Med., *107*:243, 1987.
239. Centers for Disease Control: Guidelines for prevention of transmission of human immunodeficiency virus and hepatitis B virus to health-care and public-safety workers. M.M.W.R., *38(S-6)*:1, 1989.
240. Centers for Disease Control: Recommendations for preventing transmission of human immunodeficiency virus and hepatitis B virus to patients during exposure-prone invasive procedures. M.M.W.R., *40(RR-8)*:1, 1991.
241. Kristensen, M. S., Wernberg, N. M., and Anker-Møller, E.: Healthcare workers' risk of contact with body fluids in a hospital: the effect of complying with the universal precautions policy. Infect. Control Hosp. Epidemiol., *13*:719, 1992.
242. Centers for Disease Control: Public health service statement on management of occupational exposure to human immunodeficiency virus, including considerations regarding zidovudine postexposure use. M.M.W.R., *39(RR-1)*:1, 1990.
243. Tokars, J. I. et al.: Surveillance of HIV infection and zidovudine use among health care workers after occupational exposure to HIV-infected blood. Ann. Intern. Med., *118*:913, 1993.
244. Centers for Disease Control: Guidelines for preventing the transmission of tuberculosis in health-care settings, with special focus on HIV-related issues. M.M.W.R., *39(RR-17)*:1, 1990.
245. Centers for Disease Control: Management of persons exposed to multidrug-resistant tuberculosis. M.M.W.R., *41(RR-11)*:61, 1992.
246. Glatt, A. E., Risbrook, A. T., and Jenna, R. W.: Successful implementation of a long-term care unit for patients with acquired immunodeficiency syndrome in an underserved suburban area with a high incidence of human immunodeficiency virus. Arch. Intern. Med., *152*:823, 1992.

Chapter 69

SUBSTANCE ABUSE AND OVERDOSE

JAMES DOUGHERTY
DARELL HEISELMAN

Drugs of abuse include a substance or chemical used to alter an individual's mood, sense of well-being or psychologic conception of his relation to the environment. Sometimes there is a fine line between where therapeutic use ends and abuse begins. Thus, the definition of drug or substance abuse varies but is generally defined as the use of a chemical for a desired pharmacologic effect in an inappropriate way.

HISTORY

Opioids, alcohol, and various hallucinogens have been used by humans for thousands of years to cope with enemies, anxiety, and frustration. Opium usage has been traced to the Sumerians and Egyptians over 5000 years ago. Alcohol has been used in various religious activities or in preparation for warfare, and hallucinogens have had a basic role in religious ceremonies of the South, Central, and North American Indians in the form of hallucinogenic mushrooms and peyote traced back for at least 1000 years. Drug abuse is now one of the major health problems in the United States and is implicated in many deaths, both directly from overdose and indirectly as result of injury or medical complications sustained while the individual is intoxicated.[1]

Until the nineteenth century, drugs came from unrefined plants or animal products. The usual method of administration was oral ingestion, and overdose was rare due to the low concentration of biologically active ingredients. As long ago as 1000 AD, distillation techniques were applied to fermented beverages to make the end product more potent. In the mid-1800s, morphine was isolated from opium, and in the early 1900s, cocaine was isolated from the coca leaf, and heroin was synthesized from morphine. Abuse of these purified products, which resulted in states of marked euphoria and hyperstimulation, soon followed. In the mid-1950s, the synthesis of pharmaceuticals from organic chemicals was taken one step further, and psychoactive drugs were introduced and abused.

By the late 1960s and 1970s, amphetamines and barbiturates were becoming increasingly abused, and restrictions were placed to tightly control these products. Clandestine laboratories appeared to meet the demand as pharmaceuticals became harder to obtain. In 1979 illicit drug synthesis was elevated to a new level of sophistication with the production of a new drug that was a close relative of fentanyl (Sublimaze), alpha methylfentanyl. This drug was marketed as "China White."[2]

THE SCOPE OF SUBSTANCE ABUSE AND OVERDOSE

Clearly, all sections of the community are involved in drugs of abuse. In previous years drug-related deaths increased significantly as hospitals from coast to coast were swamped with such cases, according to the latest federal government report on drug trends. *Epidemiologic Trends in Drug Abuse,* a report by the National Institute of Drug Abuse, monitors drug-related deaths, nonfatal emergencies, arrests, treatment admissions, crime, and disease in 20 metropolitan areas as part of an ongoing survey of national drug use patterns.[3]

Cocaine was the drug most frequently cited as the cause of death in nearly every major metropolitan area in the study. The most dramatic increases in emergency department admissions were seen in Philadelphia and Washington, D.C., with an 83 and 64% rise, respectively, during 1987. New York City had an estimated 690,000 substance abusers in 1988 (up 86% from 1979) and experienced a 25% jump in cocaine deaths, three quarters of whom were men. Almost half of the deaths involved a combination of cocaine and heroin.[3] As many as 38% of all hospital emergency department visits in New York City in 1987 were related to cocaine abuse.[2]

An estimated 28 million Americans used illicit drugs in 1988. Greater than 21 million Americans admitted to trying cocaine once, and almost one half used drugs in the previous calendar year according to the National Institute on Drug Abuse. Approximately 3.5 million users were in the 18- to 35-year-old age group. Studies further suggest that approximately 50% of high school seniors have tried cocaine, 7% use it daily, and 40% of seniors admit to trying another drug, usually amphetamine.[2]

The Centers for Disease Control and Prevention (CDC) reported on trends in mortality that were due to unintentional poisoning between 1980 and 1986.[4] Misuse of drugs, primarily opiates and related narcotics and cocaine, was responsible for a substantial increase in such deaths among young men during the 7-year period, according to the report. Deaths that were due to unintentional poisoning increased from 1.9 to 2.3/100,000 population during that time. This trend can be explained by a 49% increase in deaths from drug poisoning, including drugs used for medical and nonmedical purposes. Opiates and related narcotics and local anesthetics including cocaine were the leading causes of fatal unintentional drug poisoning.

The mortality rate of poisoning in males remained more than twice that for females during 1980 to 1986, and the rates for blacks for both sexes were constantly higher than those for whites. In 1986 the rate for black males was 5.4 deaths per 100,000 population, and for white males, 3.2 deaths per 100,000. The highest mortality rates of poisoning for both blacks and whites were among young adult men, 20 to 39 years of age. Men in this group accounted for 40% of all unintentional poisoning deaths and 46% of all unintentional drug poisoning deaths during 1980 to 1986.

In comparison to the entire spectrum of substance abuse, Dans et al. reported that the prevalence of diagnoses consistent with drug abuse or dependence rose in-hospital from 0.6 to 3.5% from 1983 to 1988.[5] The National Institute on Drug Abuse (NIDA) reported increases in morbidity and mortality associated with nonmedical use of both heroin-morphine and cocaine during 1985 to 1987. Through its Drug Abuse Warning Network (DAWN), NIDA monitors emergency departments and medical examiner's offices in selective locations for drug-related emergency visits and deaths. In 1987 cocaine was the most frequently reported drug involved in more than one third of the deaths reported to DAWN. According to DAWN during the year 1987, persons 20 to 39 years of age accounted for 70% of all drug abuse emergency visits and 65% of all drug abuse deaths.

In 176 suspected drug overdose cases presenting to an emergency department, Mahoney and colleagues found nearly 70% of drug detections and 80% of admissions were related to six classes of drugs: ethanol, benzodiazepines, salicylates, acetaminophen, barbiturates, and tricyclic antidepressants.[6]

Clearly, if one excludes alcohol as an abused "drug," the most abused drugs fall into major classes such as stimulants, narcotics, sedative-hypnotics, and hallucinogens. Marijuana was identified in a number of deaths in Atlanta and San Diego, but this drug is primarily used in combination with other drugs. Marijuana ranked second in emergency department visits in six cities and third in five others. Emergency departments in Miami, Philadelphia, Seattle, San Francisco, and Washington, D.C., reported increases in cases involving marijuana use of more than 70%, and it was frequently cited as a secondary drug problem among treatment admissions in other cities for the years 1985 to 1987.

In contrast to Chapter 70, this chapter focuses on the medical evaluation of those drug reactions that occur from the **intentional** use of mind-altering chemicals for the pleasurable side affects associated with these drugs, not for the intentional overdose or suicide attempt. The abused substances discussed in this chapter are the following drug classes:

- Opiates
- Sedative-hypnotics
- Alcohol
- Central nervous system (CNS) stimulants
- Hallucinogens
- Cannabis
- Volatile inhalants

GENERAL CONSIDERATIONS IN THE SUBSTANCE ABUSER: PRE-ICU PHASE

The earliest clues that one may be dealing with a problem of substance abuse may be the clinical findings related to the route of administration of the abused substance. Behavior patterns and "red flags" in the patient's history provide additional clues, prompting the clinician to seek additional help from the toxicology laboratory. Although the latter provides some diagnostic benefit, the clinician should also be aware that certain "cutting substances" can produce similar CNS and cardiovascular disruptions, mimicking those of the abused substances. Beyond toxicity, the manifestations may be those of withdrawal or overwhelming infection. Under all circumstances, the general principles of management are aimed at the stabilization of the CNS and respiratory and cardiovascular systems.

Routes of Administration

Only the imagination and the resourcefulness of the user limit how an abused drug can be consumed. A drug of abuse can be administered by any means, including orally, by insufflation ("snorting"), smoking or injected subcutaneously ("skin popping"), intramuscularly, or intravenously ("mainlining"). Administration into the web spaces of the fingers and toes, into the sublingual area, as well as by the dangerous internal jugular or subclavian route has been attempted. This last is referred to as the "pocket shot" and is an attempt to obtain venous access by injecting into one of the large veins in the neck. Because of the proximity of the apical pleura to the internal jugular vein, this approach frequently causes a pneumothorax. In nearly every case, the lure of the drug "high" supersedes common sense in dangerous situations of drug administration.

Drugs that are taken intravenously are usually heated in a spoon or bottle cap, drawn into a syringe or eye dropper through cotton or other homemade filters to remove large impurities, and then injected within the skin. Frequently, the same syringe is used by several persons, substantially increasing the risk for communicable diseases such as hepatitis, AIDS, or tetanus.

Generally, the route of administration depends on the pharmacology of the substance being consumed, the circumstances surrounding consumption, and the desire for the degree of intensity of the euphoria obtained with many of these substances. Although the easiest, the oral route involves the longest time from consumption until pleasurable symptoms, hence the intensity of these symptoms may not be satisfactory for many abusers. In addition, many of the abused chemicals are rapidly neutralized when consumed orally, negating the reason for consuming them in the first place. Oral administration, however, does not offer the "stigma" of intravenous (IV) drug injection to "soft core" users.

Injecting intravenously is the most rapid form of delivering a drug to the body and hence is preferred by many "hard-core" abusers for the intensity (albeit short-lived) of the drug response. Chemicals such as crack cocaine that are heat stable can be consumed by smoking. This is a rapid form of consumption rivaling IV use without the stigmata, problems with vascular access, or procurement of specialized equipment such as needles and syringes.[1]

If a chemical can be absorbed across membranes, the nose, rectum, or vagina offer convenient portals of entry to the systemic system. Although not offering the quick "rush" of the IV or pulmonary routes, they offer more prolonged absorption, hence duration of action, as well as relatively anonymity of consumption.[1,2]

Diagnosing Substance Abuse (The "High Risk" Patient)

The Diagnostic and Statistical Manual for Mental Disorders (DSM-III) defines two major criteria for substance abuse.[2a] First is a pattern of pathologic use. For barbiturates or similar-acting sedatives, this is characterized as the inability to reduce or discontinue use, intoxication throughout the day, frequent use of the equivalent of 600 mg of secobarbital or 60 mg of diazepam, or amnesic periods for events that occurred during intoxication. In the case of opiates, the pattern consists of the inability to stop or reduce use, intoxication throughout the day, use nearly every day, or episodes of overdose. The second major criteria for substance abuse is the impairment of social or occupational functioning. This is characterized by fights, loss of friends, family disintegration, absence from work, loss of a job, or legal difficulties. The disorder should be present for at least a month.

Drug abuse is more common among the affluent and the poor than in middle income groups, according to a survey conducted by the Media Advertising partnership for a Drug-Free America. In a survey of 4737 adults, they found that 20% consider cocaine use a status symbol, 11% feel that occasional use of cocaine is not risky, 29% think that cigarettes are worse than marijuana, and 26% think it is O.K. to smoke marijuana in private. They also found that women today are nearly identical to men in their use of marijuana and cocaine. Blacks and Hispanics are more likely to be drug abusers than the general public. About 30% of these adults aged 18 to 35 years have used cocaine at least once. About 70% of those aged 26 to 30 years have tried marijuana at least once.[7]

Although not specific for the substance abusers, some key features will help alert the astute clinician to the possibility of substance abuse. The examining physician should always keep in mind that many times the history can be elicited only by asking specifically about frequently abused drugs, quantity taken, and how consumed. Patients often will not voluntarily admit the history of substance abuse to the examining physician. Indeed, the consuming patient may not even be aware that they are abusing drugs. Some signs and symptoms that should alert one to the possibility of substance abuse are found in Table 69-1.

Once the diagnosis is suspected, key features of the substance abuse history help to define the function and the substance abused. The recent pattern of use should be obtained, including the dose and usual pattern of pill taking. Prescription drug users tend to underestimate their use, either out of shame, fear of rejection, or unawareness as a result of intoxication. Therefore, it is useful to try to obtain pill counts for the preceding week. The presence of tolerance can be assessed by a pattern of escalating doses;

Table 69-1. Clues to Identifying the Drug Abuser

Poorly kept, disheveled appearance
Abnormal mental status, particularily agitated
Highly manipulative activity
Rapid mood shifts
Drug equipment found by family, police, or emergency medical service personnel
Evasive or inconsistent answers
Chronic lack of money
Needle marks, multiple tattoos, nasal septal perforation, skin "pop"
Frequent job firings or changes
Marital or family instability
Beeper without obvious explanation
Excessive jewelry inconsistent with job status

dependence is evident by the existence of withdrawal symptoms. Indirect evidence of dependence can be seen by a pattern of regular dosing approximately equal to the half-life of the drug. A full history of other substances used should be obtained including alcohol, nicotine, caffeine, marijuana, stimulants, sedatives, hypnotics, tranquilizers, inhalants, opiates, and hallucinogens to identify possible problems of concurrent or sequential addictions. Included is the common use of sedatives to counter the effects of excess caffeine or stimulant use.[7,8] Inquiries about a history of overdose should also be obtained.

The Toxicology Laboratory in Substance Abuse

The time required for drug analysis is often longer than the critical course of an overdose, relegating the toxicology laboratory to a useful adjunct in the management of substance abusers. Clinical indicators of toxicity are almost always more useful than absolute drug concentrations with the abused drugs. A negative toxicology screen in the setting of clinical abnormalities suggesting drug ingestion should be ignored, and the clinical abnormalities treated.

Several techniques are available for drug screening.[2,6,9-11] Chemical spot tests provide quick screening for certain drugs. This is ideal for emergency department and ICU use where high drug concentrations, ease of application, and quick turnaround time make it an ideal test. Spectrometric assays were commonly used 10 years ago but were prone to interference and have been partially supplanted by immunoassays (often used as initial "screen" for drugs then confirmed by a second method) and chromatographic assays, now widely used in emergency toxicology because many drugs can be detected in a single screen.

Urine is the best sample for finding the greatest number of drugs in easily detectable quantities. Adding a blood sample to a urine specimen produces a slightly greater overall yield of positive results. Most laboratories will not report a positive drug identification unless it is present on two procedures or unless the single method used is known to be highly specific for a highly prevalent intoxicant such as ethanol by gas chromatography.

Of the 1.3 million reported cases of accidental or suicidal chemical ingestions annually causing 545 fatalities, drug ingestion accounted for 91% of these deaths. The drug categories most commonly implicated were antidepressants, analgesics (non-narcotics and narcotics), stimulants, sedative-hypnotics, cardiovascular drugs, and alcohol.[2] Although all of these drug classes are detected by commonly used comprehensive toxicology screens, it is vitally important to know what kind of drugs the laboratory is testing for. Certain commonly abused drugs such as lysergic acid diethylamide (LSD) and fentanyl cannot be identified on routine toxicology screening.

Several studies have looked at the impact of drug screening in the emergency department setting. Kellerman and associates[11] performed a prospective study and found that the diagnostic certainty of an ingestion was only increased by a mean value of 16.5% after results of a toxicology screen were obtained. Mahoney et al.[6] performed a retrospective study of 176 suspected drug overdose cases presenting to an emergency department. Qualitative serum toxicology samples were obtained in 93% of patients, and the serum screening was positive in 81% of samples. Nearly 70% of drug detections and 80% of admissions were related to six classes of drugs: ethanol, benzodiazepines, salicylates, acetaminophen, barbiturates and tricyclic antidepressants (TCAs). In only 12% of the cases were drugs found on the test that were not suspected on the basis of the history, none at toxic levels. In only 1% of the cases drug-specific treatment was initiated on the basis of the serum screen, and in 2% it was discontinued. Mahoney and co-workers[6] concluded that serum screening had no impact on treatment in 90% of cases and was responsible for medical admission or prolonged emergency department observation in only 4% of cases.

Fifty to seventy percent of toxicology screens are positive.[2] The reliability of any test is affected by prevalence of the drug or the prior probability of the test condition. Because of this observation as well as the clinical observations of Kellerman et al.[11] and Mahoney et al.,[6] the "rule-in" value of a drug screen is more valuable than its use to "rule out" a diagnosis. For this very reason, a positive drug screen may be useful in confirming a history or clinically based suspicions of a certain type of overdose or ingestion, but a negative drug screen proves nothing, particularly in the setting of a compatible toxic "syndrome."[2,6,12]

Problems Common to Substances Abusers

Septic arthritis and osteomyelitis are the third most common complications of nonalcoholic substance abuse, following hepatitis B viral infection and endocarditis.[2] Substance abusers offer the physician a plethora of potential complications related to the technical and biochemical side effects of their consumed drugs.[12-17] Dans et al. found that 42% of drug abusers in a hospital setting were positive for human immunodeficiency virus (HIV), with 7% having acquired immune deficiency syndrome (AIDS).[5] As a group, IV drug users represent the most rapidly growing source of new AIDS cases.[2] HIV-1 is believed to have been introduced into the parenteral drug-using population in the 1970s.[2] Parenteral drug users are the second largest risk group to develop AIDS in the United States. As of January 2, 1989, 22,025 cases of AIDS among IV drug users were reported to the CDC, 27% of all adult cases. Of these, IV drug use was the only risk factor for 63%. Forty-five percent of all new AIDS cases in New York City are related to IV drugs. Nationally, 17% of men and 52% of women recently diagnosed with AIDS will have IV drug use as their only identifiable risk factor.[2] Additional problems common to substance abusers can be found in Tables 69-2 and 69-3.

Table 69-2. Problems Common to Substance Abusers

Organ System	Pathologic State
Infectious	AIDS, hepatitis, tetanus, botulism, skin abscess, cellulitis, bacterial and viral infections, septic arthritis and osteomyelitis
Cardiovascular	Endocarditis, myocarditis, myocardial infarction, arrhythmia, aneurysm, sudden death
Central nervous system	Seizures, cerebral abscess, cerebrovascular accident
Pulmonary	Pulmonary hypertension, pulmonary fibrosis, pneumonia, pulmonary emboli, pneumothorax bullous emphysema
Psychiatric	Paranoia, psychosis, anxiety, depression, flashbacks, suicidal ideation
Trauma	Multisystem, isolated

Cutting Substances

Street drugs are impure substances. A dose may contain only 5 to 20% of the desired substance and 80 to 90% "cutting" substances, many of which have significant biochemical actions of their own. The use of cutting substances increases the dealer's profit but also increases the users' risk. Drugs obtained on the street are always mixed with "cutting" substances in ratios of 20:1 to 100:1, and it may be those substances that cause adverse reactions. Many agents are used as cutting substances, although caffeine, ephedrine, lidocaine, and procaine account for 80% of substitute compounds found.[1,2]

Local anesthetics may be added to simulate the expected anesthetic effect of cocaine. Procaine is by far the most common local anesthetic cutting agent followed by lidocaine, benzocaine, and tetracaine. Procaine is also the least toxic; lidocaine is about two to three times more toxic than procaine. Lidocaine is the most common adulterant (52%) in cocaine samples.[1,2]

Quinine is a bitter-tasting white powder that was first used as a heroin adulterant during an epidemic of malaria in New York City in the early 1940s. Its use has continued, and for many drug dealers it is the preferred adulterant for two reasons: (1) Its bitter taste prevents the buyer from testing the heroin content by tasting for bitterness, and (2) when injected IV, quinine produces a flush mimicking the effect of IV heroin. As much as 59 to 188 times the currently recommended safe dose for humans may be unknowingly consumed in adulterated samples. Quinine has gastrointestinal, auditory, neurologic, ophthalmic, and renal toxic effects, which alone may cause major clinical side effects and mortality.

In addition to quinine, other cutting substances include sugars, local anesthetic, baking soda, starch, stimulants (including caffeine), CNS depressants (including barbiturates), powdered milk, and easily obtainable narcotic-like substances such as propoxphene. Phencyclidine has also

Table 69-3. Complications of Drugs of Abuse

Class of Drug	Complication
CNS Stimulants	
Cocaine	Acute MI, sudden death, cardiac arrhythmias, seizures
Amphetamines	Cardiac arrhythmias, hypertensive crisis, seizures, acute renal failure from rhabdomyolysis
Look-alikes	Severe hypertension, intracranial hemorrhage, chest pain, MI, renal failure
Caffeine	Diuresis with fluid loss, hypokalemia, hyperglycemia, leukocytosis, metabolic acidosis
CNS Depressants	
Ethanol	DTs, seizures, GI bleeding, depression, trauma
Barbiturates	CNS depression with shock, coma, death mimics ethanol intoxication
Nonbarbiturates	All can cause CNS depression with hypotension
Nonbenzodiazepines	Chloral hydrate: arrhythmias, GI bleeding; Glutethimide: fluctuating LOC; Methaqualone: paradoxic CNS excitation; blisters; Ethchlorvynol: noncardiac pulmonary edema
Benzodiazepines	CNS depression
Opiates	CNS and respiratory depression with respiratory arrest. Noncardiac pulmonary edema; Meperidine: mydriasis; Propoxyphene: lethal cardiac arrhythmias
Hallucinogens	Flashbacks, terror, "bad trips"; Mydriasis, hyperthermia, altered mental status; Seizures, coma, tachycardia, hypertension; PCP: rhabdomyolysis
Volatile Inhalants	Conjunctival injection, hypersalivation, altered mental status, paranoia, GI complaints, cyanosis, weakness, euphoria, visual, auditory hallucinations, respiratory depression, seizures, sudden death
Cannabis	Symptoms usually mild, peripheral vasodilatation, mild pulmonary mucous irritation, euphoria, relaxation, mood alteration, increased sensory awareness, possible psychosis, black-outs

CNS, central nervous system; DT, delerium tremens; GI, gastrointestinal; LOC, level of consciousness; MI, myocardial infarction; PCP, phenocyclidine.

Table 69-4. Different Cutting Substances

Classes of Adulterants	Signs and Symptoms: Comment
Stimulants	
Ephedrine	Hypertension, tachycardia, seizures
Pseudoephedrine	Euphoria, tremor, irritability
Phenylpropanolamine	Hyperreflexia, insomnia, psychosis
Caffeine	Most toxic of group: PACs, PVCs
Local anesthetics	
Procaine	Procaine least toxic
Lidocaine	Lidocaine two to three times more toxic than procaine
Benzocaine	Side effects: rapid cardiac conduction
Tetracaine	Defects, arrhythmias, hypotension, cardiac arrest, central nervous system stimulation
Toxins	
Quinine and quinidine	Can produce "cinchonism:" tinnitus, headaches, visual disturbances, vertigo, nausea, vomiting, diarrhea
Arsenic	Intracellular toxin, symmetric polyneuropathy
Thallium	Colorless, odorless, tasteless, gastrointestinal tract toxicity
Stychnine	Used as cocaine adulterant; central nervous system stimulation
Hallucinogens	
Phencyclidine	One of most commonly used pharmacologically active adulterants
Others: LSD, mescaline psilocybin, MDMA (methamphetamine derivatives and MDA	Used to alter cognitive and perceptual states
Sugars	
Lactose, mannitol, dextrose inositol, sucrose	Widely available, found in cocaine and heroin samples; irritates mucous membranes
Inert compounds	
Microcrystalline cellulose	Gangrene from inadvertent arterial injection
Talc	Very common in cocaine and heroin; chronic pulmonary hypertension
Starches	Foreign body granuloma
Cotton fibers	"Cotton fever" syndrome: myalgias, fever, abdominal cramps
Miscellaneous	
Calcium and sodium salts	Used in herioin, cocaine, and LSD
Ascorbic acid	Increases bulk and sale price
Saccharin	Increases bulk and sale price
Powdered milk	"Street remedy" for opiate overdose

been used. The sugars lactose, sucrose, and inositol (an isomer of glucose) may be added as adulterants because they act as fillers and add weight. In addition to all these substances, the mixture may be contaminated with bacteria, fungi, or viruses.[1] Table 69-4 shows the large number of adulterants found in today's abused drugs.

General Treatment Principles

Drug users may have multiple complaints referable to many systems because they frequently abuse more than one substance and often adjust to large proportions of unknown diluents that are added to the abused drug without the observance of proper sterile precautions. Usually, only the most severe and dramatic complications of drug use are seen in the emergency department, and even fewer still in the ICU. They may consist of toxic, physiologic, psychologic, and behavioral manifestations such as life-threatening reactions resulting from intentional and unintentional overdose and abstinence syndromes of varying intensity.

As a general rule, only life-threatening manifestations of substance abuse need be treated emergently with CNS and cardiovascular manifestations such as seizures and arrhythmias taking precedence in treatment algorithms. Oral consumption of a drug offers the possibility of drug emptying and neutralization with gastric lavage followed by activated charcoal. Ipecac has fallen into disfavor because many of the abused drugs can cause seizures. With ipecac, aspiration can occur during a seizure that follows administration of ipecac. Other forms of drug administration by nasal, IV, or subcutaneous routes preclude these techniques. Hypotension frequently responds to IV crystalloids. Vasopressors are usually not required. Airway integrity must take precedence in any treatment schema. If there is any question of airway compromise such as hypoventilation, diminished or absent gag reflex, or excessive upper airway secretions, rapid endotracheal intubation should be performed. If orogastric lavage is contemplated in any of these settings, intubation is especially indicated.

Very few drugs of abuse have true "antidotes," so treatment revolves around the following:

- Preventing continued drug effects by gastric emptying and gastrointestinal neutralization
- Identifying potentially dangerous drugs with long half-lives that can cause delayed symptoms if missed
- Treating life-threatening complications (usually CNS or cardiovascular)
- Identifying associated disorders that are not immediately life-threatening but can cause major morbidity

Many patients who are the victims of substance abuse present to the emergency department or have side effects or major sequelae that result in a prehospital medical response. Valuable information can be obtained from the emergency medical service (EMS) squad. The EMS team is uniquely situated to obtain visual evidence of drug abuse when in the patient's home or place of illness. This includes evidence of multiple pill bottles, obvious drugs or drug paraphernalia, or other individuals using drugs at the same location. Simple "debriefing" of the paramedics when they arrive in the emergency department with the patient is usually sufficient to obtain this valuable information.

Additional History

Young men account for the highest percentage group abusing drugs. Therefore, any man in the 20- to 39-year-old category who presents usually at night, on a weekend, or on a holiday with vague complaints not easily confirmed by phone conversation with the patient's attending physician or examination (i.e., cancer in an out-of-state patient, "kidney stone" pain in a patient with dye allergy) and requesting narcotic or mood-altering drugs should be viewed with suspicion. Trusting one's "sixth sense" regarding a suspicious story is usually more often right than wrong. In addition, any young or middle-aged individual presenting with altered CNS findings without an obvious cause should be suspected of abusing drugs. Additional history valuable in identifying the drug abuser includes the following:

- Multiple emergency department (ED) visits for the same problem
- A history of multiple drug allergies to "safe" medications such as nonsteroidal anti-inflammatory drugs (NSAIDs) or acetaminophen
- A previous admission confirming illicit drug usage

Vital Signs

Careful attention to the evaluation of abnormal vital signs in the suspected drug user can give a surprising amount of information regarding the identification of the suspected drug.[18] The pulse rate is the net result of a balance between adrenergic and cholinergic tone. It follows that any drug that alters any of these parameters will change pulse rate alone illustrating that no single indicator alone can establish a toxicologic diagnosis.

Temperature is frequently overlooked in the evaluation of these patients. An accurate core temperature is an essential requirement to assist diagnosis. The respiratory vital signs should be evaluated not only for rate, because some abused drugs cause an early decrease in tidal volume, then followed by bradypnea. Therefore, the rate, pattern, and depth of respirations should all be recorded and evaluated serially. Table 69–5 shows some of the more common vital sign abnormalities in abused drugs.[18]

Reflex Diagnostics and Therapeutics

When drug abuse is suspected, certain diagnostic and therapeutic decisions can become nearly "automatic." If there is any abnormality of the initial vital signs, an IV of D5W to keep the vein open (kvo), oxygen by nasal cannula, and cardiac monitor should be placed on the patient until a more thorough evaluation of the patient can be conducted. If the patient shows sign of respiratory embarrassment such as stridor, cyanosis, tachypnea, accessory muscle use, excessive upper airway secretions or bradypnea, endotracheal intubation should be carried out immediately. A good rule is to view the "ET" like "LP." That is, if you think about doing it, you should do it. It is better to remove a tube after the airway has been cleared than to delay intubation and deal with the irreversible consequences of hypoxia. An absent gag reflex in an obtunded patient or in a patient requiring a gastric lavage is another indication for intubation.

The only rationale for a short delay in intubation is to administer 2 mg of naloxone IV. In the patient with opiate overdose, this may be sufficient to reverse respiratory depression and obviate the need for intubation. Any patient with an overdose and diminished CNS or respiratory status should receive a trial of naloxone.

A bedside finger-stick glucose should be performed in any patient with decreased level of consciousness, and 50 ml of 50% dextrose should be administered for a reading less than 100 mg%. Thiamine, 100 mg IV or intramuscularly (IM) should be given in any alcohol-consuming patient.

For hypotension not arrhythmia generated, a cautious trial of miniboluses of IV crystalloid is indicated. Careful attention for the presence or development of noncardiogenic pulmonary edema, especially in suspected opiate and CNS-depressant ingestors, is warranted.

Any patient with altered CNS status not readily explained by other means should be considered to be drug-intoxicated, and gastric emptying procedures should be instituted. A large-bore orogastric or nasogastric tube should be inserted. Our protocol is to immediately administer 50 to 100 g of activated charcoal, wait 10 minutes for drug absorption, and then remove by suction. A contin-

Table 69–5. Abnormal Vital Signs in Drug Ingestions

Blood Pressure Changes

Hypertension	Hypotension
Amphetamines	Antipsychotics
Cocaine	Ethanol
Nicotine	Opioids
PCP	Sedative-hypnotic
Sympathomimetics	Thiamine depletion
TCAs	TCAs

Respiratory Rate Changes

Tachypnea	Bradypnea
Amphetamine	Anesthetics
CO (early)	CO
Clonidine	Clonidine
CNS stimulants	Cyanide
Cocaine	Ethanol
Ethanol	Opioids
Ethylene glycol	Sedative-hypnotics
Salicylates	
Theophylline	
Withdrawal	

Temperature Changes

Hyperthermia	Hypothermia
Amphetamines	Antipsychotic
Anticholinergics	Ethanol
Antihistamines	Hypoglycemia
Cocaine	Opioids
Alcohol withdrawal	Sedative-hypnotics
LSD	Thiamine depletion
PCP	
Salicylates	
Sympathomimetics	
TCAs	

Pulse Changes

Tachycardia	Bradycardia
Amphetamines	Beta-blockers
Anticholinergics	Calcium channel blockers
Antihistamines	Clonidine
Atropine	Digoxin
Caffeine	Gasoline
CO (early)	Mushrooms
Cocaine	Opioids
Cyanide	Organophosphates
Ethanol	Sedative-hypnotics
Hypoglycemia	
Nicotine	
Salicylates	
Sympathomimetics	
TCAs	
Withdrawal	

CNS, central nervous system; CO, carbon monoxide; LSD, lysergic acid diethylamide; PCP, phencyclidine; TCA, tricyclic antidepressant.

---

uous irrigation with fluid is then performed. A minimum of 3 L is used. The type and sterility of the fluid is not as important as the manner, timing, and quantity of delivery. If the aspirate remains cloudy or particulate, continued irrigation is performed until clear. Once clear, 50 to 100 g of activated charcoal with sorbitol is placed in the stomach, and the tube is clamped for 30 minutes. Multiple-dose charcoal can be administered per tube every 2 to 4 hours until the identity of the ingested drug is known. Confirmation of stooling is critical to avoid hypermagnesia if a magnesium-containing cathartic is used repetitively. Ipecac is not used because of the risk of seizures in many abused substances and the resultant risk of aspiration during these seizures.

Certain diagnostic studies are performed on nearly every patient. A urine and serum toxicology screen, complete blood count (CBC), and a chemistry profile to include glucose and electrolytes are routine tests. In addition, a serum ethanol level is done if the patient smells or admits to alcohol. Any temperature elevation warrants at least two sets of blood cultures, a chest radiograph and urinalysis as well as a careful cardiac auscultatory exam to evaluate for endocarditis. An irregular pulse or hypotension requires an electrocardiogram (ECG) in addition to the preceding tests. Respiratory abnormalities require arterial blood gases, chest radiograph, and continuous pulse oximetry.

ICU Admission Criteria

A critical phase of the intoxicated patient's management is the "transfer" phase when responsibility for the patient's care is transferred from the emergency physician to the intensivist. Communication between these two physicians is critical to ensure optimal patient care in a critical setting. Clarification of the patient's medical history, recent events leading to their emergency department visit, type of drug(s) consumed, suspected complications of these drugs, and emergency management including treatment, laboratory, and radiographic and ECG monitoring are all issues that need to be carefully discussed and shared between these two physicians. This free exchange of critical information allows for the smooth continuation of any treatment started in the emergency department. In addition, it prevents needless duplication of diagnostic studies and allows a shared "game plan" of patient evaluation, management, and rehabilitation to be developed.

An important issue that has not been extensively studied is the topic of an appropriate admission to the ICU. Some admissions are obvious: an intubated patient, the patient requiring frequent doses of pulsed charcoal, or aggressive crystalloid support of vital signs, persistently depressed level of consciousness with poor or absent gag reflex, and recurrent or refractory major CNS complications such as grand mal seizures or drug-induced arrhythmias.

Brett et al.[19] examined parameters easily obtained in the emergency department to predict which patients suffering from intentional drug overdose did not require ICU treatment. Of the 209 patients studied, he stratified 151 patients into a low risk category on the basis of the following parameters being absent:

- Need for intubation
- Seizures
- Unresponsiveness to verbal stimuli
- Arterial P_{CO_2} greater than 45 mm Hg
- Any rhythm except sinus
- Second- or third-degree atrioventricular block
- QRS greater than 0.12 seconds
- Systolic blood pressure less than 80 mm Hg

Although cases transferred from other facilities and cases of nonintentional drug toxicity were excluded from this study, none of these 151 patients developed a high risk condition after admission, and none required intensive care management. Parameters such as these may serve as a useful guide for the emergency and intensive care physicians to base their decision on the appropriate disposition of the drug-intoxicated patient. Additional or extenuating circumstances must always take priority in the ultimate decision to admit these patients to the ICU. If there is any doubt about the stability of the drug-intoxicated patient, it is better to err on the side of patient safety and admit the patient to an ICU or intermediate care unit with the availability of sufficient nursing staff, monitoring resources such as telemetry, and expertise in caring for the critically ill patient.[19]

ICU PHASE

Central Nervous System Stimulants

Central nervous system stimulants are currently used by 30% of drug abusers.[20] The most prevalent and socially acceptable stimulants are nicotine and tobacco products and caffeine in coffee, tea, soft drinks, and combination medicines. The most toxic drugs in this group are the amphetamines, cocaine, and the so-called "look-alike" drugs, drugs that are abused because their "street name" or appearance associates with them the effects of a controlled drug.[1,2,13]

Demographic characteristics, personality traits, or features of early cocaine use do not differentiate heavy cocaine abusers from noncompulsive users.[21] NIDA has estimated that of 30,000,000 Americans who have tried cocaine intravenously, 80% have now become regular users and 95% are not addicted to the drug. Similarly, when amphetamines were prescribed in the early 1960s for millions of depressed, anergic, or overweight persons, most patients were easily weaned when restrictions were applied. Apart from co-existing psychiatric disorders, no predispositions to stimulant abuse have been identified.

Signs and Symptoms

In small doses, amphetamines are euphorogenic, elevating mood and producing feelings of well-being and excitement. Stimulants appear to produce euphoria by activating reward ("pleasure") pathways in the brain. Both large doses and rapid routes of administration result in high plasma concentrations, producing a euphoria so extreme that it is often compared to orgasm. A series of experiments over the past decade have demonstrated that activation of the neurotransmitter dopamine and mesolimbic or mesocortical pathways mediates this euphoria. Lesions of these pathways induced by either surgery or neurotoxins or dopamine-receptor blockers (e.g., haloperidol) attenuate or eliminate both the effects of stimulants and the self-administration of stimulants.[21]

All the stimulant drugs cause many similar effects on the central and peripheral nervous systems and the cardiovascular system. Some of the other effects from the stimulants include a temporary sense of exhilaration and euphoria, increased feelings of sexuality, hyperactivity, irritability, decreased fatigue, and extended wakefulness. Anorexia is also an effect of the stimulants, and it is this property that may initially attract some people to these drugs as an appetite suppressant.

Physical signs of stimulant use may include tremors, dizziness, dilated and reactive pupils, dry mouth, hyperreflexia, mild hypertension, and tachycardia. Many abusers "shoot" these drugs because with intravenous administration, the effects are greatly intensified. Shortly after injection a sudden sensation known as a "flash" or "rush" is felt. This feeling is described by users as a "total body orgasm." The protracted use of stimulants is usually followed by a period of depression that is known as "crashing." This depression can be temporarily relieved by more stimulants, thereby setting up a vicious cycle of repetitive use for the abuser.

Large doses of these drugs may result in unusual behavioral abnormalities such as repetitive grinding of the teeth, touching or picking the face and extremities, performing the same act repetitively over hours and hours, preoccupation with one's own thought processes, suspiciousness, paranoia, and auditory or visual hallucinations. Physiologic abnormalities include tachydysrhythmias, hypertensive crisis, cardiovascular collapse, renal failure, and death.[1,21]

Cocaine

As recently as 1984, cocaine was claimed to be relatively safe, nonaddicting euphoriant. Believing that the drug was safe, millions of people tried cocaine, and cocaine abuse exploded. By 1986 the NIDA estimated that 3,000,000 people abused cocaine regularly, more than 5 times the number addicted to heroin.[3] Between 1976 and 1986, emergency department visits attributed to cocaine abuse increased by more than 15-fold. By 1986 almost 15% of the US population had tried cocaine, with nearly 40% in the age range between 25 and 30 years.[21] Recent data, however, suggest that for the first time cocaine usage may be declining. Cocaine-related hospital emergencies fell 28% in 9 months and the number of teenagers who said they used cocaine in 1989 declined 44%.[2,22]

Stimulants produce a neurochemical magnification of the pleasure experienced in most activities. They produce alertness and a sense of well-being. They lower anxiety and social ambitions and heighten energy, self-esteem, sexuality, and the emotions aroused by interpersonal experiences. Because these experiences appear to be free of negative consequences, repeat users discover that higher doses are needed to intensify the pharmacologic euphoria. Unless there are self-imposed or external limits on supplies (e.g., lack of money to purchase the product), doses gradually increase. While intoxicated, the user focuses increasingly on trying to recapture the intense euphoric internal sensations of his first experience with cocaine, withdrawing over time from what began as a social experience.

Cocaine "binges," characterized by readministration of the drug up to every 10 minutes, occur because of its short euphoric state. These binges can cause rapid and frequent mood changes. Although cocaine binges can last as long as 7 consecutive days, the average length is 12 hours.

Signs and Symptoms. Systemically, cocaine stimulates the CNS from above downward. The first recognizable action is on the cortex and is manifested by excitement, euphoria, garrulousness, and restlessness. These are some of the pleasurable effects sought after by the user. There may be also an increased capacity for muscular work, nausea, vomiting, and abdominal pain. Other signs and symptoms may include headache, chills, fever, mydriasis, and formication, which is the sensation of insects crawling under the skin ("cocaine bugs"). These tactile hallucinations may lead to serious degrees of self-excoriation. Cocaine causes mydriasis indirectly by blocking the reuptake of norepinephrine. As the doses increase, lower motor centers are stimulated, causing tremors and seizures.[1,2] Signs and symptoms of cocaine intoxication are found in Table 69-6.

Typically, cocaine is distributed as a white crystalline powder cut into grams or "spoons." A spoon is considered approximately 0.5 g and may produce 15 to 20 "lines" of cocaine. The user of street cocaine usually obtains a 5% mixture that may range from 10 to 200 mg of cocaine per dose. The average "line" of cocaine is 25 mg, and 10 to 15 mg is usually administered by the IV route. The latter provides the equivalent of 10 mg of dextroamphetamine.

Cocaine is absorbed from most routes and may be injected IV, swallowed, smoked, nasally insufflated, applied to oral or genital mucosal membranes, or mixed with liquor to make a "liquid lady." The effects of IV administration are similar to those with smoking because both routes of administration demonstrate almost immediate effects.[1] Cocaine is usually not taken orally for recreational purposes, but toxic reactions and deaths have been reported from "body packing," which is ingestion of drug-filled balloons or condoms to avoid police detection.

The most common method of administration is insufflation. After insufflation, approximately 60% of the drug is absorbed, and cocaine may be detected on the nasal mucosa for as long as 3 hours after application. Cocaine administration by this route limits its own absorption by causing vasoconstriction of the nasal mucosa, and the plasma drug concentration usually rises relatively slowly. This self-titration allows drug effects beginning within 5 minutes, reaching a maximum in 20 minutes, and lasting for more than 30 to 60 minutes.

Cocaine hydrochloride is not suitable for smoking, because heat causes it to decompose. To be smoked, the cocaine hydrochloride must be made into a free base, which is then more heat stable. Cocaine hydrochloride can be converted to free base using a relatively simple chemical procedure by dissolving it in an alkaline aqueous solution followed by extraction with a solvent such as ether. This free base is absorbed from all sites but primarily from the lung. "Crack" or "rocks" are designed for individuals who wish to try free-base cocaine.[1] Free-base cocaine is called "crack" because of the sound made by crystals popping when it is heated and "rocks" because of its appearance. Crack cocaine has revolutionized the drug supply market; dealers prefer to sell crack rather than cocaine powder because of crack's high addiction potential, low unit cost, and easy means of handling. One "rock" usually provides two to three inhalations, and the effects may last approximately 20 minutes.

The major effects of cocaine are due to adrenergic stimulation and resemble the "fight, flight, or fright" reaction. Cardiovascular stimulation results in hypertension and tachycardia. Sympathetic stimulation also causes mydriasis, increased body temperature, tremors, seizures, loss of consciousness, and respiratory depression. Myocardial infarction, cerebral vascular events, mesenteric infarctions, and pulmonary edema may also be noted.[23,24]

Cocaine blocks the reuptake of dopamine and norepinephrine in the CNS, which results in euphoria, garrulousness, restlessness, and increased motor activity. The major neurochemical actions of cocaine include the following:

- CNS stimulation with release of dopamine
- Inhibition of neuronal catecholamine uptake with resultant generalized sympathetic stimulation
- Release of blockade of serotonin uptake
- Inhibition of the sodium current in neural tissue with resultant local anesthetic effects[2]

These mechanisms appear to be involved in the physical and psychologic dependence noted earlier. Cocaine causes an increase in heat production by stimulating muscular activity and decreasing heat loss through vasoconstriction. This can lead to life-threatening hyperpyrexia.

Complications. Rarely does cocaine ingestion lead to death. In a retrospective study of cocaine fatalities, more than 60% of cocaine-induced deaths were associated with IV administration of cocaine, and approximately 15% were associated with ingestion of cocaine. More than 50% of cocaine fatalities occurred within 1 hour of exposure, and nearly 75% within 2 hours. There was no correlation between survival time and the route of administration. Survival for 3 hours has been claimed to be associated with nearly complete recovery within another 3 hours.[1]

Intravenous injection sites of cocaine users are somewhat unique and may be noted to have prominent ecchymosis, sometimes with a central area of pallor. Multiple ecchymotic areas are probably due to direct cytoxic reaction of cocaine coupled with the ischemic vascular injury secondary to vasoconstriction.[1] Some cutting substances may be added to cocaine, which may add greatly to its toxicity (see Table 69-4). Adulteration of cocaine makes it impossible for cocaine users to know how much cocaine they are taking. The user may only be getting 5 to 40% pure cocaine when purchasing drugs on the street. Most active ingredients used as cutting substances for cocaine are in three major drug categories: xanthine alkaloids, local anesthetics, or decongestants.[2]

Extreme CNS stimulation, usually associated with high

Table 69-6. Signs and Symptoms of Cocaine Intoxication

Vital signs and external appearance	Hypertension, tachypnea, tachycardia mydriasis, diaphoresis, hyperthermia, agitation
Cardiovascular	Tachycardia, hypertension, arrhythmias, chest pain, myocardial ischemia
CNS	Tremulousness, irritability, agitation, seizures, headache, hyperactivity, itracranial hemorrhage, syncope, cerebral infarct
Neuropsychiatric	Anxiety, sense of doom, paranoia, depression, mood lability, insomnia
Miscellaneous	Tachypnea, pulmonary edema, pneumothorax, rhinitis, sinusitis, nausea, abdominal pain, renal failure, hepatitis

doses of cocaine, may cause generalized clonic/tonic seizures. Seizures may occur from minutes to as long as 12 hours after IV use and may be a preterminal event. Although seizures are usually associated with lactic acidosis and hyperthermia, they may also be associated with cerebral vascular infarct or hemorrhage. The first reported case of stroke related to cocaine abuse was in 1977.[2] The latency period from cocaine ingestion to CNS symptoms can be from minutes to 1 day. Other neurologic problems commonly reported include headache without intracranial bleeding and syncope that occurs minutes after injecting cocaine.[25] In general, the hypersympathetic, hypertensive, vasculitic, and vasospastic effects of cocaine appear to be likely responsible for most neurologic problems.[23,26]

Seizures and deaths have been associated with a wide range of plasma concentrations. Other direct physiologic effects may include tachypnea and tachycardia. Paradoxic respiratory depression may lead to rapid, shallow respirations or Cheyne-Stokes breathing, and death may occur from central respiratory depression.[23]

Cocaine causes pulmonary complications ranging from tachypnea to pulmonary edema. Death by respiratory arrest, independent of the route of cocaine use has been described. Other complications such as pneumomediastinum, bronchiolitis obliterans, or hypersensitivity pneumonitis are related specifically to smoking free base or crack. Chronic cough and pleuritic chest pain are the most common pulmonary complaints. Pulmonary edema that is due to cocaine intoxication is unusual. A syndrome of "crack lung" has been described. This occurs after smoking cocaine in which the user develops progressive dyspnea, cough, fever, eosinophilia, fleeting pulmonary infiltrates, and evidence of airway obstruction.[23]

Because the majority of users insufflate or "snort" cocaine intranasally, this route has lead to a variety of nasal and sinus diseases including chronic rhinitis, epistaxis, cartilaginous necrosis, and sinusitis.[23] These complications are largely due to cocaine's ability to cause marked vasoconstriction in the dense vascular bed supplying the nasal mucosa and sinuses. Early reports of cocaine abuse in the 1960s and 1970s noted nasal septal perforation as a common marker of cocaine abusers. Subsequent studies, however, reveal that this is actually uncommon. More commonly, patients complain of nasal irritation, recurrent epistaxis, nasal stuffiness, and facial pain typical of sinusitis. More severe complications such as infectious sinusitis and osteolytic sinusitis requiring drainage have been reported.[23] Two cases of staphylococcus sepsis, undoubtedly related to cocaine-induced rhinitis and sinusitis have been reported.[1,23]

Cocaine can increase the complications of pregnancy and adversely affect the newborn. Pregnant women who use cocaine have a higher rate of spontaneous abortion, abruptio placentae, and stillbirths associated with abruptio. The drug has been related to the premature onset of labor with abruptio placentae. Infants exposed to cocaine in utero have a high risk of congenital malformations, perinatal mortality, and neurobehavior impairments.[1,23]

Infectious complications related to IV cocaine use are not unique to cocaine. All IV drug users are at risk for infections such as AIDS, cellulitis, tetanus, and endocarditis which is due to nonsterile technique and shared needles.[27,28] Cocaine users are at higher risk than heroin users for developing endocarditis, possibly because the shorter half-life of cocaine requires more frequent IV injections, presumably with contaminated needles. The intensity of cocaine use, with its multiple, repeated injections, may in part cause this risk. Other factors, such as not heating the cocaine to dissolve it before injection or drug-induced valvular interstitial damage, may also be causative.

The septic cocaine user may be confused with the intoxicated user. Fever, confusion, tremor, and tachycardia may represent acute endocarditis rather than acute cocaine intoxication. Order blood cultures for all febrile IV cocaine abusers. Fever in an IV drug user is endocarditis until proven otherwise. Clinical data, especially obtained in the emergency department, is grossly inaccurate in diagnosing endocarditis in this population.[29] Contagious viruses causing hepatitis and AIDS are transmitted by sharing needles. Although cocaine may be directly hepatotoxic, test for hepatitis B if liver enzymes are elevated.[23]

With lethal doses, malignant hyperthermia, status epilepticus, ventricular dysrhythmia, and respiratory arrest can occur. Rhabdomyolysis and acute myoglobinuric renal failure have been associated with cocaine use.[30,31] Malignant hyperthermia is due to stimulation of the heat-regulatory centers in combination with increased skeletal muscle activity. Sudden death from the recreational use of cocaine may be preceded by delirium, hyperpyrexia, and convulsions.[1]

Small doses of systemically administered cocaine may paradoxically slow the heart either because of central vagal stimulation or as a reflex response to the drug-mediated hypertension. Dysrhythmia is associated with cocaine use and includes sinus tachycardia, ventricular premature contractions, ventricular tachycardia, fibrillation, and asystole. Sinus tachycardia is the most common cardiac arrhythmia in cocaine users.[2]

In addition to cardiac dysrhythmia, cocaine may precipitate other life-threatening cardiac events. Cocaine presents a potential hazard to individuals with underlying fixed coronary artery disease because it causes increases in heart rate, systolic blood pressure, and myocardial oxygen consumption. Angina pectoris and myocardial infarction that were apparently due to coronary artery constriction have also been reported in young, otherwise healthy individuals who used cocaine. It is noteworthy that myocardial infarction may develop from hours to days after the time of the last dose, probably reflecting the variable time course of the development of thrombosis as well as possibly vasospasm at the site.[1,2,32,33] Regular cocaine users may be symptom free yet have persistent ST-segment elevations during the first week of drug withdrawal.[2]

Diagnosis and Treatment. The clinical picture of cocaine poisoning can easily be confused with that of amphetamine, anticholinergic, or phencyclidine poisoning.[1,2] In most instances the distinctive clinical feature of cocaine poisoning is the more rapid return of the patient to a normal physical state. Cocaine reaction in the body is diphasic with initial sympathetic stimulation followed by abrupt generalized CNS depression. In cases of acute toxicity, if death occurs, it usually does so within 2 to 3 minutes, but sometimes there is a delay of up to 30 minutes. Deaths, although rare, have been reported after smoking, insufflation, intravenous injection, and oral use. Any sudden death or cardiac arrest in an otherwise healthy individual should evoke consideration of cocaine as a precipitant.[1]

None of the routine biochemistry-hematology determinations have been correlated with the clinical severity of cocaine intoxication. Electrocardiograms may be useful in assessing and monitoring cardiac abnormalities, and a chest radiograph should be done to rule out pulmonary edema following IV administration of free-base cocaine.[34]

The effects of acute cocaine intoxication are often not due to cocaine alone. Cocaine is commonly consumed with other drugs such as heroin, marijuana, barbiturates, and benzodiazepines. Alcohol is most often used to downward titrate the CNS stimulant effects of cocaine. In early 1980 a study in Chicago found that 25% of cocaine users regularly mixed the drug with heroin (a "speed ball"). Reports also include the concomitant use of tricyclic antidepressants (see Chap. 70). These combinations may further confuse the clinical picture and therapy. In addition, some of the side effects may be related to the chemicals with which the cocaine has been cut.[23] Because of these considerations, a urine and serum toxicology screen are mandatory on all patients suspected of cocaine ingestion.

Psychiatric complications are the most common cocaine-associated CNS disorder and cause most cocaine-related emergency department visits.[35] Both acute and chronic overdoses can cause auditory, visual, and tactile hallucinations. Users seeking euphoria often develop anxiety, agitation, and dysphoria at higher doses and with chronic use. Profound depression with suicidal ideation may also occur with chronic prolonged use.[1,2]

Decontamination procedures have no therapeutic benefit, because cocaine is absorbed rapidly from both nasal and gastrointestinal mucosa except in the special circumstances of "body packing" (see following discussion).

Management of the effects of acute cocaine intoxication is primarily directed toward attenuating or blocking hyperadrenergic signs and symptoms and treating the specific organ most severely affected. As with all toxicologic emergencies, basic principles must always be applied. Immediately secure the airway, breathing, and circulation. Rapidly treat obtundation or other alterations in mental status with one or two trials of 2 mg of IV naloxone. Give thiamine, 100 mg IV, to alcoholic or malnourished patients who are often among chronic abusers. Hypoglycemia can be ruled out with rapid methods such as finger-stick blood testing. Treat with 25 g of IV glucose as necessary. Midazolam, 5 to 10 mg IM, works quickly (3 to 5 minutes) for seizures or extreme agitation and is useful if an IV is not available.[2] Diazepam is the first-line drug of choice for treating excess sympathomimetic symptoms such as agitation, seizures, tachycardia, and hypertension. Administer diazepam in 2.5- to 5.0-mg boluses every 5 minutes while cardiopulmonary status is carefully monitored. This can be followed by the beta-adrenergic antagonist propranolol or the combined alpha- and beta-adrenergic blocker labetalol. Propranolol is used in 1-mg increments every 5 minutes in patients refractory to diazepam. Because propranolol blocks beta-adrenergic receptors, alpha receptors remain unopposed in peripherally constricted vessels and may cause a worsening of severe hypertension. The use of labetalol with its combined alpha- and beta-adrenergic blocker effect appears to have merit.[2,36] This drug can be administered in 10- to 20-mg IV boluses, increasing by 20-mg increments every 10 to 15 minutes to control severe hypertension associated with cocaine use. Labetalol (2 mg/min) can also be used like nitroprusside as a constant infusion, but unlike nitroprusside, it lacks the potential for tachycardia. In addition, although clinical experience is limited, a carefully titrated infusion of esmolol (500 μg/kg per minute) loading dose, followed by 50 μg/kg per minute for 4 minutes), a short-acting, nonselective beta blocker may also be an excellent drug in the treatment of cocaine-induced hypersympathetic states. Therapeutic end points include a decrease in resting heart rate and blood pressure to near normal values and should occur within minutes of drug administration.

Management of patients with ischemic pain should be identical to management of those with atherosclerotic cardiovascular disease. Thrombolytic therapy for patients with evidence of acute myocardial infarction should be considered but may be associated with high complication rates. Reduction of high adrenergic tone is crucial in these patients. Diazepam is the first-line agent for reducing central adrenergic effects.

An accurate core temperature should be obtained, and hyperthermia should be aggressively treated by undressing the patient and using external cooling with fans and lukewarm or cool water to the body. For patients who do not respond to routine cooling methods, diazepam and adrenergic blockade should be instituted. Because hyperthermia and excessive muscle activity with or without seizures may induce rhabdomyolysis, fluid resuscitation should be aggressive, and high urine output should be maintained using mannitol and furosemide, if necessary. In severe cases of refractory muscle activity, neuromuscular paralysis with endotracheal intubation may be necessary to prevent rhabdomyolysis.

Seizures that are due to cocaine may be difficult to control and may occur before death.[37] If the patient is refractory to diazepam, initiate preparations for intubation and general anesthesia with thiopental with or without neuromuscular blockade. Brain seizure activity can continue with paralysis, so continuous electroencephalogram (EEG) monitoring to evaluate for seizure activity is necessary. Seizures are usually brief or self-limited. Repeated seizures suggest hyperthermia, intracerebral hemorrhage, metabolic abnormalities, or massive cocaine intake (body packer).

Last, ventricular arrhythmias may be difficult to control with lidocaine. Adrenergic blockage with propranolol to block catecholamine-induced ventricular irritation may be effective in lidocaine-resistant cases.[2,23] A summary of treatment is found in Table 69-7.

Admission Criteria. Any patient suspected of ingesting cocaine should be admitted if he has any of the following symptoms:

- Suspected "body packer"
- Chest pain not explainable by musculoskeletal source

Table 69-7. Symptoms and Treatment in Cocaine and Amphetamine Intoxications

Symptoms	Treatment
General intoxication	Cooling blanket if hyperthermic Naloxone, 2 mg IV, mr × 1 Thiamine, 100 mg IV Glucose, 25 g IV Oxygen, IV D5W tko
Increased CNS activity	
Agitation	Diazepam, 2.5–5 mg IV q5 minutes, or midazolam, 5–10 mg IM or 1–2 mg IV
Seizures	As above, then phenobarbital, 1.5–2 mg/kg IV or phenytoin, 15–18 mg/kg
Cardiovascular	
Hypertension	Diazepam, 2.5–5 mg IV q5 minutes, or midazolam, 1–2 mg IV, then labetolol, 10–20 mg IV, or esmolol, 500 μg/kg loading, then 50 μg/kg/min
Ventricular arrhythmias	Lidocaine, 75–100 mg loading, 2–4 mg/min
Ischemia	Nitrates (nitroglycerin, 0.4 mg sublingually) Nitroglycerin paste, 0.5–1 inch Calcium-channel blockers Thrombolysis (t-PA, anistreptase, etc.)
Rhabdomyolysis	IV crystalloids: 500 ml/hr Consider alkalinizing urine

IV, intravenous; kvo, keep vein open; mr, may repeat; t-PA, tissue plasminogen activator.

- Dysrhythmia
- Persistently abnormal vital signs after 4 to 6 hours of observation
- Suspected CNS, cardiovascular, or neuropsychiatric complication

Particular attention should be paid to obtaining a careful history to evaluate the patient's suicidal potential. Although many cocaine abusers are depressed, active suicidal ideation requires urgent psychiatric admission in the absence of any medical complications from their cocaine abuse. Conversely, many patients will come to the hospital requesting admission for "detox." This may be from a genuine concern and willingness to discontinue cocaine but also frequently is a ploy when the abuser's money has run out and he has no food or shelter. In-hospital detoxification of cocaine addiction has not been found to be more effective than outpatient treatment. Because cocaine and other stimulant withdrawal is not associated with life-threatening complications, these patients can be referred to appropriate outpatient community facilities.

Body Packing. Smuggling cocaine across international borders by ingesting large numbers of drug-filled packets poses a unique problem for custom officials and physicians.[38] The "body packer" or "mule" carries 50 to 200 discretely and usually tightly wrapped condoms or latex bags filled with high grade cocaine. Most "body packers" are asymptomatic and are apprehended by suspicious custom officials at airport checkpoints. Some become acutely symptomatic when packets leak, resulting in massive intoxication, seizures, or sudden death. Some individuals take a substance such as diphenoxylate (Lomotil) before boarding the plane to slow gastrointestinal motility and to prevent passage of the cocaine packets before landing. They then take a laxative once they reach their destination. A similar problem may occur in "body stuffers," cocaine users or traffickers who ingest bags of cocaine when arrested. Often a radiograph will show evidence of these condoms as multiple oval soft tissue densities surrounding a gas-like halo. An abdominal radiograph combined with genital rectal examination is the best initial screening for body packers, although a negative radiograph does not exclude this condition. A biscodyl rectal suppository should be used to attempt to rapidly obtain the package(s). Female body packers may also carry packets in the vagina.

Many deaths are associated with body packing because leakage or rupture can occur in one or more of the packets. The rupture of even one packet could cause death because of the large dose of pure cocaine that is suddenly absorbed through the intestinal mucosa. Enteric septicemia caused by fecal contamination of subsequently injected cocaine has been reported.[1,2,38]

Prolonged or cyclic CNS stimulation in a patient with signs and symptoms of cocaine toxicity should raise the possibility of continued or periodic gastrointestinal leakage from these packets. Additional management strategies consists of multiple-dose oral charcoal plus repeated doses of cathartics such as sorbitol or magnesium citrate. Alternatively, a continuous infusion of polyethylene glycol electrolyte solution available commercially as Colyteb or Golytely—a solution routinely used to irrigate the bowel before surgery—can be given to accelerate gastrointestinal transit time.[39] The usual adult dose is 2 L per hour orally or by nasogastric tube.[2,29] ICU admission for these patients is mandatory, and symptomatic management is as described previously.

Amphetamines

Amphetamines became a drug of abuse 50 years ago when they were available in nasal decongestant inhalers and other over-the-counter preparations. Subsequent recognition of the limited therapeutic value and high abuse potential of amphetamines lead to a marked reduction in their medical use. Current applications include treatment for narcolepsy, appetite control, and control of hyperkinetic behavior in children.

Although a CNS stimulant like cocaine, the amphetamines are structurally dissimilar to cocaine. Their neurologic, chemical, and clinical effects, however, are quite similar. Their main difference concerns duration of action. Cocaine's plasma half-life is 90 minutes, whereas that of amphetamine is much longer. Because of its shortened half-life, cocaine's euphoria lasts less than 45 minutes, while amphetamine's duration of euphoria is four to eight times longer.

The IV injection of amphetamine produces a sudden "flash" or "rush" that is described as exhilarating. The rush is followed by a persisting, invigorating sense of euphoria, clear thinking, gregariousness, self-confidence, excitement, and invulnerability. Methamphetamine may be favored by the drug abuser for parenteral use because it is water soluble and can be injected more readily than other agents. In addition, it has more pronounced pleasurable central effects and less pronounced peripheral side effects.[1,2,21]

Signs and Symptoms. Amphetamines are structurally related to norepinephrine but have a greater central stimulant activity than norepinephrine and other catecholamines. Amphetamines are rapidly absorbed from the gastrointestinal tract. Following therapeutic doses, peak blood levels occur 1 to 2 hours after ingestion. Metabolism of 30 to 40% of the therapeutic dose occurs in the liver. The remainder of the parent drug as well as its metabolites is excreted in the urine. The mechanism of action of amphetamines on peripheral structures is thought to be due to a combination of indirect action by release of norepinephrine from stores in adrenergic nerve terminals and a direct action on both alpha- and beta-receptor sites. The main site of CNS action appears to be the cerebral cortex, where amphetamines cause a release of catecholamines into the synaptic cleft and decrease the rate of neuronal firing.[1,2,21]

At average oral dosages, amphetamines produce euphoria, a feeling of energy, extended wakefulness and alertness, and decreased appetitive. These are the desired effects of amphetamines that are sought after by the user.

Amphetamines may be taken on a short- or long-term basis by oral, respiratory, IV, or vaginal routes. The amount of amphetamine required to produce a serious overdose depends to a large extent on frequency of a previous usage and the size of the dose. The margin of safety between therapeutic and lethal dosages is relatively large. After repeatedly taking amphetamines, most users develop a tolerance to the drug, and larger amounts can be taken with each dose.

A patient who injects amphetamine in moderate amounts may become symptomatic within 30 minutes. These symptoms may last for several hours and may include tachycardia, flushing, sweating, palpitation, and headache. Continued high-dose IV use induces mental disturbances such as confusion, delirium, and acute psychosis that may be indistinguishable from schizophrenia. The individual may appear confused with disorganized behavior and may exhibit compulsive repetition of meaningless acts, such as picking at bed sheets. The patient may be irritable, fearful, or suspicious of his surroundings and experience delusions or hallucinations. Hallucinations may be both visual and auditory.[1,2,21]

Complications. A significant overdose of amphetamines may cause dilated, reactive pupils, profound anxiety, and seizures. Severe overdoses may be followed by cardiac dysrhythmia, delirium, hypertensive crisis, cerebral vascular accidents, circulatory collapse, coma or status epilepticus. Hypothermia and disseminated intravascular coagulation have also been observed. Acute renal failure associated with rhabdomyolysis is a well-recognized complication of amphetamine overdose. Clinical evidence of rhabdomyolysis and myoglobinuria usually consists of myalgia, muscle tenderness, myoedema, elevated creatinine phosphokinase concentrations, and myoglobinuria. Ischemic chest pain can occur and may be secondary to coronary artery vasospasm.[1,2,21]

Withdrawal from long-term amphetamine use causes symptoms that are the inverse of the acute effects of stimulants. They include decreased energy (anergia), limited interest in the environment, and limited ability to experience pleasure (anhedonia). Often at their mildest immediately after a so-called "crash," these symptoms increase in intensity during the next 12 to 96 hours. They fluctuate and are neither constant nor severe enough to meet psychiatric diagnostic criteria for major mood disorders. Serious depression and suicidal ideation may occur and can be quite prolonged. After long-term high dose use, abusers exhibit a profound depression, apathy, and fatigue. Precautions against suicide should be enacted for patients withdrawing from amphetamines. Because the severity of withdrawal symptoms depends on the extent of stimulant abuse, intermittent or recreational users do not experience significant withdrawal symptoms.[1,2,21]

Diagnosis and Management. The diagnosis of amphetamine abuse can be made through the use of patient history, a positive toxicology screen on urine and blood, and a predominance of excess sympathomimetic symptoms from the patient. Qualitative toxicology screens are helpful to confirm the clinical suspicion of amphetamine abuse, quantitative screens are not. Some of the newer synthetic amphetamines cannot be assayed by traditional toxicology screens.[2] Because tolerance to amphetamine effects occur, the estimation of the severity of a poisoning should be based on the clinical picture, not on the reported dose or plasma level of the drug.[1,34]

No specific antidote is available for amphetamine overdose, and most of the treatment is supportive. Fatalities are unusual following acute intoxication, and if they occur are usually attributable to CNS hemorrhage or cardiac arrhythmias. If the drug has been ingested orally, then lavage followed by the administration of activated charcoal and a cathartic should be administered. Hypertension should be managed more aggressively than in the patient with known chronic hypertension. Alpha-adrenergic blocking agents can be lifesaving in patients with hypertensive crisis. The major complications related to amphetamine abuse are virtually identical to those found in cocaine use. A description of these complications and their treatment can be found in Table 69–7.

The plasma half-life of amphetamine depends on the pH of the urine. With an alkaline urine (pH greater than 7.5), plasma half-life of amphetamine is 16 to 31 hours, whereas with an acidic urine (pH less than 6.0), the half-life is 8 to 10 hours. Acidic urine increases excretion of both the parent drug and metabolites but runs the risk of precipitating acute renal failure if myoglobinuria is present. Aggressive extracellular volume replacement in attempt to avert acute renal failure should be instituted.[34]

For treatment of acute psychotic manifestations, haloperidol or phenothiazines are commonly used but may impair heat dissipation and lower the seizure threshold. Neuroleptics should be withheld and used in those cases in which an acute psychosis persists after the acute intoxication has resolved or in the actively psychotic, intoxicated patient who is in danger of harming himself or others. Chlorpromazine is believed by some investigators to prolong the half-life of amphetamines, and thus 2 to 5 mg of haloperidol by IM injection is the preferred drug treatment of acute psychotic reactions. Diazepam can be administered by seizures and agitation.[1,2,34]

The treatment of ventricular arrhythmias or ectopy should be by beta$_1$ blockers such as esmolol by continuous IV infusion of 500 µg/kg per minute preceded by a 500 µg/kg loading dose. Lidocaine can theoretically cause seizures, so it is not a first-choice antiarrhythmic. The treatment of amphetamine-induced chest pain remains controversial, but until this issue is settled, it should be treated and evaluated similarly to cocaine-induced chest pain. Hyperthermia, if present, should not be treated with antipyretics but rather with aggressive external cooling and benzodiazepines.[2] Generally, admission criteria are the same as those for cocaine intoxication.

Special Considerations. As in cocaine, amphetamine binges also occur and often last more than 24 hours with 1 to several hours between readministrations of the drug. When the amount and duration of cocaine abuse are the same as those of high dose amphetamine, their psychiatric sequelae are indistinguishable.[21]

A new form of amphetamine, known to the Japanese as "Shabu" and to the Koreans as "Hiroppon," is present now in epidemic proportions in parts of Southeast Asia and Hawaii.[40,41] This drug is known simply as "ice" in the United States and, in contrast of the fleeting 20-minute high of crack, an "ice" buzz may last anywhere from 8 to 24 hours. Unlike cocaine, which comes from a plant indigenous to the Andes, "ice" can be cooked up in a home laboratory using easily obtained retail chemicals. So far, the spread to the United States has been largely confined to the Hawaiian Islands. The quickness with which it has overtaken that state is startling. In just over 4 years, "ice" has surpassed marijuana and cocaine and is Hawaii's number-one drug problem. "Ice" costs approximately $50 per "paper" (less than 1 g). It has a duration of action of 8 to 24 hours and causes immediate, intense euphoria and increased alertness. This pyrolized methamphetamine has significant side effects including aggressive behavior, hallucinations, paranoia, and fatal kidney failure. Its management is similar to that of cocaine and other amphetamines but may be more prolonged as a result of its longer duration of action.

The Look-Alike Drugs

The "look-alike" drugs are found in the form of tablets or capsules that resemble prescription drugs in shape, size, color, and markings but differ in the fact that they do not contact the same ingredients or have the same effectiveness as the original drug. Look-alike drugs are defined as psychoactive drugs whose "street trade" names or appearances are designed to associate them with the effects of a controlled drug. The most common over-the-counter stimulants sold as look-alikes are phenylpropanolamine (PPA), ephedrine, caffeine, and pseudoephedrine.

In contrast to amphetamine and cocaine, the so-called look-alike drugs are relatively unfamiliar to many nonprofessionals. Their prevalence in over-the-counter preparations, foods, and beverages make them readily accessible if not unavoidable. This is particularly true of caffeine, which many people use regularly to wake up in the morning, enhance concentration during the day, and stay awake at night. At least 1 billion kg of coffee are consumed annually in the United States alone.[20]

Signs and Symptoms. Although these compounds have chemical structures and actions similar to amphetamines, there are substantial differences in magnitude of response of various organ systems. Phenylpropanolamine is the most dangerous of the look-alikes and appears to have the greatest hypertensive activity. Both PPA and ephedrine have fewer CNS effects than amphetamines.[1,2,34]

The look-alikes can produce mood elevation and an alerted state of consciousness, as seen with amphetamines. Patients have a generalized feeling of well-being and experience anorexia, decreased fatigue, enhanced sensory perceptions, and improved motor skills.[42]

Orally consumed, these drugs are absorbed from the gastrointestinal tract. The timing of peak levels after overdose is unknown, but after therapeutic doses, 50% of ingested pseudoephedrine is absorbed within 1 hour. Enzymatic metabolism does occur, and a metabolite of pseudoephedrine is toxic. The majority of ephedrine and 45% of PPA is excreted unchanged in the urine. Renal excretion of ephedrine and pseudoephedrine is increased with urinary acidification. The plasma half-life at therapeutic levels is 4 hours for ephedrine and 8 hours for pseudoephedrine.

Following an overdose with any of these compounds, clinical effects rarely last longer than 8 hours. Symptoms persisting for longer periods may be attributable to secondary complications. Cardiovascular side effects include hypertension, tachycardia, palpitations, and arrhythmias (premature atrial contractions [PACs] and premature ventricular contractions [PVCs]). Reflex bradycardia has occurred after PPA ingestion. Central nervous system effects include headache, restlessness, insomnia, tremors, convulsions, hallucinations, delirium, occasionally psychoses, and intracerebral hemorrhage. Other clinical effects may occur and include nausea, vomiting, abdominal pain, and diuresis. Hypertensive crisis can result from even a single therapeutic dose of PPA.[21] Intracranial hemorrhage has occurred secondary to severe hypertension. These hypertensive effects may be potentiated by various other drugs, including monoamine oxidase inhibitors (MAO inhibitors), ephedrine, caffeine, anticholinergic drugs, amphetamines, and antihypertensive agents.[1] Chest pain with elevation of the MB (muscle band) fractions of creatine phosphokinase (CPK) have also been described.[43] Renal failure with and without rhabdomyolysis and hypertension may occur with PPA overdoses.[1]

Diagnosis and Treatment. Quantitative identification of PPA in urine can be accomplished by using thin-layer chromatography or enzyme-modified immunoassay. These techniques may not be readily available, however. Qualitative identification of the urine can also be performed but is usually not clinically useful.

The sympathomimetic abusing patient may present with a variety of findings.[2] The mildly intoxicated person will have palpitations, chest pain, headache, or a sense of impending doom. He may be upset, agitated, tremulous and have dilated pupils. The vital signs are abnormal; hypertension and tachycardia are common findings. Hyperthermia and tachypnea may be present.

Treatment of an overdose with a sympathomimetic agent consists of gastrointestinal decontamination within 2 hours of ingestion followed by supportive care. Extreme agitation may be controlled with diazepam. Tachycardia compromising cardiovascular function may respond to propranolol. Following PPA ingestion, frequent PVCs may be treated with lidocaine. Bradycardia may be treated with atropine. Severe hypertension may be treated with sodium nitroprusside or phentolamine. Although the renal excretion of ephedrine and pseudoephedrine may be enhanced by the acidification of the urine, the usefulness of this approach in the clinical setting has not been established.[34]

Treatment of patients with suspected overdose of a look-alike drug should include frequent monitoring of the vital signs for possible life-threatening sequelae such as cardiac dysrhythmia and hypertensive crisis. Most episodes of hypertension subside within 3 or 4 hours without treatment or with the addition of a mild sedative such as a benzodiazepine. Hypertension should be treated if accompanied by signs and symptoms of myocardial ischemia or hypertensive encephalopathy; sodium nitroprusside, beginning at 3 µg/kg per minute and titrated according to effect is suggested. If serious cardiac dysrhythmia is present, lidocaine should be administered. Beta-adrenergic blocking drugs, although potentially useful for the tachydysrhythmias, may be harmful if the hypertension causes vagal stimulation, which produces a reflex bradycardia that may be potentiated by the beta-adrenergic-blocking drug.

Psychosis, if not responsive to supportive care, can be managed with the use of haloperidol or diazepam. Seizures should be treated with IV diazepam.[1,2,20,34]

Caffeine

Caffeine is a widely abused drug that is often overlooked as a cause of acute reaction. Caffeine not only can be found as an adulterant of illicit stimulants but can also be purchased as an appetite suppressant or legal stimulant without a prescription. Caffeine belongs to a group of methylated xanthines found in a variety of plants throughout the world. It is widely consumed today in beverages such as coffee, tea, and cocoa and is also an ingredient in chocolate as well as many over-the-counter analgesics, headache remedies, anorectic agents, and stimulants. Soft drinks represent a major source of dietary caffeine, particularly for children. Ingestion is common for therapeutic purposes or from consumption of various beverages.[1]

Signs and Symptoms. Caffeine is absorbed rapidly after oral administration, and serum concentrations reach their peak in 30 to 60 minutes. The presence or absence of food in the stomach does not influence the absorption of caffeine. Caffeine has a plasma half-life of 3 to 4 hours in adults. It is metabolized in the liver to inactive metabolites, which are secreted in the urine. Caffeine is also metabolized to theophylline as a by-product.

Caffeine causes a translocation of intracellular calcium by increasing permeability of calcium in the sarcoplasmic reticulum, which accounts for its action of increasing the contractility of skeletal and cardiac muscle. By inhibiting the enzyme phosphodiesterase, it also causes an increased accumulation of cyclic nucleotides, particularly cyclic adenosine monophosphate (cAMP). Through this action, the metabolic effect of endogenous sympathomimetics are enhanced. Caffeine is a potent releaser of epinephrine and to a lesser extent norepinephrine from the adrenal medulla. Cardiac toxic effects as well as metabolic effects (hyperglycemia, ketosis, and metabolic acidosis) of caffeine are probably due to increasing circulating concentrations of epinephrine and norepinephrine.[1]

Caffeine has a wider therapeutic index than theophylline, resulting in lower incidences of toxicity. Toxic doses of caffeine are not well established but have been reported to be 78 mg/kg in a child and 1 g/kg in an adult. Symptoms of acute caffeine overdose often begin within 30 to 60 minutes of ingestion. Pupils are most often miotic but may be dilated. Gastrointestinal symptoms are characteristic of caffeine overdose. Abdominal cramps and vomiting usually are prominent. Neurologic symptoms may last as long as 48 hours and include alteration of behavior, tonic posturing, rigidity, coma, and convulsions. Initially, convulsions are epileptiform, but later they may resemble reflex hyperexcitability. Other neuromuscular symptoms include fasciculations and alterations in muscle tone. Changes in heart rate, paroxysmal atrial tachycardia (PAT), extrasystoles, hypertension, and hypotension have all been reported.[1,2,20,34]

Complications. The diuretic effect of caffeine may result in the loss of fluid volume and hypokalemia. Hyperglycemia, leukocytosis, and metabolic acidosis have also been reported. Fatalities from acute caffeine poisoning are unusual.[34]

Treatment and Diagnosis. Because caffeine and theophylline are both methylxanthines and because caffeine decreases the hepatic clearance of theophylline, serum concentrations of theophylline should be measured when large changes in caffeine intake are to be expected. Caffeine use can be confirmed by thin-layer chromatography.

Because there is no specific antidote, treatment of an acute overdose of caffeine usually is limited to supportive therapy and abstention from the caffeine-containing substances. Emesis or lavage followed by administration of activated charcoal and a cathartic should be performed in the acute overdose of caffeine tablets. Seizures should be controlled with a benzodiazepine such as diazepam. Although it may seem logical to use a beta-adrenergic-blocking drug to reverse the manifestations of the hyperadrenergic syndrome, unopposed alpha-adrenergic effect may result. For this reason, alpha-adrenergic block may be necessary if a beta-blocking drug has been used. Administration of lidocaine or phenytoin is recommended for treatment of cardiac dysrhythmia. Hemorrhagic gastritis may be treated with ice fluid lavage, histamine$_2$ blockers, and antacids.[1,2,34]

ICU Admission Criteria. Any patient manifesting persistent tachycardia, hypertension, or CNS excitability after 4 to 6 hours of ER observation should probably be admitted. In addition, any patient with a seizure, cardiac arrhythmia, gastrointestinal bleeding, or extreme hypertension requiring repeated or continuous pharmacologic intervention obviously should be admitted.

Special Considerations. One of the major problems associated with the look-alike drugs is the small margin of safety between therapeutic and toxic dosages of these agents. This exposes patients to potentially toxic amounts at doses barely exceeding those found in a standard pill. In addition, the inexperienced drug user may inadvertently overdose because of the mistaken idea that these drugs will produce a "high" equivalent to that of amphetamines. Such users may also wrongly assume that look-alikes are safer, less potent substances and take several pills at a time, causing even greater toxicity.[1]

Central Nervous System Depressants

Alcohol

At least 10,000,000 Americans, or the equivalent of the entire population of the entire city of New York, abuse alcohol. It is estimated that 10% of the adult population is alcoholic. As many as 40% of admissions to general medical and surgical wards are related to ethanol abuse.[44] Annual estimates suggest that greater than 20,000,000 Americans will require emergency care for trauma-related events, and 45,000 will die. Ethanol can be linked to approximately one half of these deaths.[2]

Only 3% of alcoholics are "skid row" types, while the remaining 97% are employed. Of those employed, 37% have a high school education; 25% are in white collar jobs; 30% are manual workers, and 45% are managerial or professional people.[45,46]

Ethanol is used as a solvent in many medicinal and nonmedicinal products including antiseptics. Ethyl alcohol is used externally as a solvent for many drugs as well as a skin disinfectant. Household ethanol sources include perfumes, colognes, aftershaves, mouthwashes, antiseptics, elixirs, and food abstracts.

The most frequent cause of a patient presenting to an emergency department with an altered mental status involves the acute ingestion of ethyl alcohol. Ethanol is the most widely abused "drug" and is a component of overdose in up to 70% of cases. In addition, physicians frequently encounter sequelae from the multisystem dysfunction caused by the chronic ingestion of alcohol. Alcohol substitutes consist of methanol, ethylene glycol, and isopropyl alcohol and may be consumed accidentally or if the alcoholic cannot obtain ethyl alcohol. Clinicians must be able to identify and treat acute and chronic alcohol intoxication and acute ingestion of ethylene glycol and methanol and to use serum osmolality and osmolar gap measurements in obtaining a diagnosis of a toxic or medical disorder.[1,2]

Signs and Symptoms. Because alcohol often induces an initial euphoria, it is frequently mistakenly classified as a stimulant rather than a depressant. This is because inhibitory synapses in the brain are depressed slightly earlier than are excitatory synapses with low doses of ethanol. Ethanol, however, acts as a sedative-hypnotic throughout the entire CNS. Usually, patients present with concomitant trauma or other medical problems with ethanol ingestion as an additional finding.

The acute ingestion of ethanol may result in decreased inhibitions, visual impairment, diplopia, nystagmus, muscular incoordination, slurred speech, ataxia, slowing of reaction time, tachycardia, vasodilatation, hypoglycemia (especially in children), stupor, and depression of the deep tendon reflexes. In severe stages, hypothermia, hypoventilation, hypotension, and cardiovascular collapse may be seen.

Blood ethanol concentrations after ingestion of ethanol are affected by the rate of absorption from the gastrointestinal tract, space of distribution in the body, and the rate of elimination. Ethyl alcohol is absorbed rapidly by diffusion mainly from the small intestine and to a lesser extent from the stomach and large intestine. Concentrations usually reach a peak 30 to 60 minutes after ingestion. There may be a delay if food is present in the stomach. The volume of distribution of ethanol is 0.6 L/kg, which is approximately equal to that of total body water so that ethanol diffuses freely in body tissues.

Ethanol metabolism occurs predominantly in the liver. Recent research, however, has identified the presence of alcoholic dehydrogenase in the gastric mucosa, where it acts as a first-pass mechanism.[4] Several hepatic enzyme systems participate in ethanol metabolism, converting it to acetaldehyde. The metabolism of ethanol occurs principally through oxidative metabolism in the liver by as many as three separate pathways. The alcohol dehydrogenase pathway is the predominant system and contains a number of isoenzymes that appear to account for the great variability in metabolism among individuals. The second pathway is the microsomal ethanol-oxidizing system located in the endoplasmic reticulum. The third system involves catalases located in the perioxisomes.

In most individuals, the range of metabolism of ethanol is in the range of 15 to 25 mg/dl per hour, regardless of the plasma concentration. Thirty milliliters (1 ounce) of 80-proof whiskey can be expected to raise a serum ethanol concentration by approximately 25 to 30 mg/dl in a 70-kg individual. A 12-ounce can of beer and a 4-ounce glass of wine will raise the ethanol as much as 1 ounce of liquor. In other words, it takes a 150-pound person approximately 1 hour to metabolize the amount of ethanol in 10 ounces of beer.

Because ethyl alcohol is rapidly absorbed from the stomach, its blood concentration is usually at or near maximum elevation shortly after ingestion.[1] Most authorities no longer hold that the rate of ethanol metabolism can be materially increased by the coadministration of other substances, such as fructose or other sugars, hormones, vitamins, or enzymatic co-factors. Intoxication from ethanol ingestion largely depends on how quickly a blood ethanol concentration has been achieved as well as on the length of time it has been maintained by continued oral consumption.[1,44]

Complications. Entire textbooks are devoted to the study and description of the substantial complications related to alcohol use. Some are life-threatening, many are not.[44,47] Those life-threatening complications related to alcohol abuse are delirium tremens, status epilepticus, major traumatic injuries, gastrointestinal bleeding, hepatic failure, suicidal ideation, CNS depression, alcoholic ketoacidosis, hypoglycemia, lactic acidosis, and hypomagnesemia.[44,48] All sedative-hypnotics potentiate ethanol's depressive effects, and those that the cytochrome p450 system metabolizes—such as the benzodiazepines or barbiturates—may produce fatal respiratory depression when combined with ethanol.[44]

Diagnosis and Treatment. When ethyl alcohol use is combined with multiple drug overdose, head injury, coma, major trauma, seizure, or psychosis, it is particularly important to obtain an ethanol concentration. The determination of serum ethanol concentration can be done in most hospital laboratories in 30 to 60 minutes. The most commonly used specimen for obtaining an ethanol level is the blood, although the breath and occasionally the urine may be used. Capillary and arterial blood most accurately indicate brain ethanol concentrations; venous blood lags slightly in ethanol content during the absorption distribution phase. The breath alcohol analyzer has been studied extensively and shown to be sufficiently accurate for clinical use.

Blood concentrations greater than 50 mg/dl (0.05%) may be associated with some impairment and concentrations greater than 100 mg/dl (0.1%) are generally used as a legal definition of intoxication. Interpretation of the physiologic effects of a particular blood alcohol concentration may be difficult, because there is such a wide variability among individuals. This is especially true in the individual who chronically ingests ethyl alcohol. It is not uncommon to see patients with blood alcohol levels in the range of 200 to 300 mg/dl whose impairment appears minimal on examination. This represents the typical findings in the chronic alcoholic who has built up a tolerance to ethanol. On the other hand, a low serum ethanol level (less than 50 mg/dl) is extremely useful in the evaluation of the CNS-depressed or "drunk"-appearing patient because it indicates another potentially serious cause for the CNS depression. Ethanol concentrations in the range of 100 to 250 mg/dl generally cause mental confusion, ataxia, nystagmus, exaggerated emotional state, and incoordination. The most fatal intoxications are associated with ethanol concentrations greater than 400 mg/dl, although the highest reported concentration in a survivor was 1510 mg/dl. Because alcohol is frequently consumed with other drugs for its CNS-sedating effects, a standard urine and serum toxicology screen should be obtained in any intoxicated patient with a clinical presentation or history suggesting concurrent drug consumption.

Other than hemodialysis, no proven method reverses acute ethanol intoxication despite numerous anecdotal reports of improvement with agents such as fructose, antithyroid agents, and naloxone.[44] Although the alcoholic provides the potential for a plethora of complications, the treatment of an acute ethanol ingestion is relatively straightforward. If the patient presents with an altered mental status, 2 mg of IV naloxone, 25 g of glucose and 100 mg of thiamine should be administered IM or IV. If the patient responds to the dextrose, a continuous infusion of 10% dextrose should be administered pending serum glucose results. Wernicke's encephalopathy, reversed by thiamine, has a 17% mortality rate. It consists of the triad of mental confusion, cerebellar ataxia, and oculomotor disturbances. Hypomagnesemia, common in the alcoholic, may cause thiamine resistance. Some sources therefore recommend the administration of 1 to 2 ml of 50% magnesium solution IM when thiamine is given.[44]

Unless ingestion of other drugs is suspected, gastric emptying is probably useful only if performed within 2 hours of ingestion. Conflicting reports have been made about the absorption of ethanol by charcoal. Some investigators reported no significant absorption, and others found moderate absorption.[44] If alveolar hypoventilation is present, a patent airway with supportive mechanical ventilation must be established. A diminished or absent gag reflex necessitates prophylactic intubation before gastric lavage. Correction of fluid deficits, acid/base disturbances, and hypothermia are important ancillary measures. Alcoholic ketoacidosis can be treated with glucose and saline. Insulin is not indicated, and bicarbonate therapy is usually not necessary. Status epilepticus is rare, and the differential diagnosis should include hypoglycemia, hypoxia, hyponatremia, hypomagnesemia, hypocalcemia, trauma, subdural and CNS infections, and cerebrovascular accidents.[44] Diazepam is the treatment of choice, although lorazepam may be advantageous secondary to its increased duration of action and the fact that it is not metabolized by the liver.[44] Hypotension generally responds well to volume replacement unless it is due to unsuspected causes such as occult trauma.

Admission Criteria. Most symptomatic ethanol ingestions do not require hospital admission. Once an adequate period of observation has been undertaken in the emergency department (usually 4 to 6 hours), the patient can be discharged to a responsible adult. Admission guidelines for the intoxicated patient need to be flexible. Suspected or apparent trauma, persistent CNS depression, gastrointestinal bleeding, impending delirium tremens, or abnormal vital signs are the clinical situations most often requiring admission. ICU admission is generally reserved for patients with unstable gastrointestinal bleeding, full-blown or impending delerium tremens, traumatic injuries, pulmonary aspiration, fulminant hepatic failure, or the septic, intoxicated patient.

Alcohol Withdrawal. The DSM-III lists no less than seven ethanol-induced organic brain syndromes: two intoxication disorders and five withdrawal syndromes.[44] Because of the widespread abuse of ethyl alcohol, withdrawal from chronic ethanol consumption is commonly encountered in the emergency department, in-patient unit, and ICU. Any hospitalized patient who develops altered mental status with sympathetic symptoms such as diaphoresis, tachycardia, hypertension, tachypnea, or severe tremors should be evaluated for drug withdrawal from ethanol or sedative-hypnotics. Ethanol is a cellular depressant, so with its abrupt cessation, rebound neuronal hyperexcitability occurs, the severity of which is directly related to the amount of ethyl alcohol that was regularly consumed by the alcoholic patient. These withdrawal symptoms begin within 12 to 24 hours after cessation of ethanol ingestion and may last for 48 to 72 hours.

The following independent clinical syndromes are associated with ethanol withdrawal:

- Tremors
- Hallucinations
- Seizures
- Delirium tremens[44,49]

The early stages of ethanol withdrawal are characterized by autonomic nervous system hyperactivity manifested by tachycardia and hypertension, diaphoresis, generalized tremulousness, insomnia, and irritability. Most patients experiencing acute alcohol withdrawal do not require pharmacologic intervention. In the early stages of alcohol withdrawal, patients may have a mild disorientation of their sense of time with some impairment of memory. A small percentage, however, may develop severe complications requiring treatment. Complications of severe untreated alcohol withdrawal may include significant dysrhythmia or hypertension, seizures, hallucinations, and delirium tremens. Delirium tremens is the most advanced state of alcohol withdrawal and includes hallucinatory behavior associated with severe tremors and autonomic hyperactivity. This stage occurs 2 to 3 days after cessation or marked curtailment of alcohol consumption and may last 3 to 5 days. The most significant complications occur during this phase and may include seizures, dysrhythmia, and hyperthermia and may ultimately lead to cardiovascular collapse. Table 69-8 lists the three clinical phases of the alcohol withdrawal syndrome and the treatment of these phases. Alcohol withdrawal seizures are almost always grand mal and may be solitary or recurrent and usually respond to anticonvulsant therapies such as IV benzodiazepines. Ninety percent of patients have initiation and termination of these seizures 7 to 48 hours after abstinence from alcohol. Many patients with alcohol withdrawal seizures are also treated with phenytoin, which is of questionable efficacy. The development of status epilepticus has a high morbidity, and mortality and should be aggressively treated.[44]

Benzodiazepines are now considered one of the safest classes of compounds for the treatment of alcohol withdrawal. The benzodiazepines not only are effective in suppressing the withdrawal symptoms and in treating or preventing seizures but are also exceptionally safe because of their minimal respiratory and cardiac depression.[44] Lorazepam (Ativan) can be given in a dose of 0.5 to 4.0 mg IV every 15 to 30 minutes or 0.97 mg/kg IM for excess sympathetic symptoms. Once the acute symptoms have resolved, 6 to 7 mg/kg per day can be administered orally in three divided doses. Diazepam (Valium) in a dose of 5 mg IV every 5 minutes is an alternative. Doses of the benzodiazepines in these patients is highly variable, and massive doses as high as 2335 mg per 48 hours of diazepam, have been reported in the treatment of delirium tremens. In the ICU the ultra-short-acting drug midazolam (Versed) is attractive and can be administered in doses ranging as high as 20 to 75 mg per hour for control of symptoms. Haloperidol should be used in those patients not responding to benzodiazepines. It can be given IV, IM, or orally with a total safe dose not to exceed 480 mg per 8 hours. Clonidine and beta blockers have also been used in the alcohol withdrawal syndrome but are less desirable than the benzodiazepines.[44]

Sedative-Hypnotics

The use of depressant compounds is as old as the use of alcohol. Sedative-hypnotic compounds are drugs that may have diverse chemical structures but have in common their ability to induce various degrees of behavioral depression. Hypnotics are used to produce sleep, and sedatives are used to relieve anxiety, restlessness, irritability, and tension. Often, no sharp distinction exists between the two effects, and the same drug may exhibit both actions, depending on the method of use and the dose. Other terms to describe these drugs include minor tranquilizers, anxiolytic drugs, and antianxiety drugs.

Sedative-hypnotics may be categorized into one of three main types:

- Barbiturates
- Nonbarbiturate nonbenzodiazepines
- Benzodiazepines

Drugs in the first two classes have a greater potential for serious systemic reactions than those in the last group.[1] As with narcotics, there are two areas of concern: the management of the overdose patient, and the management of the withdrawal state, which is recognized as a medical emergency more serious than that of any drug abuse.

Table 69-8. Ethanol Withdrawal Syndrome: Three Phases

	Characteristics	Treatment
Phase 1	Mild-to-moderate dependency: onset 8–24 hr after ethanol, psychomotor agitation, tremors, anxiety, apprehension, weakness, nausea, vomiting	Thiamine, 100 mg IM Lorazepam, 1–2 mg t.i.d. p.o. Phenergan, 25–50 mg IM (p.r.n, nausea/vomiting) Glucose, 25 g IV
Phase 2	Moderate-to-severe dependency: onset 12–24 hr after phase one severe tremors, fever, diaphoresis, muscle cramps, tachycardia, HBP, dramatic change to respiratory alkalosis from metabolic acidosis, insomnia, extreme agitation	Thiamine, 100 mg IV Lorazepam, 2 mg t.i.d. p.o. (taper by 20% every day) Haloperidol, 5 mg q30 minutes (p.r.n. agitation not responding to lorazepam) Glucose 25 g IV
Phase 3	Indicative of physical dependence manifestations: delirium tremens 2–4 days of cessation of drinking, severe tremors, diaphoresis, confusion disorientation, extreme agitation, panic, delusions, paranoia, hallucinations, muscle spasms, myoclonic jerks can progress to grand mal seizures	Thiamine, 100 mg IV Lorazepam, 0.5–4 mg IV (q15–30 min) or Midazolam, 1–3 mg IV Haloperidol, 5 mg q30 minutes p.r.n. Glucose, 25 g IV MVI, 5 ml/L of fluid

HBP, Hypertension; IM, intramuscular; IV, intravenous; MVI, multivitamin intravenous.

Barbiturates were first synthesized in 1864. They have had wide use as tranquilizers, anticonvulsants, and preoperative sedatives. They have also become popular drugs of abuse and are known on the street as "yellow jackets," "reds" and "barbs."[50] Patterns of abuse vary from intermittent recreational use to compulsive daily use with chronic intoxication.

The nonbarbiturate, nonbenzodiazene group comprises four major drugs:

- Chloral hydrate
- Glutethimide
- Methaqualone
- Ethchlorvynol

Of these drugs, glutethimide is popular when mixed with codeine and is known on the street in this combination as "loads," "4s and doors," or "set ups." Injected, it provides a euphoria equivalent to heroin. Although most manufacturers have suspended the manufacture of methaqualone, street forms are still available. Ethchlorvynol is known on the street as "Mr. Green Jeans," "pickles," or "jelly beans." It is a frequently abused drug with a small margin of safety. Chloral hydrate is rarely abused.[1]

The first benzodiazepine was introduced in 1960. These drugs are currently the drugs of choice for the pharmacologic treatment of anxiety because of their low lethality even when taken in massive doses and the fact that they rarely interfere with the metabolism of other drugs the patient may be taking. When alcohol or other CNS depressants are not used concomitantly, the benzodizepines are the safest of all currently available antianxiety and hypnotic drugs. Although they appear to have a low potential for abuse, these drugs are used by more Americans than any other single prescription drug. Benzodiazepines are used to treat sleep disorders, anxiety, alcohol withdrawal, and seizure disorders. They are also administered as anesthetics and before surgery. The wide margin of safety of benzodiazepines permits their use in numerous clinical situations.[1,2]

Signs and Symptoms. Low doses of the sedative-hypnotics produce mild sedation. In large amounts these drugs produce a state of intoxication similar to that induced by ethanol and, in addition, can produce sedation, tranquilization, hypnosis, and anesthesia. In high doses, it is a main cause of morbidity from resulting coma and apnea. Tolerance to the intoxicating effects develops rapidly and may lead to a progressive narrowing of the margin of safety between the intoxicating and lethal dose of the drug. Chronic drug abusers may be able to increase their daily dose up to 10 to 20 times the recommended therapeutic dose.

Toxic reactions from the sedative-hypnotics involve a general slowing of mental functions, slurred speech, ataxia, and impairment of thinking, including poor comprehension, memory disturbance, increased reaction time, poor judgment, limited attention span, labile mood, and release of aggressive impulses. In large doses, sleep, stupor, coma, and death from circulatory and respiratory depression are possible.[51]

Barbiturates can produce all levels of CNS depression from mild sedation to hypnosis to deep coma and death. Lipid solubility of the barbiturates is a dominant factor in their distribution throughout the body. The more lipid soluble the barbiturate, the more rapid the onset of its action, the shorter duration of its effects, and the greater the degree of its hypnotic activity. The degree of CNS depression depends on the dose, route of administration, and pharmacokinetics of the particular barbiturate. Mild-to-moderate barbiturate intoxication may mimic the clinical picture of alcohol intoxication. The neurologic examination may reveal general inco-ordination with nystagmus, slurred speech, dysmetria, and ataxia. Other signs and symptoms include disorientation, sleeplessness, flaccid muscles, decreased reflexes, hypotension, shock, pulmonary edema, and pneumonia. Overdose of short-acting barbiturates such as pentobarbital has the highest mortality rate. A lethal dose of barbiturates varies but is generally about 10 times greater than the hypnotic dose if it is taken within a short period, such as 3 hours.[1,2]

Special clinical features of barbiturate overdose are barbiturate blisters.[1] These were first described about 50 years ago, and although blisters do not affect the outcome of a barbiturate-intoxicated patient, they can be of considerable diagnostic importance. They can appear as early as 4 hours after ingestion and do not necessarily occur over areas of maximum pressure; rather, they most often occur where skin surfaces have been in contact with each other. These lesions are usually multiple and consist of erythematous, indurated, irregular patches progressing to bulbus lesions. Although the precise mechanism of these lesions is unknown, a local toxic effect has been postulated.[1]

All the drugs in the **nonbarbiturate-nonbenzodiazepine** group (chloral hydrate, glutethimide, methaqualone, and ethchlorvynol) share the same potential for CNS depression including drowsiness, hypotension, hypothermia, lethargy, respiratory depression, and stupor. In addition, each of the drugs has additional specific areas of organ system compromise.

A feature of the benzodiazepine class is their selective action on the CNS. The changes induced by these drugs on peripheral functions are the result of their action on the CNS. The molecular effect of benzodiazepines is indirectly to enhance or facilitate the inhibitory neuronal properties of gamma-aminobutyric acid (GABA), now recognized as the most important inhibitory neurotransmitter in the CNS. The benzodiazepines can produce all levels of CNS depression, from mild sedation to hypnosis and coma.[1,2]

In addition, the benzodiazepines suppress the spread of seizure activity but do not abolish the abnormal discharge from the seizure focus in epileptics. In therapeutic amounts, the benzodiazepines produce sedation and relief of anxiety and, at higher doses, muscle relaxation. When taken alone, massive quantities of benzodiazepines can be ingested with little or no risk of prolonged CNS depression. An overdose of benzodiazepines alone is rarely fatal, although the combination of benzodiazepines and alcohol has been lethal, however.[52]

Symptoms of overdose of the benzodiazepines include drowsiness, ataxia, dizziness, delirium, somnolence, confusion, and occasionally aggression. Hypotension and respiratory depression rarely occur. If deep coma with marked hypotension or cardiovascular collapse is clinically present, the clinician should suspect concomitant ingestion of another CNS depressant.

Complications. Overdose of the sedative-hypnotics produces CNS depression ranging from mild drowsiness and sleep to coma and death. Respiratory depression may progress to Cheyne-Stokes respiration and apnea. Hypothermia results from the depression of the temperature-regulating mechanism in the hypothalamus. Patients with a severe overdose often experience typical shock syndrome such as apnea along with circulatory collapse.

Barbiturates may have a direct toxic effect in the myocardium, but large doses are required to achieve this effect. In addition, vasomotor tone of the smaller peripheral blood vessels may be reduced, with extravasation of fluid into the extravascular space leading to hypotension and shock. Serious complications from barbiturate overdose include pulmonary complications such as aspiration, pneumonia, and pulmonary edema. In addition, acute tubular necrosis with subsequent hypotension, hypovolemia, and cerebral edema have also been reported. A severe overdose of barbiturates can also cause hypotension, profound shock and ventilatory depression, coma, and death as a result of cardioventilatory failure from depression of the vital medually centers.

Cardiac dysrhythmia in **chloral hydrate** overdose can occur and is manifested by atrial fibrillation, PVCs, torsade de pointes, and ventricular tachycardia.[1] Chloral hydrate is irritating to the gastric mucosa, and gastric necrosis with gastrointestinal hemorrhage has occurred after intoxicating doses. In addition, hepatotoxicity and renal failure may occur. **Glutethimide** overdose can manifest itself with significant anticholinergic effects such as hypotension, tachycardia, and urinary retention. A prominent feature of glutethimide is a characteristic fluctuation in level of consciousness, which may be due to the formation of metabolites but may also include further absorption of the parent compound from the gastrointestinal tract after recovery from the ileus.[1] In addition, continued enterohepatic circulation of glutethimide and its metabolites and ongoing release of the drug from body fat may contribute to the fluctuating sensorium. **Methaqualone** overdose can also cause paradoxic CNS stimulation with muscle hypertonicity, myoclonus, seizures, hyperreflexia, and restlessness. In addition, it can cause bleeding and blistering.[1] Some patients have experienced necrotizing cystitis manifested by painful hematuria after injection of methaqualone purchased on the street. This reaction is believed to be due to orthotoluidine, which is a contaminant of these street drugs. **Ethchlorvynol** overdose can cause hematologic side effects including hemolysis, pancytopenia, and thrombocytopenia. In addition, noncardiogenic pulmonary edema and peripheral neuropathy have been described with ethchlorvynol overdose. A large number of patients with ethchlorvynol overdose by either IV or oral routes have developed noncardiogenic acute pulmonary edema with marked hypotension.[53]

Diagnosis and Treatment. Serum barbiturate concentration is not regarded as an important indicator of the severity of poisoning, because it is not necessarily related to the clinical state. It also has little prognostic value in determining the depth or duration of coma. Such determinations may be of benefit, however, in determining the cause of coma and can distinguish short- from long-acting agents. In assessing the patient with suspected barbiturate poisoning, the serum concentration should always be considered in relation to the patient's history and clinical condition at the time of drug sampling. The clinical status of the patient supersedes the absolute drug level in importance when treatment decisions need to be made.

Single values of the plasma concentration of many of the benzodiazepines and the nonbarbiturate, nonbenzodiazepine class of drugs are not closely related to their therapeutic or toxin effects, because of the presence of metabolites as well as other factors. Qualitative laboratory analysis may be useful to confirm a particular ingestion, but quantitation is rarely of any benefit in the clinical management or as a predictor of outcome in these patients.

As for many of the substances of abuse, no antidote exists, so the treatment of barbiturate overdose consists mainly of supportive therapy. Because most deaths are due to respiratory causes, attention to the airway is an immediate priority. Maintenance of adequate airway, administration of oxygen and assisted respirations, if necessary, are extremely important. If you think an endotracheal tube is needed, perform the procedure if there is no improvement with 2 mg of naloxone. Analeptic agents have no role, because they may result in severe CNS and cardiac toxicity. Measures to remove the remaining material from the gastrointestinal tract by ipecac or lavage followed by administration of activated charcoal should be instituted. Fluids should be administered for blood pressure support or for diuresis, if necessary. Often, the blood pressure may return to normal after dehydration has been corrected and adequate ventilation has been restored. Vasoconstrictors are usually not necessary for blood pressure support, and fluid administration is usually adequate to correct even severe hypotension.

Multiple doses of activated charcoal are of great benefit for phenobarbital overdose by decreasing the half-life of the drug, enhancing the elimination, and shortening the duration of coma.[1] Fifty to 100 g of charcoal can be administered either orally or through a nasogastric tube every 4 to 6 hours. Activated charcoal, by absorbing phenobarbital in the gastrointestinal tract, sets up a gradient differential that causes phenobarbital to diffuse from the blood into the bowel, where it is subsequently absorbed by the charcoal. In addition to its direct absorptive properties, activated charcoal significantly shortens the elimination half-life and increases total body nonrenal clearance of the drug. The effectiveness of this procedure is comparable to forced alkaline diuresis or dialysis, and it can be promptly and safely initiated.

Urinary alkalinization promotes ionization of barbiturates, which prevents tubular reabsorption and thus traps the drug in the kidney for excretion. An alkaline diuresis may be useful in enhancing the excretion of the long-acting barbiturates (phenobarbital, barbital) and drugs that are converted to phenobarbital in the body (primodone and mephobarbital). It is ineffective for the short- or intermediate-acting barbiturates. The goal of alkaline diuresis is to obtain a urine pH of 7.5 to 8.5. It can be accomplished by administering 500 ml per hour of D5 + 0.5 NS with 20 to 30 mEq/L of sodium bicarbonate. Diuresis can be accomplished by the administration of mannitol, 20 to 100 g IV, or furosemide, 20 to 40 mg IV. Although an alkaline diuresis removes reasonable amounts of these long-acting barbiturates, it should be reserved for the severely poisoned patient, because risks are associated with this procedure.[1]

Hemodialysis and, to a lesser extent, peritoneal dialysis, also remove long-acting barbiturates in a severely poisoned patient. Hemoperfusion has also been shown to decrease the duration of coma-caused long-acting barbiturates. Indications for hemodialysis or hemoperfusion are stage 4 Coma with high plasma levels of phenobarbital (more than 10 mg/dl) or the ingestion of a short-acting barbiturate with elevated levels (more than 5 mg/dl) not responding to intensive supportive care. Extracorporeal measures should be used only if other measures are unsuccessful or in patients with impaired drug elimination that is due to renal failure. These methods should be necessary only in rare cases. Recovery time and length of obtundation are difficult, if not impossible to predict, which is due to the frequency of co-drug ingestion, especially ethanol as well as recurrent and secondary absorption from concretions and short-acting versus long-acting substances.

Treatment for overdose of the nonbarbiturate, nonbenzodiazepine class of drugs is directed toward supporting the patient and consists of attempts to remove the drug by emesis or lavage even many hours after ingestion because of the prolonged time many of these drugs can remain in the gastrointestinal tract. Concretions in the gastrointestinal tract may also form from a large amount of glutethimide and ethchlorvynol and be responsible for prolonged intoxication.[1] Because glutethimide is commonly taken in association with codeine, 2 mg of IV naloxone should be used for CNS or respiratory depression in this overdose. Lidocaine or propanol may be used to treat ventricular tachydysrhythmias. If torsade de pointes is present, overdrive pacing, isoproterenol, or atropine may be effective. Diuresis, dialysis, and hemoperfusion are not helpful. In glutethimide overdose, the question of effectiveness of multiple-dose activated charcoal remains unanswered. The known enterohepatic circulation of some of the metabolites of glutethimide suggests that continued administration of activated charcoal may be of benefit.[1] Care should be taken not to overtreat the ethchlorvynol patient with fluids, because this may increase the likelihood of pulmonary edema. Hypotension responds to cautious administration of crystalloid fluid boluses or pressors.[53]

At the present time in the United States, the treatment for benzodiazepine overdose is supportive. Even after a significant overdose of benzodiazepines, mechanical ventilation is not usually required, although, rarely, coma may persist for up to 3 days. Diuresis, dialysis, and hemoperfusion are not useful. Several "antidotes" have been found to selectively block the interaction of benzodiazepines with their specific receptors in the central nervous system. Most clinical investigations have studied the imidazo-benzodiazepine derivative called Ro 15-1788. Outside the United States, the drug has been marketed as Flumazenil. When this compound was administered in patient trials, patients whose symptoms were due to benzodiazepines only were fully awake and alert within 1 to 2 minutes.[1,54] In many of these patients, CNS depression developed 1 to 4 hours after administration because of the relatively short half-life of the compound ($t\frac{1}{2}$ = 55 minutes). No adverse effects and no acute withdrawal symptoms were observed.[1,54] The true clinical impact of these agents may be minimal, because supportive care alone is usually successful. Their greatest value may lie in their diagnostic ability to "wake up" a suspected benzodiazepine-overdosed patient when toxicologic confirmation is not available.

ICU Admission Criteria. Because of the benzodiazepines' large therapeutic margin of safety, it is extremely rare to have to admit a patient with a "pure" benzodiazepine overdose. More commonly patients with a barbiturate or glutethimide or ethchlorvynol overdose are admitted to the ICU because of the potentially serious side effects of these drugs. Clearly, patients who require airway support through mechanical ventilation, patients in whom "pulse" or frequent doses of activated charcoal are deemed necessary, or patients in renal failure that may require the sophistication of hemodialysis or peritoneal dialysis, or anyone in whom urinary alkalization or acidification is deemed necessary should be admitted. Also, persistent CNS depression after 4 to 6 hours of observation in the emergency department warrants ICU admission.

Sedative-Hypnotic Withdrawal. The abrupt cessation or reduction of high dose sedative hypnotics may result in a characteristic withdrawal syndrome that closely resembles the alcohol withdrawal syndrome.[1,2,55] This withdrawal syndrome should be recognized as a medical emergency that may be more serious than that of most other drugs of abuse.[1,2,55,56] Long-term intoxication with the equivalent of 600 to 800 mg of pentobarbital or secobarbital is sufficient to produce clinically significant physical dependency. The equivalent doses of any of the other sedatives-hypnotics may also cause a severe abstinence syndrome, ranging from tremulousness and irritability, to seizures, delirium, and death. Short-acting barbiturates, such as pentobarbital and secobarbital and the short-acting benzodiazepines such as triazolam, produce an acute withdrawal syndrome similar to that of ethanol. The long-acting barbiturates as well as benzodiazepines have a delayed onset of withdrawal symptoms, beginning 48 to 72 hours after the last dose with a prolonged clinical course of withdrawal.[1,2,56]

The first symptoms after drug withdrawal may first be seen in 12 to 16 hours with symptoms of apprehension and weakness, tremors, insomnia, diaphoresis, and restlessness composing the clinical picture. Vomiting and abdominal cramps may develop. With severe withdrawal, major symptoms and neurologic manifestations appear as well as orthostatic hypotension and seizures. Myoclonic muscular contractions, spasmodic jerking of the extremities, and grand mal seizures may develop, sometimes leading to status epilepticus. Often, after a seizure, hallucinations and delirium may develop. The hallucinations are usually auditory and may be indistinguishable from those of delirium tremors associated with alcohol withdrawal. Symptoms usually peak during the second or third day of abstinence from the short-acting barbiturates or meprobamate. This symptom peak may be delayed until the seventh or eighth day of abstinence from long-acting barbiturates or some of the benzodiazepines. During this peak period the major withdrawal symptoms usually occur. Because of the serious nature of the withdrawal from sedative-hypnotics, patients should be admitted and placed under experienced medical supervision.[1,2,55,56] Specific treatment of the withdrawal state consists of replacing the sedative-hypnotic with a short- or long-acting barbiturate and gradually tapering this dose over a time under close clinical observation. Major symptoms can be treated with diazepam, 5 to 10 mg IV every 5 to 10 minutes or pentobarbital, 120 mg IV over 20 minutes and repeated in 10 to 15 minutes if necessary. Generally, diazepam is repeated to a total of 40 mg and pentobarbital can be repeated one time to produce results. Minor symptoms can be treated with 120 mg of pentobarbital orally or 20 mg of diazepam every 2 hours until signs of intoxication (drowsiness, ataxia, nystagmus) are apparent or until 1000 mg of pentobarbital or 100 mg of diazepam is reached. The dose should then be diminished by 30 mg per day of pentobarbital or 10 mg per day of diazepam. No drug has been found to be effective in seizure prophylaxis.

Opioids

Narcotic drugs can be divided into three groups: natural, semisynthetic, and synthetic. The naturally occurring narcotics include opium, morphine, codeine, and thebaine. Of these, only morphine and codeine are of clinical significance. Narcotics are opiates that are substances that are isolated from the opium poppy. Narcotics also include the semisynthetic opium derivatives, all of which produce tolerance and can suppress narcotic withdrawal. Narcotics include any drug that can be substituted for heroin or morphine for the abuser.

The semisynthetic narcotics include heroin, hydromorphone, oxycodone, and oxymorphone. These are produced from minor chemical alterations of the poppy plant. Hydromorphone (Dilaudid) is a pure narcotic agonist and a strong analgesic used in the relief of moderate-to-severe pain. It has twice the potency of morphine and a more rapid onset and shorter duration of action than morphine. It has more sedative and less euphoriant properties than morphine. Because of its greater potency, hydromorphone is a highly abused drug that is much sought after by narcotic addicts.

Oxycodone is similar in effect to codeine but is more potent and thus has a higher dependence potential. It is available only in combination products. It is used to relieve moderate-to-moderately severe pain. Addicts take this drug orally as Percodan or Tylox or dissolve the tablets in water, filter out the insoluble material, and "mainline" the active drug by IV injection.

Meperidine (Demerol) is a pure narcotic agonist and was the first synthetic narcotic. It was initially synthesized as a substitute for atropine because of its anticholinergic effects.

Methadone (Dolophione) is a pure opiate agonist structurally similar to propoxyphene and was first synthesized by German scientists during World War II because of a shortage of morphine. It is, along with heroin, one of the most frequently abused narcotics. It is used mainly in detoxification programs for maintenance treatment of opiate addicts.

Pentazocine (Talwin) is a synthetic opiate agonist with a very weak antagonistic effect. It was initially developed with the intention of producing an analgesic with the potency of an opiate but with less potential for addiction because of its mixed agonist-antagonist properties.

Fentanyl is an opiate agonist related to the phenylpiperidines and is an ingredient in Sublimaze. It was first introduced in 1968 as an IV analgesic anesthetic. Fentanyl is estimated to be 50 to 100 times more potent as an analgesic than morphine. A methyl analog of fentanyl produced in clandestine laboratories has been sold along the West Coast as "super heroin." Methyl-fentanyl, known as "China White" is a synthetic opioid that may be as much as 200 times more potent than heroin and 2000 times more potent than morphine. It was the first of more than 10 "designer drugs" to appear on the street.[2,57]

A major use of opioids is for relief of intense pain. Typically, these drugs suppress perception of pain and reduce the response to pain without causing loss of consciousness. Opioids interact with specific receptors in the CNS to inhibit activity of pain fibers. The opioid receptors are distributed throughout the central and peripheral nervous systems and in the gastrointestinal tract. Five main receptor sites have been identified: mu, kappa, delta, sigma, and epsilon. Of these, the mu, kappa, and delta receptors mediate analgesics, with the mu receptor considered the most important for supraspinal analgesia. The toxic effects of opiates such as hypothermia, hypotension, and bradycardia are mediated through stimulation of the mu and kappa receptors.[2]

Narcotics are also used as cough suppressants by their direct suppression of the cough centers in the medulla, to treat diarrhea, and to treat cardiogenic pulmonary edema. The opioids are also used preoperatively for sedation and as a supplement to anesthesia.

Signs and Symptoms. Clinical effects of opioids include euphoria as well as drowsiness, apathy, lethargy, and sedation. In addition, nausea and vomiting, constipation, miosis, sleep, and respiratory depression are seen. Respiratory rate is an unreliable measure of intoxication because opiates cause decreases in tidal volume before the respiratory rate is affected. The presence of shallow respirations rather than bradypnea should be carefully sought.[2,17] Large doses of some opiate agonists may induce excitation and seizures. Nausea and vomiting are caused by stimulation of the chemoreceptor trigger zone in the medulla oblongata. Noncardiogenic pulmonary edema is a well-documented side effect of opiate and, in particular, heroin ingestion, occurring in as many as 48% of cases. Although the precise mechanism is unknown, pulmonary edema may occur in less than 2 hours following heroin ingestion and within 6 to 12 hours following methadone ingestion.[2]

Although codeine is a naturally occurring ingredient of raw opium, most of it is produced from morphine. Codeine is a pure opiate agonist approximately 20% as potent as morphine and is metabolized by enzymes in the liver to morphine, which then enters the brain and accounts for the pharmacologic actions of the drug. Codeine has great use as an analgesic and the relief of mild-to-moderate pain that is not alleviated by nonopioid agonists. It is also used extensively as an antitussive. It is in its role as an antitussive that codeine is most frequently abused. The most frequent adverse effects of codeine use are gastrointestinal with reported abdominal pain, cramping, constipation, and occasional nausea and vomiting. Fatal intoxications are rare but have occurred. Deaths are more common when codeine is mixed with analgesics, antihistamines, or sedatives and are usually from respiratory depression. Codeine is more stimulating to the spinal cord than other narcotics, and as a result, seizures may occur during coma.

Meperidine toxicity includes seizures, myoclonus, CNS stimulation, jitteriness, and tremors. These signs generally appear after several days of use and are due either to the anticholinergic activity of the compound or the accumulation of normeperidine, its only active metabolite. Meperidine differs from other narcotics in that it does not cause miosis and, in fact, may cause mydriasis or pupillary changes secondary to its anticholinergic effect.[1,2]

A single dose of methadone produces less sedation and euphoria than morphine but has an extended duration of action (4 to 6 hours). Because of this longer duration of action, depressant effects after overdosage may continue for 36 to 48 hours.

Propoxyphene is a pure opiate agonist that is structurally similar to methadone and contains the phenylpiperidine complex found in all narcotic analgesics. It is a weaker analgesic than codeine or salicylate in single doses and is solely available as an oral preparation. Propoxyphene is an extremely dangerous drug because only 15 or 20 capsules can cause death.[1,2] It also has the potential for inducing seizures and cardiac dysrhythmia in addition to its typical narcotic effects. Conduction defects described include transient bundle branch block, QRS prolongation, bigeminy, and nonspecific S- and ST-wave changes.[2] Acute toxicity from propoxyphene overdose may result in symptoms similarly to those of acute opium intoxication. These include miosis, coma, respiratory depression, circulatory collapse, and pulmonary edema. Seizures, dysrhythmia, and bundle branch block occur frequently shortly after ingestion with propoxyphene and can be life-threatening. Although naloxone is effective as an antidote, large dosages may be necessary. In addition, the action of propoxyphene may outlast that of naloxone, necessitating frequent repeated doses of naloxone to sustain a positive therapeutic effect. Naloxone will not reverse propoxyphene-induced cardiac toxicity that occurs secondary to local membrane anesthetic action rather than from an opioid mechanism.[2]

The most common side effect of Talwin (pentazocine) is sedation with subsequent diaphoresis and dizziness. In an abuse situation, pentazocine is often combined with an antihistamine known as tripelennamine to form a street substitute for heroin known as "Ts and Blues" that is injected intravenously. Microemboli from microcrystalline cellulose and talc from this combination can cause seizures, pulmonary hypertension, septic emboli, and CVAs.[2,16]

Fentanyl-specific mu-receptor agonists have a 90-second onset of action after injection with a 30- to 60-minute duration of effect. Because of the extreme potency of fentanyl and that of its analog, 3-methyl fentanyl, small mistakes in dilution cause near instant death from respiratory depression. Some fatal abusers have been found with the needle still in their vein.[2] The most common route of administration of fentanyl is IV; however, smoking and insufflation of fentanyl are growing in popularity. Large doses of naloxone may be required as an antidote.

Butorphanol (Stadol) is a partial agonist that is structurally related to morphine but pharmacologically similar to pentazocine. The analgesic activity of butorphanol is four to seven times that of morphine. Because the drug does not suppress the abstinence syndrome and may actually induce withdrawal in opiate-dependent patients, it cannot be substituted for an opiate agonist in the addicted individual without prior detoxification.[1,2]

Complications. The main complications of opiate abuse involve CNS and respiratory depression. Urgent airway support with intubation and mechanical ventilation may be necessary if symptoms are not reversed with 2 to 4 mg IV of naloxone. Noncardiogenic pulmonary edema can also be seen with as little as a single IV injection of an opiate.[2] Intravenous pentazocine abusers can develop type I membranoproliferative glomerulonephritis.[2] Other complications such as endocarditis, hepatitis, and AIDS as well as skin abscesses are found in the individuals favoring IV injection, particularly with shared needles.[1,2,14] Common complications of IV drug abuse can be found in Table 69-2 and 69-3. Specific medical complications associated with opiate abuse are found in Table 69-9.

Diagnosis and Treatment. There is usually no indication for determining exact serum concentrations of opiates. Quantitative acetaminophen and salicylate levels should be checked in all opiate-intoxicated patients because propoxyphene, oxycodone, and codeine preparations are frequently combined with either substance and consumed by the abuser. A qualitative drug screen can help determine which opiate is present, whether any additional unsuspected drugs were consumed, and the half-life of the narcotic drug that is useful in predicting the duration

Tabloe 69-9. Specific Medical Complications Associated With Opiate Ingestion

Noncardiogenic pulmonary edema
   Heroin
   Methadone
   Propoxyphene
Generalized seizures
   Propoxyphene (large ingestion)
   Intravenous fentanyl and sufentanil
   Prolonged use of meperidine
   Pentazocine overdose
   Neonates: opioid withdrawal
   High doses of intravenous morphine
Acute rhabdomyolysis
   Heroin
   Methadone
   Propoxyphene

of pharmacologically induced symptoms. The clinical presentation of the patient dictates the urgency of treatment.

The classic triad for acute opiate intoxication is symmetric pinpoint pupils, depressed respiratory rate, and coma.[1,2] In addition, cardiovascular effects and pulmonary edema may be present. The differential diagnosis of decreased mental status and miosis includes overdose of clonidine, organophosphates, or carbamates, phenothizines, PCP, sedative-hypnotics, and pontine hemorrhage. Clonidine ingestion, particularly in children, most closely resembles opiate overdose.[2] The onset of CNS-depressant effects may occur immediately after IV administration of the opiate. Normally, opiate-induced miosis is presumed to be due to an excitatory effect of the drug on the autonomic segment of the ocular motor nerve. This effect may be antagonized by an anticholinergic drug such as atropine and may be absent in meperidine ingestion.[1,2] Therefore, if a patient's pupils are dilated or normal, opiate ingestion cannot be ruled out. Causes of dilated or normal pupil in opiate overdose follow:[2]

- Meperidine, morphine, or propoxyphene
- Hypoxia
- Early stages of diphenoxylate hydrochloride with atropine sulfate (Lomotil) poisoning
- After naloxone use
- Co-ingestants with sympathomimetic or anticholinergic effects

Treatment of an overdose of any narcotic includes support of the patient's airway and establishing an IV line. Two milligrams of naloxone should be administered and repeated until the respiratory rate and the mental status are normal or near normal. Naloxone offers the dual advantage of providing both a diagnostic and therapeutic test. Naloxone is more potent than most agonists except when given to patients who have ingested fentanyl or one of its derivative. A given quantity of naloxone can reverse 10 to 100 times the amount of opioids. The effects of 25 mg of heroin can be blocked by as small a dose as 1 mg of naloxone.[2] Naloxone can be administered IM or sublingually or given via endotracheal tube if IV access cannot be established. As much as 4 mg/kg of naloxone has been given safely in humans.[2] If greater than the customary 2-mg dose of naloxone is required to reverse CNS and respiratory symptoms, the following drug identities should be considered: codeine, diphenoxylate, propoxyphene, pentazocine, butorphanol, buprenorphine, and nalbuphine.[2] If a continuous infusion of naloxone is required to maintain clinical effect, two thirds of the amount needed to reverse respiratory depression should be administered hourly by continuous IV infusion.[2] In an adult, 12 mg of naloxone in 1 L of D5W or crystalloid at 100 ml per hour provides a reasonable starting dose.[17]

If the offending drug is taken orally, attempts to retrieve the material should be performed. A gastric lavage should be conducted, and the patient should be prophylactically intubated if the gag reflex is absent or diminished. Treatment of noncardiogenic pulmonary edema includes support of respirations and oxygen and careful attention to fluid balance by Swan-Ganz catheterization. Positive end expiratory pressure can be added to mechanical ventilation but is seldom necessary. Minimization of IV fluids as well as supplemental oxygenation is necessary. Response is usually dramatic, and physical findings clear within 1 day with radiographic changes returning to normal within 72 to 96 hours. No evidence suggests that dialysis, diuresis, or hemoperfusion are beneficial.[1,2]

Admission Criteria. Any patient presenting with a sustained depressed level of consciousness from an opiate ingestion should be admitted. In addition, any patient requiring the administration of naloxone for therapeutic reasons such as pulmonary hypoventilation should be admitted for observation and serial airway evaluations. Coma, respiratory failure requiring intubation, suspicion of noncardiogenic pulmonary edema, or seizures are all obvious reasons justifying ICU admission.

Special Considerations. 1-Methyl-4-phenyl-4-propionoxy-piperidine (MPPP) is a little known derivative of meperidine that has been used in the manufacture of industrial chemicals. It has recently surfaced as a "designer drug" of abuse.[1,2,58] It is most often falsely sold on the street as heroin. Street names include "synthetic heroin," "new heroin," and "synthetic Demerol." Faulty synthesis of this drug can produce the compound 1-methyl-4-phenyl-1,2,3,6-tetrahydropyridine (MPTP), which has produced destructive lesions of the substantia nigra, resulting in a clinical picture similar to that of Parkinsonism. Neurologic damage of brain cells by MPTP is irreversible and worsens with time, especially if the user has repeated exposures to MPTP.[1,58]

Narcotic Withdrawal. Early signs and symptoms of narcotic withdrawal include yawning, lacrimation, rhinorrhea, and sweating; these occur about 8 to 10 hours after the last dose. Withdrawal from narcotics generally is not life-threatening. Seizures do not occur as part of opium withdrawal unless the abuser continually consumes a sedative-hypnotic as part of the narcotic "cocktail." If treatment is deemed necessary, it should be symptomatic and supportive to include the treatment of the acute physical discomfort experienced by the patient. Opiate narcotic withdrawal is never life-threatening unless the patient is co-addicted to barbiturates or short-acting sedative-hypnotics. A phenothiazine may be administered for nausea and vomiting, and a non-narcotic pain medication may be given for pain relief. Non-narcotic antidiarrheal agents can also be administered. Clonidine has been reported to be effective in narcotic withdrawal. In-hospital treatment of "pure" narcotic withdrawal is usually not indicated but may be necessary in postoperative patients admitted to the ICU or the narcotic-addicted patient admitted to the ICU for other reasons.[1,2]

Hallucinogens

Chemicals or substances used to produce changes in perception, thought, or mood have been labeled hallucinogens or less commonly, psycholytics, psychomimetics, or psychotogens. The prototype of this drug class, known also as the "psychedelics," is lysergic acid diethylamide-25 (LSD-25), which was accidentally ingested and produced hallucinations for Albert Hofmann in 1938.[59] The typical hallucinogens are consumed in pill form, gelatin squares, permeated paper, sugar cubes, or mushrooms. Phencyclidine (PCP) can be taken orally, injected, inhaled (snorted), or smoked.

Historically, the oldest recorded account of hallucinogens appears to be the ritualistic use of cannabis and mind-altering mushrooms dating back to India in nearly 5000 BC. Hallucinogens were initially investigated for the treatment of mental illness, but the final results were dismally poor. Because of the ability of hallucinogens to mimic psychosis, the earliest work attempted to discover an "endogenous hallucinogen" that would be found to be responsible for various psychoses. The recreational use of these substances in the United States intensified during the early 1960s and peaked in the early 1970s. Recreational hallucinogenic drug use has since declined at a steady rate, but intermittent resurgences of use appear to occur. Phencyclidine usage was one such resurgence, which peaked during the 1970s and early 1980s in many cities. Since then, there have been only erratic reports of its use.

The hallucinogens can be subdivided into two types: (1) indolalkylamines, which include lysergic acid diethylamide (LSD), dimethyltryptamine (DMT), psilocybin, and psilocin, and (2) phenylisopropylamines, which include mescaline, peyote, methylenedioxyamphetamine (MDA), 3,4-methylenedioxymeth-amphetamine (MDMA) and 3,4-methylenedioxyethamphetamine (MDEA). In addition, certain chemicals include or strongly resemble the clinical effects of hallucinogens, but some have additional effects such as dissociative behavior, schizophrenic reactions, opisthotonis, seizures, and violent behavior that differentiate them from the typical hallucinogens. These drugs include phencyclidine, ketamine, and delta-9-tetrahydrocannabinol (THC) (Table 69–10).

Signs and Symptoms. Although the hallucinogens are thought to affect the pons, their true mechanism of action is unknown. There appears to be some interaction with neurotransmission and serotonin synapses. Present theories postulate that they cause decreased neuronal firing and serotonin turnover on the pontine raphe nuclei.

Most commonly, hallucinogens create a distortion of stimuli; rarely, they may bring about a stimulus de novo. The hallucinations and illusions are predominantly visual and less frequently auditory, olfactory, or another atypical sensory perception. This type of atypical sensory experience involves the "tasting" of colors or "seeing" sounds or music. Additional psychologic effects include ego dissolution and detachment, a diminished sense of reality, depersonalization, slowing of subjective time, and increased sense of meaningfulness of the experience.

The predominate physical findings are sympathomimetic and include pupillary dilatation with retention of reactivity to light, increased blood pressure and heart rate, hyperreflexia, hyperthermia, piloerection, chills, tremor, and flushing. Although all of these drugs can cause nausea and vomiting, this is a predominant feature of ingestion of mescaline and peyote. Nystagmus is classically observed with both mescaline (peyote) and phencyclidine (both horizontal and vertical). Last, rigidity may dominate the clinical picture of phencyclidine and the so-called "designer drugs," MDMA, MDEA, and MDA. The different hallucinogens have variable onset of action and duration of action that may affect the timing of both the psychologic and physical findings (Table 69-11).

Complications. While a median lethal dose (LD$_{50}$) for humans is unknown, only one published article of a possible death that was due to LSD has been reported.[60] Therefore, directly fatal ingestions are extremely rare. Instead, injury and death to the patient more commonly occur from the misinterpretation of information in the intoxicated individual, either from the environment or self, such as jumping from a high building, thinking he had wings and could fly.

Grand mal seizures have been described after ingestion of LSD, phencyclidine, MDMA, MDEA, and MDA.[61] To date, chronic organ toxicity, withdrawal syndromes, or physical dependence from the purely psychedelic drug class such as LSD have not been described.[62]

An idiosyncratic syndrome observed in some hallucinogen users is the "flashback." The flashback is the recurrence of a previous illusiogenic experience days, months, or even years after the consumption of these drugs. This intermittent phenomenon has been observed most commonly with the use of LSD and PCP. Flashbacks are more commonly associated with negative hallucinogenic experiences known in street parlance as "bummers." Occasionally, flashbacks are precipitated by stress, fatigue, marijuana usage, or antihistamines. With cessation of drug usage, flashbacks usually disappear with time and continued reassurance of the patient.

Diagnosis and Treatment. The intensivist rarely sees the uncomplicated hallucinogenic experience. The unto-

Tabloe 69–10. Classification of Hallucinogenic Drugs

Indolalkylamies
  LSD (lysergic acid diethylamide)
  Psilocybin
  Psilocin
  DMT (dimethyltryptamine)
Phenylisopropylamines
  Mescaline
  Peyote
  MDA (methylenedioxyamphetamine)
  MDEA (3,4-methylenedioxyethamphetamine)
  MDMA (3,4-methylenedioxymeth-amphetamine)
Atypical hallucinogens
  Phencyclidine
  Ketamine
  THC (delta-9-tetrahydrocannabinol)

Table 69–11. Time Course of Action of Various Hallucinogens

Drug	Onset	Peak	Duration
LSD (lysergic acid diethylamide)	20 min to 1 hr	2–3 hr	8–12 hr
Psilocybin	30 min	1–2 hr	2–4 hr
Mescaline (Peyote)	1–2 hr	5–6 hr	8–12 hr
MDMA (3,4-methylenedioxymeth-amphetamine) and MDEA (3,4-methylenedioxy-ethamphetamine)	30 min	2–3 hr	4–6 hr

ward effects of the "bummer" (e.g., unpleasant illusions) that present to the emergency department most often involve psychiatric side effects such as panic attacks, anxiety, or psychosis. The management of these problems is best realized by understanding that the patient is in an increased sensitivity state to external stimuli. A darkened environment, preferably with someone in attendance familiar to the patient, can provide reassurance and allow a more thorough history and physical to be conducted. Minor sedatives, such as diazepam or lorazepam, may be used for more severe forms of anxiety or agitation not responding to gentle reassurance. Chlorpromazine or haloperidol should be reserved for the most resistant cases because the IM use of either drug may contribute to rhabdomyolysis in some patients. Additionally, chlorpromazine has both anticholinergic and alpha-blocking activity, which may make the drug relatively contraindicated in this clinical setting of increased sympathomimetic activity.[63] Severe hypotension and anticholinergic crisis have been described when treating PCP and 2,5 dimethoxy-4-methyl-amphetamine ("STP").[64]

Urine and serum drug screens should always be performed even in the mildest cases of assumed hallucinogen drug overdoses because of the common practice of "cutting" or mixing several drugs together for "special" effects. The majority of illicit drugs sold on the street as mescaline or peyote are, in fact, LSD. In addition, PCP is commonly sold for THC or can be found contaminating cannabis claimed to be from "high grade" marijuana areas such as Hawaii. In addition, cocaine and amphetamines are common contaminates of various street drug preparations. Therefore, all drug screening should test for cocaine, PCP, and amphetamines. Usually, a special laboratory is required for quantitative or qualitative determination of LSD, although quantitative levels are rarely of clinical benefit in the management of hallucinogen intoxications.

Of special note is the treatment of PCP, MDMA, MEA, and MDEA overdose. These particular hallucinogens exhibit extreme symptom complexes of increased sympathomimetic activity. Frequently, patients "high" on these drugs will display inordinate amounts of physical strength requiring extreme physical and neurochemical restraints. This is particularly true of PCP ingestions. Muscle rigidity, hyperthermia, and seizures may contribute to the development of rhabdomyolysis and acute tubular (myoglobinuric) necrosis. This poses a treatment dichotomy because the treatment/prophylaxis for rhabdomyolysis requires urinary alkalinization. PCP, however, is acidophilic, and therefore urinary acidification and gastric lavage followed by activated charcoal is most commonly used to accelerate excretion. In addition, many patients with overdoses already have a metabolic acidosis, negating the need for this process. Acidification may also impair the excretion of co-ingested drugs such as salicylates or phenobarbital. If acidification is deemed necessary, it can be accomplished by ascorbic acid, 1 g IV every 6 hours, and if this is unsuccessful, NH_3Cl 4 g every 2 hours orally or by nasogastric tube or a 1 to 2% solution in normal saline IV. Urine pH should be monitored hourly with the goal of therapy to achieve a urine pH of 5.5 to 6.5. During the acidification process, the plasma potassium must be followed closely. An alternative method of acidification is to administer 1 L of D5NS per hour with arginine or lysine hydrochloride (10 g IV over 30 minutes) then D5NS at 500 ml per hour by 2 hours. Some authors have recommended prophylactic phenytoin or diazepam for seizures in significant PCP overdoses.[65] Last, airway protection and endotracheal intubation may be more difficult secondary to induced laryngospasm.

ICU Admission Criteria. The majority of patients who present with intoxication of typical hallucinogenic drugs will require only observation for 12 to 24 hours until the panic or anxiety attack resolves. The patient should then be discharged home with a competent individual responsible for continuing observation during the next 12 to 24 hours. A psychiatric/medical follow-up should be arranged for further evaluation to determine the need for education rehabilitation.

The more dramatic psychologic disturbances involving true psychosis or prolonged anxiety reactions will require admission to the psychiatric units, usually for 1 or 2 days. A significant hallucinogen overdose with PCP, MDMA, MDEA, and MEA often requires observation in the ICU for the development of rhabdomyolysis, treatment of hyperthermia, seizures, acute paranoid psychosis, or airway management/protection.

Special Consideration. Many natural plants contain various substances with hallucinogenic potential if ingested in large enough quantities. The nut of the fruit of the tree Myristica fragrans is nutmeg, and when dried and ground to a powder form it is called mace. Nutmeg is converted in vivo to 3-methoxy-4,5 methylenedioxyamphetamine (MMDA) and 3,4,5-trimethoxyamphetamine (TMA).[65] LSD is present in morning glory seeds; ingestion of these seeds can produce a mild form of LSD ingestion with attendant hallucinations, nausea, diarrhea, and coma. Other plant sources include passion flowers, juniper berries, mandrake and, most important, jimson weed.[66] Jimson weed (Datura stramonium) grows wild throughout the United States and produces both hallucinations and an anticholinergic syndrome/crisis.[67]

Marijuana

Marijuana is the most commonly abused illegal drug in the United States today. Its use was first described in ancient China in 2737 BC both for recreational and therapeutic effects.[68] During the nineteenth century, use of marijuana was applied extensively for mental conditions, labor, and headache. Today, marijuana has legitimate medical uses in special cases for the treatment of glaucoma and nausea during oncologic chemotherapy.

The term marijuana refers to the dried leaf, flower, and stem of the hemp plant, Cannabis sativa. Besides marijuana, over 40 different substances are produced from the hemp plant. A significant number of these chemicals are referred to as the cannabinoids. The most active ingredient in marijuana is THC and is found in a concentration of approximately 1 to 2%. Hashish and hashish oil are concentrated forms of the plant resin, and THC content is approximately 10 to 15% percent.

Marijuana is usually smoked in a pipe or rolled in a cigarette paper or may be ingested orally in the form of cookies, brownies, or other food.

Signs and Symptoms. The onset of action of smoked marijuana is 5 to 10 minutes with a peak at 20 to 30 minutes and effects lasting for approximately 2 to 3 hours. Because of the delay in absorption with oral ingestion, onset of effects is 30 minutes to 1 hour with a more prolonged but less intense experience lasting 4 to 5 hours.

Marijuana appears to act on the hypothalamus and the striate bodies. Moderate doses of the drug cause euphoria, relaxation, impairment of cognition and memory, slowing of time, increased senses of smell, taste, and touch, increased appetite, and impairment of motor function.[69] A small number of marijuana users, especially those psychologically predisposed or first-time users, will experience adverse experiences. These negative reactions include panic, paranoid reactions, hallucinations, confusion, distortions of body image, and depersonalization.

Physical effects observed from marijuana are usually minimal, noted as sinus tachycardia, mild changes in blood pressure (orthostasis), decreased lacrimation, and conjunctional hyperemia.

Diagnosis and Treatment. It is extremely rare that marijuana overdose requires anything more than reassurance and emotional support. If this is inadequate, benzodiazepines can be given for their anxiolytic effects. In extreme cases of hallucinations and delusions predominating the clinical picture, haloperidol administered IM is the drug of choice. The physician should always be suspicious of other contaminants in a "marijuana overdose" whose symptom complex appears out of proportion to expectation. Qualitative drug screening of serum and urine is recommended to analyze for PCP, THC, cocaine, or other common diluents or co-consumed drugs.

A "positive" urine drug screen for THC does not necessarily indicate acute or recent consumption, because THC metabolites can be found for up to 21 days in heavy users.

As with all drug-induced psychoses, follow-up and evaluation are critical. These reactions may be the first presentation of a premorbid, unstable personality. Therefore, a physician visit in the first 5 days after discharge should be arranged. The patient should avoid any exposure to further medications until follow-up has been completed.

Special Consideration. In the mid- to late 70s, great health concerns arose from the spraying of marijuana fields with the herbicide paraquat, which in animal studies caused the development of irreversible pulmonary fibrosis. Despite these fears, because of pyrolysis of the paraquat, no significant reports of lung damage in humans have been reported from marijuana paraquat exposure.[70]

Volatile Inhalants

Volatile inhalants are substances that vaporize at ambient temperature. These chemicals are found in a wide range of categories including aliphatic hydrocarbons, aromatic hydrocarbons, anesthetic agents, fluorocarbon aerosols, esters, fuels, halogenated hydrocarbons (solvents), ketones, and nitrites.

The solvents are volatile, lipophilic, and vary considerably in their other properties. All of these substances are used for their ability to produce an altered state of consciousness or euphoric state. Some of the more commonly available substances abused by inhalation are typewriter correction fluid, paint thinner, glue, nail polish remover, gasoline, hair spray, paints, and nail polish. A more exhaustive compilation can be found in other sources.[1]

These substances easily pass through the lungs in the volatile state into the blood, bypassing first-pass metabolism via the liver. Because of their lipophilic nature, the volatile inhalants readily affect higher lipid content organs systems such as the brain, liver, and heart. The majority of excretion occurs by exhalation with minimal metabolism via the kidneys and liver.

Inhalant abuse is primarily a practice of youth, with a noted predominance in certain ethnic groups such as Mexican-Americans and Native Americans.[65,71] Adult inhalant abuse is most commonly observed in substance abusers who have restricted access to their "drugs of choice" such as those persons in prison or military service. In addition, adult male homosexuals may abuse amyl and butyl nitrite for delayed ejaculation and relaxation of the anal sphincter for receptive anal intercourse.

Several methods are used for inhalation. The easiest method involves simply inhaling the substance directly from the container (sniffing). A cloth or rag may be soaked in the inhalant and placed over the face to inhale the vapors (huffing). The most dangerous and preferred method is placing the volatile inhalant in a plastic bag, shaking it to induce more vaporization, blowing more air into the bag, and then inhaling directly with the bag placed over the face. This method, known as "bagging," is the most direct form of inhalant consumption and offers the highest concentration of vapors to the abuser, hence the highest risk of complications.

Signs and Symptoms. The acute effects during intoxication with volatile inhalants closely resemble those found in the anesthetic agents and/or ethanol. The predominant clinical manifestations involve the central nervous and cardiovascular systems. Symptoms may range from euphoria, exhilaration, ataxia, and nystagmus to CNS depression, coma, and death. A significant number of reports has been noted describing the "sudden sniffing death" syndrome.[72-74] The proposed mechanism is a presumed arrhythmia such as ventricular fibrillation because the volatile inhalants are known to sensitize the myocardium to endogenous circulating epinephrine.

Complications. In addition to the acute CNS and cardiovascular effects, the emergency and critical care physician should be aware of the chronic effects of the volatile inhalants because the patient's clinical presentation may be dominated by the long-term effects of these drugs. This population of substance abusers may present with mild cognitive dysfunction to the extremes of severe dementia. Reports of long-term sequelae have included optic atrophy, deafness, encephalopathy, cerebellar degeneration, seizures, tremor, and peripheral neuropathies.[75]

Patients who present with encephalopathy should be investigated for possible lead poisoning from gasoline abuse.[76] They may have basophilic stippling of the red blood cells on peripheral smear, increased 24-hour lead urinary excretion, and elevated erythrocyte protoporphyrin levels.

Distal renal tubular acidosis is associated with long-term abuse of toluene.[77] Electrolyte disturbances may also develop including hypokalemia, hypophosphatemia, and rhabdomyolysis. Aplastic anemia is more commonly associated with the aromatic hydrocarbon, benzene. Benzene may be a common contaminant in many of the products abused by inhalers.

A fetal solvent-inhalant syndrome has been described in pregnant women abusers.[78]

Diagnosis and Treatment. Signs of recent abuse may be evidenced on physical examination by white flecks of typing correction fluid, gold fingernail polish, or glue around the mouth, nose, hands, or clothes. In addition, corroborating history from family, friends, police, or paramedics is particularly useful. The "sudden cardiac death" or arrhythmia in a young adult or teenager should raise clinical suspicion of inhalant abuse. Cardiac arrest or arrhythmias are treated in the normal fashion. Examination of the nasal mucosa may reveal erosions, inflammation, or discharge from the sinuses.

Because the volatile inhalants affect a wide variety of organ systems, laboratory evaluation should be principally oriented toward the renal, hepatic, hematologic, pulmonary, and central nervous systems. Appropriate baseline studies include a CBC, liver and pulmonary functions, creatinine, BUN, and urinalysis. The majority of these abnormalities are reversed with time and abstinence. Psychiatric evaluation and scheduled follow-up are mandatory.[79]

Nitrite abusers may acquire methemoglobinemia. They present with cyanosis not relieved by oxygen, and their blood has a distinct brown appearance. No treatment is required unless the patient is symptomatic. Methylene blue, 1 to 2 mg/kg IV will reverse the methemoglobin to hemoglobin. The dose may be repeated or given orally, 3 to 5 mg/kg.

Long-standing abusers may develop chronic seizures requiring anticonvulsants such as diphenylhydantoin. After several months of abstinence and the EEG returning to normal, the majority of these individuals can be withdrawn safely from antiepileptic medication.

Although less prevalent than in the past because of reduced levels of lead in fuels, chronic gasoline abusers who have developed lead intoxication/poisoning should be given chelating agents (dimercaprol, penicillamine) to enhance and accelerate lead excretion.

Special Considerations. Chronic, heavy solvent abusers may exhibit signs of withdrawal. These symptoms consist of tachycardia, agitation, delusions, hallucinations, tremors, and delirium and usually begin within a few hours or days of cessation of chemical use.

Treatment should be as an in-patient and include psychologic support and long-acting sedative-hypnotics (benzodiazepines or phenobarbital) with eventual withdrawal over 7 to 10 days.

REHABILITATION PHASE

An ideal time to intervene in the disruptive cycle of drug dependency and abuse is in the hospital setting. Until the drug abuser suffers a life-threatening complication of drug use, denial supercedes common reasoning when confronted by family, friends, or co-workers. The hospital setting reinforces the serious nature of the drug abuser's dependence, unequivocally confirms their use by toxicologic testing, and offers the psychiatric and social support services necessary for proper rehabilitation of the drug abuser after medical complications have been solved.

As long as there are drugs with euphoric pleasurable side effects, there will be people who abuse those drugs. The numerous categories of preferred drugs of abuse present a diagnostic as well as a therapeutic challenge to the critical care physician. Through careful history taking a skillful examination in conjunction with an accurate sophisticated toxicology department, these complicated, challenging cases can be properly managed.

REFERENCES

1. Bryson, P.: Comprehensive Review in Toxicology. 2nd Ed. Aspen Publishers, 1989, p. 313.
2. Augenstein, W. L. (ed.): Emergency aspects of drug abuse. Emerg. Clin. North Am., 8:3, 1990.
2a. American Psychiatric Association: Diagnostic and Statistical Manual of Mental Disorders. 3rd Ed. (DSM III). Washington, D.C., 1980.
3. Epidemiologic Trends in Drug Abuse. Proceedings. Rockville, MD, U.S. Department of Health and Human Services, 1988.
4. Unintentional poisoning mortality in the United States, 1980–86. MMWR, 38:10, 1989.
5. Dans, P., Matriccian, R., Otter, S., and Reuland, D.: Intravenous drug abuse and one academic health center. JAMA, 263:23, 1990.
6. Mahoney, J. D. et al.: Quantitative serum toxic screening in the management of suspected drug overdose. Am. J. Emerg. Med. 8:16, 1990.
7. Who does, doesn't do drugs. USA Today, Dec. 6:13A, 1989.
8. Ogur, B.: Prescription drug abuse and dependence in clinical practice. South. Med. J., 80:1153, 1987.
9. Schwartz, R.: Urine testing in the detection of drugs of abuse. Arch. Intern. Med., 148:2406, 1988.
10. Gold, M., and Dackis, C.: Role of the laboratory in the evaluation of suspected drug abuse. J. Clin. Psychiatry, 47:17, 1986.
11. Kellerman, A. L. et al.: Utilization and yield of drug screening in the emergency department. Am. J. Emerg. Med., 6:14, 1988.
12. Perry, S.: Substance-induced organic mental disorders. *In* Textbook of Neurology. 4th Ed. Edited by R. E. Halls and C. S. Yadofky. Washington, D.C., American Psychiatric Press, 1987.
13. Sloan, E. P.: Toxicology screening in urban trauma patients: drug prevalence and its relationship to trauma severity and management. J. Trauma, 29:1647, 1989.
14. Glassroth, J., Adams, G. D., and Schnoll, S.: The impact of substance abuse on the respiratory system. Chest, 91:4, 1987.
15. Schoenbaum, E. E. et al.: Risk factors for human immunodeficiency virus infection in intravenous drug users. N. Engl. J. Med., 321:13, 1989.
16. Lam, D., and Goldschlager, N.: Myocardial injury associated with polysubstance abuse. Am. Heart J., 115:3, 1988.
17. Jackson, C., Hart, A., and Robinson, M.: Fatal intracranial hemorrhage associated with phenylpropanolamine, pentazocine and tripelennamine overdose. J. Emerg. Med., 3:127, 1985.

18. Goldfrank, L. R., and Kulberg, A. G.: Vital signs and toxic syndromes. *In* Goldfrank's Toxicologic Emergencies. 3rd Ed. Norwalk, CT, Appleton-Century-Crofts, 1986.
19. Brett, A. S., Rothschild, N., Gray, R., and Perry, M.: Predicting the clinical course of unintentional drug overdose. Arch. Intern. Med., *147*:133–137, 1987.
20. Lake, C. R., and Quirk, R. S.: CNS stimulants and the lookalike drugs. Psychiatr. Clin. North Am., *7*:4, 1984.
21. Gawin, F., and Ellinwood, E.: Cocaine and other stimulants. N. Engl. J. Med., *318*:18, 1988.
22. Hewlett, D., and Kelly, J.: Drug Czar: Problem is getting better. USA Today, *Sept. 5*:3A, 1990.
23. Brody, S. L., and Slovis, C. M.: Recognition and management of complications related to cocaine abuse. Emerg. Med. Rep., *9*:41, 1988.
24. Hoffman, C. K., and Goodman, P. C.: Pulmonary edema in cocaine smokers. Radiology, *172*:463, 1989.
25. Levine, S. R. et al.: Cerebrovascular complications of the use of the "crack" form of alkaloid cocaine. N. Engl. J. Med., *323*:699, 1990.
26. Derlet, R.: Emergency department presentation of cocaine intoxication. Ann. Emerg. Med., *18*:2, 1989.
27. Chaisson, R. et al.: Cocaine use and HIV infection in intravenous drug users in San Francisco. JAMA, *261*:4, 1989.
28. Tarr, J. E., and Macklin, M.: Cocaine. Pediatr. Clin. North Am., *34*:2, 1987.
29. Marantz, P. R. et al.: Inability to predict diagnosis in febrile intravenous drug abusers. Ann. Intern. Med., *106*:823, 1989.
30. Zamora-Quezada, J., Dinerman, H., Stadecker, M., and Kelly, J.: Muscle and skin infarction after free-basing cocaine (crack). Ann. Intern. Med., *108*:4, 1988.
31. Rubin, R. B., and Neugarten, J.: Cocaine-induced rhabdomyolysis masquerading as myocardial ischemia. Am. J. Med., *86*:551, 1989.
32. Valladares, B., and Lemberg, L.: The Miami vices in the CCU. Part 1. Cardiac manifestations of cocaine use. Heart Lung, *16*:4, 1987.
33. Gradman, A. H.: Cardiac effects of cocaine: a review. Yale J. Biol. Med., *61*:137, 1988.
34. McGuigan, M. A.: Toxicology of drug abuse. Emerg. Med. Clin. North Am., *2*:1, 1984.
35. Washton, A. M., Gold, M. S., and Pottash, A. C.: Cocaine abuse: techniques of assessment, diagnosis and treatment. Psychiatr. Med., *3*:185, 1987.
36. Lange, R. A. et al.: Potentiation of cocaine-induced coronary vasoconstriction by beta-adrenergic blockage. Ann. Intern. Med., *112*:897, 1990.
37. Klonoff, D., Andrews, B. T., and Obana, W. G.: Stroke associated with cocaine use. Arch. Neurol., *46*:989, 1989.
38. Roberts, J. R., Price, D., Goldfrank, L., and Hartnett, L.: The bodystuffer syndrome: a clandestine form of drug overdose. Am. J. Emerg. Med., *4*:24, 1986.
39. Rosenberg, Paul J., Livingstone, D. J., and McLellan, B. A.: Effect of whole-bowel irrigation on the antidotal efficacy of oral activated charcoal. Ann. Emerg. Med., *17*:681, 1988.
40. Lerner, M. A.: The fire of "ice." Newsweek, *Nov. 27*:37, 1989.
41. Albrecht, S.: Aloha from "ice" land. Law and Order, *December*:55, 1989.
42. Bernstein, E., and Diskant, B. M.: Phenylpropanolamine: a potentially hazardous drug. Ann. Emerg. Med., *11*:311, 1982.
43. Carson, P., Oldroyd, K., and Phadke, K.: Myocardial infarction due to amphetamine. Br. Med. J., *294*:1525, 1987.
44. Myerson, R. M., and Rubin, W.: Ethanol: Mimicry, masquerade and mayhem. Emerg. Med. Rep., *11*:111, 1990.
45. Genz, D.: Recognizing the chemical abuser. Dental Assist., *Nov/Dec*:18, 1982.
46. Schnoll, S., and Karan, L.: Substance abuse. JAMA, *263*:2682, 1990.
47. Bergman, M., and Gleckman, R.: Infectious complications in alcohol abuser. Hosp. Pract., *23*:145, 1988.
48. Williams, H. E.: Alcoholic hypoglycemia and ketoacidosis. Med. Clin. North Am., *68*:1, 1984.
49. Liskow, B., and Goodwin, D.: Pharmacological treatment of alcohol intoxication, withdrawal and dependence: a critical review. J. Stud. Alcohol, *48*:4, 1987.
50. Giannini, J. A., Price, W., and Giannini, M.: Contemporary drugs of abuse. Am. Fam. Physician, *33*:3, 1986.
51. Cushman, P.: Sedative drug interactions of clinical importance. Om. Rec. Dev. Alcohol., *4*:61, 1986.
52. Chan, A.: Effects of combined alcohol and benzodiazepine: a review. Drug Alcohol Dep., *13*:315, 1984.
53. Yell, R. P.: Ethchlorvynol overdose. Am. J. Emerg. Med., *8*:246, 1990.
54. Hofer, P., and Scollo-Lavizzari, G.: Benzodiazepine antagonist Ro 15-1788 in self-poisoning. Arch. Intern. Med., *145*:663, 1985.
55. Woods, J., Kata, J., and Winger, G.: Use and abuse of benzodiazepines. JAMA, *260*:23, 1988.
56. Treatment of acute drug abuse reactions. Med. Lett., *29*:83, 1987.
57. Henderson, G. L.: Designer drugs: past history and future prospects. J. Forensic Sci., *33*:569, 1988.
58. A growing industry and menace: makeshift laboratory's designer drugs (Medical news and perspectives). JAMA, *256*:3061, 1986.
59. Hofmann, A.: LSD: My Problem Child. Los Angeles, J. P. Tharcher, 1983.
60. Griggs, E., and Ward, M.: LSD-toxicity: a suspected cause of death. J. Ky. Med. Assoc., *75*:172, 1977.
61. Fisher, D., and Ungerleider, J.: Grand mal seizures following ingestion of LSD. Calif. Med., *106*:210, 1967.
62. Strassman, R. J.: Adverse reactions to psychedelic drugs: a review of the literature. J. Nerv. Ment. Dis., *172*:577, 1984.
63. Schwartz, C.: Paradoxical responses to chlorpromazine after LSD. Psychosomatics, *8*:210, 1967.
64. Solursh, L.: Emergency treatment of adverse reactions to hallucinogenic drugs. *In* Acute Drug Emergencies. Edited by P. Bourne. New York, Academic Press, 1976, p. 139.
65. Cohen, C.: The hallucinogens and the inhalants. Psych. Clin. North Am., *7*:681, 1984.
66. Brown, R. T., and Braden, N. J.: Hallucinogens. Pediatr. Clin. North Am., *34*:341, 1987.
67. Levy, R.: Jimson seed poisoning: a new hallucinogen on the horizon. JACEP, *6*:58, 1977.
68. Tashkin, D. et al.: Cannabis. Ann. Intern. Med., *89*:539, 1977.
69. Nicholi, A. M., Jr.: The nontherapeutic use of psychoactive drugs: a modern epidemic. N. Engl. J. Med., *308*:925, 1983.
70. Fairshter, R., and Wilson, A.: Paraquat and marijuana. Chest, *74*:357, 1978.
71. Coulehan, J. et al.: Gasoline sniffing and lead toxicity in Navajo adolescents. Pediatrics, *71*:113, 1983.
72. Kirk, L., Anderson, R., and Martin, K.: Sudden death from toluene abuse. Ann. Emerg. Med., *13*:68, 1984.
73. Boon, N.: Solvent abuse and the heart. Br. Med. J., *294*:722, 1987.
74. Reinhardt, C. et al.: Cardiac arrhythmias and aerosol "sniffing." Arch. Environ. Health, *22*:265, 1971.
75. Hormes, J., Filley, C., and Rosenberg, N.: Neurologic sequelae of chronic solvent vapor abuse. Neurology, *36*:698, 1986.
76. Moss, M., and Cooper, P.: Gasoline sniffing and lead poisoning. Acta Pharmacol. Toxicol., *59*:48, 1986.

77. Patel, R.: Renal disease associated with toluene inhalation. Clin. Toxicol., *24:*213, 1986.
78. Goodwin, J. M. et al.: Inhalant abuse, pregnancy and neglected children. (Letter.) Am. J. Psychiatry, *138:*126, 1981.
79. Heiselman, D. E., and Cannon, L. A.: Benzene and the aromatic hydrocarbons. *In* Poisoning and Drug Overdose. 2nd Ed. Edited by L. Haddad and J. Winchester. Philadelphia, W. B. Saunders, 1990, p. 1222.

SUPPLEMENTAL READINGS

Collee, G. G., and Hanson, G. C.: The management of acute poisoning. Br. J. Anaesth., *70:*562, 1993.

Dauer, J., and Geiderman, J.: The use of vasoactive agents in the treatment of refractory hypotension seen in tricyclic antidepressant overdose. J. Clin. Pharmacol., *10:*409, 1990.

Fine, J. S., and Goldfrank, L. R.: Update in medical toxicology. Pediatr. Clin. North Am., *39:*1031, 1992.

Harris, C. R., and Kingston, R.: Gastrointestinal decontamination. Which method is best? Postgrad. Med., *92:*116, 1992.

Klein-Schwartz, W., and Oderda, G. M.: Poisoning in the elderly. Drugs Aging, *1:*67, 1991.

Kulik, K.: Initial management of ingestions of toxic substances. N. Eng. J. Med., *18:*326:1677, 1992.

Lip, G. Y., Metcalfe, M. J., and Dunn, F. G.: Diagnosis and treatment of digoxin toxicity. Postgrad. Med. J., *69:*337, 1993.

Longmire, A. W., and Seger, D. L.: Topics in clinical pharmacology. Am. J. Med. Sci., *306:*49, 1993.

Su, Y. J., and Shannon, M.: Pharmacokinetics of drugs and overdose. Clin. Pharmacokinet., *23:*93, 1992.

Tenenbein, M.: Multiple doses of activated charcoal: time for reappraisal. Ann. Emerg. Med., *20:*529, 1991.

Vale, J. A.: Clinical toxicology. Postgrad. Med. J., *69:*19, 1993.

Chapter 70

TOXINS AND POISONINGS

ERIC P. BRASS

Poisonings are a major cause of morbidity and mortality in our society, and a significant cause of admissions to intensive care units (ICU). Although statistics vary between specific units, 5 to 30% of all ICU admissions are the result of poisonings, with a mortality of 0.6 to 6% in this population.[1,2] Poisonings can result from accidental ingestions or exposures, suicide attempts, or overdoses during the course of drug therapy (prescription errors, dosing errors, etc.), or as a consequence of substance abuse. Each of these etiologies has unique aspects to their presentation, diagnosis, and management. Overdoses involving drugs of abuse are discussed in detail in Chapter 69.

PRESENTATION AND INITIAL APPROACH TO THE POISONED PATIENT: PRE-ICU PHASE

The initial presentation of the poisoned patient covers a broad spectrum of scenarios depending on the poison involved and the circumstances of exposure. A comprehensive, systematic approach to the poisoned patient is essential (Table 70-1). Patients may be unresponsive at the time of presentation and thus unable to provide a history of exposure. A patient involved in a suicide attempt may give misleading or inaccurate information, confusing the assessment. Toxicity from a prescribed medication may cause nonspecific symptoms in a patient with a complex underlying medical condition, making a causal association difficult. Thus, the possibility of a toxicologic etiology must be included in the differential diagnosis of a diverse group of clinical presentations.

The history and physical examination may provide important information suggestive of potential toxic exposures. The history (in addition to any admitted recognized exposure) should include a list of medications used by the patient to establish drugs to which the patient has access, as well as suggesting possible toxicities in the course of therapy. Possible accidental exposures at home (e.g., carbon monoxide from a wood burning stove) or occupationally need to be sought in the history. Information from relatives may be particularly important in supplementing the history from adolescents, the elderly, and patients with altered mental status or psychiatric illness. A thorough review of systems may identify a symptom complex characteristic of a particular toxin.

An immediate physical examination is critical not only for evaluating cardiopulmonary status, but also for providing important information suggesting the involvement of a poison (Table 70-2). Toxins affecting the autonomic nervous system can produce alterations in pupillary diameter, salivation, perspiration, bronchial secretions, and heart rate. Muscle tone, body temperature, and deep tendon reflexes all can be affected in poisonings. Many poisons depress the nervous systems, and loss of the gag reflex places the patient at risk for aspiration. Additionally, it is important to search for evidence of trauma, focal neurologic findings, or other abnormalities indicating a nontoxicologic etiology for the patient's condition.

Routine clinical laboratory evaluation may similarly provide evidence of involvement of a specific poison in the patient's clinical presentation (Table 70-3). Metabolic acidosis is a prominent component of poisonings related to salicylates, ethylene glycol, and methanol. Hyperkalemia may be noted in digoxin poisoning. Arterial blood gas analysis permits assessment of ventilation and oxygenation, as well as acid-base status. Electrocardiography may identify drug-induced alterations such as prolongation of the QRS interval by tricyclic antidepressants.

If a poisoning is suspected, based on historical or clinical information, specific laboratory tests can be used to verify the diagnosis, and in some cases, are useful in formulating management plans. Drug screens are designed to identify the presence of a large number of potential toxins in biologic fluids. Several methods are used in clinical laboratories that differ with respect to the number of potential poisons identified and detection sensitivity. Drug screens usually are performed using urine samples, and as in most cases, the poison is present at higher concentrations in urine than in plasma. Gastric aspirates can also be evaluated using drug screen methods. Although drug screens are extremely useful in evaluating potentially poisoned patients, their limitations must be recognized. First, the drug screen is a qualitative test that detects the presence of drug, but it gives no quantitative information other than whether the concentration exceeds the detection limit of that technique. Thus, a urine drug screen that is positive for salicylate might result from a patient taking 2 aspirin to treat a headache or from a patient ingesting 30 aspirin in a suicide attempt. Second, not all poisons or drugs are detected by drug screens; lithium, ethylene glycol, cyanide, and carbon monoxide are examples. It is important that physicians be aware of the limitations of the toxicology screens used at their institutions and that they communicate with the laboratory if any specific agents are suspected. The laboratory staff can then confirm that the suspected poison is detectable and optimize the tests used to the extent possible.

Table 70-1. Steps in the Management of the Poisoned Patient

Pre-ICU Phase
  Initial stabilization
    Airway maintenance
    Respiratory support
    Hemodynamic support
  Diagnosis
    History
    Physical examination
    General laboratory testing
    Toxicology laboratory testing
  Emergency therapy
  Decontamination or gastrointestinal tract
ICU Phase
  General supportive care
  Consider enhanced elimination
  Specific antidotes
Post-ICU Phase
  Etiology of poisoning
    Prevention
    Education
  Late complications and sequelae

Table 70-2. Potential Findings on Physical Examination in Poisoned Patient

Physical Finding	Potential Agents	
Vital signs		
Hyperthermia	Anticholinergic agents	Amphetamine
	Phencylidine	Monoamine oxidase inhibitors
	Iron	
Hypothermia	Barbiturates	Opioids
	Ethanol	
Tachycardia	Anticholinergic agents	Amphetamine
	Carbon monoxide	Theophylline
	Cyanide	
Bradycardia	Digoxin	Organophosphate
	Beta-adrenergic antagonist	Amanita muscaria
Tachypnea	Salicylate	Carbon monoxide
	Ethylene glycol	Cyanide
	Methanol	
Hypoventilation	Barbiturates	Tricyclic antidepressants
	Opioids	
	Benzodiazepines	Ethanol
Hypertension	Monoamine oxidase inhibitor	Cocaine
	Amphetamine	Phencyclidine
Skin		
Sweating	Salicylate	Organophosphate
	Monoamine oxidase inhibitor	Amanita muscaria
Eyes		
Dilated pupils	Anticholinergics	Sympathomimetics
	Amphetamines	Phenothiazines
	Cocaine	Tricyclic antidepressants
Constricted pupils	Opioids	Organophosphate
Musculoskeletal		
Decreased muscle tone	Benzodiazepines	Opioids
	Barbiturates	Beta-adrenergic antagonists
	Ethanol	
Neurologic		
Hyperreflexia	Anticholinergics	Phencyclidine
	Amphetamine	Tricyclic antidepressants
	Monoamine oxidase inhibitor	Lithium
Decreased gag reflex	Barbiturates	Tricyclic antidepressants
	Benzodiazepines	
	Ethanol	

It is important to use drug screens to verify a suspected diagnosis whenever possible. A high percentage of overdoses involve multiple drugs (20 to 60% of suicides[1,3]). The patient or physician may confidently identify one drug taken, but miss one or more other potentially toxic substances. Studies suggest that as often as 30% of the time, the physician's assessment of the agent responsible for an overdose is inaccurate or incomplete, when complete toxicologic studies are performed.[3] For several types of poisonings, however, delays in instituting therapy increase the risk to the patient (e.g., cyanide, acetaminophen). In those cases, therapy must be instituted on the basis of the history and clinical impression using the laboratory for confirmation.

In addition to the qualitative information available from drug screens, quantitative assays are available for a number of compounds and can be used to determine the absolute concentration of a toxin in blood. In some cases, the plasma concentration can be useful in assessing the severity of the poisoning and the risk to the patient, as well as in planning appropriate therapy. For many compounds, however, the plasma concentration does not correlate well with risk or clinical effects, and the clinical assessment provides the best information for decision making. Examples of poisonings in which plasma concentrations are useful or provide little information are listed in Table 70-4.

Once a diagnosis of a poisoning has been established, management decisions can be based on the patient's clinical status, the pharmacology of the specific poison(s) involved, and the risk of complications from the poisoning. Admission of poisoning victims to the ICU is often necessitated because they have been intubated to ensure adequate ventilation or for airway protection. Cardiac monitoring may be indicated because of established arrhythmias or toxicities with high risk of arrhythmias. Uncontrolled seizures, shock, hypotension, or coma may necessitate ICU admission. The risk of developing serious complications in a patient who currently is stable is an important consideration. As discussed previously, plasma concentrations of the poison may be useful in risk assessment in patients who currently are asymptomatic. Knowledge of the time course of the effects of a specific poison, use of clinical indices of the chemicals' action (i.e., electrocardiographic changes in tricyclic antidepressant overdoses), and the individual patient's overall clinical status are all key components of risk assessment.

INTERVENTIONS IN THE POISONED PATIENT: ICU PHASE

General Considerations and Approach

Attentive, comprehensive supportive care is the cornerstone in the management of poisoning victims. Fundamentals, including verifying the presence and protection of an adequate airway, ensuring adequate ventilation, and assess-

Table 70-3. Laboratory Alterations in Poisoned Patients

Abnormality	Potential Agents
Arterial blood gas	
Respiratory acidosis	Barbiturates
	Benzodiazepines
	Opioids
Respiratory alkalosis	Salicylate
Metabolic acidosis	Methanol
	Ethylene glycol
	Salicylate
	Cyanide
	Carbon monoxide
Electrolytes	
Hypokalemia	Theophylline
	Salicylate
Hyperkalemia	Digoxin
Hypocalcemia	Ethylene glycol
Miscellaneous	
Hypoglycemia	Insulin
	Oral hypoglycemics
	Salicylate
Hyperglycemia	Theophylline
	Salicylate
Hyperosmolality	Ethanol
	Ethylene glycol
	Methanol

Table 70-5. Potential Interventions in Specific Poisoning

Poison	Intervention
Pharmacokinetics-enhanced elimination	
Salicylate	Sodium bicarbonate
	Hemodialysis
Carbon monoxide	Oxygen
Theophylline	Hemoperfusion
	Hemodialysis
	Repetitive oral charcoal
Lithium	Hemodialysis
Ethylene glycol	Hemodialysis
Methanol	Hemodialysis
Iron	Deferoxamine
Pharmacokinetic-Altered Metabolism	
Acetaminophen	N-Acetylcysteine
Ethylene glycol	Ethanol
Methanol	Ethanol
Pharmacodynamic and Miscellaneous Pharmacokinetic	
Tricyclic antidepressants	Alkalinization of plasma
Digoxin	Antidigoxin antibody
Cyanide	Nitrites, sodium thiosulfate
Organophosphate pesticide	2-PAM, atropine
Snake venom	Antivenin
Insulin, oral hypoglycemic	Glucose
Warfarin	Vitamin K, fresh frozen plasma
Opioids	Naloxone

ing circulatory status are critical as often they are all affected by toxins, they can deteriorate rapidly during the clinical course, and other interventions are irrelevant if they are neglected. All major organ systems may become involved, and frequent re-evaluation of the patient and a supportive management plan are an integral part of the care of the poisoned patient. If the poisoning is the result of a suicide attempt, precautions should be taken to prevent further self-inflicted injury. These considerations cannot be overemphasized despite the apparently larger effort devoted to discussion of more specific aspects of poisonings.

Interventions in poisonings and overdoses can be characterized as pharmacokinetic, in which the absorption, distribution, or elimination of the toxin is altered, or pharmacodynamic in which the biologic action of the poison is affected or countered. Several techniques used to modify a drug's pharmacokinetics are discussed in this chapter,

Table 70-4. Are Plasma Concentrations Useful?

Help Assess Risk or Guide Therapy*	Provide Little Additional Information
Acetaminophen (see Fig. 70-1)	Tricyclic antidepressants
Salicylate (see Fig. 70-2)	Benzodiazepines
Lithium (above 1.5 mEq/L)	Anticoagulants
Ethylene glycol (above 25 mg/dl)	Antihypertensives
Methanol (above 25 mg/dl)	Oral hypoglycemic
Ethanol (variable; above 200 mg/dl)	Antihistamines
Iron (above 350 mg/dl or total iron binding capacity)	Opioids
Digoxin (variable; above 2.5 ng/ml)	
Theophylline (variable; above 30 μg/ml)	

* Guidelines for interpreting toxic levels shown in parentheses.

with application to specific poisonings summarized in Table 70-5. Pharmacodynamic interventions are based on the specific characteristics of the poison and are illustrated in Table 70-5 with detailed discussion in subsequent sections.

Because the risk in most poisonings is increased with increasing dose of the poison, attempts to decrease the systemic absorption of orally ingested toxins are often initiated. The stomach can be emptied rapidly by induction of emesis. Ipecac causes emesis by both direct irritation and central nervous system stimulation, working clinically after a delay of 15 to 30 minutes. Emesis should never be attempted in a patient with an impaired gag reflex because of the risk of aspiration. Induction of emesis is also contraindicated if the ingestion involves strong acids or bases that could damage the esophagus or pharynx, or when volatile compounds (e.g., kerosene, gasoline) have been ingested, given the risk of pneumonitis. Ingestions involving central nervous system stimulants are associated with risk of seizures, and further central stimulation with ipecac should be avoided. Ipecac is usually effective in children, but the response is variable in adults. Because of the delay in inducing emesis, the unpredictable response to ipecac in adults and the risk of esophageal rupture, gastric lavage is often a preferred method for decontamination of the stomach in adults.

Gastric lavage to remove chemicals and extract pills from the stomach must be conducted with a large bore orogastric tube, with multiple large side holes to avoid clogging. Passage of the tube should not be attempted unless the patient's airway is protected, either with an adequate gag reflex or prophylactic endotracheal intubation. Aspiration or esophageal perforation are rare but serious complications of tube placement. Lavage should be conducted with saline, and repeated until the lavage return is clear (a minimum of 6 L, but 20 to 30 L total lavage may be required).

Activated charcoal administered orally prevents drug absorption by adsorbing the drug onto the charcoal where it remains until passed through the gastrointestinal tract. To be effective, the charcoal and drug must be in physical proximity within the stomach or intestine. Therefore, if gastric lavage has been conducted adequately, the added benefit of charcoal administration is questionable. Definitive data on the optimal strategy for minimizing drug absorption in the clinical overdose setting is lacking, and in most centers, thorough lavage (or induction of emesis) is favored, followed by charcoal, if tolerated. If emesis has been induced using ipecac, the patient often is unable to tolerate oral charcoal because of continued nausea. The use of cathartics to increase gastrointestinal motility, decreasing residence time, is also widely recommended. Repetitive administration of activated charcoal can also be used in some instances to enhance drug elimination (see subsequent discussion).

Decontamination of the stomach is indicated even several hours after ingestion, despite the normal 30- to 90-minute gastric emptying time. Many drugs decrease gastric emptying, and thus, their own entry into the duodenum. Additionally, several drugs have limited solubility, and in the absence of dissolution, they can be recovered as intact pills or pill fragment from the stomach hours after ingestion.

After the toxin has been absorbed, consideration should be given to strategies to enhance toxin elimination, thereby decreasing the overall exposure. Elimination of drug from the body can be described quantitatively using the drug's clearance. Analogous to creatinine clearance, drug clearance relates to the amount of drug removed from the body per unit time to the plasma drug concentration, and is conceptually the volume of plasma completely cleared of drug per unit of time (e.g., milliliters per minute). It is important to recognize that for drugs cleared by multiple routes, the individual clearances are additive to yield the total drug clearance (e.g., total clearance = hepatic clearance + renal clearance). Elimination of chemicals from the body occurs primarily by hepatic metabolism or renal elimination. Although hepatic metabolism theoretically can be accelerated by induction of the microsomal oxidation system, this change is of no practical benefit in the management of acute overdoses because of the time required for induction. For some chemicals, metabolites generated in the liver are primarily responsible for clinical toxicity (e.g., acetaminophen, ethylene glycol), and altering hepatic metabolism becomes an important component of therapy.

Renal elimination of some drugs can be increased by forced diuresis and/or ionic trapping. Forced diuresis with saline or mannitol generally is of limited value, causing no more than a 30-70% increase in drug clearance, and is associated with significant risk of fluid overload, particularly in the elderly. Most drugs are weak organic acids or bases and are present as protonated and unprotonated species at physiologic pHs. By adjusting urinary pH to keep the drugs ionized (high pH for acids, low pH for bases), reabsorption of the filtered drug by nonionic diffusion can be minimized. Alkalization of the urine to pH 8.0 can result in a threefold increase in urinary elimination of drugs such as salicylate or phenobarbital. Urinary alkalization can be achieved by administration of sodium bicarbonate (with accompanying risk of fluid overload) or by use of carbonic anhydrase inhibitors such as acetazolamide (with risk of systemic acidosis).

Drug elimination can also be enhanced by artificial measures. The ability of activated charcoal in the gastrointestinal tract to adsorb drugs can be used to trap a drug that diffuses from the systemic circulation into the gastrointestinal tract (reversible passive, nonionic diffusion). The binding of the drug to the charcoal maintains a concentration gradient for diffusion from the circulation, "drawing" drug into the gastrointestinal tract. Thus, by repetitive administration of oral charcoal, drug elimination can be increased. This effect is independent of any effects on absorption, as it is effective after intravenous drug administration. A similar mechanism results in charcoal accelerating the elimination of drugs that undergo enterohepatic circulation. To achieve maximal efficacy in enhancing drug clearance, charcoal (20 to 40 g) is given every 2 to 4 hours. This regimen should be continued until the plasma drug concentration has fallen below dangerous levels. The charcoal is administered in a sorbitol solution. The mixture often is not well tolerated, and a severe osmotic diarrhea develops. Administration of the charcoal solution can also result in aspiration, and associated morbidity. Several charcoal aspiration fatalities have been reported.[4,5] Nevertheless, in selected patients and for selected drugs (e.g., theophylline), oral charcoal administration provides an effective means for increasing drug clearance.

Hemodialysis and hemoperfusion represent additional methods for increasing toxin elimination. Both methods require the establishment of an extracorporeal circulation. In hemodialysis, blood is circulated past a semipermeable membrane. The membrane establishes a concentration gradient for drug between blood and dialysis fluid, permitting net drug removal. In hemoperfusion, blood is pumped through a cartridge containing activated charcoal or binding resin to which drug in the blood is adsorbed. The use of either method necessitates establishing high volume vascular access. In general, hemoperfusion is more effective than hemodialysis in enhancing drug elimination, but it is associated with potentially serious complications including thrombocytopenia and hypocalcemia.

Importantly, artificial methods to enhance drug elimination are not effective for all drugs, and even if effective in accelerating drug removal, they are not indicated in all clinical situations because of potential risks. Several properties of the drug or toxin predictably cause artificial methods of elimination to be ineffective. All of the available methods remove the drug from the plasma compartment. Drugs distribute, however, throughout the body. The volume of distribution of a drug relates its plasma concentration to the total body drug burden. The larger a drug's volume of distribution, the less drug (as a percentage of the total body burden) is present in the plasma. Thus, for drugs with a large volume of distribution (e.g., digoxin or tricyclic antidepressants), methods such as hemodialysis or hemoperfusion have minimal impact on total drug elimination. Similarly, if a drug is strongly protein bound in plasma, minimal free drug will be available to cross the dialysis membrane or to bind to the cartridge matrix. Finally, the drug must be able to diffuse across the hemodialysis membrane or to bind to the hemoperfusion cartridge matrix if removal by these techniques is to be effective.

Although the initial management of the poisoned patient is similar to that of any critically ill patient, the physician is faced with a series of diagnostic and therapeutic decisions unique to the overdose. The appropriate strategy varies from poison to poison and from patient to patient, making risk assessment in individual patients particularly critical. Imperative for rationalizing this decision-making process is an understanding of the pharmacology (pharmacokinetics and pharmacodynamics) and toxicology of the poisons involved, and incorporation of this understanding into the formulation of a clinical plan.

Specific Chemicals, Drugs, and Toxins

A comprehensive review of the clinical toxicology for all potential poisons and toxins is beyond the scope of this text. A relatively small list of compounds, however, are responsible for the majority of poisonings. The clinical pharmacology and toxicology of these compounds are discussed subsequently, emphasizing the interrelationships between the basic pharmacology of these agents, the associated clinical pathophysiology, and the development of a rational approach to risk assessment and clinical management. This approach to the management of the poisoned patient can then be extended to any other specific agent encountered. Additional information can be obtained from one of the several excellent textbooks available and product handbooks,[6-8] and poison control centers provide important sources of treatment guidelines and detailed references.

Acetaminophen

Acetaminophen is a non-narcotic analgesic available without a prescription in the United States. It is contained in a number of commercial preparations, both alone and in combination with other drugs. During the 1970s and 1980s, acetaminophen-containing products captured a large portion of the non-narcotic analgesic market in the United States. This wide availability has led to a corresponding increase in the incidence of acetaminophen poisoning, both accidental and in suicide attempts.

Acetaminophen (N-acetyl-p-aminophenol) normally is cleared by hepatic metabolism, and in normal therapeutic use, it has a half-life of 2 hours. After therapeutic doses, most acetaminophen is conjugated with glucuronate or sulfate and excreted in the urine.[9] Some acetaminophen, however, is oxidized by the microsomal P-450 system to form a reactive metabolite.[9,10] This metabolite is extremely reactive and normally is removed by conjugation with glutathione. Under conditions in which large amounts of the reactive metabolite are generated (i.e., acetaminophen overdose), hepatic glutathione can be depleted. The reactive intermediate can then covalently interact with hepatic proteins. This depletion of glutathione and the covalent interaction of acetaminophen metabolites with hepatic structures is directly associated with acetaminophen-induced hepatic necrosis, the major clinical toxicity in acetaminophen poisoning.[9] Thus, the chemical acetaminophen itself is not responsible for significant morbidity, but the generation of the toxic metabolite in excess of the liver's ability to remove it by conjugation with glutathione results in the clinical features of acetaminophen poisoning. An understanding of this mechanism of toxicity allows appreciation of the clinical course of acetaminophen overdoses, and permitted the development of efficacious antidotes to acetaminophen hepatoxicity.

Initial symptoms and signs following a potentially life-threatening acetaminophen ingestion may be minimal and misleading.[9] Only mild epigastric distress or nausea may be present. As the ingested acetaminophen is metabolized, the toxic metabolite is generated and hepatic damage ensues. Liver function abnormalities become apparent 12 to 24 hours after serious poisonings, and the patient may experience right upper quadrant abdominal pain. Liver failure is progressive over the next 24 to 48 hours, and the sequelae of hepatic failure dominate the clinical course. Renal failure, independent of liver failure, has also been seen in some cases of acetaminophen poisoning.[9] Because the toxic metabolite is generated from acetaminophen, the plasma acetaminophen concentration provides a measure of risk to the patient before the onset of liver failure and while intervention is still possible (Fig. 70-1).[9-11] The plasma acetaminophen concentration is reflective of the

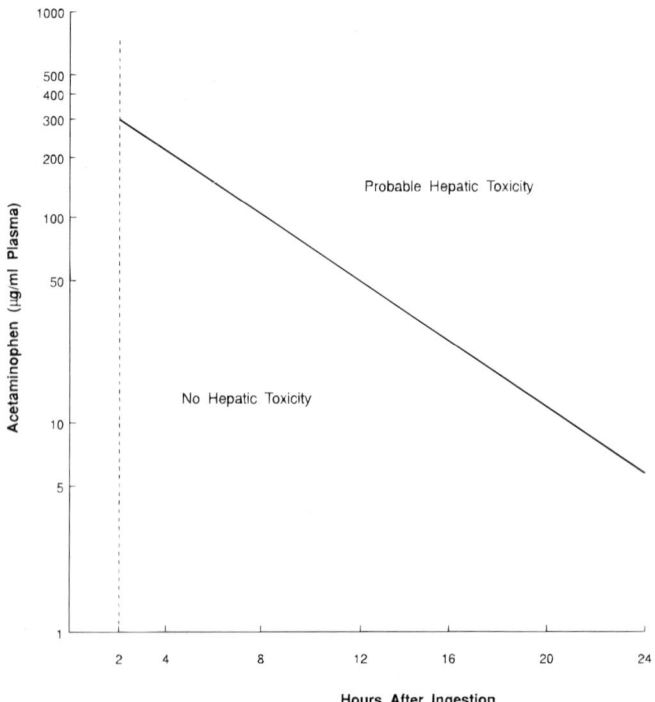

Fig. 70-1. Risk of hepatic toxicity in acetaminophen poisoning. Plasma acetaminophen concentrations measured between 4 and 24 hours after ingestion can be used to assess risk. (From Rumack, B. H., and Matthew, H.: Acetaminophen poisoning and toxicity. Pediatrics, 55:873, 1975.)

body acetaminophen burden only after the absorption and distribution phase of the pharmacokinetics is complete. Therefore, plasma acetaminophen concentrations drawn within 4 hours of ingestion may be misleading and are not clinically useful.

To prevent acetaminophen-induced hepatotoxicity, therapy must be directed toward preventing formation of the toxic metabolite and facilitating the removal of any metabolite that is formed. Minimizing systemic acetaminophen absorption by emptying the stomach is the first step in decreasing risk to the patient. To enhance removal of the toxic metabolite, sulfydryl-containing compounds are used as a substitute for the depleted hepatic glutathione.[9] N-acetylcysteine is available as an oral preparation in the United States, and has been shown to decrease the incidence of hepatic necrosis dramatically following potentially serious acetaminophen ingestions. A loading dose of N-acetylcysteine (140 mg/kg) is given orally, followed by 70 mg/kg orally every 4 hours for a total of 18 doses.[9,12] As would be expected on the basis of mechanism of toxicity, it is critical to institute N-acetylcysteine therapy as soon after ingestion as possible. Clinical studies demonstrate that efficacy is maximal when the first dose of N-acetylcysteine is administered within 8 hours of ingestion, and falls to zero if therapy is delayed until 18 to 24 hours after ingestion.[9] When the presenting history suggests a potentially serious acetaminophen poisoning, N-acetylcysteine therapy should be initiated pending the plasma acetaminophen level. The plasma acetaminophen concentration can then be used as a basis for deciding whether the full 18-dose protocol is necessary (see Fig. 70-1).

Other sulfydryl reagents, including methionine, cysteine, and cysteamine, have been used to treat acetaminophen poisoning. In many patients, vomiting is a major problem, complicating oral administration of N-acetylcysteine. Intravenous preparations of N-acetylcysteine are currently in clinical trials and have the potential to facilitate the treatment of these patients.

After the institution of appropriate gastrointestinal decontamination and N-acetylcysteine therapy, the management of patients with acetaminophen poisoning is dictated by their liver and renal function. In uncomplicated cases, liver and renal function tests can be assessed as clinically indicated. In the absence of complications, patients can be medically discharged after completion of the N-acetylcysteine therapy. If hepatic failure develops, the management is analogous to that for failure of other etiologies (see Chap. 54). As for any poisoning, steps must be taken to identify why the poisoning occurred, and to prevent recurrences.

Salicylates

Salicylates are widely used as anti-inflammatory, analgesic, or antipyretic agents. The most common salicylate product, aspirin (acetylsalicylic acid), is deacetylated rapidly after systemic absorption, generating salicylate. Salicylate is highly protein bound and is both metabolized by the liver and excreted unchanged in the urine. At high plasma salicylate concentrations, hepatic metabolism becomes saturated, and urinary elimination becomes increasingly important. Salicylate is a weak organic acid and filtered salicylate may be reabsorbed from the urine in the renal tubule by passive diffusion of the un-ionized form of the compound. Plasma protein binding of salicylate is saturated at high salicylate concentrations, resulting in an increased unbound fraction and volume of distribution.

After an oral overdose, aspirin can be recovered from the stomach for many hours after ingestion. This fact reflects in part the poor solubility of acetylsalicylic acid at the acid pH of the stomach. Solubility may be so limited that mechanical obstruction of the gastric outlet (bezoar) by aspirin tablets may result. Thus, aspirin poisoning is a situation in which late gastric lavage is indicated and gastric endoscopy may be required in extreme cases to dislodge the bezoar.

At initial presentation, patients with aspirin poisoning often complain of epigastric pain or discomfort, nausea, and vomiting.[13,14] Hyperventilation is often present, and reflects a central stimulation of ventilation by salicylate. An arterial blood gas analysis obtained during this period will demonstrate a respiratory alkalosis. In cases of severe poisoning, however, this alkalosis will evolve into a severe anion-gap metabolic acidosis. This metabolic acidosis reflects accumulation of a variety of endogenously generated organic acids secondary to disruption of cellular intermediary metabolism by salicylate. The plasma salicylate concentration is a useful predictor of risk to the patient (Fig. 70-2), and permits physicians to make management decisions before the development of severe metabolic acidosis.[13]

Other features of severe salicylate intoxication may include eighth cranial nerve toxicity (tinnitus, deafness),

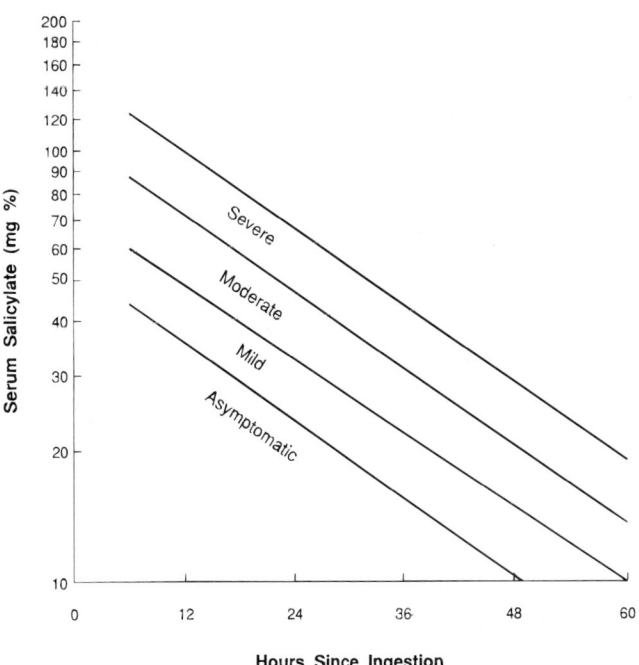

Fig. 70-2. Severity of toxicity in salicylate poisoning as related to plasma salicylate concentrations. (From Done, A. K.: Salicylate intoxication. Pediatrics, 26:805, 1960.)

fluid and electrolyte disturbances (hypokalemia, dehydration, hypo- or hypernatremia), altered glucose homeostasis (hyper- or hypoglycemia), or bleeding (decreased platelet function, hypoprothrombinemia). Pulmonary edema is a major potential problem in patients with salicylate toxicity, and results from a pulmonary capillary leak syndrome.[13,15] Central nervous system depression is a late development in severe poisonings.

Management of salicylate poisoning requires careful attention to the overall fluid and electrolyte status of the patient and an understanding of the evolution of the acid-base disturbances. Interventions to enhance salicylate elimination must be considered in potentially serious overdose cases. Alkalinization of the urine to pH 8.0 increases urinary salicylate elimination by increasing the ionized form of the drug in the tubule, thus decreasing passive diffusion out of the urine. Quantitatively, the increase in salicylate clearance is relatively small. Carbonic anhydrase inhibition should be avoided because of the risk of worsening the systemic metabolic acidosis. Intravenous administration of sodium bicarbonate can increase the urinary pH, but caution must be exercised to avoid fluid overload and subsequent leakage of fluid into the lungs if salicylate-induced pulmonary edema develops. Intravenous bicarbonate administration can correct severe systemic metabolic acidosis, and it has also been suggested as a means to decrease central nervous system toxicity from salicylate by decreasing the partitioning of the salicylate to brain across the blood-brain barrier, as well as the intracellular-extracellular salicylate concentration gradient.[16] Vitamin K administration may be useful in correcting salicylate-induced prolongation of the prothrombin time.

Definitive removal of salicylate from seriously poisoned patients requires extracorporeal elimination, and hemodialysis has been widely used.[17] On the basis of plasma salicylate concentrations, individuals at high risk for serious sequelae can be identified, and hemodialysis should be considered early in their hospital course.[13,16,17] The presence of a salicylate-induced hemorrhagic diathesis may increase the risk of bleeding during catheter placement for hemodialysis. Plasma salicylate concentrations above 100 mg/100 ml or severe, difficult to control acid-base disturbances are generally accepted as indications for hemodialysis.

Patients that can be clinically stabilized usually do not suffer relapses in their clinical course or other late sequelae. A relapse of salicylate toxicity symptoms can result from late absorption from the gastrointestinal tract, and can be avoided by adequate gastrointestinal lavage. Following resolution of the acute clinical course, necessary counseling, education, and other preventive measures should be instituted.

Tricyclic Antidepressants

Tricyclic antidepressants are widely used in patients with significant depressive disorders, and may have significant impact on the quality of life in these individuals. This patient population also is inherently at increased risk for suicide attempts and, when available, tricyclic antidepressants may be ingested in an intentional overdose. The toxicity of tricyclic antidepressants is potentially life-threatening, and recognition of overdosed patients is critical.

Tricyclic antidepressants are absorbed rapidly from the gastrointestinal tract. The tricyclic antidepressants are metabolized by the liver with a high intrinsic clearance. Therefore, they undergo first-pass elimination, which decreases their systemic bioavailability. The tricyclic antidepressants are bound to plasma proteins but also have a high volume of distribution, because they are lipophilic and bind to tissue proteins. Although tricyclic antidepressants block re-uptake of biogenic amines by nerve terminals, they also are antagonists of muscarinic, cholinergic, and alpha-adrenergic receptors. These effects on peripheral autonomic nervous system receptors contribute to the pathophysiology of tricyclic antidepressant toxicity.

Clinical symptoms and signs in patients with tricyclic antidepressant toxicity predominately reflect the actions of these drugs on the autonomic nervous system. Anticholinergic effects of the drugs cause tachycardia, mydriasis, decreased gastric motility, and urinary retention. Central nervous system toxicity also includes aspects consistent with anticholinergic effects including disorientation, agitation, hallucinations, and fever. Pyramidal signs, decreased responsiveness, myoclonic jerks, and seizures may develop in patients with severe poisonings. Cardiovascular toxicity of tricyclic antidepressants results from anticholinergic actions and direct membrane effects of the drugs.[18] The electrocardiogram demonstrates sinus tachycardia, and may also reveal nonspecific ST segment/T wave changes, prolongation of the PR and QT intervals, bundle branch blocks, and prolongation of the QRS interval. The actions of tricyclic antidepressants at toxic concentrations on cardiac excitable membranes of the heart are similar to those seen in quinidine or procainamide poisoning. In severe poisonings, ventricular tachycardia and/or ventricular fibrillation may result. Tricyclic antidepressants also have been reported to have negative inotropic effects, and cardiogenic shock has been described in cases of severe toxicity.

Because of the anticholinergic effects of tricyclic antidepressants, pills can be recovered from the stomach many hours after ingestion, and gastric lavage is, therefore, indicated even if the initial presentation is several hours after the ingestion. The gag reflex is often impaired in patients following tricyclic antidepressant poisoning and special attention must be given to ensuring adequate airway protection throughout the lavage to minimize the risk of aspiration.

Tricyclic antidepressant toxicity is known to cause life-threatening complications (arrhythmias or seizures) in some apparently stable patients many hours after initial evaluation. Thus, a method for assessing which patients are at risk would be of great clinical utility. Plasma tricyclic antidepressant concentrations are not useful in identifying high risk patients. A normal QRS interval duration (0.12 second) on the electrocardiogram has been reported to identify patients at very low risk for clinically serious medical sequelae from acute tricyclic antidepressant intoxication.[19] Although the utility of this observation has been questioned,[20] it is a readily available, inexpensive method to assist in risk assessment. Other important considerations in evaluating risk and need for monitoring include central nervous system, cardiovascular, and respiratory status; the presence of underlying medical disorders; and the length of time the patient has been clinically stable since ingestion. The presence of an arrhythmia (excluding hemodynamically stable sinus tachycardia) or the occurrence of a seizure dictate a period of close medical supervision.

In addition to supportive measures, specific therapy may be required to treat tricyclic antidepressant-induced seizures or arrhythmias. Because the action of the tricyclic antidepressants on cardiac excitable tissue is analogous to class Ia antiarrhythmics (e.g., quinidine, procainamide), these agents are contraindicated in acute therapy of tricyclic antidepressant poisoning. Lidocaine is safe and effective in suppressing ventricular ectopy under such conditions.[18] Phenytoin may shorten the QT and PR intervals in patients with tricyclic antidepressant toxicity,[21] but studies are not available on which to base a recommendation for routine or therapeutic use of phenytoin in this population. Alkalosis, induced by hyperventilation or by bicarbonate administration, is also effective in reducing ventricular ectopy in tricyclic antidepressant poisoning in animal models[22] and clinically.[23]

Seizures occurring in association with tricyclic antidepressant poisoning should acutely be treated pharmacologically like any other generalized seizure (see Chap. 6). Benzodiazepines are effective as first-line therapy. The use of cholinesterase inhibitors, like physostigmine, is logical to counteract the anticholinergic action of the tricyclic antidepressants. Physostigmine use however, has been associated with a risk of life-threatening complications, including asystole.[24] Therefore, the use of cholinesterase inhibitors should be reserved for refractory seizures and undertaken with extreme caution.

The tricyclic antidepressants have a large volume of distribution and, therefore, attempts to increase plasma clearance of the drugs would not be expected to impact the clinical course of patients poisoned with these agents. The effects of repetitive oral charcoal administration on tricyclic antidepressant pharmacokinetics are variable.[25,26] In the absence of clear clinical data, and because of the drugs' large volume of distribution, attempts to enhance tricyclic antidepressant elimination should not be pursued.

The large volume of distribution of the tricyclic antidepressants accounts for their long plasma half-life (e.g., 16 hours for amitriptyline). Thus, direct drug toxicity may persist for several days. In patients who are hospitalized for management or monitoring, a 24-hour period without serious arrhythmias or seizures indicates a low probability of subsequent complication.[27]

Nontricyclic Antidepressants

Monoamine oxidase inhibitors are used clinically as antidepressants and act by inhibiting the catabolism of catecholamines, important neurotransmitters, by the enzyme monoamine oxidase. Toxicity from monoamine oxidase inhibitors can result from overdoses as well as from drug or food interactions that cause a hypercatecholamine state. The symptoms and signs of monoamine oxidase inhibitor poisoning are, therefore, those of catecholamine excess.[28] Evidence of central nervous system toxicity includes agitation, hallucinations, hyperreflexia, hyperpyrexia, and, in severe cases, convulsions. Peripheral manifestations may include dilated pupils, muscle fasciculation, and tachycardia. Both hypertension and hypotension have been reported with monoamine oxidase inhibitor poisoning. The hypertension results from the direct actions of the catecholamine on the cardiovascular system, i.e., tachycardia, positive inotropic action, and increased systemic vascular resistance related to vasoconstriction. Hypotension often is a poor prognostic sign and usually represents a decrease in circulating volume.

Diagnosis of monoamine oxidase inhibitor poisoning is often difficult, with the clinical presentation often attributed to primary hypertensive crisis. Diagnosis is complicated further because the monoamine oxidase inhibitors usually are not detected by routine drug screens. After acute monoamine oxidase inhibitor overdose, symptom development is delayed, peaking 6 to 12 hours after ingestion.

Although monoamine oxidase inhibitors have a relatively short half-life (approximately 4 hours), their duration of action is considerably longer because they irreversibly inhibit the monoamine oxidase enzyme.[28] Because only a small percentage of total monoamine oxidase activity is required to relieve symptoms and signs, however, symptoms in overdosed patients usually resolve over 48 to 96 hours as new enzyme is synthesized. Hypertension requiring therapy usually responds to nitroprusside or phentolamine (an alpha-adrenergic antagonist). In those patients with volume depletion, antihypertensive drugs must be administered cautiously because this state predisposes them to hypotension.[29] Volume repletion should be tried first in patients who develop hypotension. The administration of alpha-adrenergic agonists (e.g., norepinephrine) to treat hypotension requires extreme caution; the use of drugs interacting directly with the postsynaptic adrenergic receptor is preferred to permit better titration of action (e.g., norepinephrine is preferable to ephedrine).

Severe hyperthermia may also occur with monoamine oxidase inhibitor poisoning. Cooling blankets and acetaminophen are often sufficient to control the body temperature. In severe cases, paralysis with curare or succinylcholine, dantrolene, and chlorpromazine have all been effective in individual patients. Chlorpromazine, which interacts with multiple receptor types, may be associated with an increased risk of hypotension in patients with monoamine oxidase inhibitor toxicity.

Because of the fluctuating, labile cardiovascular status of patients with severe monoamine oxidase inhibitor poisoning, those who require admission should be monitored until they are stable for 24 to 48 hours.

Several newer antidepressants have been introduced, the results of attempts to maintain the pharmacologic properties of the tricyclic antidepressants while minimizing the risk of toxicity (e.g., trazodone, fluoxetine, and maprotiline). Limited data and experience suggest that several of these agents may be associated with a decreased risk of central nervous system and cardiovascular toxicity when ingested in suicide attempts as compared with the tricyclic antidepressants.[30] Further data are required before broad recommendations and conclusions can be made concerning poisoning with these agents.

Carbon Monoxide

Acute and chronic monoxide poisoning is responsible for significant morbidity and mortality throughout the world.[31,32] Carbon monoxide is generated during fuel combustion, and clinically significant exposures may be associated with automobile exhausts, wood or coal burning stoves, and smoke inhalation. Carbon monoxide reversibly binds to hemoglobin to form carboxyhemoglobin with an affinity 200 times that of oxygen. As a result, in the presence of carbon monoxide, the oxygen carrying capacity of blood and oxygen delivery to tissues are reduced. Carbon monoxide bound to one or more of the heme binding sites also increases the affinity for oxygen binding at the other available sites. This shifting of the hemoglobin-oxygen dissociation curve to the left means that what oxygen reaches tissues bound to hemoglobin may not be released for use by the tissues. This impaired oxygen delivery and resultant tissue hypoxia is the dominant pathophysiologic feature of carbon monoxide poisoning. Carbon monoxide can also bind to the heme moieties of the cytochromes involved in mitochondrial electron transport, potentially further compromising tissue oxidation metabolism. Carbon monoxide does not, however, have a significantly higher affinity than oxygen for the cytochromes (in contrast to the situation for hemoglobin). Thus, effects of carbon monoxide on mitochondrial function are probably of secondary importance as compared with alterations in oxygen delivery.

The clinical presentation of carbon monoxide poisoning is influenced by several variables. The percentage of hemoglobin present as carboxyhemoglobin can be measured directly. Because some carbon monoxide is generated by endogenous metabolism and through environmental exposure, carboxyhemoglobin levels of 1 to 2% are normal in nonsmokers, and 5 to 7% carboxyhemoglobin may be present in smokers.[32] Whereas the carboxyhemoglobin level provides a measure of lost oxygen-carrying capacity, it does not reliably predict clinical status or prognosis following acute carbon monoxide poisoning.[33] This fact may in part reflect variability in the amount of carbon monoxide present in tissues and interindividual variation in sensitivity to the impairment in oxygen delivery. For example, patients with underlying cardiovascular disease may develop symptoms and signs with mild compromise of oxygen delivery to the myocardium. Metabolic acidosis, when present, is an indicator of severe poisoning.

Additionally, acute and chronic carbon monoxide poisoning generally have different presentations when initially seen and evaluated. Symptoms and signs associated with chronic carbon monoxide poisoning may be nonspecific and difficult to attribute to carbon monoxide if the source of exposure is occult.[34] Carboxyhemoglobin levels of 10 to 20% may be associated with fatigue, headache, palpitations, or gastrointestinal complaints.

The brain and heart are highly dependent on oxidative metabolism, and these organs are most sensitive to injury in acute carbon monoxide poisoning. Neurologic symptoms range from headache to coma and convulsions, and cardiovascular symptoms from palpitation or dyspnea to myocardial infarction, arrhythmias, or cardiorespiratory arrest. Thus, therapy is directed to restoring normal tissue oxidative metabolism as quickly as possible.

Because carboxyhemoglobin formation is reversible, removing the patient from the environment containing carbon monoxide permits net elimination of carbon monoxide during exhalation. When breathing room air, the half-life for carbon monoxide elimination is approximately 4 hours. With administration of 100% oxygen, the half-life for carbon monoxide is reduced to approximately 50 minutes, as more oxygen is available to compete with released carbon monoxide for hemoglobin binding.[32] The use of hyperbaric oxygen (2 to 5 atmospheres) further reduces the half-life of carbon monoxide to 20 to 25 minutes.[32] Additionally, under hyperbaric conditions, sufficient oxygen is directly dissolved in blood to permit oxygen delivery to tissues independent of hemoglobin. This direct oxygen delivery to tissues also facilitates removal of carbon monoxide associated with tissue cytochromes.

Therefore, the management of patients with acute carbon monoxide poisonings consists of removal of the patient from the carbon monoxide source and the administration of 100% oxygen. Hyperbaric oxygen is optimal therapy, but it is available at only a few medical centers, and no clear data or guidelines exist to define when hyperbaric treatment should be used. Additionally, because carbon monoxide is eliminated with a 50-minute half-life during 100% oxygen therapy, hyperbaric oxygen therapy must be instituted early in most cases to alter the clinical course significantly. If hyperbaric oxygen is available, reasonable guidelines for its use in acute carbon monoxide poisoning apply to patients with carboxyhemoglobin contents above 40%, significant neurologic defects, or cardiac symptoms or signs.[32]

When carbon monoxide poisoning results from smoke inhalation in a fire, patients must be evaluated carefully for other sequelae. Airway burns and inhalation of other toxic products of combustion, as well as external injuries or burns, may contribute to the overall clinical situation in these patients (see Chap. 18).

Once carbon monoxide has been cleared from the patient's system, the clinical course is largely dictated by the degree of hypoxic injury to the heart and central nervous system. It is also possible for neuropsychiatric problems to persist, or even to develop, weeks after the initial carbon monoxide exposure. These residual deficits are often subtle, but they are well documented,[35] and may include impairment of memory, personality changes, intellectual impairment, and motor dysfunction. Treatment with hyperbaric oxygen can decrease the neuropsychiatric sequelae of carbon monoxide poisoning, and may represent an important justification for the use of this therapy.

Theophylline

Theophylline is a bronchodilator used widely in the treatment of asthma and chronic obstructive pulmonary disease. The pharmacokinetics of this agent vary widely across the patient population and in individual patients over time. In that theophylline has a narrow therapeutic index (concentration associated with toxicity close to that required for efficacy), this variability in pharmacokinetics contributes to the high incidence of theophylline toxicity associated with its therapeutic use. Additionally, theophylline poisoning may result from accidental or suicidal ingestion of large amounts of the drug.

Symptoms and signs of theophylline intoxication range from mild (nausea, headache, diarrhea, vomiting) to serious (gastrointestinal bleeding, seizures, arrhythmias). The adverse effects of theophylline in part correlate with plasma theophylline concentrations. Theophylline concentrations less than 15 µg/ml in general are well tolerated. Mild toxicity is seen with levels of 15 to 30 µg/ml, and potentially serious toxicity is seen at concentrations above 30 µg/ml.[36] Clearly, however, variability is seen in the response of individual patients to a given theophylline concentration. Many patients tolerate theophylline concentrations of 40 to 50 µg/ml, whereas fatal seizures have been associated with theophylline concentration of 25 µg/ml. Underlying medical diseases may contribute to this variability in sensitivity.[37]

Management of the care of the patient with theophylline poisoning must initially be directed toward supportive measures. Many widely used theophylline preparations are slow release formulations, which reinforces the need for decontamination of the gastrointestinal tract using thorough lavage. The ingestion of slow release formulation may lead to a delay in the appearance of the peak plasma level. Seizures and cardiac arrhythmias are the major causes of morbidity and mortality in serious theophylline poisoning. The management approach of theophylline-induced seizures is the same as for any other such seizure disorder (see Chap. 6), with benzodiazepines considered reasonable initial therapy. Theophylline-induced cardiac arrhythmias are also approached as appropriate for the presenting arrhythmia (see Chap. 27). Supraventricular tachyarrhythmias are common with theophylline poisoning. The beta-adrenergic antagonists are generally useful in treating these tachyarrhythmias, but they must be used cautiously in patients with theophylline intoxication because of the possibility of reactive airway disease (as the basis for initiation of theophylline therapy), which would be aggravated by beta blockers. Verapamil or other calcium-channel antagonists that slow cardiac conduction can be used for rate control if treatment of the tachyarrhythmias is necessitated by hemodynamic compromise or myocardial risk.

Theophylline is eliminated by hepatic metabolism. As discussed previously, the half-life for theophylline elimination varies considerably in the population, ranging from 3 hours to as long as 20 to 30 hours.[38] Additionally, theophylline metabolism may become saturated at theophylline concentrations seen in overdosed patients.[39] This saturation of theophylline metabolism may result in zero order elimination kinetics, and slower net elimination of the drug as compared with predictions based on the half-life at therapeutic concentrations. The possibility of a prolonged period of risk because of a long drug life and life-threatening toxicity (seizures and arrhythmias) has led to intense investigation of strategies to enhance theophylline elimination.

Theophylline can be removed from the systemic circulation by hemodialysis.[39,40] The potential impact of hemodialysis on theophylline elimination can be seen by comparing the hemodialyzer theophylline clearance with the endogenous theophylline clearance (assuming the endogenous elimination kinetics are first order): total theophylline clearance will be the sum of the extracorporeal and endogenous clearances. As seen in Table 70-6, endogenous theophylline clearance may range from 20 to 100 ml per minute, depending on patient characteristics including age, liver function, presence of acute infections, heart failure, and smoking history. Hemodialysis theophylline clearances of approximately 30 to 80 ml/min can be obtained.[39,40] In a patient with high endogenous theophylline clearance, the impact of hemodialysis will be to less than double total theophylline elimination. In contrast, in a patient with low endogenous clearance, hemodialysis may result in a three- to five-fold increase in total drug removal. Thus, the decision to use hemodialysis (or any intervention) balances the probable benefit in an individual patient (recognizing the inherent delay in initiating dialysis), the risks of emergent hemodialysis, and the risk of the theophylline toxicity in the patient.

Repetitive oral administration of charcoal can result in total theophylline clearances double the endogenous value.[41] This type of therapy, therefore, has the potential to be as effective as hemodialysis for enhancing theophylline elimination and can be initiated with minimal delays. To achieve maximal theophylline clearance, charcoal must be administered frequently (every 2 to 4 hours) with associated risks of aspiration, diarrhea, and fluid/electrolyte disturbances.

Charcoal hemoperfusion is effective in removing theophylline from the circulation.[42] Approximately 80 to 100% of the theophylline present in blood is removed in a single passage through the hemoperfusion cartridge. In clinical use, charcoal hemoperfusion can be expected to yield theophylline clearances of 200 ml/min. Clearances in this range have the potential to decrease serum theophylline levels rapidly. This efficacy is potentially offset by the morbidity associated with emergent hemoperfusion, including the risks of complications from arterial access, thrombocytopenia, and hypocalcemia.

Unfortunately, no clear criteria or prospective studies permit definition of the risk of intervention versus risk of the theophylline poisoning for individual patients.[42] Individual patient characteristics influence both risks, and the serum theophylline concentration should also be used in the risk assessment. Pharmacokinetic factors potentially

Table 70-6. Clearance of Theophylline

Method	Clearance (ml/min)
Endogenous clearance	
Young, healthy, smoker	100
Average adult	60
Elderly adult with liver disease	20
Repetitive oral charcoal	60
Hemodialysis	30–80
Hemoperfusion	100–200

Clearance expresses the rate of drug removal quantitatively as the volume of plasma completely cleared of drug per unit time.

associated with high risk from theophylline poisoning include theophylline concentrations above 60 μg/ml and a documented or high probability of low endogenous clearance (liver disease, congestive heart failure). Additionally, underlying cardiovascular or central nervous system disease may enhance the risk of serious theophylline toxicity at any given serum theophylline concentration.[42]

Thus, although theophylline toxicity is potentially life-threatening, rational symptomatic and specific pharmacologic treatment can offset pharmacodynamic actions of theophylline, and options exist for pharmacokinetic intervention to enhance theophylline elimination. In patients receiving theophylline, appropriate therapeutic drug monitoring and clinical observation are important tools in preventing iatrogenic theophylline toxicity.

Digoxin

Digoxin is an antiarrhythmic and inotropic agent. Digoxin toxicity may occur at plasma concentrations only twice those required for effective therapy. Additionally, the action of digoxin on the myocardium depends on several patient characteristics, including serum potassium concentration, thyroid status, paO_2, underlying myocardial disease, and divalent cation concentrations. These parameters can also change in individual patients over time. Digoxin is eliminated primarily by renal excretion, and digoxin clearance parallels changes in creatinine clearance.[43] Thus, alterations in renal function also result in altered steady state digoxin concentrations on a fixed-dosing regimen. These pharmacodynamic and pharmacokinetic characteristics make iatrogenic digoxin toxicity common, particularly in patients with unstable or compromised renal function, adding to the digoxin poisonings resulting from accidental ingestion of large doses or suicide attempts.

The pharmacokinetics of digoxin are characterized by a large volume of distribution (6 L/kg, or approximately 400 liters in a 70-kg patient), which results from extensive binding of digoxin in skeletal and cardiac muscle, and has important implications for managing digoxin poisoning. First, even in patients with normal renal function and a high digoxin clearance, the half-life for digoxin elimination is extremely long (approximately 40 hours). This long half-life is explained by the fact that the bulk of the patient's total digoxin burden is in the tissues, and hence efficient removal of digoxin from plasma impacts only a small fraction of the total body digoxin load. This same principle limits the efficacy of any attempts to significantly enhance digoxin elimination that acts on the plasma alone.

Digoxin poisoning is associated with gastrointestinal and central nervous system symptoms, but cardiovascular toxicity is the major potentially life-threatening clinical problem.[44] Digoxin toxicity may be associated with a wide variety of cardiac arrhythmias. Actions of digoxin to impair intracardiac conduction may result in high degree atrioventricular block and bradyrhythmias. Digoxin also increases the irritability of myocardial tissue, so that ectopic foci, either atrial or ventricular, may result in tachyarrhythmias. This variability in cardiac presentation, particularly in patients with underlying cardiac disease, often makes the diagnosis of digoxin toxicity difficult to establish. The serum digoxin concentration often is not helpful in ruling in or out the presence of digoxin toxicity.[45] Although population studies demonstrate higher serum digoxin concentrations in patients with digoxin toxicity as compared to those without toxicity, considerable overlap occurs in digoxin concentrations in the two groups. This lack of adequate sensitivity and specificity, which may reflect the multiple variables influencing digoxin action on the heart, limits the utility of the digoxin concentration for diagnosing digoxin toxicity in an individual patient. Thus, although the digoxin concentration may be an adjunct to diagnosis, establishing the presence of digoxin toxicity as responsible for a given cardiac or systemic sign remains primarily a clinical exercise.

The initial objective in digoxin-toxic patients is to control any arrhythmias that may compromise hemodynamic stability. Atropine can be used to treat sinus bradyarrhythmias that result from the vagolytic effects of digoxin. Phenytoin has been reported to increase atrioventricular conduction in digoxin intoxication; however, temporary electric pacing is often required to maintain an adequate ventricular rate. Digoxin intoxication also increases ventricular irritability. Electrocardioversion of a supraventricular arrhythmia related to digoxin toxicity may lead to the development of a less stable, more difficult to control ventricular arrhythmia.[46] The approach to managing ventricular ectopy in patients with digoxin poisoning is similar to the general management of ventricular arrhythmias (see Chap. 27). Attention must also be given to correcting any electrolyte (i.e., hypokalemia) or respiratory abnormalities (i.e., hypoxia) that may aggravate digoxin cardiotoxicity. Hyperkalemia may result from inhibition of the Na-K ATPase by digoxin, and often indicates severe toxicity.

The long half-life of digoxin and the potentially life-threatening toxicity of the drug motivated the development of a digoxin-specific antibody to remove digoxin rapidly from body stores.[47,48] The Fab fragment of digoxin antibodies developed in sheep are currently available for use in life-threatening digoxin intoxication. Administration of digoxin-specific Fab by intravenous injection leads to a rapid (within 30 minutes) increase in the plasma total digoxin concentration. The plasma-free or unbound digoxin concentration approaches zero, however, because all the digoxin is bound to the Fab fragment and, thus, is unable to interact with its tissue receptor. Clinically, this rapid sequestration of the digoxin load leads to resolution of digoxin-induced arrhythmias and a decrease in the plasma potassium concentration as the Na-K ATPase is reactivated. This redistribution of the potassium tissues may unmask an underlying hypokalemia. The digoxin-Fab complex is excreted in the urine. Thus, the digoxin-specific antibody has the potential to transform a protracted, difficult management problem into an easily managed situation with the single administration of the antidote.

Dosing of the digoxin-specific antibody is based on an estimate of the patient's total body digoxin burden (in milligrams). This estimate can be based on the amount of digoxin ingested or on the plasma digoxin concentration and digoxin volume of distribution, assuming steady state. (Body burden (mg) = serum digoxin concentration (ng/

ml) × 5.6 × patient's weight (kg ÷ 1000), for digitoxin substitute 0.56 for 5.6.) Each 40 mg of the antibody (Digibind) can bind 0.6 mg of digoxin or digitoxin.

To date, experience with the Fab antibody has not demonstrated serious contraindications to its use. Because the antibody is of ovine origin, it is a foreign protein, and immunologic reactions are possible. Skin testing can be undertaken if a high risk of allergic reaction is suspected. Incidences of worsening cardiac failure after antibody administration have been reported and may relate to loss of digoxin inotropic action in patients with underlying cardiac disease. Although deposition of digoxin-Fab complexes in the vascular system is theoretically possible, no sequelae analogous to serum sickness have been reported, even after administration to patients with severe renal failure. These considerations, plus the high cost of this antibody, limit the indications for its use to patients with life-threatening digoxin toxicity.

For patients in whom digoxin therapy is continued after an episode of digoxin intoxication, educational and preventive measures are important in avoiding a recurrence. Alterations in the dosing regimen should not be undertaken without consultation with the primary physician, and conditions associated with decreased renal function such as dehydration or worsening heart failure should also be reported. For each patient, consideration must also be given to the issue of whether the clinical benefits from continued use of digoxin justify the risks associated with the medication. Particularly in a geriatric population, a significant percentage of patients show no clinical deterioration when chronic digoxin therapy is stopped.[49]

Lithium

Lithium is an elemental, monovalent cation with pharmacologic effects on the functions of a number of cellular systems. Clinically, lithium (in the form of lithium carbonate) is used in the treatment of manic-depressive illness and other psychiatric disorders. The potential toxicity of lithium has been recognized since the 1930s when lithium was used as a sodium-salt substitute.[50] The development of assay methods for measuring serum lithium concentrations on a routine basis, and recognition of lithium's narrow margin between toxic and therapeutic concentrations, permitted the widespread use of lithium in psychiatry.

Lithium toxicity may occur as a complication of routine clinical use of the drug, or as the result of intentional or accidental acute overdoses. Lithium is handled by the kidney in the proximal tubule in a manner similar to sodium, and it is excreted in the urine.[51] Lithium is readily filtered at the glomerulus, and 80% of the filtered lithium is reabsorbed in the proximal tubule.

Lithium clearance normally is 10 to 40 ml per minute, yielding a half-life of approximately 30 hours. The proximal reabsorption of lithium is increased under conditions in which proximal tubule sodium reabsorption is enhanced, as in systemic dehydration. This increased lithium reabsorption decreases lithium clearance, leading to increased serum concentrations and potential toxicity. Primary renal disease also decreases lithium clearance.

Clinical features of lithium toxicity primarily involve excitable tissue.[51-53] Severe toxicity during clinical use of the drug is often preceded by a prodromal syndrome, which includes vomiting, diarrhea, drowsiness, tremor, tinnitus, and polyuria. The polyuria is the result of lithium-induced nephrogenic diabetes insipidus, and may lead to severe hypernatremia. Neurologic symptoms and signs in lithium poisoning may include mental sluggishness, irregular tremor, weakness, ataxia, fasciculation, and hyperreflexia, progressing to stupor, convulsions, or coma in severe cases. Gastrointestinal symptoms (nausea, vomiting, diarrhea) and ECG changes (T wave flattening and ST segment depression) may also be present. In the absence of a history of lithium use, diagnosis of lithium poisoning may be difficult, and lithium is not identified in routine toxicologic screens. In general, the serum lithium concentration is predictive of the poisoning severity, with concentrations of 1.5 to 3.5 mEq/L indicating serious toxicity with concentrations above 3.5 mEq/L being potentially life-threatening.

Initial therapy in lithium intoxication must be directed toward normalizing volume status. Appropriate therapy with water and electrolytes is important, not only for hemodynamic reasons, but also to ensure normal sodium delivery to the kidney, thereby minimizing reabsorption of filtered lithium. Normal saline is the fluid of choice in most lithium poisonings. Because of the lithium-induced diabetes insipidus, intoxicated patients are at risk for hypernatremia and care in fluid administration is important. Diuretics, by inducing proximal tubule sodium reabsorption secondary to relative volume depletion, are frequent precipitants of lithium intoxication and should not be continued in patients with lithium poisoning. Abnormal fluid and electrolyte homeostasis may persist for weeks following lithium poisoning. (See Chapter 38 for detailed discussion of electrolyte abnormalities and their management.)

Lithium can be cleared effectively by hemodialysis, which is the treatment of choice for potentially severe lithium poisonings.[51] The serum lithium concentration can be used as a guide to the efficiency of the dialysis, and to monitor for possible postdialysis increases in the serum drug concentration.

Confusion exists as to the optimal duration of dialysis and to the potential need for repetitive dialysis treatments. In part, this uncertainty may result from the variable amount of lithium that has reached intracellular compartments in individual cases. Hemodialysis effectively removes lithium from the extracellular compartment, whereas intracellular lithium may contribute to symptomatology and provides a reservoir of drug to re-equilibrate with the extracellular compartment.

In most patients, signs and symptoms usually resolve gradually over 2 to 5 days after serum lithium concentrations are brought into the therapeutic range (0.4 to 1.3 mEq/L). In rare cases, residual deficits have persisted, including dementia and cerebellar or extrapyramidal signs.

Patients using lithium need to understand the potential of toxicity from the drug. Early identification of toxic symptoms, avoiding dehydration, and avoiding self-initiated dosage changes are all important steps in preventing serious lithium toxicity. The physician must be alert for signs of toxicity, and the use of therapeutic drug monitoring is an important adjunct to the safe therapeutic use of lithium.

Ethylene Glycol/Methanol

Ethylene glycol and methanol are alcohols found in a large number of household and commercial products in which they are used as solvents or antifreezes. Poisonings involving ethylene glycol or methanol result from suicide attempts or accidental ingestions, including the drinking of methanol ("wood alcohol") misidentified as ethanol. The serious toxicity of ethylene glycol and methanol is the result of metabolism of the alcohols to organic aldehydes and acids. Both ethylene glycol and methanol have direct effects on the central nervous system similar to ethanol, and in the early stages of poisonings with these solvents, the patient may appear "drunk" but without the odor of alcohol on the breath (unless ethanol has also been ingested). Neither ethylene glycol nor methanol are detected by most routine toxicologic screens, and a special, specific laboratory test (usually gas chromatographic analysis for volatile alcohols in plasma) should be ordered to exclude their presence in suspected poisonings. Clinical suspicion may arise on the basis of an anion gap metabolic acidosis (see subsequent discussion).

The first step in the metabolism of both ethylene glycol and methanol is the oxidation of the alcohol to form the corresponding aldehydes. This reaction is catalyzed by alcohol dehydrogenase. These aldehydes are, in turn, further oxidized, yielding formic acid from methanol, and a spectrum of organic acids from ethylene glycol.[54,55] The generation of these organic acids from the solvents is responsible for the characteristic anion gap metabolic acidosis seen in severe ethylene glycol or methanol poisonings. Recognition that metabolism through alcohol dehydrogenase is responsible for the generation of these toxic metabolites was key in the development of a rational therapeutic strategy for management of poisonings with methanol or ethylene glycol.[56]

Clinical presentation of methanol and ethylene glycol poisonings share many features, but characteristic differences also are present. Because of the lag in generating and accumulating the toxic metabolites, development of severe symptoms or signs may be delayed for several hours. Ingestion of ethanol at the time the solvents are taken may further delay the onset of symptoms, by inhibiting methanol and ethylene glycol metabolism (see subsequent section). Methanol poisoning is often associated with abdominal pain, nausea, vomiting, and gastrointestinal hemorrhage.[54,56] An elevation of the serum amylase value has been reported in methanol poisoning, leading to diagnostic confusion with acute pancreatitis. Ocular toxicity is a serious complication of methanol ingestion and includes blurred vision, altered visual fields, and photophobia progressing to blindness. Examination of the eye typically is normal, with abnormalities limited to dilated pupils and hyperemia of the fundus. For both methanol and ethylene glycol poisoning, the development of a severe metabolic acidosis with attempts at respiratory compensation (i.e., tachypnea, low arterial P_{CO_2}) dominate the clinical picture. Central nervous system symptoms and signs may develop earlier in ethylene glycol poisoning (slurred speech, somnolence, nystagmus, hyporeflexia), but progression to seizures and coma may occur with large ingestions of either solvent. Renal failure is a common feature of ethylene glycol poisoning,[57,58] and is attributable to both direct tubular toxicity and crystalluria (oxalate and/or hippurate). Generation of oxalate may also induce hypocalcemia in patients with ethylene glycol poisoning.

Diagnosis of ethylene glycol or methanol poisoning is accomplished by quantitation of the solvent in a blood sample. This assay often is not included in an initial evaluation, however, and it may not be readily available in all laboratories. The solvent levels may be very low or zero even in severe poisonings if the test is drawn after the methanol or ethylene glycol has been completely metabolized to the toxic metabolites.

The presence of an osmolar gap may be a useful indicator of poisoning in the absence of specific assays for the solvents.[54,58,59] Normally, the serum osmolality can be accounted for by sodium (and associated anions), glucose, and urea (calculated as Osmolality = 2× [Na] + 2× [K] + [BUN] ÷ 2.8 + [glucose] ÷ 18). A discrepancy between the measured osmolality and the osmolality calculated on the basis of these solutes indicates the presence of an unanticipated solute such as an organic alcohol. Each milligram per deciliter of methanol or ethylene glycol increases the serum osmolality by 0.34 and 0.20 mOsm/kg H_2O, respectively. The serum ethylene glycol or methanol concentration is a useful measure of risk in that it is a direct measurement of the potential to generate the toxic organic acids. Concentrations of either solvent above 25 to 50 mg/dl should be considered clinically serious.

Paramount in the management of ethylene glycol or methanol poisonings is the prevention of metabolism to the toxic metabolites by inhibition of alcohol dehydrogenase.[54,58] Alcohol dehydrogenase has a higher affinity for ethanol than either methanol or ethylene glycol, such that in the presence of 100 mg/dl ethanol, essentially no methanol or ethylene glycol will be metabolized. Thus, ethanol should be administered as soon as possible in patients with established poisonings and when a high index of suspicion exists for ethylene glycol or methanol poisoning. The latter point is key because of the possible delay in establishing a definite diagnosis, the relative safety of ethanol administration, and the importance of preventing further metabolism. A loading dose of 600 mg ethanol/kg followed by an infusion of 70 mg ethanol/kg per hour is usually sufficient to yield an ethanol concentration of 100 mg/dl, but this value should be confirmed by direct laboratory measurement. In a nonhospital setting, 125 ml of an 86-proof alcoholic beverage orally will also effectively and quickly provide the ethanol loading dose. Higher infusion rates may be necessary in regular ethanol users because of their higher ethanol disposition rates.

Once the metabolism of the poison has been inhibited, hemodialysis is used to definitively remove the ethylene glycol or methanol. Hemodialysis also removes the metabolites of the solvent that have accumulated, and may be useful in managing acid/base disturbances. Because hemodialysis also removes ethanol, the rate of the ethanol infusion should be increased, typically to approximately 7 g per hour, during dialysis. Other interventions should be directed toward controlling acid-base, fluid, and electrolyte abnormalities and hemodynamic status. Administration of folate in cases of methanol poisoning, and thiamine and pyridoxine for cases of ethylene glycol poisoning, have been advocated to accelerate the metabolism of metabolic products generated after the alcohol dehydrogenase reaction. The importance of these measures is secondary, however, to the prompt administration of ethanol and to appropriate hemodialysis.

In most cases, recovery from ethylene glycol or methanol poisoning is complete following early control of the acidosis and elimination of the solvent. Blindness from methanol poisoning may, however, be irreversible. Cerebral edema may be associated with severe cases of ethylene glycol or methanol intoxication, and may lead to a slow recovery of normal central nervous system function.

Cyanide

Cyanide is a potent, potentially lethal poison. Exposure to cyanide may result from industrial accidents, ingestion of cyanide salt, or consumption of plants containing certain glycosides that generate cyanide when eaten (including the seeds of peaches, apricots, and bitter almonds, and elderberry leaves).[60] The toxicity of cyanide results from its binding to the ferric iron of cytochrome oxidase.[60] Cytochrome oxidase, which is inactive when cyanide is bound, is essential for the functioning of the electron transport chain, and hence for aerobic energy production. The interaction of cyanide with cytochrome oxidase occurs rapidly, and hence symptoms develop soon after exposure, although absorption from the gastrointestinal tract may be slow and rate limiting following oral ingestion.

Symptoms and signs of cyanide poisoning are those expected from loss of aerobic ATP synthesis. The central nervous system and the heart, given their dependence on aerobic metabolism, are significantly affected.[60,61] Central nervous system toxicity may initially involve headache, dizziness, nausea, and drowsiness, with progression to seizures and coma in severe cases. Electrocardiographic changes characteristic of myocardial ischemia may be present. The patient will not be cyanotic, because the interaction of oxygen with hemoglobin is unaffected, and oxygen use is decreased, resulting in bright red venous blood. The detection of oxygen by the chemoreceptor depends on oxidative metabolism, and thus the cyanide-poisoned patient hyperventilates. Cyanide is not detected by a routine toxicologic screen, and special, specific assays should be requested to confirm a suspected diagnosis of cyanide poisoning.

Because of the catastrophic consequences to the central nervous system when oxidative metabolism is unable to supply ATP, intervention in cyanide poisoning must be initiated without delay. One strategy for relieving the inhibition of cytochrome oxidase is to provide alternative binding sites for the cyanide. Conversion of the iron in hemoglobin to the ferric state by generating methemoglobin provides a large number of alternative binding sites for cyanide.[60] Amyl nitrate can be administered by inhalation to generate methemoglobin, and while having the advantage of ease of rapid administration, it usually does not result in the formation of sufficient methemoglobin. Therefore, as soon as intravenous access is obtained, sodium nitrite (10 ml of 3% solution) is given. Blood pressure is monitored to avoid excessive hypotension. The degree of methemoglobinemia is monitored and maintained at less than 40% to preserve oxygen delivery capacity. Cobalt and hydroxocobalamin have also been used to bind cyanide in competition with the cytochrome oxidase.[60,61]

Cyanide is metabolized to thiocyanate, a less toxic compound, in a reaction catalyzed by the enzyme rhodanese. Thiosulfate is the second substrate in this reaction, and its availability may be rate limiting for cyanide metabolism. Therefore, sodium thiosulfate (50 ml of a 25% solution) should be administered intravenously to patients with cyanide poisoning.

Once these specific interventions have been initiated, other aspects of general care, including gastric lavage if oral ingestion is suspected, can be initiated. Although administration of 100% oxygen is of no value in overcoming cyanide's inhibition of cytochrome oxidase, clinical reports and animal studies document potential beneficial effects of oxygen therapy when used as an adjunct to the definitive measures just discussed.[58] Decisions concerning repetitive dosing with sodium nitrate and/or sodium thiosulfate can be based on the measured methemoglobin level and the individual clinical sequence and situation. Given the sensitivity of the central nervous system to the loss of aerobic energy production, neurologic deficits may not completely resolve in patients who otherwise recover.

Iron

Formulations of iron salts are widely used as dietary supplements, and thus are available for accidental or suicidal ingestion in potentially toxic doses. The most commonly used preparations, ferrous sulfate and ferrous gluconate, contain 65 mg and 37 mg of elemental iron per 325-mg tablet, respectively. Iron ingestions of 60 mg/kg or greater are potentially toxic.[62] Iron salts are directly toxic to the gastric mucosa, and symptoms of nausea, vomiting, abdominal pain, diarrhea, and hematemesis are common.

Iron that is absorbed is taken up by the liver, with hepatic toxicity resulting in severe cases. Iron interferes with a number of important metabolic processes in the liver, including mitochondrial oxidative phosphorylation. Symptoms and signs of the liver injury develop after a delay of 2 to 48 hours after ingestion, and may include a metabolic acidosis and fever, as well as evidence of hepatic necrosis. Shock may develop from excessive gastrointestinal blood loss or severe metabolic acidosis. The metabolic acidosis is the result of excess generation of lactate and other organic acids attributable to the metabolic derangements.

Because iron salts are directly toxic to the gastric mucosa and are absorbed slowly, gastric lavage is particularly important in cases of iron poisoning. Use of sodium bicarbonate in the lavage results in the formation of ferrous carbonate, which is insoluble, and this may decrease iron absorption. Abdominal radiographs can be used to assess the amount of intact iron tablets remaining in the stomach.

The amount of iron reaching the circulation can be assessed by measurement of the serum iron concentration and total iron binding capacity (TIBC). A serum iron concentration exceeding either 350 mg/dl or the TIBC, or a clinical picture consistent with severe iron toxicity (i.e., shock), are indications for initiation of chelation therapy to lower the iron burden. Most clinical laboratory toxicology screens do not detect iron. Deferoxamine, given intravenously (10 mg/kg/hr), is the chelator of choice for treating iron toxicity. Deferoxamine may induce or worsen hypotension, but it is otherwise well tolerated. The deferoxamine-iron complex has an orange appearance that can be followed in the urine as an index of iron excretion.

The gastric mucosal injury induced by iron salts may lead to scarring and gastric outlet obstruction as a late complication of iron poisoning. Although intervention has been shown to decrease the incidence of this complication, patients should be evaluated, by history and examination, to identify the development of this syndrome.

Organophosphate Pesticides

Organophosphates are major constituents in agricultural, industrial, and household pesticides (insecticides, rodenticides). Organophosphates are inhibitors of the enzyme acetylcholinesterase, the enzyme that catalyzes the breakdown of the neurotransmitter acetylcholine. Inhibition of the acetylcholinesterase by these agents involves covalent phosphorylation and is therefore not readily reversible. Thus, organophosphates cause accumulation of acetylcholine, and accentuate cholinergic effects in the poisoned patient.[63]

Most organophosphates are lipophilic and are readily absorbed from the gastrointestinal tract, skin, lungs (the agents are often used as aerosols, which can be inhaled), and mucous membranes. This lipophilicity also means the compounds cross the blood-brain barrier and affect the central nervous system.

Symptoms and signs of organophosphate poisoning are those predicted based on the distribution and function of cholinergic receptors (muscarinic, nicotinic, and neuromuscular), with the sequence and timing of appearance affected by the route of exposure (i.e., inhalation with prominent respiratory symptoms early versus oral ingestion with gastrointestinal symptoms appearing earliest).[64] Muscarinic effects include copious production of secretions including saliva, sweat, tears, and bronchial secretions. Loss of bowel and bladder control occurs, and extreme bradycardia can be seen. Cramping abdominal pain, nausea, vomiting, and diarrhea may all be present. Pupils demonstrate a severe miosis. Skeletal muscle function is affected, with weakness and fasciculations progressing to paralysis. Central nervous system manifestations include confusion, restlessness, loss of reflexes, and ataxia progressing to seizures, coma, and respiratory arrest.

Respiratory failure, because of loss of muscle function and central drive, is the greatest danger in organophosphate poisoning. Protecting the airway, clearing of secretions, and adequate ventilation, as well as decontamination to prevent further absorption, are all critical. During decontamination, care is needed to avoid exposure of health care personnel to the poison. Diagnosis of anticholinesterase poisoning can usually be made on the basis of specific history and/or the constellation of symptoms and signs. Laboratory confirmation of the diagnosis can be made by measuring red blood cell and plasma cholinesterase activities.

Specific pharmacologic intervention in organophosphate poisoning involves two strategies. First, receptor antagonists can be used to inhibit the action of the accumulating acetylcholine. Atropine competitively inhibits acetylcholine action at muscarinic receptors.[64] Because of the large amount of acetylcholine present, extremely large doses of atropine (10- to 30-mg doses are common) may be required to establish inhibition. Atropine is effective in decreasing secretions, increasing the heart rate, and decreasing bronchospasm. Repeated administration may be needed to maintain muscarinic blockade. Atropine has no effect, however, at the neuromuscular junction and does not alter the underlying acetylcholinesterase inhibition. Therefore, a second strategy involves agents that regenerate the acetylcholinesterase by interacting with the phosphate moiety from the poison bound to the enzyme. Pralidoxime, or 2-PAM (pyridine-2-aldoxime methyl chloride), was designed specifically to recognize the acetylcholinesterase active site, and to interact with the phosphate group, reactivating the enzyme. 2-PAM should be given intravenously (1 g) to severe organophosphate poisoning victims. Repetitive dosing with 2-PAM may be necessary, with the clinical response and course determining the dosing requirement. 2-PAM is a quaternary amine and thus does not cross the blood-brain barrier.

Other therapeutic interventions in organophosphate poisoning should be supportive. Given the risk of seizures, the use of medications that may further lower seizure threshold should be avoided if possible. If seizures develop, standard therapeutic strategies beginning with diazepam should be used. In the absence of central nervous system damage, patients recovering from acute organophosphate poisoning should experience no sequelae.

Snake and Spider Bites

Although snake envenomations are estimated to cause 30,000 deaths per year worldwide, snake and spider bites are less frequent causes of mortality and morbidity in the United States.[65] An estimated 8000 bites from poisonous snakes occur annually in the United States, with a mortality of approximately 0.2%.[65] In general, snake venoms are a mixture of enzymes and bioactive peptides that produce local and systemic effects.[66-68] The coral snake found in the southern United States has a bite characterized by multiple punctures. Coral snake venom contains a neurotoxin and induces a limited local reaction at the bite site. The coral snake neurotoxin may result in progressive neurologic symptoms, beginning with numbness and weakness, progressing to slurring and slowed speech, to total paralysis. Loss of ventilation (impaired respiratory muscle function) is the major danger in coral snake bites. The pit vipers (rattlesnakes, water moccasins, and copperhead) produce a severe, local reaction at the site of the bite. Local pain and swelling may be followed by development of bullae and tissue necrosis. Systemic sequelae of pit viper bites include fever, nausea and vomiting, coagulopathies (both pro- and anticoagulant properties), muscle cramping, hypotension, delirium, and seizures. An increase in capillary permeability may contribute to both the severe swelling and hypotension in pit viper envenomations.

Risk to the victim after a snake bite is related to the venom dose. Children and small adults are at increased risk, and delivered dose is influenced by the size of the snake and the depth of the fang penetration. Spread of the venom from the bite is through lymphatics. This delivery can be decreased by placing the victim at rest and immobilizing the affected area. A loose fitting tourniquet (not affecting venous drainage) can decrease lymphatic drainage from the wound area. Venom can be removed from the bite site through a small incision (straight, 1 cm in length, through depth of the skin) using a suction device. Removal of venom by mouth should only be attempted in the absence of alternative suction devices and if no oral lesions are present through which venom can enter.

Whereas symptoms from envenomation begin soon after the bite and progress without lag, an estimated 25% of all bites do not result in envenomation.[68] Thus, the clinical course provides important information as to the severity of the poisoning. Specific assays for venom are being developed, but their clinical utility have not been evaluated. All patients should receive tetanus prophylaxis and local wound care. Infection of the wound site is an important potential complication. Coagulation status should be monitored. Antivenin is available against coral snake and pit viper venoms. These preparations are prepared from horse serum, and thus administration carries a risk of anaphylaxis and serum sickness. Dosing of the antivenin is based on the clinical severity of the bite with up to 10 to 15 vials required in severe cases. Antivenin for bites from snakes not indigenous to the United States are not readily available in the United States, but the Arizona Poison and Drug Information Center in Tucson (602-626-6016) maintains a national antivenin inventory. Other supportive measures are instituted as indicated in individual envenomation victims.

Black widow spider bites are associated with envenomation.[67] The female spider is responsible for human bites, with a peak incidence from April through October. A clear history of the spider bite and physical evidence of the bite are often absent. The black widow spider venom causes diffuse activation of neurotransmitter receptors, and initially causes cramping pain and muscle spasm at the site of the bite. Symptomatology becomes more diffuse with development of hypertension and hyperreflexia. A hard, although nontender, abdomen may lead to diagnostic confusion with an intraabdominal process. A horse serum-derived antiserum for treatment of black widow spider bites is available, but its use is usually not required and the risk of allergic side effects should limit its use to clinically severe poisonings in which other supportive measures are insufficient.

Brown spider bites (Loxosceles species) cause intense local pain and tissue necrosis.[67] Although self-limiting, the local reaction may have a course of weeks and diagnostic confusion may result in the absence of a bite history. Systemic symptoms and signs have been reported in individual cases including flu-like illness, intravascular hemolysis, and disseminated intravascular coagulation. Attention to local wound care usually is sufficient, but other interventions including corticosteroids and surgical excision have been advocated by individual authors.

Mushrooms

Serious mushroom poisonings in the United States are primarily attributed to members of the Amanita species.[69,70] Two distinct syndromes are associated with Amanita poisoning. The first, associated with ingestion of Amanita muscaria, is mediated by the muscarinic agonist muscarine. The resulting parasympathetic stimulation results in the predicted symptom complex, including increased secretions (tears, sweat, salivation, bronchial), nausea, vomiting, diarrhea, bronchoconstriction, bradycardia, hypotension, and central nervous system manifestations (confusion, delirium). These symptoms typically develop within hours after mushroom ingestion. Atropine can be used in severe cases to control parasympathetic system-related symptoms.

The second form of Amanita toxicity results from the action of cytotoxic peptides, of which alpha-amanitin is the best characterized.[70] Cellular toxicity is due in part to inhibition of RNA polymerase and the consequent inability to synthesize mRNA and proteins. Liver, kidney, skeletal muscle, and brain are all targets of alpha-amanitin toxicity. The consequences of the cellular insult appear after a lag of up to 20 hours after ingestion. Initial symptoms may be severe, and include abdominal pain, vomiting, hypotension, headache, altered mental status, and seizures. Liver and renal failure may develop, with the expected consequences of failure of these key homeostatic organs. Fluid and electrolyte disturbances, hypoglycemia, and hemodynamic status require careful, aggressive support in severe alpha-amanitin poisoning. Tissue damage may be irreversible. Hemoperfusion has been shown to remove alpha-amanitin, and it may be effective if initiated early in Amanita poisoning. Administration of cytochrome c and alpha-lipoic acid have also been suggested as therapy in alpha-amanitin poisoning, but no data are available to support their general clinical use.[70,71]

Miscellaneous Pharmacologic Agents

Many drugs are widely prescribed, and are thus potentially available for accidental or intentional poisonings. In most cases, the toxicity of these compounds is that expected on the basis of their pharmacologic properties. For example, hypoglycemia is the major complication of poisoning with oral hypoglycemic drugs, and bleeding a problem with anticoagulant overdose.

Nonsalicylate nonsteroidal antiinflammatory drugs (NSAIDs) have been the subject of several overdose series.[72,73] The propionic acid derivatives cause symptoms limited to the gastrointestinal tract in most cases, but renal failure, cardiovascular shock, and coma have all been described, as well as several deaths. Poisoning with fenamates appears associated with a greater risk of muscle twitching and seizures than other NSAIDs. Overdoses with indomethacin are usually well tolerated with mild gastrointestinal (nausea, vomiting, abdominal pain) and central nervous system (headache, tinnitus, dizziness, confusion) symptoms described most commonly.

Toxicity from antiarrhythmic drugs in overdoses frequently involve disturbances in cardiac conduction.[74] The spectrum of dysrhythmias observed in such cases is broad, and an understanding of the pharmacology of the agents involved is critical for rational therapy. Similarly, antihypertensive agents have significant potential for inducing hypotension in overdoses. The mechanism of the specific antihypertensive aids the choice of optimal therapy (i.e., central versus peripheral action, direct versus indirect action).

Extensive clinical experience is lacking for many new drugs in overdose situations. Appropriate use of diagnostic, decontamination, and supportive strategies, when combined with an understanding of the pharmacology of these agents, ensures a reasoned approach to management. Manufacturers, of both pharmaceuticals and other industrial chemicals, and regional poison control centers provide important sources of supplemental and updated toxicologic information.

CONSIDERATIONS DURING THE POST-ICU PHASE FOR THE POISONED PATIENT

Despite the life-threatening nature of many poisonings and the need for intensive care, most victims survive the acute event with proper management. Complications frequently seen in the poisoned patient include pneumonia (aspiration and infectious), fever, and rhabdomyolisis.[2] A complete review of all organ systems should be made before discharge from the ICU to rule out unsuspected sequelae from the poisoning. In many cases, preexisting medical problems require stabilization in the postpoisoning phase of the hospitalization.

Considerable attention should be given to determining why the poisoning occurred and to establishing mechanisms to prevent a recurrence. As many as 90% of poisonings that necessitate admission to the ICU are the result of intentional overdoses.[2] Survivors of suicide attempts provide a challenge to the entire health care system. Psychiatric consultation should be obtained as soon as the patient is medically able to cooperate, and discharge from the ICU to an inpatient psychiatric ward is often necessary. Many patients who attempt suicide have a previous history of a suicide attempt (20 to 25% in most series), emphasizing the need for long-term management plans.[1] The safety of using psychoactive drugs that can be used in suicide attempts has been discussed in many settings. As many as 75% of patients who attempt suicide with a psychotropic drug receive a new prescription for the same or similar medication after recovery.[75] It is equally important to recognize, however, that, annually, only 0.3% of patients who are prescribed psychotropic drugs attempt to overdose with the medication.[75] Because these drugs may have dramatic benefit, a careful risk assessment is needed to formulate the optimal postsuicide attempt management plan.

Poisonings that result from accidental exposure also warrant intensive follow-up. Poisonings involving children require education of the parents or guardian concerning safety latches on cabinets, proper storage procedures, and the use of childproof seals. On rare occasions, childhood poisonings may be a manifestation of child abuse, and the physician must be alert to this possibility. Accidental poisonings also occur in the elderly.[76] These geriatric poisonings may result from misidentification of a food or medicine, or use of household products in an unsafe manner. An alarming number of geriatric poisonings occur in nursing homes,[76] where potential toxins are left in the vicinity of unsupervised patients where they can be ingested. Identification of the factors leading to the poisoning permits implementation of remedial steps. In these situations, appropriate consultation with in-hospital social services and external social agencies is an integral part of discharge planning. Similarly, poisoning in the occupational setting should result in a review of safety, storage, and emergency care procedures at the work site.

Patients in whom toxicity develops in the course of drug therapy should be evaluated for risk factors that could result in unpredictable pharmacokinetics or pharmacodynamics, such as drug-drug or nutrient-drug interactions. Patients should be educated to refrain from self-adjustment in dosage without physician approval, and in regard to potential early symptoms of mild toxicity that might forewarn more serious potential complications. Therapeutic drug monitoring might be used to evaluate the dosing regimen to identify changes in drug pharmacokinetics over time. In difficult cases, the choice of drug may be dictated by the individual patient's ratio of therapeutic to toxic drug concentrations or pharmacokinetic characteristics.

As was true for the medical management of the poisoned patient, individualizing the management plan during the post-ICU phase permits the health care provider to address the specific needs and problems of the patient. Management of the poisoned patient from the pre-ICU through the post-ICU phase requires a variety of skills from the physician, but it also provides the opportunity to formulate and implement rational therapies that will have a dramatic impact on the patient's well being.

REFERENCES

1. Stern, T. A., Mulley, A. G., Thibault, G. E.: Life-threatening drug overdose. JAMA, *251:*1983, 1984.
2. Leykin, Y., et al.: Acute poisoning treated in the intensive care unit: A case series. Isr. J. Med. Sci., *25:*98, 1989.
3. Kerr, H. D.: Self-poisoning with drugs. Wisc. Med. J., *88:*15, 1989.
4. Menzies, D. G., Busuttil, A., and Prescott, L. F.: Fatal pulmonary aspiration of oral activated charcoal. Br. Med. J., *297:*459, 1988.
5. Rau, N. R., et al.: Fatal pulmonary aspiration of oral activated charcoal. Br. Med. J., *297:*918, 1988.
6. Haddad, L. M., and Winchester, J. (Eds.): Clinical Management of Poisoning and Drug Overdose. Philadelphia, W. B. Saunders, 1983.
7. Gosselin, R. E., Smith, R. P., and Hodge, H. C. (Eds.): Clinical Toxicology of Commercial Products. 5th Ed. Baltimore, Williams & Wilkins, 1984.
8. Ellenhorn, M. J., and Barceloux, D. (Eds.): Medical Toxicology: Diagnosis and Treatment of Human Poisoning. New York, Elsevier, 1987.
9. Prescott, L. F.: Paracetamol overdosage. Drugs, *25:*290, 1983.

10. Black, M.: Acetaminophen hepatotoxicity. Gastroenterology, *78:*382, 1980.
11. Rumack, B. H., and Matthew, H.: Acetaminophen poisoning and toxicity. Pediatrics, *55:*871, 1975.
12. Smilkstein, M. D., et al.: Efficacy of oral N-acetylcysteine in the treatment of acetaminophen overdose. N. Engl. J. Med., *319:*1557, 1988.
13. Brenner, B. E., and Simon, R. R.: Management of salicylate intoxication. Drugs, *24:*335, 1982.
14. Temple, A. R.: Pathophysiology of aspirin overdosage toxicity, with implications for management. Pediatrics, *62(Suppl.):*873, 1978.
15. Heffner, J. E., and Sahn, S. A.: Salicylate-induced pulmonary edema. Ann. Intern. Med., *95:*405, 1981.
16. Done, A. K.: Aspirin overdosage: Incidence, diagnosis, and management. Pediatrics, *62(Suppl.):*890, 1978.
17. Henry, J., and Volans, G.: Analgesic poisoning. I. Salicylates. Br. Med. J., *289:*820, 1984.
18. Marshall, J. B., and Forker, A. D.: Cardiovascular effects of tricyclic antidepressant drugs: Therapeutic usage, overdose, and management of complications. Am. Heart J., *103:*401, 1982.
19. Boehnert, M. T., and Lovejoy, Jr., F. H.: Value of the QRS duration versus the serum drug level in predicting seizures and ventricular arrhythmias after an acute overdose of tricyclic antidepressants. N. Engl. J. Med., *313:*474, 1985.
20. Foulke, G. E., and Albertson, T. E.: QRS interval in tricyclic antidepressant overdosage: Inaccuracy as a toxicity indicator in emergency settings. Ann. Emerg. Med., *16:*160, 1987.
21. Hagerman, G. A., and Hanashiro, P. K.: Reversal of tricyclic-antidepressant-induced cardiac conduction abnormalities by phenytoin. Ann. Emerg. Med., *10:*82, 1981.
22. Nattel, S., and Mittleman, M.: Treatment of ventricular tachyarrhythmias resulting from amitriptyline toxicity in dogs. J. Pharmacol. Exp. Ther., *231:*430, 1984.
23. Hodes, D.: Sodium bicarbonate and hyperventilation in treating an infant with severe overdose of tricyclic antidepressant. Br. Med. J., *288:*1800, 1984.
24. Pentel, P., and Peterson, C. D.: Asystole complicating physostigmine treatment of tricyclic antidepressant overdose. Ann. Emerg. Med., *9:*588, 1980.
25. Swartz, C. M., and Sherman, A.: The treatment of tricyclic antidepressant overdose with repeated charcoal. J. Clin. Psychopharmacol., *4:*336, 1984.
26. Goldberg, M. J., et al.: Lack of effect of oral activated charcoal on imipramine clearance. Clin. Pharmacol. Ther., *38:*350, 1985.
27. Goldberg, R. J., Capone, R. J., and Hunt, J. D.: Cardiac complications following tricyclic antidepressant overdose. Issues for monitoring policy. JAMA, *254:*1772, 1985.
28. Guzzardi, L.: Monoamine oxidase inhibitors. *In* Clinical Management of Poisoning and Drug Overdose. Edited by L. M. Haddad and J. F. Winchester. Philadelphia, W. B. Saunders, 1983.
29. Breheny, F. X., Dobb, G. J., and Clarke, G. M.: Phenelzine poisoning. Anaesthesia, *41:*53, 1986.
30. Crome, P., and Ali, C.: Clinical features and management of self-poisoning with newer antidepressants. Med. Toxicol., *1:*411, 1986.
31. Carbon monoxide intoxication: a preventable environmental health hazard. MMWR, *31:*529, 1982.
32. Meredith, T., and Vale, A.: Carbon monoxide poisoning. Br. Med. J., *296:*77, 1988.
33. Norkool, D. M., and Kirkpatrick, J. N.: Treatment of acute carbon monoxide poisoning with hyperbaric oxygen: A review of 115 cases. Ann. Emerg. Med., *14:*1168, 1985.
34. Grace, T. W., and Platt, F. W.: Subacute carbon monoxide poisoning. JAMA, *246:*1698, 1981.
35. Choi, H. S.: Delayed neurologic sequelae in carbon monoxide intoxication. Arch. Neurol., *40:*433, 1983.
36. Singer, E. P., and Kolischenko, A.: Seizures due to theophylline overdose. Chest, *87:*755, 1985.
37. Hendeles, L., Weinberger, M., and Johnson, G.: Monitoring serum theophylline levels. Clin. Pharmacokinet., *3:*294, 1978.
38. Lesko, L. J.: Dose-dependent elimination kinetics of theophylline. Clin. Pharmacokinet., *4:*449, 1979.
39. Levy, G., et al.: Hemodialysis clearance of theophylline. JAMA, *237:*1466, 1977.
40. Anderson, J. R., et al.: Effects of hemodialysis on theophylline kinetics. J. Clin. Pharmacol., *23:*428, 1983.
41. Radomski, L., et al.: Model for theophylline overdose treatment with oral activated charcoal. Clin. Pharmacol. Ther., *35:*402, 1984.
42. Park, G. D., et al.: Use of hemoperfusion for treatment of theophylline intoxication. Am. J. Med., *74:*961, 1983.
43. Mooradian, A. D.: Digitalis. Clin. Pharmacokinet., *15:*165, 1988.
44. Antman, E. M., and Smith, T. W.: Digitalis toxicity. Annu. Rev. Med., *36:*357, 1985.
45. Ingelfinger, J. A., and Goldman, P.: The serum digitalis concentration—Does it diagnose digitalis toxicity? N. Engl. J. Med., *294:*867, 1976.
46. Kleiger, R., and Lown, B.: Cardioversion and digitalis. II. Clinical studies. Circulation, *33:*878, 1966.
47. Smith, T. W., et al.: Treatment of life-threatening digitalis intoxication with digoxin-specific Fab antibody fragments. N. Engl. J. Med., *307:*1357, 1982.
48. Wenger, T. L., et al.: Treatment of 63 severely digitalis-toxic patients with digoxin-specific antibody fragments. J. Am. Coll. Cardiol., *5:*118A, 1985.
49. Boman, K., Allgulander, S., and Skoglund, M.: Is maintenance digoxin necessary in geriatric patients. Acta Med. Scand., *210:*493, 1981.
50. Lydiard, R. B., and Gelenberg, A. J.: Hazards and adverse effects of lithium. Annu. Rev. Med., *33:*327, 1982.
51. Winchester, J. F.: Lithium. *In* Clinical Management of Poisoning and Drug Overdose. Edited by L. M. Haddad and J. F. Winchester. Philadelphia, W. B. Saunders, 1983.
52. Hansen, H. E., and Amdisen, A.: Lithium intoxication. Q. J. Med., *47:*123, 1978.
53. Dyson, E. H., et al.: Self-poisoning and therapeutic intoxication with lithium. Hum. Toxicol., *6:*325, 1987.
54. Becker, C. E.: Acute methanol poisoning. West. J. Med., *135:*122, 1981.
55. Gabow, P. A., et al.: Organic acids in ethylene glycol intoxication. Ann. Intern. Med., *105:*16, 1986.
56. Swartz, R. D., et al.: Epidemic methanol poisoning: Clinical and biochemical of a recent episode. Medicine, *60:*373, 1981.
57. Underwood, F., and Bennet, W. M.: Ethylene glycol intoxication: Prevention of renal failure by aggressive management. JAMA, *226:*1453, 1973.
58. Brown, C. G., Trumbull, D., and Klein-Schwartz, J. D.: Ethylene glycol poisoning. Ann. Emerg. Med., *12:*501, 1983.
59. Jacobsen, D., et al.: Anion and osmolal gaps in the diagnosis of methanol and ethylene glycol poisoning. Acta Med. Scand., *212:*17, 1982.
60. Way, J. L.: Cyanide intoxication and its mechanism of antagonism. Annu. Rev. Pharmacol. Toxicol., *24:*451, 1984.
61. Peters, C. G., Mundy, J. V. B., and Rayner, P. R.: Acute cyanide poisoning. Anaesthesia, *37:*582, 1982.

62. Robotham, J. L., and Lietman, P. S.: Acute iron poisoning: A review. Am. J. Dis. Child., *134*:875, 1980.
63. Namba, T., et al.: Poisoning due to organophosphate insecticides. Am. J. Med., *50*:475, 1971.
64. Steinhart, C. M., and Pearson-Shaver, A. L.: Poisoning. Issues Pediatr. Crit. Care, *4*:845, 1988.
65. Wallace, J. F.: Disorders caused by venoms, bites and stings. *In* Harrison's Principles of Internal Medicine. 11th Ed. Edited by E. Braunwald, et al. New York, McGraw-Hill, 1987.
66. Wasserman, G. S.: Wound care of spider and snake envenomations. Ann. Emerg. Med., *17*:1331, 1988.
67. Banner, Jr., W.: Bites and stings in the pediatric patient. Curr. Probl. Pediatr., Jan. 1988, p. 9.
68. Nelson, B. K.: Snake envenomation: Incidence, clinical presentation and management. Med. Toxicol., *4*:17, 1989.
69. Hall, A. H., Spoerke, D. G., and Rumack, B. H.: Mushroom poisoning: Identification, diagnosis, and treatment. Pediatr. Rev., *8*:291, 1987.
70. Piqueras, J.: Hepatotoxic mushroom poisoning: Diagnosis and management. Mycopathologia, *105*:99, 1989.
71. Friedman, P. A.: Poisoning and its management. *In* Harrison's Principles of Internal Medicine. 11th Ed. Edited by E. Braunwald, et al. New York, McGraw-Hill, 1987.
72. Meredith, T. J., and Vale, J. A.: Non-narcotic analgesics: Problems of overdosage. Drugs, *32(Suppl. 4)*:177, 1986.
73. Court, H., Streete, P., and Volans, G. N.: Acute poisoning with ibuprofen. Hum. Toxicol., *2*:381, 1983.
74. Hruby, K., and Missliwetz, J.: Poisoning with oral antiarrhythmic drugs. Int. J. Clin. Pharmacol. Ther. Toxicol., *23*:253, 1985.
75. Skegg, K., Skegg, D. C. G., and Richards, S. M.: Incidence of self-poisoning in patients prescribed psychotropic drugs. Br. Med. J., *286*:841, 1983.
76. Klein-Schwartz, W., Oderda, G. M., and Booze, L.: Poisoning in the elderly. J. Am. Geriatr. Soc., *31*:195, 1983.

Chapter 71

IMAGING TECHNIQUES IN THE INTENSIVE CARE UNIT

MOULAY A. MEZIANE

In the past two decades, assessment and management of the critically ill patient in the ICU have been greatly enhanced by the advent of a whole array of new diagnostic and therapeutic techniques. With the development of new imaging modalities, such as ultrasonography (US), computed tomography (CT), digital angiography, and magnetic resonance imaging (MRI), the radiologic evaluation of the patient has become more sophisticated. With the computerization and miniaturization of radiologic equipment, certain ultrasonographic, fluoroscopic, and nuclear medical examinations can be performed at the bedside. Although angiography, CT scanning, and MRI studies cannot be performed at the bedside, the angiographic and scanning suites are now designed to accommodate the critically ill with all life-support devices that may be connected to the patient. CT scanning is being used with increased frequency when intracranial, intra-abdominal, or intrathoracic pathology is suspected. Conventional radiography (plain films) using portable techniques, however, remains the main imaging modality used in the ICU. The portable chest x-ray film, obtained at the patient's bedside, remains the most common radiologic procedure performed in the ICU. Historically the few radiologic methods offered to the critically ill patient have been of a limited diagnostic value when compared with the multitude of sophisticated radiologic examinations that are available to the ambulatory patient.

It is somewhat of a paradox that the most critically ill patients, who require the best and the most sensitive radiological workup, often undergo radiologic examinations that have a limited diagnostic value. Attempts are continually being made to improve the quality and consistency of the radiographic images by improving the quality of the portable radiologic equipment available and by perfecting new technologies. New film-screen combinations and grid systems dedicated to such equipment have produced images of better diagnostic quality.[1]

Digital radiography, which uses an entirely new technology, is being considered as an alternative to conventional film-screen technologies for the bedside radiographic examination of the critically ill patient. Digital acquisition and processing have been routinely used for CT, MRI, US, and digital angiography. Early experience with high-resolution digital imaging in portable radiography using storage phosphor films showed improvement of the quality of the images over conventional radiography.[2] Chest images require a higher spatial resolution to have a diagnostic quality acceptable to both radiologists and clinicians. The wide latitude of the storage phosphor technique permits satisfactory imaging in portable radiography, in which exposure factors cannot be accurately or easily controlled. The added advantage of digital imaging is the possibility to transmit images electronically from the radiographic department to any remote site, such as ICUs.[3,4] The implementation of digital imaging will promote the development of picture archiving and communications systems (PACS), in which images can be stored, transmitted, or retrieved in a consistent, reliable, and efficient fashion.

Before digital imaging can be widely applied, further large-scale studies are necessary to evaluate the diagnostic superiority of such systems and the financial impact of such imaging procedures when switching to this new technology.

The success of the imaging procedure relies not only on the sophistication of the radiologic equipment, but also on the skill of the personnel performing the procedure. It is necessary to have a good, highly trained technology personnel that is dedicated to imaging the critically ill patient. The radiologist is a member of the ICU team working in close relationship with the referring physician through daily consultation and teaching rounds. A well-informed radiologist, knowledgeable about the condition of the patient being examined, helps eliminate unnecessary procedures and obtains the best diagnostic examination. Although plain radiographs represent the first screening imaging modality available to answer common medical problems, more complex diagnostic methods should be used to diagnose complex cases (Table 71-1).

IMAGING OF THE CHEST

The portable chest film obtained at the patient's bedside is the most commonly ordered radiographic examination in the ICU. In most large institutions, portable chest films constitute up to 80% of all portable examinations and 50% of all chest studies. For example, more than 40,000 portable chest examinations are performed every year at the Cleveland Clinic Foundation. Much information on the patient's status can be derived from the interpretation of the chest film alone. It monitors the status of two important vital functions: the patient's breathing and the cardiovascular function. It also detects abnormalities involving the lungs, heart, pleural space, and mediastinum. Information regarding the airways, diaphragms, chest wall, or subdi-

Table 71–1. Portable Imaging Modalities Available to be Performed at the Bedside

Plain Films
  Chest x-ray film (upright or supine)
    Projections
      Anteroposterior (AP)
      Posteroanterior (PA)
      Lateral
      Cross-table lateral
      Lateral decubitus
  Abdomen and pelvis
  Head and neck
  Extremities and joints
  Soft tissues
Ultrasonography
  Chest
    Pleural space
    Mediastinum
    Heart, pericardium
  Abdomen
    Liver
    Pancreas
    Spleen
    Kidneys
    Gallbladder, biliary tree
    Large veins, arteries
    Retroperitoneum
    Pelvis
Nuclear Medicine
  Lungs
  Kidneys
  Gallbladder
Fluoroscopy
  Limited application owing to poor quality of images
    Contrast studies
    Placement of monitoring and life-support devices

Table 71–2. Diagnosis and Monitoring Uses of the Portable Chest X-ray Film

Lung Parenchyma
  Edema
  Pneumonia
  Infarction
  Bleeding
  Atelectasis
  Cavitation
  Emphysema
  Tumor
  Aspiration
Pleural space
  Effusion
  Pneumothorax
Heart, vasculature
  Enlargement
  Pericardial effusion
Mediastinum
  Bleeding
  Pneumomediastinum
  Airway abnormalities (obstruction, narrowing, displacement)
  Esophageal abnormalities (obstruction, rupture, dilatation)
  Vascular abnormalities (dilatation, aneurysm)
  Adenopathy, tumor
Chest wall
  Fractures
  Hematoma, abscess
Neck and subdiaphragmatic abnormalities
Monitoring devices
  To check for placement and complications

aphragmatic organs can be derived from the same examination. It is routinely obtained after invasive instrumentation of the chest with tubes, catheters, drains, or wires to check their proper placement or the potential complications they may create (Table 71–2).

LIFE-SUPPORT AND MONITORING DEVICES

Tracheal Intubation

Portable radiographs of the chest are routinely obtained after tracheal intubation because the tubes can often be malpositioned (12%).[5] Tracheostomy tubes and endotracheal tubes, which can be inserted through the nose or mouth, are recognized radiographically through radiopaque markers seen at the tip or along the wall of the tube (Figs. 71–1 through 71–4). Proper inflation of the cuff that

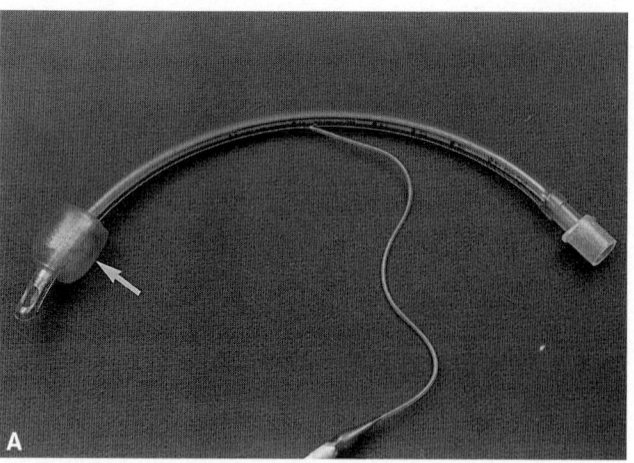
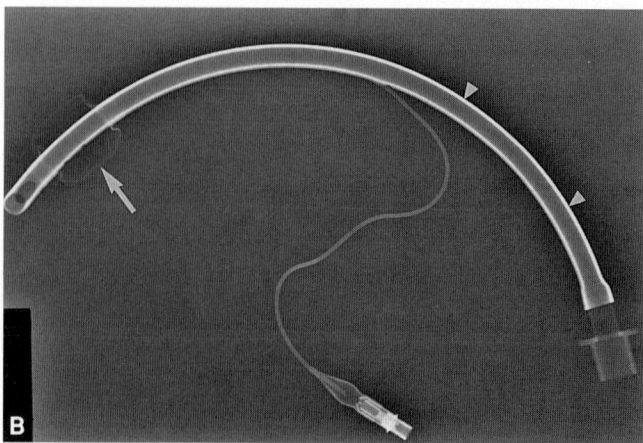

Fig. 71–1. Endotracheal tube. *A,* Photograph of the commonly used endotracheal tube seen with the cuff partially inflated (arrow). *B,* Radiograph of the endotracheal tube shown in *A* with the cuff seen partially inflated (arrow). Note the radiopaque marker identified throughout the course of the tube (arrowheads).

IMAGING TECHNIQUES IN THE INTENSIVE CARE UNIT

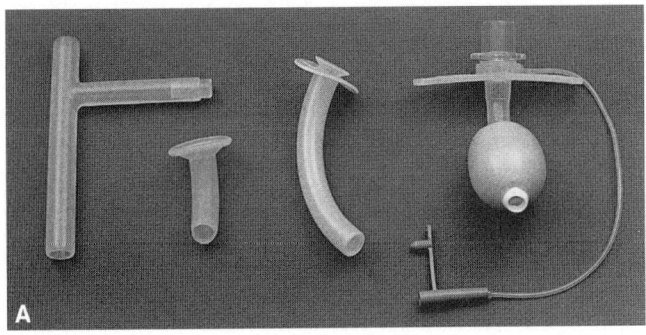 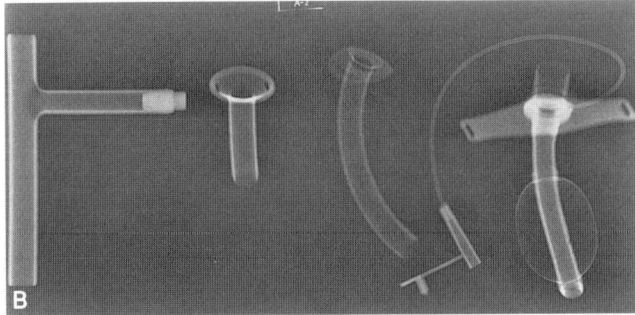

Fig. 71–2. Tracheostomy tubes. *A,* Photographs of different types of commonly used rubber tracheostomy tubes. *B,* Radiographs of the tracheostomy tubes shown in *A.*

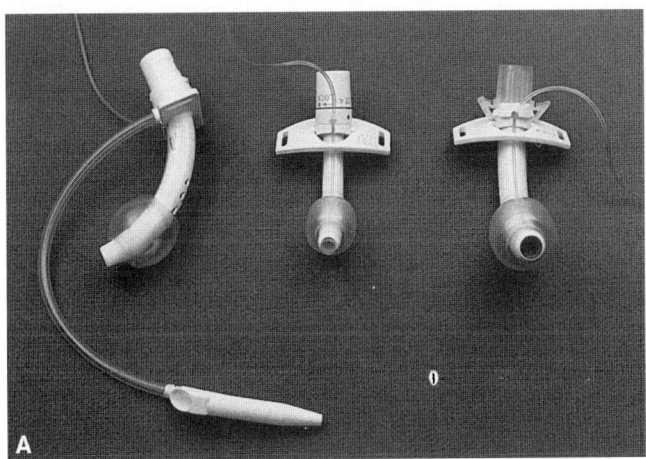 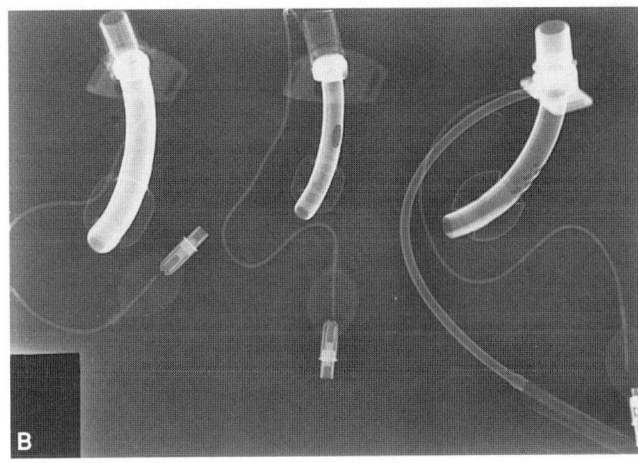

Fig. 71–3. Tracheostomy tubes. *A,* Photographs of different types of commonly used plastic tracheostomy tubes shown with the distal cuffs partially inflated. *B,* Radiographs of the tracheostomy tubes shown in *A.*

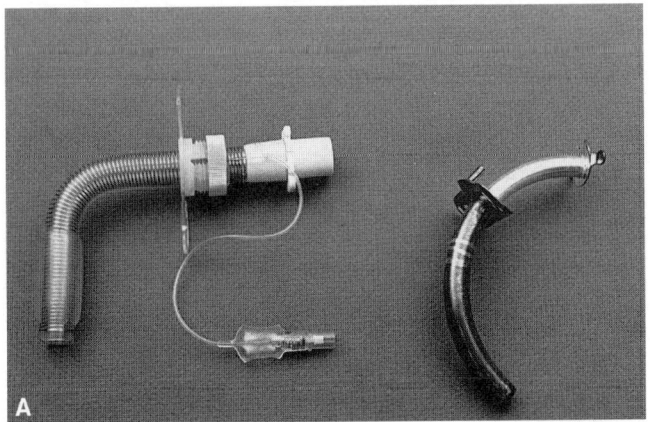

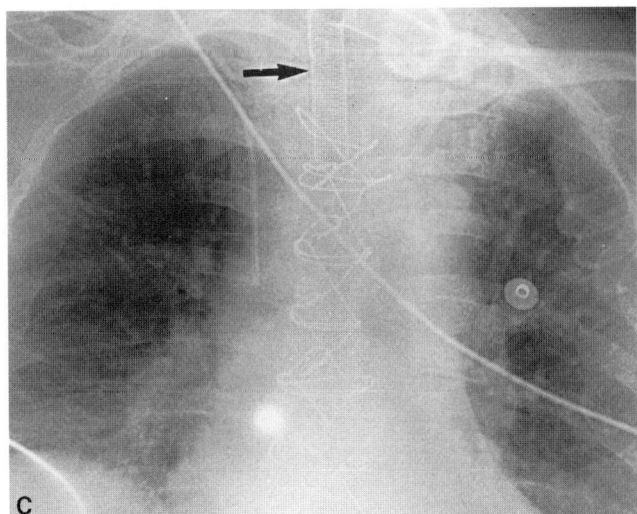

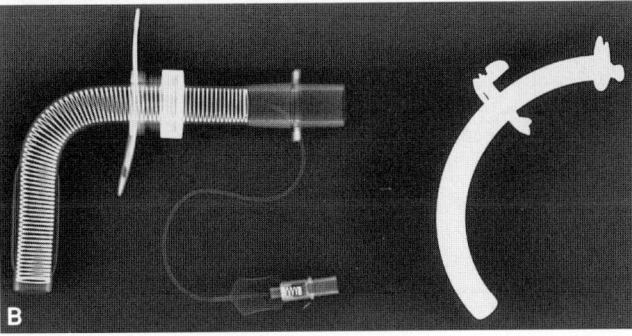

Fig. 71–4. Tracheostomy tubes. *A,* Photographs of an expandable tracheostomy tube that has a metallic coil lining (left) and a fully metallic silver tracheostomy tube (right). *B,* Radiograph of the tracheostomy tubes shown in *A. C,* The metallic coil in the tracheostomy tube offers a good radiopaque marker easy to identify when placed in the patient (arrow).

THE HIGH RISK PATIENT: MANAGEMENT OF THE CRITICALLY ILL

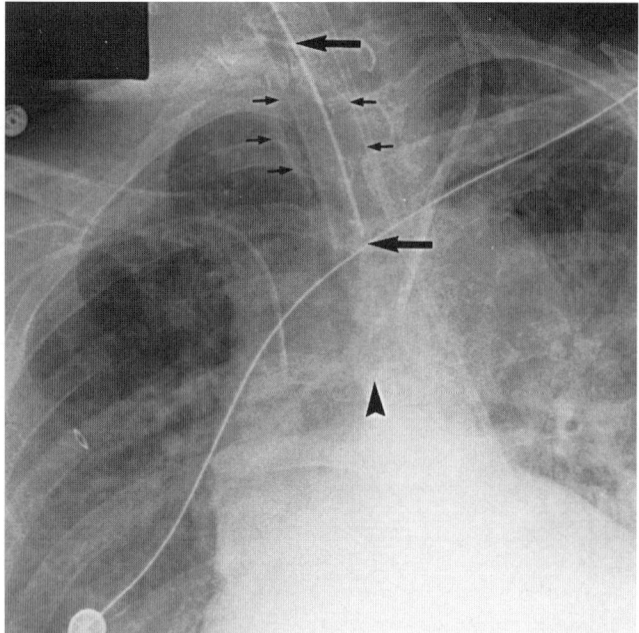

Fig. 71-5. Endotracheal tube—hyperinflated cuff. Portable chest anteroposterior film obtained supine in a patient with congestive heart failure demonstrates diffuse pulmonary vascular prominence and interstitial edema with a right pleural effusion identified as a haze projecting over the right lower chest. The cardiac-pericardiac silhouette is enlarged. An endotracheal tube is recognized by its radiopaque marker (large arrows). The tip is in normal position approximately 2 inches above the carina (arrowhead). The inflated cuff is recognized as a lucency near the tip of the endotracheal tube (small arrows) seen here bulging the right lateral wall of the trachea.

surrounds the tip of the tube seals the airway and secures the tube. The ideal location of the tip of the tube is approximately 2 to 3 inches from the carina, remembering that a neck extension will move the tip approximately 1 to 2 inches cephalad and that the tip will descend closer to the carina approximately 1 to 2 inches with flexion of the neck.[6] Hyperinflated cuffs beyond the normal tracheal diameter bulge the lateral tracheal walls and may create tracheal erosion and subsequent stricture formation (Fig. 71-5). Tracheal stricture can also be observed at the site of a previous tracheostomy (Fig. 71-6).[7] Noninflated or asymmetrically inflated cuffs may cause the tip to abut the tracheal wall leading to tracheal erosion. During intubation, tracheal or pharyngeal perforation and rarely esophageal trauma may occur. Teeth can be aspirated or ingested when they are inadvertently dislodged during intubation (Fig. 71-7). A tube can be inadvertently placed into a main stem bronchus, causing hyperinflation of the intubated lung and possibly creating a pneumothorax. It may also cause blockage of the opposite main stem bronchus with subsequent lung atelectasis (Fig. 71-8).

Thoracostomy Tubes

Pleural drainage tubes (thoracostomy or chest tubes) are faintly radiodense except for a radiopaque marker that runs along the length of the tube, interrupted only at the site of the side holes. The tip and the side holes should lie within the pleural space, ideally in an anterior location for pneumothorax drainage and posterior location for pleural effusion drainage. Appropriate placement is crucial for loculated fluid or air collections. A persistent pleural collection, despite the presence of a chest tube, should raise the

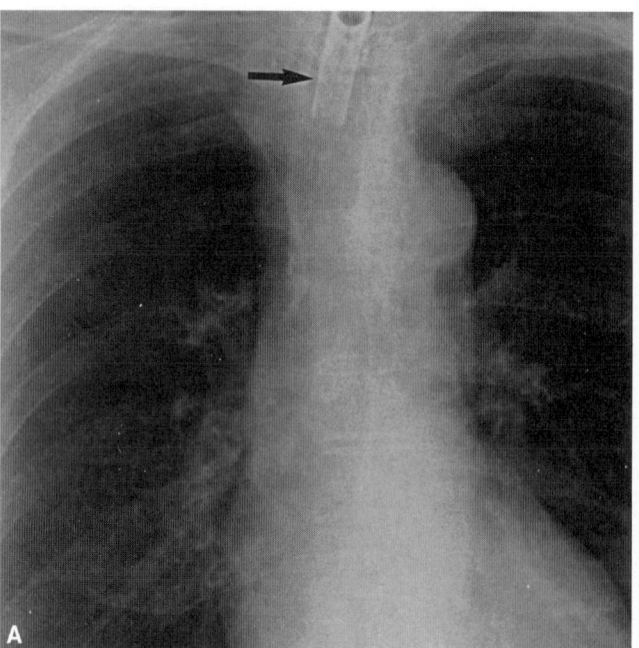
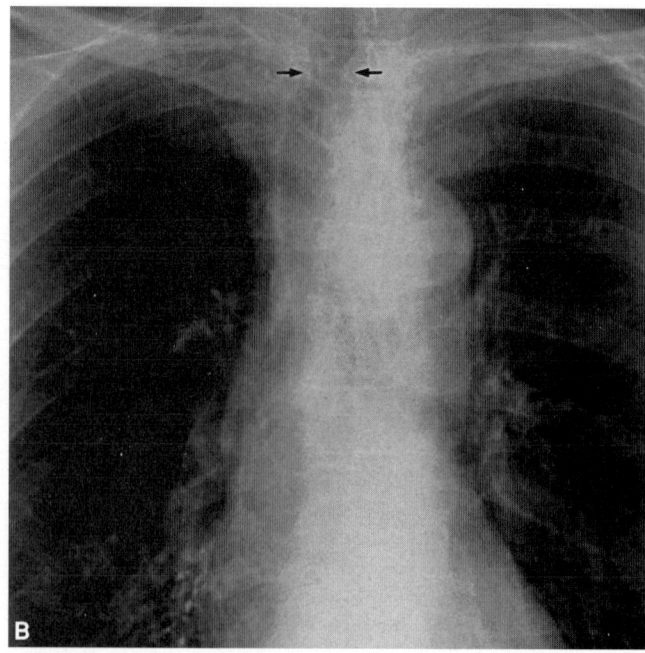

Fig. 71-6. Post-tracheostomy stricture. A, Chest posteroanterior film obtained after tracheostomy tube placement in a 59-year-old patient with history of chronic obstructive pulmonary disease. The tracheostomy tube (arrow) is in satisfactory position with the tip approximately 3 inches above the carina. B, Chest anteroposterior film obtained 1 year later after removal of the tracheostomy demonstrates an area of concentric tracheal narrowing at the site of the prior tracheostomy (arrows). There is evidence of bilateral hyperinflation of the lungs compatible with chronic obstructive pulmonary disease with bilateral lower lung dense infiltrates owing to prior aspiration of contrast material.

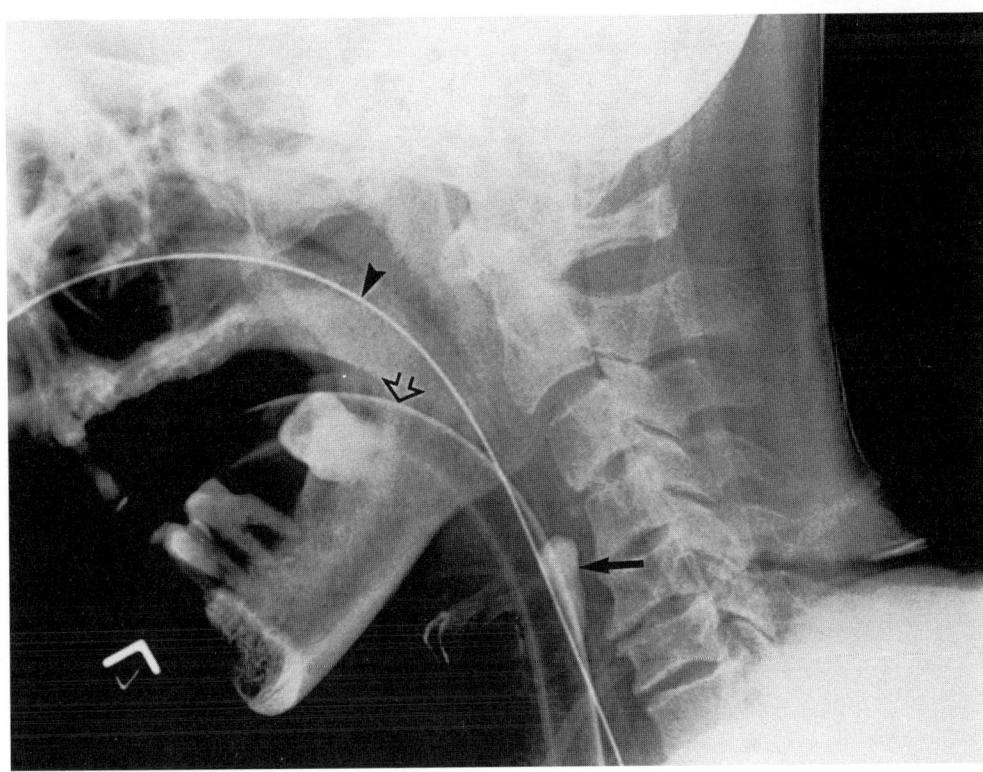

Fig. 71-7. Postintubation dental extraction. A lateral view of the neck demonstrates a tooth in the hypopharynx (arrow), which has been accidentally dislodged during intubation. A nasogastric tube (plain arrowhead) and an endotracheal tube (open arrowhead) are easily identified with the help of the radiopaque markers seen in their wall.

suspicion of a misplaced tube within the soft tissues of the chest wall or within a fissure. The improper placement of the tube can be suspected on the anteroposterior view alone, but to confirm the exact location and course, further radiographic examinations such as lateral views (Fig. 71-9) or a CT scan examination may be necessary (Fig. 71-10).[8] A tube inserted too superficially with the side hole in the chest wall may cause subcutaneous emphysema, whereas a tube inserted too deep may injure the mediastinal structures. Rarely, chest tubes may be forced into the lungs causing trauma to the lung parenchyma (Fig. 71-11).

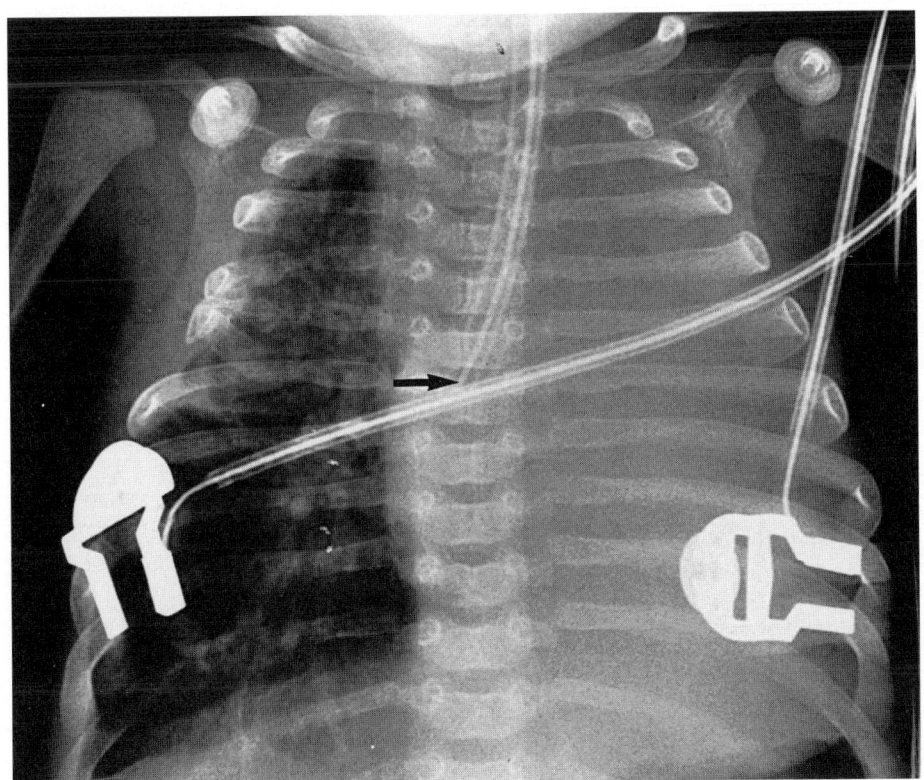

Fig. 71-8. Endotracheal tube misplacement. A chest anteroposterior portable film obtained on a 6-month-old premature infant with history of bronchopulmonary dysplasia and right chest surgery demonstrates an endotracheal tube curving at the entrance of the right main stem bronchus with the tip within the proximal right main stem bronchus (arrow). Note the complete opacification of the left hemithorax caused by the left lung atelectasis secondary to the blockage of the left main stem bronchus by the left side wall of the endotracheal tube. Note the hyperinflation of the right lower lung owing to the selective intubation of the right lung. Because of the small length of the trachea in very young patients, it is not uncommon that endotracheal tubes are placed far distally within the airways.

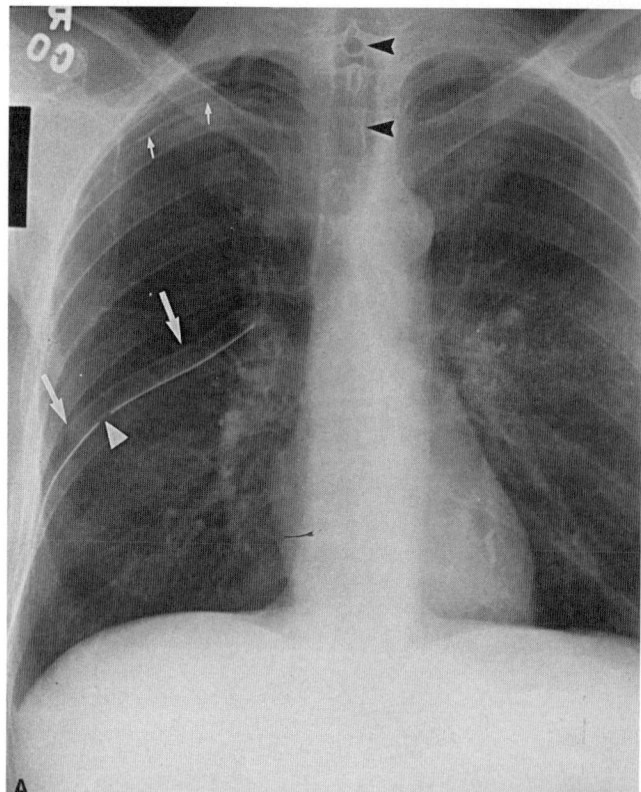
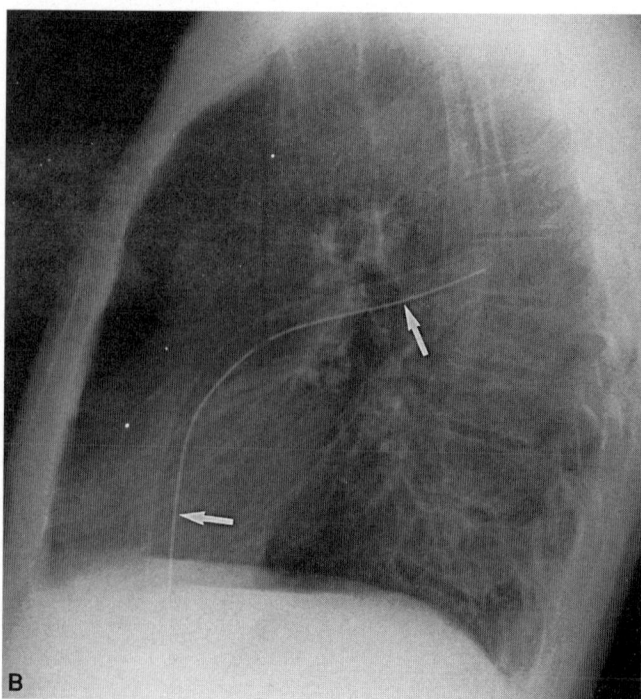

Fig. 71-9. Chest tube in the fissure. A, Chest posteroanterior film demonstrates a right chest tube entering the right lower chest and coursing toward the medial aspect of the right midchest. It follows the expected course of the right major fissure (large white arrows). The chest tube is easily identified by the radiopaque marker included throughout the length of its wall. The side hole can be visualized projecting within the right hemithorax (white arrowhead). Note the presence of a persistent right apical pneumothorax (small white arrows). Without a radiopaque marker, the tracheostomy tube is faintly visualized (black arrowheads). B, Careful examination of the lateral view shows that the chest tube is within the right major fissure. As in the posteroanterior view, the right chest tube is seen along the expected course of the major fissure (arrows).

Enteric Tubes

Except for a smaller diameter, nasogastric tubes have a similar appearance to that of chest tubes. A radiopaque marker runs throughout the course of the tube, interrupted by the side hole furthest from the catheter tip (Fig. 71-12). The tip and the side hole should lie within the stomach. Tubes can inadvertently migrate into the esophagus (Fig. 71-13) or be accidentally placed into the airways causing lung atelectasis, contusion, or aspiration (Fig. 71-14).[9] Rarely, accidental perforation of the esophagus may occur after intubation (Fig. 71-15). Feeding tubes are usually of a much smaller caliber and faintly radiopaque and are recognized by their radiopaque tip. The optimal position of the tip should be in the duodenum before feeding can be started. Fluoroscopically guided placement may be necessary in difficult cases. A radiograph of the abdomen is required to check for the position of the tube before feeding is started because potential misplacement into the upper airways or lungs is not uncommon (Fig. 71-16).

Venous Catheters

Central venous catheters used for monitoring central venous pressure or for intravenous administration of fluid or drugs are commonly inserted through a subclavian vein or jugular vein approach. They should follow a course compatible with the expected anatomy of the major mediastinal veins, with the tip placed central to the venous valves at the origin of the superior vena cava. The catheters are often incorrectly placed, misdirected cephalad toward the neck, into a contralateral vein, internal mammary vein, azygous vein (Figs. 71-17 and 71-18), hepatic veins, or in the cardiac chambers.[10] When a patient has a persistent left-sided superior vena cava, a catheter or wire placed through a left peripheral approach can mimic an arterial placement (Figs. 71-19 and 71-20). Inadvertent puncture of the pleural space may create a pneumothorax or pleural effusion. Extravascular placement may create bleeding within the mediastinum or pleural space (Figs. 71-21 and 71-22). Catheters placed deep within the cardiac chambers may create arrhythmia and therefore should be repositioned. Cardiac perforation has been reported to occur after infusion of venous catheters wedged within the wall of the cardiac chambers.[11,12] Accidental ectopic infusion of fluid into the pleural space or mediastinum, secondary to ectopic misplacement of catheters, can be recognized when there is a rapid accumulation of fluid within these spaces.

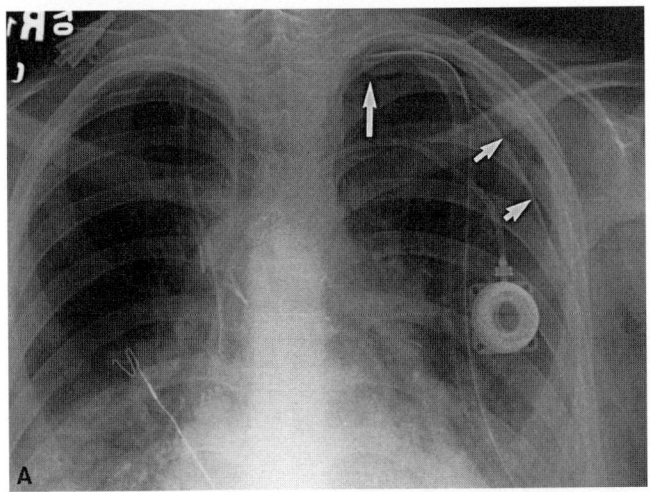
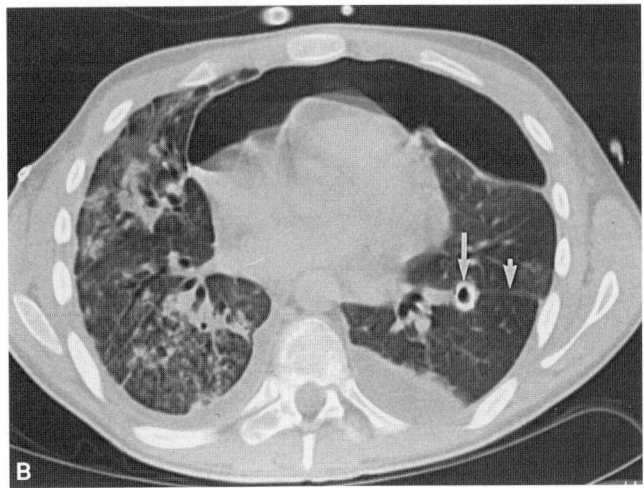
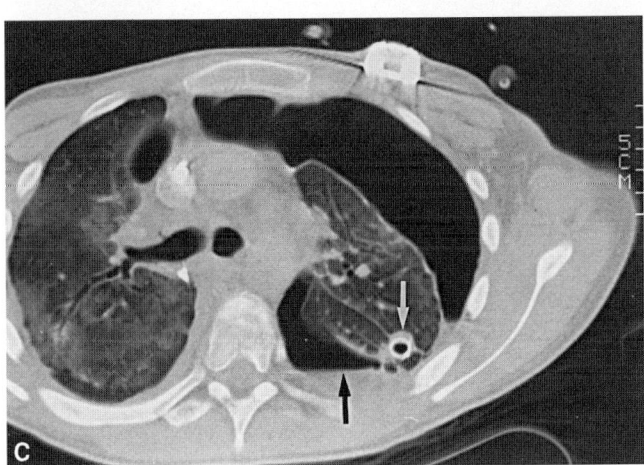

Fig. 71–10. Chest tube in the fissure. *A,* Portable chest anteroposterior film obtained in a 19-year-old patient status post bilateral lung transplant demonstrates bilateral lower lung infiltrates and a persistent left pneumothorax (short arrows). This anteroposterior view shows a left chest tube with its tip in the left apex (long arrow). *B,* A CT scan examination performed to evaluate the pleural and parenchymal changes seen on the chest films reveals the unsuspected location of the left chest tube in the left major fissure (long arrow). The left major fissure is seen as a thin line projecting lateral to the chest tube (short arrow). Note that both the pleural effusion seen collecting posteromedially and the pneumothorax seen anteriorly are better identified on the CT scan. *C,* An axial scan obtained at the level of the carina shows the course of the chest tube high up within the left major fissure (white arrow). The extent of the left hydropneumothorax (black arrow) and the diffuse right lung infiltrates are better appreciated on the CT scan examination as compared with the chest anteroposterior portable film obtained the same day (shown in *A*).

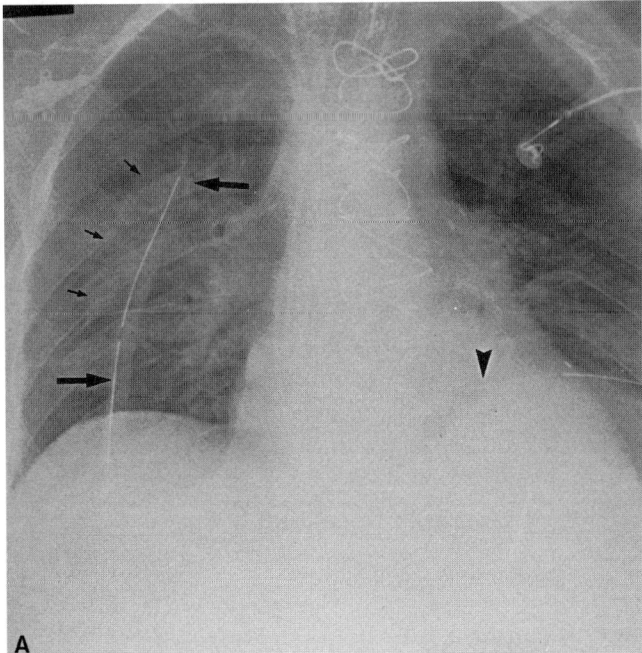
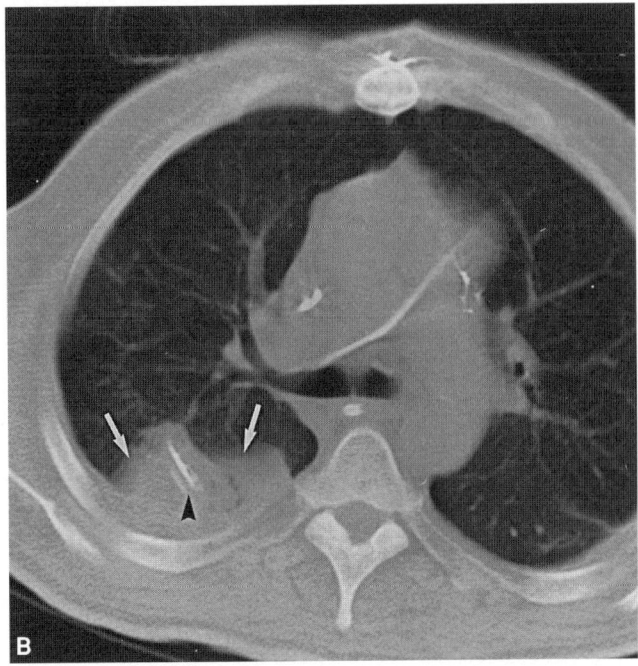

Fig. 71–11. Lung contusion post chest tube placement. *A,* A portable chest anteroposterior film examination obtained supine in a patient status post mediastinotomy for coronary artery bypass demonstrates a left lower chest tube with the tip near the left cardiophrenic angle (arrowhead) and a right chest tube projecting over the right midchest (large arrows). A vague infiltrate is seen surrounding the distal portion of the right chest tube (small arrows). *B,* A CT scan examination obtained to evaluate the chest for the source of the patient's fever demonstrates that the right chest tube is projecting in the superior segment of the right lower lobe (black arrowhead). An infiltrate caused by lung contusion and hemorrhage is seen surrounding the tube (white arrows). Images through the lower chest demonstrated that the tube was actually within the right major fissure with the tip ending intraparenchymally within the right lung.

1480   THE HIGH RISK PATIENT: MANAGEMENT OF THE CRITICALLY ILL

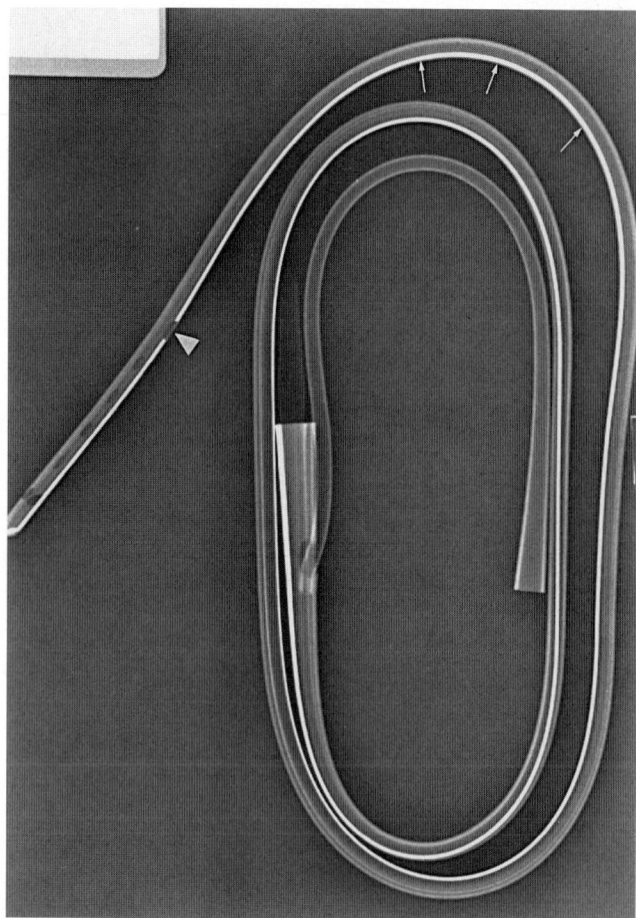

Fig. 71–12. Nasogastric tube. A radiograph of a nasogastric tube demonstrates a radiopaque marker running throughout the course of the nasogastric tube (arrows) with multiple side holes identified at the distal tip. The most proximal side hole interrupts the marker (arrowhead).

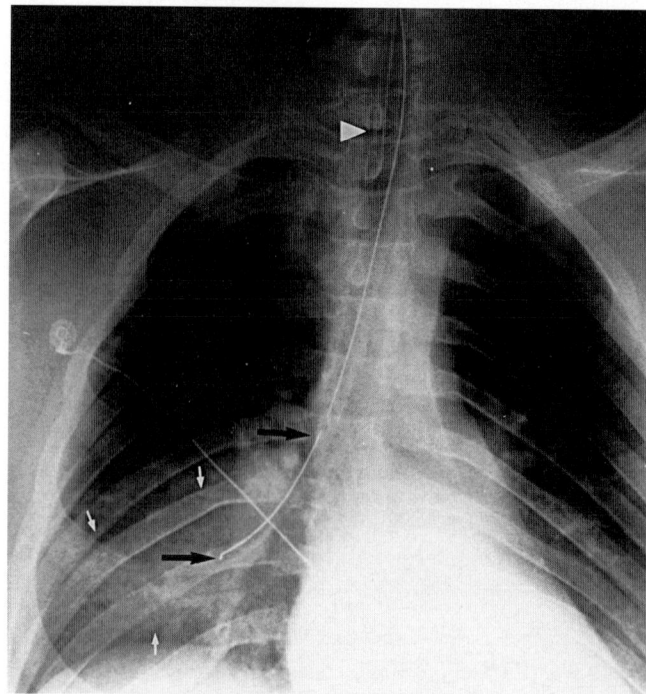

Fig. 71–14. Nasogastric tube in the airways. A chest anteroposterior film demonstrates that the nasogastric tube has been inadvertently placed into the right lower lung through the right main stem bronchus (black arrows). An acute infiltrate owing to lung contusion or aspiration is seen in the right lower lung surrounding the nasogastric tube (small white arrows). Note the endotracheal tube in the upper trachea (white arrowhead).

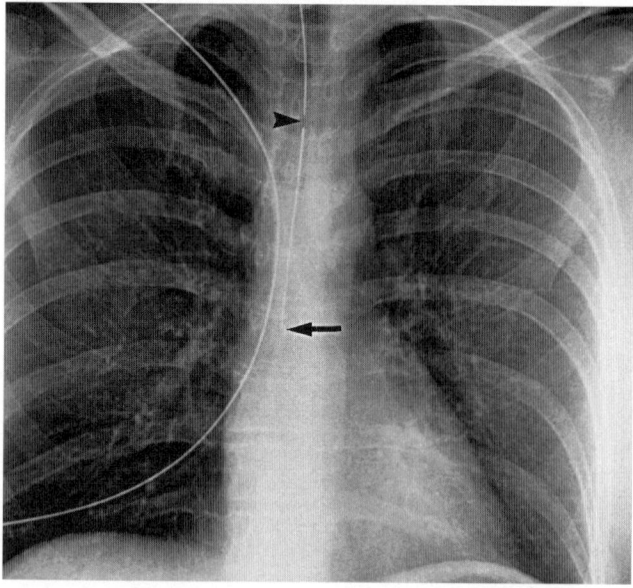

Fig. 71–13. Nasogastric tube in the esophagus. A nasogastric tube is demonstrated with its tip faintly visualized in the region of the midesophagus (arrow). The side hole near the distal portion of the tube is more easily recognized in the proximal esophagus (arrowhead).

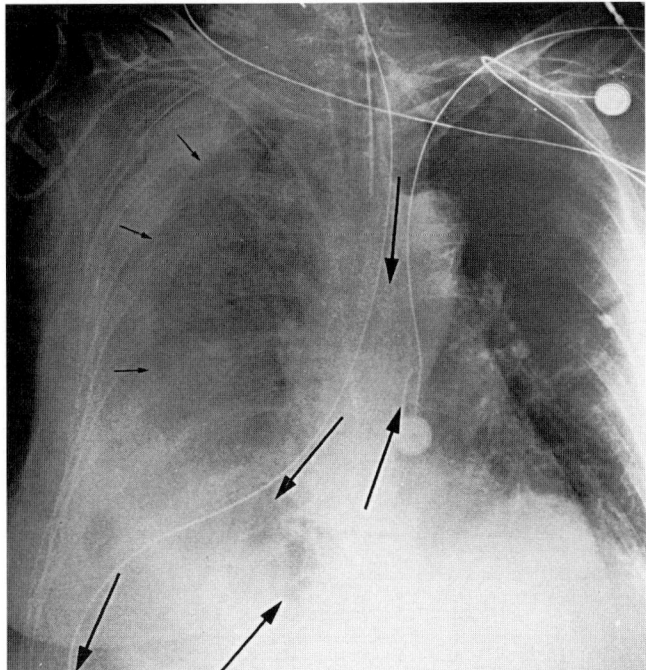

Fig. 71–15. Esophageal perforation postintubation. A portable chest film obtained in a 68-year-old patient who had multisystem failure complicating abdominal surgery demonstrates an acute large right pleural effusion (small arrows). The nasogastric tube is seen projecting over the mediastinum and right lower hemithorax in an abnormal course (arrows). Autopsy revealed perforation of the esophagus caused by nasogastric tube injury with the tube entering both the parenchymal and the pleural space in the right lower chest.

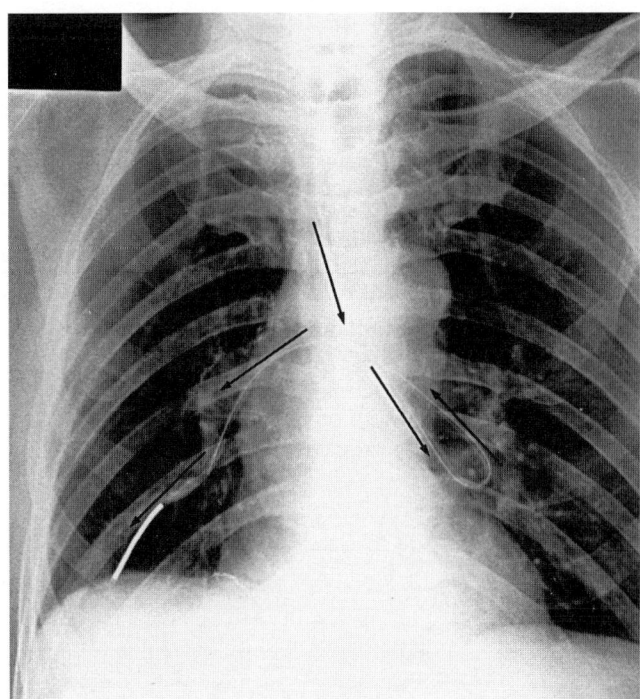

Fig. 71–16. Feeding tube in the airway. Radiographs of the abdomen are commonly obtained to check for proper placement of a feeding tube before the start of feeding. In this case, a prior radiograph of the abdomen could not demonstrate the presence of the feeding tube. A chest film demonstrates that the feeding tube has been inadvertently introduced into the airways, seen coiled with the left main stem bronchus and coursing back through the right main stem bronchus into the right lower lung (arrows).

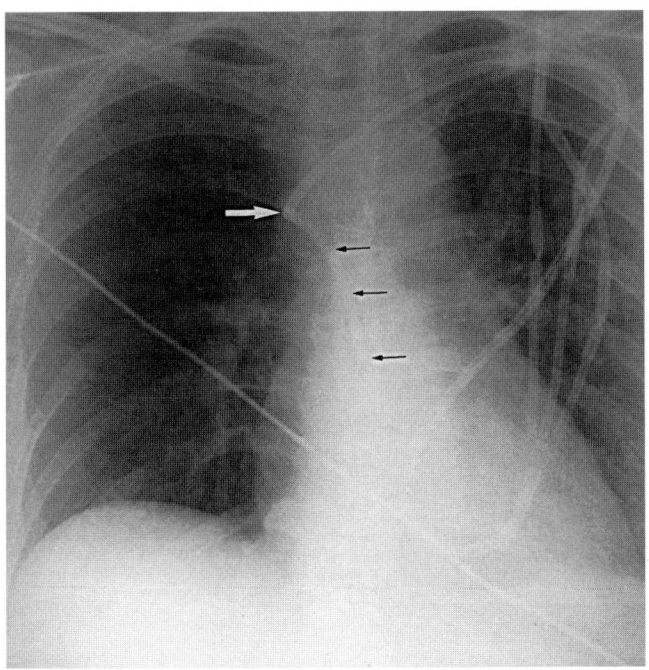

Fig. 71–17. Central venous catheter in the azygous vein. A portable chest film obtained after placement of a left subclavian line demonstrates an abnormal course of the distal portion of the venous catheter showing an abrupt angle at the level of the azygous arch (white arrow) with an abnormal course (black arrows) medial to the expected course of the superior vena cava.

THE HIGH RISK PATIENT: MANAGEMENT OF THE CRITICALLY ILL

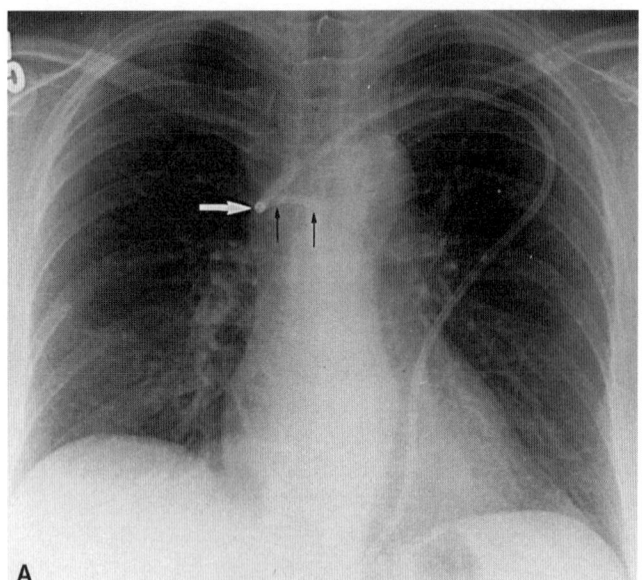
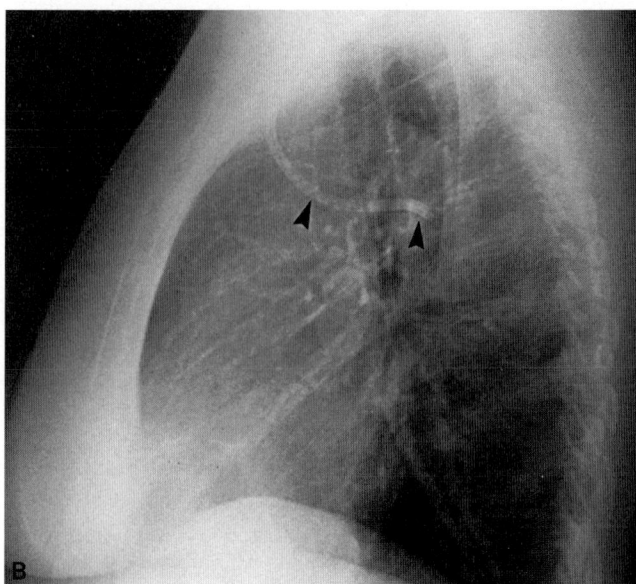

Fig. 71–18. Venous catheter in the azygous vein. *A*, Chest posteroanterior film demonstrates a left subclavian venous catheter showing an abrupt angle in its course at the level of the azygous vein (white arrow) with the distal portion of the catheter coursing in a medial direction toward the mediastinum (black arrows). *B*, The lateral view demonstrates that the catheter is coursing posteriorly in the azygous arch (arrowheads).

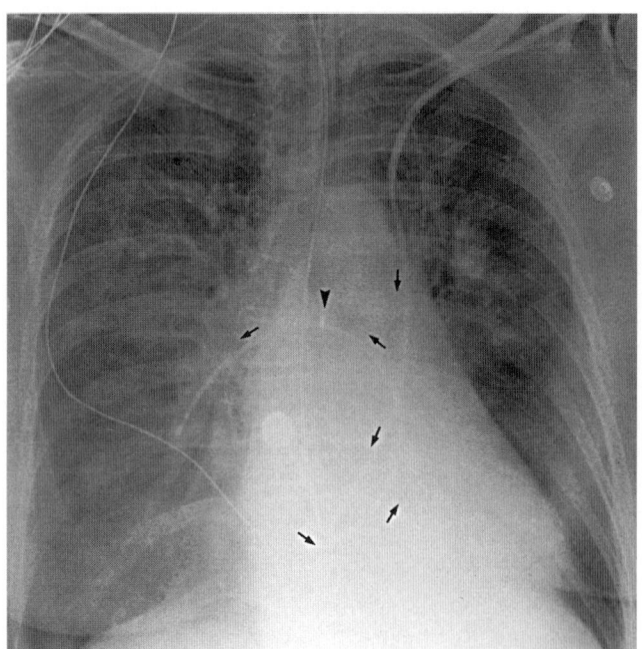

Fig. 71–19. Left-sided superior vena cava. A chest anteroposterior film obtained supine in a 52-year-old patient with history of renal failure and recent placement of a left subclavian Swan-Ganz catheter demonstrates that the catheter has entered a left-sided superior vena cava (arrows), entered the right atrium through the coronary sinus, and coursed from the right atrium into the right ventricle into the right pulmonary artery. The tip of an intra-aortic balloon pump is visualized in the proximal portion of the descending thoracic aorta (arrowhead). Both a nasogastric tube and endotracheal tube are in place. There is evidence of a right pleural effusion shown as a haze projecting over the lower right hemithorax.

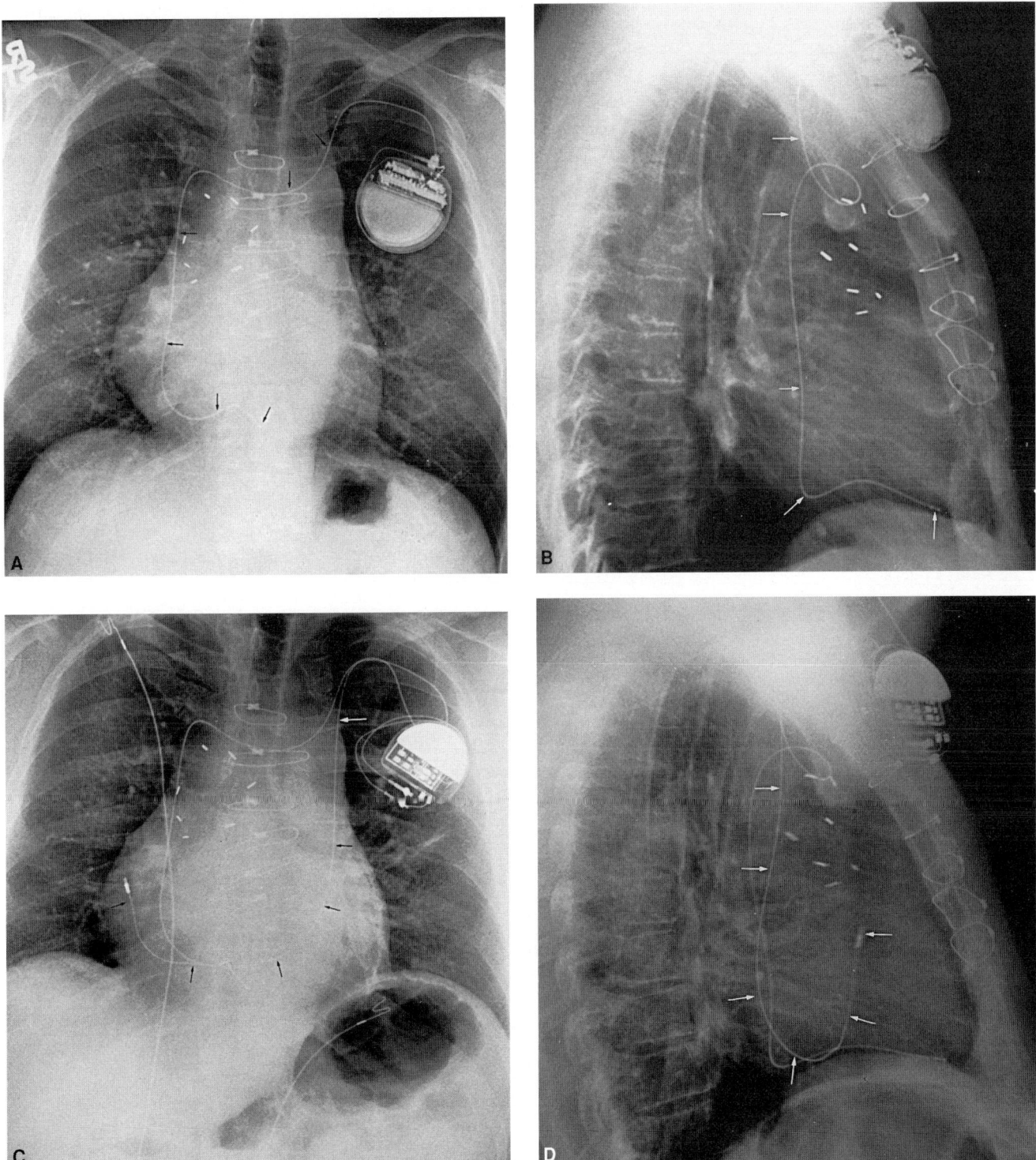

Fig. 71-20. Right and left superior vena cava. *A, B,* Chest posteroanterior *(A)* and lateral *(B)* films obtained after placement of a pacemaker show the course of the pacemaker wire through a left subclavian approach into the left brachiocephalic vein, right superior vena cava, right atrium, and right ventricle (arrows). *C, D,* Chest posteroanterior and lateral films obtained after the placement of a new pacemaker show that the additional pacemaker wire has entered the left side of the mediastinum through a left-sided superior vena cava that courses along the left side of the mediastinum entering the right atrium through the coronary sinus (arrows).

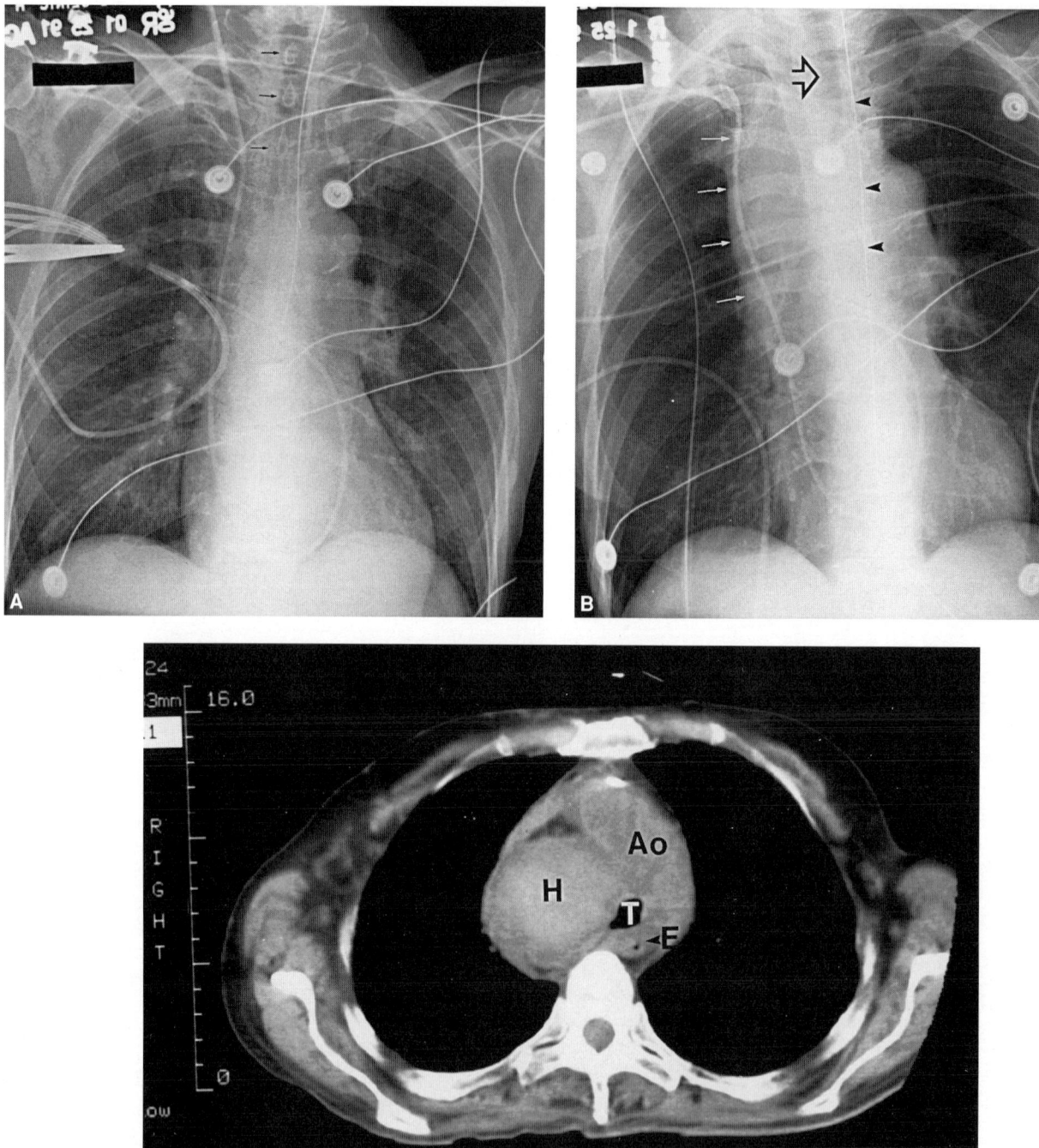

Fig. 71–21. Mediastinal hematoma. *A,* A baseline chest anteroposterior film after placement of a nasogastric tube and a Swan-Ganz catheter in a 54-year-old patient demonstrates a normal mediastinum and midline trachea (arrows). *B,* A follow-up chest anteroposterior film obtained 10 hours after the x-ray film shown in *A,* after failed attempts to place a right venous catheter, demonstrates acute widening of the upper mediastinum shown as a right paratracheal soft tissue density (white arrows). Note the displacement of the trachea (open arrowhead) and esophagus (black arrowheads) to the left. *C,* An axial scan through the upper mediastinum at the level of the aortic arch (Ao) demonstrates a large high-density fluid collection in the right paratracheal region compatible with a hematoma (H). Note the lateral displacement of the trachea (T) and esophagus (E).

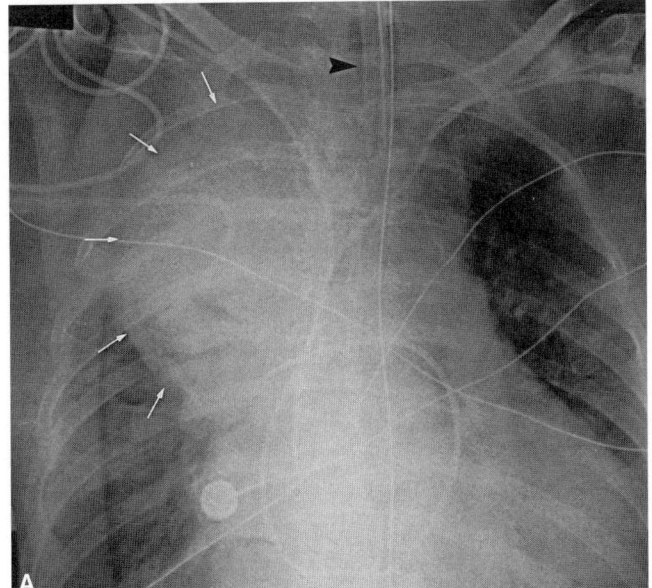
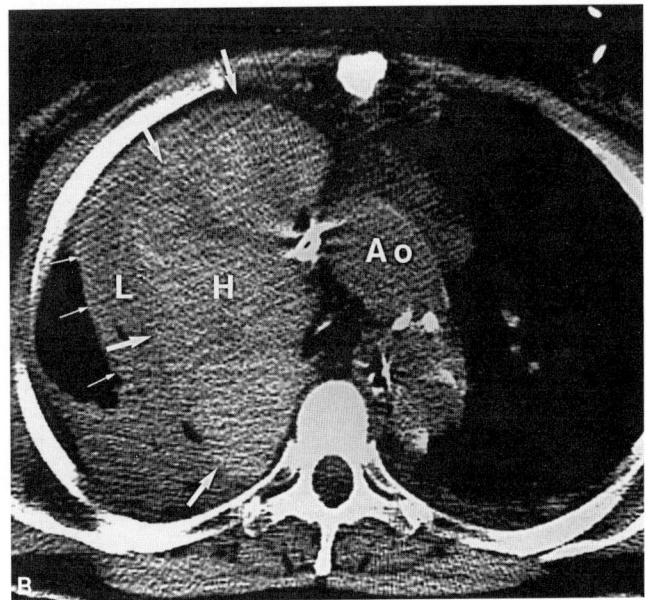
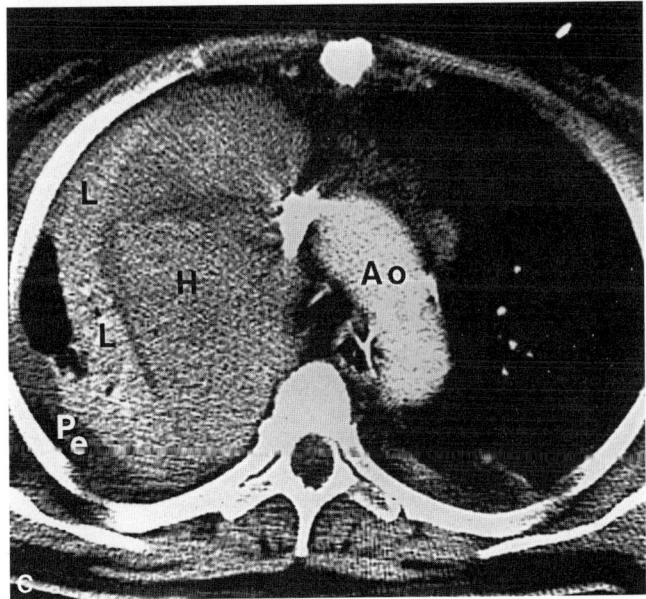

Fig. 71–22. Mediastinal hematoma secondary to superior vena cava injury after catheterization. *A,* Chest anteroposterior portable film obtained after a failed attempt to place a right venous catheter demonstrates a large radiodensity occupying the right upper hemithorax (small white arrows) with shift of the trachea to the left side (arrowhead). *B,* A nonenhanced CT scan of the chest obtained at the level of the aortic arch (Ao) demonstrates a large high-density fluid collection in the right side of the mediastinum representing a large hematoma (H, large arrows). Note the compressed lung lateral to the mediastinal hematoma (L, small arrows). *C,* A CT scan at the same level repeated after administration of intravenous contrast material demonstrates opacification of the aortic arch (Ao) and the atelectatic lung (L) lateral to the large mediastinal hematoma (H). A small pleural effusion (Pe) is better identified.

Swan-Ganz Catheter

Through a radiographically detectable sheath that is introduced through a systemic vein, the Swan-Ganz catheter is placed into the pulmonary arterial circulation to monitor cardiac function. Ideally the tip of the catheter should be within the right or left main pulmonary artery but is commonly seen spontaneously flipping from one artery to the contralateral artery. The balloon at the tip of the catheter should not be distended. When it is inflated, it can be visible as a small lucency surrounding the tip, potentially causing thrombosis or pulmonary arterial rupture when wedged in a small branch (Fig. 71-23). Peripheral placement in the lung may lead to pulmonary infarction (Fig. 71-24).[13,14]

Intra-Aortic Balloon Pump

The intra-aortic balloon pump (IABP), which is designed to improve cardiac function, is placed through a femoral artery into the thoracic aorta. It is recognizable by the radiopaque marker at the tip of the catheter, which is ideally positioned at the level of the proximal descending thoracic aorta, at the level of the aortic arch (see Fig. 71-24). The balloon, which inflates during diastole, can be recognized as a long tubular lucency at the distal portion of the catheter, measuring approximately 10 inches in length. A low placement of the tip of the IABP within the descending thoracic aorta may obstruct the renal or mesenteric arteries. A high position within the aortic arch may obstruct the left subclavian artery. Rarely, aortic injury with

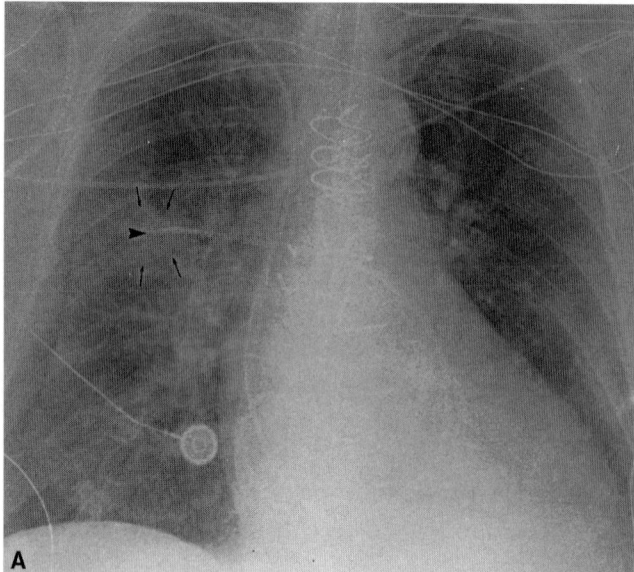
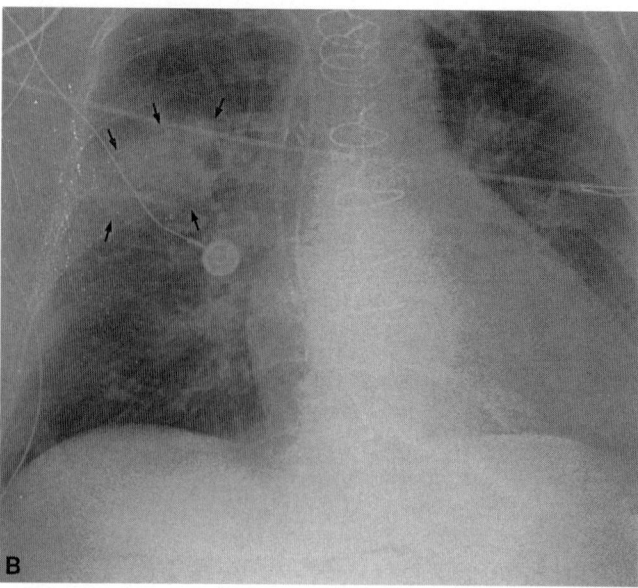

Fig. 71-23. Pulmonary artery branch rupture complicating Swan-Ganz catheter placement. *A*, A chest anteroposterior portable film obtained after placement of a Swan-Ganz catheter demonstrates that the tip of the catheter is wedged far distally within the right midlung (arrowhead). A small infiltrate is seen surrounding the tip of the catheter (arrows). *B*, A follow-up chest anteroposterior portable film obtained 2 hours later because of persistent hemoptysis demonstrates an increase of the previously seen right lung infiltrate (arrows), representing intraparenchymal hemorrhage believed due to a rupture of a small pulmonary artery branch secondary to the inflation of the balloon at the tip of the Swan-Ganz catheter. The infiltrates and hemoptysis subsided within 48 hours.

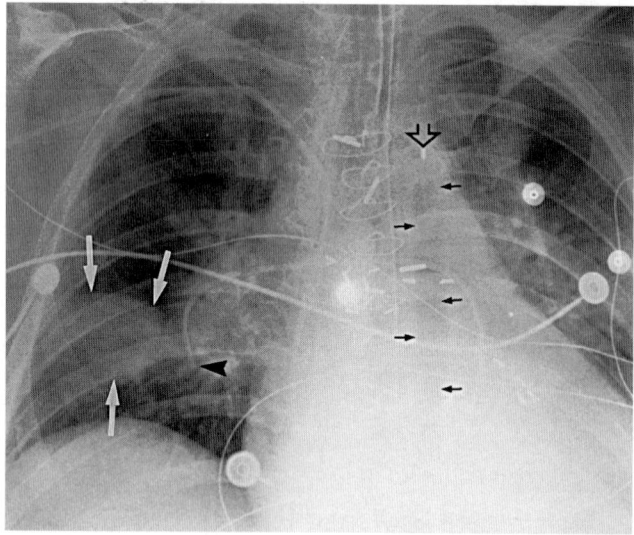

Fig. 71-24. Pulmonary infarction post Swan-Ganz catheter placement, intra-aortic balloon pump. A chest anteroposterior portable film obtained after placement of intra-aortic balloon pump demonstrates that the Swan-Ganz catheter placed earlier has been advanced far distally in an interlobar pulmonary artery branch with the tip (arrowhead) seen proximal to a newly appearing wedge-shaped peripheral infiltrate in the right lung base compatible with a focal infarction (white arrows). The intra-aortic balloon pump is recognized with the help of its radiopaque tip seen here at the level of the aortic arch (open arrowhead). During inflation at diastole, the balloon can be identified as a long tubular radiolucency (small black arrows).

dissection may be caused during the placement of the IABP.[15]

ACUTE LUNG DISEASE

Atelectasis

Pulmonary atelectasis is the most common abnormality observed on chest radiographs of patients in the ICU. Poor ventilation and inflation of the lung owing to various reasons, such as recent chest or abdominal surgery or pulmonary, pleural, abdominal, or central nervous system abnormality, may cause radiographically detectable peripheral subsegmental or linear atelectases (Fig. 71-25).[16] They have no major clinical significance and often spontaneously resolve after normal ventilation of the lungs. Segmental or lobar atelectasis is often detected in the lung bases mimicking lung infiltrates and consolidation owing to pneumonia. As seen with airway disease secondary to other causes such as infection, hemorrhage or edema, air bronchograms can be detected in the affected collapsed lung. Repeated chest films with better inflation or a lateral decubitus examination when a pleural effusion is present may show clearance of the atelectasis, helping to differentiate it from true air-space disease, such as pneumonia. The presence of large pleural effusions may render the interpretation of the underlying lung parenchyma difficult. The densely compressed lung by the pleural fluid cannot be radiographically separated from the opacity of the underlying pleural effusion unless air bronchograms are present (Fig. 71-26). Elevation of the hemidiaphragms and the cardiac silhouette may also obscure the presence of basilar atelectasis.

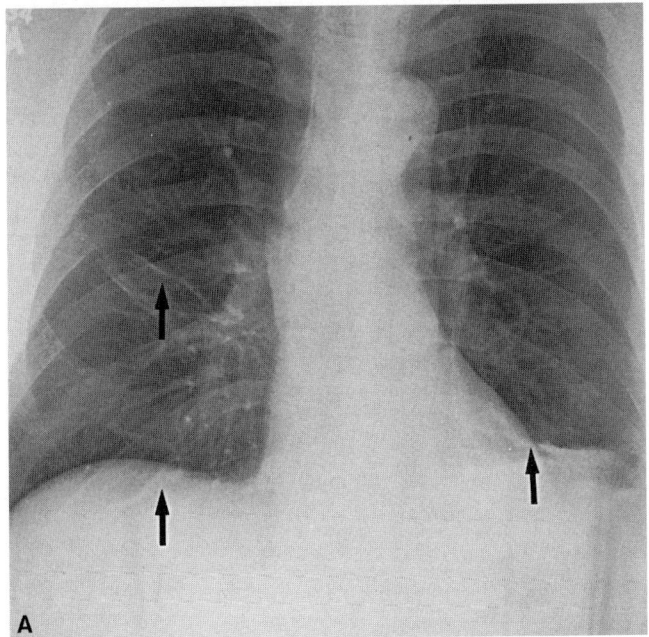 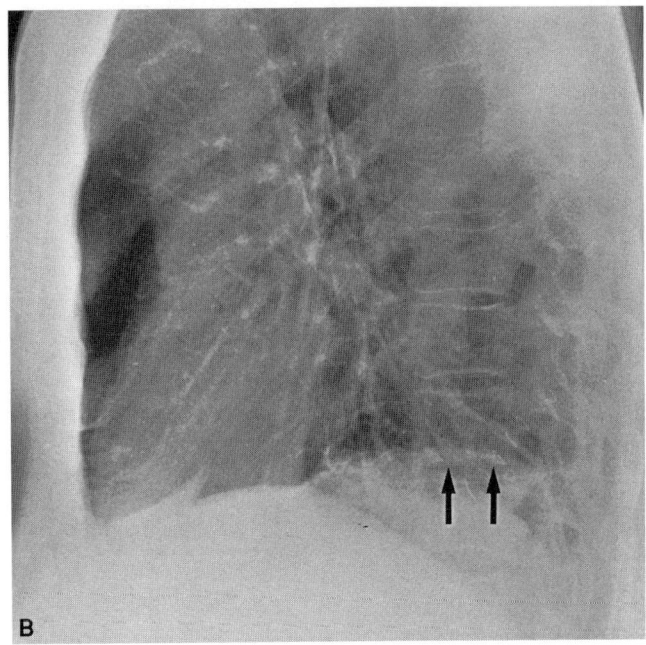

Fig. 71–25. Linear atelectasis post abdominal surgery. Chest posteroanterior (A) and lateral (B) films obtained 1 week post left flank surgery demonstrates areas of linear radiodensity in both lung bases (arrows) representing focal linear areas of nonaerated lung. They often resolve when the lungs reach their full inflating capacity.

Overpenetrated radiographs would better demonstrate the findings of basilar atelectasis. They may be shown as areas of increased parenchymal density, with crowding of the bronchovascular markings silhouetting the adjacent structures, such as diaphragms, spine, and descending thoracic aorta (see Fig. 71–26).

Atelectasis caused by a proximal bronchial obstruction, such as mucous plugging, would not create an air bronchogram but rather shows signs of segmental or lobar atelectasis and secondary signs of loss of volume, such as elevation of the hemidiaphragm and displacement of the hilum or the mediastinal structures (Fig. 71–27). Complete lobar atelectases can be difficult to detect on the portable chest film, especially when other parenchymal abnormalities, such as edema or pneumonia, are already present. They can also be obscured by underlying pleural effusions. Only careful examination of the radiograph can show the subtle changes of lobar atelectasis. When the patient's condition permits, a well-exposed posteroanterior and lateral view or a CT scan examination may be necessary to define the atelectasis better (Fig. 71–28). The left lower lung is the most common portion of the lung affected by atelectasis, often seen after cardiac surgery, and should not be mistaken for pneumonia.[17] It is believed to be due to multiple compounding factors, including the presence of underlying compressing pleural fluid and enlarged heart and the result of the phrenic nerve freezing performed at the time of surgery.

Pneumonia

The radiographic changes of pneumonia can be difficult to ascertain because they can be similar to the parenchymal changes created by atelectasis, infarction, hemorrhage, or aspiration of noninfected fluid.[18] The diagnostic task can be even more difficult when the lungs are already involved with edema or adult respiratory distress syndrome (ARDS) or when pleural effusions obscure the lung parenchyma (Fig. 71–29). Focal bacterial pneumonia, in an otherwise normal lung, can be detected as an area of patchy alveolar infiltrate in a segmental or lobar distribution (Fig. 71–30).

Viral pneumonias usually have a more diffuse distribution presenting as either interstitial or mixed interstitial and alveolar infiltrates (Fig. 71–31). Fungal pneumonias, in otherwise healthy patients, have a tendency to produce nodular infiltrates. If the patient is immunocompromised or debilitated, the fungal infiltrates manifest as alveolar consolidations or rapidly spreading nodular infiltrates. Cavitation may occur at any time during the progression of the infiltrate. Pneumocystis pneumonia can be difficult to detect, initially mimicking the appearance and distribution of early pulmonary edema.

When one clinically suspects pneumonia, but the initial radiographs are negative, CT scanning of the chest can help detect early changes of alveolar or interstitial infiltrates (Fig. 71–32). When there is rapid spread of disease to both lungs, the radiographic appearance may be similar to that of pulmonary edema or ARDS. One also needs to recognize that the diagnosis of pneumonia cannot be based on the radiographic findings alone but relies on the constellation of the radiographic, laboratory, and clinical findings. It is almost impossible to differentiate the radiographic findings of infection from those of hemorrhage, infarction, edema, proteinosis, or tumor (Figs. 71–33 and 71–34).

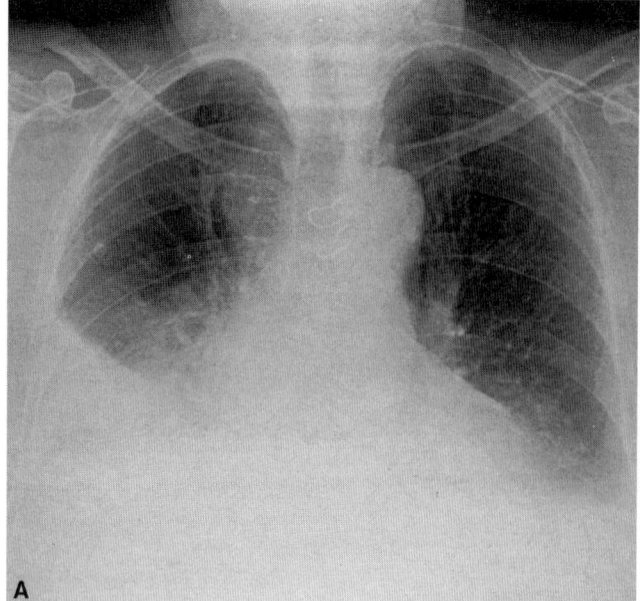
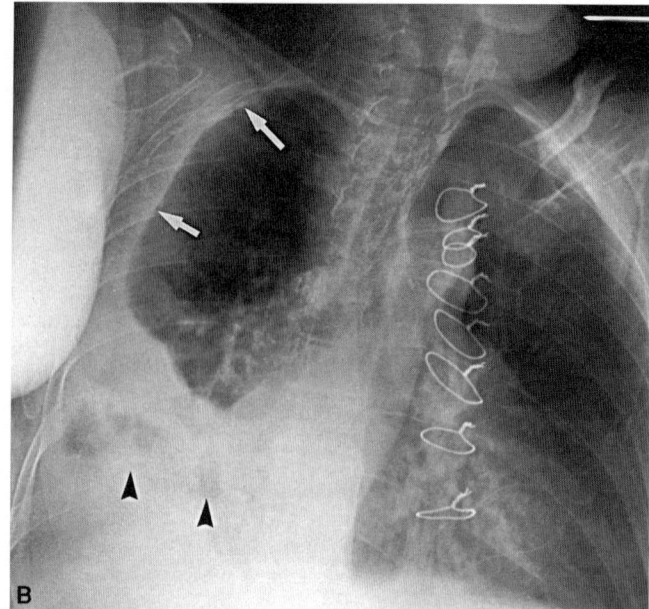
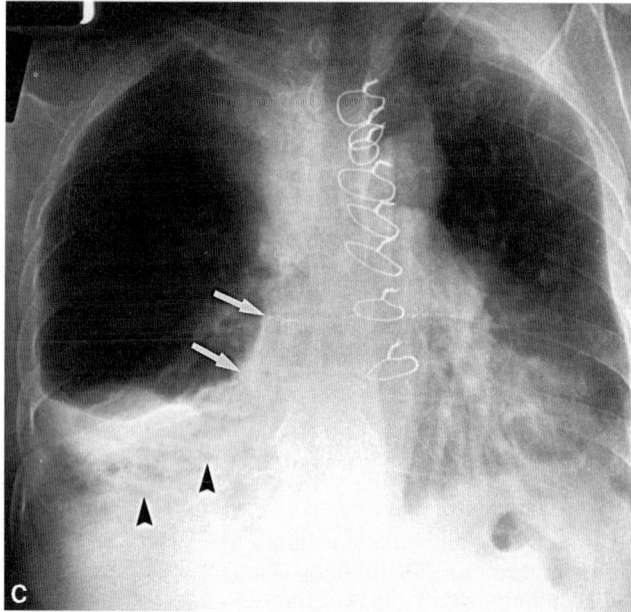

Fig. 71–26. Lung atelectasis secondary to pleural effusions. *A,* Chest anteroposterior film obtained after cardiac surgery and resolving congestive heart failure demonstrates bilateral costophrenic angle blunting owing to bilateral pleural effusions with the right bigger than the left. The lung bases cannot be well evaluated because of the underlying pleural effusions. Right lateral decubitus *(B)* and left lateral decubitus *(C)* films reveal the extent of the right lung parenchymal disease when the right pleural effusion is shifted away (white arrows). The air bronchogram (black arrowheads) identified in the right lung base represents atelectatic lung. The parenchymal changes resolved 48 hours later after clearance of the pleural effusion.

Infiltrates caused by infection are better recognized when complications such as abscess formation or empyema occur. When cavitation is suspected, CT scanning can determine with more certainty the extent of both parenchymal and pleural changes. This is also true for the detection of early septic embolic disease when radiographs are equivocal (Fig. 71–35).[19,20] In more advanced disease, septic emboli with parenchymal involvement manifests as small, ill-defined nodules or focal patchy infiltrates seen in the periphery of the lungs (Fig. 71–36). When cavitation occurs, the diagnosis becomes unequivocal. Aspiration pneumonia or pneumonitis manifests as an acute infiltrate occurring in the portion of the lungs that is gravity dependent at the time of the aspiration (Fig. 71–37). In the bedridden ICU patient, the infiltrates are observed mainly in the posterior aspect of the upper and lower lungs. The aspiration of acid gastric juice creates a chemical pneumonitis often seen as an area of consolidation, which clears in the following few days.[21] If the infiltrates fail to resolve, superimposed infection must be suspected, especially when cavitation owing to abscess formation and pleural effusions owing to empyemas are detected.

Pulmonary Edema

Pulmonary infiltrates owing to pulmonary edema are a common finding in the chest film of the ICU patient. They are recognized based on their appearance, distribution,

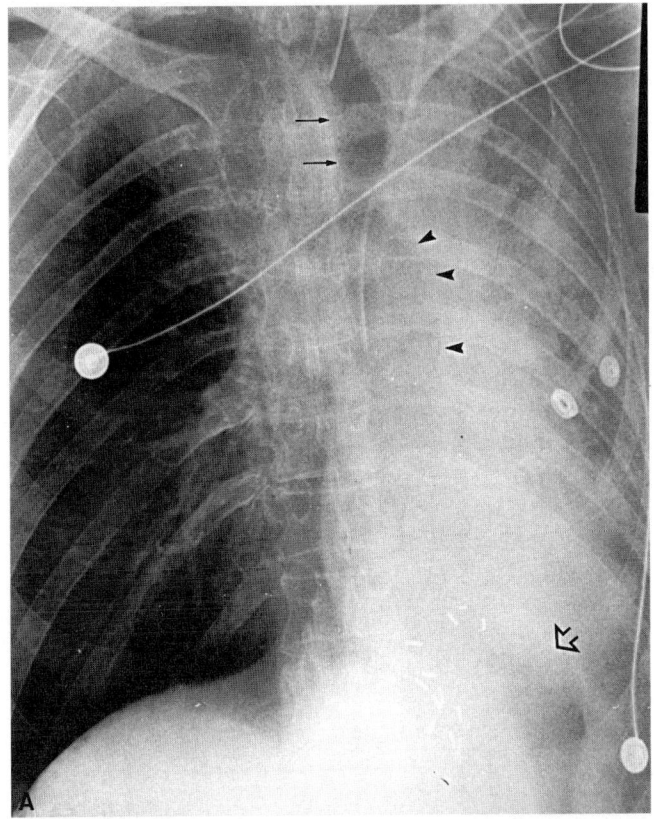

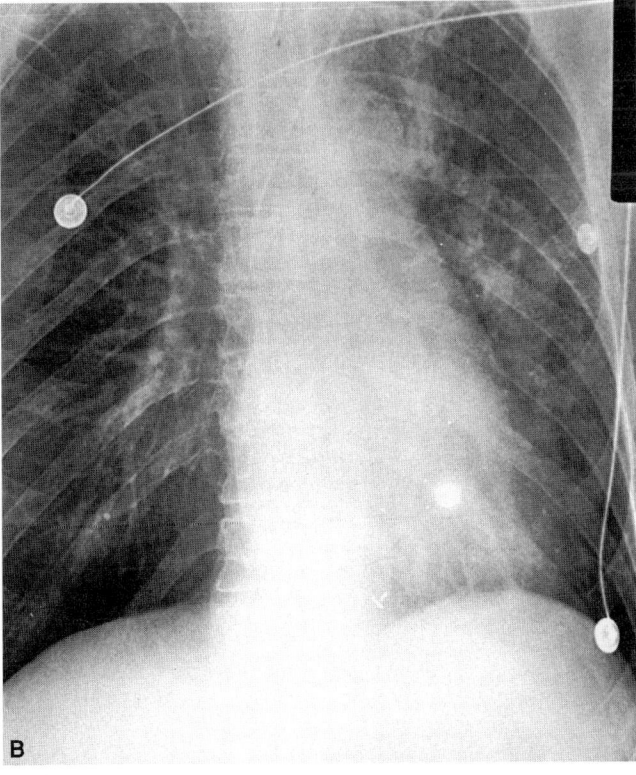

Fig. 71–27. Lung atelectasis owing to mucous plugging. *A,* Chest anteroposterior portable film obtained in a 54-year-old patient status post left upper quadrant surgery and shortness of breath demonstrates diffuse increased density of the left lung owing to atelectasis with shift of the heart and mediastinal structures to the site of the atelectasis. The trachea is shifted to the left (arrows), and the right lung is seen herniating into the left hemithorax (arrowhead). Although obscured, the hemidiaphragm is elevated, indirectly seen by the shift toward the left hemithorax of the surgical clips and gastric air bubble (open arrowhead). *B,* A follow-up chest film obtained immediately after bronchoscopy, which revealed a mucous plug in the left main stem bronchus, demonstrates almost complete resolution of the left lung atelectasis with shift of the mediastinum, heart, and left hemidiaphragm to their normal positions.

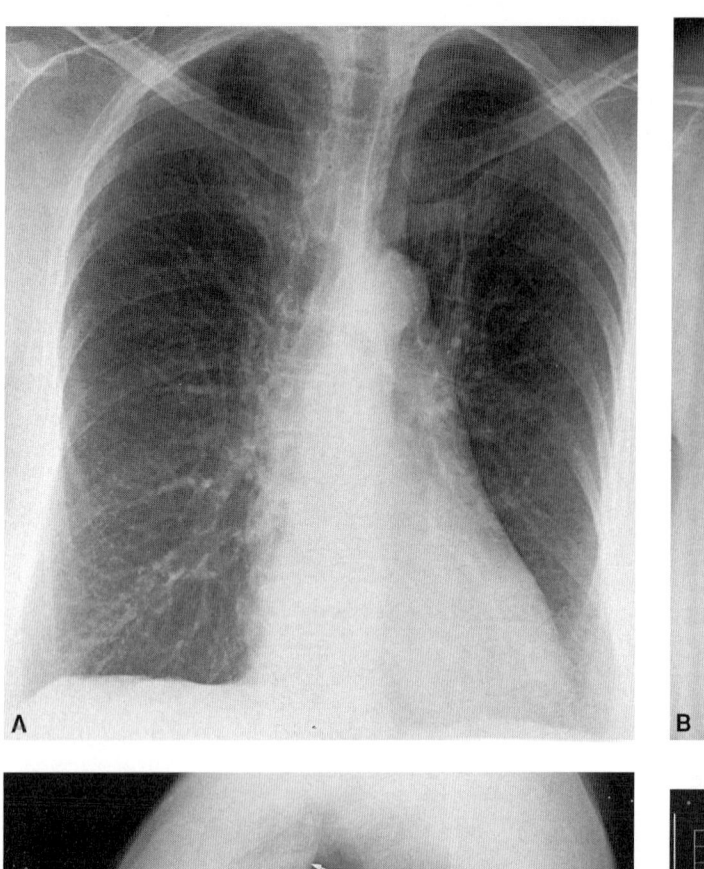
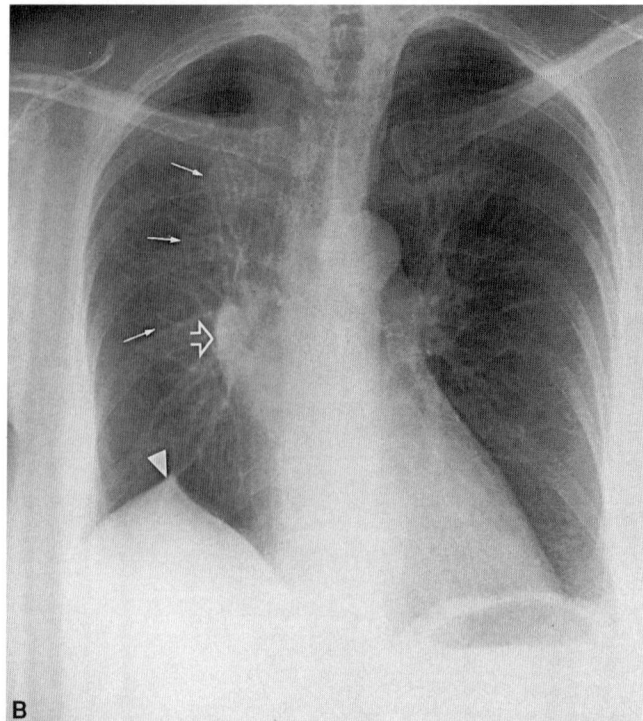
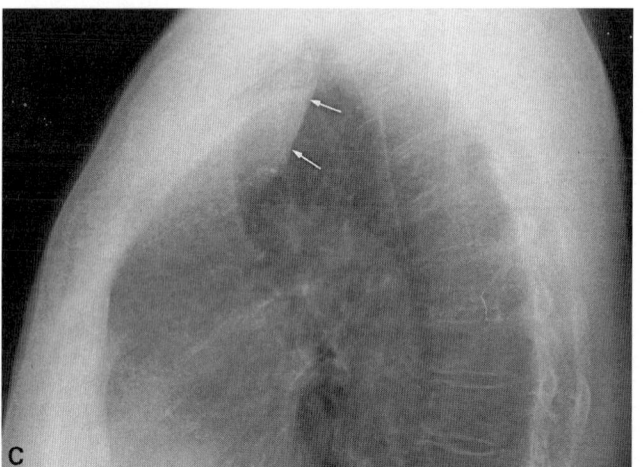
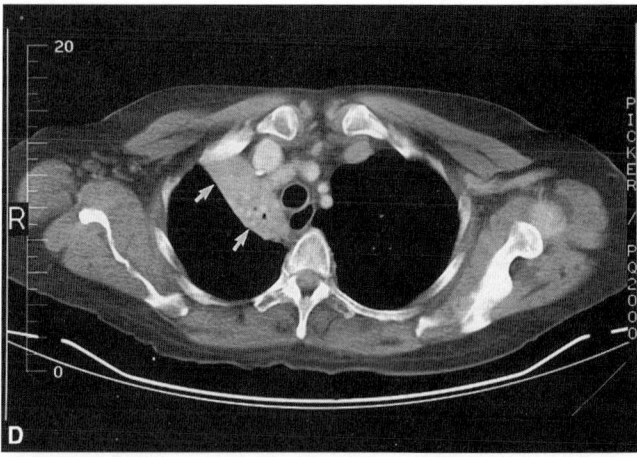
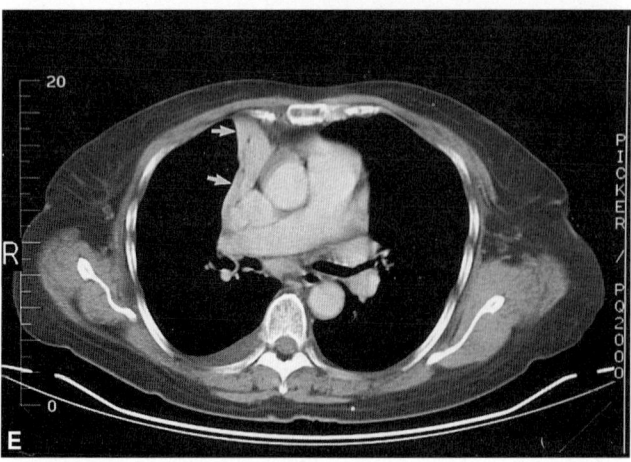

Fig. 71–28. Lobar atelectasis. Baseline chest posteroanterior (A) and follow-up chest posteroanterior (B) and lateral (C) films in a 63-year-old patient demonstrates changes of complete right upper lobe atelectasis. It is shown on the posteroanterior view as a diffuse haze projecting of the right hilum and medial portion of the right upper lung. The right hilum is displaced upward (open arrowhead), and the right hemidiaphragm is tented upward (arrowhead). The lateral view demonstrates an abnormal density projecting in the upper retrosternal region (arrows). A CT scan examination of the chest obtained after administration of intravenous contrast material with axial images obtained through the level of the apices (D) and below the carina (E) demonstrates the collapsed right upper lobe abutting anteriorly and medially against the mediastinum (arrows). The atelectatic lobe is seen smoothly marginated posteriorly by the major fissure. Small air bronchograms and enhancing vessels can be identified within the collapsed lobe.

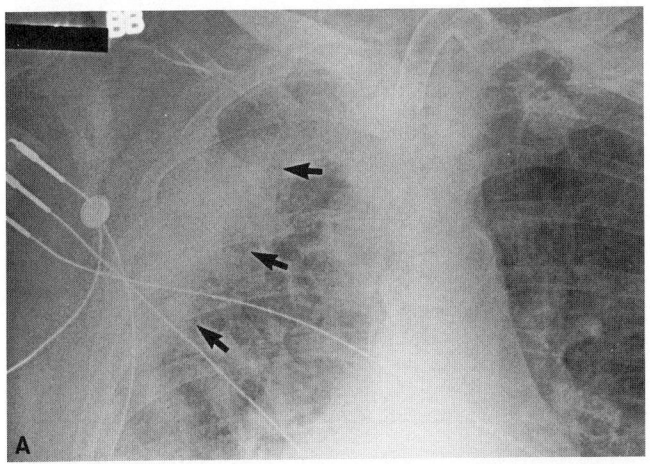
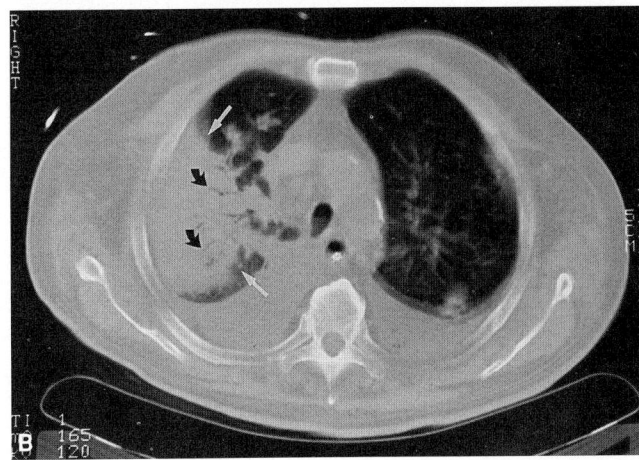
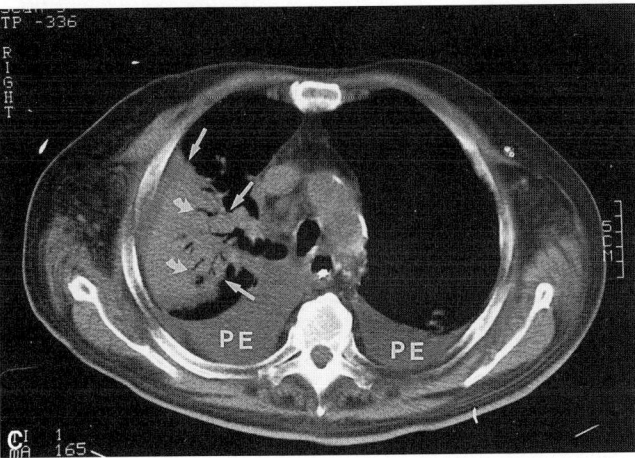

Fig. 71–29. Pneumonia: portable chest film vs. CT scan. *A,* A chest anteroposterior portable film obtained in a 77-year-old patient status post abdominal surgery and persistent fever demonstrates bilateral pleural effusions and a focal radiodensity seen in the lateral portion of the right upper chest (arrows). Based on the x-ray appearance, this may represent an area of loculated pleural fluid or a parenchymal process. The bilateral pleural effusions are obscuring the lower lung bases. *B, C,* A CT scan of the upper chest obtained the same day as the chest film shown in *A* with an axial scan imaged at lung window *(B)* and soft tissue window *(C)* demonstrates moderate-sized bilateral pleural effusions (PE) and a large parenchymal consolidation in the right upper lobe (arrows) with multiple air bronchograms (arrowheads). This is a case in which the CT scan clearly demonstrates the extent of the pleural and parenchymal changes far superiorly than what the chest film can offer.

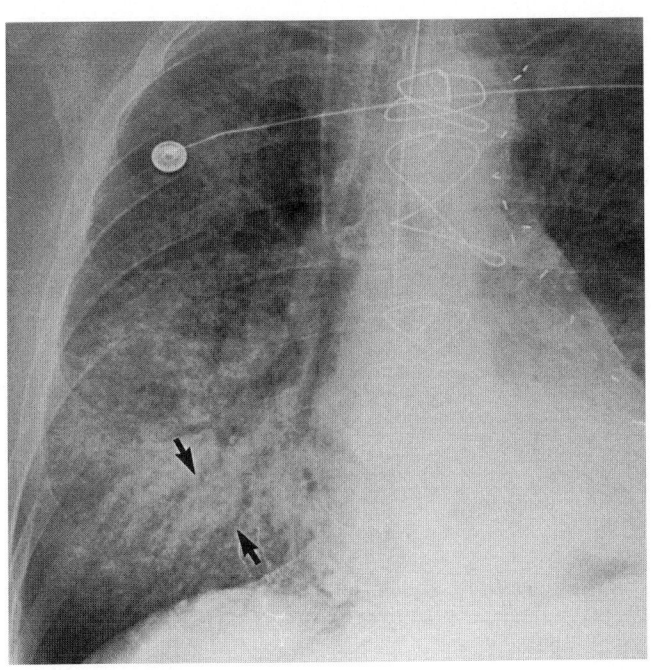

Fig. 71–30. Bacterial pneumonia. A chest anteroposterior portable film obtained in a 62-year-old patient with shortness of breath and fever 3 days post mediastinotomy for open heart surgery demonstrates bilateral diffuse alveolar infiltrates with predominance in the lung bases. Note the air bronchogram best demonstrated in the right lower lung (arrows). Sputum cultures revealed a mixed bacterial flora. The infiltrates cleared after 2 weeks of antibiotic treatment.

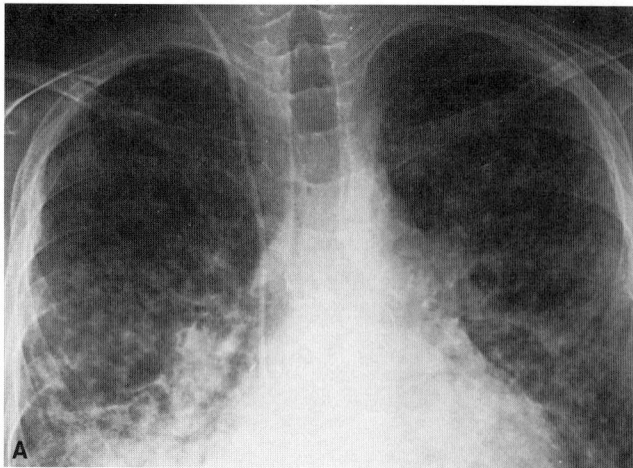
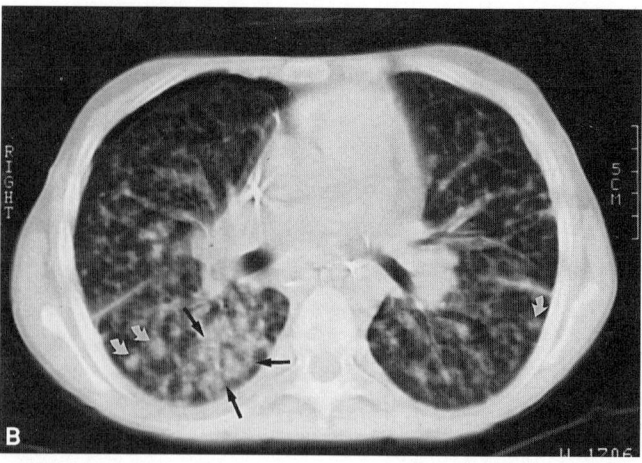

Fig. 71-31. Viral pneumonia. *A,* A chest anteroposterior film obtained in an 18-year-old patient status post bilateral lung transplant demonstrates bilateral lower and midlung reticulonodular infiltrates with dense areas of consolidation in the right lower lung. *B,* A CT scan examination of the chest with an axial image obtained below the carina demonstrates the extent and the diffuse distribution of the infiltrate throughout both lungs. The nodular appearance of the infiltrate (white curved arrows) owing to cytomegalovirus infection is better appreciated on the CT scan. Confluence of the infiltrates in the right lower lobe shows dense consolidation (black arrows) with a central air bronchogram.

and their course on serial chest films. It is often difficult, however, to recognize specific patterns to determine the cause of the pulmonary edema, which may be due to cardiogenic or noncardiogenic disturbances (fluid overload and increased capillary permeability).[22,23] In the early changes of cardiogenic pulmonary edema, accumulation of fluid in the interstitium can be detected by the presence of peribronchial cuffing, thickened interlobular septa (Kerley's lines), and fluid within the subpleural space ("thickened" fissures) (Fig. 71-38). Pleural effusions and perihilar haze are often present. Distention of the upper lung vessels, with redistribution of blood flow from the lower to the upper lungs, can be observed in the upright films if the cardiac failure persists.[24] With more accumulation of fluid, the air space is then involved, reflected by the presence of bilateral diffuse and symmetric patchy alveolar infiltrates in a perihilar distribution, which progresses toward the periphery of the lungs (Fig. 71-39). In pulmonary edema due to noncardiac origins, the alveolar infiltrates, owing to edema, have a more patchy and peripheral distri-

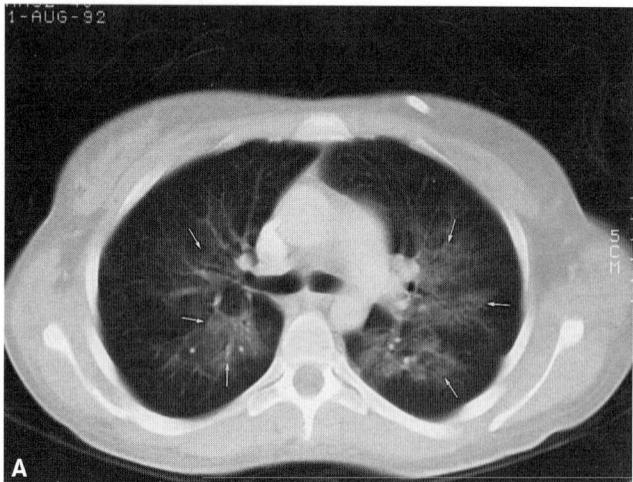
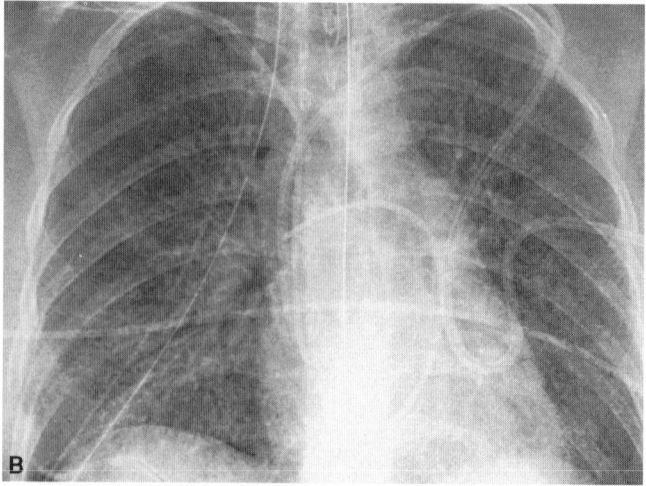

Fig. 71-32. Pneumocystis pneumonia. A 25-year-old patient with history of leukemia and shortness of breath had a nondiagnostic chest film obtained the same day as the CT scan shown in Fig. 71-30A. *A,* A CT scan with an axial image obtained at the level of the carina demonstrates early perihilar patchy infiltrate of a ground-glass appearance commonly seen in pneumocystis pneumonia (arrows). Without clinical information, the appearance of the infiltrates may mimic those of early pulmonary edema. *B,* A chest film obtained 1 week later demonstrates diffuse involvement of both lung fields owing to pneumocystis infection. The infiltrates have a diffuse hazy ground-glass appearance. The vascular markings are somewhat obscured, but there are no signs of pulmonary edema. The heart size is normal. There is no sign of pleural effusion. A right chest tube has been placed to control a spontaneous pneumothorax.

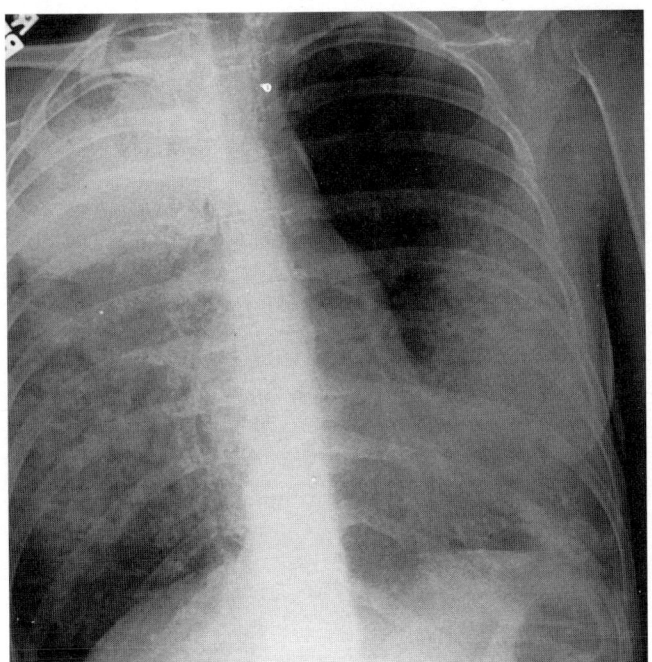

Fig. 71–33. Bronchoalveolar carcinoma. A chest anteroposterior film was obtained on admission in a 28-year-old patient who has been treated with antibiotics during a period of 8 weeks for suspected pneumonia demonstrates bilateral diffuse alveolar infiltrates with consolidations in the right upper and left lower lungs. The patient was admitted to the ICU, where she expired 48 hours later. Autopsy revealed diffuse bronchoalveolar carcinoma, which mimicked infectious infiltrates.

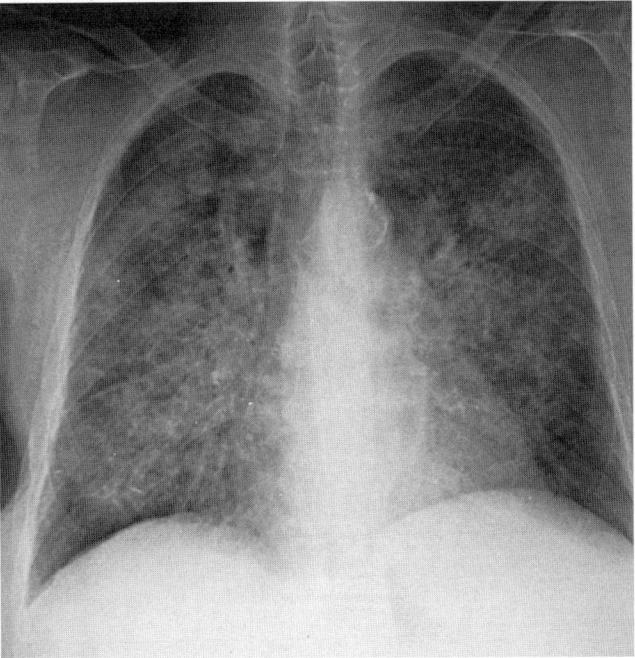

Fig. 71–34. Pulmonary alveolar proteinosis. A chest anteroposterior film obtained on a 54-year-old patient admitted to the ICU for shortness of breath demonstrates bilateral diffuse alveolar infiltrates. The infiltrates are similar to those of pneumocystis pneumonia shown in Fig. 71–32B. Open lung biopsy revealed alveolar proteinosis with no evidence of infection.

bution. The heart is usually of normal size, and pleural effusions are infrequent. The interstitium is infrequently involved (no peribronchial cuffing or Kerley lines). Infiltrates caused by pulmonary edema can sometimes be difficult to separate from those of pneumonia or hemorrhage. Rapid clearance (hours to a few days) is more characteristic of pulmonary edema. Persistent infiltrates, owing to pulmonary edema, can be seen after clinical recovery when there is a slow lymphatic clearance of a previous extensive alveolar edema.[25] Pulmonary hemorrhage, depending on its extent, is usually slower to clear than pulmonary edema but faster than infectious infiltrates. Pulmonary edema may have an asymmetric distribution mimicking infiltrates due to other causes, such as infection, in cases in which there is underlying lung disease. This is best seen in patients with pulmonary emphysema and bullous disease or end-stage fibrocystic lung disease (Fig. 71–40). Any other parenchymal process preventing the edema to have a diffuse distribution may give the edema an asymmetric patchy distribution (prior lung surgery, consolidation, atelectasis, cavities, or masses). Unilateral or focal pulmonary edema can be due to a variety of causes, including aspiration of acid gastric content in one lung, in a patient selectively lying on one side of the chest, or seen following rapid re-expansion of a collapsed lung after removal of a large amount of pleural fluid or air.[26,27] It can be seen unilaterally after single lung transplant involving the transplanted lung (Fig. 71–41).

Adults Respiratory Distress Syndrome

The radiographic diagnosis of ARDS relies on the interpretation of serial radiographs, which need to be correlated with the physiologic data and the clinical course of the patient.[28] After a latent period of 12 to 24 hours from the pulmonary symptoms, the chest radiograph demonstrates bilateral perihilar infiltrates owing to edema and pneumonitis (Fig. 71–42). Within 24 hours, the edema may progress to a fulminant course, creating diffuse opacification of both lungs (Fig. 71–43). The lack of pleural effusions and cardiomegaly helps in differentiating the infiltrates of ARDS from those of pulmonary edema as a result of cardiac failure. The diagnosis of ARDS is confirmed radiographically by the fixed appearance of the infiltrates for the next several days. Superimposed infection with cavitation or barotrauma from increased positive end-expiratory pressure (PEEP) may alter the homogeneous diffuse appearance of the infiltrates. Increased PEEP may push the intra-alveolar fluid against the wall of the alveoli, giving a false appearance of improvement of the infiltrates (Fig. 71–44). An increase in PEEP may also cause the air to leak into the mediastinum or pleural space with the subsequent formation of pneumomediastinums, pneumothoraces, pneumoretroperitoneums, and pneumoperitoneums (see Fig. 71–44). This is particularly true when there is extensive damage to the lung parenchyma with subsequent necrosis and interstitial emphysema. After recovery, and depending on the extent of lung injury, the lungs may return to a normal radiographic appearance or may show residual fibrosis (Figs. 71–45 and 71–46).

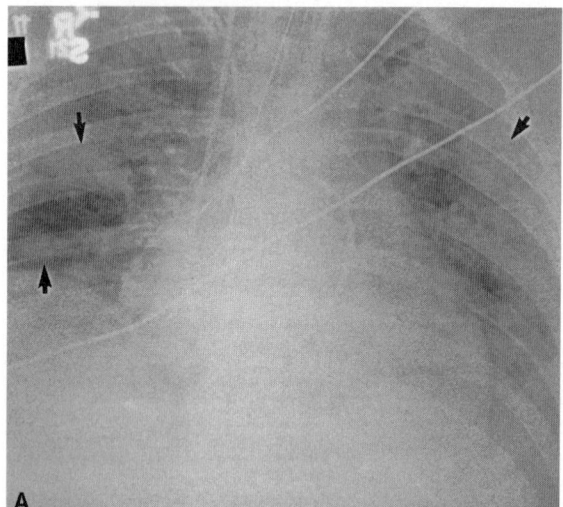
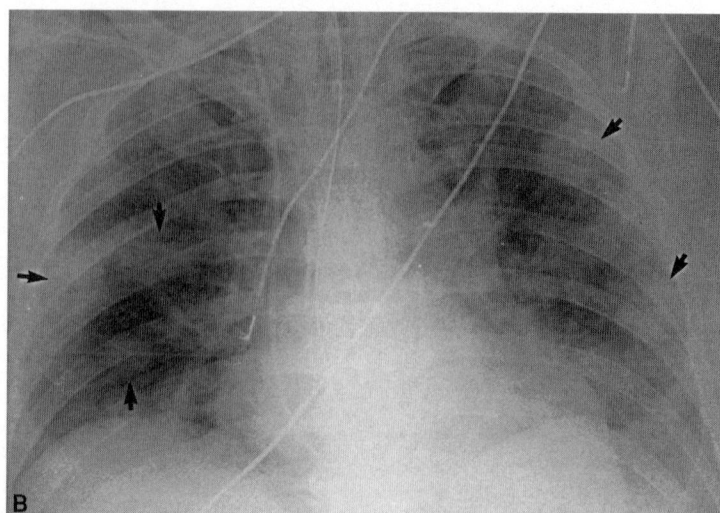
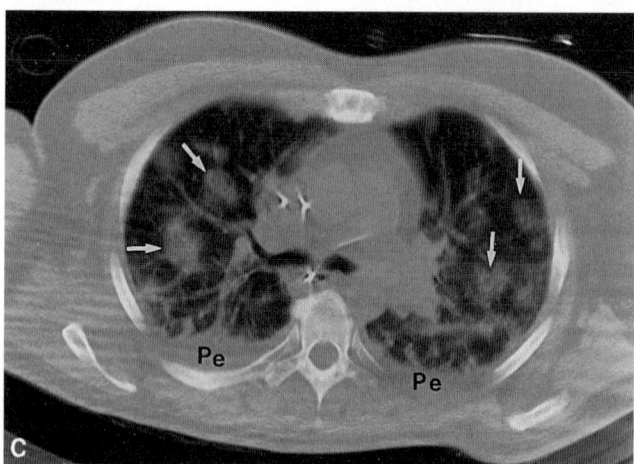
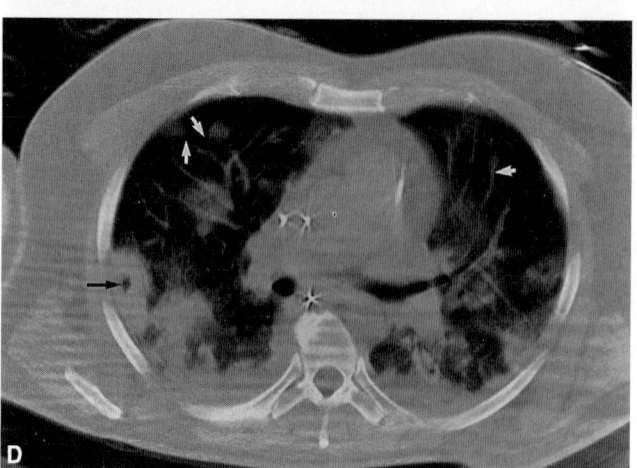

Fig. 71-35. Septic emboli. *A*, A chest anteroposterior portable film obtained on a 68-year-old patient with history of septicemia, fever, and shortness of breath demonstrates ill-defined nonspecific focal patchy infiltrates throughout both lung fields (arrows). *B*, A follow-up chest film obtained 24 hours later with better inflation reveals progression of the infiltrate organized in a nodular fashion in the periphery of both lungs (arrows). A CT scan examination of the chest obtained the same day demonstrates better the extent, location, and appearance of the infiltrate. An axial image obtained at the level of the carina *(C)* demonstrates multiple nodular infiltrates throughout both lung fields (arrows). Note the presence of small bilateral pleural effusions (Pe) unsuspected on the chest films. An axial image obtained below the carina *(D)* demonstrates early cavitation within one peripheral lung nodule in the right lung base suggestive of septic infarction (black arrow). Note that focal septic nodules can be seen connected to pulmonary vessels (white arrows) suggesting their hematogenous origin.

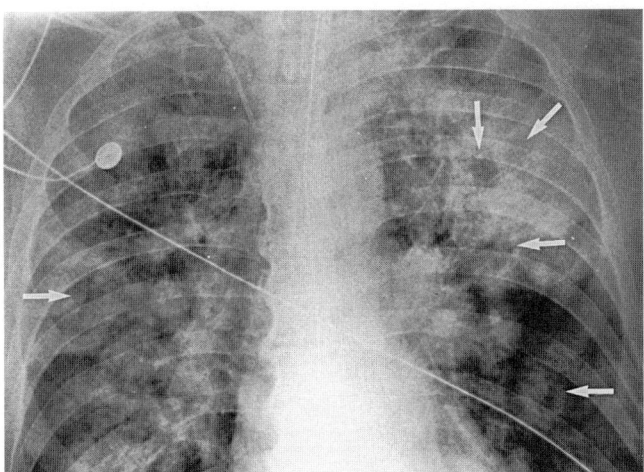

Fig. 71-36. Septic emboli. A chest anteroposterior film obtained in a 72-year-old patient with history of endocarditis, septicemia, and fever demonstrates multiple bilateral nodules with acute cavitation characteristic of lung infection owing to septic emboli. In this advanced case, cavitation is better appreciated in the left lung nodules (arrows).

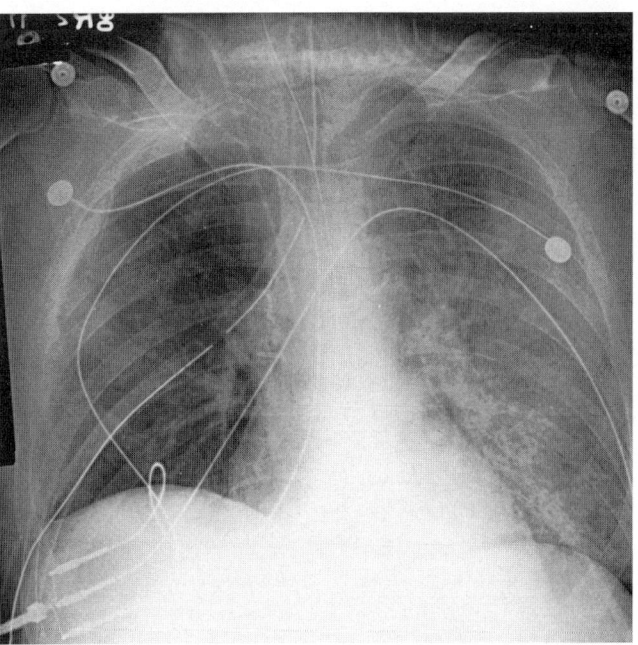

Fig. 71-37. Aspiration pneumonia. A chest film obtained after right lung surgery on a 57-year-old patient demonstrates unilateral diffuse left lung infiltrates owing to aspiration, which was believed to have happened at the time of surgery when the patient was lying with the left side down. Radiographically the infiltrates may mimic those of unilateral edema. The latter clears much faster.

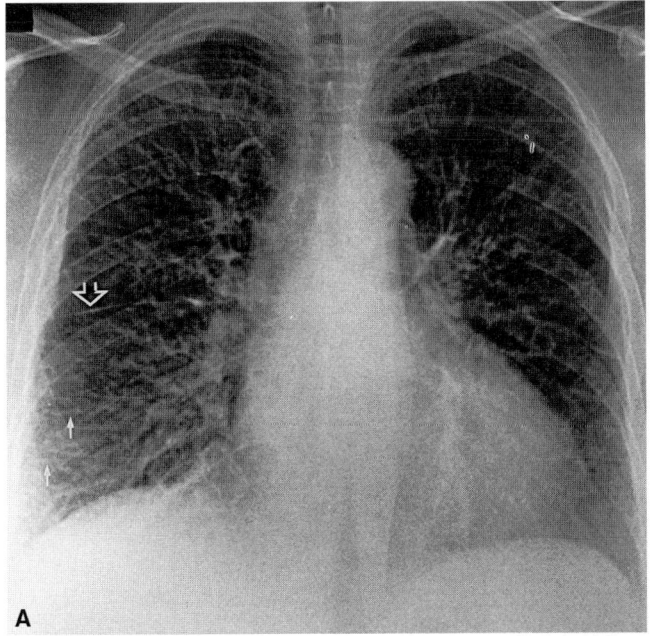

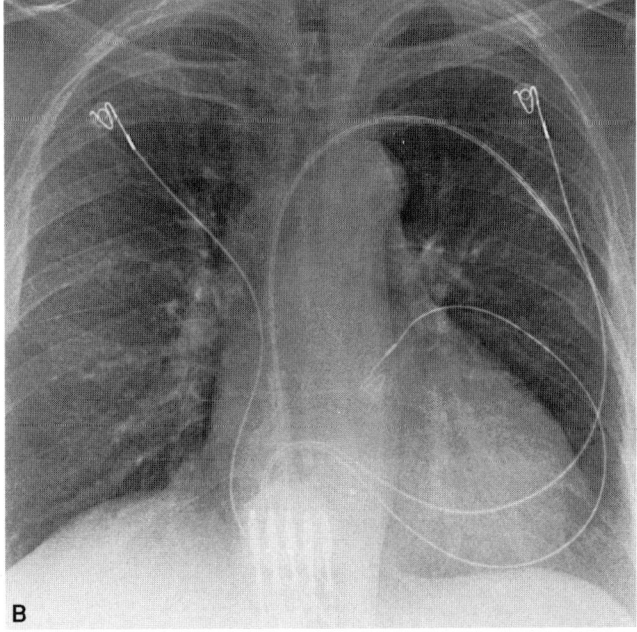

Fig. 71-38. Interstitial edema owing to congestive heart failure. *A*, Chest anteroposterior film obtained in a 58-year-old patient admitted because of acute myocardial infarction demonstrates diffuse pulmonary vascular prominence and increased interstitial lung markings seen throughout both lung fields with Kerley's B lines seen at the periphery of the lung bases (small arrows). Note the small right pleural effusion and thickening of the minor fissure on the right (arrowhead). The left ventricle is enlarged, and there are fractures involving the lateral portion of the left midribs sustained during prior cardiac resuscitation. *B*, A chest posteroanterior film obtained 24 hours later demonstrates resolution of the interstitial edema.

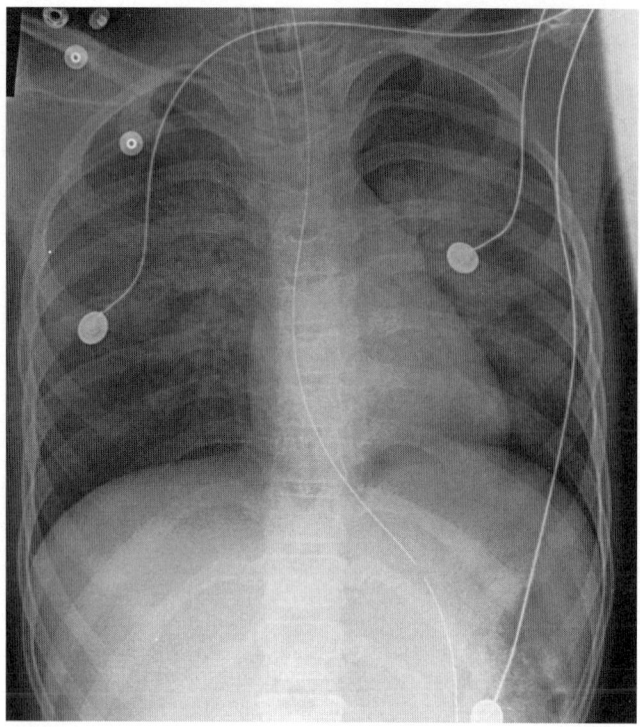

Fig. 71-39. Perihilar pulmonary edema. A chest anteroposterior portable film obtained in a 12-year-old patient with history of near-drowning demonstrates bilateral perihilar symmetric infiltrate owing to pulmonary edema. Note that the bronchovascular markings in the perihilar region are obscured by the edema.

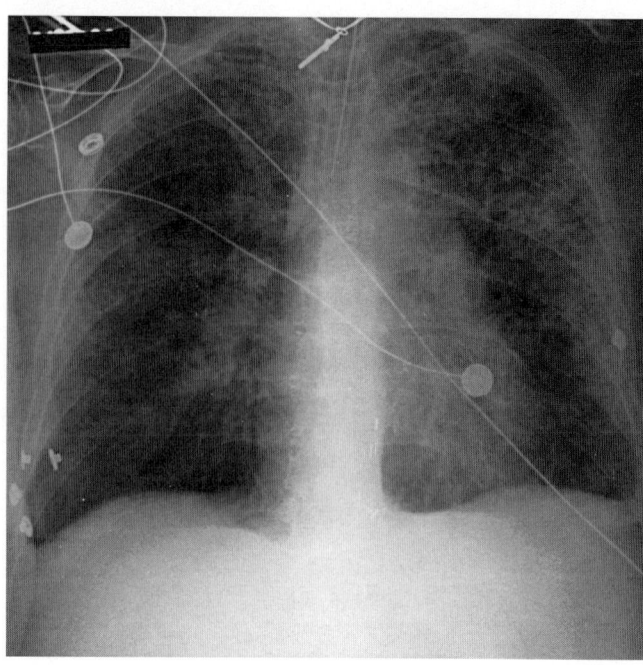

Fig. 71-40. Pulmonary edema superimposed on pulmonary emphysema. A chest anteroposterior portable film obtained in a 68-year-old patient with history of chronic pulmonary emphysema and acute congestive heart failure demonstrates bilateral ill-defined, nonuniform, patchy mixed alveolar and interstitial infiltrates. Multiple lucencies are seen throughout the lung infiltrates representing areas of underlying destroyed lung by pulmonary emphysema. The pulmonary vasculature is prominent, and small bilateral pleural effusions are present. The edema cleared within 24 hours.

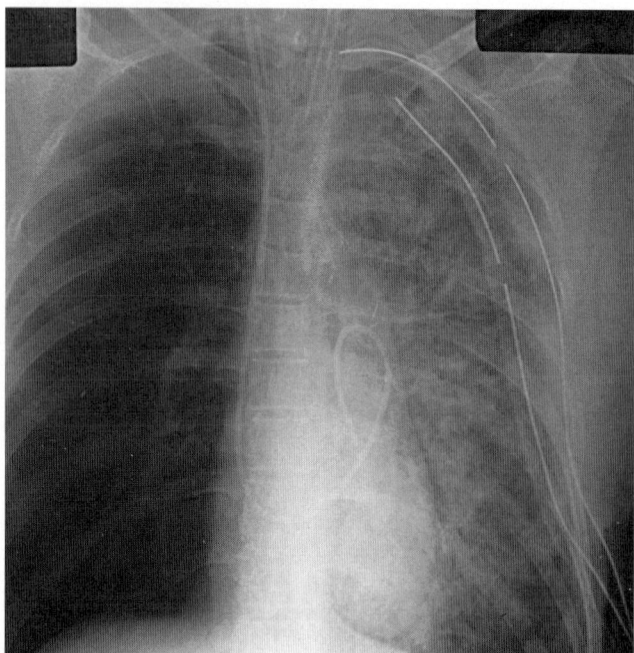

Fig. 71-41. Unilateral pulmonary edema. A chest anteroposterior film obtained in a 44-year-old patient status post left lung transplant demonstrates diffuse infiltrates involving the transplanted lung with no sign of infiltrates involving the hyperexpanded right lung. The edema resolved within 48 hours.

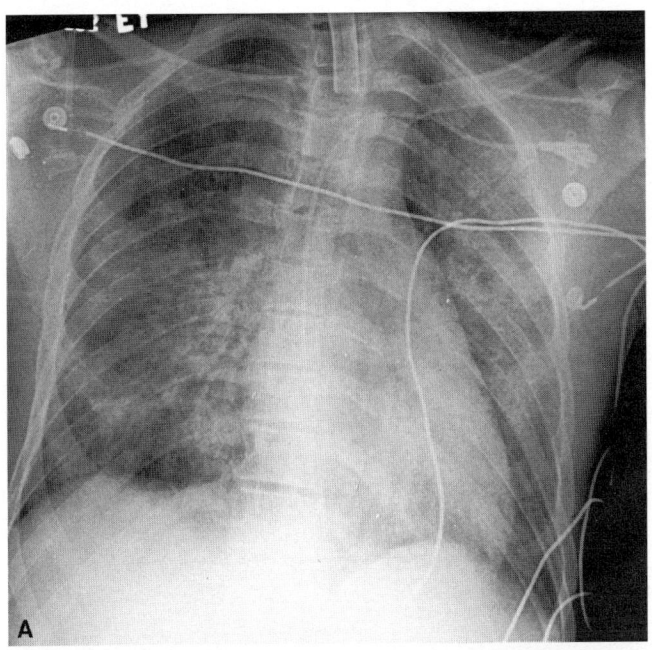
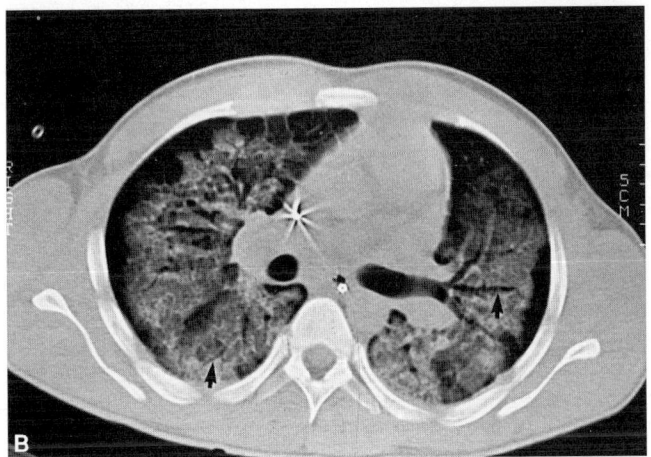
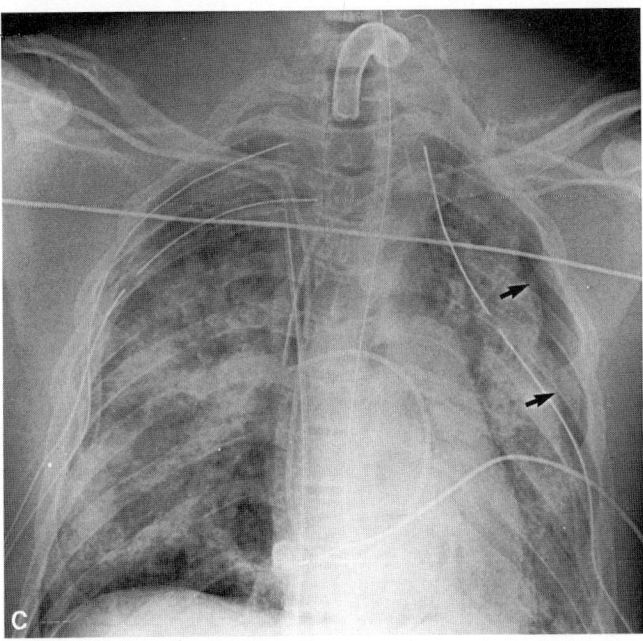

Fig. 71-42. Adult respiratory distress syndrome (ARDS). *A,* A chest anteroposterior portable film was obtained in a 19-year-old patient admitted to the ICU for shortness of breath and history of leukemia. There are bilateral diffuse perihilar infiltrates similar to that of pulmonary edema. There is no sign of pleural effusion or cardiac enlargement. *B,* A CT scan of the chest obtained the same day with an axial image at the level of the carina demonstrates bilateral diffuse alveolar infiltrates with lung consolidation better seen on the CT scan examination by the presence of well-defined air bronchograms (arrows). *C,* A chest anteroposterior portable film obtained 1 week later demonstrates progression of the infiltrates. In the interim, bilateral chest tubes have been placed to control the pneumothoraces, which occurred after increase of the positive end-expiratory pressure. Note that the left pneumothorax (arrows) has not resolved despite the placement of the left chest tube. This is believed to be due to the poor compliance and re-expansion of the lungs involved by ARDS.

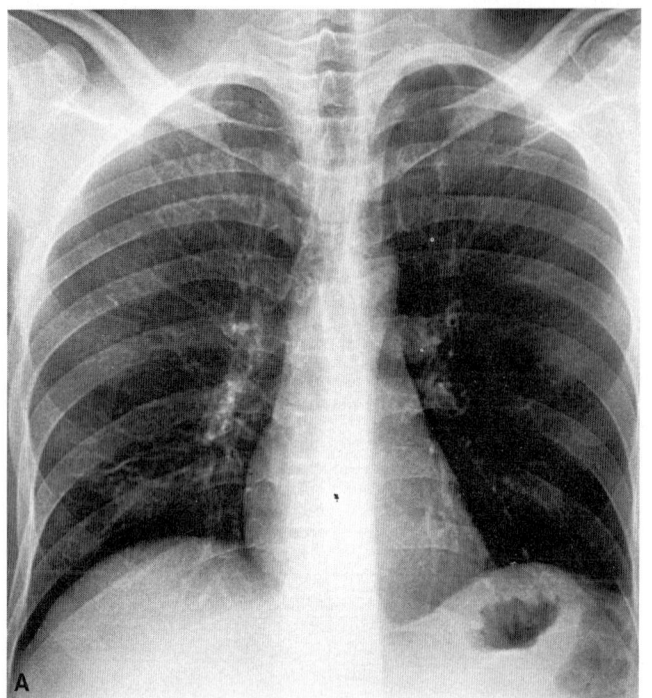
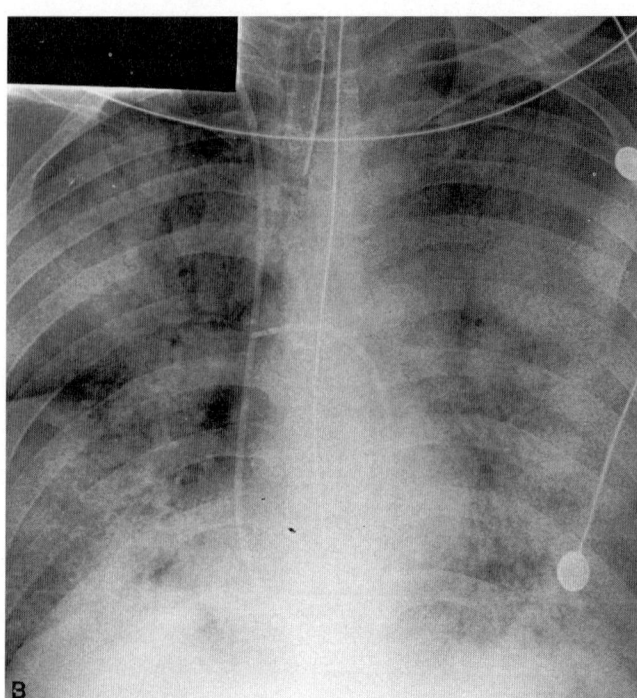
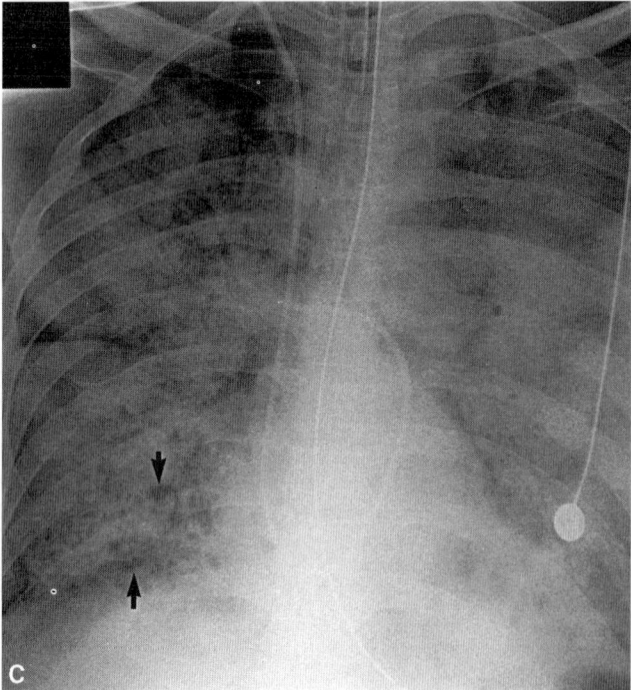

Fig. 71–43. ARDS. *A*, An admission chest posteroanterior film of a 25-year-old patient admitted for pancreatitis revealed no parenchymal or cardiovascular abnormality. *B*, The patient was admitted to the ICU 48 hours later because of acute shortness of breath. The chest anteroposterior film demonstrates extensive bilateral lung consolidation with alveolar infiltrates. Note that the cardiac size remains within normal limits, and there is no sign of pleural effusion. *C*, A chest anteroposterior portable film obtained 4 days after the x-ray films shown in *B* shows no improvement of the bilateral diffuse lung consolidation. Ill-defined areas of lucencies are now seen throughout both lung bases suggestive of lung necrosis (arrows). The patient expired 10 hours after the film was taken.

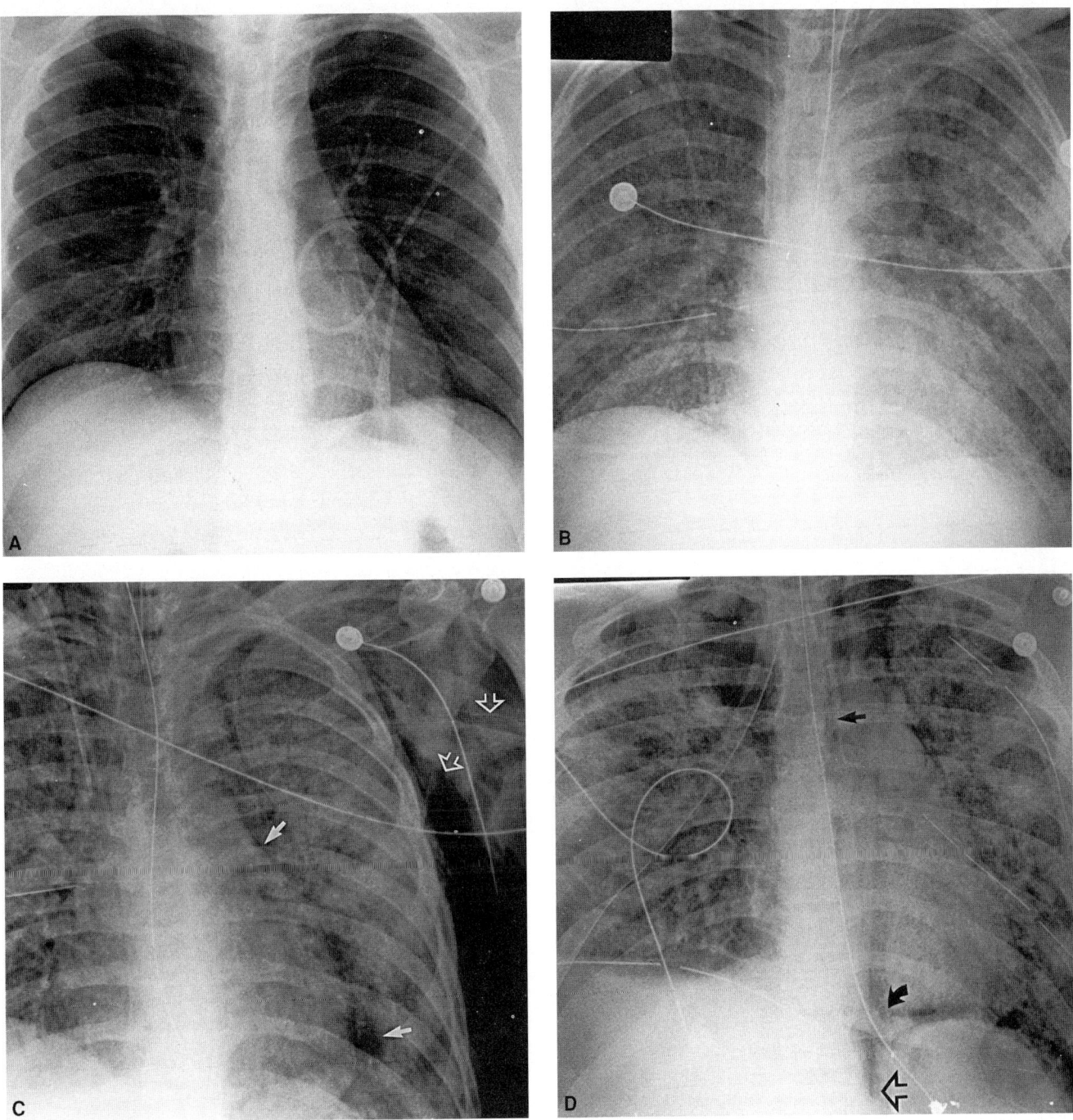

Fig. 71–44. ARDS with barotrauma owing to increased positive end-expiratory pressure. *A,* A baseline chest posteroanterior film in a 45-year-old patient with history of lymphoma shows no parenchymal abnormality. *B,* The patient was admitted to the ICU because of increasing shortness of breath and multisystem failure. The examination demonstrates bilateral diffuse new infiltrates obscuring the bronchovascular markings. There is no sign of cardiomegaly or pleural effusion. There were no clinical signs of infection. Owing to worsening of the breathing function, the positive end-expiratory pressure was subsequently increased. *C,* A chest anteroposterior portable film obtained 36 hours later demonstrates a pneumomediastinum (arrows) seen best along the left heart border and mediastinum extending into the soft tissue of the neck and bilateral subcutaneous emphysema (arrowheads). *D,* A further increase of the positive end-expiratory pressure because of continuous worsening of the respiratory function shows a relative improvement of the appearance of the lung infiltrates. Bilateral chest tubes were placed to control the bilateral spontaneous pneumothoraces, which have not completely resolved (curved arrow). The pneumomediastinum is now more extensive (straight arrow) with extension of air below the diaphragm (open arrowhead).

(Figure continues)

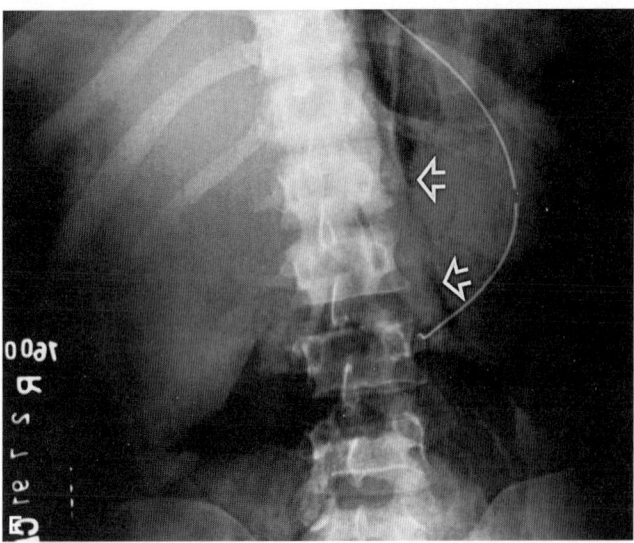
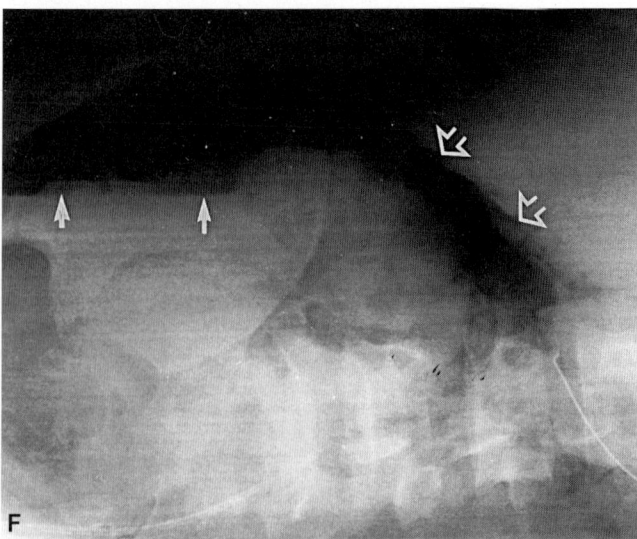

Fig. 71–44. *(Continued) E,* A portable examination of the abdomen obtained in a supine position demonstrates retroperitoneal air, which has dissected from the chest (arrowheads). *F,* A left lateral decubitus examination obtained at the bedside also demonstrates a hydropneumoperitoneum (arrows) consequent to the dissection of air from the chest. The inferior portion of the liver is outlined by air (open arrowheads).

PLEURAL SPACE

Accumulation of fluid or air within the pleural space is a common occurrence in the ICU patient. Because of the poor quality of the portable examination of the chest and the supine position of the patient, small pleural collections can be difficult to detect. Large pleural effusions or pneumothoraces that compromise the underlying lungs and become life-threatening need to be recognized.

Pneumothorax

Pneumothoraces are often detected after thoracic cardiac or lung surgery. They can be seen after trauma to the chest with or without associated rib fractures. They can complicate invasive procedures, such as thoracenteses or transbronchial and transthoracic biopsies, or after central venous catheterization (Fig. 71–47).[29] They can rarely occur after tracheal intubation.[30] They are often seen in barotrauma, complicating mechanical ventilation, or seen to complicate underlying cavitary or cystic lung processes that rupture into the pleural space (Fig. 71–48).[31] They can spontaneously occur in patients with underlying pulmonary emphysema and subpleural bullous disease and in patients with pneumocystis pneumonia.[32] Although small pneumothoraces may not have a significant impact on the patient's breathing, they may become larger in mechanically ventilated patients. The pneumothorax can be recognized easily when the thin white line representing the visceral pleura is identified and no lung markings can be seen peripheral to the line (see Fig. 71–47). Skin folds that can mimic pneumothoraces are identified as an edge of diffuse increased density against a radiolucency (Fig. 71–49). The inferior and upper margins of the skin folds are often seen to fade away or project beyond the margin of the ribs. Artifacts from tubes, wires, or dressing may overlie the patient and mimic pneumothoraces. In a supine position, small free pneumothoraces collect in the anterior-inferior portion of the chest, easily avoiding detection. Larger collections interface with the diaphragm and the heart border, rendering their margins sharp and creating an overall increased lucency, owing to the lack of lung markings ("deep sulcus sign") (Figs. 71–50 and 71–51).[33] Sometimes pneumothoraces can be confined to the medial portion of the lungs mimicking pneumomediastinums (Fig. 71–52). Cross-lateral table examination or, if necessary, CT scan of the chest can confirm the presence and the location of the abnormal air collection when the anteroposterior views of the chest are equivocal. Tension pneumothoraces can be life-threatening and are easily visualized radiographically when there is a shift of the mediastinum and heart, depression of the diaphragm, and widening of the intercostal space (Fig. 71–53; see Fig. 71–46B). In patients with fixed mediastinums, stiff lungs, or loculation of the air collections, the diagnosis of tension can be difficult to ascertain based on the radiographic findings alone.[34]

Pleural Effusions

Pleural effusions are a common finding in the chest radiographs of ICU patients. They are commonly seen after thoracic or abdominal surgery or in the patient with congestive heart failure.[35] Pneumonia and pulmonary infarction are other common causes that may be associated with pleural effusions. Small pleural fluid collections can be difficult to detect on the supine patient but are often seen during CT scan examinations of the ICU patient (Fig. 71–54).[36,37] Layering of pleural fluid in the dependent portion of the chest, on the supine patient, gives the appearance of a diffuse haze of increased density of the hemithorax (see Fig. 71–54A). Most commonly, small pleural effusions would be seen as areas of minimal increased density of the bases caused by the fluid itself or by the underly-

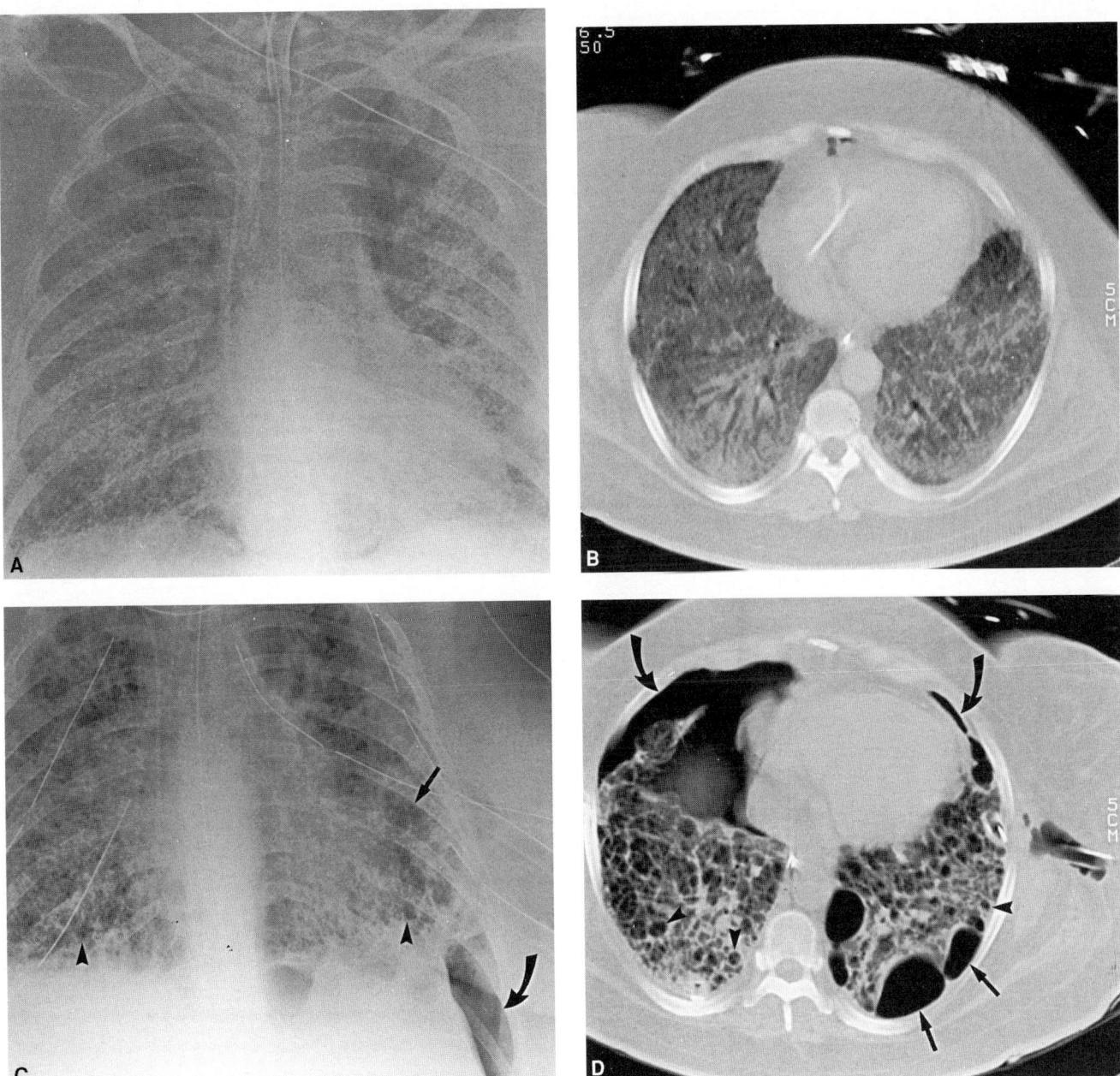

Fig. 71–45. Post-ARDS lung. *A, B,* A chest anteroposterior film *(A)* and a CT scan through the lung bases *(B)* both obtained the same day in a 44-year-old patient with a 3-week history of ARDS status post pancreatitis demonstrate bilateral diffuse infiltrates involving homogeneously both lung fields with a ground-glass appearance. *C, D,* Follow-up chest anteroposterior film *(C)* and CT scan of the chest *(D)* obtained the same day 1 month after the examinations shown in *A* and *B* demonstrate relative clearance of the bilateral infiltrates owing to the progression of the fibrocystic changes best demonstrated on the CT scan images. Multiple cystic spaces are seen throughout both lung fields (arrowheads) with coalescence into multiple subpleural blebs (arrows). Bilateral pneumothoraces are seen near both costophrenic angles (curved arrows). These findings represent progression of ARDS into end-stage fibrocystic disease of the lungs.

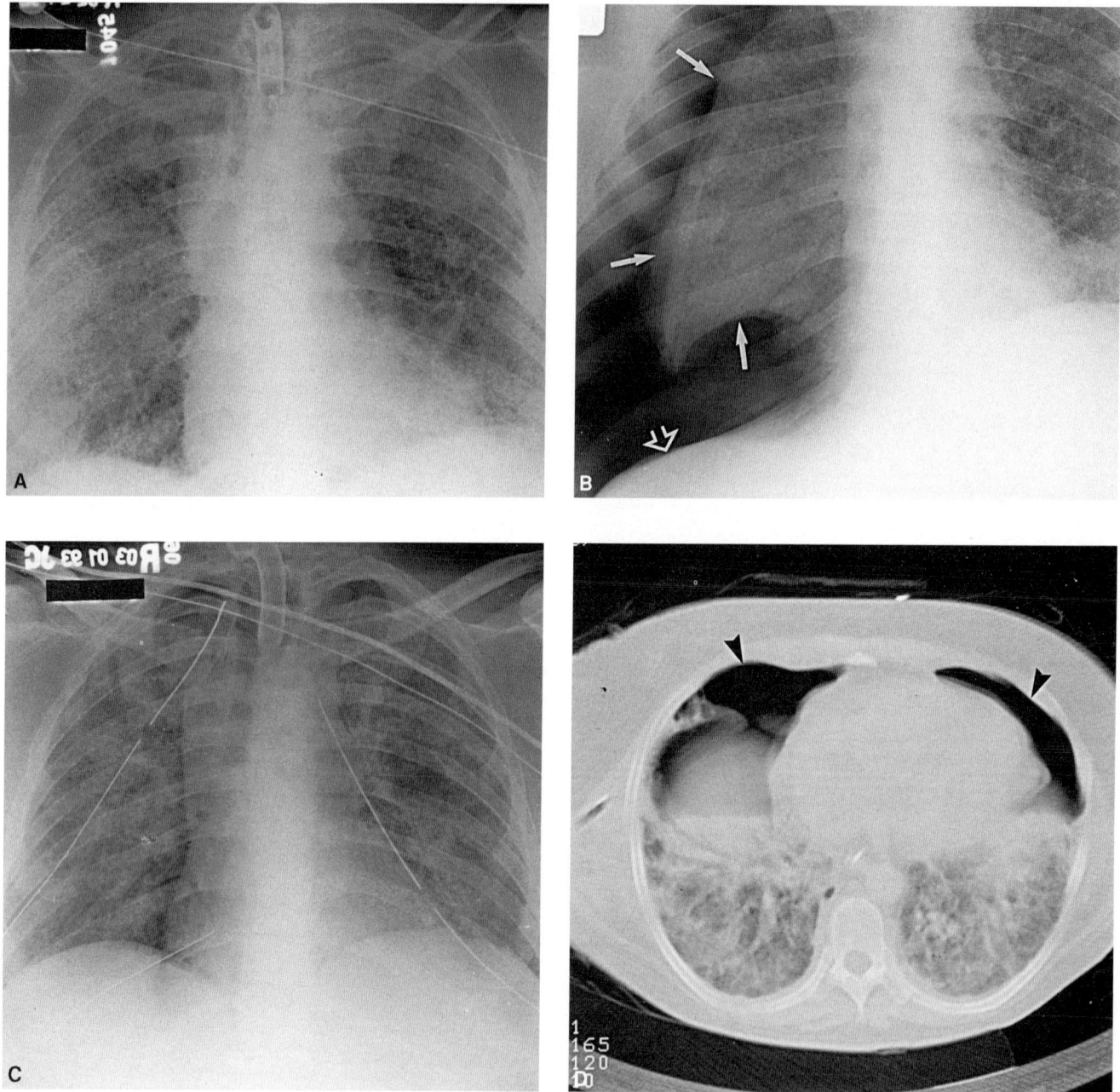

Fig. 71-46. Post-ARDS lung. *A,* A chest anteroposterior film obtained in a 26-year-old patient status post septicemia and ARDS demonstrates bilateral granular infiltrates secondary to ARDS. *B,* A follow-up chest anteroposterior film obtained 2 days later because of shortness of breath demonstrates a large right tension pneumothorax with collapse of the right lung (arrows) and lower shift of the right hemidiaphragm (arrowhead). *C, D,* A chest anteroposterior film *(C)* and a CT scan of the chest *(D)* obtained 1 week after *B* demonstrate relative improvement of the bilateral infiltrates with persistent bilateral pneumothoraces despite the presence of bilateral draining chest tubes. The pneumothoraces are better visualized on the CT scan examination (arrowheads).

(Figure continues)

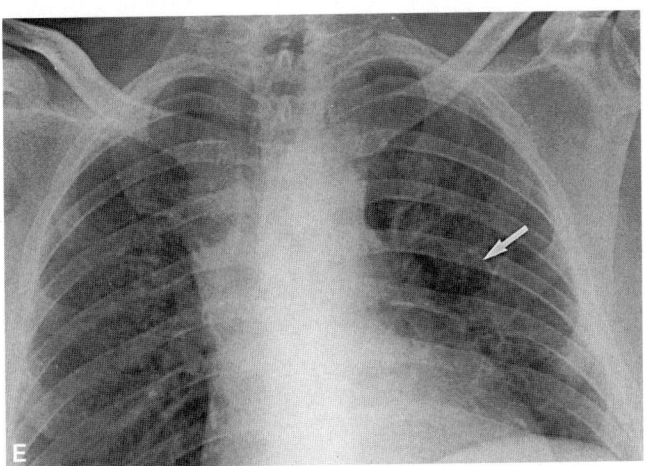 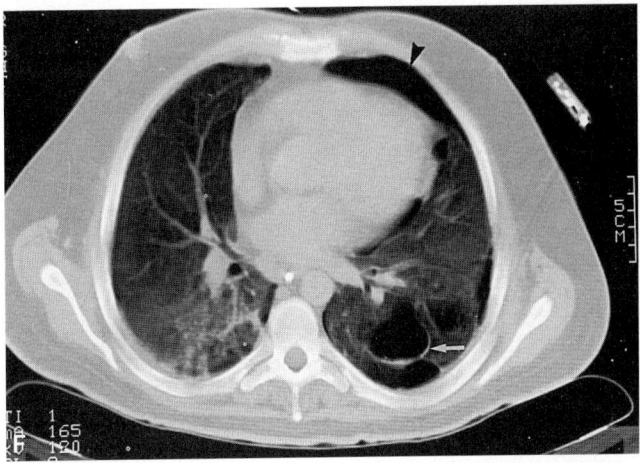

Fig. 71–46. *(Continued) E, F,* A chest anteroposterior film *(E)* and a CT scan of the chest *(F)* obtained 1 month later demonstrate almost complete resolution of the bilateral infiltrates except for residual fibrocystic changes seen best on the CT scan in the posterior aspect of both lung bases (arrows). Owing to the poor compliance of the lung involved by ARDS, pneumothoraces (arrowhead) can persist for a long time. (See *F* and *D.*) Depending on the severity of the insult to the lung, the extent of the parenchymal damage resulting in fibrocystic disease can be extensive (see Fig. 71–45) or minimal, as here.

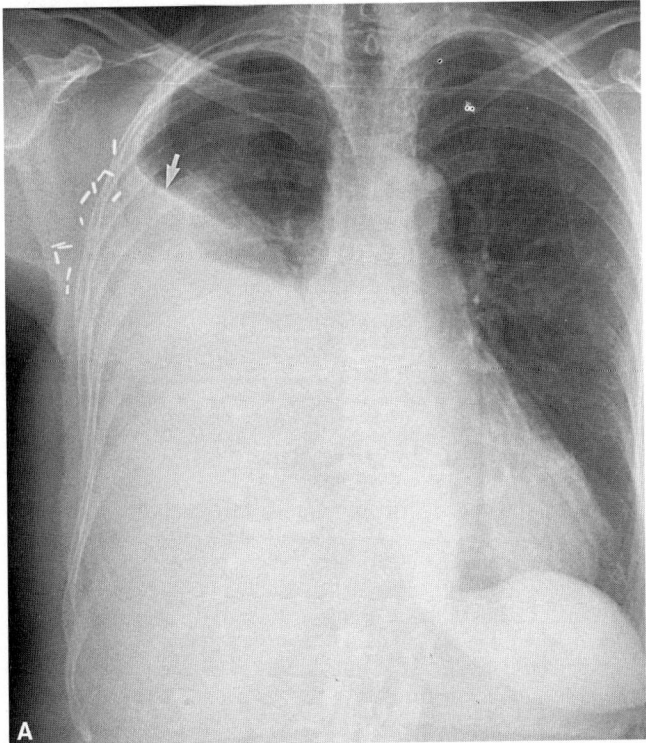 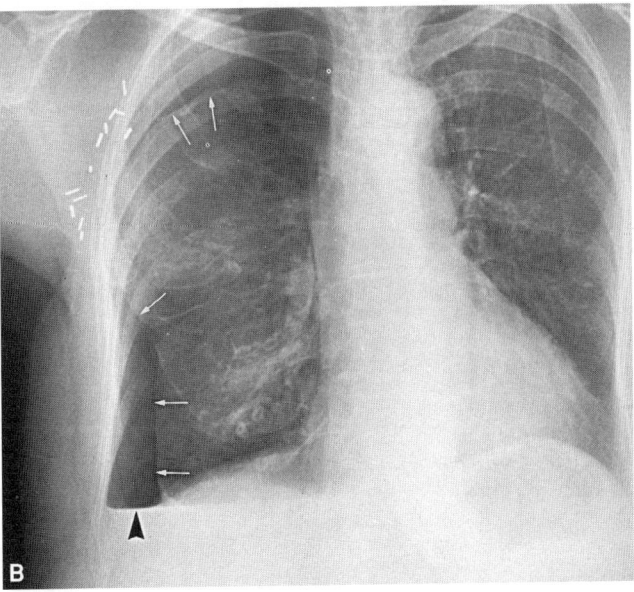

Fig. 71–47. Hydropneumothorax. *A,* A chest posteroanterior film obtained in a 78-year-old patient status post right mastectomy and shortness of breath demonstrates a large right pleural effusion (arrow). *B,* After thoracentesis and removal of 2000 ml of fluid, a chest posteroanterior fluid demonstrates a right hydropneumothorax shown as an air-fluid level at the right costophrenic angle (black arrowhead) with the collapsed lung seen demarcated by a thin white line representing the visceral pleura (white arrows). Note the absence of lung markings lateral to the collapsed lung.

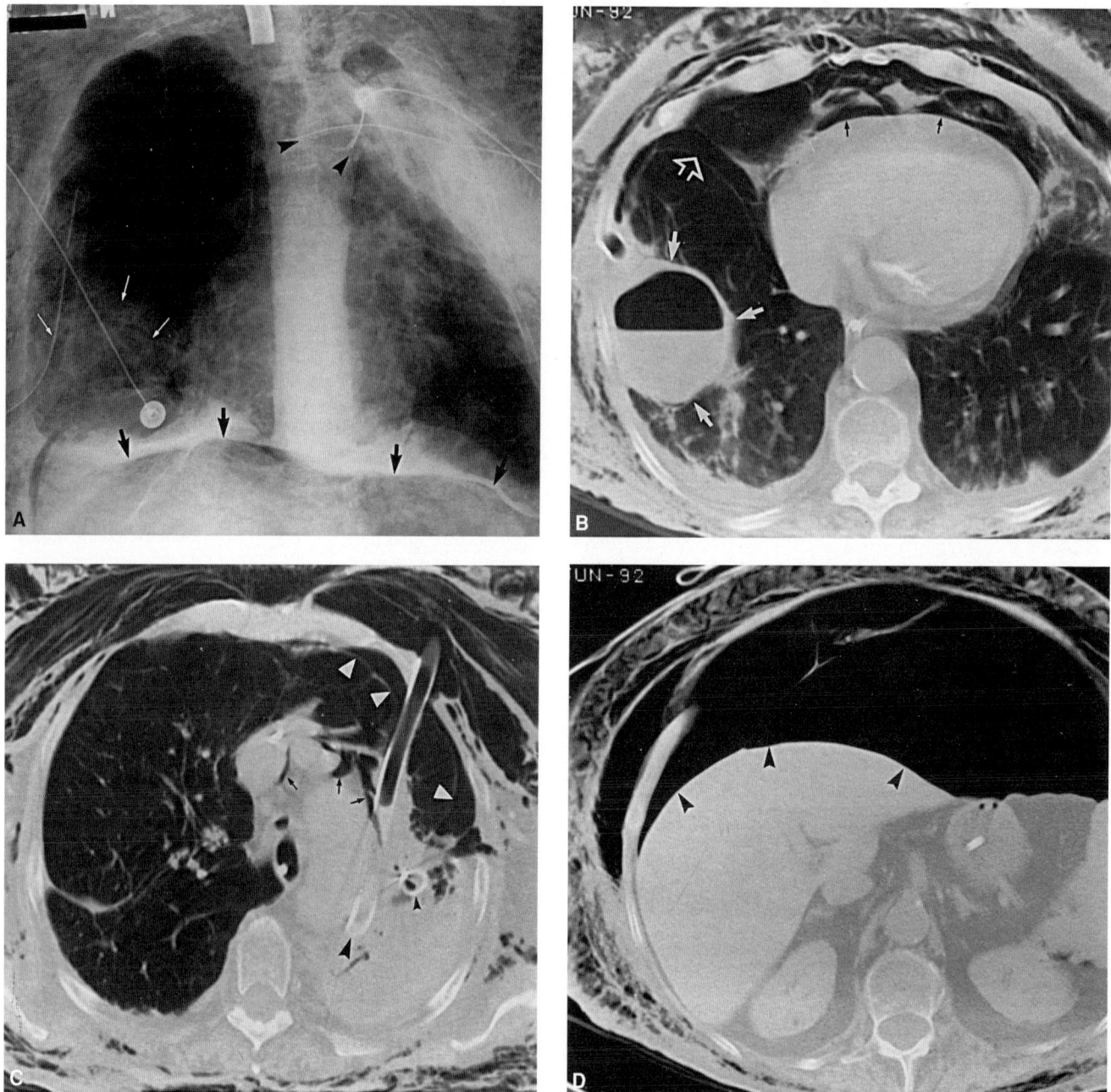

Fig. 71–48. Dissecting pneumothoraces. A 72-year-old patient with long-standing history of pulmonary emphysema was admitted to evaluate the source of acute onset of fever. During the course of his hospitalization, the patient developed bilateral pneumothoraces. A, A chest anteroposterior portable film obtained after placement of bilateral chest tubes demonstrates extensive bilateral subcutaneous emphysema rendering the interpretation of the lung parenchyma difficult. Pneumothoraces can also be difficult to detect when there is extensive subcutaneous emphysema. Note the poor positioning of the left chest tubes with the tips seen medially (black arrowheads). There is an acute infiltrate in the left apex (see C) representing lung contusion and hemorrhage. There is a large pneumoperitoneum identified as a large lucency outlining the anterior aspect of the diaphragm on this supine examination (black arrows). There is a right lung abscess identified as a vague radiodensity in the right lower chest (small white arrows). B, A CT scan of the chest obtained to evaluate the extent of pleural, parenchymal, and mediastinal disease demonstrates a 6-cm abscess in the right lower lobe (white arrows) with an air-fluid level not suspected on the supine chest film. There is a small right anterior pneumothorax (open arrowhead). There is also evidence of a pneumomediastinum seen anterior to the heart (small black arrows). There is extensive subcutaneous emphysema throughout the soft tissues of the chest wall. C, An axial image obtained at the level of the aortic arch demonstrates a left pneumothorax (white arrowheads) and a pneumomediastinum (small black arrows). One left chest tube is seen entering the major fissure and ending within the left apex (large black arrowhead). A second chest tube is seen lateral to it within the lung parenchyma (small black arrowhead). There is consolidation of the posterior aspect of the left lung believed to be due to contusion. Note again the extensive subcutaneous emphysema. D, An axial image through the upper abdomen demonstrates the large pneumoperitoneum seen as a lucency occupying the anterior third of the abdomen displacing the liver posteriorly (arrowheads). Extensive subcutaneous emphysema is seen involving the abdominal wall.

IMAGING TECHNIQUES IN THE INTENSIVE CARE UNIT 1505

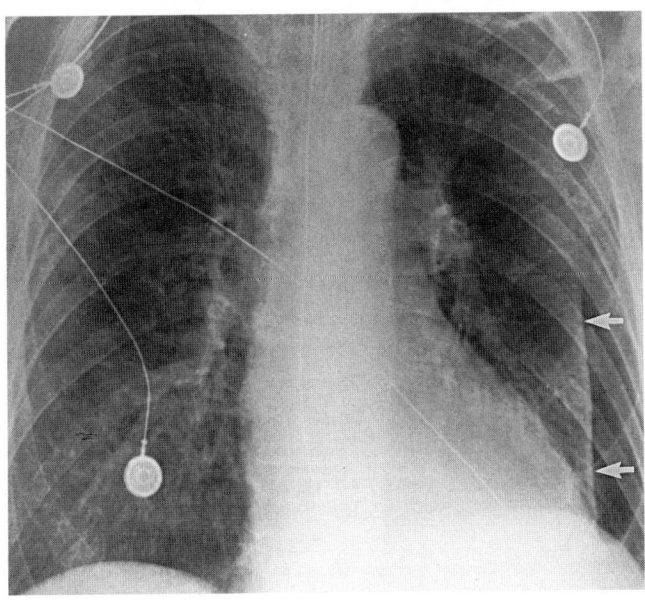

Fig. 71–49. Skin fold. A chest anteroposterior portable film obtained in a patient with a history of congestive heart failure demonstrates diffuse minimal interstitial edema. Incidentally, there is a vertical linear radiodensity overlying the left lower hemithorax (arrows). Note that there are lung markings seen lateral to the line. Note that the white radiodensity, which represents the folded skin, fades cephalad and medially. The line can often be traced outside of the rib cage.

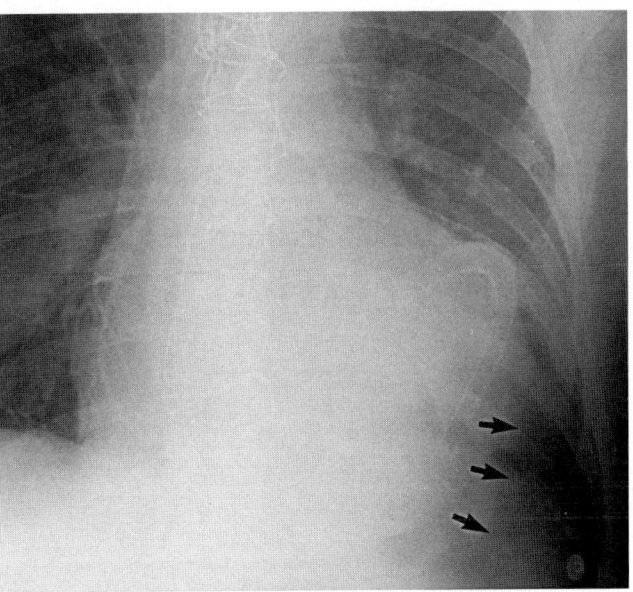

Fig. 71–50. Deep sulcus sign. A chest anteroposterior portable film obtained in a supine position after cardiac surgery demonstrates a lucency in the region of the left costophrenic angle representing a small left pneumothorax collecting in the anterior-inferior aspect of the chest (the least dependent portion) (arrows).

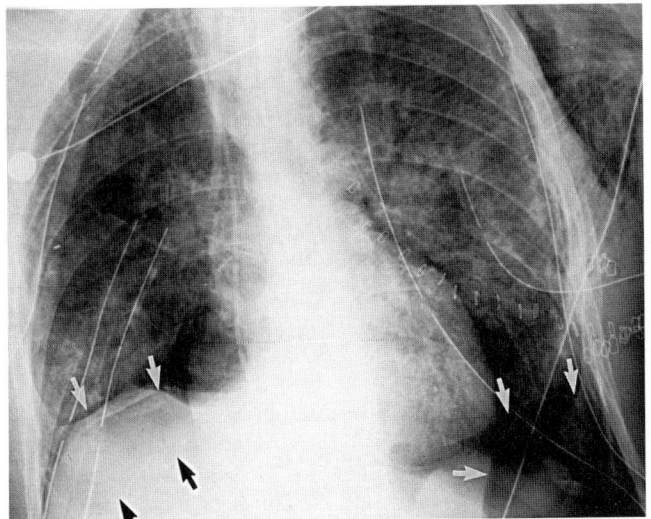

Fig. 71–51. Bilateral deep sulcus sign. In a 52-year-old patient status post bilateral lung transplant, bilateral lower chest pneumothoraces are identified as an increased lucency overlying both hemidiaphragms (arrows).

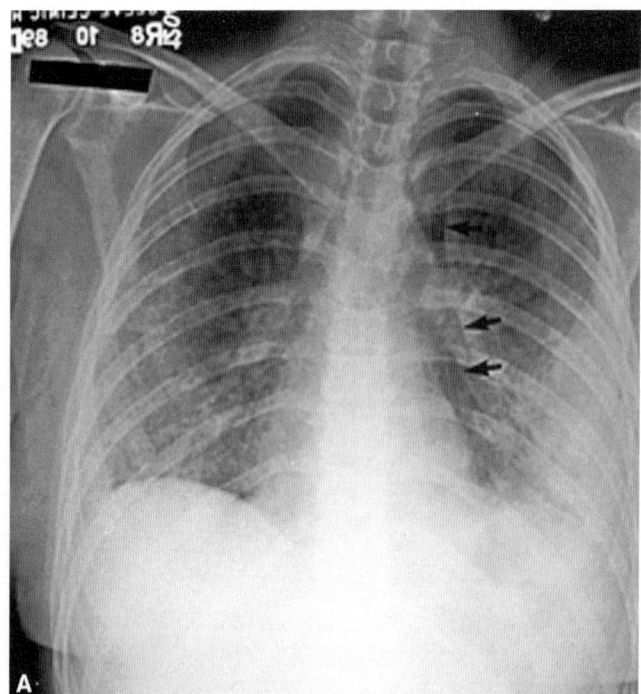

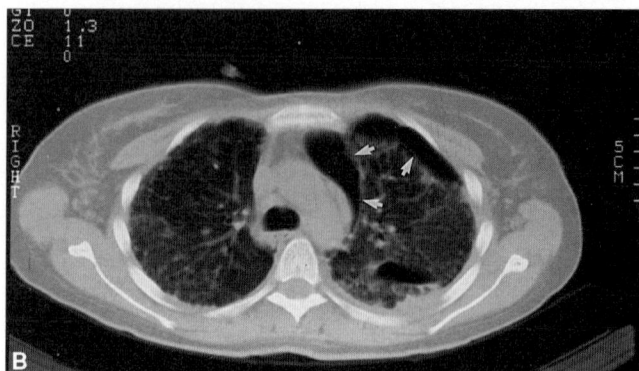

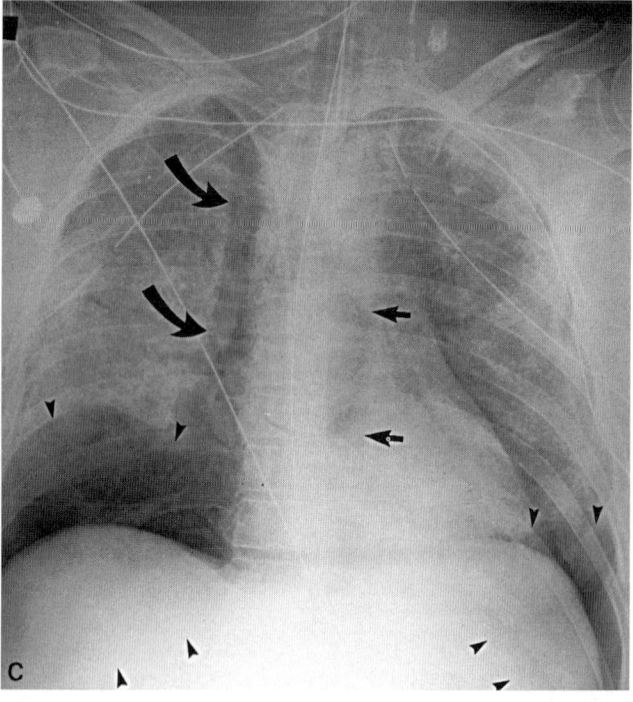

Fig. 71-52. Medial pneumothorax. *A*, A chest anteroposterior portable film obtained in a 30-year-old patient with history of varicella pneumonia demonstrates bilateral diffuse infiltrates. A left pneumothorax is barely identified in the medial aspect of the left hemithorax (arrows). *B*, A CT scan of the chest with an axial image obtained at the level of the aortic arch demonstrates better the extent and size of the left pneumothorax (arrows). The posteromedial aspect of the left lung is seen projecting posterior to the pneumothorax, rendering its detection difficult on the chest film. *C*, A follow-up chest anteroposterior film obtained a few days later demonstrates bilateral pneumothoraces despite the presence of chest tubes. There is a persistent medial left pneumothorax (arrows) and a new right medial pneumothorax (curved arrows). In this supine examination, the largest portion of the pneumothoraces is collecting in the anterior-inferior portion of the hemithoraces creating a deep sulcus sign bilaterally (arrowheads).

ing atelectatic lung obscuring the margins of the diaphragms. If the diagnosis of pleural effusion is important for the patient's management, either a left lateral decubitus examination or an ultrasound examination at the bedside can confirm the presence of pleural fluid. Subphrenic pleural effusions give the appearance of an elevated diaphragm (Fig. 71-55). Loculated pleural effusions within the fissures or the pleural space may have a confusing appearance on the chest film, mimicking parenchymal or chest wall processes (Figs. 71-56 and 71-57). Loculation is more commonly observed when the pleural fluid has a high viscosity of protein content leading to inflammation and the formation of adhesions. This is commonly seen in empyemas and hemothoraces. The appearance and nature of the pleural collection can be diagnosed more easily with CT. A hemothorax, when acute, has a high CT attenuation (Fig. 71-58). Early changes of empyema can be difficult to diagnose based on the radiographic findings alone. CT is helpful in detecting small air collections in the cases of empyemas with gas-forming organisms (Fig. 71-59). In

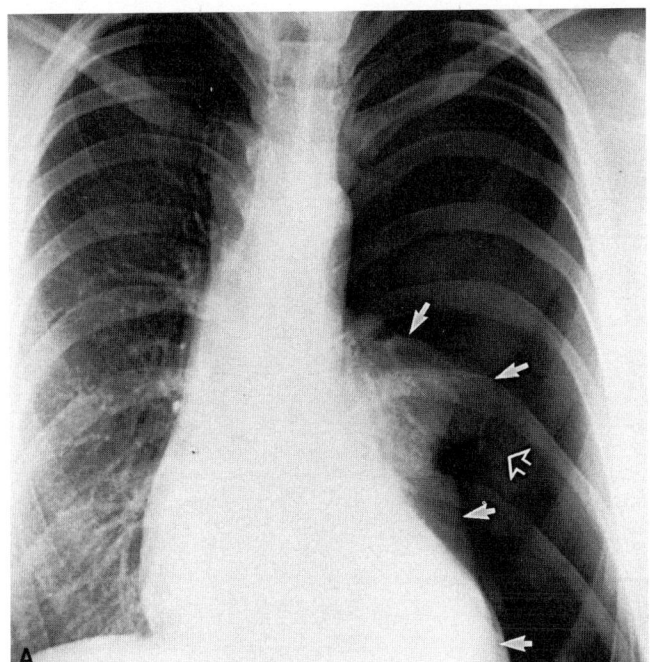
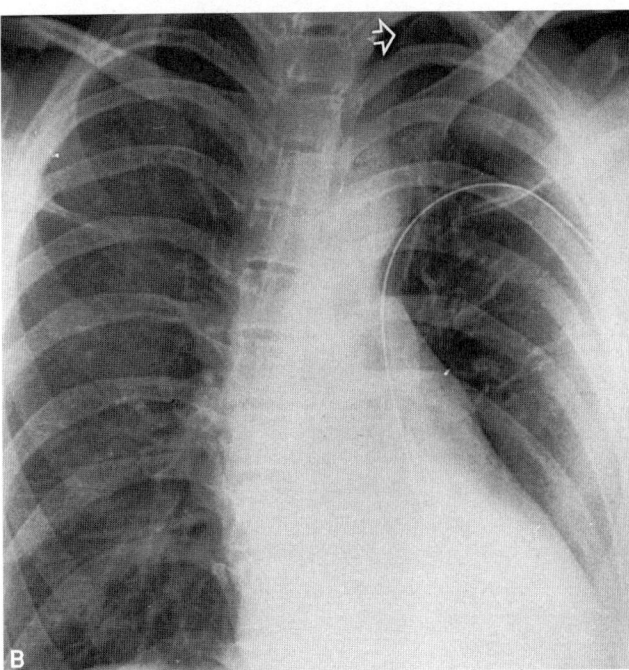

Fig. 71–53. Tension pneumothorax. *A*, A chest anteroposterior film obtained in a 20-year-old patient with history of Marfan's disease and shortness of breath shows a large left tension pneumothorax. The collapsed left lung is seen as a small soft tissue density in the medial aspect of the left lower chest and perihilar region (arrows). Note a small bleb seen in the collapsed left apex (open arrowhead). The heart and mediastinum are shifted to the right side with depression of the left hemidiaphragm and widening of the intercostal spaces. The right lower lung is minimally compressed. *B*, A chest anteroposterior film obtained after expansion of the left lung demonstrates shift of the mediastinum and heart to their normal positions. Note again the small bleb in the left apex (open arrowhead). The left lower lung remains partially collapsed, seen here as an increased density behind the heart obscuring the left hemidiaphragm. The patient has the left ventricle enlarged owing to aortic valve insufficiency.

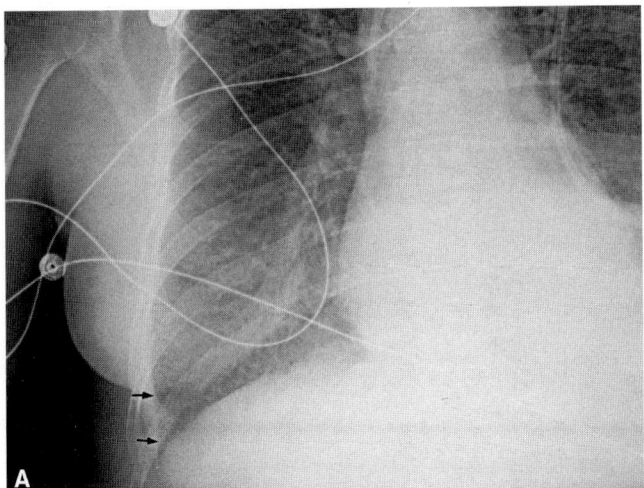
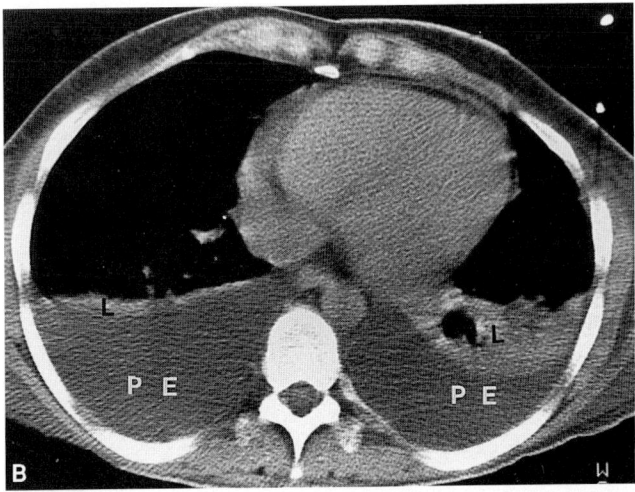

Fig. 71–54. Pleural effusions of CT scan. CT scan examinations are more sensitive than portable chest films for detecting pleural effusions. In this case, the chest anteroposterior portable film *(A)* obtained in a supine position 2 hours before the CT scan examination showed questionable pleural effusions seen as a haze in lower hemithoraces. There is blunting of the right costophrenic angle (arrows). A CT scan examination of the abdomen with images through the lower chest *(B)* demonstrated moderate-sized bilateral pleural effusions (PE). Note the areas of compression atelectasis seen involving the lung parenchyma (L) anterior to the pleural effusions.

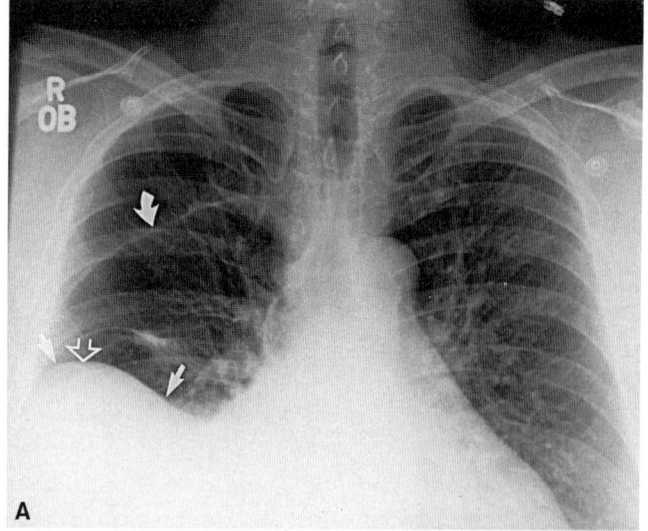
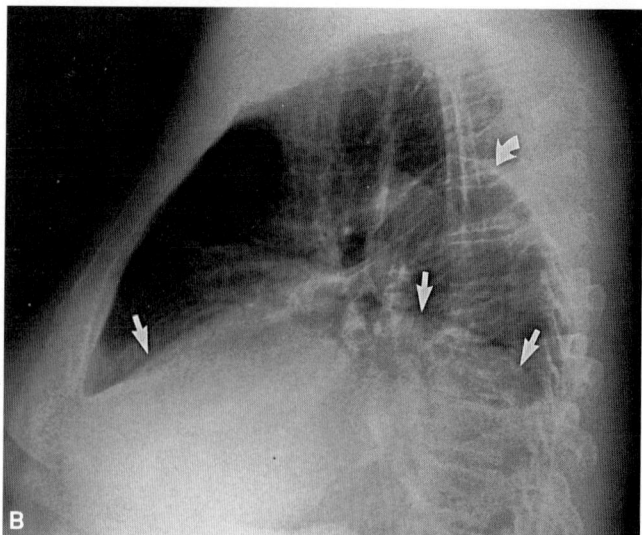
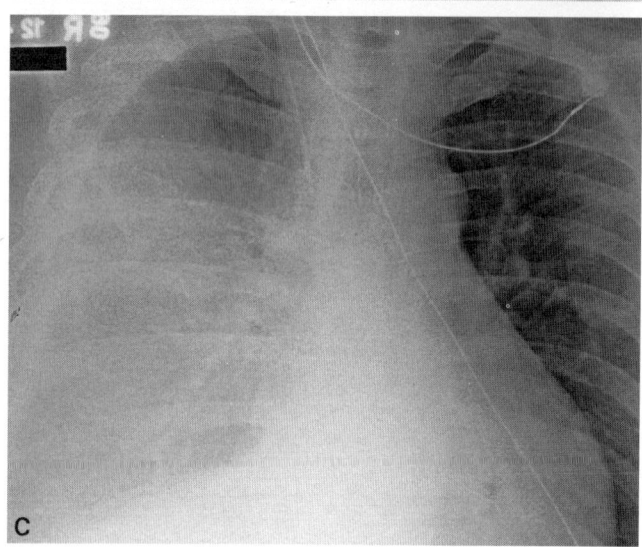

Fig. 71-55. Subpulmonic pleural effusion. *A, B,* Chest posteroanterior *(A)* and lateral *(B)* films in a 48-year-old patient status post abdominal surgery demonstrate elevation of which appears to be the right hemidiaphragm (arrows), elevation of the minor fissure, and thickening and/or fluid within the right major fissure (curved arrow). Note that on the posteroanterior view, the peak of the elevated pseudodiaphragm (open arrowhead) is not at the center but rather close to the chest wall suggestive of the interface between the lung and the subpulmonic pleural effusion. *C,* A chest anteroposterior film obtained supine demonstrates a large right pleural effusion layering in the posterior and lateral aspect of the right pleural space, opacifying the right hemithorax.

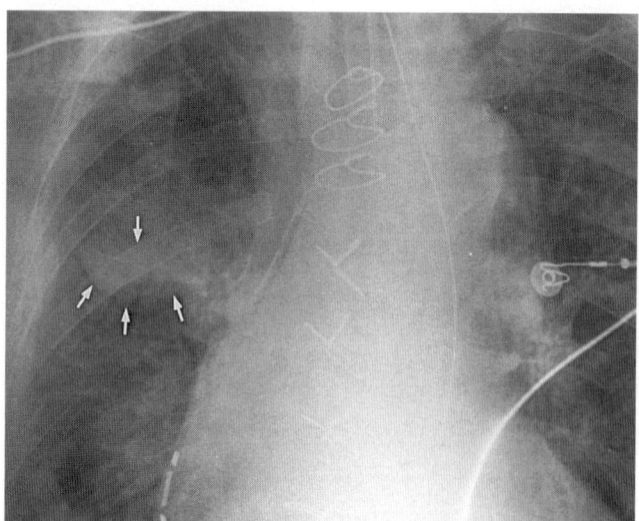

Fig. 71-56. Loculated pleural effusion in the minor fissure. A chest anteroposterior portable film obtained in a 72-year-old patient status post mediastinotomy demonstrates a vague radiodensity in the right midchest (arrows) representing a loculated effusion within the minor fissure mimicking an intraparenchymal process.

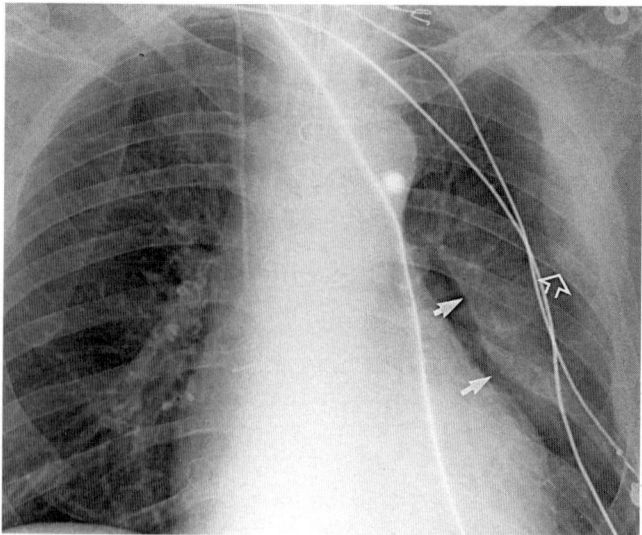

Fig. 71-57. Pleural effusion in the major fissure. Chest anteroposterior portable film obtained in a 50-year-old patient status post mediastinotomy demonstrates a vague radiodensity paralleling the left heart border (arrows) and fluid within the left major fissure. Partially loculated fluid is demonstrated in the lateral aspect of the pleural space in the left midchest (arrowhead).

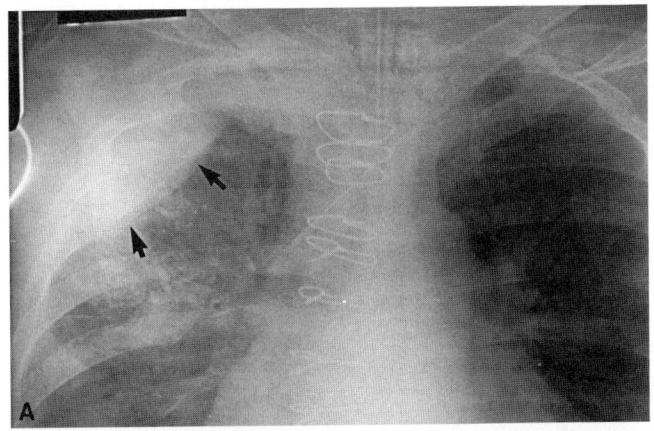
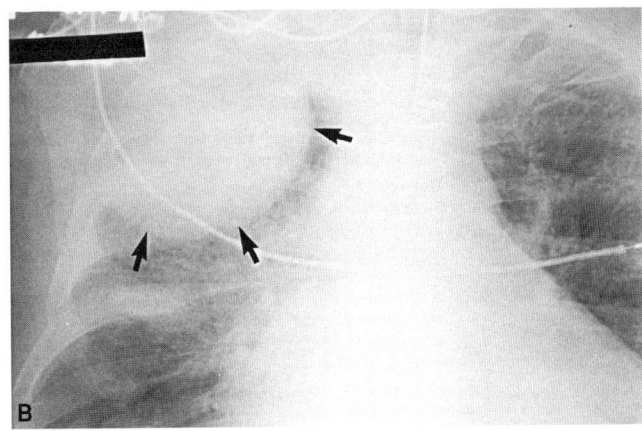

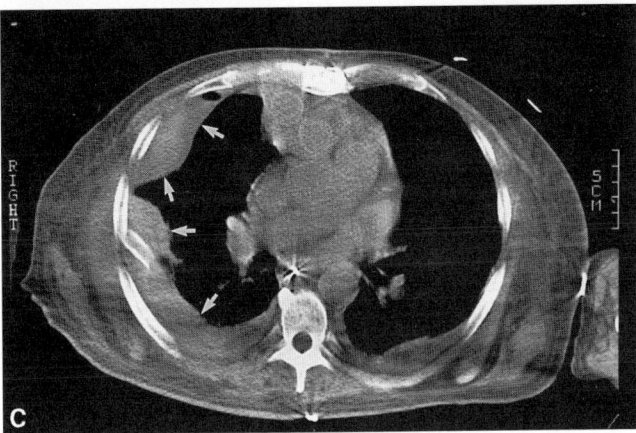

Fig. 71-58. Hemothorax. *A*, A chest anteroposterior portable film supine was obtained in a 62-year-old patient with prior open heart surgery. The x-ray film was obtained immediately after a failed attempt of placement of a right subclavian central line. It demonstrates an acute loculated fluid collection within the lateral aspect of the right upper chest (arrows). Note the conduit of the heart assist device projecting over the lower cardiac chamber. *B*, A follow-up chest film obtained 2 hours later showed a marked increase of the size of the loculated effusion within the right apex (arrows). *C*, A CT scan examination of the chest obtained 24 hours later after placement of a drainage tube demonstrates a persistent multiloculated pleural effusion with the high CT attenuation characteristic of a hemothorax (arrows).

more advanced cases, specific pleural changes of thickening and enhancement can be observed ("split pleura sign") (Figs. 71-59 and 71-60).[38]

POST-THORACOTOMY AND CARDIAC SURGERY PATIENTS

Postpneumonectomy Patients

It is important to recognize the chest radiographic findings of the postpneumonectomy patient and the chronology of the changes observed to detect any potential complication (Tables 71-3 and 71-4). Immediately after pneumonectomy, the chest film demonstrates an empty pneumonectomy space that has little or no fluid (Fig. 71-61A). The mediastinum and heart are either midline or minimally shifted toward the side of the surgery. In certain cases, irrigation fluid is put within the pneumonectomy space at the time of surgery and is visible on the initial chest film. One needs to realize that the amount of fluid is better appreciated if the x-ray film is obtained in

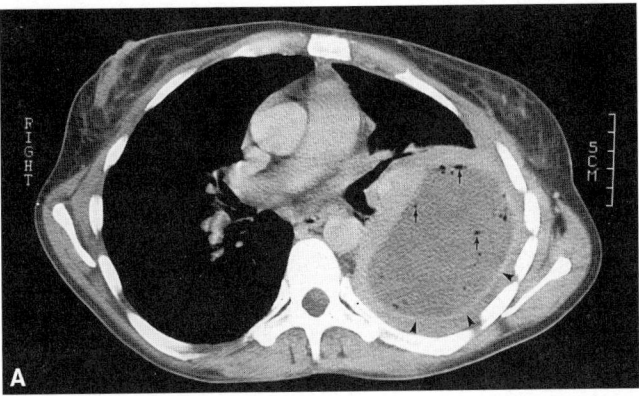
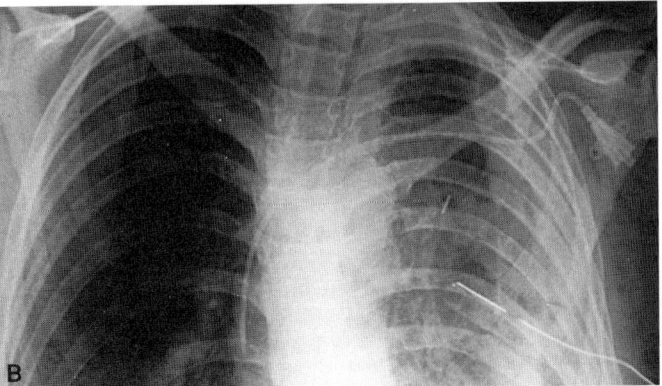

Fig. 71-59. Empyema. *A*, A CT scan of the chest in a 33-year-old patient status post left lung surgery and persistent fever demonstrates a large fluid collection in the left hemithorax with multiple small air bubbles trapped within the fluid (arrows). Note the thickened dense pleura seen split from the costal margins (arrowheads) (split pleural sign). *B*, A follow-up chest anteroposterior portable film obtained 72 hours after placement of a left drainage tube shows persistence of the left empyema in the left lower hemithorax. The patient required surgical drainage and decortication.

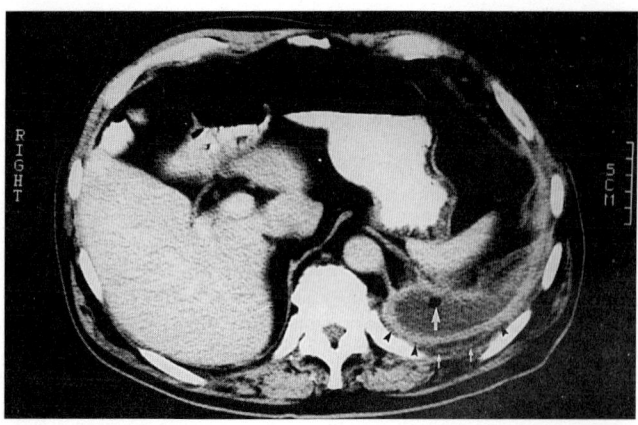

Fig. 71-60. Empyema. A CT scan of the chest that was obtained in a 70-year-old patient with progressive shortness of breath demonstrates the presence of a lenticular-shaped loculated fluid collection in the left lower pleural space. There is thickening and enhancement of the pleura (black arrowheads) with thickening of the subpleural tissues (small white arrows). A small air collection is seen within the fluid collection (large white arrow).

Table 71-3. Postpneumonectomy Changes

	24 Hours	1 Week	4 Weeks	8 Weeks
Pneumonectomy	Air, minimal fluid	Air-fluid level close to apex	Fluid (small air collection may persist in apex)	Fluid, fibrosis
Mediastinum	Midline to minimal shift to side of surgery	Shift to side of surgery	Further shift	Mediastinum and heart remain shifted

Table 71-4. Complications After Pneumonectomy

Acute

	Bleeding	Bronchopleural Fistula
Pneumonectomy space	Rapid accumulation of fluid	Persistent large collections of air
Mediastinum	No shift or shift opposite to the side of surgery	No shift or shift to opposite side

Subacute

	Bleeding	Bronchopleural Fistula	Empyema
Pneumonectomy space	Fluid* increase	Air increase (reaccumulation of air or new air collection)	Fluid* increase with or without new air collections
Mediastinum	Shift to opposite side	No shift or shift to opposite side	Shift to opposite side

Late

	Empyema	Bronchopleural Fistula	Recurrent Tumor
Pneumonectomy space	Fluid* increase with or without new air collections	New air collections	
Mediastinum	Shift to opposite side	No shift or shift to opposite side	Shift to opposite side. Displacement of surgical staples or sutures

* The increase of fluid may be difficult to detect if the pneumonectomy space is already filled with fluid.

Fig. 71-61. Normal postpneumonectomy changes. *A,* A chest anteroposterior portable film obtained in a supine position in a 53-year-old patient immediately after pneumonectomy for lung neoplasm demonstrates diffuse lucency of the right hemithorax. The changes are compatible with an empty pneumonectomy space except for minimal fluid in the right lower chest, shown here as haze projecting over the lower third of the right pneumonectomy space. Note the absence of lung markings on the right. *B,* A chest anteroposterior portable film obtained 48 hours later demonstrates opacification of the right lower hemithorax owing to accumulation of fluid within the pneumonectomy space. There is a lucency overlying the upper portion of the right pneumonectomy space owing to residual air. *C,* A chest anteroposterior portable film obtained in a supine position 1 week later demonstrates almost complete opacification of the right pneumonectomy space compatible with further accumulation of fluid and resorption of air. *D,* A chest anteroposterior portable film obtained in the upright position 10 days later demonstrates an air-fluid level within the apex of the right pneumonectomy space (arrow). Such an air-fluid level slowly and gradually moves toward the apex until complete resorption of the air. *E, F,* Bronchopleural fistula postpneumonectomy. *E,* A chest anteroposterior portable film of the same patient as shown in *A* through *D,* obtained in the supine position 2 weeks after surgery, demonstrates hyperexpansion of the right pneumonectomy space with diffuse increased lucency owing to newly collecting air within the pneumonectomy space. At this time, the primary diagnoses are of a bronchopleural fistula or possibly an empyema. *F,* A right chest tube was placed within the right pneumonectomy space seen overlying the right apex. Nonpurulent fluid was obtained from the pneumonectomy space. Note the persistent hyperexpansion of the right pneumonectomy with large amounts of air within the surgical bed. A bronchopleural fistula with failure of the bronchial stump was suspected and later confirmed during surgery.

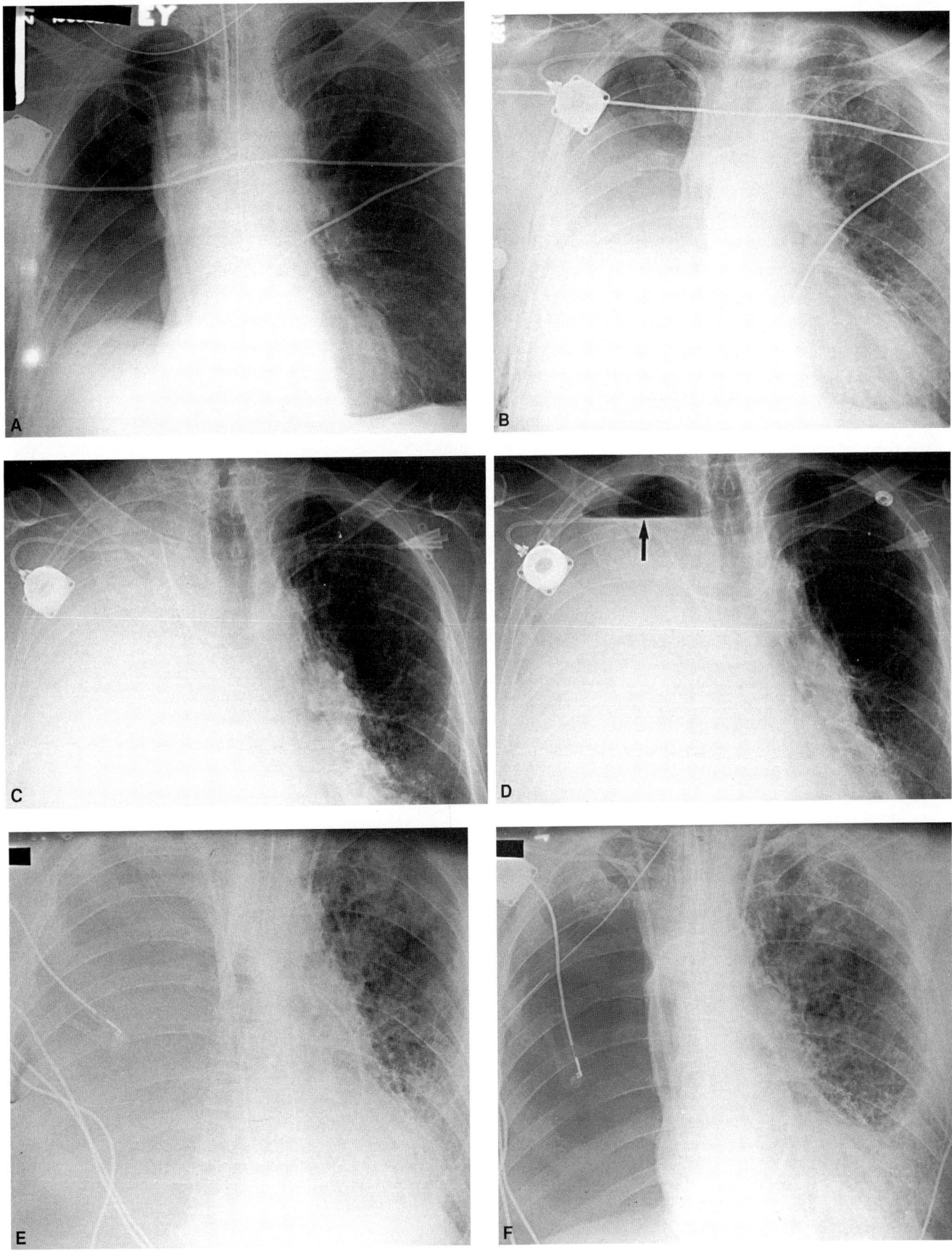

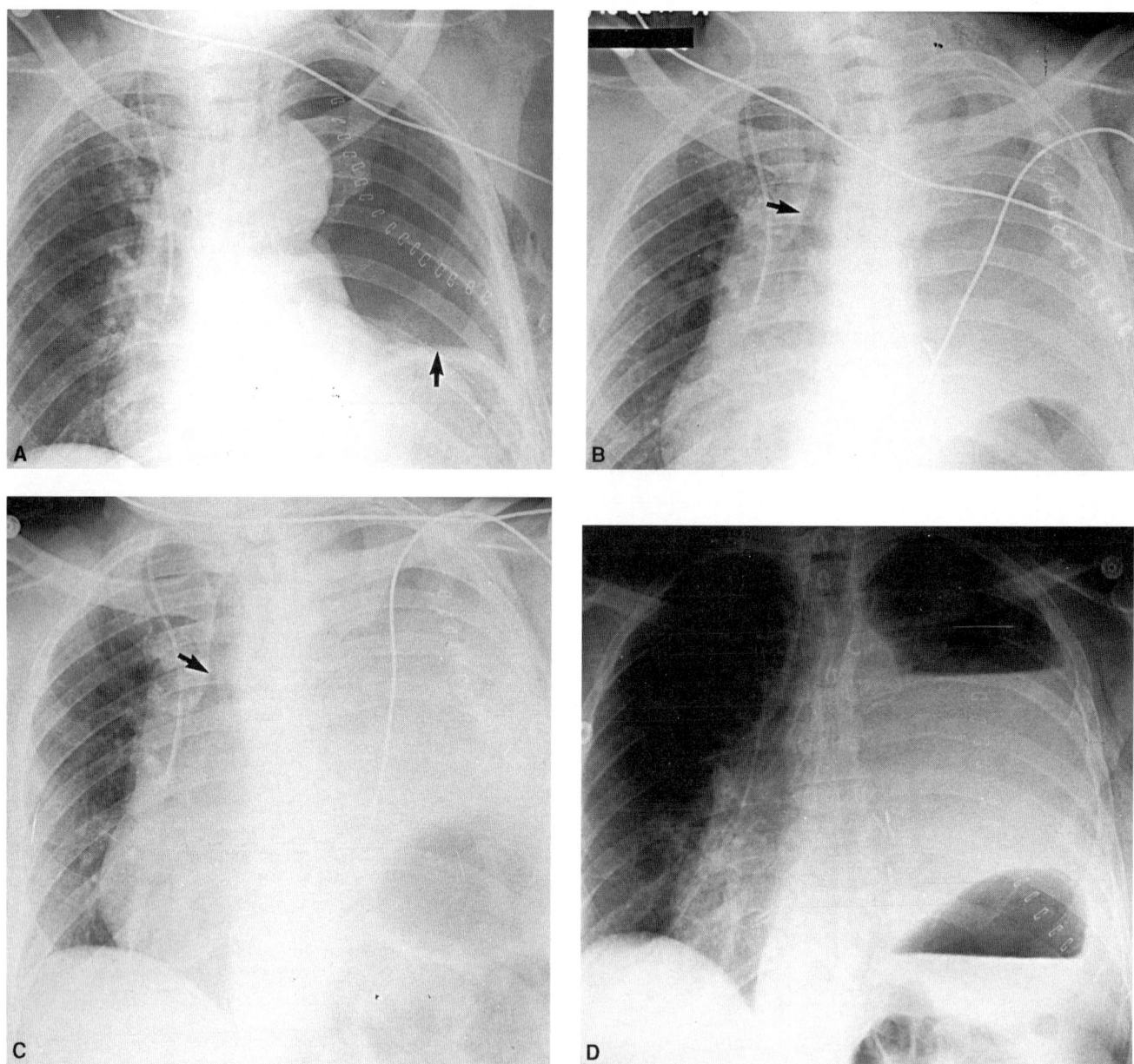

Fig. 71-62. Postpneumonectomy hemorrhage. *A,* Chest anteroposterior portable film obtained supine in a 64-year-old patient immediately after left pneumonectomy for lung neoplasm demonstrates air and minimal fluid within the left pneumonectomy space. Note the loss of volume of the left hemithorax owing to elevation of the left hemidiaphragm (arrow). The heart and mediastinal structures are midline. *B,* A supine chest anteroposterior portable film obtained 48 hours later demonstrates moderate accumulation of fluid within the pneumonectomy space. There is shift of the mediastinum and trachea, however, to the contralateral side of surgery (arrow). *C,* A chest anteroposterior portable film obtained less than 24 hours after the x-ray films shown in *B* demonstrates further, rapid accumulation of fluid within the left pneumonectomy space with further displacement of the heart, mediastinum, and trachea toward the side opposite to surgery. The patient's hematocrit markedly decreased between the time of the film shown in *B* and the one shown in *C*. A failure of the arterial stump was suspected and later confirmed and corrected at surgery. *D,* A chest posteroanterior film obtained in the upright position 1 week after the latest surgery demonstrates normal accumulation of fluid within the left pneumonectomy space with a gradual shift of the mediastinum back to the side of the surgery. *(Figure continues)*

an upright position with a recognizable air-fluid level; however, most of the immediate postoperative examinations are obtained in a supine position. During the next few days, a gradual accumulation of fluid is noted within the pneumonectomy space, with gradual resorption of air and accumulation of fluid (Fig. 71-61B,C). A more rapid accumulation is noted in the cases of extrapleural pneumonectomy. If the x-ray film is obtained in the upright position, one should expect a rise of the air-fluid level of one to two intercostal spaces per day. A persistent air-fluid level in the apex can be seen weeks after the surgery[39] (Fig. 71-61D). The lack of resorption of air from the pneumonectomy space, or rapid accumulation of air within the pneumonectomy space with shift of the mediastinum to

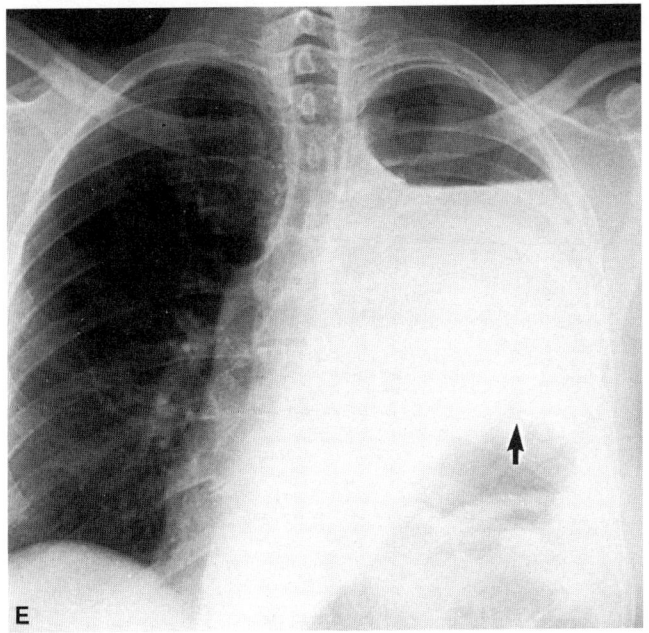 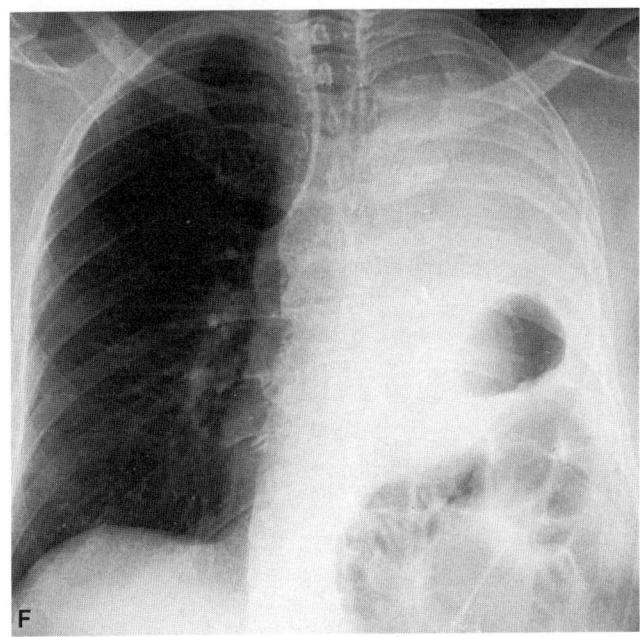

Fig. 71-62. *(Continued) E,* A follow-up chest film obtained 2 weeks later demonstrates further accumulation of fluid within the pneumonectomy space, with loss of volume of the pneumonectomy space reflected by shift of the mediastinum back to the side of the surgery and elevation of the left hemidiaphragm (arrow). *F,* A chest posteroanterior film obtained 3 months later demonstrates total obliteration of the left pneumonectomy space owing to complete resolution of the previously seen air and air-fluid level. The mediastinum and left hemidiaphragm have further shifted toward the side of the surgery.

the opposite side, should lead to the suspicion of a bronchopleural fistula or a gas-forming organism empyema (Fig. 71-61E,F). A rapid accumulation of fluid with total obliteration of the pneumonectomy space and shift of the mediastinum to the contralateral side should lead to the suspicion of hemorrhage (bleeding from intercostal vessels or lymphatics or failure of the arterial stump) (Fig. 71-62) or empyema (Fig. 71-63). In the late stages (a month to years), a sudden or gradual shift of the mediastinum to the side opposite to surgery should lead to the suspicion of a late empyema or recurrent tumor (Fig. 71-64).[40]

Post Cardiac Surgery Patient

The immediate postoperative findings seen on a chest film of the patient who has undergone a mediastinotomy for cardiac surgery (coronary artery bypass grafting and valvular replacement) are related to the results of general anesthesia, the patient's cardiac disease, and the mediastinotomy approach. As discussed earlier, atelectasis in the lung bases is the most common radiographic finding in the poststernotomy patient (Fig. 71-65).[41] It is usually more severe and persists longer in the left lung base. It is due to multiple factors, including pleural effusions, which are usually larger on the left; cardiomegaly, which compresses the left lower lung; and injury to the left phrenic nerve at the time of surgery, which may cause paresis of the left hemidiaphragm.[42] A pneumopericardium can be visualized along the left heart border and apex immediately after surgery and should resolve within the next few days (Fig. 71-66).

Pulmonary edema is commonly observed immediately after surgery and is usually related to fluid overload and cardiac dysfunction at the time of surgery (Fig. 71-67). The edema usually resolves within the next few hours. The mediastinum is somewhat difficult to evaluate in the immediate postoperative stage owing to the magnification from the anteroposterior projection and the poor inflation of the lungs, which compresses the mediastinal structures. An acute change in the mediastinal widening should lead to the suspicion of hemorrhage, either related to surgery or secondary to the placement of a central line (see Figs. 71-21 and 71-22). In the proper clinical setting, subacute mediastinal widening may be due to the formation of an abscess. CT examination would confirm the presence of abnormal fluid or air collections in the mediastinum (Fig. 71-68). Abscesses or infected hematomas may be caused during surgery or result as a complication of sternal osteomyelitis (Fig. 71-69). A pericardial effusion or hemopericardium complicating cardiac surgery may be detected by the changes in appearance of the cardiac-pericardiac silhouette on chest films but are more sensitively detected by echocardiograms or CT examinations (Figs. 71-70 and 71-71).[43,44]

IMAGING OF ACUTE AORTIC DISEASE

In the ICU population, the most common aortic abnormalities are those of trauma, aneurysms, and dissection. Traumatic injury of the thoracic or abdominal aorta has a high incidence of mortality, requiring prompt diagnosis and surgical repair.[45] In the cases of suspected thoracic aortic trauma, the chest radiograph is the first screening imaging modality available. Plain radiographs may show an abnormal widened mediastinum, displacement of the trachea or bronchi, or a pleural effusion.[46,47] In the ab-

1514   THE HIGH RISK PATIENT: MANAGEMENT OF THE CRITICALLY ILL

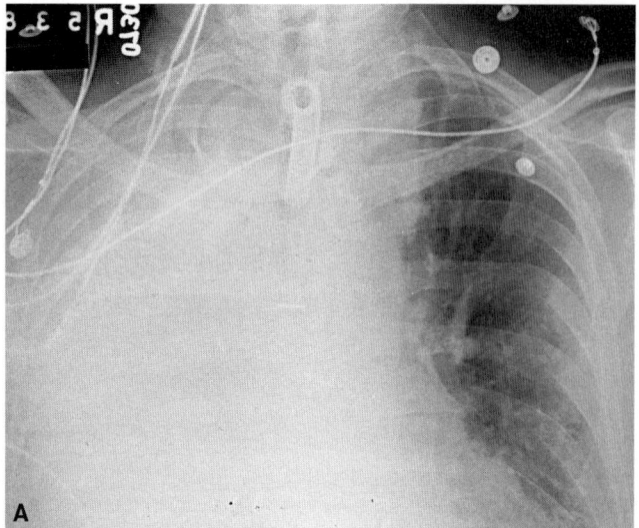
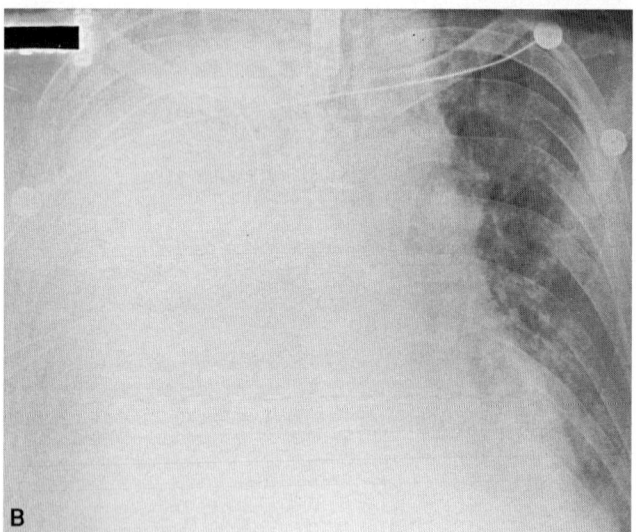
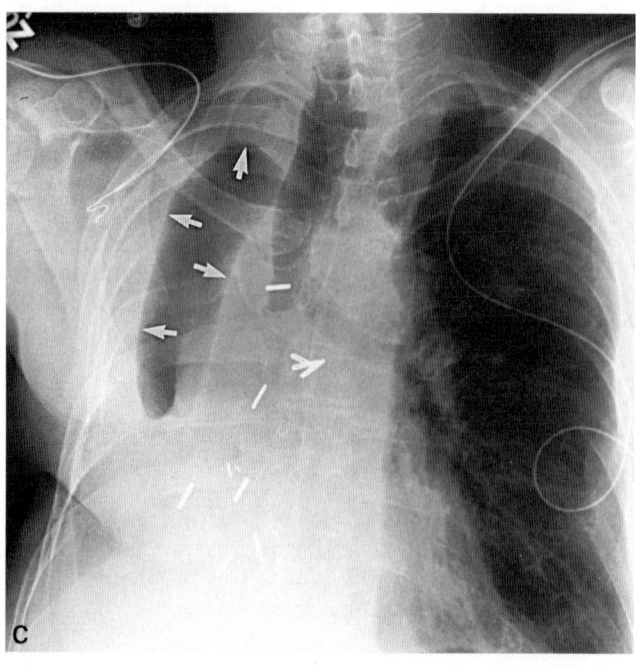

Fig. 71–63. Empyema postpneumonectomy. *A,* A supine chest anteroposterior portable film obtained in a 56-year-old patient 8 weeks after a normal postoperative course after right pneumonectomy demonstrates total opacification of the right hemithorax. *B,* The patient was readmitted 4 weeks after the date of the x-ray film shown in *A*. The film demonstrates gradual shift of the heart and mediastinum opposite to the side of the surgery, suggestive of an abnormal new accumulation of fluid within the pneumonectomy space. Note that the normal left lung now appears smaller. *C,* A chest film obtained after removal of 1200 ml of purulent material demonstrates an air collection within the pneumonectomy space outlining diffuse pleural thickening (arrows). The heart and mediastinal structures are shifted back to the side of the surgery.

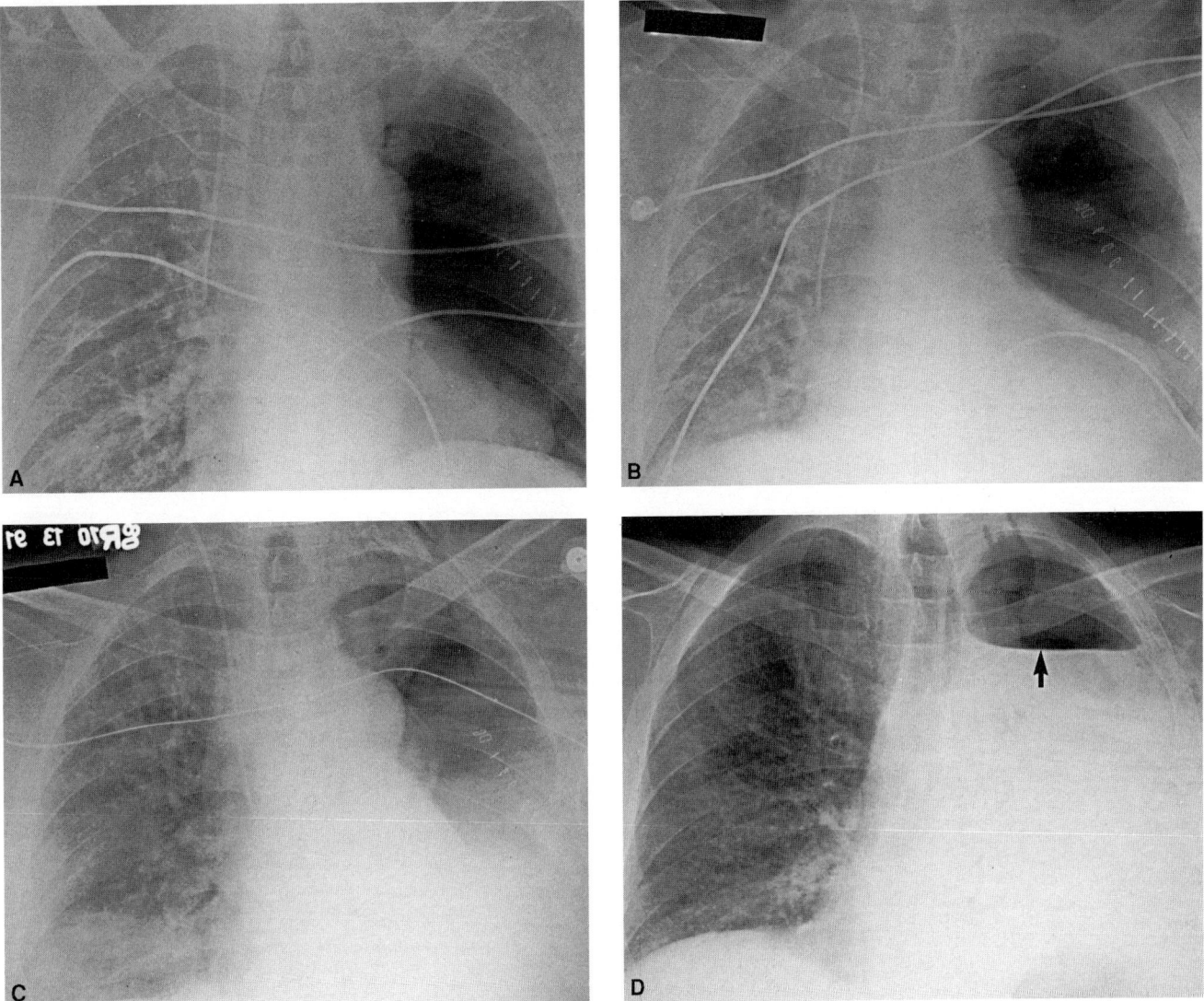

Fig. 71–64. Recurrent tumor postpneumonectomy. *A–E,* Serial normal postoperative x-ray films obtained in a 69-year-old patient status post left pneumonectomy for bronchogenic neoplasm. *A,* A chest anteroposterior film obtained supine **immediately** after left pneumonectomy demonstrates diffuse lucency of the left hemithorax compatible with an empty pneumonectomy space filled mainly with air. Note that the mediastinum and heart are midline. *B,* A follow-up chest anteroposterior obtained supine **24 hours** later demonstrates a haze of density in the left lower pneumonectomy space owing to newly accumulated fluid. The mediastinal structures remain midline. *C,* A follow-up chest anteroposterior film obtained supine **48 hours** after surgery demonstrates further accumulation of fluid and resorption of air in the left pneumonectomy space. There is minimal shift of the mediastinal structures toward the side of surgery. *D,* A chest posteroanterior film obtained upright **1 week** after surgery demonstrates an air-fluid level (arrow) within the upper portion of the left pneumonectomy space with further shift of the mediastinum and heart toward the side of surgery. *E,* Upright chest posteroanterior (E-1) and lateral (E-2) films obtained **1 month** after surgery demonstrate total opacification of the left hemithorax owing to complete obliteration of the left pneumonectomy space by fluid after the complete resorption of air. The heart and mediastinum are completely shifted toward the side of surgery. **Fifteen months** later, the patient complained of dysphasia and cough. *F,* Upright chest posteroanterior (F-1) and lateral (F-2) films were obtained **fifteen months** after surgery. Although the heart and mediastinum remain shifted toward the side of surgery, a new soft tissue mass is seen in the region of the midmediastinum projecting over the right hilum (large black arrows). Compare the appearance of the mediastinum with the chest posteroanterior and lateral views shown in *E-1.* Note the new esophageal thickening seen posterior to the tracheal wall on the lateral view (arrowheads). A vague infiltrate caused by aspiration is identified in the right lower lung on the posteroanterior view (small arrows). *G,* A chest posteroanterior film obtained after a barium swallow demonstrates an irregular collection of extravasated contrast material in the midmediastinum (arrow) with a fistula between the esophagus and right main stem bronchus (large arrowhead).

(Figure continues)

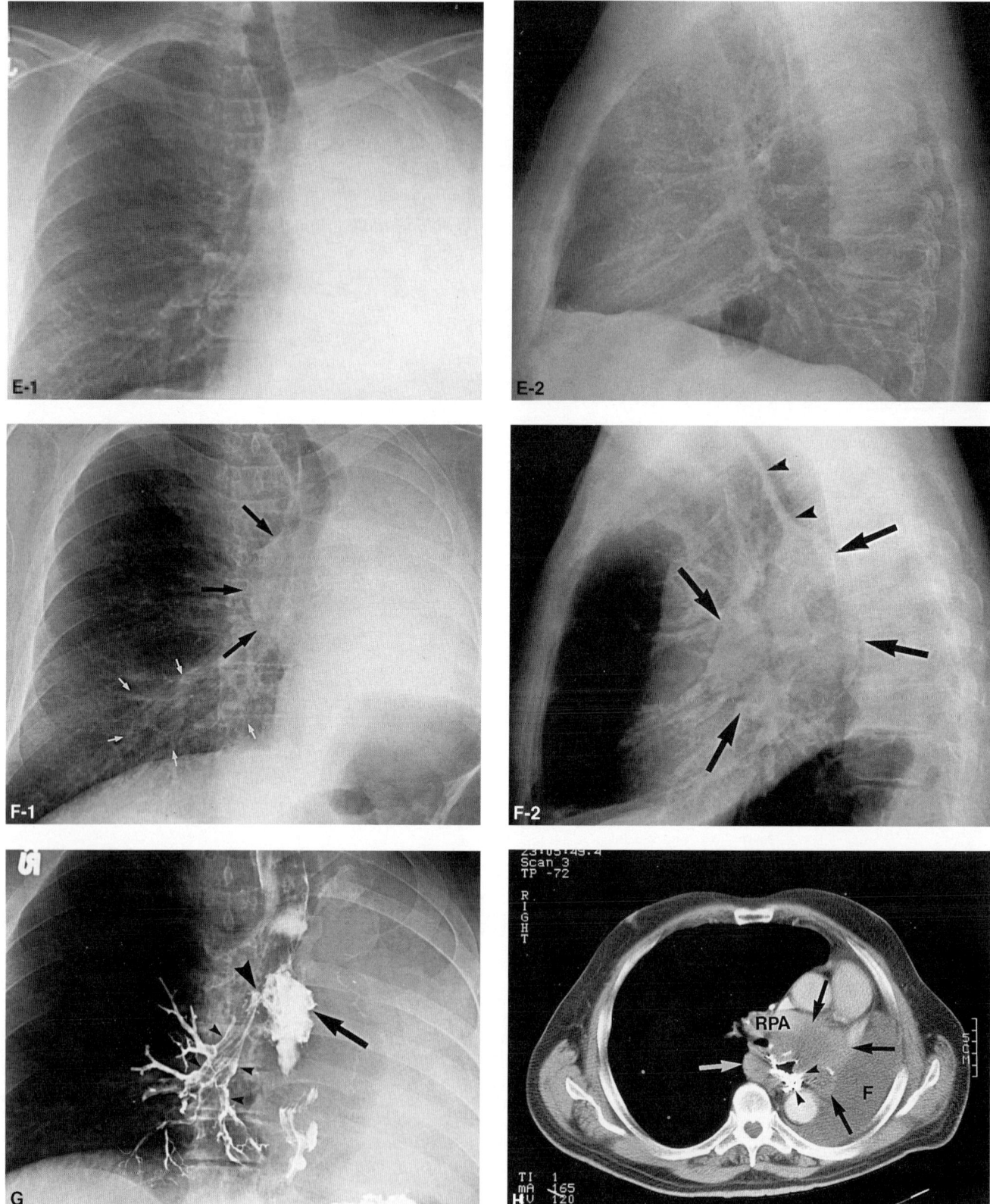

Fig. 71–64. *(Continued)* The right main stem bronchus and right lower lung bronchi are opacified (small arrowheads). *H,* A CT scan examination obtained after administration of intravenous contrast material with an axial image obtained through the midchest below the carina demonstrates a large low-density mediastinal mass at the level of the carina compatible with a necrotic recurrent tumor (arrows). Note the extravasated barium in the mediastinum (arrowheads) owing to a bronchoesophageal fistula. There is encasement of the right pulmonary artery (RPA). The mediastinal structures are shifted to the left side with a normal-appearing left pneumonectomy space filled with fluid (F).

IMAGING TECHNIQUES IN THE INTENSIVE CARE UNIT

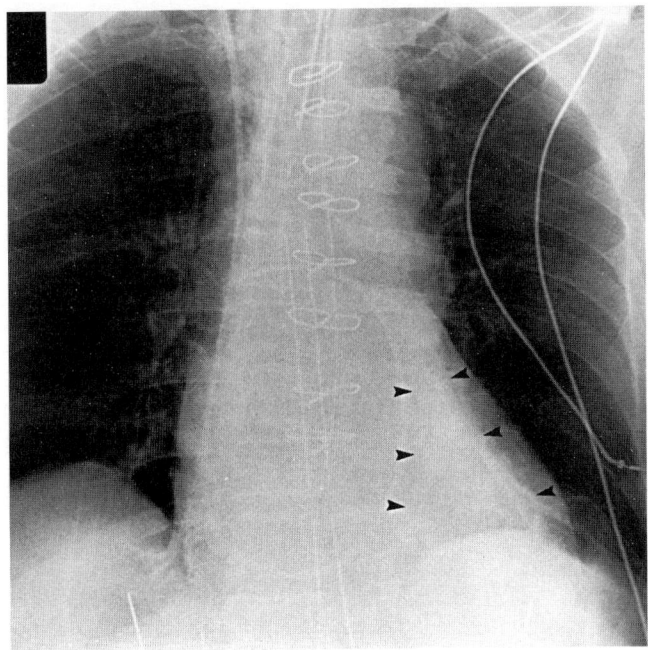

Fig. 71-65. Left lower lobe atelectasis post cardiac surgery. A chest anteroposterior portable film obtained in a 62-year-old patient status post mediastinotomy for coronary artery bypass demonstrates a wedge-shaped radiodensity projecting behind the heart representing partial atelectasis of the left lower lobe (arrowheads).

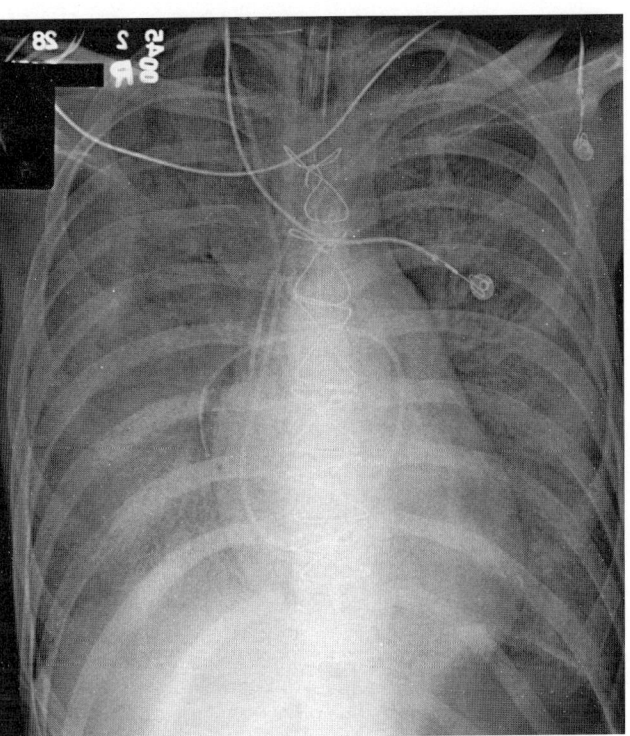

Fig. 71-67. Pulmonary edema post cardiac surgery. A supine chest anteroposterior film obtained in a 48 year-old patient immediately after cardiac surgery demonstrates bilateral diffuse homogeneous alveolar infiltrate owing to acute pulmonary edema.

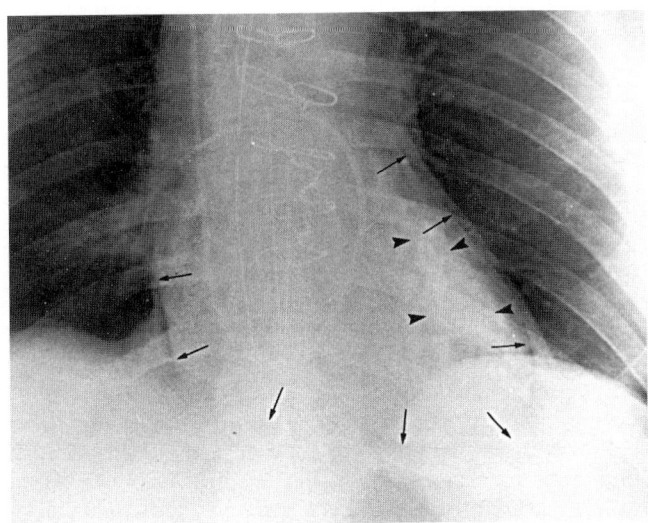

Fig. 71-66. Pneumopericardium post cardiac surgery. A chest anteroposterior portable film obtained immediately after open heart surgery on a 69-year-old patient demonstrates a lucency outlining both the left and right heart borders and the left ventricular apex owing to a pneumopericardium (arrows). Note the focal atelectasis involving the left lower lobe (arrowheads). The nasogastric tube is seen with the tip in the distal esophagus.

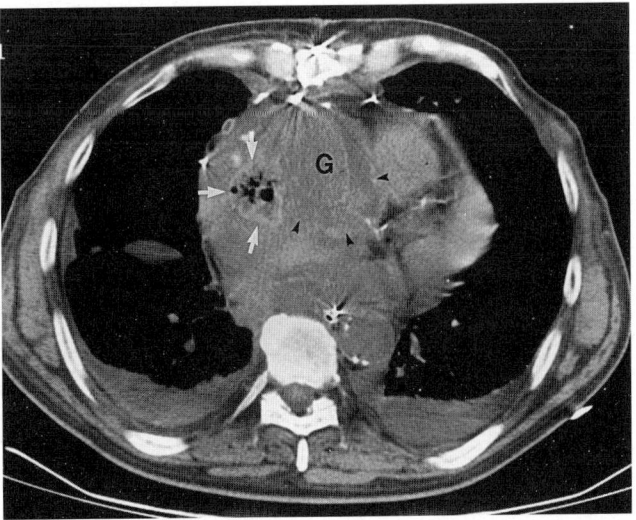

Fig. 71-68. Mediastinal abscess post cardiac surgery. A 71-year-old patient with a history of thoracic aortic aneurysm had cardiac surgery for placement of an ascending aortic graft. A chest film obtained to look for the source of persisting fever was nondiagnostic. A CT scan examination obtained with an axial image through the level of the aortic route demonstrates an abnormal air collection in the right side of the mediastinum (white arrows) seen lateral to the ascending aortic graft (G). Note the large hematoma surrounding the graft (black arrowheads). The patient was taken back to surgery to drain the abscess.

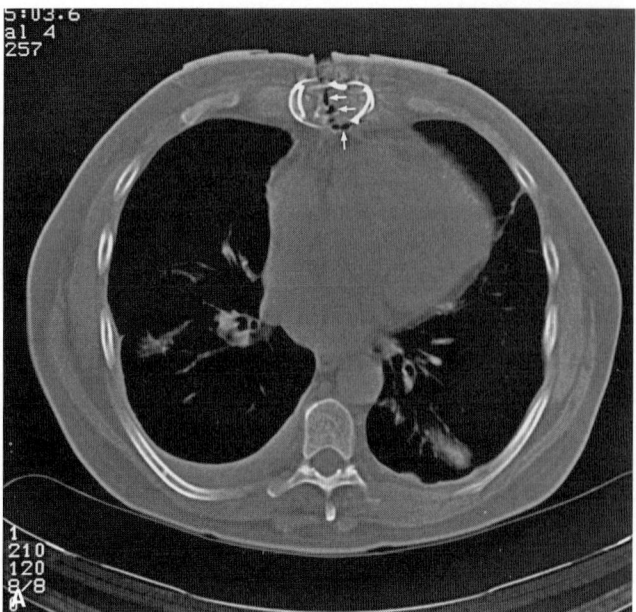
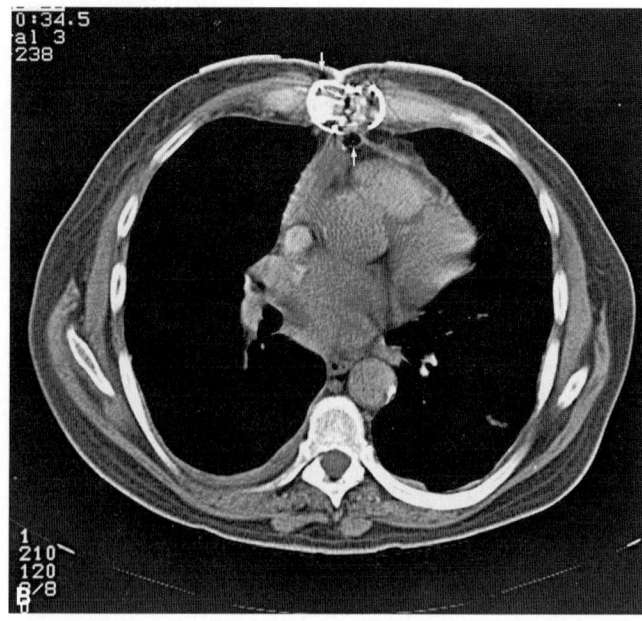

Fig. 71-69. *A, B,* Sternal osteomyelitis post median sternotomy. A CT scan of the chest was obtained on a 61-year-old patient 10 days status post mediastinotomy for cardiac surgery, with persistent fever and drainage of pus at the incision wound. The chest film could not help determine the source of the infection. An axial image obtained through the lower portion of the sternum imaged at bone windows *(A)* and midportion of the sternum imaged at soft tissue windows *(B)* demonstrates newly appearing multiple small air collections (arrows) seen between the bony fragments of the sternum and extending into the posterior mediastinum and subcutaneous tissues. Newly appearing fluid or air collections at the site of the sternal surgery are helpful for the diagnosis of infection because the bony changes of osteomyelitis can be difficult to separate from the sternal fractures and deformity occurring at the time of surgery.

sence of radiographic findings, US or, more sensitively, CT scan examinations of the chest with contrast enhancement are more helpful in detecting acute dissection of the aorta (Fig. 71-72).[48-50] Mediastinal hematomas, hemopericardiums, or hemothoraces would be more readily detected by CT. Both CT and angiography are sensitive in detecting the presence and extent of intimal flaps seen in dissections (Fig. 71-73).[51] Although MRI is sensitive in evaluating thoracoabdominal aortic abnormalities, it is of a limited value in the acute and unstable cases that are encountered in the ICU population.[52] Dissecting aneurysms or hematomas are characterized as intramural hematomas resulting from laceration of the intima. It creates an intramural channel within the media, which communicates with the true aortic lumen at the level of the primary laceration. A dissecting hematoma is due to increasing pressure within the aortic lumen and weakness of the adjacent aortic wall. It may be caused by trauma, hypertension, mycotic infection, and connective tissue disorders, such as Marfan's syndrome and Ehlers-Danlos syndrome. As classified by Debakey,[53] there are three types of dissecting aneurysms: Type I, in which the primary laceration is in the ascending aorta, with extension along the full length of the thoracic aorta; type II, in which the primary laceration is in the ascending aorta and the false lumen extends only to the level of the aortic arch. In both type I and type II, there may be bleeding within the pericardium creating tamponade. Both echocardiography and CT of the chest may be helpful in detecting such complications. Type III represents dissection of the descending thoracic aorta, in which the primary laceration is at the junction of the aortic arch and the descending thoracic aorta distal to the left subclavian artery.

The diagnosis of abdominal aortic aneurysm is difficult by plain radiography. The presence of mural calcification, detected on the plain film of the abdomen, may lead to the suspicion of such abnormality involving the abdominal aorta (Fig. 71-74). Ultrasound examinations and CT of the abdomen are more sensitive for the evaluation of the size

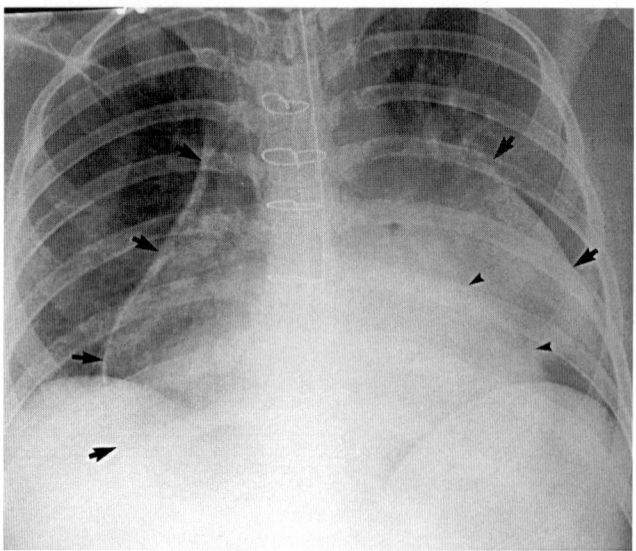

Fig. 71-70. Hydropneumopericardium post cardiac surgery. A chest anteroposterior film supine obtained in a 48-year-old patient status post open heart surgery demonstrates an unusually large hydropneumopericardium (arrows). The left heart border can be visualized outlined by air (arrowheads).

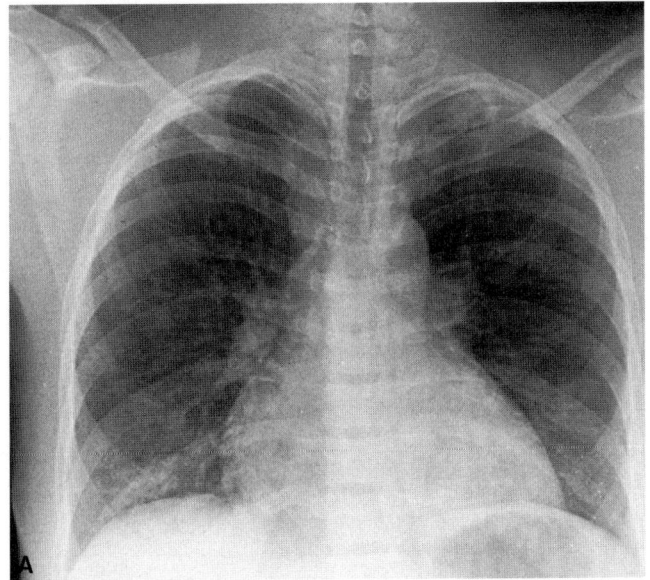
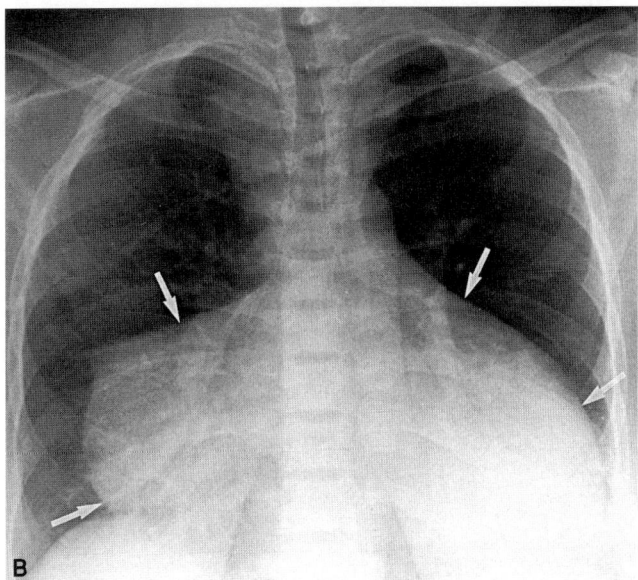
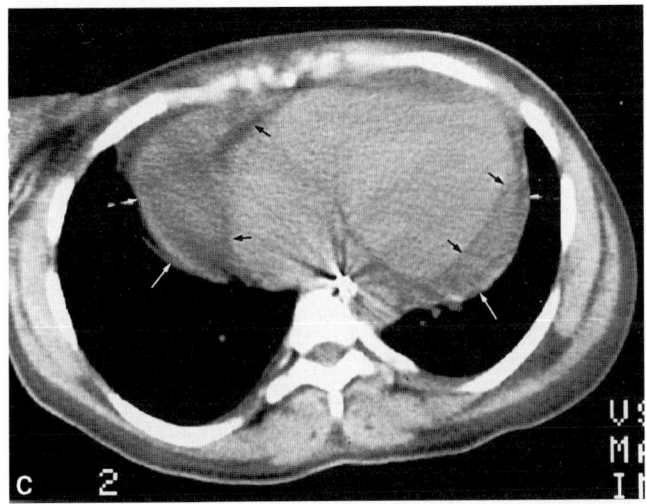

Fig. 71-71. Pericardial effusion. *A,* A baseline chest posteroanterior film obtained on a 38-year-old patient with history of chronic renal failure demonstrates minimal enlargement of the cardiac-pericardiac silhouette. *B,* A follow-up chest posteroanterior film obtained 1 week later because of history of tamponade demonstrates acute and marked globular enlargement of the cardiac-pericardiac silhouette (arrows). The acute enlargement is suggestive of a pericardial effusion. *C,* A CT examination of the lower chest demonstrates a large fluid collection surrounding the heart, characteristic of a pericardial effusion (arrows).

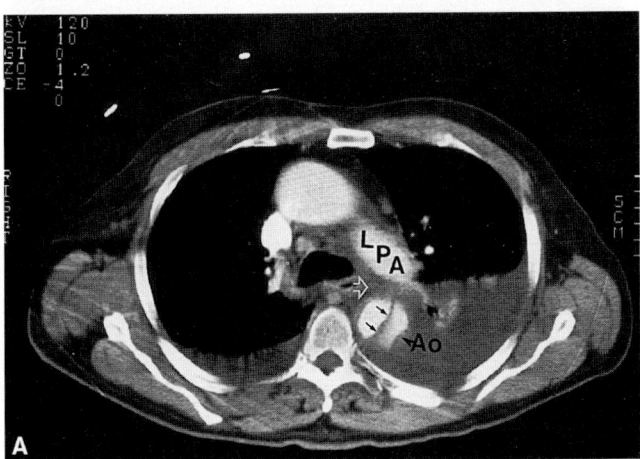
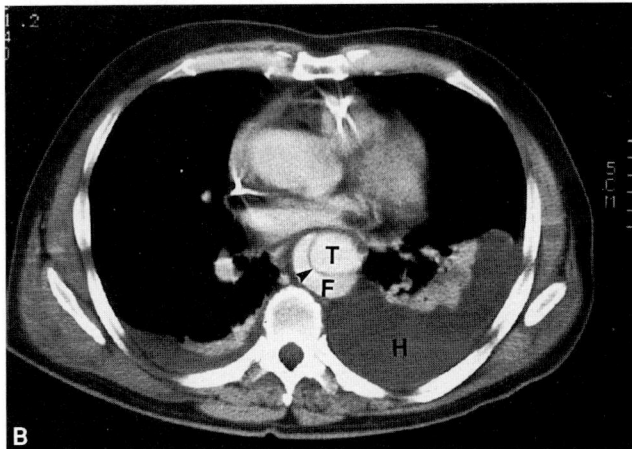

Fig. 71-72. Type III acute thoracic aortic dissection. *A,* A CT scan examination of the chest with intravenous contrast material was obtained on a 60-year-old patient with history of hypertension and chest pain. An axial image obtained at the level of the carina demonstrates a linear defect within the descending thoracic aorta representing the intimal flap (small arrows) separating the true and false lumen. There is evidence of a hematoma seen as a fluid collection (open arrowhead) between the left pulmonary artery (LPA) and descending thoracic aorta (Ao). *B,* An axial image through the level of the cardiac chambers demonstrates increase of the overall caliber of the descending thoracic aorta, with the intimal flap (arrowhead) separating the true lumen (T) and false lumen (F). The large left pleural effusion represents a hemothorax (H).

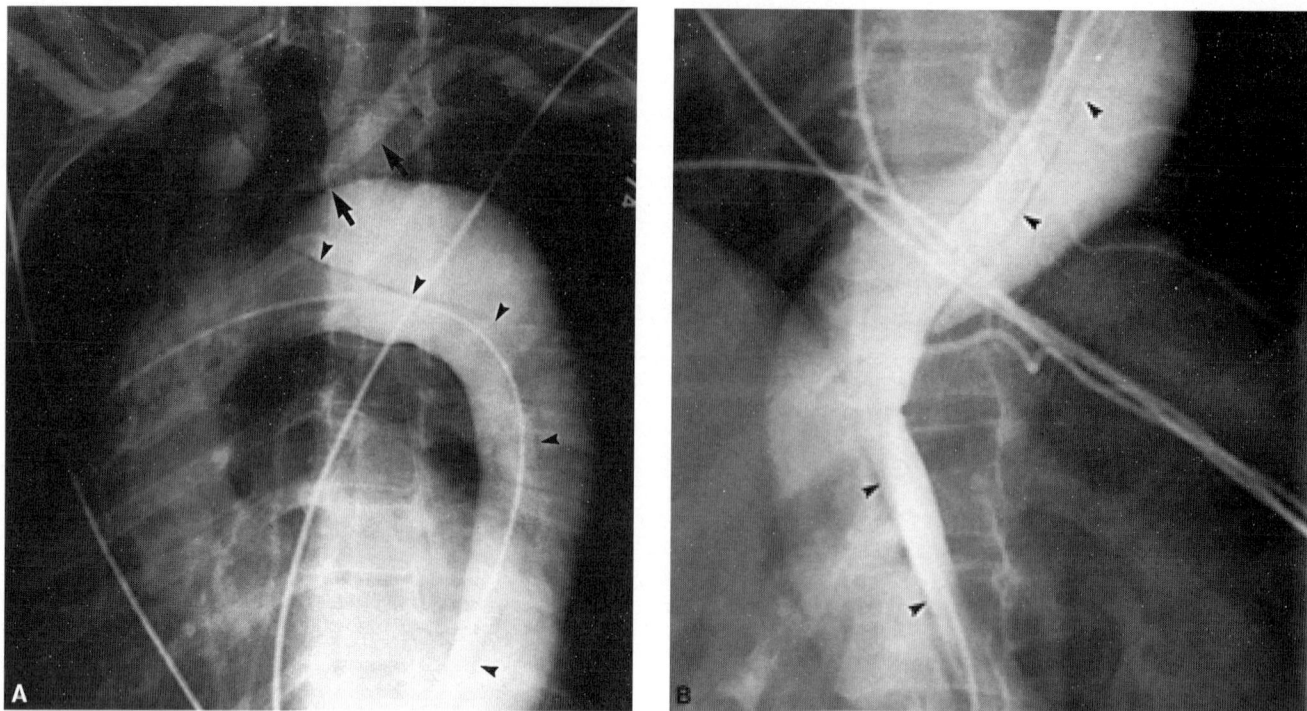

Fig. 71-73. Type III dissection, angiographic appearance. *A,* An aortogram with an oblique view obtained at the level of the aortic arch demonstrates a linear defect involving the posterior aspect of the aortic arch, representing an intimal flap (arrowheads) arising just distal to the origin of the left subclavian artery (arrows). *B,* An anteroposterior image of the descending thoracic aorta demonstrates the extent of the intimal flap into the lower thoracic and upper abdominal aorta (arrowheads). Note the marked tortuosity of the thoracoabdominal aorta.

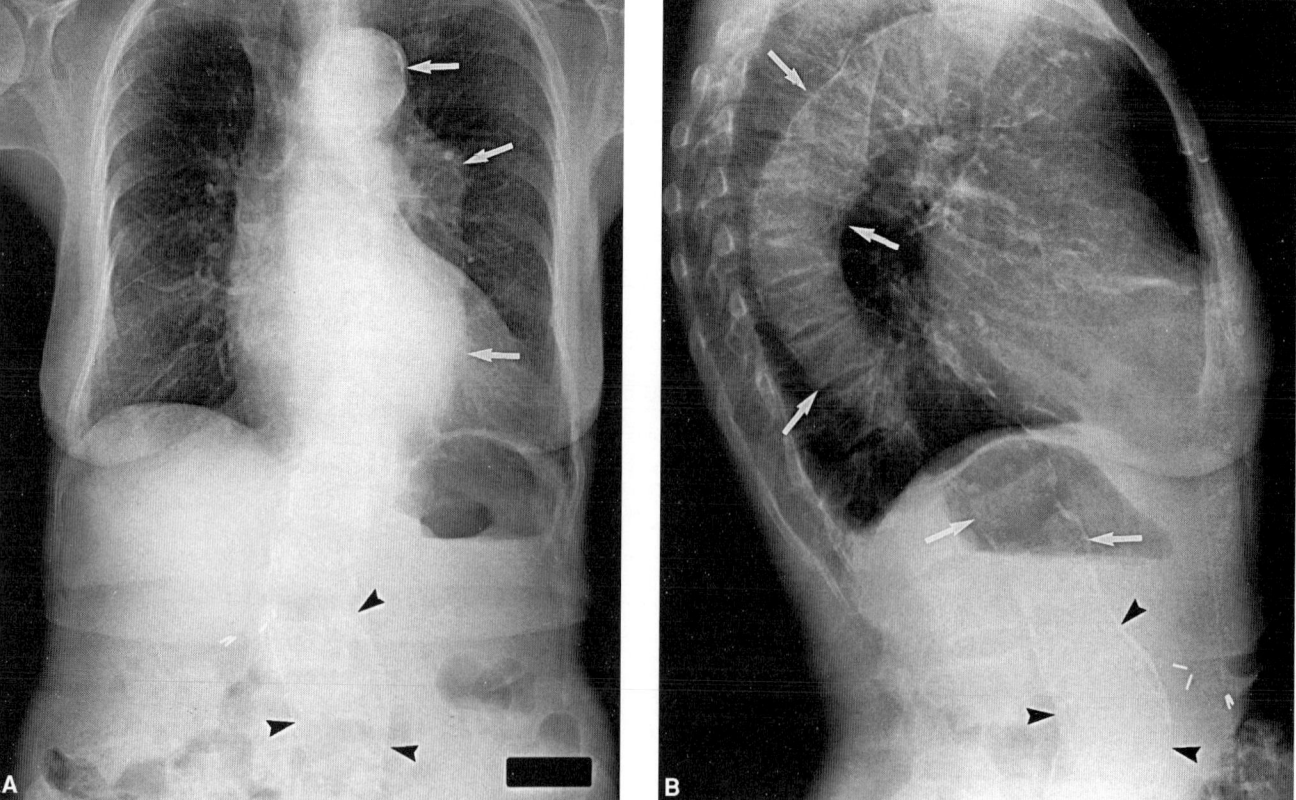

Fig. 71-74. Atherosclerotic thoracoabdominal aneurysm. Chest posteroanterior *(A)* and lateral *(B)* films with views of the upper abdomen obtained in a 75-year-old patient demonstrate extensive arteriosclerosis of the thoracoabdominal aorta (arrows). The extensive calcification outlines the entire course of the thoracoabdominal aorta and permits visualization of the aneurysmal dilatation of the lower abdominal aorta (arrowheads).

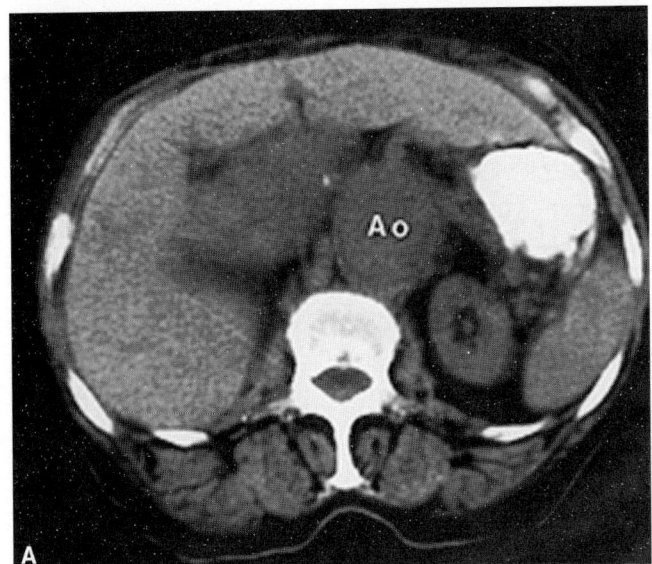
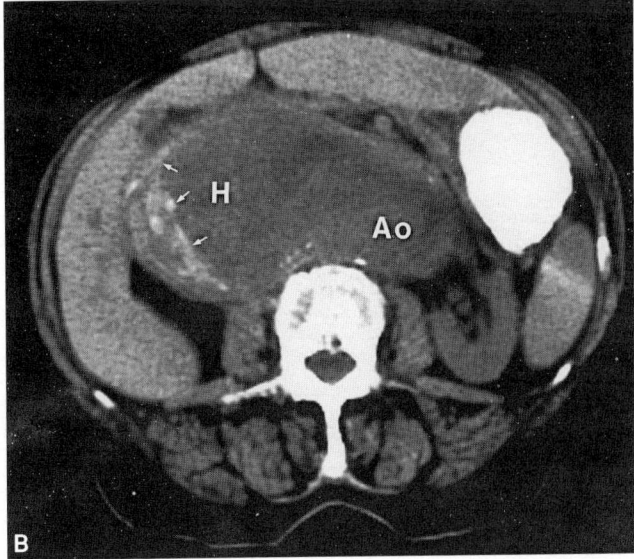
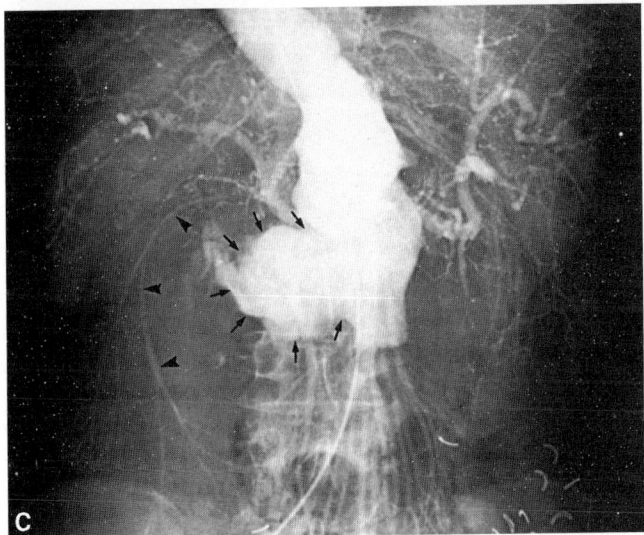

Fig. 71–75. Contained rupture of abdominal aortic aneurysm. *A*, A CT scan examination of the abdomen was obtained in a 58-year-old patient because of abdominal pain. An axial image obtained through the upper abdomen on a nonenhanced examination demonstrates enlargement of the proximal abdominal aorta measuring 5 cm in diameter (Ao). *B*, An axial image obtained 2 cm below the image shown on *A* demonstrates marked dilatation of the aorta with a large contained hematoma in the right lateral aspect of the aneurysm (H). There are calcifications seen in the infralateral aspect of the wall of the hematoma/aneurysm (arrows). *C*, An aortogram demonstrates a markedly tortuous, irregular distal thoracic aorta and proximal abdominal aorta owing to atherosclerosis. A large aneurysm begins at the level of the celiac axis and extends to the bifurcation. A contained rupture of the aneurysm, which originates from the right lateral wall of the abdominal aorta, is seen partially opacified (arrows). Note that only a portion of the aneurysm visualized on the CT scan is opacified. The most right lateral aspect of the aneurysm is not opacified but seen displacing the surrounding abdominal vessels (arrowheads).

and extent of the aneurysm.[54] The incidence of rupture varies with the size of the aneurysms. It is believed that aortic abdominal aneurysms grow at the rate of approximately ⅓ cm per year; therefore the chance of rupture increases with age. Rupture of an aortic abdominal aneurysm is expected to occur in 30 to 60% of patients who do not undergo surgical repair.[55] Rupture of an aortic abdominal aneurysm may be contained (Fig. 71–75) or may leak into the retroperitoneum or rarely into the gastrointestinal tract. In the cases of small or contained leaks, a rind of dense perivascular fibrous granulation tissue may occur later, involving the ureters, renal arteries, or duodenum (Fig. 71–76).

IMAGING OF ACUTE ABDOMINAL DISEASE

The plain film of the abdomen remains the most commonly ordered radiologic examination when acute abdominal disease is suspected (Table 71–5). Information pertaining to the status of the gastrointestinal tract can be derived from the plain films alone. Distention of the gastrointestinal tract, with either air or fluid related to ileus or obstruction, can be determined from the analysis of the plain x-ray film. Sometimes mucosal thickening, owing to either edema or ischemia, can be recognized. The plain films can demonstrate large intraperitoneal or retroperitoneal fluid collections, such as abscesses or hemorrhage when they displace adjacent organs (i.e., spleen, liver, kidneys). When acute abdominal disease is suspected to involve intra-abdominal organs, such as the hepatobiliary system, spleen, pancreas, genitourinary tract, and the gastrointestinal tract, more sophisticated studies are necessary to determine the nature and extent of disease. CT, US, and scintigraphy are now readily used for the critically ill patient. Although certain US and nuclear medicine examinations can be performed at the bedside, CT has been used with increased frequency because CT scan images can now be

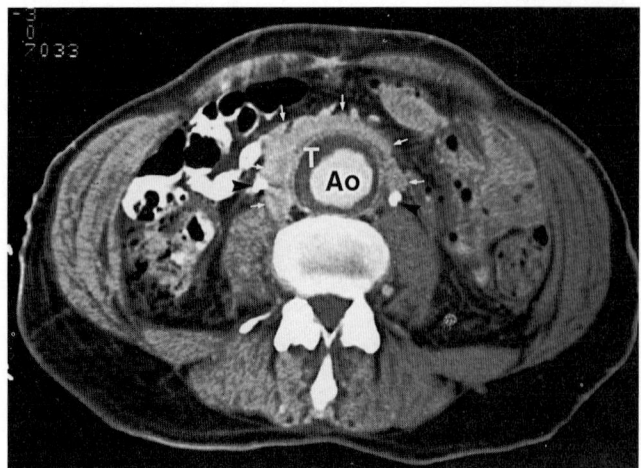

Fig. 71-76. Aortic abdominal aneurysm with retroperitoneal fibrosis. A CT scan examination of the abdomen obtained after administration of intravenous contrast material in a 65-year-old patient with history of renal failure demonstrates an approximately 5 cm infrarenal abdominal aortic aneurysm (Ao), which extends to the level of the aortic bifurcation. There is a moderate amount of thrombus within the aneurysm seen surrounding the lumen of the aorta (T). There is increased soft tissue density in the periaortic region representing fibrotic tissue (arrows). There are bilateral double J stints within the ureters to alleviate the ureteral obstruction caused by the surrounding fibrosis (arrowheads).

obtained at the subsecond level, and studies can be completed within a few minutes.

Free air within the abdomen or pneumoretroperitoneum can and should be recognized in plain radiographs. Small air collections can be difficult to detect on the portable examination of the abdomen taken supine.[56] It is not uncommon that pneumoperitoneums are incidentally detected on the chest film. They are seen as a lucency in the upper abdomen projecting below the diaphragms (Fig. 71-77). Large air collections are more easily detected on the supine films when they are seen as large lucencies collecting in the anterior portion of the abdomen ("foot-

Table 71-5. Diagnosis and Monitoring Uses of Portable Radiograph of the Abdomen and Pelvis

Gastrointestinal tract
  Ileus
  Obstruction (stomach, small and large bowel)
  Volvulus (sigmoid, cecum, stomach)
  Toxic megacolon
  Bowel edema (ischemia)
  Pneumatosis intestinalis
Abnormal air collections
  Free peritoneal air
  Retroperitoneal air
  Air in biliary tree, venous system
  Air in organs (e.g., kidney, gallbladder, pancreas, liver)
Ascites
Organomegaly
Bones and soft tissue
  Trauma
  Bleeding
  Infection

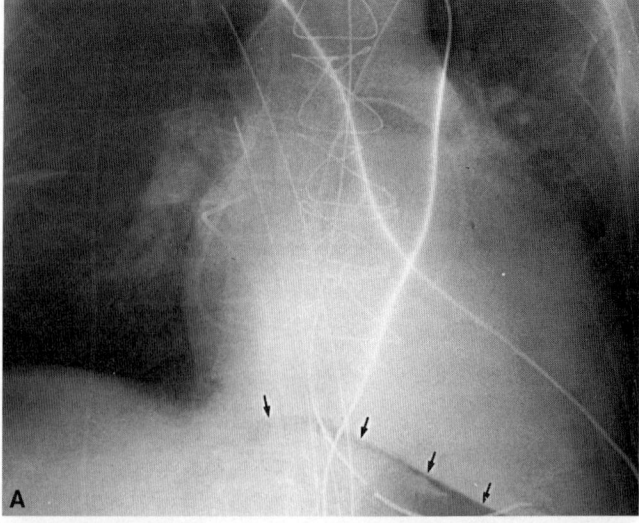

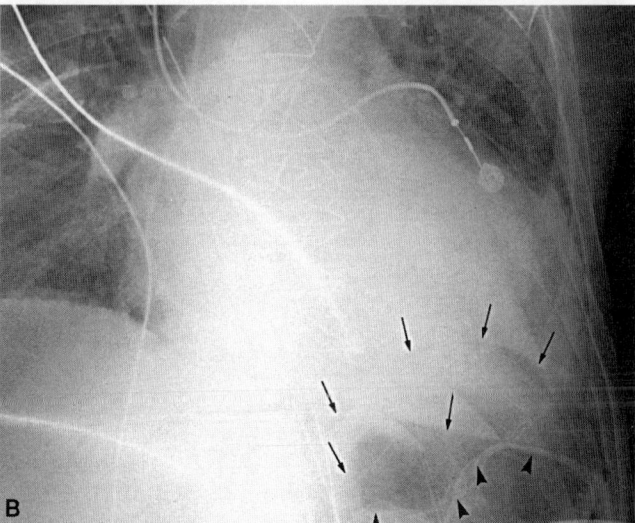

Fig. 71-77. Pneumoperitoneum post cardiac surgery (see also Fig. 71-48A). A, A portable supine chest anteroposterior film was obtained in a 63-year-old patient status post cardiac surgery for placement of an aortic valve prosthesis. It demonstrates an abnormal linear lucency projecting over the upper portion of the midabdomen and left upper quadrant (arrows). This represents a pneumoperitoneum outlining the inferior portion of the left hemidiaphragm and collecting in the anterior aspect of the upper abdomen. Note the opacification of the left lower hemithorax, which represents a combination of a left pleural effusion and partial atelectasis of the left lower lobe. B, The pneumoperitoneum went undetected for 24 hours, and a follow-up chest film obtained supine 24 hours later happened to show a larger portion of the upper abdomen. Free air is again demonstrated under the left hemidiaphragm (arrows). At this time, the wall of the large bowel at the region of the splenic flexure is visualized (arrowheads) outlined by air on both sides of the lumen (free air and intraluminal air). A perforated gastric ulcer was discovered at surgery.

ball sign"). The bowel wall becomes evident when outlined by air from both the intraluminal and extraluminal side (Fig. 71-78). An upright or left lateral decubitus examination performed at the bedside confirms the presence of free air (Figs. 71-78 and 71-79).

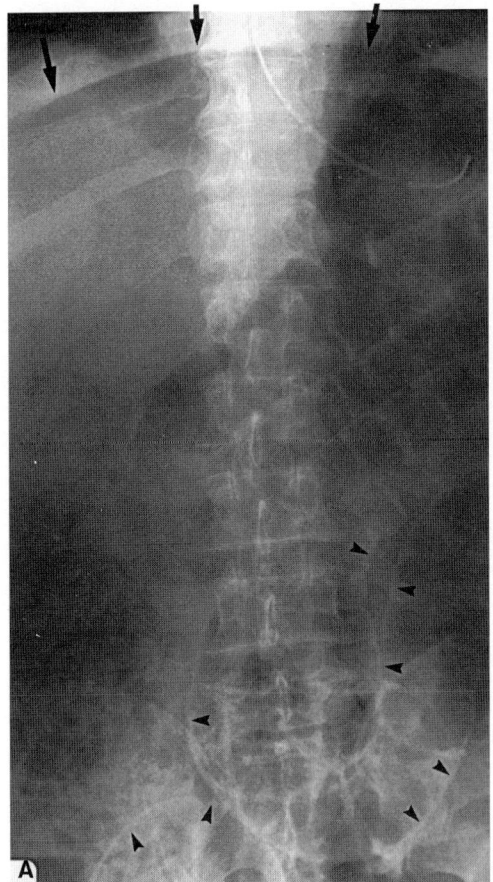
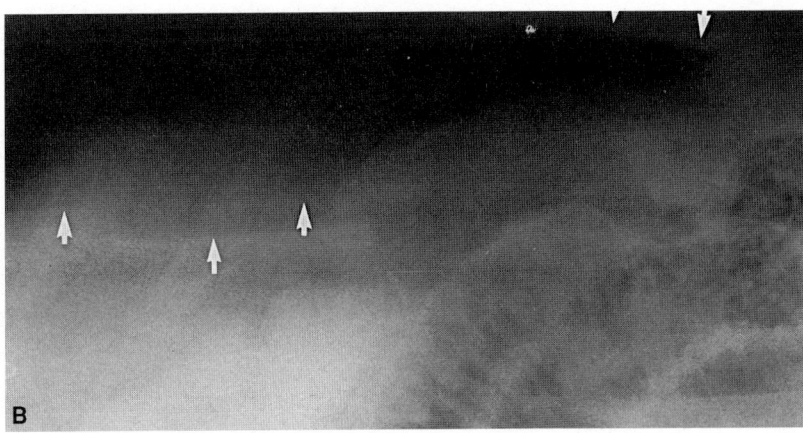

Fig. 71–78. Pneumoperitoneum. *A*, A supine film of the abdomen obtained on a 58-year-old patient who presented with abdominal pain demonstrates a large lucency overlying the abdomen with a sharp line overlying the lower midchest representing the most cephalad portion of the pneumoperitoneum, giving the appearance of a continuous diaphragm (arrows). The wall of the small bowel (arrowheads) in the left side of the abdomen is well visualized outlined by intraluminal air and free air. *B*, A left lateral decubitus examination of the abdomen obtained at the patient's bedside demonstrates a large hydropneumoperitoneum in the right upper quadrant (arrows). A perforated duodenal ulcer was found at surgery.

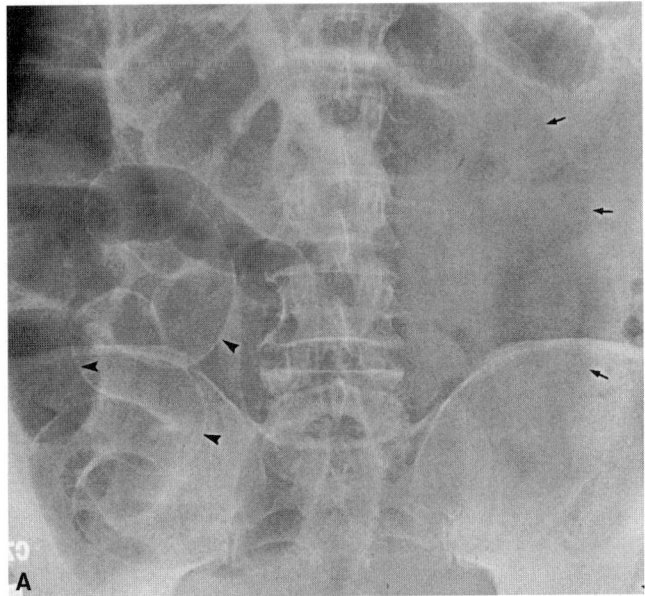
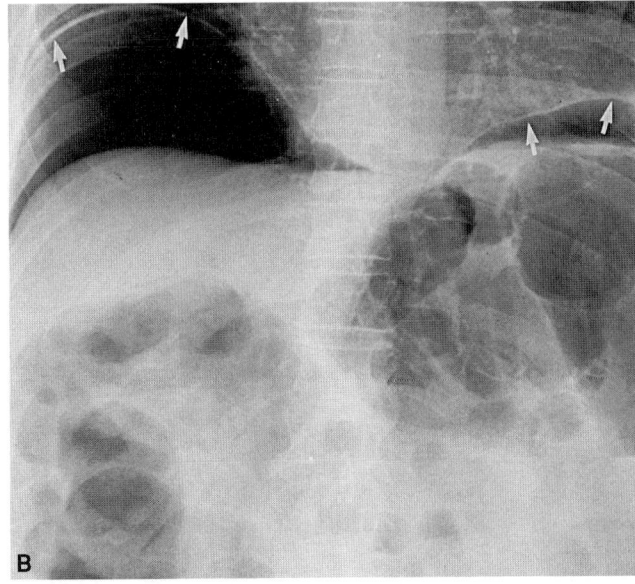

Fig. 71–79. Pneumoperitoneum. *A*, A plain film of the abdomen obtained supine in a 68-year-old patient who presented with right lower quadrant pain demonstrates a vague lucency projecting over the left side of the abdomen (arrows). The wall of the terminal ileum (arrowheads) is seen in the right lower quadrant outlined by intraluminal air and free air. *B*, An upright examination of the abdomen demonstrates the large pneumoperitoneum seen collecting under both hemidiaphragms (arrows). A perforated cecal diverticulum was found at surgery.

1524   THE HIGH RISK PATIENT: MANAGEMENT OF THE CRITICALLY ILL

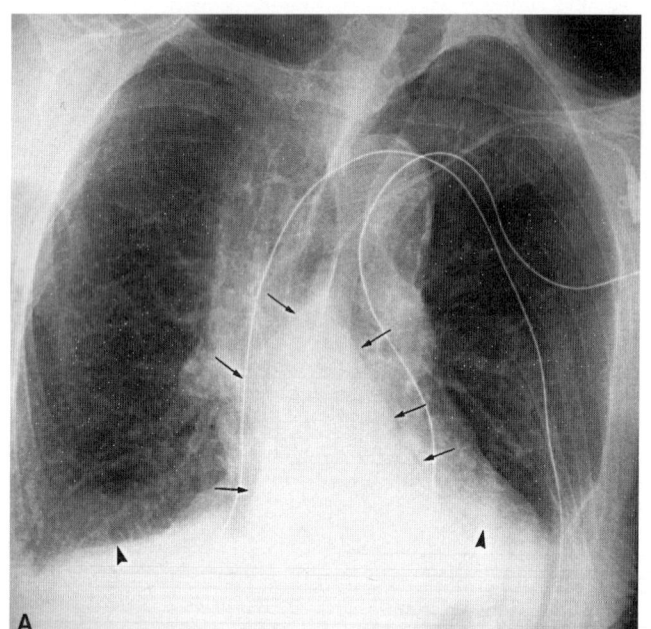

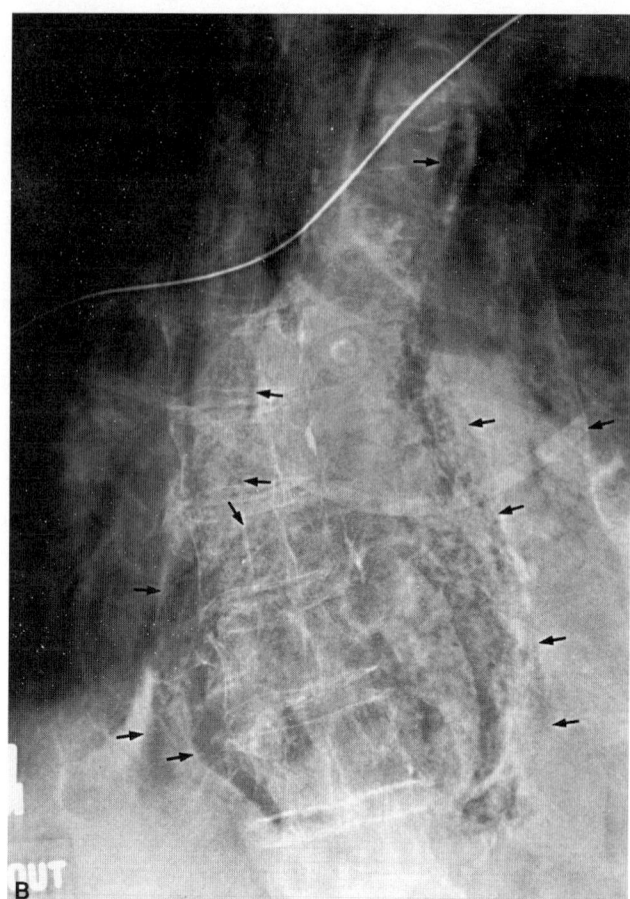

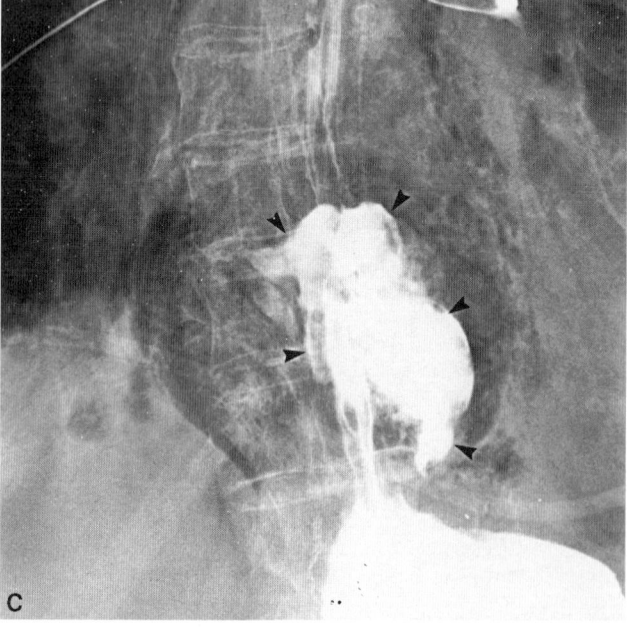

Fig. 71–80. Boerhaave's syndrome. *A,* An admission chest film obtained in an 88-year-old patient presenting with chest pain after a bout of vomiting demonstrates widening of the lower mediastinum (arrows) and bilateral pleural effusions (arrowheads). No definite sign of pneumomediastinum can be visualized on this examination. *B,* In the next few hours, the patient had worsening of the mediastinal pain. A barium swallow was ordered to evaluate the lower mediastinal widening. An overpenetrated radiograph of the chest obtained supine demonstrates an extensive pneumomediastinum (arrows). There is a left lower lobe consolidation or atelectasis. *C,* A barium swallow performed through a nasogastric tube placed in the distal esophagus demonstrates a large area of extravasated barium within the lower mediastinum (arrowheads). Aspirated barium is seen in the trachea and proximal bronchi. Note again the extensive pneumomediastinum.

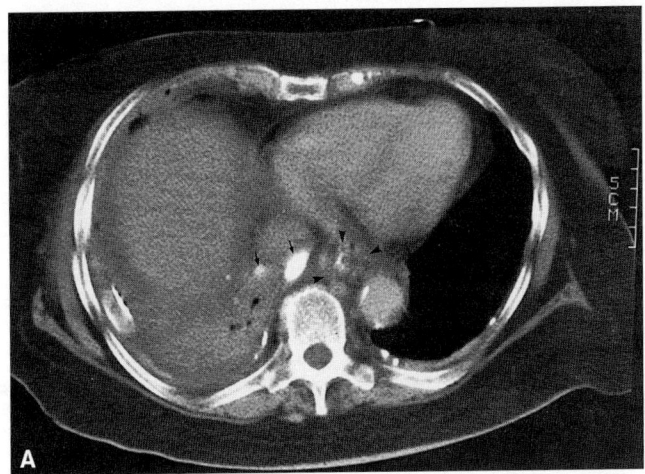 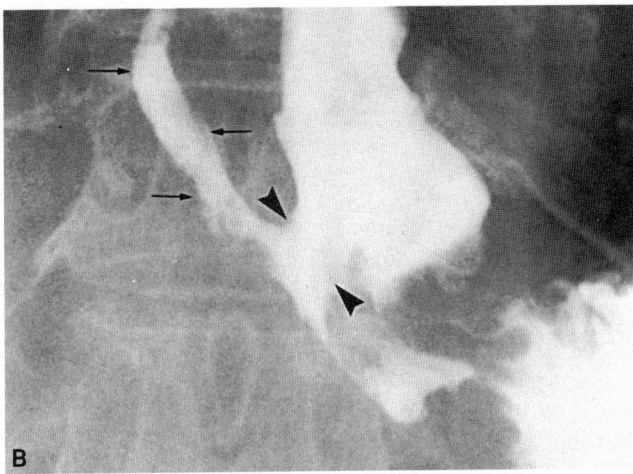

Fig. 71–81. Esophageal perforation. *A,* A CT scan examination of the chest was obtained in a 72-year-old patient who had chest pain after esophageal dilatation for an esophageal stricture. An axial image obtained through the lower mediastinum after the administration of oral and intravenous contrast material demonstrates an abnormal collection of contrast material seen in the lower mediastinum (arrows) lateral to the esophagus (arrowheads). A right chest tube is in place to treat an acute right pleural effusion. The patient later developed a right empyema. *B,* Because the CT scan examination could not help determine the exact location of the esophageal perforation, a barium swallow was performed, showing the location of the perforation (arrowheads). The collection of contrast material seen in the lower mediastinum right to the esophagus corresponds to the collection seen on the CT scan examination (arrows).

Gastrointestinal Tract

Esophagus

Most of acute esophageal disease can be screened and detected by plain x-ray films alone. Esophageal bleeding and perforation are among the most common esophageal problems seen in the ICU. Although bleeding cannot be detected by simple radiographic means, esophageal perforation is usually easily recognized. Whether iatrogenically, after endoscopy, or spontaneously, esophageal perforation can be suspected by the presence of a pneumomediastinum with or without mediastinal widening (Fig. 71–80). Often unilateral or sometimes bilateral pleural effusions and basilar infiltrates are present. Rarely pneumothoraces or pneumopericardiums can be detected. The diagnosis of perforation can be confirmed after the administration of contrast with diluted barium, which determines the site of the perforation. This can be performed under fluoroscopic control or with plain films obtained at the bedside of the patient. Often when the size of the perforation is small, the site cannot be detected with certainty. Abnormal collections of extravasated contrast material can be seen within the mediastinum or pleural space. If necessary, CT can determine the exact location of the extravasated contrast material and its relationship to the mediastinal structures (Fig. 71–81). The exact site of the esophageal perforation is, however, rarely identified on the CT examinations. In the cases of prior esophagectomy and gastric pull-through, the diagnosis of perforation and anastomotic leak can be difficult based on the plain films alone. The diagnosis of perforation complicated by a mediastinal abscess is more easily made with barium studies or CT scanning (Fig. 71–82).

Stomach and Duodenum

As with the esophagus, the most commonly encountered gastric and duodenal problems in the ICU are related to bleeding and perforation. Gastric distention is not uncommon in the postsurgical patient. Decompression of a markedly distended stomach can be monitored by plain films of the abdomen. Gastric outlet obstruction can be suspected by the visualization on serial x-ray films of a persistently distended stomach. Gastric and duodenal ulcers are relatively common in the ICU patient.[57] They may be complicated by hemorrhage and perforation. Although hemorrhage can be diagnosed with endoscopy, difficult cases may need to be confirmed by angiography or scintigraphy (Fig. 71–83). Treatment by embolization material can be performed during the angiographic examination. Small amounts of free air can be detected after gastric perforation when the x-ray films are obtained in the upright or left lateral decubitus position (see Figs. 71–77, 71–78, and 71–79). Larger amounts of free air can be detected in the supine patient. Perforation into the lesser sac or retroperitoneum, with or without abscess formation, are more readily diagnosed by CT scanning (Fig. 71–84).

Small and Large Bowel

Ischemia and distention of the bowel, owing to either ileus or obstruction, are among the most common gastrointestinal tract abnormalities encountered in the ICU patient. Although ischemia, secondary to either underlying vascular disease or resulting from obstruction, is difficult to diagnose based on plain films only, small and large bowel ileus and obstruction are easily diagnosed and monitored with plain films. When suspected, ischemia can be confirmed primarily with angiographic studies (Figs. 71–85 and

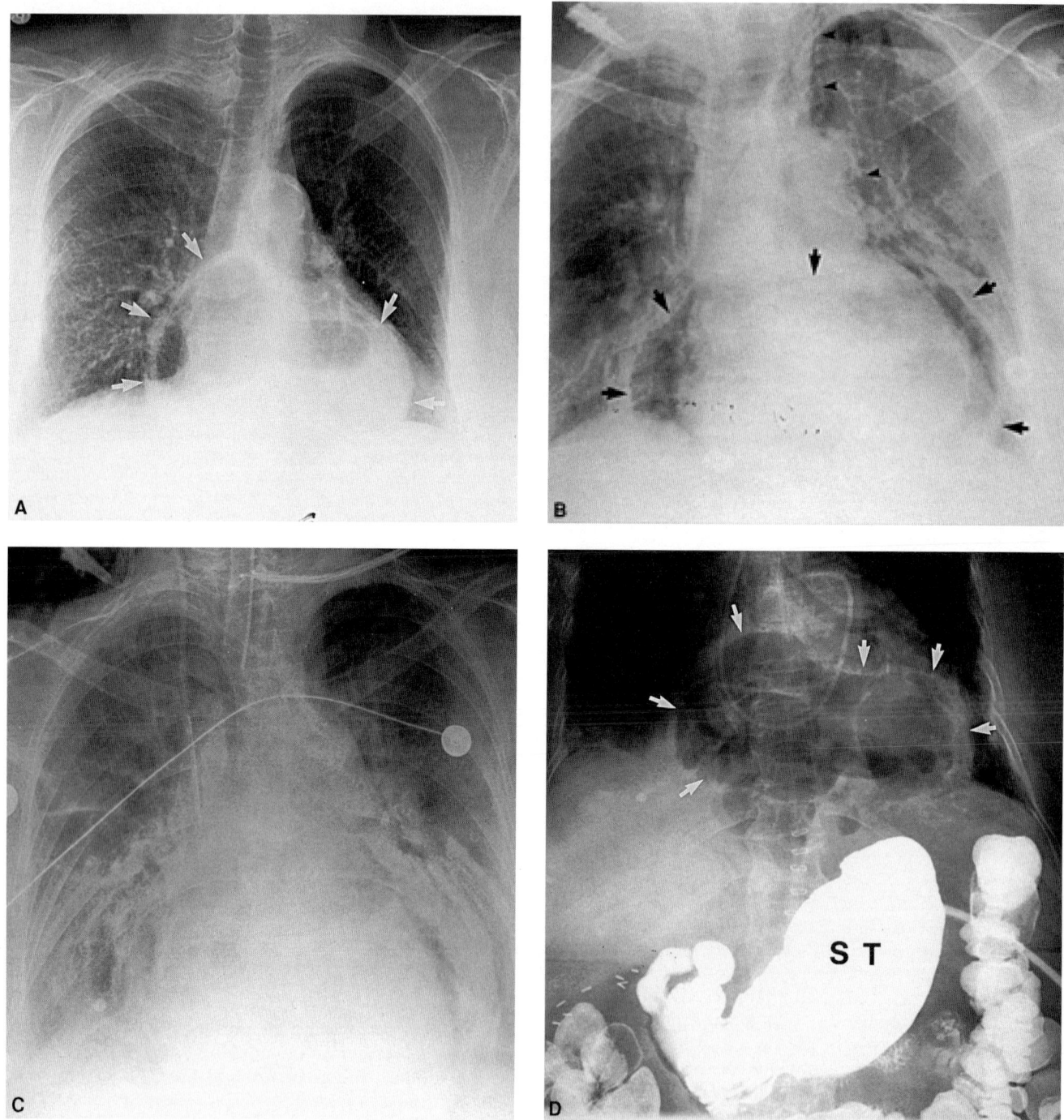

Fig. 71–82. Mediastinal abscess post hiatal hernia repair. *A*, A chest posteroanterior film obtained in a 68-year-old patient demonstrates a large hiatal hernia in the lower mediastinum (arrows). The patient underwent surgical repair of the hernia. *B*, Because of persistent fever, a follow-up portable chest anteroposterior film was obtained 3 days after surgery, which demonstrates a large air collection within the lower mediastinum (arrows) initially believed to represent recurrence of the hiatal hernia. There is an extensive pneumomediastinum seen along the upper portion of the mediastinum (arrowheads). *C*, A chest anteroposterior portable film obtained supine 24 hours later demonstrates a persistent pneumomediastinum with further accumulation of fluid within the lower mediastinum. The extent and irregularity of both the air and the fluid collection within the mediastinum do not suggest a hiatal hernia but rather a large abscess (compare with the baseline film shown in *A*). *D*, A barium study through a gastrostomy tube demonstrates that the stomach is within the abdomen (ST) and that the abnormal air and fluid collections within the lower mediastinum (arrows) represent a large abscess.

(Figure continues)

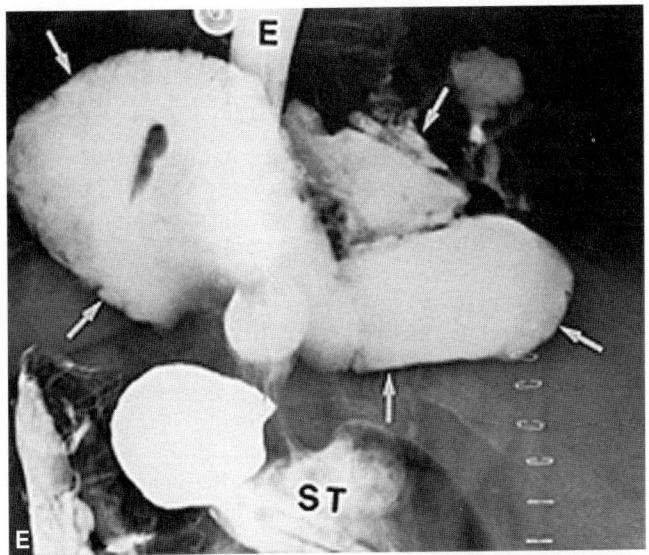

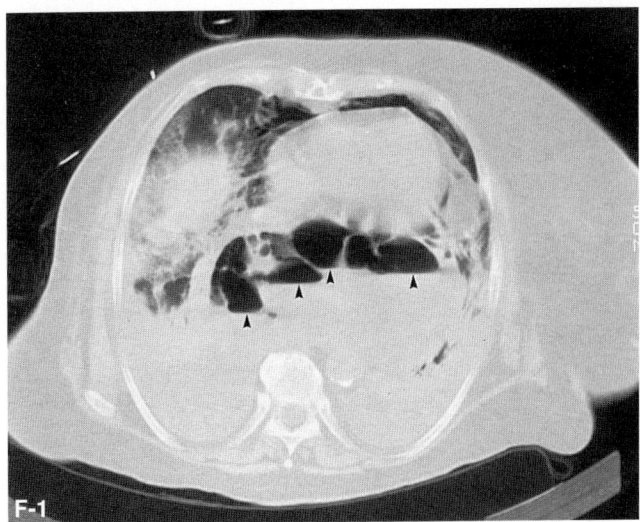

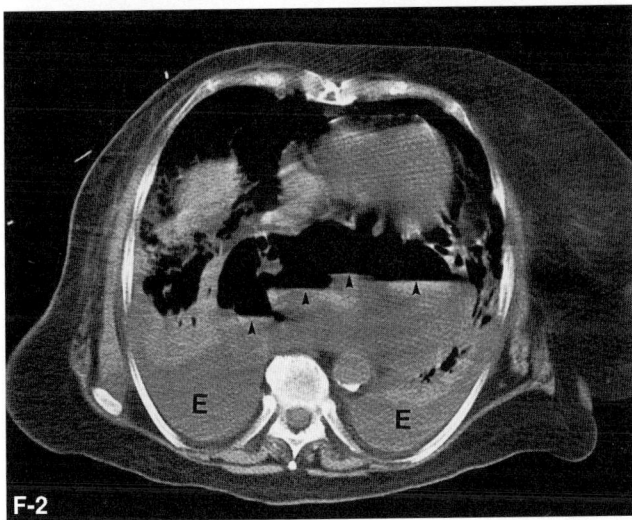

Fig. 71–82. *(Continued) E,* A follow-up barium study with contrast material ingested through the esophagus demonstrates communication between the esophagus (E) and the large mediastinal abscess (arrows) seen above the stomach (ST). *F,* A CT scan examination through the lower mediastinum imaged with parenchymal windows *(F-1)* and soft tissue windows *(F-2)* demonstrates multiple large air-fluid levels loculated throughout the posterior lower mediastinum (arrowheads), representing a mediastinal abscess secondary to rupture and necrosis of the anastomosis between the esophagus and stomach. Note the bilateral empyema (E).

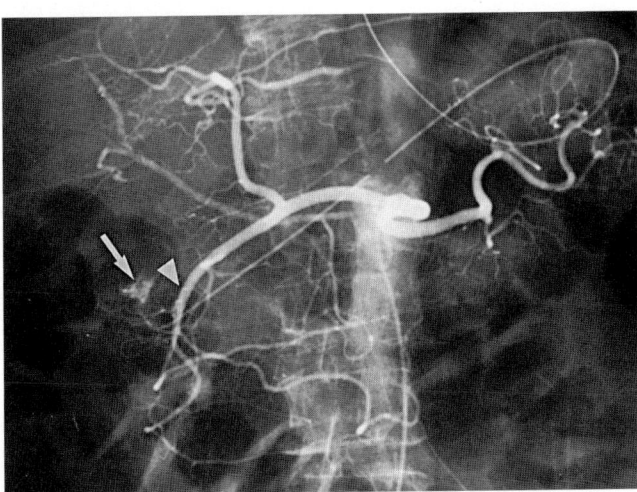

Fig. 71–83. Hemorrhagic duodenal ulcer—angiography. A celiac arteriogram obtained in a 67-year-old patient with history of hematemesis and endoscopically documented bleeding from the second and third portions of the duodenum demonstrates extravasation of contrast material (arrow) from a branch of the proximal gastroduodenal artery (arrowhead). The bleeding was successfully treated with transcatheter embolotherapy.

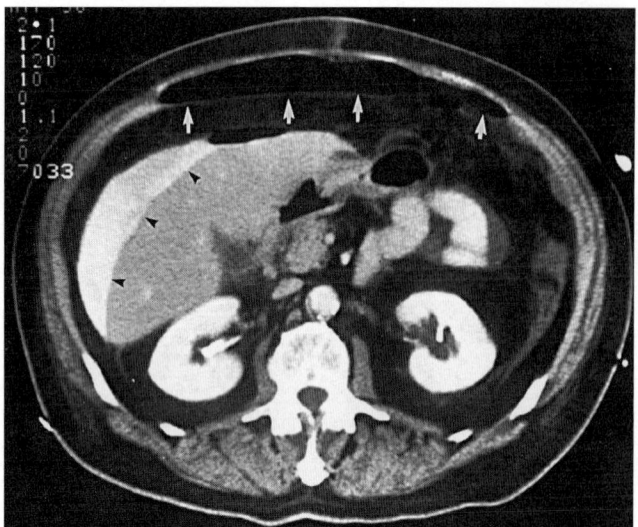

Fig. 71-84. Perforated duodenal ulcer post open heart surgery. A 72-year-old patient status post open heart surgery 2 weeks earlier complained of increasing abdominal pain. The patient was afebrile and without leukocytosis. A CT scan examination was performed to rule out an abdominal aortic aneurysm. A CT examination obtained through the upper abdomen after administration of intravenous and oral contrast material demonstrates free air within the anterior portion of the abdomen (arrows). A large collection of high-density material is noted around the right lobe of the liver (arrowheads), which represents oral contrast material that has leaked from the perforated duodenal ulcer into the peritoneum. The perforated duodenal ulcer was surgically repaired.

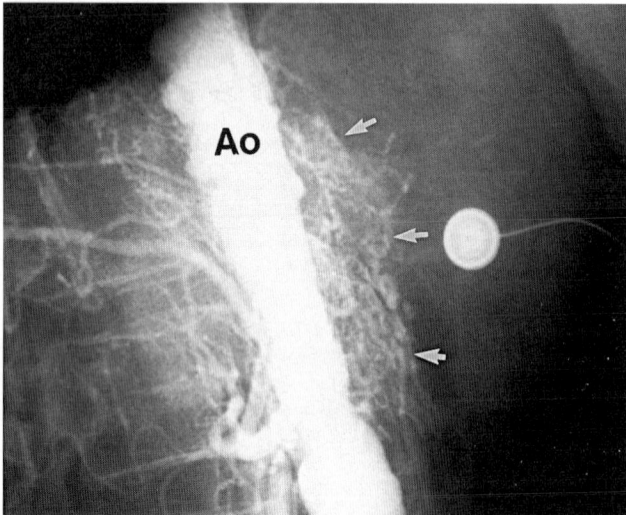

Fig. 71-85. Mesenteric ischemia. A 61-year-old patient presented with diffuse abdominal pain owing to occlusive mesenteric ischemia resulting from advanced arteriosclerotic disease. A lateral aortic angiogram shows marked arteriosclerotic irregularity of the wall of the abdominal aorta (Ao). The celiac axis and superior mesenteric and inferior mesenteric arteries are not visualized, owing to occlusion at their origins. Multiple retroperitoneal collaterals are identified (arrows).

71-86). Plain films may demonstrate bowel wall thickening or localized stricture. In advanced cases, secondary signs of necrotizing enterocolitis can be visualized on plain films by the presence of pneumatosis intestinalis and air within the portal venous system.

Pneumatosis intestinalis is a rare condition characterized by the collection of multiple intramural pockets of gas, involving the gastrointestinal tract and mesenteric attachments. Pneumatosis in adults frequently has a benign course and prognosis (Fig. 71-87) and may be seen in patients with chronic obstructive pulmonary disease, bullous disease of the lung, collagen vascular disorders, leukemia, and cystic fibrosis. It can complicate dissecting pneumomediastinums and steroid treatments. Pneumatosis, however, accompanying necrotizing enteritis (Fig. 71-88), has a more severe course and high mortality.

The adynamic ileus is usually seen after major abdominal surgery and manifests with diffuse distention of the intra-abdominal gastrointestinal tract (stomach, small and large bowel). It usually subsides in the next few days, with follow-up radiographs showing gradual improvement. Focal ileus can occur secondary to an underlying inflammation from a nearby organ (i.e., pancreatitis) and can be difficult to separate from partial bowel obstruction. In partial small bowel obstruction, air may be seen distal to the site of obstruction in the small and large bowel, however, disproportionately less than the amount of air distention proximal to the site of obstruction (Fig. 71-89). In complete small bowel obstruction (Fig. 71-90), residual air within the bowel distal to the site of obstruction usually clears within 48 hours. In equivocal cases, barium studies with serial follow-up radiographic examinations can help to confirm the diagnosis, but such studies are contraindicated when ischemia is suspected. In acute large bowel obstruction, owing to volvulus or intussusception, plain x-ray films demonstrate distention of the large bowel segment proximal to the site of obstruction.

A sigmoid volvulus occurs when there is a closed-loop obstruction of the sigmoid colon. The fixation point is over the upper pelvis, and the distended bowel loops extend upward under the right or left hemidiaphragms. It has a typical inverted U configuration (Fig. 71-91). In contrast to a colonic ileus, the distended sigmoid in volvuli may project superior to the transverse colon and may show a loss of the haustra. A cecal volvulus manifests as a distended bowel loop in the right side of the abdomen, extending toward the left or right upper quadrants (Fig. 71-92). Perforation of the large bowel can occur especially in the region of the cecum, when the diameter of the bowel exceeds 14 cm.[58] When the plain films are equivocal and the site of obstruction needs to be determined, barium enema examination can be performed. The enema examination is, however, contraindicated in the cases of suspected toxic megacolon with inflammation of the bowel wall. Toxic megacolon is one of the few life-threatening conditions in which the diagnosis can be made based on the radiographic findings alone (Fig. 71-93). Toxic megacolon is an acute dilatation of the colon, most commonly seen involving the transverse portion. The degree of distention is usually less than the one seen with obstruction or volvulus. It typically occurs in fulminating

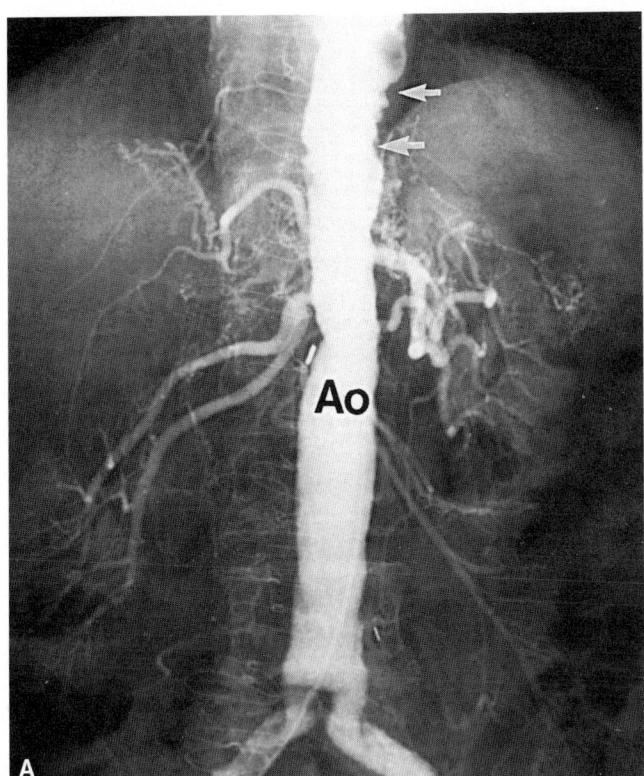 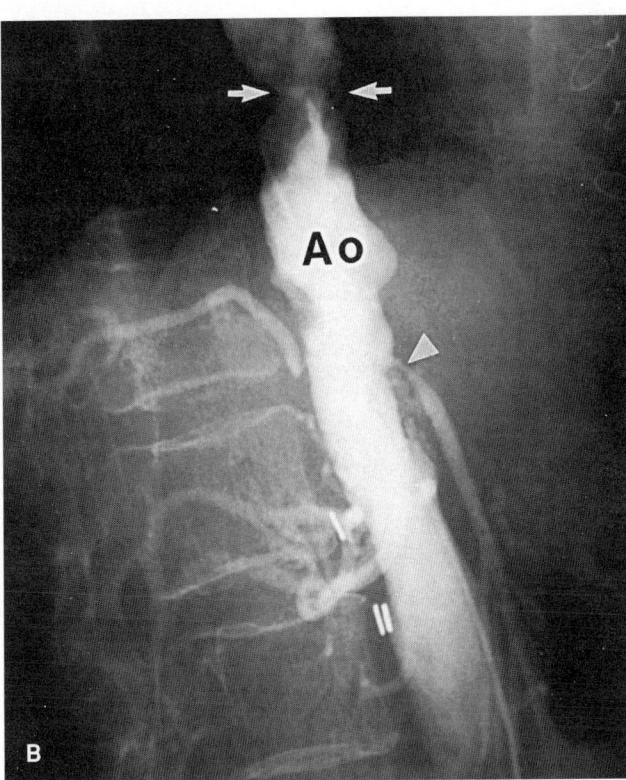

Fig. 71–86. *A, B,* Chronic mesenteric ischemia. An aortogram was obtained in an elderly patient with previous aortoiliac occlusive disease who presented with weight loss and a several month history of abdominal pain that was exacerbated by meals. Anteroposterior *(A)* and lateral *(B)* views demonstrate marked atherosclerotic changes (arrows) seen as irregularity of the lumen of the aorta (Ao). There is complete occlusion of the celiac trunk and inferior mesenteric artery. There is severe stenosis of the origin of the superior mesenteric artery (arrowhead).

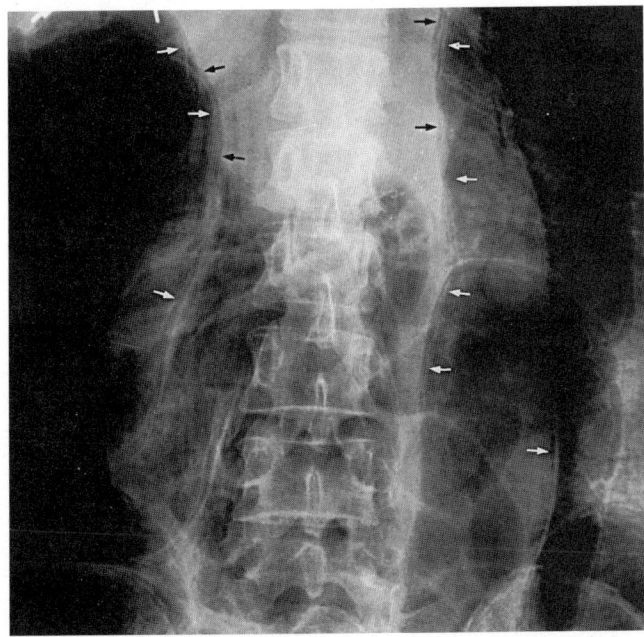

Fig. 71–87. Pneumatosis intestinalis ("benign"). A supine portable examination obtained in a 62-year-old patient who presented with abdominal distention and pain demonstrates diffuse distention with air of the large and small bowel. There is evidence of pneumatosis intestinalis diffusely involving the large bowel seen as linear lucencies in the wall of the colon (arrows). There is no evidence of portal gas in the right upper quadrant. The patient was receiving steroids, which is believed to be the cause of the pneumotosis.

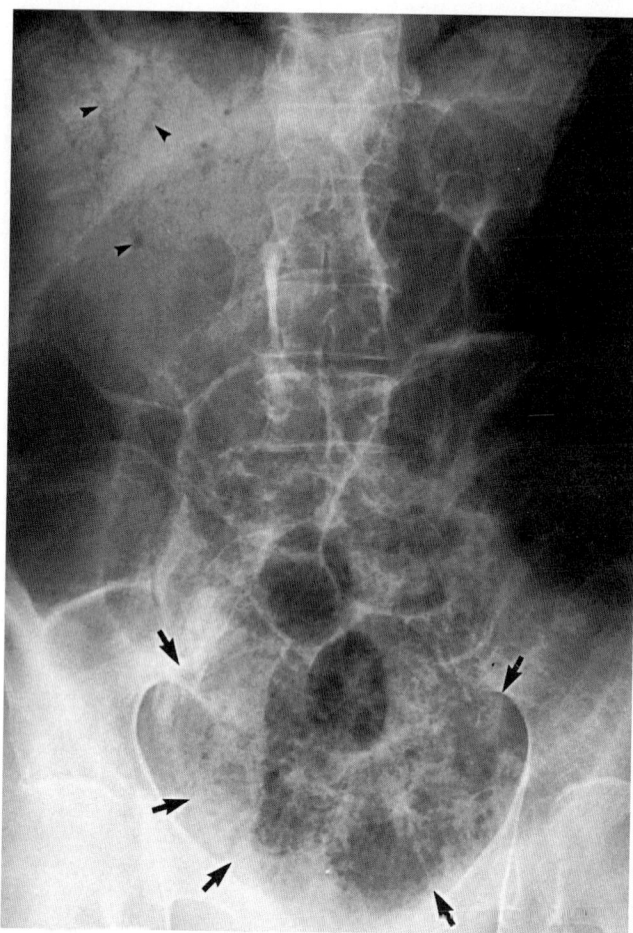

Fig. 71–88. Mesenteric infarction with portal venous gas and pneumatosis intestinalis ("malignant"). A supine view of the abdomen obtained in a 74-year-old patient with abdominal pain demonstrates diffuse distention with air of the large and small bowel. There is a mottled lucency overlying the bowel in the pelvis representing pneumatosis (arrows). Multiple branching linear lucencies are seen in the region of the liver representing portal venous gas (arrowheads). The patient died a few hours after this radiograph.

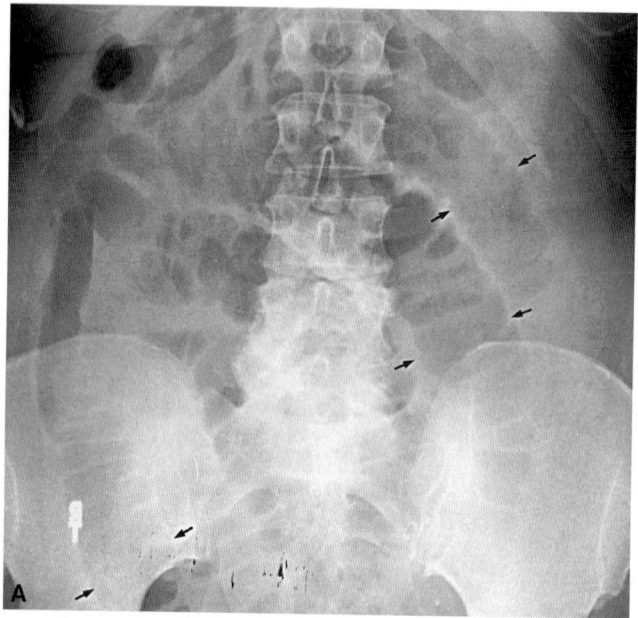
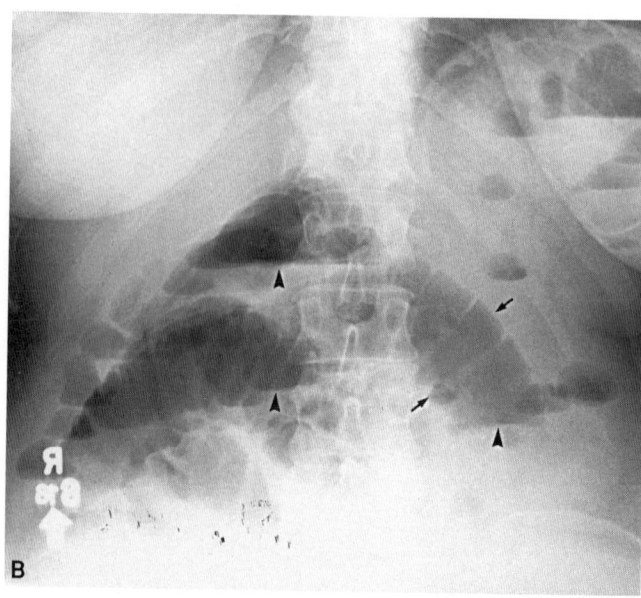

Fig. 71–89. Partial small bowel obstruction. An abdominal film obtained supine (A) and upright (B) in a 65-year-old patient with prior history of pelvic surgery and intermittent abdominal pain demonstrates distention of the small bowel (arrows) with air and fluid with multiple air-fluid levels (arrowheads) seen in the small bowel. Minimal air and fluid within the large colon is best seen in the region of both hepatic and splenic flexures.

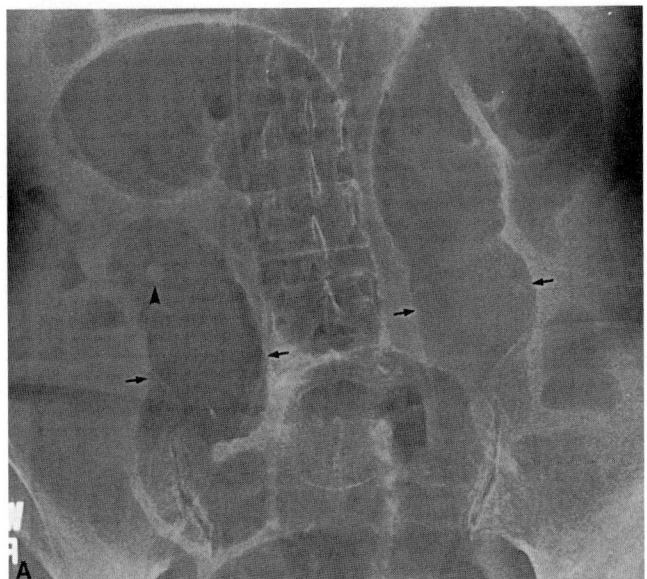
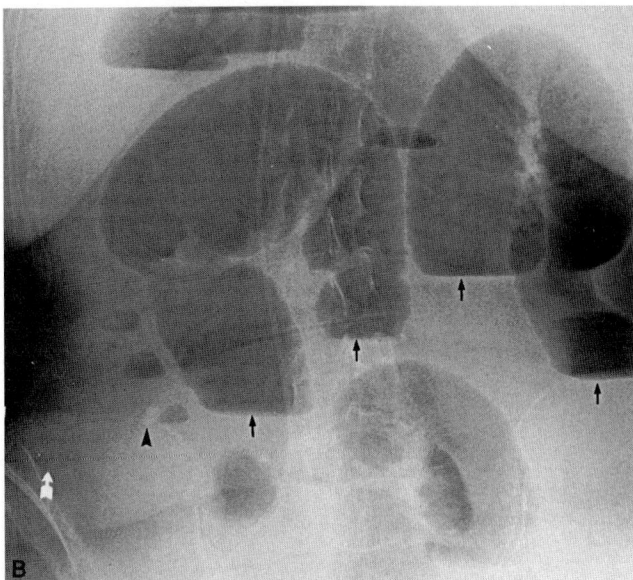

Fig. 71-90. Small bowel obstruction. An abdominal film obtained supine (A) and upright (B) in a 57-year-old patient status post pelvic surgery demonstrates multiple distended small bowel loops with air and fluid with multiple air-fluid levels (arrows). A 1-cm calcification is seen in the right lower quadrant suggestive of an appendicolith (arrowhead).

colitis, most often seen in ulcerative colitis. Changes of inflammation of the bowel are usually present. Perforation may occur spontaneously or inadvertently if a barium enema study is performed.

Pancreas

The pancreas is best imaged by CT, but US can play an important role in the screening of patients with suspected pancreatic disease. A common clinical problem is to determine the presence of acute pancreatitis. An ultrasound examination, performed at the patient's bed, can determine the presence of pancreatic enlargement or edema associated with acute pancreatitis. The ultrasound examination helps to determine the presence of pancreatic or biliary duct dilatation and the presence of hepatic, biliary, or gallbladder abnormality. In cases of acute pancreatitis, US may detect the changes of enlargement, edema (hypoechogenicity), and the presence of pseudocysts or abscesses.[59] Compared with US, CT is more sensitive for the diagnosis of pancreatitis because it can better define the pancreatic and peripancreatic anatomy, visualizing the extent of inflammation in the peritoneal and retroperitoneal spaces (Fig. 71-94).[60,61] Pseudocysts and abscesses are better visualized when they occur in areas difficult to examine by ultrasound examination (retroperitoneum, mesenteric, mediastinum) (Figs. 71-95, 71-96, and 71-97).[62] Necrotizing and hemorrhagic pancreatitis is better determined by CT because both hemorrhage and gas are best visualized by CT (Fig. 71-98). Drainage procedures for pancreatic abscesses and pseudocysts can be performed under the guidance of either US or CT. Vascular complications, such as bleeding, thrombosis, or pseudoaneurysm formation, can be detected by either US or CT. In equivocal cases, angiography may be necessary.

Gallbladder and Hepatobiliary System

The ultrasound examination, performed at the bedside, is the method of choice to evaluate the gallbladder and biliary system in the case of suspected cholecystitis.[63] Calculi within the gallbladder or common bile duct are usually easy to detect by ultrasound examination alone. Because most cases of acute cholecystitis are complications of cholelithiasis, one of the most common sonographic findings is the presence of gallstones. Nonvisualization of cholelithiasis, however, does not rule out the presence of acute cholecystitis. The sonographic signs of acute cholecystitis include thickening of the gallbladder wall and the detection of intraluminal sludge. The gangrenous cholecystitis may show a sloughed mucosa projecting in the lumen of the gallbladder. In the case of a perforated gallbladder, a pericholecystic abscess is demonstrated as a fluid collection surrounding the gallbladder wall (Fig. 71-99).[64] The size and dilatation of the common bile duct and biliary tree can be detected by the ultrasound examination alone. In equivocal cases or in cases of acalculous cholecystitis, biliary scintigraphy is helpful in determining the function of the hepatobiliary system.[65] Hepatobiliary scans are performed with technetium-99m diisopropyl imidoacetic acid (DISIDA), which allows visualization of the hepatobiliary system in patients with a bilirubin level up to 20 mg/dl. It is used for the evaluation of acute cholecystitis, biliary atresia, and postsurgical biliary leaks. In a normal study, the liver is visualized by 5 minutes, the gallbladder by 15 minutes, and the duodenum by 30 minutes. Nonvisualization of the gallbladder by 1 hour, with adequate hepatic visualization, suggests acute cholecystitis (Fig. 71-100). If there is nonvisualization of the gallbladder or bowel, common bile duct obstruction should be suspected. The normal gallbladder should become increasingly intense throughout the study, while the liver becomes less apparent. De-

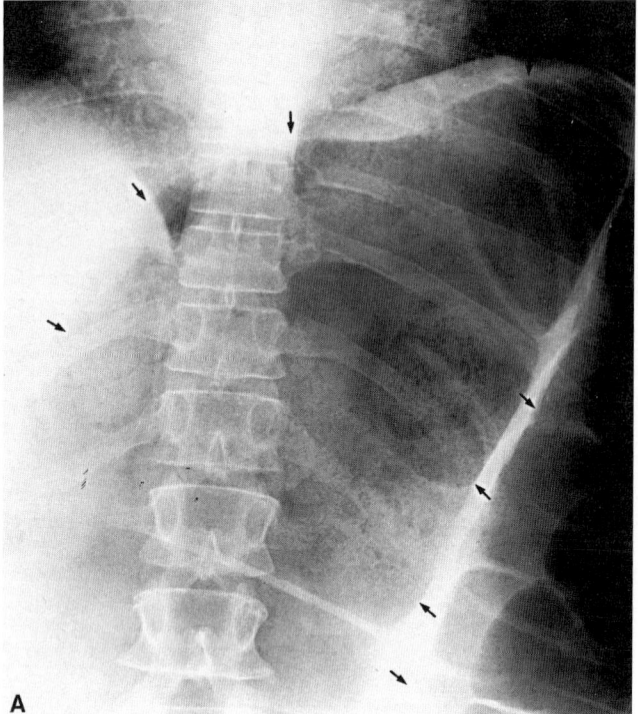
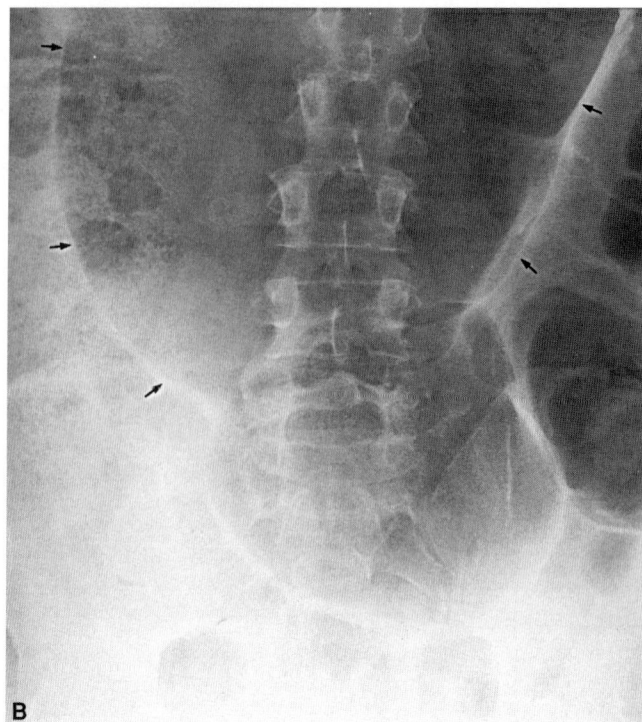
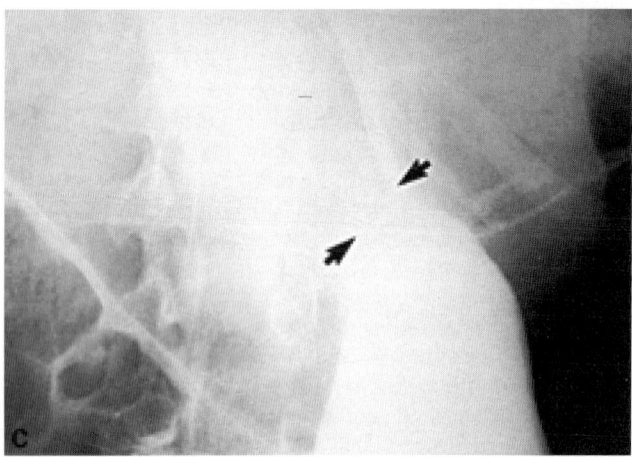

Fig. 71–91. Sigmoid volvulus. A 40-year-old patient with history of chronic constipation was admitted because of abdominal pain and distention. *A, B,* A plain film of the abdomen obtained supine with a view of the upper abdomen *(A)* and lower abdomen *(B)* demonstrates a markedly distended loop of bowel extending from the pelvis to the left upper quadrant beneath the left hemidiaphragm (arrows). The bowel loop is relatively ahaustral with the appearance of an inverted U. *C,* A single contrast barium enema examination confirms the diagnosis of sigmoid volvulus with filling of the rectum and beaking of the rectus sigmoid region at the site of the volvulus (arrows).

layed visualization of the gallbladder (1 to 4 hours) suggests chronic cholecystitis; however, acute cholecystitis cannot be totally excluded.

The liver parenchyma, in the critically ill patient, is best evaluated by US first because both morphology and texture can be evaluated. Cirrhosis, passive congestion, and fatty infiltration can be detected with a relatively high degree of sensitivity by an ultrasound examination performed at the patient's bed. Focal lesions, such as masses, hemangiomas, or abscesses, are also easily determined by the method. CT examinations can be complementary to US in complex cases, such as in the cases of liver transplantation and its complications.

Spleen and Retroperitoneum

Complications of hemorrhage and infections are the main splenic abnormalities evaluated in the ICU. Spontaneous and post-traumatic intrasplenic or subcapsular hemorrhage can be detected by both US and CT examinations. The diagnosis of splenic laceration is, however, made more sensitively by CT (Fig. 71-101).[66,67] The spleen is the intraperitoneal organ most frequently injured in blunt trauma, with patients with splenomegaly at the greatest risk. Plain films are not reliable in assessing splenic injury. Signs of rib fractures, displacement of the stomach, or splenic flexure of the colon may raise the suspicion of splenic or retroperitoneal abnormalities. Also the diagnosis of splenic abscess can be difficult even in the clinical setting of fever, leukocytosis, and left upper quadrant pain. Most cases are associated with hematogenous spread of infection and often are seen in the immunocompromised patients. CT and, to a lesser degree, US play an important role in the early diagnosis of splenic abscesses. They are detected as abnormal intrasplenic fluid collections with or without the presence of air (Fig. 71-102). As with liver and pancreatic

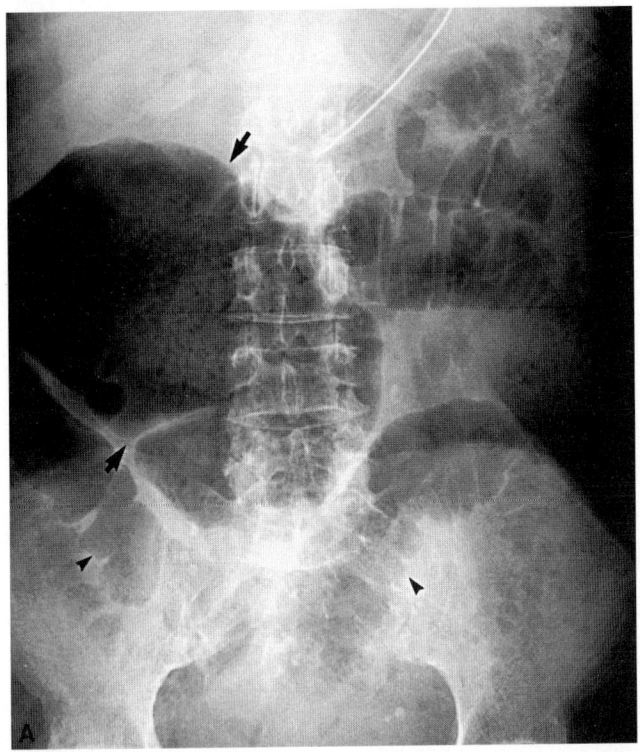

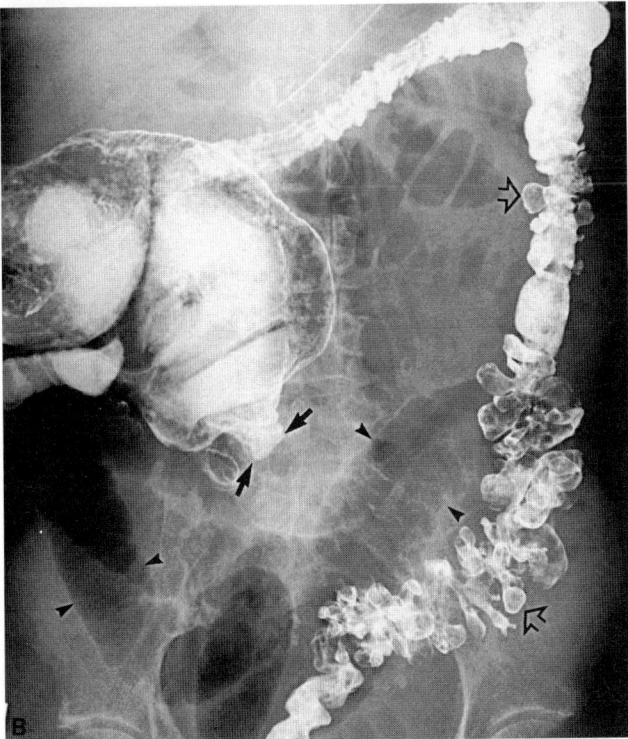

Fig. 71–92. Cecal volvulus. *A,* A plain film of the abdomen was obtained in a 71-year-old patient status post recent right inguinal surgery and abdominal pain and distention. It demonstrates marked distention of the cecum seen on the right side of the abdomen (arrows) with moderate distention of the distal small bowel near the ileocecal valve (arrowheads). *B,* A single barium enema study again demonstrates marked distention of the cecum with abrupt beaking and obstruction at the inferior portion of the cecum (arrows). Note the persistent distention of the terminal small bowel (arrowheads). Multiple diverticula are seen throughout the left and sigmoid colon (open arrowheads).

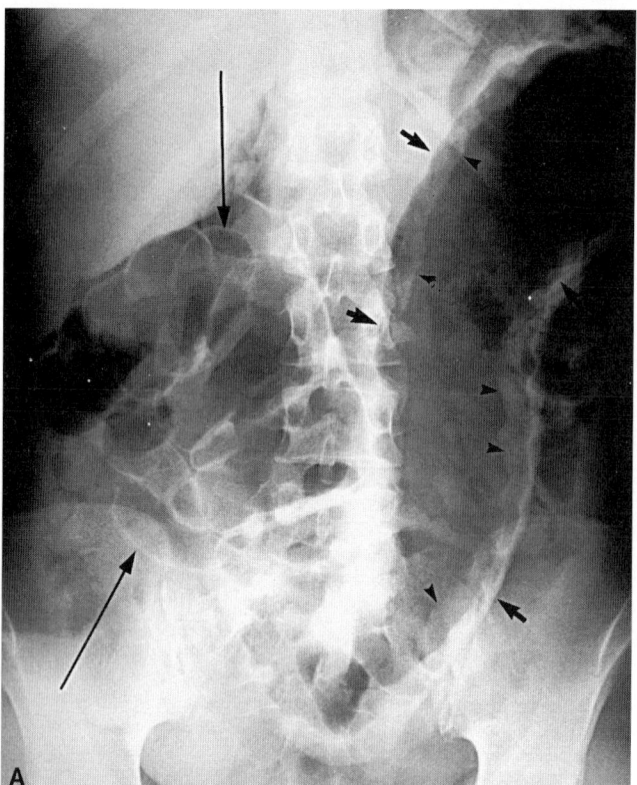
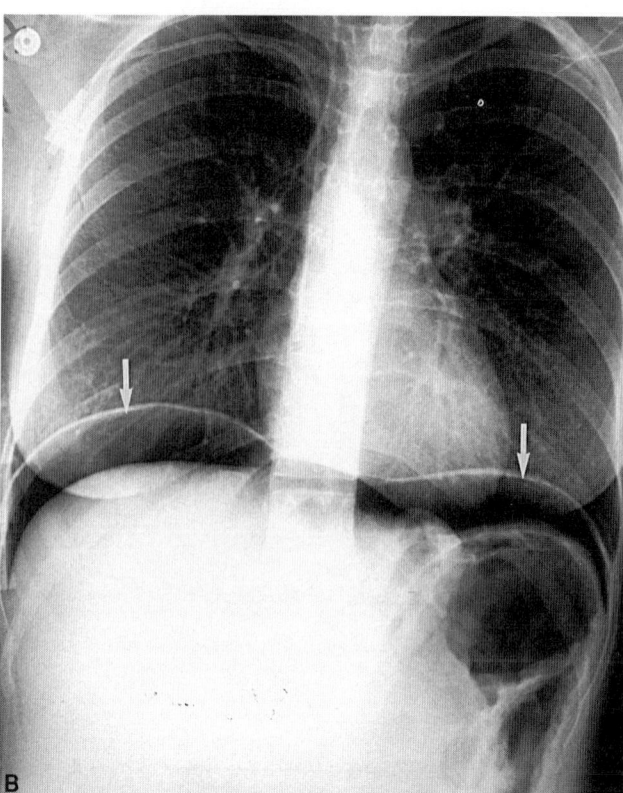

Fig. 71-93. Toxic megacolon. *A,* A supine plain film of the abdomen was obtained in a 20-year-old patient with history of ulcerative colitis and abdominal pain. The plain radiograph demonstrates distention of the transverse colon (short arrows). There is effacement of the haustral markings with diffuse wall thickening and mucosal nodularity owing to inflammation (arrowheads). A pneumoperitoneum is seen outlining bowel loops in the right upper quadrant (long arrows) with free air seen outlining the inferior border of the liver. *B,* An upright chest film demonstrates the pneumoperitoneum collecting below the hemidiaphragms (arrows).

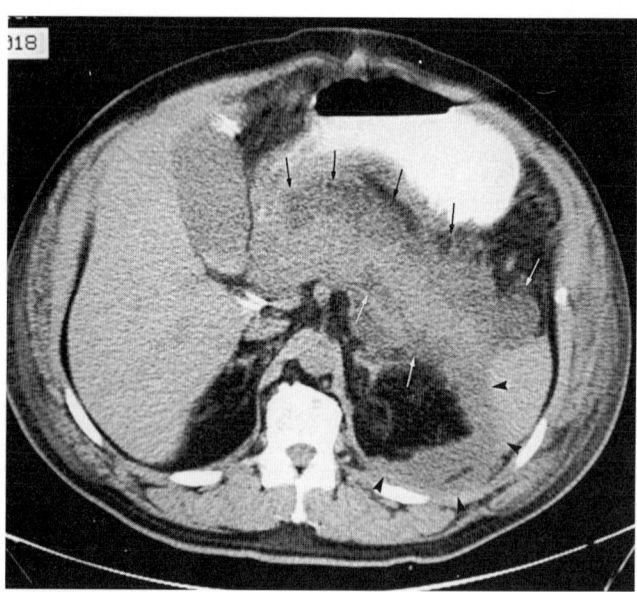

Fig. 71-94. Acute pancreatitis. A CT scan examination of the abdomen obtained in a 56-year-old patient who presented with abdominal pain demonstrates diffuse enlargement of the pancreas with areas of low attenuation caused by edema surrounding the pancreas (arrows). The peripancreatic soft tissues are obliterated by the edema with extension to the retroperitoneum in the left posterior pararenal space (arrowheads).

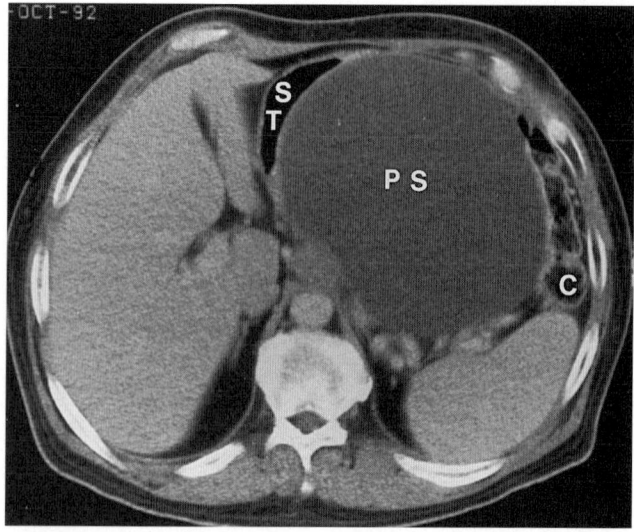

Fig. 71-95. Pancreatic pseudocyst. An axial image obtained in a 53-year-old patient with history of pancreatitis and abdominal distention demonstrates a large fluid collection in the lesser sac representing a large pancreatic pseudocyst (PS) seen to displace markedly the stomach medially (ST) and the colon laterally (C).

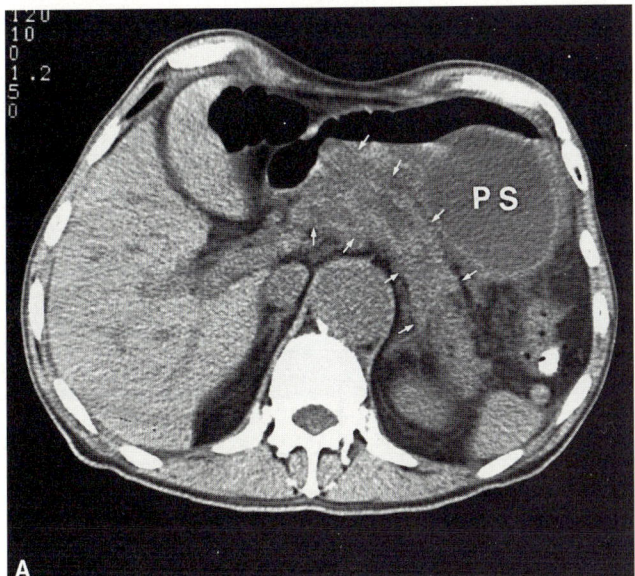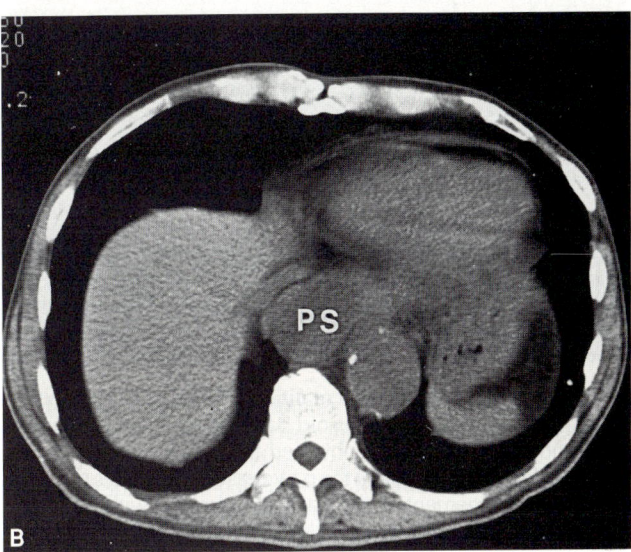

Fig. 71-96. Pancreatitis with pseudocyst in the lower mediastinum. A CT scan examination of the abdomen was performed on a 61-year-old patient with history of acute pancreatitis. *A,* An axial image obtained through the level of the pancreas demonstrates diffuse edematous enlargement of the pancreas (arrows) with a pseudocyst seen in the left upper quadrant (PS). *B,* An axial image obtained through the lower chest demonstrates an approximately 5-cm fluid collection in the lower mediastinum seen in the prevertebral region compatible with a pseudocyst (PS) dissecting in the lower mediastinum.

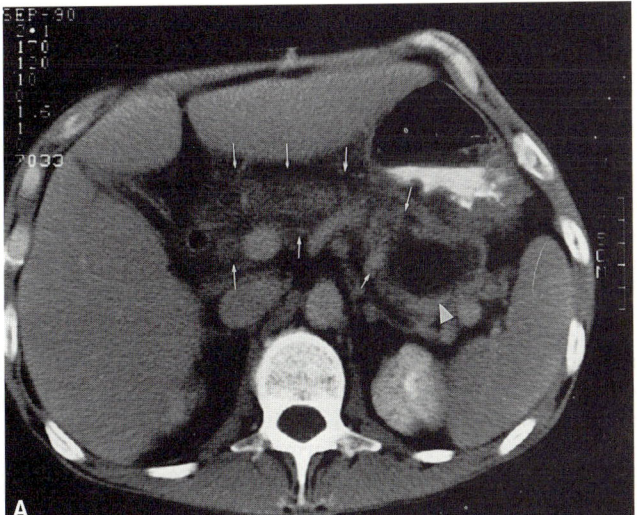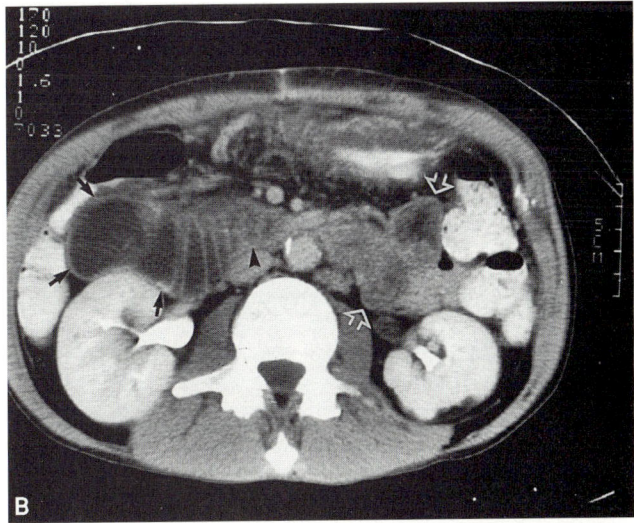

Fig. 71-97. Acute pancreatitis with pancreatic abscess. A CT examination of the abdomen was obtained in a 42-year-old patient with history of alcoholism and recurrent bouts of acute pancreatitis. The patient had a 2-day history of fever, chills, and a gram-negative bacteremia. *A,* An axial image through the upper abdomen after the administration of oral and intravenous contrast material demonstrates edema of the body of the pancreas (arrows) and the peripancreatic tissues owing to acute pancreatitis. Additionally, there is a fluid collection in the region of the tail of the pancreas with a thick wall (arrowhead) consistent with either a pseudocyst or an abscess. The fluid collection was aspirated under CT guidance, and subsequent cultures revealed gram-negative bacilli. *B,* An axial image obtained below the one shown on *A* demonstrates focal distention with fluid of the duodenum (black arrows), representing a focal ileus in reaction to the nearby inflammation of the pancreas (black arrowhead). Note the inferior extent of the abscess in the tail of pancreas (open arrowheads).

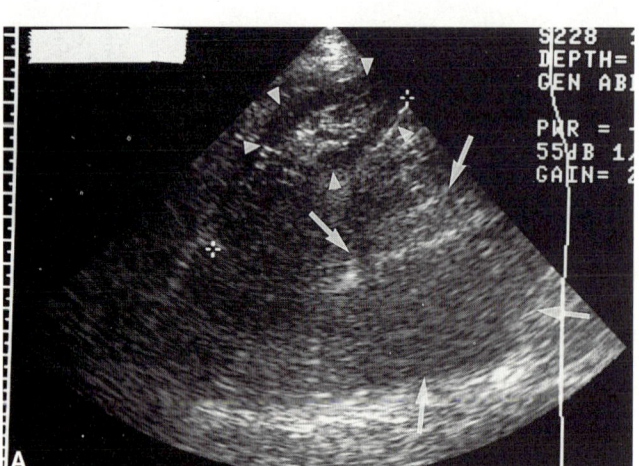
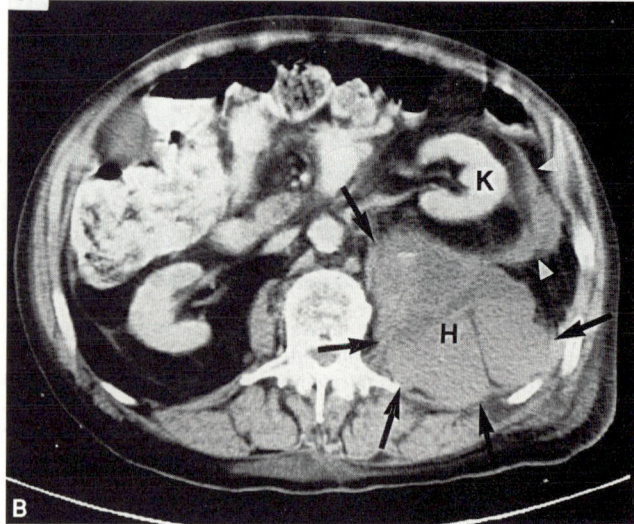

Fig. 71-103. Spontaneous retroperitoneal hematoma secondary to anticoagulation. *A,* An ultrasound examination of the left upper quadrant/retroperitoneum was obtained in a 59-year-old patient who experienced an acute decrease of his hematocrit after anticoagulative therapy for coronary catheterization. The scan demonstrates a markedly displaced left kidney anteriorly (arrowheads) by a large mass of heterogeneous echogenicity (arrows). *B,* A CT scan examination through the midabdomen obtained after the administration of oral and intravenous contrast material demonstrates a large hematoma of mixed attenuation in the left retroperitoneum (black arrows, H) surrounding the left psoas muscle and markedly displacing the left kidney (K). Note the hemorrhage in the left perirenal space (white arrowheads).

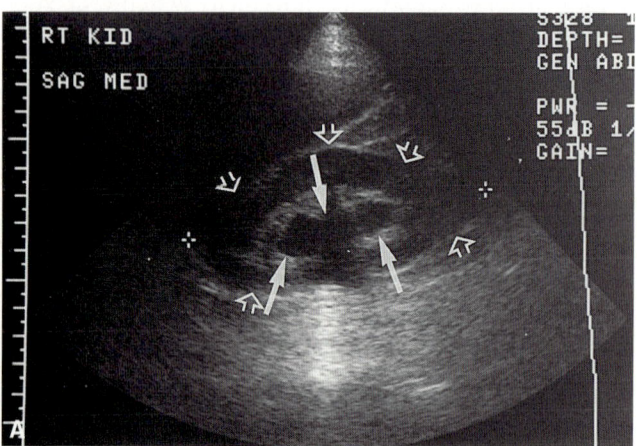
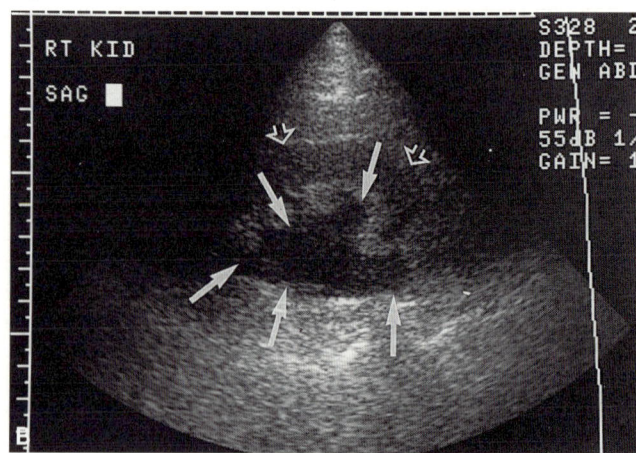

Fig. 71-104. *A, B,* Hydronephrosis. An ultrasound examination was obtained in a 78-year-old patient with history of prostate enlargement and decreased urine output. Sagittal images through the right kidney (open arrowheads) at the level of the calyces *(A)* and pelvicalyceal system *(B)* demonstrate dilatation of the calyces, pelvis, and ureter (arrows). The dilated right ureter was visualized down to the level of the ureterovesical junction and the enlarged prostate.

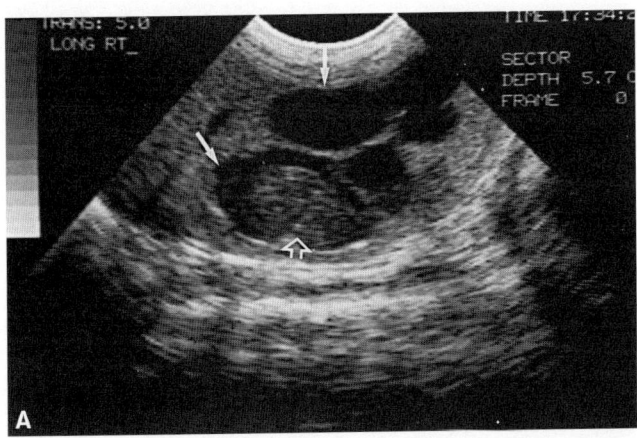
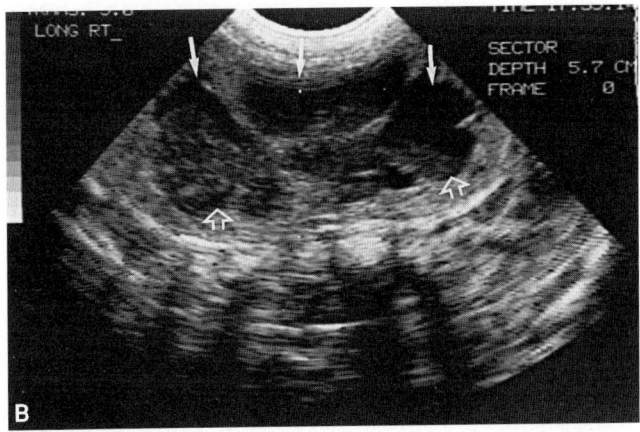

Fig. 71–105. *A, B,* Hydronephrosis owing to candida fungus balls. An ultrasound examination of the kidney was obtained in a premature infant with multiorgan failure. Longitudinal images of the right kidney demonstrate marked dilatation of the collection system (arrows) with multiple echogenic masses in the collecting system representing large mycetomas (open arrowheads).

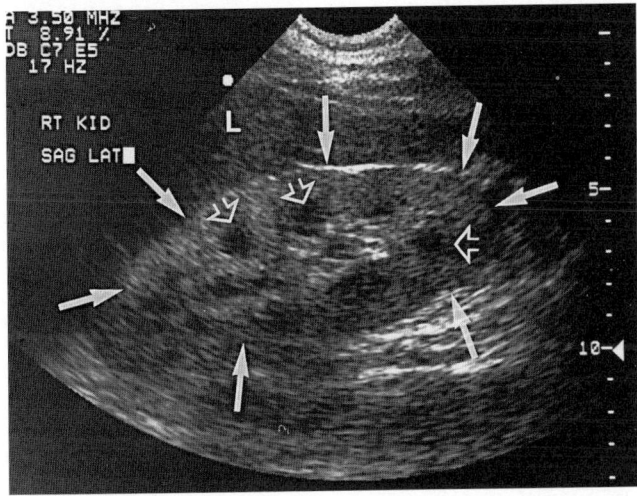

Fig. 71–106. Acute medical renal disease (membranoproliferative glomerulonephritis). An ultrasound examination of the kidneys was obtained in a 27-year-old HIV-positive patient with a history of intravenous drug abuse. A longitudinal scan of the right kidney demonstrates enlargement of the kidney (arrows) with diffuse increased cortical echogenicity (compare with the density of the liver [L], which should be more echogenic than the renal cortex). The pyramids (open arrowheads) are hypoechoic, simulating the appearance of hydronephrosis.

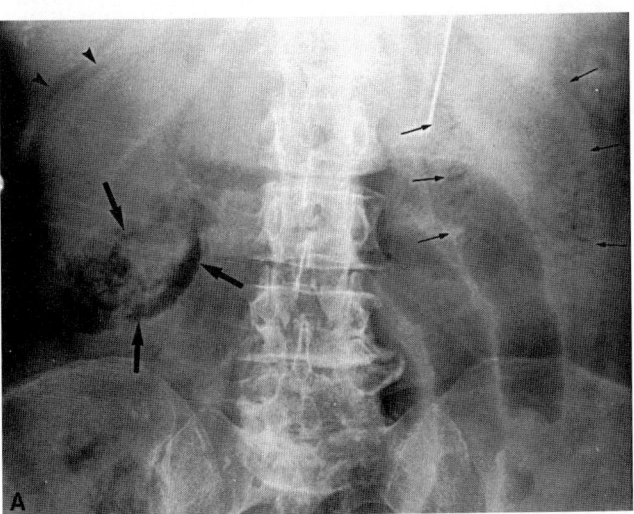
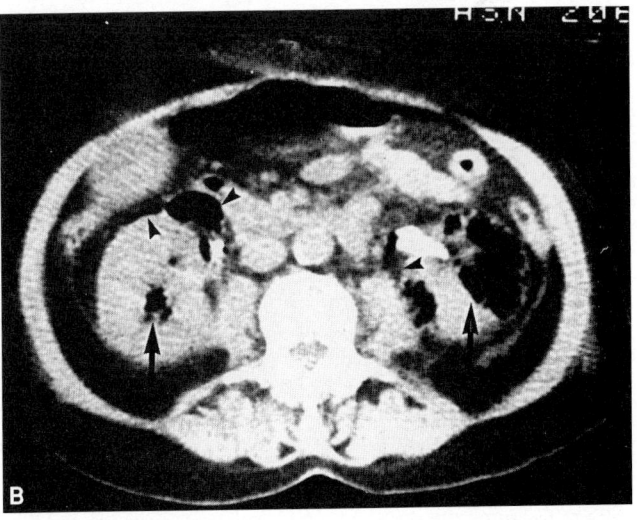

Fig. 71–107. Emphysematous pyelonephritis. *A,* A supine plain film of the abdomen obtained in a 50-year-old patient with a history of diabetes mellitus and right flank pain demonstrates mottled lucencies overlying the lower pole of the right kidney (large arrows). There is a lucent ring outlining the right kidney (arrowheads) and streaky lucencies overlying the left kidney (small arrows). *B,* A CT scan of the abdomen obtained after the administration of oral and intravenous contrast material demonstrates multiple collections of gas within the parenchyma of both kidneys (arrows) and within both perirenal spaces, indicative of emphysematous pyelonephritis (arrowheads).

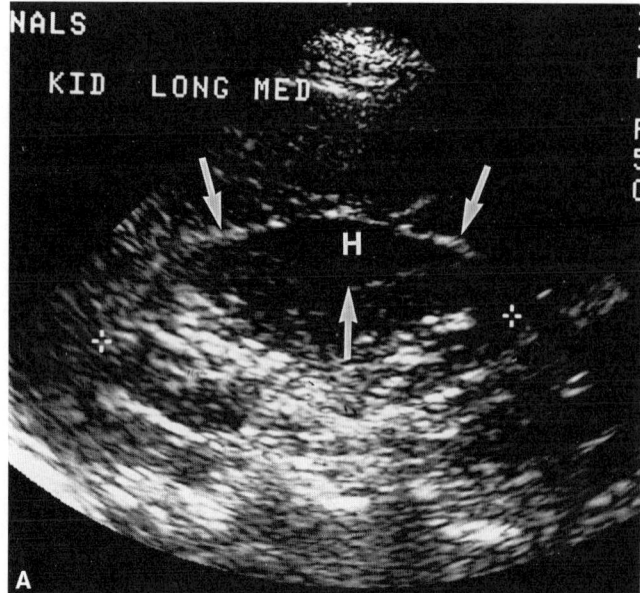
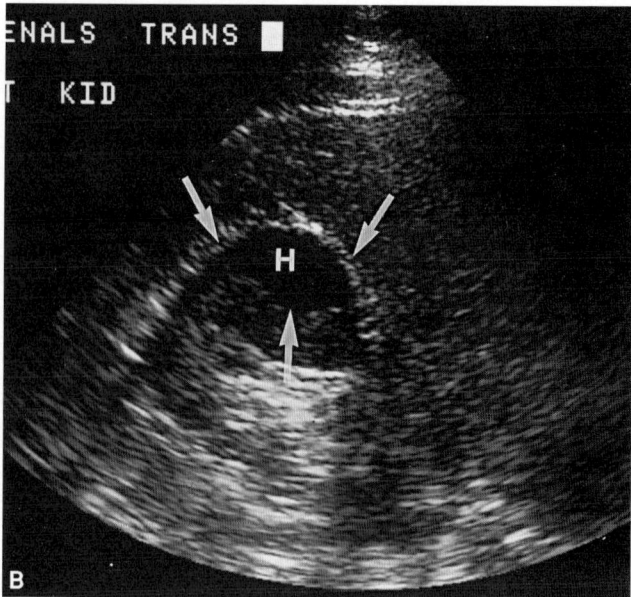

Fig. 71-108. A, B, Renal subcapsular hematoma—ultrasonography. An ultrasound examination of the right kidney was obtained in a 64-year-old patient who had received extracorporeal shock wave lithotripsy 6 weeks earlier but had persistent right flank pain. Longitudinal (A) and sagittal (B) views of the right kidney demonstrate a lenticular-shaped hypoechoic lesion in the anterior interpolar portion of the right kidney representing a subcapsular hematoma (arrows, H).

hemorrhage and hematomas may have a characteristic appearance on CT. When suspected, renal artery injury with subsequent renal infarction and renal vein thrombosis can be evaluated by ultrasound examination. CT can further help in determining the extent of renal infarction and

Fig. 71-109. Renal infarction—CT. A CT scan examination with oral and intravenous contrast material was obtained in an 88-year-old patient with history of aortic dissection and left flank pain of 3 weeks' duration. An axial image obtained through the midkidney demonstrates diffuse decreased attenuation of the left kidney (L) representing left renal infarction (arrows). There is minimal peripheral enhancement of the renal cortex secondary to capsular branches. Note the eccentric thrombus formation (open arrowhead) involving the abdominal aorta at the origin of the left renal artery. Note the normal function of the right kidney (R).

sometimes identify the site of the renal artery injury or the site of renal vein thrombosis (Fig. 71-109).[76,77] If necessary, angiographic studies are the definitive studies to confirm acute vascular abnormality involving the renal system (Fig. 71-110).

Ureter, Bladder, and Urethra

Unless dilated, the ureter is somewhat difficult to visualize ultrasonographically in its entire length. Ureteral injury, with urine extravasation, is best diagnosed with pyelography. Bladder anomalies, such as rupture, hemorrhage, or inflammation, can be first screened by US and further evaluated by CT if necessary.[78] Urethra abnormalities seen in the ICU patients are mainly related to obstructions and trauma.[79] A retrograde urethrogram is the method of choice to evaluate the urethra.

Pelvic anomalies affecting the genitourinary organs are mainly related to fluid collections in the pelvis, such as hematomas and ascites. Infection due to pelvic inflammatory disease or ruptured sigmoid diverticulitis rarely occurs in the ICU. Although US can be used as a screening method, CT is the method of choice to evaluate the nature and extent of the pelvic disease.

Renal Transplant

Ultrasound examinations can be performed at the patient's bedside to evaluate the transplanted kidney and the potential complications. US is particularly helpful in evaluating the texture of the kidney, its collecting system, and its vascular pedicles. It is used for the diagnosis of obstructive uropathy and the demonstration of perigraft collections (urinoma, hematoma, abscess, and lymphocele). Pulsed or color Doppler flow can demonstrate occlusion of the renal

IMAGING TECHNIQUES IN THE INTENSIVE CARE UNIT

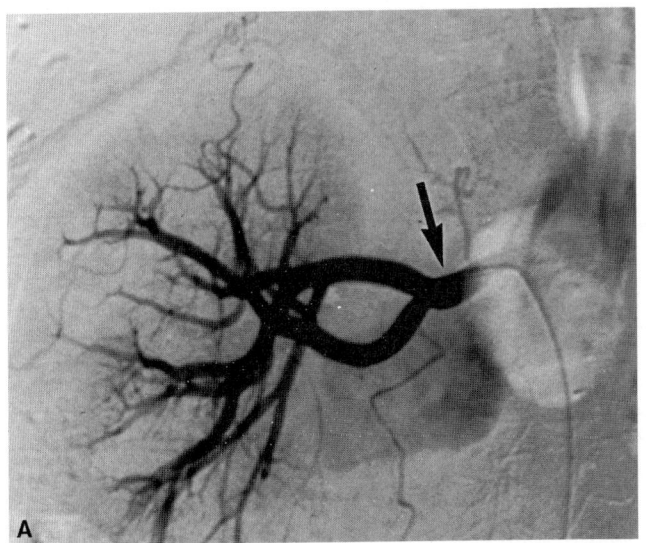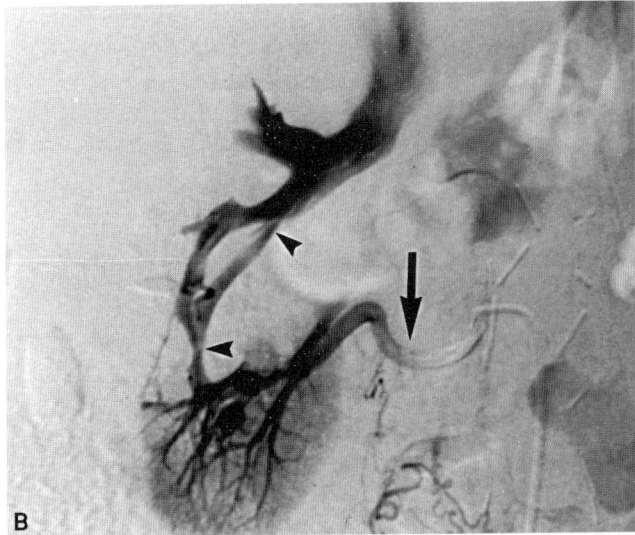

Fig. 71-110. Renal arteriovenous fistula. A renal arteriogram was performed after a renal biopsy on a 61-year-old patient with history of amyloidosis, hypotension, and hematuria. A, A selective right main renal arteriogram (arrow) shows no sign of hemorrhage. B, A selective accessory right renal artery arteriogram (arrow) demonstrates an arteriovenous fistula with the right renal vein (arrowheads). The fistula was successfully corrected with embolization material.

artery or vein that can occur immediately after surgery.[80] The loss of arterial flow owing to end-stage vascular rejection can be diagnosed by US when this shows a gradual decrease or loss of arterial flow. Loss of perfusion can also be confirmed by angiographic or scintigraphic studies (Fig. 71-111). Renal artery stenosis, a relatively common complication of transplantation (12%), can be diagnosed by duplex sonography or by scintigraphy but is usually confirmed by angiography.[81,82]

Peritransplant fluid collections are some of the complications that can be easily diagnosed and monitored radiologically. Hematomas and urinomas are among the early complications (7 to 10 days). Abscesses usually occur later (1 to 3 weeks), and lymphoceles occur 4 weeks or more after surgery. Both US and CT can detect the presence, the extent, and sometimes the nature of the fluid collections (Fig. 71-112). Plain films of the abdomen are helpful only if the fluid collections are large enough to create mass effect and displacement of the surrounding organs.

Although a renal biopsy is the definite diagnostic method for rejection, radiology can play an important role for the initial assessment of the renal morphology, texture (US), and renal function (scintigraphy). There are three major types of renal transplant rejection: a hyperacute rejection immediately after transplantation; an acute rejection that may occur within 6 to 12 months after surgery; and a chronic rejection, which is a result of a slow, progressive, and irreversible rejection. Chronic rejection may result in renal atrophy with diffuse renal calcinosis detectable by plain radiography (Fig. 71-113).

IMAGING OF ACUTE NEUROLOGIC DISEASE

The neurologic evaluation of the ICU patient can be difficult. Conditions such as a coma or a change of mental status are among the most commonly encountered clinical problems that need a prompt diagnostic investigation. Once metabolic causes are ruled out and central nervous involvement is suspected, a quick diagnosis of the intracranial abnormality is necessary to prevent high mortality and morbidity. MRI has become the method of choice for the evaluation of central and peripheral nervous pathology for

Fig. 71-111. Renal transplant infarcts. A technetium-99m glucoheptonate scan was obtained in a 46-year-old patient who had a renal transplant because of end-stage polycystic kidney disease. Early and delayed views of the pelvis demonstrate multiple wedge-shaped photopenic areas in the renal transplant compatible with infarcts (arrowheads). An arteriogram showed irregularity of the renal transplant artery but no definite stenosis.

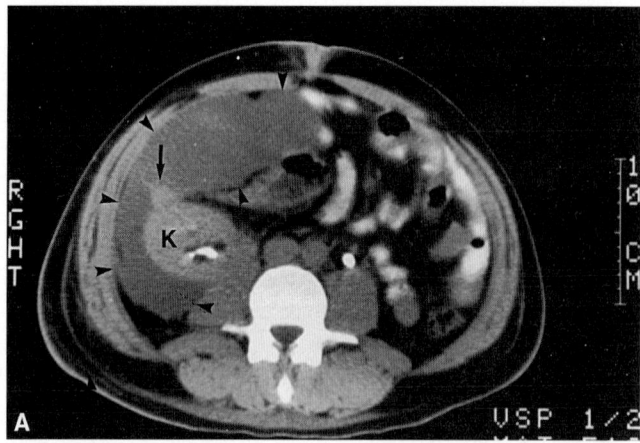 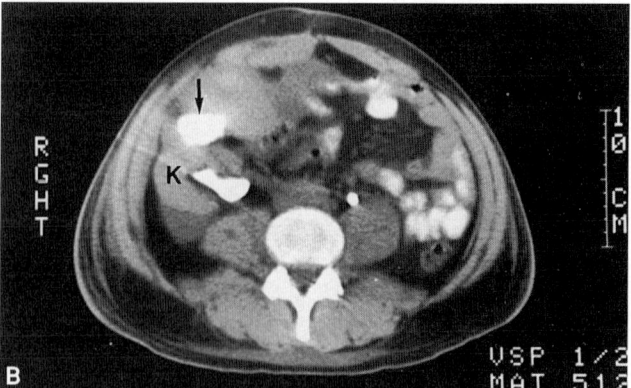

Fig. 71–112. *A, B,* Peritransplant urinoma. A CT scan examination with the administration of oral and intravenous contrast material was obtained in a 43-year-old patient who 10 days earlier had a right iliac fossa autorenal transplant. The examination was performed because of a decrease in the urine output and an increase of the serum creatinine level. An early axial image *(A)* and a delayed image *(B)* obtained through the lower abdomen demonstrate a fluid collection (arrowheads) surrounding the transplanted kidney (K). A small collection of extravasated contrast material is seen anterior to the kidney communicating with the perirenal collection, confirming the diagnosis of urinoma (arrow).

the ambulatory patient. Its use for critically ill patients, however, remains limited owing to the length of the examination and the inability of the MRI units to accommodate the extremely sick patients and their life-supporting devices. CT remains the method of choice in the initial assessment and monitoring of acute intracranial disease.

Acute infarction is one of the most common conditions that affects the brain in the ICU patient. Both acute hemorrhagic infarction and ischemic infarction, owing to the lack of blood flow to a portion of the brain, can be sensitively detected by CT.[83] The CT findings of ischemic infarcts can be divided into three categories based on the age of the cerebral changes. In the first 24 hours, the diagnosis can be difficult to ascertain by CT. During the acute phase, subtle focal areas of decreased attenuation of the brain matter, or effacement of the cortical sulci, may be seen within hours of the event representing early ischemic vasogenic edema (Fig. 71–114). Later during the acute phase (1 to 7 days), decreased attenuation of brain matter, effacement of the sulci, and mass effect become more evident, especially in large infarcts. The detection of involvement of specific central nervous system structures and compartments helps explain the clinical findings. The maximum mass effect is seen 3 to 10 days after infarction. During the subacute phase (7 to 21 days), there is resolution of the edema and mass effect, resulting in better delineation of the margins of the infarct seen on CT (Figs. 71–115 and 71–116). A CT scan after administration of intravenous

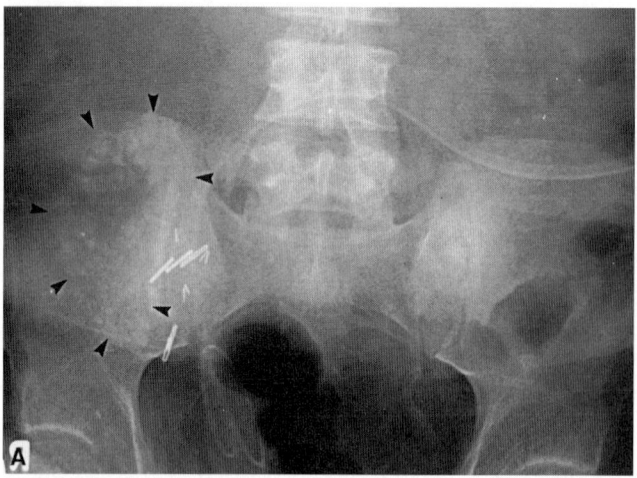 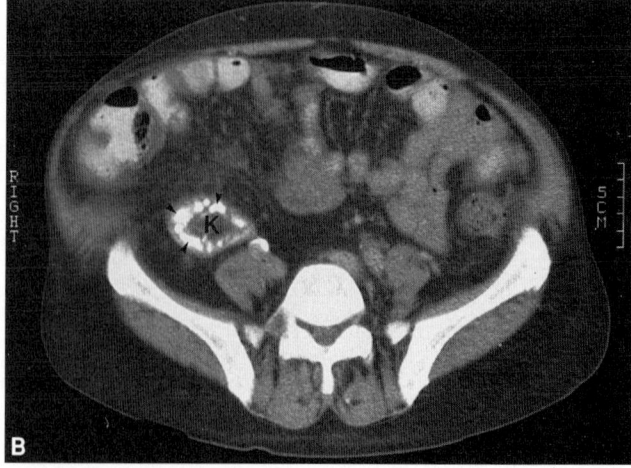

Fig. 71–113. Chronic renal transplantation rejection. *A,* A plain film of the abdomen obtained in a 46-year-old patient who is status post right iliac fossa renal transplantation demonstrates numerous amorphous calcification in a reniform distribution (arrowheads). Multiple surgical clips are seen at the site of the transplanted renal hilum. *B,* A CT scan examination obtained after the administration of oral contrast material demonstrates marked atrophy of the transplanted kidney (K) with extensive calcification throughout the cortex of the kidney (arrowheads).

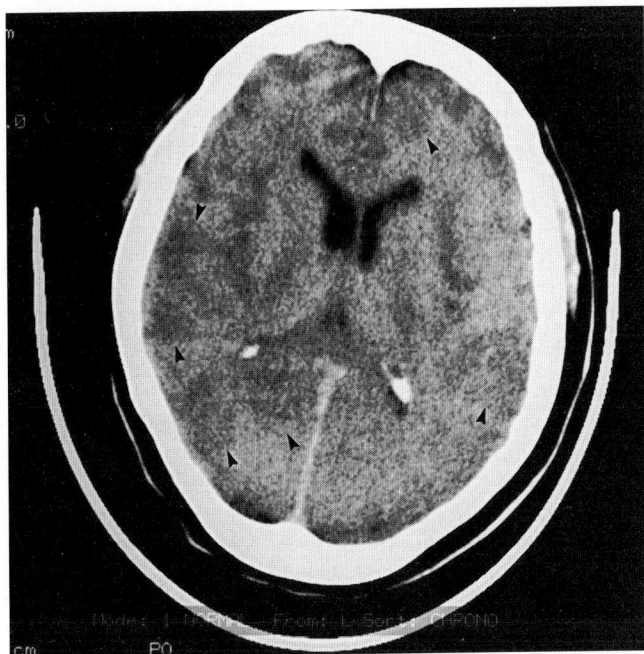

Fig. 71–114. Diffuse cerebral ischemia. An enhanced CT scan of the brain was obtained in a 71-year-old patient who had open heart surgery and a change of mental status in the postoperative period. An axial image obtained at the level of the frontal horns of the lateral ventricles demonstrates almost complete effacement of the sulci of the brain with multiple patchy areas of decreased attenuation of the cortical gray matter (arrowheads) involving both cerebral hemispheres and compatible with diffuse brain ischemia and edema. Causes of global hypoxic brain damage as seen in this patient include cardiorespiratory arrest, severe systemic hypotension, carbon monoxide poisoning, strangulation, and near-drowning.

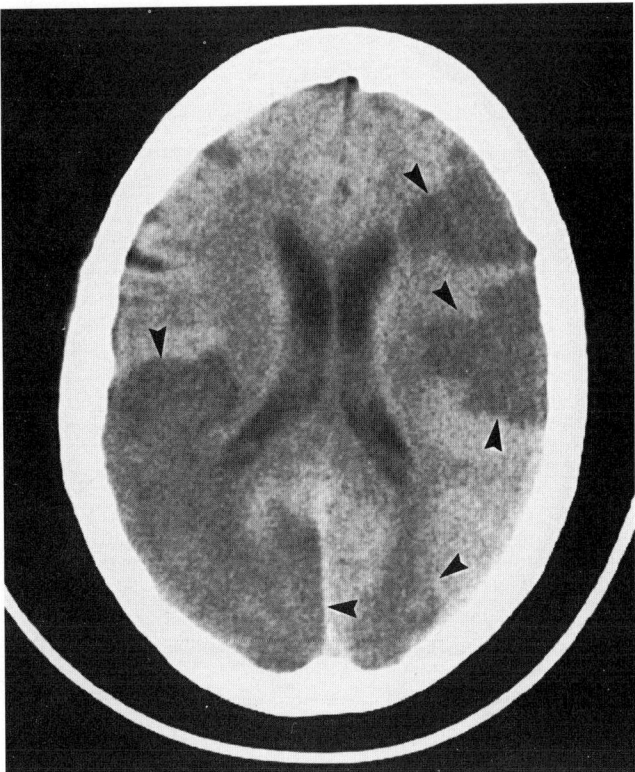

Fig. 71–115. Diffuse embolic cerebral infarctions. A nonenhanced CT scan of the brain was obtained in a 65-year-old patient who was found unresponsive. An axial image obtained at the level of the lateral ventricles demonstrates multiple areas of low attenuation throughout both hemispheres compatible with acute embolic infarcts (arrowheads). In this case, infarcts were detected both supratentorially and infratentorially. Note that there are no extra-axial fluid collections or midline shift.

contrast material may demonstrate areas of enhancement at the site of the infarct.[84] In the chronic stage, the reabsorbed necrotic tissue leaves areas of atrophy or cystic changes. In the cases of hemorrhagic infarction, nonenhanced CT scans demonstrate intraparenchymal areas of high attenuation owing to fresh bleeding in the area of infarction. Surrounding edema and mass effect are often present. The location of the hematoma, especially in the region of the basal ganglia, helps correlate the clinical findings (Fig. 71–117).

Aside from head trauma, the principal cause of intracerebral hematoma is hypertensive vascular disease. Other causes of bleeding include rupture of an aneurysm or arteriovenous malformation, postinfarction hemorrhage, collagen vascular disease, neoplasms, and anticoagulative therapy. Subarachnoid hemorrhage can be diagnosed when blood is visualized within the ventricles, cisterns, or the subarachnoid space surrounding the sulci of the brain (Fig. 71–118). The diagnosis of subarachnoid hemorrhage is important because the underlying cause, such as a ruptured aneurysm or arteriovenous malformation, needs to be corrected, preventing further complications (Fig. 71–119). Both intracranial complications (vasospasm and subsequent ischemic infarction, hydrocephalus) and extracranial complications (pulmonary edema and cardiac arrhythmias) can occur.

Subdural hematomas (SDHs) may occur in the ICU in patients with coagulopathies or who are receiving anticoagulants. Rarely, they may be seen following accidental falls while in the ICU. SDHs occur secondary to rupture of the thin-walled veins bridging the subdural space or rarely occur from bleeding of the superficial cerebral arteries. They are easily diagnosed by CT when there is active bleeding and mass effect (Fig. 71–120).[85] The characteristic CT appearance of SDH is that of a crescent-shaped collection between the skull and brain matter. Acute, subacute, and chronic SDHs have a higher, isodense, and lower attenuation than normal gray matter. A SDH that has become isodense with the brain can be difficult to diagnose but can be indirectly detected when there is displacement of the brain cortex and shift of midline structures (Fig. 71–121). The diagnosis becomes even more difficult in the presence of bilateral isodense hematomas when there is no shift of the midline structures. Epidural hematomas are less common in the ICU patient but more commonly seen associated with trauma and skull fractures (Fig. 71–122). The CT appearance of arterial epidural hematomas is of a lentiform-shaped collection often seen in the

1544   THE HIGH RISK PATIENT: MANAGEMENT OF THE CRITICALLY ILL

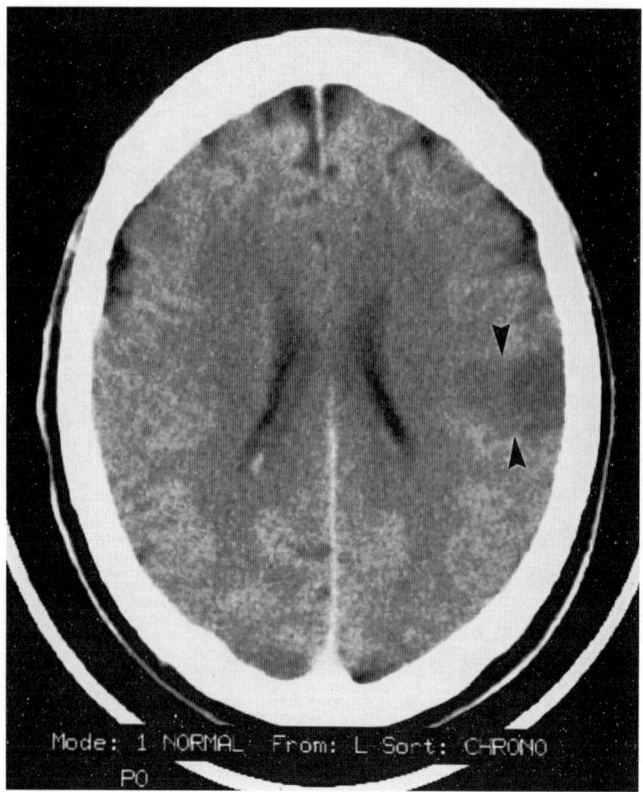

Fig. 71–116. Ischemic cerebral infarct in the left middle cerebral artery distribution. An enhanced CT scan of the brain was obtained in a 67-year-old patient who presented with right hemiparesis and aphasia after cardiac catheterization. A nonenhanced CT scan performed immediately after cardiac catheterization showed a questionable and subtle focal effacement over the left parietal convexity. The CT scan shown was obtained 2 days later. An axial image obtained at the level of the lateral ventricles shows a focal area of decreased attenuation within the cerebral cortex in the distribution of the left middle cerebral artery (arrowheads).

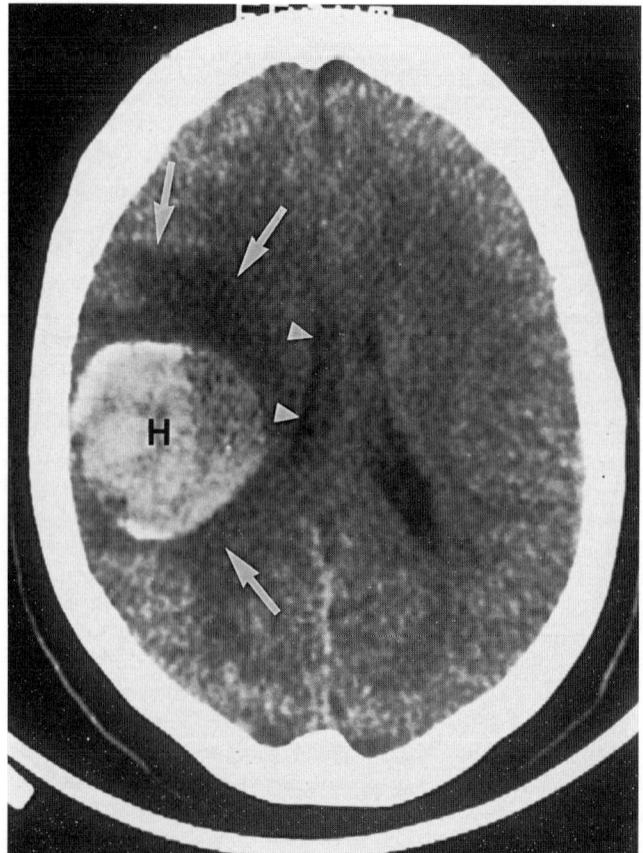

Fig. 71–117. Spontaneous cerebral hematoma owing to thrombocytopenia. A nonenhanced CT scan of the brain was obtained in a 58-year-old patient with a history of severe thrombocytopenia and a new onset of left facial droop and drooling. An axial image obtained at the level of the lateral ventricles demonstrates a large mass of high attenuation representing a hematoma (H) surrounded by low-attenuation areas caused by edema (arrows). There is a mass effect with disfacement of the right lateral ventricle (arrowheads).

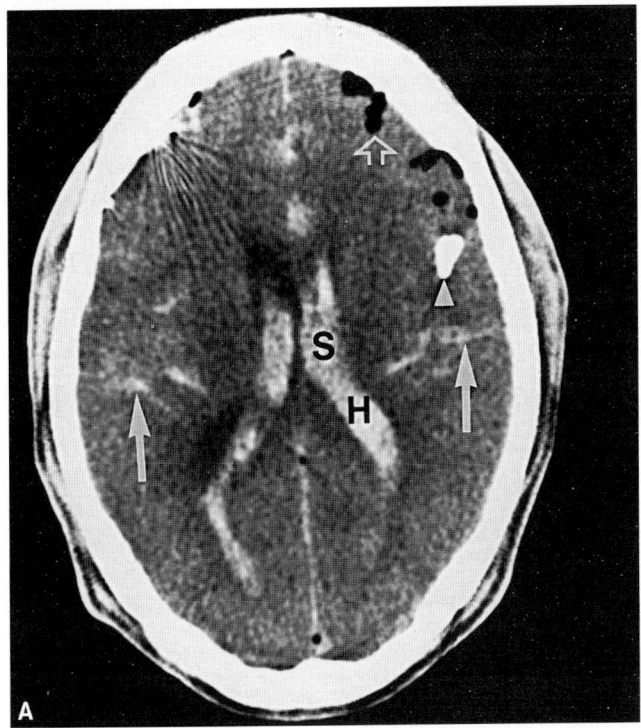
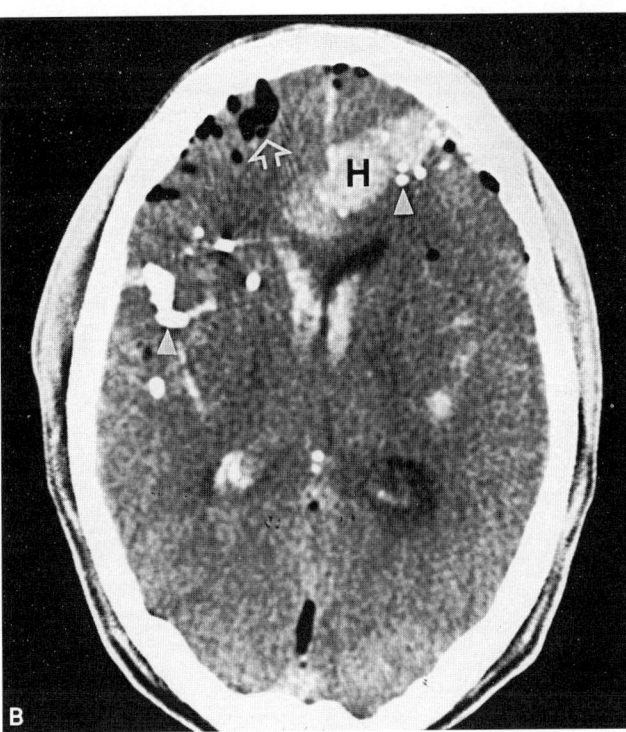

Fig. 71–118. *A, B,* Subarachnoid hemorrhage post gunshot wound. A nonenhanced CT scan of the brain was obtained in a 32-year-old patient who was unresponsive after a bullet wound to the head. Sequential images obtained through the level of the lateral ventricles *(A)* and at a slightly lower level *(B)* demonstrate extensive hemorrhage in the lateral ventricle seen as areas of high attenuation (SH) replacing the normally low-attenuation cerebrospinal fluid. Streaky bands of high attenuations are seen throughout the sulci representing hemorrhage within the subarachnoid space surrounding the sulci, best seen in the region of the sylvian fissures (arrows). A hematoma is seen in the left frontal area (H) secondary to cerebral contusion and trauma along the bullet track. Multiple bullet fragments are seen throughout the frontoparietal regions (plain arrowheads). Note also the multiple small air collections seen along the brain convexity (open arrowhead).

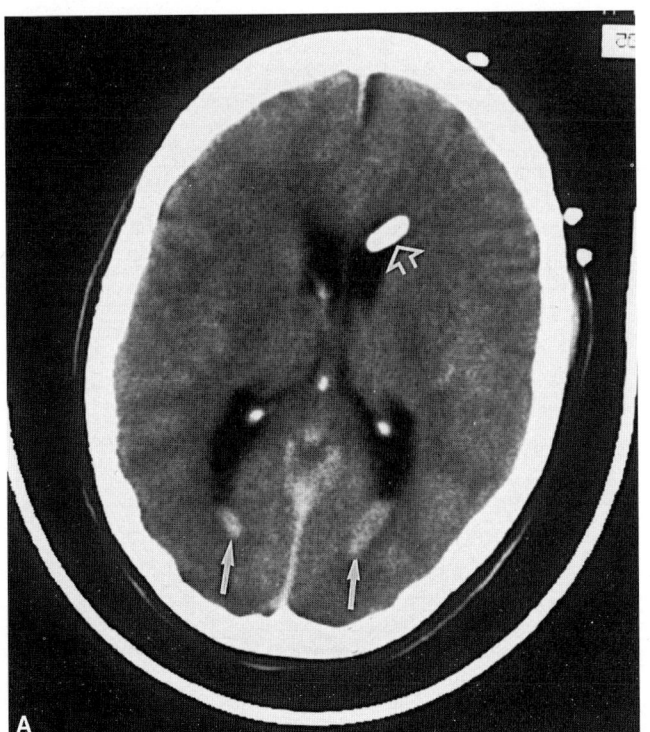
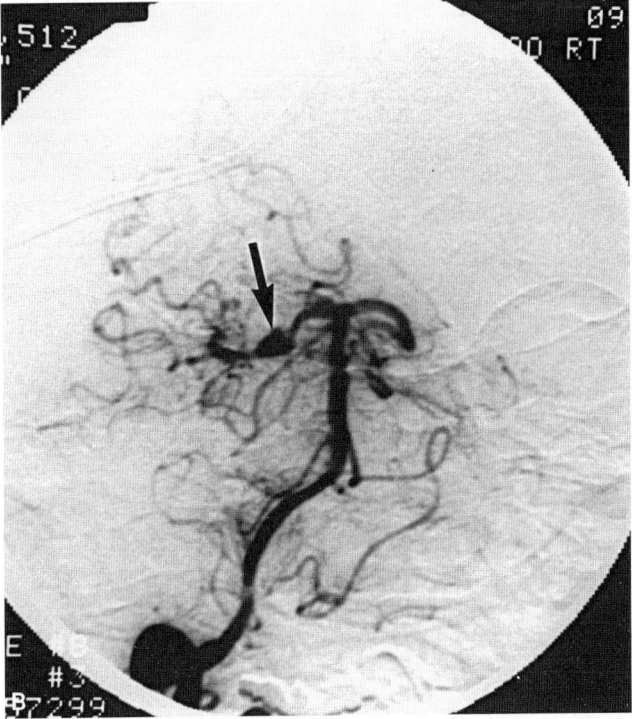

Fig. 71–119. Subarachnoid hemorrhage secondary to ruptured aneurysm. *A,* A nonenhanced CT scan of the brain was obtained in a 51-year-old patient with severe headaches and a history of prior seizures. Earlier scans demonstrated extensive subarachnoid hemorrhage and dilatation of the lateral ventricles. A ventriculoperitoneal shunting tube was placed to relieve the hydrocephalus. Following that, a nonenhanced CT scan of the brain shows residual blood within the dependent portion of the occipital horns of the lateral ventricles (arrows). The tube is in the left frontal horn of the lateral ventricles (open arrowhead). *B,* An intra-arterial digital subtraction angiogram of the vertebral arteries demonstrates a small 1-cm aneurysm (arrow) at the origin of the posterior-inferior cerebellar artery.

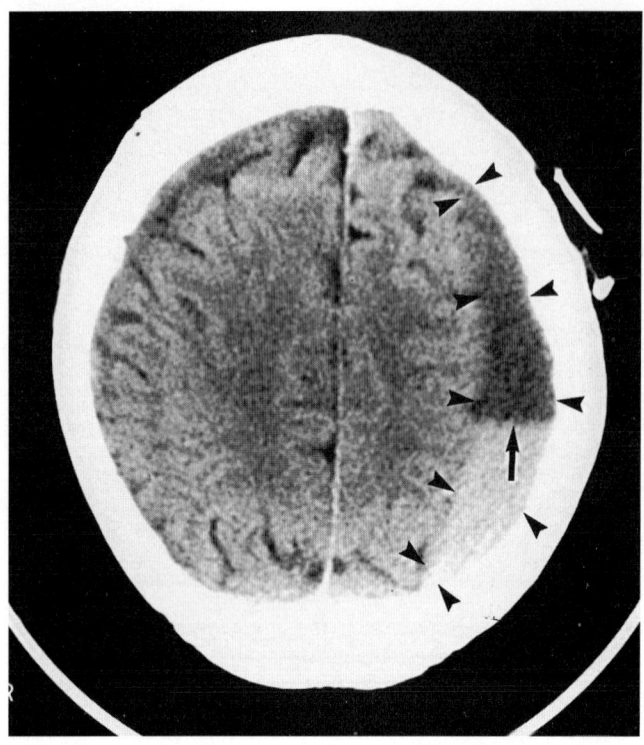

Fig. 71-120. Subdural hematoma. A nonenhanced CT scan of the brain was obtained in a 42-year-old patient with a prior history of surgery for a left frontal ganglioma and recent neurologic changes. An image obtained through the brain convexity demonstrates a crescentic-shaped extra-axial collection lateral to the occipitoparietal lobes (arrowheads). There is a red blood cell-fluid layer (arrow) within the subdural hematoma.

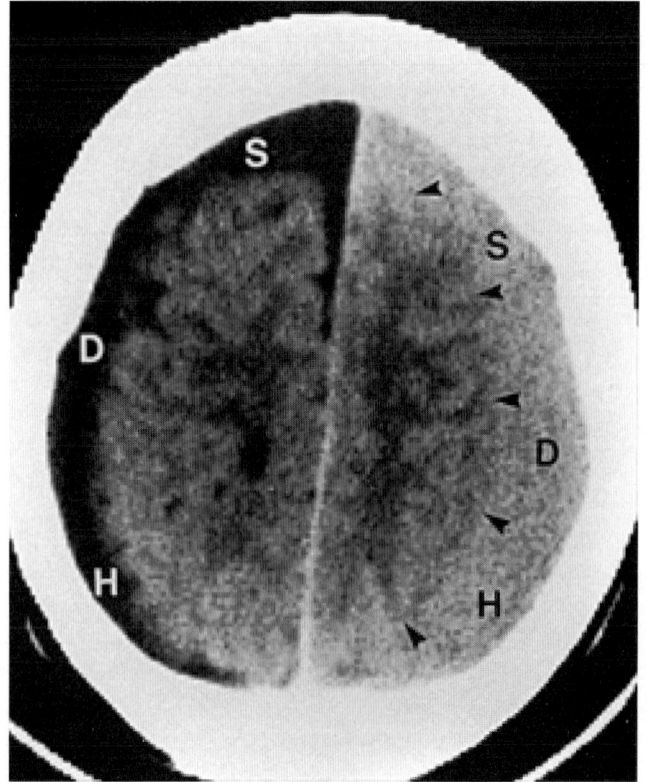

Fig. 71-121. Isodense subacute left subdural hematoma and hypodense chronic right subdural hematoma. A nonenhanced CT scan of the brain was obtained in an 81-year-old patient with a history of seizures. An image obtained through the cerebral convexity demonstrates a large left isodense subdural hematoma (SDH) causing medial displacement of the brain matter (arrowheads). A smaller, old hypodense subdural hematoma is seen on the right side (SDH).

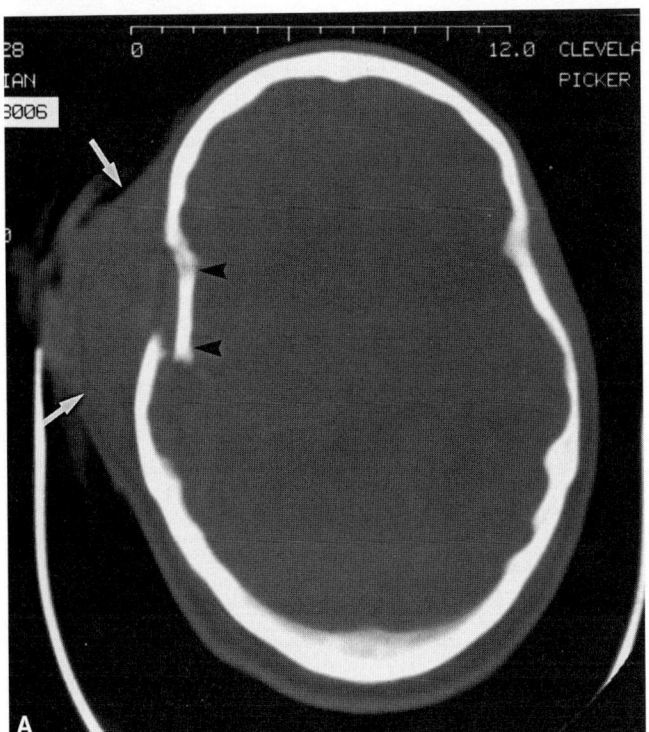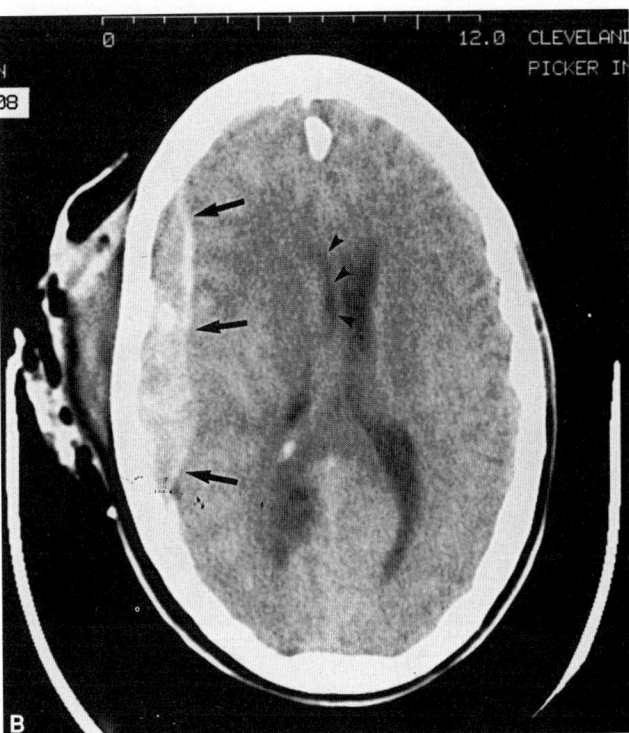

Fig. 71-122. Epidural hematoma with depressed skull fracture. An enhanced CT scan of the brain was obtained in a 32-year-old patient who was hit to the head with a brick. A, An axial image obtained through the brain with bone window settings demonstrates a depressed skull fracture in the right temporoparietal region (arrowheads) and marked soft tissue swelling (arrows). B, An axial image at a slightly higher level demonstrates a lentiform-shaped, localized extra-axial collection seen immediately adjacent to the skull fracture representing an epidural hematoma (arrows). Note the midline shift and compression of the right frontal horn of the lateral ventricles (arrowheads).

temporoparietal region. Epidural hematomas are seen after a meningeal artery tear as a result of a skull fracture. Venous epidural hematomas are seen more commonly at the skull vertex as a result of ruptured diploic veins or venous sinuses.

Infectious involvement of the brain is another clinical problem seen in the ICU, especially in the immunocompromised patient. Although abscesses can be easily diagnosed by CT, meningitis is more difficult.[86] In nonenhanced CT scans, abscesses show characteristic features. CT shows a thin isodense ring representing the fibrous capsule, a central hypodense zone composed of necrotic tissue and pus and a hypodense surrounding tissue representing reactive edema (Fig. 71-123A). On enhanced CT scans, the capsule shows a thin, ringlike, well-defined smooth enhancement (Fig. 71-123B). The appearance differs from the irregular thick enhancement seen in tumors and gyral-like enhancement in resolving hematomas. The clinical presentation and course are important to differentiate between the aforementioned entities. Meningitis is a diffuse process, more difficult to diagnose by CT because the scan often shows no abnormality. Meningitis can be suspected when there is diffuse enhancement of the meninges after administration of an intravenous contrast agent or in the presence of diffuse cerebral or cerebellar edema (Fig. 71-124).

The diagnosis of brain death is based on local established guidelines. They include cerebral and brain stem unresponsiveness for at least 24 hours, with absence of all the brain functions as evidenced by dilated unreactive pupils and absent eye movements. Electroencephalograms should demonstrate absence of electrocerebral activity. Radionuclide and contrast angiography may provide supplemental information when the brain stem cannot be evaluated. Angiogram of the brain demonstrates marked, prolonged circulation with nonvisualization of the brain circulation beyond the supracondyloid portion of the internal carotid artery (Fig. 71-125). The superior sagittal sinus is usually not visualized. One needs to put the angiographic findings with the clinical context because other clinical conditions may have a prolonged circulation time. These include marked increase of intracranial pressure, arterial thrombosis, arterial sclerosis, and arterial spasm.

APPENDIX

There is a continuous debate over the sensitivity and specificity of the different imaging modalities that are now available to clinicians. Certain complex clinical conditions can be easily diagnosed by simple, accessible imaging means, but certain conditions may need complex and costly studies to be diagnosed. Physicians have to decide on what is the most appropriate modality that will offer a

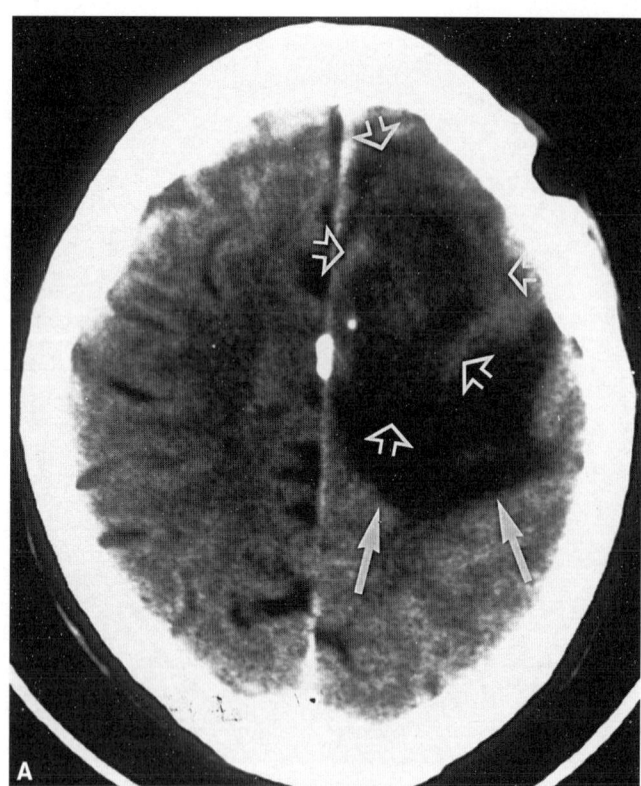
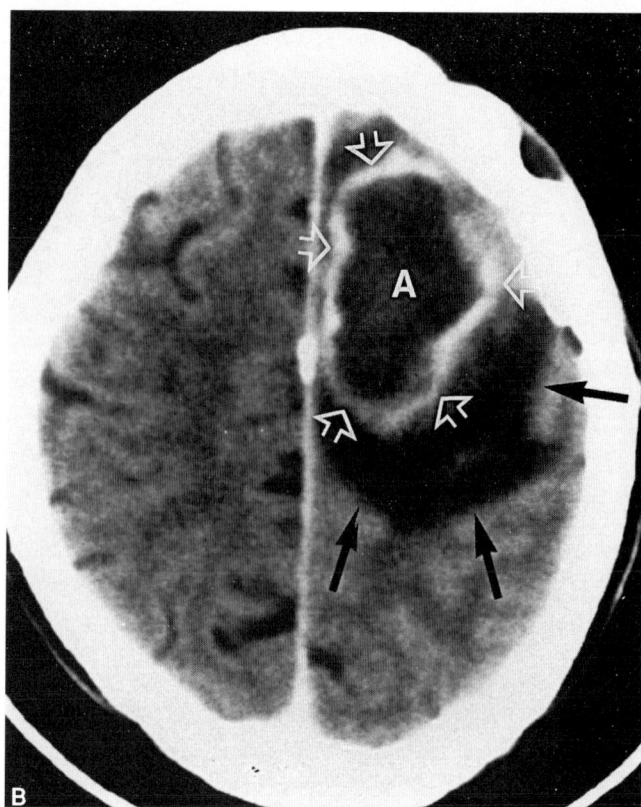

Fig. 71–123. Brain abscess. A CT scan of the brain was obtained in a 58-year-old patient with prior craniotomy for excision of meningioma 5 weeks earlier and a history of 1 week of progressive right-sided hemiparesis and expressive aphasia. *A*, An image obtained after a nonenhanced CT scan through the cerebral convexities demonstrates a large low-density lesion involving the left frontoparietal region (open arrowheads) surrounded by edema (arrows). *B*, An image obtained after the administration of intravenous contrast material demonstrates that the lesion (A) has an enhancing ring (arrowheads). Note the surrounding vasogenic edema (arrows). The culture was positive for Propionibacterium acnes.

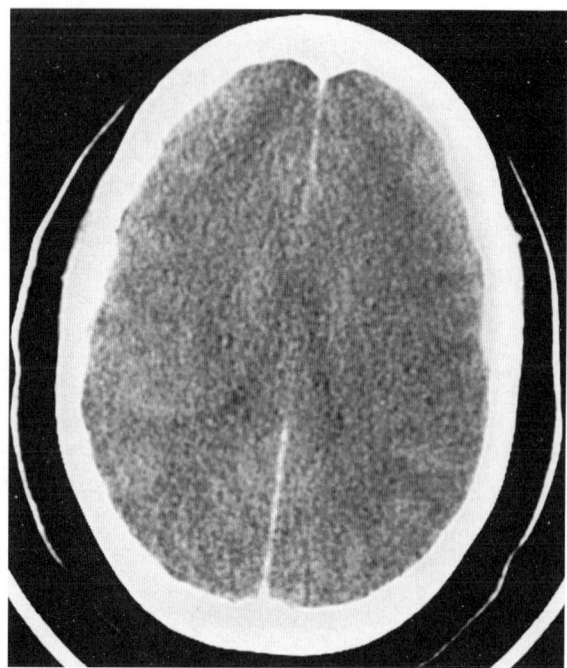

Fig. 71–124. Meningitis (cerebral edema). Axial image through the level of the lateral ventricles obtained during a nonenhanced CT scan of the brain in a 45-year-old woman with streptococcal meningitis demonstrate effacement of the cortical sulci resulting from diffuse edema.

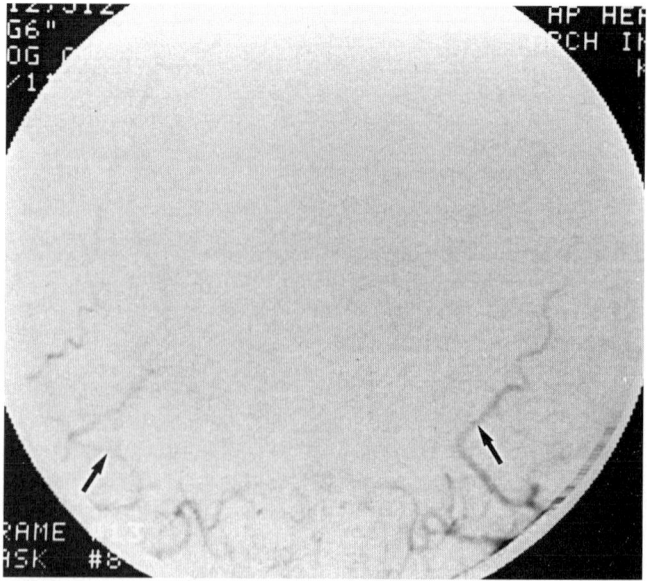

Fig. 71–125. Brain death—angiography. An angiogram of the brain was obtained in a 46-year-old patient who had brain surgery for the clipping of an aneurysm. He subsequently developed a left hemispheric infarct followed by subfalcian and transtentorial herniation. The intracranial circulation was evaluated from an aortic arch injection. The anteroposterior view demonstrates no filling of the internal carotid artery on either side. Delayed images demonstrate slight filling of both vertebral arteries (arrows) but no brain circulation.

Table 71-6. Common Clinical Conditions Encountered in the ICU

Organ	Condition	Primary Screening Imaging Modality	Secondary or Confirmatory Imaging Modality
Abdomen	Ascites	US	CT, PF abdomen
	Neoplasm	CT	US
	Pneumoperitoneum	PF abdomen	
Airways	Obstruction, narrowing, displacement, rupture	CXR	CT, PF of soft tissues
Aorta (thoracic)	Aneurysm, dilatation	CXR	CT
	Dissection, rupture	CT	Angiography, CXR
Aorta (abdominal)	Aneurysm, dilatation	US	CT, angiography
	Dissection, rupture	CT	Angiography, US
Bladder	Hemorrhage	US	CT
	Infection	US	Cystogram, CT
	Obstruction, dilatation	US	Cystogram, CT
	Neoplasm	US	CT, cystogram
Bowel (small)	Ileus	PF abdomen	
	Ischemia, hemorrhage	Angiography	
	Neoplasm	UGI	CT
	Obstruction	PF abdomen	UGI
	Perforation	PF abdomen	CT
Bowel (large)	Diverticulitis, abscess	CT	BE
	Ileus	PF abdomen	
	Ischemia, hemorrhage	Angiography	
	Neoplasm	BE	CT
	Obstruction	PF abdomen	BE
	Perforation	PF abdomen	CT
	Toxic megacolon	PF abdomen	
	Volvulus	PF abdomen	BE
Brain	Abscess, infection	CT	
	Aneurysm, arteriovenous malformation	CT	Angiography
	Hemorrhage	CT	
	Infarction	CT	
	Neoplasm	CT	
Esophagus	Dilatation	CXR	CT
	Hemorrhage	CT	Angiography
	Infection	UGI	CXR, CT
	Rupture	Barium or gastrographin swallow	CT
	Neoplasm	UGI	CT
Gallbladder	Cholecystitis	NM	US
	Gallstone	US	PF abdomen
	Obstruction	NM	US
Heart	Abscess, infection	CT	US
	Aneurysm	US	CXR, NM, CT
	Enlargement	CXR	US
	Pericardial effusion, hemopericardium	US	CT, CXR
	Infarction	NM	
	Neoplasm	CT	US
Kidney	Abscess, infection	CT	US, PF abdomen
	Cyst	US	CT
	Hemorrhage, infarction	CT	Angiography, US
	Obstruction, hydronephrosis	US, angiography	IVP, CT, cholangiogram
	Neoplasm	CT	US
	Stone, calcification	PF abdomen	US, CT, IVP
	Rejection	US	NM
Liver	Abscess, infection	CT	US
	Biliary tree abnormality	US	Cholangiogram, CT
	Neoplasm	CT	US, angiography
	Hepatic vascular or portal abnormality	US	Angiography
Lungs	Aspiration	CXR	
	Atelectasis	CXR	CT
	Cavitation, emphysema	CXR	CT
	Hemorrhage	CXR	CT
	Pneumonia, abscess, septic emboli	CXR	CT
	Pulmonary emboli, infarct	VQ scan	Angiography CXR, CT
	Neoplasm	CXR	CT
Mediastinum	Abscess, infection	CT	CXR
	Adenopathy	CT	CXR
	Hemorrhage	CT	CXR, angiography
	Pneumomediastinum	CXR	CT

(continued)

Table 71-6. Common Clinical Conditions Encountered in the ICU—*(Continued)*

Organ	Condition	Primary Screening Imaging Modality	Secondary or Confirmatory Imaging Modality
Pancreas	Acute pancreatitis	CT	US
	Pseudocyst	US	CT
	Neoplasm	CT	US
Prostate	Enlargement, neoplasm	US	CT
Retroperitoneum	Hemorrhage	CT	Angiography
	Infection, tumor	CT	US
Spleen	Abscess, hemorrhage, tumor	CT	US
Vascular	Arteriosclerosis, narrowing, obstruction	US	Angiography
	Deep venous thrombosis	US	Angiography
	Superior vena cava syndrome	CT	Angiography
Uterus	Enlargement, neoplasm	US	
	Hemorrhage, infection	US	
	Pregnancy	US	

BE, Barium enema, CXR, chest x-ray film; CT, computed tomography; IVP, intravenous pyelogram; NM, nuclear medicine scan; PF, plain films; US, ultrasound; UGI, upper gastrointestinal series; VQ, ventilation perfusion.

precise diagnosis using the most convenient, cost-efficient means. Table 71-6 lists the common clinical conditions encountered in the ICU. Certain sensitive modalities, such as MRI, have been intentionally omitted because they are not primarily designed for the acutely ill patient. The primary or screening imaging modality should be considered first. If a diagnosis cannot be attained or if the modality is not available, one needs to consider the secondary modality as either an alternative or as a final step. There are no strict guidelines to the list offered because the examinations vary greatly depending on the condition of the patient, the availability of the radiologic equipment, and the personal preference and skill level of the physicians involved in the studies.

REFERENCES

1. O'Donovan, P. B., et al.: Device for facilitating precise alignment in bedside radiography. Radiology, *184:*284, 1992.
2. Fuhrman, C. R., Gur, D., and Schaetzing, R.: High-resolution digital imaging with storage phosphors. J. Thorac. Imag., *5:*21, 1990.
3. DeSimone, D. N., et al.: Effect of a digital imaging network on physician behavior in an intensive care unit. Radiology, *169:*41, 1988.
4. Cho, P. S., et al.: Clinical evaluation of a radiologic picture archiving and communication system for a coronary care unit. Am. J. Roentgenol., *151:*823, 1988.
5. Henschke, C. I., et al.: Bedside chest radiography: diagnostic efficacy. Radiology, *149:*23, 1983.
6. Conrardy, P. A., Goodman, L. R., Lainge, R., and Singer, M. M.: Alteration of endotracheal tube position: flexion and extension of the neck. Crit. Care Med., *4:*7, 1976.
7. Arola, M. K., Inberg, M. V., and Puhakka, H.: Tracheal stenosis after tracheostomy and after orotracheal cuffed intubation. Acta Chir. Scand., *147:*183, 1981.
8. Webb, W. R., and LaBerge, J. M.: Radiographic recognition of chest tube malposition in the major fissure. Chest, *85:*81, 1984.
9. McWey, R. E., et al.: Complications of nasoenteric feeding tubes. Am. J. Surg., *155:*253, 1988.
10. Langston, C. S.: The aberrant central venous catheter and its complications. Radiology, *100:*55, 1971.
11. Kline, I. K., and Hofman, W. I.: Cardiac tamponade from CVP catheter perforation. JAMA, *206:*1794, 1968.
12. Bone, D. K., Maddrey, W. C., Eagan, J., and Cameron, J. L.: Cardiac tamponade: a fatal complication of central venous catheterization. Arch. Surg., *106:*868, 1973.
13. Sise, M. J., et al.: Complications of the flow-directed pulmonary artery catheter: a prospective analysis of 219 patients. Crit. Care Med., *9:*315, 1981.
14. McLoud, T. C., and Putman, C. E.: Radiology of the Swan-Ganz catheter and associated pulmonary complications. Radiology, *116:*19, 1975.
15. Pace, P. D., Tilney, N. L., Lesch, M., and Couch, N. P.: Peripheral arterial complications on intra-aortic balloon counterpulsation. Surgery, *82:*685, 1977.
16. Strandberg, A., et al.: Atelectasis during anesthesia and in the postoperative period. Acta Anaesthesiol. Scand., *30:*154, 1986.
17. Shevland, J., Hirleman, M. T., Huang, K. A., and Kealey, G. P.: Lobar collapse in the surgical intensive care unit. Br. J. Radiol., *56:*531, 1983.
18. Bryant, L. R., et al.: Misdiagnosis of pneumonia in patients needing mechanical respiration. Arch. Surg., *106:*286, 1973.
19. Huang, R. M., et al.: Septic pulmonary emboli: CT-radiographic correlation. Am. J. Roentgenol., *153:*41, 1989.
20. Kuhlman, J. E., Fishman, E. K., and Teigen, C.: Pulmonary septic emboli: diagnosis with CT. Radiology, *174:*211, 1990.
21. Landay, M. J., Christensen, E. E., and Bynum, L. J.: Pulmonary manifestations of acute aspiration of gastric contents. Am. J. Roentgenol., *131:*587, 1978.
22. Sivak, E. D., Richmond, B. J., O'Donovan, P. B., and Borkowski, G. P.: Valve of extravascular lung water measurements vs. portable chest x-ray in the management of pulmonary edema. Crit. Care Med., *11:*498, 1983.
23. Halperin, B. D., et al.: Evaluation of the portable chest roentgenogram for quantitating extravascular lung water in critically ill adults. Chest, *88:*649, 1985.
24. Pistolesi, M., and Giuntini, C.: Assessment of extravascular lung water. Radiol. Clin. North Am., *16:*551, 1978.
25. Nakahara, K., et al.: Dynamic insufficiency of lung lymph from the right lymph duct with acute infiltration edema. Am. Rev. Respir. Dis., *127:*67, 1983.

26. Calenoff, L., Kruglik, G., Woodruff, A.: Unilateral pulmonary edema. Radiology, *126*:19, 1978.
27. Leeming, B. W. A.: Gravitational edema of the lungs observed during assisted respiration. Chest, *64*:719, 1973.
28. Greene, R., Jantsch, H., Boggis, C., and Strauss, W.: Respiratory distress syndrome with new consideration. Radiol. Clin. North Am., *21*:699, 1983.
29. Bernard, R. W., Stahl, W. M., and Chase, R. M.: Subclavian vein catheterizations: a perspective study. II. Infectious complications. Ann. Surg., *173*:191, 1971.
30. Zwilich, C. W., et al.: Complications of assisted ventilation: a prospective study of 354 consecutive episodes. Am. J. Med., *57*:161, 1974.
31. Bone, R. C.: Complications of mechanical ventilation and positive end-expiratory pressure. Respir. Care, *27*:402, 1982.
32. Sherman, M., Levin, D., and Breidbart, D.: Pneumocystis carinii pneumonia with spontaneous pneumothorax: a report of three cases. Chest, *90*:609, 1986.
33. Gordon, R.: The deep sulcus sign. Radiology, *136*:25, 1980.
34. Gobien, R. P., Reines, H. D., and Schabel, S. J.: Localized tension pneumothorax: unrecognized form of barotrauma in adult respiratory distress syndrome. Radiology, *142*:15, 1986.
35. Light, R. W., and George, R. B.: Incidence and significance of pleural effusions after abdominal surgery. Chest, *69*:621, 1976.
36. Woodring, J. H.: Recognition of pleural effusion on supine radiographs: how much fluid is required? Am. J. Roentgenol., *142*:59, 1984.
37. Ruskin, J. A., Gurney, J. W., Thorsen, M. K., and Goodman, L. R.: Detection of pleural effusions on supine chest radiographs. Am. J. Roentgenol., *148*:681, 1987.
38. McLoud, T., and Flower, C.: Imaging of the pleura: sonography, CT and MR imaging. Am. J. Roentgenol., *156*:1145, 1991.
39. Adkins, P. C., and Slovin, A. J.: Complications of pulmonary resection. *In* Management of Surgical Complications. 3rd Ed. Edited by C. P. Artz and J. D. Hardy. Philadelphia, W. B. Saunders, 1975, p. 309.
40. Kerr, W. F.: Late-onset post-pneumonectomy empyema. Thorax, *32*:149, 1977.
41. Carter, A. R., Sostman, H. D., Curtis, A. M., and Swett, H. A.: Thoracic alterations after cardiac surgery. Am. J. Roentgenol., *140*:475, 1983.
42. Wilcox, P., et al.: Phrenic nerve function and its relationship to atelectasis after coronary artery bypass surgery. Chest, *93*:693, 1988.
43. Stevenson, L. W., Child, J. S., Laks, H., and Kern, L.: Incidence and significance of early pericardial effusions after cardiac surgery. Am. J. Cardiol., *54*:848, 1984.
44. Fyke, F. E., III, et al.: Detection of intrapericardial hematoma after open heart surgery: the roles of echocardiography and computed tomography. J. Am. Coll. Cardiol., *5*:1496, 1985.
45. Hirst, A. E., Jr., Johns, V. J., Jr., and Klime, S. W., Jr.: Dissecting aneurysm of the aorta: a review of 505 cases. Medicine, *37*:217, 1958.
46. Wyman, S. M.: Dissecting aneurysm of the thoracic aorta: its roentgen recognition. Am. J. Roentgenol., *78*:247, 1957.
47. Eyler, W. R., and Clark, M. D.: Dissecting aneurysms of the aorta: roentgen manifestations including a comparison with other types of aneurysms. Radiology, *85*:1047, 1965.
48. Victor, M. F., et al.: Two-dimensional echocardiographic diagnosis of aortic dissection. Am. J. Cardiol., *48*:1155, 1981.
49. Godwin, J. D., et al.: Evaluation of dissections and aneurysms of the thoracic aorta by conventional and dynamic CT scanning. Radiology, *136*:125, 1980.
50. Larde, D., et al.: Computed tomography of aortic dissection. Radiology, *136*:147, 1980.
51. Stein, H. L., and Steinberg, I.: Selective aortography, definitive technique for the diagnosis of dissecting aneurysm of the aorta. Am. J. Roentgenol., *102*:333, 1968.
52. Kersting-Sommerhoff, B. A., et al.: Aortic dissection: sensitivity and specificity of MR imaging. Radiology, *166*:651, 1988.
53. DeBakey, M. E., Cooley, D. A., and Creech, O., Jr.: Surgical considerations of dissecting aneurysm of the aorta. Ann. Surg., *142*:586, 1955.
54. Shuman, W. P., et al.: Suspected leaking abdominal aortic aneurysm: use of sonography in the emergency room. Radiology, *168*:117, 1988.
55. Darling, R. C., Messina, C. R., Brewster, D. C., and Ottinger, L. W.: Autopsy study of unoperated abdominal aortic aneurysms: the case for early resection. Circulation, *56*:161, 1977.
56. Levine, M. S., et al.: Diagnosis of pneumoperitoneum on supine abdominal radiographs. Am. J. Roentgenol., *156*:731, 1991.
57. Peora, D. A.: Stress-related mucosal damage: an overview. Am. J. Med., *83(Suppl. 6A)*:3, 1987.
58. Casola, G., et al.: Percutaneous cecostomy for decompression of the massively distended cecum. Radiology, *158*:793, 1986.
59. Jeffrey, R. B., Jr.: Sonography in acute pancreatitis. Radiol. Clin. North Am., *27*:5, 1989.
60. Siegelman, S. S., et al.: CT of fluid collections associated with pancreatitis. Am. J. Roentgenol., *134*:1121, 1980.
61. Jeffrey, R. B., Federle, M. P., and Laing, F. C.: Computed tomography of mesenteric involvement in fulminant pancreatitis. Radiology, *147*:185, 1983.
62. Federle, M. P., et al.: Computed tomography of pancreatic abscesses. Am. J. Roentgenol., *136*:879, 1981.
63. Ralls, P. W., et al.: Real-time sonography in suspected acute cholecystitis. Radiology, *155*:767, 1985.
64. Madrazo, B. L., et al.: Sonographic findings in perforation of the gallbladder. Radiology, *139*:491, 1982.
65. Freitas, J. E.: Cholecystintigraphy in acute and chronic cholecystis. Semin. Nucl. Med., *12*:18, 1982.
66. Wing, V. M., et al.: The clinical impact of CT for blunt abdominal trauma. Am. J. Roentgenol., *145*:1191, 1985.
67. Federle, M. P., and Jeffrey, R. B.: Hemoperitoneum studied by computed tomography. Radiology, *148*:187, 1983.
68. Lerner, R. M., and Spataro, R. F.: Splenic abscess: percutaneous drainage. Radiology, *153*:643, 1984.
69. Callen, P. W.: Computed tomographic evaluation of abdominal and pelvic abscesses. Radiology, *131*:171, 1979.
70. Crass, J. R., and Karl, R.: Bedside drainage of abscesses with sonographic guidance in the desperately ill. Am. J. Roentgenol., *139*:183, 1982.
71. Kamholtz, R. G., Cronan, J. J., and Dorfman, G. S.: Obstruction and the minimally dilated renal collecting system: US evaluation. Radiology, *170*:51, 1989.
72. Silver, T. M., et al.: The radiological spectrum of acute pyelonephritis in adults and adolescents. Radiology, *118*:65, 1976.
73. Degesys, D. E., et al.: Retroperitoneal fibrosis: use of CT in distinguishing among possible causes. Am. J. Roentgenol., *146*:57, 1986.
74. Hoddick, W., et al.: CT and sonography of severe renal and perirenal infections. Am. J. Roentgenol., *140*:517, 1983.
75. Lang, E. K.: Renal, perirenal, and perirenal abscesses: percutaneous drainage. Radiology, *174*:109, 1990.
76. Glazer, G., et al.: Computed tomography of renal infarction: clinical and experimental observations. Am. J. Roentgenol., *140*:721, 1983.
77. Hilton, S., et al.: CT findings in acute renal infarction. Urol. Radiol., *6*:158, 1984.

78. Cass, A. S., and Luxenberg, M.: Features of 164 bladder ruptures. J. Urol., *138:*743, 1987.
79. Sandler, C. M., Harris, J. H., Jr., Corriere, J. N., Jr., and Toombs, B. D.: Posterior urethral injuries after pelvic fracture. Am. J. Roentgenol., *137:*1233, 1981.
80. Taylor, K. J. W., et al.: Vascular complications in renal allografts: detection with duplex Doppler US. Radiology, *162:*31, 1987.
81. Faenza, B., et al.: Renal artery stenosis after renal transplantation. Kidney Int., *23(Suppl. 14):*S54, 1983.
82. Snider, J. F., et al.: Transplant renal artery stenosis: evaluation with duplex sonography. Radiology, *172:*1027, 1989.
83. Drayer, B., et al.: The capacity for computer tomography diagnosis of cerebral infarction. Radiology, *125:*393, 1977.
84. Weisberg, L. A.: Computerized tomographic enhancement patterns in cerebral infarction. Arch. Neurol., *37:*21, 1980.
85. Bergstrom, M., et al.: Computed tomography of cranial subdural and epidural hematomas: variations of attenuation related to time and clinical events such as rebleeding. J. Comput. Assist. Tomogr., *1:*449, 1977.
86. Britt, R. H., and Enzmann, D. R.: Clinical stages of human brain abscesses on serial CT scans after contrast infusion: computerized tomographic, neuropathological, and clinical correlations. J. Neurosurg., *59:*972, 1983.

Section Ten

MANAGERIAL AND QUALITY ASSURANCE ISSUES

Chapter 72

THE TEAM CONCEPT OF PATIENT CARE

KATHLEEN DRACUP
BART CHERNOW

Over the course of a noncritical illness, patients develop unique relationships with a variety of health care professionals. The collaborative efforts of these individuals are often less important to a good outcome than the knowledge and talent of a specific professional. For example, the diagnostic acumen and interpersonal skills of the physician may be the critical factors in a patient's recovery from an illness that does not require hospitalization. A hospice nurse may be the key to a patient's dignified dying at home. A physical therapist may be responsible for the physical recovery of a patient following a stroke. Thus, the team concept of patient care can translate in practice to a team of physicians, a team of nurses, a team of pharmacists, etc., working in a model that some have compared to toddlers in parallel play.[1]

Critical care is different. Optimal patient care in an intensive care unit (ICU) requires the intense collaborative efforts of a variety of professionals, i.e., physicians, nurses, pharmacists, social workers, dietitians, physical therapists, biomedical engineers, and respiratory therapists, among others. A critical care unit is far more than a collection of individual nurses and physicians caring for individual patients. The interdependencies that exist in the ICU team actually define the unit, with the whole being far greater than the sum of its parts.

The ICU has long been identified as a model for interdisciplinary collaboration because the demands of caring for an individual in severe physiologic crisis requires that all professionals work closely and effectively with each other.[2-4] In this discussion, we consider impediments to effective teamwork, and strategies that can be used to enhance it prior to the admission of a patient to intensive care, during his or her stay in the ICU, and during the recovery phase after ICU discharge.

PHYSICIAN-NURSE COLLABORATION

Although many of the issues surrounding collaborative practice have similar ramifications for the various professions represented on the ICU team, collaboration between medicine and nursing is highlighted in this chapter. The relationships between members of these two disciplines are important because physicians and nurses are the major players in ICU patient care and because their relationship appears to affect patient outcomes significantly.

Medicine and Nursing Central to Patient Care

Nursing and medicine play central roles in the care of the critically ill patient, and the overlap is large between the domains of the two professions in the ICU. According to Bates, "Medicine and nursing have common goals: the preservation and restoration of health. Yet, their roles in achieving these objectives are not identical and may be visualized as two overlapping circles, each with its own content but sharing a common ground."[5] In comparison, the other professions play more of a supporting role in patient care and enjoy clearer role definitions than the boundary that exists between medicine and nursing. The overlay between the professional roles of critical care physicians and nurses can have an important impact on the recovery of patients who require intensive care.

Impact on Patient Outcomes

In a study of 5030 patients hospitalized in ICUs, Knaus and colleagues[6] identified variation in nurse-physician collaboration as a primary factor in differing mortality rates in ICUs. Among the 13 hospitals studied, one hospital had 41% fewer deaths than predicted, whereas another had 58% more deaths than predicted. The researchers found that the communication patterns of the physicians and nurses working in the ICUs of the hospitals with the lowest actual-to-predicted mortality ratio were characterized by mutual respect, frequent interaction, and joint goal setting. In contrast, the relationships of physicians and nurses in the hospitals with the worst mortality statistics were characterized by difficult and incomplete communication. Based on the mortality statistics, the researchers ranked hospitals from 1 (best) to 13 (worst). As described by Knaus and colleagues, physicians and nurses in hospital 12 had problems ". . . because of personality differences and the lack of an institutional structure in which to resolve them."[7] In hospital 13, "No policy was established for routine discussion of patient treatment, and there was no direct coordination of staff capabilities with clinical demands. Frequent disagreements about the ability of the nursing staff to treat additional patients occurred, and there was an atmosphere of distrust."[8]

The findings of Knaus and colleagues reflect the reality of physician-nurse teamwork in the intensive care setting. In some units, working relationships are close to ideal and are supported by hospital administrative structures that facilitate effective communication and mutual respect.[9] In others, relationships are characterized by mistrust, disrespect, and open hostility.[11] As key members of the team, physicians and nurses most often set the tone for the working relationships of the other members of the team; therefore, an analysis that focuses on "the good, the bad, and the ugly" in physician-nurse relationships is key to understanding how to achieve optimal ICU team functioning.

Impediments to Effective Teamwork

Given the commitment of the medical and nursing professions to effective teamwork in the ICU, one might question how it could be undermined. Two potential sources of conflict exist. First, conflict can occur over the decisions related to patient care and the processes by which those decisions are made. Second, conflict is rooted in the different traditions that inspire the two professions and that provide the bases for various value judgments.

Conflict Related to Patient Care Decisions

Conflict over patient care decisions can occur when nurses and physicians do not share each others' goals for patient care and do not negotiate their differences openly and constructively. Researchers[12-14] who have examined the patterns of physician-nurse communication suggest that problems exist in both professions that impede effective communication. For example, in one study,[15] the primary means used by nurses in handling disagreements were competition (assertive and uncooperative) and accommodation (unassertive and cooperative). Neither style is effective.

Researchers[14,16,17] have found nurses hesitant to question medical recommendations, even when they did not understand them or disagreed with them, and reluctant to present their assessment of a patient's clinical status. This unwillingness to take responsibility for their own clinical judgments may in part be responsible for Prescott and Brown's[15] finding that the nurses participating in their study assumed physicians to be competent unless proved otherwise, whereas physicians assumed nurses to be incompetent unless proved otherwise. Having to prove competence with each new physician is a time-consuming and arduous process.

Ineffective conflict management is also promoted by the traditional hierarchic model of decision-making in which the physician is viewed as the head of the team and the nurse as the implementor. The hierarchic model has its roots in the history of hospitals in United States and Europe, with hospital-based schools of nursing being important sources of nurse labor. This model is similar to a military model and is based on the assumption of unquestioning obedience to orders. The vestiges of the military tradition in hospitals can be seen in the use of nursing and medical student uniforms (with ICU scrubs similar to battle fatigues), the hierarchic chain of command, and some of the terminology (e.g., doctor's orders, house officers, and chief of staff). It is reflected in a communication pattern that Stein and co-workers[18,19] labeled "the doctor-nurse game." The rules of the game dictate that the nurse must make substantive recommendations for patient care such that the recommendations appear to be initiated by the physician. Again, this tradition does not facilitate cooperation and mutual respect among physicians and nurses in the ICU. Passivity on the part of nurses should not be confused with collaboration.

Conflict Related to Differences in Professional Orientation

The second source of conflict evolves from the different educational orientation of the two professions. Although nursing and medicine share the common goal of preserving and restoring health, their educational programs prepare them to view the critically ill patient from different vantage points. Medicine focuses on the diagnosis and treatment of disease. Using infectious disease as a model, medicine has adopted an interventionist approach that focuses on the identification of a specific disease and its cure. The existence of real or presumed disease is assumed in physician-patient encounters.[20] As noted by Rosenberg, "Specialization exemplified and exacerbated a more general tendency of medicine toward the reductionist and technological; its existence helped justify and act out the powerful image of the hospital as a scientific institution."[21] The reductionist view also confuses professional expertise with moral authority, and can lead to conflicts not only with other members of the health team, but also with the patient and family.

In contrast to the interventionist orientation in medicine, nursing has retained a strong orientation to "care." The profession has its roots in the 1860s, when society at large did not expect to be "cured" from disease. At this time, nursing defined its role as supporting personal resistance to the ravages of disease and controlling the environment to maximize health and encourage recovery. Nursing was a substitute for family care and, as such, developed a tradition of organizing care around individuals rather than diseases.[20] Although the myriad tasks associated with diagnosis and therapy have dominated the interior life of hospitals and the workday of nurses in the twentieth century, nurses have held on to their ideology of holism and family-based care and continue to be oriented toward preserving relationships and giving comfort.[17,20]

The nature of the ICU environment, in which uncertainty and ambiguity about medical prognosis are combined with technology that can sustain physiologic life indefinitely, can lead to clinically important conflicts between medicine and nursing. When team members lack effective conflict management skills, the disagreements can spill over into discussions with families and patients.

Other focuses can also be identified that serve to exacerbate the sources of conflict between physicians and nurses. These forces include:

- Recent changes in health care economics
- Changes in gender role expectations
- Increased technology in the ICU
- Increased scientific base in both medicine and nursing
- Increased specialization in medicine and nursing

Many of these changes have been dramatic and not sufficiently appreciated by members of the two professions in relation to one another.

Recommendations of Professional Organizations

The importance of the physician-nurse relationship in the ICU team has been highlighted over the past 20 years. In 1971, the American Medical Association and the American Nurses Association established the National Joint Practice Commission.[20] Although its aims were not specific for the ICU, they are nonetheless appropriate for this setting. The commission established four demonstration projects with the following goals: (1) to improve role definition and decision-making for nurses; (2) to reduce the need for physicians to supervise other professionals; (3) to improve the use of professional staff and patient satisfaction; and (4) to encourage more continuous, personalized care for patients. On evaluation, the demonstration projects resulted in the following changes:

- Higher patient satisfaction
- Improved quality of care
- Reduced costs
- Increased nurse retention
- Decreased litigation

These effects were credited to an improvement in the effective working relationships of physicians and nurses and to better patient education and discharge planning.[21]

In 1982, the Society of Critical Care Medicine and the American Association of Critical-Care Nurses (SCCM-AACN) issued a joint position paper listing the principles by which critical care units could function successfully through collaboration (Table 72-1).[21] In this statement, collaboration is taken out of the realm of individual physician-nurse intention and personality by providing suggestions for unit level structure that is designed to support effective physician-nurse collaboration.

The structure suggested in 1982 received further support in 1983 at the Conference on Critical Care of the National Institutes of Health. According to the participants, "The organization or structure (of the ICU) should promote and require that nurses and physicians work together as colleagues at all levels."[23]

Finally, in 1990, the Society of Critical Care Medicine held a consensus conference entitled "Fostering More Humane Caring—Creating a Healing Environment." Approximately 30 physicians, nurses, respiratory therapists, and individuals from allied health professions convened to discuss ways in which intensive care could be delivered in the most humane way possible. They discussed the ICU environment, use of technology, and models of decision-making. Participants rejected the traditional hierarchic model of care and chose in its place a collaborative model that included all team members. The patient and family members were also identified as important members of this team. The document[24] that evolved as a result of this conference serves as a blueprint for developing and maintaining an effective team in the ICU. Its authors underscored the importance of mutual respect and open communication among physicians and nurses, and stated that "physicians and nurses have primary responsibility for diagnosis, treatment, and coordination of care, and share both the development of the plan of care and provision of care with members of their disciplines."[24]

Even an informal collaborative project can do much to bring physicians and nurses out of their respective private worlds and into closer cooperation. In 1989, the Baystate Medical Center in Springfield, Massachusetts devoted its Pride in Medicine project to the nurse-physician relationship. Nurses and physicians were asked to comment in detail on the qualities that they respected in one another. The project yielded a printed compilation of comments by the participants, a summary of findings, and suggestions for further improvement.[25] The document is an exemplar of the best of physician-nurse mutual respect and collaboration.

TEAM CONCEPT AND THE HIGH RISK PATIENT

Effective collaboration among team members is essential before a patient is admitted to the ICU, in the ICU phase, and following discharge to a less acute area. Ultimately, this collaboration requires the support of organizational factors within the hospital, management within individual ICUs, and the members of the entire ICU team (Fig. 72-1).

Pre-ICU Phase

The goals in this phase are to identify those patients who are at high risk for a critical illness and to gather appropriate assessment data for possible future use by the ICU team. It is also important that the patient and family discuss their wishes about ICU treatment before admission and to formalize advance directives.[26] Finally, relationships

Table 72-1. Summary of Joint Position Statement from the Society of Critical Care Medicine and the American Association of Critical-Care Nurses on Collaborative Practice Model: The Organization of Human Resources in Critical Care Units

1. Responsibility and accountability for effective functioning of a critical care unit must be vested in physician and nurse directors who are on an equal decision-making level.
2. These directors must be appropriately prepared and educated in patient management, management principles, resources management, and have skills in interpersonal relationships (including conflict resolution).
3. Physicians must be autonomous when dealing with issues that affect medical practice.
4. Nurses must be autonomous when dealing with issues that affect nursing practice.
5. Aspects of patient care that require interdependence between physicians and nurses must be identified and addressed jointly.
6. Care delivered by other health team members must be coordinated by the physician and nurse directors.
7. Unit support services must be organized to enable the directors to optimally carry out their responsibilities related to patient care.
8. The directors are accountable for the evaluation of the quality and efficiency of care and the financial provision of that care.
9. The directors are responsible for creating and maintaining an environment in which individuals have opportunities to realize their potentials.
10. Close collaboration between the directors is essential for successful management.

(From American Association of Critical-Care Nurses and Society of Critical Care Medicine: Postion statement: Collaborative practice model: The organization of human resources in critical care units. Newport Beach, CA, American Association of Critical-Care Nursing, 1982.)

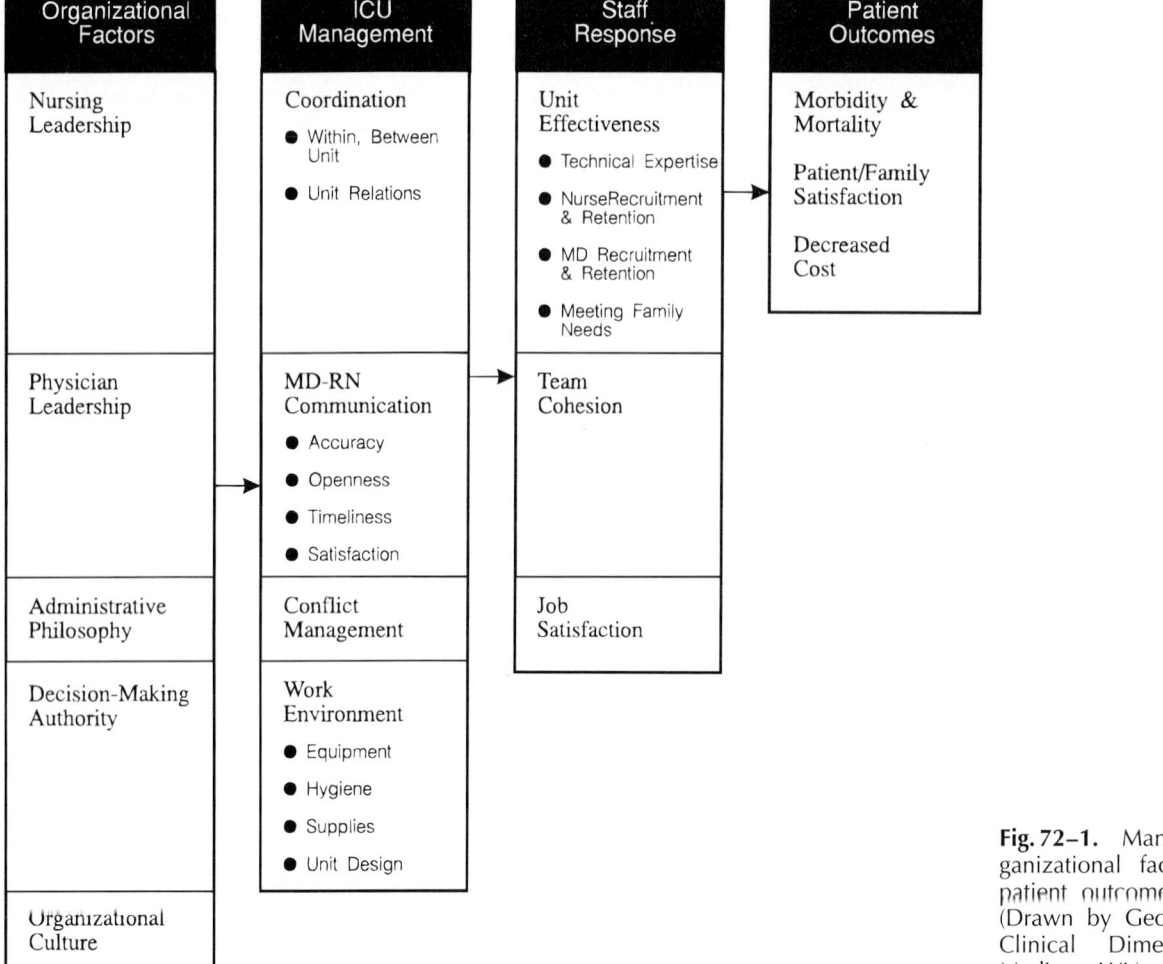

Fig. 72–1. Managerial and organizational factors affecting patient outcome in the ICU (Drawn by George Morrison, Clinical Dimensions, Inc., Madison, WI.)

with other departments need to be evaluated and any impediments to communication resolved.

Especially critical is the free sharing of information between non-ICU and ICU personnel. Pre-ICU caregivers are the best source of information for ICU personnel about the condition and disease course of a patient. From the beginning, information on the high risk patient should be recorded in such a way that it will be accessible and useful in the event of an ICU admission. And caregivers from the pre-ICU phase should share freely with the ICU staff any insights they have gleaned about the patient.

Educational programs designed for both the ICU and the non-ICU nurse and physician can facilitate better communication between ICU staff and nurses working in settings other than the ICU. These programs are somewhat necessitated by the recent increase in acuity of non-ICU patients. For example, non-ICU staff are now caring for patients on ventilators, vasoactive medications, and antiarrhythmic drugs. Educational programs can assist nurses and physicians who normally practice outside the ICU setting to identify the patient at high risk for a physiologic crisis and to care competently for patients that require more monitoring and technologic care than in times past. Joint educational programs can also be effective in bringing together ICU and non-ICU health professionals in informal discussions, which ultimately enhances communication.

Assessment

The identification of a patient who is at high risk for a critical illness event that would require hospitalization in the ICU can be made by any member of the health care team. Most often, however, it is the private physician who is aware of a disease course or of a confluence of risk factors that makes such a hospitalization likely. Information obtained prior to the patient's arrival needs to be communicated in writing as well as verbally to assure that all members of the ICU team obtain a complete picture of the physiologic and psychosocial status of the patient before his or her arrival in the ICU. It is particularly important to evaluate and to develop and implement multidisciplinary strategies for caring for patients who have challenging problems such as pain, terminal illness, or unsupportive families before their admission to an ICU.

Treatment Decisions

High risk patients can be encouraged to consider what level of medical treatment they desire in case they become acutely ill and are hospitalized in an ICU. Issues of disease prognosis and quality of life are critical to these discussions. On the basis of recent data, patients who choose that life support not be instituted can be reassured that their care in the ICU will not be compromised.[27]

All patients need to make their wishes known to family members and to discuss the feelings these wishes may engender, so that families support the decision. Such open discussions, although always difficult, have the potential of eliminating the distressing situation that occurs when the patient and family members are not in accord among themselves or with various members of the health care team about the level of therapy desired. Health care providers can be extremely helpful in supporting both patient and family during these difficult discussions, clarifying appropriate use and limitations of advanced technologies, and providing information about advanced directives for medical care (e.g., living wills and durable powers of attorney).

Once a decision has been made, it is important to convey this decision to everyone involved. If a nonhospitalized patient and family have agreed that the patient will not be resuscitated, family members need to rehearse what to do in case of an emergency, because paramedics in most states have to institute cardiopulmonary resuscitation procedures. If the physician is aware of these wishes and the patient is hospitalized in an ICU, it is important that the ICU staff be apprised of the patient's wishes as soon as possible. Unfortunately, clinical experience suggests that it is easier to not institute life support than to discontinue it once it has been started.

Relationships with Other Departments

In the pre-ICU phase, it is extremely helpful if communication with other departments is timely, accurate, and complete. In the case of scheduled ICU admissions (e.g., from the operating room or recovery room), patient/family education programs that include a visit from one of the ICU nursing staff before the operation can reduce anxiety and increase trust. In the case of unscheduled admissions (e.g., from the emergency room or less acute hospital units), the ICU and other hospital departments or wards should work together to optimize the time of the admission and to transmit all the necessary patient/family data.

ICU Phase

Strategies need to be in place at the management level to support a collaborative practice model. If such strategies are not "institutionalized," the effectiveness of the team can be jeopardized as personnel change. In the end, severe personality conflicts between key players can undermine the best of structures, but having the structures in place can often provide a degree of damage control.

The guidelines of the National Joint Practice Commission for collaborative practice[21] noted the importance of institutional support to the success of a collaborative practice program. A jealous hospital administrative staff may work against the success of such a program, because joint practice tends to give increased weight in administrative decisions to physicians and nurses, rather than to administrators. Administrative support is important to achieve, however. It lends legitimacy to collaborative practice in the view of the hospital staff in general. It also facilitates the near-simultaneous introduction of all of the various components of a joint practice program, which greatly increases the likely success of the venture. The medical and nursing coordinators in the individual ICUs play a critical role in allaying anxieties, minimizing personality conflicts, and resolving the minor crises that inevitably arise when a collaborative practice model is initiated.[21]

Medical and Nursing Co-Directors

Responsibility and accountability for effective functioning of a critical care unit must be vested in physician and nurse co-directors who have equal decision-making power in the hospital organizational structure.[22] Physicians in the unit must have autonomy when dealing with issues of medical practice, and nurses must have autonomy when dealing with issues of nursing practice. Ultimately, this autonomy is reflected in the mutually supportive but separate roles of medical and nursing unit directors.

Many aspects of care in an ICU require interdependence; for example, the formulation of clinical protocols or admission-discharge criteria. These areas of interdependence need to be identified and addressed jointly by the directors. The directors also are jointly responsible for coordinating the efforts of other members of the health team (e.g., dietitians, pharmacists, laboratory technicians, etc.).

This shared governance structure is the most effective when it reflects the philosophy of the hospital. Committee structure is one indication of a philosophic commitment to collaborative practice. Nurses and physicians need representation on all patient care (including procedures, research, and ethics) and quality assurance committees. Rules or bylaws that exclude either member of the team (physician or nurse) from chairmanship duties reflect an elitism that runs counter to a shared governance model.

Clinical Protocols

Standing clinical protocols are helpful in providing guidance to both physician and nurse members of the health care team as they deal with patients who are often in physiologic crisis and who cannot afford wasted time to treatment.[28,29] They aid physicians and other team members in following a detailed pathway that applies a consistent logic. In medical centers, they offset the confusion that exists when different faculty and house staff rotate on and off the ICU services. Appropriate use of protocols can reduce patient mortality.[6]

Clinical protocols need to be based on research findings and must have the consensus of both medical and nursing members of the team. They are best derived through interdisciplinary clinical practice committees. Protocols provide a blueprint for action based on the medical diagnosis and/or clinical status of a patient. For example, a clinical protocol for a patient arriving in the emergency room with chest pain would indicate the order in which the following activities occur: history, vital signs, electrocardiogram, placement on a cardiac monitor, cardiac enzyme samples, and institution of an intravenous line for thrombolysis.

Table 72-2. Critical Pathway for a Patient with Acute Pancreatitis

	Admission	Day 2	Day 3	Day 4
Diagnostic work-up	SMA_7, SMA_{12}, liver function tests, serum amylase and lipase, CBC, coagulation profile, chest radiograph, ECG, all available cultures, urinalysis.	*Throughout stay:* Daily SMA_7, amylase, lipase, CBC, coagulation profile, chest radiograph, ECG.	CT scan abdomen, cardiac echo, abdominal sonogram	*Through week 1:* Daily liver function tests.
Cardiovascular	Monitor vital signs q1hr until stable, Swan-Ganz catheter placement. Check hemodynamic profile q2–4hr. Low-dose dopamine infusion started.	*Through week 1:* Follow closely for evidence of hyperdynamic parameters indicating sepsis. Sequential TEDS stockings to reduce occurrence of DVTs. Monitor for pericardial effusion.		Monitor closely for myocardial depression, cardiac failure, or bleeding. Notify MD if SVO_2 <60 or >80.
Pulmonary	Elective intubation if there is excess energy expenditure related to sepsis. Chest physiotherapy q2hr. ABG q1–2hr. *Through week 1:* Assess q2hr for rales, wheezing, tubular breath sounds; check ABG for respiratory alkalosis. *Through week 2:* Follow for rising pulmonary inspiratory pressure, falling Po_2, difficulty "bagging" patient as evidence of declining compliance. Neuromuscular blocking agents may be necessary. Assess chest radiograph report daily for effusions, infiltrate, or ARDS.	*Through week 2:* Monitor closely for ARDS. Assess closely for barotrauma. Follow for change in sputum color or quantity.		
Renal	Foley catheter placed. Send urine for R/O myoglobin. *Through week 3:* Monitor for >30 ml/hr urine output. *Through week 4:* Daily weight to assess fluid balance.		24hr urine for creatinine clearance. Monitor all drugs for nephrotoxic insult.	Check urine urea nitrogen (to assess adequacy of nutrition).
Gastrointestinal/Nutritional	NPO with NG tube. Check gastric pH q2hr. Monitor for any GI bleeding. H2 blockers begun for gastric protection. *Through week 3:* Monitor blood glucose q6hr for potential hyperglycemia. *Throughout stay:* Assess daily for abdominal tenderness or pain.	TPN initiated. Adjust TPN insulin to blood glucose level. Baseline caloric measurement via metabolic cart study. Monitor for retroperitoneal bleeding. *Through week 3:* Watch GI drainage for color, clarity, odor. Assess for hiccups. Maintain strict NPO.		
Emotional/Neurologic	Orient patient/family to SICU environment. Complete family assessment tool and organize teaching accordingly. Assess for tremors or tetany. Inquire when ETOH last consumed. Monitor for withdrawal. Apply soft hand restraints to keep tubes and drains intact if needed. *Through week 3:* Assess pain medication requirements daily and medicate PRN with Demerol to promote comfort and decrease catecholamine release. Glasgow Coma Score (initially q2–4hr).	Group care activities to allow REM sleep. Begin daily updates with patient and family regarding plan of care.		Assess anxiety level. Reorient and explain all activities and diagnostic procedures.

(continued)

Table 72–2. Critical Pathway for a Patient with Acute Pancreatitis—*(Continued)*

	Admission	Day 2	Day 3	Day 4
Rehabilitative	Assess prior level of ADL and check for presence of prior contractures or foot drop. *Throughout stay:* Turn and reposition q2hr to reduce immobility complications.	*Throughout stay:* Range-of-motion therapy q2–4hr. Consult OT/PT to prevent long-term complications.		
Wound care	*Throughstay:* Wound and skin precautions. Assess wound for any drainage, granulation or odor. Monitor sump drainage and irrigation systems for patency.	Administer antibiotics per order		*Throughout stay:* Inspect abdominal wound q8hr and redress per protocol of surgeon. Report any necrotic areas or new bleeding.
Discharge planning	Establish realistic plans based on patient's acuity. Initially evaluate present support system for patient/family.		Assess for any financial or insurance problems family may be concerned about.	

(From Smith, A.: Acute pancreatitis. Am. J. Nurs., *91*:38, 1991.)

Such a protocol allows the medical and nursing team to act efficiently and swiftly and minimizes conflict about appropriate actions to take and delay to definitive treatment.

Extensive clinical protocols (termed "critical paths") have been developed for various critically ill patients to trace a patient's progress throughout the ICU hospitalization. A clinical path is a combination of clinical practices that results in the most resource efficient, clinically appropriate, and shortest length of stay for a specific medical condition or procedure. It is based on a "typical" case and reflects the consensus of physicians, nurses, and other caregivers. An example of a critical path developed for a patient with acute pancreatitis is presented in Table 72-2.

Patient Progress Rounds

Daily progress rounds with physician(s), nurses, and members of other disciplines present as appropriate enhance close collaboration and effective communication in the ICU. Medical and nursing plans of care can be discussed and decisions made so that future misunderstandings are avoided. In teaching hospitals, the most common model of patient rounds is the presentation of patient data by an intern or resident to an attending physician, followed by a discussion of the medical plan of care by the physicians in attendance. The nurse may or may not be asked for an opinion or recommendations. Because nurses are with their patients continuously and their observations are critical to the assessment of the response to therapy, a model of teaching rounds in which the nurse (rather than the house officer) provides the initial summary of patient data may be more effective to the ultimate goal of quality patient care. Nurses need to be active discussants in these rounds and to take responsibility for bringing their concerns to this forum. Nurses are often the individuals to bring up issues of discharge planning, family concerns, or ethical dilemmas. Patient rounds that occur without these discussions are incomplete at best. Because nurses in many institutions are not accustomed to this structure, they initially may need the encouragement and support of the unit directors and their physician colleagues.

Interdisciplinary Conferences

Formal and informal patient care conferences and ethics committee meetings also provide important opportunities for nurses and physicians working in ICUs to share relevant clinical information. Such meetings are essential to making optimal decisions about patient care in that they provide a forum for exchange of data, opinions, and values. Nurses and physicians often have different perspectives on patients' responses to illness and therapy and it is important to air these differences. The payment for not providing such a forum is a plan of care that is either inappropriate or not supported by the entire team. Ideally, providing for such an interchange will lead to reduced resentment on the part of formerly "underconsulted" team members, greater understanding of and respect for team members with different clinical styles, an improved overall working relationship within the team, and better patient care.

Interdisciplinary conferences need to be formalized by scheduling them on a weekly or twice weekly basis. In many institutions they are held under the aegis of discharge planning. The primary physician and nurse should present appropriate clinical and psychosocial data concerning each patient in the unit. The team can then discuss plans for care and ultimate plans for discharge from the unit. Typically, participants include the medical and nursing co-directors, nursing staff (including the clinical nurse specialist), medical staff and/or house staff, social worker, dietitian, respiratory therapist, and/or psychiatric liaison.

Integrated Patient Records

Patient charts provide an opportunity for all team members to communicate relevant information about the ICU patient. Unfortunately, many recording formats are antiquated. These systems, which usually include a log format for nurses to chart their observations and patient care activities, often are designed to withstand legal scrutiny, not to encourage effective communication. When nurses chart reams of repetitive phrases that contribute little meaningful information, everyone (including other nurses) is discouraged from reading what they have to say.

Joint progress notes are replacing the previously used nursing notes and physician progress notes in documentation systems. For each patient entering the unit, the physician and nurse develop a problem list that is a compilation of the medical and nursing diagnoses. This list is used for all charting on the patient's progress, using the problem-oriented SOAP format. For each problem identified, subjective (S) and objective (O) data are given to support the existence of the problem, the assessment (A) of the problem's etiology and current status is described, and a plan (P) of care is outlined. When combined with flow sheets for recording quantitative values, a problem-oriented system of charting can provide an important mechanism for exchange among the members of the ICU team.

An overhaul of charting will not necessarily in itself translate into improved patient care. Rather, it must be accompanied by a commitment on the part of both nurses and physicians to consult with one another frequently. In the National Joint Practice Commission report, an intern noted: "I enjoyed the fact that if [a nurse] observed something, rather than just reporting it to me and putting down in the chart 'M.D. aware,' she presented me with the data and discussed what should be done."[21] Here, the key change is the improved communication, not the improved charting.

Inclusion of Patients and Family

The integration of patient and family input into consideration of the team is essential to achieve humane care. The personal characteristics and values of the patient and family shape the critical care experience, and ICU health care providers have an obligation to recognize the patient and family as contributors to the decisions made by the team.[24] Given that people feel dehumanized when they are treated as if they have no options,[30] patients and families need to understand alternatives related to treatment. They also need to understand that the right to consent to a treatment also implies the right to refuse.

The primary physician and nurse should meet with the patient's family and loved ones on a daily basis to update them and to clarify areas of concern or misunderstanding. Research on the roles of families during critical illness uniformly supports the concept of open visiting and inclusion of family members in various aspects of care.[31-33] In all studies in which families were asked to describe their needs related to the hospitalization of a loved one in the ICU (see Hickey[34] for a review), family members identified physical access to their loved ones as a primary need. Frequent family visitation results in shorter ICU stays,[33] increased patient comfort,[31,33] and improved patient and family satisfaction.[32,33] In one study of patients hospitalized in a coronary care unit for chest pain, those patients who were allowed to contract with a nurse for unrestricted family visiting were less anxious and depressed during their stay in the unit than those patients whose families were restricted from visiting.[33] The positive outcomes documented in this study and the consistency with which families ask for open visiting serve as a challenge to the severely restricted visitation policies set in most adult ICUs in which family visiting is limited to a set schedule (for example, 10 minutes every other hour).

Table 72–3. Communication Strategies Conducive to Collaboration

Promote participation
   Actively seek out and approach other professionals caring for patient
   Ask participation of others
   Be available
Participate in interaction
   Make eye contact
   Show interest and indicate involvement
   Listen actively
   Question and enter into discussion
Give and seek opinion
   Provide and elicit opinions and recommendations
   Provide and elicit concerns
   Respond to communication
Give and seek information
   Provide and elicit facts and observations
   Provide and elicit feedback
Promote understanding
   Clarify statements and ideas
   Review known information
   Reinforce information, statements, ideas
   Communicate clearly without repetition
Focus on subject or issue
   Prepare for interaction
   Focus on problem/topic
   Accomplish task, make decisions
Modify position
   Consider needs of others
   Incorporate other ideas or information
   Alter behavior as necessary
Value self and others
   Recognize skills, knowledge, and limitations
   Recognize overlapping roles and expertise
   Promote egalitarian relationship
   Acknowledge other's contributions
   Promote positive emotional tone

(From Ray, L.: Definition and application of collaboration on nursing practice. Emphasis: Nursing (Harbor-UCLA Medical Center, Torrance, CA), 3:29, 1990.)

Communication Styles

Collaboration is reflected at the micro level in the communication styles of the team members. Communication is most effective when it reflects mutual respect, validation of feelings, and recognition of each individual's unique contribution to patient care (i.e., lack of stereotyping). Mutual respect is characterized by letting each person speak without interruption, using appropriate eye contact, and using forms of address that connote equal status.

Ray examined communication styles among nurses.[35] She identified those that encouraged collaboration, and divided them into eight categories; the categories and their descriptors appear in Table 72–3.

Post-ICU Phase

Discharge Planning

Patients and their families need to be included in planning unit or institutional transfers. In an age of shortened hospital stays, the family needs help with learning how to take care of the patient who may be discharged with critical care needs. They may also need assistance in obtaining appropriate community resources to supplement home care.

Ideally, discharge planning begins at the time of admission. Gathering the skills, psychologic resources, and community support necessary for home care can take time. More importantly, a focus to the extent possible on rehabilitation and release, even in the early stages of hospitalization, is of psychologic benefit to both the patient and the family, and helps them to work together toward those goals.

During hospitalization of a patient in the ICU, the family should sense a cohesive plan for rehabilitation and discharge on the part of the various caregivers. Unfortunately, family members sometimes experience conflicting expectations and plans among members of the health care team. For example, physicians and nurses may be in accord about the length of time required for the patient to be in ICU whereas a member of the hospital administrative staff presses for early transfer. To prevent families from experiencing conflict surrounding discharge plans, a multidisciplinary discharge conference with the family in attendance is essential. Discussions should focus on solving problems and anticipating difficulties following discharge or transfer. The weekly team conference discussed previously can provide the structure to ensure that the entire team is in accord with a specific treatment plan. A meeting with family members, physician, and primary nurse is essential, however, before the discharge of the patient from the unit or prior to making any major change in treatment plan.

Quality Assurance

Quality assurance programs should include a mechanism by which patients and families can participate in the evaluation of critical care staff and the care they receive.[24] Patient and family satisfaction is an important factor in the perceived quality of ICU care and needs to be evaluated systematically, along with mortality and cost data. Informal feedback can be obtained by the co-directors or clinical nurse specialist during the period of hospitalization, but clearly this evaluation can be biased, either negatively or positively, by the patient's and family's sense of dependency on the staff. A more systematic evaluation can be conducted using a written mailed survey or a structured telephone interview after the patient has been discharged from the hospital. Such evaluation should have support at the highest level of hospital administration, because there may be no better measure of the quality of services provided.

Patient and Family Education

Patients who are at high risk for future physiologic crises require intensive education about their risk and the ways in which they can reduce it. Unfortunately, the hospital environment is somewhat antithetic to learning. Most patient education studies conducted in the ICU or post-ICU setting have demonstrated that patients retain little of what is told them while they are hospitalized. For example, in randomized clinical trials conducted to demonstrate that in-hospital patient teaching was effective in increasing knowledge and changing behavior in postmyocardial infarction patients, no such change was identified on follow-up.[36-38] Although these studies may have been subject to type II error because of small sample size, the finding that inpatient teaching programs make no difference in knowledge or compliance is too consistent to ignore. Researchers[36-38] have hypothesized that a combination of anxiety and physiologic disequilibrium are probably responsible for the minimal effects of patient teaching.

Because patients appear generally unable to comprehend much of the information given them before discharge from the hospital, the educational process needs to include significant others and needs to be supplemented with written material and follow-up outpatient teaching. The family plays an important role in enhancing patient adherence to medical regimens,[39-41] and this fact provides further impetus to including family members in all inpatient education activities.

OUTCOMES

Documented outcomes of effective collaboration in the ICU (see Fig. 72-1) include decreased patient morbidity and mortality, increased patient and family satisfaction, and decreased cost.[6,31,33] Studies of nurse recruitment and retention also suggest that effective physician-nurse collaboration is an important strategy for attracting and keeping skilled nursing staff, which in turn translates to lower costs for the institution.[41,42] Moreover, compared with the traditional practice model, collaborative practice motivates all participants to share in efforts at controlling costs and preventing malpractice. These results make the work of physicians in the ICU easier and more effective than in the traditional practice model.

To achieve these positive outcomes, the institution must have effective leadership in hospital management, nursing, and medicine (see Fig. 72-1). A lack of leadership in any one of these areas can pose a serious threat to effective collaboration. If the leaders identify each other as potential combatants or encourage competition, it is difficult for the individuals working in individual units to escape this negative model. The institutional climate must also support a shared governance model of decision-making at the level of the individual ICU and provide medical and nursing co-directors with the autonomy required to make sound decisions.

As summarized in Figure 72-1 and in the preceding discussion, the medical and nursing co-directors must model effective communication and conflict management styles. The co-directors should be able to communicate accurately, openly, and in a timely fashion. Both should leave interchanges feeling that they have been heard by the other and that decisions in areas of interdependence will be made jointly.

Physicians and nurses who collaborate effectively require clear definitions of the professional boundaries in medicine and nursing and are able to observe these boundaries while respecting the skills and talents of other professionals on the team.[43] By virtue of their practice acts, physicians and nurses each have spheres of independent practice. Nurses also function dependently when they engage in those activities that require medical licensure (for example, initiating intravenous lidocaine for multifocal premature ventricular contractions). The majority of activities in an ICU, however, are interdependent. In a collaborative model, all physicians and nurses share in the partnership of care and decisions are made together in areas of interdependence. The physicians and nurses working in a collaborative model learn to focus on the results of the team, rather than on the contributions of the individual providers. Ultimately, the didactic training of some team members complements the clinical training of others, and the team concept of patient care benefits everyone by promoting a humane and healing environment.

REFERENCES

1. Kallish, B. and Kalish, P.: An analysis of the sources of physician-nurse conflict. J. Nurs. Admin., 7:51, 1977.
2. Hamilton, S.: Collaborative practice is necessary in ICU. Nurs. Management, 22:96J, 1991.
3. Makadon, H. J., and Gibbins, M. P.: Nurses and physicians: Prospects for collaboration. Ann. Intern. Med., 103:134, 1985.
4. Dracup, K., and Marsden, C.: Critical Care Nursing: Perspectives and Challenges. In The Nursing Profession: Turning Points. Edited by Norma Chaska. St. Louis, C. V. Mosby, 1989.
5. Bates, B.: Doctor and nurse: Changing roles and relations. N. Engl. J. Med., 283:129, 1970.
6. Knaus, W., et al.: An evaluation of outcome from intensive care in major medical centers. Ann. Intern Med., 104:410, 1986.
7. Knaus, W., et al.: An evaluation of outcome from intensive care in major medical centers. Ann. Intern. Med., 104:416, 1986.
8. Knaus, W., et al.: An evaluation of outcome from intensive care in major medical centers. Ann. Intern. Med., 104:417, 1986.
9. Allen, M. L., Jackson, D., Younger, S.: Closing the communication gap between physicians and nurses in the intensive care unit setting. Heart Lung, 9:836, 1980.
10. This reference has been deleted.
11. Cox, H.: Verbal abuse nationwide, part I: Oppressed group behavior. Nurs. Management, 22:32, 1991.
12. Weiss, S. J.: Role differentiation between nurse and physician: Implications for nursing. Nurs. Res., 32:133, 1983
13. Taylor, S. G., Pickens, J. M., Geden, E. A.: Interactional styles of nurse practitioners and physicians regarding patient decision making. Nurs. Res., 38:50, 1989.
14. Cavanagh, S. J.: The conflict management style of intensive care nurses. Intensive Care Nurs., 4:118, 1988.
15. Prescott, P. A., and Bowen, S. A.: Physician-nurse relationships. Ann. Intern. Med., 103:127, 1985.
16. Katzman, E. M., and Roberts, J. I.: Nurse-physician conflicts as barriers to the enactment of nursing roles. West. J. Nurs. Res., 10:576, 1988.
17. Lynaugh, J. E., and Fagin, C. M.: Nursing comes of age. Image, 20;184, 1988.
18. Stein, L. I.: The doctor-nurse game. Arch. Gen. Psychiatry, 16:699, 1967.
19. Stein, L. I., Watts, D. T., Howell, T.: The doctor-nurse game revisited. N. Engl. J. Med., 322:546, 1990.
20. Rosenberg, C. E. (Ed.): The Care of Strangers: The Rise of America's Hospital System. New York, Basic Books, Inc., 1987.
21. Guidelines for Establishing Joint or Collaborative Practice in Hospitals. Chicago, The National Joint Practice Commission, 1981.
22. American Association of Critical-Care Nurses and Society of Critical Care Medicine: Position statement: Collaborative practice model: The organization of human resources in critical care units. Newport Beach, CA, American Association of Critical-Care Nursing, 1982.
23. National Institutes of Health Consensus Conference on Critical Care. JAMA, 250:798, 1983.
24. Harvey, M., et al.: Results of the 1990 consensus conference on fostering more humane critical care: creating a healing environment. AACN Clin. Issues Crit. Care Nurs., 4:484, 1993.
25. Pride in Medicine Project: How We View Each Other. Springfield, MA, Baystate Medical Center, 1989.
26. McCarrick, P. M.: Living wills and durable powers of attorney: Advance directive legislation and issues. Scope Note 2. Washington, DC: National Reference Center for Bioethics Literature, Kennedy Institute of Ethics, February, 1990.
27. Lewandowski, W., et al.: Treatment and care of "do not resuscitate" patients in a medical intensive care unit. Heart Lung, 14:175, 1985.
28. Phillip, M., et al.: An algorithmic approval to diagnosis of hypoglycemia. J. Pediatr., 110:387, 1987.
29. Margolis, C. Z.: Uses of clinical algorithms. JAMA, 249:627, 1983.
30. Howard, J.: Humanization and dehumanization of health care. In Humanizing Health Care. Edited by J. Howard and A. Strauss. New York, John Wiley & Sons, 1975.
31. Kulik, J.: Social support and recovery from surgery. Health Psychol., 8:221, 1989.
32. Dracup, K., and Breu, C.: Using research findings to meet the needs of grieving spouses. Nurs. Res., 27:212, 1978.
33. Ziemann, K., and Dracup, K.: Patient-nurse contracts in critical care. A controlled trial. Prog. Cardiovasc. Nurs., 5:98, 1990.
34. Hickey, M.: What are the needs of families of critically ill patients? A review of the literature since 1976. Heart Lung, 19:401, 1990.
35. Ray, L.: Definition and application of collaboration on nursing practice. Emphasis: Nursing (Harbor-UCLA Medical Center, Torrance, CA), 3:29, 1990.
36. Sivarajan, E. S., et al.: Limited effects of outpatient teaching and counseling after myocardial infarction: A controlled study. Heart Lung, 12:65, 1983.
37. Maeland, J. G., and Havik, O. E.: The effects of an in-hospital teaching programme for myocardial infarction patients. Scand. J. Rehabil. Med., 19:57, 1987.
38. Scalzi, C. C., Burke, L. E., Greenland, S.: Evaluation of an inpatient educational program for coronary patients and families. Heart Lung, 9:846, 1980.
39. Haynes, R. B.: A critical review of the 'determinants' of patient compliance with therapeutic regimens. In Compliance with Therapeutic Regimens. Edited by D. L. Sackett and R. B. Haynes. Baltimore, The Johns Hopkins University Press, 1976.
40. Mechanic, D., and Volkart, E. A.: Illness behavior and medical diagnoses. J. Health Hum. Behav., 1:86, 1980.
41. McClure, M. L., et al. (Eds.): Magnet Hospitals: Attraction and Retention of Professional Nurses. Kansas City, American Academy of Nursing, 1983.
42. Aiken, L. H., and Mullinix, C. F.: The nurse shortage: Myth or reality? N. Engl. J. Med., 317:641, 1987.
43. Burcell, R. C., Thomas, D. A., and Smith, H. L.: Some considerations for implementing collaborative practice. Am. J. Med., 74:9, 1985.

SUPPLEMENTAL READINGS

Cerra, F. B.: Healthcare reform: The role of coordinated critical care. Crit. Care Med. *21*:457, 1993.

Dubaybo, B. A., Samson, M. K., Carlson, R. W.: The role of physician assistants in critical care units. Chest, *99*:89, 1991.

Field, M., Lohr, K. (Eds.): Guidelines for Clinical Practice: From Development to Use. Washington, D.C., Institute of Medicine, National Academy Press, 1992.

Fletcher, R. H., and Fletcher, S. W.: Clinical practice guidelines. Ann. Intern. Med., *113*:645, 1990.

Knickman, J. P.: The potential for using non-physicians to compensate for the reduced availability of residents. Acad. Med., *67*:429, 1992.

National League for Nursing: An Agenda for Nursing Education Reform. New York, 1993.

Office of Technology Assessment: Nurse Practitioners, Physician Assistants, and Certified Nurse Midwives: A Policy Analysis: Health Technology Case Study #37. Washington, D.C., Office of Technology Assessment Congress of the United States, 20510-8025, 1986.

Pearson, L. J.: 1992–93 Update: How each state stands on legislative issues affecting advanced nursing practice. Nurse Pract., *18*:23, 1993.

Record, J. (Ed.): Staffing Primary Care in 1990: Physician Replacement and Cost Savings. Vol. 6. New York, Springer, 1981.

Relman, A. S.: The healthcare industry: Where is it taking us? N. Engl. J. Med., *325*:854, 1991.

Safriet, B. J.: Healthcare dollars and regulatory sense: The role of advanced practice nursing. Yale J. Regulation, *9*:417, 1992.

United States General Accounting Office, HRD-91-102: U.S. Healthcare Spending: Trends, Contributing Factors, and Proposals for Reform, 1991.

Chapter 73

PSYCHOLOGIC STRESS IN THE CRITICALLY ILL PATIENT

SUZANNE CLARK

THE CRISIS OF CRITICAL ILLNESS

Most of us go about our daily lives trying to maintain a degree of balance or homeostasis. We use a variety of coping mechanisms to adjust to the pressures and changes that normally confront us to maintain that state of equilibrium. Some events, however, are so overwhelming that the coping mechanisms that we rely on are no longer effective, and we plummet into a state of disequilibrium, characterized by feelings of increased tension, confusion, anxiety, fear, and helplessness. This state of imbalance and dysphoria that results from life events that are not amenable to reorganization through our usual coping activities is known as a crisis.[1] An acute illness, or an exacerbation of a chronic illness, that requires an admission to a critical care unit can cause a crisis for patients and their families.

Seasoned clinicians know that not every patient who has a critical illness experiences the psychologic responses associated with a crisis. Many patients are able to adapt to the sick role and fulfill its obligations with little or no difficulty. These patients acknowledge that they are sick and they seek out technically competent help to get well. They recognize that being sick is an undesirable state and they cooperate in getting well by following the treatment plan and returning to preillness function.[2] They express gratitude for the efforts of health-care providers. The patient's response facilitates the business of providing life-saving treatment and requires little adaptation on the part of the caretaker.

Conversely, some patients react vehemently to the impact of illness and hospitalization, and responses can range from panic, noncompliance with treatment, extreme dependence, and even psychosis.[3] Their attempts at coping with the situation can be disruptive to healing and may contribute to mortality as well.[4-8] Their behavior may alienate their families who are trying to provide comfort and the staff who is attempting to provide care. The way a patient reacts to the experience of illness and hospitalization can profoundly affect the therapeutic outcome. Before the medical needs of these patients can be addressed adequately, caregivers must intervene to modify these psychologic responses.

Some patients are at greater risk than others for experiencing critical illness and subsequent hospitalization as an overwhelming situation. Are there factors that predispose some individuals to experience acute illness as a crisis whereas others retain their sense of control? Are there factors inherent in the experience of being ill or the critical care setting that contribute to a crisis state? This discussion explores the answers to these questions.

Crisis Theory

Crisis theory provides a working model to help caretakers plan appropriate interventions for patients who are having difficulty coping with their situations (Fig. 73-1).

An individual is confronted with an event, such as acute illness and admission to a critical care unit. Factors related to the illness challenge the individual and lead to uncomfortable feelings. Patients have a need to do something to resolve the crisis and restore the previous state of equilibrium. Balancing factors help to explain why some people respond to acute illness with disorganization and others are able to maintain reasonable balance. These factors, which help to determine how the crisis resolves, include the ability to perceive an event realistically, the presence or absence of an involved support system, and the coping strategies used.[9] A crisis confronts an individual with both danger and opportunity. The danger lies in the possibility that the individual will never adapt to the challenges and will function in a maladaptive way. Crises also, however, offer the opportunity for positive adaptation and growth.

PRE-ICU PHASE: PATIENTS AT RISK

An exploration of the balancing factors can help to identify which patients are at high risk for experiencing illness and hospitalization as a crisis.

Realistic Perception of the Event

The ability to perceive an event realistically, with minimal distortion, is one of the most important factors in determining whether or not an event will assume crisis proportions. Lazarus defines the complex process of evaluation of a stimulus as cognitive appraisal.[10] Some individuals are more likely than others to appraise situations in such a way as to initiate a stress response. Some factors that influence the way an individual is likely to interpret events are past experiences, personality factors, and metabolic and neurologic factors.

Past Experiences

Prior experiences with stress can have a steeling effect and aid with positive adaptation, or they may sensitize individuals, making them more vulnerable to stress.[11] Individuals who have responded to previous life stress success-

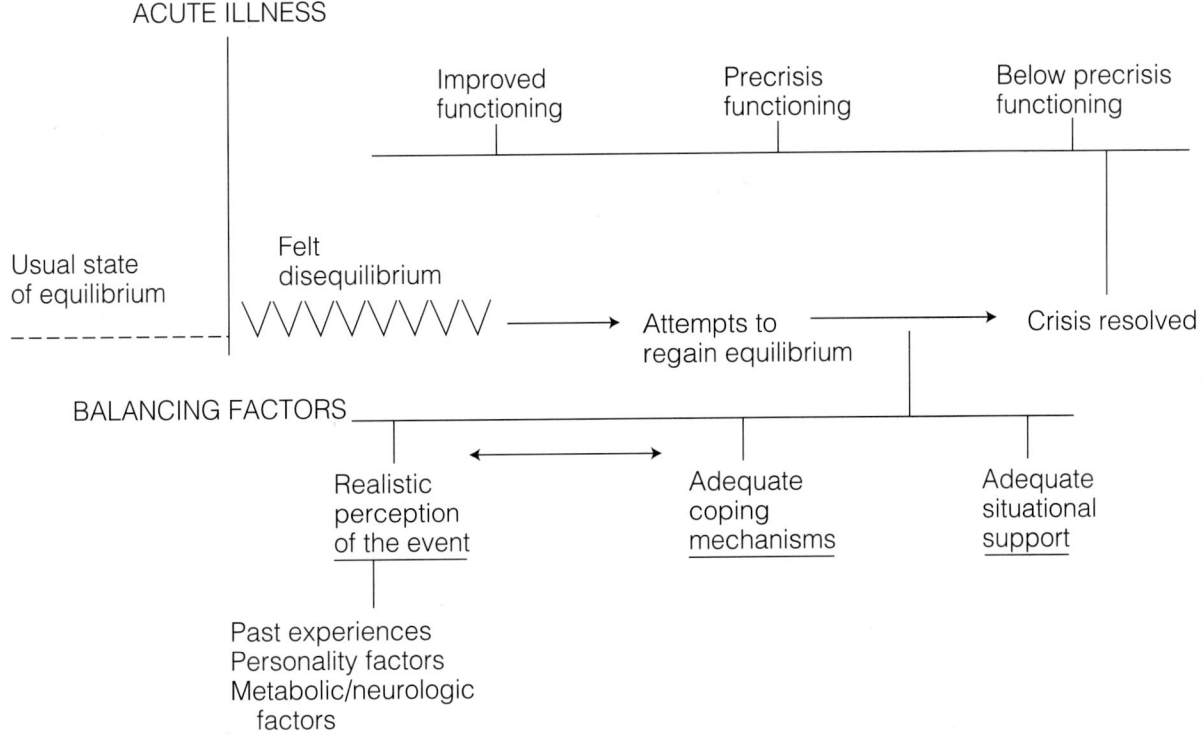

Fig. 73–1. Crisis model of an acute illness.

fully often have a general feeling of hopefulness of their ability to cope with new problems. Also, many patients have known significant others who have suffered illness and have had an opportunity to observe the outcome. A result that included permanent disability or death may color their ability to view what is happening to them realistically.

Cultural background contributes to the meaning of illness, symptoms, and body parts. For example, a woman who defines herself by her sexuality may be more disturbed by a loss of a breast than a woman who derives her self-esteem from a variety of sources. A patient who needed a heart transplant was unable to proceed because he viewed the heart as the resting place of his soul. He thought he would be judged by someone else's sins if he accepted a donor heart.

Negative past experiences with authority figures may limit patients from viewing their caretakers as helpful and caring.

Personality Factors

Individuals who seem to take life stresses in stride and recover readily from misfortune or change are said to be resilient.[11,12] They have the quality of psychologic hardiness.[13,14] Hardy and resilient individuals have several personality traits in common. They are able to forego the more primitive or regressive ego defense mechanisms such as distortion of reality, projection of one's own feelings onto others, and covertly expressing anger while appearing to be compliant.[15] Instead, they manage their anxiety with more effective regulating mechanisms, such as seeking out information, enlisting support, problem solving, distraction, and managing emotions through release.

Resilient people have a sense of self-esteem and are confident in their abilities to deal with unpredictable situations. They have a readiness to cope with stress and a belief that they can control or influence their experience. They have a sense of purpose and they value their contributions. They feel deeply involved and committed to their lives and view change as a challenge to future development.[16]

Individuals who possess psychologic hardiness tend to have a balanced perspective of life experiences, recognizing that change rather than stasis is the norm and that joy and sorrow are part of any human existence.[17]

Conversely, individuals who have difficulty coping with unexpected and intense situations generally have a sense of helplessness about their ability to influence their situations and fail to initiate action on their own behalf. They have difficulty asking for help. They find it hard to identify the salient parts of a problem and to weigh alternatives.[18]

Individuals who are at risk for experiencing physical illness as a crisis have unresolved maturational issues around dependency, trust, and self-control. These patients may exhibit a dependence on caregivers that is beyond that imposed by the actual illness. They may try to exercise control of everything and everybody, refusing medical treatment and making unrealistic demands for attention. They may react with rage that interferes with their receipt of appropriate support.[19]

For a review of metabolic and neurologic factors, see Chapters 1, 2, 5, and 7.

Adequate Situational Support

Personality factors and past experiences contribute to an individual's inner resources available to deal with stress. Situational support refers to external resources that can buffer the effects of stress. These resources include the support of powerful persons or agencies as well as economic and physical factors. Lack of support from these resources places individuals at risk for a crisis by weakening the capacity to master the threat.[10]

The importance of adequate social support to mediate the stress response and physical and mental health has been well documented. In a study of 4775 adults between the ages of 30 and 69 years, researchers developed a "social network" index that assessed four types of social ties: (1) marriage, (2) extended family/friends; (3) church membership; and (4) other formal and informal group relationships. An analysis that controlled for health, socioeconomic status, obesity, alcohol use, smoking, race, life satisfaction, activity, and use of preventative health services demonstrated that individuals with low social affiliations were twice as likely to die as those who had a greater social network.[20] Large epidemiologic studies have shown that age-adjusted mortality rates from all causes of death are higher among unmarried people.[21]

Clinical studies have also shown links between stress, illness outcome, and social support. In a study of postmyocardial infarction patients, Ruberman et al. demonstrated that those with perceived life stress and little social support had four times the risk of sudden cardiac death than those patients with lower levels of perceived stress and greater social connectedness.[22] In another study, when families were used to provide support to patients transferred from the coronary care unit, they experienced reduced stress levels and fewer number of cardiovascular complications after transfer.[23]

Social support can buffer the stress of illness in several important ways. It may influence the decision to seek treatment in the first place, the decision to submit to treatments offered, and the response to the treatment itself.[24] During hospitalization, the staff caring for the patient becomes part of the available support system and can contribute to feelings of either powerlessness or confidence to handle the potential crisis of illness. Just as "difficult patients" make the work of caring for them frustrating, "difficult caretakers" make the patient's work of healing harder.

Adequate Coping Mechanisms

Coping mechanisms are ongoing cognitive and behavioral efforts to solve the presenting problem and manage internal and external demands, and they can include the following behaviors:[18,25]

- Seeking information
- Talking with others
- Using humor
- Not thinking about the problem
- Distracting oneself through other activities
- Doing something positive to change the situation
- Redefining the meaning of the situation
- Reducing tension through eating, drugs, or alcohol
- Running away
- Blaming someone/something else for the problem
- Doing something irrational or reckless
- Hoping the problem will go away
- Accepting the inevitable

These behaviors represent the principle coping styles of attempting to solve the problem directly, avoiding the problem, attacking the harmful stimulus, or deciding that nothing can be done (apathy).

Based on studies that have examined how patients cope in specific situations, several broad generalizations about coping can be made:[26-28]

- In complex situations, most people use a combination of coping responses, some of which are directed toward the actual problem and others that are aimed at mitigating their emotional response.
- The coping response depends on the individual's appraisal—if an individual believes that something can be done, problem-focused coping will be used; but if a person feels that nothing can be done to change the situation, coping responses aimed at the dysphoric feelings predominate.
- The type of coping response can change from one situation to another and over the course of time.
- Some coping behaviors may work well in one phase of the illness and may not be useful in another phase.
- The need for coping behaviors depends on what is at stake for the individual.

Because coping behaviors are so individual, it may be difficult to determine if a patient's response is within normal limits. While trying to evaluate the adequacy of coping responses of critically ill patients who are responding to threats to body, ego, and social situation, the most important question to ask is: Does this behavior work for this person, at this time, in this context?[29] For example, patients who use denial when they experience symptoms and delay seeking treatment are coping ineffectively because the behavior has implications for their physical well-being. Patients who use denial to control their anxiety regarding the meaning of their symptoms but still seek out and accept treatment, however, are coping adequately even though they are not yet able to confront the problem directly. Patients who get angry to avoid feelings of powerlessness but are able to talk about their emotions with caregivers are coping effectively. Patients who direct their anger about their illness toward caregivers, as if they, rather than the situation, were the source of the stress, cut themselves off from support and are coping ineffectively. Adequate coping, then, is characterized by the ability to: (1) maintain supportive relationships, (2) contain anxiety to manageable levels, and (3) minimize the threat to physical well-being.[25]

Sometimes, defense mechanisms, unconscious psychologic processes, are used to control feelings of intense anxiety by permitting a person to take in only as much reality as they feel equipped to handle. Some defenses take a greater toll than others in terms of the effects on well-being, social relationships, and frame of mind. Under severe threat, more pathologic defenses may be evident.[15]

The least effective mechanisms alter reality for the person using them but appear to be "crazy" to others. Distortion involving delusions and hallucinations to reshape reality is an example of this level of defense.

Immature mechanisms, used by normal children, can be used by adults who, under extreme stress, have regressed to earlier behavior patterns. Projection, passive-aggressive behavior, and acting out are examples of this type of defense. These mechanisms generally create feelings of annoyance and irritation in the people around them. One of the most difficult type of patient is the one who uses acting out and anger characterized by verbal threats, physical aggression, and hostility that often evokes an automatic defensive reaction. Although understandable, this response escalates the patient's anger and usually leads to a no-win power struggle.[30]

Neurotic defenses are common and can be seen in most healthy adults, especially at times of acute stress. Displacement and intellectualization are examples of this level of defense mechanism.

Defense mechanisms are neither bad nor good, but serve a useful purpose as the individual's best available method for containing intense anxiety. They are unconscious and may not be specifically intended to create negative reactions in others, even though that often is the end result.[31] Defense mechanisms need to be considered, along with other coping behaviors, within the context of how they serve the patient in preventing spiraling disorganization.

People who have a level of maturity through reasonable resolution of developmental tasks, an acceptable level of self-confidence and self-esteem, an active and involved support system, and an ability to move with relative ease between dependence and independence have the lowest risk of experiencing illness as a crisis. This statement is not to imply that they are unaffected by events. They may have periods of regression during which they are unable to perceive their situations realistically, drive away supports, or select coping behaviors that prolong problem resolution. Resilient people, however, use positive coping mechanisms in a timely manner so that they never completely lose their sense of integrity and continuity.

Those at greatest risk of being overwhelmed are people who have been scarred by past experiences. They have learned that the world is a dangerous place and they generally are helpless to control or modify their situation. They have learned few coping skills and they are unable to be flexible in applying them. If one fails, they have no other to try. They have little confidence in themselves or others. These patients present the greatest challenge for those responsible for getting them well.

ICU PHASE: SUPPORT

Once a patient is admitted to the critical care setting, the experience of psychologic stress is highly dependent on the specific nature of the problem.[32] What demands confront the patient? How does the illness and hospitalization impact the psychologic balance the patient has achieved?

General Stressors

Patients in critical care units must cope with similar and predictable challenges.[32-34] Perhaps for the first time, they are confronted with the possibility of their own deaths. Thoughts of their own mortality can initiate intense anxiety that must be addressed. This serious threat to existence, often in the context of uncertainty of outcome, initiates a variety of responses, depending on individual style and how real the threat of death. Grief is mixed with hope in varying degrees—a situation to which some physicians and nurses have difficulty responding. Often, if a patient expresses sadness over the possibility of death, the caregiver feels obligated to counter with hope. If, on the other hand, the patient expresses hope for recovery, the caregiver often is fearful that the patient is in denial and feels obligated to present "reality" to the patient. A more helpful approach in this situation is to recognize the appropriateness of the range of feelings and to allow the patient opportunities to express them.

Another concern for critically ill patients is the experience of or the threat of pain.[35,36] Not only is pain a distressing sensory experience, but it contributes to sleep deprivation, leads to feelings of powerlessness, and increases susceptibility to other stimuli that might otherwise be tolerated. Ensuring pain management, either through adequate analgesia, teaching relaxation, or providing information regarding the type of discomfort to anticipate, has been shown to increase feelings of personal control, decrease the amount of analgesia required, and in some cases, shorten the hospital stay.[37,38]

Patients must also cope with a multitude of caregivers whose skills are usually unknown to them. They must submit to respiratory therapists, radiology and ECG personnel, and laboratory technicians, nurses, and physicians, all of whom are asking them to participate in procedures that may increase pain and vulnerability. It takes a great deal of interpersonal skill and energy to relate positively to the numbers of people who are privy to one's intimate body parts and emotional reactions.

Feelings of being out of control are common. Critical illness swiftly and categorically deprives one of daily routines, social roles, relationships, and control over many bodily functions. Patients must try to maintain a sense of self-control and identity in the face of what may feel like impending doom. Remembering to address the patient appropriately, offering choices regarding treatment times, and providing self-administered pain medication programs are examples of interventions that decrease feelings of powerlessness. Ordering adequate anxiolytic medication or teaching simple relaxation exercises are other ways to help patients regain a sense of control.

Disease-Specific Stressors

Each disease follows a relatively predictable course, presents unique challenges, and creates particular limitations and possibilities. The situational demands created by the illness determines, in large part, the behavioral responses and coping strategies. Patients responding to the onset of an acute illness respond differently than patients who are hospitalized for an exacerbation of a chronic illness. Anxiety may be heightened in the latter case because the patient understands the implications of the symptoms. Conversely, experienced patients may know the routine, have expectations of treatment, be familiar with caretakers, and feel relieved that they will be treated.

Different phases of an illness present different challenges. The patient who is awaiting diagnosis is faced with ambiguity and uncertainty. Once a diagnosis is made, patients then have to confront the impact of the illness and make treatment decisions. At this point, patients must cope with uncertainty while at the same time, they must cope with the reality of the illness. Thus, caregivers should expect to see different behavior patterns. A patient with an abnormal growth, who is scheduled to undergo exploratory surgery, may use denial of the potential seriousness of the diagnosis and hope that what is found will be easily removed and treated. If a diagnosis of cancer is made, the patient may enlist problem-solving skills, identifying what modifications have to be made to undergo treatment, and they may change lifestyle and diet in hopes of strengthening immune function. If a discovery of metastasis is made, the patient must confront the inadequacy of medicine to solve the problem as well as failure of his or her own coping mechanisms to provide protection. At this point, the patient may exhibit feelings of anxiety, hopelessness, or anger.

As discussed previously, the specific body part and function that is affected, and the meaning and importance that an individual attaches to it, influences individual response. This point is paramount in understanding and supporting patients. How the caretaker thinks the patient should be reacting is not the standard against which the patient's response should be judged. A study identifying the type and severity of stressors associated with coronary artery bypass surgery showed significant differences between the perceptions of nurses and those of patients. Nurse stress ratings for both hospital and illness-related factors were significantly higher than patient ratings. The situations that were ranked as more stressful by the patients than the nurses are listed in Table 73-1. The situations that were ranked more stressful by the nurses than the patients are listed in Table 73-2.[39]

Caregivers often make assumptions about the patient's experiences and base their interactions on inaccurate information. For example, the patients in the study cited in Tables 73-1 and 73-2 were concerned about increasing their activities after cardiac surgery, whereas the nurses barely gave it a second thought. Patients who are reluctant to increase their independence and take longer to engage in self-care are often labeled as dependent and unwilling to do what they have to do to get well. This conclusion may be a misperception on the part of the caregivers. These patients would benefit from a discussion of their fears related to the likelihood of another cardiac event, helping them to distinguish between postoperative pain and cardiac disease-related pain, and the suspicion that activity may cause their incision to re-open.

Finally, critically ill patients are in a precarious physiologic state and are subjected to many changes that can alter perceptual ability, mood, and energy level. They may appear restless, depressed, irritable, uncooperative, and anxious. Hypoxia, hypercapnia, electrolyte imbalance, medications, changes in pH, sleep deprivation, and sensory deprivation and overload are just some of the factors that can alter perception and behavior.

Organic brain disorders, along with anxiety and depression, are the most common types of psychiatric disturbances seen in acutely ill medical patients.[40] One evening, a patient who was recovering normally from ocular surgery, started to refuse food and would not talk to her physician. It was determined that she probably was coping poorly with the operation and hospitalization and would recover better if she were discharged. By the next morning, she was paranoid and stood at her window screaming at passersby that she was being held prisoner and needed help. She eventually needed to be restrained by security personnel and sedated with neuroleptic medication. Behavior that was initially attributed to ineffective coping was later related to a reaction to her eye drops that contained scopolamine.

Another patient with AIDS was referred for psychiatric evaluation because of increasing withdrawal from self-care activities, extreme fatigue, and feelings of wanting to die. At the time of admission to the hospital, the patient had a hemoglobin value between 5 and 6. An eventual diagnosis of thrombotic thrombocytic purpura (TTP) was made and the patient was treated with plasmapheresis. As the hemoglobin value returned to normal, the patient again began to care for himself and looked forward to resuming preillness activities.

In the critical care setting, it is particularly important to evaluate behavioral changes within the context of a biopsychosocial model. Automatically attributing behavior changes to emotional causes may delay important treatment. Ongoing mental status examinations promote early detection of delirium (see Chap. 2).

Table 73-1. Cardiac Surgery Stressors Ranked Greater by Patients than Nurses*

Stressor	Patient Ranking	Nurse Ranking
Resuming previous life style	2.0	7.0
Absence from home/business	5.0	14.0
Increasing activity	7.0	20.0
Sharing room with another patient	9.0	18.5
Needing pain medications	10.0	26.0

* Scale of 1 to 30, 1 is highest stress.

Table 73-2. Cardiac Surgery Stressors Ranked Greater by Nurses than Patients*

Stressor	Patient Ranking	Nurse Ranking
Monitors/other equipment	23.5	15.5
Call light not being answered	20.0	4.5
Explanations of hospital procedures	28.0	17.0
Loss of income	13.0	9.0

* Scale of 1 to 30, 1 is the highest stress.

Helping Patients Cope with Psychologic Stress

When critically ill patients become anxious, irritable, listless, depressed, or uncooperative, it is important to assess all possible causes. The first step in helping patients cope is to rule out organic factors. Once this cause has been eliminated with reasonable certainty, attention can be directed toward psychologic interventions.

Most patients who have had reasonable success with coping with past stressors, have some successful relationships, and have completed the transitions of life with at least partial success require relatively simple interventions that can be instituted within the context of normal interaction. Patients want to feel confident in the people in whom they are trusting their lives. Going about the business of providing care with confidence and calm efficiency will be translated to the patient. The main ways to communicate calm to others include speech content, voice tones and pacing, and body language. A sense of having the situation under control or knowing how to call on the necessary resources often is comforting.[41]

Patients also need some time to express their concerns and to receive information related to their progress. Allowing the patient to present his or her subjective view of the meaning of the illness offers opportunities to correct misconceptions and to understand the patient's responses more clearly. They need to hear a mix of reality tempered with hope.

Expert practitioners have a great deal of experience in the expected course of an illness. This information is invaluable to many patients, helping them to prepare for events and taking some of the fear out of the unknown.

Most patients feel supported with the preceding interventions and manage to cope reasonably well. Other patients, however, do not respond to these efforts. Their coping mechanisms are ineffective for the amount of stress they are experiencing, and they may begin to exhibit behaviors that interfere with effective treatment. "Difficult" patients require greater periods of time than their medical diagnosis would suggest and stimulate negative responses in their caregivers.[42]

Some of these patients, however, may be labeled difficult and uncooperative when, in fact, their behavior may reflect a clash between the cultural beliefs of the patients and caregivers. Health professionals may view behavior that would be appropriate in the patient's own culture as deviant.[43] An example of this discrepancy lies in how patients express pain. If the patient expresses pain loudly and frequently with a caretaker who believes that pain should be borne silently and stoically, it is likely that the patient will be labeled difficult. It is important to try to understand the behavior of the patient within his or her own cultural context so that care is not withheld or the patient is not made to feel guilty.

Other patients try the patience of everyone who comes in contact with them. They are likely to have the patient representative, the social worker, the psychiatric liaison clinician, and the nursing supervisor deeply involved in their care. Some of these patients are overly dependent and expect the caregiver to fill their bottomless pit of neediness. Others, in order to have their needs met, use guilt and intimidation. Still others demand help and then proceed to reject it when they get it. When caretakers are confronted with these patients, it is helpful to have outside consultation to help with negative feelings and to develop a plan that includes clear limits on what can and cannot be done (Table 73-3). Enlisting the help of a psychiatrist, psychiatric clinical nurse specialist, or social worker to defuse the patient's feelings can free the critical care team so they can treat the medical condition.

Table 73–3. Interventions for Patients Experiencing Psychologic Stress

For Patients who:
    State they are unable to cope
    Experience the stress as greater than their available resources, either internal or external
    Have behaviors that are destructive to self or others (aggression, suicide, use of alcohol/drugs)
    Are unable to solve problems
    Use defense mechanisms that interfere with getting treatment or support (acting out, rejecting help, being overly dependent, manipulation)
Interventions
    Assess mental status
        Assess memory for recent past events and immediate recall
        Observe for altered/abnormal perceptions
        Assess thought processes
        Identify potential organic causes for behavior change and order appropriate diagnostic tests
    Give short simple explanations during high levels of anxiety
        Be prepared to repeat them given decreased ability to process information
    Develop nonjudgmental attitude through use of effective communication skills
        When you are with the patient listen with undivided attention
        Offer opportunities to ask questions
        Give information to correct misconceptions
        Help clearly define the problem with the patient
        Provide anticipatory guidance related to usual course of illness and hospitalization, sensations, available help, i.e., medication, relaxation technique, counseling
        Avoid passing judgment on behavior or feelings, i.e., "Most patients don't get this upset"
        Avoid giving false reassurance, i.e., "Everything's going to be just fine"
    Set limits on unacceptable behavior
        Recognize patient's anger early
        Set clear limits with kind firmness; do not confront or challenge the patient
        Consider use of family members to help maintain control
        Consider physical or chemical restraints to prevent harm to self or others
        Involve entire team so that consistency is maintained
        Assess need for psychiatric consultation to assist with modifying patient behavior and supporting staff

Maintaining Family Relationships

As stated previously, supportive relationships bolster the ability of an individual to cope with stress. Spouses and children of patients, however, describe feelings of vulnerability, intense emotions, and uncertainty. In one study, spouse respondents used such terms as very traumatic, disheartening, devastating, and like Hell to describe the experience of having a partner in a critical care unit.[44] Family members need to help to cope with the patient's illness so that they can continue to be a source of hope for the patient.

In several studies the needs of the families of critically ill patients have been identified.[45-48] The threats to effective coping identified most frequently were as follows:

- Lack of knowledge regarding the patient's condition
- Hopelessness regarding the patient's condition
- Fear of spouse's death
- Fear that the patient would be treated in a depersonalized manner

If caregivers can respond to these concerns, families may be able to cope with the experience more effectively and therefore can provide a greater degree of support to the patient.

Relationships with Caregivers

The patient's experience is influenced also by the expectations of the staff related to how patients should be sick and get well. The psychologic and cultural "match" between the patient, the physician, and the other health professionals providing care contributes to raising or lowering the psychologic stress of the patient.

On a subjective level, patients recognize the importance of support of those providing care. According to Drew, when patients had caretakers they described as lacking emotional warmth, impatient, irritated, bored, or preoccupied, they felt more hopeless and that their recovery slowed. Conversely, patients who received care from people they perceived as caring and involved with their work felt more in control, stronger, and as if their healing had been enhanced.[49]

In a small exploratory study, patients who required mechanical ventilation were asked to identify the stressors of the experience as well as interventions that helped to reduce the stress.[50] Patients identified the following as problematic, among other things:

- Activity restriction
- Inability to communicate
- Insufficient explanations
- Discomfort of the endotracheal tube

They could not recall specific interventions that helped, but they did recall reassuring words and a "caring" manner, confirming the findings of DiMatteo that when caretakers convey psychologic support, they positively influence patient recovery.[51]

Clearly, it is not the technology of the critical care unit alone that contributes to healing. Because the staff-patient relationship is an important factor in patients' responses to illness and hospitalization, caregivers must monitor their own stress levels and use coping responses that help to avoid detachment and cynicism, the cardinal signs of "burnout."

Impact of Critical Care on the Professional Staff

Long-term exposure to multiple stressors can lead to a stress response and physical and emotional exhaustion. Members of the health team can begin to feel overwhelmed by their work and lose the ability to care. Morale and performance suffer and optimal patient care cannot be delivered.

In a plethora of studies of critical care units, investigators have identified the multiple challenges to those persons who work in critical care:[52-58]

- Working closely with dying patients
- Facing the inevitability of death
- Confronting pain and suffering
- Learning to live with unpredictability
- Accepting the responsibility of detecting early signs of instability and initiating appropriate action
- Accepting the inevitability of imperfection and error
- Environmental stress from too many interruptions; lack of support from ancillary services, such as laboratory and pharmacy; excessive noise; work load; inadequate staffing
- Conflicts with co-workers or administrative personnel

Understanding the stress inherent in a critical care unit warrants attention so that professionals can be helped to cope in effective ways. Individuals and institutions can use several strategies to manage stress more effectively.

First, individuals need to become self-aware and recognize when they are under stress and what situations are creating the problem.[59] At this stage, problems often begin, because individuals who are experiencing stress may not always recognize it in themselves. They tend to externalize problems, blame others, and fail to recognize their own part in their situation. Those who work in this setting need to acknowledge the inherent stress in the setting and develop a personal stress management plan that includes good nutrition, exercise, enough sleep, laughter, and fun.

Support groups or meaningful peer relationships that allow open communication are helpful in reducing feelings of stress.[60,61] These groups permit individuals to explore their reactions and to get help in recognizing when they may be experiencing high degrees of stress. The groups can give permission for individuals to seek help to regain their sense of control.

Although individual care providers have the responsibility of maintaining their own psychologic health, those who are responsible for administering the critical care unit bear some responsibility for creating a climate in which staff can function optimally. The leadership style of the head nurse has been shown to contribute to job stress.[62] The attention that a leader pays to organizational structure, combined with attention to relationships, can influence the stress tolerance of the staff. Leaders who have an open, fair style of leadership provide an environment with reduced stress. Leaders who emphasize structure without attention to human needs of their staff, foster higher levels of burnout.

In 1986, researchers used the APACHE II severity-of-disease classification system to study prospectively the treatment and outcome in more than 5000 ICU patients.[63,64] The results demonstrated that patients did best in units in which communication between physicians and nurses was good and reflected professional respect. Patients fared worst in an atmosphere of mistrust. Developing collaborative practice models only decreases stress in caregivers but also improves patient care outcomes.

Finally, even the hardiest, most stress-tolerant people have their limits. No amount of stress management, open leadership, or collaborative relationships will work if the real problems of increased workload, insufficient staff, and poorly trained staff are not addressed. Although personal and unit-based stress management programs are successful, planned problem-solving must be used to address larger problems created by current trends in health care.

POST-ICU PHASE: REHABILITATION

The post-ICU phase begins with transfer from the critical care setting. For the cardiac patient who has been monitored closely, this change can be traumatic, associated with an increase in cardiovascular complication. Specific interventions that have reduced subjective stress as well as cardiac complications with readmission to the critical care unit have included anticipatory guidance, reassurance of transfer as a sign of progress, involving family members to provide support during and immediately post-transfer, and providing continuity of care after transfer, either through the ICU staff making post-transfer visits or by introducing the stepdown unit nurse prior to transfer.[23,65] Other studies have revealed that patients experience nightmares for some days or weeks after transfer from an ICU.[66]

Depression is a common finding in patients who have experienced a cardiac event requiring a stay in the coronary care unit. In a study of 68 patients with myocardial infarctions, 70% were depressed throughout the 1-year follow-up and failed to return to work or previous level of sexual function.[67]

Studies of various patient populations indicate that adjustment to a critical illness involves a process that takes place over time.[68-71] Patients must come to terms with the meaning of the illness or trauma; accept residual limitations, if any; refocus attention on other aspects of their lives that may have been neglected; and attain feelings of satisfaction again. As this process takes place, patients may experience signs and symptoms of anxiety and depression, which are frightening to both patient and family. People are in a hurry to get things "back the way they were" so they often do not accept these feelings or try to minimize them. This denial delays the work of healing that must take place.

Family members, too, must go through a period of adjustment.[72] They must readjust to the patient's increasing level of wellness and resumption of preillness roles. In the period after an illness, spouses have been reported to have an increase in both psychiatric and physical symptoms.[73,74] Clearly, the aftermath of illness is a stressful time.

Preparing the Patient for Discharge

Today's economic climate demands shorter hospital stays and increases the use of extended care facilities and home health services. Transfer from a critical care unit or discharge from a hospital is not based, as a rule, on the psychologic adjustment or readiness of the patient. Unfortunately, patients may be left to make the necessary psychologic adjustments isolated from primary caretakers.

Anticipating which patients will need help in the post-ICU phase can be determined, in part, by how the patient coped with the acute phase of the illness. Some patients, however, who were cooperative and apparently nonplused by their acute experience can be overwhelmed by the long process of recovery or the need to accept permanent disability. By evaluating the patient's and family's subjective view of the illness, the potential disturbance in the ability to perform activities of daily living and the anticipated residual symptoms of illness that might be experienced, caregivers may get some guidance as to what kind of services would benefit the patient. A patient whose self-esteem has been undermined by the meaning of the illness may benefit from counseling or short-term psychotherapy. Many patient-support groups are offered by agencies like the YMCA, American Cancer Society, American Heart Association, the Lupus Foundation, etc. Patients who may have difficulty carrying out routine tasks may need a rehabilitation program to relearn skills. Patients who may continue to experience symptoms of illness need extensive education as to symptom management. Hospitals should have ready access to community resources and literature that help patients and families plan for their future.

Patients benefit from anticipatory guidance, thinking through potential problems with experts—either patients with similar problems or with health-care providers who have experience with patients and families coping with the effects of illness. The goal, at the very least, is to return the patient and family to the preillness level of psychologic functioning. Some patients, if they are able to integrate the experience and find meaning in it, are often heard to remark, "I wouldn't wish this experience on anyone, but without it, I wouldn't have grown into the person I've become."

REFERENCES

1. Rapoport, L.: The state of crisis: Some theoretical considerations. *In* Crisis Intervention: Selected Readings. Edited by H. Parad. New York, Family Service Association of America, 1967.
2. Segall, A.: The sick role concept: Understanding illness behavior. J. Health Soc. Behav., *17*:163, 1976.
3. Perry, S., and Viederman, M.: Management of emotional reactions to acute medical illness. Med. Clin. North Am., *65*:3, 1981.
4. Thomas, S. A., Lynch, J. J., Mills, M. E.: Psychological influences on heart rhythm in the coronary care unit. Heart Lung, *4*:746, 1975.
5. Lown, B., et al.: Psychophysiologic factors in sudden cardiac death. Am. J. Psychiatry, *137*:1325, 1980.
6. Krantz, D. S., Glas, D. C.: Personality, behavior patterns, and physical illness: Conceptual and methodological issues. *In* Handbook of Behavioral Medicine. Edited by W. D. Gentry. New York, Guilford Press, 1984, p. 38.
7. Borysenko, M., and Borysenko, J.: Stress, behavior and immunity: Animal models and mediating mechanisms. Gen. Hosp. Psychiatry, *4*:59, 1982.
8. Kemeny, M. E., et al.: Psychoneuroimmunology. *In* A Comprehensive Textbook of Neuroendocrinology. Edited by C. Nemeroff. Caldwell, NJ: Telford Press, In press.

9. Aguilera, D. C., Messick, J. M., Farrel, M. S.: Crisis Intervention: Theory and Methodology. St. Louis, CV Mosby, 1970, p. 52.
10. Lazarus, R. S.: Psychological Stress and the Coping Process. New York, McGraw Hill, 1966.
11. Rutter, M.: Resilience in the face of adversity. Br. J. Psychiatry, 147:598, 1985.
12. Kadner, K. D.: Resilience: Responding to adversity. J. Psychosoc. Nurs. Ment. Health Serv., 27:20, 1989.
13. Hull, J. G., VanTreuren, R. R. Virnilli, S.: Hardiness and health: A critique and alternative approach. J. Pers. Soc. Psychol., 53:518, 1987.
14. Lee, H. J.: Analysis of a concept: Hardiness. Oncol. Nurs. Forum, 10:32, 1983.
15. Vaillant, G. E.: Theoretical hierarchy of adaptive ego mechanisms. Arch. Gen. Psychiatry, 24:535, 1976.
16. Kobasa, S. C.: Stressful life events, personality and health: An inquity into hardiness. J. Pers. Soc. Psychol., 37:1, 1979.
17. Wagnild, G., and Young, H. M.: Resilience among older women. Image, 22:252, 1990.
18. Weisman, A. D.: Coping with illness. In Massachusetts General Hospital Handbook of General Hospital Psychiatry. Edited by T. Hackett and N. Cassem. Littleton, MA, PSG Publishing, 1987.
19. Geringer, E. S., and Stern, T. A.: Coping with medical illness: The impact of personality types. Psychomatics 27:251, 1986.
20. Berkman, L. F., Syme, S.: Social networks, host resistance and mortality: A nine year follow-up study of Alameda County residents. Am. J. Epidemiol., 102:186, 1979.
21. House, J. S., Landis, K. R., Umberson, D.: Social relationships and health. Science, 241:540, 1988.
22. Ruberman, W., et al.: Psychosocial influences on mortality after myocardial infarction. N. Engl. J. Med., 311:552, 1984.
23. Schwartz, L. P., Brenner, Z. R.: Critical care unit transfer: Reducing stress through nursing interventions. Heart Lung, 8:540, 1979.
24. Goodwin, J. S., et al.: The effect of marital status on stage, treatment and survival of cancer patients. JAMA, 258:3125, 1987.
25. Lazarus, R. S., and Folkman, S.: Stress, Appraisal, and Coping. New York, Springer, 1984.
26. Nyamathi, A.: Coping response of spouses of MI patients and of hemodialysis patients as measured by the Jalowiec Coping Scale. J. Cardiovasc. Nurs., 2:67, 1987.
27. King, K. B.: Measurement of coping strategies, concerns, and emotional response in patients undergoing coronary bypass grafting. Heart Lung, 14:579, 1985.
28. Sutherland, S.: Burned adolescents' descriptions of their coping strategies. Heart Lung, 17:150, 1988.
29. Clark, S.: Psychosocial needs of the critically ill patient. In Critical Care Nursing. Edited by J. Closky, C. Breu, S. Cardin, and A. Whitaker. Philadelphia, W. B. Saunders, In press.
30. Minarik, P., and Leavitt, M.: The angry, demanding, hostile response. In Psychological Aspects of Critical Care Nursing. Edited by B. Reigel and D. Ehrenreich. Rockville, MD, Aspen, 1988.
31. Clark, S.: Preoperative phase: Intervention, In Nursing Care of the Critically Ill Surgical Patient. Edited by R. G. Hathaway. Rockville, MD, Aspen, 1988.
32. Moos, R. H., and Tsu, V. D.: The crisis of physical illness: An overview. In Coping with Physical Illness. Edited by R. Moos. New York, Plenum Medical, 1979.
33. Beglinger, J. E.: Coping tasks in critical care. Dimens. Crit. Care Nurs., 2:80, 1983.
34. Keily, W. F.: Coping with severe illness. Adv. Psychosom. Med., 8:105, 1972.
35. Ballard, K.: Identification of environmental stressors for patients in a surgical intensive care unit. Issues Ment. Health Nurs., 3:89, 1981.
36. Jones, J., et al.: What patients say: A study of reactions to an intensive care unit. Intensive Care Med., 5:89, 1979.
37. Flaherty, G. G., and Fitzpatrick, J. J.: Relaxation technique to increase comfort level in postoperative patients: A preliminary study. Nurs. Res., 27:352, 1978.
38. Radwin, L. E.: Autonomous nursing interventions for treating the patient in acute pain: A standard. Heart Lung, 16:258, 1987.
39. Carr, J. A., and Powers, M. J.: Stressors associated with coronary bypass surgery. Nurs. Res., 35:243, 1986.
40. Schwab, J. J.: Psychiatric illness in medically ill patients: Why it goes undiagnosed. Psychosomatics, 23:225, 1982.
41. Proudfoot, M. H. J.: Contagious calmness: A sense of calmness in acute care settings. Top. Clin. Nurs., 4:18, 1983.
42. Groves, J. E.: Taking care of the hateful patient. N. Engl. J. Med., 298:883, 1978.
43. Podrasky, D. L., and Sexton, D. L.: Nurses' reactions to difficult patients. Image, 20:16, 1988.
44. Titler, M. G., Cohen, M. Z., Craft, M. J.: Impact of adult critical care hospitalization: Perceptions of patients, spouses, children, and nurses. Heart Lung, 20:174, 1991.
45. Rodgers, C.: Needs of relatives of cardiac surgery patients during the critical care phase. Focus Crit Care, 10:50, 1983.
46. Molter, N. C.: Needs of relatives of critically ill patients: A descriptive study. Heart Lung, 8:332, 1979.
47. Daley, L.: The perceived immediate needs of families with relatives in the intensive care setting. Heart Lung, 13:231, 1984.
48. Leske, J. S.: Needs of relatives of critically ill patients: A follow-up. Heart Lung, 15:189, 1986.
49. Drew, N.: Exclusion and confirmation: A phenomonology of patient's experience with caregivers. Image, 18:39, 1986.
50. Gries, M. L., and Fernsler, J.: Patient perceptions of the mechanical ventilation experience. Focus Crit. Care, 15:52, 1988.
51. DiMatteo, R.: A sociological-psychological analysis of the physician-patient rapport: Toward a science of the art of medicine. J. Soc. Issues, 35:112, 1979.
52. Gentry, W. D., Foster, S. B., Froehling, S.: Psychological response to situational stress in intensive care and non-intensive care nursing. Heart Lung, 1:794, 1972.
53. Gentry, W. D., and Parkes, K. R.: Psychologic stress in intensive care unit and non-intensive care unit nursing: A review of the past decade. Heart Lung, 11:43, 1982.
54. Norbeck, J. S.: Perceived job stress, job satisfaction and psychological symptoms in critical care nursing. Research in Nursing and Health, 8:253, 1985.
55. Kelly, J. G., Cross D. G.: Stress, coping behaviors, and recommendations for intensive care and medical surgical ward registered nurses. Res. Nurs. Health, 8:321, 1985.
56. Topf, M.: Personality hardiness, occupational stress and burnout in critical care nurses. Res. Nurs. Health, 12:179, 1989.
57. Topf, M., and Dillon, E.: Noise-induced stress as a predictor of burnout in critical care nurses. Heart Lung, 17:567, 1988.
58. Robinson, J. A., and Lewis, D. J.: Coping with ICU work-related stressors: A study. Crit. Care Nurse, 10:80, 1990.
59. Gardner, E. R., and Hall, R. C. W.: The professional stress syndrome. Psychosomatics, 22:672, 1981.
60. Simon, N. M., and Whitely, S.: Psychiatric consultation with MICU nurses: The consultation conference as a working group. Heart Lung, 6:497, 1977.
61. Fawzy, F. I., et al.: Preventing nursing burnout: A challenge for liaison psychiatry. Gen. Hosp. Psychiatry, 5:141, 1983.
62. Duxbury, M. L., et al.: Head nurse leadership style with staff

nurse burnout and job satisfaction in neonatal intensive care units. Nurs. Res., *33:*97, 1984.
63. Knauss, W. A., et al.: An evaluation of outcome from intensive care in major medical centers. Ann. Intern. Med., *104:*410, 1986.
64. Draper, E. A.: Effects of nurse/physician collaboration and nursing standards on ICU patient outcomes. Curr. Concepts Nurs., *1:*2, 1986.
65. Klein, R. F., et al.: Transfer from a coronary care unit: Some adverse responses. Arch. Intern. Med., *122:*104, 1968.
66. Kornfeld, D. S.: The intensive care unit in adults: Coronary care and general medical/surgical. Adv. Psychosom. Med., *10:*1, 1980.
67. Stern, M. J., Pascale, L., Ackerman, A.: Life adjustment post-myocardial infarction. Arch. Intern. Med., *137:*680, 1977.
68. Brown, J. T.: Grief response in trauma patients and their families. Adv. Psychosom. Med., *16:*93, 1986.
69. Sutherland, S.: Burned adolescents' descriptions of their coping strategies. Heart Lung, *17:*150, 1988.
70. Johnson, J. L., and Morse, J. M.: Regaining control: the process after myocardial infarction. Heart Lung, *19:*126, 1990.
71. Fife, B. L.: A model for predicting the adaptation of families to medical crisis: an analysis of role integration. Image, *17:*108, 1985.
72. Michel, M. H., and Murdaugh, C. L.: Family adjustment to heart transplantation: redesigning the dream. Nurs. Res., *36:*332, 1987.
73. Mayou, R., et al.: The psychological and social effects of myocardial infarction on wives. Br. Med. J., *1:*699, 1978.
74. Skelton, M., and Dominian, J.: Psychological stress in wives of patients with myocardial infarction. Br. Med. J., *14:*101, 1973.

SUPPLEMENTAL READINGS

Evans, S. A., and Carlson, R. C.: Nurse/physician collaboration: Solving the nursing shortage crisis. Am. J. Crit. Care, *1:*25, 1992.

Ferrando, S. J., and Eisendrath, S. J.: Adverse neuropsychiatric effects of dopamine antagonist medications: Misdiagnosis in the medical setting. Psychosomatics, *32:*426, 1991.

McNamara, M. E.: Psychological factors affecting neurological conditions. Psychosomatics, *32:*255, 1991.

Myer, J. D., and Fink, C. M.: Psychiatric symptoms from prescription medications. Professional Psychology: Research and Practice, *20:*90, 1989.

Neese, J. B.: Depression in the general hospital. Nurs. Clin. North Am., *26:*613, 1991.

Rodin, G., Craven, J., Littlefield, C.: Depression in the Medically Ill: An Intregrated Approach. New York, Brunner/Mazel, 1991.

Scwartz, J., et al.: Antidepressants in the medically ill: Prediction of benefits. Int. J. Psychiatry Med., *19:*363, 1989.

Smith, R. C., and Zimny, G. H.: Physician's emotional reactions to patients. Psychosomatics, *29:*393, 1988.

… Chapter 74

QUALITY ASSESSMENT AND ASSURANCE IN THE INTENSIVE CARE UNIT

CARL A. SIRIO
WILLIAM A. KNAUS

Intensive care units (ICUs) developed in the 1950s and 1960s concurrently with the introduction of postoperative recovery rooms and the development of effective external cardiac massage and defibrillation. The first ICUs provided state-of-the-art continuous electrocardiographic monitoring capabilities and advanced respiratory support. The positive impact of these now seemingly rudimentary efforts on preventing premature death led to a proliferation of intensive care services worldwide.[1] The aim of introducing these specialized units was to improve the overall quality of care for severely ill patients by concentrating personnel and technologic services in a centralized location.

Today, physicians admit patients to ICUs primarily for two reasons: (1) Highly technical and active treatment provided acutely ill patients may improve the chances for successful recovery, and (2) Stable patients admitted for intensive monitoring may have reduced major morbidity and mortality. The thresholds for admitting and treating patients in the ICUs vary greatly throughout the world depending on national practice styles and the availability of resources devoted to high technology critical care services.[2-5]

This variation in patient selection, as well as the diversity of medical and surgical diseases treated in ICUs, and the wide variety of critical care services provided among hospitals have made the precise evaluation of care difficult.[6] The clinical literature highlights conflicting evidence regarding the benefit of intensive care in various disease states. Several investigators have shown a reduction in mortality for respiratory failure treated with ventilatory support. Similarly, mortality rates after open heart surgery have decreased with the use of surgical critical care. Conversely, retrospective reviews of outcome from severe pneumococcal bacteremia do not show a reduction in mortality.[7-9]

To date, the outcome most commonly studied has been death. Other outcomes of clinical importance include the incidence of morbidity and the overall length and quality of survival. Examples of these outcomes are provided in Table 74-1.

Considering the lack of clear-cut evidence regarding the efficacy of intensive care therapy and the wide variation in thresholds for admitting patients to ICUs, the need for quality assessment in critical care is great. Appropriate quality assessment activities can have a direct impact on evaluating the efficacy of individual care. In addition, the efficiency and utility of overall resource use at an institutional, as well as regional or national level, can be better assessed. The demand for improved and formalized methods of monitoring quality and outcomes have increased as the cost of medical and hospital care has escalated.

As an integral component of a professional responsibility, physicians have always had an obligation to perform peer review and quality assessment. The urgency to fulfill this mandate has increased as interested third parties, including government agencies, employers, and insurance carriers, have taken a more active role in attempting to define and understand the components of effective medical care.

Despite these demands for quality assessment, minimal published information exists on reliable or efficient methods to assess quality. This deficiency is due in large part to the difficulty clinicians have had in determining the incremental value that improvements and advances in diagnostic, therapeutic, and monitoring technology have had on outcome. This problem impacts equally on both actively treated and primarily monitored ICU patients. For both groups, the fundamental questions remain: Who benefits from the higher level and intensity of care afforded in the critical care arena? and How can that care be provided most efficiently?

Analysis of these complex questions is predicated on having effective measures of patient characteristics, the process of clinical care, and outcome. Measures of patient characteristics must include adequate and appropriate appraisals of the severity of illness, prior functional status, age, major diagnosis, and the location of treatment before admission to the ICU. Evaluation of the process of care must include a consideration of both the clinical care provided to an individual and the institutional framework in which care is delivered. Assessing this framework includes scrutinizing the overall organization and management of the ICU. Outcome assessment can begin with short-term events such as hospital mortality, although this review should be expanded to include long-term morbidity and mortality.

To date, governmental and institutional efforts to evaluate quality of care using a retrospective analysis of hospital mortality and morbidity data derived from administrative discharge information have met with skepticism. This response is attributable mainly to the underlying limitations of the tools used for analysis.[10-12] Methods to control the

Table 74–1. Outcomes from Critical Care of Clinical Importance

Mortality
Morbidity
    Nosocomial infection
    Re-intubation
    Self-extubation
    Re-admission to the intensive care unit within 24 hours
Length of survival after hospital discharge
Quality of survival
    Activities of daily living
    Satisfaction with quality of life achieved
    Return to work

Table 74–2. Distinctions between Quality Assessment and Quality Assurance

Quality assessment
    Development of standards of care that change over time to incorporate new insights into illness
    Systematic monitoring of care for effectiveness
    Systematic evaluation of care using outcomes
    Comparison of care to established standards
    Identification of opportunities to continually improve care
Quality assurance
    Designation of individuals and institutional departments responsible for the evaluation of care
    Verification of adequacy of care
    Development and implementation of recommendations to improve the quality of care with an eye toward excellence

differences in patient characteristics have been ineffective and the processes of care have largely been ignored. Left unaccounted are differences in patient characteristics, notably severity of illness, that confound an analysis of care given differences in patients' potential for recovery. Similarly, traditional methods of quality assessment, including review of adverse occurrence, documentation of policies and procedures, infection control programs, and periodic focused chart audits, do not place adequate emphasis on overall improvement in the quality of care and resource utilization.

Rather than reiterate the current state of affairs, however, we focus this discussion on developing a comprehensive approach to quality in critical care. Specific developments in the area of assessing care are evaluated as they relate to the practice of medicine in an ICU. In this chapter, we incorporate an evaluation of the decision to admit a patient to the ICU, the components of care within the critical care unit, and the assessment of outcome.

QUALITY OF CARE MANAGEMENT

As terminology is currently used, quality assessment activities involve the systematic monitoring and evaluation of care with some predetermined method of confirming quality by comparisons to established standards. Substantiation of quality by individual or structured entities responsible for evaluation of care both within and outside a hospital facility constitutes quality assurance.[13] The distinctions between quality assessment and quality assurance are highlighted in Table 74–2.

The overriding focus of all quality evaluation is a continued search for excellence. The Institute of Medicine has defined quality of care as "the degree to which health services for individuals and populations increase the likelihood of desired health outcomes and are consistent with current professional knowledge." Health outcomes must reflect a broad set of health status and health-related outcomes, such as those described in Table 74–1. In addition, this broad definition of quality recognizes the importance of professional responsibility to the individual patient within the context of the public's overall health.

Within this framework, certain minimal criteria have been established to guarantee that hospitals provide adequate resources when establishing and providing critical care services. These fundamental requirements have typically been determined by consensus and are enumerated by the Society of Critical Care Medicine,[14] the Joint Commission on Accreditation of Health Care Organizations,[15] and the National Institutes of Health.[16] They emphasize the important physical aspects of providing specialized care and the special supervisory, educational, and monitoring skills required.

Beyond these lists of technologies and competencies deemed necessary for the provision of critical care, a consensus on the most appropriate use of ICU resources does not exist, in part from the paucity of data regarding the relative impact on outcome of the observations and measurements made and therapies administered in the ICU.[17] This lack of consensus has made the tasks of assessing care difficult, despite the fact that quality assessment and assurance have been the focus of scientific study.[18,19] The parameter to assess quality used and studied most widely has been the evaluation of outcome.[20–24]

HISTORY OF OUTCOME AND QUALITY EVALUATION IN CRITICAL CARE

Measurement of Patient Characteristics

Patient outcome is influenced by a variety of factors both before and during the course of therapy, as outlined in Table 74–3. Patient characteristics observed before treatment define the underlying severity of disease. Successful outcome depends on the interaction between underlying patient characteristics and therapy.

Current efforts to assess outcome and quality in critical care began with the development of disease-specific in-

Table 74–3. Determinants of Patient Outcome

Information Available	Patient and Treatment Factors

Before treatment	Type of disease (diagnosis)
	Severity of disease
	Physiologic reserve
	    Age
	    Chronic disease

After treatment	Therapy available
	Application of therapy
	    Timing of therapy
	    Process of care
	Response to therapy

dices designed to capture severity of illness. These indices served as refined measures of patient characteristics felt to impact on survival. Examples include the Killip classification system for patients with acute myocardial infarction and the Glasgow Coma Score for patients with acute neurologic injury.[25,26] These systems have been limited by their disease specificity, but they are useful tools to compare patients within and across institutions as they classify patients irrespective of the care subsequently received.

Measurement of the Process of Care

Physicians have increasingly sophisticated and complex resources from which to select diagnostic and therapeutic courses for patient care. Hospitals, as complex institutions, are structured in a multiplicity of ways to implement clinical care plans. An understanding of the processes and systems used at a unit or institutional level may be important in the complete understanding of outcome. The ability to measure the impact that these differences have on outcome currently is constrained by the lack of a full understanding of those components of the process of implementing a clinical plan that are fundamental to attaining excellent outcomes. In addition, few tools measure these components thoroughly.

The Therapeutic Intervention Scoring System (TISS) developed by Cullen et al. was designed to quantify the amount of care a patient received.[27] Seventy-six procedures or clinical situations, common in most ICUs and reflecting the process of care, are awarded numeric points. Points range from 1 to 4 and are summed over 24 hours. They reflect the intensity of nursing work required to perform a task or to monitor a clinical event. In addition to providing information on nurse staffing requirements for varying levels of patient severity, TISS can be used for an analysis of both critical care unit use and the cost of care relative to the intensity of care provided.

The application of TISS to the measurement of the process of care has several qualifications. Quantification of clinical activity presupposes that care provided is appropriate, specific, identifiable, discrete, and applied consistently. Further, the underlying model assumes that a clear correlation exists between severity of disease and the number of interventions required. Clearly, clinical care is influenced by local factors such as medical and nursing culture, protocols, and policies. Nevertheless, TISS serves as an indirect measure of the severity of illness across heterogeneous disease entities. An important limitation of TISS is its inability to allow for a direct understanding of the relationship between the specific illness of a patient and the impact of ICU care. Despite these encumbrances, TISS can provide a reasonable measure of the quantity and the nature of the therapy and the clinical process used by physicians and nurses in critical care.

As highlighted previously, an evaluation of the process of care in the ICU must include an assessment of the overall framework in which individual care is provided. Formal measures to evaluate the organization and management structure of ICUs do not currently exist. Only recently have investigators begun to describe the key components of structure and management in the ICU.[28] An important finding in this preliminary study was that improved outcomes were related most strongly to the interaction and coordination of each hospital's intensive care physician and nursing staffs. The overall administrative structure of a unit had a relatively small impact on overall unit performance as measured by improved mortality. Once the important organizational elements have been identified, the next challenge will be to develop the necessary tools to compare and contrast outcome as a consequence of these differences.

Measurement of Outcome

As highlighted in Table 74-3, a spectrum of clinical end points can be considered valuable in measuring the outcome derived from ICU care. An important step forward in the assessment of outcomes was made with the development of the Acute Physiology and Chronic Health Evaluation (APACHE) by Knaus et al.[29,30] This system was designed to risk stratify ICU patients with diverse admitting diagnoses. The APACHE is predicated on the postulate that, prior to therapy, short-term hospital mortality in critically ill adults is influenced by four patient variables: the degree of physiologic deviation from normal, age, co-morbid conditions, and disease. Analyzing the interaction of these variables using multiple logistic regression techniques yields a more accurate understanding of the interrelationships between disease, physiology, and the ability of the individual to recoup from physiologic stress. Acute physiologic abnormalities are the most important determinant of short-term risk of hospital death.

Subsequent to the development of the APACHE model, other investigators designed a variety of physiologically based severity of illness stratification systems designed to predict short-term outcome. For critically ill adults, these systems include the Simplified Acute Physiology Score (SAPS)[31] and the Mortality Prediction Models (MPM).[32] In pediatrics, the Physiologic Stability Index (PSI)[33,34] and the Pediatric Risk of Mortality Score (PRISM)[35] have been developed. To date, few studies are designed to evaluate the length and quality of life following hospitalization.

An appropriate diagnostic label is essential for careful comparisons of severity of illness between patients, because an understanding of the interaction between the underlying pathophysiologic condition and the physiologic abnormalities thereby engendered are important. These interactions play a major role in determining patient risk of death. The diagnosis is therefore an integral component in severity systems such as APACHE and improves overall explanatory power. Authors of retrospective reliability studies using APACHE have indicated that primary organ system failure and diagnosis can be credibly abstracted.[36] Others have found many inaccuracies in re-abstracting studies designed to capture diagnostic labeling errors.[37-40]

Although severity of illness measures for critically ill patients attempt to capture all important variables that affect outcome, unmeasured variability still exists. As systems designed to quantitate severity of illness become more refined and their underlying normative databases grow, the effect of these unmeasured variations will become small. As highlighted by Pollack and colleagues using the PRISM in pediatric ICUs across hospitals, the physiologically based severity systems can capture sufficient data to assess severity and to explain much variation in patient outcome.[35]

The importance of this evolution in accurate patient description and risk stratification relates to a vital issue in quality assessment. The nature, characteristics, and risks of the patient population in question must be documented reliably and accurately and well understood before useful statements regarding quality can be made.

ICU DECISION-MAKING

Decisions in the intensive care sphere center around three distinct topical areas: triage assessments, diagnostic and therapeutic determinations, and strategy for the organization, management, and structure of intensive care delivery. Triage assessments have an impact on the overall quality of care before, during, and after admission to the ICU. Diagnostic and therapeutic judgments, as well as the organization and structure of the ICU, affect the quality of care during the time spent in the critical care unit. Both triage and diagnostic and therapeutic decisions have clear immediacy regarding their impact on patient care.

Decisions regarding the structure, organization, and management of intensive care services delivered may also influence the overall delivery of quality care. They impact the care provided to all patients irrespective of the individual clinical situation. It is necessary to focus on all three areas of ICU decision-making and their potential impact on the quality of care.

Triage

Triage, derived from the French word meaning "to sort," is the medical screening of patients to determine their priority for treatment. In the critical care setting, it involves decisions that affect both the admission and discharge of patients from the unit. A central issue in triage is the allocation of resources to maximize the potential for appropriate outcomes for individuals while using total resources in the most effective overall manner. This issue can also be framed in the form of the previously stated fundamental questions. Is intensive care beneficial? If so, when is it of value and to whom?

The pressure to move patients into and out of the ICU can vary enormously between institutions depending on a variety of factors, such as the size, location, and case mix of a hospital, as well as local practice styles regarding the use of intensive care resources. Bed availability and hospital protocols influence decision to admit and discharge patients from the ICU.[41-43] In addition, physician-specific decisions based on personal heuristics or rules of thumb can influence the type of patients admitted into the critical care unit.

Concern is growing that patient outcome may be adversely affected by the selection criteria used to admit or to exclude patients from critical care services. For hospitals coping with intense triage pressure, this concern centers on how quality may be impacted when, potentially patients are discharged prematurely.[44] Conversely, delayed discharge may prevent admission of patients who might benefit from ICU care if beds were available during occasions of limited bed availability.

To evaluate these issues fully, an accurate assessment of patients' clinical characteristics is required at the time ICU admission is considered. The components of this measure should include precise diagnostic information and an assessment of acute severity of illness and chronic health status. Using such a comprehensive evaluation of patient characteristics, physicians will be better able to determine which patients are in greatest need of critical care services. The result will be a more objective determination of those most likely to benefit from admission to the ICU. These insights can help structure admission criteria for patients likely to receive active intensive care treatment as well as those likely to need solely monitoring.

Depending on the ICU examined, anywhere from 20 to 80% of admissions are for monitoring and not for acute life support. Recent work indicates that acute physiologic abnormalities are powerful predictors of patient risk for those admitted for monitoring to subsequently require active ICU therapies.[45,46]

For many of these patients for whom objective measures of physiologic status indicate they are "low risk monitor" admissions, questions as to whether they are best treated in an ICU, in a less intensive step-down unit, or on the general hospital floor are legitimate. For those instances in which a patient is admitted, it would be helpful to know when discharge can be safely considered. The accurate and reliable identification of these low risk monitor patients, and a measure of their eventual requirement for therapy, can serve as an excellent quality assessment activity.

Hospital populations also include groups of patients for whom critical care is not successful in reversing the effects of an acute illness. Some patients are at a high risk of short-term mortality despite aggressive intervention whereas others fail to respond to treatment. Patients in these circumstances may be candidates for setting therapeutic limits or withdrawal of life-sustaining therapies. The decision to forgo critical care treatment is often complex and wrought with emotion. Nevertheless, such decisions are made with increasing frequency and are legitimate areas for quality assessment and assurance activities.

The systematic collection of fundamental patient characteristics such as disease and disease severity are leading to reliable and accurate estimates of the probability of mortality for severely ill patients. The decision to forestall intensive care of these patients will be enhanced by better assessments of the attendant risk of a decision to either provide or waive intensive care. It is becoming increasingly evident that physicians will rely on physiology estimates of mortality risk as the appraisals of outcome become more accurate. As individual estimates become more universally available, they can serve as the quantitative basis for quality assessment activities regarding decisions to withhold care. Precise estimates of the likely benefit derived from aggressive care will also allow clinicians to judge objectively comparative entitlements to care.[47-49] Increasingly, physicians will be required to make clinical judgments to select patients who can significantly benefit from high technology care in an era of growing resource constraints. Although physicians are unaccustomed to, and may initially be uncomfortable with, explicit probabilities used as adjuncts and incorporated into decision-making, such probability statements could improve the overall quality of patient care.[50-53]

The crucial issue in the selection of patients for intensive care becomes assuring that we do not limit access to those who will benefit while limiting admission to patients who are unlikely to benefit from intensive care. Strategies need to be developed to monitor outcomes of those denied care to assure that they receive high quality care appropriate for their specific clinical condition and stage of illness.

Diagnostic and Therapeutic Decision-Making—The Process of Care

A tool used commonly in quality assessment is the internal or external chart audit. The standards to which such charts are held vary depending on local standards of care as well as the abilities and knowledge base of the chart reviewer. The current process of care makes little provision for objective estimation of patient risk or severity of illness, much less the efficiency and efficacy of care. Selection of charts for review typically results from the identification of important sentinel events such as the need for mechanical ventilation or inotropic support. Charts may also be "flagged" for selective analysis of iatrogenic complications, nosocomial infections, medication errors, reintubation rates, readmission to the ICU after discharge to the ward, or other suspected markers of deficient process of care. Establishing protocols and standards by which charts are evaluated is helpful, but more widely applicable benchmarks for review and evaluation are needed.

Adequate assessment of the significance on patient outcome of these and other sentinel events necessitates quantifiable, reproducible, and validated means of estimating the a priori risk of these events occurring. Any study coupling chart audit review with an objective judgment of patient risk has been limited.[54] When this is done, the outcome considered most often is mortality. The aim of this type of analysis is to search for examples of "preventable deaths."

Quantification of mortality during intensive care therapy and hospitalization for an acute illness is a useful measure of quality if lower death rates clearly reflect differences in medical care. We must also, however, be willing to consider other markers of care. For patients hospitalized with a terminal illness, death may be both the inevitable and acceptable outcome. For this subset of patients, the quality of comfort measures provided and the emotional ease, for the patient and family, with which death occurred may be paramount.[55] Extensive application of ICU technology may be inappropriate.

A fundamental issue in this evaluation of the process of individual patient care is an assessment of the efficacy of diagnostic and treatment decisions over time and their relationship to outcome. This area of research is still in its formative stages. Intuitively, patients who improve rapidly with initial ICU care are more likely to have successful outcomes. Investigators applying the Mortality Prediction Model published results suggesting that accurate predictions were available when the model was used at 48 and 72 hours into intensive care. Chang developed a dynamic conceptual framework to identify patients who are likely to die after failing to respond to initial ICU therapy. The majority of predictions were completed within the initial 5 days of ICU treatment.[56] Preliminary findings suggest that updating predictions over the course of therapy leads to improved predictive ability.

Extensive experience delineating outcome from multiple system organ failure indicates the initial 48 to 72 hours is critical for recovery.[57] A comprehensive assessment of quality would include the precise nature of the type of intensive care provided and an appraisal of its impact on the speed with which deranged physiology was stabilized. Currently available severity measures provide a mechanism to accomplish this task and work in this area is ongoing.[58]

Clinical Outcome, Mortality, and Quality of Care

As suggested in the preceding discussion, an analysis of patient mortality has been touted as a primary method to evaluate the quality of hospital care. Nevertheless, a nagging and persistent question remains. Can hospital death rates be adjusted adequately for variations in the baseline risk of death of patients to accurately reflect the quality of care? Data in this area are not convincing. Few clinically convincing data support the assertion that a large number of deaths are preventable.

Rutsein developed a conceptual model of what he labeled, "sentinel health events," events that should occur if patients were receiving high quality care. For example, deaths associated with surgical procedures that should be extremely safe, such as elective herniorrhaphy and tonsillectomy, were included in the paradigm. Unfortunately, this conceptual framework was not supported by empiric data.[59]

In a study of autopsy findings, Landefeld et al. suggested a potential for avoidable deaths.[60] In 26 of 233 consecutive, retrospective cases studied, postmortem findings uncovered information that, if known prior to death, would most likely have led to changes in therapy. These changes in therapy would have been expected to have a positive effect on outcome. Despite a strong suggestion that some deaths may be premature, this study is limited by the obvious selection bias of patients undergoing autopsy.[60] Similarly, in an analysis of asthma deaths, Eason and Markowe claimed that for 35 patients who died of an acute attack, death was preventable in 46%. Preventable deaths were attributed to inadequate patient monitoring and ineffective use of beta agonist therapy.[61] In a study of perinatal maternal mortality in New York, a sixfold difference in the maternal mortality rates was found among 67 hospitals. Review of these deaths suggested that institutional rates of preventable perinatal mortality ranged from 14 to 82%.[62]

A study by Dubois et al. also raised the possibility of differences in the process and quality of care in hospitals identified as high and low death rate outliers for patients with cerebrovascular accidents and pneumonia. Their methodology incorporated both objective and expert subjective analysis to reach conclusions regarding preventable deaths. They suggested that preventable deaths were more likely to be found in patients with an initially low risk of death when compared to those with intermediate or high risks. Although doubt remains as to the reliability with which preventable deaths can be determined, this type of research is beginning to shed light on an aspect of care that is important yet difficult to analyze.[54,63]

Results of these studies suggest some deaths are preventable. In addition, they support the theory that some hospitals have a higher preventable death rate than others. In view of these limited data, an active debate is ongoing as to the degree to which hospital mortality is a distinct marker of quality in hospital care. The intensity of this debate has been heightened by the release of mortality data based on large administrative data bases that do not accurately reflect differences in severity of illness.[64,65]

There are obstacles to making the use of risk adjusted death rate data a valid and reproducible technique in quality assessment. Even if adequate control of all relevant patient attributes that influence outcome can be achieved, several other legitimate concerns exist regarding the widespread use of mortality rates for internal institutional and broader societal review of the quality of care. First, solely as a consequence of statistical selection and random variation, a hospital could become a statistic outlier. Every patient's clinical course has some unpredictability associated with it that cannot be controlled by using even the most comprehensive case mix adjustment. Consequently, hospital adjusted overall death rates will have some degree of unpredictability. Therefore, within any given time, a hospital could have the misfortune of being a statistic outlier. This designation would be an aberration relative to the care being provided and would most likely be corrected in analyses over time.

Second, hospital discharge practices, patient and family preferences, and the selection of alternative sites, such as nursing home or hospice facilities, for death can also impact hospital mortality statistics. As a consequence, hospital mortality should be assessed within a context of postdischarge deaths. Although deaths that occur after hospitalization may not reflect entirely the quality of hospital care because of intervening medical events, they may uncover disparities in death rates because of the time selected for discharge. Similarly, the frequency with which do-not-resuscitate orders are implemented may impact the mortality rate recorded at hospitals providing care to the critically or terminally ill.

Until 1989, a national benchmark for comparison of outcomes in critical care did not exist. The completion of the APACHE III study potentially will allow for the firm establishment of a national mortality-based performance assessment standard for all hospitals greater than 200 beds.[66] This standard will be accomplished by including hospitals of varying size, location, and teaching status within the cohort of randomly selected participating study hospitals. The data base of approximately 17,500 patients will permit statistically powerful comparison of outcome between individuals and hospitals. In time, it is hoped that such a representative data base will continue to grow, bringing continued refinement in the accuracy of the outcome data as well as the incorporation of changes in clinical care as technology and knowledge evolve.

Nevertheless, in the intensive care arena, data are coming to light that suggest risk adjusted hospital mortality can be used to assess quality. Knaus et al. reviewed the outcome data for 13 hospitals in the United States in which APACHE II scores and disease were used to control for variations in patient characteristics. In this study, two hospitals were identified as having actual death rates significantly different than that predicted. One hospital had a standardized mortality ratio (observed death rate/predicted death rate) of 0.59, whereas another hospital had a ratio of 1.59. Substantial differences were noted retrospectively in the clinical and organizational process of care between the two institutions. The hospital with lower than expected mortality performance had 24-hour in-unit physician coverage, a full-time ICU director, and comprehensive nursing continuing education. In addition, patients received on average larger amounts of skilled nursing as measured by TISS. Most importantly, the hospital with a better than predicted mortality performance had open and effective communication between the nursing and medical staffs. In contrast, the hospital with worse than expected outcome did not have such clinical or organization characteristics and exhibited poor communication between physicians and nurses. This study strongly supports the hypothesis that the process of care can impact outcome in both positive and deleterious ways.[67] These findings have led to a prospective multi-institutional study evaluating the potential links between the process of care and patient outcome from critical care.

A final issue regarding the quality of ICU care remains. If mortality rates are tied to the quality of clinical care and clinical decision-making, what are the normative standards that are most appropriately applied to an institution? Should hospital outcome be compared only to outcomes for hospitals with similar characteristics such as size, geographic location, and teaching status, or should universal standards apply for all institutions? To date, no consensus to these questions has arisen.

In sum, hospital mortality date may prove over time to distinguish accurately those institutions providing better than expected care as well as those providing suboptimal care. The diagnostic and therapeutic decisions that make up the processes of care remain open to scrutiny. Current levels of sophistication regarding the interpretation of these data do not allow one to make unqualified statements pertaining to the quality of care. It is apparent that many issues need to be addressed and understood when evaluating mortality data as a marker for the quality of clinical care.

Assuring Quality of Care—The Organization and Management of the ICU

The preceding discussion concentrated on measuring and evaluating patient characteristics, their clinical care, and outcome. Critical care medicine is on the forefront of another phenomena in quality evaluation in institutional medicine. Attention is being directed toward understanding the possible correlations between outcome and the organization, structure, and management of an ICU. Providing critical care requires the effective and coordinated activity of many individuals with a diversity of clinical skills. Consequently, the quality of care delivered could depend on the smooth interactions of the health care professionals providing direct bedside care as well as ancillary support.

Although the provision of orderly and effective intensive care requires a physician team leader, the environment in which care is provided should foster a sense of individual accountability. Each provider of an aspect of critical care should be guided by an institutional commitment to continued quality improvement. The leaders of the health care team have a responsibility to instill the belief in all participants that improvement in the quality of care delivered is a continuous and evolving process. This responsibility for self-scrutiny cannot be delegated to a committee or review panel but must be embedded within the foundation of the ICU and hospital structure.

This more comprehensive and proactive approach to quality improvement is beginning to take hold in the American health care system. It is based on an industrial model of quality assurance outlined by Deming.[68] This strategy attempts to avoid or anticipate problems rather than trying to solve them after they have become unwieldy. The fundamental construct of this approach to quality is reducing variation and increasing consistency in the delivery of high technology medical service. Deming developed a common sense approach to reducing variations in the day-to-day action of complex organizations that may indeed be applicable to the critical care setting. His insights reflect the nature of the relationships that exist between individuals in organizations that successfully and consistently perform to high standards. Many of his observations and solutions may seem platitudinous, but one must consider how often large organizations fail to incorporate them into their organizational and management structure.[69]

The overriding precept of the Deming approach to quality is that people work together effectively by sharing common goals. To assure quality in patient care, the aim of providing superlative care must be stated explicitly and understood by all. Improvement in the delivery of critical care requires a commitment to continuing education. This education, however, cannot be limited to traditional programs for physician and nursing staffs. It must involve everyone who supports the process of care. In addition, it must foster a sense of participation and motivate all caregivers to devise solutions to problems in their area of responsibility. A climate with a free exchange of information leads to a better understanding by all of the specific needs and expectations of others on the health care team. It also fosters an environment in which the interest is focused on areas for improvement rather than attributing blame when difficulties arise.

Unfortunately, current efforts at quality assessment and assurance are often viewed as restrictive and punitive. They foster an attitude of contempt among physicians and sometimes defeat the stated goal of improved performance in the best interest of patients. Despite frustration, physicians cannot abrogate their leadership role in the arena of striving for excellence in critical care. In addition, the fear of retribution or criticism must not become a deterrant to seeking ways to improve the smooth functioning of the ICU. Improvement can occur in an environment in which people feel comfortable admitting mistakes, offering suggestions, and seeking counsel when difficulties arise.

In addition, communication should foster the elimination of barriers between team members both within the unit and between others who are important to the delivery of intensive care services. Open and direct communication can eliminate undercurrents of discontent. Further, the medical leadership in the unit can strengthen the cohesiveness of the health care team by effectively acknowledging that work by other providers is valued. Pride in performance remains a valuable tool to motivate people to higher levels of achievement.

Physicians often remain skeptical of institutional or organizational efforts to impact or improve the delivery of care.[70] Nevertheless, as health care delivery in the ICU has become increasingly complex, the need for continued attention to quality of care by attention to both medical and management issues has become imperative. We must promote and provide an environment that is conducive to continued improvement in care over time by constantly questioning the processes used in the delivery of that care.[71]

The preceding discussion presumes that methods that have been established in the organization and management of other large service and industrial organizations are effective in clinical quality assurance. A large multicenter evaluation of the impact of organization and management strategies on patient outcome within medical and surgical ICUs is ongoing. The APACHE III study, currently nearing completion, is explicitly evaluating the impact that diversity in setting, organization, and operating protocols of ICUs have on patient outcome. The process of care is being explored systematically to evaluate whether seven key components of organization and management interact to affect quality. These processes include perceived unit effectiveness, staff communication, coordination, conflict resolution, member satisfaction, organizational culture, and leadership. If, as hypothesized, links are established between a unit's organizational structure, management, and process of delivering care, and its risk adjusted patient outcome, evidence will be convincing that ICU quality is directly impacted by the manner in which health care professionals are organized.[72] This finding will provide the impetus to develop specific organizational strategies in intensive care that stress the importance of the interrelationships and interactions of the critical care team at the bedside.

QUALITY OF CARE, LONG-TERM SURVIVAL, AND QUALITY OF LIFE/FUTURE DIRECTIONS

The current focus of much of the scientific inquiry evaluating the quality of ICU care stresses short-term patient outcome. Current instruments measuring important patient characteristics such as severity of illness are limited by their inability to provide estimates of outcome beyond hospital discharge. In studies of post-hospital follow-up, Mundt et al. remind us that longer periods of observation and measurement of quality of life provide another important dimension to evaluating care.[73,74]

Functional status after hospitalization apparently is correlated most strongly to an individual's functional state and health status prior to admission.[75,76] It will, therefore, be difficult to assess the impact that the quality of intensive care has on post-hospital outcome when long-term status may be substantially affected by factors that are unrelated and cannot be affected by ICU care. In addition, the speed and timing of recovery may be affected by elements such as the effectiveness of rehabilitative services as well as personal economic and social factors beyond the direct control of intensive caregivers.

Despite inherent difficulties, assessing the long-term impact of critical care on survival may be facilitated by comparisons of outcome to actuarial survival data in patients with chronic diseases. Dragsted et al. reported that patients discharged from an ICU had a lower survival rate than would be expected when compared to an age- and sex-matched control group that had not required intensive care hospitalization.[77] It may be possible to combine this type of evaluation in multi-institutional comparisons that would allow for more definitive statements regarding the far-reaching impact of critical care. Quality comparisons might be inferred from differing outcomes after controlling for variables unrelated to the process of care.

Issues that impact patients and have importance include employment and functional status, social productivity, interactive and self-care capabilities, emotional state, and the ability to enjoy leisure time. Research is needed on the differing values patients place on various aspect of long-term outcome. Although a consensus regarding the precise role each of these considerations should play in a comprehensive quality of life assessment does not currently exist, research interest in this area is growing and progress is expected shortly.[78] Today, we have the capability to predict the risk of an acutely ill patient surviving treatment; tomorrow, we will predict the length and quality of that survival.[79]

IMPLEMENTING A QUALITY ASSESSMENT PROGRAM

If quality of care and continuous assessment is a worthy goal in critical care, methods for ongoing evaluation must be implemented. These methods cannot be overly labor intensive and must go beyond traditional formulas for evaluating care, such as retrospective chart reviews.[80]

Selective chart review may be of value in specific instances in which suspected lapses in the process of care led to deficient care. For example, patients determined to be at a low risk of death based on a physiologic assessment of severity who die during the course of care warrant explicit case review. If, however, the quality of care is affected primarily by the ongoing process of care, then ongoing and overall monitoring of that care is needed. The most effective way to collect the needed information is with computerized data collection. This tool facilitates analysis and may help highlight subtle deficiencies that may not otherwise be apparent from the more conventional chart review process. Having this overall portrayal of the clinical process will then allow for a more focused evaluation of individual case histories.

A model for continuous quality assurance and assessment in the critical care unit is presented in Figure 74-1. The model is predicated on the concepts developed in this chapter. Included are measurements of selected patient characteristics, an evaluation of the process of care, and outcome assessments. The goal of this model is to evaluate comprehensively all aspects of clinical ICU care, including triage, diagnostic and therapeutic decision-making, and organization and management.

Patient characteristics collected include acute disease, severity of illness, age, chronic health status, and patient location prior to ICU admission. These data are used to calculate a short-term probability of death using a represen-

---

Model for Quality Assessment and Assurance in Critical Care Medicine

Requires the reliable and validated measurement of:

Patient characteristics	Process of care	Outcomes
Disease	TISS	Short term measures:
Severity of illness	Organizational structure	—Hospital mortality
Age	Management process, policies and	Low risk deaths
Chronic health status	protocols	—Length of stay
Location of patient prior to ICU admission (e.g., ER, OR/RR, floor, another hospital)		—Sentinel events
		Morbid events
		Complications of care (expected and unexpected)
		Long term measures:
		—Mortality
		—Functional status
		—Patient satisfaction and preferences for quality of life

Fig. 74–1. The assessment of quality in critical care requires an evaluation of the patient characteristics and processes of care, which provides the information necessary to understand the implications of the measured clinical outcomes.

tative, reliable, and validated comparative data base such as that collected for APACHE III. In this manner, the observed and predicted risk adjusted mortality rates can be compared.

In addition, this physiologically based patient data can be the basis for predicting other important aspects of care, including length of stay; requirements for resource consumption, including nursing care; and complications. When these predicted outcomes are compared to observed events, a portrait of care rendered is produced. Examples of the simple formulas for producing risk adjusted outcome ratios for several outcome measurements are depicted in Figure 74-2.

Over time, it is anticipated that expanded data bases will allow for predictions of long-term outcomes that will further enhance a comprehensive evaluation of the impact and quality of ICU care. The eventual inclusion of patient preferences and satisfaction into the outcome assessment model is a goal requiring clinical instruments under development.[77]

Evaluation of the clinical process of care is accomplished concurrently with the physiologically based assessment of outcome using a measure of bedside clinical intensity. The TISS serves this function in the proposed model. In addition, an understanding of the organization and management of a critical care unit focuses on the overall process under which care is administered.

In conclusion, as part of the continued effort to improve health care delivery, the evaluation of quality remains an area of focused attention within hospitals and among other interested third parties. A commitment to excellence remains a professional responsibility. External agencies will continue to mandate organized programs of quality assessment and assurance for ICUs. If these efforts are to have meaning to physicians and be of clinical utility in the process of evaluating critical care, an assessment of each patient's relative risks for morbidity and mortality prior to therapy is essential. Incorporating accurate patient risk stratification into the quality of care assessment can help guarantee that information produced by these efforts is reliable and meaningful.

The process for achieving this form of comprehensive quality assessment and assurance in the intensive care setting is in an early but encouraging stage. Computerized programs to aid in this evaluation already exist. The evolution of well-constructed protocols for evaluating critical care continue to develop as the methods to measure appropriate and meaningful outcomes become more sophisticated. The current state of the art requires experimentation and manipulation of quality assurance models to develop information that is useful to the medical community and the public. With the continued expansion of computerized data capturing, the job of collecting important information will be facilitated, quality assessment activities will become less expensive, and the results will be more clinically meaningful.

REFERENCES

1. Oliver, M. F., Julian, D. G., Donald, K. W.: Problems in evaluating coronary care units; their responsibilities and their relation to the community. Am. J. Cardiol., *20*:465, 1967.
2. Knaus, W. A., et al.: A comparison of intensive care in the U.S.A. and France. Lancet, *2*:642, 1982.
3. Zimmerman, J. E., et al.: Patient selection for intensive care: A comparison of New Zealand and U.S. hospitals. Crit. Care Med., *16*:318, 1988.
4. Knaus, W. A., et al.: An evaluation of outcome from intensive care in major medical centers. Ann. Intern. Med., *104*:419, 1986.
5. Abizanda, R.: The facilities. In Management of the ICU—Guidelines for better use of resources. Edited by D. R. Miranda, A. Williams, and P. Loirat. Dordrecht, The Netherlands, Kluwer Academic, 1990, p. 55.
6. Knaus, W. A., et al.: An evaluation of outcome from intensive care in major medical centers. Ann. Intern Med. *104*:410, 1986.
7. Petty, T. L., et al.: Intensive respiratory care unit: Review of 10 years' experience. JAMA, *34*:322, 1975.
8. Rogers, R. M., Weiler, C., Ruppenthal, B.: Impact of the respiratory intensive care unit in survival of patients with acute respiratory failure. Chest, *77*:501, 1972.
9. Hook, E. W., Horton, C. A. Schaberg, D. R.: Failure of intensive care unit support to influence mortality from pneumococcal bacteremia. JAMA, *249*:1055, 1983.
10. Jencks, S. F., Williams, D. K., Kay, T. L.: Assessing hospital-associated deaths from discharge data; the role of length of stay and comorbidities. JAMA, *260*:2240, 1988.
11. Park, E. R., et al.: Explaining variations in hospital death rates—randomness, severity of illness, quality of care. JAMA, *264*:484, 1990.
12. Epstein, A. E.: The outcomes movement—will it get us where we want to go? N. Eng. J. Med., *323*:266, 1990.
13. Council on Medical Service, American Medical Association, Chicago, Illinois: Guidelines for quality assurance. JAMA, *259*:2572, 1988.
14. Task Force on Guidelines: Society of Critical Care Medicine. Recommendations for critical care unit design. Crit. Care Med., *16*:796, 1988.
15. Examples of monitoring and evaluation in special care units. Joint Commission on Accreditation of Healthcare Organizations. Chicago, Illinois, 1988, p. 45.
16. Parrillo, J.: NIH Consensus Development Conference on Critical Care Medicine. Crit. Care Med., *11*:466, 1983.

Risk Adjusted Outcomes Measures

$$\text{Patient Risk Adjusted Mortality Ratio} = \frac{\text{Predicted Number of Deaths*}}{\text{Observed Number of Deaths}}$$

$$\text{Patient Risk Adjusted Length of Stay} = \frac{\text{Aggregate Predicted Length of Stay*}}{\text{Aggregate Observed Length of Stay}}$$

$$\text{Patient Risk Adjusted Nursing Intensity} = \frac{\text{Aggregate Predicted TISS*}}{\text{Aggregate Observed TISS}}$$

Fig. 74-2. Selected examples of using risk adjusted severity of illness information to assess quality of care. *All predicted values are derived from a normative, comparative data base. Using the normative data base, a level of statistical significance for a particular ratio is determined, allowing for isolation of areas of potential strengths and weaknesses in an institution.

17. Dawson, N. V., and Arkes, H. R.: Systematic errors in medical decision making. J. Gen. Intern. Med., 2:183, 1987.
18. Ayers, S. M., et al.: National Institutes of Health consensus development conference summary. Critical Care Medicine. Washington, D.C., U.S. Government Printing Office, 1983.
19. U.S. Congress Office of Technology Assessment: Life-Sustaining Technologies and the Elderly, OTA-BA-306. Washington, D.C., U.S. Government Printing Office, July, 1987.
20. Chang, R. W.: Predicting deaths among ICU patients. Crit. Care Med., 16:34, 1988.
21. Edgten, E., et al.: Prediction of outcome after cardiac arrest. Crit. Care Med., 15:820, 1987.
22. Knaus, W. A., et al.: APACHE II: A severity of disease classification system. Crit. Care Med., 13:818, 1985.
23. Lemeshow, S., et al.: Refining intensive care unit outcome prediction by using changing probabilities of mortality. Crit. Care Med., 16:470, 1988.
24. Zaren, B., and Hedstrand, U.: Quality of life among long-term survivors of intensive care. Crit. Care Med., 15:743, 1987.
25. Killip, T., and Kimball, J. T.: Treatment of myocardial infarction in a coronary care unit. A two-year experience with 2150 patients. Am. J. Cardiol., 20:457, 1967.
26. Jennett, B.: Resource allocation for the severely brain damaged. Arch. Neurol., 33:595, 1976.
27. Cullen, D. J., et al.: Therapeutic Intervention Scoring System: A method for quantitative comparison of patient care. Crit. Care Med., 2:57, 1974.
28. Knaus, W. A., Draper, E. A., Wagner, D. P.: An evaluation of outcome from intensive care in major medical centers. Ann. Intern. Med., 104:410, 1986.
29. Knaus, W. A., et al.: APACHE-acute physiology and chronic health evaluation: A physiologically-based classification system. Crit. Care Med., 9:591, 1981.
30. Knaus, W. A., et al.: The APACHE III prognostic system: Risk prediction of hospital mortality for critically ill hospitalized patients. Chest, 100:1619, 1991.
31. LeGall, J. R., et al.: A simplified acute physiology score for ICU patients. Crit. Care Med., 12:975, 1984.
32. Teres, D., et al.: Validation of the Mortality Prediction Model for ICU patients. Crit. Care Med., 15:208, 1987.
33. Yeh, T. S., et al.: Validation of the physiologic stability index (PSI) for use in critically ill infants and children. Pediatr. Res., 18:445, 1984.
34. Pollack, M., Ruttimann, U. E., Getson, P. R.: Accurate prediction of the outcome of pediatric intensive care: A new quantitative method. N. Engl. J. Med., 316:134, 1987.
35. Pollack, M., Ruttimann, U. E., Getson, P. R.: Pediatric risk of mortality (PRISM) score. Crit. Care Med., 16:1110, 1988.
36. Damiano, A. M., et al.: Reliability of a measure of severity of illness: Acute physiology and chronic health evaluation III. J. Clin. Epidemiol., In press.
37. Demlo, L. K., and Campbell, P. M.: Improving hospital discharge data: Lessons from the National Hospital Discharge Survey. Med. Care, 19:1030, 1981.
38. Demlo, L. K., Campell, R. M., Brown, S. S.: Reliability of information abstracted from patient's medical records. Med. Care, 16:995, 1978.
39. Hsia, D. C., Krushat, W. M., Fagan, A. B.: Accuracy of diagnostic coding for Medicare patients under the prospective-payment system. N. Engl. J. Med., 318:352, 1988.
40. California Medical Review Inc., San Francisco, CA: Premature discharge study prepared of the Health Care Financing Administration, U.S. Department of Health and Human Services (undated).
41. Sax, F. L., Charlson, M. E.: Utilization of critical care units: A prospective study of physician triage and patient outcome. Arch. Intern. Med., 147:929, 1987.
42. Singer, D. E., et al.: Rationing intensive care: Physician responses to a resource shortage. N. Engl. J. Med., 309:1155, 1983.
43. Strauss, M. J., et al.: Rationing of intensive care unit: Identifying patients at high risk of unexpected death or unit readmission. Am. J. Med., 84:863, 1988.
44. Bloomfield, H., and Moskowitz, M. A.: Discharge decision-making in a medical intensive care unit: Identifying patients at high risk of unexpected death or unit readmission. Am. J. Med., 84:863, 1988.
45. Wagner, D. P., et al.: Identification of low-risk monitor patients within a medical-surgical intensive care unit. Med. Care, 21:425, 1983.
46. Wagner, D. P., Knaus, W. A., Draper, E. A.: Identification of low-risk monitor admissions to medical-surgical ICUs. Chest, 92:423, 1987.
47. McClish, D. K., and Powell, S.: How well can physicians estimate mortality in a medical intensive care unit? Med. Decis. Making, 9:125, 1989.
48. Brannen, A. L., Godfrey, L. J., Goetter, W. E.: Prediction of outcome from critical illness; a comparison of clinical judgement with a prediction rule. Arch. Intern. Med., 149:1083, 1989.
49. Chang, R. W., et al.: Accuracy of decisions to withdraw therapy in critically ill patients: Clinical judgement versus a computer model. Crit. Care Med., 17:1091, 1989.
50. Bion, J. F., et al.: Validation of a prognostic score in critically ill patients undergoing transport. Br. Med. J., 291:432, 1985.
51. Chang, R. W. S., Jacobs, S., Lee, B.: Use of APACHE II severity of disease classification to identify intensive-care unit patients who would not benefit from total parenteral nutrition. Lancet 2:1483, 1986.
52. Ruark, J. E., Raffin, T. A.: The Stanford University Medical Center Committee on Ethics: Initiating and withdrawing life support: Principles and practice in adult medicine. N. Engl. J. Med., 318:25, 1988.
53. Griner, P. F.: The relationship between managerial and clinical decision making in the hospital. Med. Decis. Making, 8:151, 1988.
54. Dubois, R. W., et al.: Hospital inpatient mortality: Is it a predictor of quality? N. Engl. J. Med., 317:1674, 1987.
55. Kahn, K. L., et al.: Interpreting hospital mortality data: How can we proceed? JAMA, 260:3625, 1988.
56. Chang, R. W. S.: Individual outcome prediction models for intensive care units. Lancet, 2:143, 1989.
57. Rauss, A., et al.: Prognosis for recovery from multiple organ system failure: The accuracy of objective estimates of changes for survival. Med. Decis. Making, 10:155, 1990.
58. Knaus, W. A., et al.: Development of an automated clinical information system for intensive care: The APACHE II Project. Med. Decis. Making, 20:334, 1990.
59. Rutstein, D. D., et al.: Measuring the quality of medical care: A clinical method. N. Engl. J. Med., 294:582, 1976.
60. Landefeld, C. D., et al.: Diagnostic yield of the autopsy in a university hospital and community hospital. N. Engl. J. Med., 318:1249, 1988.
61. Eason, J., Markowe, H. L.: Controlled investigation of deaths from asthma in a hospital in the Northeast Thames region. Br. Med. J., 294:1255, 1987.
62. Donabedian, A.: Explorations in Quality Assessment and Monitoring. Vol. III. The Methods and Findings of Quality Assessment and Monitoring. Ann Arbor, MI, Health Administration Press, 1985.
63. Dubois, R. W., and Brook, R. H.: preventable deaths; who, how often and why? Ann. Intern. Med., 109:582, 1988.
64. Greenfield, S., et al.: Flaws in mortality data: The hazards of ignoring comorbid disease. JAMA, 260:2253, 1988.

65. Green, J., et al.: The importance of severity of illness in assessing hospital mortality. JAMA, *263*:241, 1990.
66. Zimmerman, J. E., (Ed.): APACH III study design: Analytic plan for evaluation of severity and outcome. Crit. Care Med., *17*:S169, 1989.
67. Knaus, W. A., et al.: An evaluation of outcome from intensive care in major medical centers. Ann. Intern. Med., *104*:410, 1986.
68. Deming, W. E.: Out of the Crisis. Cambridge, MA, Massachusetts Institute of Technology, Center for Advanced Engineering Study, 1982.
69. Deming, W. E.: Out of the Crisis. Cambridge, MA, Massachusetts Institute of Technology, Center for Advanced Engineering Study, 1986.
70. Colombotos, J., and Kirshner, C.: Physicians and Social Change. New York, Oxford University Press, 1986.
71. Goldfield, N., and Nash, D.: Providing Quality Care: The Challenge to Clinicians. Vol. 159. Philadelphia, American College of Physicians, 1989, p. 452.
72. Shortell, S., Rousseau, D., Gillies, R.: APACHE III Study Design: Analytic plan for evaluation of severity and outcome. Edited by J. E. Zimmerman. Crit. Care Med., *17*:S213, 1989.
73. Mundt, D. J., et al.: Intensive care unit patient follow-up: Mortality, functional status and return to work at six months. Arch. Intern. Med., *149*:68, 1989.
74. Yinnon, A., Zimran, A., Hershko, C.: Quality of life and survival following intensive medical care. Q. J. Med., *71*:347, 1989.
75. Goldstein, R. L., et al.: Functional outcomes following medical intensive care. Crit. Care Med., *14*:783, 1986.
76. Jacobs, C. J., et al.: Mortality and quality of life after intensive care for critical illness. Intensive Care Med., *14*:217, 1988.
77. Dragsted, L., Qvist, J., Madsen, M.: Outcome from intensive care (part IV): A five-year study of 1308 patients: Long-term outcome. Eur. J. Anaesthesiol., *7*:51, 1990.
78. SUPPORT: Study to understand prognosis and preferences for outcomes and risk of treatments: Study design. Edited by D. J. Murphy and L. Cluff. J. Clin. Epidemiol., In press.
79. Knaus, W. A.: Predicting and evaluating patient outcomes. Ann. Intern. Med., *109*:521, 1988.
80. Sivak, E. D., and Perez-Trepichio, A.: Quality assessment in the medical intensive care unit: Evolution of a data model. Cleve. Clin. J. Med., *57*:273, 1990.

# Chapter 75

INFECTION CONTROL

THOMAS F. KEYS

Nosocomial infections likely complicate the hospital stay of at least 1 in every 20 patients admitted. This risk rises significantly with admission to an intensive care unit (ICU) and continues the longer the patient requires intensive support. In our experience, 20% of patients who require intensive care for longer than 72 hours develop some type of nosocomial infection, ranging in severity from asymptomatic bacteriuria to necrotizing pneumonia. Underlying diseases such as diabetes mellitus, renal failure, valvular heart disease, cirrhosis, pancreatitis, and malnutrition predispose patients to infectious complications (Table 75-1). Further compromise occurs when they are treated with various immunosuppressive drugs such as corticosteroids, azathioprine, cyclosporine, and cancer chemotherapeutic agents.

Superimposed on this setting is the likelihood (50% or more in most hospitals) that these same patients have already or are currently receiving prophylactic or therapeutic antibiotic agents prior to being transferred to the ICU. Antibiotic administration predisposes the patient to become colonized, if not infected, with relatively resistant bacteria and yeasts.

The application of basic epidemiologic methods allows for evaluation and control of hospital-associated infections. Surveillance, the collection, collation, analysis, and dissemination of data, is essential for success. Routine surveillance provides information on the cause and origin of hospital infections at an endemic level. If a potential epidemic or outbreak situation develops, this data base is available for review. Surveillance also stimulates an awareness of potential infection problems and provides a format for continuing education or physicians, nurses, and other health care providers. Studies performed by the Centers for Disease Control (CDC) suggest that effective surveillance coupled with control measures prevents one third of cases of nosocomial bacteremia, postoperative wound infections, and postoperative pneumonia.[1] Infection control practitioners (ICPs) should conduct surveillance rounds in ICUs at least two to three times per week.

A simple collection form is used to record surveillance data (Fig. 75-1). This type of form contains the following data elements:

- Patient demographics
- Hospital admission
- ICU admission data
- Patient origin
- ICU admission diagnosis
- Site of infection
- Microbiology of the infection
- Risk factors

Only those infections not present or incubating at the time of admission to the ICU should be considered ICU associated. Bacteriologic information along with the patient's name, identification number, and ICU location are entered on the card (see Fig. 75-1). Admission data, hospital service, and working diagnoses are transcribed from the medical record. After careful review, the appropriate diagnosis of nosocomial infection is listed. As shown, certain factors that predispose patients to infection may also be noted. Standard definitions for infections are adapted from those developed by the CDC.[2]

Nosocomial infection rates for an ICU should be reported at least quarterly. Included are relevant denominator data expressed as number of infected cases per number of cases at risk (total dismissals) and number of infected cases per 100 patient days. The latter is a more valuable denominator when comparing rates over time, especially for patients who have prolonged ICU stays. For example, a 10-bed ICU has a total of 300 potential patient day care days in a 30-day month (10 beds × 30 days). During 1 month, there may be 40 new admissions and another month only 25 admissions, with 5 long-term patients accounting for the bulk of patient days. A greater number of infections in the long-term patients would increase the rate of infection in 100 days of patient care. An example of an annual report, showing quarterly data arranged according to site and per 100 patient days, is shown in Table 75-2. From this report, it is possible to develop rates for specific infections according to duration of risk factors (intubation days, central vascular catheter days, bladder catheter days, and so forth). Thresholds can be established for various infection complications in the ICU using established rates over time. When an attack rate exceeds the threshold by 2 standard deviations, more intense investigation should occur and result in considerations for a change in practice. Repeating monitoring activity after an intervention provides the ICU staff with a measurement for assessing their success or failure. Infections occurring with a greater than expected frequency because of the same microorganism should trigger interest and concern for a suspected common source or even a carrier of the microbe by an ICU staff member. Infections with different microorganisms occurring in greater than expected frequency usually indicate a technical or maintenance problem related

Table 75-1. Risk Factors for Nosocomial Infections

Underlying diseases
    Malnutrition
    Diabetes mellitus
    Renal failure
    Valvular heart disease
    Cirrhosis
    Pancreatitis
Antimicrobials
    Prolonged prophylaxis
    Therapy for infections
Immunosuppressives
    Corticosteroids
    Azathioprine
    Cyclosporine
    Cancer
    Chemotherapy
Prolonged hospital stay
    Colonization with resistant bacteria and fungi

Table 75-2. ICU Surveillance by Quarter—1989*

Infection Site	First Qtr.	Second Qtr.	Third Qtr.	Fourth Qtr.	Annual
Blood	0.36	1.02	0	0.42	0.44
Respiratory	0.48	0.38	0.24	0.55	0.41
Wound	0.12	0.25	0	0.42	0.19
Urinary	0.48	0.13	0.12	0.69	0.35
Other	0.24	0	0	0.14	0.09
Overall	1.66	1.78	0.37	2.22	1.48
Patient days	841	787	819	832	3279
Patients	236	327	299	262	1124

* Incidence per 100 patient days.

to a task or procedure. Rarely is it necessary to perform a detailed statistical analysis of these data. Nevertheless, the ICP should be acquainted with basic analytic methods in problem solving, particularly when a problem can become a nonproblem simply by performing a careful analysis of surveillance data.[3]

Before formal infection control guidelines were accepted, wide variations with policies and procedures existed throughout the country. By 1970, the CDC formalized guidelines by publishing "Isolation Techniques for Use in Hospitals."[4] This manual listed seven categories of isolation precautions with specifications for barrier attire and the handling of equipment for each category (strict, respiratory, wound and skin, and so forth). Although no controlled studies had been done to show the efficacy or benefit of the system, it was soon adopted by most acute care hospitals in the United States. Although the CDC updated guidelines for isolation precautions in 1983, the system remained unwieldy, because the majority of guidelines applied to community rather than hospital-acquired (nosomial) infections. It has long been recognized that transmission of many nosocomial infections comes from unrecognized sources or undiagnosed cases of infection The landmark article by Jackson and Lynch published in 1984 provided an impetus to revise traditional infection control practices.[5] The authors stressed the need for individual patient assessment. They noted the disregard on the part of health care workers when handling body substances from "unmarked" patients and exaggerated efforts when handling body substances from "infected patients."

PATIENT NAME _____ DATE _____
HOSPITAL NO. _____ AGE _____ SEX _____
PRIMARY PHYSICIAN _____ HOSP ADMIT DATE _____
ICU ADMIT DATE _____ ADMITTED TO ICU FROM _____
REASON FOR ICU ADMISSION _____

INFECTION DIAGNOSIS
_____ Urinary   _____ Pneumonia   _____ Wound   _____ Other _____
_____ Bloodstream   Primary _____   Secondary _____   Unknown _____

MICROBIOLOGY

DATE   SOURCE   ORGANISM   ANTIBIOTIC SUSCEPTIBILITY

RISK FACTORS
_____ Urethral catheterization; Date _____
_____ Intubation; Date _____
_____ Surgery; Date _____ Type _____
_____ Vascular line; Date _____ Type _____
_____ Other _____

Fig. 75-1. Example of a data collection sheet for surveillance in an ICU.

Table 75–3. A Guide to Barrier Precautions

Clinical Situation	Barrier*
Endotracheal toilet	Gloves, masks
Bronchoscopy	Gloves, masks, eyewear
Incontinent stool and urine	Gloves
Catheter adjustments (vascular, urinary)	Gloves

* Gloves must be changed and hands washed after each encounter.

The AIDS epidemic has dramatically illustrated the inherent weakness of a diagnosis-dependent isolation system and stimulated the need for precautions with all body substances. Such awareness and application should reduce the risk of transmission of infections not only to patients, but also to health care workers.[6] All ICU personnel should wear gloves when handling blood and body fluids and, depending on the likelihood of contact with eyes, nose, and mouth, masks and protective eyewear. Gloves are an important barrier, but they are not totally impermeable and should be removed after patient contact.[7] Hands must be washed after glove removal. Table 75-3 provides a guide to barrier precautions that we use at the Cleveland Clinic.

PRE-ICU PHASE

In the pre-ICU phase of hospitalization, the clinician should be mindful that certain factors make the possibility of nosocomial infection in the ICU a self-fulfilling prophecy. These factors generally fall into the categories colonization, underlying infectious disease, and suboptimal use of antibiotics for prophylaxis and therapy.

Colonization

Hospitalized patients destined for transfer to the ICU likely are already colonized with antibiotic-resistant bacteria and fungi. Larson and colleagues[8] reported that the skin flora of hospitalized patients contained high carriage rates of Proteus, Pseudomonas, and Candida species when compared to nonhospitalized healthy adults. One example is methicillin-resistant Staphylococcus epidermidis (MRSE) found on the skin of patients after cardiac surgery.[9] Isolates containing subpopulations highly resistant to methicillin were recovered from only 3 (4%) of 80 patients before surgery, but from 43 (54%) patients 5 days after the operation. All patients received perioperative cephalosporin prophylaxis, which may have selected out resistant strains. Colonization with antibiotic-resistant bacteria may occur in hospitalized patients who have not received antibiotics. In 1972, Johansen and colleagues reported respiratory colonization with gram-negative bacteria in 21 (55%) of 38 patients with acute respiratory failure who had not been exposed to antibiotics.[10]

Broad-spectrum antibiotics may alter the composition of the intestinal microflora. Ten years later, Giuliano and colleague noted that cefoperazone reduced aerobic and anaerobic bacteria to undetectable levels.[11] These authors noted extensive overgrowth with enterococci and yeasts, organisms that are emerging now as significant ICU pathogens. Alterations in intestinal microflora seem related to loss of colonization resistance, with the normal anaerobic gut flora having a protective role. Barza and colleagues, however, were unable to confirm this hypothesis.[12]

Underlying Infectious Diseases

Patients with life-threatening infections may require admission to the ICU. Despite optimal antimicrobial therapy and life support, individuals with high APACHE scores will likely die. Stevens and colleagues[13] reported a discouraging experience. Patients with community-acquired pneumonia who received admission to their ICU had a mortality rate of 59%, higher than when pneumonia was acquired in the ICU. Postoperative pneumonia, when associated with remote organ failure, often is fatal.[14] Other factors associated with risk of death from pneumonia include prolonged hospital stay and underlying neoplastic disease.

Intraabdominal sepsis may result in a hospital death. Sinanan and colleagues[15] reviewed 100 abdominal explorations in 71 patients with suspected intraabdominal sepsis. Fifty-two (77%) patients had positive preoperative physical findings or scan evidence suggesting an intraabdominal focus. The best approach to improve survival was urgent or emergency laparotomy before the patient developed bacteremia and/or septic shock. An appropriate and timely work-up, including an abdominal CT scan, a magnetic resonance scan, a sonogram, or, if necessary, exploratory laparotomy, should avoid an unacceptably high mortality, which was 90% in the experience of these authors.

Patients with infective endocarditis and acute valvular dysfunction require urgent corrective surgery.[16] Other considerations for surgical intervention include evidence of myocardial invasion (persistent fever or conduction disturbances), resistant organisms such as Pseudomonas aeruginosa and yeasts, and large vegetation. Additionally, it should be noted that in the nonaddict population, death is more likely to result from endocarditis attributable to Staphylococcus aureus than from other causes.[17] Such patients deserve special consideration for early operative intervention. Serial echocardiography may be helpful in detecting periannular extension in native valve endocarditis.[18]

Optimal Antibiotic Prophylaxis and Therapy

Most hospital patients receive antibiotics, a significant percentage needlessly. Prophylaxis is not recommended for cardiac catheterization, endoscopy, arterial punctures, thoracentesis, or paracentesis, but it often is prescribed. Even when appropriate, prophylaxis frequently is continued longer than necessary. Empiric therapy may be continued long after initial cultures have been reported as negative and, when in retrospect, the patient did not have objective evidence of a bacterial infection. Overprescribing not only increases the cost of health care, but also it may lead to superinfection with antibiotic-resistant bacteria and fungi, and increase the likelihood for an adverse drug reaction. Monitoring of antibiotic usage with feedback to prescribing physicians tends to reduce indiscriminate prescribing and stimulates self-education. Prescribing guidelines should be developed in collaboration with in-

Table 75-4. Guidelines for Therapy of Nosocomial Infections

Infection Source	Likely Organism(s)	Therapy	Duration
Lungs	Pseudomonas aeruginosa	Antipseudomonas penicillin or cephalosporin with gentamicin	3 wk
	Staphylococcus aureus	Vancomycin*	4 wk
	Aspiration	Clindamycin with gentamicin	10–14 d
Urine	GNB†	Ampicillin with gentamicin	2 wk
Vascular catheter	Staphylococcus aureus	Vancomycin*	2–4 wk
	Staphylococcus epidermidis	Vancomycin*	
	GNB	Advanced-generation cephalosporin with gentamicin	2 wk

† GNB, Gram-negative bacilli. Switch to appropriate antibiotic based on in vitro susceptibility studies.
* Switch to oxacillin if organism methicillin-sensitive S. aureus.

fectious disease specialists familiar with the clinical and epidemiologic problems of the hospital and ICU. Selected guidelines for therapy of various nosocomial infections are shown in Table 75-4. It is important to make adjustments once results of in vitro susceptibility studies are available from the microbiology laboratory. Again, it is also possible that MRSA and MRSE may cause significant infections in the ICU. Therefore, when suspected, staphylococcal infection warrants empiric therapy with vancomycin until findings of in vitro susceptibility studies are available.

Guidelines for surgical antibiotic prophylaxis are published periodically by the *Medical Letter*.[19] A single parenteral dose of antibiotic, if given preoperatively within 30 minutes of the procedure, provides adequate tissue concentrations for most operations. If surgery is longer than 2 hours or is complicated by major blood loss, a second dose can be given intraoperatively. **Continuation of prophylaxis postoperatively is not necessary.** The antibiotic selected should reduce the number of bacteria below a critical level to prevent infection. For most operations, cefazolin, a first generation cephalosporin with a sustained serum half-life, has proven effective. Third generation cephalosporins, as well as antipseudomonas penicillins, should not be used for prophylaxis.

Guidelines for endocarditis prophylaxis have been updated by the American Heart Association.[20] Prophylaxis continues to be indicated for dental procedures known to induce gingival bleeding, tonsillectomy, adenoidectomy, rigid bronchoscopy, gastrointestinal surgery, procedures such as sclerotherapy and esophageal dilatation, and urologic procedures or operations. Patients who benefit from prophylaxis include those with prosthetic heart valves, a history of native valve endocarditis, congenital or acquired heart disease, hypertrophic cardiomyopathy, and mitral valve prolapse with regurgitation.

The standard regimen recommended for dental, oral, and upper respiratory procedures is 3 g of amoxicillin orally 1 hour before the procedure and then 1.5 g 6 hours afterward. For the penicillin-allergic patient, 800 mg of erythromycin ethylsuccinate is given orally 2 hours before the procedure, with 400 mg taken 6 hours afterward, or 300 mg of clindamycin orally 1 hour before the procedure followed by 150 mg 6 hours later. For patients undergoing genitourinary or gastrointestinal procedures or surgeries, the standard regimen recommended is 2 g of ampicillin IM or IV plus 80 mg of gentamicin IM or IV 30 minutes before the procedure and 1.5 g of amoxicillin orally 6 hours afterward, or the parenteral regimen may be repeated at 8 hours. For the penicillin-allergic patient, 1 g of vancomycin IV over 1 hour starting 1 hour before the procedure is substituted for ampicillin. No repeat dosing is necessary if vancomycin is substituted.

ICU SUPPORT PHASE

Strategies to prevent nosocomial infections in the ICU require an understanding of the types of infections one is likely to encounter, a knowledge of potential routes of transmission (such as patient-to-patient and common source), and a selection of the most appropriate infection control measures for the problem at hand.

Types of Nosocomial Infections

The types of nosocomial infections encountered in the ICU are, in part, determined by the technology used for monitoring or facilitating patient care. Generally, the techniques include vascular catheters, pressure monitors, respiratory therapy equipment, and urinary catheters.

Vascular Catheters

Vascular catheter septicemia is reported in 3 to 7% of patients who receive intravenous therapy.[21] Purulence or cellulitis at the skin entry site of the catheter is a tipoff to the diagnosis. Organisms may also gain access to the circulation, however, from contaminated infusion fluids, tubing, or remote infection sites. The microbiologic diagnosis of catheter-associated septicemia was problematic until Maki and colleagues[22] published their landmark article in 1977. These investigators described a semiquantitative culture technique performed by rolling an amputated distal catheter segment across a blood agar plate (Fig. 75-2). Catheter segments from patients with catheter-associated bloodstream infections grew 15 or more colonies on the plate. Segments with lower colony counts indicated colonization or bacteremic seeding of the catheter from another source. Such factors as catheter material (plastic versus steel), duration (days versus hours), insertion (cutdown versus puncture), and site (central versus peripheral) determine the likelihood of infection.[23] For example, peripheral cannulas continued for longer than 72 hours are more likely to result in infection. Unfortunately, few

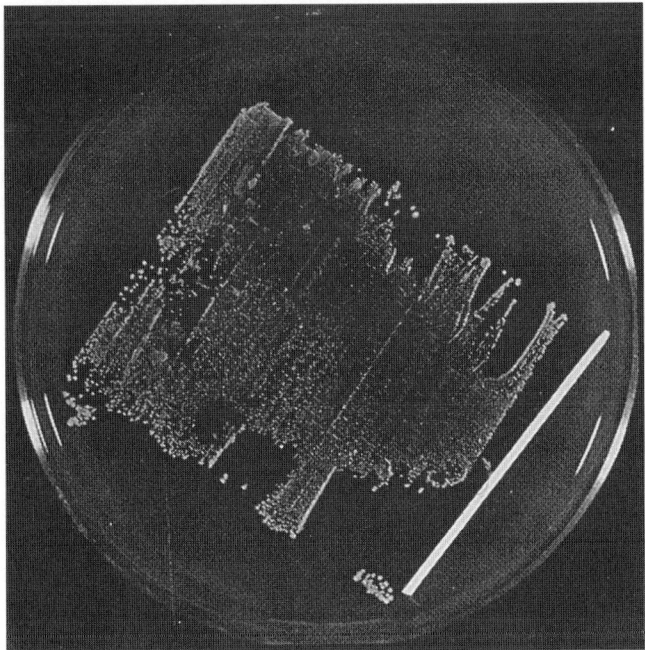

Fig. 75-2. A positive semiquantitative catheter culture. The original catheter segment has been placed on the plate for perspective. (From Maki, D. G., Weise, C. E., Sarafin, H. W.: A semiquantitative culture method of identifying intravenous-catheter-related infection. N. Engl. J. Med., *296*:1305, 1977.)

well-designed studies have been done with central venous or arterial catheters. Most vascular catheter infections are caused by Staphylococcus aureus or Staphylococcus epidermidis; however, with prolonged cannulation, especially in patients with multiple organ failure, enterococci, gram-negative bacilli, or even yeasts may cause infection.

Techniques for minimizing risks of catheter infections are listed in Table 75-5. All central lines should be inserted under sterile conditions, using an appropriate topical antiseptic and sterile gloves. Antimicrobial ointments may be applied to the skin site immediately after cannula insertion and during each dressing change. The choice of antimicrobial ointment is problematic. In a prospective study, Maki and Bond[24] noted local infection in 6.5% of patients who received nothing, 3.6% of patients dressed with an iodophor, and 2.2% dressed with polysporin (a combination of polymixin, neomycin, and bacitracin). The rate of catheter-related bacteremia was less than 1% in all three groups.

Table 75-5. Minimizing Risk of Vascular Catheter Infections

Always insert catheters under sterile conditions (gloves and masks)
Use a topical antiseptic agent before insertion
Change sterile gauze dressings every 48 hours
Apply an antimicrobial ointment with each dressing change
Replace IV administration sets every 72 hours
Consider the use of a silver-impregnated vascular cuff if duration of catheter placement will be longer than 72 hours
Remove the catheter at first sign of sepsis (purulence or cellulitis at skin entry site)

Regardless of ointment selection, skin sites should be inspected daily for evidence of infection and dressings should be replaced every 48 hours.

Gram-negative bacteria, such as Klebsiella and Enterobacter species, proliferate in IV glucose-containing solutions at room temperature. A nationwide epidemic in 1971 and 1972 caused by intrinsic contamination of IV solutions, prompted the CDC to recommend that IV therapy administration sets be changed every 24 hours.[25] The cost effectiveness of this recommendation, however, was never shown. Results of recent studies suggested that a 72-hour interval for replacing IV administration sets is perfectly safe and is less expensive. Maki and colleagues[26] estimated this change would save their hospital more than $100,000 annually.

Sterile gauze dressings have been a tradition for catheter skin-site care for years. A transparent tape dressing, which allows inspection of the catheter skin junction site without dressing removal, is now available. Findings of early studies suggested the tape reduced skin colonization adjacent to the cannula. Conly and co-authors[27] reported, however, that transparent dressings may be more hazardous when applied to central venous catheter skin sites. Patients were randomized to receive either a transparent or gauze dressing. Skin colonization was greater under transparent than under gauze dressings. Local infections developed in 62% of patients with transparent dressings and in 24% of patients with gauze dressings. More disturbing, all seven episodes of catheter-associated bacteremia occurred in patients assigned transparent dressings.

Triple-lumen catheters are associated with more infection complications than single-lumen catheters. Hilton and colleagues[28] reported an infection rate of 8% in patients who received single-lumen vascular catheters and 32% in those with triple-lumen catheters. These authors recommended that catheters may be replaced over a guide wire when catheter-associated sepsis is suspected, but no cellulitis or purulence is present at the skin site. If, however, the amputated catheter tip subsequently grows as much as or more than 15 cfu per plate, the catheter should be removed.

A more recent technical advance in central vascular catheters is the placement of a silver-impregnated cuff in the subcutaneous space. The cuff contains biodegradable collagen impregnated with silver ions that provide broad spectrum antimicrobial activity. Maki and colleagues[21] found that cuffless catheters were three times more likely to be colonized and nearly four times more likely to be associated with secondary bacteremia than were cuffed catheters. Flowers and associates[29] reported no catheter-related bloodstream infections in patients assigned cuffed catheters, but a rate of 13.8% was noted in control subjects. They noted that many catheter-associated infections were caused by Candida albicans. The reason for this tendency was unclear, but this finding prompted these authors to recommend the use of an iodophor, which has antifungal activity, instead of an antibiotic ointment with dressing changes. The most recent development in this field is a novel antiseptic central vascular catheter that is reported to reduce the risk of sepsis.[29a] The catheter is impregnated with silver-sulfadiazine and chlorhexidine. A preliminary study appears encouraging, but conclusive studies have yet to be published.

Pressure Monitors

Intravascular pressure monitoring devices are widely used in ICUs. Epidemics of bacteremia caused by contamination of transducer heads or domes have been attributed to Serratia marcescens, Klebsiella oxytoca, Acinetobacter calcoaceticus, and Pseudomonas cepacia.[30] In one outbreak, reusable transducers had been improperly disinfected or fitted with improperly sterilized domes. The space between transducer heads and dome membranes should be sterile. If lubrication is necessary, use of sterile saline, bacteriostatic water, or preferably 70% alcohol, is advised. Extrinsic contamination of devices may result from frequent manipulations by soiled hands of ICU staff. Handwashing must be done before and after handling any device. Disposable components should not be reused. Reusable transducer components should be cleaned and sterilized or subjected to high level disinfection between patient use.

Respiratory Therapy Equipment

Pneumonia is a serious complication for the intubated patient. Gram-negative bacteria colonize the endotracheal tube from the oral pharynx. Each breathing cycle can blow them into the lower airway. The trachea is further compromised because the endotracheal tube destroys the protective microvillae. Like vascular catheters, endotracheal tubes promote surface colonization because they are inert foreign bodies. Once in the lower airway, bacteria can invade the lung parenchyma. Pseudomonas aeruginosa, which secretes enzymes that enhance invasion, produces tissue hemorrhage and necrosis. Underlying obstructive airways disease, pulmonary edema, and adult respiratory distress syndrome (ARDS) further compromise the host response.

In contrast to the community-acquired form, pneumonia in the intubated patient is difficult to diagnose. White blood cell counts, sputum cultures, and chest radiographs are imprecise diagnostic studies. Although cultures of blood or empyema fluid may be helpful, most cases of pneumonia are diagnosed presumptively. Accuracy is further compromised by coexisting ARDS. In one study, the diagnosis of pneumonia was missed in 33% of cases that came to autopsy.[31] Mortality from ICU-associated pneumonia may be as high as 70% in high risk patients.

Thirty years ago, outbreaks of pneumonia from Pseudomonas aeruginosa were caused by contamination of medication nebulizers.[32] Fortunately, this problem was remedied by appropriate disinfection practices. Contamination of medication nebulizers may happen now by reflux of condensate containing oral pharyngeal flora into ventilator circuitry. Craven and associates[33] reported that 68% of nebulizer reservoirs they sampled were heavily contaminated with bacteria. The investigators produced bacterial aerosols by inoculating nebulizers with the same concentrations of organisms isolated from in-use equipment. This finding prompted the authors to clean or disinfect nebulizers after each treatment rather than at 24-hour intervals.

Table 75-6. Minimizing Infection Complications of Mechanical Ventilation

Clean medication nebulizer after each treatment
Avoid prolonged nasotracheal intubation
Replace ventilator tubing every 48 hours
Consider SDD prophylaxis in the high risk trauma patient
Consider sucralfate for antiulcer prophylaxis instead of antacids and H_2 blockers
Position patient properly to avoid aspiration

SDD, Selective digestive decontamination.

This and other strategies to minimize infection complications of mechanical ventilation are listed in Table 75-6.

Otitis media has been reported as a complication of intubation. Tympanocentesis fluid has grown Pseudomonas aeruginosa, Klebsiella oxytoca, and Enterobacter cloacae.[34] Paranasal sinusitis is another complication, first recognized in neurosurgical patients, that results from prolonged nasotracheal intubation.[35] Regular sinus radiographs may be normal. Computerized tomographic scanning is the preferred procedure to make the diagnosis (Fig. 75-3). Without removal of the nasotracheal tube, the infection persists even with antibiotic therapy.

The timing for replacement of ventilator tubing has been controversial. Years ago, authorities recommended changes every 24 hours because of fear of contamination of reservoirs by water-loving bacteria. Craven and colleagues[36] challenged this recommendation in 1982. Patients who required continuous mechanical ventilation were randomly assigned tubing changes at 24 or 48 hours. Samples of inspiratory phase gas from ventilators were cultured. The frequency of positive cultures was 30% in cases with tubing changes at 24 hours and 32% for cases with tubing changes at 48 hours. The authors recommended replacing ventilator tubing every 48 hours, which resulted in an annual savings of more than $30,000 to their hospital.

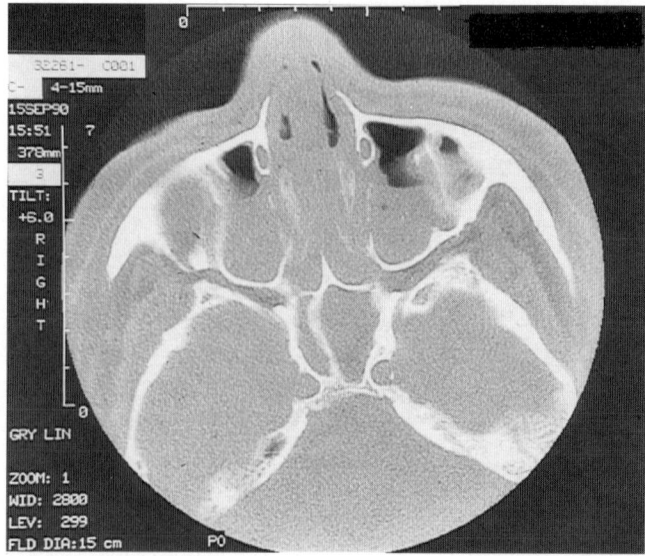

Fig. 75-3. Nasotracheally associated sinusitis in a 63-year-old man. This CT scan shows complete opacification of both ethmoid air cells, sphenoid sinuses, maxillary sinuses, and frontal sinuses.

The cascade bubbling humidifier, another potential source for contamination, may generate microaerosols of bacteria.[37] Although the significance of this finding was uncertain, Rhame and colleagues recommended changing sterile humidifier water every 24 hours. Heat and moisture exchangers within ventilator tubing might be a source of contamination. Saravolatz and associates,[38] however, were unable to generate bacterial aerosols even after contaminating the exchangers with Staphylococcus aureus and Pseudomonas aeruginosa.

With improved technology, airway contamination has shifted from equipment to the patient. In 1978, Atherton and White[39] described 10 ventilated patients with paralytic ileus, 9 of whom had microbial overgrowth in their stomachs. In 3, the stomach was implicated as the source of airway colonization. Donowitz and colleagues[40] noted that nearly one half of patients with a gastric pH of 4 or greater were heavily colonized with gram-negative bacteria. This finding was associated with antacids and H2-blocking agents used for ulcer prophylaxis.

Various antimicrobial prophylaxis programs have been studied to prevent infection of the respiratory tract (Table 75-7). Feeley and colleagues[41] gave aerosolized polymixin to chronically intubated patients. Although the frequency of pneumonia was reduced, subsequent cases of pneumonia were caused by polymixin-resistant bacteria and often were lethal. The use of selective digestive decontamination (SDD) is reportedly more successful. This technique results in the removal of transient aerobic gram-negative gut bacteria while maintaining the anaerobic component that apparently preserves colonization resistance.[42] Stoutenbeek and colleagues[43] from the Netherlands assigned trauma patients SDD (tobramycin, colistin, and amphotericin B) in an oral paste (Orabase) and in suspension through a gastric tube every 6 hours. Patients also simultaneously received cefotaxime IV for several days. In contrast to historical controls, their patients had fewer lower respiratory tract infections (8 versus 59%). Ledingham and associates[44] from the United Kingdom reported a substantial reduction in nosocomial infections, from 24% in historical controls to 10% in patients given SDD. Brun-Buisson and colleagues[45] studied SDD during an outbreak of multiple-resistant Klebsiella species. Their subjects were randomly selected to receive oral neomycin plus polymixin E plus nalidixic acid or placebo. No patients received IV antibiotics. Colonization with the multiple-resistant strain dropped from 10 to 3%, although colonization by gram-positive cocci rose. Furthermore, no difference was noted in the overall nosocomial infection rate. The authors cautioned that SDD should not be used routinely. In one other study, Godard and colleagues[46] gave patients placebo or a suspension of tobramycin, colistin, and amphotericin B through a gastric feeding tube during a study period of 8 months. Although a reduced incidence of pneumonia was claimed, hospital mortality showed no difference. Results of SDD studies have been critically reviewed by Johanson.[47] He concludes that further evaluation and careful designs of future experiments must take place before SDD should be accepted more universally.

Nasogastric tube feeding can be an important component to nutritional support of the critically ill patient. Tube feeding formulas usually are delivered by continuous infusion, which promotes gastric colonization with gram-negative bacteria. Lee and associates[48] found that intermittent nasogastric feeding resulted in a significant reduction in pneumonia compared to patients fed continuously.

Sucralfate, a chemical complex of sucrose octosulfate and aluminum hydroxide, is an effective antiulcer prophylactic agent that does not alter gastric pH. Driks and colleagues[49] noted that patients who received sucralfate had less gram-negative bacterial colonization and one half the frequency of pneumonia as compared to patients who received antacids. Sucralfate was studied further in 100 ventilated, high risk patients by Tryba and associates.[50] Patients were randomly assigned sucralfate suspension every 4 hours or antacid every 2 hours. Excluding patients with primary chest trauma, they found pneumonia in 3 (10.3%) of 29 sucralfate-treated patients and 11 (34.4%) of 32 antacid-treated patients.

Finally, a study reported the danger of the supine position in promoting aspiration in mechanically ventilated patients. Using ^{99m}technetium sulfur colloid labeling of gastric contents, Torres and co-investigators demonstrated marked uptake in endobronchial secretions after supine position versus semirecumbent position.[50a] Elevation of the head of the patient's bed may be the most cost-effective and simplest way to prevent pulmonary aspiration of gastric contents.

Table 75-7. Antimicrobial Prophylaxis to Prevent ICU Pneumonia Results in Selected Series

Year	Primary Author	Population	Program	Findings
1975	Feeley[41]	General ICU	Polymyxin aerosol prophylaxis	Antibiotic resistance; mortality from pneumonia
1987	Stoutenbeek[43]	Trauma ICU	SDD (TCA)* oral paste suspension IV† cefotaxime	Pneumonia compared to historical controls (8% vs 59%) and Mortality (3% vs 8%)
1988	Ledingham[44]	General ICU	(same)	Nosocomial infections compared to historical controls (10% vs 24%); no difference in mortality
1989	Brun-Buisson[45]	General ICU	NCNA† in oral suspension	Colonization of multiple-resistant strain of gram-negative bacilli; no difference in infection rates
1990	Godard[46]	General ICU	TCA* in oral suspension	Pneumonia compared to placebo controls (2% vs 15%); no difference in mortality

* TCA, Tobramycin, colistin, and amphotericin B.
† NCNA, Nystatin, colistin, and naladixic acid.

Urinary Catheters

Urinary tract infections (UTIs) in ICUs are invariably-associated with urethral catheterization or some other manipulation of the genitourinary tract.[51] Alternative methods for draining the bladder, such as intermittent catheterization or diapering, usually are not appropriate in the ICU setting. Suprapubic catheterization may delay the onset of bacteriuria,[52] but infection is inevitable after several weeks of catheterization. Most catheter-associated UTIs are asymptomatic. Usually no specific therapy is required unless the patient develops clinical evidence of infection. Bacteria, once established in the catheterized urinary tract, quickly proliferate to achieve concentrations of 10^5 organisms or more per milliliter of urine.[53] The same generally holds true for patients who develop candiduria, usually in association with antibacterial therapy. If, however, the threat of the patient developing systemic yeast infection is high, local instillation or irrigation of amphotericin B, using a dose of 20 mg diluted in 100 ml of sterile water, may be prescribed every 6 to 8 hours for 7 to 10 days.

Closed urinary drainage, originally described by Dukes in 1929,[54] remains the benchmark for catheter systems. The junction between the catheter and drainage system should not be violated. One study even suggested that mortality was higher for patients with broken junction seals than for patients with catheter seals that were preserved.[55] Adding antimicrobial agents to the drainage bag is of no benefit.[56] Most UTIs are caused by invasion of bacteria from the external surface of the catheter into the periurethral space. Despite this knowledge, Burke and colleagues[57] found that applying antibiotic ointment to the urethral meatus did not reduce UTIs.

Transmission of UTIs from patient to patient may occur by ICU staff. If soilage is anticipated, ICU personnel should wear gloves and wash their hands after each patient encounter. The urinary drainage bag should not be positioned above the patient's pelvis to prevent reflux of bag urine into the urinary tract.

Calvin Kunin,[58] a noted authority on UTIs, has challenged industry to produce a better drainage system for patients who require long-term catheterization. Consider a thin-walled, continuously lubricated, collapsing catheter, suspended in the bladder without a balloon and washed intermittently with physiologic fluids!

Spread of Microorganisms

To this point, risk factors that predispose individual patients to infections in the ICU have been emphasized. It is clear that the ICU environment amplifies transmission of infections more so than the regular hospital ward. Vulnerable ICU patients are assaulted by invasive therapeutic and monitoring devices that with time become colonized by nosocomial bacteria. Potential pathogens also colonize the patient's oral pharynx, skin, gut, and urinary tract. Hands of ICU staff may serve as vectors for transmission of organism from the environment to patients or from one patient to another. Spread of gram-negative bacteria through an ICU was graphically illustrated in one study reported from the United Kingdom.[59] Pseudomonas aeruginosa, Acinetobacter anitratus, and Aeromonas hydrophilia were easily cultured from tap water and the skin of the staff in the ICU. These bacteria were also noted in mouthwash, oral nutritional feeding, and fluid from nasogastric aspiration bottles. Finally, these same bacterial species were cultured from the upper airway, umbilicus, perineum, and rectum of patients. In our current era of computer technology, skin pathogens have been passed from patient to touch screens to patients (E. Sivak, personal communication).

The wrong microbe in the wrong place at the wrong time may result in lethal consequences. Craven and colleagues[60] studied large numbers of patients admitted to the medical and surgical ICUs at Boston City Hospital over a 20-month period. The relative risk of death following nosocomial infection was 3.5 times higher than for patients assigned to the general hospital ward. To avert this risk, principles of infection control must be practiced by all ICU staff. Maki[61] observed that physicians remain "blissfully unaware;" handwashing is poorly practiced "by health care professionals in nearly all hospitals." Whereas infection control principals should be incorporated into the design of the ICU,[62] conventional methods may not be as applicable as on the regular ward. Olson and colleagues[63] reported their frustrations in attempting to control spread of Pseudomonas aeruginosa in an ICU. Strains were of different serotypes, cases were not clustered, and sources were not apparent. Only 12 of 100 cases of infection appeared to have been caused by spread from readily explainable sources. The authors estimated "barrier isolation" would have prevented only 5 cases. In their study, undetected gastrointestinal carriage appeared to be the most likely source of colonization.

The anaerobic bacterial species Clostridium difficile is a normal inhabitant of the lower intestinal tract. Broad spectrum antibiotic therapy promotes overgrowth with secretion of a toxin that may result in pseudomembranous enterocolitis. Outbreaks of C. difficile diarrhea have been reported from ICUs.[64] This organism is passed easily from one patient to another by the hands of ICU staff. McFarland and colleagues[65] stress the need for handwashing and appropriate barrier precautions to prevent this problem. Generally speaking, C. difficile diarrhea, if it is not serious, will simply respond to symptomatic measures and withdrawal of systemic antibiotic therapy. It may be necessary, however, to treat the patient with a specific antibiotic agent. At present, 250 mg of metronidazole given orally four times per day for 7 days resolves most cases of C. difficile-associated diarrhea. If the problem is serious and prolonged, however, vancomycin (125 mg given orally every 6 hours), which is more expensive than metronidazole but may be more effective, can be used.

Antibiotic Control

More than 20 years ago, a disturbing outbreak of multiple-resistant Klebsiella aerogenes developed in a neurosurgical ICU in Glasgow, Scotland.[66] Nine patients developed Klebsiella meningitis after surgery. Antibiotic prescribing had been practiced without restriction in this unit for years. Investigators noted that the frequency of meningitis was directly related to the rate of respiratory tract colonization with Klebsiella. If colonization exceeded 10%, meningitis was likely. Despite all sorts of attempts to control the outbreak, it persisted until all antibiotics were stopped. This measure seemed drastic, but an immediate decrease in infections was noted. By 4 weeks, the organism no longer caused colonization or infection. The fear was raised that infections caused by more sensitive organisms would increase; however, in fact, ICU respiratory and urinary infection rates fell from 45 to 15% and 21 to 7%, respectively.

Monitoring of antibiotic use with feedback to prescribing physicians prevents the indiscriminate use of antibiotics. An example of an antibiotic order form used at the Cleveland Clinic is shown in Figure 75-4. The prescribing physician checks the indication (prophylaxis, empiric therapy, therapy for proven infection) and includes a limited amount of clinical and laboratory information. The drug, route, dose, and interval are given and the physician signs the request. The Infectious Disease Society of America[67] also recommends that automatic stop orders be in effect at 24 to 48 hours for prophylaxis, 12 to 24 hours for empiric therapy, and 5 to 7 days for therapy of a known infection. If longer duration is required, a new order must be written. Antibiotic prescribing monitoring data can be sorted to provide prescribers with information about their practice in using antibiotics for prophylaxis, empiric therapy, or therapy for proven infections. Educational material appropriate to the problem can be provided at the same time.

Special Problems

In 1980, Peacock and associates[68] reported a frightening observation. Several years earlier, a patient was admitted to their hospital with methicillin-resistant Staphylococcus aureus (MRSA) endocarditis. He had multiple skin lesions harboring MRSA. Patient-to-patient spread was traced beginning in the regular hospital ward and spreading into the ICU. Although possible, it did not appear that spread was caused by the hands of colonized ICU staff. The authors speculated that transient airborne spread may have occurred over short distances from heavily colonized or infected patients. Once the epidemic strain became established, it was difficult to eradicate, even by using strict isolation measures. Since this original article, two thirds of reported MRSA outbreaks in the United States have been in ICUs.[69] Cohorting colonized or infected MRSA patients from other patients until discharge may control an outbreak if traditional measures have failed.

For several decades, coagulase-negative staphylococci (CNS) have become respectable nosocomial pathogens. Previously, they were considered innocent bystanders. At present, a significant number of nosocomial strains are methicillin resistant. A case of continuous ambulatory peritoneal dialysis (CAPD)-associated peritonitis from vancomycin-resistant CNS was reported.[70] Initially, this strain was susceptible to vancomycin, but it became resistant during treatment of subsequent episodes of peritonitis. Enterococcus faecalis, another emerging nosocomial pathogen, was reported as resistant to gentamicin by Zervos and colleagues.[71] No combination of antibiotics was effective in vitro against this strain. Infected patients had received previous antibiotics, especially aminoglycosides and cephalosporins, during lengthy hospitalizations. Although the strain was found on hands of several ICU staff and in the environment, no common source was identified. A more recent discovery is multiple-resistant Enterococcus faecium, resistant not only to aminoglycosides, but also to the penicillins and vancomycin.[71a] Such organisms pose a significant threat to patients in the ICU because they quickly colonize the gut and can be readily transmitted to other patients by the hands of health-care workers.

Certain gram-negative bacteria contain plasmids with aminoglycoside resistance, which may spread to other bacteria. Schlaes and colleagues[72] reported that 8.2% of hospital patients were colonized with gentamicin-resistant strains, some with plasmids containing these markers. Spread of these plasmids may disseminate antibiotic resistance throughout an ICU.

After Legionella pneumophilia was found responsible for the 1976 outbreak of pneumonia in Philadelphia, it gained even more prominence by causing nosocomial infections.[73] Environmental water sources can harbor large numbers of bacteria that may be inhaled or aspirated into the lower airway, causing pneumonia. These include hospital ventilation systems, cooling tower water, and porta-

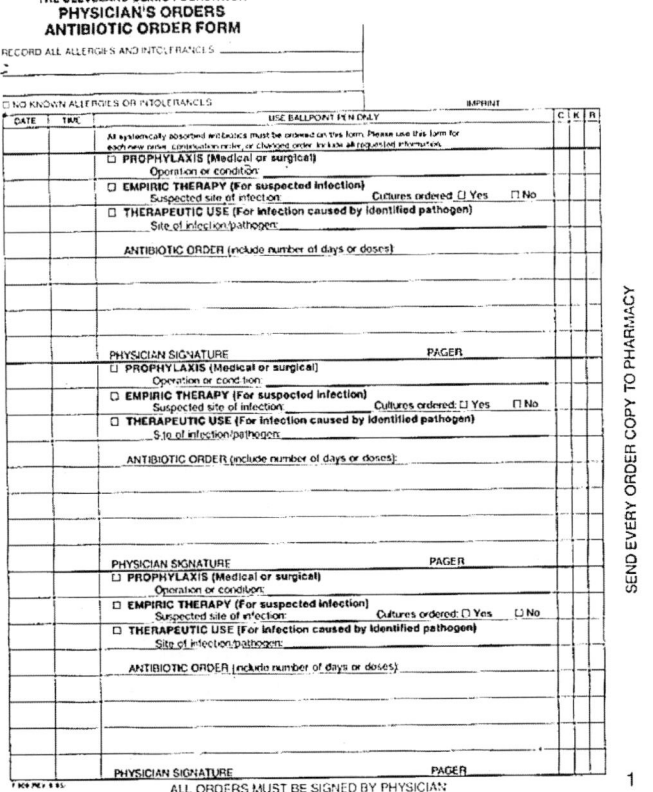

Fig. 75-4. Example of an antibiotic order form used at the Cleveland Clinic. The indication for the antibiotic is noted and a limited amount of clinical and laboratory information is requested.

ble water used for showering and drinking. Legionella macdadei (Pittsburgh pneumonia agent) has been recovered from nebulizers used for respiratory therapy.[74] Contamination of water sources is best prevented by maintaining water temperatures between 60 and 65°C. Chlorination or intermittent steam flushing of water lines can be done if this is not successful.

Of growing concern is exposure of ICU staff to Mycobacterium tuberculosis from patients with unrecognized disease. Catanzaro[75] related an experience that illustrates the problem. A critically ill patient was transferred to an ICU with uncontrolled seizures and gastrointestinal bleeding. A recent portable chest radiograph showed a right upper lobe infiltrate that was attributed to aspiration. After endothelial intubation, the patient required frequent suctioning and vigorous chest physiotherapy. Endotracheal cultures subsequently grew Mycobacterium tuberculosis. Fourteen (31%) of 45 susceptible house staff converted their tuberculin skin tests. Contact investigation was instituted in this case because one physician developed clinical pulmonary tuberculosis several months after exposure to the index patient. With the rising incidence of tuberculosis, especially in patients with AIDS, all ICU staff should have annual tuberculin testing and also participate in appropriate follow-up testing after exposure to an unrecognized case.[76]

POST-ICU PHASE

Once the diagnosis of nosocomial infection is established, patients should receive the most appropriate type and duration of antibiotic therapy. Guidelines have already been reviewed. After completing therapy, however, patient follow-up is needed to ascertain if recurrence or relapse has occurred, especially for patients with pneumonia and infection from endovascular sources. Follow-up blood cultures may be warranted, particularly if new fever or leukocytosis has developed. It should not be routine practice to repeat cultures from patients if they are responding appropriately to antimicrobial therapy. Patients with invasive candidiasis usually are treated with at least 1.0 to 1.5 g IV of amphotericin B, therapy that may continue after discharge from the ICU. Although patients with candidemia from a vascular catheter source may be cured simply by removing the catheter, our practice is to treat such ICU patients with a short course of amphotericin B therapy (total dose of 200 to 500 mg) because of our concern for dissemination.

All ICU physicians must know the limitations of microbiologic studies. Routine cultures may yield bacteria or fungi that have no clinical relevance; however, obtaining endotracheal cultures from chronically ventilated patients once or twice a week may be of some benefit. If the patient's condition deteriorates, this knowledge may assist the physician in initiating more appropriate antimicrobial therapy when pneumonia is suspected. It is important to practice clinical skills at the bedside and to treat the patient, not the culture result. Also, a point to remember is that patients may remain colonized with antibiotic-resistant organisms after completing successful therapy for an infection. Only under rare circumstances should one attempt to treat this type of colonization. Systemic antimicrobial therapy will more likely result in toxicity, superinfection, and added expense than in eradication. As the patient recovers from the ICU stay, so do their own bacteria, which again will provide the individual with a normal host defense.

REFERENCES

1. Haley, R. W., et al.: Hospital infection control. Am. J. Infect. Control, 13:97, 1985.
2. Garner, J. S., et al.: CDC definitions for nosocomial infections. Am. J. Infect. Control, 16:128, 1988.
3. Massanari, R. M., and Hierholzer, Jr., W. J.: Numbers that count. Am. J. Infect. Control, 14:149, 1986.
4. Centers for Disease Control: Isolation Techniques for Use in Hospitals. Atlanta, GA, 1970.
5. Jackson, M. M., and Lynch, P.: Infection control—too much or too little? Am. J. Nursing, 84:208, 1984.
6. Lynch, P., et al.: Rethinking the role of isolation practices in the prevention of nosocomial infections. Ann. Intern. Med., 107:243, 1987.
7. Doebbeling, B. N., et al.: Removal of nosocomial pathogens from the contaminated glove. Ann. Intern. Med., 109:394, 1988.
8. Larson, E. L., et al.: Composition and antimicrobic resistance of skin flora in hospitalized and healthy adults. J. Clin. Microbiol., 23:604, 1986.
9. Archer, G. L., and Tenenbaum, M. J.: Antibiotic-resistant Staphylococcus epidermidis in patients undergoing cardiac surgery. Antimicrob. Agents Chemother., 17:269, 1980.
10. Johanson, Jr., W. G., et al.: Nosocomial respiratory infections with gram-negative bacilli. Ann. Intern. Med., 77:701, 1972.
11. Giuliano, M., et al.: Effect of broad-spectrum parenteral antibiotics on composition of intestinal microflora of humans. Antimicrob. Agents Chemother., 31:202, 1987.
12. Barza, M., et al.: Effect of broad-spectrum parenteral antibiotics on "colonization resistance" of intestinal microflora of humans. Antimicrob. Agents Chemother., 31:723, 1987.
13. Stevens, R. M., et al.: Pneumonia in an intensive care unit. Arch. Intern. Med., 134:106, 1974.
14. Martin, L. F., et al.: Postoperative pneumonia. Arch. Surg., 119:379, 1984.
15. Sinanan, M., Maier, R. V., Carrico, J.: Laparotomy for intraabdominal sepsis in patients in an intensive care unit. Arch. Surg., 119:652, 1984.
16. Calderwood, S. B., et al.: Prosthetic valve endocarditis. J. Thorac. Cardiovasc. Surg., 92:776, 1986.
17. D'Agostino, R. S., et al.: Valve replacement in patients with native valve endocarditis: What really determines operative outcome? Ann. Thorac. Surg., 40:429, 1985.
18. Omari, B., et al.: Predictive risk factors for periannular extension of native valve endocarditis. Chest, 96:1273, 1989.
19. Antimicrobial prophylaxis in surgery. Medical Letter, 31:105, 1989.
20. Committee on Rheumatic Fever, Bacterial Endocarditis and Kawasaki Disease of the Council on Cardiovascular Disease in the Young of the American Heart Association: Prevention of bacterial endocarditis. JAMA, 264:2919, 1990.
21. Maki, D. G., et al.: An attachable silver-impregnated cuff for prevention of infection with central venous catheters: A prospective randomized multicenter trial. Am. J. Med., 85:307, 1988.
22. Maki, D. G., Weise, C. E., Sarafin, H. W.: A semiquantitative culture method of identifying intravenous-catheter-related infection. N. Engl. J. Med., 296:1305, 1977.
23. Simmons, B. P.: CDC guidelines for the prevention and con-

trol of nosocomial infections. Am. J. Infect. Control, *11*:183, 1983.
24. Maki, D. G., and Bond, J. D.: A comparative study of polyantibiotic and iodophor ointments in prevention of vascular catheter-related infection. Am. J. Med., *70*:739, 1981.
25. Nosocomial bacteremia associated with intravenous fluid therapy. MMWR, *20(Suppl. 9)*:1, 1971.
26. Maki, D. G., et al.: Prospective study of replacing administration sets for intravenous therapy at 48- vs. 72-hours intervals. JAMA, *258*:1777, 1987.
27. Conly, J. M., Grieves, K., Peters, B.: A prospective randomized study comparing transparent and dry gauze dressings for central venous catheters. J. Infect. Dis., *159*:310, 1989.
28. Hilton, E., et al.: Central catheter infections: Single- versus triple-lumen catheters. Am. J. Med., *84*:667, 1988.
29. Flowers, R. H., et al.: Efficacy of an attachable subcutaneous cuff for the prevention of intravascular catheter-related infection. JAMA, *261*:878, 1989.
29a. Maki, D. G., Wheeler, S. J., and Stolz, S. M.: Clinical trial of a novel anti-septic coated central venous catheter. (Abstract.) Thirty-first Interscience Conference on Antimicrobial Agents and Chemotherapy, October, 1991.
30. Beck-Sague, C. M., and Jarvis, W. R.: Epidemic bloodstream infections associated with pressure transducers: A persistent problem. Infect. Control Hosp. Epidemiol., *10*:54, 1989.
31. Andrews, C. P., et al.: Diagnosis of nosocomial bacterial pneumonia in acute, diffuse lung injury. Chest, *80*:254, 1981.
32. Pierce, A. K., et al.: Long-term evaluation of decontamination of inhalation-therapy equipment and the occurrence of necrotizing pneumonia. N. Engl. J. Med., *282*:528, 1970.
33. Craven, D. E., et al.: Contaminated medication nebulizers in mechanical ventilator circuits. Am. J. Med., *77*:834, 1984.
34. Lucks, D., et al.: Incidence and microbiological etiology of middle ear effusion complicating endotracheal intubation and mechanical ventilation. J. Infect. Dis., *157*:368, 1988.
35. Deutschman, C. S., et al.: Paranasal sinusitis: A common complication of nasotracheal intubation in neurosurgical patients. Neurosurgery, *17*:296, 1985.
36. Craven, D. E., et al.: Contamination of mechanical ventilators with tubing changes every 24 or 48 hours. N. Engl. J. Med., *306*:1505, 1982.
37. Rhame, R. S., et al.: Bubbling humidifiers produce microaerosols which can carry bacteria. Infect. Control Hosp. Epidemiol., *7*:403, 1986.
38. Saravolatz, L. D., et al.: Lack of bacterial aerosols associated with heat and moisture exchangers. Am. Rev. Respir. Dis., *134*:214, 1986.
39. Atherton, S. T., and White, D. J.: Stomach as source of bacteria colonizing respiratory tract during artificial ventilation. Lancet, *2*:968, 1978.
40. Donowitz, L. G., et al.: Alteration of normal gastric flora in critical care patients receiving antacid and cimetidine therapy. Infect. Control Hosp. Epidemiol., *7*:23, 1986.
41. Feeley, T. W., et al.: Aerosol polymyxin and pneumonia in seriously ill patients. N. Engl. J. Med., *293*:471, 1975.
42. Clasener, H. A. L., Vollaard, E. J., van Saene, H. K. F.: Long-term prophylaxis of infection by selective decontamination in leukopenia and in mechanical ventilation. Rev. Infect. Dis., *9*:295, 1987.
43. Stoutenbeek, C. P., et al.: The effect of oropharyngeal decontamination using topical nonabsorbable antibiotics on the incidence of nosocomial respiratory tract infections in multiple trauma patients. J. Trauma, *27*:357, 1987.
44. Ledingham, I. M., et al.: Triple regimen of selective decontamination of the digestive tract, systemic cefotaxime and microbiological surveillance for prevention of acquired infection in intensive care. Lancet, *1*:785, 1988.
45. Brun-Buisson, C., et al.: Intestinal decontamination for control of nosocomial multiresistant gram-negative bacilli. Ann. Intern. Med., *110*;873, 1989.
46. Godard, J., et al.: Intestinal decontamination in a polyvalent ICU. Intensive Care Med., *16*:307, 1990.
47. Johanson, W. G.: Infection prevention by selective decontamination in intensive care. Intensive Care Med., *15*:417, 1989.
48. Lee, B., Chang, W. S., Jacobs, S.: Intermittent nasogastric feeding. Clin. Intensive Care, *4*:100, 1990.
49. Driks, M. R., et al.: Nosocomial pneumonia in intubated patients given sucralfate as compared with antacids or histamine type 2 blockers. N. Engl. J. Med., *317*:1376, 1987.
50. Tryba, M.: Risk of acute stress bleeding and nosocomial pneumonia in ventilated intensive care unit patients: Sucralfate versus antacids. Am. J. Med., *83(Suppl. 3B)*:117, 1987.
50a. Torres, A., et al.: Pulmonary aspiration of gastric contents in patients receiving mechanical ventilation: the effect of body position. Ann. Intern. Med., *116*:540, 1992.
51. Kunin, C. M.: Genitourinary infections in the patient at risk: Extrinsic risk factors. Am. J. Med., *76(Suppl. 5A)*:131, 1984.
52. Lyon, R. P.: The use of suprapubic catheterization to prevent nosocomial UTIs. Infect. Urol., *Jan/Feb* 21, 1989.
53. Stark, R. P., and Maki, D. G.: Bacteriuria in the catheterized patient. N. Engl. J. Med., *311*:560, 1984.
54. Dukes, C.: Urinary infection after excision of the rectum, their cause and prevention. Proc. R. Soc. Med., *22*:1, 1928.
55. Platt, R., et al.: Reduction of mortality associated with nosocomial urinary tract infection. Lancet, *1*:893, 1983.
56. Thompson, R. L., et al.: Catheter-associated bacteriuria. JAMA, *251*:747, 1984.
57. Burke, J. P., et al.: Evaluation of daily meatal care with polyantibiotic ointment in prevention of urinary catheter-associated bacteriuria. J. Urol., *129*:331, 1983.
58. Kunin, C. M.: Can we build a better urinary catheter? N. Engl. J. Med. *319*:365, 1988.
59. Millership, E. E., Patel, N., Chattopadhyay, B.: The colonization of patients in an intensive treatment unit with gram-negative flora: The significance of the oral route. J. Hosp. Infect., *7*:226, 1986.
60. Craven, D. E., et al.: Nosocomial infection and fatality in medical surgical intensive care unit patients. Arch. Intern. Med., *148*:1161, 1988.
61. Maki, D. G.: Risk factors for nosocomial infection in intensive care. Arch. Intern. Med., *149*:30, 1989.
62. Wenzel, R. P., et al.: Hospital-acquired infection in intensive care unit patients: An overview with emphasis on epidemics. Infect. Control Hosp. Epidemiol., *4*:371, 1983.
63. Olson, B., et al.: Epidemiology of endemic *Pseudomonias aeruginosa:* Why infection control efforts have failed. J. Infect. Dis., *150*:808, 1984.
64. Walters, B. A. J., et al.: Contamination and crossinfection with *C. difficile* in an ICU. Aust. N.Z. J. Med., *12*:255, 1982.
65. McFarland, L. V., et al.: Nosocomial acquisition of *C. difficile* infection. N. Engl. J. Med., *320*:204, 1989.
66. Price, D. J. E., and Sleigh, J. D.: Control of infection due to *Klebsiella aerogenes* in a neurosurgical unit by withdrawal of all antibiotics. Lancet, *2*:1213, 1970.
67. Marr, J. J., Moffet, H. L., Kunin, C. M.: Guidelines for improving the use of antimicrobial agents in hospitals: A statement by the Infectious Diseases Society of America. J. Infect. Dis., *157*:869, 1988.
68. Peacock, Jr., J. E., Marsik, F. J., Wenzel, R. P.: Methicillin-resistant *Staphylococcus aureus:* Introduction and spread within a hospital. Ann. Intern. Med., *93*:526, 1980.

69. Thompson, R. L., Cabezudo, I., Wenzel, R. P.: Epidemiology of nosocomial infections caused by methicillin-resistant *Staphylococcus aureus*. Ann. Intern. Med., *97*:309, 1982.
70. Schwalbe, R. S., Stapleton, J. T., Gilligan, P. H.: Emergence of vancomycin resistance in coagulase-negative staphylococci. N. Engl. J. Med., *316*:927, 1987.
71. Zervos, M. J., et al.: Nosocomial infection by gentamicin-resistant *Streptococcus faecalis*. Ann. Intern. Med., *106*:687, 1987.
71a. Spera, R. V., and Farber, B. F.: Multiply resistant *Enterococcus faecium*: the nosocomial pathogen of the 1990's. JAMA, *268*:2563, 1992.
72. Schlaes, D. M., et al.: Gentamicin-resistance plasmids in an intensive care unit. Infect. Control Hosp. Epidemiol., *7*:355, 1986.
73. Kirby, B. D., and Harris, A. A.: Nosocomial legionnaire's disease. Semin. Resp. Infect., *2*:255, 1987.
74. Gorman, G. W., et al.: Isolation of Pittsburgh pneumonia agent from nebulizers used in respiratory therapy. Ann. Intern. Med., *93*:572, 1980.
75. Catanzaro, A.: Nosocomial tuberculosis. Am. Rev. Respir. Dis., *125*:559, 1982.
76. Nardell, E. A.: Dodging droplet nuclei. Am. Rev. Respir. Dis., *142*:501, 1990.

Chapter 76

PROCEDURES: STANDARDS, INDICATIONS, AND QUALITY

HERBERT J. ROGOVE
MARY JO FITZPATRICK

The use of invasive procedures and technology has become so commonplace in the intensive care unit (ICU) over the past 15 years that physicians must keep abreast of new indications and contraindications for these procedures. It is not difficult to develop technical ability; however, the competency, understanding, and interpretation of data, and troubleshooting of invasive procedures involves skill, experience, and good clinical judgment. The purpose of this chapter is to discuss the clinical uses and quality issues for commonly performed procedures in the critical care unit (Table 76-1).

QUALITY AND APPROPRIATENESS

As physicians, nurses, and other members of the health care team have strived for excellence in their care of patients, the Joint Commission on Accreditation of Healthcare Organizations (JCAHO) in turn has supported the development of guidelines for quality assurance. In the critical care setting, as in all other areas, the quality and appropriateness of care must be monitored. Systematic evaluation of procedures is necessary to improve care and clinical performance and to resolve identified problems. The process to initiate a quality assurance program includes the following:

- Assignment of responsibility
- Delineation of the scope of care or service
- Identification of important aspects of care or service
- Identification of indications
- Establishment of criteria to evaluate the indicators
- Evaluation of care to determine if a problem is present
- Collection and analysis of data
- Taking action to resolve identified problems
- Assessment of improvement
- Dissemination of this information to the clinical and administrative staff[1]

Additionally, safety, documentation, and proper use of analgesics are major operational concerns. Procedures must be performed in an area in which safety is maximal. Some procedures must be done emergently and therefore choice is not possible; however, procedures such as the insertion of a pulmonary artery catheter should be undertaken only in areas with the necessary equipment and experienced personnel. Experienced physician supervision is imperative in teaching hospitals. All first-year physicians in training who perform invasive procedures should be thoroughly familiar with the risks of the procedure and should be supervised until a predetermined level of competence is achieved.

Documentation of the procedure cannot be overemphasized. The recording of indications, location of device, medications used, data obtained, confirmation of position, and complications must be a part of the patient's record. The physician and nurse must communicate that the procedure went well before anything is removed, infused, or changed through a catheter or tube. If a complication occurs, even if minor, it too must be documented fully in the patient's chart. The appropriate reporting form should be completed, the patient and/or family should receive an explanation, and the hospital's risk management department should be notified.

Finally, the proper use of patient analgesia is a preeminent priority. To ensure the performance of a procedure that is pain free and stress free, it is important to emphasize that both the awake and the comatose patient need an adequate local anesthetic. It is often necessary to inject the anesthetic into deep tissue or adjacent to bone. One should allow sufficient time for the medication to work, noting whether the patient appears comfortable. Reassurance and explanation of what is to occur often allays patient fears.

ARTERY CATHETERIZATION (PERCUTANEOUS) (CPT 36620)

Since the introduction of the Seldinger technique in the 1950s, arterial blood gases and arterial lines have become important aspects in the management of critically ill patients. Often, acutely ill patients may appear to have no obtainable blood pressure or a pressure that is very low; however, the insertion of the arterial catheter reveals that auscultation may be insensitive to a very low blood pressure.[2] Likewise, in hypertensive patients, the cuff pressure may be significantly lower than the arterial measurement because of the phenomenon known as overshoot.[3] Percutaneous access has gained popularity as infection rates are less than those associated with the cutdown method.

Choosing the site of catheterization is a matter of clinical judgment often based on potential for complications as well as ease of insertion and patient comfort. Radial and femoral arteries are often used and both are equally *as safe*.[4] When both sites are not available or cannot be cannu-

Table 76–1. Commonly Performed Procedures in the ICU*

Procedure	CPT	Complication Rate	References
Artery, catheterization (percutaneous)	36620	15–40%	9
Bronchoscopy; diagnostic	31622	1–10%	15, 23
Central venous catheter	36489	Int. jugular—overall 0.1–4.2%	28
		Int. jugular—pneumothorax 0–0.2%	28
		Subclavian—Overall 1–2%	28
		Subclavian—Pneumothorax 0–5%	28
Chest tubes	32020	1–2.4%	40
Defibrillation/cardioversion	92960	1–2%	50
Dialysis catheters:			
Hemodialysis	36800, 36810,	2–20%	56, 59
Peritoneal dialysis	49420	7–17%	54
IABP (intra-aortic balloon pump) (percutaneous insertion)	93529	9% or greater	65
ICP (intracranial pressure) monitoring	61107	0–25% (up to 100%)	75
Intubation	31500	Self-extubation 10–13%	86
Lumbar puncture	62270	2–13%	90
Temporary pacing	33210	1–50%	93
Lead displacement		25–40%	94
Cardiac tamponade		1%	94
Abdominal paracentisis	49080	3%	103
Pericardiocentesis; initial	33010	0–5%	104
Pulmonary artery catheter	93503	Arrhythmia—0–5%	114, 118
		Pneumothorax—1–6%	114
		Sepsis—2%	118
Thoracentesis	32000	14% Major	130
		33% Minor	130

* Physicians' Current Procedural Terminology, 1994, Chicago, American Medical Association, 1993.

lated, the left axillary artery is an excellent alternative.[5] The right axillary artery, unlike the left, has a more direct connection through the brachiocephalic artery to the carotid artery. Consequently, air can embolize to the brain without difficulty. The brachial artery is often cited as a last choice because of poor collateral blood flow and the disastrous result if thrombosis should occur. Therefore, many clinicians avoid the brachial artery under any circumstance, whereas others find it to be both safe and extremely accurate.[6,7]

Indications

The main indication for an arterial line is for monitoring. When vasoactive agents such as dobutamine, sodium nitroprusside, dopamine, and other vasopressors are being titrated on a minute-to-minute basis, real-time monitoring is essential.

Frequent need for blood sampling is an additional indication. Over the past several years, the need for many arterial blood gases has been tempered by the use of pulse oximeters. Unfortunately, if the patient is in a low flow state and is hypotensive, blood gases are still needed because of a poorly functioning and inaccurate oximeter. Samples for other laboratory work may also be withdrawn from the arterial line. Care in pulling off enough discard before the sample is obtained is important to prevent the heparin flush from causing inaccurate coagulation values. New devices are being developed to accomplish this task by saving the discard in an attached reservoir that can be reinfused into the patient.[8] Additionally, this system protects the health care worker from needlesticks, exposure to blood, and line contamination. Finally, in the rare patient in whom cardiac outputs are being measured with indocyanine green dye, arterial samples are needed.

Contraindications

If a patient has a significant coagulopathy, the choice of a site is a most important consideration when the patient absolutely needs continuous monitoring. One should avoid deep vessels, such as the femoral or axillary artery, in which bleeding may be difficult, if not impossible, to control.

Catheters should be avoided in patients who have vasospastic disease such as Raynaud's or in whom significant peripheral vascular disease exists.

Areas for catheter insertion to avoid include draining wounds and near sites of infection. Also, in patients who have had previous vascular surgery, one should avoid placing a catheter into a graft.

The insertion of intravascular catheters is best avoided if the patient is to receive thrombolytic therapy. If a catheter is already in place, it should remain because of the likelihood of hemorrhage at the removal site.

Complications and Management

Efforts to reduce risks should be optimized to keep complications at a minimum. Estimates as to the overall complication rate range from 15 to 40%.[9] Principle complications include the following:

- Thrombosis and embolism
- Hemorrhage and hematoma
- Infection
- Peripheral neuropathy

- Skin necrosis
- Vascular complications: arteriovenous (AV) fistula and false aneurysm

Thrombosis and embolism are complications that can occur with any vessel. Therefore, proper evaluation of the artery by clinical or Doppler examination may avoid this problem. Nurses and physicians should always remove a catheter at the first sign of occlusion, such as coolness, color change, or pain at or near the site of the catheter. Choosing a catheter with the smallest diameter possible may prevent this complication. Because the right axillary artery communicates with the common carotid artery, a cerebral air embolus is always a risk; therefore, the left axillary artery should be used. Hemorrhage and hematoma may occur, but in most instances, local compression is adequate. If hemorrhage is significant, a compartment syndrome may develop. Clues to this problem are swelling, pain, and parethesias. To avoid hemorrhage from accidental disconnection, most manufacturers now use luer locks. Additionally, the use of heparin flush has caused thrombocytopenia and alteration in coagulation; therefore, the use of sodium citrate (1.4%) may be a safe alternative.[10]

Additional vigilance is necessary when swelling develops around the site of insertion, especially in the case of bronchial or femoral catheters. Pulses may be present distally but local swelling with bleeding into surrounding tissue may lead to compartment syndromes when the pressure increases on muscles and nerves within fascial planes. The awake and communicative patient will complain of pain and paresthesias in the area. The sedated patient may voice no complaints, with the end result being major muscle and nerve damage, neurosis, and possible loss of an extremity. The treatment of choice for the complication is fasciotomy. Any suspicion of such a problem necessitates consultation with an orthopedic or vascular surgeon.

A noticeable number of ICU patients who develop bacteremia may have an arterial line as the cause. Those patients who have a catheter for longer than 4 days may be at risk.[11] Some authorities think changing catheters routinely does not diminish the risk for infection.[12] If catheter sepsis is suspected, the catheter should be removed and cultured. Antibiotics may be warranted for at least 7 to 10 days, unless endocarditis is suspected and then treatment is prolonged.

Neurologic complications that may occur usually are attributable to a peripheral neuropathy. A median nerve neuropathy may be seen in patients with a radial artery catheter and a brachial plexus injury may occur with an axillary artery.[13]

Other complications include skin necrosis or AV fistula and false aneurysm formation, which may occur days to weeks after the procedure.

Data Analysis

In analyzing blood pressure measurements, a rule to remember is that the smaller the vessel and the further it is from the central aorta, the greater the gradient of pressure that may cause systolic pressure elevation. Therefore, it is possible that measurement of radial arterial pressures, because of their smaller size, may be higher than the pressure recorded at the femoral artery.

Systolic overshoot is a phenomenon in which the monitored blood pressure exceeds the auscultated pressure by as much as 50 mm Hg. Causes attributed to overshoot include increased cardiac contractility, tachycardia, recent vascular or cardiac surgery, severe atherosclerosis, small air bubbles, or excessive tubing length.[3] Following the digital mean arterial pressure off the bedside monitor may be more accurate because the systolic overshoot area under the blood pressure curve occupies a smaller portion than the mean pressure.

In contrast to overshoot, the patient's arterial waveform may appear blunted and the cuff pressure may be higher than the intraarterial pressure by more than the acceptable 5 to 15 mm Hg. In this situation, overdampening has occurred, necessitating the search for either large air bubbles, overly compliant tubing, kinking of the tubing, loose connections, blood clots, or the wrong-sized cuff.[3]

Quality Enhancement

The overall approach to ensuring the quality of arterial catheter use and data collection is minimizing the known risks associated with the technical insertion, maintenance of the catheter, and maximizing data interpretation (Table 76-2). Careful zeroing of the transducer and appropriate tubing size and length are necessary to ensure the accuracy of the data obtained. Such efforts are directed at enhancing the safety and effectiveness of the patient care process.

The timing of insertion of arterial lines should be mentioned. Placement of an arterial line before inserting a pulmonary catheter permits continuous monitoring of the patient while the sterile drapes used for the pulmonary artery catheter insertion are obstructing the clinician's view of the patient. Also, the nurse is free to help during the procedure rather than being interrupted to obtain vital signs.

Additional nursing responsibilities not mentioned include the ICU admission measurement of blood pressure by cuff in both arms. This determination is a helpful baseline, ensures adequate blood flow bilaterally, and serves as a correlate to the arterial line. Checking the patency of

Table 76–2. Quality Enhancement for Arterial Lines

Minimize Risk
  Check pulses before insertion; make sure no bruits are heard
  Use small diameter catheters (20 gauge or smaller)
  Avoid, if possible, in patients with peripheral vascular disorders
  Minimize duration (ideally less than 7 days, but clinical judgment must prevail)
  Exercise extreme care in patients with coagulation abnormalities
  Use a percutaneous method of insertion
  Insert below the inguinal ligament when using the femoral artery
  Confirm patency of the catheter before flushing
  Remove immediately if the extremity with the catheter has lost a pulse; or if color changes, temperature changes, or pain occur
  Strict asepsis of stopcocks
Maximize risk
  Use short, noncompliant tubing
  Calibrate and zero transducer properly
  Calibrate monitor properly
  Check for air bubbles in the system

the catheter is important to guarantee accuracy of measurement. If occlusion is suspected, the line is aspirated first. Flushing before aspiration may dislodge a clot and cause embolization.

BRONCHOSCOPY (CPT 31622)

The use of fiberoptic bronchoscopy in the ICU is for diagnostic, therapeutic, or both purposes. In the critical care setting, fiberoptic bronchoscopy has gained in popularity over rigid bronchoscopy. A reason for poor use of the fiberoptic bronchoscope had been unfounded fear that adequate suctioning was not possible.

Indications

One of the most frequent respiratory problems in ICU patients is atelectasis. Typically, atelectasis can be treated adequately with aggressive suctioning, bronchodilators, and chest percussion. If, however, these maneuvers are unsuccessful in re-expanding the collapsed lobe or segment, then therapeutic bronchoscopy should be used. Patients with spinal cord injuries or problems associated with inadequate pulmonary toilet may benefit from early bronchoscopy.[14] Refractory atelectasis has been treated with balloon occlusion and positive pressure ventilation through the lumen of the balloon catheter.[15] Development of the technique of wedging the bronchoscope into each segment or subsegment of the collapsed lung and insufflating the atelectatic alveoli with air after suctioning and lavage has resulted in a high rate of complete re-expansion.[16] In the trauma patient who sustains blunt chest injury, especially those with a rapid deceleration injury, one should entertain the possibility of tracheobronchial disruption. Even without signs or symptoms of airway injury, patients with fractures of the first three ribs or mediastinal injury should be considered for further evaluation, including bronchoscopy.

Massive hemoptysis, in which a patient loses several hundred milliliters of blood over 1 to 2 days, may require bronchoscopy to locate the site, control the rate of bleeding, and control the airway. For difficult-to-manage hemorrhage, balloon-tipped catheters passed through the bronchoscope may help to tamponade the bleeding.[14] Occasionally, massive and continuous bleeding cannot be managed with the fiberoptic bronchoscope. In this situation, a rigid bronchoscope may be helpful. In the future, the use of laser technology may eventually attain a place in hemorrhage management.

An increasing number of patients with pneumonias are being admitted to the ICU with a long list of etiologic possibilities. Therefore, to arrive at a more specific diagnosis, many physicians are performing diagnostic bronchoscopy with a protected specimen brush and bronchoalveolar lavage.[15] The major goal is to determine whether the process is infectious or noninfectious. Patients most likely to benefit are those who are immunosuppressed, are receiving ventilator support, have a progressive pneumonia not responding to therapy, or have necrotizing pneumonias.[14] Management of foreign body aspiration in adults is another major indication for the use of the fiberoptic bronchoscope, especially in patients with peripheral bronchial obstruction, patients on ventilators, and those whose neck is unstable from trauma.[17] It is important, however, that the value of rigid bronchoscopy lies in its speed, diversity of available complementary instruments, and control of the airway.[17] Along with the increased popularity of fiberoptic bronchoscopy comes a concomitant decrease in training and competence in rigid bronchoscopy. A convincing argument to stress the value of rigid bronchoscopy is that the foreign body removal success rate is 98% with rigid versus 60% with fiberoptic bronchoscopy.[17]

Other indications in the critical care setting include assessment of airway patency and evaluation of airway damage from an endotracheal or tracheostomy tube. Patients who are difficult to intubate, such as those with severe facial and neck burns, are best managed diagnostically and therapeutically with bronchoscopy. On rare occasions, lavage is used in patients who are failing aggressive therapies for status asthmaticus.[18]

The use of fiberoptic bronchoscopy also has a role in the management of a bronchopleural fistula (BPF). Direct visualization of the BPF or demonstration that occlusion of the fistula by the bronchoscope decreases or stops the leak are needed in the evaluation process.[19] Endobronchial occlusion can be accomplished with tissue glue, fibrin glue, gelfoam, lead plugs, balloon catheter, or an autologous blood patch.[19,20]

Diagnostic considerations also include transbronchial biopsy, bronchoalveolar lavage (BAL), and use of the protected brush catheter during bronchoscopy. Bronchoalveolar lavage has been promising in the diagnosis of infections in the immunocomprised patient. In Pneumocystis carinii, yields are close to 100%, although the addition of protected catheter brushings may or may not be more helpful than BAL alone.[15,21] For other patients, the specificity is lower. Lavage for malignancy, pulmonary hemorrhage, and drug reactions are about 40%; however, the low morbidity of the procedure still suggests some utility.[21] Because transbronchial biopsy is associated with bleeding and pneumothorax, the physician needs to decide if the diagnostic yield is worth the risk in a patient receiving mechanical ventilation. Early lavage alone is becoming the prominent diagnostic method in many ICU patients. If the risks are high or contraindications exist for bronchoscopy, then the patient should be evaluated for the risks and benefits of an open lung biopsy.

Contraindications

One of the most essential reasons to defer bronchoscopy in the critically ill individual is the inability to oxygenate the patient.[21,22] Under the best of circumstances, arterial oxygen tensions in an ICU patient can drop as much as 60 mm Hg.[21] Other contraindications include inexperienced personnel and worsening hypercarbia.[15] Patients with unstable asthma, unstable angina, lethal arrhythmias, a recent myocardial infarction, or increased intracranial pressure should be stabilized before bronchoscopy is attempted. Similarly, uncooperative or tachypneic patients are not candidates for this procedure.

Complications

The incidence of complications may vary between 0.08 and 10%.[15,23] Medications and local anesthesia in preparation for the procedure may cause respiratory depression, hypotension, laryngospasm, bronchospasm, seizures, or cardiopulmonary arrest.[23] To avoid these side effects, one must consider the age of the patient and their cardiovascular and hepatic function. For example, a patient who receives topical lidocaine may have higher than anticipated serum levels because of abnormal hepatic function.[23] Patients with asthma or bronchospastic disease are at high risk for severe airway compromise.

As mentioned previously, the procedure itself is associated with hypoxemia; therefore, the potential for arrhythmias is significant. Preoxygenation of patients before the examination may avoid or minimize the problem. Fever and aspiration pneumonia have also been reported.[23] Laryngospasm and bronchospasm may occur from both the procedure itself as well a medications given for preparation. With transbronchial biopsy, the potential for hemorrhage or pneumothorax is increased. To minimize the risk of hemorrhage, the platelet count should be greater than 50,000 L/μl.[14] Fluoroscopic guidance may lower the incidence of pneumothorax, and correcting coagulation abnormalities will help those who are predisposed to hemorrhagic complications.[15,23] For those patients with a protime of greater than 60% of control or a bleeding time greater than 15 seconds, the risk of hemorrhage may preclude elective bronchoscopy, especially if a biopsy is planned.[24] In patients who have a critical need for the procedure, the clinician should perform the bronchoscopy carefully and quickly and obtain only what is needed. Bronchoalveolar lavage poses a minimal risk in these individuals and should replace a transbronchial biopsy as the test of choice in these high risk patients.

Data Analysis

With the difficulty of distinguishing respiratory infection from colonization, quantitative bacterial cultures are valuable. Colony counts of 10^5 or greater are considered true pneumonias, whereas a colony count of no more than 10^3 has been interpreted as contamination.[21]

Quality Enhancement

Identification of high risk patients may minimize the occurrence of a complication. Patient cooperation is essential. Elderly and malnourished patients may be at increased risk for problems.[21] Patients who have a lung abscess are at risk for flooding the airway with infected material, and those with uremia are at risk for bleeding. Likewise, patients in the ICU frequently have uremia or thrombocytopenia; if the platelet count is less than 50,000/μl, the likelihood of bleeding increases and therefore biopsies should not be attempted. Individuals receiving mechanical ventilation and positive end expiratory pressure (PEEP) may be predisposed to pneumothorax. Finally, immunosuppressed patients have a higher likelihood of infection.

Preoxygenation with 100% oxygen and pulse oximetry may protect and alert the physician to episodes of hypoxemia during bronchoscopy. Additionally, complete sedation, especially in patients with adult respiratory distress syndrome (ARDS) or those who are fighting the ventilator, may minimize cardiopulmonary risk.[25]

Nonintubated patients who have marginal oxygenation or those with severe hypoxemia should be intubated electively before the procedure. Patients with hemoptysis or those undergoing a transbronchial biopsy should also be intubated. When placing an endotracheal tube, the tube should be at least an 8F to allow ample room for the bronchoscope. The patient should also receive 100% F_{IO_2} and low flow rates to minimize peak airway pressures. The physician should be aware that vigorous suctioning may allow the patient to lose up to 300 ml of tidal volume.[26]

CENTRAL VENOUS PRESSURE (CPT 36489)

In 1952, central venous access, gained by a subclavian venipuncture, was first described.[27] Shortly thereafter, Seldinger reported his percutaneous technique involving use of a guidewire for catheter placement. Of the several methods of insertion developed, the percutaneous puncture of the subclavian or of the internal jugular vein are the most popular. Currently, many physicians favor the internal jugular approach because of the lower risk for pneumothorax.[28]

Indications

With the advent of the pulmonary artery catheter, the use of central venous pressure (CVP) measurement for hemodynamic assessment is limited. Central venous pressures, however, especially if low, will confirm a clinical impression of hypovolemia. A major use of the CVP is for the administration of large volumes of fluid, especially when peripheral access is not obtainable or sufficient. Often in low flow states, the flotation of a pulmonary artery catheter is difficult; therefore, for rapid volume expansion, central venous access with a single or a multilumen catheter, a pulmonary artery catheter introducer, or a rapid infusion device will expedite fluid resuscitation. In addition to volume infusion, central access is often a means to obtain blood for laboratory tests. With the addition of a stopcock for withdrawal of blood, however, an additional entry site for infection is present. Central access also serves as an important route for certain medications that may cause phlebitis or tissue damage if extravasation occurs peripherally. The list of medications includes potassium chloride, dopamine, dobutamine, levarterenol, and hydrochloric acid infusion. Although central access may be the preferred route, good clinical judgment should prevail in those rare instances in which parenteral inotropes or vasopressors are needed emergently and central access is not obtainable or is too risky. Finally, central access is important for the infusion of total parenteral nutrition (TPN).

The cannulation of a central vein during cardiopulmonary resuscitation (CPR) should be limited to the experienced physician and the ease of access. The subclavian vein apparently is more accessible than the internal jugular vein during the performance of CPR and airway maintenance, although some clinicians may prefer the internal jugular route because of the uninterrupted and direct course into the right atrium. For situations in which a pacemaker wire is to be inserted, the latter approach may be more practical.

Contraindications

It would be difficult to establish absolute contraindications for the insertion of a central line. Therefore, it is best to define situations in which the clinician must be aware of potential problems. Patients with underlying lung disease such as interstitial fibrosis and chronic obstructive pulmonary disease (COPD) may not tolerate a pneumothorax; therefore, use of an insertion site with minimal risk should be entertained. Another consideration is to insert the catheter on the side of the chest that already has a chest tube, in which a pneumonectomy was performed or in which large pleural effusion or tumor mass may be present.

Patients with a coagulopathy are at risk for hemorrhagic complications, particularly those with underlying liver disease or uremia, and those receiving systemic anticoagulation. Caution must be exercised in patients with platelet counts below 50,000/μl if the CVP is considered a necessity. It is preferable to correct the underlying abnormality and to consider replacement of platelets if urgency is not a major concern. In those patients with liver disease, correction of the protime to 3 seconds above baseline would be helpful.[28]

Occasionally, patients have suspected or known venous thrombosis in the vessel to be cannulated. In this situation, selection of an alternative site is recommended. One should also avoid catheter insertion near areas of recent surgical intervention. Finally, catheterization of patients with a pacemaker or a Broviac, Hickman, or other catheter already in place should be done carefully and meticulously. In these patients, it is more important to be aware of the potential for dislodgement or knotting of the catheter.

Data Analysis

Before any catheter value is accepted, health-care personnel should always verify that the number is determined accurately. Checking the height of the transducer, the waveform, the catheter position, and calibration are imperative.

The major cause for a low CVP is hypovolemia. Searching for other causes should always include a review of medications that may cause venodilatation, such as nitrates, phentolamine, nitroprusside, prazosin, captopril, and nifedipine. Additionally, placement of the catheter in the pleural space may result in falsely low values.

On the other hand, patients in whom the CVP is elevated should be evaluated for the following:

- Right ventricular failure
- Increased venous return
- Pericardial tamponade
- Right ventricular infarct
- Positive pressure ventilation
- Pneumothorax
- Advanced COPD
- Severe bronchospasm

Right atrial waveforms may also be helpful if they demonstrate mechanical flutter wave or cannon waves. These pressure contours may aid in the diagnosis of atrial flutter, ventricular tachycardia, and supraventricular tachycardia.[29]

Complications and Management

Complications are best understood in the context of those that are local and those that are systemic.

Local Complications

Daily inspection of the catheter site for signs of infection, including erythema, induration, or purulence is mandatory. If these signs are noted, the catheter should be removed or exchanged over a guidewire followed by culture of the catheter tip and blood. Pain or extremity edema occurs on the same side as the catheter is suggestive of the development of phlebitis or thrombosis. Venography should be considered and the catheter should be removed. Bleeding and hematoma formation may occur in patients with abnormal coagulation studies. In those patients at risk, the use of an 18- or 20-gauge "search" needle is a good suggestion. Both the carotid and subclavian arteries are the more common vessels that are punctured inadvertently, and therefore, one should be alert to the formation of a hematoma. The health care team should also be cognizant of the potential of AV fistula or pseudoaneurysm development in catheterized vessels.

A sudden leak around an endotracheal tube or hemoptysis should alert the physician to the possibility of tracheal puncture or rupture of the endotracheal tube cuff. The endotracheal tube is changed carefully if the cuff is damaged and the patient has a significant loss of tidal volume.

Systemic Complications

One of the systemic complications seen most frequently is pneumothorax. The average occurrence for this complication in catheters inserted by the internal jugular or subclavian vein approach is 0 to 0.2% and 1 to 2%, respectively.[28]

Air embolism is a complication that may occur not only during insertion, but also during removal.[30] Clinical suspicion should arise when the patient suddenly develops dyspnea and respiratory distress during these times. Cardiac auscultation may reveal a coarse "mill wheel murmur" indicating air. The patient is placed immediately on the left side, in Trendelenburg position, and air is aspirated through the catheter.

Pericardial tamponade has been reported in association with almost every type of central venous catheter.[31] Strict guidelines, especially proper location of the distal tip in the proximal superior vena cava or distal innominate vein, should minimize this problem. If any patient with a central catheter should experience a sudden drop in blood pressure or sustain a cardiac arrest, immediate attention is directed to excluding catheter perforation and pericardial tamponade. Placement is also important to prevent migration into the inferior vena cava or hepatic vein.[7]

Fever often alerts the ICU team that catheter infection may be present. This diagnosis may be difficult to confirm, but, by definition, most catheter infections are diagnosed by culturing the same organism from both the blood and the catheter tip. Most infections are from skin flora; therefore, staphylococcus may be a leading but certainly is not the only offender. All fevers do not necessitate the removal of a catheter; however, if sepsis is clinically suspected, especially if supported by a positive culture, then the catheter should be removed. Peripheral access is then obtained, if possible, or a new site for central access is chosen. Areas of study that require further clarification and consensus are duration of catheter in one site and the role of the guidewire in changing a catheter to minimize infection.[32] Total agreement is still lacking as to whether duration of the catheter plays a significant role in catheter sepsis.[33] If a guidewire is used to remove an old and place a new catheter, the use of a semiquantitative culture of the catheter tip may elucidate if the catheter is a source of infection.[34] The concern for an extraordinarily high rate of sepsis in ICU patients with malignancies or AIDS has not always been substantiated.[35]

A topic of considerable discussion is whether triple-lumen catheters have a higher incidence of infection. Several major studies and our own experience support that this may not be the case and that the incidence of catheter-related sepsis in these patients is about 2%.[33]

Other complications associated with central venous catheters include carotid and subclavian artery puncture, catheter embolism, cerebrovascular accident, neurologic syndromes, and arrhythmias.[28,36]

Quality Enhancement

Measures to maintain low complication rates are directed at potential problems that might occur with significant frequency (Table 76-3). The development of infection is a serious potential problem; therefore, quality enhancement in this area should be directed toward prevention. Duration of catheter use is an area to observe closely. Catheters should be maintained only to aid in diagnostic efforts or for treatment purposes. When these criteria have been satisfied, the catheter should be removed.

Table 76-3. Quality Enhancement for Central Venous Catheters

Be aware of clinical signs of complications during both insertion as well as removal of the catheter
Verify position radiologically
Minimize risk of air embolus; the atrium should be lower than the insertion site
Exchange the old catheter by guidewire exchange if parenteral nutrition is to be instituted
Avoid sepsis
  Insert under asepsis
  Remove when the clinical goal is accomplished
  Consider removal if local signs of inflammation are present and the source of sepsis is unknown
  Use a percutaneous route
  Change tubing and dressings every 48 hours (dressing may require more frequent change if patient diaphoretic)
  Change the catheter if inserted on an emergency basis and asepsis was not maintained
  Guidewire exchange may be used for prolonged use and in diagnosing catheter-related infection
  Experienced personnel should insert or assist in insertion of catheter
  Minimize blood sampling and manipulation

Several studies have shown that duration directly increases the chance for systemic sepsis, but total agreement on this point has not been reached.[34] In fact, other factors such as number of hospital days prior to catheter insertion, underlying disease, immunologic status, and whether a patient is already septic may be just as important. Aseptic technique during insertion, dressing changes every 48 hours, and the use of iodophor ointment have had a favorable impact on rates of infection. Monitoring infection rates by the infection control department is a helpful quality enhancement mechanism. Additional important factors to avoid infection include the percutaneous method of insertion as opposed to cutdown, strict care of transducers and tubing, catheters inserted at sites distant from draining wounds, and supervision by experienced physicians. During emergency conditions, such as CPR, catheters inserted under less than ideal aseptic conditions should be changed as soon as possible. The clinician who decides to use TPN in a patient who has a central line in place should carefully change to a new catheter before the institution of TPN. The use of a subcutaneous cuff of biodegradable collagen and bactericidal silver (VitaCuff, Vitaphore Corp., San Carlos, CA) requires additional clinical trials to validate its importance in the prevention of sepsis.[33]

In preparing the patient for catheter insertion, it is important that the site of insertion is below the right atrium to minimize the occurrence of an air embolus. While using the guidewire or connecting intravenous tubing to a port, the port should not be exposed to air for any longer than the time needed for connection. These practices should minimize the occurrence of an air embolus, both during insertion and after removal of the catheter.

After securing the catheter, radiologic confirmation of proper placement is important. Working together with the radiologist adds a further safety mechanism by providing verification of appropriate placement. Steps to avoid placement of the catheter into the right atrium should minimize the potential for perforation.

Use of the central line to obtain blood cultures to diagnose catheter-related infection should only occur if peripheral access is not available, if quantitative cultures are performed, and the clinician knows exactly how the cultures are obtained.[33]

Critical care nursing skills have also helped to minimize complications (see Table 76-3). Foremost in nursing responsibility is the verification of catheter patency, which ensures that medications and fluids are being infused properly. Monitoring the patient's cardiopulmonary status postinsertion for subtle signs of hypoperfusion or respiratory embarrassment may be the first clues to a vascular tear or tension pneumothorax. Checking the catheter site for edema, hemorrhage, erythema, or purulence may alert the ICU team to local complications. Finally, dressing changes at least every 48 hours with a sterile occlusive dressing is also an important strategy for quality catheter care. Opinions vary concerning the use of transparent occlusive dressings and the reported enhancement of bacterial colonization compared to dry gauze dressings. This issue needs further elucidation.[33]

CHEST TUBES (CPT 32020)

Critically ill patients in need of mechanical ventilators, especially those with positive end expiratory pressure (PEEP), are at an increased risk for the development of a pneumothorax. Occasionally, patients develop a tension pneumothorax that requires the emergency insertion of a chest tube. The insertion and management of chest tubes, including small-catheter pleural aspiration tubes, should be included in the scope of practice for the critical care physician.[37]

Indications (Table 76–4)

Patients at risk for the development of a pneumothorax include mechanically ventilated patients who have high airway pressures, usually exceeding 60 cm H_2O. Patients who have central venous catheters, especially if insertion was by the subclavian approach, are also at risk for a pneumothorax.

Hemothorax, if it restricts the patient's ability to ventilate, should be an indication for a chest tube. Also, if large enough, a hemothorax may adversely affect hemodynamics by decreasing venous return. Clot in the pleural space may also predispose to a coagulopathy as fibrinolytic substances are released. If the patient remains unstable despite a chest tube, if 1500 to 2000 ml are immediately drained, or if drainage is greater than 100 ml/hour for a 6-hour period, one should consider a thoracotomy.[38] Other authors think that if bleeding exceeds 250 ml/hour for more than 2 hours, a thoracotomy is indicated.[39]

In all patients who sustain a penetrating chest injury, chest tube placement should be a serious consideration prophylactically if immediate surgery is required. This step should adequately avoid the chance of a tension pneumothorax that might occur during the operation.

Additional indications for chest tubes include empyema, chylothorax, and bronchopleural fistulas.[40]

Contraindications

For life-threatening needs, chest tubes are always inserted cautiously; however, extreme care must be observed in patients with coagulopathies and platelet defects.

Complications

More of a problem than a complication is failure of the lung to reexpand after insertion. Consideration for amelio-

Table 76–4. Chest Tube Indications

Pneumothorax: spontaneous and iatropgenic
Tension pneumothorax
Penetrating chest injuries, especially before nonthoracic surgery
Hemothorax
Empyema
Sclerotherapy for malignancy
Chylothorax
Post-thoracic surgery
Bronchopleural fistula
Recurrent pleural effusions
---

rating this difficulty should include the possibilities of inadequate tube location, less than satisfactory suction, a significant air leak, and causes unrelated to the tube itself, such as a mucous plug causing airway obstruction and atelectasis or pulmonary fibrosis. The difficulty of an air leak is often self-limited, but on occasion, it may be corrected by placement of an additional chest tube and removal of the old chest tube if it is nonfunctional.

Massive subcutaneous emphysema may be encountered and, in most cases, is mostly cosmetic and resolves spontaneously. Likewise, pneumomediastinum is often seen radiographically and may remain clinically insignificant. Both, however, are the result of barotrauma and may serve as a warning that continued or further increases in peak airway pressure may be fraught with hazard.

Pain after insertion accompanies chest tube placement, and it frequently does not subside with time. Therefore, adequate analgesia as well as intercostal nerve blocks are important to ensure patient comfort, thus allowing for adequate lung expansion.

Insertion of chest tubes always carries the potential for structural damage to the lung or even abdominal organs. Bleeding from a laceration of the lung and diaphragm can be troublesome. To minimize this risk, one might avoid the use of a trocar or insertion lower than the sixth rib laterally, where the incidence of organ damage may be higher than generally appreciated.[41]

Infection is always a potential problem. Therefore, strict aseptic techniques with dressing policies should be maintained.

Finally, unilateral pulmonary edema may suddenly occur because of the rapid removal of a large effusion or re-expansion of a pneumothorax.[40] Therefore, the recommendation of slowly draining fluid and limiting the total amount to no more than 1000 ml during the first 30 minutes may be preventative.

Quality Enhancement

In critically ill patients, the value of daily chest radiographs is important and is further substantiated by the need to verify the initial tube placement and whether the chest tube continues to function adequately. The need for daily radiographic assessment is justified because moving patients in bed for various purposes creates the potential for movement or dislodgment of the tube.

The decision to use antibiotics prophylactically is without total consensus. A realistic approach would consist of not including antibiotics in the nontrauma patient and practicing good aseptic technique in the ICU.

Some ICU patients require transport to other areas of the hospital for diagnostic tests. For patients with chest tubes, a serious risk is the occurrence of a simple or tension pneumothorax if the chest tube is clamped for transport. Therefore, the chest tube should be connected to underwater seal to prevent major compromise to the patient. Additionally, the use of pulse oximetry may provide an early indication of desaturation.

The decision to remove a chest tube is a clinical judgment that may find variation. If the drainage is less than 100 ml per day, most clinicians feel comfortable in removing the tube. Difficulty arises when the patient is receiving positive pressure ventilation. Because of the fear of recurrent pneumothorax, many of our patients have chest tubes until they are weaned off the ventilator. This sequence may present a problem because the pain from the tube impairs spontaneous tidal volume and cough, all of which may retard the weaning process as well as predispose the patient to infection.

Alternatives to chest tubes may include the use of minithoracostomy tubes and modified pigtail catheters. The minithoracostomy tube is well tolerated and is more comfortable to the patient.[42] Others have used redesigned vascular catheters to provide a simple, safe, effective, and less traumatic system in infants and children.[43] The use of these techniques in mechanically ventilated patients may be limited and therefore cannot be recommended for all patients.

Goals for nursing management of chest tubes include optimizing ventilation and oxygenation, prevention of complications, and evaluation of response to therapy. Careful inspection of the water seal system and the drainage collection device is important. Maintenance of patency entails that connection points are secured and the suction is functioning properly. Attention to bubbling in the water seal chamber is a priority, indicating the presence of an air leak in the system. If a padded Kelly clamp placed between the tube insertion site and the drainage system causes the bubbling to stop, the origin of the leak is within the patient's thorax or the eyelet port of the tube is too close to the exit site. If the leak continues despite clamping, the problem is with the connection or the system itself.

Milking or "stripping" of the chest tube is indicated only for thick drainage or suspected obstruction. Excessive negative pressure using stripping devices may traumatize healing pleural tissue.[44]

DEFIBRILLATION AND CARDIOVERSION (CPT 92960)

Factors that may adversely affect successful defibrillation and cardioversion must be corrected before these procedures are performed.[45] Metabolic alterations such as hypoxemia, acidemia, and hypoglycemia should be addressed. Also, delay in defibrillation should be avoided to maximize success of defibrillation. Because of this correlation, early defibrillation is being taught to all individuals trained in basic life support (BLS).

Automated external defibrillators (AEDs) are becoming a part of emergency medical personnel equipment.[46] Attention to these details will lead to optimal therapy of the sudden death patient or elective cardioversion of a hemodynamically unstable patient.

Indications

Use of unsynchronized defibrillation is warranted for unstable ventricular tachycardia and ventricular fibrillation, including asystole, which may masquerade as ventricular fibrillation.

Urgent synchronized cardioversion is suited for the patient who initially presents with stable ventricular tachycardia but who has failed medical therapy with either one or more antiarrhythmic medications. Patients with unstable tachycardia may also be best served with cardioversion as a first line of therapy. Critically ill patients with supraventricular tachyarrhythmias who are hemodynamically unstable, in pulmonary edema, or experiencing angina should be considered for immediate cardioversion. Recommended initial energy for atrial fibrillation is 200 J for the first and 360 J for the second shock.[47] The initial dose for supraventricular tachycardia should be 75 to 100 J, and the dose for ventricular tachycardia or atrial flutter is 50 J.[47]

Complications and Management

The problem of superficial burns from defibrillation can be avoided by providing an adequate interface between the paddles and skin. Treatment of the burns is accomplished by local therapy.

Unless defibrillation is repeated frequently at high levels, the CPK elevation is primarily skeletal muscle and the CK-MB fraction is normal. If ischemia is occurring, then CK-MB will likely be positive.[48] Other authors, however, have reported a positive CK-MB after countershock alone.[49]

Transient arrhythmias may occur after cardioversion. Cause for concern and caution should occur in patients with electrolyte abnormalities and high digitalis levels.[50]

Systemic embolization is a complication that appears to be limited to atrial fibrillation. The incidence of this problem has been reported to be 1 to 2%.[50] If the patient has had chronic atrial fibrillation for more than 2 days, cardioversion should be delayed until the patient has been adequately anticoagulated for at least 3 weeks.

Pulmonary edema and unexplained, prolonged hypotension are complications that are not common but may be encountered.[50,51] Possible mechanisms for the edema are a delay in return of left atrial function or a pulmonary embolism. The hypotension usually resolves without therapy.

In the presence of an oxygen-enriched environment, the potential exists for a fire during the defibrillation procedure.[52] Steps to minimize this risk are outlined in the following section.

Quality Enhancement

A few pertinent guidelines may enable defibrillation and cardioversion to remain a safe treatment method:

- Ensure routine maintenance by the biomedical department
- Check for signs of digitalis toxicity; use lidocaine before cardioversion if toxicity is suspected (50–100 mg)
- If patient has a pacemaker, keep paddles at least 5 inches apart
- Use adequate sedation and amnesia
- Use anterior-posterior paddle placement which optimizes energy conduction and safety

Anticoagulation guidelines were discussed previously. Unfortunately, aspirin and dipyridamole cannot serve as substitutes for warfarin.

Medical personnel should be made aware of the risk of

fire associated with defibrillation and cardioversion. Steps to minimize this occurrence include removing oxygen sources from the patient, applying defibrillator paddles firmly, applying adequate gel or conductive pads to prevent arcing, avoiding defibrillation if a gel or saline bridge connects the paddles, never placing the paddles on top of an ECG electrode, removing nitroglycerin patches or ointment, and if a gel is used, making sure that it is specifically manufactured for defibrillation.[52,53]

With the institution of AEDs, it is imperative that performance of the equipment, personnel, and effectiveness of the systems are reviewed.[45] The American Heart Association suggests establishing performance goals and a system to determine whether the goals are being met by reviewing individual patient case reports.[45]

DIALYSIS ACCESS (CPT 36145, 36800, 36810, 49420)

Hemodialysis

Access for hemodialysis has evolved from the surgically placed Scribner shunt to the percutaneously inserted Shaldon femoral vein catheter and, most recently, the double-lumen subclavian vein catheter. Dialysis can be started virtually within minutes after insertion and verification of the percutaneously inserted catheter position. The focus of this discussion is on the percutaneous catheter.

Indications

Institution of both hemodialysis as well as peritoneal dialysis includes decompensated pulmonary edema, uremia, severe acidosis, hyperkalemia, hypercalcemia, hyperuricemia, hypothermia, and uremic pericarditis. An additional group of patients that may benefit from hemoperfusion or hemodialysis are those patients who have intentionally ingested toxic amounts of medications or illicit drugs such as phenobarbital, glutethimide, methaqualone, salicylates, acetaminophen, theophylline, lithium, methanol, ethylene glycol, paraquat, phenothiazines, and tricyclic antidepressants.[54]

Contraindications

Two types of patients may not tolerate dialysis. The first major group comprises those who have sustained a recent acute myocardial infarction, especially if associated with hemodynamic instability. In these patients, if dialysis is needed, either peritoneal dialysis or continuous arteriovenous hemofiltration may cause less stress on cardiovascular status than hemodialysis. The second major group are those patients who suffer an intracranial hemorrhage. The use of heparin for the dialysis itself obviously is contraindicated in these patients.

Complications

Femoral Vein. This catheter is inserted into the femoral vein and may be associated with significant hemorrhage, hematomas (including retroperitoneal), and compartment syndromes. Therefore, if a patient has uremia-associated coagulopathy of clinical significance, this approach should be abandoned in favor of a procedure with less risk. A second major complication is thrombosis, which may extend from the femoral vein into the iliac vein. Ultimately, the thrombus could fragment and embolize to the pulmonary circulation. If the catheter is used for only several days as was the original purpose, this complication is seen rarely. Other complications that may occur are perforation of the cannulated vessel and the inferior vena cava. With prolonged use, infection is also a major contributor to morbidity and mortality.

Subclavian and Internal Jugular Vein. The complications associated with these sites are essentially the same as they are for any central venous catheter. Of particular importance and frequency is thrombosis of the superior vena cava and the subclavian vein. In one study, the incidence of thrombosis proven by venography was 23% and was related to duration of the catheter.[55] This complication may also occur months after removal of the catheter and consists mainly of painless swelling of the ipsilateral arm of the cannulated site.[56] Several patients have experienced painful arm edema if further dialysis access was obtained on the same side that a subclavian vein dialysis catheter had been inserted previously.[57] A new dacron cuffed hemodialysis catheter has been evaluated and found to be safe, reliable, low in complications, and with a longer life span.[58] With further use, we will be able to evaluate its acceptance as a primary catheter. Catheter-related septicemia occurs in association with between 2 and 20% or more of the dialysis catheters used.[59] The most common organisms are skin flora such as Staphylococcus aureus and epidermis.

Quality Enhancement

On the basis of the most potentially dangerous complications, care is needed when deciding both the type as well as the site for access. Coagulation abnormalities, if clinically apparent, may best be treated with the appropriate medical therapies, such as desmopressin or cryoprecipitate, before the insertion of a catheter. In certain circumstances, time may not allow this measure, and therefore the safest approach may be the best that can be offered.

Duration of catheter access raises the same questions discussed previously in regard to ways to curtail catheter-related sepsis. Measures to reduce the chances for sepsis include aseptic insertion technique, meticulous care of occlusive dressings, avoidance of infusing any solutions other than dialysate through the access, maintenance of the exit site with povidone-iodine soaks, and avoidance of replacing functioning catheters.[54] Of additional importance is not only sepsis, but also the risk of phlebitis and thrombosis. Subclavian vein thrombosis may occur in 20 to 50% of the patients.[59]

The potential for complications may involve multiple organ systems. Vigilance and communication among the nursing and physician team emphasizes the importance of collaborative practice. Daily assessment and aseptic technique at the site will invariably have a positive impact on the prevention of infection. Likewise, alterations in mental status from the disequilibrium syndrome in which the patient presents with confusion and obtundation necessitates continuous evaluation to assure patient safety. It is best to keep the bedside rails up and to have emergency airway equipment at bedside. Because ICU patients often have multiple sites with intravenous solutions, such as parenteral nutrition, antibiotics, and other medications, strict recording of intake and fluid removal cannot be stressed enough. In this realm of patient monitoring, communication of fluid balance, including preestablished goals, is imperative as a means to prevent fluid overload. Because most patients are already on monitors, close observation for arrhythmias, especially during dialysis, hopefully will prevent infrequent arrhythmias from deteriorating into a more lethal problem. For the ICU patient who already has access with either a shunt or AV fistula, the staff must be vigilant for disturbances in tissue perfusion. Assessment includes palpation of a thrill, auscultation of a bruit, and visualization of blood flow. Episodes of hypotension predispose toward compromising patency; therefore, close observation and evaluation may preclude loss of access. Assessment also includes those pulses distal to the access site, which will ensure the viability of the entire limb. Finally, knowledge and suspicion of an air embolism should be emphasized, because this problem may occur from disruption of the access device.

Peritoneal Dialysis

Insertion of a peritoneal catheter can be accomplished immediately at the bedside with a rigid stylet catheter, or the catheter can be inserted surgically with direct visualization. The method chosen is a function of clinical preference, skill, and availability of the surgical team.

Indications

The need for peritoneal dialysis is similar to that discussed in the preceding section on hemodialysis.

Contraindications

Unless the patient has had recent abdominal surgery or has had multiple adhesions produced from past operations, most patients can undergo peritoneal dialysis.

Complications

The three major complications are pericatheter leak, outflow failure, and infection. With the Tenckhoff double cuff catheter, the incidence of these three complications is 7%, 17% and 14%, respectively, within the first year.[54]

Leakage is manifest by fluid leaking at the exit site, edema, weight gain, and a decrease in outflow volume. Most often, leaks resolve spontaneously and are aided by alteration of the exchange program.[54]

If the amount of outflow is substantially less than inflow, the following approach may be helpful. Steps include checking for catheter kinking, improving bowel motility, adding heparin to the dialysate, infusing thrombolytics into the catheter, repositioning or replacing the catheter, and searching for and treating peritonitis.[54]

Bowel perforation is a dreaded complication that fortunately occurs with a low incidence.[60] Clinical manifestations include cloudy, malodorous dialysate, and watery diarrhea. Although surgical intervention is needed only occasionally, peritonitis may occur, associated with fever, abdominal pain, significant protein loss, and septic shock. Confirmation can occur if the dialysate has greater than 300 white cells per cubic millimeter, especially if the neutrophil count is high.[54] Antibiotic therapy usually is sufficient without removing the catheter; however, with Pseudomonas aeruginosa and Candida infections, many clinicians remove the catheter.[54,61]

Cardiovascular complications with peritoneal dialysis are usually related to a decrease in cardiac output as a result of an increase in intraabdominal pressure from the instillation of the dialysate or to hypovolemia from excess removal of fluids. The second cause can be corrected easily with a fluid challenge to reestablish a normovolemic state.

Often, ICU patients are also receiving mechanical ventilation, and therefore dialysis may actually restrict diaphragmatic movement and impede weaning.

Hyperglycemia is another problem that may occur with regularity because of the high glucose content of the dialysate. If hyperglycemia remains difficult to control, alternating the percentage of dextrose in the solution or even stopping the TPN may be helpful. Also, dextrose should be removed from all other infusions.

Finally, some patients may also experience cuff erosion through the skin, pain during dialysate inflow, and abdominal wall hernias from the procedure.[62]

INTRA-AORTIC BALLOON PUMP (PERCUTANEOUS, INSERTION) (CPT 33970)

The clinical use of intra-aortic balloon counterpulsation began with the work of Kantrowitz in 1968.[63] One of the basic principles in using the pump was to reduce myocardial work and, ultimately, ischemia. Physiologically, aortic pressure or afterload is reduced and cardiac output increases and preload decreases. During diastole, aortic diastolic pressure increases and coronary artery perfusion pressure also increases. Because of these important physiologic changes, it is anticipated that myocardial oxygen demand is diminished and oxygen supply is increased. Noncardiac effects are also noted and include an increase in cerebral blood flow and preservation of renal perfusion.

Indications

Use of the pump has increased since 1968, and several indications for balloon insertion are now standard, foremost of which is earlier insertion for refractory myocardial ischemia. Another common use is for patients with low cardiac output during or after cardiac surgery.[64] The balloon is also used for unstable angina in which optimal medical management has failed. In patients who sustain a myocardial infarction and subsequently develop cardiogenic shock or intractable heart failure, the pump may be useful in the event of little or no response to vasopressors and inotropes. Thus, unstable angina or shock in a patient who is in the catheterization laboratory can be stabilized rapidly with the use of the intra-aortic balloon pump (IABP). Similarly, patients who have had unsuccessful angioplasty associated with an abrupt closure of the artery can be maintained on the IABP until the time for emergent open heart surgery.[65]

Complications of an acute myocardial infarction associated with mechanical defects such as acute mitral regurgitation and ventricular septal defect may be responsive to early use of IABP.[66]

Preoperative use of the IABP in high risk patients, such as patients with left main coronary artery disease, critical triple vessel disease, and depressed ejection fraction undergoing both cardiac as well as noncardiac surgery, has been described.[67]

Other less common uses for counterpulsation have included refractory ventricular arrhythmias, cardiac arrest, and septic shock.[68] Less than consistent results in these categories prevents routine use of the balloon for these problems.

Patients who have the best chance for survival in whom the IABP is used include those with good left ventricular function prior to use of the balloon, those for whom insertion occurs early in the disease process, and individuals undergoing coronary revascularization or valve replacement.[69]

Contraindications

The major contraindications to its use include major occlusive vascular disease, such as aortic and iliac arterial occlusion. Aortic valvular regurgitation may be worsened and therefore counterpulsation should not be used. Likewise, patients with aortic dissection or an aortic aneurysm should not receive an intra-aortic balloon. Finally, in patients who have clinically significant thrombocytopenia or a bleeding diathesis, the clinician should weigh the risks in relation to the benefit, especially because anticoagulation will be required for this procedure.

Complications

The overall complication rate may be as low as 9%.[65] The more significant problems associated with the IABP include thrombosis, ischemia, hemorrhage, and sepsis of major arteries, such as in the mesenteric, renal, and spinal vascular distribution.[65] Strict and frequent attention to distal pulses will identify this problem early, when it is still reversible. Other complications include aortic dissection and perforation and limb ischemia from either thrombosis or embolization. Severe hemorrhage occurs in less than 5% of patients.[70] Hemolysis, platelet consumption, arterial embolism, and balloon rupture are rare.[70]

Data Analysis (Figs. 76–1 to 76–4)

The timing of balloon inflation is often achieved by use of the R wave of the ECG as the trigger.[71] Inflation occurs at the onset of diastole, the dicrotic notch of the arterial pressure curve. Reinflation occurs before the next systole. A therapeutic waveform has the following four qualities:

- The presence of an augmentation wave
- A V-shaped notch between the augmentation wave and the systolic wave immediately preceding it
- "Assisted systole" wave is lower than the unassisted one
- A presystolic dip or a difference of 5 to 15 mm Hg between the end diastolic pressure following an augmentation wave and the end diastolic pressure following an unaugmented wave

Once the balloon is properly placed, timing is established so that each pulse wave is augmented as the balloon inflates, establishing a 1 to 1 ratio. As the patient is being weaned, the order is reversed so that every other (1:2), then every third pulse (1:3), is augmented. Proper timing of the pressure waveform or ECG is imperative. If the balloon inflates too early or deflates too late, the ventricle will have to eject blood against a higher resistance and therefore cardiac output may drop significantly. Late inflation is also detrimental, because the timing of diastole is reduced, causing a decrease in coronary artery perfusion.

Quality Enhancement

Perhaps one of the more difficult decisions associated with the IABP involves the ethical dilemma of its use when chances for survival with and without it are poor. Honest discussion with the patient and family cannot be overemphasized. In cases that are complex or unclear, the hospital

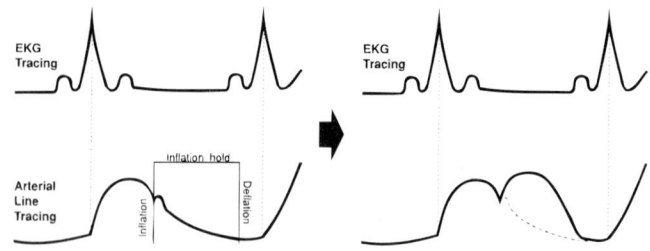

Fig. 76–1. Intra-aortic balloon pump timing mechanism and the resultant effect on the arterial wave. When a trigger is sensed, i.e. the R wave of the ECG, the mechanism is activated to suspend inflation until the onset of diastole (the dichrotic notch on the arterial waveform). The resulting waveform is illustrated on the right. (Drawn by: M.J. Fitzpatrick, courtesy of George Morrison, Clinical Dimensions, Inc., Madison, WI.)

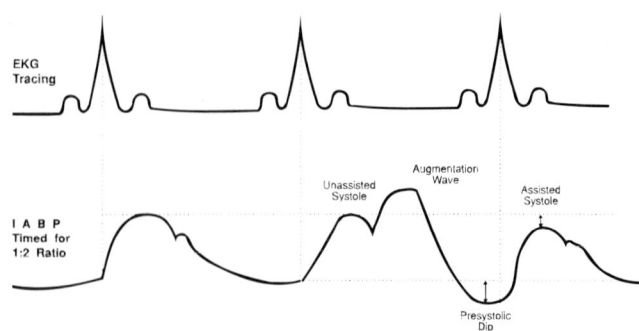

Fig. 76–2. Intra-aortic balloon pump in a 1:2 ratio. The systole preceding the augmentation wave is "unassisted," whereas the systole following it is "assisted." The presystolic dip is the calculated difference between the two end diastolic pressures. (Drawn by: M.J. Fitzpatrick, courtesy of George Morrison, Clinical Dimensions, Inc., Madison, WI.)

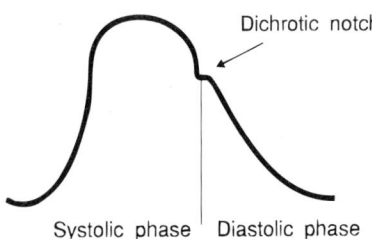

List: 1 Normal arterial wave.

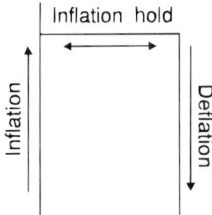

2 Timing Marker

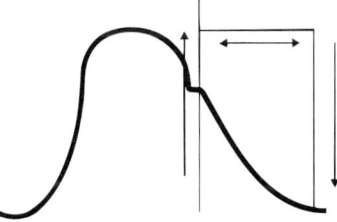

3 Timing marker super-imposed upon the arterial wave.

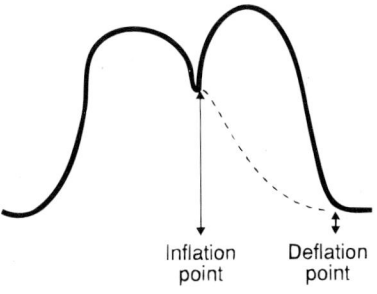

4 An augmentation wave is produced.

Fig. 76–3. Correct timing of the intra-aortic balloon pump. Note that the augmentation wave begins at the point of the dichrotic notch, at the beginning of diastole. This results in an increase in pressure along the aortic root, thus enhancing perfusion along the aortic arch and into the coronary arteries. By deflating immediately prior to the next systole, the pressure is reduced at the point of the aortic valve, creating a reduction in impedance to flow. Correct timing accomplishes: improvement in coronary artery perfusion to the myocardium; reduction of afterload and enhancement of cardiac output. (Drawn by: M.J. Fitzpatrick, courtesy of George Morrison, Clinical Dimensions, Inc., Madison, WI.)

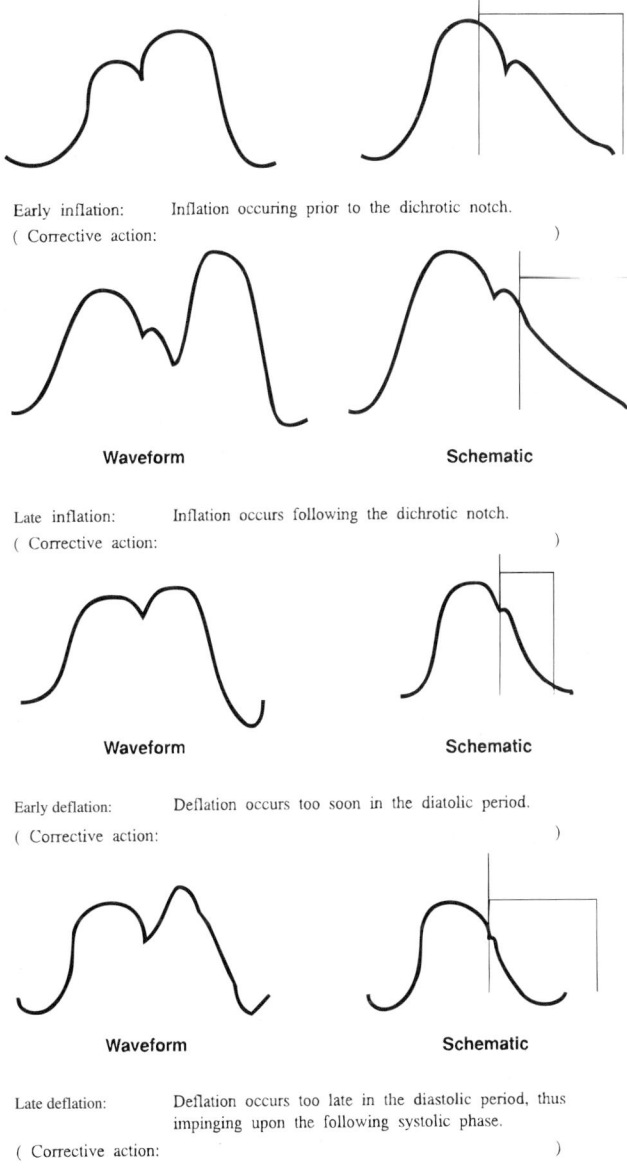

Fig. 76–4. Alterations in timing of the intra-aortic balloon pump (IABP). (Drawn by: M.J. Fitzpatrick, courtesy of George Morrison, Clinical Dimensions, Inc., Madison, WI.)

ethics committee may be an acceptable alternative for discussion.

It is essential to weigh the incidence of complications with the benefit in patients with severe peripheral vascular disease. In every patient, the monitoring of distal pulses should occur at least every 2 to 4 hours by palpation or Doppler measurement.[70] At the first sign of loss of pulse, the catheter should be removed. Anticoagulation with heparin will prevent arterial embolism and the potential for stroke and peripheral and visceral infarction.[70] Patients at high risk other than those with peripheral vascular disease include individuals with diabetes mellitus and hypertension.[70]

Timing the removal of the device has not been established. Some authors have suggested that in postoperative patients, 3 to 4 days are needed because the peak for a postoperative myocardial infarction occurs during this interval.[65] In the cardiac surgical patient, the balloon has been used until clinical hemodynamics reveal stabilization and improvement.

To assess the clinical status of a patient, such as the evaluation of heart, breath, and bowel sounds it is important to suspend the IABP. If the patient is unable to tolerate this maneuver hemodynamically, the evaluation must be deferred temporarily.

During weaning, the neurologic status is observed because it is often one of the first systems to fail. On the other hand, a decline of ectopy or control of tachyarrhythmias may reflect clinical improvement. The new onset of back pain may indicate diminishing renal flow and necessitate radiography to check for balloon placement.

To avoid change in catheter position, it is important to keep the involved extremity as straight as possible and to maintain the head at an angle no greater than 30°. Daily chest radiographs document correct position of the balloon.

The success of IABP use depends on the knowledge and experience of the team, including the nurse, perfusionist, and physicians. Technical support should be available in the hospital 24 hours a day.

INTRACRANIAL PRESSURE MONITORING (CPT 61107)

It has been about 30 years since the introduction of the bedside measurement of intracranial pressure (ICP) by ventriculostomy. The purpose of this method has been to maintain maximal cerebral perfusion and to alert medical personnel to the potential for cerebral herniation. Several types of monitoring devices are available. The first is the ventricular catheter, which is advantageous because high quality tracings are obtainable, access is available for withdrawal of cerebrospinal fluid (CSF), and it serves as a route for instillation of antibiotics. Also, the subarachnoid screw or bolt can be inserted quickly, has a low rate of infection, and is good for patients with distorted anatomy. Extradural devices also have a low infection rate but suffer technical problems such as drift.[72] A new fiberoptic device can be inserted into the ventricular system, brain parenchyma, or the subdural space providing safe, accurate, and reliable information.[73]

Indications

To justify whether the benefits outweigh the risks, one must determine whether the procedure will influence outcome. Those clinical situations in which ICP monitoring has been beneficial include closed head injuries, acute noncommunicating hydrocephalus, and Reye's syndrome.[72] Those who have sustained a head injury and have a Glasgow coma score of less than 8 need some means to assess their neurologic status, because the clinical evaluation may not be sensitive to subtle change. For those patients with an intracerebral hemorrhage, ICP monitoring may help to determine the severity of cerebral edema, mass effect, or even the need for surgery. Others may use ICP monitoring to assess the adequacy of decompression in a patient who had preoperative intracranial hypertension.[74]

Two specific indications for ICP measurement by ventriculostomy include hemorrhage and occlusion of CSF drainage or block. For the patient who sustains an intraventricular hemorrhage, vasospasm may be prevented by draining off CSF. Also, in cases of purulent meningitis or tumor in which a temporary blockage of CSF flow occurs, CSF can be drained to prevent hydrocephalus and intracranial hypertension.

For some conditions, case reports have supported the use of ICP techniques, but the question of whether it benefits all patients with the same disease is yet to be answered. Examples of these problems include patients with fulminant hepatic failure, near drowning, cardiac arrest, meningitis, encephalitis, tumor, and abscess.

Contraindications

Patients with a coagulopathy or significant thrombocytopenia should not undergo this procedure. For those patients who are immunosuppressed, one should be confident that the patient is at risk of dying or sustaining a major complication without it.

Complications and Management

A frequent and major complication is infection. The incidence varies from institution to institution and ranges from zero to as high as 25 to 100%.[75]

It appears that ventriculostomy catheters have a higher rate of infection compared to the subarachnoid bolt or epidural space. The major risk factor appears to be duration of monitoring. Infections rarely develop if the monitoring is confined to 4 days or less.[69] If meticulous care of the site is maintained and duration of the monitoring is limited, even the infection rate of ventricular catheters can be reduced to about 2%.[74] Although many physicians prescribe prophylactic antibiotic therapy, its impact on decreasing the incidence of sepsis is yet to be resolved.

A second but rare complication of monitoring is intracranial hemorrhage. Clinically, significant hemorrhage occurs in less than 1% of cases.[74]

In patients with an ICP cannula, one must be alert to the potential of system failure from occlusion.[74] This problem can be prevented by proper positioning and securing of the catheter. Ventricular collapse, another problem, may be minimized by restricting fluid withdrawal in patients with small ventricles.[74]

Data Analysis

The normal ICP is 5 to 10 mm Hg. When pressures begin to increase, a generally accepted upper limit of normal is 15 mm Hg. Cerebral perfusion pressure (CPP) is equal to the mean arterial pressure minus the ICP. Normally, the CPP is 80 to 90 mm Hg and it should be maintained above 60 mm Hg. As cerebral blood flow begins to decrease, poor perfusion occurs at 40 mm Hg and irreversible tissue hypoxia may occur at less than 30 mm Hg. Sudden rises in ICP to levels greater than 50 to 100 mm Hg may occur and are known as plateau waves. These waves may be

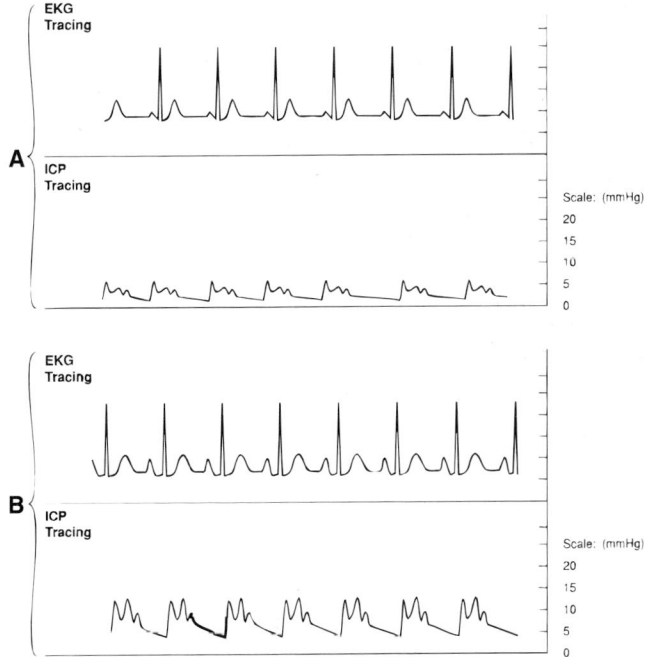

Fig. 76–5. Changes in intracranial pressure tracings to reflect an increase in the intracranial pressure (ICP) and a decrease in the intraventricular compliance. *A,* A normal tracing with the corresponding EKG. Note that p2 is less than (lower than) p1. *B,* p2 is higher than p1, indicating a decrease in compliance and an increase in mean ICP. (Drawn by: M.J. Fitzpatrick, courtesy of George Morrison, Clinical Dimensions, Inc., Madison, WI.)

provoked by hypercapnia or hypotension and therefore search for a correctable cause is warranted.

In addition to measurement of ICP, attention should also focus on compliance. In a brain with poor compliance, significantly smaller volume changes will cause elevations in ICP. As a result, tissue ischemia, hypoxemia, or herniation may occur.[76]

The three components of the ICP pulse wave are P_1 (percussion wave), P_2 (tidal wave), and P_3 (dicrotic wave)[76] (Fig. 76-5A). When P_2 reveals a progressive rise in relation to the other waves, the mean ICP is usually increasing and cerebral compliance is decreasing.[76] If this wave remains elevated despite treatment, a poor prognosis can be anticipated.[76]

Quality Enhancement

It is always best to weigh the benefits against the risks. By choosing the best site, selecting the best monitoring device, and limiting the duration, the risks are minimized.

The ICU staff should record pressure measurements in relation to the patient position. Likewise, trends, not isolated numbers, are reviewed. Results are interpreted in light of other variables, such as volume status and positive pressure mechanical ventilation.

Ways to minimize iatrogenic problems are as follows:

- Keep the head up at 30°
- Avoid the Trendelenburg position
- Do not flex the neck
- Use intravenous lidocaine prior to suctioning
- Avoid hypercapnia
- Try to avoid the use of intracranial blood volume expanders such as nitroglycerin and sodium nitroprusside[77]

Nursing policy must be developed to train the staff in the early recognition of pressure wave patterns. Measurement of ICP allows the team to institute therapy before a rise in ICP. For example, if the initial reading of P_2 is already high, attempts should be made to drain off fluid or to hyperventilate the patient.

For most patients requiring ICP measurements, an experienced physician should be available on site 24 hours a day. In hospitals without in-house physicians, using intraparenchymal and epidural fiberoptic devices may be the safest method.

INTUBATION (CPT 31500)

One of the most vital aspects of intensive care practice is airway management. The ICU team must be thoroughly conversant with lifesaving procedures to ensure a patent airway. The simple jaw thrust taught in all American Heart Association Advanced Cardiac Life Support (ACLS) CPR courses must be a learned reflex for ICU nurses and physicians. Additionally, a basic understanding of anatomy is imperative to minimize the risk of intubation to the patient.

Before any attempt at intubation, the proper equipment is assembled so that the procedure can occur rapidly and without interruption. One can always adequately ventilate and oxygenate a patient with an artificial airway in place and use of bag-valve resuscitation equipment.

Indications

Consensus has been reached concerning the major reasons in which intubation is needed.[78,79] The indications are maintenance of airway patency, protection from aspiration, help in clearing secretions, and mechanical ventilatory support.

Oral intubation offers the advantage of direct visualization and is quick. Often the critical care specialist may wish to inspect the upper airway for signs of obstruction or tissue damage. The oral route is also preferred in instances in which coagulation abnormalities exist or if the patient has nasopharyngeal deformities or trauma.

Nasal intubation may be preferred for the awake patient or for one who has a suspected cervical injury. Other advantages for its use include the awake agitated patient who may bite or clamp down on an oral endotracheal tube. The addition of an oral airway or bite block is possible, but it often adds to patient discomfort. With the tube out of the oral cavity, nursing care of the mouth and proper hygiene may be accomplished.

A major concern for the intensive care specialist is when and if the ICU patient should undergo tracheostomy. Ideal timing for a tracheostomy is a clinical decision made on the basis of a case-by-case analysis in conjunction with the expertise of those surgeons called on to perform the procedure. At a minimum, up to 2 weeks of intubation is generally acceptable.[80] Some general guidelines for tracheostomy indications include[79]:

- Minimizing further damage from translaryngeal intubation
- Improving suctioning and mouth care
- Allowing for patient mobility
- Enhancing the psychologic state
- Allowing for transfer to an intermediate care area
- Permitting speech by the use of a fenestrated or talking tracheostomy

At the same time, these advantages must be weighed against the complications and costs of the procedure. It would then seem reasonable that after about 2 to 3 weeks of intubation, one should raise the question of possibility and anticipated time to extubation and also the ultimate chances for recovery. If more than several days of further mechanical ventilatory support can be clearly established, tracheostomy should be seriously considered. For those patients who are hopelessly and terminally ill, the risks and cost are enough to postpone the tracheostomy.

Contraindications

Nasotracheal Intubation

It is prudent to avoid nasotracheal intubation in patients with coagulopathies. The risks of hemorrhage can be minimized by direct visualization and endotracheal intubation. The same rule applies for patients with anatomic defects that would preclude rapid and nontraumatic nasal intubations. This group would include patients with nasopharyngeal trauma or anatomic defects such as nasal polyps, nasal septal abnormalities, sinusitis, or CSF leaks.

Endotracheal Intubation

Movement of the head and neck in a patient with a suspected spinal cord injury may be best served by using the nasotracheal route, if no nasotracheal trauma has occurred, or even better, intubation over a fiberoptic bronchoscope in which the head may remain stationary. Similarly, in patients with severe degenerative cervical spine disorders, extreme care and possible bronchoscopically guided intubation to avoid dislocation of the odontoid process may be a reasonable alternative. For those patients with suspected severe epiglottis, intubation is best performed in a well-controlled environment, such as the operating room. In these patients, the need for emergency tracheostomy is rare; nevertheless, one should be prepared if the procedure is needed.

Complications and Management

Early Phase

If, during the procedure of intubation, hypoxemia is not corrected quickly, cardiac arrest and death may occur. Associated with a hypoxic event is cerebral anoxia and permanent neurologic damage. Preoxygenation of the patient and a good seal and adequate ventilation with a bag-valve resuscitation mask might decrease the risk of these complications.

Hasty and overly aggressive attempts at intubation may result in oropharyngeal, septal, or turbinate lacerations and broken teeth. Gentle pressure is the usual approach to avoid epistaxis and other damage that may require surgical correction. During the procedure itself, maintaining pressure on the trachea, the Sellick maneuver may prevent aspiration. In elderly patients, especially those with degenerative joint disease, spinal cord injury can be prevented by not flexing the neck too vigorously or perhaps using the nasotracheal site. Special attention is warranted for patients with a history of severe cervical spondylosis, with spinal cord or vertebral artery symptoms with movement. Also, patients with rheumatoid arthritis may have atlantoaxial subluxation.[81] Bronchospasm can be precipitated by an endotracheal tube by irritant receptor stimulation.[79] This problem may be attributed erroneously to either underlying pulmonary or even cardiac disease, and therefore proper diagnosis will avoid unnecessary therapy.

Late Phase

Some of the problems that may be encountered later in the course of a patient being supported by mechanical ventilation include obstruction of the tube itself, cuff leak, and self-extubation. By maintaining humidification and aseptic suctioning, chances for obstruction of the tube are minimized. Cuff leaks necessitate a changing of the tube. Self-extubation may occur despite arm restraints, secure taping of the tube, and sedation. To minimize dislodgement, these measures must be rechecked at frequent intervals and emergency airway equipment should be immediately available. Otitis media and sinusitis may occur and cause fever and signs of an occult infection.

Postextubation

One of the most serious clinical problems is tracheal stenosis, which may occur weeks to months after extubation. Anatomically, it appears that the larynx is the site of most of the major complications.[82] A clinical goal in all intubated patients is to minimize mucosal injury by keeping the cuff pressure below 25 mm Hg to ensure mucosal capillary blood flow. Duration and tube size may also have an impact on the rate of complications, although some studies have shown that duration has little impact on injury.[83] It is also important to realize the poor correlation between extent of laryngeal injury and its clinical correlate. Consequently, direct examination of the tissue by laryngoscopy at specified intervals is not helpful.[82] Symptoms of tracheal injury usually do not occur until the lumen diameter is about 5 mm or greater.[84]

Other complications, although rare, are tracheomalacia, posterior laryngeal abscess, laryngospasm, vocal cord paralysis, lip and tongue ulcers, and stomatitis.

Quality Enhancement (Table 76–5)

The duration of intubation remains controversial. At this time, meticulous attention is needed to minimize cuff pressures in an effort to avoid laryngeal injury. It has been

Table 76-5. Quality Enhancement for Intubation

Anticipate problems in the high risk patient
Familiarize all personnel with airway procedures
Check the airway equipment cart routinely
Ensure meticulous preparation for intubation
Choose proper tube size, for adequate management and least risk
Provide rigorous credentialling and supervision of physicians
Develop suctioning policies conjointly by physicians and nurses
Monitor infection control
Address the issue of self-extubation prevention in a unit policy
Base the duration of intubation on a case-by-case evaluation
Develop extubation procedures
Establish procedures for changing an airway tube that may minimize potential for problems
Practice universal precautions among the entire staff

suggested that women with diabetes mellitus are at particular risk for laryngeal complications.[85]

Measures should be developed to prevent self-extubation. The incidence is usually about 10 to 13%, which might serve as a threshold to maintain as an acceptable occurrence.[86] If the consequences associated with even brief extubation are respiratory arrest and subsequent death, consideration for a tracheostomy may be reasonable as an early intervention. Patients in this category may be those who are severely hypoxemic or PEEP dependent or those who have respiratory failure from neuromuscular disease or significant cardiovascular decompensation.

Because of the possibility of glottic incompetence after extubation, the patient should avoid oral intake for 24 hours to allow for improvement of this protective mechanism.[80]

Anticipation of the difficult airway may ultimately diminish the frequency of complications by at least allowing the ICU to prepare for a worst case scenario. Patients with the following criteria are at high risk for difficult airway management:

- Anatomic variations
- Congenital abnormalities
- Upper airway infections
- Tumors
- Postirradiation
- Head and neck trauma
- Degenerative joint disease
- Obesity
- Goiter
- Acromegaly
- Recent extubation

The ICU staff should consider emergency airway management as a procedure that must be accomplished with great facility and precision. Foremost in this process is maintaining a cart that contains all the necessary equipment. Just as the cardiac arrest or "code" cart is checked each shift, then so should the airway equipment cart.

Problem prevention includes preoxygenating the patient so they can withstand a brief interruption in oxygen supply during the actual intubation, and considering the use of lidocaine (1.5 mg/kg) if the patient may be adversely affected by a sudden increase in ICP.[87]

Several considerations are involved in choosing the size of an airway tube. Although smaller tubes cause less damage, they also increase airway resistance to gas flow and more cuff inflation may be required. Larger tubes, however, facilitate suctioning, can accommodate bronchoscopy, tend to be less obstructed by secretions, and allow for lower cuff pressures.[79]

Attending physicians fully conversant with critical care procedures should be available during intubation and extubation as well. It is important to emphasize that junior residents need at least a more experienced senior resident and, preferably an attending physician, before attempting to intubate. Requiring credentials for attending physicians in this as well as other ICU procedures is already occurring at many hospitals.

Suctioning policies should be developed conjointly by nursing and physician staff to determine indications, contraindications, and the appropriate handling of complications, as well as the need for premedication. A policy should also address those patients at risk for arrhythmias, bleeding, hypotension, and intracranial hypertension.

The ICU team, in conjunction with those concerned with infection control, need to monitor infections in patients receiving mechanical ventilation. This task also includes education of the staff to wear protective gloves and goggles for those patients who are risk to the ICU staff, such as patients with suspected or confirmed AIDS. Adaptation of universal precautions is a more realistic approach and improves safety to the staff.

Guidelines to address the issue of self-extubation are needed. This problem appears to be one that no one can totally eradicate, although everyone should strive for perfection.

Duration of intubation is a confusing issue. The timing of tracheostomy is an individual or case-by-case decision. Some direction should be sought as the patient reaches the end of the second to third week. For those patients with almost no chance for weaning, such as a patient with a high cervical spinal injury and quadriplegia, an earlier tracheostomy should be considered.

Elective extubation of the patient should be accompanied by a physical examination to ensure that stridor is not present and airway patency is confirmed. The patient should refrain from eating for at least 8 hours and perhaps up to 24 hours to prevent aspiration.[80]

For those patients requiring a change in their endotracheal tube, again the proper equipment is mandatory. If the potential for difficulty exists, a flexible fiberoptic bronchoscope should be at the bedside. A rigid endotracheal tube changer has been used, but its potential for injury and the fact that no visualization occurs are its limitations. A new device, the lighted stylet, is an alternative that may be an effective adjunct to intubation.[88]

LUMBAR PUNCTURE (CPT 62270)

The introduction of the lumbar puncture for clinical purposes occurred about 100 years ago. Controversy concerning its value has yielded conflicting data, including indications for its use. With the publication of two excellent consensus articles about the spinal tap, this established diagnostic procedure has been evaluated for its benefits, risks and costs.[89,90]

Indications

Four major indications for performing a lumbar puncture include (1) suspicion of central nervous system infection, (2) subarachnoid hemorrhage, (3) central nervous system malignancy, and (4) demyelinating disorders, such as multiple sclerosis and Guillain-Barré syndrome.

For certain diseases, other tests with a high degree of accuracy and safety may be used in place of a lumbar puncture. Among these disorders are cerebral abscess, systemic lupus erythematosus of the central nervous system, some primary brain tumors, solid metastatic tumors, subdural and epidural hematomas, a spinal epidural abscess, and dementia.[89,90]

Lumbar puncture may still have value in stroke patients for whom anticoagulation is considered. Also, in some patients who may have central nervous system hemorrhage after the CT was done, the lumbar puncture often provides the needed help in making this diagnosis.

Contraindications

The risk of cerebral herniation certainly exceeds the potential benefit if, on physical examination, the patient has papilledema or focal neurologic findings. The possibility of significant hemorrhage, pain, paresthesias, or hematomas exists if the patient has a coagulation disorder or severe thrombocytopenia. Therefore, the test should be deferred until after a full discussion of alternatives or if the benefit exceeds the risk. When in doubt, a CT scan of the head should rule out the presence of increased ICP of mass lesion.

Complications

One of the more frequent side effects encountered with a spinal tap is headache. By using a 20-gauge or smaller spinal needle and placing the patient prone after the procedure, these complications may be minimized.[90] Painful paresthesias occur in as many as 13% of the patients and may remain for as long as 1 year.[90] Although uncommon, the risk of meningitis is still a possibility. The potential always exists for cerebral herniation if ICP is elevated, although this occurrence has been reported to be less than 2%.[90] Finally, a spinal hematoma can be avoided by correction of coagulation abnormalities before embarking on this procedure.

Data Analysis

The analysis of spinal fluid can be obtained from most major medical textbooks (Table 76-6); however, certain laboratory values deserve emphasis.[84]

Bacterial. A leukocyte count of greater than 5 cells/mm approaches 100% sensitivity in most patients (Table 76-7); however, in patients with overwhelming Streptococcus pneumoniae or listeria meningitis, this may not occur.[90] Causes of CSF hypoglycemia may include subarachnoid hemorrhage as well as meningitis; therefore, a ratio of CSF to serum glucose of less than 0.31 suggests a bacterial cause.[90] Finally, lymphocytosis can occur in bacterial meningitis as well as in viral meningitis.

Fungal. Isolating fungal organisms from spinal fluid is difficult (see Table 76-7). To optimize the chances for recovery, at least a 5- to 10-ml, fluid-filled tube should be sent for culture. The sensitivity of the India ink smear for cryptococcus is only 26%, whereas that for the latex agglutination test for cryptococcal antigens is 58 to 90%.[90]

Table 76-6. Recommended Tests on Cerebrospinal Fluid

Routine
  Cell count (total and differential)
  Glucose level determination
When indicated
  Protein level determination
  Cell count on more than one tube
  VDRL test for syphilis
  Protein electrophoresis
  Assay for fungal antigens
  Cultures
    Bacteria
    Fungi
    Viruses
    Mycobacterium tuberculosis
  Stains
    Gram stain for bacteria
    Smear for acid-fast organisms
    Cytologic examination
Specialized (limit availability)
  Spectrophotometry (for pigment detection)
  Assay for bacterial antigens
  Assay for myelin basic protein

(From Marton, K. I., and Gean, A. D.: The spinal tap: A new look at an old test. Ann. Inter. Med., *104*:841, 1986.)

Table 76-7. Diseases Detected by the Spinal Tap*

High sensitivity, high specificity
  Bacterial meningitis
  Tuberculous meningitis
  Fungal meningitis
High sensitivity, moderate specificity
  Viral meningitis
  Subarachnoid hemorrhage
  Multiple sclerosis
  Central nervous system syphilis
  Infectious polyneuritis
  Paraspinal abscess
Moderate sensitivity, high specificity
  Meningeal malignancy
Moderate sensitivity, moderate specificity
  Intracranial hemorrhage
  Viral encephalitis
  Subdural hematoma

* Sensitivity, the ability of a test to detect disease when it is present; specificity, the ability of a test to exclude disease when it is not present. (From Health & Public Policy Committee: The diagnostic spinal tap. Ann. Intern. Med., *104*:881, 1986.)

Viral. Pleocytosis is primarily mononuclear, with normal glucose and normal to elevated protein levels. It is entirely possible that the initial predominant cell type is the polymorphonuclear cell, which may decrease in number with a subsequent puncture. Making the diagnosis of a viral process is difficult and the use of serum antibody titers for the large array of existent viruses is impractical and expensive (see Table 76-7). Future work in detecting viral glycoproteins may provide us more information.[89,90]

Subarachnoid Hemorrhage. Traumatic taps may occur in as many as 20% of the patients; therefore, it is important to distinguish trauma from underlying hemorrhage. Xanthochromia usually signifies central nervous system hemorrhage at least several hours old, but it may be seen in up to 32% of traumatic taps (see Table 76-7).[89,90] Similarly, the decrease in erythrocyte count from the first to last tube has a low specificity (56%) for traumatic tap; therefore, it is not always conclusive for that diagnosis.[90] A potentially useful test on the horizon includes spectrophotometry to test for blood pigment to enable a diagnosis of hemorrhage.[90] A second test is a cytologic examination for erythrophages, which would be negative with a traumatic tap.[90] At least for now, we continue to use clinical judgment along with nonspecific laboratory results.

Malignancy. Spinal fluid cytology often is not accurate; however, if the CSF is normal, malignancy can often be excluded. Patients with leukemia and lymphomas frequently have the highest yield for diagnosis of meningeal involvement of malignancy. Use of monoclonal antibodies may be helpful for increasing the diagnostic accuracy.[90]

Demyelinating Disease. Lumbar puncture itself cannot diagnose either Guillain-Barré syndrome or multiple sclerosis. An elevated IgG level and oligoclonal banding, however, are frequently but not exclusively seen in patients with multiple sclerosis. Likewise, a spinal fluid protein level of greater than 200 mg/dl without other abnormalities is suggestive of Guillain-Barré.

Quality Enhancement

With the slightest suspicion of intracranial hypertension, it is judicious to obtain a CT scan before a lumbar puncture. For situations in which an infectious process may exist, however, cautious puncture of the spinal canal with a 20-gauge or smaller needle may be required.

Attention should be directed toward patient comfort. Careful positioning of the patient is important, especially for elderly individuals who may have arthritic changes. As mentioned previously, placing the patient in a prone position after the procedure may lessen the risk for an ensuing headache.

Avoidance of sites that are near infected sources will help to control infection. This rule would apply especially to patients who may have chronic decubitus, burn patients, and those who have recently had an operative procedure in close proximity to the puncture site.

Cost of the procedure can be kept at a reasonable level by ordering only those tests that are applicable and have a high enough sensitivity and specificity to justify the cost.

For patients in whom subarachnoid hemorrhage is clinically suspected, the lumbar puncture is still an accurate test in light of a negative CT scan.

Again, we emphasize the need to protect the patient with thrombocytopenia or other coagulation abnormalities or those receiving anticoagulants from the risk of this procedure. Also, patients who have just completed dialysis and received heparin should have the procedure postponed for several hours. Good clinical judgment concerning the benefit-to-risk ratio as well as the use of the appropriate blood products must be a priority in the decision-making process.

TEMPORARY PACING (CPT 33210)

Temporary pacing in the critically ill patient can be accomplished by several approaches. The transvenous method is achieved through accessing the internal jugular, subclavian, basilic, or femoral vein. Skill and use of fluoroscopy often are required. Pulmonary artery catheters have been developed that have a right ventricular port so that a pacing wire can be inserted quickly. Transcutaneous temporary pacing is achievable and can be used appropriately and safely in the prehospital care setting as well as in the hospital. Transthoracic pacing has been used in the past for cardiac arrests, but it is associated with significant complications. Epicardial wires often are placed at the time of cardiac surgery and provide for a safe and immediate means for pacing. Transesophageal pacing is also a well-tolerated approach, but it is not frequently recommended for emergency situations.

Temporary cardiac pacing in the ICU setting requires both the clinical knowledge of when pacing is indicated as well as the technical skills of insertion. Because several safer and quicker alternatives are available, transthoracic pacing is used rarely.

Transcutaneous pacing has gained in popularity because of the ease of use and the noninvasive mode of function.[91] It serves well in the prehospital setting, the emergency department, and the critical care unit. It is an excellent device to have at the bedside for a patient who has a preexisting left bundle branch block and is to have a pulmonary artery catheter inserted. If a complete heart block develops, pacing capabilities can then be instituted rapidly. Postoperative cardiac surgical patients have epicardial wires that are available for hemodynamically significant bradyarrhythmias, complete atrioventricular block, or tachyarrhythmias, such as atrial flutter, that may respond to overdrive pacing. Many ICU patients have a pulmonary artery catheter; therefore, our policy is to use a pulmonary artery catheter that has a right ventricular lumen allowing for access to insert a pacing wire. Use of this type of catheter obviates the need for inserting a special pacing introducer or transporting the patient to a fluoroscopy suite.[91]

Indications

The major settings in which a critically ill patient may require a pacemaker include patients with an acute myocardial infarction and patients with bradyarrhythmias and tachyarrhythmias that have the potential for adversely affecting the hemodynamic state. For a comprehensive list of

Table 76-8. Temporary Cardiac Pacing Indications[88,92]

Acute Myocardial Infarction—Prophylactic and Therapeutic
Hemodynamically significant bradyarrhythmias (associated angina, hypotension, or heart failure)
    Sinus bradycardia, sinoatrial block, and sinus arrest unresponsive to pharmacologic therapy
    Wide complex QRS escape rhythm
    Idioventricular rhythm
Asystole
Complete atrioventricular (AV) block and wide complex QRS
New onset type II second-degree AV block
Alternating right and left bundle branch block (RBBB, LBBB)
New onset bifascicular block
    RBBB + left atrial hemibloc
    RBBB + left posterior hemibloc
Bifascicular block (new or old) with new prolongation of P-R interval
Bradyarrhythmias
Sinus node depression caused by the following drugs needed by the patient:
    Digitalis
    Antiarrhythmic agents (i.e., quinidine)
    Beta blocking agents
    Calcium antagonists (i.e., verapamil/diltiazem)
    Certain antihypertensives
Atrial fibrillation with AV node disease causing a ventricular rate of less than 45 beats per minute
Pulmonary artery catheterization in a patient with LBBB
Symptomatic clinical problems (with bradycardia and/or syncope):
    Sick sinus syndrome
    Carotid sinus hypersensitivity
    Cough
    Pharyngeal, esophageal, or gastric manipulation or distention
    Increased intracranial pressure
Tachyarrhythmias
Reentry tachycardias
    Sinus
    Intra-AV nodal
    Atrial
    WPW
Bradycardia, dependent ventricular tachycardia
    Ischemia
    Infarction
    Acquired long QT, especially from type 1 antiarrhythmics, hypokalemia, hypomagnesemia
Atrial flutter (**not** atrial fibrillation)
    Most effective if flutter rate is 230 to 350
Recurrent or refractory ventricular tachycardia
Miscellaneous
Emergency use if a permanent pacemaker fails

(Adapted from Escher, D. T.: Use of cardiac pacemakers. Hosp. Pract., 16:49, 1981; Silver, M. D., and Goldschlager, N.: Temporary transvenous cardiac pacing in the critical care setting. Chest, 93:607, 1988.)

potential indications in the critical care setting, see Table 76-8.

Contraindications

Because of the increasing popularity of transcutaneous pacing, it is important to mention that this method should be avoided in patients with suspected cervical spine injury or flail chest.[91] Although these problems are the only contraindications, it is important to realize that in other clinical situations, such as a dilated cardiomyopathy, obesity, hyperinflated lungs, pleural or pericardial effusions, or poor electrode application to the skin, transcutaneous pacing may be ineffective.[91] Patients who develop significant bradycardia in the setting of hypothermia should not be paced.[92]

Complications and Management of Transvenous Pacemakers

A brief overview of the complications is best served by reviewing three major areas in which problems occur (Table 76-9): during the insertion process, the pacemaker system itself, and direct cardiac problems.

Because complications associated with insertion are similar to the insertion of central venous catheters, the reader is referred to the section on central catheters.

Major problems with the pacemaker system include failure to pace, loss of pacing artifact, oversensing, and failure to sense (Fig. 76-6).[93,94] Of these problems, both lead displacement and failure to sense appear to be the more common system complications occurring 25 to 40% of the time.[95] Failure to sense can be treated by repositioning the pacing wire.[94,95] Oversensing, in which the pacer is inhibited by other signals such as a T wave, can be treated by decreasing the sensitivity of the pulse generator. Noncapture can be approached by increasing the output of the pacemaker or repositioning the wire.

Direct cardiac problems include arrhythmias, perforation, and tamponade. The tachyarrhythmias usually resolve on their own or with a cough. If no resolution occurs, the catheter position is assessed. Myocardial perforation should be suspected if the patient suddenly develops the pain of pericarditis or shoulder pain, he or she has a pericardial rub, a change in paced QRS configuration is noted, and the pacer fails to pace or sense.[94] The incidence of cardiac tamponade is about 1%, and it may occur as long as 24 hours after the pacing wire or catheter is removed. Therefore, sudden hypotension in this setting should raise

Table 76-9. Potential Complications of Temporary Transvenous Cardiac Pacing*

Complication	Incidence (%)
During Insertion	
Pneumothorax	1
Arterial trauma (carotid or subclavian artery)	1 to 2
Air embolism	1
Venous complications	
Phlebitis	1 to 5
Thrombosis	10
Embolism	1
Bacteremia	1 to 50†
Cardiac complications	
Myocardial perforation or penetration	2 to 30‡
Pericarditis	5
Cardiac tamponade	1
Catheter-induced arrhythmias	2 to 11
Transient right bundle branch block	1
Lead dislodgment	27

* Mortality associated with temporary transvenous pacing is less than 1%.
† Incidence of bacteremia rises significantly with time after catheter insertion and may be as high as 35 to 50% after the third day. Therefore, a sterile technique during insertion and meticulous local skin care after insertion are mandatory.
‡ Incidence varies with the method used to diagnose its presence.

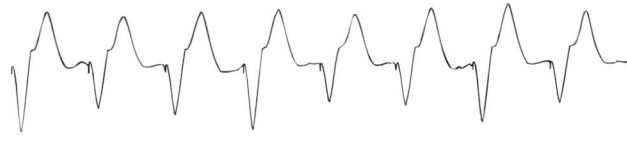

A. Noncapture

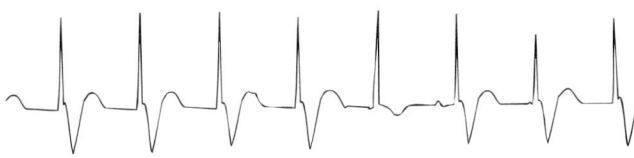

B. Undersensing

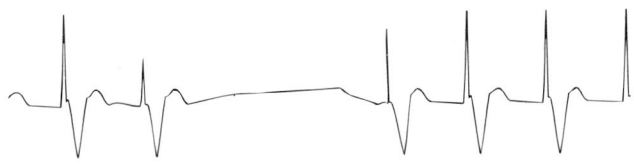

C. Oversensing

Fig. 76–6. *A,* Noncapture. Pacemaker fails to depolarize because of lead displacement, increased threshold, low battery, or electrolyte imbalance. *B,* Undersensing. Pacemaker fails to sense a spontaneous depolarization because of lead displacement, asynchronous setting, battery depletion, or a broken lead. *C,* Oversensing. Pacemaker sees another sequel and causes a pacing interval that is prolonged. Causes include magnetic interference, broken lead, incorrect setting of the sensitivity, or sensing P or T waves. (Drawn by: M.J. Fitzpatrick, courtesy of George Morrison, Clinical Dimensions, Inc., Madison, WI.)

the suspicion of tamponade.[93,94] Hypotension may also be the result of the pacemaker syndrome in which patients also develop a low cardiac output state, congestive heart failure, neurologic symptoms, and arrhythmias.[96] This syndrome is seen most often in patients with implanted ventricular pacemakers and is treated by slowing the ventricular rate to permit the native rhythm to dominate or by providing A + V sequential pacing.[96]

Additional complications of transvenous pacing include those associated with obtaining any central line: pneumothorax, arterial trauma, air embolism, phlebitis, thrombosis, embolization, and sepsis.[93] Most complications have an incidence of about 1% with the exception of sepsis; if the catheter is left in place for longer than 4 days, the occurrence is closer to 35 to 50%.[93] Finally, although rare, the runaway pacemaker seen with permanent pacers may also occur in patients with temporary pacemakers.[97]

Quality Enhancement

The ICU nursing and physician staff should be oriented and conversant with insertion and maintenance of pacemakers. The pacemaker itself should be checked preferably each shift or at least daily to ensure that battery and overall function is optimal. Information about the following should be documented in the patient's chart:

- All connections are checked for tightness of fit and electrical isolation.
- Postinsertion electrocardiography and chest radiography are important for verification.
- Daily assessment should include inspection of the skin and entry site, daily ECG or rhythm strip, and chest radiography.
- Evaluation should include inspecting the amplitude of the sensed signal and the myocardial stimulation threshold.[94]

Duration of a pacemaker should be discussed routinely, including when and if a permanent pacemaker is needed. Antibiotic prophylaxis usually is not indicated for temporary transvenous pacemakers.[91]

Pacemaker insertion should be done with extreme care in patients with a coagulopathy or thrombocytopenia. Choice of access site with the least risk should be a priority.

ABDOMINAL PARACENTESIS (CPT 49080)

Indications

The paracentesis is a procedure used for both diagnostic and therapeutic purposes. The trauma patient who suffers from blunt or even a penetrating abdominal or chest injury may require a diagnostic peritoneal lavage. Often the patient is obtunded as a result of a head injury, alcohol, or drugs. Consequently, the diagnostic lavage may be the only method to secure an expedient diagnosis. Patients in the ICU setting may have an "acute abdomen" from an infection, pancreatitis, ruptured viscus, or vascular catastrophe, and their instability may preclude their transport for diagnostic tests. These patients may benefit from bedside paracentesis. If positive, appropriate therapy, including an exploratory laparotomy, may be urgently undertaken. The patient with severe acute pancreatitis often has a relentless process that may progress to death. In an attempt to improve survival, therapeutic peritoneal lavage has been used, although results are often conflicting.[98,99]

The use of paracentesis in patients with alcoholic liver disease and ascites has been the source of much discussion. Until now, the mainstay of therapy has been bedrest, diuretics, and sodium restriction. Large volume (up to 5 liters) paracentesis with albumen infusion has been found to be safe and effective in the alcoholic population.[100,101] Patients with tense ascites are ideal candidates for paracentesis, especially if the ascites may be impairing adequate respiratory excursions and causing failure to wean from mechanical ventilation. In rare instances, paracentesis has substantially improved cardiac output to allow for the titration of pressor therapy.[102]

Contraindications and Risks

Essentially, most contraindications may be considered as relative rather than absolute. Foremost is the uncooperative patient who may inadvertently predispose themselves to a complication. Sedation, if appropriate, might be indicated. A coagulopathy should be corrected before the procedure, especially in the alcoholic patient. Extreme care

Table 76-10. Paracentesis Data

Transudate (Protein <2.5 g/dl)	Exudate (Protein >2.5 g/dl)
Cirrhosis	Carcinomatosis
Congestive heart failure	Chylous ascites
Hepatocellular carcinoma	Congestive heart failure
Nephrotic syndrome	Hepatic vein thrombus
Spontaneous bacterial peritonitis	Myxedema
	Pancreatitis
	Secondary bacterial peritonitis

Leukocytes		
WBC >500 mm³	WBC <500 mm³	Variable WBC
Bacterial tuberculosis	Chylous	Carcinomatosis
	Hepatic thrombosis	Cirrhosis
	Hepatocellular carcinoma	Congestive heart failure
	Myxedema	Pancreatitis
	Nephrotic syndrome	

is needed for the patient who has had abdominal surgery who truly needs this procedure. Likewise, if the patient is suspected of having a bowel obstruction, alternative tests should be considered. Hepatic echinococcal or a giant ovarian cyst may appear like ascites but should not be tapped.[103] If a patient has an abdominal wall infection or gravid uterus, the paracentesis should also be avoided.

Data Analysis (Table 76-10)

The routine laboratory tests that are ordered should be based on clinical suspicion. Most physicians consider the following as essential: leukocyte count and differential, glucose, total fluid and serum protein and LDH, gram stain and culture, pH, and cytology. Special tests for specific diagnosis include triglycerides for chyle, CEA and alpha-fetoprotein for malignancy, amylase for pancreatitis, and lactate or pH (less than 7.31) for suspected infection.

The ratio of protein in the ascitic fluid to that in serum can be found to be less than 0.5 to 1.0 in uncompensated cirrhosis. If the ratio is greater than 1.0, a search for infection, cancer, or pancreatitis may be in order.

Complications and Management

The incidence of complications is rare, about 3%, and they usually do not present as a major clinical problem.[103] For example, a bowel perforation usually seals quickly and peritonitis is extremely rare. Pneumoperitoneum occurs more frequently, but the hospital course is rarely affected. Dissection of air may appear in the scrotum or labial area and is best avoided by using a small needle for the procedure. Hemorrhage may occur and is one of the more frequent complications in the alcoholic population. It is imperative to correct any coagulation abnormality, thus minimizing the chance for peritoneal hemorrhage. Similarly, by emptying the bladder before surgery, one will avoid a bladder puncture.

Hypotension may occur if the volume removed is excessive and it is done too quickly. More of a nuisance is persistent leakage of ascites after the procedure. Again, prevention is best achieved by using a Z track method and removing only the needed amount of fluid.

Quality Enhancement

To minimize risks and complications, the procedure is performed only in the well-evaluated patient and at the appropriate site. Coagulation studies are checked before the procedure is performed. If the platelet count is less than 50,000/µl or the prothrombin time is greater than 5 seconds above control, replacement therapy is considered.[103] Complications that develop are addressed immediately. To avoid infection, aseptic technique is an absolute requirement. For the potentially difficult and high risk patient, either a minilaparoscopy or a bedside abdominal sonogram is helpful.[103]

PERICARDIOCENTESIS (CPT 33010)

The pericardial space may be composed of serum-like fluid, up to 50 ml, without clinical or echocardiographic changes. When the amount of pericardial fluid causes hemodynamic abnormalities such as low cardiac output and hypotension, a clinical diagnosis suggests the diastolic abnormality known as pericardial tamponade.

Indications

Because pericardial tamponade is a process necessitating urgent therapy, one cannot question the need once the diagnosis is made, but rather the method by which fluid is drained. When a patient in the proper clinical setting acutely develops hypotension, respiratory distress, and circulatory compromise, needle pericardiocentesis by the experienced physician is indicated. When urgency is not the principal factor, surgical open drainage is preferred. Under these circumstances, a safe and more effective drainage may occur. An additional benefit of surgical drainage is the option of obtaining a pericardial biopsy. Conditions for which open drainage will most likely be of benefit include constrictive pericarditis, infection, and trauma. Surgery in the trauma patient often is heeded when clotted blood cannot be aspirated effectively.

Contraindications

As an emergency procedure for a life-threatening condition, there are no contraindications. Extreme care should be observed at all times, especially in the setting of a coagulopathy.

Data Analysis and Interpretation

Normal pericardial fluid is clear and pale yellow. Fluid should undergo analysis for protein, amylase, glucose, cholesterol, hematocrit, white cell count, culture (including aerobic and anaerobic bacteria, tuberculosis, and fungi), and cytology.[104,105] Interpretation of data is similar to that for pleural fluid. Some clinical correlates in analyzing the pericardial fluid include: considering tuberculosis as a cause for tamponade in a dialysis patient and rupture or dissection of an aortic aneurysm when a large hemorrhagic effusion is obtained; when all diagnostic tests on the fluid are negative in a patient with AIDS, biopsy may reveal Kaposi's sarcoma.[106-108]

Successful pericardiocentesis is clinically documented by a decrease in elevated right atrial pressure, disappearance of pulsus paradoxus, improved blood pressure, improvement in cardiac output, and increased urine output.[104] Unsuccessful attempts may occur in traumatic hemopericardium because of the quick accumulation of blood after aspiration, the absence of an anterior effusion, or the presence of a loculated effusion or clotted blood.[104]

If the aspirated blood is from the cardiac chamber, ST segment elevation should occur and the blood should clot. A sample of blood from the cardiac chamber should spread out homogeneously on filter paper as opposed to pericardial blood, which may separate into a central deep red area and a less bloody peripheral halo.[109] Unlike blood from the cardiac chamber, pericardial blood may not clot.

Complications of Needle Pericardiocentesis

One major complication is laceration of the heart or coronary artery, which may cause tamponade when the pericardiocentesis needle is withdrawn. Other complications that occur include infection, arrhythmia, cardiac arrest, pneumothorax, and rarely, acute pulmonary edema.[110]

Quality Enhancement

Only experienced physicians should attempt pericardiocentesis for relief of the unstable patient with pericardial tamponade. The procedure is then associated with only a 0 to 5% risk of a life-threatening complication.[104]

Echocardiography may be helpful diagnostically as well as therapeutically, although in some postcardiac surgical patients, the patient may have a hemodynamically significant effusion without substantial echocardiographic changes. Therefore, the diagnosis of tamponade is primarily a clinical decision with the support of an echocardiogram and hemodynamic data from a pulmonary artery catheter.

To maintain perfusion in the patient with tamponade, one should consider volume resuscitation while preparing and performing the pericardiocentesis. This maneuver may help to stabilize the patient. At the same time, it is best to avoid the indiscriminate use of vasodilators and to minimize positive pressure ventilation if possible. Coagulation abnormalities are corrected and anticoagulants are discontinued if pericardiocentesis is to be attempted.

It is important to remember that failure to obtain fluid from a pericardiocentesis does not rule out an effusion, especially if the index of suspicion is high. Also, in any critically ill patient with a central venous catheter or pulmonary artery catheter who becomes hypotensive, tamponade from the catheter should always be considered in the differential diagnosis.

Patients should be closely observed for 24 hours after a pericardiocentesis in case of recurrence.[104]

PULMONARY ARTERY CATHETER (CPT 93503)

Bedside use of the pulmonary artery catheter for assessment of cardiac function was introduced in 1970.[111] A double-lumen catheter was used. Today, a triple-lumen pulmonary artery catheter is used for measurement of cardiac output and access for a pacing wire. At the same time, placement of this catheter through an introducer adds a fourth port for venous access.

The technology itself has stimulated such controversy that some authors have labeled its use "cultism" and have asked for a moratorium on its use.[112] Most clinicians who deal with critically ill patients realize its value in the context of complex patients and have adapted a less radical philosophy. One of the more important aspects of evaluating the catheter's use is to establish its clinical predictive value. In several studies, a significant number of inaccuracies in clinically predicting cardiac output and pulmonary artery wedge pressure have been documented.[113] It is therefore possible to have patients with a low cardiac index without clinical signs of hypoperfusion. Likewise, difficulty may exist in the bedside diagnostic distinction between cardiogenic and noncardiogenic pulmonary edema. The pulmonary artery catheter is of value diagnostically and therapeutically in the following critical situations:[114,115] acute myocardial infarction, chronic heart failure, septic shock, acute pulmonary edema, and high risk surgical patients.

Despite continued use of the pulmonary artery catheter in disease states such as ARDS and septic shock, we have not been able to affect the ultimate mortality rates associated with either disease process. If we maintain that the use of this procedure is to facilitate monitoring and response to therapy as our priority, then perhaps we can understand its true value in the proper context.

Indications

Pulmonary artery catheter placement is indicated for the following:

- Volume assessment
- Differential diagnosis of (cardiac versus noncardiac) pulmonary edema
- Diagnosis of ventricular septal defect (VSD), acute mitral regurgitation, and pericardial tamponade
- Assessing the effects of mechanical ventilation and PEEP
- Assessing the effects of therapies on hemodynamics (cardiac output, oxygen delivery, and oxygen consumption)
- Assessing high risk surgical patients
- Guiding fluid therapy in neurosurgical patients
- Monitoring high risk pregnant patients

One of the most common uses for a pulmonary artery catheter is in the assessment of the intravascular volume status in critically ill patients. Caution is imperative in patients with a poor left ventricle because compliance problems may interfere with the interpretation of volume assessment. In these patients, a seemingly high pressure may be acceptable for that patient's ventricular function. Distinguishing cardiac from noncardiac causes of pulmonary edema may be aided by the initial pulmonary artery occlusion pressure measurement. A pressure of less than 18 mm Hg may suggest a noncardiac cause. The staff should always check to see if the measurement is before or after a diuretic is given, because diuresis influences the value. Complications of an acute myocardial infarction, such as VSD, acute mitral regurgitation, and pericardial tamponade may be diagnosed at the bedside with the pulmonary artery catheter. Both mitral regurgitation and VSD are capable of producing V waves, as can the mechanical movement of the catheter produce pseudo-V waves. Assessment of hemodynamics (oxygen transport) and shunt (Qs/Qt) is helpful in assessing the therapies of patients receiving mechanical ventilation, particularly as levels of PEEP are increased. The effects of medications, especially vasopressor and inotropic agents, are measured by changes in the hemodynamic parameters of patients in septic shock, and after coronary artery bypass surgery. High risk surgical patients with prior medical problems as well as those undergoing major operations such as an abdominal aneurysm resection may benefit from both preoperative as well as intraoperative hemodynamic monitoring. Patients who are most likely to benefit from this type of monitoring are those who have incipient heart failure that may not be clinically obvious or those who have received chronic diuretic use and are mildly intravascularly depleted. Neurosurgeons have relied on capillary wedge pressures to ensure volume repletion in patients who suffer subarachnoid hemorrhage in an attempt to minimize the dreaded complication of vasospasm.[116] Finally, the critically ill pregnant patient with preeclampsia may be managed best with a minute-to-minute appreciation of hemodynamic response to the disease and its therapy. Although these indications are the more common, the practitioner may also use a pulmonary artery catheter on the basis of other clinical needs.[117]

Contraindications

Because the high risk patient is often the one who receives a pulmonary artery catheter, it would be more reasonable to advise caution in its use rather than list contraindications. Those conditions that increase the risk of the procedure include severe coagulopathy, in which risk may outweigh benefit, particularly if the site chosen is the suclavian vein, an area in which bleeding cannot be controlled easily by compression. Irritability of the myocardium must always be considered potentially dangerous; therefore, in patients with myocarditis or electrolyte abnormalities, extreme care, preparation, and modification of correctable abnormalities should occur before and during catheter insertion.

Complications and Management

Major and frequent complications include arrhythmias, pneumothorax, pulmonary artery rupture (Fig. 76-7) or infarction, and venous thrombosis.

Major complications often are addressed in terms of problems associated with the actual insertion and those occurring during use of the catheter. The process of insertion must be followed carefully to avoid lethal dysrhythmias or a pneumothorax. Most arrhythmias are not serious and the incidence of ventricular arrhythmias is usually less than 3% of those who are catheterized.[114] One of the re-

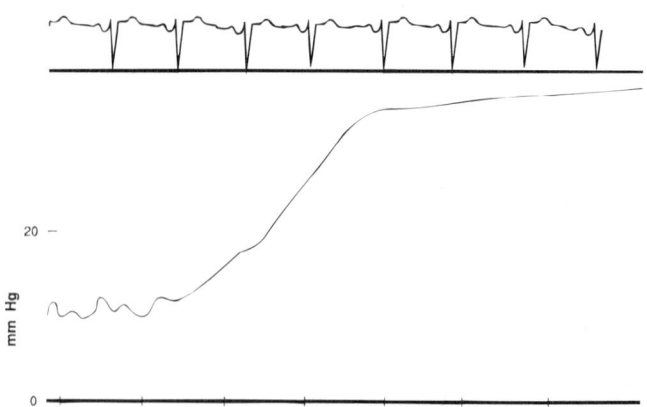

Fig. 76-7. Swan-Ganz tracing depicting overwedging or the migration of the catheter into a distal branch of the pulmonary artery that is too narrow for accurate pressure determination. Notice the abrupt plateau of the waveforms. (Drawn by: M.J. Fitzpatrick, courtesy of George Morrison, Clinical Dimensions, Inc., Madison, WI.)

ported concerns of placing a pulmonary artery catheter in a patient with a preexisting left bundle branch block (LBBB) has been the development of a right bundle branch block (RBBB) and ultimately complete heart block. Several studies have revealed an incidence of 0 to 5% as a more realistic estimate.[118] Many of the new catheters have a right ventricular port into which a pacing wire can be introduced quickly should complete heart block occur. Correction of metabolic, electrolyte, and oxygenation abnormalities may decrease this problem.

With the use of the internal jugular vein approach, pneumothorax may occur in less than 1% of patients. This statistic compares favorably with the potential of pneumothorax in 6% of patients with a subclavian vein site.[114] Once the catheter is inserted, physicians and nurses must be cognizant of additional complications. An inconvenience requiring the insertion of a new catheter may occur when the balloon ruptures as a result of frequent inflations and prolonged use.[114] Another concern is thrombosis that occurs soon after insertion of the catheter, but usually is asymptomatic.[119]

The sudden onset of hemoptysis is a life-threatening emergency that may be caused by pulmonary artery rupture or infarction. Those persons at risk for rupture include patients with pulmonary artery hypertension or hypothermia, patients receiving anticoagulants, and individuals who have undergone cardiopulmonary bypass.[118] To prevent this potentially lethal occurrence, overwedging overinflation, and overutilization should be avoided, especially in high risk patients. Should rupture occur, the following steps may be helpful:

- If the patient is receiving anticoagulation, attempt to reverse it.
- Use the catheter for embolization.
- Consider using a double-lumen endobronchial tube to protect the airway.
- Increase levels of PEEP to reduce or stop hemorrhage.
- Consider emergency thoracic surgery.[118]

The problem of catheter-associated sepsis is actually associated with an incidence of 2% or less in most ICUs.[118] Defining sepsis usually includes the documentation of the same organism isolated both from the blood and the catheter tip using semiquantitative cultures. Removing or replacing the catheter at the first suggestion of unexplained fever or sepsis is a most prudent approach only after all other possible sources have been eliminated. A variable that may affect the incidence of infection is the time the catheter is in place. Several studies have determined that after 72 hours, the incidence of infection increases.[118] One should accept this fact with caution, because debate remains as to whether this is accurate or whether duration is the only important factor to affect risk. Duration may be important, but one must also weigh the risks of inserting a catheter at a new site. Changing a catheter over a guidewire at the same site is currently used and is receiving further evaluation. Guidewire exchange and culturing the tip of the old catheter is a reasonable approach to the patient who is in need of a catheter for vascular access. If the culture proves to be positive, the catheter should then be removed and a new access site found. For the clinician, it is most important to remove the catheter when it no longer can provide help in making diagnostic or therapeutic decisions.

Additional complications include knotting, kinking, hematoma formation, aberrant position, right atrial penetration, cerebral air embolism during removal, and other less frequent problems.[118,120]

Future Use

To predict future directions for the use of pulmonary artery technology would be no less than a guess. Catheters used for oximetry provide real-time monitoring, which is an optimal goal for assessing ICU patients. Continued evaluation of its use to determine if the catheter affects decision-making and the cost of patient care, however, are vexing questions that need to be answered.[121] Specific questions include: Will the cost be offset by other tests being eliminated? Can we institute therapy sooner based on the achieved data? Will following its data trends warn of impending problems? How accurate will the oximeters remain over time? Will this technology impact morbidity and mortality?

In the continuing stages of clinical assessment and need is a catheter that allows measurement of the right ventricular ejection fraction.[122] Also, the combined use of pulse arterial oximetry and pulmonary artery oximetry, known as dual oximetry, has been studied.[123,124] Future clinical trials may help to determine new directions with pulmonary artery catheterization.

Data Analysis (Table 76–11)

To ensure optimal interpretation of hemodynamic data, simultaneous recording of the pulmonary artery catheter pressures and the electrocardiogram is needed. There are, however, limitations in data acquisition. Significant tachycardia may cause distortion in the quality of waveform acquisition and hence interpretation. In most cases, A, C, and V waveforms and the X and Y descent are more prominent using right atrial rather than pulmonary artery waveforms,[125] because of the dampened transmission of left atrial mechanics to the distal lumen of the catheter. Atrial waveforms may help in arrhythmia clarification, such as with atrial flutter. The presence of irregular cannon waves may suggest ventricular tachycardia and thus is helpful in those patients in whom it is difficult to distinguish a ventricular from a supraventricular focus.[125] Response of the mean right atrial pressure or CVP to inspiration will help in the diagnosis of tamponade. Analysis of V waves from the pulmonary artery may suggest acute mitral regurgitation or VSD, whereas V waves from the right atrial port suggest tricuspid regurgitation. A narrow pulmonary artery pulse pressure, especially when the mean right atrial pressure equals or exceeds the mean wedge pressure, suggests severe right ventricular infarct.[125] At the first sign of dampening, the clinician should immediately suspect migration of the catheter and take corrective action by pulling the catheter back.

The clinical diagnosis of an acute pulmonary embolus is often difficult. Pulmonary hypertension is seen in about

Table 76–11. Data Analysis: Pulmonary Artery Catheter Waveforms

Disorder	Interpretation
Arrhythmia	Flutter waves (300/min) confirms atrial flutter
	Regular cannon A waves may aid in diagnosis of supraventricular tachycardia
	Irregular cannon A waves suggest ventricular tachycardia
	Intermittent cannon A waves with a pacemaker suggests pacemaker syndrome when arterial blood pressure fluctuates
Acute mitral insufficiency	Large V waves
	PAEDP < PAOP
Acute tricuspid insufficiency	Right atrial V wave
	Steep Y descent
	Increased RA pressure
Acute ventricular septal defect	Pulmonary-to-systemic flow ratio >2:1
	Increased oxygen saturation ≥10% between RA and PA pressures
	V wave
	Increase RA, PA, PAOP pressures
	True systemic cardiac output is one quarter to one half of thermodilution
Right ventricular infarct	RA pressure ≥PAOP
	Y descent exceeds X descent
	Kussmauls sign (increase RA pressure with inspiration)
	Narrow PA pulse pressure
Acute pulmonary embolus	Increase in PA pressure
	Increase in RA pressure when PA pressure exceeds 35 mm Hg
	PAEDP > PAOP
	No A or V waves
Acute pericardial tamponade	Decrease in RA pressure with inspiration (opposite occurs with right ventricular infarct and constrictive pericarditis)
	Dominant X descent
	No Y descent

RA, right atrial; PA, pulmonary artery; PAOP, pulmonary artery occlusive pressure; PAEDP, pulmonary artery end-diastolic pressure.
(Adapted from Sharkey, S. W.: Beyond the wedge: Clinical physiology and the Swan-Ganz catheter. Am. J. Med., *83*:111, 1987.)

70% of the patients and usually occurs when obstruction involves 30% or more of the pulmonary vasculature.[125] With an acute embolus, the mean pulmonary artery pressure rarely exceeds 40 mm Hg; therefore, when the pressure is higher than 40 mm Hg, it may imply chronic or recurrent embolism.[125]

Because many critically ill patients are assisted by mechanical ventilators, data must take into account the effects of positive pressure on the numbers attained. At times, mechanical ventilation causes direct pressure transmission to the heart and blood vasculature. Additionally, it alters pulmonary blood flow. The classic three zones defined by West establish the relationship of lung perfusion as it is affected by pulmonary arterial, pulmonary venous, and alveolar pressures (Fig. 76-8) (see Chaps. 16 and 77). When alveolar pressure exceeds both arterial and venous pressures (zone 1), there is no perfusion. In contrast, when both arterial and venous pressures exceed alveolar pressure (zone 3), the arterial pressure gradient determines the degree of lung perfusion. Because of the forces of gravity and blood flow, most pulmonary artery catheters do flow to zone 3, which is the location in which a pulmonary artery occluded pressure approximates the pulmonary venous pressure. If the possibility that this situation may not be occurring is of clinical concern, a lateral chest radiograph will help to confirm. Suspicion should arise when a or v waves are no longer present and there is significant baseline variation of the pulmonary artery occluded pressure tracing with ventilation.[126] The clinician should also consider the effects of PEEP as it exceeds the alveolar and arterial pressure. This situation may convert zone 2 into a zone 1, especially in those patients who are hypovolemic. The clinician must then ask whether the pulmonary artery occluded pressure truly reflects the pulmonary venous pressure.

The pulmonary artery catheter is also used for the bedside diagnosis of pulmonary embolism. Since 1975, balloon occlusion pulmonary angiography has been used in critical care units.[127] Interpretation of data from this procedure must be cautious because PEEP levels of greater than 15 cm of water can artifactually decrease pulmonary artery caliber.[127]

Table 76-12. Pulmonary Artery Catheter: Quality Enhancement

Identify patient at risk for complications
Correct reversible risk factors
Verify catheter position (chest radiogaph and wave pattern analysis)
Verify accuracy of data
Establish sepsis precaution guidelines
Preparation for dealing with complications
Ensure adequate supervision/credentialing
Determine when to discontinue catheter

Quality Enhancement (Table 76-12)

The use of invasive vascular procedures necessitates the establishment of a standard whereby all practitioners in each ICU have guidelines to ensure patient safety. Issues such as catheter duration, site of insertion, and prevention of sepsis have been discussed and should be part of that quality enhancement program. Verification of catheter placement and correct "wedging" is important and can be accomplished by chest radiography, wave pattern assessment, obtaining mixed venous blood gases with the balloon inflated, or observing the "arterialization" of the digital display of an oximetry equipped pulmonary artery catheter. Data analysis often provides information for clinical decision-making; therefore, verification of accurate measurements is important. The physician must always work closely with the nursing staff to ensure accuracy of waveforms, digital values, transducers, and cardiac output analysis. By simply tapping the catheter with a finger and observing the monitor screen before insertion, one can efficiently test all connections and waveform response. Dampening, a common problem, is easily avoided by verifying that the stopcock is open, the pressure bag is adequately filled, and the catheter lumen is free of clot. A major priority of the nursing professional should be validating the accuracy of waveform interpretation. A checklist for each catheter insertion should answer the following questions:

- Is the waveform quality good?
- What effect is respiration playing on the waveform?
- Is the correct scale being used for continuous monitoring?
- Is patient position consistent for every measurement?
- Is the transducer consistently calibrated and zeroed at the phlebostatic axis?
- Is air in the transducer dome?
- Is blood backing into the transducer?
- Is patient data such as age, weight, and height accurate?

Confirming the items on this list hopefully will allow for safe and uninterrupted hemodynamic monitoring.

Although pulmonary artery catheterization generally is safe, certain types of patients may be at risk for complications. Close attention and extra care should be observed

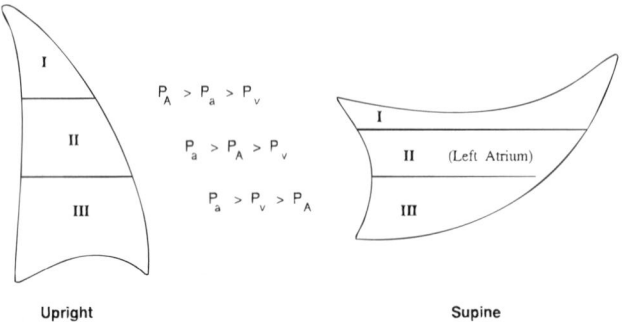

Fig. 76-8. The three zones of the lung revealing the relationships between alveolar pressure (PA), pulmonary arterial pressure (Pa), and pulmonary venous pressure (Pv). Mechanical ventilation may impact PA, causing spurious reading of the pulmonary artery occluded pressure (see text). (Drawn by: M.J. Fitzpatrick, courtesy of George Morrison, Clinical Dimensions, Inc., Madison, WI.)

if the following concurrent problems exist: hypoxia, acidosis, hypokalemia, hypomagnesemia, digitalis toxicity, left bundle branch block, fever, neutropenia, recent or recurrent ventricular tachycardia, a pacemaker in place, and predisposition for myocardial irritability, as might occur in patients with a myocarditis or cardiomyopathy. For those patients who are unstable, it may be wise to insert an arterial line before inserting the pulmonary artery catheter, enabling completion of the catheter insertion without interruption to assess vital signs. For patients with a preexistent left bundle branch block, we attach a transcutaneous pacing electrode before insertion of the catheter to be prepared in case complete heart block develops.

A frequent oversight in many discussions concerning use of the pulmonary artery catheter involves where the procedure occurs and who will supervise. Major considerations in deciding where to place the catheter should include equipment needed, sterility, and competence and familiarity of both the nursing and medical staff. The pulmonary artery catheter plays a role in the management of critically ill patients, but it is rarely considered a life or death intervention. Therefore, it is best inserted in the operating suite and critical care unit, the most likely areas in which personnel can best manage this procedure.

As to who should insert the catheter is a matter that needs to be determined at each institution. The procedure itself is usually not technically difficult, but it does require skill, experience, and the ability to intervene quickly and efficiently should a problem arise. For physicians in training, this procedure most importantly deserves an experienced physician in attendance.

Finally, the clinician should assess daily whether the catheter continues to provide needed information. When all goals have been met, it is time to consider removal of the catheter.

THORACENTESIS (CPT 32000)

Pleural effusions are a common finding in ICU patients. They may present radiographically as diffuse haziness with fluid collections at basilar, interlobar, or subpulmonic locations. Sometimes, the amount or distribution of the effusion is difficult to estimate with portable chest radiography; therefore, if this information is critical to patient management, a chest CT scan may be helpful.[128,129]

Indications

In the ICU patient with a suspected pneumonia or sepsis, the potential for pleural space infection is always a concern. Therefore, diagnostically, a thoracentesis may be indicated. Trauma patients with an effusion must always be considered for a hemothorax. Failure to provide adequate drainage in these patients may predispose them to infection and the potential for developing a fibrothorax.

The patient who may be difficult to wean with a significant unilateral effusion or bilateral effusions may need drainage. The clinical dilemma occurs when the patient is receiving mechanical ventilation, especially with PEEP. At this juncture, a clinical decision must weigh the benefit of fluid drainage and less restriction of ventilation against the risk of a pneumothorax if thoracentesis is attempted. Recurrent effusions should be approached by inserting a chest tube.

Contraindications

For those patients receiving anticoagulants, with a coagulopathy, or thrombocytopenia, only life-threatening effusions should be drained by thoracentesis. The decision to perform a thoracentesis while a patient is mechanically ventilated, especially with PEEP, is not without risk. As stated previously, clinical judgment helps to determine if the risk far exceeds the potential yield.

Data Analysis

Evaluation of the sample itself is important so that the distinction between hemorrhage, transudate, and exudate will help to determine its etiology. Hemorrhagic effusions are seen with pulmonary infarctions, tuberculosis, neoplasm, pulmonary embolism, trauma, cirrhosis, and heart failure.

The data supporting an exudate include an LDH greater than 200 units, a protein value greater than 3 g, an LDH ratio (pleural to serum) greater than 0.6, and a protein ratio (pleural to serum) greater than 0.5. The major etiologies of an exudative effusion include, but are not limited to infections, neoplasia, collagen vascular disease, and drug exposure (Table 76-13).

The pH of the pleural sample may help diagnostically. The normal pH is 7.40. When the pH begins to drop, tuberculosis, malignancy, empyema, rheumatoid arthritis, or collagen vascular disease should be considered. A lower pH should entertain the possibility of an esophageal rupture and requires urgent treatment. An elevated amylase level may point to esophageal rupture or pancreatic disease. If the pH is at 7.20 or less, and especially if the glucose is low, a chest tube is required to treat a suspected empyema.

Measurement of both serum and pleural glucose levels is helpful. A low glucose value may be seen with bacterial infections and tuberculosis as well as with rheumatoid arthritis. Gram stain and culture, especially anaerobic culture, are essential. Cytology also may reveal either a lung carcinoma or distant metastasis. Finally, cell counts may be helpful in the diagnosis of infections, leukemias, tuberculosis, and lymphomas (see Table 76-13).

Complications and Management

The incidence of complications, both minor and major, has been reported to be as high as 46%.[130] Major complications include pneumothorax, laceration of the lung and spleen, hemorrhage, reexpansion pulmonary edema, shearing of the catheter, and hypotension. Minor complications include pain, cough, subcutaneous emphysema, and a dry tap.[130] Some of the morbidity associated with the procedure may be attributed to poor technique, inability to identify landmarks, and improper use of the equipment.[123]

Steps in the management of these complications include a chest tube if the pneumothorax was 50% or greater or if the patient was receiving mechanical ventilation. Lacerations are best managed by blood replacement, unless the

Table 76-13. Diagnostic Characteristics of Pleural Fluid

Disorder	Transudate (T) or Exudate (E)	Appearance	Predominant Cell Type	Glucose (mg/100 ml)	pH	LDH (PF:S)*	Protein (PF:S)*	Amylase (PF:S)*
Pulmonary embolism								
Atelectasis	T	Serous	Mononuclear	>60	≥7.30	<0.6	<0.5	≤1
Ischemia/necrosis	E	Serosanguineous	Polymorphonuclear	>60	≥7.30	>0.6	>0.5	≤1
Congestive heart failure	T	Serous	Lymphocytes: mesothelial	>60	>7.40	<0.6	<0.5	≤1
Cirrhosis	T	Serous	Lymphocytes	>60	>7.40	<0.6	<0.5	≤1
Pneumonia	E	Turbid	Polymorphonuclear	>60	≥7.30	>0.6	>0.5	≤1
Empyema	E	Purulent	Polymorphonuclear	<60 (0–59)	<7.30 (5.50–7.29)	>0.6	>0.5	≤1
Systemic lupus erythematosus	E	Serous to turbid	Acute: polymorphonuclear; chronic: mononuclear	<60 (in 30%)	<7.30 (in 30%)	>0.6	>0.5	≤1
Rheumatoid arthritis	E	Serous to turbid	Acute: polymorphonuclear; chronic: mononuclear	<30 (0–30 in 95%)	<7.30 (usually ~7.00)	>0.6 (usually >500 IU)	>0.5	≤1
Cancer	E	Serous to bloody	Lymphocytes	<60 (in 30%)	<7.30 (7.00–7.29) (in 30%)	>0.6	>0.5	≤1
Tuberculosis	E	Serous	Lymphocytes	30–60 (in 20%)	≤7.30 (in 20%)	>0.6	>0.5	≤1
Esophageal rupture	E	Purulent	Polymorphonuclear	Normal or decreased	6.00	>0.6	>0.5	>2
Pancreatic disease	E	Serous to turbid	Acute: polymorphonuclear; chronic: mononuclear	>60	≥7.30	>0.6	>0.5	>2

*Pleural fluid to serum ratio. (From Sahn, S. A.: Pleural manifestations of pulmonary disease. Hosp. Pract., March, 1981, p. 78.)

surgeon mandates surgical intervention. If part of the catheter is sheared off and remains in the pleural space, a thoracotomy may be required. Cough usually is self-limited and treatment is not required. Pain is best managed with adequate analgesia.

Because splenic hemorrhage may occur slowly, its diagnosis may be delayed for days or even longer. Therefore any patient who has significant hemodynamic changes up to 1 week after a thoracentesis should be evaluated for a suspected splenic injury.

Quality Enhancement

Minimizing complications requires proper instruction and supervision of physicians in training, because they are the ones who frequently perform this procedure. Ultrasound-directed thoracentesis is a safe approach for patients with small amounts of fluid or who cannot be positioned properly, and when fluid does not layer out on a decubitus radiograph or the prothrombin time is elevated.[123] For patients receiving mechanical ventilation, the physician must be certain that the diagnostic and therapeutic value of the procedure will enhance the patient's ability to wean. Diagnostic thoracentesis may aid in alteration or addition of therapy and ultimately may impact chances for recovery.

Because the intensive care practitioner often deals with multiple system disease, organ systems other than the cardiovascular system should be considered etiologically. For example, the kidney may be the cause for an obscure effusion,[124] such as with the nephrotic syndrome, uremia, urinothorax, peritoneal dialysis, perinephric abscess, and acute glomerulonephritis.[131]

Before an insertion site is determined, the skin of ICU patients is evaluated to ensure the absence of skin infections such as herpes zoster.

Care should be the rule in performing a thoracentesis in an uncooperative patient or in a patient with only one lung. Agitated patients who are unable to remain still are at risk of tissue damage during the needle insertion. For those patients who have had a pneumonectomy, the degree of respiratory embarrassment from a pneumothorax might be lethal.

REFERENCES

1. Staff of the Division of Education and the Division of Accreditation: Monitoring and evaluation of the quality and appropriateness of care: An ambulatory health care example. QRB, 13:26, 1987.
2. Cohn, J. N.: Blood pressure measurement in shock. JAMA, 199:118, 1967.
3. Veremakis, C., and Halloran, T. H.: The technique of monitoring arterial blood pressure. J. Crit. Illness, 4:82, 1989.
4. Russell, J. A., et al.: Prospective evaluation of radial and femoral artery catheterization sites in critically ill adults. Crit. Care Med., 11:936, 1983.
5. DeAngelis, J.: Axillary arterial monitoring. Crit. Care Med., 4:205, 1976.
6. Bazaral, M. G., et al.: Comparison of brachial and radial arterial pressure monitoring in patients undergoing coronary artery bypass surgery. Anesthesiology, 73:38, 1990.
7. Campagna, A. C., and Matthay, M. A.: Complications of invasive monitoring in the intensive care unit. Pulm. Crit. Care Update, Lesson 18, 6:1, 1991.
8. Chernow, B., Salem, M., Stacey, J.: Blood conservation-A critical care imperative. Crit. Care Med., 19:313, 1991.
9. Liebowitz, R. S., and Rippe, J. M.: Arterial line placement and care. In Intensive Care Medicine. Edited by J. M. Rippe, R. S. Irwin, J. S. Alpert, J. E. Dalen. Boston, Little, Brown, 1985.
10. Branson, P. K., et al.: Efficacy of 1.4 percent sodium citrate in maintaining arterial catheter patency in patients in a medical ICU. Chest, 103:882, 1993.
11. Kaye, W., Wheaton, M., Potter-Bynoe, G.: Radial and pulmonary catheter-related sepsis. Crit. Care Med., 11:249, 1983.
12. Eyer, S. et al.: Catheter-related sepsis: Prospective, randomized study of three methods of long-term catheter maintenance. Crit. Care Med., 18:1073, 1990.

13. Gurman, G. M., and Kriemerman, S.: Cannulation of big arteries in critically ill patients. Crit. Care Med., 13:217, 1985.
14. Hefner, J. E.: When to consider fiberoptic bronchoscopy in the ICU. J. Crit. Illness, 3:69, 1988.
15. Olopade, C. O., and Prakash, U. B. S.: Bronchoscopy in the critical-care unit. Mayo Clin. Proc., 64:1255, 1989.
16. Tsao, T. C., et al.: Treatment for collapsed lung in critically ill patients. Chest, 97:431, 1990.
17. Limper, A. H., and Prakash, U. B. S.: Tracheobronchial foreign bodies in adults. Ann. Intern. Med., 112:604, 1990.
18. Jederlinic, P. J., and Irwin, R. S.: Status asthmaticus. J. Intensive Care Med., 4:166, 1989.
19. McManigle, J. E., Fletcher, G. L., Tenholder, M. F.: Bronchoscopy in the management of bronchopleural fistula. Chest, 5:1235, 1990.
20. York, E. L., et al.: Endoscopic diagnosis and treatment of postoperative bronchopleural fistula. Chest, 97:1390, 1990.
21. Krell, W. S.: Pulmonary diagnostic procedures in the critically ill. Crit. Care Clin., 4:393, 1988.
22. Hertz, M. I.: Minimizing the risk of bronchoscopy during mechanical ventilation. Chest, 104:1319, 1993.
23. Fulkerson, W. J.: Fiberoptic bronchoscopy. N. Engl. J. Med., 311:511, 1984.
24. Haponik, E. F., Kvale, and Wang, K.: Bronchoscopy and related procedures. In Pulmonary Diseases and Disorders. 2nd Ed. Edited by A. P. Fishman. New York, McGraw-Hill Book, 1988, p. 460.
25. Trouillet, J. L., et al.: Fiberoptic bronchoscopy in ventilated patients. Chest, 97:927, 1990.
26. Ognibene, F. P., and Shelhamer, J. H.: Bronchoscopy. In Current Therapy in Critical Care Medicine. Edited by J. E. Parrillo. Toronto, B. C. Decker, Inc., 1987, pp. 11–14.
27. Senoff, M. G.: Central venous catheterization: A comprehensive review. Part I. J. Intensive Care Med., 2:163, 1987.
28. Senoff, M. G.: Central venous catheterization: A comprehensive review. Part II. J. Intensive Care Med., 2:218, 1987.
29. Sharkey, S. W.: Beyond the wedge: Clinical physiology and the Swan-Ganz catheter. Am. J. Med., 83:111, 1987.
30. Hanley, P. C., Click, R. L., Tancredi, R. G.: Delayed air embolism after removal of venous catheters. Ann. Intern. Med., 101:401, 1984.
31. Maschke, S., and Rogove, H.: Cardiac tamponade associated with a multi-lumen venous catheter. Crit. Care Med., 12, 1984.
32. Snyder, R. H.: Catheter infection. A comparison of two catheter maintenance techniques. Ann. Surg., 208:651, 1988.
33. Norwood, S., et al.: Catheter-related infections and associated septicemia. Chest, 99:968, 1991.
34. Pilt, M. L., et al.: Catheter-relaxed infection. A plea for consensus with review and guidelines. Intensive Care Med., 14:503, 1988.
35. Henry, K., Thurn, J. R., Johnson, S.: Experience with central venous catheters in patients with AIDS. N. Engl. J. Med., 320:1496, 1989.
36. Oishi, A. J., Zietlow, S. P., and Sarr, M. G.: Erroneous arterial placement of a central venous catheter. Mayo Clin. Proc., 69:287, 1994.
37. Bone, R. C.: The technique of small-catheter pleural aspiration. J. Crit. Illness, 8:827, 1993.
38. King, T. C., and Smith, C. R.: Chest wall, pleural, lung and mediastinum. In Principles of Surgery. 5th Ed. Edited by S. I. Selwartz. New York, McGraw-Hill, 1989.
39. Eiseman, B., and Swan, K.: Military strategy in trauma. In Trauma. Edited by K. L. Mattox, E. E. Moore, and D. V. Feliciano. Norwalk, CT, Appleton and Lange, 1988.
40. Miller, K. S., and Sahn, S. A.: Chest tubes. Chest, 91:258, 1987.
41. Fraser, R. S.: Lung perforation complicating tube thoracostomy: Pathological description of three cases. Hum. Pathol., 19:518, 1988.
42. Guyton, S. W., Paull, D. L., Anderson, R. P.: Introducer insertion of mini-thoracostomy tubes. Am. J. Surg., 155:693, 1988.
43. Fuhrman, B. P., et al.: Pleural drainage using modified pigtail catheters. Crit. Care Med., 14:575, 1986.
44. Duncan, C., and Erickson, R.: Pressure associated with chest tube stripping. Heart Lung, 11:166, 1982.
45. Importance of automated external defibrillation. In Textbook of Advanced Cardiac Life Support. Dallas, American Heart Association, 1990. 2nd Ed. 287–299.
46. Cummins, R. O., Chesemore, K., White, R. D., and the Defibrillator Working Group: Defibrillator failures: causes of problems and recommendations for improvement. JAMA, 264:1019, 1990.
47. Jaffe, A. S.: Textbook of Advanced Cardiac Life Support. Dallas, American Heart Association, 1987.
48. Reiftel, J. A., et al.: Direct current cardioversion. JAMA, 239:122, 1978.
49. Pauletto, P., et al.: Myocardial damage after D.C. countershock: Myoglobin and CK-MB radioimmunoassay evaluation. Acta Cardiol., 39:115, 1984.
50. Hurst, T. W., Lown, B., DeSilva, R. A. (Eds.): The Heart, Cardioversion and Defibrillation. New York, McGraw-Hill, 1990.
51. Sutton, R. B., and Theofilos, J. T.: Pulmonary edema following direct current cardioversion. Chest, 57:191, 1970.
52. Hummel, R. S., et al.: Spark-generating properties of electrode gels used during defibrillation. JAMA, 260:3021, 1988.
53. ECRI Staff Report: Defibrillation in oxygen-enriched environments. Health Devices, 16:113, 1987.
54. Winchester, J. F.: Use of dialysis and hemoperfusion in treatment of poisoning. In Handbook of Dialysis. Edited by J. T. Daugirdas and T. S. Ingl. Boston, Little, Brown, 1988.
55. Wanscher, M., Frifelt, J. J., Smith-Sivertsen, C.: Thrombosis caused by polyurethane double-lumen subclavian superior vena cava catheter and hemodialysis. Crit. Care Med., 16:624, 1988.
56. Fant, G. F., Dennis, V. W., Quarles, L. D.: Late vascular complications of the subclavian dialysis catheter. Am. J. Kidney Dis., 7:225, 1986.
57. Coates, G. R., et al.: Painful edema of the arm after insertion of single-needle subclavian vein dialysis catheters: Pathogenesis and treatment. South. Med. J., 81:303, 1988.
58. Schwab, S. J., et al.: Prospective evaluation of a dacron cuffed hemodialysis for prolonged use. Am. J. Kidney Dis., 11:166, 1988.
59. Daugirdas, J. T., and Ingl, T. S. (Eds.): Handbook of Dialysis. Boston, Little, Brown, 1988.
60. Rigolosi, R. S., Maher, J. F., Schreiner, G. E.: Intestinal perforation during peritoneal dialysis. Ann. Intern. Med., 70:1013, 1969.
61. Bernardini, J., Paraino, B., Sorkin, M.: Analysis of continuous ambulatory peritoneal dialysis-related pseudomonas aeruginosa infections. Am. J. Med., 83:829, 1987.
62. Ash, S. R., and Daugirdas, J. T.: Peritoneal access devices. In Handbook of Dialysis. Edited by J. T. Daugirdas and T. S. Ingl. Boston, Little, Brown, 1988.
63. Kantrowitz, A., et al.: Initial clinical experience with intraaortic balloon pumping in cardiogenic shock. JAMA, 203:1113, 1968.
64. Sturm, J. T., et al.: Treatment of postoperative low output

syndrome with intraaortic balloon pumping: Experience with 419 patients. Am. J. Cardiol., 45:1033, 1980.
65. Grotz, R. L., and Yerton, N. S.: Intra-aortic balloon counterpulsation in high risk cardiac patients undergoing noncardiac surgery. Surgery, 106:1, 1989.
66. Bourdarias, J. P., Gourgas, R., Bardet, J.: Mechanical circulatory assistance by intraaortic balloon pumping for the treatment of cardiogenic shock. Intensive Care Med., 4:29, 1978.
67. Cooper, G. N., et al.: Preoperative intraaortic balloon support in surgery for left main coronary stenosis. Ann. Surg., 185:242, 1977.
68. Ito, Y., et al.: Temporary cardiopulmonary bypass for the treatment of endotoxic shock. Am. J. Surg., 136:80, 1978.
69. Alcan, K. E., Stertzer, S. H., Wallsh, E.: Current status of intra-aortic balloon counterpulsation in critical care cardiology. Crit. Care Med., 12:489, 1984.
70. Starksen, N. F., and Ports, T. A.: Intra-aortic balloon pump therapy. Pulm. Crit. Care Update, Lesson 10, 6:1, 1990.
71. Sorrentino, M., and Feldman, T.: Techniques for IABP timing, use and discontinuance. J. Crit. Illness, 7:597, 1992.
72. Borel, C., and Hanley, D.: Neurologic intensive care unit monitoring. In Critical Care Clinics. Vol. 1, No. 2. Edited by M. C. Rogers and R. J. Traystman. Philadelphia, W. B. Saunders, 1985, p. 223.
73. Ostrup, R. C., et al.: Continuous monitoring of intracranial pressure with a miniaturized fiberoptic device. J. Neurosurg., 67:206, 1987.
74. Weiss, M. H.: The technique of intracranial pressure monitoring. J. Crit. Illness, 2:85, 1987.
75. Aucoin, P. I., et al.: Intracranial pressure monitors. Am. J. Med., 80:369, 1986.
76. Germon, K.: Interpretation of ICP pulse waves to determine intracerebral compliance. J. Neurosci. Nurs., 20:344, 1988.
77. White, P. F., Schlobohm, R. M., Pitts, L. H.: A randomized study of drugs for preventing increases in intracranial pressure during endotracheal suctioning. Anesthesiology, 57:242, 1982.
78. Hee, M. K. J., Plevak, D. J., and Peters, S. G.: Intubation of critically ill patients. Mayo Clin. Proc., 67:569, 1992.
79. Consensus conference on artificial airways in patients receiving mechanical ventilation. Chest, 96:178, 1989.
80. Bishop, M. J., Weymuller, E. A., Fink, R. B.: Laryngeal effects of prolonged intubation. Anesth. Analg., 63:335, 1985.
81. Stone, D. J., and Gal, T. J.: Airway management. In Anesthesia. 3rd Ed. Edited by R. D. Miller. New York, Churchill Livingstone, Inc., 1990.
82. Colice, G. L.: Prolonged intubation versus tracheostomy in the adult. J. Intensive Care, 2:85, 1987.
83. Rashkin, M. C., and Davis, T.: Acute complications of endotracheal intubation. Relationship to reintubation, route, urgency, and duration. Chest, 89:165, 1986.
84. Gammage, G. W.: Airway management. In Critical Care. Edited by J. M. Civetta, R. W. Taylor, and R. R. Kirby. Philadelphia, J. B. Lippincott, 1988.
85. Marsh, H. M., Gillespie, D. J., Baumgartner, A. E.: Timing of tracheostomy in the critically ill patient. Chest, 96:190, 1989.
86. Heffner, J. E.: Medical indications for tracheostomy. Chest, 96:186, 1989.
87. Borland, L. M., Swan, D. M., Leff, S.: Difficult pediatric endotracheal intubation: A new approach to the retrograde technique. Anesthesiology, 55:577, 1981.
88. Ellis, D. G., et al.: Guided orotracheal intubation in the operating room using a lighted stylet: A comparison with direct laryngoscopic technique. Anesthesiology, 64:823, 1986.
89. Marton, K. I., and Glean, A. D.: The spinal tap: A new look for an old test. Ann. Intern. Med., 104:840, 1986.
90. American College of Physicians, Health and Public Policy Committee. The diagnostic spinal tap. Ann. Intern. Med., 104:880, 1986.
91. Guzy, P. M.: Emergency cardiac pacing. Emerg. Med. Clin. North Am., 4:745, 1986.
92. Syverud, S.: Cardiac pacing. Emerg. Med. Clin. North Am., 6:197, 1988.
93. Morelli, R. L., and Goldschlager, N.: Temporary transvenous pacing: Resolving postinsertion problems. J. Crit. Illness, 2:73, 1987.
94. Silver, M. D., and Goldschlager, N.: Temporary transvenous pacing in the critical care setting. Chest, 93:607, 1988.
95. Lumia, F. J., and Rios, J. C.: Temporary transvenous pacemaker therapy: An analysis of complications. Chest 64:604, 1973.
96. Ausubel, K., and Furman, S.: The pacemaker syndrome. Ann. Intern. Med., 103:420, 1985.
97. Tilden, S. J., et al.: Runaway temporary pacemaker caused by a component defect. Crit. Care Med., 17:1231, 1989.
98. Mayer, A. O.: Controlled clinical trial of peritoneal lavage for the treatment of severe acute pancreatitis. N. Engl. J. Med., 312:399, 1985.
99. Rattner, D. W., and Warshaw, A. L.: Surgical intervention in acute pancreatitis. Crit. Care Med., 16:89, 1988.
100. Kellerman, P. S., and Lirras, S. L.: Large volume paracentesis in the treatment of ascites. Ann. Intern. Med., 112:889, 1990.
101. Kao, H. W., et al.: The effect of large volume paracentesis on plasma volume-A cause of hypovolemia? Hepatology, 5:403, 1985.
102. McCullough, K. I., et al.: Circulatory shock due to ascites and responsive to paracentesis. Am. J. Cardiol., 56:500, 1985.
103. Koffel, K. K., and Reed, J. S.: The technique of abdominal paracentesis. J. Crit. Illness, 1:45, 1986.
104. Lorrel, B. H., and Braunwald, E. (Eds.): Pericardial disease in heart disease. Philadelphia, W. B. Saunders, 1988.
105. Henry, J. B. (Ed.): Clinical diagnosis and management by laboratory method. 17th Ed. Philadelphia, W. B. Saunders, 1984.
106. Kudoh, Y., et al.: Tuberculosis on regular hemodialysis-a case for pericardial tamponade. Jpn. Circ. J., 53:416, 1989.
107. Punzengruber, C., Pachinger, O., Haidenthaler, A.: Atypical clinical cause of thoracic aortic dissection with subacute pericardial hemorrhage. Z. Kardiol., 77:811, 1988.
108. Storka, J. L., et al.: Pericardial effusion and tamponade due to Kaposi's sarcoma in acquired immunodeficiency syndrome. Chest, 95:1359, 1989.
109. Hancock, E. W.: Cardiac tamponade. In Cardiac Emergencies. Edited by M. M. Scheinman. Philadelphia, W. B. Saunders, 1984.
110. Vandyke, W. H., Cure, J., Chakko, C. S.: Pulmonary edema after pericardiocentesis for cardiac tamponade. N. Engl. J. Med., 309:595, 1983.
111. Swan, H. J. C., et al.: Catheterization of the heart in man with the use of a flow-directed balloon catheter. N. Engl. J. Med., 283:447, 1970.
112. Robin, E. D.: The cult of the Swan-Ganz catheter: Overuse and abuse of pulmonary flow catheters. Ann. Intern. Med., 103:445, 1985.
113. Connors, A. F., McCaffree, D. R., Gray, B. A.: Evaluation of right-heart catheterization in the critically ill patient without acute myocardial infarction. N. Engl. J. Med., 308:263, 1983.
114. Matthay, M. A., and Chatterjee, K.: Bedside catheterization of the pulmonary artery: Risks compared to benefits. Ann. Intern. Med., 109:826, 1988.

115. Amin, D. K., Shah, P. K., and Swan, H. J. C.: Deciding when hemodynamic monitoring is appropriate. J. Crit. Illness, *8:* 1053, 1993.
116. Finn, S. S., et al.: Observations on the perioperative management of aneurysmal subarachnoid hemorrhage. J. Neurosurg., *65:*48, 1986.
117. Naylor, C. D., et al.: Pulmonary artery catheterization. Can there be an integrated strategy for guideline development and research promotion? JAMA, *269:*2407, 1993.
118. Putterman, C.: The Swan-Ganz catheter: A decade of hemodynamic monitoring. J. Crit. Care, *4:*127, 1989.
119. Chastre, J., et al.: Thrombosis as a complication of pulmonary artery catheterization via the internal jugular vein: Prospective evaluations by phlebography. N. Engl. J. Med., *306:* 278, 1982.
120. Moorthy, S. S., et al.: Cerebral air embolism during removal of a pulmonary artery catheter. Crit. Care Med., *19:*981, 1991.
121. Jastremski, M. S., et al.: Analysis of the effects of continuous on-line monitoring of mixed venous oxygen saturation on patient outcome and cost-effectiveness. Crit. Care Med., *17:* 148, 1989.
122. Hurford, W. E.: Thermodilution right ventricular ejection fraction: Remaining questions. Chest, *98:*1055, 1990.
123. Vincent, J. L., et al.: Thermodilution measurement of right ventricular ejection fraction with a modified pulmonary artery catheter. Intensive Care Med., *12:*33, 1986.
124. Räsänen, J., et al.: Estimation of oxygen utilization by dual oximetry. Ann. Surg., *206:*621, 1987.
125. Sharkey, S. W.: Beyond the wedge: Clinical physiology and the Swan-Ganz catheter. Am. J. Med., *83:*111, 1987.
126. Wiedemann, H. P., Matthay, M. A., Matthay, R. A.: Cardiovascular-pulmonary monitoring in the intensive care unit (Part 1). Chest, *85:*537, 1984.
127. Rocco, M., et al.: Balloon occlusion pulmonary angiography during mechanical ventilation with positive end-expiratory pressure in patients with acute respiratory failure. J. Crit. Care, *6:*89, 1991.
128. Peruzzi, W., et al.: Portable chest roentgenography and computed tomography in critically ill patients. Chest, *93:* 722, 1988.
129. Snow, N., Bergin, K. T., Horrigan, T. P.: Thoracic CT scanning in critically ill patients. Chest, *97:*1467, 1990.
130. Senoff, M. G., et al.: Complications associated with thoracentesis. Chest, *90:*97, 1986.
131. Sahn, S. A., and Miller, K. S.: Obscure pleural effusion. Chest, *90:*631, 1986.

Chapter 77

PITFALLS IN HEMODYNAMIC AND RESPIRATORY MONITORING

JEAN-PIERRE YARED

Monitoring of the critically ill patient is an essential diagnostic and therapeutic tool that allows early identification of evolving physiologic disturbances and assessment of their severity and response to treatment. It requires the repeated and often continuous measurement of physiologic parameters reflecting organ function either in the laboratory or at the bedside. The list of parameters monitored in the intensive care unit (ICU) is expanding continuously with the availability of simple to use, reliable measuring instruments. Unfortunately, these techniques can be affected by numerous errors that range from the readily identifiable to the subtle, and may adversely affect outcome. When such hazards are added to those resulting from misinterpretation of accurate data and to the physical risks inherent to the use of monitoring equipment, it becomes essential to learn to identify sources of error and to evaluate the risks and benefits of monitoring prior to its use.[1]

BASIS OF CLINICAL MEASUREMENTS

The human body being different from most mechanical models, it is not surprising to find that application of physical laws to clinical measurements often requires several assumptions and approximations to facilitate understanding of the physiologic mechanisms, as well as the calculations involved in those measurements. Although this process of simplification is usually sufficient for clinical application,[2] it sometimes leads to wrong conclusions, particularly when it is combined with the multiple sources of error inherent to clinical measurements.

The Measuring Instrument

The characteristics of the measuring instrument that must be known before obtained values are used to diagnose a problem or dictate a therapeutic intervention include resolution, accuracy, repeatability, and reproducibility.[3] The need for this information is illustrated by the commonly asked questions concerning the accuracy of cardiac output measurement, the magnitude of change that must occur before it is considered significant, as well as the sources of variability and error. In general, the more a measurement is repeated, the more random errors tend to sum to zero. The practicality of repeating measurements differs, however, according to the instrument and to the parameter being measured: an ECG monitor measures heart rate continuously and random errors are minimal, whereas thermodilution cardiac output measurement can be repeated only a finite number of times with, therefore, a larger margin of error. Moreover, the observer sometimes rejects readings that he or she subjectively considers incorrect, although the differences between measurements might be real and reflect differences in the phase of respiration, heart rate irregularities, or variable degrees of sedation or agitation. At the beginning of this century, a sampling interval of 5 minutes was advocated by Codman and Cushing for monitoring heart rate and blood pressure during anesthesia.[4] Only recently was a model developed to define the sampling interval for clinical monitoring of variables during anesthesia to facilitate detection of disturbances such as hypercapnia, hypoxia, and hypotension.[5] When measurements are obtained intermittently, one can only hope that they reflect a steady state that is maintained between measurements.

Operator Errors

Operator errors can result from the same operator repeating the same error in sampling or measuring or from different operators using different techniques. Significant changes in pressure recording often are noted after a shift change in nursing staff when the level and calibration of the transducers are routinely checked. User or programming error can result in incorrect labeling of the values displayed on the monitor whereby the values and tracings of the systemic and pulmonary blood pressures are interchanged. Although this switch would be readily identifiable in the normal patient, it could be missed in the presence of severe pulmonary hypertension when both pressures are similar, hence leading to major management problems. Nonlinearity of some instruments, including pulse oximeters, is associated with an adequate performance within the normal range and significant error outside that range. Similarly, respiratory equipment including pressure transducers, flow meters, and gas analysis devices need to be calibrated over the entire range of expected measurements, and calibration must be repeated at regular intervals to account for the effect of wear and tear.[3] Some techniques of measurement require a great deal of precision and expertise and may yield incorrect value with the occasional or unscrupulous user.

Signal Processing

In the past, most data were obtained as an analog signal and displayed as such on a cathode ray tube (CRT). Modern monitors, however, process the original signal through an analog to digital (A/D) converter to obtain a digital display of the information and simultaneously reconvert the digital information into an analog signal that is displayed in real time and in a nonfading pattern. The analog format, although more tedious to read, is more precise in terms of beat-to-beat variation and allows the identification of some of the sources of error in measurement. The algorithms used for D/A and A/D conversion differ between manufacturers and can introduce error in measurement.[6] Digital processing usually averages the values obtained during the last cardiac cycles (usually three) to avoid the continuous change in the displayed value that would otherwise occur. The accuracy of the analog display is affected by the inertia of the writing instrument. Modern thermal array printing devices and CRTs have minimal distortion and an excellent frequency response; however, fidelity and accuracy are usually more difficult to obtain when the analog output has to move a mechanical part like a needle particularly with high frequency signals. Fortunately, most physiologic signals have a low frequency and filters have been used to eliminate high frequency noise (low pass filters). Some information may be lost in the process, however, and some artifacts may be added.[6]

Error in Interpretation

Measurement errors theoretically are amenable to correction with improving technology and elimination of human interference in the process; however, error in interpretation of accurate data is often insidious and difficult to identify. The data may be incomplete or the expected range of a variable can be modified by disease to the extent that it becomes difficult to define the optimal value of a variable, such as what the left ventricular end diastolic pressure should be in a hypertrophic heart or the maximum heart rate acceptable in a patient with coronary artery disease. The increasing complexity of monitoring equipment mandates the availability of competent engineers and technicians able to ensure its proper functioning and to perform the required maintenance and quality checks, as well as to instruct the medical personnel about the optimal way to use the device to obtain accurate results and a lasting satisfactory performance.

Routine Clinical Assessment

Although routine clinical assessment has been shown to be a poor predictor of hemodynamic status,[7,8] monitoring cannot replace it. Close observation of the critically ill patient by nurses and physicians often uncovers impending catastrophic events that may not have resulted in a detectable change in the monitored parameters or that occur at a time the patient is not monitored appropriately to detect such changes. For example, impending septic shock often manifests by a change in the patient's mental status, skin temperature, cardiac output, or the quality of the peripheral pulses at a time the blood pressure may still be well maintained. Such observations may indicate the need to initiate more extensive monitoring techniques and diagnostic procedures that can help confirm or reject the presumptive diagnosis. Monitoring provides the medical team with early warning signals that should prompt immediate corrective action (sudden decrease in oxygen saturation, end tidal carbon dioxide concentration, blood pressure, etc.). The multitude of numbers provided should be correlated with the clinical impression and help tailor patient management. They should not replace clinical judgment. The potential for diverting the attention of the clinician away from the patient is significant, particularly when too much unnecessary information is presented or when the instrument fails to perform adequately, requiring multiple interventions to keep the information it provides accurate.

Invasive versus Noninvasive Monitoring

It is often difficult to set criteria for the type of monitoring devices necessary in a particular clinical situation. Invasive monitoring should be limited to situations in which noninvasive monitoring cannot supply the necessary information and the potential benefit outweighs the potential risk associated to its use. The decision to implement or to discontinue a monitoring method could be influenced by nonmedical factors such as cost containment, reimbursement, fear of litigation, quality control, and limited availability of a monitor. More and more, it is becoming the duty of the physician to use technology that may provide patients with extra procedure,[9] and the use of quantitative methods of assessing clinical signs is encouraged.[10] In anesthesia, many argue that improved monitoring has resulted in a significant decrease in anesthesia-related mortality and has decreased the cost of malpractice premiums.[11] In an update on Standards of Postanesthesia Care,[12] The American Society of Anesthesiologists requires the use of "a quantitative method for assessing oxygenation in the initial phase of recovery." The Standards for Basic Intraoperative Monitoring mandate that the correct positioning of an endotracheal tube should be "verified by clinical assessment and by identification of carbon dioxide in the expired gas."

The purpose of this chapter is to review the most common cardiovascular and respiratory monitoring methods used in the ICU and to evaluate their accuracy and dependability, as well as the common causes of errors in measurement and interpretation associated with their use. Techniques and complications related to line placement and indications for monitoring are addressed elsewhere in this book.

HEMODYNAMIC MONITORING AND RESPIRATORY MONITORING

The ultimate aim of hemodynamic and respiratory monitoring is to assess the balance between tissue oxygen needs and delivery, as well as the adequacy of removal of metabolic by-products. It must therefore provide information on global as well as regional oxygen requirements, delivery, and utilization. Information on organ function can be obtained directly (e.g., cardiac output, oxygen saturation) or indirectly (e.g., blood pressure, urine output). Adequacy of global as well as regional perfusion and function of the heart can, if needed, be monitored continuously and with great detail by electrocardiography and measurement of cardiac output, stroke volume, ejection fraction, and wall motion studies. Unfortunately, the EEG has not been useful in detecting cerebral oxygen deficiency, and it is often necessary to wait for tissue damage to occur before seeing evidence of end organ dysfunction when perfusion of the kidney, liver, or gastrointestinal tract are affected. Consequently, therapy is directed at optimizing determinants of global perfusion with the hope that, as a result, regional perfusion will be optimized.

Electrocardiographic (ECG) Monitoring

Electrocardiographic monitoring is used routinely anytime close observation of a patient is required. Technical advances have produced a sensitive and accurate diagnostic instrument comparable to the most sophisticated 12-lead ECG. The fidelity of the tracing is influenced by many factors including motion artifacts, electrical interference, quality of the patient-monitor interface, as well as the monitoring equipment (Table 77-1).

Heart Rate

The analog ECG signal is processed to obtain a digital readout of the heart rate and a nonfading display of the ECG tracing. The QRS is identified by recognition of the upward then downward deflection of the signal and the rate usually is obtained by averaging three or more RR intevals. Errors in heart rate measurement occur when the amplitude of the QRS complex is variable or so low that it is not recognized by the monitor, leading to misdiagnosis of asystole or bradycardia and activation of the corresponding alarms (Fig. 77-1A). Conversely, failure to differentiate a peaked P or T wave or a high amplitude pacemaker spike from a QRS complex leads to doubling of the value of the heart rate (Fig. 77-1B).

Rhythm

Identification of changes in RR intervals allows monitoring of supraventricular arrhythmias, whereas recognition of QRS complexes different form the baseline complex allows detection of ventricular arrhythmias. Misdiagnosis of ventricular arrhythmias occurs, however, when the QRS complex becomes wider as a result of intermittent conduction blocks.

Ischemia

Manifestations of myocardial ischemia include ST-segment changes, decreased ventricular wall thickening, abnormal wall motion, and decreased compliance. As a result, many monitoring techniques with variable sensitivity and specificity have been developed for early detection of myocardial ischemia. Transesophageal echocardiography (TEE) allows early detection of ischemia during surgery and angioplasty,[13,14] although its specificity can be affected by changes in loading conditions. Its use in the ICU is expanding, although it is sometimes impractical because of the need for a specialist at the bedside who is able to identify and interpret the changes. Elevation of the pulmonary capillary wedge pressure can occur during ischemia when the latter results in global ventricular dysfunction.[15] This technique, however, has a low sensitivity when ischemia is regional and its specificity can also be affected by changes in loading conditions. The 12-lead ECG remains the standard in diagnosing ischemia in terms of having both a high sensitivity and a high specificity. Modern ECG monitors are able to provide ST-segment analysis with comparable accuracy. Many algorithms measure the ST-segment deflection from the isoelectric point (PQ segment) 60 to 80 msecs after the J point (junction between QRS and the ST segment),[16] and some monitors allow manual fine adjustment of the isoelectric and ST segments to be analyzed. This feature is useful when the QRS complex is so wide that the segment analyzed by the monitor is, in fact, part of the QRS and not the ST segment (see Fig. 77-1C and D).

For ST-segment analysis to be an accurate diagnostic tool for ischemia, its use must be limited to the population with coronary artery disease, because it is nonspecific when applied to the population at large.[17] Hyperventilation and mitral valve prolapse can be associated with ECG signs of ischemia.[18] One study revealed a high incidence of ST-segment changes suggestive of ischemia in patients undergoing caesarean section under regional anesthesia.[19] The mechanism of these changes is unclear, but the authors suggested that they indicate true ischemia when they are accompanied by anginal pain. Even in patients at increased risk of coronary artery disease the high risk group, sensitivity and specificity are affected by medications like digoxin, as well as electrolytic and metabolic disturbances, left ventricular hypertrophy, and conduction abnormalities. In the absence of such abnormalities, ST-segment depression greater than 1 mm is a specific marker for ischemia, particularly as the number of diseased vessels increases (40 to 84% with one vessel and 79 to 100% with three vessel disease).[17,20] Patients with unstable angina are more likely to have ST-segment elevation (severe transmural ischemia), whereas ST segment depression is more common with stable angina.[21,22] A prerequisite for detection of ischemia is monitoring the lead or combination of

Table 77-1. Factors Affecting the Fidelity of the ECG Tracing

Patient related
   Motion artifact
   Respiratory movements
   Muscle twitches, shivering
   Wet, oily, or hairy skin
Leads and cables
   Bad connection
   Broken wire
   Inadequate shielding
   Motion
Electrode related
   Dry gel
   Poor adherence to skin
Monitoring equipment
   Susceptibility to interference
   Frequency response
   Internal noise
Environment
   Electrocautery
   Power lines (60 Hz)
   Motors
   Intravenous pumps

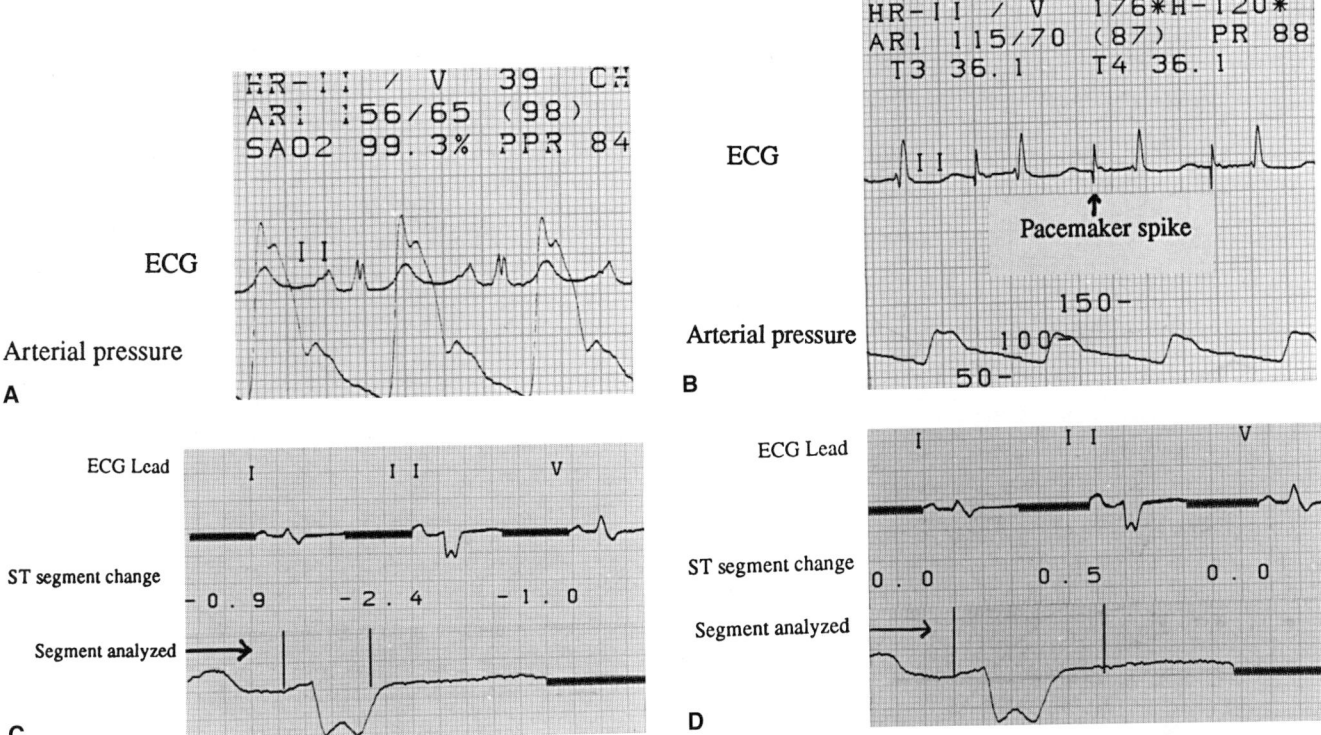

Fig. 77-1. *A*, The low amplitude QRS is detected intermittently. The QRS rate is 39 beats per minute and the pulse rate is 84 beats per minute. *B*, The atrial pacing spike is falsely identified as a QRS. Heart rate (HR) is 176 beats per minute and pulse rate is 88 beats per minute. The high rate alarm is flashing. *C*, Computerized ST segment analysis: wide QRS complex. The segment being analyzed is part of the QRS. *D*, Same as *C* after manual adjustment of the segment to be analyzed.

leads that look at the area at risk. For example, monitoring of V4R lead is highly sensitive and highly specific for detection of right ventricular ischemia, whereas monitoring of lead II and V is inadequate for this purpose.[23,24]

Depression of the J point with exercise is common in normal individuals and is followed by a steep upslope of the ST segment, which then merges with the T wave. With ischemia, the J point depression is usually followed by a flat or downsloping ST segment.[25] As a result, measuring ST-segment deflection 60 msec after the J point would be expected to improve the diagnostic accuracy. The ECG is probably insensitive when the decrease in myocardial perfusion does not cause frank ischemia.[26] In one review, five ECG monitoring systems used in the operating room[16] were compared and were found to be more sensitive and as specific as the standard 12-lead ECG and the Holter monitor when an ST-segment deviation of more than 1 mm 60 msec after the J point was used as the criterion for ischemia. All systems had comparable sensitivity, however, when a deviation greater than 0.25 mm was taken as evidence of ischemia. Conversely, other studies have shown a decrease in specificity of the 12-lead ECG for diagnosis of ischemia when using a depression of less than 1 mm.[25] Transient ECG changes compatible with ischemia occur during the immediate postcardiopulmonary bypass period in patients undergoing coronary artery bypass grafting. They may reflect either heterogeneity of intraventricular conduction because of the uneven cardioplegic protection and reperfusion of the myocardium[2] or real ischemic events.[27] If J point depression occurring with tachycardia is misinterpreted as ischemia, administration of beta blockers moves the ST segment to its previous position merely by slowing the heart rate, and false conclusions about tachycardia-induced ischemia and its reversal with beta blockade may be drawn.

Blood Pressure Monitoring

Blood pressure (BP) can be measured by invasive and noninvasive methods. Pressure per se is not, however, the ultimate goal of hemodynamic monitoring. Systemic and pulmonary artery BP are the result of the interaction between the output generated by the cardiac pump and the status of the systemic or pulmonary circulations. When pressure alone is measured, assessment of the adequacy of perfusion requires that the observer make assumptions regarding blood volume, vascular resistance, as well as regional blood flow. Accurate pressure measurement is essential to most monitoring techniques and the problems encountered in obtaining such measurements are discussed subsequently.

Systemic Pressure Measurement

Noninvasive Techniques

The most common noninvasive methods of systemic BP measurement are occlusive and intermittent. They rely on auscultation or oscillometry. Auscultation is based on the detection of the Korotkoff sounds during deflation of a cuff placed around an extremity.[28] The accuracy of these techniques is controversial. The American Heart Association defines systolic pressure as the onset of phase 1 when a snappy sound becomes audible and diastolic pressure in adults as the onset of phase 5 when all sounds disappear. The size of the cuff should be about 20% larger than the diameter of the extremity, and the bladder should be placed over the artery and cover at least one half of the circumference of the extremity. Falsely high BP measurements occur when a cuff is too small or too loosely placed around the extremity. Falsely low BP measurements are obtained with a cuff that is too large. Auscultatory methods are least reliable in hypotensive patients, because some blood flows past the cuff before a sound is generated.[29] The systolic pressure can be underestimated by as much as 34% in hypotensive patients and 64% in patients with heart failure.[30] Accuracy is affected also by the hearing ability of the person performing the measurement.

Oscillometric determinations are controversial too, but systole usually is considered the point at which oscillations increase and diastole where they first become slurred. A good correlation was found between the Dinamap 845 and intra-arterial pressure movements; however, the Dinamap overestimated the systolic and diastolic pressure in hypotensive patients and underestimated the systolic pressure in hypertensive individuals.[31] Oscillometric methods also overestimate diastolic pressure by 10% in at least 70% of elderly subjects.[32] Overall correlation with intra-arterial pressure measurement is good, despite large individual variations.[33] Measurement errors can result from changes in the blood volume in the extremity during inflation,[34] and underestimation of systolic BP can occur during cuff deflation in a bradycardic patient. When used adequately, oscillometric methods are useful in monitoring the BP of patients who are stable or recovering. Their use in hypotensive states can be hazardous and, the measurements being intermittent, beat-to-beat variation in pressure cannot be observed. Reported physical complications from automatic occlusive methods include skin avulsion, ischemia, ulnar neuropathy, and venostasis,[34-36] particularly when monitoring the unconscious patient who is unable to complain of pain and in situations in which the cuff is applied inadequately and inflations are too close to each other.

Invasive Techniques

These methods rely on converting a mechanical signal applied to a transducer into electric impulses processed digitally to obtain a digital readout of the systolic, diastolic, and mean pressures and a nonfading waveform. The instrument looks at the point at which the slope changes direction, and some devices time the measurement according to the previously detected QRS complex. The mean pressure is measured by calculating the area under the pressure curve. As with ECG signal processing, the heart rate measurement, the digital readout does not reveal beat-to-beat variations and averages the most recent pressure curves (usually three). Moreover, some monitors display mean pressures that are average weighted toward the previous running mean so that the numeric value of the pressure does not fluctuate greatly with artifacts related to motion or brief flushing.

Invasive pressure monitoring can be subject to errors related to the site of measurement, the tubing, the transducer, the operator, and the way the signal is handled before it is displayed in analog or digital form. Pressure wave reflection in the peripheral arteries causes the systolic pressure in the dorsalis pedis or radial arteries to be significantly higher than that in more proximal arteries, whereas the diastolic pressure is lower and the mean pressure is unchanged (Fig. 77-2).[37,38] Systolic pressure can increase by 10 to 20 mm Hg as it travels distally.[39] Radial artery pressure monitoring has been shown to underestimate the brachial artery pressure following rewarming on cardiopulmonary bypass, probably because of the arteriovenous shunts in the hand. This pressure gradient can also be exaggerated in the presence of lesions limiting blood flow through the subclavian and axillary arteries.[40] Presence of air bubbles in the tubing and the use of compliant tubes with multiple connections reduce damping in the system and produce artifactual oscillations that result in systolic overshoot,[41,42] particularly when the arterial upstroke is brisk and hence rich in high frequency components. When tubings of different lengths were compared (180 versus 15 cm), the additional error was 3% only.[38] The adequacy of the dynamic response of a transducer-tubing system can be checked by the response after a rapid flush.[41]

Pressure transducers must be calibrated at zero input, obtained by opening the transducer to the atmosphere and at a calibration input. Improper zero calibration adds a constant error to all readings from that instrument; spontaneous drift adds a variable error. Incorrect setting of the gain adds a proportional error to the measurement, i.e., the error will be greater with greater input values.[6] Newer transducers require only zero calibration, and spontaneous drift, as well as variation in gain, are of small magnitude.

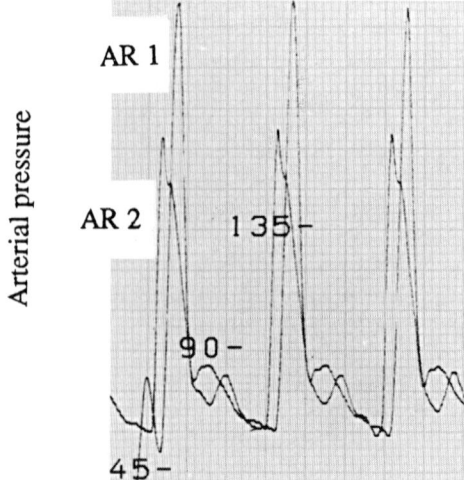

Fig. 77-2. Simultaneous radial (AR1) and brachial (AR2) artery tracings. AR1 is 205/53 (mean = 81). AR2 is 160/56 (mean = 83). (Courtesy of M. Bazaral.)

Artifactual hypertension related to transducer cable malfunction has been reported.[96] The problem was caused by an embedded pin in the cable end causing a short circuit between two pin sockets.

Central Venous and Pulmonary Artery Pressure Monitoring

Central venous and pulmonary artery thermodilution catheters are used for determination and monitoring of right (RV) and left (LV) ventricular preload, pulmonary artery pressure (PAP), RV ejection fraction, sampling of mixed venous or pulmonary capillary blood for gas analysis, and cardiac output (CO).

Many other physiologic parameters can be derived mathematically from integration of the measured values with information obtained from the ECG, arterial blood gas analysis, and systemic pressure measurements. Although it is well documented that central venous pressure (CVP) is a poor predictor of left ventricular end diastolic pressure (LVEDP), particularly in elderly patients and those with cardiopulmonary disease,[43-45] CVP monitoring is useful in assessing RV filling pressure in diseases causing increased RV afterload (e.g. pulmonary hypertension or mitral valve disease). The following discussion concentrates on evaluation of the left side of the heart, but similar principles apply to the right side.

Pulmonary Artery Occlusive Pressure (PAOP)

The PAOP obtained after inflating a balloon placed near the tip of the pulmonary artery catheter has been used to assess left atrial pressure (LAP) and the LVEDP. It measures the pressure of a static column of blood between the balloon and the left atrium, and the tracing has a venous pressure pattern (Fig. 77-3). The a wave reflects atrial contraction and follows the P wave on a simultaneously recorded ECG. It is absent in atrial fibrillation, whereas nodal rhythm with retrograde conduction results in a prominent a wave following the QRS. The X descent represents atrial relaxation and the C wave indicates the onset of ventricular systole. The v wave occurs during atrial filling while the atrioventricular valve is closed and reflects bulging of the atrioventricular valve in the atrium. It must, therefore, follow the onset of ventricular contraction and the QRS com-

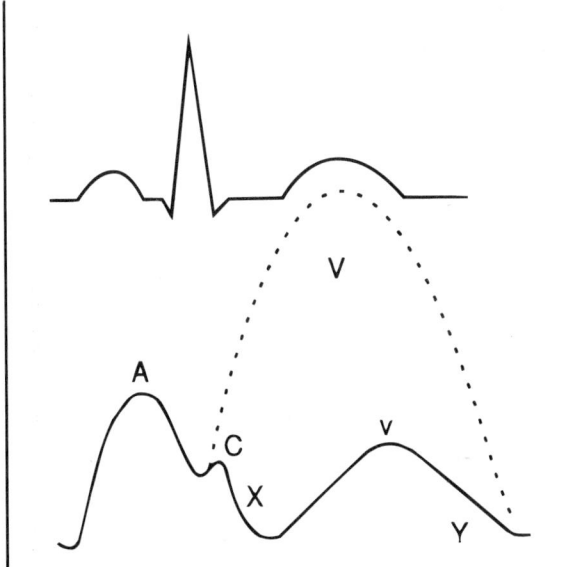

Fig. 77-4. Venous waveform is relation to the ECG.

plex on the ECG. Lastly, the Y descent represents atrial emptying during ventricular diastole (Fig. 77-4). The inference that PAOP = LAP = LVEDP implies that pulmonary vascular resistance (PVR) is low, airway pressure is low (i.e., no external forces are applied to the fluid column), LV compliance is normal, and the mitral and aortic valves are normal. The inference that change in LVEDP reflects similar change in left ventricular end diastolic volume (LVEDV) assumes that LV compliance is constant. The factors affecting the fidelity of PAOP as a representation of LV preload are discussed subsequently.

Ventricular preload should be expressed in terms of presystolic fiber length, of which LVEDV is an acceptable reflection.[46] Although CVP and PAOP do not measure blood volume and can be affected by variations in vascular tone, changes in their value reflect changes in blood volume if ventricular compliance and vascular tone are kept constant.[47] After coronary artery bypass grafting, however, changes in PAOP have been shown to correlate poorly with LVEDV.[48] Because the relationship between LVEDP and LVEDV is a function of compliance, the latter must be known before interventions based on LVEDP measurements are made. Unfortunately, compliance varies between individuals, as well as with physiologic and therapeutic alterations in the same individual (Table 77-2).[49-52]

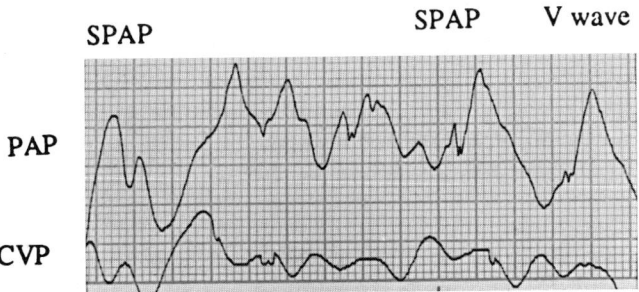

Fig. 77-3. Slow inflation of the balloon shows the progressive disappearance of the systolic pulmonary artery pressure (SPAP). Note that the V wave, previously embedded in the dicrotic notch, is now apparent.

Table 77-2. Factors Affecting Left Ventricular Compliance

Decreased Compliance	Increased Compliance
Myocardial ischemia	Vasodilators
Constrictive pericarditis	Lusitropes (amrinone)
Pericardial effusion	Calcium-channel blockers
Pericardial tamponade	Mitral insufficiency
Myocardial fibrosis	Aortic insufficiency
Left ventricular hypertrophy	Dilated cardiomyopathy
Right ventricular failure with septal shift	
Inotropes	

Table 77-3. Causes of Discrepancy between Left Atrial Pressure (LAP) and Left Ventricular End Diastolic Pressure (LVEDP)

LVEDP < mean LAP	LVEDP > mean LAP
Mitral stenosis Nodal rhythm ? Mitral insufficiency	Severe aortic insufficiency Noncompliant LV

LVEDP < a wave	LVEDP > a wave
Mitral stenosis Nodal rhythm	Severe aortic insufficiency

In the absence of gradient across the mitral valve, the LVEDP is equal to the systolic pressure generated by the left atrium (LA), i.e., the peak a wave.[53-55] The amplitude of the a wave is small in the normal heart, and in most clinical situations, it is customary to use the mean LAP as a measure of LVEDP. Several conditions associated with a discrepancy between LVEDP and mean LAP are described in Table 77-3. In mitral stenosis, a gradient exists between LAP and LVEDP and neither the a wave nor the mean LAP correlate with LVEDP. In nodal rhythm, the a wave, although not contributing to LV filling, can be large because of the contraction of the LA against a closed mitral valve. In that situation, both a and mean LAP can overestimate LVEDP. When the LV is noncompliant, the LAP can increase significantly during atrial contraction and the mean LAP underestimates the a wave and LVEDP (Fig. 77-5). Severe aortic insufficiency is associated with premature closure of the mitral valve, and LVEDP can be significantly higher than the a wave and the mean LAP.[52] With severe mitral insufficiency, the a wave is equal to LVEDP, but the large regurgitant V wave makes it difficult to identify,

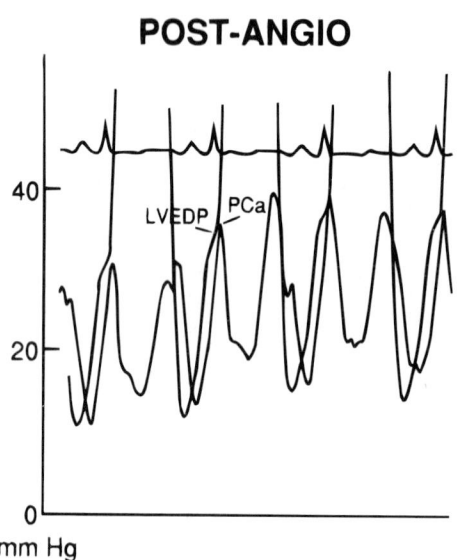

Fig. 77-5. Large a wave and "true" left ventricular end diastolic pressure (LVEDP) in a noncompliant left ventricle. (From Fisher M. L., et al.: Assessing left ventricular filling pressure with flow-directed (Swan Ganz) catheters. Chest, 66:544, 1975.)

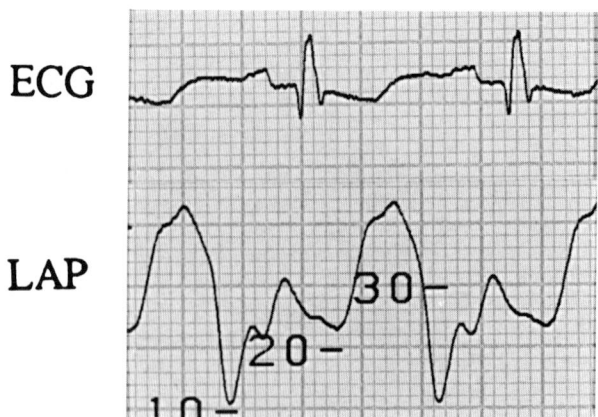

Fig. 77-6. Mitral insufficiency with prominent V wave on the left atrial pressure (LAP) tracing.

possibly resulting in a mean LAP that exceeds the a wave and overestimates LVEDP (Fig. 77-6). The V wave of regurgitation, sometimes called c-v wave, differs from the normal v wave in that it starts with ventricular contraction and thus follows the QRS complex. Although a V wave suggests the presence of mitral insufficiency, its magnitude is not a quantitative measure of the severity of the regurgitation, and its presence is not diagnostic, because it may be present even in the absence of mitral insufficiency.[56,57] The size of the V wave depends on both the regurgitant volume and left atrial compliance. Large V waves are also seen with LA enlargement and high pulmonary blood low (VSD).

Integration of information generated by the ECG with that generated by pressure monitoring helps to determine whether a rhythm disturbance is hemodynamically significant and sometimes whether indeed it occurred, in that ECG artifacts are common (Fig. 77-7).

Pulmonary venous pressure (PVP) and LAP usually are equal. Rarely, tumors compress or obstruct the pulmonary veins as they enter the left atrium, creating a gradient between them.

For PAOP to be a true reflection of LAP, it must be assumed that a static column of fluid exists between the inflated balloon and the LA. Application of internal and external forces to the fluid column will decrease the fidelity with which PAOP reflects LAP. Normally, pulmonary vascular resistance is low and PAOP is close to LAP.[58] A gradient between PAOP and LAP has been reported, however, in certain situations, including primary or secondary pulmonary vascular disease, acidosis, pulmonary embolism, sepsis, endotoxemia, and vasoactive drugs.[59-61] Accuracy in PAOP measurement requires that the fluid column between the catheter tip and the LAP is continuous, that is, the tip must be in zone III of the lung.[62] In normal subjects, the tip must be below the LA to ensure placement in zone III, and zeroing should be done with the transducer open to atmospheric pressure at the midleft atrial level.

Pulmonary Arterial End Diastolic Pressure (PAEDP)

Normally, this value is close to PAOP.[63] When PVR increases, however, a gradient across the pulmonary vessels

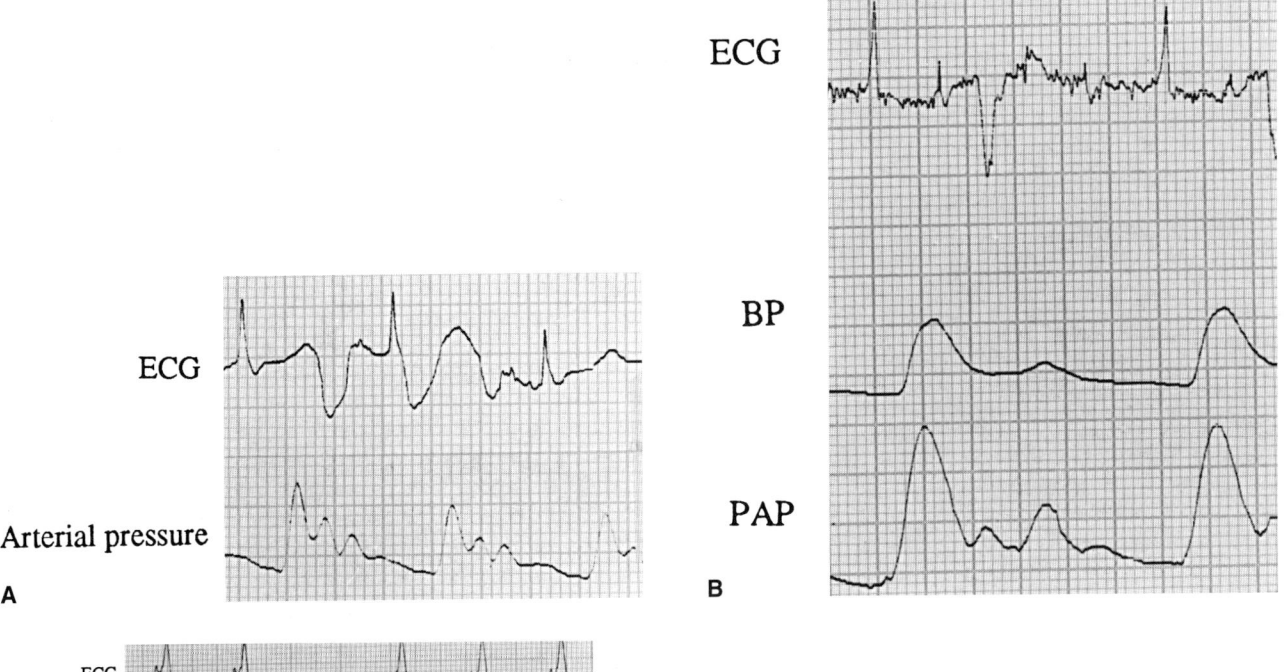

Fig. 77-7. A, ECG artifact. An extrasystole is unlikely because of the regularity of the arterial tracing. B, Bigeminy with minimal ejection with the ectopic beats on the systemic pressure tracing. BP, blood pressure; PAP, pulmonary artery pressure. C, Atrioventricular sequential pacing with intermittent capture of the atria and ventricles. First two beats: No atrial contraction after pacemaker spike; absent a wave on the central venous pressure (CVP) tracing; blood pressure (BP) is 90/60 mm Hg. Third beat: Atrial pacing spike (AS); no atrial contraction; no ventricular spike (VS) or contraction. Last three beats: Atrial contraction following the atrial pacemaker spike; a wave present. Mean systemic arterial pressure increases to 115/70 because of the atrial kick.

results, and PAEDP exceeds PAOP.[64,65] The difference becomes larger with faster heart rates because of less time for diastolic emptying into the LA.[66] If PAOP is greater than PAEDP, one must suspect overwedging, zone I placement in the presence of high airway pressure, or catheter "fling" with diastolic overshoot. In the latter situation, the numeric value of the diastolic pressure underestimates the true diastolic pressure (Fig. 77-8).

Respiratory Variations

The causes of increased external forces applied to the heart include pericardial effusion, tamponade, constrictive pericarditis, hemothorax, pneumothorax, and positive airway pressure. The most common source of such forces is the airway. Changes in airway pressure are reflected by corresponding changes in pleural pressure that in turn affect pressures in all four chambers of the heart, as well as the intrathoracic vessels. The actual distending pressure or transmural pressure of these structures is equal to the intracavitary pressure minus the intrapleural pressure. Significant errors in PAOP measurement can occur with posi-

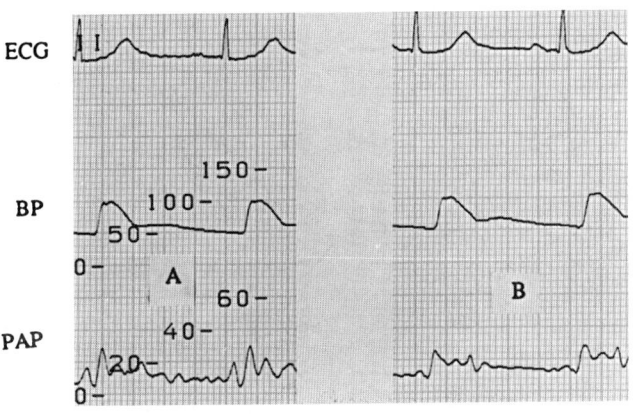

Fig. 77-8. A, Diastolic overshoot from catheter fling. B, After repositioning.

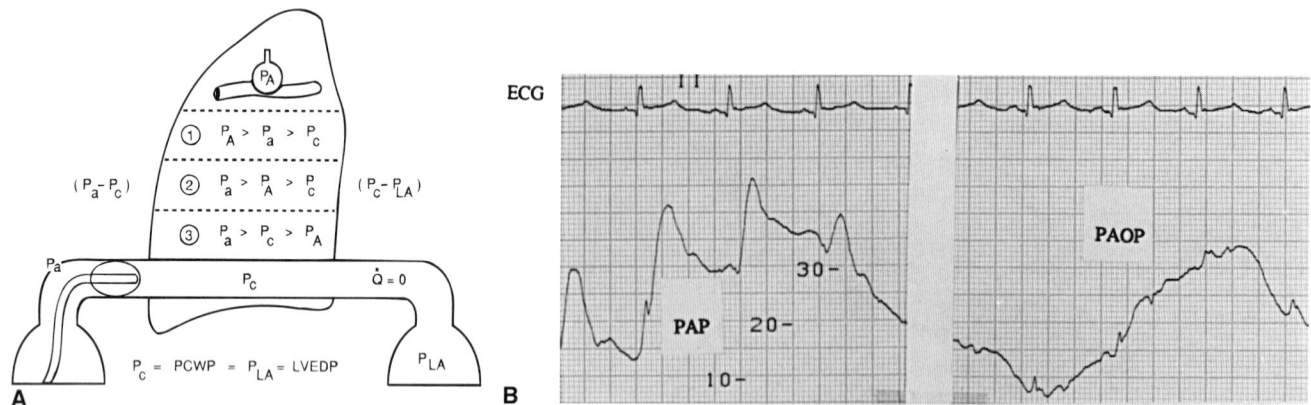

Fig. 77–9. A, The principle of the wedge pressure measurement. The lung is partitioned into three zones based on the relationship between the alveolar pressure (P_A), the mean pulmonary artery pressure (P_a), and the pulmonary capillary pressure (P_c). PAOP is an accurate measure of LAP only when P_c) exceeds P_A (zone III). (From Marino, P.: The ICU Book. Philadelphia, Lea & Febiger, 1991, p. 112.) B, Non-zone III placement of the PA catheter tip in a patient with peak airway pressure (PAP) of 50 cm H_2O and PEEP of 10 cm H_2O. PAP and PAOP increase during inspiration. Catheter was placed prior to the onset of ARDS.

tive pressure ventilation, particularly if the tip of the PA catheter is in zone I,[62] where the intraalveolar pressure exceeds the pulmonary arterial and venous pressures (Palv > Pa > Pv) and thus PAOP reflects intra-alveolar pressure during inspiration. In zone II, the PAP exceeds the alveolar pressure, which in turn exceeds the pulmonary venous pressure (Pa > Palv > Pv). Only in zone III are the intravascular pressures always larger than the intra-alveolar pressures (Pa > Pv > Palv), and thus PAOP reflects pulmonary venous pressure and LAP (Fig. 77–9). Normally, because PA catheters are flow directed, they tend to go to zone III during placement; however, subsequent hypovolemia or the addition of high level of PEEP can change zone III or zone II or I. A catheter tip placed in zone I or II should be suspected when the venous waves are absent, PAOP exceeds PAEDP, or the respiratory variations in PAOP are greater than 50% of the change in alveolar pressure.[67]

Positive airway pressure affects the relationship between LVEDP and LVEDV because it increases pericardial pressure limits LV distensibility. It also decreases venous return and, as a result, LVEDP increases while LVEDV decreases. The more compliant the lung, the more airway pressure is transmitted.[68] Thus, to maintain transmural pressure, which is the determinant of LV filling, LVEDP has to increase (Fig. 77–10). High levels of PEEP and RV failure also can shift the interventricular septum to the left, decreasing LVEDV and compliance and increasing LVEDP.[52] As a guide to the estimation of transmural pressure, it has been recommended to subtract 50% of the value of PEEP from the LVEDP with compliant lungs and 25% with noncompliant lungs.[52,54,69] During unobstructed spontaneous ventilation, pleural pressure is equal to atmospheric pressure at end expiration and measured LVEDP is equal to transmural LVEDP.[51,54] In patients with noncompliant lungs or with partial inspiratory obstruction, intrapleural pressure is negative during inspiration and the PAOP and CVP can be underestimated significantly if determinations are made during inspiration or averaged during an entire respiratory cycle, giving a false impression of hypovolemia. In patients with airway obstruction during expiration, however, particularly if they are tachypneic and have air trapping, auto PEEP can occur and falsely elevate end expiratory PAOP, giving a false impression of hypervolemia (Fig. 77–11 and 77–12). To minimize the effect of respiratory variations on PAOP, measurements are taken at the end of expiration, i.e., the highest PAOP during spontaneous ventilation without auto PEEP and the minimum PAOP during positive pressure ventilation (Fig. 77–13). The digital display usually gives an average value of the pressure during the entire respiratory cycle, and it is necessary to identify the phases of respiration on the analog display before reading the value of the pressure. When both inspiratory and expiratory obstruction are present, it becomes practically impossible to identify the

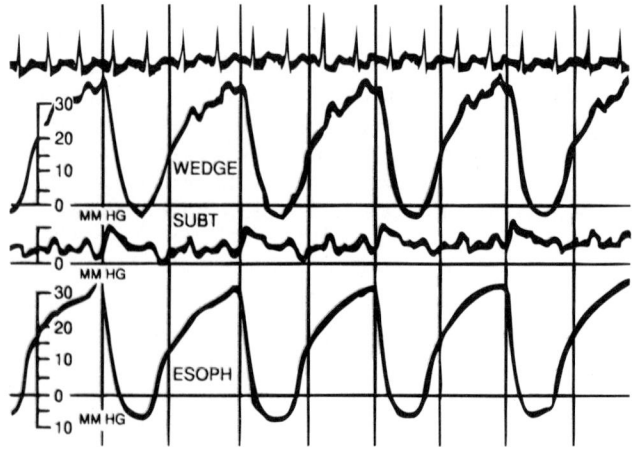

Fig. 77–10. Simultaneous tracing of the measured pulmonary artery occlusive pressure (PAOP) and esophageal pressure. Electrical subtraction demonstrates actual transmural pressure with airway obstruction. (From Rice D. L., et al.: Wedge pressure measurement in obstructive pulmonary disease. Chest 66:628, 1974.)

PITFALLS IN HEMODYNAMIC AND RESPIRATORY MONITORING

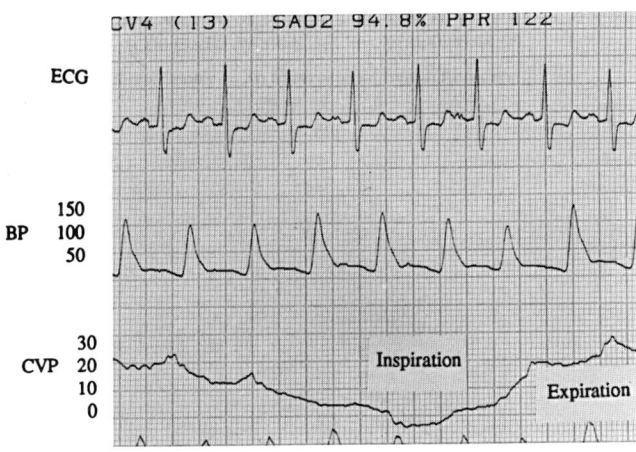

Fig. 77-11. Central venous pressure (CVP) variation in a spontaneously breathing patient with both inspiratory and expiratory obstruction. The CVP varies between −6 and +24 mm Hg. The monitor reads CVP of 13 mm Hg. BP, blood pressure.

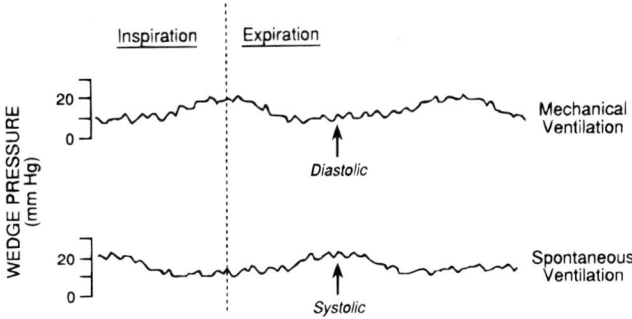

Fig. 77-13. Respiratory variations in pulmonary artery occlusive pressure tracing during spontaneous ventilation and positive pressure ventilation. The true transmural pressure is at the end of expiration, which corresponds to the systolic recording during spontaneous breathing, and diastolic recording mechanical ventilation. (From Marino, P.: The ICU Book. Philadelphia, Lea & Febiger, 1991, p. 117.)

point at which intrapleural pressure is equal to atmospheric pressure.

Technical Problems

Several technical difficulties may arise during the use of a PA catheter. Kinking of the catheter can occur where it exits from the introducer sheath, particularly when the right subclavian of left internal jugular veins are used for access. This problem is caused by the relative stiffness of the sheath and its excessive length when used in the shorter patient. Other than the appearance on chest radio-

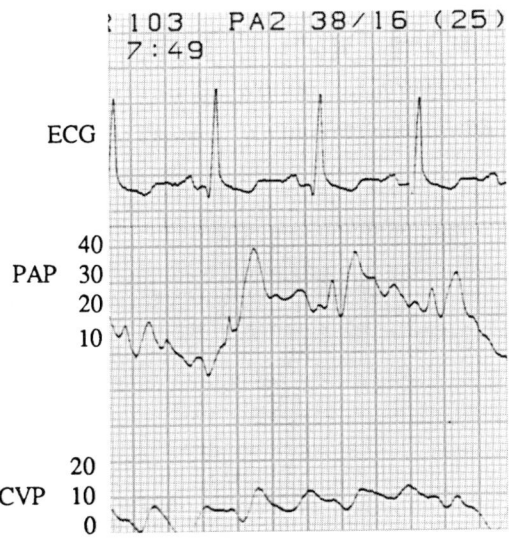

Fig. 77-12. Spontaneously breathing patient with inspiratory retractions due to noncompliant lungs. The variations in pulmonary artery (PA) pressure and central venous pressure (CVP) are parallel. PA pressure at end expiration (real filling pressure in the absence of air trapping) is 38/20, compatible with fluid overload. PA pressure during inspiration is 20/8. The average pressure given by the monitor is 38/16.

graphs, a clue to this problem is a damped pressure tracing and difficulty injecting through or aspirating from the PA or CVP ports. This situation results in overestimation of CVP, PAP, and PAOP, so that fluid overload may be incorrectly diagnosed.

Large fluctuations in pressure reading may simply reflect catheter fling with each cardiac contraction,[66] and may be decreased in magnitude by repositioning the catheter. The catheter tip may also be against the wall of the PA, resulting in a damped PAP and hindering of backflow. Distal placement of the catheter may totally occlude the arteriole where it is located, resulting in a permanent wedge tracing while the balloon is deflated and/or difficulty in aspirating blood from the PA lumen. Keeping the catheter in this position predisposes to pulmonary infarction or PA perforation, particularly if the balloon is inflated.

Overwedging can occur when the diameter of the inflated balloon exceeds the diameter of the vessel in which it is located, resulting in occlusion of the catheter tip by the wall of the pulmonary artery or the overinflated balloon. Because the catheter usually is connected to a continuous flushing device, the pressure in the catheter lumen gradually rises, resulting in a steadily rising pressure wave on the screen and a falsely elevated PAOP. To avoid this problem, it is helpful to confirm that the pressure tracing is a PAP tracing by timing the PAP waves relative to the ECG before slow inflation of the balloon. Inflation should stop if there is resistance or as soon as the shape of the PAP curve changes to either a venous waveform (see Fig. 77-3) or a straight, usually ascending line indicating overwedging. In the latter case, the catheter should be withdrawn 2 to 3 cm before subsequent inflation.

When the diameter of the inflated balloon is slightly smaller than that of the arteriole in which it is located, incomplete wedging occurs, giving falsely high readings. This problem can be avoided by making sure that the systolic peak of the PA pressure disappears completely at maximal balloon inflation. A large peak that persists beyond the normal position of the PA systolic peak is not attributable to incomplete wedging, but results from un-

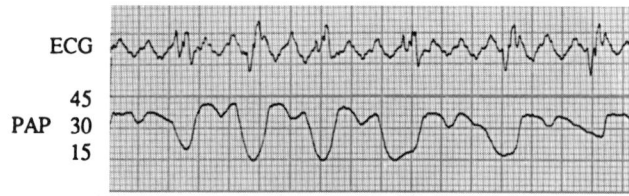

Fig. 77-14. Tracing from patient in cardiorespiratory failure. The pulmonary artery catheter tip falls in the right ventricle with each breath during intermittent positive-pressure ventilation (IPPV). PAP at the end of expiration is 36/30. The monitor reads 36/15. Note the atrial flutter.

masking of prominent a or V waves. With rapid heart rate, if the P wave is not apparent on the ECG, the V and a wave can be difficult to distinguish.

Misplacement of the catheter tip in the RV should be suspected when the PAEDP is lower than the mean CVP (Fig. 77-14). Arrhythmias secondary to direct stimulation of the RV tend to occur and hypovolemia may be diagnosed erroneously while cardiac output measurements are likely to be incorrect. Spontaneous migration of the PA catheter tip in the RV is not uncommon in patients with pulmonary hypertension and dilated pulmonary arteries, but it can also occur anytime the catheter is pulled back inadvertently.

Pulmonary artery occlusive pressure is sometimes used as a measure of pulmonary capillary hydrostatic pressure (Pc). Even in zone III, however, PAOP is not a measure of Pc because during flow, Pc is greater than LAP or PAOP. The gradient between Pc and PAOP depends on flow and resistance to flow in the pulmonary veins (Rv), which contributes about 40% of total PVR in animals.[70] In normal subjects, Rv is low and PAOP is nearly equal to Pc. Transmural pressure is the determinant of preload dependent edema formation. In ARDS, Pc can be more than twice the PAOP, and therapy should be tailored accordingly.[71]

With the numerous sources of error associated with PAOP measurement, it is not surprising to find that such errors are reported in 30% of cases.[71,72] Similarly, errors in interpretation are reported 20% of the time.[65] Because of the susceptibility of PAOP to error, a change of more than 4 mm Hg must occur before it is considered significant.[73]

Mechanical complications associated with placement of PA catheters are addressed elsewhere in this book. Complications that may not necessarily be related to catheter insertion but are included here for completion are pulmonary infarction, sepsis, arrhythmias, and thrombocytopenia. Continuous attention to the pulmonary artery pressure waveform, particularly during balloon inflation, as well as avoidance of prolonged inflation are essential to minimize catheter-related complications. When reviewing chest radiographs, it is important to check the position of the tip of the pulmonary catheter to avoid misplacement.

Thermodilution Cardiac Output Measurement

Contrary to continuous invasive BP monitoring, the common thermodilution cardiac output (TDCO) techniques are intermittent, and frequent measurements are time consuming and can possibly result in fluid overload. Although new methods of continuous CO measurement have been described,[124] they are not widely available at present. Thus, a major associated source of error comes from lack of awareness of the changes in CO that occur in between measurements. Any indirect indication of change in CO (change in heart rhythm, blood pressure, urine output, etc.) should prompt a repetition of the measurement. Accuracy is the relationship between measured CO and the actual CO obtained by another technique known to be the gold standard, although precision or reproducibility determines the number of times a CO measurement must be repeated for the average to be accurate. It also determines how much difference should be between two measurements to achieve significance.

The TDCO measurement depends on the ability of the instrument to determine a baseline blood temperature and the magnitude and rate of temperature change following the rapid injection of a bolus of fluid of known volume and temperature. The thermistor must be floating freely in the lumen; if it is stuck against the wall of the PA, it might not sense changes in temperature occurring in the blood, giving a falsely elevated CO determination. In principle, ice water injectates increase the accuracy and precision of CO measurement. They may, however, induce changes in heart rate causing acute and brief changes in CO, and the value obtained nay not be representative of the steady state.[74,75] Some studies did not show that iced saline improved accuracy,[64] and there is presently no advantage in using it in adults.[76] The injectate temperature must be entered accurately in the CO computer, and in-line temperature measurement is superior to that of a water bath kept under the same conditions as the injectate, because it eliminates the effect of warming that occurs while the operator is holding the injectate syringe awaiting the signal to inject. If the temperature probe is in ice and the injectate is allowed to warm up, the CO will increase by 3% for each degree of change.

An injectate volume larger than the programmed volume results in a falsely low CO and vice versa.[74] Because accuracy depends on a stable baseline blood temperature,[2,77] measurement of CO during rapid infusion of a fluid at a temperature different from the blood temperature through the sideport or even a peripheral intravenous line may affect accuracy, particularly if the rate of infusion varies during the measurement period.[78] Similar changes in baseline temperature occur in the immediate postcardiopulmonary bypass period.[2,79] When such changes occur after the signal to inject is given, the computer may spontaneously initiate a CO measurement that will obviously be wrong.

When a four-lumen PA catheter is placed through a standard 15-cm sheath in a short patient, both the CVP and infusion ports may be inside the sheath. As a result, rapid infusion of fluids in the sideport or infusion port increases the pressure within the sheath and thus in the CVP lumen, causing falsely elevated CVP readings[2] (Figs. 77-15 and 77-16). Also, when a CO measurement is performed, some retrograde flow of the injectate may occur in the sideport, resulting in a smaller amount of indicator reaching the

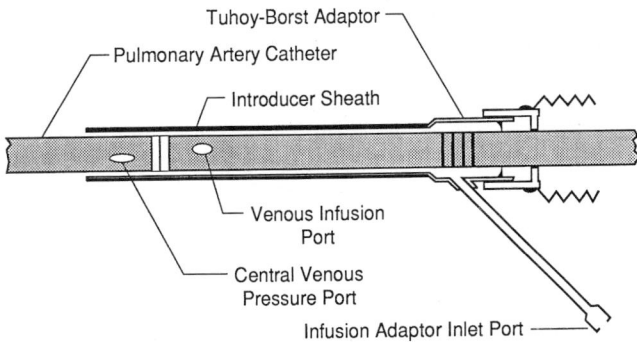

Fig. 77–15. Pulmonary artery catheter with the central venous pressure and infusion ports within the introducer sheath. (Courtesy of M. Bazaral.)

Table 77–4. Sources of Error in Thermodilution (TD) Cardiac Output (CO)

TDCO < True CO	TDCO > True CO
Tricuspid insufficiency	Right-to-left shunt
Injectate volume > volume	Left-to-right shunt
Used for calculation	Injectate volume < volume used for calculation
? Low CO	Thermistor stuck to the wall of the pulmonary artery
	Temperature of injectate > temperature used for calculation
	Injectate lumen within the sheath

thermistor, hence, overestimating CO.[80] A falsely low CO is obtained when mixing of indicator fluid is inadequate, such as occurs in tricuspid regurgitation, in which the peak is low because a small amount of indicator reaches the thermistor, but washout is prolonged because of delayed appearance of the indicator.[81] Conversely, both right-to-left and left-to-right intracardiac shunts are associated with falsely high CO.[76] Some studies have shown that very low CO states can cause a long delay before the indicator reaches the thermistor, sometimes resulting in an underestimate of the already low CO.[80,82] The results are inconsistent, however, and low output values should be treated as such, although the value of the CO may be inaccurate.

Stroke volume changes with the phases of the respiratory cycle and CO measurements performed at different phases[83] give different results, each of which is accurate within the limits described previously at the time it is measured. Respiratory variations result in 10 to 50% change in CO. Repeating measurements at the same point of the respiratory cycle improves reproducibility at the expense of accuracy.[84] Accuracy is improved by averaging measurements taken at various phases of the respiratory cycle.

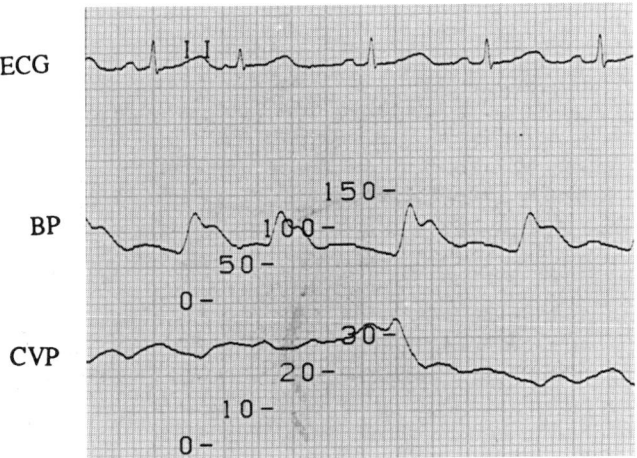

Fig. 77–16. Decrease in central venous pressure (CVP) occurs after stopping the infusion of 5 ml per minute through the sideport. (Courtesy of M. Bazaral.)

Using probability calculus, it was found that the average of two injections has a 50% chance of being within 5% of the true CO. Three injections have an 89% chance to be within 10% and a 70% chance to be within 5% of the true CO.[85]

From the clinical point of view, it may be better to inject the indicator at the same point in the respiratory cycle in order to improve reproducibility and follow trends. Variations in stroke volume and heart rate also occur with many arrhythmias (atrial fibrillation or flutter with variable atrioventricular block, premature ventricular or atrial contractions, etc.), and the measured CO reflects the heart rate and stroke volume at the time the measurement was made rather than the actual average CO. These conditions are characterized by poor reproducibility.

The first CO measurement, as well as serial measurements differing by more than 10 to 15%, should be disregarded because they often are unreliable.[75,86] A minimum of 13% change needs to occur between the average of three determinations for the difference to be significant (Table 77-4).[87]

Derived Parameters

The error on values derived mathematically from pressure, heart rate, and CO measurements usually is greater than the error made on each of the factors used in the calculation. An important physiologic parameter that is estimated in part by reading pressures and in part by calculation is afterload. By definition, afterload is the force resisting muscle shortening during contraction.[88] It is altered by factors affecting the peripheral circulation, as well as the left ventricle. Vascular resistance, an important determinant of afterload, is calculated from Ohm's law. The arterial diameter changes, however, with each systole and diastole, and thus, resistance to flow changes continuously. In the pulmonary circulation, recruitment of blood vessels can result from increases in blood flow or pressure resulting in an overall decrease in pulmonary vascular resistance (PVR). Because resistance is calculated and not measured, errors in pressure and output measurement affect its accuracy. To obtain systemic vascular resistance (SVR), the pressure gradient is between the mean systemic arterial pressure (MAP) and CVP. Normally, MAP is much larger than CVP and a small error in either one results only in a small error in SVR. When PVR is calculated, however, the pressure gradient is between mean PAP and PAOP, both

Table 77-5. Vascular Resistance in Three Patients

	Patient A	Patient B	Patient C
Body surface area (m^2)	1.73	2.25	1.35
Systemic vascular resistance (SVR) (dyne/cm/sec^{-5})	1067	820	1367
SVR index (SVR × m^2)	1846	1846	1846
Pulmonary vascular resistance (dyne/cm/sec^{-5})	142	109	182
PVR index (SVR × m^2)	246	246	246

of which normally are low. An error in measuring either pressure, particularly the more sensitive PAOP (incomplete wedge, overwedge, tip in zone I) results in large error in PVR. With respiratory variations or when the transducer connected to the tip of the PA catheter is incorrectly zeroed or leveled, PAP and PAOP are affected equally and the calculated PVR is not affected.

In some medical centers, absolute values of physiologic parameters are used instead of indices. A problem of interpretation arises anytime the patient being evaluated is significantly smaller or larger than average. To illustrate this point, we consider three hypothetic patients with identical hemodynamic profiles but with different body surface areas (BSA). Assuming that all three patients have the following: cardiac index (CI) is 2.6; MAP is 70; PAP is 23; and PAOP is 15, the standard formulae below give the resistance values shown in Table 77-5.

$$SVR = (MAP - CVP) : CO \times 80$$
$$SVRI = SVR \times BSA$$
$$PVR = (PAP - PAOP) CO \times 80$$
$$PVRI = PVR \times BSA$$

All three patients have the same CI and pressures and thus identical resistance indices. The absolute value of resistance, however, gives the false impression that patient A is more vasoconstricted than patient B and more dilated than patient C. Patient B and C could, therefore, be treated inappropriately if interventions are based on SVR and PVR.

New technologies are being developed to allow continuous measurement of CO without the need for operator intervention.[127] Their availability for clinical use will enhance the ability to identify early changes in the hemodynamic function and to intervene in a timely fashion.

Mixed Venous Oxygen Saturation

It is important to remember that normal ranges for pressure and CI are only for reference. A CI within the normal range does not necessarily indicate adequate myocardial function, because it may be obtained at the expense of high filling pressures or tachycardia, whereas peripheral distribution of blood flow may not match regional needs resulting in regional hypoxia. Mixed venous O$_2$ saturation (Svo$_2$) has been used as an indicator of adequacy of oxygen delivery to peripheral tissues.[89] Normally, 25% of the delivered oxygen is extracted, resulting, under normal pH, temperature, and hemoglobin concentration, in an Svo$_2$ of 75% and Pvo$_2$ of 40 mm Hg. A decrease in CI is accompanied by an increase in oxygen extraction and a decrease in Svo$_2$.[89,90] The Svo$_2$ value, however, reflects global oxygen utilization and is insensitive to regional imbalance in O$_2$ supply and demand, so that a normal Svo$_2$ does not rule out regional ischemia. Moreover, the critically ill patient may be unable to increase oxygen extraction when CI decreases, making oxygen consumption delivery dependent.[91,92] Other indicators of organ function, including measurement of blood lactic acid concentration, may help in this determination, but similar limitations also apply. If a region of the body is totally ischemic, lactic acid is produced but is not released in the circulation and therefore goes undetected. It actually starts appearing in the venous blood when blood flow to that area improves. Moreover, when ischemia involves only a small amount of tissues, the amount of lactic acid released in the venous blood draining those tissues is diluted by blood draining nonischemic areas, resulting in a nondetectable increase in the overall lactic acid level.[76]

When changes in Svo$_2$ are used to indicate changes in CI, it must be assumed that arterial oxygen content and oxygen consumption are constant. A mixed venous sample must be obtained from the PA, not from the RA,[93] and presence of a ventricular or atrial septal defect invalidates the results. Errors in determination of Svo$_2$ occur when blood is withdrawn quickly from a catheter advanced too peripherally, resulting in aspiration of partially arterialized blood retrograde from the pulmonary capillaries.[89] Some PA catheters include a fiberoptic bundle that allows continuous measurement of Svo$_2$. Once properly calibrated, such devices correlate highly with in vitro saturation measurement (R = 95%) and drift about 2% per day. Accuracy is not affected by hemoglobin concentration, temperature, or CO.[94] As with other physiologic indicators, looking at trends is at least as important as looking at absolute values. Slow aspiration of blood from the catheter tip during wedging allows recovery of arterialized blood that can be used to determine alveolar Po$_2$ in that particular area of the lung. This determination is not, however, a valid indicator of overall lung function if the lungs are nonhomogeneous.[60]

Right Ventricular Ejection Fraction

Pulmonary artery catheters with a fast response thermistor are used to measure right ventricular ejection fraction (RVEF). Improper positioning of the injection port in the RA and thermistor in the PA can affect the accuracy of this technique.[95] Underestimation of RVEF occurs with hypovolemia and when the distance between the injection lumen and the tricuspid value is greater than 5 cm. An increased distance between the thermistor and the pulmonic valve seems less crucial in large hearts,[96] but it can give falsely low values with smaller hearts. With tricuspid regurgitation, error results from the fact that only forward flow is measured.[97] Arrhythmias, pacemakers,[98] or low amplitude QRS complexes that are not recognized by the RVEF computer can also invalidate the results. A correlation factor of r = 0.74 was found between RVEF and the ejection fraction obtained by biplane ventriculography.

Noninvasive Blood Gas Measurement

Assessment of gas exchange is an integral part of monitoring in the critical care unit. Until recently, such measurements required collection of a blood sample and were done only at intervals that ranged from several minutes to hours depending on the acuity of the situation and therapeutic interventions. Recent technical advances allow continuous measurement of blood gases invasively (see section on mixed venous oxygen saturation) or noninvasively by oximetry and capnography. Optode technology has facilitated the development of devices that continuously measure arterial blood gases.

Oximetry

Although transcutaneous oximetry ($TcPo_2$) has proven reliable in the neonate, it yields variable results in adults because the thickness of the epidermis limits diffusion of oxygen. When the electrode is placed on a well-perfused area of the skin in patients with normal CI, $TcPo_2$ is a reasonably accurate reflection of Pao_2.[99,100] Diffusion and thus accuracy in adults improves when heat is applied to the skin around the electrode, but this technique introduces the risk of burn injury. Because of its dependence on skin perfusion, a decrease in CI below 2.0 L/min/m² causes $TcPo_2$ to underestimate Pao_2[100] and to vary directly with the CI.

Pulse oximetry (Spo_2) has achieved more widespread success and has been considered by Severinghaus and Astrup as "the most significant technologic advance ever made in monitoring the well being and safety of patients during anesthesia, recovery, and critical care."[101] It has, however, its own limitations and sources of error. Commercially available pulse oximeters measure absorption of light at two wavelengths by oxygenated and reduced hemoglobin. Arterial blood is identified by its pulsatile nature and continuous signals are assumed to come from venous blood or pigments in the tissues[102] and are thus rejected. To improve rejection of signals related artifacts, several pulsations have to be sensed by the instrument before it gives a reading, requiring usually 5 to 8 seconds.

The choice of a gold standard for comparison of results obtained from various pulse oximeters is important. Blood gas analyzers, which measure Po_2 and then calculate So_2 based on pH and temperature, are subject to errors. In vitro measurements with multiwavelength oximeters should be used instead for that purpose.[103] When blood gas analyzers are compared to Co-oximeter in healthy volunteers, an accuracy of 1 to 2% and a precision of 1 to 3% are obtained.[103,104] The Sao_2 value, however, can be significantly lower than Spo_2 if oxygen consumption occurs to a significant degree before the sample is analyzed.[105] Accuracy of pulse oximeters compared to in vitro Co-oximeters has been found to be within 2 to 3% (SD),[106,107] provided Sao_2 is kept above 70%.[108,109] Inaccuracy at low levels of saturation is attributable to the fact that pulse oximeters are calibrated by inducing hypoxia down to a saturation of 70% in normal volunteers. Because it is unsafe to use lower levels of saturation to complete the calibration, the curve is extrapolated. Oximeters have a nonlinear output, however, and therefore errors are introduced in the process of extrapolation. Inaccuracy at low levels of Sao_2 is not a major problem during normal use in adults, because such levels are not acceptable and corrective steps are taken to increase Sao_2 before they are reached. The use of pulse oximeters in neonates and patients with cyanotic heart disease may, however, mandate a greater degree of accuracy and precision at low levels of saturation.

Two common determinants of accuracy in the evaluation of pulse oximeters are bias, i.e., the mean difference between Sao_2 and Spo_2, and precision, i.e., the standard deviation of the bias. Study of nonhomogeneous adult population found the overall bias was 2.7%. A great deal of variation occurred, however, under certain circumstances, and bias increased to 5.1% at Sao_2 lower than 90% compared to 1.7% above 90%. Bias was 3.3% in blacks compared to 2.2% in whites, and errors larger than 4% occurred more frequently in blacks (27%) compared to whites (11%). Overall, it is necessary for Spo_2 to be greater than 92% in whites and 95% in blacks to predict an adequate Sao_2 reliably. Inaccurate readings were not associated with hypotension, hypothermia, or acid base abnormality.[110] Although in some studies pigmentation was not a cause of inaccuracy,[111] in others, more technical problems were noted with darker pigmentation.[112] A more important limitation of pulse oximeters relates to the shape of the oxygen-hemoglobin dissociation curve, which is almost flat above a Pao_2 of 90 mm Hg or an Sao_2 of 90%. As a result, large changes in Pao_2 can occur with minimal changes in Sao_2. Thus, important changes in pulmonary gas exchanges, as well as hyperoxia, can go unnoticed. The presence of significant amounts of abnormal hemoglobin interfere with accuracy. Carboxyhemoglobin has light absorption characteristics similar to oxyhemoglobin and leads to overestimation of Sao_2, whereas methemoglobin absorbs equal amounts of light at each of the two commonly used wavelengths, resulting in a saturation reading of 85%, which underestimates the true Sao_2.

A serious problem can result from the response time of pulse oximeters, which is longer during desaturation than resaturation, and some instruments continue to show near normal Spo_2 values when Sao_2 is 40 to 70%.[113] The same instrument was also slower to respond and less accurate when a finger probe was used instead of an ear probe, suggesting a problem with the signal from the finger (slower circulation, vasoconstriction) or the probe rather than with the instrument itself. When severe hypoxemia is produced acutely in normal volunteers, 10 to 20 seconds are necessary for detection by an ear probe and 24 to 35 seconds by a finger probe. This response is significantly faster, however, than that recorded with transcutaneous oximetry (57 seconds).[114]

A more frequent complaint is that pulse oximeters are unable to interpret a signal at the most inopportune moment, including low flow states, vasoconstriction, severe hypoxemia, and agitation. Artifact can be introduced by repetitive motion or vibration during patient transport,[115] electrocautery, and ambient light, particularly when it flickers.[116] To compensate for the variable intensity of the pulsatile signal, automatic amplification of the signal occurs. Thus, the lower the signal, the more the amplification, the more the noise and possibility of error. When the

Capnography

Capnography is the continuous, noninvasive measurement and recording of carbon dioxide in expired gas. In patients with normal pulmonary function, the early part of exhalation consists of dead space gases, usually free of CO_2. As exhalation progresses, CO_2 starts to appear, and at the end of expiration, the exhaled gas is assumed to consist entirely of alveolar gases (Fig. 77-17).[118] The Pa_{CO_2} reflects the overall CO_2 elimination process irrespective of spatial and temporal variations, whereas Pet_{CO_2} reflects Pa_{CO_2} in the alveoli that empty last and reach the sensor right before the initiation of the next breath. In patients with normal pulmonary function, the normal gradient between Pa_{O_2} and Pet_{CO_2} is 3 to 5 mmHg.[119]

The two methods by which exhaled carbon dioxide is measured are mass spectrometry and infrared spectroscopy. The sampling of gases is either by mainstream or sidestream (Fig. 77-18).[120] Table 77-6 reviews the advantages and disadvantages of each method and device.

The use of capnography as a monitoring tool is limited by lack of correlation between Pa_{CO_2} and Pet_{CO_2}. The gradient between Pa_{CO_2} and Pet_{CO_2} is widened in situations in which ventilation/perfusion abnormalities are found, including chronic obstructive pulmonary disease, ARDS, asthma, hypovolemia, low CO states, pneumothorax, and right-to-left shunt. The gradient is also increased when the exhaled tidal volume is too small or the anatomic and apparatus dead space is too large. The exhaled volume is inadequate to washout the dead space gas. The gradient between true Pet_{CO_2} and measured Pet_{CO_2} increases with leaks in the gas sampling lines and with analyzers that are miscalibrated or have a slow response time.

In addition to these findings, Hess and colleagues dem-

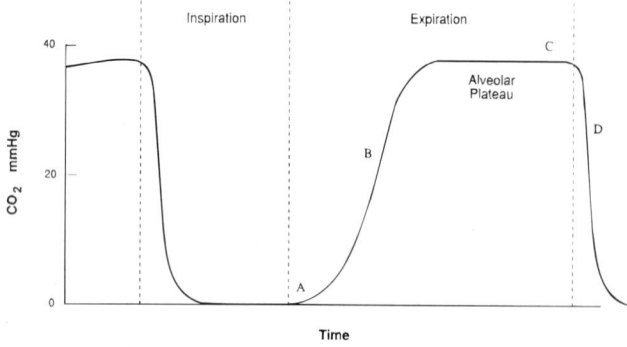

Fig. 77-17. The characteristics of the capnograph. Segment A contains air in the anatomic dead space with negligible CO_2 tension. Segment B represents a mix of dead space air and alveolar gas, also called the rapid rise segment. Segment C or "plateau phase" represents the exhalation of mixed alveolar gas. Segment D is the rapid fall off that represents the end of expiration. (Redrawn by George Morrison: Clinical Dimensions, Inc., Madison, WI, from Morley, T.: Capnography in the intensive care unit. J. Intensive Care Med., 5:209, 1990.)

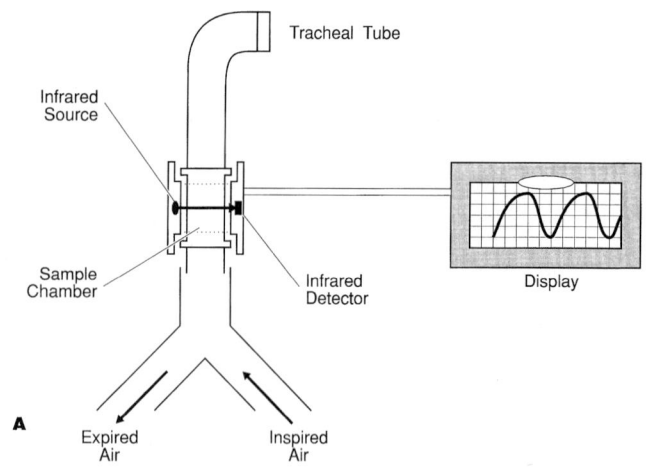

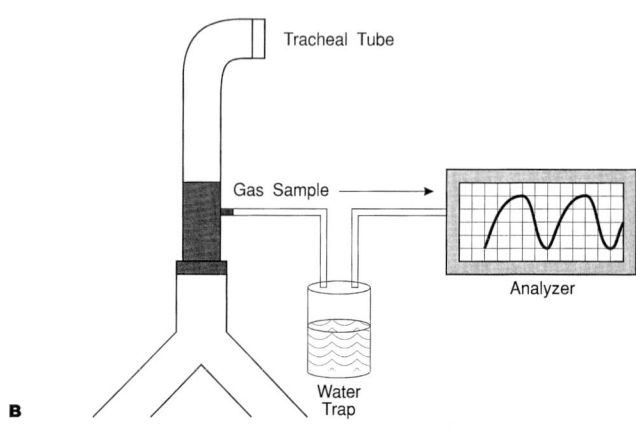

Fig. 77-18. Types of capnographs. A, A mainstream system. B, A sidestream system in which respired gases are removed at a constant rate and condensed water is removed by a trap. The gas sample is then analyzed at a site remote from the patient. (Redrawn by George Morrison: Clinical Dimensions, Inc., Madison, WI, from Morley, T.: Capnography in the intensive care unit. J. Intensive Care Med., 5:209, 1990.)

Table 77-6. Comparison of Mass Spectrometry and Infrared Capnography

Method and Device	Advantages	Disadvantages
Mass spectrometer	Central installation Oxygen as well as carbon dioxide sampling Multiple monitoring Expanded application to measure metabolic rate No correction required for water vapor when determining peak expired CO_2	Installation cost Maintenance cost Blocking of sampling lines
Infrared capnograph	Less expensive Fewer problems with secretions blocking sensor	Stand alone application Correction required for water vapor Single gas sampling

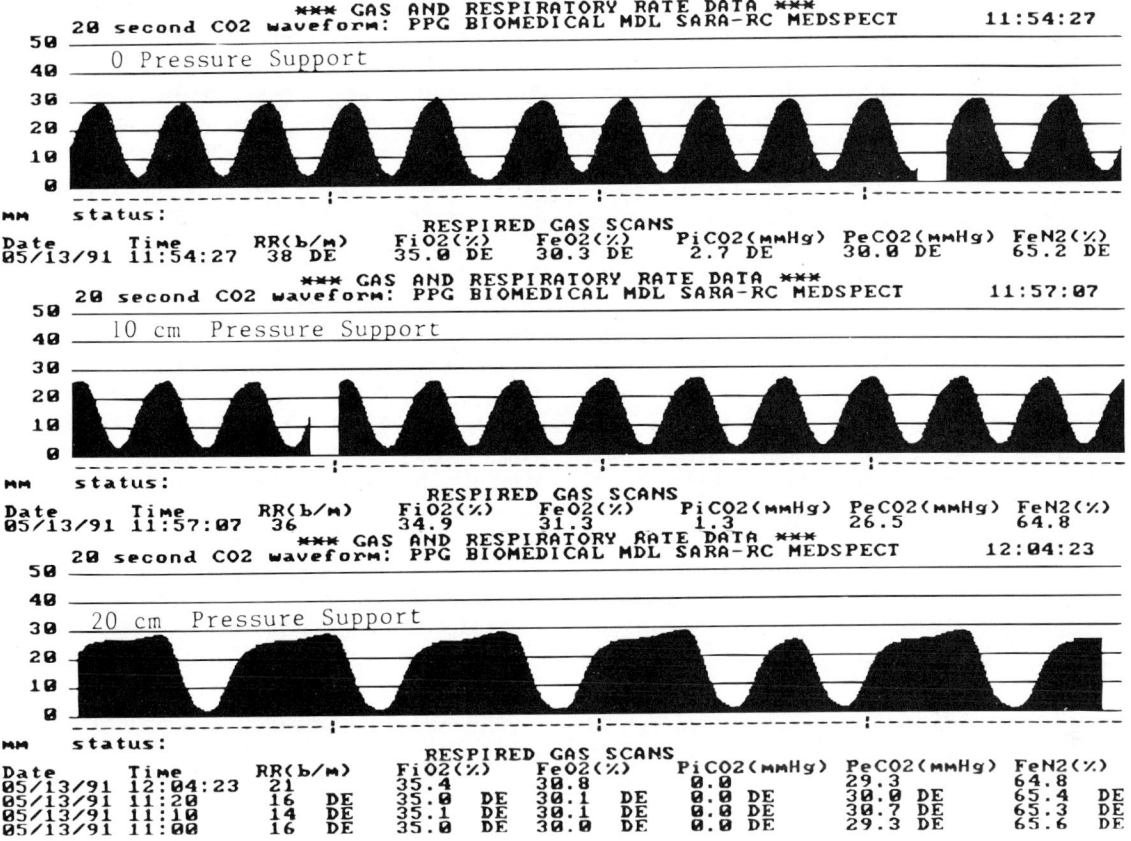

Fig. 77–19. Three different capnographic waveforms from a patient being weaned from mechanical ventilation. In the top wave, the respiratory rate (RR) is 38 breaths per minute, the P_{ICO_2} is 2.7 mm Hg, and pressure support has been increased to 0 cm. In the middle wave, the pressure support has been increased to 10 cm and the P_{ICO_2} is 1.3 mm Hg. When the pressure support was increased to 20, the respiratory rate slowed to 21 breaths per minute and the P_{ICO_2} decreased to zero.

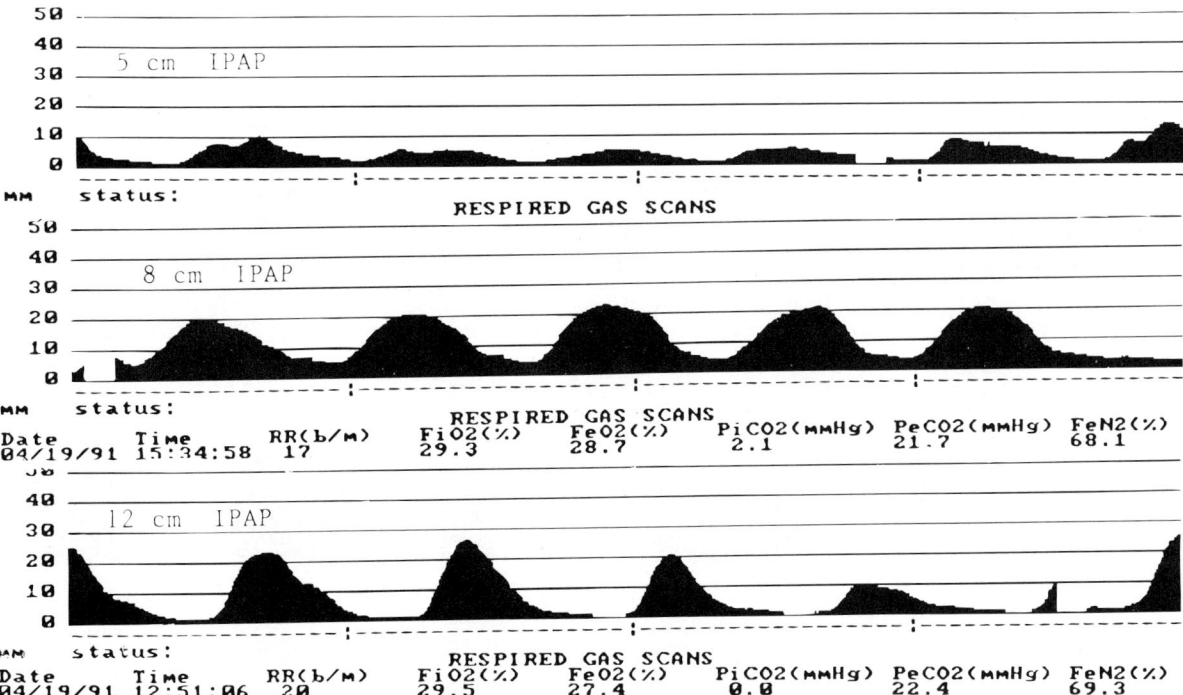

Fig. 77–20. Three waveforms from a patient with postoperative respiratory insufficiency. Biphasic positive airway pressure was administered by nasal mask. Note the poor quality of the waveform with 5 cm inspiratory pressure (top). When the inspiratory pressure was increased to 8 cm, the waveforms improved, but P_{ICO_2} was 2.1 mm Hg. When 12 cm inspiratory pressure was added, the P_{ICO_2} fell to zero. (Courtesy of E. D. Sivak, M.D.)

onstrated that although the magnitude of change in Pet_{CO_2} does correlate with the change in Pa_{CO_2}, the direction of the change does not correlate.[121]

In spite of the lack of correlation between expired and arterial P_{CO_2}, capnography has a place in the analysis of clinical conditions, including the following:

- Assessment of endotracheal tube placement and integrity
- Assessment of the adequacy of cardiopulmonary resuscitation (CPR)
- Monitoring for venous gas embolism
- Assessment of the efficiency of ventilation
- Adjustment of PEEP
- Adjustment of pressure support ventilation
- Adjustment of mask/nasal ventilation
- Detection of problems with the upper airway

The application of capnography to these situations requires clinical correlation with capnographic patterns, as well as Pet_{CO_2} values. For example, a misplaced endotracheal tube results in absent capnographic wave patterns with ventilation. A rapid fall in Pet_{CO_2} values in a presumed steady state of ventilation can be the result of a leaky airway or circuit, pulmonary embolus, decreasing CO, or pneumothorax. Adequacy of CPR can be determined by the amplitude of capnographic wave forms.[122] A rapid rise in Pet_{CO_2} can result from hypoventilation or increased CO_2 production (e.g., shivering, hyperthermia). In dogs with normal lungs, the gradient between Pa_{CO_2} and Pet_{CO_2} increases as the ventilatory mode is changed from spontaneous breathing (0.3 ± 0.04 mm Hg) to intermittent positive pressure ventilation (3.7 ± 1 mm Hg), to low frequency jet ventilation (12.6 ± 5.0 mm Hg), and lastly to high frequency jet ventilation (24.3 ± 8 mm Hg).[123] Conversely, Pet_{CO_2} may show no change at all when mixed disturbances like hypoventilation and hypovolemia occur simultaneously.[124]

The efficiency of the ventilatory process can be defined by measurement of the dead space to tidal volume ratio V_D/V_T. Obviously, the higher the ratio, the more inefficient the process of ventilation. Numerous studies have demonstrated a correlation between V_D/V_T and the difference between Pa_{CO_2} and Pet_{CO_2}.[119,125,126] A widened gradient implies inefficiency. This same logic has been applied to certain patients to adjust end expiratory pressure. In this situation, the requirement of correlation is the presence of a point of inflection on the pressure-volume curve. The "best level" of PEEP will correlate with the narrowest Pa_{CO_2}-Pet_{CO_2}.[126]

Beyond quantitation of ventilatory efficiency and adjustment of PEEP, the capnograph wave pattern is useful. Fig-

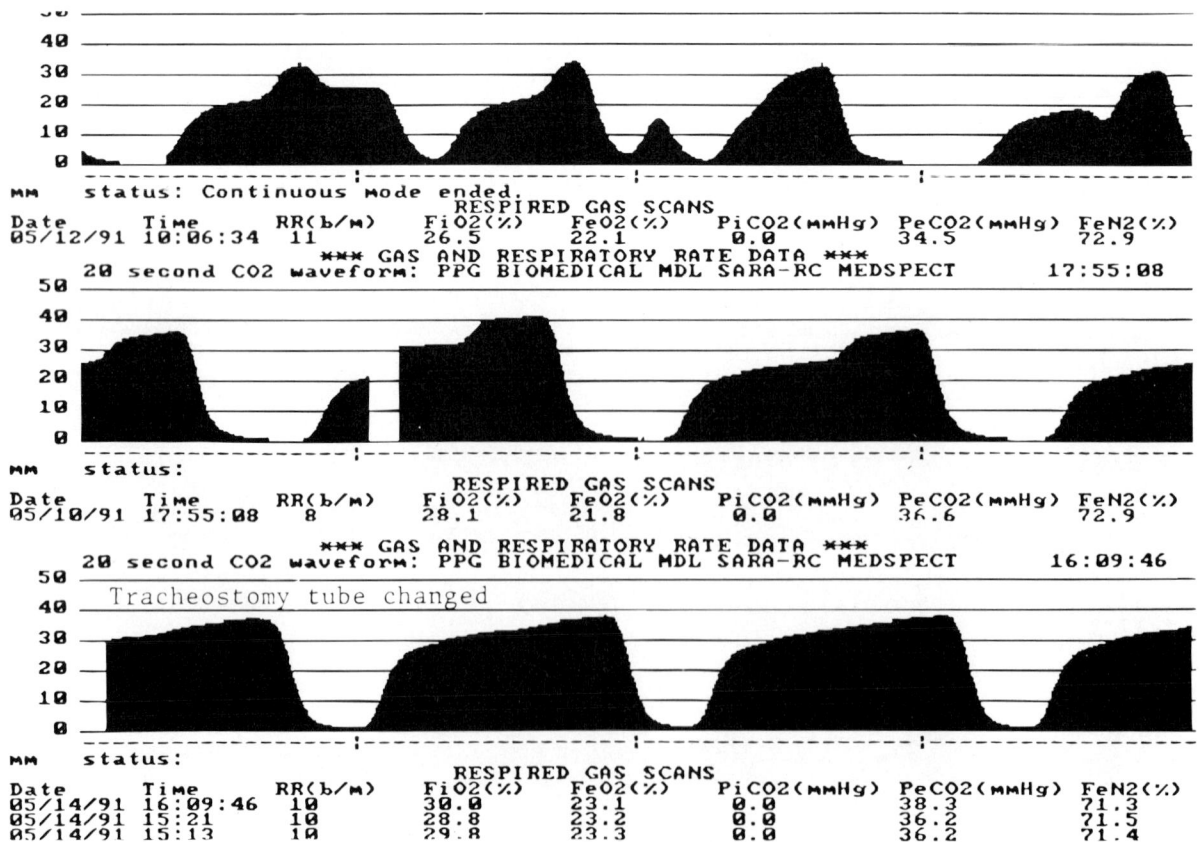

Fig. 77–21. Capnographic waveforms from a 59-year-old ventilator-dependent patient with chronic obstructive pulmonary disease. Bronchoscopy revealed narrowing of the airway distal to the end of the tracheostomy tube. Placement of a longer tube resulted in even waveforms shown in the bottom tracing. (Courtesy of E. D. Sivak, M.D.)

ure 77-19 shows three different waveforms with varying levels of pressure support. With an increase in pressure support, respiratory rate slows, but more importantly, the inspired CO_2 level decreases to zero. Similarly, the capnograph can also be used to adjust mask ventilation. In these situations, the inspiratory ventilation should be increased until CO_2 decreases to zero. Figure 77-20 shows similar effects on Pi_{CO_2} and Pet_{CO_2} with increasing inspiratory pressure delivered by nasal mask.

Problems of the upper airway can be detected in the capnographic waveform. Figure 77-21 shows a characteristic wave pattern in a patient with tracheomalacia before and after a longer tracheostomy tube was placed to bypass the area that would narrow on expiration. Figure 77-22 shows additional capnographic waveform patterns.

The principal objection to extensive use of the capnograph has been the lack of correlation between Pa_{CO_2} and Pet_{CO_2}. The foregoing discussion, however, suggests that the magnitude of the gradient, as well as proper analysis of the clinical situation, allows the clinician to evaluate the efficiency of the ventilatory process, to detect problems of leaky circuits and partial airway obstruction, and to adjust pressure support ventilation by elimination of rebreathing of carbon dioxide.

In conclusion, the ability to quantify a multitude of physiologic variables and to follow their trends has allowed the medical team to diagnose and document acute alterations in the patient's homeostasis, as well as response to therapy rapidly and efficiently. Errors in data collection, whether from equipment or operator failure, as well as erroneous interpretation of accurate data have created new sources of hazard and remain the weak link in efforts toward providing better care for critically ill patients.

REFERENCES

1. Forbes, A. D.: Medical measurement perils. J. Clin. Monit., 4:75, 1988.
2. Bazaral, M. G.: Heterogeneity of monitored parameters. In Anesthesia and the Heart Patient. Edited by G. Estafanous. Boston, Butterworth, 1989, p. 277.
3. Chatburn, R. L.: Fundamentals of metrology: Evaluation of instrument error and method agreement. Respir. Care, 35: 520, 1990.
4. Cushing, H. W.: On routine determinations of arterial tension in operating room and clinic. Boston Med. Surg. J., 148:250, 1903.
5. Gravenstein, J. S., deVries, Jr., A., Beneken, J. E. W.: Sampling intervals or clinical monitoring of variables during anesthesia. J. Clin. Monit., 5:17, 1989.
6. Horrow, J. C., and Seitman, D. T.: Electrical safety and device calibration. Anesth. Clin. North Am., 6:699, 1988.
7. Connors, A. F., McCaffree, D. R., Gray, B. A.: Evaluation of right heart catheterization in the critically ill patients without acute myocardial infarction. N. Engl. J. Med., 308:263, 1983.
8. Del Guercio, L. R. M., and Cohn, J. D.: Monitoring operative risk in the elderly. JAMA, 243:1350, 1980.
9. Rubsamen, D. S.: Continuous blood gas monitoring during cardiopulmonary bypass—How soon will it be the standard of care? (Editorial) J. Cardio. Anesth., 4:1, 1990.
10. American Society of Anesthesiologists, Director of Members: Standards of Postanesthesia Care, 1990, p. 644.
11. Pierce, E. C.: Monitoring instruments have significantly reduced anesthetic mishaps. J. Clin. Monit., 4:111, 1988.
12. Epstein, B. S.: Update-Standards of care. American Society of Anesthesiologist Newsletter, 6:18, 1991.
13. Roizen, M. F., et al.: Monitoring with two-dimensional transesophageal echocardiography. Comparison of myocardial function in patients undergoing supraceliac, suprarenal, infraceliac or infrarenal aortic occlusion. J. Vasc. Surg., 1:300, 1984.
14. Hauser, A. M., et al.: Sequence of mechanical, electrocardiographic and clinical effects of repeated coronary artery occlusion in human beings: Echocardiographic observations during coronary angioplasty. J. Am. Coll. Cardiol., 2:193, 1985.
15. Kaplan, J. A., and Wells, P. H.: Early diagnosis of myocardial ischemia using the pulmonary artery catheter. Anesth. Analg., 63:789, 1981.
16. Slogoff, S., et al.: Incidence of perioperative myocardial ischemia detected by different electrocardiographic systems. Anesthesiology, 73:1074, 1990.
17. Chaitman, B. R.: The changing role of the exercise electrocardiogram as a diagnostic and prognostic test for chronic ischemic heart disease. J. Am. Coll. Cardiol., 8:1195, 1986.

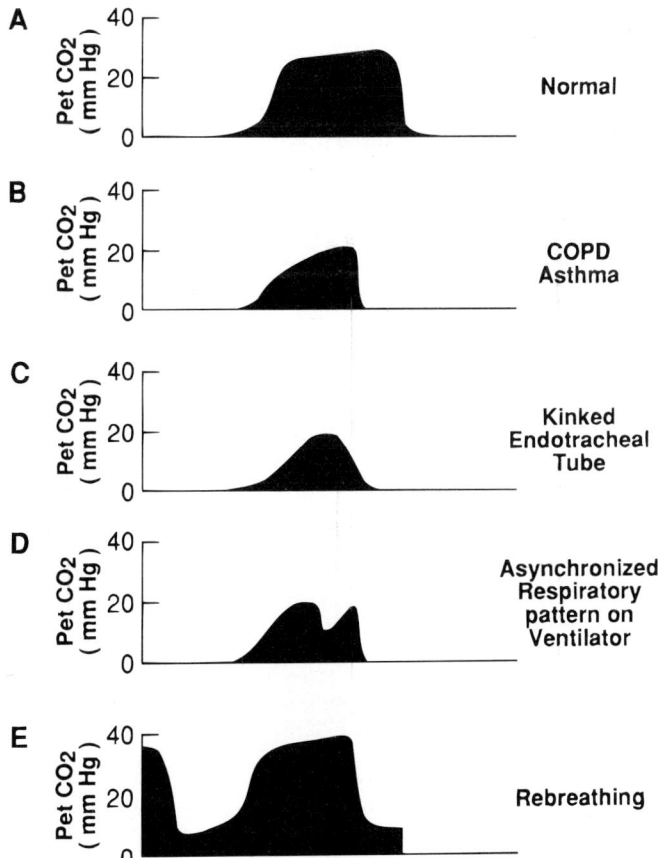

Fig. 77-22. Various capnographic waveforms are redrawn. A, A normal pattern. B, Variable emptying of alveolar units is seen with airway obstruction, as in chronic obstructive pulmonary disease or bronchospasm. C, A "kinked" endotracheal tube produces a sine wave pattern. D, Asynchronized breathing on mechanical ventilation. E, Rebreathing of CO_2 through the ventilator circuit. This pattern is seen when using pressure support at a level too low to allow full expiration and in acute bronchospasm with lower inspiratory flow rates.

18. Te-Chuan, C.: Electrocardiography in Clinical Practice. Orlando, Grune & Stratton, 1986, p. 586.
19. Palmer, C. M., et al.: Incidence of electrocardiographic changes during cesarean delivery under regional anesthesia. Anesth. Analg., 70:36, 1990.
20. Chaitman, B. R., and Hanson, J. S.: Comparative sensitivity and specificity of exercise electrocardiographic lead systems. Am. J. Cardiol., 47:1335, 1981.
21. Biagini, A., et al.: Vasospastic ischemic mechanism of frequent asymptomatic transient ST-T changes during continuous electrocardiographic monitoring in selected unstable angina patients. Am. Heart J., 103:13, 1982.
22. Chierchia, S., et al.: Impairment of myocardial perfusion and function during painless myocardial ischemia. J. Am. Coll. Cardiol., 1:924, 1983.
23. Reddy, G. V., and Schamroty, L.: The electrocardiology of right ventricular myocardial infarction. Chest, 90:756, 1987.
24. Klein, H. O., et al.: The early recognition of ventricular infarction. Diagnostic accuracy of the electrcardiographic V_4R lead. Circulation, 67:558, 1983.
25. Sheffield, L. T.: Exercise stress testing. In Heart Disease. Vol. 1. Edited by E. Braunwald. Philadelphia, W. B. Saunders, 1980, p. 257.
26. Moffitt, E.: Effects of anesthetics on intraoperative ischemia. (Abstract) Proceedings of the Annual Meeting of the Society of Cardiovascular Anesthesiologists, Montreal, April 27-30, 1986, p. 37.
27. Pichard, A. D., et al.: Coronary artery spasm and perioperative cardiac arrest. J. Thorac. Cardiovasc. Surg., 80:249, 1980.
28. Sanford, Jr., T. J., Jones, B. R., Smith, N. T.: Noninvasive blood pressure measurement. Anesth. Clin. North Am., 6:721, 1988.
29. Finnie, K. J. C., Watts, D. G., Armstrong, P. W.: Biases in the measurement of arterial pressure. Crit. Care Med., 12:965, 1984.
30. Cohn, J. N.: Blood pressure measurement in shock. Mechanism of inaccuracy in auscultatory and palpatory methods. JAMA, 199:972, 1981.
31. Hutton, P., Dye, J., Prys-Roberts, C.: An assessment of the Dinamap 845. Anesthesiology, 39:261, 1984.
32. Hla, K. M., Vokaty, K. A., Feussner, J. R.: Overestimation of diastolic blood pressure in the elderly. J. Am. Geriatr. Soc., 33:659, 1985.
33. Yelderman, M., and Ream, A. K.: Indirect measurement of mean blood pressure in the anesthetized patient. Anesthesiology, 50:253, 1979.
34. Bruner, J. M. R., et al.: Comparison of direct and indirect methods of measuring arterial blood pressure. Med. Instr., 15:11, 1981.
35. Showman, A., and Belts, E. K.: Hazard of automatic noninvasive blood pressure monitoring. Anesthesiology, 55:717, 1981.
36. Sy, W. P.: Ulnar nerve palsy possibly related to use of automatically cycled blood pressure cuff. Anesth. Analg. 60:687, 1981.
37. Boutros, A., and Albert, S.: Effect of the dynamic response of transducer-tubing system on accuracy of direct pressure measurement in patients. Crit. Care. Med., 11:124, 1983.
38. Bazaral, M. G., Nacht, A., Estafanous, F. G.: Radial artery pressures compared to subclavian artery pressure during coronary artery surgery. Cleve. Clin. J. Med., 55:448, 1988.
39. Rushmer, R. F.: Cardiovascular dynamics. Philadelphia, W. B. Saunders, 1976, p. 179.
40. Bazaral, M. G., et al.: Comparison of brachial and radial arterial pressure monitoring in patients undergoing coronary artery bypass surgery. Anesthesiology, 73:38, 1990.
41. Gardner, R. M.: Direct blood pressure measurement—dynamic response requirements. Anesthesiology, 54:227, 1981.
42. Rothe, C. F., and Kim, K. C.: Measuring systolic arterial blood pressure. Crit. Care Med., 8:683, 1988.
43. Swan, H. J. C.: Central venous pressure monitoring is an outmoded procedure of limited practical value. In Ingelfinger, F. J., et al. (Eds.): Controversies in Internal Medicine. Philadelphia, W. B. Saunders, 1974, p. 185.
44. Forrester, J. S., et al.: Filling pressures in right and left sides of the heart in acute myocardial infarction. A reappraisal of central venous pressure monitoring. N. Engl. J. Med., 285:190, 1971.
45. Samii, K., Conseiller, C., Viars, P.: Central venous pressure and pulmonary wedge pressure. Arch. Surg., 111:1122, 1976.
46. Braunwald, E., Ross, J., Sonnenblick, E. H.: Mechanisms of Contraction of the Normal and Failing Heart. 2nd Ed. Boston, Little, Brown, 1976.
47. Beaupre, P. N., et al.: Does pulmonary artery occlusion pressure adequately reflect left ventricular filling during anesthesia and surgery. Anesthesiology, 59:A3, 1983.
48. Hansen, M. D., et al.: Poor correlation between pulmonary wedge pressure and left ventricular end diastolic volume after coronary artery bypass graft surgery. Anesthesiology, 64:764, 1986.
49. Harizi, R. C., Bianco, J. A., Alpert, J. S.: Diastolic function of the heart in clinical cardiology. Arch. Intern. Med., 148:99, 1988.
50. Benumof, J. L.: Anesthesia for Thoracic Surgery. 1st Ed. Philadelphia, W. B. Saunders, 1987.
51. Carlile, P. V.: Pitfalls in the interpretation of hemodynamic data. Prog. Crit. Care Med., 2:69, 1985.
52. Jardin, F., et al.: Influence of positive end-expiratory pressure on left ventricular performance. N. Engl. J. Med., 304:387, 1981.
53. Donovan, K. L.: Invasive monitoring and support of the circulation. Clin. Anesth., 3:909, 1985.
54. O'Quin, R., and Marini, J. J.: Pulmonary artery occlusion pressure: Clinical physiology, measurement, and interpretation. Am. Rev. Respir. Dis., 128:319, 1983.
55. Rahimtoola, S. H., et al.: Relationship of pulmonary artery to left ventricular diastolic pressures in acute myocardial infarction. Circulation, 46:283, 1972.
56. Fuchs, R. M.: Part I. Limitations of pulmonary wedge V-waves in diagnosing mitral regurgitation. Am. J. Cardiol., 49:849, 1982.
57. Pichard, A. D.: Part II. Large V-waves in the pulmonary capillary wedge pressure tracing without mitral regurgitation. The influence of the pressure/volume relationship in the V-wave size. Clin. Cardiol., 6:534, 1983.
58. Hessel, II, E. A., et al.: Pulmonary artery wedge pressure compared to left atrial pressure in cardiac surgical patients. (abstract) Anesthesiology, 61:3A, 1984.
59. Fretschner, R., et al.: Pulmonary artery occlusion-left atrial pressure gradient: An important factor in determining pulmonary venous vascular resistance in acute pulmonary failure. Crit. Care Med., 19:399, 1991.
60. Henriquez, A. H., et al.: Local variations of pulmonary arterial wedge pressure and wedge angiograms in patients with chronic lung disease. Chest, 94:491, 1988.
61. Marini, J. J.: Hemodynamic monitoring with the pulmonary artery catheter. Crit. Care Clin., 2:551, 1986.
62. West, J. B., Dollery, C. T., Naimark, A.: Distribution of blood

flow in isolated lung; relation to vascular and alveolar pressures. J. Appl. Physiol., *19*:713, 1964.
63. Falicov, R. E., and Resnekov, L.: Relationship of pulmonary artery end-diastolic pressure to left ventricular end-diastolic and mean filling pressures in patients with and without left ventricular dysfunction. Circulation, *42*:65, 1970.
64. Petty, T. L.: Adult respiratory distress syndrome. Semin. Respir. Med., *3*:219, 1982.
65. Wilson, R. F., and Resnekov, L.: Relationship of pulmonary artery diastolic and wedge pressure relationships in critically ill patients. Arch. Surg., *123*:933, 1988.
66. Vender, J. S.: Pulmonary artery catheter monitoring. Anesth. Clin. North Am., *6*:743, 1988.
67. Marini, J. J.: Obtaining meaningful data from the Swan-Ganz catheter. Respir. Care, *30*:572, 1988.
68. Berryhill, R. E., and Benumof, J. L.: PEEP-induced discrepancy between pulmonary arterial wedge pressure and left atrial pressure. The influence of controlled vs. spontaneous ventilation and compliant vs. non-compliant lungs. Anesthesiology, *46*:383, 1979.
69. Chapin, J. C., et al.: Lung expansion, airway pressure transmission and positive end-expiratory pressure. Arch. Surg., *114*:1193, 1979.
70. Michel, R. P., Hakim, T. S., Chang, H. K.: Pulmonary arterial and venous pressures measured with small catheters. J. Appl. Physiol., *57*:309, 1984.
71. Morris, A. H., Chapman, R. H., Gardner, R. M.: Frequency of technical problems encountered in the measurement of the pulmonary artery wedge pressure. Crit. Care Med., *12*:164, 1984.
72. Morris, A. H., Chapman, R. H., Gardner, R. M.: Frequency of wedge pressure errors in the ICU. Crit. Care Med., *30*:705, 1985.
73. Niemens, E. J., and Woods, S. L.: Normal fluctuations in the pulmonary artery wedge pressure in acutely ill patients. Heart Lung, *11*:393, 1982.
74. Riedinger, M. S., and Shellock, F. G.: Technical aspects of the thermodilution method for measuring cardiac output. Heart Lung, *13*:215, 1984.
75. Nishikawa, T., and Namiki, A.: Mechanism for slowing of heart rate and associated changes in pulmonary circulation elicited by cold injectate during thermodilution cardiac output determinations in dogs. Anesthesiology, *68*:221, 1988.
76. Marino, P.: The ICU Book. Philadelphia, Lea & Febiger, 1991, p. 125.
77. Fegler, G.: Measurement of cardiac output in an anesthetized animal by a thermodilution method. Q. J. Exp. Physiol., *39*:153, 1954.
78. Wetzel, R. C., and Latson, T. W.: Major errors in thermodilution cardiac output measurement during rapid volume infusion. Anesthesiology, *62*:684, 1985.
79. Merrick, S. H., Hessel, II, E. A., Dillard, D. H.: Determination of cardiac output by thermodilution during hypothermia. Am. J. Cardiol., *46*:419, 1980.
80. Stoller, J. K., et al.: Spuriously high output from injecting thermal indicator through an ensheathed port. Crit. Care Med., *14*:1064, 1986.
81. Nadeau, S., and Noble, W. H.: Limitations of cardiac output measurement by thermodilution. Can. J. Anaesth., *33*:780, 1986.
82. Hillis, L. D., Firth, B. G., Winniford, M. D.: Analysis of factors affecting the variability of Fick versus indicator dilution measurements of cardiac output. Am. J. Cardiol., *56*:764, 1985.
83. Snyder, J. V., and Powner, D. J.: Effects of mechanical ventilation on the measurement of cardiac output by thermodilution. Crit. Care Med., *10*:677, 1982.
84. Armengol, J., et al.: Effects of respiratory cycle on cardiac output measurements: Reproducibility of data enhanced by timing of thermodilution injections in dogs. Crit. Care Med., *9*:852, 1981.
85. Hoel, B. L.: Some aspects of the clinical use of thermodilution in measuring cardiac output. Scand. J. Clin. Lab. Invest., *38*:383, 1978.
86. Kadota, L. T.: Theory and application of thermodilution cardiac output measurement: A review. Heart Lung, *14*:605, 1985.
87. Stetz, C. W., et al.: Reliability of the thermodilution method in the determination of cardiac output in clinical practice. Am. Rev. Respir. Dis., *126*:1001, 1982.
88. Milnor, W. R.: Arterial impedance as ventricular afterload. Circ. Res., *36*:565, 1975.
89. Kandel, G., and Aberman, A.: Mixed venous oxygen saturation; its role in the assessment of the critically ill patient. Arch. Intern. Med., *143*:1400, 1983.
90. Birman, H., et al.: Continuous monitoring of mixed venous oxygen saturation in hemodynamically unstable patients. Chest, *86*:753, 1984.
91. Mohsinifar, Z., et al.: Relationship between O_2 delivery and O_2 consumption in the adult respiratory distress syndrome. Chest, *84*:267, 1983.
92. Danek, S. J., et al.: The dependency of oxygen uptake on oxygen delivery in the adult respiratory distress syndrome. Am. Rev. Respir. Dis. *122*:387, 1980.
93. Dongre, S. S., McAslan, T. C., Shin, B.: Selection of the source of mixed venous blood samples in severely traumatized patients. Anesth. Analg., *56*:527, 1977.
94. Schweiss, J. F.: Clinical usefulness of continued mixed oxygen saturation monitoring system. Proceedings of the 9th Annual Meeting of The Society of Cardiovascular Anesthesiology, 1987, p. 39.
95. Spinale, F. G., et al.: Right ventricular function computed by thermodilution and ventriculography. A comparison of methods. J. Thorac. Cardiovasc. Surg., *99*:141, 1990.
96. Raines, D. E., et al.: Artifactual hypertension due to transducer cable malfunction. Anesthesiology, *74*:1149, 1991.
97. Hines, R.: Monitoring right ventricular function. Anesth. Clin. North Am., *6*:851, 1988.
98. Dhainaut, J. F., Brunet, F., Villemant, D.: Evaluation of right ventricular function by thermodilution techniques. Update in intensive care and emergency medicine 2. *In* Cardiopulmonary Interactions in Acute Respiratory Failure. Edited by J. L. Vincent and P. M. Suter. Berlin, Springer, 1987, p. 95.
99. Tremper, K. K., and Barker, S. J.: Transcutaneous oxygen measurement. Experimental studies and adult applications. Anesthesiol. Clin., *25*:67, 1987.
100. Tremper, K. K., et al.: Continuous transcutaneous oxygen monitoring during respiratory failure, cardiac decompensation, cardiac arrest, and CPR. Crit. Care Med., *8*:377, 1980.
101. Severinghaus, J. W., and Astrup, P. B.: History of blood gas analysis. VI. Oximetry. J. Clin. Monit., *2*:270, 1986.
102. Chaudhary, B. A., and Burki, N. K.: Ear oximetry in clinical practice. Am. Rev. Respir. Dis., *17*:173, 1978.
103. Kelleher, J. F.: Pulse oximetry. J. Clin. Monit., *5*:37, 1989.
104. Nickerson, B. G., Sarkisian, C., Tremper, K.: Bias and precision of pulse oximeters and arterial oximeters. Chest, *93*:515, 1988.
105. Weingarten, A. E., et al.: Pulse oximetry to determine oxygenation in a patient with pseudohypoxemia. (Letter) Anesth. Analg., *67*:711, 1988.
106. Tremper, K. K., and Barker, S. J.: Pulse oximetry. Anesthesiology, *70*:98, 1989.
107. Wukitsch, M. W., et al.: Pulse oximetry: Analysis of theory, technology, and practice. J. Clin. Monit., *4*:290, 1988.

108. Fanconi, S.: Reliability of pulse oximetry in hypoxic infants. Pediatrics, *112*:424, 1988.
109. Sendak, M. J., Harris, A. P., Donham, R. T.: Accuracy of pulse oximetry during arterial oxyhemoglobin desaturation in dogs. Anesthesiology, *68*:111, 1988.
110. Jubran, A., and Tobin, M. J.: Reliability of pulse oximetry in titrating supplemental oxygen therapy in ventilator-dependent patients. Chest, *97*:1420, 1990.
111. Saunders, N. A., Powles, A. C. P., Rebuck, A. S.: Ear oximetry: Accuracy and practicability in the assessment of arterial oxygenation. Am. Rev. Respir. Dis., *113*:745, 1976.
112. Ries, A. L., Prewitt, L. M., Johnson, J. J.: Skin color and ear oximetry. Chest, *96*:287, 1989.
113. Severinghaus, J. W., and Naifeh, K. H.: Accuracy of response six pulse oximeters to profound hypoxia. Anesthesiology, *67*:551, 1987.
114. Fallenstein, F., Baeckert, P., Huch, R.: Comparison of in vivo response times between pulse oximetry and transcutaneous PO_2 monitoring. Adv. Exp. Med. Biol., *220*:191, 1987.
115. Langton, J. A., and Hanning, C. D.: Effect of motion artifact on pulse oximeters: Evaluation of four instruments and finger probes. Br. J. Anaesth., *65*:564, 1990.
116. Block, F. E.: Interference in a pulse oximeter from a fiberoptic light source. J. Clin. Monit., *3*:210, 1987.
117. Falconer, R. J., and Robinson, B. J.: Comparison of pulse oximeters: Accuracy at low arterial pressure in volunteers. Br. J. Anaesth., *65*:552, 1990.
118. Morley, T.: Capnography in the intensive care unit. J. Intensive Care Med., *5*:209, 1990.
119. Nunn, J. F., and Hill, D. W.: Respiratory dead space and arterial to end tidal CO_2 tension difference in anesthetized man. J. Appl. Physiol., *15*:383, 1960.
120. Heard, S. O.: Is capnography useful in the intensive care unit? J. Intensive Care Med., *5*:199, 1990.
121. Hess, D., et al.: An evaluation of the usefulness of end-tidal PCO_2 to aid weaning from mechanical ventilation following cardiac surgery. Respir. Care *136*:837, 1991.
122. Saunders, A. B., et al.: End-tidal carbon dioxide monitoring during cardiopulmonary resuscitation. A prognostic indicator for survival. JAMA, *262*:1347, 1989.
123. Capan, L., et al.: Arterial to end-tidal CO_2 gradients during spontaneous breathing, intermittent positive-pressure ventilation, and jet ventilation. Crit. Care Med., *13*:810, 1985.
124. Good, M. L.: Capnography: Uses, interpretation and pitfalls. *In* Refresher Course Lectures. Park Ridge, Illinois, American Society of Anesthesiologists, 1989.
125. Yamanake, M. K., and Sue, D. Y.: Comparison of arterial-end-tidal PCO_2 difference and dead space/tidal volume ratio in respiratory failure. Chest, *92*:832, 1987.
126. Blanch, L., et al.: Effect of PEEP on the arterial minus end-tidal carbon dioxide gradient. Chest, *92*:451, 1987.
127. Yelderman, M. L., et al.: Continuous cardiac output measurement in ICU patients. Anesthesiology, *73*:A421, 1990.

Chapter 78

THE ROLE OF THE BIOMEDICAL ENGINEER

JOHN H. PETRE

New technology has been an integral part of advances in patient management in critical care areas. Advances in technology, such as the microprocessor computer chip, have made it possible to measure and display physiologic parameters previously accessible only to the researcher. Higher expectations for patient success have fueled the demand for new instrumentation. In some instances, technologic tools have been made available before research was sufficient to justify their application.

Critical care clinicians have been deluged with a variety of specialty products, each having unique and elaborate operational requirements. New equipment has created intellectual problems with information overload, and physical problems such as where to locate additional signal acquisition devices and displays. Often, more patient data than can be reasonably digested are available. Similarly measured patient information from several different instruments may give conflicting results. Instrumentation interaction can distort data with little warning. Automated software routines, hardware filters, and other data manipulating processes operating within medical instrumentation are designed to be transparent to the user, but they may also function or fail in ways that are not obvious, producing inaccurate but believable information. Constant financial and budgetary limitations may reduce the ability of institutions to purchase adequate quantities of clinical instruments, may necessitate "triage" decisions such as which patient is more critical, or force older equipment to remain in service beyond its expected performance life.

Clinicians routinely face these problems and related instrumentation issues, and with notable exceptions, come poorly prepared to test evaluate and troubleshoot state-of-the-art equipment. The technical nature of these problems call for the input of specialists in medical engineering. These specialists can help with the selection, operation, and maintenance of equipment essential to the modern intensive care unit (ICU). They are the resource when technical modifications are needed, or new ideas are used to improve the performance of existing instrumentation systems. Engineering personnel can save time, money, and frustration when they are involved in discussing and planning equipment acquisition and implementation. Close work with the medical engineer can resolve problems and prevent potential conflicts before they occur.

Two primary types of engineering personnel work in the medical field: biomedical and clinical engineers. Often these titles are used interchangeably with little regard to any distinction between the two job classifications. Historically, the biomedical engineer with a technically trained individual who provided engineering expertise to medical researchers. Biomedical engineers worked primarily on long-term projects, such as the development of artificial organs, limbs, and other technically sophisticated experimental instrumentation. Rarely, however, was this person involved with the day-to-day clinical activities of a medical institution. In the early 1970s, more sophisticated medical devices were introduced routinely in clinical practice. Technical support was needed to assist in the development, operation, service, and refinement of these devices. Thus, the arrival of the clinical engineer, whose training emphasized clinical equipment rather than the research and development of new equipment. In the early 1980s, the International Certification Commission defined a clinical engineer as: "A professional who brings to health care facilities a level of education, experience and accomplishment which will enable him to responsibly, effectively and safely manage and interface with medical devices, instruments, and other systems and the use thereof during patient care, and who can, because of this level of competence, responsibly and directly serve the patient and physician, nurse, and other health care professionals relative to their use of and other contact with medical instrumentation."[1]

The Association for the Advancement of Medical Instrumentation (AAMI), the official society for clinical engineering, in conjunction with the American College of Clinical Engineering, adopted a simplified definition of the term clinical engineer:[2-3] "A clinical engineer is a professional who supports and advances patient care by applying engineering and managerial skills to healthcare technology."

Although the formal training and education differ between the two classes of engineers, both groups are well versed in the basic engineering skills needed in a special care area. The desire of the individual to partake in daily instrumentation issues and problems is the most significant distinguishing characteristic. Whether the engineer considers himself or herself a biomedical or clinical engineer is of little consequence. Realistically, biomedical and clinical engineers have and continue to work side by side with minimal job classification differences. One might rather think of the biomedical or clinical engineer who works closely with clinicians and instrumentation based in the intensive care areas as a critical care engineer. Such a classification would truly denote the direct application of personnel with technical expertise to the critical care area.

Clinical engineers and biomedical engineers practicing

in the field today come from one of many formal training programs. Most such individuals received extensive education in the fields of electrical engineering, mechanical engineering, computer science, and general physiology. The length and content of their training programs vary. Most engineers complete 4-year undergraduate programs and lengthier graduate programs. Additional training typically is obtained through research activities or speciality training. Postdoctoral work is not uncommon and many students develop their specialty during this time. The AAMI also sponsors training programs as well as scientific presentations that encourage further individual development.

Like many other specialties, on-the-job experience may be the most important qualification. Technology changes so rapidly in this field that the learning process must be ongoing. Furthermore, clinically related tasks often are institution specific and only a good understanding of the processes involved will permit the application of basic engineering principles for productive interaction.

As mentioned previously, the clinical/biomedical engineer may have duties specific and limited to a single or multiple critical care patient area(s). If his or her role is part of an institution-wide engineering team, the level of service available to the area may be more limited. In either case, their work involves specific administrative, equipment support, and clinical obligations that must be clearly defined and routinely provided to critical care patient areas.

The size of the institution typically dictates how the engineering support is provided. Larger health care facilities have the financial justification for localized support. Smaller institutions generally have a more centralized distribution. Locally based support personnel have the opportunity to be more clinically involved, whereas centrally located personnel have logistic difficulty in actively participating at the bedside.

Both local and central technical support personnel have administrative roles, which include operational as well as personnel responsibilities. Furthermore, active involvement in specific projects such as new construction, equipment purchases, instrumentation interfacing, equipment design and development, clinical research, or other projects directly related to medical instrumentation are expected.

The clinical/biomedical engineer is well suited to act as a technical consultant for the medical staff regarding issues that extend outside the critical care area or outside the medical facility. As an example, the clinical/biomedical engineer often acts as a liaison with equipment developers and manufacturers. It is their responsibility to present to the vendor the clinical needs of the critical care area in a technical fashion that can be evaluated easily. System development regarding technical issues within the institution but outside the critical care area also can be pursued. For instance, clinical engineering assistance would be beneficial during the development and implementation of an automated system for delivering test samples to an in-house laboratory and the method to provide quickly and accurately the results to the clinical staff. Figure 78-1 diagramatically presents such a system, an Automated Blood Gas Acquisition and Reporting System (ABGARS) that was

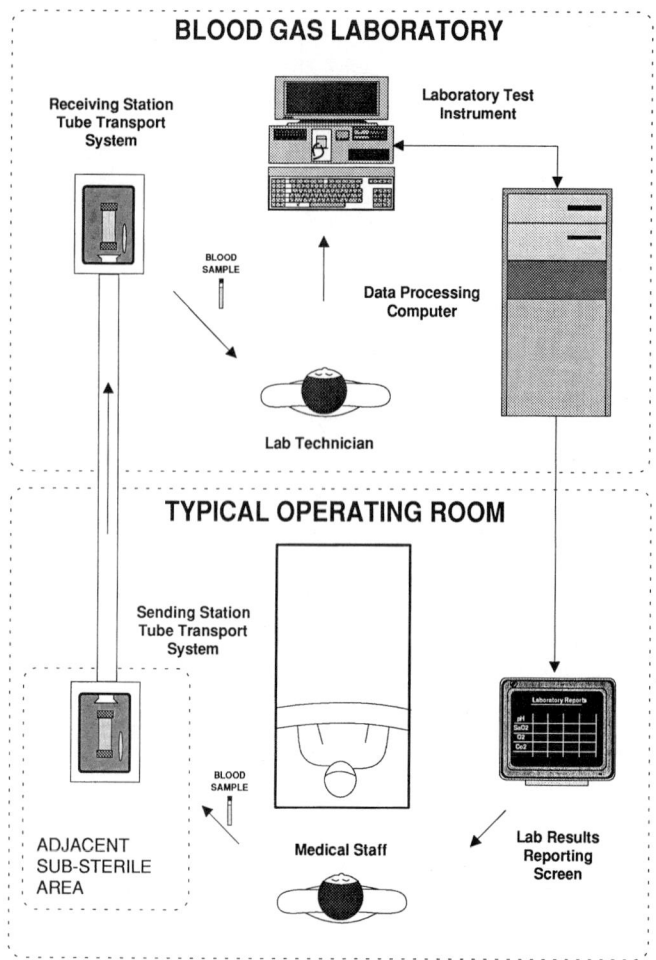

Fig. 78-1. A block diagram of the Automated Blood Gas Acquisition and Reporting System (ABGARS). The acquisition portion uses a tube system to transport the blood sample to the laboratory. A computer network links the laboratory instruments with a computer that records the test results and automatically reports the information back to the appropriate operating room.

developed and has been in daily use at the Cleveland Clinic Foundation since 1985.[4]

HISTORICAL TRENDS IN BIOMEDICAL EQUIPMENT

The treatment of critically ill patients requires rapid and accurate patient assessment to provide continuous diagnosis and treatment. Modern technology has paved the way to provide continual streams of patient information by means of sophisticated electronic monitors and diagnostic equipment. Unfortunately, the complexity of these devices and performance variability can contribute to incorrect diagnoses and improper patient care.

Instrumentation in various forms has always assisted clinicians in diagnosing health problems and administering clinical care. Early devices were simple, but they were based on the technologic and engineering principles that were well understood during their development. As new technology created more effective means to obtain patient information, the complexity of operation of these systems also increased. As a result, the average clinician may not understand fully how the equipment works and how it may fail, thus increasing the importance of good engineering surveillance and testing.

Consider the measurement of blood pressure. Early clinical blood pressure measurements were accomplished using noninvasive techniques such as the auscultatory and palpatory methods. Invasive techniques, such as direct connection to mercury or sterile water columns, were crude and cumbersome and extremely difficult to set up and use in a clinical situation. As technology brought new concepts and ideas to medicine, the pressure transducer developed into a viable mechanism to measure blood pressures continuously. The transducer has evolved over several years into a quality product that can be afforded financially as a disposable, single-use item. An older reusable transducer and a newer disposable transducer are pictured in Figure 78-2.

Financial considerations have affected the implementation of instrumentation in the special care area. Technology that has a direct positive impact on patient care is more easily justified when operational or capital equipment budgets are severely limited. Patient monitors, ventilators, and other life support equipment have always had priority over computerized data systems that can provide trending, record keeping, charting, or other semiautomated features. Technologic advances have allowed medical instrumentation to operate with improved performance, decreased size and weight, and additional functions, but they have failed to reduce equipment costs, a critical concern in today's health care field.

As new patient care procedures are developed, new support equipment must also be designed. Clinicians have raised their equipment expectation levels, demanding instrumentation that provides continuous, highly accurate patient information in a form that can be analyzed easily. Product or system performance often dictates whether the device becomes a clinical standard. If one examines the parameters monitored routinely, one finds that those instruments with proven track records are used universally, whereas those devices with questionable or inconsistent performance are limited to operation by only a few (often the sites at which initial development or beta testing was accomplished!)

In the early 1960s, electronic equipment began to appear in the operating rooms and ICUs. These devices were powered by tubes and transistors and were capable of displaying ECG information but rarely more. Most instruments were diagnostic tools and had little impact on the long-term stability of a patient. As their operation became standardized and more understandable, however, their use escalated. NASA contributed by sponsoring the development of transmitted patient information or telemetry signals. Additional parameters including temperature and blood pressure were monitored. Once these devices were used in quantity, concerns over patient safety and signal quality directed the development of future medical devices.

As instrumentation evolved in the 1970s, the capabilities and operational features of medical instrumentation expanded. Integrated circuit technology permitted increased capability at the bedside in relatively small packages. The availability of immediate patient information had a direct impact on medical intervention. The ICUs adjusted to the concept of monitored bed spaces, and central stations, nonfade displays, and multichannel recording became popular. Fiscal budgets at medical institutions were expanded to handle the cost of the new devices. Invasive blood pressure monitoring became an accepted procedure in larger institutions, whereas ECG monitoring was considered routine at all patient care facilities.

During the early 1980s, many single-purpose devices began to evolve. Automated noninvasive blood pressure instruments, pulse oximeters, mass spectrometers, capnographs, cardiac output machines, and other specialty devices were introduced. A stand-alone pulse oximeter is shown in Figure 78-3. Bed spaces became crowded with numerous stand-alone devices requiring more power receptacles than were available. Regulatory demands and the threat of malpractice often dictated the use of this instrumentation, forcing once well-planned bedspaces to become cluttered with additional equipment. Capital equipment budgets had difficulty in keeping pace with the increased equipment costs, and the new technology failed to provide any reduced costs for medical instrumentation.

During the middle of the 1980s, the development of microprocessor technology greatly influenced the medical instrumentation field. New instruments were capable of performing rapid calculations and processing tremendous quantities of patient information. The idea of a multipurpose device that could accomplish multiple tasks was now possible. A single patient monitor could easily handle multichannel ECG, multiple blood pressure channels, cardiac output, temperature monitoring, respiration, noninvasive blood pressure, capnography, and other patient parameters.

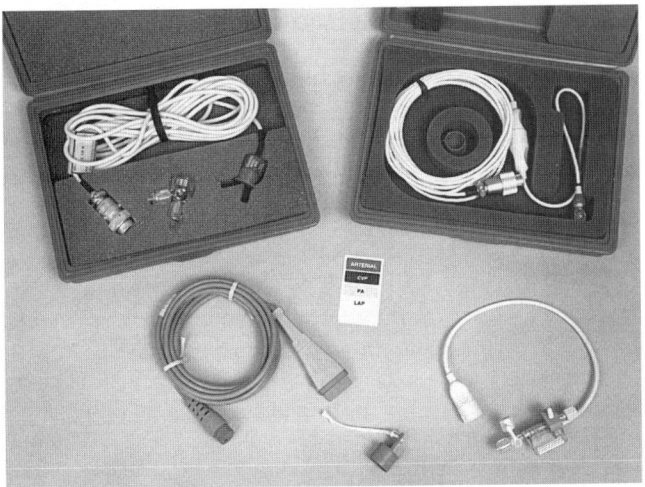

Fig. 78-2. Reusable Bentley Trantec and Spectramed P-50 Transducers and a Viggo-Spectramed disposable transducer. The Trantec and P-50 required gas sterilization or the use of a presterilized disposable dome (with diaphragm). The Trantec and P-50 required calibration whereas the disposable transducer is purchased precalibrated. (Courtesy of American Bentley, Irvine, CA, and Ohmeda, Oxnard, CA.)

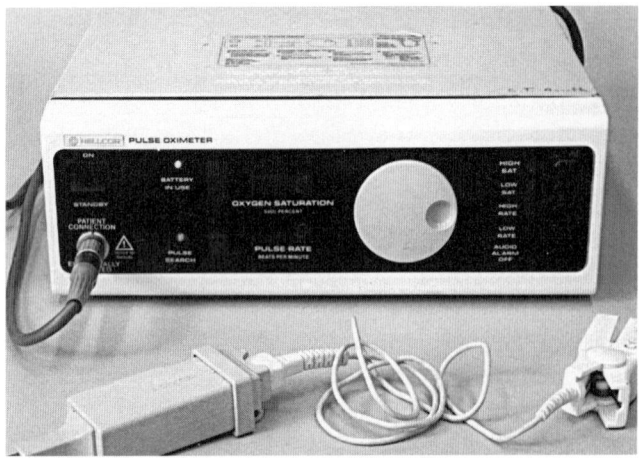

Fig. 78-3. An example of a single-purpose stand-alone medical instrument, a Nelcor pulse oximeter. At the bedside, similar devices occupy valuable space and limited electrical outlets, making access to the patient more difficult. (Courtesy of Nellcor, Pleasanton, CA.)

The versatility of these instruments brought with them user complexity. Much of the development time was directed at methods and techniques that could simplify the use and operation of these sophisticated devices. Terms such as "operator interface" and "user friendly" began to emerge as important features. The availability of mass quantities of data began to overwhelm the clinician, and new methods of storing, reducing, prioritizing, and displaying patient-generated data became important.

The 1990s look to be a time for increasing the use of patient information. A "systems" approach to disseminating information in a quickly understandable form, such as provided by a patient data management system, is essential to digest the quantity of information that is continuously available. The ability to close the loop and automatically regulate functions, such as the delivery of medications or the adjustment of a ventilator, is now in practice or development.[5-8] Truly, a medical interface for data organization and review is on the way. Reduced size continues to encourage the development of smaller packages for patient monitoring. Financial limitations require more for the dollar, and such phrases as cost containment and long-term relationships are being used to help control expenses.

INSTRUMENTATION

Critical care instrumentation has developed in conjunction with industrial developments and technologic progressions. Ideas developed for the aerospace field have had a great impact. The need to monitor physiologic parameters in early manned space flights fostered the development of instruments that could be applied in clinical situations. The development of the microprocessor-based patient monitor in the early 1980s brought vast new capabilities directly to the bedside that were never before available. Patient monitors using the same intelligent components found in an Apple personal computer brought patient information processing capabilities into the operating rooms and ICUs. Sophisticated disposable products such as blood pressure transducers and temperature sensing electrodes began to be used extensively. The terms hardware and software were introduced to clinical personnel as manufacturers began to use the benefits of such technology in their instrumentation designs in an attempt to reduce or minimize equipment obsolescence. Mass spectrometry permitted on-line analysis of inspired and expired gases. Capnography and pulse oximetry are now used routinely as safety monitoring devices that warn of possible operational problems of ventilator systems. Even manually operated measurement procedures (such as the measurement of noninvasive blood pressure) were automated to improve reliability and to reduce operational and staffing requirements. Computers have also permitted the mass storage of patient information for documentation, charting, and research purposes.

These overwhelming technologic advancements have not been accepted without some degree of concern. When introduced, many of the new features had operational problems that discouraged furthering their development. Manufacturers rushing to bring their products to market occasionally failed to consult knowledgeable medical professionals as to their clinical needs, which resulted in products with varying degrees of operational accuracy. Many products, such as pulse oximetry, noninvasive blood pressure, capnography, multilead arrhythmia analysis, and spectral EEG monitoring were developed over several years as more clinical experience with the products refined their reliability. Without question, instrumentation boasting new technology in the intensive care setting has historically been well received on a short-term basis, but only a few products have proven over time to be significant contributors to improving patient care.

The financial considerations regarding technologically advanced instrumentation is more of an issue as funding for such systems have become more difficult to obtain. Additionally, medical equipment manufacturers have not emphasized the need to use new technologic tools to help reduce manufacturing costs. New microchip and electronic hybrid technology has contributed to significantly reducing the physical size of equipment, improving portability, and lowering operational space requirements. Unfortunately, these advancements have failed to reduce costs. Despite improved and concentrated package design, or a per function basis, the cost of new medical systems (such as patient monitors, ventilators, etc.) continues to increase. In fact, most equipment that employs new technologic principles is more expensive than its less sophisticated predecessor.

Several key issues have directed the design and development of medical instrumentation over the past several decades. Initially, advances in the areas of electronics and biosensors provided the impetus to develop on-line real-time processing of patient information. These devices were minimally reliable, prone to high degrees of operator error, and generally difficult to use; however, they began to provide the clinician with a source of continuous information regarding the status of their patients. With the development of this first stage of instrumentation came the second major driving force for equipment development, the concern for patient and operator safety.

Most early instrumentation minimally protected the patient (or operator) from the effects of microshock, electrical burns, fire, explosion, or electrocution. The next generation of instrumentation featured numerous designs, including patient isolation and current limiting features, to minimize the potential for electrical mishaps. Grounding techniques and special power distribution systems minimized the concerns regarding explosion and fire, although these events were eliminated primarily by the eventual use of nonflammable anesthetic agents. Equipment was made more "user friendly" and was more rugged and resistant to environmental hazards such as fluid and physical abuse. Such devices also used new technologic developments to improve signal-to-noise ratios and thus the quality of the patient information gathered. These instruments were truly the first devices to consistently provide continuous and reliable patient information.

Technologic improvements are now concentrated in the area of miniaturization. Extremely sophisticated instruments have been designed and built with the benefit of microchip technology, including hybrid design, surface mount, and other electronic compacting processes. An example is shown in Figure 78-4. These designs have helped to reduce the space required for use in already limited bedside facilities. Small packaging has also permitted the development of multifunctional instruments sharing common data acquisition, processing, and display capabilities, which has helped to stabilize the increase in medical equipment costs.

The next phase of development is expected to focus on the reduction of expenditures for medical instrumentation. It is anticipated that cost reduction measures will take advantage of new manufacturing and component packaging techniques. The savings realized from these new techniques can be used to reduce the costs to develop and manufacture such specialized instrumentation.

Clinicians have also contributed significantly to the advancement of medical instrumentation. Until recently, the development of new equipment was solely in the hands of the manufacturer. Now, driven by the success and vast capabilities inherent to microprocessor-controlled instruments, clinical personnel have become important members of the product development path. Most manufacturers now develop new products in conjunction with one or more clinical groups. These groups or test locations are often referred to as beta sites. The design process is influenced greatly by the ideas and suggestions generated by clinical experts familiar with the function and operation of the specialized instruments. Clinicians are learning more about the limitations and capabilities of the systems and demanding that the engineered designs pay close attention to the operational needs of the users.

Patients and families now have an expectation level for the use of medical instrumentation. An ICU by its own name implies the use of sophisticated medical equipment to permit "intense and appropriate patient care." Legal concerns and the cost of malpractice insurance have also led clinicians to the routine and required use of some equipment, including capnography and pulse oximetry.[9] In the mid-1980s, the "Harvard Standards" (Department of Anaesthesia Standards of Practice 1—Minimal Monitoring) were established to help minimize intraoperative anesthesia-related patient injuries.[10] These institutional standards became patterns for national standards, such as those developed by the American Society of Anesthesiologists (ASA) Standards for basic Intra-Operative Monitoring, which became effective January 1, 1991.[11] These guidelines, which defined minimum monitoring practices for patients receiving an anesthetic, are summarized in Table 78-1. Patient safety issues addressed by these standards have effected the development of new instrumentation and helped to influence their evolution cycle.

The use of computer technology within the designs of medical instrumentation has led to the development of highly sophisticated multifunction instruments. At the bedside, these devices are used to provide immediate patient data regarding clinical status and the results of medical intervention. Away from the bedside, information gathered by diagnostic devices can be reviewed and tabulated for analysis and documentation. Additionally, this technology can be used to rapidly process data and information generated off site, such as at a laboratory facility. Similar information can be restructured for immediate display or

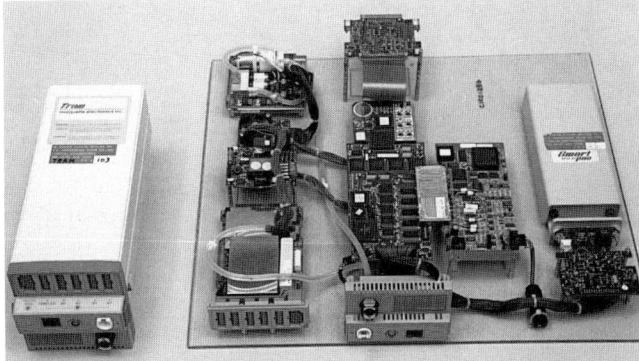

Fig. 78-4. A Marquette TRAM 300 module that monitors multiple parameters simultaneously. The electronic components used are an example of size reduction in medical instrumentation. (Courtesy of Marquette Electronics, Milwaukee, WI.)

Table 78-1. Summary of Minimal Monitoring Standards—Department of Anesthesia, Harvard Medical School, 1985

Anesthesiologist or nurse anesthetist present in operating room
Blood pressure and heart rate every 5 minutes
Electrocardiogram
Continuous monitoring
    For ventilation: reservoir bag, auscultation, expired gas flow, end-tidal CO_2
    For circulation: pulse, auscultation, arterial trace, oximetry
Breathing system disconnect alarm
Oxygen analyzer
Ability to measure temperature

(From Eichorn, J. H., et al.: Standards for patient monitoring during anesthesia at Harvard Medical School. JAMA, 256:1017, 1986.)

future retrieval. Thus, instrumentation can now be used to gather, process, organize, document, and display patient information rapidly and continuously.

The operational complexity of technically sophisticated instrumentation has increased as a result of design compactness and the availability to recall patient information rapidly. The techniques and methods required to present such a vast array of data have also become more elaborate, requiring clinical users to have higher levels of expertise in equipment operation Manufacturers have introduced concepts such as soft keys and trim knobs to facilitate the operation of their equipment. Within newer devices, a number of automated computational and logical tasks are routinely completed, resulting in the development of patient data that has been manipulated by software routines. Under adverse conditions, these data can be corrupted by algorithms that analyze the data inappropriately, creating misleading results. These types of hidden problems (software "bugs") are difficult to discover as well as solve and are one of the disadvantages associated with new technology. Within new instrumentation, other automated functions have been designed that can be helpful in self-diagnosing equipment malfunctions. These routines, however, which generally are transparent to the operator, do not totally guarantee fault-free operational performance.

Although technologic advances have provided clinicians with the benefits of reduced equipment size, additional patient data, self-testing, and automated processing, they have also contributed to the problems of operational complexity and rising instrumentation costs.

A variety of medical instrumentation is now used in most critical care areas. General categories of this equipment include: patient monitoring, infusion control, patient ventilation, patient management, patient intervention, and clinical accessories. Each group comprises a multitude of specialty devices with specific capabilities and operational features. Table 78-2 categorizes the most common critical care instruments.

The level of sophistication associated with each type of instrumentation depends on the complexity of the measurement technique, the rate of change of the monitored parameter, the calculations or data processing required, and the speed at which this information must be displayed.

Table 78-2. Critical Care Instruments

Patient monitoring: ECG, respiration, blood pressure (invasive and noninvasive), pulse oximetry, metabolic carts, capnography, cardiac output, compressed EEG displays, temperature, mass spectrometry, central monitoring stations
Infusion control: Infusion controllers, infusion pumps, closed delivery loop systems, PCA pumps
Patient ventilation: Ventilators (adult and pediatric), humidifiers, jet ventilators, IPPB machines, portable ventilators, gas concentration monitors
Patient management: Automated charting systems, data acquisition systems, patient management systems
Patient intervention: Pacemakers, defibrillators, intra-aortic balloon pumps, dialysis machines, ventricular assist devices, patient temperature control system
Clinical accessories: Disposable transducers, catheters, electrodes, nerve stimulators, flow Dopplers

Almost all instruments today make use of microprocessors to perform their required tasks. The advantages of such devices are numerous, with processing speed and flexibility to change being the most significant.

A core of medical instrumentation is typically found in almost all critical care areas. These items may vary by manufacturer, but are universally considered essential components for continually assessing patient status. A patient monitor equipped with ECG, respiration, temperature, blood pressure, and cardiac output monitoring capabilities is an example. In addition, other instruments may be available, depending on clinical practice and financial support. These systems typically are nonessential, but they help to organize, verify, and coordinate operational procedures. Examples of these include patient data management systems, automated charting, local area networks, mass spectrometers, and data acquisition systems.

Operationally and functionally, the level of sophistication of medical instrumentation varies tremendously. As stated previously, most equipment now makes use of microprocessor technology, even simplistic monitoring devices such as temperature-measuring equipment. Signal processing as well as alarm functions are always handled more effectively by such technically sophisticated devices. With these additional capabilities, however, comes the requirement for a higher level of operational interaction with the medical staff. Manufacturers have worked to reduce these problems by organizing and simplifying their interactive operational mode. Push-button menus, pop-up screens, multifunctional controls, and touch screens are used to simplify the user interface to these technically complicated devices. In most cases, medical personnel have adapted to these unique operational characteristics.

CURRENT PROBLEMS AND THE METHODS FOR DEVELOPING SOLUTIONS

The clinical engineer is involved daily with basic issues such as electrical safety, microshock, isolated power, equipotential grounding, the measurement of physiologic variables, fundamental electric principles, medical instrumentation, and technically sophisticated medical instrumentation. When problems or questions arise regarding these issues, the clinical engineer is contacted and is relied on to provide solutions. Additionally, questions regarding the physical plant, gas services, specialty systems (such as a tube/sample transport system), grounding, or power availability may be directed to the clinical engineer. Operational issues concerning patient transport equipment, new construction, equipment purchase, or equipment management also are typically a responsibility of the clinical engineer. Table 78-3 categorizes these major responsibilities.

A clinical engineer often acts as a technical resource for clinical and administrative personnel. Such activities revolve around medical instrumentation, but they may also venture into other classes of instrumentation, such as computers and devices for office automation. This range of expertise is available because of the design similarities of all microprocessor-based equipment.

Technical support is especially useful in the area of

Table 78-3. Major Responsibilities of the Clinical Engineer

Equipment Management: Clinical engineers (CEs) develop, implement, and direct equipment management programs. The primary concern is to provide cost-effective, safe, and reliable technology for healthcare delivery.

Construction and Renovation: CEs develop and manage building renovation and construction projects, coordinating equipment needs and budgetary requirements.

Consulting: The specialized skills of the CE are ideal for providing technical and operational consultation to clinical and administrative personnel.

Manufacturing: Having clinical and technical knowledge, CEs consult with equipment manufacturers regarding clinical needs, advancements in technology, and the development of medical instrumentation.

Radiation Safety: In some institutions, CEs use their radiation physics training to manage quality assurance programs and to ensure compliance with federal regulatory agencies.

Teaching: CEs provide training to numerous clinical personnel. They participate in formal training programs, teach accredited courses, and hold academic appointments.

Research: CEs, independently or in collaboration with physicians and other practitioners, perform research in the clinical environment.

Design: CEs frequently design or improve medical devices because they understand the clinical workplace, the principles of the equipment, and how the equipment is used. Their collaboration with the clinical staff is vital in medical device design and development.

Technology Assessment: CEs evaluate the costs, benefits, and risks associated with acquiring new technology.

(From CE certification information provided by AAMI, The Association for the Advancement of Medical Instrumentation, Arlington, VA, June, 1992.)

Table 78-4. Steps for New Equipment Evaluation

1. Determine performance specifications for the product
2. Determine annual usage (if a disposable) or life expectancy
3. Request quotations based on supplied usage figures
4. Check the product for significant improvements to present practice
5. Clinically evaluate only those products that meet the specifications and provide either an improvement over previous products or are equivalent but provide a cost savings to the institution
6. Verify the vendors' ability to supply quantities as needed
7. Clinically evaluate the product using multiple clinical trials
8. Request product modifications if clinical practice indicates a need for change in the design or manufacturing techniques of the product
9. Consider long-term agreements to reduce cost and minimize the time required for product evaluations
10. Select only those products that clearly are clinically acceptable to the medical staff.
11. Include in the agreement any other components required to make the desired product work properly
12. Determine prior to purchase support needed from the manufacturer to ensure proper product performance
13. Include in the agreement the costs for any training required for the operation or servicing of the product
14. If appropriate, consider the cost required to maintain, service, or repair the device
15. If on use any of the product is faulty, a full refund is appropriate
16. All contracts must have a termination clause based on product performance or the failure to support or deliver the product

equipment purchases. Purchasing agents have limited technical training and few understand the clinical concerns regarding the purchase of products. A clinical engineer can bridge this gap by providing a mix of both technical and clinical knowledge. Steps taken to evaluate the potential value of a proposed new product are outlined in Table 78-4. The complexity of new medical instrumentation is such that it is difficult and time consuming to obtain equipment that meets the specialized needs of each ICU. Technical assistance can be useful during the process of product specification, cost evaluation, and technology equivalence review, as well as during the setup and installation of the clinical instrumentation.

One of the primary responsibilities of a clinical engineer is to ensure the operational integrity of medical instrumentation. Scheduled programs must be in place to check the performance characteristics of all patient-connected medical devices routinely. A daily checklist often is used to verify equipment performance before its actual clinical use. An example of a checklist (for a patient monitor) is shown in Table 78-5. Documentation is required and preventative maintenance programs must be implemented to meet regulatory requirements. Computer data bases can be used to provide an organized approach and to permit a statistical review of equipment performance characteristics. Figure 78-5 shows an example of a database form used for equipment preventative maintenance documentation. In addition to the general checking of equipment, calibration, service, and repair are provided for medical instrumentation. Critical care equipment that fails while in use must be repaired or replaced quickly and the technical expertise of the clinical engineer is useful in resolving such problems. Equipment maintenance is clearly the work area in which a true financial saving can be seen. Normally, cost justification for a clinical engineering group can be merited merely on the funds saved with in-house service versus outside organizations.

Operational problems concerning the use of instrumentation routinely occur that directly or indirectly impact patient care. These problems usually are tolerated because of the limited technical training and time limitations of the involved medical personnel. Formulating solutions to these undesirable situations requires a mix of both technical and clinical understanding. The clinical engineer is well suited for developing solutions to such operational problems. Knowledge of both the clinical and technical aspects of any problem as well as the ability to design devices, interfaces, brackets, circuits, etc. provides the clinical engineer with the skills to resolve such issues.

Special instrumentation can be developed that involves new equipment, existing devices, or a combination of

Table 78-5. Patient Monitor Checklist

Verify proper power-up sequence of patient monitor
Verify proper initialization of default parameters (gains, calibrations, etc.)
Clear out any old patient data
Register new patient
Connect all appropriate cables, transducers, and sensors
Verify their performance using precalibrated simulators or testers
Adjust display as desired; set and verify parameter labels
Set alarm limits and verify operation; adjust audible alarms
Register patient characteristics (height, weight, etc.) for derived calculations
Set-up special functions, such as arrhythmia detect or ST changes

Annual Ohmeda Maintenance
Cleveland Clinic Foundation
Department of Cardiothoracic Anesthesiology

Location: _____

Absorber
(serial number _____) Date: _____

Maintenance Item	Comments	Init.
Inspect Interior manifold		
Change cup seals on selector valve		
Clean PEEP valve		
Inspect absorber mount		
Replace return tube		
Replace flow transducer		
Replace ventilator to Absorber tubing		

7800 Ventilator
(serial number _____) Date: _____

Maintenance Item	Comments	Init.
Replace bellows		
Perform system check		
Replace parts - Pneumatic + gas inlet		
Perform Electric safety test (Bio-med)		

Modulus II Gas Machine
(serial number _____) Date: _____

Maintenance Item	Comments	Init.
Cylinder regulator check		
Pressure sensor and low alarm system test		
Proportioning system and flowmeter		
Check and clean waste gas interface		
Check vaporizers with Riken		
Check hard lines for build-up		
Perform electrical safety tests (Bio-med)		

Note:
The data from this sheet should be transferred to the computer Superbase file 'ohmedav' for the permanent record keeping. This hard copy should also be part of a permanent record.

Fig. 78-5. A sample printout of a ventilator preventative maintenance form. Documented information is minimized to reduce unnecessary paperwork. The results are further simplified and placed into an equipment database for future referencing. Performance statistics as well as other equipment management information can be obtained.

both. Interfacing two instruments together, or connecting a computer to many devices, are examples of using existing equipment to perform a requested task. On the other hand, specialty devices may be developed in conjunction with an equipment manufacturer. A clinical engineering area may prototype a device and, after clinical acceptance, use an outside source to manufacture multiple quantities of the instrument. This process has grown significantly in the area of disposable products. Transducers, tubing sets, containers, lines, special kits, etc. have required notable in-house efforts to commercialize the clinical ideas into useful products.

Clinical engineers can be helpful in reducing the costs associated with capital equipment purchases and disposables. An understanding of both the clinical and technical requirements of a product allows more thorough evaluation and selection processes. Lower cost substitutions or equivalents can be determined more accurately. Only products that satisfy the clinical needs and demonstrate reliable performance through good technical design can be considered. The end result is a selected product that is cost effective yet provides the proper level of clinical performance.

The operational characteristics of the physical plant are extremely important to the quality of patient care delivered. The clinical engineer can be an important contributor in the development of new ideas and concepts for improved operation and function of the physical environment. New construction or remodeling plans should be reviewed by a clinical engineer to assist in the optimization of the design. Because the combination of technical and clinical knowledge is not common among architects and building consultants, the clinical engineer can offer a unique and beneficial view not available from any other single source. Specifically, assistance can be provided for the special care units, operating rooms, and other areas containing large numbers of sophisticated equipment.[12-14]

The clinical engineer is responsible for educating medical personnel in the fundamental operating principles of instrumentation, equipment operation, and electrical safety. This process occurs in the form of scheduled lectures, seminars, formal demonstrations, and one-on-one inservices. Some of these lectures are required or highly recommended by organizations that have certification concerns (such as JCAHO) or by formal educational training programs (such as a residency program, a certified registered nurse anesthetist (CRNA) school, a school for perfusionists, etc.). In our practice, engineering personnel provide extensive inservicing for patient monitoring equipment, anesthesia machines, ventilators, and transport equipment for all new residents. A formal accredited course in medical instrumentation is taught each year to student perfusionists, and CRNA students receive several lectures on electrical safety and invasive blood pressure measurement.

Because these conferences deal with highly technical material, it is the responsibility of the clinical engineer to present the information in terms that are easily understood by clinically trained operators. Technical information regarding the theory of device operation provides insight into the operational characteristics of the clinical instrumentation. Such knowledge fosters and enhances the ability to troubleshoot failed devices and to minimize operational problems. The benefits associated with understanding the correct operation of sophisticated medical devices are significant; some are listed in Table 78-6.

Electrical safety is also an important issue addressed by the clinical engineer. Because almost all diagnostic, therapeutic, and clinical instruments are powered electrically, the need to understand the hazards associated with such devices is essential. Additionally, patients in the critical care unit are more susceptible to micro and macro shock, because their first line of defense, the high resistance of their skin tissue, has been effectively by-passed. Catheters, electrodes, and other invasive probes make these patients vulnerable to any electric current. The potential hazards of micro and macroshock are demonstrated in Figure 78-6. Fortunately, equipment manufacturers have taken many steps to minimize the likelihood of such currents flowing.

Table 78-6. Benefits of Proper Equipment Operation

Reduces the possibility of obtaining incorrect patient information
Reduces the incidence of improperly identified equipment malfunction
Minimizes the need for constant on-site technical support
Minimizes damage to equipment
Shortens the length of time required for setup, use, or removal of instrumentation
Reduces the number of devices required
Reduces downtime from equipment operational problems, real and operator perceived
Minimizes unnecessary service and repair costs
Permits better interaction with other instrumentation
Improves the ability to identify and quickly resolve "real equipment problems"
Reduces the electrical hazard risk associated with AC-powered equipment to both the operator and the patient
Reduces costs associated with disposables and other accessories used with the medical devices
Minimizes the time required to operate or correct operational problems
Provides reinforcement and increased confidence in the patient information obtained or controlled
Improves patient care!

Nevertheless, the potential does exist and knowledge about the condition is essential to minimize the chances of electrically induced shock. Because manufacturers use special circuits, concepts, and mechanisms to improve electrical safety in the critical care area, it is reasonable to assume that some additional understanding of these systems is required.

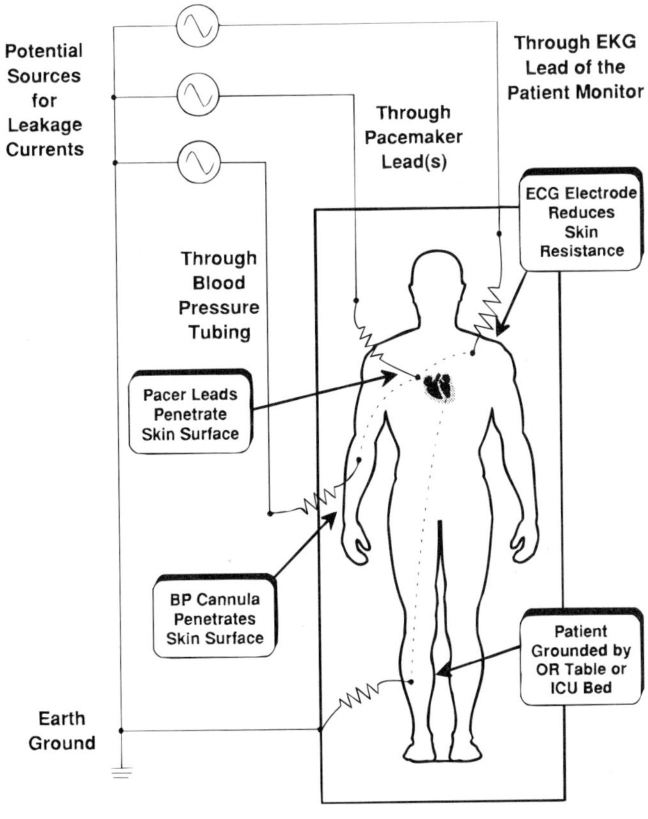

Although clinical engineers concentrate most of their efforts on applications that have a direct effect on daily activities, most also participate, in some form, in clinical research. Technical assistance is generally provided for any medical instrumentation to be used in the research study. Clinical research often requires equipment for gathering, storing, or processing patient information. Special devices may be designed and constructed, software programs to perform calculations or to store data may be developed, or equipment may be interconnected to form a specialized system. All of these equipment-related processes can be handled by a clinical engineer. Additionally, a clinical engineer can participate directly in a clinical research project as an assistant or as an operator of the developed instrumentation system.

CLINICAL ENGINEERING—RESOURCE REQUIREMENTS

Critically ill and unstable patients require continuous evaluation so their medical care can be adjusted according to their changing conditions. Events that affect the short- and long-term status of the patient must be monitored continuously. The information obtained must be processed quickly and presented back to the attending medical staff for their use. These clinical demands often dictate the minimum levels at which the equipment must be capable of performing.

During a clinical procedure, a biomedical or clinical engineer may participate directly to reduce the technical or operational responsibilities of the clinician. The engineer serves as a technical authority performing those tasks that require understanding and knowledge about the technical issues. Engineers often set up blood pressure monitoring systems or interface computers and monitors for data acquisition. The engineer may also assist in specific measurement practices that require some special knowledge of the measuring equipment.

This participation encourages the establishment of a working relationship between the technical support personnel and the medical staff. As part of the team, engineering personnel can monitor closely the performance of equipment and contribute directly to the improved operation of the device. Still, this direct interaction provides a first hand opportunity for communication regarding operational problems or possible improvements to the performance of the instrumentation. Engineering personnel often are physically located within the confines of the critical care area. This closeness can further reinforce a camaraderie between medical and technical personnel as well as permit rapid problemsolving of technical malfunctions.

Engineering personnel familiar with the daily operational routines and problems regarding equipment usage are more capable of participating in the solution process. Specifically, engineers are trained to approach equipment problems systematically by applying basic engineering principles. A thorough understanding of both the technical limitations and the operational requirements often results

Fig. 78-6. Examples of how leakage current can pass from instrumentation through a patient to ground. Once the skin is penetrated, leakage currents as small as 10 microamperes have been shown experimentally to induce ventricular defibrillation.

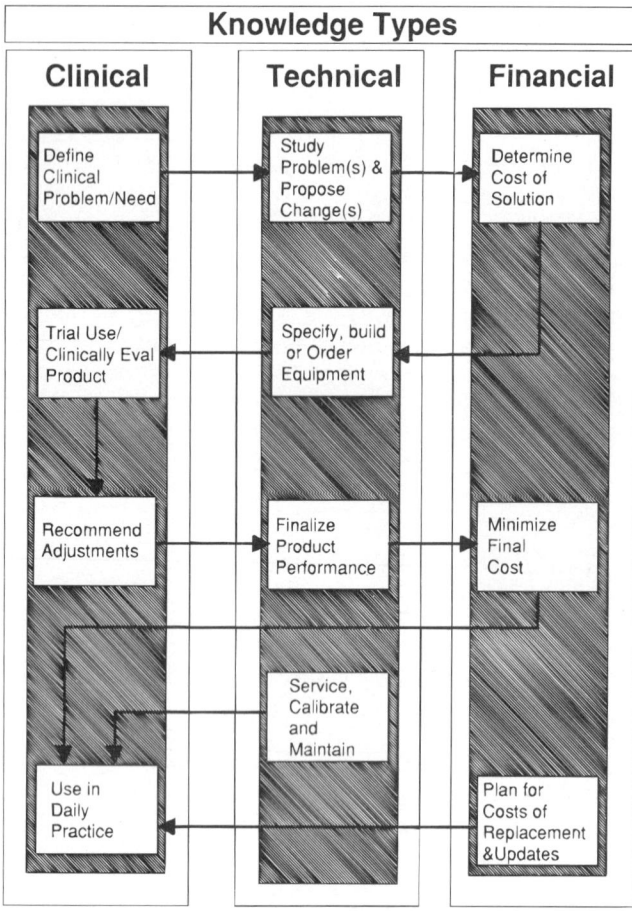

Fig. 78-7. Logic for combining knowledge from different specialties to develop a solution to a problem involving medical instrumentation.

in appropriate and practical solutions. Figure 78-7 shows how knowledge from different specialities can be combined to develop a solution to a problem involving medical instrumentation.

Without question, a working relationship between technical and medical personnel offers tremendous benefits. The development of such relationships must grow as each group realizes the other's expertise, skills, and limitations. Often, smaller joint projects lead to more significant contributions, including solutions to longstanding and historical problems.

The primary limitation to the development of this type of team approach is the cost involved. Most large institutions provide indirect technical support to their critical care units through a centralized biomedical engineering department. Few, however, have locally based technical expertise. The centralized method of distributing technical assistance can be effective provided a substantial resource commitment is arranged. The preferred course, however, is the team approach, in which physical proximity is essential to the development of a working relationship.

At the Cleveland Clinic Foundation, we have developed, in conjunction with physician expertise, several devices that have directly impacted clinical practice. A closed loop infusion control device, the Titrator (commercially manufactured by Ivac Corporation, see Fig. 78-8) was developed and is now used routinely in our cardiovascular ICUs.[15] Operating rooms and ICUs are equipped with a unique IV transport system developed completely in-house.[16-18] An automated blood gas reporting and sample tube delivery system for the operating rooms was designed and is in daily use.[4]

The expenses involved to implement a localized area of technical support for a critical care area can be classified into two specific areas: support services and labor costs. The support costs include laboratory space, test and service equipment, and general overhead to maintain the laboratory. The initial startup cost may range from $30,000 to $50,000,* depending on the size of the area. Yearly operational costs range from $15,000 to $30,000* relative to the level of responsibilities assigned to the area. Labor expenses depend greatly on the level of expertise desired and the numbers of support personnel required. Salaries for biomedical/clinical engineers range from a low of $30,000* annually upward. Additional technical support personnel, such as biomedical equipment technicians (BMETs), have yearly compensation ranges that start about 30% lower and cap off at $45,000.*

Most expenses for such an area can be justified by examining the cost of an outside service contract to maintain the instrumentation found within the critical care area. Most yearly service contracts are between 7 and 13% of the purchase price of the instrumentation they cover. The level of support provided for that fee varies among service organizations. Most service groups now limit their support to normal working hours and charge more for weekend or evening coverage. More detailed information about the costs associated with the operation of a clinical engineering area are available.[19,20]

The average purchase price of the medical equipment found at a typical critical care bed space is over $50,000. For each critical care bedspace, $5,000 (using a 10% average) per year could be justified as the minimal per bed service equipment cost. Thus, to support a 12-bed unit, $60,000 would be required for an outside service contract. On the basis of these figures, it is easy to determine the level of technical support that could be justified based solely on projected service contract costs.

The engineer is responsible for developing, implementing, and overseeing a complete equipment management program. Such a program should address operational issues that relate to equipment servicing, calibration, and repair. Guidelines for proper equipment performance are established and compared routinely to actual test data to determine the operational condition of each instrument. Documentation of the testing is maintained and all equipment is adjusted to operate within manufacturer specifications. Additionally, all instruments are continuously updated to the latest hardware and software revisions as recommended by the manufacturer. Records of the instrument analysis are maintained in conformance with JCAHO requirements. Table 78-7 contains an outline of these requirements. Quality assurance reports regarding equip-

---

* Note: Salary numbers will be affected by region.

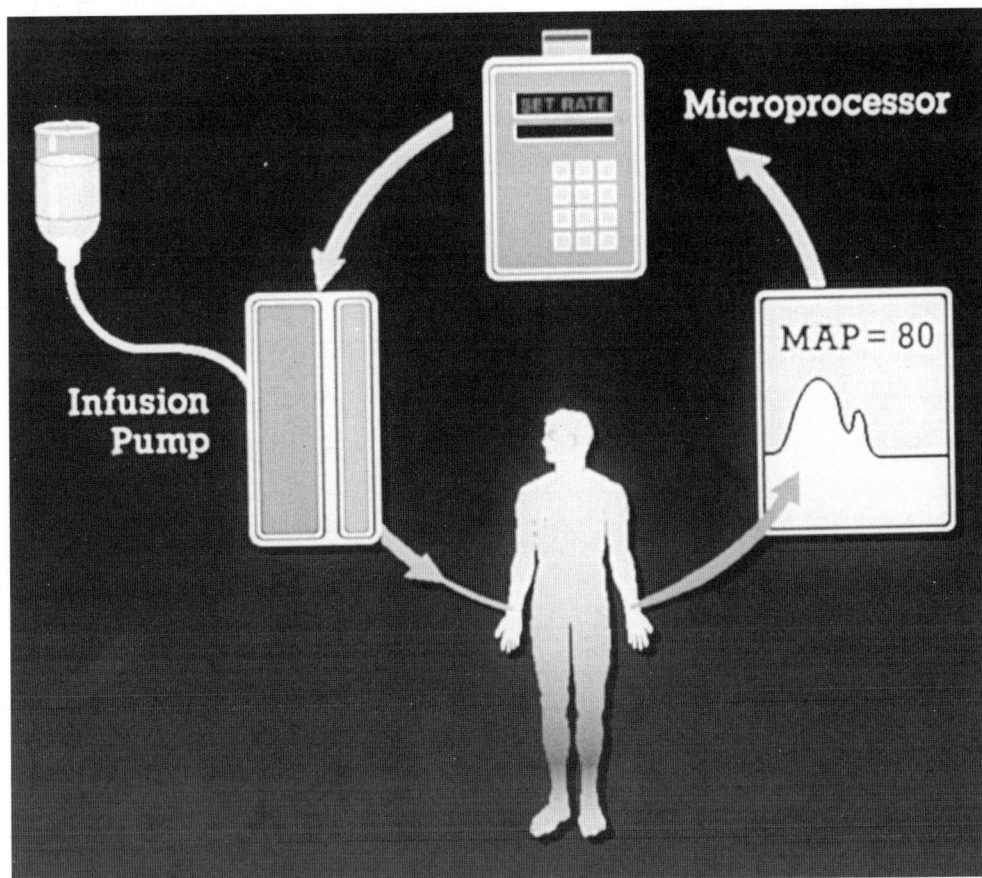

Fig. 78-8. How the Closed Loop Titrator System (IVAC, San Diego, CA) performs automated control. Blood pressure signals from the patient are used by the Titrator to determine an appropriate infusion rate. The rate is fed to the infusion pump, which delivers sodium nitroprusside to the patient at this rate. The patient's blood pressure is affected and the process repeats itself over and over until the pressure is controlled to a desired value.

ment performance can also be developed from this data base of records. Such information can be useful in determining instrument failure patterns, establishing replacement part inventories, and developing preventive maintenance schedules.

New clinical equipment is electrically safety checked, performance verified, and registered into the equipment data base. Operational and performance verification tests are developed and the device is placed on a routine preventive maintenance schedule. Equipment that fails an initial checkout process is returned to the manufacturer for corrective action.

Table 78-7. Outline of JCAHO Record Requirements for Medical Equipment

The following records or manuals must be maintained:
  Equipment operation manuals
  Procedures for performing electrical safety testing
  Records of incoming (new equipment) electrical safety testing
  Schedule for periodic electrical safety testing
  Records of periodic electrical safety testing
  Procedures for performing periodic maintenance
  Schedule for periodic maintenance
  Records of all periodic maintenance performed
  Records of any equipment service performed
  A procedure for performing quality assurance (QA) reviews
  Documentation of any adjustments to procedures made based on the QA reviews
  Records of any provided operational training or equipment inservicing

The number of personnel necessary to support a specialized ICU area depends on the type of support expected. If coverage is required for more than 8 hours per day, multiple technical personnel are needed. Typically, a single clinical engineer can supervise up to five biomedical technicians without much difficulty; however, this supervision in itself requires time. A typical 16-bed ICU area could be staffed by one clinical engineer and one technician providing coverage for 16 hours daily (7:00 A.M. to 11:00 P.M.), depending on their requested clinical involvement (research, procedures, etc.). These conditions, however, probably would not allow time for many specialty projects. Staffing is a difficult parameter to suggest because levels vary dramatically depending on the service provided. Table 78-8 presents information in the form of a guideline chart for technical staffing of a typical ICU.

WHAT DOES THE FUTURE HOLD?

It is difficult to determine the direct and indirect effects of new technology on the quality and cost associated with patient care in the critical care area. Undoubtedly, however, new technology has led to the development and modification of numerous technically advanced critical care instruments. The requirement for proper operation of these devices has increased the level of operational skills needed by clinicians. The availability of vast quantities of real-time patient data has further complicated the process of patient assessment.

Table 78-8. Technical Support Staffing*

	Daily Hours of Coverage		
	8	16	16 + Call
No. of ICU Beds	Number of FTEs required:		
1–16	1	2	2
17–32	1	2+	2+
33–48	1	2+	3
49+	2	3	3+

*Numbers are based on minimal routine practices. Coverage during employee time-off is not included. FTEs, full-time employees.

The support level required to maintain these devices has also grown. Increased levels of both functional understanding and operational knowledge is required to support new, technologically advanced equipment adequately. Education and training is required to maintain necessary skill levels. The clinical/biomedical engineering group is capable of providing support service for technically sophisticated equipment. To accomplish this task, engineering personnel must constantly update their knowledge.

As more and more technically advanced instrumentation is developed and placed into service, the need to provide skilled support personnel will grow. Additional and continuous training will be required for the existing clinical staff as well as any new personnel. In some instances, the complexity of operation of the instrumentation may require direct assistance by technical personnel.

Purchase cost will continue to rise, making product selection even more significant. The instruments selected will be expected to have longer functional lives. Ten years of use for hardware before replacement will be the accepted guideline. Service and operational costs will be scrutinized. Reimbursement from third parties for use of the devices will be reduced or, in some instances, not approved. Because technologic advancement is improving performance so rapidly, the useful lifespan of new equipment could be effectively reduced, thus shortening the payback period. All of these financial concerns dictate that significant organization and planning are essential to prevent fiscal distress.

The clinical/biomedical engineer can be a key player in organizing an effort to improve all phases of equipment management. This improvement may be accomplished as an institutional effort or as a representative of a specialized critical care service. In either case, engineering personnel must apply their technical and clinical understanding to improve the overall performance capabilities of equipment purchased.

Clearly, medical practice and methods of patient care have been influenced directly by technologic advancements. The capabilities offered by new medical instrumentation provide either more effective methods for obtaining patient information or new or additional patient information that was not available previously. In either case, the information must be presented in a form that is easily understood.

As technology continues to advance, the costs associated with medical care continue to climb, third-party reimbursement continues to fall, and the expectations of health care recipients rise, more and more pressure is brought to bear by medical institutions to provide quality care at reduced expense. This task will be difficult because the skills required to select, operate, and service highly sophisticated medical instrumentation will also continue to increase. Health care institutions will be forced to do a better overall job of medical equipment management to survive financially. The role of the clinical/biomedical engineer is to assist in this task and to promote the benefits and advantages that new technology offers to the critical care environment.

REFERENCES

1. International Certification Commission, Clinical Engineering Board of Examiners, Certification Booklet/Application, 1984.
2. American College of Clinical Engineering (ACCE), Board of Examiners: The Definition of a Clinical Engineer, May, 1991.
3. Shaffer, M. J., and Shaffer, M. D.: What is a clinical engineer? Issues in definition. Biomed. Instrum. Technol., 26:277, 1992.
4. Chou, D., and Van Lente, F.: The design and implementation of a laboratory system to service the critical care environment. Informatics Path, 1:102, 1986.
5. Mckinley, S., et al.: Clinical evaluation of closed-loop control of blood pressure in seriously ill patients. Crit. Care Med., 19:166, 1991.
6. Westenskow, D. R., and Wallroth, C.: Closed loop control for anesthesia breathing systems. J. Clin. Monit., 6:249, 1990.
7. Sebald, A. V., et al.: Engineering implications of closed loop control during cardiac surgery. J. Clin. Monit., 6:241, July.
8. Morozoff, P. E., and Evan, R. W.: Closed loop control of SaO2 in the neonate. Biomed. Instrum. Technol., 26:117, 1992.
9. Eichorn, J. H.: Prevention of intraoperative anesthesia accidents and related severe injury through safety monitoring. Anesthesiology, 70:572, 1989.
10. Eichorn, J. H., et al.: Standards for patient monitoring during anesthesia at Harvard Medical School. JAMA, 256:1017, 1986.
11. American Society of Anesthesiologists (ASA), 1992, Directory of Members, pgs. 675–676.
12. Kerr, D. R., and Malhotra, I. V.: Electrical design and safety in the operating room and intensive care unit. Int. Anesthesiol. Clin., 27:48, 1981.
13. Schmid, J. M.: ICU design. J. Oper. Res. Inst., 2:43, 1982.
14. Piegeorge, A. R., Cesarno, F. L., Casanova, D. M.: Designing the critical care unit: A multidisciplinary approach. Crit. Care Med., 11:541, 1983.
15. Cosgrove III, D. M., et al.: Automated control of postoperative hypertension: A prospective, randomized multicenter trial. Ann. Thorac. Surg., 47:678, 1989.
16. Petre, J., Bazaral, M. G., Estafanous, F. G.: Patient transport: An organized method with direct clinical benefits. Biomed. Instrum. Technol. 100:107, 1989.
17. Bazaral, M. G., et al.: Operating room design at the Cleveland Clinic Foundation. Cleve. Clin. J. Med., 55:267, 1988.
18. Weinfurt, P. T.: TRAM: A new concept in transport monitoring. Int. J. Clin. Monit. Comput., 4:149, 1987.
19. Frize, M.: Results of an International Survey of Clinical Engineering Departments. Part 2. Budgets, staffing, resources and financial strategies. Med. Biol. Eng. Comput. 28:160, 1990.
20. Staewen, W. S.: In-house service contracts. Biomed. Instrum. Technol., 24:266, 1990.

SUPPLEMENTAL READINGS

Anonymous: Central station monitors and networks. Health Devices, 21:83, 1992.

Bray, K. A., and Hearn, K.: Critical care unit design. Part III: Establishing operations. Nursing Management, 24:64A, 64F, 64H, 1993.

Cohen, T.: Computerized maintenance management systems for clinical engineering. Biomed. Instrum. Technol. 26:191, 1992.

Crawford, M. E., Sorensen, M. B., and Dahl, J. B.: International standards for intensive care unit safety. Lancet. 341:1061, 1993.

Cromwell, L., et al. (Eds.): Medical Instrumentation for Health Care. Englewood Cliffs, NJ, Prentice-Hall, 1976.

Cromwell, L., Weibell, F., and Pfeiffer, E.: Biomedical Instrumentation and Measurements. Englewood Cliffs, NJ, Prentice-Hall, 1980.

Cywinski, J., and Tardieu, B. (Eds.): The Essentials in Pressure Monitoring. Boston, Martinus Nijhoff Medical Division, 1980.

Doerr, D. F.: Biomedical engineering. A means to add new dimension to medicine and research. J. Fla. Med. Assoc., 79:530, 1992.

Dulock, H. L., and Breslin, E. H.: Collaboration between nurse researchers and biomedical engineers. Biomed. Instrum. Technol., 26:28, 1992.

Fielder, J.: The bioengineer's obligations to patients. J. Invest. Surg., 5:201, 1992.

Gardner, R. M., and Huff, S. M.: Computers in the ICU: Why? What? And so what? [editorial]. Int. J. Clin. Monit. Comput., 9:199, 1992.

Geddes, L. A., and Baker, L. E. (Eds.): Applied Biomedical Instrumentation. New York, John Wiley, 1975.

Gomolka, M.: The importance of an instrument specialist in an intensive care unit. Krankenpflege J., 30:422, 1992.

Guerin, T. B.: Materials management considerations in critical care areas. Crit. Care Nurs. Q., 15:56, 1992.

Halpern, N. A., Thompson, R. E., and Greenstein, R. J.: A computerized intensive care unit order-writing protocol. Ann. Pharmacother., 26:251, 1992.

Henneman, B.: Building the model ICU. Crit. Care Nurs., 12:112, 1992.

Meyer, C.: Visions of tomorrow's ICU. Am. J. Nurs., 93:26, 1993.

Piehler, H. R.: Innovation and change in medical technology: Interactions between physicians and engineers. J. Invest. Surg., 5:179, 1992.

Rithalia, S. V.: Role of the clinical engineer in patient monitoring services. J. Med. Eng. Technol. 15:239, 1991.

Shaffer, M. J., and Shaffer, M. D.: What is a clinical engineer? Issues in definition. (Published erratum appears in Biomed. Instrum. Technol., 26:378, 1992.) Biomed. Instrum. Technol., 26:277, 1992.

Sibbald, W. J., and Inman, K. J.: Problems in assessing the technology of critical care medicine. Int. J. Technol. Assess. Health Care, 8:419, 1992.

Simpson, R. L.: Automating the ICU: Facing the realities. Nurs. Management, 23:24, 26, 1992.

Stock, J., and Ball, J.: The role of nurses and technicians in intensive care. Intensive Crit. Care Nurs. 9:67, 1993.

Chapter 79

DISEASE CLASSIFICATION, SEVERITY OF ILLNESS, QUANTITATION OF THERAPEUTIC INTERVENTION, AND PREDICTION OF OUTCOME OF PATIENT CARE

EDWARD D. SIVAK
GEORGE E. THIBAULT

Physicians and nurses as well as hospital administrators are increasingly concerned about appropriate application of medical technology with the expectation of a good outcome in the face of declining resources and cost constraints. At the same time, quality of care has become a societal concern.[1] To address issues surrounding these circumstances, it is important to characterize patient populations within the intensive care unit (ICU).[2] This characterization could be accomplished in the generic sense by use of a case mix manager, which is a "classification system for characterizing," literally, a mixture of cases. It typically can be used for inpatients to predict costs of patient-related expenditures, to assess quality of care, or to predict outcome.[3]

Although the critical care practitioner may focus on a segment of illness that necessitates ICU admission, a large percentage of ICU patients are hospitalized before actual ICU care is delivered. Under these circumstances, less physiologically based classifications may be used and applied to either the pre-ICU phase of illness or the entire course of hospitalization. Gonnella and colleagues provide insight into non-ICU case mix measurement through a system known as Disease Staging.[4] Less physiologically based, it defines severity as the likelihood of death or residual impairment from disease irrespective of therapy. Severity scales are suggested to be useful in evaluation of physician efficiency, prognostic measures, therapeutic effectiveness, use of health-care resources, designing clinical trials, and developing systems for equitable reimbursement of health-care services.[4]

A classical example of an ICU case mix manager resulted from the APACHE system development.[5] Knaus and colleagues developed this physiologically based classification to make adjustments for severity of illness when comparing outcome of intensive care among institutions across large populations of patients. It was expected to facilitate the assessment of the efficacy of ICUs, to evaluate new therapies, and to study the use of resources.[5]

The two perspectives exemplified by Disease Staging and APACHE systems emphasize that physicians need to become familiar with a variety of classification systems for specific definition of patient populations before, during, and after ICU care. Table 79-1 is a summary of additional reasons for classifying patient populations. Along with these reasons, each system classification should be viewed for its potential application to the various phases of illness (the pre-ICU, ICU, and post-ICU phase) (see Table 79-2).

EVALUATION OF SEVERITY INDICES AND PATIENT CLASSIFICATION SYSTEMS

The validity of a classification system must be questioned before it is applied to patient populations. In other words, does a system measure what it is supposed to measure? A classification may be designed to classify patients according to severity of illness, resource consumption, or outcome. This point is easily understood when one asks, How validly does the Diagnosis-Related Groupings (DRGs) predict use of resource and cost of care? Several studies have demonstrated inequity in reimbursement for service because of lack of adjustment for severity of illness.[6,7] Logically, increased severity requires increased use of resources. Thus, one might argue that the validity of the DRG system for resource consumption measurement is questionable.

Questioning whether or not one classification system produces results similar to those of another is referred to as construct validity. The importance of this process was shown by Lemeshow and colleagues who demonstrated similarity of outcome predictions among the Mortality Prediction Model (MPM), Simplified Acute Physiology Score (SAPS), and Acute Physiology Score (APS).[8] Although similarities might exist, the state of patient classification has not yet evolved to the extent that any particular "gold standard" exists.

Predictive validity means the correlation of a predicted outcome. This concept has been studied most widely with APACHE II. Refinements in APACHE II allow assignment of a patient with a particular severity score to a specific category, which allows for prediction of survival or death for groups of patients.[9] Similar prediction is possible with the MPM.[8] Comparison of actual to predicted survival may enable quality assessment in that a better than predicted survival could be related to better quality and less than predicted survival may mean lesser quality of care. With respect to classification of severity of illness, accurate predictions of outcome for patient groups is a highly desirable

Table 79-1. Some Purposes of Patient Classification Systems

Divide large numbers of patients into homogeneous groups for analysis
Stratify patient populations for comparisons among different institutions
Group patients for reimbursement of services
Quantitate therapeutic intervention
Analyze resource consumptions by various populations
Objectively classify patients for comparison of therapeutic methods
Make adjustments for severity of illness for reimbursement of services
Make adjustments for severity of illness for outcome analysis
Analyze efficiency of care (comparison of severity of illness to quantity of therapeutic intervention)
Predict outcome of illness in patient population
Analyze the quality of patient care by comparing actual outcome to predicted outcome in patient populations

---

Table 79-3. Technical Points of Evaluation of Patient Classification, Severity of Illness Indices, and Outcome Quantitation

Validity: Does a system measure what it was designed to measure
Construct validity: Do other classifications of measurement produce similar results
Predictive validity: How accurately does a classification predict outcome
Content validity: Is there medical meaningfulness to the classification
Attribution validity: Can a classification distinguish between "bad outcomes" and patients who get worse because of their disease progression as opposed to ineffective, inappropriate, or negligent care.
Reproducibility: How accurate are results for similar patients when different raters derive a code or calculate a score.
Freedom from manipulation: How difficult or easy is it to alter a code or score for final assignment of that code or score.
Cost of measurement: What is the cost to an institution for the derivation of a code/s or score.

---

attribute, but only if all differences in patient determinants of survival have been taken into account. It is also important to realize that statistical validation of prediction models on different patient populations across many institutions is the true test of predictive validity.[10,11]

Medical meaningfulness (content validity) is another way of saying that a severity index or outcome quantitation should make sense. It should be logical, credible to clinicians, and correlate with prognosis.[12] Considering outcome of a critical illness, measurement of severity should include physiologic variables that are readily accessible and used by clinicians to assess the physiologic reserve of the patient.[13] An index that is to quantitate outcome beyond ICU survival must identify variables that correlate with physical, mental, and social well-being.[14]

Table 79-2. Patient Classification Systems for Entire Patient Populations*

Pre-ICU—Entire Hospitalization	ICU Indices	Post-ICU Quality Evaluation
Diagnosis-Related Groups	APACHE and APACHE II	Activities of Daily Living (ADL)
International Classification of Diseases (ICD-9-CM)	Simplified Acute Physiology Score (SAPS)	Karnofsky Performance Status Scale
		Sickness Impact Profile
Physician's Current Procedural Terminology (CPT)	Mortality Prediction Model (MPM)	Nottingham Health Profile
Disease Staging	APACHE III	Functional Status Questionnaire
Severity of Illness Index	Therapeutic Intervention Scoring System (TISS)	Quality Adjusted Life Years
Medical Illness Severity Grouping System (MEDISGRPS)	(See Table 79-15 for specific ICU indices)	

* Pre-ICU indices often are applied to patient populations throughout the entire course of hospitalization. ICU indices are applied to specific portions of hospitalization. Post-ICU indices are used to quantitate the long-term outcome of the patient care process.

Table 79-3 contains additional elements that must be reviewed when using any classification system. Some systems demand that some elements be evaluated more closely than others. For example, prediction of survival has different meanings than prediction of resource consumption. Medical meaningfulness may have less bearing on resource consumption. Reproducibility, on the other hand, is important for both survival prediction and resource consumption. Most importantly, the users of the classification must remember that validity is multifaceted. The application of the classification should be based on user requirements and definitions of elements to be classified.

PRE-ICU INDICES AND OTHER CLASSIFICATIONS THAT APPLY TO THE ENTIRE COURSE OF HOSPITALIZATION

Diagnosis-Related Groups (DRGs)

Historically, the development of severity of illness indices, patient classification for resource consumption analysis, and case mix managers were perceived to be of little clinical importance to most clinicians until the enactment of the Social Security Amendments of 1983.[15] Subsequently, the system that evolved for classifying patients into payment groups is the so-called DRGs which was developed in the 1970s by researchers at Yale University.[16] It is a metric that is within the public domain and is used as the basis for a prospective payment system to reimburse hospitals for Medicare patients.[17] Reimbursement is based on diagnosis and/or procedure rather than cost.

Originally, this classification system was intended to relate "the demographic, diagnostic and therapeutic characteristics of patients to the output they are provided so that cases are differentiated by only those variables related to the condition of the patient (e.g., operations) that affect this utilization of the hospital's facilities."[16] The principal deficiencies are "the inherent limitations of any classification system; the inadequacy of the data on which DRG assignments are made; the failure of DRGs to adequately show differences in 'intensity' and 'severity' within a given diagnostic category and the degree to which DRGs represent a classification based on existing prevailing patterns of medical practice of defined diagnostic entities..."[18] These shortcomings make it difficult to apply this classification system to quality assessment or efficiency of operation.[19]

If this type of payment results in reduced number of ICU beds or reduced length of ICU stay for patients who would benefit from ICU care, it could adversely affect follow-up mortality rates after ICU discharge.[20] For these reasons, physicians involved in the care of critically ill patients should familiarize themselves with the methodology of DRG application. In addition, they should also seek access to aggregate information about their own patient populations to understand better economic issues in the operations of their ICUs.[21]

Methodologically, the assignment of a DRG number is made retrospectively from data derived from the hospital discharge abstract, but prospective assignment with revision and change after discharge is possible. Assignment to a DRG requires an accounting of diagnoses, procedures, complications, comorbidities (preexisting conditions), and signs and symptoms.[22] Originally, 467 classes were identified, but presently 492 classes are included that demonstrate similar resource consumption and length of stay patterns within each class.[22,23] The method of scoring is illustrated in Figure 79-1. Patients initially are placed into one of 25 major categories on the basis of organ systems involved, clinical diagnoses, and procedures (Table 79-4). Subsequent to initial assignment, patients are further divided on the basis of diagnosis relative to length of stay, with further splitting on the basis of age, comorbid or complicating conditions, and discharge status (dead or alive).[18] From this final coding, adjustments are made for location in an urban or rural area, the extent of graduate education, relative wage rates in the labor market, the percentage of patients receiving supplemental security income, the DRG to which the case is assigned at hospital discharge, and outlier status at discharge.[17,18,24]

The basis of assignment to DRGs is the Uniform Hospital Discharge Data Set. These data elements are listed in Table 79-5. The primary diagnosis and secondary diagnoses are recorded using ICD-9-CM codes (see following section) and similar assignment is made for procedures. Such assignment, however, as noted by Iezzoni and Moskowitz, provides only a limited description of clinical conditions.[25] This information usually is computerized by hospital billing departments and may be readily available in computerized form for those wishing to review patient characteristics and hospital discharge status for patients who have received ICU care.

International Classification of Diseases (ICD-9-CM)

The International Classification of Diseases, Ninth Revision, Clinical Modification is based on a World Health Organization method for "the classification of morbidity and mortality information for statistical purposes and for the indexing of hospital records by disease and operation, for data storage and retrieval.[26] It represents the clinical modification of the World Health Organization's International Classification of Disease, Ninth Revision. The modification's intent is "to serve as a useful tool in the area of classification of morbidity data for indexing of medical rec-

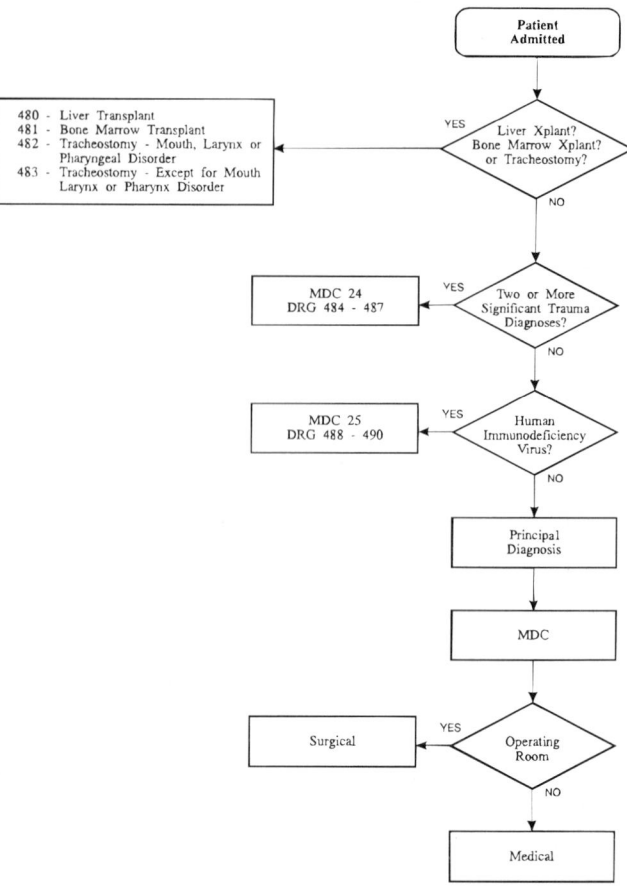

Fig. 79–1. Algorithm with the steps taken to assign a DRG. Liver transplant, bone marrow transplant, tracheostomy patients, and trauma patients are sorted out first. Patients with human immunodeficiency are then grouped, and then a principal diagnosis is used to assign a major diagnostic category (DC). Final steps include assignment to medical or surgical divisions within the category based on type of diagnosis or surgical procedure performed. Age, secondary diagnoses, nonsurgical procedures, and discharge status affect final DRG assignment. (Modified by George Morrison, Clinical Dimensions, Inc., from St. Anthony's DRG Working Guidebook, 1992. Alexandria, VA, St. Anthony's Publishing, 1991, p. iv.)

ords, medical care review and ambulatory and other medical care programs, as well as for basic health statistics."[27] The entire classification is published in three volumes (Volume 1—Diseases: Tubular List; Volume 2—Diseases: Alphabetical Index; and, Volume 3—Procedures: Tubular List and Alphabetical Index). All coding is done by four- or five-digit codes that are listed under three digit headings as shown in Table 79-6. Additional supplementary classification of factors influencing health status and contact with health services is provided. This supplement is of benefit in coding outcome of care for additional services for clinical conditions that might be required after hospital discharge. This portion of the system comprises the so-called V codes. Finally, further supplementary classifications of external causes of injury and poisoning range from railway accidents to injury resulting from operations of war.[28]

Although one may find that this system has many inher-

Table 79-4. Major Diagnostic Categories and Diagnosis-Related Groups

Major Diagnostic Category	Diagnosis-Related Groups by Range	Category Description
1	1–35	Diseases and disorders of the nervous system
2	36–48	Diseases and disorders of the eye
3	49–74	Diseases and disorders of the ear, nose, and throat (includes 168, 169, 185, 186, 187)
4	75–102	Diseases and disorders of the respiratory system (excludes 473 and includes 474)
5	103–145	Diseases and disorders of the circulatory system (includes 478, 479)
6	146–190	Diseases and disorders of the digestive system
7	191–208	Diseases and disorders of the hepatobiliary system and pancreas
8	209–256	Diseases and disorders of the musculoskeletal system and connective tissue (includes 471, 491)
9	257–284	Diseases and disorders of the skin, subcutaneous tissue, and breast
10	285–301	Endocrine, nutritional, and metabolic diseases
11	302–333	Diseases and disorders of the kidney and urinary tract
12	334–352	Diseases and disorders of the male reproductive system
13	353–369	Diseases and disorders of the female reproductive system
14	370–384	Pregnancy, childbirth, and the puerperium (includes 469)
15	385–391	Normal newborns and other neonates with certain conditions originating in the perinatal period (includes 470)
16	392–399	Diseases and disorders of the blood and blood-forming organs and immunologic disorders
17	400–414	Myeloproliferative disorders and poorly differentiated neoplasms (includes 473, 429)
18	415–423	Infectious and parasitic diseases
19	424–432	Mental disorders
20	433–438	Substance-use disorders and substance-induced organic disorders (excludes 438)
21	439–455	Injury, poisoning, and toxic effects of drugs
22	456–460	Burns (includes 472)
23	461–467*	Factors influencing health status and other contacts with health services
24	484–487	Multiple significant trauma
25	488–490	Human immunodeficiency virus infections

* Groups 468, 476, 477, 480, 481, 482, and 483 are not associated with any major diagnostic category.

ent problems, it serves as a common language for comparison of disease states around the world. The codes used are qualifiers of disease states and emphasize that quantitation is required by other methods. Because this classification is a significant component of DRGs, the clinician is well served to familiarize him or herself with the major categories in which care is delivered. With an eye to the future computerization of the ICU, data captured within the unit should be organized so that it could be passed automatically through a hospital information system to the medical records department for abstraction and coding for administrative purposes.

The DRGs and ICD-9-CM are methods of classification for financial purposes and description of clinical conditions respectively. Such classification may provide a demographic snapshot of a patient population but does not provide information about variation in cost, medical practice, or quality. They are, however, useful from an epidemiologic point of view. When beginning any type of research on resource consumption or quality assurance in the ICU, caregivers should be aware that this information may be available in computerized data bases in medical records departments.

As of this writing, ICD-10 codes are likely to replace ICD-9 codes, with further emphasis on the requirements for continued medical care following hospital discharge. The tenth revision has a new title, International Statistical Classification of Diseases and Related Health Problems, em-

Table 79-5. Uniform Hospital Discharge Data Set

Age
Sex
Date of admission, date of discharge
Principal diagnosis
Secondary diagnoses
Primary procedure
Secondary procedures
Place to where patient is discharged
Discharge status

Table 79-6. ICD-9-CM: List of Three-Digit Categories

(001–009)	Infectious and parasitic diseases
(140–239)	Neoplasms
(240–246)	Endocrine, nutritional, and metabolic diseases, and immunity disorders
(280–289)	Diseases of the blood and blood-forming organs
(290–319)	Mental disorders
(320–389)	Diseases of the nervous system and sense organs
(390–392)	Diseases of the circulatory system
(460–519)	Diseases of the respiratory system
(520–579)	Diseases of the digestive system
(580–629)	Diseases of the digestive system
(630–676)	Complications of pregnancy, childbirth, and the puerperium
(680–709)	Diseases of the skin and subcutaneous tissue
(710–739)	Diseases of the musculoskeletal system and connective tissue
(740–759)	Congenital anomalies
(760–779)	Certain conditions originating in the perinatal period
(780–799)	Symptoms, signs, and ill-defined conditions
(800–999)	Injury and poisoning

phasizing its statistical purpose and widened scope. Its principal innovation is the use of an alphanumeric coding scheme of one letter followed by 3 or 4 digits. This change has more than doubled the size of the coding frame. The 3 character categories are divided into 21 chapters. More specifically, Chapter 9 includes diseases of the circulatory system with coding of I00 to I99 rather than 390 to 392. Chapter 10 includes diseases of the respiratory system with coding of J00 to J99 rather than 460 to 519. Left ventricular failure has a code of I50.1. Pneumonia due to Klebsiella pneumoniae has a code of J15.1.[29] Volume 1 of ICD-10, International Statistical Classification of Diseases and Related Health Problems, Tenth Revision is available for educational purposes.[29] Volume 2 is an instructional manual for use of the volume, on tabulations and on planning for the use of ICD. Volume 3 is an alphabetical index that contains expanded instructions on its use. Delays in the implementation of the new coding system are likely to result from requirements for reprogramming computers used in determining reimbursement.

Current Procedural Terminology, Fourth Edition (CPT-4)

Physicians' Current Procedural Terminology is a listing rather than a classification system of... "descriptive terms and identifying codes for reporting medical services and procedures performed by physicians."[30] It is intended to provide a uniform language for accurate description of medical, surgical, and diagnostic services, thus serving as a means of communication among physicians, patients, and third party payors." In the United States, it is the most widely accepted nomenclature for the reporting of physician procedures and services to government and health carriers. As with other systems, it was devised by a panel of physicians representing all specialties of medicine with periodic revisions done in similar fashion.

More recently, this list is published annually by the American Medical Association.[30] The publication contains instructions for use and methods of modification and is also available in computerized form. The main body of material is listed in five sections as shown in Table 79-7. Definition of levels of service is provided for both outpatient and inpatient services and procedures. The listing is suitably indexed with guidelines for the reader to search by procedure or service, organ, condition, synonyms, eponyms, or abbreviations. The critical care practitioner should become familiar with these codes in the United States because reimbursement is tied to the level of service provided as well as to supporting diagnoses coded by ICD-

Table 79-7. CPT-4 Coding: Five Major Sections

Medicine (except Anesthesiology)	90000 to 99999
Anesthesiology	00100 to 01999, 99100 to 99140
Surgery	10000 to 69999
Radiology (Including nuclear medicine and diagnostic ultrasound)	70000 to 79999
Pathology and laboratory	80000 to 89999

Table 79-8. Descriptors of Critical Care Services in Medical Emergencies

Code	Description
99291*	Critical care, initial, including the diagnostic and therapeutic services and direction of care of the critically ill or multiple injured or comatose patient, requring the prolonged presence of the physician, first hour
99292*	Each additional 30 minutes
	Services for patients who are not critically ill but in the ICU
99231	Subsequent hospital care with two of the following three: problem-focused interval history; problem-focused examination; straightforward medical decision-making.
	Counseling and/or coordination of care with other agencies or providers
	Typically requires 15 minutes at the bedside
99232	Subsequent hospital care per day for evaluation and management requiring two of the following three: an expanded problem-focused interval history; an expanded problem-focused examination; medical decision-making of moderate complexity.
	Counseling and coordination as in 99231.
	Typically requires 25 minutes at the bedside.
99233	Subsequent hospital care per day as in 99231 and 99232 but with two of the following three: a detailed interval history; a detailed examination; decision-making of high complexity.
	Counseling and coordination commensurate with nature of the problem.
	Typically requires 35 minutes at the bedside.

* These descriptors may be used in lieu of those listed in Table 79-9 when the time described is used to perform the procedures described in Table 79-9. Editor's note: These codes are likely to change with yearly revisions.[30]

9-CM codes. Tables 79-7 to 79-9 illustrate the principal methods of classification and subcoding. Codes may change on a yearly basis; thus, a periodic review by the physician is necessary.

Although the principal purpose of this listing is to provide uniform language for reimbursement of services, it may also serve as a system to gather information about the process of patient care. Procedures usually are performed for diagnostic or therapeutic purposes. Coding usually is done in chronological order and should allow for at least a limited understanding of the longitudinal aspects of the care that is delivered. Billing systems are computerized and may serve as sources of information that could facilitate research, education, and quality assurance activities in the ICU.

Disease Staging

Disease Staging was developed by Gonnella on the basis of a concept developed by the National Cancer Institute to classify oncology patients. Basically, the courses of neoplastic diseases were divided into stages that can be discretely defined and detected clinically to reflect the severity of the disease. These stages are significant in that they can prognosticate as well as define levels of therapeutic intervention. As a case mix measurement system, Disease Staging is intended to evaluate diagnostic efficiency of physicians, refine measures of prognosis, assess therapeutic effectiveness, analyze utilization of health care resources,

Table 79-9. Descriptors of Commonly Performed Procedures in the ICU: CPT-4 Codes

Code	Description
31500	Intubation, endotracheal, emergency procedure
32000	Thoracentesis, puncture of pleural cavity for aspiration, initial or subsequent
36489	Placement of central venous catheter (subclavian, jugular, or other vein) (e.g., for central venous pressure, hyperalimentation, hemodialysis or chemotherapy; percutaneous, over the age of 2 years)
36620	Includes arterial catheterization or cannulation for sampling, monitoring, or transfusion; percutaneous.
36625	Includes arterial catheterization or cannulation for sampling, monitoring, or transfusion; cutdown.
49080	Peritoneocentesis, abdominal paracentesis, or peritoneal lavage; initial
62270	Spinal puncture, lumbar, diagnostic
92953	Temporary transcutaneous pacing
92950	Cardiopulmonary resuscitation
93503	Insertion and placement of flow-directed catheter (e.g., Swan-Ganz) for monitoring purposes
93561	Indicator dilution studies such as dye or thermal dilution, including arterial and/or venous catheterization; with cardiac output measurement (separate procedure)
93562	Same description as 93561, except that it designates subsequent measurement of cardiac output
94681	Oxygen uptake, expired gas analysis; including CO_2 output, percentage oxygen extracted
94690	Oxygen uptake, expired gas analysis; rest, indirect (separate procedure)
94770	Carbon dioxide, expired gas determination by infrared analyzer
95857	Tensilon test for myasthenia gravis

Editor's note: These codes may change with yearly revisions.[30]

and provide a method of equitable reimbursement for patient care services.[4]

A panel of 23 medical consultants assisted in specification of the staging criteria. Four hundred twenty categories were defined. Severity in this classification is the likelihood of death or residual impairment from disease "without consideration of treatment."[4] Each of the stages listed in Table 79-10 can be further subdivided into subcategories. Stages are defined in terms of complications only, such as infection, perforation, obstruction, hemorrhage, paralysis, shock, etc. Social disability, level of functioning, or state of health, however, are not considered.

As a classification system, Disease Staging is a method of refining traditional diagnostic classifications.[19] The emphasis is on clinical criteria of disease progression rather than on direct measures of resource utilization.[31] The system itself has been computerized and uses data derived from the hospital discharge abstract (see Table 79-5). Table 79-11 illustrates definition of the severity of diabetes mellitus. Note that ICD-9-CM codes are used to define the stage of disease. It can be used for case mix reimbursement and has the potential to account for variance in resource consumption within DRGs.[31]

A computerized algorithm that uses logic to order discharge diagnoses for derivation of severity is commercially available. Because data are gathered retrospectively from the hospital discharge abstract, this system may have inherent problems, from lack of specificity of a primary diagnosis and possible omission of relevant data from the discharge abstract.[3] In spite of these shortcomings, however, computerized staging can provide more detailed assessments of hospitalized patients than DRGs and ICD-9-CM codes alone or in combination.[3]

Severity of Illness Index (SII)

The Severity of Illness Index (SII) evolved as a case mix classification system that would reflect the total burden of a patient's illness. It takes into account severity of illness to produce groups that are more homogeneous with respect to total charges, length of stay, routine charges, and laboratory charges.[32] In contrast to systems that assign classification codes based on diagnosis (ICD-9-CM codes), SII assigns codes based on the seven dimensions of severity in Table 79-12.[33] Although assignment is a complex disease, specific criteria are the basis for each of the four levels within each of the seven dimensions listed in Table 79-12. It is conceptually more descriptive of the state of the disease than the disease itself.

The content validity for the severity levels in SII was assessed by a panel of medical experts who examined the definitions of severity levels and came to a consensus.[33] Assignment of severity level in contrast to Disease Staging is from the medical record rather than from the hospital discharge abstract (see Table 79-5). Levels of severity are based on clinical descriptions of diseases. The levels of severity, however, are ordinal and are controversial in the definition of the trim points from one level of severity of illness to another.[33] In addition, distinction between severity related to illness and severity related to poor quality of care is not made.

In spite of perceived shortcomings, this system has been used to demonstrate that differences in total charges, total costs, and length of stay across various types of hospitals frequently disappear when adjustments are made for severity of illness.[34,35] Further evaluation of its validity as a measurement of severity of illness, however, must be undertaken. One principal concern is that this index quantitates the severity over the entire course of hospitalization rather than at a single point in time, such as at the time of admission or after a certain number of days in the hospital. It may be a valid instrument to measure the impact of the burden of illness on utilization of resources.[36] Further study is necessary, however, to assess its accuracy as a predictor of outcome. This fact was emphasized by Green

Table 79-10. Disease Staging: Categories of Increasing Levels of Severity

Stage 1:	Conditions with no complications or problems of minimal severity
Stage 2:	Problems limited to an organ or organ systems; significantly increased risk of complications.
Stage 3:	Multiple site involvement; generalized systemic involvement; poor prognosis.
Stage 4:	Death

(From Gonnella, J. S., Hornbrook, M. C., Louis, D. Z.: Staging of disease. A case-mix measurement. JAMA, 251:637, 1984.)

Table 79-11. Medical and Coded Criteria for Disease Staging

Diagnosis: Diabetes Mellitus. Etiology: Metabolic

Stage	Common Description or Name of Condition	Alternate Description or Synonym	Some ICD-9-CM Codes That Define Each Stage and Substage
0	Diabetes mellitus	Hyperglycemia, "sugar diabetes"	775.10, 790.20, 250.00–250.01, 250.80–250.91
2.1	Diabetes mellitus	Diabetes mellitus with complications of infectious nature: pyoderma, impetigo, furunculosis, monilial vulvitis, monilial skin infection, cystitis, urethritis, epididymitis, prostatitis, pyelonephritis	Stage 1.01 + 320.00–342.90, 289.30, 429.89, 510.00–510.90, 513.00–513.10, 569.50, 580.81, 595.40, 597.80, 601.00–601.90, 604.99, 608.00, 614.00, 680.00, 728.00, 730.80–730.99
2.2	Diabetes mellitus with septicemia	Diabetes mellitus, infection, and associated toxins of bacteria in bloodstream	Stage 1.0 + 038.00–038.90
2.3	Diabetes mellitus with acidosis	Diabetic acidosis or ketosis; Diabetes with ketonemia or ketonuria	Stage 1.0 + 588.80, 791.60, 276.20–276.40; 250.10–250.11
2.4	Diabetes mellitus with retinopathy but without loss of vision, or glomerulosclerosis (without azotemia) or neuropathy (peripheral or autonomic), or gangrene (tissue breakdown)	Microangiopathy; Kimmelstiel-Wilson disease; Arterial insufficiency with associated tissue breakdown	Stages 1.0–2.3 + 337.10, 362,18, 443.81, 443.90, 446.60, 447.10, 581.81, 785.40, 354.00–356.90; 357.20, 362.01, 250.40–250.74
3.1	Diabetes mellitus with acidosis and coma, or retinopathy and loss of vision or necrotizing papillitis, or azotemia	Diabetic coma with ketosis or acidosis; Proliferative retinopathy; Papillary necrosis, medullary necrosis	Stage 2.4 + 276.20, 369.00–369.90; Stages 1.0–2.4 + 583.70, 780.00, 790.60, 584.50–586.00, 590.80–590.81; 362.02, 250.30–250.31
3.2	Diabetes mellitus with hyperosmolar coma	Nonketotic, hyperosmolar hyperglycemic coma	250.20–251.21
3.3	Shock		Stages 1.0–3.2 + 458.90, 785.50–785,59, 788.50, 994.00, 994.80, 995.00, 995.40, 958.40, 998.00, 999.40, 669.10–669.14, 639.50
4.0	Death		Stages 2.2–3.3 + Death

Editor's note: Since publication of this table, a number of revisions have been made. Current classification is available through Center for Research in Medical Education and Health Care, Philadelphia, PA. (Modified from Gonnella, J. S., Hornbrook, M. C., Louis, D. Z.: Staging of disease. A case-mix measurement. JAMA, *251*:637, 1984.)

and colleagues who studied 34,252 Medicare patients discharged from hospitals in 1986.[37] The diagnostic categories of cancer, severe acute heart disease, stroke, pulmonary disease, and low risk heart disease were selected. Using SII, they demonstrated an eightfold increase in accuracy of the Health Care Financial Administration (HCFA) mortality prediction model when taking into account severity of illness over the course of hospital illness. The system has been computerized and is commercially available as a case mix management system.[38]

Table 79-12. Severity of Illness Instrument

Characteristic	Levels			
	1	2	3	4
Stage of principal diagnosis	Asymptomatic	Moderate manifestations	Major manifestations	Catastrophic
Interactions	None	Low	Moderate	Major
Response to therapy (rate)	Prompt	Moderate delay	Serious delay	No response
Residual	None	Minor	Moderate	Major
Complications	None or very minor	Moderate (less important than principal diagnosis)	Major (as or more important than principal diagnosis)	Catastrophic
Dependency	Low	Moderate	Major	Extreme
Procedures (non OR)	Noninvasive diagnostic	Therapeutic or invasive	Nonemergency life sustaining	Emergency life sustaining

(Modified from Horn, S. D., Horn, R. A., Sharkey, P. D.: The severity of illness index as a severity adjustment to diagnosis-related groups. Health Care Fin. Rev., *6*(Suppl.):34, 1984.)

Table 79-13. Meaning of MEDISGROUPS Scores

MEDISGRPS Score	At First Review	At Second Review
0	No significant findings	No significant morbidity
1	Minimal findings, indicating a low potential for organ failure	
2	Either acute findings connoting a short time course with an unclear potential organ failure, or severe findings with high potential for future organ failure	Morbid
3	Both acute and severe findings indicating a high potential for imminent organ failure	
4	Clinical findings indicating the presence of organ failure	Major morbidity

(Modified from Iezzoni, L. I., et al: Admission MedisGroups Score and the cost of hospitalizations. Medical Care. 26:1068, 1988.)

MEDISGRPS-Medical Illness Severity Grouping System

The Medical Illness Severity Grouping System or MEDISGRPS is an admission-oriented patient severity grouping system that used objective key clinical findings to place patients in one of five severity groupings.[39] This system is in contrast to Disease Staging, derived from the hospital discharge record, and SII derived from the hospital discharge abstract and hospital record after discharge. It is "generic" insofar as severity of disease is assigned according to key clinical findings (KCF) rather than from diagnostic codes or descriptors of stage of disease. Conceptually, it is similar to the SII as opposed to DRGs, which are assigned according to ICD-9-CM codes. The severity group assignments or scores are made entirely from KCF, which include laboratory, radiologic, pathologic, and physical examination results. Severity is defined as the potential for organ failure and is quantitated in the manner displayed in Table 79-13. Methodologically, a review of the medical record is conducted within the first 48 hours and a second review is conducted between days 3 and 7.[39,40] Figure 79-2 illustrates the method of review. An improvement in the level of severity during hospitalization is expected, but worsening severity may indicate either progression disease or poor quality of patient care.

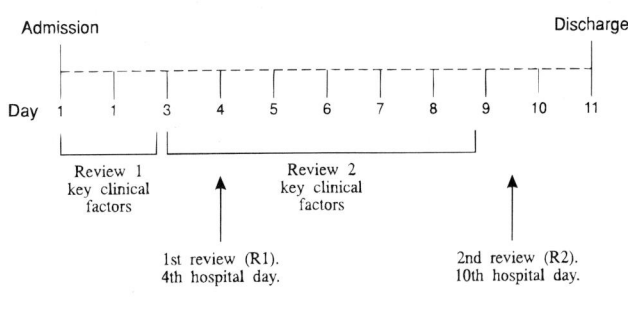

Fig. 79-2. An example of a MEDISGRPS severity review time table. The medical service admission had an 11-day length of stay. The first review done on day 4 examines severity factors from the first 48 hours. The second review, on day 9 examines factors from days 3 through 9. Worsening of severity between the two reviews may imply an issue for improvement in quality, whereas improving severity implies improvement in the illness. (Redrawn by George Morrison, Clinical Dimensions, Inc., from Brewster, A. C., et al.: MEDISGRPS (r): a clinically based approach to classifying hospital patients at admission. Inquiry, 22: 377, 1985.)

The evolution of this system was based on an empiric approach. The key clinical findings were identified by Brewster and Karlin from observations made from "morning reports" given by residents at St. Vincent Hospital in Worcester, MA.[40] These findings revealed that the information transfer between residents included a brief description of a patient's chief complaint; findings on physical examination, including vital signs; results of diagnostic studies, including laboratory results and other diagnostic or therapeutic interventions; and a management plan. The KCF focused the resident's attention on the patient's illness severity. Clinical chiefs of service were consulted to validate the appropriateness of these observations and their application to the level of severity as shown in Table 79-13. Table 79-14 is an example of how some KCF are applied to define severity of acute myocardial infarction. The final list of KCF evolved over several years.[39] The developers designed the system to serve as a screening mech-

Table 79-14. Representative Key Clinical Findings and Their Assigned MEDISGRPS Severity Group for Principal Diagnosis or Acute Myocardial Infarction

KCF-Category	1	2	3	4
ECG	Ischemia Atrial fibrillation	Myocardial infarction (acute) (extension)	Third degree block	
Chest radiograph	Cardiomegaly		Congestive heart failure	
Physical examination	Rales			Coma
Cardiac catheterization		Cardiomyopathy		
Laboratory	P_{O_2} 60–69 CPK 121–239	P_{O_2} 45–59 CPK 240+	P_{O_2} <45	
Vital signs	Respirations 25–32	Respirations >32		

(Modified from Iezzoni, L. I., et al: Admission MedisGroups Score and the cost of hospitalizations. Medical Care. 26:1068, 1988.)

anism for the identification of outliers in terms of length of stay or resource consumption as determined by the severity of illness. As expected, a correlation exists between severity and KCF.[41]

Summary of Indices

The aforementioned instruments have evolved with purposes in mind. All have been developed by health-care professionals for case mix management, whether for analysis of utilization of resources, quality assessment, or reimbursement. The choice of index depends on the questions asked, the availability of data in a given institution, and the familiarity of the user with the strength and weaknesses of each instrument. Further reference to these indices and the development of new indices in the near future are expected. One measure of the usefulness of these indices in the ICU population may be how accurately they predict need for ICU care and/or outcome of subsequent ICU care. It will also be important to determine the presence or absence of correlation with severity indices used in the ICU and after discharge from the ICU.

CASE MIX MANAGEMENT SYSTEMS WITHIN THE ICU

The previous discussion was devoted to case mix management systems for entire hospital populations. The ICU classification systems are designed to define the severity of illness and to predict the outcomes of care, including resource allocation for patients admitted to ICUs. Some indices are intended to be applied across all types of patients within the ICU and others apply to only specific disease entities. Table 79-15 outlines these two types of ICU classification systems. The subsequent discussion reviews the two types of systems in chronologic order of development to reflect the evolution of this methodology.

Table 79-15. Classification Systems for the ICU

Applied across entire ICU populations
1. Severity of illness
   Apache
   APACHE II (using Acute Physiology Score and Chronic Health Status)
   SAPS (Simplified Acute Physiology Score)
   APACHE III
2. Prediction of outcome
   MPM (Mortality Prediction Model)
   APACHE II (Application of Acute Physiology Status and Chronic Health Status to prediction model)
   APACHE III
3. Quantitation of resources or effort in care
   TISS (Therapeutic Intervention Scoring System)
4. Prediction of resource utilization
   APACHE III

Applied to specific disease or clinical states
1. Glasgow coma score, initially for classification of clinical state of head trauma victims
2. Prediction of outcome of the application of mechanical ventilation; adult respiratory distress syndrome.
3. Prediction of outcome for cardiopulmonary resuscitation
4. Prediction of outcome of acute myocardial infarction
5. Prediction of outcome from clinical shock states
6. Prognostication of patients with cirrhosis, chronic liver disease, chronic hepatitis, and variceal bleeding
7. Prediction of outcome from acute renal failure

Classifications for Application Across Entire ICU Populations

APACHE

The acronym APACHE stands for Acute Physiology and Chronic Health Evaluation.[5] It is a physiologically based classification system developed by Knaus, Zimmerman, and colleagues at George Washington University Medical Center. This consensus-generated system was first published in 1981. Initially, it called for the accumulation of 34 data points, which include physiologic status, laboratory results, and preadmission health status. As a prototypical severity of illness classification system, its authors intended it as a case mix management system for ICUs. It was expected to facilitate the assessment of the efficacy of ICUs, to evaluate new therapies, and to study the use of resources.[5]

This classification system was based on several assumptions. To begin, the authors assumed that if a measurement is important for severity of illness, it will appear in the patient record, which is the sole source of data. If data are not recorded, the value is considered normal. The parameters specified were assigned weights by the consensus of critical care experts. The scores from the addition of these weights determine the severity of illness. A worsening score implies a greater degree of illness and also correlates with increased need for therapy. A higher score is expected to correlate with a greater mortality. Figure 79-3, which is derived from validation studies of 805 patients using APACHE, illustrates this point.

The deficiencies of the APACHE score were that it underestimated the severity of illness because clinical modifiers of acute physiologic status inadequately reflected health status before ICU admission and the requirement for a large number of data points left some data fields empty.[9]

Simplified Acute Physiology Score (SAPS)

The deficiencies of APACHE were addressed indirectly by LeGall and colleagues in a simplified physiology score system that would have similar correlations with mortality as in the APACHE system itself. The number of data points was reduced to 13. The data included age, heart rate, systolic blood pressure, spontaneous respiratory rate, ventilation or CPAP, urine output in 24 hours, BUN, hematocrit, white blood cell count, serum glucose, serum sodium, serum potassium, serum bicarbonate, and the Glasgow coma score.[42] The variables in this system are assigned values of 0 to 4, depending on the degree of variation from a specified normal range. Evaluation was originally done on 679 consecutive patients admitted to 8 multidisciplinary ICUs in France. Scores ranged from 4 to more than 21 and correlated directly with an increasing mortality.[42] The developers of this system were concerned about simplifying the process of collecting variables for determination of severity of illness as compared to the original APACHE, which contained 34 variables.

A New Simplified Acute Physiology Score (SAPS II)

Further study of SAPS suggested a principal deficiency in the method was that the model predicted ICU mortality

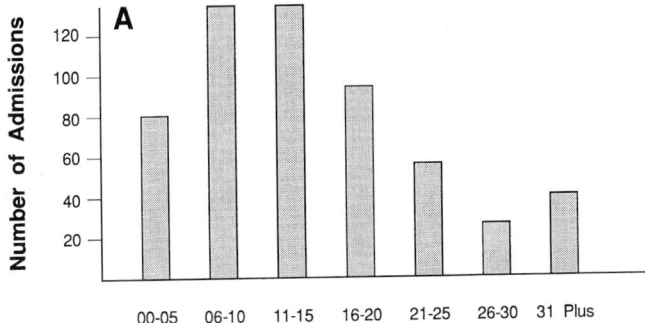
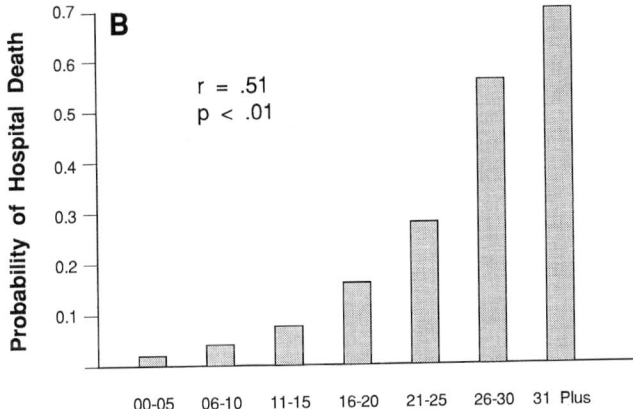
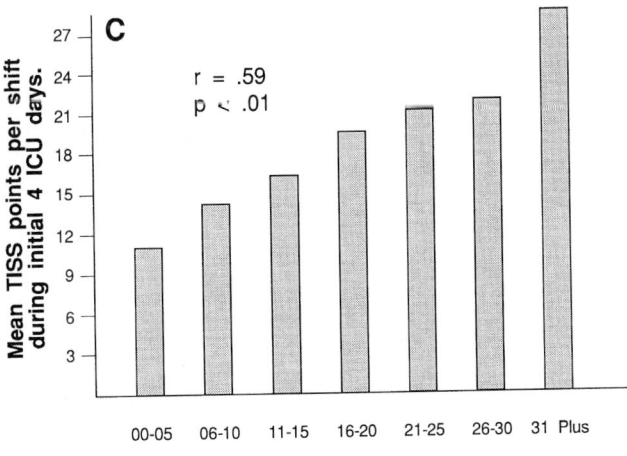

Fig. 79-3. *A,* A distribution of ICU admissions by Physiology Score (APACHE II). *B,* The relationship between physiology score and probability of hospital death is seen with increasing score and increasing probability of death. *C,* The relationship between increasing physiology score and increasing therapeutic effort. (Redrawn by George Morrison, Clinical Dimensions, Inc., from Knaus, W. A., Zimmerman, J. E., Wagner, D. P.: APACHE—acute physiology and chronic health evaluation: A physiologically based classification system. Crit. Care Med., 9:591, 1981.

rather than hospital mortality.[43] Thus, between September 30, 1991 and February 28, 1992, a large European/North American study was undertaken to propose a new simplified acute physiology score, the SAPS II, to develop a method of converting the score to a probability of hospital mortality.[44] Statistical techniques using logistic regression analysis were used to assist in:

- Selecting the variables that would constitute SAPS II
- Deciding on appropriate groupings and point assignments for each variable
- Converting the SAPS II score to a probability of hospital mortality

The study involved 137 medical, surgical, or mixed ICUs in 12 countries, including the United States. It included 13,152 patients, randomly divided into developmental (65%) and validation (35%) samples, which excluded patients less than 18 years, burn patients, coronary care patients, and cardiac surgery patients. The number of variables was enlarged to 17 (Table 79-16), and the weights assigned to the variables increased with ranges varying from 0 to 26 (Table 79-17). From the scores obtained, the probability of hospital mortality is calculated.[44]

The model performed well in the developmental sample ($P = .883$) and the validation sample ($P = .104$) with areas under the receiver operating characteristic curves of 0.88 for the developmental sample and 0.86 for the validation sample. The developers of SAPS II indicated that the area under the ROC curve was higher than the original SAPS when the comparisons were made in the validation sample (0.80 for SAPS and 0.86 for SAPS II). This system now provides methodology for estimating the risk of hospital death without the requirement to assign a specific diagnostic category.[44]

APACHE II

Knaus and colleagues refined the APACHE system to a second version—APACHE II. Data points were reduced to 12 and include temperature, mean blood pressure, heart rate, respiratory rate, oxygenation, arterial pH, serum sodium, serum potassium, serum creatinine, hematocrit, white blood count, and the Glasgow coma scale. Additional consideration was given to the age of the patient and the presence of chronic illness.[9] The worst values in the first 24 hours of ICU illness are recorded for calculation of the score. Figure 79-4 illustrates the collection form and the method by which a score is calculated.

A nominal group process was again used to choose and weigh the physiologic variables just listed. Weights of 0 to 4 were assigned to each variable, depending on the degree of physiologic derangement. The correlation of increasing score with mortality has been validated at multiple sites. As a scoring system, APACHE II is the ICU scoring system used most widely, both nationally and internationally.[45,46]

The additional utility of the APACHE system has been its predictive power for mortality in patient groups. The assignment of a patient to a category listed in Table 79-18 allows for prediction of mortality based on the diagnostic

Table 79-16. Variables and Definitions for SAPS II

Variable	Definition
Age	Use the patient's age (in years) at last birthday
Heart rate	Use the worst value in 24 hours, either low or high heart rate; if it varied from cardiac arrest (11 points) to extreme tachycardia (7 points), assign 11 points
Systolic blood pressure	Use the same method as for heart rate: e.g., if it varied from 60 to 205 mm Hg, assign 13 points
Body temperature	Use the highest temperature in degrees centigrade or Fahrenheit
PaO_2/FIO_2 ratio	If ventilated or continuous pulmonary artery pressure, use the lowest value of the ratio
Urinary output	If the patient is in the intensive care unit for less than 24 hours, make the calculation for 24 hours: e.g., 1 L in 8 hours = 3 L in 24 hours
Serum urea or serum urea nitrogen level	Use the highest value in mmol/L or g/L for serum urea, in mg/dl for serum urea nitrogen
WBC count	Use the worst (high or low) WBC count according to the scoring sheet
Serum potassium level	Use the worst (high or low) value in mmol/L, according to the scoring sheet
Serum sodium level	Use the worst (high or low) value in mmol/L, according to the scoring sheet
Serum bicarbonate level	Use the lowest value in mEq/L
Bilirubin level	Use the highest value in umol/L or mg/dL
Glasgow coma score	Use the lowest value; if the patient is sedated, record the estimated Glasgow coma score before sedation
Type of admission	Unscheduled surgical,* scheduled surgical,† or medical‡
AIDS	Yes, if HIV-positive with clinical complications such as Pneumocystis carinii pneumonia, Kaposi's sarcoma, lymphoma, tuberculosis, or toxoplasma infection
Hematologic malignancy	Yes, if lymphoma, acute leukemia, or multiple myeloma
Metastatic cancer	Yes, if proven metastasis by surgery, computed tomographic scan, or any other method

SAPS, Simplified Acute Physiology Score; FIO_2, fraction of inspired oxygen; WBC, white blood cell; AIDS, acquired immunodeficiency syndrome; HIV, human immunodeficiency virus.
* Patients added to operating room schedule within 24 hours of the operation.
† Patients whose surgery was scheduled at least 24 hours in advance.
‡ Patients having no surgery within 1 week of admission to intensive care unit.
(From Le Gall, J. R., Lemeshow, S., and Saulnier, F.: A new Simplified Acute Physiology Score (SAPS II) based on a European/North American multicenter study. JAMA, 270:2957, 1993.)

category. The correlation between predicted and observed is good in most diagnostic categories. The principal exceptions include diabetic ketoacidosis and pulmonary edema resulting from cardiac dysfunction.[47,48] The lack of correlation in a given diagnostic category may mean either that specific physiologic variables important for prognosis in the disease are not included in the model or that the model has not accounted for the efficiency of interventions for correcting physiologic abnormalities in that disease. These possibilities introduce opportunities for important ICU-based research.

Mortality Prediction Model (MPM)

The APACHE system started as a severity-of-illness classification system intended to facilitate the description of utilization patterns and to compare the efficacy of ICUs. It evolved to a quality assessment tool for predicting the outcome of intensive care. The MPM was intended to be a prediction model from its first description.[49] Its authors, Lemeshow, Teres, and colleagues, selected parameters to determine a score for outcome prediction. In contrast to the APACHE development, which involved use of the opinion of experts to select and weigh parameters used to determine the score, MPM was developed from parameters derived from statistical techniques using an extensive ICU data base. The 11 variables that proved to be predictive of mortality were as follows:

- Level of consciousness (stupor or coma)
- Type of admission (emergency or elective)
- CPR prior to admission
- Cancer
- History of chronic renal failure
- Probable and definite infection
- Age
- Previous ICU admission (within 6 months)
- Heart rate
- Surgical service admission
- Systolic blood pressure

These parameters are collected at the time of admission to the ICU.[49]

An additional difference between APACHE II and MPM is that the latter does not require the identification of a cause of major organ system failure for prediction of outcome. With APACHE, the prediction of mortality for a high severity score in a patient with hypotension requires an additional assignment to an appropriate diagnostic category (cardiogenic shock, congestive heart failure, gastrointestinal bleeding, etc).[9] Neither model has sufficient sensitivity to predict correctly those individual patients who will ultimately die. Each model estimates the probability of death and can be used to compare observed and expected mortality rates in comparable groups of patients.

Mortality Probability Models (MPM II)

Since the development of MPM, ICU technology, practices, and populations have changed. Because of these circumstances, Lemeshow, Teres, and colleagues further developed the MPM into MPM II with the goal of a valid simple system for estimating the probability of hospital mortality among ICU patients that could be used to compare quality of care within an ICU.[50] They recognized that the MPM, developed at a single site hospital, was not so robust as a model developed and validated at multiple sites.

Table 79-17. Point (pts) Assignment for Calculation of SAPS II Score*

Age (yr)	<40, 0 pts	40–59, 7 pts	60–69, 12 pts	70–79, 16 pts	>80, 18 pts
Heart rate (beats/min)	<40, 11 pts	40–69, 2 pts	10–119, 0 pts	120–159, 4 pts	>160, 7 pts
Systolic blood pressure (mm Hg)	<70, 13 pts	70–99, 5 pts	100–199, 0 pts	>200, 2 pts	
Body Temperature (C [F])	<39 (102.2), 0 pts	>39 (102.2), 3 pts			
Only if ventilated or continuous pulmonary artery pressure (PaO_2 mm Hg/FiO_2)	<100, 11 pts	100–199, 9 pts	>200, 6 pts		
Urine output (L/d)	<0.500, 11 pts	0.500–0.999, 9 pts	>1.00, 0 pts		
Serum urea level (mmol/L) or serum urea nitrogen level (mg/L)	<10.0, 0 pts <28, 0 pts	10.0–29.9, 6 pts 28–83, 6 pts			
WBC count (10^3/mm^3)	<1.0, 12 pts	1.0–19.9, 0 pts	>20.0, 3 pts		
Serum potassium (mmol/dL)	<3.0, 4 pts	3.0–4.9, 0 pts	>5.0, 3 pts		
Serum sodium (mmol/dL)	<125, 5 pts	125–144, 0 pts	>145, 1 pt		
Serum bicarbonate (meq/L)	<15, 6 pts	15–19, 3 pts	>20, 0 pts		
Bilirubin level (mg/dL)	<4.0, 0 pts	4.0–5.9, 4 pts	>6.0, 9 pts		
Glasgow coma score	<6, 26 pts	6–8, 13 pts	9–10, 7 pts	11–13, 5 pts	14–15, 0 pts
Chronic diseases	Metastatic cancer, 9 pts	Hematologic malignancy, 10 pts	AIDS, 17 pts		
Type of admission	Scheduled surgery, 0 pts	Medical diagnosis, 6 pts	Unscheduled surgery, 8 pts		

pts, Points assigned; FiO_2, fraction of inspired oxygen; WBC, white blood cell; AIDS, acquired immunodeficiency syndrome.
(From Le Gall, J. R., Lemeshow, S., and Saulnier, F.: A new Simplified Acute Physiology Score (SAPS II) based on a European/North American multicenter study. JAMA, 270:2957, 1993.)

Therefore, 2 sets of data were assembled for development and validation of a refined prediction model with an outcome measure of vital status at hospital discharge. One set was collected at 6 adult medical and surgical ICUs in 4 teaching hospitals in the northeastern United States. Data for the second set were collected at 137 medical and surgical ICUs in hospitals in 12 different countries including the United States.

The MPM II was expanded to include not only mortality prediction upon admission to the ICU (MPM_0), but also mortality prediction at 24 hours for patients staying longer than 24 hours in the ICU (MPM_{24}). Both models calibrated well (goodness of fit tests) and discriminated well (area under the receiver operator curve), as shown in Table 79-19. Data from 12,610 patients was used for the developmental model and data from 6514 patients was used for the validation model. Data from 10,357 patients remaining in the ICU at 24 hours was used for the 24-hour model (MPM_{24}).

Fifteen variables are included in the admission model (MPM_0), and an additional 8 variables are included in the 24-hour model (MPM_{24}). Table 79-20 summarizes these variables. The developers of these models intend that they be used as quality assessment tools. The principle of comparison of actual to predicted mortality is applied. A ratio of greater than 1 would suggest a need to examine circumstances that might lead to improved quality of care, whereas a ratio of less than 1 would suggest a need to examine circumstances responsible for the good quality of care and application to problem areas. The models are not intended to be triage tools that would deny a patient access to ICU care because they were not designed to predict mortality if ICU care were denied to patients.[50]

As of this writing, the MPM_0 remains the only prediction model that can be applied on admission to the ICU. Its developers plan further refinement for prediction for patients who remain longer than 24 hours in the ICU.[50]

Therapeutic Intervention Scoring System (TISS)

In contrast to the APACHE system, APACHE II, MPM, and SAPS, Therapeutic Intervention Scoring System (TISS) evolved to allow quantitative comparison of patient care requirements of different ICUs. Items of therapeutic intervention are scored according to the intensity of the process of patient care. The points per item are summated per patient per 24 hours (Table 79-21).[51] Cullen and colleagues intended this system to be used to determine the appropriate use of intensive care facilities; provide information on nurse staffing ratios for various patient care areas; quantitatively validate critically ill patients into care categories; and analyze the cost of intensive care relative to the extent of care offered.

This system was developed in 1974 and was revalidated in 1983.[51,52] Interestingly, little change occurred between the two validation years, suggesting that technology may not have changed that much. Treatments may have changed, but the methods of administration probably have not. Again, contrasting the APACHE and MPM systems, TISS is a measure of process of care rather than outcome or severity of illness. Use of this scoring system itself is labor intensive. Seventy-six variables must be verified as being used or not.

In addition to labor intensity, this system is based on assumptions that may not necessarily be true for all ICUs. The first assumption is that intervention is specific and appropriate. Care is assumed to be discrete, identifiable, and applied consistently. The second assumption is that the degree of illness is related to the number of types of interventions. This assumption implies that the philosophies of treatment are comparable among all ICUs, but experience tells us that this is not the case. The true utility of this system, however, is that, in combination with severity of other measurements, it can provide insight into efficiency of patient care.

THE APACHE II SEVERITY OF DISEASE CLASSIFICATION SYSTEM

PHYSIOLOGIC VARIABLE	HIGH ABNORMAL RANGE				0	LOW ABNORMAL RANGE			
	+4	+3	+2	+1	0	+1	+2	+3	+4
TEMPERATURE - rectal (°C)	≥ 41°	39°-40.9°		38.5°-38.9°	36°-38.4°	34°-35.9°	32°-33.9°	30°-31.9°	≤ 29.9°
MEAN ARTERIAL PRESSURE - mm Hg	≥ 180	130-159	110-129		70-109		50-69		≤ 49
HEART RATE (ventricular response)	≥ 180	140-179	110-139		70-109		55-69	40-54	≤ 39
RESPIRATORY RATE - (nonventilated or ventilated)	≥ 50	35-49		25-34	12-24	10-11	6-9		≤ 5
OXYGENATION: A-aDO$_2$ or PaO$_2$ (mm Hg) a. FIO$_2$ ≥ 0.5 record A-aDO$_2$	≥ 500	350-499	200-349		< 200				
b. FIO$_2$ < 0.5 record only PaO$_2$					PO$_2$ > 70	PO$_2$ 61-70		PO$_2$ 55-60	PO$_2$ < 55
ARTERIAL pH	≥ 7.7	7.6-7.69		7.5-7.59	7.33-7.49		7.25-7.32	7.15-7.24	< 7.15
SERUM SODIUM (mmol/L)	≥ 180	160-179	155-159	150-154	130-149		120-129	111-119	≤ 110
SERUM POTASSIUM (mmol/L)	≥ 7	6-6.9		5.5-5.9	3.5-5.4	3-3.4	2.5-2.9		< 2.5
SERUM CREATININE (mg/100 ml) (Double point score for acute renal failure)	≥ 3.5	2-3.4	1.5-1.9		0.6-1.4		< 0.6		
HEMATOCRIT (%)	≥ 60		50-59.9	46-49.9	30-45.9		20-29.9		< 20
WHITE BLOOD COUNT (total/mm³) (in 1,000s)	≥ 40		20-39.9	15-19.9	3-14.9		1-2.9		< 1
GLASGOW COMA SCORE (GCS): Score = 15 minus actual GCS									
[A] total ACUTE PHYSIOLOGY SCORE (APS): Sum of the 12 individual variable points									
Serum HCO$_2$ (venous-mmol/L) (Not preferred, use if no ABGs)	≥ 52	41-51.9		32-40.9	22-31.9		18-21.9	15-17.9	< 15

[B] AGE POINTS:
Assign points to age as follows:

AGE(yrs)	Points
≤44	0
45-54	2
55-64	3
65-74	5
≥75	6

[C] CHRONIC HEALTH POINTS
If the patient has a history of severe organ system insufficiency or is immunocompromised assign points as follows:
a. For nonoperative or emergency postoperative patients - 5 points
or
b. For elective postoperative patients - 2 points

DEFINITIONS
Organ insufficiency or immunocompromised state must have been evident prior to this hospital admission and conform to the following criteria:

LIVER: Biopsy proven cirrhosis and documented portal hypertension; episodes of past upper GI bleeding attributed to portal hypertension; or prior episodes of hepatic failure/encephalopathy/coma.

CARDIOVASCULAR: New York Heart Association class IV.

RESPIRATORY: Chronic restrictive, obstructive, or vascular disease resulting in severe exercise restriction, i.e., unable to climb stairs or perform household duties; or documented chronic hypoxia, hypercapnia, secondary, polycythemia, severe pulmonary hypertension (>40 mmHg), or respirator dependency.

RENAL: Receiving chronic dialysis.

IMMUNO-COMPROMISED: The patient has received therapy that suppresses resistance to infection, e.g., immunosuppression, chemotherapy, radiation, long term or recent high dose steroids, or has a disease that is sufficiently advanced to suppress resistance to infection, e.g., leukemia, lymphoma, AIDS.

APACHE II SCORE
Sum of [A] + [B] + [C]:

[A] APS points _____
[B] Age points _____
[C] Chronic Health points _____
Total APACHE II _____

Fig. 79-4. Method of assigning the APACHE II severity of disease score. The physiologic variables are listed along with weights to determine APS (lower right). Age points (B) are assigned according to the table (lower left). Chronic health points are assigned as item C. (From Knaus, W. A., et al.: APACHE II: A severity of disease classification system. Crit. Care Med., *13*:818, 1985.

APACHE III

The APACHE system has undergone certain evolutionary changes. Initially, it was a case mix management system for use in comparisons made across many ICUs. It subsequently evolved into a prediction model for quality assurance purposes. Most recently, the quality of a risk management system has been included.[53] In the APACHE III system, the overall severity of illness score ranges from 0 to 299 (Acute Physiology Score, 0 to 252 points; age, 0 to 24 points; and Chronic Health Evaluation, 0 to 23 points) (see Table 79-22). The system comprises 212 potential diagnostic categories, but 78 categories represent the majority. The weights for physiologic variables have been revalued to increase the explanatory power for patient outcome (compare Figs. 79-4 and 79-5). Further explanatory power for patient outcome also increased when the relationship between pH and P_{CO_2} was analyzed (Fig. 79-6). The Glasgow coma scale was also reformatted to account for "neurological abnormalities according to presence or absence of eye opening" (Fig. 79-7).[53]

This latest revision of APACHE was done to improve risk prediction for individual patients, examine issues of timing of ICU admission and location of treatment, and create objectivity in quality assurance and resource utilization.[53] When using this system, the limitations and proper applications should be considered. The focal point of clinical application is that a difference exists between the APACHE III score and risk prediction. When used alone, the

Table 79-18. Principal Diagnostic Categories for APACHE II

Nonoperative	Weight	Operative	Weight
Respiratory failure of insufficiency from:		Multiple trauma	−1.684
Asthma/allergy	−2.108	Admission because of chronic cardiovascular disease	−1.376
COPD	−0.367	Peripheral vascular surgery	−1.315
Pulmonary edema (noncardiogenic)	−0.251	Heart valve surgery	−1.261
Postrespiratory arrest	−0.168	Craniotomy for neoplasm	−1.245
Aspiration/poisoning/toxic	−0.142	Renal surgery for neoplasm	−1.245
Pulmonary embolus	−0.128	Renal transplant	−1.042
Infection	0	Head trauma	−0.995
Neoplasm	0.891	Thoracic surgery for neoplasm	−0.802
Cardiovascular failure or insufficiency from:		Craniotomy for ICH/SDH/SAH	−0.788
Hypertension	−1.798	Laminectomy and other spinal cord surgery	−0.699
Rhythm disturbance	−1.368	Hemorrhagic shock	−0.682
Congestive heart failure	−0.424	GI bleeding	−0.617
Hemorrhagic shock/hypovolemia	0.493	GI surgery for neoplasm	−0.480
Coronary artery disease	−0.191	Respiratory insufficiency after surgery	−0.140
Sepsis	0.113	GI perforation/obstruction	0.060
Postcardiac arrest	0.393	For postoperative patients admitted to the ICU for sepsis or postarrest, use the corresponding weights for nonoperative patients.	
Cardiogenic shock	−0.259		
Dissecting thoracic/abdominal aneurysm	0.731		
Trauma		If not in one of the above, which major vital organ system led to ICU admission postsurgery?	
Multiple trauma	−1.228		
Head trauma	−0.517	Neurologic	01.150
Neurologic		Cardiovascular	−0.797
Seizure disorder	−0.584	Respiratory	−0.610
ICH/SDH/SAH	0.723	Gastrointestinal	−0.613
Other		Metabolic/renal	−0.196
Drug overdose	−3.353		
Diabetic ketoacidosis	−1.507		
GI bleeding	0.334		
If not one of the specific groups above, then which major vital organ system was the principal reason for admission?			
Metabolic/renal	−0.885		
Respiratory	−0.890		
Neurologic	−0.759		
Cardiovascular	0.470		
Gastrointestinal	0.501		

(From Knaus, W. A., et al.: APACHE II: A severity of disease classification system. Crit. Care Med., 13:818, 1985.)

APACHE III score applies only to homogeneous categories and severity stratification (not risk prediction). The first day, APACHE III equation is calibrated on all patients selected for ICU admission without requirements for additional selection criteria. The first day equation for risk prediction cannot be applied beyond the first 24 hours. Additional equations exist for prediction of risk out to seven (7) days of ICU care.[53] In spite of improved risk prediction, the clinician should still be mindful that this science requires further clinical study. Estimate of risk of mortality should not override experience or clinical judgment and, most importantly, patient and family directives.

Classifications for Application To Specific Situations or Disease States

These classification systems were developed for application to specific organ system failure of specific disease entities. Each lends further definition to clinical situations and may enhance the individual predictive powers of some

Table 79-19. Statistical Analysis of MPM II

	MPM$_0$		MPM$_{24}$	
	Developmental	Validated	Developmental	Validated
Goodness of fit*	P = 0.623	P = 0.327	P = 0.764	P = 0.231
Area under the receiver operating characteristic curve (ROC)†	0.837	0.824	0.844	0.836

* The correspondence between observed and expected mortality (calibration).
† Evaluation of how well the model distinguished between patients who lived from those who died.
(Adapted from: Lemeshow, S., et al.: Mortality probability models (MPM II): based on an international cohort of intensive care unit patients. JAMA, 270:2478, 1993.)

Table 79-20. Variables in the MPM II

MPM₀	MPM₂₄
Physiology	Physiology
Coma or deep stupor	Coma or deep stupor at 24 hours
Heart rate greater or equal to 150 beats/minute	
Systolic blood pressure greater or equal 90 mmHg	
Chronic diagnoses	Chronic diagnoses
Chronic renal insufficiency	Cirrhosis
Cirrhosis	Metastatic neoplasm
Metastatic neoplasm	
Acute diagnoses	Acute diagnoses
Acute renal failure	Intracranial mass effect
Cardiac dysrhythmia	
Cerebrovascular incident	
Gastrointestinal bleeding	
Intracranial mass effect	
Other	Other
Age (10-year odds ratio)	Age (10-year odds ratio)
Cardiopulmonary resuscitation prior to admission	Medical or nonscheduled surgical admission
Mechanical ventilation	
Medical or nonscheduled surgical admission	Additional 24 hour assessments
	Creatinine > (2.0 mg/dl)
	Confirmed infection
	Mechanical ventilation
	PaO₂ <60 mm Hg
	Prothrombin time >3 sec above standard
	Urine output <150 ml in 8 hr
	Vasoactive drugs, more than 1/hr IV

(Adapted from: Lemeshow, S., et al.: Mortality probability models (MPM II): based on an international cohort of intensive care unit patients. JAMA, *270*:2478, 1993.)

of the more generalized classifications listed previously. Some of these more specific indices are listed in Table 79-15. As classification systems, not all have been validated to the same extent as APACHE (I-III), MPM and SAPs.

Glasgow Coma Scale

The Glasgow coma scale and prediction model was developed by Teasdale and Jennett as a means of stratifying outcomes for head trauma victims because of their concern about the requirements for expensive long-term care of these patients.[54] These authors defined outcome status, which ranges from death to good recovery (Table 79-23). A coma score ranged from a score of 3 (lowest function) to 15 (highest function) (Table 79-24).[55] The scores were assessed at different times in the patients' course and compared to outcomes.

The value of the Glasgow outcome scale (see Table 79-23) as a predictive model is not perfect. Teasdale and Jennett specified that no application should be made until 6 hours after admission, because of a high confidence rate for death or survival, probability greater than 0.97 in 44% of cases in 6 hours after hospitalization and 52 in 61% of cases in 3 days.[55] What is most important about this scale is that it is a milestone in the formulation of predictive indices and has been incorporated into most generalized severity classifications for the ICU, affecting the general prognostic significance of coma in all critical illness.[56]

Patients with Cardiac Disease and Myocardial Infarction

Perhaps the best known generic classification for patients with cardiac disease is the New York Heart Association Classification, which defines the level of symptoms experienced as a result of cardiac disease of any cause. The four classes are summarized in Table 79-25. Even though this classification is not an acute severity of illness index, it is of some utility in the ICU because the mortality risk is influenced by the patient's premorbid clinical status.[57,58]

Myocardial infarction (MI) is the most important single cardiac event that is responsible for ICU admission. Since the early days of coronary care units, attempts have been made to stratify MI patients for purposes of comparing outcomes and efficacy of intervention in comparable patients. Early on, it was clear this was not a homogenous group of patients and that the diagnostic label alone was insufficient as a stratification tool. The first widely used clinical stratification tool was developed by Killip,[59] in which he defines four strata based on the clinical assessment of the severity of left ventricular dysfunction (Table 79-26). This classification system was able to distinguish MI patients with hospital mortality rates as low as 6% in Killip class I and those with mortality rates as high as 81% in Killip class IV (classes II and III have intermediate values). This system was used widely because of its simplicity and reproducibility. Forrester and colleagues[60,61] refined this tool a decade later, when the Swan-Ganz catheter came into wide use, enabling rapid assessment of hemodynamics at the bedside in the ICU. This classification system combined clinical and hemodynamic assessment to yield four clinical subsets (Table 79-27), which have been used to define appropriate therapy and to make comparisons of interventions in comparable patients.

Table 79-21. Therapeutic Intervention Scoring System—1983

4 Points
a. Cardiac arrest and/or countershock within past 48 hr
b. Controlled ventilation with or without PEEP
c. Controlled ventilation with intermittent or continuous muscle relaxants
d. Balloon tamponade of varices
e. Continuous arterial infusion
f. Pulmonary artery catheter
g. Atrial and/or ventricular pacing
h. Hemodialysis in unstable patient
i. Peritoneal dialysis
j. Induced hypothermia
k. Pressure-activated blood infusion
l. G-suit
m. Intracranial pressure monitoring
n. Platelet transfusion
o. IABA (intra-aortic balloon assist)
p. Emergency operative procedures (within past 24 hrs)
q. Lavage of acute GI bleeding
r. Emergency endoscopy or bronchoscopy
s. Vasoactive drug infusion (less than one drug)

3 Points
a. Central versus hyperalimentation (includes renal, cardiac, hepatic failure fluid)
b. Pacemaker on standby
c. Chest tubes
d. Intermittent mandatory ventilation (IMV) or assisted ventilation
e. Continuous positive airway pressure (CPAP)
f. Concentrated K+ infusion via central catheter
g. Nasotracheal or orotracheal intubation
h. Blind intratracheal suctioning
i. Complex metabolic balance (frequent intake and output)
j. Multiple ABG, bleeding, and/or stat studies (greater than four per shift)
k. Frequent infusions of blood products (greater than 5 units/24 hr)
l. Bolus IV medication (nonscheduled)
m. Vasoactive drug infusion (one drug)
n. Continuous antiarrhythmia infusions
o. Cardioversion for arrhythmia (not defibrillation)
p. Hypothermia blanket
q. Arterial line
r. Acute digitalization, within 48 hr
s. Measurement of cardiac output by any method

t. Active diuresis for fluid overload
u. Active Rx for metabolic alkalosis
v. Active Rx for metabolic acidosis
w. Emergency thora-, para-, and pericardiocenteses
x. Active anticoagulation (initial 48 hr)
y. Phlebotomy for volume overload
z. Coverage with more than 2 IV antibiotics
aa. Rx of seizures or metabolic encephalopathy (within 48 hr of onset)
bb. Complicated orthopedic traction

2 Points
a. CVP (central venous pressure)
b. Two peripheral IV catheters
c. Hemodialysis-stable patient
d. Fresh tracheostomy (less than 48 hr)
e. Spontaneous respiration via endotracheal tube or tracheostomy (T-piece or trach mask)
f. GI feedings
g. Replacement of excess fluid loss
h. Parenteral chemotherapy
i. Hourly neurologic vital signs
j. Multiple dressing changes
k. Pitressin infusion

1 Point
a. ECG monitoring
b. Hourly vital signs
c. One peripheral IV catheter
d. Chronic anticoagulation
e. Standard intake and output (q24 hr)
f. Stat blood tests
g. Intermittent scheduled IV medications
h. Routine dressing changes
i. Standard orthopedic traction
j. Tracheostomy care
k. Decubitus ulcer
l. Urinary catheter
m. Supplemental oxygen (nasal or mask)
n. Antibiotics IV (two or less)
o. Chest physiotherapy
p. Extensive irrigations, packings, or debridement of wound, fistula, or colostomy
q. GI decompression
r. Peripheral hyperalimentation/intralipid therapy

(From Keene, A. R., and Cullen, R. T.: Therapeutic intervention scoring system: Update 1983. Crit. Care Med., *11*:213, 1983.)

The Multicenter Post-Infarction Research Group stratified risk factors for death at 2 years in patients who survived the ICU phase of an acute MI.[58] In 866 patients, the four factors were independent predictors of morbidity, as shown in Table 79-28. Various combinations of these risk factors identified five subgroups with progressively increasing mortality rates, as shown in Figure 79-8.[58]

Outcome and Severity of Illness Based on Frequency Distribution of Cardiorespiratory Variables

Shoemaker and colleagues developed a classification system based on the achievement of therapeutic goals.[62] The logic of the system evolved over a 6-year period and is based on the fact that survivors of "surgical trauma" can be differentiated from nonsurvivors by analysis of "cardiopulmonary variables."[62] These criteria for separation of data (cardiopulmonary variables) are listed in Table 79-29. In early studies, these investigators found that nonsurvivors had greater reductions in flow, greater elevations in peripheral and pulmonary vascular resistance and central blood volume, and greater decreases in stroke index, left and right ventricular stroke work, oxygen availability, pH, hemoglobin, and blood volume. By the same token, the survivors and nonsurvivors were not distinguishable by lack of neurohormonal responsiveness.[62] The logic of this analysis is illustrated in Figure 79-9.

Having elucidated these differences, Shoemaker and colleagues proceeded further with nonparametric analysis to identify survivors and nonsurvivors in the early and late periods of shock or circulatory instability. In a series of 98 patients, 94% of survivors were ultimately identified with one or more variables. Of those patients who die in shock, 78% were identified with one variable. This method provided a high percentage of accurate classification in the early and late periods of circulatory instability. These investigators sought to define physiologic limits for survival while seeking more sensitive criteria for early warning of cardiorespiratory failure.[63]

Table 79-22. APACHE III Points for Age and Chronic Health Evaluation

	Points
Age (yr)	
≤44	0
45–59	5
60–64	11
65–69	13
70–74	16
75–84	17
$85	24
Comorbid condition*	
AIDS	23
Hepatic failure	16
Lymphoma	13
Metastatic cancer	11
Leukemia/multiple myeloma	10
Immunosuppression	10
Cirrhosis	4

* Excluded for elective surgery patients.
(From: Knaus, W. A., et al.: The APACHE III Prognostic System. Risk prediction of hospitalized mortality for critically ill hospitalized adults. Chest 100: 1619, 1991.)

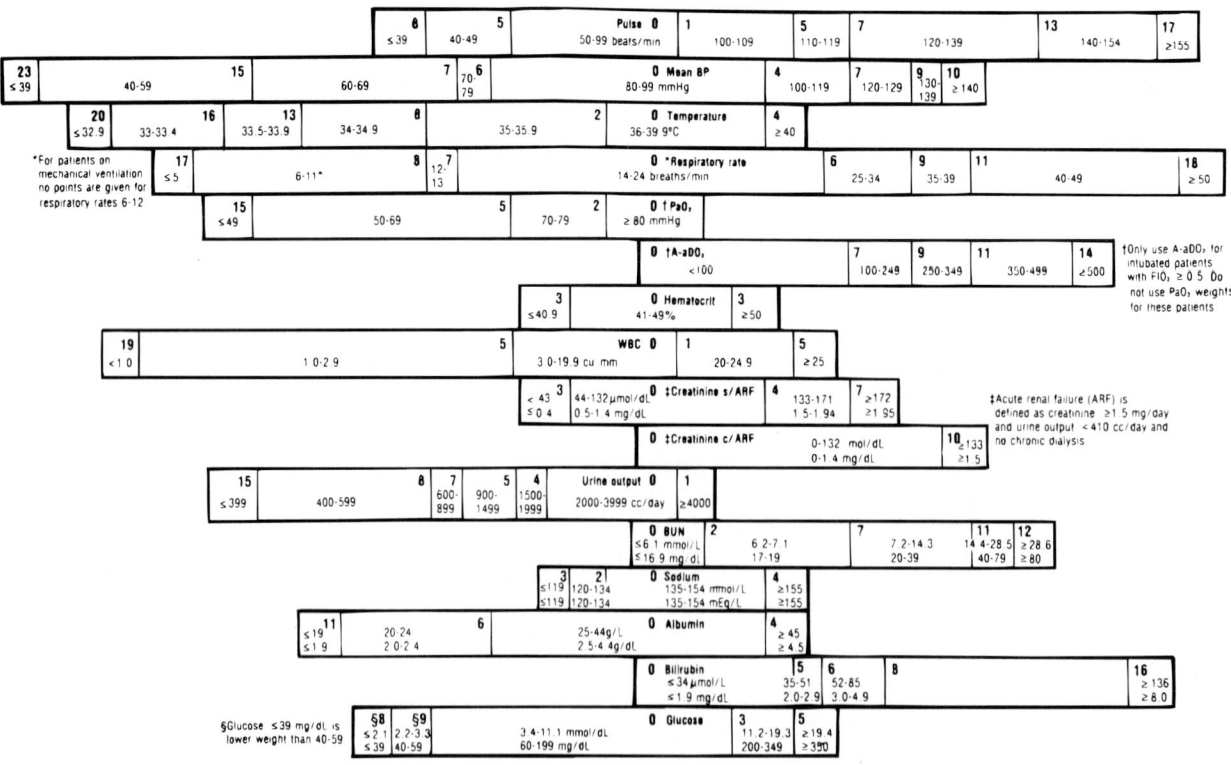

Fig. 79-6. Increased explanatory power in the APACHE III system was also gained by examination of arterial pH and PCO_2. Weights are assigned according to the relationship between pH and PCO_2. (From Knaus, W. A., et al.: The APACHE III prognostic system. Risk prediction of hospitalized mortality for critically ill hospitalized adults. Chest, 100:1619, 1991.)

Fig. 79-5. Assignment of values for physiologic variables for physiologic scoring by APACHE III. Note the higher numbers and narrower ranges of numbers for APACHE III as compared to APACHE II (Fig. 79-3). This change resulted in an increased explanatory power for APACHE III. Additional variables of BUN, urine output, serum albumin, bilirubin, and glucose increase explanatory power. (From Knaus, W. A., et al.: The APACHE III prognostic system. Risk prediction of hospitalized mortality for critically ill hospitalized adults. Chest, 100:1619, 1991.)

Eyes open spontaneously or to painful/verbal stimulation

verbal motor	oriented converses	confused conversation	inappropriate words and incomprehensible sounds	no response
obeys verbal command	0	3	10	15
localizes pain	3	8	13	15
flexion withdrawal/ decorticate rigidity	3	13	24	24
decerebrate rigidity/ no response	3	13	29	29

Eyes do not open spontaneously or to painful/verbal stimulation

verbal motor	oriented converses	confused conversation	inappropriate words and incomprehensible sounds	no response
obeys verbal command				16
localizes pain				16
flexion withdrawal/ decorticate rigidity			24	33
decerebrate rigidity/ no response			29	48

Fig. 79-7. APACHE III scoring for neurologic abnormalities according to presence or absence of eye opening. Glasgow coma variables were reformatted to eliminate similar scores with different presentations by eliminating the distinctions between incomprehensible words and inappropriate sounds, flexion withdrawal and decorticate rigidity and decerebrate rigidity, and no responses by simplifying the evaluation of eye opening. (From Knaus, W. A., et al.: The APACHE III prognostic system. Risk prediction of hospitalized mortality for critically ill hospitalized adults. Chest, 100:1619, 1991.)

Shoemaker and colleagues went on to analyze the predictive powers of cardiopulmonary parameters, which were classified into volume-related variables; flow-related variables; bodily responses; oxygen transport-related variables; and perfusion indices.[64] From this analysis, these investigators found that the clinician might be able to predict lethal aspects of circulatory failure in an early stage; measure severity of illness; quantify the relative effectiveness of therapy; quantitate the degree of physiologic deficit; and determine when effective therapy initially ceases to be effective.[64] Further analysis led to a determination that the same cardiopulmonary parameters could be re-

Table 79-23. Glasgow Outcome Scale

1. **Death:** Ascribable to primary brain damage
2. **Persistent vegetative state:** Patients who remain unresponsive and speechless for weeks or months until death after acute brain damage
3. **Severe disability** (conscious but disabled): Patients who are dependent for daily support by reason of mental or physical disability, usually a combination of both
4. **Moderate disability** (disabled but independent): Such patients can travel by public transport and can work in a sheltered environment, and therefore are independent in so far as daily life is concerned.
5. **Good recovery:** Implies the resumption of normal life despite minor neurologic and physiologic deficit.

(Modified from Jennett, B., and Teasdale, G.: Predicting outcome in individual patients after severe head injury. Lancet, 5:1031, 1976.)

Table 79-24. Glasgow Coma Scale

Parameter	Response	Score
Eyes open	Spontaneously	4
	To verbal command	3
	To pain	2
Eyes, no response		1
Best motor response to verbal command	Obeys	6
Best motor response to painful stimulus	Localizes pain	5
	Flexion (withdrawal)	4
	Flexion, abnormal (decorticate rigidity)	3
	Extension (decerebrate rigidity)	2
	No response	1
Best verbal response	Oriented and converses	5
	Disoriented and converses	4
	Inappropriate words	3
	Incomprehensible sounds	2
	No response	1
Total		3-15

(From Jennett, B., and Teasdale, G.: Predicting outcome in individual patients after severe head injury. Lancet, 5:1031, 1976.)

Table 79-25. Physical Capacity with Heart Disease: NYHA Functional Classification

Class	Description
I	Patients with cardiac disease but without resulting limitations of physical activity. Ordinary physical activity does not cause undue fatigue, palpitation, dyspnea, or anginal pain.
II	Patients with cardiac disease resulting in slight limitation of physical activity. They are comfortable at rest. Ordinary physical activity results in fatigue, palpitation, dyspnea, or anginal pain.
III	Patients with cardiac disease resulting in limitation of physical activity. They are comfortable at rest. Less than ordinary physical activity causes fatigue, palpitation, dyspnea, or anginal pain.
IV	Patients with cardiac disease resulting in inability to carry on any physical activity without discomfort. Symptoms present even at rest. If any physical activity is undertaken, discomfort is increased.

(Modified from The Critical Committee of The New York Heart Association: Diseases of the Heart and Blood Vessels. 6th Ed. Boston, Little, Brown, 1964, p. 112.)

Table 79-26. Clinical Severity in Acute Myocardial Infarction

I. No heart failure
II. Heart failure
III. Pulmonary edema
IV. Cardiogenic shock

(Adapted from Killip, T., and Kimball, J. T.: Treatment of myocardial infarction in a coronary care unit: A two-year experience with 250 patients. Am. J. Cardiol., 20:457, 1967.)

Table 79–27. Correlative Classification of Clinical and Hemodynamic Function after Acute Myocardial Infarction

Subset	Cardiac Index (L/min/m²)	Pulmonary Capillary Pressure (mm Hg)
I. No pulmonary congestion or peripheral hypoperfusion	2.7 ± 0.5	12 ± 7
II. Isolated pulmonary congestion	2.3 ± 0.4	23 ± 5
III. Isolated peripheral hypoperfusion	1.9 ± 0.4	12 ± 5
IV. Both pulmonary congestion and hypoperfusion	1.6 ± 0.6	27 ± 8

(From Forrester, J. S., Diamond, G. A., Swan, H. J. C.: Correlative classification of clinical and hemodynamic function after acute myocardial infarction. Am. J. Cardiol., *39*:137, 1977.)

Table 79–28. Independent Risk Variables for Death at 2 Years after Myocardial Infarction

Ejection fraction less than 40% 1 week after infarction
Ventricular ectopic depolarization equal or greater than 10 per hour
Pulmonary rales while the patient is in coronary care unit
New York Heart Association class II–IV 1 month before entry

(Adapted from The multicenter research group: Risk stratification and survival after myocardial infarction. N. Engl. J. Med., *309*:331, 1983.)

Table 79–29. Sequential Cardiorespiratory Variables in Defining Criteria for Therapeutic Goals and Early Warning of Death

Stage	Description
A	The control period. The preoperative period. Similar but not identical to healthy volunteer subjects.
B	The initial period of falling arterial pressure immediately after the causative event. The lowest recorded blood pressure (stage low) separates stage B from stage C.
C	The middle period. Substages C1 and C2 are separated by the point when the arterial blood pressure has returned half way to control values.
D	The late or recovery period for surviving patients. Starts when arterial blood pressure has returned to normal values.
E	The preterminal period in patients who subsequently die, stage C to about 1 or 2 hours prior to death
F	Final agonal, terminal event

(Adapted from Shoemaker, W. C., et al.: Physiologic patterns in surviving and nonsurviving shock patients. Arch. Surg., *106*:630, 1973.)

fined into a predictive index with a sensitivity of 70 to 93% depending on the stage of shock and a specificity of 76 to 92%. This severity index evolved as a process measure and an instrument to evaluate the efficacy of alternative therapies. This measure is distinctly different from APACHE, SAPS, and MPM, which are designed more to assess and quantitate outcome.[65] Assessment of cardiopulmonary parameters evolved from severity of illness indicators to therapeutic goals, which would be desirable to achieve in an effort to increase likelihood of survival.[66,67]

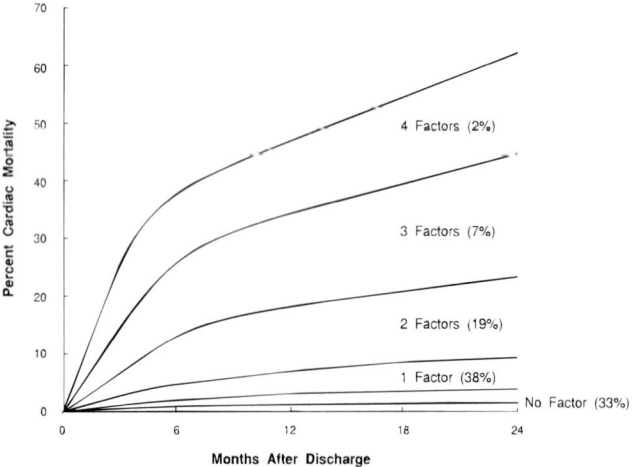

Fig. 79–8. Mortality curves after discharge and zones of risk according to number of risk factors. Risk factors in this study were New York Heart Association functional class II through IV before admission, pulmonary rales, occurrence of 10 or more ventricular extopic depolarizations per hour, and a radionuclide ejection fraction below 0.40. The variation of risk within each zone (ranging from no factor to 4 factors) reflects the spectrum of relative risk for individual factors as well as the range of multiplicative risks for combinations of two and three factors. Numbers in parentheses denote the percentage of the population with the specified number of factors (see reference 55 for details). (Redrawn by George Morrison, Clinical Dimensions, Inc., from The Multicenter Postinfarction Research Group: Risk stratification and survival after myocardial infarction. N. Engl. J. Med., *309*:331, 1983.)

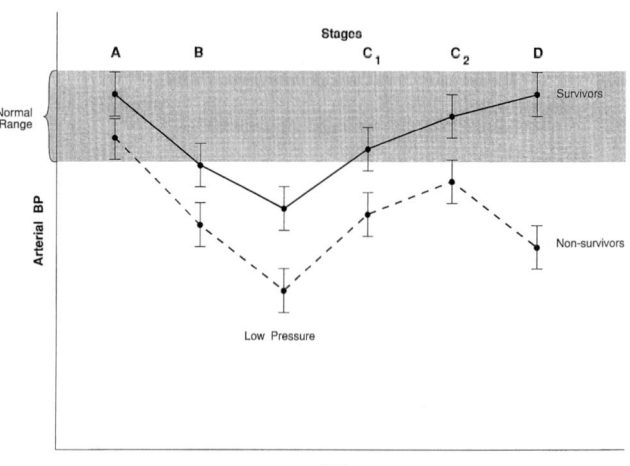

Fig. 79–9. Logic of analysis of cardiorespiratory variables by Shoemaker and colleagues. The variable of blood pressure is examined. The stages of altered blood pressure and listed in Table 79–25. Survivors tend to have a blood pressure fluctuation within a "normal range." Nonsurvivors have a more severe derangement and do not achieve a blood pressure within the normal range. (Adapted by George Morrison, Clinical Dimensions, Inc., from Shoemaker, W. C., et al.: Physiologic patterns in surviving and nonsurviving shock patients. Arch. Surg., *106*:630, 1973; Shoemaker, W. C., et al.: Comparison of hemodynamic and oxygen transport effects of dopamine and dobutamine in critically ill surgical patients. Chest, *96*:120, 1989.)

Patients with Respiratory Failure

A few systems classify patients with respiratory failure according to risk of mortality. Generally, one could find indices that predict risk of mortality for adult respiratory distress syndrome, chronic obstructive lung disease (see Chapter 15), or ability to wean from mechanical ventilation. Bartlett and colleagues formulated a Pulmonary Insufficiency Index (PII), which based mortality prediction directly on the time in days which patients with respiratory failure had an A-aO$_2$ that exceeded 300 mmHg.[68] The method by which this index is determined is illustrated in Figure 79-10. For example, an index of 1.0 is equivalent to an A-aO$_2$ gradient of 400 for 24 hours or one of 600 for 8 hours.[68] In a series of 45 patients, survivors had a mean PII of 84 and in nonsurvivors, the mean was 11.3.[68] Of interest is the inclusion of the concept of widening A-aO$_2$ gradient into APACHE II[9] and directly into SAPS.[42] Table 79-30 demonstrates stratification of patients according to PII.

Bartlett and colleagues further identified predictions of mortality in 713 patients with acute hypoxic respiratory failure in a collaborative NIH study.[69] Mortality increased with increasing number of organ failures: One organ (lung), 40%; two organs, 54%; three organs, 72%; four organs, 84%; and five organs, 100%.[69] The basic premise of this study is that mortality is more influenced by the degree of systemic damage than by the degree of alteration in lung function.

Fowler and colleagues studied 88 patients in an effort to identify predictors of mortality in patients with adult respiratory distress syndrome.[70] Of clinical, laboratory, cardiopulmonary, and demographic data collected, only four variables taken singly were significantly associated with mortality:[70] the presence of less than 10% band forms on the initial peripheral blood smear; the persistence of arterial pH below 7.40, a calculated HCO$_3$ less than 20 mg/dl, and BUN of greater than 65 mg/dl.

Again, these findings suggest that systemic effects are more powerful determinants of mortality than are measures of pulmonary function. Bone and colleagues noted a correlation between initial response to conventional therapy (antibiotics, drainage of abscess, fluid resuscitation, and PEEP) and survival.[71] After initiation of conventional therapy in a group of 82 patients, survival correlated with the maintenance of PaO$_2$/FiO$_2$ ratio of 200 or greater, whereas in nonsurvivors, the ratio did not rise above 150. Additional systemic factors were not analyzed in this study.

In contrast to the limited predictive ability of investigators in forecasting survivorship in adult respiratory distress syndrome, the degree of lung damage as determined by highest peak airway pressure, maximum pulmonary artery pressure, and lowest lung compliance was found by Ghio and colleagues to correlate with the degree of pulmonary impairment among survivors of adult respiratory distress syndrome.[72] Peters and colleagues made similar observations, but they found that higher levels of PEEP predicted better lung function, as opposed to Ghio, who found the reverse.[73]

The value of standard parameters of negative inspiratory force, minute ventilation, and maximum voluntary minute ventilation have limitations in predicting the ability to wean long-term ventilator-dependent patients.[74,75] These parameters generally were applied to specific points in time in patients who were relatively healthy after acute events, such as a surgical procedure. Ventilator dependency and impediments to weaning suggest that certain factors must be reversed before complete weaning can take place.[76,77] From a retrospective review of 11 cases of respiratory failure and ventilator dependency, Morganroth and colleagues derived a ventilator score (VS) (Table 79-31), which defined the degree of dependency, and an adverse factor score (AFS) (Table 79-32), which quantitated the factors responsible for the ventilator dependency. The VS quantitated requirements for supplemental oxygen (FiO$_2$ and PEEP) and chest wall and lung compliance as proxies for expected work of breathing. The AFS assigns points based on the severity of respiratory abnormalities and many nonrespiratory factors (e.g., hemody-

Table 79-30. Group Stratification According to Pulmonary Insufficiency Index (PII)

Type	Derangement	Description	Percent Mortality
1	A-a over 500 at 24 to 48 hours	Rapid onset, progressive aspiration, drowning; require FiO$_2$ of 1.0	100%
2	A-a over 500 in first 24 hours but less than 500 at 24 to 48 hours	Rapid onset, rapid improvement	0%
3	A-a less than 500 in the first 48 hours but over 300 in first 7 days	Gradual onset, fat embolism, past shock, viral pneumonitis.	50%
4	A-a never over 300 in first 7 days	Not truly acute respiratory insufficiency; generally managed with FiO$_2$ less than 0.5	41%

(From Bartlett, R. H., et al.: Mortality prediction in adult respiratory failure. Chest, 67:680, 1975.)

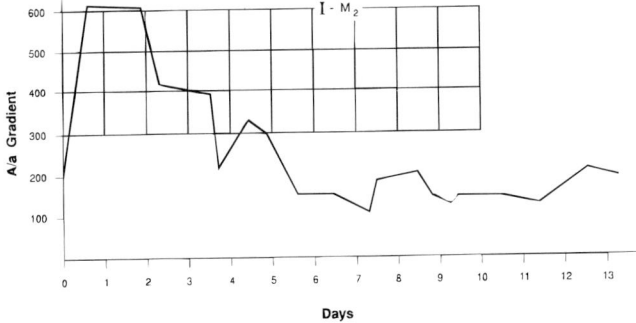

Fig. 79-10. Fluctuation in the A-a gradient over time for a typical patient with respiratory failure. Patient type 1 (A-a > 500 at 24-48 hours, M2 (died after the lungs recovered), with pulmonary insufficiency index of 6.6 (area under curve—A-a gradient/time). (Redrawn by George Morrison, Clinical Dimensions, Inc., from Bartlett, R. H., et al.: Mortality prediction in adult respiratory failure. Chest, 67:680, 1975.)

Table 79-31. Ventilator Score: Component Factors and Point Assignments*

Factor	Stratification	Score
Fraction of inspired oxygen (%)	≤40	0
	41–50	1
	51–60	2
	≥61	4
Positive end-expiratory pressure, (cm H$_2$O)	0	0
	1–5	2
	6–10	4
	11–15	6
	>15	10
Static compliance (ml/cm H$_2$O)	≥60	0
	50–59	1
	40–49	2
	30–39	3
	<30	4
Dynamic compliance	≥40	0
	30–39	1
	21–29	2
	≤20	3
Delivered ventilator-minute	≤10	0
	10.1–15	1
	15.1–20	2
	20.1–25	3
	25.1–30	4
	>30	5
Triggered respiratory rate (breaths per minute ventilation, L/min)	≤20	0
	>20	1

* Total points possible is 27. (From Morganroth, M. L., et al.: Criteria for weaning from prolonged mechanical ventilation. Arch. Intern. Med., 144:1012, 1984.)

namics, infection, mental status); the maximum VS is 27 and the maximum AFS is 48. If the combination of VS and AFS was less than 55, the chance of successful weaning was 96%. If the total score was greater than 55, the probability of unsuccessful weaning was 86%. These authors recognized that further validation of their observation was necessary and that additional consideration of the prior health status must also be recognized.[77]

Patients with Disorders of the Gastrointestinal Tract

Child and Turcolte devised a classification system for patients who had undergone shunt surgery for management of portal hypertension.[78] They used serum bilirubin and albumin values and the degree of ascites as a method of presence or absence of coma, we well as estimation of nutritional status (Table 79-33). These variables were used to define three clinical classes (A, B, and C). Conn[79] and Shellman et al.[80] considered this classification with the additional clinical parameters of respiratory and renal failure to predict survival of patients with cirrhosis. Each author found that the Child classification was reasonable in estimating degree of hepatic damage and reserve but had limited predictive power for survival after ICU admission. An increasing mortality associated with change of class from A to C was noted. Shellman also found, in a group of 100 patients, that an elevated serum creatinine was associated with decreased survival (class A, 82.5%; class B, 55.2%; and class C, 25%). The additional factor of a requirement for mechanical ventilation has a similar effect (class A, 23%; class B, 7.2%; and class C, 2%).[80] In another study of 100 patients, Goldfarb and colleagues found that the presence of severe cirrhosis, septic shock, and hepatic coma were predictive of mortality.[81] All of these authors found that requirements for mechanical ventilation were somewhat predictive of mortality when other clinical parameters were included in the analysis. Zimmerman and Knaus suggested that the incorporation of severity factors along with the Child classification might help guide physicians in decisions to institute mechanical ventilation in the face of a poor overall prognosis.[13] These observations are summarized in Table 79-34.

The Ranson classification for severity of pancreatitis was developed as a means by which surgeons might make decisions about surgical intervention for the treatment of pancreatitis.[82,83] The principal concern of Ranson and colleagues was the fact that some patients with pancreatitis could be managed with conservative therapy of nasogastric suctioning and intravenous fluids, whereas others required treatment for the serious associated factors of respiratory and kidney failure and surgical drainage of intraabdominal abscesses.[83] Initially, in 100 consecutive patients, 43 parameters were statistically analyzed. Table 79-35 is a list of the 11 variables that were of significant prognostic value. The listed values correlated with death or serious illness (serious illness was defined as a requirement for 7 days or more in the ICU). Sixty-two percent of patients with more than three of these signs died, and an additional 33% were seriously ill.[83] In similar fashion, Imrie and colleagues devised a severity classification that included most of the parameters of the Ranson classification.[84] A comparison of the two systems is in Table 79-35. These two systems provide coarse differentiation between degrees of illness but do not provide information on increasing severity and correlation with increasing mortality, probably because they were devised originally to direct therapy rather than to quantitate outcome from a disease process itself.

McMahon and co-workers were concerned that the Ranson and Imrie criteria took 48 hours to define the severity of illness.[85] Therefore, they devised a more direct method of assessing severity based on the physical characteristics of peritoneal lavage fluid, which represented a more direct method of assessing the severity of the intraabdominal inflammatory process.[85] Table 79-36 is a summary of the predictive powers of clinical assessment, peritoneal lavage, and the Ransom and Imrie criteria for severe acute pancreatitis. Direct assessment of peritoneal aspirate and/or lavage was considerably more predictive (73 versus 39%) than clinical assessments 8 hours after hospitalization. Such findings are logical given that lavage represents a direct assessment and the clinical assessment represents the effects of the inflammation on more global bodily functions. These studies underscore the difficulty with classification systems that are intended to represent severity of a single disease process that may adversely affect many other organ systems. Assessments of the body's physiologic processes seems more appropriate.

Patients with Renal Failure

McMurray and co-workers stratified patients according to three categories of predictor variables: cause, complica-

Table 79–32. Adverse Factor Score: Component Factors and Point Assignments*

Factor	Stratification	Score
Heart rate mode	<100	0
	100–120	1
	121–150	2
	>150	3
Blood pressure, minimum (mm Hg)	>100	0
	90–100	1
	61–89	3
	≤60	6
Temperature, maximum (°C)	36.1–38.2	0
	38.3–39.9	1
	≥40	3
	≤36	3
Central venous pressure (cm H_2O) or pulmonary capillary wedge (mm Hg)	<15, <18	0
	≥15, ≥18	2
Arrhythmias	Supraventricular tachycardia	1
	Supraventricular tachycardia with cardioversion	2
	Premature ventricular beats, (>6/min)	1
	Ventricular tachycardia, nonsustained	2
	Ventricular tachycardia, sustained	4
Postural drainage and clapping	Yes	0
	No	1
Secretion, quantity (frequency of suctioning, hr)	< Every 4	0
	Every 2–4	1
	> Every 2	3
Secretion, quality	Thin	0
	Mucousy	1
	Thick	2
Level of consciousness	Alert and oriented	0
	Lethargic, easily aroused	1
	Lethargic, difficult to arouse	3
	Comatose	4
Communication	Follows commands	0
	Does not follow commmands	1
Emotional status	Calm	0
	Depressed and/or anxious	1
	Agitated	2
Mobility	Ambulating or up in chair	0
	Bed rest	1
Calories/24 hr	>2,000	0
	1,001–2,000	1
	<1,000	2
Vasopressors	No	0
	Yes	2
Intravenously or intramuscularly administered antibiotics, (number of drugs)	0–1	0
	2	1
	≥3	2
Orally administered antibiotics (number of drugs)	0–1	0
	≥2	1
Sedatives (Number of doses/24 hr)	0–1	0
	2–3	1
	>3	3
Pain medication (Number of doses/24 hr)	0–2	0
	3	1
	4–5	2
	>6	3
Steroids, dosage	None	0
	<1 g every day	1
	≥1 g every day	2
Aminophylline	Yes	0
	No	1
Nebulized bronchodilators	Yes	0
	No	1

* Total points possible is 48. (From Morganroth, M. L., et al.: Criteria for weaning from prolonged mechanical ventilation. Arch. Intern. Med., *144*: 1012, 1984.)

Table 79-33. Child's Classification of Hepatic Insufficiency

Child's Class	Total Bilirubin	Albumin	Ascites	Nutrition	Encephalopathy
A	Less than 2.0 mg/dl	3.5 mg/dl	None	Good	Absent
B	2.0–3.5 mg/dl	2.0–3.5 mg/dl	Easily controlled	Fair	Absent
C	Greater than 3.5 mg/dl	Less than 2.0 mg/dl	Poorly controlled	Poor	Present at same time

(From Child, C. G., and Turcotte, J. G.: Surgery and portal hypertension. *In* The Liver and Portal Hypertension. Edited by C. G. Child. Philadelphia, W.B. Saunders, 1964, p. 50.)

tions, and miscellaneous conditions (Table 79-37).[86] In a review of 276 patients receiving care between 1967 and 1975, 63% survived. The causes of death for 102 patients were most commonly infection (54%), irreversible central nervous system damage (13%), and cardiovascular collapse (11%). No single variables correlated with death. Acute tubular necrosis caused by nephrotoxins such as antibiotics or contrast materials was associated with an 86% survival. As the number of complications listed in Table 79-37 increased, there was inverse correlation with survival (Fig. 79-11). With no complications, total parenteral nutrition had no effect on survival. If three or more complications occurred, however, survival was significantly improved with parenteral nutrition.[86] Increasing age had inverse correlation with survival. Finally, the nonoliguric state was associated with a better prognosis (80% of 69 patients) than the oliguric state (59% of 207 patients). In this study, patients were stratified according to cause of renal failure and associated complications. No variables could quantitatively define severity of renal failure other than the oliguric or nonoliguric state.

Rasmussen and Ibels analyzed 143 patients with acute tubular necrosis and found an additive interaction between acute insults and severity of renal failure.[87] Acute insults that had increased risk of mortality included aminoglycoside use, pigmenturia, dehydration, and preexisting renal disease. The severity of the acute renal failure was related to the number and severity of the acute insults. Risk factors, however, were not quantitated in a fashion such that increasing severity had an increased correlation with death. Rasmussen and others studied the prediction of outcome further by discriminant analysis of clinical variables.[88] Table 79-38 is a list of the predictor variables in order of decreasing function coefficient. A score generated by their equation may be useful in comparing severity of illness among patients, but a large multicenter study would be required for further validation.

Cioffi and co-workers studied the probability of surviving postoperative acute renal failure.[89] Table 79-39 separates significant and nonsignificant factors that differentiated survivors from nonsurvivors of 300 patients whose charts were reviewed retrospectively over a 9-year period beginning in 1973. Of 83 patients from the group that developed perioperative renal failure, the data from the first 65 patients were used to derive a prognostic index that was validated in successive study of similar patients. Linear discriminant function (LDF) variable codes and coefficient constants are listed in Table 79-40. In the group studied retrospectively, a score of less than 0.669 was associated with greater than a 50% chance of dying and classified a patient as a nonsurvivor. Patients with a score of greater than 0.669 had a greater than 50% chance of being a survivor and were classified accordingly. The accuracy of the linear discriminant function (LDF) score in predicting survival and nonsurvival is shown in Table 79-41. Ultimately, these authors suggested that their index allows segregation of patients into those with little chance

Table 79-34. Results of Statistical Model with Child's Class, Mechanical Ventilation, and Elevated Creatinine to Predict Survival

Child's Class	Mechanical Ventilation	Elevated Creatinine	Survival (%)
	−	−	95
	−	+	82.5
A	+	−	55
	+	+	23
	−	−	83.5
	−	+	55.2
B	+	−	24.3
	+	+	7.2
	−	−	57
	−	+	25
C	+	−	7.7
	+	+	2

(From Goldfarb, G., et al.: Efficacy of respiratory assistance in cirrhotic patients with liver failure. Intensive Care Med., 9:271, 1983.)

Table 79-35. Multiple Criteria for Prediction of Severe Acute Pancreatitis*

Ranson et al.[80]	Imrie et al.[81]

On admission:
  Age >55 years
  Blood glucose >11 mmol/L
  White blood count >16,000
  SGOT >120 IU/L
  LDH >350 IU/L
	During the first 48 hours:
	  Arterial P_{O_2} <56 mm Hg
	  Serum albumin <3.2 g/ml
	  Serum calcium <2.0 mmol/L
	  White cell count 15,000
	  SGOT >100 IU/L
	  LDH >600 IU/L

During the first 48 hours:
  Fall in Hct >10%
  Serum calcium <2 mmol/L
  Base deficit >4.0 mmol/L
  BUN increase >1.0 mmol/L
  Fluid sequestration >6l
  Arterial P_{O_2} <56 mm Hg
	Blood glucose >10 mmol/L
	Plasma urea >16 mmol/L
	Age >55 years

* Severe disease is indicated by the presence of three or more factors in each case. (Modified from McMahon, M. J., Playforth, M. J., Pickford, I. R.: A comparative study of methods for the prediction of severity of attacks of acute pancreatitis. Br. J. Surg., 67:22, 1980.)

Table 79–36. Relative Accuracy of Different Methods for the Prediction of Severity of Acute Pancreatitis*

Classification	Admission	8 Hours		24 Hours		48 Hours	(Ranson)†	(Imrie)
	Calcium 2 mmol/L = severe	CA‡	Lavage§	CA	CA	Methalbumin in serum = severe		
Severe (n = 18)‖	56	39	73	73	83	29	82	71
Mild	83	100	95	95	98	100	78	83

* Percentage of attacks correctly predicted after admission by using method listed.
† In neither system using multiple criteria was LDH measurement used. Severity was based on the presence of 3 of 10 positive criteria of the Ranson et al. system[80] or 3 of 8 using the Imrie et al. system.[81]
‡ CA, Clinical assessment based on physicians' opinion of an attack being mild or severe.
§ Severe attacks were based on one or more of three physical characteristics of lavage fluid: aspiration of more than 10 ml of free peritoneal fluid irrespective of its color prior to running in saline; free fluid of a dark color (prune juice); a midstraw or darker color lavage return fluid.
‖ Severity was determined retrospectively from chart review to include any of the following: more than 14 days hospitalization because of pancreatitis (recurrent attacks excluded); presence of severe complications such as renal or respiratory failure, pancreatic abscess, etc.; death. (Modified from McMahon, M. J., Playforth, M. J., Pickford, I. R.: A comparative study of methods for the prediction of severity of attacks of pancreatitis. Br. J. Surg., 67:22, 1980.)

of survival (LDF score of less than −0.423) and those with an intermediate chance of survival (LDF greater than +1.76).[89] This index requires further validation across large groups of patients and was specifically developed for patients who developed perioperative renal failure. The renal failure predictive indices were derived from retrospective review.

QUANTITATION OF OUTCOME IN THE POST-ICU PHASE

In a review of the literature from 1975 to 1979, Najman and Levine found 23 published studies on the impact of medical care or technology on the quality of life.[90] Between 1980 and 1988, Hollandsworth found 69 empirically based studies of the impact of medical treatment on the quality of life.[91] Even though none of these investigations applied specifically to the post-ICU phase of critical illness, it is important for the ICU physician to be familiar with these studies, because outcome of intensive care cannot be defined only on status at the time of discharge from the ICU. As emphasized by Zaren and Hedstrand, survival and quality of life in the first post-ICU year of life are better measures of outcome.[92] Sage and colleagues evaluated 337 mixed medical-surgical ICU patients for severity of illness, intensity of therapy, survival, and quality of life 16 to 20 months after discharge.[93] The APACHE II system was used for classification of severity of illness, the TISS for definition of intensity of therapy, and the Sickness Impact Profile (SIP) for quantitation of the quality of life after hospital discharge. Of interest is that in this study, survivors had less disability based on SIP scores than patients with chronic obstructive pulmonary disease, rheumatoid arthritis, or chronic depression or pain.[93] As social and economic pressures dictate that the costs and benefits of intensive care become defined better, clinicians will be expected to quantitate survival of patients with some objective index. Table 79–42 includes some of the scales, scores, and in-

Table 79–37. Potential Predictor Variables for Survival with Acute Tubular Necrosis

Cause	Complications	Miscellaneous
Toxin	Myocardial infarction	Age
Trauma	Pulmonary emboli	Sex
Sepsis	Gastrointestinal bleeding	Starting BUN level
Miscellaneous	Atrial tachycardia	Starting creatinine level
Surgery	Ventricular tachycardia	Maximum BUN level
	Complete heart block	Maximum creatinine level
	Bleeding dyscrasia	Lowest CO₂ content
	Wound dehiscence	Nonoliguric acute tubular necrosis
	Peritonitis	Duration of oliguria
	Pneumonia	Total parenteral nutrition
	Septicemia	
	Abscess	
	Urinary tract infection	

(From McMurray, S. D., et al.: Prevailing patterns and predictor variables in patients with acute tubular necrosis. Arch. Intern. Med., 138:950, 1978.)

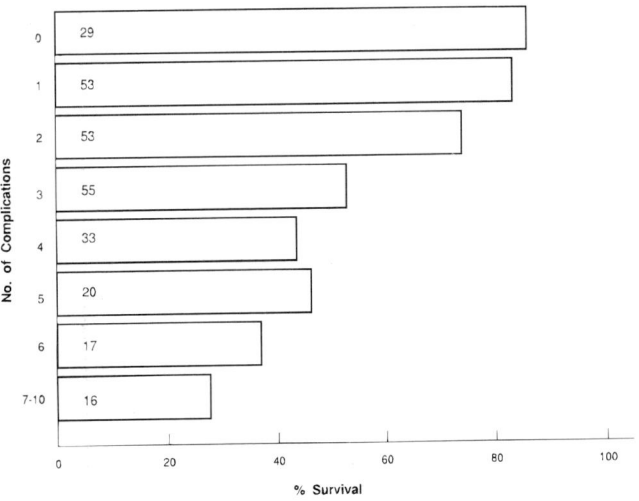

Fig. 79–11. As the number of complications associated with acute tubular necrosis (as listed in Table 79–33) increase, McMurray and colleagues found inverse correlation with survival (r = .35, p < .05). (Redrawn by George Morrison, Clinical Dimensions, Inc., from McMurray, S. D., et al.: Prevailing patterns and predictor variables in patients with acute tubular necrosis. Arch. Intern. Med., 138:950, 1978.)

Table 79-38. Predictor Variables in Acute Renal Failure in Order of Decreasing Function Coefficient*

Predictor	Survivors	Non-survivors	Univariate Probability (P)	Function Coefficient
Acute cardiac illness	2	13	0.02	0.4248
Neoplastic disease	5	21	0.005	0.3957
Oliguria	15	53	0.0005	0.3746
Acute pancreatitis	3	5	NS	0.3498
Trauma	3	9	NS	0.3170
Preexisting renal disease	10	12	NS	0.2117
"Other surgery"	12	22	NS	0.2086
CNS damage	1	6	NS	0.1977
Respiratory failure	8	29	0.005	0.1960
Preexisting heart disease	29	29	NS	0.1371

* A discriminant score for a patient is derived by the addition of functional coefficients of the relevant predictor variables and the constant term (−0.5194). When the score of 0.21 was used as the cutoff point, a positive predictive value of 100% and a sensitivity of 58% were achieved for 45 of 78 nonsurvivors. NS, not significant. (From Rasmussen, H. H., et al.: Prediction of outcome in acute renal failure by discriminate analysis of clinical variables. Arch. Intern. Med., *145*:2015, 1985.)

Table 79-39. Levels of Significance of Variables that Separate Survivors from Nonsurvivors in Postoperative Acute Renal Failure (Initial Screening by Chi-Square Method)

Variable	Alive	Dead	Significance*
Cardiac failure	25%	66%	0.02
Number of systems failed	3.0	3.8	0.03
Number of transfusions	10 (50%)	10 (87%)	0.03
Noncavitary surgery	17%	2%	0.05
Age	41.2 ′ 24	57.0 ′ 17	0.05
Injury severity score	28.5 ′ 8	42.0 ′ 11	0.02
Creatinine prior to first hemodialysis	6.6 ′ 1.7	8.2 ′ 3.2	0.02
Interval acute renal failure (ARF) to hemodialysis	6.6 ′ 2.8	8.6 ′ 7.8	0.06
Aortic surgery	0%	25%	0.13
Preoperative chronic renal insufficiency	8%	3%	NS
Sepsis	66%	66%	NS
Emergent surgery	42%	45%	NS
Perioperative myocardial infarction	8%	5%	NS
Cardiovascular disease	33%	18%	NS
Number of hemodialysis	5.7 ′ 4.8	7.5 ′ 7.8	NS
Interval from surgery to ARF	5.2 ′ 4.6	3.9 ′ 7.2	NS

* NS, not significant. (From Cioffi, W. G., Ashikaga, T., Gamelli, R. L.: Probability of surviving postoperative acute renal failure. Development of a prognostic index. Ann. Surg., *200*:205, 1984.)

dices that may be applicable in the post-ICU phase of illness.

Activities of Daily Living

Katz and colleagues developed the Index of Independence in Activities of Daily Living (Index of ADL) as a measurement of function for the aged and the chronically ill.[94] These authors expected that this index might be used to evaluate results of treatment, to quantitate natural changes in function in the ill and well, and perhaps to assess the needs for care in health care facilities.

The index was developed from observations made by physicians, nurses, sociologists, and other professional observers in the care of the aged and chronically ill. It "permits ranking of individuals according to adequacy of performance."[94] Overall performance is summarized as a grade (A through G and other) based on six functions: bathing, dressing, going to toilet, transferring, continence, and feeding. A reduction in grade results from a loss of independence in a particular area of function (Table 79-43).

The principle application of this index to outcome assessment might be its application to quantitating the speed of recovery in the late ICU phase of illness and the post-ICU phase of rehabilitation. Along these lines, the most severely ill patients, particularly those who require prolonged periods of mechanical ventilation, likely begin recovery with a grade of G (see Table 79-43). Some similarity is noted in the sequence of recovery between the chronically ill, the aged, and the recovering critically ill. In the former groups, Katz and co-workers noted that independence in feeding was the first function to return in their study population. Continence was the second func-

tion to return, and transferring and going to the toilet were the next functions to return. Recovery of complete independence in bathing and dressing were last to return.[94] This index could be used over time to quantitate the speed of recovery. From a research standpoint, various patient populations stratified according to severity of illness could

Table 79-40. Linear Discriminant Function Variable Codes and Coefficient Constants (REF)*

Variable	Significance
Age, actual age in years	0.0089
Number of transfusions: 5 = 1, 5–10 = 2, 11–20 = 3, 20 = 4	0.0006
Cardiac surgery; No = 0, Yes = 1	0.0002
Cardiac failure; No = 0, Yes = 1	0.0000
Sex; male = 1, female = 0	0.0000
Vascular surgery; † No = 0, Yes = 1	0.0001
Interval in days from onset acute renal failure to dialysis	0.0001
Preoperative hypotension; No = 0, Yes = 1	0.0001

* Significance level addition of variable adds to function.
† Other than abdominal aortic surgery. (Modified from Cioffi, W. G., Ashikaga, T., Gamelli, R. L.: Probability of surviving postoperative acute renal failure. Development of a prognostic index. Ann. Surg., *200*:205, 1984.)

Table 79-41. Accuracy of the Linear Discriminant Function (LDF) Score in Predicting Survival or Nonsurvival of Acute Renal Failure Patients

		Predicted Status	
Group	Actual Status	Alive*	Dead†
1	Alive (12)‡	83%§ (10)	17% (2)
	Dead (53)	19% (10)	81% (43)
2	Alive (5)	80% (4)	20% (1)
	Dead (13)	0% (0)	100% (13)

* Patients with a LDF score greater than 0.669. This score represents the average of the mean scores for alive and dead patients.
† Patients with a LDF score less than 0.669.
‡ Actual number of patients in each group.
§ Percentage of actually alive or dead patients predicted to be alive or dead. (From Cioffi, W. G., Ashikaga, T., Gamelli, R. L.: Probability of surviving postoperative acute renal failure. Development of a prognostic index. Ann. Surg., *200*:205, 1984.)

Table 79-43. Index of Independence in Activities of Daily Living

Category	Definition of Functional Independence or Dependence*
A	Independent in feeding, continence, transferring, going to toilet, dressing, and bathing
B	Independent in all but one of these functions
C	Independent in all but bathing and one additional function
D	Independent in all but bathing, dressing, and one additional function
E	Independent in all but bathing, dressing, going to toilet, and one additional function
F	Independent in all but bathing, dressing, going to toilet, transferring, and one additional function
G	Dependent in all six functions
Other	Dependent in at least two functions, but not classifiable as C, D, E, or F.

* Specific definition of independence and dependence in each of the six areas is available.[90] (From Katz, S., et al.: Studies of illness in the aged. The index of ADL: A standardized measure of biological and psychosocial function. JAMA, *185*:914, 1963.)

be studied to determine the speed of recovery. In addition, the resources required during recovery could be quantitated. Similar utility exists in the Langley-Porter Physical Self-Maintenance Scale (PSMS) and the Instrumental Activities of Daily Living (IADL).[95]

Karnofsky Performance Status Scale

This scale is used to quantitate the functional status of cancer patients. As with other utilities, its reliability and validity has limited documentation.[96] It has some potential application to classification of ICU patients. On one hand, it is likely that patients with cancer constitute a subpopulation of ICU patients. Some quantitation of the functional status of these patients may guide the patients, their families, and the patient caregivers in formulating aggressive or conservative, more palliative care plans. Some utility to this index is gained when categories, as listed in Table 79-44, are reviewed with respect to patient longevity. In an unspecified number of cases reviewed, Mor and colleagues found that most patients with indices of 10 to 50 die within 18 days of admission to hospice programs, whereas most (70.4%) with indices of 50 or greater live longer than 36 days.[97]

Sickness Impact Profile

The Sickness Impact Profile is a generic instrument that measures different aspects of quality of life. It takes into account not only the physical aspects of dysfunction, but also the psychosocial aspects. Originally, it was a questionnaire of 300 items that has been refined to 136 questions. The categories of this profile are displayed in Table 79-45. Each question or item within the categories is given a scale value. The values for the items checked off on the questionnaire are summed and divided by the sum of the total possible items. This value is then multiplied by 100 to express a score as a percentage. A low score of 0 would represent no health-related impairment, whereas a score of 100 would represent complete impairment. The addition of psychosocial aspects to this profile adds a dimension that is not measured by ADL and an additional aspect to the concept of quality of life.

In spite of its potential application, further research and validation is necessary. Sage and colleagues studied the long-term outcome of survivors of intensive care (140 patients of 465 total) at 16 to 20 months after ICU discharge.

Table 79-42. Scales, Scores, and Indices for Quantitation of Outcome after ICU Discharge

Instrument	Intended Application	Potential Application
Activities of Daily Living (ADL)[90]	Measurement of function for the aged and chronically ill	Application of measurement over time could quantitate the recovery process
Karnofsky Performance Scale (KPS)[91]	Quality of life of cancer patients	Possible assistance in establishing limits of therapeutic intervention for some patients
Sickness Impact Profile (SIP)[92]	Generic in that it was intended to measure the function and psychosocial impact of illness across different illnesses	Assessment of the long-term effect of critical illness on physical as well as psychologic health
Nottingham Health Profile (NHP)[93,94]	Similar in application to SIP. Additional assessment of effect of health status on occupation	Technology assessment; refinement of single index allows for quantitation of economic impact on survival of critical illness when combined with QALY
Functional Status Questionnaire (FSQ)[95]	Assessment of physical, psychologic, social, and role function of ambulatory patients	Quantitation of dysfunction or disability following illness; identification of new problems.
Quality Adjusted Life Years (QALY)[96]	Integration within an individual of the health improvements from changes in quality of life	Facilitation of decision-making concerned with the adoption and utilization of health care technologies

Table 79-44. The Karnofsky Performance Status Scale

General Category	Index	Specific Criteria
A. Able to carry on normal activity; no special care needed	100	Normal, no complaints, no evidence of disease
	90	Able to carry on normal activity, minor signs or symptoms of disease
	80	Normal activity with effort, some signs or symptoms of disease
B. Unable to work, able to live at home and care for most	70	Cares for self, unable to carry on normal activity or to do work
	60	Requires occasional assistance from others but able to care for most needs
	50	Requires considerable assistance from others and frequent medical care.
C. Unable to care for self, requires institutional or hospital care or equivalent, disease may be rapidly progressing	40	Disabled, requires special care and assistance
	30	Severely disabled, hospitalization indicated, death not imminent
	20	Very sick, hospitalization necessary, active supportive treatment necessary.
	10	Moribund.
	0	Dead.

(From Karnofsky, D. A., et al.: The use of the nitrogen mustards in the palliative treatment of carcinoma. Cancer, 1:634, 1948.)

Table 79-45. Categories and Selected Items of the Sickness Impact Profile

Category	Items Describing Behaviors Involved in or Related to	Selected Items	Scale Values
A	Social interaction	I make many demands, for example, insist that people do things for me, tell them how to do things	7.7
B	Ambulation or locomotion activity	I am walking shorter distances	3.3
		I do not walk at all	9.2
C	Sleep and rest activity	I lie down to rest more often during the day	4.6
		I sit around half asleep	8.1
D	Taking nutrition	I am eating no food at all, nutrition is taken through tubes or intravenous fluids	12.3
		I am eating special or different food, for example, soft food, bland diet, low-salt, low-fat foods	5.6
E	Usual daily work	I often act irritable toward my work associates, for example, snap at them, give sharp answers, criticize easily	7.1
		I am not working at all	8.6
F	Household management	I have given up taking care of personal or household business affairs, for example, paying bills, banking, working on budget	6.9
		I am doing less of the regular daily work around the house that I usually do	3.9
G	Mobility and confinement	I stay within one room	9.9
		I stop often when traveling because of health problems	4.2
H	Movement of the body	I am in a restricted position all the time	13.6
		I sit down, lie down, or get up only with help	10.4
I	Communication activity	I communicate only by gestures, for example, moving head, pointing, sign language	11.3
		I often lose control of my voice when I talk, for example, my voice gets louder, starts trembling, changes pitch	6.4
J	Leisure pastimes	I am doing more physically inactive pastimes instead of my other usual activities	3.9
		I am going out for entertainment less often	2.8
K	Intellectual functioning	I have difficulty reasoning and solving problems, for example, making plans, making decisions, learning new things	8.3
		I sometimes behave as if I were confused or disoriented in place or time, for example, where I am, who is around, directions, what day it is	11.2
L	Interaction with family members	I isolate myself as much as I can from the rest of the family	8.9
		I am not doing the things I usually do to take care of my children or family	6.8
M	Emotions, feelings, and sensations	I act irritable and impatient with myself, for example, talk badly about myself, swear at myself, blame myself for things that happen	5.4
		I laugh and cry suddenly for no reason	8.1
N	Personal hygiene	I dress myself, but do so very slowly	4.6
		I do not have control of my bowels	11.2

(From Bergner, M., et al.: The sickness impact profile: Validation of a health status measure. Med. Care, 14:57, 1976.)

The average SIP score was 6.8 ± 0.7%.[93] The extensiveness of this profile may be limited, because high dysfunction scores in certain areas may be offset by low scores for dysfunction because of illness. Potentially, the ability to detect subtle differences in quality of life could be limited.

Nottingham Health Profile

This profile is similar in scope to the SIP. It has been applied extensively and is currently the subject of study for refinement and retesting by The European Group for the Nottingham Health Profile (NHP).[98] It is of particular interest in that at least some "normal values" are obtained by applications to the general population presumed to be in good health (Table 79-46).[99] This profile has two components. Part I or the subjective component measures 6 dimensions: physical mobility, pain, sleep, energy, social isolation, and emotional reactions. It consists of 38 questions that have yes or no answers. Answers are weighed relative to each other, with the total score ranging from 0 for best to 100 for worst quality. Part II is more objective in the assessment of task performance affected by health. Assessment areas include occupation, ability to perform jobs around the home, social life, sexual life, home life, hobbies, and holidays. A yes answer indicates that the state of health is causing problems in a particular area. No weights are applied and the score is determined as a percentage of affirmative answers to total.

This profile by itself could further quantitate outcome of intensive care. It has been refined into a single index and combined with life expectancy gains to produce estimates of Quality Adjusted Life Years (QALYs) for evaluation of the United Kingdom heart transplant programs.[100] For this evaluation, O'Brien and colleagues chose NHP because they considered it sensitive to a wide range of health states, comparison population NHP scores were available, it could be administered by interview or by mail, and it made relatively small demands on patient time and effort. O'Brien and other colleagues applied the same profile to 48 patients before and after combined heart and lung transplantation (see Table 79-46).[101] The study itself demonstrated large and statistically significant improvements in quality of life after transplantation. Additionally, the profile itself was easy to use as either an interview during assessment for transplantation or as a postal follow-up postoperatively. This instrument could be applied widely before and after transplantation, cardiovascular surgery, thoracic surgery, and other vital operations. Its application may be limited in patients with unscheduled medical illness regarding ICU care, unless a baseline population survey of the rehabilitation phase of illness was available.

Functional Status Questionnaire

This questionnaire was designed for the comprehensive assessment of physical, psychologic, social, and comprehensive assessment of ambulatory patients. It can be self-administered with the intention of screening for disability and to monitor clinical change in function.[102] It is divided into five sections, which are summarized in Table 79-47. The section on activity is divided into basic and intermediate activities. Thirty-seven items are computed and scored to produce six summary scale scores and six single item scores. Transformed scale scores range from 0 to 100, with 100 representing maximum function. Warning zones that appear on a visual report to indicate functional disabilities were defined by a panel of experienced clinicians.[103] A review of the definitions outlined in Table 79-47 suggests that this questionnaire would be appropriate for long-term follow-up beyond hospital discharge. A sample report is

Table 79-46. Pre- and Postoperative Mean NHP Dimension Scores for Patients Undergoing Combined Heart and Lung Transplantation

	Pretransplant Assessment (n = 48)	3 Months Post-Transplant (n = 28)	6 Months Post-Transplant (n = 24)	12 Months Post-Transplant (n = 13)	"Normal" Population* Males	"Normal" Population* Females
Section I: Mean dimension score						
Energy	76.0	14.5	6.2	4.7	8.6	20.0
Pain	17.8	8.7	2.7	2.3	1.6	2.8
Emotional reactions	39.2	6.5	3.3	1.2	10.3	14.7
Sleep	38.9	13.6	4.2	6.6	8.6	9.7
Social isolation	32.1	10.3	5.0	3.1	5.6	6.9
Physical mobility	51.2	13.4	3.3	3.4	1.6	2.0
Section II: Percentage of patients experiencing problems related to their health						
Occupation	76.6	42.9	20.8	15.4	7.0	6.3
Jobs around the home	76.6	28.6	16.7	0	6.2	13.2
Social life	77.1	17.9	12.5	0	8.6	11.3
Home life	40.4	14.3	8.3	0	8.6	16.3
Sex life	65.9	28.6	8.3	15.4	6.2	23.2
Hobbies	77.1	21.4	20.8	15.4	14.1	10.1
Holidays	70.8	17.9	20.8	7.7	6.2	5.0

* Population normals for age range 25 to 29 years taken from a random sample of 2173 individuals in Nottingham.[95] Wilcoson test for repeated measures: $p < 0.05$ on all dimensions of section I for patients who completed profiles at assessment and 3 months post-transplant. McNemar Test for repeated measures: $p < 0.05$ in all dimensions of section II for patients who completed profiles at assessment and 3 months post-transplant. (From O'Brien, B. J., et al.: The Nottingham health profile as a measure of quality of life following combined heart and lung transplantation. J. Epidemiol. Comm. Health, 42:232, 1988.)

Table 79-47. Operational Definitions for Functional Status Scale Scores[101]

Item	Definition	Warning
Physical function		
Basic activities of daily living	A standardized (0–100) scale (three items) that indicates the degree to which the person has limitations in self-care, transfer from bed or chairs, or walking around the house. A high score indicates better performance.	89
Intermediate activities of daily living	A standardized (0–100) scale (six items) that indicates the degree to which the person has limitations in walking, doing house or yard work, doing errands, driving or using public transportation, or participating in vigorous recreational activities. A high score indicates better performance.	72
Psychologic function		
Mental health	A standardized (0–100) scale (five items) that indicates the frequency with which the person feels anxious, depressed, or generally happy over 1 month. A high score indicates greater well-being.	66
Role function		
Employment status	A standardized (0–100) scale (six items) that indicates the degree to which the person has limitations in working at his or her job, if employed. A high score indicates better performance.	75
Work performance		
Social function		
Social activity	A standardized (0–100) scale (three items) that indicates the degree to which the person was limited in visiting relatives or friends, participating in community activities, or taking care of other people. A high score indicates greater social activity.	78
Quality of interaction	A standardized (0–100) scale (five items) that indicates the degree to which the person has been irritable toward others, affectionate, isolated, demanding, or getting along well. A high score indicates better interactions.	61
Frequency of social contact	Single item ranging from 1 (not at all) to 6 (every day).	
Bed days	Single item	
Sexual satisfaction	A single item indicating how satisfied the person was with sexual relationships or whether the person had none. Possible responses range from 0 (did not have sexual relationships) to 5 (very satisfactory).	
Satisfaction with health	Single item. Possible responses range from 1 (very dissatisfied) to 5 (very satisfied).	

(Modified from Rubenstein, L. V., et al.: Improving patient function: A randomized trial of functional disability screening. Ann. Intern. Med., *111*: 836, 1989.)

shown in Figure 79-12. As intended, such reports might serve as a screen for clinical problems for which further analysis and quantitation would be appropriate with more specific instruments and laboratory and diagnostic techniques. Use of this tool would be of particular interest in efforts to determine if dysfunction or disability is attributable to chronic illness or to new illness.

Quality Adjusted Life Years (QALYs)

The foregoing indices and profiles were designed to quantitate the quality of life from a number of different viewpoints. Beyond this quality, however, is the perception that this quality must be measured over time. In other words, how would one quantitate this quality as a measurement of improvement in life or trade off for more freedom from chronic illness or impairment? On one hand, outcome could be quantitated by years of life gained, but some years gained might be better than others. On the other hand, simultaneous capture of the impact of the quantity and quality of life might provide better assessment. The concept of quality adjusted life years gained is shown in Figure 79-13.

"Consider a single individual whose quality of life is reduced by 0.03 for 30 years by hypertension drug therapy to gain 10 years of life extension at a quality level of 0.90. The QALYs gained for such an individual would be $10 \times 0.9 - 30 \times 0.03 = 8.8$. As a second example, consider a program that extends the life of one individual by 2 years at a quality level of 0.50 and improves the quality of life for another individual from 0.50 to 0.75 also for 2 years. The QALYs gained by the group of two individuals is $2 \times 0.50 + 2 \times 0.25 = 1.5$."[104]

Several concepts must be considered when using QALYs for quantitation of outcome. To begin, this type of quantitation of outcome is best applied to procedures or to technologic tools that intervene in an altered state of health, such as cardiac surgery, organ transplantation, hemodialysis, joint replacement, and so forth. The assessment or quantitation of quality of life before and after intervention is implicit. Beyond quantitation of quality of life is the necessity for reduction of the measurement of multiple parameters (as in the NHP and SIP) into a single number or index that can be obtained at different points in time. Then comes the requirement to validate this index as a predictive factor such that a particular intervention would improve quality of life and add life years. The final consideration is the need to create large data bases of patient information that will allow one to determine life years gained with and without intervention. Obviously, this type of measurement is best reserved for technology assessment or determining the cost of a year of life with improved quality.

In summary, the foregoing discussion was designed with a focus that patients have preexisting states of health and levels or severity of illness prior to critical illness. Many general and specific instruments are available by which

PATIENT CARE

FUNCTION STATUS REPORT FOR: Daisy Mae

PHYSICIAN Mark Reed

ID 6789   AGE 62   DATE OF QUESTIONNAIRE 01/19/84

BASIC ACTIVITY: +++++++++++++33++------

INTERMEDIATE: ++++++++28+++-------------

MENTAL HEALTH: ++++++++++++++++++++++++++++++48++++++++++++++++++++++++++++++------------------

SOCIAL ACTIVITY: ++++++++++++++++++++++++++++++44+++++++++++++++++++++++++++++++++-------------

INTERACTION: +++-----------------100

EMPLOYMENT: RETIRED BECAUSE OF HEALTH

Major Problems: doing self-care, moving to a chair, climbing stairs.
Minor Problems: visiting friends, participating in outside activities.
Last month: days in bed = 3; restricted days = 7
The above problems are chronic.

Mostly: nervous, happy, affectionate, amiable
Seldom: peaceful, downhearted, depressed, isolated, irritable, demanding
Social contact: once a month (friends = 0).
Did not have any sexual relationships.

Fig. 79-12. Sample report generated from the Functional Status Questionnaire. Categories listed are defined in Table 79-43. Warning values in each category are also listed in the table. (From Rubenstein, L. V., et al.: Improving patients function: A randomized trial of functional disability screening. Ann. Intern. Med., 111:836, 1989.)

preexisting health status can be defined. The shortcoming of each is that the medical record is not suitably equipped to facilitate capture of the data to make such definition. If one would ever attempt to truthfully answer the question of who would benefit from ICU care and who would not, objective classification systems would be necessary. With the growing emphasis on quality of patient care and responsible application of technology, various classification systems will become part of the medical record. With such an event, the critical care practitioner will have further information to facilitate decisions to apply increasingly complex technologic practices to the care of the critically ill patient. Such classification systems might be validated by their predictability of requirements for care as compared to the severity of illness at the time of admission to the ICU.

Beyond the initial focus point of illness before ICU admission is an added dimension created by objective definition of severity of illness and consumption of resources in the ICU. Such specifically applied definitions take on an element of quality assurance when one compares the prediction of outcome based on severity of illness to the actual outcome of ICU care. A less favorable outcome than that predicted for a group of patients should alert caregivers to investigate the process of patient care. Excess resource consumption in relation to severity of illness should also alert caregivers. Excess intervention may be costly and detrimental to the patient. Patient classification will become essential to the delivery of patient care.

Subsequent to survival of critical illness are additional elements of long-term survival, rehabilitation and quality of life. The post-ICU phase of illness can be prolonged and

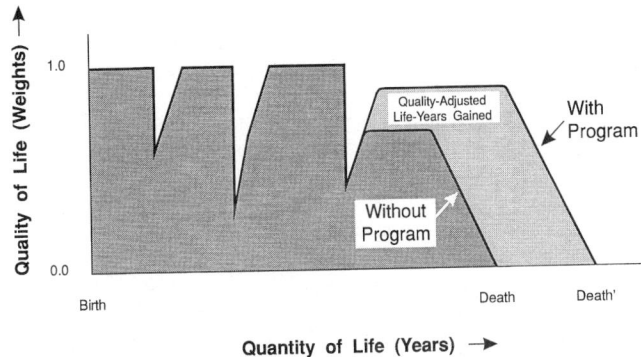

Fig. 79-13. Concept of quality adjusted life years gained. The y-axis quantifies quality of life and the x-axis represents years of life. The right side of the graph represents added quality of life from the addition of a procedure, medical program, or technology. See reference 97 for detailed explanation. (Redrawn by George Morrison, Clinical Dimensions, Inc., from Torrance, G. W., and Feeny, D.: Utilities and quality-adjusted life years. Int. J. Tech. Asses. Health Care, 5:559, 1989.)

perhaps associated with a quality of life that is less desirable to the patient. For this reason, further quantitation of outcome in terms of quality of life will become important in decisions to implement ICU admission. Many excellent reviews are available on the subject of quality. The critical care practitioner should study these reviews and seek innovative ways to quantitate outcome beyond survival of intensive care and hospital discharge for a true assessment of the technologies used in the care of critically ill patients.[105] Proper selection of quality of life measurements will facilitate the creation of data bases providing information for outcome assessment of existing and new technologic tools. Most importantly, critical illness has three phases—pre-ICU, ICU, and post-ICU. Proper quantitation of health status, severity of illness, and outcome will provide better understanding of the benefits of intensive care for the critically ill patient.

REFERENCES

1. U.S. Congress, Office of Technology Assessment, The Quality of Medical Care: Information for Consumers, OTS-H-386. Library of Congress, Catalog Card Number 88-60037, 1987.
2. Sivak, E. D., and Perez-Trepichio, A.: Quality assessment in the medical intensive care unit: Evolution of a data model Cleve. Clin. J. Med., 57:273, 1990.
3. Hornbrook, M. C.: Hospital case mix: Its definition, measurement, and use. Part II, A review of alternative measures. Med. Care Rev., 39:75, 1982.
4. Gonnella, J. S., Hornbrook, M. C., Louis, D. Z.: Staging of disease. A case-mix measurement. JAMA, 251:637, 1984.
5. Knaus, W. A., Zimmerman, J. E., Wagner, D. P.: APACHE—acute physiology and chronic health evaluation: A physiologically based classification system. Crit. Care Med., 9:591, 1981.
6. Horn, S. D., et al.: Severity of illness within DRGs: Impact on prospective payment. Am. J. Public Health, 75:1195, 1985.
7. Horn, S. D., Horn, R. A., Moses, H.: Profiles of physician practice and patient severity of illness. Am. J. Public Health, 76:532, 1986.
8. Lemeshow, S., et al.: A method of predicting survival and mortality of ICU patients using objectively derived weights. Crit. Care Med., 13:59, 1985.
9. Knaus, W. A., et al.: APACHE II: A severity of disease classification system. Crit. Care Med., 13:818, 1985.
10. Wagner, D. P., Knaus, W. A., Draper, E. A.: Statistical validation of a severity of illness measure. Am. J. Public Health, 73:878, 1983.
11. Knaus, W. A., et al.: An evaluation of outcome from intensive care in major medical centers. Ann. Intern. Med., 104: 410, 1986.
12. Thomas, J. W., Ashcraft, M. L. F., Zimmerman, J.: An evaluation of alternative severity of illness measures for use by university hospitals. In Management Summary. Ann Arbor Department of Health Services, Management and Policy, School of Public Health. Vol. I. University of Michigan, 1986.
13. Zimmerman, J. E., and Knaus, W. A.: Outcome of prediction in adult intensive care. In Textbook of Critical Care. 2nd Ed. Edited by W. C. Shoemaker, et al. Philadelphia, W. B. Saunders, 1989, p. 1447.
14. Breslow, L.: A quantitative approach to the World Health Organization definition of health: Physical, mental and social well-being. Int. J. Epidemiol., 1:347, 1972.
15. Inglehard, J. K.: Medicare begins prospective payment of hospitals. N. Engl. J. Med., 308:428, 1983.
16. Fetter, R. B., et al. Case mix definition of diagnosis-related groups. Med. Care, 18(Suppl.): 1, 1980.
17. The Medicare Prospective Payment System. Implementing Regulations—Their Implications of Hospitals. Ernst & Whinney, E & W No. J58475, 1983.
18. Vladeck, B. C.: Medicare hospital payment by diagnosis-related groups. Ann. Intern. Med., 100:576, 1984.
19. Hornbrook, M. C.: Hospital case mix: Its definition, measurement and use. Part II. Review of alternative measures. Med. Care Rev., 39:73, 1982.
20. Mayer-Oakes, S. A., et al. The early effect of medicare's prospective payment system on the use of medical intensive care services in three community hospitals. JAMA, 260: 3146, 1988.
21. Sivak, E. D., and Perez-Trepechio, A.: Quality assessment in the medical intensive care unit: Continued evolution of a data model. Quality Assurance Utilization Review, 7:42, 1992.
22. St. Anthony's DRG Working Guidebook, 992. Alexandria, VA, St. Anthony's Publishing, 1991.
23. Lichtig, L. K.: New Jersey Evaluation of ICD-9-CM DRGs. Trenton, New Jersey State Department of Health, 1981, p. 1.
24. Jencks, S. F., and Dobson, A.: Refining case-mix adjustment. The research evidence. N. Engl. J. Med., 317:679, 1987.
25. Iezzoni, L. I., and Moskowitz, M. A.: Clinical overlap among medical diagnosis-related groups. JAMA, 255:927, 1986.
26. The International Classification of Diseases, 9th revision, Clinical Modification. ICD-9-CM. U.S. Department of Health and Human Services, Public Health Service—HCFA. Publ. No. 80-126. Vol. 1, 2nd Ed. 1980, XV.
27. The International Classification of Diseases, 9th revision, Clinical Modification. ICD-9-CM. U.S. Department of Health and Human Services, Public Health Service—HCFA. Publ. No. 80-1260. Vol. 2, 2nd Ed. 1980, XVII.
28. The International Classification of Diseases, 9th revision, Clinical Modification. ICD-9-CM. U.S. Department of Health and Human Services, Public Health Service—HCFA. Publ. No. 80-1260. Vol. 1, 2nd Ed. 1980, XVII.
29. ICD-10 International Statistical Classification of Diseases and Related Health Problems. 10th rev. Geneva, World Health Organization, 1992.
30. CPT-1994. Physicians' Current Procedural Terminology. Chicago, American Medical Association, 1993.
31. Conklin, J. E., et al. Disease staging: Implications for hospital reimbursement and management. Health Care Fin. Rev., 6:(Suppl.):13, 1984.
32. Horn, S. D., Sharkey, P. D., Bertram, D. A.: Measuring severity of illness: Homogeneous case mix groups. Med. Care, 21:14, 1983.
33. Horn, S. D., Horn, R. A., Sharkey, P. D.: The severity of illness index as a severity adjustment to diagnosis-related groups. Health Care Fin. Rev., 6(Suppl.).:34, 1984.
34. Horn, S. D., et al.: Interhospital differences in severity of illness. Problems for prospective payment based on diagnosis-related groups (DRGs). N. Engl. J. Med., 313:20, 1985.
35. Horn, S. D., et al.: Severity of illness within DRGs. Homogeneity study. Med. Care, 24:225, 1986.
36. Horn, S. D., and Horn, R. A.: Reliability and validity of the severity of illness index. Med. Care, 24:159, 1986.
37. Green, J., et al.: The importance of severity of illness in assessing hospital mortality. JAMA, 235:241, 1990.
38. Horn, S. D., and Horn, R. A.: The computerized severity index: A new tool for case-mix management. J. Med. Sys., 10:73, 1986.

39. Iezzoni, L. I., et al.: Admission MEDISGRPS Score and the cost of hospitalizations. Med. Care, 26:1068, 1988.
40. Brewster, A. C., et al.: MEDISGRPS(r): A clinically based approach to classifying hospital patients at admission. Inquiry, 22:377, 1985.
41. Iezzoni, L. I., and Moskowitz, M. A.: A clinical assessment of MedisGroups. JAMA, 260:3159, 1988.
42. LeGall, J. R., et al.: A simplified acute physiology score for ICU patients. Crit. Care Med., 12:975, 1984.
43. French Multicenter Group of ICU Research, INSERM Unit 169 of Statistical and Epidemiological Studies: Factors relate to outcome in intensive care: French multicenter study. Crit. Care Med., 17:305, 1989.
44. LeGall, J. R., Lemeshow, S., and Saulnier, F.: A new simplified acute physiology score (SAPS II) based on a European/North American Multicenter Study. JAMA, 270:2953, 1993.
45. Knaus, W. A., et al.: An evaluation of outcome from intensive care in major medical centers. Ann. Intern. Med., 104:410, 1986.
46. Zimmerman, J. E., et al.: Patient selection for intensive care: A comparison of New Zealand and United States hospitals. Crit. Care Med., 16:318, 1988.
47. Zimmerman, J. E., Knaus, W. A., Draper, E. A.: Physiologic abnormalities and outcome from acute disease. Evidence for a predictable relationship. Arch. Intern. Med., 146:1389, 1986.
48. Fedullo, A. J., et al.: APACHE II score and mortality in respiratory failure due to cardiogenic pulmonary edema. Crit. Care Med., 16:1218, 1988.
49. Lemeshow, S., et al.: A method for predicting survival and mortality of ICU patients using objectively derived weights. Crit. Care Med., 13:519, 1985.
50. Lemeshow, S., et al.: Mortality probability models (MPM II): based on an international cohort of intensive care unit patients. JAMA, 270:2478, 1993.
51. Cullen, D. J., et al.: Therapeutic intervention scoring system: A method for quantitative comparison of patient care. Crit. Care Med., 2:57, 1974.
52. Keene, A. R., and Cullen, D. J.: Therapeutic intervention scoring system: Update 1983. Crit. Care Med., 11:213, 1983.
53. Knaus, W. A., et al.: The Apache III Prognostic System. Risk prediction of hospitalized mortality for critically ill hospitalized adults. Chest, 100:1619, 1991.
54. Teasdale, G., and Jennett, B.: Assessment of coma and impaired consciousness: A practical scale. Lancet, 2:81, 1974.
55. Jennett, B., and Teasdale, G.: Predicting outcome in individual patients after severe head injury. Lancet, 5:1031, 1976.
56. Teres, D., Brown, R. B., Lemeshow, S.: Predicting mortality of intensive care unit patients. The importance of coma. Crit. Care Med., 10:86, 1982.
57. The Critical Committee of the New York Heart Association: Diseases of the Heart and Blood Vessels. 6th Ed. Boston, Little, Brown, 1964, p. 112.
58. The Multicenter Postinfarction Research Group. Risk stratification and survival after myocardial infarction. N. Engl. J. Med., 309:331, 1983.
59. Killip, T., and Kimball, J. T.: Treatment of myocardial infarction in a coronary care unit: A two year experience with 250 patients. Am. J. Cardiol., 20:457, 1967.
60. Forrester, J. S., Diamond, G. A., Swan, H. J. C.: Correlative classification of clinical and hemodynamic function after acute myocardial infarction. Am. J. Cardiol., 39:137, 1977.
61. Forrester, J. S., et al.: Medical therapy of acute myocardial infarction by application of hemodynamic subsets. N. Engl. J. Med., 295:1356, 1976.
62. Shoemaker, W. C., et al.: Physiologic patterns in surviving and nonsurviving shock patients. Arch. Surg., 106:630, 1973.
63. Shoemaker, W. C., et al.: Use of nonparametric analysis of cardiorespiratory variables as early predictors of death and survival in postoperative patients. J. Surg. Res., 17:301, 1974.
64. Shoemaker, W. C., et al.: Prediction of outcome and severity of illness by analysis of the frequency distributions of cardiorespiratory variables. Crit. Care Med., 5:82, 1977.
65. Shoemaker, W. C., et al.: Cardiorespiratory monitoring in postoperative patients. I. Prediction of outcome and severity of illness. Crit. Care Med., 7:237, 1979.
66. Shoemaker, W. C., et al.: Cardiorespiratory monitoring in postoperative patients. II. Quantitative therapeutic indices as guides to therapy. Crit. Care Med., 7:243, 1979.
67. Shoemaker, W. C., et al.: Comparison of hemodynamic and oxygen transport effects of dopamine and dobutamine in critically ill surgical patients. Chest, 96:120, 1989.
68. Bartlett, R. H., et al.: Mortality prediction in adult respiratory failure. Chest, 67:680, 1975.
69. Bartlett, R. H., et al.: A prospective study of acute hypoxic respiratory failure. Chest, 89:684, 1986.
70. Fowler, A. A., et al.: Adult respiratory distress syndrome. Prognosis after onset. Am. Rev. Respir. Dis., 132:472, 1985.
71. Bone, R. C., et al.: An early test of survival in patients with the adult respiratory distress syndrome. The PaO_2/FiO_2 ratio and its differential response to conventional therapy. Chest, 96:849, 1989.
72. Ghio, A. J., et al.: Impairment after adult respiratory distress syndrome. An evaluation base on American Thoracic Society recommendations. Am. Rev. Respir. Dis., 139:1158, 1989.
73. Peters, J. I., et al.: Clinical determinants of abnormalities in pulmonary functions in survivors of the adult respiratory distress syndrome. Am. Rev. Respir. Dis., 139:1163, 1989.
74. Sahn, S. A., Lakshminarayan, S., Petty, T.: Weaning from mechanical ventilation. JAMA, 235:2208, 1976.
75. Scoggin, C. H.: Weaning respiratory patients from mechanical support. J. Respir. Dis., 1:13, 1980.
76. Sivak, E. D.: Prolonged mechanical ventilation: An approach to weaning. Cleve. Clin. Q., 47:89, 1980.
77. Morganroth, M. L., et al.: Criteria for weaning from prolonged mechanical ventilation. Arch. Intern. Med., 144:1012, 1984.
78. Child, C. G., and Turcotte, J. G.: Surgery and portal hypertension. In The Liver and Portal Hypertension. Edited by C. G. Child. Philadelphia, W. B. Saunders, 1964, p. 50.
79. Conn, H. O.: A peek at the Child-Turcotte classification. Hepatology, 1:673, 1984.
80. Shellman, R. G., et al.: Prognosis of patients with cirrhosis and chronic liver disease admitted to the medical intensive care unit. Crit. Care Med., 16:671, 1988.
81. Goldfarb, G., et al.: Efficacy of respiratory assistance in cirrhotic patients with liver failure. Intensive Care Med., 9:271, 1983.
82. Ranson, J. H. C., et al.: Prognostic signs and the role of operative management of acute pancreatitis. Surg. Gynecol. Obstet., 136:69, 1974.
83. Ranson, J. H. C., Rifkind, K. M., Turner, J. W.: Prognostic signs and nonoperative acute pancreatitis. Surg. Gynecol. Obstet., 143:209, 1976.
84. Imrie, C. W., et al.: A single-center double trial of trasylol therapy in primary acute pancreatitis. Br. J. Surg., 65:337, 1978.
85. McMahon, M. J., Playforth, M. J., Pickford, I. R.: A comparative study of methods for the prediction of severity of attacks of acute pancreatitis. Br. J. Surg., 67:22, 1980.

86. McMurray, S. D., et al.: Prevailing patterns and predictor variables in patients with acute tubular necrosis. Arch. Intern. Med., *138*:950, 1978.
87. Rasmussen, H. H., and Ibels, L. S.: Acute renal failure. Multivariate analysis of causes and risk factors. Am. J. Med., *73:*211, 1982.
88. Rasmussen, H. H., et al.: Prediction of outcome in acute renal failure by discriminate analysis of clinical variables. Arch. Intern. Med., *145:*2015, 1985.
89. Cioffi, W. G., Ashikaga, T., Gamelli, R. L.: Probability of surviving postoperative acute renal failure. Development of a prognostic index. Ann. Surg., *200:*205, 1984.
90. Najman, J. M., and Levine, S.: Evaluating the impact of medical care and technologies on the quality of life: A review and critique. Soc. Sci. Med., *15:*107, 1981.
91. Hollandsworth, Jr., J. G.: Evaluating the impact of medical treatment on the quality of life; a five year update. Soc. Sci. Med., *26:*425, 1988.
92. Zaren, B., and Hedstrand, U.: Quality of life among long-term survivors of intensive care. Crit. Care Med., *15:*743, 1987.
93. Sage, W. M., Rosenthal, M. H., Silverman, J. F.: Is intensive care worth it? An assessment of input and outcome for the critically ill. Crit. Care Med., *14:*777, 1986.
94. Katz, S., et al.: Studies of illness in the aged. The index of ADL: A standardized measure of biological and psychosocial function. JAMA, *185:*914, 1963.
95. Lawton, M. P., and Brody, E. M.: Assessment of older people: Self-maintaining and instrumental activities of daily living. Gerontologist, *9:*179, 1969.
96. Karnofksy, D. A., et al.: The use of the nitrogen mustards in the palliative treatment of carcinoma. Cancer, *1:*634, 1948.
97. Mor, V., et al.: The Karnofsky performance status scale. An examination of its reliability and validity in a research setting. Cancer, *53:*2002, 1984.
98. Announcement: Health-related quality of life: The European Group for the Nottingham Health Profile. JAMA, *263:*1132, 1990.
99. Hunt, S. M., McEwen, J., McKenna, S. P.: Perceived health, age and sex comparisons in community. J. Epidemiol. Comm. Health, *38:*156, 1984.
100. O'Brien, B. J., Buxton, M. J., Ferguson, B. A.: Measuring the effectiveness of heart transplant programs: Quality of life data and their relationship to survival analysis. J. Chron. Dis., *40:*(Suppl. 1):137s, 1987.
101. O'Brien, B. J., et al.: The Nottingham health profile as a measure of quality of life following combined heart and lung transplantation. J. Epidemiol. Comm. Health, *42:*232, 1988.
102. Rubenstein, L. V., et al.: Improving patient function: A randomized trial of functional disability screening. Ann. Intern. Med., *111:*836, 1989.
103. Jette, A. M., et al.: The functional status questionnaire: Reliability and validity when used in primary care. J. Gen. Intern. Med., *1:*143, 1986.
104. Torrance, G. W., and Feeny, D.: Utilities and quality-adjusted life years. Int. J. Tech. Assess. Health Care, *5:*559, 1989.
105. Mosteller, F., and Falotico-Taylor, J. (Eds.): Quality of Life and Technology Assessment. Monograph of the Council on Health Care Technology. Washington, National Academy Press, 1989.

Chapter 80

COMPUTERIZED PATIENT MANAGEMENT SYSTEMS FOR THE INTENSIVE CARE UNIT

JOEL S. GOCHBERG
EDWARD D. SIVAK

The acquisition of knowledge and the advancement of technology have proceeded at a furious pace in many disciplines in the last 20 years, with medicine being no different than any other service-related activity. The modern ICU has become a place where a tremendous amount of data must be assimilated, managed, and acted on. In parallel to this information explosion, a new generation of clinical information systems (CIS) has emerged that promises to control the information overload. As one looks to the future, the perspective that the ICU represents a concert of activities interdependent on ancillary resources in the entire hospital should be emphasized. In similar fashion, the computerized patient management system in the ICU represents only one component of an entire hospital information system (HIS). Just as the ICU requires teamwork from the entire hospital staff, the ICU information system requires the access to the entire HIS. It cannot stand alone and function efficiently. The following case summary represents a scenario that can develop in the computerized ICU.

Case Summary. A 73-year-old woman has enjoyed good health except for minor problems with degenerative joint disease of her knees until 10 months before the present admission. She presents to the emergency room complaining of fever and chills with vital signs as follows: pulse, 110; blood pressure (BP), 110/70; respiratory rate (RR), 22; and temperature 38.2°C. Additional history reveals that she has had a previous hospitalization for gastrointestinal bleeding. She is not sure of the details but states that her deteriorating health started with that admission. A review of systems reveals that she has had urinary frequency and dysuria for approximately 10 days. Physical examination is unremarkable except for the vital signs listed. A urine culture, complete blood count (CBC), and serum electrolytes studies are obtained. The results will be sent to her family physician. (His address is listed in the HIS.) She is given a prescription for trimethoprim/sulfamethoxazole and instructed to take the medication twice daily and drink extra fluids. Four days later, she is brought to the emergency room by a daughter who was not aware of the details of the last emergency room visit. No other history is available. The vital signs are pulse, 122; BP, 95/60; RR, 29; temperature 39.0°C. The emergency room physician retrieves the following information from the HIS:

- Attending physician and phone number
- Laboratory data from emergency room visit of 4 days ago: urine culture positive for enterococcus group D; white blood count (WBC), 13500; blood urea nitrogen (BUN), 28; and creatinine, 1.7
- Uniform hospital discharge abstracts from two previous hospitalizations within the past year: 10 months prior—upper gastrointestinal tract bleeding secondary to nonsteroidal anti-inflammatory medications, degenerative joint disease of both knees, urinary tract infection; 4 months prior—urinary retention, urinary tract infection. An intravenous pyelogram done at that time revealed a small left kidney

Intravenous fluids are started, and broad-spectrum antibiotics are started. Because of her altered mental status, she is admitted to the ICU for further observation. The bedside nurse reviews orders on the bedside computer, which indicates that the first doses of antibiotics were given in the emergency room and that among the usual ICU care guidelines are additional orders for the following:

- Intravenous fluids: D5W/normal saline (NS) at 150 ml/hour
- Dopamine infusion 250 mg in 500 ml of NS—start @ 3 µg/kg/min—titrate to systolic BP of 100 mm Hg
- Vital signs every 30 minutes

Over the next 6 hours, urine output remains low, vital signs remain altered (pulse, 130; BP, 90/60; RR, 38; temperature 39.5°C). Pulse oximetry has been monitored (initial saturation was 97% on oxygen at 3 L/min by nasal cannula). A review of the trends on the bedside computer reveal:

- Urine volume less than 30 ml/hour for the last 2 hours
- Upward trend in RR, downward trend in BP, and increasing requirements for dopamine to 12 µg/kg/min
- Downward trend in pulse oximetry from 94 to 84% in the last 30 minutes
- Automatic calculation of the severity of illness score reveals that the initial predicted risk of hospital death has risen from 15 to 65%

A diagnosis of septic shock is made, and because of persistent hypoxemia and tachypnea, the patient is intubated and started on mechanical ventilation. A flow-directed catheter and arterial line are placed to facilitate hemodynamic monitoring. Over the next 24 hours, the CIS is used for the following:

- Automatic retrieval of data from bedside monitor of heart rate, BP, pulmonary artery pressure every 30 minutes
- Calculations of infusion rates of dopamine and dobutamine
- Automatic recording of pulse oximetry every 15 minutes
- Automatic sampling of ventilator setting and parameters every hour (respiratory therapist verifies data at time of sampling)
- Calculation of fluid balance each shift from the nurse's recording of initial starting volumes of infusions and end of shift volumes remaining
- Automatic calculations of hemodynamic indices, including oxygen extraction ratio, oxygen consumption with each measurement of cardiac output, and arterial and mixed venous blood gases (blood gas values are returned to bedside computer automatically via HIS)
- Patient assessments recorded by the bedside nurse each shift (included are automatic calculations of the Glasgow Coma Score)
- Infusion changes recorded
- Laboratory data automatically sent back to the bedside computer

Over the next day, the patient's hemodynamic and respiratory status have improved. The bedside computer facilitates retrieval of the following information:

- Trend displays of improving hourly urine volume, increasing cardiac output, decreasing requirements for dopamine, increasing oxygen consumption
- A positive fluid balance of 4 L
- Downward trend in fever; a fall in WBC to 14,400
- An improving Glasgow Coma Score

Additional laboratory information shown as an alert on the computer screen reveals that the urine and blood cultures are positive for enterococcus species. The initial antibiotics started were gentamicin and ampicillin. The gentamicin levels for peak and trough values are 3.5 and less than 2.0. The antibiotic dosing calculator that is operating on the bedside computer suggests that the dose of gentamicin be increased to 55 mg every 8 hours.

By the fourth hospital day, the patient is awake and has no requirements for vasoactive agents, and the requirements for supplemental oxygen have been lowered to 35%. Hospital risk of death has fallen to 3%. Spontaneous RR is 18 per minute, vital capacity 900 ml, and spontaneous minute ventilation 12 L/min. The patient is placed on a pressure support of 7 cm H_2O. The bedside computer is set to sample minute ventilation, RR, and tidal volume. Over the next 2 hours, the ratio of the RR to the average tidal volume each minute remains less than 70. Pulse oximetry remains above 98%. Based on these observations, the patient is extubated and placed on a 40% ventimask.

Ultimately the patient is discharged from the hospital to home on the 12th hospital day. Additional administrative information reveals that the patient was discharged 2 days earlier than the national hospital average for the patient's physiology and predicted risk of death as determined by the APACHE III workstation connected to the CIS. The days of mechanical ventilation; days of hemodynamic monitoring; antibiotic utilization; and days of ICU care, hospital care, and pre-ICU and post-ICU days of care are also calculated. Therapeutic Intervention Scoring System (TISS) points are calculated automatically and passed to the hospital finance database to build information to link acuity and therapeutic intervention to cost of care.

This case is meant to illustrate the clinical as well as the administrative benefits of a computerized information system for the ICU.

Central to the issue of a computerized patient care management system (or a CIS) for the ICU is definition of links of the ICU to the entire operation of a modern hospital. From a clinical viewpoint, it represents an area in which patients with real or potential alterations in mental status, hemodynamic status, or respiratory status are admitted for monitoring and life support until these physiologic embarrassments are corrected. From an administrative viewpoint, the ICU represents a support service for an emergency room and surgical and medical services. Recognizing that such a support service requires vast amounts of data for clinical and administrative decision making, advancement into the 21st century will require efficient management of data.[1] It is only logical that computerization of the ICU is the responsibility of the entire hospital staff rather than the ICU staff by itself. To this end, the patient care management system for the ICU can be discussed in the form of the three components of critical illness: pre-ICU, ICU, and post-ICU considerations.

Pre-ICU considerations are administrative and include hospital information management strategy, executive commitment to clinical computerization of the ICU as well as the hospital, the existence of a mature information system within the hospital, and adequate administrative and clinical personnel for successful development and implementation of a system. ICU considerations are clinical as well as administrative and include equipment, the physical plant, the selection of a vendor, a development and implementation team, and definition of tasks of patient care. Post-ICU considerations become more administrative in nature and center around data abstraction and organization, quality assessment, quantitation of severity of illness, and utilization of data for outcomes research. This entire perspective is outlined in Table 80–1.

PRE-ICU CONSIDERATIONS

The usual route to computerization of an ICU is through the patient caregivers to hospital executives. The former group is only too aware of the excessive burden of data acquisition and recording in the flow sheet at the patient bedside. These individuals also must convince hospital administrators that computerization may ease their burdens. Unfortunately, such efforts are impeded by the fact that HIS have traditionally centered around the financial office

Table 80-1. Clinical and Administrative Considerations in Computerization of the ICU

Pre-ICU Considerations	ICU Considerations	Post-ICU Considerations
Hospital information strategy Executive commitment Maturity of hospital information system Adequate administrative and clinical personnel	Microprocessor-based equipment ICU physical plant Vendor selection Development and implementation team Definition of tasks of patient care	Data storage, transmission, and abstraction Quality assessment Severity of illness and outcome prediction Utilization review Quantitation of resources Outcome research

and materials handling.[1] The focus has usually been on charge capture. Thus, patient care teams are at a disadvantage if they request CIS to be added on to existing information systems. The focus of payment for hospital services being based on diagnosis related groups (DRGs) for reimbursement rather than charges may, however, become an advantage for the caregiver.[2] The emphasis is now on quality demonstrated by data derived from the clinical record.[3] From an administrative standpoint, either more personnel are employed to derive data from the medical record, or information systems are created to make administrative data a byproduct of patient care. Nonetheless, caregivers are still faced with the burden of providing cost justification for computerization of the ICU. Table 80-2 summarizes such cost justification.[4]

Information Services Policy

The modern-day hospital cannot function without some components of computerization. The most essential component of an HIS remains the admission/discharge and transfer utility. All patients who receive any service, regardless of whether it is merely a chest film or coronary artery bypass surgery, are assigned hospital numbers that are attached to any service, supplies, or queries about laboratory tests. It is through such identifying numbers that patients and services are tracked throughout the hospital. By the same token, large-volume services, such as radiology, electrocardiogram (ECG), laboratory, operating room scheduling, and admissions and discharges, are activities that are usually computerized. If a hospital's information services policy is merely to keep track of these activities administratively and ignore requirements to make computerized data retrieval available to all its caregivers, clinical application of the data becomes cumbersome. Information is only available through hard copy printout on the patient chart or by telephone conversation. Conversely, if policy dictates that clinicians must have data available in an easily retrievable fashion on computer terminals distributed throughout the hospital, the proper strategy may exist for computerization of the ICU. For ICU systems to be successful, there must be a strategy in place to permit transfer of patient demographics, laboratory data, and radiology reports. Table 80-3 summarizes the flow of data required for admission to a hospital.

Other provisions for order entry are also helpful. Electronic links from information systems within the laboratory, radiology department, pharmacy, and admission office must be made to the ICU system so it becomes an integrated component of the entire HIS. More discussion follows on this point under ICU considerations. As HIS mature, hardware and software must permit such links so ICU systems do not stand alone. Hospital executives must also realize that data derived from bedside monitors, cardiac output computers, ventilators, oximeters, infusion pumps, and other bedside devices are so abundant that it

Table 80-2. Cost-Justification of Commercial ICU Computer Systems

Category Data	Impact of Computer Systems	Documented Effects
Staffing	Reduced charting time	Reduced FTEs
Personnel retention	Reduced documentation burden	Increased nursing satisfaction Lower turnover Less training costs
Record management	Complete, detailed, and legible record that is easily searched	Less time spent on QA Better risk management Better insurance audits (fewer lost charges) More complete billing information DRG management Automated assignment of diagnosis
Supply and resource waste	Elimination of paper record and reduction in errors in medication calculations and duplication of laboratory test orders	Less cost for paper forms Less wasted medication Fewer duplicate laboratory tests
Improved quality of care	Better-quality charts Automated data entry Automated calculations Extensive error checking	Impact on length of stay Questionable outcome Questionable morbidity Questionable quality of care

FTE, Full-time equivalents (i.e., staff positions); QA, quality assurance; DRG, diagnosis-related groups.
(From East, T. D.: Computers in the ICU: panacea or plague? Respir. Care, *37*:170, 1992.)

Table 80-3. The Flow of Data Required for Admission to an ICU

Data elements authorize a patient to receive care
   A patient has an assigned identity within a community
     (Name, social security number, date of birth, gender)
     (Address, employer, health insurance policy number)
     (Admitting physician)
   The patient becomes a customer within the hosptial on admission
   Verification of identity required for delivery of care
     (Laboratory studies, x-ray, medication, administration)
Verification allows for new data files to be created
   Information is created in multiple databases
     (Laboratory studies, x-ray files, clinical narrative)
The patient record becomes a depository for information required for decision making
   Decisions include medications, surgical procedures, patient care plans, monitoring frequency, patient orders
     (All decisions are authorized by the attending physician based on the clinical needs of the patient)
The medical record becomes a depository for documentation of outcome of decisions, therapy, and quality of outcome
   The medical record is abstracted for clinical as well as administrative documentation
     (ICD-9-CM coding, DRG classification, UHDA, billing, utilization uniform clinical data sets [UCDS], QA, marketing, education, research)

is impossible to collect all of it on a central host computer. ICU data are frequently editorialized before final recording to ensure accuracy and elimination of artifact. Thus, information services policy must make provisions for distributed processing of data within the ICU. An information services policy that dictates that all processing of data must be done on a mainframe computer precludes successful computerization of the ICU.[5] Finally, the strategy must include benefits on nursing, physician, and administrative levels, as summarized in Table 80-4.

Executive Commitment to Computerization of the ICU

Financially speaking, there are two budgets—capital and operational—to consider when computerizing the ICU. Each requires executive sponsorship. The capital budget is used to purchase equipment and is usually derived from funds obtained by external means, such as contributions, grants, sale of bonds, excess funds from previous operations, and so forth. Operational funds must be derived from yearly cash flow derived from patient services. Table 80-5 summarizes capital and operational considerations for computerization of the ICU. Funding of both components is necessary for success and thus requires executive commitment of funds. Additional commitment is required when the ICU system is completed to define a time when changeover from the traditional handwritten record to the computerized record must take place. Finally, after successful implementation, further commitment is necessary for maintenance of the unit's information system.

Hospital Information System

Although it is possible to operate a CIS in a stand-alone fashion, an ICU system yields substantially greater benefits if it is integrated with other information systems within the hospital. The characteristics of the HIS are listed in Table 80-6. In particular, the admitting/discharge/transfer (ADT) system and laboratory information system should exist within a hospital before any consideration is given to computerizing the ICU. Data from each of the components of a HIS are required for the ICU system. Patient demographics—name, age, sex, hospital number, bed space location—are necessary for any patient to receive hospital services. The assignment of this information is made on admission to the hospital. In similar fashion, for an ICU information system to begin to acquire from bedside monitors or ventilators automatically or for electronically generated flow sheets to receive laboratory data, an electronic file to receive this data must be made within the ICU CIS. The assignment of demographics to the ICU system from the HIS triggers the ICU system to create this file (see Table 80-3). Conversely, to assign the demograph-

Table 80-4. Benefits to Various Organizational Levels

Level	Benefit	Definition
Nursing	Time saving	Reduction in repetitive tasks
		Automatic calculation
		Automatic acuity assessment
		Bedside acquisition of data
	Charting time	No duplication of information
		Charting by exception
	Data retrieval	Multiuser access to data
	Consistency	Standardization of formats, assessments, data entry
	Legibility (accuracy)	Handwriting is not a factor
		Calculations are automatic and performed routinely
	Safety	Patient alerts for allergies, drug interaction
	Orientation	Features that improve charting consistency decrease time for orientation of new nurses
Physician	Data access	Multiple terminals in unit and in remote locations
	Review of data	Graphic and tabular display (individually customized)
	Timeliness	Chart is always updated. No requriement for data to be filled in later
Administrator	Charge capture	Point of care charting documents utilization of supplies
	Less overtime	Reduced charting time and calculation time
	Liability	Legibility, completeness, consistency, accuracy reduce issues of uncharted data
	Retention	Facilitated charting tasks decrease time in the less attractive duties of nursing
	Image	Recruitment and marketing tool

Table 80-5. Capital and Operational Considerations in Computerization of the ICU

Capital Expenditures	Operational Expenditures
Microprocessor-based equipment (monitors, ventilators, oximeters)	Wages for development team's time
Modifications to physical resources of the ICU	Wages for clinical personnel during training and implementation
Placement of cables for beside devices	Programming of hospital information system for ICU system interface
Physical connections to hospital information system	Wages for biomedical engineering time for physical connections of bedside equipment
Bedside microcomputers, terminals	System maintenance after installation
Printers for the ICU	Wages for ongoing training for new unit personnel
Network interface cards for bedside monitors	Paper and printer maintenance
Additional interface cards for digital outputs from bedside devices such as ventilators	

ics to the system by manually entering the information into a bedside computer system is an excess burden to the caregiver and almost guarantees failure. Without automatic retrieval of laboratory data, caregivers, particularly physicians, will find the system of limited usefulness, severely inhibiting the acceptance of it into everyday practice.

As clinicians assimilate the ICU information system into everyday practice, interfaces to other systems' databases enhance the value not only of the ICU information system, but also other systems. Such systems include the pharmacy information system, radiology, order entry, and financial systems. To this end, connections must exist to permit interfaces from systems outside of the ICU to the ICU system itself. Sufficient computer processing power must be available to transmit data on a real-time basis and to permit real-time inquiries to non-ICU computer databases.

Administrative and Clinical Personnel

The importance of strategic planning has already been outlined. Following executive decisions to proceed with computerization of ICUs, the definition of resources required to accomplish the task must be made. The importance of an existing HIS has been emphasized. In addition to physical resources, such as bedside computers and hardwire for computer links, human resources are essential for development, implementation, and operation.

Information Services Personnel

Just as interfaces are required between HIS computers and the ICU information system, personnel from a hospi-

Table 80-6. Components of a Hospital Information System

Core
   (Registration—ADTR, order entry, results reporting)
Business and financial
   (Accounts receivable/payable, payroll)
Medical documentation
   (Medical record, quality assurance, utilization review, infection control, nursing, discharge planning)
Department management
   (Pathology, radiology, pharmacy, laboratory, anesthesia)
Medical support
   (Treatment protocols, pharmacokinetic dosing)
Communications/networking
   (Connecting all of the above components)

(Adapted from Friedman, B. A., and Martin, J. B.: Hospital information systems. The physician's role. JAMA, *257*:1792, 1987.)

tal's information services department may serve as liaison between patient caregivers and the vendor who will supply the system to the ICU. These individuals are the human component of the interface between systems. During development, they must familiarize themselves with the HIS operating system as well as the operating system of the ICU system. Schedules for development and definition of goals along the way to completion are in part the responsibility of the information services department. Its representatives must assist the vendor in creating interfaces to other components of the HIS and to educate the clinical development team about the potential usefulness and limitations of computerization. When the system is fully operational, information services personnel are responsible for maintenance and upgrading of the system.

Clinical Personnel

The actual definition of the computerized utilities within the ICU information system remains the responsibility of the caregivers themselves. Vendors' representatives and information services personnel are responsible only for helping caregivers translate the tasks of patient care into computerized utilities to facilitate the tasks of patient care. The development team must be afforded ample opportunity to discuss the goals of computerization, to learn about the tools of computerization, and to define formats for computer screens and logic of flow sheets. The team should never approach the system as one that will gather data for which they have needs. On the contrary, because the information system is to emulate the tasks of patient data collection and organization, the caregivers should define the tasks of patient care. The logic for design and development is outlined in Table 80-7.

Vendor Representatives

When a hospital makes a commitment to purchase an information system from a vendor, two levels of responsibility should be defined. The vendor's first responsibility to information services is to define necessary protocols for interface into the HIS to facilitate transfer of demographic data and laboratory data. Additional information should be furnished on the ICU system's operating system, database management system, and application software (terminology explained subsequently). The CIS overhead in terms of processing power required from mainframe computers, maintenance, and expandability should be outlined. Existing ICU equipment should be inventoried by the vendor

Table 80-7. A Design and Development Theme for Clinical Information Systems

Patient illnesses dictate tasks of patient care
Such tasks generate data
True requirements are for systems that facilitate data capture, organization, analysis, and calculation of data and augmentation of decision making
The data is the byproduct of patient care
End users (caregivers) should define tasks of patient care, which identify data
Methods of data capture, analysis, and so forth follow naturally

(Adapted from Sivak, E. D., Gochberg, J. S., Fronek, R., and Scott, D.: Lessons to be learned from the design, development and implementation of a computerized patient care management system for the intensive care unit. *In* Proceedings of the 11th Annual Symposium on Computer Applications in Medical Care. Washington, D.C., IEEE Press, 1987, p. 614.)

to determine if additional communication utilities to send data from bedside devices are necessary. The vendor should establish discussions with the biomedical engineering department to ensure that proper hardwire connection from bedside devices to the unit's information system can be established.

The second level of responsibility is to the patient caregivers and their representatives on the development team. Commercially available ICU information systems have utilities that permit designing computer screens to accept manually entered data, to display data in tabular or graphic format and to create hard copy printouts of data in a format that emulates the existing written record. For a development team to create these screens and formats, its members must be educated by the vendor's representatives as to how to proceed. For example, patient assessments are usually done by the bedside nurse. Computer screens should be designed to accept the nurse's observations in simplified, rapid fashion. Figure 80-1 represents several data entry screens for the physical examination. The order of screens for the assessments and the data to be entered must be defined by the care team around the logic of the screens. The vendor can educate the caregivers in the logic of the system, but the caregiver must do the actual design and definition of data. Another example is the definition of a menu for selection of respiratory therapy services delivered to a patient. Figure 80-2 represents such a menu. The therapists must define the order of the menu items in the order of the most frequently selected items. On this same theme, for example, the therapist must define the order of ventilator data elements to be displayed on a computer screen as shown on the list in Figure 80-3. Figure 80-4 is an example of a defined flow sheet.

Thus the administrative responsibility of the vendor is to HIS personnel, and the clinical responsibility is to the patient care team. The vendor must educate the caregivers in the development process, and the caregivers must educate the vendor in the methods of care delivered to their critically ill patients as defined by their practice patterns. Table 80-8 further summarizes vendor responsibilities to clients.

ICU CONSIDERATIONS

The focus of computerization begins to change to a clinical orientation as one moves from preliminary discussions handled on an administrative level to the actual project. Broadly speaking, the key issues to be considered are:

- Equipment inventory
- The unit's physical plant
- Vendor selection
- Selection of a development and implementation team
- Definition of the tasks of patient care

Equipment Inventory

The benefits of computerization of the ICU have been outlined in Table 80-4. For the bedside caregiver, automatic acquisition of data from bedside devices reduces the administrative burden of writing analog and digital data into a flow sheet. Essential to this data acquisition is the appropriate bedside equipment capable of delivering electronic signals to the computerized system. Bedside devices must be capable of delivering these signals in appropriate communications protocols for the CIS to record them into its database management system. On initial inspection of many devices, such as ventilators and monitors, communication ports are readily visible. In reality, many require the placement of additional interface cards within their enclosures to permit the CIS to acquire data from the device. Appropriate discussion between the system vendor and biomedical engineers should clarify this point. Minimal data acquisition should be from ventilators, bedside hemodynamic monitors, and oximeters. Infusion pumps and urometers provide additional information but are not essential to realize the full benefit of computerization. Similarly, for the neurosurgical ICU, intracranial pressure monitors should be interfaced. With respect to interfaces themselves, equipment must be of recent vintage with digital outputs in the form of numbers rather than the analog signals delivered in waveforms.

Unit's Physical Plant

Few ICUs have been designed to accommodate computer terminals, and few new units will be built only because of a need for computerization. For this reason, ingenuity and flexibility are essential for effective ergonomics. Ergonomics essentially means the effective placement of a computer terminal so access is easy, a comfortable placement so the caregiver is able to interface with the system without eye strain or physical discomfort from stooping or bending, and ease of connecting the system to bedside devices and HIS. Besides bedside placement, additional placement of peripheral terminals must permit access to bedside information.

Hardwire connection between the bedside devices (e.g., monitors and ventilators) must be done in such a fashion that long wires that represent safety hazards are eliminated. Bedside computer terminals must have additional connections to file servers and the HIS. Placement of these wires necessitates reviewing unit construction blueprints for avenues and conduits through which they can be strung.

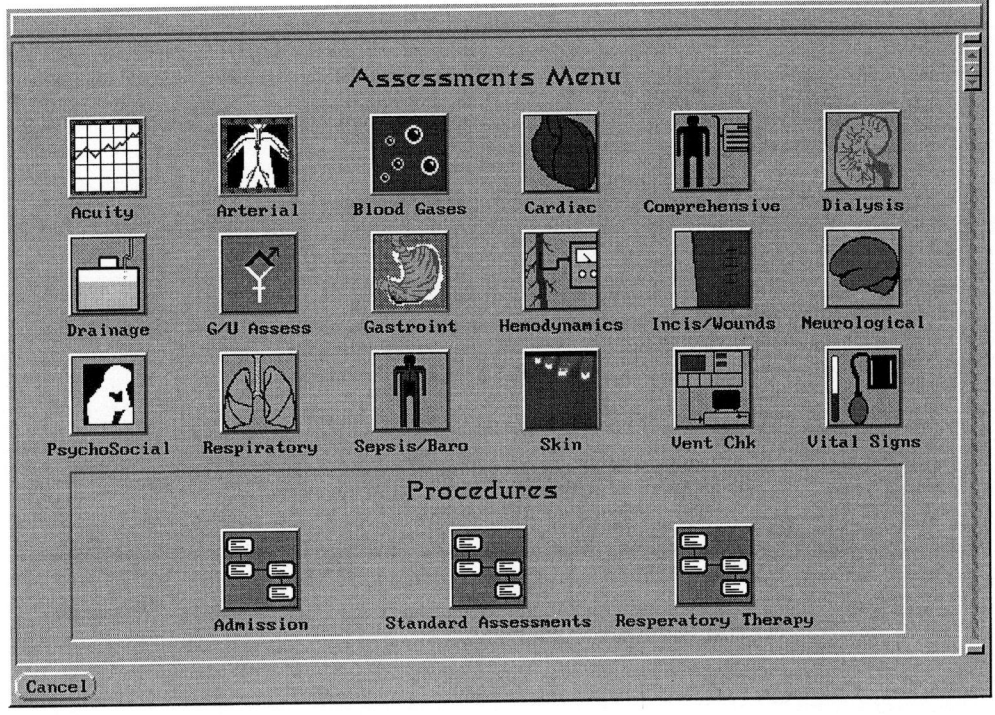

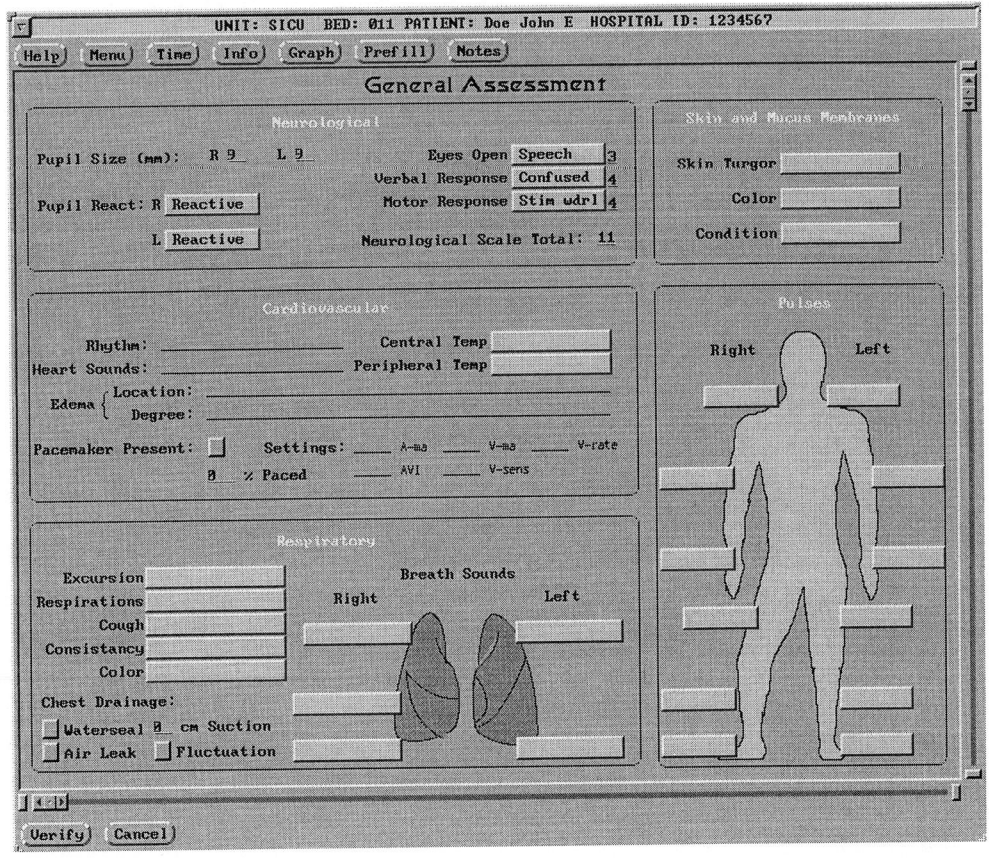

Fig. 80–1. *A*, A computer screen of an assessment menu from CarePoint (Clinical Dimensions, Inc., Madison, WI). An icon is selected via the use of a "mouse" rather than a particular utility being selected from a text menu. One can conceptualize that the user can rapidly select an item by visual inspection of the icons on the menu. This particular screen is customized to make selections to document administrative utilities, such as activity, as well as clinical utilities, such as laboratory data (arterial blood gases), bedside device data (hemodynamic monitors, ventilators), and for input of various clinical observations (gastrointestinal, neurologic, psychosocial). *B*, A customized general assessment screen for data input. Each of the highlighted areas for data contains a user text menu to prompt the user in using uniform terminology for assessments. Neurologic assessment has already been filled in with terminology compatible with the Glasgow Coma Scale. (Courtesy of George Morrison, Clinical Dimensions, Inc., Madison, WI.)

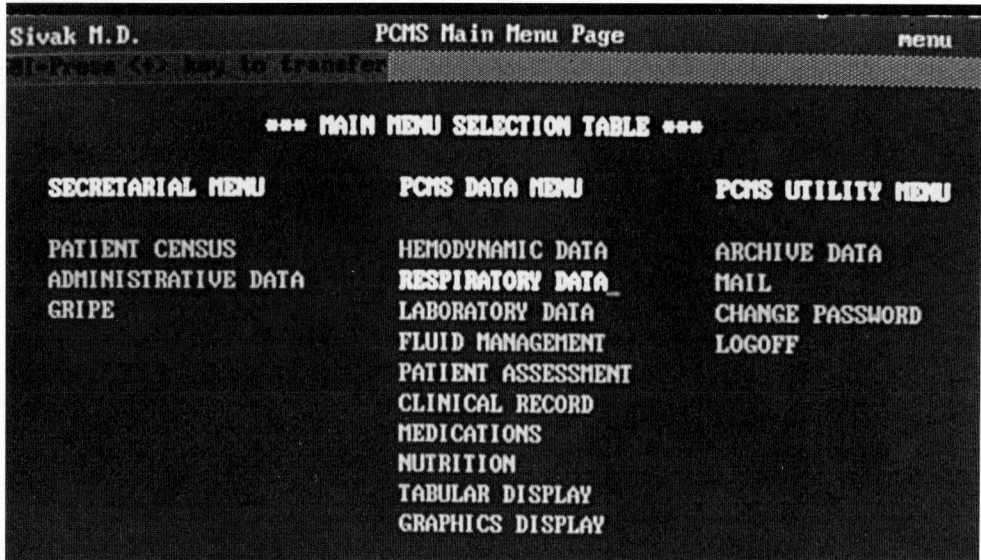

Fig. 80-2. A text menu from a prototype patient care management system (PCMS). Note the arbitrary breakdown of secretarial menu on the left, clinical utilities in the center, and utility menu on the right. One can conceptualize that it is easier to select icons from the menu in Figure 80-1 than to read items from the menu in this figure.

Clinical Information System Architecture

Commercially available systems presently come in two basic arrangements: central and distributed architecture. Central architecture features a central minicomputer with one or more terminals attached to it. Data from the monitoring system and other bedside devices is fed directly into the central host computer (Fig. 80-5). Distributed architecture is the most prevalent and has certain advantages over the centralized architecture, not the least of which is greater fault tolerance and higher performance. High performance microcomputers (Workstations) are placed at bedsides and central locations as the need dictates (Fig. 80-6). The various workstations are interconnected by a local area network. The characteristics of each type of architecture are summarized in Table 80-9. Databases within these systems have a similar configuration as shown in Figure 80-7.

Vendor Selection

There are no specific rules for selection of a vendor to supply a computerized information system to an ICU. The key individual members in the selection process are HIS executive; a designated attending physician with a keen interest in the use of computers, a nurse with a similar interest and who has the ability to build a consensus for computerization of the ICU, a respiratory therapist, and an executive representing nursing services. It is assumed that these individuals have leadership ability and talent for consensus building. These individuals should study their hospital's information services policies and determine if the conditions for pre-ICU considerations can be met. Next, a checklist should be assembled that contains questions along the following lines:

- Can the vendor make suitable interfaces between its system and the HIS? (Is two-way communication possible?)
- Can HIS personnel learn to support the system installation? (Is the software totally proprietary?)
- Do application programs permit flexibility in user interface design and input devices?
- Can existing bedside monitors and ventilators provide digital output signals for automatic data acquisition? (Will additional purchases of more contemporary bedside devices be necessary?)
- Is the database management system organized to permit easy retrieval and display of data (tabular, print and graphics display)?
- Can data be exported to other media, such as a commercially available spread sheet (e.g., Lotus 123, Excel)?
- Can executive reports be created? (See post-ICU considerations.)
- Can the system be expanded for additional interfaces to new bedside equipment, additional storage, and protocol-driven decision support systems? (Does a protocol engine exist to permit protocol development and implementation? Can user interactive decision support systems be created?)

Useful Terminology

The previous checklist contains terminology with which the decision makers should be familiar. Briefly, computers are controlled by an **operating system,** which is one or more software programs that manage the various resources that the computer offers. Taking advantage of the services of the operating system is usually a **database management system (DBMS),** which is designed to facilitate the easy storage and rapid retrieval of information. **Application programs** request services from the operation system and the DBMS to fulfill their function to the caregiver using the program (Fig. 80-8). Some additional characteristics and requirements for ICU systems are listed in Table 80-10.

User Interface

The means by which a caregiver (or any user of any computer program) interacts with the computer programs

Category	Metaschema Name	Class	Type	Description
vent	analyzeO2percent	ASSESS	I	O2 percent analyzed
vent	apneaalarmrate	ASSESS	I	Breaths per minute rate-apnea alarm
vent	apneainterval	ASSESS	I	Interval between breaths/seconds-apnea alarm
vent	apneapeakflow	ASSESS	I	Peak flow - apnea alarm
vent	apneavt	ASSESS	I	Apnea Vt
vent	cpaplevel	ASSESS	I	CPAP level
vent	cuffpress	ASSESS	I	Cuff pressure
vent	devicerr	ASSESS	I	Machine set breaths per minute
vent	endexpirpress	ASSESS	I	Patient CPAP level end expiratory pressure
vent	expirminutevolume	ASSESS	R	Patient expiratory minute volume total
vent	expirvt	ASSESS	I	Patient expired (tidal volume) Vt
vent	fiO2	ASSESS	I	O2 concentration setting
vent	flowbylevel	ASSESS	I	Flow by level
vent	himinutevolumealarm	ASSESS	R	Upper alarm setting for minute volume limit
vent	hiO2alarm	ASSESS	I	Upper alarm setting for O2
vent	hipressalarm	ASSESS	I	High pressure limit
vent	hirralarm	ASSESS	I	High respiratory rate
vent	ieratio	ASSESS	R	I E ratio
vent	insptime	ASSESS	I	Inspiratory time percent
vent	inspvt	ASSESS	I	Calculated inspiratory tidal volume
vent	loexpirvolume	ASSESS	I	Inspiratory pressure level - pressure control ventilator
vent	loexpirvolumeml	ASSESS	I	Low exhaled volume ml
vent	lominutevolmealarme	ASSESS	R	Lower limit for minute volume alarm setting
vent	loO2alarm	ASSESS	I	Lower limit for O2 alarm setting
vent	lopressalm	ASSESS	I	Low pressure alarm limit
vent	meanairwaypress	ASSESS	R	Mean airway pressure
vent	minutevolume	ASSESS	R	Machine setting minute volume
vent	pausplatpress	ASSESS	I	Pause pressure/plateau pressure
vent	paustimepercent	ASSESS	I	Pause time percent
vent	peakinspflow	ASSESS	I	Peak inspiratory flow
vent	peep	ASSESS	R	Level of PEEP setting
vent	pip	ASSESS	I	Peak inspiratory pressure
vent	presssupportlevel	ASSESS	I	Pressure support level
vent	ptparalyze	ASSESS	B	Patient paralyzed
vent	ptpeep	ASSESS	I	Patient's end expiratory pressure
vent	pulseoxispO2	ASSESS	I	Pulse oximeter SPO2
vent	rr	ASSESS	I	Total breaths per minute - patient
vent	sighmult	ASSESS	I	Sigh multiple
vent	sighrate	ASSESS	I	Sigh rate/breaths per minute
vent	sighvolume	ASSESS	I	Sigh volume
vent	sponexpiremenutevolume	ASSESS	R	Patient's spontaneous expiratory minute volume
vent	sponexpirvt	ASSESS	I	Patient's spontaneous expiratory Vt
vent	ventcircuitchngd	ASSESS	B	Circuit changed
vent	ventcircuittemp	ASSESS	R	Circuit temperature
vent	ventdevicevt	ASSESS	I	(Tidal volume) Vt machine setting
vent	ventmode	ASSESS	C	Mode of the vent being used
vent	ventpresent	ASSESS	B	Vent present
vent	ventratesimv	ASSESS	I	SIMV breaths
vent	ventriggersens	ASSESS	I	Sensitivity
vent	venttype	ASSESS	C	Type of vent being used
vent	ventworkpress	ASSESS	I	Ventilator setting for working pressure

Fig. 80-3. A "metaschema" used in the production of an ICU system. Basically it represents a list of items that might be charged on a respiratory flow sheet. The category pertains to the ventilator (vent). A metaschema name is listed, and the class of data is that of "assessment." Much of the data can be automatically derived from microprocessor-based ventilators. The description of each data element is shown in the right-hand column. (Courtesy of George Morrison, Clinical Dimensions, Inc., Madison, WI.)

1706 THE HIGH RISK PATIENT: MANAGEMENT OF THE CRITICALLY ILL

Ventilator Flowsheet

	04/01 15:00*	04/01 15:26^	04/01 15:36^	04/01 16:00*	04/01 16:10^	04/01 16:18^	04/01 17:00*	04/01 17:23^
TYPE		Servo 90	Servo 90		Servo 90	Servo 90	Servo 90	Servo 90
MODE		Vol Ctr	Vol Ctr		Vol Ctr	Vol Ctr	Vol Ctr	Vol Ctr
InspMinVol		16.0	12.0		9.2	9.2	9.2	9.2
ExpMinVol		15.9	15.9		9.0	9.0	9.0	9.0
SponExMinVol								
InspVt		750	750		625	625	625	625
ExpVt		740	740		611	611	611	611
SponExpVt								
RRMech		25	25		19	19	19	19
SIMVrate								
TotalRR		25	25		20	20	20	20
InspTime%		25	25		25	25	25	25
PauseTime%		5	5		5	5	5	5
PIP		45	45		39	39	39	39
Mean Airway Press		18	18		14	14	14	14
Pause		40	40		33	33	33	33
InsPresLev								
WorkPress		90	90		90	90	90	90
PEEP/CPAP		10	10		10	10	12	12
End Exp Lung Press		12	12		10	10	10	10
DynComp		19	19		18	18	18	18
StatComp		23	23		23	23	23	23
FIO2		65	45		40	50	70	80

A

Fig. 80–4. *A*, A computer screen of a possible version of a ventilator flow sheet. Note that data elements have been selected from the listing in Figure 80–3.

Table 80–8. Vendor Responsibilities to Uses of Clinical Information Systems for the ICU

Recognize individual and regional differences in utilization of data derived from patient care
Select flexible software tools that permit development of utilities that can facilitate patient care and allow user modification
Provide software updates at nominal fees to permit conservation of operating funds
Participate in joint development projects
Create user groups for further enhancement of the system
Define timetables for implementation
Provide training to end users and engineering and informational support personnel

(Adapted from Sivak, E. D., and Gochberg, J. S.: Lessons to be learned from implementation and maintenance of a computerized patient care management system for the ICU. In Proceedings of the 12th Annual Symposium on Computer Applications in Medical Care. Washington, D.C., IEEE Press, 1988, p. 768.)

is through the **user interface.** The user interface is a combination of hardware and software. The user interface is bidirectional. The reader is probably familiar with the two most prevalent user interface hardware components: the CRT display and the computer keyboard. The user types information on the keyboard, as the computer normally echoes the information back on the screen. Certain keystrokes or combinations of keys are meaningful commands to the computer to perform some action. The results of the action are conveyed to the user on the screen. There are a whole range of other types of input and output devices that can be used to construct the hardware portion of the user interface, ranging from the conventional (e.g., mouse or touch screen) to the esoteric (e.g., data glove and artificial reality). The user interface should be simple, friendly, and efficient. Computer screens for data entry should not be excessively crowded with useless information. Keystrokes to access the various components of the CIS should be minimal. Whenever possible, text entry of data should be minimized.

The software components of the user interface usually contain two basic components. The **driver** converts the

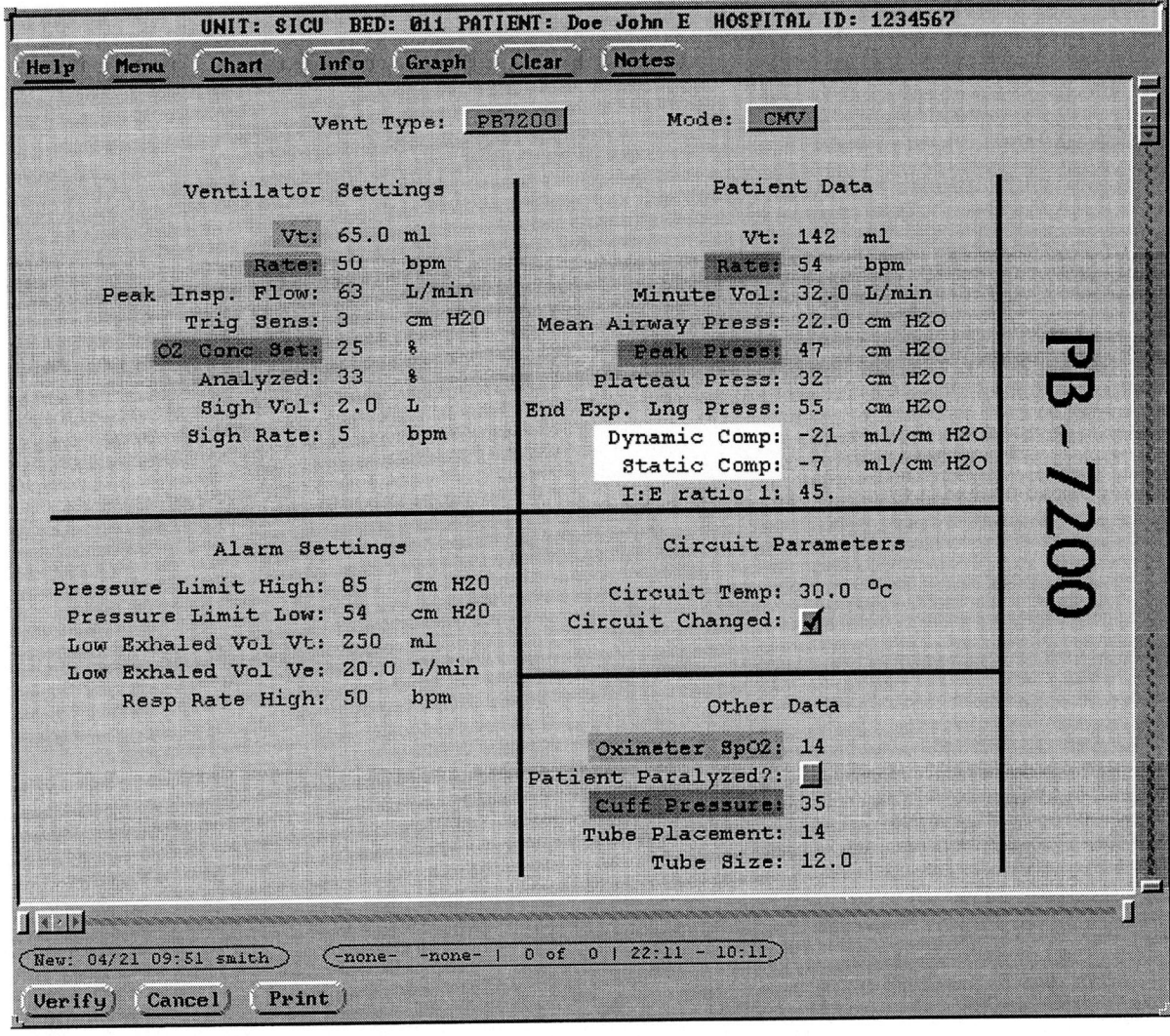

Fig. 80-4. *(Continued) B,* A computer screen used to sample and verify data derived automatically from a ventilator. Ventilator type (Puritan Bennett, 7200) and mode of ventilation (CMV) are shown on the top line. Ventilator settings, patient data, and alarm settings are shown in different sections of the screen. Note at the bottom of the figure the "please wait" prompt. This message appears as the system is commanded to sample ventilator data by the user. Data from the sample and verify screen is sent to the database from where it can be recalled in flow sheet or graphic format.

signals from the input device into a data stream that is fed into a computer **program,** which facilitates an interaction that the user can understand. The program then processes the input and may respond with some output. For example, in systems that are controlled by a mouse, a **cursor** is maintained on the screen. As the mouse is moved, the mouse driver communicates coordinate change information to the cursor, and the cursor is seen to move on the screen in a fashion analogous to the physical movement of the mouse. Commands can be sent to the computer program by pressing the buttons on the mouse.

The look and feel of the application programs can be as varied as the types of input devices. There are systems that are **menu driven** (see Fig. 80-2), and there are those that offer a visual paradigm that is familiar to the clinician; for example, a flow sheet can be drawn on the display screen that is much like, or even identical to, the paper flow sheet of a particular ICU (Figs. 80-1 and 80-9).

Selection of a Development and Implementation Team

The most essential element of the development and implementation is the closeness of fit of the computerized patient care system to the tasks of patient care and the delivery of that care. A CIS in itself is not a solution to the problems of information management but a tool that can be used in solving the problems. For successful implementation to take place, careful attention must be paid to several critical factors, all within a well-defined framework for implementation. Although a detailed discussion of such a framework and critical success factors is beyond the scope of this chapter, there are a few items worthy of discussion—notably institutional support and integration

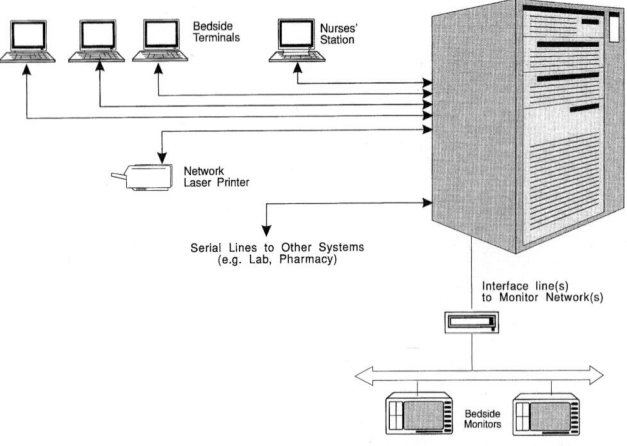

Fig. 80–5. The architecture of a centrally based CIS for the ICU. Note that each bedside terminal has no processing power. All utilities for calculations, data storage, and sampling data from bedside devices exist in the central host computer. (Courtesy of George Morrison, Clinical Dimensions, Inc., Madison, WI.)

Table 80–9. Centralized versus Distributed Architecture

Centralized	Distributed
User outlines requirements	User performs definition
User controls source documents	User manages independent database
User gets training from others	User is responsible for training
All data files are central	User has independent local files
Central report printing	User prints out reports
Priorities set by central unit	User sets priorities
User does not decide data access	User sets privileges for data access
User keys in data	User responsible for data integrity
User is not involved in evaluation	User evaluates system performance
Hardware is usually a large mainframe	Hardware is micro/mini computer
Operating system is complex	Operation and programming possible by user

(Adapted from Ahituv, N., and Neumann, S.: Distributed information systems. *In* Principles of Information Systems for Management. 2nd Ed. Dubuque, IA, Wm. C. Brown Publishers. 1986, p. 328.)

of the CIS within the context of other information systems within a hospital. The development team should contain experienced caregivers from the major disciplines providing patient care. The actual team should consist of:

- Nurses from each nursing shift
- Respiratory therapists
- A dietitian
- A pharmacist
- An information services representative
- A vendor representative
- An executive representative from nursing
- An executive representative from information services
- A physician representative of the attending physicians' groups

Most essential to development and implementation is the commitment of these individuals to computerization of the ICU record. Each individual should be articulate within his or her own discipline to recognize the similari-

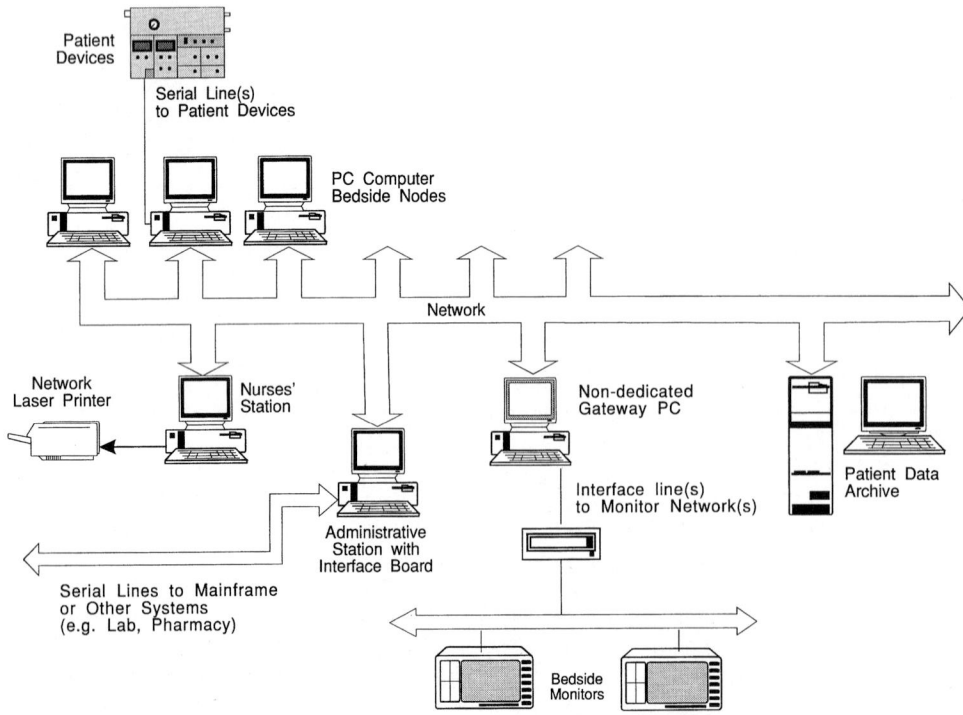

Fig. 80–6. The architecture of a distributed CIS. Each bedside computer contains the utilities for calculations, sampling of data, and the ability to store data locally. In addition, if the bedside processor is "busy" performing certain tasks, such as calculation of data, an idle processor located at another bed space can perform the sampling of data from monitor or ventilator through the network. A typical ICU network contains bedside microprocessors (PC computers); a gateway PC, which provides the physical link to a hemodynamic monitor network; an administrative work station with interface board to the HIS; and some type of storage facility for patient archive data. Bedside devices are connected to bedside nodes through serial ports. (Courtesy of George Morrison, Clinical Dimensions, Inc., Madison, WI.)

PATIENT MANAGEMENT SYSTEMS FOR THE INTENSIVE CARE UNIT

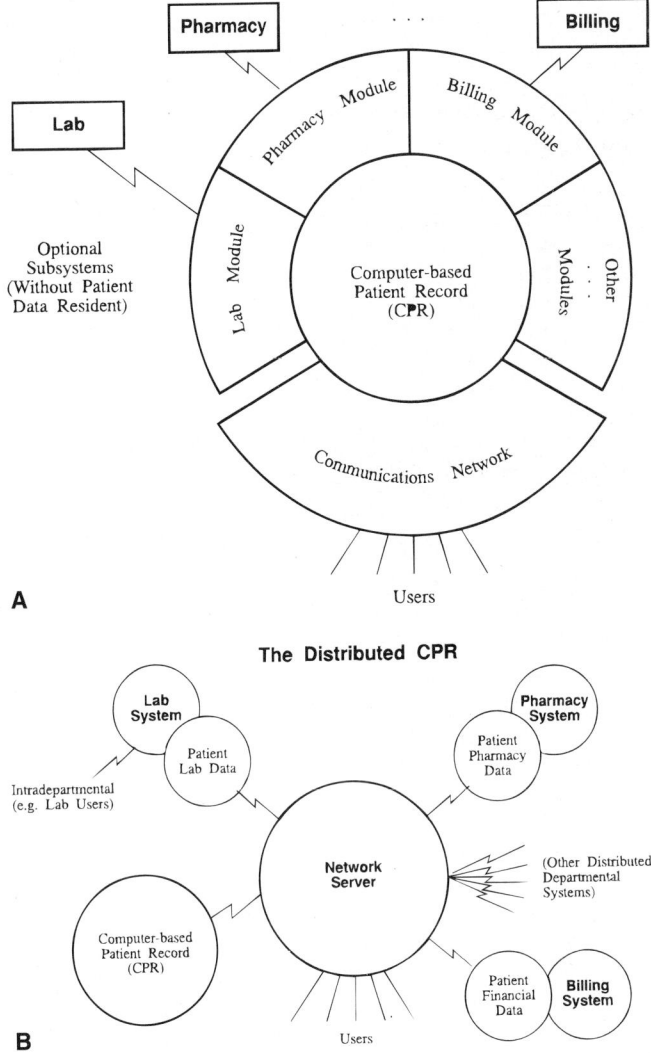

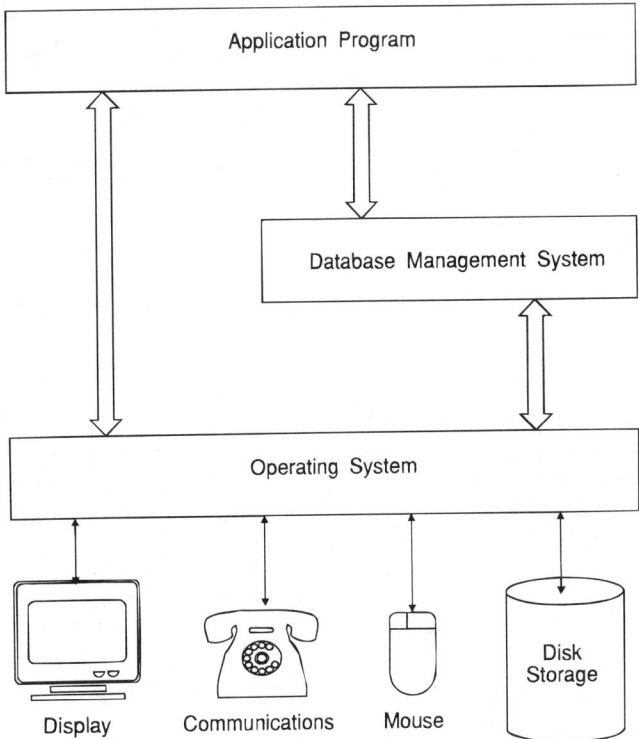

Fig. 80–8. Layers of software for a clinical information system. See text for description. (Courtesy of George Morrison, Clinical Dimensions, Inc., Madison, WI.)

Fig. 80–7. *A,* In the centralized computerized patient record (CPR), all patient data are stored in the central CPR, which is the core of the CPR system. The CPR system may be complete, supporting laboratory and nearly all other departmental functions, or it may receive data from remote distributed department subsystems for purposes of maintaining a complete CPR. *B,* In the distributed CPR, patient data are distributed in departmental systems or subsystems. Consequently the complete CPR does not exist in any one place; rather, portions of the record are distributed among several computer systems. A node on the network might regularly gather data from the distributed computers to present a view of the patient's complete CPR. (From Dick, R. S., and Steen, E. B. (Eds.): The Computer-Based Patient Record: An Essential Technology for Health Care. Washington, D.C., National Academy Press, 1991.)

ties between the written record and the computerized record. Development should focus on a theme that is outlined in Table 80–7. The same individuals responsible for development should also be involved in the implementation process. The principal reason is their familiarity with the logic of the system and its similarities to the existing manually generated record. Each computer screen is designed with a specific reason in mind, whether it be designed to enter data, retrieve data, or calculate data. Mem-

bers of the development team are best suited to pass this logic on to the future users of the system.

Definition of the Tasks of Patient Care

A development theme has been outlined in Table 80–7. It is most important to emphasize that definition of needs for data is an administrative approach to the problem of handling patient data—it is best to assume that data is a byproduct of the tasks of patient care.[7] This being the

Table 80–10. Characteristics and Requirements for Clinical Information Systems for the ICU

Multitasking, multiuser operating system
Operating system must support local area networking
Data security
Fault tolerance
Automatic restarting if bedside computers fail
Database management system must support the sharing of data
Application software must allow manual as well as automatic data entry
Displays possible in textual, tabular, and graphic form
Calculations must be performed automatically
Easy accessibility (bedside rather than central locations)
System must emulate the culture of the ICU (methods of delivery of patient care of the unit)
Hospital information system must be accessible from bedside

(Adapted from Sivak, E. D., and Gochberg, J. S.: Lessons to be learned from implementation and maintenance of a computerized patient care management system for the ICU. *In* Proceedings of the 12th Annual Symposium on Computer Applications in Medical Care. Washington, D.C., IEEE Press, 1988, p. 768.)

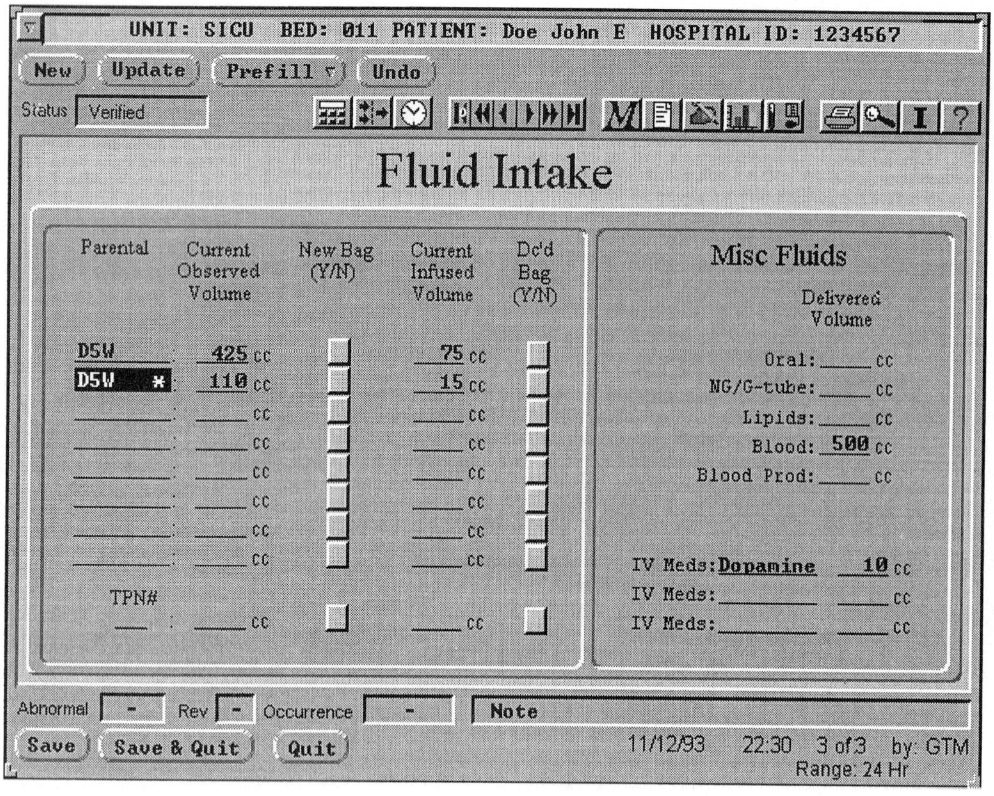

Fig. 80-9. *A*, A fluid intake screen. Note the type of infusion (D-5-W) and the observed volumes in current infusion. The rate of infusion is also listed. In the lower right-hand corner, the date and time are listed. When the caregiver reviews the fluids at the end of a shift or completion of infusion, the volume remaining is observed and recorded. The computer program automatically records the volume infused. Provisions are also made for other types of infusions, such as medications, blood, and total parenteral nutrition.

case, the care of patients should be viewed as an iterative process involving three basic steps:

- Observation
- Interpretation
- Intervention

Documentation activities occur for all three steps, and the process is repeated continuously until the patient is discharged. Although this process description is simplistic (e.g., in the ICU observation occurs continuously), it is useful as a framework to discuss the use of computer systems in the ICU to facilitate management of patients.

Observation

Before the patient is admitted to the ICU, the usual forms of observation are discussions with the patient and family, physical examination, occasional sampling of a few vital signs, laboratory work, and radiologic studies. Response to medication and other therapies are other forms of observation. Objectivity is maintained by using standard values and ranges of normal for vital sign values (temperature, pulse, respiration, BP), laboratory values (e.g., pH, P_{CO_2}, P_{O_2}, Na, K, Cl, HCO_3), the radiologist's interpretation of abnormalities, and so forth. These data become the standard language of communication within the handwritten record in chronologic fashion. Observations made by the bedside caregiver are also recorded. Sampling frequencies for all observations are relatively low in the non-ICU setting with a resultant low volume of data.

Once a patient is admitted to the ICU, sampling frequencies increase greatly, as the bedside nurse is frequently required to follow ICU protocols for higher sampling frequencies for vital signs and observations. The number of data sources also increase greatly owing to the use of bedside monitors, ventilators, oximeters, infusion pumps for vasoactive agents, and other monitoring devices depending on the instability of the patient. Laboratory tests are run more frequently, with the entire process of patient care resulting in large volumes of data. Table 80-11 lists data that is derived from the tasks of patient care.

Interpretation

The process of interpreting the various observational data acquired on the patient is essentially the same regardless of whether the patient is in the ICU or on the general floor. The difference already reviewed is the large volume of data in the ICU. The purpose of the medical record under these circumstances is to organize and display data to facilitate the task of interpretation. Studies of human cognition have shown that the average person can assimilate between four and seven objects in short-term memory at one time. Yet caregivers are routinely expected to deal with hundreds of data elements about a patient simultaneously to arrive at their interpretations. It is at this level that one begins to appreciate that logic of thought process should be the primary rule for data capture and flow sheet development and data display. The well-organized flow sheet helps the caregiver think logically when interpreting data. The addition of graphic display of data provides the

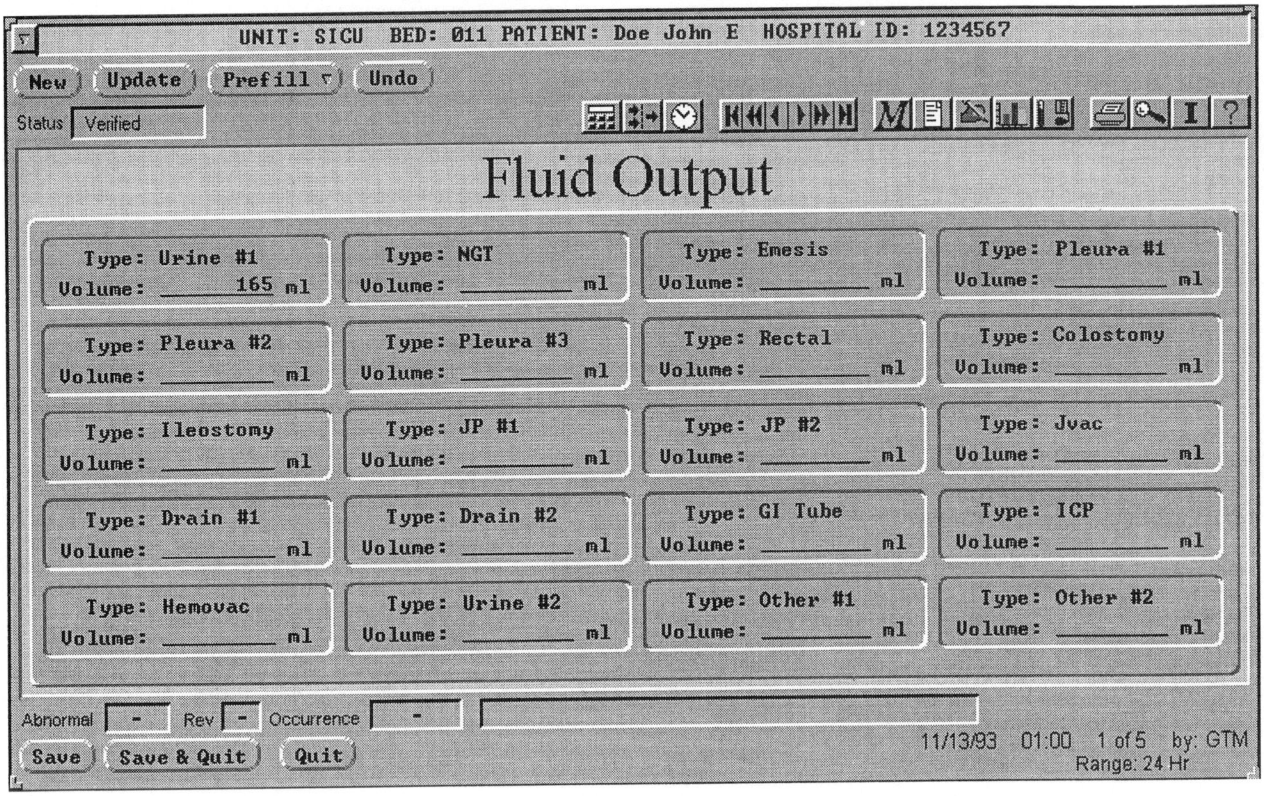

Fig. 80-9. *(Continued) B,* A fluid output screen. Note that provisions are made for output from multiple sites and sources. Volumes are recorded and added to the database according to the time of observation. Quantitation of outputs is transparent to the user because the addition to the database automatically updates totals.

ability to see change over time, particularly when assessing therapeutic intervention. These points are discussed further.

Intervention

Based on the interpretations of the patient data, the clinician may decide to intervene to affect the condition of a patient. The CIS not only acquires data, but also provides tools that facilitate analysis, such as interactive graphics, flowsheets and in some cases automatic processing of medical logic modules.

Translation of the Tasks of Patient Care into an Information System

The translation of the tasks of patient care into a computerized information system for the ICU begins with:

- Reviewing of existing flow sheets (hemodynamic, respiratory, nursing)
- Listing of data recorded on sheets
- Grouping of data elements into categories related to patient care tasks
- Defining computer screens according to tasks
- Defining flow sheet displays (ordering of data for tabular display)
- Defining hard copy printout of flow sheets
- Defining data elements for customized graphic display according to unit practice patterns

A review of existing flow sheets might reveal that vital signs are listed in columns on the left of the sheet, followed by hemodynamic parameters (cardiac output, systemic vascular resistance, pulmonary capillary wedge pressure, and so forth), followed by infusions, followed by fluid balance, and so forth, according to unit practice patterns. Respiratory parameters might follow the hemodynamic values or be placed after fluid balance. The order is not so important as the actual data elements listed on the sheets. A listing of the data gives way to logical groupings of data, which may be automatically retrieved from monitors or ventilators. These groupings lend themselves to specific information about physiology or patient situation. At the same time, they also represent data derived from the tasks of patient care—hemodynamic observation, a change in status based on therapeutic intervention or worsening of physiologic abnormalities, and so forth. These groupings lend themselves to computer screens, which correspond to the acquisition of data documenting the various tasks and observations (See Table 80-12).

Subsequent to identifying data elements and designing computer screens that facilitate the acquisition of data, the ordering of data elements for tabular display on flow sheets begins to give logic to the purpose of the unit's information

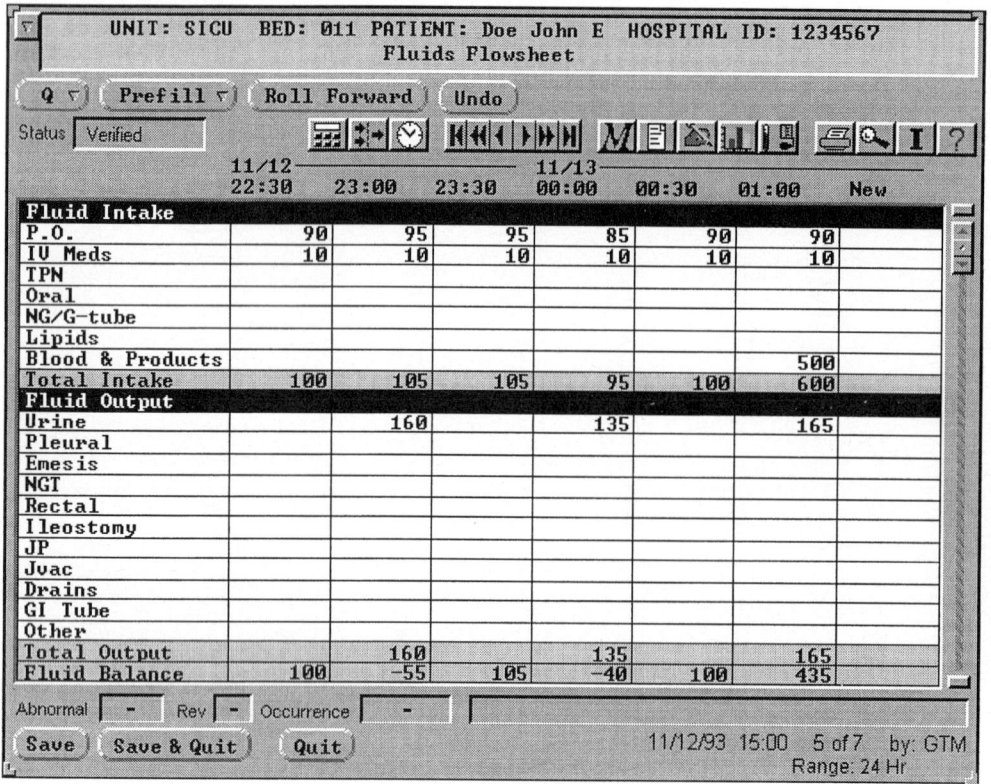

Fig. 80-9. (Continued) C, A flow sheet that derives data from the database, which has been created by the accumulation of data inputted into the system via the caregiver entry through the computer screens shown in parts A and B. Note the cumulative values listed as either positive or negative balance at the bottom of each column. The task of making such calculations is completed by the clinical information system rather than the caregiver. (Courtesy of Clinical Dimensions, Inc., Madison, WI.)

system. These same displays can be adapted to a hard copy printout of data to form the patient record or chart. Finally, from the grouping of data, customized graphic displays of data can be created for trend analysis, decision making about therapeutic intervention, and education purposes. Figure 80-10 illustrates the entire process of design and development of respiratory utilities for Meridia Huron Hospital in Cleveland, Ohio.

Decision Support Systems

Decision support systems come in a variety of packages. They may be transparent to the user and require little interaction during decision making. Simplistically, automatic calculation of data, organization of flow sheets from data entered automatically from monitors or ventilators, or the ability to create graphic displays from the data entered on flow sheets can facilitate tasks of patient care. Ordinarily cardiac index, stroke volume, systemic vascular resistance, and oxygen consumption might not be calculated until there is a free moment in a caregiver's routine or not at all. Therapeutic intervention may be changed based on these calculations in the face of seemingly stable vital signs. The automatic calculation of these values would facilitate the decision to intervene further. A graphic display of spontaneous respiratory rate and tidal volume along with the calculation of the rapid breathing index would facilitate the weaning process in ventilator-dependent patients.[9] The graphic display of data would show trends in a fashion that would allow rapid assimilation of the trend rather than the assimilation of numbers from the flow sheet into a trend. Automatic formation of flow sheets enhances the decision-making process at the bedside by pooling data from multiple databases, which might not ordinarily be accessed because of time constraints or difficulty in obtaining data.

A second type and more complex decision support system requires a higher level of caregiver interaction. Such systems are usually based on protocols for therapeutic intervention. The basic premise for computerized protocols is that the number of data elements required in complex decision making has multiplied to the point where the human mind can no longer comprehend the complexity and interactions of the processes responsible for the observations being made.[10] The HELP system at the LDS Hospital in Salt Lake City, Utah, is the most extensively described decision support system in the United States. User interactive protocols for antibiotic use, nutritional support, and mechanical ventilation for respiratory distress syndrome are available.[11-14] CarePoint (Clinical Dimensions, Inc., Madison, WI) is a commercially available product that possesses protocol capability. Computerized patient care protocols enhance decision making and may improve the quality of patient care through:

- Use of uniform logic in decision making
- Use of a uniform database for decision making
- Equal frequency of monitoring
- Equal intensity of care for all patients[15-16]

Implementation of the System into Use

A CIS affects more people than those who manage and operate an ICU. The manner in which the ICU operates

Table 80–11. Examples of Data Derived from the Tasks of Patient Care

Tasks	Data
Clinical assessment	Provisional/final diagnoses
Physical examination	Documented findings
Patient orders	
Laboratory studies	Hematology, chemistry, microbiology, arterial blood gases
Radiology	Confirmation of diagnosis; new diagnoses; therapeutic assessment
Monitoring	Hemodynamic, respiratory, mental status, therapeutic response, ventilator status
Fluid management	Fluid intake/output (balance)
Nutrition	Amount and type of caloric intake
Medications	Date, time, type, name, dosage
Respiratory management	Ventilator settings, oxygen delivery systems, therapeutic intervention
Nutritional assessment	Caloric intake/nutritional deficiency
Patient care plan	Goals of care/impediments to achievement of the goals
Calculations	Therapeutic response, clinical deterioration
Fluid balance	Trends in hemodynamic and respiratory status
Hemodynamic indices	
Respiratory indices	Trends in electrolytes, glucose, hemoglobin
Nutritional requirements	
Flow sheet generation	Trends in fluid balance, requirements for vasoactive drugs
	Changes in neurologic status if Glasgow Coma Scale is used
Procedures	Indications, patient tolerance to procedure, technique, complications
Quality assurance	Abstraction and documentation of sentinel events

Table 80–12. Examples of Information from Data Derived from the Tasks of Patient Care

Data	Information
Provisional diagnosis	DRG assignment, billing category, complexity, comorbid condition, complications
Final diagnosis	ICD-9-CM assignment
Procedures	Confirmation of diagnosis, therapeutic response, cause of pathophysiologic process, nutritional status, severity of illness
Flow sheet	Therapeutic response, clinical deterioration, severity of illness (APACHE II and III, SAPS, MPM when combined with laboratory data), requirements for fluids
Goals of care	Utilization of resources, quality of care, background for ethical decision making in limiting therapeutic intervention
Medication documentation	Medication errors, drug-drug interaction, utilization of resources
Sentinel events	Deficiency in patient care process
	Identification of opportunities to improve patient care

DRG, Diagnosis-related groups; APACHE, acute physiology and chronic health evaluation; SAPS, simplified acute physiology score; MPM, mortality prediction model.[5,6,15,16]

---

changes when a CIS is brought on line. These changes are seen in the laboratory, pharmacy, and radiology departments. Allied health professionals, such as respiratory therapists, physical therapists, social workers, and dietitians, find their work routines changing in response to the automation as well. Finally, departments managing information systems and biomedical electronics are asked to provide support and maintenance services, which require administrative assumption of the cost of the support.

With the assumption that there is administrative endorsement of the entire development of the ICU information system, the actual task of implementation begins with the translation of the tasks of patient care into the system itself. The development team establishes the logic of the system, the ordering of data, the computer screens themselves, and the displays of data. Once the system is actually available, the team becomes responsible for teaching the use of the system to the entire patient care team within the unit. This education process is time-consuming and requires the undivided attention of the caregiver for defined periods of the day. Attempting to teach the use of the system during the actual patient care process will almost certainly result in failure. Similarly, caregivers will require compensation during the learning process, so budgets should be established to all caregivers for suitable hourly reimbursement just as if they were delivering patient care.

Specific implementation plans should be made. For example, hemodynamic and respiratory flow sheets should be computerized and implemented first. This might be followed by patient assessment, medication administration, and fluid balance. Clinical notes might be implemented at any time during the implementation process. Paramount to the success of the entire process is executive directive to switch from written to computerized record. There cannot be two charting systems in effect. Definite milestones must be established and the components of the system implemented and the handwritten record eliminated according to the milestones.

POST-ICU CONSIDERATIONS

As mentioned earlier, pre-ICU considerations are generally administrative, and ICU considerations are clinical in nature. As expected, the post-ICU considerations become more administrative in nature. Issues include:

- Transfer of patient information to storage and to nursing floor
- Capture of data to calculate severity of illness for outcome adjustment
- Combination of unit data with other databases for utilization review, outcome research, quality assessment, and so forth
- Connection of the CIS to other computerized databases

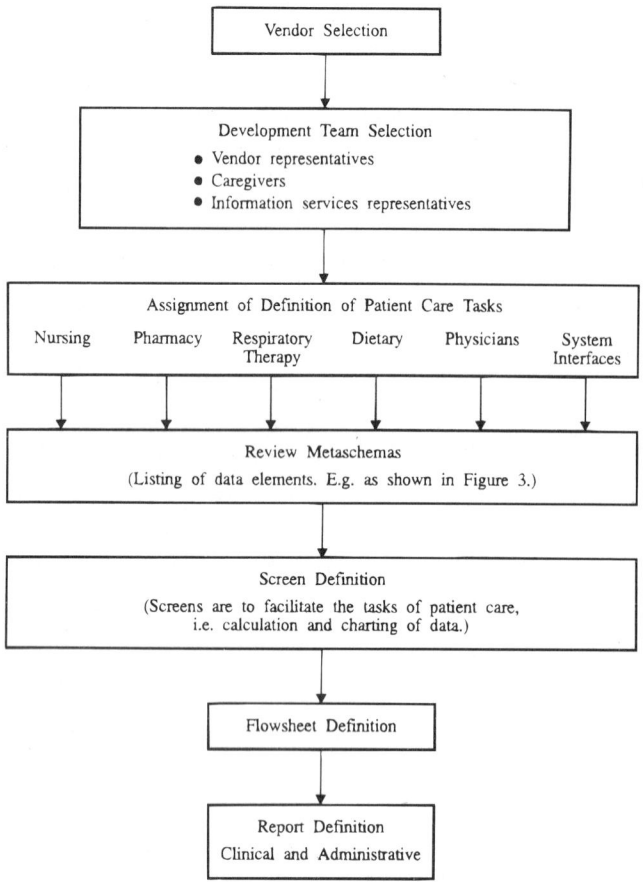

Fig. 80-10. The entire process of selecting data elements, defining computer screens, and listing orders of elements to appear on flow sheets. (Courtesy of George Morrison, Clinical Dimensions, Inc., Madison, WI.)

Transfer of Patient Information

There are two aspects of transfer of patient information. The first concerns long-term storage of information captured (automatically and manually) by the unit's CIS. Previous discussion and figures demonstrate the display of stored data. As patients are discharged from the unit, data can be stored in electronic medium for future review for outcome studies, utilization review, medical-legal problems, and so forth. Although hard copy printout would be the principal method for maintaining the patient record, over time, long-term electronic storage for easy retrieval would make the medical record much more flexible and make retrieval and review time much shorter. Current methods for this storage include optical disc and digital audiotape systems. Both provide the necessary capacity at reasonable cost today. In the future, other optical technologies, such as holographic memories, may offer near-infinite storage capacities at reasonable cost.

The second aspect of storage requires the existence of a rather extensive HIS and the availability of similar CIS on non-ICU nursing units where patients would be transferred after ICU discharge. When entire hospital records become computerized, appropriate databases exist into which the ICU record can be integrated.

Capture of Data to Document Severity of Illness

At present, numerous utilities are used to adjust for severity of illness (see Chap. 79). For the most part, these utilities are used for quality assessment to adjust outcome for severity of illness. As discussed in Chapter 79, although the data elements required for calculation of severity and prediction are of limited number, their capture is labor intensive, and calculation of prediction of outcome is often done by computer program. Additionally, these predictions may be based on formulas that are proprietary in nature (e.g., APACHE III). In the interest of preserving the processing power of the ICU system, provisions for the transfer of data to specific administrative workstations for calculation of severity and prediction of outcome may be practical, particularly in the case of proprietary utilities. Figure 80-11 illustrates such connections. Vital signs, laboratory data, patient observation (including Glasgow Coma Scale), and specific historical data could be transferred automatically from the point of capture (the bedside workstation) to an administrative workstation at a location more peripheral to the areas of patient care. As the information system within a unit would mature, daily severity and prediction of outcome could become available to the bedside caregiver. Over time, the true utility of such information could be realized and implemented into daily practice patterns.

In addition to determining individual severity of illness, there is an additional requirement to create administrative reports that define the scope of service, the average severity of illness, and length of stay for the entire unit population as well as specific groups of patients. Table 80-12 lists examples of administrative information derived from the tasks of patient care. Table 80-13 represents an algorithm for breakdown of data derived from an administrative workstation using APACHE III (Apache Medical Systems, Washington, D.C.).[17]

Combining Unit Data with Other Databases

The combination of ICU data with other databases provides insight into utilization of resources, short-term and long-term outcomes (survival, death), cost, efficacy, and efficiency of ICU organizations.[18] The difficulty with such aspirations is the availability and format of other databases. Theoretically, data from the Uniform Hospital Discharge Abstract (UHDA) (required for all hospitals accredited by the Joint Commission for the Accreditation of Health Care Organizations) provides information abstracted from the clinical record (Table 80-14). Discharge status (alive, dead, nursing home, and so forth) provides the beginning of outcome information. The National Death Index provides information on date of death, state of death, and death certificate number by matching social security number, name, date of birth, and so forth (Table 80-15). Long-term cost of care beyond ICU use is also available through access to the Medicare Automated Data Retrieval System (MADRS).[19]

The dilemma with access to these databases is the format used to make the combinations of data from the various sources. For typical ICU management, inexpensive media are available by using a personal computer that con-

Table 80-13. Total ICU Population*

Number = N
% Hospital Admissions = N
Total Hospital Days for ICU Patients = N
% of Total Days by ICU Patients = N
Total ICU Days = N
% of Total Days Used in ICU = N

MEDICAL PATIENTS (separate by diagnosis)	SURGICAL PATIENTS (separate by diagnosis)
Total ICU days	Total ICU days
% ICU days	% ICU days
Total admissions	Total admissions
% of Total ICU admissions	% of Total ICU admissions
Demographics (age, gender)	Demographics (age, gender)
Length of Stay	Length of Stay
Pre-ICU	Pre-ICU
ICU	ICU
Post-ICU	Post-ICU
Mortality	Mortality
Actual mortality	Actual mortality
Adjusted mortality (by APACHE III)	Adjusted mortality (by APACHE III)
Separation by diagnosis (APACHE III categories)	Separation by diagnosis (APACHE III categories)
Congestive heart failure	Gastrointestinal bleed requiring surgery
Pneumonia	Gastrointestinal cancer requiring surgery
Pulmonary embolism	Cholecystectomy
Gastrointestinal bleeding	Gastrointestinal obstruction requiring surgery
Myocardial infarction	Gastrointestinal surgery for perforation
Rhythm disturbances	Carotid artery surgery
Drug overdose	Femoral-popliteal artery surgery
Sepsis (pulmonary)	Laminectomy
Sepsis (gastrointestinal)	Neurosurgery for intracranial malignancy
Sepsis (urinary tract)	Surgery for renal cancer
Cardiogenic shock	Surgery for respiratory cancer
Chronic obstructive pulmonary disease	Surgery for head trauma
Asthma	Surgery for multiple trauma

* The analysis of total patient days, % ICU days, % of admissions, demographics, length of stays (pre-ICU, ICU, and post-ICU), and mortality for each diagnostic category is performed for further definition of scope of service of the ICU.[17]

tains software for spreadsheet construction (Lotus or Excel).[20] ASCII files can be constructed from various databases and inserted into appropriate columns within the ICU spreadsheet. Figure 80-11 demonstrates the various possibilities for database combinations. It is important that the ICU system provide utilities to down load data elements, which the ICU manager or researcher can specify according to information desired. These individuals can

Table 80-14. Uniform Hospital Discharge Data Sets

Patient name
Hospital number
Date of birth
Age
Gender
Admission date
Discharge date
Discharge status
Medical diagnostic category
Diagnosis related group
Principal diagnosis and description
Secondary diagnoses and description
Primary procedure and description (date and surgeon)
Secondary procedures and descriptions (date and surgeon)

then customize spreadsheets, which allow for sorting and manipulation of data to answer specific questions or speculate on unit operation.[20,21]

In summary, the algorithm for computerization is administratively and clinically complex. Just as the care of the critically ill patient involves administrative and clinical teamwork, the process of creating a computerized ICU patient care system requires a team with clinical, administrative, and vendor representation. Subsequent to formation of such a team, a plan must be outlined with definite goals for the system. If there is a major administrative focus, such as controlling cost, defining staffing, facilitating quality assurance, or tracking caregiver performance, the clinical staff will be polarized into passive participation. If there is too much clinical emphasis without focus on the necessity of making administrative data the byproduct of patient care, administrators will not permit funding of such a project. Finally, if there is no vendor accountability for meeting defined goals, a workable system will not evolve.

Planning for computerization should be done on three levels. **Strategic planning** should involve the definition of the exact goals for computerization of the ICU. Most practically the system should be designed to facilitate the

1716   THE HIGH RISK PATIENT: MANAGEMENT OF THE CRITICALLY ILL

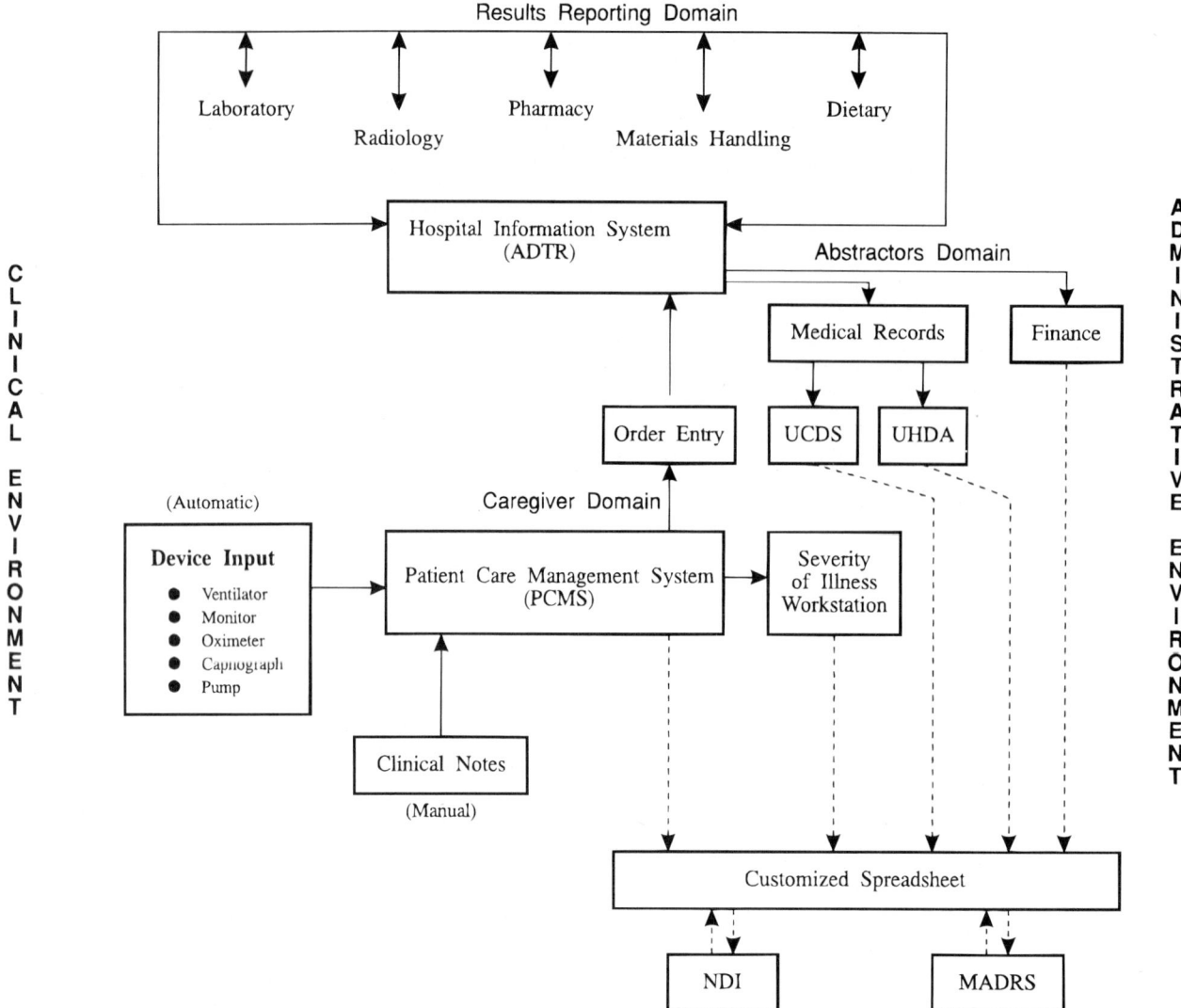

Fig. 80–11. The information domain of the ICU. Authorization for collection of data is provided by the hospital information system through the admission/discharge transfer (ADTR) module. Patient data are collected through the CIS located at the point of patient care. Data input into the CIS is both automatic and manual. Peripheral to the CIS is an administrative workstation for calculation of severity of illness. Information for the clinical environment is listed to the left and information from the administrative environment is listed to the right. The solid lines represent real-time flow of information, and the dashed lines represent the exchange of information through a medium such as magnetic disc (floppy) or tape. The latter information is used for administrative purposes, such as quality assessment, utilization review, technology assessment, and research. There is usually no requirement for real-time capture of this data because its analysis does not contribute directly to patient care. Customization of data retrieval for creation of files for accessing the national death index (NDI) and Medicare Automated Data Retrieval System (MADRS) facilitates creation of information that can be fed back into a stand-alone spreadsheet to allow the ICU practitioner to perform independent analysis. Information exchange by disc or tape is considerably less expensive than retrieval electronically. The dashed lines represent this indirect derivation of data. UCDS, Uniform clinical data sets; UHDA, uniform hospital discharge abstract. (Drawn by: George Morrison, Clinical Dimensions, Inc., Madison, WI.)

tasks of patient care. Administrative data for quality assurance, severity of illness definition, resource consumption, staffing, and so forth should be a byproduct of the delivery of patient care, not the purpose of it. **Tactical planning** should take into account the resources required for the project. Existing resources as well as those that need to be acquired should be defined. Resources include equipment as well as personnel. Following the formulation of the resources, **operations planning** should include the development of a budget for equipment purchases and for payment of the personnel who will be involved in the development and implementation of the system.

Table 80-15. National Death Index Data Set Items

Data Element	Tape Position	Descriptors
Name*		
Last	1–20	First and last names required
First	21–35	
Middle i.	36	
Social security no.*	37–45	All nine digits required
Date of birth*		
Month	46–47	May be sufficient with first and last names without social security no.
Day	48–49	
Year	50–51	
Father's surname*	52–71	
Age at death	72–74	
Sex*	75	
Race	76	
Marital status	77	
State of residence	78–79	
State of birth	80–81	
Control no.	82–91	Users identification
Optional data	92–97	(e.g., hospital record no.)
Blank	98–100	

* Data sets for possible NDI record match. Data output includes: State of death, death certificate no., first name, middle i., last name, father's surname, social security no., date of birth, age, sex, race, marital status, state of residence, state of birth, user ID.
(From National Death Index User's Manual. Hyattsville, MD, U.S. Department of Health and Human Services. Public Health Service. Centers for Disease Control. National Center for Health Statistics. DHHS Publication No. (PHS) 90-1148, 1990.)

REFERENCES

1. Friedman, B. A., and Martin, J. B.: Hospital information systems. The physician's role. JAMA, *257*:1792, 1987.
2. Vladeck, B. C.: Medicare hospital payment by diagnosis-related groups. Ann. Intern. Med., *100*:576, 1984.
3. Sivak, E. D.: Management of information as a resource. *In* Business of Critical Care. Edited by W. J. Sibbald and T. A. Massaro. Mount Kisco, NY, Futura Publishing. In press.
4. East, T. D.: Computers in the ICU: panacea or plague? Respir. Care, *37*:170, 1992.
5. Sivak, E. D., Gochberg, J., and Frank, D. M.: Lessons to be learned from the continuing epic of computerizing the intensive care unit. *In* Proceedings of the 13th Annual Symposium on Computer Applications in Medical Care. Washington, D.C., IEEE Press, 1989, p. 605.
6. Sivak, E. D., Gochberg, J. S., Fronek, R., and Scott, D.: Lessons to be learned from the design, development and implementation of a computerized patient care management system for the intensive care unit. *In* Proceedings of the 11th Annual Symposium on Computer Applications in Medical Care. Washington, D.C., IEEE Press, 1987, p. 614.
7. Sivak, E. D., and Gochberg, J. S.: Lessons to be learned from implementation and maintenance of a computerized patient care management system for the ICU. *In* Proceedings of the 12th Annual Symposium on Computer Applications in Medical Care. Washington, D.C., IEEE Press, 1988, p. 768.
8. Dick, R. S., and Steen, E. B. (Eds.): The Computer-Based Patient Record. An Essential Technology for Health Care. Washington, D.C., National Academy Press, 1991.
9. Yang, K. L., and Tobin, M. J.: A prospective study of indexes predicting the outcome of trials of weaning from mechanical ventilation. N. Engl. J. Med., *324*:1445, 1991.
10. Eddy, D. M.: Clinical decision making. JAMA, *263*:1265, 1990.
11. Pestotnik, S. L., et al.: Therapeutic antibiotic monitoring: surveillance using a computerized expert system. Am. J. Med., *88*:43, 1990.
12. Bradshaw, K. E., et al.: Computer-based data entry for nurses in the ICU. MD Computing, *6*:274, 1989.
13. East, T. D., Yank, W., Tariq, H., and Gardner, R. M.: The IEEE medical information bus of respiratory care. Crit. Care Med., *17*:580, 1989.
14. Sittig, D. F., Gardner, R. M., Morris, A. H., and Wallace, C. J.: Clinical evaluation of computer-based respiratory care algorithms. Int. J. Clin. Monit. Comput., *7*:177, 1990.
15. East, T. D., et al.: A successful computerized protocol for clinical management of pressure control inverse ratio ventilation in ARDS patients. Chest, *101*:697, 1992.
16. Morris, A. H., et al.: A controlled clinical trial of a new 3-step therapy that includes extracorporeal CO_2 removal for ARDS. Trans. Am. Soc. Artif. Intern. Organs, *11*:48, 1988.
17. Knaus, W. A., et al.: The APACHE III prognostic system. Risk prediction of hospitalized mortality for critically ill hospitalized adults. Chest, *100*:1619, 1991.
18. Sibbald, W. J., and Inman, K. J.: Problems in assessing the technology of critical care medicine. Int. J. Technol. Assess. Health Care, *8*:410, 1992.
19. Sneen, M.: Linked A/B files—Medicare Automated Data Retrieval System (MADRS). *In* Conference Proceedings—1989 Data Users Conference. Baltimore, N.C.F.A., U.S. Department of Health and Human Services, 1989, p. 79.
20. Sivak, E. D., and Perez-Trepichio, A.: Quality assessment in the medical intensive care unit: evolution of a data model. Cleve. Clin. J. Med., *57*:273, 1990.
21. Sivak, E. D., and Perez-Trepichio, A.: Quality assurance in the medical intensive care unit. Continued evolution of a data model. Quality Assurance and Utilization Review, *7*:81, 1992.

Chapter 81

MINIMIZING THE RISK OF LIABILITY

RUSSELL C. KLEIN
DONNA GUINN KLEIN

Few incidents in a physician's professional career cause more distress than becoming a defendant in a medical malpractice suit. Available data indicate that most physicians are sued at least once during their professional career. Precise statistics are not available concerning the risk of a malpractice suit in every area of the hospital, but we know that many actions involve emergency care, surgical and postoperative care, and cardiovascular diseases. With this in mind, the ICU, where desperate illness meets high technology, would appear to be a fertile field for potential litigation. A Rand Corporation study indicates that most malpractice claims are disposed of without any payment.[1] When payment is made, it is usually through the insurance claims settlement process and not through court proceedings. If the parties cannot agree on a settlement, however, the case is resolved in court. Physicians, to minimize their risks, must understand the legal basis for malpractice claims, what may occur during a malpractice suit, and what they can do to lessen the possibility of suit or increase their chance of successful defense. Minimizing risk of liability begins with an understanding that the basis of negligence is the deviation from the standards of care applicable to a particular medical specialty. For a plaintiff to prevail in a medical malpractice case, he or she must prove that the physician defendant deviated from the applicable standards of care.

BASICS OF NEGLIGENCE LIABILITY

"Negligence" is the legal term on which the theory of medical malpractice is built. The elements of negligence in a malpractice action are based on the following:

- Physicians have a legal duty to patients to act or to refrain from acting in certain ways (i.e., adhering to the "standard of care").
- A breach of that duty occurs when the physician fails to conform his or her conduct to the required standard (in other words, "negligence").
- A sufficient causal connection exists between the negligent conduct and the patient's injury.
- There is actual provable harm, harm that the law says is measurable and compensable in money damages.[2]

Standard of Care

Negligence is conduct that falls below the standard established by law for the protection of others against an unreasonable risk of harm.[3] Thus, the test for negligence is objective. It does not focus on such subjective factors as whether the physician intended to exercise due care or whether the physician did the best he or she could to be careful. Rather, the test focuses on whether the physician's conduct was that of a hypothetic "reasonably prudent physician" placed in the same or similar circumstances. In constructing the hypothetic physician, courts once commonly limited the standard of care, skill, and knowledge required of medical doctors to that customarily possessed and exercised by other reasonably well-qualified professionals in the same or a similar locality. This "locality rule" has gradually been abolished. Specialists are held to the "national" standards of that specialty.

Unreasonable Risk

The reasonably prudent physician need only protect patients against unreasonable risks of harm.[4] Under the classic legal formulation, a risk is unreasonable when the foreseeable probability and gravity of the harm outweigh the burden to the physician of alternative conduct that would have prevented the harm.[5]

Proof of Negligence/Causation

To prevail in most medical malpractice actions, plaintiffs must introduce sufficient evidence to prove that the physician's failure to adhere to the standard of care caused the injury to the patient. In some cases, courts allow circumstantial proof of causation under the doctrine of *res ipsa loquitur* (the thing speaks for itself). This doctrine is applied in the following situations:

- It is highly probable that the injury would not have occurred in the absence of someone's negligence; for example, a rongeur is left in the patient following hip replacement, or a patient awakens from surgery paralyzed in one limb with no plausible explanation.
- The indicated source of negligence is within the scope of duty owed by the defendant to the plaintiff; for example, the surgeon owes the patient a duty to ensure that such instruments are removed from the operative field or to have disclosed material risks adequately.
- Neither the plaintiff nor any third party appears to have contributed to or is able to offer an explanation

for the plaintiff's injury; for example, neither the plaintiff nor anyone else present used the rongeur or performed any act that could have resulted in the paralysis.

In such a case, there is a presumption that the defendant was negligent without any direct proof of negligence, and the defendant has the burden of going forward and introducing evidence to refute this inference.[6]

PRE-SUIT PHASE

Risk of Suit in the ICU Environment

It is estimated that 80% of all malpractice claims arise from incidents that occur in the hospital setting.[1] Data collected during 1986 and 1987 indicate that surgical issues accounted for the highest number of claims filed against physicians, but diagnostic issues accounted for the largest percentage of medical liability costs.[8] The three leading claim groups were:

- Surgery (29.3% of claims; 25.5% of costs)
- "Failure to diagnose" (28.1% of claims; 33.5% of costs)
- "Improper treatment" (27.1% of claims; 30.9% of costs)

Within the group of surgery-related allegations, the following represented 87% of the total claims: postoperative complications, inadvertent acts, inappropriate procedures, postoperative deaths, and delayed complications. In the "failure to diagnose" category, the following represented 58% of the total claims: cancer, fractures-dislocations, infection, pregnancy-related problems, and myocardial infarction. In the "improper treatment" allegations, the following represented 65% of claims: birth related, fractures-dislocations, drug side effects, infections, and insufficient therapy.[1]

Patients and Families Who Initiate Suit and Their Reasons for Doing So

It is impossible to know with certainty why the number of malpractice suits has been increasing, but some possible reasons include:

- Deterioration in the patient/physician relationship
- Patient belief that modern medicine can work miracles
- We live in a litigious society
- The need to blame when something goes wrong patient demographics

Patients once had a traditional warm relationship with their family physician, who was able to handle all problems and whose judgment was seldom questioned. In our age of specialization and highly sophisticated instruments, a patient is often seen by a battery of physicians, paraprofessionals, nurses, and technicians. Often the traditional relationship they once had with one physician is gone. Patients' self-imposed restraint against suing a "friend" has sharply diminished, and they conceptualize their relationships with health-care institutions and physicians in terms of their "rights."

Unrealistic expectations of what modern medicine can accomplish, often engendered by physicians themselves, provoke anger when things do not go as expected. Even if modern medicine could work miracles, patients are unwilling to accept the unavoidable bad outcomes when it does not.[1]

There has been a sharp rise in the amount of litigation and in the severity of awards in other areas of negligence law. The "crisis" of medical malpractice may be part of an increasing trend to file a lawsuit as a result of any perceived wrong. Health care services are commonly viewed like any other service or commodity: If something goes wrong, patients, like other consumers of goods and services, are more likely than ever to sue.[1]

In today's highly specialized, sophisticated environment, patients increasingly look to hospitals and physicians as the focus of their complaints and grievances and as someone to blame.[7]

In a large survey of suing patients, certain demographic patterns stand out. The elderly (age 65 and older) are less likely to sue than younger patients. The unemployed are much more likely to sue than the employed. Those with a brief doctor/patient relationship (less than 6 months) are much more likely to sue. Suing patients almost always view themselves as blameless in causing the illness or injury involved in the suit.[8]

SITUATIONS THAT MAY GIVE RISE TO A MALPRACTICE SUIT

Large studies of adverse events in hospitalized patients and "closed" malpractice claims reveal certain common threads.[9-11] Drug-related problems are common. They include allergic reactions; overdosage or underdosage; confusion over "sound-alike" drugs; failure to monitor therapy, especially drug levels; using an inappropriate drug or failing to use an indicated drug; and problems with drug interactions. A particularly disquieting fact related to allergic reactions was a clear prior history in most patients of allergy to the administered drug or closely related compounds.

Evidence indicates that the majority of diagnostic errors involve a relatively small number of problems or complaints. These included chest or abdominal pain, wounds and fractures, fever/meningitis, aortic aneurysm, bleeding into the central nervous system, and acute epiglottitis in one large series. Diagnostic errors often involved failure to use an indicated test, avoidable delays, and failure to act on test results. Technical errors occurring in surgical patients, infections, and inadequate monitoring following procedures are also commonly cited. Inadequate training or supervision and practice outside an area of expertise have also been cited as potential problem areas.

Theories of Negligence: The Physician's Relationship to the Hospital, Its Employees, and Other Physicians

Because an estimated 80% of all malpractice claims stem from incidents that occur in a hospital, hospitals have a primary role in preventing medical injury. Plaintiffs often name both the hospital and the physician in a malpractice lawsuit. Also, hospitals may be found liable for the negligent acts of staff physicians. Thus, the two types of providers must assist each other in minimizing the risk of liability.

Hospitals, to be accredited and licensed, must have an approved quality-assurance program. Quality assurance committees have authority to investigate complaints about the performance of staff physicians and to recommend suspension of privileges or other restriction of physicians found to be negligent or incompetent. Physicians participating in peer review activities are often reluctant to take action against medical staff members, fearing they in turn will be sued by the disciplined physician.[1] Most states, however, have statutes that provide immunity to physicians who participate in peer review. Similarly the Health Care Quality Improvement Act of 1986 offers immunity under state and federal laws, including antitrust immunity. More often than not, hospitals agree to defend and indemnify medical staff members who are sued in connection with good faith peer review activities.

Because Congress recognized the importance of peer review, it enacted the Health Care Quality Improvement Act of 1986, which provides for a qualified immunity from liability for physicians and others participating in official peer review activities in hospitals and other medical groups. The Act immunizes only peer review actions performed in good faith after a reasonable attempt to ascertain the true facts. It provides physicians, who are the subject of peer review actions, with procedural due process rights, such as hearings and appeals.

Imputed Negligence

In certain situations, the negligent act of an individual or a group of individuals may be imputed to a hospital or physician, so they are held **vicariously liable,** even though the hospital or physician is otherwise without fault. The most common doctrine imposing vicarious liability is known as *respondeat superior,* in which wrongful acts of an employee resulting in injury to a third party are imputed to the employer, who is otherwise without fault, simply because of the existence of the employment relationship. For this theory to apply, the employee must have been acting within the scope of his or her employment.[12] This doctrine is based on the theory that an employer has the duty to control and direct the conduct of its employee. Therefore the hospital or physician is said to be responsible, along with the employee who negligently performs an act, for injury to the patient.

There are times, however, when a hospital is said to have relinquished its duty to direct and control the activities of its employees and to have transferred these duties to another person, such as the staff physician. In such a circumstance, the employee is said to be a "borrowed servant" of the physician, and the doctrine of respondeat superior does not apply liability to the hospital, although it may apply liability to the physician.

The "Captain of the Ship Doctrine," once a popular theory of liability, has been eroded. This doctrine provides that a physician who exercises control and authority over nurses or other health care professionals should be held liable for their negligence on the theory of "borrowed servants." For example, under this doctrine, the surgeon in an operating room may be held responsible for the acts of the staff within, including hospital employees, residents, or assisting physicians. If the surgeon is held liable under this theory, the hospital would not be because the theory holds that the surgeon is in complete control of the operating room and all those within.[13]

As a general principle, a hospital is not vicariously liable for the negligent acts of a physician staff member. Traditionally, physicians merely used the hospital's facilities to house and provide treatment to the patient. In other instances, the relationship of a physician to the hospital has been characterized as that of an independent contractor, rather than an employee. Even though a physician may be characterized as an independent contractor by a document describing a contractual relationship between the physician and the hospital, however, courts may still find an employment or agency relationship exists.[13]

Historically, hospitals were considered charitable institutions. As such, they were exempt from the general rule that a corporation was responsible for the acts of its employees. The doctrine of charitable immunity, coupled with the general relationship of the physician as an independent contractor and not an employee, protected hospitals from most forms of liability through the 1940s. In the 1950s, however, courts began to observe the increasing importance of the hospital in providing health care and in supervising their staffs.

As medical care evolved, physicians became increasingly dependent on hospital affiliation. By 1975, few physicians could consider practicing without the resources that a hospital offered, and 25% of the 330,000 active physicians in that year practiced full-time in a hospital.[13] Although the hospitals may have been protected from liability by independent contractor relationships or under the "Captain of the Ship Doctrine," there are three theories under which a hospital may still be found vicariously liable for the negligent acts of the physician resulting in injury to a patient:

- The control test
- The ostensible agency test
- The inherent function test

In the **control test,** a court simply determines whether the physician is subject to the control of the hospital, applying a number of standard criteria for evaluating the existence of a master/servant relationship. If a contract between the hospital and the physician gave the hospital substantial control over the physician's hours of work or choice of patients or if the hospital furnished equipment or employees or did the physician's billing, an employment relationship might be found. The higher the degree of control a hospital exerts over a physician's earnings or activities, the more likely it will be found that the physician is an employee or an agent of the hospital, and liability will attach to the hospital.[14,15]

Under the **ostensible agency test,** courts have concluded that in some settings, such as an emergency room or a radiology department, the hospital "holds itself out" as offering services to the patient through a physician, even though the physician who renders the services is not a hospital employee. In this situation, the physician is an "ostensible agent" of the hospital, and liability attaches to the hospital for the physician's actions.[16,17]

Under the **inherent function test,** a court may find a hospital liable for the actions of the physician who performs services that are an inherent function of the hospital, a function without which the hospital could not properly achieve its purpose. An example of this would be a pathologist or a radiologist performing procedures within a hospital-based department where the technicians and equipment were furnished and controlled by the hospital.[18]

Joint and Several Liability

Joint and several liability allows a successful plaintiff to recover damages from any defendant in a lawsuit if any other defendant could not pay. Many states have abolished this as part of tort reform. For example, a patient is seriously injured by a large air embolus introduced into the bloodstream by a rupture in a defective intra-aortic balloon pump catheter. The patient sues not only the hospital, but also the admitting physician, the consulting cardiologist, the balloon pump manufacturer, and the catheter manufacturer. If the catheter manufacturer had gone bankrupt, under joint and several liability, the successful plaintiff in a malpractice action could recover the awarded damages from the pump manufacturer, the hospital, or the physicians.

Other Liability

Rarely, physicians face criminal prosecution for their acts. When they do, the principal situations involve right to die/do not resuscitate issues or battery (unauthorized touching of another person). The latter may occur if the physician performs a nonemergency procedure without proper consent. Battery, even if it results only in civil liability, may not be covered by insurance. Criminal conduct of any type is also rarely covered by malpractice policies, so physicians should abide by their applicable state laws. Informed consent demands that the physician use appropriate forms, follow state law as applicable, and personally obtain the consent. Only the most foolhardy delegate this responsibility to paraprofessionals. Physicians and hospitals also face severe federal civil money penalties and exclusion from Medicare or Medicaid for failing to provide emergency care for certain serious or life-threatening emergencies.

SUIT PHASE

Pretrial Activities/Notification and Filing

Plaintiffs set forth their complaints in court documents called pleading. Most malpractice lawsuits are filed in state courts. If the plaintiff and physician live in different states, however, it is possible to file the suit in federal court. In most state courts, the pleadings provide detailed facts supporting the plaintiff's allegations in addition to simply notice of a claim.

The pleading stage begins with the plaintiff's filing of the complaint or petition. This document informs the court and the defendant of the plaintiff's criticisms of the physician, the damages suffered, and request for compensation. A defendant must respond to a plaintiff's complaint with an answer. A physician should notify his or her insurer as soon as notice that a suit has been filed is received. The physician should also act immediately to protect any records, x-ray films, and so forth. The risk management office of the hospital or clinic should be notified if appropriate. A physician should not ignore the notice of a suit or speak with the plaintiff's attorney or the parties who filed the suit.

The defendant, through his or her attorney, may answer the suit by denying some or all of the plaintiff's allegations. The answer may be in the form of a specific denial of designated portions of the complaint or a qualified general denial that denies everything not expressly admitted. The defendant may also assert affirmative defenses at this stage, a basis on which the defendant would legally avoid liability even if the plaintiff's allegations were true. The pleading stage in state court may require a more detailed factual description in the petition. A hallmark of the federal pleading process is that it permits amendments to the maximum extent consistent with the purpose of pleading. Thus a party can normally correct its pleading mistakes or amend them based on newly learned information.[19] The Federal Rules of Civil Procedure as well as the procedural rules of many states provide for sanctions for frivolous or baseless allegations. As a result, greater care is taken when making factual allegations in those jurisdictions.

Preparation for Litigation

Several guidelines assist a physician in preparation for testifying in a malpractice case. Before a physician says a word "under oath," he or she should:

- Learn the applicable law
- Know all the pertinent facts
- Be aware of the legal process and the rules that apply

Most physicians have a poor idea about what laws apply to a medical malpractice case. A physician's anxiety about a case may decrease and his or her effectiveness increase when he or she realizes that "malpractice" is defined simply as "a departure from accepted standards of medical practice." There is a critical distinction between a "departure from accepted practice" and the exercise of judgment in selecting one of several available forms of treatment. A physician may testify that he or she departed from accepted practice (which means the physician is negligent) when the physician really meant that he or she selected a standard form of therapy that is less popular than available alternatives. Other important legal principles may be applicable, such as the elements of informed consent. Physicians should attempt to gain a thorough understanding of all relevant law by review of the case with the attorney.

Physicians commonly limit their prelitigation review to their own notes and may ignore other critical entries in the medical records and may fail to anticipate inconsistencies in the medical record. Physicians should read and analyze every part of the medical record, including the laboratory reports, nurse's reports, anesthesia records, recovery room records, medication charts, vital signs, and every other scrap of paper related to the patient's care. Physicians should try to search for and reconcile inconsistencies before they testify.

Physicians should understand the legal process, including how trial and pretrial activities actually operate, the role of physicians as witnesses, and the basic rules of evidence that apply to their testimony.

Medical Review Panels or Arbitration Boards

The use of screening panels and arbitration boards as a means of resolving malpractice disputes is permitted, or required, in many states. There is variation from state to state in the composition, function, and procedures that these panels and boards employ. Screening panels are designed to provide both sides with an impartial, nonbinding assessment of the validity of the plaintiff's claim. When a malpractice action is filed, the dispute is generally immediately referred to a panel, most often composed of physicians, for review of the facts and an evaluation of the merits of the claim. The majority of states allow the panel's finding to be introduced into evidence at the subsequent trial. Screening panels' findings are never binding; they merely encourage the settlement of claims or discourage the future filing of a lawsuit. There has been mixed success for state statutes creating such screening panels or arbitration boards. Constitutional challenges have been based on the right to a jury trial, separation of powers, and equal protection of the laws. These panels function as a prerequisite to a trial, not a substitute for it.[1]

Insured-Insurer Conflicts

Under some conditions of insurance, the insurance company has the power to settle malpractice suits without the defendant physician's consent. A physician must remember that the attorney named to defend him or her is paid by the insurance company and that the progress of the case is monitored by an insurance adjuster. Although the attorney has an ethical obligation to represent the physician defendant competently, conflict of interest situations may arise, especially if multiple defendants and multiple insurance companies are involved. Physicians should be cautious when a single attorney represents multiple parties. Some physicians choose to have their personal attorney monitor the case to ensure protection of their rights. Physicians have a right to competent defense and should insist that an experienced attorney be assigned.

Meeting the Attorney Assigned for Defense

Most insurers require defense counsel to meet with the physician defendant within a short period of time from the filing of the claim or suit. In preparation, the physician should gather all documents and medical records related to the case and prepare a narrative of the care provided to the patient. Ample uninterrupted time should be allowed for this meeting.

Discovery

Discovery is a process that allows either party to expand on the notice given by the pleading. It allows requests for production of documents, answers to written questions (interrogatories), admission of certain facts, and depositions of witnesses (including the opposing party). Discovery clarifies the issues and allows the parties to investigate facts and explore evidence before trial. Each party builds his or her own case and evaluates that of his or her opponent. The discovery process is intended to avoid an incorrect or unfair outcome, which might otherwise be determined by the ability of one party to pursue private investigation and the other to survive a blind trial. Discovery also facilitates settlement or dismissal of the claim, allows the tried case to proceed more efficiently, and permits a more predictable and orderly trial. The scope of discovery is wide. Generally a party may discover any matter that is relevant to the subject matter in the pending action and that is not privileged.[20]

Protecting Medical Records

Although medical records are generally relevant and therefore discoverable, some documents are privileged and protected from discovery. Quality assurance information and information gathered in peer review proceedings are granted a privilege under many state statutes, protecting this material from discovery. Without the statutes, quality assurance information would more than likely be discoverable. Quality assurance proceedings, however, are not absolutely privileged. The immunity is qualified, based on the good faith actions of the individuals involved, and because privileges can be waived, it is important for those involved in peer review to maintain confidentiality. The underlying reason to privilege quality assurance or peer review proceedings is to provide the confidentiality needed for effective peer review. Discoverability would have a chilling effect on peer review.

Discovery is further limited when the material sought was prepared by or for a party in anticipation of litigation or for trial. This "work product" doctrine may protect incident reports as long as they are kept confidential within the hospital or office and truly in anticipation of litigation. Incident reports may also be privileged as records of peer review committees. Circulation or discussion of such data outside official committee meetings leaves an incident report vulnerable to discovery. The work-product protection may not extend to prevent normal discovery of facts that happen to be embodied in an otherwise undiscoverable work product.

Discussions between a physician and his or her attorney are privileged and protected from discovery under the "attorney-client privilege," a broader protection than the work-product safeguard.

Because medical records are so important, the wise physician makes entries in the record accordingly, documenting informed consent, discussions with patients and family members, and other important findings. Unnecessary and irrelevant information should be excluded. Statements of fact should be clear and unequivocal, leaving no room for ambiguity in later interpretation. Follow-up instructions and return visits should be documented. All operating room or ICU flow sheets, anesthesia records, and other logs should be checked for accuracy. The physician should read all clinical interpretations of diagnostic tests before signing them. The physician should never write anything in a record that he or she would not want read out loud in court. The time and date of entries should be noted. If the physician makes an error in the record, he or she should line it out and initial it. A record should never be altered after suit has been filed. The medical record should not be used as a vehicle to document the errors and shortcomings of fellow physicians or paraprofessionals.

Admissibility, at trial, is a different matter from discoverability. Documents may be discoverable whether or not they will be admissible at trial. If the plaintiff inadvertently discovers a document that should have been privileged, it may become admissible at trial. Hospital and medical records are generally considered business records and are therefore admissible.[21] Such discovered documents might also be admitted as admissions against the hospital.[22] Also, an expert could examine such records even if they were nonadmissible.[23]

Interrogatories

Interrogatories are written questions, which the responding party must answer in writing, under oath, unless his or her attorney objects to the question with reasons in writing.[24] Answers to interrogatories tend to be artfully evasive, but they often provide a simple, inexpensive way to clarify issues and obtain evidence.

Expert Witnesses

Because of the technical nature of the medical care, experts are often introduced at trial to provide valid and at least ostensibly nonpartisan fact or opinion. Of course, the attorney calling the expert will have thoroughly discussed testimony with that expert beforehand. Qualifications and guidelines for experts have been promulgated[25] in an effort to curb the reprehensible practice of physicians testifying in areas well outside of their field of competence.

Unfortunately, some jurisdictions are permissive when deciding what constitutes an expert. This is particularly dangerous because experts, in contrast to other witnesses, are allowed to state opinions. Although a physician's fitness to testify is explored at trial through a process called "qualification," the judge ultimately decides who is an expert and who is not.

Pretrial Depositions

Pretrial depositions involve giving testimony in response to questions by the attorney for the opposing party in an attempt to preview trial testimony. Physicians commonly treat depositions as a necessary nuisance that they squeeze into their hectic schedule. They may think if they just answer what they perceive the central question to be, it will put the matter to rest. Answers may become long lists of reasons why the lawsuit should be dropped, and the testimony becomes a fertile source of inconsistency at trial. Physicians do not realize that depositions commit them to facts and opinions with which they will have to live at trial. Accuracy is essential. Even false impressions or incomplete answers may jeopardize credibility at trial. Physicians must remember that they swear to tell the truth, but they do not take an oath to be overly informative. Questions should be answered as briefly and with as little specificity as possible. The physician should ask that questions be rephrased if he or she does not understand them. It is quite permissible to say "I do not remember at this time" during a deposition if memory is hazy. Generally physicians should keep answers short and simple and avoid speculation. A physician should not guess. The attorney will be present and will make objections if appropriate. These are made in the hope that a judge will rule favorably on them later. The physician should not expect his or her attorney to attempt to rehabilitate or otherwise question him or her once direct deposition testimony has been taken. Defense attorneys rarely do this, preferring to save the presentation of their case for trial. Plaintiffs' attorneys often take long argumentative depositions in hopes of producing information useful to their case.

Depositions are of two types: discovery and perpetuation. Discovery depositions simply attempt to elicit facts. Perpetuation depositions are taken as a substitute for live testimony at trial. This is especially common if the plaintiff is expected to die or a witness is unavailable for trial. Videotaping depositions, especially for perpetuation, is popular and is legal in most jurisdictions.

Conduct of the Trial

The procedural conduct of most trials is virtually identical, notwithstanding whether the case is tried in federal or state court. Physicians should anticipate the order of trial, particularly because the plaintiff proceeds first. The general order of a trial is as follows:

- Jury selection
- Opening statements (plaintiff then defendant)
- Plaintiff's case is presented (defendant cross-examines)
- Defendant's motion for directed verdict (defendant submits the plaintiff failed to prove his or her claim in his or her case)
- Defendant's case is presented (if defendant's motion is denied, plaintiff cross-examines)
- Plaintiff's motion for directed verdict
- Plaintiff's closing argument
- Defendant's closing argument
- Plaintiff's rebuttal (depending on the jurisdiction)
- Judge's charges of the law to jury (if a judge trial, the matter is usually taken under advisement, and a written judgment is later issued)
- Jury deliberations
- Verdict
- Judgment on the verdict

Testimony at Trial

If physicians are not familiar with trial procedure, there is a tendency to overreact to the situation. Generally the plaintiff's witnesses testify before the physician's witnesses, unless the physician/defendant is called as part of the plaintiff's case.

In answering questions in the courtroom, physicians must consider what is being asked: whether the question is general or specific, whether it seeks a recitation of medical records or a statement of opinions, and whether it refers to a specific patient or a group of patients. They should also know whether they are being asked for an expert opinion or for factual information. The physician and the attorney should reach an understanding beforehand concerning such things as when to elaborate in answering questions; whether facts documented in medical records should be answered by verbatim reading or simply summarized; and how to respond when the question asks for facts not documented in the medical records or to questions that involve statements of opinion, especially those that appear in authoritative medical books and journals.

It is critical that the physician learn from the defense attorney the difference between direct examination and cross-examination. On direct examination, attorneys are limited to general open-ended questions that do not lead the witness to a simple yes or no answer to the question. The astute physician uses the opportunity to include all pertinent information favorable to the case.

Because physicians are trained to raise their own questions about medical treatment, they have a tendency to ignore the examiner's question and answer the question they think should have been asked. Many physicians give answers before the questions have even been completed and may therefore give an answer totally unrelated to the question, opening new avenues for opposing counsel.

Physicians may think that there is some consolation in at least hastening the proceedings. They should instead consciously pause and reflect before answering questions, particularly at trial, because if one question elicits a pregnant pause after five questions have been answered quickly, the answer may be suspect, whatever it may be.

Although attorneys can object to improper questions, many objections are overruled. Nevertheless, most defense attorneys do make objections, and the physician should always pause to allow for such objections. Even if the objection be overruled, the physician should keep in mind the nature of the attorney's objection and consider whether the question is compound, ambiguous, or assumes a false fact to be true. If the question is defective or unclear, the physician should ask for clarification rather than give an inappropriate or misleading answer.

POSSIBLE OUTCOMES

Dismissal

A trial may be avoided by a voluntary dismissal of the defendant by the plaintiff. A defendant may also obtain a dismissal of the claim by filing a motion for summary judgment early in the case or by all parties signing a stipulation of dismissal. When a defendant asks for summary judgment, he or she in effect argues that the plaintiff's contentions are baseless on their face or that the plaintiff has failed utterly to prove a case. This tactic is generally unsuccessful. An involuntary dismissal may be obtained by a defending party against the plaintiff on the grounds that the plaintiff has failed to prosecute or failed to comply with a court order or rule.[26]

Settlement

The parties may agree to a settlement and dismissal of the claim. Payment can be either lump sum or structured. A structured settlement is a negotiated settlement of a claim, either before the lawsuit is filed, during litigation or trial, or even after a verdict is rendered, by which the defendant or his or her insurer agrees to make payments periodically to the plaintiff.[1] It is a formal contract between the parties to a dispute by which the defendant or his or her insurer agrees to perform certain financial acts and the plaintiff agrees to release the claim. Releases may also be obtained to protect the physician from future claims involving the same incident. In negotiating the settlement of claims with married plaintiffs, one should include the spouse so that claims such as loss of consortium are also extinguished. Both the husband and the wife must sign the settlement documents.

Jury Verdict

After hearing the evidence, the closing arguments, and the jury instructions, the jury retires to reach a verdict. The verdict decides the contested factual issues under the applicable law. A general verdict is simply a finding by the jury that the defendant either is or is not liable. A special verdict requires a special written finding on each issue. After the verdict, the judge normally enters a judgment in conformity with the verdict.[26] A judge, however, may enter a judgment adverse to the verdict and therefore set aside the verdict against the defendant. This is called "judgment notwithstanding the verdict."[28] This also rarely occurs.

Damages

There are two kinds of relief a judge may grant to the plaintiff. The traditional legal relief is in the form of money damages, including actual damages, punitive damages, and interest on the damages. Equitable relief is a discretionary remedy available to the court when legal remedies are inadequate. Under equitable relief, a court can order the defendant to do or not to do something, as in issuing an injunction or an order for specific performance. A court normally awards costs to the prevailing party as part of any judgment. Costs are taxed by the court clerk, whose determinations may, on motion, be reviewed by the judge. Costs normally include certain litigation fees and expenses but generally not attorney's fees, which are usually by far the largest expenses. This rule, however, is subject to some significant exceptions when statutes, court rules, and judicial doctrines call for reimbursement of attorney's fees. If the plaintiff does not prevail, and the verdict and judgment find that the physician was not liable for the plaintiff's injuries, no damages are awarded to the plaintiff.

POST-SUIT PHASE

Appeals

An appealable decision is one that can receive appellate review during which time the payment of the judgment (i.e., money damages) is generally suspended until the appeal is decided. There are two levels of appeal. First, there is an appeal to the appropriate Court of Appeals. The primary function of this appeal is "correctness review," which strives to satisfy a litigant's desire for a correct result. Second, there may be review by the Supreme Court. The primary function here is "institutional review," which strives to serve the systemic need for overview of the judicial law-making branch. This largely discretionary review in a single court is granted only in important cases. Appeal does not entail a retrial of the case but rather an academic reconsideration of the reviewable issues in search of prejudicial error.

A reviewable issue is one that the appellate court considers on appeal from the trial court decision. Ordinarily, to be reviewable, an act by the trial court that supposedly affected the decision must have been objected to at the time of the act, must appear in the record, and must be asserted on appeal. There are some issues that the appellate court does not review. The alleged error must not have been harmless.

Returning to Normal

The stress of a malpractice suit, whatever the outcome, cannot be underestimated.[28] The physician often believes that the practice of medicine is less rewarding and more burdensome. Time usually lessens the bitterness. If it persists, professional help should be considered. If the suit uncovers gaps in a physician's knowledge, continuing education is indicated.

Prevention of Future Suits

A study[29] of hundreds of professional negligence cases handled by the Michigan Physicians Mutual Liability Company and other data[8] suggest that certain physician attitudes and behaviors may trigger suits. Modification of inappropriate behavior and correction of certain attitudes should go far to lessen the possibility of suit.

The physician must concentrate on the task at hand. Whether it is diagnosis, treatment, recordkeeping, or follow-up, concentration may be the best way to avoid a bad result or a lawsuit. It is certainly the most obvious way. Many malpractice suits lost by physicians involved adequate care but inadequate, illegible, or incomplete records.

Concern for patients and families is critical. People seldom sue their friends. It is important that a physician show interest in the whole person rather than just the clinical aspects of the case. Physicians should be especially cognizant of their attitudes and actions if the patient/family expresses unhappiness or if an obviously bad result has occurred.

Good communication is essential. Surveys suggest that this is the single thing that patients and family want more of. Good communication with nursing and ancillary staff also helps a physician avoid the misunderstandings and hurt feelings that have on occasion prompted some staff members to suggest litigation to patients. The most important flow of information in the intensive care setting is between physicians, especially when one consults or signs out to another.

Obtaining informed consent is essential for physicians. Obtaining informed consent means spelling out the proposed course of action, potential complications, alternative therapies, and the consequences of simply refusing care. All explanations must be conducted in a manner that enables the individual or family to understand and participate in the decision-making process. This is not a job that can be left to a nurse. After agreeing on a clinical course of action, the patient's informed consent should be documented in writing. Remember that the failure to obtain consent before proceeding with treatment may result in a battery.

A consultant should be obtained in difficult cases. No physician should undertake a case for which he or she is inadequately trained, and a wise physician seeks competent consultation early. Contrary to what some physicians believe, calling on a consultant for help can reinforce the patient's good feeling for the physician.

Courage in the face of adversity is mandatory. The physician cannot "withdraw" when an untoward result occurs. A poor result does not necessarily guarantee a lawsuit, which will be less likely if the physician continues to do his or her utmost for the patient. Try to avoid the development of an adversarial relationship. If a suit is filed and a patient's injuries do arise from physician negligence, the more practical approach may be to cooperate with the insurance company to dispose of the matter quickly, fairly, and economically. Insisting on the defense of an indefensible lawsuit serves no purpose. Admitting liability out of a sense of remorse, guilt, or panic is equally unwise. An error in judgment, choosing one course of action over another, is not necessarily malpractice. Medicine is an inexact science, and only some bad outcomes are preventable.

Personal Survival Strategy

The physician faced with a threatened or actual malpractice suit generally experiences anger, frustration, a loss of self-esteem, and occasionally significant clinical depression.[28] The physician must expect interruptions, often extended, for conferences, depositions, and the trial itself if one takes place. Adequate preparation is essential at all stages, and preparation takes time. The physician must make it available to himself or herself, using associates to cover his or her schedule as needed. Candor with associates is helpful. Malpractice suits do not stay secret, so it is useless to expend much effort to keep people from finding out. The physician should take advantage of family support and peer support, especially if organized support exists in his or her institution or medical community. The physician should seek psychiatric help if his or her emotional state becomes significantly compromised. Physicians who take an active assertive approach to the problem seem to fare better emotionally.[30]

In summary, because it is estimated that 80% of all malpractice claims arise from incidents that occur in the hospital setting, physicians, to minimize the risk of liability, should exercise special care in their treatment of hospitalized patients, especially those with critical illness. Patients seldom sue their friends and may forgive even the most egregious error if the physician is someone they like and trust.

Carefully worded, complete, and accurate medical records are essential both for recording and communicating important and relevant clinical data to hospital personnel and other physicians and for having an accurate medical record to use in any subsequent legal proceeding. A good medical record is a fine defensive weapon. Care also should be taken to communicate information to patients and family members in a thorough, sensitive manner, allowing ample time for explanation and questions. Consent should be documented in writing. Candor and empathy are important, especially if things are going badly. Avoid the promise of success, and record what you say and do.

Continuing medical education for the physician, appropriate consultation, and documented follow-up are also important. Physicians should not attempt to render care beyond their capability.

Once suit is filed, physicians may minimize the intrusion and impact on their lives by working closely with their insurance companies and attorneys. They should review every aspect of the medical record, resolve discrepancies in their own mind, and prepare extensively for all depositions. They should not contact the plaintiff or the family or volunteer any information to the plaintiff's attorney. They must give all matters ample attention and remain involved. They must expect a suit to have a significant emotional impact on them and deal with that.

Finally, once a litigation matter has been resolved, whether through dismissal, settlement, or judgment, physicians can minimize the risk of future liability by reflecting on the treatment of the patient and the nature of the proceedings and either by altering future conduct or by continuing to be vigilant to those factors that increase the likelihood of litigation. The quality assessment and risk management capabilities of the institution should be used to the fullest in defending against and preventing lawsuits.

REFERENCES*

1. Malpractice. *In* Hospital Legal Forms, Checklists and Guidelines. Edited by H. Rowland and B. Rowland. Gaithersburg, MD, Aspen, 1986.

* Because the legal reference system is so different from the medical reference system, the reader is advised to go to a law librarian for assistance in locating resources.

2. Restatement (2d) of Torts at 281.
3. Restatement (2d) of Torts at 282.
4. Restatement (2d) of Torts at 298.
5. *United States v. Carroll Towing Company* (2nd Cir. 1947).
6. *Anderson v. Somberg,* 338 A. 2d 1 (Supreme Court of New Jersey, 1974).
7. *Report of the Commission on Medical Professional Liability,* 102 ABA Annual Report 786 (1977).
8. Shapiro, R., et al.: A survey of sued and nonsued physicians and suing patients. Arch. Intern. Med., *149:*2190, 1989.
9. Karcz, A., et al.: Preventability of malpractice claims in emergency medicine: a closed claims study. Ann. Emerg. Med., *19:*865, 1990.
10. Leape, L., et al.: The nature of adverse events in hospitalized patients. N. Engl. J. Med., *324:*377, 1991.
11. Kuehm, S., and Doyle, M.: Medication errors: 1977-88. Experience in medical malpractice claims. N. J. Med., *87:*27, 1990.
12. Younger, I., et al. (Eds.): Hospital Law Manual. Gaithersburg, MD, Aspen, 1983.
13. Furrow, B., et al. (Eds.): Health Law: Cases, Materials and Problems. St. Paul, MN, West, 1987.
14. *Mduba v. Benedicten Hospital,* 384 N.Y.S. 2d 527 (3rd Dept. 1976).
15. *Kober v. Stewart,* 417 P. 2d 476 (1966).
16. *Porter v. Sisters of St. Mary,* 756 F. 2d 669 (8th Circ., 1985).
17. *Hardy v. Brantley,* 471 So. 2d 358 (Supreme Court of Mississippi 1985).
18. *Beeck v. Tucson General Hospital,* 500 P. 2d 1153 (Supreme Court of Arizona 1972).
19. F.R. Civ. P. 8(a)(2) and Rule 12 (a).
20. F.R. Civ. P. 26(b)(1).
21. F.R.E. Rule 803.
22. F.R.E. 801(b)(2)(D).
23. F.R.E. 703.
24. F.R. Civ. P. 33.
25. Guidelines for the physician expert witness. Ann. Intern. Med., *113:*789, 1990.
26. F.R. Civ. P. 41 (a) and 41 (b).
27. F.R. Civ. P. 49(a)(b) and 52 (a).
28. F.R. Civ. P. 50(b).
29. Charles, S., Wilbert, J., and Kennedy, E.: Physicians self reports of reactions to malpractice litigation. Am. J. Psychiatry, *141:*563, 1984.
30. Leitch, R.: There are six basic steps to avoiding a malpractice suit. Med. Econ., March 19, 1984.
31. Wilbert, J., et al.: Coping with the stress of malpractice litigation. Ill. Med. J., *171:*23, 1987.

Chapter 82

FOREGOING LIFE-SUPPORTING OR DEATH-PROLONGING THERAPY

JAMES P. ORLOWSKI

One of the guiding philosophies of medicine is that the health and well-being of the individual patient is of paramount consideration. In keeping with this philosophy, there is a legitimate moral and legal presumption in favor of preserving life and providing beneficial medical care with the patient's informed consent.[1] Clearly, however, avoiding death should not always be the preeminent goal.[1,2] Not all technologically possible means of prolonging life need be or should be used in every case. For the gravely ill patient and for his or her family, friends, and health-care providers, decisions about the use of life-sustaining treatment have profound consequences. These decisions, to some extent, hasten or forestall the time of death. They also shape the patient's experience of his or her remaining life, where it is lived, with whom, and with what degree of comfort or suffering.[1] This chapter deals with the moral and ethical aspects of withdrawing or withholding life-sustaining therapy when the patient does not desire the treatment or when continuing to treat is equivalent to prolonging the dying process rather than sustaining or preserving meaningful life. Table 82-1 reviews basic terminology for discussion of foregoing life-supporting or death-prolonging therapy.

LIFE-SUSTAINING TREATMENT

Life-sustaining treatment is medical intervention, technology, procedure, or medication that forestalls the moment of death, whether or not the treatment affects the underlying life-threatening diseases or biologic processes.[1,2] Examples include ventilators, dialysis, cardiopulmonary resuscitation, acute surgical intervention, amputation, antibiotics, transfusions, nutrition, and hydration. Discussions about foregoing life-sustaining treatment are often raised when death is the predictable or unavoidable outcome of the patient's underlying medical condition. A patient need not be terminally ill or imminently dying, however, for these discussions to be held.

WITHHOLDING LIFE-SUSTAINING TREATMENT

A great deal of confusion and anxiety surround the differences between withholding life-sustaining treatment, which many consider morally permissible, and withdrawing treatment that has already been instituted, which some consider morally wrong. Ethically, there is no difference between withholding or withdrawing a treatment. Treatment can be ethically withdrawn whenever it can ethically be withheld.[1,2] There are, however, pyschologic and sociologic differences between withholding and withdrawing treatment. It is sometimes psychologically more difficult to withdraw treatment than to withhold it, for withdrawal may be perceived as violating a special commitment that the health care professional has made to the patient. Likewise, society may find it less intrusive never to start a therapy than to withdraw a treatment, especially when the withdrawal of the treatment may have more obvious consequences than never having started the treatment. From a medical standpoint, however, it is usually better to initiate a treatment provisionally with a plan for stopping if it proves ineffective or unduly burdensome to the patient. This approach is in contrast to withholding a treatment altogether for fear that stopping will be impossible.[1] When it is unclear whether the burdens or benefits are overwhelming, it is appropriate to choose on the side of life and provide the treatment. If a treatment is clearly futile in the sense that it will not achieve its physiologic objective and so offers no benefit to the patient, there is no obligation to provide the treatment. It is both ethically and morally preferable to try a treatment and to withdraw it if it fails than not to try it at all in appropriate situations.

EXTRAORDINARY VERSUS ORDINARY

The terms extraordinary and ordinary are often used in an attempt to distinguish a class of treatments that may be ethically withheld or withdrawn from a class of treatments that may not. Unfortunately, these terms are a source of great confusion. People sometimes distinguish ordinary from extraordinary by appealing to the prevalence of a treatment or its level of technologic complexity. No treatment is intrinsically ordinary or extraordinary.[1] Instead, decisions should be based on a balancing of the potential benefits of the therapy with the burdens to the patient of the technology needed to provide the therapy.

AUTONOMY VERSUS SELF-DETERMINATION

Patients have a right to control what happens to their bodies, so the decision about whether to use life-sustaining treatment should, in the final analysis, be theirs. This is often referred to as the principle of self-determination or autonomy. When a patient's request for specific therapy conflicts with the physician's judgment, there is no obligation either to render useless care or to violate an established community standard of practice.[1,2] Rather physicians should decide how much to do according to what they perceive is best for that patient. A physician is entitled

Table 82–1. Definition and Terminology

Life-Sustaining Treatment: Any medical intervention, technology, procedure, or medication that forestalls the moment of death, whether or not the treatment affects the underlying life-threatening diseases or biologic processes

Withholding versus Withdrawing Life-Sustaining Therapy: Withholding is never instituting, whereas withdrawing is removing or discontinuing a treatment

Extraordinary versus Ordinary Treatments: A now obsolete method for distinguishing treatments that might be ethically withheld or withdrawn from therapies that may not, based on the prevalence or technologic complexity of the treatments. Extraordinary treatments were therapies that went beyond what was usual or customary, which therefore could be withdrawn or withheld

Autonomy or Self-Determination: The right of an individual to decide on treatments or therapies and to exercise control over their destiny in accordance with their own plan for their life

Living Wills and Advance Directives: Statements documenting an individual's desires for treatments or therapies or designating a surrogate to make these decisions if the patient lacks capacity

Durable Power of Attorney: For health care, an individual's written designation of another person to act on his or her behalf in health matters. The designation is authorized by a state's durable power of attorney statute

Capacity versus Competency: Competency and incompetency are legal terms restricted to specific situations in which a formal judicial determination has been made about the decision-making ability or rights of an individual to make informed decisions in accordance with their personal values

Surrogate Decision-Maker: An individual or group of individuals designated to make the ultimate decisions for an incapacitated patient in terms of consent or refusal for a treatment plan or therapy

Ethics Committee: Groups of individuals who convene to provide consultation in difficult or complicated care or health care cases

Persistent Vegetative State: A neurologic diagnosis of permanent unconsciousness in which the patient may demonstrate periods of wakefulness and physiologic sleep, but is not aware of self or the environment

Brain Death: A diagnosis of death based on irreversible destruction of the cerebrum and brain stem, in which artificial support of ventilation may preserve peripheral organ function for a time and give the appearance of a live body because cardiac activity and peripheral organ function persist as long as mechanical ventilation is continued

---

to decline providing any treatment that he or she believes to be nonbeneficial. There is, however, a distinction between treatment a physician believes to be detrimental to a patient's best interest and treatment to which a physician has a conscientious objection. A physician must not allow the decision as to what is in the best interest of the patient to be influenced by his or her own personal beliefs. When the patient opts for a course of action that violates the health care professional's personal, ethical, or religious convictions, the professional should discuss the problem with the patient. Under the circumstances, it may be necessary to transfer the patient to another professional's care with the patient's consent.[1,2]

LIVING WILLS AND ADVANCE DIRECTIVES

Living wills and advance directives do have a legal standing in almost every state. Even in states without such laws, advance directives are useful in documenting a patient's desires in terms of terminal treatment and have the endorsement of the American Medical Association (AMA), American College of Physicians, and the American Geriatrics Society. The Joint Commission for Accreditation of Healthcare Organizations (JCAHO) is considering requiring accredited institutions to have policies concerning advance directives. Living wills and advance directives endorse the right of a patient with decision-making capacity or a designated surrogate for a patient who lacks capacity to decide to forego any life-sustaining medical treatment. Health-care professionals must in many ways be advocates for life, even as they are willing to honor decisions to forego life-sustaining therapy or to administer necessary treatment to alleviate pain that may at the same time hasten death. Physicians, however, should not participate in outright killing, either as active euthanasia or assisting in suicide.[3-5]

As part of the Omnibus Budget Reconciliation Act of 1990, the United States Congress passed The Patient Self-Determination Act, which became effective December 1, 1991. It was the intent of Congress to further patient self-determination by increasing public awareness and use of advance directives. Unfortunately, as part of the budget reconciliation process, the Act was also designed to reduce Medicare expenditures, and the intent of Congress also may have been to assume that many patients, especially the elderly, would opt to limit the expensive, intensive treatment they may receive in hospitals. Nevertheless, as of December 1, 1991, all "covered" providers participating in Medicare or Medicaid programs are required to inform patients of their right to written advance directives under the applicable state laws and to document in the medical record whether the patient has executed an advance directive. Providers must also guarantee that they will not condition care or discriminate against any patient based on whether or not the patient has executed an advance directive and must provide education on advance directives to their staff and the community.

CAPACITY VERSUS COMPETENCE

Proper determination of capacity is crucial to an ethical decision-making process. Caregivers have a duty to respect the wishes of a patient with decision-making capacity. Capacity differs from competence. Competence and incompetence are legal terms and are restricted to situations in which a formal judicial determination has been made. Decision-making capacity refers to a patient's functional ability to make informed health care decisions in accordance with the patient's personal values. The key elements to a decision-making capacity are:

- The ability to comprehend information relevant to the decision
- The ability to deliberate about the choices in accordance with personal values and goals
- The ability to communicate either verbally or nonverbally with the caregivers[1,2]

SURROGATE DECISION MAKER

When a patient lacks decision-making capacity and attempts to restore the capacity fail (rectifying reversible causes such as overmedication, pain, or dehydration) or are not possible, a surrogate must be identified who will be the ultimate source of consent or refusal to the health care team's plan of action. In identifying such an individual, the physician should first honor any surrogate the patient has chosen in advance or a court-appointed surrogate if such exists and has medical decision-making powers. In the absence of the aforementioned the goal is to find the person who is most involved with the patient and most knowledgeable about the patient's present and past feelings and preferences. This person may be the spouse, parent, adult son or daughter, adult brother or sister, legal guardian, or a close friend. A family member is generally the best choice. In the absence of an available or willing surrogate, one may need to be appointed and his or her decisions reviewed by an ethics committee. Alternatively, an ethics committee in its role as a neutral, third party may function as a surrogate. The primary function of the surrogate is to make choices as the patient would if he or she were able, also known as the substituted judgment or best interest of the patient standards of surrogate decision making.[1,2]

By law and custom, parents usually act as the surrogate decision makers for their child, but in the rare case when the treatment choice the parents are making is considered contrary to the child's best interest, an ethics committee may be consulted. Referral to a court of law should be used only as the last resort.[1,2]

PERSISTENT VEGETATIVE STATE

The persistent vegetative state (PVS) is a state of permanent unconsciousness in which patients are unaware of themselves or their environment. They exhibit no voluntary actions or behaviors, although they may exhibit periods of eyes-open wakefulness alternating with periods of sleep. The capability to demonstrate sleep/awake cycles and yet be totally unaware is the result of a functioning brain stem in the face of total loss of cerebral cortical functioning. PVS patients are generally able to breathe spontaneously and exhibit primitive reflexes and vegetative functions controlled by the brain stem but do not have the capacity to experience pain or suffering because of the absence of cerebral cortical functioning. Patients in a PVS can survive for prolonged periods of time as long as nutrition and hydration are provided artificially.[70]

BRAIN DEATH

Brain death results from brain damage that is so severe and extensive that the brain has no potential for recovery. Breathing has irreversibly ceased, owing to structural brain damage and absence of brain stem function, but circulation is maintained because of artificial ventilation. There is general agreement in the medical profession that death of the brain is an appropriate determination of death of a human being. The concept that death can be determined based on irreversible cessation of all functions of the brain is recognized through statutes or judicial decisions in most states in the United States. The model statute states that an individual is dead if he or she has sustained either irreversible cessation of circulatory and respiratory functions or irreversible cessation of the entire brain, including the brain stem, with the determination of death being made in accordance with accepted medical standards. Because the individual is dead, the concepts of life-sustaining or death-prolonging therapies becomes immaterial.

ETHICS COMMITTEES

Ethics committees have been established to provide consultation in difficult or complicated cases. Legal, medical, and ethical decisions are explored, and conflicts among family members or with the health care team are mediated. Different views regarding prognosis and indications for treatment can also be exposed. Committee review can provide assurance that full and impartial consideration has been given to a difficult ethical decision.

A number of medical and ethical organizations, including the AMA, the Hastings Center, the President's Commission for the Study of Ethical Problems in Medicine and Biomedical and Behavioral Research, the American College of Physicians, and the Society of Critical Care Medicine, have published statements or reports on foregoing life-sustaining or death-prolonging therapy.[1-3,16,29,59,70,71]

SPECIFIC TREATMENT TERMINATION GUIDELINES

Steps in withdrawing or withholding life-sustaining or death-prolonging therapy are listed in Table 82-2. Specific issues that should be addressed include:

- Cardiopulmonary resuscitation
- ICU admission
- Mechanical ventilation
- Dialysis
- Transfusion
- Antibiotics and other medications
- Nutrition and hydration
- Pain relief

Cardiopulmonary Resuscitation

Cardiopulmonary resuscitation (CPR) refers to those measures used to restore ventilation and circulation in victims in whom these functions have been interrupted. These techniques represent the pinnacle of life support because they have the potential of reversing death. Resus-

Table 82-2. Steps in Withdrawing or Witholding Life-Supporting or Death-Prolonging Therapy

Establish the medical facts and factors influencing prognosis, the benefits and burdens of treatment, and the likely outcomes of foregoing therapy

Ascertain the patient's preferences, either directly if capable or via a surrogate if incapacitated

Agree on a course of action, with potential complications anticipated and discussed when possible; agree on primacy of comfort measures, level of consciousness, pain relief, and other factors of concern to patient, family, and health care providers

Involve all health-care providers and patient's significant others in discussion and decision making as much as possible

Obtain ethics consultation in difficult cases, uncertain cases, or where a conflict exists

Proceed with plan for withholding or withdrawing treatment

citation techniques have no value in the management of irreversible or terminal disease states. They are intended to revive otherwise healthy individuals who experience some reversible catastrophe that interrupts breathing and circulation.[6] Because of the emergency character of CPR, a patient or surrogate should be consulted in advance whenever possible about whether to begin resuscitation in the event of cardiac or respiratory arrest. Any patient who is at increased risk for cardiopulmonary arrest should be given the opportunity to make a decision about CPR while still capable of making the decision. In the absence of a do not resuscitate (DNR) order, resuscitation should be attempted, and if any doubt exists over whether a decision to forego treatment has been properly made, treatment to preserve life should be given. "Show codes" or "slow codes" should be avoided—any code should be a full code. At the time of cardiac or respiratory arrest, if the health-care professional summoned to direct resuscitation realizes that CPR cannot restore cardiac and respiratory function, the professional may call off the effort.[6] Likewise, when a patient is receiving full but ineffective treatment for failure of other organ systems in an ICU and then irreversible hemodynamic or respiratory failure develops, it is appropriate not to institute cardiopulmonary resuscitation.

ICU Admission

The following patients are candidates for admission to ICUs when it is consistent with their treatment preference and goals:

- Critically ill patients who require life support for organ system failure that may be reversible or remedial
- Patients with irreversible organ system who cannot be treated appropriately in another setting
- Patients at risk of life-threatening complications who require monitoring or treatment
- Patients who are receiving a trial period of monitoring or treatment when there is doubt about the prognosis or the effectiveness of therapy.[1]

A decision to forego some forms of life-sustaining treatment such as CPR should not preclude other forms of treatment and admission to the ICU.[1,2] The intent of ICU admission is usually to employ treatment that potentially will avoid the necessity to apply CPR. Admission should be subject to the constraints imposed by the availability of space, equipment, and personnel; the needs of patients already in the unit; and the needs of others who are also candidates for admission. Patients who generally should not be admitted to the ICU include:

- Patients with documented irreversible cessation of all functions of the entire brain
- Patients who have been firmly diagnosed as irreversibly unconscious
- Patients with irreversible illness who are near death
- Patients who, while capable of making decisions, have requested that they not receive intensive care or its equivalent.[1]

Patients are entitled to refuse admission to an ICU even when doing so puts them at risk of death. Patients should not, however, be able to demand admission to an ICU. Such a request by a patient or a surrogate may be denied if admission would be medically inappropriate for the patient, detrimental to patients already in the unit, or contrary to the admission criteria.[1] Patients should be transferred from the ICU to another setting within the hospital or to another institution when intensive care will no longer benefit them, either because they have improved to a point at which intensive care is no longer necessary or because they have deteriorated to a point at which it no longer offers reasonable promise of benefit. Such triage is ethically appropriate.[1]

Mechanical Ventilation

It is important to emphasize again that treatment can ethically be withdrawn whenever it can be ethically withheld. It is not appropriate, however, to remove a ventilator-dependent patient from a ventilator without the permission of the patient or surrogate or to pretend to use the ventilator properly while intentionally using it inadequately. If inspired oxygen concentration or minute ventilation is decreased, the intent of withdrawing therapy should be stated. The responsible health care professional should not request other health care personnel to carry out a decision that he or she would not personally carry out. In the situation of a decision by a patient or a surrogate to forego ventilation, it is ethically acceptable to sedate the patient if necessary to ensure comfort. Supplemental oxygen can be used to relieve dyspnea from hypoxemia. If relieving the patient's dyspnea or other discomfort requires sedation to the point of unconsciousness, it is ethically acceptable to do so with the consent of the patient or surrogate. A patient may also decline to be weaned from a ventilator and may wish to be simply disconnected from mechanical ventilation as part of a fundamental decision to forego any life-sustaining treatment. In such a case, it is permissible to disconnect the ventilator without weaning.[1] Under these circumstances, careful attention should be given to supplemental oxygen, sedation, and analgesia.

Dialysis

A vital part of the discussion of whether to forego dialysis concerns the patient's organ transplantation options or the possibility of recovery of renal function. To make an informed decision about whether to forego dialysis in chronic renal failure, the patient or surrogate must receive an evaluation of whether the patient could receive a kidney transplant and, if so, what the transplant possibilities are and what transplantation involves. Because dialysis is frequently supervised most directly by personnel other than the health care professional responsible, it is important that all such personnel participate in the evaluation process. It is important to explore with patients already on dialysis why they wish to stop the treatment. It may be that their discomforts can be ameliorated without stopping the treatment entirely. Another important aspect of the discussion should be the question of where death will occur when the decision has been made to forego dialysis. Often a patient will wish to die in the hospital, where supportive and palliative care are readily available. If the patient wishes to die at home, the health-care professional should inform the patient and caregivers of the risks and burdens. The patient's preference concerning the place of death should ordinarily prevail as long as adequate care can be arranged.[1]

Transfusion

Among the treatments a patient may choose to forego is the administration of blood and blood products. This refusal arises most frequently on religious grounds, usually asserted by a Jehovah's Witness. An individual's freedom to act in accord with personal religious values is one aspect of autonomy, and the right of Jehovah's Witnesses to refuse blood should be recognized. As with nonreligious aspects of autonomy, however, the right of self-determination is not absolute. These exceptions include parents making decisions for a child or when the patient is pregnant or has dependent children. This is because the right to forego treatment may sometimes be restricted on the grounds that it will cause harm to specific others. To patients who are not Jehovah's Witnesses, the decision-making process may occur when serious bleeding is expected but has not yet started, when such bleeding occurs if there is time to go through the entire decision-making process, or when treatment for bleeding has started and the question is whether to continue. All patients should receive treatment for bleeding in an emergency except when the patient, while capable of making decisions, has given directions refusing blood and blood products under all circumstances.[1]

Antibiotics and Other Medications

Some patients who are terminally ill or in a severely debilitated, irreversible condition may determine that treatment with antibiotics or other medications will only prolong their pain and suffering. Decisions about using antibiotics and other medications, similar to decisions about other forms of life-sustaining treatment, require patients or other surrogates to balance carefully the potential burdens against the benefits. Respecting the considered choice of the patient or the patient's surrogate to forego life-sustaining medication does not violate the ethical mandates of the health care professionals. Only in cases in which it is necessary to override a patient's refusal of antibiotics or other life-sustaining medications for public health reasons should a patient's wishes not be upheld.[1]

Nutrition and Hydration

Medical procedures for supplying nutrition and hydration treat malnutrition and dehydration; they may or may not relieve the hunger and thirst that can occur. Conversely, hunger and thirst can be treated without necessarily using medical nutrition and hydration techniques. For instance, dehydrated patients may have their thirst relieved by having their lips and mouth moistened with ice chips or lubricants. Patients in their last days before death may spontaneously reduce their intake without experiencing hunger or thirst. Indeed, clinical experience indicates that dehydration may offer benefits for certain dying patients. Dehydration can reduce secretions and excretions, thus producing a sedative effect on the brain, making death more tolerable. Foregoing nutrition and hydration is one of the most difficult treatment decisions because of the association of nutrition and hydration with basic needs and human caring. Individual cases should be decided by balancing these basic human needs and their potential benefits with the burden to the individual of the technology needed to provide artificial nutrition and intravenous hydration. The artificial provision of nutrition and hydration is a form of medical treatment and may be foregone when requested by a patient.[1]

Pain Relief

Pain relief is an extremely important aspect of providing humane care to dying individuals. Although the majority of dying patients do not feel substantial pain, most fear the possibility of pain—perhaps more than death itself. Because the primary goal of caring for dying patients is to relieve pain and suffering unless the patient chooses otherwise, measures involving substantial risk may be considered, although they might not be undertaken to relieve the discomfort of patients with a reasonable chance of survival. Examples of such measures include percutaneous cordotomy or neurolytic blocks. The proper and adequate use of analgesics, especially narcotics, is critically important to alleviate pain for patients who are dying. Concerns about addiction or physical dependence are irrelevant to the dying patient. Likewise, psychologic dependence on narcotics is most often the result of undermedication rather than overmedication. Patients are less likely to become psychologically dependent when narcotic agents are given on a prophylactic schedule to prevent pain rather than in response to request after pain is experienced. The health-care professional should ordinarily seek to give sufficient medication to relieve pain while enabling the patient to remain as mentally alert as the patient wishes. The continuous intravenous infusion of narcotics is appropriate therapy to alleviate pain and suffering in a dying patient, even to the point of unconsciousness, with the consent of the patient or surrogate and even though alleviation of the pain and the suffering may hasten death.[1,2]

PRE-ICU PHASE

The pre-ICU time period is important in terms of foregoing life-sustaining therapy because it is the one period of time when the patient is most likely to be capable of making decisions regarding life-supporting or death-prolonging therapy.[7] Because the patient is the only person with a clear-cut legal, moral, and ethical right to make treatment decisions and is the individual most directly affected by these treatment decisions, it becomes paramount to know the wishes of the patient.[8] Unfortunately, treatment decisions regarding future occurrences are rarely discussed or recorded, even in patients with known terminal or hopeless illnesses in which the course of the disease is predictable.

The fault does not lie just with the medical profession. Few members of the public have ever discussed their feelings or wishes for life-supporting therapy with family members or friends, and even fewer have committed their desires to writing. It is estimated that fewer than 10% of the public have a living will, durable power of attorney for health care document, or advance directive.[9] Various suggestions for improving this knowledge gap have been made but with little measurable improvements to date.[9,10]

Opportunities to discuss and record treatment choices need to be made available to all individuals, regardless of health status. It is even more imperative that patients with hopeless disease states associated with a risk of sudden catastrophe or cardiopulmonary arrest be encouraged to discuss and document their desires for life-sustaining therapy while they are still capable of participating in these discussions.[7] Discussions should include not only CPR, admission to the ICU, and mechanical ventilation, but also issues of dialysis, blood product transfusions, antibiotics, and nutrition and hydration. Assurances of adequate pain control and relief of suffering should be provided to the patient because most people fear suffering and pain much more than the medical technology. At the least, the patient should designate someone to make health care decisions for them, if they become incapable of making treatment choices.

Advance directives are written documents detailing a patient's desires for future medical treatment. They include a "health care proxy" and "durable power of attorney for health care" with which a patient appoints an agent or surrogate to make health care decisions on the patient's behalf in the event the patient is unable to make or communicate these decisions as well as living wills, which are usually applicable only when the patient is terminally ill or near death.

My personal feeling is that proxies or powers of attorney are far better than a living will.[11] Living wills are often too vague and apply only when the patient is in a terminal condition or death is imminent. Living wills are also inadequate because they generally address only a single issue, the withholding or withdrawing of life-sustaining measures or the failure to take extraordinary measures to sustain a patient's life. Living wills fail to address most healthcare decisions made by a patient of surrogate.

Although patients have a right to make treatment decisions and to forego life-sustaining treatment even when medically feasible or indicated, they do not have the right to demand futile or medically contraindicated therapy. With the privilege of autonomy comes certain responsibilities, not the least of which is to use medical technology appropriately and not to abuse its availability. Therefore a patient with end-stage malignant cancer who has exhausted all treatment modalities can refuse experimental therapy but cannot demand intensive care admission and life support, or cryogenic preservation in the hope of surviving until a cure is found.

These caveats concerning rights versus responsibilities are especially pertinent to CPR. CPR was originally developed to revive otherwise healthy individuals who had suffered some unexpected catastrophe that interrupted breathing or circulation. It was never intended to be applied to individuals with irreversible or terminal disease states.[6] It has become a therapy that is applied indiscriminately to anyone except where a DNR order has been appropriately recorded.[12] CPR has been characterized as the only medical therapy that can be administered without a physician's order and, in fact, requires a physician's order to withhold its application. This has created the deplorable situation of CPR being instituted in patients with known hopeless and terminal disease states, only because the appropriate DNR order is lacking.[13-15] This has created serious ethical quandaries not only for emergency room and hospitalized patients, but also for patients with terminal diseases who desire to die at home. Home-care hospice services and emergency medical services are beginning to address the best way to handle cardiopulmonary arrests in hopelessly ill patients and patients who are DNR but outside the medical environment.[16]

Family members do not have the right to override the wishes of a competent patient, regardless of their relationship.[16] If a legally effective request to forego resuscitation has been made by a patient, that request should be honored, regardless of the wishes of the family to the contrary. In general, the wishes of family members are legally effective only when the patient is incompetent and a relative is authorized by statute or case law to act on behalf of the patient.[17] Legal precedence for family members to make treatment decisions for a patient who is or has become incompetent is lacking in most states.[18,19]

There are studies supporting the concepts of substituted judgment by family members and physicians and other studies that suggest that potential surrogate decision makers, such as health-care workers or family members, do not always decide as the patient would decide. One study supporting substituted judgment by families and physicians found no difference between 66 competent patients who decided to forego dialysis and 66 incompetent patients for whom families and physicians decided.[20] There was also no important difference between the 17 incompetent patients for whom families decided to terminate dialysis and the 47 incompetent patients for whom the physician decided.[20] In contrast are 3 studies examining patient and family preference for intensive care and comparing them with nurse or physician assessment of the value of intensive care. Neither nurses'[21] nor physicians'[22] assessments correlated strongly with patient or family decisions.[23] Patients believed that quality of life was a less important factor of judging the usefulness of intensive care than did their nurses, and physicians' evaluations of intensive care for patients under ideal life circumstances were strongly correlated with the physicians' personal preferences for intensive care. Evidence that family members do not always decide as a patient would comes from the care of Carrie Coons.[24] Mrs. Coons entered a PVS after a massive stroke and intracerebral hemorrhage. Afterwards, a sister with whom she lived and other relatives testified that Mrs. Coons had expressed a desire for more than 50 years not to be kept alive artificially. Six months after entering PVS, the New York State Supreme Court ruled that her gastrostomy feeding tube could be removed. Approximately 1 week later, she unexpectedly regained consciousness. When asked what she wanted done about the feeding tube, she replied, "That's a very difficult decision to make" and that she would like to wait on any decision about removing the gastrostomy tube.[24]

Most appropriate decisions to forego life-support occur in the pre-ICU phase. Patients who decide to forego CPR will generally not be admitted to an ICU, although there is nothing intrinsic in a DNR order prohibiting ICU admission. Many patients gain admission to the ICU because of a cardiopulmonary arrest or impending arrest. Patients who decide to forego CPR will exclude this avenue of ICU admission. A patient can be DNR without precluding other forms of treatment, including ICU admission, especially if the ICU is necessary or the most appropriate area for other therapies. Patients who choose a DNR status often desire and choose to forego ICU admission and its technology, including mechanical ventilation.

Although pretending to resuscitate a patient effectively while purposely and knowingly making an ineffective or partial attempt is to be avoided, agreements with a patient for limited resuscitation attempts are occasionally appropriate.[25] For example, a patient might request only pharmacologic therapy for an arrhythmia, without progressing to use cardiac massage or intubation. Or a patient might request only a limited attempt at bag-and-mask ventilation, without proceeding to intubation or cardiac massage. Such limited resuscitation attempts are appropriate when agreed to by physician and patient.

At the time of cardiac or respiratory arrest, the physician directing the resuscitation may terminate the effort if and when he or she realizes that CPR cannot restore cardiac and respiratory function.[6,12,26]

Patients may also choose to forego ICU admission, often as a component of foregoing life-support therapy. Although it is possible to decide to forego CPR but still desire intensive care monitoring and therapy, the opposite is usually not possible. A patient who desires CPR generally requires ICU admission if CPR is successful except perhaps in the most limited of CPR attempts. Some combinations of patient desires to forego life-support therapy may be inappropriate, such as desiring CPR but refusing ICU admission, and the physician needs to clarify these inconsistencies.

Patients may be denied access to intensive care when ICU care is unnecessary or offers no benefit. Such triage is medically and ethically appropriate.[1,2]

Patients may decide to forego mechanical ventilation and its usually required ICU admission as part of a desire to forego life-sustaining or death-prolonging therapy. When such a decision has been made capably and competently, it is appropriate to discuss and decide on therapy for sedation and to blunt air hunger and dyspnea. If the patient concurs, it is acceptable to provide adequate analgesia and sedation to alleviate distress, even to the point of possible respiratory depression and even though the therapy to relieve distress of suffering compassionately may hasten death.[13] Only the rare patient desires to remain conscious during ensuing respiratory failure, and fortunately carbon dioxide narcosis usually produces unconsciousness.

A not uncommon occurrence in the pre-ICU phase is the patient who decides to withdraw from dialysis therapy. Certain caveats that are important in any situation in which a patient desires to forego life-sustaining therapy become even more important in the patient with renal failure who decides to withdraw from dialysis.[27] One is confirmation, usually by psychiatric evaluations, that the patient is competent to make the decision.[28] Various chemical imbalances and toxicities can create organic brain syndromes, which could alter the patient's capability to decide rationally. Another is the reasons behind the decision to stop treatment. Discomforts or depression can be ameliorated without resorting to a permanent solution to a temporary problem. Still another important aspect is the participation of all health care providers, ancillary personnel, and family members in some phases of the discussion. Although the ultimate decision rests with the patient,[29] other caregivers may have important observations and data to contribute, and many individuals will be affected to various degrees by the patient's decisions. All have a right to be heard, even though none has the right to overrule a competent patient's decision.[29]

Refusal of blood products used to be made almost exclusively on religious grounds, but in this time of the acquired immunodeficiency syndrome (AIDS) crisis, more patients are refusing blood transfusions out of fear of contracting this deadly disease. This creates a difficult dilemma for physicians because a patient has the right to refuse, but if the decision is based on misconceptions and irrational fears, the refusal may not be based on truly informed dissent. There is greater ethical and legal support for foregoing transfusion because of religious beliefs than for accepting a written document or oral statement from someone other than the patient refusing transfusion when the basis for the decision is questionable or ill-informed. As in all situations involving foregoing life-supporting treatment, if questions exist about the validity or appropriateness of a decision in an emergency situation in which the patient is incapable of clarifying or reaffirming his or her stance, it is better to err on the side of life and provide treatment, pending clarification.

Decisions concerning treatment with antibiotics, chemotherapeutic agents, and other medications are an important part of the checklist of specific therapies that should be discussed with and decided on by any patient wishing to forego life-sustaining or death-prolonging interventions. The potential or likely results of withholding or administering these agents should be conjectured and the patient's wishes recorded.

Foregoing nutrition and hydration is one of the most heavily debated issues on medical care and medical ethics at present. Clearly, a competent patient has the right to forego nutrition and hydration and its artificial provision as part of wishes to forego life-sustaining and death-prolonging therapies. What is heavily contested is whether others, such as family members or physicians, can make the decision to withdraw or withhold the artificial provision of nutrition and hydration from incompetent patients when the patient's desires are unknown or uncertain.[30–32] Various states have enacted living will and power of attorney for health-care legislation that specifically excludes the refusal or discontinuation of nutrition or hydration unless provision of nutrition or hydration would shorten the patient's life, could not be assimilated, would not provide comfort, or lack of hydration or nutrition would not result in death by dehydration or malnutrition. The official stance of the AMA[3,30] and the position taken by the President's Commission[2] and the Hastings Center[1] is that the artificial provision of nutrition and hydration, that is, other than eating and drinking by mouth, is a medical therapy and can be withheld or withdrawn when it is no longer a benefit or when the burdens exceed the benefits.

Pain management is central to the compassionate medical care of any patient and becomes the primary goal of caring for dying patients. Decisions concerning the degree of mental alertness and the adequacy of pain relief should involve the patient whenever possible. It is now an accepted standard of medical care that therapy to alleviate pain and suffering in the dying patient is not only appropriate, but also desirable, even though alleviation of pain and suffering as a primary goal may hasten death.[1,2]

Whenever possible, discussions with patients should occur and decisions be documented concerning their wishes before critical illness or deterioration occurs that will compromise their ability to express their decisions.[33-36] Certain illnesses have highly predictable courses and outcomes that permit informed discussions and decisions to be made while the patient is still capable.[37-40] Medical personnel occasionally hesitate to broach these topics for fear of distressing or depressing the patient. Studies have shown that most patients want and need open discussion of prognosis and treatment options.[39,40] The appropriate time for these discussions to occur is in the pre-ICU phase.

ICU PHASE

The ICU phase of foregoing life-supporting or death-prolonging therapy takes on an entirely different perspective from the pre-ICU phase because the majority of patients in an ICU are no longer conscious or capable of expressing their wishes and participating in decision making.[41,42] The occasional conscious and capable patient may forego therapy, if that is their wish.[43] These unique ICU patients include ventilator-dependent patients with neuromuscular diseases who are intact cerebrally and acute burn patients. Compassionate studies of massive third-degree burn patients with unprecedented survival odds being given the opportunity to forego aggressive therapy and opt for comfort measures only have been published.[44,45] Of 24 patients diagnosed on admission to have injuries without precedent of survival, 21 chose nonheroic medical care.

Unfortunately, the reality of the ICU is that most patients cannot participate in decision making. Even those patients who are conscious are so overwhelmed psychologically and physiologically that their decision-making capacity may be overwhelmed and unreliable.

A health-care proxy or durable power of attorney for health care is only effective as long as the patient is incapacitated. The power is automatically revoked if the patient regains the ability to communicate or make decisions on his or her own. Physicians are required to comply with the directions given by a valid health-care agent. A physician may decline on moral or religious grounds to honor a health-care decision made by an agent if the physician would not honor the same request if made by the patient. In such a circumstance, the physician must transfer the patient to another physician, either in the same facility or an equivalent facility, who will honor the decision. If a physician believes that a proxy is not valid or is acting in bad faith or contrary to the patient's wishes, the physician or institution must seek judicial review. The existence of a proxy does not prevent a physician from performing procedures necessary for comfort care or pain alleviation. Most states give physicians the right to administer sedatives and painkillers regardless of the directions of the agents.

Because of patients' incapacity, decisions will have to be made for many patients in the ICU. The question becomes who is best able to make decisions for the patient when the patient is incapable. It is generally assumed that in the absence of advance directives or a durable power of attorney for health care, a spouse, close family member, or close friend might substitute judgment for the patient. Unfortunately, legal precedence for such decision making is lacking in most states. Nevertheless, it is both ethically and morally sound to have the family participate in decision making when the patient is incapable and to express the wishes of the patient as they understand them.[46] If there are questions about the motives of family or friends wanting to withdraw support and such a decision is contrary to medical opinion, one should err on the side of life. Such a situation is rare.

More common problems develop when family members desire to continue all heroic measures despite a medical opinion that the situation is hopeless. As stated previously, there is no obligation to provide futile therapy.[1,2,47] In such a situation, it is advisable to get at least one other supporting medical opinion of futility and to work with the family as much as possible to help them see the reality of the situation.[48] An ethics committee or neutral third party can sometimes help in resolving an impasse.[41]

Another common occurrence is the critically ill patient in the ICU who has no identifiable next of kin to participate in decision making. If the patient is incapable of decision making, a surrogate decision maker may need to be appointed.[31,42] An ethics committee can frequently help in this situation by assisting in finding a surrogate or acting as one.[41] Unfortunately, there is no legal precedence for such action, and in many states one may need to resort to the courts for the formal appointment of an individual to act as the guardian or conservator for the patient.

Who and how one defines futility are controversial.[49-51] Scoring systems now exist that can assign a risk of mortality based on objective data gathered on admission to the ICU.[51,53] Studies have shown that experienced clinicians and nurses are as accurate in predicting mortality,[54] but the scoring system adds an air of objectivity and precision. There are also published data stating that survival with simultaneous failure of three or more organ systems for 5 or more days is unprecedented.[55,56] These data permit an objective quantification of futility.

There are also data on in-hospital and ICU performance of CPR both in terms of immediate survival and survival to hospital discharge as well as the quality of that survival.[12,26,57-59] Various studies have documented a 2 to 3% incidence of chronic PVS after CPR.[57,59] These studies have prompted some experts to define in-hospital CPR as a "desperate technique that works relatively infrequently and, in many types of patients, virtually never."[12]

There are also disease states in which if the patient progresses to cardiopulmonary arrest, the chances of recovery are nil or near nil. These include severe, chronic congestive heart failure and treatment for refractory malignancies.[37,38,60,61]

In the absence of patient or family consent, there are situations in the ICU in which withholding CPR is appropriate.[12,60,61] A physician responsible for and knowledgeable about the care of a patient may legitimately decide that CPR is futile and may withhold instituting CPR.[6,47,62] An example of such a situation is the patient who has been undergoing an "ongoing chemical code" consisting of progressive, massive escalations of pressors and inotropes and continues to deteriorate to the point of cardiac arrest. The institution of cardiac compressions is clearly futile and inappropriate, especially if the disease is known and the progression is not unexpected. This is no different than the standard policy of a physician ceasing CPR efforts when it is clear that the efforts are futile.[6]

Triage of patients into and out of the ICU is a reality of the practice of critical care medicine and is ethically appropriate. The availability of space and personnel as well as cost factors dictates that patients are discharged out of the ICU when intensive care will no longer benefit them or when a more ill patient or a patient with a greater chance of benefit is in need of admission and space or personnel are limited. Lack of benefit from intensive care not only occurs when a patient has improved to a point at which intensive care is no longer necessary, but also when a patient has deteriorated to a point at which intensive care no longer offers a reasonable expectation of benefit.[63]

Mechanical ventilation is usually not withdrawn from an ICU patient without the permission of the patient or surrogate, unless the patient is being weaned from mechanical ventilation therapeutically.[64] An exception to this statement is the patient who has fulfilled the criteria for a diagnosis of brain death. Except to maintain organ viability for transplantation, there is no requirement to continue to ventilate a brain-dead patient.[1,2] Ventilator-dependent patients can be transferred out of an ICU when a step-down unit for ventilator-dependent patients exists, regular nursing floor provisions for such patients exist, or transfer to a chronic care facility or home program has been arranged, and ICU care is no longer needed.

In the situation in which a decision has been made by a patient or surrogate to forego mechanical ventilation in the ICU, decisions about weaning versus disconnection should be worked out in advance as well as decisions about sedation to ensure comfort.[64] If agreed to by patient or surrogate, it is appropriate to sedate to the point of unconsciousness to relieve dyspnea or discomfort.[1,2]

As part of a concerted effort to forego futile therapy in a hopeless situation, it is appropriate to discontinue oxygen therapy, positive airway pressure therapy, and even mechanical ventilation. In such a situation, the medical attention should be directed to alleviating pain and suffering and providing comfort.

In the ICU setting, decisions to forego dialysis, either by not instituting the therapy or discontinuing its use, can be made by patients or surrogates as a conscious decision to forego life-supporting or death-prolonging therapy[27,42] or by physicians when it is clear that the therapy is futile and will not achieve the desired treatment goals.[1,2]

Patient and surrogates may elect to forego transfusions of blood and blood products. When such decisions are made as a therapeutic restriction rather than a choice to forego life-sustaining therapy, it can cause significant limitations on therapeutic options, especially because currently available blood substitutes have not proved effective. In the acutely and critically bleeding situation, such a decision may mean certain death. Nevertheless, the legal precedence is clearly in favor of supporting a competent adult's right to make such a decision.[1,2,42] Blood salvage and retransfusion is an available option in only a severely restricted number of circumstances and is usually not feasible in the typical ICU patient. In circumstances of slow bleeds or chronic anemias, various options are available to patients who refuse transfusions, including erythropoietin and intravenous iron infusion. These therapies require 7 to 10 days to produce a noticeable effect and therefore are not usually effective in the typical ICU patient. Blood and blood product transfusions can also be foregone by patients or families when withdrawing or withholding therapies or by physicians when the transfusions prove futile and will not attain a physiologic goal.

A patient or surrogate may choose to forego any medication as part of withdrawing or withholding life-sustaining or death-prolonging therapy. Overriding such a decision may rarely be necessary, such as instituting or continuing antibiotics for infection control purposes.[1,2] Specific medicines that are often foregone in ICUs include vasopressors, inotropes, antiarrhythmics, and antibiotics. These medicines can also be withdrawn by physicians when their continued use is futile and will not achieve the desired goals. As a general principle, these medicines can also be withheld when their use would be futile, although in many cases it is better to try the agent and withdraw it if it fails to achieve its physiologic objective than not to try it at all.[1] Clinical judgment usually dictates the best course of action.

Nutrition and hydration are usually not forgone in the ICU except as part of an overall decision to withhold or withdraw all life-supporting measures.[32]

Pain relief or control is an important aspect of intensive care, and its provision in adequate doses or measures takes on a paramount role when a decision has been reached to forego life-sustaining or death-prolonging therapies. When medicine can no longer cure, it has a duty to comfort. Although most dying patients probably do not feel substantial pain, in the absence of known or assured absence of pain, it is better to err on the side of comfort and provide adequate analgesia. The continuous intravenous infusion of narcotics is appropriate therapy to alleviate pain and suffering in the dying patient.[1,2] Patients who fulfill the criteria for a diagnosis of brain death are medically and legally dead, and all technology and therapies can be withdrawn. On occasion, a brain-dead patient may be maintained on medical therapies, usually to harvest organs for organ donation and sometimes to permit family and loved ones time to accept the diagnosis. There is no obligation or necessity to maintain a dead body by technologies or therapies if triage dictates that a living patient could benefit from the bed space, personnel, or technology. In fact, maintaining a dead body by technologic means is potentially harmful to the public image of medicine.

POST-ICU PHASE

The post-ICU phase is important because the recent admission to the ICU may portend a different course for the primary illness than had been expected, and the ICU experience may influence the patient's decisions concerning life-supporting therapy in the future. Some patients fear the technology less after experiencing intensive care, whereas others find the loss of control and autonomy even more intolerable.[65,66] The ICU admission and discharge should be used as an opportunity to discuss and clarify further patient desires for life-support treatments in the future.[67,68]

Functional capacity and physiologic status may have improved as a result of intensive care, may be relatively unchanged, may have deteriorated somewhat with the potential for some regain, or may be significantly worse. These factors can have impact on the decision-making process.[69,70]

Patients may choose to forego CPR and request a DNR status as part of a purposeful decision to avoid heroic life-sustaining or death-prolonging therapy. Alternatively a surrogate decision maker in consultation with physicians may decide that CPR would be contrary to the wishes of the patient and unlikely to benefit the patient and request a DNR status.[70,71]

Patients may decide against future ICU admissions based on their prognosis and experience with previous ICU admissions. Surrogates for incompetent patients may also choose to forego ICU admissions when, in consultation with the physicians involved, it is decided that ICU care would not benefit the patient and would be inconsistent with the desires of the patient as expressed when the patient was competent.

Some patients are discharged from the ICU while still requiring mechanical ventilation. Mechanical ventilation is provided either continually or intermittently in a step-down unit, regular nursing floor, chronic care facility, or at home. The intent is usually to wean the patient from mechanical ventilation eventually, although some patients, because of neuromuscular diseases, will never be able to be weaned. Patients receiving mechanical ventilation outside of the ICU environment may elect to be DNR in the event of cardiac arrest and may choose not to be readmitted to the ICU if their condition worsens. Surrogates may also choose such options based on the medical prognosis and their knowledge of the patient's preferences.

An interesting dilemma that can develop is the patient who is DNR at his or her request but then develops an iatrogenic complication or accident that results in a cardiopulmonary arrest. The question is whether or not the patient should be resuscitated. Examples are a patient on mechanical ventilation who is DNR and suffers a cardiac arrest because of a power failure or disconnection and an oncology patient with bone marrow depression receiving amphotericin B therapy for fever of unknown origin who suffers a cardiac arrest because of hypokalemia but is DNR. The best resolution of these ethical dilemmas is to analyze why the patient is DNR and to discuss these possibilities with the patient in advance and ascertain his or her wishes. If the patient was DNR because he or she did not wish to be resuscitated from the expected downhill course of disease, but an iatrogenic complication occurs unrelated to the normal progression of the primary disease and there is still a possibility of cure or improvement of the primary disease, then one should err on the side of life and resuscitate. If the complication is not unexpected as part of the progression of the primary disease or the patient had already expressed that he or she would prefer to die quickly as a result of a complication rather than slowly from the primary disease, then the DNR status should be respected. Whenever possible, the patient's desires should be ascertained, although most complications are unexpected and therefore will not have been anticipated and discussed in advance.

Patients receiving mechanical ventilation outside of the ICU may choose to withdraw or discontinue the therapy.[64] Such a decision may be difficult for health-care providers and families to accept, but if the patient is competent and capable of making the decision and is not being adversely influenced by psychiatric, family, financial, or social concerns, the decision should be respected. Withdrawing a therapy such as mechanical ventilation is often more difficult to accept psychosocially than withholding the same treatment. Nevertheless, there is no difference from the ethical standpoint, and any therapy that could be withheld can be withdrawn.[1,2]

If the patient desires, it is ethically acceptable to sedate the patient even to the point of unconsciousness and even if sedation may hasten death to ensure comfort.

Patients may choose to discontinue hemodialysis in the post-ICU phase, and this decision may be reached once the time course makes it clear that spontaneous renal function will not be regained and dialysis therapy will need to be chronic. This decision may be reached in concert with the medical opinion that transplantation is not an alternative because of coexisting medical problems or contraindications. If the decision is medically and ethically supportable, the emphasis switches to patient comfort and care.

The decision to withdraw dialysis may also be made for incompetent patients by surrogates in consultation with the patient's health-care providers. This decision is appropriate when the therapy will not achieve a physiologic goal, is much more of a burden than benefit to the patient, and the patient had previously expressed a desire not to be maintained alive in this way.[1,2]

Patients may choose to forego other therapies in the post-ICU phase, including transfusions, antibiotics, and other medications. When these choices are made by a psychologically sound and competent patient, they should be respected.

Patients may also choose to forego nutrition and hydration by artificial means. The more difficult situation is when a surrogate wishes to forego the artificial provision of nutrition and hydration. Again, the ethically most appropriate course of action is to balance the benefits versus burdens of the treatment and the expressed or assumed wishes of the patient. The artificial provision of nutrition and hydration is a form of medical treatment and may be foregone when requested by a patient. Whether a family member or surrogate can substitute judgment for the patient remains to be determined legally. Ethically, it is appropriate if the family member or surrogate is speaking on behalf of the patient and has only the patient's best interests and concerns in mind.[1,2]

Pain relief and pain management remain important in the post-ICU phase, especially for patients foregoing life-sustaining or death-prolonging therapy.

In conclusion, death is a difficult concept for any of us to accept. Despite most religions in the world professing a belief in life after death, most humans have difficulty conceptualizing an afterlife and prefer to cling to life as they know it. Physicians are no different. Their education and training are directed at preserving and prolonging life, and as a corollary, they equate the death of a patient with a failure to meet their goals and expectations. This chapter has dealt with the moral and ethical aspects of withdrawing or withholding life-sustaining therapy when the patient does not desire the treatment or when continuing to treat is equivalent to prolonging the dying process rather than sustaining or preserving a meaningful life. In many ways, the medical profession was more simple in days past when the physician could only rarely cure and spent most of his or her time comforting and caring. Modern technology has equipped us with the capabilities to maintain the living organism for prolonged periods of time, so now we must grapple with the concepts of quality of life, the potential for restoration of cognizant functioning, the PVS, and the prolongation of the dying process.

REFERENCES

1. Hastings Center: Guidelines on the Termination of Life-Sustaining Treatment and the Care of the Dying. Hastings Center, 1987.
2. Presidents Commission for the Study of Ethical Problems in Medicine and Biomedical and Behavioral Research: Deciding to forego life-sustaining treatment—a report on the ethical, medical, and legal issues in treatment decisions. Washington, D.C., U.S. Government Printing Office, 1983.
3. The Council on Ethical and Judicial Affairs of the American Medical Association. AMA Council Report C/A-88. Chicago, American Medical Association, 1988.
4. Orentlicher, D.: Physician participation in assisted suicide. JAMA, 262:1844, 1989.
5. American College of Physicians: American College of Physicians Ethics Manual. Part 2: The Physician and Society; research; life-sustaining treatment; other issues. Ann. Intern. Med., 111:327, 1989.
6. Standards and Guidelines for Cardiopulmonary Resuscitation (CPR) and Emergency Cardiac Care (ECC). JAMA, 255:2979, 1986.
7. Amchin, J., et al.: Interview assessment of critically ill patients regarding resuscitation decisions. Gen. Hosp. Psychiatry, 11:103, 1989.
8. Kass, L.: Ethical dilemmas in the care of the ill. JAMA, 244:1946, 1980.
9. Emanuel, L. L., and Emanuel, E. J.: The medical directive. JAMA, 261:3288, 1989.
10. Vinicky, J. K., and Kanoti, G. A.: Informed consent, bioethics, and patient value histories. Phys. Assist., 8:87, 1987.
11. Orlowski, J. P.: Ethical principles in critical care medicine. Crit. Care Clin., 2:13, 1986.
12. Blackhall, L. J.: Must we always use CPR? N. Engl. J. Med., 317:1281, 1987.
13. Jonsson, P. A., McNamee, M., and Campion, E. W.: The "Do Not Resuscitate" order. Arch. Intern. Med., 148:2373, 1988.
14. Petty, T. L.: Don't just do something—stand there! Arch. Intern. Med., 139:920, 1979.
15. Annas, G. J.: CPR: when the beat should stop. The Hastings Center Report, 12:30, 1982.
16. Ayres, R. J.: Current controversies in prehospital resuscitation of the terminally ill patient. Prehosp. Dist. Med., 5:49, 1990.
17. Stanley, J. M.: The Appleton Consensus: suggested international guidelines for decisions to forego medical treatment. J. Med. Ethics, 15:129, 1989.
18. Nelson, L. J., and Golenski, J. D.: Surrogate decision making for mentally incapacitated adults. Clin. Ethics Report, 1:1, 1987.
19. Suber, D. G., and Tabor, W. J.: Withholding of life-sustaining treatment from the terminally ill, incompetent patient: who decides? JAMA, 248:2431, 1982.
20. Silva, J. E., and Kjellstrand, C. M.: Withdrawing life support. Nephron, 48:201, 1988.
21. Danis, M., et al.: A comparison of patient, family, and nurse evaluation of the usefulness of intensive care. Crit. Care Med., 15:138, 1987.
22. Danis, M., Gerrity, M. S., Southerland, L. I., and Patrick, D. L.: A comparison of patient, family, and physician assessments of the value of medical intensive care. Crit. Care Med., 16:594, 1988.
23. Danis, M., Patrick, D. L., Southerland, L. I., and Green, M. L.: Patients' and families' preferences for medical intensive care. JAMA, 260:797, 1988.
24. Steinbock, B.: Recovery from persistent vegetative state? The case of Carrie Coons. Hastings Center Report, 19:14, 1989.
25. Wilson, J., and Pugh, D.: Limited cardiopulmonary resuscitation: the ethics of partial codes. Q. Rev. Bioethics, 1:4, 1988.
26. Taffet, G. E., Teasdale, T. A., and Luchi, R. J.: In-hospital cardiopulmonary resuscitation. JAMA, 260:2069, 1988.
27. Lowance, D. C., Singer, P. A., and Siegler, M.: Withdrawal from dialysis: an ethical perspective. Kidney Int., 34:124, 1988.
28. Drane, J. F.: Competency to give an informed consent. JAMA, 252:925, 1984.
29. Abrams, F. R.: Withholding treatment when death is not imminent. Geriatrics, 42:77, 1987.
30. Council on Scientific Affairs and Council on Ethical and Judicial Affairs: Persistent vegetative state and the decision to withdraw or withhold life support. JAMA, 263:426, 1990.
31. Areen, J.: The legal status of consent obtained from families of adult patients to withhold or withdraw treatment. JAMA, 258:229, 1987.
32. Steinbrook, R., and Lo, B.: Artificial feeding—solid ground, not slippery slope. N. Engl. J. Med., 318:286, 1988.
33. Evans, A. L., and Brody, B. A.: The Do-Not-Resuscitate order in teaching hospitals. JAMA, 253:2236, 1985.
34. Youngner, S. J., et al.: "Do Not Resuscitate" orders. JAMA, 253:54, 1985.
35. Bedell, S. E., Pelle, D., Maher, P. L., and Cleary, P. D.: Do-

Not-Resuscitate orders for the critically ill patients in hospital. JAMA, 256:233, 1986.
36. Lipton Levens, H.: Do-Not-Resuscitate decisions in a community hospital. JAMA, 256:1164, 1986.
37. Lawrence, V. A., and Clark, G. M.: Cancer and resuscitation. Arch. Intern. Med., 147:1637, 1987.
38. Wachter, R. M., Luce, J. M., Hearst, N., and Lo, B.: Decisions about resuscitation: inequities among patients with different diseases but similar prognoses. Ann. Intern. Med., 111:525, 1989.
39. Wanzer, S. H., et al.: The physician's responsibility toward hopelessly ill patients. N. Engl. J. Med., 310:955, 1984.
40. Wanzer, S. H., et al.: The physician's responsibility toward hopelessly ill patients. A second look. N. Engl. J. Med., 320:844, 1989.
41. Brennan, T. A.: Incompetent patients with limited care in the absence of family consent. Ann. Intern. Med., 109:819, 1988.
42. Luce, J. M., and Raffin, T. A.: Withholding and withdrawal of life support from critically ill patient. Chest, 94:621, 1988.
43. Cassell, E. J.: Autonomy in the intensive care unit: the refusal of treatment. Crit. Care Clin., 2:27, 1986.
44. Imbus, S. H., and Zawacki, B. E.: Autonomy for burn patients when survival is unprecedented. N. Engl. J. Med., 297:308, 1977.
45. Imbus, S. H., and Zawacki, B. E.: Encouraging dialogue and autonomy in the burn intensive care unit. Crit. Care Clin., 2:53, 1986.
46. Luce, J. M.: Ethical principles in critical care. JAMA, 263:696, 1990.
47. Ramos, T., and Reagan, J. E.: "No" when the family says "go": resisting families' requests for futile CPR. Ann. Emerg. Med., 18:898, 1989.
48. Mackillop, W. J., et al.: Clinical trials in cancer: the role of surrogate patients in defining what constitutes an ethically acceptable clinical experiment. Br. J. Cancer, 59:388, 1989.
49. Youngner, S. J.: Who defines futility? JAMA, 260:2094, 1988.
50. Lantos, J. D., et al.: The illusion of futility in clinical practice. Am. J. Med., 87:81, 1989.
51. Lantos, J. D., Miles, S. H., Silverstein, M. D., and Stocking, C. B.: Survival after cardiopulmonary resuscitation in babies of very low birth weight—is CPR futile therapy? N. Engl. J. Med., 318:91, 1988.
52. Knaus, W. A., et al.: APACHE—acute physiology and chronic health evaluation: a physiologically based classification system. Crit. Care Med., 9:591, 1981.
53. Knaus, W. A., Draper, A., Wagner, D. P., and Zimmerman, J. E.: An evaluation of outcome from intensive care in major medical centers. Ann. Intern. Med., 104:410, 1986.
54. Kruse, J. A., Thill-Baharozian, M. C., and Carlson, R. W.: Comparison of clinical assessment with APACHE II for predicting mortality risk in patients admitted to a medical intensive care unit. JAMA, 260:1739, 1988.
55. Knaus, W. A., Draper, E. A., and Wagner, D. P.: Prognosis in acute organ-system failure. Ann. Surg., 202:685, 1985.
56. Knaus, W., and Wagner, D.: Individual patient decisions. Crit. Care Med., 17:S204, 1989.
57. Bedell, S., Delbanco, T. L., Cook, E. F., and Epstein, F. H.: Survival after cardiopulmonary resuscitation in the hospital. N. Engl. J. Med., 309:569, 1983.
58. Camarata, S. J. et al.: Cardiac arrest in the critically ill. Circulation, 44:688, 1971.
59. Johnson, A. L., et al.: Results of cardiac resuscitation in 552 patients. Am. J. Cardiol., 20:831, 1967.
60. Bioethics Committee for the American College of Emergency Physicians: Medical, moral, legal and ethical aspects of resuscitation for the patient who will have minimal ability to function or ultimately survive. Ann. Emerg. Med., 14:919, 1985.
61. Hassett, J. M., and Wear, S. E.: An ethical challenge in critical care: the severely injured patient. J. Crit. Care, 2:194, 1987.
62. Stanley, D. P., and Reid, D. P.: Withholding cardiopulmonary resuscitation: one hospital's policy. Med. J. Aust., 151:257, 1989.
63. Zimmerman, J. E., et al.: The use and implications of Do Not Resuscitate orders in intensive care units. JAMA, 255:351, 1986.
64. Schneiderman, L. J., and Spragg, R. G.: Ethical decisions in discontinuing mechanical ventilation. N. Engl. J. Med., 318:984, 1988.
65. Bergbom-Enberg, I., and Haljamae, H.: Assessment of patients' experience of discomforts during respiratory therapy. Crit. Care Med., 78:1068, 1989.
66. Cassel, E. J.: The nature of suffering and the goals of medicine. N. Engl. J. Med., 306:639, 1982.
67. La Puma, J., et al.: Life-sustaining treatment. Arch. Intern. Med., 148:2193, 1988.
68. Everhart, M. A., and Pearlman, R. A.: Stability of patient preferences regarding life-sustaining treatment. Chest, 97:159, 1990.
69. Cranford, R. E.: Termination of treatment in the persistent vegetative state. Semin. Neurol., 4:36, 1984.
70. Youngner, S. J.: Do Not Resuscitate orders: no longer secret, but still a problem. Hastings Center Report, 17:24, 1987.
71. Position of the American Academy of Neurology on certain aspects of the care and management of the persistent vegetative state patient. Neurology, 39:125, 1989.
72. Task Force on Ethics of the Society of Critical Care Medicine: Consensus Report on the Ethics of Foregoing Life-Sustaining Treatment in the Critically Ill. Crit. Care Med., 18:1435, 1990.

SUPPLEMENTAL READINGS

Council on Ethical and Judicial Affairs of the AMA: Decisions near the end of life. JAMA, 267:2229, 1992.

Orlowski, J. P., and Vinicky, J. K.: The implications of DNR orders for critical care medicine. Clin. Pulm. Med., 1:39, 1994.

Orlowski, J. P., Collins, R. L., and Cancian, S. N.: Foregoing life-supporting or death-prolonging therapy: a policy statement. Cleve. Clin. J. Med., 60:81, 1993.

Stanley, J. M.: The Appelton International Conference: Developing guidelines for decisions to forego life-prolonging medical treatment. J. Clin. Ethics, 18(Suppl.):1, 1992.

Appendix

CLINICAL EPIDEMIOLOGY AND BIOSTATISTICS FOR THE INTENSIVE CARE PHYSICIAN

JOHN C. MARSHALL
AVERY B. NATHENS

The clinician should use statistics as a drunk uses a lamppost—for support rather than for illumination.
—Anonymous

Before this century, the knowledge base of clinical medicine was largely derived from tradition and the persuasive powers of its most eminent practitioners. Systematic scientific observation played a relatively minor role in understanding biologic mechanisms or in evaluating new therapies. With the transformation of medicine to a scientific discipline came a change in the way that medical knowledge is generated and evaluated. The contemporary clinician places less emphasis on the counsel of the older, more experienced clinician and more emphasis on scientific data derived from clinical and laboratory study.

The practice of contemporary critical care medicine raises innumerable questions:

- When is it safe to extubate a mechanically ventilated patient?
- What is the most effective method of diagnosing pneumonia?
- Should selective digestive tract decontamination be used to prevent pneumonia?
- What is the role of tumor necrosis factor in septic shock?
- When is withdrawal of life support appropriate?

Clinical decisions in the individual patient are categorical—to extubate or not, to start antibiotics or not, to stop therapy or to continue. The answers to such questions, however, are derived from studies of populations, and the results of these studies may be inconclusive or even contradictory; certainly they are never definitive, and they may not apply to the particular circumstances of an individual patient. The process of making a clinical decision involves the assessment of probabilities: What is the likelihood that a given action will lead to a more favorable outcome for a particular patient? The data used to evaluate probabilities come from many sources: published studies of the outcome of patients with similar problems managed by differing approaches, the clinician's experience of the outcomes of other similar patients, and the experience and expectations of other members of the health-care team and of the patient and his or her family. The latter two sources are commonly referred to as the "art" of medicine, whereas the former is the science. The science of medicine, similar to its application to clinical decision making, depends on the analysis of probabilities—the field of biostatistics. The application of this analysis is the focus of the emerging field of clinical epidemiology.

The need for a formal discipline of clinical epidemiology arises because of the inherent uncertainty that underlies clinical decision making. If we could know in advance that an intervention used in one patient would have precisely the same consequences when used in all subsequent patients, there would be no need for clinical study, and mechanistic data derived from the laboratory could be readily applied to patient care. Variability is the hallmark of living things, however, and the more complex the problem, the greater the potential for variability and the greater the need for a method of understanding its implications. Variability in biology in turn gives rise to **error** in clinical studies—the misinterpretation of data leading to a conclusion that is inconsistent with the true state of affairs. Error can arise randomly or systematically. **Random error** arises because of intrinsic differences between individuals and intrinsic inaccuracies in the techniques used to measure outcomes; systematic error or **bias** arises because of the influence of a confounding factor. Random error alters the precision of an observation; bias alters its applicability. The influence of random error can be determined by the use of biostatistics; the more subtle influence of bias can be controlled only by adherence to principles of optimal study designed that are being defined by the discipline of clinical epidemiology.

For many of us, the formal study of epidemiology and biostatistics was little more than an arcane rite of passage whose language and precepts evoked disinterest and frustration with its apparent irrelevance. It has taken the persistent efforts of a small number of pioneers of clinical epidemiology and critical appraisal (see in particular the publications in the annotated Suggested Readings) to establish the importance of these principles to the daily challenges of clinical decision making. In the ICU setting, where the clinical problems are especially complex and where a given decision may have significant implications for both cost and survival, the need for an understanding of the field is particularly important. We provide here an overview—conceptual and of necessity superficial—of biostatistics and clinical epidemiology and their uses and abuses in the study of the critically ill.

BASIC CONCEPTS IN BIOSTATISTICS
Populations, Samples, and Distribution of Data

It is a fundamental assumption of the scientific method that individual events occur in a **random** fashion, but the distribution of many random events is predictable. Statistical techniques detect deviations from randomness. Just as a pattern that deviates from randomness during a coin toss suggests that the toss is somehow rigged, deviations from those expected based on random clinical chance suggest the intervention of some other factor. This factor may be the experimental intervention of interest, or it may be an unrecognized extraneous influence resulting in bias.

A scientific investigation is undertaken to elucidate principles that apply to a particular **population**—all patients with adult respiratory distress syndrome, for example—the investigator, however, cannot study the entire population of interest but only a representative **sample**. Thus the sample must accurately reflect the larger population from which it is drawn and to which the findings of the study will be generalized. It must include only those patients who are part of the larger population and must also be large enough to reflect the intrinsic variability present in the larger population.

Comparisons between two populations are performed using numerical data derived from the study of those populations. These data may be **continuous** or **categorical**. **Continuous** data are those whose variables can assume any value, the discrimination between two adjacent values depending only on the sensitivity of the measuring device. Age, weight, duration of ICU stay, Do_2, and white blood cell count are examples of continuous variables. **Categorical** data are those that describe categories that are mutually exclusive with no intervening mean value; examples of categorical variables include gender, ICU survival, and use of antibiotics. Categorical variables representing a series of ordered categories (e.g., incremental increases in APACHE II score, for example) are known as **ordinal** variables. A continuous variable can be expressed as an average; a categorical variable can be expressed as a percentage. Differing statistical tests are used for continuous variables and categorical variables. Of course, some variables may be expressed either as continuous or categorical data—mean APACHE scores versus the number of patients within a given APACHE increment. In general, tests based on the use of a continuous variable are more sensitive to differences, and therefore studies in which the outcome of interest is a continuous variable are more likely to demonstrate an effect for a given number of patients. Categorical outcomes, however, are generally more definitive and easier to interpret (e.g., survival, discharge from hospital within 28 days).

If a sufficient number of observations are made of a continuous variable whose outcome is random (the height of a group of people or the age of a group of ICU patients), the distribution of these observations assumes the classic bell shape of a normal distribution. Normally distributed data are analyzed using a **parametric** test. If the data are not normally distributed, a **nonparametric** test must be used.

Sample and Population Descriptors

Populations and samples are described by their **central tendency** and **variability**. The common descriptors of central tendency are the **mean** and **median**. The **sample mean** is defined as the sum of the measurements divided by the total number of measurements and is used to approximate the **population mean**, denoted by the Greek letter, μ. (By convention, descriptors of the sample are denoted by English letters and descriptors of the population by Greek letters). The **median** is defined as that value for which 50% of the observations are larger and 50% of observations are smaller. In contrast to the mean, it is not affected by extreme measurements. If the data are normally distributed, the mean and the median should be roughly equal; however, this will not be the case if the data are skewed.

Measures of population variability provide an indication of the degree of spread of the individual data and include **variance** (σ^2) and **standard deviation** (σ), or s^2 and s, for sample variability. The variance is calculated by summing the squares of the differences between the individual data points and the sample mean and dividing by the number in the sample:

$$\text{Variance} = \frac{\Sigma(x_i - \bar{x})^2}{n}$$

The standard deviation is the square root of the variance.

Variability in the data from a series of observations can arise from many sources, including inherent biologic variability between differing individuals, the confounding effects of other biologic influences, and inaccuracies in the measurement itself. The standard deviation provides a measure of the variability of the data and is independent of the size of the population. The **standard error of the mean** provides a measure of the certainty with which the mean of a sample represents the true mean of the population from which the sample was drawn; it is, in essence, the variability of a group of means. It is calculated by dividing the standard deviation by the square root of the number of observations:

$$\text{SEM} = \sigma/\sqrt{n}$$

It is a common but erroneous practice for authors to use the standard error rather than the standard deviation when reporting the variability in experimental data because the standard error, being smaller, makes the difference between two means look more impressive when displayed in graphic or tabular form. Categorical data are commonly presented as rates, proportions, or percentages.

P Values, Significance, α and β Errors, and Sample Sizes

A scientific study tests an hypothesis; statistical analysis provides a method of determining whether the data generated by the study support or refute the hypothesis. Although the investigator hypothesizes that a particular experimental manipulation will produce a particular effect, statistical analysis evaluates the probability that no effect is present, that the samples of data are drawn from the same population. Thus a statistical analysis does not prove that an effect is present but rather evaluates the probability that the observed results occurred by chance. The investigator gains support for the study hypothesis by rejecting the null hypothesis, by demonstrating that the likelihood of the observed results occurring based on random error is small.

The probability that two samples are derived from the same population (the probability that there is no difference between two or more results) is denoted by the letter P and is referred to as the α level of an analysis. In practice, the investigator is not interested in a continuous probability estimate but in a categorical conclusion—whether or not an effect is present. Thus an arbitrary cutoff must be set for the α level, below which the investigator will conclude that any difference is too great to be accounted for by chance alone. For most studies, and by convention, this cutoff is set at P values less than 0.05, in other words, when there is less than 1 chance in 20 that the observed results can be explained based on random chance. The level of statistical significance reflects numeric probability, not biologic relevance. Differences that are statistically significant may not be of sufficient magnitude to alter clinical behavior, and, conversely, results that are statistically insignificant may be of considerable clinical relevance.

The α level is affected by the magnitude of the difference between the two groups, the degree of variability within each group (i.e., the standard deviation of the data), and the number of observations within each group. If the magnitude of the difference is small, the variability of the data large, or the number of observations small, the α level will be higher, and thus it is possible that an experimenter may incorrectly conclude that there is no difference between the two groups, when in fact there is. Thus the researcher is interested not only in the probability that an observed difference is likely to be an actual difference (the α value of a study), but also in the probability that an observed absence of a difference reflects the true absence of a difference. This latter probability is denoted as the β level of a study and is more commonly expressed as $1 - \beta$, or the **power** of a study to conclude that a negative experimental result reflects the true absence of an effect.

An investigation attempts to draw conclusions about a population by an analysis of a sample of that population. Findings derived from a sample, however, may not truly reflect the population, and two possible errors may occur: rejecting the null hypothesis when it is actually true (assuming an effect when none is present) and accepting the null hypothesis when it is actually false (concluding that there is no effect when one is present). The former is referred to as a **type I error** and is the α level of the analysis; the latter is called a **type II error** and is the β level of the analysis (Appendix Table-1).

When the magnitude of the expected result and the variability of the observations can be determined, the number

Appendix Table-1.

		Actual Biologic Effect	
	Effect	Effect	No Effect
Conclusion of Statistical test	Effect	True-positive ($1-\beta$)	False-positive (α) Type 1 error
	No effect	False-negative (β) Type II error	True-negative ($1-\alpha$)

of observations necessary to establish significance at a given α level with a specified power can be determined from readily available tables. For example, Ziegler and coworkers[1] conducted a study to assess the efficacy of monoclonal antiendotoxin antibody therapy in patients with sepsis and a presumed diagnosis of gram-negative infection. They hypothesized that antibody therapy would reduce mortality by 50% compared with placebo for patients with gram-negative infection and estimated that the 14-day mortality for patients in the placebo arm would be 30%. They set the α level at $P < 0.05$ and the β level at 0.20 (in other words, the study would have an 80% chance of demonstrating an effect if one was present and less than a 5% chance of assuming an effect to be present if in fact there was none). Based on these assumptions, they calculated a sample size of approximately 250 patients in each group. The sample size depends on the incidence of the end point in the population studied (in this case, 14-day mortality of 30%), the magnitude of the effect size anticipated in the study group (15%, i.e., a 50% reduction from baseline), and the α and β levels established for the study.

Relative Risk, Odds Ratios, and Confidence Intervals

Categorical data can be expressed as proportions or percentages; however, an alternate method of expressing differences between categorical variables is through the calculation of **relative risk** or **odds ratios.** Odds ratios are readily calculated from a standard 2×2 table, as shown here. Cockerill and colleagues[2] undertook a study to evaluate the effects of selective digestive tract decontamination (SDD) on ICU mortality and obtained the following results:

	Outcome	
	Lived	Died
Control	59 (a)	16 (b)
SDD	64 (c)	11 (d)

Mortality for patients in the control arm was 16/75 or 21.3%, and mortality for the SDD patients was 11/75 or 14.7%. The odds ratio for mortality for patients receiving SDD is calculated from this 2×2 table as:

$$\text{Odds Ratio (OR)} = (a \times d)/(b \times c)$$
$$= (59 \times 11)/(64 \times 16)$$
$$= (59 \times 11)/(64 \times 16)$$
$$= 0.64$$

The relative risk describes the ratio of the events in the two groups or:

$$\text{Relative Risk (RR)} = (d/c + d)/b/(a + b)$$
$$= 11/75/\ 16/75$$
$$= .69$$

Odds ratios permit an estimate of the risk reduction associated with the intervention, and because they express the reduction relative to a contemporaneous control, they have become a popular way of expressing data in meta-analyses, which combine the results of different studies. The odds ratio provides an estimate of the effect size but gives no information regarding the degree of variability in the population and therefore no indication of the significance of the effect.

An alternate approach to the analysis of data that is becoming increasingly popular is the use of **confidence intervals.**[3] Confidence intervals provide an estimate of the spread of the data, or the range of values that are plausible for a population. Typically, 95% confidence intervals are employed (in other words, there is a 95% chance that a value in this range reflects the true value of the population from which it is drawn). The value of the confidence interval depends in part on the sample size and emphasizes the magnitude of the effect rather than the calculated probability, although values for a result that lie outside the 95% confidence interval correspond to values of $P < 0.05$.

Confidence intervals are somewhat more complex to calculate but can be calculated for both means and proportions.[3] An approximation of the confidence interval for the comparison of two proportions is given by:

$$CI = \exp[(1 \pm 1.96/\sqrt{\chi^2}) \ln \psi$$

where 1.96 is the value of Z corresponding to $P = 0.05$ in the normal distribution, χ^2 is the chi square value for the 2 × 2 table resulting from the data, and ψ is the odds ratio.

For the example quoted, the 95% confidence interval is 0.22 to 1.80. Because the range includes 1, the result is not statistically significant at an α level of less than 0.05, and although the odds ratio indicates a reduction of approximately one third, the potential range of values for the true effect in the entire population is broad.

CLINICAL EPIDEMIOLOGY

The discipline of clinical epidemiology concerns the application of epidemiology and biostatistics to the study of problems encountered in clinical medicine. Its focus is the process of asking clinical questions and the critical evaluation of the answers obtained. An offshoot of that focus has been an approach to the appraisal of the medical literature that is transforming the way the literature is written and read. Principles of critical appraisal form the basis for journal clubs in many university centers, and the development of a more rigorous approach to the evaluation of study design has been directly responsible for the emergence of the structured abstract as the preferred method of data summary in the medical literature.[4]

An understanding of clinical epidemiology, therefore, is of value not primarily as a tool for the researcher, but as an instrument for the evaluation of published work and for the continuing education of the practicing intensivist. The principles of critical appraisal have been articulated in a highly recommended book by Sackett and associates;[5] these form the basis for the discussion of the essentials of research design and critical appraisal that follows.

Hypothesis and Study Question

All good research begins with an hypothesis, which gives rise to one or more questions; careful articulation of the hypothesis and the study question, in turn, determines the most appropriate study design. A study that lacks an hypothesis can generate data but not information. For example, a study undertaken to determine the mortality for all patients with closed head injuries admitted to a given ICU will yield a number, but this number is unlikely to be of any interest unless it can be compared with that derived from another population—another hospital or another group of patients managed in a different manner—or related to some other feature of that patient population.

An **hypothesis** is an assumption or set of assumptions about a problem. In formulating an hypothesis, the investigator synthesizes existing knowledge into a new model or assumption that can be tested experimentally. The testing of an hypothesis results in the generation of new hypotheses; indeed the entire body of medical literature can be seen as a series of contingent hypotheses, some of which are generally accepted and others of which are controversial or unproven. A good hypothesis must be consistent with existing biologic knowledge and must be amenable to scientific proof or rejection. An hypothesis can never be definitively proved or rejected but only supported or contradicted.

A carefully articulated hypothesis leads to the generation of one or more study **questions,** the answers to which either support or contradict the original hypothesis. An integrated series of questions and the experiments or analyses needed to answer these questions form the basis for the design of a study and the report that arises from it. A well-formulated study provides useful information whether the hypothesis is supported or rejected.

Research Designs

Clinical research is undertaken to answer questions that arise in the course of making clinical decisions in patient management. It may be possible to address these questions by the use of a simple observational study (for example, if one is primarily interested in determining the prevalence or natural history of a disease), but more commonly the investigator is interested in understanding the biology of a disease process or in determining which of two or more differing approaches to diagnosis, monitoring, or therapy is better. The best way to answer such a question would be to vary the variable of interest (and only that variable) between two or more groups of subjects who are otherwise identical at the outset of the study: Any differences in outcome over time arising under these circumstances can be attributed to the effects of the study variable. In the real world, however, intrinsic variability in patients, diseases, and measuring tools results in a large number of potential sources of error or **bias** that must somehow be eliminated through the study design. **Randomization** is the optimal method of minimizing systematic bias resulting from variability between individual patients and in the disease process of interest, whereas **blinding** minimizes bias in measurements of the outcomes of interest.

Bias to the clinical epidemiologist is the presence of a source of error that is systematic rather than random. Bias can arise from a number of sources and may be difficult to recognize. For example, the study of Ziegler and coworkers[1] to evaluate the efficacy of monoclonal antibody to endotoxin in the treatment of gram-negative infection has generated considerable discussion and controversy (not to mention a further negative trial and a financial crisis) in part because of concerns of the generalizability of the initial data. Because the antibody targets endotoxin, it would be predicted to be of benefit only to patients with gram-negative bacterial infection. Entry into the trial, however, was based on the presence of clinical sepsis syndrome, on the assumption that sepsis syndrome identified a patient population with a high prevalence of gram-negative infection. Review of data from the trial showed site-specific differences both in the prevalence of gram-negative bacteremia and in the efficacy of the therapy. Concern that the results could not be generalized to all ICU patients led the Food and Drug Administration (FDA) to require the undertaking of a second trial that was suspended prematurely when an interim analysis demonstrated increased mortality in patients without gram-negative bacteremia.[6] Here bias resulted from varying patterns of disease prevalence (and possibly varying patterns of practice) and affected the generalizability of the conclusions.

Randomization provides the best method of minimizing bias, particularly bias that might result from an unrecognized source. Randomization must be performed blindly, so the investigator is unable to influence the therapy that the patient will receive. Unblinded randomization (e.g., by birth date, initial of last name, day of the week) allows the investigator to determine which patients will be enrolled in the trial and so results in the introduction of bias. For example, Shoemaker and associates[7] suggested a beneficial role for colloid resuscitation by demonstrating an improved outcome in patients managed by one surgical service that used colloids over a second team that used crystalloid. In addition to the potential for bias introduced by the nonrandom selection of patients, bias in this study may have arisen through the use of a protocol in one group of patients, an approach that can improve outcome independent of the nature of the therapy.

Blinding ensures that patient selection and management are not systematically altered. Blinding of outcome evaluation is also crucial because the determination of many outcomes in critical care hinges on clinical judgment (the diagnosis of pneumonia, for example). Even apparently definitive outcomes such as mortality are susceptible to bias: The antiendotoxin monoclonal antibody study demonstrated improved survival at 28 days but not at 14 days.[6]

Studies to Characterize Natural History and Prognosis

Studies of natural history and prognosis are by definition longitudinal and involve two components: serial assessment of the outcomes of interest over time and analysis of the factors that differ between those patients who attain the outcome of interest and those who do not. The information derived from such studies depends on three factors:

1. Definition of end points
2. Analysis of an inception cohort
3. Accomplishment of complete follow-up

Studies of the natural history and risk factors for stress-induced gastrointestinal hemorrhage yield divergent results in part because of differences in definitions of gastrointestinal bleeding, from occult blood positivity to visible bleeding with hemodynamic instability. It is intuitively evident that prognosis will be a function of the severity of the process, but risk factors too may vary with varying definitions. A definition of gastrointestinal bleeding based on the demonstration of occult blood in the nasogastric aspirate requires that all patients have nasogastric tubes and is potentially contaminated by bleeding resulting from trauma from the tube. A definition that requires bleeding in association with hemodynamic instability results in the inclusion of patients with other sources of blood loss, such as esophageal varices. Qualification of the definition with a criterion requiring clinical judgment (e.g., "thought to be a consequence of stress ulceration") may not solve the problem because it assumes that the clinician is able to differentiate sources of bleeding reliably.

Vagaries of definition bedevil clinical trials in critical care. For many of the end points of greatest interest to the intensivist—sepsis, multiple organ failure, pneumonia, to name a few—consensus on definition is lacking, with the result that published studies display considerable variability with respect to natural history and prognosis. Even mortality as an end point may be controversial. The mortality associated with septic shock varies depending on whether one assesses 3-day mortality, 14-day mortality, 28-day mortality, ICU mortality, or hospital mortality. On the one hand, the use of an early time point for a definition of mortality avoids the inclusion of patients in whom mortality might be attributable to other causes; on the other hand, an early time point may miss deaths occurring later but biologically attributable to the process of interest.

The description of the natural history of a disease process requires that the patients be identified either before they develop the disease or at some early, consistent point in the course of the disease; such a population is termed an *inception cohort*. Cook and colleagues[8] undertook a multicenter descriptive study to determine the incidence of and risk factors for clinically important bleeding in the contemporary ICU. Such an analysis meant eliminating from consideration any patient with active bleeding at the time of admission and any patient in whom the outcome of interest could not be reliably ascertained (for example, patients with facial trauma in whom the site of bleeding might be difficult to diagnose). They found respiratory failure and coagulopathy to be independent risk factors for significant bleeding. Rates of bleeding were low (less than 4%) but ironically were significantly higher in patients receiving prophylaxis than in those not receiving prophylaxis. There are two possible explanations for this finding. First, the attending clinicians may have recognized risk factors intuitively and started a higher risk population on prophylaxis. Alternatively, and less likely, prophylaxis itself may cause bleeding. The inception cohort was appropriate, but it would appear that nonrandom assignment of patients to receive prophylaxis introduced bias that could affect the interpretation of the results.

Finally, follow-up of patients in a natural history study must be as complete as possible, to eliminate any potential bias resulting from a systematic variable leading to a dropout of study subjects.

A well-designed study of natural history and prognosis provides information on the progression of a disease process in a patient population. Beyond this, however, by the use of multivariate techniques to compare risk factors in patients developing the disease with those who remain disease-free, such studies can shed light on factors of importance in the pathogenesis of the process. Validated studies of natural history form the basis for the development of prognostic scores, which can be used as clinical tools to predict outcome in other patients. Scores are discussed more fully later.

Studies to Determine Cause

Cause is established by association; however, association is by no means proof of cause. An association between two variables implies that they are linked; however, the linkage may be that both are manifestations of a third unidentified factor. For example, the demonstration by Gutierrez and associates[9] that mucosal acidosis as measured by tonometry predicts mortality in critically ill patients does not mean that splanchnic hypoperfusion is the cause; an alternate explanation is that reduced splanchnic blood flow is simply one manifestation of generalized tissue hypoperfusion.[10] Similarly, studies demonstrating improved survival with supranormal Do_2[11] may not reflect a causal relationship between augmented Do_2 and survival but rather identify a subset of patients with an improved prognosis as a consequence of some other factor that manifests as the ability to augment Do_2 in response to therapy. Equally, however, it must be recognized that the availability of an alternate explanation for an association in no way disproves a causal relationship. Proof of cause is difficult because a given process or disease may have multiple causes, and multiple clinical associations may be present; however, evidence for causation is based on data demonstrating:

1. A significant association between the presence of the putative cause or risk factor and the development of the disease
2. The temporal presence of the risk factor before the development of the disease
3. Prevention (or at least a reduced prevalence) of the disease by removal of the risk factor
4. Reproduction of the disease under controlled circumstances in an animal model by exposure to the risk factor and prevention of the disease by antagonism of that risk factor

The potential pitfalls associated with the reproduction of the disorders of critical illness in humans and in animal models are beyond the scope of this discussion. Animal models provide the most controlled circumstances to study mechanisms of disease; however, they may not reliably model the clinical problems seen in the ICU. Nonetheless, reproduction of a disease process in an animal by exposure to a risk factor and prevention by reversal of that risk factor provide compelling proof of cause. For example, the demonstration that tumor necrosis factor is a proximate mediator of endotoxin lethality was convincingly established in studies by Tracey and colleagues[12] showing that the clinical manifestations of endotoxemia in mice could be reproduced by infusion of tumor necrosis factor and that antibody to tumor necrosis factor could block the development of these changes following endotoxin administration.

Although a randomized clinical trial would provide the most reliable evidence of causation, randomization of two groups to a risk factor for a disease is not ethically acceptable. Evidence of modulation of the course of a disease by modulation of the risk factor may provide evidence of causality. In practice, preliminary evidence for cause derives either from **cohort** studies, in which a group of patients, some of whom have the risk factor and others of whom do not, is followed for subsequent development of disease, or from **case-control** studies.

Cohort studies provide the best design for the determination of causation; however, they are expensive, time-consuming (because cases must be followed prospectively from before the onset of the outcome of interest), and subject to potential bias because they are not randomized. Case-control studies have become a standard model for the epidemiologist to investigate cause. The design involves matching each of a group of individuals (cases) who share the outcome of interest with a group of controls who do not, then evaluating the two groups for systematic differences with respect to potential etiologic factors. The influence of potential confounding variables is minimized by matching cases and controls based on these variables. Bias in a case-control study can arise as a result either of failing to match for an important confounding variable or of matching for a variable that is in fact important etiologically. The case-control design has the advantage of being

Appendix Table–2. Risk Factors for Nosocomial Candidemia

Independent Variable	Odds Ratio	95% Confidence Interval	P
Number of antibiotics	1.73	1.23–2.43	0.0017
Other site of candida infection	10.37	2.33–46.16	0.0021
Hickman catheter	7.23	1.14–46.06	0.0362
Hemodialysis	18.13	1.48–221.84	0.0234

(From Wey, S. B., et al.: Risk factors for hospital-acquired Candidemia. A matched case-control study. Arch. Intern. Med., 149:2349, 1989.)

inexpensive and relatively simple to undertake and is particularly suited to the study of uncommon disorders.

For example, Wey and associates[13] studied risk factors for nosocomial *candidemia* by studying 88 patients with *candidemia* matched based on potential confounding variables—age, sex, underlying disease, surgery, duration of hospitalization, and year of admission—with an equal number of patients who did not develop *candidemia*. The results of a stepwise multivariate analysis are shown in Appendix Table–2. Although studies such as this can define risk factors, they cannot establish a causal relationship. Is the elevated risk associated with a Hickman catheter a result of fungal colonization of an indwelling foreign body or of the underlying disease that necessitated the insertion of the catheter? And if the latter, does risk arise from the disease itself or from another confounding variable associated with the diagnosis or management of that disease? Results of case-control studies are usually, as in the present example, expressed as odds ratios and confidence intervals (see later), with univariate and multivariate analyses to establish independent risk factors.

A variant of the case-control study is the **matched cohort study,** used to define attributable morbidity and mortality. In this study, as in the case-control study, matching is used to minimize the influence of potential confounding variables, but cases are studied prospectively to quantitate attributable morbidity and mortality resulting from the presence of the risk factor of interest. For example, Leu and co-workers[14] evaluated the attributable morbidity and mortality of nosocomial pneumonia by matching a group of patients with nosocomial pneumonia to a comparable group of patients without pneumonia, then comparing the outcome of the two groups with respect to mortality and length of hospital stay.

The weakest, but also the most common, study design used to infer causality is the case series, in which the prevalence of a risk factor and an outcome is quantitated in a group of patients. Multiple studies, for example, have shown that patients with clinical evidence of sepsis have elevated circulating levels of such cytokines as tumor necrosis factor and interleukin 6; however, association here is no more proof of causality than is the observation that these same patients also have elevated lactate levels. The importance of demonstrating association should not be trivialized; however, it is only the first step in generating more compelling designs to establish causality.

Studies to Evaluate a Diagnostic Test

A diagnostic test predicts the presence of a disease or process. Ideally the test should identify that process in all the patients in whom it is present and rule out its presence in all patients in whom the test is negative. In reality, even the best of tests fail to meet this criterion, and therefore **false-positive** and **false-negative** results occur. The relationship of the results of the test to the actual state of affairs is described through the concepts of the **sensitivity** and **specificity** of a test as well as the concepts of **positive** and **negative predictive value** (Appendix Table–3).

The **sensitivity** of a test describes the ability of the test to detect the disease of interest when it is present and is calculated as the number of patients identified by the test as having the disease, divided by the number of patients who actually have the disease, both those whom the test identifies (true-positives) and those whom the test misses (false-negatives). A test that lacks sensitivity fails to identify patients who actually have the disease. Conversely the **specificity** describes the ability of the test to rule out a disease in patients who do not have that disease and is calculated as the number of patients who do not have the disease according to the test divided by the number of patients who really do not have the disease—those identified by the test (true-negatives) and those inaccurately identified by the test as having the disease (false-positives). A test that lacks specificity incorrectly identifies patients as having a disease, when in fact they do not. In practice, the concern of the clinician is not with sensitivity and specificity—concepts that relate the test to a gold standard—but with whether a positive or negative test result correctly classifies patients with or without the disease. These features are called the **positive** and **negative predictive values** of a test (see Appendix Table–3). The **positive predictive value** of a test is the number of patients who have the disease and are correctly identified by the test, divided by the total number of patients whom the test identifies as having the disease, both those identified correctly by the test (true-positives) and those incorrectly identified by the test (false-positives). The **negative predictive value** is the converse—the number of true-negatives, divided by the total number of negatives identified by the test, both true and false negatives.

Appendix Table–3. Relationship of a Test to the Presence of Disease

Conclusion of Test	Disease Present	Disease Absent
Patient has disease	True-positive (a)	False-positive (b)
Patient does not have disease	False-negative (c)	True-negative (d)

Sensitivity = a/(a + c)
Specificity = d/(b + d)

Positive predictive value = a/(a = b)
Negative predictive value = d/(d = c)

Accuracy = (a + d/(a + b + c + d)
Prevalence = (a + c)/(a + b + c + d)

A diagnostic test is used to make a categorical clinical decision—to extubate or not to extubate, to operate or not to operate, to start a therapy or not start a therapy, to stop treatment or to continue treatment. Most tests, however, do not yield categorical information but rather continuous information that must be converted to a categorical conclusion. For example, quantitative culture of a vascular catheter tip or of a brochoalveolar lavage specimen can yield any number of bacteria; however, a cutoff for a positive result is arbitrarily defined and used to make treatment decisions. An increasingly popular method of assessing the performance of a test across a continuous range of values is the use of **receiver-operating-characteristic** (ROC) curves. A ROC curve plots the proportion of true-positive results against the proportion of false-positive results for each ordinal value of the test (Appendix Fig.-1). If the test is no better than random chance, a diagonal line with a slope of 45° results; as the discriminatory value of the test increases, so does the area under the curve.

Yang and Tobin[16] evaluated the ability of a number of objective indicators of ventilatory function to predict successful weaning from mechanical ventilation (Appendix Table-4). They found that the ratio of frequency to tidal volume (f/V$_T$ ratio) was the best predictor of successful

Appendix Table-4. Accuracy of Indicators of Successful Weaning from Mechanical Ventilation

Parameter	Sensitivity	Specificity	Positive Predictive Value	Negative Predictive Value
Minute ventilation	0.78	0.18	0.55	0.38
Respiratory frequency	0.92	0.36	0.65	0.77
Tidal volume	0.97	0.54	0.73	0.94
Maximal inspiratory pressure	1.00	0.11	0.59	1.00
Po$_2$/Fio$_2$ ratio	0.81	0.29	0.59	0.53
Frequency/V$_T$ ratio	0.97	0.64	0.78	0.95
CROP index	0.81	0.57	0.71	0.70

(From Yang, K. L., and Tobin, M. J.: A prospective study of indexes predicting the outcome of trials of weaning from mechanical ventilation. N. Engl. J. Med., *324*:1445, 1991.)

weaning (reflected in a positive predictive value of 0.78), whereas the maximal inspiratory pressure and the f/V$_T$ ratio were the best predictors of failure of weaning. The area under the ROC curve was greatest for the f/V$_T$ ratio. Although information derived from a ROC curve can assist in the evaluation of a test, the use of the test in clinical practice depends on the consequences of a false-positive or false-negative result. A false-positive result of a human immunodeficiency virus (HIV) screening test may have serious consequences for an individual tested for AIDS, whereas a false-negative result has equally disastrous results when the test is used to screen banked blood. In general, as sensitivity increases, specificity decreases, and vice versa (thus the characteristic shape of the ROC curve). In the present example of criteria for extubation (and assuming that a true-positive value for f/V$_T$ is one that correctly identifies the patient who will be successfully extubated), the clinician would likely prefer to err on the side of leaving intubated a patient who might tolerate extubation (false-negative) and therefore would select a value for the f/V$_T$ ratio that favored specificity at the expense of sensitivity.

A **score** or **index** is a form of test that combines two or more variables to produce a single measure of the severity of a disease or process. The evaluation of a score therefore involves the same considerations as the evaluation of any other test, and ROC curves can be constructed to reflect the ability of the score to predict the outcome of interest (see Appendix Fig.-1). Variable weights can be established by multivariate techniques. A score merely combines information derived from several tests; it does not provide new information and is subject to the same strengths and weaknesses as the tests that compose it.

Studies to Evaluate Therapy

The gold standard for the evaluation of therapy is the **randomized, controlled clinical trial,** in which experimental therapy or placebo is allocated randomly between two groups, and outcome is evaluated with the investiga-

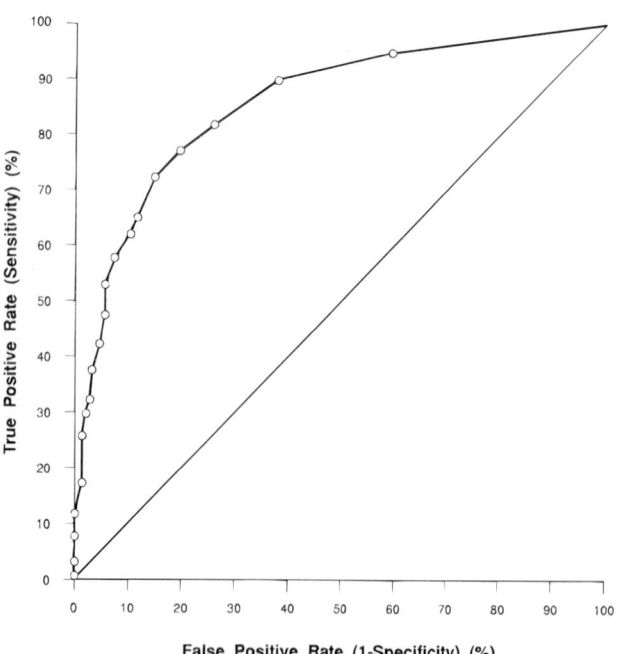

Appendix Fig.-1. A receiver-operating-characteristic (ROC) curve. The **sensitivity** of a test (Y axis) is plotted against **1-specificity** (X axis) for a range of test values. In this example, the capacity of the APACHE II score to predict mortality correctly at differing levels of APACHE II score is plotted. A test that performs no better than random chance yields a straight line at an angle of 45 degrees; as the sensitivity and specificity of the test across a range of values increase, so does the area under the ROC curve. (Redrawn courtesy of George Morrison, Clinical Dimensions, Inc., Madison, WI, from Knaus, W. A., Draper, E. A., Wagner, D. P., and Zimmerman, J. E.: APACHE II: a severity of disease classification system. Crit. Care Med., *13*:818, 1985.)

Appendix Table–5. Critical Issues in the Design of a Randomized, Controlled Trial

Study Design
  Are the primary and secondary end points defined in the methods?
  Are there adequate definitions for all important outcomes?
  Are the sample size calculations described and justified—the levels of α and β as well as whether tests are one or two tailed?
  If subgroup analyses are to be used, do the sample size calculations provide enough power to perform secondary analyses?
Study Conduct
  Is the method of randomization truly random?
  Is an intent-to-treat design used?
  Is the study multicenter?
  Are all patients accounted for at the end of the trial?
  Is there a log of all eligible but not studied patients?
Study Monitoring
  Are all outcomes assessed blindly?
  Is there a data monitoring committee?
  Is there a safety and adverse events committee?

tor blinded to the therapy each patient receives. Randomization serves to prevent bias resulting from the presence of a systematic confounding variable in one of the groups, whereas blinding prevents bias in outcome evaluation.

The principles for the conduct of a successful randomized, controlled trial have become well established (Appendix Table–5). The success of a trial rests not so much in its findings but in its design: A properly designed trial yields clinically important information, regardless of whether or not it succeeds in supporting the hypothesis that gave rise to the study.

The objective of a randomized controlled trial is to determine whether an unproven therapy is truly efficacious. Like a diagnostic test, therefore, a trial may yield results that are either falsely positive or falsely negative. Such erroneous conclusions arise as a result of inherent differences between study subjects in the severity or nature of their disease, in their response to therapy, and in the intervention of unanticipated confounding factors. Estimation of the anticipated influence of these sources of variability is a critical step in trial design because it permits the investigator to estimate how many patients must be studied to detect statistically significant differences between groups at a given α level while maintaining the probability for a type II error at an appropriately low level. The sample size necessary to detect a statistically significant difference at a given α and β level depends on the prevalence of the end point in the control group and the magnitude of the expected reduction in the study group. Because clinical trials are expensive, the number of patients to be enrolled is the minimum number required to demonstrate significance at a stated β level.

A corollary of the considerations that establish a minimum sample size for a trial is that in a given study, only one primary end point can be evaluated with confidence. The probability of demonstrating a statistically significant effect increases with the number of analyses performed, and secondary or subgroup analyses not incorporated into the original statistical design must be viewed with great suspicion. A striking example of the importance of this principle was provided by Lee and associates,[17] who reported a simulated randomized trial of a nontherapy for coronary artery disease. From a database of 1073 consecutive patients receiving medical therapy for coronary artery disease, they randomized patients to two separate groups that could be shown to be well matched with respect to important demographic and baseline variables. Yet when the investigators undertook a series of subgroup analyses on these two comparable groups, they were able to uncover statistically significant differences that, had the therapy differed, would have been concluded to represent a therapeutic effect. In actuality, the differences were simply the consequence of random variation across a large number of subgroup analyses; if 10 separate analyses are performed at an α level of 0.05, there is a 40% chance that one would be positive by chance alone.

The preliminary power calculations establish the ground rules for a study, and the resulting investigation either supports or rejects the study hypothesis. Because the research design establishes a framework to answer a categorical question, the answer must be either yes or no; a study that approaches significance is a negative study from a biostatistical perspective, although the findings may have clinical or biologic significance in the absence of statistical significance.

All patients who are randomized into a trial should be included in the final data analysis. This approach is termed an **intention to treat** design and provides maximal protection against the inadvertent introduction of bias into a trial. With an intention to treat model, the outcomes of all patients randomized are included in the final analysis, even those who may not have received the experimental intervention or whose participation in the trial may have been prematurely terminated. If such events are unrelated to therapy, they should be equally distributed between study groups and therefore not influence the study outcome. Removal of patients from analysis introduces the potential for bias because the reason for removal may have actually reflected an adverse consequence of therapy. Moreover, in the real world of clinical practice, medication errors and other similar problems do occur, and it is important that an intervention be evaluated in the conditions under which it will be applied.

Randomization of patients for a clinical trial must be accomplished in such a manner that there is no potential for bias. Randomization by techniques such as date, patient initials, or admitting service introduces bias because, at the least, the investigator will know which group the patient will be randomized to and can therefore decide to enter or exclude the patient based on the study group to which the patient has been randomized. The importance of blinding in the randomization process was evaluated by Chalmers and colleagues,[18] who showed, in a review of 145 studies of therapy for acute myocardial infarction, a striking difference in the findings of trials based on the methods of randomization. Significant treatment effects were found in 8.8% of blinded, randomized trials; in 24.4% of unblinded, randomized trials; and in 58.1% of unrandomized studies.

Although the randomized control trial is the best study design for evaluating therapy, it has drawbacks. These studies are inherently expensive and time-consuming. For uncommon diseases, it may not be possible to recruit a large enough sample of patients to meet the statistical requirements of the study design. An innovative approach to this latter problem has been the development of the N of 1 trial, in which the treatment given to a single patient is altered randomly over time between one of two therapies, and the responses during the times on each of the two therapies are compared.[19] Such studies are feasible only in a disease that is stable over time and in which the therapy alters the expression of the disease without effecting a cure.

Meta-analysis

A single clinical trial is rarely sufficiently convincing that the clinician can feel confident about incorporating its recommendations unreservedly into clinical practice. Despite the best efforts of the investigator to optimize trial design, the final results are often less than definitive because of such factors as patient heterogeneity, unanticipated variations in rates of the end point of interest, or lack of funds to complete the study. Moreover, it is common that several groups may independently embark on studies to address a common question and that differences in the formulation of that question, the patients studied, or the end point may cause the studies to yield divergent or even contradictory results. The technique of **meta-analysis** arose as a means of pooling data from two or more studies to garner information that was not evident in the individual studies and to reconcile differences between trials.

A meta-analysis is essentially a study of studies. Liberati and co-workers,[20] performed a meta-analysis of published studies of SDD (selective decontamination of the digestive tract) in an attempt to determine the effects of SDD on ICU morbidity (particularly nosocomial pneumonia) and mortality. Such a process begins with the identification of studies for potential inclusion in the meta-analysis. In addition to a review of published trials in the medical literature, these authors sought out completed trials that had been presented but not published (or published in abstract form only), identifying 25 trials in total—17 published and 8 unpublished. These trials evaluated heterogeneous populations, used different methods to achieve digestive tract decontamination, and were highly variable in the quality of the study design. Thus the authors had to establish criteria to include or exclude studies that would not introduce bias. They reviewed only randomized, controlled trials and excluded three further studies—one because contact with the authors revealed that the design was not truly random and two because of study of highly specific patient groups (esophageal resection and fulminant hepatic failure). The results of a meta-analysis are typically presented by graphing the odds ratios and 95% confidence intervals of the studies, as depicted in Appendix Figure-2. A significant effect is evident when the confidence intervals exclude 1.0 (see later).

Although there is consensus that a meta-analysis should include only randomized trials, performed using an intention-to-treat design with complete follow-up and blinded outcome assessment, the methodology is still in evolution, and a number of controversies remain unresolved.[21] For example, if the investigator includes only published stud-

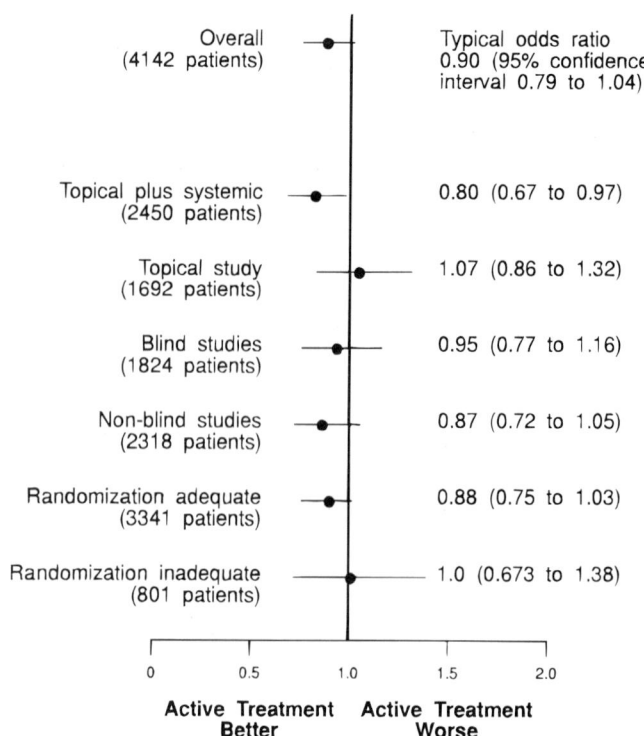

Appendix Fig.–2. Results of a meta-analysis of the effects of selective digestive tract decontamination on mortality. Odds ratios and 95% confidence intervals are plotted for varying subgroup analyses. Because the confidence interval for the entire group includes 1.0, the results are not statistically significant; however, it is apparent that mortality is significantly reduced for patients receiving both topical and systemic therapy as well as that the adequacy of randomization has an impact on the results obtained. (Redrawn courtesy of George Morrison, Clinical Dimensions, Inc., Madison, WI, from Liberati, A., et al.: Selective Decontamination of the Digestive Tract Trialists' Collaborative Group. Meta-analysis of randomised controlled trials of selective decontamination of the digestive tract. Br. Med. J., *307*:525, 1993.)

ies, there is a risk of a false-positive conclusion because negative studies are less likely to be submitted by the investigators and less likely to be published by editors. Unpublished work has not been subjected to peer review, and significant methodologic deficiencies may be the reason that the work remains unpublished. Few published studies are without significant flaws to the critical methodologist; at what level do these flaws justify exclusion of the study from consideration? Because the studies are published, their conclusions are known, and it is difficult if not impossible for the investigator to make decisions about study inclusion blindly.

BIOSTATISTICS: BASIC PRINCIPLES

Selecting the Appropriate Statistical Test

The appropriate technique of statistical analysis for a given set of data depends on a number of factors, including the nature of the dependent and independent variables (categorical versus continuous), the number of groups

Appendix Table-6. Statistical Testing for Continuous and Categorical Variables

Dependent Variable	Independent Variable	
	Categorical	Continuous
Categorical	X^2	Logistic regression
Continuous	T test	Linear regression

being analyzed, whether the distribution of the data is parametric or nonparametric, whether the data represent paired observations (for example, preintervention and postintervention values from the same individual), whether there is one or more than one independent variables, and whether data are being analyzed over time. The optimal test for a given situation is best determined in conjunction with a statistician; however, certain generalizations can be made, based on the nature of the dependent and independent variables (Appendix Table-6).

Continuous Dependent Variable, Categorical Independent Variable

The comparison of the mean values of a particular variable between two or more groups is a common objective in clinical studies. For example, Fisher and colleagues[22] evaluated the effects of the administration of a monoclonal antibody to tumor necrosis factor on circulating cytokine levels in patients with sepsis syndrome. In this study, the dependent variable is the mean plasma cytokine level, a continuous variable, and the independent variable, the dosage of anti-tumor necrosis factor antibody administered. (Note that the hypothesis is that cytokine levels depend on the dose of antibody and that the dosage groups are discrete, nonoverlapping entities).

Nonsurvivors were found to have significantly higher levels of interleukin 6 than survivors. For this analysis, there are two discrete groups for the independent variable (survival and nonsurvival), and the dependent variable; interleukin 6 is assumed to be normally distributed. The comparison of the two means is accomplished using Student's t-test. The t-test, however, is appropriate only for the comparison of two groups and only if the two groups are normally distributed.

Comparison of the means of more than two groups is accomplished by the use of **analysis of variance** (ANOVA), which analyzes multiple groups differing by only one factor and tests the hypothesis that all samples are derived from a single population. The analysis provides no indication of which mean or means is different. Only if results are statistically significant by ANOVA is it appropriate to compare any two of the groups with each other, and then the comparison is performed not with a t-test but with a post hoc test, such as the Bonferroni test, the Neuman-Keuls test, or Dunnett's t-test. Each of these post hoc tests makes adjustments for the fact that the performance of multiple comparisons increases the likelihood that one of the comparisons will be significant simply based on chance. For example, if the means of three groups—a, b, and c—are being compared, there are three different combinations of two-way comparisons—a with b, b with c, and a with c. The probability of a significant result being observed based on chance alone increases to $(1 - 0.95 \times 0.95 \times 0.95)$% or 12%. One method of correcting for the effects of multiple comparisons is to divide the P value by the number of possible combinations of comparisons and set that new value as the α level; this is the essence of the Bonferroni adjustment.

The t-test compares the means of two groups; whether a given comparison attains significance depends on the magnitude of the difference between the means, the variability of the data (the standard deviation), and the number of observations. To minimize the likelihood of a type II error, it is in the investigator's interest to use a study design that minimizes the variability of the data. When a study involves the use of before and after data (for example, a study assessing the effects of an inotrope on cardiac output might measure cardiac output before and during infusion of the agent), the paired t-test provides a more sensitive analysis of the presence or absence of an effect. The paired t-test compares the means of the differences between before and after measurements and therefore minimizes that component of variability arising from the intrinsic biologic differences between study subjects.

The use of either a t-test or an ANOVA is appropriate only when the data are normally distributed. If that assumption cannot be made, a nonparametric test must be used. The Mann-Whitney test is the nonparametric equivalent of the unpaired t-test; the nonparametric equivalent of the paired t-test is the Wilcoxon signed rank test. The nonparametric equivalent of ANOVA is the Kruskal-Wallis test, a generalization of the Mann-Whitney test. If the Kruskal-Wallis tests yields a significant P value, post hoc tests can be performed. If the groups are of equivalent sizes, a variant of the Student-Neuman-Keuls test or Dunnett's test is used; if not, Dunn's test is employed for both multiple comparisons between groups and comparisons against a single control.

Categorical Dependent Variable, Categorical Independent Variable

Mortality, a categorical variable, is an important clinical end point for studies of critically ill patients; thus techniques to analyze the distribution of a categorical variable among two or more groups are commonly encountered in the critical care literature. For example, Clemmer and associates[23] studied the impact of hypothermia on mortality in patients with sepsis syndrome. The raw data can be displayed in the form of a **contingency table** (Appendix Table-7) or as frequencies or proportions.

Appendix Table-7. Impact of Hypothermia on Outcome in Sepsis Syndrome

	Lived	Died	Total
Hypothermia	13	21	34
No hypothermia	256	92	348
Total	269	113	382

(From Clemmer, T. P., et al., and the Methylprednisolone Severe Sepsis Study Group: Hypothermia in the sepsis syndrome and clinical outcome. Crit. Care Med., *20*:1395, 1992.)

The most commonly used test in the analysis of proportions or frequencies is the **Chi-square (χ^2) test.** In this example, if the null hypothesis were true, that hypothermia has no effect on outcome, one would expect a similar proportion of nonhypothermic and hypothermic patients to die. Nonsurvivors comprise 29.6% of the total sample population (113/382); therefore the expected number of deaths in patients with hypothermia should be 29.6% of 34, or 10; similarly, 103 (29.6% of 348) nonhypothermic patients would be expected to die. The χ^2 statistic is calculated as the sum of the squares of the observed minus the expected frequencies, divided by the expected frequency:

$$\chi^2 = \sum \frac{(O - E)^2}{E}$$

Probabilities associated with differing values of the χ^2 statistic can be obtained from standard tables. The χ^2 statistic can be used to analyze differences in proportions of two or more groups; as the number of groups increases, the distribution approaches a normal distribution. Certain restrictions apply to the use of the χ^2 test. At least 80% of the cells in the table should have expected frequencies of more than 5, and all cells should have expected frequencies of more than 1. In the special case of a 2 × 2 table with an expected cell frequency of less than 5, **Fisher's exact test** can be used to provide a P value. In contrast to the χ^2 test, Fisher's exact test can yield a P value that is either one tailed or two tailed. The χ^2 test is based on a normal approximation of a binomial distribution. As the former distribution is continuous, whereas the latter represents discrete variables, the χ^2 test tends to underestimate the P value, leading to a type I error. For this reason, **Yates' continuity correction** should be used to provide a more accurate P value when using 2 × 2 contingency tables. If the groups of subjects are paired, such as in a matched cohort study or when comparing a variable before or after therapy in the same group of patients, McNemar's test for 2 × 2 tables or a modification thereof for larger contingency tables should be used.

Often an investigator is interested in knowing not only if there is a difference in rates between experimental groups at a particular point in time, but also whether rates between groups vary at multiple points over a time interval. In Ziegler's study[1] of the efficacy of monoclonal antiendotoxin antibody (HA-1A) in sepsis, for example, the authors were interested not only in how many patients in each group had died on day 14, but also in assessing how survival rates changed over time in the two groups and in determining the impact of the initial severity of illness on the final outcome. Such analyses require more complex statistical techniques. The **Mantel-Haenzel** chi square statistic permits the simultaneous analysis of two categorical independent variables (in this case, whether the patient received HA-1A and whether he or she had a low or high APACHE II score). Analysis of survival over time can be accomplished by the construction of **Kaplan-Meier** survival curves and the influence of more than one variable analyzed using a **Cox proportional hazards model.** The details of these techniques are beyond the scope of this overview.

Analyses of Continuous Independent Variables

The statistical techniques described previously can be used when the independent variable is a categorical one; however, a different approach is used when analyzing a continuous dependent variable. If both the dependent and independent variables are continuous, **linear regression analysis** and **correlation** are used.

The **correlation coefficient (r)** provides a measure of the degree of association between the values of two continuous variables. Its value ranges from -1 to $+1$; the closer **r** is to 1 or -1, the stronger the degree of association. The sign of **r** indicates whether the correlation between the two variables is a direct ($+$) or inverse ($-$) one. If data points are plotted on a graph in the form of a scatter plot, linear regression methods determine the line of best fit, and the value of **r** is a measure of the scatter of the points about the linear trend. The **Pearson product-moment correlation coefficient** is used for quantitating the strength of association between two variables that are normally distributed. In contrast, the **Spearman rank correlation coefficient** is a nonparametric test and thus places no such restriction on the population distribution of the variables.

Although correlation provides a measure of the degree of association between variables, linear regression analysis uses that information to predict the value of the dependent variable, based on that of the independent variable. In its simplest form, linear regression relates a single independent (X), or predictor, variable to a dependent (Y), or outcome, variable. The method of least squares or **least-squares regression** allows the fitting of a regression line that represents the line of best fit through the data, yielding a regression line with equation:

$$y = a + bx$$

where **a** represents the y intercept and **b** the slope of the line. The assumptions in this process are that the values of Y have a normal distribution and equal variances for each value of X and that their relationship is linear.

In practice, there is often more than one independent variable. **Multiple regression analysis** is a technique that permits the evaluation of the influences of more than one variable and is represented by the general model:

$$y = \alpha + \beta_1 x_1 + \beta_2 x_2 \ldots + \beta_n x_n$$

where $\beta_1, \beta_2, \ldots \beta_n$ represent the regression coefficients for the independent variables $x_1, x_2, \ldots x_n$. The regression coefficients represent the estimated increase in the outcome variable for every unit in the predictor variable. In **forward stepwise regression,** the unique relationship between each independent variable and the outcome variable is determined, a process termed **univariate analysis.** Those that attain statistical significance are then entered into a model in a stepwise fashion—the variable that is most strongly correlated with the dependent variable is entered first and the resulting independent influences of the remaining variables recalculated, entering the next strongest predictor variable into the regression equation.

Appendix Table–8. Factors Associated with Mortality from Nosocomial Pneumonia by Univariate Analysis

Variable	Odds Ratio for Death	P
Age >60	2.8	0.008
Service		
Medicine	7.1	<0.00001
ICU	12	<0.00001
Rapidly fatal underlying disease	3.1	0.01
High risk microorganism	72.4	<0.00001
Previous antibiotic therapy	4.3	0.0009
Bilateral chest film changes	7.4	<0.00001
Shock	13.9	<0.00001
Respiratory failure	4.3	<0.0001
Inappropriate antibiotic therapy	25	<0.00001

(From Celis, R., et al.: Nosocomial pneumonia. A multivariate analysis of risk and prognosis. Chest, *93*:318, 1988.)

This process is continued until the remaining variables no longer attain significance in the recalculated equation and is termed a multivariate analysis. Stepwise regression analysis allows the investigator to determine which variables contribute to an outcome and to gain an impression of the magnitude of the contribution of each.

Linear regression techniques assume both the dependent and the independent variables to be normally distributed and therefore cannot be used when the dependent variable is categorical. The solution is to effect a transformation of the categorical data called a **logistic function**, which then assumes a normal distribution. This technique is known as **logistic regression analysis** and, similar to linear regression, can be used to analyze the effects of more than one independent variable. For example, Celis and associates[24] studied factors influencing the prognosis of ICU-acquired pneumonia. The presence or absence of pneumonia according to predetermined criteria (a categorical variable) was the dependent variable, whereas multiple potential independent variables, both continuous and categorical, were evaluated to determine their independent contribution to that outcome. As shown in Appendix Table-8, in a univariate analysis, a number of variables were identified as being significantly predictive of mortality. In the multivariate analysis (Appendix Table-9), how-ever, only three remained significant at an α level of <0.01. The multivariate analysis suggests that the apparent contribution of certain variables identified in the univariate analysis can be accounted for by the actual contribution of other variables. For example, in the univariate analysis, the attending service (medicine or ICU) correlated strongly with outcome. In the multivariate analysis, however, this effect disappears, suggesting that what was being measured was differences in age or underlying condition, for example, between patients on medical and surgical services.

Logistic techniques such as this are potent tools for evaluating associations and inferring causation. They are critically dependent on the variables selected, however, and on the way in which those variables are defined, and one must be careful not to allow the complexities of the analytic technique to hide inadequacies of data accumulation. Moreover, association does not necessarily imply causation.

In conclusion, the continued evolution of research methods has given rise to the discipline of clinical epidemiology, whose focus is the process of the generation of medical knowledge. Although clinical epidemiology has had a significant effect on how both editors and clinicians respond to published studies, it has inadvertently alienated the clinician by creating a method and a jargon that are unfamiliar. It is an inescapable truth of the late twentieth century that the educated clinician must pay attention not only to what the clinical literature says, but also how adequately it makes its case. Fortunately, although the biostatistical underpinnings of that process are complex, the conceptual principles are not, and a series of books and monographs are available to clarify concepts of fundamental importance to the acquisition of new knowledge.

REFERENCES

1. Ziegler, E. J., et al.: Treatment of gram-negative bacteremia and septic shock with HA-1A human monoclonal antibody against endotoxin. N. Engl. J. Med., *324*:429, 1991.
2. Cockerill, F. R., III, et al.: Prevention of infection in critically ill patients by selective decontamination of the digestive tract. Ann. Intern. Med., *117*:545, 1992.
3. Gardner, M. J., and Altman, D. G.: Confidence intervals rather than P values: estimation rather than hypothesis testing. Br. Med. J., *292*:746, 1986.
4. Ad Hoc Working Group for Critical Appraisal of the Medical Literature: A proposal for more informative abstracts of clinical articles. Ann. Intern. Med., *106*:598, 1987.
5. Sackett, D. L., Haynes, R. B., and Tugwell, P.: Clinical Epidemiology. A Basic Science for Clinical Medicine. Boston, Little, Brown, 1985.
6. Luce, J. M.: Introduction of new technology into critical care practice: a history of HA-1A human monoclonal antibody against endotoxin. Crit. Care Med., *21*:1233, 1993.
7. Shoemaker, W. C., et al.: Comparison of the relative effectiveness of colloids and crystalloids in emergency resuscitation. Am. J. Surg., *142*:73, 1981.
8. Cook, D. J., et al.: Risk factors for gastrointestinal bleeding in critically ill patients. N. Engl. J. Med., *330*:377, 1994.
9. Gutierrez, G., et al.: Gastric intramucosal pH as a therapeutic index of tissue oxygenation in critically ill patients. Lancet, *339*:195, 1992.
10. Boyd, O., et al.: Comparison of clinical information obtained

Appendix Table–9. Independent Predictors of Mortality from Nosocomial Pneumonia, Multivariate Model

Variable	Odds Ratio	95% Confidence Interval	P
High risk microorganism	8.2	4.4–15.2	0.0007
Bilateral chest film changes	6.3	2.5–6.1	0.008
Respiratory failure	14.8	7.4–28.2	0.005
Inappropriate antibiotic therapy	32.5	7.8–135.6	0.02
Age >60	4.6	2.5–8.5	0.02
Fatal underlying condition	4.8	2.5–9.2	0.02

(From Celis, R., et al.: Nosocomial pneumonia. A multivariate analysis of risk and prognosis. Chest, *93*:318, 1988.)

from routine blood-gas analysis and from gastric tonometry for intramural pH. Lancet, *1:*142, 1993.
11. Shoemaker, W. C., et al.: Prospective trial of supranormal values of survivors as therapeutic goals in high-risk surgical patients. Chest, *94:*1176, 1988.
12. Tracey, K. J., et al.: Anti-cachectin/TNF monoclonal antibodies prevent septic shock during lethal bacteremia. Nature, *330:*662, 1987.
13. Wey, S. B., et al.: Risk factors for hospital-acquired Candidemia. A matched case-control study. Arch. Intern. Med., *149:*2349, 1989.
14. Leu, H.-S., et al.: Hospital-acquired pneumonia. Attributable mortality and morbidity. Am. J. Epidemiol., *129:*1258, 1989.
15. Knaus, W. A., Draper, E. A., Wagner, D. P., and Zimmerman, J. E.: APACHE II: a severity of disease classification system. Crit. Care Med., *13:*818, 1985.
16. Yang, K. L., and Tobin, M. J.: A prospective study of indexes predicting the outcome of trials of weaning from mechanical ventilation. N. Engl. J. Med., *324:*1445, 1991.
17. Lee, K. L., et al.: Lessons from a simulated trial in coronary artery disease. Circulation, *61:*508, 1980.
18. Chalmers, T. C., Celano, P., Sacks, H. S., and Smith, H.: Bias in treatment assignment in controlled clinical trials. N. Engl. J. Med., *309:*1358, 1983.
19. Guyatt, G., et al.: Determining optimal therapy—randomized trials in individual patients. N. Engl. J. Med., *314:*889, 1986.
20. Liberati, A., et al.: Selective decontamination of the digestive tract trialists' collaborative group. Meta-analysis of randomised controlled trials of selective decontamination of the digestive tract. Br. Med. J., *307:*525, 1993.
21. Thompson, S. G., and Pocock, S. J.: Can meta-analyses be trusted? Lancet, *2:*1127, 1991.
22. Fisher, C. J., et al., and the CB0006 Sepsis Syndrome Study Group: Influence of an anti-tumor necrosis factor monoclonal antibody on cytokine levels in patients with sepsis. Crit. Care Med., *21:*318, 1993.
23. Clemmer, T. P., et al., and the Methylprednisolone Severe Sepsis Study Group: Hypothermia in the sepsis syndrome and clinical outcome. Crit. Care Med., *20:*1395, 1992.
24. Celis, R., et al.: Nosocomial pneumonia. A multivariate analysis of risk and prognosis. Chest, *93:*318, 1988.

SUPPLEMENTAL READINGS

There are now available a number of concise, nonmathematical overviews of the principles discussed in this review, and the interested reader is referred to them for a more comprehensive introduction to clinical epidemiology and biostatistics.

Fletcher, R. H., Fletcher, S. W., and Wagner, E. H.: Clinical Epidemiology. The Essentials. Baltimore, Williams & Wilkins, 1988.

A concise overview of the field of clinical epidemiology, long on concepts and illustrative cases and short on incomprehensible mathematics. This book was one of the first to provide a comprehensive framework for the evolving field of clinical epidemiology.

Norman, G. R., and Streiner, D. L.: PDQ Statistics. Toronto, B.C. Decker, 1986.

A primer of the application of statistical methodology to problems in clinical medicine. The approach is lighthearted and conceptual and requires little or no knowledge of the mathematical underpinnings of biostatistics.

Sackett, D. L., Haynes, R. B., and Tugwell, P.: Clinical Epidemiology. A Basic Science for Clinical Medicine. Boston, Little, Brown, 1985.

An excellent, comprehensive discussion of the application of the principles of clinical epidemiology to the practice of clinical medicine. The authors are pioneers of clinical epidemiology and critical appraisal, and the book is a readable classic.

Troidl, H., et al.: Principles and Practice of Research. Strategies for Surgical Investigators. New York, Springer-Verlag, 1991.

Oriented toward the needs of the neophyte surgical investigator, this text is in fact a comprehensive overview of the process of research from the initial idea to publication and presentation. It includes good chapters on biostatistics and the principles of study design and execution and is unusual in the international perspective afforded by its authors.

INDEX

Abdomen
  open, management of, *1012,* 1012–1013
  veins in, in hepatic disorders, 1059–1060, *1061*
Abdominal disorders
  imaging studies in, 1521–1522, *1522,* 1522t, *1523,* 1524–1536
  infectious. *See* Intra-abdominal infection
Abdominal films, plain, in hepatic disorders, *1066,* 1066–1067, *1067*
Abdominal surgery, as risk factor for neurologic surgical complications, 1220
Abducens nerve palsy, intracranial hypertension and, 66
Abortion, septic, antimicrobial therapy for, 1382
Abscesses. *See specific sites*
Acalculous cholecystitis, 1050–1051, *1051*
Accessory bypass tract tachycardia, 537, *540, 541*
Acclimatization
  to cold stress, 52
  to heat stress, 53
Acetaminophen intoxication, *1458,* 1458–1459
Acetazolamide, for metabolic alkalosis, 769
N-Acetylcysteine, for acetaminophen intoxication, 1459
Acid maltase deficiency (AMD), adult onset, 141–142
Acid/base disorders, 755–769. *See also* Metabolic acidosis; Metabolic alkalosis; Respiratory alkalosis
  identification of, 755–757
    compensatory responses in, 755–757, 756t, 757t
  in fulminant hepatic failure, 1089
Acid/base metabolism, normal, 755
Acidosis
  lactic, metabolic acidosis associated with, treatment of, 763
  metabolic. *See* Metabolic acidosis
  renal. *See* Renal tubular acidosis (RTA)
Acquired immunodeficiency syndrome (AIDS). *See* HIV infection/AIDS
Activated charcoal, 1457
  for substance abuse/overdose, 1429–1430
    with sedative/hypnotic, 1443
  for theophylline intoxication, 1463, 1463t
Activities of daily living, measurement of outcome and, 1688–1689, 1689t
Acute Physiology and Chronic Health Evaluation (APACHE). *See* APACHE II; APACHE; APACHE III
Acute renal failure (ARF), 783–798
  during ICU phase, 787–791

cause and presentation of, 789, *789,* 790t, 791
diagnosis of, 787–789, 788t
during post-ICU phase, 797–798
  renal support for, 797–798
during pre-ICU phase, 783–787, *784,* 784t
  drug adjustment and addition in, 785–787, 786t, *787*
  fluid therapy and balance in, 784–785, *785*
in chronic renal failure, 819–821
  risk phase of, 819–821, 820t
  support/rehabilitative phase of, 821
in patients awaiting liver transplantation
  cerebral edema and, 1139–1140
  coagulopathy and, 1139
  hepatic encephalopathy and, 1139
  metabolic disorders and, 1140
  sepsis and, 1139
  treatment of, 1138–1140
treatment of, 791–797
  mechanical support in, 792t, 792–797, *793–795*
    therapy selection and patient outcome and, 792–797, *796,* 796t, 797
  medical, 791–792
Acute tubular necrosis (ATN)
  in diffuse alveolar hemorrhage, 346
  in HIV infection/AIDS, 1414
Acyclovir
  dosing adjustment for renal or hepatic dysfunction, 1350t
  dosing during hemofiltration and hemodialysis, 1352t
  for eczema herpeticum, 950
  for herpes simplex encephalitis, 949
  for varicella-zoster virus infections, 953
  prophylactic
    following cardiac transplantation, 651
    for pneumonia, 413t
Addison's disease, 1175t, 1175–1176
  coma and, 13
  during post-ICU phase, 1181
Adenosine
  for supraventricular tachycardia, 543t
  in cardiopulmonary resuscitation, 556t
Adjustment disorder, with depressed mood, 33
Adrenal crisis, during ICU phase, 1179–1180
Adrenal disorders. *See also specific disorders*
  during ICU phase, 1179–1180
  failure. *See* Addison's disease
  in HIV infection/AIDS, 1414
  insufficiency, following renal surgery, 847–848
  tumors, hypertension with. *See* Hypertension, with adrenal tumors

Adrenergic receptors, shock and. *See* Shock
Adrenocorticotropic hormone (ACTH), deficiency of, 1177, 1180
Adrenoleukodystrophy, coma and, 12
Adult respiratory distress syndrome (ARDS), 164–167, *165, 166,* 302–310, 1004
  definition of, 302–303
  diagnostic criteria for, 303, 303t
  diffuse alveolar hemorrhage versus, 345–346
  during ICU phase, 304–310
    alveolar macrophage in, *306,* 306–307
    bronchoalveolar lavage markers of, 306–307
    clinical findings and criteria for admission to special units and, 307, 307t
    as systemic illness and prognostic indicator, 309–310
  pathogenesis of, 304–306
    complement-mediated neutrophil activation phase in, 305
    cytokine network phase in, 305–306
    permeability phase in, 304–305
  pathophysiology of, 304
  pharmacologic treatment for, 309
  supportive treatment for, 307t, 307–309
    fluid management in, 308
    infection surveillance in, 308–309
    nutritional interventions in, 308
    positive end-expiratory pressure in, 307–308
  during post-ICU phase, pulmonary sequelae and, 310
  during pre-ICU phase, risk factors, host factors, and clinical setting and, 303–304
  imaging studies in, 1493, *1497–1502*
  in disseminated intravascular coagulation, 875
  in necrotizing pancreatitis, 1020–1021
  therapeutic strategy for, 167, 167t
Advance directives, 1728, 1732
Adverse factor score, for ventilatory weaning, 443
Aerosol therapy
  during post-ICU phase, 491–492, 493–494
  during pre-ICU phase, 471–475, *472,* 472t, *473,* 473t
    anticholinergics and, 474
    anti-inflammatory agents and, 474
    antimicrobials and, 474, *475*
    antiviral agents and, 474–475, *475*
    beta-adrenergic agents and, 474
    bland aerosols and, 472–473
    mucolytic aerosols and, 473–474
Affect, in mental status examination, 30

1753

INDEX

Afterload, 509-511, *510*, 511t
Age. *See also* Elderly patients
  as surgical risk factor
    for neurologic complications, 1217
    for pulmonary complications, 1202
  pulmonary function and, 242, *243*
Agitation, 43-44
  etiology of, 43
  pharmacologic treatment of, 43-44
    benzodiazepines in, 44
    intravenous haloperidol in, 43t, 43-44
    muscle relaxants in, 44
    other neuroleptics in, 44
AIDS. *See* HIV infection/AIDS
Air, in pleural space, following thoracic surgery, 376-377
Air embolism, as complication of nutritional support, 1261
Airway management, 483-484, *484*, 484t
  following head and neck surgery, 213-214, *214*
  following thoracic surgery. *See* Thoracic surgical patients
  in brain injuries, 82
  in inhalation injury, 322-323, *323*
  in spinal cord injury, 147
  in upper airway obstruction. *See* Upper airway obstruction (UAO)
  initial, in upper airway obstruction, 194
  intracranial hypertension and, 67
Airway obstruction
  by malignant disease, 869-871, 870t
    during ICU phase, 870
    during post-ICU phase, 870-871
    during pre-ICU phase, 870
  of upper airway. *See* Upper airway obstruction (UAO)
Airway secretions, following thoracic surgery, 373-374
Albumin
  deficiency of
    as complication of nutritional support, 1263
    in brain injury, 86
  in hepatic disorders, 1064
Alcohol abuse/overdose, 1439-1441
  admission criteria in, 1440
  alcohol withdrawal and, 1440-1441, 1441t
  as predisposing condition to infection, 400
  coma and, 11
  complications of, 1439-1440
  diagnosis and treatment of, 1440
  hepatitis caused by, in cirrhosis, 1104-1107, 1105t, *1106*
  hypomagnesemia caused by, 1186
  pancreatitis due to, 1017, 1023, 1024
  signs and symptoms of, 1439
Aldosteronoma, hypertension and
  during ICU phase, 835-836
  during post-ICU phase, 836
  during pre-ICU phase, 835
Alkali administration, metabolic alkalosis associated with, 766
Alkaline phosphatase, in hepatic disorders, 1065
Alkalosis. *See* Metabolic alkalosis; Respiratory alkalosis
Allergic reactions
  shock and, 1315, 1315t
  to chemotherapy drugs, 892-893
    during ICU phase, 893
    during post-ICU phase, 893
    during pre-ICU phase, 892-893

Allopurinol, interaction with azathioprine, 1148
Alpha blockers, for hypertension, postoperative, 747
Alpha-methyldopa, for hypertension, 692t-694t
Alveolar hypoventilation. *See* Hypoventilation syndromes
Alveolar macrophage, in adult respiratory distress syndrome, *306*, 306-307
Amanita toxicity, 1469
Amantadine
  dosing adjustment for renal or hepatic dysfunction, 1350t
  dosing during hemofiltration and hemodialysis, 1352t
Ambulation, postoperative, pulmonary function and, 1207
Amdinocillin
  dosing adjustment for renal or hepatic dysfunction, 1350t
  dosing during hemofiltration and hemodialysis, 1352t
Amikacin
  for intra-abdominal infections, 1378
  for pneumonia, 1375
    nosocomial, 394
Amino acids, for total parenteral nutrition, 1259, 1261t
Aminoglycosides. *See also specific drugs*
  computer programs for dosing with, 1355-1359
    in anuric renal failure and hemodialysis, 1357, *1358*, 1359
    in good renal function, 1355-1357, *1356, 1357*
  dosing adjustment for renal or hepatic dysfunction, 1350t
  dosing during hemofiltration and hemodialysis, 1352t
  for intra-abdominal infections, 1378
  pharmacokinetics of, 1342-1347, 1343t
    distribution volume and, 1343-1344
    high-dose therapy and, 1346-1347
    in hemodialysis, dosage and, 1344-1345
    infection-induced renal dysfunction and, 1345
    large-dose once-a-day dosing and, 1347
    renal function and, 1344
    toxicities and, 1345-1346
  resistance to, 1386-1387
    patterns of, application to ICU phase of patient management, 1391-1393, *1391-1393*, 1393t
Aminophylline, in cardiopulmonary resuscitation, 556t
Aminotransferases, in hepatic disorders, 1064-1065
Amiodarone
  for supraventricular tachycardia, 543t
  for ventricular tachycardia, 544t, 544-545
  in cardiopulmonary resuscitation, 558
Ammonia, inhalation injury caused by, 319
Ammonium chloride, for hallucinogen abuse/overdose, 1449
Amnesia, concussive head injury and, 77
Amphetamine abuse/overdose, 1435-1437
  complications of, 1436
  diagnosis and management of, 1436-1437
  signs and symptoms of, 1436
  special considerations in, 1437
Amphotericin B
  dosing adjustment for renal or hepatic dysfunction, 1350t

  dosing during hemofiltration and hemodialysis, 1352t
  for line sepsis, 1384
  for pneumonia, in granulocytopenic hosts, 409-410
  for urinary tract infections, 1381
Ampicillin
  dosing adjustment for renal or hepatic dysfunction, 1350t
  dosing during hemofiltration and hemodialysis, 1352t
  for central nervous system infections, 1372
  for meningococcemia, 1382
Amrinone
  during weaning from cardiopulmonary bypass, 648
  for shock, 1325t, 1328
Amylase, serum level of, in pancreatitis, 1022-1023
Amyloid angiopathy, 79
Amyotrophic lateral sclerosis (ALS), 136-138, 137t
  during ICU phase, 137
  during post-ICU phase, 137-138
  during pre-ICU phase, 137
Analgesia, 1283-1286. *See also* Analgesics; *specific drugs and procedures*
  administration routes for, 1283
  epidural, postoperative, for thoracic surgery patients, 371
  indications for, 1279
  intercostal nerve blocks for, 1285-1286
  parenteral narcotics for, 1283t, 1283-1285, 1284t
  patient-controlled, 1284
  peridural narcotics for, 1285, 1285t
  postoperative, for thoracic surgery patients, *371*, 371-372, *372*
  termination guidelines for, 1731, 1734, 1735-1736, 1737
Analgesics. *See also* Analgesia; *specific drugs*
  following head and neck surgery, 223
  for elevated intracranial pressure, in comatose patient, 19
  for pancreatitis, 1033
Analysis of variance, 1749
Anaphylactic reactions, shock and, 1315, 1315t
Anaphylactoid reactions, shock and, 1315, 1315t
Anaphylaxis, upper airway obstruction and, during pre-ICU phase, 192, 193
Anemia, 877-878
  coma and, 9
  during ICU phase, 878
  during post-ICU phase, 878
  during pre-ICU phase, 878
  erythropoietin deficiency causing, 901-902
  following vascular surgery, 724
  hemolytic. *See* Hemolytic anemia
  in diffuse alveolar hemorrhage, 342
  in HIV infection/AIDS, 1412
  iron deficiency, 901
  megaloblastic, 901
  of chronic renal failure, 807-808
Anesthesia. *See also* Anesthetics
  as surgical risk factor, for pulmonary complications, 1201-1202
  for cardiac transplantation, 646
  for thoracic surgery, 363
  malignant hyperthermia caused by. *See* Malignant hyperthermia (MH)
  recovery from, following cardiac surgery, 596

INDEX

Anesthetics. *See also* Anesthesia
   as cutting substances in street drugs, 1427, 1428t
   hypertension caused by, 740
   in bronchospastic disease, 237
   inhalation, for elevated intracranial pressure, in comatose patient, 19
   peridural, for pain control, 1285, 1285t
Aneurysm(s)
   aortic, resection of, hypertension following, 736
   thoracic, 709-712
     false, 709-710
       clinical situation and diagnosis of, 709-710, *710*
     true, 710-711
       ascending, clinical presentations of, 710-711
       descending and thoracoabdominal, 711-712
Aneurysmal subarachnoid hemorrhage, 88
Angina
   as indication for surgery, 587, 588t
   Ludwig's, during pre-ICU phase, 192
   stable, surgical indications in, 587, 588t
Angioedema, during pre-ICU phase, 192-193, 193t
Angiography
   cerebral
     in brain injury, 85
     in intracranial hypertension, 68
   coronary, preoperative, 1210
   following vascular surgery, during pre-ICU phase, 714
   in focal pulmonary hemorrhage, 352
   in gastrointestinal bleeding, 996-997
     constrictive technique for, 997
     occlusive technique for, 997
   in hepatic disorders, 1073-1074, *1074*
   in mitral regurgitation, 665
   magnetic resonance, in brain injury, 85
   pulmonary, in pulmonary embolism, 425
Angiomas, spider, in hepatic disorders, 1059, *1060*
Angiomatosis, bacillary, cutaneous, in HIV infection/AIDS, 1410
Angiopathy, amyloid, 79
Angiotensin-converting enzyme (ACE) inhibitors. *See also specific drugs*
   for acute myocardial infarction, 577
   for hypertension, 692t-694t
     postoperative, 749
   for mitral regurgitation, 666t
Anhydrides, inhalation injury caused by, 320
Anion gap, in metabolic acidosis, 758
Antagonist narcotic agents, for pain control, 1284-1285
Anterior SCI syndrome, 149-150
Anterograde amnesia, concussive head injury and, 77
Anthropometric measurements, in nutrition assessment, 1251
Antiarrhythmic drugs. *See also specific drugs and drug types*
   for hypothermia, 56
   intoxication by, 1470
Antibasement membrane antibody (ABMA) disease, diffuse alveolar hemorrhage and, 343-344, 344t, 347
Antibiotic(s), 1368t. *See also specific drugs and drug types*
   control of, 1594-1595, *1595*
   pharmacokinetics of, 1338-1359
     dosing in renal and/or hepatic dysfunction and, 1349-1354, 1350t-1354t
     in multiple organ system failure, 1349, 1353-1354
     interdependency with disease states, 1340-1342
       during ICU phase, 1341-1342, 1342t
       during post-ICU phase, 1342
       during pre-ICU phase, 1340-1341, 1341t
     of aminoglycosides. *See* Aminoglycosides, pharmacokinetics of
     of antifungals, 1355
     of antivirals, 1355
     of beta-lactams. *See* Beta-lactams, pharmacokinetics of
     of vancomycin, 1347-1349
       dosing in elderly patients and, 1348
       dosing in hemodialysis patients and, 1348-1349
     pharmacokinetic models and, 1338-1340, *1339, 1340*
     mode of action and, 1340, 1340t
Antibiotic prophylaxis
   following cardiac transplantation, 651
   following vascular surgery, 720
   for infection control, 1589-1590
   for multiple organ system failure, 1302
   for thoracic surgery, 366
Antibiotic resistance, 1385-1387
   application to ICU phase of patient management, 1387-1395
   aminoglycosides and, 1391-1393, *1391-1393*, 1393t
   beta-lactams and, 1387-1391, *1388, 1389t, 1390,* 1391t
   fluoroquinolones and, 1393, *1394, 1395, 1395*
   to aminoglycosides, 1386-1387
   to beta-lactams, 1385-1386, *1386*
   to fluoroquinolones, 1387
Antibiotic therapy, 1365-1396. *See also* Antibiotic prophylaxis; Antibiotic therapy; *specific drugs*
   as predisposing condition to infection, 401
   during ICU phase, 1370-1385
     for febrile patients, 1370t, 1370-1371
     with infections complicating special aspects of critical care, 1383-1384
     with infections usually incidental to critical care, 1385
     with localized infections, 1372-1383
     with nonlocalized infections, 1371t, 1371-1372
     with nosocomial infections, 1383
     with parasitic, tropical, exotic, and travelers' infections, 1384-1385
   during post-ICU phase, 1395-1396
   during pre-ICU phase, 1369-1370
   effective, 1366, 1368-1369, 1369t
   following head and neck surgery, 223
   following liver transplantation, 1148
   for bone marrow transplantation, 881-882
   for bronchospastic disease, 235
   for cellulitis, 927
   for chronic obstructive pulmonary disease, 252
   for erysipelas, 925
   for infection control, 1589-1590, 1590t
   for intra-abdominal infection, 1010-1011
   for leukopenia, 877
   for meningococcal infections, cutaneous, 944
   for necrotizing fasciitis, 935
   for pancreatitis, 1033-1034, 1034t
   for patients awaiting liver transplantation, 1137
   for pneumonia
     community-acquired, 391t, 391-392
     during post-ICU phase, 395-396
     in granulocytopenic hosts, 409-410
     nosocomial, 393t, 393-394
     with B-cell host defects, 410
     with cell-mediated host defects, 410
     with solid tumors, 410-411
   for pseudomonal infections, cutaneous, 941
   for spontaneous bacterial peritonitis, 1110
   for staphylococcal scalded skin syndrome, 930
   for toxic epidermal necrolysis, 963-964
   for toxic shock syndrome, 933
   hypomagnesemia caused by, 1186
   in aerosol therapy, 474, *475*
   in renal failure, adjustment of, 785
   selection of drugs for, 1365-1366, 1366t-1369t
   termination guidelines for, 1731, 1733
Antibody-mediated hemolytic anemia, 904-905
Anticholinergics. *See also specific drugs*
   for bronchospastic disease, 233t, 234
   for chronic obstructive pulmonary disease, 249
   in aerosol therapy, 474
Anticoagulants. *See also specific drugs*
   calcium binding and, 1190
   circulating, acquired, 913-914
   following vascular surgery, 719-720
   for aortic regurgitation, during post-ICU phase, 679
   for atrial fibrillation, 540
   for disseminated intravascular coagulation, 875
   for mitral regurgitation, 669
   for prevention of myocardial infarction, 581, 582
   for pulmonary embolism, 421-422, 429-431, 430t, 431t
     long-term, 433
   necrosis induced by, *968*, 968-969
   oral, for thrombotic disorders, 915-916, 916t
Antidepressants. *See also specific drugs*
   newer, 37
   nontricyclic, poisoning by, 1461-1462
   tricyclic. *See* Tricyclic antidepressants (TCAs)
Antidotes, in inhalation injury, 323-324
Antifungals, 1368t. *See also specific drugs*
   pharmacokinetics of, 1355
Antihypertensive agents. *See also specific drugs and drug types*
   centrally acting, for hypertension, postoperative, 748-749
Anti-inflammatory agents. *See also specific drugs*
   in aerosol therapy, 474
Antilymphocyte globulin (ALG)
   following renal transplantation, 829
   for bone marrow transplantation, 881t
Antimicrobials. *See* Antibiotic *entries*
Antimyosin scanning, in cardiac trauma, nonpenetrating, 632-633
Antiparasitic agents, 1368t
Antiplatelet agents. *See also specific drugs*
   following vascular surgery, 720
   for prevention of myocardial infarction, 581-582

INDEX

Antiretroviral therapies, for HIV infection, 1403–1404
Antithyroid drugs. *See also specific drugs*
 for thyroid storm, 1177
Antivenin, for snake bites, 1469
Antiviral agents, 1368t. *See also specific drugs*
 for HIV infection, 1403–1404
 in aerosol therapy, 474–475, *475*
 pharmacokinetics of, 1355
Anuria
 following cardiac surgery, 600–601
 management of, 853–854, *854*
Anxiety, 32–33
 diagnostic and clinical characteristics of, 32, 32t
 etiologic and predisposing factors for, 32, 33t
 treatment of, 32–33, 33t
Aortic coarctation, thoracic, resection of, hypertension following, 736–737
Aortic disorders. *See also specific disorders*
 aneurysmal. *See* Aneurysm(s)
 following renal revascularization, 833–834, 834t
 imaging studies in, 1513, 1518, *1519–1522,* 1521
Aortic dissection, 700–709, *701*
 anatomy and pathophysiology of, 700–701, 701t
 aortic regurgitation and, 670–671, *672*
 classification of, 702
 during ICU phase, 703–709
  ascending
   definitive therapy of, 705–707, *706, 707*
   late follow-up of, 709
   postoperative management and, 707–708, *708*
  definitive diagnosis of, 703–704, *705*
  treatment of, 704–709, 705t
 during post-ICU phase, 709
  descending, 709
 during pre-ICU phase, 702–703
  clinical syndromes and natural history of, 702, 702t
  diagnosis of, 702–703
  indications for ICU admission and, 703
Aortic regurgitation, 670–680
 during ICU phase, 677–679
  surgical management of, 678–679, *679*
 during post-ICU phase, 679–680
  anticoagulation and, 680
  endocarditis prophylaxis and, 679–680
  management of underlying disorder and, 680
  postoperative recovery and evaluation and, 679
 during pre-ICU phase, 670–677
  auscultation in, 671–673
  cause of, 670t, 670–671
   aortic root dilatation as, 671
   cusp abnormality as, 670, *671*
   loss of commissural support as, 670–671, *672*
   prosthetic valve dysfunction as, 671
  clinical manifestations of, 671, 672t
  laboratory studies in, 673–677
   cardiac catheterization, 677
   chest radiography, 673
   echocardiography, 673–676, *674–676*
   electrocardiography, 673, 673t
   prosthetic valve assessment, 676–677
   radionuclide imaging, 677
  pathophysiology of, 671

Aortic root dilatation, aortic regurgitation and, 671
Aortic sclerosis, as risk factor for neurologic surgical complications, 1218
Aortic valvuloplasty, of aortic regurgitation, 678–679, *679*
Aortography, in aortic dissection, 704
APACHE, 1672–1673, *1673*
APACHE II, 1673–1674, *1676,* 1677t
 evaluation of, 1664–1665, 1665t
 in pancreatitis, 1025–1027, *1026*
APACHE III, *1676,* 1676–1677, *1680,* 1680t, *1681*
Appeals, of verdict, 1724–1725
Appearance, in mental status examination, 29
Appendix, imaging studies of, 1547, 1549t–1550t, 1550
Application programs, 1704
Arbitration boards, 1722
Arginine hydrochloride, for hallucinogen abuse/overdose, 1449
Arrhythmias, 530–551
 cocaine abuse/overdose causing, 1433
  treatment of, 1434
 digoxin causing, 1464
 during ICU phase, 534–538, 535t
  bradyarrhythmias, 545–548, 546t, *547–550*
  following vascular surgery, 717
  supraventricular, 535–538, *536–542*
   treatment of, 539–542, 543t
  ventricular, 542–545, 543t, 544t, *545, 546*
 during post-ICU phase, 548–549, 551
 during pre-ICU phase, 530–534, *531, 533*
 following thoracic surgery, 378
 monitoring for, in acute myocardial infarction, 577–578
 pre-cardiac transplantation, 642
 refractory, in hypomagnesemia, 1187
 supraventricular, following cardiac surgery, 597
 theophylline causing, 1463
 treatment of, preoperative, for prevention of cardiovascular complications, 1215
 ventricular, following cardiac surgery, 597
Arterial blood gases (ABGs)
 following vascular surgery, during ICU phase, 716
 for monitoring respiratory insufficiency, 479
 in adult respiratory distress syndrome, 165
 in bronchospastic disease, 230
 noninvasive measurement of, 1643–1647
  capnography for, 1644, 1644t, *1644–1647,* 1646–1647
  oximetry for, 1643–1644
Arterial catheterization, 1599–1602. *See also* Pulmonary artery catheterization
 complications and management of, 1600–1601
 contraindications to, 1600
 data analysis for, 1601
 indications for, 1600
 quality enhancement for, 1601t, 1601–1602
Arterial pulse recordings, indirect, ventricular function evaluation using, 518
Arteriosclerosis, following cardiac transplantation, 652–653
Arteriovenous access. *See* Hemodialysis, access for

Arteriovenous malformations (AVMs), hemorrhagic stroke and, 80
Arthritis, septic, intracranial, pre-ICU evaluation of, 105
Arthroplasty, as risk factor for neurologic surgical complications, 1219–1220
Ascites
 in cirrhosis, 1107t, 1107–1116
  ascitic fluid analysis in, 1108–1109, 1109t
  causes of, 1108
  clinical evaluation of, 1108
  complications of, *1109,* 1109–1113
   culture-negative neutrocytic ascites, 1111
   hepatic hydrothorax, 1112–1113
   hernia, 1112
   monomicrobial neutrocytic bacterascites, 1111–1112
   spontaneous bacterial peritonitis, 1109–1111, 1110t
  pathogenesis of, 1107–1108
  treatment of, 1113–1116
   diuretics in, 1113–1114
   in patients awaiting liver transplantation, 1136–1137
   paracentesis in, 1114
   peritoneovenous shunts in, 1114–1116, *1115, 1116*
 malignant, 873
  during ICU phase, 873
  during post-ICU phase, 873
  during pre-ICU phase, 873
Ascorbic acid, for hallucinogen abuse/overdose, 1449
Aseptic meningitis, pre-ICU evaluation of, 107
Aspartate aminotransferase (AST), serum levels of, in acute myocardial infarction, 571, *571*
Aspiration pneumonitis, in brain injury, 86
Aspirin
 following vascular surgery, 720
 for prevention of myocardial infarction, 581–582
 for thrombotic disorders, 916
 platelet disorders related to, 910–911
 poisoning by, *1459,* 1459–1460
Assist ventilation, 485
Assist-control ventilation (AMV). *See* Mechanical ventilation, assist/control mode
Asthma, 242. *See also* Bronchospastic disease; Chronic obstructive pulmonary disease (COPD)
 as surgical risk factor, for pulmonary complications, 1203
 factitious, during pre-ICU phase, 194
 pulmonary function testing in, 464–465, *466*
Atelectasis
 following thoracic surgery, 375
 following vascular surgery, 720–721
 imaging studies in, 1486–1487, *1487–1490*
 monitoring for, during mechanical ventilation, 293–294, 294t
 prevention and treatment of, 467–468, *468*
Atenolol, for thyroid storm, 1178
Atherosclerosis
 coronary, prevention of, 603
 following vascular surgery, during pre-ICU phase, 714

INDEX

Atracurium, 1287t, 1287-1288
   during mechanical ventilation, during ICU phase, 290
Atrial electrogram, in arrhythmias, 532-533, *533*
Atrial fibrillation, 536, *536*
   in acute myocardial infarction, 578
   treatment of, 539-540, 543t
Atrial flutter, 536, *537*
   treatment of, 540-541
Atrial premature complexes (APCs), 535-536
   treatment of, 543t
Atrial tachycardia, multifocal, 538
   treatment of, 542
Atropine
   for organophosphate intoxication, 1468
   in cardiopulmonary resuscitation, 556t, 558
Attorneys. *See* Liability
Attribution validity, 1665t
Auscultation, in aortic regurgitation, 671-673
Austin Flint murmur, in aortic regurgitation, 672
Autoimmune hemolytic anemia, drug-related, 905
Autologous blood donation (ABD) programs, 1240-1241
Autonomic hyperreflexia, hypertension following, postoperative, 737
Autonomy
   definition of, 1728t
   patients' rights to, 1727-1728
Autotransfusion, intraoperative, 1241
Axillary vein thrombosis, management of, 434
Azathioprine
   following cardiac transplantation, 650-651
   following renal transplantation, 829
   interaction with allopurinol, 1148
Azidothymidine (AZT; Retrovir; zidovudine), for HIV infection, 1403-1404
Azlocillin
   dosing adjustment for renal or hepatic dysfunction, 1350t
   dosing during hemofiltration and hemodialysis, 1352t
Azotemia, 802
Aztreonam
   dosing adjustment for renal or hepatic dysfunction, 1350t
   dosing during hemofiltration and hemodialysis, 1352t
   for pneumonia, 1375

Bacillary peliosis hepatitis, in HIV infection/AIDS, 1410
Bacteremia
   antimicrobial therapy for, 1382-1383
   in hepatic artery thrombosis, following liver transplantation, 1146
   in HIV infection/AIDS, 1409
   shock and, 1314-1315
   systemic inflammatory response syndrome and, 1003
Bacteria
   anaerobic, antimicrobials effective against, 1379
   in cerebrospinal fluid, analysis of, 1616
Bacterial endocarditis, coma and, 10

Bacterial infections. *See* Infection, bacterial; *specific infections*
Balloon tamponade
   for esophageal varices, 1097-1098, *1098*
   for gastrointestinal bleeding, in patients awaiting liver transplantation, 1135-1136, 1136t
Barbiturate(s). *See also* Sedative/hypnotic(s); *specific drugs*
   for delirium, 1283
   for elevated intracranial pressure, in comatose patient, 19-20
   for intracranial hypertension, 73
   intoxication by, coma and, 11
Barbiturate coma, 1283
   for status epilepticus, 99, *99*, 99t
Barotrauma, monitoring for, during mechanical ventilation, 293
Basal energy expenditure (BEE), for estimation of energy requirements, 1254
Basilar skull fracture, 78
Basophils, 899
BCNU, for bone marrow transplantation, 881t
Bedside screening devices, for monitoring and detection of respiratory insufficiency, 464, *465*
Bedside spirometry, for monitoring and detection of respiratory insufficiency, 462, 464, 464t, 479-480
Behavior, in mental status examination, 29
Behavioral problems, 44-45
Behavioral responses
   to cold stress, 52
   to heat stress, 52
Benzodiazepines, 1280t, 1280-1281
   for agitation, 44
   intoxication by, coma and, 11
Benzyl penicillin, for meningococcal infections, cutaneous, 944
Beta agonists. *See also specific drugs*
   for chronic obstructive pulmonary disease, 249
   in bronchospastic disease, 233t, 233-234
Beta blockers. *See also specific drugs*
   adrenergic response and, 1322
   following cardiac surgery, 603-604
   for acute myocardial infarction, 576, 576t
   for hypertension, 692t-694t
   postoperative, 747-748
   for prevention of myocardial infarction, 581
Beta-adrenergic agents. *See also specific drugs*
   in aerosol therapy, 474
Beta-lactams. *See also specific drugs*
   pharmacokinetics of, 1354-1355
      antistaphylococcal penicillins, 1354
      cephalosporins, 1354-1355
      penicillins, carbapenems, and monobactams, 1354
   resistance to, 1385-1386, *1386*
   patterns of, application to ICU phase of patient management, 1387-1391, *1388*, 1389t, *1390*, 1391t
Bias, in research, 1739, 1743
BICAP probe, for therapeutic endoscopy, 993
Bicarbonate. *See* Sodium bicarbonate
Biliary obstruction, extrahepatic, jaundice and, postoperative, 1120-1121
Biliary sepsis. *See* Gallstone(s)
Biliary stents, *1054*, 1054-1055, *1055*

Biliary tract disease. *See also specific disorders*
   in HIV infection/AIDS, 1408-1409
Bilirubin, in hepatic disorders, 1062-1064, 1063t
   jaundice, postoperative, 1119
Biomedical engineering, 1651-1662, *1652*
   future of, 1661-1662
   historical background of, 1652-1654, *1653*, *1654*
   instrumentation and, 1654-1656, *1655*, 1655t, 1656t
   problems and solutions in, 1656-1659, 1657t, *1658*, *1659*, 1659t
   resource requirements for, 1659-1661, *1660*, *1661*, 1661t, 1662t
Biomedicus centrifugal pump, 593
Biostatistics. *See* Clinical epidemiology, biostatistics and
Bites, of snakes and spiders, 1468-1469
Bladder disorders, imaging studies in, 1540
Blinding, 1743
Blood. *See also* Hematologic *entries*; Hemoglobin *entries*; Red cells; White cells; *specific disorders*
   autologous donation of, 1240-1241
   replacement of. *See* Transfusion therapy
Blood conservation techniques, 1240
Blood flow, cerebral, in traumatic brain injury, 87
Blood gases. *See* Arterial blood gases (ABGs)
Blood pressure. *See also* Hypertension; Hypotension
   intermediate-term regulation of, 730-732, *731*
   long-term regulation of, *732*, 732-733, *733*
   short-term regulation of, 729-730, *730*
   systemic. *See* Systemic blood pressure
Blood pressure limits, postcraniotomy, 89
Blood pressure monitoring, 1633-1640. *See also* Central venous pressure monitoring; Pulmonary artery pressure monitoring
   systemic, 1633-1635
      invasive techniques for, *1634*, 1634-1635
      noninvasive techniques for, 1633-1634
Blood urea nitrogen (BUN), in renal failure, 788
Blood vessels, infection of, antimicrobial therapy for, 1377
Body mass index (BMI), in nutrition assessment, 1250-1251
Body packing, 1435
Body temperature, 51. *See also* Thermoregulation; *specific thermoregulatory disorders*
   measurement of, 51
Bone marrow transplantation, 880-883, 881t
   allogenic, 881
   autologous, 881
   during ICU phase, 882-883
   during post-ICU phase, 883
   during pre-ICU phase, 881t, 881-882
   syngenic, 881
Botulism, 135-136
   during ICU phase, 136
   during post-ICU phase, 136
   during pre-ICU phase, 135-136
Bradyarrhythmias, treatment of, 545-548, 546t, *547*-550
Bradycardia
   sinus, in acute myocardial infarction, 578
   ventricular arrhythmias and, 534

INDEX

Brain
  abscess of, 80-81, *81*, 89
    coma and, 8
    during ICU phase, 120t, 120-122, 121t, 123
    pre-ICU evaluation of, 113-114
  coma and. *See* Coma
  edema of, postcraniotomy, 89
  tumors of, 81, 89
Brain death, 1729
  definition of, 1728t
  establishment of, 22
  in intracranial hypertension, 73, 74
Brain injury, 76-90, 77t. *See also specific injuries*
  acute, 76-80
    hemorrhagic stroke, 79-80
    traumatic brain injury, 76-79
  during ICU phase, 86-89
    hemorrhagic stroke, 88-89
    intracranial pressure and, 86
    systemic management and assessment and, 86-87
    traumatic brain injury, 87-88
  during post-ICU phase, 89-90
    ICU readmission and, 89
    placement and rehabilitation and, 89-90
  during pre-ICU phase, 81-85
    assessment and, 83-85
    patient stabilization and, 82-83
    triage and, 85, 85t, 86t
  localization of lesions and, 76, 77t
  mass lesions, progressive, 80-81
    abscesses, 80-81
    tumors, 81
  presentation of, 76
  traumatic. *See* Traumatic brain injury
Brain stem auditory evoked potentials (BAEPs), in comatose patient, 21
Breathing
  in spinal cord injury, 147
  work of
    effort of breathing contrasted with, 170, *170*
    ventilatory failure and, 168-172, 168-173
      ability to accomplish, 172-173
      mechanical output and, 168-170, *169, 170*
      oxygen consumption and, 168
      partially assisted breathing cycles and, 171-172, *172*
      spontaneous breathing cycles and, 170-171, *171*
Bretylium
  for ventricular tachycardia, 544, 544t
  in cardiopulmonary resuscitation, 556t, 558
Bridging veins, 78
Bronchiectasis, 242. *See also* Chronic obstructive pulmonary disease (COPD)
Bronchiolitis obliterans organizing pneumonia (BOOP), 395
Bronchitis
  acute, during ICU phase, 253
  antimicrobial therapy for, 1374
  chronic, 242. *See also* Chronic obstructive pulmonary disease (COPD)
Bronchoalveolar lavage (BAL)
  adult respiratory distress syndrome markers and, 306-307
  during mechanical ventilation, 296
  in bronchospastic disease, 237-238

in diffuse alveolar hemorrhage, 343
  in pneumonia, 412
    nosocomial, 393
Bronchodilators. *See also specific drugs*
  for inhalation injury, 333
  pulmonary surgery and, 1208
Bronchopleural fistula, following thoracic surgery, 374
Bronchopulmonary hygiene therapy, during pre-ICU phase, 475-476
  chest percussion and vibration and, 475
  cough and deep breathing exercises and, 475
  postural drainage therapy and, 475-476, *476, 477,* 478t
Bronchoscopy, 1602-1603
  complications of, 1602-1603
  contraindications to, 1602
  data analysis for, 1603
  during mechanical ventilation, 295-296
  in focal pulmonary hemorrhage, 350, 351
  in pneumonia, 408, 412
    nosocomial, 393
  indications for, 1602
  quality enhancement for, 1603
  therapeutic, 482
Bronchospastic disease, 228-239, *229*. *See also* Asthma
  during ICU phase, 233-238
    drug therapy and, 233t, 233-235
    heroic measures and, 237-238
    monitoring of response and, 238
    ventilation and, 235-237, *237*
  during post-ICU phase, 238-239
  during pre-ICU phase, 228-233
    history and physical examination and, 228-230, *229*, 229t
    in special patient populations, 231t, 231-233
    pulmonary function and blood gases and, 230, 230t
    routine laboratory studies and, 230-231
Brown-Sequard syndrome, 150
Budd-Chiari syndrome, 1079-1080
  imaging in, 1067, *1068*
Bullectomy, following thoracic surgery, 378
Bullous drug eruptions, 967
Bupivacaine, peridural, for pain control, 1285, 1285t
Busulfan, for bone marrow transplantation, 881t
Butorphanol (Stadol), abuse/overdose of, 1446
Butyrophenones, for delirium, 1282-1283

Caffeine abuse/overdose, 1438-1439
  complications of, 1438
  diagnosis and treatment of, 1438
  ICU admission criteria in, 1438
  signs and symptoms of, 1438
  special considerations in, 1439
Calcitonin, for hypercalcemia, 884, 1193, 1193t
Calcium, 1189-1193
  balance of, 1190. *See also* Hypercalcemia; Hypocalcemia
  for shock, 1329
  in cardiopulmonary resuscitation, 556t, 557-558
  ionized, 1190
  plasma, 1189-1190
Calcium channel blockers
  for acute myocardial infarction, 577

for elevated intracranial pressure, in comatose patient, 20
  for hypertension, 692t-694t
    postoperative, 748
Calcium chloride, in cardiopulmonary resuscitation, 561-562
Calcium deposition, in spinal cord injury, 156
Calcium gluconate
  for hyperkalemia, 779t, 779-780
  for hypermagnesemia, 1189
Calf vein thrombosis, management of, 433
Camino ICP system, 70, *70*
Cancer. *See* Malignancy; Mass lesions; Oncologic emergencies; *specific cancers*
Candidiasis, oral, in HIV infection/AIDS, 1408
Capacity, 1728
  definition of, 1728t
Capnography, 1644, 1644t, *1644-1647*, 1646-1647
  for monitoring respiratory insufficiency, 480-481, *481*
Captopril
  for hypertension, 692t-694t
  for mitral regurgitation, 666t
Carbapenems, pharmacokinetics of, 1354
Carbenicillin
  dosing adjustment for renal or hepatic dysfunction, 1350t
  dosing during hemofiltration and hemodialysis, 1352t
Carbon dioxide, minute ventilation and, 265, 265t
Carbon monoxide
  diffusing capacity for, in diffuse alveolar hemorrhage, 343
  inhalation injury caused by, 318-319
  intoxication by, 1462
    coma and, 9-10
Carboplatin, for bone marrow transplantation, 881t
Carcinoid tumors, resection of, hypertension following, 738
Cardiac arrhythmias. *See* Arrhythmias
Cardiac catheterization
  in aortic regurgitation, 677
  in mitral regurgitation, 663
Cardiac disorders. *See also specific disorders*
  chemotherapy-induced, 892
    during ICU phase, 892
    during post-ICU phase, 892
    during pre-ICU phase, 892
  classification systems for, 1678-1679, 1681t, *1682*, 1682t
  in fulminant hepatic failure, 1086-1087
  in HIV infection/AIDS, 1414
  shock and, adrenergic response and, 1322-1323
Cardiac function, 507-526
  determinants of, 507-514
    afterload, 509-511, *510*, 511t
    inotropy, *511*, 511-512, 512t
      descending limb of Starling curve and, 512
    of right ventricular function, 512-514, *514*, 514t
    preload, 507-509, *508*
      disease states influencing, 508-509, 509t
  follow-up of critically ill patient and, 522-526, 524t, *526*
  intrinsic contractility and, 507
  ventricular. *See* Ventricular function

Cardiac hemolytic anemia, traumatic, 904
Cardiac massage
  external
    closed chest, complications of, 562
    in cardiopulmonary resuscitation, 561
    open-chest, in cardiopulmonary resuscitation, 561-562
Cardiac output. *See also* Heart failure, high output
  thermodilution cardiac output measurement and, 1640-1642, *1641,* 1641t
    derived parameters and, 1641-1642, 1642t
Cardiac pacing
  for bradyarrhythmias, 545-548, 546t, *547-550*
  in cardiopulmonary resuscitation, 562
  temporary, 1617-1619
    complications and management of transvenous pacemakers and, 1618t, 1618-1619, *1619*
    contraindications to, 1618
    indications for, 1617-1618, 1618t
    quality enhancement for, 1619
Cardiac surgery
  coma and, 9
  imaging studies following, 1513, *1517-1519*
Cardiac tamponade, following cardiac surgery, 598
Cardiac transplantation, 640-653
  candidates for, 640-641
    contraindications and, 640, 641t
    evaluation of, 640-641, 641t
    indications and, 640
  during post-ICU phase, 652-653
    discharged patients and, 652
      surgical procedures on, 652
    graft arteriosclerosis of transplanted heart and, 652-653
    hospitalized patients and, 652
    infections and, 653
    malignant disease and, 653
  operative phase of, 645-648
    donor during, 645-646
    recipient during, 646-648
      cardiopulmonary bypass, cardiectomy, and implantation and, 646-647
      drugs and anesthesia for, 646
      induction, preparation and cannulation of, 646
      myocardial preservation and, 647
      weaning from cardiopulmonary bypass, 647-648
      timing of surgery and, 645
  postoperative ICU phase of, 648-652
    early, 648-651
      cardiac considerations during, 649
      central nervous system considerations during, 649
      coagulation during, 649
      gastrointestinal considerations during, 649-650
      infection prophylaxis during, 651
      metabolic considerations during, 650
      pulmonary considerations during, 649
      rejection prophylaxis, monitoring, and therapy during, 650t, 650-651, 651t
      renal considerations during, 649
    late, 652
      hypertension during, 652, 736
  pretransplant period and, 641-645

before donor identification, 641-652
donor during, 643t, 643-645
matching during, 643
recipient during, 643
Cardiac trauma, 627-634
  nonpenetrating, 629-634, 630t, *631*
    during ICU phase, 630-633
      diagnostic evaluation of, 630-633
      hemodynamic features of, 633, *633*
      treatment of, 633, *634*
    during post-ICU phase, 633-634
    during pre-ICU phase, 630, 632t
  penetrating, 627-629
    during ICU phase, *628,* 628-629, *629*
    during post-ICU phase, 629
    during pre-ICU phase, 627-628, *628*
Cardiectomy, for cardiac transplantation, 647
Cardiogenic shock, 1314
  in acute myocardial infarction, 578
  percutaneous transluminal coronary angioplasty for, 575
Cardiomyopathy
  dilated, 618-622, 619t
    during ICU phase, 619-620
      diagnostic evaluation of, 619
      endomyopathy biopsy in, 619, *620,* 621t
      hemodynamic features of, 619
      treatment of, 619-620
    during post-ICU phase, 621-622
    during pre-ICU phase, 618
  hypertrophic, 622-625
    during ICU phase, 622-625
      diagnostic evaluation of, 622-623
      hemodynamic features of, 623, *624*
      treatment of, 623-625, 624t
    during post-ICU phase, 625
    during pre-ICU phase, 622
  treatment of, preoperative, for prevention of cardiovascular complications, 1216
  in HIV infection/AIDS, 1414
Cardioplegia, as surgical risk factor, for pulmonary complications, 1202
Cardiopulmonary bypass
  for cardiac transplantation, 646
  weaning from, 647-648
Cardiopulmonary bypass (CPB), pathophysiology of, *594,* 594-595, *595*
Cardiopulmonary disorders. *See also specific disorders*
  in brain injury, 86
Cardiopulmonary resuscitation (CPR), 553-566, *554*
  airway in, 553-554
  circulation in, 554-555
  complications of, 562-563, 563t
  defibrillation in, 560-561
  drugs used in, 555-560, 556t
    amiodarone, 558
    atropine, 556t, 558
    bretylium, 556t, 558
    calcium, 556t, 557-558
    calcium chloride, 562
    dopamine, 556t, 559
    epinephrine, 555-556, 556t, 560
      high dose, 561
    isoproterenol, 556t, 559-560
    lidocaine, 556t, 557, 560
    nitroprusside, 556t, 560
    norepinephrine, 556t, 560
    oxygen, 555, 556t
    sodium bicarbonate, 556t, 557, 562

during ICU phase, 565-566
during post-ICU phase, 566
during pre-ICU phase, 563t, 563-564
external cardiac massage in, 561
external pacemakers in, 562
in emergency department, 564-565, *565*
in HIV infection/AIDS, 1415
in hypothermia, 56
open-chest cardiac massage in, 561-562
P$_{ETCO_2}$ monitoring in, 561
termination guidelines for, 1729-1730, 1733, 1735, 1736
ventilation in, 554
Cardiopulmonary support, in intra-abdominal infections, 1008
Cardiorespiratory variables, classification systems for, 1679, 1681-1682, *1682,* 1682t
Cardiovascular disorders. *See also specific disorders*
  following vascular surgery, 721-722
    during pre-ICU phase, 714
  in chronic renal failure, 808-813
  in hypocalcemia, 1191
  preload conditions affected by, 508-509, 509t
Cardiovascular management, in spinal cord injury, 152-153
Cardiovascular surgical complications, 1208-1216
  during ICU phase, 1214t, 1214-1216
    arrhythmia control and, 1215
    hemodynamic management and, 1215
    hypertension control and, 1215
    hypertrophic cardiomyopathy and, 1216
    identification of high risk patients and, 1214-1215
    valvular heart disease and, 1215-1216
  during pre-ICU phase, 1208-1224
    risk factors for
      laboratory studies defining, 1208-1211, 1209t, 1210t, *1211*
      quantification of, 1211-1214
Cardioversion, 1607-1608
  complications and management of, 1607
  for supraventricular tachycardia, 539-540, 541, 543t
  indications for, 1607
  quality enhancement for, 1607-1608
Care process, decision making and, 1580-1581
Caregivers, relationships with, 1572
Carotid artery, rupture of, following head and neck surgery, 221
Carotid body tumors, resection of, hypertension following, 738
Carotid endarterectomy, hypertension following, 736
Carotid sinus massage, in arrhythmias, 532
Case mix management systems, 1672t, 1672-1673
  APACHE, 1672-1673, *1673*
  APACHE II, 1673-1674, *1676,* 1677t
    evaluation of, 1664-1665, 1665t
    in pancreatitis, 1025-1027, *1026*
  APACHE III, *1676,* 1676-1677, *1680,* 1680t, *1681*
  for specific situations or disease states, 1677-1687
    cardiac disease and myocardial infarction, 1678-1679, 1681t, *1682,* 1682t
    cardiorespiratory variables and, 1679, 1681-1682, *1682,* 1682t

Case mix management systems (Continued)
  gastrointestinal disorders, 1684, 1686t, 1687t
  Glasgow Coma Scale, 83, 83t, 1678, 1681t
  renal failure, 1684, 1686-1687, *1687*, 1687t-1689t
  respiratory failure, *1683*, 1683t-1685t, 1683-1684
  Mortality Prediction Model, 1674
  Mortality Probability Models, 1674t, 1674-1675, 1678t
  New Simplified Acute Physiology Score, 1672-1673, 1674t, 1675t
  Simplified Acute Physiology Score (SAPS), 1672
  Therapeutic Intervention Scoring System, 1675, 1679t
Case-control studies, 1744
Catecholamines, circulating, in brain injury, 86
Categorical variables, 1740, 1749t, 1749-1750
Catheter(s)
  infection related to, 1383-1384
  placement of, as risk factor for neurologic surgical complications, 1219
  urinary
    infection related to, 1594
    antimicrobial therapy for, 1381
    placement of. *See* Urologic management, catheter placement in
  vascular, infection related to, 1590-1592, *1591*, 1591t
  venous, imaging studies and, 1478, *1481-1485*
  ventricular, for intracranial pressure monitoring, 69-70, *70*
Catheterization. *See* Arterial catheterization; Cardiac catheterization; Peripheral artery catheterization; Pulmonary artery catheterization
Cauda equina injuries, 150
Cause, studies to determine, 1744-1745, 1745t
Cavernous sinus, septic thrombosis of, pre-ICU evaluation of, 105
Cefamandole
  dosing adjustment for renal or hepatic dysfunction, 1350t
  dosing during hemofiltration and hemodialysis, 1352t
Cefazolin
  dosing adjustment for renal or hepatic dysfunction, 1350t
  dosing during hemofiltration and hemodialysis, 1352t
  for pneumonia, nosocomial, 393t
Cefmetazole
  dosing adjustment for renal or hepatic dysfunction, 1350t
  dosing during hemofiltration and hemodialysis, 1352t
Cefonicid
  dosing adjustment for renal or hepatic dysfunction, 1350t
  dosing during hemofiltration and hemodialysis, 1352t
Cefoperazone
  dosing adjustment for renal or hepatic dysfunction, 1350t
  dosing during hemofiltration and hemodialysis, 1352t
Ceforanide
  dosing adjustment for renal or hepatic dysfunction, 1350t

  dosing during hemofiltration and hemodialysis, 1352t
Cefotaxime
  dosing adjustment for renal or hepatic dysfunction, 1350t
  dosing during hemofiltration and hemodialysis, 1352t
  for central nervous system infections, 1372
  for pancreatitis, 1034t
Cefotetan
  dosing adjustment for renal or hepatic dysfunction, 1350t
  dosing during hemofiltration and hemodialysis, 1352t
  for intra-abdominal infections, 1379
Cefoxitin
  dosing adjustment for renal or hepatic dysfunction, 1350t
  dosing during hemofiltration and hemodialysis, 1352t
  for intra-abdominal infections, 1379
Ceftazidime
  dosing adjustment for renal or hepatic dysfunction, 1350t
  dosing during hemofiltration and hemodialysis, 1352t
Ceftizoxime
  dosing adjustment for renal or hepatic dysfunction, 1350t
  dosing during hemofiltration and hemodialysis, 1352t
  for pancreatitis, 1034t
Ceftriaxone
  dosing adjustment for renal or hepatic dysfunction, 1350t
  dosing during hemofiltration and hemodialysis, 1352t
  for central nervous system infections, 1372
  for meningococcal infections, cutaneous, 944
Cefuroxime
  dosing adjustment for renal or hepatic dysfunction, 1350t
  dosing during hemofiltration and hemodialysis, 1352t
  prophylactic, following cardiac transplantation, 651
Cellular damage, coma and, 4
Cellulitis, 926-928
  clinical presentation and differential diagnosis of, *926*, 926-927, *927*, 927t
  laboratory studies in, 927
  pathophysiology and risk factors for, 926
  pseudomonal, 940
  recovery from, 927-928
  treatment of, 927
Central cord syndrome, 149
Central herniation, coma and, 5-6
Central line sepsis, following vascular surgery, 725
Central nervous system, following cardiac transplantation, 649
Central nervous system depressants, abuse/overdose of, 1439-1445. *See also specific drugs*
Central nervous system disorders. *See also specific disorders*
  in multiple organ system failure, 1293t
  infectious
    antimicrobial therapy in, 1372t, 1372-1373
    in HIV infection/AIDS, 1407, *1407*
    prophylaxis and treatment of, 1405

Central nervous system stimulants, abuse/overdose of, 1431-1439. *See also specific drugs*
  signs and symptoms of, 1431
Central tendency, 1740
Central venous pressure monitoring, 1603-1605
  complications and management of, 1604-1605
    local complications, 1604
    systemic complications, 1604-1605
  contraindications to, 1604
  data analysis for, 1604
  indications for, 1603
  quality enhancement for, 1605, 1605t
Cephalosporins
  for pneumonia, 1375
    community-acquired, 391, 391t
    nosocomial, 393t, 394
  pharmacokinetics of, 1354-1355
Cephalothin
  dosing adjustment for renal or hepatic dysfunction, 1350t
  dosing during hemofiltration and hemodialysis, 1352t
Cephapirin
  dosing adjustment for renal or hepatic dysfunction, 1350t
  dosing during hemofiltration and hemodialysis, 1352t
Cephradine
  dosing adjustment for renal or hepatic dysfunction, 1350t
  dosing during hemofiltration and hemodialysis, 1352t
Cerebellar artery ischemia, coma and, 8
Cerebral angiography
  in brain injury, 85
  in intracranial hypertension, 68
Cerebral blood flow, in traumatic brain injury, 87
Cerebral edema
  cardiopulmonary resuscitation and, 562-563
  hepatic coma and, 1083-1084
  in acute renal failure, in patients awaiting liver transplantation, 1139-1140
Cerebral hemispheres, coma and, 3
Cerebral hemorrhage, coma and, 6
Cerebral infarcts, coma and, 6
Cerebral protection, in traumatic head injury, 87
Cerebral vascular disease, as risk factor for neurologic surgical complications, 1217-1218
Cerebral vasospasm, subarachnoid hemorrhage and, 80, 81t, 88
Cerebral vein occlusion, coma and, 6
Cerebrospinal fluid (CSF) otorrhea/rhinorrhea, in traumatic brain injury, 87
Cervical esophagostomy, following head and neck surgery, 222
Cervical spine radiographs, in brain injuries, 84
Charcoal. *See* Activated charcoal
Chemical warfare agents, inhalation injury caused by, 320
Chemicals. *See also specific chemicals*
  hepatic failure induced by, 1079
Chemotherapy
  as predisposing condition to infection, 401
  emergencies induced by, 886-893
    allergic reactions to chemotherapy drugs, 892-893

cardiac, 892
  gastrointestinal, 890–892
  neurologic, 889–890, 890t
  renal and electrolyte complications, 886–888
  respiratory, 888t, 888–889
 for bone marrow transplantation, 881t
 for hypercalcemia, 1193, 1193t
 hemolytic uremic syndrome associated with, 861
Chest, imaging of, 1473–1474, 1474t
 in aortic regurgitation, 673
 in cardiomyopathy, dilated, 619
 in heart failure, high output, 626
 in hypertrophic cardiomyopathy, 623
 in pericardial effusion, 612
Chest physical therapy, 475
 preoperative, 1208
Chest radiography, in constrictive pericarditis, 617
Chest tubes, 1606–1607
 complications of, 1606
 contraindications to, 1606
 following renal surgery, 848
 indications for, 1606, 1606t
 quality enhancement for, 1606–1607
Chest wall diseases, restrictive, mechanical ventilation in, elective use of, 439–440
Child-Turcotte classification, of hepatic disorders, 1062, 1063t
Chi-square test, 1750
Chloral hydrate abuse/overdose, 1443
Chloramphenicol
 dosing adjustment for renal or hepatic dysfunction, 1350t
 dosing during hemofiltration and hemodialysis, 1352t
 for central nervous system infections, 1372
 for intra-abdominal infections, 1379
 for Rocky Mountain spotted fever, 946
Chlordiazepoxide (Librium), for sedation, 1280t, 1281
Chloride, for metabolic alkalosis, 767–769
Chlorine, inhalation injury caused by, 319
Chlorpromazine (Thorazine), for delirium, 1282
Chlorpropamide, hypoglycemia caused by, 1168–1169
Cholangiography, 1071–1073, 1072, 1073
Cholangitis
 acute, 1051–1052, 1052
 sclerosing, 1053–1054, 1054
Cholecystectomy, 1054
 concomitant, 1046
Cholecystitis, acalculous, 1050–1051, 1051
 jaundice and, postoperative, 1121–1122
Cholescintigraphy, 1068, 1069
Cholestasis, in jaundice, postoperative, 1120
Cholinergic crisis, in myasthenia gravis, 134–135
Chordae tendineae, mitral regurgitation and, 657–658, 659
Chronic obstructive pulmonary disease (COPD), 242–273
 aerosol therapy in, 491–492, 493–494
 airway management in, 493–494
  aerosol therapy in, 493–494
  bronchopulmonary hygiene therapy in, 493
  mucolytic agents in, 494
 arrhythmias in, 534
 as surgical risk factor, for pulmonary complications, 1202–1203

 during ICU phase, 183, 253–269
  acute respiratory insufficiency and, 253t, 253–254
  for maintenance of hemodynamic status, 262–263
  hemodynamic status maintenance and, 261–263
  nutrition and, 263–265
  oxygen therapy and, 258–259
  pathophysiology of respiratory failure and, 255, 255–256, 256, 256t
  pharmacotherapy and, 256–258, 257, 257t, 258t, 259, 262–263, 263
   diaphragmatic inotropic agents in, 259
   inotropic agents in, 262–263, 263
   vasodilators in, 262, 262t
  respiratory mechanics assessment and, 268t, 268–269
  rest versus exercise and, 267–268
  ventilatory capacity and, 266t, 266–267
  ventilatory mode and, 268
  ventilatory support and, 259–260
  ventilatory weaning and, 265t, 265–266
 during post-ICU phase, 183–184, 269–273, 491–494
  home ventilation and, 272
  lung transplantation and, 272–273
  nutritional support and, 271–272
  oxygen therapy and, 272
  rehabilitation and, 270–271
  smoking cessation and, 269–270
  ventilatory muscle rest and, 271
 during pre-ICU phase, 179, 180, 180, 242–253
  course and prognosis and, 245t, 245–246, 246t, 247, 248, 248, 248t
  epidemiology and, 244
  etiology and pathogenesis and, 242–244
  pharmacologic therapy and, 249–252
   antibiotics in, 252
   anticholinergics in, 249
   beta agonists in, 249
   corticosteroids in, 250–251, 251t
   digoxin in, 252
   influenza vaccine in, 252
   mucolytic agents in, 252
   theophylline in, 249–250, 250
  prediction of outcome and, 252–253
  symptoms and signs and, 248–249
 mechanical ventilation in, 259–260
  elective use of, 439–440
  home, 272
 oxygen therapy in, 258–259, 272, 492t, 492–493
  outpatient, 492–493, 493t
  oxygen delivery devices for, 492
 pulmonary function testing in, 464–465, 466
 pulse oximetry in, 493
 surgical management of myocardial ischemia and infarction and, 590
Chronic renal failure (CRF), 802–821, 803, 804, 805t. See also End-stage renal disease (ESRD)
 anemia of, 807–808
 cardiovascular disease in, 808–813. See also specific disorders
 gastrointestinal disease in, 818–819
 immune consequences of, 814t, 814–815
 infectious diseases in, 814–818. See also specific disorders
 pulmonary disease in, 813–814
Chyle fistulas, following head and neck surgery, 220–221

Chylothorax, following thoracic surgery, 377
Cigarette smoking. See Smoking
Cilastin
 dosing adjustment for renal or hepatic dysfunction, 1350t
 dosing during hemofiltration and hemodialysis, 1352t
Cimetidine, for pancreatitis, 1035
Cingulate herniation, coma and, 5
Ciprofloxacin
 dosing adjustment for renal or hepatic dysfunction, 1350t
 dosing during hemofiltration and hemodialysis, 1352t
 for pneumonia, 1375
 prophylactic, for pneumonia, 413t
Circulatory disorders
 in multiple organ system failure, 1299–1300
 in spinal cord injury, 147
Circulatory support, pre-cardiac transplantation, 642
Cirrhosis, 1093t, 1093–1117
 alcoholic, imaging in, 1067, 1068
 clinical presentation of, 1093–1094
 complications of, 1094–1117
  alcoholic hepatitis, 1104–1107, 1105t, 1106
  ascites. See Ascites, in cirrhosis
  esophageal varices. See Varices, esophageal
  gastropathy, 1103, 1103
  hepatorenal syndrome, 1116–1117
  portal hypertension. See Portal hypertension, in cirrhosis
 gallstones in, during pre-ICU phase, 1048
 prognosis of, 1117
 surgery in, 1117–1119
Cisplatin, for bone marrow transplantation, 881t
Clavulanic acid
 dosing adjustment for renal or hepatic dysfunction, 1350t
 dosing during hemofiltration and hemodialysis, 1352t
Clearance, 1338
Clindamycin
 dosing adjustment for renal or hepatic dysfunction, 1350t
 dosing during hemofiltration and hemodialysis, 1352t
 for intra-abdominal infections, 1379
 for pneumonia
  community-acquired, 391, 391t, 392
  nosocomial, 393t
Clinical epidemiology, 1739–1751
 biostatistics and, 1740–1742, 1748–1751
  categorical dependent variables and independent variables and, 1749t, 1749–1750
  continuous and categorical dependent variables and, 1749
  P values, significance, errors, and sample sizes and, 1740–1741, 1741t
  populations, samples, and distribution of data and, 1740
  relative risk, odds ratios, and confidence intervals and, 1741–1742
  sample and population descriptors and, 1740
  selection of appropriate statistical test and, 1748–1749, 1749t
 hypothesis and study question and, 1742
 meta-analysis and, 1748, 1748

INDEX

Clinical epidemiology *(Continued)*
  research designs and, 1742-1748
    for studies to characterize natural history and prognosis, 1743-1744
    for studies to determine cause, 1744-1745, 1745t
    for studies to evaluate diagnostic tests, 1745t, 1745-1746, *1746*, 1746t
    for studies to evaluate therapy, 1746-1748, 1747t
Clinical personnel, computerized patient management system and, 1701, 1702t
Clinical protocols, 1559, 1560t-1561t, 1561
Clinical trials, 1746-1747
Clonidine, for hypertension, postoperative, 745t, 748-749
Closed chest external cardiac massage, complications of, 562
Clotrimazole, prophylactic, following cardiac transplantation, 651
Coagulation
  following cardiac transplantation, 649
  inhibitors of, circulating, acquired, 913-914
Coagulation factors, *900*, 900-901, 901t
  disorders of. *See* Coagulopathies; *specific disorders*
  transfusions of, 920
Coagulopathies, *911*, 911-914. *See also specific disorders*
  acquired, 912-914
  congenital, 911-912
  fibrinolytic, 914
  following vascular surgery, 724
  gastrointestinal bleeding and, correction of, 992
  in acute renal failure, in patients awaiting liver transplantation, 1139
  in brain injury, 87
  in fulminant hepatic failure, 1089-1090
  in necrotizing pancreatitis, 1022
Cocaine abuse/overdose, 1431-1435
  admission criteria in, 1434-1435
  body packing and, 1435
  coma and, 11
  complications of, 1432-1433
  diagnosis and treatment of, 1433-1434, 1435t
  signs and symptoms of, 1431-1432, 1432t
Cohort studies, 1744-1745
Cold stress, thermoregulatory response to, 52
Cold-reactive antibodies, 905
Colindine, for hypertension, 692t-694t
Colonic disorders
  bleeding, endoscopic treatment of, 996
  chemotherapy-induced, 891-892
  imaging studies in, 1525, 1528, *1528-1534*, 1531
  ischemic, following vascular surgery, 722-723
Colonization, 1589
Color flow mapping, in aortic regurgitation, 674-676, *675*, *676*
Colostomy, closure of, following pancreatitis, 1039
Coma, 3-23
  barbiturate, 1283
    for status epilepticus, 99, *99*, 99t
  brain death and, establishment of, 22
  hepatic, 1080-1086
    cerebral edema and, 1083-1084
    chronic hepatic encephalopathy and, 1082
    clinical picture in, 1080-1082, 1081t, 1082t
      prodromal stage, 1081
    pathogenesis of, 1082-1083
    stage II, 1081
    stage III (stupor), 1081
    stage IV (coma), 1081
    treatment of, 1084-1086, *1086*
  hyperglycemic hyperosmolar nonketotic. *See* Hyperglycemic hyperosmolar nonketotic coma (HHNK)
  management of, 14-22, 15t
    electrophysiologic monitoring in, *20*, 20-21, *21*
    elevated intracranial pressure and, 18-20
    gastrointestinal aspiration in, 16-17
    gastrointestinal complications and, 21
    general physical examination for, 17
    hemodynamic, 16
    metabolic, 15-16
    neurologic examination for, 17t, 17-18
    neuro-ophthalmologic examination for, 18
    nutrition in, 21-22
    radiologic imaging in, 18
    seizure control in, 16
    temperature regulation in, 16
    urologic care in, 17
    ventilation in, 14-15
  myxedema, 1178-1179
  pathophysiology of, 3-4
    cellular mechanisms in, 4
    structural mechanisms in, 3-4
  prognosis following, 22-23
    in nontraumatic coma, 22-23
    in toxic/metabolic coma, 23
    in traumatic coma, 23, 23t
  risk factors for, 4-14
    demyelinating disease as, 12
    drug intoxication as, 10-12
    endocrine disease as, 12-13
    infection as, 10
    metabolic disease as, 8-10
      hypoglycemia and, 8-10
      hypoxia and, 8-10
    seizures as, 14
    subtentorial lesions as, 7t, 7-8, *8*
    supratentorial lesions as, 4-7
      extracerebral versus intracerebral, 6-7
      mass effect and, *5*, 5-6
      pathophysiology of, 5, *5*
    systemic disease as, 13-14
Communication
  in upper airway obstruction, 205-206, *206*
  inhalation injury and, 326
Communication styles, team concept and, 1562, 1562t
Competency, 1728
  definition of, 1728t
Computed tomography (CT)
  in aortic dissection, 703
  in brain injuries, 84t, 84-85
  in hepatic disorders, 1070, *1071*, *1072*
  in intracranial hypertension, 67, 68t
  in pancreatitis, 1027, *1028*
  in pericardial effusion, 612
  of comatose patient, 18
Computerized patient management systems, 1697-1716
  during pre-ICU phase, 1698-1702, 1699t
    administrative and clinical personnel and, 1701-1702
    clinical personnel and, 1701, 1702t
    information services personnel, 1701
    vendor representatives and, 1701-1702, *1703-1707*, 1706t
  executive commitment to, 1700, 1701t
  hospital information system and, 1700-1701
  information services policy and, 1699-1700, 1700t
  ICU considerations and, 1702, 1704, 1706-1713
    decision support systems, 1712
    definition of patient care tasks, 1709-1711
      interpretation and, 1710-1711
      intervention and, 1711
      observation and, 1710, 1713t
    development and implementation team selection, 1707-1709
    equipment inventory, 1702
    implementation of system, 1712-1713
    physical plant, 1702, 1704
      clinical information system architecture and, 1704, *1708*, 1708t, *1709*
    translation of patient care tasks into information system, 1711-1712, 1713t, *1714*
    vendor selection, 1704, 1706-1707
    terminology and, 1704, *1709*, 1709t
    user interface and, 1704, 1706-1707, *1710-1712*
  post-ICU considerations and, 1713-1716
    capture of data to document severity of illness, 1714, 1715t, *1716*
    combining unit data with other databases, 1714-1716, 1715t, 1717t
    transfer of patient information, 1714
Concussive head injury, 77
Conduction disturbances. *See also* Arrhythmias
  in acute myocardial infarction, 578
Conductive heat transfer, 51
Confidence intervals, 1742
Conflict, among team members, 1556
  related to differences in professional orientation, 1556
  related to patient care decisions, 1556
Confusional state, 3. *See also* Delirium
Congestive heart failure, in chronic renal failure, 809-811
  rehabilitative phase of, 810-811
  risk phase of, 810
  support phase of, 810
Consciousness level
  alterations of, 3. *See also* Coma
  intracranial hypertension and, 66
Constrictive pericarditis. *See* Pericarditis, constrictive
Construct validity, 1665t
Content validity, 1665t
Contingency table, 1749, 1749t
Continuous positive airway pressure (CPAP), 486
  in atelectasis, 468-469, *469*
  in chronic obstructive pulmonary disease, 259-260
  nasal, 496, *496*
    bilevel, 498
Continuous quality improvement (CQI), respiratory care services and, *499*, 499-500
Continuous variables, 1740, 1749, 1750-1751, 1751t

INDEX

Contractility
  augmentation of, following vascular surgery, 717–718
  intrinsic, 507
    inotropy and, *511*, 511–512, 512t
Control test, for imputed negligence, 1720
Control ventilation, 485
Contusions, brain injury and, 77
Conus medullaris syndrome, 150
Convective heat loss, 51
Convulsions. *See* Seizures
Coping mechanisms, 1568–1569
  helping patients develop, 1571, 1571t
Coronary angiography, preoperative, 1210
Coronary artery bypass grafting (CABG), 587–604
  during ICU phase, 593–602
    intraoperative care and, 593–594
    operative technique for, 594
    pathophysiology of cardiopulmonary bypass and, *594*, 594–595, *595*
    postoperative care and, 595–602, 596t
    preoperative considerations for, 593
  during post-ICU phase, *602*, 602–604, *603*
    delayed complications in, 603
    long-term preventive goals for, 603–604
  during pre-ICU phase, 587–593
    in acute myocardial infarction, indications for, 588–589
    in unstable angina, indications for, 587
    profile of candidate for myocardial revascularization and, 587, *588*, 588t
    risk factors for, 589t, 589–593
      intra-aortic balloon pump to reduce, 591–592
      peripheral vascular and renal disease, 591
      scoring systems for, 590–591, *591*, 591t
      ventricular assist devices to reduce, 592–593
      ventricular dysfunction, 591
  emergency, 590
  for acute myocardial infarction, 575–576
  postoperative care and, 595–602, 596t
    early ICU concerns for, 595–599
    late ICU concerns for, 599–602
  reoperation, 590
Coronary artery disease, atherosclerotic, prevention of, 603
Coronary artery disease (CAD)
  as risk factor for neurologic surgical complications, 1216–1217
  in chronic renal failure, 811–812
    rehabilitative phase of, 812
    risk phase of, 811
    support phase of, 811
Correlation, 1750
Correlation coefficient, 1750
Corticosteroids. *See also specific corticosteroids; specific drugs*
  catecholamines, for shock, 1324–1325, 1325t
  following cardiac transplantation, 650, 651t
  for adult respiratory distress syndrome, 309
  for chronic obstructive pulmonary disease, 250–251
    in hospitalized patients with acute respiratory failure, 251
    in mild exacerbations, 251
    in stable outpatients, 250–251, 251t
  for inhalation injury, 333
  for myasthenia gravis, 133
  for shock, 1330
  for Stevens-Johnson syndrome, 961
  for toxic epidermal necrolysis, 964
  in bronchospastic disease, 235
Cortisol, stress and, 1173–1174
Cost, of measurement, 1665t
Costal arch, infection of, following thoracic surgery, 378
Costal cartilage, infection of, following thoracic surgery, 378
Co-trimoxazole
  dosing adjustment for renal or hepatic dysfunction, 1351t
  dosing during hemofiltration and hemodialysis, 1352t
Cough, in bronchopulmonary hygiene therapy, 475
Coumarin, necrosis induced by, *968*, *968*
Cox proportional hazards model, 1750
Cramps, heat, 57
Cranial nerve deficits. *See also specific nerves*
  following head and neck surgery, 224–226
Craniotomy, postoperative care and, 88–89
Creatine kinase (CK)
  isoenzymes of, in acute myocardial infarction, 571
  serum level of, in acute myocardial infarction, 571, *571*
Creatinine
  serum level of, in renal failure, 788
  urinary rate of excretion of, in nutrition assessment, 1252
Creatinine phosphokinase (CPK)
  in cardiac trauma, nonpenetrating, 630
  isoenzymes of, in cardiac trauma, nonpenetrating, 630–632
Creutzfeldt-Jakob disease, contagion of, 1373
Criminal prosecution, 1721
Cromolyn sodium (Intal), in aerosol therapy, 474
CROP Index, 448–449, 450t
Culture-negative neutrocytic ascites (CNNA), in cirrhosis, 1111
Current Procedural Terminology (CPT-4), 1668, 1668t, 1669t
Cursor, 1707
Cushing response, intracranial hypertension and, 66
Cushing's syndrome. *See* Hyperadrenalism
Cushing's ulcer. *See* Stress ulcer
Cutaneous bacillary angiomatosis, in HIV infection/AIDS, 1410
Cutaneous disorders. *See also specific disorders*
  in HIV infection/AIDS, 1411
  infections. *See also specific infections*
    antimicrobial therapy for, 1382–1383
    during ICU phase, 982–983, *983*, *984*
    during post-ICU phase, 985
    during pre-ICU phase, 982
  Cutaneous reactions, life-threatening, 958–972. *See also specific disorders*
Cutaneous trauma
  during ICU phase, 983
  during post-ICU phase, 985
  during pre-ICU phase, 982
Cyanide
  inhalation injury caused by, 319
  intoxication by, 1467
Cyclophosphamide, for bone marrow transplantation, 881t
Cyclosporine
  following cardiac transplantation, 650
  following liver transplantation, 1148, 1149t
  following renal transplantation, 829–830
Cystectomy, radical
  during ICU phase, 843
  during post-ICU phase, 844
  during pre-ICU phase, 840
    preoperative preparation for, 841
    technique for, 842, 842t
Cystic fibrosis, 242. *See also* Chronic obstructive pulmonary disease (COPD)
Cytomegalovirus (CMV) infections
  following bone marrow transplantation, 882
  following liver transplantation, 1147
  in HIV infection/AIDS, 1406, 1411
  retinitis and, 1411
Cytosine arabinoside, for bone marrow transplantation, 881t

Damages, in lawsuits, 1724
Database management system (DBMS), 1704
Dead space, minute ventilation and, 265–266, 266t
Death. *See also* Mortality; Survival
  attitudes toward, 1737
Death-prolonging therapy, withholding. *See* Life-sustaining treatment, withholding
Decision making
  quality assessment/assurance and. *See* Quality assessment/assurance, decision making and
  surrogate decision maker and, 1728–1729, 1732–1733, 1734
    definition of, 1728t
  team concept and, 1558–1559
Decision support systems, 1712
Decontamination
  gastric, for poisonings, 1457
  in inhalation injury, 322
Decubitus ulcers. *See* Pressure sores
Deep breathing exercises, 475
Deep vein thrombosis
  in spinal cord injury, 152
  objective testing for, role of, 425–426
Defense mechanisms
  in immunocompromised host, 399
  pulmonary, 401–403, 402t, *403*
Defibrillation, 1607–1608
  complications and management of, 1607
  electrical, in hypothermia, 56
  in cardiopulmonary resuscitation, 560–561
  indications for, 1607
  quality enhancement for, 1607–1608
Dehydration, antibiotic pharmacokinetics and, 1341
Delirium, 3, 37–43, 1281–1283, 1282t
  diagnostic and clinical features of, 38t, 38–39, 39t
  evaluation of, 39
  pharmacologic control of, 1282–1283
    barbiturates for, 1283
    butyrophenones for, 1282–1283
    phenothiazines for, 1282
  treatment of, 39–43
    drug toxicity and, 39–40
    drug withdrawal and, 40–41, 41t
    in nonspecific delirium, 41–42, 42t
    neuroleptic agents in, 41–42, 42t
    nonpharmacologic, 43

Demyelinating disorders
  coma and, 12
  lumbar puncture in, data analysis for, 1617
Depositions, 1723
Depressants, abuse/overdose of, 1439–1445. *See also specific drugs*
Depressed skull fracture, 79, *79*
Depression, 33–37
  diagnosis and clinical characteristics of, 33–34
  differential diagnosis of, 34–35, 35t
  evaluation of, 35
  incidence of, 34
  major, in critically ill patient, 33
  treatment of, 35–37, 36t
    lithium in, 37
    monoamine oxidase inhibitors in, 37
    newer antidepressants in, 37
    psychostimulants in, 37
    tricyclic antidepressants in, 36–37
Dermatologic disorders. *See Cutaneous disorders; Skin; specific disorders*
Development and implementation team, for computerized patient management system, 1707–1709
Dexamethasone, for spinal cord compression, 869
Dextran, for thrombotic disorders, 916
Dextrose, for total parenteral nutrition, 1259, 1261t
Diabetes mellitus, 1157–1170. *See also Diabetic ketoacidosis (DKA); Hyperglycemic hyperosmolar nonketotic coma (HHNK)*
  as predisposing condition to infection, 400
  comorbid conditions in, 806t, 806–807
  during ICU phase, 1170
  end-stage renal disease associated with, 803–806
  following vascular surgery, 719, 723
  gallstones in, during pre-ICU phase, 1047–1048, *1048*, 1048t
  hyperglycemia in surgical patients in, 1165–1168
    during ICU phase, 1166t, 1166–1168, 1167t
    during post-ICU phase, 1168, 1168t
    during pre-ICU phase, 1165t, 1165–1166
  hypoglycemia in, 1168–1170
    during ICU phase, 1169, 1169t
    during post-ICU phase, 1169t, 1169–1170
    during pre-ICU phase, 1168t, 1168–1169
  hypomagnesemia caused by, 1186
  in necrotizing pancreatitis, 1021
  neuropathy in, 806
  retinopathy in, 806
  surgical management of myocardial ischemia and infarction and, 590
  vasculopathy in, 806–807
Diabetic ketoacidosis (DKA), 1157–1163
  coma and, 12
  during ICU phase, 1160, 1162t, 1162–1163
  during post-ICU phase, 1163, 1163t
  during pre-ICU phase, 1158t, 1158–1159
    etiology of, assessment of, 1158
    hydration in, assessment of, 1159
    metabolic status in, assessment of, 1159
    risk factors for, 1158

  in surgical patients, 1166
  initial treatment of, 1159–1160, *1161*
Diagnosis-related groups (DRGs), 1665–1666, *1666*, 1667t
Diagnostic tests. *See also specific tests*
  sensitivity of, 1745, 1745t
  studies to evaluate, *1745*, 1745t, 1745–1746, 1746t
Dialysis. *See Hemodialysis; Peritoneal dialysis*
Diaphragmatic dysfunction, rehabilitation of ventilator-dependent patients and, 445
Diarrhea
  antimicrobial therapy for, 1380–1381
  as complication of nutritional support, 1263–1264
  in HIV infection/AIDS, 1408
  metabolic acidosis associated with, treatment of, 763, 764
  secretory, hypomagnesemia caused by, 1186
Diastolic function, assessment of, 521–522, *523*, *524*
Diazepam (Valium)
  as premedication, for thoracic surgery, 362
  during mechanical ventilation, during ICU phase, 290
  for alcohol withdrawal, 1441, 1441t
  for cocaine abuse/overdose, 1434, 1435t
  for sedation, 1280t, 1281
  for sedative/hypnotic withdrawal, 1445
Diazoxide, for hypertension, 692t, 693t
  postoperative, 745t, 746
Dichloroacetate (DCA), for metabolic acidosis, 763
Diffuse alveolar hemorrhage (DAH), 341–347, 342t
  adult respiratory distress syndrome versus, 345–346
  during ICU phase, 345–347
  during post-ICU phase, 347
  during pre-ICU phase, 341–345
    clinical and roentgenographic features of, 341–342
    diagnostic approach to, 342–345
      defining presence of diffuse alveolar hemorrhage and, 342–343
      immune and nonimmune diffuse alveolar hemorrhage and, 343–345, 344t
Diffusing capacity for carbon monoxide (DLCO), in diffuse alveolar hemorrhage, 343
Diffusion capacity, measurement of, 1204–1205
Diffusion limitation, in parenchymal respiratory failure, 164
Digitalis, cardiotoxicity of, in hypomagnesemia, 1187
Digoxin
  for shock, 1329
  for supraventricular tachycardia, 539, 543
  intoxication by, 1464–1465
Digoxin-specific antibody, for digoxin poisoning, 1464–1465
Dihydropyridines, for hypertension, 692t–694t
Dilated cardiomyopathy. *See Cardiomyopathy, dilated*
Diltiazem
  for hypertension, 693t, 694t
  for renal failure, 786t
Dimethylsulfoxide (DMSO), for inhalation injury, 333

Dipstix testing, in renal failure, 788
Dipyridamole thallium testing, preoperative, 1213t, 1213–1214
Discharge, preparing patient for, 1573
Discharge planning, 1562–1563
Discovery, 1722
Disease staging, 1668–1669, 1669t, 1670t
Dismissal, of liability claim, 1724
Disopyramide, for ventricular tachycardia, 544t
Disseminated intravascular coagulation (DIC), 874t, 874–875, 914, 969–972
  cardiopulmonary resuscitation and, 562, 563
  clinical presentation of, 970–971
  coma and, 9
  diagnosis of, 971
  during ICU phase, 875
  during post-ICU phase, 875
  during pre-ICU phase, 875
  following vascular surgery, 724
  outcome of, 972
  pathogenesis of, 969–970, 970t
  treatment of, 971–972
Distributional fluid losses, hypovolemia caused by, fluid resuscitation for, 1236–1237
Distributive shock, 1314
Diuretics. *See also specific drugs*
  for cirrhosis, 1113–1114
  for hyperkalemia, 779t
  for hypertension, 692t–694t
  for intracranial hypertension, 72–73
  hypomagnesemia caused by, 1185
  metabolic alkalosis associated with, 766
Dobutamine
  during weaning from cardiopulmonary bypass, 648
  following vascular surgery, 718
  for intra-abdominal infection, 1009
  for shock, 1325t, 1326
  in cardiopulmonary resuscitation, 556t, 559
Documentation, inhalation injury and, 326
Dopamine
  during weaning from cardiopulmonary bypass, 648
  following vascular surgery, 718
  for renal failure, 786t, 787
  for shock, 1325t, 1325–1326, *1326*
  in cardiopulmonary resuscitation, 556t, 559
Dopexamine, for shock, 1327
Doxacurium, 1287t, 1288
Doxycycline
  dosing adjustment for renal or hepatic dysfunction, 1351t
  dosing during hemofiltration and hemodialysis, 1352t
  for intra-abdominal infections, 1379
  for pneumonia, community-acquired, 391t
Drainage systems, closed, following head and neck surgery, assessment of, 216–217, *217*
Driver, 1707
Droperidol (Inapsine)
  for delirium, 1283
  for sedation, 1280t
Drug(s). *See also specific drugs*
  allergy to, shock and, 1315, 1315t
  autoimmune hemolytic anemia caused by, 905
  chronic obstructive pulmonary disease related to, 254

INDEX

elimination of, enhancement of, 1457-1458
exacerbating myasthenia gravis, 132t, 132-133
fever induced by, 1371
hepatic failure induced by, 1079
hypertension caused by, postoperative, 740-741
intoxication by. *See also* Substance abuse/overdose; *specific drugs*
   coma and, 10-12
   delirium and, 39-40
lupus-like reaction induced by, 969, 969t
necrosis induced by, *968*, 968-969
neutropenia caused by, 906-907
   evaluation and treatment of, 906-907
   increased destruction in, 906
pharmacokinetics of, 1338-1340, *1339, 1340*
platelet disorders related to, 910-911
thermoregulatory disorders and, 53, 53t
thrombocytopenia caused by, 909t, 909-910
Drug abuse/overdose. *See* Substance abuse/overdose; *specific substances*
Drug eruptions, 964t, 964-967
   bullous, 967
   erythema multiforme, 967
   morbilliform, *966*, 966-967
   type I (immediate hypersensitivity), 965
   type II (cytotoxic antibody reactions), 965
   type III (immune complex-mediated), 965
   type IV (delayed-type hypersensitivity), 965
   urticaria, 965-966, *966*
Drug interactions
   hypertension caused by, postoperative, 741
   of allopurinol and azathioprine, 1148
   of cyclosporine, 1148, 1149t
   seizure patients and, 99-100, 100t
Drug reactions, antimicrobial therapy for, 1383
Drug therapy. *See also specific drugs and drug types*
   as predisposing condition to infection, 400
   during mechanical ventilation, during ICU phase, 290
   during weaning from cardiopulmonary bypass, 648
   following cardiac transplantation, 650t, 650-651, 651t
   following head and neck surgery, 223
   following liver transplantation, 1148, 1149t
   following vascular surgery, 720
   for acute myocardial infarction, 576t, 576-577, 577t
   for Addison's disease, 1176
   for adult respiratory distress syndrome, 309
   for agitation, 43t, 43-44
   for airway obstruction, 870
   for anxiety, 33, 34t
   for aortic dissection, 704-705, 705t
   for aortic regurgitation, 677-678
   for botulism, 136
   for brain abscess, 120t, 120-122, 121t
   for bronchospastic disease, 233t, 233-235, 238-239
   for cardiac transplantation, 646
   for cerebral protection, in brain injury, 87
   for chronic obstructive pulmonary disease. *See* Chronic obstructive pulmonary disease (COPD)
   for delirium, 40-42, 41t, 42t
   for depression, 36t, 36-37
   for diffuse alveolar hemorrhage, 345
   for dural venous sinus phlebitis, 115-116
   for epidural empyema, 116-117
   for esophageal varices, 1097, 1134-1135, 1135t
   for HIV encephalopathy, 47
   for hypercalcemia, 884, 884t
   for hyperkalemia, 779t, 779-780
   for hypertension, 691, 692t-694t, 695, 697-698
   for hypothermia, 56
   for inhalation injury, 333-334
   for intracranial hypertension, 19-20, 68, 71, 71t, 72-73
   for leukopenia, 877
   for malignant hyperthermia, 60, 61
   for meningitides, 117-119
   for meningoencephalitis, 112, 119-120
   for mitral regurgitation, 665-667, 666t
   for myasthenia gravis, 133, 134, 135
   for neuroleptic malignant syndrome, 62
   for parameningeal infections, 114-117
   for Rocky Mountain spotted fever, 946
   for seizures, 96t, 96-97, 97t, 99, *99*, 99t
      drug interactions and, 99-100, 100t
   for shock, 1324-1331
      weaning from, 1330-1331
   for skeletal infections, parameningeal, 115
   for soft tissue infections, parameningeal, 115
   for spinal cord compression, 869
   for subdural empyema, 116-117
   for supraglottitis, 191
   for supraventricular tachycardia, 538-539, 540, 541, 542, 543t
   for tetanus, 141
   for thrombocytosis, 879
   for thrombotic disorders, 915-917
   for upper airway obstruction, 194-195
   for vascular infections, parameningeal, 115
   hypoglycemia caused by, 1168-1169
   in renal failure, adjustment and addition of, 785-787, 786t, 787
   termination guidelines for, 1731, 1733, 1735
Drug withdrawal. *See also* Medication withdrawal
   delirium and, 40-41, 41t
   from alcohol, 1440-1441, 1441t
   from amphetamines, 1436
   from narcotics, 1447
   from sedative/hypnotics, 1444-1445
DSRS shunt, for esophageal varices, 1101-1102, *1102*
Duodenal disorders, imaging studies in, 1525, *1527, 1528*
Durable power of attorney, 1732, 1734
   definition of, 1728t
Dural venous sinus phlebitis, septic
   during ICU phase, 115-116
   pre-ICU evaluation of, 105-106
Dysphagia, in HIV infection/AIDS, 1408

Echocardiography
   Doppler, ventricular function evaluation using, 517-518
   in aortic dissection, 703, 704
   in aortic regurgitation, 673-677, *674-676*
   in cardiac trauma, nonpenetrating, 633
   in cardiomyopathy, dilated, 619, *621*
   in constrictive pericarditis, 617
   in heart failure, high output, 626
   in hypertrophic cardiomyopathy, 623, *623, 624*
   in mitral regurgitation, 661-662, *663, 664*
   in pericardial effusion, 612, *613, 614*
   two-dimensional, ventricular function evaluation using, 517, *517, 518*
Eczema herpeticum, 949-950
   clinical manifestations and differential diagnosis of, 949-950, *950*
   laboratory studies in, 950
   pathophysiology of, 949
   treatment and outcome of, 950
Edema
   cerebral. *See* Cerebral edema
   of brain, postcraniotomy, 89
   pulmonary. *See* Pulmonary edema
Edrophonium chloride test, in myasthenia gravis, 132, 132t, 135
Eicosanoids, in shock, 1316, *1318*
Ejection fraction, 519
Elderly patients
   bronchospastic disease in, 231t, 231-232, 235
   gallstones in, 1047
   vancomycin dosing in, 1348
Electrocardiographic (ECG) monitoring, 1632t, 1632-1633
   in ischemia, 1632-1633
   of heart rate, 1632, *1633*
   of rhythm, 1632
Electrocardiography (ECG)
   in acute myocardial infarction, 571-572, *572*
   in aortic regurgitation, 673, 673t
   in bronchospastic disease, 231
   in cardiac trauma, nonpenetrating, 630, 632t
   in cardiomyopathy, dilated, 619
   in heart failure, high output, 626
   in hypertrophic cardiomyopathy, 622-623
   in mitral regurgitation, 661, 662t
   in pericardial effusion, 612
Electrocoagulation, for gastrointestinal bleeding, 993
Electroencephalography (EEG)
   in comatose patient, 20, *20*, 21
   in seizures, 95
Electrogram (EGM), atrial, in arrhythmias, 532-533, *533*
Electrolyte disorders. *See also specific disorders*
   as complication of nutritional support, 1263-1264
   chemotherapy-induced, 886-888
   in fulminant hepatic failure, 1089
   in HIV infection/AIDS, 1413-1414
   shock and, adrenergic response and, 1323-1324
Electrolyte requirements, 1256, 1256t
Electrophysiologic monitoring. *See also* Electroencephalography (EEG)
   in traumatic brain injury, 87
   of comatose patient, *20*, 20-21, *21*
Embolism, air, as complication of nutritional support, 1261
Embolization
   coma and, 6
   following vascular surgery, 722
Emesis, for poisonings, 1456
Emphysema, 242. *See also* Chronic obstructive pulmonary disease (COPD)
   subcutaneous, following thoracic surgery, 378

Empyema
  epidural
    during ICU phase, 116-117, 122
    pre-ICU evaluation of, 106-107
  following thoracic surgery, 374-375
  in pneumonia, 394-395
  subdural, 81, 82
    during ICU phase, 116-117
    pre-ICU evaluation of, 106-107
Enalapril
  for hypertension, 693t, 694t
  for mitral regurgitation, 666t
Enalaprilat
  for hypertension, 692t
    postoperative, 745t, 749
  for mitral regurgitation, 666t
Encephalitis
  coma and, 10
  HSV. See Herpes simplex encephalitis (HSE)
Encephalopathy
  hepatic (portosystemic). See also Coma, hepatic
    chronic, 1082
    coma and, 13
    in acute renal failure, in patients awaiting liver transplantation, 1139
    in patients awaiting liver transplantation, treatment of, 1138, 1138t
    with shunt procedures, 1100
  HIV, 46-47, 1406
  hypertensive, coma and, 9
  in multiple organ system failure, 1305-1306
Endobronchial intubation, for thoracic surgery, 363, 363t, 365, 365
Endocarditis
  infective
    antimicrobial therapy for, 1376-1377
    aortic regurgitation and, 670, 671
    coma and, 10
    intracranial
      during ICU phase, 115
      pre-ICU evaluation of, 104-105
    prophylaxis of
      in aortic regurgitation, during post-ICU phase, 679-680
      in mitral regurgitation, 669
  prosthetic valve, 658
Endocrine disorders. See also specific disorders, hormones and glands
  coma and, 12-13
  in HIV infection/AIDS, 1414
  in multiple organ system failure, 1293t
  necrotizing pancreatitis and
    assessment of, 1039
    long-term changes in, 1039t, 1040
Endomyopathy biopsy, in cardiomyopathy, dilated, 619
Endoscopic retrograde cholangiopancreatography (ERCP)
  in hepatic disorders, 1072, 1073
  in pancreatitis, 1027
  pancreatitis due to, 1015, 1016t
Endoscopy
  in gastrointestinal bleeding
    emergency, 992
    lower, 996
      technique for, 996
      therapeutic, 996
    therapeutic, 993
      for colonic bleeding, 996
      variceal ligation and, 994, 1098, 1136

  upper
    interpretation of, 992-993
    technique for, 992
  in inhalation injury, 328-330, 330
Endotoxin, in multiple organ system failure, 1306-1307
Endotracheal intubation, 484-485
  contraindications to, 1614
End-stage renal disease (ESRD), diabetes mellitus as cause of, 802, 803-806
Enoximine, for shock, 1329
Enteral feeding, following head and neck surgery, 223, 223t
Enteral formulas, 1259, 1261
Enteric tubes, imaging studies and, 1478, 1480, 1481
Envenomations, 1468-1469
Environmental factors, chronic obstructive pulmonary disease related to, pathogenesis of, 243-244
Enzyme-linked immunosorbent assay (ELISA), for HIV infection, 1402
Epidemiology. See Clinical epidemiology
Epidural analgesia, postoperative, for thoracic surgery patients, 371
Epidural empyema
  during ICU phase, 116-117, 122
  pre-ICU evaluation of, 106-107
Epilepsy. See Seizures
Epinephrine
  for shock, 1325t, 1327
  for urticaria, 966
  in cardiopulmonary resuscitation, 555-556, 556t, 560
    high dose, 561
Equipment inventory, for computerized patient management system, 1702
Error, statistical, 1739
  α and β, 1741, 1741t
Erysipelas, 925-926
  clinical presentation and differential diagnosis of, 925, 926
  laboratory studies in, 925
  pathophysiology and risk factors for, 925
  treatment and recovery from, 925-926
Erythema multiforme, 967
Erythromycin
  dosing adjustment for renal or hepatic dysfunction, 1351t
  dosing during hemofiltration and hemodialysis, 1352t
  for pneumonia, 1375
    community-acquired, 391t, 391-392
    nosocomial, 393t
Erythropoiesis, acceleration of, 1241
Erythropoietin (EPO), deficiency of, anemia due to, 901-902
Esmolol (Brevibloc)
  following vascular surgery, 718
  for amphetamine abuse/overdose, 1437
  for aortic dissection, 705t
  for cocaine abuse/overdose, 1434, 1435t
  for hypertension, postoperative, 745t, 747-748
  for supraventricular tachycardia, 539, 543
Esophageal disorders. See also Varices
  following thoracic surgery, 379
  imaging studies in, 1525, 1534-1537
  in HIV infection/AIDS, 1408
Esophagostomy, cervical, following head and neck surgery, 222
Ethanol. See also Alcohol abuse/overdose
  for ethylene glycol/methanol poisoning, 1466
  injection of, for bleeding ulcers, 993

Ethchlorvynol abuse/overdose, 1443
Ethics committee, 1729, 1734
  definition of, 1728t
Ethylene glycol intoxication, 1466-1467
  coma and, 12
  metabolic acidosis associated with, treatment of, 763
Etidronate, for hypercalcemia, 884, 1193
Euthyroid sick syndrome, 1174-1175, 1175t
  during ICU phase, 1177
  during post-ICU phase, 1180-1181
Euvolemic hyponatremia, 770-771, 771t
Evacuation, in inhalation injury, 322
Evaporative heat loss, 51
Evoked potentials, in comatose patient, 20-21
Executive commitment, to computerization, 1700, 1701t
Exercise testing, preoperative, 1206, 1212t, 1212-1213
Exertional heat stroke, 57
  clinical features of, 58
Exocrine function, necrotizing pancreatitis and
  assessment of, 1039
  long-term changes in, 1038t, 1039
Experiences, perception of events and, 1566-1567
Expert witnesses, 1723
Expiratory pressure, in hypoventilation syndromes, 181
External cardiac massage
  closed chest, complications of, 562
  in cardiopulmonary resuscitation, 561
Extracorporeal membrane oxygenation (ECMO)
  for inhalation injury, 332-333
  pre-cardiac transplantation, 642
Extradural hematoma, 78, 79
Extraordinary treatments, 1727
  definition of, 1728t
Extremity surgery, hypertension following, 739
Extubation, 490
  complications and management of, 1614
  of thoracic surgery patients, 367
Eye infections, pseudomonal, 941
Eye movements, in neuro-ophthalmologic examination, of comatose patient, 18

Factitious asthma, during pre-ICU phase, 194
Failure to thrive, pancreatitis and, 1038
Falciparum malaris, antimicrobial therapy for, 1385
False-negative results, 1745, 1745t
False-positive results, 1745, 1745t
Family members
  as surrogate decision makers, 1732-1733, 1734
  as team members, 1562
  education of, 1563
  initiating lawsuits, 1719
  maintaining interest of, rehabilitation of ventilator-dependent patients and, 444
  maintaining relationships in, 1571-1572
  rights of, 1732
Famotidine, for pancreatitis, 1034t
Fat embolism, coma and, 9
Fatigue, muscular. See Respiratory muscles
Fatty liver, of pregnancy, 1080
Feedings, transitional, 1269-1270, 1270
Fenoldapam, for shock, 1327

INDEX

Fentanyl
  abuse/overdose of, 1445, 1446
  for pain control, 1283t, 1284
  peridural, for pain control, 1285, 1285t
Fever
  antimicrobial therapy and. See Antibiotic therapy, during ICU phase
  drug-induced, 1371
  in HIV infection/AIDS, 1416
  in shock, 1317
Fibrillation
  atrial, 536, *536*
    in acute myocardial infarction, 578
    treatment of, 54t, 539–540
  ventricular, in acute myocardial infarction, 577–578
Fibrinolysis
  disorders of, 914. *See also specific disorders*
  primary, 914
Fibrinolytic agents. *See* Thrombolytic therapy; *specific drugs*
Filing, of suit, 1721
Filling pressures, optimization of, following vascular surgery, 717
Fisher's exact test, 1750
Fistulas
  bronchopleural, following thoracic surgery, 374
  chyle, following head and neck surgery, 220–221
  graft-enteric, following vascular surgery, 725
  nephrocutaneous, following renal surgery, 848
  pancreatic, pancreatitis and, 1039
    surgery for, 1037
  tracheoesophageal, 870–871
Flashbacks, hallucinogens causing, 1448
Flecainide, for ventricular tachycardia, 544t
Fluconazole
  dosing adjustment for renal or hepatic dysfunction, 1351t
  dosing during hemofiltration and hemodialysis, 1352t
  prophylactic, for pneumonia, 413t
Flucytosine
  dosing adjustment for renal or hepatic dysfunction, 1351t
  dosing during hemofiltration and hemodialysis, 1352t
Fluid
  pleural, following thoracic surgery, 376–377
  requirements for, 1256
  restriction of, for elevated intracranial pressure, in comatose patient, 19
Fluid disorders
  as complication of nutritional support, 1263–1264
  in HIV infection/AIDS, 1413–1414
Fluid elimination, for elevated intracranial pressure, in comatose patient, 19
Fluid management. *See also* Fluid resuscitation; Hydration therapy
  following vascular surgery, 718
  for lithium intoxication, 1465
  for renal failure, 784–785, *785*, 791
  for thoracic surgery patients, 368–369
  for toxic shock syndrome, 933
  in adult respiratory distress syndrome, 308
  in diabetic ketoacidosis, 1159
  in gastrointestinal bleeding, 992
  in hyperglycemic hyperosmolar nonketotic coma, 1164, 1165
  in pancreatitis, 1031–1032

Fluid resuscitation, 1226–1238
  during ICU phase, 1231–1237, 1233t
    for hypovolemia, 1233–1237, 1234t
      distributional fluid losses and, 1236–1237
      gastrointestinal fluid loss and, 1234
      hemorrhage and, 1233–1234
      sensible and insensible fluid losses and, 1235–1236, *1236*
      urinary fluid losses and, 1234–1235, 1235t
    monitoring of, 1231–1233, *1232*, 1232t
  during post-ICU phase, 1237–1238
    home venous access for, 1238
    recovery and, 1237–1238
  during pre-ICU phase, 1227–1231, *1230*, 1231t
    fluids for, 1228–1230, 1229t
    history and, 1227, 1227t
    initial monitoring and, 1228
    laboratory and diagnostic studies and, 1228
    physical examination and, 1227t, 1227–1228
Flumazenil, for sedation, 1281
Fluoroquinolones. *See also specific drugs*
  resistance to, 1387
  patterns of, application to ICU phase of patient management, 1393, *1394*, 1395, *1395*
Fluoroscopy, in hypoventilation syndromes, 181–182
Fluosol, for anemia, 878
Flurocortisone, for Addison's disease, 1176
Flutter, atrial, 536, *537*
Focal demyelination, coma and, 12
Focal pulmonary hemorrhage (FPH), 347–352
  during ICU phase, 350–352
    airway measurement and, 350
    angiographic localization and embolization for, 352
    diagnosis of specific causes and, 351
    localization of bleeding and, 350–351
    surgical repair and excision for, 351–352
  during post-ICU phase, 352
  during pre-ICU phase, 348–350
    risk assessment and, 348t, 348–349, *349*
    triage and, 349–350
Forced diuresis, for poisonings, 1457
Forward stepwise regression, 1750–1751
Foscarnet
  dosing adjustment for renal or hepatic dysfunction, 1351t
  dosing during hemofiltration and hemodialysis, 1352t
Fractures. *See specific sites*
Freedom from manipulation, 1665t
Fresh-frozen plasma, transfusions of, 1245–1246, 1247t
Friends, maintaining interest of, rehabilitation of ventilator-dependent patients and, 444
Frontal limbic system, coma and, 3
Fulminant hepatic failure (FHF), 1076–1093
  causes of, 1076t, 1076–1080
    acute viral hepatitis, 1077t, 1077–1079, *1078*, 1078t
    chemicals and poisons, 1079
    drugs, 1079
    ischemia and hypoxia, 1079–1080
    metabolic, 1080
    metastatic liver disease, 1080

  complications of, 1080–1091
    acid/base abnormalities, 1089
    coagulopathy, 1089–1090
    electrolyte abnormalities, 1089
    hemodynamic, 1086–1087
    hepatic coma. *See* Coma, hepatic
    infection, 1089, *1089*
    metabolic, 1090–1091
    pancreatitis, 1091
    portal hypertension, 1091
    pulmonary, 1087, *1087*
    renal failure, 1087–1089, *1088*
  prognosis of, 1091–1093, 1092t
Functional abnormalities, thermoregulatory disorders and, 53
Functional Status Questionnaire, 1691–1692, 1692t, *1693*
Functional tests, in nutrition assessment, 1252, 1253t
Fundi, in neuro-ophthalmologic examination, of comatose patient, 18
Fungal infections. *See* Infection, fungal; *specific infections*
Fungi, in cerebrospinal fluid, analysis of, 1616
Furosemide (Bumex; Lasix)
  following vascular surgery, 717
  for cirrhosis, 1113
  for hypercalcemia, 1192–1193, 1193t
  for renal failure, 786t, 787
Futility, defining, 1734–1735

Gaeltec ICP monitor, 70
Gallbladder
  disorders of, imaging studies in, 1531–1532, *1536*
  in hepatic disorders, 1061–1062, *1062*
  on plain abdominal radiographs, *1066*, 1066–1067, *1067*
Gallium nitrate, for hypercalcemia, 884
Gallstone(s), 1046–1055
  during ICU phase, 1049–1054
    acalculous cholecystitis and, 1050–1051, *1051*
    acute cholangitis and, 1051–1052, *1052*
    hepatic abscess and, 1052–1053, *1053*
    jaundice and, 1050, *1050*
    sclerosing cholangitis and, 1053–1054, *1054*
    total parenteral nutrition and, 1053
  during post-ICU phase, *1054*, 1054–1055, *1055*
  during pre-ICU phase, 1046–1049
    asymptomatic, 1046
    cholecystectomy concomitant with, 1046
    microbiology of, 1048–1049
    morbidity and mortality and, 1046–1047, 1047t
    special risk groups for, 1047–1048
      cirrhotic patients, 1048
      diabetic patients, 1047–1048, *1048*, 1048t
      elderly patients, 1047
      jaundiced patients, 1048
  on plain abdominal radiographs, 1066, *1066*
Gallstone pancreatitis, 1023–1024
Ganciclovir
  dosing adjustment for renal or hepatic dysfunction, 1351t
  dosing during hemofiltration and hemodialysis, 1353t
  prophylactic, following cardiac transplantation, 651

Gangrene, scrotal, 851
Gastric decontamination, for poisonings, 1457
Gastric disorders, imaging studies in, 1525, *1527, 1528*
Gastric emptying, delayed, pancreatitis and, 1039
Gastric lavage, for poisonings, 1456–1457
Gastrointestinal aspiration, in comatose patient, 16–17
Gastrointestinal bleeding, 989–998
   during ICU phase, 991–997
     angiography in, 996–997
     correction of coagulopathy in, 992
     endoscopy in, 992–993
      emergency, 992
      in lower gastrointestinal bleeding, 996
      in upper gastrointestinal bleeding, 992–993
     lower gastrointestinal bleeding, 996
      endoscopy in, 996
     monitoring parameters and, 991–992
     upper gastrointestinal bleeding, 992–993
     variceal bleeding in portal hypertension, 994–996
      sclerotherapy for, 994, 996
      Sengstaken-Blakemore balloon tamponade in, 994, *995*
     volume replacement in, 992
   during post-ICU phase, 998
   in cirrhosis. See Portal hypertension, gastropathy in; Varices
   integrated care in, 998
   monitoring for, during mechanical ventilation, 294
   natural history of, 989–990, 990t
     risk stratification and, 989–990
   nutritional support in, 997–998
   pre-ICU assessment of, 990–991
     indications for ICU admission and management of, 991, 991t
     of bleeding activity, 990
     of source of, 990
     search for source of bleeding in, 991, 991t
   surgical management of, 997
Gastrointestinal disorders. *See also specific disorders*
   chemotherapy-induced, 890–892
     of large bowel, 891–892
     of midgut and liver, 891
     of upper digestive tract, 890–891
   classification systems for, 1684, 1686t, 1687t
   following cardiac surgery, 602
   following renal surgery, 848–849
   following vascular surgery, 722–723
   in chronic renal failure, 818–819
     rehabilitative phase of, 810
     risk phase of, 818–819
     support phase of, 810
   in comatose patient, 21
   in HIV infection/AIDS, 1408–1409
     esophageal, 1408
     hepatic, biliary, and pancreatic, 1408–1409
     oral, 1408
   in multiple organ system failure, 1293t, 1300–1302
   infections, antimicrobial therapy for, 1380–1381
Gastrointestinal management, in spinal cord injury, 154–155

Gastrointestinal tract
   fluid loss from, hypovolemia caused by, fluid resuscitation for, 1234
   following cardiac transplantation, 649–650
   in disseminated intravascular coagulation, 875
Gastropathy, portal hypertensive, 1103, *1103*
Gastrostomy, following head and neck surgery, 222–223
Genitourinary disorders. *See also specific disorders*
   infections of. *See also* Urinary tract infection (UTI)
     antimicrobial therapy for, 1381–1382
   management of, in spinal cord injury, 155
Gentamicin
   for intra-abdominal infections, 1378
   for pneumonia, nosocomial, 394
   in hemodialysis, 1345
Geriatric patients. *See* Elderly patients
Glasgow Coma Scale, 1678, 1681t
Glasgow Coma Scale (GCS), in brain injuries, 83, 83t
Glottic dysfunction, rehabilitation of ventilator-dependent patients and, 445
Glucagon, for shock, 1325t, 1329
Glucose. *See also* Hyperglycemia; Hypoglycemia
   for alcohol withdrawal, 1441t
   for cocaine abuse/overdose, 1434, 1435t
   for hyperkalemia, 779t
   for shock, 1330
Glutethimide abuse/overdose, 1443
Glyburide, hypoglycemia caused by, 1169
Graft dysfunction
   following liver transplantation, 1145t, 1145–1146, 1146t
   late, 1149–1150
   graft-enteric erosion, following vascular surgery, 725
   graft-enteric fistula, following vascular surgery, 725
Graft rejection
   following cardiac transplantation, prophylaxis of, 650t, 650–651, 651t
   following liver transplantation, 1146
   following renal transplantation, 828t, 828–829, 829t
Graft versus host disease (GVHD), following bone marrow transplantation, 882, 883
Gram-negative organisms, antibiotic resistance of, to beta-lactams, 1385–1386
Gram-positive organisms, antibiotic resistance of, to beta-lactams, 1385
Granulocytopenia
   as predisposing condition to infection, 400–401
   pneumonia with, treatment of, 409–410
Graves' disease, during pre-ICU phase, 1176
Growth hormone, secretion of, 1173
Guanethidine, for hypertension, 692t–694t
Guillain-Barré syndrome (GBS), 127–131
   during ICU phase, 129–130
     general support and, 129–130
     intravenous immunoglobulin treatment and, 130
     plasmapheresis and, 130
   during post-ICU phase, 130–131
   during pre-ICU phase, 128t, 128–129, 129t

   pathogenesis of, 128, 128t
   pathology of, 128
Gynecologic disorders, in HIV infection/AIDS, 1411–1412
Gynecologic surgery, as risk factor for neurologic surgical complications, 1220

Hairy leukoplakia, oral, 1408
Half-life, of drugs, 1338
Hallucinogen abuse/overdose, 1447–1449, 1448t
   complications of, 1448
   diagnosis and treatment of, 1448–1449
   ICU admission criteria in, 1449
   signs and symptoms of, 1448, 1448t
   special considerations in, 1449
Halo orthosis, in spinal cord injury, 152
Haloperidol (Haldol)
   for agitation, 43t, 43–44
   for alcohol withdrawal, 1441, 1441t
   for amphetamine abuse/overdose, 1436–1437
   for delirium, 1282–1283
   for sedation, 1280t
Halothane, hepatitis induced by, 1119–1120
Head and neck surgery, postoperative management following, 212–226
   during ICU phase, 213–223
     airway management and, 213–214, *214*
     medications and, 223
     nutritional management and, 221–223
     patient positioning and, 213
     total laryngectomy and, 214–215, *215, 216*
     wound management and, 215–221
   during post-ICU phase, 223–226
     cranial nerve deficits and, 224–226
     laryngeal surgery and, 224
     oral cavity surgery and, 224
     speech and swallowing and, 224
   during pre-ICU phase, 212–213
Headaches, migraine, coma and, 9
Heart. *See also* Cardiac *entries*
   following cardiac transplantation, 649
Heart disease, valvular, treatment of, preoperative, for prevention of cardiovascular complications, 1215–1216
Heart failure
   congestive. *See* Congestive heart failure
   high-output, 625t, 625–627
     during ICU phase, 626
      diagnostic evaluation of, 626
      hemodynamic features of, 626
      treatment of, 626
     during post-ICU phase, 626
     during pre-ICU phase, 625–626
   in multiple organ system failure, 1299
Heart rate
   electrocardiographic monitoring of, 1632, *1633*
   following cardiac surgery, 597
Heart rhythm, electrocardiographic monitoring of, 1632
Heart sounds
   first (S_1), 531
   in aortic regurgitation, 671–673
   second (S_2), 531
Heat cramps, 57
Heat exhaustion, 57
   salt-depletion, 57
   water-depletion, 57

INDEX

Heat loss
  convective, 51
  evaporative, 51
Heat stress, thermoregulatory response to, 52-53
Heat stroke, 57t, 57-59
  classic, 57
    clinical features of, 57-58
    during ICU phase, 58-59
    during post-ICU phase, 59
    during pre-ICU phase, 57t, 57-58
      clinical features of, 57-58, 58t
      treatment of, 58
  exertional, 57
    clinical features of, 58
Heat transfer
  conductive, 51
  radiative, 51
Heater probe, for therapeutic endoscopy, 993
Hematologic disorders. *See also specific disorders*
  following vascular surgery, 724
  in HIV infection/AIDS, 1412
  in multiple organ system failure, 1293t, 1302-1303
Hematologic emergencies, 873-883. *See also specific disorders*
Hematologic function, normal, 899-901
  coagulation factors and, *900*, 900-901, 901t
  platelets and, 900
  red cells and, 899
  white cells and, 899-900
Hematologic studies, in inhalation injury, 327-328
Hematoma
  extradural, 78, *79*
  following head and neck surgery, 219-220
  subdural, 78, *78*
Hematuria, management of, 853
Hemilaryngectomy, postoperative care for, 224
Hemodialysis
  access for, 792, 1608-1609
    complications of, 1608
      of femoral vein, 1608
      of subclavian and internal jugular veins, 1608
    contraindications to, 1608
    indications for, 1608
    quality enhancement for, 1608-1609
  aminoglycosides and, 1344-1345
    dosage of, 1344-1345, 1357, *1358*, 1359
  continuous arterial venous
    aminoglycosides and, 1344
    vancomycin dosing and, 1348
  for ethylene glycol/methanol intoxication, 1466-1467
  for hypercalcemia, 1193
  for lithium intoxication, 1465
  for multiple organ system failure, 1304
  for poisonings, 1457
  for renal failure
    during ICU phase, 792t, 792-797, *793-795*
    during post-ICU phase, 797-798
  for salicylate intoxication, 1460
  for sedative/hypnotic abuse/overdose, 1444
  for theophylline intoxication, 1463, 1463t
  termination guidelines for, 1730-1731, 1733, 1735, 1736

vancomycin dosing in, 1348-1349, 1357, *1358*, 1359
Hemodilution, 1241
Hemodynamic disorders
  in fulminant hepatic failure, 1086-1087
  shock and, 1315
Hemodynamic management
  following cardiac surgery, 597
  in chronic obstructive pulmonary disease, 261-263
    assessment and, 261
    therapy for, 262-263
  in pulmonary embolism, 421
  of comatose patient, 16
  preoperative, for prevention of cardiovascular complications, 1215
Hemodynamic monitoring, 1630-1647. *See also specific types of hemodynamic monitoring*
  basis of clinical measurements and, 1630-1631
  during mechanical ventilation, 292t, 292-293
  errors in interpretation and, 1631
  for respiratory insufficiency, 479
  for routine clinical assessment, 1631
  in pulmonary embolism, 421
  invasive versus noninvasive, 1631
  operator errors and, 1630-1631
  signal processing and, 1630-1631
Hemodynamic support, for multiple organ system failure, 1307
Hemodynamics
  in cardiac trauma, nonpenetrating, 633, *633*
  in cardiomyopathy, dilated, 619
  in constrictive pericarditis, 617, *617*
  in heart failure, high output, 626
  in hypertrophic cardiomyopathy, 623, *624*
  in mitral regurgitation, 663, 665
  in necrotizing pancreatitis, 1017-1019, 1018t, *1019*
  in pericardial effusion, 612-615, *615*
  in renal failure, 788
  in sepsis-related myocardial dysfunction, *636*, 636-637
Hemofiltration
  continuous arterial venous
    aminoglycosides and, 1344
    vancomycin dosing and, 1348
  for multiorgan dysfunction, 797-798
  for poisonings, 1457
  for renal failure, 792
Hemoglobin, abnormalities of, 903-904. *See also specific abnormalities*
Hemoglobin solutions, as red blood cell substitute, 1248
Hemoglobin test, in renal failure, 788
Hemoglobinuria, nocturnal, paroxysmal, 904
Hemolytic anemia, 902, 903t
  antibody-mediated, 904-905
  autoimmune, drug-related, 905
  macroangiopathic, 904
  microangiopathic, 904
Hemolytic uremic syndrome (HUS), 861, 908
  chemotherapy-associated, 861, 887-888
    during ICU phase, 887-888
    during post-ICU phase, 888
    during pre-ICU phase, 887
Hemoperfusion, for hepatic coma, 1085
Hemophilia, 911-912
Hemoptysis, in diffuse alveolar hemorrhage, 341-342
Hemorrhage. *See also Diffuse alveolar hemorrhage (DAH)*

  cerebral, coma and, 6
  following cardiac surgery, 598, *598*
  following renal surgery, 847
  following thoracic surgery, 375
  following transurethral prostatectomy, 850
  gastrointestinal. *See Gastrointestinal bleeding*
  hypovolemia caused by, fluid resuscitation for, 1233-1234
  in following renal revascularization, 833
  intracerebral, 79-80, *80*, 88
    hypertensive, 79
  intracranial. *See Intracranial hypertension*
  intraventricular, 80
  pulmonary, 341-352. *See also Diffuse alveolar hemorrhage (DAH); Focal pulmonary hemorrhage (FPH)*
  reperfusion, postcraniotomy, 89
  retroperitoneal, following vascular surgery, 722
  subarachnoid, 80, 81t
Hemorrhagic stroke, 79-80, 88-89
  aneurysmal subarachnoid hemorrhage and, 80, 81t, 88
  intracerebral hemorrhage and, 79-80, *80*, 88
  intraventricular hemorrhage and, 80
  postcraniotomy care and, 88-89
Hemoximetry, for monitoring respiratory insufficiency, 479
Heparin
  following vascular surgery, 720, 722
  for cardiac transplantation, 646
  for disseminated intravascular coagulation, 875, 971-972
  for inhalation injury, 333-334
  for prevention of myocardial infarction, 581, 582
  for pulmonary embolism, 421-422, 429-431
    continuous intravenous therapy with, 430, 430t, 431t
    low molecular weight, 430-431
  for thrombotic disorders, 914
  necrosis induced by, 969
  thrombocytopenia induced by, 909-910
Heparin-induced thrombocytopenia and thrombosis syndrome (HITT), 909-910
Hepatic abscess, gallstones and, 1052-1053, *1053*
Hepatic artery thrombosis (HAT), following liver transplantation, 1146
Hepatic coma. *See Coma, hepatic*
Hepatic disorders, 1058t, 1058-1122. *See also specific disorders*
  antibiotic dosing in, 1349-1354, 1350t-1354t
  chemotherapy-induced, 891
  coagulopathy in, 913
  evaluation of, 1058-1076
    history in, 1058-1059, 1059t
    imaging in, 1066-1074
      abdominal radiography, *1066*, 1066-1067, *1067*
      angiography, 1073-1074, *1074*
      cholangiography, 1071-1073, *1072, 1073*
      cholescintigraphy, 1068, *1069*
      computed tomography, 1070, *1071, 1072*
      magnetic resonance imaging, 1070
      scintigraphy, 1067-1068, *1068*
      ultrasonography, 1068-1070, *1070*

1769

Hepatic disorders *(Continued)*
  laboratory studies in, 1062-1066, 1063t
    of albumin, 1064
    of alkaline phosphatase, 1065
    of aminotransferases, 1064-1065
    of bilirubin, 1062-1064, 1063t
    of miscellaneous markers, 1065-1066
    of prothrombin time, 1064
    routine, 1065
  liver biopsy in, 1074-1076, *1075,* 1076t
  physical examination in, 1059-1062, *1059-1062*
  imaging studies in, 1536-1537, *1538-1541,* 1540
  in HIV infection/AIDS, 1408-1409
  in multiple organ system failure, 1293t, 1301
  in necrotizing pancreatitis, 1021
Hepatic encephalopathy. *See* Coma, hepatic; Encephalopathy, hepatic (portosystemic)
Hepatic failure
  fulminant. *See* Fulminant hepatic failure (FHF)
  nutritional support in, 1268
Hepatitis
  alcoholic, in cirrhosis, 1104-1107, 1105t, *1106*
  drug-induced, by halothane, 1119-1120
  ischemic, 1120
  peliosis, bacillary, in HIV infection/AIDS, 1410
  viral, 1066
    fulminant hepatic failure caused by, 1077t, 1077-1079, *1078,* 1078t
    hepatitis A, 1077, *1078*
    hepatitis B, 1077
    hepatitis C, 1077-1078, 1078t
    hepatitis D, 1077
    hepatitis E, 1078-1079
Hepatobiliary disorders, imaging studies in, 1531-1532, *1536*
Hepatocellular dysfunction, in jaundice, postoperative, 1119-1120
Hepatorenal syndrome, in cirrhosis, 1116-1117
Hernia
  in cirrhosis, 1112
  repair of, as risk factor for neurologic surgical complications, 1220
Herniation, supratentorial, coma and, 5, 5-6
Heroin intoxication, coma and, 11
Herpes simplex encephalitis (HSE), 948-949
  clinical manifestations and differential diagnosis of, 948
  during ICU phase, 119-120, 122-123
  laboratory studies in, 948-949
  pathophysiology of, 948
  pre-ICU evaluation of, 111t, 111-113
  treatment and outcome of, 949
Herpes simplex virus (HSV) infections, *947,* 947-954. *See also specific infections*
Herpesvirus infections, cutaneous, 946-965. *See also specific infections*
H-graft, for esophageal varices, 1102, *1102*
High frequency jet ventilation (HFJV), 288t, 288-290, 289t
  for thoracic surgery patients, 370
HIV infection/AIDS, 1399-1417
  diarrhea in, antimicrobial therapy for, 1380
  during ICU phase, 1416-1417
    diagnostic and support measures and, 1416

infection control and, 1416-1417
reassessment and decision making and, 1417
during post-ICU phase, 1417
  psychosocial and ethical issues and, 1417
  recovery and, 1417
  site of care and, 1417
during pre-ICU phase, 1400-1416
  classification of, 1402t, 1402-1403, 1403t
  epidemiology of, 1400
  immunopathogenesis of, 1401, 1401t
  influence on ICU admission, 1414-1416
    patient preferences and, 1415-1416
    prognosis of conditions leading to ICU care and, 1414-1415
  natural history of, 1401-1402
  sequelae of, 1405-1414
    cardiac, 1414
    dermatologic, 1411
    disseminated infections, 1409t, 1409-1411
    gastrointestinal, 1408-1409
    gynecologic, 1411-1412
    hematologic, 1412
    metabolic and endocrinologic, 1413-1414
    musculoskeletal and rheumatologic, 1414
    neoplastic, 1412-1413
    neurologic, 1406-1408, *1407*
    ophthalmologic, 1411
    renal, 1414
    respiratory, 1405-1406
  testing for, 1402
  transmission of, 1400-1401
  treatment of, 1403t, 1403-1405
    antiretroviral therapies in, 1403-1404
    prophylaxis and treatment of opportunistic infections in, 1404t, 1404-1405
neuropsychiatric manifestations of, 46-47
  encephalopathy, 46-47
  etiology of, 46
  treatment of, 47
respiratory infections in, antimicrobial therapy for, 1373
substance abuse and, 1427
Home total parenteral nutrition, 1271
Home venous access, for fluid resuscitation, 1238
Home ventilation. *See* Mechanical ventilation, long-term use of
Hormones. *See also specific hormones*
  hypothalamic, 1173, 1174t
  pituitary, 1173, 1174t
Hospital information system, 1700-1701, 1701t
Hospital prognostic index (HPI), 1253, 1254t
Human immunodeficiency virus (HIV) infection. *See* HIV infection/AIDS
Humidity therapy, 481
Hydralazine
  for hypertension, 692t-694t
    postoperative, 745t, 746
  for mitral regurgitation, 666t
Hydration therapy. *See also* Fluid management
  in diabetic ketoacidosis, assessment of, 1159
  termination guidelines for, 1731, 1733-1734, 1735, 1737

Hydrocephalus, subarachnoid hemorrhage and, 80, 81t, 88
Hydrochloric acid, for metabolic alkalosis, 768
Hydrocortisone
  for Addison's disease, 1176
  for adrenal crisis, 1179
Hydrogen fluoride, inhalation injury caused by, 319
Hydrogen sulfide, inhalation injury caused by, 319
Hydromorphone (Dilaudid), abuse/overdose of, 1445
Hydrothorax, hepatic, in cirrhosis, 1112-1113
Hyperadrenalism, coma and, 13
Hyperaldosteronism, hypertension and, 834
Hyperalimentation. *See also* Total parenteral nutrition (TPN)
  in brain injury, 86
Hyperbaric oxygen therapy, for carbon monoxide intoxication, 1462
Hypercalcemia, 883-884, 1192-1193
  during ICU phase, 884, 884t, 1192-1193
    maintenance therapy for, 1193
    management of, *1192,* 1192-1193, 1193t
    phosphonates for, 1193, 1193t
  during post-ICU phase, 884
  during pre-ICU phase, 883t, 883-884, 1192
    clinical appearance of, 1192
Hypercapnia, chronic, metabolic alkalosis associated with, 766-767
Hyperglycemia
  in brain injury, 86
  in diabetes mellitus. *See* Diabetes mellitus
Hyperglycemic hyperosmolar nonketotic coma (HHNK), 12-13, 1163-1165
  during ICU phase, 1164t, 1164-1165
  during post-ICU phase, 1165, 1165t
  during pre-ICU phase, 1163t, 1163-1164
    evaluation and treatment of, 1164
    risk factors for, 1163-1164
Hyperinflation, in ventilatory failure, 172-173, *173*
Hyperkalemia, 778-780
  as complication of nutritional support, 1262
  during ICU phase, 779t, 779-780
  during post-ICU phase, 780
  during pre-ICU phase, 778-779
    differential diagnosis of, 778t, 778-779
    laboratory studies in, 779
    signs and symptoms of, 779
Hyperleukocytosis, with malignant disease, 875-876
  during ICU phase, 876
  during post-ICU phase, 876
  during pre-ICU phase, 875-876
Hypermagnesemia, 1189
  as complication of nutritional support, 1263
  during ICU phase, 1189
  during pre-ICU phase, 1189
Hypermetabolic state, 1264-1265
  nutritional needs in
    defining, 1264, 1264t
    problems with meeting, 1264-1265
Hypernatremia, 773-774
  during ICU phase, 773-774
    diagnosis of, 773-774
    treatment of, 774, 774t
  during post-ICU phase, 774
  during pre-ICU phase, 773

laboratory studies in, 773, 773t
signs and symptoms of, 773
Hyperphosphatemia, as complication of nutritional support, 1263
Hyperreflexia, autonomic, hypertension following, postoperative, 737
Hypertension
  arterial, following cardiac surgery, 596-597
  following cardiac transplantation, 652
  following vascular surgery, 719
  in chronic renal failure, 808-809
    rehabilitative phase of, 809
    risk phase of, 808-809
    support phase of, 809
  intracerebral, in brain injury, 86
  intracranial. See Intracranial hypertension
  malignant, during pre-ICU phase, 689-690, 690t
  management of, in brain injuries, 82-83
  portal. See Portal hypertension
  postoperative, 728-749
    causes of, 733t-735t, 733-741
      anesthesia, 740
      aortic aneurysm resection, 736
      autonomic hyperreflexia, 737
      cardiac transplantation, 736
      carotid endarterectomy, 736
      drug interactions, 741
      endocrine-secreting tumor resection, 738-739
      extremity surgery, 739
      intracranial hypertension, 737
      liver transplantation, 740
      medication withdrawal, 740-741
      myocardial revascularization, 735
      neurovascular surgery, 737
      obstetric surgery, 739
      radical neck dissection, 740
      renal surgery, 739
      thoracic aortic coarctation resection, 736-737
      urologic surgery, 739-740
      valvular heart surgery, 735-736
    definition of, 728
    management of, 741, 741-749, 742, 742t, 743t, 744, 745t
      alpha blockers in, 747
      angiotensin-converting enzyme inhibitors in, 749
      autonomic ganglia blockers in, 746-747
      beta blockers in, 747-748
      calcium channel blockers in, 748
      centrally acting antihypertensive agents in, 748-749
      combined alpha and beta blockers in, 747
      vascular smooth muscle relaxers in, 746
    pathophysiology of, 728-733, 729t
      intermediate-term blood pressure regulation and, 730-732, 731
      long-term blood pressure regulation and, 732, 732-733, 733
      short-term blood pressure regulation and, 729-730, 730
    preoperative, postoperative hypertension and, 734, 734t
    treatment of, preoperative, for prevention of cardiovascular complications, 1215
    with adrenal tumors, 834-836
      during post-ICU phase, 836
      during pre-ICU phase, 834-835
        aldosteronoma and, 835

hyperaldosteronism and, 834
intraoperative considerations and, 835
pheochromocytoma and, 835
postoperative monitoring during ICU phase and, 835-836
  aldosteronoma and, 835-836
  pheochromocytoma and, 835
Hypertensive emergencies, 686-698, 687t
  during ICU phase, 696
    circumstances of management and, 696
    data acquisition and, 696, 697t
    outcome and, 696-697, 697t
  during post-ICU phase, therapy and management of, 697-698
  during pre-ICU phase, 686-696
    approach to, 689t, 689-690, 690t
    circumstances of, 686-687, 887t
    initial data acquisition and, 687-689, 688t
    outcome and, 690-691, 692t-695t, 695-696
Hypertensive encephalopathy, coma and, 9
Hypertensive intracerebral hemorrhage, 79
Hyperthermia
  malignant. See Malignant hyperthermia (MH)
  monoamine oxidase inhibitors causing, 1461
  treatment of, in cocaine abuse/overdose, 1434
Hyperthyroidism
  during post-ICU phase, 1180-1181
  during pre-ICU phase, 1176
Hypertrophic cardiomyopathy. See Cardiomyopathy, hypertrophic
Hyperventilation
  for elevated intracranial pressure, in comatose patient, 19
  for intracranial hypertension, 72
Hyperviscosity, 873-874, 874t
  during ICU phase, 874
  during post-ICU phase, 874
  during pre-ICU phase, 873-874
Hypervolemia, hypertension and, postoperative, 734
Hypnotics, 1280t, 1280-1281
Hypoadrenalism
  coma and, 13
  during post-ICU phase, 1181
Hypoalbuminemia
  as complication of nutritional support, 1263
  in brain injury, 86
Hypocalcemia, 1190-1192
  during ICU phase, 1191-1192
    calcium replacement for, 1191-1192
      intravenous, 1191-1192, 1192t
      no-reflow phenomenon and, 1191
      postresuscitation syndrome and, 1191
      reperfusion injury and, 1191
    clinical signs of, 1191
      cardiovascular, 1191
      neuromuscular, 1191
  during pre-ICU phase, 1190-1191
    alkalosis as cause of, 1190
    hypomagnesemia as cause of, 1190
    renal failure as cause of, 1190-1191
    sepsis as cause of, 1190
  in fulminant hepatic failure, 1089
  in hypomagnesemia, 1186
  in necrotizing pancreatitis, 1021-1022
  shock and, adrenergic response and, 1323
Hypoglycemia, 886
  coma and, 10

during ICU phase, 886
during post-ICU phase, 886
during pre-ICU phase, 886
in diabetes mellitus. See Diabetes mellitus
in fulminant hepatic failure, 1090-1091
in sepsis, 1323
Hypokalemia, 775-778
  as complication of nutritional support, 1262
  during ICU phase, 776-778
  during post-ICU phase, 778
  during pre-ICU phase, 775-776
    differential diagnosis of, 775-776
    laboratory studies in, 776, 777t
    signs and symptoms of, 776
  following vascular surgery, 723
  in cirrhosis, 1114
  in fulminant hepatic failure, 1089
  in hypomagnesemia, 1186
Hypomagnesemia, 1185-1189
  as complication of nutritional support, 1263
  during ICU phase, 1187-1188
    cardiac manifestations of, 1187
    diagnosis of, 1187-1188
    magnesium replacement therapy and, 1188, 1188t
    monitoring of, 1188
    protocols for, 1188, 1188t
  during post-ICU phase, 1188-1189
    maintenance therapy and, 1188
    nutritional support and, 1188-1189
    oral supplements and, 1189
  during pre-ICU phase, 1185-1187
    clinical markers of, 1186-1187
      hypocalcemia, 1186-1187
      hypokalemia, 1186-1187
      hypophosphatemia, 1186-1187
      neurologic syndromes, 1187
    predisposing conditions for, 1185
      alcohol-related illnesses, 1186
      antibiotic therapy, 1186
      diabetes mellitus, 1186
      diuretic therapy, 1186, 1186
      secretory diarrhea, 1186
  hypocalcemia caused by, 1190
  in fulminant hepatic failure, 1089
  shock and, adrenergic response and, 1323-1324
Hyponatremia, 770-773, 885t, 885-886
  during ICU phase, 771-772, 772t, 885
  during post-ICU phase, 772-773, 885-886
  during pre-ICU phase, 770t, 770-771, 771t, 885
    euvolemic, 770-771, 771t
    hypovolemic, 770
    laboratory studies in, 771
    signs and symptoms of, 771
  in cirrhosis, 1114
  in fulminant hepatic failure, 1089
  in traumatic brain injury, 88
Hypophosphatemia
  as complication of nutritional support, 1262-1263
  in fulminant hepatic failure, 1089
  in hypomagnesemia, 1186
  shock and, adrenergic response and, 1323
Hypopituitarism, 1177
  during ICU phase, 1180
  during post-ICU phase, 1181
Hypotension
  intraoperative, as risk factor for neurologic surgical complications, 1218
  management of, in brain injuries, 82

Hypothalamic pituitary-endocrine axis, normal function of, 1173, 1174t
Hypothalamic-pituitary-peripheral gland unit, response to stress of illness, 1173–1175
  cortisol output and, 1173–1174
  euthyroid sick syndromes and, 1174–1175, 1175t
  pituitary-gonadal axis and, 1175
Hypothalamus, coma and, 4
Hypothermia
  accidental, 54t, 54–57
    during ICU phase, 56–57
    during post-ICU phase, 57
    during pre-ICU phase, 54–56
      clinical features of, 55, 55t
      treatment of, 55–56
  following cardiac surgery, 596
  following vascular surgery, 719
  hypertension and, postoperative, 734
  induced
    for intracranial hypertension, 73
    for respiratory failure, 1288–1289
Hypothesis, 1742
Hypothyroidism
  coma and, 13
  during post-ICU phase, 1180–1181
  during pre-ICU phase, 1176–1177
Hypoventilation
  as surgical risk factor, for pulmonary complications, 1201
  coma and, 14
  in parenchymal respiratory failure, 163–164
  mechanical, controlled, in bronchospastic disease, 236–237
  voluntary, in hypoventilation syndromes, 180–181
Hypoventilation syndromes, 178–186
  during ICU phase, 182–183
  during post-ICU phase, 183–185
  during pre-ICU phase, 178–182, 179, 179t
    history and physical examination and, 180
    laboratory evaluation and, 180, 180–182, 181
Hypovolemia
  fluid resuscitation for. See Fluid resuscitation, during ICU phase
  hyponatremia and, 770
  hypovolemic shock and, 1313–1314
  with diuretics, 1113–1114
Hypoxia
  coma and, 8–10
  hepatic failure induced by, 1079–1080
  tissue, in multiple organ system failure, 1295–1296
Hysterical conversion, spinal cord injury and, 150

Ibuprofen
  for adult respiratory distress syndrome, 309
  for shock, 1329–1330
  intoxication by, coma and, 12
ICU organization and management, quality of care and, 1581–1582
Idiopathic hypertrophic subaortic stenosis (IHSS). See Cardiomyopathy, hypertrophic
Idiopathic thrombocytopenic purpura (ITP), 908–909
Ileus, paralytic, following vascular surgery, 722

Illegal drugs. See Substance abuse/overdose; specific substances
Illness, hypothalamic-pituitary-peripheral gland unit response to. See Hypothalamic-pituitary-peripheral gland unit
Imaging studies, 1473–1550, 1474t. See also specific modalities
  enteric tubes and, 1478, 1480, 1481
  in abdominal disease, 1521–1522, 1522, 1522t, 1523, 1524–1536
    esophageal, 1525, 1534–1537
    gastric and duodenal, 1525, 1527, 1528
    of gallbladder and hepatobiliary system, 1531–1532, 1536
    of small and large bowel, 1525, 1528, 1528–1534, 1531
    of spleen and retroperitoneum, 1532, 1536, 1537, 1538
    pancreatic, 1531, 1534–1536
  in acute myocardial infarction, 572
  in adult respiratory distress syndrome, 1493, 1497–1502
  in aortic disease, 1513, 1518, 1519–1522, 1521
  in aortic dissection, 703–704, 705
  in atelectasis, 1486–1487, 1487–1490
  in brain injuries, 83–85, 84t
  in diffuse alveolar hemorrhage, 342
  in hepatic disease, 1536–1537, 1538–1541, 1540
  in inhalation injury, 328, 329
  in intracranial hypertension, 67–68, 68t
  in mitral regurgitation, 661
  in neurologic diseases, 1541–1543, 1543–1548, 1547
  in pleural effusions, 1500, 1506, 1507–1510, 1509
  in pneumonia, 406, 406t, 1487–1488, 1491–1495
  in pneumothorax, 1500, 1503–1507
  in post cardiac surgery patients, 1513, 1517–1519
  in postpneumonectomy patients, 1509, 1510t, 1511, 1512–1513, 1512–1516
  in pulmonary edema, 1488, 1492–1493, 1495, 1496
  in renal failure, 788–789
  in renal transplantation, 1540–1541, 1541, 1542
  in ureteral, bladder, and urethral diseases, 1540
  intra-aortic balloon pump and, 1485–1486
  of appendix, 1547, 1549t–1550t, 1550
  of chest, 1473–1474, 1474t
  of comatose patient, 18
  Swan-Ganz catheter and, 1485, 1486
  thoracostomy tubes and, 1476–1477, 1478, 1479
  tracheal intubation and, 1474, 1474–1477, 1476
  venous catheters and, 1478, 1481–1485
Imipenem
  dosing adjustment for renal or hepatic dysfunction, 1351t
  dosing during hemofiltration and hemodialysis, 1353t
Imipenem/cilastin, for pancreatitis, 1034t
Immobilization, in spinal cord injury, 147, 156
Immune response, in necrotizing pancreatitis, 1022
Immunocompromised patients
  human immunodeficiency virus infection and. See HIV infection/AIDS

pneumonia in. See Pneumonia, in immunocompromised host
Immunologic disorders. See also specific disorders
  diffuse alveolar hemorrhage and, 343–344, 344t
  in chronic renal failure, 814t, 814–815. See also specific infections
  in multiple organ system failure, 1293t
Immunologic tests, in pneumonia, 406
Immunosuppression, as predisposing condition to infection, 401
Immunosuppressive therapy, following renal transplantation, 829–830
  complications of, 830
Impedance plethysmography, in pulmonary embolism, 427–428
Imputed negligence, 1720–1721
Incentive spirometry
  in atelectasis, 467–468, 468
  preoperative, 1207
Inception cohort, 1744
Incisions, as surgical risk factor, for pulmonary complications, 1202
Index, 1746
Index of Activities of Daily Living (Index of ADL), 1688–1689, 1689t
Infarcts, cerebral, coma and, 6
Infection. See also Antibiotic entries; Sepsis; specific sites and types and specific infections
  as predisposing condition to further infection, 400
  bacterial
    antimicrobial choice for, 1368t
    disseminated, in HIV infection/AIDS, 1409–1410, 1410t
    gram-negative, cutaneous, 939–944. See also specific infections
    gram-positive, cutaneous, 925–936. See also specific infections
  cocaine abuse/overdose causing, 1433
  coma and, 10
  following bone marrow transplantation, 882
  following cardiac transplantation, 653
  following head and neck surgery, 220
  following liver transplantation, 1147t, 1147–1148
  following vascular surgery, 724
  fungal
    antimicrobial choice for, 1368t
    disseminated, in HIV infection/AIDS, 1410–1411
    in HIV infection/AIDS, 1406
    in fulminant hepatic failure, 1089, 1090
    in multiple organ system failure, 1302
    in patients awaiting liver transplantation, treatment of, 1137t, 1137–1138
  multiple organ system failure and, 1292–1294
  nosocomial. See also Pneumonia, nosocomial
    antibiotic therapy for, 1383
    infection control and. See Infection control, during ICU phase
    shock and, 1314–1315
  opportunistic, in HIV infection/AIDS, prophylaxis and treatment of, 1404t, 1404–1405
  parasitic, antimicrobial therapy for, 1368t, 1384–1385
  predisposing conditions to, 399–401
    neoplastic, 400–401
    non-neoplastic, 399–400

INDEX

prophylaxis of, following cardiac transplantation, 651
rickettsial, cutaneous, 944-945. *See also specific infections*
viral, cutaneous, 946-954. *See also specific infections*
Infection control, 1587-1596, *1588*, 1588t, 1589t
  during ICU phase, 1590-1596
    antibiotic control and, 1594-1595, *1595*
    special problems in, 1595-1596
    spread of microorganisms and, 1594
    types of nosocomial infections and, 1590-1594
      pressure monitors and, 1592
      respiratory therapy equipment and, *1592*, 1592t, 1592-1593, 1593t
      urinary catheters and, 1594
      vascular catheters and, 1590-1592, *1591*, 1591t
  during post-ICU phase, 1596
  during pre-ICU phase, 1589-1590
    antibiotic prophylaxis and therapy for, 1589-1590, 1590t
    colonization and, 1589
    underlying infectious diseases and, 1589
  HIV infection/AIDS and, 1416-1417
  pneumonia and, 411-412
Infection surveillance, in adult respiratory distress syndrome, 308-309
Infections, viral
  antimicrobial choice for, 1368t
  disseminated, in HIV infection/AIDS, 1411
Infective endocarditis. *See Endocarditis, infective*
Infiltrations, 984-985, *984-986*
Inflammation, controlled versus malignant, in multiple organ system failure, 1294-1295, *1295*, *1296*
Information services personnel, computerized patient management system and, 1701
Information services policy, 1699-1700, 1700t
Inhalants, volatile. *See Volatile inhalant abuse/overdose*
Inhalation anesthetics, for elevated intracranial pressure, in comatose patient, 19
Inhalation injury, 315-335, *316*
  acute outcomes of, 334
  clinical presentation of, 320-322, *321*, 321t
  exposures causing, 318t, 318-320
    ammonia, 319
    anhydrides, 320
    carbon monoxide, 318-319
    chemical warfare agents, 320
    chlorine, 319
    cyanide, 319
    hydrogen fluoride, 319
    hydrogen sulfide, 319
    isocyanates, 320
    metallic compounds, 320
    nitrogen oxides, 319
    ozone, 319
    phosgene, 319
    smoke, 320, 320t
    sulfur dioxide, 319
  hospital confirmation of, 326t, 326-331
    endoscopic procedures for, 328-330, *330*
    general diagnostic approaches for, 331
    hematologic studies for, 327-328

physiologic measurements for, 330-331
    radiologic tests for, 328, *329*
  hospital management of, 331-334, 332t
  long-term sequelae of, 334, *335*
  pathogenesis of, 315-318
    cellular events in, 317
    major physiologic sequelae and, 317-318
    primary mechanisms of injury and, 315-317, *316*
  prehospital assessment and management of, 322-326
    antidote administration in, 323-324
    communication and documentation in, 326
    evacuation and decontamination in, 322
    general risk appraisal in, 324
    triage in, 325t, 325-326
    upper airway management in, 322-323, *323*
  prevention of, 334-335
Inherent function test, for imputed negligence, 1721
Inotropic agents. *See also specific drugs*
  during weaning from cardiopulmonary bypass, 648
  for chronic obstructive pulmonary disease, 262-263, *263*
Inotropy, *511*, 511-512, 512t
  descending limb of Starling curve and, 512
Insensible fluid losses, hypovolemia caused by, fluid resuscitation for, 1235-1236, *1236*
Inspiratory pressure, in hypoventilation syndromes, 181
Insulin therapy
  for hyperkalemia, 779t
  for shock, 1330
  hypoglycemia caused by, 1169-1170
  in cardiopulmonary resuscitation, 556t
  in diabetic ketoacidosis, 1159-1160, 1162-1163
  in hyperglycemia, 1166, 1167-1168
  in hyperglycemic hyperosmolar nonketotic coma, 1165
  in hypoglycemia, 1168
Insurance, insured-insurer conflicts and, 1722
Integrated patient records, 1561-1562
Intention to treat, 1747
Intercostal nerve blocks, 1285-1286
  postoperative, for thoracic surgery patients, *371*, 371-372
Interdisciplinary conferences, 1561
Interleukins, in shock, 1317, 1317t
Intermittent mandatory ventilation (IMV), 287-288, 486, 486t
Intermittent positive pressure breathing, preoperative, 1207-1208
Intermittent positive pressure breathing (IPPB), in atelectasis, 468
International Classification of Diseases (ICD-9-CM), 1666-1668, 1667t
Interpersonal problems, 44-45
Interrogatories, 1723
Intra-abdominal infections, 1000-1013
  antimicrobial therapy for, 1377-1380, 1378t
  during ICU phase, *1007*, 1007-1011
    antibiotic therapy and, 1010-1011
    cardiopulmonary support and oxygen transport and, 1008-1009
    nutritional support and, 1009-1010
    ongoing infection and, 1011

prevention and, 1007
  renal dysfunction and, 1010
  source control and, 1007-1008
  during post-ICU phase, 1011-1012
  during pre-ICU phase, 1000-1007, 1001t
    indications for ICU admission and, 1002-1003
    pathophysiology of sepsis and, *1003*, 1003t, 1003-1007, *1005*, *1006*, 1006t
  open abdomen management and, *1012*, 1012-1013
Intra-aortic balloon pump (IABP), 1609-1612
  complications of, 1610
  contraindications to, 1610
  data analysis for, 1610, *1610*, *1611*
  for mitral regurgitation, 667
  imaging studies and, 1485-1486
  indications for, 1609-1610
  pre-cardiac transplantation, 642
  preoperative, 591-592
  quality enhancement for, 1610-1612
Intracerebral hemorrhage (ICH), 79-80, *80*, 88
  hypertensive, 79
Intracerebral hypertension, in brain injury, 86
Intracerebral lesions, coma and, 6-7
Intracranial hemorrhage
  acute, diagnosis of, 85
  coma and, 7-8
  traumatic, 87
Intracranial hypertension, 65-74
  brain death and, 73, *74*
  during ICU phase, 68-73
    aggressive measures for, 72-73
    systemic stabilization and, 73
    basic measures for, 71-72
    ICP monitoring and, 68-70, *69*, *70*
    management principles for, 70-71, 71t
      medical treatment and, 71
      surgical treatment and, 71
  during post-ICU phase, 74
  during pre-ICU phase, 66-68
    airway and ventilation and, 67
    criteria for ICP monitoring and, 68
    institution of ICP therapy and, 68, 68t
    neurologic assessment and, 67
    normalization of systemic blood pressure and, 67
    patient stabilization and, 67
    radiographic examination and, 67-68, 68t
    triage and, 68
  hepatic coma and, 1083-1084
  management of, in comatose patient, 18-20
  pathophysiology of, 65, *66*
  postoperative hypertension following, 737
  signs of, 65-66
  tapering of therapy for, 73, 73t
Intracranial infections, 102-123, 103t
  during ICU phase, 114-122
    meningitides and, 117-119
    parameningeal infections and, 114-117
    parenchymal infections and, 119-122
  during post-ICU phase, 122t, 122-123
  pre-ICU evaluation of, 103-114
    in meningitides, 107-111, 108t
    in parameningeal infections, 103-107
    in parenchymal infections, 111-114
Intracranial pressure (ICP), elevated. *See Intracranial hypertension*

INDEX

Intracranial pressure (ICP) monitoring, 68–70, 1612–1613
  complications and management of, 1612
  contraindications to, 1612
  criteria for, 68
  data analysis for, 1612–1613, *1613*
  indications for, 1612
  nonfluid coupled systems for, 69–70, *70*
  quality enhancement for, 1613
  role of, 68–69, *69*
  techniques for, 69
Intrapulmonary shunting, in fulminant hepatic failure, 1087, *1087*
Intravenous immunoglobulin (IVIG), for Guillain-Barré syndrome, 130
Intraventricular hemorrhage, 80
Intrinsic contractility, 507
  inotropy and, *511*, 511–512, 512t
Intubation, 1613–1615. *See also specific types of intubation*
  complications and management of, 1614
    during early phase, 1614
    during late phase, 1614
    postextubation, 1614
  contraindications to, 1614
  in substance abuse/overdose, 1429
  indications for, 1613–1614
  need for, 282–283
  quality enhancement for, 1614–1615, 1615t
Invasive procedures, in pneumonia, 407–408
Inverse ratio ventilation, 286–287
  during ICU phase, 286–287
Ipecac, for poisonings, 1456
Ipratropium bromide (Atrovent)
  for chronic obstructive pulmonary disease, 249
  in aerosol therapy, 474
Iron deficiency anemia, 901
Iron intoxication, 1467–1468
Ischemia
  following vascular surgery, 722
  hepatic failure induced by, 1079–1080
  myocardial. *See* Myocardial ischemia
  of cerebellar artery, coma and, 8
  of vertebral artery, coma and, 8
Ischemic colitis, following vascular surgery, 722–723
Ischemic hepatitis, 1120
Isocyanates, inhalation injury caused by, 320
Isoniazid
  dosing adjustment for renal or hepatic dysfunction, 1351t
  dosing during hemofiltration and hemodialysis, 1353t
Isoproterenol
  during weaning from cardiopulmonary bypass, 648
  for bronchospastic disease, 233t, 234
  for shock, 1325t, 1327
  in cardiopulmonary resuscitation, 556t, 559–560

Jaundice
  bilirubin in, 1062–1064, 1063t
  gallstones in
    during ICU phase, 1050, *1050*
    during pre-ICU phase, 1048
  postoperative, 1119–1122
    acute acalculous cholecystitis and, 1121–1122
    bilirubin metabolism in, 1119
    cholestasis and, 1120

    extrahepatic biliary obstruction and, 1120–1121
    hepatocellular dysfunction in, 1119–1120
Jejunostomy, following head and neck surgery, 223
Joint and several liability, 1721
Judgment, in mental status examination, 31–32
Jugular venous pulse, 531
Jury verdict, 1724
  appeal of, 1724–1725

Kaplan-Meier survival curves, 1750
Kaposi's sarcoma, in HIV infection/AIDS, 1411, 1412–1413
Karnofsky Performance Status Scale, 1689, 1690t
Kawasaki's disease, 932–933
Keratitis, in HIV infection/AIDS, 1411
Ketoacidosis
  diabetic. *See* Diabetic ketoacidosis (DKA)
  metabolic acidosis associated with, treatment of, 762–763
Ketorolac tromethamine, for pain control, 1286
Kidney stones, surgical treatment of, 846
Kidneys. *See also* Renal *entries*
  following cardiac transplantation, 649

Labetalol (Normodyne)
  for aortic dissection, 705t
  for cocaine abuse/overdose, 1434, 1435t
  for hypertension, 692t–694t
    postoperative, 745t, 747
Lactate dehydrogenase, serum levels of, in acute myocardial infarction, 571, *571*
Lactic acidosis, metabolic acidosis associated with, treatment of, 763
Lactitol, for hepatic coma, 1084–1085
Lactulose
  for hepatic coma, 1084
  for thyroid storm, 1178
Lambert-Eaton myasthenic syndrome (LEMS), 135
Language, in mental status examination, 29–30
Laryngectomy
  supraglottic, postoperative care for, 224
  total, postoperative care and, 214–215, *215, 216,* 224, *225*
Laser photocoagulation, for gastrointestinal bleeding, 993
Lateral sinus thrombosis, septic, pre-ICU evaluation of, 105
Lawsuits. *See* Liability
Least-squares regression, 1750
Left ventricular failure, in acute myocardial infarction, 578t, 578–579, *580*
Left ventricular function, preoperative evaluation of, 1211t, 1211–1212
Left ventricular thrombi, as risk factor for neurologic surgical complications, 1218
Legionellosis, for pneumonia, 1375–1376
Leukocytosis. *See* Hyperleukocytosis
Leukoencephalopathy
  multifocal, progressive, in HIV infection/AIDS, 1407
  progressive multifocal, coma and, 12
Leukopenia, 876t, 876–877
  during ICU phase, 877
  during pre-ICU phase, 876–877

Leukoplakia, hairy, oral, 1408
Liability, 1718–1726
  basis of, 1718–1719
    proof of negligence/causation and, 1718–1719
    standard of care and, 1718
    unreasonable risk and, 1718
  outcomes of suits and, 1724
    damages and, 1724
    dismissal, 1724
    jury verdicts, 1724
    settlement, 1724
  post-suit phase and, 1724–1726
    appeals and, 1724–1725
    personal survival strategy and, 1725–1726
    prevention of future suits and, 1725
    returning to normal and, 1725
  pre-suit phase and, 1719
    patients and families initiating suits and, 1719
    risk of suit in ICU environment and, 1719
  situations giving rise to suits and, 1719–1721
    imputed negligence and, 1720–1721
    joint and several liability and, 1721
    physician's relationship to hospital, its employees, and other physicians and, 1719–1720
  suit phase and, 1721–1724
    conduct of trials and, 1723
    depositions and, 1723
    discovery and, 1722
    expert witnesses and, 1723
    insured-insurer conflicts and, 1722
    interrogatories and, 1723
    medical review panels and arbitration boards and, 1722
    meeting defense attorney and, 1722
    preparation for litigation and, 1721–1722
    pretrial activities and, 1721
    protecting medical records and, 1722–1723
    testimony and, 1723–1724
Lidocaine
  for cocaine abuse/overdose, 1435t
  for ventricular tachycardia, 544, 544t
  in cardiopulmonary resuscitation, 556t, 557, 560
  peridural, for pain control, 1285, 1285t
Life-sustaining treatment, 1727
  definition of, 1728t
  withdrawing, definition of, 1728t
  withholding, 1727–1737, 1728t
    autonomy versus self-determination and, 1727–1728
    brain death and, 1729
    capacity versus competence and, 1728
    definition of, 1728t
    during ICU phase, 1734–1736
    during post-ICU phase, 1736–1737
    during pre-ICU phase, 1731–1734
    ethics committees and, 1729
    extraordinary versus ordinary treatments and, 1727
    ICU admission and, 1730
    living wills and advance directives and, 1728
    of cardiopulmonary resuscitation, 1729–1730
    of dialysis, 1730–1731
    of mechanical ventilation, 1730
    of medications, 1731

INDEX

of nutrition and hydration, 1731
of pain relief, 1731
of transfusion therapy, 1731
persistent vegetative state and, 1729
surrogate decision makers and, 1728–1729
Limbic system, coma and, 3
Line sepsis, 1383–1384
Linear regression analysis, 1750
Lipids, for total parenteral nutrition, 1259
Lisinopril, for hypertension, 693t, 694t
Listeriosis, in HIV infection/AIDS, 1410
Lithium
  for depression, 37
  intoxication by, 1465–1466
    coma and, 12
Litigation. *See* Liability
Liver. *See also* Hepatic *entries*
  shock, 1120
Liver biopsy, 1074–1076, *1075*, 1076t
Liver transplantation, 1134–1150, 1135t
  during ICU phase, 1141t, 1141–1145
    immediate postoperative monitoring and care and, 1143–1144
    intraoperative monitoring and, 1142
    intraoperative predictors of survival and, 1142
    operative procedure for, 1142–1143, *1143*, *1144*
    postoperative course and, 1144–1145
    preoperative preparation for, 1142
    timing of recipient procedure and, 1142
  during post-ICU phase, 1145–1150, 1149t
    postoperative complications of, 1145–1148
      graft dysfunction, 1145t, 1145–1146, 1146t, 1149–1150
      infectious, 1147t, 1147–1148
      malignancy, 1148
      neurologic toxicity, 1148
      renal dysfunction, 1148
      surgical, 1146–1147
    postoperative course and, 1145
    quality of life and, 1150
    retransplantation and, 1149, 1149t
    survival and, 1149, 1149t
  for hepatic coma, 1085
  hypertension following, 740
  in cirrhosis, 1103–1104
  pretransplant period and, 1134–1140
    acute liver failure during, 1138–1140
    ascites during, 1136–1137
    gastrointestinal bleeding during, 1134–1136
      tamponade for, 1135–1136, 1136t
      variceal obliteration for, 1136
      vasoactive therapy for, 1134–1135, 1135t
    hepatic encephalopathy during, 1138, 1138t
    infections during, 1137t, 1137–1138
    search for liver during, 1140, 1140t, 1141t
    reoperation and, 1146–1147, 1149, 1149t
Living wills, 1728
Lobar collapse, following thoracic surgery, 375
Lobar torsion, following thoracic surgery, 376
Logistic function, 1751, 1751t
Logistic regression analysis, 1751, 1751t
Look-alike drugs, 1437–1438
  diagnosis and treatment of, 1437–1438
  signs and symptoms of, 1437

Lorazepam (Ativan)
  during mechanical ventilation, during ICU phase, 290
  for alcohol withdrawal, 1441, 1441t
  for sedation, 1280t, 1281
Lucid interval, extradural hematoma and, 78
Ludwig's angina, during pre-ICU phase, 192
Lumbar puncture, 1615–1617
  complications of, 1616
  contraindications to, 1616
  data analysis for, 1616t, 1616–1617
    bacterial, 1616
    demyelinating disease and, 1617
    fungal, 1616
    malignancy and, 1617
    subarachnoid hemorrhage and, 1617
    viral, 1617
  indications for, 1616
  quality enhancement for, 1617
Lung(s)
  defense mechanisms of, 401–403, 402t, *403*
  following cardiac transplantation, 649
Lung parenchyma, functional status of, rehabilitation of ventilator-dependent patients and, 446
Lung scanning, in pulmonary embolism, *422*, 422–424, 423t, *424*
Lung transplantation
  complications following, 379–381
    during first 48 hours, 379–381, *380*
    from 48 hours to 2 weeks, 381
  in chronic obstructive pulmonary disease, 272–273
  preoperative considerations with, 359t, 359–360, *360*, 360t
Lupus, drug-induced, 969, 969t
Lupus anticoagulant, 913–914
Lymphocytes, 899
Lymphomas
  in HIV infection/AIDS, 1413
  non-Hodgkin's
    following cardiac transplantation, 653
    in HIV infection/AIDS, 1413
Lysergic acid diethylamide (LSD), 1447–1448
Lysine hydrochloride, for hallucinogen abuse/overdose, 1449

Macroangiopathic hemolytic anemia, 904
Magnesium, 1183–1189
  balance of, 1183–1184, 1184t. *See also* Hypermagnesemia; Hypomagnesemia
  in plasma, 1183–1184, *1184*
  regulatory mechanisms for, 1184, *1184*, 1184t
  infusions of, in bronchospastic disease, 237
  laboratory tests for, 1185
Magnesium sulfate, in cardiopulmonary resuscitation, 556t
Magnetic resonance angiography (MRA), in brain injury, 85
Magnetic resonance imaging (MRI)
  cine, in mitral regurgitation, 662–663
  in aortic dissection, 703–704
  in aortic regurgitation, 677
  in brain injuries, 85
  in constrictive pericarditis, 617
  in hepatic disorders, 1070
  in intracranial hypertension, 67–68
  in pericardial effusion, 612
  of comatose patient, 18
Major depression, 33

Malaria, antimicrobial therapy for, 1384–1385
Malignancy. *See also* Mass lesions; Oncologic emergencies; *specific malignancies*
  ascites and. *See* Ascites, malignant
  following cardiac transplantation, 653
  following liver transplantation, 1148
  in cholangitis, 1052, *1052*
  lumbar puncture in, data analysis for, 1617
Malignant hyperthermia (MH), 59–61
  during ICU phase, 61
  during post-ICU phase, 61
  during pre-ICU phase, 59t, 59–61
    clinical features of, 60
    treatment of, 60
Malnutrition. *See also* Nutritional support; Total parenteral nutrition (TPN)
  as predisposing condition to infection, 399–400
  diagnosis of, 1249, 1250t
  pulmonary function and, 494–495, 495t
Malpractice suits. *See* Liability
Mandatory minute ventilation (MMV), 486
Mannitol
  for elevated intracranial pressure, in comatose patient, 19
  for intracranial hypertension, 1084
  for renal failure, 786t, 787
Mantel-Haenzel chi-square statistic, 1750
Marijuana abuse/overdose, 1449–1450
  diagnosis and treatment of, 1450
  signs and symptoms of, 1450
  special considerations in, 1450
Mass lesions. *See also* Malignancy; Oncologic emergencies; *specific lesions and disorders*
  as predisposing condition to infection, 400–401
  coma and, 8
  in HIV infection/AIDS, 1412–1413
  intracranial, in HIV infection/AIDS, 1407–1408
  of brain, 81, 89
  pneumonia with, treatment of, 410–411
  supratentorial, 5, 5–6
Matched cohort studies, 1745
Mean, 1740
Measurement, cost of, 1665t
Measuring instruments, for monitoring, 1630
Mechanical ventilation, 280–298, *485*, 485–490. *See also* Ventilatory support
  assist mode, 485
  assist/control mode, 485–486
    continuous positive airway pressure, 486
    for ventilatory failure, 171
    intermittent mandatory ventilation/synchronized intermittent mandatory ventilation, 287, 486, 486t
    mandatory minute ventilation, 486
    pressure control, 486
  control mode, 485
  during ICU phase, 284–296
    initial ventilatory settings for, 284t, 284–285
    inverse ratio ventilation and, 286–287
    options for, 287–290
      assist-control mode as, 287
      high frequency ventilation as, 288t, 288–290, 289t
      intermittent mandatory ventilation mode as, 287–288

1775

Mechanical ventilation *(Continued)*
    pressure support ventilation as, 288
    oxygen administration and, 285
    patient monitoring during, 290–295
        for atelectasis, 293–294, 294t
        for barotrauma, 293
        for gastrointestinal hemorrhage, 294
        for hemodynamic instability, 292t, 292–293
        for nosocomial pneumonia, 294–295
        for pulmonary embolism, 294
        ventilatory monitoring and, 291t, 291–292
    pharmacologic interventions during, 290
    positive end-expiratory pressure and, 285–286, *286*
    procedures during, 295–296
        bronchoalveolar lavage, 296
        bronchoscopy, 295–296
        open lung biopsy, 296
        tracheostomy, 295
        transbronchial biopsy, 296
    during post-ICU phase, 296–298
        failure of mechanical ventilation and, 297–298
        preparation for weaning and, 296–297
        prognosis and, 297
    during pre-ICU phase, 280–284
        alternatives to ICU admission and, 283t, 283–284
        appropriateness of instituting, 283
        clinical considerations in implementing, 438–439
        decision to institute, 441, 441t
        elective use of, 439–440
            in chronic obstructive pulmonary disease, 440
            in neuromuscular disease, 439–440
            in restrictive chest wall disease, 440
        need for intubation and, 282–283
        nonelective use of, 440, 440t
        noninvasive methods of, 440, 441t
        risk factors for requiring, 280–281, 281t
        signs and symptoms of acute respiratory failure and, 281–282, 282t
    following vascular surgery, 718–719
    for thoracic surgery, 363, 363t, 365, *365*, 369–370
    in adult respiratory distress syndrome, 307–308
    inverse ratio, 167, *167*
    pressure and, 165–167, *166*
    in brain injuries, 82
    in diffuse alveolar hemorrhage, 346–347
    in hypoventilation syndromes, 183
    in intra-abdominal infection, 1008, 1011
    in non-ICU settings, 496–498, 497t
        discharge planning for, 498
        technical aspects of, 497–498
    in pancreatitis, 1032–1033
    in spinal cord injury, 151–152
    in ventilatory failure, 171–172, *172*
        assist-control (AMV), 171
        pressure support ventilation (PSV), 171–172
        synchronized intermittent mandatory ventilation (SIMV), 171
    intracranial hypertension and, 67
    long-term use of, 453–457
        equipment selection for home care and, 455–456
        home going prescription for, 456–457, 457t

        noninvasive respiratory ICU and, 454, 455t
        patient selection for, 455, 455t
    nasal continuous positive airway pressure, in hypoventilation syndromes, 184
    nasally applied positive pressure ventilation, in hypoventilation syndromes, 185
    negative pressure, in hypoventilation syndromes, 185
    of comatose patient, 14–15
    positive end-expiratory pressure. *See* Positive end-expiratory pressure (PEEP)
    positive expiratory pressure, in atelectasis, 468–469, *469*
    positive pressure, in hypoventilation syndromes, 185
    prolonged, following cardiac surgery, 599–600, 600t
    termination guidelines for, 1730, 1733, 1735, 1736
    with neuromuscular blocking agents, 1286
Median, 1740
Mediastinitis, following cardiac surgery, 602
Medical co-director, 1559
Medical records
    integrated, 1561–1562
    protection of, 1722–1723
    transfer of, 1714
Medical review panels, 1722
Medication withdrawal, hypertension caused by, postoperative, 740–741
MEDISGRPS index, *1671*, 1671t, 1671–1672
Megaloblastic anemia, 901
Melphalan, for bone marrow transplantation, 881t
Meningitides. *See also specific disorders*
    during ICU phase, 117–119
    pre-ICU evaluation of, 107–111, 108t
Meningitis. *See also* Meningitides
    aseptic, pre-ICU evaluation of, 107
    bacterial
        coma and, 10
        during ICU phase, 117–119, 122
        pre-ICU evaluation of, 107–111
    cryptococcal, in HIV infection/AIDS, 1410–1411
    opportunistic, in HIV infection/AIDS, prophylaxis and treatment of, 1404–1405
    tuberculous, in HIV infection/AIDS, 1407
    viral, pre-ICU evaluation of, 109, 111
Meningococcal infections, cutaneous, 941–944
    clinical features and differential diagnosis of, *942*, 942–943
    laboratory studies in, 943–944
    outcome of, 944, 944t
    pathophysiology of, 941–942
    treatment of, 944
Meningoencephalitis
    during ICU phase, 119–120
    pre-ICU evaluation of, 111t, 111–113
Mental status examination (MSE), 29–32
    appearance in, 29
    behavior in, 29
    judgment in, 31–32
    mood and affect in, 30
    perceptions in, 30–31
    sensorium in, 31, 31t
    speech and language in, 29–30
    thinking in, 30
Menu driven systems, 1707

Meperidine (Demerol)
    abuse/overdose of, 1445, 1446
    for pain control, 1283t, 1284
Mesocaval shunt, interposition, for esophageal varices, 1102, *1102*
Meta-analysis, 1748, *1748*
Metabolic acidosis, 757–764
    during ICU phase, 758–763
        differential diagnosis of, 758–759, 759t
        signs and symptoms of, 760
        treatment of, 760t, 760–761
        treatment of disorders causing, 761–763
            bicarbonate loss, 762
            intoxication, 762
            ketoacidosis, 762–763
            lactic acidosis, 763
            renal disease, 761–762
    during post-ICU phase, 763–764
        diarrhea and, 764
        renal acidosis and, 764
    during pre-ICU phase, 757–758
    risk factors for, 757–758
Metabolic alkalosis, 764–769
    during ICU phase, 767–769
        evaluation of, 767
        treatment of, 767–769
            for chloride-resistant metabolic alkalosis, 769
            for chloride-responsive metabolic alkalosis, 767–769
    during post-ICU phase, 769
    during pre-ICU phase, 764–767
        consequences of, 765
        mechanisms of, 764–765
        risk factors for, 765–767, 766t
            alkali administration, 766
            diuretics, 766
            hypercapnia, 766–767
            mineralocorticoid excess, 767
            nasogastric suction, 765–766
            vomiting, 765
    hypocalcemia caused by, 1190
Metabolic disorders. *See also* Acid/base disorders; Metabolic acidosis; Metabolic alkalosis
    as complication of nutritional support, 1261–1262
    coma and, 8–10
    following vascular surgery, 723
    hepatic failure caused by, 1080
    in acute renal failure, in patients awaiting liver transplantation, 1140
    in fulminant hepatic failure, 1090–1091
    in HIV infection/AIDS, 1413–1414
    in multiple organ system failure, 1293t
Metabolic management, of comatose patient, 15–16
Metabolic rate, minute ventilation and, 265
Metabolic status, in diabetic ketoacidosis, assessment of, 1159
Metabolism
    acid/base, normal, 755
    following cardiac transplantation, 650
Metallic compounds, inhalation injury caused by, 320
Metastatic disease, hepatic, hepatic failure caused by, 1080
Metered dose inhalers (MDIs), in bronchospastic disease, 233–234
Methadone (Dolophine), abuse/overdose of, 1445, 1446
Methanol intoxication, 1466–1467
    coma and, 12
    metabolic acidosis associated with, treatment of, 763

INDEX

Methaqualone abuse/overdose, 1443
Methicillin
   dosing adjustment for renal or hepatic dysfunction, 1351t
   dosing during hemofiltration and hemodialysis, 1353t
Methimazole, for thyroid storm, 1178
Methyldopa, for hypertension, postoperative, 745t, 749
Methylene blue, for volatile inhalant abuse/overdose, 1451
3-Methylhistidine (3-MEH), urinary, in nutrition assessment, 1252
1-Methyl-4-phenyl-1,2,3,6-tetrahydropyridine (MPTP), 1447
1-Methyl-4-phenyl-4-propionoxy-piperidine (MPPP), 1447
Methylprednisolone
   following cardiac transplantation, 650, 651t
   for diffuse alveolar hemorrhage, 345
Methylxanthines, in bronchospastic disease, 233t, 234-235
Metocurine, 1287t, 1288
Metronidazole
   dosing adjustment for renal or hepatic dysfunction, 1351t
   dosing during hemofiltration and hemodialysis, 1353t
   for cutaneous infections, 1383
   for intra-abdominal infections, 1379
Mexiletine, for ventricular tachycardia, 544t
Mezlocillin
   dosing adjustment for renal or hepatic dysfunction, 1351t
   dosing during hemofiltration and hemodialysis, 1353t
   for pancreatitis, 1034t
Miami Acute Collar (MAC), 153, *153*
Miami J collar, 153, *154*
Miconazole
   dosing adjustment for renal or hepatic dysfunction, 1351t
   dosing during hemofiltration and hemodialysis, 1353t
Microangiopathic hemolytic anemia, 904
Microbiologic tests, in pneumonia, 406-407
Microbiology
   of gallstones, 1048-1049
   of infections affecting specific organ systems, 1367t
   of pneumonia, 385-387, 386t
Microorganisms, spread of, 1594
Midarm circumference (MAC) measurement, in nutrition assessment, 1251
Midazolam (Versed)
   during mechanical ventilation, during ICU phase, 290
   for alcohol withdrawal, 1441, 1441t
   for cocaine abuse/overdose, 1435t
   for sedation, 1280t, 1281
   for seizures, cocaine abuse/overdose causing, 1434
Midbrain, coma and, 4
Migraine headaches, coma and, 9
Milrinone, for shock, 1325t, 1328-1329
Mineral(s), requirements for, 1256, 1256t
Mineralocorticoids, excess of, metabolic alkalosis associated with, 767
Mini-Mental State Examination (MMSE), 31, 31t
Minocycline
   dosing adjustment for renal or hepatic dysfunction, 1351t
   dosing during hemofiltration and hemodialysis, 1353t

Minoxidil, for hypertension, 692t-694t
Minute ventilation, requirements for, 265-266
   increased CO_2 production, 265, 265t
   increased dead space, 265-266, 266t
   increased metabolic rate, 265
   increased muscular activity, 265
   substrate utilization, 265
Mithramycin, for hypercalcemia, 1193, 1193t
Mitral regurgitation (MR), 656-670
   during ICU phase, 665-669
     mechanical support and, 667
     medical management of, 665-667, 666t
     surgical management of, 667-669, *668*
   during post-ICU phase, 669-670
     anticoagulation and, 669
     endocarditis prophylaxis and, 669
     management of underlying disorder and, 669-670
   during pre-ICU phase, 656-665
     cause of, 656-659, 657t
       chordae tendineae as, 657-658, *659*
       mitral valve leaflets as, 656-657, *657, 658*
       papillary muscle dysfunction as, 658
       prosthetic valve dysfunction as, 658-659, *660*
     clinical characteristics of, 660-661
       physical examination, 660-661, 661t
       presentation, 660
     laboratory evaluation of, 661-665
       angiography in, 665
       cardiac catheterization in, 663
       cine magnetic resonance imaging in, 662-663
       echocardiography in, 661-662, *663, 664*
       electrocardiography in, 661, 662t
       hemodynamics in, 663, 665
       radiologic studies in, 661
     pathophysiology of, 659-660
Mitral valve leaflets, mitral regurgitation and, 656-657, *657, 658*
Mivacurium, 1287t
Mixed venous oxygen saturation, 1642
Monitoring. *See* Patient monitoring; *specific types of monitoring*
Monoamine oxidase inhibitors (MAOIs)
   for depression, 37
   intoxication by, 1461
Monobactams, pharmacokinetics of, 1354
Monoclonal antibodies
   following renal transplantation, 830
   for endotoxin, 1306-1307
Monocytes, 899
Monomicrobial neutrocytic bacterascites (MNB), in cirrhosis, 1111-1112
Monro-Kellie doctrine, 65
Mood, in mental status examination, 30
Morbidity
   in chronic obstructive pulmonary disease, 244
   with gallstones, 1046-1047, 1047t
Morbilliform eruption, *966*, 966-967
Moricizine, for ventricular tachycardia, 544t
Morphine
   abuse/overdose of, 1445-1446
   during mechanical ventilation, during ICU phase, 290
   for pain control, 1283t, 1283-1284
   following vascular surgery, 720
   peridural, 1285, 1285t

Mortality. *See also* Death; Survival
   in chronic obstructive pulmonary disease, 244, *244*
   quality of care and, 1580-1581
Mortality Prediction Model (MPM), 1674
Mortality Probability Models (MPM II), 1674t, 1674-1675, 1678t
Motor neuron disorders, 136-141. *See also specific disorders*
Moxalactam
   dosing adjustment for renal or hepatic dysfunction, 1351t
   dosing during hemofiltration and hemodialysis, 1353t
Mucolytic agents, in aerosol therapy, 473-474
   in chronic obstructive pulmonary disease, 494
Mucous membranes, in disseminated intravascular coagulation, 875
Multifocal atrial tachycardia, 538
   treatment of, 542
Multiple organ system failure (MOF), 1291-1307
   antibiotic pharmacokinetics in, 1349, 1353-1354
   clinical management issues in, 1306-1307
     general support, 1306-1307
     hemodynamic support, 1307
     metabolic support, 1306
   during ICU phase, 1298-1306, *1299*
     circulatory dysfunction in, 1299-1300
     hematologic dysfunction in, 1302-1303
     neurologic dysfunction in, 1304-1306
       encephalopathy, 1305-1306
       peripheral neuropathy, 1304-1305
     renal dysfunction in, 1303-1304
     respiratory dysfunction in, 1303
     splanchnic organ dysfunction in, 1300-1302
   during pre-ICU phase, 1296-1298
     concurrent risk factors for, *1297*, 1297-1298, *1298*
     preexisting risk factors for, 1296-1297, *1297*
     propagating risk factors for, 1298, *1298*
   epidemiology of, 1291-1292, 1292t-1294t
   hemofiltration for, 798
   in brain injury, 87
   necrotizing pancreatitis and. *See* Pancreatitis, necrotizing
   pathogenesis of, 1292-1296, 1294t
     controlled versus malignant inflammation in, 1294-1295, *1295, 1296*
     infection and host septic response in, 1292-1294
     tissue hypoxia in, 1295-1296
Multiple regression analysis, 1750-1751
Muromonab-CD3, following cardiac transplantation, 650, 651, 651t
Muscle disorders, 141-142
Muscle relaxants. *See* Neuromuscular blocking agents; *specific agents*
Musculoskeletal disorders, in HIV infection/AIDS, 1414
Musculoskeletal management, in spinal cord injury, 155, 156
Mushroom poisoning, 1469
Myasthenia gravis (MG), 131-135
   during ICU phase, 134-135
     cholinergic crisis and, 134-135
     myasthenic crisis and, 134
     postoperative patients and, 135

Myasthenia gravis (MG) *(Continued)*
   during pre-ICU phase, 131t, 131–134, 132t
     general management considerations for, 133
     new-onset MG and, 133t, 133–134
     preoperative patients and, 134, 134t
   following thoracic surgery, 378
Myasthenic crisis, 134
Mycobacterial infections, in HIV infection/AIDS, 1409, 1410t
Myocardial dysfunction
   nonischemic, 610–637. *See also* Cardiac trauma; Cardiomyopathy; Heart failure; Pericardial disease; Pericardial effusion
   sepsis-related, 634–637, *635*
     during ICU phase, 636–637
       diagnostic evaluation of, 636
       hemodynamic features of, *636*, 636–637
       treatment of, 637
     during post-ICU phase, 637
     during pre-ICU phase, 635t, 635–636
   shock and, 1315
Myocardial infarction
   acute, 570–582
     during ICU phase, 576–579
       arrhythmia monitoring in, 577–578
       drug therapy for, 576–577
       left ventricular failure in, 578t, 578–579, *580*
     during post-ICU phase, 579–582
       alteration of coronary risk factors in, 582
       anticoagulants and antiplatelet agents in, 581–582
       beta blockers in, 581
       secondary prevention of myocardial infarction and, 580–581, 581t
       transfer from ICU and, 579–580
     during pre-ICU phase, 570–576
       coronary artery bypass surgery for, 575–576
       laboratory studies in, *571*, 571–572, *572*
       percutaneous transluminal angioplasty for, 575, 575t
       physical examination in, 570–571
       thrombolytic therapy for, *573*, 573–575, 574t
   in hypomagnesemia, 1187
   as indication for surgery, 587, 588t
   classification systems for, 1678–1679, 1681t, *1682*, 1682t
   following cardiac surgery, 597
   prevention of, 580–581, 581t
   surgical treatment of. *See* Coronary artery bypass grafting (CABG)
Myocardial ischemia
   acute, surgical indications in, 588–589
   arrhythmias associated with, 534
   electrocardiographic monitoring in, 1632–1633
   hypertension and, postoperative, 734
   surgical treatment of. *See* Coronary artery bypass grafting (CABG)
Myocardial oxygen consumption, reduction of, following vascular surgery, 718–720
Myocardial preservation, during cardiac transplantation, 647
Myocardial revascularization, hypertension following, 735

Myopathy, 141–142
Myxedema coma, 1178–1179

Nafcillin
   dosing adjustment for renal or hepatic dysfunction, 1351t
   dosing during hemofiltration and hemodialysis, 1353t
   for pneumonia
     community-acquired, 391, 391t
     nosocomial, 393t
Naloxone
   for alcohol abuse/overdose, 1440
   for cocaine abuse/overdose, 1434, 1435t
   for narcotic abuse/overdose, 1447
   for sedative/hypnotic abuse/overdose, 1443, 1444
   for shock, 1325t, 1329
   for substance abuse/overdose, 1429
Narcotic(s)
   abuse/overdose of, 1445–1447
     coma and, 11
     complications of, 1446, 1446t
     diagnosis and treatment of, 1446–1447
     during ICU phase, 1445–1447
       admission criteria and, 1447
       complications of, 1446, 1446t
       diagnosis and treatment of, 1446–1447
       narcotic withdrawal and, 1447
       signs and symptoms of, 1445–1446
     ICU admission criteria in, 1447
     signs and symptoms of, 1445–1446
     special considerations in, 1447
     withdrawal and, 1447
   parenteral, for pain control, 1283t, 1283–1285, 1284t
   peridural, for pain control, 1285, 1285t
Narcotic agonists. *See also specific drugs*
   for pain control, 1284–1285
Nasal continuous positive airway pressure (NCPAP), in hypoventilation syndromes, 184
Nasal disorders, cocaine abuse/overdose causing, 1433
Nasally applied positive pressure ventilation (NPPV), in hypoventilation syndromes, 185
Nasoenteric tube feeding, in upper airway obstruction, 203
Nasogastric intubation, following head and neck surgery, 222
Nasogastric suction
   in pancreatitis, 1034–1035
   metabolic alkalosis associated with, 765–766
Nasogastric tubes, as surgical risk factor, for pulmonary complications, 1202
Nasotracheal intubation, contraindications to, 1614
Natural history, studies characterizing, 1743–1744
Near drowning, coma and, 10
Neck dissection, radical, hypertension following, 740
Necrosis. *See also* Acute tubular necrosis (ATN)
   anticoagulant-induced, *968*, 968–969
   development of, in pancreatitis, 1017
   tubular
     in diffuse alveolar hemorrhage, 346
     in HIV infection/AIDS, 1414
Necrotizing fasciitis, 934–936
   clinical presentation of, *934*, 934–935

   differential diagnosis of, 935
   pathophysiology and risk factors for, 934
   recovery from, 936
   treatment of, *935*, 935–936
Needle aspiration, in pneumonia, 407
Negative predictive value, 1745, 1745t
Negative pressure ventilation (NPV), in hypoventilation syndromes, 185
Negligence suits. *See* Liability
Neoplastic disease. *See* Malignancy; Mass lesions; Oncologic emergencies; *specific malignancies*
Neostigmine, for reversal of neuromuscular blockade, 1288
Nephrectomy
   bilateral, 846
   partial, 846
   radical, 845–846
   simple, 846–847
Nephrocutaneous fistulas, following renal surgery, 848
Nephrologic injury, in chronic renal failure, 819–821
   acute renal failure as, 819–821
     risk phase of, 819–821, 820t
     support/rehabilitative phase of, 821
Nephropathy, in HIV infection/AIDS, 1414
Nephrotoxicity, of aminoglycosides, 1345–1346
Nephroureterectomy, 846
Nerve blocks, intercostal, 1285–1286
   postoperative, for thoracic surgery patients, *371*, 371–372
Netilmicin
   for pancreatitis, 1034t
   large-dose once-a-day dosing with, 1347
Neurochecks, postcraniotomy, 88–89
Neurogenic pulmonary embolism, in brain injury, 86
Neuroleptic agents. *See also specific drugs*
   for agitation, 43t, 43–44
   for delirium, 41–42, 42t
Neuroleptic malignant syndrome (NMS), 61–63
   during ICU phase, 62–63
   during post-ICU phase, 63
   during pre-ICU phase, 61–62
     clinical features of, 62
     treatment of, 62
Neurologic assessment
   in brain injuries, 83–85
     examination in, 83, 83t, 84t
     history in, 83, 83t
     neuroimaging in, 83–85, 84t
     triage in, 85, 85t, 86t
   in disseminated intravascular coagulation, 875
   in intracranial hypertension, 67–68
   in spinal cord injury, 148–150, 149t
   of comatose patient, 17t, 17–18
Neurologic disorders. *See also specific disorders*
   chemotherapy-induced, 889–890, 890t
   following cardiac surgery, *601*, 601–602
   following liver transplantation, 1148
   following vascular surgery, 723–724
   during pre-ICU phase, 714–715
   imaging studies in, 1541–1543, *1543–1548*, 1547
   in HIV infection/AIDS, 1406–1408, *1407*
   in hypomagnesemia, 1187
   in multiple organ system failure, 1304–1306
     encephalopathy, 1305–1306
     peripheral neuropathy, 1304–1305
   nutritional support in, 1269

INDEX

Neurologic management, in spinal cord injury, 153, 153–154, *154*
Neurologic surgical complications, 1216–1220
  cerebrovascular risk factors for, 1216t, 1216–1219
    during ICU phase, 1218t, 1218–1219
    during pre-ICU phase, 1216–1218
      age, 1217
      aortic sclerosis, 1218
      cerebral vascular disease, 1217–1218
      coronary artery disease, 1216–1217
      hypotension, intraoperative, 1218
      left ventricular thrombi, 1218
  peripheral nerve risk factors for, 1219t, 1219–1220
    during pre-ICU phase, 1219–1220
      positioning, 1219
      procedures, 1219–1220
    recovery from nerve injury and, 1220
  spinal cord risk factors for, 1220, 1220t
Neuromuscular blocking agents, 1286t, 1286–1288, 1287t
  depolarizing, 1287, 1287t
  during mechanical ventilation, during ICU phase, 290
  for elevated intracranial pressure, in comatose patient, 19
  nondepolarizing, 1287–1288, 1288t
    for agitation, 44
    potentiation of effects of, 1288, 1288t
    reversal of effect of, 1288
Neuromuscular disorders, 127–142. *See also specific disorders*
  in hypocalcemia, 1191
  in hypoventilation syndromes, *181*, 181–182
  mechanical ventilation in, elective use of, 439–440
  motor neuron, 136–141
  of muscles, 141–142
  of neuromuscular junction transmission, 131–136
Neuro-ophthalmologic examination, of comatose patient, 18
Neuropathy, diabetic, 806
Neuropsychiatric disorders, 29–48
  agitation, 43–44
  anxiety, 32–33
  behavioral problems, 44–45
  delirium. *See* Delirium
  depression, 33–37
  following transfer from ICU, 47–48
  HIV infection and AIDS, 46–47
  interpersonal problems, 44–45
  mental status examination and, 29–32
  noncompliance and, 45
  threat to sign out and, 45
  weaning from ventilator and, 45–46
Neurovascular surgery, hypertension following, 737
Neutropenia, 905–907
  decreased production in, 905
  drug-induced, 906–907
    evaluation and treatment of, 906–907
    increased destruction in, 906
  increased destruction in, 906
Neutrophilia, 907, 907t
New Simplified Acute Physiology Score (SAPS II), 1672–1673, 1674t, 1675t
Nicardipine (Cardene), for hypertension, postoperative, 745t, 748
Nifedipine
  for hypertension, 692t
  postoperative, 745t, 748

for mitral regurgitation, 666t
for renal failure, 786t
Nimbus Hemopump, 592–593
Nimodipine, for hypertension, postoperative, 745t, 748
Nitrates, for acute myocardial infarction, 576–577, 577t
Nitrogen balance, in nutrition assessment, 1251–1252
Nitrogen oxides, inhalation injury caused by, 319
Nitroglycerin
  for cocaine abuse/overdose, 1435t
  for esophageal varices, 1097
  for gastrointestinal bleeding, in patients awaiting liver transplantation, 1135t
  for hypertension, 692t–694t
    postoperative, 745t, 746
Nitroglycerine, for mitral regurgitation, 666t
Nitroprusside. *See* Sodium nitroprusside
Noncompliance, 45
Nonfluid coupled systems, for intracranial pressure monitoring, 69–70, *70*
Non-Hodgkin's lymphomas
  following cardiac transplantation, 653
  in HIV infection/AIDS, 1413
Nonketotic hyperglycemic hyperosmolality, coma and, 12–13
Nonparametric tests, 1740
Nonshivering thermogenesis, 52
Nonsteroidal anti-inflammatory drugs (NSAIDs). *See also specific drugs*
  for adult respiratory distress syndrome, 309
  intoxication by, 1469–1470
  platelet disorders related to, 910–911
No-reflow phenomenon, in hypocalcemia, 1191
Norepinephrine
  for shock, 1325t, 1327
  in cardiopulmonary resuscitation, 556t, 560
Normal perfusion pressure breakthrough syndrome, postcraniotomy, 89
Nosocomial infections. *See also* Pneumonia, nosocomial
  antimicrobial therapy for, 1383
  infection control and. *See* Infection control, during ICU phase
Notification, of suit, 1721
Nottingham Health Profile (NHP), 1691, 1691t
Nurses, collaboration with physicians. *See* Team concept, physician-nurse collaboration and
Nursing co-director, 1559
Nutrients. *See* Nutritional support; *specific types of nutritional support*
Nutrition assessment. *See* Nutritional support, during pre-ICU phase
Nutrition risk index (NRI), 1254t
Nutritional status, rehabilitation of ventilator-dependent patients and, 444
Nutritional support, 1249–1271. *See also* Total parenteral nutrition (TPN)
  during ICU phase, 1264–1269
    determination of nutrient needs for, 1264, 1264t
    hypermetabolic state and, 1264–1265
    determining nutrient needs for, 1264, 1264t
    problems with meeting nutrient needs in, 1264–1265
    normal nutritional biochemistry and physiology and, 1264

  reassessment of nutritional status for, 1265
  specialized, 1267–1269
    in hepatic failure, 1268
    in neurologic disease, 1269
    in pulmonary failure, 1268–1269
    in renal failure, 1267–1268
    in sepsis, 1269
    with postoperative complications, 1269
  total parenteral nutrition prescription for, 1265–1267
during post-ICU phase, 1269–1271
  during post-ICU phase, effect on gut function, 1270
  home parenteral nutrition and, 1271
  prolonged enteral and parenteral nutrition and, 1270–1271
  transitional feedings for, 1269–1270, *1270*
during pre-ICU phase, 1249–1264
  complications of, 1259, 1261t, 1261–1264, *1262*
  determination of nutrient needs for, 1254–1257, 1255t
    protein requirements and, 1255t, 1255–1257, 1256t, *1257*, *1258*
  diagnosis of malnutrition and, 1249, 1250t
  methods of, *1258*, 1258–1259, 1260t
  total parenteral nutrition prescription and, 1259, *1261*, 1261t
  nutrition assessment and, 1249–1252
    anthropometric measurements in, 1251
    history and physical examination in, 1249–1251, 1250t
    laboratory studies in, 1251–1252, 1252t, 1253t
  prognostic use of nutrition assessment parameters for, 1253–1254, 1254t
following head and neck surgery, 221–223
  cervical esophagostomy and, 222
  enteral feeding and, 223, 223t
  gastrostomy and, 222–223
  jejunostomy and, 223
  nasogastric intubation and, 222
  nutritional assessment and, 221–222
  pharyngotomy and, 222
  total parenteral nutrition and, 223
following vascular surgery, 723
for comatose patient, 21–22
in adult respiratory distress syndrome, 308
in brain injury, 86
in chronic obstructive pulmonary disease, 263–265, 271–272
in gastrointestinal bleeding, 997–998
in hypomagnesemia, 1188–1189
in intra-abdominal infection, 1009–1010
in multiple organ system failure, 1306
in spinal cord injury, 154
in toxic epidermal necrolysis, 964
in upper airway obstruction, 203
termination guidelines for, 1731, 1733–1734, 1735, 1737

Obesity
  as surgical risk factor, for pulmonary complications, 1201
  pulmonary function and, 495–496
Obesity-hypoventilation syndrome (OHS), 179, 184

Obstetric surgery, hypertension following, 739
Obstructive cardiomyopathy, hypertrophic. See Cardiomyopathy, hypertrophic
Obstructive shock, 1314
Obstructive sleep apnea (OSA)
  as surgical risk factor, for pulmonary complications, 1201
  during post-ICU phase, 184
  during pre-ICU phase, 179, 182
Obtundation, 3
Oculomotor palsy, intracranial hypertension and, 66
Odds ratios, 1741–1742
Ofloxacin, for pancreatitis, 1034t
Oliguria, following cardiac surgery, 600–601
Oncologic emergencies, structural, 866–873. See also specific disorders
Open lung biopsy
  during mechanical ventilation, 296
  in diffuse alveolar hemorrhage, 343
  in pneumonia, 408, 412
Open skull fracture, 79
Open-chest cardiac massage, in cardiopulmonary resuscitation, 561–562
Operating system, 1704
Operations planning, 1716
Operator errors, in monitoring, 1630
Ophthalmologic disorders, in HIV infection/AIDS, 1411
Opiate receptors, 1283
Opioid(s). See Narcotic(s)
Opportunistic infections, in HIV infection/AIDS, prophylaxis and treatment of, 1404t, 1404–1405
Oral cavity
  intraoral incision care and, 217, 218
  surgery of, postoperative care for, 224
Ordinal variables, 1740
Ordinary treatments, 1727
  definition of, 1728t
Organophosphate intoxication, 1468
Oropharyngeal colonization, in pneumonia, 403–405
Orthotopic liver transplantation (OLT). See Liver transplantation
Osmolal gap, in ethylene glycol/methanol intoxication, 1466
Ostensible agency test, for imputed negligence, 1720–1721
Otitis externa, pseudomonal, 940–941
Otorrhea, CSF, in traumatic brain injury, 87
Ototoxicity, of aminoglycosides, 1346
Overdoses. See Substance abuse/overdose; specific substances
Oxacillin
  dosing adjustment for renal or hepatic dysfunction, 1351t
  dosing during hemofiltration and hemodialysis, 1353t
  for pneumonia
    community-acquired, 391, 391t
    nosocomial, 393t
Oxazepam, for sedation, 1281
Oximetry, 1643–1644
Oxycodone, abuse/overdose of, 1445
Oxygen
  for cocaine abuse/overdose, 1434, 1435t
  for mechanical ventilation, 285
  in cardiopulmonary resuscitation, 555, 556t
  inspired, reduced fraction of, in parenchymal respiratory failure, 163

venous, partial pressure of, in multiple organ system failure, 1299–1300
Oxygen consumption
  in ventilatory respiratory failure, 168
  myocardial, reduction of, following vascular surgery, 718–720
  red cell transfusions and, 1242
Oxygen delivery, red cell transfusions and, 1242
Oxygen saturation, mixed venous, 1642
Oxygen tension, venous, mixed, in parenchymal respiratory failure, 164
Oxygen therapy, 469t, 469–471, 470t
  delivery systems for, 469–470, 470, 492
    low flow, 471
    mask oxygen and, 471, 471
    nasal oxygen and, 471, 471
    partial rebreathing mask and nonrebreathing mask, 471, 472
  during pre-ICU phase, 469t, 469–471, 470t
    delivery systems for, 469–470, 470
    flow generating devices for, 470–471
    low flow oxygen delivery systems for, 471
  flow generating devices for, 470–471
  hyperbaric, for carbon monoxide intoxication, 1462
  in chronic obstructive pulmonary disease. See Chronic obstructive pulmonary disease (COPD), oxygen therapy in
  outpatient, 492–493, 493t
Oxygen transport, 1008–1009
  monitoring, red cell transfusions and, 1242–1245, 1243
Oxygen-free radicals, pancreatitis and, 1015–1016
Ozone, inhalation injury caused by, 319

p24 antigen, for HIV infection, 1402
P value, 1741
Pacing. See Cardiac pacing
Pain, 1278–1283
  control of. See Analgesia; Analgesics; specific drugs and procedures
  patterns of, 1283
  population differences affecting pain response and, 1278–1279, 1279t
Pancreatic disorders. See also specific disorders
  imaging studies in, 1531, 1534–1536
  in multiple organ system failure, 1301
Pancreatitis, 1015–1020
  alcoholic, 1017, 1023, 1024
  coma and, 14
  critical pathway for patient with, 1560t–1561t
  during ICU phase, 1030–1035
    admissions criteria for surgical ICU and, 1030–1031
    antibiotics and, 1033–1034, 1034t
    discharge criteria for, 1038
    fluid management and, 1031–1032
    mechanical ventilation and, 1032–1033
    nasogastric suction and, 1034–1035
    necrotizing, comprehensive management of, 1035–1036
      infected pancreatic and panpancreatic necrosis and, 1035–1036
      operative, 1036
      uninfected pancreatic and panpancreatic necrosis and, 1035
    pain control and, 1033

peritoneal lavage and, 1032
pre- and postoperative complications and, 1036–1038, 1037t
total parenteral nutrition and, 1035
unresolved issues regarding, 1038
during post-ICU phase, 1038–1040
  assessment of exocrine and endocrine functions and, 1039
  colostomy closure and biliary surgery and, 1039
  delayed gastric emptying and, 1039
  failure to thrive and, 1038
  long-term changes in endocrine function and, 1039t, 1040
  long-term changes in exocrine function and, 1038t, 1039
  long-term morphologic changes and, 1038t, 1039
  pancreatic fistulas and pseudocysts and, 1039
  splenic vein thrombosis and, 1039
during pre-ICU phase, 1022–1030
  assessment of etiology of, 1023–1024
  assessment of severity of, 1025t, 1025–1030
    anatomic predictors for, 1027, 1027t, 1028–1030, 1029
    assessment of infection in pancreatic necrosis and, 1029–1030, 1030t
    physiologic indices for, 1025t, 1025–1027, 1026
  confirmation of diagnosis of, 1022–1023
    ancillary studies and, 1022
    history and, 1022
    physical examination and, 1022
    serum amylase and, 1022–1023
edematous, 1016–1017
etiology of, 1015, 1016t
gallstone, 1023–1024
hemorrhagic, 1016–1017
hyperstimulation-cerulein induced, 1016–1017
hypovolemia caused by, fluid resuscitation for, 1236–1237
in fulminant hepatic failure, 1091
in HIV infection/AIDS, 1409
necrotizing
  assessment of infection in, 1029–1030, 1030t
  endocrine function and
    assessment of, 1039
    long-term changes in, 1039t, 1040
  exocrine function and
    assessment of, 1039
    long-term changes in, 1038t, 1039
  infected, surgical ICU management of, 1035–1036
pathophysiology of, 1017–1022, 1018
  coagulation response in, 1022
  diabetes mellitus in, 1021
  hemodynamic changes in, 1017–1019, 1018t, 1019
  hypocalcemia in, 1021–1022
  immune response in, 1022
  liver function and morphologic alterations in, 1021
  renal failure in, 1019–1020
  respiratory complications in, 1020t, 1020–1021
  uninfected, surgical ICU management of, 1035
pathogenesis of, 1015–1017
  initiators and mediators of injury in

INDEX

intracellular, 1016-1017
    vascular, 1015-1016
    progression of edema to necrosis in, 1017
Pancuronium, 1287t, 1288
    during mechanical ventilation, during ICU phase, 290
Panhypopituitarism, 1177
Papillary muscle dysfunction, mitral regurgitation and, 658
Paracentesis, 1619-1620
    complications and management of, 1620
    contraindications and risks of, 1619-1620
    data analysis for, 1620, 1620t
    for ascites, in cirrhosis, 1114
    indications for, 1619
    quality enhancement for, 1620
Paralytic ileus, following vascular surgery, 722
Parameningeal infections
    during ICU phase, 114-117, 122
        epidural and subdural empyema and, 116-117
        septic dural venous sinus phlebitis and, 115-116
        skeletal and soft tissue infections and, 115
        vascular infections and, 115
    pre-ICU evaluation of, 103-107
        in epidural and subdural empyema, 106-107
        in septic dural venous sinus phlebitis, 105-106
        in skeletal and soft tissue infections, 103-104
        in vascular infections, 104-105
Parametric tests, 1740
Parasitic infections, antimicrobial therapy for, 1368t, 1384-1385
Parenchymal infections, intracranial
    during ICU phase, 119-122
        brain abscess, 120t, 120-122, 121t
        meningoencephalitis, 119-120
    pre-ICU evaluation of, 111-114
        in brain abscess, 113-114
        in meningoencephalitis, 111t, 111-113
Parenteral nutrition. *See* Nutritional support; Total parenteral nutrition (TPN)
Paroxysmal nocturnal hemoglobinuria (PNH), 904
Paroxysmal supraventricular tachycardia (PST), 536-537, *538*, *539*
    treatment of, 543t
Patient(s)
    as team members, 1562
    assessment of, team concept and, 1558
    autonomy and self-determination of, 1727-1728
    initiating lawsuits, 1719
    rights of, responsibilities versus, 1732
    stress experienced by. *See* Psychological stress
Patient care
    tasks of, computerized patient management system and. *See* Computerized patient management system
    team concept of. *See* Team concept
Patient classification systems, evaluation of, 1664-1665, 1665t
Patient education, 1563
Patient information. *See* Medical records
Patient management systems, computerized. *See* Computerized patient management systems

Patient monitoring. *See also specific types of monitoring*
    during cardiac surgery, 593-594
    during liver transplantation, 1142
    during mechanical ventilation. *See* Mechanical ventilation, during ICU phase
    following cardiac transplantation, 651
    following liver transplantation, 1143-1144
    following renal transplantation, 826-827
    following vascular surgery, during ICU phase, 715t, 715-717
    for thoracic surgery, 362, 362t, *363*
    in gastrointestinal bleeding, 991-992
    invasive versus noninvasive, 1631
    of magnesium replacement therapy, 1188
    of oxygen transport, red cell transfusions and, 1242-1245, *1243*
Patient positioning
    as risk factor for neurologic surgical complications, 1219
    following cardiac surgery, 599
    following head and neck surgery, 213
Patient progress rounds, 1561
Patient records. *See* Medical records
Patient stabilization. *See also* Airway management; Hypertension; Hypotension; Ventilation
    in brain injuries, 82-83
    in intracranial hypertension, 73
    intracranial hypertension and, 67
Patient-controlled analgesia (PCA), 1284
Pearson product-moment correlation coefficient, 1750
Peliosis hepatitis, bacillary, in HIV infection/AIDS, 1410
Pelvic surgery. *See specific procedures*
Pemphigus, antimicrobial therapy for, 1383
Penetrating trauma, to brain, 87
Penicillin(s)
    antistaphylococcal, pharmacokinetics of, 1354
    pharmacokinetics of, 1354
Penicillin G
    dosing adjustment for renal or hepatic dysfunction, 1351t
    dosing during hemofiltration and hemodialysis, 1353t
    for central nervous system infections, 1372
    for cutaneous infections, 1383
    for erysipelas, 925
    for meningococcemia, 1382
    for pneumonia, community-acquired, 391, 391t
    for tetanus, 1384
Pentamidine
    dosing adjustment for renal or hepatic dysfunction, 1351t
    dosing during hemofiltration and hemodialysis, 1353t
    for pneumonia, community-acquired, 392
Pentazocine (Talwin), abuse/overdose of, 1445, 1446
Pentobarbital (Nembutal)
    for delirium, 1283
    for intracranial hypertension, 1084
    for sedative/hypnotic withdrawal, 1445
Pentobarbital tolerance test, 41, 41t
Perceptions
    in mental status examination, 30-31
    of events. *See* Psychological stress, during pre-ICU phase
Percutaneous transhepatic cholangiography (PTHC), in hepatic disorders, 1071-1073, *1072*, 1073

Percutaneous transluminal coronary angioplasty (PTCA), for acute myocardial infarction, 575
    immediately following thrombolytic therapy, 575, 575t
    in patients failing thrombolytic therapy, 575
    with cardiogenic shock, 575
    with contraindications to thrombolytic therapy, 575
Perfluorochemical emulsions, as red blood cell substitute, 1246-1247
Pericardial disease, 610-618. *See also specific disorders*
    anatomy and physiology of, 610, *611*
    in chronic renal failure, 812-813
        risk phase of, 812, *813*
        support phase of, 812-813
Pericardial effusion, 610-616, 611t, *612*
    during ICU phase, 612-616
        diagnostic evaluation in, 612
        differential diagnosis of, 615
        hemodynamic features in, 612-615, *615*
        treatment of, *615*, 615-616
    during post-ICU phase, 616
    during pre-ICU phase, 611-612
Pericardial tamponade, with malignant disease, 871t, 871-872
    during ICU phase, 871-872
    during post-ICU phase, 872
    during pre-ICU phase, 871, *871*
Pericardiocentesis, 1620-1621
    contraindications to, 1620
    data analysis and interpretation of, 1620-1621
    for pericardial effusion, 615-616
    indications for, 1620
    needle, complications of, 1621
    quality enhancement for, 1621
Pericarditis
    constrictive, 616t, 616-618
        during ICU phase, 617-618
            diagnostic evaluation of, 617
            differential diagnosis of, 617, 618t
            hemodynamic features of, 617, *617*
            treatment of, 617-618
        during post-ICU phase, 618
        during pre-ICU phase, 616-617
    in HIV infection/AIDS, 1414
Peripheral artery catheterization, for monitoring respiratory insufficiency, 477-479
Peripheral neuropathy
    in HIV infection/AIDS, 1406
    in multiple organ system failure, 1304-1305
Peripheral vascular disease, as risk factor for cardiac surgery, 591
Peritoneal dialysis
    access for, 1609
    complications of, 1609
    contraindications to, 1609
    indications for, 1609
    for sedative/hypnotic abuse/overdose, 1444
Peritoneal lavage, in pancreatitis, 1027, 1029, *1029*, *1030*, 1032
Peritoneovenous shunts, for ascites, in cirrhosis, 1114-1116, *1115*, *1116*
Peritonitis, bacterial
    secondary to cirrhosis, 1112
    spontaneous. *See* Spontaneous bacterial peritonitis (SBP)
Persistent vegetative state (PVS), 1729
    definition of, 1728t

Personality, perception of events and, 1567
Personnel. *See also* Physician(s); Professional staff
  computerized patient management system and. *See* Computerized patient management system
  team concept and. *See* Team concept
P$_{ETCO_2}$ monitoring, in cardiopulmonary resuscitation, 561
pH. *See also* Acid/base disorders; Acid/base metabolism
  of blood, calcium binding and, 1190
  of urine, in renal failure, 788
Pharyngeal surgery, postoperative care for, 224
Pharyngitis, antimicrobial therapy for, 1373
Pharyngotomy, following head and neck surgery, 222
Phenergan, for alcohol withdrawal, 1441t
Phenobarbital
  for delirium, 1283
  for seizures, in cocaine abuse/overdose, 1435t
Phenothiazines, for delirium, 1282
Phenoxybenzamine, for hypertension, 692t, 693t
Phentolamine, for hypertension, 692t, 693t
  postoperative, 745t, 747
Phenylephrine, for shock, 1325t
Phenytoin
  for seizures, in cocaine abuse/overdose, 1435t
  for ventricular tachycardia, 544t
Phenytoin hypersensitivity syndrome, 967-968
Pheochromocytomas, hypertension and
  during ICU phase, 835
  during post-ICU phase, 836
  during pre-ICU phase, 690, 835
  following resection, 738
Phlebitis, of dural venous sinus, septic
  during ICU phase, 115-116
  pre-ICU evaluation of, 105-106
Phosgene, inhalation injury caused by, 319
Phosphodiesterase inhibitors. *See also specific drugs*
  for shock, 1327-1329, *1328*
Phosphonates, for hypercalcemia, 1193, 1193t
Physical examination, of comatose patient, 17
Physical plant, computerized patient management system and, 1702, 1704
  clinical information system architecture and, 1704, *1708*, 1708t, *1709*
Physician(s)
  criminal prosecution of, 1721
  liability suits and. *See* Liability
Physician-nurse collaboration. *See* Team concept, physician-nurse collaboration and
Physiologic monitoring, in traumatic brain injury, 87
Pickwickian syndrome, 184
Piloerection, 52
Pipecuronium, 1287t, 1288
Piperacillin
  dosing adjustment for renal or hepatic dysfunction, 1351t
  dosing during hemofiltration and hemodialysis, 1353t
  for intra-abdominal infections, 1379
  for pancreatitis, 1034t
Pituitary. *See also* Hypothalamic-pituitary-peripheral gland unit
  disorders of. *See also specific disorders*
  coma and, 13
Pituitary-gonadal axis, normal function of, 1175
Plain abdominal films, in hepatic disorders, *1066*, 1066-1067, *1067*
Plasma, fresh-frozen, transfusions of, 1245-1246, 1247t
Plasma osmolality disorders. *See* Hypernatremia; Hyponatremia; Sodium balance disorders
Plasmapheresis
  for Guillain-Barré syndrome, 130
  for myasthenia gravis, 133-134
Plasmids, 1387
Plasmodium falciparum, coma and, 10
Platelet(s)
  normal function of, 900
  transfusions of, 919-920, 1245-1246, 1246t
Platelet activating factor (PAF), for inhalation injury, 334
Platelet disorders, *907*, 907-911. *See also specific disorders*
  functional, 910-911
    acquired, 910t, 910-911
    congenital, 910
    uremia and, 911
Pleading, 1721
Pleural effusions
  following vascular surgery, 721
  imaging studies in, 1500, 1506, *1507-1510*, 1509
  in pneumonia, 394
  with malignant disease, 872-873
    during ICU phase, 872
    during post-ICU phase, 872-873
    during pre-ICU phase, 872
Pleural fluid, persistent drainage of, following thoracic surgery, 377
Plicamycin (mithramycin), for hypercalcemia, 884
Pneumonectomy, imaging studies following, 1509, 1510t, *1511*, 1512-1513, *1512-1516*
Pneumonia
  community-acquired
    during ICU phase, therapy of, 391t, 391-392
    during pre-ICU phase, diagnosis of, 388-389
  following vascular surgery, 721, 724
  imaging studies in, 1487-1488, *1491-1495*
  in chronic obstructive pulmonary disease, during ICU phase, 254
  in chronic renal failure, 815-816
    rehabilitative phase of, 816
    risk phase of, 815
    support phase of, 815-816
  in HIV infection/AIDS, 1405-1406
    prognosis of, 1415
  in immunocompromised host, 385-396, 399-413
    conditions predisposing to infection and, 399-401
      neoplastic, 400-401
      non-neoplastic, 399-400
    defense mechanisms and, 399, 400t
    during ICU phase, 391-395, 411-413
      clinical re-evaluation and, 412
      diagnosis of nosocomial pneumonia and, 392-393
      discharge criteria and, 395
      infection control and, 411-412
      management of complications and, 394-395
      superinfection and, 413
      therapy of community-acquired pneumonia and, 391t, 391-392
      therapy of nosocomial pneumonia and, 393t, 393-394
    during post-ICU phase, 395-396, 413, 413t
    during pre-ICU phase, 385-391, 410-411
      assessment of need for hospitalization and transfer to ICU and, 389-391, 390t
      clinical manifestations of, 387t, 387-388
      community-acquired, diagnosis of, 388-389
      diagnosis of, 405-408
      in granulocytopenic hosts, 409-410
      microbiology and epidemiology of, 385-387, 396t
      oropharyngeal colonization and, 403-405
      pathogenesis of, 403, 404t
      pulmonary defense mechanisms and, 401-403, 402t, *403*
      treatment of, 408-411, 409t
      with B-cell host defects, 410
      with cell-mediated host defects, 410
      with solid tumors, 410-411
    ICU admission for, 411
  nosocomial
    antimicrobial therapy for, 1374-1376, *1375*, 1375t
    monitoring for, during mechanical ventilation, 294-295
    tracheal intubation and, 202-203
  opportunistic, in HIV infection/AIDS, prophylaxis and treatment of, 1404, 1405
  staphylococcal, antimicrobial therapy for, 1376
Pneumonitis, aspiration, in brain injury, 86
Pneumothorax
  as complication of nutritional support, 1259, 1261
  following renal surgery, 848
  following thoracic surgery, 377
  imaging studies in, 1500, *1503-1507*
  in chronic obstructive pulmonary disease, during ICU phase, 254
Poisonings, 1454-1470. *See also specific substances*
  during ICU phase, 1455-1470
    acetaminophen and, *1458*, 1458-1459
    antiarrhythmic agents and, 1470
    carbon monoxide and, 1462
    cyanide and, 1467
    digoxin and, 1464-1465
    ethylene glycol and, 1466-1467
    general considerations and approach for, 1455-1458, 1456t
    iron and, 1467-1468
    lithium and, 1465-1466
    methanol and, 1466-1467
    mushrooms and, 1469
    nonsteroidal anti-inflammatory drugs and, 1469-1470
    nontricyclic antidepressants and, 1461-1462
    organophsophate pesticides and, 1468
    salicylates and, *1459*, 1459-1460
    snake bites and, 1468-1469
    spider bites and, 1468-1469
    theophylline and, 1462-1464, 1463t

INDEX

tricyclic antidepressants and, 1460-1461
  during post-ICU phase, 1470
  during pre-ICU phase, 1454-1455, 1455t, 1456t
  hepatic failure induced by, 1079
Poliomyelitis, 138-140
  during ICU phase, 139
  during post-ICU phase, 139-140
  during pre-ICU phase, 139
Polycythemia, 877
  during ICU phase, 877
  during post-ICU phase, 877
  during pre-ICU phase, 877
Polyneuropathy, of critical illness, 1304-1305
Polysomnography, nocturnal, in hypoventilation syndromes, 182
Pons, coma and, 4
Population, 1740
Population mean, 1740
Portacaval shunt
  end-to-side, for esophageal varices, 1101, *1101*
  side-to-side, for esophageal varices, 1101, *1101*
Portal decompression, partial, for esophageal varices, 1102
Portal hypertension
  gastropathy in, 1103, *1103*
    bleeding and, in patients awaiting liver transplantation, treatment of, 1134-1136
  in cirrhosis, 1094
    bleeding in, treatment of, 1096-1097
    diagnosis of, 1094-1095, 1096t
  in fulminant hepatic failure, 1091
  variceal bleeding in, 994-996
    sclerotherapy for, 994, 996
    Sengstaken-Blakemore balloon tamponade for, 994, *995*
  varices in. *See* varices
Portal systemic encephalopathy (PSE). *See* Coma, hepatic; Encephalopathy, hepatic (portosystemic)
Positive end-expiratory pressure (PEEP)
  antibiotic pharmacokinetics and, 1353-1354
  during ICU phase, 285-286, *286*
  following cardiac surgery, 598, 599t
  for inhalation injury, 332
  for thoracic surgery, 365, *365*, 369-370
  in adult respiratory distress syndrome, 307-308
  in intra-abdominal infection, 1008
Positive expiratory pressure (PEP), in atelectasis, 468-469, *469*
Positive predictive value, 1745, 1745t
Positive pressure ventilation (PPV), in hypoventilation syndromes, 185
Posterior cord syndrome, 150
Postoperative hypertension (POH). *See* Hypertension, postoperative
Postpolio syndrome, 139
Postresuscitation syndrome, in hypocalcemia, 1191
Post-transfusion purpura (PTP), 909
Post-TURP syndrome, 850
Postural drainage therapy (PDT), 475-476, *476*, *477*, 478t
Potassium, for shock, 1330
Potassium balance disorders, 774-780. *See also* Hyperkalemia; Hypokalemia
Potassium cyanide intoxication, coma and, 12

Power, statistical, 1741
Power of attorney, durable, 1732, 1734
  definition of, 1728t
Pralidoxime (2-PAM), for organophosphate intoxication, 1468
Prazosin, for mitral regurgitation, 666t
Predictive validity, 1665t
Predictive value
  negative, 1745, 1745t
  positive, 1745, 1745t
Prednisone
  following cardiac transplantation, 650, 651t
  for diffuse alveolar hemorrhage, 345
  for erythema multiforme, 967
  for morbilliform eruptions, 967
  for toxic epidermal necrolysis, 964
Pregnancy
  bronchospastic disease during, 231, 231t
  complications of, cocaine abuse/overdose causing, 1433
  fatty liver of, 1080
  hypertension during, during pre-ICU phase, 690, 690t
  pulmonary embolism during, 434
Preload, 507-509, *508*
  disease states influencing, 508-509, 509t
  following cardiac surgery, 597
Premature ventricular depolarizations (PVDs), treatment of, 542-544, 543t, 544t
Premedication, for thoracic surgery, 362
Pressure control ventilation, 486
Pressure gradients, 65
Pressure monitors, infection related to, 1592
Pressure sores, 976-982
  during ICU phase, 981
  during post-ICU phase, *981*, 981-982, *982*
  during pre-ICU phase, 976-980
    risk factors for, 976-978, 977t, *977-979*
    staging of, 978, *979*, *980*
    treatment of, 978, 980
  prevention of, in spinal cord injury, 155-156
Pressure support ventilation (PSV), 288
  in ventilatory failure, 171-172
Pressure waves, in intracranial hypertension, 68
Procainamide, for ventricular tachycardia, 544, 544t
Procaine, as cutting substance in street drugs, 1427
Prochlorperazine (Compazine), for delirium, 1282
Professional staff. *See also* Physician(s); Team concept
  impact of critical care on, 1572-1573
  liability and. *See* Liability
Prognosis. *See also specific disorders*
  studies characterizing, 1743-1744
Prognostic nutritional index (PNI), 1253, 1254t
Programs, 1704, 1707
Progressive multifocal leukoencephalopathy (PML)
  coma and, 12
  in HIV infection/AIDS, 1407
Prolactin (PRL), 1173
Proof, of negligence/causation, 1718-1719
Propafenone, for ventricular tachycardia, 544
Propofol, for sedation, 1280t, 1281
Propoxyphene, abuse/overdose of, 1446

Propranolol
  for aortic dissection, 705t
  for cocaine abuse/overdose, 1434
  for esophageal varices, 1102-1103
  for supraventricular tachycardia, 539, 543
Propylthiouracil (PTU), for thyroid storm, 1177
Prostaglandin E_2, for shock, 1330
Prostaglandin inhibitors. *See also specific drugs*
  for shock, 1329-1330
Prostate, perforations of, transurethral prostatectomy and, 850
Prostatectomy
  radical
    during ICU phase, 842-843
    during post-ICU phase, 843-844
    during pre-ICU phase, 839-840
    preoperative preparation for, 840-841
    technique for, 841, 842t
  transurethral. *See* Transurethral prostatectomy (TURP)
Prosthetic valves
  assessment of, in aortic regurgitation, 676-677
  dysfunction of
    aortic regurgitation and, 671
    mitral regurgitation and, 658-659, *660*
Prosthetic vascular grafts, infection of, following vascular surgery, 724-725
Protein
  requirements for, 1255-1256
  visceral, in nutrition assessment, 1251, 1252t
Prothrombin time, in hepatic disorders, 1064
Protozoal infections, disseminated, in HIV infection/AIDS, 1411
Pseudocysts, pancreatic, pancreatitis and, 1039
Pseudomonal infections, cutaneous, 939-941
  clinical features and differential diagnosis of, 939-941, *940*
  laboratory studies in, 941
  outcome of, 941
  pathophysiology of, 939
  treatment of, 941
Pseudothrombocytopenia, 879
Psychedelic drugs. *See* Hallucinogen abuse/overdose
Psychiatric disorders, cocaine abuse/overdose causing, 1434
Psychologic management, in spinal cord injury, 156-157
Psychologic management of, following thoracic surgery, 381-382
Psychological stress, 1566-1573
  crisis of critical illness and, 1566
  crisis theory and, 1566, *1567*
  during ICU phase, 1569-1573
    disease-specific stressors and, 1569-1570, 1570t
    general stressors and, 1569
    helping patients cope with, 1571, 1571t
    impact of critical care on professional staff and, 1572-1573
    maintaining family relationships and, 1571-1572
    relationships with caregivers and, 1572
  during post-ICU phase, 1573
    preparing patients for discharge and, 1573

Psychological stress *(Continued)*
  during pre-ICU phase, 1566-1569
    coping mechanisms and, 1568-1569
    realistic perception of event and, 1566-1567
      past experiences and, 1566-1567
      personality factors and, 1567
    situational support and, 1568
Psychostimulants, for depression, 37
Pulmonary alveolar hypoventilation (PAH), 179, 182
Pulmonary angiography, in pulmonary embolism, 425
Pulmonary artery catheterization, 1621-1625
  complications and management of, *1622*, 1622-1623
  contraindications to, 1622
  data analysis for, 1623t, 1623-1624, *1624*
  following vascular surgery, during ICU phase, 716
  future use of, 1623
  indications for, 1621-1622
  quality enhancement for, 1624t, 1624-1625
Pulmonary artery end diastolic pressure (PAEDP), 1636-1637, *1637*
Pulmonary artery occlusive pressure (PAOP), 1635t, 1635-1636, *1635-1637*, 1636t
Pulmonary artery pressure monitoring, 1635-1640
  pulmonary artery end diastolic pressure and, 1636-1637, *1637*
  pulmonary artery occlusive pressure and, 1635t, 1635-1636, *1635-1637*, 1636t
  respiratory variations and, 1637-1639, *1638, 1639*
  technical problems in, 1639-1640, *1640*
Pulmonary aspiration, as complication of nutritional support, 1263
Pulmonary disorders. *See also* Respiratory disorders; *specific disorders*
  following vascular surgery, 720-721
  in chronic renal failure, 813-814
  in fulminant hepatic failure, 1087, *1087*
  infectious, focal pulmonary hemorrhage and, 351
  systemic inflammatory response syndrome and, 1004
Pulmonary edema
  hydrostatic, during ICU phase, 253-254, *254*, 254t
  imaging studies in, 1488, 1492-1493, *1495, 1496*
  in chronic renal failure, 809-811
    rehabilitative phase of, 810-811
    risk phase of, 810
    support phase of, 810
  reexpansion, following thoracic surgery, 376
  reperfusion, following lung transplantation, 379, *380*
Pulmonary embolism, 417-434, 418t
  brain injury and, 89
  coma and, 9
  during ICU phase, 419-433
    diagnosis of venous thrombosis and, 426-429
      clinical features and differential diagnosis and, 426-427
      noninvasive testing in, 427-428
      practical approach to, *428*, 428-429
      venography in, 427

general considerations for, 419-420, 420t
in hemodynamically stable patients, 422-426
  lung scanning and, *422*, 422-424, 423t, *424*
  practical diagnostic approach for, 426, *426*
  pulmonary angiography and, 425
  role of objective testing for venous thrombosis and, 425-426
in hemodynamically unstable patients, 420-422
  initial physiologic support for, 420-421
  specific therapy and clinical course of, 421-422
initial treatment of venous thromboembolism in, 429t, 429-433
  anticoagulant therapy in, 429-431
  thrombolytic therapy in, 431-433
during post-ICU phase, 433-434
  axillary vein thrombosis in, 434
  calf-vein thrombosis in, 433
  suspected pulmonary embolism during pregnancy and, 434
during pre-ICU phase, 417-419
  natural history and clinical course of venous thromboembolism and, 417-418
  prevention of venous thromboembolism and, 418-419, 419t
  risk factors and classification of risk and, 418, 418t
following thoracic surgery, 375
following vascular surgery, 722
monitoring for, during mechanical ventilation, 294
neurogenic, in brain injury, 86
Pulmonary function, age-related changes in, 242, *243*
Pulmonary function testing
  in bronchospastic disease, 230, 230t
  in chronic obstructive pulmonary disease and asthma, 464-465, *466*
  in hypoventilation syndromes, 180, *180*
  in inhalation injury, 330-331
  invasive, preoperative, 1205t, 1205-1206, 1207, *1207*
  noninvasive, preoperative, 1203-1205, 1204t
  prior to thoracic surgery, 356-357, 357t
Pulmonary hemorrhage, 341-352. *See also* Diffuse alveolar hemorrhage (DAH); Focal pulmonary hemorrhage (FPH)
Pulmonary management, in spinal cord injury, 150-152, *151*
Pulmonary monitoring, following vascular surgery, during ICU phase, 716
Pulmonary surgical complications, 1199-1208, *1200*, 1200t
  during ICU phase, 1207t, 1207-1208
  during pre-ICU phase, 1201-1207
    invasive pulmonary vascular studies and exercise testing and, 1205t, 1205-1207, *1207*
    noninvasive pulmonary studies and, 1203-1205, 1204t
    nonpulmonary surgical risk factors for, 1201t, 1201-1202
      age, 1202
      anesthesia, 1201-1202
      cardioplegia, 1202
      incisions, 1202

nasogastric tubes, 1202
obesity, 1201
sleep apnea/hypoventilation, 1201
smoking, 1201
pulmonary surgical risk factors for, *1202*, 1202t, 1202-1203
  asthma, 1203
  chronic obstructive pulmonary disease, 1202-1203
Pulse, venous, jugular, 531
Pulse oximetry
  for monitoring and detection of respiratory insufficiency, 465-467, 466t, *467*
    clinical application and considerations with, 466-467
    technical considerations with, 466, *467, 468*
  for monitoring respiratory insufficiency, 479-480
  in chronic obstructive pulmonary disease, 493
Pulse recordings, arterial, indirect, ventricular function evaluation using, 518
Pupils, in neuro-ophthalmologic examination, of comatose patient, 18
Purpura. *See* Idiopathic thrombocytopenic purpura (ITP); Post-transfusion purpura (PTP); Thrombotic thrombocytopenic purpura (TTP)

QT interval, prolongation of, arrhythmias and, 534-535
Quality Adjusted Life Years (QALYs), 1692-1694, *1693*
Quality assessment/assurance, 1563, 1576-1584
  decision making and, 1579-1582
    ICU organization and management and, 1581-1582
    process of care and, 1580-1581
      clinical outcome, mortality, and quality of care and, 1580-1581
    triage and, 1579-1580
  for arterial catheterization, 1601t, 1601-1602
  for bronchoscopy, 1603
  for cardioversion, 1607-1608
  for central venous pressure monitoring, 1605, 1605t
  for chest tubes, 1606-1607
  for defibrillation, 1607-1608
  for dialysis access, 809
  for intra-aortic balloon pump, 1610-1612
  for intracranial pressure monitoring, 1613
  for intubation, 1614-1615, 1615t
  for lumbar puncture, 1617
  for paracentesis, 1620
  for pericardiocentesis, 1621
  for pulmonary artery catheterization, 1624t, 1624-1625
  for temporary pacing, 1619
  for thoracentesis, 1626
  implementing programs for, *1583*, 1583-1584, *1584*
  measurement of outcome and, 1578-1579
  measurement of patient characteristics and, 1577t, 1577-1578
  measurement of process of care and, 1578
  quality of care, long-term survival, and quality of life and, 1582-1583
  quality of care management and, 1577, 1577t
  standards and guidelines for, 1599

INDEX

Quality of life
  following liver transplantation, 1150
  quality of care and, 1583
  quantification of outcome and, 1687–1694, 1689t
    activities of daily living and, 1688–1689, 1689t
    Functional Status Questionnaire for, 1691–1692, 1692t, *1693*
    Karnofsky Performance Status Scale for, 1689, 1690t
    Nottingham Health Profile for, 1691, 1691t
    Quality Adjusted Life Years for, 1692–1694, *1693*
    Sickness Impact Profile for, 1689, 1690t, 1691
Quinidine
  for malaria, 1385
  for ventricular tachycardia, 544t
Quinine, as cutting substance in street drugs, 1427

Rabies, contagion of, 1373
Radiation, as predisposing condition to infection, 400
Radiative heat transfer, 51
Radiologic imaging. *See* Imaging studies; *specific modalities*
Radionuclide imaging
  in aortic regurgitation, 677
  in cardiac trauma, nonpenetrating, 632
  in focal pulmonary hemorrhage, 351
  in hepatic disorders, 1067–1068, *1068*
Radionuclide ventriculography (RVG), 515, 515–517, *516*
  ejection fraction and, 519
  in cardiac trauma, nonpenetrating, 632
Random error, 1739
Randomization, 1743
Randomized, controlled clinical trial, 1746–1747
Randomness, 1740
Ranitidine, for pancreatitis, 1035
Ranson's signs, in pancreatitis, 1025, 1025t
Rapid latex agglutination test, for HIV infection, 1402
Receiver-operating characteristic (ROC) curve, 1746, *1746*
Recombinant tissue plasminogen activator (rt-PA)
  for pulmonary embolism, 433
  for thrombotic disorders, 917
Reconstruction flaps
  free, following head and neck surgery, 218–219
  pedicled, following head and neck surgery, 218, *219*
Red cells
  disorders of, 901–905. *See also* Anemia; Hemolytic anemia
    extrinsic abnormalities and, 904–905
    intrinsic abnormalities and, 902–904
      enzyme deficiencies, 904
      hemoglobin abnormalities, 903–904
      paroxysmal nocturnal hemoglobinuria, 904
      primary membrane disorders, 902–903
    of inadequate production, 901–902
    of increased destruction, 902
    of increased production, 905
  normal function of, 899
  transfusions of. *See* Transfusion therapy

Reflex vasodilation, 52
Rehabilitation
  following brain injury, 89–90
  following pneumonia, 413
  following thoracic surgery, 381–382
  in arrhythmias, 548–549, 551
  in chronic obstructive pulmonary disease, 270–271
  in spinal cord injury, 158
  pulmonary, 498–499
Rehemorrhage, subarachnoid, 80, 81t, 88
Relative risk, 1741
Renal arterial thrombosis, in following renal revascularization, 833
Renal biopsy
  following renal transplantation, 829
  in renal failure, 789
Renal disorders. *See also specific disorders*
  antibiotic dosing in, 1349–1354, 1350t–1354t
  as risk factor for cardiac surgery, 591
  chemotherapy-induced, 886–888
    hemolytic-uremic syndrome, 887–888
    tumor lysis syndrome, 886–887, 886–888
  following liver transplantation, 1148
  following vascular surgery, 723
  in HIV infection/AIDS, 1414
  in multiple organ system failure, 1293t, 1303–1304
  infection-related, 1345
    gram-negative-related, mechanism of, 1345
  metabolic acidosis associated with, treatment of, 761–762, 764
Renal failure. *See also* Acute renal failure (ARF); Chronic renal failure (CRF); End-stage renal disease (ESRD)
  anuric
    aminoglycoside dosing in, 1357, *1358*, 1359
    following cardiac surgery, 600–601
    vancomycin dosing in, 1357, *1358*, 1359
  classification systems for, 1684, 1686–1687, *1687*, 1687t–1689t
  coma and, 13
  following renal surgery, 848
  following vascular surgery, 723
  hypocalcemia caused by, 1190–1191
  in fulminant hepatic failure, 1087–1089, *1088*
  in intra-abdominal infection, 1010
  in necrotizing pancreatitis, 1019–1020
  nutritional support in, 1267–1268
  oliguric, following cardiac surgery, 600–601
Renal function, aminoglycosides and, 1344
Renal function studies, in metabolic acidosis, 758–759, 759t
Renal insufficiency, hypermagnesemia caused by, 1189
Renal monitoring, following vascular surgery, during ICU phase, 716
Renal surgery, 845–849. *See also* Renal transplantation
  during ICU phase, 847–849
    adrenal insufficiency and, 847–848
    fistulas and, 848
    gastrointestinal complications of, 848–849
    hemorrhage and, 847
    pneumothorax and chest tube management and, 848

renal failure and, 848
urinary leak and, 848
  during post-ICU phase, 849
  during pre-ICU phase, 845t, 845–847
    bilateral nephrectomy, 846
    for kidney stones, 846
    nephroureterectomy, 846
    partial nephrectomy, 846
    radical nephrectomy, 845–846
    simple nephrectomy, 846–847
  hypertension following, 739
Renal system, in disseminated intravascular coagulation, 875
Renal toxicity, of aminoglycosides, 1345–1346
Renal transplantation, 825–831
  during ICU phase, 826–830
    intraoperative considerations and, 826
    postoperative monitoring and, 826–827
    post-transplantation complications and, 827t, 827–830
      immunosuppression, 829–830
      lymphocele, 828
      rejection, 828t, 828–829, 829t
      surgical, 827
      urologic, 827–828
  during post-ICU phase, 830–831
  during pre-ICU phase, 825–826
    donor candidate identification for, 826, 826t
    recipient candidate identification for, 825–826, 826t
  imaging studies in, 1540–1541, *1541*, *1542*
Renal tubular acidosis (RTA)
  in diabetes mellitus, 805
  treatment of, 761–762
Renovascular disease, 831–834
  during ICU phase, 833–834
    postoperative complications and, 833–834
    postoperative monitoring and, 833
  during post-ICU phase, 834
  during pre-ICU phase, 831–833
    candidate identification and, 831–832
    intraoperative considerations and, 832–833
    preoperative preparation and, 832
Reperfusion hemorrhage, postcraniotomy, 89
Reperfusion injury, in hypocalcemia, 1191
Reproducibility, 1665t
Res ipsa loquitur doctrine, 1718–1719
Research design. *See* Clinical epidemiology, research designs and
Reserpine, for hypertension, 692t, 693t
Respirations, alterations in, intracranial hypertension and, 66
Respiratory alkalosis, hypocalcemia caused by, 1190
Respiratory care services, 461–500, 462t
  bilevel nasal continuous positive airway pressure and, 498
  consequences of malnutrition for pulmonary function and, 494–495, 495t
  continuous quality improvement and, *499*, 499–500
  during ICU phase, 476–491, 478t
    airway management and, 483–484, *484*, 484t
    endotracheal intubation and, 484–485
    mechanical ventilation and. *See* Mechanical ventilation; Ventilatory weaning

1785

Respiratory care services *(Continued)*
  modalities commonly used in, 481–483
    aerosol therapy, 481
    aerosolized pharmacologic agents, 482, 482t
    bronchopulmonary hygiene therapy, 481–482
    for prevention and treatment of atelectasis, 483, *483*, 483t
    humidity therapy, 481
    therapeutic bronchoscopy, 482
    monitoring of respiratory insufficiency and. *See* Respiratory insufficiency
  preparation for discharge and, 490–491
  during post-ICU phase, 491–494
    aerosol therapy in, 491–492, 493–494
    airway management in, 493–494
    bronchopulmonary hygiene therapy in, 493
    goals of management and, 491, 491t
    in chronic obstructive pulmonary disease. *See* Chronic obstructive pulmonary disease (COPD)
    oxygen therapy in, 492t, 492–493, 493t
    pulse oximetry in, 493
  during pre-ICU phase, 461–476
    aerosol therapy in. *See* Aerosol therapy
    bronchopulmonary hygiene therapy in. *See* Bronchopulmonary hygiene therapy
    monitoring and detection of respiratory insufficiency and. *See* Respiratory insufficiency
    oxygen therapy in. *See* Oxygen therapy
    patient assessment and evaluation for, 462, *463*
    prevention and treatment of atelectasis and, 467–469
      continuous positive airway pressure and positive expiratory pressure in, 468–469, *469*
      incentive spirometry in, 467–468, *468*
      intermittent positive pressure breathing in, 468
  for obese patients, 495–496
  for prevention and treatment of postoperative complications, 494, *495*
  for ventilator-dependent patients in non-ICU settings, 496–498, 497t
    discharge planning and, 498
    technical aspects of, 497–498
    in obstructive sleep apnea, 496, *496*
    pulmonary rehabilitation and, 498–499
Respiratory depression, benzodiazepine-induced, 1280–1281
Respiratory disorders. *See also* Pulmonary disorders; *specific disorders*
  chemotherapy-induced, 888t, 888–889
  during ICU phase, 889
  during post-ICU phase, 889
  during pre-ICU phase, 888–889, *889*
  cocaine abuse/overdose causing, 1433
  in multiple organ system failure, 1293t, 1303
  in necrotizing pancreatitis, 1020t, 1020–1021
  infectious. *See also specific respiratory tract infections*
    in HIV infection/AIDS, 1405–1406
    of chest and lower respiratory tract, antimicrobial therapy for, 1374–1376, *1375*, 1375t
    of upper respiratory tract, antimicrobial therapy for, 1373–1374
Respiratory failure, 163–175, *164*
  classification systems for, *1683*, 1683t–1685t, 1683–1684
  in acid maltase deficiency, 141–142
  in diffuse alveolar hemorrhage, 346
  in HIV infection/AIDS, prognosis of, 1415
  in organophosphate intoxication, 1468
  induced hypothermia for, 1288–1289
  nutritional support in, 1268–1269
  parenchymal, 163–164
    diffusion limitation and, 164
    during ICU phase, 164–167, *165*, *166*
      duty cycle and inverse ratio ventilation and, 167, *167*
      therapeutic strategy for, 167, 167t
    during post-ICU phase, 167–168
    during pre-ICU phase, 163–164
    general approach to, 164
    hypoventilation and, 163–164
    low mixed venous oxygen tension and, 164
    reduced fraction of inspired oxygen and, 163
    shunt and, 164
    ventilation-perfusion mismatching and, 164
  pathophysiology of, *255*, 255–256, *256*, 256t
  signs and symptoms of, 281–282, 282t
  ventilatory (pump), 168–175
    during ICU phase, 168–173
      ability to accomplish ventilatory workload and, 172–173
      work of breathing and, 168–172
    during post-ICU phase, 173–175
      adjunctive ventilatory support and, 175
      muscle training and, 175
      weaning from mechanical ventilation and, 173–175, 174t, *175*
Respiratory insufficiency
  acute, in chronic obstructive pulmonary disease, during ICU phase, 253t, 253–254
  during ICU phase, monitoring of, 477–481
    arterial blood gases and hemoximetry for, 479
    bedside spirometry for, 479–480
    capnography for, 480–481, *481*
    hemodynamic monitoring for, 479
    peripheral artery catheterization for, 477–479
    pulse oximetry for, 480, 480t
  during pre-ICU phase, monitoring and detection of, 462, 464–467
    bedside screening device for, 464, *465*
    bedside spirometry in, 462, 464, 464t
    preoperative assessment and, 464
    pulmonary function assessment in chronic obstructive pulmonary disease and asthma and, 464–465, *466*
    pulse oximetry for, 465–467, 466t, *467*
  following thoracic surgery, 376
Respiratory management, following cardiac surgery, 598–599, 599t
Respiratory monitoring, 1630–1647. *See also specific types of respiratory monitoring*
  basis of clinical measurements and, 1630–1631
  errors in interpretation and, 1631
  for routine clinical assessment, 1631
  invasive versus noninvasive, 1631
  operator errors and, 1630–1631
  signal processing and, 1630–1631
Respiratory muscles
  activity of, minute ventilation and, 265
  endurance of, rehabilitation of ventilator-dependent patients and, 445–446, *447*, 447–448, *448*
  exercise of, in chronic obstructive pulmonary disease, rest versus, 267–268
  fatigue of
    in chronic obstructive pulmonary disease, 266–267
    in ventilatory failure, 173
  rest of, in chronic obstructive pulmonary disease, 271
  strength of, rehabilitation of ventilator-dependent patients and, 445–447
  training of
    in chronic obstructive pulmonary disease, 183–184
    in ventilatory failure, 175
Respiratory quotient (RQ), for estimation of energy requirements, 1255, 1255t
Respiratory therapy. *See also* Respiratory care services
  following thoracic surgery, 381
  for thoracic surgery patients, 370
Respiratory therapy equipment, infection related to, *1592*, 1592t, 1592–1593, 1593t
Respondeat superior doctrine, 1720–1721
Rest, in chronic obstructive pulmonary disease, exercise versus, 267–268
Resting energy expenditure (REE), for estimation of energy requirements, 1254–1255
Resuscitation, for shock, 1324
Retinitis, in HIV infection/AIDS, 1411
Retinopathy, diabetic, 806
Retrograde amnesia, concussive head injury and, 77
Retroperitoneal disorders, imaging studies in, 1532, 1536, *1537*, *1538*
Rewarming, in hypothermia, 55–56
Rheumatic disorders, as predisposing condition to infection, 400
Rheumatologic disorders, in HIV infection/AIDS, 1414
Rhinorrhea, CSF, in traumatic brain injury, 87
Rib resection, as risk factor for neurologic surgical complications, 1219
Rickettsial infections, cutaneous, 944–946. *See also specific infections*
Rifampin, for pneumonia, community-acquired, 391t, 392
Right ventricular ejection fraction (RVEF), 1642
Right ventricular function, 512–514, *514*, 514t
Risk
  of lawsuits, 1719
  relative, 1741
  unreasonable, 1718
Risk factors. *See specific disorders*
Rocky Mountain spotted fever, 944–946
  antimicrobial therapy for, 1382
  clinical features and diagnosis of, 945
  laboratory studies in, 945–946
  outcome of, 946
  pathophysiology of, 945
  treatment of, 946
Rotorest treatment table, 150, *151*

Salicylate intoxication, *1459*, 1459-1460
    coma and, 12
    metabolic acidosis associated with, treatment of, 763
Saline infusions, for hypercalcemia, 1192
Salt-depletion heat exhaustion, 57
Sample, 1740
Sample mean, 1740
Sclerosing cholangitis, 1053-1054, *1054*
Sclerotherapy, for variceal bleeding, 994, 996, 1098, 1100-1101, 1103-1104
    emergency surgery and, 994
    endoscopic ligation and, 994
    in patients awaiting liver transplantation, 1136
Scopolamine, as premedication, for thoracic surgery, 362
Score, 1746
Scrotal gangrene, 851
    during ICU phase, 851
    during post-ICU phase, 851
    during pre-ICU phase, 851
Sedation. *See also specific drugs and drug types*
    benzodiazepines for, 1280t, 1280-1281
    during mechanical ventilation, during ICU phase, 290
    indications for, 1279-1280, 1280t
    population differences affecting pain response and, 1278-1279, 1279t
Sedative/hypnotic(s), 1280t, 1280-1281
    abuse/overdose of, 1441-1445
        complications of, 1443
        diagnosis and treatment of, 1443-1444
        ICU admission criteria in, 1444
        signs and symptoms of, 1442-1443
        withdrawal and, 1444-1445
Sedative-hypnotic abstinence syndrome, rehabilitation of ventilator-dependent patients and, 444
Seizures, 94-100, 95t
    cocaine abuse/overdose causing, 1433
        treatment of, 1434
    coma and, 14
    during ICU phase, 98t, 98-100
        barbiturate coma and, 99, *99,* 99t
        complications of status epilepticus and, 98, 98t
        pharmacokinetic interactions and, 99-100, 100t
    during post-ICU phase, 100
    during pre-ICU phase, 95-97, 96t, 97t
    hallucinogens causing, 1448
    in comatose patient, management of, 16
    status epilepticus and, 94-95, 95t
        complications of, 98, 98t
    theophylline causing, 1463
    tricyclic antidepressants causing, 1461
Self-determination
    definition of, 1728t
    patients' rights to, 1727-1728
Sengstaken-Blakemore balloon tamponade, for variceal bleeding, 994, *995*
Sensible fluid losses, hypovolemia caused by, fluid resuscitation for, 1235-1236, *1236*
Sensitivity, of tests, 1745, 1745t
Sensorium, in mental status examination, 31, 31t
Sepsis, 1003. *See also Infection*
    abdominal. *See Intra-abdominal infections*
    as complication of nutritional support, 1259
    biliary. *See Gallstone(s)*
    central line, following vascular surgery, 725

definition of, 1294
hypocalcemia caused by, 1190
hypovolemia caused by, fluid resuscitation for, 1237
in acute renal failure, in patients awaiting liver transplantation, 1139
in brain injury, 87
in febrile patients, 1371
in multiple organ system failure, 1300
intracranial
    during ICU phase, 115
    pre-ICU evaluation of, 104
line, 1383-1384
myocardial dysfunction associated with. *See Myocardial dysfunction, sepsis-related*
nutritional support in, 1269
pathophysiology of, *1003,* 1003t, 1003-1007, *1005, 1006,* 1006t
pseudomonal, cutaneous, 939-940, *940*
shock and, adrenergic response and, 1323
Septic abortion, antimicrobial therapy for, 1382
Septic arthritis, intracranial, pre-ICU evaluation of, 105
Septic response, multiple organ system failure and, 1292-1294
Septic shock, definition of, 1294
Septicemia, in chronic renal failure, 816-818
    rehabilitative phase of, 817-818
    risk phase of, 817
    support phase of, 817
Seroma, following head and neck surgery, 220
Serum alanine aminotransferase (ALT), in hepatic disorders, 1064-1065
Serum aspartate aminotransferase (AST), in hepatic disorders, 1064-1065
Settlement, of suit, 1724
Severity indices
    evaluation of, 1664-1665, 1665t
    in pancreatitis, 1025-1027, *1026*
    MEDISGRPS, 1671, 1671t, 1671-1672
    Severity of Illness Index (SII), 1669-1670, 1670t
Severity of illness, capture of data to document, 1714, 1715t, *1716*
Severity of Illness Index (SII), 1669-1670, 1670t
Shear injuries, concussive head injury and, 77
Shivering, following cardiac surgery, 596
Shivering thermogenesis, 52
Shock, 1313-1331
    cardiogenic, 1314
        in acute myocardial infarction, 578
        percutaneous transluminal angioplasty for, 575
    clinical presentation of, 1313, 1314t
    definition of, 1313
    distributive, 1314
    during ICU phase, 1324-1329
        calcium for, 1329
        catecholamines for, 1324-1325, 1325t
        diagnosis of, 1324
        dobutamine for, 1326
        dopamine for, 1325-1326, *1326*
        dopexamine for, 1327
        epinephrine for, 1327
        fenoldapam for, 1327
        isoproterenol for, 1327
        norepinephrine for, 1327
        phosphodiesterase inhibitors for, 1327-1329, *1328*
        resuscitation for, 1324

during post resuscitation phase, 1330-1331
    ICU discharge criteria and, 1331
    weaning pharmacologic support and, 1330-1331
during pre-ICU phase, 1314-1325
    adrenergic receptors in, 1317-1321, 1319t
        activation of adrenergic system and, 1318-1319, *1320,* 1321, *1321*
        receptor subtypes and, 1318
    anaphylactic and anaphylactoid reactions as risk factors for, 1315, 1315t
    bacteremia and nosocomial infections as risk factors for, 1314-1315
    blood flow limitations as risk factors for, 1315
    factors affecting adrenergic responses and, 1321t, 1321-1324
        cardiac disease, 1322-1323
        electrolyte disorders, 1323-1324
        individual differences, 1322
        sepsis, 1323
    mediators in, 1315-1317, *1316,* 1317t
        eicosanoids, 1316, *1318*
    myocardial dysfunction as risk factor for, 1315
hypovolemic, 1313-1314
in pulmonary embolism, management of, 420
obstructive, 1314
septic, definition of, 1294
unconventional therapeutic approaches for, 1329-1330
    corticosteroids, 1330
    digoxin, 1329
    glucagon, 1329
    naloxone, 1329
    prostaglandin E$_2$, 1330
    prostaglandin inhibitors, 1329-1330
Shock liver, 1120
Shunt procedures
    for ascites, in cirrhosis, 1114-1116, *1115, 1116*
    for esophageal varices, 1098-1099, *1101,* 1101-1102, *1102*
    for parenchymal respiratory failure, 164
Sickle cell disease, 903
Sickness Impact Profile, 1689, 1690t, 1691
Signal processing, in monitoring, 1630-1631
Significance, statistical, 1741
Simplified Acute Physiology Score (SAPS), 1672
Single photon emission computed tomography (SPECT), in hepatic disorders, 1067-1068
Sinus bradycardia, in acute myocardial infarction, 578
Sinus disorders, cocaine abuse/overdose causing, 1433
Sinus node reentry, 537-538, *542*
Sinus tachycardia, 535
    treatment of, 543t
Sinusitis
    antimicrobial therapy for, 1373-1374
    in HIV infection/AIDS, 1406
Sitting, postoperative, pulmonary function and, 1207-1208
Situational support, 1568
Skeletal infections, intracranial
    during ICU phase, 115
    pre-ICU evaluation of, 103-104
Skeletal muscle, properties of fibers of, ventilatory workload and, 172

Skin. *See also* Cutaneous disorders; *specific disorders*
  in disseminated intravascular coagulation, 875
  infections of. *See specific infections*
  management of, in spinal cord injury, 155–156
  trauma to, antimicrobial therapy for, 1383
Skin grafting, split-thickness, following head and neck surgery, 217–218
Skull fracture, 78–79, *79*
  basilar, 78
  depressed, 79, *79*
  open, 79
Skull radiographs, in brain injuries, 83–84, *84*
Sleep apnea. *See* Obstructive sleep apnea (OSA)
Sleep studies, in hypoventilation syndromes, 182
Small bowel disorders, imaging studies in, 1525, 1528, *1528–1534*, 1531
Smoke, inhalation injury caused by, 320, 320t
Smoking
  as surgical risk factor, for pulmonary complications, 1201
  cessation of
    following cardiac surgery, 603
    in chronic obstructive pulmonary disease, 269–270
    preoperative, 1208
    surgical management of myocardial ischemia and infarction and, 590
  chronic obstructive pulmonary disease related to, pathogenesis of, 243
Snake bites, 1468–1469
Sodium
  hypertonic, for hyperkalemia, 779t
  plasma level of, calcium binding and, 1190
Sodium balance disorders, 769–774. *See also* Hypernatremia; Hyponatremia
Sodium bicarbonate
  for hyperkalemia, 779t
  for metabolic acidosis, 760t, 760–761, 763
  in cardiopulmonary resuscitation, 556t, 557, 561–562
Sodium carbonate, for metabolic acidosis, 763
Sodium nitroprusside
  following vascular surgery, 717
  for aortic dissection, 704, 705t
  for aortic regurgitation, 677–678
  for hypertension, 692t, 693t
    postoperative, 745t, 746
  for look-alike drug abuse/overdose, 1438
  for mitral regurgitation, 666t
  in cardiopulmonary resuscitation, 556t, 560
  intoxication by, coma and, 12
Sodium polystyrene sulfonate (Kayexalate), for hyperkalemia, 779t, 780
Sodium thiosulfate, for cyanide poisoning, 1467
Soft tissue infections
  intracerebral, during ICU phase, 122
  intracranial
    during ICU phase, 115
    pre-ICU evaluation of, 103–104
Somatosensory evoked potentials (SEPs), in comatose patient, 20–21
Spearman rank correlation coefficient, 1750
Specific gravity, of urine, in renal failure, 788

Specificity, of tests, 1745, 1745t
Speech
  following head and neck surgery, 224
  in mental status examination, 29–30
Spider angiomas, in hepatic disorders, 1059, *1060*
Spider bites, 1468–1469
Spinal cord
  compression of, by malignant disease, *868*, 868–869
  risk factors for surgical complications and, 1220, 1220t
Spinal cord compression, by malignant disease
  during ICU phase, 869
  during post-ICU phase, 869
  during pre-ICU phase, 868–869, *869*
Spinal cord injury (SCI), 146–158
  anterior SCI syndrome, 149–150
  Brown-Sequard syndrome, 150
  cauda equina injuries and, 150
  central cord syndrome, 149
  complete, 148
  conus medullaris syndrome, 150
  during ICU phase, 150–157
    cardiovascular management and, 152–153
    gastrointestinal and nutritional management and, 154–155
    genitourinary management and, 155
    musculoskeletal and skin protocol and, 155–156
    neurologic management and, *153*, 153–154, *154*
    psychologic protocol and, 156–157
    pulmonary management and, 150–152, *151*
  during post-ICU phase, 157t, 157–158
  during pre-ICU phase, 146–147
    airway management and, 147
    breathing and, 147
    circulation and, 147
    immobilization and, 147
    transportation and, 147
  emergency room management of, 147–150
    neurologic evaluation in, 148–150, 149t
  hysterical conversion and, 150
  incomplete, 148–149, 149t
  posterior cord syndrome, 150
  vascular surgery and, 723–724
Spirometry
  bedside, for monitoring and detection of respiratory insufficiency, 462, 464, 464t, 479–480
  incentive
    in atelectasis, 467–468, *468*
    preoperative, 1207–1208
Spironolactone, for cirrhosis, 1113
Splanchnic organ dysfunction, in multiple organ system failure, 1300–1302
Splenectomy, as predisposing condition to infection, 399
Splenic disorders, imaging studies in, 1532, 1536, *1537*, *1538*
Splenic vein thrombosis, pancreatitis and, 1039
Spontaneous bacterial peritonitis (SBP)
  in cirrhosis, 1109–1111, 1110t
    clinical picture in, 1109–1110
    mortality in, 1110–1111
    pathogenesis of, 1110
    recurrence of, 1111
    treatment of, 1110
  in patients awaiting liver transplantation, 1137t, 1137–1138

Stabilization. *See* Patient stabilization
Staff. *See* Personnel; Physician(s); Professional staff; Team concept
Standard deviation, 1740
Standard error of the mean, 1740
Standard of care, 1718
Staphylococcal scalded skin syndrome (SSSS), 928–931
  clinical presentation of, 928–929, *929*
  differential diagnosis and laboratory studies in, 929–930, 930t
  pathophysiology of, 928
  recovery from, 930–931
  risk factors for, 928
  treatment of, 930
Statistical tests, selection of, 1748–1749, 1749t
Statistics. *See* Clinical epidemiology, biostatistics and
Status epilepticus, 94–95, 95t
  complications of, 98, 98t
Steritek ICP monitoring system, 70
Sternal dehiscence, following cardiac surgery, 602
Sternotomy, median, as risk factor for neurologic surgical complications, 1219
Steroids. *See also specific steroids and types of steroids*
  following renal transplantation, 829
  for elevated intracranial pressure, in comatose patient, 19
Stevens-Johnson syndrome, 958–961
  clinical presentation of, 958–959, *959*, *960*, 960t
  diagnosis of, 959–960
  laboratory studies in, 960
  outcome of, 961
  pathophysiology and risk factors for, 958, 959t
  recovery from, 961
  treatment of, 960–961
Stimulants, abuse/overdose of, 1431–1439. *See also specific drugs*
  signs and symptoms of, 1431
Strategic planning, 1715–1716
Street drugs. *See* Substance abuse/overdose; *specific substances*
Streptokinase
  for pulmonary embolism, 432–433
  for thrombotic disorders, 916–917
Stress
  of illness, hypothalamic-pituitary-peripheral gland unit response to. *See* Hypothalamic-pituitary-peripheral gland unit
  psychological. *See* Psychological stress
Stress ulcers, prophylaxis of, in brain injury, 86–87
Stroke
  heat. *See* Heat stroke
  hemorrhagic. *See* Hemorrhagic stroke
Structural lesions. *See also* Coma, risk factors for
  thermoregulatory disorders and, 53
Study questions, 1742
Subaortic stenosis, hypertrophic, idiopathic. *See* Cardiomyopathy, hypertrophic
Subarachnoid bolt, for intracranial pressure monitoring, 69–70, *70*
Subarachnoid hemorrhage (SAH), 80, 81t
  aneurysmal, 88
  lumbar puncture in, data analysis for, 1617

INDEX

Subclavian artery
  laceration of, as complication of nutritional support, 1261
  thrombosis of, as complication of nutritional support, 1261
Subcutaneous emphysema, following thoracic surgery, 378
Subdural empyema, 81, 82
  during ICU phase, 116-117
  pre-ICU evaluation of, 106-107
Subdural hematoma (SDH), 78, 78
  acute, 78
  chronic, 78
Substance abuse/overdose, 1424-1451
  during ICU phase, 1431-1451
    central nervous system depressants and, 1439-1445. See also specific drugs
    central nervous system stimulants and, 1431-1439. See also specific substances
    look-alike drugs, 1437-1438
    signs and symptoms of, 1431
    hallucinogens and, 1447-1449, 1448t
    marijuana and, 1449-1450
    opioids and, 1445-1447
    volatile inhalants and, 1450-1451
  during pre-ICU phase, 1425-1431
    administration routes and, 1425-1426
    common problems in, 1427t, 1427-1428, 1428t
    cutting substances, 1427-1428, 1428t
    diagnosis of, 1426t, 1426-1427
    toxicology laboratory and, 1426-1427
    general treatment principles for, 1428-1429
    history taking and, 1429
    ICU admission criteria for, 1430-1431
    reflex diagnostics and therapeutics for, 1429-1430
    vital signs in, 1429, 1430t
  historical background of, 1424
  rehabilitation phase in, 1451
  scope of, 1424-1425
Substrate utilization
  for estimation of energy requirements, 1255, 1255t
  minute ventilation and, 265
Subtentorial lesions, coma and. See Coma, risk factors for
Succinylcholine, 1287, 1287t
Sufentanil, for pain control, 1283t, 1284
Suit. See Liability
Sulbactam
  dosing adjustment for renal or hepatic dysfunction, 1351t
  dosing during hemofiltration and hemodialysis, 1353t
Sulfamethoxazole
  dosing adjustment for renal or hepatic dysfunction, 1351t
  dosing during hemofiltration and hemodialysis, 1353t
Sulfur dioxide, inhalation injury caused by, 319
Superinfection, in pneumonia, 413
Superior sagittal sinus, septic thrombosis of, pre-ICU evaluation of, 105-106
Superior vena cava, obstruction of, by malignant disease, 866-868, 867t
  during ICU phase, 867
  during post-ICU phase, 868
  during pre-ICU phase, 866-867, 867, 867t
Support, situational, 1568
Supraglottic laryngectomy, postoperative care for, 224

Supraglottitis, during pre-ICU phase, 189-192
Supratentorial lesions, coma and. See Coma, risk factors for
Supraventricular arrhythmias
  following cardiac surgery, 597
  paroxysmal tachycardia, 536-537, 538, 539, 543
  treatment of, 538-542, 543t
Surgery. See also specific sites and procedures
  as risk factor for neurologic surgical complications, 1219-1220
  following cardiac transplantation, 652
  hypertension following. See Hypertension, postoperative
  in cirrhosis, 1117-1119
  in myasthenia gravis patients, 134, 134t
    postoperative care and, 135
  jaundice following. See Jaundice, postoperative
  nutritional support following, 1269
  pulmonary complications of, prevention and treatment of, 494, 495
Surgical management
  for aortic dissection
    ascending, 705-708, 706, 707
      postoperative management and, 707-708, 708
    descending, 708-709
      postoperative care and, 708-709
  for focal pulmonary hemorrhage, 351-352
  for intracranial hypertension, 71
  for mitral regurgitation, 667-669, 668
  for myocardial ischemia and infarction. See Coronary artery bypass grafting (CABG)
  for necrotizing fasciitis, 935, 935
  for pancreatitis, 1036
    complications of, 1036-1038, 1037t
  of aortic regurgitation, 678-679, 679
  of gastrointestinal bleeding, 997
Surrogate decision maker, 1728-1729, 1732-1733, 1734
  definition of, 1728t
Survival, quality of care and, 1582-1583
Swallowing, following head and neck surgery, 224
Swan-Ganz catheter, imaging studies and, 1485, 1486
Sweating, 52
Sympathetic activity, increased, arrhythmias associated with, 534
Sympatholytics, for hypertension, 692t-694t
Synchronized intermittent mandatory ventilation (SIMV), 486, 486t
  in ventilatory failure, 171
Syndrome of inappropriate antidiuretic hormone (SIADH)
  during pre-ICU phase, 885
  during post-ICU phase, 885-886
  hyponatremia and, 770-771, 771t
  in HIV infection/AIDS, 1413-1414
  with malignancy, 885-886
Syphilis
  in HIV infection/AIDS, 1409-1410
  neurologic disorders caused by, in HIV infection/AIDS, 1407
Systemic blood pressure, normalization of, intracranial hypertension and, 67
Systemic disorders. See also specific disorders
  coma and, 13-14
  thermoregulatory disorders and, 53-54, 54t

Systemic hypertension, intracranial hypertension and, 66
Systemic inflammatory response syndrome (SIRS), 1000, 1003, 1003-1004, 1005. See also Intra-abdominal infections
Systemic lupus erythematosus (SLE), diffuse alveolar hemorrhage and, 344, 344t
Systolic function, assessment of, 518-521, 519t, 520

Tachycardia
  accessory bypass tract, 537, 540, 541
  atrial, multifocal, 538
    treatment of, 542
  sinus, 535
    treatment of, 543t
  supraventricular
    paroxysmal, 536-537, 538, 539
      treatment of, 543t
    treatment of, 538-542, 543t
  ventricular
    in acute myocardial infarction, 577
    sustained, treatment of, 543t, 543-545, 544t, 545, 546
Tachyphylaxis, 1323
Tactical planning, 1716
Tamponade, following cardiac surgery, 598
Tazobactam, for intra-abdominal infections, 1379
Team concept, 1555-1564
  high risk patients and, 1557-1563
    during ICU phase, 1559-1562
      clinical protocols and, 1559, 1560t-1561t, 1561
      communication styles and, 1562, 1562t
      inclusion of patients and family and, 1562
      integrated patient records and, 1561-1562
      interdisciplinary conferences and, 1561
      medical and nursing co-directors and, 1559
      patient progress rounds and, 1561
    during post-ICU phase, 1562-1563
      discharge planning and, 1562-1563
      patient and family education and, 1563
      quality assurance and, 1563
    during pre-ICU phase, 1557-1559
      assessment and, 1558
      relationships with other departments and, 1559
      treatment decisions and, 1558-1559
  outcomes and, 1563-1564
  physician-nurse collaboration and, 1555-1557
    centrality to patient care, 1555
    impact on patient outcomes, 1555-1556
    impediments to, 1556
      conflict related to differences in professional orientation and, 1556
      conflict related to patient care decisions and, 1556
    professional organizations' recommendations regarding, 1557, 1557t
Teicoplanin
  dosing adjustment for renal or hepatic dysfunction, 1351t

Teicoplanin *(Continued)*
    dosing during hemofiltration and hemodialysis, 1353t
Temperature, of blood, calcium binding and, 1190
Temporary pacing. *See* Cardiac pacing, temporary
Tensilon test, in myasthenia gravis, 132, 132t, 135
Test dose, of peridural narcotics, 1285
Testicular cancer, surgery for, 844–845
    during ICU phase, 844
    during post-ICU phase, 844–845
    during pre-ICU phase, 844
Testimony, 1723–1724
Tetanus, 140–141
    antimicrobial therapy for, 1384
    during ICU phase, 141, 141t
    during post-ICU phase, 141
    during pre-ICU phase, 140t, 140–141
Tetracycline
    dosing adjustment for renal or hepatic dysfunction, 1351t
    dosing during hemofiltration and hemodialysis, 1353t
    for Rocky Mountain spotted fever, 946
Thalamus
    bilateral medial infarction of, coma and, 6
    coma and, 3–4
Thalassemia, 903–904
Theophylline
    for chronic obstructive pulmonary disease, 249–250, *250*
    intoxication by, 1462–1464, 1463t
Therapeutic Intervention Scoring System (TISS), 1675, 1679t
Therapies. *See* Treatment; *specific treatment modalities*
Thermodilution cardiac output (TDCO) measurement, 1640–1642, *1641*, 1641t
    derived parameters and, 1641–1642, 1642t
Thermogenesis
    nonshivering, 52
    shivering, 52
Thermoregulation, 51–63
    anatomy and physiology of, 51–52
    body temperature and, 51
    disorders of, 53–63. *See also specific disorders*
        general mechanisms of, 53t, 53–54, 54t
    in comatose patient, 16
    response to cold stress and, 52
    response to heat stress and, 52–53
    temperature measurement and, 51
Thiamine
    for alcohol withdrawal, 1441t
    for cocaine abuse/overdose, 1434, 1435t
    for substance abuse/overdose, 1429
Thiethylperazine (Torecan), for delirium, 1282
Thinking, in mental status examination, 30
Thiopental sodium (Pentothal), for delirium, 1283
Thiotepa, for bone marrow transplantation, 881t
Thoracentesis, 1625–1626
    complications and management of, 1625–1626
    contraindications to, 1625
    data analysis for, 1625, 1626t
    indications for, 1625
    quality enhancement for, 1626

Thoracic surgical patients, 356–382
    operative considerations with, 362–366
        airway obstruction, 362–363, *364*
        anesthetic choice, 363
        antibiotic prophylaxis, 366
        endobronchial intubation, 363, 363t, 365, *365*
        monitoring and invasive devices, 362, 362t, *363*
        premedication, 362
    postoperative considerations with, *366*, 366–381, *367*, 372t, 373t
        airway complications, 372–375
            bronchopleural fistula, 374
            empyema, 374–375
            retained secretions and blood in airway and, 373–374
        analgesia, *371*, 371–372, *372*
        bullectomy, 378
        cardiac dysrhythmias, 378
        chest wall complications, 377–378
            infection of incisions, 377–378
            infections of costal cartilage and costal arch, 378
            subcutaneous emphysema, 378
        esophageal complications, 379
        extubation and airway, 367–368, *368*
        fluids, 368–369
        following lung transplantation, 379–381
            during first 48 hours, 379–381, *380*
            from 48 hours to 2 weeks, 381
        mediastinal complications, 378
        pleural complications, 376–377
            chylothorax, 377
            fluid and air, 376–377
            pleural fluid drainage, 377
            pneumothorax, 377
        pulmonary parenchymal complications, 375–376
            atelectasis, 375
            lobar collapse, 375
            lobar torsion, 376
            pre-expansion pulmonary edema, 376
            respiratory insufficiency, 376
        respiratory therapy, 370
        vascular complications, 375
            hemorrhage, 375
            pulmonary emboli, 375
            systemic tumor emboli, 375
        ventilator support, 369–370
    preoperative considerations with, 356–362
        in lung transplantation patients, 359t, 359–360, *360*, 360t
        outcome assessment as, 360–362
            staging for, 361t, 361–362, 362t
        preoperative evaluation and, 356–357, 357t, 358t
        severity of illness scoring as, 357–359, 358t, 359t
    rehabilitation/post-ICU care for, 381–382
        discharge considerations and, 381
        psychologic support and, 381–382
        respiratory therapy in, 381
Thoracostomy tubes, imaging studies and, 1476–1477, *1478*, *1479*
Thrombocytopenia, 879–880, 907–910. *See also* Hemolytic uremic syndrome (HUS); Idiopathic thrombocytopenic purpura (ITP); Post-transfusion purpura (PTP); Thrombotic thrombocytopenic purpura (TTP)
    decreased production in, 907–908
    decreased survival in, 908, 908t
    dilution in, 880

    drug-induced, 909t, 909–910
    enhanced destruction in, 880
        during ICU phase, 880
        during pre-ICU phase, 880, 880t
    in HIV infection/AIDS, 1412
    poor production in, 879–880
    pseudothrombocytopenia and, 879
    sequestration in, 880
Thrombocytosis, 878–879, 910, 910t
    during ICU phase, 879
    during post-ICU phase, 879
    during pre-ICU phase, 878–879
    essential, 878
    reactive, 878
Thromboembolic disorders
    in chronic obstructive pulmonary disease, during ICU phase, 254
    venous. *See* Pulmonary embolism
Thrombolytic therapy, 916–917. *See also specific drugs*
    for acute myocardial infarction, *573*, 573–575, *574*
    for pulmonary embolism, 431–433
        protocol for, 432
        recombinant tissue plasminogen activator in, 433
        streptokinase in, 432–433
        urokinase in, 433
Thrombotic disorders. *See also specific disorders*
    deep vein thrombosis
        in spinal cord injury, 152
        objective testing for, role of, 425–426
    of hepatic artery, following liver transplantation, 1146
    of renal arteries, following renal revascularization, 833
    of splenic vein, pancreatitis and, 1039
    of subclavian artery, as complication of nutritional support, 1261
    treatment of, 914–917
        aspirin in, 916
        dextran in, 916
        fibrinolytic agents in, 916–917
        heparin in, 915
        oral anticoagulants in, 915–916, 916t
Thrombotic thrombocytopenic purpura (TTP), 859–863, 908
    during ICU phase, 862–863
        treatment of, 862–863
    during post-ICU phase, 863
    during pre-ICU phase, 859–862
        clinical course of, 861–862
        clinical presentation of, 860, 860t
        differential diagnosis of, 860t, 860–861, 861t
        etiology and pathogenesis of, 859–860, 860t
        laboratory studies in, 860, 860t
Thrush, in HIV infection/AIDS, 1408
Thyroid disorders. *See also specific disorders*
    during ICU phase, 1177–1180
    during post-ICU phase, 1180–1181
    during pre-ICU phase, 1176–1177
    in HIV infection/AIDS, 1414
Thyroid storm
    during ICU phase, 1177–1178
    hypertension following, postoperative, 738–739
Thyroid-stimulating hormone (TSH), deficiency of, 1177
Thyrotoxicosis
    coma and, 13
    hypertension following, postoperative, 738–739

INDEX

L-Thyroxine
  for euthyroid sick syndrome, 1177
  for hypothyroidism, 1180–1181
  for myxedema coma, 1179
Thyroxine (T₄), in euthyroid sick syndrome, 1174–1175, 1175t
Ticarcillin
  dosing adjustment for renal or hepatic dysfunction, 1351t
  dosing during hemofiltration and hemodialysis, 1353t
Ticarcillin-clavulanate, for pneumonia
  community-acquired, 391t
  nosocomial, 393t
Tissue hypoxia, in multiple organ system failure, 1295–1296
Tobacco. *See* Smoking
Tobramycin
  for intra-abdominal infections, 1378
  for pancreatitis, 1034t
  for pneumonia, nosocomial, 394
  in hemodialysis, 1345
  large-dose once-a-day dosing with, 1347
Tocainide, for ventricular tachycardia, 544t
Total energy expenditure (TEE), for estimation of energy requirements, 1254–1255
Total parenteral nutrition (TPN)
  at home, 1271
  following head and neck surgery, 223, 223t
  following vascular surgery, 723
  for multiple organ system failure, 1302
  for renal failure, 791
  gallstones and, 1053
  in borderline malnourished patients, 1253
  in hyperglycemic patients, 1167, 1167t, 1168
  in pancreatitis, 1035
  in spinal cord injury, 154
  prescription for, 1259, 1265–1267
    amino acids in, 1259, 1261t
    dextrose in, 1259, 1261t
    enteral formulas and, 1259, 1261
    lipids in, 1259
Toxic epidermal necrolysis (TEN), 961–964
  antimicrobial therapy for, 1383
  clinical presentation of, 962, 962, 963, 963t
  differential diagnosis of, 962
  outcome of, 964
  pathogenesis of, 961–962, 962t
  recovery from, 964
  treatment of, 962–964
Toxic shock syndrome (TSS), 931–934
  antimicrobial therapy for, 1383
  clinical presentation and laboratory studies in, 931–932
  diagnosis of, 932t, 932–933
  pathophysiology and risk factors for, 931, 931t
  recovery from, 933–934
  treatment of, 933
Toxicology laboratory, in substance abuse, 1426–1427
Toxins. *See* Poisonings; *specific substances*
Toxoplasma retinitis, in HIV infection/AIDS, 1411
Toxoplasmosis, in HIV infection/AIDS, 1407, 1407
Trace minerals, requirements for, 1256, 1256t
Tracheal intubation
  imaging studies and, 1474, 1474–1477, 1476
  nosocomial pneumonia and, 202–203

Tracheal malacia, post-tracheostomy, 207–208
  management of, 208
Tracheal stenosis, post-tracheostomy, 207–208
  management of, 208, 208
Tracheoesophageal fistula, 870–871
Tracheostomy
  during mechanical ventilation, 295
  in brain injury, 86
  in upper airway obstruction
    communication and, 205–206
    decannulation and, 206–207, 207
    late complications of, 207–208, 208
    long-term, 206
    nutrition and, 203
  percutaneous, for thoracic surgery patients, 367–368, 368
  timing of placement of, rehabilitation of ventilator-dependent patients and, 444–445
Tracheotomy, in upper airway obstruction, 199–202, 200t–202t, 201–203
Transbronchial biopsy
  during mechanical ventilation, 296
  in pneumonia, 408
Transfusion therapy, 917–920, 1240–1248, 1241t
  coagulation factors in, 920
  during ICU phase, 1241–1248
    platelets and fresh-frozen plasma for, 1245–1246, 1246t, 1247t
    red blood cell substitutes for, 1246–1248
      hemoglobin solutions, 1248
      perfluorochemical emulsions, 1246–1247
    red blood cells for, 917–918, 918t, 1241–1245
      monitoring oxygen transport and, 1242–1245, 1243
      oxygen delivery/oxygen consumption and, 1242
    white blood cells in, 918–919
  during post-ICU phase, 1248
  during pre-ICU phase, 1240–1241
    autologous blood donation and, 1240–1241
    autotransfusion and, intraoperative, 1241
    blood conservation techniques and, 1240
    erythropoiesis and, acceleration of, 1241
    hemodilution and, 1241
  platelets in, 919–920
  termination guidelines for, 1731, 1733, 1735
Transitional feedings, 1269–1270, 1270
Transjugular intrahepatic portal system shunt (TIPS), for esophageal varices, 1099, 1099–1100, 1100
Translaryngeal intubation, in upper airway obstruction, 195–199, 196t, 197–199, 199t
Transport
  of critically ill patients, 488, 490
  of spinal cord injured patients, 147
Transurethral prostatectomy (TURP), 849–850
  during ICU phase, 850
    hemorrhage and, 850
    perforations and, 850

post-TURP syndrome and, 850
  during post-ICU phase, 850
  during pre-ICU phase, 849–850
Trauma. *See specific site*
Traumatic brain injury, 76–79, 87–88
  cerebral protection in, 87
  concussive, 77
  contusions and, 77
  delayed neurologic deterioration in, 88
  electrophysiologic monitoring in, 87
  extradural hematoma and, 78, 79
  intracranial hemorrhage in, 87
  open, 87
  physiologic monitoring in, 87
  skull fracture and, 78–79, 79
  subdural hematoma and, 78, 78
Traumatic cardiac hemolytic anemia, 904
Treatment. *See also specific treatment modalities*
  studies to evaluate, 1746–1748, 1747t
  withdrawing, definition of, 1728t
  withholding. *See also* Life-sustaining treatment, withholding
    definition of, 1728t
Treatment decisions. *See* Decision making
Triage, 1735
  in brain injury, 85, 85t, 86t
  in focal pulmonary hemorrhage, 349–350
  in inhalation injury, 325t, 325–326
  in intracranial hypertension, 68
  quality assessment/assurance and, 1579–1580
Trials. *See* Liability
Triceps skinfold (TSF) measurement, in nutrition assessment, 1251
Tricyclic antidepressants (TCAs)
  for depression, 36–37
  intoxication by, 1460–1461
    coma and, 11–12
  poisoning by, 1460–1461
Triiodothyronine (T₃), in euthyroid sick syndrome, 1174–1175, 1175t
Trimethaphan (Arfonad)
  for aortic dissection, 704–705, 705t
  for hypertension, 692t, 693t
    postoperative, 745t, 746–747
Trimethoprim
  dosing adjustment for renal or hepatic dysfunction, 1351t
  dosing during hemofiltration and hemodialysis, 1353t
Trimethoprim-sulfamethoxazole (TMP-SMX)
  for pneumonia
    community-acquired, 391t, 392
    in granulocytopenic hosts, 410
    prophylactic, for pneumonia, 413t
T-tube, for upper airway obstruction, 208, 208
Tube misplacement/perforation, as complication of nutritional support, 1263
Tuberculosis
  antimicrobial therapy for, 1376
  extrapulmonary, in HIV infection/AIDS, 1409
  in HIV infection/AIDS, 1406
  opportunistic, in HIV infection/AIDS, prophylaxis and treatment of, 1405
D-Tubocurarine, 1287t, 1288
Tumor(s). *See* Malignancy; Mass lesions; Oncologic emergencies; *specific malignancies*
Tumor emboli, systemic, following thoracic surgery, 375

1791

INDEX

Tumor lysis syndrome, 886–887
    during ICU phase, 887
    during post-ICU phase, 887
    during pre-ICU phase, 887
Tumor necrosis factor (TNF), in shock, 1316
Type I error, 1741, 1741t
Type II error, 1741, 1741t

Ulcers
    bleeding from. *See* Gastrointestinal bleeding
    decubitus. *See* Pressure sores
    stress, prophylaxis of, in brain injury, 86–87
Ultrafiltration, for renal failure, during ICU phase, 792t, 792–797, *793–795*
Ultrasonography
    in hepatic disorders, 1068–1070, *1070*
    in pneumonia, 406, 406t
    in pulmonary embolism, 428
Uncal herniation, coma and, 6
Univariate analysis, 1750–1751
Unreasonable risk, 1718
Upper airway dysfunction, rehabilitation of ventilator-dependent patients and, 445, 445t
Upper airway management, in inhalation injury, 322–323, *323*
Upper airway obstruction (UAO), 189–208. *See also* Airway obstruction
    during ICU phase, 195–204
        extubation and, 203–204
        nutrition and, 203
        tracheal intubation-related pneumonia and, 202–203
        tracheotomy and, 199–202, 200t–202t, *201–203*
        translaryngeal intubation and, 195–199, 196t, *197–199,* 199t
    during post-ICU phase, 204–208
        communication and, 205–206, *206*
        decannulation and, 206–207, *207*
        tracheostomy and
            late complications of, 207–208, *208*
            long-term, 206
    during pre-ICU phase, 189–195, *190*
        dynamic vocal cord paralysis and, 193–194
        infectious/inflammatory disorders and, 189–193
        symptoms and diagnosis and, 189, *191, 192*
        treatment and, 194–195
Urapadil, for hypertension, postoperative, 747
Uremia, 802
    as predisposing condition to infection, 400
    metabolic acidosis associated with, treatment of, 761
    platelet disorders related to, 911
Ureteral disorders, imaging studies in, 1540
Urethral disorders, imaging studies in, 1540
Urinalysis, in renal failure, 788, 788t
Urinary catheters, infection related to, 1594
Urinary leak, following renal surgery, 848
Urinary tract infection (UTI)
    antimicrobial therapy for, 1381–1382
    following vascular surgery, 724
    management of, 854–855
Urine
    acidification of, for hallucinogen abuse/overdose, 1449

alkalinization of
    for salicylate intoxication, 1460
    for sedative/hypnotic abuse/overdose, 1443–1444
fluid loss in, hypovolemia caused by, fluid resuscitation for, 1234–1235, 1235t
volume of, in renal failure, 787
Urobilinogen, urinary, in hepatic disorders, 1065
Urokinase
    for pulmonary embolism, 433
    for thrombotic disorders, 917
Urologic disorders. *See also specific disorders*
    following renal transplantation, 827–828
Urologic management, 851–855
    catheter placement in, 851–852
        during ICU phase, 852, *852,* 853
        during post-ICU phase, 852
        during pre-ICU phase, 851–852
    for anuria, 853–854, *854*
    for hematuria, 853
    for urinary tract infection, 854–855
    of comatose patient, 17
Urologic surgery, hypertension following, 739–740
Urticaria, drug-induced, 965–966, *966*
User interface, 1704, 1706–1707, *1710–1712*

Vagal stimulation, in arrhythmias, 531–532
Validity, 1665t
Valproate intoxication, coma and, 12
Valvular heart disease, treatment of, preoperative, for prevention of cardiovascular complications, 1215–1216
Valvular heart surgery, hypertension following, 735–736
Valvular regurgitation. *See* Aortic regurgitation; Mitral regurgitation (MR)
Valvuloplasty, aortic, of aortic regurgitation, 678–679, *679*
Vancomycin
    computer programs for dosing with, 1355–1359
    in anuric renal failure and hemodialysis, 1357, *1358,* 1359
    in good renal function, 1355–1357, *1356, 1357*
    dosing adjustment for renal or hepatic dysfunction, 1351t
    dosing during hemofiltration and hemodialysis, 1353t
    for diarrhea, 1381
    for endocarditis, 1376–1377
    for pneumonia, community-acquired, 391t
    pharmacokinetics of, 1347–1349
        dosing in elderly patients and, 1348
        dosing in hemodialysis patients and, 1348–1349
Variability, 1740
Variance, 1740
Varicella-zoster immune globulin (VZIG), for varicella-zoster virus infections, 953
Varicella-zoster virus (VZV) infections, 950–954
    clinical manifestations, differential diagnosis, and laboratory studies in
        in primary infection, 950–952, *951*
        in recrudescent infection, *952,* 952–953
    outcome of, 953t, 953–954, *954*
    treatment of, 953

Varices, esophageal
    in cirrhosis, 1094
    diagnosis of, 1094, *1095, 1096*
    in patients awaiting liver transplantation, treatment of, 1134–1136
    recurrent bleeding from, 1100–1103
    rupture of, 1095–1096
        acute, 1097–1100
        treatment of, 1097–1103
            balloon tamponade in, 1097–1098, *1098*
            drug therapy in, 1097, 1102–1103
            sclerotherapy in, 1098, 1100–1101
            shunt procedures in, 1098–1099, *1101,* 1101–1102, *1102*
    in portal hypertension. *See* Portal hypertension, variceal bleeding in
Vascular catheter, infection related to, 1590–1592, *1591,* 1591t
Vascular disorders. *See also specific disorders*
    extracardiac, surgical management of myocardial ischemia and infarction and, 590
    following renal transplantation, 828
Vascular infections, intracranial
    during ICU phase, 115
    pre-ICU evaluation of, 104–105
Vascular resistance, reduction of, following vascular surgery, 717
Vascular surgery, postoperative care and, 713–726
    during ICU phase, 715–725
        arrhythmias and, identification and correction of, 717
        augmentation of poor contractility and, 717–718
        cardiovascular complications and, 721–722
        gastrointestinal complications and, 722–723
        hematologic complications and, 724
        infectious complications and, 724–725
        intraoperative considerations in, 715, *715*
        metabolic complications and, 723
        neurologic complications and, 723–724
        optimization of filling pressures and, 717
        patient monitoring and, 715t, 715–717
        pulmonary complications and, 720–721
        reduction of elevated vascular resistances and, 717
        reduction of excessive myocardial oxygen consumption and, 718–720
        renal complications and, 723
    during post-ICU phase, 725–726
    during pre-ICU phase, 713–715, 714t
        angiography in, 714
        cardiovascular considerations in, 714
        neurologic considerations in, 714–715
Vasculopathy, diabetic, 806–807
Vasoconstriction, 52
Vasodilation, reflex, 52
Vasodilators
    for chronic obstructive pulmonary disease, 262, 262t
    for hypertension, 692t–694t
Vasopressin
    for esophageal varices, 1097
    for gastrointestinal bleeding, in patients awaiting liver transplantation, 1134–1135, 1135t

Vasospasm, cerebral, subarachnoid hemorrhage and, 88
Vecuronium, 1287, 1287t
Vegetative state, 3
Vendor representatives, computerized patient management system and. *See* Computerized patient management system
Venography, in pulmonary embolism, 427
Veno-occlusive disease, hepatic failure caused by, 1080
Venous access
 for fluid resuscitation, at home, 1238
 for hemodialysis. *See* Hemodialysis, access for
Venous catheters, imaging studies and, 1478, *1481-1485*
Venous oxygen, partial pressure of, in multiple organ system failure, 1299-1300
Venous sinus occlusion, coma and, 6
Venous thromboembolism. *See* Pulmonary embolism
Venous thrombosis, following vascular surgery, 722
Venovenous access, for hemodialysis, 792
Ventilation-perfusion lung scanning
 in pulmonary embolism, *422*, 422-424, 423t, *424*
 preoperative, 1204
Ventilation-perfusion mismatching, in parenchymal respiratory failure, 164
Ventilator score, for ventilatory weaning, 443
Ventilators, 486-488
 graphics and waveforms and, 488, *489*
 monitoring of, 291t, 291-292
 respiratory mechanics and, 487-488
 weaning from. *See* Ventilatory weaning
 with continuous flow, 487
 with inverse I:E ratio, 487, *487*
 with multiple flow patterns, 486-487, 487t
 with pressure support, 487
Ventilatory capacity, in chronic obstructive pulmonary disease, 266t, 266-267
 respiratory muscle fatigue and, 266-267
Ventilatory control
 disorders of. *See* Hypoventilation syndromes
 rehabilitation of ventilator-dependent patients and, 445
Ventilatory drive, in ventilatory failure, 172, 172t
Ventilatory failure. *See* Respiratory failure, ventilatory (pump)
Ventilatory support. *See also* Mechanical ventilation; Ventilatory weaning
 adjunctive, in ventilatory failure, 175
 in acid maltase deficiency, 142
 in amyotrophic lateral sclerosis
  during ICU phase, 137
  during post-ICU phase, 137-138
 in bronchospastic disease, 235-237, *237*
  controlled mechanical hypoventilation and, 236-237
  volume-cycled ventilators and, 236
 in chronic obstructive pulmonary disease, 259-260
  continuous positive airway pressure in, 259-260

home ventilation, 272
 mechanical, 260, 260t
 noninvasive, 260
 in hypoventilation syndromes, 184-185
 in spinal cord injury, 147-148, 151-152
 in tetanus, 141
Ventilatory weaning, 45-46, 438-457, 439t, 488, 490
 adverse factor score for, 443
 during ICU phase, 441-453
  clinical protocol for, 449-450, *451-453*, 453
  common impediments to, 443t, 443-444, 444t
  critical success factors in, 443
  magnitude of dependence and, 441-442, 442t
  patient management theme for weaning and rehabilitation and, 442t, 442-443, 443t
  physiologic considerations for, 445-453, 446t
  CROP Index and Weaning Index, 448-449, 450t
  endurance, *447*, 447-448, *448*
  strength, 446-447
  preparation for ICU discharge and, 453, 454t
  special considerations for, 444-445, 445t
 during pre-ICU phase, 438-441
 in chronic obstructive pulmonary disease, 265t, 265-266
  requirements for minute ventilation and, 265t, 265-266, 266t
  respiratory mechanics and, 268t, 268-269
  ventilatory mode and, 268
 in diffuse alveolar hemorrhage, 347
 in intra-abdominal infection, 1011
 in spinal cord injury, 152
 in upper airway obstruction, 203-204
 in ventilatory failure, 173-175, 174t, *175*
 of thoracic surgery patients, 367-368, *368*
 parameters for predicting acceptability of, 446t
 preparation for, 296-297
 ventilator score for, 443
Ventricular arrhythmias
 following cardiac surgery, 597
 treatment of, 542-545, 543t, 544t, *545, 546*
Ventricular assist devices (VAD), 592-593
 pre-cardiac transplantation, 642
Ventricular catheter, for intracranial pressure monitoring, 69-70, *70*
Ventricular depolarizations, premature, treatment of, 542-544, 543t, 544t
Ventricular dysfunction, as risk factor for cardiac surgery, 591
Ventricular ejection, afterload and, 509-511, *510*, 511t
Ventricular failure, left, in acute myocardial infarction, 578t, 578-579, *580*
Ventricular fibrillation, in acute myocardial infarction, 577-578
Ventricular function
 evaluation of, in ICU setting, 514-522
  diastolic function assessment in, 521-522, *523, 524*
  indirect pulse recordings in, 518
  radionuclide ventriculography in, *515*, 515-517, *516*

systolic function measurement in, 518-521, 519t, *520*
 two-dimensional and Doppler echocardiography in, *517*, 517-518, *518*
 right, determinants of, 512-514, *514*, 514t
Ventricular pressure tracings, in constrictive pericarditis, 617, *617*
Ventricular tachycardia
 in acute myocardial infarction, 577
 sustained, treatment of, 543t, 543-545, 544t, *545, 546*
Ventriculography, radionuclide, *515*, 515-517, *516*
 ejection fraction and, 519
 in cardiac trauma, nonpenetrating, 632
Verapamil
 for hypertension, 692t-694t
 for supraventricular tachycardia, 538, 543t
Verdict, 1724
 appeal of, 1724-1725
Vertebral artery ischemia, coma and, 8
Vicarious liability, 1720-1721
Vidarabine
 dosing adjustment for renal or hepatic dysfunction, 1351t
 dosing during hemofiltration and hemodialysis, 1353t
 for varicella-zoster virus infections, 953
Viral infections. *See* Infection, viral; *specific viral infections*
Viral meningitis, pre-ICU evaluation of, 109, 111
Viruses, in cerebrospinal fluid, analysis of, 1617
Visceral disorders, following renal revascularization, 834, 834t
Vital signs, in substance abuse/overdose, 1429, 1430t
Vitamin(s), requirements for, 1256, 1256t
Vitamin K, deficiency of, coagulopathy related to, 912-913
Vocal cord paralysis (VCP), during pre-ICU phase, 193-194
Volatile inhalant abuse/overdose, 1450-1451
 complications of, 1450-1451
 diagnosis and treatment of, 1451
 signs and symptoms of, 1450
 special considerations in, 1451
Volume depletion. *See* Hypovolemia
Volume excess, hypertension and, postoperative, 734
Vomiting, metabolic alkalosis associated with, 765
Von Willebrand's disease (vWD), 912
VP-16, for bone marrow transplantation, 881t

Warfarin
 following vascular surgery, 719
 for thrombotic disorders, 915
Warm-reactive antibodies, 904-905
Warren shunt, for esophageal varices, 1101-1102, *1102*
Wasting, in HIV infection/AIDS, 1413
Water-depletion heat exhaustion, 57
Weaning
 from cardiopulmonary bypass, 647-648
 from ventilator. *See* Ventilatory weaning
Weaning Index, 448-449, 450t
Wegener's granulomatosis, diffuse alveolar hemorrhage and, 344, 344t
Weight loss, in HIV infection/AIDS, 1413

INDEX

Western blot test, for HIV infection, 1402
White cells
    disorders of, 905-907, *906*. See also Neutropenia
        neutrophilia, 907, 907t
    normal function of, 899-900
    transfusions of, 918-919
White nails of Terry, in hepatic disorders, 1059, *1060*
Wilson's disease, hepatic failure caused by, 1080
Withdrawal syndromes. *See* Drug withdrawal
Withdrawing treatment, definition of, 1728t
Withholding treatment. *See also* Life-sustaining treatment, withholding
    definition of, 1728t

Witnesses, expert, 1723
Wound dehiscence, following head and neck surgery, 220
Wound healing, in multiple organ system failure, 1293t
Wound infection, following thoracic surgery, 377-378
Wound management, following head and neck surgery, 215-221
    closed drainage system assessment and, 216-217, *217*
    intraoral incision care and, 217, *218*
    reconstruction flaps and, 218-219, *219*
    split-thickness skin grafts and, 217-218
    wound assessment and, 216
    wound complications and, 219-221

Xanthelasma, in hepatic disorders, 1059, *1059*
X-ray studies, in intracranial hypertension, 67

Yates' continuity correction, 1750

Zidovudine
    dosing adjustment for renal or hepatic dysfunction, 1351t
    dosing during hemofiltration and hemodialysis, 1353t

GERALD E. SWANSON, M.D.
ROAD
MN 55431
TEL: 881-9869